The Family Physician's Compendium of Drug Therapy

Compendium of Drug Therapy

The Family Physician's

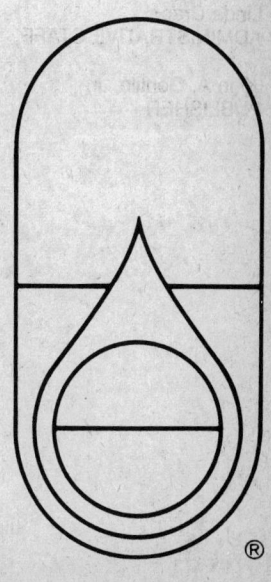

McGRAW-HILL BOOK COMPANY
New York   St. Louis   San Francisco   Hamburg
London   Mexico   Montreal   Sydney   Toronto

Edwin S. Geffner
EDITOR-IN-CHIEF

Marie-Louise Best,
Michael Mittman
SENIOR EDITORS

Bobbi Mark
EDITOR, CONSUMER EDITION

Cecilia Rosenblatt
ASSISTANT EDITOR

Pauline Harris
COPY EDITOR

Jeanette Griffith
EDITORIAL ASSISTANT

Joan Simpson
EXECUTIVE ART DIRECTOR

Robert Mancuso
SENIOR ART DIRECTOR

Peter Dov Varga
ASSISTANT ART DIRECTOR

Patricia Catlett, Randi Cheng,
Yuen Cheng, Gwendolyn Dixon,
Karen Gutwirth, Corina Igin,
Thomas F. Mahoney, Bart Slomkowski
ART STAFF

Ira Friedman
VICE PRESIDENT,
PRODUCTION AND PURCHASING

Jay Soltz
PRODUCTION MANAGER

Valerie Yenolevage
TRAFFIC COORDINATOR

Steve Blackwelder
FULFILLMENT

Dwan Tolbert
ASSISTANT DIRECTOR OF
PLANNING AND OPERATIONS

Thomas E. Bucks
COMPTROLLER

Linda Crape
ADMINISTRATIVE STAFF

John A. Gentile, Jr.
PUBLISHER

NOTICE

Medicine is an ever-changing science. As new research and clinical experience broaden our knowledge, changes in treatment and drug therapy are required. The editors and the publisher of this work have checked with sources believed to be reliable in their efforts to provide drug dosage schedules that are complete and in accord with the standards accepted at the time of publication. However, readers are advised to check the product information sheet included in the package of each drug they plan to administer to be certain that the information contained in these schedules is accurate and that changes have not been made in the recommended dose or in the contraindications for administration. This recommendation is of particular importance in connection with new or infrequently used drugs.

COMPENDIUM OF DRUG THERAPY

Copyright © 1987 by McGraw-Hill, Inc. All rights reserved. Printed in the United States of America. Except as permitted under the United States Copyright Act of 1976, no part of this publication may be reproduced or distributed in any form or by any means, or stored in a data base or retrieval system, without the prior written permission of the publisher.

ISBN 0-07-023237-7

Controlled circulation edition to health-care practitioners published by BMI/McGraw-Hill, 800 Second Avenue, New York, NY 10017.

Consumer edition published by McGraw-Hill General Books Division, 11 West 19th Street, New York, NY 10011.

Printed in the United States of America.

Robert L. Kennett
PRESIDENT

John A. Gentile, Jr.
SENIOR VICE PRESIDENT
GENERAL MANAGER,
COMPENDIUM DIVISION

Editorial Advisory Board

ALLERGY

Stanley Goldstein, MD
Attending Physician
Nassau County Medical Center
East Meadow, NY
Nassau Hospital
Mineola, NY

CARDIOLOGY

Mark A. Goodman, MD
Director, Coronary Care Unit
Nassau Hospital
Mineola, New York
Assistant Professor of Medicine
State University of New York at Stony Brook
Stony Brook, New York

Ernesto Jonas, MD
Chief, Division of Cardiology
Department of Medicine
Nassau County Medical Center
East Meadow, New York
Assistant Professor of Medicine
State University of New York at Stony Brook
Stony Brook, New York

DERMATOLOGY

Joel Jack Kassimir, MD
Clinical Instructor of Dermatology
New York University Hospital
New York, New York

FAMILY PRACTICE

John H. Renner, MD
Director, Family Practice Residency Program
St. Mary's Hospital
Kansas City, Missouri

GASTROENTEROLOGY

Charles S. Winans, MD
Professor of Medicine
Co-Director, Section of Gastroenterology
University of Chicago
Pritzker School of Medicine
Chicago, Illinois

GENERAL SURGERY

Robert E. Hermann, MD
Head, Department of General Surgery
Cleveland Clinic Foundation
Cleveland, Ohio

G. Thomas Shires, MD
Surgeon-in-Chief
New York Hospital
Professor and Chairman
Department of Surgery
Cornell University Medical College
New York, New York

HOSPITAL PHARMACY

John R. Coppola, RPh

INFECTIOUS DISEASES

Edmund C. Tramont, MD
Professor of Medicine
Chief, Department of Bacterial Disease
Walter Reed Army Institute of Research
Washington, D.C.

INTERNAL MEDICINE

Morton D. Bogdonoff, MD
Professor of Medicine
Cornell University Medical College
New York, New York

Rubin R. Bressler, MD
Professor and Head, Internal Medicine
Professor of Pharmacology and
  Chief, Clinical Pharmacy
University of Arizona
Health Sciences Center
Tucson, Arizona

Marvin Moser, MD
Clinical Professor of Medicine
New York Medical College
White Plains, New York

NUTRITION

Jules Hirsch, MD
Professor and Senior Physician
The Rockefeller University Hospital
New York, New York

OBSTETRICS AND GYNECOLOGY

Gary S. Berger, MD
Assistant Clinical Professor
  of Obstetrics and Gynecology
Duke University
Durham, North Carolina
Director, Center for Advancement
  of Reproductive Health
Chapel Hill, North Carolina

Arnold N. Fenton, MD
Chairman, Gynecology Department
North Shore Universtiy Hospital
Manhasset, New York

Louis G. Keith, MD
Professor of Obstetrics and Gynecology
Northwestern University Medical School
Chicago, Illinois

William J. Ledger, MD
Chairman, Department of
  Obstetrics and Gynecology
Cornell University Medical College
New York, New York

OPHTHALMOLOGY

Jules L. Baum, MD
Senior Ophthalmologist
New England Center Hospitals
Professor of Ophthalmology
Tufts University School of Medicine
Boston, Massachusetts

Lawrence A. Yannuzzi, MD
Surgeon Director in Ophthalmology
Manhattan Eye, Ear and Throat Hospital
Associate Clinical Professor of
  Ophthalmology
Cornell University Medical College
New York, New York

ORTHOPEDIC SURGERY

Stephen C. Allen, MD
Attending Staff
St. Luke's–Roosevelt Hospital Center
Physician to the Outpatient Department
  for Orthopedics
Hospital for Special Surgery
New York, New York

Bernard Jacobs, MD
Attending Orthopedic Surgeon
Hospital for Special Surgery
Clinical Professor of Orthopedic Surgery
Cornell University Medical College
New York, New York

OSTEOPATHIC MEDICINE

Robert E. Mancini, PhD, DO
Chairman, Department of Phamacology
  and Toxicology
Associate Professor of Pharmacology
  and Medicine
New York College of Osteopathic Medicine
Old Westbury, New York

OTOLARYNGOLOGY

David N. F. Fairbanks, MD
Professor and Chairman,
  Division of Otolaryngology
The George Washington University
  School of Medicine and Health Sciences
Bethesda, Maryland

Kenneth Francis Mattucci, MD
Chief, Department of Otolaryngolgy
North Shore University Hospital
Manhasset, New York
Associate Professor, Clinical Otolarynogology
Cornell University Medical College
New York, New York

PEDIATRICS

Vincent J. Fontana, MD
Pediatrician-in-Chief and Medical Director
New York Foundling Hospital
Professor of Clinical Pediatrics
New York University College of Medicine
New York, New York

Roy Horowitz, MD
Attending Physician, Nassau Hospital
Mineola, New York
Clinical Instructor of Pediatrics
State University of New York at Stony Brook
Stony Brook, New York

Sumner J. Yaffe, MD
Director, Center for Research
  for Mothers and Children
National Institute of Child Health
  and Human Development
National Institutes of Health
Bethesda, Maryland

PHYSICIAN ASSISTANTS

Ronald Nelson, PA-C
President, American Academy of
  Physician Assistants
White Cloud, Michigan

PSYCHIATRY

William A. Frosch, MD
Attending Psychiatrist and Medical Director
Payne Whitney Clinic
New York Hospital
Professor and Vice Chairman
Department of Psychiatry
Cornell University Medical College
New York, New York

Leo E. Hollister, MD
Professor of Medicine, Psychiatry,
  and Pharmacology
Stanford University School of Medicine
Palo Alto, California

PULMONARY DISEASES

Richard Gordon, MD

RHEUMATOLOGY

Joseph A. Markenson, MD
Assistant Attending Physician
Hospital of Special Surgery
Assistant Professor of Medicine
Cornell University Medical College
New York, New York

TOXICOLOGY

Anthony R. Temple, MD
President, American Association
  of Poison Control Centers
Adjunct Associate Professor of Pediatrics
University of Pennsylvania School of
  Medicine
Philadelphia, Pennsylvania

UROLOGY

E. Everett Anderson, MD
Professor of Urology
Duke University Medical Center
Durham, North Carolina

Preface

The drugs described in detail in this Compendium represent nearly all medications routinely prescribed or recommended by family physicians. Brand and generic names, dosage forms and strengths, and dosage recommendations for less frequently prescribed drugs are presented in summary tables following the table of contents of each chapter. The drug information is arranged by therapeutic categories. You can locate any product either by finding the brand or generic name in the general index in the front of the book or by looking for it on the contents page of the particular chapter.

CHART FORMAT AND INFORMATION

The drug information in this book is based on the official labeling supplied by the manufacturer and includes all indications currently approved by the US Food & Drug Administration. The top of each chart lists the brand name and composition of the drug, the manufacturer, and the various dosage forms and strengths available. When a drug can be given by more than one route, separate dosage recommendations for each mode of delivery appear side by side next to the indication. The dosages offered next to each indication are those recommended by the manufacturer for patients with normal kidney and liver function. Recommended adjusted dosages for patients with impaired kidney or liver function or other special-risk conditions, the preparation and delivery of solutions, and other essential administration and dosage information is provided in the "Administration/Dosage Adjustments" section of the chart.

All contraindications (indicating patients who should *not* take the drug), warnings, and precautions mentioned by the manufacturer in the package literature have been edited for conciseness and easy access to important points. The reason for shortening this material was to limit it to the information necessary for the safe and effective use of the drug described. Additional precautions concerning proper use of the drug in children and pregnant or nursing women may be found within boxes at the end of each chart. In some cases, precautions not mentioned in the package insert, but relevant to the use of the drug in special groups of patients (such as those with liver damage or an allergy of some type), have been included and appropriately referenced.

All of the adverse reactions reported by the manufacturer are listed according to the organ system they affect. Where known, the reactions that occur most frequently and those observed in 1% or more of patients are printed in *italics;* in some cases, the actual incidence of a reaction, as reported by the manufacturer, has been included in parentheses. It must be stressed, however, that the reactions listed include all adverse effects that have been observed in a great number of patients who have used the particular drug. There is no reason to assume that any one patient will experience any of these reactions.

When a specific frequency is mentioned after a series of reactions, it refers to each reaction in the series and not to just the last. Reactions pertaining to special groups of patients, such as children or elderly patients, and rare reactions are noted parenthetically following the mention of the specific reaction.

In addition, the charts supply information on the signs and symptoms of overdosage and its management. This is followed by a summary of drugs that interact with the particular drug. Once again, these drug interactions are provided to alert a physician to a potential problem in using two drugs together; the reactions described include both those reported in a great many patients and those occurring in just one patient. In addition, alterations in blood/serum and urinary laboratory values are offered toward the bottom of each chart; information on these values is often supplemented with data from the current medical and pharmacologic literature. This type of information is invaluable to certain patients, such as diabetics who may get falsely elevated glucose determinations when performing daily blood or urine tests after beginning therapy with a particular drug.

OTHER FEATURES OF THE COMPENDIUM

The *Compendium of Drug Therapy* contains several other features designed to meet specific drug information needs:

☐ The index lists products alphabetically by both brand name and generic name for quick access to information on specific drugs.

☐ A full-color drug identification guide (Chapter 1) is provided to help identify an unfamiliar tablet or capsule by its color, size, shape, and imprint code number. Color reproductions of oral contraceptive compacts and transdermal products appear immediately preceding a complete alphabetical index containing the descriptions and locations of over 1,800 drugs.

☐ A directory of pharmaceutical manufacturers and their emergency telephone numbers for obtaining further drug information appears in Chapter 2. A section listing the product imprint codes of all tablets and capsules manufactured by a number of major pharmaceutical companies appears at the end of this chapter.

☐ A directory of over 800 drug information centers, poison control centers, pain clinics, voluntary health organizations, and other patient counseling and referral services is provided in Chapter 3 under the heading "Information Resources."

☐ "Essential Pharmacokinetic Data," found in Chapter 4, contains specific information on how drugs work within the body. "Diagnostics," Chapter 35, explains how certain in-office tests are used by physicians, and offers information on some retail tests used by patients, such as pregnancy, ovulation, and occult blood tests.

☐ Chapter 5 covers significant new drugs, as well as last-minute changes in prescribing information received at press time. Consult this section for the most recent information regarding indications, dosages, new formulations, drug interactions, and other important changes. This chapter also includes full charts on a number of important agents — including psychostimulants, vaccines, and drugs used for treating addiction — that do not fit within the therapeutic categories used in the rest of the book.

☐ A glossary of over 1,300 medical and pharmaceutical terms commonly used within the drug charts has been included at the end of this volume for easy reference and familiarization with medical terminology.

Contents

Index of Product and Generic Names   XIII

CHAPTER 1
Drug Identification Guide and Index   1
Color Reproduction Section   1
Drug Identification Index   49

CHAPTER 2
Directory of Manufacturers   69
Product Imprint Codes   73

CHAPTER 3
Information Resources   87
Drug Information Centers   87
Poison Control Centers   89
Comprehensive Cancer Centers   95
Comprehensive Pain Centers   95
Sleep Disorders Centers   97
Voluntary Health Organizations   97

CHAPTER 4
Essential Pharmacokinetic Data   100
Pharmacokinetics of Commonly Used Drugs   101
Pharmacokinetic Data for Drug Monitoring   112

CHAPTER 5
New Products/Revised Drug Information/Other Agents   128
New Products   130
   Antiarrhythmics   134
   Antihypertensive Agents   138
   Antiviral Agents   139
   Bone/Calcium Metabolism Regulators   141
   Cephalosporins   142
   Fertility Inducers   143
   Miscellaneous Antibiotics   145
   Monobactam Antibiotics   148
   Ophthalmic Agents   150
   Oral Corticosteroids   151
   Penicillins   154
   Psoriasis Preparations   155
   Vaccines   158
Revised Drug Information   132
Other Agents   134
   Alcohol-Abuse Deterrents   159
   Antidotes   161
   Antiplatelet Agents   164
   Bone/Calcium Metabolism Regulators   165
   Chemonucleolytic Enzymes   168
   Gallstone-Dissolving Agents   172
   Patent Ductus Arteriosus Therapy   174
   Psychostimulants   176
   Smoking Deterrents   181
   Vaccines   183

CHAPTER 6
Acne Preparations/Antidandruff Shampoos   197
Acne Preparations   200
Antidandruff Shampoos   222

CHAPTER 7
Controlled Analgesics   228

CHAPTER 8
Nonnarcotic Analgesics/Antipyretics   276

CHAPTER 9
Antacids/Antiflatulents/Digestants   330
Antacids/Antiflatulents   334
Digestants   344

CHAPTER 10
Anthelmintics/Scabicides/Pediculicides   348
Anthelmintics   349
Scabicides/Pediculicides   353

CHAPTER 11
Antianginal Agents   357
Beta-Adrenergic Blockers   358
Calcium Antagonists   368
Nitrates   379

continued

Contents continued

CHAPTER 12
Antianxiety Agents   **404**
Benzodiazepines   405
Nonbenzodiazepines   417

CHAPTER 13
Antiarrhythmics   **428**

CHAPTER 14
Antiarthritic Agents   **474**

CHAPTER 15
Anticoagulants/Thrombolytic   **529**
Agents/Other Blood Modifiers
Anticoagulants   530
Thrombolytic Agents   541
Antifibrinolytic Agents   547
Hemorheologic Agents   548
Antiplatelet Agents   549
Hemostatic Agents   558

CHAPTER 16
Anticonvulsants/Antiparkinson   **560**
Agents
Barbiturates   562
Hydantoins   573
Succinimides   580
Miscellaneous Anticonvulsants   583
Antiparkinson Agents   597

CHAPTER 17
Antidepressants   **614**
Antidepressants   615
Antidepressant Combinations   644

CHAPTER 18
Antidiarrheal Agents/Oral   **653**
Electrolyte Solutions
Antidiarrheal Agents   654
Oral Electrolyte Solutions   665

CHAPTER 19
Antifungal/Antitrichomonal/   **668**
Antiviral Agents/Other
Topicals
Topical Agents   673
Vaginal Preparations   685
Systemic Agents   692

CHAPTER 20
Antigout Agents   **716**

CHAPTER 21
Antihistamines/Antipruritics/   **727**
Mast-Cell Stabilizers
Antihistamines/Antipruritics   729
Mast-Cell Stabilizers   749

CHAPTER 22
Antihypertensive Agents   **754**
Alpha-and Beta-Adrenergic Blockers   758
Angiotensin-Converting Enzyme Inhibitors   763
Beta-Adrenergic Blockers   767
Calcium Antagonists   783
Central Alpha$_2$-Adrenergic Agonists   788
Indolines   794
Peripheral Vasodilators   795
Sympatholytics   805
Antihypertensives with Diuretics   811

CHAPTER 23
Anti-Infectives: 1   **862**
Aminoglycosides   867
Sulfonamides   880
Miscellaneous Anti-Infective Agents   888

CHAPTER 24
Anti-Infectives: 2   **914**
Cephalosporins   920
Penicillins   966

CHAPTER 25
Anti-Infectives: 3   **1014**
Erythromycins   1016
Tetracyclines   1034

CHAPTER 26
Antimigraine Agents — 1048

CHAPTER 27
Antinauseants/Antiemetics — 1058

CHAPTER 28
Antineoplastic Agents — 1085
- Alkylating Agents — 1088
- Antimetabolites — 1098
- Antineoplastic Antibodies — 1103
- Hormones — 1111
- Interferons — 1114
- Miscellaneous Antineoplastic Agents — 1118

CHAPTER 29
Antiulcer/Antireflux/Antispasmodic Agents — 1126
- Antiulcer/Antireflux Agents — 1130
- Antispasmodics — 1138

CHAPTER 30
Bronchodilators/Antiasthmatic Agents — 1152
- Inhalant Bronchodilators/Antiasthmatic Agents — 1156
- Systemic Bronchodilators/Antiasthmatic Agents — 1178

CHAPTER 31
Cardiac Agents — 1231
- Angiotensin-Converting Enzyme Inhibitors — 1232
- Cardiac Glycosides — 1234
- Sympathomimetic Agents — 1241
- Miscellaneous Inotropic Agents — 1249

CHAPTER 32
Contraceptives — 1252

CHAPTER 33
Corticosteroids — 1309
- Oral and Injectable Corticosteroids — 1314
- Topical Corticosteroids — 1339
- Inhalant Corticosteroids — 1372
- Nasal Corticosteroids — 1380
- Rectal Corticosteroids/Hemorrhoidals — 1384

CHAPTER 34
Cough/Cold/Other Upper Respiratory Medications — 1394
- Summary Table — 1401
- Antitussives — 1409
- Antitussive Combinations — 1409
- Decongestants/Upper Respiratory Combinations — 1443
- Expectorants — 1462

CHAPTER 35
Diagnostics — 1464
- Blood Chemistry Tests — 1467
- Urine Chemistry Tests — 1469
- Fecal Occult Blood Tests — 1474
- Ovulation Tests — 1477
- Pregnancy Tests — 1480
- Bacterial Screening Tests — 1495
- Culture Tests — 1501
- Mononucleosis Tests — 1504
- Rubella Tests — 1508
- Rheumatoid Factor Tests — 1508
- Home Pregnancy Tests — 1466

CHAPTER 36
Diuretics — 1512
- Thiazide-Type Diuretics — 1515
- Loop Diuretics — 1526
- Potassium-Sparing Diuretics — 1530
- Carbonic Anhydrase Inhibitors — 1536
- Diuretic Combinations — 1537

CHAPTER 37
Hormones — 1546
- Androgens — 1550
- Estrogens — 1554
- Progestins — 1570
- Fertility Inducers — 1573
- Prolactin Inhibitors — 1581
- Growth Hormones — 1584
- Thyroid Hormones — 1585

CHAPTER 38
Hypoglycemic Agents — 1599
- Insulin — 1600
- Oral Hypoglycemic Agents — 1603

continued

Contents continued

CHAPTER 39	
Hypolipidemic Agents	**1615**

CHAPTER 40	
Laxatives/Stool Softeners	**1626**

CHAPTER 41	
Major Tranquilizers	**1646**
Antimanic Agents	1647
Butyrophenones	1654
Dibenzoxazepines	1657
Dihydroindolones	1659
Phenothiazines	1661
Thioxanthenes	1692

CHAPTER 42	
Muscle Relaxants	**1698**
Muscle Relaxants	1699
Muscle Relaxants with Analgesics	1712

CHAPTER 43	
Ophthalmic/Otic Preparations	**1720**
Antiglaucoma Agents/Miotics	1722
Mydriatics/Cycloplegics	1736
Ophthalmic Anti-Infectives	1738
Ophthalmic Corticosteroids	1755
Ophthalmic Decongestants/Antiallergic Agents	1759
Otic Analgesics/Anesthetics	1763
Otic Anti-Infectives	1765
Cerumen Softeners	1770

CHAPTER 44	
Potassium Supplements	**1773**

CHAPTER 45	
Sedatives/Hypnotics	**1792**
Barbiturates	1793
Nonbarbiturates	1807

CHAPTER 46	
Urinary Anti-Infectives/Other Urinary Agents	**1821**
Urinary Anti-Infectives	1823
Urinary Analgesics	1848
Urinary Antispasmodics	1850
Parasympathomimetics	1853

CHAPTER 47	
Vitamins/Minerals/Infant Formulas/Nutritionals	**1856**
Multivitamins/Multivitamins with Minerals	1857
B-Complex Vitamins/B-Complex with C Vitamins	1859
Hematinics	1861
Pediatric Vitamins	1863
Prenatal Vitamins with Minerals	1866
Calcium Supplements	1867
Nutritionals	1868
Infant Formulas	1871

Glossary	**1873**

Index

This index lists the brand and generic names of all products included in this Compendium. Brand names appear in CAPITAL LETTERS, whereas generic names are printed in upper- and lowercase letters.

A

ABBOKINASE, p. 541
ABBOKINASE OPEN-CATH, p. 541
ABDEC, p. 1863
ACCUTANE, p. 200
Acebutolol hydrochloride, p. 465, 778
Acetaminophen, p. 279, 280, 282, 283, 286, 293, 314, 315, 321, 326, 328
Acetaminophen, aspirin, and caffeine, p. 279
Acetaminophen and codeine phosphate, p. 229, 243, 257, 268
Acetaminophen and diphenhydramine citrate, p. 279
Acetaminophen and hydrocodone bitartrate, p. 229
Acetaminophen, pamabrom, and pyrilamine maleate, p. 279
Acetaminophen, phenylpropanolamine hydrochloride, and phenyltoloxamine citrate, p. 1456
Acetaminophen and phenyltoloxamine citrate, p. 315
Acetaminophen, phenyltoloxamine citrate, and caffeine, p. 279
Acetazolamide, p. 1536, 1724
ACETEST, p. 1467, 1469
Acetic acid, p. 1769
Acetophenazine maleate, p. 1684
Acetylcysteine, p. 161, 1170
ACHROMYCIN, p. 202, 1034
ACHROMYCIN Ointment, p. 671
ACHROMYCIN V, p. 202, 1034
ACLOVATE, p. 1339
ACTIDIL, p. 728
ACTIFED, p. 1401
ACTIFED with Codeine, p. 1409
ACTOL, p. 1401
Acyclovir, p. 685, 708
Acyclovir sodium, p. 709
ADALAT, p. 368
ADAPIN, p. 615
ADRENALIN, p. 1178
ADRIAMYCIN, p. 1103
ADVANCE, p. 1871
ADVANCE Pregnancy Test, p. 1466
ADVIL, p. 281
AEROBID, p. 1156, 1372
AEROLONE, p. 1154
AEROSEB-DEX, p. 1340
AEROSEB-HC, p. 1341
AEROSPORIN, p. 864
AFRIN, p. 1401
AFRINOL, p. 1401
AFTATE, p. 669
AGORAL, p. 1627
AGORAL Plain, p. 1627
A-HYDROCORT, p. 1311
AKINETON, p. 597
ALBUSTIX, p. 1469

Albuterol, p. 1172, 1177
Albuterol sulfate, p. 1199, 1200, 1229
Alclometasone dipropionate, p. 1339
ALCONEFRIN, p. 1401
ALDACTAZIDE, p. 1537
ALDACTONE, p. 1530
ALDEFLOR, p. 1863
ALDEFLOR Drops, p. 1863
ALDEFLOR M, p. 1863
ALDOCLOR, p. 811
ALDOMET, p. 788
ALDORIL, p. 813
ALGICON, p. 334
ALKA MINTS, p. 331, 1867
ALKA-SELTZER, p. 331, 334
ALKA-SELTZER PLUS, p. 1401
ALKERAN, p. 1088
ALKETS, p. 331
ALLBEE C-800, p. 1859
ALLBEE C-800 plus Iron, p. 1859
ALLBEE with C, p. 1859
ALLBEE-T, p. 1859
ALLEREST, p. 1401
Allopurinol, p. 722, 724
Alprazolam, p. 416
Alseroxylon, p. 756
ALternaGEL, p. 334
ALU-CAP, p. 332
ALUDROX, p. 332
Aluminum carbonate gel, basic, p. 335
Aluminum hydroxide, p. 334
Aluminum hydroxide and magnesium carbonate, p. 332, 336
Aluminum hydroxide/magnesium carbonate gel and magnesium carbonate, p. 334
Aluminum hydroxide and magnesium hydroxide, p. 332, 333
Aluminum hydroxide, magnesium hydroxide, and simethicone, p. 333, 337, 339
Aluminum hydroxide and magnesium trisilicate, p. 336
Aluminum hydroxide gel, p. 332
Aluminum hydroxide gel and magnesium hydroxide, p. 332
Aluminum hydroxide gel, magnesium hydroxide, and simethicone, p. 342
ALUPENT, p. 1180
ALUPENT Inhalant Solution, p. 1157
ALUPENT Metered Dose Inhaler, p. 1158
ALURATE, p. 1792
ALU-TAB, p. 332
Amantadine hydrochloride, p. 612, 704
AMBENYL, p. 1411
AMBENYL-D, p. 1401
AMCILL, p. 966
Amcinonide, p. 1351
Amdinocillin, p. 974, 1831
AMEN, p. 1549
AMERICAINE-Otic, p. 1763
A-METHAPRED, p. 1311
AMICAR, p. 547
Amikacin, p. 113
Amikacin sulfate, p. 867
AMIKIN, p. 867
Amiloride hydrochloride, p. 1534
Amiloride hydrochloride and

hydrochlorothiazide, p. 1543
9-Aminoacridine hydrochloride, polyoxyethylene nonyl phenol, sodium edetate, and sodium dioctyl sulfosuccinate, p. 691
Aminocaproic acid, p. 547
AMINOPHYLLIN, p. 1181
AMINOPHYLLIN Injection, p. 1154
Aminophylline, p. 1154, 1181
Aminophylline, anhydrous, p. 1211
Aminophylline and guaifenesin, p. 1155
Amiodarone, p. 434
Amitryptiline, p. 113
Amitriptyline hydrochloride, p. 620, 622
Amobarbital, p. 562, 1793
Amobarbital sodium, p. 562, 1793
Amoxapine, p. 616
Amoxicillin, p. 967, 979, 995, 1010
Amoxicillin and clavulanate potassium, p. 968
Amoxicillin trihydrate, p. 918
AMOXIL, p. 967
AMPHOJEL, p. 332
Amphotericin B, p. 696
Ampicillin, p. 966, 983, 993, 996, 1001, 1009, 1010
Ampicillin and probenecid, p. 916
Ampicillin sodium, p. 983, 993, 1009
Ampicillin sodium and sulbactam sodium, p. 154
Amrinone lactate, p. 1249
Amyl nitrite, p. 357
AMYTAL, p. 562, 1793
AMYTAL Sodium, p. 562, 1793
ANACIN, p. 281, 476
ANACIN-3, p. 282
ANAPROX, p. 284, 477
ANASPAZ, p. 1128
ANCEF, p. 920
ANCOBON, p. 692
ANDROID, p. 1547
ANHYDRON, p. 1513
Anisotropine methylbromide, p. 1129
ANSPOR, p. 921
ANTABUSE, p. 159
ANTIMINTH, p. 349
Antipyrine and benzocaine, p. 1764
ANTIVERT, p. 1060
ANTRENYL, p. 1128
ANTROCOL, p. 1128
ANTURANE, p. 717
ANUSOL, p. 1384
ANUSOL-HC, p. 1385
APF ARTHRITIS PAIN FORMULA, p. 286
APRESAZIDE, p. 815
APRESOLINE, p. 795
APRESOLINE-ESIDRIX, p. 756
Aprobarbital, p. 1792
AQUATENSEN, p. 1513
ARAMINE, p. 1241
ARFONAD, p. 756, 805
ARISTOCORT, p. 1314
ARISTOCORT A Cream and Ointment, p. 1342
ARISTOCORT Cream and Ointment, p. 1342
ARISTOSPAN, p. 1311
A.R.M., p. 1401

COMPENDIUM OF DRUG THERAPY

ARM-A-MED Isoetharine Hydrochloride, p. 1158
ARMOUR Thyroid, p. 1585
ARTANE, p. 598
ARTHRITIS PAIN FORMULA, p. 286, 479
ARTHROPAN, p. 287, 479
ASBRON G, p. 1154
ASCRIPTIN, p. 288, 289, 480, 549
ASCRIPTIN A/D, p. 288, 481, 550
ASCRIPTIN with Codeine, p. 229
ASENDIN, p. 616
Asparaginase, p. 1086
Aspirin, p. 114, 279, 280, 290, 296, 297, 320, 482, 498, 500, 551, 554, 556
Aspirin and acetaminophen, p. 300
Aspirin, acetaminophen, caffeine, dried aluminum hydroxide gel, and magnesium hydroxide, p. 280
Aspirin, aluminum glycinate, and magnesium carbonate, p. 292, 484, 553
Aspirin, aluminum hydroxide, and magnesium hydroxide, p. 286, 479
Aspirin and caffeine, p. 281, 325, 476, 524
Aspirin, caffeine, magnesium hydroxide, and dried aluminum hydroxide gel, p. 279
Aspirin, cinnamedrine hydrochloride, and caffeine, p. 279
Aspirin and codeine phosphate, p. 241
Aspirin, magnesium hydroxide, and aluminum hydroxide, p. 288, 480, 481, 549, 550
Aspirin, magnesium oxide, and dried aluminum hydroxide gel, p. 279
Aspirin, magnesium-aluminum hydroxide, and codeine phosphate, p. 229
Aspirin and phenyltoloxamine citrate, p. 279
Aspirin, sodium bicarbonate, and citric acid, p. 331
ATARAX, p. 417, 729
ATARAX 100, p. 417, 729
Atenolol, p. 366, 779
Atenolol and chlorthalidone, p. 853
ATIVAN, p. 405
ATIVAN Injection, p. 406
ATROMID-S, p. 1616
Atropine methyl nitrate and pancreatic enzymes, p. 333
Atropine sulfate, p. 1128
Atropine sulfate and phenobarbital, p. 1128
Atropine sulfate, scopolamine hydrobromide, hyoscyamine sulfate, and phenobarbital, p. 1129
A/T/S, p. 204
Attapulgite, p. 654, 658, 664
AUGMENTIN, p. 968
AURALGAN Otic Solution, p. 1764
Auranofin, p. 519
AUREOMYCIN Ointment, p. 671
Aurothioglucose, p. 522
AVAIL, p. 1867
AVC, p. 685
AVITENE, p. 558
AXOTAL, p. 279
AYGESTIN, p. 1549
AZACTAM, p. 148
Azatadine maleate, p. 735
Azatadine maleate and pseudoephedrine sulfate, p. 1460
Azathioprine, p. 503
AZLIN, p. 970
Azlocillin sodium, p. 970
AZMACORT, p. 1159, 1374

AZO GANTANOL, p. 1823
AZO GANTRISIN, p. 1824
AZOLID, p. 475
AZOSTIX, p. 1467
Aztreonam, p. 148
AZULFIDINE, p. 880

B

Bacampicillin hydrochloride, p. 1002
BACID, p. 653
BACIGUENT, p. 671
Bacitracin, p. 671
Bacitracin, neomycin sulfate, and polymyxin B sulfate, p. 672
Baclofen, p. 1701
BACTIGEN Group A *Streptococcus*, p. 1495
BACTIGEN *H. influenzae*, p. 1495
BACTIGEN *N. meningitidis*, p. 1496
BACTIGEN *S. pneumoniae*, p. 1496
BACTRIM, p. 888, 1826
BACTRIM DS, p. 888, 1826
BACTRIM I.V. Infusion, p. 890, 1828
BACTURCULT, p. 1501
BANCAP HC, p. 229
BANTHINE, p. 1128
BARBIDONNA, p. 1128
BASALJEL, p. 335
BAYER Aspirin, p. 290, 482, 551
BAYER Children's Cold Tablets, p. 1401
BAYER Cough Syrup for Children, p. 1401
b-CAPSA I, p. 183
Beclomethasone dipropionate, p. 1161, 1176, 1376, 1379, 1380, 1383
BECLOVENT, p. 1161, 1376
BECONASE, p. 1380
BECOTIN, p. 1859
BECOTIN with Vitamin C, p. 1859
BECOTIN-T, p. 1859
Beef insulin, p. 1600, 1601
Beef and pork insulin, p. 1600, 1601
BELAP, p. 1128
BELLADENAL, p. 1138
BELLADENAL-S, p. 1138
Belladonna and opium, p. 229
Belladonna alkaloids, levorotatory, p. 1128
Belladonna alkaloids and phenobarbital, p. 1138
Belladonna extract and butabarbital sodium, p. 1128
Belladonna extract and phenobarbital, p. 1129
Belladonna tincture, p. 1128
BELLAFOLINE, p. 1128
BELLERGAL-S, p. 1139
BEMINAL 500, p. 1859
BEMINAL Forte, p. 1859
BEMINAL STRESS PLUS with Iron, p. 1859
BEMINAL STRESS PLUS with Zinc, p. 1859
BENADRYL, p. 599, 600, 730, 1058, 1401
BENADRYL Cream, p. 728
Bendroflumethiazide, p. 1513
BENEMID, p. 717
BENTYL, p. 1141
BENYLIN, p. 1401
BENYLIN DM, p. 1401
BENYLIN DME, p. 1401
BENZAC, p. 204
BENZAC W, p. 204
BENZAC W Wash, p. 204
BENZAGEL, p. 205
BENZAMYCIN, p. 206

BENZEDREX, p. 1401
Benzocaine, p. 1763
Benzocaine, 8-hydroxyquinoline sulfate, menthol, zinc oxide, and balsam Peru, p. 1389
Benzonatate, p. 1409
Benzoyl peroxide, p. 198, 199, 204, 205, 206, 208, 209, 211, 214, 215, 216, 217, 219
Benzoyl peroxide and hydrocortisone, p. 221
Benzquinamide hydrochloride, p. 1065
Benzthiazide, p. 1513
Benztropine mesylate, p. 601
Benzyl benzoate, Peruvian balsam, zinc oxide, and pramoxine hydrochloride, p. 1384
BEROCCA, p. 1859
BEROCCA Parenteral Nutrition, p. 1857
BEROCCA Plus, p. 1857
BETADINE, p. 671
BETAGAN, p. 1722
Betamethasone, p. 1317
Betamethasone benzoate, p. 1313
Betamethasone dipropionate, p. 1353, 1354
Betamethasone sodium phosphate, p. 1317
Betamethasone sodium phosphate and betamethasone acetate, p. 1317
Betamethasone valerate, p. 1369
BETAPEN-VK, p. 915
Betaxolol hydrochloride, p. 1723
Bethanechol chloride, p. 1853, 1854
BETOPTIC, p. 1723
βhCG-ROCHE EIA, p. 1480
BICILLIN C-R, p. 971
BICILLIN C-R 900/300, p. 971
BICILLIN L-A, p. 972
BiCNU, p. 1089
Bi-K, p. 1773
BILI-LABSTIX, p. 1469
BILI-LABSTIX SG, p. 1469
BILTRICIDE, p. 348
BIOCAL Chewable, p. 1867
BIOCAL Swallowable, p. 1867
BIOZYME-C, p. 711
Biperiden, p. 597
Bisacodyl, p. 1627, 1633
Bisacodyl tannex, p. 1627
Bismuth subgallate, bismuth resorcin compound, benzyl benzoate, Peruvian balsam, and zinc oxide, p. 1384
Bismuth subsalicylate, p. 663, 1068
Bitolterol mesylate, p. 1175
BLENOXANE, p. 1105
Bleomycin sulfate, p. 1105
BLEPH-10, p. 1738
BLEPHAMIDE, p. 1739
BLOCADREN, p. 767
β-NEOCEPT 30, p. 1482
B&O, p. 229
BONINE, p. 1058
BQ, p. 1401
BREONESIN, p. 1401
BRETHAIRE, p. 1162
BRETHINE, p. 1182
Bretylium tosylate, p. 429
BRETYLOL, p. 429
BREVIBLOC, p. 134
BREVICON 21-DAY, p. 1255
BREVICON 28-DAY, p. 1255
BRICANYL, p. 1183
Bromocriptine mesylate, p. 607, 1574, 1581
Bromodiphenhydramine hydrochloride and codeine phosphate, p. 1411

Brompheniramine maleate, p. 733
Brompheniramine maleate, phenylpropanolamine hydrochloride, and codeine phosphate, p. 1414
Brompheniramine maleate, pseudoephedrine hydrochloride, and dextromethorphan hydrobromide, p. 1416
BRONDECON, p. 1184
BRONKAID MIST, p. 1154
BRONKEPHRINE, p. 1154
BRONKODYL, p. 1185
BRONKOLIXIR, p. 1154
BRONKOMETER, p. 1163
BRONKOSOL, p. 1163
BUCLADIN-S, p. 1058
Buclazine hydrochloride, p. 1058
BUFFERIN, p. 292, 484, 553
BUGS BUNNY, p. 1863
BUGS BUNNY plus Iron, p. 1863
BUGS BUNNY + Minerals, p. 1863
BUGS BUNNY with Extra C, p. 1863
Bumetanide, p. 1526
BUMEX, p. 1526
BUMINTEST, p. 1471
BUPRENEX, p. 231
Buprenorphine hydrochloride, p. 231
BUSPAR, p. 418
Buspirone hydrochloride, p. 418
Busulfan, p. 1087
Butabarbital, sodium, p. 1794
Butalbital, acetaminophen, and caffeine, p. 299
Butalbital and aspirin, p. 279
Butalbital, aspirin, and caffeine, p. 246
Butalbital, aspirin, caffeine, and codeine phosphate, p. 247
Butalbital, caffeine, and acetaminophen, p. 279
BUTAZOLIDIN, p. 485
BUTIBEL, p. 1128
BUTICAPS, p. 1794
BUTISOL Sodium, p. 1794
Butoconazole nitrate, p. 686
Butorphanol tartrate, p. 322

C

CAFERGOT, p. 1049
CAFERGOT P-B, p. 1049
CALADRYL, p. 728
Calamine and diphenhydramine hydrochloride, p. 728
CALAN, p. 370, 430, 783
CALAN SR, p. 370, 430, 783
CALAN Injection, p. 432
CALCIDRINE, p. 1412
CALCIMAR, p. 165
CALCIPARINE, p. 530
Calcitonin-human, p. 141
Calcitonin-salmon, p. 165
CALCITREL, p. 332
Calcium carbonate, p. 331, 332, 343
Calcium carbonate, aluminum hydroxide, magnesium hydroxide, and simethicone, p. 333
Calcium carbonate, magnesium carbonate, and magnesium oxide, p. 331
Calcium carbonate and magnesium hydroxide, p. 332, 333
Calcium polycarbophil, p. 661, 1638
CALEL-D, p. 1867
CAL SUP 300, p. 1867
CAL SUP 600, p. 1867
CAL SUP 600 Plus, p. 1867
CAL SUP Instant 1000, p. 1867

CALTRATE 600, p. 1867
CALTRATE 600 + Iron and Vitamin D, p. 1867
CALTRATE 600 + Vitamin D, p. 1867
CAMA, p. 279
CAMALOX, p. 336
Camphorated tincture of opium, p. 661
CANTIL, p. 1128
CAPITAL with Codeine, p. 229
CAPOTEN, p. 763, 1232
CAPOZIDE, p. 818
Captopril, p. 763, 1232
Captopril and hydrochlorothiazide, p. 818
CARAFATE, p. 1130
Caramiphen edisylate and phenylpropanolamine hydrochloride, p. 1442
Carbamazepine, p. 114, 589
Carbamide peroxide, p. 1771, 1772
Carbenicillin disodium, p. 977, 999
Carbenicillin indanyl sodium, p. 976, 1834
Carbetapentane tannate, chlorpheniramine tannate, ephedrine tannate, and phenylephrine tannate, p. 1433
Carbidopa and levodopa, p. 610
Carbinoxamine maleate, p. 728
Carbinoxamine maleate and pseudoephedrine hydrochloride, p. 1453
Carbinoxamine maleate, pseudoephedrine hydrochloride, and dextromethorphan hydrobromide, p. 1429
CARDILATE, p. 379
CARDIZEM, p. 372
Carisoprodol, p. 1708
Carisoprodol and aspirin, p. 1716
Carisoprodol, aspirin, and codeine phosphate, p. 1717
CARMOL HC, p. 1343
Carmustine (BCNU), p. 1089
CAROID, p. 1627
Casanthranol and docusate sodium, p. 1641
Cascara sagrada extract and phenolphthalein, p. 1627
CATAPRES, p. 789
CATAPRES-TTS, p. 791
CEBENASE, p. 1860
CECLOR, p. 923
CEDILANID-D, p. 1231
CeeNU, p. 1090
Cefaclor, p. 923
Cefadroxil, p. 933, 960
CEFADYL, p. 924
Cefamandole nafate, p. 944
Cefazolin sodium, p. 920, 942
CEFIZOX, p. 926
CEFOBID, p. 927
CEFOL, p. 1860
Cefonicid sodium, p. 948
Cefoperazone sodium, p. 927
Ceforanide, p. 952
CEFOTAN, p. 929
Cefotaxime sodium, p. 931
Cefotetan disodium, p. 929
Cefoxitin sodium, p. 946
Ceftazidime, p. 934, 956, 958
Ceftizoxime sodium, p. 926
Ceftriaxone sodium, p. 954
Cefuroxime sodium, p. 940, 964
CELESTONE, p. 1317
CELESTONE Phosphate, p. 1317
CELESTONE SOLUSPAN, p. 1317
Cellulase, pancreatin, glutamic acid hydrochloride, ox bile extract, and pepsin, p. 345

CELONTIN, p. 580
CENTRAX, p. 407
CENTRUM, p. 1857
CENTRUM, Jr., p. 1864
CENTRUM, Jr. + Extra C, p. 1864
CENTRUM, Jr. + Extra Calcium, p. 1864
CENTRUM, Jr. + Iron, p. 1864
Cephalexin, p. 142, 936
Cephalothin sodium, p. 919, 938
Cephapirin sodium, p. 924
Cephradine, p. 921, 961
CEROSE-DM, p. 1401
CERUBIDINE, p. 1106
CERUMENEX, p. 1770
CE-VI-SOL, p. 1864
CHARDONNA-2, p. 1129
CHEMSTRIP 3, p. 1472
CHEMSTRIP 4, p. 1472
CHEMSTRIP 5, p. 1472
CHEMSTRIP 5L, p. 1472
CHEMSTRIP 6, p. 1472
CHEMSTRIP 6L, p. 1472
CHEMSTRIP 7, p. 1472
CHEMSTRIP 7L, p. 1472
CHEMSTRIP 8, p. 1472
CHEMSTRIP 9, p. 1472
CHEMSTRIP bG, p. 1467
CHEMSTRIP uG, p. 1472
CHEMSTRIP uGK, p. 1472
CHEMSTRIP GP, p. 1472
CHEMSTRIP K, p. 1472
CHEMSTRIP L, p. 1472
CHEMSTRIP LN, p. 1472
CHENIX, p. 172
Chenodiol, p. 172
CHERACOL, p. 1396
CHERACOL D, p. 1401
CHERACOL PLUS, p. 1401
CHEXIT, p. 1401
Chloral hydrate, p. 1811
Chlorambucil, p. 1094
Chloramphenicol, p. 115, 672, 892, 1765
Chloramphenicol and polymyxin B sulfate, p. 1742
Chloramphenicol palmitate, p. 892
Chloramphenicol sodium succinate, p. 892
Chlorcyclizine hydrochloride and hydrocortisone acetate, p. 1313
Chlordiazepoxide and amitriptyline hydrochloride, p. 647
Chlordiazepoxide and esterified estrogens, p. 1549
Chlordiazepoxide hydrochloride, p. 408
Chlordiazepoxide hydrochloride and clidinium bromide, p. 1147
Chlorhexidine gluconate, p. 672
Chlormezanone, p. 424
CHLOROMYCETIN, p. 892
CHLOROMYCETIN Cream, p. 672
CHLOROMYCETIN Otic, p. 1765
CHLOROMYCETIN Palmitate, p. 892
CHLOROMYCETIN Sodium Succinate, p. 892
CHLOROMYXIN, p. 1742
Chlorothiazide, p. 1516
Chlorothiazide and reserpine, p. 825
Chlorothiazide sodium, p. 1516
Chlorotrianisene, p. 1569
Chlorphenesin carbamate, p. 1703
Chlorpheniramine maleate, p. 731, 732, 746
Chlorpheniramine maleate and phenylephrine hydrochloride, p. 1399
Chlorpheniramine maleate, phenylephrine hydrochloride, and methscopolamine

COMPENDIUM OF DRUG THERAPY

nitrate, p. 1399
Chlorpheniramine maleate and phenylpropanolamine hydrochloride, p. 1449
Chlorpheniramine maleate, phenyltoloxamine citrate, and phenylephrine hydrochloride, p. 1443
Chlorpheniramine maleate and pseudoephedrine hydrochloride, p. 1398, 1399, 1444
Chlorpheniramine maleate, pseudoephedrine hydrochloride, and dextromethorphan hydrobromide, p. 1397
Chlorpromazine hydrochloride, p. 1075, 1680
Chlorpropamide, p. 1605
Chlorprothixene, p. 1694
Chlortetracycline hydrochloride, p. 671
Chlorthalidone, p. 1513, 1523
Chlorthalidone and reserpine, p. 845
CHLOR-TRIMETON, p. 731
CHLOR-TRIMETON Decongestant, p. 1401
CHLOR-TRIMETON Injection, p. 732
Chlorzoxazone, p. 1704
Chlorzoxazone and acetaminophen, p. 1714
CHOLEDYL, p. 1188
CHOLEDYL SA, p. 1188
Cholestyramine, p. 1623
Choline magnesium trisalicylate, p. 527
Choline salicylate, p. 287, 479
CHOLOXIN, p. 1617
Chorionic gonadotropin, human (HCG), p. 1579
CHRONULAC, p. 1629
CHYMODIACTIN, p. 168
Chymopapain, p. 168, 170
CIBACALCIN, p. 141
CIBALITH-S, p. 1647
Ciclopirox olamine, p. 674
Cimetidine, p. 1135
CINOBAC, p. 1830
Cinoxacin, p. 1830
Cisplatin, p. 1123
CITRUCEL, p. 1629
CLAFORAN, p. 931
CLEARASIL, p. 206
CLEARBLUE, p. 1466
Clemastine fumarate, p. 744, 745
Clemastine fumarate and phenylpropanolamine hydrochloride, p. 1457
CLEOCIN HCl, p. 894
CLEOCIN PEDIATRIC, p. 894
CLEOCIN PHOSPHATE, p. 894
CLEOCIN T, p. 207
Clidinium bromide, p. 1129
Clindamycin hydrochloride, p. 894
Clindamycin palmitate hydrochloride, p. 894
Clindamycin phosphate, p. 207, 894
CLINISTIX, p. 1469
CLINITEST, p. 1473
CLINORIL, p. 488
Clioquinol, p. 670
Clioquinol and hydrocortisone, p. 1370
CLISTIN, p. 728
Clobetasol propionate, p. 1366
Clocortolone pivalate, p. 1344
CLODERM, p. 1344
Clofibrate, p. 1616
CLOMID, p. 1573
Clomiphene citrate, p. 1573, 1580
Clonazepam, p. 585
Clonidine, p. 791

Clonidine hydrochloride, p. 789
Clonidine hydrochloride and chlorthalidone, p. 821
Clorazepate dipotassium, p. 413, 592
Clotrimazole, p. 675, 677, 678, 687, 688
Clotrimazole and betamethasone dipropionate, p. 676
Cloxacillin sodium, p. 1004
CLUVISOL, p. 1857
CLUVISOL 130, p. 1857
CLYSODRAST, p. 1627
COACTIN, p. 974, 1831
Coal tar, p. 226
Coal tar, menthol, and alcohol, p. 222
Coal tar and parachlorometaxylenol, p. 227
Cocoa butter, zinc oxide, and bismuth subgallate, p. 1390
Codeine and calcium iodide, p. 1412
Codeine phosphate, p. 232
Codeine phosphate, carbetapentane citrate, chlorpheniramine maleate, guaifenesin, sodium citrate, and citric acid, p. 1398
Codeine phosphate and guaifenesin, p. 1396
Codeine phosphate, phenylephrine hydrochloride, chlorpheniramine maleate, and potassium iodide, p. 1398
Codeine phosphate, phenylpropanolamine hydrochloride, and guaifenesin, p. 1434
Codeine phosphate, pseudoephedrine hydrochloride, and chlorpheniramine maleate, p. 1419, 1431
Codeine phosphate, pseudoephedrine hydrochloride, and guaifenesin, p. 1397, 1398, 1420, 1432
Codeine polistirex and chlorpheniramine polistirex, p. 1421
Codeine sulfate, p. 232, 1397
Codeine sulfate and papaverine hydrochloride, p. 1397
Codeine sulfate and terpin hydrate, p. 1398
COGENTIN, p. 601
CO-GESIC, p. 229
COLACE, p. 1630
ColBENEMID, p. 719
Colchicine, p. 721
COLESTID, p. 1618
Colestipol hydrochloride, p. 1618
Colistimethate sodium, p. 896
Colistin sulfate, p. 897
Colistin sulfate, neomycin sulfate, thonzonium bromide, and hydrocortisone acetate, p. 1766
Collagenase, p. 711, 713
COLOGEL, p. 1627
COLOSCREEN Self Test (CS-T), p. 1474
COLREX, p. 1401
COLREX Compound, p. 1397
COLY-MYCIN M, p. 896
COLY-MYCIN S, p. 897
COLY-MYCIN S Otic, p. 1766
COMBIPRES, p. 821
COMBISTIX, p. 1469
COMHIST, p. 1443
COMHIST LA, p. 1443
COMOXOL, p. 1822
COMPAZINE, p. 1060, 1661
COMTREX, p. 1402
COMTREX A/S, p. 1402
CONAR, p. 1402
CONAR-A, p. 1402
CONCEPTROL, p. 1254
CONEX, p. 1402

CONEX with Codeine, p. 1397
CONGESPIRIN, p. 1402
CONGESPIRIN Aspirin Free, p. 1402
CONGESTAC, p. 1402
CONSTANT-T, p. 1190
CONTAC, p. 1402
CONTAC Jr., p. 1402
COPAVIN, p. 1397
COPE, p. 279
CO-PYRONIL 2, p. 1402
CORDARONE, p. 434
CORDRAN, p. 1345
CORDRAN SP, p. 1345
CORDRAN-N, p. 1347
CORGARD, p. 358, 769
CORICIDIN, p. 1402
CORICIDIN 'D', p. 1402
CORILIN, p. 1402
CORRECTOL, p. 1627
CORTAID, p. 1312
CORT-DOME Cream and Lotion, p. 1348
CORT-DOME Suppositories, p. 1386
CORTEF, p. 1320
CORTEF ACETATE, p. 1320
CORTEF ACETATE Ointment, p. 1348
CORTEF Feminine Itch Cream, p. 1312
CORTEF Oral Suspension, p. 1320
CORTENEMA, p. 1386
CORTICAINE, p. 1388
Cortisone acetate, p. 1323
CORTISPORIN Cream, p. 1349
CORTISPORIN Ointment, p. 1350
CORTISPORIN Ophthalmic Ointment, p. 1740
CORTISPORIN Ophthalmic Suspension, p. 1741
CORTISPORIN Otic Solution, p. 1767
CORTISPORIN Otic Suspension, p. 1767
CORTRIL, p. 1312
CORYBAN-D, p. 1402
CORZIDE, p. 823
COSMEGEN, p. 1086
COTAZYM, p. 344
COTAZYM-S, p. 344
COTRIM, p. 1822
CoTYLENOL, p. 1402
COUMADIN, p. 532
COVANGESIC, p. 1402
CREMACOAT, p. 1402, 1403
CREAMALIN, p. 332
CRITICARE HN, p. 1868
Cromolyn sodium, p. 749, 750, 752, 1165, 1166, 1762
Cryptenamine tannate and methyclothiazide, p. 756
CRYSTODIGIN, p. 437, 1234
CULTURETTE 10-Minute Group A Strep ID, p. 1497
CUPRIMINE, p. 490
CUTICURA, p. 208
Cyclacillin, p. 975
CYCLAPEN-W, p. 975
Cyclizine, p. 1059
Cyclobenzaprine hydrochloride, p. 1700
CYCLOCORT, p. 1351
CYCLOGYL, p. 1736
Cyclopentolate hydrochloride, p. 1736
Cyclophosphamide, p. 1091
Cyclothiazide, p. 1513
CYLERT, p. 176
Cyproheptadine hydrochloride, p. 737
CYSTOSPAZ, p. 1850
CYSTOSPAZ-M, p. 1850
Cytarabine (ara-C), p. 1098
CYTOMEL, p. 1587
CYTOSAR-U, p. 1098
CYTOXAN, p. 1091

D

Dacarbazine, p. 1093
Dactinomycin, p. 1086
DAISY 2, p. 1466
DALMANE, p. 1807
Danazol, p. 1550
DANOCRINE, p. 1550
Danthron, p. 1638
Danthron and docusate sodium, p. 1628, 1631
DANTRIUM, p. 1699
Dantrolene sodium, p. 1699
DARBID, p. 1129
DARICON, p. 1129
DARVOCET-N 50, p. 233
DARVOCET-N 100, p. 233
DARVON, p. 235
DARVON Compound, p. 236
DARVON Compound-65, p. 236
DARVON with A.S.A., p. 229
DARVON-N, p. 235
DARVON-N with A.S.A., p. 229
DATRIL, Extra-Strength, p. 293
Daunorubicin hydrochloride, p. 1106
DAYALETS, p. 1857
DAYALETS + Iron, p. 1857
DAYCARE, p. 1403
DEBROX, p. 1771
DECADERM, p. 1352
DECADRON, p. 1325
DECADRON Phosphate, p. 1325, 1352
DECADRON Phosphate Ophthalmic, p. 1755
DECADRON-LA Suspension, p. 1325
DECASPRAY, p. 1352
DECHOLIN, p. 1627
DECLOMYCIN, p. 1036
DECONAMINE, p. 1444
DECONAMINE SR, p. 1444
DECONGEST, p. 1403
Dehydrocholic acid, p. 1627
DELATESTRYL, p. 1547
DELCID, p. 332
DELESTROGEN, p. 1548
DELFEN, p. 1254
DELSYM, p. 1403
DELTA-CORTEF, p. 1312
DELTASONE, p. 1328
DEMAZIN, p. 1403
Demeclocycline hydrochloride, p. 1036
DEMEROL, p. 238
DEMEROL APAP, p. 229
Demi-REGROTON, p. 845
DEMULEN 1/35-21, p. 1257
DEMULEN 1/35-28, p. 1257
DEMULEN 1/50-21, p. 1260
DEMULEN 1/50-28, p. 1260
DENOREX, p. 222
DEPAKENE, p. 583
DEPAKOTE, p. 583
DEPEN, p. 492
DEPO-ESTRADIOL, p. 1548
DEPO-MEDROL, p. 1330
DEPONIT, p. 379
DEPO-PROVERA, p. 1549
DEPO-Testosterone, p. 1551
DEPROL, p. 614
DERMOLATE, p. 1312
DESENEX, p. 670
Deserpidine, p. 756
Desipramine, p. 115
Desipramine hydrochloride, p. 614, 629
Deslanoside, p. 1231
Desonide, p. 1368
Desonide and acetic acid, p. 1768
Desoximetasone, p. 1367
DESQUAM-X, p. 209

DESQUAM-X Wash, p. 209
DESYREL, p. 618
DETECT-A-STREP, p. 1497
Dexamethasone, p. 1312, 1325, 1340, 1352
Dexamethasone, neomycin sulfate, and polymyxin B sulfate, p. 1745
Dexamethasone acetate, p. 1325
Dexamethasone sodium phosphate, p. 1173, 1312, 1325, 1352, 1377, 1755
Dexamethasone sodium phosphate and neomycin sulfate, p. 1313
Dexbrompheniramine maleate and pseudoephedrine sulfate, p. 1398
Dexchlorpheniramine maleate, p. 742
Dexchlorpheniramine maleate, pseudoephedrine sulfate, and guaifenesin, p. 1399
DEXEDRINE, p. 178
Dexpanthenol and choline bitartrate, p. 337
Dextroamphetamine sulfate, p. 178
Dextromethorphan hydrobromide and guaifenesin, p. 1398
Dextromethorphan hydrobromide, pseudoephedrine hydrochloride, and guaifenesin, p. 1398
Dextrose, levulose, and phosphoric acid, p. 1066
DEXTROSTIX, p. 1468
Dextrothyroxine sodium, p. 1617
D.H.E. 45, p. 1048
DIAβETA, p. 1603
DIABINESE, p. 1605
DIALOSE, p. 1630
DIALOSE Plus, p. 1631
DIAMOX, p. 1536, 1724
DIASORB, p. 654
DIASTIX, p. 1469
Diazepam, p. 414, 415, 594, 1709, 1710
Diazoxide, p. 797
DIBENZYLINE, p. 756
Dibucaine, p. 1390
DICAL-D, p. 1867
DICAL-D Wafers, p. 1867
DICARBOSIL, p. 332
Dicloxacillin sodium, p. 916
Dicumarol, p. 529
Dicyclomine hydrochloride, p. 1141
DIDRONEL, p. 167
Dienestrol, p. 1548, 1564
Diethylstilbestrol, p. 1554
Diflorasone diacetate, p. 1313, 1355, 1363
Diflunisal, p. 294, 496
DI-GEL, p. 332
Digitalis, p. 1231
Digitoxin, p. 116, 437, 1234
Digoxin, p. 116, 446, 447, 1237
Dihydrocodeine bitartrate, aspirin, and caffeine, p. 261
Dihydroergotamine mesylate, p. 1048
Dihydroxyaluminum sodium carbonate, p. 333
p-Diisobutylphenoxypolyethoxyethanol, p. 1254
DILANTIN, p. 573
DILANTIN Parenteral, p. 575
DILANTIN with Phenobarbital, p. 561
DILATRATE-SR, p. 380
DILAUDID, p. 240
DILAUDID Cough Syrup, p. 1413
DILAUDID-HP, p. 229
DILONE, p. 279
DILOR-G, p. 1154
Diltiazem hydrochloride, p. 372
DIMACOL, p. 1403

Dimenhydrinate, p. 1064
DIMENSYN, p. 279
DIMETANE, p. 733
DIMETANE Decongestant, p. 1403
DIMETANE-DC, p. 1414
DIMETANE-DX, p. 1416
DIMETANE-TEN, p. 733
DIMETAPP, p. 1403
DIOSTATE-D, p. 1867
Diphenhydramine hydrochloride, p. 599, 600, 728, 730, 1058
Diphenidol, p. 1059
Diphenoxylate hydrochloride and atropine sulfate, p. 659
Diphenylpyraline hydrochloride, p. 728
Diphtheria and tetanus toxoids and pertussis vaccine, adsorbed, p. 183, 196
Dipivefrin hydrochloride, p. 1733
DIPROLENE, p. 1353
DIPROSONE, p. 1354
Dipyridamole, p. 164
DISALCID, p. 495
DISCASE, p. 170
DISIPAL, p. 561
DISOPHROL, p. 1398
Disopyramide, p. 117
Disopyramide phosphate, p. 453
Disulfiram, p. 159
DITROPAN, p. 1851
DIUCARDIN, p. 1513
DIULO, p. 1515
DIUPRES, p. 825
DIURIL, p. 1516
DIURIL, Sodium, p. 1516
DIUTENSEN, p. 756
DIUTENSEN-R, p. 756
Divalproex sodium, p. 583
Dobutamine hydrochloride, p. 1242
DOBUTREX, p. 1242
Docusate calcium, p. 1644
Docusate calcium and danthron, p. 1632
Docusate potassium, p. 1627, 1630
Docusate potassium and casanthranol, p. 1631
Docusate sodium, p. 1630, 1632, 1643
Docusate sodium and yellow phenolphthalein, p. 1635
DOLOBID, p. 294, 496
DONNAGEL, p. 654
DONNAGEL-PG, p. 655
DONNATAL, p. 1142
DONNAZYME, p. 333
Dopamine hydrochloride, p. 1244
DOPAR, p. 603
DORBANTYL, p. 1631
DORBANTYL Forte, p. 1631
DORCOL Children's Cough Syrup, p. 1403
DORCOL Children's Decongestant Liquid, p. 1403
DORCOL Children's Fever and Pain Reducer, p. 279
DORCOL Children's Liquid Cold Formula, p. 1403
DORIDEN, p. 1808
DORYX, p. 1037
Doxepin hydrochloride, p. 615, 635
DOXIDAN, p. 1632
DOXINATE, p. 1632
Doxorubicin hydrochloride, p. 1103
Doxycycline, p. 1046
Doxycycline hyclate, p. 1015, 1037, 1046
DRAMAMINE, p. 1064
DRAMAMINE Injection, p. 1064
DRISTAN, p. 1403
DRISTAN-AF, p. 1403

DRIXORAL, p. 1403
Dronabinol, p. 1067
Droperidol, p. 421
DTIC-Dome, p. 1093
DUADACIN, p. 1403
DULCOLAX, p. 1633
DUO-MEDIHALER, p. 1164
DURAPHYL, p. 1192
DURATION, p. 1403
DURICEF, p. 933
DUVOID, p. 1853
DV Cream, p. 1548
DYAZIDE, p. 1539
DYNAPEN, p. 916
Dyphylline, p. 1196
Dyphylline and guaifenesin, p. 1154, 1155
Dyphylline, guaifenesin, ephedrine hydrochloride, and phenobarbital, p. 1155
DYRENIUM, p. 1532

E

EARLY DETECTOR, p. 1475
EASPRIN, p. 279
Echothiophate iodide, p. 1730
Econazole nitrate, p. 683
ECOTRIN, p. 296, 498, 554
EDECRIN, p. 1514
EDECRIN, Sodium, p. 1514
E.E.S., p. 1016
EFFER-SYLLIUM, p. 1634
EFUDEX, p. 1099
ELASE, p. 712
ELASE-CHLOROMYCETIN, p. 712
ELAVIL, p. 620
ELDEC, p. 1857
ELIXOPHYLLIN, p. 1194
ELIXOPHYLLIN SR, p. 1194
ELSPAR, p. 1086
EMBOLEX, p. 534
EMCYT, p. 1118
EMETE-CON, p. 1065
EMETROL, p. 1066
EMKO, p. 1254
EMKO BECAUSE, p. 1254
EMKO PRE-FIL, p. 1254
EMPIRIN, p. 297, 500, 556
EMPIRIN with Codeine, p. 241
EMPRACET with Codeine, p. 243
E-MYCIN, p. 1017
E-MYCIN E, p. 1017
Enalapril maleate, p. 765
Enalapril maleate and hydrochlorothiazide, p. 858
Encainide hydrochloride, p. 135
ENCAPRIN, p. 279
ENCARE, p. 1254
EN-CEBRIN, p. 1866
EN-CEBRIN F, p. 1866
ENDECON, p. 1403
ENDEP, p. 622
ENDURON, p. 1518
ENDURONYL, p. 827
ENDURONYL Forte, p. 827
ENFAMIL, p. 1871
ENFAMIL with Iron, p. 1871
ENKAID, p. 135
ENOVID 5 mg, p. 1254
ENOVID 10 mg, p. 1548
ENOVID-E 21, p. 1254
ENRICH, p. 1868
ENSURE, p. 1868
ENSURE HN, p. 1868
ENSURE PLUS, p. 1869
ENSURE PLUS HN, p. 1869
ENSURE PUDDING, p. 1869

ENTEX, p. 1445
ENTEX LA, p. 1445
ENTOZYME, p. 333
Ephedrine hydrochloride, phenobarbital, theophylline calcium salicylate, and potassium iodide, p. 1201
Ephedrine sulfate, guaifenesin, theophylline, and phenobarbital, p. 1154
Ephedrine sulfate, theophylline, and hydroxyzine hydrochloride, p. 1197
EPIFRIN, p. 1726
Epinephrine, p. 1154, 1155
Epinephrine bitartrate, p. 1154
Epinephrine hydrochloride, p. 1178
EPT PLUS, p. 1466
EQUAGESIC, p. 244
EQUANIL, p. 420
ERGOSTAT, p. 1048
Ergotamine tartrate, p. 1048
Ergotamine tartrate and caffeine, p. 1049, 1056
Ergotamine tartrate, caffeine, belladonna alkaloids, and pentobarbital, p. 1049
ERYC, p. 1019
ERYC 125, p.1019
ERYCETTE, p. 209
ERYDERM, p. 210
ERYMAX, p. 198
EryPed, p. 1021
ERY-TAB, p. 1023
Erythrityl tetranitrate, p. 379
ERYTHROCIN Lactobionate-I.V., p. 1024
ERYTHROCIN Piggyback, p. 1024
ERYTHROCIN Stearate, p. 1024
Erythromycin, p. 198, 199, 204, 209, 210, 218, 1017, 1019, 1023, 1028, 1744
Erythromycin and benzoyl peroxide, p. 206
Erythromycin estolate, p. 1026
Erythromycin ethylsuccinate, p. 1016, 1017, 1021, 1030, 1032
Erythromycin ethylsuccinate and sulfisoxazole acetyl, p. 901
Erythromycin lactobionate, p. 1024
Erythromycin stearate, p. 1024, 1032
ESGIC, p. 279
ESIDRIX, p. 1519
ESIMIL, p. 829
ESKALITH, p. 1648
ESKALITH CR, p. 1648
Esmolol hydrochloride, p. 134
ESTINYL, p. 1548
ESTRACE, p. 1556
ESTRACE Vaginal Cream, p. 1556
ESTRADERM, p. 1558
Estradiol, p. 1556, 1558
Estradiol cypionate, p. 1548
Estradiol valerate, p. 1548
Estramustine phosphate sodium, p. 1118
Estrogens, conjugated, p. 1566, 1567
Estrogens, esterified, p. 1548
Estropipate, p. 1562
ESTROVIS, p. 1560
Ethacrynate sodium, p. 1514
Ethacrynic acid, p. 1514
Ethchlorvynol, p. 1814
Ethinamate, p. 1816
Ethinyl estradiol, p. 1548
Ethopropazine hydrochloride, p. 561
Ethosuximide, p. 118, 582
Ethotoin, p. 579
Ethylnorepinephrine hydrochloride, p. 1154
Ethynodiol diacetate and ethinyl estradiol, p. 1257, 1260
Ethynodiol diacetate and mestranol, p. 1297
Etidronate disodium, p. 167
Etoposide, p. 1125
ETRAFON, p. 644
Etretinate, p. 155
EUTHROID, p. 1590
EUTONYL, p. 756
EUTRON, p. 756
EXCEDRIN, p. 279
EXCEDRIN P.M., p. 279
EX-LAX, p. 1635
EXNA, p. 1513
EXSEL, p. 222
EZ-DETECT, p. 1475

F

FACT, p. 1466
Famotidine, p. 1131
FEDAHIST, p. 1398
FEDRAZIL, p. 1403
FELDENE, p. 501
FEMIRON, p. 1861
FEMIRON Multivitamins and Iron, p. 1857
FEMSTAT, p. 686
Fenoprofen calcium, p. 308, 513
Fentanyl citrate, p. 259
FEOSOL, p. 1861
FEOSOL Elixir, p. 1861
FERANCEE, p. 1861
FERANCEE-HP, p. 1861
FERGON, p. 1861
FERGON Plus, p. 1861
FERMALOX, p. 1861
FERO-FOLIC-500, p. 1861
FERO-GRAD-500, p. 1861
FERO-GRADUMET, p. 1861
FERRO-SEQUELS, p. 1861
FESTAL II, p. 333
FESTALAN, p. 333
Fibrinolysin and desoxyribonuclease, combined (bovine), p. 712
Fibrinolysin and desoxyribonuclease, combined (bovine), and chloramphenicol, p. 712
FILIBON, p. 1866
FILIBON F.A., p. 1866
FILIBON Forte, p. 1866
FIOGESIC, p. 1404
FIORICET, p. 299
FIORINAL, p. 246
FIORINAL with Codeine, p. 247
FIRST RESPONSE Ovulation Predictor Test, p. 1477
FIRST RESPONSE Pregnancy Test, p. 1466
FLAGYL, p. 693, 897
FLAGYL I.V., p. 899
FLAGYL I.V. RTU, p. 899
Flavoxate hydrochloride, p. 1852
Flecainide acetate, p. 467
FLEET Bisacodyl Enema, p. 1627
FLEET DETECATEST, p. 1475
FLEET Enema, p. 1635
FLEET Mineral Oil Enema, p. 1627
FLEXERIL, p. 1700
FLINT SSD, p. 672
FLINTSTONES, p. 1864
FLINTSTONES Complete, p. 1864
FLINTSTONES plus Extra C, p. 1864
FLINSTONES plus Iron, p. 1864
FLORINEF Acetate, p. 1312
FLORONE, p. 1355
Floxuridine, p. 1086
Flucytosine, p. 118, 692
Fludrocortisone acetate, p. 1312
Flunisolide, p. 1156, 1372, 1382

Fluocinolone acetonide, p. 1364, 1365
Fluocinonide, p. 1360
Fluorometholone, p. 1756, 1757
FLUOR-OP, p. 1756
Fluorouracil, p. 1099, 1100
Fluoxymesterone, p. 1547, 1553
Fluphenazine decanoate, p. 1669
Fluphenazine enanthate, p. 1670
Fluphenazine hydrochloride, p. 1666, 1669
Flurandrenolide, p. 1345
Flurandrenolide and neomycin sulfate, p. 1347
Flurazepam hydrochloride, p. 1807
Flurbiprofen sodium, p. 150
FML, p. 1757
FORMULA 44, p. 1404
FORMULA 44D, p. 1404
FORMULA 44M, p. 1404
FORTAZ, p. 934
FOSTEX, p. 198
FOSTRIL, p. 198
FUDR, p. 1086
FULVICIN P/G 165 and 330, p. 695
FULVICIN-U/F, p. 695
FUNGIZONE, p. 696
FURACIN, p. 672
FURADANTIN, p. 1832
Furazolidone, p. 653
Furosemide, p. 1528
FUROXONE, p. 653

G

GANTANOL, p. 882
GANTANOL DS, p. 882
GANTRISIN, p. 884
GARAMYCIN, p. 869
GARAMYCIN Cream and Ointment, p. 673
GARAMYCIN Ophthalmic, p. 1743
GASTROLYTE, p. 665
GAS-X, p. 332
GAVISCON, p. 336
GAVISCON-2, p. 336
GELUSIL, p. 337
GELUSIL-II, p. 337
GELUSIL-M, p. 337
Gemfibrozil, p. 1620
GEMNISYN, p. 300
GEMONIL, p. 563
GENTACIDIN, p. 1744
Gentamicin, p. 119
Gentamicin sulfate, p. 673, 869, 1743, 1744
GENTLE NATURE, p. 1627
GEOCILLIN, p. 976, 1834
GEOPEN, p. 977
GERIPLEX-FS, p. 1857, 1860
GERITOL COMPLETE, p. 1857
GERITOL High Potency Tonic, p. 1860
GERIX, p. 1860
GEVRABON, p. 1860
GEVRAL, p. 1857
GEVRAL Protein, p. 1869
GEVRAL-T, p. 1857
Glipizide, p. 1607
GLUCOSTIX, p. 1468
GLUCOTROL, p. 1607
Glutethimide, p. 1808
Glyburide, p. 1603, 1609
Glycerin and sodium stearate, p. 1636
Glycerin suppositories, p. 1636
Glycopyrrolate, p. 1129
Gold sodium thiomalate, p. 511
GONODECTEN, p. 1497
GRIFULVIN V, p. 670

GRISACTIN, p. 670
GRISACTIN Ultra, p. 670
Griseofulvin, microsize, p. 670, 695
Griseofulvin, ultramicrosize, p. 670, 695
Gris-PEG, p. 670
Guaifenesin and codeine phosphate, p. 1428
Guaifenesin, pseudoephedrine hydrochloride, and codeine phosphate, p. 1428
Guanabenz acetate, p. 792
Guanadrel sulfate, p. 806
Guanethidine monosulfate, p. 807
Guanethidine monosulfate and hydrochlorothiazide, p. 829
Guanfacine hydrochloride, p. 138
GYNE-LOTRIMIN, p. 687
GYNOL II, p. 1254

H

Halazepam, p. 410
HALCIDERM, p. 1356
Halcinonide, p. 1356, 1357
HALCION, p. 1810
HALDOL, p. 1654
HALDOL Decanoate, p. 1654
HALDRONE, p. 1312
HALOG, p. 1357
HALOG-E, p. 1357
Haloperidol, p. 1654
Haloperidol decanoate, p. 1654
Haloprogin, p. 674
HALOTESTIN, p. 1553
HALOTEX, p. 674
HALTRAN, p. 301
HARMONYL, p. 756
HEAD & CHEST, p. 1404
HEAD & SHOULDERS, p. 222
HEMA-CHEK, p. 1476
HEMA-COMBISTIX, p. 1469
HEMASTIX, p. 1469
HEMATEST, p. 1476
HEMOCCULT, p. 1476
Hemophilus b polysaccharide vaccine, p. 183, 186, 187
Heparin, p. 119
Heparin calcium, p. 530
Heparin sodium, p. 536
Heparin sodium and dihydroergotamine mesylate, p. 534
Hepatitis B vaccine, p. 184
Hepatitis B vaccine (recombinant), p. 158
HEPICEBRIN, p. 1857
HEPTAVAX-B, p. 184
HEPTUNA Plus, p. 1862
HEXADROL, p. 1312
HEXADROL Phosphate Injection, p. 1312
HIBICLENS, p. 672
HIB-IMUNE, p. 186
HIBISTAT, p. 672
HIBVAX, p. 187
HIPREX, p. 1834
HISPRIL, p. 728
HISTABID, p.1398
HISTADYL and A.S.A., p. 1404
HISTADYL E.C., p.1404
HISTALET, p. 1398
HISTALET DM, p. 1397
HISTALET Forte, p. 1398
HISTALET X, p. 1399
HISTASPAN-D, p. 1399
HISTASPAN-Plus, p. 1399
HISTATAPP, p. 1404
HOLD, p. 1404
HOMICEBRiN, p. 1857
Human insulin, p. 1600, 1601

HUMATIN, p. 863
HUMULIN BR, p. 1600
HUMULIN L, p. 1601
HUMULIN N, p. 1600
HUMULIN R, p. 1600
HYBEPHEN, p. 1129
HYCODAN, p. 1417
HYCOMINE, p. 1418
HYCOMINE Compound, p. 1397
HYCOTUSS, p. 1397
Hydralazine hydrochloride, p. 795
Hydralazine hydrochloride and hydrochlorothiazide, p. 756, 815
HYDREA, p. 1120
Hydrochlorothiazide, p. 1519, 1521
Hydrochlorothiazide and deserpidine, p. 757
Hydrochlorothiazide and reserpine, p. 832
Hydrocodone and phenyltoloxamine, p. 1439
Hydrocodone bitartrate and acetaminophen, p. 267, 271, 274
Hydrocodone bitartrate and guaifenesin, p. 1397
Hydrocodone bitartrate and homatropine methylbromide, p. 1417
Hydrocodone bitartrate, phenindamine tartrate, and guaifenesin, p. 1400
Hydrocodone bitartrate, phenylephrine hydrochloride, phenylpropanolamine hydrochloride, pheniramine maleate, and pyrilamine maleate, p. 1399
Hydrocodone bitartrate, phenylephrine hydrochloride, pyrilamine maleate, chlorpheniramine maleate, phenindamine tartrate, and ammonium chloride, p. 1400
Hydrocodone bitartrate and phenylpropanolamine hydrochloride, p. 1418
Hydrocodone bitartrate, phenylpropanolamine hydrochloride, pheniramine maleate, pyrilamine maleate, and guaifenesin, p. 1435
Hydrocodone bitartrate and pseudoephedrine hydrochloride, p. 1437
Hydrocodone bitartrate, pseudoephedrine hydrochloride, and guaifenesin, p. 1438
Hydrocortisone, p. 1312, 1313, 1320, 1341, 1348, 1358
Hydrocortisone and acetic acid, p. 1770
Hydrocortisone acetate, p. 1312, 1313, 1343, 1348, 1386
Hydrocortisone acetate, benzocaine, 8-hydroxyquinoline sulfate, ephedrine hydrochloride, menthol, ichthammol, and zinc oxide, p. 1313
Hydrocortisone acetate, bismuth subgallate, bismuth resorcin compound, benzyl benzoate, Peruvian balsam, and zinc oxide, p. 1385
Hydrocortisone acetate and dibucaine, p. 1388
Hydrocortisone acetate and lidocaine, p. 1313
Hydrocortisone acetate and neomycin sulfate, p. 1313
Hydrocortisone acetate and pramoxine hydrochloride, p. 1391
Hydrocortisone acetate, sodium thiosulfate, salicylic acid, and isopropyl alcohol, p. 1313
Hydrocortisone acetate suspension, p. 1320
Hydrocortisone cypionate, p. 1320
Hydrocortisone retention enema, p. 1386

Hydrocortisone sodium succinate, p. 1311, 1320
Hydrocortisone valerate, p. 1371
HYDROCORTONE, p. 1313
HydroDIURIL, p. 1521
Hydroflumethiazide, p. 1513
Hydroflumethiazide and reserpine, p. 847
Hydromorphone hydrochloride, p. 229, 240
Hydromorphone hydrochloride and guaifenesin, p. 1413
HYDROMOX, p. 1513
HYDROMOX R, p. 756
HYDROPRES, p. 832
Hydroxyurea, p. 1120
Hydroxyzine hydrochloride, p. 417, 426, 729, 1083
Hydroxyzine pamoate, p. 425, 749
HYGROTON, p. 1523
HYLOREL, p. 806
Hyoscyamine, p. 1850
Hyoscyamine sulfate, p. 1128, 1145, 1146, 1850
HYPERSTAT I.V., p. 797
HY-PHEN, p. 229
HYTONE, p. 1358

I

IBERET, p. 1862
IBERET-500, p. 1862
IBERET Liquid, p. 1862
IBERET-500 Liquid, p. 1862
IBERET-FOLIC-500, p. 1862
Ibuprofen, p. 281, 301, 305, 306, 313, 318, 327, 510, 520
ICTOTEST, p. 1474
ILOPAN-CHOLINE, p. 337
ILOSONE, p. 1026
ILOTYCIN, p. 1744
ILOZYME, p. 344
IMFERON, p. 1862
Imipenem and cilastatin sodium, p. 903
Imipramine hydrochloride, p. 638
Imipramine pamoate, p. 640
IMODIUM, p. 656
IMURAN, p. 503
INAPSINE, p. 421
INCREMIN with Iron, p. 1862
Indapamide, p. 794
INDERAL, p. 359, 439, 771, 1050
INDERAL LA, p. 362, 773, 1053
INDERIDE, p. 834
INDERIDE LA, p. 836
INDOCIN, p. 504
INDOCIN I.V., p. 174
INDOCIN SR, p. 504
Indomethacin, p. 504
Indomethacin sodium trihydrate, p. 174
INFALYTE, p. 665
INFLAMASE, p. 1758
INFLAMASE Forte, p. 1758
Influenza virus vaccine, monovalent, subvirion, p. 189
Influenza virus vaccine, trivalent, subvirion, p. 188
INOCOR, p. 1249
INSTA KIT for Group A Strep ID, p. 1498
INSULATARD NPH, p. 1600
INSULATARD NPH Human, p. 1601
Insulin, p. 1600
INTAL Capsules, p. 749, 1165
INTAL Inhaler, p. 750, 1166
INTAL Nebulizer Solution, p. 750, 1165
INTERCEPT, p. 1254
Interferon alfa-2a, recombinant, p. 1116
Interferon alfa-2b, recombinant, p. 1114

INTRON A, p. 1114
INTROPIN, p. 1244
Iodinated glycerol, p. 1462
Iodinated glycerol and codeine phosphate, p. 1440
Iodinated glycerol and dextromethorphan hydrobromide, p. 1441
Iodoquinol and hydrocortisone, p. 1313
IRCON-FA, p. 1862
ISMELIN, p. 807
Isocarboxazid, p. 626
ISOCAL, p. 1869
ISOCAL HCN, p. 1869
ISOCLOR, p. 1399
ISOCLOR Expectorant, p. 1397
ISOCULT Culture Test for Bacteriuria, p. 1501
ISOCULT Culture Test for Candida (Monilia), p. 1501
ISOCULT Culture Test for Neisseria gonorrhoeae, p. 1502
ISOCULT Culture Test for Pseudomonas aeruginosa, p. 1502
ISOCULT Culture Test for Staphylococcus aureus, p. 1502
ISOCULT Culture Test for Throat Streptococci, p. 1503
ISOCULT Culture Test for Trichomonas vaginalis, p. 1503
Isoetharine hydrochloride, p. 1158, 1163
Isoetharine mesylate, p. 1163, 1168
Isometheptene mucate, dichloralphenazone, and acetaminophen, p. 1054
ISOMIL, p. 1871
ISOMIL SF, p. 1872
Isopropamide iodide, p. 1129
Isoproterenol hydrochloride, p. 1154, 1167, 1245
Isoproterenol hydrochloride and phenylephrine bitartrate, p. 1164
Isoproterenol sulfate, p. 1168
Isoproterenol sulfate and calcium iodide, p. 1400
ISOPTIN, p. 374, 442, 785
ISOPTIN SR, p. 374, 442, 786
ISOPTIN Injection, p. 444
ISORDIL, p. 382
Isosorbide dinitrate, p. 380, 382, 399
Isotretinoin, p. 200
I-SOYALAC, p. 1872
ISUPREL, p. 1154, 1245
ISUPREL MISTOMETER, p. 1167

K

KABIKINASE, p. 543
Kanamycin sulfate, p. 871
KANTREX, p. 871
KANULASE, p. 345
KAOCHLOR 10% Liquid, p. 1774
KAOCHLOR S-F 10% Liquid, p. 1774
KAOCHLOR-EFF, p. 1774
Kaolin and pectin, p. 658
Kaolin, pectin, hyoscyamine sulfate, atropine sulfate, and scopolamine hydrobromide, p. 654
KAON, p. 1775
KAON CL-10, p. 1776
KAON-CL, p. 1776
KAON-CL 20%, p. 1776
KAOPECTATE, p. 658
KAOPECTATE Concentrate, p. 658
KAOPECTATE Tablets, p. 658
KASOF, p. 1627
KAY CIEL, p. 1778
K-DUR, p. 1779

KEFLET, p. 142
KEFLEX, p. 936
KEFLIN, p. 938
KEFUROX, p. 940
KEFZOL, p. 942
KEMADRIN, p. 604
KENALOG, p. 1359
KENALOG-10, p. 1333
KENALOG-40, p. 1334
KENALOG-H, p. 1359
Ketoconazole, p. 681, 700
KETO-DIASTIX, p. 1469
Ketoprofen, p. 517
KETOSTIX, p. 1469
KINESED, p. 1144
KLONOPIN, p. 585
K-LOR, p. 1780
KLORVESS, p. 1781
KLOTRIX, p. 1782
K-LYTE, p. 1784
K-LYTE DS, p. 1784
K-LYTE/CL, p. 1784
K-LYTE/CL 50, p. 1784
KOLANTYL, p. 332
KOLYUM, p. 1773
KOMED, p. 211
KOMED-HC, p. 1313
KORO-FLEX, p. 1254
KOROMEX, p. 1254
K•TAB, p. 1785
KWELL, p. 353

L

Labetalol hydrochloride, p. 758, 760
LABSTIX, p. 1469
LACTAID, p. 333
Lactase, p. 333
LACTINEX, p. 659
Lactobacillus acidophilus and L bulgaricus cultures, p. 659
Lactobacillus acidophilus and sodium carboxymethylcellulose, p. 653
LACTRASE, p. 333
Lactulose, p. 1629
LANOXICAPS, p. 446, 1237
LANOXIN, p. 447, 1237
LAROBEC, p. 1860
LARODOPA, p. 605
LAROTID, p. 979
LASIX, p. 1528
LAtest-RF, p. 1508
LAXCAPS, p. 1627
LEDERCILLIN VK, p. 980
LEDERPLEX, p. 1860
Lente ILETIN I, p. 1601
Lente ILETIN II, p. 1601
Lente Insulin, p. 1601
Lente Purified Insulin, p. 1601
Leucovorin calcium, p. 1087
LEUKERAN, p. 1094
Leuprolide acetate, p. 1111
LEVLEN 21, p. 1263
LEVLEN 28, p. 1263
Levobunolol hydrochloride, p. 1722
Levodopa, p. 603, 605
LEVO-DROMORAN, p. 230
Levo-epinephrine hydrochloride, p. 1726
Levonorgestrel and ethinyl estradiol, p. 1263, 1272, 1300, 1305
LEVOPHED, p. 1246
LEVOPROME, p. 302
Levorphanol tartrate, p. 230
LEVOTHROID, p. 1591
Levothyroxine sodium, p. 1594
LEVSIN, p. 1145
LEVSINEX, p. 1146

LIBRAX, p. 1147
LIBRITABS, p. 408
LIBRIUM, p. 408
LIDA-MANTLE-HC, p. 1313
LIDEX, p. 1360
LIDEX-E, p. 1360
Lidocaine, p. 120
Lidocaine hydrochloride, p. 472
LIMBITROL, p. 647
LIMBITROL DS, p. 647
Lime, sulfurated, p. 222
LINCOCIN, p. 865
Lincomycin hydrochloride, p. 865
Lindane, p. 353
LIORESAL, p. 1701
Liothyronine sodium, p. 1587
Liotrix, p. 1590
LIQUIPRIN, p. 279
LITHANE, p. 1646
Lithium, p. 120
Lithium carbonate, p. 1646, 1647, 1648, 1651, 1652
Lithium citrate, p. 1647, 1651
LITHOBID, p. 1647
LITHONATE, p. 1652
LITHOTABS, p. 1652
LOESTRIN 21 1/20, p. 1265
LOESTRIN 21 1.5/30, p. 1265
LOESTRIN Fe 1/20, p. 1265
LOESTRIN Fe 1.5/30, p. 1265
LOFENALAC, p. 1872
LOMOTIL, p. 659
Lomustine (CCNU), p. 1090
LONITEN, p. 799
LO/OVRAL, p. 1268
LO/OVRAL-28, p. 1268
Loperamide hydrochloride, p. 656
LOPID, p. 1620
LOPRESSOR, p. 363, 775
LOPRESSOR HCT, p. 839
LOPROX, p. 674
LOPURIN, p. 722
Lorazepam, p. 405, 406
LORELCO, p. 1621
LOROXIDE, p. 211
LOTRIMIN, p. 675
LOTRISONE, p. 676
LOTUSATE, p. 1796
Loxapine hydrochloride, p. 1657
Loxapine succinate, p. 1657
LOXITANE, p. 1657
LOXITANE C, p. 1657
LOXITANE IM, p. 1657
LOZOL, p. 794
LUDIOMIL, p. 624
LUFYLLIN, p. 1196
LUFYLLIN-EPG, p. 1155
LUFYLLIN-GG, p. 1155
LUPRON, p. 1111
LURIDE, p. 1864
LURIDE 0.25 mg F, p. 1864
LURIDE 0.5 mg F, p. 1864
LURIDE 1.0 mg F, p. 1864
LURIDE-SF 1.0 mg F, p. 1864
LYSODREN, p. 1086
LYTREN, p. 666

M

MAALOX, p. 338
MAALOX Plus, p. 338
MAALOX TC, p. 338
MACRODANTIN, p. 1835
Magaldrate, p. 342
Magaldrate and simethicone, p. 342
MAGAN, p. 303, 507
Magnesium hydroxide, p. 1642
Magnesium hydroxide and aluminum hydroxide, p. 338
Magnesium hydroxide, aluminum hydroxide, and calcium carbonate, p. 336
Magnesium hydroxide, aluminum hydroxide, and simethicone, p. 338
Magnesium salicylate, p. 303, 507
Malt soup extract, p. 1628
MALTSUPEX, p. 1628
MANDELAMINE, p. 1837
MANDOL, p. 944
Mannitol, p. 1514
MANTADIL, p. 1313
MAOLATE, p. 1703
Maprotiline hydrochloride, p. 624
MARAX, p. 1197
MARAX-DF, p. 1197
MAREZINE, p. 1059
MARINOL, p. 1067
MARPLAN, p. 626
MATERNA 1•60, p. 1866
MATULANE, p. 1086
MAXIFLOR, p. 1313
MAXITROL, p. 1745
MAXZIDE, p. 1541
Measles, mumps, and rubella live virus vaccine, p. 190
MEBARAL, p. 564, 1797
Mebendazole, p. 352
Mechlorethamine hydrochloride, p. 1087
MECLAN, p. 212
Meclizine hydrochloride, p. 1058, 1059, 1060
Meclocycline sulfosalicylate, p. 212
Meclofenamate sodium, p. 508
MECLOMEN, p. 508
MEDICONE, p. 1389
MEDICONE DERMA-HC, p. 1313
MEDIHALER-EPI, p. 1154
MEDIHALER ERGOTAMINE, p. 1048
MEDIHALER-ISO, p. 1168
MEDIPREN, p. 305
MEDIQUELL, p. 1404
MEDROL, p. 1330
MEDROL Acetate, p. 1313
Medroxyprogesterone acetate, p. 1549, 1572
Mefenamic acid, p. 316
MEFOXIN, p. 946
MEGACE, p. 1112
Megestrol acetate, p. 1112
MELLARIL, p. 1665
MELLARIL-S, p. 1665
Melphalan, p. 1088
MENEST, p. 1548
Menotropins, p. 1577
MENRIUM, p. 1549
Mepenzolate bromide, p. 1128
MEPERGAN, p. 248
MEPERGAN Fortis, p. 249
Meperidine hydrochloride, p. 238
Meperidine hydrochloride and acetaminophen, p. 229
Meperidine hydrochloride and promethazine hydrochloride, p. 248, 249
Mephenytoin, p. 578
Mephobarbital, p. 564, 1797
Meprobamate, p. 404, 420, 423
Meprobamate and aspirin, p. 244, 250
Meprobamate and benactyzine hydrochloride, p. 614
Meprobamate and conjugated estrogens, p. 1549
MEPROSPAN, p. 404
Mercaptopurine, p. 1087
MESANTOIN, p. 578
Mesoridazine besylate, p. 1672
METAHYDRIN, p. 1513
METAMUCIL, p. 1637
METAMUCIL, Instant Fiber Mix, p. 1637
METANDREN, p. 1547
METAPREL, p. 1199
METAPREL Inhalant Solution, p. 1169
METAPREL Metered Dose Inhaler, p. 1169
Metaproterenol sulfate, p. 1157, 1158, 1169, 1180, 1199
Metaraminol bitartrate, p. 1241
METATENSIN, p. 757
Metaxalone, p. 1708
Methacycline hydrochloride, p. 1015
Methantheline bromide, p. 1128
Metharbital, p. 563
Methdilazine hydrochloride, p. 728
Methenamine, methylene blue, phenyl salicylate, benzoic acid, atropine sulfate, and hyoscyamine, p. 1847
Methenamine hippurate, p. 1834
Methenamine mandelate, p. 1837
Methicillin sodium, p. 917
Methocarbamol, p. 1707
Methocarbamol and aspirin, p. 1715
Methotrexate, p. 121, 1101
Methotrexate sodium, p. 1086, 1087
Methotrimeprazine, p. 302
Methscopolamine bromide, p. 1129
Methsuximide, p. 580
Methyclothiazide, p. 1513, 1518
Methyclothiazide and deserpidine, p. 827
Methyclothiazide and reserpine, p. 756
Methylcellulose, p. 1627, 1629
Methyldopa, p. 788
Methyldopa and chlorothiazide, p. 811
Methyldopa and hydrochlorothiazide, p. 813
Methylphenidate hydrochloride, p. 179
Methylprednisolone, p. 1330
Methylprednisolone acetate, p. 1313
Methylprednisolone acetate suspension, p. 1330
Methylprednisolone sodium succinate, p. 1311, 1330
Methyltestosterone, p. 1547, 1548
Methyprylon, p. 1813
Methysergide maleate, p. 1055
Metoclopramide hydrochloride, p. 1073, 1132
Metolazone, p. 1515, 1524
Metoprolol tartrate, p. 363, 775
Metoprolol tartrate and hydrochlorothiazide, p. 839
METRODIN, p. 143
Metronidazole, p. 693, 702, 897, 899, 905
Metronidazole hydrochloride, p. 899
MEXATE, p. 1086
MEXATE-AQ, p. 1087
Mexiletine hydrochloride, p. 451
MEXITIL, p. 451
MEZLIN, p. 981
Mezlocillin sodium, p. 981
MICATIN, p. 670
MI-CEBRIN, p. 1857
MI-CEBRIN T, p. 1857
Miconazole, p. 698
Miconazole nitrate, p. 670, 677, 687
MICRAININ, p. 250
MICROCULT-GC, p. 1503
Microfibrillar collagen hemostat (MCH), p. 558
MICRO-K, p. 1786
MICRONASE, p. 1609
MICRONOR, p. 1254

MICROSTIX-3, p. 1504
MICROSTIX-CANDIDA, p. 1504
MICROSTIX-Nitrite, p. 1498
MICROTRAK *Chlamydia trachomatis*, p. 1498
MIDAMOR, p. 1534
Midazolam hydrochloride, p. 1817
MIDOL, p. 279
MIDOL 200, p. 305
MIDOL PMS, p. 279
MIDRIN, p. 1054
Milk of magnesia, p. 332
MILONTIN, p. 581
MILPREM, p. 1549
MILTOWN, p. 423
MILTOWN 600, p. 423
Mineral oil, p. 1627, 1628
Mineral oil and phenolphthalein, p. 1627
MINIPRESS, p. 800
MINIZIDE, p. 841
MINOCIN p. 213, 1039
Minocycline hydrochloride, p. 213, 1039
Minoxidil, p. 799
MINTEZOL, p. 349
MITHRACIN, p. 1108
Mitomycin, p. 1109
Mitotane, p. 1086
MITROLAN, p. 661, 1638
MIXTARD, p. 1600
M-M-R II, p. 190
MOBAN, p. 1659
MOCTANIN, p. 173
MODANE, p. 1638
MODANE Plus, p. 1628
MODERIL, p. 756
MODICON 21, p. 1270
MODICON 28, p. 1270
MODURETIC, p. 1543
Molindone hydrochloride, p. 1659
MOL-IRON, p. 1862
MOL-IRON with Vitamin C, p. 1862
MOMENTUM, p. 279
MONISTAT 3, p. 687
MONISTAT 7, p. 687
MONISTAT i.v., p. 698
MONISTAT-DERM, p. 677
MONISTAT DUAL-PAK, p. 687
MONOCID, p. 948
MONO-DIFF, p. 1504
MONOLATEX, p. 1505
Monooctanoin, p. 173
MONOSPOT, p. 1505
MONOSTICON, p. 1506
MONOSTICON DRI-DOT, p. 1506
MONO-SURE, p. 1506
MONO-TEST, p. 1507
MONO-TEST (FTB), p. 1507
Morphine sulfate, p. 230
Morphine sulfate injection, p. 252
MOTRIN, p. 306, 510
Moxalactam disodium, p. 950
MOXAM, p. 950
MS CONTIN, p. 230
MSIR, p. 230
MUCOMYST, p. 161, 1170
MUDRANE-2, p. 1155
MUDRANE GG, p. 1155
MUDRANE GG-2, p. 1155
MULTICEBRIN, p. 1858
MULTISTIX, p. 1469
MULTISTIX SG, p. 1470
MULVIDREN-F, p. 1864
MURINE, p. 1772
MUSTARGEN, p. 1087
MUTAMYCIN, p. 1109
M.V.I.-12, p. 1858
M.V.I. Pediatric, p. 1858

MYADEC, p. 1858
MYCELEX, p. 677
MYCELEX Troche, p. 678
MYCELEX TWIN PACK, p. 688
MYCELEX-G, p. 688
MYCIFRADIN, p. 873
MYCIGUENT, p. 672
MYCITRACIN, p. 672
MYCOLOG-II, p. 679, 1361
MYCOSTATIN, p. 700
MYCOSTATIN Cream, Ointment, and Powder, p. 680
MYCOSTATIN Vaginal Tablets, p. 689
MYDRIACYL, p. 1737
MYLANTA, p. 339
MYLANTA-II, p. 339
MYLERAN, p. 1087
MYLICON, p. 340
MYLICON-80, p. 340
MYOCHRYSINE, p. 511
MYSOLINE, p. 587
MYSTECLIN-F, p. 1040

N

Nadolol, p. 358, 769
Nadolol and bendroflumethiazide, p. 823
NAFCIL, p. 916
Nafcillin sodium, p. 916, 1011
Nalbuphine hydrochloride, p. 312
NALDECON, p. 1446
NALDECON-CX, p. 1397
NALDECON-DX, p. 1404
NALDECON-EX, p. 1404
NALDEGESIC, p. 1404
NALFON, p. 308, 513
Nalidixic acid, p. 1837
Naloxone hydrochloride, p. 163
Naphazoline hydrochloride and antazoline phosphate, p. 1762
Naphazoline hydrochloride and pheniramine maleate, p. 1759
NAPHCON-A, p. 1759
NAPROSYN, p. 310, 515
Naproxen, p. 310, 515
Naproxen sodium, p. 284, 477
NAQUA, p. 1513
NAQUIVAL, p. 757
NARCAN, p. 163
NARDIL, p. 627
NASALCROM, p. 752
NASALIDE, p. 1382
NATABEC, p. 1866
NATABEC Rx, p. 1866
NATABEC with Fluoride, p. 1866
NATAFORT, p. 1866
NATALINS, p. 1866
NATALINS Rx, p. 1866
NATURACIL, p. 1628
NATURETIN, p. 1513
NAVANE, p. 1692
NEBCIN, p. 875
NegGram, p. 1837
NEMBUTAL, p. 566, 1799
NEMBUTAL Sodium, p. 566, 567, 1799, 1800
NEO-CALGLUCON, p. 1867
NEO-CORT-DOME, p. 1313
NEO-CORTEF, p. 1313
NeoDECADRON, p. 1313
NeoDECADRON Ophthalmic, p. 1746
NEO-DELTA-CORTEF, p. 1313
NEO-MEDROL, p. 1313
Neomycin sulfate, p. 672, 873
Neomycin sulfate and dexamethasone sodium phosphate, p. 1746
Neomycin sulfate and fluocinolone acetonide, p. 1362
Neomycin sulfate and hydrocortisone, p. 1313
Neomycin sulfate and methylprednisolone acetate, p. 1313
Neomycin sulfate, polymyxin B sulfate, and bacitracin zinc, p. 672
NEO-PLANOTEST DUOCLON, p. 1481
NEO-POLYCIN, p. 672
NEO-PREGNOSTICON DUOCLON, p. 1481
NEOSPORIN, p. 680
NEOSPORIN Ophthalmic, p. 1748
NEO-SYNALAR, p. 1362
NEO-SYNEPHRINE, p. 1404
NEO-SYNEPHRINE Injection, p. 1248
NEO-SYNEPHRINE Ophthalmic, p. 1760
NEO-SYNEPHRINE II, p. 1405
NEOTEP, p. 1399
Netilmicin sulfate, p. 877
NETROMYCIN, p. 877
NEUTROGENA, p. 199
Niacin, p. 1622
NICLOCIDE, p. 351
Niclosamide, p. 351
NICORETTE, p. 181
Nicotine polacrilex, p. 181
NICOLAR, p. 1622
Nifedipine, p. 368, 376
NILSTAT, p. 670
NIMBUS, p. 1483
NIPRIDE, p. 802
NITRO-BID, p. 383
NITRO-BID IV, p. 385
NITRO-BID Ointment, p. 384
NITRODISC, p. 387
NITRO-DUR, p. 386
NITRO-DUR II, p. 386
Nitrofurantoin, p. 1832
Nitrofurantoin macrocrystals, p. 1835
Nitrofurazone, p. 672
NITROGARD, p. 388
Nitroglycerin, p. 379, 383, 384, 385, 386, 387, 388, 390, 391, 393, 394, 395, 397, 400, 402
Nitroprusside, sodium, p. 802
NITROL Ointment, p. 390
NITROL IV, p. 391
NITROLINGUAL, p. 393
NITROPRESS, p. 756
NITROSTAT, p. 394
NITROSTAT Ointment, p. 394
NITROSTAT IV, p. 395
NIX, p. 354
NIZORAL, p. 700
NIZORAL Cream, p. 681
N-MULTISTIX, p. 1470
N-MULTISTIX SG, p. 1470
NOCTEC, p. 1811
NOLAHIST, p. 728
NOLAMINE, p. 1399
NOLUDAR, p. 1813
NOLUDAR 300, p. 1813
NOLVADEX, p. 1112
Nonoxynol-9, p. 1254
NORDETTE-21, p. 1272
NORDETTE-28, p. 1272
Norepinephrine bitartrate, p. 1246
Norethindrone, p. 1254, 1570
Norethindrone and ethinyl estradiol, p. 1255, 1270, 1275, 1283, 1287, 1290, 1292, 1302
Norethindrone and mestranol, p. 1254, 1277, 1285
Norethindrone acetate, p. 1549, 1570
Norethindrone acetate and ethinyl estradiol, p. 1265, 1280

Norethindrone acetate and ethinyl estradiol; ferrous fumarate, p. 1265, 1280
Norethynodrel and mestranol, p. 1254, 1548
NORFLEX, p. 1703
Norfloxacin, p. 1839
NORGESIC, p. 1712
NORGESIC Forte, p. 1712
Norgestrel, p. 1254
Norgestrel and ethinyl estradiol, p. 1268, 1295
NORINYL 1 + 35 21-DAY, p. 1275
NORINYL 1 + 35 28-DAY, p. 1275
NORINYL 1 + 50 21-DAY, p. 1277
NORINYL 1 + 50 28-DAY, p. 1277
NORINYL 1 + 80 21-DAY, p. 1277
NORINYL 1 + 80 28-DAY, p. 1277
NORINYL 2 mg, p. 1254
NORISODRINE with Calcium Iodide, p. 1400
NORLESTRIN 21 1/50, p. 1280
NORLESTRIN 21 2.5/50, p. 1280
NORLESTRIN 28 1/50, p. 1280
NORLESTRIN Fe 1/50, p. 1280
NORLESTRIN Fe 2.5/50, p. 1280
NORLUTATE, p. 1570
NORLUTIN, p. 1570
NORMODYNE, p. 758
NOROXIN, p. 1839
NORPACE, p. 453
NORPACE CR, p. 453
NORPRAMIN, p. 629
NOR-Q.D., p. 1254
Nortriptyline, p. 121
Nortriptyline hydrochloride, p. 631
NÖSTRIL, p. 1405
NÖSTRILLA, p. 1405
NOVAFED, p. 1447
NOVAFED A, p. 1448
NOVAHISTINE, p. 1405
NOVAHISTINE DH, p. 1419
NOVAHISTINE DMX, p. 1405
NOVAHISTINE Expectorant, p. 1420
NOVOLIN 70/30, p. 1600
NOVOLIN L, p. 1601
NOVOLIN N, p. 1601
NOVOLIN R, p. 1600
NPH ILETIN I, p. 1601
NPH ILETIN II, p. 1601
NPH Insulin, p. 1601
NPH Purified Insulin, p. 1601
NTS, p. 397
NTZ, p. 1405
NUBAIN, p. 312
NUCOFED, p. 1397
NUCOFED Expectorant, p. 1397
NUCOFED Expectorant, Pediatric, p. 1398
NUMORPHAN, p. 254
NUPERCAINAL, p. 1390
NUPRIN, p. 313
N-URISTIX, p. 1470
NURSOY, p. 1872
NUTRAMIGEN, p. 1872
NYQUIL, p. 1405
Nystatin, p. 670, 680, 689, 700
Nystatin and triamcinolone acetonide, p. 679, 1361

O

Octoxynol, p. 1254
OCUFEN, p. 150
OCUSERT, p. 1727
OGEN, p. 1562
OGEN Vaginal Cream, p. 1562

OMNIPEN, p. 983
OMNIPEN-N, p. 983
ONCOVIN, p. 1121
ONE-A-DAY Essential, p. 1858
ONE-A-DAY Maximum Formula, p. 1858
ONE-A-DAY Plus Extra C, p. 1858
Opium, kaolin, pectin, hyoscyamine sulfate, atropine sulfate, and scopolamine hydrobromide, p. 655
OPTICROM, p. 752, 1762
OPTILETS-500, p. 1858
OPTILETS-M-500, p. 1858
OPTIMINE, p. 735
ORAP, p. 1646
ORA-TESTRYL, p. 1548
ORETICYL, p. 757
ORETO Methyl, p. 1548
OREXIN, p. 1860
ORGANIDIN, p. 1462
ORIMUNE, p. 192
ORINASE, p. 1611
ORNADE, p. 1449
ORNEX, p. 1405
Orphenadrine citrate, p. 1703
Orphenadrine citrate, aspirin, and caffeine, p. 1712
Orphenadrine hydrochloride, p. 561
ORTHO β-HCG, p. 1483
ORTHO Diaphragm Kit, p. 1254
ORTHO Diaphragm Kit-ALL FLEX, p. 1254
ORTHO Dienestrol Cream, p. 1564
ORTHO-CREME, p. 1254
ORTHO-GYNOL, p. 1254
ORTHO-NOVUM 1/35 □ 21, p. 1283
ORTHO-NOVUM 1/35 □ 28, p. 1283
ORTHO-NOVUM 1/50 □ 21, p. 1285
ORTHO-NOVUM 1/50 □ 28, p. 1285
ORTHO-NOVUM 1/80 □ 21, p. 1285
ORTHO-NOVUM 1/80 □ 28, p. 1285
ORTHO-NOVUM 7/7/7 □ 21, p. 1287
ORTHO-NOVUM 7/7/7 □ 28, p. 1287
ORTHO-NOVUM 10/11 □ 21, p. 1290
ORTHO-NOVUM 10/11 □ 28, p. 1290
ORTHO-WHITE, p. 1254
ORTHOXICOL, p. 1405
ORUDIS, p. 517
OS-CAL 250, p. 1868
OS-CAL 500, p. 1868
OS-CAL Forte, p. 1868
OS-CAL Plus, p. 1868
OSMITROL, p. 1514
OSMOLITE, p. 1869
OSMOLITE HN, p. 1869
OTOBIOTIC, p. 1769
OTRIVIN, p. 1405
OVCON-35, p. 1292
OVCON-50, p. 1292
OVRAL, p. 1295
OVRAL-28, p. 1295
OVRETTE, p. 1254
OVULEN-21, p. 1297
OVULEN-28, p. 1297
OVUSTICK, p. 1478
Oxacillin sodium, p. 997
Oxamniquine, p. 348
Oxazepam, p. 411
Oxtriphylline, p. 1188
Oxtriphylline and guaifenesin, p. 1184
OXY-5, p. 214
OXY-10, p. 214, 215
Oxybutynin chloride, p. 1851
Oxycodone hydrochloride and acetaminophen, p. 255, 270
Oxycodone hydrochloride, oxycodone terephthalate, and aspirin, p. 256
Oxymorphone hydrochloride, p. 254

Oxyphencyclimine hydrochloride, p. 1129
Oxyphencyclimine hydrochloride and hydroxyzine hydrochloride, p. 1129
Oxyphenonium bromide, p. 1128
Oxytetracycline, p. 1044
Oxytetracyline hydrochloride, p. 1044
Oxytetracycline hydrochloride, sulfamethizole, and phenazopyridine hydrochloride, p. 1822

P

P_1E_1, P_2E_1, P_3E_1, P_4E_1, P_5E_1, and P_6E_1, p. 1729
PABALATE, p. 280
PABALATE-SF, p. 280
PAMELOR, p. 631
PAMINE, p. 1129
PANADOL, p. 314, 315
PANCREASE, p. 346
Pancreatic enzymes, p. 333
Pancreatin, pepsin, and bile salts, p. 333
Pancreatin, pepsin, bile salts, hyoscyamine sulfate, atropine sulfate, scopolamine hydrobromide, and phenobarbital, p. 333
Pancrelipase, p. 344, 346
PANMYCIN, p. 1015
PanOxyl, p. 215
PanOxyl AQ, p. 215
PANWARFIN, p. 539
PARADIONE, p. 561
PARAFLEX, p. 1704
PARAFON FORTE, p. 1714
Paramethadione, p. 561
Paramethasone acetate, p. 1312
Paregoric, p. 661
Paregoric, pectin, and kaolin, p. 663
PAREPECTOLIN, p. 663
Pargyline hydrochloride, p. 756
Pargyline hydrochloride and methyclothiazide, p. 756
PARLODEL, p. 607, 1574, 1581
PARNATE, p. 633
Paromomycin sulfate, p. 863
PARSIDOL, p. 561
PATHIBAMATE, p. 1148
PATHILON, p. 1129
PATHODX Strep A, p. 1499
PAXIPAM, p. 410
PBZ, p. 736
PBZ-SR, p. 736
PCE, p. 1028
PEDIACARE, p. 1405
PEDIACOF, p. 1398
PEDIALYTE, p. 666
PEDIALYTE RS, p. 666
PEDIAPRED, p. 151
PEDIAMYCIN, p. 1030
PEDIAZOLE, p. 901
PEGANONE, p. 579
Pemoline, p. 176
Penicillamine, p. 490, 492
Penicillin G benzathine, p. 972, 988
Penicillin G benzathine and penicillin G procaine, p. 971
Penicillin G potassium, p. 916, 985
Penicillin G procaine, p. 918, 989
Penicillin V potassium, p. 915, 917, 980, 986, 1012
PENNTUSS, p. 1421
Pentaerythritol tetranitrate, p. 398
PENTAM 300, p. 865
Pentamidine isoethionate, p. 865
Pentazocine hydrochloride and acetaminophen, p. 262
Pentazocine hydrochloride and aspirin,

p. 230
Pentazocine hydrochloride and naloxone hydrochloride, p. 265
Pentazocine lactate, p. 264
PENTIDS, p. 985
Pentobarbital, p. 566, 1799
Pentobarbital sodium, p. 566, 567, 1799, 1800
Pentoxifylline, p. 548
PEN•VEE K, p. 986
PEPCID, p. 1131
PEPCID I.V., p. 1131
PEPTO-BISMOL, p. 663, 1068
PERCOCET, p. 255
PERCODAN, p. 256
PERCODAN-Demi, p. 256
PERCOGESIC, p. 315
PERDIEM, p. 1639
PERDIEM Plain, p. 1640
PERGONAL, p. 1577
PERIACTIN, p. 737
PERI-COLACE, p. 1641
PERIHEMIN, p. 1862
PERITINIC, p. 1862
PERITRATE, p. 398
PERITRATE SA, p. 398
PERMAPEN, p. 988
Permethrin, p. 354
PERMITIL, p. 1666
PERNOX, p. 199
Perphenazine, p. 1059, 1687
Perphenazine and amitriptyline hydrochloride, p. 644, 649
PERSA-GEL, p. 216
PERSA-GEL W, p. 216
PERSANTINE, p. 164
PERTOFRANE, p. 614
PERTUSSIN, p. 1405, 1406
PFIZERPEN, p. 916
PFIZERPEN-AS, p. 989
PHAZYME, p. 340
PHAZYME 95, p. 340
PHAZYME 125, p. 340
PHAZYME-PB, p. 341
Phenacemide, p. 588
PHENAPHEN, p. 280
PHENAPHEN with Codeine, p. 257
PHENAPHEN-650 with Codeine, p. 257
Phenazopyridine hydrochloride, p. 1848
Phenazopyridine hydrochloride, hyoscyamine hydrobromide, and butabarbital, p. 1849
Phenelzine sulfate, p. 627
PHENERGAN, p. 739, 1069
PHENERGAN Injection, p. 740, 1071
PHENERGAN VC, p. 1451
PHENERGAN VC with Codeine, p. 1425
PHENERGAN with Codeine, p. 1422
PHENERGAN with Dextromethorphan, p. 1424
PHENERGAN-D, p. 1399
Phenindamine tartrate, p. 728
Phenindamine tartrate, chlorpheniramine maleate, and phenylpropanolamine hydrochloride, p. 1399
PHENISTIX, p. 1470
Phenobarbital, p. 122, 569, 1802
Phenobarbital and belladonna extract, p. 1128
Phenobarbital, ergotamine tartrate, and belladonna alkaloids, p. 1139
Phenobarbital, hyoscyamine sulfate, atropine sulfate, and hyoscine hydrobromide, p. 1142
Phenobarbital, hyoscyamine sulfate, atropine sulfate, and scopolamine hydrobromide, p. 1128, 1144

Phenobarbital sodium, p. 569, 1802
Phenolphthalein and docusate sodium, p. 1627
Phenoxybenzamine hydrochloride, p. 756
Phensuximide, p. 581
Phentolamine mesylate, p. 756, 803
PHENURONE, p. 588
Phenylbutazone, p. 475, 485
Phenylephrine hydrochloride, p. 1248, 1760
Phenylephrine hydrochloride, antipyrine, and benzocaine, p. 1764
Phenylephrine hydrochloride and chlorpheniramine maleate, p. 1398, 1399
Phenylephrine hydrochloride, chlorpheniramine maleate, codeine phosphate, and acetaminophen, p. 1397
Phenylephrine hydrochloride, chlorpheniramine maleate, hydrocodone bitartrate, acetaminophen, and caffeine, p. 1397
Phenylephrine hydrochloride, phenylpropanolamine hydrochloride, chlorpheniramine maleate, hyoscyamine sulfate, atropine sulfate, and scopolamine hydrobromide, p. 1454
Phenylephrine hydrochloride, phenylpropanolamine hydrochloride, and guaifenesin, p. 1445
Phenylephrine tannate, chlorpheniramine tannate, and pyrilamine tannate, p. 1399, 1455
Phenylpropanolamine hydrochloride and chlorpheniramine maleate, p. 1398
Phenylpropanolamine hydrochloride, chlorpheniramine maleate, acetaminophen, and salicylamide, p. 1399
Phenylpropanolamine hydrochloride, codeine phosphate, and guaifenesin, p. 1397
Phenylpropanolamine hydrochloride and guaifenesin, p. 1445
Phenylpropanolamine hydrochloride, guaifenesin, and codeine phosphate, p. 1397
Phenylpropanolamine hydrochloride, pheniramine maleate, and pyrilamine maleate, p. 1459
Phenylpropanolamine hydrochloride, phenylephrine hydrochloride, phenyltoloxamine citrate, and chlorpheniramine maleate, p. 1446
Phenylpropanolamine hydrochloride, pyrilamine maleate, chlorpheniramine maleate, and phenylephrine hydrochloride, p. 1398
Phenytoin, p. 122, 573
Phenytoin sodium, p. 575
Phenytoin sodium, extended, p. 573
Phenytoin sodium and phenobarbital, p. 561
PHILLIPS' Milk of Magnesia, p. 1642
pHisoAc BP, p. 217
PHOSPHOLINE IODIDE, p. 1730
PHOSPHO-SODA, p. 1628
Pilocarpine, p. 1727
Pilocarpine hydrochloride, p. 1732
Pilocarpine hydrochloride and epinephrine bitartrate, p. 1729
PILOPINE HS, p. 1732
Pimozide, p. 1646
Pindolol, p. 781
Piperacillin sodium, p. 991

PIPRACIL, p. 991
Piroxicam, p. 501
PLACIDYL, p. 1814
PLATINOL, p. 1123
Plicamycin, p. 1108
PMB, p. 1549
Pneumococcal vaccine, polyvalent, p. 194, 195
PNEUMOVAX 23, p. 194
PNU-IMUNE 23, p. 195
POLARAMINE, p. 742
POLARAMINE Expectorant, p. 1399
Poliovirus vaccine, live, trivalent, p. 192
POLYCILLIN, p. 993
POLYCILLIN-N, p. 993
POLYMOX, p. 995
Polymyxin B sulfate, p. 864, 865
Polymyxin B sulfate and bacitracin zinc, p. 682
Polymyxin B sulfate, bacitracin zinc, and neomycin sulfate, p. 680, 1748
Polymyxin B sulfate, bacitracin zinc, neomycin sulfate, and hydrocortisone, p. 1350, 1740
Polymyxin B sulfate and hydrocortisone, p. 1769
Polymyxin B sulfate and neomycin sulfate, p. 680
Polymyxin B sulfate, neomycin sulfate, and gramicidin, p. 1748
Polymyxin B sulfate, neomycin sulfate, and hydrocortisone acetate, p. 1349
Polymyxin B sulfate, neomycin sulfate, and hydrocortisone, p. 1741, 1767
Polyoxyethylene nonyl phenol, sodium edetate, and sodium dioctyl sulfosuccinate, p. 691
POLY-PRED, p. 1748
POLYSPORIN, p. 682
Polythiazide, p. 1513
Polythiazide and reserpine, p. 757
POLY-VI-FLOR 0.25 mg, p. 1864
POLY-VI-FLOR 0.5 mg Drops, p. 1864
POLY-VI-FLOR 0.5 mg Tablets, p. 1864
POLY-VI-FLOR 1.0 mg, p. 1864
POLY-VI-FLOR 0.25 mg with Iron, p. 1864
POLY-VI-FLOR 0.5 mg with Iron Drops, p. 1864
POLY-VI-FLOR 0.5 mg with Iron Tablets, p. 1864
POLY-VI-FLOR 1.0 mg with Iron, p. 1865
POLY-VI-SOL Drops, p. 1865
POLY-VI-SOL Tablets, p. 1865
POLY-VI-SOL with Iron, p. 1865
POLY-VI-SOL with Iron and Zinc, p. 1865
PONSTEL, p. 316
Pork insulin, p. 1600
PORTAGEN, p. 1869
POSTURE, p. 1868
POSTURE-D, p. 1868
Potassium acetate, potassium bicarbonate, and potassium citrate, p. 1773
Potassium bicarbonate, p.1784
Potassium bicarbonate and potassium citrate, p. 1784
Potassium chloride, p. 1774, 1776, 1778, 1779, 1780, 1781, 1782, 1784, 1785, 1786, 1788, 1789
Potassium chloride, potassium bicarbonate, and L-lysine monohydrochloride, p. 1781, 1784
Potassium chloride, potassium citrate, potassium bicarbonate, and betaine hydrochloride, p. 1774
Potassium gluconate, p. 1775
Potassium gluconate and potassium

citrate, p. 1773
Potassium gluconate, potassium citrate, and ammonium chloride, p. 1773
Potassium gluconate and potassium chloride, p. 1773
Potassium iodide, p. 1400
Potassium iodide and aminophylline, p. 1155
Potassium salicylate and potassium aminobenzoate, p. 280
POVAN, p. 352
Povidone-iodine, p. 671
PRAMET FA, p. 1867
PRAMILET FA, p. 1867
Pramoxine hydrochloride, p. 1392
Prazepam, p. 407
Praziquantel, p. 348
Prazosin hydrochloride, p. 800
Prazosin hydrochloride and polythiazide, p. 841
PRECEF, p. 952
PRECISION HIGH NITROGEN DIET, p. 1869
PRECISION ISOTONIC DIET, p. 1869
PRECISION LR DIET, p. 1870
Prednisolone, p. 1312
Prednisolone acetate, p. 1337
Prednisolone acetate and neomycin sulfate, p. 1313
Prednisolone acetate, neomycin sulfate, and polymyxin B sulfate, p. 1748
Prednisolone sodium phosphate, p. 151, 1337, 1758
Prednisone, p. 1328
PREGESTIMIL, p. 1872
PREGNACLONE Slide, p. 1484
PREGNACLONE Tube, p. 1485
PREGNAZYME, p. 1485
PREGNOLISA, p. 1486
PREGNOSIS, p. 1487
PREGNOSPIA, p. 1488
PREGNOSTICON, p. 1489
PREGNOSTICON DRI-DOT, p. 1488
PREMARIN, p. 1566
PREMARIN Vaginal Cream, p. 1567
PREPARATION H, p. 1390
PRIMATENE Mist, p. 1154
PRIMATENE Mist Suspension, p. 1154
PRIMATENE Tablets, p. 1155
PRIMAXIN, p. 903
Primidone, p. 123, 587
PRINCIPEN, p. 996
PRINCIPEN with Probenecid, p. 916
PRIVINE, p. 1406
PRO-BANTHINE, p. 1150
PROBEC-T, p. 1860
Probenecid, p. 717
Probenecid and colchicine, p. 719
Probucol, p. 1621
Procainamide, p. 124
Procainamide hydrochloride, p. 455, 457, 458
PROCAN SR, p. 455
Procarbazine hydrochloride, p. 1086
PROCARDIA, p. 376
Prochlorperazine, p. 1060, 1661
PROCTOFOAM-HC, p. 1391
Procyclidine hydrochloride, p. 604
PROFASI HP, p. 1579
PROGESTASERT, p. 1254
PROLIXIN, p. 1669
PROLIXIN Decanoate, p. 1669
PROLIXIN Enanthate, p. 1670
PROLOID, p. 1593
PROLOPRIM, p. 1840
Promazine hydrochloride, p. 1674
Promethazine hydrochloride, p. 739, 740, 1069, 1071
Promethazine hydrochloride and codeine phosphate, p. 1422
Promethazine hydrochloride and dextromethorphan hydrobromide, p. 1424
Promethazine hydrochloride and phenylephrine hydrochloride, p. 1451
Promethazine hydrochloride, phenylephrine hydrochloride, and codeine phosphate, p. 1425
PRONEMIA, p. 1862
PRONESTYL, p. 457
PRONESTYL-SR, p. 458
PROPAGEST, p. 1406
Propantheline bromide, p. 1150
PROPINE, p. 1733
Propoxyphene hydrochloride, p. 235
Propoxyphene hydrochloride and acetaminophen, p. 273
Propoxyphene hydrochloride and aspirin, p. 229
Propoxyphene hydrochloride, aspirin, and caffeine, p. 236
Propoxyphene napsylate, p. 235
Propoxyphene napsylate and aspirin, p. 229
Propoxyphene napsylate and acetaminophen, p. 233
Propranolol hydrochloride, p. 359, 362, 439, 771, 773, 1050, 1053
Propranolol hydrochloride and hydrochlorothiazide, p. 834, 836
PROSOBEE, p. 1872
PROSTAPHLIN, p. 997
Protamine, Zinc & ILETIN I, p. 1601
Protamine, Zinc & ILETIN II, p. 1601
PROTOSTAT, p. 702, 905
Protriptyline hydrochloride, p. 642
PROTROPIN, p. 1584
PROVENTIL, p. 1199, 1200
PROVENTIL Inhaler, p. 1172
PROVERA, p. 1572
PRUNICODEINE, p. 1398
Pseudoephedrine hydrochloride, p. 1447
Pseudoephedrine hydrochloride and chlorpheniramine maleate, p. 1398, 1448
Pseudoephedrine hydrochloride and codeine phosphate, p. 1397
Pseudoephedrine hydrochloride and guaifenesin, p. 1399
Pseudoephedrine hydrochloride and promethazine hydrochloride, p. 1399
Pseudoephedrine hydrochloride and triprolidine hydrochloride, p. 1399
PSORCON, p. 1363
Psyllium, p. 1627,1628, 1634, 1637, 1640
Psyllium and senna, p. 1639
PULMOCARE, p. 1870
Purified beef insulin, p. 1600, 1601, 1602
Purified pork insulin, p. 1600, 1601, 1602
PURINETHOL, p. 1087
P-V-TUSSIN, p. 1400
PYOPEN, p. 999
Pyrantel pamoate, p. 349
Pyrethrins, piperonyl butoxide, and petroleum distillate, p. 355
Pyrethrins, piperonyl butoxide, petroleum distillate, and benzyl alcohol, p. 356
PYRIDIUM, p. 1848
PYRIDIUM Plus, p. 1849
Pyrithione zinc, p. 227
PYRROXATE, p. 1406
Pyrvinium pamoate, p. 352

Q

QTEST Group A Strep Test, p. 1499
QTEST Ovulation Test, p. 1479
QTEST Pregnancy Test, p. 1490
QUADRINAL, p. 1201
QUARZAN, p. 1129
QUELIDRINE, p. 1406
QUELTUSS, p. 1406
QUESTRAN, p. 1623
QUIBRON, p. 1204
QUIBRON-300, p. 1204
QUIBRON PLUS, p. 1155
QUIBRON-T, p. 1204
QUIBRON-T/SR, p. 1204
QUINAGLUTE, p. 460
QUINAMM, p. 1705
Quinestrol, p. 1560
Quinethazone, p. 1513
Quinethazone and reserpine, p. 756
QUINIDEX, p. 462
Quinidine, p. 124
Quinidine gluconate, p. 460
Quinidine sulfate, p. 462, 463
Quinine sulfate, p. 1705

R

R&C SHAMPOO, p. 355
RAMP, p. 1491
RAMSES, p. 1254
RAMSES BENDEX, p. 1254
Ranitidine hydrochloride, p. 1137
RAPIDTEST-STREP, p. 1500
RAUDIXIN, p. 756
RAUTRAX, p. 757
RAUWILOID, p. 756
Rauwolfia serpentina and bendroflumethiazide, p. 843
Rauwolfia serpentina, flumethiazide, and potassium chloride, p. 757
Rauwolfia serpentina (whole root), p. 756
RAUZIDE, p. 843
RCF, p. 1872
RECOMBIVAX HB, p. 158
REGITINE, p. 756, 803
REGLAN, p. 1073, 1132
REGROTON, p. 845
Regular ILETIN I, p. 1600
Regular ILETIN II, p. 1600
Regular (Concentrated) ILETIN II, p. 1602
Regular Insulin, p. 1600
Regular Purified Insulin, p. 1600
REGUTOL, p. 1643
REMEGEL, p. 332
RENESE, p. 1513
RENESE-R, p. 757
RENOQUID, p. 885
Rescinnamine, p. 756
Reserpine, p. 809
Reserpine and hydralazine hydrochloride, p. 757
Reserpine, hydralazine hydrochloride, and hydrochlorothiazide, p. 850
Reserpine and hydrochlorothiazide, p. 757
RESPBID, p. 1206
RESPIHALER DECADRON Phosphate, p. 1173, 1377
RESTORIL, p. 1815
RETIN-A, p. 217
RETROVIR, p. 139
RHEABAN, p. 664
RHEUMANOSTICON, p. 1509
RHEUMANOSTICON DRI-DOT, p. 1509
RHEUMATEX, p. 1510
RHEUMATON, p. 1510
RHINEX D•LAY, p. 1399

Ribavirin, p. 707
RID, p. 356
RIDAURA, p. 519
RIFADIN, p. 865
Rifampin, p. 865, 866
RIMACTANE, p. 866
RIOPAN, p. 341
RIOPAN PLUS, p. 342
RITALIN, p. 179
RITALIN-SR, p. 179
RMS, p. 230
ROBAXIN, p. 1707
ROBAXISAL, p. 1715
ROBICILLIN VK, p. 917
ROBINUL, p. 1129
ROBINUL Forte, p. 1129
ROBITET, p. 1015
ROBITUSSIN, p. 1406
ROBITUSSIN A-C, p. 1428
ROBITUSSIN-CF, p. 1406
ROBITUSSIN-DAC, p. 1428
ROBITUSSIN-DM, p. 1406
ROBITUSSIN NIGHT RELIEF, p. 1406
ROBITUSSIN-PE, p. 1406
ROCEPHIN, p. 954
ROFERON-A, p. 1116
ROLAIDS, p. 333
RONDEC, p. 1453
RONDEC-DM, p. 1429
RONDEC-TR, p. 1453
RONDOMYCIN, p. 1015
ROSS SLD, p. 1870
ROXANOL, p. 230
ROXANOL SR, p. 230
R₃-SCREEN TEST, p. 1509
RUBACELL II, p. 1508
RUBAQUICK, p. 1508
RUFEN, p. 318, 520
RU-TUSS, p. 1454
RU-TUSS Expectorant, p. 1398
RU-TUSS Liquid, p. 1406
RU-TUSS with Hydrocodone, p. 1399
RU-TUSS II, p. 1406
RU-VERT-M, p. 1059
RYNA, p. 1406
RYNA-C, p. 1431
RYNA-CX, p. 1432
RYNATAN, p. 1399, 1455
RYNATUSS, p. 1433

S

Salsalate, p. 495
SALURON, p. 1513
SALUTENSIN, p. 847
SALUTENSIN-Demi, p. 847
SANSERT, p. 1055
SANTYL, p. 713
Scopolamine, p. 1082
Scopolamine hydrobromide, p. 1129
SEBULEX, p. 224
Secobarbital sodium, p. 571, 1804
Secobarbital sodium and amobarbital sodium, p. 1806
SECONAL Sodium, p. 571, 1804
SECTRAL, p. 465, 778
SEFFIN, p. 919
SELDANE, p. 743
Selenium sulfide, p. 222, 225
SELSUN, p. 225
SELSUN BLUE, p. 225
SEMICID, p. 1254
Semilente ILETIN I, p. 1600
Semilente Insulin, p. 1600
Semilente Purified Insulin, p. 1600
Senna, p. 1643
Senna concentrate and docusate sodium, p. 1628
Senna extract, p. 1628
Sennosides, p. 1627
SENOKAP DSS, p. 1628
SENOKOT, p. 1643
SENOKOT-S, p. 1628
SEPTRA, p. 907, 1841
SEPTRA DS, p. 907, 1841
SEPTRA I.V. Infusion, p. 909, 1843
SER-AP-ES, p. 850
SERAX, p. 411
SERENTIL, p. 1672
SEROPHENE, p. 1580
SERPASIL, p. 809
SERPASIL-APRESOLINE, p. 757
SERPASIL-ESIDRIX, p. 757
SIGTAB, p. 1858
SILAIN-GEL, p. 333
SILVADENE, p. 682
Silver sulfadiazine, p. 672, 682
SIMECO, p. 342
Simethicone, p. 332, 340
Simethicone, aluminum hydroxide, and magnesium hydroxide, p. 332
Simethicone, calcium carbonate, and magnesium hydroxide, p. 332
Simethicone and phenobarbital, p. 341
SIMILAC, p. 1872
SIMILAC PM 60/40, p. 1872
SIMILAC with Iron, p. 1872
SIMRON, p. 1862
SIMRON PLUS, p. 1862
SINAREST, p. 1407
SINE-AID, p. 1407
SINEMET, p. 610
SINE-OFF, p. 1407
SINEQUAN, p. 635
SINEX, p. 1407
SINGLET, p. 1407
SINUBID, p. 1456
SINULIN, p. 1407
SINUTAB, p. 1407
SINUTAB II, p. 1407
SK-AMPICILLIN, p. 1001
SKELAXIN, p. 1708
SLO-BID, p. 1208
SLO-PHYLLIN, p. 1208
SLO-PHYLLIN GG, p. 1155
SLOW FE, p. 1862
SLOW-K, p. 1788
SMA, p. 1872
SMURF, p. 1865
SMURF with Iron and Zinc, p. 1865
Sodium bicarbonate, p. 333
Sodium bicarbonate, citric acid, and potassium bicarbonate, p. 334
Sodium nitroprusside, p. 756, 802
Sodium phosphate and sodium biphosphate, p. 1628, 1635
Sodium salicylate, p. 280
Sodium salicylate and sodium aminobenzoate, p. 280
Sodium sulfacetamide and sulfur, p. 220
Sodium thiosalicylate, p. 280
Sodium thiosulfate, salicylic acid, and isopropyl alcohol, p. 211
SOLGANAL, p. 522
SOLU-CORTEF, p. 1320
SOLU-MEDROL, p. 1330
SOMA, p. 1708
SOMA Compound, p. 1716
SOMA Compound with Codeine, p. 1717
Somatrem, p. 1584
SOMOPHYLLIN, p. 1211
SOMOPHYLLIN Rectal Solution, p. 1211
SOMOPHYLLIN-CRT, p. 1212
SOMOPHYLLIN-DF, p. 1211
SOMOPHYLLIN-T, p. 1211
SORBITRATE, p. 399
SOYALAC, p. 1872
SPARINE, p. 1674
SPARTUS, p. 1858
SPARTUS + Iron, p. 1858
SPEC-T, p. 1407
SPECTAZOLE, p. 683
Spectinomycin hydrochloride, p. 866
SPECTROBID, p. 1002
Spironolactone, p. 1530
Spironolactone and hydrochlorothiazide, p. 1537
ST. JOSEPH Aspirin, p. 320
ST. JOSEPH, Aspirin-Free, p. 321
ST. JOSEPH Cold Tablets, p. 1407
ST. JOSEPH Cough Syrup, p. 1407
STADOL, p. 322
STAPHCILLIN, p. 917
STATICIN, p. 218
STELAZINE, p. 1676
STREPTASE, p. 545
Streptokinase, p. 543, 545
Streptomycin sulfate, p. 863
Streptozocin, p. 1096
STREPTOZYME, p. 1500
STRESSCAPS, p. 1860
STRESSGARD, p. 1858
STRESSTABS 600, p. 1860
STRESSTABS 600 + Iron, p. 1860
STRESSTABS 600 + Zinc, p. 1860
STRI-DEX, p. 219
STUART FORMULA, p. 1858
STUART PRENATAL, p. 1867
STUARTINIC, p. 1862
STUARTNATAL 1 + 1, p. 1867
SUBLIMAZE, p. 259
Sucralfate, p. 1130
SUCRETS, p. 1407
SUDAFED, p. 1407
SUDAFED Plus, p. 1407
SUDAFED S.A., p. 1407
SULAMYD, Sodium, p. 1749
Sulfacetamide sodium, p. 1738, 1749
Sulfacetamide sodium and prednisolone acetate, p. 1739, 1751
Sulfacetamide sodium and prednisolone sodium phosphate, p. 1752
SULFACET-R, p. 220
Sulfacytine, p. 885
Sulfadiazine, p. 864
Sulfadiazine, sulfamerazine, and sulfamethazine, p. 864
Sulfamethizole, p. 886
Sulfamethizole and phenazopyridine hydrochloride, p. 1822
Sulfamethoxazole, p. 882
Sulfamethoxazole and phenazopyridine hydrochloride, p. 1823
Sulfamethoxazole and trimethoprim, p. 1822
Sulfanilamide, p. 692
Sulfanilamide, aminacrine hydrochloride, and allantoin, p. 685
Sulfapyridine, p. 864
Sulfasalazine, p. 880
Sulfathiazole, sulfacetamide, and sulfabenzamide, p. 690
Sulfinpyrazone, p. 717
Sulfisoxazole, p. 884
Sulfisoxazole and phenazopyridine hydrochloride, p. 1824
Sulfur, p. 198
Sulfur and salicylic acid, p. 198, 199, 224
Sulindac, p. 488
SULTRIN, p. 690
SUMYCIN, p. 1042

SUPLICAL, p. 1868
SUPLICAL Chewable, p. 1868
Suprofen, p. 323
SUPROL, p. 323
SURBEX, p. 1860
SURBEX with C, p. 1860
SURBEX-750 with Iron, p. 1860
SURBEX-750 with Zinc, p. 1860
SURBEX-T, p. 1860
SURFAK, p. 1644
SURMONTIL, p. 636
SUS-PHRINE, p. 1155
SUSTACAL HC, p. 1870
SUSTACAL Liquid, p. 1870
SUSTACAL Powder, p. 1870
SUSTACAL Pudding, p. 1870
SUSTAGEN, p. 1870
Sutilains, p. 714
SYMMETREL, p. 612, 704
SYNACORT, p. 1313
SYNALAR, p. 1364
SYNALAR-HP, p. 1364
SYNALGOS, p. 325, 524
SYNALGOS-DC, p. 261
SYNEMOL, p. 1365
SYNTHROID, p. 1594

T

T_3/T_4 liotrix, p. 1596
T_4 thyroxine sodium, p. 1591
TABRON, p. 1862
TACARYL, p. 728
TACE, p. 1569
TAGAMET, p. 1135
TALACEN, p. 262
Talbutal, p. 1796
TALWIN Compound, p. 230
TALWIN Injection, p. 264
TALWIN Nx, p. 265
TAMBOCOR, p. 467
Tamoxifen citrate, p. 1112
TAO, p. 866
TARACTAN, p. 1694
TAVIST, p. 744
TAVIST Syrup, p. 745
TAVIST-1, p. 745
TAVIST-D, p. 1457
TAZICEF, p. 956
TAZIDIME, p. 958
TEDRAL, p. 1214
TEDRAL SA, p. 1214
TEGISON, p. 155
TEGOPEN, p. 1004
TEGRETOL, p. 589
TEGRIN, p. 226
TELDRIN, p. 746
TEMARIL, p. 747
Temazepam, p. 1815
TEMOVATE, p. 1366
TEMPO, p. 333
TEMPRA, p. 326
TENEX, p. 138
TEN-K, p. 1789
TENORETIC, p. 853
TENORMIN, p. 366, 779
Terbutaline sulfate, p. 1162, 1182, 1183
Terfenadine, p. 743
TERFONYL, p. 864
Terpin hydrate with codeine, p. 1434
Terpin hydrate with dextromethorphan, p. 1407
TERRAMYCIN, p. 1044
TERRAMYCIN Intramuscular Solution, p. 1044
TERRAMYCIN Intravenous, p. 1044
TESLAC, p. 1114

TESSALON, p. 1409
TESTPACK hCG-Serum Test, p. 1491
TESTPACK hCG-Urine Test, p. 1492
TESTPACK Strep A Test, p. 1500
TES-TAPE, p. 1474
Testolactone, p. 1114
Testosterone cypionate, p. 1553
Testosterone enanthate, p. 1547
Tetracycline and amphotericin B, p. 1040
Tetracycline hydrochloride, p. 202, 220, 671, 1015, 1034, 1042
Tetrahydrozoline hydrochloride, p. 1400
THALITONE, p. 1513
THEO-24, p. 1215
THEOBID, p. 1218
THEOBID Jr., p. 1218
THEO-DUR, p. 1220
THEO-DUR Sprinkle, p. 1220
THEOLAIR, p. 1222
THEOLAIR-SR, p. 1222
THEO-ORGANIDIN, p. 1155
THEOPHYL-SR, p. 1225
Theophylline, anhydrous, p. 125, 1185, 1190, 1192, 1194, 1204, 1206, 1208, 1211, 1212, 1215, 1218, 1220, 1222, 1225, 1227
Theophylline or aminophylline, ephedrine hydrochloride, phenobarbital, and guaifenesin, p. 1155
Theophylline, ephedrine hydrochloride, and phenobarbital, p. 1214
Theophylline, ephedrine hydrochloride, and phenobarbital or pyrilamine maleate, p. 1155
Theophylline and guaifenesin, p. 1155, 1204
Theophylline, guaifenesin, ephedrine hydrochloride, and butabarbital, p. 1155
Theophylline and iodinated glycerol, p. 1155
Theophylline sodium glycinate and guaifenesin, p. 1154
THEOPHYL-SR, p. 1225
THERACAL Chewable, p. 1868
THERACEBRIN, p. 1858
THERA-COMBEX H-P, p. 1860
THERAGRAN, p. 1858
THERAGRAN HEMATINIC, p. 1862
THERAGRAN Liquid, p. 1858
THERAGRAN Stress Formula, p. 1860
THERAGRAN-M, p. 1858
Thiabendazole, p. 349
Thiethylperazine maleate, p. 1081
Thioguanine, p. 1087
Thioridazine, p. 1665
Thioridazine hydrochloride, p. 1665
THIOSULFIL, p. 886
THIOSULFIL Forte, p. 886
THIOSULFIL-A, p. 1822
Thiotepa, p. 1095
Thiothixene, p. 1692
THORAZINE, p. 1075, 1680
Thrombin, p. 559
THROMBOSTAT, p. 559
Thyroglobulin, p. 1593
Thyroid, p. 1585
THYROLAR, p. 1596
TICAR, p. 1005
Ticarcillin disodium, p. 1005
Ticarcillin disodium and clavulanate potassium, p. 1007
TIGAN, p. 1080
TIMENTIN, p. 1007
TIMOLIDE, p. 855
Timolo maleate, p. 767, 1734
Timolol maleate and hydrochlorothiazide, p. 855
TIMOPTIC, p. 1734
TINACTIN, p. 684
TINDAL, p. 1684
TITRALAC, p. 343
Tobramycin, p. 126, 1750
Tobramycin sulfate, p. 875
TOBREX, p. 1750
Tocainide hydrochloride, p. 470
TODAY, p. 1254
TOFRANIL, p. 638
TOFRANIL-PM, p. 640
Tolazamide, p. 1612
Tolbutamide, p. 1611
TOLECTIN 200, p. 525
TOLECTIN DS, p. 525
TOLINASE, p. 1612
Tolmetin sodium, p. 525
Tolnaftate, p. 669, 684
TONOCARD, p. 470
TOPEX, p. 199
TOPICORT, p. 1367
TOPICORT LP, p. 1367
TOPICYCLINE, p. 220
TORECAN, p. 1081
TORNALATE, p. 1175
TOTACILLIN, p. 1009
TOTACILLIN-N, p. 1009
TRANCOPAL, p. 424
TRANDATE, p. 760
TRANSDERM SCŌP, p. 1082
TRANSDERM-Nitro, p. 400
TRANXENE, p. 413, 592
TRANXENE-SD, p. 413, 592
Tranylcypromine sulfate, p. 633
TRAUMA-AID HBC, p. 1870
TRAUMACAL, p. 1870
TRAVASE, p. 714
Trazodone hydrochloride, p. 618
TRENDAR, p. 327
TRENTAL, p. 548
Tretinoin, p. 217
Triamcinolone, p. 1314
Triamcinolone acetonide, p. 1159, 1333, 1334, 1342, 1359, 1374
Triamcinolone diacetate, p. 1314
Triamcinolone hexacetonide, p. 1311
TRIAMINIC Allergy Tablets, p. 1407
TRIAMINIC Cold Tablets and Syrup, p. 1407
TRIAMINIC Chewable Tablets, p. 1407
TRIAMINIC Expectorant, p. 1407
TRIAMINIC Expectorant DH, p. 1435
TRIAMINIC Expectorant with Codeine, p. 1434
TRIAMINIC Pediatric Drops, p. 1459
TRIAMINIC TR, p. 1459
TRIAMINIC-12, p. 1408
TRIAMINIC-DM, p. 1408
TRIAMINICIN, p. 1408
TRIAMINICOL, p. 1408
Triamterene, p. 1532
Triamterene and hydrochlorothiazide, p. 1539, 1541
TRIAVIL, p. 649
Triazolam, p. 1810
TRI-B-PLEX, p. 1860
Trichlormethiazide, p. 1513
Trichlormethiazide and reserpine, p. 757
Triclocarban, p. 208
TRIDESILON, p. 1368
TRIDESILON, Otic, p. 1768
Tridihexethyl chloride, p. 1129
Tridihexethyl chloride and meprobamate, p. 1148
TRIDIL, p. 402
TRIDIONE, p. 593

Triethanolamine polypeptide oleate-condensate, p. 1770
Trifluoperazine hydrochloride, p. 1676
Triflupromazine hydrochloride, p. 1059, 1690
Trifluridine, p. 1754
TriHEMIC 600, p. 1863
Trihexyphenidyl hydrochloride, p. 598
TRI-IMMUNOL, p. 196
TRIKATES, p. 1773
TRILAFON, p. 1059, 1687
TRI-LEVLEN 21, p. 1300
TRI-LEVLEN 28, p. 1300
TRILISATE, p. 527
Trimeprazine tartrate, p. 747
Trimethadione, p. 593
Trimethaphan camsylate, p. 756, 805
Trimethobenzamide hydrochloride, p. 1080
Trimethoprim, p. 1840, 1845
Trimethoprim and sulfamethoxazole, p. 888, 890, 907, 909, 1826, 1828, 1841, 1843
Trimipramine maleate, p. 636
TRIMOX, p. 1010
TRIMPEX, p. 1845
TRINALIN, p. 1460
TRIND, p. 1408
TRIND-DM, p. 1408
TRI-NORINYL 21-DAY, p. 1302
TRI-NORINYL 28-DAY, p. 1302
TRINSICON, p. 1863
TRINSICON M, p. 1863
Tripelennamine, p. 736
Tripelennamine hydrochloride, p. 736
TRIPHASIL-21, p. 1305
TRIPHASIL-28, p. 1305
TRIPHED, p. 1399
Triple sulfa, p. 864
Triprolidine hydrochloride, p. 728
Triprolidine hydrochloride, pseudoephedrine hydrochloride, and codeine phosphate, p. 1409
TRI-VI-FLOR 0.25 mg, p. 1865
TRI-VI-FLOR 0.5 mg, p. 1865
TRI-VI-FLOR 1.0 mg, p. 1865
TRI-VI-FLOR 0.25 mg with Iron, p. 1865
TRI-VI-SOL, p. 1865
TRI-VI-SOL with Iron, p. 1865
TROBICIN, p. 866
Troleandomycin, p. 866
TRONOLANE, p. 1392
TROPH-IRON, p. 1860
TROPHITE, p. 1861
Tropicamide, p. 1737
T-STAT, p. 199
TUCKS, p. 1393
TUINAL, p. 1806
TUMS, p. 343, 1868
TUMS E-X, p. 343, 1868
TUSSAGESIC, p. 1408
TUSSAR-2, p. 1398
TUSSAR DM, p. 1408
TUSSAR SF, p. 1398
TUSSEND, p. 1437
TUSSEND Expectorant, p. 1438
TUSSIONEX, p. 1439
TUSSI-ORGANIDIN, p. 1440
TUSSI-ORGANIDIN DM, p. 1441
TUSS-ORNADE, p. 1442
TWIN-K, p. 1773
TWIN-K-CI, p. 1773
TwoCal HN, p. 1870
TYCOLET, p. 267
TYCOPAN, p. 1858
TYLENOL, p. 328
TYLENOL Sinus Medication, p. 1408

TYLENOL with Codeine, p. 268
TYLOX, p. 270
TYMPAGESIC Otic Solution, p. 1764
TYZINE, p. 1400

U

UCG-BETA SLIDE, p. 1492
UCG-BETA STAT, p. 1493
UCG-LYPHOTEST, p. 1494
UCG-Slide, p. 1494
ULTRACEF, p. 960
Ultralente ILETIN I, p. 1601
Ultralente Insulin, p. 1601
Ultralente Purified Insulin, p. 1602
UNASYN, p. 154
Undecylenate, p. 670
UNICAP, p. 1858
UNICAP Jr, p. 1865
UNICAP M, p. 1859
UNICAP Plus Iron, p. 1859
UNICAP Senior, p. 1859
UNICAP T, p. 1859
UNIPEN, p. 1011
UNIPHYL, p. 1227
UNPROCO, p. 1398
Urea, p. 1514
UREAPHIL, p. 1514
URECHOLINE, p. 1854
URISED, p. 1847
URISPAS, p. 1852
URISTIX, p. 1470
UROBILISTIX, p. 1470
UROBIOTIC-250, p. 1822
Urofollitropin, p. 143
Urokinase, p. 541
URSINUS, p. 1408
UTICILLIN VK, p. 917
UTICORT, p. 1313

V

VAGESIC, p. 691
VAGISEC PLUS, p. 691
VAGITROL, p. 692
VALISONE, p. 1369
VALIUM, p. 414, 594, 1709
VALMID, p. 1816
VALPIN 50, p. 1129
Valproic acid, p. 126, 583
VALRELEASE, p. 415, 595, 1710
VANCENASE, p. 1383
VANCERIL Inhaler, p. 1176, 1379
VANCOCIN HCl, p. 911
VANCOCIN HCl IntraVenous, p. 911
VANCOLED, p. 145
Vancomycin, p. 127
Vancomycin hydrochloride, p. 145, 911
VANOXIDE, p. 211
VANOXIDE-HC, p. 221
VANQUISH, p. 280
VANSIL, p. 348
VASERETIC, p. 858
VASOCON-A, p. 1762
VASOCIDIN Ophthalmic Ointment, p. 1751
VASOCIDIN Ophthalmic Solution, p. 1752
VASOTEC, p. 765
VATRONOL, p. 1408
V-CILLIN K, p. 1012
VEETIDS, p. 917
VELBAN, p. 1087
VELOSEF, p. 961
VELOSULIN, p. 1600
VELOSULIN Human, p. 1600
VENTOLIN, p. 1229
VENTOLIN Inhaler, p. 1177

VEPESID, p. 1125
Verapamil hydrochloride, p. 370, 374, 430, 432, 442, 444, 783, 785, 786
VERMOX, p. 352
VERSED, p. 1817
VESPRIN, p. 1059, 1690
VIBRAMYCIN, p. 1046
VIBRAMYCIN Intravenous, p. 1046
VIBRA-TABS, p. 1046
VICKS, p. 1408
VICODIN, p. 271
VICON FORTE, p. 1859
VICON Plus, p. 1859
VICON-C, p. 1861
Vidarabine monohydrate, p. 705
VI-DAYLIN ADC Drops, p. 1865
VI-DAYLIN Chewable, p. 1865
VI-DAYLIN Drops, p. 1865
VI-DAYLIN Liquid, p. 1865
VI-DAYLIN ADC + Iron Drops, p. 1865
VI-DAYLIN + Iron Chewable, p. 1865
VI-DAYLIN + Iron Drops, p. 1865
VI-DAYLIN + Iron Liquid, p. 1865
VI-DAYLIN/F ADC Drops, p. 1865
VI-DAYLIN/F ADC + Iron Drops, p. 1866
VI-DAYLIN/F Chewable, p. 1865
VI-DAYLIN/F Drops, p. 1866
VI-DAYLIN/F + Iron Chewable, p. 1866
VI-DAYLIN/F + Iron Drops, p. 1866
VIGRAN, p. 1859
Vinblastine sulfate, p. 1087
Vincristine sulfate, p. 1121
VIOFORM, p. 670
VIOFORM-Hydrocortisone, p. 1370
VIOKASE, p. 346
VI-PENTA Infant Drops, p. 1866
VI-PENTA Multivitamin Drops, p. 1866
VI-PENTA F Chewable, p. 1866
VI-PENTA F Infant Drops, p. 1866
VI-PENTA F Multivitamin Drops, p. 1866
VIRA-A, p. 705
VIRAZOLE, p. 707
VIROGEN Rubella, p. 1508
VIRO-MED, p. 1408
VIROPTIC, p. 1754
VISIDEX II, p. 1468
VISKEN, p. 781
VISTARIL, p. 425, 749
VISTARIL Intramuscular Solution, p. 426, 1083
VISTRAX, p. 1129
VITA-KAPS, p. 1859
VITAKAPS-M, p. 1859
VITAL High Nitrogen, p. 1870
VITRON-C, p. 1863
VITRON-C-PLUS, p. 1863
VIVACTIL, p. 642
VIVONEX, HIGH NITROGEN, p. 1871
VIVONEX, STANDARD, p. 1871
VIVONEX T.E.N., p. 1871
VIVOX, p. 1015
VI-ZAC, p. 1859
VLEMASQUE, p. 222
VONTROL, p. 1059
VōSoL HC Otic Solution, p. 1770
VōSoL Otic Solution, p. 1769
VYTONE, p. 1313

W

Warfarin sodium, p. 539
Warfarin sodium, crystalline, p. 532
4-WAY, p. 1408
WELLCOVORIN, p. 1087
WESTCORT, p. 1371
WIGRAINE, p. 1056
WinGel, p. 333

Witch hazel, p. 1393
Witch hazel and glycerin, p. 1393
Witch hazel and isopropyl alcohol, p. 199
WITHIN, p. 1859
WYAMYCIN E, p. 1032
WYAMYCIN S, p. 1032
WYCILLIN, p. 918
WYGESIC, p. 273
WYMOX, p. 918
WYTENSIN, p. 792

X

XANAX, p. 416
X-PREP, p. 1628

XYLOCAINE for Ventricular Arrhythmias, p. 472

Y

Yeast cell derivative (live) and shark liver oil, p. 1390
Yellow phenolphthalein, p. 1627, 1635
Yellow phenolphthalein and docusate sodium, p. 1627

Z

ZANOSAR, p. 1096
ZANTAC, p. 1137
ZARONTIN, p. 582
ZAROXOLYN, p. 1524
Z-BEC, p. 1861
ZETAR, p. 227
Zidovudine, p. 139
ZINACEF, p. 964
ZINCON, p. 227
Zinc pyrithione, p. 223
ZORPRIN, p. 280
ZOVIRAX Capsules, p. 708
ZOVIRAX Ointment, p. 685
ZOVIRAX Sterile Powder, p. 709
ZYDONE, p. 274
ZYLOPRIM, p. 724
ZYMACAP, p. 1859

Drug Identification

COMPENDIUM OF DRUG THERAPY

Chapter 1

Drug Identification Guide and Index

This chapter contains color photographs and physical descriptions of over 1,800 prescription and over-the-counter medications. The products were selected on the basis of frequency of use and general availability. Not all dosage forms or strengths of a particular product may be shown; therefore, the reader is urged to consult the corresponding drug chart in subsequent sections for information concerning other dosage forms, particularly liquid and parenteral preparations.

COLOR REPRODUCTIONS

For quick visual identification of an unfamiliar capsule or tablet, products are arranged according to color — pink, red, purple, blue, green, yellow, orange, peach, tan, brown, gray, black, multicolored, and white — and by size and shape within each color grouping. (See below for the pages of a particular color grouping.) Two-colored capsules are grouped according to the color of the *outer* capsule shell (or cap); layered tablets are arranged according to the color of the side bearing the name of the product or manufacturer. Round tablets are shown first, followed by oval tablets, capsule-shaped tablets, capsules, and miscellaneous tablet shapes (triangles, squares, pentagons, etc.). Each product is identified by brand name, dosage strength, manufacturer, and, where applicable, manufacturer code number or other markings. All preparations appear in their actual size, except for the oral contraceptive compacts and transdermal patches at the end of the section.

Although great care has been taken to reproduce the appearance of each product, slight color deviations may occur due to limitations of the printing process. When comparing the product illustrations with the appearance of the actual capsules or tablets, remember that colors may vary from batch to batch and are affected by the light under which they are viewed. Other factors inherent in the photography process, such as exposure to light, heat, moisture, and handling (especially of sugar-coated tablets), might alter the drug's appearance slightly. Also, very small or faint markings may not reproduce well because of printing limitations.

Please also remember that manufacturers periodically change the appearance of a pill. Should identification of a certain drug prescribed years ago be in question because it does not match the representation on the following pages, contact the manufacturer for substantiation of the drug's identity (see "Directory of Manufacturers" in Chapter 2 for telephone numbers).

For these reasons, this section should be regarded only as a quick reference guide to drug identification and, except in an emergency situation, should not substitute for a comprehensive chemical analysis when the identity of a particular product is in question.

DRUG IDENTIFICATION GUIDE AND INDEX

Drugs are listed alphabetically by brand name, followed by the name of the manufacturer, dosage strength (unless the drug is a combination product), color, shape, scoring, and manufacturer's code number or other distinguishing marks (indicated by *italics*). The number and letter printed at the end of each description identify the page and row on which the product photograph may be found. The location of oral contraceptive compacts and wallets immediately follows the description and page numbers of the individual contraceptive formulations.

CONTENTS OF COLOR REPRODUCTION SECTION

Capsules and Tablets	**1–41**
Pink	1–4
Red	5–7
Purple	8
Blue	9–11
Green	12–14
Green/Yellow	15
Yellow	16–19
Yellow/Orange	20
Orange	21–23
Peach	24–25
Tan	26
Brown	27–28
Gray/Black	29
Multicolored	30
White	31–41
Oral Contraceptive Compacts	**42–46**
Transdermal Products	**47–48**

Compendium of Drug Therapy

PINK

a SORBITRATE Sublingual 5 mg — Stuart 760	REDISOL 50 μg — Merck Sharp & Dohme	DILAUDID 3 mg — Knoll	FLORINEF Acetate 0.1 mg — Squibb 429	LEVOTHROID 200 μg — Rorer LR	DIULO 2½ mg — Searle 501
b NORLUTATE 5 mg — Parke-Davis 918	DELTASONE 2.5 mg — Upjohn 32	METHERGINE 0.2 mg — Sandoz Pharmaceuticals 78-54	PROLIXIN 1 mg — Princeton 863	TINDAL 20 mg — Schering 968	DARICON-PB — Beecham Laboratories 146
c SYNTHROID 200 μg — Flint	FEMINONE 50 μg — Upjohn	DICUMAROL 50 mg — Abbott AO	HALODRIN — Upjohn 38	ESIDRIX 25 mg — CIBA 22	MODANE Mild 37.5 mg — Adria 13 502
d ENOVID-E — Searle 131	THYROLAR-1 — Rorer YE	EUTONYL 10 mg — Abbott NA	ETRAFON 2-25 — Schering 598	DARBID 5 mg — Smith Kline & French D62	ESTINYL 0.05 mg — Schering 070
e DIUTENSEN-R — Wallace 274	ISORDIL Oral Titradose 5 mg — Wyeth 4152	OREXIN — Stuart	ROBINUL 1 mg — Robins 7824	CELESTONE 0.6 mg — Schering 011	TROPHITE — SmithKline Consumer Products
f MICRONASE 2.5 mg — Upjohn	MESANTOIN 100 mg — Sandoz Pharmaceuticals 78-52	ANASPAZ PB — Ascher 225/300	LEVSIN/PHENOBARBITAL — Kremers-Urban 534	TRIAMINICOL — Sandoz Consumer	NOLAMINE — Carnrick 86204
g SER-AP-ES — CIBA 71	PARNATE 10 mg — Smith Kline & French	PROLIXIN 10 mg — Princeton 956	ST. JOSEPH Aspirin-Free Children's Chewable 80 mg — Plough fruit flavored	ALLEREST Children's Chewable — Pharmacraft	CORRECTOL — Plough
h SPARINE 100 mg — Wyeth 200	NALDECON — Bristol Laboratories N1	ROBINUL Forte 2 mg — Robins 7840	DIUPRES-250 — Merck Sharp & Dohme 230	PHENERGAN 50 mg — Wyeth 227	METAHYDRIN 2 mg — Merrell Dow 62
i NILSTAT Oral 500,000 U — Lederle N5	LARODOPA 250 mg — Roche	ESTRATAB 2.5 mg — Reid-Rowell 1025	DIMETANE Extentabs 8 mg — Robins 1868	Children's ANACIN-3 Chewable 80 mg — Whitehall	Children's PANADOL 80 mg — Glenbrook

COMPENDIUM OF DRUG THERAPY

Compendium of Drug Therapy

PINK

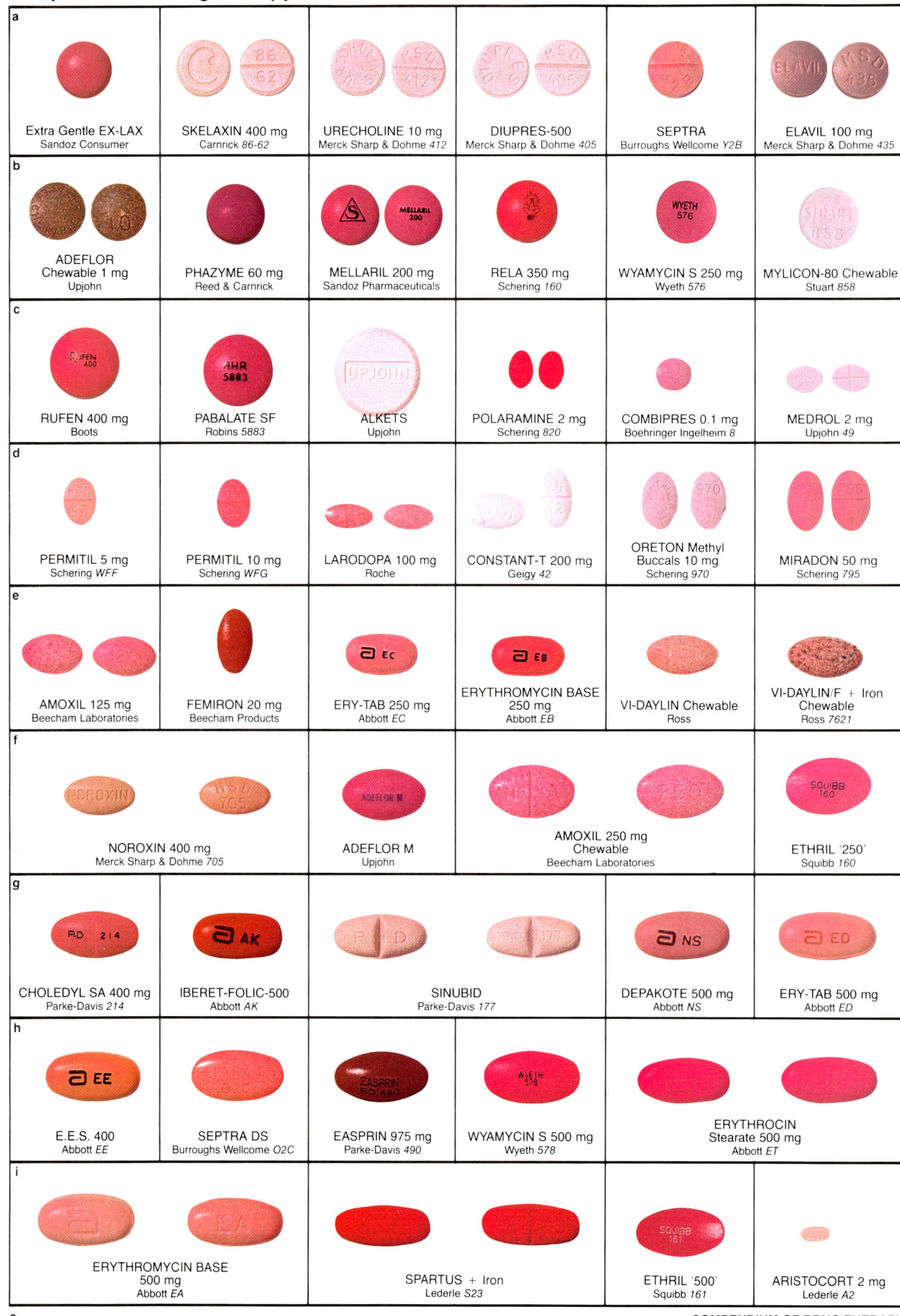

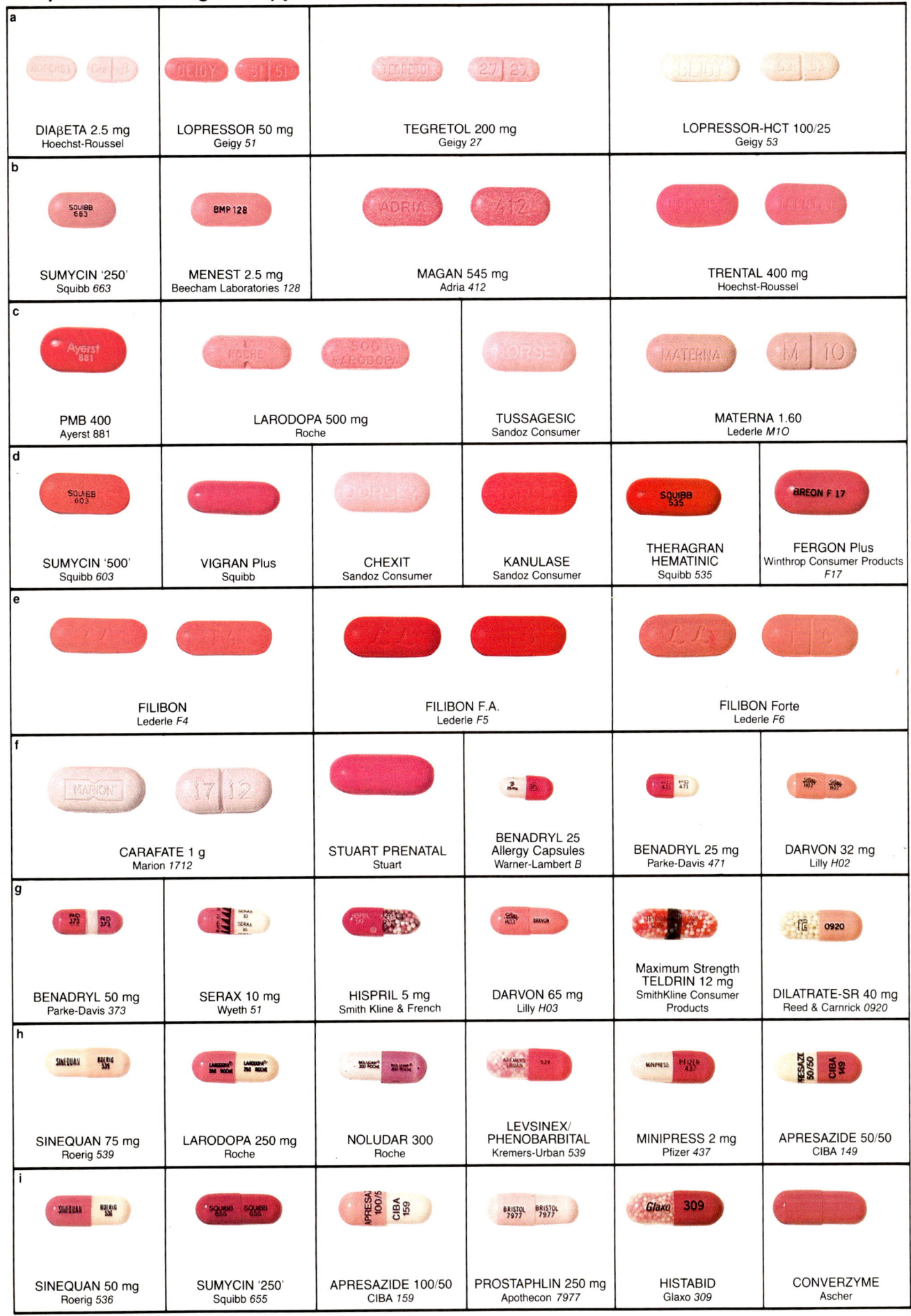

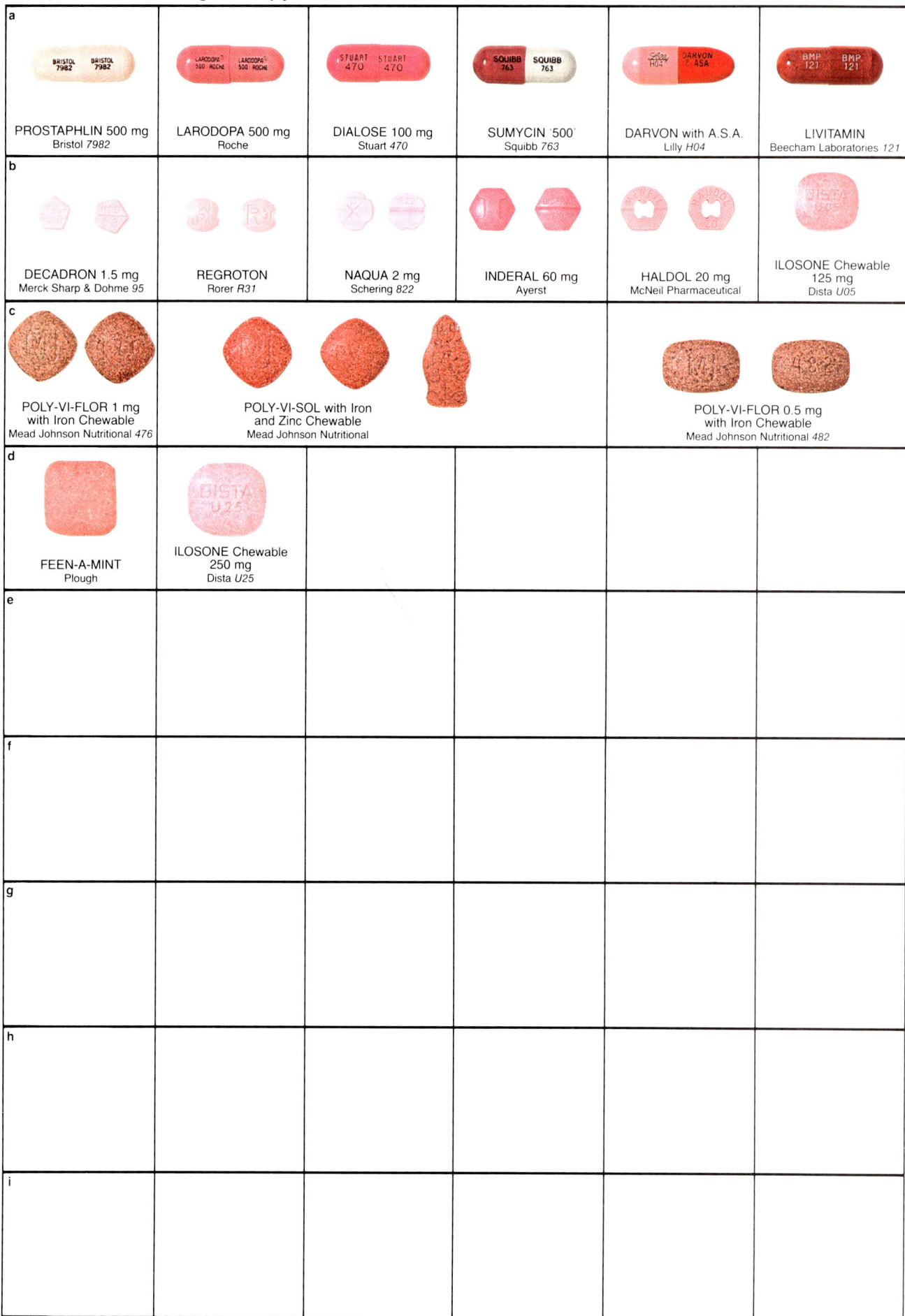

Compendium of Drug Therapy

RED

	1	2	3	4	5	6
a	ETRAFON-FORTE 4-25 Schering 720	SUDAFED 30 mg Burroughs Wellcome	SERENTIL 10 mg Boehringer Ingelheim	BUTAZOLIDIN 100 mg Geigy 14	SERENTIL 25 mg Boehringer Ingelheim	PREMARIN with Methyl-testosterone 0.625/5 Ayerst 878
b	PYRIDIUM 100 mg Parke-Davis 180	CHOLEDYL 100 mg Parke-Davis 210	RAUDIXIN 50 mg Princeton 713	DECLOMYCIN 150 mg Lederle D11	SERENTIL 50 mg Boehringer Ingelheim	ONE-A-DAY Essential Miles Laboratories
c	RAUDIXIN 100 mg Princeton 776	TUSSEND Merrell Dow 42	TEDRAL SA Parke-Davis 231	MOL-IRON with Vitamin C Schering	SERENTIL 100 mg Boehringer Ingelheim	PYRIDIUM 200 mg Parke-Davis 181
d	THIOSULFIL-A Ayerst 784	DECLOMYCIN 300 mg Lederle D12	CORICIDIN Schering 522	AZO GANTANOL Roche	AZO GANTRISIN Roche	Children's HOLD Beecham Products
e	K-LYTE/CL 25 mEq Bristol Laboratories *fruit-punch flavored*					
f			K-LYTE/CL 50 mEq Bristol Laboratories *fruit-punch flavored*			
g	POLARAMINE 4 mg Schering 095	POLARAMINE 6 mg Schering 148	MOL-IRON Schering	PREMARIN 0.625 mg Ayerst	UNICAP Plus Iron Upjohn	FEMIRON Beecham Products
h	SIGTAB Upjohn	FERANCEE-HP Stuart	ALLBEE C-800 + Iron Robins 0678		DEPAKOTE 125 mg Abbott NT	MEDIATRIC Ayerst 752
i	FERO-FOLIC-500 Abbott AJ	FERO-GRAD-500 Abbott	PHAZYME-95 Reed & Carnrick	IBERET-500 Abbott	PERITINIC Lederle P8	

COMPENDIUM OF DRUG THERAPY

Compendium of Drug Therapy

RED

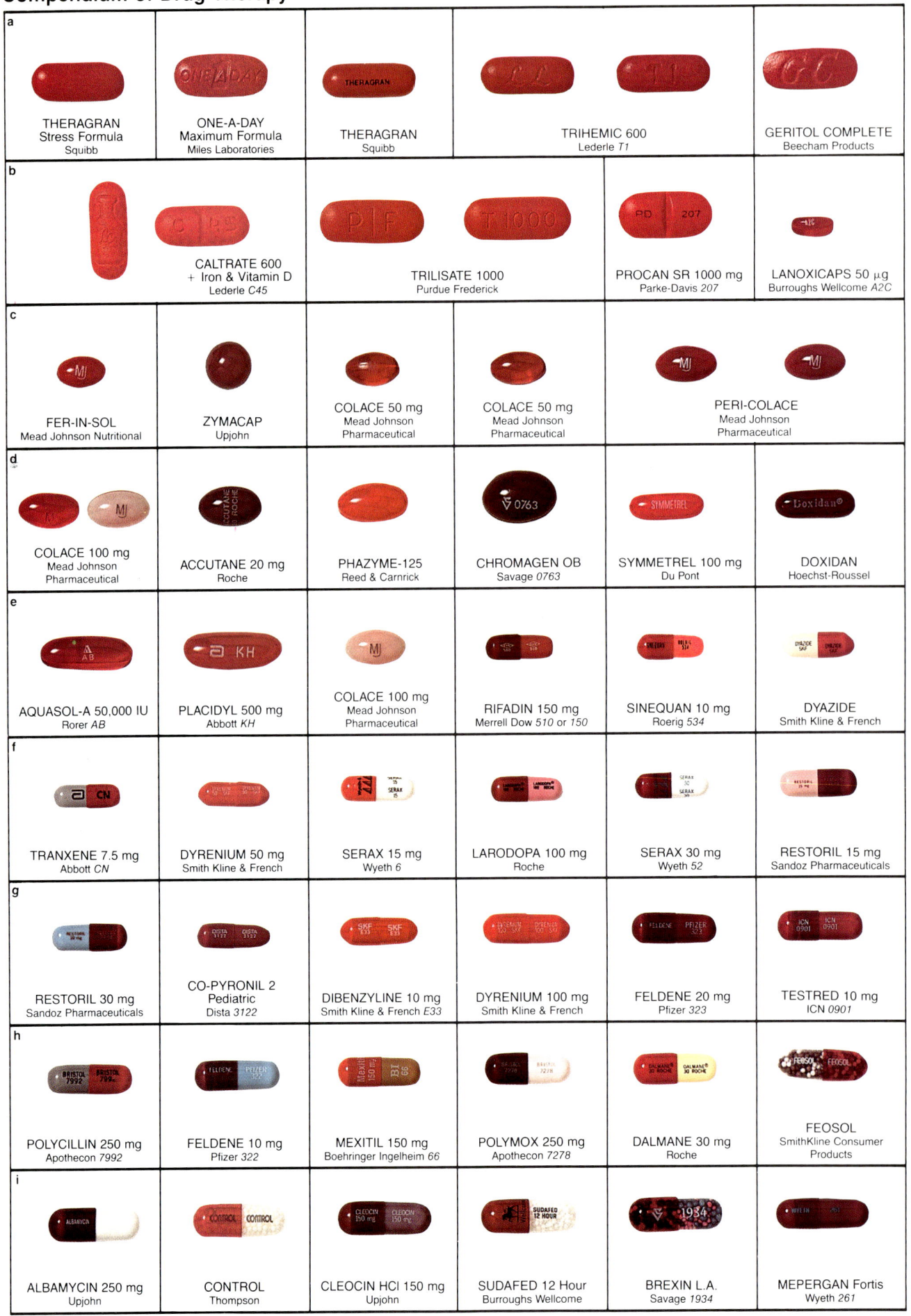

Compendium of Drug Therapy

RED

a VICON-Plus — Glaxo	MEXITIL 200 mg — Boehringer Ingelheim 67	RIFADIN 300 mg — Merrell Dow 508 or 300	THEO-24 300 mg — Searle 2852	DURICEF 500 mg — Mead Johnson 784	DIALUME — Rorer RD
b NICO-400 — Marion 1575	POLYMOX 500 mg — Apothecon 7279	MEXITIL 250 mg — Boehringer Ingelheim 68	NOVAFED-A — Merrell Dow 106	TYLENOL with Codeine No. 4 — McNeil Pharmaceutical	Extra Strength Aspirin-Free SINE-OFF — SmithKline Consumer Products
c RIFAMATE — Merrell Dow 509	DEXATRIM Extra Strength with Vitamin C — Thompson	MIDRIN — Carnrick 86120	POLYCILLIN 500 mg — Apothecon 7993	FIORINAL with Codeine No. 1 — Sandoz Pharmaceuticals 78-105	SURFAK 240 mg — Hoechst-Roussel
d HEPTUNA Plus — Roerig 504	TRINSICON — Glaxo	TRINSICON M — Glaxo	BASALJEL — Wyeth 472	FERGON 435 mg — Winthrop-Breon	CHROMAGEN — Savage 4285
e VASERETIC — Merck Sharp & Dohme 720	ASPERGUM — Plough cherry flavored	SPEC-T Anesthetic Lozenges — Squibb			

Compendium of Drug Therapy

PURPLE

a ESTRACE 1 mg Mead Johnson Laboratories 755	LEVOTHROID 125 µg Rorer *LH*	ZAROXOLYN 2½ mg Pennwalt	MELLARIL 15 mg Sandoz Pharmaceuticals *78-8*	MENRIUM 10-4 Roche	SYNTHROID 75 µg Flint
b THYROLAR-¼ Rorer *YC*	CHLORTHALIDONE 50 mg Abbott *AB*	PBZ-SR 100 mg Geigy *48*	MS CONTIN 30 mg Purdue Frederick *M30*	MOBAN 10 mg Du Pont	PANWARFIN 2 mg Abbott *LM*
c URISED Alcon *W-2183*	COUMADIN 2 mg Du Pont	METATENSIN No. 4 Merrell Dow *65*	ALLEREST Chewable Pharmacraft	TEMPRA Chewable 80 mg Mead Johnson Nutritional	PERCODAN-Demi Du Pont *136*
d PHRENILIN Carnrick *8650*	HALCION 0.125 mg Upjohn	XANAX 1 mg Upjohn	OS-CAL Plus Marion	PREMARIN 2.5 mg Ayerst	EUTRON Abbott *NK*
e PRAMILET FA Ross *121*	MANDELAMINE 1 g Parke-Davis *167*	MEDIATRIC Ayerst *252*	KAON 5 mEq Adria *312*		NITRO-BID 2.5 mg Marion *1550*
f CECLOR 250 mg Lilly *3061*	SECTRAL 200 mg Wyeth *4177*	MINOCIN 100 mg Lederle *M4*	PATHOCIL 250 mg Wyeth *360*	OMNIPEN 250 mg Wyeth *53*	ACHROMYCIN V 250 mg Lederle *A3*
g AMOXIL 250 mg Beecham Laboratories	PHRENILIN with Codeine No. 3 Carnrick *8655*	SLO-PHYLLIN 250 mg Rorer *1356*	OMNIPEN 500 mg Wyeth *309*	PATHOCIL 500 mg Wyeth *593*	PHRENILIN Forte Carnrick *8656*
h CECLOR 500 mg Lilly *3062*	ACHROMYCIN V 500 mg Lederle *A5*	AMOXIL 500 mg Beecham Laboratories	HALDOL 2 mg McNeil Pharmaceutical	INDERAL 90 mg Ayerst	
i					

Compendium of Drug Therapy

BLUE

a						
	NORPRAMIN 10 mg Merrell Dow 68-7	NYTILAX 12 mg Mentholatum	LEVOTHROID 150 µg Rorer LN	CYSTOSPAZ 0.15 mg Alcon 2225	BLOCADREN 5 mg Merck Sharp & Dohme 59	ZAROXOLYN 5 mg Pennwalt
b	DIULO 5 mg Searle 511	BREVICON Syntex 110	TRI-NORINYL Syntex 110	ELAVIL 10 mg Merck Sharp & Dohme 23	RITALIN 10 mg CIBA 3	STELAZINE 1 mg Smith Kline & French S03
c	MAXOLON 10 mg Beecham Laboratories 192	RENESE-R Pfizer 446	ESTROVIS 100 µg Parke-Davis 437	SYNTHROID 150 µg Flint	BENTYL 20 mg Lakeside 123 or 20	STELAZINE 2 mg Smith Kline & French S04
d	DIUTENSEN Wallace 272	MICRONASE 5 mg Upjohn	DISOPHROL Schering WBS	BLOCADREN 10 mg Merck Sharp & Dohme 136	DITROPAN 5 mg Marion 1375	CHLOR-TRIMETON Decongestant Tablets Schering 901
e	MOBAN 50 mg Du Pont	KLONOPIN 1 mg Roche	APRESOLINE 25 mg CIBA 39	ALLEREST Allergy and Hay Fever Tablets Pharmacraft		FLAGYL 250 mg Searle 1831
f	STELAZINE 5 mg Smith Kline & French S06	DEMAZIN Schering 133	APRESOLINE 50 mg CIBA 73	REMSED 50 mg Du Pont 051	METAHYDRIN 4 mg Merrell Dow 63	ESIDRIX 100 mg CIBA 192
g	DIMETAPP Robins 2254	LIMBITROL Roche	STELAZINE 10 mg Smith Kline & French S07	CORGARD 40 mg Princeton 207	ESTRATAB 0.3 mg Reid-Rowell 1014	AFRINOL 120 mg Schering
h	FIORICET Sandoz Pharmaceuticals	CORGARD 80 mg Princeton 241	DIMETAPP Robins	DISALCID 500 mg Riker	NORMODYNE 300 mg Schering 438	COMBIPRES 0.2 mg Boehringer Ingelheim 9
i	HALCION 0.25 mg Upjohn	UNISOM Dual Relief Leeming	SORBITRATE Oral 40 mg Stuart 774	SORBITRATE Oral 20 mg Stuart 820	SINEMET 10-100 Merck Sharp & Dohme 647	OGEN 2.5 Abbott LX

COMPENDIUM OF DRUG THERAPY

Compendium of Drug Therapy

BLUE

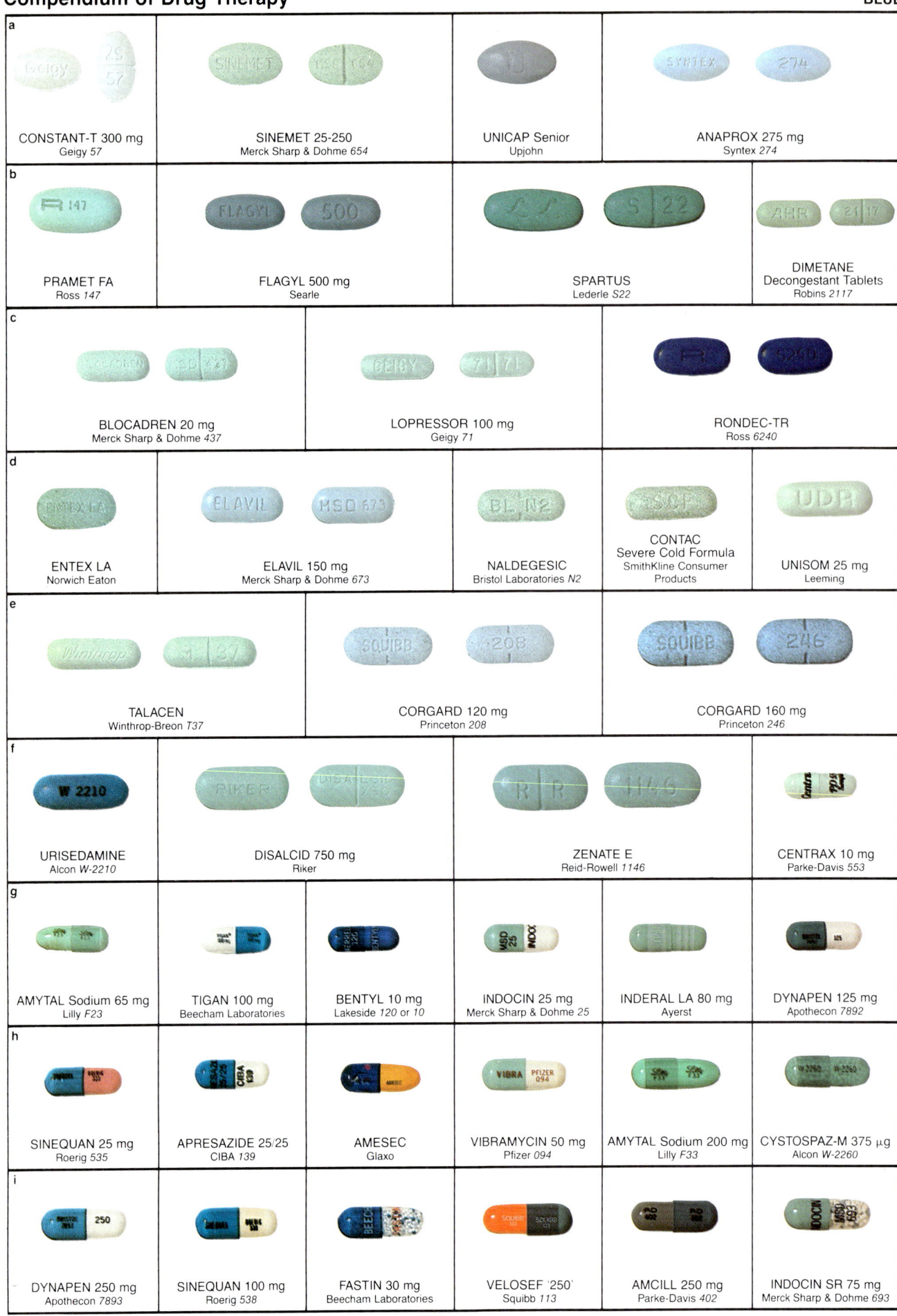

Compendium of Drug Therapy

BLUE

a BENADRYL Decongestant Allergy Capsules — Warner-Lambert *D*	VALRELEASE 15 mg — Roche	SURMONTIL 25 mg — Wyeth *4132*	THEOBID Jr. 130 mg — Glaxo *295*	DORYX 100 mg — Parke-Davis	RONDOMYCIN 150 mg — Wallace *37-4001*
b INDERAL LA 120 mg — Ayerst	INDERAL LA 160 mg — Ayerst	TIGAN 250 mg — Beecham Laboratories	TUSS-ORNADE — Smith Kline & French	INDOCIN 50 mg — Merck Sharp & Dohme *50*	ZOVIRAX 200 mg — Burroughs Wellcome
c LINCOCIN 250 mg — Upjohn	SUPROL 200 mg — McNeil/Ortho Pharmaceutical *1500*	NAVANE 20 mg — Roerig *577*	Tetracycline 250 mg — Wyeth *389*	CORYBAN-D — Leeming *369*	SYNALGOS-DC — Wyeth *4191*
d DYCILL 250 mg — Beecham Laboratories *165*	RONDOMYCIN 300 mg — Wallace *37-4101*	ORNEX — SmithKline Consumer Products	VIBRAMYCIN 100 mg — Pfizer *095*	HEAD & CHEST — Richardson-Vicks Health Care *NE 036*	DYNAPEN 500 mg — Apothecon *7658*
e AMCILL 500 mg — Parke-Davis *404*	DYCILL 500 mg — Beecham Laboratories *166*	DEMSER 250 mg — Merck Sharp & Dohme *690*	MINIPRESS 5 mg — Pfizer *438*	HYDROCET — Carnrick *8657*	SINEQUAN 150 mg — Roerig *537*
f VELOSEF '500' — Squibb *114*	VALMID 500 mg — Dista *H74*	THEOBID 260 mg — Glaxo *268*	FIORINAL with Codeine No. 3 — Sandoz Pharmaceuticals *78-107*	Tetracycline 500 mg — Wyeth *471*	LINCOCIN 500 mg — Upjohn
g DECONAMINE SR — Berlex *181*	NICOBID 500 mg — Rorer *2841*	INDERAL 20 mg — Ayerst	DECADRON 0.75 mg — Merck Sharp & Dohme *63*	DIABINESE 100 mg — Pfizer *393*	HYGROTON 50 mg — Rorer *20*
h TRANXENE 3.75 mg — Abbott *TL*	TIMOLIDE 10-25 — Merck Sharp & Dohme *67*	TRIAVIL 2-10 — Merck Sharp & Dohme *914*	VALIUM 10 mg — Roche	HALDOL 10 mg — McNeil Pharmaceutical	DIABINESE 250 mg — Pfizer *394*
i					

COMPENDIUM OF DRUG THERAPY

Compendium of Drug Therapy

GREEN

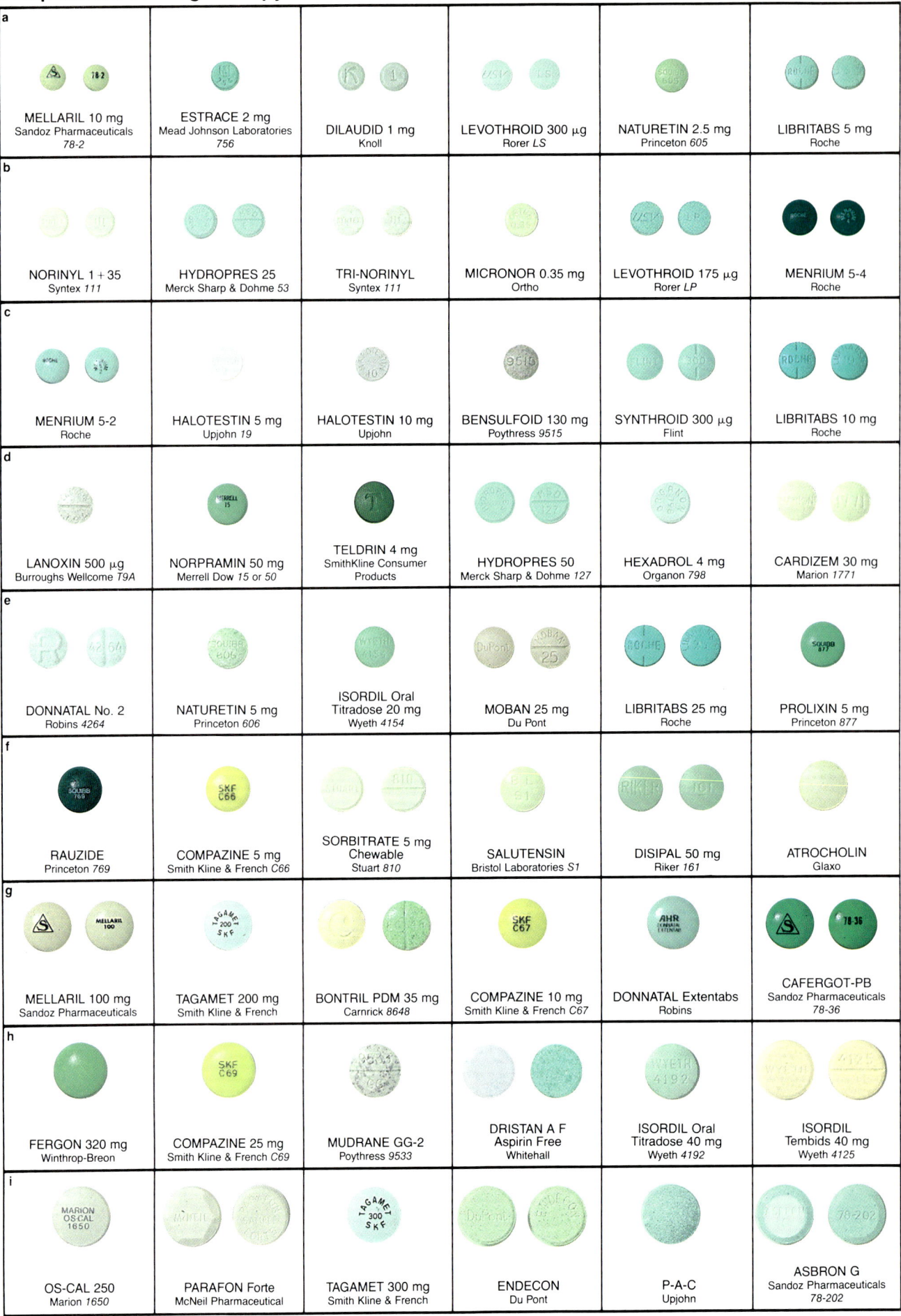

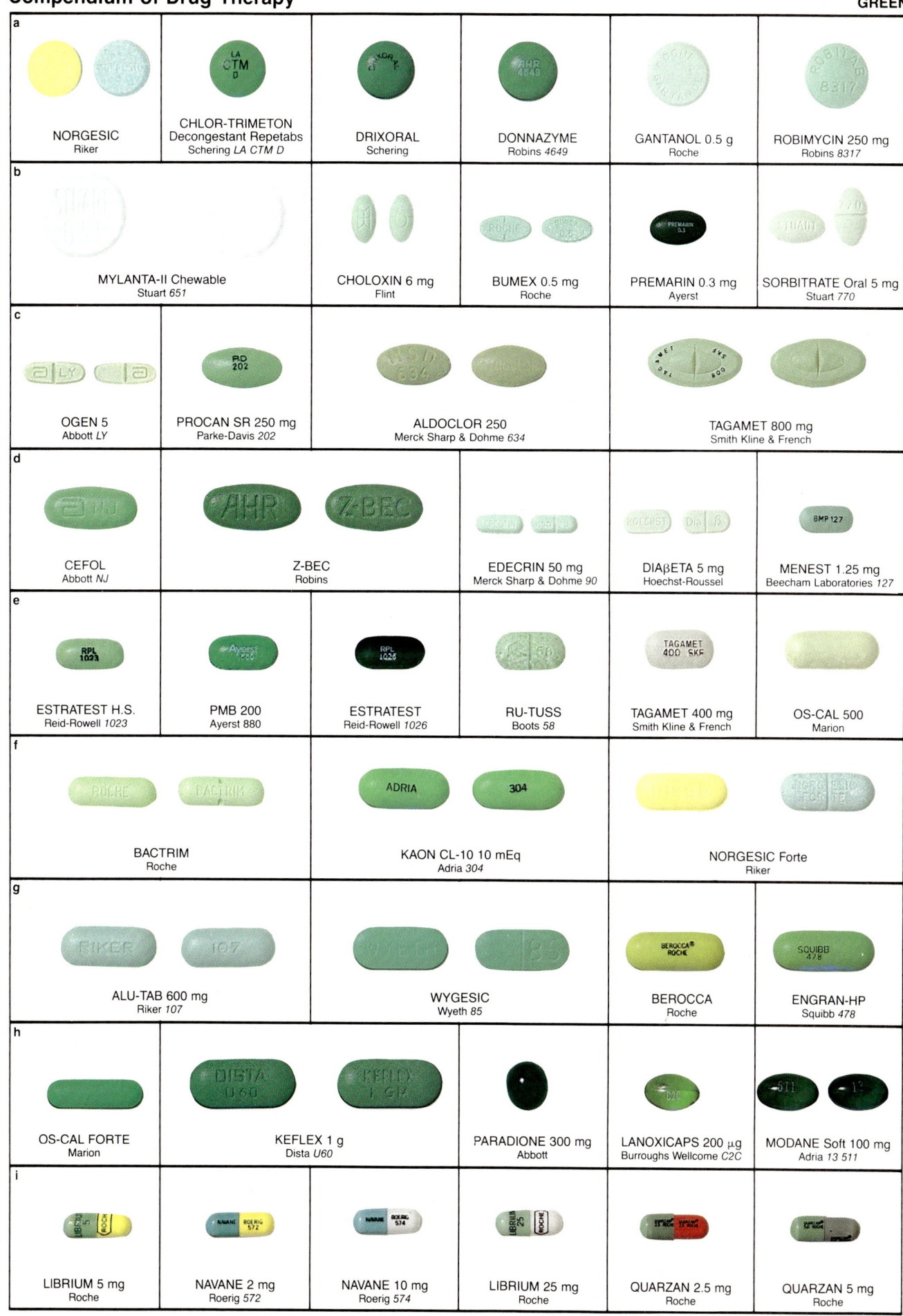

Compendium of Drug Therapy

GREEN

a VISTARIL 25 mg — Pfizer 541	VISTARIL 50 mg — Pfizer 542	IMODIUM 2 mg — Janssen	CENTRAX 5 mg — Parke-Davis 552	ANTROCOL — Poythress	DONNATAL — Robins 4207
b LIBRAX — Roche	ADAPIN 25 mg — Pennwalt	CO-PYRONIL 2 — Dista 3123	TUSSIONEX — Pennwalt	VISTARIL 100 mg — Pfizer 543	CLOXAPEN 250 mg — Beecham Laboratories 169
c NORPACE CR 100 mg — Searle 2732	CINOBAC 250 mg — Dista 3055	MINIZIDE 2 — Pfizer 432	MINIZIDE 1 — Pfizer 430	ADAPIN 50 mg — Pennwalt	THEOVENT 125 mg — Schering 402
d ORUDIS 75 mg — Wyeth 4187	ANCOBON 250 mg — Roche	ORUDIS 50 mg — Wyeth 4181	COMPAL — Reid-Rowell 1290	AQUASOL-E 100 IU — Rorer	TRIMOX '250' — Squibb 230
e ALLBEE with C — Robins 0674	RU-TUSS II — Boots 31	PRELU-2 105 mg — Boehringer Ingelheim 64	KUTRASE — Kremers-Urban 475	ADAPIN 100 mg — Pennwalt	FERRO-Sequels — Lederle F2
f BONTRIL 105 mg — Carnrick 8647	DIMACOL — Robins 1652	ANTURANE 200 mg — CIBA 168	VANSIL 250 mg — Pfizer 641	QUIBRON PLUS — Bristol Laboratories 518	MINIZIDE 5 — Pfizer 436
g DISALCID 500 mg — Riker	HYDREA 500 mg — Squibb 830	CLOXAPEN 500 mg — Beecham Laboratories 170	FIORINAL — Sandoz Pharmaceuticals 78-103	LIVITAMIN with Intrinsic Factor — Beecham Laboratories 122	THEOVENT 250 mg — Schering 753
h NICOBID 250 mg — Rorer 2840	PHENAPHEN with Codeine No. 4 — Robins 6274	KEFLEX 250 mg — Dista H69	TACE 25 mg — Merrell Dow 691	NITRO-BID 9 mg — Marion 1553	COTAZYM 25 mg — Organon 381
i SOLATENE 30 mg — Roche	TRIMOX '500' — Squibb 231	UNIPEN 250 mg — Wyeth 57	ALU-CAP 475 mg — Riker	CINOBAC 500 mg — Dista 3056	KEFLEX 500 mg — Dista H71

Compendium of Drug Therapy

GREEN/YELLOW

a TACE 12 mg Merrell Dow 690	ATARAX 25 mg Roerig	FEOSOL SmithKline Consumer Products	DECADRON 6 mg Merck Sharp & Dohme 147	NAQUA 4 mg Schering 547	HALDOL 5 mg McNeil Pharmaceutical
b INDERAL 40 mg Ayerst	ANDROID-10 Brown 958		SPEC-T Decongestant Lozenges Squibb		
c					
d					
e ISORDIL 2.5 mg Sublingual Wyeth	NORINYL 1+80 Syntex 3	OVRETTE 0.075 mg Wyeth 62	TRIPHASIL Wyeth 643	ANTROCOL Poythress 9540	TRI-LEVLEN Berlex 97
f SANSERT 2 mg Sandoz Pharmaceuticals 78-58	NORLESTRIN 1/50 Parke-Davis 904	DULCOLAX 5 mg Boehringer Ingelheim 12	SORBITRATE Sublingual 10 mg Stuart 761	DILAUDID 4 mg Knoll	OVCON-50 Mead Johnson Laboratories 584
g DIULO 10 mg Searle 521	INVERSINE 2.5 mg Merck Sharp & Dohme 52	LANOXIN 125 μg Burroughs Wellcome Y3B	MEPHYTON 5 mg Merck Sharp & Dohme 43	RITALIN 5 mg CIBA 7	NOR Q.D. 0.35 mg Syntex 2107
h CANTIL 25 mg Merrell Dow 37	DARANIDE 50 mg Merck Sharp & Dohme 49	ORTHO-NOVUM 1/50 Ortho 150	ZAROXOLYN 10 mg Pennwalt	ELAVIL 25 mg Merck Sharp & Dohme 45	JANIMINE 25 mg Abbott NE
i TORECAN 10 mg Boehringer Ingelheim 28	SPARINE 25 mg Wyeth 29	SYNTHROID 100 μg Flint	PLEGINE 35 mg Ayerst	NAQUIVAL Schering 394	THYROLAR-3 Rorer YH

Compendium of Drug Therapy

YELLOW

a ETRAFON 2-10 Schering 287	NORPRAMIN 25 mg Merrell Dow 11 or 25	RITALIN 20 mg CIBA 34	HEXADROL 0.5 mg Organon 792	SERPASIL-APRESOLINE No. 1 CIBA 40	APRESOLINE 10 mg CIBA 37
b TRIAMINIC Allergy Sandoz Consumer	CHLOR-TRIMETON 4 mg Schering 080	PRIMATENE P-Formula Whitehall	BUCLADIN-S Stuart 864	PANWARFIN 7½ mg Abbott LR	ALDOMET 125 mg Merck Sharp & Dohme 135
c ISORDIL 10 mg Chewable Wyeth 4164	PRIMATENE M-Formula Whitehall	PROLIXIN 2.5 mg Princeton 864	ANASPAZ O.125 mg Ascher 225/295	FEDRAZIL Burroughs Wellcome	PROLOPRIM 200 mg Burroughs Wellcome
d ISMELIN 10 mg CIBA 49	METATENSIN No. 2 Merrell Dow 64	HYDROMOX R Lederle	SALUTENSIN-Demi Bristol Laboratories S3	RENESE 2 mg Pfizer 376	CHLOR-TRIMETON Repetabs 8 mg Schering 374
e COUMADIN 7½ mg Du Pont	SORBITRATE 10 mg Chewable Stuart 815	ISOPTIN 80 mg Knoll	PURINETHOL 50 mg Burroughs Wellcome O4A	REGUTOL 100 mg Plough	PREMARIN with Methyl-testosterone 1.25/10 Ayerst 879
f CARDIZEM 60 mg Marion 1772	MUDRANE Poythress 9550	DRISTAN Whitehall	ESTRATAB 0.625 mg Reid-Rowell 1022	MUDRANE GG Poythress 9551	ENDEP 75 mg Roche
g ALDOMET 250 mg Merck Sharp & Dohme 401	MODANE 75 mg Adria 13 501	MELLARIL 150 mg Sandoz Pharmaceuticals	PERCODAN Du Pont	COMHIST Norwich Eaton 0444-0149	EQUANIL Wyseals 400 mg Wyeth 33
h Cod Liver Oil Concentrate Schering	NAPROSYN 250 mg Syntex 272	LUFYLLIN-GG Wallace 541	SORBITRATE SA 40 mg Stuart 880	TRIAMINIC TR Sandoz Consumer	SINAREST Sinus Relief Pharmacraft
i URECHOLINE 25 mg Merck Sharp & Dohme 457	Regular Strength SINE-OFF with Aspirin SmithKline Consumer Products	KAON-CL 6.7 mEq Adria 307	MI-CEBRIN Dista C19	UNILAX Ascher	PANMYCIN 500 mg Upjohn

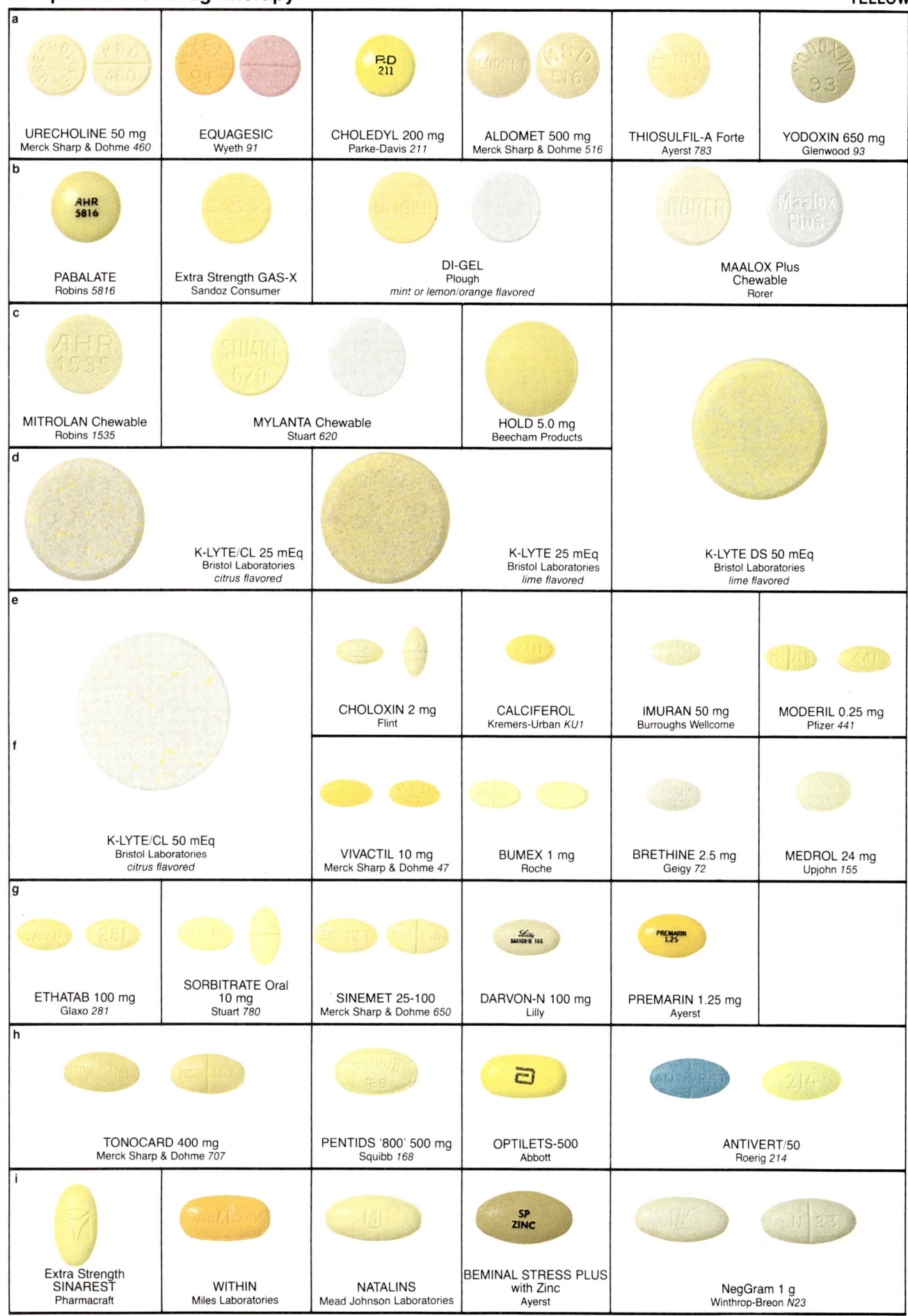

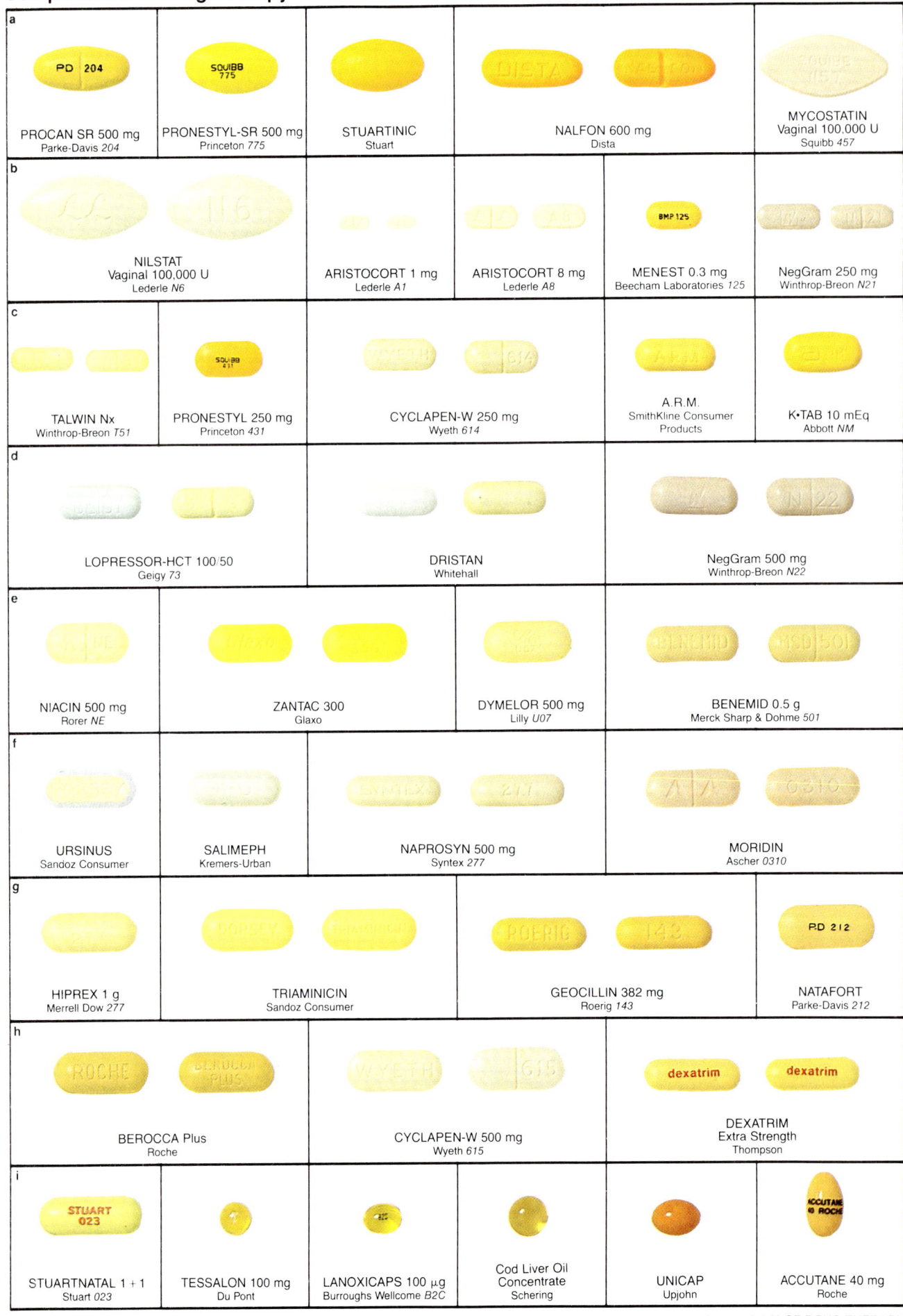

Compendium of Drug Therapy

YELLOW

a CELONTIN 150 mg — Parke-Davis 537	CENTRAX 20 mg — Parke-Davis 554	NEMBUTAL Sodium — Abbott CH	ADAPIN 10 mg — Pennwalt	IONAMIN 30 mg — Pennwalt	MACRODANTIN 50 mg — Norwich Eaton 0149-0008
b AVENTYL HCl 10 mg — Lilly H17	ACTIFED — Burroughs Wellcome	CELONTIN 300 mg — Parke-Davis 525	MATULANE 50 mg — Roche	PRONESTYL 250 mg — Princeton 758	DANOCRINE 100 mg — Winthrop-Breon DO4
c ADAPIN 75 mg — Pennwalt	MACRODANTIN 100 mg — Norwich Eaton 0149-0009	CUPRIMINE 250 mg — Merck Sharp & Dohme 602	PONSTEL 250 mg — Parke-Davis 540	FEDAHIST — Kremers-Urban 1053	COMHIST LA — Norwich Eaton 0149-0446
d ACTIFED 12-Hour — Burroughs Wellcome	KU-ZYME — Kremers-Urban 522	ANACIN — Whitehall	AVENTYL HCl 25 mg — Lilly H19	ELIXOPHYLLIN 200 mg — Forest	QUIBRON — Bristol Laboratories 516
e QUIBRON — Bristol Laboratories 516	DIALOSE Plus — Stuart 475	UROBIOTIC-250 — Roerig 092	Extra Strength Aspirin-Free SINE-OFF — SmithKline Consumer Products	GRISACTIN 250 mg — Ayerst	TERRAMYCIN 250 mg — Pfizer 073
f QUIBRON-300 — Bristol Laboratories 515		TACE 72 mg — Merrell Dow 692		DECADRON 0.5 mg — Merck Sharp & Dohme 41	HALDOL 1 mg — McNeil Pharmaceutical
g MIDAMOR 5 mg — Merck Sharp & Dohme 92	ENDURONYL — Abbott LS	ATARAX 50 mg — Roerig	DILANTIN INFATABS 50 mg — Parke-Davis 007	SERAX 15 mg — Wyeth 317	FLEXERIL 10 mg — Merck Sharp & Dohme 931
h OCTAMIDE 10 mg — Adria 230	TRIAVIL 4-25 — Merck Sharp & Dohme 946	VALIUM 5 mg — Roche	INDERAL 80 mg — Ayerst	CLINORIL 150 mg — Merck Sharp & Dohme 941	CLINORIL 200 mg — Merck Sharp & Dohme 942
i TRIAMINIC Chewable — Sandoz Consumer	KENACORT 8 mg — Squibb 518	MAXZIDE — Lederle M8	QUIBRON-T 300 mg — Bristol Laboratories 512	TONOCARD 600 mg — Merck Sharp & Dohme 709	

COMPENDIUM OF DRUG THERAPY

Compendium of Drug Therapy

YELLOW/ORANGE

a SPEC-T Cough Suppressant Lozenges — Squibb					
b					
c					
d PERSANTINE 25 mg — Boehringer Ingelheim 17	NORDETTE — Wyeth 75	ERGOSTAT Sublingual 2 mg — Parke-Davis 111	DILAUDID 2 mg — Knoll	JANIMINE 10 mg — Abbott ND	MINOCIN 50 mg — Lederle M3
e LEVOTHROID 25 μg — Rorer LK	ENDEP 10 mg — Roche	LUDIOMIL 50 mg — CIBA 26	EUTONYL 25 mg — Abbott NB	VONTROL 25 mg — Smith Kline & French	ETRAFON-A 4-10 — Schering 119
f PERSANTINE 50 mg — Boehringer Ingelheim 18	THYROLAR-½ — Rorer YD	MOBAN 5 mg — Du Pont	VIGRAN — Squibb	PONDIMIN 20 mg — Robins 6447	HEXADROL 1.5 mg — Organon 790
g PHENERGAN-D — Wyeth 434	KLONOPIN 0.5 mg — Roche	TRIAMINIC Cold Tablets — Sandoz Consumer	MINOCIN 100 mg — Lederle M5	TARACTAN 50 mg — Roche	ENOVID 5 mg — Searle 51
h LODOSYN — Merck Sharp & Dohme 129	PANWARFIN 2½ mg — Abbott LN	ENDEP 25 mg — Roche	PHENERGAN 12.5 mg — Wyeth 19	ST. JOSEPH Chewable Aspirin 81 mg — Plough orange flavored	TEDRAL-25 — Parke-Davis 238
i MARPLAN 10 mg — Roche	PAXIPAM 20 mg — Schering 251	PERSANTINE 75 mg — Boehringer Ingelheim 19	CHLOR-TRIMETON Repetabs 12 mg — Schering 009	NORPRAMIN 75 mg — Merrell Dow 19 or 75	SPARINE 50 mg — Wyeth 28

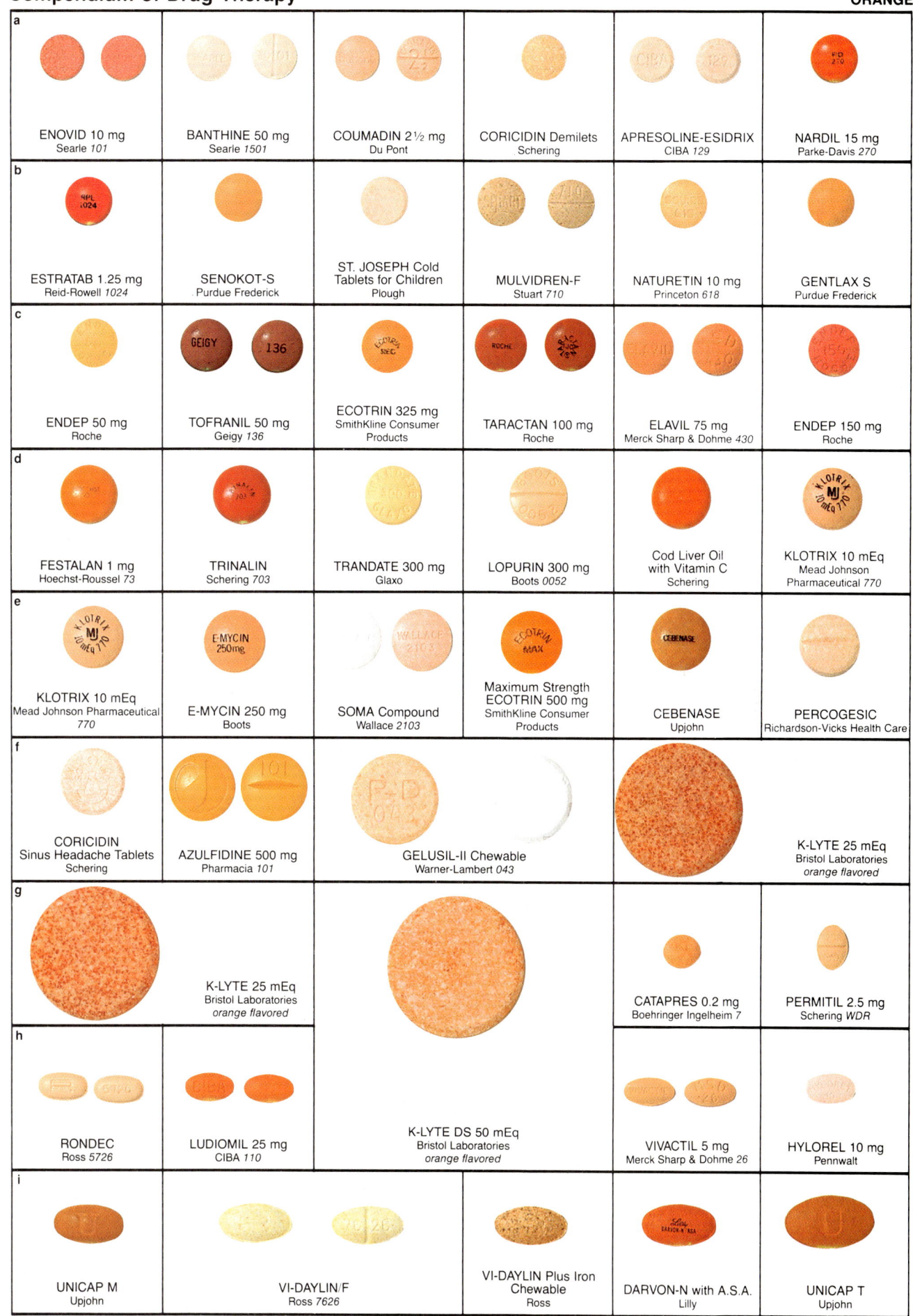

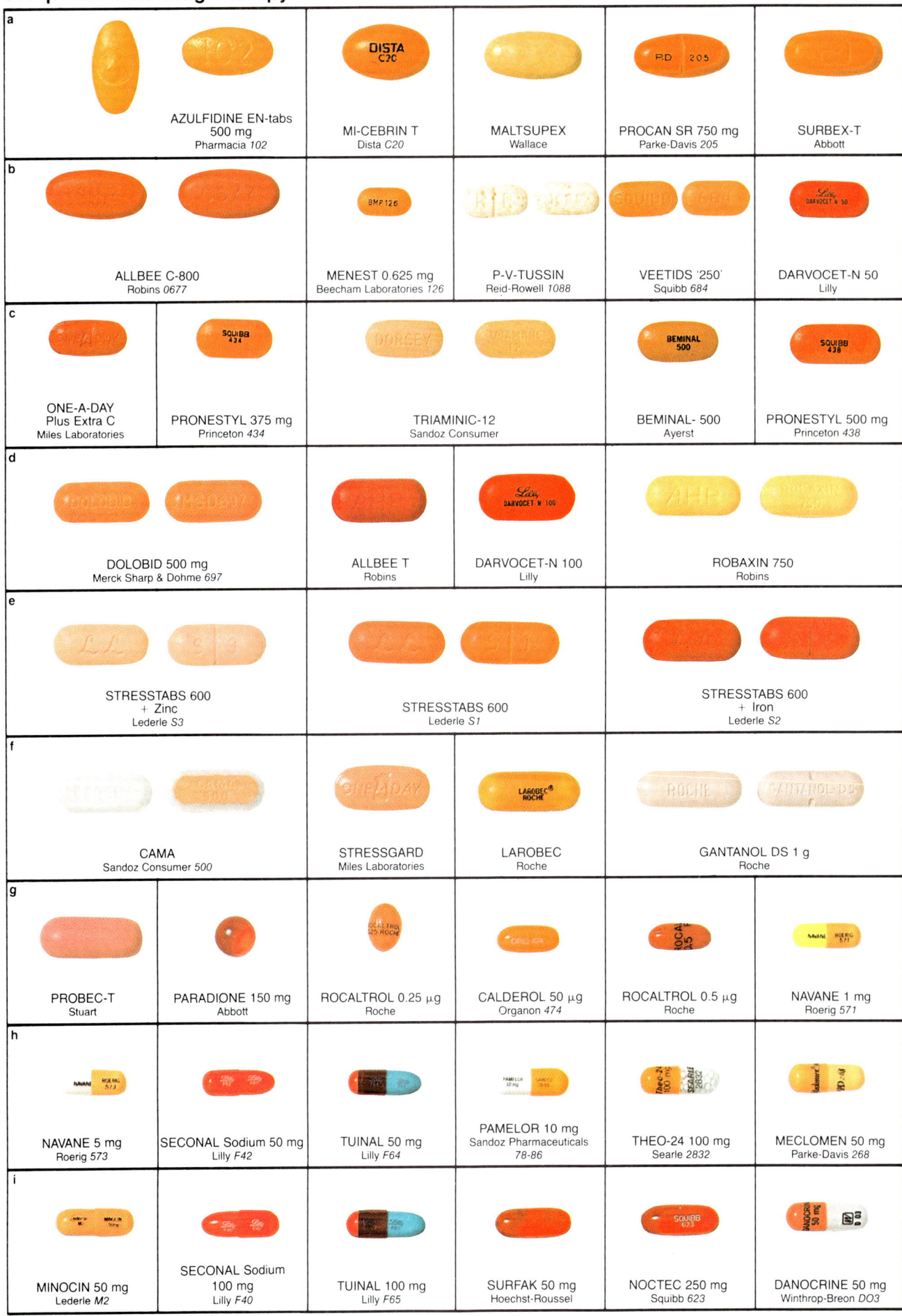

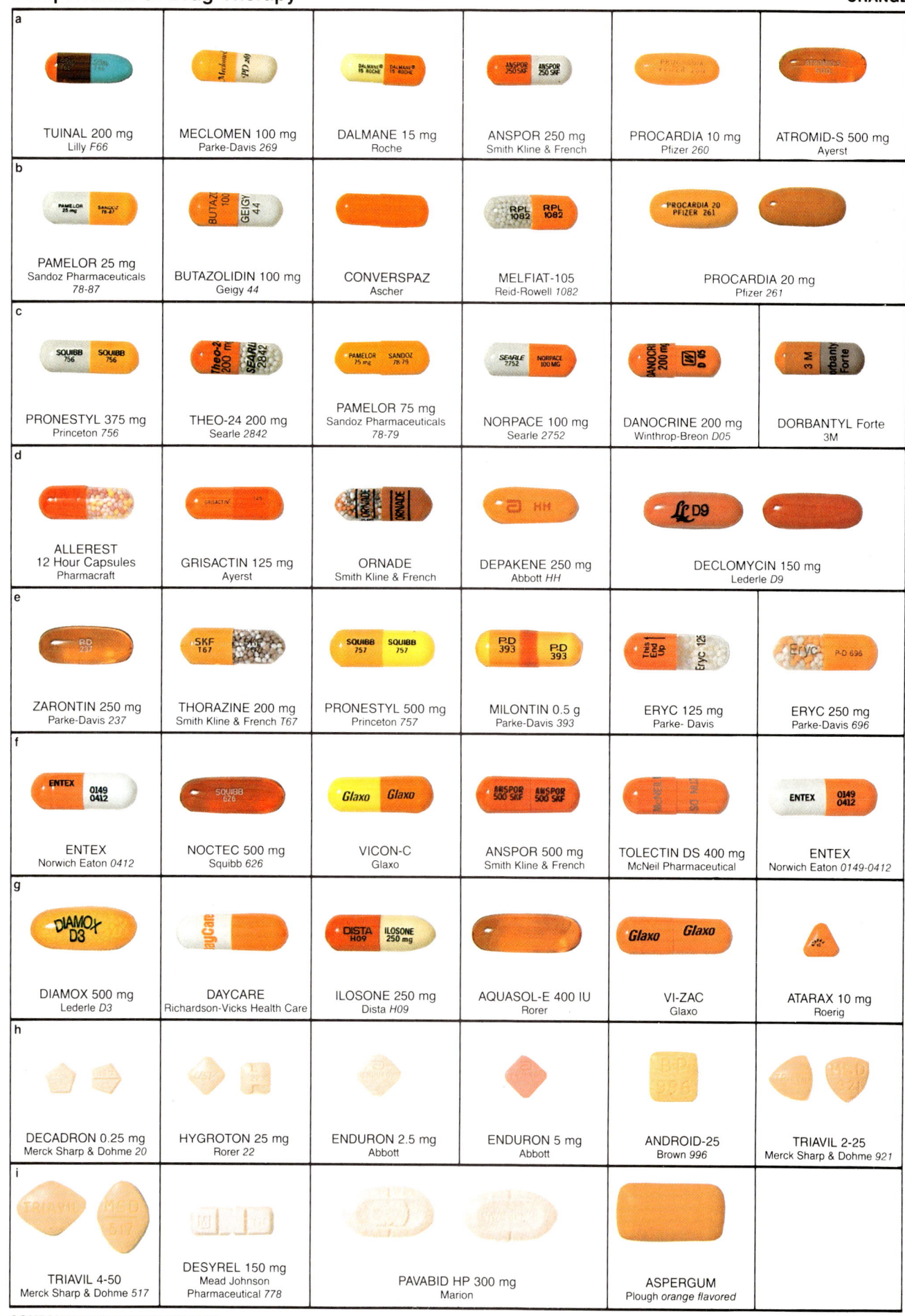

Compendium of Drug Therapy

PEACH

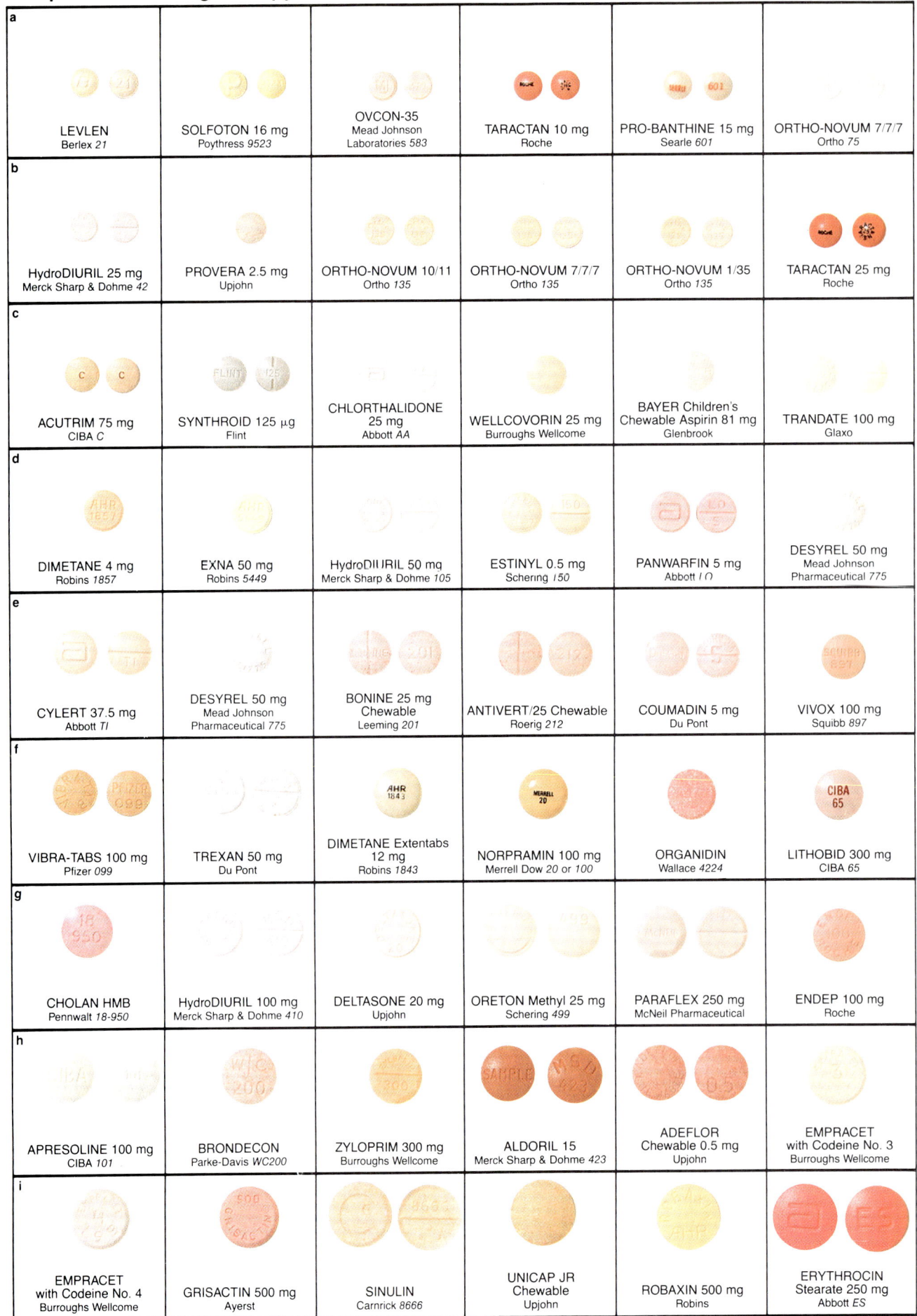

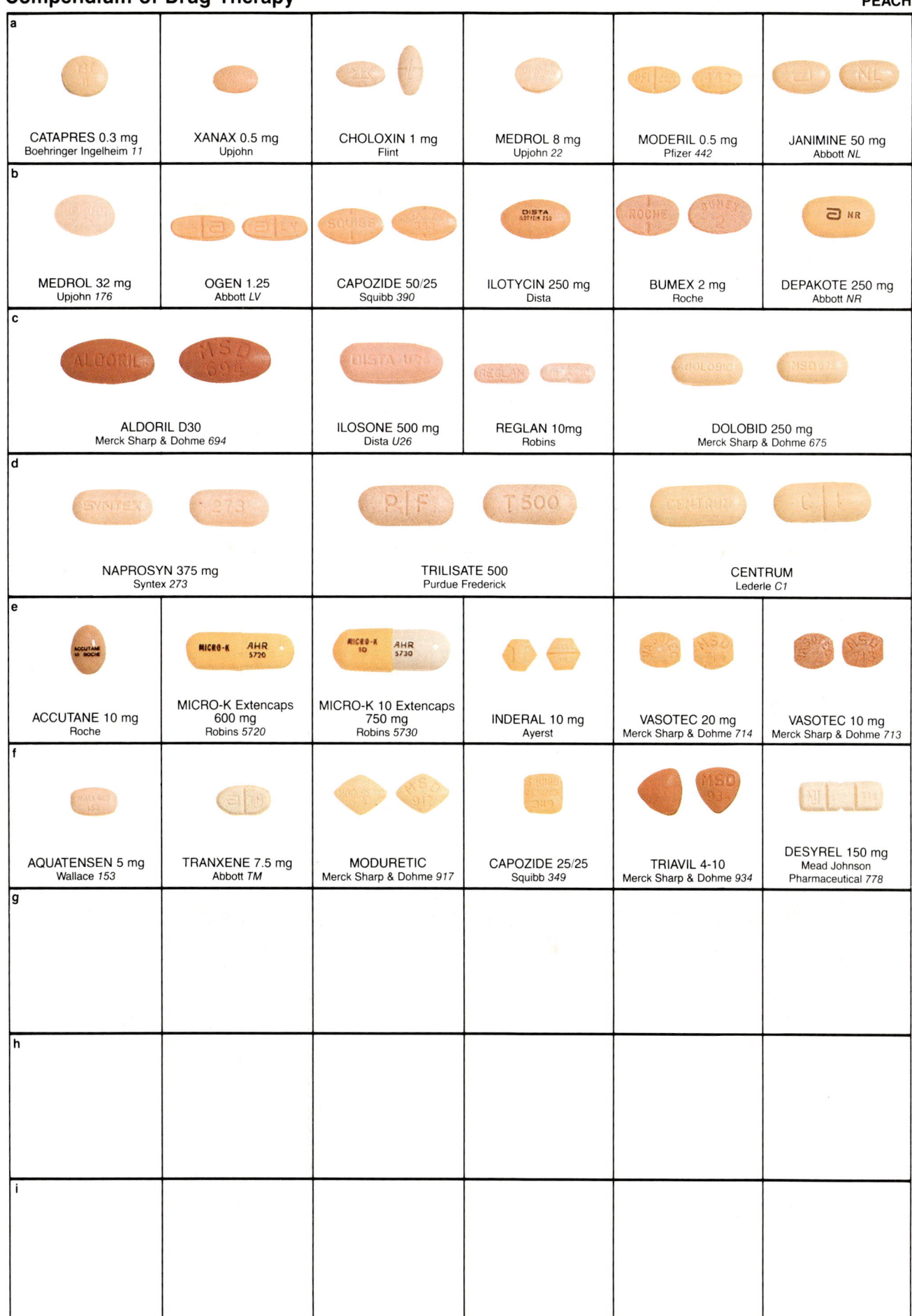

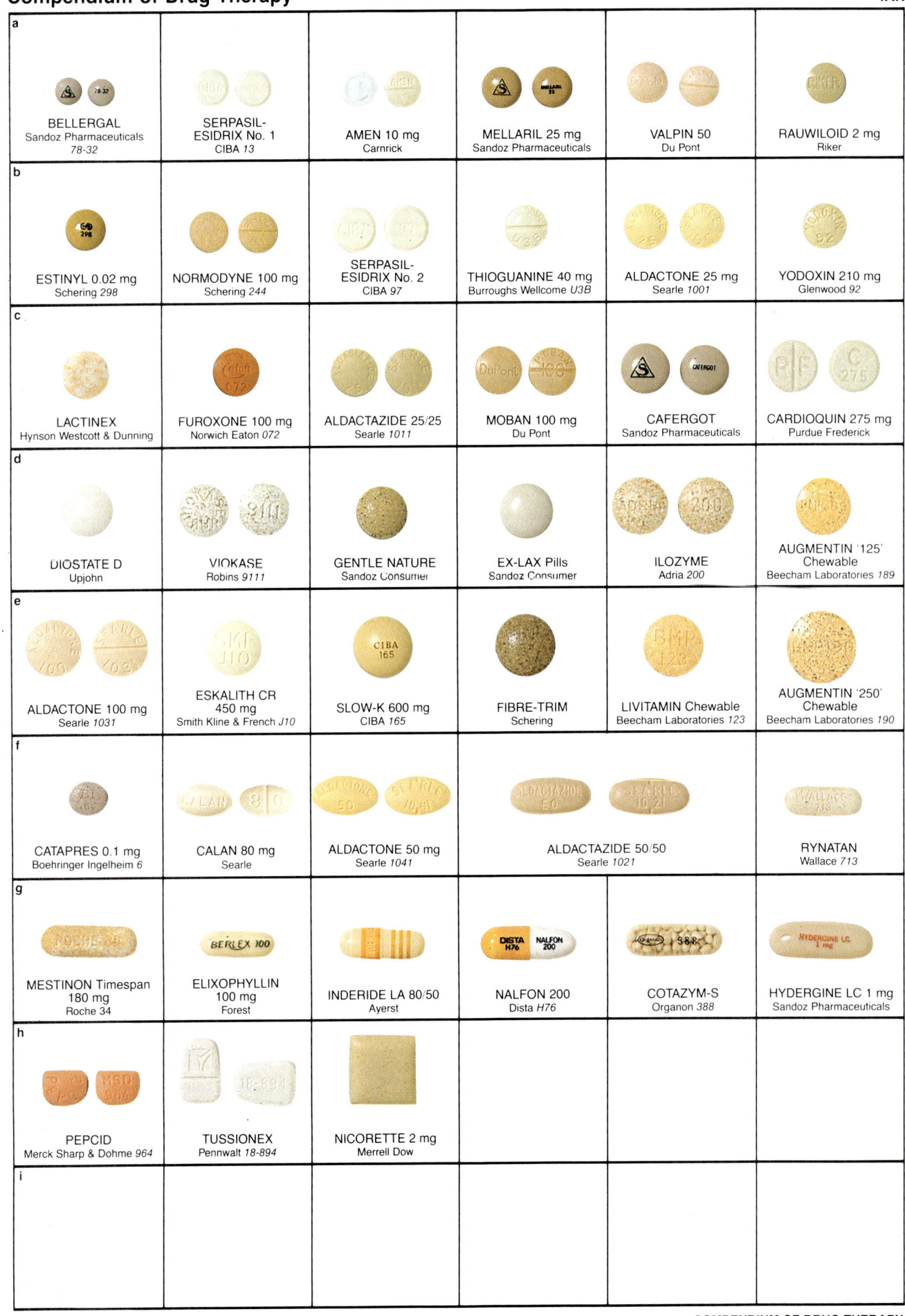

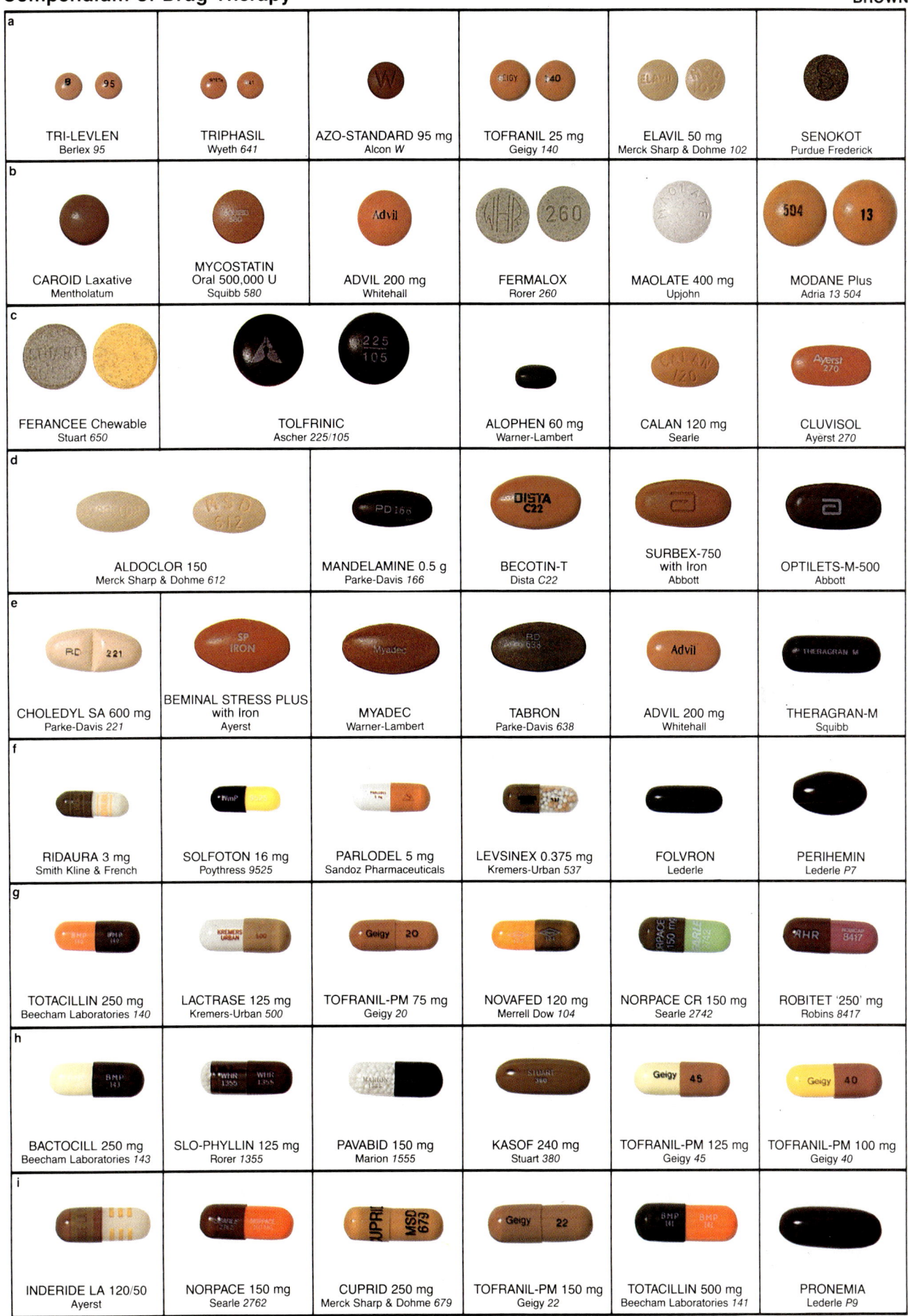

Compendium of Drug Therapy

BROWN

a ROBITET '500' Robins *8427*	NALFON 300 mg Dista *H77*	INDERIDE LA 160/50 Ayerst	BACTOCILL 500 mg Beecham Laboratories *144*	MYSTECLIN-F Squibb *779*	SECTRAL 400 mg Wyeth *4179*
b CLUVISOL Ayerst *293*	TOFRANIL 10 mg Geigy *32*				
c					
d					
e					
f					
g					
h					
i					

Compendium of Drug Therapy

GRAY/BLACK

a					
LEVOTHROID 75 μg Rorer *LT*	TRILAFON 4 mg Schering *940*	TRILAFON 2 mg Schering *705*	TEMARIL 2.5 mg Smith Kline & French *HL T41*	CHARDONNA-2 Kremers-Urban *202*	TRILAFON 16 mg Schering *077*

b					
TRILAFON 8 mg Schering *313*	ESKALITH 300 mg Smith Kline & French *J09*	RYNATUSS Wallace *717*	SURBEX-750 with Zinc Abbott		CALTRATE 600 + Vitamin D Lederle *C40*

c					
TRANXENE 3.75 mg Abbott *CI*	TEMARIL 5 mg Smith Kline & French *HL T50*	CUPRIMINE 125 mg Merck Sharp & Dohme *672*	IONAMIN 15 mg Pennwalt	TRANXENE 15 mg Abbott *CK*	WYMOX 250 mg Wyeth *559*

d					
PRINCIPEN '250' Squibb *971*	ESKALITH 300 mg Smith Kline & French	PANMYCIN 250 mg Upjohn	ANCOBON 500 mg Roche	FIORINAL with Codeine No. 2 Sandoz Pharmaceuticals *78-106*	DARVON Compound Lilly *3110*

e					
DARVON Compound-65 Lilly *3111*	PRINCIPEN '500' Squibb *974*	WYMOX 500 mg Wyeth *560*	ENDURONYL Forte Abbott *LT*		

f					

g					
LIBRIUM 10 mg Roche	COMPAZINE 10 mg Smith Kline & French *C44*	COMPAZINE 15 mg Smith Kline & French *C46*	BIPHETAMINE '12½' Pennwalt *18-878*	NICOBID 125 mg Rorer *2835*	TEGOPEN 250 mg Apothecon *7935*

h					
COMPAZINE 30 mg Smith Kline & French *C47*	DEXATRIM Regular Strength Thompson	NITRO-BID 6.5 mg Marion *1551*	PHENAPHEN with Codeine No. 3 Robins *6257*	PHENAPHEN with Codeine No. 2 Robins *6242*	VICON Forte Glaxo *316*

i					
TEGOPEN 500 mg Apothecon *7496*	ULTRACEF 500 mg Bristol Laboratories *7271*				

Compendium of Drug Therapy

MULTICOLORED

a	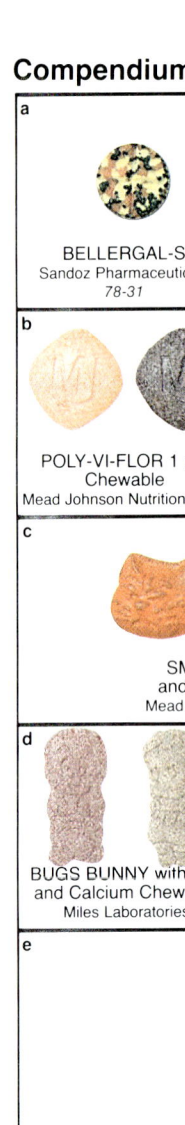 BELLERGAL-S Sandoz Pharmaceuticals 78-31	BELLADENAL-S Sandoz Pharmaceuticals 78-27	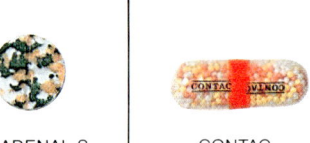 CONTAC SmithKline Consumer Products	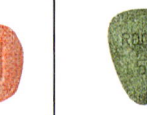 TRI-VI-FLOR 1 mg Chewable Mead Johnson Nutritional 477	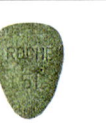 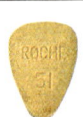 VI-PENTA F Chewable Roche 51
b	POLY-VI-FLOR 1 mg Chewable Mead Johnson Nutritional 474	POLY-VI-SOL Chewable Mead Johnson Nutritional	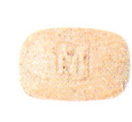 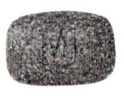 POLY-VI-FLOR 0.5 mg Chewable Mead Johnson Nutritional 468	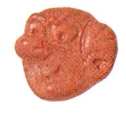 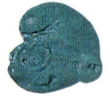 SMURF Chewable Mead Johnson Nutritional	
c	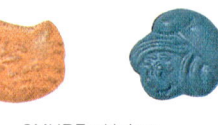 SMURF with Iron and Zinc Chewable Mead Johnson Nutrtitional	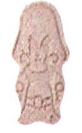 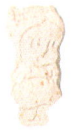 BUGS BUNNY Chewable Miles Laboratories	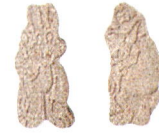 BUGS BUNNY Plus Iron Chewable Miles Laboratories	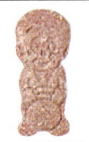 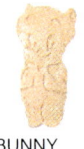 BUGS BUNNY with Extra C Chewable Miles Laboratories	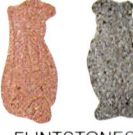 FLINTSTONES Plus Iron Chewable Miles Laboratories
d	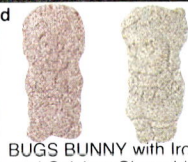 BUGS BUNNY with Iron and Calcium Chewable Miles Laboratories	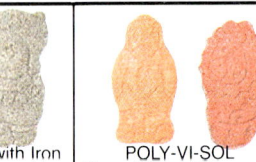 POLY-VI-SOL Circus-Shaped Chewable Mead Johnson Nutritional	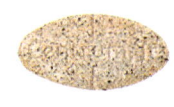 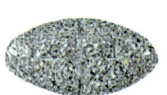 CENTRUM Jr. & Iron Chewable Lederle C2	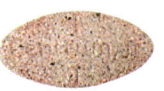 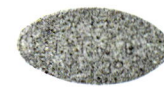 CENTRUM Jr. & Extra C Chewable Lederle C39	

Compendium of Drug Therapy

WHITE

a SORBITRATE Sublingual 2.5 mg — Stuart 853	ARMOUR Thyroid 15 mg (¼ gr) — Rorer TC	NITROGARD Transmucosal 1 mg — Parke-Davis	NORINYL 1 + 50 — Syntex 1	NITROGARD Transmucosal 2 mg — Parke-Davis	TRI-LEVLEN — Berlex 96
b DICUMAROL 25 mg — Abbott AN	ORETIC 25 mg — Abbott	ISORDIL 10 mg Sublingual — Wyeth	NITROGARD Transmucosal 3 mg — Parke-Davis	LO/OVRAL — Wyeth 78	CYTOMEL 5 μG — Smith Kline & French D14
c ARMOUR Thyroid 30 mg (½ gr) — Rorer TD	LOMOTIL — Searle 61	PARSIDOL 10 mg — Parke-Davis 320	TRIPHASIL — Wyeth 642	PRO-BANTHINE 7½ mg — Searle 611	NORLUTIN 5 mg — Parke-Davis 882
d ISUPREL Glossets 15 mg — Winthrop-Breon J77	ANTRENYL 5 mg — CIBA 15	MAZANOR 1 mg — Wyeth 71	ORTHO-NOVUM 10/11 — Ortho 535	NOLUDAR 50 mg — Roche 16	ARLIDIN 6 mg — Rorer 45
e METICORTEN 1 mg — Schering 843	ISUPREL Glossets 10 mg — Winthrop-Breon J75	COGENTIN 0.5 mg — Merck Sharp & Dohme 21	DEMULEN 1/50 — Searle 71	ORTHO-NOVUM 7/7/7 — Ortho 535	ORTHO-NOVUM 1/80 — Ortho 1
f ORTHO-NOVUM 2 mg — Ortho	ORTHO-NOVUM 10/11 — Ortho 535	PROVENTIL 2 mg — Schering 252	LEVOTHROID 50 μg — Rorer LL	DELTA-CORTEF 5 mg — Upjohn 25	DEMEROL 50 mg — Winthrop-Breon D35
g MODICON — Ortho 535	DELTASONE 5 mg — Upjohn	CARDILATE 5 mg — Burroughs Wellcome P2B	OVRAL — Wyeth 56	VISKEN 5 mg — Sandoz Pharmaceuticals 78-111	MYLERAN 2 mg — Burroughs Wellcome K2A
h VENTOLIN 2 mg — Glaxo	NORINYL 2 mg — Syntex	PAMINE 2.5 mg — Upjohn	DEMULEN 1/35 — Searle 151	PARLODEL 2½ mg — Sandoz Pharmaceuticals	TAVIST 2.68 mg — Sandoz Pharmaceuticals 78-72
i PBZ 25 mg — Geigy 111	LEUKERAN 2 mg — Burroughs Wellcome	KEMADRIN 5 mg — Burroughs Wellcome S3A	BELLAFOLINE 0.25 mg — Sandoz Pharmaceuticals 78-30	PERIACTIN 4 mg — Merck Sharp & Dohme 62	LOZOL 2.5 mg — Rorer 82

Compendium of Drug Therapy

WHITE

a CYTOMEL 25 μG Smith Kline & French D16	HYGROTON 100 mg Rorer 21	Morphine Sulfate 15 mg Purdue Frederick MI15	CURRETAB 10 mg Reid-Rowell 1007	RENESE 1 mg Pfizer 375	COGENTIN 2 mg Merck Sharp & Dohme 60
b ANADROL-50 Syntex 2902	LONITEN 10 mg Upjohn	SYNTHROID 50 μg Flint	MYSOLINE 50 mg Ayerst	LONITEN 2.5 mg Upjohn 121	PROVERA 10 mg Upjohn
c CYLERT 18.75 mg Abbott TH	SUDAFED Plus Burroughs Wellcome	LANOXIN 250 μg Burroughs Wellcome X3A	ACTIDIL 25 mg Burroughs Wellcome L2A	DARICON 10 mg Beecham Laboratories 145	ARMOUR Thyroid 60 mg (1 gr) Rorer TE
d DARAPRIM 25 mg Burroughs Wellcome A3A	TENORMIN 50 Stuart 105	NEPTAZANE 50 mg Lederle N1	MAREZINE 50 mg Burroughs Wellcome T4A	ACTIFED Burroughs Wellcome M2A	ALKERAN 2 mg Burroughs Wellcome A2A
e SYNKAVITE 5 mg Roche	SALURON 50 mg Bristol Laboratories S2	HEXADROL 0.75 mg Organon 791	HYDERGINE 1 mg Sandoz Pharmaceuticals	ALUPENT 10 mg Boehringer Ingelheim 74	TENORETIC 50 Stuart 115
f DEMEROL 100 mg Winthrop-Breon D37	LEUCOVORIN Calcium 5 mg Lederle C33	LASIX 40 mg Hoechst-Roussel	LEVSIN 0.125 mg Kremers-Urban 531	BRICANYL 5 mg Lakeside 750 or 5	BRICANYL 2.5 mg Lakeside 725 or 2½
g BRETHINE 5 mg Geigy 105	SLOW FE 50 mg CIBA NR	WELLCOVORIN 5 mg Burroughs Wellcome R3C	ORETIC 50 mg Abbott	FUROSE Ascher 225/425	PANWARFIN 10 mg Abbott LF
h METANDREN 10 mg CIBA 30	SERPASIL 0.25 mg CIBA 36	ARLIDIN 12 mg Rorer 46	PBZ 50 mg Geigy 117	DONNATAL Robins 4250	KLONOPIN 2 mg Roche
i ANDROID-F 10 mg Brown 998	SLO-PHYLLIN 100 mg Rorer 351	PHENERGAN 25 mg Wyeth 27	SLO-PHYLLIN 200 mg Rorer 352	TEDRAL Parke-Davis 230	SERPASIL 0.1 mg CIBA 35

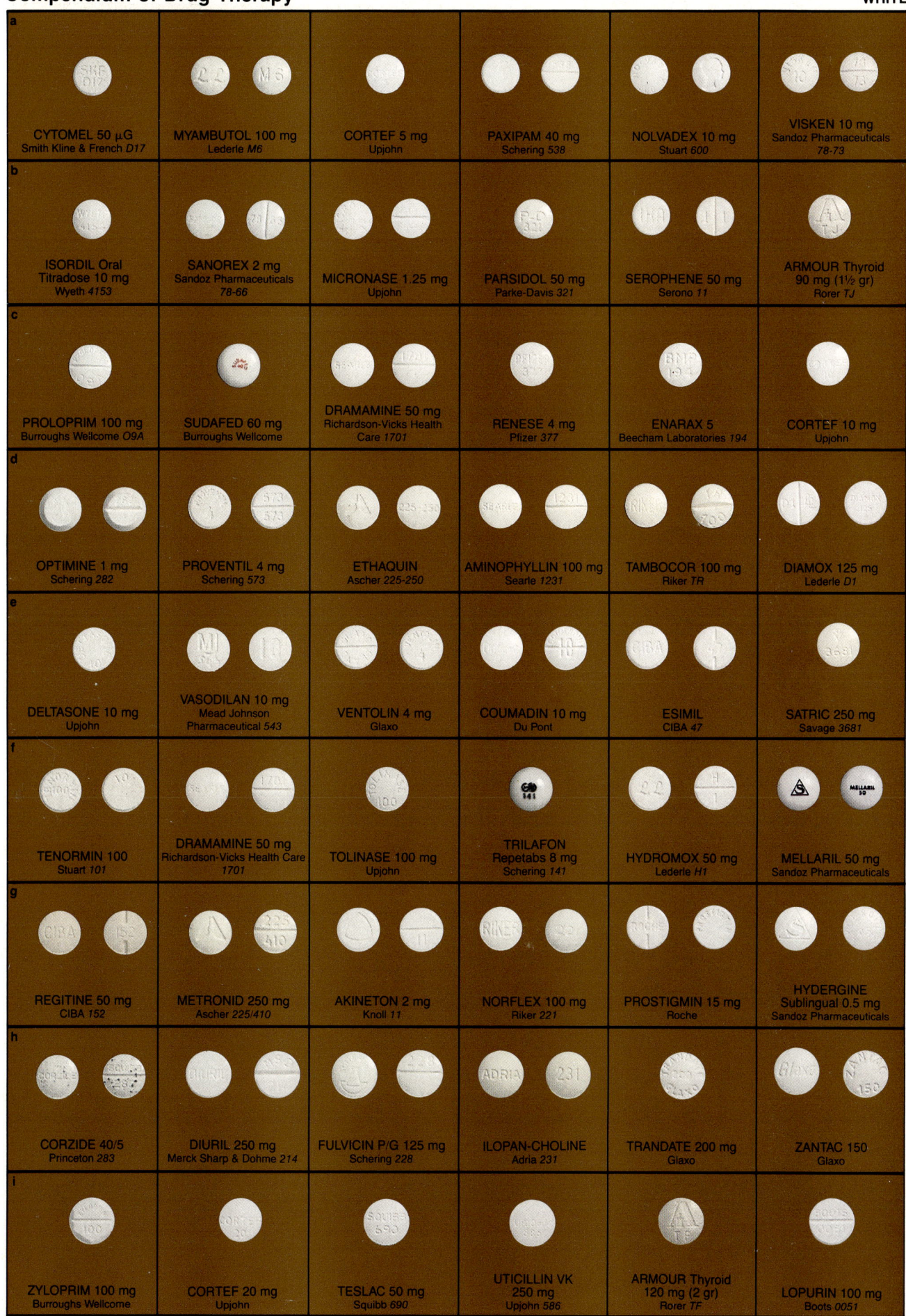

Compendium of Drug Therapy

WHITE

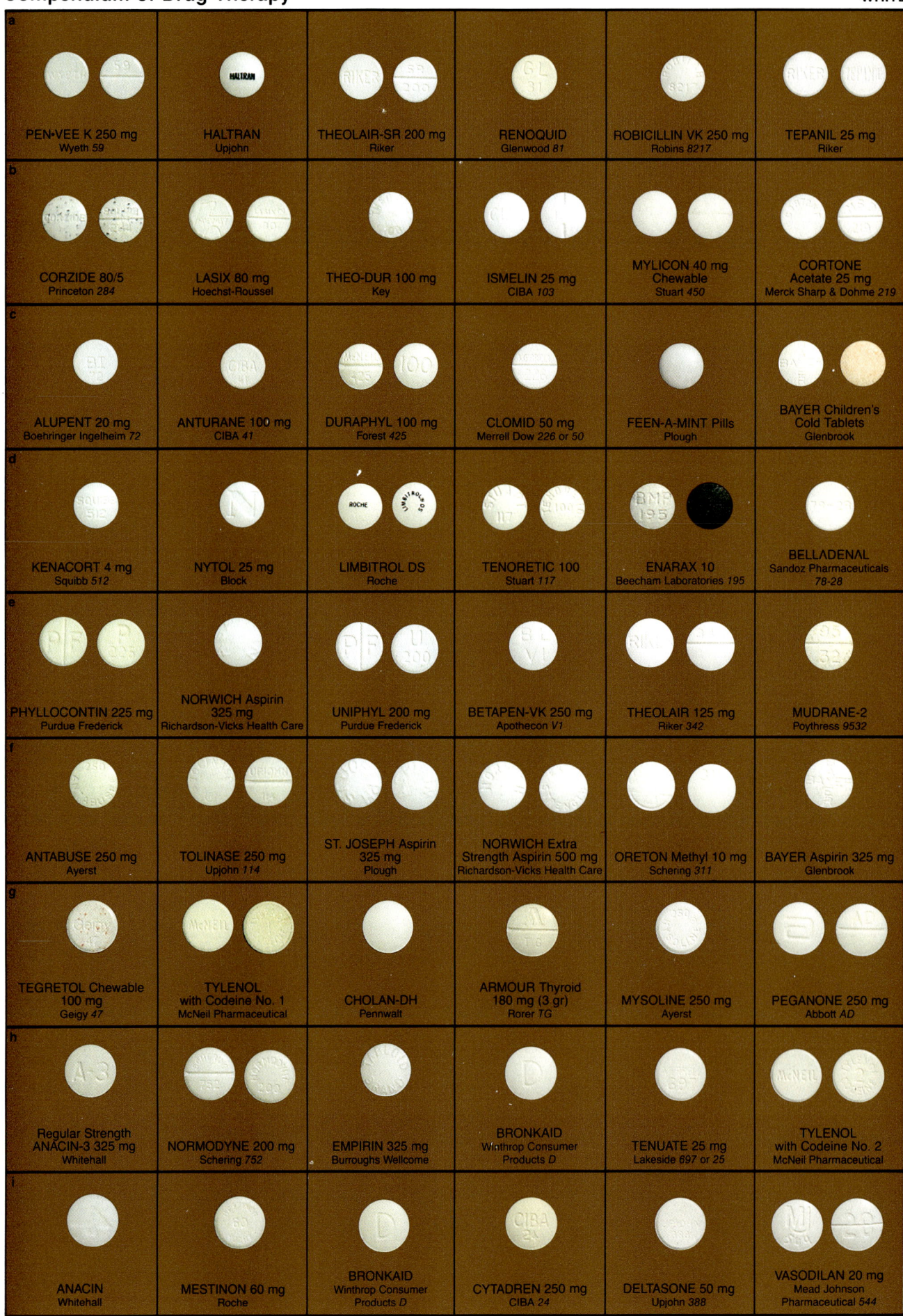

Compendium of Drug Therapy

WHITE

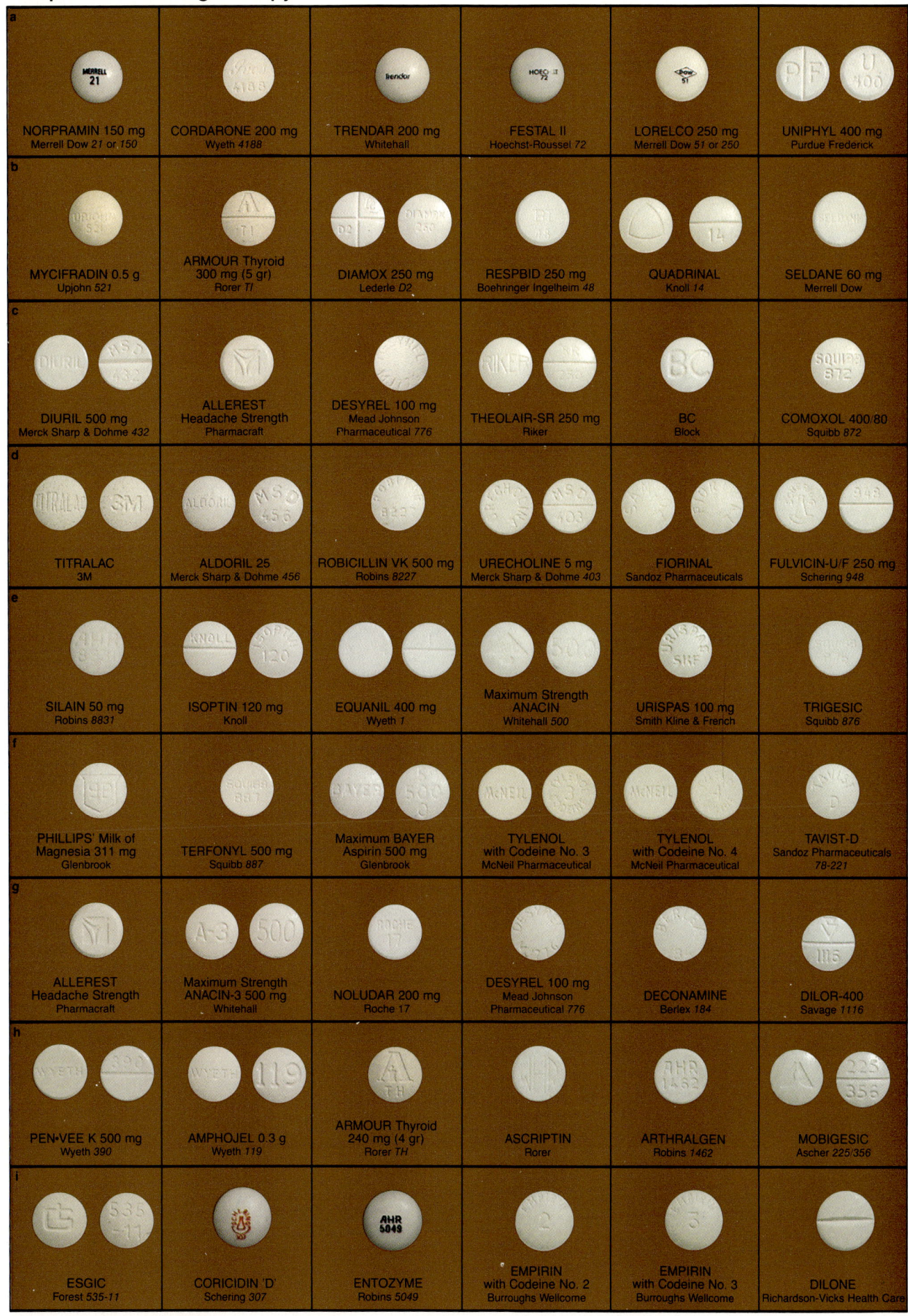

35

Compendium of Drug Therapy

WHITE

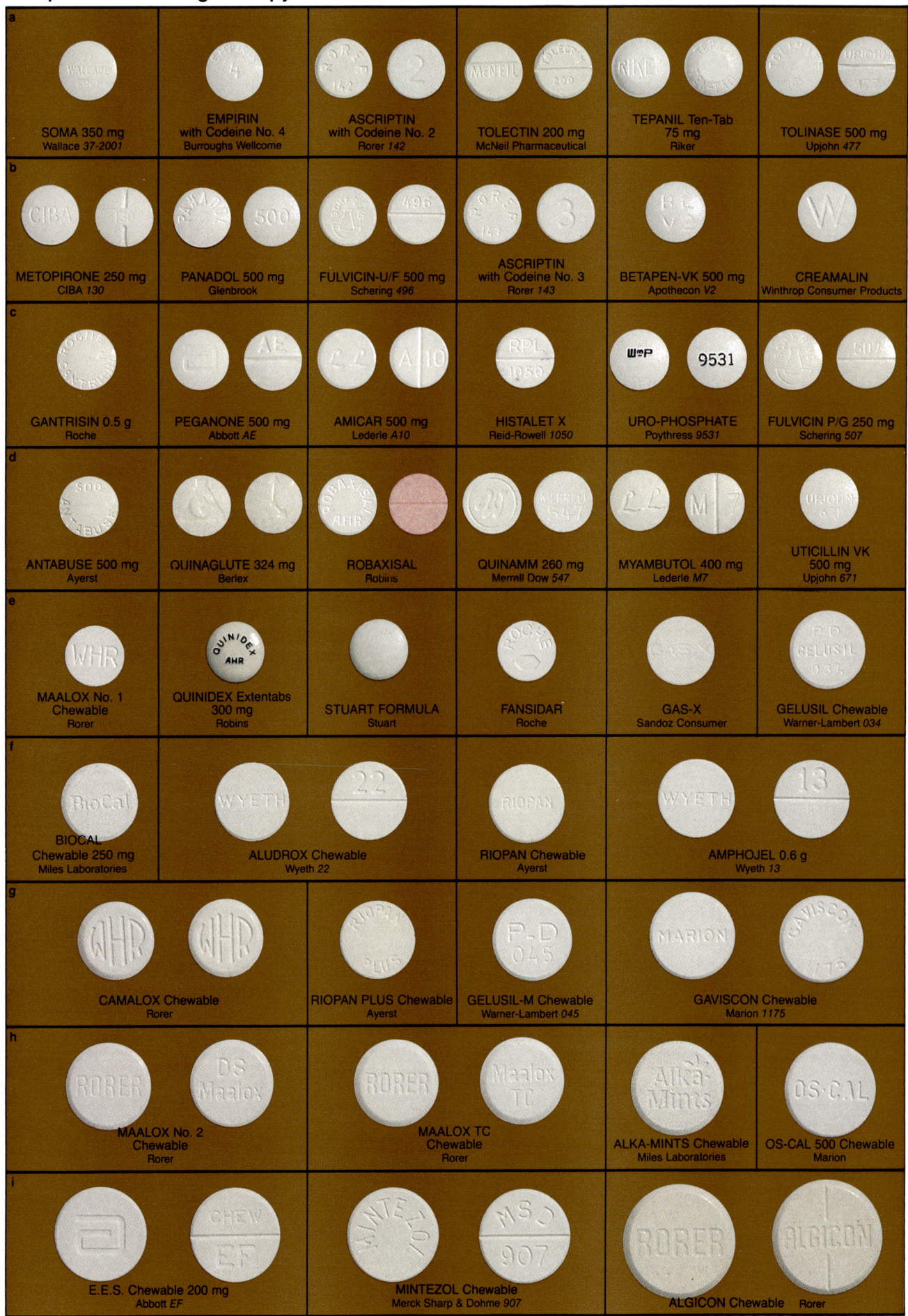

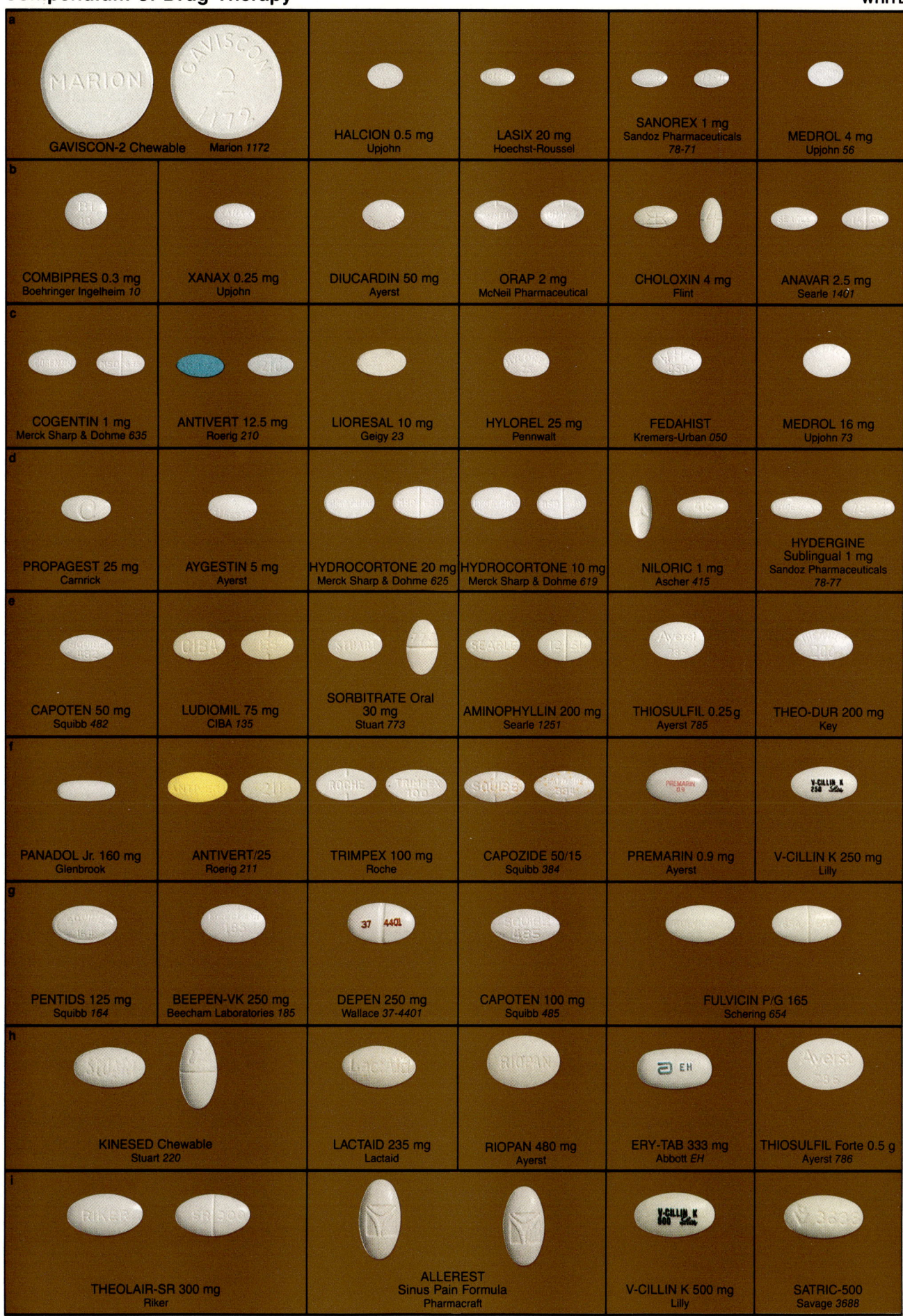

Compendium of Drug Therapy

WHITE

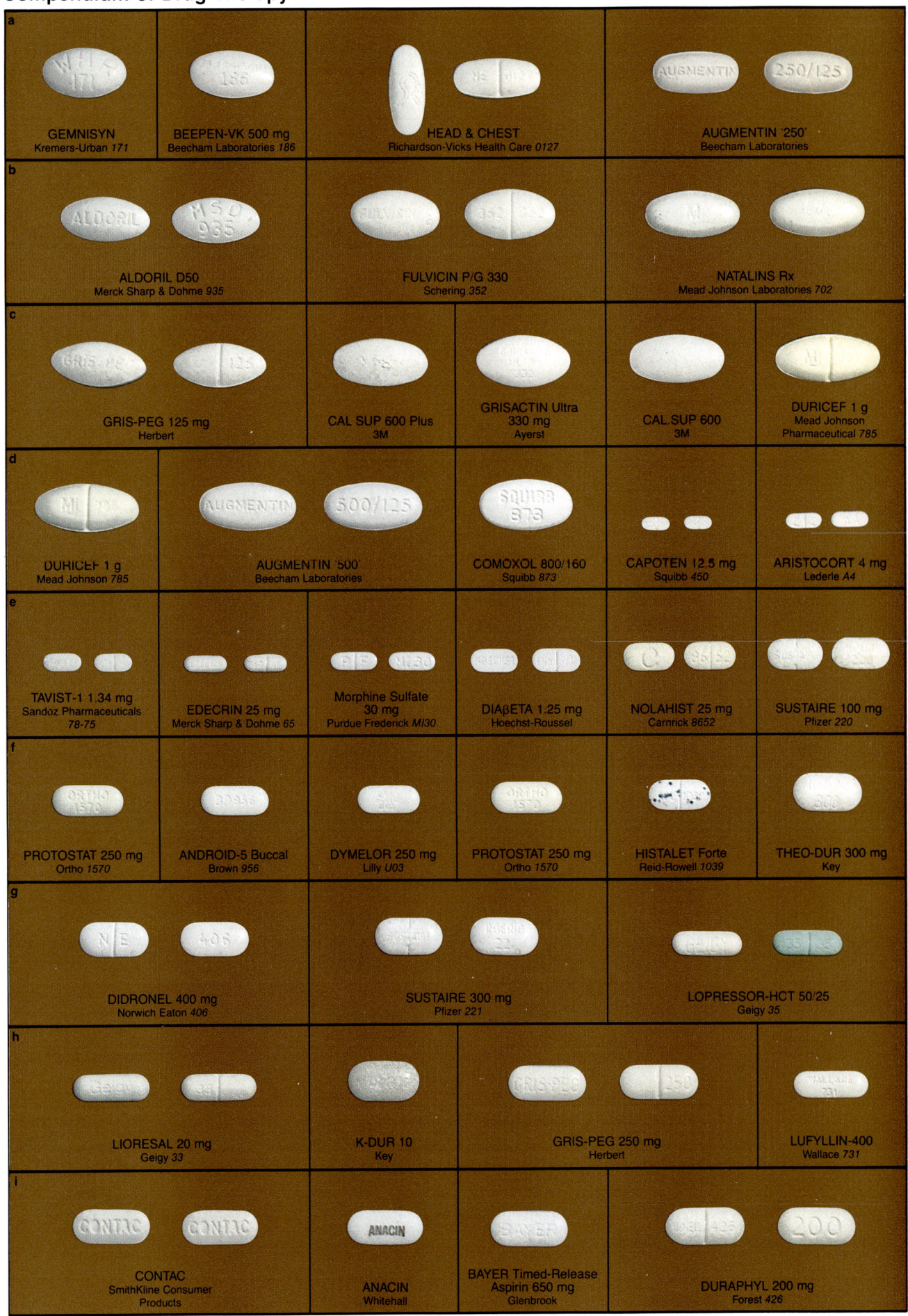

38

COMPENDIUM OF DRUG THERAPY

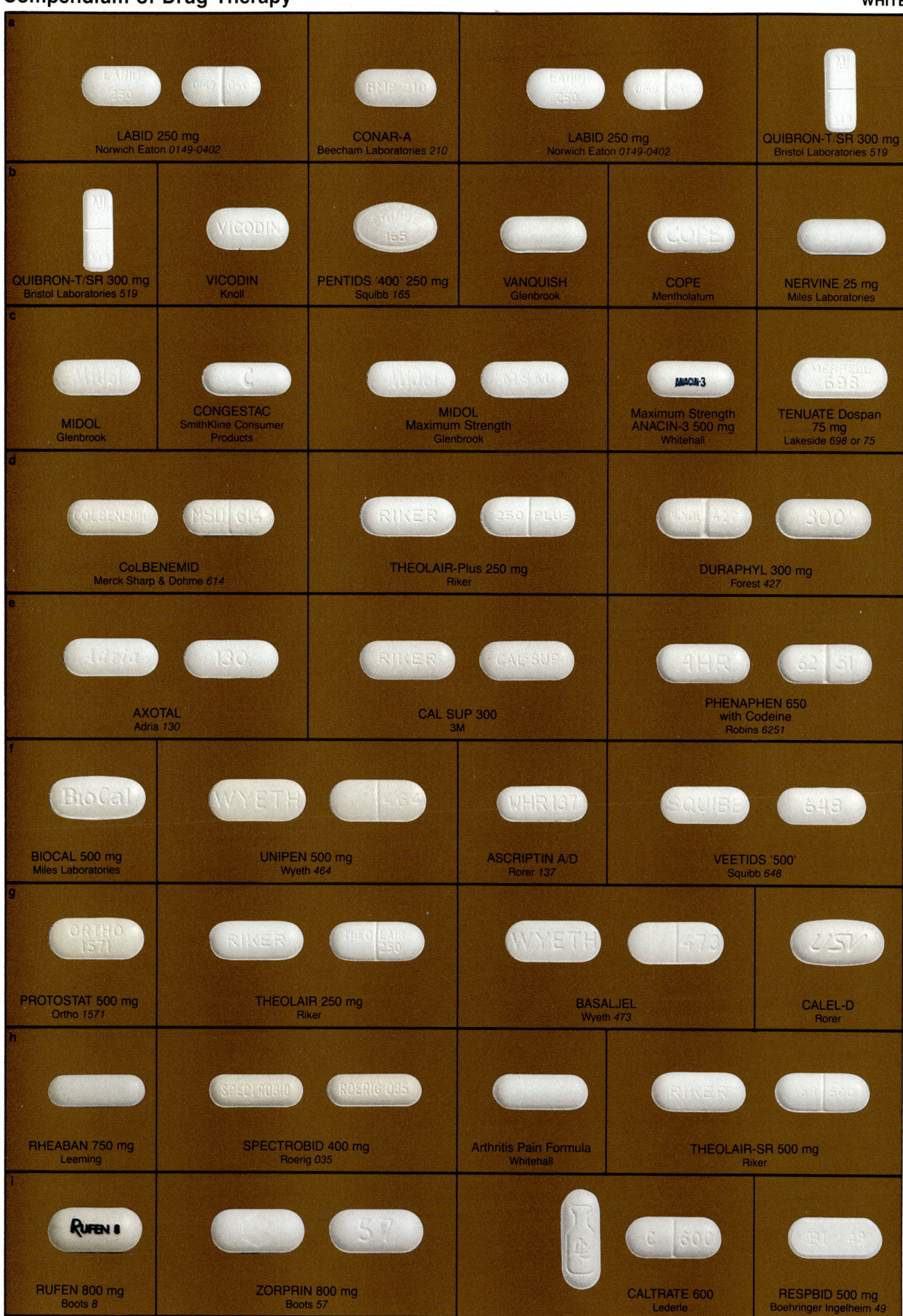

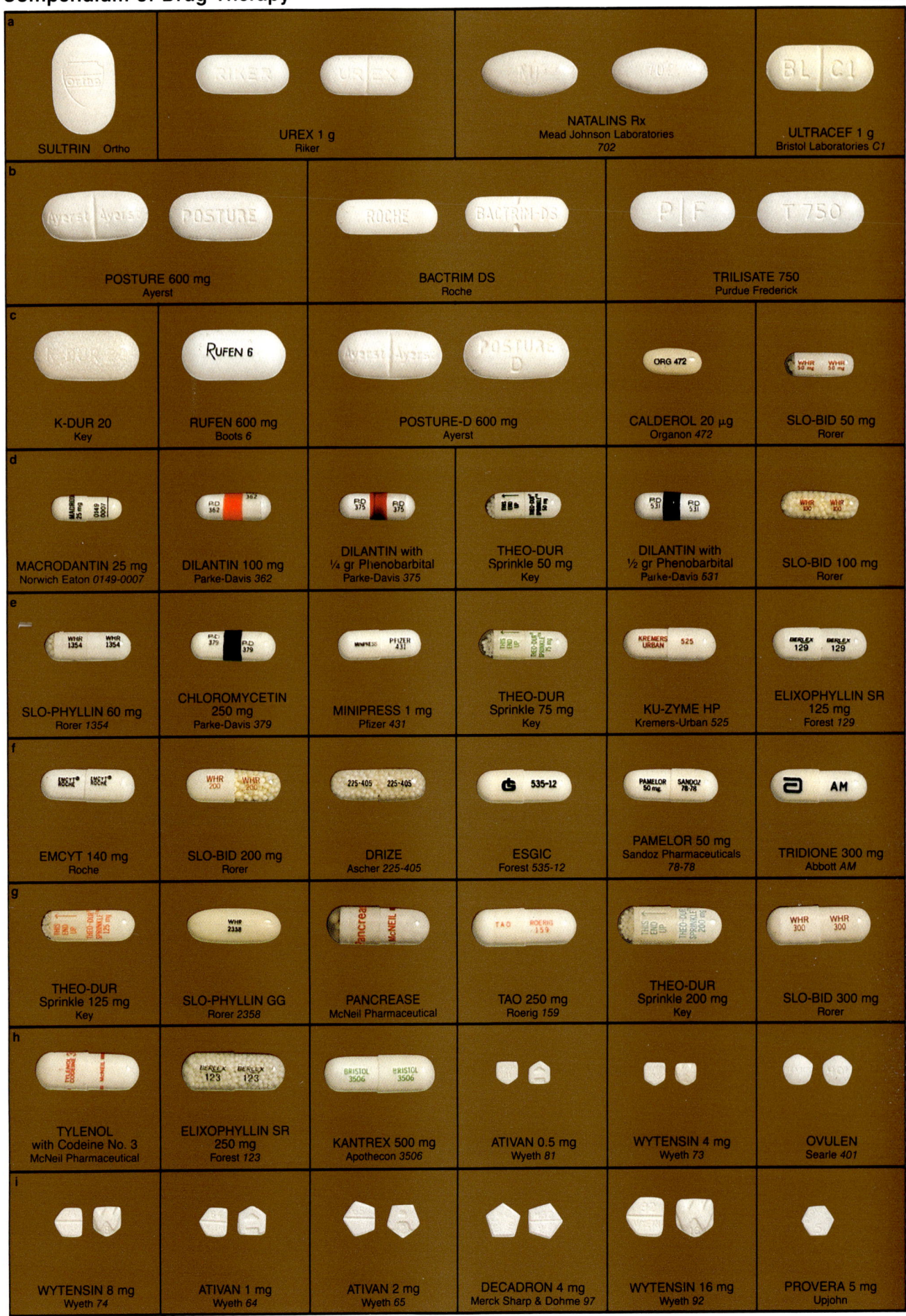

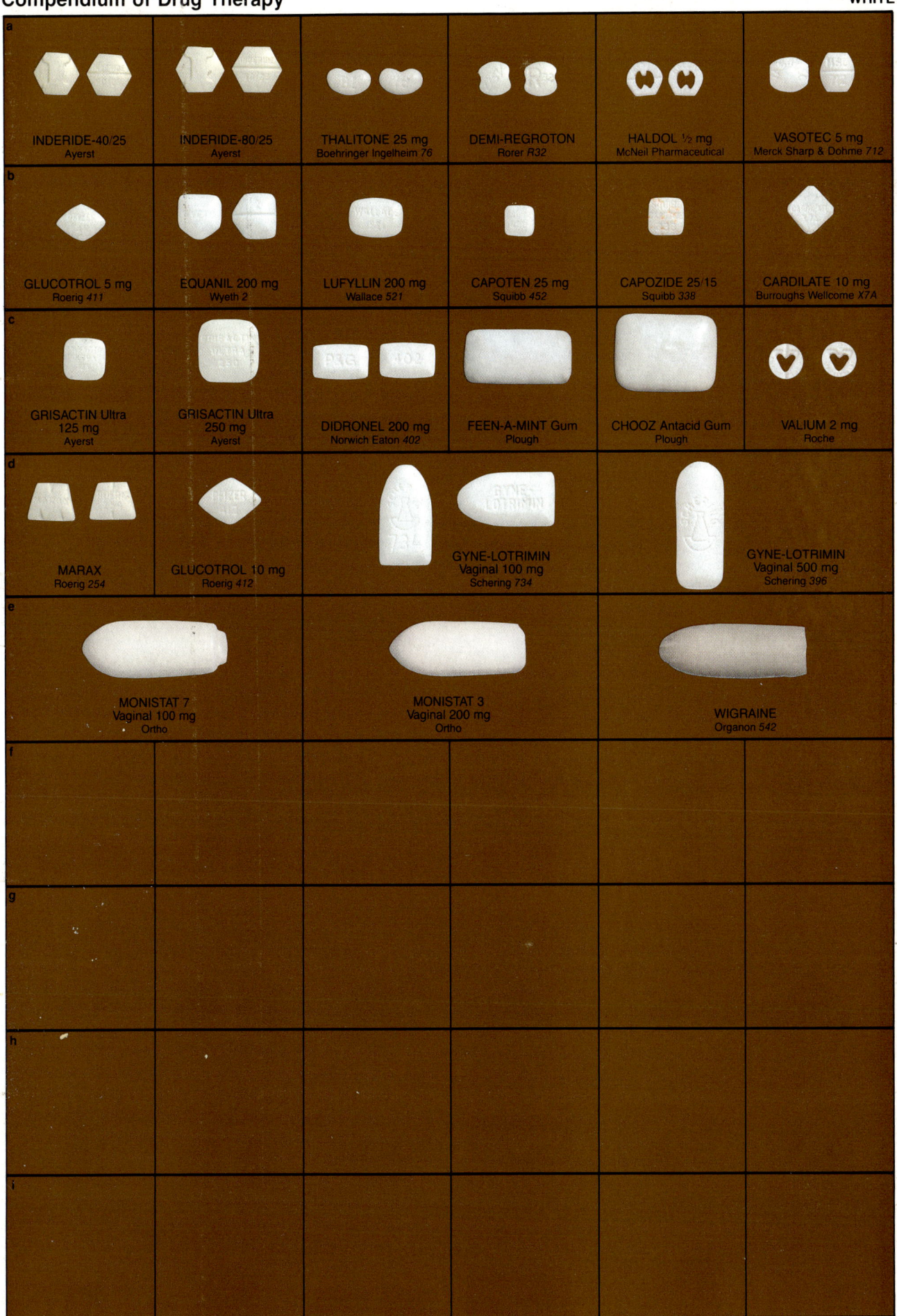

Compendium of Drug Therapy

ORAL CONTRACEPTIVE COMPACTS

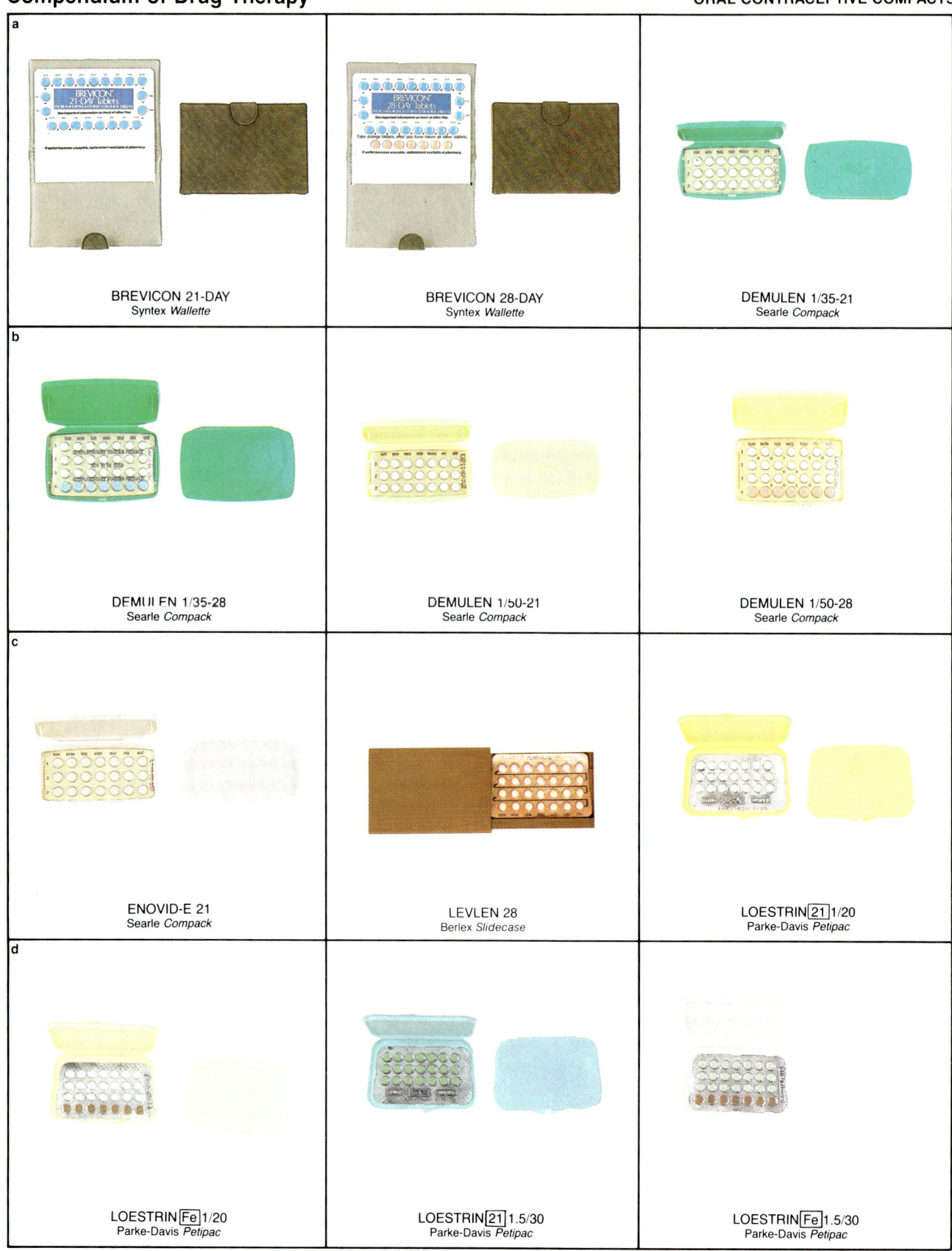

Compendium of Drug Therapy

ORAL CONTRACEPTIVE COMPACTS

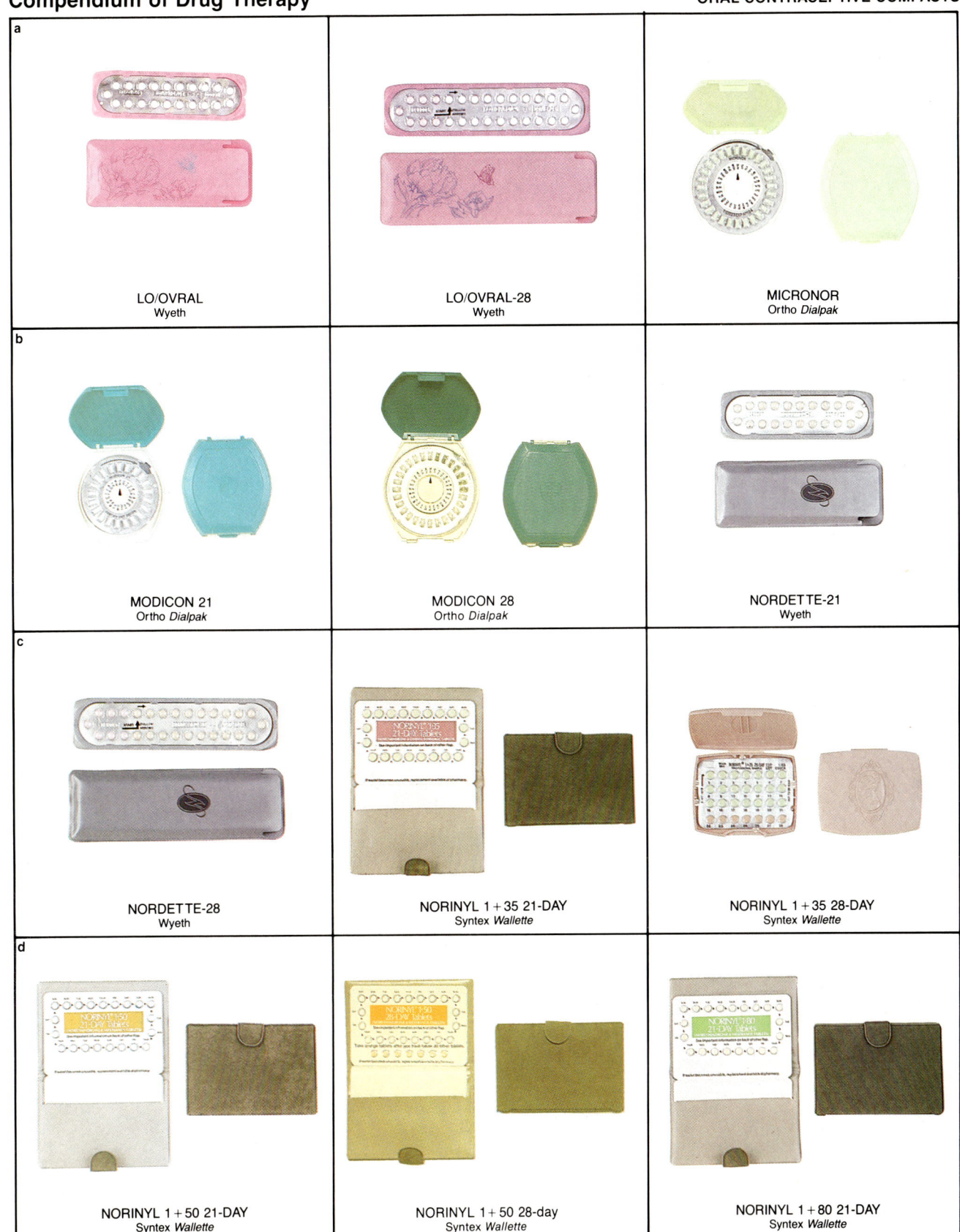

Compendium of Drug Therapy

ORAL CONTRACEPTIVE COMPACTS

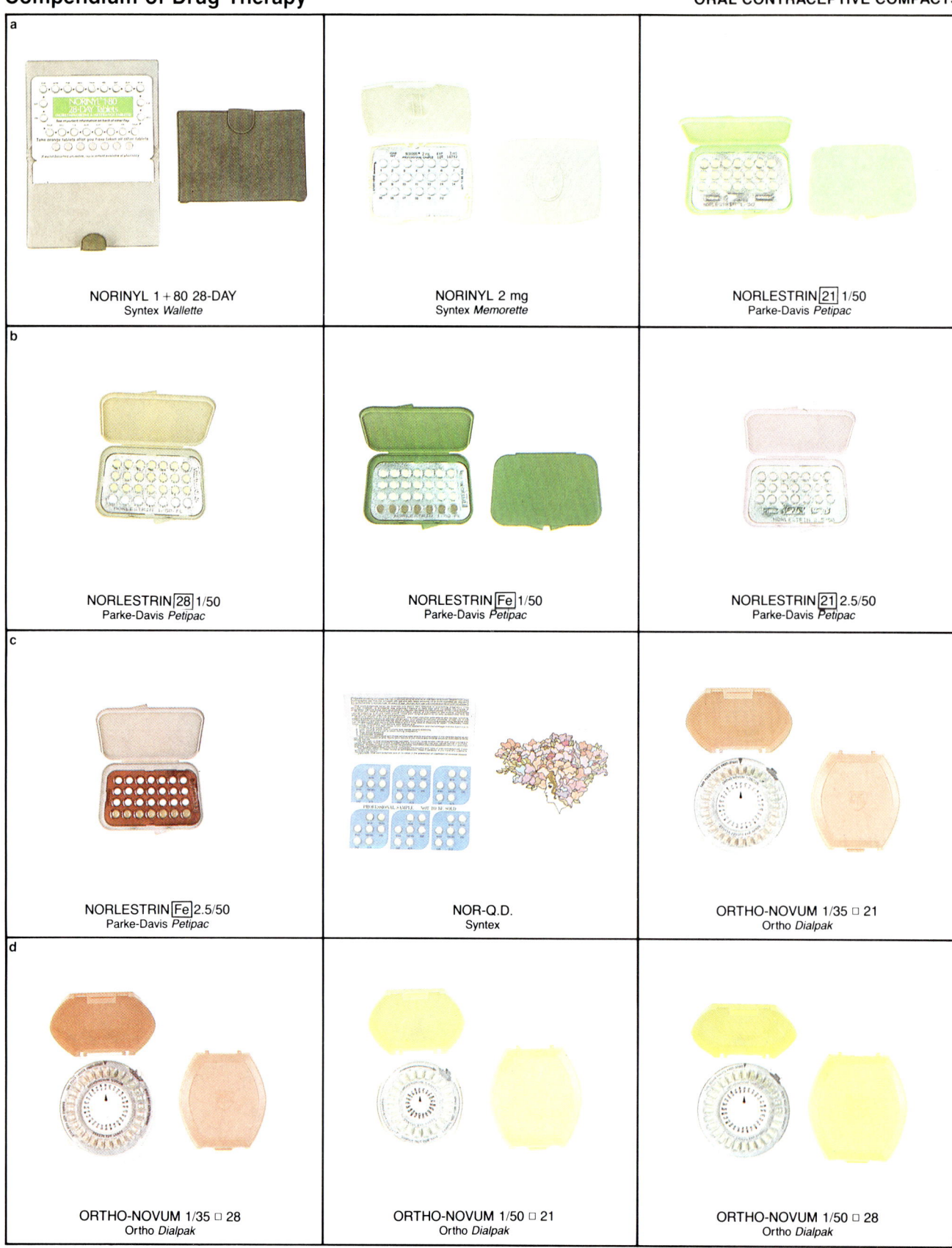

Compendium of Drug Therapy

ORAL CONTRACEPTIVE COMPACTS

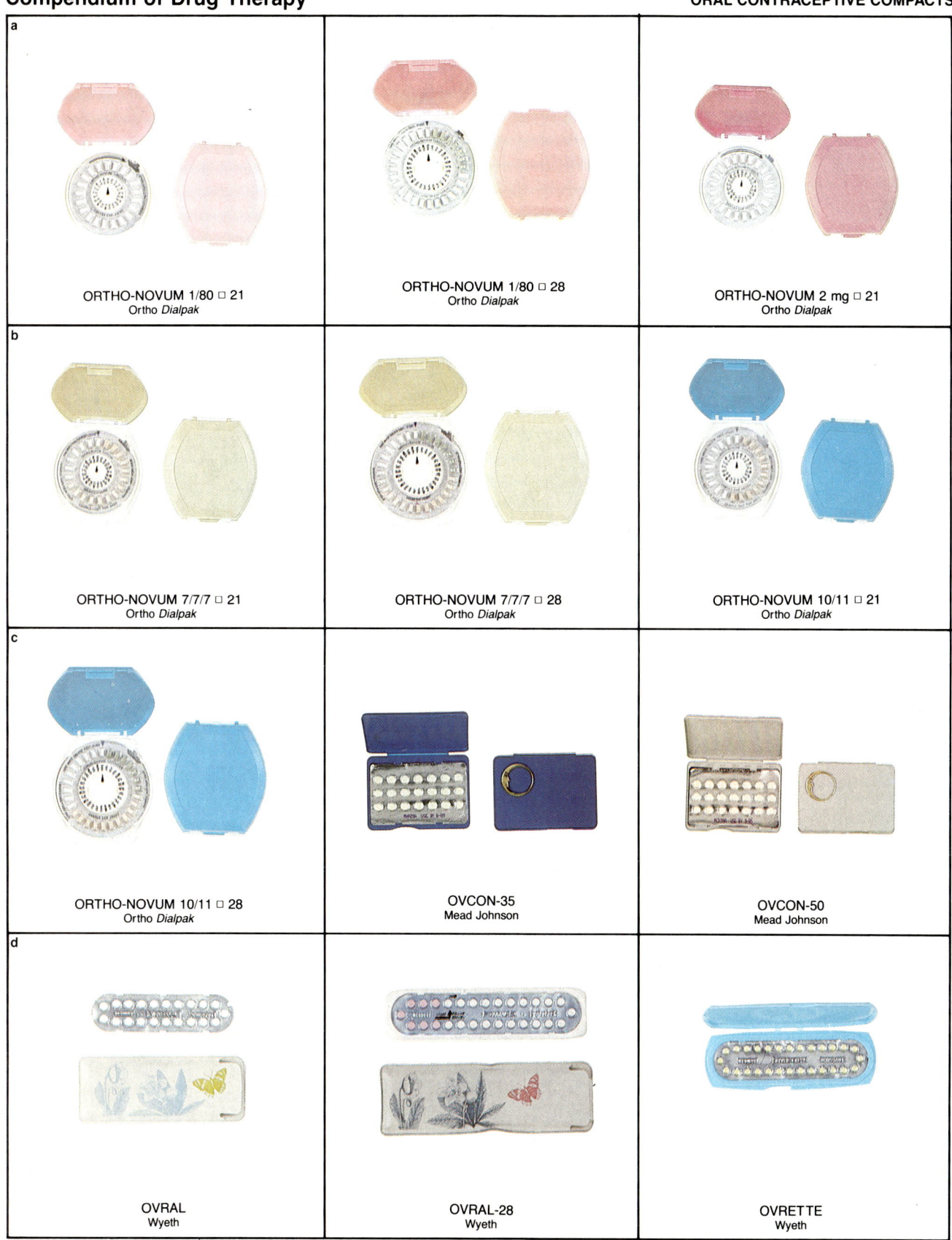

Compendium of Drug Therapy

ORAL CONTRACEPTIVE COMPACTS

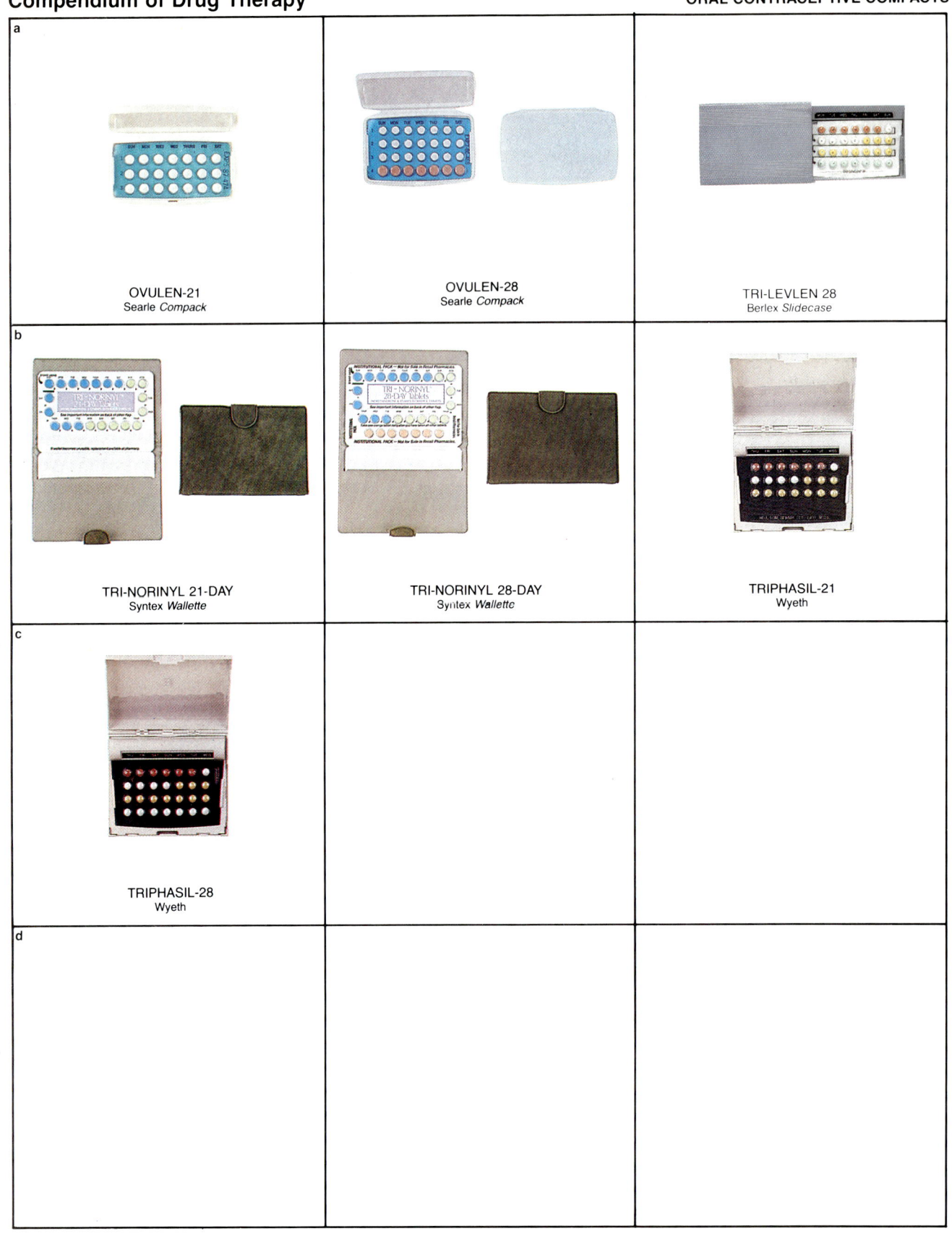

Compendium of Drug Therapy

TRANSDERMAL PRODUCTS

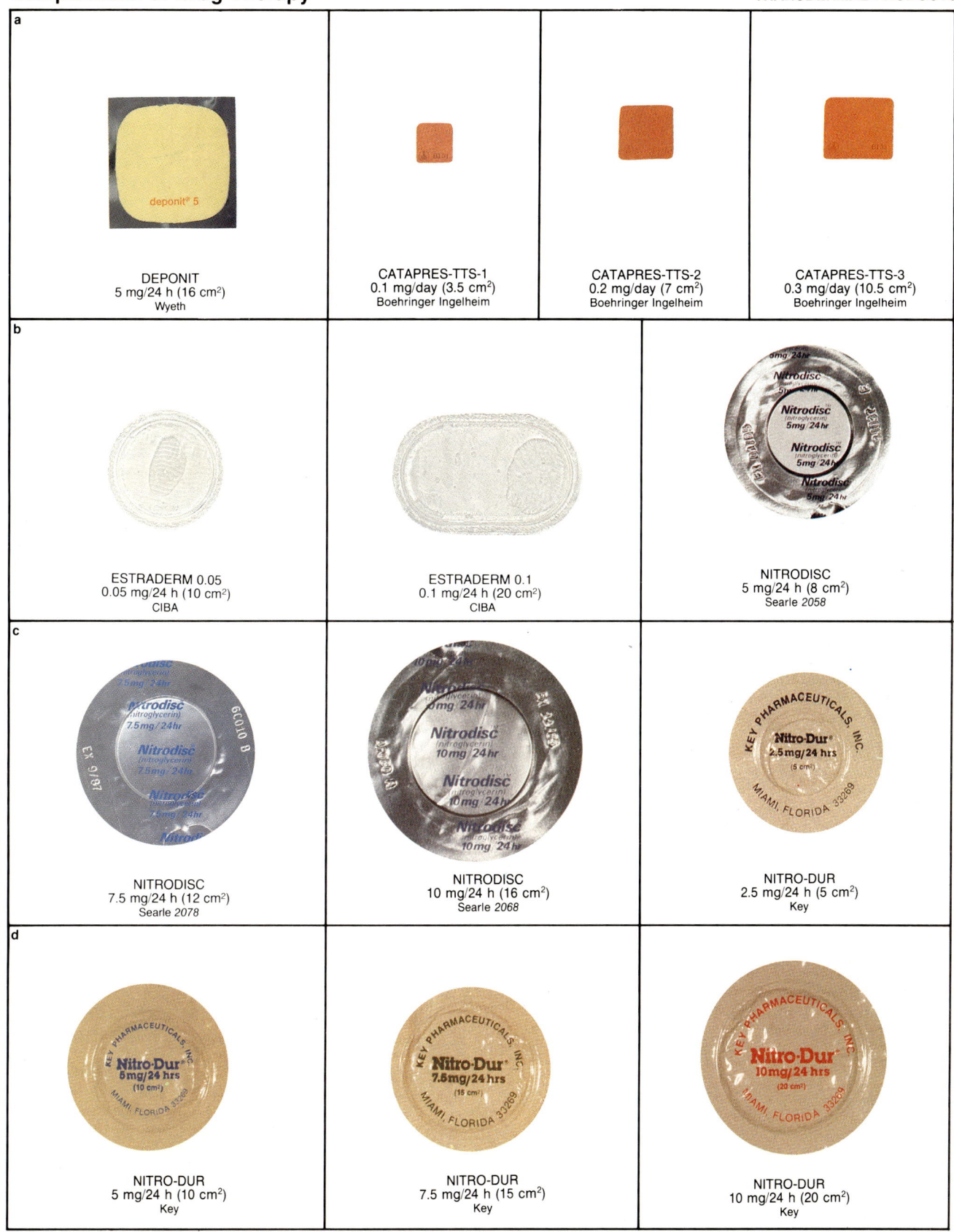

Compendium of Drug Therapy

TRANSDERMAL PRODUCTS

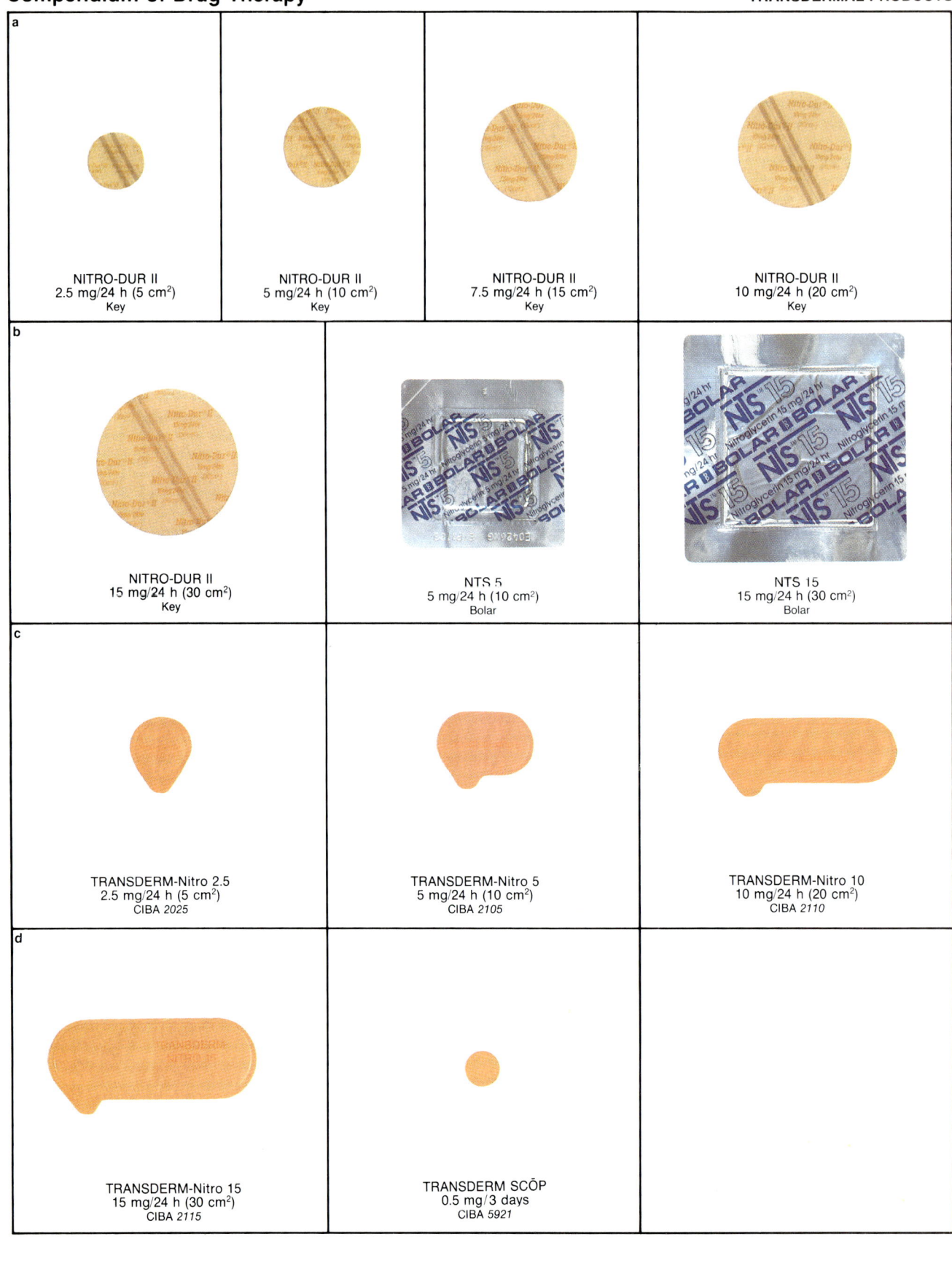

Drug Identification Index

A

ACCUTANE Capsules (Roche)
10 mg, light pink, p. 25e
20 mg, maroon, p. 6d
40 mg, yellow, p. 18i

ACHROMYCIN V Capsules (Lederle)
250 mg, blue and yellow, *A3*, p. 8f
500 mg, blue and yellow, *A5*, p. 8h

ACTIDIL Tablets (Burroughs Wellcome)
25 mg, white, round, scored, *L2A*, p. 32c

ACTIFED Capsules (Burroughs Wellcome)
yellow, p. 19b

ACTIFED 12-Hour Capsules (Burroughs Wellcome)
yellow and clear with yellow and white beads, p. 19d

ACTIFED Tablets (Burroughs Wellcome)
white, round, scored, *M2A*, p. 32d

ACUTRIM Precision Release Tablets (CIBA)
75 mg, pale peach, round, *C*, p. 24c

ADAPIN Capsules (Pennwalt)
10 mg, gold, p. 19a
25 mg, lime and gold, p. 14b
50 mg, lime, p. 14c
75 mg, gold and white, p. 19c
100 mg, lime and white, p. 14e

ADEFLOR Chewable Tablets (Upjohn)
0.5 mg, pink, mottled, round, p. 24h
1 mg, lilac, mottled, round, p. 2b

ADEFLOR M Tablets (Upjohn)
hot pink, oval, p. 2f

ADVIL Caplets (Whitehall)
200 mg, brown, oval, p. 27e

ADVIL Tablets (Whitehall)
200 mg, brown, round, p. 27b

AFRINOL Repetabs (Schering)
120 mg, blue, round, p. 9g

AKINETON Tablets (Knoll)
2 mg, white, round, scored, *11*, p. 33g

ALBAMYCIN Capsules (Upjohn)
250 mg, dark maroon and white, p. 6i

ALDACTAZIDE 25/25 Tablets (Searle)
tan, round, *1011*, p. 26c

ALDACTAZIDE 50/50 Tablets (Searle)
tan, capsule-shaped, scored, *1021*, p. 26f

ALDACTONE Tablets (Searle)
25 mg, light yellow, round, *1001*, p. 26b
50 mg, tan, oval, scored, *1041*, p. 26f
100 mg, tan, round, scored, *1031*, p. 26e

ALDOCLOR 150 Tablets (Merck Sharp & Dohme)
beige, oval, *612*, p. 27d

ALDOCLOR 250 Tablets (Merck Sharp & Dohme)
green, oval, *634*, p. 13c

ALDOMET Tablets (Merck Sharp & Dohme)
125 mg, yellow, round, *135*, p. 16b
250 mg, yellow, round, *401*, p. 16g
500 mg, yellow, round, *516*, p. 17a

ALDORIL 15 Tablets (Merck Sharp & Dohme)
salmon, round, *423*, p. 24h

ALDORIL 25 Tablets (Merck Sharp & Dohme)
white, round, *456*, p. 35d

ALDORIL D30 Tablets (Merck Sharp & Dohme)
salmon, oval, *694*, p. 25c

ALDORIL D50 Tablets (Merck Sharp & Dohme)
white, oval, *935*, p. 38b

ALGICON Chewable Tablets (Rorer)
white, round, scored, p. 36i

ALKA-MINTS Chewable Tablets (Miles Laboratories)
white, round, p. 36h

ALKERAN Tablets (Burroughs Wellcome)
2 mg, white, round, scored, *A2A*, p. 32d

ALKETS Tablets (Upjohn)
pale pink, round, p. 2c

ALLBEE C-800 Tablets (Robins)
orange, oval, *0677*, p. 22b

ALLBEE C-800 + Iron Tablets (Robins)
red, oval, *0678*, p. 5h

ALLBEE T Tablets (Robins)
orange, capsule-shaped, p. 22d

ALLBEE with C Capsules (Robins)
green and yellow, *0674*, p. 14e

ALLEREST Allergy and Hay Fever Tablets (Pharmacraft)
blue, round, p. 9e

ALLEREST Children's Chewable Tablets (Pharmacraft)
pink, mottled, round, p. 1g

ALLEREST Headache Strength Tablets (Pharmacraft)
white, round, p. 35c

ALLEREST Sinus Pain Formula Tablets (Pharmacraft)
white, oval, p. 37i

ALLEREST 12 Hour Capsules (Pharmacraft)
orange and clear with pink, yellow, and white beads, p. 23d

ALOPHEN Tablets (Warner-Lambert)
60 mg, brown, oval, p. 27c

ALU-CAP Capsules (Riker)
475 mg, green and red, p. 14i

ALU-TAB Tablets (Riker)
600 mg, green, capsule-shaped, *107*, p. 13g

ALUDROX Chewable Tablets (Wyeth)
white, round, scored, *22*, p. 36f

ALUPENT Tablets (Boehringer Ingelheim)
10 mg, white, round, scored, *74*, p. 32e
20 mg, white, round, scored, *72*, p. 34c

AMCILL Capsules (Parke-Davis)
250 mg, blue and gray, *402*, p. 10i
500 mg, blue and gray, *404*, p. 11e

AMEN Tablets (Carnrick)
10 mg, peach and white, layered, round, scored, p. 26a

AMESEC Capsules (Glaxo)
blue and orange, p. 10h

AMICAR Tablets (Lederle)
500 mg, white, round, scored, *A10*, p. 36c

AMINOPHYLLIN Tablets (Searle)
100 mg, white, round, scored, *1231*, p. 33d
200 mg, white, oval, scored, *1251*, p. 37e

AMOXIL Capsules (Beecham Laboratories)
250 mg, dark blue and pink, p. 8g
500 mg, dark blue and pink, p. 8h

AMOXIL Chewable Tablets (Beecham Laboratories)
250 mg, pink, oval, scored, p. 2f

AMOXIL Tablets (Beecham Laboratories)
125 mg, pink, oval, p. 2e

AMPHOJEL Tablets (Wyeth)
0.3 g, white, round, *119*, p. 35h
0.6 g, white, round, scored, *13*, p. 36f

AMYTAL Sodium Capsules (Lilly)
200 mg, blue, *F33*, p. 10h

AMYTAL Sodium Pulvules (Lilly)
65 mg, blue, *F23*, p. 10g

ANACIN Caplets (Whitehall)
white, capsule-shaped, p. 38i

ANACIN Capsules (Whitehall)
yellow and white, p. 19d

ANACIN Maximum Strength Tablets (Whitehall)
white, round, *500*, p. 35e

ANACIN Tablets (Whitehall)
white, round, p. 34i

ANACIN-3 Children's Chewable Tablets (Whitehall)
80 mg, pink, round, scored, p. 1i

ANACIN-3 Maximum Strength Caplets (Whitehall)
500 mg, white, capsule-shaped, p. 39c

ANACIN-3 Maximum Strength Tablets (Whitehall)
500 mg, white, round, p. 35g

ANACIN-3 Regular Strength Tablets (Whitehall)
325 mg, white, round, scored, p. 34h

ANADROL-50 Tablets (Syntex)
50 mg, white, round, scored, *2902*, p. 32b

ANAPROX Tablets (Syntex)
275 mg, light blue, oval, *274*, p. 10a

ANASPAZ Tablets (Ascher)
0.125 mg, yellow, round, scored, *225/295*, p. 16c

ANASPAZ PB Tablets (Ascher)
pink, round, scored, *225/300*, p. 1f

ANAVAR Tablets (Searle)
2.5 mg, white, oval, scored, *1401*, p. 37b

ANCOBON Capsules (Roche)
250 mg, green and gray, p. 14d
500 mg, gray and white, p. 29d

ANDROID-5 Buccal Tablets (Brown)
5 mg, white, capsule-shaped, *956*, p. 38f

ANDROID-10 Tablets (Brown)

COMPENDIUM OF DRUG THERAPY

DRUG IDENTIFICATION INDEX

10 mg, green, square, *958*, p. 15b
ANDROID-25 Tablets (Brown)
   25 mg, yellow, square, *996*, p. 23h
ANDROID-F Tablets (Brown)
   10 mg, white, round, scored, *998*, p. 32i
ANSPOR Capsules (Smith Kline & French)
   250 mg, orange and white, p. 23a
   500 mg, orange, p. 23f
ANTABUSE Tablets (Ayerst)
   250 mg, white, round, scored, p. 34f
   500 mg, white, round, scored, p. 36d
ANTIVERT Tablets (Roerig)
   12.5 mg, white and turquoise, layered, oval, *210*, p. 37c
ANTIVERT/25 Chewable Tablets (Roerig)
   25 mg, pink, round, scored, *212*, p. 24e
ANTIVERT/25 Tablets (Roerig)
   25 mg, white and yellow, layered, oval, *211*, p. 37f
ANTIVERT/50 Tablets (Roerig)
   50 mg, yellow and blue, layered, oval, *214*, p. 17f
ANTRENYL Tablets (CIBA)
   5 mg, white, round, scored, *15*, p. 31d
ANTROCOL Capsules (Poythress)
   green, p. 14a
ANTROCOL Tablets (Poythress)
   yellow, round, *9540*, p. 15e
ANTURANE Capsules (CIBA)
   200 mg, green, *168*, p. 14f
ANTURANE Tablets (CIBA)
   100 mg, white, round, scored, *41*, p. 34c
APRESAZIDE 25/25 Capsules (CIBA)
   light blue and white, *139*, p. 10h
APRESAZIDE 50/50 Capsules (CIBA)
   pink and white, *149*, p. 3h
APRESAZIDE 100/50 Capsules (CIBA)
   flesh pink and white, *159*, p. 3i
APRESOLINE Tablets (CIBA)
   10 mg, pale yellow, round, *37*, p. 16a
   25 mg, deep blue, round, *39*, p. 9e
   50 mg, light blue, round, *73*, p. 9f
   100 mg, peach, round, *101*, p. 24h
APRESOLINE-ESIDRIX Tablets (CIBA)
   orange, round, *129*, p. 21a
AQUASOL-A Capsules (Rorer)
   50,000 IU, red, clear, *AB*, p. 6e
AQUASOL-E Capsules (Rorer)
   100 IU, green, clear, p. 14d
   400 IU, orange, clear, p. 23g
AQUATENSEN Tablets (Wallace)
   5 mg, peach, rectangular, scored, *153*, p. 25f
ARISTOCORT Tablets (Lederle)
   1 mg, yellow, capsule-shaped, scored, *A1*, p. 18b
   2 mg, pink, capsule-shaped, scored, *A2*, p. 2i
   4 mg, white, capsule-shaped, scored, *A4*, p. 38d
   8 mg, yellow, capsule-shaped, scored, *A8*, p. 18b
ARLIDIN Tablets (Rorer)
   6 mg, white, round, scored, *45*, p. 31d
   12 mg, white, round, scored, *46*, p. 32h
A.R.M. Tablets (SmithKline Consumer Products)
   yellow, capsule-shaped, p. 18c
ARMOUR Thyroid Tablets (Rorer)
   15 mg (¼ gr), off-white, round, *TC*, p. 31a
   30 mg (½ gr), off-white, round, *TD*, p. 31c
   60 mg (1 gr), off-white, round, *TE*, p. 32c
   90 mg (1½ gr), off-white, round, *TJ*, p. 33b
   120 mg (2 gr), off-white, round, *TF*, p. 33i
   180 mg (3 gr), off-white, round, *TG*, p. 34g
   240 mg (4 gr), off-white, round, *TH*, p. 35g
   300 mg (5 gr), off-white, round, *TI*, p. 35b
ARTHRALGEN Tablets (Robins)
   white, round, scored, *1462*, p. 35h
ARTHRITIS PAIN FORMULA Caplets (Whitehall)
   white, capsule-shaped, scored, p. 39h
ASBRON G Tablets (Sandoz Pharmaceuticals)
   green with white inlay, round *78-202*, p. 12i
ASCRIPTIN Tablets (Rorer)
   white, round, p. 35h
ASCRIPTIN with Codeine No. 2 Tablets (Rorer)
   white, round, *142*, p. 36a
ASCRIPTIN with Codeine No. 3 Tablets (Rorer)
   white, round, *143*, p. 36b
ASCRIPTIN A/D Tablets (Rorer)
   white, capsule-shaped, *137*, p. 39f
ASPERGUM Gum (Plough)
   orange, oblong, *orange flavored*, p. 23i
   red, oblong, *cherry flavored*, p. 7e
ATARAX Tablets (Roerig)
   10 mg, orange, triangular, p. 23g
   25 mg, dark green, triangular, p. 15a
   50 mg, yellow, triangular, p. 19g
ATIVAN Tablets (Wyeth)
   0.5 mg, white, five-sided, *81*, p. 40h
   1 mg, white, five-sided, scored, *64*, p. 40i
   2 mg, white, five-sided, scored, *65*, p. 40i
ATROCHOLIN Tablets (Glaxo)
   light green, round, scored, p. 12f
ATROMID-S Capsules (Ayerst)
   500 mg, clear orange, p. 23a
AUGMENTIN '125' Chewable Tablets (Beecham Laboratories)
   yellow, oval, *189*, p. 26d
AUGMENTIN '250' Chewable Tablets (Beecham Laboratories)
   yellow, mottled, round, *190*, p. 26e
AUGMENTIN '250' Tablets (Beecham Laboratories)
   white, oval, p. 38a
AUGMENTIN '500' (Beecham Laboratories)
   white, oval, p. 38d
AVENTYL HCl Pulvules (Lilly)
   10 mg, yellow and white, *H17*, p. 19b
   25 mg, yellow and white, *H19*, p. 19d
AXOTAL Tablets (Adria)
   white, capsule-shaped, *130*, p. 39e
AYGESTIN Tablets (Ayerst)
   5 mg, white, oval, scored, p. 37d
AZO GANTANOL Tablets (Roche)
   red, round, p. 5d
AZO GANTRISIN Tablets (Roche)
   red, round, p. 5d
AZO-STANDARD Tablets (Alcon)
   95 mg, brown, round, *W*, p. 27a
AZULFIDINE EN-tabs (Pharmacia)
   500 mg, orange-yellow, oval, *102*, p. 22a
AZULFIDINE Tablets (Pharmacia)
   500 mg, orange-yellow, round, scored, *101*, p. 21f

B

BACTOCILL Capsules (Beecham Laboratories)
   250 mg, brown and pale yellow, *143*, p. 27h
   500 mg, brown and pale yellow, *144*, p. 28a
BACTRIM Tablets (Roche)
   light green, capsule-shaped, scored, p. 13f
BACTRIM DS Tablets (Roche)
   white, capsule-shaped, scored, p. 40b
BANTHINE Tablets (Searle)
   50 mg, pale orange, round, scored, *1501*, p. 21a
BASALJEL Capsules (Wyeth)
   maroon and yellow, *472*, p. 7d
BASALJEL Tablets (Wyeth)
   white, capsule-shaped, scored, *473*, p. 39g
BAYER Aspirin Tablets (Glenbrook)
   325 mg, white, round, p. 34f
BAYER Aspirin Tablets, Maximum (Glenbrook)
   500 mg, white, round, p. 35f
BAYER Children's Chewable Aspirin Tablets (Glenbrook)
   81 mg, orange, round, p. 24c
BAYER Children's Cold Tablets (Glenbrook)
   white and peach, layered, round, p. 34c
BAYER Timed-Release Aspirin Tablets, 8-Hour (Glenbrook)
   650 mg, white, oblong, scored, p. 38i
BC Tablets (Block)
   white, round, p. 35c
BECOTIN-T Tablets (Dista)
   cinnamon brown, oval, *C22*, p. 27d
BEEPEN-VK Tablets (Beecham Laboratories)
   250 mg, white, oval, *185*, p. 37g
   500 mg, white, oval, *186*, p. 38a
BELLADENAL Tablets (Sandoz Pharmaceuticals)
   white, round, scored, *78-28*, p. 34d
BELLADENAL-S Tablets (Sandoz Pharmaceuticals)
   salmon pink, emerald green, and white, mottled, round, scored, *78-27*, p. 30a
BELLAFOLINE Tablets (Sandoz Pharmaceuticals)
   0.25 mg, white, round, scored, *78-30*, p. 31i
BELLERGAL Tablets (Sandoz Pharmaceuticals)
   shell pink, round, *78-32*, p. 26a
BELLERGAL-S Tablets (Sandoz Pharmaceuticals)
   dark green, orange, light lemon yellow, mottled, round, scored, *78-31*, p. 30a
BEMINAL STRESS PLUS with Iron Tablets (Ayerst)
   burnt orange, oval, p. 27e
BEMINAL STRESS PLUS with Zinc Tablets (Ayerst)

DRUG IDENTIFICATION INDEX

buff, oval, p. 17i
BEMINAL-500 Tablets (Ayerst)
  orange, capsule-shaped, p. 22c
BENADRYL 25 Allergy Capsules
  (Warner-Lambert)
  25 mg, pink and white, *B*, p. 3f
BENADRYL Capsules (Parke-Davis)
  25 mg, pink and white, *471*, p. 3f
BENADRYL Decongestant Allergy
  Capsules (Warner-Lambert)
  powder blue, *D*, p. 11a
BENADRYL Kapseals (Parke-Davis)
  50 mg, pink with white band, *373*, p. 3g
BENEMID Tablets (Merck Sharp &
  Dohme)
  0.5 g, yellow, capsule-shaped, *501*, p. 18e
BENSULFOID Tablets (Poythress)
  130 mg, gray-green, round, *9515*, p. 12c
BENTYL Capsules (Lakeside)
  10 mg, blue, *120* or *10*, p. 10g
BENTYL Tablets (Lakeside)
  20 mg, blue, round, *123* or *20*, p. 9c
BEROCCA Tablets (Roche)
  light green, capsule-shaped, p. 13g
BEROCCA Plus Tablets (Roche)
  golden yellow, capsule-shaped, p. 18h
BETAPEN-VK Tablets (Apothecon)
  250 mg, white, round, *V1*, p. 34e
  500 mg, white, round, *V2*, p. 36b
BIOCAL Chewable Tablets (Miles
  Laboratories)
  250 mg, white, round, p. 36f
BIOCAL Tablets (Miles Laboratories)
  500 mg, white, capsule-shaped, p. 39f
BIPHETAMINE 12½ Capsules
  (Pennwalt)
  black and white, *18-878*, p. 29g
BLOCADREN Tablets (Merck Sharp &
  Dohme)
  5 mg, light blue, round, *59*, p. 9a
  10 mg, light blue, round, scored, *136*, p. 9d
  20 mg, light blue, capsule-shaped, scored, *437*, p. 10c
BONINE Chewable Tablets (Leeming)
  25 mg, light peach, mottled, round, scored, *201*, p. 24e
BONTRIL PDM Tablets (Carnrick)
  35 mg, green, white, and yellow, layered, round, scored, *8648*, p. 12g
BONTRIL Slow Release Capsules
  (Carnrick)
  105 mg, opaque green and clear yellow, *8647*, p. 14f
BRETHINE Tablets (Geigy)
  2.5 mg, yellow, oval, scored, *72*, p. 17f
  5 mg, white, round, scored, *105*, p. 32g
BREVICON Tablets (Syntex)
  blue, round, *110*, p. 9b
  21-day *Wallette*, p. 42a
  28-day *Wallette*, p. 42a
BREXIN L.A. Capsules (Savage)
  red and clear with blue and pink beads, *1934*, p. 6i
BRICANYL Tablets (Lakeside)
  2.5 mg, white, round, scored, *725* or *2½*, p. 32f
  5 mg, white, round, scored, *750*, or white, square, scored, *5*, p. 32f
BRONDECON Tablets (Parke-Davis)
  salmon pink, mottled, round, *WC200*, p. 24h
BRONKAID Tablets (Winthrop
  Consumer Products)
  white, round, scored, *D*, p. 34h
BUCLADIN-S Tablets (Stuart)
  yellow, round, scored, *864*, p. 16b
BUGS BUNNY Chewable Tablets
  (Miles Laboratories)
  various colors and cartoon character shapes, p. 30c
BUGS BUNNY Plus Iron Chewable
  Tablets (Miles Laboratories)
  various colors and cartoon character shapes, p. 30c
BUGS BUNNY with Extra C Chewable
  Tablets (Miles Laboratories)
  various colors and cartoon character shapes, p. 30c
BUGS BUNNY with Iron and Calcium
  Chewable Tablets (Miles
  Laboratories)
  various colors and cartoon character shapes, p. 30d
BUMEX Tablets (Roche)
  0.5 mg, light green, oval, scored, p. 13b
  1 mg, yellow, oval, scored, p. 17f
  2 mg, pink, oval, scored, p. 25b
BUTAZOLIDIN Capsules (Geigy)
  100 mg, orange and white, *44*, p. 23b
BUTAZOLIDIN Tablets (Geigy)
  100 mg, red, round, *14*, p. 5a

C

CAFERGOT Tablets (Sandoz
  Pharmaceuticals)
  shell pink, round, p. 26c
CAFERGOT-PB Tablets (Sandoz
  Pharmaceuticals)
  bright green, round, *78-36*, p. 12g
CALAN Tablets (Searle)
  80 mg, peach, oval, scored, p. 26f
  120 mg, brown, oval, scored, p. 27c
CALCIFEROL Tablets (Kremers-Urban)
  yellow, oval, *KU1*, p. 17e
CALDEROL Capsules (Organon)
  20 μg, white, *472*, p. 40c
  50 μg, orange, *474*, p. 22g
CALEL-D Tablets (Rorer)
  white, capsule-shaped, scored, p. 39g
CAL SUP 300 Tablets (3M)
  300 mg, white, capsule-shaped, p. 39e
CAL SUP 600 Tablets (3M)
  white, oval, p. 38c
CAL SUP 600 Plus Tablets (3M)
  white, oval, p. 38c
CALTRATE 600 Tablets (Lederle)
  600 mg, white, capsule-shaped, scored, p. 39i
CALTRATE 600 + Iron & Vitamin D
  Tablets (Lederle)
  red, capsule-shaped, scored, *C45*, p. 6b
CALTRATE 600 + Vitamin D Tablets
  (Lederle)
  pale gray, capsule-shaped, scored, *C40*, p. 29b
CAMA Tablets (Sandoz Consumer)
  white with orange inlay, capsule-shaped, *500*, p. 22f
CAMALOX Chewable Tablets (Rorer)
  white, round, p. 36g
CANTIL Tablets (Merrell Dow)
  25 mg, yellow, round, *37*, p. 15h
CAPOTEN Tablets (Squibb)
  12.5 mg, white, oblong, scored, *450*, p. 38d
  25 mg, white, square, scored, *452*, p. 41b
  50 mg, white, oval, scored, *482*, p. 37e
  100 mg, white, oval, scored, *485*, p. 37g
CAPOZIDE 25/15 Tablets (Squibb)
  white with orange specks, square, scored, *338*, p. 41b
CAPOZIDE 25/25 Tablets (Squibb)
  peach, square, scored, *349*, p. 25f
CAPOZIDE 50/15 Tablets (Squibb)
  white with orange specks, oval, scored, *384*, p. 37f
CAPOZIDE 50/25 Tablets (Squibb)
  peach, oval, scored, *390*, p. 25b
CARAFATE Tablets (Marion)
  1 g, light pink, capsule-shaped, *1712*, p. 3f
CARDILATE Tablets (Burroughs
  Wellcome)
  5 mg, white, round, scored, *P2B*, p. 31g
  10 mg, white, square, scored, *X7A*, p. 41b
CARDIOQUIN Tablets (Purdue
  Frederick)
  275 mg, beige, round, scored, p. 26c
CARDIZEM Tablets (Marion)
  30 mg, green, round, *1771*, p. 12d
  60 mg, yellow, round, scored, *1772*, p. 16f
CAROID Laxative Tablets
  (Mentholatum)
  brown, round, p. 27b
CATAPRES Tablets (Boehringer
  Ingelheim)
  0.1 mg, tan, oval, scored, *6*, p. 26f
  0.2 mg, orange, oval, scored, *7*, p. 21g
  0.3 mg, peach, oval, scored, *11*, p. 25a
CATAPRES-TTS Transdermal
  Therapeutic Systems (Boehringer
  Ingelheim)
  0.1 mg/day (3.5 cm^2), p. 47a
  0.2 mg/day (7 cm^2), p. 47a
  0.3 mg/day (10.5 cm^2), p. 47a
CEBENASE Tablets (Upjohn)
  pale orange, round, p. 21e
CECLOR Pulvules (Lilly)
  250 mg, purple and white, *3061*, p. 8f
  500 mg, purple and gray, *3062*, p. 8h
CEFOL Filmtabs (Abbott)
  green, capsule-shaped, *NJ*, p. 13d
CELESTONE Tablets (Schering)
  0.6 mg, pink, round, scored, *011*, p. 1e
CELONTIN Kapseals (Parke-Davis)
  150 mg, yellow with brown band, *537*, p. 19a
  300 mg, yellow with orange band, *525*, p. 19b
CENTRAX Capsules (Parke-Davis)
  5 mg, lime green, *552*, p. 14a
  10 mg, aqua, *553*, p. 10f
  20 mg, yellow, *554*, p. 19a
CENTRUM Tablets (Lederle)
  light peach, capsule-shaped, scored, *C1*, p. 25d
CENTRUM Jr. & Extra C Chewable
  Tablets (Lederle)
  various colors, mottled, oval, scored,

DRUG IDENTIFICATION INDEX

C39, p. 30d
CENTRUM Jr. & Iron Chewable Tablets (Lederle)
  various colors, oval, scored, *C2*, p. 30d
CHARDONNA-2 Tablets (Kremers-Urban)
  dark gray, round, *202*, p. 29a
CHEXIT Tablets (Sandoz Consumer)
  pale pink, capsule-shaped, p. 3d
CHLOROMYCETIN Kapseals (Parke-Davis)
  250 mg, white with gray band, *379*, p. 40e
CHLORTHALIDONE Tablets (Abbott)
  25 mg, peach, round, scored, *AA*, p. 24c
  50 mg, lavender, round, scored, *AB*, p. 8b
CHLOR-TRIMETON Allergy Tablets (Schering)
  4 mg, yellow, round, scored, *080*, p. 16b
CHLOR-TRIMETON Decongestant Tablets (Schering)
  blue, round, scored, *901*, p. 9d
CHLOR-TRIMETON Long Acting Allergy Repetabs (Schering)
  8 mg, yellow, round, *374*, p. 16d
  12 mg, orange, round, *009*, p. 20i
CHLOR-TRIMETON Long Acting Decongestant Repetabs (Schering)
  green, round, *LA CTM D*, p. 13a
CHOLAN-DH Tablets (Pennwalt)
  white, round, p. 34g
CHOLAN HMB Tablets (Pennwalt)
  flesh pink, round, *18-950*, p. 24g
CHOLEDYL Tablets (Parke-Davis)
  100 mg, red, round, *210*, p. 5b
  200 mg, yellow, round, *211*, p. 17a
CHOLEDYL SA Tablets (Parke-Davis)
  400 mg, pink, oval, scored, *214*, p. 2g
  600 mg, tan, oval, scored, *221*, p. 27e
CHOLOXIN Tablets (Flint)
  1 mg, orange, oval, scored, p. 25a
  2 mg, yellow, oval, scored, p. 17e
  4 mg, white, oval, scored, p. 37b
  6 mg, green, oval, scored, p. 13b
CHOOZ Antacid Gum (Plough)
  white, chiclet-shaped, p. 41c
CHROMAGEN Capsules (Savage)
  maroon, *4285*, p. 7d
CHROMAGEN OB Capsules (Savage)
  maroon, *0763*, p. 6d
CINOBAC Pulvules (Dista)
  250 mg, green and orange, *3055*, p. 14c
  500 mg, green and orange, *3056*, p. 14i
CLEOCIN HCl Capsules (Upjohn)
  150 mg, maroon and lavender, p. 6i
CLINORIL Tablets (Merck Sharp & Dohme)
  150 mg, yellow, hexagonal, *941*, p. 19h
  200 mg, yellow, hexagonal, *942*, p. 19h
CLOMID Tablets (Merrell Dow)
  50 mg, white, round, scored, *226* or *50*, p. 34c
CLOXAPEN Capsules (Beecham Laboratories)
  250 mg, lime green and beige, *169*, p. 14b
  500 mg, lime green and peach, *170*, p. 14g
CLUVISOL Capsules (Ayerst)
  dark brown, *293*, p. 28b
CLUVISOL Tablets (Ayerst)
  burnt orange, capsule-shaped, *270*, p. 27c
Cod Liver Oil Concentrate Capsules (Schering)
  yellow, clear, round, p. 18i
Cod Liver Oil Concentrate Tablets (Schering)
  yellow, round, p. 16h
Cod Liver Oil Concentrate with Vitamin C Tablets (Schering)
  orange, round, p. 21d
COGENTIN Tablets (Merck Sharp & Dohme)
  0.5 mg, white, round, scored, *21*, p. 31e
  1 mg, white, oval, scored, *635*, p. 37c
  2 mg, white, round, scored, *60*, p. 32a
COLACE Capsules (Mead Johnson Pharmaceuticals)
  50 mg, dark red, oval, p. 6c
  100 mg, dark red and off-white, oval, p. 6d
CoLBENEMID Tablets (Merck Sharp & Dohme)
  white, capsule-shaped, scored, *614*, p. 39d
COMBIPRES Tablets (Boehringer Ingelheim)
  0.1 mg, pink, oval, scored, *8*, p. 2c
  0.2 mg, blue, oval, scored, *9*, p. 9h
  0.3 mg, white, oval, scored, *10*, p. 37b
COMHIST Tablets (Norwich Eaton)
  yellow, round, scored, *0149-0444*, p. 16g
COMHIST LA Capsules (Norwich Eaton)
  yellow and clear with yellow and white beads, *0149-0446*, p. 19c
COMOXOL 400/80 Tablets (Squibb)
  white, round, scored, *872*, p. 35c
COMOXOL 800/160 Tablets (Squibb)
  white, oval, scored, *873*, p. 38d
COMPAL Capsules (Reid-Rowell)
  bluish-green and light aqua, *1290*, p. 14d
COMPAZINE Spansules (Smith Kline & French)
  10 mg, black and clear with light green beads, *C44*, p. 29g
  15 mg, black and clear with light green beads, *C46*, p. 29g
  30 mg, black and clear with light green beads, *C47*, p. 29h
COMPAZINE Tablets (Smith Kline & French)
  5 mg, yellow-green, round, *C66*, p. 12f
  10 mg, yellow-green, round, *C67*, p. 12g
  25 mg, yellow-green, round, *C69*, p. 12h
CONAR-A Tablets (Beecham Laboratories)
  white, capsule-shaped, *210*, p. 39a
CONGESTAC Tablets (SmithKline Consumer Products)
  white, capsule-shaped, scored, *C*, p. 39c
CONSTANT-T Tablets (Geigy)
  200 mg, light pink, oval, scored, *42*, p. 2d
  300 mg, light blue, oval, scored, *57*, p. 10a
CONTAC Continuous Action Decongestant Caplets (SmithKline Consumer Products)
  white, capsule-shaped, p. 38h
CONTAC Continuous Action Decongestant Capsules (SmithKline Consumer Products)
  clear with red band and colored beads, p. 30a
CONTAC Severe Cold Formula Caplets (SmithKline Consumer Products)
  light blue, mottled, capsule-shaped, p. 10d
CONTROL Capsules (Thompson)
  red and clear with white beads, p. 6i
CONVERSPAZ Capsules (Ascher)
  orange, p. 23b
CONVERZYME Capsules (Ascher)
  pink, p. 3i
COPE Tablets (Mentholatum)
  white, capsule-shaped, p. 39b
CO-PYRONIL 2 Pulvules (Dista)
  green and yellow, *3123*, p. 14b
CO-PYRONIL 2 Pediatric Pulvules (Dista)
  maroon, *3122*, p. 6g
CORDARONE Tablets (Wyeth)
  200 mg, white, round, scored, *4188*, p. 35a
CORGARD Tablets (Princeton)
  40 mg, sky blue, round, scored, *207*, p. 9g
  80 mg, light blue, round, scored, *241*, p. 9h
  120 mg, powder blue, capsule-shaped, scored, *208*, p. 10e
  160 mg, sky blue, capsule-shaped, scored, *246*, p. 10e
CORICIDIN 'D' Decongestant Tablets (Schering)
  white, round, *307*, p. 35i
CORICIDIN Demilets (Schering)
  orange, mottled, round, scored, p. 21a
CORICIDIN Extra Strength Sinus Headache Tablets (Schering)
  orange, mottled, round, scored, p. 21f
CORICIDIN Tablets (Schering)
  dark red, round, *522*, p. 5d
CORRECTOL Tablets (Plough)
  deep pink, round, p. 1g
CORTEF Tablets (Upjohn)
  5 mg, white, round, scored, p. 33a
  10 mg, white, round, scored, p. 33c
  20 mg, white, round, scored, p. 33i
CORTONE Acetate Tablets (Merck Sharp & Dohme)
  25 mg, white, round, scored, *219*, p. 34b
CORYBAN-D Capsules (Leeming)
  dark blue and blue, *369*, p. 11c
CORZIDE 40/5 Tablets (Princeton)
  white with blue specks, round, scored, *283*, p. 33h
CORZIDE 80/5 Tablets (Princeton)
  white with blue specks, round, scored, *284*, p. 34b
COTAZYM Capsules (Organon)
  25 mg, green, *381*, p. 14h
COTAZYM-S Capsules (Organon)
  clear with white beads, *388*, p. 26g
COUMADIN Tablets (Du Pont)
  2 mg, lavender, round, scored, p. 8c
  2½ mg, orange, round, scored, p. 21a
  5 mg, peach, round, scored, p. 24e
  7½ mg, yellow, round, scored, p. 16e
  10 mg, white, round, scored, p. 33e

DRUG IDENTIFICATION INDEX

CREAMALIN Tablets (Winthrop Consumer Products)
white, round, p. 36b

CUPRID Capsules (Merck Sharp & Dohme)
250 mg, light brown, *679*, p. 27i

CUPRIMINE Capsules (Merck Sharp & Dohme)
125 mg, gray and yellow, *672*, p. 29c
250 mg, ivory, *602*, p. 19c

CURRETAB Tablets (Reid-Rowell)
10 mg, white, round, scored, *1007*, p. 32a

CYCLAPEN-W (Wyeth)
250 mg, yellow, capsule-shaped, scored, *614*, p. 18c
500 mg, yellow, capsule-shaped, scored, *615*, p. 18h

CYLERT Tablets (Abbott)
18.75 mg, white, round, scored, *TH*, p. 32c
37.5 mg, peach, round, scored, *TI*, p. 24e

CYSTOSPAZ Tablets (Alcon)
0.15 mg, light blue, round, *2225*, p. 9a

CYSTOSPAZ-M Timed-Release Capsules (Alcon)
375 µg, light blue and clear with white beads, *W-2260*, p. 10h

CYTADREN Tablets (CIBA)
250 mg, white, round, quarter-scored, *24*, p. 34i

CYTOMEL Tablets (Smith Kline & French)
5 µg, white, round, *D14*, p. 31b
25 µg, white, round, scored, *D16*, p. 32a
50 µg, white, round, scored, *D17*, p. 33a

D

DALMANE Capsules (Roche)
15 mg, orange and ivory, p. 23a
30 mg, red and ivory, p. 6h

DANOCRINE Capsules (Winthrop Pharmaceuticals)
50 mg, orange and white, *DO3*, p. 22i
100 mg, yellow, *D04*, p. 19b
200 mg, orange, *D05*, p. 23c

DARANIDE Tablets (Merck Sharp & Dohme)
50 mg, yellow, round, scored, *49*, p. 15h

DARAPRIM Tablets (Burroughs Wellcome)
25 mg, white, round, scored, *A3A*, p. 32d

DARBID Tablets (Smith Kline & French)
5 mg, pink, round, *D62*, p. 1d

DARICON Tablets (Beecham Laboratories)
10 mg, white, round, scored, *145*, p. 32c

DARICON-PB Tablets (Beecham Laboratories)
pink, round, scored, *146*, p. 1b

DARVOCET-N 50 Tablets (Lilly)
orange, oblong, p. 22b

DARVOCET-N 100 Tablets (Lilly)
orange, oblong, p. 22d

DARVON Pulvules (Lilly)
32 mg, light pink, *H02*, p. 3f
65 mg, light pink, *H03*, p. 3g

DARVON Compound Pulvules (Lilly)
light gray and light pink, *3110*, p. 29d

DARVON Compound-65 Pulvules (Lilly)
light gray and red, *3111*, p. 29e

DARVON with A.S.A. Pulvules (Lilly)
light pink and red, *H04*, p. 4a

DARVON-N Tablets (Lilly)
100 mg, buff, oval, p. 17g

DARVON-N with A.S.A. Tablets (Lilly)
orange, oval, p. 21i

DAYCARE Capsules (Richardson-Vicks Health Care)
orange and off-white, p. 23g

DECADRON Tablets (Merck Sharp & Dohme)
0.25 mg, orange, pentagonal, scored, *20*, p. 23h
0.5 mg, yellow, pentagonal, scored, *41*, p. 19f
0.75 mg, bluish-green, pentagonal, scored, *63*, p. 11g
1.5 mg, pink, pentagonal, scored, *95*, p. 4b
4 mg, white, pentagonal, scored, *97*, p. 40i
6 mg, green, pentagonal, scored, *147*, p. 15a

DECLOMYCIN Capsules (Lederle)
150 mg, two-tone coral, *D9*, p. 23d

DECLOMYCIN Tablets (Lederle)
150 mg, red, round, *D11*, p. 5b
300 mg, red, round, *D12*, p. 5d

DECONAMINE Tablets (Berlex)
white, round, scored, *184*, p. 35g

DECONAMINE SR Capsules (Berlex)
blue and yellow, *181*, p. 11g

DELTA-CORTEF Tablets (Upjohn)
5 mg, white, round, scored, *25*, p. 31f

DELTASONE Tablets (Upjohn)
2.5 mg, pink, round, scored, *32*, p. 1b
5 mg, white, round, scored, p. 31g
10 mg, white, round, scored, p. 33e
20 mg, peach, round, scored, p. 24g
50 mg, white, round, scored, *388*, p. 34i

DEMAZIN Repetabs (Schering)
blue, round, *133*, p. 9f

DEMEROL Tablets (Winthrop Pharmaceuticals)
50 mg, white, round, scored, *D35*, p. 31f
100 mg, white, round, *D37*, p. 32f

DEMI-REGROTON Tablets (Rorer)
white, uniquely-shaped, *R32*, p. 41a

DEMSER Capsules (Merck Sharp & Dohme)
250 mg, dark blue and light blue, *690*, p. 11e

DEMULEN 1/35 Tablets (Searle)
white, round, *151*, p. 31h
21-day *Compack*, p. 42a
28-day *Compack*, p. 42b

DEMULEN 1/50 Tablets (Searle)
white, round, *71*, p. 31e
21-day *Compack*, p. 42b
28-day *Compack*, p. 42b

DEPAKENE Capsules (Abbott)
250 mg, orange, *HH*, p. 23d

DEPAKOTE Tablets (Abbott)
125 mg, salmon pink, oval, *NT*, p. 5h
250 mg, peach, oval, *NR*, p. 25b
500 mg, lavender, oval, *NS*, p. 2g

DEPEN Tablets (Wallace)
250 mg, white, oval, scored, *37-4401*, p. 37g

DEPONIT Transdermal Delivery Systems (Wyeth)
5 mg/24 h (16 cm^2), p. 47a

DESYREL Dividose Tablets (Mead Johnson Pharmaceuticals)
150 mg, orange, oblong, triple-scored, *778*, p. 23i

DESYREL Tablets (Mead Johnson Pharmaceuticals)
50 mg, peach, round, scored, *775*, p. 24d
100 mg, white, round, scored, *776*, p. 35c

DEXATRIM Extra Strength Capsules (Thompson)
yellow, oval, p. 18h

DEXATRIM Extra Strength with Vitamin C Capsules (Thompson)
dark red and clear with red and yellow beads, p. 7c

DEXATRIM Regular Strength Capsules (Thompson)
black and clear with red and yellow beads, p. 29h

DIAβETA Tablets (Hoechst-Roussel)
1.25 mg, white, oblong, scored, p. 38e
2.5 mg, pink, oblong, scored, p. 3a
5 mg, light green, oblong, scored, p. 13d

DIABINESE Tablets (Pfizer)
100 mg, blue, D-shaped, scored, *393*, p. 11g
250 mg, blue, D-shaped, scored, *394*, p. 11h

DIALOSE Capsules (Stuart)
100 mg, pink, *470*, p. 4a

DIALOSE Plus Capsules (Stuart)
yellow, *475*, p. 19e

DIALUME Capsules (Rorer)
maroon and white, *RD*, p. 7a

DIAMOX Sequels (Lederle)
500 mg, orange, *D3*, p. 23g

DIAMOX Tablets (Lederle)
125 mg, white, round, scored, *D1*, p. 33d
250 mg, white, round, double-scored, *D2*, p. 35b

DIBENZYLINE Capsules (Smith Kline & French)
10 mg, red, *E33*, p. 6g

DICUMAROL Tablets (Abbott)
25 mg, white, round, *AN*, p. 31b
50 mg, pink, round, scored, *AO*, p. 1c

DIDRONEL Tablets (Norwich Eaton)
200 mg, white, rectangular, *402*, p. 41c
400 mg, white, capsule-shaped, scored, *406*, p. 38g

DI-GEL Tablets (Plough)
yellow and white, layered, round, *mint or lemon/orange flavored*, p. 17b

DILANTIN Infatabs (Parke-Davis)
50 mg, yellow, triangular, scored, *007*, p. 19g

DILANTIN Kapseals (Parke-Davis)
100 mg, white with orange band, *362*, p. 40d

DILANTIN with ¼ gr Phenobarbital Kapseals (Parke-Davis)
white with red band, *375*, p. 40d

DILANTIN with ½ gr Phenobarbital Kapseals (Parke-Davis)
white with black band, *531*, p. 40d

DILATRATE-SR Capsules (Reed & Carnrick)
40 mg, flesh pink and clear with white beads, *0920*, p. 3g

DILAUDID Tablets (Knoll)
1 mg, green, round, p. 12a
2 mg, orange, round, p. 20d

DRUG IDENTIFICATION INDEX

3 mg, pink, round, p. 1a
4 mg, yellow, round, p. 15f
DILONE Tablets (Richardson-Vicks Health Care)
white, round, scored, p. 35i
DILOR-400 Tablets (Savage)
400 mg, white, round, scored, *1116*, p. 35g
DIMACOL Capsules (Robins)
green and orange, *1652*, p. 14f
DIMETANE Decongestant Tablets (Robins)
light blue, capsule-shaped, scored, *2117*, p. 10b
DIMETANE Extentabs (Robins)
4 mg, orange, round, scored, *1857*, p. 24d
8 mg, pink, round, *1868*, p. 1i
12 mg, peach, round, *1843*, p. 24f
DIMETAPP Extentabs (Robins)
light blue, round, p. 9h
DIMETAPP Tablets (Robins)
light blue, round, *2254*, p. 9g
DIOSTATE D Tablets (Upjohn)
cream, round, p. 26d
DISALCID Capsules (Riker)
500 mg, aqua and white, p. 14g
DISALCID Tablets (Riker)
500 mg, light blue, round, p. 9h
750 mg, light blue, capsule-shaped, scored, p. 10f
DISIPAL Tablets (Riker)
50 mg, green, round, *161*, p. 12f
DISOPHROL Tablets (Schering)
blue and white, mottled, round, scored, *WBS*, p. 9d
DITROPAN Tablets (Marion)
5 mg, blue, round, scored, *1375*, p. 9d
DIUCARDIN Tablets (Ayerst)
50 mg, white, oval, scored, p. 37b
DIULO Tablets (Searle)
2½ mg, pink, round, *501*, p. 1a
5 mg, blue, round, *511*, p. 9b
10 mg, yellow, round, *521*, p. 15g
DIUPRES-250 Tablets (Merck Sharp & Dohme)
pink, round, scored, *230*, p. 1h
DIUPRES-500 Tablets (Merck Sharp & Dohme)
pink, round, scored, *405*, p. 2a
DIURIL Tablets (Merck Sharp & Dohme)
250 mg, white, round, scored, *214*, p. 33h
500 mg, white, round, scored, *432*, p. 35c
DIUTENSEN Tablets (Wallace)
white with blue specks, round, scored, *272*, p. 9d
DIUTENSEN-R Tablets (Wallace)
white with pink specks, round, scored, *274*, p. 1e
DOLOBID Tablets (Merck Sharp & Dohme)
250 mg, peach, capsule-shaped, *675*, p. 25c
500 mg, orange, capsule-shaped, *697*, p. 22d
DONNATAL Capsules (Robins)
green and white, *4207*, p. 14a
DONNATAL Extentabs (Robins)
pale green, round, p. 12g
DONNATAL Tablets (Robins)
white, round, scored, *4250*, p. 32h
DONNATAL No. 2 Tablets (Robins)
green, round, scored, *4264*, p. 12e
DONNAZYME Tablets (Robins)
Kelly green, round, *4649*, p. 13a

DORBANTYL Forte Capsules (3M)
orange and gray, p. 23c
DORYX Capsules (Parke-Davis)
100 mg, blue and clear with yellow beads, p. 11a
DOXIDAN Capsules (Hoechst-Roussel)
clear maroon, p. 6d
DRAMAMINE Tablets (Richardson-Vicks Health Care)
50 mg, white, round, scored *1701*, p. 33c
DRISTAN Caplets (Whitehall)
yellow and white, layered, capsule-shaped, p. 18d
DRISTAN Tablets (Whitehall)
white and yellow, layered, round, p. 16f
DRISTAN AF Aspirin Free Tablets (Whitehall)
green and white, layered, round, p. 12h
DRIXORAL Sustained-Action Tablets (Schering)
green, round, p. 13a
DRIZE Slow Release Capsules (Ascher)
clear with white beads, *225-405*, p. 40f
DULCOLAX Tablets (Boehringer Ingelheim)
5 mg, yellow, round, *12*, p. 15f
DURAPHYL Tablets (Forest)
100 mg, white, round, scored, *425*, p. 34c
200 mg, white, capsule-shaped, scored, *426*, p. 38i
300 mg, white, capsule-shaped, scored, *427*, p. 39d
DURICEF Capsules (Mead Johnson Pharmaceuticals)
500 mg, red and white, *784*, p. 7a
DURICEF Tablets (Mead Johnson Pharmaceuticals)
1 g, off-white, oval, scored, *785*, p. 38c
DYAZIDE Capsules (Smith Kline & French)
red and white, p. 6e
DYCILL Capsules (Beecham Laboratories)
250 mg, blue and peach, *165*, p. 11d
500 mg, blue and peach, *166*, p. 11e
DYMELOR Tablets (Lilly)
250 mg, white, capsule-shaped, scored, *U03*, p. 38f
500 mg, yellow, capsule-shaped, scored, *U07*, p. 18e
DYNAPEN Capsules (Apothecon)
125 mg, blue and white, *7892*, p. 10g
250 mg, blue and white, *7893*, p. 10i
500 mg, blue and white, *7658*, p. 11d
DYRENIUM Capsules (Smith Kline & French)
50 mg, maroon, p. 6f
100 mg, maroon, p. 6g

E

E.E.S. Chewable Tablets (Abbott)
200 mg, white, round, scored, *EF*, p. 36i
E.E.S. 400 Filmtabs (Abbott)
400 mg, pink, oval, *EE*, p. 2h
EASPRIN Tablets (Parke-Davis)
975 mg, salmon pink, oval, *490*, p. 2h
ECOTRIN Tablets (SmithKline Consumer Products)

325 mg, orange, round, p. 21c
ECOTRIN Tablets, Maximum Strength (SmithKline Consumer Products)
500 mg, orange, round, p. 21e
EDECRIN Tablets (Merck Sharp & Dohme)
25 mg, white, capsule-shaped, scored, *65*, p. 38e
50 mg, green, capsule-shaped, scored, *90*, p. 13d
ELAVIL Tablets (Merck Sharp & Dohme)
10 mg, blue, round, *23*, p. 9b
25 mg, yellow, round, *45*, p. 15h
50 mg, beige, round, *102*, p. 27a
75 mg, orange, round, *430*, p. 21c
100 mg, mauve, round, *435*, p. 2a
150 mg, blue, capsule-shaped, *673*, p. 10d
ELIXOPHYLLIN Capsules (Forest)
100 mg, off-white, p. 26g
200 mg, off-white, p. 19d
ELIXOPHYLLIN SR Capsules (Forest)
125 mg, white, *129*, p. 40e
250 mg, clear with white beads, *123*, p. 40h
EMCYT Capsules (Roche)
140 mg, white, p. 40f
EMPIRIN Tablets (Burroughs Wellcome)
325 mg, white, round, p. 34h
EMPIRIN with Codeine No. 2 Tablets (Burroughs Wellcome)
white, round, p. 35i
EMPIRIN with Codeine No. 3 Tablets (Burroughs Wellcome)
white, round, p. 35i
EMPIRIN with Codeine No. 4 Tablets (Burroughs Wellcome)
white, round, p. 36a
EMPRACET with Codeine No. 3 Tablets (Burroughs Wellcome)
peach, round, p. 24h
EMPRACET with Codeine No. 4 Tablets (Burroughs Wellcome)
peach, round, p. 24i
E-MYCIN Tablets (Upjohn)
250 mg, orange, round, p. 21e
ENARAX 5 Tablets (Beecham Laboratories)
white, round, scored, *194*, p. 33c
ENARAX 10 Tablets (Beecham Laboratories)
black and white, layered, round, scored, *195*, p. 34d
ENDECON Tablets (Du Pont)
light green, mottled, round, p. 12i
ENDEP Tablets (Roche)
10 mg, orange, round, scored, p. 20e
25 mg, orange, round, scored, p. 20h
50 mg, orange, round, scored, p. 21c
75 mg, yellow, round, p. 16f
100 mg, peach, round, scored, p. 24g
150 mg, salmon, round, scored, p. 21c
ENDURON Tablets (Abbott)
2.5 mg, orange, square, scored, p. 23h
5 mg, salmon, square, scored, p. 23h
ENDURONYL Tablets (Abbott)
yellow, square, scored, *LS*, p. 19g
ENDURONYL Forte Tablets (Abbott)
gray, square, scored, *LT*, p. 29e
ENGRAN-HP Tablets (Squibb)
green, capsule-shaped, *478*, p. 13g
ENOVID Tablets (Searle)
5 mg, light orange, round, *51*, p. 20g

DRUG IDENTIFICATION INDEX

10 mg, coral, mottled, round, *101*, p. 21a
ENOVID-E Tablets (Searle)
 pale pink, round, *131*, p. 1d
 21-day *Compack*, p. 42c
ENTEX Capsules (Norwich Eaton)
 orange and white, *0412*, p. 23f
ENTEX LA Tablets (Norwich Eaton)
 blue, oval, scored, p. 10d
ENTOZYME Tablets (Robins)
 white, round, *5049*, p. 35i
EQUAGESIC Tablets (Wyeth)
 yellow and pink, layered, round, scored, *91*, p. 17a
EQUANIL Tablets (Wyeth)
 200 mg, white, five-sided, scored, *2*, p. 41b
 400 mg, white, round, scored, *1*, p. 35d
EQUANIL Wyseals (Wyeth)
 400 mg, yellow, round, *33*, p. 16g
ERGOSTAT Sublingual Tablets (Parke-Davis)
 2 mg, orange, round, *111*, p. 20d
ERYC Capsules (Parke-Davis)
 125 mg, orange and clear with white beads, p. 23e
 250 mg, orange and clear with orange and white beads, *696*, p. 23e
ERY-TAB Tablets (Abbott)
 250 mg, pink, capsule-shaped, *EC*, p. 2e
 333 mg, white, capsule-shaped, *EH*, p. 37h
 500 mg, pink, capsule-shaped, *ED*, p. 2g
ERYTHROCIN Stearate Filmtabs (Abbott)
 250 mg, salmon, round, *ES*, p. 24i
 500 mg, hot pink, capsule-shaped, *ET*, p. 2h
ERYTHROMYCIN BASE Filmtabs (Abbott)
 250 mg, pink, capsule-shaped, *EB*, p. 2e
 500 mg, pink, capsule-shaped, *EA*, p. 2i
ESGIC Capsules (Forest)
 white, *535-12*, p. 40f
ESGIC Tablets (Forest)
 white, round, *535-11*, p. 35i
ESIDRIX Tablets (CIBA)
 25 mg, pink, round, scored, *22*, p. 1c
 100 mg, blue, round, scored, *192*, p. 9f
ESIMIL Tablets (CIBA)
 white, round, scored, *47*, p. 33e
ESKALITH Capsules (Smith Kline & French)
 300 mg, gray and yellow, p. 29d
ESKALITH Tablets (Smith Kline & French)
 300 mg, gray, round, scored, *J09*, p. 29b
ESKALITH CR Tablets (Smith Kline & French)
 450 mg, buff, round, scored, *J10*, p. 26e
ESTINYL Tablets (Schering)
 0.02 mg, beige, round, *298*, p. 26b
 0.05 mg, pink, round, *070*, p. 1d
 0.5 mg, peach, round, scored, *150*, p. 24d
ESTRACE Tablets (Mead Johnson Laboratories)
 1 mg, lavender, round, scored, *755*, p. 8a

2 mg, turquoise, round, scored, *756*, p. 12a
ESTRADERM Transdermal Systems (CIBA)
 0.05 mg/24 h (10 cm^2), p. 47b
 0.1 mg/24 h (20 cm^2), p. 47b
ESTRATAB Tablets (Reid-Rowell)
 0.3 mg, bright blue, round, *1014*, p. 9g
 0.625 mg, yellow, round, *1022*, p. 16f
 1.25 mg, red-orange, round, *1024*, p. 21b
 2.5 mg, sugar pink, round, *1025*, p. 1i
ESTRATEST Tablets (Reid-Rowell)
 dark green, oval, *1026*, p. 13e
ESTRATEST H.S. Tablets (Reid-Rowell)
 light green, oval, *1023*, p. 13e
ESTROVIS Tablets (Parke-Davis)
 100 µg, blue, round, *437*, p. 9c
ETHAQUIN Tablets (Ascher)
 white, round, *225-250*, p. 33d
ETHATAB Tablets (Glaxo)
 100 mg, yellow, oval, *281*, p. 17g
ETHRIL '250' Tablets (Squibb)
 250 mg, hot pink, oval, *160*, p. 2f
ETHRIL '500' Tablets (Squibb)
 500 mg, dark pink, oval, *161*, p. 2i
ETRAFON 2-10 Tablets (Schering)
 deep yellow, round, *287*, p. 16a
ETRAFON 2-25 Tablets (Schering)
 pink, round, *598*, p. 1d
ETRAFON-A 4-10 Tablets (Schering)
 orange, round, *119*, p. 20e
ETRAFON-FORTE 4-25 Tablets (Schering)
 red, round, *720*, p. 5a
EUTONYL Filmtabs (Abbott)
 10 mg, pink, round, *NA*, p. 1d
 25 mg, apricot, round, *NB*, p. 20e
EUTRON Filmtabs (Abbott)
 lilac, capsule-shaped, scored, *NK*, p. 8d
EX-LAX Pills (Sandoz Consumer)
 beige, round, p. 26d
EX-LAX Tablets, Extra Gentle (Sandoz Consumer)
 pink, round, p. 2a
EXNA Tablets (Robins)
 50 mg, yellow, round, scored, *5449*, p. 24d

F

FANSIDAR Tablets (Roche)
 white, round, scored, p. 36e
FASTIN Capsules (Beecham Laboratories)
 30 mg, blue and clear with blue and white beads, p. 10i
FEDAHIST Gyrocaps (Kremers-Urban)
 clear yellow and white with yellow and green beads, *1053*, p. 19c
FEDAHIST Tablets (Kremers-Urban)
 white, oval, scored, *050*, p. 37c
FEDRAZIL Tablets (Burroughs Wellcome)
 yellow, round, p. 16c
FEEN-A-MINT Gum (Plough)
 white, oblong, p. 41c
FEEN-A-MINT Pills (Plough)
 white, round, p. 34c
FEEN-A-MINT Tablets (Plough)
 rose pink, mottled, square, scored, p. 4d
FELDENE Capsules (Pfizer)
 10 mg, maroon and blue, *322*, p. 6h
 20 mg, maroon, *323*, p. 6g

FEMINONE Tablets (Upjohn)
 50 µg, pink, round, scored, p. 1c
FEMIRON Multivitamins and Iron Tablets (Beecham Products)
 dark pink, oval, p. 5g
FEMIRON Tablets (Beecham Products)
 20 mg, hot pink, oval, p. 2e
FEOSOL Capsules (SmithKline Consumer Products)
 red and clear with maroon and light pink beads, p. 6h
FEOSOL Tablets (SmithKline Consumer Products)
 dark green, triangular, p. 15a
FER-IN-SOL Capsules (Mead Johnson Nutritional)
 red, oval, p. 6c
FERANCEE Chewable Tablets (Stuart)
 brown and yellow, layered, round, *650*, p. 27c
FERANCEE-HP Tablets (Stuart)
 red, oval, p. 5h
FERGON Capsules (Winthrop Consumer Products)
 435 mg, dark-red and clear with red and gray beads, p. 7d
FERGON Tablets (Winthrop Consumer Products)
 320 mg, green, round, p. 12h
FERGON Plus Caplets (Winthrop Consumer Products)
 pink, oblong, *F17*, p. 3d
FERMALOX Tablets (Rorer)
 light brown, round, *260*, p. 27b
FERO-FOLIC-500 Filmtabs (Abbott)
 red, capsule-shaped, *AJ*, p. 5i
FERO-GRAD-500 Filmtabs (Abbott)
 dark red, capsule-shaped, p. 5i
FERRO-Sequels (Lederle)
 green, *F2*, p. 14e
FESTAL II Tablets (Hoechst-Roussel)
 white, round, *72*, p. 35a
FESTALAN Tablets (Hoechst-Roussel)
 1 mg, orange, round, *73*, p. 21d
FIBRE-TRIM Tablets (Schering)
 khaki, mottled, round, p. 26e
FILIBON Tablets (Lederle)
 pink, capsule-shaped, *F4*, p. 3e
FILIBON F.A. Tablets (Lederle)
 pink, capsule-shaped, *F5*, p. 3e
FILIBON Forte Tablets (Lederle)
 pink, capsule-shaped, scored, *F6*, p. 3e
FIORICET Tablets (Sandoz Pharmaceuticals)
 light blue, round, p. 9h
FIORINAL Capsules (Sandoz Pharmaceuticals)
 bright Kelly green and lime green, *78-103*, p. 14g
FIORINAL Tablets (Sandoz Pharmaceuticals)
 white, round, p. 35d
FIORINAL with Codeine No. 1 Capsules (Sandoz Pharmaceuticals)
 red and yellow, *78-105*, p. 7c
FIORINAL with Codeine No. 2 Capsules (Sandoz Pharmaceuticals)
 gray and yellow, *78-106*, p. 29d
FIORINAL with Codeine No. 3 Capsules (Sandoz Pharmaceuticals)
 blue and yellow, *78-107*, p. 11f
FLAGYL Tablets (Searle)
 250 mg, blue, round, *1831*, p. 9e
 500 mg, blue, oblong, p. 10b
FLEXERIL Tablets (Merck Sharp & Dohme)

DRUG IDENTIFICATION INDEX

10 mg, butterscotch yellow, D-shaped, *931*, p. 19g

FLINTSTONES Plus Iron Chewable Tablets (Miles Laboratories)
various colors and cartoon character shapes, p. 30c

FLORINEF Acetate Tablets (Squibb)
0.1 mg, light pink, round, scored, *429*, p. 1a

FOLVRON Capsules (Lederle)
brown, p. 27f

FULVICIN P/G Tablets (Schering)
125 mg, off-white, round, scored, *228*, p. 33h
250 mg, off-white, round, scored, *507*, p. 36c

FULVICIN P/G 165 Tablets (Schering)
165 mg, off-white, oval, scored, *654*, p. 37g

FULVICIN P/G 330 Tablets (Schering)
330 mg, off-white, oval, scored, *352*, p. 38b

FULVICIN-U/F Tablets (Schering)
250 mg, white, round, scored, *948*, p. 35d
500 mg, white, round, scored, *496*, p. 36b

FUROSE Tablets (Ascher)
white, round, scored, *225/425*, p. 32g

FUROXONE Tablets (Norwich Eaton)
100 mg, tan, round, scored, *072*, p. 26c

G

GANTANOL Tablets (Roche)
0.5 g, green, round, scored, p. 13a

GANTANOL DS Tablets (Roche)
1 g, light orange, capsule-shaped, scored, p. 22f

GANTRISIN Tablets (Roche)
0.5 g, white, round, scored, p. 36c

GAS-X Tablets (Sandoz Consumer)
white, round, scored, p. 36e

GAS-X Tablets, Extra Strength (Sandoz Consumer)
yellow, round, scored. p. 17b

GAVISCON Chewable Tablets (Marion)
white, round, *1175*, p. 36g

GAVISCON-2 Chewable Tablets (Marion)
white, round, *1172*, p. 37a

GELUSIL Chewable Tablets (Warner-Lambert)
white, round, *034*, p. 36e

GELUSIL-II Chewable Tablets (Warner-Lambert)
mottled orange and white, layered, round, *043*, p. 21f

GELUSIL-M Chewable Tablets (Warner-Lambert)
white, round, *045*, p. 36g

GEMNISYN Tablets (Kremers-Urban)
white, oval, scored, *171*, p. 38a

GENTLAX S Tablets (Purdue Frederick)
orange, round, p. 21b

GENTLE NATURE Tablets (Sandoz Consumer)
tan with black specks, round, p. 26d

GEOCILLIN Tablets (Roerig)
382 mg, yellow, capsule-shaped, *143*, p. 18g

GERITOL COMPLETE Tablets (Beecham Products)
dark red, capsule-shaped, p. 6a

GLUCOTROL Tablets (Roerig)
5 mg, white, diamond-shaped, scored, *411*, p. 41b
10 mg, white diamond-shaped, scored, *412*, p. 41d

GRIS-PEG Tablets (Herbert)
125 mg, white, oval, scored, p. 38c
250 mg, white, capsule-shaped, scored, p. 38h

GRISACTIN Capsules (Ayerst)
125 mg, orange, p. 23d
250 mg, yellow, p. 19e

GRISACTIN Tablets (Ayerst)
500 mg, flesh pink, round, scored, p. 24i

GRISACTIN Ultra Tablets (Ayerst)
125 mg, white, square, p. 41c
250 mg, white, square, p. 41c
330 mg, white, oval, scored, p. 38c

GYNE-LOTRIMIN Vaginal Tablets (Schering)
100 mg, white, half oval-shaped, *734*, p. 41d
500 mg, white, oblong, *396*, p. 41d

H

HALCION Tablets (Upjohn)
0.125 mg, pale lavender, oval, p. 8d
0.25 mg, powder blue, oval, scored, p. 9i
0.5 mg, white, oval, scored, p. 37a

HALDOL Tablets (McNeil Pharmaceutical)
½ mg, white, irregularly shaped with H-shaped cutout, scored, p. 41a
1 mg, yellow, irregularly shaped with H-shaped cutout, scored, p. 19f
2 mg, pink, irregularly shaped with H-shaped cutout, scored, p. 8h
5 mg, green, irregularly shaped with H-shaped cutout, scored, p. 15a
10 mg, aqua, irregularly shaped with H-shaped cutout, scored, p. 11h
20 mg, salmon, irregularly shaped with H-shaped cutout, scored, p. 4b

HALODRIN Tablets (Upjohn)
pale pink, round, scored, *38*, p. 1c

HALOTESTIN Tablets (Upjohn)
5 mg, light green, round, scored, *19*, p. 12c
10 mg, green, round, scored, p. 12c

HALTRAN Tablets (Upjohn)
white, round, p. 34a

HEAD & CHEST Capsules (Richardson-Vicks Health Care)
blue and white, *NE 036*, p. 11d

HEAD & CHEST Tablets (Richardson-Vicks Health Care)
white, oval, scored, *0127*, p. 38a

HEPTUNA Plus Capsules (Roerig)
red and white, *504*, p. 7d

HEXADROL Tablets (Organon)
0.5 mg, yellow, round, scored, *792*, p. 16a
0.75 mg, white, round, scored, *791*, p. 32e
1.5 mg, peach, round, scored, *790*, p. 20f
4 mg, green, round, scored, *798*, p. 12d

HIPREX Tablets (Merrell Dow)
1 g, yellow, capsule-shaped, scored, *277*, p. 18g

HISPRIL Spansules (Smith Kline & French)
5 mg, pink and clear with pink, white, and purple beads, p. 3g

HISTABID Capsules (Glaxo)
pink and clear with pink and white beads, *309*, p. 3i

HISTALET Forte Tablets (Reid-Rowell)
white with blue specks, capsule-shaped, scored, *1039*, p. 38f

HISTALET X Tablets (Reid-Rowell)
white with green specks, round, scored, *1050*, p. 36c

HOLD Children's Lozenges (Beecham Products)
red, round, p. 5d

HOLD Lozenges (Beecham Products)
5.0 mg, yellow, round, p. 17c

HYDERGINE Tablets (Sandoz Pharmaceuticals)
1 mg, white, round, p. 32e

HYDERGINE LC Capsules (Sandoz Pharmaceuticals)
1 mg, off-white, p. 26g

HYDERGINE Sublingual Tablets (Sandoz Pharmaceuticals)
0.5 mg, white, round, p. 33g
1 mg, white, oval, *78-77*, p. 37d

HYDREA Capsules (Squibb)
500 mg, green and pink, *830*, p. 14g

HYDROCET Capsules (Carnrick)
blue and white, *8657*, p. 11e

HYDROCORTONE Tablets (Merck Sharp & Dohme)
10 mg, white, oval, scored, *619*, p. 37d
20 mg, white, oval, scored, *625*, p. 37d

HydroDIURIL Tablets (Merck Sharp & Dohme)
25 mg, peach, round, scored, *42*, p. 24b
50 mg, peach, round, scored, *105*, p. 24d
100 mg, peach, round, scored, *410*, p. 24g

HYDROMOX Tablets (Lederle)
50 mg, white, round, scored, *H1*, p. 33f

HYDROMOX R Tablets (Lederle)
yellow, round, scored, p. 16d

HYDROPRES 25 Tablets (Merck Sharp & Dohme)
green, round, scored, *53*, p. 12b

HYDROPRES 50 Tablets (Merck Sharp & Dohme)
green, round, scored, *127*, p. 12d

HYGROTON Tablets (Rorer)
25 mg, peach, H-shaped, *22*, p. 23h
50 mg, aqua, H-shaped, *20*, p. 11g
100 mg, white, round, scored, *21*, p. 32a

HYLOREL Tablets (Pennwalt)
10 mg, light orange, elliptical, scored, p. 21h
25 mg, white, elliptical, scored, p. 37c

I

IBERET-500 Filmtabs (Abbott)
red, capsule-shaped, p. 5i

IBERET-FOLIC-500 Filmtabs (Abbott)
dark pink, capsule-shaped, *AK*, p. 2g

ILOPAN-CHOLINE Tablets (Adria)
cream, round, *231*, p. 33h

ILOSONE Chewable Tablets (Dista)
125 mg, light pink, square, *U05*, p. 4b
250 mg, light pink, square, *U25*, p. 4d

ILOSONE Pulvules (Dista)
250 mg, red and ivory, *H09*, p. 23g

DRUG IDENTIFICATION INDEX

ILOSONE Tablets (Dista)
500 mg, light pink, capsule-shaped, scored, *U26*, p. 25c
ILOTYCIN Tablets (Dista)
250 mg, orange, oval, p. 25b
ILOZYME Tablets (Adria)
beige, mottled, round, *200*, p. 26d
IMODIUM Capsules (Janssen)
2 mg, dark green and light green, p. 14a
IMURAN Tablets (Burroughs Wellcome)
50 mg, yellow, oval, scored, p. 17e
INDERAL Tablets (Ayerst)
10 mg, orange, hexagonal, scored, p. 25e
20 mg, blue, hexagonal, scored, p. 11g
40 mg, green, hexagonal, scored, p. 15b
60 mg, pink, hexagonal, scored, p. 4b
80 mg, yellow, hexagonal, scored, p. 19h
90 mg, lavender, hexagonal, scored, p. 8h
INDERAL LA Capsules (Ayerst)
80 mg, light blue, p. 10g
120 mg, dark blue and light blue, p. 11b
160 mg, dark blue, p. 11b
INDERIDE-40/25 Tablets (Ayerst)
off-white, hexagonal, scored, p. 41a
INDERIDE-80/25 Tablets (Ayerst)
off-white, hexagonal, scored, p. 41a
INDERIDE LA 80/50 Capsules (Ayerst)
beige with gold bands, p. 26g
INDERIDE LA 120/50 Capsules (Ayerst)
beige and brown with gold bands, p. 27i
INDERIDE LA 160/50 Capsules (Ayerst)
brown with gold bands, p. 28a
INDOCIN Capsules (Merck Sharp & Dohme)
25 mg, blue and white, p. 10g
50 mg, blue and white, p. 11b
INDOCIN SR Capsules (Merck Sharp & Dohme)
75 mg, blue and clear with blue and white beads, *693*, p. 10i
INVERSINE Tablets (Merck Sharp & Dohme)
2.5 mg, yellow, round, scored, *52*, p. 15g
IONAMIN Capsules (Pennwalt)
15 mg, gray and yellow, p. 29c
30 mg, yellow, p. 19a
ISMELIN Tablets (CIBA)
10 mg, pale yellow, round, scored, *49*, p. 16d
25 mg, white, round, scored, *103*, p. 34a
ISOPTIN Tablets (Knoll)
80 mg, yellow, round, scored, p. 16e
120 mg, white, round, scored, p. 35e
ISORDIL Chewable Tablets (Wyeth)
10 mg, yellow, round, scored, *4164*, p. 16c
ISORDIL Oral Titradose Tablets (Wyeth)
5 mg, pink, round, scored, *4152*, p. 1e
10 mg, white, round, scored, *4153*, p. 33b
20 mg, green, round, scored, *4154*, p. 12e
40 mg, light green, round, scored, *4192*, p. 12h
ISORDIL Sublingual Tablets (Wyeth)
2.5 mg, yellow, round, p. 15e
10 mg, white, round, p. 31b
ISORDIL Tembids Tablets (Wyeth)
40 mg, green, round, scored, *4125*, p. 12h
ISUPREL Glossets Sublingual Tablets (Winthrop Pharmaceuticals)
10 mg, white, round, scored, *J75*, p. 31e
15 mg, white, round, scored, *J77*, p. 31d

J

JANIMINE Filmtabs (Abbott)
10 mg, orange, round, *ND*, p. 20d
25 mg, yellow, round, *NE*, p. 15h
50 mg, peach, oval, *NL*, p. 25a

K

KANTREX Capsules (Apothecon)
500 mg, white, *3506*, p. 40h
KANULASE Tablets (Sandoz Consumer)
rose pink, capsule-shaped, p. 3d
KAON Tablets (Adria)
5 mEq, purple, capsule-shaped, *312*, p. 8e
KAON-CL Controlled-Release Tablets (Adria)
6.7 mEq, yellow, round, *307*, p. 16i
KAON CL-10 Controlled-Release Tablets (Adria)
10 mEq, green, capsule-shaped, *304*, p. 13f
KASOF Capsules (Stuart)
240 mg, brown, *380*, p. 27h
K-DUR 10 Sustained-Release Tablets (Key)
10 mEq, grayish-white, mottled, oblong, p. 38h
K-DUR 20 Sustained-Release Tablets (Key)
20 mEq, grayish-white, mottled, oblong, scored, p. 40c
KEFLEX Pulvules (Dista)
250 mg, dark green and white, *H69*, p. 14h
500 mg, dark green and light green, *H71*, p. 14i
KEFLEX Tablets (Dista)
1 g, green, capsule-shaped, *U60*, p. 13h
KEMADRIN Tablets (Burroughs Wellcome)
5 mg, white, round, scored, *S3A*, p. 31i
KENACORT Tablets (Squibb)
4 mg, white, round, scored, *512*,, p. 34a
8 mg, buff, octagonal, scored, *518*, p. 19i
KINESED Chewable Tablets (Stuart)
white, oval, scored, *220*, p. 37h
KLONOPIN Tablets (Roche)
0.5 mg, orange, round, scored, p. 20g
1 mg, blue, round, scored, p. 9e
2 mg, white, round, scored, p. 32h
KLOTRIX Slow-Release Tablets (Mead Johnson Pharmaceuticals)
10 mEq, light orange, round, *770*, p. 21d
K-LYTE Effervescent Tablets (Bristol Laboratories)
25 mEq, orange, mottled, round, *orange flavored*, p. 21f
25 mEq, yellow, mottled, round, *lime flavored*, p. 17d
K-LYTE DS Effervescent Tablets (Bristol Laboratories)
50 mEq, yellow, mottled, round, *lime flavored*, p. 17c
50 mEq, orange, mottled, round, *orange flavored*, p. 21g
K-LYTE/CL Effervescent Tablets (Bristol Laboratories)
25 mEq, pale yellow, mottled, round, *citrus flavored*, p. 17d
25 mEq, pale red, mottled, round, *fruit-punch flavored*, p. 5e
50 mEq, pale yellow, mottled, round, *citrus flavored*, p. 17e
50 mEq, pale red, mottled, round, *fruit-punch flavored*, p. 5f
K•Tab Extended Release Tablets (Abbott)
10 mEq, yellow, capsule-shaped, *NM*, p. 18c
KU-ZYME Capsules (Kremers-Urban)
yellow and white, *522*, p. 19d
KU-ZYME HP Capsules (Kremers-Urban)
white, *525*, p. 40e
KUTRASE Capsules (Kremers-Urban)
green and white, *475*, p. 14e

L

LABID Tablets (Norwich Eaton)
250 mg, white, capsule-shaped, scored, *0149-0402*, p. 39a
LACTAID Tablets (Lactaid)
235 mg, white, oval, p. 37h
LACTINEX Tablets (Hynson Westcott & Dunning)
yellow, mottled, round, p. 26c
LACTRASE Capsules (Kremers-Urban)
125 mg, brown and white, *500*, p. 27g
LANOXICAPS Capsules (Burroughs Wellcome)
50 μg, red, *A2C*, p. 6b
100 μg, yellow, *B2C*, p. 18i
200 μg, green, *C2C*, p. 13h
LANOXIN Tablets (Burroughs Wellcome)
125 μg, yellow, round, scored, *Y3B*, p. 15g
250 μg, white, round, scored, *X3A*, p. 32c
500 μg, green, round, scored, *T9A*, p. 12d
LAROBEC Tablets (Roche)
orange, capsule-shaped, p. 22f
LARODOPA Capsules (Roche)
100 mg, scarlet and pink, p. 6f
250 mg, pink and beige, p. 3h
500 mg, pink, p. 4a
LARODOPA Tablets (Roche)
100 mg, pink, oval, scored, p. 2d
250 mg, pink, round, scored, p. 1i
500 mg, pink, capsule-shaped, scored, p. 3c
LASIX Tablets (Hoechst-Roussel)
20 mg, white, oval, p. 37a
40 mg, white, round, scored, p. 32f
80 mg, white, round, scored, p. 34b
LEUCOVORIN Calcium Tablets (Lederle)
5 mg, off-white, round, *C33*, p. 32f
LEUKERAN Tablets (Burroughs Wellcome)
2 mg, white, round, p. 31i
LEVLEN Tablets (Berlex)

DRUG IDENTIFICATION INDEX

peach, round, *21*, p. 24a
28-day *Slidecase*, p. 42c
LEVOTHROID Tablets (Rorer)
  25 μg, orange, round, *LK*, p. 20e
  50 μg, white, round, *LL*, p. 31f
  75 μg, gray, round, *LT*, p. 29a
  125 μg, purple, round, *LH*, p. 8a
  150 μg, blue, round, *LN*, p. 9a
  175 μg, turquoise, round, *LP*, p. 12b
  200 μg, pink, round, *LR*, p. 1a
  300 μg, green, round, *LS*, p. 12a
LEVSIN Tablets (Kremers-Urban)
  0.125 mg, white, round, scored, *531*, p. 32f
LEVSIN/PHENOBARBITAL Tablets (Kremers-Urban)
  pink, round, scored, *534*, p. 1f
LEVSINEX Timecaps (Kremers-Urban)
  0.375 mg, brown and clear with brown and white beads, *537*, p. 27f
LEVSINEX/PHENOBARBITAL Timecaps (Kremers-Urban)
  pink and clear with pink and white beads, *539*, p. 3h
LIBRAX Capsules (Roche)
  green, p. 14b
LIBRITABS Tablets (Roche)
  5 mg, turquoise green, round, scored, p. 12a
  10 mg, turquoise green, round, scored, p. 12c
  25 mg, turquoise green, round, scored, p. 12e
LIBRIUM Capsules (Roche)
  5 mg, green and yellow, p. 13i
  10 mg, black and green, p. 29g
  25 mg, green and white, p. 13i
LIMBITROL Tablets (Roche)
  blue, round, p. 9g
LIMBITROL DS Tablets (Roche)
  white, round, p. 34d
LINCOCIN Capsules (Upjohn)
  250 mg, powder blue, p. 11c
  500 mg, dark blue and powder blue, p. 11f
LIORESAL Tablets (Geigy)
  10 mg, white, oval, scored, *23*, p. 37c
  20 mg, white, capsule-shaped, scored, *33*, p. 38h
LITHOBID Slow-Release Tablets (CIBA)
  300 mg, peach, round, *65*, p. 24f
LIVITAMIN Capsules (Beecham Laboratories)
  red, *121*, p. 4a
LIVITAMIN Chewable Tablets (Beecham Laboratories)
  yellow, round, *123*, p. 26e
LIVITAMIN with Intrinsic Factor Capsules (Beecham Laboratories)
  green, *122*, p. 14g
LODOSYN Tablets (Merck Sharp & Dohme)
  orange, round, scored, *129*, p. 20h
LOESTRIN 21 1/20 (Parke-Davis)
  21-day *Petipac*, p. 42c
LOESTRIN Fe 1/20 (Parke-Davis)
  28-day *Petipac*, p. 42d
LOESTRIN 21 1.5/30 (Parke-Davis)
  21-day *Petipac*, p. 42d
LOESTRIN Fe 1.5/30 (Parke-Davis)
  28-day *Petipac*, p. 42d
LOMOTIL Tablets (Searle)
  white, round, *61*, p. 31c
LONITEN Tablets (Upjohn)
  2.5 mg, white, round, scored, *121*, p. 32b
  10 mg, white, round, scored, p. 32b

LO/OVRAL Tablets (Wyeth)
  white, round, *78*, p. 31b
  21-day compact, p. 43a
  28-day compact, p. 43a
LOPRESSOR Tablets (Geigy)
  50 mg, light red, capsule-shaped, scored, *51*, p. 3a
  100 mg, light blue, capsule-shaped, scored, *71*, p. 10c
LOPRESSOR-HCT 50/25 Tablets (Geigy)
  blue and white, layered, capsule-shaped, scored, *35*, p. 38g
LOPRESSOR-HCT 100/25 Tablets (Geigy)
  pink and white, layered, capsule-shaped, scored, *53*, p. 3a
LOPRESSOR-HCT 100/50 Tablets (Geigy)
  yellow and white, layered, capsule-shaped, scored, *73*, p. 18d
LOPURIN Tablets (Boots)
  100 mg, white, round, scored, *0051*, p. 33i
  300 mg, peach, round, scored, *0052*, p. 21d
LORELCO Tablets (Merrell Dow)
  250 mg, white, round, *51* or *250*, p. 35a
LOZOL Tablets (Rorer)
  2.5 mg, white, round, *82*, p. 31i
LUDIOMIL Tablets (CIBA)
  25 mg, dark orange, oval, scored, *110*, p. 21h
  50 mg, orange, round, scored, *26*, p. 20e
  75 mg, off-white, oval, scored, *135*, p. 37e
LUFYLLIN Tablets (Wallace)
  200 mg, white, rectangular, scored, *521*, p. 41b
LUFYLLIN-400 Tablets (Wallace)
  400 mg, white, capsule-shaped, scored, *731*, p. 38h
LUFYLLIN-GG Tablets (Wallace)
  light yellow, round, scored, *541*, p. 16h

M

MAALOX No. 1 Chewable Tablets (Rorer)
  white, round, p. 36e
MAALOX No. 2 Chewable Tablets (Rorer)
  white, round, p. 36h
MAALOX Plus Chewable Tablets (Rorer)
  yellow and white, layered, round, p. 17b
MAALOX TC Chewable Tablets (Rorer)
  white, round, p. 36h
MACRODANTIN Capsules (Norwich Eaton)
  25 mg, white, *0149-0007*, p. 40d
  50 mg, yellow and white, *0149-0008*, p. 19a
  100 mg, yellow, *0149-0009*, p. 19c
MAGAN Tablets (Adria)
  545 mg, pink, capsule-shaped, *412*, p. 3b
MALTSUPEX Tablets (Wallace)
  light orange, capsule-shaped, p. 22a
MANDELAMINE Tablets (Parke-Davis)
  0.5 g, brown, oval, *166*, p. 27d
  1 g, purple, oval, *167*, p. 8e
MAOLATE Tablets (Upjohn)

400 mg, light coffee-colored, round, scored, p. 27b
MARAX Tablets (Roerig)
  white, M-shaped, *254*, p. 41d
MAREZINE Tablets (Burroughs Wellcome)
  50 mg, white, round, scored, *T4A*, p. 32d
MARPLAN Tablets (Roche)
  10 mg, peach, round, scored, p. 20i
MATERNA 1•60 Tablets (Lederle)
  pink, capsule-shaped, scored, *M10*, p. 3c
MATULANE Capsules (Roche)
  50 mg, ivory, p. 19b
MAXOLON Tablets (Beecham Laboratories)
  10 mg, light blue, round, scored, *192*, p. 9c
MAXZIDE Tablets (Lederle)
  light yellow, bow tie-shaped, scored, *M8*, p. 19i
MAZANOR Tablets (Wyeth)
  1 mg, white, round, scored, *71*, p. 31d
MECLOMEN Capsules (Parke-Davis)
  50 mg, orange and light orange, *268*, p. 22h
  100 mg, orange and beige, *269*, p. 23a
MEDIATRIC Capsules (Ayerst)
  purple-brown, *252*, p. 8e
MEDIATRIC Tablets (Ayerst)
  red, capsule-shaped, *752*, p. 5h
MEDROL Tablets (Upjohn)
  2 mg, pink, oval, scored, *49*, p. 2c
  4 mg, white, oval, scored, *56*, p. 37a
  8 mg, peach, oval, scored, *22*, p. 25a
  16 mg, white, oval, scored, *73*, p. 37c
  24 mg, light yellow, oval, scored, *155*, p. 17f
  32 mg, peach, oval, scored, *176*, p. 25b
MELFIAT-105 Slow Release Unicelles (Reid-Rowell)
  105 mg, orange and clear, *1082*, p. 23b
MELLARIL Tablets (Sandoz Pharmaceuticals)
  10 mg, lime green, round, *78-2*, p. 12a
  15 mg, pink, round, *78-8*, p. 8a
  25 mg, light brown, round, p. 26a
  50 mg, white, round, p. 33f
  100 mg, light green, round, p. 12g
  150 mg, yellow, round, p. 16g
  200 mg, pink, round, p. 2b
MENEST Tablets (Beecham Laboratories)
  0.3 mg, yellow, oval, *125*, p. 18b
  0.625 mg, orange, oval, *126*, p. 22b
  1.25 mg, aqua, oval, *127*, p. 13d
  2.5 mg, pink, capsule-shaped, *128*, p. 3b
MENRIUM 5-2 Tablets (Roche)
  light green, round, p. 12c
MENRIUM 5-4 Tablets (Roche)
  dark green, round, p. 12b
MENRIUM 10-4 Tablets (Roche)
  purple, round, p. 8a
MEPERGAN Fortis Capsules (Wyeth)
  maroon, *261*, p. 6i
MEPHYTON Tablets (Merck Sharp & Dohme)
  5 mg, yellow, round, scored, *43*, p. 15g
MESANTOIN Tablets (Sandoz Pharmaceuticals)
  100 mg, pale pink, round, scored,

DRUG IDENTIFICATION INDEX

78-52, p. 1f
MESTINON Tablets (Roche)
60 mg, white, round, scored, p. 34i
180 mg, gold, mottled, capsule-shaped, scored, 34, p. 26g
METAHYDRIN Tablets (Merrell Dow)
2 mg, pink, round, 62, p. 1h
4 mg, aqua, round, 63, p. 9f
METANDREN Tablets (CIBA)
10 mg, white, round, scored, 30, p. 32h
METATENSIN No. 2 Tablets (Merrell Dow)
yellow, round, 64, p. 16d
METATENSIN No. 4 Tablets (Merrell Dow)
lavender, round, 65, p. 8c
METHERGINE Tablets (Sandoz Pharmaceuticals)
0.2 mg, rose, round, 78-54, p. 1b
METICORTEN Tablets (Schering)
1 mg, white, round, 843, p. 31e
METOPIRONE Tablets (CIBA)
250 mg, white, round, scored, 130, p. 36b
METRONID Tablets (Ascher)
250 mg, white, round, scored, 225/410, p. 33g
MEXITIL Capsules (Boehringer Ingelheim)
150 mg, red and light brown, 66, p. 6h
200 mg, red, 67, p. 7a
250 mg, red and green, 68, p. 7b
MI-CEBRIN Tablets (Dista)
yellow, round, C19, p. 16i
MI-CEBRIN T Tablets (Dista)
orange, oval, C20, p. 22a
MICRO-K 10 Extencaps (Robins)
600 mg, pale orange, 5720, p. 25e
750 mg, pale orange and white, 5730, p. 25e
MICRONASE Tablets (Upjohn)
1.25 mg, white, round, scored, p. 33b
2.5 mg, dark pink, round, scored, p. 1f
5 mg, blue, round, scored, p. 9d
MICRONOR Tablets (Ortho)
0.35 mg, green, round, p. 12b
Dialpak, p. 43a
MIDAMOR Tablets (Merck Sharp & Dohme)
5 mg, yellow, diamond-shaped, 92, p. 19g
MIDOL Caplets (Glenbrook)
white, capsule-shaped, p. 39c
MIDOL Maximum Strength Tablets (Glenbrook)
white, capsule-shaped, p. 39c
MIDRIN Capsules (Carnrick)
red with pink band, 86120, p. 7c
MILONTIN Kapseals (Parke-Davis)
orange with dark orange band, 393, p. 23e
MINIPRESS Capsules (Pfizer)
1 mg, white, 431, p. 40e
2 mg, pink and white, 437, p. 3h
5 mg, blue and white, 438, p. 11e
MINIZIDE 1 Capsules (Pfizer)
blue-green, 430, p. 14c
MINIZIDE 2 Capsules (Pfizer)
blue-green and pink, 432, p. 14c
MINIZIDE 5 Capsules (Pfizer)
blue-green and blue, 436, p. 14f
MINOCIN Capsules (Lederle)
50 mg, orange, M2, p. 22i
100 mg, purple and orange, M4, p. 8f
MINOCIN Tablets (Lederle)
50 mg, orange, round, M3, p. 20d
100 mg, orange, round, scored, M5, p. 20g
MINTEZOL Chewable Tablets (Merck Sharp & Dohme)
500 mg, white, round, scored, 907, p. 36i
MIRADON Tablets (Schering)
50 mg, pink, oval, scored, 795, p. 2d
MITROLAN Chewable Tablets (Robins)
yellow, round, 1535, p. 17c
MOBAN Tablets (Du Pont)
5 mg, orange, round, p. 20f
10 mg, lavender, round, p. 8b
25 mg, light green, round, scored, p. 12e
50 mg, blue, round, scored, p. 9e
100 mg, tan, round, scored, p. 26c
MOBIGESIC Tablets (Ascher)
white, round, scored, 225/356, p. 35h
MODANE Soft Capsules (Adria)
100 mg, green, 13 511, p. 13h
MODANE Tablets (Adria)
75 mg, yellow, round, 13 501, p. 16g
MODANE Mild Tablets (Adria)
37.5 mg, pink, round, 13 502, p. 1c
MODANE Plus Tablets (Adria)
brown, round, 13 504, p. 27b
MODERIL Tablets (Pfizer)
0.25 mg, yellow, oval, scored, 441, p. 17e
0.5 mg, peach, oval, scored, 442, p. 25a
MODICON Tablets (Ortho)
white, round, 535 (0.5 mg norethindrone and 35 µg ethinyl estradiol), p. 31g
21-day Dialpak, p. 43b
28-day Dialpak, p. 43b
MODURETIC Tablets (Merck Sharp & Dohme)
peach, diamond-shaped, 917, p. 25f
MOL-IRON Tablets (Schering)
dark maroon, oval, p. 5g
MOL-IRON with Vitamin C Tablets (Schering)
dark maroon, round, p. 5c
MONISTAT 3 Vaginal Suppositories (Ortho)
200 mg, white, bullet-shaped, p. 41e
MONISTAT 7 Vaginal Suppositories (Ortho)
100 mg, white, bullet-shaped, p. 41e
MORIDIN Tablets (Ascher)
yellow, capsule-shaped, scored, 0310, p. 18f
Morphine Sulfate Tablets (Purdue Frederick)
15 mg, white, round, scored, MI15, p. 32a
30 mg, white, oblong, scored, MI30, p. 38e
MS CONTIN Controlled Release Tablets (Purdue Frederick)
30 mg, lavender, round, M30, p. 8b
MUDRANE Tablets (Poythress)
pale yellow, round, scored, 9550, p. 16f
MUDRANE-2 Tablets (Poythress)
white, mottled, round, scored, 9532, p. 34e
MUDRANE GG Tablets (Poythress)
yellow, mottled, round, scored, 9551, p. 16f
MUDRANE GG-2 Tablets (Poythress)
green, mottled, round, 9533, p. 12h
MULVIDREN-F Tablets (Stuart)
orange, mottled, round, scored, 710, p. 21b
MYADEC Tablets (Warner-Lambert)
red-brown, oval, p. 27e
MYAMBUTOL Tablets (Lederle)
100 mg, white, round, M6, p. 33a
400 mg, white, round, scored, M7, p. 36d
MYCIFRADIN Tablets (Upjohn)
0.5 g, off-white, round, 521, p. 35b
MYCOSTATIN Oral Tablets (Squibb)
500,000 U, light brown, round, 580, p. 27b
MYCOSTATIN Vaginal Tablets (Squibb)
100,000 U, pale yellow, diamond-shaped, 457, p. 18a
MYLANTA Chewable Tablets (Stuart)
yellow and white, layered, round, 620, p. 17c
MYLANTA-II Chewable Tablets (Stuart)
green and white, layered, round, 651, p. 13b
MYLERAN Tablets (Burroughs Wellcome)
2 mg, white, round, scored, K2A, p. 31g
MYLICON Chewable Tablets (Stuart)
40 mg, white, round, scored, 450, p. 34b
MYLICON-80 Chewable Tablets (Stuart)
80 mg, pink, round, scored, 858, p. 2b
MYSOLINE Tablets (Ayerst)
50 mg, white, round, scored, p. 32b
250 mg, white, round, scored, p. 34g
MYSTECLIN-F Capsules (Squibb)
brown and yellow, 779, p. 28a

N

NALDECON Tablets (Bristol Laboratories)
white with pink flecks, round, scored, N1, p. 1h
NALDEGESIC Tablets (Bristol Laboratories)
light blue, capsule-shaped, scored, N2, p. 10d
NALFON Pulvules (Dista)
300 mg, ocher and yellow, H77, p. 28a
NALFON Tablets (Dista)
600 mg, yellow, capsule-shaped, scored, p. 18a
NALFON 200 Pulvules (Dista)
200 mg, ocher and white, H76, p. 26g
NAPROSYN Tablets (Syntex)
250 mg, yellow, round, scored, 272, p. 16h
375 mg, peach, capsule-shaped, 273, p. 25d
500 mg, yellow, capsule-shaped, 277, p. 18f
NAQUA Tablets (Schering)
2 mg, pink, clover-shaped, scored, 822, p. 4b
4 mg, aqua, clover-shaped, scored, 547, p. 15a
NAQUIVAL Tablets (Schering)
yellow, round, scored, 394, p. 15i
NARDIL Tablets (Parke-Davis)
15 mg, orange, round, 270, p. 21a
NATAFORT Filmseal Tablets (Parke-Davis)
yellow, capsule-shaped, 212, p. 18g
NATALINS Tablets (Mead Johnson Laboratories)

DRUG IDENTIFICATION INDEX

yellow, oval, p. 17i
NATALINS Rx Tablets (Mead Johnson Laboratories)
  white, oval, *702*, p. 38b
NATURETIN Tablets (Princeton)
  2.5 mg, green, round, *605*, p. 12a
  5 mg, green, mottled, round, scored, *606*, p. 12e
  10 mg, orange, round, scored, *618*, p. 21b
NAVANE Capsules (Roerig)
  1 mg, orange and yellow, *571*, p. 22g
  2 mg, turquoise and yellow, *572*, p. 13i
  5 mg, orange and white, *573*, p. 22h
  10 mg, turquoise and white, *574*, p. 13i
  20 mg, blue and green, *577*, p. 11c
NegGram Caplets (Winthrop Pharmaceuticals)
  250 mg, ivory, capsule-shaped, scored, *N21*, p. 18b
  500 mg, ivory, capsule-shaped, scored, *N22*, p. 18d
  1 g, ivory, oval, scored, *N23*, p. 17i
NEMBUTAL Sodium Capsules (Abbott)
  yellow, *CH*, p. 19a
NEPTAZANE Tablets (Lederle)
  50 mg, white, round, scored, *N1*, p. 32d
NERVINE Tablets (Miles Laboratories)
  25 mg, white, capsule-shaped, p. 39b
Niacin Tablets (Rorer)
  500 mg, yellow, capsule-shaped, scored, *NE*, p. 18e
NICO-400 Capsules (Marion)
  400 mg, maroon and bright pink, *1575*, p. 7b
NICOBID Tempules (Rorer)
  125 mg, black and clear with yellow, green, and white beads, *2835*, p. 29g
  250 mg, green and clear with yellow, green, and white beads, *2840*, p. 14h
  500 mg, blue and white, *2841*, p. 11g
NICORETTE Chewing Gum (Merrell Dow)
  2 mg, beige, square, p. 26h
NILORIC Tablets (Ascher)
  1 mg, white, oval, *415*, p. 37d
NILSTAT Oral Tablets (Lederle)
  500,000 U, pink, round, *N5*, p. 1i
NILSTAT Vaginal Tablets (Lederle)
  100,000 U, pale yellow, oblong, *N6*, p. 18b
NITRO-BID Capsules (Marion)
  2.5 mg, light purple and clear with white beads, *1550*, p. 8e
  6.5 mg, dark blue and yellow with white beads, *1551*, p. 29h
  9 mg, green and yellow with white beads, *1553*, p. 14h
NITRODISC Transcutaneous Discs (Searle)
  5 mg/24 h (8 cm^2), *2058*, p. 47b
  7.5 mg/24 h (12 cm^2), *2078*, p. 47c
  10 mg/24 h (16 cm^2), *2068*, p. 47c
NITRO-DUR Transdermal Infusion Systems (Key)
  2.5 mg/24 h (5 cm^2), p. 47c
  5 mg/24 h (10 cm^2), p. 47d
  7.5 mg/24 h (15 cm^2), p. 47d
  10 mg/24 h (20 cm^2), p. 47d
NITRO-DUR II Transdermal Infusion Systems (Key)
  2.5 mg/24 h (5 cm^2), p. 48a
  5 mg/24 h (10 cm^2), p. 48a
  7.5 mg/24 h (15 cm^2), p. 48a
  10 mg/24 h (20 cm^2), p. 48a
  15 mg/24 h (30 cm^2), p. 48b
NITROGARD Transmucosal Controlled Release Tablets (Parke-Davis)
  1 mg, off-white, round, p. 31a
  2 mg, white, round, p. 31a
  3 mg, white, round, p. 31b
NOCTEC Capsules (Squibb)
  250 mg, orange, clear, *623*, p. 22i
  500 mg, orange, clear, *626*, p. 23f
NOLAHIST Tablets (Carnrick)
  25 mg, white, capsule-shaped, scored, *8652*, p. 38e
NOLAMINE Tablets (Carnrick)
  pink, round, *86204*, p. 1f
NOLUDAR Tablets (Roche)
  50 mg, white, round, scored, *16*, p. 31d
  200 mg, white, round, scored, *17*, p. 35g
NOLUDAR 300 Capsules (Roche)
  300 mg, amethyst and white, p. 3h
NOLVADEX Tablets (Stuart)
  10 mg, white, round, cameo-debossed, *600*, p. 33a
NORDETTE Tablets (Wyeth)
  light orange, round, *75*, p. 20d
  21-day compact, p. 43b
  28-day compact, p. 43c
NORFLEX Tablets (Riker)
  100 mg, white, round, *221*, p. 33g
NORGESIC Tablets (Riker)
  light green, white, and yellow, layered, round, p. 13a
NORGESIC Forte Tablets (Riker)
  light green, white, and yellow, layered, capsule-shaped, scored, p. 13f
NORINYL Tablets (Syntex)
  2 mg, white, round, p. 31h
  Memorette, p. 44a
NORINYL 1+35 Tablets (Syntex)
  green, round, *111*, p. 12b
  21-day *Wallette*, p. 43c
  28-day *Wallette*, p. 43c
NORINYL 1+50 Tablets (Syntex)
  white, round, *1*, p. 31a
  21-day *Wallette*, p. 43d
  28-day *Wallette*, p. 43d
NORINYL 1+80 Tablets (Syntex)
  yellow, round, *3*, p. 15e
  21-day *Wallette*, p. 43d
  28-day *Wallette*, p. 44a
NORLESTRIN 1/50 Tablets (Parke-Davis)
  yellow, round, *904*, p. 15f
  21 *Petipac*, p. 44a
  28 *Petipac*, p. 44b
  Fe *Petipac*, p. 44b
NORLESTRIN 2.5/50 (Parke-Davis)
  21 *Petipac*, p. 44b
  Fe *Petipac*, p. 44c
NORLUTATE Tablets (Parke-Davis)
  5 mg, pink, round, scored, *918*, p. 1b
NORLUTIN Tablets (Parke-Davis)
  5 mg, white, round, scored, *882*, p. 31c
NORMODYNE Tablets (Schering)
  100 mg, light brown, round, scored, *244*, p. 26b
  200 mg, white, round, scored, *752*, p. 34h
  300 mg, blue, round, *438*, p. 9h
NOROXIN Tablets (Merck Sharp & Dohme)
  400 mg, dark pink, oval, *705*, p. 2f
NORPACE Capsules (Searle)
  100 mg, orange and white, *2752*, p. 23c
  150 mg, brown, and orange, *2762*, p. 27i
NORPACE CR Capsules (Searle)
  100 mg, light green and white, *2732*, p. 14c
  150 mg, brown and light green, *2742*, p. 27g
NOR Q.D. Tablets (Syntex)
  0.35 mg, yellow, round, *2107*, p. 15g
  compact, p. 44c
NORPRAMIN Tablets (Merrell Dow)
  10 mg, blue, round, *68-7*, p. 9a
  25 mg, yellow, round, *11* or *25*, p. 16a
  50 mg, green, round, *15* or *50*, p. 12d
  75 mg, orange, round, *19* or *75*, p. 20i
  100 mg, peach, round, *20* or *100*, p. 24f
  150 mg, white, round, *21* or *150*, p. 35a
NORWICH Aspirin Tablets (Richardson-Vicks Health Care)
  325 mg, white, round, p. 34e
NORWICH Extra Strength Aspirin Tablets (Richardson-Vicks Health Care)
  500 mg, white, round, p. 34f
NOVAFED Controlled-Release Capsules (Merrell Dow)
  120 mg, brown and orange, *104*, p. 27g
NOVAFED-A Controlled-Release Capsules (Merrell Dow)
  red and orange, *106*, p. 7b
NTS 5 Transdermal Delivery Systems (Bolar)
  5 mg/24 h (10 cm^2), p. 48b
NTS 15 Transdermal Delivery Systems (Bolar)
  15 mg/24 h (30 cm^2), p. 48b
NYTILAX Tablets (Mentholatum)
  12 mg, light blue, round, p. 9a
NYTOL Tablets (Block)
  25 mg, white, round, p. 34d

O

OCTAMIDE Tablets (Adria)
  10 mg, yellow, octagonal, scored, *230*, p. 19h
OGEN 1.25 Tablets (Abbott)
  1.5 mg, peach, oval, scored, *LV*, p. 25b
OGEN 2.5 Tablets (Abbott)
  3 mg, blue, oval, scored, *LX*, p. 9i
OGEN 5 Tablets (Abbott)
  5 mg, light green, oval, scored, *LY*, p. 13c
OMNIPEN Capsules (Wyeth)
  250 mg, purple and pink, *53*, p. 8f
  500 mg, purple and pink, *309*, p. 8g
ONE-A-DAY Essential Tablets (Miles Laboratories)
  dark red, round, p. 5b
ONE-A-DAY Maximum Formula Tablets (Miles Laboratories)
  dark red, oval, p. 6a
ONE-A-DAY Plus Extra C Tablets (Miles Laboratories)
  orange, capsule-shaped, p. 22c
OPTILETS-500 Tablets (Abbott)
  yellow, oval, p. 17h
OPTILETS-M-500 Tablets (Abbott)
  brown, capsule-shaped, p. 27d
OPTIMINE Tablets (Schering)
  1 mg, white, round, scored, *282*, p.

DRUG IDENTIFICATION INDEX

33d
ORAP Tablets (McNeil Pharmaceutical)
2 mg, white, oval, scored, p. 37b
ORETIC Tablets (Abbott)
25 mg, white, round, p. 31b
50 mg, white, round, scored, p. 32g
ORETON Methyl Buccal Tablets (Schering)
10 mg, lavender, oval, *970*, p. 2d
ORETON Methyl Tablets (Schering)
10 mg, white, round, *311*, p. 34f
25 mg, peach, round, *499*, p. 24g
OREXIN Tablets (Stuart)
pale pink, mottled, round, p. 1e
ORGANIDIN Tablets (Wallace)
rose, mottled, round, scored, *4224*, p. 24f
ORNADE Spansules (Smith Kline & French)
orange and clear with multi-colored beads, p. 23d
ORNEX Capsules (SmithKline Consumer Products)
royal blue and white, p. 11d
ORTHO-NOVUM 1/35 Tablets (Ortho)
peach, round, *135*, p. 24b
21-day *Dialpak*, p. 44c
28-day *Dialpak*, p. 44d
ORTHO-NOVUM 1/50 Tablets (Ortho)
yellow, round, *150*, p. 15h
21-day *Dialpak*, p. 44d
28-day *Dialpak*, p. 44d
ORTHO-NOVUM 1/80 Tablets (Ortho)
white, round, *1*, p. 31e
21-day *Dialpak*, p. 45a
28-day *Dialpak*, p. 45a
ORTHO-NOVUM 2 mg Tablets (Ortho)
white, round (2 mg norethindrone and 100 µg mestranol), p. 31f
21-day *Dialpak*, p. 45a
ORTHO-NOVUM 7/7/7 Tablets (Ortho)
light peach, round, *75* (0.75 mg norethindrone and 35 µg ethinyl estradiol), p. 24a
peach, round, *135* (1 mg norethindrone and 35 µg ethinyl estradiol), p. 24b
white, round, *535* (0.5 mg norethindrone and 35 µg ethinyl estradiol), p. 31e
21-day *Dialpak*, p. 45b
28-day *Dialpak*, p. 45b
ORTHO-NOVUM 10/11 Tablets (Ortho)
white, round, *535* (0.5 mg norethindrone and 35 µg ethinyl estradiol), p. 31d
peach, round, *135* (1 mg norethindrone and 35 µg ethinyl estradiol), p. 24b
21-day *Dialpak*, p. 45b
28-day *Dialpak*, p. 45c
ORUDIS Capsules (Wyeth)
50 mg, dark green and light green, *4181*, p. 14d
75 mg, dark green and white, *4187*, p. 14d
OS-CAL 250 Tablets (Marion)
light green, round, *1650*, p. 12i
OS-CAL 500 Chewable Tablets (Marion)
500 mg, white, round, p. 36h
OS-CAL 500 Tablets (Marion)
500 mg, light green, capsule-shaped, p. 13e
OS-CAL Forte Tablets (Marion)
green, capsule-shaped, p. 13h
OS-CAL Plus Tablets (Marion)

lavender, oval, p. 8d
OVCON-35 Tablets (Mead Johnson Laboratories)
peach, round, *583*, p. 24a
compact, p. 45c
OVCON-50 Tablets (Mead Johnson Laboratories)
yellow, round, *584*, p. 15f
compact, p. 45c
OVRAL Tablets (Wyeth)
white, round, *56*, p. 31g
21-day compact, p. 45d
28-day compact, p. 45d
OVRETTE Tablets (Wyeth)
0.075 mg, yellow, round, *62*, p. 15e
compact, p. 45d
OVULEN Tablets (Searle)
white, pentagonal, *401*, p. 40h
21-day *Compack*, p. 46a
28-day *Compack*, p. 46a

P

PABALATE Tablets (Robins)
yellow, round, *5816*, p. 17b
PABALATE SF Tablets (Robins)
Persian rose, round, *5883*, p. 2c
P-A-C Tablets (Upjohn)
light green, mottled, round, p. 12i
PAMELOR Capsules (Sandoz Pharmaceuticals)
10 mg, orange and off-white, *78-86*, p. 22h
25 mg, orange and off-white, *78-87*, p. 23b
50 mg, off-white, *78-78*, p. 40f
75 mg, orange, *78-79*, p. 23c
PAMINE Tablets (Upjohn)
2.5 mg, white, round, p. 31h
PANADOL Children's Tablets (Glenbrook)
80 mg, pink, round, scored, p. 1i
PANADOL Jr. Caplets (Glenbrook)
160 mg, white, oval, scored, p. 37f
PANADOL Tablets (Glenbrook)
500 mg, white, round, p. 36b
PANCREASE Capsules (McNeil Pharmaceutical)
clear and white with red bands and white beads, p. 40g
PANMYCIN Capsules (Upjohn)
250 mg, dark gray and yellow, p. 29d
PANMYCIN Tablets (Upjohn)
500 mg, mustard, round, p. 16i
PANWARFIN Tablets (Abbott)
2 mg, lavender, round, scored, *LM*, p. 8b
2½ mg, orange, round, scored, *LN*, p. 20h
5 mg, peach, round, scored, *LO*, p. 24d
7½ mg, yellow, round, scored, *LR*, p. 16b
10 mg, white, round, scored, *LF*, p. 32g
PARADIONE Capsules (Abbott)
150 mg, orange, clear, round, p. 22g
300 mg, green, clear, round, p. 13h
PARAFLEX Tablets (McNeil Pharmaceutical)
250 mg, light orange, round, bevelled, scored, p. 24g
PARAFON Forte (McNeil Pharmaceutical)
green, bevelled, round, p. 12h
PARLODEL Capsules (Sandoz Pharmaceuticals)

5 mg, caramel and white, p. 27f
PARLODEL Tablets (Sandoz Pharmaceuticals)
2½ mg, white, round, scored, p. 31h
PARNATE Tablets (Smith Kline & French)
10 mg, rose-red, round, p. 1g
PARSIDOL Tablets (Parke-Davis)
10 mg, white, round, *320*, p. 31c
50 mg, white, round, scored, *321*, p. 33b
PATHOCIL Capsules (Wyeth)
250 mg, purple and white, *360*, p. 8f
500 mg, purple and white, *593*, p. 8g
PAVABID Capsules (Marion)
150 mg, brown and clear with white beads, *1555*, p. 27h
PAVABID HP Capsulet Tablets (Marion)
300 mg, pale orange, capsule-shaped, p. 23i
PAXIPAM Tablets (Schering)
20 mg, orange, round, scored, *251*, p. 20i
40 mg, white, round, scored, *538*, p. 33a
PBZ Tablets (Geigy)
25 mg, white, round, scored, *111*, p. 31i
50 mg, white, round, scored, *117*, p. 32h
PBZ-SR Tablets (Geigy)
100 mg, lavender, round, *48*, p. 8b
PEGANONE Tablets (Abbott)
250 mg, white, round, scored, *AD*, p. 34g
500 mg, white, round, scored, *AE*, p. 36c
PEN•VEE K Tablets (Wyeth)
250 mg, white, round, scored, *59*, p. 34a
500 mg, white, round, scored, *390*, p. 35h
PENTIDS Tablets (Squibb)
125 mg, white, oval, scored, *164*, p. 37g
PENTIDS '400' Tablets (Squibb)
250 mg, white, oval, scored, *165*, p. 39b
PENTIDS '800' Tablets (Squibb)
500 mg, yellow, oval, scored, *168*, p. 17h
PEPCID Tablets (Merck Sharp & Dohme)
light tan, D-shaped, *964*, p. 26h
PERCODAN Tablets (Du Pont)
yellow, round, scored, p. 16g
PERCODAN-Demi Tablets (Du Pont)
pink, round, scored, *136*, p. 8c
PERCOGESIC Tablets (Richardson-Vicks Health Care)
light orange, mottled, round, scored, p. 21e
PERIACTIN Tablets (Merck Sharp & Dohme)
4 mg, white, round, scored, *62*, p. 31i
PERI-COLACE Capsules (Mead Johnson Pharmaceuticals)
dark red, oval, p. 6c
PERIHEMIN Capsules (Lederle)
red-brown, oval, *P7*, p. 27f
PERITINIC Tablets (Lederle)
maroon, capsule-shaped, *P8*, p. 5i
PERMITIL Tablets (Schering)
2.5 mg, light orange, oval, scored, *WDR*, p. 21g
5 mg, light pink, oval, scored, *WFF*, p. 2d

COMPENDIUM OF DRUG THERAPY

DRUG IDENTIFICATION INDEX

10 mg, pink, oval, scored, *WFG*, p. 2d
PERSANTINE Tablets (Boehringer Ingelheim)
  25 mg, orange, round, *17*, p. 20d
  50 mg, orange, round, *18*, p. 20f
  75 mg, orange, round, *19*, p. 20i
PHAZYME Tablets (Reed & Carnrick)
  60 mg, pink, round, p. 2b
PHAZYME-95 Tablets (Reed & Carnrick)
  95 mg, red, oval, p. 5i
PHAZYME-125 Capsules (Reed & Carnrick)
  125 mg, red, oval, p. 6d
PHENAPHEN 650 with Codeine Tablets (Robins)
  white, capsule-shaped, scored, *6251*, p. 39e
PHENAPHEN with Codeine No. 2 Capsules (Robins)
  black and yellow, *6242*, p. 29h
PHENAPHEN with Codeine No. 3 Capsules (Robins)
  black and green, *6257*, p. 29h
PHENAPHEN with Codeine No. 4 Capsules (Robins)
  green and white, *6274*, p. 14h
PHENERGAN Tablets (Wyeth)
  12.5 mg, orange, round, scored, *19*, p. 20h
  25 mg, white, round, quarter-scored, *27*, p. 32i
  50 mg, pink, round, *227*, p. 1h
PHENERGAN-D Tablets (Wyeth)
  white and orange, layered, round, scored, *434*, p. 20g
PHILLIPS' Milk of Magnesia Tablets (Glenbrook)
  311 mg, white, round, p. 35f
PHRENILIN Tablets (Carnrick)
  pale violet, round, scored, *8650*, p. 8d
PHRENILIN Forte Capsules (Carnrick)
  amethyst, *8656*, p. 8i
PHRENILIN with Codeine No. 3 Capsules (Carnrick)
  amethyst and white, *8655*, p. 8g
PHYLLOCONTIN Controlled Release Tablets (Purdue Frederick)
  225 mg, off-white, round, scored, p. 34e
PLACIDYL Capsules (Abbott)
  500 mg, red, *KH*, p. 6e
PLEGINE Tablets (Ayerst)
  35 mg, yellow, round, scored, p. 15i
PMB 200 Tablets (Ayerst)
  green, capsule-shaped, *880*, p. 13e
PMB 400 Tablets (Ayerst)
  pink, capsule-shaped, *881*, p. 3c
POLARAMINE Repetabs (Schering)
  2 mg, hot pink, oval, *820*, p. 2c
  4 mg, light red, oval, *095*, p. 5g
  6 mg, bright red, oval, *148*, P. 5g
POLY-VI-FLOR Chewable Tablets (Mead Johnson Nutritional)
  0.5 mg, various colors, mottled, oblong, *468*, p. 30b
  1 mg, various colors, mottled, diamond-shaped, *474*, p. 30b
POLY-VI-FLOR with Iron Chewable Tablets (Mead Johnson Nutritional)
  0.5 mg, brownish-pink, mottled, oblong, *482*, p. 4c
  1 mg, brownish-pink, mottled, diamond-shaped, *476*, p. 4c
POLY-VI-SOL Chewable Tablets (Mead Johnson Nutritional)
  various colors, mottled, diamond-shaped, p. 30b
  various colors, various circus shapes, p. 30d
POLY-VI-SOL with Iron and Zinc Chewable Tablets (Mead Johnson Nutritional)
  brownish-pink, mottled, diamond-shaped, p. 4c
  brownish-pink, various circus shapes, p. 4c
POLYCILLIN Capsules (Apothecon)
  250 mg, red and gray, *7992*, p. 6h
  500 mg, red and gray, *7993*, p. 7c
POLYMOX Capsules (Apothecon)
  250 mg, maroon and flesh pink, *7278*, p. 6h
  500 mg, maroon and flesh pink, *7279*, p. 7b
PONDIMIN Tablets (Robins)
  20 mg, orange, round, scored, *6447*, p. 20f
PONSTEL Kapseals (Parke-Davis)
  250 mg, yellow with blue band, *540*, p. 19c
POSTURE Tablets (Ayerst)
  600 mg, white, capsule-shaped, scored, p. 40b
POSTURE-D Tablets (Ayerst)
  600 mg, white, capsule-shaped, scored, p. 40c
PRAMET FA Tablets (Ross)
  aqua, capsule-shaped, *147*, p. 10b
PRAMILET FA Tablets (Ross)
  lavender, oval, *121*, p. 8e
PRELU-2 Capsules (Boehringer Ingelheim)
  105 mg, celery and green, *64*, p. 14e
PREMARIN Tablets (Ayerst)
  0.3 mg, green, oval, p. 13b
  0.625 mg, maroon, oval, p. 5g
  0.9 mg, white, oval, p. 37f
  1.25 mg, yellow, oval, p. 17g
  2.5 mg, purple, oval, p. 8d
PREMARIN with Methyltestosterone Tablets (Ayerst)
  0.625 mg conjugated estrogens and 5 mg methyltestosterone, maroon, round, *878*, p. 5a
  1.25 mg conjugated estrogens and 10 mg methyltestosterone, yellow, round, *879*, p. 16e
PRIMATENE M-Formula Tablets (Whitehall)
  yellow, round, scored, p. 16c
PRIMATENE P-Formula Tablets (Whitehall)
  yellow, round, scored, p. 16b
PRINCIPEN Capsules (Squibb)
  250 mg, light gray, *971*, p. 29d
  500 mg, dark gray and light gray, *974*, p. 29e
PRO-BANTHINE Tablets (Searle)
  7½ mg, white, round, *611*, p. 31c
  15 mg, peach, round, *601*, p. 24a
PROBEC-T Tablets (Stuart)
  salmon, capsule-shaped, p. 22g
PROCAN SR Tablets (Parke-Davis)
  250 mg, green, elliptical, *202*, p. 13c
  500 mg, yellow, elliptical, scored, *204*, p. 18a
  750 mg, orange, elliptical, scored, *205*, p. 22a
  1,000 mg, red, oblong, scored, *207*, p. 6b
PROCARDIA Capsules (Pfizer)
  10 mg, orange, *260*, p. 23a
  20 mg, two-tone orange, oval, *261*, p. 23b
PROLIXIN Tablets (Princeton)
  1 mg, bright pink, round, *863*, p. 1b
  2.5 mg, bright yellow, round, *864*, p. 16c
  5 mg, green, round, *877*, p. 12e
  10 mg, salmon pink, round, *956*, p. 1g
PROLOPRIM Tablets (Burroughs Wellcome)
  100 mg, white, round, scored, *09A*, p. 33c
  200 mg, yellow, round, scored, p. 16c
PRONEMIA Capsules (Lederle)
  red-brown, *P9*, p. 27i
PRONESTYL Capsules (Princeton)
  250 mg, bright yellow, *758*, p. 19b
  375 mg, orange and white, *756*, p. 23c
  500 mg, orange and yellow, *757*, p. 23e
PRONESTYL Tablets (Princeton)
  250 mg, bright yellow, capsule-shaped, *431*, p. 18c
  375 mg, bright orange, capsule-shaped, *434*, p. 22c
  500 mg, dark orange, capsule-shaped, *438*, p. 22c
PRONESTYL-SR Tablets (Princeton)
  500 mg, lemon yellow, oval, *775*, p. 18a
PROPAGEST Tablets (Carnrick)
  25 mg, white, oval, scored, p. 37d
PROSTAPHLIN Capsules (Apothecon)
  250 mg, flesh pink, *7977*, p. 3i
  500 mg, flesh pink, *7982*, p. 4a
PROSTIGMIN Tablets (Roche)
  15 mg, white, round, scored, p. 33g
PROTOSTAT Tablets (Ortho)
  250 mg, white, capsule-shaped, scored, *1570*, p. 38f
  500 mg, white, capsule-shaped, scored, *1571*, p. 39g
PROVENTIL Tablets (Schering)
  2 mg, white, round, scored, *252*, p. 31f
  4 mg, white, round, scored, *573*, p. 33d
PROVERA Tablets (Upjohn)
  2.5 mg, peach, round, scored, p. 24b
  5 mg, white, hexagonal, scored, p. 40i
  10 mg, white, round, scored, p. 32b
PURINETHOL Tablets (Burroughs Wellcome)
  50 mg, cream, round, scored, *04A*, p. 16e
P-V-TUSSIN Tablets (Reid Rowell)
  light orange with dark orange specks, capsule-shaped, p. 22b
PYRIDIUM Tablets (Parke-Davis)
  100 mg, dark maroon, round, *180*, p. 5b
  200 mg, dark maroon, round, *181*, p. 5c

Q

QUADRINAL Tablets (Knoll)
  white, round, scored, *14*, p. 35b
QUARZAN Capsules (Roche)
  2.5 mg, green and red, p. 13i
  5 mg, green and gray, p. 13i
QUIBRON Capsules (Bristol Laboratories)
  yellow, *516*, p. 19d
QUIBRON-300 Capsules (Bristol Laboratories)

DRUG IDENTIFICATION INDEX

yellow and white, *515*, p. 19f
QUIBRON PLUS Capsules (Bristol Laboratories)
  green, *518*, p. 14f
QUIBRON-T Dividose Tablets (Bristol Laboratories)
  300 mg, ivory, oblong, triple-scored, *512*, p. 19i
QUIBRON-T/SR Sustained-Release Dividose Tablets (Bristol Laboratories)
  300 mg, white, oblong, triple-scored, *519*, p. 39a
QUINAGLUTE Sustained-Release Tablets (Berlex)
  324 mg, white, mottled, round, p. 36d
QUINAMM Tablets (Merrell Dow)
  260 mg, round, white, *547*, p. 36d
QUINIDEX Extentabs (Robins)
  300 mg, white, round, p. 36e

R

RAUDIXIN Tablets (Princeton)
  50 mg, red, round, *713*, p. 5b
  100 mg, red, round, *776*, p. 5c
RAUWILOID Tablets (Riker)
  2 mg, beige, round, p. 26a
RAUZIDE Tablets (Princeton)
  dark green, round, *769*, p. 12f
REDISOL Tablets (Merck Sharp & Dohme)
  50 µg, pink, mottled, round, p. 1a
REGITINE Tablets (CIBA)
  50 mg, off-white, round, scored, *152*, p. 33g
REGLAN Tablets (Robins)
  10 mg, pink, capsule-shaped, scored, p. 25c
REGROTON Tablets (Rorer)
  pink, uniquely-shaped, *R31*, p. 4b
REGUTOL Tablets (Plough)
  100 mg, yellow, round, p. 16e
RELA Tablets (Schering)
  350 mg, salmon pink, round, *160*, p. 2b
REMSED Tablets (Du Pont)
  50 mg, light blue, round, scored, *051*, p. 9f
RENESE Tablets (Pfizer)
  1 mg, white, round, scored, *375*, p. 32a
  2 mg, yellow, round, scored, *376*, p. 16d
  4 mg, white, round, scored, *377*, p. 33c
RENESE-R Tablets (Pfizer)
  blue, round, scored, *446*, p. 9c
RENOQUID Tablets (Glenwood)
  white, round, scored, *81*, p. 34a
RESPBID Tablets (Boehringer Ingelheim)
  250 mg, white, round, scored, *48*, p. 35b
  500 mg, white, capsule-shaped, scored, *49*, p. 39i
RESTORIL Capsules (Sandoz Pharmaceuticals)
  15 mg, maroon and pink, p. 6f
  30 mg, maroon and blue, p. 6g
RHEABAN Tablets (Leeming)
  750 mg, white, oblong, p. 39h
RIDAURA Capsules (Smith Kline & French)
  3 mg, tan and brown, p. 27f
RIFADIN Capsules (Merrell Dow)
  150 mg, maroon and red, *510* or *150*, p. 6e
  300 mg, maroon and red, *508* or *300*, p. 7a
RIFAMATE Capsules (Merrell Dow)
  red, *509*, p. 7c
RIOPAN Chewable Tablets (Ayerst)
  480 mg, white, round, p. 36f
RIOPAN Tablets (Ayerst)
  480 mg, white, oval, p. 37h
RIOPAN PLUS Chewable Tablets (Ayerst)
  white, round, p. 36g
RITALIN Tablets (CIBA)
  5 mg, yellow, round, *7*, p. 15g
  10 mg, pale green, round, scored, *3*, p. 9b
  20 mg, pale yellow, round, scored, *34*, p. 16a
ROBAXIN Tablets (Robins)
  500 mg, light orange, round, scored, p. 24i
ROBAXIN 750 Tablets (Robins)
  750 mg, orange, capsule-shaped, p. 22d
ROBAXISAL Tablets (Robins)
  white and pink, layered, round, scored, p. 36d
ROBICILLIN VK Tablets (Robins)
  250 mg, white, round, scored, *8217*, p. 34a
  500 mg, white, round, scored, *8227*, p. 35d
ROBIMYCIN Tablets (Robins)
  250 mg, light green, round, *8317*, p. 13a
ROBINUL Tablets (Robins)
  1 mg, pink, round, scored, *7824*, p. 1e
ROBINUL Forte Tablets (Robins)
  2 mg, pink, round, scored, *7840*, p. 1h
ROBITET Capsules (Robins)
  250 mg, brown and pink, *8417*, p. 27g
  500 mg, maroon and tan, *8427*, p. 28a
ROCALTROL Capsules (Roche)
  0.25 µg, light orange, p. 22g
  0.5 µg, dark orange, p. 22g
RONDEC Tablets (Ross)
  orange, oval, *5726*, p. 21h
RONDEC-TR Tablets (Ross)
  dark blue, oval, *6240*, p. 10c
RONDOMYCIN Capsules (Wallace)
  150 mg, blue and white, *37-4001*, p. 11a
  300 mg, blue and white, *37-4101*, p. 11d
RU-TUSS Tablets (Boots)
  green, mottled, oblong, scored, *58*, p. 13e
RU-TUSS II Capsules (Boots)
  green and clear with green and white beads, *31*, p. 14e
RUFEN Tablets (Boots)
  400 mg, magenta, round, p. 2c
  600 mg, white, oblong, *6*, p. 40c
  800 mg, white, oblong, *8*, p. 39i
RYNATAN Tablets (Wallace)
  buff, capsule-shaped, scored, *713*, p. 26f
RYNATUSS Tablets (Wallace)
  mauve, capsule-shaped, scored, *717*, p. 29b

S

SALIMEPH Tablets (Kremers-Urban)
  light yellow, capsule-shaped, p. 18f
SALURON Tablets (Bristol Laboratories)
  50 mg, white, round, scored, *S2*, p. 32e
SALUTENSIN Tablets (Bristol Laboratories)
  lime green, round, scored, *S1*, p. 12f
SALUTENSIN-Demi Tablets (Bristol Laboratories)
  yellow, round, scored, *S3*, p. 16d
SANOREX Tablets (Sandoz Pharmaceuticals)
  1 mg, white, oval, *78-71*, p. 37a
  2 mg, white, round, scored, *78-66*, p. 33b
SANSERT Tablets (Sandoz Pharmaceuticals)
  2 mg, yellow, round, *78-58*, p. 15f
SATRIC Tablets (Savage)
  250 mg, white, round, *3681*, p. 33e
SATRIC-500 Tablets (Savage)
  500 mg, white, oval, *3688*, p. 37i
SECONAL Sodium Pulvules (Lilly)
  50 mg, orange, *F42*, p. 22h
  100 mg, orange, *F40*, p. 22i
SECTRAL Capsules (Wyeth)
  200 mg, purple and orange, *4177*, p. 8f
  400 mg, brown and orange, *4179*, p. 28a
SELDANE Tablets (Merrell Dow)
  60 mg, white, round, p. 35b
SENOKOT Tablets (Purdue Frederick)
  khaki brown, round, p. 27a
SENOKOT-S Tablets (Purdue Frederick)
  light orange, round, p. 21b
SEPTRA Tablets (Burroughs Wellcome)
  pink, round, scored, *Y2B*, p. 2a
SEPTRA DS Tablets (Burroughs Wellcome)
  pink, oval, scored, *O2C*, p. 2h
SER-AP-ES Tablets (CIBA)
  light salmon pink, round, *71*, p. 1g
SERAX Capsules (Wyeth)
  10 mg, pink and white, *51*, p. 3g
  15 mg, red and white, *6*, p. 6f
  30 mg, maroon and white, *52*, p. 6f
SERAX Tablets (Wyeth)
  15 mg, yellow, five-sided with raised S, *317*, p. 19g
SERENTIL Tablets (Boehringer Ingelheim)
  10 mg, red, round, p. 5a
  25 mg, red, round, p. 5a
  50 mg, red, round, p. 5b
  100 mg, red, round, p. 5c
SEROPHENE Tablets (Serono)
  50 mg, white, round, scored, *11*, p. 33b
SERPASIL Tablets (CIBA)
  0.1 mg, white, round, *35*, p. 32i
  0.25 mg, white, round, scored, *36*, p. 32h
SERPASIL-APRESOLINE No. 1 Tablets (CIBA)
  yellow, round, *40*, p. 16a
SERPASIL-ESIDRIX No. 1 Tablets (CIBA)
  light orange, round, *13*, p. 26a
SERPASIL-ESIDRIX No. 2 Tablets (CIBA)
  light orange, round, *97*, p. 26b
SIGTAB Tablets (Upjohn)
  red, oval, p. 5h
SILAIN Tablets (Robins)
  50 mg, white, round, *8831*, p. 35e
SINAREST Extra Strength Tablets (Pharmacraft)
  yellow, oval, p. 17i

DRUG IDENTIFICATION INDEX

SINAREST Sinus Relief Tablets (Pharmacraft)
yellow, round, p. 16h
SINE-OFF Extra Strength, Aspirin-Free Capsules (SmithKline Consumer Products)
yellow, p. 19e
SINE-OFF Extra Strength, No Drowsiness Aspirin-Free Capsules (SmithKline Consumer Products)
red, p. 7b
SINE-OFF Regular Strength with Aspirin Tablets (SmithKline Consumer Products)
yellow, round, p. 16i
SINEMET 10-100 Tablets (Merck Sharp & Dohme)
dark dapple blue, oval, scored, 647, p. 9i
SINEMET 25-100 Tablets (Merck Sharp & Dohme)
yellow, oval, scored, 650, p. 17g
SINEMET 25-250 Tablets (Merck Sharp & Dohme)
light dapple blue, oval, scored, 654, p. 10a
SINEQUAN Capsules (Roerig)
10 mg, red and pink, 534, p. 6e
25 mg, blue and pink, 535, p. 10h
50 mg, pink and light pink, 536, p. 3i
75 mg, light pink, 539, p. 3h
100 mg, blue and light pink, 538, p. 10i
150 mg, blue, 537, p. 11e
SINUBID Tablets (Parke-Davis)
pink and light pink, layered, ellipsoid, scored, 177, p. 2g
SINULIN Tablets (Carnrick)
peach, round, scored, 8666, p. 24i
SKELAXIN Tablets (Carnrick)
400 mg, pale rose, round, scored, 86-62, p. 2a
SLO-BID Gyrocaps (Rorer)
50 mg, white and clear with white beads, p. 40c
100 mg, clear with white beads, p. 40d
200 mg, white and clear with white beads, p. 40f
300 mg, white, p. 40g
SLO-PHYLLIN Gyrocaps (Rorer)
60 mg, white and clear with white beads, 1354, p. 40e
125 mg, brown and clear with white beads, 1355, p. 27h
250 mg, purple and clear with white beads, 1356, p. 8g
SLO-PHYLLIN Tablets (Rorer)
100 mg, white, round, scored, 351, p. 32i
200 mg, white, round, scored, 352, p. 32i
SLO-PHYLLIN GG Capsules (Rorer)
off-white, 2358, p. 40g
SLOW FE Tablets (CIBA)
50 mg, ivory, round, NR, p. 32g
SLOW-K Tablets (CIBA)
600 mg, buff, round, 165, p. 26e
SMURF Chewable Tablets (Mead Johnson Nutritional)
various colors and Smurf shapes, p. 30b
SMURF with Iron and Zinc Chewable Tablets (Mead Johnson Nutritional)
various colors and Smurf shapes, p. 30c
SOLATENE Capsules (Roche)
30 mg, green and blue, p. 14i
SOLFOTON Capsules (Poythress)
16 mg, brown and yellow, 9525, p. 27f
SOLFOTON Tablets (Poythress)
16 mg, yellow, round, 9523, p. 24a
SOMA Tablets (Wallace)
350 mg, white, round, 37-2001, p. 36a
SOMA Compound Tablets (Wallace)
white and orange, layered, round, 2103, p. 21e
SORBITRATE Chewable Tablets (Stuart)
5 mg, green, round, scored, 810, p. 12f
10 mg, yellow, round, scored, 815, p. 16e
SORBITRATE Oral Tablets (Stuart)
5 mg, green, oval, scored, 770, p. 13b
10 mg, yellow, oval, scored, 780, p. 17g
20 mg, blue, oval, scored, 820, p. 9i
30 mg, white, oval, scored, 773, p. 37e
40 mg, light blue, oval, scored, 774, p. 9i
SORBITRATE Sublingual Tablets (Stuart)
2.5 mg, white, round, 853, p. 31a
5 mg, pink, round, 760, p. 1a
10 mg, yellow, round, 761, p. 15f
SORBITRATE SA Tablets (Stuart)
40 mg, yellow, round, 880, p. 16h
SPARINE Tablets (Wyeth)
25 mg, yellow, round, 29, p. 15i
50 mg, orange, round, 28, p. 20i
100 mg, pink, round, 200, p. 1h
SPARTUS + Iron Tablets (Lederle)
pink, capsule-shaped, scored, S23, p. 2i
SPARTUS Tablets (Lederle)
blue, capsule-shaped, scored, S22, p. 10b
SPEC-T Anesthetic Lozenges (Squibb)
red, square, p. 7e
SPEC-T Cough Suppressant Lozenges (Squibb)
yellow, square, p. 20a
SPEC-T Decongestant Lozenges (Squibb)
green, square, p. 15b
SPECTROBID Tablets (Roerig)
400 mg, white, oblong, 035, p. 39h
ST. JOSEPH Aspirin Tablets (Plough)
325 mg, white, round, p. 34f
ST. JOSEPH Aspirin-Free Children's Chewable Tablets (Plough)
80 mg, pink, round, fruit flavored, p. 1g
ST. JOSEPH Chewable Aspirin for Children (Plough)
81 mg, light orange, round, orange flavored, p. 20h
ST. JOSEPH Cold Tablets for Children (Plough)
orange and white, layered, round, p. 21b
STELAZINE Tablets (Smith Kline & French)
1 mg, blue, round, S03, p. 9b
2 mg, blue, round, S04, p. 9c
5 mg, blue, round, S06, p. 9f
10 mg, blue, round, S07, p. 9g
STRESSGARD Tablets (Miles Laboratories)
pumpkin orange, capsule-shaped, p. 22f
STRESSTABS 600 Tablets (Lederle)
orange, capsule-shaped, scored, S1, p. 22e
STRESSTABS 600 + Iron Tablets (Lederle)
burnt-orange, capsule-shaped, scored, S2, p. 22e
STRESSTABS 600 + Zinc Tablets (Lederle)
light orange, capsule-shaped, scored, S3, p. 22e
STUART FORMULA Tablets (Stuart)
white, round, p. 36e
STUART PRENATAL Tablets (Stuart)
sugar pink, capsule-shaped, p. 3f
STUARTINIC Tablets (Stuart)
yellow, oval, p. 18a
STUARTNATAL 1 + 1 Tablets (Stuart)
light yellow, capsule-shaped, 023, p. 18i
SUDAFED Tablets (Burroughs Wellcome)
30 mg, red, round, p. 5a
60 mg, white, round, p. 33c
SUDAFED 12 Hour Capsules (Burroughs Wellcome)
red and clear with white beads, p. 6i
SUDAFED Plus Tablets (Burroughs Wellcome)
white, round, scored, p. 32c
SULTRIN Vaginal Tablets (Ortho)
white, oval, p. 40a
SUMYCIN '250' Capsules (Squibb)
250 mg, dark pink, 655, p. 3i
SUMYCIN '500' Capsules (Squibb)
500 mg, dark pink and white, 763, p. 4a
SUMYCIN '250' Tablets (Squibb)
250 mg, light pink, capsule-shaped, 663, p. 3b
SUMYCIN '500' Tablets (Squibb)
500 mg, rose pink, capsule-shaped, 603, p. 3d
SUPROL Capsules (McNeil/Ortho Pharmaceutical)
200 mg, blue and yellow, 1500, p. 11c
SURBEX-750 with Iron Tablets (Abbott)
rust brown, capsule-shaped, p. 27d
SURBEX-750 with Zinc Tablets (Abbott)
light gray, capsule-shaped, p. 29b
SURBEX-T Tablets (Abbott)
orange, capsule-shaped, p. 22a
SURFAK Capsules (Hoechst-Roussel)
50 mg, clear orange, p. 22i
240 mg, clear red, p. 7c
SURMONTIL Capsules (Wyeth)
25 mg, blue and yellow, 4132, p. 11a
SUSTAIRE Tablets (Pfizer)
100 mg, white, oval, scored, 220, p. 38e
300 mg, white, oval, scored, 221, p. 38g
SYMMETREL Capsules (Du Pont)
100 mg, red, p. 6d
SYNALGOS-DC Capsules (Wyeth)
blue and gray, 4191, p. 11c
SYNKAVITE Tablets (Roche)
5 mg, white, round, p. 32e
SYNTHROID Tablets (Flint)
50 μg, white, round, scored, p. 32b
75 μg, violet, round, scored, p. 8a
100 μg, yellow, round, scored, p: 15i
125 μg, brown, round, scored, p. 24c
150 μg, blue, round, scored, p. 9c
200 μg, pink, round, scored, p. 1c
300 μg, green, round, scored, p. 12c

DRUG IDENTIFICATION INDEX

T

TABRON Filmseal Tablets (Parke-Davis)
  pinkish-brown, mottled, elliptical, *638*, p. 27e
TACE Capsules (Merrell Dow)
  12 mg, green, *690*, p. 15a
  25 mg, two-tone green, *691*, p. 14h
  72 mg, green and yellow, *692*, p. 19f
TAGAMET Tablets (Smith Kline & French)
  200 mg, pale green, round, p. 12g
  300 mg, pale green, round, p. 12i
  400 mg, pale green, oblong, p. 13e
  800 mg, pale green, oval, scored, p. 13c
TALACEN Caplets (Winthrop Pharmaceuticals)
  pale blue, capsule-shaped, scored, *T37*, p. 10e
TALWIN Nx Tablets (Winthrop Pharmaceuticals)
  yellow, oblong, scored, *T51*, p. 18c
TAMBOCOR Tablets (Riker)
  100 mg, white, round, scored, p. 33d
TAO Capsules (Roerig)
  250 mg, white, *159*, p. 40g
TARACTAN Tablets (Roche)
  10 mg, peach, round, p. 24a
  25 mg, peach, round, p. 24b
  50 mg, orange, round, p. 20g
  100 mg, orange, round, p. 21c
TAVIST Tablets (Sandoz Pharmaceuticals)
  2.68 mg, white, round, scored, *78-72*, p. 31h
TAVIST-1 Tablets (Sandoz Pharmaceuticals)
  1.34 mg, white, oval, scored, *78-75*, p. 38e
TAVIST-D Tablets (Sandoz Pharmaceuticals)
  white, round, *78-221*, p. 35f
TEDRAL Tablets (Parke-Davis)
  white, round, scored, *230*, p. 32i
TEDRAL SA Tablets (Parke-Davis)
  coral and mottled white, layered, round, scored, *231*, p. 5c
TEDRAL-25 Tablets (Parke-Davis)
  orange, round, scored, *238*, p. 20h
TEGOPEN Capsules (Apothecon)
  250 mg, black and orange, *7935*, p. 29g
  500 mg, black and orange, *7496*, p. 29i
TEGRETOL Chewable Tablets (Geigy)
  100 mg, red-speckled, round, scored, *47*, p. 34g
TEGRETOL Tablets (Geigy)
  200 mg, pink, capsule-shaped, scored, *27*, p. 3a
TELDRIN Sustained-Release Capsules, Maximum Strength (SmithKline Consumer Products)
  12 mg, clear with turquoise band and pink, red, and white beads, p. 3g
TELDRIN Tablets (SmithKline Consumer Products)
  4 mg, green, round, p. 12d
TEMARIL Spansules (Smith Kline & French)
  5 mg, gray and clear with gray and white beads, *HL T50*, p. 29c
TEMARIL Tablets (Smith Kline & French)
  2.5 mg, gray, round, *HL T41*, p. 29a
TEMPRA Chewable Tablets (Mead Johnson Nutritional)
  80 mg, purple, mottled, round, scored, p. 8c
TENORETIC 50 Tablets (Stuart)
  white, round, *115*, p. 32e
TENORETIC 100 Tablets (Stuart)
  white, round, *117*, p. 34d
TENORMIN 50 Tablets (Stuart)
  50 mg, white, round, scored, *105*, p. 32d
TENORMIN 100 Tablets (Stuart)
  100 mg, white, round, *101*, p. 33f
TENUATE Dospan Tablets (Lakeside)
  75 mg, white, capsule-shaped, *698* or *75*, p. 39c
TENUATE Tablets (Lakeside)
  25 mg, white, round, *697* or *25*, p. 34h
TEPANIL Tablets (Riker)
  25 mg, white, round, p. 34a
TEPANIL Ten-Tab (Riker)
  75 mg, white, round, p. 36a
TERFONYL Tablets (Squibb)
  500 mg, white, round, scored, *887*, p. 35f
TERRAMYCIN Capsules (Pfizer)
  250 mg, yellow, *073*, p. 19e
TESLAC Tablets (Squibb)
  50 mg, white, round, *690*, p. 33i
TESSALON Perles (Du Pont)
  100 mg, yellow, clear, round, p. 18i
TESTRED Capsules (ICN)
  10 mg, red, *0901*, p. 6g
Tetracycline Capsules (Wyeth)
  250 mg, blue and yellow, *389*, p. 11c
  500 mg, blue and yellow, *471*, p. 11f
THALITONE Tablets (Boehringer Ingelheim)
  25 mg, white, kidney-shaped, *76*, p. 41a
THEO-24 Controlled Release Capsules (Searle)
  100 mg, gold and clear with white beads, *2832*, p. 22h
  200 mg, orange and clear with white beads, *2842*, p. 23c
  300 mg, red and clear with white beads, *2852*, p. 7a
THEOBID Duracaps (Glaxo)
  260 mg, blue and clear with white beads, *268*, p. 11f
THEOBID Jr. Duracaps (Glaxo)
  130 mg, blue and clear with white beads, *295*, p. 11a
THEO-DUR Sprinkle Sustained-Action Capsules (Key)
  50 mg, white and clear with white beads, p. 40d
  75 mg, white and clear with white beads, p. 40e
  125 mg, white and clear with white beads, p. 40g
  200 mg, white and clear with white beads, p. 40g
THEO-DUR Sustained-Action Tablets (Key)
  100 mg, white, round, scored, p. 34b
  200 mg, white, oval, scored, p. 37e
  300 mg, white, oblong, scored, p. 38f
THEOLAIR Tablets (Riker)
  125 mg, white, round, scored, *342*, p. 34e
  250 mg, white, capsule-shaped, scored, p. 39g
THEOLAIR-Plus Tablets (Riker)
  250 mg, white, capsule-shaped, scored, p. 39d
THEOLAIR-SR Tablets (Riker)
  200 mg, white, round, scored, p. 34a
  250 mg, white, round, scored, p. 35c
  300 mg, white, oval, scored, p. 37i
  500 mg, white, capsule-shaped, scored, p. 39h
THEOVENT Long-Acting Capsules (Schering)
  125 mg, dark green and yellow, *402*, p. 14c
  250 mg, dark green and clear, *753*, p. 14g
THERAGRAN HEMATINIC Tablets (Squibb)
  salmon pink, capsule-shaped, *535*, p. 3d
THERAGRAN-M Tablets (Squibb)
  brown, capsule-shaped, p. 27e
THERAGRAN Stress Formula Tablets (Squibb)
  rust, capsule-shaped, p. 6a
THERAGRAN Tablets (Squibb)
  rust, capsule-shaped, p. 6a
THIOGUANINE Tablets (Burroughs Wellcome)
  40 mg, greenish-yellow, round, scored, *U3B*, p. 26b
THIOSULFIL Tablets (Ayerst)
  0.25 g, white, oval, scored, *785*, p. 37e
THIOSULFIL Forte Tablets (Ayerst)
  0.5 g, white, oval, scored, *786*, p. 37h
THIOSULFIL-A Tablets (Ayerst)
  red, round, *784*, p. 5d
THIOSULFIL-A Forte Tablets (Ayerst)
  yellow, round, *783*, p. 17a
THORAZINE Spansules (Smith Kline & French)
  200 mg, orange and clear with pale pink and white beads, *T67*, p. 23e
THYROLAR-¼ Tablets (Rorer)
  violet and white, layered, round, *YC*, p. 8b
THYROLAR-½ Tablets (Rorer)
  peach and white, layered, round, *YD*, p. 20f
THYROLAR-1 Tablets (Rorer)
  pink and white, layered, round, *YE*, p. 1d
THYROLAR-3 Tablets (Rorer)
  yellow and white, layered, round, *YH*, p. 15i
TIGAN Capsules (Beecham Laboratories)
  100 mg, blue and white, p. 10g
  250 mg, blue, p. 11b
TIMOLIDE 10-25 Tablets (Merck Sharp & Dohme)
  light blue, hexagonal, *67*, p. 11h
TINDAL Tablets (Schering)
  20 mg, flesh pink, round, *968*, p. 1b
TITRALAC Tablets (3M)
  white, round, p. 35d
TOFRANIL Tablets (Geigy)
  10 mg, coral, triangular, *32*, p. 28b
  25 mg, coral, round, *140*, p. 27a
  50 mg, coral, round, *136*, p. 21c
TOFRANIL-PM Capsules (Geigy)
  75 mg, coral, *20*, p. 27g
  100 mg, coral and dark yellow, *40*, p. 27h
  125 mg, coral and light yellow, *45*, p. 27h
  150 mg, coral, *22*, p. 27i
TOLECTIN Tablets (McNeil Pharmaceutical)
  200 mg, white, round, scored, p. 36a
TOLECTIN DS Capsules (McNeil

DRUG IDENTIFICATION INDEX

Pharmaceutical)
400 mg, orange with purple-gray parallel bands, p. 23f
TOLFRINIC Tablets (Ascher)
brown, round, *225/105*, p. 27c
TOLINASE Tablets (Upjohn)
100 mg, white, round, scored, p. 33f
250 mg, white, round, scored, *114*, p. 34f
500 mg, white, round, scored, *477*, p. 36a
TONOCARD Tablets (Merck Sharp & Dohme)
400 mg, yellow, oval, scored, *707*, p. 17h
600 mg, yellow, oblong, scored, *709*, p. 19i
TORECAN Tablets (Boehringer Ingelheim)
10 mg, yellow, round, *28*, p. 15i
TOTACILLIN Capsules (Beecham Laboratories)
250 mg, brown and orange, *140*, p. 27g
500 mg, brown and orange, *141*, p. 27i
TRANDATE Tablets (Glaxo)
100 mg, peach, round, scored, p. 24c
200 mg, white, round, scored, p. 33h
300 mg, peach, round, scored, p. 21d
TRANSDERM-NITRO Transdermal Therapeutic Systems (CIBA)
2.5 mg/24 h (5 cm^2), *2025*, p. 48c
5 mg/24 h (10 cm^2), *2015*, p. 48c
10 mg/24 h (20 cm^2), *2110*, p. 48c
15 mg/24 h (30 cm^2), *2115*, p. 48d
TRANSDERM SCOP Tranderdmal Therapeutic Systems (CIBA)
0.5 mg/3 days, *5921*, p. 48d
TRANXENE Capsules (Abbott)
3.75 mg, gray and white, *Cl*, p. 29c
7.5 mg, maroon and gray, *CN*, p. 6f
15 mg, gray, *CK*, p. 29c
TRANXENE Tablets (Abbott)
3.75 mg, blue, oval, bevelled, scored, *TL*, p. 11h
7.5 mg, peach, oval, bevelled, scored, *TM*, p. 25f
TRENDAR Tablets (Whitehall)
200 mg, white, round, p. 35a
TRENTAL Tablets (Hoechst-Roussel)
400 mg, pink, oblong, p. 3b
TREXAN Tablets (Du Pont)
50 mg, pale peach, mottled, round, scored, p. 24f
TRIAMINIC Allergy Tablets (Sandoz Consumer)
yellow, round, scored. p. 16b
TRIAMINIC Chewable Tablets (Sandoz Consumer)
yellow, octagonal, p. 19i
TRIAMINIC Cold Tablets (Sandoz Consumer)
orange, round, p. 20g
TRIAMINIC TR Tablets (Sandoz Consumer)
yellow, round, p. 16h
TRIAMINIC-12 Sustained-Release Tablets (Sandoz Consumer)
orange, capsule-shaped, p. 22c
TRIAMINICIN Tablets (Sandoz Consumer)
yellow, capsule-shaped, p. 18g
TRIAMINICOL Tablets (Sandoz Consumer)
pink, round, p. 1f
TRIAVIL 2-10 Tablets (Merck Sharp & Dohme)
blue, triangular, *914*, p. 11h
TRIAVIL 2-25 Tablets (Merck Sharp & Dohme)
orange, triangular, *921*, p. 23h
TRIAVIL 4-10 Tablets (Merck Sharp & Dohme)
salmon, triangular, *934*, p. 25f
TRIAVIL 4-25 Tablets (Merck Sharp & Dohme)
yellow, triangular, *946*, p. 19h
TRIAVIL 4-50 Tablets (Merck Sharp & Dohme)
orange, diamond-shaped, *517*, p. 23i
TRIDIONE Capsules (Abbott)
300 mg, white, *AM*, p. 40f
TRIGESIC Tablets (Squibb)
white, round, scored, *876*, p. 35e
TRIHEMIC 600 Tablets (Lederle)
red, capsule-shaped, *T1*, p. 6a
TRILAFON Repetabs (Schering)
8 mg, white, round, *141*, p. 33f
TRILAFON Tablets (Schering)
2 mg, gray, round, *705*, p. 29a
4 mg, gray, round, *940*, p. 29a
8 mg, gray, round, *313*, p. 29b
16 mg, gray, round, *077*, p. 29a
TRI-LEVLEN Tablets (Berlex)
brown, round, *95* (0.050 mg levonorgestrel and 30 μg ethinyl estradiol), p. 27a
white, round, *96* (0.075 mg levonorgestrel and 40 μg ethinyl estradiol), p. 31a
yellow, round, *97* (0.125 mg levonorgestrel and 30 μg ethinyl estradiol), p. 15e
28-day *Slidecase*, p. 46a
TRILISATE 500 Tablets (Purdue Frederick)
500 mg, pale pink, capsule-shaped, scored, p. 25d
TRILISATE 750 Tablets (Purdue Frederick)
750 mg, white, capsule-shaped, scored, p. 40b
TRILISATE 1000 Tablets (Purdue Frederick)
1,000 mg, red, capsule-shaped, scored, p. 6b
TRIMOX '250' Capsules (Squibb)
250 mg, dark green, *230*, p. 14d
TRIMOX '500' Capsules (Squibb)
500 mg, dark green and light green, *231*, p. 14i
TRIMPEX Tablets (Roche)
100 mg, white, elliptical, scored, p. 37f
TRINALIN Long-Acting Repetabs (Schering)
coral, round, *703*, p. 21d
TRI-NORINYL Tablets (Syntex)
blue, round, *110* (0.5 mg norethindrone and 35 μg ethinyl estradiol), p. 9b
green, round, *111* (1 mg norethindrone and 35 μg ethinyl estradiol), p. 12b
21-day *Wallette*, p. 46b
28-day *Wallette*, p. 46b
TRINSICON Capsules (Glaxo)
dark red and dark pink, p. 7d
TRINSICON M Capsules (Glaxo)
dark red and dark pink, p. 7d
TRIPHASIL Tablets (Wyeth)
brown, round, *641* (0.050 mg levonorgestrel and 30 μg ethinyl estradiol), p. 27a
white, round, *642* (0.075 mg levonorgestrel and 40 μg ethinyl estradiol), p. 31c
light yellow, round, *643* (0.125 mg levonorgestrel and 30 μg ethinyl estradiol), p. 15e
21-day compact, p. 46b
28-day compact, p. 46c
TRI-VI-FLOR Chewable Tablets (Mead Johnson Nutritional)
1 mg, various colors, mottled, square, *477*, p. 30a
TROPHITE Tablets (SmithKline Consumer Products)
pink, round, p. 1e
TUINAL Pulvules (Lilly)
50 mg, orange and blue, *F64*, p. 22h
100 mg, orange and blue, *F65*, *p. 22i*
200 mg, orange and blue, *F66*, p. 23a
TUSS-ORNADE Spansules (Smith Kline & French)
light blue and clear with pink, white, and blue beads, p. 11b
TUSSAGESIC Tablets (Sandoz Consumer)
light pink, capsule-shaped, p. 3c
TUSSEND Tablets (Merrell Dow)
red, round, *42*, p. 5c
TUSSIONEX Capsules (Pennwalt)
green and white, p. 14b
TUSSIONEX Tablets (Pennwalt)
light brown, trapezoidal-shaped, scored, *18-894*, p. 26h
TYLENOL with Codeine No 3 Capsules (McNeil Pharmaceutical)
white with red bands, p. 40h
TYLENOL with Codeine No. 4 Capsules (McNeil Pharmaceutical)
red, p. 7b
TYLENOL with Codeine No. 1 Tablets (McNeil Pharmaceutical)
white, round, p. 34g
TYLENOL with Codeine No. 2 Tablets (McNeil Pharmaceutical)
white, round, p. 34h
TYLENOL with Codeine No. 3 Tablets (McNeil Pharmaceutical)
white, round, p. 35f
TYLENOL with Codeine No. 4 Tablets (McNeil Pharmaceutical)
white, round, p. 35f

U

ULTRACEF Capsules (Bristol Laboratories)
500 mg, black and blue, *7271*, p. 29i
ULTRACEF Tablets (Bristol Laboratories)
1 g, off-white, capsule-shaped, scored, *C1*, p. 40a
UNICAP Capsules (Upjohn)
gold, p. 18i
UNICAP Jr Chewable Tablets (Upjohn)
peach, mottled, round, p. 24i
UNICAP M Tablets (Upjohn)
orange, oval, p. 21i
UNICAP Plus Iron Tablets (Upjohn)
red, oval, p. 5g
UNICAP Senior Tablets (Upjohn)
powder blue, oval, p. 10a
UNICAP T Tablets (Upjohn)
orange, oval, p. 21i
UNILAX Tablets (Ascher)
gold, round, p. 16i
UNIPEN Capsules (Wyeth)

DRUG IDENTIFICATION INDEX

250 mg, green and yellow, *57*, p. 14i
UNIPEN Tablets (Wyeth)
500 mg, white, capsule-shaped, scored, *464*, p. 39f
UNIPHYL Tablets (Purdue Frederick)
200 mg, white, round, scored, p. 34d
400 mg, white, round, scored, p. 35a
UNISOM Dual Relief Tablets (Leeming)
pale blue, capsule-shaped, p. 9i
UNISOM Tablets (Leeming)
25 mg, pale blue, oval, scored, p. 10d
URECHOLINE Tablets (Merck Sharp & Dohme)
5 mg, white, round, scored, *403*, p. 35d
10 mg, pink, round, scored, *412*, p. 2a
25 mg, yellow, round, scored, *457*, p. 16i
50 mg, yellow, round, scored, *460*, p. 17a
UREX Tablets (Riker)
1 g, white, oval, scored, p. 40a
URISED Tablets (Alcon)
purple, round, *W-2183*, p. 8c
URISEDAMINE Tablets (Alcon)
blue, capsule-shaped, *W-2210*, p. 10f
URISPAS Tablets (Smith Kline & French)
100 mg, white, round, p. 35e
UROBIOTIC-250 Capsules (Roerig)
yellow and green, *092*, p. 19e
URO-PHOSPHATE Tablets (Poythress)
white, round, *9531*, p. 36c
URSINUS Tablets (Sandoz Consumer)
white with yellow inlay, capsule-shaped, p. 18f
UTICILLIN VK Tablets (Upjohn)
250 mg, white, round, scored, *586*, p. 33i
500 mg, white, round, scored, *671*, p. 36d

V

VALIUM Tablets (Roche)
2 mg, white, round with V-shaped cutout, scored, p. 41c
5 mg, yellow, round with V-shaped cutout, scored, p. 19h
10 mg, blue, round with V-shaped cutout, scored, p. 11h
VALMID Pulvules (Dista)
500 mg, blue and light blue, *H74*, p. 11f
VALPIN 50 Tablets (Du Pont)
50 mg, beige, round, scored, p. 26a
VALRELEASE Capsules (Roche)
15 mg, blue and yellow, p. 11a
VANQUISH Caplets (Glenbrook)
white, capsule-shaped, p. 39b
VANSIL Capsules (Pfizer)
250 mg, green and yellow, *641*, p. 14f
VASERETIC Tablets (Merck Sharp Dohme)
red, capsule-shaped, square, *720*, p. 7e
VASODILAN Tablets (Mead Johnson Pharmaceuticals)
10 mg, white, round, *543*, p. 33e
20 mg, white, round, scored, *544*, p. 34i
VASOTEC Tablets (Merck Sharp & Dohme)
5 mg, white, barrel-shaped, scored, *712*, p. 41a
10 mg, red, barrel-shaped, *713*, p. 25e
20 mg, peach, barrel-shaped, *714*, p. 25e
V-CILLIN K Tablets (Lilly)
250 mg, white, oval, p. 37f
500 mg, white, oval, p. 37i
VEETIDS '250' Tablets (Squibb)
250 mg, orange, capsule-shaped, *684*, p. 22b
VEETIDS '500' Tablets (Squibb)
500 mg, white, capsule-shaped, *648*, p. 39f
VELOSEF '250' Capsules (Squibb)
250 mg, blue and orange, *113*, p. 10i
VELOSEF '500' Capsules (Squibb)
500 mg, blue, *114*, p. 11f
VENTOLIN Tablets (Glaxo)
2 mg, white, round, scored, p. 31h
4 mg, white, round, scored, p. 33e
VIBRAMYCIN Capsules (Pfizer)
50 mg, blue and white, *094*, p. 10h
100 mg, blue, *095*, p. 11d
VIBRA-TABS (Pfizer)
100 mg, peach, round, *099*, p. 24f
VICODIN Tablets (Knoll)
white, capsule-shaped, scored, p. 39b
VICON-C Capsules (Glaxo)
orange and yellow, p. 23f
VICON Forte Capsules (Glaxo)
black and orange, *316*, p. 29h
VICON-Plus Capsules (Glaxo)
red and beige, p. 7a
VI-DAYLIN Chewable Tablets (Ross)
pink, mottled, oval, p. 2e
VI-DAYLIN Plus Iron Chewable Tablets (Ross)
orange with brown specks, oval, p. 21i
VI-DAYLIN/F Tablets (Ross)
yellow with orange specks, oval, scored, *7626*, p. 21i
VI-DAYLIN/F + Iron Chewable Tablets (Ross)
pink, mottled, oval, scored, *7621*, p. 2e
VIGRAN Plus Tablets (Squibb)
bright pink, capsule-shaped, p. 3d
VIGRAN Tablets (Squibb)
dark orange, round, p. 20f
VIOKASE Tablets (Robins)
tan, round, *9111*, p. 26d
VI-PENTA F Chewable Tablets (Roche)
orange, green, pink, yellow, or purple, triangular, *51*, p. 30a
VISKEN Tablets (Sandoz Pharmaceuticals)
5 mg, white, round, scored, *78-111*, p. 31g
10 mg, white, round, scored, *78-73*, p. 33a
VISTARIL Capsules (Pfizer)
25 mg, dark green and light green, *541*, p. 14a
50 mg, green and white, *542*, p. 14a
100 mg, gray and green, *543*, p. 14b
VIVACTIL Tablets (Merck Sharp & Dohme)
5 mg, orange, oval, *26*, p. 21h
10 mg, yellow, oval, *47*, p. 17f
VIVOX Tablets (Squibb)
100 mg, peach, round, *897*, p. 24e
VI-ZAC Capsules (Glaxo)
orange, p. 23g
VONTROL Tablets (Smith Kline & French)
25 mg, dark yellow, round, p. 20e

W

WELLCOVORIN Tablets (Burroughs Wellcome)
5 mg, off-white, round, *R3C*, p. 32g
25 mg, peach, round, p. 24c
WIGRAINE Rectal Suppositories (Organon)
white, oval, *542*, p. 41e
WITHIN Tablets (Miles Laboratories)
gold, capsule-shaped, p. 17i
WYAMYCIN S Tablets (Wyeth)
250 mg, pink, round, *576*, p. 2b
500 mg, pink, oval, *578*, p. 2h
WYGESIC Tablets (Wyeth)
green, capsule-shaped, scored, *85*, p. 13g
WYMOX Capsules (Wyeth)
250 mg, gray and green, *559*, p. 29c
500 mg, gray and green, *560*, p. 29e
WYTENSIN Tablets (Wyeth)
4 mg, white, five-sided with raised W, *73*, p. 40h
8 mg, white, five-sided with raised W, scored, *74*, p. 40i
16 mg, white, five-sided with raised W, scored, *92*, p. 40i

X

XANAX Tablets (Upjohn)
0.25 mg, white, oval, scored, p. 37b
0.5 mg, peach, oval, scored, p. 25a
1 mg, lavender, oval, scored, p. 8d

Y

YODOXIN Tablets (Glenwood)
210 mg, light yellow-tan, round, *92*, p. 26b
650 mg, yellow, round, *93*, p. 17a

Z

ZANTAC 150 Tablets (Glaxo)
150 mg, white, round, p. 33h
ZANTAC 300 Tablets (Glaxo)
300 mg, yellow, capsule-shaped, p. 18e
ZARONTIN Capsules (Parke-Davis)
250 mg, clear orange, *237*, p. 23e
ZAROXOLYN Tablets (Pennwalt)
2½ mg, pink, round, p. 8a
5 mg, blue, round, p. 9a
10 mg, yellow, round, p. 15h
Z-BEC Tablets (Robins)
dark green, oval, p. 13d
ZENATE E Tablets (Reid-Rowell)
baby blue, capsule-shaped, scored, *1146*, p. 10f
ZORPRIN Tablets (Boots)
800 mg, white, capsule-shaped, *57*, p. 39i
ZOVIRAX Capsules (Burroughs Wellcome)
200 mg, blue, p. 11b
ZYLOPRIM Tablets (Burroughs Wellcome)
100 mg, white, round with raised hexagonal, scored, p. 33i
300 mg, peach, round with raised hexagonal, scored, p. 24h
ZYMACAP Capsules (Upjohn)
dark red, p. 6c

Chapter 2

Directory of Pharmaceutical Manufacturers

Key

BH = Business hours
N = Nights (after business hours)
H = Holidays
W = Weekends
A = All times (including nights, holidays, and weekends)

Abbott Laboratories, 1400 Sheridan Road, North Chicago, IL 60064 Tel: 312/937-7069 (8 am-5:15 pm Mon-Fri)

Adria Laboratories, Division of Erbamont Inc., PO Box 16529, Columbus, OH 43216 Tel: 614/764-8100 (A)

Advanced Care Products, Division of Ortho Pharmaceutical Corporation, Route 202, Raritan, NJ 08869 Tel: 201/524-5211

Akorn, Inc., 100 Akorn Drive, Abita Springs, LA 70420 Tel: 800/535-7155 (8 am-5 pm Mon-Fri) (outside LA), 800/344-2291 (8 am-5 pm Mon-Fri) (in LA), 504/893-9300

Alcon Laboratories, Inc., 6201 South Freeway, Fort Worth, TX 76134 Tel: 817/293-0450 (BH), 817/921-0884 (N,H,W)

Allergan Pharmaceuticals, Inc., 2525 Dupont Drive, Irvine, CA 92715 Tel: 714/752-4500 ext 4281, 4586, or 4959 (BH); 714/752-4335 or 714/752-4244 (N,H,W)

Alza Corporation, 950 Page Mill Road, Palo Alto, CA 94303-0802 Tel: 415/494-5000; 415/948-2242, James L. Strand, MD (A, emergencies)

American Chicle Group, Warner-Lambert Company, 201 Tabor Road, Morris Plains, NJ 07950 Tel: 201/540-2000

American Dermal Corporation, 12-L World's Fair Drive, Somerset, NJ 08873 Tel: 800/526-0199 (BH) (outside NJ), 201/356-5544 (A)

Ames Division, Miles Laboratories, Inc., 1127 Myrtle Street, Elkhart, IN 46515 Tel: 219/264-8444 (BH), 219/264-8111 (N,H,W)

Anaquest, Division of BOC Inc., 2005 West Beltline Highway, Madison, WI 53713-2318 Tel: 1-800/ANA-DRUG (BH), 608/273-0019

Apothecon, Division of Bristol-Myers Company, 2404 Pennsylvania Street, Evansville, IN 47721-0001 Tel: 812/429-5000 (A)

Armour Pharmaceutical Company, Suite 4000, One Sentry Parkway, Blue Bell, PA 19422 Tel: 215/834-3850

B.F. Ascher & Company, Inc., 15501 West 109th Street, Lenexa, KS 66219 Tel: 913/888-1880 (8 am-4:30 pm Mon-Fri)

Astra Pharmaceutical Products Inc., 50 Otis Street, Westborough, MA 01581-4428 Tel: 617/366-1100 (BH), 1-800/225-4803 (N,H,W) (outside MA), 1-800/451-2512 (N,H,W) (in MA)

Ayerst Laboratories, Division of American Home Products Corporation, 685 Third Avenue, New York, NY 10017-4071 Tel: 212/878-5900 (9 am-5 pm Mon-Fri); 212/986-1000, 212/878-5000, or 212/878-5900 (N,H,W)

Barnes-Hind Inc., 895 Kifer Road, Sunnyvale, CA 94086 Tel: 1-800/538-1680 or 1-800/854-2790 (outside CA), 1-800/542-6000 (in CA), 408/736-5462

Beecham Laboratories, Division of Beecham, Inc., 501 Fifth Street, Bristol, TN 37620 Tel: 615/764-5141 (A)

Beecham Products, Division of Beecham, Inc., PO Box 1467, Pittsburgh, PA 15230 Tel: 800/245-1040 (A) (outside PA), 800/242-1718 (A) (in PA)

Berlex Laboratories, Inc., Professional Services, 110 East Hanover Avenue, Cedar Knolls, NJ 07927 Tel: 201/292-3007 (A)

Block Drug Company Inc., 257 Cornelison Avenue, Jersey City, NJ 07302 Tel: 201/434-3000 (A)

Boehringer Ingelheim Pharmaceuticals, Inc., 90 East Ridge, PO Box 368, Ridgefield, CT 06877 Tel: 203/ 438-0311 (A)

Boehringer Mannheim Diagnostics, A Division of Boehringer Mannheim Corporation, 9115 Hague Road, Indianapolis, IN 46250 Tel: 800/428-5074

Bolar Pharmaceutical Co., Inc., 33 Ralph Avenue, Copiague, NY 11726 Tel: 516/842-8383

Boots Pharmaceuticals, Inc., 8800 Ellerbe Road, PO Box 6750, Shreveport, LA 71136-6750 Tel: 318/861-8200 (8 am-4:30 pm Mon-Fri)

Bristol Laboratories, Division of Bristol-Myers Company, 2404 Pennsylvania Street, Evansville, IN 47721-0001 Tel: 812/429-5000 (A)

Bristol-Myers Oncology Division, Division of Bristol-Myers Company, 2404 Pennsylvania Street, Evansville, IN 47721-0001 Tel: 812/429-5000 (A)

Bristol-Myers Products, Division of Bristol-Myers Company, 1350 Liberty Avenue, Hillside, NJ 07207 Tel: 212/546-4616 (9 am-5 pm Mon-Fri), 212/546-4700 (N,H,W)

The Brown Pharmaceutical Company, Inc., 2500 West Sixth Street, Los Angeles, CA 90057 Tel: 213/389-1394 or 213/389-1395 (BH)

Burroughs Wellcome Company, 3030 Cornwallis Road, Research Triangle Park, NC 27709 Tel: 919/248-3000 (A)

Canaan Laboratories Ltd., 50 Locust Avenue, New Canaan, CT 06840 Tel: 800/222-0830 (9 am-5:30 pm Mon-Fri) (outside CT), 203/966-6700 (9 am-5:30 pm Mon-Fri)

Carnrick Laboratories, Inc., 65 Horse Hill Road, Cedar Knolls, NJ 07927 Tel: 201/267-2670

Central Pharmaceuticals, Inc., 120 East Third Street, Seymour, IN 47274 Tel: 812/522-3915

CIBA Pharmaceutical Company, Division of CIBA-GEIGY Corporation, 556 Morris Avenue, Summit, NJ 07901 Tel: 201/277-5000 (A), 201/277-5342

Clay Adams, 299 Webro Road, Parsippany, NJ 07054 Tel: 201/887-4800

Colgate-Hoyt Laboratories, Division of Colgate-Palmolive Company, 1 Colgate Way, Canton, MA 02021 Tel: 800/225-3756 (8:30 am-4:15 pm)

Connaught Laboratories, Route 611, Box 187, Swiftwater, PA 18370 Tel: 800/VACCINE (8 am-8 pm Mon-Fri), 717/839-7187 (A)

CooperVision Ophthalmic Products, 2610 Orchard Parkway, San Jose, CA 95134 Tel: 800/538-7834 (BH), 408/434-7000 (BH), 415/948-9563 (for information on solutions) (N,H,W)

Danker Laboratories, Inc., 6805 33rd Street East, PO Box 1899, Sarasota, FL 33578 Tel: 800/237-9641 (8:30 am-5:30 pm Mon-Fri) (outside FL), 800/282-9661 (8:30 am-5:30 pm Mon-Fri) (in FL), 813/758-7711 (8:30 am-5:30 pm Mon-Fri) (local)

Dermik Laboratories, Inc., Division of William H. Rorer, Inc., 790 Penllyn Pike, Blue Bell, PA 19422 Tel: 215/283-2000 (8:30 am-4:30 pm Mon-Fri)

Dista Products Company, Division of Eli Lilly and Company, Lilly Corporate Center, Indianapolis, IN 46285 Tel: 317/261-3714 (BH), 317/261-4000 (N,H,W)

Du Pont Critical Care, Subsidiary of E.I. du Pont de Nemours & Co., 1600 Waukegan Road, Waukegan, IL 60085 Tel: 800/323-4980 (A), 312/473-3000 (A)

Du Pont Pharmaceuticals, E.I. du Pont de Nemours & Co., Barley Mill Plaza, Caverly Mill, Building 26, Wilmington, DE 19898 Tel: 1-800/441-8961 (A) (outside DE), 800/441-3273 (A) (in DE)

Elkins-Sinn, Inc., Subsidiary of A.H. Robins Company, Two Esterbrook Lane, Cherry Hill, NJ 08003-4099 Tel: 800/257-8349

Ethitek Pharmaceuticals Company, 8104 North Lawndale Avenue, Skokie, IL 60076 Tel: 312/675-6616 (A)

Fisher Medical Division, Division of Fisher Scientific Group Inc., 526 Route 303, Orangeburg, NY 10962 Tel:

COMPENDIUM OF DRUG THERAPY

69

DIRECTORY OF MANUFACTURERS

Key

BH = Business hours
N = Nights (after business hours)
H = Holidays
W = Weekends
A = All times (including nights, holidays, and weekends)

800/431-1861 (8 am-5 pm Mon-Fri) (outside NY), 914/359-9200 (A)

Fisons Corporation, Pharmaceutical Division, Two Preston Court, Bedford, MA 01730   Tel: 617/275-1000 ext 352 (BH), 617/275-3037 (N,H,W), 617/275-1000 ext 341 (emergencies)

C.B. Fleet Company, Inc., 4615 Murray Place, Lynchburg, VA 24506   Tel: 800/446-0991, 804/528-4000 (BH)

Flint Laboratories, Inc., 1425 Lake Cook Road, Deerfield, IL 60015   Tel: 1-800/323-1817 (7:30 am-4:30 pm Mon-Fri) (outside IL), 312/940-5220 (7:30 am-4:30 pm Mon-Fri)

Forest Pharmaceuticals, Inc., Subsidiary of Forest Laboratories, Inc., 2510 Metro Boulevard, Maryland Heights, MO 63043-9979   Tel: 314/569-3610 (A)

Geigy Pharmaceuticals, Division of CIBA-GEIGY Corporation, 556 Morris Avenue, Summit, NJ 07901   Tel: 201/277-5000 (A)

Genentech, Inc., 460 Point San Bruno Boulevard, South San Francisco, CA 94080   Tel: 800/821-8590 (A)

Gilbert Laboratories, Affiliate of Forest Pharmaceuticals, Inc., 31 Fairmont Avenue, Chester, NJ 07930   Tel: 201/879-7374

Glaxo Inc., Five Moore Drive, Research Triangle Park, NC 27709   Tel: 1-800/334-0089 (A), 919/248-2100 (A)

Glenbrook Laboratories, Division of Sterling Drug Inc., 90 Park Avenue, New York, NY 10016   Tel: 212/907-2790 (BH), 212/907-2000 (N,H,W)

Glenwood Inc., 83 North Summit Street, Tenafly, NJ 07670   Tel: 201/569-0050 (8 am-5 pm Mon-Fri)

Gray Pharmaceutical Co., Affiliate of The Purdue Frederick Company, 100 Connecticut Avenue, Norwalk, CT 06856   Tel: 203/853-0123

Herbert Laboratories, Dermatology Division of Allergan Pharmaceuticals, Inc., 2525 Dupont Drive, Irvine, CA 92715   Tel: 714/752-4500 ext 4281, 4586, or 4959 (BH); 714/752-4335 or 714/752-4244 (N,H,W)

Hermal Pharmaceutical Laboratories, Route 145, Oak Hill, NY 12460   Tel: 518/239-4714 (8 am-4:30 pm Mon-Fri)

Hoechst-Roussel Pharmaceuticals Inc., Route 202-206 North, Somerville, NJ 08876   Tel: 201/231-2611 (8:30 am-5 pm Mon-Fri), 201/231-2000 (A)

Hynson, Westcott & Dunning Products, BBL Microbiology Systems, Division of Becton Dickinson and Company, 250 Schilling Circle, Cockeysville, MD 21030   Tel: 301/584-7177

ICI Pharma, Division of ICI Americas Inc., Concord Pike and New Murphy Road, Wilmington, DE 19897   Tel: 800/441-7758 (8:15 am-4:30 pm Mon-Fri) (outside DE), 302/576-3000 (A)

ICN Pharmaceuticals, Inc., 3300 Hyland Avenue, Costa Mesa, CA 92626   Tel: 800/556-1937 (outside CA), 800/331-2331 (in CA), 714/545-0100 (A)

Iolab Pharmaceuticals, Division of Johnson & Johnson Company, 861 South Village Oaks Drive, Covina, CA 91724   Tel: 800/423-1871 (outside CA), 800/352-1891 (in CA), 818/915-7681 (A)

Janssen Pharmaceutica Inc., Division of Johnson & Johnson Company, 40 Kingsbridge Road, Piscataway, NJ 08854-3998   Tel: 201/524-9881 (A)

Jeffrey Martin Inc., 410 Clermont Terrace, Union, NJ 07083   Tel: 201/687-4000

KabiVitrum, Inc., 1311 Harbor Bay Parkway, Alameda, CA 94501   Tel: 1-800/227-1518, 1-800/526-5224, 415/769-4600 (A) (in CA)

Kendall McGaw Laboratories, Inc., 2525 McGaw Avenue, Irvine, CA 92714-5895   Tel: 800/854-8651 (A)

Key Pharmaceuticals, Division of Schering-Plough Corporation, Galloping Hill Road, Kenilworth, NJ 07033   Tel: 201/558-4908 (BH), 201/558-4000 (N,H,W)

Knoll Pharmaceuticals, A Unit of BASF K&F Corporation, c/o Medical Affairs Department, 30 North Jefferson Road, Whippany, NJ 07981   Tel: 800/526-0221 (outside NJ), 201/428-8250 (A)

Kremers Urban Company, PO Box 2038, Milwaukee, WI 53201   Tel: 800/558-5114 (7:30 am-4 pm Mon-Fri) (outside WI), 414/354-4300

Lactaid Inc., 600 Fire Road, PO Box 111, Pleasantville, NJ 08232-0111   Tel: 609/645-7500

Lakeside Pharmaceuticals Inc., Division of Merrell Dow Pharmaceuticals Inc., 10123 Alliance Road, Cincinnati, OH 45242-9553   Tel: 513/948-6040 (8:15 am-5 pm), 513/948-9111 (N,W)

Lederle Laboratories, A Division of American Cyanamid Company, Middletown Road, Pearl River, NY 10965   Tel: 914/735-5000 (A)

Leeming Division, Pfizer Inc., 100 Jefferson Road, Parsippany, NJ 07054   Tel: 201/887-2100

Lemmon Company, 850 Cathill Road, Sellersville, PA 18960   Tel: 800/523-6542 (8 am-5 pm Mon-Fri) (outside PA), 215/723-5544 (8 am-5 pm Mon-Fri)

Eli Lilly and Company, Lilly Corporate Center, Indianapolis, IN 46285   Tel: 317/261-3704 (BH), 317/261-2000 (N,H,W)

Loma Linda Foods, Inc., 11503 Pierce Street, Riverside, CA 92515   Tel: 1-800/932-5525 (8 am-5 pm Mon-Thurs, 8 am-2 pm Fri) (outside CA), 800/442-4917 (8 am-5 pm Mon-Thurs, 8 am-2 pm Fri) (in CA), 714/687-7800 (8 am-5 pm Mon-Thurs, 8 am-2 pm Fri)

Marion Laboratories, Inc., Medical Information, Park A, PO Box 9627, Kansas City, MO 64134   Tel: 800/821-2130 (A) (outside MO), 816/966-5000 (A)

McNeil Consumer Products Company, Camp Hill Road, Fort Washington, PA 19034   Tel: 215/233-7000

McNeil Pharmaceutical, Welsh Road, Spring House, PA 19477   Tel: 215/628-5000 (A)

Mead Johnson Nutritionals, Bristol-Myers U.S. Pharmaceutical and Nutritional Group, 2404 West Pennsylvania Street, Evansville, IN 47721-0001   Tel: 812/429-7983 (BH), 812/ 429-5000 (A)

Mead Johnson Laboratories, Bristol-Myers U.S. Pharmaceutical and Nutritional Group, 2404 West Pennsylvania Street, Evansville, IN 47721-0001   Tel: 812/429-5000 (7:30 am-4 pm Mon-Fri), 812/429-7500 (N,H,W)

Mead Johnson Pharmaceuticals, Bristol-Myers U.S. Pharmaceutical and Nutritional Group, 2404 West Pennsylvania Street, Evansville, IN 47721-0001   Tel: 812/429-5000 (7:30 am-4 pm Mon-Fri), 812/429-7500 (N,H,W)

Medicone Company, 225 Varick Street, New York, NY 10014   Tel: 212/924-5166

The Mentholatum Company, 1360 Niagara Street, Buffalo, NY 14213   Tel: 800/822-1400 (outside NY), 716/882-7660 (8:45 am-5:15 pm)

Merck Sharp & Dohme, Division of Merck & Co., Inc., Building 35-9, Sumneytown Pike, West Point, PA 19486   Tel: 215/661-7300 (8:30 am-4:45 pm Mon-Fri), 215/661-5000 (N,H,W, emergencies)

Merrell Dow Pharmaceuticals Inc., Subsidiary of The Dow Chemical Company, 10123 Alliance Road, Cincinnati, OH 45242-9553   Tel: 513/948-6040 (8:15 am-5 pm), 513/948-9111 (N,W, emergencies)

Miles Laboratories, Inc., Consumer Healthcare Division, 1127 Myrtle Street, Elkhart, IN 46515   Tel: 219/264-8955 (8 am-5 pm Mon-Fri), 219/264-8111 (N,H,W)

Miles Pharmaceuticals, Division of Miles Laboratories, Inc., 400 Morgan Lane, West Haven, CT 06516   Tel: 203/937-2000 (A)

Monoclonal Antibodies, Inc., 2319 Charleston Road, Mountain View, CA 94043   Tel: 800/227-8855 (outside CA), 415/960-1320

Neutrogena Corporation, 5755 West 96th Street, Los Angeles, CA 90045   Tel: 800/421-6857 (8:30 am-5 pm Mon-Fri) (in CA), 213/642-1150 (8:30 am-5 pm Mon-Fri)

NMS Pharmaceuticals, Inc., 1533 Monrovia Avenue, Newport Beach, CA 92663   Tel: 800/854-3002 (outside CA), 800/367-4200 (in CA), 714/645-2111

Norcliff Thayer Inc., 303 South Broadway, Tarrytown, NY 10591   Tel: 914/631-0033

Nordisk-USA, Affiliate of Nordisk

DIRECTORY OF MANUFACTURERS

Gentofte, 3202 Monroe Street, Suite 100, Rockville, MD 20852 Tel: 301/770-4400 (BH)

Norwich Eaton Pharmaceuticals, Inc., A Procter & Gamble Company, PO Box 231, Norwich, NY 13815-0231 Tel: 607/335-2565 (A)

Organon Inc., 375 Mount Pleasant Avenue, West Orange, NJ 07052 Tel: 800/631-1253 (8 am-5 pm Mon-Fri) (outside NJ), 201/325-4500 (8 am-5 pm Mon-Fri)

Organon Teknika Inc., 800 Capitol Drive, Durham, NC 27713 Tel: 919/361-1995

Ortho Dermatological Division, Ortho Pharmaceutical Corporation, Route 202, PO Box 300, Raritan, NJ 08869-0602 Tel: 201/524-0400

Ortho Diagnostic Systems, Inc., Route 202, Raritan, NJ 08869 Tel: 800/526-3875 (outside NJ), 201/218-8152

Ortho Pharmaceutical Corporation, Route 202, PO Box 300, Raritan, NJ 08869-0602 Tel: 201/218-6000 (BH), 201/524-0400 (N,H,W)

Owen Laboratories, Division of Alcon Laboratories, Inc., 6201 South Freeway, Fort Worth, TX 76134 Tel: 817/293-0450

Parke-Davis, Division of Warner-Lambert Company, 201 Tabor Road, Morris Plains, NJ 07950 Tel: 800/223-0432 (9 am-5 pm Mon-Fri) (outside NJ), 201/540-2000 (A)

Parke-Davis Consumer Health Products Group, Warner-Lambert Company, 201 Tabor Road, Morris Plains, NJ 07950 Tel: 201/540-2000

Pennwalt Prescription Division, Pennwalt Corporation, 755 Jefferson Road, Rochester, NY 14623 Tel: 716/475-9000 (A)

Pfizer Laboratories Division, Pfizer Inc., 235 East 42nd Street, New York, NY 10017 Tel: 212/573-2422 (A)

Pharmacia Laboratories, Division of Pharmacia Inc., 800 Centennial Avenue, Piscataway, NJ 08854 Tel: 1-800/526-3619 (8:30 am-4:45 pm Mon-Fri) (outside NJ), 201/457-8000 (8:30 am-4:45 pm Mon-Fri), 201/457-0571 (N,H,W)

Pharmacraft Division, Pennwalt Corporation, 755 Jefferson Road, Rochester, NY 14623 Tel: 716/475-9000 ext 2375 (8 am-4:45 pm) (BH), 716/475-9000 (N,H,W)

Plough, Inc., 3030 Jackson Avenue, Memphis, TN 38151-0377 Tel: 901/320-2386 (BH), 901/320-2011 (emergencies)

Polymer Technology Corporation, 100 Research Drive, Wilmington, MA 01887 Tel: 800/343-1445 (A) (outside MA), 617/658-6111 (A)

Poythress Laboratories, Inc., 16 North 22nd Street, Richmond, VA 23261 Tel: 804/644-8591 (8 am-4:30 pm Mon-Fri)

Princeton Pharmaceutical Products, Subsidiary of E.R. Squibb & Sons, Inc., PO Box 4000, Princeton, NJ 08543-4000 Tel: 609/921-4006 (A)

The Procter & Gamble Company, 11511 Reed Hartman Highway, Cincinnati, OH 45241 Tel: 513/530-2154 (BH) (in OH), 513/751-5525 (N,H,W) (call collect)

The Purdue Frederick Company, 100 Connecticut Avenue, Norwalk, CT 06856 Tel: 203/853-0123

Reed & Carnrick Pharmaceuticals, Division of Block Drug Company, One New England Avenue, Piscataway, NJ 08854 Tel: 201/981-0070

Reid-Rowell, 901 Sawyer Road, Marietta, GA 30062 Tel: 404/898-1040 (BH), 404/973-1982 (N,H,W)

Richardson-Vicks Inc. Health Care Products Division, One Far Mill Crossing, Shelton, CT 06484 Tel: 203/929-2500 (A)

Richardson-Vicks Inc. Personal Care Products Division, One Far Mill Crossing, Shelton, CT 06484 Tel: 203/929-2500 (8:30 am-4:30 pm Mon-Fri), 301/328-2425 (N,W, emergencies)

Riker Laboratories, Inc., Subsidiary of 3M Company, Building 225-1N-07, 3M Center, St. Paul, MN 55144-1000 Tel: 612/736-4930 (A)

A.H. Robins Company, 1407 Cummings Drive, Richmond, VA 23220 Tel: 804/257-2000 (A), 804/257-7788 (N,H,W)

Roche Diagnostic Systems, Division of Hoffmann-La Roche Inc., 11 Franklin Avenue, Belleville, NJ 07109 Tel: 1-800/526-1247 (BH), 1-201/235-5000 (N,H,W emergencies)

Roche Laboratories, Division of Hoffman-La Roche Inc., Professional Services Department, 340 Kingsland Street, Nutley, NJ 07110 Tel: 201/235-2355 (8:30 am-5 pm Mon-Fri) (emergencies)

Roerig, A Division of Pfizer Pharmaceuticals, 235 East 42nd Street, New York, NY 10017 Tel: 212/573-2187 (A)

Rorer Pharmaceutical Corporation, 500 Virginia Drive, Fort Washington, PA 19034 Tel: 215/628-6159 (8:15 am-4:45 pm Mon-Fri), 215/628-6671 (8:15 am-4:45 pm Mon-Fri) (N,H,W), 215/628-6200 (emergencies)

Ross Laboratories, A Division of Abbott Laboratories, 625 Cleveland Avenue, Columbus, OH 43216 Tel: 614/227-3333 (A)

Roxane Laboratories, Inc., PO Box 16532, Columbus, OH 43216 Tel: 800/848-0120 (BH) (outside OH), 614/276-4000 (BH), 614/261-6563 (N,H,W)

Sandoz Consumer Health Care Group, One Upper Pond Road, Parsippany, NJ 07054 Tel: 201/386-7764 (BH), 201/386-7500 (N,H,W)

Sandoz Nutrition Corporation, Clinical Products Division, 5320 West 23rd Street, Minneapolis, MN 55440 Tel: 800/328-7874, 612/925-2100

Sandoz Pharmaceuticals Corporation, 59 Route 10, East Hanover, NJ 07936 Tel: 201/386-7764 (BH), 201/386-7500 (N,H,W)

Savage Laboratories, Division of Atlanta Inc., 60 Baylis Road, Melville, NY 11747 Tel: 800/213-0206 (8:45 am-4:45 pm Mon-Fri) (outside NY), 516/454-9071 (8:45 am-4:45 pm Mon-Fri)

Schering Corporation, Galloping Hill Road, Kenilworth, NJ 07033 Tel: 201/558-4908 (BH), 201/558-4000 (N,H,W)

Schmid Laboratories, Inc., Route 46 West, Little Falls, NJ 07424-0415 Tel: 201/256-5500 (BH)

Searle Pharmaceuticals Inc., Subsidiary of G.D. Searle & Co., 4901 Searle Parkway, Skokie, IL 60077 Tel: 800/323-4204 (BH) (outside IL), 312/982-7000 (A)

Self Care Systems, Inc., 1527 Monrovia Avenue, Newport Beach, CA 92663 Tel: 800/854-3002 (outside CA), 800/367-4200 (in CA), 714/645-4244

Serono Laboratories, Inc., 280 Pond Street, Randolph, MA 02368 Tel: 800/225-5185 (A) (outside MA), 617/963-8154 (A)

Smith Kline & French Laboratories, A SmithKline Beckman Company, 1500 Spring Garden Street, Philadelphia, PA 19101 Tel: 800/523-4835 (A) (outside PA), 215/751-5231 (BH), 215/751-5900 (N,H,W)

SmithKline Consumer Products, A SmithKline Beckman Company, 680 Allendale Road, King of Prussia, PA 19406 Tel: 215/768-3600 (BH), 215/751-5000 (N,H,W)

SmithKline Diagnostics, Inc., A SmithKline Beckman Company, 485 Potrero Avenue, PO Box 3947, Sunnyvale, CA 94008-3947 Tel: 800/538-1581, 408/732-6000

E.R. Squibb & Sons, Inc., PO Box 4000, Princeton, NJ 08543-4000 Tel: 609/921-4006 (A)

Squibb-Novo, Inc., 211 Carnegie Center, Princeton, NJ 08540-6213 Tel: 609/987-5800 (8:30 am-5 pm), 609/987-5800 (N,H,W)

Stiefel Laboratories, Route 145, Oak Hill, NY 12460 Tel: 518/239-6901 (8:30 am-5 pm Mon-Fri)

Stuart Pharmaceuticals, Division of ICI Americas Inc., Concord Pike and New Murphy Road, Wilmington, DE 19897 Tel: 800/441-7758 (8:15 am-4:30 pm Mon-Fri) (outside DE), 302/575-3000 (A)

Syntex Laboratories, Inc., 3401 Hillview Avenue, Palo Alto, CA 94304 Tel: 415/855-5545 or 415/852-1384 (BH), 415/855-5050 (A)

Syntex Medical Diagnostics, 900 Arastradero Road, Palo Alto, CA 94304 Tel: 800/821-1131 (outside CA), 800/367-7633 (in CA), 415/494-1086

Syva Company, 900 Arastradero Road, Palo Alto, CA 94304 Tel: 800/227-8994 (outside CA), 800/982-6006 (in CA)

Tambrands Inc., One Marcus Avenue, Lake Success, NY 11042 Tel: 516/437-8800

TAP Pharmaceuticals, 1400 Sheridan Road, North Chicago, IL 60064 Tel: 1-800/622-2011 (A)

Thompson Medical Company, Inc., 919 Third Avenue, New York, NY 10022 Tel: 212/688-4420 (A)

3M Company, Consumer Specialties

DIRECTORY OF MANUFACTURERS

Key

BH = Business hours
N = Nights (after business hours)
H = Holidays
W = Weekends
A = All times (including nights, holidays, and weekends)

Division—Personal Care Products/ 3M, 3M Center, St. Paul, MN 55144-1000 Tel: 612/733-1110

Travenol Laboratories, Inc., Wilson Road at Route 120, Round Lake, IL 60073 Tel: 312/546-6311

United States Packaging Corporation, 506 Clay Street, La Porte, IN 46350 Tel: 219/362-9782

The Upjohn Company, 7000 Portage Road, Kalamazoo, MI 49001 Tel: 616/323-6615 (A)

Upsher-Smith Laboratories, Inc., 14905 23rd Avenue North, Minneapolis, MN 55441 Tel: 612/473-4412 (8 am–5 pm Mon–Fri)

VLI Corporation, 2031 Main Street, Irvine, CA 92714 Tel: 800/223-2329 (8 am–4 pm Mon–Fri) (outside CA), 800/222-2329 (8 am–4 pm Mon–Fri) (in CA), 714/863-9511

Wallace Laboratories, Division of Carter-Wallace, Inc., Half Acre Road, Cranbury, NJ 08512 Tel: 609/655-6000 (BH), 609/799-1167 (N,H,W)

Wampole Laboratories, Division of Carter-Wallace, Inc., Half Acre Road, Cranbury, NJ 08512 Tel: 800/257-9525 (outside NJ), 609/655-6000

Warner-Lambert Consumer Health Products Group, Warner-Lambert Company, 201 Tabor Road, Morris Plains, NJ 07950 Tel: 201/540-2000

Webcon Pharmaceuticals, Division of Alcon Laboratories, Inc., 6201 South Freeway, Fort Worth, TX 76134 Tel: 817/293-0450 (BH), 817/921-0884 (N,H,W)

Westwood Pharmaceuticals Inc., 100 Forest Avenue, Buffalo, NY 14213 Tel: 716/887-3400

Whitehall Laboratories, Division of American Home Products Corporation, 685 Third Avenue, New York, NY 10017-4076 Tel: 212/878-5508

Winthrop Consumer Products, Division of Sterling Drug Inc., 90 Park Avenue, New York, NY 10016 Tel: 212/907-2525, 212/907-2000

Winthrop Pharmaceuticals, Division of Sterling Drug Inc., 90 Park Avenue, New York, NY 10016 Tel: 800/446-6267 (BH), 212/907-2525 (BH), 212/907-2000 (A)

Winthrop-Breon, see Winthrop Pharmaceuticals

Wyeth Laboratories, Division of American Home Products Corporation, King of Prussia Road and Lancaster Avenue, Radnor, PA 19087 Tel: 215/688-4400 (A)

Product Imprint Codes

Symbols and Abbreviations

ⓐ	Abbott
▲	Ascher
BMP	Beecham
BI	Boehringer Ingelheim
◯	Knoll
KU	Kremers Urban
ℒℒ	Lederle
MJ	Mead Johnson
MSD	Merck Sharp & Dohme
P-D	Parke-Davis
◑	Pharmacia
AHR	Robins
WHR	Rorer
ᴙ	Ross
S	Sandoz Pharmaceuticals
▽	Savage
Schering	Schering
SKF	Smith Kline & French
W	Winthrop Pharmaceuticals

Abbott

AA	Chlorthalidone, 25 mg
AB	Chlorthalidone, 50 mg
AD	PEGANONE (ethotoin), 250 mg
AE	PEGANONE (ethotoin), 500 mg
AF	Colchicine, 0.6 mg
AH	ORETICYL 25 (hydrochlorothiazide and deserpidine)
AI	ORETICYL 50 (hydrochlorothiazide and deserpidine)
AJ	FERO-FOLIC-500 (iron, folic acid, and vitamin C)
AK	IBERET-FOLIC-500 (multivitamin)
AM	TRIDIONE (trimethadione), 300 mg
AN	Dicumarol, 25 mg
AO	Dicumarol, 50 mg
AT	VERCYTE (pipobroman), 25 mg
CF	NEMBUTAL (pentobarbital), 50 mg
CH	NEMBUTAL (pentobarbital), 100 mg
EA	Erythromycin, 500 mg
EB	Erythromycin, 250 mg
EC	ERY-TAB (erythromycin), 250 mg
ED	ERY-TAB (erythromycin), 500 mg
EE	E.E.S. 400 (erythromycin), 400 mg
EF	E.E.S. (erythromycin), 200 mg
EH	ERY-TAB (erythromycin), 333 mg
ES	ERYTHROCIN (erythromycin), 250 mg
ET	ERYTHROCIN (erythromycin), 500 mg
HH	DEPAKENE (valproic acid), 250 mg
II	PHENURONE (phenacemide), 500 mg
KH	PLACIDYL (ethchlorvynol), 500 mg
KN	PLACIDYL (ethchlorvynol), 750 mg
LE	TRIDIONE (trimethadione), 150 mg
LF	PANWARFIN (warfarin), 10 mg
LK	HARMONYL (deserpidine), 0.25 mg
LL	ORETICYL Forte (hydrochlorothiazide and deserpidine)
LM	PANWARFIN (warfarin), 2 mg
LN	PANWARFIN (warfarin), 2.5 mg
LO	PANWARFIN (warfarin), 5 mg
LR	PANWARFIN (warfarin), 7.5 mg
LS	ENDURONYL (methyclothiazide and deserpidine)
LT	ENDURONYL FORTE (methyclothiazide and deserpidine)
LU	OGEN (estropipate), 0.75 mg
LV	OGEN (estropipate), 1.5 mg
LX	OGEN (estropipate), 3 mg
LY	OGEN (estropipate), 6 mg
MC	DESOXYN (methamphetamine), 5 mg (sustained-release tablets)
ME	DESOXYN (methamphetamine), 10 mg
MF	DESOXYN (methamphetamine), 15 mg
NA	EUTONYL (pargyline), 10 mg
NB	EUTONYL (pargyline), 25 mg
ND	JANIMINE (imipramine), 10 mg
NE	JANIMINE (imipramine), 25 mg
NF	TRAL (hexocyclium), 25 mg
NJ	CEFOL (multivitamin), 25 mg
NK	EUTRON (pargyline and methyclothiazide)
NL	JANIMINE (imipramine), 50 mg
NM	K-TAB (potassium), 10 mEq
NR	DEPAKOTE (divalproex), 250 mg
NS	DEPAKOTE (divalproex), 500 mg
NT	DEPAKOTE (divalproex), 125 mg
TE	DESOXYN (methamphetamine), 5 mg
TF	GEMONIL (metharbital), 100 mg
TH	CYLERT (pemoline), 18.75 mg
TI	CYLERT (pemoline), 37.5 mg
TJ	CYLERT (pemoline), 75 mg

continued

COMPENDIUM OF DRUG THERAPY

PRODUCT IMPRINT CODES

TK	CYLERT (pemoline), 37.5 mg (chewable tablets)	8	COMBIPRES 0.1 (clonidine and chlorthalidone)
TL	TRANXENE (clorazepate), 3.75 mg	9	COMBIPRES 0.2 (clonidine and chlorthalidone)
TM	TRANXENE (clorazepate), 7.5 mg	10	COMBIPRES 0.3 (clonidine and chlorthalidone)
TN	TRANXENE (clorazepate), 15 mg	11	CATAPRES (clonidine), 0.3 mg
TX	TRANXENE-SD (clorazepate), 11.25 mg	12	DULCOLAX (bisacodyl), 5 mg
TY	TRANXENE-SD (clorazepate), 22.5 mg	17	PERSANTINE (dipyridamole), 25 mg
		18	PERSANTINE (dipyridamole), 50 mg
		19	PERSANTINE (dipyridamole), 75 mg

Adria

130	AXOTAL (aspirin and butalbital)	28	TORECAN (thiethylperazine), 10 mg
200	ILOZYME (pancrelipase)	31	CATAPRES TTS-1 (clonidine), 0.1 mg
217	EVAC-Q-TABS (phenolphthalein), 130 mg	32	CATAPRES TTS-2 (clonidine), 0.2 mg
231	ILOPAN-CHOLINE (dexpanthenol and choline)	33	CATAPRES TTS-3 (clonidine), 0.3 mg
239	OCTAMIDE (metoclopramide), 10 mg	48	RESPBID (theophylline), 250 mg
304	KAON CL-10 (potassium chloride), 10 mEq	49	RESPBID (theophylline), 500 mg
307	KAON-CL (potassium chloride), 6.7 mEq	62	PRELUDIN (phenmetrazine), 75 mg
312	KAON (potassium), 5 mEq	64	PRELU-2 (phendimetrazine), 105 mg
412	MAGAN (magnesium salicylate), 545 mg	66	MEXITIL (mexiletine), 150 mg
501	MODANE (danthron), 75 mg	67	MEXITIL (mexiletine), 200 mg
502	MODANE Mild (danthron), 37.5 mg	68	MEXITIL (mexiletine), 250 mg
503	MODANE Soft (docusate), 120 mg	72	ALUPENT (metaproterenol), 20 mg
504	MODANE Plus (danthron and docusate)	74	ALUPENT (metaproterenol), 10 mg
		76	THALITONE (chlorthalidone), 25 mg

Ascher

CIBA

0310	MOBIDIN (magnesium salicylate), 600 mg	3	RITALIN (methylphenidate), 10 mg
225/105	TOLFRINIC (iron, cyanocobalamin, and vitamin C)	7	RITALIN (methylphenidate), 5 mg
225/250	ETHAQUIN (ethaverine), 100 mg	13	SERPASIL-ESIDRIX No. 1 (reserpine and hydrochlorothiazide)
225/295	ANASPAZ (hyoscyamine), 0.125 mg	15	ANTRENYL (oxyphenonium), 5 mg
225/300	ANASPAZ PB (hyoscyamine and phenobarbital)	16	RITALIN-SR (methylphenidate), 20 mg
225/356	MOBIGESIC (magnesium salicylate and phenyltoloxamine)	22	ESIDRIX (hydrochlorothiazide), 25 mg
225/400	ADIPOST (phendimetrazine), 105 mg	24	CYTADREN (aminoglutethimide), 250 mg
225/410	METRONID (metronidazole), 250 mg	26	LUDIOMIL (maprotiline), 50 mg
225/450	FUROSE (furosemide), 40 mg	30	METANDREN (methyltestosterone), 10 mg (tablets)
225/450	HY-PHEN (hydrocodone and acetaminophen)	32	METANDREN (methyltestosterone), 25 mg
		34	RITALIN (methylphenidate), 20 mg

Beecham Laboratories

105	ANEXSIA with CODEINE (aspirin, caffeine, and codeine)	35	SERPASIL (reserpine), 0.1 mg
106	ANEXSIA-D (aspirin and hydrocodone)	36	SERPASIL (reserpine), 0.25 mg
112	DASIN (aspirin, caffeine, and atropine)	37	APRESOLINE (hydralazine), 10 mg
119	HYBEPHEN (belladonna alkaloids and phenobarbital)	39	APRESOLINE (hydralazine), 25 mg
121	LIVITAMIN (multivitamin)	40	SERPASIL-APRESOLINE No. 1 (reserpine and hydralazine)
122	LIVITAMIN with Intrinsic Factor (multivitamin)	41	ANTURANE (sulfinpyrazone), 100 mg
123	LIVITAMIN Chewable (multivitamin)	46	ESIDRIX (hydrochlorothiazide), 50 mg
125	MENEST (esterified estrogens), 0.3 mg	47	ESIMIL (guanethidine and hydrochlorothiazide)
126	MENEST (esterified estrogens), 0.625 mg	49	ISMELIN (guanethidine), 10 mg
127	MENEST (esterified estrogens), 1.25 mg	51	METANDREN (methyltestosterone), 5 mg
128	MENEST (esterified estrogens), 2.5 mg	64	METANDREN (methyltestosterone), 10 mg (caplets)
135	SEMETS (benzocaine and cetylpyridium)	65	LITHOBID (lithium), 300 mg
140	TOTACILLIN (ampicillin), 250 mg	71	SER-AP-ES (reserpine, hydralazine, and hydrochlorothiazide)
141	TOTACILLIN (ampicillin), 500 mg	73	APRESOLINE (hydralazine), 50 mg
143	BACTOCILL (oxacillin), 250 mg	97	SERPASIL-ESIDRIX No. 2 (reserpine and hydrochlorothiazide)
144	BACTOCILL (oxacillin), 500 mg	101	APRESOLINE (hydralazine), 100 mg
145	DARICON (oxphencylimine), 10 mg	103	ISMELIN (guanethidine), 25 mg
146	DARICON-PB (oxphencylimine and phenobarbital)	104	SERPASIL-APRESOLINE No. 2 (reserpine and hydralazine)
156	TIGAN (trimethobenzamide), 100 mg	110	LUDIOMIL (maprotiline), 25 mg
157	TIGAN (trimethobenzamide), 250 mg	129	APRESOLINE-ESIDRIX (hydralazine and hydrochlorothiazide)
165	DYCILL (dicloxacillin), 250 mg	130	METOPIRONE (metyrapone), 250 mg
166	DYCILL (dicloxacillin), 500 mg	135	LUDIOMIL (maprotiline), 75 mg
169	CLOXAPEN (cloxacillin), 250 mg	139	APRESAZIDE 25/25 (hydralazine and hydrochlorothiazide)
170	CLOXAPEN (cloxacillin), 500 mg	149	APRESAZIDE 50/50 (hydralazine and hydrochlorothiazide)
182	NUCOFED (pseudoephedrine and codeine)	154	RIMACTANE (rifampin), 300 mg
185	BEEPEN-VK (penicillin V), 250 mg	159	APRESAZIDE 100/50 (hydralazine and hydrochlorothiazide)
186	BEEPEN-VK (penicillin V), 500 mg	165	SLOW-K (potassium chloride), 600 mg
189	AUGMENTIN 125 (amoxicillin and clavulanate)	168	ANTURANE (sulfinpyrazone), 200 mg
190	AUGMENTIN 250 (amoxicillin and clavulanate)	192	ESIDRIX (hydrochlorothiazide), 100 mg
194	ENARAX 5 (oxphencylimine and hydroxyzine)	2025	TRANSDERM-NITRO (nitroglycerin), 5 cm^2
195	ENARAX 10 (oxphencyclimine and hydroxyzine)	2105	TRANSDERM-NITRO (nitroglycerin), 10 cm^2
210	CONAR-A (phenylephrine, dextromethorphan, acetaminophen, and guaifenesin)		

Boehringer Ingelheim

6	CATAPRES (clonidine), 0.1 mg
7	CATAPRES (clonidine), 0.2 mg

PRODUCT IMPRINT CODES

2110	TRANSDERM-NITRO (nitroglycerin), 20 cm^2
2115	TRANSDERM-NITRO (nitroglycerin), 30 cm^2
4345	TRANSDERM SCOP (nitroglycerin), 2.5 cm^2

Dista

C03	ILOTYCIN (erythromycin), 250 mg
C19	MI-CEBRIN (multivitamin)
C20	MI-CEBRIN T (multivitamin)
C22	BECOTIN-T (multivitamin)
F62	BECOTIN (multivitamin)
F77	BECOTIN with Vitamin C (multivitamin)
H07	ILOSONE (erythromycin), 125 mg
H09	ILOSONE (erythromycin), 250 mg
H69	KEFLEX (cephalexin), 250 mg
H71	KEFLEX (cephalexin), 500 mg
H74	VALMID (ethinamate), 500 mg
H76	NALFON (fenoprofen), 200 mg
H77	NALFON (fenoprofen), 300 mg
U05	ILOSONE (erythromycin), 125 mg
U25	ILOSONE (erythromycin), 250 mg
U26	ILOSONE (erythromycin), 500 mg
U59	NALFON (fenoprofen), 600 mg
U60	KEFLEX (cephalexin), 1 g
3055	CINOBAC (cinoxacin), 250 mg
3056	CINOBAC (cinoxacin), 500 mg
3122	CO-PYRONIL 2 Pediatric (chlorpheniramine and pseudoephedrine)
3123	CO-PYRONIL 2 (chlorpheniramine and pseudoephedrine)

Du Pont

0072	MOBAN (molindone), 5 mg
0073	MOBAN (molindone), 10 mg
0074	MOBAN (molindone), 25 mg
0076	MOBAN (molindone), 50 mg
0077	MOBAN (molindone), 100 mg
0056/0010	TESSALON (benzonatate), 100 mg
0056/0080	TREXAN (naltrexone), 50 mg
0060/0127	PERCOCET (oxycodone and acetaminophen)
0060/0135	PERCODAN (oxycodone and aspirin)
0060/0136	PERCODAN-DEMI (oxycodone and aspirin)

Geigy

14	BUTAZOLIDIN (phenylbutazone), 100 mg (tablets)
20	TOFRANIL-PM (imipramine), 75 mg
22	TOFRANIL-PM (imipramine), 150 mg
23	LIORESAL (baclofen), 10 mg
32	TOFRANIL (imipramine), 10 mg
33	LIORESAL (baclofen), 20 mg
40	TOFRANIL-PM (imipramine), 100 mg
42	CONSTANT-T (theophylline), 200 mg
44	BUTAZOLIDIN (phenylbutazone), 100 mg (capsules)
45	TOFRANIL-PM (imipramine), 125 mg
48	PBZ-SR (tripelennamine), 100 mg
51	LOPRESSOR (metoprolol), 50 mg
52	TEGRETOL (carbamazepine), 100 mg
57	CONSTANT-T (theophylline), 300 mg
67	TEGRETOL (carbamazepine), 200 mg
71	LOPRESSOR (metoprolol), 100 mg
72	BRETHINE (terbutaline), 2.5 mg
105	BRETHINE (terbutaline), 5 mg
111	PBZ (tripelennamine), 25 mg
117	PBZ (tripelennamine), 50 mg
136	TOFRANIL (imipramine), 50 mg
140	TOFRANIL (imipramine), 25 mg

Glaxo

232	ATHEMOL (theobromine and nicotinate)
255	ATHEMOL-N (theobromine and nicotinate)
268	THEOBID (theophylline), 260 mg
281	ETHATAB (ethaverine), 100 mg
295	THEOBID Jr. (theophylline), 130 mg
309	HISTABID (phenylpropanolamine and chlorpheniramine)
316	VICON FORTE (multivitamin)

Hoechst-Roussel

72	FESTAL II (digestive enzymes)
73	FESTALAN (atropine and digestive enzymes)

ICN

0901	TESTRED (methyltestosterone), 10 mg

Knoll

11	AKINETON (biperiden), 2 mg
14	QUADRINAL (ephedrine and phenobarbital)
24	VICODIN (hydrocodone and acetaminophen)

Kremers Urban

1	CALCIFEROL (ergocalciferol), 1.25 mg
050	FEDAHIST (chlorpheniramine and pseudoephedrine)
171	GEMNISYN (aspirin and acetaminophen)
202	CHARDONNA-2 (belladonna and phenobarbital)
475	KUTRASE (hyoscyamine, phenyltoloxamine, and digestive enzymes)
500	LACTRASE (lactase), 125 mg
522	KU-ZYME (digestive enzymes)
525	KU-ZYME HP (pancrelipase)
531	LEVSIN (hyoscyamine), 0.125 mg
534	LEVSIN with Phenobarbital (hyoscyamine and phenobarbital)
537	LEVSINEX (hyoscyamine), 0.375 mg
539	LEVSINEX with Phenobarbital (hyoscyamine and phenobarbital)
1053	FEDAHIST Gyrocaps (chlorpheniramine and pseudoephedrine)

Lederle

A1	ARISTOCORT (triamcinolone), 1 mg
A2	ARISTOCORT (triamcinolone), 2 mg
A3	ACHROMYCIN V (tetracycline), 250 mg
A4	ARISTOCORT (triamcinolone), 4 mg
A5	ACHROMYCIN V (triamcinolone), 500 mg
A8	ARISTOCORT (triamcinolone), 8 mg
A9	ARTANE (trihexyphenidyl), 5 mg
A10	AMICAR (aminocaproic acid), 500 mg
A11	ARTANE (trihexyphenidyl), 2 mg
A12	ARTANE (trihexyphenidyl), 5 mg
A13	ASENDIN (amoxapine), 25 mg
A15	ASENDIN (amoxapine), 50 mg
A17	ASENDIN (amoxapine), 100 mg
A18	ASENDIN (amoxapine), 150 mg
A19	Acetaminophen, 500 mg (tablets)
A20	Acetaminophen, 500 mg (capsules)
A21	Acetaminophen, 325 mg
A23	Acetaminophen and codeine
A24	Amitriptyline, 10 mg
A25	Amitriptyline, 25 mg
A26	Amitriptyline, 50 mg
A27	Amitriptyline, 75 mg
A28	Amitriptyline, 100 mg
A31	Ampicillin, 250 mg
A32	Ampicillin, 500 mg
A33	Amoxicillin, 250 mg
A34	Amoxicillin, 500 mg
A36	Ascorbic acid, 250 mg
A37	Ascorbic acid, 500 mg
A39	Acetaminophen and codeine
A43	Allopurinol, 100 mg
A44	Allopurinol, 300 mg
B10	Benztropine, 1 mg
B11	Benztropine, 2 mg
C1	CENTRUM (multivitamin)
C2	CENTRUM, Jr. (multivitamin)
C7	Chlorthalidone, 25 mg
C9	Chlordiazepoxide, 5 mg
C10	Chlordiazepoxide, 10 mg

continued

PRODUCT IMPRINT CODES

C11	Chlordiazepoxide, 25 mg
C13	Chlorothiazide, 250 mg
C14	Chlorothiazide, 500 mg
C15	Chlorthalidone, 50 mg
C16	Chlorpheniramine, 4 mg
C17	Chlorpheniramine, 8 mg
C18	Chlorpheniramine, 12 mg
C19	Chlorzoxazone and acetaminophen
C22	Chlorpromazine, 25 mg
C23	Chlorpromazine, 50 mg
C24	Chlorpromazine, 100 mg
C25	Chlorpromazine, 200 mg
C30	Cloxacillin, 250 mg
C31	Cloxacillin, 500 mg
C33	Leucovorin, 5 mg
C37	Chlorpropamide, 100 mg
C38	Chlorpropamide, 250 mg
C39	CENTRUM, Jr. + Extra C (multivitamin)
C40	CALTRATE 600 + D (calcium carbonate and vitamin D)
C42	Clonidine, 0.1 mg
C43	Clonidine, 0.2 mg
C44	Clonidine, 0.3 mg
C45	CALTRATE 600 + Iron (calcium carbonate and iron)
C600	CALTRATE 600 (calcium carbonate)
D1	DIAMOX (acetazolamide), 125 mg
D2	DIAMOX (acetazolamide), 250 mg
D3	DIAMOX (acetazolamide), 500 mg
D9	DECLOMYCIN (demeclocycline), 150 mg (capsules)
D11	DECLOMYCIN (demeclocycline), 150 mg (tablets)
D12	DECLOMYCIN (demeclocycline), 300 mg
D16	Dicloxacillin, 250 mg
D17	Dicloxacillin, 500 mg
D22	Doxycycline, 50 mg
D23	Dicyclomine, 10 mg
D24	Dicyclomine, 20 mg
D25	Doxycycline, 100 mg (capsules)
D27	Ergoloid mesylates, 0.5 mg
D28	Ergoloid mesylates, 1 mg (sublingual)
D31	Diphenoxylate and atropine sulfate
D32	Docusate, 100 mg
D33	Docusate, 250 mg
D34	Docusate and casanthranol
D35	DOLENE AP-65 (propoxyphene and acetaminophen)
D36	DOLENE (propoxyphene), 65 mg
D41	Doxycycline, 100 mg (tablets)
D42	DOLENE COMPOUND-65 (propoxyphene, aspirin, and caffeine)
D43	Disopyramide, 150 mg
D44	Dipyridamole, 25 mg
D45	Dipyridamole, 50 mg
D46	Dipyridamole, 75 mg
D51	Diazepam, 2 mg
D52	Diazepam, 5 mg
D53	Diazepam, 10 mg
D62	Disopyramide, 100 mg
E2	Erythromycin, 250 mg
E3	Ergoloid mesylates, 1 mg (oral)
E5	Erythromycin, 500 mg
E10	Erythromycin, 400 mg
F1	FOLVITE (folic acid), 1 mg
F2	FERRO-SEQUELS (ferrous fumarate and docusate)
F4	FILIBON (multivitamin)
F5	FILIBON F.A. (multivitamin)
F6	FILIBON Forte (multivitamin)
F11	Furosemide, 20 mg
F12	Furosemide, 40 mg
F13	Furosemide, 80 mg
F15	Flurazepam, 30 mg
F20	Ferrous sulfate, 300 mg
F21	Ferrous gluconate, 300 mg
F30	Flurazepam, 30 mg
G1	GEVRAL (multivitamin)
G2	GEVRAL T (multivitamin)
H1	HYDROMOX (quinethazone), 50 mg
H2	HYDROMOX R (quinethazone and reserpine)
H11	Hydralazine, 25 mg
H12	Hydralazine, 50 mg
H14	Hydrochlorothiazide, 25 mg
H15	Hydrochlorothiazide, 50 mg
H17	Hydroxyzine, 10 mg
H18	Hydroxyzine, 25 mg
H22	Reserpine, hydralazine, and hydrochlorothiazide
I11	Imipramine, 10 mg
I12	Imipramine, 25 mg
I13	Imipramine, 50 mg
I15	Isosorbide dinitrate, 5 mg (oral)
I16	Isosorbide dinitrate, 10 mg (oral)
I17	Isosorbide dinitrate, 2.5 mg (sublingual)
I18	Isosorbide dinitrate, 5 mg (sublingual)
I19	Indomethacin, 25 mg
I20	Indomethacin, 50 mg
I21	Isoxsuprine, 10 mg
I22	Isoxsuprine, 20 mg
I23	Isosorbide dinitrate S.A., 40 mg (oral)
I24	Isosorbide dinitrate, 20 mg (oral)
I28	Ibuprofen, 400 mg
I29	Ibuprofen, 600 mg
L1	LOXITANE (loxapine), 5 mg
L2	LOXITANE (loxapine), 10 mg
L3	LOXITANE (loxapine), 25 mg
L4	LOXITANE (loxapine), 50 mg
L6	LEDERPLEX (multivitamin)
L9	LEDERCILLIN VK (penicillin V), 500 mg
L10	LEDERCILLIN VK (penicillin V), 250 mg
L11	Levothyroxine, 0.1 mg
L12	Levothyroxine, 0.2 mg
L13	Levothyroxine, 0.3 mg
L15	Brompheniramine, phenylephrine, and phenylpropanolamine
L17	Levothyroxine, 0.15 mg
L30	Lorazepam, 0.5 mg
L31	Lorazepam, 1 mg
L32	Lorazepam, 2 mg
M1	Methotrexate, 2.5 mg
M2	MINOCIN (minocycline), 50 mg (capsules)
M3	MINOCIN (minocycline), 50 mg (tablets)
M4	MINOCIN (minocycline), 100 mg (capsules)
M5	MINOCIN (minocycline), 100 mg (tablets)
M6	MYAMBUTOL (ethambutol), 100 mg
M7	MYAMBUTOL (ethambutol), 400 mg
M8	MAXZIDE (triamterene and hydrochlorothiazide)
M10	MATERNA 1•60 (multivitamin)
M12	Meclizine, 12.5 mg
M13	Meclizine, 25 mg
M19	Methocarbamol, 500 mg
M20	Methocarbamol, 750 mg
M21	Methyldopa, 125 mg
M22	Methyldopa, 250 mg
M23	Methyldopa, 500 mg
M25	Methyclothiazide, 5 mg
M26	Metronidazole, 250 mg
M27	Metronidazole, 500 mg
M28	Metoclopramide, 10 mg
M35	Medroxyprogesterone, 10 mg
N1	NEPTAZANE, 50 mg
N5	NILSTAT (nystatin), 500,000 units (oral tablets)
N6	NILSTAT (nystatin), 100,000 units (vaginal tablets)
N10	Neomycin, 500 mg
N20	Nitroglycerin, 2.5 mg
N21	Nitroglycerin, 6.5 mg
N22	Nitroglycerin, 9 mg
N23	Nylidrin, 6 mg
N24	Nylidrin, 12 mg
P1	PATHIBAMATE 200 (tridihexethyl chloride and meprobamate)
P2	PATHIBAMATE 400 (tridihexethyl chloride and meprobamate)

PRODUCT IMPRINT CODES

P4	PATHILON (tridihexethyl chloride), 25 mg	A16	Thyroid, 120 mg
P7	PERIHEMIN (hematinic)	A17	Thyroid, 200 mg
P8	PERITINIC (hematinic)	A19	Diethylstilbestrol, 0.1 mg
P9	PRONEMIA (hematinic)	A20	Diethylstilbestrol, 0.25 mg
P11	Papaverine, 150 mg	A21	Diethylstilbestrol, 0.5 mg
P13	Papaverine, 100 mg	A22	Diethylstilbestrol, 1 mg
P17	Penicillin G potassium, 400,000 units	A24	SECONAL Sodium (secobarbital), 100 mg
P21	Phenobarbital, 30 mg	A25	A.S.A. (aspirin), 324 mg
P24	Prednisone, 5 mg	A26	Ox bile extract, 324 mg
P25	Probenecid, 500 mg	A30	Aminosalicylic acid, 500 mg
P26	Probenecid and colchicine	A31	Potassium chloride, 1 g
P29	Procainamide, 250 mg (capsules)	A32	A.S.A. (aspirin), 648 mg
P30	Procainamide, 375 mg	A33	Diethylstilbestrol, 5 mg
P31	Procainamide, 500 mg (capsules)	A36	Ferrous sulfate, 324 mg
P33	Propylthiouracil, 50 mg	C06	Cascara, 324 mg
P34	Pseudoephedrine, 60 mg	C07	Cascara Compound (cascara, aloin, podophyllum, and belladonna alkaloids)
P35	Pseudoephedrine, 30 mg		
P36	Pyrazinamide, 500 mg	C09	DIGIGLUSIN (digitalis), 1 USP unit
P37	Pyridoxine, 25 mg	C11	RHINITIS (camphor, quinine, and belladonna)
P38	Pyridoxine, 50 mg	C13	Ferrous sulfate, 324 mg
P39	Propoxyphene and acetaminophen	C16	PAGITANE (cycrimine), 1.25 mg
P44	Propranolol, 10 mg	C17	PAGITANE (cycrimine), 2.5 mg
P45	Propranolol, 20 mg	C27	V-CILLIN K (penicillin V), 125 mg
P46	Propranolol, 40 mg	C29	V-CILLIN K (penicillin V), 250 mg
P47	Propranolol, 80 mg	C36	Quinine, 324 mg
P48	Procainamide, 250 mg (tablets)	C46	V-CILLIN K (penicillin V), 500 mg
P49	Procainamide, 500 mg (tablets)	C47	HEPICEBRIN (multivitamin)
P50	Procainamide, 750 mg	C51	DARVOCET-N 50 (propoxyphene and acetaminophen)
Q11	Quinidine sulfate, 200 mg		
Q13	Quinidine gluconate, 324 mg	C53	DARVON-N (propoxyphene), 100 mg
Q15	Quinine, 325 mg	C54	DARVON-N with A.S.A. (propoxyphene and aspirin)
S1	STRESSTABS 600 (multivitamin)		
S2	STRESSTABS 600 w/Iron (multivitamin)	C63	DARVOCET-N 100 (propoxyphene and acetaminophen)
S3	STRESSTABS 600 w/Zinc (multivitamin)		
S5	STRESSTABS (multivitamin)	C71	MULTICEBRIN (multivitamin)
S12	Spironolactone and hydrochlorothiazide	F03	ZENTINIC (multivitamin)
S13	Spironolactone, 25 mg	F04	SEROMYCIN (cycloserine), 250 mg
S14	Sulfasalazine, 0.5 g	F11	A.S.A. (aspirin), 324 mg (clear)
S22	SPARTUS (multivitamin)	F12	A.S.A. (aspirin), 324 mg (pink)
S23	SPARTUS + Iron (multivitamin)	F14	Ephedrine and AMYTAL (ephedrine and amobarbital)
T1	TriHEMIC 600 (hematinic)		
T10	Thioridazine, 10 mg	F15	LEXTRON (multivitamin)
T11	Thiamine, 50 mg	F16	LEXTRON Ferrous (multivitamin)
T12	Thiamine, 100 mg	F19	EXTRALIN (liver-stomach concentrate), 50 mg
T13	Sulfamethoxazole and trimethoprim	F21	EXTRALIN B (multivitamin)
T14	Thyroid, 60 mg	F22	LEXTRON F.G. (multivitamin)
T16	Sulfamethoxazole and trimethoprim	F23	AMYTAL Sodium (amobarbital), 65 mg
T17	Tolbutamide, 500 mg	F24	Ephedrine, 25 mg
T19	Tolazamide, 100 mg	F25	Ephedrine, 50 mg
T20	Tolazamide, 250 mg	F26	Quinine, 130 mg
T22	Tolazamide, 500 mg	F27	Quinine, 194 mg
T23	Triprolidine and pseudoephedrine	F29	Quinine, 324 mg
T25	Thioridazine, 25 mg	F31	ACIDULIN (glutamic acid), 340 mg
T27	Thioridazine, 50 mg	F32	Digitalis, 100 mg
T28	Thioridazine, 100 mg	F33	AMYTAL Sodium (amobarbital), 200 mg
V11	Vitamin A, 25,000 IU	F34	Carbarsone, 250 mg
V14	Vitamin C, 250 mg	F36	COPAVIN (codeine and papaverine)
V15	Vitamin C, 500 mg	F39	Quinidine, 200 mg
V19	Vitamin E, natural, 400 IU	F40	SECONAL Sodium (secobarbital), 100 mg
V21	Vitamin E, 200 IU	F41	BILRON (iron bile salts), 300 mg
V22	Vitamin E, 400 IU	F42	SECONAL Sodium (secobarbital), 50 mg
V23	Vitamin E, 600 IU	F43	BETALIN Compound (multivitamin)
V24	Vitamin E, 1,000 IU	F44	Ferrous gluconate, 324 mg
		F52	Dibasic calcium phosphate and vitamin D

Lilly

A01	Ammonium chloride, 486 mg	F54	Dicumarol, 50 mg
A02	Ferrous sulfate, 324 mg	F56	Calcium gluconate with vitamin D
A04	Pancreatin, 1 g	F61	BILRON (iron bile salts), 150 mg
A05	Potassium chloride, 300 mg	F63	Dibasic calcium phosphate with vitamin D and iron
A06	Potassium iodide, 300 mg	F64	TUINAL (secobarbital and amobarbital), 25 mg/25 mg
A09	Sodium chloride, 1.004 g		
A10	Sodium salicylate, 324 mg	F65	TUINAL (secobarbital and amobarbital), 50 mg/50 mg
A11	Sodium salicylate, 648 mg		
A12	Ammonium chloride, 972 mg	F66	TUINAL (secobarbital and amobarbital), 100 mg/100 mg
A14	Thyroid, 30 mg		
A15	Thyroid, 60 mg	F71	Dicumarol, 25 mg
		F72	SECONAL Sodium (secobarbital), 30 mg

continued

PRODUCT IMPRINT CODES

F74	TYCOPAN (multivitamin)		T37	AMYTAL (amobarbital), 50 mg
F92	EXTRALIN F (hematinic)		T39	Calcium gluconate, 486 mg
F96	RETICULEX (hematinic)		T40	AMYTAL (amobarbital), 15 mg
H02	DARVON (propoxyphene), 32 mg		T44	Calcium gluconate with vitamin D
H03	DARVON (propoxyphene), 65 mg		T45	CEVALIN (ascorbic acid), 100 mg
H04	DARVON with A.S.A. (propoxyphene and aspirin)		T46	Sulfapyridine, 0.5 mg
H10	EN-CEBRIN-F (multivitamin)		T52	BETALIN S (thiamine), 10 mg
H12	EN-CEBRIN (multivitamin)		T53	Niacinamide, 100 mg
H17	AVENTYL HCl (nortriptyline), 10 mg		T54	Sulfadiazine, 0.5 g
H19	AVENTYL HCl (nortriptyline), 25 mg		T55	Papaverine, 100 mg
H72	THERACEBRIN (multivitamin)		T56	AMYTAL (amobarbital), 30 mg
J02	Atropine, 0.4 mg		T59	BETALIN S (thiamine), 25 mg
J03	Belladonna extract, 15 mg		T60	CEVALIN (ascorbic acid), 250 mg
J04	Bismuth subcarbonate, 324 mg		T61	Dibasic calcium phosphate, 486 mg
J05	Citrated caffeine, 64.8 mg		T62	BETALIN S (thiamine), 50 mg
J09	Codeine sulfate, 15 mg		T63	BETALIN S (thiamine), 100 mg
J10	Codeine sulfate, 30 mg		T67	CEVALIN (ascorbic acid), 500 mg
J11	Codeine sulfate, 60 mg		T72	HEXA-BETALIN (pyridoxine), 50 mg
J13	Colchicine, 0.6 mg		T73	Papaverine, 200 mg
J20	Quinidine, 200 mg		T75	NEOTRIZINE (sulfadiazine, sulfamerazine, and sulfamethazine)
J23	SODA MINT (bicarbonate), 324 mg			
J24	Bicarbonate, 324 mg		T91	PAVERIL (dioxyline), 200 mg
J25	Thyroid, 60 mg		T93	Isoniazid, 100 mg
J26	Thyroid, 120 mg		T96	Neomycin, 500 mg
J29	Thyroid, 30 mg		T99	HALDRONE (paramethasone), 1 mg
J30	Thyroid, 15 mg		U01	HALDRONE (paramethasone), 2 mg
J31	Phenobarbital, 15 mg		U03	DYMELOR (acetohexamide), 250 mg
J32	Phenobarbital, 30 mg		U07	DYMELOR (acetohexamide), 500 mg
J33	Phenobarbital, 100 mg		U09	ANHYDRON (cyclothiazide), 2 mg
J36	ERGOTRATE Maleate (ergonovine), 0.2 mg		U23	Isoniazid, 300 mg
J37	Phenobarbital, 60 mg		U29	SANDRIL (reserpine), 0.25 mg
J41	Niacin, 20 mg		U53	Methadone, 40 mg
J42	Niacin, 100 mg		U56	Folic acid, 1 mg
J43	Niacin, 50 mg			
J45	HEXA-BETALIN (pyridoxine), 25 mg		3061	CECLOR (cefaclor), 250 mg
J46	Niacinamide, 50 mg		3062	CECLOR (cefaclor), 500 mg
J47	Riboflavin, 5 mg		3075	HISTADYL and A.S.A. (chlorpheniramine and aspirin)
J49	Diethylstilbestrol, 0.1 mg			
J50	Diethylstilbestrol, 0.25 mg		3110	DARVON COMPOUND (propoxyphene, aspirin, and caffeine)
J51	Diethylstilbestrol, 0.5 mg			
J52	Diethylstilbestrol, 1 mg		3111	DARVON COMPOUND-65 (propoxyphene, aspirin, and caffeine)
J53	PANTHOLIN (pantothenate), 10 mg			
J54	Diethylstilbestrol, 5 mg		3113	A.S.A. and Codeine Compound No. 3 (codeine, aspirin, and caffeine)
J56	HEXA-BETALIN (pyridoxine), 10 mg			
J57	CRYSTODIGIN (digitoxin), 0.2 mg		4067	A.S.A. and Codeine Compound No. 3 (codeine, aspirin, and caffeine)
J60	CRYSTODIGIN (digitoxin), 0.1 mg			
J61	Papaverine, 30 mg			
J62	Papaverine, 60 mg			
J63	Riboflavin, 10 mg			

Marion

1375	DITROPAN (oxybutynin chloride)
1550	NITRO-BID (nitroglycerin), 2.5 mg
1551	NITRO-BID (nitroglycerin), 6.5 mg
1553	NITRO-BID (nitroglycerin), 9 mg
1555	PAVABID (papaverine), 150 mg
1712	CARAFATE (sucralfate), 1 gm
1771	CARDIZEM (diltiazem), 30 mg
1772	CARDIZEM (diltiazem), 60 mg

J64	DOLOPHINE (methadone), 5 mg
J69	Propylthiouracil, 50 mg
J72	DOLOPHINE (methadone), 10 mg
J73	Methyltestosterone, 10 mg
J74	Methyltestosterone, 25 mg
J75	CRYSTODIGIN (digitoxin), 0.05 mg
J76	CRYSTODIGIN (digitoxin), 0.15 mg
J94	TAPAZOLE (methimazole), 5 mg
J95	TAPAZOLE (methimazole), 10 mg
J96	TYLOSTERONE (diethylstilbestrol and methyltestosterone)

Mead Johnson Laboratories

512	QUIBRON-T (theophylline), 300 mg
516	QUIBRON (theophylline and guaifenesin)
519	QUIBRON-T/SR (theophylline), 300 mg
583	OVCON-35 (norethindrone and ethinyl estradiol)
584	OVCON-50 (norethindrone and ethinyl estradiol)
702	NATALINS Rx (multivitamin)
755	ESTRACE (estradiol), 1 mg
756	ESTRACE (estradiol), 2 mg

J97	PAVERIL (dioxyline), 100 mg
J99	SANDRIL (reserpine), 0.1 mg
T01	ZENTRON (multivitamin)
T05	A.S.A. (aspirin), 324 mg
T06	A.S.A. (aspirin), 324 mg
T13	Calcium lactate, 324 mg
T14	Calcium lactate, 648 mg
T20	Methenamine, 500 mg
T21	Methenamine and sodium biphosphate

Mead Johnson Pharmaceuticals

770	KLOTRIX (potassium chloride), 10 mEq
775	DESYREL (trazodone), 50 mg
776	DESYREL (trazodone), 100 mg
778	DESYREL (trazodone), 150 mg
784	DURICEF (cefadroxil), 500 mg
785	DURICEF (cefadroxil), 1 g

T23	Sodium chloride, 2.25 g
T24	Sodium chloride, 1 g
T26	Pancreatin, 325 mg
T29	Bicarbonate, 648 mg
T32	AMYTAL (amobarbital), 100 mg
T35	Calcium carbonate, 648 mg
T36	Calcium gluconate, 1 g

PRODUCT IMPRINT CODES

Merck Sharp & Dohme

20	DECADRON (dexamethasone), 0.25 mg
21	COGENTIN (benztropine), 0.5 mg
23	ELAVIL (amitriptyline), 10 mg
25	INDOCIN (indomethacin), 25 mg
26	VIVACTIL (protriptyline), 5 mg
41	DECADRON (dexamethasone), 0.5 mg
42	HYDRO-DIURIL (hydrochlorothiazide), 25 mg
43	MEPHYTON (phytonadione), 5 mg
45	ELAVIL (amitriptyline), 25 mg
47	VIVACTIL (protriptyline), 10 mg
49	DARANIDE (dichlorphenamide), 50 mg
50	INDOCIN (indomethacin), 50 mg
52	INVERSINE (mecamylamine), 2.5 mg
53	HYDROPRES 25 (reserpine and hydrochlorothiazide)
59	BLOCADREN (timolol), 5 mg
60	COGENTIN (benztropine), 2 mg
62	PERIACTIN (cyproheptadine), 4 mg
63	DECADRON (dexamethasone), 0.75 mg
65	EDECRIN (ethacrynic acid), 25 mg
67	TIMOLIDE 10–25 (timolol and hydrochlorothiazide)
90	EDECRIN (ethacrynic acid), 50 mg
92	MIDAMOR (amiloride), 5 mg
95	DECADRON (dexamethasone), 1.5 mg
97	DECADRON (dexamethasone), 4 mg
102	ELAVIL (amitriptyline), 50 mg
105	HYDRO-DIURIL (hydrochlorothiazide), 50 mg
127	HYDROPRES 50 (reserpine and hydrochlorothiazide)
135	ALDOMET (methyldopa), 125 mg
136	BLOCADREN (timolol), 10 mg
147	DECADRON (dexamethasone), 6 mg
214	DIURIL (chlorothiazide), 250 mg
219	CORTONE (cortisone), 25 mg
230	DIUPRES 250 (reserpine and chlorothiazide)
401	ALDOMET (methyldopa), 250 mg
403	URECHOLINE (bethanechol), 5 mg
405	DIUPRES 500 (reserpine and chlorothiazide)
410	HYDRODIURIL (hydrochlorothiazide), 100 mg
412	URECHOLINE (bethanechol), 10 mg
423	ALDORIL 15 (methyldopa and hydrochlorothiazide)
430	ELAVIL (amitriptyline), 75 mg
432	DIURIL (chlorothiazide), 500 mg
435	ELAVIL (amitriptyline), 100 mg
437	BLOCADREN (timolol), 20 mg
456	ALDORIL 25 (methyldopa and hydrochlorothiazide)
457	URECHOLINE (bethanechol), 25 mg
460	URECHOLINE (bethanechol), 50 mg
501	BENEMID (probenecid), 0.5 g
516	ALDOMET (methyldopa), 500 mg
517	TRIAVIL 4–50 (perphenazine and amitriptyline)
602	CUPRIMINE (penicillamine), 250 mg
612	ALDOCLOR 150 (methyldopa and chlorothiazide)
614	COLBENEMID (probenecid and colchicine)
619	HYDROCORTONE (hydrocortisone), 10 mg
625	HYDROCORTONE (hydrocortisone), 20 mg
634	ALDOCLOR 250 (methyldopa and chlorothiazide)
635	COGENTIN (benztropine), 1 mg
647	SINEMET 10–100 (carbidopa and levodopa)
650	SINEMET 25–100 (carbidopa and levodopa)
654	SINEMET 25–250 (carbidopa and levodopa)
672	CUPRIMINE (penicillamine), 125 mg
673	ELAVIL (amitriptyline), 150 mg
675	DOLOBID (diflunisal), 250 mg
679	CUPRID (trientine), 250 mg
690	DEMSER (metyrosine), 250 mg
693	INDOCIN (indomethacin), 250 mg
694	ALDORIL D30 (methyldopa and hydrochlorothiazide)
697	DOLOBID (diflunisal), 500 mg
705	NOROXIN (norfloxacin), 400 mg
707	TONOCARD (tocainide), 400 mg
709	TONOCARD (tocainide), 600 mg
712	VASOTEC (enalapril), 5 mg
713	VASOTEC (enalapril), 10 mg
714	VASOTEC (enalapril), 20 mg
720	VASERETIC 10-25 (enalapril and hydrochlorothiazide)
907	MINTEZOL (thiabendazole), 500 mg
914	TRIAVIL 2–10 (perphenazine and amitriptyline)
917	MODURETIC (amiloride and hydrochlorothiazide)
921	TRIAVIL 2–25 (perphenazine and amitriptyline)
931	FLEXERIL (cyclobenzaprine), 10 mg
934	TRIAVIL 4–10 (perphenazine and amitriptyline)
935	ALDORIL D50 (methyldopa and hydrochlorothiazide)
941	CLINORIL (sulindac), 150 mg
942	CLINORIL (sulindac), 200 mg
946	TRIAVIL 4–25 (perphenazine and amitriptyline)
963	PEPCID (famotidine), 20 mg
964	PEPCID (famotidine), 40 mg

Merrell Dow

37	CANTIL (mepenzolate), 25 mg
62	METAHYDRIN (trichlormethiazide), 2 mg
63	METAHYDRIN (trichlormethiazide), 4 mg
277	HIPREX (methenamine), 1 g
547	QUINAMM (quinine), 260 mg
690	TACE (chlorotrianisene), 12 mg
691	TACE (chlorotrianisene), 25 mg
692	TACE (chlorotrianisene), 72 mg

Miles Pharmaceuticals

093	MYCELEX-G (clotrimazole), 100 mg
095	MYCELEX Troche (clotrimazole), 10 mg
097	MYCELEX-G (clotrimazole), 500 mg
121	DECHOLIN (dehydrocholic acid), 250 mg
132	STILPHOSTROL (diethylstilbestrol), 50 mg
411	DOMEBORO (aluminum sulfate and calcium)
521	BILTRICIDE (praziquantel), 600 mg
721	NICLOCIDE (niclosamide), 500 mg
811	ADALAT (nifedipine), 10 mg
821	ADALAT (nifedipine), 20 mg
951	LITHANE (lithium), 300 mg

Norwich Eaton

036	FURADANTIN (nitrofurantoin), 50 mg
037	FURADANTIN (nitrofurantoin), 100 mg
045	DUVOID (bethanechol), 10 mg
046	DUVOID (bethanechol), 25 mg
047	DUVOID (bethanechol), 50 mg
072	FUROXONE (furazolidone), 100 mg
402	DIDRONEL (etidronate), 200 mg
406	DIDRONEL (etidronate), 400 mg
0149 0412	ENTEX (phenylephrine, phenylpropanolamine, and guaifenesin)
0149 0007	MACRODANTIN (nitrofurantoin macrocrystals), 25 mg
0149 0008	MACRODANTIN (nitrofurantoin macrocrystals), 50 mg
0149 0009	MACRODANTIN (nitrofurantoin macrocrystals), 100 mg

Organon

381	COTAZYM (pancrelipase)
388	COTAZYM-S (pancrelipase)
472	CALDEROL (calcifediol), 0.02 mg
474	CALDEROL (calcifediol), 0.05 mg
542	WIGRAINE (ergotamine tartrate and caffeine)
790	HEXADROL (dexamethasone), 1.5 mg
791	HEXADROL (dexamethasone), 0.75 mg
792	HEXADROL (dexamethasone), 0.5 mg
798	HEXADROL (dexamethasone), 4.0 mg

Ortho Pharmaceutical

1570	PROTOSTAT (metronidazole), 250 mg
1571	PROTOSTAT (metronidazole), 500 mg

continued

PRODUCT IMPRINT CODES

Parke-Davis

001	PERITRATE (pentaerythritol tetranitrate), 20 mg
004	PERITRATE SA (pentaerythritol tetranitrate), 80 mg
007	DILANTIN (phenytoin), 50 mg
008	PERITRATE (pentaerythritol tetranitrate), 40 mg
010	PROMAPAR (chlorpromazine), 10 mg
013	PERITRATE (pentaerythritol tetranitrate), 10 mg
025	PROMAPAR (chlorpromazine), 25 mg
037	Ferrous sulfate, 325 mg
050	PROMAPAR (chlorpromazine), 50 mg
100	PROMAPAR (chlorpromazine), 100 mg
111	ERGOSTAT (ergotamine), 2 mg
117	Diphenoxylate and atropine
121	Chlorthalidone, 50 mg
123	Chlorthalidone, 25 mg
141	Diazepam, 2 mg
142	Diazepam, 5 mg
143	Diazepam, 10 mg
166	MANDELAMINE (methenamine), 0.5 g
167	MANDELAMINE (methenamine), 1 g
177	SINUBID (acetaminophen, phenylpropanolamine, and phenyltoloxamine)
180	PYRIDIUM (phenazopyridine), 100 mg
181	PYRIDIUM (phenazopyridine), 200 mg
182	PYRIDIUM Plus (phenazopyridine, hyoscyamine, and butabarbital)
200	BRONDECON (oxtriphylline and guaifenesin)
201	PROMAPAR (chlorpromazine), 200 mg
202	PROCAN SR (procainamide), 250 mg
204	PROCAN SR (procainamide), 500 mg
205	PROCAN SR (procainamide), 750 mg
207	PROCAN SR (procainamide), 1,000 mg
210	CHOLEDYL (oxtriphylline), 100 mg
211	CHOLEDYL (oxtriphylline), 200 mg
214	CHOLEDYL SA (oxtriphylline), 400 mg
221	CHOLEDYL SA (oxtriphylline), 600 mg
230	TEDRAL (theophylline, ephedrine, and phenobarbital)
231	TEDRAL SA (theophylline, ephedrine, and phenobarbital)
237	ZARONTIN (ethosuximide), 250 mg
247	D-S-S (docusate), 100 mg
248	D-S-S Plus (docusate and casanthranol)
251	PROLOID (thyroglobulin), ½ gr
252	PROLOID (thyroglobulin), 1 gr
253	PROLOID (thyroglobulin), 1½ gr
254	PROLOID (thyroglobulin), 3 gr
257	PROLOID (thyroglobulin), 2 gr
260	EUTHROID-½ (levothyroxine and liothyronine)
261	EUTHROID-1 (levothyroxine and liothyronine)
262	EUTHROID-2 (levothyroxine and liothyronine)
263	EUTHROID-3 (levothyroxine and liothyronine)
268	MECLOMEN (meclofenamate), 50 mg
269	MECLOMEN (meclofenamate), 100 mg
270	NARDIL (phenelzine), 15 mg
271	Amitriptyline, 100 mg
272	Amitriptyline, 10 mg
273	Amitriptyline, 25 mg
274	Amitriptyline, 50 mg
275	Amitriptyline, 75 mg
276	CENTRAX (prazepam), 10 mg
278	Amitriptyline, 150 mg
282	NATAFORT (multivitamin)
320	PARSIDOL (ethopropazine), 10 mg
321	PARSIDOL (ethopropazine), 50 mg
337	ELDEC (multivitamin)
362	DILANTIN (phenytoin), 100 mg
365	DILANTIN (phenytoin), 30 mg
373	BENADRYL (diphenhydramine), 50 mg
375	DILANTIN with ¼ gr Phenobarbital (phenytoin and phenobarbital)
379	CHLOROMYCETIN (chloramphenicol), 250 mg
390	NATABEC (multivitamin)
393	MILONTIN (phensuximide), 500 mg
402	AMCILL (ampicillin), 250 mg
404	AMCILL (ampicillin), 500 mg
407	CYCLOPAR (tetracycline), 250 mg
420	Quinine, 5 gr
437	ESTROVIS (quinestrol), 0.1 mg
440	Furosemide, 20 mg
441	Furosemide, 40 mg
442	Furosemide, 80 mg
471	BENADRYL (diphenhydramine), 25 mg
490	EASPRIN (aspirin), 975 mg
525	CELONTIN (methsuximide), 300 mg
529	HUMATIN (paromomycin), 250 mg
531	DILANTIN with ½ gr Phenobarbital (phenytoin and phenobarbital)
533	Calcium lactate, 325 mg
534	NATABEC with Fluoride (multivitamin)
537	CELONTIN (methsuximide), 150 mg
540	PONSTEL (mefenamic acid), 250 mg
541	NATABEC-FA (multivitamin)
544	GERIPLEX-FS (multivitamin)
547	NATABEC Rx (multivitamin)
552	CENTRAX (prazepam), 5 mg
553	CENTRAX (prazepam), 10 mg
554	CENTRAX (prazepam), 20 mg
604	Calcium lactate, 650 mg
606	Aspirin, 325 mg
607	Phenobarbital, 60 mg
618	NORLESTRIN 28 1/50 placebo tablet
622	Ferrous fumarate, 75 mg
634	Acetaminophen and Codeine Phosphate No. 2
635	Acetaminophen and Codeine Phosphate No. 3
637	Acetaminophen and Codeine Phosphate No. 4
638	TABRON (multivitamin)
640	TAPAR (acetaminophen), 325 mg
648	PENAPAR VK (penicillin V), 250 mg
669	LOPID (gemfibrozil), 300 mg
672	ERYPAR (erythromycin), 250 mg
673	PENAPAR VK (penicillin V), 500 mg
692	Propoxyphene, 65 mg
696	ERYC (erythromycin), 250 mg
697	CYCLOPAR 500 (tetracycline), 500 mg
698	Phenobarbital, 100 mg
699	Phenobarbital, 15 mg
700	Phenobarbital, 30 mg
702	THIURETIC (hydrochlorothiazide), 25 mg
710	THIURETIC (hydrochlorothiazide), 50 mg
712	Spironolactone with Hydrochlorothiazide
713	Spironolactone, 25 mg
725	Aspirin and Codeine Phosphate No. 2
726	Aspirin and Codeine Phosphate No. 3
727	Aspirin and Codeine Phosphate No. 4
730	UTIMOX (amoxicillin), 250 mg
731	UTIMOX (amoxicillin), 500 mg
800	Chlordiazepoxide, 5 mg
801	Chlordiazepoxide, 10 mg
802	Chlordiazepoxide, 25 mg
813	Doxycycline, 100 mg (tablets)
829	Doxycycline, 50 mg
830	Doxycycline, 100 mg (capsules)
849	Quinidine, 200 mg
850	DURAQUIN (quinidine), 330 mg
865	Methyldopa, 250 mg
866	Methyldopa, 500 mg
882	NORLUTIN (norethindrone), 5 mg
887	Indomethacin, 25 mg
888	Indomethacin, 50 mg
901	NORLESTRIN 2.5/50 (norethindrone and ethinyl estradiol)
904	NORLESTRIN 1/50 (norethindrone and ethinyl estradiol)
915	LOESTRIN 1/20 (norethindrone and ethinyl estradiol)
916	LOESTRIN 1.5/30 (norethindrone and ethinyl estradiol)
918	NORLUTATE (norethindrone), 5 mg
919	Erythromycin, 500 mg

PRODUCT IMPRINT CODES

Pfizer

073	TERRAMYCIN (oxytetracycline), 250 mg (capsules)
084	TERRAMYCIN (oxytetracycline), 250 mg (tablets)
094	VIBRAMYCIN (doxycycline), 50 mg
095	VIBRAMYCIN (doxycycline), 100 mg (capsules)
099	VIBRAMYCIN (doxycycline), 100 mg (tablets)
220	SUSTAIRE (theophylline), 100 mg
221	SUSTAIRE (theophylline), 300 mg
260	PROCARDIA (nifedipine), 10 mg
261	PROCARDIA (nifedipine), 20 mg
322	FELDENE (piroxicam), 10 mg
323	FELDENE (piroxicam), 20 mg
375	RENESE (polythiazide), 1 mg
376	RENESE (polythiazide), 2 mg
377	RENESE (polythiazide), 4 mg
393	DIABINESE (chlorpropamide), 100 mg
394	DIABINESE (chlorpropamide), 250 mg
430	MINIZIDE 1 (prazosin and polythiazide)
431	MINIPRESS (prazosin), 1 mg
432	MINIZIDE 2 (prazosin and polythiazide)
436	MINIZIDE 5 (prazosin and polythiazide)
437	MINIPRESS (prazosin), 2 mg
438	MINIPRESS (prazosin), 5 mg
441	MODERIL (rescinnamine), 0.25 mg
442	MODERIL (rescinnamine), 0.5 mg
446	RENESE-R (reserpine and polythiazide)
541	VISTARIL (hydroxyzine), 25 mg
542	VISTARIL (hydroxyzine), 50 mg
543	VISTARIL (hydroxyzine), 100 mg
641	VANSIL (oxamniquine), 250 mg

Pharmacia

101	AZULFIDINE (sulfasalazine), 500 mg
102	AZULFIDINE EN-tabs (sulfasalazine), 500 mg

Poythress

9523	SOLFOTON (phenobarbital), 16 mg (capsules)
9525	SOLFOTON (phenobarbital), 16 mg (tablets)
9531	URO-PHOSPHATE (methenamine and sodium biphosphate)
9532	MUDRANE-2 (potassium iodide and aminophylline)
9533	MUDRANE GG-2 (aminophylline and guaifenesin)
9540	ANTROCOL Capsules (atropine and phenobarbital)
9541	ANTROCOL Tablets (atropine and phenobarbital)
9550	MUDRANE (potassium iodide, aminophylline, and phenobarbital)
9551	MUDRANE GG (aminophylline, ephedrine, phenobarbital, and guaifenesin)

Princeton

207	CORGARD (nadolol), 40 mg
208	CORGARD (nadolol), 120 mg
232	CORGARD (nadolol), 20 mg
241	CORGARD (nadolol), 80 mg
246	CORGARD (nadolol), 160 mg
283	CORZIDE 40/5 (nadolol and bendroflumethiazide)
284	CORZIDE 80/5 (nadolol and bendroflumethiazide)
431	PRONESTYL (procainamide), 250 mg (tablets)
434	PRONESTYL (procainamide), 375 mg (tablets)
438	PRONESTYL (procainamide), 500 mg (tablets)
539	RAUTRAX N (rauwolfia serpentina, bendroflumethiazide, and potassium chloride)
602	NATURETIN c̄K 2.5/500 (bendroflumethiazide and potassium chloride)
605	NATURETIN-2.5 (bendroflumethiazide), 2.5 mg
606	NATURETIN-5 (bendroflumethiazide), 5 mg
608	NATURETIN c̄K 5/500 (bendroflumethiazide and potassium chloride)
618	NATURETIN-10 (bendroflumethiazide), 10 mg
685	RAUTRAX (bendroflumethiazide), 10 mg
713	RAUDIXIN (rauwolfia serpentina), 50 mg
756	PRONESTYL (procainamide), 375 mg (capsules)
757	PRONESTYL (procainamide), 500 mg (capsules)
758	PRONESTYL (procainamide), 250 mg (capsules)
769	RAUZIDE (rauwolfia serpentina and bendroflumethiazide)
775	PRONESTYL-SR (procainamide), 500 mg
776	RAUDIXIN (rauwolfia serpentina), 100 mg
863	PROLIXIN (fluphenazine), 1 mg
864	PROLIXIN (fluphenazine), 2.5 mg
877	PROLIXIN (fluphenazine), 5 mg
956	PROLIXIN (fluphenazine), 10 mg

Reid-Rowell

1007	CURRETAB (medroxyprogesterone), 10 mg
1014	ESTRATAB (esterified estrogens), 0.3 mg
1022	ESTRATAB (esterified estrogens), 0.625 mg
1023	ESTRATEST H.S. (esterified estrogens and methyltestosterone)
1024	ESTRATAB (esterified estrogens), 1.25 mg
1025	ESTRATAB (esterified estrogens), 2.5 mg
1026	ESTRATEST (esterified estrogens and methyltestosterone)
1039	HISTALET Forte (phenylephrine, phenylpropanolamine, pyrilamine, and chlorpheniramine)
1050	HISTALET X (pseudoephedrine and guaifenesin)
1082	MELFIAT-105 (phendimetrazine), 105 mg
1088	P-V-TUSSIN (hydrocodone, phenindamine, and guaifenesin)
1146	ZENATE (multivitamin)
1290	COMPAL (dihydrocodeine, acetaminophen, and caffeine)
7720	CHENIX (chenodiol), 250 mg

Robins

1535	MITROLAN (calcium polycarbophil)
4207	DONNATAL Capsules (phenobarbital, hyoscyamine, atropine, and scopolamine)
4250	DONNATAL Tablets (phenobarbital, hyoscyamine, atropine, and scopolamine)
4649	DONNAZYME (pancreatin, pepsin, bile salts, hyoscyamine, atropine, scopolamine, and phenobarbital)
5049	ENTOZYME (pancreatin, pepsin, and bile salts)
5449	EXNA (benzthiazide), 50 mg
5720	MICRO-K (potassium chloride), 600 mg
5730	MICRO-K 10 (potassium chloride), 750 mg
5816	PABALATE (sodium salicylate and sodium aminobenzoate)
5883	PABALATE-SF (potassium salicylate and potassium aminobenzoate)
6207	PHENAPHEN (acetaminophen), 325 mg
6242	PHENAPHEN with Codeine No. 2 (acetaminophen and codeine)
6257	PHENAPHEN with Codeine No. 3 (acetaminophen and codeine)
6274	PHENAPHEN with Codeine No. 4 (acetaminophen and codeine)
6447	PONDIMIN (fenfluramine), 20 mg

Roche

16	NOLUDAR (methyprylon), 50 mg
17	NOLUDAR (methyprylon), 200 mg
34	MESTINON (pyridostigmine), 180 mg
51	VI-PENTA F (multivitamin)

Roerig

035	SPECTROBID (bacampicillin), 400 mg
092	UROBIOTIC-250 (oxytetracycline, sulfamethizole, and phenazopyridine)
143	GEOCILLIN (carbenicillin), 382 mg
159	TAO (troleandomycin), 250 mg
210	ANTIVERT (meclizine), 12.5 mg
211	ANTIVERT/25 (meclizine), 25 mg
212	ANTIVERT/25 (meclizine), 25 mg (chewable)
214	ANTIVERT/50 (meclizine), 50 mg
254	MARAX (ephedrine, theophylline, and hydroxyzine)
411	GLUCOTROL (glipizide), 5 mg
412	GLUCOTROL (glipizide), 10 mg

continued

PRODUCT IMPRINT CODES

504	HEPTUNA PLUS (multivitamin)
534	SINEQUAN (doxepin), 10 mg
535	SINEQUAN (doxepin), 25 mg
536	SINEQUAN (doxepin), 50 mg
537	SINEQUAN (doxepin), 150 mg
538	SINEQUAN (doxepin), 100 mg
539	SINEQUAN (doxepin), 75 mg
560	ATARAX (hydroxyzine), 10 mg
561	ATARAX (hydroxyzine), 25 mg
562	ATARAX (hydroxyzine), 50 mg
563	ATARAX (hydroxyzine), 100 mg
571	NAVANE (thiothixene), 1 mg
572	NAVANE (thiothixene), 2 mg
573	NAVANE (thiothixene), 5 mg
574	NAVANE (thiothixene), 10 mg
577	NAVANE (thiothixene), 20 mg

Rorer

LH	LEVOTHROID (T$_4$ thyroxine), 0.125 mg
LK	LEVOTHROID (T$_4$ thyroxine), 0.025 mg
LL	LEVOTHROID (T$_4$ thyroxine), 0.050 mg
LM	LEVOTHROID (T$_4$ thyroxine), 0.100 mg
LN	LEVOTHROID (T$_4$ thyroxine), 0.150 mg
LP	LEVOTHROID (T$_4$ thyroxine), 0.175 mg
LR	LEVOTHROID (T$_4$ thyroxine), 0.200 mg
LS	LEVOTHROID (T$_4$ thyroxine), 0.300 mg
LT	LEVOTHROID (T$_4$ thyroxine), 0.075 mg
NE	NICOLAR (niacin), 500 mg
TC	ARMOUR Thyroid (thyroid), ¼ gr
TD	ARMOUR Thyroid (thyroid), ½ gr
TE	ARMOUR Thyroid (thyroid), 1 gr
TJ	ARMOUR Thyroid (thyroid), 1½ gr
TF	ARMOUR Thyroid (thyroid), 2 gr
TG	ARMOUR Thyroid (thyroid), 3 gr
TH	ARMOUR Thyroid (thyroid), 5 gr
TI	ARMOUR Thyroid (thyroid), 5 gr
YC	THYROLAR-¼ (T$_3$/T$_4$ liotrix)
YD	THYROLAR-½ (T$_3$/T$_4$ liotrix)
YE	THYROLAR-1 (T$_3$/T$_4$ liotrix)
YF	THYROLAR-2 (T$_3$/T$_4$ liotrix)
YH	THYROLAR-3 (T$_3$/T$_4$ liotrix)
20	HYGROTON (chlorthalidone), 50 mg
21	HYGROTON (chlorthalidone), 100 mg
22	HYGROTON (chlorthalidone), 25 mg
31	REGROTON (chlorthalidone and reserpine)
32	DEMI-REGROTON (chlorthalidone and reserpine)
45	ARLIDIN (nylidrin), 6 mg
46	ARLIDIN (nylidrin), 12 mg
50	SLO-BID (theophylline), 50 mg
82	LOZOL (indapamide), 2.5 mg
100	SLO-BID (theophylline), 100 mg
136	Extra Strength ASCRIPTIN (aspirin, magnesium hydroxide, and aluminum hydroxide)
137	ASCRIPTIN A-D (aspirin, magnesium hydroxide, and aluminum hydroxide)
142	ASCRIPTIN with Codeine No. 2 (aspirin, magnesium hydroxide, aluminum hydroxide, and codeine)
143	ASCRIPTIN with Codeine No. 3 (aspirin, magnesium hydroxide, aluminum hydroxide, and codeine)
160	PERTOFRANE (desipramine), 25 mg
161	PERTOFRANE (desipramine), 50 mg
200	SLO-BID (theophylline), 200 mg
300	SLO-BID (theophylline), 300 mg
351	SLO-PHYLLIN (theophylline), 100 mg
352	SLO-PHYLLIN (theophylline), 200 mg
1354	SLO-PHYLLIN (theophylline), 60 mg
1355	SLO-PHYLLIN (theophylline), 125 mg
1356	SLO-PHYLLIN (theophylline), 250 mg
2358	SLO-PHYLLIN GG (theophylline and guaifenesin)
2835	NICOBID (niacin), 125 mg
2840	NICOBID (niacin), 250 mg
2841	NICOBID (niacin), 500 mg

Ross

121	PRAMILET FA (multivitamin)
147	PRAMET FA (multivitamin)
5726	RONDEC (carbinoxamine and pseudoephedrine)
6240	RONDEC-TR (carbinoxamine and pseudoephedrine)

Roxane

UM	MARINOL (dronabinol), 2.5, 5, and 10 mg
54 090	ROXANOL SR (morphine sulfate), 30 mg
54 213	Lithium carbonate, 150 mg
54 452	Lithium carbonate, 300 mg (tablets)
54 463	Lithium carbonate, 300 mg (capsules)
54 582	ROXICODONE (oxycodone), 5 mg
54 702	Lithium carbonate, 600 mg

Sandoz Phamaceuticals

78–2	MELLARIL (thioridazine), 10 mg
78–8	MELLARIL (thioridazine), 15 mg
78–27	BELLADENAL-S (belladonna alkaloids and phenobarbital)
78–28	BELLADENAL (belladonna alkaloids and phenobarbital)
78–30	BELLAFOLINE (belladonna alkaloids), 0.25 mg
78–31	BELLERGAL-S (belladonna alkaloids, ergotamine, and phenobarbital)
78–36	CAFERGOT P-B (ergotamine, caffeine, belladonna alkaloids, and pentobarbital)
78–52	MESANTOIN (mephenytoin), 100 mg
78–54	METHERGINE (methylergonovine), 0.2 mg
78–58	SANSERT (methysergide), 2 mg
78–66	SANOREX (mazindol), 2 mg
78–71	SANOREX (mazindol), 1 mg
78–72	TAVIST (clemastine), 2.68 mg
78–73	VISKEN (pindolol), 10 mg
78–75	TAVIST-1 (clemastine), 1.34 mg
78–77	HYDERGINE (ergoloid mesylates), 1 mg
78–78	PAMELOR (nortriptyline), 50 mg
78–79	PAMELOR (nortriptyline), 75 mg
78–86	PAMELOR (nortriptyline), 10 mg
78–87	PAMELOR (nortriptyline), 25 mg
78–105	FIORINAL with Codeine No. 1 (butalbital, aspirin, caffeine, and codeine)
78–106	FIORINAL with Codeine No. 2 (butalbital, aspirin, caffeine, and codeine)
78–107	FIORINAL with Codeine No. 3 (butalbital, aspirin, caffeine, and codeine)
78–111	VISKEN (pindolol), 5 mg
78–202	ASBRON G (theophylline and guaifenesin)
78–212	METAPREL (metaproterenol), 10 mg
78–213	METAPREL (metaproterenol), 20 mg
78–221	TAVIST-D (clemastine and phenylpropanolamine)

Savage

0762	CHROMAGEN OB (multivitamin)
1115	DILOR (dyphylline), 200 mg
1116	DILOR-400 (dyphylline), 400 mg
1124	DILOR-G (dyphylline), 400 mg
1934	BREXIN L.A. (chlorpheniramine and pseudoephedrine)
3681	SATRIC (metronidazole), 250 mg
3688	SATRIC (metronidazole), 500 mg
4285	CHROMAGEN (hematinic)

Schering

009	CHLOR-TRIMETON (chlorpheniramine), 12 mg
011	CELESTONE (betamethasone), 0.6 mg
070	ESTINYL (ethinyl estradiol), 0.05 mg
077	TRILAFON (perphenazine), 16 mg
080	CHLOR-TRIMETON (chlorpheniramine), 4 mg
095	POLARAMINE (dexchlorpheniramine), 4 mg
119	ETRAFON-A 4–10 (perphenazine and amitriptyline)
141	TRILAFON (perphenazine), 8 mg (sustained-release tablets)

PRODUCT IMPRINT CODES

148	POLARAMINE (dexchlorpheniramine), 6 mg	571	Furosemide, 20 mg
150	ESTINYL (ethinyl estradiol), 0.5 mg	581	Furosemide, 40 mg
160	RELA (carisoprodol), 350 mg	601	PRO-BANTHINE (propantheline), 15 mg
228	FULVICIN P/G (ultramicrosize griseofulvin), 125 mg	611	PRO-BANTHINE (propantheline), 7.5 mg
231	DISOPHROL Chronotabs (pseudoephedrine and dexbrompheniramine)	831	Haloperidol, 0.5 mg
		841	Haloperidol, 1 mg
		851	Haloperidol, 2 mg
244	NORMODYNE (labetalol), 100 mg	861	Haloperidol, 5 mg
251	PAXIPAM (halazepam), 20 mg	871	Haloperidol, 10 mg
252	PROVENTIL (albuterol), 2 mg	1001	ALDACTONE (spironolactone), 25 mg
258	AFRINOL (pseudoephedrine), 120 mg	1011	ALDACTAZIDE (spironolactone and hydrochlorothiazide), 25 mg/25 mg
282	OPTIMINE (azatadine), 1 mg		
287	ETRAFON 2–10 (perphenazine and amitriptyline)	1021	ALDACTAZIDE (spironolactone and hydrochlorothiazide), 50 mg/50 mg
298	ESTINYL (ethinyl estradiol), 0.02 mg		
307	CORICIDIN 'D' (chlorpheniramine and phenylpropanolamine)	1031	ALDACTONE (spironolactone), 100 mg
		1041	ALDACTONE (spironolactone), 50 mg
311	ORETON Methyl (methyltestosterone), 10 mg	1231	AMINOPHYLLIN (aminophylline), 100 mg
313	TRILAFON (perphenazine), 8 mg	1251	AMINOPHYLLIN (aminophylline), 200 mg
316	PERMITIL (fluphenazine), 10 mg	1401	ANAVAR (oxandrolone), 2.5 mg
352	FULVICIN P/G (ultramicrosize griseofulvin), 330 mg	1501	BANTHINE (methantheline), 50 mg
		1701	DRAMAMINE (dimenhydrinate), 50 mg
374	CHLOR-TRIMETON (chlorpheniramine), 8 mg	1831	FLAGYL (metronidazole), 250 mg
394	NAQUIVAL (trichlormethiazide and reserpine)	1851	CALAN (verapamil), 80 mg
396	GYNE-LOTRIMIN (clotrimazole), 500 mg	1861	CALAN (verapamil), 120 mg
402	THEOVENT (theophylline), 125 mg	2732	NORPACE CR (disopyramide), 100 mg
438	NORMODYNE (labetalol), 300 mg	2742	NORPACE CR (disopyramide), 150 mg
442	PERMITIL (fluphenazine), 2.5 mg	2752	NORPACE (disopyramide), 100 mg
445	DRIXORAL (dexbrompheniramine and pseudoephedrine)	2762	NORPACE (disopyramide), 150 mg
		2832	THEO-24 (theophylline), 100 mg
496	FULVICIN-U/F (griseofulvin), 500 mg	2842	THEO-24 (theophylline), 200 mg
499	ORETON Methyl (methyltestosterone), 25 mg	2852	THEO-24 (theophylline), 300 mg
507	FULVICIN P/G (ultramicrosize griseofulvin), 250 mg		

Smith Kline & French

522	CORICIDIN (chlorpheniramine), 325 mg	C44	COMPAZINE (prochlorperazine), 10 mg (capsules)
538	PAXIPAM (halazepam), 40 mg	C46	COMPAZINE (prochlorperazine), 15 mg
547	NAQUA (trichlormethiazide), 4 mg	C47	COMPAZINE (prochlorperazine), 30 mg
550	PERMITIL (fluphenazine), 5 mg	C66	COMPAZINE (prochlorperazine), 5 mg
573	PROVENTIL (albuterol), 4 mg	C67	COMPAZINE (prochlorperazine), 10 mg (tablets)
598	ETRAFON 2–25 (perphenazine and amitriptyline)	C69	COMPAZINE (prochlorperazine), 25 mg
654	FULVICIN P/G (ultramicrosize griseofulvin), 165 mg	D14	CYTOMEL (liothyronine), 0.005 mg
		D16	CYTOMEL (liothyronine), 0.025 mg
703	TRINALIN (azatadine and pseudoephedrine)	D17	CYTOMEL (liothyronine), 0.050 mg
705	TRILAFON (perphenazine), 2 mg	D62	DARBID (isopropamide), 5 mg
720	ETRAFON-FORTE 4–25 (perphenazine and amitriptyline)	E12	DEXEDRINE (dextroamphetamine), 5 mg (capsules)
734	GYNE-LOTRIMIN (clotrimazole), 100 mg	E13	DEXEDRINE (dextroamphetamine), 10 mg
751	DEMAZIN (chlorpheniramine and phenylephrine)	E14	DEXEDRINE (dextroamphetamine), 15 mg
752	NORMODYNE (labetalol), 200 mg	E19	DEXEDRINE (dextroamphetamine), 5 mg (tablets)
753	THEOVENT (theophylline), 250 mg	E33	DIBENZYLINE (phenoxybenzamine), 10 mg
795	MIRADON (anisindione), 50 mg	J09	ESKALITH (lithium), 300 mg
820	POLARAMINE (dexchlorpheniramine), 2 mg	J10	ESKALITH CR (lithium), 450 mg
822	NAQUA (trichlormethiazide), 2 mg	S03	STELAZINE (trifluoperazine), 1 mg
843	METICORTEN (prednisone), 1 mg	S04	STELAZINE (trifluoperazine), 2 mg
866	DISOPHROL (dexbrompheniramine and pseudoephedrine)	S04	STELAZINE (trifluoperazine), 5 mg
		S06	STELAZINE (trifluoperazine), 10 mg
901	CHLOR-TRIMETON Decongestant (chlorpheniramine and pseudoephedrine)	T63	THORAZINE (chlorpromazine), 30 mg
		T64	THORAZINE (chlorpromazine), 75 mg
940	TRILAFON (perphenazine), 4 mg	T66	THORAZINE (chlorpromazine), 150 mg
948	FULVICIN-U/F (griseofulvin), 250 mg	T67	THORAZINE (chlorpromazine), 200 mg (capsules)
968	TINDAL (acetophenazine), 20 mg	T69	THORAZINE (chlorpromazine), 300 mg
970	ORETON Methyl Buccal (methyltestosterone), 10 mg	T73	THORAZINE (chlorpromazine), 10 mg
		T74	THORAZINE (chlorpromazine), 25 mg
		T76	THORAZINE (chlorpromazine), 50 mg
		T77	THORAZINE (chlorpromazine), 100 mg
		T79	THORAZINE (chlorpromazine), 200 mg (tablets)

Searle

51	ENOVID (norethynodrel and mestranol)
71	DEMULEN 1/50 (ethynodiol and ethinyl estradiol)
101	ENOVID (norethynodrel and mestranol)
131	ENOVID-E (norethynodrel and mestranol)
151	DEMULEN 1/35 (ethynodiol and ethinyl estradiol)
401	OVULEN (ethynodiol and mestranol)
500	FLAGYL (metronidazole), 500 mg
501	DIULO (metolazone), 2.5 mg
511	DIULO (metolazone), 5 mg
521	DIULO (metolazone), 10 mg
531	Chlorthalidone, 25 mg
541	Chlorthalidone, 50 mg

Squibb

F16	PRINCIPEN with Probenecid (ampicillin and probenecid)
113	VELOSEF '250' (cephradine), 250 mg
114	VELOSEF '500' (cephradine), 500 mg
160	ETHRIL '250' (erythromycin), 250 mg
161	ETHRIL '500' (erythromycin), 500 mg
164	PENTIDS (penicillin G), 200,000 units
165	PENTIDS '400' (penicillin G), 400,000 units

continued

PRODUCT IMPRINT CODES

168	PENTIDS '800' (penicillin G), 800,000 units		hydroxide, and simethicone)
196	Vitamin C, 250 mg	710	MULVIDREN-F (multivitamin)
197	Vitamin C, 500 mg	760	SORBITRATE (isosorbide dinitrate), 5 mg (sublingual)
201	Aspirin, 324 mg		
230	TRIMOX '250' (amoxicillin), 250 mg	761	SORBITRATE (isosorbide dinitrate), 10 mg (sublingual)
231	TRIMOX '500' (amoxicillin), 500 mg		
338	CAPOZIDE 25/15 (captopril and hydrochlorothiazide)	770	SORBITRATE (isosorbide dinitrate), 5 mg (oral)
		773	SORBITRATE (isosorbide dinitrate), 30 mg (oral)
349	CAPOZIDE 25/25 (captopril and hydrochlorothiazide)	774	SORBITRATE (isosorbide dinitrate), 40 mg (oral)
355	VALADOL (acetaminophen), 325 mg	780	SORBITRATE (isosorbide dinitrate), 10 mg (oral)
384	CAPOZIDE 50/15 (captopril and hydrochlorothiazide)	810	SORBITRATE (isosorbide dinitrate), 5 mg (chewable)
390	CAPOZIDE 50/25 (captopril and hydrochlorothiazide)	815	SORBITRATE (isosorbide dinitrate), 10 mg (chewable)
429	FLORINEF (fludrocortisone), 0.1 mg	820	SORBITRATE (isosorbide dinitrate), 20 mg (oral)
450	CAPOTEN (captopril), 12.5 mg	853	SORBITRATE (isosorbide dinitrate), 2.5 mg (sublingual)
452	CAPOTEN (captopril), 25 mg		
455	ORAGRAFIN (ipodate), 500 mg	858	MYLICON-80 (simethicone), 80 mg
457	MYCOSTATIN (nystatin), 100,000 units	864	BUCLADIN-S (buclizine), 50 mg
470	CAPOTEN (captopril), 37.5 mg	880	SORBITRATE SA (isosorbide dinitrate), 40 mg
478	ENGRAN-HP (multivitamin)		
482	CAPOTEN (captopril), 50 mg		
485	CAPOTEN (captopril), 100 mg		

Syntex

1	NORINYL 1+50 (norethindrone and mestranol)
2	NORINYL (norethindrone and mestranol)
3	NORINYL 1+80 (norethindrone and mestranol)
11	NORINYL 1+35 (norethindrone and ethinyl estradiol)
110	TRI-NORINYL (norethindrone and ethinyl estradiol), 0.5 mg/0.035 mg
111	TRI-NORINYL (norethindrone and ethinyl estradiol), 1.0 mg/0.035 mg
272	NAPROSYN (naproxen), 250 mg
273	NAPROSYN (naproxen), 375 mg
274	ANAPROX (naproxen sodium), 275 mg
277	NAPROSYN (naproxen), 500 mg
2110	BREVICON (norethindrone and ethinyl estradiol)
2902	ANADROL-50 (oxymetholone), 50 mg

512	KENACORT (triamcinolone), 4 mg
518	KENACORT (triamcinolone), 8 mg
535	THERAGRAN Hematinic (multivitamin)
537	Niacin, 500 mg
549	Iron and vitamin C
573	ORA-TESTRYL (fluoxymesterone), 5 mg
580	MYCOSTATIN (nystatin), 500,000 units
603	SUMYCIN '500' (tetracycline), 500 mg
610	Niacin, 25 mg
611	Niacin, 50 mg
612	Niacin, 100 mg
623	NOCTEC (chloral hydrate), 250 mg
626	NOCTEC (chloral hydrate), 500 mg
637	NYDRAZID (isoniazid), 100 mg
648	VEETIDS '500' (penicillin V), 500 mg
655	SUMYCIN '250' (tetracycline), 250 mg (capsules)
663	SUMYCIN '250' (tetracycline), 250 mg (tablets)
684	VEETIDS '250' (penicillin V), 250 mg
690	TESLAC (testolactone), 50 mg
763	SUMYCIN '500' (tetracycline), 500 mg
779	MYSTECLIN-F (tetracycline and amphotericin B)
830	HYDREA (hydroxyurea), 500 mg
872	COMOXOL 400/80 (sulfamethoxazole and trimethoprim)
873	COMOXOL 800/160 (sulfamethoxazole and trimethoprim)
876	TRIGESIC (acetaminophen, aspirin, and caffeine)
883	VIVOX (doxycycline), 50 mg
884	VIVOX (doxycycline), 100 mg (capsules)
887	TERFONYL (trisulfapyrimidines), 500 mg
897	VIVOX (doxycycline), 100 mg (tablets)
915	Thiamine, 50 mg
916	Thiamine, 100 mg
971	PRINCIPEN '250' (ampicillin), 250 mg
974	PRINCIPEN '500' (ampicillin), 500 mg

Upjohn

10	HALCION (triazolam), 0.125 mg
11	FEMINONE (ethinyl estradiol), 0.05 mg
12	CORTEF (hydrocortisone), 5 mg
14	HALOTESTIN (fluoxymesterone), 2 mg
15	Cortisone, 5 mg
17	HALCION (triazolam), 0.25 mg
18	DIDREX (benzphetamine), 25 mg
19	HALOTESTIN (fluoxymesterone), 5 mg
22	MEDROL (methylprednisolone), 8 mg
23	Cortisone, 10 mg
24	DIDREX (benzphetamine), 50 mg
25	DELTA-CORTEF (prednisolone), 5 mg
27	HALCION (triazolam), 0.5 mg
29	XANAX (alprazolam), 0.25 mg
31	CORTEF (hydrocortisone), 10 mg
32	DELTASONE (prednisone), 2.5 mg
34	Cortisone, 25 mg
36	HALOTESTIN (fluoxymesterone), 10 mg
38	HALODRIN (fluoxymesterone and ethinyl estradiol)
44	CORTEF (hydrocortisone), 20 mg
45	DELTASONE (prednisone), 5 mg
49	MEDROL (methylprednisolone), 2 mg
50	PROVERA (medroxyprogesterone), 10 mg
55	XANAX (alprazolam), 0.5 mg
56	MEDROL (methylprednisolone), 4 mg
61	PAMINE (methscopolamine), 2.5 mg
64	PROVERA (medroxyprogesterone), 2.5 mg
70	TOLINASE (tolazamide), 100 mg
73	MEDROL (methylprednisolone), 16 mg
81	ADEFLOR (multivitamin), 0.5 mg
90	XANAX (alprazolam), 1 mg
92	ADEFLOR (multivitamin), 1 mg
100	ORINASE (tolbutamide), 0.5 mg
101	ALBAMYCIN (novobiocin), 250 mg
103	E-MYCIN (erythromycin), 250 mg
106	DIOSTATE-D (multivitamin)
114	TOLINASE (tolazamide), 250 mg

Stuart

023	STUARTNATAL 1+1 (multivitamin)
101	TENORMIN (atenolol), 100 mg
105	TENORMIN (atenolol), 50 mg
115	TENORETIC-50 (atenolol and chlorthalidone)
117	TENORETIC-100 (atenolol and chlorthalidone)
220	KINESED (belladonna alkaloids and phenobarbital)
380	KASOF (docusate), 240 mg
450	MYLICON (simethicone), 40 mg
470	DIALOSE (docusate), 100 mg
475	DIALOSE Plus (casanthranol and docusate)
600	NOLVADEX (tamoxifen), 10 mg
620	MYLANTA (aluminum hydroxide, magnesium hydroxide, and simethicone)
650	FERANCEE (ferrous fumarate and vitamin C)
651	MYLANTA-II (aluminum hydroxide, magnesium

PRODUCT IMPRINT CODES

115	ADEFLOR-M (multivitamin)		13	AMPHOJEL (aluminum hydroxide), 0.6 g
121	LONITEN (minoxidil), 2.5 mg		19	PHENERGAN (promethazine), 12.5 mg
122	CEBENASE (multivitamin)		22	ALUDROX (alumina and magnesia)
131	MICRONASE (glyburide), 1.25 mg		27	PHENERGAN (promethazine), 25 mg
137	LONITEN (minoxidil), 10 mg		28	SPARINE (promazine), 50 mg
138	UNICAP (multivitamin)		29	SPARINE (promazine), 25 mg
141	MICRONASE (glyburide), 2.5 mg		33	EQUANIL (meprobamate), 400 mg
155	MEDROL (methylprednisolone), 24 mg		51	SERAX (oxazepam), 10 mg
165	DELTASONE (prednisone), 20 mg		52	SERAX (oxazepam), 30 mg
171	MICRONASE (glyburide), 2.5 mg		53	OMNIPEN (ampicillin), 250 mg
176	MEDROL (methylprednisolone), 32 mg		56	OVRAL (norgestrel and ethinyl estradiol)
193	DELTASONE (prednisone), 10 mg		57	UNIPEN (nafcillin), 250 mg
198	UNICAP Jr (multivitamin)		59	PEN-VEE K (penicillin V), 250 mg
225	CLEOCIN HCl (clindamycin), 150 mg		62	OVRETTE (norgestrel), 0.075 mg
243	ALKETS (calcium carbonate, magnesium oxide, and magnesium carbonate)		64	ATIVAN (lorazepam), 1 mg
			65	ATIVAN (lorazepam), 2 mg
251	Calcium gluconate, 975 mg		71	MAZANOR (mazindol), 1 mg
272	Calcium lactate, 650 mg		73	WYTENSIN (guanabenz), 4 mg
285	UNICAP (multivitamin)		74	WYTENSIN (guanabenz), 8 mg
286	PROVERA (medroxyprogesterone), 5 mg		75	NORDETTE-21 (levonorgestrel and ethinyl estradiol)
331	CLEOCIN HCl (clindamycin), 75 mg			
336	LINCOCIN (lincomycin), 250 mg		78	LO/OVRAL (norgestrel and ethinyl estradiol)
363	ZYMACAP (multivitamin)		81	ATIVAN (lorazepam), 0.5 mg
388	DELTASONE (prednisone), 50 mg		85	WYGESIC (propoxyphene and acetaminophen)
412	MAOLATE (chlorphenesin), 400 mg		91	EQUAGESIC (meprobamate and aspirin)
461	SIGTAB (multivitamin)		92	WYTENSIN (guanabenz), 16 mg
477	TOLINASE (tolazamide), 500 mg		119	AMPHOJEL (aluminum hydroxide), 0.3 g
500	LINCOCIN (lincomycin), 500 mg		165	BICILLIN (penicillin G), 200,000 units
521	MYCIFRADIN (neomycin), 0.5 g		200	SPARINE (promazine), 100 mg
586	UTICILLIN VK (penicillin V), 250 mg		227	PHENERGAN (promethazine), 50 mg
671	UTICILLIN VK (penicillin V), 500 mg		261	MEPERGAN FORTIS (meperidine and promethazine)
701	ORINASE (tolbutamide), 250 mg			
725	MOTRIN (ibuprofen), 800 mg		267	Phenobarbital, 15 mg
730	PHENOLAX (phenolphthalein)		268	Phenobarbital, 30 mg
733	MOTRIN (ibuprofen), 300 mg		269	Phenobarbital, 100 mg
742	MOTRIN (ibuprofen), 600 mg		308	Meperidine, 50 mg
750	MOTRIN (ibuprofen), 400 mg		309	OMNIPEN (ampicillin), 500 mg
782	PANMYCIN (tetracycline), 250 mg		313	Aspirin, 300 mg
873	SUPER D (vitamins A and D)		317	SERAX (oxazepam), 15 mg
949	Uracil, 1 mg		320	Phenobarbital, 60 mg
3176	E-MYCIN (erythromycin), 333 mg		326	Codeine, 30 mg
3212	PYRROXATE (chlorpheniramine, phenylpropanolamine, and acetaminophen)		327	Codeine, 60 mg
			360	PATHOCIL (dicloxacillin), 250 mg
3293	KAOPECTATE (attapulgite), 600 mg		389	Tetracycline, 250 mg
3300	P-A-C (aspirin and caffeine)		390	PEN-VEE K (penicillin V), 500 mg
3336	UNICAP M (multivitamin)		434	PHENERGAN-D (promethazine and pseudoephedrine)
3338	UNICAP T (multivitamin)			
3340	UNICAP Senior (multivitamin)		445	OVRAL-28 pink inert tablet
3342	UNICAP (multivitamin)		464	UNIPEN (nafcillin), 500 mg
3402	HALTRAN (ibuprofen), 200 mg		471	Tetracycline, 500 mg
			472	BASALJEL (aluminum carbonate), 608 mg (capsules)

Winthrop Pharmaceuticals

			473	BASALJEL (aluminum carbonate), 608 mg (tablets)
A77	ARALEN (chloroquine), 500 mg		486	NORDETTE-28 and LO/OVRAL-28 pink inert tablet
B34	BILOPAQUE (tyropanoate), 750 mg		559	WYMOX (amoxicillin), 250 mg
D03	DANOCRINE (danazol), 50 mg		560	WYMOX (amoxicillin), 500 mg
D04	DANOCRINE (danazol), 100 mg		576	WYAMYCIN-S (erythromycin), 250 mg
D05	DANOCRINE (danazol), 200 mg		578	WYAMYCIN-S (erythromycin), 500 mg
D35	DEMEROL (meperidine), 50 mg		593	PATHOCIL (dicloxacillin), 500 mg
D37	DEMEROL (meperidine), 100 mg		614	CYCLAPEN-W (cyclacillin), 250 mg
M90	MODRASTANE (trilostane), 60 mg		615	CYCLAPEN-W (cyclacillin), 500 mg
M91	MODRASTANE (trilostane), 30 mg		2511	OVRAL-28 (norgestrel and ethinyl estradiol)
N21	NegGram (nalidixic acid), 250 mg		2514	LO/OVRAL-28 (norgestrel and ethinyl estradiol)
N22	NegGram (nalidixic acid), 500 mg		2533	NORDETTE-28 (levonorgestrel and ethinyl estradiol)
N23	NegGram (nalidixic acid), 1 g			
P61	PLAQUENIL (hydroxychloroquine), 200 mg		2535	TRIPHASIL-21 (levonorgestrel and ethinyl estradiol)
T31	TELEPAQUE (iopanoic acid), 500 mg			
T37	TALACEN (pentazocine and acetaminophen)		2536	TRIPHASIL-28 (levonorgestrel and ethinyl estradiol)
T51	TALWIN Nx (pentazocine and naloxone)			
T100	TRANCOPAL (chlormezanone), 100 mg		4120	CYCLOSPASMOL (cyclandelate), 100 mg
T200	TRANCOPAL (chlormezanone), 200 mg		4124	CYCLOSPASMOL (cyclandelate), 200 mg
W53	WINSTROL (stanozolol), 2 mg		4125	ISORDIL (isosorbide dinitrate), 40 mg (controlled-release tablets)

Wyeth

			4126	ISORDIL (isosorbide dinitrate), 5 mg (sublingual)
1	EQUANIL (meprobamate), 400 mg		4130	TRECATOR-SC (ethionamide), 250 mg
2	EQUANIL (meprobamate), 200 mg		4132	SURMONTIL (trimipramine), 25 mg
6	SERAX (oxazepam), 15 mg		4133	SURMONTIL (trimipramine), 50 mg *continued*

PRODUCT IMPRINT CODES

4139	ISORDIL (isosorbide dinitrate), 2.5 mg (sublingual)
4140	ISORDIL (isosorbide dinitrate), 40 mg (controlled-release capsules)
4148	CYCLOSPASMOL (cyclandelate), 400 mg
4152	ISORDIL (isosorbide dinitrate), 5 mg (oral)
4153	ISORDIL (isosorbide dinitrate), 10 mg (oral)
4154	ISORDIL (isosorbide dinitrate), 20 mg (oral)
4158	SURMONTIL (trimipramine), 100 mg
4159	ISORDIL (isosorbide dinitrate), 30 mg (oral)
4161	ISORDIL (isosorbide dinitrate), 10 mg (sublingual)
4164	ISORDIL (isosorbide dinitrate), 10 mg (chewable)
4177	SECTRAL (acebutolol), 200 mg
4179	SECTRAL (acebutolol), 400 mg
4181	ORUDIS (ketoprofen), 50 mg
4187	ORUDIS (ketoprofen), 75 mg
4188	CORDARONE (amiodarone), 200 mg
4190	SYNALGOS (aspirin and caffeine)
4191	SYNALGOS-DC (hydrocodone, aspirin, and caffeine)
4192	ISORDIL (isosorbide dinitrate), 40 mg (oral)

Chapter 3

Information Resources

Drug Information Centers

The following centers provide answers by telephone to routine questions about drugs—identification, availability, therapeutic uses, dosage, side effects, drug interactions, etc— and can offer advice on specific therapeutic problems. In addition, many centers follow up verbal communications with written reports, provide comprehensive evaluations of new drugs and information on investigational compounds and uses, publish newsletters and bulletins, and serve as regional poison control centers. These services are usually available free of charge to all health-care professionals in the region served by the center.

Alabama
Auburn University Drug Information Center
School of Pharmacy
Auburn University
Auburn, AL 36849
205/826-4037 (8 am-5 pm Mon-Fri)

Drug Communication Service
Department of Pharmacy
University of Alabama Hospitals
619 South 19th Street
Birmingham, AL 35233
205/934-2162 (24 hours)

Arkansas
Arkansas Poison Control
Drug Information Center
4301 West Markham Street
Little Rock, AR 72201
501/666-5532, 800/482-8948
(24 hours)

Arizona
Arizona Poison and
Drug Information Center
Arizona Health Sciences Center
University of Arizona
Tucson, AZ 85724
602/626-6016, 800/362-0101
(Arizona only) (24 hours)

California
Drug Information Service
Alta Bates Hospital
3001 Colby Street at Ashby
Berkeley, CA 94705
415/540-1503 (9 am-4 pm Mon-Fri)

Kaiser-Permanente Drug Information Center
9521 Dalen Street
Downey, CA 90242
213/803-2134 (9 am-5 pm Mon-Fri and after hours)

Drug Information Service
El Cajon Valley Hospital
1688 East Main Street
El Cajon, CA 92021
714/440-1122 ext 333 (8 am-4:30 pm)

Drug Information Analysis Center
Valley Medical Center
445 South Cedar Avenue
Fresno, CA 93702
209/453-4596 (8 am-5 pm Mon-Fri)

Drug Information Service
Memorial Hospital Medical Center
PO Box 1428, 2801 Atlantic Avenue
Long Beach, CA 90801
213/595-2303 (24 hours)

Drug Information Center, Room 1107
Los Angeles County-University of Southern California Medical Center
1200 North State Street
Los Angeles, CA 90033
213/226-7741 (8 am-4 pm Mon-Fri)

Drug Information Analysis Service
VA Medical Center
3350 La Jolla Village Drive
San Diego, CA 92161
619/453-7500 ext 3026 (8 am-4 pm Mon-Fri), 619/453-7500
pager 649 (evenings, weekends, and holidays)

Drug Information Analysis Service
Division of Clinical Pharmacy (C152)
University of California
Hospitals and Clinics
Third and Parnassus Avenues
San Francisco, CA 94143
415/476-4346 (8 am-6 pm Mon-Fri),
415/476-2845 (after hours)

Drug Information Center
Department of Pharmacy Services
Stanford University Hospital
Stanford, CA 94305
415/497-6422 (7:30 am-11 pm)

Colorado
Rocky Mountain Drug Consultation Center
Denver General Hospital
645 Bannock Street
Denver, CO 80204-4507
303/893-DRUG, 800/332-6475
(Colorado only)

Connecticut
Drug Information Center
University of Connecticut Health Center
Farmington, CT 06032
203/674-2782 (8 am-5 pm Mon-Fri)

Drug Information Service
Hartford Hospital
80 Seymour Street
Hartford, CT 06115
203/524-2221 (8:30 am-5 pm Mon-Fri)

Drug Information Service
Yale-New Haven Hospital
20 York Street
New Haven, CT 06504
203/785-2248 (24 hours)

District of Columbia
Drug Information Center
Department of Pharmacy Services
Children's Hospital National Medical Center
111 Michigan Avenue
Washington, DC 20010
202/745-2055 (8 am-4 pm Mon-Fri)

Drug Information Service
Howard University Hospital
2041 Georgia Avenue NW
Washington, DC 20060
202/745-1325 (9 am-5 pm Mon-Fri and after hours)

Washington Hospital Center
110 Irving Street NW
Washington, DC 20010
202/541-6646 (8 hours Mon-Fri),
202/541-6745 (emergencies)

Florida
Drug Information and Pharmacy Resource Center
Box J-4, College of Pharmacy
J. Hillis Miller Health Center
University of Florida
Gainesville, FL 32610
904/392-3576 (9 am-5 pm Mon-Fri),
800/342-1106 (in Florida) (9 am-5 pm Mon-Fri)

Up Front Drug Information
5701 Biscayne Boulevard #602
Miami, FL 33137
305/757-2566, 800/432-8255 (Florida only) (9 am-5 pm Mon-Fri)

Georgia
Drug Information Center
Mercer University School of Pharmacy
345 Boulevard NE
Atlanta, GA 30312
404/688-6291 (8 am-4 pm Mon-Fri)

Drug Information Center
Pharmacy Department
Medical College of Georgia
Augusta, GA 30912
404/828-2887 (8:30 am-5 pm)

Idaho
Idaho Drug Information and Regional Poison Control Center
755 Hospital Way, Suite F2
Pocatello, ID 83201
208/234-0777 ext 5019, 5029, or 5039;
800/632-9490 (Idaho only)

Illinois
Drug Information Center
Rush-Presbyterian-St. Luke's Medical Center
1753 West Congress Parkway
Chicago, IL 60612
312/942-6525 (9 am-5 pm Mon-Fri)

Drug Information Service
Box 434, University of Chicago Medical Center
5841 South Maryland Avenue
Chicago, IL 60637
312/962-1388 (8 am-5 pm Mon-Fri),
312/962-1387 (24 hours)

Drug Information Center
Room C-300, Department of Pharmacy Service
University of Illinois Hospital
1740 West Taylor Street
Chicago, IL 60612
312/996-0209 (7 am-6 pm),
312/996-0209 (after hours)

Drug Information-Poison Control Center
Brokaw Hospital
Virginia at Franklin Streets
Normal, IL 61761
309/454-1400 ext 178
(6:30 am-11:30 pm)

Northern Illinois Poison Control Center
1400 Charles Street
Rockford, IL 61101
815/968-6000 (24 hours)

Drug Information Service
Department of Pharmacy
Illini Hospital
801 Hospital Road
Silvis, IL 61282
309/792-9363 ext 306 (24 hours)

Indiana
Drug Information Services
Room N109A, Department of Pharmacy
Indiana University Hospitals
1100 West Michigan Street
Indianapolis, IN 46223
317/264-3581 (8 am-5 pm Mon-Fri and after hours)

Iowa
Drug Information Center
Mercy Hospital Medical Center
Sixth and University Avenues
Des Moines, IA 50314
515/247-3286 (24 hours)

Variety Club Poison and Drug Information Service
1200 Pleasant Street
Des Moines, IA 50308
515/283-6254 (24 hours),
800/362-2327 (Iowa only)

Drug Information Service
Department of Pharmacy
Trinity Regional Hospital
Kenyon Road
Fort Dodge, IA 50501
515/573-7211 (24 hours)

Drug Information and Poison Control Center
University of Iowa Hospitals and Clinics
Iowa City, IA 52242
319/356-2600 (8 am-5 pm Mon-Fri and after hours)

Kentucky
Drug Information Center
University of Kentucky Medical Center
Lexington, KY 40536
606/233-5320 (8 am-5 pm)

Louisiana
St. Francis Hospital Drug Information and Poison Control Center
309 Jackson Street
Monroe, LA 71201
318/325-6454 (24 hours)

Xavier University Drug Information Center at Tulane Medical Center
1415 Tulane Avenue
New Orleans, LA 70112
504/588-5670 (9 am-5 pm Mon-Fri)

COMPENDIUM OF DRUG THERAPY

INFORMATION RESOURCES

Maryland
Drug Information Services
Anne Arundel General Hospital
Franklin and Cathedral Streets
Annapolis, MD 21401
301/267-1126 or 301/267-1130,
301/267-1000 (after hours)

Drug Information Center
Osler, Room 526
Department of Pharmacy Services
Division of Clinical Pharmacology
The Johns Hopkins Hospital
600 North Wolfe Street
Baltimore, MD 21205
301/955-6348 (8 am-5 pm)

Drug Information Center
Room NIW89
Department of Pharmacy Services
University of Maryland Medical
Systems
22 South Greene Street
Baltimore, MD 21201
301/528-5668 (8:30 am-5 pm)

Drug Information Services
Malcolm Grow USAF Medical Center
Andrews AFB
Camp Springs, MD 20331
301/981-2997 (8 am-5 pm Mon-Fri)

Drug Information Center
Department of Pharmacy
Memorial Hospital
South Washington Street
Easton, MD 21601
301/822-1000 ext 5645 (7 am-7:30 pm
and after hours)

Massachusetts
Drug Information Center at Brigham
and Women's Hospital
75 Francis Street
Boston, MA 02115
617/732-7166 (7 am-5 pm Mon-Fri
and after hours)

New England Drug Information
Consultation Service
Massachusetts College of Pharmacy
and Allied Health Sciences
179 Longwood Avenue
Boston, MA 02115
617/732-2818 (9 am-5 pm Mon-Fri)

Northeastern University College of
Pharmacy and Allied Health
Professions
Mugar Health Professions Resource
Center
Room 203 Mugar
360 Huntington Avenue
Boston, MA 02115
617/437-3213 (9 am-5 pm Mon-Fri)

Michigan
Drug Information Service
Room B1C255
University of Michigan
Adult General Hospital
East Medical Center Drive
Ann Arbor, MI 48109
313/936-6020 (8 am-5 pm Mon-Fri)

Drug Information Center
Harper-Grace Hospitals
3990 John Road
Detroit, MI 48201
313/494-9477 (8 am-4:30 pm and
after hours)

Drug Information Service
Department of Pharmacy
Henry Ford Hospital
2799 West Grand Boulevard
Detroit, MI 48202
313/876-3324 (after hours)

Drug and Poison Information Center
Bronson Methodist Hospital
252 East Lovell Street
Kalamazoo, MI 49006
616/383-6409 (24 hours)

Drug Information Center
St. Lawrence Hospital
1210 West Saginaw Street
Lansing, MI 48915
517/377-0408 (24 hours)

Drug Information Center
St. Joseph Mercy Hospital
900 Woodward Avenue
Pontiac, MI 48053
313/858-3055 (8 am-5 pm Mon-Fri
and after hours)

Drug Information Center
William Beaumont Hospital
3601 West 13 Mile Road
Royal Oak, MI 48072
313/288-8000 or 313/288-7114
(24 hours)

Saginaw Region Poison Center and
Drug Information
Saginaw General Hospital
1447 North Harrison Avenue
Saginaw, MI 48602
517/771-4076 (7 am-10 pm)

Drug Information Service
Providence Hospital
16001 West Nine Mile Road
Southfield, MI 48037
313/424-3125 (8 am-5 pm)

Minnesota
Drug Information Center
University of Minnesota Hospital
Box 611, Mayo Memorial Building
420 Delaware Street SE
Minneapolis, MN 55455
612/373-8888 (8 am-4:30 pm Mon-Fri)

Drug Information Service
Department of Pharmacy
Saint Mary's Hospital of Rochester
1216 SW Second Street
Rochester, MN 55901
507/285-5062 (8 am-5 pm Mon-Fri)

Mississippi
University of Mississippi
Medical Drug Information Service
Department of Pharmacy
University Medical Center
2500 North State Street
Jackson, MS 39216
601/987-3608 (8 am-5 pm Mon-Fri)

Missouri
Drug Information Center
Freeman Hospital
1102 West 32nd Street
Joplin, MO 64801
417/623-2081 ext 276 (7 am-11 pm)

Drug Information Center
Department of Pharmacy Services
St. John's Regional Medical Center
2727 McClelland Boulevard
Joplin, MO 64801
417/781-2727 ext 2452 (24 hours)

Drug Information Center
Lakeside Hospital
8701 Troost Avenue
Kansas City, MO 64131
816/995-2260 (7 am-9 pm Mon-Fri)

Drug Information Service
Room H5,D28
University of Missouri
Kansas City School of Pharmacy
Truman Medical Center
2301 Holmes Street
Kansas City, MO 64108
816/471-1895 (8 am-5 pm Mon-Fri)

Medication Information Service
Heartland Hospital West
801 Faraon Street
St. Joseph, MO 64501
816/271-7583 (24 hours)

Substance Abuse Center
St. Joseph's State Hospital
3400 Frederick Avenue
St. Joseph, MO 64502
816/232-8431 (24 hours)

St. Louis Drug Information Center
St. Louis College of Pharmacy
4588 Parkview Place
St. Louis, MO 63110
314/454-8399 (24 hours)

Drug Information Center
St. John's Regional Health Center
1235 East Cherokee Street
Springfield, MO 65802
417/885-3488 (24 hours)

Drug Information Service
Johnson County Memorial Hospital
Burkarth Road and East Gay Street
Warrensburg, MO 64093
816/747-3181 ext 233 (6:45 am-5 pm)

Nebraska
Drug Information Center
St. Joseph Hospital
601 North 30th Street
Omaha, NE 68131
402/449-5800 (8 am-4:30 pm Mon-Fri)

Drug Information Services
Room 2370
University of Nebraska Medical Center
University Hospital
42nd and Dewey Streets
Omaha, NE 68105
402/559-4114

New Jersey
Pharmaceutical Extension Service
Rutgers University
College of Pharmacy
Piscataway, NJ 08854
201/932-2677 (8:30 am-4:30 pm)

New Mexico
New Mexico Poison and
Drug Information Center
University of New Mexico
Albuquerque, NM 87131
505/843-2551 (24 hours),
800/432-6866 (New Mexico only)
(24 hours)

New York
Drug Information Service
Montefiore Medical Center
111 East 210th Street
Bronx, NY 10467
212/920-4511 (8:30 am-5 pm Mon-
Fri), 212/920-4103 (after-hours
emergency service)

Arnold and Marie Schwartz
International Pharmaceutical
and Therapeutic Drug Information
Center
81 DeKalb Avenue
Brooklyn, NY 11201
212/403-1064 (9 am-5 pm Mon-Fri)

Drug Information Service
119A Veterans Administration Medical
Center
Canandaigua, NY 14424
716/394-2000 ext 174 (8 am-4:30 pm
Mon-Fri)

Drug Information Center
Lenox Hill Hospital
100 East 77th Street
New York, NY 10021
212/794-4284 (9 am-5 pm Mon-Fri)

Drug Information Service
Mercy Hospital
1000 North Village Avenue
Rockville Centre, NY 11570
516/255-2407 (24 hours)

North Carolina
Drug Information Service
Pharmacy Department
North Carolina Memorial Hospital
University of North Carolina
Chapel Hill, NC 27514
919/966-2373 (8 am-5 pm Mon-Fri),
pager 3866 (24 hours)

North Dakota
Drug Information Center
College of Pharmacy
North Dakota State University
Fargo, ND 58105
701/237-7609 (8 am-5 pm Mon-Fri)

Ohio
Drug Information Center
Raabe College of Pharmacy
and Health Sciences
Ohio Northern University
Ada, OH 45810
419/772-2307 (8 am-5 pm Mon-Fri
and after hours)

Drug and Poison Information Center
Room 7701
University of Cincinnati
Medical Center
231 Bethesda Avenue, ML #144
Cincinnati, OH 45267
513/872-5111 (24 hours)

Drug Information Center
Department of Pharmacy
Room 368
The Ohio State University Hospitals
410 West 10th Avenue
Columbus, OH 43210-1228
614/421-8679 (8 am-5 pm Mon-Fri),
614/421-8470 (after hours)

Drug Information Center
Pharmacy Department
Bethesda Hospital
2951 North Maple Avenue
Zanesville, OH 43701
614/454-4223 (7:30 am-11 pm
Mon-Fri, 8 am-10 pm Sat, Sun, and
holidays)

Oklahoma
Drug Information Center
Presbyterian Hospital
NE 13th at Lincoln Boulevard
Oklahoma City, OK 73104
405/271-6226 (8 am-4:30 pm Mon-Fri)

Drug Information Service
St. Francis Hospital
6161 South Yale Avenue
Tulsa, OK 74136
918/494-1167 (9:30 am-5:30 pm
Mon-Fri)

Oregon
Oregon Poison Control and Drug
Information Center
Oregon Health Sciences University
3181 SW Sam Jackson Park Road
Portland, OR 97201
503/225-8968, 800/452-7165
(24 hours)

Pennsylvania
Drug Information Service
Geisinger Medical Center
North Academy Avenue
Danville, PA 17822
717/271-8176 (8 am-4:30 pm Mon-Fri
and after hours)

Drug Information Center
Hamot Medical Center
201 State Street
Erie, PA 16550
814/870-6022

Drug Information Service
Hospital of the University of
Pennsylvania
3400 Spruce Street
Philadelphia, PA 19104
215/662-2903 (8 am-5 pm Mon-Fri)
215/662-2907 (after hours)

Drug Information Center
Pharmacy Department
Temple University Hospital
3401 North Broad Street
Philadelphia, PA 19140
215/221-4644 (8 am-4 pm Mon-Fri)

Drug Information Center
Pharmacy Department
Thomas Jefferson University Hospital
11th and Walnut Streets
Philadelphia, PA 19107
215/928-8877 (8 am-5 pm)

Drug Information Center
Mercy Hospital
Pride and Locust Streets
Pittsburgh, PA 15219
412/232-7903, 412/232-7907
(24 hours)

Drug Information Center
School of Pharmacy
University of Pittsburgh
239-B Victoria Building
Pittsburgh, PA 15261
412/624-DRUG (9 am-5 pm Mon-Fri
and after hours)

INFORMATION RESOURCES

Susquehanna Pharmaceutical Profile
Center
The Williamsport Hospital
777 Rural Avenue
Williamsport, PA 17701
717/322-7861 ext 2158 (8 am-5 pm
Mon-Fri), pager (24 hours)

Rhode Island
Drug Information Service
Rhode Island Hospital
Department of Pharmacy
593 Eddy Street
Providence, RI 02902
401/277-5547 or 401/277-8320
(8:30 am-5 pm daily),
401/277-8172 (emergencies)

URI Drug Information Center
Roger Williams General Hospital
825 Chalkstone Avenue
Providence, RI 02908
401/456-2260 (9 am-5 pm Mon-Fri
and after hours)

South Carolina
Drug Information Service
Medical University of South Carolina
171 Ashley Avenue
Charleston, SC 29425
803/792-3896 (8 am-5 pm Mon- Fri)
(answering machine 5 pm-8 am)

Drug Information Service
School of Medicine Library
University of South Carolina
Columbia, SC 29208
803/733-3170 (7:30 am-4:30 pm
Mon-Fri)

South Dakota
Drug Information Service
Department of Pharmacy
McKennan Hospital
800 East 21st Street
Sioux Falls, SD 57101
605/339-8062 (24 hours)

Drug Information Service
Department of Pharmacy
Sacred Heart Hospital
1000 West Fourth Street
Yankton, SD 57078
605/665-9371 (7 am-11 pm Mon-Fri)

Tennessee
Drug Information Center
College of Pharmacy/Health Sciences
Library
University of Tennessee-Memphis
877 Madison Avenue, Suite 210
Memphis, TN 38163
901/528-5555 (8 am-5 pm Mon-Fri)

Texas
Drug Information Center
Department of Pharmacy
M.D. Anderson Hospital and Tumor
Institute
6723 Bertner Avenue
Houston, TX 77030
713/792-2858 (7 am-5 pm Mon-Fri)

The Hermann Drug Information
Center
Hermann Hospital
5484 Jones Pavilion
1203 Ross Sterling
Houston, TX 77030
713/797-2073 (8 am-5:30 pm) (in
Houston), 1-800/392-1741 (8 am-
5:30 pm) (in Texas)

Turner Drug Information Center
University of Houston
College of Pharmacy
1441 Moursund Street
Houston, TX 77030
713/749-4011 (9 am-5 pm Mon-Fri
and after hours [emergencies only])

UTHSCSA-Drug Information Service
Department of Pharmacology
7703 Floyd Curl Drive
San Antonio, TX 78284
512/691-6419 (8 am-5 pm Mon-Fri)

Utah
Drug Information Center
Room A-050
Department of Pharmacy Services
University of Utah Hospital
50 North Medical Drive
Salt Lake City, UT 84132
801/581-2073 (8 am-4:30 pm Mon-Fri
and after hours)

Virginia
Drug Information Center
Drawer 640, Hampton General
Hospital
3120 Victoria Boulevard
Hampton, VA 23669
804/727-7185 (8 am-5 pm)

ADAPTS, Inc.
932 West Franklin Street
Richmond, VA 23220
804/358-0408 (9 am-5 pm Mon-Fri)

Clinical Pharmacy and Drug
Information Services
St. Mary's of Richmond
Department of Pharmacy
5801 Bremo Road
Richmond, VA 23226
804/281-8213 (24 hours)

Drug Information Service
Medical College of Virginia Hospitals
Box 42, MCV Station
Richmond, VA 23298
804/786-0754 (8 am-5 pm Mon-Fri
and after hours) (health
professionals only)

Drug Information Service
Waynesboro Community Hospital
501 Oak Avenue
Waynesboro, VA 22980
703/943-3101 ext 440 (8 am-11 pm)

Washington
Drug Information Center
Washington State University
College of Pharmacy
Pullman, WA 99164-6510
509/335-1402 (8 am-5 pm Mon-Fri)

Drug Information Service
Hospital Pharmacy, SB-55
University of Washington
Seattle, WA 98195
206/543-9487 (8 am-5 pm Mon-Fri)

West Virginia
Drug Information Center
School of Pharmacy
West Virginia University
Medical Center
Morgantown, WV 26506
800/352-2501 (West Virginia only),
304/293-5101 (8 am-9 pm and
after hours)

Wisconsin
Drug Information and Poison Control
Center
Pharmacy Department
University of Wisconsin Hospital and
Clinics
600 Highland Avenue
Madison, WI 53792
608/262-1315 (24 hours)

Wyoming
Drug Information Center
School of Pharmacy
University of Wyoming
PO Box 3375, University Station
Laramie, WY 82071
307/766-6128 (8 am-5 pm Mon-Fri)

Poison Control Centers

The following directory of poison
control centers was compiled from
information furnished by the National
Clearinghouse for Poison Control
Centers, US Department of Health and
Human Services. Facilities designated
by the American Association of
Poison Control Centers as regional
centers are indicated by an asterisk.

Alabama
Northeast Alabama Regional Medical
Center
400 East 10th Street
Anniston, AL 36201
205/236-2210

The Children's Hospital of Alabama
1600 Seventh Avenue South
Birmingham, AL 35233
205/933-4050, 800/292-6678

Southeast Alabama Medical Center
PO Drawer 6987, Highway 84 East
Dothan, AL 36301
205/793-8111

University of South Alabama
Medical Center
2451 Fillingim Street
Mobile, AL 33617
205/471-7100

Alabama Poison Center
809 University Boulevard East
Tuscaloosa, AL 35401
205/345-0600, 800/462-0800
(24 hours)

John A. Andrews Hospital
Emergency Room
Tuskegee University
Tuskegee, AL 36088
205/727-8495/8490

Alaska
Anchorage Poison Center
Providence Hospital
PO Box 196604
Anchorage, AK 99519-6604
907/562-2211

Fairbanks Poison Center
Fairbanks Memorial Hospital
1650 Cowles Street
Fairbanks, AK 99701
907/456-7182

Arizona
Flagstaff Hospital and Medical Center
of Northern Arizona
1215 North Beaver Street
Flagstaff, AZ 86001
602/779-0555

Central Arizona Regional Poison
Management Center
St. Lukes Hospital
525 North 18th Street
Phoenix, AZ 85006
602/253-3334 (24 hours)

Arizona Poison and Drug Information
Center*
Arizona Health Sciences Center
University of Arizona
Tucson, AZ 85724
602/626-6016, 800/362-0101 (Arizona
only) (24 hours)

Yuma Regional Medical Center
Avenue A and 24th Street
Yuma, AZ 85364
602/344-2000

Arkansas
Warner Brown Hospital
Emergency Department
460 West Oak Street
El Dorado, AR 71730
501/863-2266, 501/863-2000

Sparks Regional Medical Center
1311 South 'I' Street
Fort Smith, AR 72901
501/441-5011

St. Edward's Mercy Medical Center
7301 Rogers Avenue
Fort Smith, AR 72903
501/452-5100 ext 2401

Boone County Hospital Emergency
Room
620 North Willow Street
Harrison, AR 72601
501/741-6141 ext 275 or 276

Helena Hospital
Newman Drive
Helena, AR 72342
501/338-6411 ext 340

University of Arkansas
for Medical Sciences
College of Pharmacy
Slot 522
4301 West Markham Street
Little Rock, AR 72205
501/661-5544, 800/482-8948

Osceola Memorial Hospital
611 Lee Avenue West
Osceola, AR 72370
501/563-7180

Jefferson Regional Medical Center
1515 West 42nd Avenue
Pine Bluff, AR 71603
501/541-7111

California
Central-Coast Counties Regional
Poison Center
Fresno Regional Poison Control
Center of Fresno Community
Hospital and Medical Center
PO Box 1232, Fresno and R Streets
Fresno, CA 93715
209/442-6408, 209-445-1222
(emergencies)

Los Angeles County
Medical Association
Poison Information Center
1925 Wilshire Boulevard
Los Angeles, CA 90057
213/664-2121 (professional),
213/484-5151 (public)

Children's Hospital Medical Center
of Northern California
51st and Grove Streets
Oakland, CA 94609
415/428-3248

University of California
Irvine Medical Center
Regional Poison Center
101 The City Drive, Route 32
Orange, CA 92688
714/634-5988

Redding Medical Center
1450 Liberty Street
Redding, CA 96099
916/243-4043

Regional Poison Center
University of California
Davis Medical Center
2315 Stockton Boulevard
Sacramento, CA 95817
916/453-3414, 916/453-3692
(emergency)

San Diego Regional Poison Center*
University of California
Medical Center
225 Dickinson Street
San Diego, CA 92103
619/294-6000 (24 hours)

San Francisco Bay Area
Regional Poison Control Center*
1001 Potrero Avenue
San Francisco, CA 94110
415/476-6600

Santa Clara Valley Medical Center
751 South Bascom Avenue
San Jose, CA 95128
408/299-5112

Colorado
Rocky Mountain Poison Center*
Denver General Hospital
645 Bannock Street
Denver, CO 80204-4507
303/629-1123, 800/332-3073
(Colorado only)

Connecticut
Bridgeport Hospital
267 Grant Street
Bridgeport, CT 06602
203/384-3566

St. Vincent's Medical Center
2800 Main Street
Bridgeport, CT 06606
203/576-5178

Danbury Hospital
24 Hospital Avenue
Danbury, CT 06810
203/797-7300

INFORMATION RESOURCES

Connecticut Poison Center
University of Connecticut
  Health Center
Farmington, CT 06032
203/674-3456

Middlesex Memorial Hospital
28 Crescent Street
Middletown, CT 06457
203/347-9471

The Hospital of St. Raphael
1450 Chapel Street
New Haven, CT 06511
203/789-3464

Department of Pediatrics
Yale-New Haven Hospital
789 Howard Avenue
New Haven, CT 06504
203/785-2222

Norwalk Hospital
Maple Street
Norwalk, CT 06856
203/852-2160

St. Mary's Hospital
56 Franklin Street
Waterbury, CT 06702
203/574-6011

Delaware
Wilmington Medical Center
Delaware Division
501 West 14th Street
Wilmington, DE 19899
302/655-3389

District of Columbia
National Capital Poison Center*
Georgetown University Hospital
3800 Reservoir Road
Washington, DC 20007
202/625-3333

Florida
George E. Weems Memorial Hospital
PO Box 610, Franklin Square
Apalachicola, FL 32320
904/653-8853

Manatee Memorial Hospital
206 Second Street East
Bradenton, FL 33505
813/746-5111 ext 466

Tampa Bay Regional Poison Control
  Center
Tampa General Hospital
PO Box 18582
Davis Island, FL 33606
813/253-0711 ext 4444

Halifax Hospital Medical Center
Emergency Department
PO Box 1990
Daytona Beach, FL 32015
904/258-1513

Broward General Medical Center
Emergency Department
1600 South Andrews Avenue
Fort Lauderdale, FL 33316
305/463-3131 ext 1955, 1956

Lee Memorial Hospital
PO Drawer 2218, 2776 Cleveland
  Avenue
Fort Meyers, FL 33902
813/332-1111 ext 5287

Humana Hospital Fort Walton Beach
Pharmacy Department
1000 Mar-Walt Drive
Fort Walton Beach, FL 32548
904/862-1111 ext 571

Shands Teaching Hospital and Clinics
University of Florida
Gainesville, FL 32610
904/395-0333

Citrus Memorial Hospital
502 Highland Boulevard
Inverness, FL 32650
904/726-2800

Department of Pharmacy Services
St. Vincent's Medical Center
PO Box 2982
Jacksonville, FL 32203
904/387-7500, 904/387-7499

Leesburg Regional Medical Center
600 East Dixie Avenue
Leesburg, FL 32748
904/787-9900

James E. Holmes Regional
  Medical Center
1350 South Hickory Street
Melbourne, FL 32901
305/676-7307

Naples Community Hospital
350 Seventh Street North
Naples, FL 33940
813/262-3131 ext 2222

Munroe Regional Medical Center
PO Box 6000
Ocala, FL 32678
904/351-7607

Orlando Regional Medical Center
Orange Division
1414 South Kuhl Avenue
Orlando, FL 32806-2093
305/841-5111

Medical Center Hospital
809 East Marion Avenue
Punta Gorda, FL 33950
813/637-2597

Wuesthoff Memorial Hospital
110 Longwood Avenue
Rockledge, FL 32955
305/636-2211 ext 3107

Memorial Hospital
1700 South Tamiami Trail
Sarasota, FL 33579-9990
813/953-1332

Tallahassee Memorial Regional
  Medical Center
1300 Miccosukee Road
Tallahassee, FL 32308-8257
904/681-5411

Tampa Bay Regional
Poison Control Center
Davis Island
Tampa, FL 33606
813/253-0711 ext 4444

Jess Parrish Memorial Hospital
PO Drawer W
941 North Washington Avenue
Titusville, FL 32781-1104
305/268-6260

Good Samaritan Hospital
Palm Beach Lakes Boulevard
West Palm Beach, FL 33402
305/655-5511 ext 4250

Winter Haven Hospital
691 Avenue F NE
Winter Haven, FL 33880
813/299-9701

Georgia
Phoebe Putney Memorial Hospital
417 Third Avenue
Albany, GA 31702
912/888-4150

Athens General Hospital
1199 Prince Avenue
Athens, GA 30613
404/543-5215

Georgia Poison Control Center*
Grady Memorial Hospital
80 Butler Street SE
Atlanta, GA 30335
404/589-4400, 404/525-3323 (deaf
  only), 1-800/282-5846
  (Georgia only)

University Hospital
1350 Walton Way
Augusta, GA 30902
404/722-9011 ext 2440

The Medical Center
710 Center Street
Columbus, GA 31994
404/571-1080

Medical Center of Central Georgia
777 Hemlock Street
Macon, GA 31201
912/744-1427

Floyd Medical Center
Turner McCall Boulevard, PO Box 233
Rome, GA 31061
404/295-5500

Savannah Regional Poison Center
Department of Emergency Medicine
Memorial Medical Center
PO Box 23089
Savannah, GA 31403
912/355-5228

John D. Archbold Memorial Hospital
900 Gordon Avenue at Mimosa Drive
Thomasville, GA 31792
912/228-2000, 912/228-2837

South Georgia Medical Center
PO Box 1727, Pendleton Park
Valdosta, GA 31601
912/333-1110

Memorial Hospital
410 Darling Avenue
Waycross, GA 31501
912/283-3030

Hawaii
Kapiolani/Children's Medical Center
1319 Punahou Street
Honolulu, HI 96826
808/941-4411, 1-800/362-3585
  (Hawaii only) (24 hours)

Idaho
Idaho Poison Center
St. Alphonsus Regional
  Medical Center
1055 North Curtis Road
Boise, ID 83705
208/334-2241, 800/632-8000
  (Idaho only)

Eastern Idaho Regional Medical
  Center
Emergency Department
900 Memorial Drive
Idaho Falls, ID 83402
208/522-3600

Idaho Drug Information and Regional
  Poison Control Center
Pocatello Regional Medical Center
777 Hospital Way
Pocatello, ID 83201
208/234-0777 ext 2019 or 2029,
  800/632-9490 (Idaho only)

Illinois
Rush-Presbyterian-St. Luke's
  Medical Center
1753 West Congress Parkway
Chicago, IL 60612
312/942-5969, 800/942-5969

Peoria Poison Center
Saint Francis Medical Center
530 Northeast Glen Oak Avenue
Peoria, IL 61637
309/672-2334, 800/322-5330
  (Illinois only)

St. John's Hospital Central and
  Southern Illinois Regional Poison
  Resource Center*
800 East Carpenter Street
Springfield, IL 62769
217/753-3330, 800/252-2022

Indiana
Community Hospital
1515 North Madison Avenue
Anderson, IN 46012
317/646-5143

St. John's Medical Center
2015 Jackson Street
Anderson, IN 46014
317/646-8220

Cameron Memorial Hospital
416 East Maumee Street
Angola, IN 46703
219/665-2141 ext 146

Bartholomew County Hospital
2400 East 17th Street
Columbus, IN 47201
812/376-5277

St. Anthony Medical Center
Main Street and Franciscan Road
Crown Point, IN 46307
219/738-2100

St. Catherine's Hospital
4321 Fir Street
East Chicago, IN 46312
219/392-1700, 219/392-7203

Elkhart General Hospital
600 East Boulevard
Elkhart, IN 46514
219/294-2621, 1-800/382-9097
  (Indiana only), 1-800/442-4571
  (Michigan only)

Deaconess Hospital
600 Mary Street
Evansville, IN 47747
812/426-3333

Welborn Memorial Baptist Hospital
401 Southeast Sixth Street
Evansville, IN 47713
812/426-8336

Lutheran Hospital
3024 Fairfield Avenue
Fort Wayne, IN 46807
219/458-2211

Parkview Memorial Hospital
2200 Randalia Drive
Fort Wayne, IN 46805
219/484-6636 ext 6000

St. Joseph's Hospital
700 Broadway
Fort Wayne, IN 46802
219/425-3765

Clinton County Hospital
1300 South Jackson Street
Frankfort, IN 46041
317/659-4731

Methodist Hospital of Gary
600 Grant Street
Gary, IN 46402
219/886-4710

Goshen General Hospital
200 High Park Avenue
Goshen, IN 46526
219/533-2141

St. Margaret Hospital
5454 Hohman Avenue
Hammond, IN 46320
219/932-2300, 219/931-4477 ext 4139

Indiana Poison Center*
1001 West 10th Street
Indianapolis, IN 46202
317/630-7351 (24 hours),
  800/382-9097 (Indiana only)
  (24 hours)

Methodist Hospital of Indiana
1604 North Capitol Avenue
Indianapolis, IN 46202
317/929-3521

McCray Memorial Hospital
PO Box 249, Hospital Drive
Kendallville, IN 46755
219/347-1100

Howard Community Hospital
3500 South LaFountain Street
Kokomo, IN 46902
317/453-8444

Lafayette Home Hospital
2400 South Street
Lafayette, IN 47902
317/447-6811 (24 hours)

St. Elizabeth Hospital
Medical Center
1501 Hartford Street
Lafayette, IN 47902
317/423-6699

LaGrange Hospital
Route Five, Box 79
LaGrange, IN 46761
219/463-2143

LaPorte Hospital
Box 250, State and Madison Streets
LaPorte, IN 46350
219/326-1234

Witham Memorial Hospital
1124 North Lebanon Street
Lebanon, IN 46052
317/482-2700 ext 241

King's Daughter's Hospital
112 Presbyterian Avenue, PO Box 447
Madison, IN 47250
812/265-5211 ext 131

Marion General Hospital
Wabash and Euclid Avenues
Marion, IN 46952
317/662-4693

INFORMATION RESOURCES

Ball Memorial Hospital
2401 University Avenue
Muncie, IN 47303
317/747-3241

Jay County Hospital
500 West Votaw Street
Portland, IN 47371
219/726-7131

Reid Memorial Hospital
1401 Chester Boulevard
Richmond, IN 47374
317/983-3148

William S. Major Hospital
150 West Washington Street
Shelbyville, IN 46176
317/392-3211 ext 52

St. Joseph's Medical Center
811 East Madison Street
South Bend, IN 46634
219/237-7264

Union Hospital
1606 North Seventh Street
Terre Haute, IN 47804
812/238-7000 ext 7523

Porter Memorial Hospital
814 LaPorte Avenue
Valparaiso, IN 46383
219/464-8611 ext 232, 312, 334

The Good Samaritan Hospital
520 South Seventh Street
Vincennes, IN 47591
812/885-3348

Iowa
Variety Club Poison and Drug
 Information Center
Iowa Methodist Medical Center
1200 Pleasant Street
Des Moines, IA 50308
515/283-6254, 1-800/362-2327

Trinity Regional Hospital
Kenyon Road
Fort Dodge, IA 50501
515/573-7211, 515/573-3101

University of Iowa Hospital
Poison Information Center*
Iowa City, IA 52242
319/356-2922, 800/272-6477

Allen Memorial Hospital
Emergency Department
1825 Logan Avenue
Waterloo, IA 50703
319/235-3893 (24 hours)

Kansas
Atchison Hospital
1301 North Second Street
Atchinson, KS 66002
913/367-2131

Humana Hospital Dodge City
Ross and Avenue A, PO Box 1478
Dodge City, KS 67801
316/225-9050 ext 381

Newman Memorial Hospital
12th and Chestnut Streets
Emporia, KS 66801
316/343-6800 ext 545

Irwin Army Hospital Emergency Room
Fort Riley, KS 66442
913/239-7777, 913/239-7778

Mercy Hospital
821 Burke Street
Fort Scott, KS 66701
316/223-2200

Central Kansas Medical Center
3515 Broadway
Great Bend, KS 67530
316/792-2511 ext 115

Hadley Regional Medical Center
201 East Seventh Street
Hays, KS 67601
913/628-8251 (24 hours)

Mid-America Poison Center
University of Kansas Medical Center
39th Street and Rainbow Boulevard
Kansas City, KS 66103
913/588-6633, 800/332-6633
 (Kansas only)

Lawrence Memorial Hospital
325 Maine Street
Lawrence, KS 66044
913/749-6100 ext 162, 163

St. John's Hospital
139 North Penn Street
Salina, KS 67401
913/827-3187

Northeast Kansas Poison Center
St. Francis Hospital and Medical
 Center
1700 West Seventh Street
Topeka, KS 66606
913/295-8095 (24 hours)

Stormont-Vail Regional Medical
 Center
10th and Washburn Streets
Topeka, KS 66606
913/354-6100

Wesley Medical Center
550 North Hillside Avenue
Wichita, KS 67214
316/688-2277

Kentucky
St. Luke's Hospital
85 North Grand Avenue
Fort Thomas, KY 41075
606/572-3215

Williamson Appalachian
 Regional Hospital
Central Pharmaceutical Service
Central Baptist Hospital
1740 South Limestone Street
Lexington, KY 40503
606/278-3411 ext 363

Kentucky Regional Poison Center
of Kosair Children's Hospital
PO Box 35070
Louisville, KY 40232-5070
502/589-8222, 1-800/722-5725

Murray-Calloway County Hospital
803 Poplar Street
Murray, KY 42071
502/753-7588

Owensboro-Daviess County Hospital
811 Hospital Court
Owensboro, KY 42301
502/926-3030 ext 180, 186

Western Baptist Hospital
2501 Kentucky Avenue
Paducah, KY 42001
502/575-2105, 502/575-2180

Poison Control Center
Highlands Regional Medical Center
Prestonburg, KY 41653
606/886-8511 ext 174, 135

Emergency Department
2000 Central Avenue
South Williamson, KY 41503
606/237-1010

Louisiana
Rapides General Hospital
Box 30101, 301 Fourth Street
Alexandria, LA 71301-7887
318/487-8111

Our Lady of Lourdes Regional
 Medical Center
PO Box 4027-C
Lafayette, LA 70502
318/231-2910

Lake Charles Memorial Hospital
PO Drawer M, 1701 Oak Park
 Boulevard
Lake Charles, LA 70601
318/478-6800

School of Pharmacy
Northeast Louisiana University
700 University Avenue
Monroe, LA 71209
318/342-3008

St. Francis Medical Center
PO Box 1901, 309 Jackson Street
Monroe, LA 71210-1901
318/325-6454

LSU Medical Center
PO Box 33932, 1501 Kings Highway
Shreveport, LA 71130
318/425-1524, 800/535-0525
 (Louisiana only)

Maine
Maine Poison Control Center
Emergency Department
Maine Medical Center
22 Bramhall Street
Portland, ME 04102
207/871-2950, 800/442-6305
 (24 hours)

Maryland
Maryland Poison Center*
University of Maryland
 School of Pharmacy
20 North Pine Street
Baltimore, MD 21201
301/528-7701, 1-800/492-2414
 (24 hours)

Tri-State Poison Center
Sacred Heart Hospital
900 Seton Drive
Cumberland, MD 21502
301/722-6677

Massachusetts
Massachusetts Poison Control System
300 Longwood Avenue
Boston, MA 02115
617/232-2120 or 1-800/682-9211
 (24 hours)

Michigan
Emma L. Bixby Hospital
818 Riverside Avenue
Adrian, MI 49221
517/263-2412

University of Michigan Adult
 General Hospital
East Medical Center Drive, Room
 B1C255
Ann Arbor, MI 48109
313/936-6020, 313/936-6666
 (24 hours)

Community Hospital
Pharmacy Department
183 West Street
Battle Creek, MI 49016
616/963-5521

Bay Medical Center
1900 Columbus Avenue
Bay City, MI 48706
517/894-3131

Berrien General Hospital
Dean's Hill Road
Berrien Center, MI 49102
616/471-7761

Community Health Center
of Branch County
274 East Chicago Street
Coldwater, MI 49036
517/278-7361

Poison Control Center
Children's Hospital of Michigan
3901 Beaubien Boulevard
Detroit, MI 48201
313/745-5711, 800/462-6642 (outside
 metro area 313), 800/572-1655
 (rest of Michigan) (24 hours)

Mount Carmel Mercy Hospital
Pharmacy Department
6071 West Outer Drive
Detroit, MI 48235
313/927-7000 (8:30 am-5 pm)

Blodgett Regional Poison Center*
Blodgett Memorial Medical Center
1840 Wealthy SE
Grand Rapids, MI 49506
616/774-7854, 800/632-2727
 (Michigan only)

St. Mary's Hospital
201 Lafayette SE
Grand Rapids, MI 49503
616/774-6794

W.A. Foote Memorial Hospital
205 North East Street
Jackson, MI 49201
517/788-4816

Great Lakes Poison Center
Bronson Methodist Hospital
252 East Lovell Street
Kalamazoo, MI 49007
616/383-6409, 1-800/442-4112
 (24 hours)

Midwest Poison Center
Borgess Medical Center
1521 Gull Road
Kalamazoo, MI 49001
616/383-7070, 1-800/632-4177

St. Lawrence Hospital
1210 West Saginaw Street
Lansing, MI 48915
517/372-5112 or 517/372-5113
 (24 hours)

Upper Peninsula Regional
 Poison Center
Marquette General Hospital
420 West Magnetic Street
Marquette, MI 49855
906/228-9440, 1-800/562-9781
 (24 hours)

Midland Hospital Center
Poison Control
4005 Orchard Drive
Midland, MI 48640
517/631-8100 (24 hours)

Poison Information Center
St. Joseph Mercy Hospital
900 South Woodward Avenue
Pontiac, MI 48053
313/858-7373, 313/858-7374

Port Huron Hospital
1001 Kearney Street
Port Huron, MI 48060
313/987-5555, 313/987-5000

Saginaw Region Poison Center
Saginaw General Hospital
1447 North Harrison Avenue
Saginaw, MI 48602
517/755-1111

Westland Medical Center
2345 Merriman Road
Westland, MI 48185
313/467-2650, 313/467-2300

Minnesota
St. Luke's Hospital
Emergency Department
915 East First Street
Duluth, MN 55805
218/726-5466

St. Mary's Medical Center
Poison Information
 and Treatment Center
407 East Third Street
Duluth, MN 55805
218/726-4500, 800/862-1174
 (Minnesota only), 1-800/328-1858
 (out-of-state)

Fairview-Southdale Hospital
6401 France Avenue South
Edina, MN 55435
612/924-5000

Unity Medical Center
550 Osborne Road
Fridley, MN 55432
612/786-2200

Immanuel-St. Joseph's Hospital
325 Garden Boulevard
Mankato, MN 56001
507/625-4031

Fairview and St. Mary's Emergency
 Center
2312 South Sixth Street
Minneapolis, MN 55454
612/371-6402

Hennepin Poison Center*
Hennepin County Medical Center
701 Park Avenue
Minneapolis, MN 55415
612/347-3141

Stevens Community Memorial Hospital
Morris, MN 56267
612/589-1313 ext 231

Poison Center
Saint Mary's Hospital
1216 Second Street SW
Rochester, MN 55902
507/285-5123 (professional only)

INFORMATION RESOURCES

St. Cloud Hospital
Emergency Trauma Unit/
 Minnesota Poison Control Center
1406 Sixth Avenue North
St. Cloud, MN 56301
612/255-5656 (poison
 information/education),
 1-800/222-1222 (poison
 control/management)

Bethesda Lutheran Hospital
559 Capitol Boulevard
St. Paul, MN 55103
612/221-2301

Minnesota Poison Control System
St. Paul-Ramsey Hospital
640 Jackson Street
St. Paul, MN 55101
612/221-2113, 1-800/222-1222

St. John's Hospital
403 Maria Avenue
St. Paul, MN 55106
612/228-3132 (24 hours)

Rice Memorial Hospital
301 Becker Avenue SW
Willmar, MN 56201
612/235-4543

Worthington Regional Hospital
1018 Sixth Avenue
Worthington, MN 56187
507/372-2941

Mississippi
Gulf Coast Community Hospital
4642 West Beach Boulevard
Biloxi, MS 39531
601/388-1919

USAF Hospital Keesler
Keesler Air Force Base
Biloxi, MS 39534
601/377-6555, 601/377-6556

Rankin General Hospital
Emergency Room
350 Crossgates Boulevard
Brandon, MS 39042
601/825-2811 ext 405 or 406

Marion County General Hospital
Sumrall Road
Columbia, MS 39429
601/736-6303 ext 217

Greenwood-Leflore Hospital
River Road
Greenwood, MS 38930
601/459-2633

Forrest County General Hospital
400 South 28th Avenue
Hattiesburg, MS 39401
601/264-4235

St. Dominic-Jackson Memorial
 Hospital
969 Lakeland Drive
Jackson, MS 39216
601/982-0121 ext 2345

University Medical Center
2500 North State Street
Jackson, MS 39216
601/354-7660

Jones County Community Hospital
Jefferson Street and 13th Avenue
Laurel, MS 39440
601/649-4000 ext 630, 631, or 632

Meridian Regional Hospital
Highway 39 North
Meridian, MS 39301
601/483-6211 ext 440

Singing River Hospital
Emergency Department
2809 Denny Avenue
Pascagoula, MS 39567
601/938-5162

University of Mississippi
School of Pharmacy
University, MS 38677
601/234-1522

Missouri
St. Francis Medical Center
St. Francis Drive
Cape Girardeau, MO 63701
314/651-6235

University of Missouri-Columbia
 Hospital and Clinics
One Hospital Drive
Columbia, MO 65212
314/882-1000

St. Elizabeth's Hospital
109 Virginia Street
Hannibal, MO 63401
314/221-0414 ext 101

Charles E. Still Osteopathic Hospital
1125 Madison Street
Jefferson City, MO 65101
314/635-7141 ext 215

St. John's Regional Medical Center
2727 McClelland Boulevard
Joplin, MO 64801
417/781-2727 ext 2305

Children's Mercy Hospital
24th and Gillham Road
Kansas City, MO 64108
816/234-3000

Kirksville Osteopathic Health Center
Box 949, One Osteopathy Avenue
Kirksville, MO 63501
816/626-2266

Lucy Lee Hospital
2620 North Westwood Boulevard
Poplar Bluff, MO 63901
314/785-7721

Phelps County Memorial Hospital
1000 West Tenth Street
Rolla, MO 65401
314/364-1322

Methodist Medical Center
Seventh to Ninth on Faraon Street
St. Joseph, MO 64501
816/271-7580, 816/232-8481

Cardinal Glennon Children's Hospital
Regional Poison Center
1465 South Grand Boulevard
St. Louis, MO 63104
314/772-5200, 1-800/392-9111
 (Missouri only)

Ozark Poison Center
Lester E. Cox Medical Center
1423 North Jefferson Street
Springfield, MO 65802
417/831-9746 (call collect)

St. John's Regional Health Center
1235 East Cherokee Street
Springfield, MO 65802
417/885-2115

Ozarks Medical Center
1103 Alaska Avenue
West Plains, MO 65775
417/256-9111 ext 6600

Montana
Montana Poison Control System
Cogswell Building
Helena, MT 59620
406/444-3895 (office hours),
 1-800/525-5042 (24 hours)

Nebraska
Mid-Plains Regional Poison Center
Children's Memorial Hospital
8301 Dodge Street
Omaha, NE 68114
402/390-5400, 800/642-9999
 (Nebraska only), 800/228-9515
 (surrounding states)

Nevada
Humana Hospital Sunrise
3186 South Maryland Parkway
Las Vegas, NV 89109
702/731-8000

Southern Nevada Memorial Hospital
1800 West Charleston Boulevard
Las Vegas, NV 89102
702/383-2000 ext 2211

St. Mary's Hospital
235 West Sixth Street
Reno, NV 89503
702/789-3013

Washoe Medical Center
77 Pringle Way
Reno, NV 89502
702/785-4129

New Hampshire
New Hampshire Poison Information
 Center
2 Maynard Street
Hanover, NH 03756
603/646-5000, 1-800/562-8236

New Jersey
Atlantic City Medical Center
1925 Pacific Avenue
Atlantic City, NJ 08401
609/344-4081 ext 2359

Clara Maass Medical Center
1A Franklin Avenue
Belleville, NJ 07109
201/450-2100

Camden County Poison Control
 Center
West Jersey Health System
Southern Division
White Horse Pike and Townsend
 Avenue
Berlin, NJ 08009
609/768-6666 (24 hours)

Riverside Hospital
Powerville Road
Boonton, NJ 07055
201/334-5000 ext 186 or 187

St. Clare's Hospital/Riverside
 Medical Center
Pocono Road
Denville, NJ 07834
201/625-6063

East Orange General Hospital
300 Central Avenue
East Orange, NJ 07019
201/672-8400 ext 223

St. Elizabeth's Hospital
225 Williamson Street
Elizabeth, NJ 07207
201/527-5059

Englewood Hospital
350 Engle Street
Englewood, NJ 07631
201/894-3440

Monmouth Medical Center
Emergency Department
Dunbar and Second Avenue
Long Branch, NJ 07740
201/222-2210

Mountainside Hospital
Bay and Highland Avenues
Montclair, NJ 07042
201/429-6100

Memorial Hospital of Burlington
 County
175 Madison Avenue
Mount Holly, NJ 08060
609/267-7877

Jersey Shore Medical Center
1945 Corlies Avenue
Neptune, NJ 07753
201/775-5500, 800/962-1253

New Jersey Poison Information
 and Education System
201 Lyons Avenue
Newark, NJ 07112
201/926-8005, 800/962-1253 (New
 Jersey only), 201/926-8008 (TTY)
 (24 hours)

Middlesex General-University Hospital
180 Somerset Street
New Brunswick, NJ 08903
201/937-8583

St. Peter's Medical Center
245 Easton Avenue
New Brunswick, NJ 08903
201/745-8527

Newton Memorial Hospital
Emergency Room
175 High Street
Newton, NJ 07860
201/383-2121 ext 270, 271, or 273

Hospital Center at Orange
Emergency Department
188 South Essex Avenue
Orange, NJ 07051
201/266-2120

St. Mary's Hospital
211 Pennington Avenue
Passaic, NJ 07055
201/470-3035

Raritan Bay Medical Center
530 New Brunswick Avenue
Perth Amboy, NJ 08861
201/442-3700 ext 2501

Warren Hospital
185 Rosenberry Street
Phillipsburg, NJ 08865
201/859-6768

The Northern Ocean Hospital System
Point Pleasant Division
Osborn Avenue and River Front
Point Pleasant, NJ 08742
201/926-8005, 1-800/962-1253

The Medical Center at Princeton
253 Witherspoon Street
Princeton, NJ 08540
609/734-4554

Saddle Brook General Hospital
300 Market Street
Saddle Brook, NJ 07662
201/368-6025

Somerset Medical Center
Rehill Avenue
Somerville, NJ 08876
201/685-2921

Overlook Hospital
193 Morris Avenue
Summit, NJ 07901
201/522-2232

Holy Name Hospital
718 Teaneck Road
Teaneck, NJ 07666
201/833-3000

Helene Fuld Medical Center
750 Brunswick Avenue
Trenton, NJ 08638
609/396-1077

Memorial General Hospital
1000 Galloping Hill Road
Union, NJ 07083
201/687-1900 ext 3700

New Mexico
New Mexico Poison and
 Drug Information Center*
University of New Mexico
Albuquerque, NM 87131
505/843-2551, 1-800/432-6866 (New
 Mexico only)

New York
Our Lady of Lourdes Memorial
 Hospital
169 Riverside Drive
Binghamton, NY 13905
607/798-5231

Southern Tier Poison Center
United Health Services
Mitchell Avenue
Binghamton, NY 13903
607/723-8929

Western New York Poison Control
 Center
Children's Hospital of Buffalo
219 Bryant Street
Buffalo, NY 14222
716/878-7654, 716/878-7655

Brooks Memorial Hospital
529 Central Avenue
Dunkirk, NY 14048
716/366-1111 ext 414 or 415

Long Island Regional Poison
 Control Center*
Nassau County Medical Center
2201 Hempstead Turnpike
East Meadow, NY 11554
516/542-2323 (TTY), 516/542-2324,
 516/542-2325

Arnot Ogden Memorial Hospital
Roe Avenue and Grove Street
Elmira, NY 14901
607/737-4100

St. Joseph's Hospital Health Center
555 East Market Street
Elmira, NY 14901
607/734-2662

INFORMATION RESOURCES

Ideal Hospital
600 High Avenue
Endicott, NY 13760
607/754-7171 (24 hours)

Glens Falls Hospital
100 Park Street
Glens Falls, NY 12801
518/761-5261

Women's Christian Association
  Hospital
207 Foote Avenue
Jamestown, NY 14701
716/487-0141, 716/484-8648

Wilson Memorial Hospital
33-57 Harrison Street
Johnson City, NY 13790
607/773-6611

New York City Poison Center*
Department of Health
Bureau of Laboratories
455 First Avenue
New York, NY 10016
212/340-4494, 212/764-7667

Hudson Valley Poison Center
Nyack Hospital
North Midland Avenue
Nyack, NY 10960
914/353-1000

Finger Lakes Regional Poison
  Control Center LIFE LINE*
University of Rochester
Medical Center
Rochester, NY 14642
716/275-5151 (24 hours),
  716/275-2700 (TTY)

Ellis Hospital
1101 Nott Street
Schenectady, NY 12308
518/382-4039, 518/382-4309

Central New York Regional Poison
  Control Center
750 East Adams Street
Syracuse, NY 13210
315/476-4766, 315/473-5831

St. Mary's Hospital
1300 Massachusetts Avenue
Troy, NY 12180
518/272-5792

St. Luke's Hospital Center
PO Box 479
Utica, NY 13502
315/798-6200, 315/798-6223

Watertown Poison Information Center
House of the Good Samaritan
  Hospital
Washington and Pratt Streets
Watertown, NY 13602
315/788-8700

North Carolina
Western North Carolina Poison
  Control Center
509 Biltmore Avenue
Asheville, NC 28801
704/255-4490

Mercy Hospital
2001 Vail Avenue
Charlotte, NC 28207
704/379-5827

Duke University Medical Center
Poison Control Center
PO Box 3007
Durham, NC 27710
1-800/672-1697 (North Carolina only),
  919/684-8111 (24 hours)

Triad Poison Center
Moses H. Cone Memorial Hospital
1200 North Elm Street
Greensboro, NC 27401-1020
919/379-4105, 1-800/722-2222
  (24 hours)

Margaret R. Pardee Memorial Hospital
Fleming Street
Hendersonville, NC 28739
704/693-6522 ext 555 or 556

Catawba Memorial Hospital
810 Fairgrove Church Road SE
Hickory, NC 28602
704/322-6649 (24 hours)

Onslow Memorial Hospital
Western Boulevard
Jacksonville, NC 28540
919/577-2555

New Hanover Memorial Hospital
2131 South 17th Street
Wilmington, NC 28402
919/343-7046

North Dakota
MedCenter One
Emergency/Trauma Center
300 North Seventh Street
Bismarck, ND 58501
701/223-4357

St. Luke's Hospitals*
Fifth Street and Mills Avenue
Fargo, ND 58122
701/280-5575, 1-800/732-2200
  (24 hours)

United Hospital
1200 South Columbia Road
Grand Forks, ND 58201
701/780-5000

St. Joseph's Hospital
Third Street and Fourth Avenue SE
Minot, ND 58701
701/857-2553

Mercy Hospital
1301 15th Avenue
West Williston, ND 58801
701/572-7661

Ohio
Children's Hospital
Medical Center of Akron
281 Locust Street
Akron, OH 44308
216/379-8562, 1-800/362-9922

Aultman Hospital Emergency Room
Emergency/Trauma Center
2600 Sixth Street SW
Canton, OH 44710
216/438-6203

Drug and Poison Information Center
Southwest Ohio Regional Poison
  Control System
University of Cincinnati Medical
  Center
Room 7701
231 Bethesda Avenue, ML 144
Cincinnati, OH 45267
513/872-5111 (24 hours),
  800/872-5111

Greater Cleveland Poison Control
  Center
2101 Adelbert Road
Cleveland, OH 44106
216/231-4455 (24 hours)

Central Ohio Poison Control Center
Children's Hospital
700 Children's Drive
Columbus, OH 43205
614/228-1323, 800/682-7625

Western Ohio Regional Poison and
  Drug Information Center
Children's Medical Center
One Children's Plaza
Dayton, OH 45404
513/222-2227, 1-800/762-0727
  (Ohio only)

Lorain Community Hospital
3700 Kolbe Road
Lorain, OH 44053
216/282-2220

Mansfield General Hospital
335 Glessner Avenue
Mansfield, OH 44903
419/526-8200

Community Hospital
2615 East High Street
Springfield, OH 44501
513/325-1255

Poison Information Center
Medical College of Ohio
PO Box 6190, 3001 Arlington Avenue
Toledo, OH 43614
419/381-3897

Mahoning Valley Poison Center
St. Elizabeth Hospital Medical Center
1044 Belmont Avenue
Youngstown, OH 44501
216/746-2222, 216/746-5510 (TTY)

Poison Control Center
Bethesda Hospital
2951 Maple Avenue
Zanesville, OH 43701
614/454-4221 (24 hours)

Oklahoma
Valley View Hospital
1300 East Sixth Street
Ada, OK 74820
405/322-2323 ext 200

Memorial Hospital of Southern
  Oklahoma
1011 14th Avenue
Ardmore, OK 73401
405/223-5400

Comanche County Memorial Hospital
3401 Gore Boulevard
Lawton, OK 73501
405/355-8620

McAlester Regional Hospital
PO Box 669, One Clark Bass
  Boulevard
McAlester, OK 74501
918/426-1800 ext 7705

Oklahoma Poison Control Center
Oklahoma Children's Memorial
  Hospital
PO Box 26307, 940 NE 13th Street
Oklahoma City, OK 73126
405/271-5454, 800/522-4611

St. Joseph Medical Center
Emergency Room
14th Street and Hartford Avenue
Ponca City, OK 74601
405/765-0584

Oregon
Oregon Poison Control and Drug
  Information Center
The Oregon Health Services
  University
3181 SW Sam Jackson Park Road
Portland, OR 97201
503/225-8968, 1-800/452-7165
  (Oregon only)

Pennsylvania
Lehigh Valley Poison Center
17th and Chew Streets
Allentown, PA 18102
215/433-2311

Keystone Region Poison Center
2500 Seventh Avenue
Altoona, PA 16603
814/946-3711

The Bloomsburg Hospital
549 East Fair Street
Bloomsburg, PA 17815
717/784-4241

Bradford Hospital
Interstate Parkway
Bradford, PA 16701
814/368-4143 ext 274

The Bryn Mawr Hospital
Bryn Mawr Avenue
Bryn Mawr, PA 19010
215/896-3577

Sacred Heart Medical Center
Ninth and Wilson Streets
Chester, PA 19013
215/494-4400

Clearfield Hospital
809 Turnpike Avenue
Clearfield, PA 16830
814/765-5341

Coaldale State General Hospital
Seventh Street
Coaldale, PA 18218
717/645-2131

Charles Cole Memorial Hospital
RD Three, US Route Six
Coudersport, PA 16915
814/274-9300

Susquehanna Poison Center
Geisinger Medical Center
North Academy Avenue
Danville,, PA 17821
717/275-6116 or 717/271-6116
  (24 hours)

Doylestown Hospital
595 West State Street
Doylestown, PA 18901
215/345-2283

Pocono Hospital
206 East Brown Street
East Stroudsburg, PA 18301
717/421-4000

Easton Hospital
21st and Lehigh Streets
Easton, PA 18042
215/250-4000

Metro Health Center
252 West 11th Street
Erie, PA 16501
814/454-2120

Millcreek Community Hospital
5515 Peach Street
Erie, PA 16509
814/864-4031 ext 442

Poison Control Center
Hamot Medical Center
201 State Street
Erie, PA 16550
814/870-6111

Northwest Poison Center
Saint Vincent Health Center
232 West 25th Street
Erie, Pa 16544
814/452-3232

The Gettysburg Hospital
147 Gettys Street
Gettysburg, PA 17324
717/334-9155

Westmoreland Hospital
532 West Pittsburgh Street
Greensburg, PA 15601
412/832-4355

Hanover General Hospital
300 Highland Avenue
Hanover, PA 17331
717/637-3711

Polyclinic Hospital
Third and Polyclinic Avenues
Harrisburg, PA 17105
717/782-4141 ext 4132

Capital Area Poison Center
The University Hospital
The Milton S. Hershey Medical Center
University Drive
Hershey, PA 17033
717/534-6111, 717/534-6039

Jeanette District Memorial Hospital
600 Jefferson Avenue
Jeannette, PA 15644
412/527-9300

Jersey Shore Hospital
Thompson Street
Jersey Shore, PA 17740
717/398-0100 ext 225

Conemaugh Valley Memorial Hospital
1086 Franklin Street
Johnstown, PA 15905
814/535-5351

Mercy Hospital
1020 Franklin Street
Johnstown, PA 15905
814/535-5353

Lancaster General Hospital
PO Box 3555, 555 North Duke Street
Lancaster, PA 17603
717/299-5511 or 717/295-8322
  (24 hours)

St. Joseph's Hospital
250 College Avenue
Lancaster, PA 17604
717/299-4546 (24 hours)

North Penn Hospital
100 Medical Campus Drive
Lansdale, PA 19446
215/368-2100

Good Samaritan Hospital
Fourth and Walnut Streets
Lebanon, PA 17042
717/272-7611

Gnaden-Huetten Memorial Hospital
11th and Hamilton Streets
Lehighton, PA 18235
215/377-1300 ext 552

INFORMATION RESOURCES

Lewistown Hospital
Highland Avenue
Lewistown, PA 17044
717/248-5411

Muncy Valley Hospital
215 East Water Street
Muncy, PA 17756
717/546-8282, 717/327-8137

Nanticoke State General Hospital
North Washington Street
Nanticoke, PA 18643
717/735-5000 ext 261

Paoli Memorial Hospital
Lancaster Pike
Paoli, PA 19301
215/648-1043

Delaware Valley Regional Poison
 Control Center
One Children's Center
34th Street and Civic Center
 Boulevard
Philadelphia, PA 19104
215/386-2100, 215/386-2066

Philipsburg State General Hospital
Locklomond Road
Philipsburg, PA 16866
814/342-3320 ext 293

Pittsburgh Poison Center
Children's Hospital of Pittsburgh
One Children's Place
3705 Fifth Avenue at DeSoto Street
Pittsburgh, PA 15213
412/681-6669 (emergencies),
 412/647/5600 (consultation)

Pottstown Memorial Medical Center
1600 East High Street
Pottstown, PA 19464
215/327-7100

Good Samaritan Hospital
East Norwegian and Tremont Streets
Pottsville, PA 17901
717/622-3400 ext 270

Community General Hospital
145 North Sixth Street
Reading, PA 19601
215/375-9115 (24 hours)

The Robert Packer Hospital
Guthrie Square
Sayre, PA 18840
717/888-6666

Grand View Hospital
Lawn Avenue
Sellersville, PA 18960
215/257-5955

Somerset Community Hospital
225 South Center Avenue
Somerset, PA 15501
814/443-2626

Centre Community Hospital
Orchard Road
State College, PA 16803
814/238-4351

Titusville Hospital
406 West Oak Street
Titusville, PA 16354
814/827-1851

Tyler Memorial Hospital
RD 1
Tunkhannock, PA 18657
717/836-2161 ext 180

NPW-Medical Center
1000 E. Mountain Boulevard
Wilkes-Barre, PA 18704
717/826-7762

Memorial Hospital
325 South Belmont Street
York, PA 17405
717/843-8623

York Hospital
1001 South George Street
York, PA 17405
717/771-2311

Rhode Island
Rhode Island Poison Center
Rhode Island Hospital
593 Eddy Street
Providence, RI 02902
401/277-5727

South Carolina
Palmetto Poison Center
University of South Carolina
 College of Pharmacy
Columbia, SC 29208
803/765-7359, 1-800/922-1117

South Dakota
The Dakota Midland Poison Control
 Center
Dakota Midland Hospital
1400 15th Avenue NW
Aberdeen, SD 57401
605/225-1880, 800/592-1889 (South
 Dakota only) (24 hours)

Rapid City Regional Poison Center
353 Fairmont Boulevard
Rapid City, SD 57701
605/341-3333

McKennan Hospital Poison Center
800 East 21st Street, PO Box 5045
Sioux Falls, SD 57117-5045
605/336-3894, 1-800/952-0123 (South
 Dakota only), 1-800/843-0505 (Iowa,
 Nebraska, and Minnesota)

Tennessee
T.C. Thompson Children's Hospital
910 Blackford Street
Chattanooga, TN 37403
615/778-6100

Maury County Hospital
1224 Trotwood Avenue
Columbia, TN 38401
615/381-4500 ext 405

Cookeville General Hospital
142 West Fifth Street
Cookeville, TN 38501
615/526-4818

Jackson-Madison County
 General Hospital
708 West Forest Avenue
Jackson, TN 38301
901/425-6000

Johnson City Medical Center Hospital
Poison Control Center
400 State of Franklin Road
Johnson City, TN 37601
615/461-6572

University of Tennessee Memorial
Research Center and Hospital
1924 Alcoa Highway
Knoxville, TN 37920
615/544-9400

Southern Poison Center
848 Adams Avenue
Memphis, TN 38103
901/528-6048

Vanderbilt University Medical Center
Poison Control Center
1161 21st Avenue South
Nashville, TN 37232
615/322-6435 (adult, pediatric, or
 night line)

Texas
Hendrick Medical Center
19th and Hickory Streets
Abilene, TX 79601
915/677-7762

Amarillo Emergency Receiving Center
Amarillo Hospital District
PO Box 1110, 1501 Coulter Drive
Amarillo, TX 79106
806/376-4292

Baptist Hospital of Southeast Texas
PO Box 1591
Beaumont, TX 77704
409/833-7409

Memorial Medical Center
PO Box 5280, 2606 Hospital
 Boulevard
Corpus Christi, TX 78405
512/881-4559

El Paso County Poison Control Center
R.E. Thomason General Hospital
4815 Alameda Avenue
El Paso, TX 79905
915/533-1244

W.I. Cook Children's Hospital
Cook Poison Center-Fort Worth
1212 West Lancaster Street
Fort Worth, TX 76102
817/336-6611 (24 hours)

Texas State Poison Center
University of Texas Medical Branch
Eighth and Mechanic Streets
Galveston, TX 77550
800/392-8548, 409/765-1420
 (Galveston), 713/654-1701
 (Houston), 512/478-4490 (Austin)

Valley Baptist Hospital
PO Box 2588, 2000 Peace Street
Harlingen, TX 78550
512/421-1860, 512/421-1859

Mercy Hospital
1515 Logan Street
Laredo, TX 78040
512/724-6247

Methodist Hospital Poison Control
 Center
3615 19th Street
Lubbock, TX 79410
806/793-4366

Midland Memorial Hospital
2200 West Illinois Avenue
Midland, TX 79701
915/685-1558

Medical Center Hospital
Poison Control Center
PO Box 7239, Fourth and Allegheny
 Streets
Odessa, TX 79760
915/333-1231

Central Plains Regional Hospital*
2601 Dimmitt Road
Plainview, TX 79072
806/296-9601

Shannon West Texas Memorial
 Hospital
PO Box 1879, 120 East Harris
San Angelo, TX 76902
915/655-5330

East Texas Poison Center
Medical Center Hospital
1000 South Beckham Street
Tyler, TX 75701
214/597-8884

Hillcrest Baptist Medical Center
3000 Herring Avenue
Waco, TX 76708
817/753-1412

Wichita Falls General Hospital
1600 Eighth Street
Wichita Falls, TX 76301
817/322-6771

Utah
Intermountain Regional Poison
 Control Center*
50 North Medical Drive
Salt Lake City, UT 84132
801/581-2151, 800/662-0062

Vermont
Vermont Poison Center
Medical Center Hospital
Colchester Avenue
Burlington, VT 06401
802/658-3456

Virginia
Alexandria Hospital
4320 Seminary Road
Alexandria, VA 22314
703/379-3070

Arlington Hospital
1701 North George Mason Drive
Arlington, VA 22205
703/558-6161

Montgomery County Community
 Hospital
Route 460 South
Blacksburg, VA 24060
703/951-1111 ext 140

Blue Ridge Poison Center
University of Virginia Medical Center
PO Box 484
Charlottesville, VA 22908
804/924-5543 (collect calls accepted)
 (24 hours), 800/552-3723 (TTY:
 Virginia only), 800/446-9876 (TTY:
 out of state)

Danville Memorial Hospital
142 South Main Street
Danville, VA 24541
804/799-2222, 804/799-3869

Poison Control Center
Fairfax Hospital
3300 Gallows Road
Falls Church, VA 22046
703/698-2900, 703/698-3111

Hampton General Hospital
3120 Victoria Boulevard
Hampton, VA 23669
804/722-1131

Rockingham Memorial Hospital
235 Cantrell Avenue
Harrisonburg, VA 22801
703/433-9706

Stonewall Jackson Hospital
Spotswood Drive
Lexington, VA 24450
703/463-1492

Lynchburg General Marshall Lodge
 Hospital
Tate Springs Road
Lynchburg, VA 24504
804/528-2066

Northampton-Accomack Memorial
 Hospital
Nassawadox, VA 23413
804/442-8700

Riverside Hospital
500 J. Clyde Morris Boulevard
Newport News, VA 23601
804/599-2050

Tidewater Poison Center
DePaul Hospital
Granby Street and Kingsley Lane
Norfolk, VA 23505
804/489-5288

Petersburg General Hospital
801 South Adams Street
Petersburg, VA 23803
804/861-2992

Naval Hospital
Portsmouth, VA 23708
804/398-5898 (24 hours)

Access Emergency Center
11900 Baron Cameron Avenue
Reston, VA 22091
703/437-5992

Central Virginia Poison Center
Medical College of Virginia
PO Box 522 MCV Station
Richmond, VA 23298
804/786-4780 (24 hours)

Southwest Virginia Poison Center
Roanoke Memorial Hospital
PO Box 13367, Belleview and
 Jefferson Street
Roanoke, VA 24033
703/981-7336

King's Daughter's Hospital
PO Box 3000, 1410 North Augusta
 Street
Staunton, VA 24401
703/887-2525

Waynesboro Community Hospital
501 Oak Avenue
Waynesboro, VA 22980
703/942-4096

Williamsburg Community Hospital
Drawer H, 1238 Mount Vernon
 Avenue
Williamsburg, VA 23185
804/253-6005

INFORMATION RESOURCES

Washington
Seattle Poison Center
Children's Orthopedic Hospital
  and Medical Center*
4800 Sandpoint Way NE,
  PO Box 5371
Seattle, WA 98105
206/526-2121, 1-800/732-6985
  (Washington only) (24 hours)

Spokane Poison Center*
Deaconess Medical Center
West 800 Fifth Avenue
Spokane, WA 99210
509/747-1077 (TTY), 1-800/572-5842
  (Washington only), 1-800/541-5624
  (northern Idaho and western
  Montana)

Mary Bridge Children's Hospital
311 South L Street
Tacoma, WA 98405-0588
206/594-1414, 800/542-6319
  (Washington only)

Central Washington Poison Center
Yakima Valley Memorial Hospital
2811 Tieton Drive
Yakima, WA 98902
509/248-4400, 1-800/572-9176
  (Washington only)

West Virginia
West Virginia Poison Center
West Virginia University
School of Pharmacy
3110 MacCorkle Avenue SE
Charleston, WV 25304
1-800/642-3625, 304/348-4211

Wisconsin
Luther Hospital
310 Chestnut Street
Eau Claire, WI 54701
715/835-1515

Green Bay Poison Control Center
St. Vincent Hospital
PO Box 13508
Green Bay, WI 54307-3508
414/433-8100

St. Francis Medical Center
700 West Avenue South
LaCrosse, WI 54601
608/784-3971

Madison Area Poison Center
University Hospital and Clinic
600 Highland Avenue
Madison, WI 53792
608/262-3702

Milwaukee Poison Center
Children's Hospital of Wisconsin
1700 West Wisconsin Avenue
Milwaukee, WI 53233
414/931-4114

Wyoming
Wyoming Poison Center
DePaul Hospital
2600 East 18th Street
Cheyenne, WY 82001
307/777-7955

Comprehensive Cancer Centers

The following institutions have been designated as Comprehensive Cancer Centers by the National Cancer Institute. To earn this designation, the institution must meet certain criteria, including support of a strong research program in the prevention, diagnosis, and treatment of cancer; an ability to participate in integrated, nationwide clinical trials; and the capacity to perform advanced diagnostic techniques and treatment modalities.

Alabama
Comprehensive Cancer Center
University of Alabama in Birmingham
University Station
Birmingham, AL 35294
205/934-6612

California
UCLA Jonsson Comprehensive
  Cancer Center
UCLA Center for Health Sciences
10833 Leconte Avenue
Los Angeles, CA 90024
213/825-5268 (professional),
  213/206-6017 (public)

University of Southern California
Comprehensive Cancer Center
2025 Zonal Avenue
Los Angeles, CA 90033
213/224-6600

Connecticut
Yale University Comprehensive
  Cancer Center
333 Cedar Street
New Haven, CT 06510
203/785-4098

District of Columbia
Vincent T. Lombardi Cancer Research
  Center
Georgetown University Medical Center
3800 Reservoir Road NW
Washington, DC 20007
202/625-7066

Howard University Cancer Center
2041 Georgia Avenue NW
Washington, DC 20060
202/636-7697

Florida
Papanicolaou Comprehensive Cancer
  Center
University of Miami
School of Medicine
PO Box 016960 (D8-4)
Miami, FL 33101
305/548-4800

Illinois
Illinois Cancer Council
36 South Wabash Avenue, Suite 700
Chicago, IL 60603
312/346-9813, 1-800/4-CANCER

Northwestern University Cancer
  Center
Health Sciences Building
303 East Chicago Avenue
Chicago, IL 60611
312/908-5250

Rush Cancer Center
Rush-Presbyterian-St. Luke's Medical
  Center
1753 West Congress Parkway
Chicago, IL 60612
312/942-6028

Cancer Research Center
University of Chicago
5841 South Maryland Avenue,
  Box 444
Chicago, IL 60637
312/962-6180

University of Illinois
PO Box 6998
Chicago, IL 60608
312/996-8843, 312/996-6666

Maryland
The Johns Hopkins Oncology Center
600 North Wolfe Street
Baltimore, MD 21205
301/955-3636

Massachusetts
Dana-Farber Cancer Institute
44 Binney Street
Boston, MA 02115
617/732-3000

Michigan
Comprehensive Cancer Center
  of Metropolitan Detroit
110 East Warren Avenue
Detroit, MI 48201
313/833-0710 ext 356 or 393

Minnesota
Mayo Comprehensive Cancer Center
200 First Street SW
Rochester, MN 55901
507/284-8285

New York
Roswell Park Memorial Institute
666 Elm Street
Buffalo, NY 14263
716/845-2300

Columbia University
Comprehensive Cancer Center
College of Physicians and Surgeons
701 West 168th Street
New York, NY 10032
212/694-6900

Memorial Sloan-Kettering Cancer
  Center
1275 York Avenue
New York, NY 10021
212/794-7984

North Carolina
Duke Comprehensive Cancer Center
Duke University Medical Center
PO Box 3814
Durham, NC 27710
919/684-2282

Ohio
The Ohio State University
Comprehensive Cancer Center
Suite 302, 410 West 12th Avenue
Columbus, OH 43210
614/422-5022

Pennsylvania
Fox Chase/University of Pennsylvania
Comprehensive Cancer Center
7701 Burholme Avenue
Philadelphia, PA 19111
215/728-6900

Texas
The University of Texas Health
  System
Cancer Center
M.D. Anderson Hospital and Tumor
  Institute
Box 90, 6723 Bertner Avenue
Houston, TX 77030
713/792-3030

Washington
Fred Hutchinson Cancer Research
  Center
1124 Columbia Street
Seattle, WA 98104
206/292-6301

Wisconsin
The University of Wisconsin
Clinical Cancer Center
600 Highland Avenue
Madison, WI 53706
608/263-8600

Comprehensive Pain Centers and Clinics

The following list of pain centers and clinics, compiled by the Committee on Pain Therapy of the American Society of Anesthesiologists, offers a broad range of diagnostic and therapeutic modalities.

Alabama
Brookwood Medical Center
Pain Management Center
2022 Brookwood Medical Center Drive
Birmingham, AL 35209
205/877-1569

Pain Management Center
University of Alabama in Birmingham
Kracke Building
1920 Seventh Avenue South
Birmingham, AL 35233
205/934-6174

Arizona
St. Joseph's Hospital Pain Program
PO Box 2071
Phoenix, AZ 85001-2071
602/285-3474

Pain Clinic
University of Arizona Hospital
University of Arizona
Health Sciences Center
1501 North Campbell Avenue
Tucson, AZ 85724
602/626-6239

California
Lawrence Pain Control Group
28240 West Agoura Road, Suite 101
Agoura, CA 91301
818/991-6740

New Hope Pain Center
  Medical Group, Inc.
100 South Raymond Avenue
Alhambra, CA 91801
213/570-1607

Pain Treatment Center
Scripps Clinic & Research Foundation
10666 North Torrey Pines Road
La Jolla, CA 92037
619/455-8898

Pain Control and Health
  Support Services
Loma Linda Anesthesiology
  Medical Group, Inc.
PO Box 962
Loma Linda, CA 92354
714/796-0231

Pain Management Program
VA Medical Center
5901 East Seventh Street
Long Beach, CA 90822
213/498-6233

Pain Management Center
AR-200 Center for Health Sciences
UCLA School of Medicine
Los Angeles, CA 90024
213/825-4291

Los Medanos Community Hospital
Pain Management Center
2311 Loveridge Road
Pittsburg, CA 94565
415/432-2200 ext 236

The Center for Behavioral Medicine
1884 Business Center Drive
San Bernardino, CA 92408
714/889-0526

Pain Unit, San Diego VA Medical
  Center
3350 La Jolla Drive
San Diego, CA 92161
714/453-7500

Saint Francis Memorial Hospital
900 Hyde Street
San Francisco, CA 94109
415/775-4321

St. Mary's Hospital
450 Stanyan Street
San Francisco, CA 94117
415/668-1000

Orthopaedic Pain Center of San Jose
Cambrian Park Plaza
14438 Union Avenue
San Jose, CA 95124
408/371-2137

Walnut Creek Hospital
175 La Casa Vista
Walnut Creek, CA 94598
415/933-7990

Colorado
Boulder Memorial Hospital
Pain Control Center
311 Mapleton Avenue
Boulder, CO 80302
303/441-0507

Pain Clinic, University of Colorado
  Medical Center
4200 East Ninth Avenue, Box B113
Denver, CO 80262
303/394-7078

Connecticut
Arthur Taub, MD, PhD
60 Temple Street
New Haven, CT 06510
203/789-2151

Delaware
Delaware Pain Clinic
249 East Main Street
Newark, DE 19711
302/738-0262

District of Columbia
Georgetown University Medical Center
Department of Anethesia
3800 Reservoir Road, NW
Washington, DC 20007
202/625-7163

INFORMATION RESOURCES

Florida
Pain Treatment Center
Baptist Hospital of Miami
8900 North Kendall Drive
Miami, FL 33176
305/596-6552

The Pain Center
Mount Sinai Medical Center
4300 Alton Road
Miami Beach, FL 33140
305/674-2070

University of Miami
School of Medicine
Comprehensive Pain and
 Rehabilitation Center at South
 Shore Hospital and Medical Center
600 Alton Road
Miami Beach, FL 33139
305/672-2100, ext 3525

Georgia
Atlanta Pain Control and
 Rehabilitation Center, Inc.
315 Boulevard NE, Suite 100
Atlanta, GA 30312
404/653-4632

Pain Control and Rehabilitation
 Institute of Georgia, Inc.
350 Winn Way
Decatur, GA 30030
404/297-1400

The Pain Rehabilitation and
 Biofeedback Center of West
 Georgia, Inc.
6128 F Prestley Mill Road
Douglasville, GA 30134
404/949-1222

Savannah Pain Control and
 Rehabilitation Center
5354 Reynolds Street, Suite 518
Savannah, GA 31405
912/355-4568

Illinois
The Center for Pain Studies
Rehabilitation Institute of Chicago
345 East Superior Street
Chicago, IL 60611
312/908-6011

Chronic Pain and Headache
 Treatment Center
Illinois Masonic Medical Center
836 West Wellington Street
Chicago, IL 60657
312/883-7036 (9 am-5 pm Mon-Fri)

Rush Pain Center
1725 West Harrison Street
Chicago, IL 60612
312/942-6631

The Pain Treatment Center
Lake Forest Hospital
660 North Westmoreland
Lake Forest, IL 60045
312/234-5600 ext 5561

Pain Management Clinic
Methodist Medical Center
221 NE Glen Oak
Peoria, IL 61636
309/672-5950

Pain Center
Marianjoy Rehabilitation Hospital
26 West 171 Roosevelt Road
Wheaton, IL 60187
312/462-4132

Indiana
Rehabilitation Center for Pain
Community Hospital Rehabilitation
1500 North Ritter Avenue
Indianapolis, IN 46219
317/353-5987

Pain Rehabilitation Center
St. Joseph's Medical Center
PO Box 1935 811 East Madison
South Bend, IN 46634
219/237-7360

Kentucky
Louisville Pain Clinic
326 Medical Towers South
Louisville, KY 40202
502/587-6523

Louisiana
Hotel Dieu Pain Rehabilitation Unit
2021 Perdido Street
New Orleans, LA 70112
504/588-3477

Shreveport Pain and Rehabilitation
 Center, Inc.
1805 Line Avenue
Shreveport, LA 71101-4611
318/227-2780

Maryland
Pain Treatment Center
The Johns Hopkins Hospital
600 North Wolfe Street, Meyer 279
Baltimore, MD 21205
301/955-3270

Sinai Hospital of Baltimore
Belvedere and Greenspring Avenues
Baltimore, MD 21215
301/367-7800

Clinical Pain Section, Neurobiology
 and Anesthesiology Branch
National Institute of Dental Research
National Institutes of Health
Building 30, Room B18
Bethesda, MD 20205
301/496-6804

Associated Pain Consultants
8808 Cameron Street
Silver Spring, MD 20910
301/565-2633

Massachusetts
Boston Pain Center
Spaulding Rehabilitation Hospital
125 Nashua Street
Boston, MA 02114
617/720-6669

New England Rehabilitation Hospital
Two Rehabilitation Way
Woburn, MA 01801
617/935-5050

University of Massachusetts Medical
 Center
55 Lake Avenue
Worcester, MA 01605
617/856-0011

Michigan
Ingham Medical Center
Back and Pain Clinic
401 West Greenlawn Avenue
Lansing, MI 48909
517/374-2465

Minnesota
Golden Valley Health Center
4101 Golden Valley Road
Golden Valley, MN 55422
612/588-2771

Parkview Treatment Center
3705 Park Center Boulevard
Minneapolis, MN 55416
612/929-5531

Pilling Pain Clinic
825 South Eighth Street
Minneapolis, MN 55404-1289
612/347-4548

Mayo Clinic Pain Management Center
St. Mary's Hospital
5DE 1216 Second Street SW
Rochester, MN 55902
507/285-5921

Mayo Pain Clinic
200 Second Street SW
Rochester, MN 55901
507/284-8311

Midway Hospital
1700 University Avenue
St. Paul, MN 55104
612/641-5610

Nebraska
Nebraska Pain Management Center
University of Nebraska Hospital
42nd and Dewey Avenue
Omaha, NE 68105
402/559-4364

New Jersey
Kim Rehabilitation Institute, PA
405 Northfield Avenue
West Orange, NJ 07052
201/736-3434

New York
Pain Management Center
Lourdes Hospital
169 Riverside Drive
Binghamton, NY 13905
607/798-5358

Pain Treatment Center
Montefiore Medical Center
111 East 210th Street
Bronx, NY 10467
212/920-4440

Department of Rehabilitation Medicine
Kingsbrook Jewish Medical Center
585 Schenectady Avenue
Brooklyn, NY 11203
718/604-5341

Pain Therapy Center
Maimonides Medical Center
931 48th Street
Brooklyn, NY 11219
718/270-7182

Anesthesiology Pain Treatment
 Service
Department of Anesthesiology
Columbia-Presbyterian Medical Center
622 West 168th Street
New York, NY 10032
212/305-7114

Hospital for Joint Diseases
1919 Madison Avenue
New York, NY 10035
212/650-4570

Upstate Medical Center
State University Hospital
750 East Adams Street
Syracuse, NY 13210
315/473-4720

North Carolina
Pain Center
University of North Carolina
North Carolina Memorial Hospital
NCMH Box 106
Chapel Hill, NC 27514
919/966-5216

Pain Clinic
Duke University Medical Center
Department of Anesthesiology
Box 3060
Durham, NC 27710
919/684-6542

North Dakota
T.N.I. Pain Clinic
700 First Avenue South
Fargo, ND 58103
701/235-5354 ext 65

Ohio
Pain Control Center
University of Cincinnati
Medical Center
234 Goodman Street, ML 586
Cincinnati, OH 45267
513/872-5664

The Ohio Pain and Stress
 Treatment Center
1460 West Lane Avenue
Columbia, OH 43221
614/488-5971

Medical College of Ohio Hospital
3000 Arlington Avenue, CS 10008
Toledo, OH 43699
419/391-4106

Youngstown Osteopathic Hospital
1319 Florencedale Street
Youngstown, OH 44505
216/744-9200

Oregon
Sacred Heart General Hospital
1200 Alder Street
Eugene, OR 97401
503/686-6854

Pain Clinic
Good Samaritan Hospital and Medical
 Center
Suite 319 2222 NW Lovejoy
Portland, OR 97210
503/229-7461

Northwest Pain Center Associates
10615 SE Cherry Blossom Drive
Portland, OR 97216
503/256-1930

Pennsylvania
Pain Control Clinic
Charles Cole Memorial Hospital
Coudersport, PA 16915
814/274-9527

Pain Control Center of Temple
 University
Temple University Hospital
3401 North Broad Street
Philadelphia, PA 19140
215/221-2100

Pain Control Center, Suite 9408
Presbyterian University Hospital
Desoto at O'Hara Streets
Pittsburgh, PA 15213
412/647-3680

Veterans Administration Medical
 Center
University Drive "C"
Pittsburgh, PA 15240
412/683-3000

South Carolina
Veterans Administration Medical
 Center
Garner's Ferry Road
Columbia, SC 29201
803/776-4000

Texas
University of Texas Medical Branch
301 University Avenue
Galveston, TX 77550
409/761-2930

Chronic Pain Treatment Program of
B.C.M. at the Methodist Hospital
6516 Bertner Boulevard
Houston, TX 77030
713/468-8967

Behavioral Medicine Service
Medical Center Del Oro Hospital
8081 Greenbriar Street
Houston, TX 77054
713/790-8550

Pain Control and Biofeedback Clinic
6560 Fannin, Scurlock Tower, Suite
 900
Houston, TX 77030
713/799-5796

The University of Texas Medical
 School
Division of Neurosurgery
6431 Fannin Street
Houston, TX 77030
713/792-5760

Wilford Hall USAF Medical Center
Lackland AFB, TX 78236
512/670-7100

Texas Tech University
School of Medicine
Health Sciences Center Hospital
3601 Fourth Street
Lubbock, TX 79430
806/743-3111

Anesthesia Pain Clinic
Suite 306 4499 Medical Drive
San Antonio, TX 78229
512/692-0101

Anesthesia Pain Clinic
The University of Texas Health
 Science Center
7703 Floyd Curl Drive
San Antonio, TX 78284
512/691-6664

Scott and White Clinic
Scott and White Hospital
2401 South 31st Street
Temple, TX 76508
817/774-2111

Hohf Clinic and Hospital
1404 East Hiller Street
Victoria, TX 77901
512/573-7468

Utah
Stewart Rehabilitation Center
McKay-Dee Hospital
3939 Harrison Boulevard
Ogden, UT 84409
801/393-1300

INFORMATION RESOURCES

Virginia
Department of Anethesiology
Pain Management Center
University of Virginia Medical Center
Box 293
Charlottesville, VA 22908
804/924-5581

Medical College of Virginia
Virginia Commonwealth University
1200 East Broad Street
Richmond, VA 23298
804/786-9000

Washington
The Pain Center
Swedish Hospital Medical Center
747 Summit Avenue
Seattle, WA 98104
206/292-2013

Pain Clinic, RC-76
University of Washington
1959 NE Pacific Street
Seattle, WA 98195
206/548-4282

West Virginia
Pain Clinic
Department of Anesthesiology
West Virginia University Hospital Inc.
Morgantown, WV 26506
304/293-5411

Wisconsin
Pain Clinic, University of Wisconsin
  Clinical Science Center
600 Highland Avenue, F6-5
Madison, WI 53792
608/263-9551, 608/263-6385

Chronic Pain Management Program
Mt. Sinai Medical Center
950 North 12th Street
Milwaukee, WI 53233
414/289-8653

Curative Rehabilitation Center
9001 West Watertown Plank Road
Milwaukee, WI 53226
414/259-1414

Sleep Disorders Centers

The following centers and clinics specialize in the management of sleep disorders and will answer questions related to particular therapeutic problems.

California
Sleep Disorders Center
Holy Cross Hospital
15031 Rinaldi Street
Mission Hills, CA 91345
818/898-4639

Sleep Disorders Center
University of California
Irvine Medical Center
101 City Drive South
Orange, CA 92688
714/634-5776

Sleep Disorders Center
Stanford University Medical Center
Building TD, Room 114
Stanford, CA 94305
415/497-8131

Florida
Sleep Disorders Center
Mt. Sinai Medical Center
4300 Alton Road
Miami Beach, FL 33140
305/674-2613

Illinois
Sleep Disorders Center
Northwestern Memorial Hospital
10th Floor, Passvant Pavillion
303 East Superior Street
Chicago, IL 60611
312/649-2458, 312/649-2650

Sleep Disorders Center
Rush-Presbyterian-St. Luke's Medical
  Center
1753 Congress Parkway
Chicago, IL 60612
312/942-5440

Louisiana
Tulane Sleep Disorders Center
Tulane Medical Center
New Orleans, LA 70112
504/587-7457

Maryland
The Johns Hopkins University
Sleep Disorders Center
4940 Eastern Avenue
Baltimore, MD 21224
301/955-0571

Massachusetts
Sleep Disorders Center
Department of Neurology
University of Massachusetts Medical
  Center
Worcester, MA 01605
617/856-3968

Michigan
Sleep Disorders Center
Henry Ford Hospital
2799 West Grand Boulevard
Detroit, MI 48202
313/876-2233

Minnesota
Minnesota Regional Sleep Disorders
  Center
Hennepin County Medical Center
701 Park Avenue South
Minneapolis, MN 55415
612/347-6289

New Hampshire
Dartmouth-Hitchcock Sleep Disorders
  Center
Dartmouth Medical School
703 Remsen Building
Hanover, NH 03756
603/646-7534

New York
Sleep-Wake Disorders Center
Montefiore Medical Center
111 East 210th Street
Bronx, NY 10467
212/920-4841

Sleep Disorders Center
Department of Psychiatry
University Hospital
SUNY at Stony Brook
Stony Brook, NY 11794-7139
516/444-2916

Ohio
Sleep Disorders Laboratory
of the Jewish Hospital
1275 East Kemper Road
Cincinnati, OH 45246
513/671-3101

Sleep Disorders Center
Mt. Sinai Medical Center
University Circle
Cleveland, OH 44106
216/421-3678

Sleep Disorders Center
Department of Psychiatry
Ohio State University
Columbus, OH 43210
614/421-8260

Sleep Wake Disorders Unit
Miami Valley Hospital
Dayton, OH 45409
513/220-2515

Oklahoma
Sleep Disorders Center
Presbyterian Hospital
NE 13th at Lincoln Boulevard
Oklahoma City, OK 73104
405/271-6312

Pennsylvania
Sleep Evaluation Center
Western Psychiatric Institute and
  Clinic
3811 O'Hara Street
Pittsburgh, PA 15213
412/624-2246, 412/624-2040 (night
  line)

Sleep Disorders Center
Department of Neurology
Crozer-Chester Medical Center
Upland-Chester, PA 19013
215/447-2689

Tennessee
BMH Sleep Disorders Center
Baptist Memorial Hospital
Memphis, TN 38146
901/522-5651

Texas
Sleep Disorder and Research Center
Baylor College of Medicine
Houston, TX 77030
713/799-4886

Sleep Disorders Center
Humana Hospital Metropolitan
1303 McCullough Street
San Antonio, TX 78212
512/223-4057

Voluntary Health Organizations

The following organizations and agencies provide educational materials to health-care professionals, conduct seminars and workshops, and support education and research in their field of interest. Many also provide information to the lay public, conduct patient counseling and support groups, and offer a variety of rehabilitation services.

Aging
American Geriatrics Society
10 Columbus Circle, Suite 1470
New York, NY 10019
212/582-1333

The Gerontological Society of
  America
1411 K Street NW, Suite 300
Washington, DC 20005
202/393-1411

National Clearinghouse on Aging
330 Independence Avenue SW
Washington, DC 20201
202/245-2158

National Council on the Aging
600 Maryland Avenue SW,
  West Wing 100
Washington, DC 20024
202/479-1200 (9 am-5 pm Mon-Fri)

National Council of Senior Citizens,
  Inc.
925 15th Street NW
Washington, DC 20005
202/347-8800

Alcoholism
Al-Anon Family Group Headquarters
PO Box 862, Midtown Station
New York, NY 10018-0862
212/302-7240

Alcoholics Anonymous, Inc.
Room 219, 175 Fifth Avenue
New York, NY 10010
212/473-6200

National Clearinghouse for Alcoholism
  Information
PO Box 2345
Rockville, MD 20852
301/468-2600

National Council on Alcoholism, Inc.
12 West 21st Street, Seventh Floor
New York, NY 10010
212/206-6770

National Council on Alcoholism, Inc.
1511 K Street NW, Suite 320
Washington, DC 20005
202/737-8122

Anorexia Nervosa
National Association of Anorexia
  Nervosa and Associated Disorders
PO Box 7
Highland Park, IL 60035
312/831-3438

Arthritis
The Arthritis Foundation
1314 Spring Street NW
Atlanta, GA 30309
404/872-7100 (9 am-5 pm)

Asthma and Allergy
American Lung Association
1740 Broadway
New York, NY 10019
212/245-8000

Asthma and Allergy Foundation of
  America
1835 K Street NW, Suite P-900
Washington, DC 20006
202/293-2950 (8:30 am-5:30 pm
  Mon-Fri)

Blood Diseases
National Hemophilia Foundation
19 West 34th Street
New York, NY 10001
212/563-0211

National Sickle Cell Disease Program
Division of Blood Diseases and
  Resources
National Heart, Lung, and Blood
  Institute
National Institutes of Health
Room 504, Federal Building
7550 Wisconsin Avenue
Bethesda, MD 20205
301/496-6931

Cancer
American Cancer Society, Inc.
90 Park Avenue
New York, NY 10016
212/599-8200, 212/595-4490 (night
  line)

Cancer Counseling and Research
  Center
6060 North Central Expressway,
  Suite 140
Dallas, TX 75206
214/373-7744

Damon Runyon-Walter Winchell
  Cancer Fund
33 West 56th Street
New York, NY 10019
212/582-5400

Leukemia Society of America, Inc.
733 Third Avenue
New York, NY 10017
212/573-8484

Living with Cancer, Inc.
PO Box 3060
Long Island City, NY 11101
718/241-4100

National Cancer Institute
Cancer Information Service
Office of Cancer Communications
Building 31, Room 10A18
9000 Rockville Pike
Bethesda, MD 20892
1-800/4-CANCER, 1-800/638-6070 (in
  Alaska), 808/524-1234 (in Hawaii)

Cerebral Palsy
United Cerebral Palsy Association
66 East 34th Street
New York, NY 10016
212/481-6347

Child Abuse and Neglect
American Humane Association
9725 East Hampden
Denver, CO 80231
303/695-0811

CALM, Child Abuse Listening
  Mediation, Inc.
PO Box 718
Santa Barbara, CA 93102
805/682-1366, 805/569-2255 (hot
  line)

Clearinghouse on Child Abuse and
  Neglect Information
PO Box 1182
Washington, DC 20013
202/245-2856

Childbirth/Maternity Care
International Childbirth Education
  Association, Inc.
PO Box 20048
Minneapolis, MN 55420
612/854-8660

Maternity Center Association
48 East 92nd Street
New York, NY 10128
212/369-7300

INFORMATION RESOURCES

Childhood Life-Threatening Illnesses
The Candlelighters
Childhood Cancer Foundation
2025 Eye Street NW
Washington, DC 20006
202/659-5136

The Compassionate Friends, Inc.
PO Box 3696
Oak Brook, IL 60521
312/323-5010

Cystic Fibrosis
Cystic Fibrosis Foundation
6000 Executive Boulevard, Suite 309
Rockville, MD 20852
301/881-9130

Diabetes
American Diabetes Association, Inc.
National Service Center
1660 Duke Street, PO Box 25757
Alexandria, VA 22313
703/549-1500

Joslin Diabetes Center
One Joslin Place
Boston, MA 02215
617/732-2400

The Juvenile Diabetes Foundation
60 Madison Avenue
New York, NY 10010
212/889-7575

National Diabetes Information
  Clearinghouse
Box NDIC
Bethesda, MD 20892
301/468-2162

Digestive Diseases
American Digestive Disease Society, Inc.
7720 Wisconsin Avenue
Bethesda, MD 20814
301/652-9293

National Digestive Diseases
  Information Clearinghouse
1255 23rd Street NW, Suite 275
Washington, DC 20037
202/296-1138

National Foundation for Ileitis and
  Colitis, Inc.
444 Park Avenue South
New York, NY 10016
212/685-3440

Drug Abuse and Narcotic Addiction
Do It Now Foundation
PO Box 5115
Phoenix, AZ 85010-5115
602/257-0797

Drug Abuse Clearinghouse
PO Box 416
Kensington, MD 20795
301/443-6500

Narcotics Education, Inc.
6830 Laurel Street NW
Washington, DC 20012
202/722-6740

Epilepsy
Epilepsy Foundation of America
4351 Garden City Drive
Landover, MD 20785
301/459-3700

The Epilepsy Institute
67 Irving Place
New York, NY 10003
212/677-8550

Family Planning/Sex Information
The Alan Guttmacher Institute
2010 Massachusetts Avenue NW
Washington, DC 20036
202/296-4012

The Alan Guttmacher Institute
360 Park Avenue South
New York, NY 10010
212/685-5858

American Social Health Association
260 Sheridan Avenue
Palo Alto, CA 94306
415/327-6465

Emory University-Grady Memorial
  Hospital
Family Planning Program
80 Butler Street SE
Atlanta, GA 90303
404/588-3680

Human Life International
418 C Street NE
Washington, DC 20002
202/546-2257

National Clearinghouse for Family
  Planning Information
PO Box 12921
Arlington, VA 22209
703/558-7932

Planned Parenthood Federation of
  America, Inc.
810 Seventh Avenue
New York, NY 10017
212/541-7800

Population Council, Inc.
One Dag Hammerskjold Plaza
New York, NY 10017
212/644-1300

Sex Information and Education
  Council of the United States
80 Fifth Avenue, Suite 801
New York, NY 10011
212/929-2300

Fertility
The American Fertility Society
2131 Magnolia Avenue, Suite 201
Birmingham, AL 35256
205/251-9764

Resolve, Inc.
PO Box 474
Belmont, MA 02178
617/484-2424

Genetic Diseases
American Genetic Association
1028 Connecticut Avenue NW
Washington, DC 20036
202/659-2096

Friedreich's Ataxia Group in America, Inc.
PO Box 11116
Oakland, CA 94611
Tel: 415/655-0833

March of Dimes Birth Defects
  Foundation
1275 Mamaroneck Avenue
White Plains, NY 10605
914/428-7100

National Center for Education
  in Maternal and Child Health
38th and R Streets NW
Washington, DC 20057
202/625-8400

National Genetics Foundation
555 West 57th Street
New York, NY 10019
212/586-5800

National Huntington's Disease
  Association
1182 Broadway, Suite 402
New York, NY 10001
212/684-2781

National Tay-Sachs and Allied
  Diseases Association, Inc.
92 Washington Avenue
Cedarhurst, NY 11516
516/569-4300 (8:30 am-4:30 pm Mon-Fri)

The RP Foundation
1401 Mount Royal Avenue, 4th Floor
Baltimore, MD 21217
301/225-9400, 800/638-2300, TDD 301/225-9409

Handicapped/Rehabilitation
American Coalition of Citizens With
  Disabilities, Inc.
1200 15th Street NW, Suite 201
Washington, DC 20005
202/785-4265

The National Information Center for
  Handicapped Children and Youth
PO Box 1492
Washington, DC 20013
703/522-3332

Federation of the Handicapped
211 West 14th Street
New York, NY 10011
212/242-9050

Goodwill Industries of America, Inc.
9200 Wisconsin Avenue
Bethesda, MD 20814
301/530-6500

March of Dimes Birth Defects
  Foundation
1275 Mamaroneck Avenue
White Plains, NY 10605
914/428-7100

The National Easter Seal Society
2023 West Ogden Avenue
Chicago, IL 60612
312/243-8400

National Rehabilitation Information
  Center
Catholic University of America
4407 Eighth Street NE
Washington, DC 20017
202/635-5822

National Spinal Cord Injury
  Association
149 California Street
Newton, MA 02158
617/964-0521

People-to-People Committee for the
  Handicapped
Vanguard Building, Sixth Floor
1111 20th Street NW
Washington, DC 20036
202/653-5007

Rehabilitation International, U.S.A.
1123 Broadway, Suite 704
New York, NY 10010
212/620-4040 (9 am-5 pm)

The Sister Kenny Institute
800 East 28th Street
Minneapolis, MN 55407

Spina Bifida Association of America
343 South Dearborn Street
Chicago, IL 60604
312/663-1562

Health Information
American Red Cross
17th and D Streets NW
Washington, DC 20006
202/737-8300

National Health Information
  Clearinghouse
PO Box 1133
Washington DC, 20013
800/336-4797, 703/522-2590 (collect
  in Virginia) (8:30 am-5 pm)

Hearing and Speech Disorders
Alexander Graham Bell Association
  for the Deaf
3417 Volta NW
Washington DC, 20007
202/337-5220 (voice or TTY)

American Speech-Language-Hearing
  Association
10801 Rockville Pike
Rockville MD, 20852
301/897-5700

The Better Hearing Institute
1430 K Street North, Suite 600
Washington DC 20005
202/638-7577

Deafness Research Foundation
55 East 34th Street
New York, NY 10016
212/684-6556

National Association of the Deaf
814 Thayer Avenue
Silver Spring, MD 20910
301/587-1788

National Association for Hearing and
  Speech Action
10801 Rockville Pike
Rockville, MD 20852
301/897-8682 (in Maryland),
  800/638-8255 (help-line)

Heart Disease
American Heart Association
7320 Greenville Avenue
Dallas, TX 75231
214/750-5300

The Mended Hearts, Inc.
7320 Greenville Avenue
Dallas, TX 75231
214/750-5442

Kidney Disease
National Association of Patients on
  Hemodialysis and Transplantation,
  Inc.
150 Nassau Street, Suite 1305
New York, NY 10038
212/619-2727

National Kidney Foundation, Inc.
Two Park Avenue
New York, NY 10016
212/889-2210

Learning Disabilities
Association for Children and Adults
  With Learning Disabilities
4156 Library Road
Pittsburgh, PA 15234
412/341-1515

Federation for Children with Special
  Needs
120 Boylston Street, Suite 338
Boston, MA 02116
617/482-2915

National Society for Autistic Children
Suite 1017
1234 Massachusetts Avenue NW
Washington, DC 20005
202/783-0125

Lupus Erythematosus
National Lupus Erythematosus
  Foundation, Inc.
5430 Van Nuys Boulevard, Suite 206
Van Nuys, CA 91401
213/88-LUPUS

Medical Alert
Medic Alert Foundation International
PO Box 1009
Turlock, CA 95380
209/668-3333

Mental Health/Retardation
Alzheimer's Disease and Related
  Disorders Association, Inc.
70 East Lake Street, Suite 600
Chicago, IL 60601
312/853-3060 (8 am-5:30 pm Mon-
  Fri), 800/621-0379, 800/572-6037
  (Illinois only)

American Mental Health Foundation
Two East 86th Street
New York, NY 10028
212/737-9027

Association for Alzheimer's and
  Related Diseases
360 North Michigan Avenue
Chicago, IL 60601
800/621-0379

Association for Children with
  Retarded Mental Development
817 Broadway
New York, NY 10003
212/475-7200

Association for Retarded Citizens
2501 Avenue J
Arlington, TX 76011
817/640-0204

Kennedy Child Study Center
151 East 67th Street
New York, NY 10021
212/988-9500

National Society for Autistic Children
Suite 1017
1234 Massachusetts Avenue NW
Washington, DC 20005
202/783-0125

Neurotics Anonymous International
  Liason, Inc.
PO Box 4866, Cleveland Park Station
Washington, DC 20008
202/628-4379

INFORMATION RESOURCES

President's Committee on Mental Retardation
330 Independence Avenue SW
Washington, DC 20210
202/245-7634

Multiple Sclerosis
National Multiple Sclerosis Society
205 East 42nd Street
New York, NY 10017
212/986-3240

Muscular Dystrophy
Muscular Dystrophy Association
810 Seventh Avenue
New York, NY 10019
212/586-0808

Myasthenia Gravis
Myasthenia Gravis Foundation, Inc.
225 Park Avenue South
New York, NY 10003
212/777-5000 ext 190 (10 am-4 pm)

Parkinson's Disease
American Parkinson's Disease Association
116 John Street
New York, NY 10038
212/732-9550

Parkinson's Disease Foundation
Columbia Presbyterian Medical Center
650 West 168th Street
New York, NY 10032
212/923-4700

Psoriasis
The National Psoriasis Foundation
6443 SW Beaverton Highway, Suite 210
Portland, OR 97221
503/297-1545

Respiratory Diseases
American Lung Association
1740 Broadway
New York, NY 10019
212/245-8000

Reye's Syndrome
National Reye's Syndrome Foundation
PO Box 829
Bryan, OH 43506
419/636-2679

Stroke
National Stroke Association
1420 Ogden Street
Denver, CO 80218
303/839-1992

Vision Disorders/Blindness
American Council of the Blind
1211 Connecticut Avenue NW
Washington, DC 20036
800/424-8666

American Foundation for the Blind, Inc.
15 West 16th Street
New York, NY 10011
212/620-2000

American Humane Association
National Hearing Dog Project
PO Box 1266
Denver, CO 80201
303/695-0811 (voice/TTY)

American Printing House for the Blind
1839 Frankfort Avenue
Louisville, KY 40206
502/895-2405

Associated Blind, Inc.
135 West 23rd Street
New York, NY 10011
212/255-1122

Association for Education and Rehabilitation of the Blind and Visually Impaired
206 North Washington Street, Suite 320
Alexandria, VA 22314
703/548-1884

Better Vision Institute, Inc.
230 Park Avenue
New York, NY 10169
212/682-1731

Fight for Sight, Inc.
139 East 57th Street
New York, NY 10022
212/751-1118

Guiding Eyes for the Blind, Inc.
611 Granite Springs Road
Yorktown Heights, NY 10598
914/245-4024

National Association for the Visually Handicapped
3201 Balboa Street
San Francisco, CA 94121
415/221-3201, 415/221-8753

National Library Service for the Blind and Physically Handicapped
The Library of Congress
1291 Taylor Street NW
Washington, DC 20542
202/287-5100

National Society to Prevent Blindness
79 Madison Avenue
New York, NY 10016
212/684-3505

Recording for the Blind, Inc.
20 Roszel Road
Princeton, NJ 08540
609/452-0606

COMPENDIUM OF DRUG THERAPY

Chapter 4

Essential Pharmacokinetic Data

Pharmacokinetics of Commonly Used Drugs — 101
Victor Lampasona, PharmD
Donna S. Carr, PharmD
Timothy A. Poole, PharmD

Introduction	101
Androgens	102
Antianginal Agents	102
Antianxiety Agents	102
Antiarrhythmics	103
Antiasthmatic Agents	108
Antibacterial Agents	103
Anticoagulants	104
Anticonvulsants	104
Antidepressants	105
Antiemetics	107
Antifungal Agents	105
Antigout Agents	105
Antihistamines	105
Antihypertensive Agents	106
Antimanic Agents	107
Antimigraine Agents	107
Antinauseants	107
Antipsychotic Agents	107
Antipruritics	107
Antireflux Agents	107
Antiulcer Agents	107
Antiviral Agents	108
Bronchodilators	108
Diuretics	108
Gold Compounds	108
Hypnotics	110
Hypoglycemic Agents	109
Hypolipidemic Agents	109
Inotropic Agents	109
Muscle Relaxants	109
Narcotic Analgesics	109
Nonnarcotic Analgesics	110
Nonsteroidal Anti-inflammatory Agents	110
Sedatives	110
Thyroid Hormones	111

Pharmacokinetic Data for Drug Monitoring — 112
Ray R. Maddox, PharmD
Victor Lampasona, PharmD

Introduction	112
Amikacin	113
Amitriptyline	113
Aspirin	114
Carbamazepine	114
Chloramphenicol	115
Desipramine	115
Digitoxin	116
Digoxin	116
Disopyramide	117
Ethosuximide	118
Flucytosine	118
Gentamicin	119
Heparin	119
Lidocaine	120
Lithium	120
Methotrexate	121
Nortriptyline	121
Phenobarbital	122
Phenytoin	122
Primidone	123
Procainamide	124
Quinidine	124
Theophylline	125
Tobramycin	126
Valproic acid	126
Vancomycin	127

Pharmacokinetics of Commonly Used Drugs

Victor Lampasona, PharmD
Donna S. Carr, PharmD
Timothy A. Poole, PharmD

Emory University Hospital, Atlanta, GA

This section is a compilation of selected pharmacologic and pharmacokinetic information on many commonly used drugs. The sources used to ascertain this information include the manufacturer's package insert; however, in many cases, more clinically appropriate data were found in reference texts or review articles and, consequently, were included.

The information given in the table reflects only values that correspond to pharmacokinetic processes in adult patients with normal organ function. The reader can, however, utilize these data to anticipate which drugs may require dosage adjustments in certain disease states because of changes in drug clearance. The column entitled **Excreted unchanged** indicates how much of a particular compound is eliminated as parent drug. If a drug is not 100% eliminated as the parent compound, it is assumed that the drug is metabolized to active or inactive compounds. The column headed **Route of elimination** indicates which processes are responsible for eliminating the unchanged parent drug and the active and inactive metabolites. Disease states that interfere with drug metabolic processes in the liver may alter the disposition of compounds that depend highly on hepatic metabolism for elimination, ie, those compounds represented with low percent "excreted unchanged." On the other hand, the clearance of drugs that are largely excreted unchanged may be affected by renal disease. Please refer to the complete drug chart elsewhere in this volume for appropriate dosage modifications. Other column headings are defined as follows:

- **Route** indicates the usual method of drug administration; however, other routes may occasionally be utilized. In this column, PO, SC, IM, and IV have their usual meanings, SL indicates sublingual administration, "Inhal" means oral inhalation, and an asterisk placed after PO indicates oral administration of the sustained-, controlled-, or extended-release dosage form.
- **Dosing interval** describes the manufacturer's recommended interval between doses for patients with normal organ function. As mentioned above, this may be extended for patients with hepatic or renal impairment.
- **Onset of action** indicates the average time after dosage administration that the pharmacologic or clinical effect of the drug can be anticipated in most patients. It is assumed for most antibiotics that this time coincides with the attainment of therapeutic serum levels.
- **Duration of action** indicates the average period of therapeutic effectiveness in patients with normal organ function.
- **Protein binding** indicates the percentage of drug bound to plasma proteins, principally albumin. Protein binding has clinically significant implications if a drug is at least 85% bound. In these cases, changes in drug binding due to alterations in binding-receptor affinity, competition from other substances, or a decreased concentration of plasma proteins can affect the pharmacologic response exhibited by the patient.
- **Elimination half-life** is the time required to decrease the blood concentration of the drug by 50%; values given in parentheses are the half-lives of the active metabolites, if any.

The drugs are arranged according to their therapeutic class to allow the reader to compare the pharmacokinetic parameters of drugs used for similar clinical situations. Unfortunately, data could not be found for each parameter for every drug; where no data were available, a dash was placed in the column. For other information regarding these drugs, consult the appropriate full drug chart.

PHARMACOKINETICS

Drug	Route	Dosing interval	Onset of action	Duration of action	Protein binding	Excreted unchanged	Elimination half-life	Route of elimination
ANDROGENS								
Danazol	PO	12 h	1 mo	2–3 mo	—	5%	29 h	Renal
Fluoxymesterone	PO	6–24 h	1 mo	6 mo	98%	5%	9.2 h	Renal
Methyltestosterone	PO	24 h	1 mo	6 mo	98%	<10%	2.5–3 h	Renal/biliary
Testosterone cypionate	IM	2–4 wk	1 mo	2–4 wk	98%	<4%	10–100 min	Renal
Testosterone enanthate	IM	2–4 wk	1 mo	2–4 wk	98%	<4%	10–100 min	Renal
ANTIANGINAL AGENTS								
Beta Blockers								
Atenolol	PO	24 h	—	24 h	10%	85%	6–7 h	Renal
Metoprolol	PO	8–12 h	12 h	—	12%	<5%	3–7 h	Renal
Nadolol	PO	24 h	—	24 h	25%	70%	20–24 h	Renal
Propranolol	PO	6–8 h	1–1.5 h	—	90%	1%	4 h	Renal
	PO*	24 h	—	—				
Calcium Antagonists								
Diltiazem	PO	6–8 h	30 min	—	80%	2–4%	3.5 h	Renal/biliary
Nifedipine	PO	8 h	—	6–12 h	92–98%	0%	4 h	80% Renal/ 15% fecal
Verapamil	PO	6–8 h	<2 h	6–8 h	90%	<3%	2.8–12 h	70% Renal/ 16% biliary
Nitrates								
Erythrityl tetranitrate	SL	prn	5 min	2 h	—	—	—	Renal
	PO	3–4 h	15–30 min	4 h				
Isosorbide dinitrate	SL	2–3 h	3–15 min	45 min–2 h	28%	<1%	30 min–1.5 h	Renal
	PO	6 h	30–60 min	3–6 h				
	PO*	8–12 h	30–60 min	6–10 h				
Nitroglycerin	Buccal	prn	2–5 min	3–5 h	60%	<1%	1.7–2.9 min	Renal
	Lingual	prn	2–5 min	10–30 min				
	SL	prn	2–5 min	10–30 min				
	PO*	8–12 h	30–45 min	2–8 h				
	Paste	4–8 h	20–60 min	2–8 h				
	Patch	24 h	30–60 min	24 h				
	IV	3–5 min	Immediate	Transient				
Pentaerythritol tetranitrate	PO	6 h	30 min	3–6 h	—	<10%	10 min	Renal/fecal
	PO*	12 h	0.5–2 h	6–10 h				
ANTIANXIETY AGENTS								
Benzodiazepines								
Alprazolam	PO	8 h	—	—	80%	20%	12–15 h	Renal
Chlordiazepoxide	PO	6–8 h	1 h	—	96–97%	<1%	7–13 h (5–10 h; 48–76 h)	Renal
	IM	6–8 h	—	—				
	IV	6–8 h	1–5 min	15–60 min				
Clorazepate	PO	6–24 h	—	—	97.5%	<1%	1–3 h (5–10 h; 48–76 h)	Renal
Diazepam	PO	6–12 h	15–45 min	—	97–99%	<1%	30–56 h (5–10 h; 48–76 h)	Renal
	IM	3–4 h	15–30 min	—				
	IV	3–4 h	1–5 min	15–60 min				
Halazepam	PO	6–8 h	—	—	97%	<1%	14 h (5–10 h; 48–76 h)	Renal
Lorazepam	PO	8–12 h	—	—	85%	<1%	12–18 h	Renal
	IM	—	15–30 min	12–24 h				
	IV	—	15–20 min	6–8 h				
Oxazepam	PO	6–8 h	—	—	97.8%	<1%	5–10 h	Renal
Prazepam	PO	8–24 h	—	—	97.5%	<1%	1–2 h (5–10 h; 48–76 h)	Renal
Miscellaneous								
Buspirone	PO	8 h	—	—	95%	1%	2–3 h	29–63% Renal/18–38% fecal
Chlormezanone	PO	6–8 h	15–30 min	—	48%	—	24 h	Renal/biliary
Hydroxyzine	PO	6 h	15–30 min	4–6 h	—	<1%	3 h	Biliary
	IM	4–6 h	—	—				
Meprobamate	PO	6–8 h	1–3 h	—	20%	10–12%	6–16 h	Renal

*Sustained, controlled, or extended-release form

PHARMACOKINETICS

Drug	Route	Dosing interval	Onset of action	Duration of action	Protein binding	Excreted unchanged	Elimination half-life	Route of elimination
ANTIARRHYTHMICS								
Acebutolol	PO	12–24 h	1.5 h	—	26%	40%	3–4 h (8–13 h)	30–40% Renal/50–60% fecal
Amiodarone	PO	12–24 h	1–3 wk	Weeks to months	96%	0%	40–55 days	Biliary
Bretylium	IM, IV	6 h	20 min–6 h	6–24 h	0–8%	70–85%	6.9–8.1 h	Renal
Digoxin	PO	6–8 h	30 min–2 h	3–4 days	20–25%	50–70%	1.5–2 days	Renal
	IM	—	30 min–2 h	3–4 days				
	IV	4–8 h	5–30 min	3–4 days				
Disopyramide	PO	6 h	30 min–3.5 h	1.5–8.5 h	50–65%	50%	5–10 h	Renal
	PO*	12 h	—	—			7.5–16 h	
Encainide	PO	8 h	1–2 h	12–14 h	90%	0%	2–4 h (3–4 h; 6–12 h)	50% Renal/50% biliary
Esmolol	IV	—	<5 min	10–20 min	55%	<2%	9 min	Renal
Flecainide	PO	12 h	3–5 days	8–24 h	40–50%	10–50%	12–27 h	Renal
Lidocaine	IM	—	5–15 min	<3 h	60–80%	2%	1.5–2 h	Renal
	IV	—	Immediate	10–20 min				
Mexiletine	PO	8–12 h	2–4 h	12–24 h	50–60%	10%	10–12 h	Renal
Procainamide	PO	3 h	45 min–2.5 h	3–6 h	16%	50%	2.4–3.6 h	Renal
	PO*	6 h	—	3–6 h			(4–15 h)	
	IM	3–6 h	10–30 min	—				
	IV	—	5–10 min	—				
Propranolol	PO	6–8 h	1–1.5 h	—	90%	1%	4 h	Renal
	IV	—	<5 min	—				
Quinidine	PO	2–12 h	1–3 h	6–8 h	70–95%	10–20%	4.4–8 h	Renal
Tocainide	PO	8 h	2 h	—	10–50%	40%	11–15 h	Renal
Verapamil	PO	6–8 h	<2 h	6–8 h	90%	<3%	2.8–12 h	70% Renal/16% biliary
	IV	—	1 min	10–20 min			2–5 h	
ANTIBACTERIAL AGENTS								
Aminoglycosides								
Amikacin	IM	8 h	1–2 h	8 h	<30%	100%	2–3 h	Renal
	IV	8 h	30 min	8 h				
Gentamicin	IM	8 h	1–2 h	8 h	<30%	100%	2–3 h	Renal
	IV	8 h	30 min	8 h				
Netilmicin	IM	8 h	1–2 h	8 h	<30%	100%	2–3 h	Renal
	IV	8 h	30 min	8 h				
Tobramycin	IM	8 h	1–2 h	8 h	<30%	100%	2–3 h	Renal
	IV	8 h	30 min	8 h				
Cephalosporins								
Cefaclor	PO	8 h	30 min–1 h	8 h	25%	>90%	0.8–1.3 h	Renal
Cefadroxil	PO	6–12 h	75–90 min	6–12 h	20%	>90%	1.5–2 h	Renal
Cefamandole	IM, IV	6–8 h	30 min–2 h	6–8 h	75%	>90%	0.5–1.2 h	Renal/biliary
Cefazolin	IM, IV	8–12 h	1–2 h	8–12 h	80%	>90%	1.4–1.8 h	Renal
Cefonicid	IM, IV	24 h	1 h	24 h	90%	99%	3.5–5.8 h	Renal
Cefoperazone	IM, IV	12 h	1 h	12 h	90%	99%	1.6–2.6 h	Biliary/renal
Ceforanide	IM, IV	12 h	1 h	12 h	80–90%	80–93%	2.6–3.3 h	Renal
Cefotaxime	IM, IV	6–8 h	30 min	6–8 h	35%	50–60%	1 h	Renal
Cefotetan	IM, IV	12 h	30 min	12 h	88%	100%	3–4.6 h	Renal/biliary
Cefoxitin	IM, IV	6–8 h	15–30 min	6–8 h	50–60%	85%	0.7–1.1 h	Renal
Ceftazidime	IM, IV	8–12 h	45 min	8–12 h	17%	90%	1.8 h	Renal
Ceftizoxime	IM, IV	8–12 h	30 min	8–12 h	40%	95%	1.7 h	Renal
Ceftriaxone	IM, IV	12–24 h	2 h	12–24 h	95%	>95%	5.8–8.7 h	Renal/biliary
Cefuroxime	IM, IV	8 h	1 h	8 h	33%	90%	1.5 h	Renal
Cephalexin	PO	6–12 h	1 h	6–12 h	6–15%	>90%	0.9–1.2 h	Renal
Cephalothin	IM, IV	4–6 h	30 min	4 h	65%	60–70%	0.5–0.8 h	Renal
Cephapirin	IM, IV	4–6 h	30 min	4 h	45%	50–70%	0.7 h	Renal
Cephradine	PO	6–12 h	1 h	6–12 h	6–20%	>90%	0.8–1.3 h	Renal
Moxalactam	IM, IV	8–12 h	1–2 h	8–12 h	45–60%	90%	2.1–2.3 h	Renal
Penicillins								
Amdinocillin	IM, IV	4 h	25–50 min	4 h	5–15%	70%	0.8–0.9 h	Renal
Amoxicillin	PO	8 h	2 h	8 h	17–20%	68%	1–1.3 h	Renal
Ampicillin	PO	6 h	1.5–2 h	6 h	15–25%	90%	0.5–1 h	Renal/biliary
	IM, IV	4–6 h	1 h	6 h		50–85%		
Azlocillin	IV	6 h	—	6 h	20–46%	50–70%	0.8–1.3 h	Renal
Bacampicillin	PO	12 h	30 min–1 h	12 h	20%	75%	0.5–1 h	Renal
Carbenicillin	PO	6 h	30 min–2 h	6 h	29–60%	90%	1–1.5 h	Renal
	IM, IV	4–6 h	30 min–2 h	4–6 h				
Cloxacillin	PO	6 h	30 min–2 h	6 h	90–96%	90%	0.4–0.8 h	Renal/biliary
Cyclacillin	PO	6–8 h	30 min–1 h	6–8 h	18–25%	85%	0.5–0.7 h	Renal

*Sustained, controlled, or extended-release form

continued

PHARMACOKINETICS

Drug	Route	Dosing interval	Onset of action	Duration of action	Protein binding	Excreted unchanged	Elimination half-life	Route of elimination
Methicillin	IV	4–6 h	30 min–1 h	4–6 h	35–45%	65–85%	0.5–1 h	Renal
Mezlocillin	IM, IV	4–6 h	50–75 min	4–6 h	25–50%	39–72%	0.7–1.3 h	Renal
Nafcillin	PO	4–6 h	30 min–2 h	4–6 h	90–96%	40%	0.5–1.5 h	Renal/biliary
	IM, IV	4–6 h	—	4–6 h				
Oxacillin	PO	4–6 h	30 min–1 h	4–6 h	90%	40–70%	0.5–0.7 h	Renal
	IM, IV	4–6 h	0.5 h	4–6 h				
Penicillin G	IM	—	13–24 h	6 h	45–68%	90%	0.4–0.9 h	Renal
Penicillin V	PO	6–8 h	30 min–1 h	6–8 h	75–89%	90%	0.5–1 h	Renal
Piperacillin	IM, IV	4–8 h	30–50 min	4–8 h	16–22%	42–90%	0.6–1.3 h	Renal/biliary
Ticarcillin	IV	3–6 h	30–80 min	3–6 h	45–65%	80–93%	0.9–1.3 h	Renal
Quinolones								
Cinoxacin	PO	6–12 h	—	6 h	60–70%	60%	2.5 h	Renal
Nalidixic acid	PO	6 h	1–2 h	6 h	82–97%	10–20%	1–2 h	Renal
Norfloxacin	PO	12 h	1 h	12 h	10–15%	—	3–4 h	Renal/biliary
Sulfonamides								
Sulfacytine	PO	6 h	2–3 h	6 h	85–90%	—	4–4.5 h	Renal
Sulfamethizole	PO	6–8 h	2 h	6–8 h	90%	90–95%	—	Renal
Sulfamethoxazole	PO	8–12 h	2–4 h	8–12 h	60%	50%	8–10 h	Renal
Sulfisoxazole	PO	4–6 h	1–4 h	4–6 h	85%	50%	5–6 h	Renal
Tetracyclines								
Doxycycline	PO	12 h	2–4 h	12 h	25–93%	35%	12–22 h	Biliary/renal
	IV	12–24 h	—	12–24 h				
Minocycline	PO	12 h	2–4 h	12 h	55–88%	5–10%	11–23 h	Biliary/renal
	IV	12 h	—	12 h				
Oxytetracycline	PO	6 h	2–4 h	6 h	10–40%	60%	6–10 h	Renal/biliary
	IM	8–12 h	—	8–12 h				
Tetracycline	PO	6–12 h	2–4 h	6–12 h	60%	40–60%	6–11 h	Renal/biliary
	IM, IV	8–12 h	—	8–12 h				
Miscellaneous								
Aztreonam	IM, IV	6–12 h	1 h	8 h	56%	94%	1.5–2 h	Renal/biliary
Chloramphenicol	PO	6 h	1–3 h	6 h	60%	—	1.5–4 h	Renal
	IV	6 h	<1 h	6 h		30%		
Clindamycin	PO	4–6 h	30 min–1 h	6 h	93%	10%	2–4 h	Renal
	IM, IV	6–12 h	3 h	6 h				
Erythromycin	PO	6 h	3–4 h	4–6 h	80%	2–5%	1.5–2.5 h	Biliary
	IV	6 h	<1 h	4–6 h		12–15%		
Imipenem	IV	6 h	<1 h	4–6 h	20%	—	1 h	Renal
Methenamine	PO	12 h	<2 h	12 h	—	45–75%	3–6 h	Renal
Metronidazole	PO	6–8 h	1–3 h	6–8 h	20%	15–40%	6–10 h	Renal
	IV	6 h	—	6 h				
Nitrofurantoin	PO	6 h	30 min	6 h	60%	30–50%	0.5 h	Renal
Trimethoprim	PO	12–24 h	1–4 h	12–24 h	40–70%	65–85%	10–12 h	Renal
Vancomycin	PO	6–8 h	1 h	6–8 h	10–55%	100%	6 h	Fecal
	IV	6–12 h	1 h	6–12 h				Renal

ANTICOAGULANTS

Drug	Route	Dosing interval	Onset of action	Duration of action	Protein binding	Excreted unchanged	Elimination half-life	Route of elimination
Heparin	SC	8–12 h	20–60 min	8–12 h	>85%	<10%	1–2 h	Renal/RE system
	IV	4–6 h	Immediate	4–6 h				
Warfarin	PO	24 h	2–7 days	2–5 days	97%	0%	12–72 h	Renal
	IM, IV	24 h	2–7 days	2–5 days				

ANTICONVULSANTS

Barbiturates

Drug	Route	Dosing interval	Onset of action	Duration of action	Protein binding	Excreted unchanged	Elimination half-life	Route of elimination
Amobarbital sodium	IM	—	—	—	—	<1%	20–25 h	Renal
	IV	—	—	3–6 h				
Mephobarbital	PO	24 h	—	10–16 h	—	—	11–67 h (81–117 h)	Renal
Pentobarbital sodium	IM	—	10–25 min	—	35–45%	<1%	35–50 h	Renal
	IV	—	1 min	15 min				
Phenobarbital	PO	8–12 h	2–3 wk	—	20–45%	24%	81–117 h	Renal
	IM	—	—	—				
	IV	—	5 min	4–6 h				
Primidone	PO	6–8 h	—	—	51%	15–25%	3–13 h (81–117 h)	Renal
Secobarbital	IM	3–4 h	<7–10 min	—	30–45%	5%	30 h	Renal
	IV	3–4 h	<1–3 min	15 min				

COMPENDIUM OF DRUG THERAPY

PHARMACOKINETICS

Drug	Route	Dosing interval	Onset of action	Duration of action	Protein binding	Excreted unchanged	Elimination half-life	Route of elimination
Benzodiazepines								
Clonazepam	PO	8 h	1–2 h	6–12 h	86%	<1%	18–50 h	Renal
Diazepam	PO	6–12 h	15–45 min	—	97–99%	<1%	30–56 h (5–10 h; 48–76 h)	Renal
	IM	3–4 h	15–30 min	—				
	IV	3–4 h	1–5 min	15–60 min				
Hydantoins								
Ethotoin	PO	4–6 h	—	—	—	<5%	3–9 h	Renal/fecal
Mephenytoin	PO	24 h	30 min	24–48 h	—	<20%	—	Renal
Phenytoin	PO	6–24 h	2–24 h	—	89%	1–5%	7–29 h	Renal
	PO*	6–24 h	2–24 h	—			7–42 h	
	IV	—	1–2 h	—			10–15 h	
Oxazolidinediones								
Paramethadione	PO	6–8 h	—	—	—	<5%	24 h	Renal
Trimethadione	PO	24 h	—	—	—	3%	5–10 days	Renal
Succinimides								
Ethosuximide	PO	24 h	4–7 days	—	0%	25%	37–53 h	Renal
Methsuximide	PO	24 h	—	—	—	<1%	2 h (40 h)	Renal
Phensuximide	PO	8–12 h	—	—	—	—	4 h (8 h)	Renal
Miscellaneous								
Carbamazepine	PO	6–12 h	5–7 days	12–24 h	76%	3%	12–17 h	72% Renal/ 28% fecal
Valproic acid, divalproex	PO	8–12 h	Few days to > 1 wk	—	90%	2–7%	6–16 h	Renal
ANTIDEPRESSANTS								
Tricyclics								
Amitriptyline	PO	8–24 h	2 wk	—	94.8%	<2%	6–22 h (18–44 h)	Renal
Amoxapine	PO	24 h	<2 wk	—	90%	—	8 h (30 h)	Renal
Desipramine	PO	8–24 h	<2–3 wk	—	90%	3%	12–24 h	Renal
Doxepin	PO	8–24 h	2 wk	—	90%	0%	11–23 h (34–68 h)	Renal
Imipramine	PO	6–24 h	2 wk	—	94.8%	<2%	11–25 h (12–24 h)	Renal
	IM	6–24 h	—	—				
Nortriptyline	PO	8–24 h	2 wk	—	92%	2%	18–93 h	Renal
Protriptyline	PO	6–8 h	2 wk	—	92%	—	67–89 h	Renal
Trimipramine	PO	6–24 h	≥2 wk	1–2 days	>85%	<20%	9.1 h	Renal/fecal
Miscellaneous								
Maprotiline	PO	8–24 h	6–10 days	—	88%	0%	27–58 h	60% Renal/ 30% fecal
Trazodone	PO	6 h	1–4 wk	—	89–95%	<1%	5–9 h	70–75% Renal/20–25% biliary
ANTIFUNGAL AGENTS								
Amphotericin	IV	24 h	—	—	90%	—	24–48 h	30% Renal
Flucytosine	PO	6 h	1 h	—	10%	>95%	3–4 h	Renal
Griseofulvin	PO	6–24 h	4–8 h	1 day	—	<1%	9–24 h	Renal/fecal
Ketoconazole	PO	24 h	—	—	99%	<10%	2–8 h	Renal/fecal
Miconazole	IV	8 h	—	—	80–90%	<10%	4–24 h	Renal/fecal
Nystatin	PO	6–8 h	12–24 h	—	—	100%	—	Fecal
ANTIGOUT AGENTS								
Allopurinol	PO	24 h	2–3 days	24 h	0%	5–7%	1–2 h (15 h)	80% Renal/ 20% biliary
Colchicine	PO	1–24 h	—	—	31%	—	1 h	Renal/biliary
	IV	6–24 h	—	—				
Probenicid	PO	12 h	<30 min	—	83–95%	5%	2–11 h	Renal
Sulfinpyrazone	PO	12 h	—	4–6 h	98%	45%	1–9 h	Renal
ANTIHISTAMINES/ANTIPRURITICS								
Azatadine	PO	12 h	1–4 h	8–12 h	Minimal	20%	9–12 h	Renal
Brompheniramine	PO	4–6 h	1–5 h	4–48 h	—	5–10%	11.8–34.7 h	Renal
	PO*	8–12 h	—	—				
Chlorpheniramine	PO	4–6 h	30 min–1 h	4–24 h	69–72%	3–7%	12–43 h	Renal
	PO*	12 h	—	—				
Clemastine	PO	8–24 h	2–4 h	10–24 h	—	—	—	Renal

*Sustained, controlled, or extended-release form

continued

PHARMACOKINETICS

Drug	Route	Dosing interval	Onset of action	Duration of action	Protein binding	Excreted unchanged	Elimination half-life	Route of elimination
Cyproheptadine	PO	8 h	30 min–1 h	8–12 h	—	0%	—	65–75% Renal/25–35% fecal
Dexchlorpheniramine	PO PO*	4–6 h 8–12 h	30 min–1 h —	4–24 h —	69–72%	3–7%	12–43 h	Renal
Diphenhydramine	PO IM IV	4–6 h — —	<1 h — —	4–6 h — —	82%	1%	2.4–7 h	Renal
Hydroxyzine	PO	6 h	15–30 min	4–6 h	—	<1%	3 h	Biliary
Promethazine	PO IM IV	4–6 h — —	20 min — 3–5 min	4–12 h — —	—	<10%	—	Renal/fecal
Terfenadine	PO	12 h	1–2 h	>12 h	97%	0%	16–23 h	60% Biliary/40% renal
Trimeprazine	PO PO*	6 h 12 h	1 h 1 h	6–12 h 12 h	—	—	—	—
Tripelennamine	PO	4–12 h	30 min–1 h	4–6 h	—	<10%	—	Renal

ANTIHYPERTENSIVE AGENTS

ACE Inhibitors

Drug	Route	Dosing interval	Onset of action	Duration of action	Protein binding	Excreted unchanged	Elimination half-life	Route of elimination
Captopril	PO	8–12 h	<15 min	2–6 h	25–30%	38%	1.9 h	Renal
Enalapril	PO	12–24 h	1 h	24 h	—	—	11 h	Renal

Beta Blockers

Drug	Route	Dosing interval	Onset of action	Duration of action	Protein binding	Excreted unchanged	Elimination half-life	Route of elimination
Acebutolol	PO	12–24 h	1.5 h	—	26%	40%	3–4 h (8–13 h)	30–40% Renal/50–60% fecal
Atenolol	PO	24 h	1 h	24 h	10%	85%	6–7 h	Renal
Metoprolol	PO	8 h	12 h	—	10%	<5%	3–7 h	Renal
Nadolol	PO	24 h	—	24 h	25%	70%	20–24 h	Renal
Pindolol	PO	12 h	1–2 h	24 h	55%	40%	3–4 h	Renal
Propranolol	PO PO*	12 h 24 h	1–1.5 h —	— —	90%	1%	4 h	Renal
Timolol	PO	12 h	Few days	—	10–60%	20%	4 h	Renal

Calcium Antagonists

Drug	Route	Dosing interval	Onset of action	Duration of action	Protein binding	Excreted unchanged	Elimination half-life	Route of elimination
Verapamil	PO PO*	6–8 h 12–24 h	1–2 h 1–2 h	6–8 h 12–24 h	90%	<3%	2.8–12 h	70% Renal/16% biliary

Central Alpha-Adrenergic Agonists

Drug	Route	Dosing interval	Onset of action	Duration of action	Protein binding	Excreted unchanged	Elimination half-life	Route of elimination
Clonidine	PO Patch	8–12 h 7 days	30 min–1 h 2–3 days	6–8 h 7 days	—	32%	7–20 h	65% Renal/20% biliary
Guanabenz	PO	12 h	<1 h	6–8 h	90%	<1%	6 h	Renal
Guanfacine	PO	24 h	2 h	24–36 h	70%	50%	10–30 h	Renal
Methyldopa	PO IV	6–12 h 6 h	<4–6 h 3–5 h	— 6–12 h	1–16%	28%	2 h	Renal

Peripheral Vasodilators

Drug	Route	Dosing interval	Onset of action	Duration of action	Protein binding	Excreted unchanged	Elimination half-life	Route of elimination
Diazoxide	IV	4–24 h	2 min	<12 h	>90%	20%	20–36 h	Renal
Hydralazine	PO IM IV	6 h — —	1 h 20–40 min 10–20 min	2–30 h 3–8 h 3–8 h	90%	<10%	2–8 h	Renal
Minoxidil	PO	12–24 h	30 min	2–5 days	0%	10%	2.8–4.2 h	Renal
Nitroprusside	IV	—	30–60 s	3–5 min	—	<1%	2–7 days	Renal
Prazosin	PO	8–12 h	1.5 h	<24 h	95%	4%	2–3 h	>90% Biliary/<10% renal

Sympatholytics

Drug	Route	Dosing interval	Onset of action	Duration of action	Protein binding	Excreted unchanged	Elimination half-life	Route of elimination
Guanadrel	PO	6–12 h	30 min–2 h	4–14 h	20%	40–50%	10 h	Renal
Guanethidine	PO	24 h	1–3 wk	—	—	—	4–8 days	Renal
Reserpine	PO IM	24 h 3 h	<2–3 wk 2 h	6–24 h —	96%	—	11.3 h	Renal/fecal
Trimethaphan	IV	—	Immed	<10 min	—	—	—	Renal

Miscellaneous

Drug	Route	Dosing interval	Onset of action	Duration of action	Protein binding	Excreted unchanged	Elimination half-life	Route of elimination
Indapamide	PO	24 h	—	—	71–79%	7%	14 h	70% Renal/23% biliary
Labetalol	PO IV	12 h 10 min	2–4 h 5 min	8–12 h 2–4 h	50%	<5%	6–8 h 5.5 h	55–60% Renal/30% biliary

*Sustained, controlled, or extended-release form

PHARMACOKINETICS

Drug	Route	Dosing interval	Onset of action	Duration of action	Protein binding	Excreted unchanged	Elimination half-life	Route of elimination
ANTIMANIC AGENTS								
Lithium	PO	6–8 h	5–7 days	—	0%	95%	14–30 h	Renal
ANTIMIGRAINE AGENTS								
Ergotamine	PO, SL	0.5 h	5 h	—	—	<10%	21 h	Fecal
	Inhal	5 min	—					
Dihydroergotamine	IM	1 h	15–30 min	3–4 h	90%	<10%	21–32 h	90% Biliary/ 10% renal
	IV	1 h	5–10 min					
Methysergide	PO	24 h	1–2 days	1–2 days	—	56%	10 h	Renal
Propranolol	PO	12 h	—	—	90%	1%	4 h	Renal
	PO*	24 h	—	—				
ANTINAUSEANTS/ANTIEMETICS								
Dimenhydrinate	PO	4–6 h	15–30 min	3–6 h	—	2–5%	4 h	Renal
	IM	4 h	20–30 min	—				
	IV	4 h	Immediate					
Hydroxyzine	IM	—	—	—	—	<1%	3 h	Biliary
Meclizine	PO	24 h	1 h	8–24 h	—	0–5%	6 h	Renal
Metoclopramide	IV	2–3 h	1–3 min	1–2 h	13–22%	Up to 25%	5–6 h	80% Renal
Prochlorperazine	PO	6–8 h	30–40 min	3–4 h	80–90%	—	—	Renal/fecal
	PO*	12–24 h	30–40 min	10–12 h				
	Rectal	12 h	60 min	—				
	IM	3–4 h	10–20 min	3–4 h				
Promethazine	PO	4–6 h	20 min	4–12 h	—	<10%	—	Renal/fecal
	IM	4 h	—	—				
	IV	4 h	3–5 min	—				
Scopolamine	Patch	72 h	4 h	up to 72 h	—	4–5%	—	Renal
Thiethylperazine	PO	8–24 h	30 min	4 h	High	0%	20–40% h	Renal/biliary
Trimethobenzamide	PO	6–8 h	10–40 min	3–4 h	—	30–50%	—	Renal/biliary
	IM	6–8 h	15–35 min	2–3 h				
ANTIPSYCHOTIC AGENTS								
Phenothiazines								
Chlorpromazine	PO	6–8 h	30 min–1 h	4–6 h	95–98%	<1%	23–37 h	Renal/fecal
	PO*	12–24 h	30 min–1 h	10–12 h				
	IM	3–4 h	—	—				
Fluphenazine decanoate	SC, IM	4–6 wk	24–72 h	1–6 wk	>80%	—	6.8–9.6 days	Renal/fecal
Fluphenazine enanthate	SC, IM	1–3 wk	24–72 h	—	>80%	—	3.6–3.7 days	Renal/fecal
Fluphenazine hydrochloride	PO	6–8 h	1 h	1 h	>80%	—	14.7–15.3 h	Renal/fecal
	IM	6–8 h	1 h	6–8 h				
Mesoridazine	PO	8 h	—	—	High	—	24–84 h	Renal/fecal
	IM	—	—	—				
Perphenazine	PO	6–12 h	—	—	High	—	—	Renal/fecal
	PO*	12 h	—	—				
	IM	6 h	—	—				
Thioridazine	PO	6–12 h	—	—	>80%	—	—	Renal/fecal
Trifluoperazine	PO	12 h	2–3 wk	—	>80%	—	—	Renal/fecal
	IM	4–6 h	—	—				
Miscellaneous								
Chlorprothixene	PO	6–8 h	—	—	—	—	—	Renal/fecal
	IM	6–8 h	10–30 min	—				
Haloperidol	PO	8–12 h	—	—	92%	<5%	11.5–24.3 h	Renal/fecal
	IM	1–8 h	<30–45 min	—				
Haloperidol decanoate	IM	—	6–7 days	—	92%	<5%	3 wk	Renal/fecal
Loxapine	PO	6–12 h	20–30 min	12 h	—	<10%	19 h	Renal/fecal
	IM	4–12 h						
Molindone	PO	6–8 h	—	24–36 h	—	<2–3%	1.5 h	Renal/fecal
Thiothixene	PO	8–12 h	Few days to several wk	—	—	—	—	Biliary
	IM	6–12 h	1–6 h	—				
ANTIULCER/ANTIREFLUX AGENTS								
Cimetidine	PO	24 h	45–90 min	4–5 h	13–25%	77%	2 h	Renal
	IM	6 h	—	—				
	IV	6 h	—	—				
Famotidine	PO	12–24 h	<1 h	10–12 h	15–20%	25–30%	2.5–3.5 h	Renal/fecal
	IV	12 h	<30 min	10–12 h		65–70%		

*Sustained, controlled, or extended-release form

continued

PHARMACOKINETICS

Drug	Route	Dosing interval	Onset of action	Duration of action	Protein binding	Excreted unchanged	Elimination half-life	Route of elimination
Metoclopramide	PO	6 h	30–60 min	1–2 h	13–22%	Up to 25%	5–6 h	80% Renal
	IM	6 h	10–15 min	1–2 h				
	IV	6 h	1–3 min	1–2 h				
Ranitidine	PO	12 h	1–3 h	8–12 h	15%	30%	2–3 h	Renal
	IM	6–8 h	—	—		—		
	IV	6–8 h	15 min	—		70%		

ANTIVIRAL AGENTS

Drug	Route	Dosing interval	Onset of action	Duration of action	Protein binding	Excreted unchanged	Elimination half-life	Route of elimination
Acyclovir	PO	4 h	2 h	5–6 h	15%	95%	2.5–3.5 h	Renal
	IV	8 h	—	—				
Amantadine	PO	12–24 h	1–4 h	—	—	>90%	9–37 h	Renal
Vidarabine	IV	—	<5 days	—	20–30%	1–3%	1.5 (3.3 h)	Renal

BRONCHODILATORS/ANTIASTHMATIC AGENTS

Drug	Route	Dosing interval	Onset of action	Duration of action	Protein binding	Excreted unchanged	Elimination half-life	Route of elimination
Albuterol	Inhal	4–6 h	<15 min	3–4 h	—	28%	3.8 h	Renal
	PO	6–8 h	<30 min	4–6 h		30%	5 h	
Bitolterol	Inhal	4–8 h	3–4 min	5–8 h	—	0%	3 h	Renal
Cromolyn	Inhal	6 h	1 min	>5 h	—	100%	81 min	50% Renal/ 50% biliary
Ipratropium	Inhal	6 h	<15 min	3–6 h	—	>80%	2 h	Fecal
Isoetharine	Inhal	4 h	<5–15 min	1–4 h	—	10%	—	Renal
Isoproterenol	Inhal	3–4 h	Immediate	30–60 min	—	5–15%	—	Renal/fecal
Metaproterenol	Inhal	4–8 h	1–30 min	1–6 h	—	<10%	—	Renal/fecal
	PO	6–8 h	15 min	4 h				
Terbutaline	Inhal	4–6 h	5–30 min	3–4 h	—	60%	—	Renal
	PO	6 h	1–2 h	4–8 h				
	SC	—	15 min	1.5–4 h				
Theophylline	PO	6–8 h	<1–2 h	4–6 h	56%	13%	6.9–11.1 h	Renal
	PO*	8–12 h	<4 h	8–12 h				
	IV	—	15 min	—				

DIURETICS

Loop

Drug	Route	Dosing interval	Onset of action	Duration of action	Protein binding	Excreted unchanged	Elimination half-life	Route of elimination
Bumetanide	PO	24 h	30–60 min	4 h	94–96%	45%	1–1.5 h	80% Renal/ 20% fecal
	IM	24 h	40 min	5–6 h			1–1.5 h	
	IV	24 h	Few minutes	2–3 h			3.1–3.4 h	
Ethacrynic acid	PO	12–24 h	30 min	6–8 h	—	30–40%	—	Biliary/renal
	IV	24 h	5 min	2 h				
Furosemide	PO	12–24 h	<1 h	6–8 h	91–98%	66%	50 min	Renal
	IM	12–24 h	—	—				
	IV	12–24 h	<5 min	2 h				

Potassium-sparing

Drug	Route	Dosing interval	Onset of action	Duration of action	Protein binding	Excreted unchanged	Elimination half-life	Route of elimination
Amiloride	PO	24 h	<2 h	24 h	—	50%	6–9 h	50% Renal/ 40% fecal
Spironolactone	PO	24 h	2 days	2–3 days	90%	<10%	9–26 h	Renal
Triamterene	PO	12 h	2–4 h	7–9 h	43–53%	21%	2–4 h	Renal/biliary

Thiazides

Drug	Route	Dosing interval	Onset of action	Duration of action	Protein binding	Excreted unchanged	Elimination half-life	Route of elimination
Bendroflumethiazide	PO	12–24 h	<2 h	18–24 h	—	0%	—	Renal
Benzthiazide	PO	12–24 h	<2 h	12–18 h	—	0%	—	Renal
Chlorothiazide	PO	12–24 h	<2 h	6–12 h	94.6%	92%	1.3–1.7 h	Renal
	IV	12–24 h	<15 min	2 h				
Chlorthalidone	PO	24 h	2 h	48–72 h	75%	65%	35–54 h	Renal
Hydrochlorothiazide	PO	24 h	<2 h	6–12 h	40–64%	>95%	6–15 h	Renal
Hydroflumethiazide	PO	12–24 h	<2 h	10–12 h	—	0%	17 h	Renal
Metolazone	PO	24 h	<1 h	12–24 h	33%	70–95%	5.3 h	Renal
Methyclothiazide	PO	24 h	<2 h	24 h	—	0%	—	Renal
Polythiazide	PO	24 h	2 h	24–36 h	—	60%	—	Renal/fecal
Quinethazone	PO	24 h	<2 h	18–24 h	—	—	—	—
Trichlormethiazide	PO	24 h	<2 h	24 h	—	<10%	—	Renal

GOLD COMPOUNDS

Drug	Route	Dosing interval	Onset of action	Duration of action	Protein binding	Excreted unchanged	Elimination half-life	Route of elimination
Auranofin	PO	24 h	3–4 mo	—	60%	100%	17–26 days	60% Fecal/ 40% renal
Aurothioglucose	IM	1 wk	6–8 wk	—	95%	100%	6 days	70% Renal/ 30% fecal
Gold sodium thiomalate	IM	1–4 wk	6–8 wk	—	95%	100%	5–6 days	70% Renal/ 30% fecal

*Sustained, controlled, or extended-release form

PHARMACOKINETICS

Drug	Route	Dosing interval	Onset of action	Duration of action	Protein binding	Excreted unchanged	Elimination half-life	Route of elimination
HYPOGLYCEMIC AGENTS								
Insulins								
Extended insulin zinc	SC	24 h	4–8 h	>36 h	—	<2%	—	Renal
Insulin zinc	SC	12–24 h	1–2.5 h	24 h	—	<2%	—	Renal
Isophane insulin (NPH)	SC	12–24 h	1–1.5 h	24 h	—	<2%	—	Renal
70% Isophane insulin and 30% regular insulin	SC	24 h	30 min	24 h	—	<2%	—	Renal
Prompt insulin zinc	SC	8–24 h	30 min–1 h	6–8 h	—	<2%	—	Renal
Protamine zinc insulin	SC	24 h	4–8 h	36 h	—	<2%	—	Renal
Regular insulin	SC	6–8 h	30 min–1 h	6–8 h	—	<2%	—	Renal
Sulfonylureas								
Acetohexamide	PO	12–24 h	<3 h	12–24 h	>80%	40%	2–5 h	Renal
Chlorpropamide	PO	24 h	<1 h	24–72 h	87%	20%	36 h	Renal
Glipizide	PO	24 h	<30 min	6–12 h	98–99%	<10%	2–4 h	Renal
Glyburide	PO	12–24 h	15–60 min	24 h	>99%	0%	10 h	50% Renal/ 50% biliary
Tolazamide	PO	12–24 h	20–60 min	14–16 h	>80%	<10%	7 h	Renal
Tolbutamide	PO	8–24 h	<1 h	6–12 h	95%	0%	4.5–6.5 h	Renal/fecal
HYPOLIPIDEMIC AGENTS								
Clofibrate	PO	6–12 h	2–6 h	6 h	96.5%	10–20%	6–25 h	Renal
Dextrothyroxine	PO	24 h	—	—	99%	—	18 h	Renal/fecal
Gemfibrozil	PO	12 h	1–2 h	3 h	95%	70%	1.3–1.5 h	70% Renal/ 6% fecal
Probucol	PO	12 h	2–4 wk	—	—	—	20 days	Fecal
INOTROPIC AGENTS								
Amrinone	IV	—	2–5 min	30 min–2 h	10–49%	51%	3.6 h	Renal
Digoxin	PO	6–8 h	30 min–2 h	3–4 days	20–25%	50–70%	1.5–2 days	Renal
	IV	4–8 h	5–30 min	—				
MUSCLE RELAXANTS								
Baclofen	PO	8 h	Hours to weeks	8 h	30%	85%	2.5–4 h	70–80% Renal/ 20–30% fecal
Carisoprodol	PO	8 h	<30 min	4–6 h	—	Trace	8 h	Renal
Chlorphenesin	PO	8 h	1–3 h	6–12 h	—	0%	2.3–5.1 h	Renal
Chlorzoxazone	PO	6–8 h	1 h	3–4 h	—	0%	1 h	Renal
Cyclobenzaprine	PO	8 h	1 h	12–24 h	93%	0%	1–3 days	Renal
Dantrolene	PO	6–12 h	1 wk	—	High	5%	8.7 h	Renal
	IV	6–8 h	Immediate	—				
Diazepam	PO	6–12 h	15–45 min	—	97–99%	<1%	30–56 h (3–21 h; 30–200 h)	Renal
	IM	3–4 h	15–30 min	—				
	IV	3–4 h	1–5 min	15–60 min				
Metaxalone	PO	6–8 h	<1 h	4–6 h	—	0%	2–3 h	Renal
Methocarbamol	PO	6–8 h	<30 min	6–8 h	—	0–5%	0.9–2.2 h	Renal/fecal
	IM	8 h	<30 min	—				
	IV	8 h	Immediate	—				
Orphenadrine	PO	12 h	1 h	4–6 h	—	5%	14 h	Renal
	IM, IV	12 h	—	—				
Quinine	PO	24 h	1–3 h	8–24 h	70%	5%	4–21 h	Renal
NARCOTIC ANALGESICS								
Buprenorphine	IM	6 h	15 min	1–6 h	96%	<20%	1.2–7.2 h	Renal
	IV	6 h	<15 min	<6 h				
Butorphanol	IM	3–4 h	<10 min	3–4 h	80%	<5%	3–4 h	60–80% Renal/ 11–14% fecal
	IV	3–4 h	1 min	2–4 h				
Codeine	PO	4–6 h	15–30 min	4–6 h	<50%	7%	2.5–4 h	Renal
	IM, SC	4–6 h	15–30 min	4–6 h				
Fentanyl	IM	1–2 h	7–8 min	1–2 h	80%	<10%	3.6 h	75% Renal/ 9% fecal
	IV	1–2 h	1–2 min	30 min–1 h				
Hydrocodone	PO	4–6 h	10–30 min	4–6 h	—	—	3.8 h	Renal
Hydromorphone	PO	4–6 h	30 min	4–5 h	—	<10%	1.8–3.5 h	Renal
	IM, SC	4–6 h	15–30 min	4–5 h				
	IV	—	<15 min	4–5 h				

continued

PHARMACOKINETICS

Drug	Route	Dosing interval	Onset of action	Duration of action	Protein binding	Excreted unchanged	Elimination half-life	Route of elimination
Levorphanol	PO	6–8 h	10–60 min	6–8 h	—	<10%	11 h	Renal
	SC	6–8 h	60–90 min	6–8 h				
	IV	6–8 h	20 min	6–8 h				
Meperidine	PO	3–4 h	15 min	2–4 h	60%	1–25%	2.4–4 h	Renal
	IM, SC	3–4 h	10–15 min	2–4 h				
	IV	—	1 min	2–4 h				
Methadone	PO	3–4 h	30–60 min	4–6 h	90%	<10%	13–47 h	Renal/fecal
	IM, SC	3–4 h	10–20 min	4–6 h				
Morphine	PO	4 h	<60 min	4–5 h	33%	6–10%	1.5–2 h	85–90% Renal/ 7–10% fecal
	PO*	8–12 h	<60 min	8–12 h				
	SC	4 h	<50–90 min	4–5 h				
	IM	4 h	<30–60 min	4–5 h				
	IV	—	<20 min	4–5 h				
	Rectal	4 h	<20–60 min	4–5 h				
Nalbuphine	IM, SC	3–6 h	<15 min	3–6 h	<60%	7%	5 h	Biliary/renal
	IV	3–6 h	2–3 min	3–6 h				
Oxycodone	PO	6 h	10–15 min	3–6 h	—	—	2–3 h	Renal
Oxymorphone	IM, SC	4–6 h	10–15 min	3–6 h	—	<10%	—	Renal
	IV	4–6 h	5–10 min	3–6 h				
	Rectal	4–6 h	15–30 min	3–6 h				
Pentazocine	PO	4 h	15–30 min	3–4 h	60%	<13%	2–3 h	Renal
	IM, SC	3–4 h	15–20 min	2 h				
	IV	3–4 h	2–3 min	1 h				
Propoxyphene	PO	4 h	15–60 min	4–6 h	—	25%	6–12 h	Renal

NONNARCOTIC ANALGESICS/NONSTEROIDAL ANTI-INFLAMMATORY AGENTS

Drug	Route	Dosing interval	Onset of action	Duration of action	Protein binding	Excreted unchanged	Elimination half-life	Route of elimination
Acetaminophen	PO	4–6 h	10–60 min	4–6 h	<50%	3%	1.6–2.4 h	Renal
Diflunisal	PO	8–12 h	1 h	8–12 h	>99%	10%	8–12 h	Renal
Fenoprofen	PO	6–8 h	15–30 min	4–6 h	99%	10%	3 h	Renal
Ibuprofen	PO	4–6 h	30 min	4–6 h	90–99%	<10%	1.8–2 h	Renal
Indomethacin	PO	8–12 h	7–14 days	—	90%	30%	4.5 h	60% Renal/ 33% fecal
Ketoprofen	PO	6–8 h	—	—	99%	—	2–4 h	60% Renal/ 40% fecal
Meclofenamate	PO	6–8 h	—	—	99.8%	<5%	3.3 h	66% Renal/ 33% fecal
Mefenamic acid	PO	6 h	—	—	>80%	67%	2 h	67% Renal/ 20–25% fecal
Naproxen	PO	12 h	2 h	<7 h	>99%	<1%	13 h	Renal
Naproxen sodium	PO	6–8 h	1 h	<7 h	>99%	<1%	13 h	Renal
Phenylbutazone	PO	6–8 h	3–4 days	—	98%	1%	54–99 h	61% Renal/ 27% fecal
Piroxicam	PO	24 h	—	—	99.3%	<5%	30–86 h	66% Renal/ 33% fecal
Salicylates	PO	4 h	<30 min	3–6 h	75–90%	2–80%	2–19 h	Renal
Sulindac	PO	12 h	—	—	93%	—	16.4 h	50% Renal/ 25% fecal
Suprofen	PO	4–6 h	1–2 h	4–6 h	>99%	<15%	2–4 h	85–95% Renal/5–10% fecal
Tolmetin	PO	6–8 h	—	—	99%	20%	5 h	Renal

SEDATIVES/HYPNOTICS

Barbiturates

Drug	Route	Dosing interval	Onset of action	Duration of action	Protein binding	Excreted unchanged	Elimination half-life	Route of elimination
Amobarbital	PO	6–12 h	10–30 min	3–11 h	—	<1%	20–25 h	Renal
Aprobarbital	PO	8 h	20–60 min	6–8 h	20%	25–50%	14–40 h	Renal
Butabarbital	PO	6–8 h	10–30 min	6–8 h	—	1–2%	34–42 h	Renal
Mephobarbital	PO	6–8 h	20–60 min	10–16 h	—	—	11–67 h (81–117 h)	Renal
Pentobarbital	PO	6–8 h	15–60 min	1–4 h	35–45%	<1%	35–50 h	Renal
	IM	—	10–25 min	—				
	IV	—	1 min	15 min				
Phenobarbital	PO	8–12 h	1 h	10–12 h	20–45%	24%	81–117 h	Renal
	IM	8–12 h	—	—				
	IV	8–12 h	5 min	4–6 h				
Secobarbital	PO	24 h	<15 min	1–4 h	30–45%	5%	30 h	Renal
	IM	—	<7–10 min	—				
	IV	—	<1–3 min	15 min				

*Sustained, controlled, or extended-release form

PHARMACOKINETICS

Drug	Route	Dosing interval	Onset of action	Duration of action	Protein binding	Excreted unchanged	Elimination half-life	Route of elimination
Benzodiazepines								
Flurazepam	PO	24 h	15–45 min	7–8 h	96.6%	<1%	2–3 h (47–100 h)	Renal
Midazolam	IM	4–6 h	15 min	Several hours	97%	<1%	1.2–12.3 h	Renal
	IV	4–6 h	3–5 min					
Temazepam	PO	24 h	1–3 h	10 h	96%	10%	9.5–12.4 h	90% Renal
Triazolam	PO	24 h	—	—	47–85%	2%	1.6–5.4 h	Renal
Miscellaneous								
Chloral hydrate	PO	8–24 h	30–60 min	4–8 h	—	0%	8–11 h	Renal/biliary
Ethchlorvynol	PO	24 h	15–60 min	5 h	—	10%	10–20 h	Renal
Ethinamate	PO	24 h	20 min	3–8 h	—	0%	2.5 h	Renal
Glutethimide	PO	24 h	<30 min	4–8 h	50%	<2%	10–12 h	Renal
Methyprylon	PO	24 h	<45 min	5–8 h	40–60%	1–3%	4 h	Renal
THYROID HORMONES								
Liothyronine	PO	24 h	12–36 h	3–5 days	99%	0%	1–2 days	Renal/biliary
Thyroxine	PO	24 h	3–5 days	7–10 days	99%	Some	6–7 days	Renal/biliary

Pharmacokinetic Data for Drug Monitoring

Ray R. Maddox, PharmD
Victor Lampasona, PharmD

Emory University Hospital, Atlanta, GA

This section provides pharmacologic and pharmacokinetic information on a select group of drugs for which there is a clear relationship between serum concentration and clinical response; it does not include every drug for which pharmacokinetic data exist. The tables are intended for use by clinicians and other health-care professionals who already have some knowledge of clinical pharmacokinetics, enabling them to make informed decisions when designing and manipulating drug dosage schedules for individual patients.

Many factors influence serum drug concentrations and the response of patients to drug therapy. These factors include the concomitant use of other drugs, the presence of coexisting disease states, and genetic and environmental influences. They increase the complexity of prescribing and dispensing drugs and, if not taken into account, introduce errors in fixed dosage regimens. Often, the patient's clinical condition and metabolic functions may change quickly, necessitating a continual reappraisal of drug dosage to ensure safe and effective therapy. For these patients in particular, frequent monitoring of serum drug levels, coupled with close clinical observation, offers an ideal approach to dosage adjustment.

The data in the tables were accumulated from various published sources and do not necessarily coincide with package insert data. The pharmacokinetic values listed are averages observed in normal, healthy individuals, unless indicated otherwise. The half-life ($t_{1/2}$) and elimination rate constant (K_e) values are for the terminal elimination phase, or β-phase (ie, after distribution of the drug). Except for aspirin, heparin, and phenytoin, a linear elimination process is assumed; ie, serum drug concentrations can be expected to change in direct proportion to the dose. Most dosages are expressed in terms of kilograms of *total* body weight, except where noted. These dosages should be considered as rough guidelines; for more complete information, consult the appropriate full drug chart.

Abbreviations

H	Hemodialysis	ACT	Activated Clotting Time
P	Peritoneal dialysis	APTT	Activated Partial Thromboplastin Time
		WBAPTT	Whole Blood Activated Partial Thromboplastin Time
EMIT	Enzyme Multiplied Immunoassay Technique		
FPI	Fluorescence Polarization Immunoassay	WBCT	Whole Blood Clotting Time
HPLC	High Performance Liquid Chromatography		
RIA	Radioimmunoassay	n/a	Not available

PHARMACOKINETICS

Amikacin

Oral bioavailability (%)	Serum protein binding (%)	Renal excretion (% unchanged)	Active metabolites	V_d (liters/kg)	$t_{1/2}$ (h)	K_e (h^{-1})
—	< 10	> 95	None known	**Adult:** 0.25 (0.17–0.45) **Child:** 0.45 (0.25–0.70) **Neonate:** 0.70 0.45–0.90)	**Adult:** 2.0 (0.5–3.0) **Child:** 1.3 (0.5–2.0) **Neonate:** 7.0 (2.0–9.0)	**Adult:** 0.3465 **Child:** 0.5330 **Neonate:** 0.0990

Clinical considerations: obesity, extensive burns, ascites, cystic fibrosis: ⇧ V_d; renal impairment: ⇧ $t_{1/2}$ ⇩ K_e

Distribution in body	Time to reach steady state (h)	Sampling times for measurement of serum drug concentrations	Assay methods used	Therapeutic range (μg/ml)	Toxic serum level (μg/ml)
Extracellular fluid, renal cortex; crosses placenta	9 (6–18)	**Peak:** 60 min after IM injection; 15–30 min after 30-min IV infusion; 15 min after 60-min IV infusion **Trough:** immediately before the next dose	RIA, EMIT, FPI	**Peak:** 20.0–30.0 **Trough:** < 10.0	**Peak:** > 35.0 **Trough:** > 10.0

Clinical considerations: sustained trough levels > 10.0 μg/ml are associated with nephrotoxicity; sustained peak levels > 35.0 μg/ml may be associated with ototoxicity

Usual route of administration	Initial loading dose (mg/kg)	Maintenance dosage (mg/kg/day)	Usual dosing interval (h)	Adjustment for hepatic failure	Adjustment for renal failure	Removed by dialysis
IM, intermittent IV infusion	**Adult:** 7.5 **Child:** 7.5 **Neonate:** 10.0	**Adult:** 10.0–15.0 **Child:** 10.0–15.0 **Neonate:** 10.0–15.0	**Adult:** 6–8 **Child:** 6–8 **Neonate:** 12–24	None	Reduce dosage; see Sarubbi FA, Hull JH: *Ann Intern Med* 89:612–618, 1978	Yes: H, P

Clinical considerations: not absorbed by adipose tissue; use ideal (lean) body weight to calculate dosage and V_d

Amitriptyline

Oral bioavailability (%)	Serum protein binding (%)	Renal excretion (% unchanged)	Active metabolites	V_d (liters/kg)	$t_{1/2}$ (h)	K_e (h^{-1})
60–70	> 95	< 10	Nortriptyline, 10-hydroxy-nortriptyline	**Adult:** 8.3 (6–36)	**Adult:** 17 (9–46)	**Adult:** 0.0408

Clinical considerations: protein binding exhibits significant interindividual variation and may be altered by malignancy and hepatic or renal disease

Distribution in body	Time to reach steady state (h)	Sampling times for measurement of serum drug concentrations	Assay methods used	Therapeutic range (ng/ml)[1]	Toxic serum level (ng/ml)
Most tissues, erythrocytes	100	Immediately before the next dose	HPLC, FPI[2]	80–200	≥ 1,000

Clinical considerations: concentration-response relationship is not as well defined as with some other drugs; consequently, use clinical response as the major determinant of drug dosage

Usual route of administration	Initial loading dose (mg)	Maintenance dosage (mg/day)	Usual dosing interval (h)	Adjustment for hepatic failure	Adjustment for renal failure	Removed by dialysis
Oral	**Adult:** 75–150	**Adult:** 50–100	8–12	Dosage reduction may be necessary, depending on clinical response	None	No

Clinical considerations: adolescent and elderly patients may respond to lower doses

[1] Range includes parent drug concentration plus the concentration of the hydroxy metabolite
[2] FPI is not specific for individual agents

continued

PHARMACOKINETICS

Aspirin[1]

Oral bioavailability (%)	Serum protein binding (%)	Renal excretion (% unchanged)	Active metabolites	V_d (liters/kg)	$t_{1/2}$ (h)	K_e (h^{-1})
85–95	75–90	2–80	Several metabolites with unknown activity	Adult: 0.15–0.20 Child: 0.16–0.35	Adult: 2–19 Child: 2–19	See clinical considerations

Clinical considerations: all pharmacokinetic parameters are dose dependent (⇧ dose: ⇩ protein binding ⇩ renal excretion ⇧ V_d ⇧ $t_{1/2}$ ⇩ K_e); ⇧ urine pH: ⇧ renal excretion

Distribution in body	Time to reach steady state (h)	Sampling times for measurement of serum drug concentrations	Assay methods used	Therapeutic range (μg/ml)	Toxic serum level (μg/ml)
Most tissues and transcellular fluids, including synovial, spinal, and peritoneal fluids; crosses placenta readily	10–105	Peak: 1–2 h after the last dose Trough: immediately before the next dose	Colorimetric, fluorometric, FPI	Analgesia: 0–100 Anti-inflammatory: 150–300 Rheumatic fever: 250–400	> 200

Clinical considerations: time to reach steady-state serum levels is dose dependent

Usual route of administration	Initial loading dose (mg/kg)	Maintenance dosage (mg/kg/day)	Usual dosing interval (h)	Adjustment for hepatic failure	Adjustment for renal failure	Removed by dialysis
Oral	—	Adult: 45–60 Child: 45–60	4	Dosage reduction probably necessary, depending on serum level	Increase dosing interval to 6–8 h	Yes: H, P

Clinical considerations: dosages given here should produce anti-inflammatory serum levels of salicylic acid and may be adjusted on the basis of the actual serum levels obtained

[1] Values given in this table are for salicylic acid, to which aspirin is rapidly hydrolyzed

Carbamazepine

Oral bioavailability (%)	Serum protein binding (%)	Renal excretion (% unchanged)	Active metabolites	V_d (liters/kg)	$t_{1/2}$ (h)	K_e (h^{-1})
79 (fasting) to 95 (after meals)	75 (54–78)	< 5	Carbamazepine 10,11-epoxide (CBZ-E)	Adult: 1.2 (0.8–1.9) Child: 1.9 (1.2–2.5) Neonate: 1.5 (1.1–1.5)	Adult: 35[1] (21–60) Child: 10[2] (5–18) Neonate: 10[2] (8–28)	Adult: 0.0198[1] Child: 0.0693[2] Neonate: 0.0693[2]

Clinical considerations: concomitant anticonvulsant therapy will influence carbamazepine pharmacokinetics; pediatric patients may have increased free concentrations of carbamazepine; CBZ-E is 50% bound to serum protein, with a range of 25–59%

Distribution in body	Time to reach steady state (h)	Sampling times for measurement of serum drug concentrations	Assay methods used	Therapeutic range (μg/ml)	Toxic serum level (μg/ml)
Most tissues and fluids, including brain, liver, kidneys, salivary glands, and milk; crosses placenta	200 (60–360)[3]	Peak: 2–12 h after the last dose Trough: immediately before the next dose	Gas chromatography, EMIT, HPLC, FPI	5–10	> 16

Clinical considerations: because of the variation in time to peak concentration, trough levels are suggested for routine monitoring; some patients may exhibit side effects at serum levels < 16 μg/ml

COMPENDIUM OF DRUG THERAPY

PHARMACOKINETICS

Usual route of administration	Initial loading dose (mg/kg)	Maintenance dosage (mg/kg/day)	Usual dosing interval (h)	Adjustment for hepatic failure	Adjustment for renal failure	Removed by dialysis
Oral	Start with a low dose and titrate upward according to clinical response and patient tolerance	Adult: 12–16 Child: ≤ 25 (usually not to exceed 1 g/day)	8–12	Dosage reduction probably necessary, depending on serum level	None	Unknown

[1] Value obtained after a single dose; since carbamazepine exhibits autoinduction, expect $t_{1/2}$ to decline to about 10–20 h after about 2 wk of multiple dosing
[2] Value obtained after multiple dosing ($t_{1/2}$ after a single dose may be expected to be longer)
[3] Value based on experience with single doses; multiple dosing shortens the time to reach steady state

Chloramphenicol

Oral bioavailability (%)	Serum protein binding (%)	Renal excretion (% unchanged)	Active metabolites	V_d (liters/kg)	$t_{1/2}$ (h)	K_e (h^{-1})
100[1]	53	13.6 (2.1–56.3)	None known	Adult: 0.6 (0.4–1.0) Child: 1.4 (0.8–2.1) Neonate: 1.4 (0.8–2.1)	Adult: 5.1 (3.1–8.1) Child: 4.0 (2.1–8.3) Neonate: 10 to > 48	Adult: 0.14 (0.09–0.22) Child: 0.20 (0.08–0.33) Neonate: < 0.01 to 0.07

Clinical considerations: cirrhosis: ▽ protein binding; severe liver disease with jaundice: △ $t_{1/2}$ ▽ K_e

Distribution in body	Time to reach steady state (h)	Sampling times for measurement of serum drug concentrations	Assay methods used	Therapeutic range (μg/ml)	Toxic serum level (μg/ml)
Most body fluids and tissues, including brain	Adult: 17–45 Child: 12–46 Neonate: ≥ 55	Peak: 1½–2 h after completion of intermittent IV infusion Trough: immediately before the next dose	HPLC, microbiological	10–20	> 25

Clinical considerations: serum levels > 25 μg/ml are associated with an increased risk of hematological toxicity; serum levels > 50 μg/ml have been measured in premature infants and newborns with "gray syndrome"

Usual route of administration	Initial loading dose (mg/kg)	Maintenance dosage (mg/kg/day)	Usual dosing interval (h)	Adjustment for hepatic failure	Adjustment for renal failure	Removed by dialysis
Oral, IM, intermittent IV infusion	—	Adult: 50–100 Child: 50–75 Neonate: 25–50	Adult: 6 Child: 6–8 Neonate: 6–8	Reduce dosage, depending on serum level	Dosage reduction may be considered, depending on serum level	Yes: H

Clinical considerations: absorption following IM injection is poor; renal failure may result in the accumulation of metabolites or the parent drug

[1] Bioavailability of oral palmitate ester exceeds that of the parenteral succinate ester because a significant amount of the latter (~ 20%) is excreted unchanged in the urine

Desipramine

Oral bioavailability (%)	Serum protein binding (%)	Renal excretion (% unchanged)	Active metabolites	V_d (liters/kg)	$t_{1/2}$ (h)	K_e (h^{-1})
33–51	83 (73–92)	< 10	2-Hydroxy-desipramine	Adult: 34 (24–60)	Adult: 17 (12–28)	Adult: 0.0408

Clinical considerations: protein binding exhibits significant interindividual variation and may be altered by malignancy and hepatic or renal impairment

Distribution in body	Time to reach steady state (h)	Sampling times for measurement of serum drug concentrations	Assay methods used	Therapeutic range (ng/ml)	Toxic serum level (ng/ml)
Most tissues, erythrocytes	100	Immediately before the next dose	HPLC, FPI[1]	75–160	≥ 1,000

continued

PHARMACOKINETICS

Usual route of administration	Initial loading dose	Maintenance dosage (mg/day)	Usual dosing interval (h)	Adjustment for hepatic failure	Adjustment for renal failure	Removed by dialysis
Oral	Start low and titrate upward, depending on clinical response	**Adult:** 100–300	12–24	Dosage reduction may be necessary, depending on clinical response	None	No

Clinical considerations: adolescent and elderly patients may respond to lower doses and should not be given > 150 mg/day

[1] FPI is not specific for individual agents

Digitoxin

Oral bioavailability (%)	Serum protein binding (%)	Renal excretion (% unchanged)	Active metabolites	V_d (liters/kg)	$t_{1/2}$ (h)	K_e (h^{-1})
90–100	> 90	32 (26–48)	Digoxin	**Adult:** 0.60 (0.45–0.82)	**Adult:** 180 (60–390)[1]	**Adult:** 0.0039

Clinical considerations: nephrotic syndrome: ▽ protein binding △ V_d ▽ $t_{1/2}$ △ K_e; although digitoxin is metabolized by the liver, hepatic disease does not appreciably affect $t_{1/2}$

Distribution in body	Time to reach steady state (h)	Sampling times for measurement of serum drug concentrations	Assay methods used	Therapeutic range (ng/ml)	Toxic serum level (ng/ml)
Most body tissues, including erythrocytes, skeletal muscle, and heart; crosses placenta	540 (360–1,070)	**Peak:** ~ 6 h after the last dose **Trough:** immediately before the next dose	RIA, FPI	15–25[2]	> 40

Clinical considerations: because of the difficulty in obtaining appropriate blood samples for measuring peak serum levels, trough samples are suggested for routine monitoring

Usual route of administration	Initial loading dose	Maintenance dosage (mg/day)	Usual dosing interval (h)	Adjustment for hepatic failure	Adjustment for renal failure	Removed by dialysis
Oral, IM, IV bolus injection	See Crystodigin drug chart	**Adult:** 0.05–0.3 **Child:** 10% of loading dose	24	Reduce dosage depending on serum level	Reduce dosage if failure is severe; see Bennett WM, et al: *Am J Kidney Dis* 3:155-193, 1983	No

Clinical considerations: because of the long $t_{1/2}$ of this drug, a loading dose is essential (the dose should be divided and given over 1–2 days); concurrent treatment with quinidine may increase serum digitoxin levels, requiring a reduction in digitoxin dosage

[1] The wide variation in $t_{1/2}$ is due to interindividual differences in hepatic metabolism of this drug
[2] Concentrations > 25 µg/ml may be required for atrial fibrillation or flutter; dosage should be guided by clinical response

Digoxin

Oral bioavailability (%)	Serum protein binding (%)	Renal excretion (% unchanged)	Active metabolites	V_d (liters/kg)	$t_{1/2}$ (h)	K_e (h^{-1})
Capsules: 90–100 **Elixir:** 70–80 **Tablets:** 60–70	< 25	75–85	Digoxigenin monodigitoxiside, digoxigenin didigitoxiside	**Adult:** 6.5 (5.1–8.1) **Child:** 12.8 (9.7–16.3) **Neonate:** 11.0 (9.9–11.1)	**Adult:** 36 (26–44) **Child:** 24 (18–24) **Neonate:** 48 (35–69)	**Adult:** 0.019 **Child:** 0.029 **Neonate:** 0.014

Clinical considerations: renal impairment: ▽ renal excretion ▽ V_d △ $t_{1/2}$ ▽ K_e; concurrent treatment with quinidine or verapamil: ▽ V_d

PHARMACOKINETICS

Distribution in body	Time to reach steady state (h)	Sampling times for measurement of serum drug concentrations	Assay methods used	Therapeutic range (ng/ml)	Toxic serum level (ng/ml)
Most body tissues, including erythrocytes, skeletal muscle, and heart; crosses placenta	Adult: 143–242 Child: 99–132 Neonate: 193–380	Peak: 6–8 h after the last dose Trough: immediately before the next dose	RIA, FPI	Congestive heart failure: 0.9–2.0 Atrial flutter or fibrillation: > 2.0	> 2.0

Clinical considerations: serum levels > 1.5 ng/ml are associated with an increased incidence of side effects, but concentrations of serum electrolytes dramatically influence both the therapeutic effect and toxicity of digoxin

Usual route of administration	Initial loading dose (mg/kg)	Maintenance dosage (mg/kg/day)	Usual dosing interval (h)	Adjustment for hepatic failure	Adjustment for renal failure	Removed by dialysis
Oral, IV bolus injection	See Lanoxin drug chart	See Lanoxin drug chart	24	None	See Lanoxin drug chart	No

Clinical considerations: poorly distributed in adipose tissue; use ideal (lean) body weight to calculate dosage and V_d

Disopyramide

Oral bioavailability (%)	Serum protein binding (%)	Renal excretion (% unchanged)	Active metabolites	V_d (liters/kg)	$t_{1/2}$ (h)	K_e (h^{-1})
83 (60–91)	55–80[1]	40–60	Mono-N-dealkylated disopyramide	Adult: 0.80	Adult: 7 (4–10)	Adult: 0.099

Clinical considerations: acute myocardial infarction, renal impairment: ⇧ $t_{1/2}$ ⇩ K_e; ⇧ serum drug level; ⇩ protein binding

Distribution in body	Time to reach steady state (h)	Sampling times for measurement of serum drug concentrations	Assay methods used	Therapeutic range (µg/ml)	Toxic serum level (µg/ml)
Extracellular fluid, erythrocytes; may cross placenta	42 (24–60)	Peak: 2–3 h after administration of immediate-release preparation Trough: immediately before the next dose	EMIT, HPLC, FPI	2–4	> 5

Usual route of administration	Initial loading dose (mg)	Maintenance dosage (mg/day)	Usual dosing interval (h)	Adjustment for hepatic failure	Adjustment for renal failure	Removed by dialysis
Oral	Adult: 300	Adult: 600 (400–800)	Immediate-release preparation: 6 Controlled-release preparation: 12	Reduce dosage to 400 mg/day	Reduce dosage; see Bennett WM, et al: *Am J Kidney Dis* 3:155-193, 1983; if failure is severe, use only the immediate-release preparation	Yes: H

Clinical considerations: patients < 50 kg: limit maintenance dosage to 400 mg/day (with a loading dose of 200 mg, if needed); patients with cardiomyopathy or possible cardiac decompensation: omit loading dose and limit maintenance dosage to 400 mg/day

[1] Range observed at therapeutic serum levels

continued

PHARMACOKINETICS

Ethosuximide

Oral bioavail-ability (%)	Serum protein binding (%)	Renal excretion (% unchanged)	Active metabolites	V_d (liters/kg)	$t_{1/2}$ (h)	K_e (h^{-1})
Unknown, but presumed to be 100%	0	20	None known	Adult: 0.62 Child: 0.69 Neonate: n/a	Adult: 60 (50–60) Child: 30 (29–33) Neonate: 41[1]	Adult: 0.0116 Child: 0.0231 Neonate: 0.0169[1]

Clinical considerations: limited data suggest that serum concentrations of this drug may vary disproportionately with dosage in some patients

Distribution in body	Time to reach steady state (h)	Sampling times for measurement of serum drug concentrations	Assay methods used	Therapeutic range (µg/ml)	Toxic serum level (µg/ml)
Total body water, placenta, milk	Adult: 180[2] Child: 90[2]	Peak: 3–7 h after the last dose Trough: immediately before the next dose	Gas chromatography, EMIT, HPLC, FPI	40–80	> 80 to 100

Usual route of administration	Initial loading dose (mg/kg)	Maintenance dosage (mg/kg/day)	Usual dosing interval (h)	Adjustment for hepatic failure	Adjustment for renal failure	Removed by dialysis
Oral	—	Adult: 20 Child: 20	12–24	Dosage reduction may be necessary, depending on serum level	Reduce dosage if failure is severe; see Bennett WM, et al: *Am J Kidney Dis* 3:155-193, 1983	Yes: H

Clinical considerations: begin with low maintenance doses and increase the dosage as tolerated to achieve the desired clinical response and to attain therapeutic serum levels; some patients may require > 20 mg/kg/day

[1] Value based on a single case report of a child who was exposed to primidone and ethosuximide in utero
[2] Some variation may be expected due to the usual interindividual variability in $t_{1/2}$

Flucytosine

Oral bioavail-ability (%)	Serum protein binding (%)	Renal excretion (% unchanged)	Active metabolites	V_d (liters/kg)	$t_{1/2}$ (h)	K_e (h^{-1})
85	< 5	> 95	5-Fluorouracil	Adult: 0.6 (0.5–0.8)	Adult: 3.5 (1.8–7.9)	Adult: 0.384

Clinical considerations: renal impairment: ↑ $t_{1/2}$ ↓ K_e

Distribution in body	Time to reach steady state (h)	Sampling times for measurement of serum drug concentrations	Assay methods used	Therapeutic range (µg/ml)	Toxic serum level (µg/ml)
Most tissues and transcellular fluids, including pleural, cerebrospinal, peritoneal, and synovial fluids	19 (10–43)	Peak: 1–1½ h after oral dose Trough: immediately before the next dose	HPLC, microbiological	50–100	> 100

Clinical considerations: serum levels > 100 µg/ml are associated with hematological and hepatic toxicity, possibly due to accumulation of 5-fluorouracil, which occurs more commonly in patients with renal dysfunction

Usual route of administration	Initial loading dose (mg/kg)	Maintenance dosage (mg/kg/day)	Usual dosing interval (h)	Adjustment for hepatic failure	Adjustment for renal failure	Removed by dialysis
Oral	—	Adult: 50–150	6	None	Increase dosing interval to 12–24 h if CCr = 10–50 ml/min or 24–48 h if < 10 ml/min	Yes: H, P; give a reloading dose of 20–30 mg/kg after hemodialysis

PHARMACOKINETICS

Gentamicin

Oral bioavailability (%)	Serum protein binding (%)	Renal excretion (% unchanged)	Active metabolites	V_d (liters/kg)	$t_{1/2}$ (h)	K_e (h^{-1})
—	0–30	> 95	None known	**Adult:** 0.25 (0.07–0.70) **Child:** 0.45 (0.25–0.70) **Neonate:** 0.70 (0.45–0.90)	**Adult:** 1.7 (0.5–3.0) **Child:** 1.3 (0.5–2.0) **Neonate:** 6.0 (2.0–9.0)	**Adult:** 0.396 **Child:** 0.554 **Neonate:** 0.116

Clinical considerations: obesity, extensive burns, ascites, cystic fibrosis: ⇧ V_d; renal impairment: ⇧ $t_{1/2}$ ⇩ K_e

Distribution in body	Time to reach steady state (h)	Sampling times for measurement of serum drug concentrations	Assay methods used	Therapeutic range (µg/ml)	Toxic serum level (µg/ml)
Extracellular fluid, renal cortex; crosses placenta	9 (6–18)	**Peak:** 60 min after IM injection; 15–30 min after 30-min IV infusion; 15 min after 60-min IV infusion **Trough:** immediately before the next dose	RIA, EMIT, FPI	**Peak:** 5.0–10.0 **Trough:** < 2.0	**Peak:** > 12.0 **Trough:** > 2.0

Clinical considerations: sustained trough levels > 2.0 µg/ml are associated with nephrotoxicity; sustained peak levels > 12.0 µg/ml may be associated with ototoxicity

Usual route of administration	Initial loading dose (mg/kg)	Maintenance dosage (mg/kg/day)	Usual dosing interval (h)	Adjustment for hepatic failure	Adjustment for renal failure	Removed by dialysis
IM, intermittent IV infusion	**Adult:** 2.5–3.0 **Child:** 2.5–3.0 **Neonate:** 2.0–3.0	**Adult:** 3.0–5.0 **Child:** 6.0–7.5 **Neonate:** up to 5.0	**Adult:** 6–8 **Child:** 6–8 **Neonate:** 12–24	None	Reduce dosage; see Sarubbi FA, Hull JH: *Ann Intern Med* 89:612–618, 1978	Yes: H, P

Clinical considerations: not absorbed by adipose tissue; use ideal (lean) body weight to calculate dosage and V_d

Heparin

Oral bioavailability (%)	Serum protein binding (%)	Renal excretion (% unchanged)	Active metabolites	V_d (liters/kg)	$t_{1/2}$ (min)	K_e (min^{-1})
—	> 95	< 2	Uroheparin (?)	**Adult:** 0.07 (0.04–0.13) **Child:** n/a	**Adult:** 90 (12–355) **Child:** n/a	**Adult:** 0.008 **Child:** n/a

Clinical considerations: elimination rate is dose dependent (⇧ dose: ⇧ $t_{1/2}$ ⇩ K_e)

Distribution in body	Time to reach steady state (h)	Sampling times for measurement of serum drug concentrations	Assay methods used[1]	Therapeutic range	Toxic serum level
Primarily plasma; not found in milk; does not cross placenta	1–33	**SC, IM, or IV bolus injection, intermittent IV infusion:** immediately before the next dose **Continuous IV infusion:** anytime during administration	ACT, APTT, WBAPTT, WBCT	1½–3 times the normal clotting time	Hemorrhagic complications may occur at any level

Usual route of administration	Initial loading dose (units/kg)[2]	Maintenance dosage (units/kg/24 h)[2]	Usual dosing interval (h)	Adjustment for hepatic failure	Adjustment for renal failure	Removed by dialysis
SC, IM, IV bolus injection, intermittent or continuous IV infusion	**Adult:** 50–70 **Child:** 50	**Adult:** 400 **Child:** 600	If not given by continuous IV infusion, then 4–12, depending on route of administration	Adjust dosage as indicated by results of coagulation tests	None	Yes: H (insignificant)

[1] These assays measure heparin activity and are not true measurements of concentration
[2] Doses necessary for "therapeutic" anticoagulation

continued

PHARMACOKINETICS

Lidocaine

Oral bioavailability (%)	Serum protein binding (%)	Renal excretion (% unchanged)	Active metabolites	V_d (liters/kg)	$t_{1/2}$ (h)	K_e (h^{-1})
30–40 (insufficient to produce therapeutic serum levels)	70 (60–80)	< 10	Monoethylglycinexylidide, glycinexylidide	Adult: 1.7 (1.1–2.2) Child: n/a Neonate: 2.7[2]	Adult: 1.5 (1.2–2.3)[1] Child: n/a Neonate: 3.16 (3.0–3.5)[2]	Adult: 0.462[1] Child: n/a Neonate: 0.2193[2]

Clinical considerations: cardiac failure, cirrhosis: ⇧ $t_{1/2}$ ⇩ K_e; acute myocardial infarction: ⇧ binding of lidocaine to α-1-glycoprotein

Distribution in body	Time to reach steady state (h)	Sampling times for measurement of serum drug concentrations	Assay methods used	Therapeutic range (μg/ml)	Toxic serum level (μg/ml)
Most tissues, including adipose tissue, erythrocytes; crosses placenta	6–12[3]	Anytime during maintenance therapy (continuous IV infusion)	EMIT, HPLC, FPI	1.5–5.0	> 5.0

Clinical considerations: serum levels > 5.0 μg/ml are associated with hypotension and CNS symptoms

Usual route of administration	Initial loading dose (mg/kg)	Maintenance dosage (mg/min)	Usual dosing interval (h)	Adjustment for hepatic failure	Adjustment for renal failure	Removed by dialysis
IM or IV bolus injection, continuous IV infusion	Adult: 4.3 (IM) or 1 (IV)	Adult: 1.5–3.0 (= serum level of 3.0 μg/ml in patients without CHF or hepatic failure)	—	Reduce maintenance infusion rate, depending on serum level and clinical response	None	No

Clinical considerations: giving the loading dose in a two-step infusion will obviate the "first-hour gap" in attaining therapeutic serum levels; the loading dose should be given in a bolus slowly over a period of 1–2 min; titrate maintenance dosage to clinical response

[1] Average values in healthy adult patients
[2] Average values obtained in four neonates after SC administration
[3] Range observed in healthy patients

Lithium

Oral bioavailability (%)	Serum protein binding (%)	Renal excretion (% unchanged)	Active metabolites	V_d (liters/kg)	$t_{1/2}$ (h)	K_e (h^{-1})
85–90	0	> 95	None known	Adult: 0.7 (0.4–1.4)	Adult: 24 (14–33)	Adult: 0.0289

Clinical considerations: renal impairment: ⇧ $t_{1/2}$ ⇩ K_e; use with caution in the elderly

Distribution in body	Time to reach steady state (h)	Sampling times for measurement of serum drug concentrations	Assay methods used	Therapeutic range (mEq/liter)	Toxic serum level (mEq/liter)
Total body water, erythrocytes, salivary glands, milk; crosses placenta	144 (84–198)	Immediate-release preparations: 12 h after the last dose Slow- or sustained-release preparations: immediately before the next dose	Flame photometry	Acute manic phase: 1.0–1.5[1] Maintenance phase: 0.6–1.2[1]	> 2.0

Clinical considerations: samples obtained < 12 h after last dose may show significant fluctuations due to distribution characteristics of the drug; during the acute manic phase, some patients may require serum concentrations exceeding the usual therapeutic range

PHARMACOKINETICS

Usual route of administration	Initial loading dose (mg)	Maintenance dosage (mg/day)	Usual dosing interval (h)	Adjustment for hepatic failure	Adjustment for renal failure	Removed by dialysis
Oral	Adult: 600	Adult: 900–1,200	6–12, depending on type of preparation and phase of illness	None	Lithium is not recommended for patients with severe renal failure (CCr $\leq$ 30 ml/min)	Yes: H, P

Clinical considerations: after an acute manic phase, dosage should be reduced for long-term maintenance

[1] Based on standardized 12-h serum lithium concentrations

Methotrexate

Oral bioavailability (%)	Serum protein binding (%)	Renal excretion (% unchanged)	Active metabolites	V_d (liters/kg)	$t_{1/2}$ (h)[1]	K_e (h^{-1})[2]
50–85 at doses $\leq$ 30 mg/m²; 50–70 at doses > 80 mg/m²	50	94	7-Hydroxy-methotrexate; 4-amino-4-deoxy-N^{10}-methylpteroic acid	Adult: 0.75 (0.70–0.80) Child: 0.75 (0.70–0.80)	Adult: 9.5 (8.0–15.0) Child: 9.5 (8.0–15.0)	Adult: 0.0729 Child: 0.0729

Clinical considerations: prior or concurrent treatment with nonabsorbable antibiotics: ⇧ oral absorption of methotrexate; concurrent treatment with salicylates, sulfonamides, or phenytoin: ⇩ serum binding of methotrexate; pleural effusions, ascites, renal impairment, gastrointestinal obstruction: ⇩ clearance of methotrexate

Distribution in body	Time to reach steady state (h)	Sampling times for measurement of serum drug concentrations	Assay methods used	Therapeutic range (M)	Toxic serum level (M)
Most body fluids and tissues, except CSF	75[2]	May vary depending on protocol; if patient is at risk, monitor serum concentration until level < 0.01 × 10^{-6} M	EMIT, HPLC, RIA, FPI	> 0.01 × 10^{-6} (minimum cytotoxic serum concentration)	> 5 × 10^{-6}, measured 24 h after high-dose methotrexate infusion

Clinical considerations: therapeutic response depends on factors other than the action of the drug, and therefore a simple relationship between clinical response and serum concentration should not be expected; clinical toxicity resulting from high-dose infusion of the drug may be obviated in some patients by continuing leucovorin until serum methotrexate level < 0.01 × 10^{-6} M

Usual route of administration	Initial loading dose (mg/kg)	Maintenance dosage (mg/kg/day)	Usual dosing interval (h)	Adjustment for hepatic failure	Adjustment for renal failure	Removed by dialysis
Oral, IM, intermittent IV infusion	Varies depending on protocol	Varies depending on protocol	Varies depending on protocol	None	Reduce dosage or discontinue medication to avoid further damage	Yes, but poorly: H, P

[1] Terminal $t_{1/2}$ (> 30 h after infusion); when measured 0–24 h after infusion in patients with normal renal function, $t_{1/2}$ = 2–3 h
[2] Based on terminal $t_{1/2}$ (> 30 h after infusion)

Nortriptyline

Oral bioavailability (%)	Serum protein binding (%)	Renal excretion (% unchanged)	Active metabolites	V_d (liters/kg)	$t_{1/2}$ (h)	K_e (h^{-1})
46–70	94 (87–95)	< 10	10-Hydroxy-nortriptyline	Adult: 18 (15–23)	Adult: 23 (18–56)	Adult: 0.0301

Clinical considerations: protein binding exhibits significant interindividual variation and may be altered by malignancy and hepatic or renal disease

continued

PHARMACOKINETICS

Distribution in body	Time to reach steady state (h)	Sampling times for measurement of serum drug concentrations	Assay methods used	Therapeutic range (ng/ml)	Toxic serum level (ng/ml)
Most tissues, erythrocytes	130	Immediately before the next dose	HPLC, FPI[1]	50–150	≥ 1,000

Clinical considerations: serum levels > 150 ng/ml do not result in further improvement of depression

Usual route of administration	Initial loading dose	Maintainance dosage (mg/day)	Usual dosing interval (h)	Adjustment for hepatic failure	Adjustment for renal failure	Removed by dialysis
Oral	Start low and titrate upward, depending on clinical response	Adult: 25–100	6–8	Dosage reduction may be necessary, depending on clinical response	None	No

Clinical considerations: adolescent and elderly patients may respond to lower doses and should not be given > 50 mg/day

[1] FPI is not specific for individual agents

Phenobarbital

Oral bioavail-ability (%)	Serum protein binding (%)	Renal excretion (% unchanged)	Active metabolites	V_d (liters/kg)	$t_{1/2}$ (h)	K_e (h^{-1})
> 80[1]	45	20–30	None known	Adult: 0.7 (0.7–1.0) Child: 0.8 (0.5–0.9) Neonate: 0.8 (0.7–1.0)	Adult: 80 (50–110) Child: 65 (60–70) Neonate: 110 (43–217)	Adult: 0.009 Child: 0.011 Neonate: 0.006

Clinical considerations: ⇑ urine pH: ⇑ renal excretion; autoinduction during maintenance therapy increases the drug's metabolism and accelerates its clearance

Distribution in body	Time to reach steady state (h)	Sampling times for measurement of serum drug concentrations	Assay methods used	Therapeutic range (µg/ml)	Toxic serum level (µg/ml)
Most tissues and fluids, including CSF; crosses placenta	Adult: 275–605 Child: 330–385 Neonate: 240–1,194	Immediately before the first maintenance dose of the day	EMIT, gas chromatography	10–35	> 35

Clinical considerations: serum levels of 35–80 µg/ml may be reflected by slowness and ataxia; levels of 65–110 µg/ml may be manifested by coma but intact reflexes; areflexia may occur at serum levels > 100 µg/ml

Usual route of administration	Initial loading dose (mg/kg)	Maintenance dosage (mg/kg/day)	Usual dosing interval (h)	Adjustment for hepatic failure	Adjustment for renal failure	Removed by dialysis
Oral, IM, IV bolus injection	Adult: 10 Child: 10 Neonate: 15	Adult: 2–5 Child: 3–8 Neonate: 1–3	12–24	Lengthen interval between doses, depending on serum level	Lengthen interval between doses, depending on serum level	Yes: H, P

[1] Absolute bioavailability has not been established, but both oral and IM administration result in good absorption

Phenytoin

Oral bioavail-ability (%)	Serum protein binding (%)	Renal excretion (% unchanged)	Active metabolites	V_d (liters/kg)	$t_{1/2}$ (h)	K_e (h^{-1})
20–90	88–92	< 5	None known	Adult: 0.7 (0.6–1.2) Child: 0.7 (0.6–1.2) Neonate: 1.2	Adult: 23 (8–60) Child: 23 (8–60) Neonate: 30	Adult: 0.0301 Child: 0.0301 Neonate: 0.0231

Clinical considerations: oral bioavailability depends on preparation used; hypoalbuminemia, uremia, cirrhosis, other disease states that alter drug binding to albumin: ⇓ protein binding[1]; uremia: ⇑ V_d ⇓ $t_{1/2}$ ⇑ K_e; $t_{1/2}$ is dependent on serum concentration and dose and can vary significantly in patients with normal liver and kidney function

122 COMPENDIUM OF DRUG THERAPY

PHARMACOKINETICS

Distribution in body	Time to reach steady state (h)	Sampling times for measurement of serum drug concentrations	Assay methods used	Therapeutic range (μg/ml)	Toxic serum level (μg/ml)
Most tissues and fluids, including brain, liver, salivary glands, and milk; crosses placenta	130 (120–240)	**Peak:** ~ 6 h after the last dose **Trough:** immediately before the next dose	Gas chromatography, EMIT, HPLC, FPI	10–20	> 20

Clinical considerations: because the time to peak after oral administration varies and is dependent on the product used, trough levels are recommended for routine monitoring; patients may exhibit signs of toxicity at therapeutic serum levels; conditions that affect phenytoin protein binding (see above) may force an adjustment of the therapeutic range

Usual route of administration	Initial loading dose (mg/kg)	Maintenance dosage (mg/kg/day)	Usual dosing interval (h)	Adjustment for hepatic failure	Adjustment for renal failure	Removed by dialysis
Oral, IM, IV bolus injection	**Adult:** 20 (oral) or 10 (IV) **Child:** 15–20 (oral) or 10 (IV) **Neonate:** 15–20 (oral) or 10 (IV)	**Adult:** 5 **Child:** 5–15 **Neonate:** 3–5	8–12, except if extended phenytoin sodium capsules are used	Dosage reduction usually necessary, depending on serum level	None	No

Clinical considerations: IM injection results in slow, erratic absorption and should be avoided if possible; IV injection must not exceed 50 mg/min

[1] Protein binding of phenytoin is also decreased in neonates

Primidone

Oral bioavailability (%)	Serum protein binding (%)	Renal excretion (% unchanged)	Active metabolites	V_d (liters/kg)	$t_{1/2}$ (h)	K_e (h^{-1})
Unknown, but presumed to be 100%	0–20	20 (10–40)	Phenobarbital (5–25%), phenylethylmalonamide (45%)	**Adult:** 0.6 **Child:** 0.6	**Adult:** 11 (10–12) **Child:** 8.7 (4.5–11.0)	**Adult:** 0.063 **Child:** 0.0797

Clinical considerations: because primidone is partly metabolized to phenobarbital, serum levels of both drugs should be monitored; concurrent anticonvulsant therapy may alter $t_{1/2}$

Distribution in body	Time to reach steady state (h)	Sampling times for measurement of serum drug concentrations	Assay methods used	Therapeutic range (μg/ml)	Toxic serum level (μg/ml)
Most tissues and fluids, including milk; crosses placenta	60 (50–72)	**Peak:** 3–9 h after the last dose **Trough:** immediately before the next dose	Gas chromatography, EMIT HPLC, FPI	5–12	> 12

Clinical considerations: because the time to peak varies, trough levels are recommended for routine monitoring

Usual route of administration	Initial loading dose (mg/kg)	Maintenance dosage	Usual dosing interval (h)	Adjustment for hepatic failure	Adjustment for renal failure	Removed by dialysis
Oral	—	**Adult:** 1.0–1.5 g/day (not to exceed 2 g/day) **Child:** 10–25 mg/kg/day	6–8	Dosage reduction may be necessary, depending on serum level	Reduce dosage; see Bennett WM, et al: *Am J Kidney Dis* 3:155-193, 1983	Yes: H

Clinical considerations: increase maintenance dosage gradually based on clinical response, tolerance, and serum drug levels

continued

PHARMACOKINETICS

Procainamide

Oral bioavailability (%)	Serum protein binding (%)	Renal excretion (% unchanged)	Active metabolites	V_d (liters/kg)	$t_{1/2}$ (h)	K_e (h^{-1})
80 (75–90)	15 (14–23)	50	N-acetyl-procainamide (NAPA; $t_{1/2}$ = 6 h)	Adult: 2.7 Child: n/a	Adult: 3.0 (2.5–4.7) Child: n/a	Adult: 0.231 Child: n/a

Clinical considerations: NAPA concentration depends on patient's acetylator phenotype (rapid acetylators have a higher concentration of NAPA than of procainamide); renal disease: ⇧ NAPA serum level

Distribution in body	Time to reach steady state (h)	Sampling times for measurement of serum drug concentrations	Assay methods used	Therapeutic range (μg/ml)	Toxic serum level (μg/ml)
Most tissues, except brain	18 (13–25)	Peak: 1–2 h after administration of immediate-release preparation Trough: immediately before the next dose	Gas chromatography, EMIT, HPLC, FPI	4–10	> 10

Clinical considerations: therapeutic range for sum of procainamide and NAPA concentrations in serum is 10–30 μg/ml; some assays can quantitate procainamide and NAPA serum levels

Usual route of administration	Initial loading dose (mg/kg)	Maintenance dosage (mg/kg/day)	Usual dosing interval (h)	Adjustment for hepatic failure	Adjustment for renal failure	Removed by dialysis
Oral, IM, intermittent IV infusion (≤ 50 mg/min)	Adult: twice the maintenance dose orally or 14–17 IV Child: n/a	Adult: 50 (oral) Child: 50 (oral)	Immediate-release preparations: 4–8 Sustained-release preparations: 6–8	Dosage reduction may be necessary, depending on serum level and clinical response	Reduce dosage; see Coyle JD, et al, in Evans WE, et al (eds): *Applied Pharmacokinetics*, 2nd Ed. San Francisco, Applied Therapeutics Inc., 1986, pp 682–711	Yes: H, P

Quinidine

Oral bioavailability (%)	Serum protein binding (%)	Renal excretion (% unchanged)	Active metabolites	V_d (liters/kg)	$t_{1/2}$ (h)	K_e (h^{-1})
80 (70–87)	70–80	10–20	3-Hydroxyquinidine, 2-oxyquinidinone, o-desmethylquinidine	Adult: 3.0 (2.0–3.5) Child: n/a	Adult: 6.5 (5–12) Child: n/a	Adult: 0.1066 Child: n/a

Clinical considerations: cirrhosis, other disease states affecting albumin and α-1-acid glycoprotein concentrations: ⇩ protein binding; congestive heart failure: ⇩ V_d, possibly requiring a reduction in quinidine maintenance dose; ⇧ urine pH: ⇩ renal excretion

Distribution in body	Time to reach steady state (h)	Sampling times for measurement of serum drug concentrations	Assay methods used	Therapeutic range (μg/ml)	Toxic serum level (μg/ml)
Most tissues, except brain	24–48	Peak: 1½ h after oral administration of an immediate-release preparation; 3–4 h after oral administration of a sustained-release preparation Trough: immediately before the next dose	Fluorometric, EMIT, HPLC, FPI	2.0–5.0[1] 4.0–8.0[2]	> 5.0[1] 10.0[2]

PHARMACOKINETICS

Usual route of administration	Initial loading dose (mg/kg)	Maintenance dosage (mg/kg/day)	Usual dosing interval (h)	Adjustment for hepatic failure	Adjustment for renal failure	Removed by dialysis
Oral, IM, intermittent IV infusion	Adult: twice the maintenance dose orally or 0.2–0.3 IV Child: n/a	Adult: 14 Child: 3–22	6–12, depending on type of preparation administered	Dosage reduction may be necessary, depending on serum level and clinical response	Reduce dosage by ~ 50%	Yes: H, P

Clinical considerations: dosages given here are quinidine base requirements to achieve a steady-state serum concentration of 1.5 µg/ml when assayed by specific procedures (EMIT, FPI, HPLC); in some patients, IM administration may result in erratic, nonlinear absorption

[1] Values obtained by use of assay methods specfic for quinidine (EMIT, FPI, HPLC)
[2] Values obtained by use of nonspecific (fluorometric) assay methods, which include quinidine and its metabolites

Theophylline

Oral bioavailability (%)	Serum protein binding (%)	Renal excretion (% unchanged)	Active metabolites	V_d (liters/kg)	$t_{1/2}$ (h)	K_e (h^{-1})
100	55 (50–60)	< 10	3-Methyl-xanthine (in neonates: caffeine, theobromine)	Adult: 0.5 (0.3–0.7) Child: 0.5 (0.1–0.7) Neonate: 0.9 (0.7–2.9)	Adult: 8.7 (3.6–20.7) Child: 3.5 (1.4–7.9) Neonate: 30 (15.0–57.7)	Adult: 0.080 Child: 0.198 Neonate: 0.023

Clinical considerations: cirrhosis: ▽ protein binding △ V_d △ $t_{1/2}$ ▽ K_e; cigarette smoking: ▽ $t_{1/2}$ △ K_e; neonates: ▽ protein binding; elimination rate may be nonlinear in young children

Distribution in body	Time to reach steady state (h)	Sampling times for measurement of serum drug concentrations	Assay methods used	Therapeutic range (µg/ml)	Toxic serum level (µg/ml)
All tissues and fluids, except adipose tissue; crosses placenta	Adult: 20–114 Child: 8–43 Neonate: 83–317	**Oral:** for peak values, 1 h after administration of an immediate-release product or 4–5 h after administration of a sustained-release product; for trough values, immediately before the next dose **Intermittent IV infusion:** for peak values, immediately after completing the infusion; for trough values, immediately before the next dose **Continuous IV infusion:** anytime during administration	EMIT, HPLC, FPI	Asthma: 10–20 Neonatal apnea: 4–12	> 20

Clinical considerations: for adjusting dosage, blood should be sampled immediately before giving a dose when using oral or intermittent IV therapy

Usual route of administration	Initial loading dose (mg/kg)	Maintenance dosage (mg/kg/day)	Usual dosing interval (h)	Adjustment for hepatic failure	Adjustment for renal failure	Removed by dialysis
Oral, intermittent or continuous IV infusion, rectal enema	Adult: 5 Child: 5 Neonate: 5	Adult: 10–15 Child: 20–24 Neonate: 1–5	Immediate-release preparations: 6–8 Sustained-release preparations: 8–12	Reduce dosage depending on serum level	None	Yes: H, P

Clinical considerations: use ideal (lean) body weight to calculate dosage; patients with congestive heart failure, liver disease, or cor pulmonale may require a smaller maintenance dose; adults who smoke may require a larger maintenance dose

continued

Tobramycin

Oral bioavailability (%)	Serum protein binding (%)	Renal excretion (% unchanged)	Active metabolites	V_d (liters/kg)	$t_{1/2}$ (h)	K_e (h^{-1})
—	0–30	> 95	None known	Adult: 0.25 (0.07–0.70) Child: 0.45 (0.25–0.70) Neonate: 0.70 (0.45–0.90)	Adult: 1.7 (0.5–3.0) Child: 1.3 (0.5–2.0) Neonate: 6.0 (2.0–9.0)	Adult: 0.396 Child: 0.554 Neonate: 0.116

Clinical considerations: obesity, extensive burns, ascites, cystic fibrosis: ⇑ V_d; renal impairment: ⇑ $t_{1/2}$ ⇓ K_e

Distribution in body	Time to reach steady state (h)	Sampling times for measurement of serum drug concentrations	Assay methods used	Therapeutic range (µg/ml)	Toxic serum level (µg/ml)
Extracellular fluid, renal cortex; crosses placenta	9 (6–18)	**Peak:** 60 min after IM injection; 15–30 min after 30-min IV infusion; 15 min after 60-min IV infusion **Trough:** immediately before the next dose	RIA, EMIT, FPI	Peak: 5.0–10.0 Trough: < 2.0	Peak: > 12.0 Trough: > 2.0

Clinical considerations: sustained trough levels > 2.0 µg/ml are associated with nephrotoxicity; sustained peak levels > 12.0 µg/ml may be associated with ototoxicity

Usual route of administration	Initial loading dose (mg/kg)	Maintenance dosage (mg/kg/day)	Usual dosing interval (h)	Adjustment for hepatic failure	Adjustment for renal failure	Removed by dialysis
IM, intermittent IV infusion	Adult: 2.5–3.0 Child: 2.5–3.0 Neonate: 2.0–3.0	Adult: 3.0–5.0 Child: 6.0–7.5 Neonate: up to 4.0	Adult: 6–8 Child: 6–8 Neonate: 12–24	None	Reduce dosage; see Sarubbi FA, Hull JH: *Ann Intern Med* 89:612–618, 1978	Yes: H, P

Clinical considerations: not absorbed by adipose tissue; use ideal (lean) body weight to calculate dosage and V_d

Valproic Acid

Oral bioavailability (%)	Serum protein binding (%)	Renal excretion (% unchanged)	Active metabolites	V_d (liters/kg)	$t_{1/2}$ (h)	K_e (h^{-1})
100	90 (80–95)	< 5	3-Oxo-valproic acid, succinic acid	Adult: 0.2 (0.1–0.4) Child: 0.14–0.41 Neonate: n/a	Adult: 8–15 Child: 8–11 Neonate: 10–67	Adult: 0.087–0.046 Child: 0.087–0.063 Neonate: 0.069–0.01

Clinical considerations: protein binding is dependent on drug and protein concentration and may be altered by hepatic or renal failure and by concomitant therapy with drugs that are highly bound to serum proteins

Distribution in body	Time to reach steady state (h)	Sampling times for measurement of serum drug concentrations	Assay methods used	Therapeutic range (µg/ml)	Toxic serum level (µg/ml)
Plasma and rapidly exchangeable ECF, CSF, saliva, milk; crosses placenta	20–85	Immediately before the first maintenance dose of the day	Gas chromatography, EMIT, FPI	50–100	> 100

Clinical considerations: toxicity may occur in the therapeutic range if combination therapy is used or a condition resulting in abnormal protein binding exists

PHARMACOKINETICS

Usual route of administration	Initial loading dose (mg/kg)	Maintenance dosage (mg/kg/day)	Usual dosing interval (h)	Adjustment for hepatic failure	Adjustment for renal failure	Removed by dialysis
Oral	—	**Adult:** 10–45 **Child:** 15–100	6–12	Unknown; adjust dosage depending on serum level	None	Unknown

Clinical considerations: the maximum dosage approved by the FDA is 60 mg/kg/day; use of dosages exceeding this limit should be governed by measurement of serum drug concentrations

Vancomycin

Oral bioavailability (%)	Serum protein binding (%)	Renal excretion (% unchanged)	Active metabolites	V_d (liters/kg)	$t_{1/2}$ (h)	K_e (h^{-1})
Poor	10–55[1]	80–90	None known	**Adult:** 0.8 (0.4–1.3) **Child:** 0.4–0.8	**Adult:** 6 (4–11) **Child:** 3–7	**Adult:** 0.1155 **Child:** n/a

Clinical considerations: renal impairment: ⇧ $t_{1/2}$ ⇩ K_e

Distribution in body	Time to reach steady state (h)	Sampling times for measurement of serum drug concentrations	Assay methods used	Therapeutic range ($\mu g/ml$)	Toxic serum level ($\mu g/ml$)
Most body fluids and tissues, except CSF and bile	36 (24–66)	**Peak:** 2 h after 1-h IV infusion (4–6 h for renally impaired patients) **Trough:** immediately before the next dose	RIA, FPI	2.5–40	> 50

Clinical considerations: most authorities suggest an arbitrary maximum peak serum level of 40–50 $\mu g/ml$; serum levels > 80 $\mu g/ml$ are consistently associated with ototoxicity; desired serum level depends on sensitivity of infecting organism

Usual route of administration	Initial loading dose (mg/kg)	Maintenance dosage	Usual dosing interval (h)	Adjustment for hepatic failure	Adjustment for renal failure	Removed by dialysis
Oral, intermittent IV infusion	—	**Adult:** 2 g/day **Child:** 44 mg/kg/day	6–12	None	Reduce dosage; see Bennett WM, et al: *Am J Kidney Dis* 3:155-193, 1983	Yes: P[2]

Clinical considerations: uremic patients being treated orally for staphylococcal enterocolitis or antibiotic-associated pseudomembranous colitis may be given the full dosage, as absorption from the gastrointestinal tract is negligible

[1] Only one study has shown that 55% of the drug is protein bound; other studies indicate that < 10% is bound
[2] In one study, serum levels were reduced by 35%

Chapter 5

New Products/Revised Drug Information/Other Agents

New Products — 130
A brief description of the new products introduced in this edition of the Compendium, immediately following this table of contents.

Revised Drug Information — 132
Important changes in formulations, indications, dosages, precautions, and drug interactions received at press time.

Antiarrhythmics — 134
BREVIBLOC (Du Pont Critical Care) — 134
Esmolol hydrochloride *Rx*

ENKAID (Bristol Laboratories) — 135
Encainide hydrochloride *Rx*

Antihypertensive Agents — 138
TENEX (Robins) — 138
Guanfacine hydrochloride *Rx*

Antiviral Agents — 139
RETROVIR (Burroughs Wellcome) — 139
Zidovudine *Rx*

Bone/Calcium Metabolism Regulators — 141
CIBACALCIN (CIBA) — 141
Calcitonin-human *Rx*

Cephalosporins — 142
KEFLET (Dista) — 142
Cephalexin *Rx*

Fertility Inducers — 143
METRODIN (Serono) — 143
Urofollitropin *Rx*

Miscellaneous Antibiotics — 145
VANCOLED (Lederle) — 145
Vancomycin hydrochloride *Rx*

Monobactam Antiobiotics — 148
AZACTAM (Squibb) — 148
Aztreonam *Rx*

Ophthalmic Agents — 150
OCUFEN (Allergan) — 150
Flurbiprofen sodium *Rx*

Oral Corticosteroids — 151
PEDIAPRED (Fisons) — 151
Prednisone sodium phosphate *Rx*

Penicillins — 154
UNASYN (Roerig) — 154
Ampicillin sodium and sulbactam sodium *Rx*

Psoriasis Preparations — 155
TEGISON (Roche) — 155
Etretinate *Rx*

Vaccines
RECOMBIVAX HB (Merck Sharp & Dohme) — 158
Hepatitis B vaccine (recombinant) *Rx*

Other Agents — 159

Alcohol-Abuse Deterrents — 159
ANTABUSE (Ayerst) — 159
Disulfiram *Rx*

Antidotes — 161
MUCOMYST (Bristol) — 161
Acetylcysteine *Rx*

NARCAN (Du Pont) — 163
Naloxone hydrochloride *Rx*

Antiplatelet Agents — 164
PERSANTINE (Boehringer Ingelheim) — 164
Dipyridamole *Rx*

Bone/Calcium Metabolism Regulators — 165
CALCIMAR (Rorer) — 165
Calcitonin-salmon *Rx*

DIDRONEL (Norwich Eaton) — 167
Etidronate disodium *Rx*

Chemonucleolytic Enzymes — 168
CHYMODIACTIN (Flint) — 168
Chymopapain *Rx*

DISCASE (Flint) — 170
Chymopapain *Rx*

Gallstone-Dissolving Agents — 172
CHENIX (Reid-Rowell) — 172
Chenodiol *Rx*

MOCTANIN (Ethitek) — 173
Monooctanoin *Rx*

Patent Ductus Arteriosus Therapy — 174
INDOCIN I.V. (Merck Sharp & Dohme) — 174
Indomethacin sodium trihydrate *Rx*

Psychostimulants — 176
CYLERT (Abbott) — 176
Pemoline *C-IV*

DEXEDRINE (Smith Kline & French) — 178
Dextroamphetamine sulfate *C-II*

RITALIN (CIBA) 179
Methylphenidate hydrochloride C-II

RITALIN-SR (CIBA) 179
Methylphenidate hydrochloride C-II

Smoking Deterrents 181

NICORETTE (Lakeside) 181
Nicotine polacrilex Rx

Vaccines 183

b-CAPSA I (Mead Johnson) 183
Hemophilus b polysaccharide vaccine Rx

Diphtheria and tetanus toxoids and pertussis vaccine, 183
adsorbed (Connaught) Rx

HEPTAVAX-B (Merck Sharp & Dohme) 184
Hepatitis B vaccine Rx

HIB-IMUNE (Lederle) 186
Hemophilus b polysaccharide vaccine Rx

HIBVAX (Connaught) 187
Hemophilus b polysaccharide vaccine Rx

Influenza virus vaccine, monovalent, subvirion 189
(Wyeth) Rx

Influenza virus vaccine, trivalent, subvirion 188
(Wyeth) Rx

M-M-R II (Merck Sharp & Dohme) 190
Measles, mumps, and rubella live virus vaccine Rx

ORIMUNE (Lederle) 192
Poliovirus vaccine, live, trivalent Rx

PNEUMOVAX 23 (Merck Sharp & Dohme) 194
Pneumococcal vaccine, polyvalent Rx

PNU-IMUNE (Lederle) 195
Pneumococcal vaccine, polyvalent Rx

TRI-IMMUNOL (Lederle) 196
Diphtheria and tetanus toxoids and pertussis
vaccine, adsorbed Rx

New Products

The following recently introduced products represent significant new additions to the Compendium. Please refer to the index for the appropriate chapter and page number for further information. This list does not include diagnostics or nutritional products, new dosage forms or strengths, or new indications for existing products. The reader is urged to consult the individual drug charts and the following supplement for the latest information on each drug.

ACLOVATE (alclometasone diproprionate) Glaxo
A topical corticosteroid for *inflammatory and pruritic manifestations of corticosteroid-responsive dermatoses.*

AZACTAM (aztreonam) Squibb
A parenteral monobactam antibiotic for *septicemia* and *lower respiratory tract, skin, skin structure, intraabdominal, gynecological,* and *urinary tract infections.*

BREVIBLOC (esmolol hydrochloride) Du Pont Critical Care
A parenteral beta$_1$-selective adrenergic receptor blocker for short-term, rapid control of ventricular rate in patients with *atrial fibrillation* or *atrial flutter,* as well as *noncompensatory sinus tachycardia* requiring specific intervention.

BUSPAR (buspirone hydrochloride) Mead Johnson Pharmaceuticals
An oral nonbenzodiazepine anxiolytic for *anxiety disorders* and short-term relief of *symptoms of anxiety.*

CIBACALCIN (calcitonin-human) CIBA
A parenteral synthetic polypeptide hormone for symptomatic *Paget's disease of bone.*

DEPONIT (nitroglycerin) Wyeth
A transdermal nitroglycerin delivery system for prevention and treatment of *angina pectoris* due to coronary artery disease.

DIASORB (attapulgite) Key
An oral, nonsystemic adsorbent for *diarrhea.*

DORYX (doxycycline hyclate) Parke-Davis
An oral tetracycline capsule for treatment of *gram-positive and gram-negative bacterial infections, gonorrhea, chlamydial infections, mycoplasmal pneumonia, syphilis, severe acne,* and other infections caused by tetracycline-susceptible organisms.

ENKAID (encainide hydrochloride) Bristol
A class 1C oral antiarrhythmic agent for *life-threatening ventricular arrhythmias, symptomatic nonsustained ventricular tachycardia,* and *frequent premature ventricular complexes.*

ESTRADERM (estradiol) CIBA
A transdermal estradiol delivery system for moderate to severe *menopausal vasomotor symptoms, female hypogonadism or castration, primary ovarian failure,* and atrophic conditions such as *atrophic vaginitis* and *kraurosis vulvae* caused by deficient endogenous estrogen production.

GASTROLYTE Rorer
An oral electrolyte concentrate for *maintenance of water and electrolyte levels* and *replacement of mild-to-moderate fluid losses,* particularly in mild to moderate diarrhea.

HALTRAN (ibuprofen) Upjohn
An oral analgesic/antipyretic for *headache, toothache, backache, muscular ache, menstrual pain, minor pain of arthritis, minor ache and pain of colds,* and *fever.*

HIB-IMUNE (hemophilus b polysaccharide vaccine) Lederle
A parenteral vaccine for *prevention of Hemophilus influenzae type b diseases* in children.

HibVAX (hemophilus b polysaccharide vaccine) Connaught
A parenteral vaccine for *prevention of Hemophilus influenzae type b diseases* in children.

HUMULIN BR (human insulin) Lilly
A synthetic human insulin product for *diabetes mellitus* uncontrollable by diet alone.

INSULATARD NPH Human (human insulin) Nordisk-USA
A synthetic human insulin product for *diabetes mellitus* uncontrollable by diet alone.

INTRON A (interferon alfa-2b, recombinant) Schering
A synthetic human leukocyte interferon for *hairy cell leukemia* in splenectomized and nonsplenectomized patients.

K-DUR (potassium chloride) Key
An oral, sustained-release potassium supplement for prevention and treatment of *hypokalemia, digitalis intoxication,* and *hypokalemic familial periodic paralysis.*

KEFLET (cephalexin) Dista
An oral cephalosporin for *otitis media* and *respiratory tract, bone, genitourinary tract, skin,* and *skin structure infections.*

KEFUROX (cefuroxime sodium) Lilly
A parenteral cephalosporin for *prevention of postoperative infection* and treatment of *lower respiratory tract, urinary tract, skin,* and *skin structure infections, septicemia, meningitis, uncomplicated gonorrhea,* and *disseminated gonococcal infections.*

MARINOL (dronabinol) Roxane
An oral cannabinoid antiemetic for *nausea and vomiting associated with cancer chemotherapy* in patients unresponsive to conventional antiemetic therapy.

MEDIPREN (ibuprofen) McNeil Consumer Products
An oral analgesic/antipyretic for *headache, toothache, backache, muscular ache, menstrual pain, minor pain of arthritis, minor ache and pain of colds,* and *fever.*

METRODIN (urofollitropin) Serono
A parenteral gonadotropin for *induction of ovulation* in patients with ovarian disease with an elevated LH/FSH ratio who are unresponsive to clomiphene therapy.

MIDOL 200 (ibuprofen) Glenbrook
An oral analgesic/antipyretic for *headache, toothache, backache, muscular ache, menstrual pain, minor pain of arthritis, minor ache and pain of colds,* and *fever.*

MONISTAT DUAL-PAK (miconazole nitrate) Ortho
A combination of three 200-mg Monistat 3 vaginal suppositories with 3% Monistat-Derm dermatological cream for *concomitant vaginal and dermatological candidal infections.*

MYCELEX TWIN PACK (clotrimazole) **Miles Pharmaceuticals**

A combination of one 500-mg Mycelex-G vaginal tablet with 1% Mycelex dermatological cream for *concomitant vaginal and dermatological candidal infections.*

NITROGARD (nitroglycerin) **Parke-Davis**

A transmucosal, controlled-release nitrate preparation for *prevention of anticipated acute angina pectoris* and *treatment of acute angina pectoris.*

NOROXIN (norofloxacin) **Merck Sharp & Dohme**

A synthetic, oral, broad-spectrum antibiotic for *urinary tract infections.*

NOVOLIN 70/30 (human insulin) **Squibb-Novo**

A synthetic human insulin product for *diabetes mellitus* uncontrollable by diet alone.

OCUFEN (flurbiprofen sodium) **Allergan**

An ophthalmic prostaglandin inhibitor agent for *inhibition of intraoperative miosis.*

PCE (erythromycin) **Abbott**

An oral tablet for *mild-to-moderate respiratory tract, skin, and skin structure infections, chlamydial infections, acute pelvic inflammatory disease,* and other infections caused by erythromycin-susceptible organisms.

PEDIAPRED (prednisolone sodium phosphate) **Fisons**

An oral solution of prednisolone formulated specifically for pediatric use for *conditions requiring corticosteroid therapy.*

PEPCID/PEPCID I.V. (famotidine) **Merck Sharp & Dohme**

An oral and parenteral histamine H_2-receptor antagonist for *active duodenal ulcers, maintenance therapy of acute healed duodenal ulcers,* and *pathological hypersecretory conditions.*

PSORCON (diflorasone diacetate) **Dermik**

A topical corticosteroid for *inflammatory and pruritic manifestations of corticosteroid-responsive dermatoses.*

RECOMBIVAX HB (hepatitis B vaccine [recombinant]) **Merck Sharp & Dohme**

A parenteral vaccine for *prevention of type B hepatitis* in persons at risk or following exposure to the hepatitis B antigen.

RETROVIR (zidovudine) **Burroughs Wellcome**

An oral antiviral agent for management of *symptomatic HIV infection (AIDS and advanced ARC)* in certain adult patients who have a history of cytologically confirmed *Pneumocystis carinii* pneumonia or an absolute T4 (CD4) lymphocyte count of less than 200 mm[3] in the peripheral blood.

ROFERON-A (interferon alfa-2a, recombinant) **Roche**

A synthetic human leukocyte interferon for *hairy cell leukemia* in splenectomized and nonsplenectomized patients.

TEGISON (etretinate) **Roche**

An oral retinoid for *severe recalcitrant psoriasis.*

TENEX (guanfacine hydrochloride) **Robins**

An oral, central alpha$_2$-receptor agonist for *hypertension* in patients already receiving a thiazide-type diuretic.

TRENDAR (ibuprofen) **Whitehall**

An oral analgesic for *dysmenorrhea, headaches, backaches,* and *neuromuscular aches and pains* associated with premenstrual syndrome.

TYCOLET (hydrocodone bitartrate and acetaminophen) **McNeil Pharmaceutical**

An oral controlled analgesic combination for *mild-to-moderately severe pain.*

UNASYN (ampicillin sodium and sulbactam sodium) **Roerig**

A parenteral combination of ampicillin with a beta-lactamase inhibitor for *skin, skin structure, intraabdominal,* and *gynecological infections.*

VANCOLED (vancomycin hydrochloride) **Lederle**

A parenteral broad-spectrum antibiotic for *enterocolitis, antibiotic-associated pseudomembranous colitis,* and *serious or severe staphylococcal infections,* as well as *prevention of bacterial endocarditis.*

VASERETIC (enalapril maleate and hydrochlorothiazide) **Merck Sharp & Dohme**

An oral antihypertensive product combining an angiotensin converting enzyme inhibitor with a diuretic for *essential hypertension.*

VELOSULIN (human insulin) **Nordisk-USA**

A synthetic human insulin product for *diabetes mellitus* uncontrollable by diet alone.

ZYDONE (hydrocodone bitartrate and acetaminophen) **Du Pont**

An oral controlled analgesic for *moderate to moderately severe pain.*

continued

Revised Drug Information

The following information supplements the drug information presented elsewhere in this volume. The information includes important changes in formulations, indications, dosages, precautions, adverse reactions, and drug interactions received at press time.

ACCUTANE (isotretinoin) Roche
Warn patient that night vision may decrease suddenly and to exercise caution when operating vehicles at night; follow visual problems closely. Mild-to-moderate increases in hepatic enzyme levels have occurred in 15% of patients, and hepatitis has been associated with administration of isotretinoin; treatment should be discontinued if such hepatic changes occur.

ALUPENT Inhalant Solution (metaproterenol sulfate) Boehringer Ingelheim
Now available as a 0.4% solution in 2.5-ml vials; indications and dosage remain the same.

AVC (sulfanilamide) Merrell Dow
This antifungal agent has been reformulated without aminacrine or allantoin and is now solely indicated for *candidal vulvovaginitis*; available as a 1% vaginal cream in 4-oz tubes and vaginal suppositories containing 1.05 g of sulfanilamide. Recommended adult dosage: one applicatorful of cream or one suppository once or twice daily for 30 days.

BUSPAR (buspirone hydrochloride) Mead Johnson Pharmaceuticals
Concomitant administration of buspirone with haloperidol has been found to increase haloperidol serum levels; in addition, four occurrences of elevated blood pressure have been reported in patients taking buspirone and an MAO inhibitor. Consequently, concomitant use of this drug with either haloperidol or an MAO inhibitor is not recommended.

CARDIZEM (diltiazem hydrochloride) Marion
Now available in 90- and 120-mg tablet strengths; indications and dosage remain the same.

CLEOCIN T (clindamycin phosphate) Upjohn
Now available as a gel containing clindamycin phosphate equivalent to 10 mg/ml of clindamycin and packaged in 7.5-g and 30-g tubes; indications and dosage remain the same.

CORGARD (nadolol) Princeton
Now available in a 20-mg tablet strength; indications and dosage remain the same.

DILANTIN Parenteral (phenytoin sodium) Parke-Davis
Now available in 2- and 5-ml vials containing 50 mg/ml of phenytoin sodium; indications and dosage remain the same.

FML Forte Ophthalmic Suspension (fluorometholone) Allergan
Now available in a 2-ml plastic dropper bottle.

INAPSINE (droperidol) Janssen
Now available in 1-ml vials containing 2.5 mg/ml of droperidol; indications and dosage remain the same.

ISUPREL Injection (isoproterenol hydrochloride) Winthrop Pharmaceuticals
This sympathomimetic amine is now specifically indicated for mild or transient episodes of heart block that do not require electroshock or pacemaker therapy, serious episodes of heart block and Adams-Stokes attacks (except when caused by ventricular tachycardia or fibrillation), cardiac arrest (until electroshock or pacemaker therapy can be instituted), and bronchospasm occurring during anesthesia, and as adjunctive therapy of low cardiac output states, congestive heart failure, and hypovolemic, cardiogenic, and septic shock. The contraindications have been extended to include tachyarrhythmias, digitalis-induced tachycardia or heart block, ventricular arrhythmias requiring inotropic therapy, and angina pectoris. Recommended dosages and directions for use remain the same except for a new pediatric dosage, based on American Heart Association guidelines, for heart block, Adams-Stokes attacks, and cardiac arrest: 0.1 µg/kg/min, given by infusion to start, followed, if necessary, by up to 1.0 µg/kg/min.

Use of another agent initially for cardiogenic shock owing to myocardial infarction is now recommended, with isoproterenol being given only after arterial pressure has been restored. Additional adverse reactions include weakness, dizziness, angina, hyper- and hypotension, ventricular arrhythmias, tachyarrhythmias, and, in a few patients, paradoxical exacerbation of heart block and precipitation of Adams-Stokes attacks. Isoproterenol is now listed as a Pregnancy Category C drug, to be used during pregnancy only if clearly needed. It should be used with caution in nursing mothers.

KENALOG (triamcinolone acetonide) Squibb
The 0.025% ointment is no longer available in 60-g tubes.

LARGON (propiomazine hydrochloride) Wyeth
This sedative-hypnotic is no longer supplied in cartridge-needle units (Tubex).

NAPROSYN (naproxen) Syntex
Now available as an orange/pineapple-flavored suspension containing 125 mg of naproxen per 5 ml; a measuring cup is supplied with the suspension. The recommended dosage for adults with rheumatoid arthritis, osteoarthritis, or ankylosing spondylitis is 10–20 ml (2–4 tsp) bid (morning and evening); for acute gout, 30 ml (6 tsp) to start, followed by 10 ml (2 tsp) q8h until attack has subsided; and for mild-to-moderate pain, primary dysmenorrhea, and acute tendinitis and bursitis, 20 ml (4 tsp) to start, followed by 10 ml (2 tsp) q6–8h, as needed.

Patients with rheumatoid arthritis, osteoarthritis, and ankylosing spondylitis who tolerate lower doses well may now be given up to 1,500 mg/day for limited periods. Such patients should be observed to ensure that the clinical benefit obtained justifies the potential increased risk of adverse reactions.

Naproxen is also now indicated for juvenile rheumatoid arthritis. The recommended dosage is 5 mg/kg bid. Children weighing 13 kg should be given 2.5 ml (½ tsp) of the suspension bid; those weighing 25 kg, 5 ml (1 tsp) bid; and those weighing 38 kg, 7.5 ml (1½ tsp) bid. The scored 250-mg tablets may also be used to approximate the daily dose. Safety and effectiveness in children under the age of 2 yr have not been established.

Because the plasma fraction of naproxen that is unbound is increased in the elderly and in patients with chronic alcoholic liver disease and probably other forms of cirrhosis, the manufacturer now recommends using the lowest effective dose in these patients. It is also recommended that ophthalmic studies be carried out if any change or disturbance in vision occurs. The sodium content of the suspension (20 mg/ml) should be taken into consideration in treating patients whose sodium intake must be restricted.

NORLESTRIN (norethindrone acetate and ethinyl estradiol) Parke-Davis

Hemolytic uremic syndrome has been associated with use of oral contraceptives, but no causal relationship has been established. A new regimen starting on Sunday has been added, in which a patient begins taking light-colored tablets on the first Sunday after menstrual flow begins (if menstrual flow begins on Sunday, the first tablet is taken that day); all the light-colored pills are taken in 21 days, followed by a seven-day period in which no pills are taken or the iron pills or placebos are taken, depending on the dispenser used. The next course then resumes on a Sunday.

NORLUTIN (norethindrone) Parke-Davis

Concomitant administration of rifampin may decrease the efficacy of norethindrone and increase the incidence of breakthrough bleeding.

PEPCID (famotidine) Merck Sharp & Dohme

Now available as a cherry/banana/mint-flavored oral suspension containing 40 mg of famotidine per 5 ml after constitution; this suspension may be substituted for Pepcid tablets in patients who have difficulty swallowing solid medications. The recommended adult dosage for duodenal ulcer is 40 mg (5 ml), given once daily at bedtime, or 20 mg (2.5 ml), given twice daily; for maintenance therapy, give 20 mg (2.5 ml) once daily at bedtime. For pathological hypersecretory conditions, give 20 mg every 6 hours to start, up to 160 mg every 6 hours.

PRED FORTE/PRED MILD (prednisolone acetate) Allergan

The 1.0% suspension is now available in 1-ml dropper bottles. In cases of accidental ingestion, instruct patient to drink fluids. Safety and effectiveness for use in children have not been established; guidelines for pediatric use have been deleted. Classified as Pregnancy Category C; use during pregnancy only if the expected benefits justify the potential risk to the fetus. Use with caution in nursing women.

PROVENTIL Solution for Inhalation (albuterol) Schering

This selective beta$_2$-adrenergic bronchodilator is now available as a nebulizer solution for *relief of bronchospasm* in patients with reversible obstructive airway disease and *acute attacks of bronchospasm;* available as a 0.5% solution in 20-ml bottles and as a 0.083%-solution in 3-ml unit-dose bottles. Recommended dosage for adults and children over 12 yr of age: 2.5 mg administered 3–4 times/day by nebulization, continued, as needed, to control recurring bronchospastic episodes.

ROFERON-A (interferon alfa-2a, recombinant) Roche

Now available as a sterile powder in 3-ml vials containing 18 million IU of interferon alfa-2a (6 million IU/ml after reconstitution). Decreases in serum estradiol and progesterone levels have been seen in women given human leukocyte interferon.

SELDANE (terfenadine) Merrell Dow

Confusion, arrhythmias, rash, urticaria, and pruritus have been reported. Signs and symptoms of overdosage include headache, nausea, and confusion, with torsades de pointes followed by ventricular fibrillation; for treatment, remove unabsorbed drug, institute appropriate symptomatic and supportive measures, and monitor cardiac function for at least 24 h.

TAGAMET (cimetidine) Smith Kline & French

Now available in 2-ml single-dose ADD-Vantage vials containing 300 mg of cimetidine; indications and dosage remain the same.

THORAZINE (chlorpromazine hydrochloride) Smith Kline & French

No longer indicated for nonpsychotic anxiety.

VENTOLIN Solution for Inhalation (albuterol) Glaxo

This selective beta$_2$-adrenergic bronchodilator is now available as a nebulizer solution for *relief of bronchospasm* in patients with reversible obstructive airway disease and *acute attacks of bronchospasm;* available as a 0.5% solution in 20-ml bottles. Recommended dosage for adults and children over 12 yr of age: 2.5 mg administered 3–4 times/day by nebulization, continued, as needed, to control recurring bronchospastic episodes.

VEPESID (etoposide) Bristol-Myers Oncology

Now available in 50-mg capsules for oral administration in cases of small-cell lung carcinoma. Recommended oral dosage for adults is 70 mg/m^2/day, given for 4 days, to 100 mg/m^2/day, given for 5 days, every 3–4 wk with other appropriate therapy after adequate recovery from toxicity. Dosage should be modified by taking the myelosuppressive effects of concomitantly used drugs and prior chemotherapy or irradiation into consideration. Etoposide is mutagenic and genotoxic in mammalian cells. New adverse reactions have been reported, particularly hematological effects.

VERSED (midazolam hydrochloride) Roche

When using midazolam for conscious sedation prior to diagnostic studies or endoscopy, start with 2–2.5 mg (0.035 mg/kg), injected IV over a 2- to 3-min period; if necessary, small increments in dosage may be given after 1–2 min until speech becomes slurred. Elderly, debilitated, or chronically ill patients should be given approximately 1–1.5 mg to start; reduce the rate of injection and decrease the size of any dosage increments in these patients, since the risk of underventilation and apnea is increased and the peak effect of the drug may be delayed. Patients who are elderly or chronically ill or who have been given other cardiorespiratory depressants simultaneously may suffer serious or even fatal cardiorespiratory reactions if the dose used for conscious sedation is excessive, given rapidly, or administered as a single bolus. If narcotics or other CNS depressants are given concomitantly, reduce the dosage of midazolam by about 25–30% for patients who are healthy and by 50–60% for debilitated, chronically ill, or elderly patients (to facilitate titration, the drug solution may be diluted to 2–5 times the original volume with 0.9% sodium chloride or 5% dextrose in water). Monitor patient response continuously for early signs of hypoventilation or apnea, since they may progress to hypoxia and/or cardiac arrest. Neurological reactions, including hyperactivity, combativeness, agitation, and involuntary movements (including muscle tremor and tonic/clonic movements) have been reported; should such reactions occur, exercise caution before continuing administration.

XANAX (alprazolam) Upjohn

To avoid withdrawal seizures, reduce the daily dose by not more than 0.5 mg every 3 days. For hypotension associated with overdosage, give a vasopressor. Concomitant use of alprazolam with imipramine may increase the plasma level of imipramine and its active metabolite, desipramine. Withdrawal reactions, flaccidity, and respiratory problems may occur in neonates whose mothers received benzodiazepines during pregnancy; avoid use during the first trimester (use during the second and third trimesters is not recommended).

ZANTAC Injection (ranitidine hydrochloride) Glaxo

Now available in 100-ml plastic containers containing 0.5 mg/ml of ranitidine hydrochloride (for IV infusion only); indications and dosage remain the same.

ANTIARRHYTHMICS

BREVIBLOC (esmolol hydrochloride) Du Pont Critical Care Rx

Ampuls: 250 mg/ml (10 ml)

INDICATIONS

Short-term treatment of **atrial fibrillation or atrial flutter** when rapid control of ventricular rate is indicated
Noncompensatory sinus tachycardia requiring specific intervention

PARENTERAL DOSAGE

Adult: 500 µg/kg/min by IV infusion for 1 min, followed by a maintenance infusion of 50 µg/kg/min over a period of 4 min; if an adequate response is not obtained within 5 min, give 500 µg/kg/min by IV infusion for 1 min, followed by a maintenance infusion of 100 µg/kg/min over a period of 4 min. Continue titration by repeating the loading infusion (500 µg/kg/min over 1 min) and increasing the maintenance infusion by increments of 50 µg/kg/min (for 4 min), up to 200 µg/kg/min; when the desired heart rate or safety end-point (eg, lowered blood pressure) is approached, omit the loading infusion, reduce the incremental dose in the maintenance infusion from 50 µg/kg/min to 25 µg/kg/min or lower, and increase the interval between titration steps from 5 to 10 min.

CONTRAINDICATIONS

Sinus bradycardia   Heart block greater than first degree   Cardiogenic shock
Overt heart failure

ADMINISTRATION/DOSAGE ADJUSTMENTS

Preparation of infusion	Aseptically remove 20 ml from a 500-ml container of 5% dextrose injection USP, 5% dextrose in Ringer's injection, 5% dextrose and 0.45% sodium chloride injection USP, 5% dextrose and 0.9% sodium chloride injection USP, lactated Ringer's injection USP, 0.45% sodium chloride injection USP, or 0.9% sodium chloride injection USP and add the contents of 2 ampuls to the remaining 480 ml, yielding a final concentration of 10 mg/ml. Esmolol is *not* compatible with 5% sodium bicarbonate injection USP.
Switching to alternative antiarrhythmics	Once the heart rate is adequately controlled and a stable clinical status has been achieved, the patient may be transferred to an alternative antiarrhythmic agent, such as propranolol, digoxin, or verapamil. Give the first dose of the alternative agent, wait 30 min, and then reduce the infusion rate of esmolol by 50%; esmolol may be discontinued following the second dose of the alternative agent if satisfactory control is maintained for the first hour. Recommended doses for alternative agents are: 10–20 mg of propranolol q4–6h, 0.125–0.5 mg of digoxin PO or IV, or 80 mg of verapamil q6h; however, carefully consider the labeling instructions for the alternative agent.
Concomitant use of other agents	Titrate the dose of esmolol with caution in patients being treated concurrently with digoxin, morphine, succinylcholine, or warfarin

WARNINGS/PRECAUTIONS

Hypotension	In clinical trials, hypotension (systolic pressure < 90 mm Hg and/or diastolic pressure < 50 mm Hg) has occurred in 20–50% of patients; approximately 12% of patients have experienced symptoms, mainly diaphoresis or dizziness. Although hypotension may occur at any dose, it has proven to be dose-related; doses beyond 200 µg/kg/min are therefore not recommended. Closely monitor patients, especially if the blood pressure was low prior to treatment; hypotension may be reversed within 30 min by decreasing the dose or discontinuing the infusion.
Cardiac failure	Beta blockade may further depress myocardial contractility and precipitate more severe failure; continued myocardial depression by beta-blocking agents may, over time, lead to cardiac failure. Reduce dosage or withdraw esmolol at the first sign or symptom of impending cardiac failure; more specific treatment may be needed if withdrawal is not sufficient (see OVERDOSAGE).
Patients with bronchospastic disease	In general, patients with bronchospastic disease should not receive beta blockers. However, esmolol may be used with caution in these patients because of its relative selectivity for beta$_1$ receptors. For these patients, esmolol should be given at the lowest possible effective dose; if bronchospasm occurs, discontinue the infusion immediately. A beta$_2$ agonist may be administered if indicated, but it should be used with particular caution, since patients already have rapid ventricular rates.
Diabetic patients	Beta blockade may mask certain manifestations of hypoglycemia, such as tachycardia; however, in most cases, symptomatic dizziness and sweating are not significantly affected. Use with caution in diabetics.
Patients with renal impairment	Use with caution in patients with impaired renal function
Venous irritation, thrombophlebitis	Because infusion concentrations of 20 mg/ml have been associated with more venous irritation and thrombophlebitis than have concentrations of 10 mg/ml, do not use a concentration greater than 10 mg/ml (see ADMINISTRATION/DOSAGE ADJUSTMENTS for instructions on preparing suitable infusions)
Carcinogenicity, mutagenicity, effect on fertility	No studies have been performed to evaluate the carcinogenic or mutagenic potential of esmolol or its effect, if any, on fertility

ADVERSE REACTIONS

Frequent reactions (incidence ≥ 1%) are printed in *italics*

Cardiovascular	*Asymptomatic hypotension (25%), symptomatic hypotension, including diaphoresis and dizziness (12%); peripheral ischemia (1%),* pallor, flushing, bradycardia (heart rate < 50 beats/min), chest pain, syncope, pulmonary edema, heart block; severe bradycardia/sinus pause/asystole (in two patients without supraventricular tachycardia but with serious coronary artery disease)
Central nervous system	*Dizziness, somnolence (3%); confusion, headache, agitation (2%); fatigue (1%);* paresthesia, asthenia, depression, abnormal thinking, anxiety, anorexia, lightheadedness; grand mal seizure (1 case)
Respiratory	Bronchospasm, wheezing, dyspnea, nasal congestion, rhonchi, rales
Gastrointestinal	*Nausea (7%), vomiting (1%),* dyspepsia, constipation, dry mouth, abdominal discomfort, taste perversion
Local	*Inflammation and induration at infusion site (8%),* edema, erythema, skin discoloration, burning at the infusion site
Other	Urinary retention, speech disorder, abnormal vision, midscapular pain, rigors, fever

OVERDOSAGE

Signs and symptoms	Marked bradycardia and hypotension, drowsiness
Treatment	Discontinue administration. For bradycardia, administer atropine or another anticholinergic drug IV. For bronchospasm, administer a beta$_2$ stimulating drug and/or a theophylline derivative. For cardiac failure, administer a diuretic and/or a digitalis glycoside IV; if shock results from inadequate cardiac contractility, administer dopamine, dobutamine, isoproterenol, or amrinone IV.

DRUG INTERACTIONS

Reserpine, other catecholamine-depleting drugs	⚠ Risk of marked bradycardia and hypotension; watch carefully for vertigo, syncope, and other manifestations of orthostatic hypotension
Morphine (IV), warfarin	⚠ Blood level of esmolol; although clinical significance is probably small, titrate esmolol dosage carefully if morphine or warfarin has been given
Digoxin (IV)	⚠ Plasma level of digoxin; although clinical significance is probably small, titrate esmolol dosage carefully if digoxin has been given
Succinylcholine	⚠ Duration of neuromuscular blockade; although clinical significance is probably small, titrate esmolol dosage carefully if succinylcholine has been given

ALTERED LABORATORY VALUES

No clinically significant alterations in blood/serum or urinary values occur at therapeutic dosages

USE IN CHILDREN

Safety and effectiveness for use in children have not been established

USE IN PREGNANT AND NURSING WOMEN

Pregnancy Category C: reproduction studies in rats and rabbits given esmolol at dosages up to 3,000 and 1,000 µg/kg/min IV, respectively, for 30 min/day have shown no evidence of maternal toxicity, embryotoxicity, or teratogenicity; however, dosages of 10,000 µg/kg/min IV given to rats for 30 min/day have produced maternal toxicity and lethality, and dosages of 2,500 µg/kg/min IV given to rabbits for 30 min/day have caused minimal maternal toxicity and increased fetal resorptions. No adequate, well-controlled studies have been performed in pregnant women; use during pregnancy only if the expected benefit justifies the potential risk to the fetus. It is not known whether esmolol is excreted in human milk; because many drugs are excreted in human milk, use with caution in nursing mothers.

ANTIARRHYTHMICS

ENKAID (encainide hydrochloride) Bristol   Rx

Capsules: 25, 35, 50 mg

INDICATIONS

Life-threatening ventricular arrhythmias, such as sustained ventricular tachycardia
Symptomatic, nonsustained ventricular tachycardia
Frequent premature ventricular complexes

ORAL DOSAGE

Adult: 25 mg q8h to start, followed by an increase to 35 mg tid after 3–5 days, if needed; if the desired response is not achieved after an additional 3–5 days, 50 mg tid may be given. For maintenance dosage, see ADMINISTRATION/DOSAGE ADJUSTMENTS. Do not give a loading dose or increase the dose rapidly.

ENKAID

CONTRAINDICATIONS

Preexisting second- or third-degree AV block

Hypersensitivity to encainide

Right bundle branch block associated with left hemiblock (bifascicular block), unless a pacemaker is present

Cardiogenic shock

ADMINISTRATION/DOSAGE ADJUSTMENTS

Limitations of treatment	The effects of encainide in patients with supraventricular arrhythmias and in patients with a recent acute myocardial infarction have not been adequately studied; encainide, like other antiarrhythmics, has not been shown to have a favorable effect on survival or sudden death
High-dose therapy	Occasionally, patients with ventricular ectopic activity may require up to 50 mg qid to achieve the desired therapeutic response; higher doses are not normally recommended. However, if careful dosage titration up to 50 mg tid has failed in hospitalized patients with documented life-threatening arrhythmias, up to 75 mg qid may be given. Once the desired response is achieved, patients may be adequately maintained at doses lower than the maximum achieved during titration.
Maintenance therapy	Patients with malignant arrhythmias who have achieved an adequate therapeutic response as judged by objective criteria (eg, Holter monitoring, programmed electrical stimulation, exercise testing) may be maintained on chronic encainide therapy. Patients with arrhythmias well-controlled with dosages of 50 mg tid or less may be given the drug q12h to increase convenience and help assure compliance; during 12-h dosing, monitor patient to ensure that an adequate suppression of ventricular ectopy is maintained. The maximum single dose should not exceed 75 mg.
Hospitalization	Because of the relatively high frequency of arrhythmogenic events in patients with sustained ventricular tachycardia, therapy should be initiated in the hospital to permit close clinical observation and ECG monitoring. Hospitalization is also advisable for other patients at risk of proarrhythmia, including patients with symptomatic congestive heart failure, cardiomyopathy, sinus node dysfunction, or nonsustained ventricular tachycardia (depending on cardiac status and underlying cardiac disease), and when dosages are increased to 200 mg/day or above.
Timing of dosage adjustments	Allow 3–5 days between dosing increments, since this interval will allow all patients to achieve steady-state blood levels of encainide and its active metabolites before the dosage is increased and will help avoid use of unnecessarily high doses, which may increase the risk of proarrhythmic events.
Patients with hepatic impairment	Patients with hepatic impairment eliminate encainide more slowly, probably due to a decreased rate of metabolism; although there are insufficient data to be certain about the need for altering the dose and/or dosing intervals in these patients, increase doses cautiously.
Patients with renal impairment	Because significant accumulation of encainide and its active metabolites can occur in patients with severe renal impairment (serum creatinine > 3.5 mg/dl or creatinine clearance < 20 ml/min), give 25 mg/day to start, followed, if necessary after 7 days, by 25 mg bid, and then 35 mg tid after an additional 7 days, if indicated; do not exceed a dosage of 150 mg/day. If renal function deteriorates significantly, consider reducing the dosage.
Transferring patients from other antiarrhythmic agents	Allow at least 2–4 plasma half-lives to elapse for the drug being discontinued before starting encainide therapy; when withdrawal of a previous antiarrhythmic agent may produce life-threatening arrhythmias, consider hospitalization of the patient

WARNINGS/PRECAUTIONS

Proarrhythmia	Encainide can cause new arrhythmias or worsen existing arrhythmias, ranging from an increased frequency of premature ventricular contractions to development of more severe and potentially fatal ventricular tachycardia (eg, tachycardia that is more sustained or resistant to conversion to sinus rhythm). Provocation or aggravation of existing arrhythmias occurred most frequently in patients with a history of sustained ventricular tachycardia, cardiomyopathy, congestive heart failure, or sustained ventricular tachycardia with cardiomyopathy or congestive heart failure. Proarrhythmic events have occurred most commonly during the first week of therapy, and have been much more common at doses exceeding 200 mg/day; the risk of proarrhythmia is reduced when therapy is initiated at 75 mg/day and doses are adjusted gradually.
Congestive heart failure	New or worsened congestive heart failure has occurred infrequently during encainide therapy; use with caution in patients with congestive heart failure or congestive cardiomyopathy
Hepatic impairment	Elevated alkaline phosphatase and serum transaminase levels, jaundice, and hepatitis have been reported rarely during encainide therapy; although no causal relationship has been established, use with caution in patients who develop unexplained jaundice or signs of hepatic dysfunction and, if indicated, discontinue therapy
Sick sinus syndrome	Encainide may cause sinus bradycardia, sinus pause, or sinus arrest in patients with sick sinus syndrome; use with extreme caution in such patients
Potassium imbalance	Hypokalemia or hyperkalemia may alter the effects of Class I antiarrhythmic drugs; correct any preexisting potassium imbalance before instituting encainide therapy
Diabetic patients	Elevated blood glucose levels or increased insulin requirements have been reported rarely during encainide therapy; although no causal relationship has been established, use with caution in patients with hyperglycemia and, if indicated, discontinue use

ENKAID

ECG changes	Encainide slows conduction and produces dose-related changes in the P-R and QRS intervals, which increase linearly at doses ranging from 30 to 225 mg/day. The J-T interval does not change consistently; the Q-Tc interval increases, but only to the extent of the QRS interval increase. These ECG changes do not in themselves, indicate effectiveness, toxicity, or overdosage, nor can they routinely be used to predict efficacy. Sinus bradycardia, sinus pause, or sinus arrest has occurred in 1% of patients; prolongation of the QRS interval $\geq$ 20 s has been experienced by about 7% of patients; and second- or third-AV block has occurred in 0.5% and 0.2% of patients, respectively.
Carcinogenicity	Studies in rats and mice fed doses up to 300 mg/kg/day and 135 mg/kg/day, respectively, have found no drug-related increase in tumor incidence
Mutagenicity	The results of bacterial and mammalian mutagenicity tests conducted with encainide have been negative
Impairment of fertility	Studies in male and female rats simultaneously fed 28 mg/kg/day of encainide prior to mating showed a reduction in fertility; however, no reduction was evident when each sex was treated separately with the same dose

ADVERSE REACTIONS

Frequent reactions (incidence $\geq$ 1%) are printed in *italics*

Cardiovascular	*Palpitations, ventricular tachycardia, prolonged QRS interval ($\geq$ 0.20 s), congestive heart failure, syncope,* premature ventricular contractions, increased or decreased blood pressure
Gastrointestinal	*Nausea, constipation, diarrhea, dyspepsia, abdominal pain, dry mouth, anorexia, taste perversion, vomiting,* elevated alkaline phosphatase, SGOT, and SGPT levels, hepatitis, and jaundice (rare)
Central nervous system	*Dizziness, asthenia, insomnia, nervousness, headache, upper/lower extremity pain, paresthesia, somnolence,* tremor, pain, confusion, ataxia, abnormal gait, abnormal sensation, abnormal dreams
Respiratory	*Dyspnea, chest pain,* increased cough
Dermatological	*Rash*
Ophthalmic	*Abnormal/blurred vision,* diplopia, photophobia, periorbital edema
Metabolic	Elevated blood glucose levels or increased insulin requirements in diabetic patients

OVERDOSAGE

Signs and symptoms	Excessive widening of the QRS complex and Q-T interval, AV dissociation, hypotension, bradycardia, asystole, conduction disturbances, convulsions
Treatment	Empty stomach contents by gastric lavage and then administer activated charcoal. Hypertonic sodium bicarbonate may be useful in managing cardiac toxicity. Patient should be hospitalized and provided with cardiac monitoring and advanced life-support systems. Supportive measures may be necessary.

DRUG INTERACTIONS

Other antiarrhythmic agents, drugs affecting cardiac conduction (diuretics, beta blockers, calcium channel blockers)	△ Pharmacologic effects of encainide (theoretically); exercise caution
Cimetidine	△ Plasma level of encainide and its active metabolites; exercise caution when using encainide in combination with cimetidine, and reduce the dosage of cimetidine when instituting encainide therapy

ALTERED LABORATORY VALUES

Blood/serum values	△ Alkaline phosphatase △ SGOT △ SGPT △ Glucose

No clinically significant alterations in urinary values occur at therapeutic dosages

---

USE IN CHILDREN

Safety and effectiveness for use in children under 18 yr of age have not been established

USE IN PREGNANT AND NURSING WOMEN

Pregnancy Category B: reproduction studies performed in rats and rabbits at doses up to 13 and 9 times the average human dose of encainide, respectively, have revealed no fetal harm. No adequate, well-controlled studies have been performed in pregnant women; use during pregnancy only if clearly needed. Encainide is excreted in the milk of laboratory animals and has been reported in human milk. Decreased pup weight has been observed in rodent studies at doses of 28 mg/kg/day; no other overt postnatal effects have been observed. However, the potential for serious adverse effects in nursing infants from encainide is unknown. Patient should not nurse while taking this drug.

ANTIHYPERTENSIVE AGENTS

TENEX (guanfacine hydrochloride) Robins   Rx

Tablets: 1 mg

INDICATIONS	**ORAL DOSAGE**
Hypertension in patients who are already receiving a thiazide-type diuretic	**Adult:** 1 mg/day, given at bedtime, to start; if satisfactory results are not obtained after 3–4 wk of therapy, doses of 2 mg and then 3 mg may be given. If a rise in blood pressure occurs toward the end of the dosing interval, the daily dose may be divided.

CONTRAINDICATIONS

Hypersensitivity to guanfacine

ADMINISTRATION/DOSAGE ADJUSTMENTS

High-dose therapy	Although higher daily doses (up to 40 mg/day, given in divided doses) have been used rarely, adverse reactions increase significantly with doses above 3 mg/day with no increase in efficacy
Therapy with guanfacine alone	No studies have established an appropriate dose or dosing interval when guanfacine is given as the sole antihypertensive agent; therefore, use only in patients already receiving a thiazide-type diuretic

WARNINGS/PRECAUTIONS

Discontinuation of therapy	Caution patients against discontinuing therapy abruptly; increased plasma and urinary catecholamine levels, nervousness and anxiety, and, less commonly, increased blood pressure to a level significantly greater than that recorded prior to initiation of therapy may occur. Although the frequency of rebound hypertension is low, it may occur 2–4 days after discontinuation of the drug; in most cases, blood pressure returns to pretreatment levels slowly (within 2–4 days) with no untoward effects.
Mental impairment	Caution patients to be careful driving or engaging in other activities requiring mental alertness until it is determined that they do not become drowsy or dizzy while taking this drug, especially during initiation of therapy; patients should also be warned that their tolerance of alcohol and other CNS depressants may be diminished (see DRUG INTERACTIONS)
Special-risk patients	Use with caution in patients with severe coronary insufficiency, recent myocardial infarction, cerebrovascular disease, or chronic renal or hepatic failure
Drug abuse and dependence	Dependence and abuse have not been associated with use of this drug
Carcinogenicity, mutagenicity, effect on fertility	No evidence of carcinogenicity has been observed in mice given doses more than 150 times the maximum recommended human dose for 78 wk or in rats given more than 100 times the maximum recommended human dose for 102 wk; guanfacine has shown no evidence of mutagenicity in a variety of test models. Fertility studies in male and female rats have shown no impairment of fertility.

ADVERSE REACTIONS[1]

The most frequent reactions, regardless of incidence, are printed in *italics*

Central nervous system, neuromuscular	*Weakness/asthenia, dizziness, headache, insomnia, fatigue, somnolence,* amnesia, confusion, depression, malaise, paresthesia, leg cramps, hypokinesia, paresis
Gastrointestinal	*Constipation,* abdominal pain, diarrhea, dyspepsia, dysphagia, nausea
Cardiovascular	Bradycardia, palpitations, substernal pain
Ophthalmic	Conjunctivitis, iritis, vision disturbance
Respiratory	Dyspnea
Dermatological	Dermatitis, pruritus, purpura, sweating
Genitourinary	Impotence (with doses of 3 mg/day), decreased libido, testicular disorder, urinary incontinence
Other	*Dry mouth,* rhinitis, taste perversion, tinnitus

OVERDOSAGE

Signs and symptoms	Severe drowsiness, bradycardia (45 beats/min)
Treatment	Empty stomach by gastric lavage, and administer 0.8 mg of isoproterenol by infusion over 12 h

DRUG INTERACTIONS

Alcohol, phenothiazines, barbiturates, benzodiazepines, and other CNS depressants	⬔ CNS depression

ALTERED LABORATORY VALUES

No clinically significant alterations in blood/serum or urinary values occur at therapeutic dosages

USE IN CHILDREN

Safety and effectiveness for use in children under 12 yr of age have not been established; use of guanfacine in this age group is not recommended

USE IN PREGNANT AND NURSING WOMEN

Pregnancy Category B: studies in rats and rabbits given 70 and 20 times the maximum recommended human dose, respectively, have shown no evidence of impaired fertility or fetal harm; higher doses (100 and 200 times the maximum recommended human dose in rabbits and rats, respectively) have resulted in reduced fetal survival and maternal toxicity. Guanfacine crosses the placental barrier. Use of this drug is not recommended for treatment of acute hypertension associated with toxemia of pregnancy. No adequate, well-controlled studies have been performed in pregnant women; use during pregnancy only if clearly needed. Guanfacine is excreted in the milk of lactating rats. It is not known whether this drug is excreted in human milk; because many drugs are excreted in human milk, use with caution in nursing mothers.

[1] Most reactions are mild and disappear with continued administration; reasons for dropouts among subjects enrolled in clinical trials included somnolence, headache, weakness, dry mouth, dizziness, impotence, insomnia, constipation, syncope, urinary incontinence, conjunctivitis, paresthesia, dermatitis, confusion, depression, palpitations, nausea, orthostatic hypotension, and nightmares.

ANTIVIRAL AGENTS

RETROVIR (zidovudine) Burroughs Wellcome   Rx

Capsules: 100 mg

INDICATIONS

Management of certain adult patients with **symptomatic HIV infection** (AIDS and advanced AIDS-related complex [ARC]) who have a history of cytologically confirmed *Pneumocystis carinii* pneumonia or an absolute peripheral T4 (CD4) lymphocyte count of less than 200/mm^3

ORAL DOSAGE

Adult: 200 mg q4h (including at night) to start

CONTRAINDICATIONS

Potentially life-threatening allergic reaction to any component

WARNINGS/PRECAUTIONS

Hematological toxicity — **Description:** Zidovudine can cause severe anemia and granulocytopenia in a significant proportion of patients. A reduction in hemoglobin (Hb) level may occur as early as 2–4 wk after the start of therapy, with significant anemia developing after 4–6 wk. Granulocytopenia usually occurs after 6–8 wk. The risk appears to be directly related to dose and duration of therapy and inversely proportional to pretreatment T4 lymphocyte count, Hb level, and granulocyte count. The frequency of severe anemia in patients with initial T4 lymphocyte counts of 200/mm^3 or less was 30% when judged by an absolute Hb level of less than 7.5 g/dl and 45% when judged by a reduction of more than 25% from the initial Hb level; the corresponding frequencies in patients with higher initial T4 lymphocyte counts were 3% and 10%, respectively. The frequency of severe granulocytopenia in the former group was 47% as determined by a granulocyte count of less than 750/mm^3 and 55% as determined by a reduction of more than 50% from the initial baseline level; the corresponding frequencies in patients with pretreatment T4 lymphocyte counts exceeding 200/mm^3 were 10% and 40%, respectively.

Prevention: Obtain blood counts at least every 2 wk for all patients. Use with extreme caution in patients with a granulocyte count of less than 1,000/mm^3 or a hemoglobin level of less than 9.5 g/dl.

Management: If the hemoglobin level decreases below 7.5 mg/dl or by more than 25% or if the granulocyte count drops below 750/mm^3 or by more than 50%, it may be necessary to discontinue therapy until some evidence of bone marrow recovery is seen; for treatment of significant anemia, blood transfusions may also be required. If less severe anemia or granulocytopenia develops, a reduction in dosage may be adequate; once bone marrow recovery occurs, the dose may be gradually increased, depending on clinical and hematological response.

Safety and efficacy — Careful studies have only been done in patients who were seriously ill and received this drug for a limited period; the full safety and effectiveness of this drug has not been determined, especially for long-term use or patients with less advanced disease

Patients with renal or hepatic disorders — No data on use in patients with functional renal or hepatic impairment is currently available; however, since zidovudine is metabolized in the liver and eliminated mainly by the kidney, there may be a greater risk of toxicity when this drug is used in these patients

RETROVIR

Opportunistic infections	Zidovudine does not eliminate the risk of opportunistic infections or other types of infection associated with AIDS or ARC
Carcinogenicity, mutagenicity	An in vitro mammalian cell transformation assay has shown zidovudine to be carcinogenic at concentrations of 0.5 g/ml and higher. (In patients given 250 mg q4h, the trough plasma level is 0.16 μg/ml and the peak plasma level is 0.62 μg/ml.) No evidence of mutagenicity has been found in the Ames *Salmonella* test; however, the drug has been shown to be weakly mutagenic in cultured mouse lymphoma cells, and structural chromosomal abnormalities have been detected in cultured human lymphocytes at concentrations of 3 μg/ml and higher, but not at 0.3 or 1 μg/ml. In vivo, no effect on chromosome number or structure has been seen in rats given single IV doses of 37.5–300 mg/kg, despite peak plasma levels reaching as high as 453 μg/ml 5 min after injection.
Effect on fertility	The effect of zidovudine on fertility has not been studied
Patient information	Patients should be advised that treatment with zidovudine will not cure AIDS or ARC and that they may continue to develop opportunistic infections and other complications of HIV infection. The importance of taking this drug exactly as prescribed, every 4 h around the clock, even if it interferes with sleep, should be emphasized, as well as the importance of seeking medical attention for any change in health. Patients should be informed about the hematological toxicity of zidovudine, the extreme importance of biweekly blood tests, the necessity to avoid such drugs as acetaminophen or aspirin, and, should toxicity occur, the possibility that dosage adjustments, discontinuation of therapy, and/or transfusions may be needed. Patients should also be advised that zidovudine therapy has not been shown to reduce the risk of transmission of HIV through sexual contact or blood contamination.

ADVERSE REACTIONS

Frequent reactions (incidence >5%) are printed in *italics*

Hematological	*Granulocytopenia and/or anemia* (see warning, above, regarding hematological toxicity)
Gastrointestinal	*Nausea (46%), GI pain (20%), diarrhea (12%), anorexia (11%), vomiting (6%), dyspepsia (5%)*, constipation, dysphagia, eructation, flatulence, rectal hemorrhage
Central nervous system	*Headache (42%), asthenia (19%), somnolence and malaise (8%), paresthesias and dizziness (6%), insomnia (5%)*, anxiety, confusion, depression, emotional lability, nervousness, loss of mental acuity, vertigo, hyperalgesia, back or chest pain, hearing loss
Dermatological	*Rash (17%)*, acne, pruritus, urticaria
Musculoskeletal	*Myalgia (8%)*, arthralgia, muscle spasm, tremor, twitch
Respiratory	*Dyspnea (5%)*, cough, epistaxis, pharyngitis, rhinitis, sinusitis, hoarseness
Oral	*Perversion of taste (5%)*, edema of the lip or tongue, bleeding gums, mouth ulcer
Ophthalmic	Amblyopia, photophobia
Cardiovascular	Vasodilation, syncope
Urinary	Dysuria, polyuria, urinary frequency or hesitancy
Other	*Fever (16%), diaphoresis (5%)*, body odor, flu syndrome, lymphadenopathy

OVERDOSAGE

Signs and symptoms	No cases of overdose have been reported
Treatment	Watch carefully for evidence of bone marrow suppression; transfusions and other appropriate measures may be necessary. Although other nucleoside analogs have been partially removed from the blood by hemodialysis or peritoneal dialysis, it is not known whether these procedures would be effective in removing zidovudine.

DRUG INTERACTIONS

Drugs metabolized by glucuronidation, (eg, acetaminophen, aspirin, or indomethacin); nephrotoxic or cytotoxic drugs and agents that interfere with blood cell development or function (eg, dapsone, pentamidine, amphotericin B, flucytosine, vincristine, vinblastine, doxorubicin, or interferon)	⇧ Risk of zidovudine toxicity; avoid concomitant use
Experimental nucleoside analogs affecting DNA replication	⇩ Antiviral effect of zidovudine; avoid concomitant use

RETROVIR ■ CIBACALCIN

| Acyclovir | ⚠ Risk of neurotoxicity[1] |

ALTERED LABORATORY VALUES

| Blood/serum values | See warning, above, concerning hematological toxicity |
| Urinary values | No clinically significant alterations in urinary values occur at therapeutic dosages |

USE IN CHILDREN

Safety and effectiveness for use in children have not been established

---

USE IN PREGNANT AND NURSING WOMEN

Pregnant women: No evidence of harm to the fetus has been seen in rats given up to 20 times the human dose; however, other reproduction studies have not been completed. It is not known whether zidovudine can cause harm to the human fetus. Use during pregnancy only if clearly needed. **Nursing mothers:** It is not known whether zidovudine is excreted in human milk; because of the potential for serious adverse reactions in nursing infants, women should not nurse during therapy.

---

[1] One case of seizures and one case of profound lethargy have been reported following concomitant use; however, in controlled studies, no increase in acyclovir-related neurotoxicity has occurred

---

BONE/CALCIUM METABOLISM REGULATORS

CIBACALCIN (calcitonin-human) CIBA   Rx

Syringes (double-chambered): 0.5 mg, with 1-ml of mannitol and water for injection in separate chamber

INDICATIONS

Symptomatic Paget's disease of bone

PARENTERAL DOSAGE

Adult: 0.5 mg/day SC to start; sufficient improvement in some cases may occur with 0.5 mg given 2–3 times weekly or 0.25 mg/day. For severe cases (eg, evidence of mechanically weak bones with osteolytic lesions), up to 0.5 mg bid may be given. Adjust dosage according to clinical and radiologic evidence, as well as changes in serum alkaline phosphatase levels and urinary hydroxyproline excretion.

CONTRAINDICATIONS

None known

ADMINISTRATION/DOSAGE ADJUSTMENTS

Paget's disease	In patients with moderate to severe disease, characterized by multiple bone involvement and elevated serum alkaline phosphatase and urinary hydroxyproline levels, calcitonin has been shown to subjectively relieve bone pain and tenderness and reduce elevated skin temperature over affected skeletal areas in some patients
Monitoring of therapy	Determine serum alkaline phosphatase level and urinary hydroxyproline excretion prior to initiation of therapy, during the first 3 mo, and at 3- to 6-mo intervals during chronic treatment. Although reduction of serum alkaline phosphatase and urinary hydroxyproline levels usually occurs within 3 mo of treatment initiation, maximum reductions may not occur until after 6–24 mo of continuous treatment.
Duration of therapy	Continue treatment for 6 mo; if symptoms have been relieved, discontinue therapy until symptoms or radiologic signs recur. However, biochemical parameters will relapse after discontinuation of therapy and should not be relied upon as the basis for reinitiation of therapy.
Administration	This product is primarily intended for patient self-injection; carefully instruct patients in sterile-injection techniques. Reconstituted solution should be used within 6 h.
Adverse effects	Side effects, such as nausea and flushing, may be minimized by administration at bedtime and usually improve with continued therapy; if necessary, adjust dosage

WARNINGS/PRECAUTIONS

Systemic allergic reactions	The possibility of systemic allergic reactions to calcitonin should not be disregarded; institute appropriate emergency measures if hypersensitivity reactions occur
Osteogenic sarcoma	The incidence of osteogenic sarcoma is increased in patients with Paget's disease. Pagetic lesions, with or without therapy, may appear to progress markedly by x-ray examination, and some loss of definition of periosteal margins may be evident. Evaluate such lesions carefully to differentiate them from osteogenic sarcoma.
Hypocalcemic tetany	Calcitonin may cause hypocalcemic tetany under special circumstances; have parenteral calcium available during the first few administrations

COMPENDIUM OF DRUG THERAPY

CIBACALCIN ■ KEFLET

Carcinogenicity	No long-term studies have been performed to evaluate the carcinogenic potential of this drug

ADVERSE REACTIONS[1] Frequent reactions (incidence ≥ 1%) are printed in *italics*

Gastrointestinal	*Nausea, with or without vomiting (14–21%)*, anorexia, diarrhea, epigastric discomfort, abdominal pain
Dermatological, hypersensitivity	*Flushing of face, ears, or hands (16–21%)*, skin rash (rare)
Genitourinary	*Increased frequency of urination (5–10%)*
Other	Mild tetanic symptoms, chills, chest pressure, weakness, headache, tenderness of palms and soles, dizziness, nasal congestion, shortness of breath, metallic taste, and paresthesia (rare); asymptomatic mild hypercalcemia (one case)

OVERDOSAGE

No cases of human overdosage have been reported; no evidence of toxicity has been observed in animals given as much as 1,000 mg/kg in a single dose

DRUG INTERACTIONS

No clinically significant drug interactions have been identified

ALTERED LABORATORY VALUES

Blood/serum values	▽ Alkaline phosphatase ▽ Calcium
Urinary values	△ Sodium △ Phosphorus △ Calcium

USE IN CHILDREN

Human calcitonin has been used in children for the treatment of "juvenile Paget's disease"; however, safety and effectiveness for use in children have not been established

USE IN PREGNANT AND NURSING WOMEN

Pregnancy Category C: no animal reproduction studies have been performed with human calcitonin; however, a decrease in fetal birth weight has been observed in rabbits fed 14–56 times the recommended human dose, possibly due to the drug's metabolic effects on the mother (calcitonin does not cross the placental barrier). It is not known whether calcitonin can cause fetal harm or affect reproductive capacity in humans; use during pregnancy only if clearly needed. Calcitonin inhibits lactation in animals and, although it is unlikely that active calcitonin would be absorbed by a nursing infant, it is not known whether the drug is excreted in human milk; because many drugs are excreted in human milk, use with caution in nursing mothers.

[1] The adverse reaction rates listed here derive from studies that included a large proportion of patients with a history of unresponsiveness to nonhuman calcitonins; a number of these patients were unable to tolerate such preparations

---

CEPHALOSPORINS

KEFLET (cephalexin) Dista   Rx

Tablets: 250, 500 mg; 1 g

INDICATIONS

Respiratory tract infections caused by susceptible strains of *Streptococcus pneumoniae* and Group A beta-hemolytic streptococci
Bone infections caused by susceptible strains of staphylococci and/or *Proteus mirabilis*
Genitourinary tract infections caused by susceptible strains of *Escherichia coli, Proteus mirabilis,* and *Klebsiella*
Skin and skin structure infections caused by susceptible strains of staphylococci and/or streptococci

Otitis media caused by susceptible strains of *Streptococcus pneumoniae, Hemophilus influenzae,* staphylococci, streptococci, and *Neisseria catarrhalis*

ORAL DOSAGE

Adult: for streptococcal pharyngitis, uncomplicated cystitis in patients over 15 yr of age, and skin and skin-structure infections, 500 mg q12h; for other infections, 250 mg q6h. Dosages of up to 4 g/day may be necessary for infections that are more severe or are caused by less susceptible organisms; if a dosage exceeding 4 g/day is required, parenteral cephalosporin therapy should be considered.
Infant and child: 25–50 mg/kg/day, given in 2 divided doses q12h (for streptoccocal pharyngitis in patients over 1 yr of age and for skin and skin-structure infections) or given in 4 divided doses (for other infections); dosage may be doubled for severe infections

Infant and child: 75–100 mg/kg/day, given in 4 divided doses

CONTRAINDICATIONS

Hypersensitivity to cephalosporins

KEFLET ■ METRODIN

ADMINISTRATION/DOSAGE ADJUSTMENTS

Duration of treatment	Cystitis should be treated for 7–14 days and infections caused by beta-hemolytic streptococci for at least 10 days

WARNINGS/PRECAUTIONS

Cross-allergenicity	Use with caution in penicillin-allergic patients
Hypersensitivity	Serious anaphylactic reactions may occur, most likely in patients with a history of allergy, necessitating administration of epinephrine, pressor amines, antihistamines, or corticosteroids
Pseudomembranous colitis	May occur due to alteration of the normal intestinal flora and should be considered in any patient who develops diarrhea during or after therapy. Mild cases may respond to withdrawal of the drug alone. Moderate to severe cases should be managed by sigmoidoscopy, appropriate bacteriological studies, fluid and electrolyte replacement, and protein supplementation, as needed. Oral vancomycin is the treatment of choice for severe or refractory colitis associated with the overgrowth of *Clostridium difficile*; however, other possible causes should also be considered.
Superinfection	Overgrowth of nonsusceptible organisms may occur with prolonged use; careful clinical observation is essential
Special-risk patients	Patients with markedly impaired renal function should be carefully monitored during therapy, as lower than usual dosage may be required; use with caution in patients with a history of GI disease, particularly colitis

ADVERSE REACTIONS

Frequent reactions (incidence ≥ 1%) are printed in *italics*

Gastrointestinal	*Diarrhea,* dyspepsia, abdominal pain, pseudomembranous colitis; nausea and vomiting (rare)
Hepatic	Slight increase in SGOT and SGPT levels; transient hepatitis and cholestatic jaundice (rare)
Hypersensitivity	Rash, urticaria, angioedema, anaphylaxis; erythema multiforme, Stevens-Johnson syndrome, and toxic epidermal necrolysis (rare)
Renal	Reversible interstitial nephritis (rare)
Genitourinary	Genital and anal pruritus, genital moniliasis, vaginitis, vaginal discharge
Central nervous system	Dizziness, fatigue, headache
Hematological	Eosinophilia, neutropenia, thrombocytopenia

OVERDOSAGE

Signs and symptoms	See ADVERSE REACTIONS
Treatment	Discontinue medication; treat symptomatically and institute supportive measures, as required

DRUG INTERACTIONS

Probenecid	⇧ Cephalexin blood level and/or toxicity

ALTERED LABORATORY VALUES

Blood/serum values	⇧ Alkaline phosphatase ⇧ SGOT ⇧ SGPT + Coombs' test
Urinary values	⇧ Glucose (with Clinitest tablets)

USE IN CHILDREN

See INDICATIONS; adjust dosage according to body weight and severity of infection

USE IN PREGNANT AND NURSING WOMEN

Pregnancy Category B: use during pregnancy only if clearly needed. Reproduction studies in mice and rats have shown no adverse effects on fertility, fetal viability, fetal weight, or litter size; however, the safety of cephalexin has not been established in pregnant women. Although enhanced toxicity has not been observed in newborn or weanling rats, clinical studies have not ruled out the possibility of harm. Positive Coombs' tests have been reported in newborns of mothers who received cephalosporins prior to delivery. Cephalexin is excreted in human milk; use with caution in nursing mothers.

FERTILITY INDUCERS

METRODIN (urofollitropin) Serono   Rx

Ampuls: 75 IU follicle-stimulating hormone (FSH); for IM use only

INDICATIONS

Induction of ovulation in patients with polycystic ovarian disease who have an elevated LH/FSH ratio and have failed to respond to adequate clomiphene therapy

PARENTERAL DOSAGE

Adult: 75 IU/day IM for 7–12 days, followed, when sufficient follicular maturation has occurred, by 5,000–10,000 USP units of human chorionic gonadotropin (hCG) 1 day after the last dose. If there are signs of ovulation, but pregnancy does not ensue, repeat the same course at least twice before increasing the dosage to 150 IU/day. If necessary, repeat the higher-dosage course twice. If inadequate follicle development is indicated by estrogen and/or ultrasound measurement, urofollitropin administration may exceed 12 days.

CONTRAINDICATIONS

Elevated levels of *both* LH and FSH, indicating primary ovarian failure	Overt thyroid or adrenal dysfunction	Organic intracranial lesion (eg, pituitary tumor)
Infertility not caused by anovulation	Abnormal bleeding of undetermined origin	Ovarian cysts or enlargement not due to polycystic ovary syndrome
Pregnancy		

ADMINISTRATION/DOSAGE ADJUSTMENTS

Pretreatment evaluation	Document anovulation; rule out endometrial carcinoma (particularly in older patients), uterine and tubal pathology, primary ovarian failure, and early pregnancy; evaluate the male partner's fertility potential
Monitoring of therapy	Follicular growth and development may be monitored by ultrasonography, increases in serum and 24-h urinary estrogen levels, and changes in vaginal and cervical smears; when examining cervical mucus, note volume, appearance, and spinnbarkeit and look for ferning. For confirmation of ovulation, watch for the following: (1) increases in basal body temperature and urinary pregnanediol level, (2) change in the cervical mucus from a fern pattern to a cellular pattern, (3) vaginal cytology characteristic of the luteal phase, and (4) menstruation after the shift in basal body temperature.
Preparation of parenteral solution and IM administration	Reconstitute with sterile saline solution, using 1–2 ml per ampul; administer IM immediately, and discard any unused reconstituted material

WARNINGS/PRECAUTIONS

Ovarian overstimulation	Mild to moderate uncomplicated ovarian enlargement, possibly with abdominal distention and/or pain, occurs in ~ 20% of patients and generally regresses without treatment in 2–3 wk. The hyperstimulation syndrome has occurred in 6% of patients given the recommended dose; this syndrome, characterized by sudden ovarian enlargement and ascites and sometimes accompanied by pain and/or pleural effusion, develops rapidly over a period of 3–4 days, generally within the first 2 wk following treatment. Excessive ovarian stimulation is most evident 7–10 days after ovulation. During therapy and the 2-wk period after hCG administration, examine all patients at least every other day for signs of overstimulation and perform appropriate tests and procedures (see "Monitoring of therapy," above). If the ovaries become abnormally enlarged or abdominal pain occurs, stop therapy and hospitalize the patient; for treatment of the hyperstimulation syndrome, see OVERDOSAGE.
Hemoperitoneum	During therapy, hemoperitoneum from ruptured ovarian cysts can occur, usually as a result of pelvic examination. If bleeding necessitates surgery, perform a partial resection of the enlarged ovary or ovaries. To lessen the danger of hemoperitoneum, instruct patients with significant postovulatory ovarian enlargement not to engage in intercourse
Multiple births	Before beginning treatment, advise patient and her husband of the frequency and potential hazards of multiple births; 17% of pregnancies following urofollitropin-hCG therapy have resulted in multiple births, including triplets and quintuplets
Arterial thromboembolism	Although there have been no such reports associated with urofollitropin therapy, arterial thromboembolism has been reported following menotropins therapy
Birth defects	In clinical studies of urofollitropin in infertile women, birth defects were seen in three completed pregnancies; however, these defects were not considered to be drug-related, and the incidence did not exceed that found in the general population[1]
Fever	Febrile reactions, possibly accompanied by chills, musculoskeletal aches or pain, malaise, and fatigue, have occurred after administration of urofollitropin; however, it is not clear whether they are pyrogenic responses or possible allergic reactions
Carcinogenicity	No long-term studies have been done to determine the carcinogenic potential of this preparation

ADVERSE REACTIONS[2]

Frequent reactions (incidence ≥ 1%) are printed in *italics*

Genitourinary	*Mild to moderate uncomplicated ovarian enlargement, possibly with abdominal distention and/or pain (~ 20%); hyperstimulation syndrome (10%):* sudden ovarian enlargement and ascites, possibly with pain and/or pleural effusion; ectopic pregnancy
Gastrointestinal	*Abdominal pain (10%),* nausea, vomiting, diarrhea, abdominal cramps, bloating
Dermatological, hypersensitivity	*Pain, rash, swelling, and/or irritation at injection site (10%),* dry skin, body rash, hair loss, urticaria
Central nervous system	Headache
Endocrinological	Breast tenderness
Other	Fever, birth defects[1]

OVERDOSAGE

Signs and symptoms	Hyperstimulation syndrome (see "Ovarian overstimulation," above)
Treatment	Stop therapy, hospitalize patient, and determine if hemoconcentration associated with fluid loss into the abdominal cavity has occurred by evaluating fluid intake and output, weight, hematocrit, serum and urinary electrolytes, and urine specific gravity daily or more often, if necessary. Treat symptomatically with bed rest, fluid and electrolyte replacement, and analgesics, as needed. *Do not remove ascitic fluid.*

DRUG INTERACTIONS

No clinically significant drug interactions have been identified

ALTERED LABORATORY VALUES

Blood/serum values — ⇧ Estrogen

Urinary values — ⇧ Estrogen ⇧ Estriol ⇧ Pregnanediol

USE IN CHILDREN
Not indicated for use in children

USE IN PREGNANT AND NURSING WOMEN
Pregnant women: Pregnancy Category X: urofollitropin is contraindicated for use during pregnancy. **Nursing mothers:** It is not known whether this drug is excreted in human milk; because many drugs are excreted in human milk, use with caution in nursing women.

---

[1] The following chromosomal abnormalities and congenital anomalies have been observed in clinical studies: one trisomy 13, one trisomy 18, one meningocele, one external ear defect, and one dislocated hip and ankle

[2] Arterial thromboembolism and hemoperitoneum have occurred during menotropins therapy, but have not been reported during trials with urofollitropin

---

MISCELLANEOUS ANTIBIOTICS

VANCOLED (vancomycin hydrochloride) Lederle Rx

Vials: 500 mg (10 ml)

INDICATIONS	ORAL DOSAGE	PARENTERAL DOSAGE
Enterocolitis caused by staphylococci **Antibiotic-associated pseudomembranous colitis (AAPC)** caused by *Clostridium difficile*	**Adult:** 0.5–2 g/day, given in 3–4 divided doses; for AAPC, administer for 7–10 days **Child:** 40 mg/kg/day, up to 2 g/day, given in 4 divided doses; for AAPC, administer for 7–10 days	
Serious or severe infections caused by susceptible strains of **methicillin-resistant staphylococci** **Serious or severe infections** caused by susceptible strains of **other staphylococci** when other anti-infectives, including penicillins and cephalosporins, are ineffective or contraindicated	—	**Adult:** 500 mg IV q6h or 1 g IV q12h **Neonate (0–7 days):** 15 mg/kg IV to start, followed by 10 mg/kg IV q12h **Neonate (8 days to 1 mo):** 15 mg/kg IV to start, followed by 10 mg/kg IV q8h **Infant (> 1 mo) and child:** 40 mg/kg/day, given IV in divided doses
Prevention of bacterial endocarditis in penicillin-allergic patients who have prosthetic heart valves or other particularly high-risk conditions and are undergoing **dental procedures or upper respiratory tract surgery or instrumentation**[1]	—	**Adult:** 1 g IV over a period of 1 h, beginning 1 h before the procedure **Child:** 20 mg/kg, up to 1 g, IV over a period of 1 h, beginning 1 h before the procedure
Prevention of bacterial endocarditis in penicillin-allergic patients at risk who are undergoing **GI or genitourinary tract surgery or instrumentation**[1]	—	**Adult:** 1 g IV over a period of 1 h, beginning 1 h before the procedure, plus 1.5 mg/kg gentamicin IM or IV 1 h before the procedure; these doses may be repeated once 8–12 h after the initial dose **Child:** 20 mg/kg, up to 1 g, IV over a period of 1 h, beginning 1 h before the procedure, plus 2 mg/kg gentamicin IM or IV 1 h before the procedure; these doses may be repeated once 8–12 h after the initial dose

CONTRAINDICATIONS

Hypersensitivity to vancomycin

ADMINISTRATION/DOSAGE ADJUSTMENTS

When used orally

Preparation of oral solution — To reconstitute the solution, add 1 fl oz of water to the vial. Solutions may be given orally (with common flavoring syrups) or via a nasogastric tube.

When used parenterally

VANCOLED

Staphylococcal infections	Vancomycin has been shown to be an effective antistaphylococcal agent in the treatment of endocarditis, septicemia, and infections of the bone, skin, skin structure, and lower respiratory tract. This drug may be given for *initial* therapy when methicillin-resistant staphylococci are suspected.
Nonstaphylococcal endocarditis	Vancomycin has been reported to be effective in the treatment of endocarditis caused by diphtheroids, enterococci such as *Streptococcus faecalis* (when used in combination with an aminoglycoside), viridans streptococci, and *Streptococcus bovis;* this drug has been used successfully in combination with rifampin, an aminoglycoside, or both agents to treat early-onset prosthetic valve endocarditis caused by *Streptococcus epidermidis* or diphtheroids
Preparation of IV solution	Add 10 ml of sterile water for injection to the 500-mg vial. Dilute solution with at least 100 ml of a compatible diluent. The following diluents are compatible with vancomycin: 5% dextrose injection USP, 0.9% sodium chloride injection USP, 5% dextrose injection and 0.9% sodium chloride injection USP, Isolyte E, lactated Ringer's injection USP, acetated Ringer's injection, and 5% dextrose injection with either lactated Ringer's injection or Normosol-M.
Intravenous administration	Adverse effects, including exaggerated hypotension, wheezing, dyspnea, urticaria, pruritus, flushing of the upper body ("red neck"), pain and spasm of the chest and back, and, in rare cases, cardiac arrest, can occur during or soon after IV infusion, particularly when the rate of administration is rapid; these effects usually disappear within 20 min after cessation of infusion, but they may persist for several hours. To minimize the risk of these reactions, administer each dose by slow IV infusion over a period of at least 60 min. Since concomitant administration of anesthetics reportedly increases this risk, infusion of vancomycin should be completed before induction of anesthesia. Inadvertent extravasation or IM injection may produce pain, tenderness, and necrosis; therefore, make sure that IV route is secure. To avoid thrombophlebitis, dilute solution (see "Preparation of solution") and rotate sites of infusion.
Obese patients	Adjustment of usual dosage may be necessary for patients who are obese
Elderly patients	A dosage adjustment will be necessary for elderly patients since GFR and renal function decrease with age; see recommendations for patients with renal impairment, below
Patients with renal impairment	If renal function is impaired, give an initial IV dose of at least 15 mg/kg. For maintenance of therapeutic plasma levels when the creatinine clearance is 10–100 ml/min, use the table below. For functionally anephric patients, a maintenance dose may be given every several days; the dose should be the equivalent of 1.9 mg/kg/24 h. If the patient is anuric, give 1 g every 7–10 days. Measurement of the plasma drug level can be helpful in determining the optimal dosage, especially when renal function is changing. Creatinine clearance can be estimated if the serum creatinine level is known and renal function is stable. For adult men, use the following formula: (weight [kg])(140 − age [yr])/(72) (serum creatinine level [mg/dl]); for adult women, multiply this quotient by 0.85. This formula should *not* be used if one of the following conditions is present: (1) shock, severe heart failure, oliguria, or other disorders associated with a progressive decline in renal function or (2) obesity, liver disease, edema, ascites, debilitation, malnutrition, inactivity, or other conditions in which the normal relationship between muscle mass and total body weight is distorted.

Creatinine clearance (ml/min)	Dosage (mg/24 h)	Creatinine clearance (ml/min)	Dosage (mg/24 h)
10	155	60	925
20	310	70	1,080
30	465	80	1,235
40	620	90	1,390
50	770	100	1,545

Measurement of plasma drug level	Microbiologic assay, RIA, HPLC, fluorescence immunoassay, or fluorescence polarization immunoassay may be used to measure the plasma level of vancomycin
Intrathecal administration	Safety and effectiveness of intralumbar or intraventricular administration have not been established

WARNINGS/PRECAUTIONS

When used orally

Risks of oral therapy	In general, vancomycin is poorly absorbed after oral administration; however, in some patients, the plasma drug level may be clinically significant and the systemic reactions seen with IV administration may develop. Renal function should be monitored serially in patients who are elderly, receiving aminoglycosides, or have renal impairment; serial tests of auditory function may be helpful in minimizing the risk of ototoxicity.

When used parenterally

Ototoxicity	Transient or permanent ototoxicity may occur, particularly in patients who are elderly, receiving excessive doses or ototoxic drugs, or have renal impairment or an underlying hearing loss; serial tests of auditory function may be helpful in minimizing the risk of ototoxicity

VANCOLED

Nephrotoxicity	Azotemia, characterized by increases in BUN or serum creatinine level, may occur, particularly in patients who are elderly, receiving aminoglycosides, or have renal impairment; azotemia is usually reversed by discontinuation of therapy. To minimize the risk of nephrotoxicity, monitor renal function serially in patients who are elderly, receiving aminoglycosides, or have renal impairment and carefully adhere to dosing schedules recommended for patients with renal dysfunction (see ADMINISTRATION/DOSAGE ADJUSTMENTS).
Neutropenia	Reversible neutropenia may develop, usually after a cumulative dose of 25 g has been given or after at least 1 wk of therapy has elapsed; periodically monitor WBC count in patients undergoing prolonged therapy or receiving other drugs associated with neutropenia

ADVERSE REACTIONS

Otic	Hearing loss, vertigo, dizziness, tinnitus
Renal	Azotemia
Hematological	Neutropenia, thrombocytopenia
Cardiovascular	Hypotension, flushing of the upper body, cardiac arrest
Respiratory	Wheezing, dyspnea
Musculoskeletal	Pain and muscle spasm of the chest and back
Other	Anaphylaxis, drug fever, chills, rash, urticaria, pruritus, thrombophlebitis at injection site

OVERDOSAGE

Signs and symptoms	See reactions associated with IV therapy
Treatment	Maintain renal function; institute other supportive measures. Hemoperfusion with Amberlite XAD-4 resin may be of limited benefit in removing vancomycin from the blood; the drug is poorly removed by dialysis.

DRUG INTERACTIONS

Aminoglycosides, amphotericin B, bacitracin, polymyxin B, colistin, viomycin, cisplatin	⇧ Risk of ototoxicity or nephrotoxicity; carefully monitor clinical response and appropriate parameters when vancomycin and any of these drugs is given sequentially or concomitantly
Anesthetics	⇧ Risk of adverse effects associated with IV infusion (see "Intravenous administration")

ALTERED LABORATORY VALUES

Blood/serum values	⇧ BUN ⇧ Creatinine

No clinically significant alterations in urinary values occur at therapeutic dosages

---

USE IN CHILDREN

See INDICATIONS and dosage recommendations; closely monitor plasma drug level in neonates and young infants given IV doses

USE IN PREGNANT AND NURSING WOMEN

Pregnancy Category C: reproduction studies have not been done; it is not known whether vancomycin can cause harm to the fetus or affect reproductive capacity. Use during pregnancy only if clearly needed. It is not known whether this drug is excreted in human milk; use with caution in nursing mothers. Bear in mind that even if this drug were to appear in human milk, it is unlikely that a nursing infant with a normal GI tract would absorb a significant amount.

---

[1] Dosage is based on recommendations of the American Heart Association (*Circulation* 70:1123A–1127A, 1984)

MONOBACTAM ANTIBIOTICS

AZACTAM (aztreonam) Squibb   Rx

Vials (single-dose): 500 mg; 1, 2 g (15-ml fill)   **Infusion bottles:** 500 mg; 1, 2 g (100-ml fill)

INDICATIONS

Lower respiratory tract infections, including pneumonia and bronchitis, caused by susceptible strains of *Escherichia coli, Klebsiella pneumoniae, Pseudomonas aeruginosa, Hemophilus influenzae, Proteus mirabilis, Enterobacter,* and *Serratia marcescens*

Septicemia caused by susceptible strains of *Escherichia coli, Klebsiella pneumoniae, Pseudomonas aeruginosa, Proteus mirabilis, Serratia marcescens,* and *Enterobacter*

Skin and skin structure infections, including those associated with postoperative wounds, ulcers, and burns, caused by susceptible strains of *Escherichia coli, Proteus mirabilis, Serratia marcescens, Enterobacter, Pseudomonas aeruginosa, Klebsiella pneumoniae,* and *Citrobacter*

Intraabdominal infections, including peritonitis, caused by susceptible strains of *Escherichia coli, Klebsiella* (including *K pneumoniae*), *Enterobacter* (including *E cloacae*), *Pseudomonas aeruginosa, Citrobacter* (including *C freundii*), and *Serratia* (including *S marcescens*)

Gynecological infections, including endometritis and pelvic cellulitis, caused by susceptible strains of *Escherichia coli, Klebsiella pneumoniae, Enterobacter* (including *E cloacae*), and *Proteus mirabilis*

Urinary tract infections, including pyelonephritis and initial and recurrent cystitis, caused by susceptible strains of *Escherichia coli, Klebsiella pneumoniae, Proteus mirabilis, Pseudomonas aeruginosa, Enterobacter cloacae, Klebsiella oxytoca, Citrobacter,* and *Serratia marcescens*

PARENTERAL DOSAGE

Adult: for moderately severe systemic infections, 1 or 2 g, given IM or IV at 8- or 12-h intervals; for severe or life-threatening systemic infections, 2 g, given IV at 6- or 8-h intervals. Maximum recommended dose: 8 g/day.

Adult: 500 mg or 1 g, given IM or IV at 8- or 12-h intervals; maximum recommended dose: 8 g/day

CONTRAINDICATIONS

Hypersensitivity to aztreonam

ADMINISTRATION/DOSAGE ADJUSTMENTS

Route of administration	The IV route is recommended for patients requiring single doses exceeding 1 g or those with bacterial septicemia, localized parenchymal abscess (eg, intraabdominal abscess), peritonitis, or other severe systemic or life-threatening infections
Pseudomonal infections	Because of the seriousness of systemic infections caused by *Pseudomonas aeruginosa*, 2 g given at 6- or 8-h intervals is recommended, at least upon initiation of therapy
Adjunctive therapy	Aztreonam is indicated as an adjunct to surgery in the management of infections caused by susceptible organisms, including abscesses, infections complicating hollow viscous perforations, cutaneous infections, and infections of serous surfaces; aztreonam is effective against most common gram-negative aerobic pathogens encountered during general surgery
Intravenous bolus injection	Reconstitute the contents of a single-dose 15-ml vial with 6–10 ml of sterile water for injection USP; upon adding the diluent to the container, shake the contents immediately and vigorously. A bolus injection may then be used to initiate therapy. Slowly inject the required dose directly into a vein or the tubing of a suitable administration set over a period of 3–5 min. Should the entire volume not be used for a single dose, discard the unused solution.

AZACTAM

Preparation of IV infusion	Reconstitute the contents of a single-dose 100-ml bottle using at least 50 ml of an appropriate IV infusion solution for each gram of aztreonam. Any of the following solutions may be used: 0.9% sodium chloride injection USP, Ringer's injection USP, lactated Ringer's injection USP, 5% or 10% dextrose injection USP, 5% dextrose and 0.9% sodium chloride injection USP, 5% dextrose and 0.45% sodium chloride injection USP, 5% dextrose and 0.2% sodium chloride injection USP, sodium lactate injection USP, Ionosol B and 5% dextrose, Isolyte E, Isolyte E with 5% dextrose, Isolyte M with 5% dextrose, Normosol-R, Normosol-R and 5% dextrose, Normosol-M and 5% dextrose, 5% or 10% mannitol injection USP, lactated Ringer's and 5% dextrose injection, Plasma-Lyte M and 5% dextrose, 10% Travert injection, 10% Travert and Electrolyte No. 1 injection, 10% Travert and Electrolyte No. 2 injection, and 10% Travert and Electrolyte No. 3 injection. If the contents of a 15-ml capacity vial are to be transferred to an appropriate infusion solution, initially reconstitute each gram of aztreonam with at least 3 ml of sterile water for injection USP and then further dilute with an appropriate infusion solution. Upon adding the diluent to the container, shake the contents immediately and vigorously; should the entire volume not be used for a single dose, discard the unused solution.
Administration of IV infusion	Any infusion of aztreonam should be completed within 20–60 min. When using a Y-type administration set, give careful attention to the calculated volume of solution so that the entire dose is infused. A volume control administration set may be used to deliver an initial dilution of aztreonam into a compatible infusion solution during administration; when this mode is used, the final dilution of aztreonam should have a concentration not exceeding 2% w/v.
Intramuscular administration	Reconstitute the contents of a single-dose 15-ml vial using at least 3 ml of an appropriate diluent for each gram of aztreonam. Any of the following solutions may be used: sterile water for injection USP, bacteriostatic water for injection USP (with benzyl alcohol or with methyl- and propylparabens), 0.9% sodium chloride injection, or bacteriostatic sodium chloride injection USP (with benzyl alcohol or with methyl- and propylparabens). Upon adding the diluent to the container, shake the contents immediately and vigorously; should the entire volume not be used for a single dose, discard the unused solution. Inject deeply into a large muscle mass, such as the upper outer quadrant of the gluteus maximus or the lateral aspect of the thigh; do not admix aztreonam with any local anesthetic agent.
Patients with renal impairment	If creatinine clearance (Ccr) = 10–30 ml/min, administer an initial loading dose of 1 or 2 g and reduce subsequent doses by one half. In patients with severe renal failure (Ccr < 10 ml/min), such as those supported by hemodialysis, give the usual dose to start and reduce subsequent doses by three fourths. For serious or life-threatening infections, give one-eighth of the initial dose after each dialysis session in addition to the maintenance dosage. If necessary, the Ccr for males may be calculated from the serum creatinine concentration by use of the following formula: Ccr = [weight (kg) × (140 − age)]/[72 × creatinine concentration]; for female patients, multiply this value by 0.85.
Elderly patients	Obtain estimates of creatinine clearance (serum creatinine may not accurately portray renal status) and modify dosage, if necessary; renal status is the major dosage determinant, since elderly patients may have diminished renal function
Admixtures with other antibiotics	Intravenous infusions of aztreonam prepared with 0.9% sodium chloride injection USP or 5% dextrose injection USP to which clindamycin phosphate, gentamicin sulfate, tombramycin sulfate, or cefazolin sodium have been added are stable for up to 48 h at room temperature or 7 days under refrigeration. Ampicillin sodium admixtures with aztreonam in 0.9% sodium chloride injection USP are stable for 24 h at room temperature and 48 h under refrigeration; stability of this admixture in 5% dextrose injection is 2 h at room temperature and 8 h under refrigeration. Admixtures of aztreonam and cloxacillin sodium or vancomycin hydrochloride are stable in Dianeal 137 with 4.25% dextrose for up to 24 h at room temperature. Axtreonam is incompatible with nafcillin sodium, cephradine, and metronidazole.
Concurrent therapy	Concurrent initial therapy with other antimicrobial agents and aztreonam is recommended before the causative organism(s) have been identified in seriously ill patients who may have an infection due to gram-positive aerobic pathogens; if anaerobic organisms are also suspected, initiate therapy using an antianaerobic agent concurrently with aztreonam. Do not use beta-lactamase-inducing antibiotics concurrently with aztreonam. Continue appropriate antibiotic therapy following identification and susceptibility testing of the causative organisms.
Duration of therapy	Although the duration of therapy depends on the severity of infection, aztreonam should be continued for at least 48 h after the patient becomes asymptomatic or evidence of bacterial eradication has been obtained; persistent infections may require treatment for several weeks

WARNINGS/PRECAUTIONS

Hypersensitivity	Prior to initiating therapy, determine whether the patient has a history of hypersensitivity to any antibiotic or other drugs. Use with caution in any patient who has had some form of allergy, particularly to drugs; patients who have had anaphylactic or urticarial reactions to penicillins and/or cephalosporins should be followed carefully. If an allergic reaction to aztreonam occurs, discontinue use and institute appropriate supportive measures, including maintenance of ventilation and administration of pressor amines, antihistamines, and corticosteroids, as warranted. Serious hypersensitivity reactions may require use of epinephrine and other emergency measures.

AZACTAM ■ OCUFEN

Patients with impaired renal or hepatic function	Appropriate monitoring is recommended during aztreonam therapy for patients with renal or hepatic dysfunction
Concomitant use of aminoglycosides	If an aminoglycoside antibiotic is used concurrently with aztreonam, especially if the aminoglycoside dosage is high or therapy is prolonged, renal function should be monitored because of the potential nephrotoxicity and ototoxicity of aminoglycosides
Superinfection	Overgrowth of nonsusceptible organisms, including gram-positive organisms (eg, *Staphylococcus aureus, Streptococcus faecalis*) and fungi, may occur during aztreonam therapy; institute appropriate measures if superinfection occurs
Carcinogenicity	No studies have been performed to evaluate the carcinogenic potential of this drug
Mutagenicity	Studies in several standard laboratory models, both in vivo and in vitro, have revealed no evidence of mutagenic potential at the chromosomal or genic level
Effect on fertility	Studies in two generations of rats at daily doses up to 20 times the maximum recommended human dose prior to and during gestation and lactation have revealed no evidence of impaired fertility; although a slightly reduced survival rate occurred during the lactation period in the offspring of rats receiving the highest dosage, no such effect occurred in the offspring of rats receiving 5 times the maximum recommended human dose of aztreonam

ADVERSE REACTIONS

Frequent reactions (incidence ≥ 1%) are printed in *italics*

Local	*Discomfort/swelling at the injection site (with IM use) (3.9%), phlebitis/thrombophlebitis (with IV use) (1.9%)*
Hematological	Pancytopenia, neutropenia, thrombocytopenia, anemia, leukocytosis, thrombocytosis, eosinophilia
Gastrointestinal	*Diarrhea, nausea and/or vomiting (1–1.3%)*, abdominal cramps; *Clostridium difficile*-associated diarrhea or gastrointestinal bleeding (rare)
Cardiovascular	Hypotension, transient ECG changes (ventricular bigeminy and PVC)
Respiratory	Flushing, chest pain, and dyspnea (one patient)
Hepatic	Hepatitis, jaundice
Central nervous system, neuromuscular	Seizure, confusion, vertigo, paresthesia, insomnia, dizziness, tinnitus, diplopia, weakness, headache, muscular aches
Dermatological, hypersensitivity	*Rash (1–1.3%)*, purpura, erythema multiforme, urticaria, exfoliative dermatitis, petechiae, pruritus, diaphoresis, anaphylaxis
Other	Mouth ulcer, altered taste, numb tongue, sneezing and nasal congestion, halitosis, vaginal candidiasis, vaginitis, breast tenderness, fever, malaise

OVERDOSAGE

Signs and symptoms	See ADVERSE REACTIONS
Treatment	Discontinue use and institute supportive treatment, if needed; aztreonam may be cleared from the serum by hemodialysis or peritoneal dialysis

DRUG INTERACTIONS

Beta-lactamase-inducing antibiotics (eg, cefoxitin, imipenem)	▽ Antibacterial effect of aztreonam; do not use concurrently

ALTERED LABORATORY VALUES

Blood/serum values	△ SGOT △ SGPT △ Alkaline phosphatase △ Creatinine △ Prothrombin time △ Partial thromboplastin time + Coombs test

No clinically significant alterations in urinary values occur at therapeutic dosages

---

USE IN CHILDREN

Safety and effectiveness for use in infants and children have not been established

USE IN PREGNANT AND NURSING WOMEN

Pregnancy Category B: no evidence of embryotoxicity, fetotoxicity, or teratogenicity has been found in rabbits and rats given daily doses of up to 5 and 15 times, respectively, the maximum recommended human dose; no drug-induced changes were seen in any maternal, fetal, or neonatal parameters monitored in rats given 15 times the maximum recommended human dose of aztreonam during late gestation and lactation. Aztreonam crosses the placental barrier and enters the fetal circulation. No adequate, well-controlled studies have been performed in pregnant women; use during pregnancy only if clearly needed. Aztreonam is excreted in breast milk in concentrations that are less than 1% of the maternal serum level; temporarily discontinuing nursing during therapy should be considered.

OPHTHALMIC AGENTS

OCUFEN (flurbiprofen sodium) Allergan   Rx
Solution: 0.03% (2.5, 5, 10 ml)

INDICATIONS	TOPICAL DOSAGE
Inhibition of intraoperative miosis	Adult: 1 drop instilled every 30 min, beginning 2 h before surgery, for a total of 4 drops

CONTRAINDICATIONS

Epithelial herpes simplex keratitis (dendritic keratitis)	Hypersensitivity to any component

WARNINGS/PRECAUTIONS

Cross-sensitivity	Use with caution in patients who have previously exhibited hypersensitivity to acetylsalicylic acid (aspirin) and other nonsteroidal anti-inflammatory drugs
Patients with a history of herpes simplex keratitis	Closely monitor patients with a history of herpes simplex keratitis
Delayed wound healing	Flurbiprofen may delay wound healing
Patients with bleeding tendencies	Use with caution in patients with bleeding tendencies[1]
Carcinogenicity, mutagenicity	No evidence of carcinogenicity has been found in long-term studies in mice and/or rats; no studies have been performed to evaluate the mutagenic potential of this drug
Effect on fertility	No impairment of fertility has been found in long-term studies in mice and/or rats

ADVERSE REACTIONS

Local	Transient burning and stinging upon instillation, minor symptoms of ocular irritation

USE IN CHILDREN
Safety and effectiveness for use in children have not been established

USE IN PREGNANT AND NURSING WOMEN
Pregnancy Category C: flurbiprofen has been shown to be embryocidal, delay parturition, prolong gestation, reduce weight, and/or slightly retard fetal growth in rats fed 0.4 mg/kg/day or more (approximately 185 times the recommended human dose). No adequate, well-controlled studies have been performed in pregnant women; use during pregnancy only if the expected benefit justifies the potential risk to the fetus. It is no known whether flurbiprofen is excreted in human milk; because many drugs are excreted in human milk, patient should not nurse during therapy.

VEHICLE/BASE
Solution: 1.4% polyvinyl alcohol (Liquifilm), 0.005% thimerosal, edetate disodium, potassium chloride, sodium chloride, sodium citrate, citric acid, hydrochloric acid and/or sodium hydroxide (to adjust pH), and purified water

[1] Systemic absorption may occur with some ocularly applied drugs, and nonsteroidal anti-inflammatory drugs have been shown to increase bleeding time by interfering with platelet aggregation; however, no effect on bleeding time has been reported with ocularly applied flurbiprofen

---

ORAL CORTICOSTEROIDS

PEDIAPRED (prednisolone sodium phosphate) Fisons Rx
Oral liquid (per 5 ml): 5 mg (4 fl oz) *raspberry flavored*

INDICATIONS
Endocrine disorders, including primary or secondary adrenocortical insufficiency, congenital adrenal hyperplasia, hypercalcemia associated with cancer, and nonsuppurative thyroiditis
Adjunctive, short-term treatment of **rheumatic disorders,** including psoriatic arthritis, rheumatoid arthritis, juvenile rheumatoid arthritis, ankylosing spondylitis, acute and subacute bursitis, acute nonspecific tenosynovitis, acute gouty arthritis, posttraumatic osteoarthritis, synovitis of osteoarthritis, and epicondylitis
Collagen diseases, including selected cases of systemic lupus erythematosus, systemic dermatomyositis (polymyositis), and acute rheumatic carditis
Dermatologic diseases, including pemphigus, bullous dermatitis herpetiformis, severe erythema multiforme (Stevens-Johnson syndrome), exfoliative dermatitis, mycosis fungoides, severe psoriasis, and severe sebborheic dermatitis
Allergic conditions, including seasonal or perennial allergic rhinitis, bronchial asthma, contact dermatitis, atopic dermatitis, serum sickness, and drug hypersensitivity reactions, when these conditions are severe or incapacitating and do not respond to adequate conventional therapy
Severe acute and chronic **allergic and inflammatory ophthalmic conditions involving the eye and its adnexa,** including allergic conjunctivitis, keratitis, allergic corneal marginal ulcers, herpes zoster ophthalmicus, iritis and iridocyclitis, chorioretinitis, anterior segment inflammation, diffuse posterior uveitis and choroiditis, optic neuritis, and sympathetic ophthalmia
Respiratory diseases, including symptomatic sarcoidosis, Loeffler's syndrome not manageable by other means, berylliosis, fulminating or disseminated pulmonary tuberculosis (when used concurrently with appropriate antituberculous chemotherapy), and aspiration pneumonitis
Hematological disorders, including idiopathic thrombocytopenic purpura or secondary thrombocytopenia in adults, acquired (autoimmune) hemolytic anemia, erythroblastopenia (RBC anemia), and congenital (erythroid) hypoplastic anemia
Palliative management of **leukemias and lymphomas** in adults and **acute leukemia** in childhood
Induction of diuresis or remission of proteinuria in **the nephrotic syndrome,** when this syndrome is nonuremic and either idiopathic or due to lupus erythematosus
Gastrointestinal diseases, including ulcerative colitis and regional enteritis
Tuberculous meningitis with subarachnoid block or impending block (when used concurrently with appropriate antituberculous chemotherapy)
Trichinosis with neurological or myocardial involvement

ORAL DOSAGE
Adult and child: 5–60 mg/day to start, depending on the disease, initial patient response, and duration of relief

PEDIAPRED

Acute exacerbations of **multiple sclerosis**	**Adult and child:** 200 mg/day for 1 wk, followed by 80 mg every other day or 4–8 mg of dexamethasone every other day for 1 mo

CONTRAINDICATIONS

Systemic fungal infections

ADMINISTRATION/DOSAGE ADJUSTMENTS

Maintenance therapy	Once an adequate response has been obtained, reduce dosage gradually and in small increments to the lowest effective level. Keep patient under supervision during maintenance therapy; dosage adjustments may be necessary because of certain conditions, such as stress, change in response to the drug, and remission or progression of the disease. Continue supervision following termination of therapy since acute adrenocortical insufficiency may develop and severe manifestations of the treated disease may suddenly recur at that time.
Duration of treatment	Complications of glucocorticoid treatment depend upon the size of the dose and duration of treatment; consider each individual case to determine the dose and duration of treatment, and whether daily or intermittent therapy should be used
Decreasing dosage	To minimize the risk of acute adrenocortical insufficiency, reduce dosage gradually rather than abruptly whenever possible
Adrenocortical insufficiency	Mineralocorticoid supplementation may be necessary in patients treated for primary or secondary adrenocortical insufficiency, particularly in infants
Juvenile rheumatoid arthritis	Selected patients may require low-dose maintenance therapy

WARNINGS/PRECAUTIONS

Stress	If unusual stress occurs during therapy, give a rapid-acting corticosteroid before, during, and after the stressful situation; it may also be necessary to increase the dosage of prednisolone. If a stressful situation, such as trauma, surgery, or severe illness, occurs in the months after discontinuation of prednisolone, glucocorticoid therapy should be reinstituted in combination with administration of sodium chloride and/or a mineralocorticoid.
Infection	During therapy, some signs of infection may be masked, and new infections may appear. Resistance may be decreased, and an infection may be difficult to localize; watch for evidence of intercurrent infection.
Ocular damage	Prolonged use may cause posterior subcapsular cataracts and glaucoma, with possible optic nerve damage, and may enhance development of secondary fungal or viral infections of the eye. Use with caution in patients with ocular herpes simplex because of possible corneal perforation.
Electrolyte imbalance	Prednisolone can elevate blood pressure, cause retention of salt and water, and increase potassium and calcium excretion; dietary salt restriction and potassium supplementation may be necessary during therapy
Psychological effects	Corticosteroids can cause psychic disturbances, including euphoria, insomnia, mood swings, personality changes, severe depression, and overt psychosis, and may exacerbate preexisting emotional instability or psychotic tendencies
Menstrual irregularities	Caution women past menarche that menstrual irregularities may occur
Hypothyroidism, hepatic cirrhosis	Corticosteroid effects are enhanced in patients with hypothyroidism or hepatic cirrhosis
Special-risk patients	When using this drug in patients with nonspecific ulcerative colitis, exercise caution if there is a probability of impending perforation, abscess, or other pyogenic infection. Use with caution in patients with hypoprothrombinemia, diverticulitis, fresh intestinal anastomoses, active or latent peptic ulcer, renal insufficiency, hypertension, osteoporosis, or myasthenia gravis
Immunization	Vaccination, including immunization against smallpox, should not be undertaken during therapy, particularly when high corticosteroid doses have been given, because neurological complications may develop and antibody response may fail to occur
Skin tests	Corticosteroids may suppress response to skin tests
Tuberculosis	Corticosteroids may be used as an adjunct to antituberculous therapy, but only for fulminating or disseminated forms of the active disease (see also DRUG INTERACTIONS). When using corticosteroids in patients with latent tuberculosis or tuberculin reactivity, observe patient closely since tuberculosis may be reactivated; during prolonged therapy, institute chemoprophylactic measures.
Multiple sclerosis	Although corticosteroids have proven effective in speeding the resolution of acute exacerbations of multiple sclerosis during controlled clinical trials, there is no evidence that they affect the ultimate outcome or natural history of the disease; relatively high doses are indicated to demonstrate a significant effect

ADVERSE REACTIONS

Cardiovascular	Sodium and fluid retention, congestive heart failure in susceptible patients, hypokalemic alkalosis, hypertension

PEDIAPRED

Musculoskeletal	Muscle weakness, steroid myopathy, loss of muscle mass, osteoporosis, vertebral compression fractures, aseptic necrosis of femoral and humeral heads, pathologic fracture of long bones
Gastrointestinal	Peptic ulcer with possible perforation and hemorrhage, pancreatitis, abdominal distention, ulcerative esophagitis
Dermatological	Impaired wound healing, thin fragile skin, petechiae, ecchymoses, facial erythema, increased sweating, suppressed reactions to skin tests
Central nervous system	Convulsions, increased intracranial pressure with papilledema (pseudomotor cerebri; usually after therapy), vertigo, headache
Endocrinological	Menstrual irregularities, development of cushingoid state, secondary adrenocortical and pituitary unresponsiveness (particularly with stress), suppression of growth in children, decreased carbohydrate tolerance, manifestations of latent diabetes mellitus, increased requirements for insulin or oral hypoglycemic agents in diabetic patients
Ophthalmic	Posterior subcapsular cataracts, increased intraocular pressure, glaucoma, exophthalmos
Metabolic	Negative nitrogen balance due to protein catabolism, hypokalemia

OVERDOSAGE

Signs and symptoms	Mental symptoms, moon face, abnormal fat deposits, fluid retention, excessive appetite, weight gain, hypertrichosis, acne, striae, ecchymosis, increased sweating, pigmentation, dry scaly skin, thinning scalp hair, increased blood pressure, tachycardia, thrombophlebitis, decreased resistance to infection, negative nitrogen balance with delayed bone and wound healing, headache, weakness, menstrual disorders, accentuated menopausal symptoms, neuropathy, fractures, osteoporosis, peptic ulcer, decreased glucose tolerance, hypokalemia, and adrenal insufficiency; hepatomegaly and abdominal distention (in children)
Treatment	Immediately perform gastric lavage or induce emesis; for chronic overdosage in the face of severe disease requiring continuous steroid therapy, reduce dosage temporarily or introduce alternate-day treatment

DRUG INTERACTIONS

Isoniazid	▽ Antitubercular effectiveness of isoniazid; higher doses of isoniazid may be needed during corticosteroid therapy
Oral contraceptives	△ Pharmacologic effects of prednisolone; monitor patient for signs of corticosteroid toxicity and reduce dosage, if needed
Rifampin	▽ Pharmacologic effects of prednisolone; adjust dosage accordingly
Salicylates	▽ Serum level of salicylates; adjust dosage accordingly
Barbiturates	▽ Pharmacologic effects of prednisolone; adjust dosage accordingly
Hydantoins	▽ Pharmacologic effects of prednisolone; adjust dosage accordingly
Cardiac glycosides	△ Risk of digitalis toxicity
Vaccines	▽ Antibody response △ Risk of neurological effects of vaccines △ Risk of viral infection (with live virus vaccines)
Amphotericin B	△ Risk of hypokalemia
Oral anticoagulants	△ Risk of hemorrhage and GI ulceration ▽ Hypoprothrombinemic effect
Anticholinesterase agents	▽ Pharmacologic effects of anticholinesterase agents
Pancuronium, tubocurarine	▽ Neuromuscular blockade

ALTERED LABORATORY VALUES

Blood/serum values	△ Glucose ▽ Calcium △ Cholesterol ▽ Potassium ▽ PBI ▽ Thyroxine (T_4) △ Sodium △ Uric acid ▽ ^{131}I thyroid uptake
Urine values	△ Glucose ▽ 17-OHCS ▽ 17-KS

USE IN CHILDREN

See INDICATIONS and ORAL DOSAGE; growth and development should be carefully observed in children undergoing prolonged therapy

USE IN PREGNANT AND NURSING WOMEN

Pregnancy Category C: prednisolone has been shown to be teratogenic in many species given doses equivalent to the human dose; studies in mice, rats, and rabbits given prednisolone have shown an increased incidence of cleft palate in offspring. No adequate, well-controlled studies have been done in pregnant women; use during pregnancy only if the expected benefit justifies the potential risk to the fetus. Prednisolone is excreted in breast milk in small (and probably clinically insignificant) amounts; use with caution in nursing mothers.

PENICILLINS

UNASYN (ampicillin sodium and sulbactam sodium) Roerig — Rx

Vials: 1 g ampicillin[1] and 0.5 g sulbactam[1] (1.5 g); 2 g ampicillin[1] and 1 g sulbactam[1] (3 g)   **Piggyback bottles:** 1 g ampicillin[1] and 0.5 g sulbactam[1] (1.5 g); 2 g ampicillin[1] and 1 g sulbactam[1] (3 g)

INDICATIONS	**PARENTERAL DOSAGE**

Skin and skin-structure infections caused by beta-lactamase producing strains of *Staphylococcus aureus, Escherichia coli, Klebsiella* (including *K pneumoniae*), *Proteus mirabilis, Bacteroides fragilis, Enterobacter,* and *Acinetobacter calcoaceticus*
Intraabdominal infections caused by beta-lactamase-producing strains of *Escherichia coli, Klebsiella* (including *K pneumoniae*), *Bacteroides* (including *B fragilis*), and *Enterobacter*
Gynecological infections caused by beta-lactamase producing strains of *Escherichia coli* and *Bacteroides* (including *B fragilis*)

Adult: 1.5–3 g of Unasyn IM or IV q6h; maximum sulbactam dosage: 4 g/day

CONTRAINDICATIONS

Hypersensitivity to penicillins

ADMINISTRATION/DOSAGE ADJUSTMENTS

Intravenous administration	To prepare the solution for IV administration, add the required amount of an appropriate diluent to either of the piggyback units. Alternatively, reconstitute the contents of a vial with sterile water for injection to yield a solution of 375 mg of Unasyn per ml; immediately dilute an appropriate volume with a suitable diluent to yield a solution containing 3–45 mg of Unasyn per ml. Any of the following diluents may be used: sterile water for injection, 0.9% sodium chloride injection, 5% dextrose injection, lactated Ringer's injection, M/6 sodium lactate injection, 5% dextrose in 0.45% saline, and 10% invert sugar. Allow solution to stand after dissolution to allow any foaming to dissipate. Give by slow IV injection over a period of at least 10–25 min or, in greater dilutions with 50–100 ml of an appropriate diluent, by IV infusion over a period of 15–30 min.
Intravenous admixtures	When concomitant treatment with a parenteral aminoglycoside is indicated, reconstitute and administer Unasyn and the aminoglycoside separately to avoid in vitro inactivation
Intramuscular administration	For IM use, reconstitute the contents of a vial with sterile water for injection, 0.5% lidocaine hydrochloride injection, or 2% lidocaine hydrochloride injection; use 3.2 ml for the 1.5-g vial and 6.4 ml for the 3-g vial (final concentration: 375 mg of Unasyn per ml). Administer by deep IM injection within 1 h after preparation of the solution.
Patients with renal impairment	If creatinine clearance (Ccr) $\geq$ 30 ml/min, give 1.5–3 g q6–8h; if Ccr = 15–29 ml/min, give 1.5–3 g q12h; if Ccr = 5–14 ml/min, give 1.5–3 g q24h. The Ccr of patients with stable renal function may be estimated from serum creatinine levels if a measured value cannot be obtained; for adult men, use the following formula (weight [kg]) (140 − age [yr])/(72) (serum creatinine level [mg/dl]), for adult women, multiply this quotient by 0.85.
Cultures and susceptibility testing	Perform cultures and susceptibility testing prior to treatment to identify the causative organism and determine its susceptibility to this drug; therapy may be initiated before the test results are known when there is reason to believe that the organism is susceptible to Unasyn. Therapy may be adjusted, if appropriate, once the results of testing are known.
Mixed infections	Infections caused by ampicillin-susceptible organisms and beta-lactamase-producing organisms susceptible to this drug should not require addition of another anti-infective agent

WARNINGS/PRECAUTIONS

Hypersensitivity	Serious and occasionally fatal anaphylactic reactions have occurred in patients taking penicillins, generally in those with a history of penicillin hypersensitivity or sensitivity to multiple allergens. Urticaria, erythema multiforme, and exfoliative dermatitis may be controlled with antihistamines and, if necessary, systemic corticosteroids. As a rule, use of this drug should be discontinued if such reactions occur; however, this should be decided individually. Serious anaphylactoid reactions may necessitate emergency measures, such as immediate use of epinephrine, oxygen, IV corticosteroids, and airway management, including intubation. Use with caution in patients who have experienced allergic reactions to cephalosporins.
Patients with mononucleosis	Ampicillin should not be given to patients with infectious mononucleosis; a high percentage of such patients develop a skin rash after receiving ampicillin
Superinfection	Overgrowth of mycotic or bacterial pathogens may occur during therapy; if superinfection occurs (usually involving *Pseudomonas* or *Candida*), discontinue use and/or institute appropriate therapy
Carcinogenicity, mutagenicity	No long-term studies have been performed to evaluate the carcinogenic or mutagenic potential of this formulation

UNASYN ■ TEGISON

ADVERSE REACTIONS[2]	Frequent reactions (incidence ≥ 1%) are printed in *italics*
Local	*Pain at IM injection site (16%), pain at IV injection site and thrombophlebitis (3%)*
Gastrointestinal	*Diarrhea (3%)*, nausea, vomiting, flatulence, glossitis, gastritis, stomatitis, abdominal distension, black hairy tongue, enterocolitis, pseudomembranous colitis
Hypersensitivity	*Rash (< 2%)*, itching, erythema, urticaria, erythema multiforme, exfoliative dermatitis; anaphylaxis (rare)
Central nervous system	Fatigue, malaise, headache
Genitourinary	Urinary retention, dysuria, presence of RBCs and hyaline casts in urine
Hematological	Decreased hemoglobin, hematocrit, RBC count, WBC count, and neutrophils; increased monocytes, basophils, and eosinophils; increased or decreased lymphocytes and platelets, agranulocytosis
Other	Chills, candidiasis, tightness in the throat, chest/substernal pain, edema, facial swelling, epistaxis, mucosal bleeding
OVERDOSAGE	
Signs and symptoms	Neurological reactions, including convulsions
Treatment	Discontinue use; treat symptomatically. Hemodialysis may be helpful in removing the drug from the circulation.
DRUG INTERACTIONS	
Probenecid	↑ Blood level of ampicillin and sulbactam
Allopurinol	↑ Risk of rash due to potential interaction with ampicillin component
ALTERED LABORATORY VALUES	
Blood/serum values	↑ SGOT ↑ SGPT ↑ Alkaline phosphatase ↑ LDH ↓ Albumin ↓ Total proteins ↑ BUN ↑ Creatinine
Urinary values	False-positive glucose reaction with Clinitest tablets and Benedict's or Fehling's solution; use glucose tests based on enzymatic glucose oxidase reactions (eg, Clinistix, Tes-Tape)

USE IN CHILDREN
Safety and effectiveness for use in children under 12 yr of age have not been established

USE IN PREGNANT AND NURSING WOMEN
Pregnancy Category B: reproduction studies in rats, mice, and rabbits at up to 10 times the human dose have revealed no evidence of impaired fertility or fetal harm. No adequate, well-controlled studies have been performed in pregnant women; use during pregnancy only if clearly needed.[3] IV administration of ampicillin to guinea pigs has been shown to decrease uterine tone and the frequency, height, and duration of uterine contractions; however, it is not known if these reactions are predictive of human response. Low concentrations of ampicillin and sulbactam are excreted in human milk; use with caution in nursing mothers.

[1] As the sodium salt
[2] Includes reactions common to ampicillins in general
[3] Plasma levels of total conjugated estriol, estriol-glucuronide, conjugated estrone, and estradiol may decrease temporarily following administration of ampicillin to pregnant women

---

PSORIASIS PREPARATIONS

TEGISON (etretinate) Roche   Rx
Capsules: 10, 25 mg

INDICATIONS	**ORAL DOSAGE**
Severe recalcitrant psoriasis, including erythrodermic and generalized postular types, unresponsive to conventional therapy (including topical tar plus UVB light, psoralens plus UVA light, systemic corticosteroids, and methotrexate) or in patients who cannot tolerate such treatment	**Adult:** 0.75–1 mg/kg/day to start, given in divided doses with meals; erythrodermic psoriasis may respond to an initial dosage of 0.25 mg/kg/day, with weekly increases of 0.25 mg/kg/day until an optimal response is achieved. Maximum dose: 1.5 mg/kg/day.
CONTRAINDICATIONS	
Pregnancy (see WARNINGS/PRECAUTIONS)	

TEGISON

ADMINISTRATION/DOSAGE ADJUSTMENTS

Maintenance therapy — Following an initial response (generally after 8–16 wk of therapy), maintenance therapy may be initiated at a level of 0.5–0.75 mg/kg/day; discontinue treatment in patients whose lesions have sufficiently resolved

Relapses — Relapses may be treated as outlined for initial therapy (see ORAL DOSAGE)

WARNINGS/PRECAUTIONS

Women of childbearing potential — Etretinate can cause major human fetal abnormalities (see USE IN PREGNANT AND NURSING WOMEN); this drug must not be used by women who are pregnant, who may become pregnant, or who may not use reliable contraception during treatment. Test for pregnancy within 2 wk before the start of therapy and begin treatment on the second or third day of the next normal menstrual period. An effective form of contraception must be used for at least 1 mo before the onset of therapy and continued for an indefinite period after the end of treatment. Patients should be fully informed of the serious risks associated with the use of etretinate during pregnancy.

Ophthalmic and neurologic disorders — Pseudotumor cerebri and corneal erosion, abrasion, irregularity, and punctate staining have occurred during etretinate therapy; these effects disappeared or improved following discontinuation of therapy. Decreased visual acuity, blurring of vision, minimal posterior subcapsular cataract formation, iritis, blot retinal hemorrhage, scotoma, and photophobia have also been reported. Night vision may decrease, sometimes suddenly; advise patient to exercise caution when driving or operating any vehicle at night. If visual disturbances occur, discontinue use and perform or refer patient for an ophthalmologic examination. Check for papilledema if patient experiences nausea, vomiting, headache, or visual disturbances; if papilledema is detected, discontinue use and refer patient to a neurologist. Caution patients that during and after treatment they may experience decreased tolerance to contact lenses.

Hepatotoxicity — Elevations in SGOT, SGPT, and LDH levels, as well as clinical and histologic evidence of hepatitis and pathologic findings of hepatic fibrosis, necrosis, and/or cirrhosis, have occurred in individuals treated with etretinate and may have been related to the drug; four cases of hepatitis-related deaths in patients taking etretinate have been reported worldwide. Liver function has returned to normal in the majority of patients affected after the drug was withdrawn. If hepatotoxicity is suspected during therapy, discontinue use and investigate the cause.

Skeletal changes — Development of hyperostosis is very likely during etretinate therapy; involvement has tended to be bilateral and multifocal, with the most common sites being the ankles, pelvis, and knees. Spinal changes have been uncommon, and no bone or joint symptoms were evident at the sites of radiographic abnormalities in 47% of the patients examined. Ossification of interosseous ligaments and tendons of the extremities has been reported in children; in addition, two children have shown x-ray changes suggestive of premature epiphyseal closure during etretinate therapy. Although it is not known whether these effects occur more commonly in children, it is of concern because of the growth process; perform pretreatment x-rays for bone age, including x-rays of the knees, and follow with yearly monitoring. Pain or limitation of motion should be evaluated with appropriate radiological examination.

Hypertriglyceridemia — Increased triglyceride levels may occur during therapy, especially in patients at risk because of diabetes mellitus, obesity, increased alcohol intake, or a family history of hypertriglyceridemia. Serum triglyceride levels exceeding 800 mg/dl have been associated with acute pancreatitis. Plasma triglycerides increase in approximately 45% of patients and cholesterol in about 16%, and a decrease in high-density lipoproteins occurs in approximately 37%; these changes are reversible upon discontinuation of therapy. Some patients have been able to continue on etretinate while reversing the hypertriglyceridemia, hypercholesterolemia, and decreased HDL levels by weight reduction and restriction of dietary fat and alcohol. Blood-lipid determinations should be performed before initiating etretinate therapy and then weekly or biweekly until the lipid response to the drug is established (this usually takes up to 4–8 wk). These tests should be obtained under fasting conditions; if alcohol has been consumed before the test, wait at least 36 h before drawing blood for the determination.

Cardiovascular effects — Hypertriglyceridemia, hypercholesterolemia, and decreased HDL levels may increase a patient's cardiovascular risk status; significant cardiovascular accidents not considered to be related to etretinate therapy have occurred in patients with a strong history of cardiovascular risk. However, two cases of myocardial infarction possibly related to etretinate therapy have been reported.

Vitamin supplementation — Caution patient to avoid taking vitamin supplements containing vitamin A (see DRUG INTERACTIONS)

Exacerbation of psoriasis — Inform patients that a transient exacerbation of psoriasis may occur, especially during the initial period of treatment

Food-drug interactions — Concomitant consumption of milk with etretinate results in increased etretinate absorption

Carcinogenicity — An increased incidence of blood-vessel tumors (hemangiomas and hemangiosarcomas in several different tissue sites) has been observed in male Crl:CD-1 (ICR) BR mice fed 4–5 mg/kg/day of etretinate for 80 wk; however, no such effect was observed in female rats. No increase in tumor incidence was observed in male or female Sprague-Dawley rats fed up to 3 mg/kg/day of etretinate for 2 yr.

TEGISON

Mutagenicity	Except for a weakly positive response in the Ames test using the tester strain TA 100, no evidence of genotoxicity has been observed in standard laboratory tests for mutagenicity; no differences in the rate of sister chromatid exchange have been noted in lymphocytes of patients before and after 4 wk of treatment with therapeutic doses of etretinate
Impairment of fertility	The readiness of rats to copulate was reduced in rats fed 5 mg/kg/day (approximately 3 times the maximum recommended human dose) of etretinate, but the pregnancy rate was unaffected; the number of viable young at birth, postnatal weight gain, and survival were also adversely affected, and the pregnancy rate of untreated first-generation animals and postnatal weight gain of untreated second-generation animals were also reduced. Testicular atrophy has been noted in subchronic and chronic rat studies and in a chronic dog study, in some cases at doses approaching the recommended human dose; decreased sperm counts have been reported in dogs fed 3 mg/kg/day of etretinate for 13 wk, and spermatogenic arrest has been reported following chronic administration of the all-*trans* metabolite to dogs. However, no adverse effects on sperm production have been noted in 12 psoraiatic patients given 75 mg/kg/day of etretinate for 1 mo and 50 mg/day for an additional 2 mo.

ADVERSE REACTIONS

Frequent reactions (incidence ≥ 1%) are printed in *italics*

Dermatological	*Loss of hair, palm/sole/fingertip bleeding (> 75%); dry skin, itching, rash, red scaly face, skin fragility (50-75%); bruising, sunburn (25-50%); nail disorder, skin peeling (10-25%); hair abnormalities, bullous eruption, cold/clammy skin, onycholysis, paronchyia, pyogenic granuloma, changes in perspiration (1-10%);* abnormal skin odor, granulation tissue, healing impairment, herpes simplex, hirsutism, increased pore size, sensory skin changes; skin atrophy, fissures, infection, nodule, or ulceration; urticaria
Musculoskeletal	*Hyperostosis (> 75%), bone/joint pain (50-75%), muscle cramps (25-50%), myalgia (1-10%),* gout, hyperkinesia, hypertonia
Central nervous system	*Fatigue (50-75%), headache (25-50%), fever (10-25%); dizziness, lethargy, changes in sensation, pain, rigors (1-10%);* abnormal thinking, amnesia, anxiety, depression, pseudotumor cerebri, emotional lability, faint feeling, flu-like symptoms
Ophthalmic	*Irritation of eyes (50-75%); eyeball pain, eyelid abnormalities (25-50%); conjuctivitis, decrease in visual acuity, double vision, abnormalities of the conjunctiva, cornea, lens, or retina (10-25%); abnormal lacrimation or vision, abnormalities of extraocular musculature, ocular tension, pupil, and vitreous (1-10%);* night vision decrease, photophobia, visual change, scotomata
Otic	*Earache, otitis externa (1-10%);* ear drainage, infection, hearing decrease
Gastrointestinal	*Abdominal pain, changes in appetite (25-50%); nausea (10-25%);* constipation, diarrhea, melena, flatulence, weight loss, oral ulcers, taste perversion, tooth caries
Hepatic	*Increased triglycerides (25-50%); increased SGOT, SGPT, GGTP, alkaline phosphatase, globulin, and cholesterol (10-25%); increased bilirubin, increased or decreased total protein and albumin, hepatitis (1-10%)*
Cardiovascular	*Cardiovascular thrombotic or obstructive events, edema (1-10%);* atrial fibrillation, chest pain, coagulation disorder, phlebitis, postural hypotension, syncope
Respiratory	*Dyspnea (1-10%),* coughing, increased sputum, dysphonia, pharyngitis
Renal	Kidney stones
Hematological, electrolyte balance	*Increased MCHC (60%); increased MCH, reticulocyte count, PTT, and ESR, increased or decreased potassium, increased or decreased calcium or phosphorus (25-50%); decreased hemoglobin/HCT, RBC count, and MCV, increased platelets, increased or decreased WBC and component count, prothrombin time, venous CO$_2$, sodium, chloride, and FBS (10-25%); decreased platelets, MCH, MCHC, PTT; increased hemoglobin/HCT, RBC count, and bilirubin (1-10%)*
Genitourinary	*WBCs in urine (10-25%); proteinuria, glycosuria, microscopic hematuria, casts in urine, acetonuria, hemoglobinuria, increased BUN, increased creatinine (1-10%);* abnormal menses, atrophic vaginitis, dysuria, polyuria, urinary retention
Other	*Dry nose, chapped lips (> 75%); excessive thirst, sore mouth (50-75%); nosebleed (25-50%); cheilitis, sore tongue (10-25%); dry eyes, mucous membrane abnormalities, dry mouth, gingival bleeding/inflammation, malignant neoplasms (1-10%);* decreased mucus secretion, rhinorrhea

OVERDOSAGE

Signs and symptoms	See ADVERSE REACTIONS (generally resemble manifestations of hypervitaminosis A)
Treatment	There has been no experience with acute overdosage in humans

DRUG INTERACTIONS

Vitamin A	⇧ Risk of toxicity due to chemical similarity

ALTERED LABORATORY VALUES

Blood/serum values — △ Triglycerides △ Cholesterol ▽ High-density lipoproteins △ Alkaline phosphatase △ SGOT △ SGPT △ GGTP △ LDH △ Globulin △ or ▽ Potassium △ or ▽ Venous CO₂ △ or ▽ Sodium △ or ▽ Chloride △ or ▽ Calcium △ or ▽ Phosphorus △ or ▽ FBS △ CPK △ BUN △ Creatinine △ or ▽ Total protein △ or ▽ Albumin △ or ▽ Venous CO₂

Urinary values — + WBC + Protein + Glucose + Blood + Acetone + Hemoglobin

USE IN CHILDREN

No clinical studies have been performed in the US using etretinate in children; because of the lack of data in children, the possibility of their being more sensitive to the effects of this drug, and the observation of skeletal changes in children (see WARNINGS/PRECAUTIONS), etretinate should be used only when all alternative therapies have been exhausted

USE IN PREGNANT AND NURSING WOMEN

Pregnancy Category C: major fetal abnormalities, including meningomyelocele, meningoencephalocele, multiple synostoses, facial dysmorphia, syndactylies, absence of terminal phalanges, malformations of the hip, ankle, and forearm; low-set ears, high palate, decreased cranial volume, and alterations of the skull and cervical vertebrae have been associated with use of etretinate by pregnant women; although no adverse effects on parameters of late gestation and lactation have been observed in rats at doses of up to 4 mg/kg/day, doses of 8 mg/kg/day resulted in an increased rate of stillbirths and reduced neonatal weight gain and survival rate. Do not administer to women who are or who plan to become pregnant (see warning, above, concerning use in women of childbearing potential). Etretinate is excreted in the milk of lactating rats. It is not known whether this drug is excreted in human milk; because many drugs are excreted in human milk, etretinate should not be given to nursing women.

VACCINES

RECOMBIVAX HB (hepatitis B vaccine [recombinant]) Merck Sharp & Dohme Rx

Vials: 10 µg/ml hepatitis B surface antigen, recombinant (0.5, 3 ml)

INDICATIONS

Prevention of type B hepatitis in persons at risk, particularly (1) health-care practitioners, paraprofessionals, and staff members (including blood bank, laboratory, and plasma fractionation workers), (2) medical, dental, and nursing students, (3) staff in hemodialysis or hematology/oncology units, (4) patients with hemophilia, thalassemia, or other conditions necessitating frequent or large-volume blood transfusions or clotting factor concentrates, (5) users of illicit parenteral drugs, (6) residents and staff of institutions for the mentally handicapped, (7) classroom contacts of aggressive, mentally handicapped persons having persistent hepatitis B antigenemia, (8) household or other intimate contacts of persons having persistent hepatitis B antigenemia, (9) persons who repeatedly contract sexually transmitted diseases, (10) prostitutes, (11) homosexually active males, (12) prisoners, (13) military personnel at risk, (14) morticians and embalmers, (15) Indochinese and Haitian refugees, (16) Alaskan Eskimos, and (17) infants born to carriers of the hepatitis B surface antigen, whether positive or negative for the hepatitis B e antigen

Prevention of type B hepatitis following (1) percutaneous, ocular, or mucous membrane exposure to blood known or presumed to contain hepatitis B antigen, (2) percutaneous bites by known or presumed human carriers of the antigen, or (3) intimate sexual contact with known or presumed carriers of the antigen

PARENTERAL DOSAGE

Adult and older child: 3 IM doses of 1 ml each, the first two given 1 mo apart and the third 6 mo after the first

Child (birth to 10 yr): 3 IM doses of 0.5 ml each, the first two given 1 mo apart and the third 6 mo after the first. For infants born to carriers of the hepatitis B surface antigen, give 3 IM doses of 0.5 ml each, the first within 7 days of birth, the second 1 mo later, and the third 6 mo after the first; in addition, give 0.5 ml of hepatitis B immune globulin at birth.

Adult: 3 IM doses of 1 ml each, the first given within 7 days of exposure, the second 1 mo later, and the third 6 mo after the first; in addition, give 0.06 ml/kg of hepatitis B immune globulin as soon as possible after exposure (preferably within 24 h)

CONTRAINDICATIONS

Hypersensitivity to yeast or to any component

ADMINISTRATION/DOSAGE ADJUSTMENTS

Parenteral administration — Administer IM or, if necessary, SC; do not inject IV or intradermally. For IM administration in adults, use the deltoid muscle; for IM injection in children, use an anterolateral thigh muscle. If the vaccine and hepatitis B immune globulin are to be given to an infant at the same time, inject the vaccine in one thigh and the globulin in the opposite thigh. The buttocks are generally not recommended as a site because the vaccine may be inadvertently injected into adipose tissue and, as a result, absorption and antibody response may be reduced. Subcutaneous administration should be reserved for patients in whom IM injection poses a risk of hemorrhage (eg, hemophiliacs); although IM and SC use of this vaccine have been shown to produce a similar immune response and comparable clinical reactions, SC administration of other aluminum-absorbed vaccines has been associated with an increased incidence of local reactions, including subcutaneous nodules. Before withdrawing a dose, thoroughly agitate the vial to suspend the vaccine. To prevent transmission of infection (eg, serum hepatitis), for each patient use a separate, sterile syringe and needle; the syringe should be free of preservatives, antiseptics, and detergents. Store the vaccine at 2–8°C; do not freeze.

RECOMBIVAX HB ■ ANTABUSE

Immunogenicity	Antibody response depends on age; the seroconversion rate is 100% for children 1–20 yr of age, 95–99% for adults 20–39 yr of age, and 91% of adults 40 yr of age or older. Prophylactic treatment of infants born to carriers of the hepatitis B surface and e antigens has been effective in 94% of infants at 6 mo of age and 93% of infants at 9 mo of age.
Immune status after vaccination	To determine immune status, measure antibody to the hepatitis B surface antigen (HBsAg) by radioimmunoassay (RIA) or enzyme immunoassay (EIA); active immunity is characterized by 10 or more RIA sample ratio units or a positive EIA response. Infants born to carriers of HBsAg should be tested at 12–15 mo of age; protective immunity is indicated by the absence of HBsAg and the presence of antibodies to this antigen.
Revaccination	The duration of immunity and the need for booster doses have not yet been determined. The antibody level in patients at high risk of exposure to hepatitis B virus may be checked periodically after vaccination; if the sample falls below 10 RIA sample ratio units or no antibody is detectable, administration of a booster dose should be considered.

WARNINGS/PRECAUTIONS

Hypersensitivity	Although not observed with this product, hypersensitivity reactions, including urticaria, angioedema, and pruritus, may occur within the first few hours after vaccination; an apparent hypersensitivity syndrome, characterized by transient arthritis, fever, and dermatological reactions (eg, urticaria, ecchymoses, erythema multiforme), may have been seen days or weeks after vaccination. Although no serious hypersensitivity reactions have been reported, epinephrine should be available during administration for immediate use. If symptoms suggestive of hypersensitivity develop after an injection, the regimen should be discontinued.
Patients with active infection	If possible, delay use in patients with any serious active infection
Other special-risk patients	Use with caution and appropriate care in patients in whom a systemic reaction (including fever) could pose a significant risk, such as in patients with severely compromised cardiopulmonary functions
Vaccination of patients with unrecognized hepatitis B infections	Because of the long incubation period for hepatitis B (6 wk to 6 mo), unrecognized infection may be present when this vaccine is given; under such circumstances, the vaccine may not prevent the subsequent development of clinical infection

ADVERSE REACTIONS[1]

Frequent reactions (incidence ≥ 1%) are printed in *italics*

Central nervous system	*Fatigue/weakness, headache,* achiness, lightheadedness, vertigo/dizziness, paresthesia, insomnia/disturbed sleep
Musculoskeletal	Arthralgia, including monoarticular, myalgia, back pain, neck pain, shoulder pain, and stiffness
Gastrointestinal	*Nausea, diarrhea,* vomiting, abdominal pains/cramps, dyspepsia, diminished appetite
Local	*Injection site reactions, including soreness, pain, tenderness, pruritus, erythema, ecchymosis, swelling, warmth, and nodule formation*
Hypersensitivity	Pruritus, nonspecifies rash, angioedema, urticaria
Respiratory	*Pharyngitis, upper respiratory tract infections,* rhinitis, influenza, cough
Hematological	Lymphadenopathy
Other	*Fever ≥ 100°F, malaise,* earache, dysuria, hypotension

USE IN CHILDREN
See INDICATIONS and PARENTERAL DOSAGE

USE IN PREGNANT AND NURSING WOMEN
Pregnancy Category C: reproduction studies have not been performed in animals or humans to determine whether this vaccine can adversely affect fetal development or reproductive capacity. Use during pregnancy only if clearly needed. It is not known whether this drug is excreted in human milk; because many drugs are excreted in human milk, use with caution in nursing mothers.

[1] Although the following reactions have not been reported with use of this product, they have been reported with use of other hepatitis B vaccines and, therefore, are considered potential reactions: delayed hypersensitivity syndrome of arthritis (usually transient), fever, and dermatological reactions (including urticaria, erythema multiforme, and ecchymoses); optic neuritis, myelitis (including transverse myelitis), acute radiculoneuropathy (including Guillain-Barré syndrome), peripheral neuropathy (including Bell's Palsy and herpes zoster), thrombocytopenia, tinnitus, and visual disturbances

---

ALCOHOL-ABUSE DETERRENTS

ANTABUSE (disulfiram) Ayerst   Rx

Tablets: 250, 500 mg

INDICATIONS
Alcoholism, as an adjunct to supportive and psychotherapeutic treatment in patients who want to remain in a state of enforced sobriety

ORAL DOSAGE
Adult: up to 500 mg/day in a single daily dose for 1–2 wk, followed by 125–500 mg/day for maintenance; average maintenance dosage: 250 mg/day

ANTABUSE

CONTRAINDICATIONS

Recent or current use of metronidazole, paraldehyde, alcohol, or alcohol-containing preparations	Severe myocardial disease	Coronary occlusion
	Hypersensitivity to disulfiram or other thiuram derivatives used in pesticides and rubber vulcanization	Alcohol intoxication
Psychoses		

ADMINISTRATION/DOSAGE ADJUSTMENTS

Initiation of therapy	Requires that patient has abstained from alcohol at least 12 h beforehand
Duration of therapy	Maintenance therapy is required until the patient is fully recovered socially and a basis for permanent self-control is established
Timing of administration	Although usually taken in the morning, daily dose may be taken upon retiring if patient experiences sedation
Trial with alcohol	If test reaction is deemed necessary, slowly give 15 ml (1/2 oz) of 100-proof whiskey or equivalent after the first 1–2 wk of therapy with 500 mg/day; repeat test dose of alcoholic beverage once only. Once reaction develops, no more alcohol should be consumed. Conduct test in hospital or, alternatively, wherever comparable supervision and facilities, including oxygen, are available. Do not test reaction in patients over 50 yr of age.

WARNINGS/PRECAUTIONS

Disulfiram-alcohol reaction	Caution patients that this will occur with even small amounts of alcohol, up to 14 days after ingesting disulfiram, and may produce flushing, throbbing in head and neck, throbbing headache, respiratory difficulty, nausea, copious vomiting, sweating, thirst, chest pain, palpitation, dyspnea, hyperventilation, tachycardia, hypotension, syncope, marked uneasiness, weakness, vertigo, blurred vision, and confusion; in severe reactions, there may be respiratory depression, cardiovascular collapse, arrhythmias, myocardial infarction, acute congestive heart failure, unconsciousness, convulsions, and death. For severe reactions, restore blood pressure and treat shock. Administer oxygen, carbogen (95% oxygen and 5% carbon dioxide), massive IV doses (1 g) of vitamin C, and ephedrine sulfate. Antihistamines have been used intravenously. Hypokalemia has been reported; monitor potassium levels, particularly in digitalized patients.
Alcohol-containing substances	Warn patients taking disulfiram to avoid alcohol in disguised forms; eg, in sauces, vinegars, cough mixtures, aftershave lotions, and back rubs
Alcohol intoxication	Do not administer to intoxicated patient or without patient's full knowledge; inform relatives accordingly
Concomitant use of phenytoin or its congeners	May lead to phenytoin intoxication; use disulfiram with caution. Obtain serum levels of phenytoin prior to and after initiating disulfiram therapy and adjust phenytoin dosage as needed.
Concomitant use of oral anticoagulants	May increase prothrombin time; adjust anticoagulant dosage as necessary when initiating or stopping disulfiram
Concomitant use of isoniazid	May produce unsteady gait or marked changes in mental status; discontinue disulfiram if such signs appear
Concomitant ingestion of nitrites	Has been reported to cause tumors in rats; significance of this finding in humans is not known
Special-risk patients	Use with extreme caution in patients with diabetes mellitus, hypothyroidism, epilepsy, cerebral damage, chronic and acute nephritis, or hepatic cirrhosis or insufficiency
Patients with rubber contact dermatitis	Should be evaluated for hypersensitivity to thiuram derivatives before receiving disulfiram (see CONTRAINDICATIONS)
Patient identification card	Should be carried by the patient, stating that patient is receiving disulfiram, and describing symptoms most likely to occur as a result of the disulfiram-alcohol reaction; the card should also indicate the physician or institution to be contacted in an emergency. (Cards may be obtained from the manufacturer upon request.)
Skin eruptions	May occur; if troublesome, add an antihistamine
Concomitant use of barbiturates	Possibility of initiating a new abuse should be considered
Hepatic dysfunction	May occur; perform baseline and follow-up transaminase tests every 10–14 days, as well as a complete blood count and a sequential multiple analysis-12 (SMA-12) test every 6 mo
Exposure to ethylene dibromide or its vapors	Has resulted in a higher incidence of tumors and mortality in disulfiram-treated rats; although correlation of this finding to humans has not been demonstrated, caution patients against exposure to this substance
Metallic or garlicky aftertaste	May occur during first 2 wk of therapy

ADVERSE REACTIONS

Central nervous system	Optic neuritis, peripheral neuritis, polyneuritis, transient mild drowsiness, fatigability, headache; psychotic reactions[1]
Dermatological	Skin eruptions, acneform eruptions, allergic dermatitis
Genitourinary	Impotence

ANTABUSE ■ MUCOMYST

| Gastrointestinal | Metallic or garlicky aftertaste |
| Hepatic | Cholestatic and fulminant hepatitis |

OVERDOSAGE

| Signs and symptoms | See ADVERSE REACTIONS |
| Treatment | Treat symptomatically |

DRUG INTERACTIONS

Oral anticoagulants	⇧ Anticoagulant effect
Isoniazid	Unsteady gait, mental changes, psychosis
Metronidazole	Psychosis
Paraldehyde	⇧ Adverse reactions
Phenytoin and its congeners	⇧ Serum phenytoin level

ALTERED LABORATORY VALUES

| Blood/serum values | ⇧ Cholesterol |
| Urinary values | ⇩ VMA |

USE IN CHILDREN

Consult manufacturer

USE IN PREGNANT AND NURSING WOMEN

Safety for use during pregnancy has not been established; use in pregnant women only when the probable benefits outweigh the possible risks. Consult manufacturer for use in nursing women.

---

[1] In most cases attributable to high doses, concomitant use of metronidazole or isoniazid, or unmasking of underlying psychoses

---

ANTIDOTES

MUCOMYST (acetylcysteine) Bristol   Rx

Vials: 10% (Mucomyst-10) (4, 10, 30 ml), 20% (4, 10, 30 ml)

INDICATIONS

Abnormal, viscid, or inspissated mucous secretions associated with or resulting from bronchopulmonary disease, cystic fibrosis, surgery, anesthesia, post-traumatic chest conditions, atelectasis, tracheostomy, and similar conditions

Abnormal, viscid, or inspissated mucous secretions that may interfere with diagnostic bronchial studies, eg, bronchograms, bronchospirometry, and bronchial wedge catheterization

Prevention or reduction of hepatotoxicity associated with **acetaminophen overdose**

INHALANT DOSAGE

Adult and child: for nebulization into a face mask, mouth piece, or tracheostomy, 1–10 ml of the 20% solution or 2–20 ml of the 10% solution q2–6h (usual dosage: 3–5 ml of the 20% solution or 6–10 ml of the 10% solution tid or qid); for nebulization into a tent or Croupette, use a sufficient volume of the 10% or 20% solution (up to 300 ml) to maintain a very heavy mist for the desired period

Adult and child: 1–2 ml of the 20% solution or 2–4 ml of the 10% solution given by nebulization 2–3 times before the procedure

ORAL DOSAGE

Adult and child: 140 mg/kg, given as a loading dose within 24 h of ingestion, followed by 70 mg/kg, starting 4 h after the loading dose and repeated q4h for 17 doses (unless the serum acetaminophen level indicates minimal risk of hepatotoxicity [see table in ADMINISTRATION/DOSAGE ADJUSTMENTS])

INTRATRACHEAL DOSAGE

Adult and child: for direct instillation, 1–2 ml of the 10% or 20% solution given as frequently as once every hour; for instillation in the routine care of patients with a tracheostomy, 1–2 ml of the 10% or 20% solution q1–4h; for instillation into a particular bronchopulmonary segment with an intratracheal catheter, 2–5 ml of the 20% solution; for instillation with a percutaneous intratracheal catheter, 1–2 ml of the 20% solution or 2–4 ml of the 10% solution q1–4h

Adult and child: 1–2 ml of the 20% solution or 2–4 ml of the 10% solution instilled 2–3 times before the procedure

CONTRAINDICATIONS

Hypersensitivity to acetylcysteine (when used as a mucolytic agent)

ADMINISTRATION/DOSAGE ADJUSTMENTS

When used as a mucolytic agent

COMPENDIUM OF DRUG THERAPY

MUCOMYST

Preparation of solution	The 20% solution may be diluted with sterile normal saline or sterile water for injection USP; the 10% solution may be used undiluted. Do not mix either solution with amphotericin B, tetracycline, oxytetracycline, chlortetracycline, ampicillin, erythromycin lactobionate, iodized oil, trypsin, chymotrypsin, or hydrogen peroxide. After a vial is opened, the solution may turn light purple; this change will not significantly affect the safety or effectiveness of the drug. Unused portions should be stored under refrigeration and used within 96 h.
Nebulizing equipment	For aerosol administration, use a conventional mechanical nebulizer made of plastic or glass that produces a high proportion of particles less than 10 μ in diameter; the parts that come into contact with the solution may contain plain or anodized aluminum, chromed metal, tantalum, sterling silver, or stainless steel, but should not contain any other material (especially rubber, iron, or copper). Although hand bulbs may also be used, they are not recommended for routine administration, since their output is generally too low and, in some cases, the particles they produce are too large. For delivery of the solution, compressed tank air or an air compressor is recommended (oxygen may also be used, but with caution in patients with severe respiratory disease and CO_2 retention). To provide a warm mist, add the solution to a separate unheated nebulizer that is attached to an apparatus containing a heated nebulizer; do not place the solution directly into the chamber of a heated nebulizer. Nebulizing equipment should be cleaned immediately after use to avoid accumulation of residues that may clog the fine orifices or corrode the metal parts.
Prolonged nebulization	Delivery of the drug may be impeded during prolonged nebulization because of an increase in concentration of the solution as the solvent evaporates; after 75% of the initial volume of solution has been given, dilute the remaining volume 1 : 1 with sterile water for injection USP

When used as an antidote

Initial treatment of acetaminophen overdose	Promptly empty stomach by performing gastric lavage or inducing emesis with syrup of ipecac (15–30 ml for children, 30–45 ml for adults). Give ipecac with copious quantities of water; if emesis does not occur within 20 min, repeat the dose. Activated charcoal may be given if acetaminophen has been ingested with certain other drugs, but should be removed by lavage prior to administration of acetylcysteine. Avoid forced diuresis or use of diuretics when treating acetaminophen overdose.
Preparation of acetylcysteine	Dilute the 20% solution 1 : 4 with cola, Fresca, or other soft drink (water may be used as a diluent for administration by gastric tube or Miller-Abbott tube); use the solution within 1 h of preparation
Administration	Start treatment as soon as possible; each dose should be given orally. If vomiting occurs within 1 h of administration, repeat the dose. If the patient persistently fails to retain the antidote after oral administration, the diluted solution may be given by duodenal intubation.
Laboratory testing	Measure the serum level of *unconjugated* acetaminophen as early as possible, but no sooner than 4 h after an acute overdose; when possible, this should be done by gas-liquid or high-pressure liquid chromatography, although a colorimetric assay may also be used. Do not wait for laboratory results to become available before starting acetylcysteine. If the serum level equals or exceeds the value listed in the table below (or if the serum level cannot be obtained), continue giving the entire 18-dose course; if the serum level is less than the value listed below, administration can be stopped.

Time after ingestion (h)	Plasma acetaminophen level (μg/ml)	Time after ingestion (h)	Plasma acetaminophen level (μg/ml)
4.0	150.0	14.0	25.5
4.5	135.0	15.0	21.5
5.0	125.0	16.0	18.0
6.0	105.0	17.0	15.0
7.0	88.0	18.0	12.5
8.0	74.0	19.0	10.5
9.0	62.0	20.0	8.8
10.0	52.0	21.0	7.4
11.0	46.0	22.0	6.3
12.0	36.0	23.0	5.2
13.0	30.5	24.0	4.4

To monitor hepatic and renal function and electrolyte and fluid balance, determine the prothrombin time, SGOT and SGPT levels, and serum concentrations of bilirubin, creatinine, BUN, glucose, and electrolytes q24h. If the prothrombin time exceeds 1.5 times the control value, give vitamin K_1; if the prothrombin time exceeds 3 times the control value, give fresh frozen plasma. Institute appropriate measures to treat hypoglycemia and electrolyte and fluid imbalance.

WARNINGS/PRECAUTIONS

When used as a mucolytic agent

Airway obstruction	Acetylcysteine may block the airway by causing an increase in the volume of liquefied bronchial secretions. If local accumulation cannot be removed by coughing, provide mechanical suction; if a large mechanical block develops (owing to local accumulation or the presence of a foreign body), clear the airway by endotracheal aspiration, with or without bronchoscopy.

MUCOMYST ■ NARCAN

Bronchospasm	Carefully monitor asthmatic patients; if bronchospasm occurs, immediately discontinue acetylcysteine and administer a bronchodilator
Odor, stickiness	A slight transient odor may be detected when beginning administration; stickiness may develop with use of a face mask, but can be easily removed with water

When used as an antidote

Hypersensitivity	If generalized urticaria or other allergic reactions occur, discontinue acetylcysteine unless the drug is essential and the reaction can be controlled
Encephalopathy	Acetylcysteine can theoretically exacerbate hepatic failure; if encephalopathy owing to hepatic failure becomes evident, the drug should be discontinued
Upper GI reactions	Acetylcysteine can exacerbate acetaminophen-induced vomiting; the benefit of preventing or lessening hepatic injury should be weighed against the risk of inducing GI bleeding before administering acetylcysteine to patients susceptible to upper GI hemorrhage (eg, patients with peptic ulcers or esophageal varices)

ADVERSE REACTIONS

When used as a mucolytic agent

Respiratory	Bronchospasm, rhinorrhea
Other	Stomatitis, nausea, sensitivity, sensitization

When used as an antidote

Gastrointestinal	Nausea, vomiting, other GI reactions
Hypersensitivity	Rash with or without mild fever (rare)

DRUG INTERACTIONS

Activated charcoal	▽ Bioavailability of oral acetylcysteine
Amphotericin B, tetracycline, oxytetracycline, chlortetracycline, ampicillin, erythromycin lactobionate, iodized oil, trypsin, chymotrypsin, hydrogen peroxide	Physical incompatibility (with mucolytic solutions of acetylcysteine)

ALTERED LABORATORY VALUES

No clinically significant alterations in blood/serum or urinary values occur at therapeutic dosages

---

USE IN CHILDREN	USE IN PREGNANT AND NURSING WOMEN
See INDICATIONS and dosage recommendations	Consult manufacturer

---

ANTIDOTES

NARCAN (naloxone hydrochloride) Du Pont   Rx

Ampuls: 0.02 mg/ml[1] (2 ml), 0.4 mg/ml[1] (1 ml), 1 mg/ml (1, 2 ml)   **Vials:** 0.4 mg/ml (10 ml), 1 mg/ml (10 ml)   **Prefilled syringes:** 0.4 mg/ml (1 ml)

INDICATIONS	PARENTERAL DOSAGE
Postoperative narcotic depression	**Adult:** 0.1–0.2 mg, given IV at 2- to 3-min intervals; if necessary, repeat q1–2h **Neonate:** 0.01 mg/kg, given IV, IM, or SC at 2- to 3-min intervals; if necessary, repeat q1–2h **Child:** 0.005–0.01 mg, given IV at 2- to 3-min intervals; if necessary, repeat q1–2h
Acute narcotic overdosage (known or suspected)	**Adult:** 0.4–2 mg IV or, if necessary, IM or SC; repeat at 2- to 3-min intervals, as needed **Child:** 0.01 mg/kg IV, followed, if necessary, by 0.1 mg/kg IV; if IV administration is not feasible, administer IM or SC in divided doses

CONTRAINDICATIONS

Hypersensitivity to naloxone

ADMINISTRATION/DOSAGE ADJUSTMENTS

Narcotic depression	Repeat appropriate dose at 2- to 3-min intervals until adequate ventilation and alertness occur without significant pain or discomfort. If supplemental doses are given IM (q1–2h), a more prolonged effect will be produced.
Narcotic overdosage	Diagnosis should be questioned if no response is observed after a total of 10 mg (for an adult) has been administered

NARCAN ■ PERSANTINE

Preparation for IV infusion	Naloxone may be diluted in normal saline or 5% dextrose solutions; if necessary, Sterile Water for Injection may be used as a diluent in cases of pediatric overdosage. Naloxone should not be mixed with solutions having an alkaline pH, agents whose effects on the stability of naloxone-containing solutions have not been established, or preparations containing bisulfite, metabisulfite, or long-chain or high-molecular-weight anions. Solutions should be used within 24 h.
Onset of action	Administer by IV route in emergency situations; onset of action is generally apparent within 2 min of injection and is only slightly less rapid by IM or SC route

WARNINGS/PRECAUTIONS

Withdrawal symptoms	May be precipitated in the presence of physical dependence on narcotics; administer with caution to persons who are physically dependent on narcotics, including newborns of physically dependent mothers; abrupt and complete reversal of narcotic effects may precipitate an acute abstinence syndrome in such cases
Patient monitoring/repeat dosing	Continued surveillance of patients who have responded satisfactorily to naloxone is essential; administer repeated doses as needed, since the duration of action of some narcotics may exceed that of naloxone
Nonopioid-induced respiratory depression	Should not be treated with naloxone, as it is not effective against respiratory depression caused by nonnarcotic drugs
Additional measures to counteract acute narcotic overdosage	Other resuscitative measures (eg, maintenance of a free airway, artificial ventilation, cardiac massage, and vasopressor therapy) should be available and used when needed
Special-risk patients	Use with caution in patients with cardiac disease and in patients who have received potentially cardiotoxic drugs, because cardiovascular reactions[2] have occurred with postoperative use, and most of the cases have involved such patients
Carcinogenicity, mutagenicity	The carcinogenic and mutagenic potential of this drug has not been studied
Effect on fertility	Reproduction studies in mice and rats have shown no evidence of impaired fertility

ADVERSE REACTIONS[3]

Gastrointestinal	Nausea and vomiting (with abrupt reversal)
Cardiovascular	Tachycardia and increased blood pressure (with abrupt reversal)[2]
Other	Sweating and tremulousness (with abrupt reversal)

OVERDOSAGE

Signs and symptoms	Significant reversal of analgesia, excitement, and increased blood pressure may occur when naloxone is used in larger than necessary dosage to reverse postoperative narcotic depression; acute overdosage in humans has not been reported
Treatment	Discontinue use; treat symptomatically and institute supportive measures, as needed

DRUG INTERACTIONS

Narcotic analgesics	Reversal of narcotic depression

ALTERED LABORATORY VALUES

No clinically significant alterations in blood/serum or urinary values occur at therapeutic dosages

---

USE IN CHILDREN	USE IN PREGNANT AND NURSING WOMEN
See INDICATIONS and PARENTERAL DOSAGE	Pregnancy Category B: use during pregnancy only if clearly needed. Reproduction studies in mice and rats given up to 1,000 times the human dose have shown no evidence of harm to the fetus. No adequate, well-controlled studies have been performed in pregnant women. It is not known whether naloxone is excreted in human milk; use with caution in nursing mothers, because many drugs are excreted in human milk.

[1] Supplied with and without methyl- and propylparaben
[2] Ventricular tachycardia and fibrillation, hypotension, hypertension, and pulmonary edema have occurred after postoperative use; however, a causal relationship has not been established
[3] Seizures have occurred (infrequently) with use of naloxone; however, a causal relationship has not been established

---

ANTIPLATELET AGENTS

PERSANTINE (dipyridamole) Boehringer Ingelheim   Rx

Tablets: 25, 50, 75 mg

INDICATIONS	ORAL DOSAGE
Prevention of postoperative thromboembolism after cardiac valve replacement when used as an adjunct to coumarin anticoagulants	Adult: 75–100 mg qid

PERSANTINE ■ CALCIMAR

CONTRAINDICATIONS
None known

ADMINISTRATION/DOSAGE ADJUSTMENTS
Concomitant use of warfarin — This drug is intended for use with warfarin and other coumarin anticoagulants; no greater frequency or severity of bleeding has been observed during concomitant therapy with dipyridamole and warfarin than with warfarin alone

WARNINGS/PRECAUTIONS
Peripheral vasodilation — Use with caution in patients with hypotension, since peripheral vasodilation may be produced

Adverse effects — At therapeutic doses, adverse effects are usually minimal and transient, and initial reactions usually disappear after long-term therapy; discontinue use if reactions become persistent or intolerable

Carcinogenicity — No carcinogenic effects have been found in mice given 8, 25, and 75 mg/kg of dipyridamole orally for 111 wk or in rats that were fed these doses for 128–142 wk

Mutagenicity — The results of mutagenicity studies have been negative

Effect on fertility — No evidence of impaired fertility has been found in animal reproduction studies

ADVERSE REACTIONS[1]
Frequent reactions (incidence ≥ 1%) are printed in *italics*

Central nervous system — *Dizziness (13.6%), headache (2.3%)*

Cardiovascular — Flushing, angina pectoris (rare)

Gastrointestinal — *Abdominal distress (6.1%)*, diarrhea, vomiting

Dermatological — *Rash (2.3%)*, pruritus

OVERDOSAGE
Signs and symptoms — Hypotension (of short duration)

Treatment — Administer a vasopressor, if necessary. Dipyridamole is highly protein bound; dialysis is not likely to be of benefit.

DRUG INTERACTIONS
Aspirin — ⇧ Risk of bleeding and hemorrhage

ALTERED LABORATORY VALUES
No clinically significant alterations in blood/serum or urinary values occur at therapeutic dosages

---

USE IN CHILDREN

Safety and effectiveness for use in children under 12 yr of age have not been established

USE IN PREGNANT AND NURSING WOMEN

Pregnancy Category B: reproduction studies in mice, rats, and rabbits at doses up to 125 mg/kg have shown no evidence of impaired fertility or fetal harm. No adequate, well-controlled studies have been performed in pregnant women; use during pregnancy only if clearly needed. Dipyridamole is excreted in human milk; use with caution in nursing women.

---

[1] Includes reactions reported during concomitant therapy with dipyridamole and warfarin

---

BONE/CALCIUM METABOLISM REGULATORS

CALCIMAR (calcitonin-salmon) Rorer   Rx

Vials: 200 IU/ml (2 ml)

INDICATIONS	PARENTERAL DOSAGE
Symptomatic Paget's disease of bone	Adult: 100 IU/day SC or IM to start; for maintenance, 50 IU may be given daily or every other day. If a patient has a serious deformity or a neurological complication, the initial dose should not be reduced, since it is not known whether 50 IU will be as effective as 100 IU in promoting the formation of more normal bone structure.
Hypercalcemia	Adult: 4 IU/kg q12h SC or IM to start; if response is inadequate after 1–2 days, increase dosage to 8 IU/kg q12h (doses > 2 ml in volume should be given IM into multiple sites); if response remains unsatisfactory after 2 more days, increase dosage to 8 IU/kg q6h

COMPENDIUM OF DRUG THERAPY

CALCIMAR

Postmenopausal osteoporosis — **Adult:** for treatment, 100 IU/day SC or IM in conjunction with a vitamin D intake of at least 400 units/day, calcium supplementation (eg, 1.5 g/day of calcium carbonate), and a diet containing adequate amounts of other nutrients

CONTRAINDICATIONS
Clinical allergy to synthetic salmon calcitonin

ADMINISTRATION/DOSAGE ADJUSTMENTS

Pretreatment skin test — Prepare a dilution of 10 IU/ml by withdrawing 0.05 ml in a tuberculin syringe and filling it to 1.0 ml with Sodium Chloride Injection USP. Mix well, discard 0.9 ml, and inject 0.1 ml intracutaneously on the inner side of the forearm. Check 15 min later; more than mild erythema or a wheal constitutes a positive response (see WARNINGS/PRECAUTIONS)

Paget's disease — *Therapeutic use:* In patients with moderate to severe disease, characterized by polyostotic involvement and increases in serum alkaline phosphatase and urinary hydroxyproline levels, calcitonin has been shown to reduce both the biochemical abnormalities and bone pain. Although elevated cardiac output has also been reduced and, in some cases, neurological complications have been reversed (auditory improvement has been seen in 4 of 29 patients with hearing loss), the likelihood that these particular effects will occur cannot be predicted since clinical experience is limited. Mild symptoms of Paget's disease can usually be managed with analgesics. Prophylactic use of calcitonin in asymptomatic patients has not been shown to be beneficial; however, such use may be considered if there is extensive involvement of the skull or spinal cord and a risk of irreversible neurological damage. *Monitoring of therapy:* Evaluate clinical symptoms, and periodically measure serum alkaline phosphatase and 24-h urinary hydroxyproline levels; bone pain and elevated laboratory values usually decrease within the first few months of therapy, whereas neurological improvement, if it occurs, often is not evident until after 1 yr. *Relapse:* Assess patient compliance. Look for laboratory or clinical evidence of antibody formation. An increase in dosage above 100 IU/day does not usually enhance response.

WARNINGS/PRECAUTIONS

Systemic allergic reactions — May occur; institute appropriate emergency measures. Do not begin treatment in patients with positive skin tests (see ADMINISTRATION/DOSAGE ADJUSTMENTS).

Pagetic lesions — Should be carefully distinguished from osteogenic sarcoma, the incidence of which is increased in Paget's disease

Hypocalcemic tetany — May occur, although no cases have been reported; have parenteral calcium available during first several administrations

Urine sediment abnormalities — May occur and may include coarse granular casts and casts containing renal tubular epithelial cells; examine urine sediment periodically during prolonged therapy

Carcinogenicity — The carcinogenic potential of this drug has not been evaluated

ADVERSE REACTIONS

Frequent reactions (incidence ≥ 1%) are printed in *italics*

Dermatological — Rash

Gastrointestinal — *Nausea (10%), vomiting*

Other — *Inflammation at injection site (10%), flushing of face or hands (2–5%)*

OVERDOSAGE

Signs and symptoms — Nausea, vomiting

Treatment — Discontinue use; treat symptomatically, if needed

DRUG INTERACTIONS
No clinically significant drug interactions have been identified

ALTERED LABORATORY VALUES

Blood/serum values — ⇑ PTH (transient) ⇓ Calcium ⇓ Alkaline phosphatase

Urinary values — ⇑ Sodium ⇑ Potassium ⇑ Magnesium ⇑ Chloride ⇑ Phosphate ⇑ or ⇓ Calcium ⇓ Hydroxyproline

---

USE IN CHILDREN
There are no adequate data to support the use of this drug in children

USE IN PREGNANT AND NURSING WOMEN
Pregnancy Category C: administration to rabbits of 14–56 times the human dose has caused a decrease in fetal birth weights, possibly as a result of the drug's metabolic effects (calcitonin does not cross the placental barrier); use during pregnancy only if the expected benefit justifies the potential risk to the fetus. This drug inhibits lactation in animals; it is not known whether it is excreted in human milk. Because many drugs are excreted in breast milk, patient should not nurse if this drug is prescribed.

BONE/CALCIUM METABOLISM REGULATORS

DIDRONEL (etidronate disodium) Norwich Eaton   Rx

Tablets: 200, 400 mg

INDICATIONS	ORAL DOSAGE
Symptomatic Paget's disease of bone[1]	**Adult:** 5 mg/kg/day, given in a single daily dose for up to 6 mo. After cessation of therapy, therapeutic effects may continue for months (in many patients, for at least 1 yr); check condition of patients every 3–6 mo. Repeat the course of treatment only if, after a drug-free period of at least 90 days, there is evidence of disease; administer initial dosage or, if necessary, up to 20 mg/kg/day (see ADMINISTRATION/DOSAGE ADJUSTMENTS).
Prevention and treatment of **heterotopic ossification complicating total hip replacement**	**Adult:** 20 mg/kg/day, given in a single daily dose for 1 mo preoperatively and for 3 mo postoperatively
Prevention and treatment of **heterotopic ossification due to spinal cord injury**	**Adult:** 20 mg/kg/day, given in a single daily dose for 2 wk, followed by 10 mg/kg/day for 10 wk

CONTRAINDICATIONS

None known

ADMINISTRATION/DOSAGE ADJUSTMENTS

Administration	Instruct patients not to consume food (especially milk, milk products, or other foods with a high calcium content) or vitamins with mineral supplements or antacids with high levels of calcium, iron, magnesium, aluminum, or other metals within a period of 2 h before or after administration. Divide the total daily dose if GI discomfort occurs.
Dosage increases in Paget's disease	Onset of therapeutic response may be slow; avoid premature dose increase. Dosages greater than 10 mg/kg/day should be used with caution, for no longer than 3 mo, and only when lower dosages are ineffective or when there is an overriding need to suppress rapid bone turnover (eg, when irreversible neurologic damage is possible) or reduce elevated cardiac output. Do not exceed 20 mg/kg/day.
Initiation of therapy after spinal cord injury	Begin treatment as soon after the injury as is medically feasible, preferably prior to any radiographic evidence of heterotopic ossification
Retreatment of heterotopic ossification	Has not been studied; there is no evidence that etidronate disodium affects mature heterotopic bone

WARNINGS/PRECAUTIONS

Nutritional status	Instruct patients to consume an adequate amount of nutrients, especially calcium and vitamin D
Patients with enterocolitis	Diarrhea may occur in such patients, particularly at higher dosages; consider withholding therapy
Patients with renal impairment	Closely observe patients with renal insufficiency, and reduce the dosage if the glomerular filtration rate is decreased; etidronate is excreted by the kidney
Patients with fractures	It may be advisable to delay or interrupt use of this drug in patients with fractures (particularly fractures of the long bones) until callus is evident, because etidronate may retard mineralization of osteoid. In clinical studies, etidronate did not inhibit fracture healing or stabilization of the spine.
Carcinogenicity	Long-term studies in rats have shown no evidence of carcinogenicity

ADVERSE REACTIONS

Frequent reactions (incidence $\geq$ 1%) are printed in *italics*

Gastrointestinal	*Diarrhea and nausea (7–30%, depending on dosage)*
Skeletal	*Increased or recurrent bone pain at pagetic sites and/or pain at previously asymptomatic sites (10–20%, depending on dosage)*
Hypersensitivity	Angioedema/urticaria, rash, and pruritus (rare)

OVERDOSAGE

Signs and symptoms	Hypocalcemia (theoretical effect)
Treatment	Discontinue use; drug is rapidly cleared by the kidneys

DRUG INTERACTIONS

No clinically significant drug interactions have been identified

ALTERED LABORATORY VALUES

Blood/serum values	△ Phosphate ▽ Alkaline phosphatase
Urinary values	▽ Hydroxyproline

USE IN CHILDREN	USE IN PREGNANT AND NURSING WOMEN
Safety and efficacy have not been established for use in children	Pregnancy Category B: reproduction studies in rats and rabbits given up to 5 times the maximum human dose have shown no evidence of impaired fertility or harm to the fetus; in rats, a decrease in live fetuses was seen at 22 times the maximum human dose, and skeletal malformations were detected at exaggerated parenteral doses. No adequate, well-controlled studies have been performed in pregnant women; use during pregnancy only if clearly needed. It is not known whether etidronate disodium is excreted in human milk; use with caution in nursing mothers.

[1] Although use in patients with asymptomatic Paget's disease has not been studied, such use may be warranted if major joints or major weight-bearing bones are threatened or if irreversible neurologic damage is possible

---

CHEMONUCLEOLYTIC ENZYMES

CHYMODIACTIN (chymopapain) Flint
Rx

Vials: 4,000 pKat (2 ml), 10,000 pKat (5 ml)

INDICATIONS

Herniated lumbar intervertebral disks when signs and symptoms, particularly sciatica, are unresponsive to conservative therapy

INTRADISCAL DOSAGE

Adult: 2,000–4,000 pKat/disk (usual dose: 3,000 pKat/disk); maximum total dose for a single patient with multiple-disk herniation: 8,000 pKat

CONTRAINDICATIONS

Severe, progressing paralysis indicated by rapidly progressing neurologic dysfunction

Severe spondylolisthesis

Significant spinal stenosis

Use in any spinal region other than the lumbar area

Spinal cord tumor, cauda equina lesion, or other lesions producing spinal motor or sensory dysfunction

Hypersensitivity to chymopapain, papaya, or papaya derivatives (including contact lens cleaners and meat tenderizers that contain papain)

Previous injection with any form of chymopapain

ADMINISTRATION/DOSAGE ADJUSTMENTS

Requirements for use	Chymopapain should be used only by surgeons who have extensive training and experience in diagnosing and treating spinal disorders and who have been specially trained and licensed to perform chemonucleolysis. The diagnosis must be established precisely since nerve root compression can result from causes other than a herniated disk. The drug should be administered only in a hospital setting, with personnel and facilities available for the immediate treatment of any potential complication.
Preparation of solution	Add 2 ml of sterile water for injection USP (supplied) to the 2-ml vial or 5 ml to the 5-ml vial; do not reconstitute with bacteriostatic water for injection since it may inactivate the enzyme. Alcohol used to cleanse the vial stopper may also inactivate the enzyme and therefore should be allowed to air dry before insertion of the needle into the vial. To reduce the possibility of coring the stopper, exercise care in the selection and use of needles; do not use automatic filling syringes because the powder is in a vacuum. Administer solution within 2 h of reconstitution; discard the unused portion.
Anesthesia	Use local or supplemented local anesthesia rather than general anesthesia whenever possible because anaphylaxis and neurological reactions are more likely to occur with general anesthesia. During local anesthesia, the patient can complain if the needle impinges on nerve tissue and object to repeated attempts to place the needle; the patient can also report premonitory symptoms of anaphylaxis. Moreover, when the patient is awake, it may be possible to establish a correlation between sciatic pain and a specific disk. General anesthesia, while not recommended, offers the following advantages: ease of airway management in cases of anaphylaxis, more precise positioning of the body, and less discomfort for the patient. Keep in mind that ventricular tachycardia or fibrillation may occur during halothane anesthesia if epinephrine is used for treatment of anaphylaxis.
Needle placement	To avoid puncture of the dura mater, use the lateral approach for needle placement; the posterior or transdural approach must be avoided because of the risk of serious neurological reactions. Take great care to assure that the dura is not penetrated and that chymopapain and contrast agents do not enter the subarachnoid space; chymopapain and some contrast agents are extremely toxic when injected intrathecally. Before injection, verify the exact location of the needle tip by evaluating intensified x-ray images of both the anteroposterior and lateral views; chemonucleolysis should not be performed if high quality x-ray equipment, including an image intensifier, are not available. If there is any question about the location of the needle tip within the nucleus of the disk, terminate this procedure and do not inject chymopapain.

CHYMODIACTIN

Discography	Since discography appears to increase the risk of serious neurological reactions, the procedure should generally not be performed in conjunction with chemonucleolysis; to determine whether a disk is abnormal and to correlate that abnormality with sciatic pain, use a water or saline acceptance test in place of discography. A contrast agent may be administered if, in a particular case, it is deemed essential and benefits outweigh risks. After injection of a contrast agent, observe response for at least 15 min before giving chymopapain; if the contrast agent enters the subarachnoid space, terminate the procedure and do not inject chymopapain.
Prevention of anaphylaxis	Before using this drug, determine whether the patient has a history of multiple allergies and consider using a preoperative screening test for chymopapain-specific IgE antibody. An H_1- and an H_2-antagonist should be administered before chemonucleolysis; in one widely used regimen, 300 mg of cimetidine and 50 mg of diphenhydramine are given orally q6h for a period of 24 h prior to the procedure. To ensure that the patient is well-hydrated and thereby reduce the potential effect of anaphylactic-induced hypotension, give oral or IV liquids before administration. For a period of 3 min before injection, 100% oxygen may be administered as a prophylactic measure. Since rapid management of anaphylaxis is critical, keep at least one open IV line in place when using this drug. To identify those patients who are most sensitive to this drug, give a test dose of 400 pKat 10–15 min before the injection of the full therapeutic dose; if signs or symptoms of anaphylaxis are seen, do not administer the full dose. Bear in mind that a negative response to a test dose does not rule out the possibility of anaphylaxis since the reaction can subsequently occur in less sensitive patients following the therapeutic dose.

WARNINGS/PRECAUTIONS

Anaphylaxis	Life-threatening anaphylaxis can occur immediately or up to 2 h after injection and can vary in duration from a few minutes to several hours or longer; bronchospasm, hypotension (the more common effect), or both reactions may develop initially and can be followed by laryngeal edema, arrhythmia, cardiac arrest, coma, and death. Anaphylaxis is more likely to occur in women (especially black women) and patients receiving a general anesthetic. The frequency of anaphylaxis is 0.8% in women and 0.3% in men; it is 0.5% with general anesthesia and 0.4% with local anesthesia. For preoperative measures to prevent anaphylaxis, see ADMINISTRATION/DOSAGE ADJUSTMENTS. After administration, watch for signs and symptoms of an allergic response, including erythema, pilomotor erection, rash, pruritic urticaria, conjunctivitis, vasomotor rhinitis, angioedema, and GI disturbances. Rapid diagnosis and treatment of anaphylaxis is critical since signs, severity, progression, and duration of the reaction are highly unpredictable. Epinephrine is the drug of choice for the immediate treatment of anaphylaxis; reserve use of corticosteroids and other drugs for cases where epinephrine is inappropriate. Bear in mind that epinephrine may be ineffective if the patient is receiving a beta blocker.
Delayed hypersensitivity reactions	Rash, urticaria, or pruritus may develop as late as 15 days after injection; instruct patients to report these reactions
Neurotoxicity	Serious neurological effects, including paraparesis, paraplegia, seizures, and subarachnoid and intracerebral hemorrhage, have occurred in 0.05% of patients. Hemorrhage has been severe, extensive, or fatal in a number of patients with a cerebrovascular anomaly, a history of hypertension, or a personal or strong family history of cerebrovascular accident. Signs and symptoms of neurological reactions are generally seen within hours or days; however, manifestations of acute transverse myelitis or acute transverse myelopathy are not evident until 2–3 wk after the procedure. The frequency of acute transverse myelitis and myelopathy, 1 in 18,000, is higher than the rate seen in the general population. However, no causal relationship has been established between proper *intradiscal* administration of chymopapain and myelitis, myelopathy, or any other neurological effect. In some instances, neurological reactions may be due to needle trauma or intrathecal injection of the drug and contrast agents (see ADMINISTRATION/DOSAGE ADJUSTMENTS.)
	The risk of neurological reactions appears to be increased by discography, general anesthesia, injection in more than one disk, and a history of lumbar spine surgery. If possible, avoid discography and general anesthesia. Inject the drug in more than one disk only if such action is indicated by definitive signs, symptoms, and diagnostic procedures. Use in patients with a history of lumbar spine surgery only after carefully weighing the risks and benefits.
Back pain	Inform patients that after the injection they may experience lower back pain or spasm for several days and residual lower back stiffness or soreness for several months

ADVERSE REACTIONS[1]

	Frequent reactions (incidence ≥ 1%) are printed in *italics*
Central nervous system	*Back pain/stiffness/soreness (50%), back spasm (30%)*, paraplegia and paraparesis (including paralysis associated with the cauda equina syndrome), subarachnoid and intracerebral hemorrhage, seizures, acute transverse myelitis, acute transverse myelopathy, sacral burning, leg pain, hypalgesia, leg weakness, foot drop, cramping in both calves, pain in the opposite leg, paresthesia, tingling in legs, numbness of legs/toes, headache, dizziness
Gastrointestinal	Nausea, paralytic ileus

CHYMODIACTIN ■ DISCASE

Hypersensitivity	Anaphylaxis, rash, pruritus, urticaria
Other	Urinary retention, bacterial and aseptic discitis

OVERDOSAGE

Overdosage has not been reported

DRUG INTERACTIONS

No clinically significant drug interactions have been identified

ALTERED LABORATORY VALUES

No clinically significant alterations in blood/serum or urinary values occur at therapeutic dosages

---

USE IN CHILDREN

Chymopapain should not be used in children since safety and effectiveness for use in these patients have not been established

USE IN PREGNANT AND NURSING WOMEN

Pregnancy Category C: no reproduction studies have been performed in animals. It is not known whether chymopapain can cause harm to the human fetus or affect reproductive capacity. Use during pregnancy only if clearly needed. Consult manufacturer for use in nursing mothers.

---

[1] Overall mortality associated with chemonucleolysis is approximately 0.02%

CHEMONUCLEOLYTIC ENZYMES

DISCASE (chymopapain) Flint　　　　　　　　　　　　　　　　　　　　Rx

Vials: 12,500 pKat (5 ml)

INDICATIONS

Herniated lumbar intervertebral disks that are unresponsive to conservative therapy

INTRADISCAL DOSAGE

Adult: 5,000 pKat/disk; maximum total dose for a single patient with multiple-disk herniation: 10,000 pKat

CONTRAINDICATIONS

Severe, progressing paralysis indicated by rapidly progressing neurologic dysfunction

Severe spondylolisthesis

Spinal cord tumor or a cauda equina lesion

Use in any spinal region other than the lumbar area

Previous injection with any form of chymopapain

Hypersensitivity to chymopapain, papaya, or papaya derivatives (including contact lens cleaners and meat tenderizers that contain papain)

ADMINISTRATION/DOSAGE ADJUSTMENTS

Requirements for use	Chymopapain should be used only by surgeons who have extensive training and experience in diagnosing and treating spinal disorders and who have been specially trained and licensed to perform chemonucleolysis. The diagnosis must be established precisely since nerve root compression can result from causes other than a herniated disk. The drug should be administered only in a hospital setting, with personnel and facilities available for the immediate treatment of any potential complication.
Preparation of solution	Add 5 ml of sterile water for injection USP to the vial; do not reconstitute with bacteriostatic water for injection since it may inactivate the enzyme. Alcohol used to cleanse the vial stopper may also inactivate the enzyme and therefore should be allowed to air dry before insertion of the needle into the vial. To reduce the possibility of coring the stopper, exercise care in the selection and use of needles. Administer solution within 2 h of reconstitution; discard the unused portion.
Anesthesia	Use supplemented local anesthesia rather than general anesthesia whenever possible because anaphylaxis and neurological reactions are more likely to occur with general anesthesia. During local anesthesia, the patient can complain if the needle impinges on nerve tissue and object to repeated attempts to place the needle; the patient can also report premonitory symptoms of anaphylaxis. Moreover, when the patient is awake, it may be possible to establish a correlation between sciatic pain and a specific disk. During halothane anesthesia, ventricular tachycardia or fibrillation may occur if epinephrine is used for treatment of anaphylaxis.

DISEASE

Needle placement — To avoid puncture of the dura mater, use the lateral approach for needle placement; the posterior approach must be avoided because of the risk of serious neurological reactions. Take great care to assure that the dura is not penetrated and that chymopapain and contrast agents do not enter the subarachnoid space; chymopapain and some contrast agents are extremely toxic when injected intrathecally. Before injection, verify the exact location of the needle tip by evaluating intensified x-ray images obtained at right angles to each other; chemonucleolysis should not be performed if high quality x-ray equipment, including an image intensifier, are not available. If there is any question about the location of the needle tip within the nucleus of the disk or if needle placement is difficult and repeated attempts are necessary, terminate this procedure and do not inject chymopapain.

Discography — Since discography appears to increase the risk of serious neurological reactions, the procedure should generally not be performed in conjunction with chemonucleolysis; to determine whether a disk is abnormal and to correlate that abnormality with sciatic pain, perform a water or saline acceptance test or discometry in place of discography. A contrast agent may be administered if, in a particular case, it is deemed essential. After injection of a contrast agent, observe response for at least 15 min before giving chymopapain; if the contrast agent enters the subarachnoid space, terminate the procedure and do not inject chymopapain.

WARNINGS/PRECAUTIONS

Anaphylaxis — Life-threatening anaphylaxis can occur immediately or up to 1 h after injection and can vary in duration from a few minutes to several hours or longer; bronchospasm, hypotension (the more common effect), or both reactions may develop initially and can be followed by laryngeal edema, arrhythmia, cardiac arrest, coma, and death. Anaphylaxis is more likely to occur if the patient is female or receiving a general anesthetic. In one study, the frequency of anaphylaxis was 0.69% in women and 0.3% in men; it was 0.48% with general anesthesia and 0.2% with local anesthesia. A statistically significant difference between local and general anesthesia was not shown in this study, but has been demonstrated in another study.

Before using this drug, determine whether the patient has a history of multiple allergies. Since signs, severity, progression, and duration of anaphylaxis are highly unpredictable, diagnosis and treatment must be done rapidly. When using this drug, keep at least one open IV line in place. After administration, watch for signs and symptoms of an allergic response, including erythema, pilomotor erection, rash, pruritic urticaria, conjunctivitis, vasomotor rhinitis, angioedema, and GI disturbances. Epinephrine is the drug of choice for the immediate treatment of anaphylaxis; reserve use of corticosteroids and other drugs for cases where epinephrine is inappropriate. Bear in mind that epinephrine may be ineffective if the patient is receiving a beta blocker.

Delayed hypersensitivity reactions — Rash, urticaria, or pruritus may develop as late as 15 days after injection

Neurotoxicity — Serious neurological effects, including paraplegia and cerebral hemorrhage, have occurred in a number of patients. Signs and symptoms of neurological reactions are generally seen within hours or days; however, manifestations of acute transverse myelitis or acute transverse myelopathy are not evident until 2–3 wk after the procedure. The frequency of acute transverse myelitis and myelopathy, 1 in 18,000, is higher than the rate seen in the general population. However, no causal relationship has been established between proper *intradiscal* administration of chymopapain and myelitis, myelopathy, or any other neurological effect. In some instances, neurological reactions may be due to needle trauma or intrathecal injection of the drug and contrast agents (see ADMINISTRATION/DOSAGE ADJUSTMENTS.)

The risk of neurological reactions appears to be increased by discography, general anesthesia, injection in more than one disk, and a history of lumbar spine surgery. If possible, avoid discography and general anesthesia. Inject the drug in more than one disk only if such action is indicated by definitive signs, symptoms, and diagnostic procedures. Use in patients with a history of lumbar spine surgery only after carefully weighing the risks and benefits.

Back pain — Inform patients that after the injection they may experience lower back pain or spasm for several days and residual lower back stiffness or soreness for several months

ADVERSE REACTIONS

Frequent reactions (incidence ≥ 1%) are printed in *italics*

Central nervous system — *Back pain/stiffness/soreness (50%), back spasm (30%),* paraplegia, cerebral hemorrhage, acute transverse myelitis, acute transverse myelopathy, sacral burning, leg pain, hypalgesia, leg weakness, cramping in both calves, pain in the opposite leg, paresthesia, tingling in legs, numbness of legs/toes, headache, dizziness

Gastrointestinal — Nausea, paralytic ileus

Genitourinary — Urinary retention

Hypersensitivity — Anaphylaxis, rash, pruritus, urticaria

OVERDOSAGE

Hypersensitivity reactions may be dose-related and therefore may be more likely to occur following an overdose; however, no cases of overdosage have been reported

DRUG INTERACTIONS

No clinically significant drug interactions have been identified

ALTERED LABORATORY VALUES

No clinically significant alterations in blood/serum or urinary values occur at therapeutic dosages

---

USE IN CHILDREN

Chymopapain should not be used in children since safety and effectiveness for use in these patients have not been established

USE IN PREGNANT AND NURSING WOMEN

Pregnancy Category C: no reproduction studies have been performed in animals. It is not known whether chymopapain can cause harm to the human fetus or affect reproductive capacity. Use during pregnancy only if clearly needed. Consult manufacturer for use in nursing mothers.

GALLSTONE-DISSOLVING AGENTS

CHENIX (chenodiol) Reid-Rowell   Rx

Tablets: 250 mg

INDICATIONS

Dissolution of radiolucent cholesterol stones in a well-opacifying gallbladder, when systemic disease or age precludes surgery

ORAL DOSAGE

Adult: 250 mg bid for the first 2 wk, followed, as tolerated, by weekly increases of 250 mg/day, up to 13–16 mg/kg/day (the recommended dosage range) for a period of up to 24 mo

CONTRAINDICATIONS

Gallstone complications or other conditions that mandate surgery (eg, unremitting acute cholecystitis, cholangitis, biliary obstruction, gallstone pancreatitis, biliary GI fistula)

Radiopaque stones

Nonvisualization of the gallbladder after two consecutive doses of dye

Pregnancy

Hepatocellular dysfunction

Bile duct abnormalities (eg, intrahepatic cholestasis, primary biliary cirrhosis)

ADMINISTRATION/DOSAGE ADJUSTMENTS

Selection of patients — Chenodiol is particularly effective in the dissolution of small, floatable gallstones; nonfloatable stones are less likely to respond to therapy. For patients with nonfloatable stones, there is a greater risk that the condition will deteriorate during therapy and that a more urgent form of surgery will eventually be required. Chenodiol will not dissolve bile pigment stones, calcified radiopaque stones, or partially calcified radiolucent stones.

Minimum dosage — The final, titrated dosage should not be less than 10 mg/kg/day; lower dosages are usually ineffective and may increase the likelihood of cholecystectomy

Management of diarrhea — Diarrhea may be expected in 30–40% of patients, usually when therapy is started. If the diarrhea is intolerable, reduce the dosage until the symptoms abate; antidiarrheal agents may be helpful. The dosage usually can then be increased to the previous level; however, some patients may require a permanent reduction in dosage. For 3% of patients, diarrhea can be controlled only by discontinuing use of chenodiol.

Monitoring of gallstone dissolution — Obtain an oral cholecystogram or ultrasonogram every 6–9 mo. Continue treatment for 1–3 mo after dissolution appears to be complete and then repeat the test. Once dissolution has been confirmed, therapy generally should be stopped; however, serial cholecystograms or ultrasonograms are recommended because gallstones can be expected to recur within 5 yr in 50% of patients. Guidelines and safety for use in repeated courses of therapy have not been established. If partial dissolution is not evident within 9–12 mo, the likelihood of successful treatment is greatly reduced; discontinue use if no therapeutic response occurs within 18 mo. Caution patients to report any symptoms indicating gallstone complications.

WARNINGS/PRECAUTIONS

Liver function abnormalities — Minor, transient elevations in serum transaminase levels (mainly SGPT) have occurred in 30% of patients; the elevations usually return to normal during the following 6 mo of continued treatment. In 2–3% of patients, however, SGPT levels rose to more than 3 times the upper normal limit and necessitated discontinuation of chenodiol therapy. Drug-induced hepatitis has been suspected in three patients and confirmed by biopsy in a fourth; chenodiol may have contributed to the death of a fifth patient with preexisting hepatobiliary disease. An increased incidence of intrahepatic cholestasis has also been observed in patients treated with chenodiol. Although fulminant lesions have not been reported, the possibility remains that an occasional patient may develop serious hepatic disease during therapy. Chenodiol should not be administered to patients with preexisting hepatic or biliary disorders (see CONTRAINDICATIONS). Monitor serum transaminase levels monthly for the first 3 mo and thereafter every 3 mo; discontinue use immediately if serum levels exceed 3 times the upper limit of normal. During clinical studies, minor elevations (1.5–3 times the upper limit of normal) were allowed to persist for 3–6 mo before therapy was interrupted; the safety of this practice has not been established.

CHENIX ■ MOCTANIN

Changes in serum lipid values	Serum low-density lipoprotein (LDL) and total cholesterol values may increase by 10% or more; changes in the high-density lipoprotein (HDL) fraction have not been reported. Small decreases in serum triglyceride levels have been seen in women. Check serum cholesterol values every 6 mo; if these values exceed the level acceptable for the patient's age, it may be advisable to discontinue use.
Carcinogenicity	Epidemiological studies have suggested that bile acids may contribute to the development of colon cancer, but there has been no direct evidence. Bile acids, including chenodiol and its major metabolite, lithocholic acid, are not carcinogenic in animals but can augment the tumor-producing potential of certain carcinogens.

ADVERSE REACTIONS
The most frequent reactions, regardless of incidence, are printed in *italics*

Gastrointestinal	*Diarrhea (30–40%);* urgency, cramps, heartburn, constipation, nausea, vomiting, anorexia, epigastric distress, dyspepsia, flatulence, nonspecific abdominal pain
Other	*Hepatic enzyme elevations and other changes* (see WARNINGS/PRECAUTIONS), hypercholesterolemia, decreases in WBC count (but not below 3,000/mm³)

OVERDOSAGE
One patient received 58 mg/kg/day (4 g/day) for 6 mo without incident; accidental or intentional overdosage has not been reported

DRUG INTERACTIONS

Cholestyramine, colestipol, aluminum-based antacids	▽ Absorption of chenodiol
Estrogens, oral contraceptives; clofibrate, other hypolipidemic drugs	▽ Therapeutic effect of chenodiol

ALTERED LABORATORY VALUES

Blood/serum values	△ SGPT △ SGOT △ Cholesterol (total and LDL fraction) ▽ Triglycerides (in women)

No clinically significant alterations in urinary values occur at therapeutic dosages

---

USE IN CHILDREN

Safety and effectiveness for use in children have not been established

---

USE IN PREGNANT AND NURSING WOMEN

Pregnancy Category X: chenodiol may cause harm to the fetus. Use of chenodiol in women who are or may become pregnant is contraindicated; pregnant patients who are taking this drug should be apprised of the potential hazard to the fetus. Serious hepatic, renal, and adrenal lesions have been seen in the fetuses of Rhesus monkeys after administration of 60–90 mg/kg/day, and hepatic lesions have been found in baboons born to mothers who received 18–38 mg/kg/day. Teratogenic effects have not been observed in these species. Reproduction studies in rats and hamsters have shown no evidence of fetal liver damage or abnormal development. No information on clinical use during pregnancy is available. It is not known whether chenodiol is excreted in human milk; use with caution in nursing mothers.

GALLSTONE-DISSOLVING AGENTS

MOCTANIN (monooctanoin) Ethitek   Rx

Perfusion fluid: 80–85% glyceryl-1-mono-octanoate, 10–15% glyceryl-1-mono-decanoate and glyceryl-1-2-di-octanoate, and up to 2.5% free glycerol (120 ml)

INDICATIONS

Dissolution of cholesterol (radiolucent) gallstones retained in the biliary tract following cholecystectomy, when other means of removal have failed or cannot be undertaken[1]

DOSAGE

Adult: 3–5 ml/h, administered by continuous perfusion through a catheter inserted into the common bile duct at an optimal pressure of 10 cm H$_2$O; *do not administer IV or IM*

CONTRAINDICATIONS

Clinical jaundice	Significant biliary tract infection	Recent duodenal ulcer or jejunitis

ADMINISTRATION/DOSAGE ADJUSTMENTS

Pretreatment analysis	Stones must be radiolucent and readily accessible to the perfusate. Recently removed stones should be analyzed for composition or incubated in monooctanoin at body temperature; do not use this preparation if the stone proves not to be made of cholesterol or if no dissolution is observed after 72 h of incubation with stirring.

MOCTANIN ■ INDOCIN I.V.

Administration	Administer monooctanoin through a catheter inserted directly into the common bile duct via a T-tube or a nasobiliary tube placed by endoscopy. Warm the fluid to 70–80°F prior to administration and take care not to let the temperature fall below 65°F during perfusion. An overflow manometer, peristaltic pump, or similar means of keeping the perfusion pressure below 15 cm H_2O is essential for the procedure. The manometer may be connected directly to the T-tube or nasobiliary tube and should be securely positioned at an appropriate height to assure accurate measurement of biliary tract pressure. Perfusion is best regulated by a peristaltic pump; a battery operated pump may be used with outpatients. Administration may be interrupted during meals.
Duration of therapy	The average duration of monooctanoin perfusion is 9.4 days; discontinue therapy if endoscopy or x-ray examination shows no elimination or reduction in size of stones after 10 days

WARNINGS/PRECAUTIONS

GI irritation	Monooctanoin is irritating to the gastrointestinal and biliary tracts of animals and humans. Closely monitor perfusion pressure and rate of administration since a close relationship between these factors and irritation seems to exist; to minimize gastrointestinal and/or biliary irritation, do not give more than 5 ml/h at a pressure of 10 cm H_2O. Reducing the perfusion rate and discontinuing the perfusion during meals may help diminish GI symptoms. Ascending cholangitis, possibly related to obstruction in the common bile duct, may occur; discontinue treatment if fever, chills, leukocytosis, severe right upper quadrant abdominal pain, or jaundice occurs. Duodenal irritation is reversible and disappears 2–7 days after therapy is completed.
Metabolic acidosis	Routine liver function tests are advisable before starting treatment since patients with impaired hepatic function may develop metabolic acidosis

ADVERSE REACTIONS

Frequent reactions (incidence ≥ 1%) are printed in *italics*

Gastrointestinal	*Abdominal pain or distress (43%), nausea (32%), vomiting (20%), diarrhea (19%), discomfort (7.3%), anorexia (3.0%), loose stools (1.5%), indigestion (1.2%),* "burning" epigastrium, increased drainage from fistula; irritation of duodenal mucosa (reversible); hematemesis due to multiple duodenal ulcerations (one case)
Hepatic	Increased serum amylase concentration, bile shock; acute, fatal pancreatitis and cholangitis (one case)
Hematological	Persistent leukopenia
Central nervous system	Fatigue/lethargy, depression, headache
Hypersensitivity	Pruritus, allergic reaction
Other	*Fever (6.3%)*, hypokalemia, intolerance, chills, diaphoresis; reversible upper right quadrant abdominal pain, dyspnea, and hypotension with hyperventilation (one case, in a patient with lupus erythematosus)

DRUG INTERACTIONS
None identified

ALTERED LABORATORY VALUES

Blood/serum values	△ Amylase ▽ Potassium

No clinically significant alterations in urinary values occur at therapeutic dosages

---

USE IN CHILDREN

Safety and effectiveness for use in children have not been established

USE IN PREGNANT AND NURSING WOMEN

Pregnancy Category C: no reproductive studies have been done in laboratory animals; it is not known whether monooctanoin can cause fetal harm when administered to a pregnant woman or can affect reproductive capacity. Use during pregnancy only if clearly needed. It is not known whether this drug is excreted in human milk; because many drugs are excreted in human milk, use with caution in nursing women.

---

[1] Complete stone dissolution occurs in about one-third of patients and is more likely for single stones than multiple stones; it is uncommon in diabetic patients. A reduction in stone size occurs in approximately another one-third of patients; these smaller stones may pass spontaneously or may be more easily extracted.

PATENT DUCTUS ARTERIOSUS THERAPY

INDOCIN I. V. (indomethacin sodium trihydrate) Merck Sharp & Dohme   Rx

Vials: 1 mg indomethacin[1]

INDICATIONS	PARENTERAL DOSAGE
Hemodynamically significant **patent ductus arteriosus** in premature infants weighing 500–1,750 g, when use of conventional measures for 48 h has been ineffective	**Neonate (<48 h):** 0.2 mg/kg IV, followed by 2 IV doses of 0.1 mg/kg each at intervals of 12–24 h **Neonate (2–7 days):** 0.2 mg/kg IV q12–24h for a total of 3 doses **Neonate (>7 days):** 0.2 mg/kg IV, followed by 2 IV doses of 0.25 mg/kg each at intervals of 12–24 h

INDOCIN I.V.

CONTRAINDICATIONS

Congenital heart diseases that can be exacerbated by closure of the ductus arteriosus (eg, pulmonary atresia, severe tetralogy of Fallot, severe coarctation of the aorta)

Bleeding, especially active intracranial hemorrhage or GI bleeding

Thrombocytopenia

Significant renal impairment

Untreated infection

Necrotizing enterocolitis

Coagulation defects

ADMINISTRATION/DOSAGE ADJUSTMENTS

Selection of patients	This drug should be reserved for use in neonates with cardiomegaly, respiratory distress, continuous murmur, precordial hyperactivity, pulmonary plethora (in a chest x-ray), or other clear-cut clinical evidence of a hemodynamically significant patent ductus arteriosus. Before considering this drug, treat condition with conventional measures such as fluid restriction, diuretics, digitalis, and respiratory support.
Preparation of solution	Add 1–2 ml of preservative-free 0.9% sodium chloride injection or preservative-free sterile water for injection to the vial. Prepare a fresh solution for each dose; do not save any unused portion.
Intravenous administration	Inject solution over a period of 5–10 s; avoid extravascular injection and leakage, which may cause irritation
Additional doses	If the size of the ductus arteriosus is not significantly reduced 48 h or more after the last dose, 1–3 additional doses may be given at intervals of 12–24 h. These additional doses may also be given if the ductus arteriosus reopens; however, in 70% of cases of reopening seen in clinical studies, the ductus arteriosus closed again without recourse to a second set of doses. If closure does not occur after a total of 6 doses has been given, surgery may be necessary.

WARNINGS/PRECAUTIONS

Adverse effects	Stop treatment if severe adverse effects occur
Nephrotoxicity	This product may cause marked oliguria, anuria, or acute renal failure. Renal dysfunction, seen in 41% of patients, has usually been transient. It is especially likely to occur in conjunction with conditions that can affect renal function, such as hypovolemia, cardiac failure, sepsis, hepatic impairment, and use of nephrotoxic drugs. Carefully monitor urinary output after each dose; if output is less than 0.6 ml/kg/h at the scheduled time of a dose, delay administration until laboratory results show that renal function has returned to normal. A study in 19 infants receiving IV indomethacin has shown that concomitant use of furosemide enhances GFR, urinary output, and excretion of sodium and chloride; these results suggest that furosemide can help maintain renal function during indomethacin therapy. Because indomethacin may reduce renal function, this should be taken into account when coadministering drugs that require adequate renal function for their elimination, particularly digitalis.
Hyponatremia, hyperkalemia	Monitor serum electrolyte levels since dilutional hyponatremia and elevation of the serum potassium level may occur during therapy
Gastrointestinal effects	In a placebo-controlled study, this product caused an increase in minor, but not major, GI bleeding; severe GI effects have occurred with use of oral indomethacin
Bleeding	Reversible, grossly abnormal platelet aggregation has been seen in premature infants given oral indomethacin; watch for signs of bleeding during therapy. Although indomethacin can theoretically increase the risk of spontaneous CNS intraventricular hemorrhage associated with prematurity, such an effect has not been observed in controlled studies.
Infection	Keep in mind throughout treatment that indomethacin can mask signs and symptoms of infection. Use with particular care in infants with infections; do not give this drug if the infection has not yet been treated.
Hepatic effects	Chronic oral therapy in adults has caused severe hepatic reactions; IV therapy should be discontinued if clinical signs and symptoms of liver disease occur or secondary systemic manifestations develop
Neuronal necrosis	In rats and mice, oral administration of 4 mg/kg/day during the last 3 days of gestation has caused an increase in neuronal necrosis in the diencephalon, a reduction in maternal weight gain, and maternal and fetal deaths; no increase in neuronal necrosis has been seen in rats and mice following administration of 0.5 or 4 mg/kg/day during the first 3 days of life
Pulmonary hypertension	In rats, administration of 2 and 4 mg/kg/day during the last trimester of gestation has produced an excessive amount of muscular tissue in pulmonary blood vessels and reduced the number of pulmonary vessels that were formed; these findings are similar to those characteristic of neonatal, persistent pulmonary hypertension
Circulatory dysfunction	Administration of indomethacin to adult patients with severe heart failure and hyponatremia has produced a significant deterioration in circulatory function, presumably due to inhibition of prostaglandin-dependent compensatory mechanisms
Carcinogenicity, mutagenicity, and effect on fertility	No carcinogenic effects have been seen in rats given up to 1 mg/kg/day for 81 wk or in mice and rats given up to 1.5 mg/kg/day throughout their lives. No evidence of mutagenicity has been detected in a host-mediated assay or in the Ames, mouse micronucleus, and *Drosophila* tests. Reproduction studies in rats and mice have shown no adverse effect on fertility.

INDOCIN I.V. ■ CYLERT

ADVERSE REACTIONS[2]

Renal	Renal dysfunction (41%), including oliguria, uremia, increases in BUN and serum creatinine levels, and decreases in GFR, free water clearance, urinary output and osmolality, and urinary levels of sodium, chloride, and potassium
Gastrointestinal	Gross or microscopic GI bleeding (3–9%); vomiting, abdominal distention, transient ileus, and localized perforation(s) of the small and/or large intestine (1–3%)
Hematological	Decreased platelet aggregation (1–3%), disseminated intravascular coagulation
Respiratory	Pulmonary hemorrhage
Local	Oozing from the skin after needle stick
Other	Hyponatremia and elevated potassium level (3–9%); hypoglycemia and fluid retention (1–3%)

OVERDOSAGE

No information on overdose has been reported

DRUG INTERACTIONS

Digitalis	△ Risk of digitalis toxicity; during combination therapy, observe infant closely and, if necessary, check ECG and serum digitalis level frequently
Gentamicin, amikacin	△ Peak and trough serum levels of gentamicin and amikacin

ALTERED LABORATORY VALUES

Blood/serum values	△ Creatinine △ BUN ▽ Sodium △ Potassium ▽ Glucose
Urinary values	▽ Sodium ▽ Chloride ▽ Potassium

USE IN CHILDREN
See INDICATIONS and PARENTERAL DOSAGE

USE IN PREGNANT AND NURSING WOMEN
This product is not indicated for use in pregnant or nursing women

[1] As the sodium salt
[2] Reactions for which a causal relationship has not been established include intracranial bleeding, bradycardia, apnea, exacerbation of pulmonary infection, metabolic acidosis or alkalosis, necrotizing enterocolitis, and retrolental fibroplasia; reactions seen to date only with oral indomethacin should be considered potential effects of IV therapy (see package insert)

PSYCHOSTIMULANTS

CYLERT (pemoline) Abbott   C-IV
Tablets: 18.75, 37.5, 75 mg   **Chewable tablets:** 37.5 mg

INDICATIONS	ORAL DOSAGE
Attention deficit disorder with hyperactivity	Child (≥6 yr): 37.5 mg/day, given in a single morning dose, to start, followed by weekly increments of 18.75 mg/day until the desired clinical response is achieved (usual dosage: 56.25–75 mg/day); do not exceed 112.5 mg/day

CONTRAINDICATIONS

Hepatic impairment	Hypersensitivity or idiosyncratic reaction to pemoline

ADMINISTRATION/DOSAGE ADJUSTMENTS

Selection of patients	The following symptoms, seen in a developmentally inappropriate context, characterize the attention deficit syndrome: moderate to severe distractability, short attention span, hyperactivity, emotional lability, and impulsiveness; signs of CNS dysfunction, such as nonlocalizing (soft) neurological signs, learning disability, and abnormal EEG, may or may not be evident. If the onset of symptoms is comparatively recent, the diagnosis should be considered tentative. The decision to use pemoline should not rest solely on the presence of symptoms, but rather should be based on an assessment of the chronicity and severity of symptoms and their appropriateness for the child's age; drug therapy may not be necessary in all cases of attention deficit syndrome. Use of pemoline, when indicated, should be viewed as an integral part of a treatment program that also includes psychological, social, and educational measures.
Onset of action	Significant clinical improvement may not be evident until the third or fourth week of therapy
Discontinuation of therapy	If possible, interrupt therapy occasionally to determine whether therapy is still necessary

CYLERT

Management of adverse reactions	Mild effects seen early in treatment are often transient; if reactions are significant or protracted, reduce dosage or discontinue use

WARNINGS/PRECAUTIONS

Weight loss, suppression of growth	During the first weeks of therapy, anorexia and weight loss may occur; reactions are usually transient, and normal weight gain is generally seen within 3–6 mo. However, long-term use may cause a reduction in the rate of weight gain or linear growth; during long-term therapy, monitor patient carefully.
Psychotic children	Pemoline may exacerbate symptoms of behavior disturbance and thought disorder in psychotic children
Patients with renal impairment	Use with caution in patients with significant renal impairment since pemoline is excreted mainly by the kidneys
Hepatotoxicity	Elevated liver enzyme levels, hepatitis, and jaundice have been seen in patients given pemoline. Perform liver function tests before starting therapy and periodically thereafter; if abnormalities are detected and then subsequently confirmed, discontinue use.
Insomnia	The most frequent reaction to pemoline is insomnia; this reaction usually occurs during the first weeks of therapy, before an optimal clinical response has been attained, and generally disappears with continued use or a reduction in dosage
Concomitant therapy	Carefully monitor patients receiving other drugs, especially those with CNS activity (see DRUG INTERACTIONS)
Tics, Tourette's syndrome	Pemoline may precipitate motor and phonic tics and Tourette's syndrome; patients and their families should be evaluated clinically for evidence of tics and Tourette's syndrome before the start of therapy
Drug abuse and dependence	Long-term use in adults at excessive dosages has resulted in transient psychosis. Although studies in primates given pemoline have failed to demonstrate dependence, the pharmacologic similarity of this drug to other psychostimulants suggests a risk of psychological or physical dependence. Use with caution in emotionally unstable patients since they may increase the dosage on their own.
Carcinogenicity, mutagenicity	No evidence of carcinogenicity has been seen in rats given up to 150 mg/kg/day for 18 mo; tests have not been done to evaluate the mutagenic potential of pemoline
Effect on fertility	No evidence of impaired fertility has been seen in rats given 18.75 or 37.5 mg/kg/day

ADVERSE REACTIONS

Central nervous system	Convulsive seizures, insomnia, mild depression, dizziness, increased irritability, headache, drowsiness, Tourette's syndrome, hallucinations; abnormal oculomotor function (including nystagmus and oculogyric crisis); dyskinetic movements of the tongue, lips, face, and extremities
Gastrointestinal	Anorexia, weight loss, stomachache, nausea
Hepatic	Elevated liver enzyme levels, hepatitis, jaundice
Other	Rash, suppression of growth, aplastic anemia

OVERDOSAGE

Signs and symptoms	Vomiting, agitation, tremors, hyperreflexia, muscle twitching, convulsions, coma, euphoria, confusion, hallucinations, delirium, sweating, flushing, headache, hyperpyrexia, tachycardia, hypertension, mydriasis
Treatment	If patient is alert and signs and symptoms are not too severe, empty stomach. Institute supportive measures as needed. Protect patient from self-injury and any external stimuli that can exacerbate condition. Chlorpromazine may be useful in treating symptoms. The effectiveness of dialysis has not been established.

DRUG INTERACTIONS

Anticonvulsants	▽ Seizure threshold

ALTERED LABORATORY VALUES

Blood/serum	△ SGOT △ SGPT △ LDH

No clinically significant alterations in urinary values occur at therapeutic dosages

---

USE IN CHILDREN

Safety and effectiveness for use in children under 6 yr of age have not been established

USE IN PREGNANT AND NURSING WOMEN

Pregnancy Category B: in rats, an increase in stillbirths and cannibalization has been seen at 37.5 mg/kg/day and a reduction in surviving offspring has been observed at 18.75 and 37.5 mg/kg/day; use during pregnancy only if clearly needed. It is not known whether pemoline is excreted in human milk; use with caution in nursing mothers.

DEXEDRINE

PSYCHOSTIMULANTS

DEXEDRINE (dextroamphetamine sulfate) Smith Kline & French — C-II

Capsules (sustained release): 5, 10, 15 mg **Tablets:** 5 mg **Elixir (per 5 ml):** 5 mg[1] (16 fl oz) *orange flavored*

INDICATIONS	ORAL DOSAGE
Narcolepsy	**Adult:** 5–60 mg/day, given in divided doses **Child (6–12 yr):** 5 mg/day to start, followed by weekly increments of 5 mg/day until optimal response is obtained; if sustained-release capsules are used, 5 mg once daily, followed by weekly increments of 5 mg/day, where appropriate **Child (> 12 yr):** 10 mg/day to start, followed by weekly increments of 10 mg/day until optimal response is obtained; if sustained-release capsules are used, 10 mg once daily, followed by weekly increments of 10 mg/day, where appropriate
Attention deficit disorder accompanied by hyperactivity	**Child (3–5 yr):** 2.5 mg/day to start, followed by weekly increments of 2.5 mg/day until optimal response is obtained **Child (6–12 yr):** 5 mg 1–2 times/day to start, followed by weekly increments of 5 mg/day until optimal response is obtained; if sustained-release capsules are used, 5–10 mg once daily to start, followed by weekly increments of 5 mg/day, where appropriate; maximum dosage: 40 mg/day, except in rare cases
Exogenous obesity, as a short-term adjunct to caloric restriction in patients refractory to alternative therapy	**Adult:** up to 30 mg/day, given in divided doses of 5–10 mg 30–60 min before meals; if sustained-release capsules are used, 10–15 mg once daily (AM)

CONTRAINDICATIONS

Hypersensitivity or idiosyncratic reaction to sympathomimetic amines	Advanced arteriosclerosis	Hyperthyroidism
	Symptomatic cardiovascular disease	Glaucoma
MAO inhibitor therapy (see WARNINGS/PRECAUTIONS)	Moderate to severe hypertension	Agitated states
History of drug abuse		

ADMINISTRATION/DOSAGE ADJUSTMENTS

Insomnia or anorexia	Dosage should be reduced if bothersome adverse reactions appear; late-evening doses tend to cause insomnia, particularly with capsules, and should be avoided
Child dosage intervals	With tablets or elixir, give 1st dose on awakening and 1–2 additional doses at intervals of 4–6 h
Duration of therapy for attention deficit disorder	Interrupt therapy occasionally to determine whether symptoms recur, warranting continued administration

WARNINGS/PRECAUTIONS

Mental impairment	Caution patients that their ability to drive or perform other potentially hazardous activities may be impaired
Drug dependence	When tolerance to the anorectic effect develops, discontinue use rather than increase the dosage, because extreme psychological dependence and severe social disability may otherwise occur. Chronic toxicity may be manifested by severe dermatoses, marked insomnia, irritability, hyperactivity, personality changes, or psychosis; withdrawal reactions include extreme fatigue, mental depression, and changes in the sleep EEG.
Hypertension	May worsen; use with caution in patients with even mild hypertension
MAO inhibitor therapy	Wait at least 14 days after discontinuing MAO inhibitors before instituting treatment with this drug (see DRUG INTERACTIONS)
Tartrazine sensitivity	Presence of FD&C Yellow No. 5 (tartrazine) in all dosage forms may cause allergic-type reactions, including bronchial asthma, in susceptible individuals
Carcinogenicity, mutagenicity	No studies evaluating the carcinogenic or mutagenic potential of this drug have been performed

ADVERSE REACTIONS

Cardiovascular	Palpitations, tachycardia, hypertension
Central nervous system	Overstimulation, restlessness, dizziness, insomnia, euphoria, dyskinesia, dysphoria, tremor, headache, exacerbation of motor and phonic tics, Tourette's syndrome; psychotic disturbances (rare)
Gastrointestinal	Dry mouth, unpleasant taste, diarrhea, constipation, anorexia, other disturbances
Dermatological	Urticaria
Endocrinological	Impotence, altered libido, weight loss

DEXEDRINE ■ RITALIN

OVERDOSAGE

Signs and symptoms	Restlessness, tremor, hyperreflexia, rapid respiration, confusion, assaultiveness, hallucinations, panic, fatigue, depression, arrhythmias, hypertension, hypotension, circulatory collapse, nausea, vomiting, diarrhea, abdominal cramps, convulsions, coma, death
Treatment	Empty stomach by gastric lavage. Use saline cathartics to hasten evacuation of sustained-release capsules. Administer a barbiturate to provide sedation; chlorpromazine can also be given to reduce CNS stimulation. Acidify the urine to promote excretion of the drug. For acute, severe hypertension, administer IV phentolamine.

DRUG INTERACTIONS

Urinary and GI acidifiers, lithium	▽ Pharmacologic effects of dextroamphetamine
Urinary and GI alkalinizers	△ Pharmacologic effects of dextroamphetamine
MAO inhibitors	△ Risk of hypertensive crisis
Chlorpromazine, haloperidol	▽ Central stimulant effects of dextroamphetamine
Tricyclic antidepressants	△ Antidepressant effects and pharmacologic activity of dextroamphetamine
Meperidine	△ Analgesia
Antihistamines	▽ Sedation
Norepinephrine, sympathomimetic agents	△ Adrenergic effects
Adrenergic blockers	▽ Adrenergic blockade
Reserpine, guanethidine	▽ Antihypertensive effects and pharmacologic effects of dextroamphetamine
Veratrum alkaloids, other antihypertensive agents	▽ Antihypertensive effects
Phenobarbital, phenytoin	Delayed intestinal absorption of phenobarbital and phenytoin △ Anticonvulsant effects
Ethosuximide	Delayed intestinal absorption of ethosuximide
Propoxyphene	△ Risk of convulsions (when administered in cases of propoxyphene overdosage)

ALTERED LABORATORY VALUES

Blood/serum values	△ Corticosteroids
Urinary values	Interference with steroid determinations

USE IN CHILDREN

See INDICATIONS and ORAL DOSAGE; prescription of this drug for attention deficit disorder should take into account the chronicity and severity of the child's symptoms and their appropriateness for his or her age. A clinical evaluation for motor and phonic tics and Gilles de la Tourette's syndrome should be done before beginning therapy because amphetamines can exacerbate these disorders. Dextroamphetamine should not be used in children under 3 yr of age or, in most cases, for symptoms associated with acute stress reactions. The drug is also not recommended for use as an anorectic in children under 12 yr of age. In psychotic children, use of amphetamines may exacerbate behavior disturbances and thought disorder. Growth should be monitored during treatment. Long-term effects in children are unknown.

USE IN PREGNANT AND NURSING WOMEN

Pregnancy Category C: embryotoxic and teratogenic effects have been observed in mice given 41 times the maximum human dose; however, embryotoxic effects have not been seen in rabbits given 7 times the human dose nor in rats given 12.5 times the maximum human dose. No adequate, well-controlled teratogenicity studies have been performed in pregnant women. Premature delivery, low birth weight, and neonatal withdrawal reactions (dysphoria, lassitude) are more likely if pregnant patients are dependent on amphetamines. Use during pregnancy only if the expected benefit justifies the potential risk to the fetus. It is not known whether this drug is excreted in breast milk; use with caution in nursing mothers.

[1] Contains 10% alcohol

PSYCHOSTIMULANTS

RITALIN (methylphenidate hydrochloride) CIBA C-II
Tablets: 5, 10, 20 mg

RITALIN-SR (methylphenidate hydrochloride) CIBA C-II
Tablets (sustained release): 20 mg

INDICATIONS
Attention deficit disorder (minimal brain dysfunction, hyperkinetic child syndrome, minimal brain damage, minimal cerebral dysfunction, minor cerebral dysfunction)
Narcolepsy

ORAL DOSAGE
Adult: 20–30 mg/day, given in 2–3 divided doses, preferably 30–45 min before meals; some patients may need only 10–15 mg/day, while others may require 40–60 mg/day
Child ($\geq$ 6 yr): 5 mg given before breakfast and lunch to start, followed by gradual increases of 5–10 mg/wk up to 60 mg/day; if no improvement is observed after 1 mo, discontinue therapy

RITALIN

CONTRAINDICATIONS

Marked anxiety, tension, and agitation	Motor tics	Glaucoma
Severe exogenous or endogenous depression	Gilles de la Tourette's syndrome	
Hypersensitivity to methylphenidate	Family history of Gilles de la Tourette's syndrome	

ADMINISTRATION/DOSAGE ADJUSTMENTS

Management of insomnia	Instruct patient to take last dose before 6 PM
Paradoxical aggravation of symptoms	Reduce dosage or, if necessary, discontinue drug
Use of sustained-release tablets	Ritalin-SR may be given q8h in place of Ritalin if a single dose of Ritalin-SR corresponds to the titrated 8-h dose of Ritalin; sustained-release tablets must be swallowed whole, not chewed or crushed
Duration of therapy in children	Interrupt therapy periodically to assess the child's condition. Therapy should not be indefinite and may usually be discontinued in children after puberty.

WARNINGS/PRECAUTIONS

Growth suppression	May occur with long-term therapy; weight gain and growth rate in children should be carefully monitored
Agitated patients	May react adversely; discontinue therapy if necessary
Psychotic children	Symptoms of behavior disturbance and thought disorder may be exacerbated
Seizures	May occur in patients with a history of seizures or EEG abnormalities or, rarely, with neither; discontinue therapy
Blood pressure	Should be monitored, especially in hypertensive patients; use with caution in the presence of hypertension
Drug dependence	Marked tolerance and psychic dependence may develop with chronic abuse; use with caution in emotionally unstable individuals or where there is a history of drug dependence or alcoholism. Drug withdrawal may precipitate severe depression or unmask the effects of chronic overactivity; provide close supervision.
Prolonged therapy	Obtain a CBC, differential count, and platelet count periodically

ADVERSE REACTIONS[1]

Central nervous system	Nervousness, insomnia, dizziness, headache, dyskinesia, drowsiness, toxic psychosis, Gilles de la Tourette's syndrome (rare)
Ophthalmic	Accommodation difficulties and blurred vision (rare)
Gastrointestinal	Anorexia, nausea, abdominal pain, weight loss during prolonged therapy
Cardiovascular	Palpitations, blood pressure and pulse changes, tachycardia, angina, arrhythmias
Hypersensitivity	Skin rash, urticaria, fever, arthralgia, exfoliative dermatitis, erythema multiforme with histopathologic findings of necrotizing vasculitis, thrombocytopenic purpura

OVERDOSAGE

Signs and symptoms	Vomiting, agitation, tremors, hyperreflexia, muscle twitching, convulsions (may be followed by coma), euphoria, confusion, hallucinations, delirium, sweating, flushing, headache, hyperpyrexia, tachycardia, palpitations, cardiac arrhythmias, hypertension, mydriasis, dryness of mucous membranes
Treatment	Institute appropriate supportive measures. Protect patient against self-injury and against external stimuli that would aggravate overstimulation. If signs and symptoms are not too severe and patient is conscious, induce emesis or perform gastric lavage to empty stomach. If severe, administer a carefully titrated dose of a *short-acting* barbiturate before performing gastric lavage. Maintain adequate circulation and respiratory exchange. External cooling procedures may be required for hyperpyrexia. Efficacy of hemodialysis or peritoneal dialysis has not been established.

DRUG INTERACTIONS

Guanethidine	▽ Antihypertensive effect
Vasopressors	△ Pressor effect
MAO inhibitors	△ Risk of hypertensive crisis
Oral anticoagulants	△ Prothrombin time
Phenobarbital, phenytoin, primidone	△ Anticonvulsant blood levels
Imipramine, desipramine	△ Antidepressant blood levels

ALTERED LABORATORY VALUES

No clinically significant alterations in blood/serum or urinary values occur at therapeutic dosages

USE IN CHILDREN

See INDICATIONS and ORAL DOSAGE; prescription of this drug should take into account the chronicity and severity of the child's symptoms and their appropriateness for his or her age. Methylphenidate should not be used in children under 6 yr of age or, in most cases, for symptoms associated with acute stress reactions. Long-term effects in children are unknown. Anorexia, abdominal pain, weight loss (with prolonged use), insomnia, and tachycardia are the reactions that are most likely to occur in children.

USE IN PREGNANT AND NURSING WOMEN

Safety for use during pregnancy has not been established. It is not known whether methylphenidate is excreted in human milk; use with caution in nursing mothers, because many drugs are excreted in human milk.

[1] Other reactions for which a causal relationship has not been established include scalp hair loss and leukopenia and/or anemia

---

SMOKING DETERRENTS

NICORETTE (nicotine polacrilex) Lakeside   Rx

Chewing gum: nicotine polacrilex equivalent to 2 mg nicotine/piece of gum *sugar-free*

INDICATIONS

Pharmacologic substitute for the nicotine contained in cigarettes for patients who have ceased smoking completely and are participating in a medically supervised behavior modification program that provides education, counseling, and psychological support

ORAL DOSAGE

Adult: 2 mg (1 piece) whenever the urge to smoke arises, not to exceed 60 mg (30 pieces)/day; usual dosage during the first month of therapy: 20 mg (10 pieces)/day

CONTRAINDICATIONS

Severe or worsening angina	Life-threatening arrhythmias	Pregnancy
Period immediately following myocardial infarction	Active temporomandibular joint disease	Nonsmokers

ADMINISTRATION/DOSAGE ADJUSTMENTS

Selection of patients	In general, patients who are most likely to benefit from use of this preparation have a strong physical dependence on nicotine; such patients tend to (1) smoke more than 15 cigarettes/day, (2) prefer cigarette brands with nicotine levels greater than 0.9 mg/cigarette, (3) usually inhale the smoke, (4) smoke the first cigarette of the day within 30 min after arising, (5) find this first cigarette the hardest one to give up, (6) smoke more frequently in the morning, (7) find it difficult to refrain from smoking in places where it is forbidden, or (8) smoke even when they are so ill that they are bedridden most of the day
Administration	Instruct the patient to chew each piece slowly and intermittently for about 30 min, stopping whenever the gum can be tasted or a slight tingling sensation can be felt in the mouth; chewing may be resumed when the taste or sensation is about to disappear. Chewing the gum too fast may cause light-headedness, nausea, vomiting, mouth or throat irritation, hiccups, upset stomach, or other toxic reactions, which may be controlled by chewing more slowly. Local reactions, such as traumatic injury to the oral mucosa or teeth, jaw ache, and eructation owing to aerophagia may be minimized by chewing the gum in a different manner.
Monitoring of therapy	Assess the patient's progress at least monthly. Patients who have successfully abstained from cigarette smoking after 3 mo should be encouraged to stop using the gum, as administration for longer periods has *not* been shown to increase the likelihood of smoking cessation and, furthermore, may increase the risk of dependence on this product. Nevertheless, use for up to 6 mo may be considered after weighing the risks of dependence and toxicity against the potential benefit of preventing relapse; administration for more than 6 mo is not recommended. Withdrawal should be gradual if the patient has used this preparation for more than 3 mo.

NICORETTE

WARNINGS/PRECAUTIONS

Patients with cardiovascular disease	Carefully weigh the risks and benefits before prescribing this preparation to patients with a history of myocardial infarction and/or angina pectoris, serious cardiac arrhythmias, systemic hypertension, or vasospastic diseases (eg, Buerger's disease, Prinzmetal [variant] angina)
Patients with catecholamine-sensitive conditions	Since nicotine can release catecholamines from the adrenal medulla, even after tolerance to other effects have developed, use with caution in patients with hyperthyroidism, pheochromocytoma, or insulin-dependent diabetes
Patients with GI disorders	Use in patients with inactive peptic ulcer only when the benefits outweigh the risks; use with caution in patients with a history of peptic ulcer or esophagitis
Patients with oropharyngeal conditions	Use with caution in patients with oral or pharyngeal inflammation. Exercise caution in patients who have dental problems that may be exacerbated by chewing gum. If the gum becomes excessively sticky, it may damage dental work (caps, dentures, bridges); the degree of stickiness depends upon such factors as dryness of the mouth, amount and composition of saliva, type of dental material, possible interaction with dental adhesives, and use of denture-cleaning compounds. Instruct patient to discontinue use and consult a physician or dentist if damage occurs.
Carcinogenicity, mutagenicity, effect on fertility	Inconclusive evidence suggests that conitine, a metabolite of nicotine, may be carcinogenic in rats; nicotine has not been reported to cause or promote the growth of tumors in mice. No mutagenic effects have been detected with use of nicotine in the Ames test. Studies in rats given nicotine have shown a decrease in litter size.

ADVERSE REACTIONS

Frequent reactions are italicized

Central nervous system	*Dizziness/light-headedness (2.1%); insomnia, irritability/fussiness, and headache (1.1%)*, euphoria
Gastrointestinal	*Nausea/vomiting (18.1%), nonspecific GI distress (9.6%), eructation (6.4%), anorexia (1.1%)*, laxative effect, constipation, gas pains
Cardiovascular	Flush; atrial fibrillation (one case)
Oropharyngeal	*Mouth or throat soreness (37.2%), aching jaw muscle (18.1%), hiccups (14.9%), excessive salivation (2.1%)*, hoarseness, dry mouth, cough
Other	Sneezing; acute nicotine toxicity (one case)

OVERDOSAGE

Signs and symptoms	Nausea, salivation, abdominal pain, vomiting, diarrhea, cold sweat, headache, dizziness, disturbed hearing and vision, mental confusion, and marked weakness, followed, in more severe cases, by faintness, prostration, hypotension, dyspnea, abnormal pulse, cardiovascular collapse, convulsions, and respiratory paralysis; acute toxicity is unlikely to result from swallowing of the gum, but may occur if many pieces of gum are chewed either simultaneously or in rapid succession
Treatment	If the patient is conscious and has not vomited, induce emesis with ipecac syrup; if the patient is unconscious, perform gastric lavage, and then administer a suspension containing activated charcoal. To hasten evacuation of the gum, use a saline cathartic. For severe toxicity, provide mechanical ventilation and treat cardiovascular reactions vigorously.

DRUG INTERACTIONS

Cessation of smoking, with or without substitution of nicotine, may produce increases in the serum level of theophylline, caffeine, imipramine, pentazocine, and propoxyphene and a decrease in the serum level of glutethimide; cessation may also increase the blood pressure-lowering effect of propranolol, alter the therapeutic response to other adrenergic agents, and enhance the diuretic effect of furosemide

ALTERED LABORATORY VALUES

Blood/serum values	⇧ Catecholamines ⇧ Cortisol
Urinary values	⇧ Catecholamines ⇧ Cortisol

USE IN CHILDREN

Safety and effectiveness for use in children have not been established

USE IN PREGNANT AND NURSING WOMEN

Pregnancy Category X: nicotine may cause harm to the fetus. Use of this drug during the third trimester has been associated with a decrease in fetal breathing movements and, in one case, may have been partly responsible for a miscarriage; studies in rhesus monkeys have shown that this drug can cause acidosis, hypoxia, and hypercaphea in the fetus. Teratogenicity has been demonstrated in mice given SC 300 times the human buccal dose, but has not been shown in rats or monkeys at doses that would be produced by cigarette smoking. Use of this drug in women who are or may become pregnant is contraindicated. Before beginning therapy, instruct the patient to take adequate contraceptive measures, and consider performing a pregnancy test. If a patient becomes pregnant during therapy, she should be apprised of the potential risk to the fetus. Nicotine is excreted in human milk; because of the potential for serious adverse reactions in nursing infants, patients should not nurse while taking this drug.

VACCINES

b-CAPSA I (hemophilus b polysaccharide vaccine) Mead Johnson   Rx

Vials (per 0.5-ml dose): 25 μg purified capsular polysaccharide from *Hemophilus influenzae* b (10 doses)

INDICATIONS

Prevention of *Hemophilus influenzae* b diseases in any child who is 2–6 yr of age and in any high-risk child, such as one attending a daycare center, who is 18–23 mo of age

PARENTERAL DOSAGE

Child (18 mo to 6 yr): 25 μg (0.5 ml), given in a single SC dose

CONTRAINDICATIONS

Hypersensitivity to any component

ADMINISTRATION/DOSAGE ADJUSTMENTS

Preparation and administration — Use a sterile needle and syringe free of preservatives, antiseptics, and detergents when preparing and administering the solution. For reconstitution, add 6 ml of the supplied diluent to the powder-filled vial; mix to dissolve contents. Administer solution by withdrawing 0.5 ml and injecting it SC (*not* IV or intradermally); to prevent transmission of infection, use a separate syringe and needle for each patient.

Revaccination — The need and timing for revaccination, particularly for children 18–23 mo of age, is now under study

WARNINGS/PRECAUTIONS

Impaired immune response — In patients with antibody deficiency, whether owing to genetic defect or immunosuppressive therapy, vaccination may not produce the expected immune response. Clinically protective antibody titers (≥ 1 μg/ml) have been attained in 76% of children 18–20 mo of age, 96% of children 24–29 mo of age, and 100% of children 30 mo of age or older; caution parents that this vaccine is not likely to be completely effective in children who are under 24 mo of age.

Hypersensitivity reactions — Make sure that 0.1% epinephrine injection is available for immediate treatment of an anaphylactoid reaction

Fever, infection — Delay vaccination if the child has fever or an active infection

ADVERSE REACTIONS

Frequent reactions (incidence $\geq$ 1%) are printed in *italics*

Local — *Swelling and erythema (1.5%)*

Systemic — Fever ($>$ 101° F)

USE IN CHILDREN

See prescribing information above; do not use in infants under 18 mo of age

USE IN PREGNANT AND NURSING WOMEN

Pregnancy Category C: reproduction studies have not been done; it is not known whether this vaccine can cause harm to the fetus or affect reproductive capacity. No available data justify use during pregnancy. This product is not indicated for use by nursing mothers.

VEHICLE/BASE
Vials: 0.01% thimerosal, lactose, and sodium chloride (after reconstitution)

VACCINES

Diphtheria and tetanus toxoids and pertussis vaccine, adsorbed Connaught   Rx

Vials (per 0.5-ml dose): 6.7 flocculating units (Lf) diphtheria toxoid, 5 Lf tetanus toxoid, and 4 units pertussis vaccine (7.5 ml)

INDICATIONS

Prevention of diphtheria, tetanus, and pertussis

PARENTERAL DOSAGE

Child (2 mo to 6 yr): 3 IM doses of 0.5 ml each at intervals of 4–6 wk, followed by a fourth IM dose of 0.5 ml approximately 1 yr after the third dose; the first dose should be given at 2–3 mo of age or during a 6-wk checkup

DTP ■ HEPTAVAX-B

CONTRAINDICATIONS

History of shock, collapse, neurological signs or symptoms, high fever (> 39°C), or development of "excessive screaming syndrome" following administration	Evolving or changing neurological disorder	Anaphylactoid and/or allergic reaction following prior administration
Hypersensitivity to any component	Personal or family history of CNS disorders or convulsions	Acute illness (except for minor illness not associated with fever)
Age ≥ 7 yr	Outbreak of poliomyelitis (if the child is over 6 mo of age)	Concomitant use of other vaccines not proven effective during concurrent use
Immunosuppressive therapy or immunodeficiency disorder	Recent gammaglobulin injection or plasma or blood transfusion	Leukemia, lymphoma, or generalized malignancy

ADMINISTRATION/DOSAGE ADJUSTMENTS

Administration — Shake the vial vigorously before withdrawing each dose. Administer by deep IM injection, preferably into a midlateral thigh muscle (vastus lateralis); avoid injection into a blood vessel. To prevent transmission of hepatitis virus and other infectious agents, use a separate sterile syringe and needle for each patient. Do not give more than one inoculation at the same site.

Booster dose — Administer a booster dose of 0.5 ml when the child is 4–6 yr of age, preferably before the child enters kindergarten or elementary school; thereafter, administer booster doses every 10 yr with tetanus and diphtheria toxoids, adsorbed (for adult use)

WARNINGS/PRECAUTIONS

Life-threatening reactions — In rare cases, pertussis vaccine can cause high fever (> 39°C), transient shocklike episode, excessive screaming, somnolence, convulsions, encephalopathy, thrombocytopenia, and hemolytic anemia; neurological disorders such as encephalopathy may be fatal or result in permanent CNS damage. These reactions almost always appear within 24–48 h after injection but may develop as much as 7 days later. If a neurological sign or symptom or one of the above reactions is seen after administration of this product, discontinue use. Bear in mind that tetanus toxoid has also been associated with neurological complications, including cochlear lesion, brachial plexus neuropathy, paralysis of radial or recurrent nerve, difficulty in swallowing, accommodation paresis, EEG disturbances, and polyradiculoneuropathy.

Special-risk patients — Carefully weigh the relative benefits and risks of routine immunization with this product if the child has an active infection or a personal or family history of neurological disturbances

Hypersensitivity — Systemic anaphylactoid and/or allergic reactions can occur; before administering this product, make sure that epinephrine 1:1,000 is available for immediate use. Should such reactions occur, do not readminister.

Sudden infant death syndrome (SIDS) — Although SIDS has been reported rarely following administration of DTP vaccine, a causal relationship has not been established

ADVERSE REACTIONS

Central nervous system — Transient shocklike episode, excessive screaming, somnolence, convulsions, encephalopathy, irritability, cochlear lesion, brachial plexus neuropathies, paralysis of radial or recurrent nerve, accommodation paresis, EEG disturbances, polyradiculoneuropathy; swallowing difficulty (one case)

Local — Pain, erythema, tenderness, heat, edema, and induration at injection site; nodule formation, sterile abscess

Hematological — Thrombocytopenia, hemolytic anemia

Other — High fever (> 39°C), moderate transient fever, chills, malaise

---

USE IN CHILDREN

See INDICATIONS and ORAL DOSAGE; do not give this product to children who have reached 7 yr of age

USE IN PREGNANT AND NURSING WOMEN

This product is not indicated for use in pregnant or nursing women

---

VACCINES

HEPTAVAX-B (hepatitis B vaccine) Merck Sharp & Dohme   Rx

Vials: 20 μg/ml hepatitis B surface antigen (0.5, 3 ml)

INDICATIONS

Prevention of type B hepatitis in persons at risk, particularly (1) health-care practitioners, paraprofessionals, and staff members (including blood bank, laboratory, and plasma fractionation workers), (2) medical, dental, and nursing students, (3) patients and staff in hemodialysis or hematology/oncology units, (4) patients with hemophilia, thalassemia, or other conditions necessitating frequent or large-volume blood transfusions or clotting factor concentrates, (5) users of illicit parenteral drugs, (6) residents and staff of institutions for the mentally handicapped, (7) classroom contacts of aggressive, mentally handicapped persons having persistent hepatitis B antigenemia, (8) household or other intimate contacts of persons having persistent hepatitis B antigenemia, (9) persons who repeatedly contract sexually transmitted diseases, (10) prostitutes, (11) homosexually active males, (12) prisoners, (13) military personnel at risk, (14) morticians and embalmers, (15) Indochinese and Haitian refugees, (16) Alaskan Eskimos, and (17) infants born to carriers of the hepatitis B surface antigen

PARENTERAL DOSAGE

Adult and older child: 3 IM doses of 1 ml each, the first two given 1 mo apart and the third 6 mo after the first

Child (birth to 10 yr): 3 IM doses of 0.5 ml each, the first two given 1 mo apart and the third 6 mo after the first. For infants born to carriers of the hepatitis B surface antigen, give 3 IM doses of 0.5 ml each, the first within 7 days of birth, the second 1 mo later, and the third 6 mo after the first; in addition, give 0.5 ml of hepatitis B immune globulin at birth.

HEPTAVAX-B

Prevention of type B hepatitis following (1) percutaneous, ocular, or mucous membrane exposure to blood known or presumed to contain hepatitis B antigen, (2) percutaneous bites by known or presumed human carriers of the antigen, or (3) intimate sexual contact with known or presumed carriers of the antigen

Adult: 3 IM doses of 1 ml each, the first given within 7 days of exposure, the second 1 mo later, and the third 6 mo after the first; in addition, give 0.06 ml/kg of hepatitis B immune globulin as soon as possible after exposure (preferably within 24 h)

CONTRAINDICATIONS

Hypersensitivity to any component

ADMINISTRATION/DOSAGE ADJUSTMENTS

Parenteral administration	Administer IM or, if necessary, SC; do not inject IV or intradermally. For IM administration in adults, use the deltoid muscle; for IM injection in children, use an anterolateral thigh muscle. If the vaccine and hepatitis B immune globulin are to be given to an infant at the same time, inject the vaccine in one thigh and the globulin in the opposite thigh. The buttocks are generally not recommended as a site because the vaccine may be inadvertently injected into adipose tissue and, as a result, absorption and antibody response may be reduced. Subcutaneous administration should be reserved for patients in whom IM injection poses a risk of hemorrhage (eg, hemophiliacs); although IM and SC use of this vaccine have been shown to produce a similar immune response and comparable clinical reactions, SC administration of other aluminum-adsorbed vaccines has been associated with an increased incidence of local reactions, including subcutaneous nodules. Before withdrawing a dose, thoroughly agitate the vial to suspend the vaccine. To prevent transmission of infection (eg, serum hepatitis), for each patient use a separate, sterile syringe and needle; the syringe should be free of preservatives, antiseptics, and detergents. Store the vaccine at 2–8°C; do not freeze.
Dialysis and immunocompromised patients	Patients undergoing dialysis or immunosuppressive therapy or with immunodeficiency disease require larger doses. Initially give 2 ml IM in two 1-ml doses at different sites; repeat the injections 1 mo later and then again 6 mo after the initial administration. Immunocompromised patients do not respond as well to this vaccine as healthy patients.
Immunogenicity	Antibody response depends on age; the seroconversion rate is 100% for children 1–10 yr of age, 92–96% for adults 20–49 yr of age, and 77% for adults 50 yr of age or older. Immunocompromised and hemodialysis patients do not respond as well as healthy persons. Antibody can be detected in approximately 60% of hemodialysis patients after completion of the 3-dose series; the antibody levels in these patients, in comparison to those of healthy persons, is lower and tends to remain at protective levels for shorter periods. Prophylactic treatment of infants born to carriers of the hepatitis B surface and e antigens has been effective in 85–93% of cases.
Immune status after vaccination	Routine testing for immunity after vaccination is advised only for the following: (1) persons whose immune status will affect how they will be managed (eg, patients and members of staff in dialysis units), (2) persons in whom a suboptimal response may be anticipated (eg, persons over 50 yr of age, immunocompromised patients), and (3) infants born to carriers of the hepatitis B surface antigen (HBsAg). To determine immune status, measure antibody to HBsAg by radioimmunoassay (RIA) or enzyme immunoassay (EIA); active immunity is characterized by 10 or more RIA sample ratio units or a positive EIA response. Infants born to carriers of HBsAg should be tested at 12–15 mo of age; protective immunity is indicated by the absence of HBsAg and the presence of antibodies to this antigen. Revaccination of persons who do not respond to the 3-dose primary series results in immunity in only one third of cases and is therefore not recommended as a routine practice.
Revaccination	The duration of immunity and the need for booster doses have not yet been determined. Over a period of 3–4 yr, the level of antibody to hepatitis B surface antigen may fall below the minimum protective level of 10 RIA sample ratio units in some patients. In one study, protection against chronic antigenemia and hepatitis appeared to persist despite a drop below 10 RIA sample ratio units. The antibody level in individuals at high risk of exposure to hepatitis B virus may be checked periodically after vaccination; if the level falls below 10 RIA sample ratio units, administration of a booster dose should be considered.

WARNINGS/PRECAUTIONS

Hypersensitivity	Hypersensitivity reactions, including urticaria, angioedema, and pruritus, have occurred within the first few hours after vaccination; an apparent hypersensitivity syndrome, characterized by arthritis, fever, and dermatological reactions (eg, urticaria, ecchymoses, erythema multiforme), has been seen days or weeks after vaccination. Although hypersensitivity reactions occur rarely, epinephrine should be available during administration for immediate use. If symptoms suggestive of hypersensitivity develop after an injection, the regimen should be discontinued.
Patients with active infection	If possible, delay use in patients with any serious active infection
Other special-risk patients	Use with caution and appropriate care in patients in whom a systemic reaction (including fever) could pose a significant risk, such as in patients with severely compromised cardiopulmonary function

Vaccination of patients with unrecognized hepatitis B infections	Because of the long incubation period for hepatitis B (6 wk to 6 mo), unrecognized infection may be present when this vaccine is given; under such circumstances the vaccine may not prevent the subsequent development of clinical infection

ADVERSE REACTIONS[1]

Frequent reactions (incidence $\geq$ 1%) are printed in *italics*

Central nervous system	*Headache (3.1%), fatigue/asthenia (1.9%)*, optic neuritis; myelitis (including transverse myelitis); acute radiculoneuropathy (including Guillain-Barré syndrome); peripheral neuropathy (including Bell's palsy and herpes zoster); malaise, dizziness, disturbed sleep, paresthesia, irritability
Musculoskeletal	*Myalgia (1.2%)*, arthralgia
Gastrointestinal	*Gastrointestinal illness (2%), including anorexia, nausea, vomiting, abdominal pain, and diarrhea;* abdominal cramps
Hypersensitivity	Urticaria, angioedema, pruritus, arthritis, fever, ecchymoses, and erythema multiforme (rare)
Hematological	Thrombocytopenia
Local	*Injection site reactions (12.3%), including soreness, erythema, swelling, warmth, and induration*
Other	*Upper respiratory tract illness (2.5%), fever $\geq 100°$ F (1.8%)*, chills, sensation of warmth, diaphoresis, rash, adenitis, tinnitus, visual disturbances, flushing

USE IN CHILDREN

See INDICATIONS and PARENTERAL DOSAGE

USE IN PREGNANT AND NURSING WOMEN

Pregnancy Category C: use during pregnancy only if clearly needed. Reproduction studies have not been performed in animals or humans to determine whether this vaccine can adversely affect fetal development or reproductive capacity. Studies in 12 nursing mothers have shown no evidence that the vaccine is excreted in human milk.

[1] Although liver function abnormalities have been reported in clinical use, no causal relationship has been established; moreover, a controlled study has shown no significant difference between placebo and vaccine in the frequency of increased SGPT levels

---

VACCINES

HIB-IMUNE (hemophilus b polysaccharide vaccine) Lederle Rx

Vials (per 0.5-ml dose): 25 µg purified capsular polysaccharide from *Hemophilus influenzae* type b (1 dose)

INDICATIONS

Prevention of *Hemophilus influenzae* type b diseases in all children who are 2-5 yr of age and in certain children who are 18-23 mo of age

PARENTERAL DOSAGE

Child (18 mo to 5 yr): 25 µg (0.5 ml), given in a single IM or SC dose

CONTRAINDICATIONS

Hypersensitivity to any component

ADMINISTRATION/DOSAGE ADJUSTMENTS

Children 2-5 yr of age	Hemophilus b polysaccharide vaccine should generally be given at 24 mo of age. The decision to immunize children who have not been vaccinated by 24 mo of age should be based on an assessment of the risk of *Hemophilus influenzae* type b disease since this risk declines with age. When considering immunization of children whose ages vary from 2 to 5 yr, give priority to the younger children in the group.[1]
Immunization at 18 mo of age	Administration of this vaccine at 18 mo of age may be considered, especially for children in high-risk groups, since the likelihood of infection is greater at 18 mo than at 24 mo. Among those particularly susceptible to *Hemophilus influenzae* type b disease are the following[1]: (1) children who attend daycare facilities, (2) children with antibody deficiency syndrome, functional or anatomical asplenia (eg, sickle cell disease, splenectomy), or a malignancy such as Hodgkin's disease that necessitated immunosuppressive therapy, (3) children of American Indians, Eskimos, or blacks, and (4) children from a lower socioeconomic class. Bear in mind that this vaccine is not likely to be as effective in children aged 18-23 mo as in older children; a second dose may be necessary within 18 mo after the first dose if this vaccine is given at 18-23 mo of age. Inform parents about this age-related difference in immunogenicity.
Concomitant administration of DTP vaccine	This vaccine can be given at the same time as DTP vaccine, with a separate site for each vaccine, since frequency of adverse reactions and immune response to each antigen are not affected by simultaneous administration

HIB-IMUNE ■ HibVAX

Preparation and administration	For reconstitution, add 0.6 ml of the supplied diluent to the powder-filled vial; shake vial gently to dissolve contents. Withdraw 0.5 ml and administer IM or SC (*not* IV). To prevent transmission of infection, use a separate, sterile needle and syringe for each patient.

WARNINGS/PRECAUTIONS

Impaired immune response	This vaccine may fail to induce the expected antibody response in immunocompromised patients; nevertheless, children with chronic conditions such as asplenia or treated Hodgkin's disease should receive this vaccine (see above "Immunization at 18 mo of age")
Neurological effects	Seizures have occurred with use of this vaccine, and other neurological disorders have been seen following injection of many other biological products; although no causal relationship has been established in these instances, the possibility of such reactions should always be carefully considered. This vaccine has produced sleep disturbances.
Hypersensitivity reactions	Make sure that 0.1% epinephrine injection is available for immediate treatment of anaphylaxis and other allergic reactions
Fever, infection	Delay vaccination if the child has fever or an acute infection
Local reactions	In general, local reactions are mild; they occur most frequently about 6 h after injection and usually disappear within 24 h
Febrile reactions	Fever exceeding 101.3° F has been seen within 24 h after vaccination in 1.5% of patients; this grade of fever occurred only in patients who were 18–23 mo of age

ADVERSE REACTIONS[2]

Local	Erythema, warmth, swelling, tenderness
Systemic	Fever > 101.3° F, irritability, anorexia, sleep disturbances

USE IN CHILDREN	USE IN PREGNANT AND NURSING WOMEN
See prescribing information above; do not use in infants under 18 mo of age	**Pregnant women:** Pregnancy Category C: reproduction studies have not been done; it is not known whether this vaccine can cause harm to the fetus or affect reproductive capacity. Do not use in pregnant women. **Nursing mothers:** It is not known whether this vaccine is excreted in human milk; do not use in nursing mothers.

VEHICLE/BASE
Vials: 0.01% thimerosal, sucrose, and phosphate-buffered sodium chloride (after reconstitution)

[1] *MMWR* 34:201–205, 1985
[2] Seizures and rashes have been reported with use of hemophilus b polysaccharide vaccine in the US; however, a causal relationship has not been established

---

VACCINES

HibVAX (hemophilus b polysaccharide vaccine) Connaught Rx

Vials (per 0.5-ml dose): 25 µg purified capsular polysaccharide from *Hemophilus influenzae* type b (1, 5, 10 doses)

INDICATIONS	PARENTERAL DOSAGE
Prevention of *Hemophilus influenzae* type b diseases in all children who are 2–5 yr of age and in certain children who are 18–23 mo of age	**Child (18 mo to 5 yr):** 25 µg (0.5 ml), given in a single IM or SC dose

CONTRAINDICATIONS
Hypersensitivity to any component

ADMINISTRATION/DOSAGE ADJUSTMENTS

Children 2–5 yr of age	Hemophilus b polysaccharide vaccine should generally be given at 24 mo of age. The decision to immunize children who have not been vaccinated by 24 mo of age should be based on an assessment of the risk of *Hemophilus influenzae* type b disease since this risk declines with age. When considering immunization of children whose ages vary from 2 to 5 yr, give priority to the younger children in the group.[1]
Immunization at 18 mo of age	Administration of this vaccine at 18 mo of age may be considered, especially for children in high-risk groups, since the likelihood of infection is greater at 18 mo than at 24 mo. Among those particularly susceptible to *Hemophilus influenzae* type b disease are the following: (1) children who attend daycare facilities, (2) children with antibody deficiency syndrome, functional or anatomical asplenia (eg, sickle cell disease, splenectomy), or a malignancy such as Hodgkin's disease that necessitated immunosuppressive therapy, (3) children of American Indians, Eskimos, or blacks, and (4) children from a lower socioeconomic class. Bear in mind that this vaccine is not likely to be as effective in children aged 18–23 mo as in older children; a second dose may be necessary within 18 mo after the first dose if this vaccine is given at 18–23 mo of age. Inform parents about this age-related difference in immunogenicity.
Concomitant administration of DTP vaccine	This vaccine can be given at the same time as DTP vaccine, with a separate site for each vaccine, since the frequency of adverse reactions and the immune response to each antigen are not affected by simultaneous administration

HibVAX ■ Influenza virus vaccine

Preparation and administration	For reconstitution, add the appropriate amount of the supplied diluent to the powder-filled vial; shake vial to dissolve contents. Withdraw 0.5 ml and administer SC or IM (*not* IV) in the midthigh or deltoid areas; aspirate before injection in order to ensure that the needle has not entered a blood vessel. To prevent transmission of infection, use a separate, sterile needle and syringe (or disposable unit) for each patient.

WARNINGS/PRECAUTIONS

Impaired immune response	This vaccine may fail to induce the expected antibody response in immunocompromised patients; moreover, it may not be effective in all healthy children. Nevertheless, children with chronic conditions such as asplenia or treated Hodgkin's disease should receive this vaccine (see above "Immunization at 18 mo of age").
Hypersensitivity reactions	Make sure that 0.1% epinephrine injection is available for immediate treatment of anaphylaxis and other allergic reactions
Fever, infection	Delay vaccination if the child has fever or an acute infection
Local reactions	Transient erythema, induration, and tenderness have been seen 24 h after injection
Recurrent upper respiratory tract disease	This vaccine does not protect against diseases caused by nonencapsulated (nontypeable) strains of *Hemophilus influenzae* and, therefore, should not be used to prevent recurrences of sinusitis, otitis media, or other upper respiratory tract diseases, since these disorders are generally due to nonencapsulated strains. (The type b strain accounts for only 5–10% of cases of *H influenzae*-caused otitis media.)
Epidemiological effect	This vaccine is unlikely to be of substantial benefit in reducing the frequency of secondary cases of *Hemophilus influenzae* type b disease in the general population since it is not effective in children who are most susceptible to this disease, namely, those under 18 mo of age

ADVERSE REACTIONS[2]

	Frequent reactions (incidence ≥ 1%) are printed in *italics*
Local	*Transient local reactions (10%), including erythema, induration, and tenderness*
Systemic	*Fever > 101° F (2%)*

USE IN CHILDREN

See prescribing information above; do not use in infants under 18 mo of age

USE IN PREGNANT AND NURSING WOMEN

Pregnant women: Pregnancy Category C: reproduction studies have not been done; it is not known whether this vaccine can cause harm to the fetus or affect reproductive capacity. Do not use in pregnant women. **Nursing mothers:** This product is not indicated for use in nursing mothers.

VEHICLE/BASE
Vials: 0.01% thimerosal, lactose, and isotonic sodium chloride (after reconstitution)

[1] *MMWR* 34:203, 1985
[2] Seizures, rashes, and vomiting have been reported with use of hemophilus b polysaccharide vaccine in the US; however, a causal relationship has not been established

---

VACCINES

Influenza virus vaccine, trivalent, subvirion Wyeth Rx

Vials (per 0.5-ml dose):[1] not less than 15 μg hemagglutinin antigen each of A/Chile/1/83 (H1N1), A/Mississippi/1/85 (H3N2), and B/Ann Arbor/1/86 (5 ml) **Cartridge-needle units (per 0.5-ml dose):**[1] not less than 15 μg hemagglutinin antigen each of A/Chile/1/83 (H1N1), A/Mississippi/1/85 (H3N2), and B/Ann Arbor/1/86 (0.5 ml)

INDICATIONS

Prevention of influenza in the following groups: (1) high-risk patients, ie, (a) those with chronic cardiovascular or pulmonary disorders sufficiently severe to require regular medical supervision or hospitalization within a year before anticipated time of vaccination and (b) residents of chronic-care facilities; (2) moderate-risk patients, ie, (a) individuals 65 yr of age or older, (b) patients with renal impairment, anemia, chronic metabolic diseases (including diabetes), immunosuppressive disorders, or asthma sufficiently severe to require regular medical supervision or hospitalization within a year before anticipated time of vaccination, and (c) children undergoing long-term aspirin therapy (influenza infection in these children may result in Reye's syndrome); (3) persons capable of transmitting influenza infection to high-risk patients, ie, (a) medical personnel who have extensive contact with high-risk patients and (b) persons who care for high-risk patients at home; and (4) individuals who wish to reduce their risk of infection

PARENTERAL DOSAGE

Adult (≥ 13 yr): 0.5 ml IM
Child (6–35 mo; never received an influenza vaccine from 1978–79 to 1985–86 seasons): 2 IM doses of 0.25 ml each, given 4 or more weeks apart
Child (6–35 mo; received 1 or more doses of an influenza vaccine from 1978–79 to 1985–86 seasons): 0.25 ml IM
Child (3–12 yr): same as younger child, except dose is 0.5 ml

Influenza virus vaccine

Influenza virus vaccine, monovalent, subvirion Wyeth   Rx

Vials (per 0.5-ml dose):[1] not less than 15 μg hemagglutinin antigen of A/Taiwan/1/86 (H1N1) (5 ml)   **Cartridge-needle units (per 0.5-ml dose):**[1] not less than 15 μg hemagglutinin antigen of A/Taiwan/1/86 (H1N1) (0.5 ml)

INDICATIONS

Prevention of influenza in the following groups: (1) high-risk patients under 35 yr of age, ie, those with chronic cardiovascular or pulmonary disorders sufficiently severe to require regular medical supervision or hospitalization within a year before anticipated time of vaccination; (2) moderate-risk patients under 35 yr of age, ie, (a) patients with chronic metabolic diseases (including diabetes), renal impairment, anemia, immunosuppressive disorders, or asthma sufficiently severe to require regular medical supervision or hospitalization within a year before anticipated time of vaccination and (b) children undergoing long-term aspirin therapy (influenza infection in these children may result in Reye's syndrome); (3) persons under 35 yr of age capable of transmitting influenza infection to high-risk patients, ie, (a) medical personnel who have extensive contact with high-risk patients and (b) persons who care for high-risk patients at home; and (4) individuals of any age who wish to reduce their risk of infection

PARENTERAL DOSAGE

Adult (≥ 13 yr): for persons who received the 1986–87 trivalent vaccine, 0.5 ml IM 4 or more weeks after the trivalent dose; for persons who did not receive the 1986–87 trivalent vaccine, 0.5 ml IM with 1 dose of the 1986–87 trivalent vaccine

Child (6–35 mo; never received an influenza vaccine from 1978–79 to 1985–86 seasons): for those who received 2 doses of the 1986–87 trivalent vaccine, 0.25 ml IM 4 or more weeks after the second trivalent dose; for those who received 1 dose of the trivalent vaccine, 0.25 ml IM with 1 dose of the trivalent vaccine 4 or more weeks after the first trivalent dose; for those who did not receive the 1986–87 trivalent vaccine, 0.25 ml IM, with 1 dose of the 1986–87 trivalent vaccine, on each of 2 visits 4 or more weeks apart

Child (6–35 mo; received at least 1 dose of an influenza vaccine from 1978–79 to 1985–86 seasons): for those who also received the 1986–87 trivalent vaccine, 0.25 ml IM 4 or more weeks after the trivalent dose; for those who did not receive the 1986–87 trivalent vaccine, 0.25 ml with 1 dose of the trivalent vaccine

Child (3–12 yr): same as younger child, except dose is 0.5 ml

CONTRAINDICATIONS

Hypersensitivity to chicken egg   History of Guillain-Barré syndrome

ADMINISTRATION/DOSAGE ADJUSTMENTS

Parenteral administration	Inject solution into the deltoid muscle of an adult or older child or into the anterolateral thigh muscle of an infant or young child; do not give IV. If a second vaccine is given simultaneously, administer it at a separate site. To help prevent inadvertent intravascular injection, aspirate the needle after insertion. Use a separate, heat-sterilized syringe and needle for each patient to avoid transmission of hepatitis B or other infections.
Time of administration	For most areas in the US, November is the optimal time for administration of these vaccines; however, immunization in September or October should be considered under certain circumstances, such as the following: (1) where the regional pattern (as in Alaska) varies from the national pattern, (2) when a high-risk patient leaves a hospital during that time, or (3) when a patient comes for a routine visit at that time and a return visit is unlikely. Children who require 2 doses should be given the second dose before December. Do not delay administration of the trivalent vaccine because the monovalent vaccine is not available; give the monovalent vaccine either with the second trivalent dose or 4 or more weeks after the last trivalent dose. Although this vaccine may be given during the period of influenza activity, temporary chemoprophylaxis may be indicated in such a situation.
Effectiveness	In most individuals, this vaccine is effective only against those strains of influenza virus from which it is prepared and closely related strains; it is not effective against all possible influenza strains. Immunity declines within a year after vaccination; for optimal protection, the vaccine must be given annually.
Use with other vaccines	Influenza vaccine may be given simultaneously with a pneumococcal or routine pediatric vaccine (at different sites); no increase in adverse effects should result

WARNINGS/PRECAUTIONS

Hypersensitivity	This vaccine is prepared from the allantoic fluids of chick embryos. Before vaccinating any patient, make sure that epinephrine 1:1,000 is available for immediate treatment of possible acute anaphylactic reactions. If the patient may be hypersensitive to eggs, perform a skin test or other appropriate allergy test with this vaccine before administration; if reaction is positive, do not vaccinate the patient. Do not give this vaccine to patients who are undergoing acute respiratory distress or circulatory collapse or who have experienced an anaphylactic reaction (including swelling around the lips or tongue) following ingestion of eggs. This vaccine contains up to 0.25 μg of gentamicin per 0.5-ml dose; persons with sensitivity to gentamicin or other aminoglycosides should not receive this vaccine.
Common systemic effects	Fever, malaise, and myalgia may occur 6–12 h after injection and persist for 1–2 days; these effects occur more frequently in children and others who have not been exposed to the antigens in this vaccine

Guillain-Barré syndrome	In 1976, the Guillain-Barré syndrome (GBS) developed within 10 wk after administration of the A/New Jersey/76 influenza. The frequency, 1 case per 100,000, was 5–6 times higher than that of nonrecipients; the syndrome was more commonly seen among those over 25 yr of age. Although surveillance of individuals given the 1978–79, 1979–80, and 1980–81 formulations showed no association between GBS and the vaccine, patients should be cautioned about the potential risk of this syndrome.
Febrile illness	Wait until temporary signs and symptoms of acute febrile illness abate before giving this vaccine
Immunosuppressive therapy	The expected antibody response may not occur in patients undergoing immunosuppressive therapy
Concomitant use of warfarin or theophylline	Influenza vaccination has been reported to increase the pharmacological effects of warfarin and theophylline; although most studies have failed to confirm this report, the risk of toxicity should be considered

ADVERSE REACTIONS

Local	Slight-to-moderate tenderness, erythema, and induration at injection site, lasting 1–2 days (33%)
Systemic	Fever, malaise, myalgia, Guillain-Barré syndrome[2]
Hypersensitivity	Flare, wheal, and respiratory impairment (rare)

USE IN CHILDREN

See INDICATIONS and PARENTERAL DOSAGE; adverse effects may be particularly common in children

USE IN PREGNANT AND NURSING WOMEN

Pregnant women: Pregnancy Category C: no evidence of risk to the fetus has been reported or suggested; nevertheless, since reproduction studies have not been done, vaccination, when clearly needed, should generally be delayed until the second or third trimester. However, bear in mind that such a delay may be undesirable if a pregnant woman has a high-risk condition and influenza activity will begin during her first trimester. **Nursing mothers:** consult manufacturer.

[1] Vaccine prepared for the 1986–87 season contained the viral antigens listed here; since the antigen content of influenza vaccines is reviewed annually by the US Public Health Service, the formulation may be different for the 1987–88 season. The vaccine also contains 0.01% thimerosal and 0.5 μg/ml of gentamicin sulfate.
[2] Other neurologic disorders, including encephalopathies, have been temporally associated with influenza vaccination

---

VACCINES

M-M-R II (measles, mumps, and rubella live virus vaccine) Merck Sharp & Dohme   Rx

Vials (per 0.5-ml dose): 1,000 tissue culture infective doses ($TCID_{50}$) of measles virus, 5,000 $TCID_{50}$ of mumps virus, and 1,000 $TCID_{50}$ of rubella virus (1, 10 doses)

INDICATIONS	PARENTERAL DOSAGE
Prevention of **measles, mumps, and rubella** infections	**Adult and child ($\geq$15 mo):** 0.5 ml SC, preferably in the outer aspect of the upper arm

CONTRAINDICATIONS

Pregnancy	History of anaphylactoid reaction to eggs or neomycin[1]	Immunosuppressive therapy
Febrile respiratory illness or other active febrile infection	Active untreated tuberculosis	Blood dyscrasias, leukemia, lymphomas, or other malignant neoplasia affecting the bone marrow or lymphatic system
Primary immunodeficiencies, including cellular immunodeficiency, hypogammaglobulinemia, and dysgammaglobulinemia	Family history of congenital or hereditary immunodeficiency (unless immunocompetence of patient is demonstrated)	

ADMINISTRATION/DOSAGE ADJUSTMENTS

Preparation, administration, storage	Use a sterile syringe with a 25-gauge, ⅝″-long needle for preparation and administration; the syringe and needle should be free of preservatives, antiseptics, detergents, and other substances that might inactivate the vaccine. Reconstitute solution only with the supplied diluent, since it contains no antiviral products. To prevent transmission of hepatitis B virus and other infectious agents, use a separate sterile syringe and needle for each patient. Store reconstituted solutions in a dark place at 2–8° C; administer within 8 h. If the multidose vial is used, exercise particular care in maintaining the sterility and potency of the solution; bear in mind that the diluent does not contain any preservatives.
Transfusions, immune globulin	Do not give this vaccine to a patient who received within the past 3 mo or is currently receiving immune globulin or a blood or plasma transfusion

M-M-R II

Concomitant immunization	This vaccine should generally not be given within 1 mo before or after administration of other virus vaccines because information on concomitant immunization is inadequate; however, in some cases, especially when the patient may not return for another visit, this vaccine may be administered with diphtheria, tetanus, and pertussis (DTP) vaccine and/or oral poliovirus vaccine. If DTP and this vaccine are given at the same time, separate sites and syringes should be used.
Tuberculin test	This vaccine may reduce skin sensitivity to tuberculin; administer a tuberculin test before vaccination or at the same time

WARNINGS/PRECAUTIONS

Infants under 15 mo of age	It may be desirable to vaccinate a child less than 15 mo of age under the following circumstances: (1) if the child is a member of a population group in which measles may occur in a significant proportion of infants under 15 mo of age or (2) if the child lives in a relatively inaccessible area and timely immunization is logistically difficult. However, since the measles component of this vaccine may fail to produce an antibody response in a child under 15 mo of age because of the presence of maternal antibodies, a child given this vaccine at less than 12 mo of age should be revaccinated after reaching 15 mo of age. Bear in mind that there is some evidence to suggest that immunization at less than 1 yr of age may preclude development of sustained antibody levels following vaccination at 15 mo of age; therefore, before using this product in children under 15 mo of age, carefully weigh the advantage of early protection against the risk of an inadequate response following revaccination.
Children in contact with pregnant women	To reduce risk of rubella during pregnancy, vaccinate unimmunized children who are living with a susceptible pregnant woman
Women of childbearing age	Do not give this vaccine during pregnancy. Before using it in nonpregnant women of childbearing age, determine their susceptibility to rubella by performing appropriate serologic tests; if the rubella antibody titer with hemagglutination inhibition is 1:8 or more, the vaccine should not be given since it is unnecessary. (Bear in mind that the Immunization Practices Advisory Committee does not require serologic testing for nonpregnant women who have no history of vaccination.) It may be convenient to administer the vaccine to women immediately after they have given birth; however, bear in mind that the attenuated virus may be excreted into breast milk (see USE IN PREGNANT AND NURSING MOTHERS). After vaccination, instruct women not to become pregnant for at least 3 mo.
Hypersensitivity	The measles and mumps vaccines are produced in chick embryo cell cultures; do not use this preparation in patients who have experienced immediate-type allergic reactions, such as anaphylaxis, urticaria, swelling of the mouth and throat, dyspnea, hypotension, or shock, after ingestion of eggs. Patients who have an egg allergy that is not characterized by anaphylactoid reactions do not appear to be at increased risk. Before administering this vaccine, make sure that epinephrine 1:1,000 is available for immediate use.
Neurological disorders	Serious CNS reactions, such as encephalitis, encephalopathy, and subacute sclerosing panencephalitis, may occur on very rare occasions; the frequency of significant CNS reactions following use of attenuated measles vaccine is one case per million doses. Encephalitis and encephalopathy have been seen within 30 days after vaccination. Rubella vaccine can produce polyneuritis; the reaction occurs most frequently and with greatest severity in adult women. Polyneuropathy, including the Guillain-Barré syndrome, has occurred following use of measles and rubella vaccines
Fever	A temperature of 101.0–102.9° F occurs occasionally, while high fever (>103° F) is seen less commonly; measles vaccine has caused prolonged high fever. Febrile convulsions occur on rare occasions. Watch for evidence of an increase in temperature following vaccination. Use with caution in patients with a history of febrile convulsions, cerebral injury, or any other condition that can be precipitated or exacerbated by fever.
Musculoskeletal effects	Attenuated rubella virus can cause arthritis and arthralgia. The frequency of joint reactions is high in adult women, low in children, and moderate in adolescent women (0–3% in children and 12–20% in postpubertal women). Joint reactions tend to be more severe and last longer in postpubertal women than in children; symptoms initially occur 2–4 wk after vaccination and may persist for months or, on rare occasions, for years. These reactions are generally well tolerated, even in women 35–45 yr of age, and rarely interfere with normal activities. Caution postpubertal women about the risk of arthritis and arthralgia.
Ophthalmic effects	Optic neuritis, including retrobulbar neuritis, papillitis, and retinitis, has occurred 1–3 wk after administration of some live virus vaccines. Ocular palsies have been seen 3–24 days after vaccination with attenuated measles virus, but a definite causal relationship has not been established.
Generalized rash	Rash occurs infrequently, and the effect is usually minimal; however, on rare occasions, a generalized rash can occur
Measles infection	Attenuated measles virus vaccine has caused atypical measles in patients who had previously received a killed measles virus vaccine
Local effects	This vaccine can cause injection-site reactions (see ADVERSE REACTIONS); administration of attenuated measles virus vaccine has produced extensive local reactions and, in patients who had previously received a killed measles virus vaccine, has caused marked swelling, erythema, and vesiculation

M-M-R II ■ ORIMUNE

Close personal contact	Although small amounts of the attenuated rubella virus are usually excreted from the nose or throat 7–28 days after vaccination, there is no confirmed evidence that the virus is transmitted to susceptible individuals through close personal contact with vaccinees; transmission of attenuated mumps or measles virus from vaccinees to susceptible contacts has not been reported
Effectiveness	Not all patients respond to this vaccine; in clinical studies, this vaccine induced measles hemagglutination-inhibiting (HI) antibodies in 95% of patients, mumps neutralizing antibodies in 96% of patients, and rubella HI antibodies in 99% of patients

ADVERSE REACTIONS

Central nervous system	Headache, malaise, nerve deafness, polyneuritis, polyneuropathy, Guillain-Barré syndrome, encephalitis, encephalopathy, subacute sclerosing panencephalitis
Ophthalmic	Optic neuritis, including retrobulbar neuritis, papillitis, and retinitis; ocular palsy
Musculoskeletal	Arthritis, arthralgia
Hematological	Thrombocytopenia, purpura
Hypersensitivity	Wheal and flare at injection site, urticaria
Local	Burning, stinging, erythema, induration, tenderness, wheal and flare, regional lymphadenopathy
Other	Sore throat, fever, rash, parotitis, orchitis, panniculitis

USE IN CHILDREN

See INDICATIONS and PARENTERAL DOSAGE. Children under 12 mo of age should be routinely revaccinated; children given this vaccine at 12 mo of age or later should be revaccinated only if there is evidence to suggest that the initial vaccination was not effective.

USE IN PREGNANT AND NURSING WOMEN

Pregnancy Category C: measles infection has caused increases in spontaneous abortion, stillbirth, congenital defects, and premature birth; although use of attenuated measles virus during pregnancy has not been adequately studied, it is prudent to assume that the attenuated virus can also produce these effects. The mumps virus can infect the placenta and fetus; however, there is no good evidence that it is teratogenic in humans. The attenuated mumps virus has been detected in the placenta, but not in fetal tissue. No evidence of congenital rubella syndrome has been seen in a survey of infants born to women who received rubella vaccine within 3 mo before or after conception. Do not use M-M-R II during pregnancy or within 3 mo before conception (see warning above concerning women of childbearing age). Attenuated rubella virus can be excreted in human milk and transmitted to nursing infants; a mild infection has occurred in one infant. It is not known whether attenuated measles or mumps virus is excreted in human milk. Use M-M-R II with caution in nursing mothers.

[1] Each 0.5-ml dose contains 25 µg of neomycin

VACCINES

ORIMUNE (poliovirus vaccine, live, trivalent) Lederle Rx

Prefilled pipettes (per 0.5-ml dose): $10^{5.4}$–$10^{6.4}$ tissue culture infective doses (TCID$_{50}$) of poliovirus Type 1, $10^{4.5}$–$10^{5.5}$ TCID$_{50}$ of poliovirus Type 2, and $10^{5.2}$–$10^{6.2}$ TCID$_{50}$ of poliovirus Type 3 (0.5 ml) for oral use only

INDICATIONS

Prevention of poliomyelitis in (1) children and (2) adults at increased risk due to contact with or travel to epidemic or endemic areas or due to occupation (eg, medical personnel and sanitation workers)

ORAL DOSAGE

Adult: for previously immunized patients, 0.5 ml, given in a single dose (see ADMINISTRATION/DOSAGE ADJUSTMENTS concerning use in unimmunized patients)
Infant: 3 doses of 0.5 ml each, beginning at 6–12 wk of age; give the second dose not less than 6 and preferably 8 wk after the first, followed by a third dose 8–12 mo later (alternatively, the 3 doses may be given at 2, 4, and approximately 18 mo of age, with an optional fourth dose at 6 mo in areas where poliomyelitis is endemic)
Child and adolescent ($\leq$ 18 yr): 3 doses of 0.5 ml each, the first two given not less than 6 and preferably 8 wk apart and the third 6–12 mo after the second

CONTRAINDICATIONS

Acute illness	Advanced, debilitated conditions	Persistent vomiting or diarrhea
Compromised immune function (see WARNINGS/PRECAUTIONS)		

ADMINISTRATION/DOSAGE ADJUSTMENTS

Oral administration	The vaccine may be administered directly from the pipette, mixed with distilled water, unchlorinated tap water, simple syrup, or milk, or adsorbed on bread, cake, or cube sugar; if the vaccine was frozen, it must be completely thawed before use
Unimmunized adults	Basic immunization with inactivated poliovirus vaccine (IPV) is recommended for unimmunized adults at increased risk. If immunological protection is required in less than 4 wk, administer a single 0.5-ml dose of Orimune; IPV should be used for additional doses if the patient remains at increased risk.

Chapter 6

Acne Preparations/Antidandruff Shampoos

Acne Preparations — 200

ACCUTANE (Roche) — 200
Isotretinoin *Rx*

ACHROMYCIN (Lederle) — 202
Tetracycline hydrochloride *Rx*

ACHROMYCIN V (Lederle) — 202
Tetracycline hydrochloride *Rx*

A/T/S (Hoechst-Roussel) — 204
Erythromycin *Rx*

BENZAC (Owen) — 204
Benzoyl peroxide *Rx*

BENZAC W (Owen) — 204
Benzoyl peroxide *Rx*

BENZAC W Wash (Owen) — 204
Benzoyl peroxide *Rx*

BENZAGEL (Dermik) — 205
Benzoyl peroxide *Rx*

BENZAMYCIN (Dermik) — 206
Erythromycin and benzoyl peroxide *Rx*

CLEARASIL (Richardson-Vicks Health Care Products) — 206
Benzoyl peroxide *OTC*

CLEOCIN T (Upjohn) — 207
Clindamycin phosphate *Rx*

CUTICURA Acne Cream (Jeffrey Martin) — 208
Benzoyl peroxide *OTC*

CUTICURA Medicated Soap (Jeffrey Martin) — 208
Triclocarban *OTC*

DESQUAM-X (Westwood) — 209
Benzoyl peroxide *Rx*

DESQUAM-X Wash (Westwood) — 209
Benzoyl peroxide *Rx*

ERYCETTE (Ortho) — 209
Erythromycin *Rx*

ERYDERM (Abbott) — 210
Erythromycin *Rx*

KOMED (Barnes-Hind) — 211
Sodium thiosulfate, salicylic acid, and isopropyl alcohol *OTC*

LOROXIDE (Dermik) — 211
Benzoyl peroxide *OTC*

MECLAN (Ortho) — 212
Meclocycline sulfosalicylate *Rx*

MINOCIN (Lederle) — 213
Minocycline hydrochloride *Rx*

OXY-5 (Norcliff Thayer) — 214
Benzoyl peroxide *OTC*

OXY-10 (Norcliff Thayer) — 214
Benzoyl peroxide *OTC*

OXY-10 Cover (Norcliff Thayer) — 214
Benzoyl peroxide *OTC*

OXY-10 Wash (Norcliff Thayer) — 215
Benzoyl peroxide *OTC*

PanOxyl (Stiefel) — 215
Benzoyl peroxide *Rx*

PanOxyl AQ (Stiefel) — 215
Benzoyl peroxide *Rx*

PERSA-GEL (Ortho) — 216
Benzoyl peroxide *Rx*

PERSA-GEL W (Ortho) — 216
Benzoyl peroxide *Rx*

pHisoAc BP (Winthrop Consumer Products) — 217
Benzoyl peroxide *OTC*

RETIN-A (Ortho) — 217
Tretinoin *Rx*

STATICIN (Westwood) — 218
Erythromycin *Rx*

STRI-DEX (Glenbrook) — 219
Benzoyl peroxide *OTC*

SULFACET-R (Dermik) — 220
Sodium sulfacetamide and sulfur *Rx*

TOPICYCLINE (Norwich Eaton) — 220
Tetracycline hydrochloride *Rx*

VANOXIDE (Dermik) — 211
Benzoyl peroxide *OTC*

VANOXIDE-HC (Dermik) — 221
Benzoyl peroxide and hydrocortisone *Rx*

VLEMASQUE (Dermik) — 222
Lime, sulfurated *OTC*

Antidandruff Shampoos — 222

DENOREX (Whitehall) — 222
Coal tar, menthol, and alcohol *OTC*

EXSEL (Herbert) — 222
Selenium sulfide *Rx*

HEAD & SHOULDERS (Procter & Gamble) — 223
Zinc pyrithione *OTC*

SEBULEX (Westwood) — 224
Sulfur and salicylic acid *OTC*

SEBULEX with Protein (Westwood) — 224
Sulfur and salicylic acid *OTC*

SELSUN (Abbott) — 225
Selenium sulfide *Rx*

SELSUN BLUE (Ross) — 225
Selenium sulfide *OTC*

TEGRIN Medicated Shampoo (Block) — 226
Coal tar *OTC*

ZETAR (Dermik) — 227
Coal tar and parachlorometaxylenol *OTC*

ZINCON (Lederle) — 227
Pyrithione zinc *OTC*

COMPENDIUM OF DRUG THERAPY

Acne Preparations/Antidandruff Shampoos continued

Other Acne Preparations — 198

ERYMAX (Herbert) — 198
Erythromycin *Rx*

FOSTEX 5% Benzoyl Peroxide Gel (Westwood) — 198
Benzoyl peroxide *OTC*

FOSTEX Medicated Cleansing Bar and Cream (Westwood) — 198
Sulfur and salicylic acid *OTC*

FOSTEX 10% Benzoyl Peroxide Cleansing Bar and Wash (Westwood) — 198
Benzoyl peroxide *OTC*

FOSTEX 10% Benzoyl Peroxide Cream and Gel (Westwood) — 198
Benzoyl peroxide *OTC*

FOSTRIL (Westwood) — 198
Sulfur *OTC*

NEUTROGENA Acne-Drying Gel (Neutrogena) — 199
Witch hazel and isopropyl alcohol *OTC*

PERNOX Medicated Lathering Scrub Cleanser and Lotion (Westwood) — 199
Sulfur and salicylic acid *OTC*

TOPEX (Richardson-Vicks Health Care Products) — 199
Benzoyl peroxide *OTC*

T-STAT (Westwood) — 199
Erythromycin *Rx*

OTHER ACNE PREPARATIONS

DRUG	HOW SUPPLIED	USUAL DOSAGE[1]
ERYMAX (Herbert) Erythromycin *Rx*	Solution: 2% (4 fl oz)	**Adult:** apply lightly to affected area bid (morning and evening); wash and dry skin before each application
FOSTEX 5% Benzoyl Peroxide Gel (Westwood) Benzoyl peroxide *OTC*	Gel: 5% (1.5 oz)	**Adult:** after washing, rub into affected areas bid, avoiding contact with eyes, lips, and mouth; those living in dry climates or with fair skin should start with 1 daily application; to adjust degree of drying or peeling, increase or decrease frequency of use
FOSTEX Medicated Cleansing Bar and Cream (Westwood) Sulfur and salicylic acid *OTC*	Bar: 2% sulfur and 2% salicylic acid (3¾ oz) Cream: 2% sulfur and 2% salicylic acid (4 oz)	**Adult:** use instead of soap to wash face and other affected areas, followed by a thorough rinse, bid or tid, or according to desired degree of drying; for use as a shampoo: after wetting scalp and hair, apply cream liberally and massage into scalp, rinse, and repeat, using as often as needed
FOSTEX 10% Benzoyl Peroxide Cleansing Bar and Wash (Westwood) Benzoyl peroxide *OTC*	Bar: 10% (3¾ oz) Wash: 10% (5 fl oz)	**Adult:** use instead of soap to wash face and other affected areas for 1–2 min bid or tid, avoiding contact with eyes, lips, and mucous membranes; rinse well; to adjust degree of drying or peeling, increase or decrease frequency of use
FOSTEX 10% Benzoyl Peroxide Cream and Gel (Westwood) Benzoyl peroxide *OTC*	Cream: 10% (1.5 oz) Gel: 10% (1.5 oz)	**Adult:** after washing, rub into affected area bid, avoiding contact with eyes, lips, and mucous membranes; those living in dry climates or with fair skin should start with 1 daily application; to adjust degree of drying or peeling, increase or decrease frequency of use
FOSTRIL (Westwood) Sulfur *OTC*	Lotion: 2% (1 fl oz)	**Adult:** apply a thin film to affected area 1–2 times/day

[1] Where pediatric dosages are not given, consult manufacturer

continued

COMPENDIUM OF DRUG THERAPY

OTHER ACNE PREPARATIONS continued

DRUG	HOW SUPPLIED	USUAL DOSAGE[1]
NEUTROGENA Acne-Drying Gel (Neutrogena) Witch hazel and isopropyl alcohol *OTC*	**Gel:** (¾ oz)	**Adult:** after washing, apply a small amount of gel directly to affected areas with fingers or cotton as often as necessary, depending upon degree of drying desired
PERNOX Medicated Lathering Scrub Cleanser and Lotion (Westwood) Sulfur and salicylic acid *OTC*	**Cleanser:** 2% sulfur and 1.5% salicylic acid (2, 4 oz) *plain or lemon-scented* **Lotion:** 2% sulfur and 1.5% salicylic acid (5 fl oz)	**Adult:** use instead of soap to wash skin, applying with fingertips and massaging into skin up to 1 min, then rinse thoroughly, 1–2 times/day, or as needed
TOPEX (Richardson-Vicks Health Care Products) Benzoyl peroxide *OTC*	**Lotion:** 10% (1 fl oz)	**Adult:** following normal cleansing routine, for first 3 days, apply sparingly with fingers to an affected area; if no discomfort or reaction occurs, apply bid to areas where acne lesions normally appear, rubbing in lotion until it disappears; to adjust degree of drying or flaking, decrease frequency of use
T-STAT (Westwood) Erythromycin *Rx*	**Solution:** 2% (60 ml)	**Adult:** apply to affected area bid (morning and evening); wash and dry skin before each application

[1] Where pediatric dosages are not given, consult manufacturer

COMPENDIUM OF DRUG THERAPY

ACNE PREPARATIONS

ACCUTANE (isotretinoin) Roche   Rx
Capsules: 10, 20, 40 mg

INDICATIONS	**ORAL DOSAGE**
Severe cystic acne unresponsive to conventional therapy, including systemic antibiotics	**Adult:** 0.5-1 mg/kg/day to start; for acne that is very severe or that occurs mainly on the body, up to 2 mg/kg/day to start. Adjust dosage during therapy, as needed and tolerated (cheilitis and hypertriglyceridemia are usually dose-related). Give daily dose in 2 divided doses. Treatment should generally be continued for 15-20 wk; however, if the total cyst count has been reduced by more than 70% before the fifteenth week, therapy can be discontinued at that time. If cystic acne is severe or recurrent, a second course of therapy may be started 2 mo or more after the end of the first course.

CONTRAINDICATIONS

Pregnancy (see WARNINGS/PRECAUTIONS)	Sensitivity to parabens (used as preservatives in the formulation)

ADMINISTRATION/DOSAGE ADJUSTMENTS

Dosage individualization	Adjust dose after 2 or more weeks of therapy if clinical side effects appear (see ADVERSE REACTIONS) and/or the patient's response to treatment warrants an adjustment; inform patients that transient exacerbation of acne may occur, generally during the initial period of therapy
Reinitiation of therapy	After 2 mo off therapy, a second course may be given if warranted by the persistence of severe cystic acne

WARNINGS/PRECAUTIONS

Women of childbearing potential	To avoid major teratogenic effects (see USE IN PREGNANT AND NURSING WOMEN), test for pregnancy within 2 wk before the start of therapy and begin treatment on the second or third day of the next normal menstrual period. An effective form of contraception should be used for a period beginning at least 1 mo before the onset of therapy and continuing until 1 mo after the end of treatment. Patients should be fully informed of the serious risks associated with use of isotretinoin during pregnancy.
Ophthalmic and neurologic disorders	Pseudotumor cerebri and corneal opacities have been associated with use of isotretinoin. If visual disturbances occur, discontinue administration and perform an ophthalmological examination. Check for papilledema if patient experiences nausea, vomiting, or headache; if papilledema is detected, discontinue use and refer patient to a neurologist. Dry eyes and decreased night vision have occurred during treatment and, in rare instances, have persisted despite cessation of therapy. Caution patients that during and after treatment they may experience decreased tolerance to contact lenses.
Intestinal disorders	Inflammatory bowel disease, including regional ileitis, has been temporally associated with use of isotretinoin; if patient experiences abdominal pain, rectal bleeding, or severe diarrhea, discontinue administration immediately
Hypertriglyceridemia	May occur during therapy, especially in patients at risk because of diabetes mellitus, obesity, increased alcohol intake, or a family history of hypertriglyceridemia. Serum triglyceride levels exceeding 800 mg/dl have been associated with acute pancreatitis. Plasma triglycerides increase in approximately 25% of patients and cholesterol in about 7%, and a decrease in high-density lipoproteins occurs in approximately 15%; these changes are reversible upon discontinuation of therapy. Some patients have been able to continue on isotretinoin while reversing the hypertriglyceridemia by weight reduction, restriction of dietary fat and alcohol, and a decrease in dosage. Blood lipid determinations should be done before initiating isotretinoin therapy and repeated weekly or biweekly until the lipid response to the drug is established (this usually takes up to 4 wk). These tests should be obtained under fasting conditions; if alcohol has been consumed before the test, wait at least 36 h before drawing blood for the determination.
Vitamin supplementation	Caution patient to avoid using vitamin supplements containing vitamin A (see DRUG INTERACTIONS)
Exaggerated healing response	May occur, manifested by exuberant granulation tissue with crusting
Skeletal changes	Minimal skeletal hyperostosis has been detected during cystic acne therapy; treatment of keratinization disorders has resulted in a high incidence of skeletal hyperostosis and, in two children, premature closure of the epiphysis
Exacerbation of acne	Inform patients that transient exacerbation of acne may occur, especially during the initial period of treatment
Hyperglycemia	Elevation of fasting blood glucose level has been seen during therapy; periodically measure serum glucose level in known or suspected diabetics
Depression	This drug has caused depression in some patients
Thinning of hair	In rare cases, thinning of hair has persisted despite cessation of therapy

ACCUTANE

Increased CPK level	Elevation of the CPK level has occurred in some patients who were undergoing vigorous physical activity; the clinical significance of this reaction is not known
Carcinogenicity	An increased incidence of pheochromocytoma and adrenal medullary hyperplasia has been observed in Fischer 344 rats following more than 18 mo of treatment with isotretinoin. The clinical relevance of these findings is unclear, however, since this strain normally shows a high level of spontaneous pheochromocytoma, and the same dosages of isotretinoin decreased the incidence of hepatic adenomas and angiomas and leukemias in these animals.
Mutagenicity	No evidence of mutagenicity has been observed in Chinese hamster cells, the mouse micronucleus test, or in *Salmonella cerevisiae;* the Ames test produced negative results in one laboratory and a weakly positive effect (with one particular strain) in another laboratory
Effect on fertility	No adverse effects on gonadal function, fertility, conception rate, gestation, or parturition have been observed in male and female rats given 2, 8, and 32 mg/kg of isotretinoin daily. Although daily administration of 20 and 60 mg/kg to dogs for approximately 30 wk resulted in decreased spermatogenesis and testicular atrophy, human males treated with isotretinoin have shown no significant changes in sperm count or motility in the ejaculate.
Animal toxicity studies	Long-bone fractures have been observed in rats given 32 mg/kg/day for approximately 15 wk. Rats treated with 8 or 32 mg/kg/day for 18 mo or more exhibited an increase in the incidence of focal calcification, fibrosis and inflammation of the myocardium, calcification of the coronary, pulmonary, and mesenteric arteries, and metastatic calcification of the gastric mucosa. Focal endocardial and myocardial calcifications associated with coronary artery calcification have also been observed in two dogs after approximately 6–7 mo of treatment at 60–120 mg/kg/day. Chronic administration of 60 mg/kg/day has also produced corneal ulcers and opacities in dogs (patients treated with isotretinoin have also developed corneal opacities).

ADVERSE REACTIONS[1]

Frequent reactions (incidence $\geq$ 1%) are printed in *italics*

Dermatological	*Cheilitis ($>$ 90%); dry skin, skin fragility, and pruritus ($\leq$ 80%); rash and thinning of hair ($<$ 10%); peeling of palms and soles, skin infections, and increased susceptibility to sunburn (5%);* exuberant granulation tissue with crusting
Ophthalmic and neurological	*Conjunctivitis (38%),* pseudotumor cerebri, corneal opacities, dry eyes, diminished night vision, cataracts, visual disturbances
Hematological	*Increased erythrocyte sedimentation rate (40%), decreased RBC parameters and WBC counts and increased platelet counts (10–20%)*
Genitourinary	*WBC in urine (10–20%), microscopic or gross hematuria ($<$ 10%), nonspecific urogenital findings (5%)*
Gastrointestinal	*Nonspecific GI symptoms (5%),* inflammatory bowel disease
Other	*Dry nose, dry mouth, and epistaxis ($\leq$ 80%); reversible musculoskeletal symptoms (16%); fatigue and headache (5%),* skeletal hyperostosis, transient chest pain, depression

OVERDOSAGE

Signs and symptoms	Vomiting, facial flushing, cheilosis, abdominal pain, headache, dizziness, ataxia
Treatment	Symptoms quickly resolve without apparent residual effects

DRUG INTERACTIONS

Vitamin A	△ Risk of toxicity due to chemical similarity

ALTERED LABORATORY VALUES

Blood/serum values	△ Triglycerides △ Cholesterol ▽ High-density lipoprotein △ Alkaline phosphatase △ SGOT △ SGPT △ GGTP △ LDH △ Glucose (fasting) △ CPK △ Uric acid
Urinary values	+ Protein

USE IN CHILDREN

See INDICATIONS and ORAL DOSAGE

USE IN PREGNANT AND NURSING WOMEN

Pregnancy Category X: major fetal abnormalities, including hydrocephalus, microcephalus, abnormalities of the external ear (micropinna, small or absent external auditory canals), microphthalmia, and cardiovascular abnormalities have been associated with use of isotretinoin by pregnant women; do not administer to women who are or who plan to become pregnant (see precaution, above, concerning use in women of childbearing potential). Excretion in human milk is unknown; because of the potential for adverse effects, isotretinoin should not be given to nursing women.

---

[1] Other reactions for which a causal relationship has not been established include seizures, emotional instability, dizziness, nervousness, drowsiness, malaise, weakness, insomnia, lethargy, paresthesias, hypopigmentation, hyperpigmentation, urticaria, bruising, disseminated herpes simplex, edema, hair problems (other than thinning), hirsutism, respiratory infections, weight loss, erythema nodosum, paronychia, nail dystrophy, bleeding and inflammation of gums, abnormal menses, optic neuritis, and Wegener's granulomatosis. Eruptive xanthomas have occurred in an obese male patient with Darier's disease.

ACNE PREPARATIONS

ACHROMYCIN (tetracycline hydrochloride) Lederle   Rx
Vials: 100, 250 mg (for IM use); 250, 500 mg (for IV use)

ACHROMYCIN V (tetracycline hydrochloride) Lederle   Rx
Capsules: 250, 500 mg   **Suspension (per 5 ml):** 125 mg (2, 16 fl oz) *cherry flavored*

INDICATIONS

Gram-negative bacterial infections caused by *Hemophilus ducreyi* (chancroid), *Calymmatobacterium granulomatis* (granuloma inguinale), *Yersinia pestis* (plague), *Francisella tularensis* (tularemia), *Bartonella bacilliformis* (bartonellosis), *Bacteroides, Vibrio cholerae* (cholera), and *Campylobacter fetus* (vibriosis), as well as susceptible strains of *Escherichia coli, Enterobacter aerogenes, Shigella, Acinetobacter, Hemophilus influenzae* (respiratory tract infections only), and *Klebsiella* (respiratory and urinary tract infections only)

Mycoplasmal pneumonia (primary atypical pneumonia)

Streptococcal infections caused by susceptible strains[1]

Skin and soft tissue infections caused by susceptible strains of *Staphylococcus aureus*[2]

Rickettsial infections

Psittacosis (ornithosis)

Lymphogranuloma venereum, trachoma, and (when given orally) **inclusion conjunctivitis** and uncomplicated adult **urethral, endocervical, and rectal infections** caused by *Chlamydia trachomatis*

Relapsing fever

As an adjunct to amebicides for **acute intestinal amebiasis**

As an alternative to penicillin for **gonococcal and clostridial infections, listeriosis, yaws, anthrax, Vincent's infection, actinomycosis,** and (when given IV) **meningococcal infections**

Severe acne (oral therapy only)

Syphilis in cases where penicillin is contraindicated

Brucellosis

ORAL DOSAGE

Adult: 1–2 g/day, given in 2 or 4 equally divided doses, depending on the severity of the infection; for acute gonococcal infections, 1.5 g to start, followed by 500 mg q6h for 4 days, for a total of 9 g; for chlamydial urethral, endocervical, and rectal infections, 500 mg qid for at least 7 days

Child (> 8 yr): 25–50 mg/kg/day, given in 2 or 4 equally divided doses

Adult: 30–40 g total, given in equally divided doses over a period of 10–15 days

Adult: 500 mg qid for 3 wk (with 1 g streptomycin IM bid 1st wk and once daily 2nd wk)

PARENTERAL DOSAGE

Adult: 250 mg, given in a single IM dose q24h, or 300 mg/day, given in 2 or 3 divided IM doses q8–12h; if rapid, high blood levels are needed, give 250–500 mg IV q12h, or up to 500 mg IV q6h if necessary

Child (> 8 yr): 15–25 mg/kg/day, up to 250 mg/day, given in a single daily IM dose or 2 or 3 divided IM doses q8–12h; if rapid, high blood levels are needed, give 10–20 mg/kg/day IV, depending on the severity of the infection (usual dosage: 6 mg/kg bid)

CONTRAINDICATIONS
Hypersensitivity to tetracyclines

ADMINISTRATION/DOSAGE ADJUSTMENTS

Duration of treatment — Unless otherwise indicated, continue treatment for at least 24–48 h after symptoms and fever have subsided; infections caused by Group A beta-hemolytic streptococci should be treated for at least 10 days. If patient is started on parenteral therapy, institute oral therapy as soon as possible.

Intramuscular administration — Reserve for situations in which oral therapy is not feasible. Add 2 ml of sterile water for injection or sodium chloride injection to 100- or 250-mg vial, withdraw required dose, and inject deeply into a large muscle mass, such as the gluteus. Use the reconstituted solution within 24 h. IM administration produces lower blood levels than oral administration at recommended dosages.

Intravenous administration — Use only when rapidly attained, high blood levels are needed and oral therapy is not adequate or tolerated. To reconstitute the solution, add 5 ml of sterile water for injection to the 250-mg vial or 10 ml to the 500-mg vial; use within 12 h. Immediately before administration, dilute the solution to a final volume of 100–1,000 ml with 5% dextrose injection USP, sodium chloride injection USP (alone or with 5% dextrose), or 5% protein hydrolysate (low sodium) injection USP (alone, with 5% dextrose, or with 10% invert sugar). Solutions containing calcium generally should be avoided, unless necessary, as they tend to precipitate tetracycline; Ringer's and lactated Ringer's injection USP may be used with caution, however, because their calcium ion content does not normally precipitate tetracycline at acid pH. Prolonged IV administration may cause thrombophlebitis. Avoid rapid administration.

ACHROMYCIN

Timing of oral administration	Food and some dairy products interfere with absorption; give oral forms 1 h before or 2 h after meals

WARNINGS/PRECAUTIONS

Patients with renal impairment	Usual doses may lead to excessive drug accumulation and possible hepatic toxicity. If impairment is significant, azotemia, hyperphosphatemia, and acidosis may occur due to antianabolic action of drug. Reduce dosage by lowering individual doses and/or lengthening interval between doses, monitor kidney and liver function both before and during therapy, and follow serum tetracycline levels periodically (particularly if therapy is prolonged).
Pregnant and postpartum patients with pyelonephritis	Potentially fatal hepatic failure may occur with parenteral administration; do not allow serum level to exceed 15 µg/ml, monitor liver function frequently, and avoid concomitant use of other potentially hepatotoxic drugs
Superinfection	Overgrowth of nonsusceptible organisms, including fungi, may occur
Suspected syphilitic lesions	If syphilis is suspected, perform a dark-field examination before instituting therapy and monthly serology tests for at least 4 mo thereafter
Long-term therapy	Perform hemapoietic, renal, and hepatic studies periodically
Photosensitivity (exaggerated sunburn)	May occur; caution patients likely to be exposed to direct sunlight or UV light and discontinue use of tetracycline at first sign of skin erythema

ADVERSE REACTIONS

Gastrointestinal	Anorexia, nausea, vomiting, diarrhea, glossitis, dysphagia, enterocolitis, inflammatory lesions (with monilial overgrowth) in the anogenital region
Dermatological	Maculopapular and erythematous rashes, exfoliative dermatitis (rare), photosensitivity
Hypersensitivity	Urticaria, angioneurotic edema, anaphylaxis, anaphylactoid purpura, pericarditis, exacerbation of systemic lupus erythematosus
Hematological	Hemolytic anemia, thrombocytopenia, neutropenia, eosinophilia
Other	Microscopic discoloration of thyroid glands, bulging fontanels in infants, local irritation after IM injection

OVERDOSAGE

Signs and symptoms	See ADVERSE REACTIONS
Treatment	Discontinue medication, treat symptomatically, and institute supportive measures, as required

DRUG INTERACTIONS

Oral anticoagulants	△ Prothrombin time
Penicillin	▽ Bactericidal activity of penicillin; avoid concomitant use
Antacids, sodium bicarbonate, iron supplements	▽ Absorption of oral tetracycline; antacids containing aluminum, calcium, or magnesium should not be administered concomitantly
Methoxyflurane	△ Risk of nephrotoxicity

ALTERED LABORATORY VALUES

Blood/serum values	△ Alkaline phosphatase △ BUN △ Amylase △ Bilirubin △ SGOT △ SGPT ▽ Prothrombin activity
Urinary values	△ Catecholamines (with Hingerty fluorometric method)

USE IN CHILDREN

Not recommended for use during infancy through 8 yr of age unless other drugs are not likely to be effective or are contraindicated; use in this age group may cause permanent discoloration of teeth or enamel hypoplasia. A reversible decrease in fibula growth rate has been observed in premature infants given oral tetracycline (100 mg/kg/day).

USE IN PREGNANT AND NURSING WOMEN

Use during latter half of pregnancy (fetal tooth development) may cause permanent discoloration of teeth or enamel hypoplasia. Animal studies indicate that tetracyclines cross the placental barrier, are found in fetal tissues, and can cause both embryotoxicity and fetal toxicity, including retardation of skeletal development. Tetracyclines are excreted in breast milk; if drug is essential, patient should not nurse.

---

[1] Tetracyclines should not be used for streptococcal disease unless bacterial susceptibility has been demonstrated
[2] Tetracyclines are not the drug of choice for treating any staphylococcal infection

ACNE PREPARATIONS

A/T/S (erythromycin) Hoechst-Roussel   Rx

Solution: 2% (60 ml)

INDICATIONS	TOPICAL DOSAGE
Acne vulgaris	**Adult:** apply with applicator or pad to affected areas bid after areas have been washed thoroughly with soap and warm water, rinsed well, and patted dry

CONTRAINDICATIONS

Hypersensitivity to any component

WARNINGS/PRECAUTIONS

Sensitive surfaces	Avoid contact with eyes, nose, mouth, and other mucous membranes
Superinfection	Overgrowth of nonsusceptible organisms may occur; if reaction occurs, discontinue administration
Carcinogenicity, mutagenicity, effect on fertility	No studies have been done to evaluate the carcinogenic or mutagenic potential of this preparation or its effect on fertility

ADVERSE REACTIONS

Local	Dryness, tenderness, pruritus, desquamation, erythema, oiliness, burning, ocular irritation
Systemic	Generalized urticaria (one case)

DRUG INTERACTIONS

Other topical acne preparations, especially peeling, desquamating, and abrasive agents	△ Irritation; exercise caution during concomitant therapy

---

USE IN CHILDREN

Not indicated for use in children

USE IN PREGNANT AND NURSING WOMEN

Pregnancy Category C: reproduction studies have not been done; it is not known whether erythromycin can cause harm to the fetus or affect reproductive capacity. Use during pregnancy only when clearly needed. Erythromycin is excreted in human milk; use with caution in nursing mothers.

VEHICLE/BASE
Solution: 66% alcohol, propylene glycol, and citric acid

ACNE PREPARATIONS

BENZAC (benzoyl peroxide) Owen   Rx

Gel (alcohol base): 5% (60 g) (benzac 5), 10% (60 g) (benzac 10)

INDICATIONS	TOPICAL DOSAGE
Acne vulgaris (adjunctive therapy)	**Adult:** apply 1–2 times/day after washing with a mild cleanser and water; modify dosage schedule to obtain desired degree of drying and peeling

BENZAC W (benzoyl peroxide) Owen   Rx

Gel (water base): 2.5% (60, 90 g) (benzac w 2½), 5% (60, 90 g) (benzac w 5), 10% (60, 90 g) (benzac w 10)

INDICATIONS	TOPICAL DOSAGE
Acne vulgaris (adjunctive therapy)	**Adult:** apply 1–2 times/day after washing with a mild cleanser and water; modify dosage schedule to obtain desired degree of drying and peeling

BENZAC W Wash (benzoyl peroxide) Owen   Rx

Solution: 5% (4, 8 fl oz) (benzac w WASH 5), 10% (8 fl oz) (benzac w WASH 10)

INDICATIONS	TOPICAL DOSAGE
Mild to moderate acne vulgaris Severe, complicated acne vulgaris, as an adjunct to other treatment regimens	**Adult:** after wetting area of application, apply to hands and wash affected area 1–2 times/day; rinse with water and dry; modify dosage schedule to obtain desired degree of drying and peeling

BENZAC/BENZAC W ■ BENZAGEL

CONTRAINDICATIONS

Hypersensitivity to any component

WARNINGS/PRECAUTIONS

Sensitive surfaces	Contact with eyes, eyelids, lips, and mucous membranes should be avoided; if accidental contact occurs, rinse with water
Bleaching	May occur; avoid contact with hair and colored fabrics
Severe irritation	May occur; discontinue use and institute appropriate therapy
Carcinogenicity, mutagenicity, and effect on fertility	There is no evidence that benzoyl peroxide is carcinogenic or mutagenic or that it impairs fertility

ADVERSE REACTIONS

Local	Allergic contact dermatitis

USE IN CHILDREN

Safety and effectiveness for use in children have not been established

USE IN PREGNANT AND NURSING WOMEN

Pregnancy Category C: use during pregnancy only if clearly needed. It is not known whether this drug causes fetal harm or teratogenicity, nor are data available on the effect of benzoyl peroxide on the later growth, development, and functional maturation of the unborn child. Excretion of this drug in breast milk is unknown; use with caution in nursing mothers.

VEHICLE/BASE
Benzac: 12% alcohol, 6% polyoxyethylene lauryl ether, dimethicone, carbomer-940, fragrance, and purified water; may also contain sodium hydroxide and/or citric acid to adjust pH
Benzac W: dioctyl sodium sulfosuccinate, edetate disodium, poloxamer 182, carbomer-940, propylene glycol, silicon dioxide, and purified water; may also contain sodium hydroxide and/or citric acid to adjust pH
Benzac W Wash solution: sodium C14-16 olefin sulfonate, carbomer-940, and purified water

---

ACNE PREPARATIONS

BENZAGEL (benzoyl peroxide) Dermik Rx

Gel: 5% (1½, 3 oz) (5 Benzagel), 10% (1½, 3 oz) (10 Benzagel)

INDICATIONS

Mild to moderate acne, alone or as an adjunct to other treatment regimens, including retinoic acid products, systemic antibiotics, and sulfur- and salicylic acid-containing preparations

TOPICAL DOSAGE

Adult: after washing and drying affected areas, apply sparingly once or more daily; if patient is very fair, start with a single application at bedtime

CONTRAINDICATIONS

Hypersensitivity to benzoyl peroxide or any other component

WARNINGS/PRECAUTIONS

Sensitive surfaces	Avoid contact with eyes and mucosae
Local reactions	If itching, redness, burning, swelling, or undue dryness occurs, discontinue use
Bleaching	May occur; avoid contact with colored fabrics

ADVERSE REACTIONS

Local	Irritation, contact dermatitis

USE IN CHILDREN

Safety and effectiveness have not been established for use in children under 12 yr of age

USE IN PREGNANT AND NURSING WOMEN

Pregnancy Category C: use during pregnancy only if clearly needed. No animal reproductive studies have been done, nor is it known whether administration to pregnant women can cause fetal harm or whether this drug can affect reproductive capacity. It is not known whether benzoyl peroxide is excreted in human milk; use with caution in nursing mothers.

VEHICLE/BASE
Gel: purified water, carbomer 940, 14% alcohol, sodium hydroxide, dioctyl sodium sulfosuccinate, alkyl polyglycol ether, and fragrance

COMPENDIUM OF DRUG THERAPY

ACNE PREPARATIONS

BENZAMYCIN (erythromycin and benzoyl peroxide) Dermik Rx

Gel: 3% erythromycin and 5% benzoyl peroxide (23.3 g)

INDICATIONS	**TOPICAL DOSAGE**
Acne vulgaris	**Adult:** after skin has been thoroughly washed, rinsed with warm water, and patted dry, apply gel to affected area; administer bid, morning and evening

CONTRAINDICATIONS

Hypersensitivity to erythromycin, benzoyl peroxide, or any other component

ADMINISTRATION/DOSAGE ADJUSTMENTS

Preparation and storage	Add 3 ml of ethanol to the vial containing erythromycin powder and shake well; then, add this solution to the supplied benzoyl peroxide gel and stir until the preparation appears homogeneous (approximately 1–1½ min). Refrigerate Benzamycin gel after it has been prepared; use within 3 mo.

WARNINGS/PRECAUTIONS

Sensitive surfaces	Avoid contact with eyes and other mucous membranes
Local irritation	If severe irritation or dryness develops, discontinue use and institute appropriate therapy
Superinfection	Overgrowth of nonsusceptible organisms may occur; if reaction is seen, discontinue use and take appropriate measures
Bleaching	This preparation may bleach hair or colored fabric
Carcinogenicity, effect on fertility	No long-term studies have been done to evaluate the carcinogenic potential of this preparation or its effect on fertility

ADVERSE REACTIONS The most frequent reaction is italicized

Hypersensitivity	*Dryness (3%)*, erythema, pruritus, urticaria

DRUG INTERACTIONS

Other topical acne preparations	⇧ Irritation; exercise caution during concomitant therapy

---

USE IN CHILDREN

Safety and effectiveness for use in children under 12 yr of age have not been established

USE IN PREGNANT AND NURSING WOMEN

Pregnancy Category C: no reproduction studies have been done with this preparation; it is not known whether it can cause harm to the fetus or affect reproductive capacity. Use during pregnancy only if clearly needed. It is also not known whether this preparation is excreted in human milk; use with caution in nursing mothers.

VEHICLE/BASE

Gel: carbomer 940, 22% alcohol, sodium hydroxide, docusate sodium, fragrance, and purified water

---

ACNE PREPARATIONS

CLEARASIL (benzoyl peroxide) Richardson-Vicks Personal Care Products OTC

Cream: 10% (0.65, 1 oz) clear, tinted **Lotion:** 10% (1 fl oz)

INDICATIONS	**TOPICAL DOSAGE**
Acne vulgaris	**Adult and child:** after thoroughly washing affected area, apply cream or lotion; administer up to twice daily

CONTRAINDICATIONS

Sensitivity to benzoyl peroxide

ADMINISTRATION/DOSAGE ADJUSTMENTS

Sensitivity test	Apply cream or lotion sparingly to a small affected area; if no discomfort occurs, preparation may be used

WARNINGS/PRECAUTIONS

Local reactions	Excessive dryness or peeling may occur especially in patients with unusually dry, sensitive, or maturing skin. If itching, redness, burning, swelling, or undue dryness occurs, discontinue use or reduce dosage. Patients should report persistent reactions.

Sensitive membranes	Avoid contact with eyes, lips, mouth, and sensitive areas of the neck
Bleaching	Benzoyl peroxide may bleach hair and dyed fabrics

DRUG INTERACTIONS

Other topical acne preparations	⇧ Irritation and dryness

USE IN CHILDREN	USE IN PREGNANT AND NURSING WOMEN
See INDICATIONS and TOPICAL DOSAGE	Consult manufacturer

VEHICLE/BASE
Cream (clear): propylene glycol, aluminum hydroxide, bentonite, glyceryl stearate SE, isopropyl myristate, cellulose gum, dimethicone, PEG-12, potassium carbomer-940, methylparaben, propylparaben, and water
Cream (tinted): propylene glycol, aluminum hydroxide, bentonite, glyceryl stearate SE, isopropyl myristate, cellulose gum, dimethicone, PEG-12, potassium carbomer-940, methylparaben, propylparaben, titanium dioxide, iron oxides, and water
Lotion: aluminum hydroxide, isopropyl stearate, PEG-100 stearate, glyceryl stearate, cetyl alcohol, glycereth-26, isocetyl stearate, glycerin, dimethicone copolyol, sodium citrate, citric acid, methylparaben, propylparaben, fragrance, and water

---

ACNE PREPARATIONS

CLEOCIN T (clindamycin phosphate) Upjohn   Rx

Solution: clindamycin phosphate equivalent to 10 mg/ml clindamycin (30, 60, 473 ml)

INDICATIONS	TOPICAL DOSAGE
Acne vulgaris[1]	**Adult:** apply a thin film to affected areas bid

CONTRAINDICATIONS

Hypersensitivity to clindamycin or lincomycin	History of regional enteritis or ulcerative colitis	History of antibiotic-associated colitis

WARNINGS/PRECAUTIONS

Drug-induced colitis (including pseudomembranous colitis)	Has been reported with use of topical clindamycin (severe colitis, followed by death, has been associated with systemic use); symptoms can occur within a few days, weeks, or months after start of clindamycin therapy, or up to several weeks after cessation of therapy, and usually consist of severe persistent diarrhea, severe abdominal cramps, and possibly, the passage of blood and mucus. If significant diarrhea occurs, discontinue use; if the diarrhea is severe, consider performing a large bowel endoscopic examination, which may reveal pseudomembranous colitis. Mild cases of colitis may respond to withdrawal of the drug alone. Moderate to severe cases should be managed by fluid and electrolyte replacement and protein supplementation, as indicated. Cholestyramine and colestipol resins have been shown to bind the toxin in vitro. Systemic corticosteroids and corticosteroid retention enemas may be helpful. For pseudomembranous colitis produced by *Clostridium difficile,* administer vancomycin, 0.5–2 g/day orally in 3–4 divided doses for 7–10 days. (If both vancomycin and a resin are to be administered concurrently, it may be advisable to separate the time of administration of each drug.) Antiperistaltic agents, such as opiates and diphenoxylate with atropine, may prolong or worsen the condition.
Contact with eyes, abraded skin, or mucous membranes	Will cause burning and irritation, due to alcohol base; bathe with large amounts of cool tap water
Atopic patients	Use with caution
Unpleasant taste	Advise patients to exercise caution when applying clindamycin around the mouth

ADVERSE REACTIONS

The most frequent reaction is italicized

Gastrointestinal	Diarrhea, bloody diarrhea, colitis (including pseudomembranous colitis), abdominal pain, other GI disturbances
Local	*Dryness,* contact dermatitis, oiliness, sensitization, irritation
Other	Stinging of the eyes, gram-negative folliculitis

DRUG INTERACTIONS

Neuromuscular blocking agents	⇧ Neuromuscular blockade
Chloramphenicol, erythromycin	⇩ Pharmacologic effects of clindamycin

ALTERED LABORATORY VALUES

No clinically significant alterations in blood/serum or urinary values occur at therapeutic dosages

USE IN CHILDREN
Consult manufacturer

USE IN PREGNANT AND NURSING WOMEN
Pregnancy Category B: use during pregnancy only if clearly indicated. Reproductive studies in animals have shown no evidence of fetal harm or impaired fertility. No adequate, well-controlled studies have been done in pregnant women. Whether topical clindamycin is excreted in human milk is unknown; oral and parenteral clindamycin do appear in breast milk. As a rule, nursing should not be undertaken during therapy.

VEHICLE/BASE
Solution: 50% isopropyl alcohol, propylene glycol, and water

[1] In view of the potential for diarrhea, bloody diarrhea, and pseudomembranous colitis, the physician should consider whether other agents are more appropriate

---

ACNE PREPARATIONS

CUTICURA Acne Cream (benzoyl peroxide) Jeffrey Martin — OTC
Cream: 5% (1 oz)

INDICATIONS	TOPICAL DOSAGE
Acne vulgaris	**Adult:** apply a thin layer to affected areas after thorough washing, once daily to start, then bid or tid

CONTRAINDICATIONS	
Extreme skin sensitivity	Hypersensitivity to benzoyl peroxide

CUTICURA Medicated Soap (triclocarban) Jeffrey Martin — OTC
Soap: 1% (3.25, 5 oz bars)

INDICATIONS	TOPICAL DOSAGE
Unwanted oil, dirt, makeup, and impurities	**Adult:** work up lather with warm water and apply to affected areas at least bid; rinse thoroughly with cool water
Excess oil	**Infant ($\geq$ 6 mo) and child:** same as adult

WARNINGS/PRECAUTIONS

Skin irritation	If irritation or excessive dryness and/or peeling occurs with use of the cream, reduce frequency of application or amount used per application; discontinue use if excessive itching, redness, burning, or swelling occurs
Sensitive surfaces	Avoid contact of cream with eyes, lips, and other mucous membranes
Bleaching	May occur; avoid contact with hair or colored or dyed fabrics
Concomitant use of cream with other medications	Other topical acne preparations should not be used at the same time as the cream

ADVERSE REACTIONS

Local	Irritation, dryness, peeling, itching, redness, burning, swelling (with cream)

USE IN CHILDREN
Use according to medical judgment; do not use soap in infants under 6 mo of age

USE IN PREGNANT AND NURSING WOMEN
Consult manufacturer

VEHICLE/BASE
Cream: water, stearyl alcohol, PEG-40 stearate, diisopropyl adipate, titanium dioxide, bentonite, phenoxyethanol, PPG-9-buteth-12, dimethicone, SD-40 alcohol, allantoin, iron oxides, and fragrance
Soap: sodium tallowate, sodium cocoate, water, glycerin, fragrance, petrolatum, mineral oil, sodium chloride, magnesium silicate, tetrasodium EDTA, sodium bicarbonate, ultramarine blue, and iron oxides

ACNE PREPARATIONS

DESQUAM-X (benzoyl peroxide) Westwood — Rx

Gel: 2.5% (1.5 oz) (Desquam-X 2.5 Gel); 5% (1.5, 3 oz) (Desquam-X 5 Gel); 10% (1.5, 3 oz) (Desquam-X 10 Gel)

INDICATIONS	TOPICAL DOSAGE
Mild to moderate acne vulgaris **Severe acne vulgaris,** as an adjunct to other treatment regimens, including antibiotics, retinoic acid products, and sulfur/salicylic acid-containing preparations	**Adult:** rub gently into affected areas 1–2 times/day after washing; modify dosage schedule or drug concentration to obtain desired degree of drying and peeling. If patient is fair skinned or atmospheric conditions are very dry, apply once daily to start.

DESQUAM-X Wash (benzoyl peroxide) Westwood — Rx

Solution: 5% (5 fl oz) (Desquam-X 5 Wash); 10% (5 fl oz) (Desquam-X 10 Wash)

INDICATIONS	TOPICAL DOSAGE
Same as Desquam-X	**Adult:** after wetting skin areas to be treated, apply solution, lather, rinse thoroughly, and pat dry 1–2 times/day; modify dosage schedule or drug concentration to obtain desired degree of drying and peeling

CONTRAINDICATIONS

Sensitivity to any component

WARNINGS/PRECAUTIONS

Sensitive surfaces	Avoid contact with eyes or mucous membranes
Bleaching	May occur; avoid contact with hair or colored fabrics
Sensitivity reactions	May occur in patients sensitive to benzoic acid derivatives (including certain topical anesthetics) and cinnamon
Concomitant use of PABA-containing sunscreens	May result in transient skin discoloration
Excessive scaling, erythema, or edema	May occur; discontinue use and apply emollients, cool compresses, and/or topical corticosteroids to hasten resolution; if excessive use and not allergenicity is suspected, reinstitute therapy at a reduced dosage after signs and symptoms subside
Carcinogenicity, mutagenicity, effect on fertility	Benzoyl peroxide is not considered to be a carcinogen, even though one study in mice who were highly susceptible to cancer has shown evidence of tumor promotion. Mutagenicity has not been observed in the Ames test or other assays; the dominant lethal mutation test showed no effect on spermatogenesis in mice.

ADVERSE REACTIONS

Frequent reactions (incidence $\geq$ 1%) are printed in *italics*

Local	*Excessive drying, manifested by marked peeling, erythema, and possibly edema (4%);* allergic contact sensitization

USE IN CHILDREN

Safety and effectiveness have not been established for use in children under 12 yr of age

USE IN PREGNANT AND NURSING WOMEN

Pregnancy Category C: use during pregnancy only when clearly needed. Animal reproductive studies have not been done. It is not known whether fetal harm can occur when administered to pregnant women. Excretion of this drug in human milk is unknown; use with caution in nursing mothers.

VEHICLE/BASE
Gel: carbomer 940, diisopropanolamine, disodium edetate, 6% laureth-4, and water
Solution: sodium octoxynol-3 sulfonate, dioctyl sodium sulfosuccinate, sodium lauryl sulfoacetate, magnesium aluminum silicate, methylcellulose, EDTA, and water

---

ACNE PREPARATIONS

ERYCETTE (erythromycin) Ortho — Rx

Solution: 2%

INDICATIONS	TOPICAL DOSAGE
Acne vulgaris	**Adult:** after thorough washing with soap and water and patting dry, rub 1 or more saturated swabs, as needed, over affected area; administer bid

ERYCETTE ■ ERYDERM

CONTRAINDICATIONS
Hypersensitivity to any component

WARNINGS/PRECAUTIONS
Sensitive surfaces	Avoid contact with the eyes, nose, mouth, and other mucous membranes
Superinfection	Overgrowth of nonsusceptible organisms may occur; if reaction is seen, discontinue use and take appropriate measures

ADVERSE REACTIONS
Local	Dryness, tenderness, pruritus, desquamation, erythema, oiliness, burning, ocular irritation
Systemic	Generalized urticaria (one case)

DRUG INTERACTIONS
Other topical acne preparations	⚠ Irritation; exercise caution during concomitant therapy

USE IN CHILDREN
Consult manufacturer

USE IN PREGNANT AND NURSING WOMEN
Safety for use in pregnant or nursing women has not been established

VEHICLE/BASE
Solution: 66% alcohol, propylene glycol, and citric acid

ACNE PREPARATIONS

ERYDERM (erythromycin) Abbott   Rx
Solution: 2% (60 ml)

INDICATIONS
Acne vulgaris

TOPICAL DOSAGE
Adult: apply lightly with applicator or pad to affected areas bid, after thorough washing with soap and water; if the applicator is used, apply with a dabbing action

CONTRAINDICATIONS
Hypersensitivity to any component

WARNINGS/PRECAUTIONS
Sensitive surfaces	Avoid contact of solution with eyes and mucous membranes, including those of the nose and mouth
Staining of fabrics	May occur; avoid contact of solution with clothing or furniture
Concomitant topical acne therapy	Use with caution, since a cumulative irritant effect may occur, especially if peeling, desquamating, or abrasive agents are used concurrently
Superinfection	Overgrowth of antibiotic-resistant organisms may occur; discontinue administration and institute appropriate measures

ADVERSE REACTIONS
Local	Dryness, pruritus, erythema, desquamation, burning sensation

USE IN CHILDREN
Consult manufacturer

USE IN PREGNANT AND NURSING WOMEN
Safety for use during pregnancy or by nursing mothers has not been established

VEHICLE/BASE
Solution: polyethylene glycol, acetone, and 77% alcohol

ACNE PREPARATIONS

KOMED (sodium thiosulfate, salicylic acid, and isopropyl alcohol) Barnes-Hind — OTC

Lotion: 8% sodium thiosulfate, 2% salicylic acid, and 25% isopropyl alcohol (52.5 ml)

INDICATIONS	TOPICAL DOSAGE
Acne vulgaris associated with oily skin	**Adult:** apply a thin film 2 or more times daily, after washing affected areas thoroughly **Child:** use according to medical judgment

CONTRAINDICATIONS

Hypersensitivity to any component	Ophthalmic use

WARNINGS/PRECAUTIONS

Persistent acne, skin irritation	Package label advises patient to discontinue use and consult a physician if acne persists or skin irritation occurs
Sensitive surfaces	Do not use on or near the eyes

ADVERSE REACTIONS

Local	Irritation

USE IN CHILDREN	USE IN PREGNANT AND NURSING WOMEN
Use according to medical judgment	Consult manufacturer

VEHICLE/BASE
Lotion (greaseless, vanishing): colloidal alumina, menthol, camphor, edetate disodium, and purified water

---

ACNE PREPARATIONS

LOROXIDE (benzoyl peroxide) Dermik — OTC

Lotion: 5.5% (25 g) *flesh tinted*

VANOXIDE (benzoyl peroxide) Dermik — OTC

Lotion: 5% (25, 50 g) *clear*

INDICATIONS	TOPICAL DOSAGE
Acne vulgaris and oily skin	**Adult:** apply a small amount to affected areas, massaging lightly, 1–2 times/day or according to medical judgment **Child:** use according to medical judgment

CONTRAINDICATIONS

Hypersensitivity to benzoyl peroxide or any other component

ADMINISTRATION/DOSAGE ADJUSTMENTS

Excessive redness or peeling	May be controlled by reducing amount and frequency of application

WARNINGS/PRECAUTIONS

Sensitive surfaces	Avoid contact with eyes; apply with caution on neck and other sensitive areas
Transient stinging or burning sensation	May occur upon initial application but invariably disappears with continued use
Local irritation and sensitization	May occur during long-term therapy; observe patient carefully. If irritation or sensitivity occurs, discontinue use. Harsh, abrasive cleansers should not be used simultaneously with these lotions.
UV irradiation	Reduce exposure to ultraviolet or cold quartz light, due to keratolytic and drying effect
Bleaching	May occur; avoid contact with colored or dyed fabrics
Addition of other substances	Advise patient not to add any other medicaments or substances to these products unless specifically directed to do so

ADVERSE REACTIONS

Local	Erythema, peeling, allergic reactions

LOROXIDE/VANOXIDE ■ MECLAN

USE IN CHILDREN	USE IN PREGNANT AND NURSING WOMEN
Use according to medical judgment	Consult manufacturer

VEHICLE/BASE

Loroxide Lotion (water-washable, flesh-tinted): purified water, propylene glycol, hydroxyethylcellulose, caramel color, cholesterol-sterol, cetyl alcohol, propylene glycol monostearate, polysorbate 20, lanolin alcohol, propylparaben, decyl oleate, stearyl heptanoate, antioxidants, vegetable oil, methylparaben, tetrasodium EDTA, buffers, cyclohexanediamine tetraacetic acid, calcium phosphate, silicone emulsion, silica, kaolin, talc, and titanium dioxide

Vanoxide Lotion (water-washable, clear): purified water, propylene glycol, hydroxyethylcellulose, FD&C color, cholesterol-sterol, cetyl alcohol, propylene glycol monostearate, polysorbate 20, lanolin alcohol, propylparaben, decyl oleate, stearyl heptanoate, antioxidants, vegetable oil, methylparaben, tetrasodium EDTA, buffers, cyclohexanediamine tetraacetic acid, calcium phosphate, silicone emulsion, and silica

ACNE PREPARATIONS

MECLAN (meclocycline sulfosalicylate) Ortho   Rx

Cream: 1% (20, 45 g)

INDICATIONS	TOPICAL DOSAGE
Acne vulgaris	**Adult:** apply to affected areas bid (AM and PM); less frequent application may be needed, depending upon patient response

CONTRAINDICATIONS

Hypersensitivity to tetracyclines or any other component

WARNINGS/PRECAUTIONS

Hepatic or renal dysfunction	Administer with caution; percutaneous absorption may result from prolonged use
Sensitive surfaces	Avoid contact with eyes, nose, and mouth
Sensitivity to formaldehyde	Use with caution
Staining of fabrics	May result from excessive use

ADVERSE REACTIONS

Local	Skin irritation, acute contact dermatitis (one case), temporary follicular staining (with excessive application)

USE IN CHILDREN	USE IN PREGNANT AND NURSING WOMEN
Not indicated for use in children under 12 yr of age	Pregnancy Category B: use during pregnancy only if clearly needed. Reproductive studies in rats and rabbits at oral dosages of up to 10 g/day of meclocycline have shown no evidence of impaired fertility or fetal harm; topical meclocycline caused a slight delay in ossification in rabbits. No adequate, well-controlled studies have been done in pregnant women. It is not known whether topical meclocycline is excreted in human milk; use with caution in nursing mothers.

VEHICLE/BASE

Cream (aqueous): glyceryl stearate, propylene glycol stearate, caprylic/capric triglyceride, paraffin, trihydroxystearin, polysorbate 40, sorbitol solution, propyl gallate, sorbic acid, sodium formaldehyde sulfoxylate, perfume, and water

ACNE PREPARATIONS

MINOCIN (minocycline hydrochloride) Lederle   Rx

Capsules: minocycline hydrochloride equivalent to 50 and 100 mg minocycline   **Tablets:** minocycline hydrochloride equivalent to 50 and 100 mg minocycline   **Suspension (per 5 ml):** minocycline hydrochloride equivalent to 50 mg minocycline[1] (2 fl oz) custard-flavored   **Vials:** 100 mg

INDICATIONS

Gram-negative bacterial infections caused by *Hemophilus ducreyi* (chancroid), *Calymmatobacterium granulomatis* (granuloma inguinale), *Yersinia pestis* (plague), *Francisella tularensis* (tularemia), *Bartonella bacilliformis* (bartonellosis), *Bacteroides, Brucella* (when combined with streptomycin), *Vibrio cholerae* (cholera), and *Campylobacter fetus* (vibriosis), as well as susceptible strains of *Escherichia coli, Enterobacter aerogenes, Shigella, Acinetobacter, Hemophilus influenzae* (respiratory tract infections only), and *Klebsiella* (respiratory and urinary tract infections only)

Mycoplasmal pneumonia (primary atypical pneumonia)

Streptococcal infections caused by susceptible strains[2]

Skin and soft tissue infections caused by susceptible strains of *Staphylococcus aureus*[3]

Rickettsial infections

Psittacosis (ornithosis)

Lymphogranuloma venereum, trachoma, and (when given orally) **inclusion conjunctivitis** and uncomplicated adult **urethral, endocervical, and rectal infections** caused by *Chlamydia trachomatis* or *Ureaplasma urealyticum*

Relapsing fever

As an adjunct to amebicides for **acute intestinal amebiasis**

As an alternative to penicillin for **gonococcal and clostridial infections, listeriosis, syphilis, yaws, anthrax, Vincent's infection, actinomycosis,** and (when given IV) **meningococcal infections**

Severe acne (oral therapy only)

Mycobacterium marinum **infections**

Eradication of **meningococcal carrier state**

ORAL DOSAGE

Adult: 200 mg to start, followed by 100 mg q12h, or 100–200 mg to start, followed by 50 mg qid; for gonorrhea, 200 mg to start, followed by 100 mg q12h for at least 4 days; for gonococcal urethritis in men, 100 mg bid for 5 days; for nongonococcal urethritis in men and women and endocervical and rectal infections caused by *Chlamydia trachomatis* or *Ureaplasma urealyticum,* 100 mg bid for at least 7 days

Child (> 8 yr): 4 mg/kg to start, followed by 2 mg/kg q12h

Adult: 100 mg bid for 6–8 wk

Adult: 100 mg q12h for 5 days

PARENTERAL DOSAGE

Adult: 200 mg IV to start, followed by 100 mg IV q12h, or up to 400 mg/24 h if needed

Child (> 8 yr): 4 mg/kg IV to start, followed by 2 mg/kg IV q12h

CONTRAINDICATIONS
Hypersensitivity to tetracyclines

ADMINISTRATION/DOSAGE ADJUSTMENTS

Duration of treatment	Unless otherwise indicated, continue treatment for at least 24–48 h after symptoms and fever have subsided; infections caused by Group A beta-hemolytic streptococci should be treated for at least 10 days, and syphilis for 10–15 days. If patient is started on parenteral therapy, institute oral therapy as soon as possible.
Intravenous administration	Use only when rapidly attained, high blood levels are needed and oral therapy is not adequate or tolerated. To reconstitute the solution, dissolve the powder and then, just before administration, further dilute the solution to a final volume of 500–1,000 ml with 5% dextrose injection USP or 5% sodium chloride injection USP (with or without 5% dextrose); Ringer's and lactated Ringer's injection USP may also be used, but other diluents containing calcium should not in order to avoid formation of a precipitate. Use the reconstituted solution within 24 h. Prolonged IV administration may cause thrombophlebitis. Avoid rapid administration.
Timing of oral administration	May be administered with food or milk, if desired

WARNINGS/PRECAUTIONS

Patients with renal impairment	Usual doses may lead to excessive drug accumulation and possible hepatic toxicity. If impairment is significant, azotemia, hyperphosphatemia, and acidosis may occur due to antianabolic action of drug. Reduce dosage by lowering individual doses and/or lengthening interval between doses, monitor kidney and liver function both before and during therapy, and follow serum tetracycline levels periodically (particularly if therapy is prolonged).

Pregnant and postpartum patients with pyelonephritis	Potentially fatal hepatic failure may occur with parenteral administration; do not allow serum level to exceed 15 µg/ml, monitor liver function frequently, and avoid concomitant use of other potentially hepatotoxic drugs
Superinfection	Overgrowth of nonsusceptible organisms, including fungi, may occur
Suspected syphilitic lesions	If syphilis is suspected, perform a dark-field examination before instituting therapy and monthly serology tests for at least 4 mo theraffer
Long-term therapy	Perform hemapoietic, renal, and hepatic studies periodically
Photosensitivity (exaggerated sunburn)	May occur; caution patients likely to be exposed to direct sunlight or UV light and discontinue use of minocycline at first sign of skin erythema
Light-headedness, dizziness, and/or vertigo	May occur; caution patients about driving or engaging in other potentially hazardous activities requiring mental alertness or physical coordination. CNS symptoms may disappear during treatment and usually disappear rapidly upon discontinuation of therapy.
Thrombophlebitis	May result from prolonged IV administration; switch to oral form as soon as possible

ADVERSE REACTIONS

Gastrointestinal	Anorexia, nausea, vomiting, diarrhea, glossitis, dysphagia, enterocolitis, inflammatory lesions (with monilial overgrowth) in the anogenital region, increase in liver enzyme levels; hepatitis (rare)
Dermatological	Maculopapular and erythematous rashes, exfoliative dermatitis (rare), photosensitivity (rare), pigmentation of skin and mucous membranes
Hypersensitivity	Urticaria, angioneurotic edema, anaphylaxis, anaphylactoid purpura, pericarditis, exacerbation of systemic lupus erythmatosus; pulmonary infiltrates with eosinophilia (rare)
Hematological	Hemolytic anemia, thrombocytopenia, neutropenia, eosinophilia
Central nervous system	Light-headedness, dizziness, vertigo; pseudotumor cerebri (rare)
Other	Microscopic discoloration of thyroid glands, bulging fontanels in infants

OVERDOSAGE

Signs and symptoms	See ADVERSE REACTIONS
Treatment	Discontinue medication; treat symptomatically and institute supportive measures, as required

DRUG INTERACTIONS

Oral anticoagulants	△ Prothrombin time
Penicillin	▽ Bactericidal activity of penicillin; avoid concomitant use
Antacids, sodium bicarbonate, iron supplements	▽ Absorption of minocycline; antacids containing aluminum, calcium, or magnesium should not be administered concomitantly
Methoxyflurane	△ Risk of nephrotoxicity

ALTERED LABORATORY VALUES

Blood/serum values	△ Alkaline phosphatase △ BUN △ Amylase △ Bilirubin △ SGOT △ SGPT ▽ Prothrombin activity
Urinary values	△ Catecholamines (with Hingerty fluorometric method)

USE IN CHILDREN

Not recommended for use during infancy through 8 yr of age unless other drugs are not likely to be effective or are contraindicated; use in this age group may cause permanent discoloration of teeth or enamel hypoplasia. A reversible decrease in fibula growth rate has been observed in premature infants given oral tetracycline (100 mg/kg/day).

USE IN PREGNANT AND NURSING WOMEN

Use during latter half of pregnancy (fetal tooth development) may cause permanent discoloration of teeth or enamel hypoplasia. Animal studies indicate that tetracyclines cross the placental barrier, are found in fetal tissues, and can cause both embryotoxicity and fetal toxicity, including retardation of skeletal development. Tetracyclines are excreted in breast milk; if drug is essential, patient should not nurse.

[1] Contains 5% alcohol
[2] Tetracyclines should not be used for streptococcal disease unless bacterial susceptibility has been demonstrated
[3] Tetracyclines are not the drug of choice for treating any staphylococcal infection

---

ACNE PREPARATIONS

OXY-5 (benzoyl peroxide) Norcliff Thayer   OTC
Lotion: 5% (1 fl oz) *clear*

OXY-10 (benzoyl peroxide) Norcliff Thayer   OTC
Lotion: 10% (1 fl oz) *clear*

OXY-10 Cover (benzoyl peroxide) Norcliff Thayer   OTC
Lotion: 10% (1 fl oz) *flesh-tinted*

INDICATIONS Acne vulgaris	**TOPICAL DOSAGE** **Adult and child:** after thoroughly washing and drying affected area, apply lotion in dabs and then spread it out evenly; to treat particularly troublesome areas with the flesh-tinted lotion, apply an extra dab. Use the lotion once daily to start, then bid or tid.

OXY-10 Wash (benzoyl peroxide) Norcliff Thayer OTC

Solution: 10% (4 fl oz)

INDICATIONS
Acne vulgaris

TOPICAL DOSAGE
Adult and child: wet affected area, apply solution, massage gently for 1-2 min, and then rinse thoroughly; use bid or tid

CONTRAINDICATIONS
Sensitivity to benzoyl peroxide

ADMINISTRATION/DOSAGE ADJUSTMENTS
Sensitivity test	Test sensitivity to benzoyl peroxide by applying lotion or solution to a small affected area once daily for 2 days; if excessive dryness or undue irritation develops, do not use

WARNINGS/PRECAUTIONS
Sensitive membranes	Avoid contact with eyes, lips, and mouth
Bleaching	Benzoyl peroxide may bleach hair or dyed fabrics
Local reactions	If discomforting irritation or undue dryness occurs during treatment, reduce frequency of use or dose; if excessive itching, redness, burning, swelling, irritation, or dryness occurs, discontinue administration

---

USE IN CHILDREN
See INDICATIONS and TOPICAL DOSAGE

USE IN PREGNANT AND NURSING WOMEN
Consult manufacturer

VEHICLE/BASE
Clear lotion: water, cetyl alcohol, silica (Sorboxyl), propylene glycol, citric acid, sodium citrate, sodium lauryl sulfate, methylparaben, and propylparaben
Flesh-tinted lotion: water, titanium dioxide, cetyl alcohol, silica (Sorboxyl), glyceryl stearate, propylene glycol, stearic acid, iron oxides, sodium lauryl sulfate, citric acid, sodium citrate, methylparaben, and propylparaben
Solution: water, cetyl alcohol, citric acid, propylene glycol, sodium citrate, sodium lauryl sulfate, methylparaben, and propylparaben

---

ACNE PREPARATIONS

PanOxyl (benzoyl peroxide) Stiefel Rx
Gel: 5% (PanOxyl 5), 10% (PanOxyl 10) (2, 4 oz)

PanOxyl AQ (benzoyl peroxide) Stiefel Rx
Gel (aqueous, nonalcoholic): 2.5% (PanOxyl AQ 2½), 5% (PanOxyl AQ 5), 10% (PanOxyl AQ 10) (2, 4 oz)

INDICATIONS
Acne vulgaris

TOPICAL DOSAGE
Adult: apply to affected areas bid, as tolerated, after washing with nonmedicated soap and water

CONTRAINDICATIONS
Hypersensitivity to any component

ADMINISTRATION/DOSAGE ADJUSTMENTS
Initiation of therapy	During the first week apply PanOxyl 5 or PanOxyl AQ 2½ once a day; thereafter, apply bid, as tolerated. If accommodation occurs, use a higher concentration of benzoyl peroxide.

WARNINGS/PRECAUTIONS
Sensitive surfaces	Avoid contact with eyes or mucous membranes
Bleaching	May occur; avoid contact with hair, colored linens, towels, or apparel
Excessive erythema and peeling	Occur most often during initial phase of therapy and may be controlled normally by reducing the frequency of use
Carcinogenicity	No evidence of carcinogenicity has been detected in long-term studies on mice and rats treated with benzoyl peroxide

PanOxyl/PanOxyl AQ ■ PERSA-GEL

ADVERSE REACTIONS	Frequent reactions (incidence ≥ 1%) are printed in *italics*
Local	*Excessive erythema and peeling (5%)*, allergic contact sensitization (1–2.5%)

USE IN CHILDREN
Use according to medical judgment

USE IN PREGNANT AND NURSING WOMEN
Pregnancy Category C: use during pregnancy only when clearly needed. Animal reproductive studies have not been done. It is not known whether fetal harm can occur when administered to pregnant women or if reproductive capacity is affected in humans. Benzoyl peroxide excretion in human milk is unknown; use with caution in nursing mothers.

VEHICLE/BASE
Gel: 20% ethyl alcohol, polyoxyethylene lauryl ether, colloidal magnesium aluminum silicate, hydroxypropylmethylcellulose, citric acid, and purified water
Aqueous gel (2.5%): purified water, polyoxyethylene lauryl ether, carbomer, sodium hydroxide, and methylparaben
Aqueous gel (5% and 10%): purified water, polyoxyethylene lauryl ether, carbomer, sodium hydroxide, and methylparaben

---

ACNE PREPARATIONS

PERSA-GEL (benzoyl peroxide) Ortho — Rx
Gel (acetone-based): 5%, 10% (1.5, 3 oz)

PERSA-GEL W (benzoyl peroxide) Ortho — Rx
Gel (water-based): 5%, 10% (1.5, 3 oz)

INDICATIONS	TOPICAL DOSAGE
Acne vulgaris	**Adult:** apply to affected areas 1–2 times/day after washing with a mild cleanser and water; modify dosage schedule to obtain desired degree of drying and peeling

CONTRAINDICATIONS
Hypersensitivity to any component

WARNINGS/PRECAUTIONS

Severe irritation	May occur; discontinue use and institute appropriate therapy. After reaction clears, treatment may often be resumed with less frequent application.
Sensitive surfaces	Contact with eyes, eyelids, lips, and mucous membranes should be avoided; if accidental contact occurs, rinse with water
Bleaching	May occur; avoid contact with hair and colored fabrics
Carcinogenicity, mutagenicity, and effect on fertility	There is no evidence that benzoyl peroxide is carcinogenic or mutagenic or that it impairs fertility

ADVERSE REACTIONS

Local	Severe irritation, allergic contact dermatitis

USE IN CHILDREN
Safety and effectiveness for use in children have not been established

USE IN PREGNANT AND NURSING WOMEN
Pregnancy Category C: use during pregnancy only when clearly needed. Animal reproductive studies have not been done. It is not known whether fetal harm can result from administration of benzoyl peroxide to pregnant women. Excretion of this drug in human milk is unknown; use with caution in nursing mothers.

VEHICLE/BASE
Persa-Gel: acetone, carbomer 940, trolamine, sodium lauryl sulfate, propylene glycol, and purified water
Persa-Gel W: carbomer, sodium hydroxide, hydroxypropyl methylcellulose 2906, laureth-4, and purified water

ACNE PREPARATIONS

pHisoAc BP (benzoyl peroxide) Winthrop Consumer Products — OTC

Cream: 10% (1 oz)

INDICATIONS	**TOPICAL DOSAGE**
Acne vulgaris	**Adult and child:** after thoroughly washing and drying affected area, apply a thin layer; use once daily to start and then, if necessary, bid or tid

CONTRAINDICATIONS	
Extreme skin sensitivity	Sensitivity to benzoyl peroxide

ADMINISTRATION/DOSAGE ADJUSTMENTS

Sensitivity test	Test sensitivity to benzoyl peroxide by applying cream to a small affected area once daily for 1 or 2 days; if excessive dryness or undue irritation develops, do not use

WARNINGS/PRECAUTIONS

Sensitive surfaces	Avoid contact with eyes, lips, mouth, and sensitive areas of the neck
Skin irritation	If mild irritation occurs, use less frequently or apply a smaller amount to affected areas; if severe irritation occurs, discontinue use. Persistent signs and symptoms should be reported.
Bleaching	To prevent bleaching, avoid contact with hair and dyed fabrics

ADVERSE REACTIONS

Local	Redness, burning, itching, peeling, swelling

USE IN CHILDREN
See TOPICAL DOSAGE

USE IN PREGNANT AND NURSING WOMEN
Consult manufacturer

VEHICLE/BASE
Cream (colorless, greaseless, odorless): mineral oil, white petrolatum, and glyceryl stearate

---

ACNE PREPARATIONS

RETIN-A (tretinoin) Ortho — Rx

Cream: 0.05% (20, 45 g), 0.1% (20 g)   **Gel:** 0.025%, 0.01% (15, 45 g)   **Liquid:** 0.05% (28 ml)

INDICATIONS	**TOPICAL DOSAGE**
Acne vulgaris	**Adult:** apply lightly to affected area once daily, at bedtime, to start

CONTRAINDICATIONS	
Hypersensitivity to any component	

ADMINISTRATION/DOSAGE ADJUSTMENTS

Administration	Transitory warmth or slight stinging may occur after application; to minimize possible irritation, wait 20–30 min after washing, until skin is completely dry, before applying this preparation. Use of large amounts will not improve the results of therapy and may cause marked redness, peeling, or discomfort; the risk of excessive medication can be minimized if the gel is used, because overapplication of the gel results in dry flaking, or "pilling." Apply the liquid with a fingertip, gauze pad, or cotton swab; do not oversaturate the gauze or cotton to the extent that the medication would run into areas where it is not wanted.
Monitoring of therapy	Changes in dosage form or frequency of application may be necessary during initial therapy. Do not discontinue use if an apparent exacerbation of inflammatory lesions, caused by the action of tretinoin on deep, previously unseen lesions, occurs during the early weeks of therapy. Although therapeutic effects should be evident after 2–3 wk, definite results may not be seen until after 6 wk or more; when a satisfactory response has been obtained, the preparation may be given less frequently.

WARNINGS/PRECAUTIONS

Sensitive surfaces	Avoid contact with eyes, mouth, angles of the nose, and mucous membranes

COMPENDIUM OF DRUG THERAPY

RETIN-A ■ STATICIN

Irritation	If the skin becomes excessively red, edematous, blistered, or encrusted, reduce dosage or discontinue use temporarily; if these reactions result from hypersensitivity, discontinue use permanently. Use with extreme caution in patients with eczema; severe irritation may occur in such patients.
Use of other topical products	Allow the skin to recover from the effects of other topical preparations before beginning tretinoin therapy; thoroughly cleanse affected areas before each application if cosmetics are used during treatment. If topical products, including medicated or abrasive soaps and cleansers, soaps and cosmetics with a strong drying effect, astringents, and products with spices, lime, or a high concentration of alcohol, are given concomitantly, exercise caution; preparations containing sulfur, resorcinol, or salicylic acid should be used with particular caution.
Carcinogenicity	Long-term studies to determine the carcinogenic potential of tretinoin have not been performed; however, 30-wk studies in hairless albino mice suggest that tretinoin may accelerate the tumorigenic potential of ultraviolet radiation. Caution patients to avoid or minimize exposure to sunlight (including sunlamps), especially if they are inherently sensitive to sunlight. If exposure is unavoidable, sunscreen products and protective clothing should be used over treated areas. Patients with sunburn should not use tretinoin until fully recovered. Weather extremes (eg, wind or cold) may also cause irritation.

ADVERSE REACTIONS[1]

Local	Excessively red, edematous, blistered, and/or crusted skin; temporary hypopigmentation or hyperpigmentation; increased susceptibility to sunlight; contact allergy (rare)

USE IN CHILDREN
Consult manufacturer

USE IN PREGNANT AND NURSING WOMEN
Pregnancy Category B: reproduction studies in rats and rabbits given topically up to 50 times the human dose have shown no evidence of impaired fertility or harm to the fetus; however, a slightly higher incidence of irregularly contoured or partially ossified skull bones has been observed in some of these studies. No adequate, well-controlled studies have been performed in pregnant women; use during pregnancy only if clearly needed. It is not known whether tretinoin is excreted in human milk; use with caution in nursing mothers.

VEHICLE/BASE
Gel: butylated hydroxytoluene, hydroxypropyl cellulose, and 90% alcohol
Cream (hydrophilic): stearic acid, isopropyl myristate, polyoxyl 40 stearate, stearyl alcohol, xanthan gum, sorbic acid, butylated hydroxytoluene, and purified water
Liquid: polyethylene glycol 400, butylated hydroxytoluene, and 55% alcohol

[1] To date, all adverse reactions have been reversible upon discontinuation of therapy

---

ACNE PREPARATIONS

STATICIN (erythromycin) Westwood Rx
Solution: 1.5% (60 ml)

INDICATIONS	TOPICAL DOSAGE
Control of **acne vulgaris** and prevention of new inflammatory acne lesions	**Adult:** apply with applicator to affected areas bid, in the morning and evening, after areas have been washed, rinsed well, and patted dry. If solution is applied with fingertips, wash hands afterwards. To control drying and peeling, reduce frequency of application.

CONTRAINDICATIONS
Hypersensitivity to any component

WARNINGS/PRECAUTIONS

Sensitive surfaces	Avoid contact with eyes, mouth, and other mucous membranes
Superinfection	Overgrowth of nonsusceptible organisms may occur with prolonged use; if superinfection occurs, discontinue administration
Accidental ingestion	Nausea and vomiting may occur following accidental ingestion; in small children, sedation or inebriation can also occur. For treatment, determine amount ingested and time since ingestion and then induce emesis, perform gastric lavage, or give demulcent liquids, as required; institute appropriate supportive measures.
Carcinogenicity, mutagenicity	No long-term studies have been done to evaluate the carcinogenic potential of this product; it has been shown to be nonmutagenic in the Ames test

STATICIN ■ STRI-DEX

ADVERSE REACTIONS

Local	Dryness, peeling, erythema, irritation

DRUG INTERACTIONS

Other topical acne preparations, especially peeling, desquamating, and abrasive agents	△ Irritation; exercise caution during concomitant therapy
Sodium alginate, pectin, bentonite, calamine, silica, polysorbate 80; solutions with a pH of less than 7 or more than 10.5	▽ Pharmacologic effect of erythromycin

---

USE IN CHILDREN

Safety and effectiveness for use in children under 12 yr of age have not been established

USE IN PREGNANT AND NURSING WOMEN

Pregnancy Category B: no evidence of impaired fertility or harm to the fetus has been seen in rats and rabbits given 1.5, 4, and 13 times the estimated human dose of erythromycin; use during pregnancy only if clearly needed. Consult manufacturer for use in nursing mothers.

VEHICLE/BASE
Solution: 55% alcohol, propylene glycol, laureth-4, and fragrance

---

ACNE PREPARATIONS

STRI-DEX (benzoyl peroxide) Glenbrook   OTC

Cream: 10% (1 oz) *clear*

INDICATIONS	TOPICAL DOSAGE
Acne vulgaris	**Adult and child:** after thoroughly washing affected area, apply cream once daily to start; if necessary, gradually increase frequency to bid or tid

CONTRAINDICATIONS	
Sensitivity to benzoyl peroxide	Very sensitive skin

WARNINGS/PRECAUTIONS

Sensitive membranes	Avoid contact with eyes, lips, and mouth
Bleaching	Benzoyl peroxide may bleach hair or dyed fabrics
Local reactions	This product may cause irritation, characterized by redness, burning, itching, peeling, or possible swelling; more frequent use or higher concentrations may aggravate the condition. If mild irritation occurs, reduce frequency of use or substitute a lower concentration; if irritation becomes severe, discontinue use. Patients should report persistent reactions.

DRUG INTERACTIONS

Other topical acne preparations	△ Irritation and dryness; if reactions occur during combination therapy, discontinue other preparations

---

USE IN CHILDREN

See INDICATIONS and TOPICAL DOSAGE

USE IN PREGNANT AND NURSING WOMEN

Consult manufacturer

VEHICLE/BASE
Cream (clear): bronopol, cellulose, dimethicone, docusate sodium solution, glyceryl stearate, PEG–100 stearate, laureth–4, light mineral oil, purified water, stearamide MEA–stearate, and white petrolatum

COMPENDIUM OF DRUG THERAPY

ACNE PREPARATIONS

SULFACET-R (sodium sulfacetamide and sulfur) Dermik   Rx

Lotion: 10% sodium sulfacetamide and 5% sulfur (1 fl oz) *flesh-tinted*

INDICATIONS	TOPICAL DOSAGE
Acne vulgaris, acne rosacea, and seborrheic dermatitis	**Adult:** apply a thin film 1–3 times/day with light massaging to blend into skin

CONTRAINDICATIONS	
Kidney disease	Hypersensitivity to sulfonamides,[1] sulfur, or any other component

WARNINGS/PRECAUTIONS	
Sensitivity to sulfacetamide	May occur; prescribe with caution to patients who may be prone to topical sulfonamide hypersensitivity, particularly if denuded or abraded skin areas are involved. Therapy in such individuals should be carefully supervised.
Long-term therapy	Observe patient closely for local irritation or sensitization; discontinue medication if irritation occurs
Reddening, epidermal scaling	May occur in the treatment of acne vulgaris and, alone, are not a cause of concern; caution patient of this possibility
Carcinogenicity	The long-term carcinogenic potential of this drug is unknown

ADVERSE REACTIONS	
Local	Reddening, scaling, irritation

USE IN CHILDREN
Safety and effectiveness have not been established for use in children under 12 yr of age

USE IN PREGNANT AND NURSING WOMEN
Pregnancy Category C: use during pregnancy only if clearly needed. Reproductive studies have not been done in animals, nor is it known whether this drug can cause fetal harm or affect reproductive capacity in humans. It is not known whether this drug is excreted in human milk; however, small amounts of orally administered sulfonamides have been found in human milk. In view of this, and because many drugs are excreted in human milk, use with caution in nursing mothers.

VEHICLE/BASE
Lotion: purified water, alkylaryl sulfonic acid salts, hydroxyethylcellulose, propylene glycol, xanthan gum, lauric myristic diethanolamide, polyoxyethylene laurate, butylparaben, methylparaben, silicone emulsion, talc, zinc oxide, titanium dioxide, attapulgite, iron oxides, pH buffers, and 2-bromo-2-nitropropane-1,3-diol

[1] Sulfonamide sensitivity may have been manifested by agranulocytosis, acute hemolytic anemia, purpura hemorrhagica, drug fever, jaundice, contact dermatitis, or other previous systemic toxic reactions

---

ACNE PREPARATIONS

TOPICYCLINE (tetracycline hydrochloride) Norwich Eaton   Rx

Solution: 2.2 mg/ml after reconstitution (70 ml)

INDICATIONS	TOPICAL DOSAGE
Acne vulgaris	**Adult:** apply generously bid to affected areas (not just individual lesions) until the skin is thoroughly wet

CONTRAINDICATIONS	
Hypersensitivity to any component or other tetracyclines	

ADMINISTRATION/DOSAGE ADJUSTMENTS	
Preparation of solution and storage	Prior to dispensing, mix powder and liquid together, following the instructions contained in the package; reconstituted solution will provide about an 8-wk supply for patients treating the face and neck and about a 4-wk supply if additional areas are to be treated. Store the solution at or below room temperature.
Use of cosmetics	Advise patient that cosmetics may be worn, as usual

WARNINGS/PRECAUTIONS	
Sensitive surfaces	Avoid contact with eyes, nose, and mouth

TOPICYCLINE ■ VANOXIDE-HC

Sulfite sensitivity	Sodium bisulfite in this product may cause urticaria, pruritus, wheezing, anaphylaxis, or other allergic-type reactions in susceptible patients, such as those with asthma or atopy
Carcinogenicity	No evidence of carcinogenicity has been observed in mice after topical application for a period of 2 yr
Effect on fertility	No evidence of impaired fertility has been observed in animal studies

ADVERSE REACTIONS
Frequent reactions (incidence ≥ 1%) are printed in *italics*

Local	*Transient stinging or burning upon application (33%);* severe dermatitis (rare)

USE IN CHILDREN
Safety and effectiveness for use in children under 11 yr of age have not been established

USE IN PREGNANT AND NURSING WOMEN
Pregnancy Category B: use during pregnancy only if clearly needed. Reproduction studies performed in rats and rabbits at doses up to 246 times the human dose (estimated to be 1.3 ml/40 kg/day, or 0.072 mg/kg/day) have shown no evidence of impaired fertility or harm to the fetus; however, no adequate, well-controlled studies have been done in pregnant women. It is not known whether tetracycline or other components of this preparation are excreted in human milk after topical application; use with caution in nursing mothers because many drugs are excreted in human milk.

VEHICLE/BASE
Solution (aqueous): 4-epitetracycline hydrochloride, sodium bisulfite, 40% alcohol, n-decyl methyl sulfoxide, and citric acid

---

ACNE PREPARATIONS

VANOXIDE-HC (benzoyl peroxide and hydrocortisone) Dermik   Rx
Lotion: 5% benzoyl peroxide and 0.5% hydrocortisone (25 g) *clear*

INDICATIONS
Acne vulgaris and oily skin

TOPICAL DOSAGE
Adult: apply a thin film to affected areas 1–3 times/day, with gentle massaging to blend into skin, or use according to medical judgment; if patient is very fair skinned, start with a single application at bedtime

CONTRAINDICATIONS
Hypersensitivity to benzoyl peroxide, hydrocortisone, or any other component

Viral skin diseases, such as varicella and vaccinia

WARNINGS/PRECAUTIONS

Sensitive surfaces	Avoid contact with eyes and mucosae
Local reactions	If itching, redness, swelling, or undue dryness occurs, discontinue use
Bleaching	May occur; avoid contact with colored fabrics

ADVERSE REACTIONS

Local[1]	Burning, itching, irritation, dryness, folliculitis, hypertrichosis, acneform eruptions, hypopigmentation, perioral dermatitis, allergic contact dermatitis, maceration, secondary infection, skin atrophy, striae, miliaria

USE IN CHILDREN
Safety and effectiveness have not been established for use in children under 12 yr of age

USE IN PREGNANT AND NURSING WOMEN
Pregnancy Category C: use during pregnancy only if clearly needed. Reproductive studies have not been done in animals, nor is it known whether this preparation can cause fetal harm or affect reproductive capacity in humans. It is not known whether either active component is excreted in human milk following topical application; use with caution in nursing mothers.

VEHICLE/BASE
Lotion (water-washable, clear): purified water, calcium phosphate, propylene glycol, caprylic/capric triglyceride, propylene glycol monostearate, laneth-10 acetate, decyl oleate, polysorbate 20, cetyl alcohol, mineral oil, lanolin alcohol, sodium phosphate, sodium biphosphate, stearyl heptanoate, hydroxyethylcellulose, tetrasodium EDTA, cyclohexanediamine tetraacetic acid, propylparaben, methylparaben, vegetable oil, monoglyceride citrate, simethicone, BHT, sodium hydroxide, BHA, propyl gallate, and FD&C colors

[1] Includes reactions common to topical corticosteroids in general; irritation and contact dermatitis are the most frequent side effects of the benzoyl peroxide component of this preparation

ACNE PREPARATIONS

VLEMASQUE (lime, sulfurated) Dermik — OTC
Mask: 6% (4 oz)

INDICATIONS	TOPICAL DOSAGE
Acne vulgaris	**Adult:** apply a generous layer to face and neck, avoiding eyes, nostrils, and lips, and leave on for 20–25 min; remove with lukewarm water, using a gentle circular motion, and pat dry; repeat daily **Child:** use according to medical judgment

WARNINGS/PRECAUTIONS

Contact with eyes	If contact occurs, flush eyes thoroughly
Irritation	If any irritation occurs, discontinue use

ADVERSE REACTIONS

Local	Irritation

USE IN CHILDREN	USE IN PREGNANT AND NURSING WOMEN
Use according to medical judgment	Consult manufacturer

VEHICLE/BASE
Mask: clay and 7% alcohol

ANTIDANDRUFF SHAMPOOS

DENOREX (coal tar, menthol, and alcohol) Whitehall — Rx
Lotion: 9.0% coal tar, 1.5% menthol, and 7.5% alcohol (4, 8, 12 oz) *regular, mountain-fresh herbal scent shampoo, and shampoo/conditioner formulation* Gel: 9.0% coal tar, 1.5% menthol, and 7.5% alcohol (2, 4 oz) *regular scent*

INDICATIONS	TOPICAL DOSAGE
Dandruff; flaking, itching, and scaling associated with **eczema, seborrhea, and psoriasis**	**Adult:** wet hair thoroughly, briskly massage shampoo into hair to form a rich lather, rinse thoroughly, and repeat application

CONTRAINDICATIONS
None known

ADMINISTRATION/DOSAGE ADJUSTMENTS

Frequency of use	For optimal results, use every other day; for severe scalp problems, use daily

WARNINGS/PRECAUTIONS

Contact with eyes	Avoid contact with the eyes
Irritation	Discontinue use if irritation occurs
Internal use	Ingestion may be harmful; keep out of reach of children

ADVERSE REACTIONS

Local	Irritation (see WARNINGS/PRECAUTIONS)

USE IN CHILDREN	USE IN PREGNANT AND NURSING WOMEN
Use according to medical judgment	Consult manufacturer

VEHICLE/BASE
Lotion (shampoo): TEA-lauryl sulfate, lauramide DEA, stearic acid, chloroxylenol, and water
Lotion (shampoo-conditioner): TEA-lauryl sulfate, lauramide DEA, PEG-27 lanolin, quaterium 23, fragrance, chloroxylenol, hydroxypropyl methylcellulose, citric acid, and water
Gel: TEA-lauryl sulfate, hydroxypropyl methylcellulose, chloroxylenol, and water

---

ANTIDANDRUFF SHAMPOOS

EXSEL (selenium sulfide) Herbert — Rx
Lotion: 2.5% (4 fl oz)

INDICATIONS	TOPICAL DOSAGE
Dandruff and seborrheic dermatitis of the scalp	**Adult:** wet scalp, massage 5–10 ml (1–2 tsp) into scalp, wait 2–3 min, and then rinse thoroughly; repeat application, rinse thoroughly, and wash hands

EXSEL ■ HEAD & SHOULDERS

| Tinea versicolor | **Adult:** apply to affected areas, lather well, wait 10 min, and then rinse body thoroughly and wash hands |

CONTRAINDICATIONS

Hypersensitivity to any component

ADMINISTRATION/DOSAGE ADJUSTMENTS

| Frequency of application | For dandruff and seborrheic dermatitis, apply twice a week for 2 wk, then reduce frequency to once a week or as seldom as once every 4 wk, as needed, to maintain control of symptoms. For tinea versicolor, apply once daily for a period of 7 days; if infection persists or recurs, course can be repeated. |

WARNINGS/PRECAUTIONS

Contact with eyes	Should be avoided; chemical conjunctivitis may result if this preparation enters the eyes
Acute inflammation or exudation	Use with caution in patients with acute inflammation or exudation since absorption may be increased in these patients
Cutaneous sensitization or irritation	If sensitivity reactions occur, discontinue use. During treatment of tinea versicolor, skin irritation may occur, especially in the genital region and other places with skin folds; these areas should be rinsed thoroughly after each application.
Hair discoloration	To avoid or minimize hair discoloration, rinse thoroughly after each application
Jewelry damage	To avoid possible damage from this product, remove jewelry before use
Accidental oral ingestion	Evacuation of the stomach contents should be considered; although there have been no reports of serious toxicity in humans after acute ingestion of this product, acute toxicity studies in animals suggest that ingestion of large amounts could result in human toxicity
Carcinogenicity	No evidence of carcinogenicity has been observed in mice after topical application of 0.63% and 1.25% solutions over a period of 88 wk

ADVERSE REACTIONS

| Local | Cutaneous irritation, increase in normal hair loss, hair discoloration, oiliness or dryness of hair and scalp, cutaneous sensitization |

USE IN CHILDREN

Safety and effectiveness for use on children have not been established

USE IN PREGNANT AND NURSING WOMEN

Pregnancy Category C: no reproduction studies have been performed to determine whether topical application can adversely affect reproductive capacity or fetal development; under ordinary circumstances, this preparation should not be used during pregnancy for the treatment of tinea versicolor

VEHICLE/BASE
Lotion: edetate disodium, bentonite, sodium dodecylbenzene sulfonate, sodium C14-16 olefin sulfonate, glyceryl ricinoleate, dimethicone copolyol, titanium dioxide, citric acid monohydrate, sodium phosphate (monobasic) monohydrate, fragrance, and purified water

---

ANTIDANDRUFF SHAMPOOS

HEAD & SHOULDERS (zinc pyrithione) Procter & Gamble   OTC

Cream: 1% (5.5 oz) **Lotion:** 1% (4, 7, 11, 15 fl oz)

INDICATIONS	TOPICAL DOSAGE
Dandruff and seborrheic dermatitis of the scalp	**Adult:** use as often as needed, depending upon severity of scalp condition; a minimum of four shampooings are recommended before full effect may be expected **Child:** use according to medical judgment

CONTRAINDICATIONS

Consult manufacturer

WARNINGS/PRECAUTIONS

| Contact with eyes | Should be avoided: in case of contact, rinse eyes with water |
| Internal use | Ingestion of this product may be harmful; keep out of reach of children |

HEAD & SHOULDERS ■ SEBULEX

ADVERSE REACTIONS
Consult manufacturer

USE IN CHILDREN	USE IN PREGNANT AND NURSING WOMEN
Use according to medical judgment	Consult manufacturer

VEHICLE/BASE
Cream (normal to oily formula): water, sodium cocoglyceryl ether sulfonate, sodium chloride, sodium lauroyl sarcosinate, cocamide DEA, cocoyl sarcosine, fragrance, and FD&C Blue No. 1
Cream (normal to dry formula): propylene glycol and ingredients of normal to oily formula
Lotion (normal to oily formula): water, ammonium lauryl sulfate, ammonium laureth sulfate, cocamide MEA, glycol distearate, ammonium xylenesulfonate, fragrance, citric acid, methylchloroisothiazolinone, methylisothiazolinone, and FD&C Blue No. 1
Lotion (normal to dry formula): propylene glycol and ingredients of normal to oily formula

---

ANTIDANDRUFF SHAMPOOS

SEBULEX (sulfur and salicylic acid) Westwood   OTC
Cream: 2% sulfur and 2% salicylic acid (4 oz)   Lotion: 2% sulfur and 2% salicylic acid (4, 8 fl oz)

INDICATIONS	TOPICAL DOSAGE
Dandruff	**Adult:** massage shampoo into wet scalp, allowing lather to remain on scalp for 5 min before rinsing and repeating application. Use daily or every other day to start, depending upon condition; once symptoms are controlled, shampoo once or twice weekly (may also be used daily, if desired). **Child:** use according to medical judgment

SEBULEX with Protein (sulfur and salicylic acid) Westwood   OTC
Lotion: 2% sulfur and 2% salicylic acid (4, 8 fl oz)

INDICATIONS	TOPICAL DOSAGE
Dandruff and seborrheic dermatitis	**Adult:** massage shampoo into wet scalp, allowing lather to remain on scalp for 5 min before rinsing and repeating application. Use daily to start; once symptoms are controlled, shampoo 2–3 times/wk (may also be used daily, if desired). **Child:** use according to medical judgment

CONTRAINDICATIONS
None known

WARNINGS/PRECAUTIONS
Skin irritation	May occur or increase; discontinue use
Contact with eyes	Should be avoided; in case of contact, flush eyes thoroughly with water

ADVERSE REACTIONS
Local	Irritation (see WARNINGS/PRECAUTIONS)

USE IN CHILDREN	USE IN PREGNANT AND NURSING WOMEN
There are no contraindications for use in children	There are no contraindications for use in pregnant and nursing women

VEHICLE/BASE
Cream: same as regular-formula lotion plus ceteareth-20, dextrin, magnesium aluminum silicate, and stearyl alcohol
Lotion (regular formula): D&C Yellow No. 10, docusate sodium, EDTA, FD&C Blue No. 1, fragrance, PEG-6 lauramide, PEG-14 M, sodium dodecyl benzene sulfonate, sodium octoxynol-2 ethane sulfonate, and water
Lotion (protein formula): water, sodium octoxynol-3 sulfonate, sodium lauryl sulfate, lauramide DEA, acetamide MEA, amphoteric-2, hydrolyzed animal protein, magnesium aluminum silicate, propylene glycol, methylcellulose, PEG-14 M, fragrance, disodium EDTA, dioctyl sodium sulfosuccinate, FD&C Blue No. 1, D&C Yellow No. 10

ANTIDANDRUFF SHAMPOOS

SELSUN (selenium sulfide) Abbott Rx

Lotion: 2.5% (4 fl oz)

INDICATIONS	TOPICAL DOSAGE
Dandruff and seborrheic dermatitis of the scalp	**Adult:** wet scalp, massage 5–10 ml (1–2 tsp) into scalp, wait 2–3 min, and then rinse thoroughly; repeat application, rinse thoroughly, and wash hands
Tinea versicolor	**Adult:** apply to affected areas, lather with a small amount of water, wait 10 min, and then rinse body thoroughly

CONTRAINDICATIONS

Hypersensitivity to any component — Acute inflammation or exudation

ADMINISTRATION/DOSAGE ADJUSTMENTS

Frequency of application	For dandruff and seborrheic dermatitis, apply twice a week for 2 wk, then reduce frequency to once a week or as seldom as once every 4 wk, as needed to maintain control of symptoms; for tinea versicolor, apply once daily for a period of 7 days

WARNINGS/PRECAUTIONS

Contact with eyes	Should be avoided; irritation of mucous membranes may result if this preparation enters the eyes
Cutaneous sensitization or irritation	Discontinue use if sensitivity reactions occur. During treatment of tinea versicolor, skin irritation may occur, especially in the genital region and other places with skin folds; these areas should be rinsed thoroughly after each application.
Hair discoloration	Can be avoided or minimized by thorough rinsing of the hair after treatment
Jewelry damage	To avoid possible damage from this product, remove jewelry before shampooing
Accidental oral ingestion	Evacuation of the stomach contents should be considered; although there have been no reports of serious toxicity in humans after acute ingestion of this product, acute toxicity studies in animals suggest that ingestion of large amounts could result in human toxicity
Carcinogenicity	No evidence of carcinogenicity has been observed in mice after topical application of 0.68% and 1.25% solutions over a period of 88 wk

ADVERSE REACTIONS

Local	Cutaneous irritation, increase in normal hair loss, hair discoloration, oiliness or dryness of hair and scalp, cutaneous sensitization

---

USE IN CHILDREN

See INDICATIONS and TOPICAL DOSAGE; safety and effectiveness for use on infants have not been established

USE IN PREGNANT AND NURSING WOMEN

Pregnancy Category C: no reproduction studies have been performed to determine whether topical application can adversely affect reproductive capacity or fetal development; under ordinary circumstances, this preparation should not be used during pregnancy for the treatment of tinea versicolor

---

VEHICLE/BASE
Lotion: bentonite, lauric diethanolamide, ethylene glycol monostearate, titanium dioxide, amphoteric-2, sodium lauryl sulfate, sodium phosphate (monobasic), glyceryl monoricinoleate, citric acid, captan, perfume, and water

---

ANTIDANDRUFF SHAMPOOS

SELSUN BLUE (selenium sulfide) Ross OTC

Lotion: 1% (4, 7, 11 fl oz)[1]

INDICATIONS	TOPICAL DOSAGE
Dandruff	**Adult:** lather, rinse thoroughly, and repeat application; use once or twice weekly **Child:** use according to medical judgment

CONTRAINDICATIONS

None

SELSUN BLUE ■ TEGRIN

ADMINISTRATION/DOSAGE ADJUSTMENTS

Bleaching, tinting, or permanent waving	Rinse hair with cool water for at least 5 min when shampoo is used before or after bleaching, tinting, or permanent waving

WARNINGS/PRECAUTIONS

Contact with eyes	Avoid contact with the eyes; if contact occurs, rinse eyes thoroughly with water
Irritation	Discontinue use if irritation occurs

ADVERSE REACTIONS

Local	Irritation (see WARNINGS/PRECAUTIONS)

USE IN CHILDREN
Use according to medical judgment

USE IN PREGNANT AND NURSING WOMEN
Consult manufacturer

---

[1] This product is available in formulations for normal, oily, and dry hair and in an extra-conditioning formula

VEHICLE/BASE
Lotion (dry formula): acetylated lanolin alcohol, ammonium laureth sulfate, ammonium lauryl sulfate, cetyl acetate, citric acid, cocamide DEA, cocamidopropyl betaine, DMDM hydantoin, FD&C Blue No. 1, fragrance, hydroxypropyl methylcellulose, magnesium aluminium silicate, polysorbate 80, titanium dioxide, TEA-lauryl sulfate, water, and other ingredients
Lotion (normal formula): ammonium laureth sulfate, ammonium lauryl sulfate, bentonite, citric acid, cocamide DEA, cocamidopropyl betaine, DMDM hydantoin, FD&C Blue No. 1, fragrance, magnesium aluminum silicate, titanium dioxide, TEA-lauryl sulfate, water, and other ingredients
Lotion (oily formula): ammonium laureth sulfate, ammonium lauryl sulfate, bentonite, citric acid, cocamide DEA, cocamidopropyl betaine, DMDM hydantoin, FD&C Blue No. 1, fragrance, magnesium aluminum silicate, sodium lauryl sulfate, titanium dioxide, TEA-lauryl sulfate, water, and other ingredients
Lotion (extra conditioning formula): acetylated lanolin alcohol, aloe, ammonium laureth sulfate, ammonium lauryl sulfate, cetyl acetate, citric acid, cocamide DEA, cocamidopropyl betaine, DMDM hydantoin, FD&C Blue No. 1, fragrance, glycol distearate, hydroxypropyl methylcellulose, magnesium aluminum silicate, polysorbate 80, propylene glycol, sodium chloride, TEA-lauryl sulfate, titanium dioxide, water, and other ingredients

---

ANTIDANDRUFF SHAMPOOS

TEGRIN Medicated Shampoo (coal tar) Block

OTC

Cream: 5% coal tar (2 oz) *regular and herbal fragrances* **Gel:** 5% coal tar (2.5 oz) **Lotion:** 5% coal tar (3.75, 6.6 fl oz) *regular and herbal fragrances*

INDICATIONS	TOPICAL DOSAGE
Moderate to severe **dandruff**; flaking, itching, and scaling associated with **eczema**, **seborrhea**, and **psoriasis**	**Adult:** wet hair, rub shampoo liberally into hair and scalp, rinse thoroughly, reapply, briskly massage scalp to form lather, and rinse thoroughly
Child: use according to medical judgment

CONTRAINDICATIONS

None known

ADMINISTRATION/DOSAGE ADJUSTMENTS

Frequency of use	Use at least twice a week for the first 2 wk and, thereafter, at least once a week or more often, if needed

WARNINGS/PRECAUTIONS

Contact with eyes	Should be avoided; if necessary, rinse eyes with warm water
Irritation	May occur; discontinue use
Internal use	May be harmful; keep out of reach of children

ADVERSE REACTIONS

Local	Irritation (see WARNINGS/PRECAUTIONS)

USE IN CHILDREN
Use according to medical judgment

USE IN PREGNANT AND NURSING WOMEN
Consult manufacturer

VEHICLE/BASE
Cream (regular formula): 3% SD alcohol 23-A, water, sodium lauryl sulfate, amphoteric-2, stearic acid, glycol stearate and other ingredients, propylene glycol, emulsifying wax NF, hydroxyethylcellulose, sodium hydroxide, lanolin, fragrance, methylparaben, and propylparaben
Cream (herbal formula): 3% SD alcohol 23-A, water, sodium lauryl sulfate, amphoteric-2, stearic acid, glycol stearate and other ingredients, propylene glycol, emulsifying wax NF, hydroxyethylcellulose, fragrance, sodium hydroxide, lanolin, methylparaben, propylparaben, and FD&C Blue No. 1
Gel: 4.6% SD alcohol 23-A, water, sodium lauryl sulfate, ammonium lauryl sulfate, cocamide DEA, hydroxypropyl methylcellulose, fragrance, sodium phosphate, disodium phosphate, phosphoric acid, methylparaben, D&C Green No. 8, propylparaben, FD&C Blue No. 1
Lotion (regular formula): 4.6% SD alcohol 23-A, water, sodium lauryl sulfate, lauramide DEA, sodium styrene/acrylates/divinylbenzene copolymer (and) ammonium nonoxynol-4 sulfate, sodium chloride, fragrance, citric acid, methylparaben, and propylparaben
Lotion (herbal formula): 4.6% SD alcohol 23-A, water, sodium lauryl sulfate, cocamide DEA, sodium styrene/acrylates/divinylbenzene copolymer (and) ammonium nonoxynol-4 sulfate, fragrance, citric acid, methylparaben, propylparaben, and FD&C Blue No. 1

ANTIDANDRUFF SHAMPOOS

ZETAR (coal tar and parachlorometaxylenol) Dermik   OTC

Foam: 1% whole coal tar and 0.5% parachlorometaxylenol (6 fl oz)

INDICATIONS	TOPICAL DOSAGE
Oily, itchy skin conditions, including **psoriasis, seborrhea, dandruff, and cradle cap**	**Adult:** massage into moistened scalp, rinse, reapply, and rinse thoroughly after 5 min

CONTRAINDICATIONS	
Acute inflammation	Open or infected lesions

WARNINGS/PRECAUTIONS	
Contact with eyes	Should be avoided
Irritation	Patients should discontinue use and seek medical attention if undue irritation occurs or increases
Hair discoloration	Temporary discoloration of blond, bleached, or tinted hair may occur

ADVERSE REACTIONS	
Local	Irritation; hair discoloration (rare)

USE IN CHILDREN	USE IN PREGNANT AND NURSING WOMEN
Consult manufacturer	Consult manufacturer

ANTIDANDRUFF SHAMPOOS

ZINCON (pyrithione zinc) Lederle   OTC

Liquid: 1% (4, 8 fl oz)

INDICATIONS	TOPICAL DOSAGE
Dandruff	**Adult:** wet hair, apply to scalp, massage vigorously, rinse, and repeat application; for optimum results, use twice a week **Child (≥ 2 yr):** same as adult

CONTRAINDICATIONS
Consult manufacturer

WARNINGS/PRECAUTIONS	
Contact with eyes	Should be avoided; if contact occurs, rinse eyes with water

ADVERSE REACTIONS
Consult manufacturer

USE IN CHILDREN	USE IN PREGNANT AND NURSING WOMEN
See INDICATIONS and TOPICAL DOSAGE; do not use in children under 2 yr of age	Consult manufacturer

VEHICLE/BASE
Liquid: water, sodium methyl cocoyl taurate, cocamide MEA, sodium chloride, magnesium aluminum silicate, sodium cocoyl isethionate, fragrance, glutaraldehyde, and D&C Green No. 5, plus citric acid or sodium hydroxide to adjust pH

Chapter 7

Controlled Analgesics

BUPRENEX (Norwich Eaton) Buprenorphine hydrochloride *C-V*	231
Codeine phosphate (Lilly) *C-II*	232
Codeine sulfate (Lilly) *C-II*	232
DARVOCET-N 50 (Lilly) Propoxyphene napsylate and acetaminophen *C-IV*	233
DARVOCET-N 100 (Lilly) Propoxyphene napsylate and acetaminophen *C-IV*	233
DARVON (Lilly) Propoxyphene hydrochloride *C-IV*	235
DARVON-N (Lilly) Propoxyphene napsylate *C-IV*	235
DARVON Compound (Lilly) Propoxyphene hydrochloride, aspirin, and caffeine *C-IV*	236
DARVON Compound-65 (Lilly) Propoxyphene hydrochloride, aspirin, and caffeine *C-IV*	236
DEMEROL (Winthrop-Breon) Meperidine hydrochloride *C-II*	238
DILAUDID (Knoll) Hydromorphone hydrochloride *C-II*	240
EMPIRIN with Codeine (Burroughs Wellcome) Aspirin and codeine phosphate *C-III*	241
EMPRACET with Codeine (Burroughs Wellcome) Acetaminophen and codeine phosphate *C-III*	243
EQUAGESIC (Wyeth) Meprobamate and aspirin *C-IV*	244
FIORINAL (Sandoz Pharmaceuticals) Butalbital, aspirin, and caffeine *C-III*	246
FIORINAL with Codeine (Sandoz Pharmaceuticals) Butalbital, aspirin, caffeine, and codeine phosphate *C-III*	247
MEPERGAN (Wyeth) Meperidine hydrochloride and promethazine hydrochloride *C-II*	248
MEPERGAN Fortis (Wyeth) Meperidine hydrochloride and promethazine hydrochloride *C-II*	249
MICRAININ (Wallace) Meprobamate and aspirin *C-IV*	250
Morphine sulfate injection *C-II*	252
NUMORPHAN (Du Pont) Oxymorphone hydrochloride *C-II*	254
PERCOCET (Du Pont) Oxycodone hydrochloride and acetaminophen *C-II*	255
PERCODAN (Du Pont) Oxycodone hydrochloride, oxycodone terephthalate, and aspirin *C-II*	256
PERCODAN-Demi (Du Pont) Oxycodone hydrochloride, oxycodone terephthalate, and aspirin *C-II*	256
PHENAPHEN with Codeine (Robins) Acetaminophen and codeine phosphate *C-III*	257
PHENAPHEN-650 with Codeine (Robins) Acetaminophen and codeine phosphate *C-III*	257
SUBLIMAZE (Janssen) Fentanyl citrate *C-II*	259
SYNALGOS-DC (Wyeth) Dihydrocodeine bitartrate, aspirin, and caffeine *C-III*	261
TALACEN (Winthrop-Breon) Pentazocine hydrochloride and acetaminophen *C-IV*	262
TALWIN Injection (Winthrop-Breon) Pentazocine lactate *C-IV*	264
TALWIN Nx (Winthrop-Breon) Pentazocine hydrochloride and naloxone hydrochloride *C-IV*	265
TYCOLET (McNeil Pharmaceutical) Hydrocodone bitartrate and acetaminophen *C-III*	267
TYLENOL with Codeine (McNeil Pharmaceutical) Acetaminophen and codeine phosphate *C-III*	268
TYLENOL with Codeine Elixir (McNeil Pharmaceutical) Acetaminophen and codeine phosphate *C-V*	268
TYLOX (McNeil Pharmaceutical) Oxycodone hydrochloride and acetaminophen *C-II*	270
VICODIN (Knoll) Hydrocodone bitartrate and acetaminophen *C-III*	271
WYGESIC (Wyeth) Propoxyphene hydrochloride and acetaminophen *C-IV*	273
ZYDONE (Du Pont) Hydrocodone bitratrate and acetaminophen *C-III*	274

Other Controlled Analgesics 229

ASCRIPTIN with Codeine (Rorer) Aspirin, magnesium-aluminum hydroxide, and codeine phosphate *C-III*	229
BANCAP HC (Forest) Acetaminophen and hydrocodone bitartrate *C-III*	229
B&O (Webcon) Belladonna and opium *C-II*	229
CAPITAL with Codeine (Carnrick) Acetaminophen and codeine phosphate *C-III, C-V*	229
CO-GESIC (Central) Acetaminophen with hydrocodone bitartrate *C-III*	229
DARVON with A.S.A. (Lilly) Propoxyphene hydrochloride and aspirin *C-IV*	229

DARVON-N with A.S.A. (Lilly) Propoxyphene napsylate and aspirin *C-IV*	229	**MS CONTIN** (Purdue Frederick) Morphine sulfate *C-II*	230
DEMEROL APAP (Winthrop-Breon) Meperidine hydrochloride and acetaminophen *C-II*	229	**MSIR** (Purdue Frederick) Morphine sulfate *C-II*	230
DILAUDID-HP (Knoll) Hydromorphone hydrochloride *C-II*	229	**RMS** (Upsher-Smith) Morphine sulfate *C-II*	230
HY-PHEN (Ascher) Acetaminophen and hydrocodone bitartrate *C-III*	229	**ROXANOL** (Roxane) Morphine sulfate *C-II*	230
LEVO-DROMORAN (Roche) Levorphanol tartrate *C-II*	230	**ROXANOL SR** (Roxane) Morphine sulfate *C-II*	230
Morphine sulfate (Roxane) *C-II*	230	**TALWIN Compound** (Winthrop-Breon) Pentazocine hydrochloride and aspirin *C-IV*	230

OTHER CONTROLLED ANALGESICS

DRUG	HOW SUPPLIED	USUAL DOSAGE[1]
ASCRIPTIN with Codeine (Rorer) Aspirin, magnesium-aluminum hydroxide, and codeine phosphate *C-III*	**Tablets:** 325 mg aspirin, 150 mg magnesium-aluminum hydroxide, and 15 mg (No. 2) or 30 mg (No. 3) codeine phosphate	**Adult:** 2 No. 2 tabs or 1–2 No. 3 tabs q3–4h, as needed
BANCAP HC (Forest) Acetaminophen and hydrocodone bitartrate *C-III*	**Capsules:** 500 mg acetaminophen and 5 mg hydrocodone bitartrate	**Adult:** 1 cap q4–6h, as needed; for more severe pain, 2 caps q6h
B&O (Webcon) Belladonna and opium *C-II*	**Suppositories:** 16.2 mg belladonna extract and 30 mg (No. 15A) or 60 mg (No. 16A) opium	**Adult:** 1 suppository 1–2 times/day
CAPITAL with Codeine (Carnrick) Acetaminophen and codeine phosphate *C-III, C-V*	**Tablets:** 325 mg acetaminophen and 30 mg codeine phosphate *(C-III)* **Suspension (per 5 ml):** 120 mg acetaminophen and 12 mg codeine phosphate *(C-V)* (16 fl oz)	**Adult:** 1–2 tabs or 15 ml (1 tbsp) q4h, as needed **Child (3–6 yr):** 5 ml (1 tsp) tid or qid **Child (7–12 yr):** 10 ml (2 tsp) tid or qid
CO-GESIC (Central) Acetaminophen and hydrocodone bitartrate *C-III*	**Tablets:** 500 mg acetaminophen and 5 mg hydrocodone bitartrate	**Adult:** 1 tab q4–6h, as needed; for more severe pain, 2 tabs q6h
DARVON with A.S.A. (Lilly) Propoxyphene hydrochloride and aspirin *C-IV*	**Capsules:** 65 mg propoxyphene hydrochloride and 325 mg aspirin	**Adult:** 1 cap q4h, as needed, up to 6 caps/day
DARVON-N with A.S.A. (Lilly) Propoxyphene napsylate and aspirin *C-IV*	**Tablets:** 100 mg propoxyphene napsylate and 325 mg aspirin	**Adult:** 1 tab q4h, as needed
DEMEROL APAP (Winthrop-Breon) Meperidine hydrochloride and acetaminophen *C-II*	**Tablets:** 50 mg meperidine hydrochloride and 300 mg acetaminophen	**Adult:** 1–2 tabs q3–4h, as needed
DILAUDID-HP (Knoll) Hydromorphone hydrochloride *C-II*	**Ampuls:** 10 mg/ml	**Adult:** 1–14 mg IM or SC
HY-PHEN (Ascher) Acetaminophen and hydrocodone bitartrate *C-III*	**Tablets:** 500 mg acetaminophen and 5 mg hydrocodone bitartrate	**Adult:** 1 tab q4–6h, as needed; for more severe pain, 2 tabs q6h

[1] Where pediatric dosages are not given, consult manufacturer

continued

OTHER CONTROLLED ANALGESICS continued

DRUG	HOW SUPPLIED	USUAL DOSAGE[1]
LEVO-DROMORAN (Roche) Levorphanol tartrate C-II	**Tablets:** 2 mg **Ampuls:** 2 mg/ml (1 ml) **Vials:** 2 mg/ml (10 ml)	**Adult:** 2 mg PO or SC, or up to 3 mg PO or SC, if needed
Morphine sulfate (Roxane) C-II	**Oral solution:** 2 mg/ml (5, 10, 500 ml); 4 mg/ml (100, 500 ml) **Tablets:** 15, 30 mg	**Adult:** 10–20 mg (solution) or 15–30 mg (tablets) q4h
MS CONTIN (Purdue Frederick) Morphine sulfate C-II	**Tablets (controlled release):** 30 mg	**Adult:** 30 mg q12h
MSIR (Purdue Frederick) Morphine sulfate C-II	**Tablets:** 15, 30 mg	**Adult:** 15–30 mg q4h
RMS (Upsher-Smith) Morphine sulfate C-II	**Suppositories:** 5, 10, 20 mg	**Adult:** 10–20 mg q4h
ROXANOL (Roxane) Morphine sulfate C-II	**Oral solution (per 1 ml dropperful:** 20 mg (30, 120 ml) (Roxanol) **Oral solution (per 5 ml):** 100 mg (240 ml) (Roxanol 100)	**Adult:** 10–30 mg q4h
ROXANOL SR (Roxane) Morphine sulfate C-II	**Tablets (sustained release):** 30 mg	**Adult:** 30 mg q8h to start
TALWIN Compound (Winthrop-Breon) Pentazocine hydrochloride and aspirin C-IV	**Tablets:** 12.5 mg pentazocine hydrochloride and 325 mg aspirin	**Adult:** 2 tabs tid or qid

[1] Where pediatric dosages are not given, consult manufacturer

CONTROLLED ANALGESICS

BUPRENEX (buprenorphine hydrochloride) Norwich Eaton C-V
Ampuls: 0.3 mg buprenorphine[1] (1 ml)

INDICATIONS	**PARENTERAL DOSAGE**
Moderate to severe pain	Adult and child ($\geq$ 13 yr): 0.3 mg or, if necessary, up to 0.6 mg, given by IM or slow IV injection at intervals of up to 6 h, as needed; during long-term therapy, dose should not exceed 0.6 mg
CONTRAINDICATIONS	
Hypersensitivity to buprenorphine	
WARNINGS/PRECAUTIONS	
Drug dependence	Buprenorphine has opioid properties that may lead to psychic dependence; however, withdrawal studies have shown that the drug produces a low level of physical dependence. Exercise caution when prescribing this agent to drug abusers or ex-narcotic addicts.
Narcotic antagonist effect	Do not use buprenorphine in narcotic-dependent patients since the drug has narcotic antagonist properties and can therefore induce withdrawal reactions in these patients
Respiratory depression	Buprenorphine can precipitate respiratory depression; use with caution in patients with compromised respiratory function, such as those with chronic obstructive pulmonary disease, cor pulmonale, decreased respiratory reserve, hypoxia, hypercapnia, or preexisting respiratory depression. For treatment of respiratory depression, see OVERDOSAGE.
Biliary tract dysfunction	Buprenorphine can cause an increase in intracholedochal pressure; use with caution in patients with dysfunction of the biliary tract
Ambulatory patients	Caution patients to avoid driving or any other potentially hazardous activity requiring mental alertness or physical coordination; warn patients that they must refrain from these activities if alcohol or any other CNS depressant is taken during therapy (see DRUG INTERACTIONS)
Patients with head injuries or other intracranial lesions	Buprenorphine can increase CSF pressure; use with caution in patients with head injuries, intracranial lesions, or other conditions that may be associated with increased CSF pressure. Bear in mind that this drug can interfere with clinical evaluation of these conditions by causing miosis and altering the level of consciousness.
Patients with hepatic impairment	Use with caution in patients with hepatic impairment because buprenorphine is metabolized by the liver
Other special-risk patients	Exercise caution if the patient is elderly or debilitated, is in a state of CNS depression or coma, or has myxedema, hyperthyroidism, adrenal cortical insufficiency (eg, Addison's disease), severe renal impairment, toxic psychosis, prostatic hypertrophy, urethral stricture, acute alcoholism, delirium tremens, or kyphoscoliosis
Effect on fertility	No evidence of impaired fertility has been seen in rats following SC or IM administration of 10–1,000 times the human dose
ADVERSE REACTIONS	Frequent reactions (incidence $\geq$ 1%) are printed in *italics*
Central nervous system	*Sedation (66%); dizziness/vertigo (5–10%), headache (1–5%)*, confusion, euphoria, weakness/fatigue, dry mouth, nervousness, depression, slurred speech, paresthesias, dreaming, psychosis, malaise, hallucinations, depersonalization, coma, tremor; dysphoria/agitation and convulsions/lack of muscle coordination (one case)
Ophthalmic	*Miosis (1–5%)*, diplopia, visual abnormalities, blurred vision, conjunctivitis, amblyopia
Cardiovascular	*Hypotension (1–5%)*, hypertension, tachycardia, bradycardia, Wenckebach block
Gastrointestinal	*Nausea (5–10%), vomiting (1–5%)*, constipation, dyspepsia, flatulence; loss of appetite (rare), diarrhea (one case)
Respiratory	*Hypoventilation (1–5%)*, dyspnea, cyanosis, apnea
Dermatological	Pruritus, rash; urticaria (one case)
Other	*Sweating (1–5%)*, injection site reactions, urinary retention, flushing/warmth, chills/cold, tinnitus, pallor
OVERDOSAGE	
Signs and symptoms	Respiratory depression, miosis, extreme somnolence progressing to stupor or coma, skeletal-muscle flaccidity, cold and clammy skin, bradycardia, hypotension, and, in severe cases, apnea, circulatory collapse, and cardiac arrest
Treatment	Carefully monitor respiratory and cardiovascular response. Give primary attention to reestablishing adequate respiratory exchange through provision of an adequate airway and through assisted or controlled ventilation; if pulmonary edema is present, positive-pressure respiration may be desirable. Oxygen, IV fluids, vasopressors, and other supportive measures should be employed, as needed. Although naloxone or doxapram may be helpful, these drugs are only partially effective in reversing respiratory depression. *Do not use analeptic agents.*

BUPRENEX ■ Codeine

DRUG INTERACTIONS

Other CNS depressants, including alcohol; MAO inhibitors	◇ CNS depression; there have been isolated reports of respiratory and cardiovascular collapse in patients given buprenorphine and diazepam. If buprenorphine and another CNS depressant are to be used concomitantly, the dosage of one or both agents should be reduced; see also warning above for ambulatory patients.
Phenprocoumon	◇ Risk of purpura

ALTERED LABORATORY VALUES

Blood/serum values — ◇ Amylase ◇ Lipase

No clinically significant alterations in urinary values occur at therapeutic dosages

---

USE IN CHILDREN

Safety and effectiveness for use in children under 13 yr of age have not been established

USE IN PREGNANT AND NURSING WOMEN

Pregnancy Category C: in rats, IM administration at 10 and 100 times the human dose (but not at 1,000 times the human dose) has caused mild postimplantation losses and early fetal deaths, and IV administration at 40 and 160 times the human dose has produced a slight increase in postimplantation losses; in rabbits, extra rib formation has been seen following IM administration at 1,000 times the human dose. Dystocia has occurred in rats given SC or IM doses that were 1,000 times the human dose. No adequate, well-controlled studies have been performed in pregnant women; safety for use during labor and delivery has not been established. Use during pregnancy only if the expected benefit justifies the potential risk to the fetus. It is not known whether buprenorphine is excreted in human milk; use with caution in nursing mothers.

[1] As the hydrochloride salt

CONTROLLED ANALGESICS

Codeine phosphate Lilly   C-II
Soluble hypodermic tablets: 15, 30, 60 mg   Vials: 30 mg/ml (20 ml)

Codeine sulfate Lilly   C-II
Tablets: 15, 30, 60 mg   Soluble hypodermic tablets: 15, 30, 60 mg

INDICATIONS	ORAL DOSAGE	PARENTERAL DOSAGE
Mild to moderate pain	**Adult:** 15–60 mg q4h, as needed **Child (≥ 1 yr):** 0.5 mg/kg (15 mg/m²) q4–6h, as needed	**Adult:** 15–60 mg IM or SC q4h, as needed **Child (≥ 1 yr):** 0.5 mg/kg (15 mg/m²) IM or SC q4–6h, as needed

CONTRAINDICATIONS
Hypersensitivity to codeine

WARNINGS/PRECAUTIONS

Drug dependence	Psychic and/or physical dependence and tolerance may develop, especially in addiction-prone individuals
Ambulatory patients	Caution patients not to engage in potentially hazardous activities requiring full mental alertness or physical coordination and to avoid alcohol and other CNS depressants, which may produce additional CNS depression
Patients with head injuries or other intracranial lesions	The respiratory depressant effects of this drug and its capacity to elevate CSF pressure may be markedly exaggerated in such patients; side effects may also interfere with the clinical evaluation of head injuries. Administer with extreme caution and only if use of this drug is deemed essential.
Patients with acute abdominal conditions	Use of this drug may obscure the diagnosis or clinical course of acute abdominal conditions
Patients with hepatic or renal dysfunction	Codeine may have a prolonged cumulative effect in such patients
Other special-risk patients	Use with caution in the elderly or debilitated and in patients with severe hepatic or renal impairment, hypothyroidism, Addison's disease, prostatic hypertrophy, or urethral stricture

ADVERSE REACTIONS
Frequent reactions (incidence ≥ 1%) are printed in *italics*

Central nervous system	*Light-headedness, dizziness, sedation,* euphoria, dysphoria

Codeine ■ DARVOCET-N

Gastrointestinal	*Nausea, vomiting,* constipation
Dermatological	Pruritus

OVERDOSAGE

Signs and symptoms	Respiratory depression, miosis, extreme somnolence progressing to stupor or coma, skeletal-muscle flaccidity, cold and clammy skin, hypotension, bradycardia, and, in severe cases, apnea, circulatory collapse, and cardiac arrest
Treatment	Give primary attention to reestablishing adequate respiratory exchange through provision of an adequate airway and assisted or controlled ventilation; positive-pressure respiration may be desirable if pulmonary edema is present. If respiratory depression is significant, promptly administer naloxone (adult, 0.4 mg; child, 0.01 mg/kg), preferably IV, and repeat at 2- to 3-min intervals until satisfactory breathing is restored. *Do not use analeptic agents.* Oxygen, IV fluids, vasopressors, and other supportive measures should be employed, as needed. Gastric lavage, followed by instillation of activated charcoal, may be useful; dialysis is of little value unless other, dialyzable substances (such as barbiturates) have been simultaneously ingested.

DRUG INTERACTIONS

Other narcotic analgesics; sedative-hypnotics, antianxiety agents, phenothiazines, general anesthetics, and other CNS depressants (including alcohol); MAO inhibitors; tricyclic antidepressants	△ CNS depression; reduce dose of one or both agents if used concomitantly or in close succession
Anticholinergic agents	△ Risk of paralytic ileus

ALTERED LABORATORY VALUES

Blood/serum values	△ Amylase △ Lipase

No clinically significant alterations in urinary values occur at therapeutic dosages

---

USE IN CHILDREN

See INDICATIONS and ORAL DOSAGE

USE IN PREGNANT AND NURSING WOMEN

Pregnancy Category C: use during pregnancy only if clearly needed. Reproduction studies have not been done in animals. It is also not known whether codeine can adversely affect human fetal development or reproductive capacity; however, clinical use of codeine in all stages of pregnancy has not been associated historically with fetal abnormalities. If used in obstetrics, codeine may prolong labor and produce respiratory depression in the newborn, possibly necessitating administration of a narcotic antagonist. Codeine is excreted in human milk; use with caution in nursing mothers.

CONTROLLED ANALGESICS

DARVOCET-N 50 (propoxyphene napsylate and acetaminophen) Lilly   C-IV

Tablets: 50 mg propoxyphene napsylate and 325 mg acetaminophen

DARVOCET-N 100 (propoxyphene napsylate and acetaminophen) Lilly   C-IV

Tablets: 100 mg propoxyphene napsylate and 650 mg acetaminophen

INDICATIONS

Mild to moderate pain alone or accompanied by fever

ORAL DOSAGE

Adult: 2 Darvocet-N 50 tabs or 1 Darvocet-N 100 tab q4h, as needed, not to exceed 600 mg of propoxyphene napsylate daily

CONTRAINDICATIONS

Suicidal or addiction-prone individuals	Hypersensitivity to propoxyphene or acetaminophen

ADMINISTRATION/DOSAGE ADJUSTMENTS

Patients with renal or hepatic impairment	Consider reducing the daily dose if the patient has renal or hepatic impairment since the serum level or half-life of propoxyphene may be increased in such a patient

WARNINGS/PRECAUTIONS

Drug dependence	Psychic dependence and, less often, physical dependence and tolerance may develop when taken in higher-than-recommended doses for prolonged periods, especially in addiction-prone individuals

DARVOCET-N

Overdosage	Excessive doses of propoxyphene, either alone or in combination with other CNS depressants, including alcohol (see DRUG INTERACTIONS), are a major cause of drug-related deaths; caution patients not to exceed recommended dosage and to limit their alcohol intake, and that the concomitant use of other CNS depressants can cause additional CNS depression
Ambulatory patients	Caution patients that their ability to engage in potentially hazardous activities requiring full mental alertness or physical coordination may be impaired and that alcohol and other CNS depressants may produce additional CNS depression
Hepatotoxicity	Propoxyphene has been associated with abnormal liver function tests and, more rarely, with reversible jaundice. Fatal hepatic necrosis has occurred in rare instances following short-term administration of 2.5–10 g/day of acetaminophen to alcoholics; necrosis has also been seen after acute acetaminophen overdose.

ADVERSE REACTIONS

The most frequent reactions, regardless of incidence, are printed in *italics*

Central nervous system	*Dizziness, sedation,* light-headedness, euphoria, dysphoria, minor visual disturbances, weakness, headache
Gastrointestinal	*Nausea, vomiting,* constipation, abdominal pain
Hepatic	Jaundice, abnormal liver function values
Dermatological	Rash

OVERDOSAGE

Signs and symptoms	*Propoxyphene-related effects:* CNS depression, ranging from somnolence (usually) to stupor and coma; respiratory depression, progressing to Cheyne-Stokes respiration, cyanosis, hypoxia, and apnea; pinpoint pupils, becoming dilated as hypoxia increases, fall in blood pressure and deterioration in cardiac performance, culminating in pulmonary edema and circulatory collapse; respiratory and metabolic acidosis; cardiac conduction delay and arrhythmias; convulsions; *acetaminophen-related effects:* nausea, anorexia, vomiting, abdominal pain, diarrhea, diaphoresis, malaise during the first 24 h; prolonged prothrombin time, elevated serum levels of SGOT, SGPT, LDH, and bilirubin, and signs of acute renal failure during the next 24–48 h (renal toxicity is usually more apparent 6–9 days after overdose)
Treatment	Give primary attention to reestablishing adequate respiratory exchange through provision of adequate airway and assisted or controlled ventilation; positive-pressure respiration may be desirable if pulmonary edema is present. If respiratory depression is significant, promptly administer naloxone. For adults, give 0.4–2 mg IV (or, if necessary, IM or SC) at intervals of 2–3 min, as needed; for children, give 0.01 mg/kg IV and then, if dose is not adequate, 0.1 mg/kg IV (if IV administration is not feasible, divide each dose and give IM or SC). Naloxone may also be administered by continuous IV infusion. Reevaluate diagnosis if no response is seen after giving 10 mg of naloxone. *Do not use analeptic agents.* Monitor blood gases, pH, and electrolytes and promptly correct any acid-base or electrolyte abnormalities present (lactic acidosis may require IV sodium bicarbonate for prompt correction). Administer an anticonvulsant in carefully titrated doses if seizures occur. Oxygen, IV fluids, vasopressors, and other supportive measures should be employed, as needed. ECG monitoring is essential since ventricular fibrillation or cardiac arrest can occur.
	Promptly empty stomach by performing gastric lavage or inducing emesis; activated charcoal may also be used to remove propoxyphene. Administer oral acetylcysteine as soon as possible (no later than 24 h after ingestion); give a loading dose of 140 mg/kg and then, at 4-h intervals, 17 maintenance doses of 70 mg/kg. (Charcoal, if used, should be removed before acetylcysteine is given.) Measure the plasma level of unconjugated acetaminophen as early as possible, but no sooner than 4 h after ingestion. Determine prothrombin time, SGOT and SGPT levels, and serum concentrations of bilirubin, creatinine, BUN, glucose, and electrolytes every 24 h. If the prothrombin time exceeds 1.5 times the control value, give vitamin K_1; if the prothrombin time exceeds 3 times this value, give fresh frozen plasma. Institute appropriate measures to treat hypoglycemia and electrolyte and fluid imbalance. Avoid forced diuresis or use of diuretics when treating an acetaminophen overdose. For additional information on use of acetylcysteine and interpretation of the plasma acetaminophen level, see Mucomyst chart.

DRUG INTERACTIONS

Other narcotic analgesics; sedative-hypnotics, antianxiety agents, phenothiazines, general anesthetics, muscle relaxants, and other CNS depresssants; MAO inhibitors; tricyclic antidepressants	△ CNS depression; use with caution in patients who require concomitant administration of other CNS depressants
Alcohol	△ CNS depression; use with caution in patients who consume excessive amounts of alcohol
Carbamazepine, tricyclic antidepressants, barbiturates, oral anticoagulants	△ Pharmacologic effect of interacting drug

ALTERED LABORATORY VALUES

Blood/serum values — ▽ Glucose (with glucose oxidase/peroxidase tests) Abnormal liver function values

Urinary values — △ 5-HIAA (with nitrosonaphthol reagent test)

USE IN CHILDREN
Not recommended for use in children

USE IN PREGNANT AND NURSING WOMEN
Safety for use during pregnancy has not been established in regard to fetal development; neonatal withdrawal symptoms have been reported following propoxyphene usage during pregnancy. Use in pregnant women only if the expected therapeutic benefit outweighs the possible hazards. Although low levels of propoxyphene have been found in human milk, no adverse effects have been noted in nursing infants.

CONTROLLED ANALGESICS

DARVON (propoxyphene hydrochloride) Lilly — C-IV
Capsules: 32, 65 mg

INDICATIONS	ORAL DOSAGE
Mild to moderate pain	**Adult:** 65 mg q4h, as needed, up to 390 mg/day

DARVON-N (propoxyphene napsylate) Lilly — C-IV
Tablets: 100 mg **Suspension (per 5 ml):** 50 mg (16 fl oz)

INDICATIONS	ORAL DOSAGE
Mild to moderate pain	**Adult:** 100 mg or 10 ml (2 tsp) q4h, as needed, up to 600 mg/day

CONTRAINDICATIONS	
Suicidal or addiction-prone individuals	Hypersensitivity to propoxyphene

ADMINISTRATION/DOSAGE ADJUSTMENTS

Patients with renal or hepatic impairment — Consider reducing the daily dose if the patient has renal or hepatic impairment since the serum level or half-life of propoxyphene may be increased in such a patient

WARNINGS/PRECAUTIONS

Drug dependence — Psychic dependence and, less often, physical dependence and tolerance may develop when taken in higher-than-recommended doses for prolonged periods, especially in addiction-prone individuals

Overdosage — Excessive doses of propoxyphene, either alone or in combination with other CNS depressants, including alcohol (see DRUG INTERACTIONS), are a major cause of drug-related deaths; caution patients not to exceed recommended dosage, to limit their alcohol intake, and that the concomitant use of other CNS depressants can cause additional CNS depression

Ambulatory patients — Caution patients that their ability to engage in potentially hazardous activities requiring full mental alertness or physical coordination may be impaired and that alcohol and other CNS depressants may produce additional CNS depression

ADVERSE REACTIONS

The most frequent reactions, regardless of incidence, are printed in *italics*

Central nervous system — *Dizziness, sedation,* light-headedness, headache, weakness, euphoria, dysphoria, minor visual disturbances

Gastrointestinal — *Nausea, vomiting,* constipation, abdominal pain, liver dysfunction

Dermatological — Rash

OVERDOSAGE

Signs and symptoms — CNS depression, ranging from somnolence (usually) to stupor and coma; respiratory depression, progressing to Cheyne-Stokes respiration, cyanosis, hypoxia, and apnea; pinpoint pupils, becoming dilated as hypoxia increases; fall in blood pressure and deterioration in cardiac performance, culminating in pulmonary edema and circulatory collapse; respiratory and metabolic acidosis; cardiac conduction delay and arrhythmias; convulsions

DARVON/DARVON-N ■ DARVON Compound

Treatment	Give primary attention to reestablishing adequate respiratory exchange through provision of an adequate airway and assisted or controlled ventilation; positive-pressure respiration may be desirable if pulmonary edema is present. If respiratory depression is significant, promptly administer naloxone. For adults, give 0.4–2 mg IV (or, if necessary, IM or SC) at intervals of 2–3 min, as needed; for children, give 0.01 mg/kg IV and then, if dose is not adequate, 0.1 mg/kg IV (if IV administration is not feasible, divide each dose and give IM or SC). Naloxone may also be administered by continuous IV infusion. Reevaluate diagnosis if no response is seen after giving 10 mg of naloxone. *Do not use analeptic agents.* Monitor blood gases, pH, and electrolytes and promptly correct any acid-base or electrolyte abnormalities present (lactic acidosis may require IV sodium bicarbonate for prompt correction). Administer an anticonvulsant in carefully titrated doses if seizures occur. Oxygen, IV fluids, vasopressors, and other supportive measures should be employed, as needed. ECG monitoring is essential since ventricular fibrillation or cardiac arrest can occur. Gastric lavage, followed by instillation of activated charcoal, may be useful. Dialysis is of little value in propoxyphene poisoning. If possible, determine whether the patient has ingested other agents, such as alcohol, barbiturates, tranquilizers, or other CNS depressants, since these increase CNS depression as well as cause specific toxic effects.

DRUG INTERACTIONS

Other narcotic analgesics; sedative-hypnotics, antianxiety agents, phenothiazines, general anesthetics, muscle relaxants, and other CNS depressants; MAO inhibitors; tricyclic antidepressants	△ CNS depression; use with caution in patients who require concomitant administration of other CNS depressants
Alcohol	△ CNS depression; use with caution in patients who consume excessive amounts of alcohol
Carbamazepine, tricyclic antidepressants, barbiturates, oral anticoagulants	△ Pharmacologic effect of interacting drug

ALTERED LABORATORY VALUES

No clinically significant alterations in blood/serum or urinary values occur at therapeutic dosages

USE IN CHILDREN	USE IN PREGNANT AND NURSING WOMEN
Not recommended for use in children	Safety for use during pregnancy has not been established in regard to fetal development; neonatal withdrawal symptoms have been reported following propoxyphene usage during pregnancy. Use in pregnant women only if the expected therapeutic benefit outweighs the possible hazards. Although low levels of propoxyphene have been found in human milk, no adverse effects have been noted in nursing infants.

CONTROLLED ANALGESICS

DARVON Compound (propoxyphene hydrochloride, aspirin, and caffeine) Lilly   C-IV

Capsules: 32 mg propoxyphene hydrochloride, 389 mg aspirin, and 32.4 mg caffeine

DARVON Compound-65 (propoxyphene hydrochloride, aspirin, and caffeine) Lilly   C-IV

Capsules: 65 mg propoxyphene hydrochloride, 389 mg aspirin, and 32.4 mg caffeine

INDICATIONS	ORAL DOSAGE
Mild to moderate pain alone or accompanied by fever	**Adult:** 1 cap q4h, as needed, not to exceed 390 mg of propoxyphene hydrochloride daily

CONTRAINDICATIONS

Suicidal or addiction-prone individuals	Hypersensitivity to propoxyphene, aspirin, or caffeine

ADMINISTRATION/DOSAGE ADJUSTMENTS

Patients with renal or hepatic impairment	Consider reducing the daily dose if the patient has renal or hepatic impairment since the serum level or half-life of propoxyphene may be increased in such a patient

WARNINGS/PRECAUTIONS

Drug dependence	Psychic dependence and, less often, physical dependence and tolerance may develop when taken in higher-than-recommended doses for prolonged periods, especially in addiction-prone individuals

DARVON Compound

Overdosage	Excessive doses of propoxyphene, either alone or in combination with other CNS depressants, including alcohol (see DRUG INTERACTIONS), are a major cause of drug-related deaths; caution patients not to exceed recommended dosage, to limit their alcohol intake, and that the concomitant use of other CNS depressants can cause additional CNS depression
Ambulatory patients	Caution patients that their ability to engage in potentially hazardous activities requiring full mental alertness or physical coordination may be impaired and that alcohol and other CNS depressants may produce additional CNS depression
Other special-risk patients	Use with extreme caution in patients with peptic ulcer or coagulation abnormalities
Reye's syndrome	Some reports claim that use of aspirin in children or adolescents with influenza or chickenpox increases the likelihood that Reye's syndrome will subsequently develop

ADVERSE REACTIONS

The most frequent reactions, regardless of incidence, are printed in *italics*

Central nervous system	*Dizziness, sedation,* light-headedness, euphoria, dysphoria, headache, weakness, minor visual disturbances
Gastrointestinal	*Nausea, vomiting,* constipation, abdominal pain, liver dysfunction
Dermatological	Rash

OVERDOSAGE

Signs and symptoms	*Propoxyphene-related effects:* CNS depression, ranging from somnolence (usually) to stupor and coma; respiratory depression, progressing to Cheyne-Stokes respiration, cyanosis, hypoxia, and apnea; pinpoint pupils, becoming dilated as hypoxia increases; fall in blood pressure and deterioration in cardiac performance, culminating in pulmonary edema and circulatory collapse; respiratory and metabolic acidosis; cardiac conduction delay and arrhythmias; convulsions; *aspirin-related effects:* hyperpnea, nausea, vomiting, vertigo, tinnitus, flushing, sweating, thirst, headache, drowsiness, diarrhea, and tachycardia, progressing to hyperthermia, hemorrhage, acid-base disturbances, restlessness, confusion, convulsions, vasomotor depression, coma, and respiratory failure; *caffeine-related effects:* insomnia, restlessness, and excitement progressing to mild delirium, dehydration, fever, tachycardia, extrasystoles, tremor, and convulsions
Treatment	Give primary attention to reestablishing adequate respiratory exchange through provision of an adequate airway and assisted or controlled ventilation; positive-pressure respiration may be desirable if pulmonary edema is present. If respiratory depression is significant, promptly administer naloxone. For adults, give 0.4–2 mg IV (or, if necessary, IM or SC) at intervals of 2–3 min, as needed; for children, give 0.01 mg/kg IV and then, if dose is not adequate, 0.1 mg/kg IV (if IV administration is not feasible, divide each dose and give IM or SC). Naloxone may also be administered by continuous IV infusion. Reevaluate diagnosis if no response is seen after giving 10 mg of naloxone. *Do not use analeptic agents.* Monitor blood gases, pH, and electrolytes and promptly correct any acid-base or electrolyte abnormalities present (lactic acidosis may require IV sodium bicarbonate for prompt correction). Administer an anticonvulsant in carefully titrated doses if seizures occur. Oxygen, IV fluids, vasopressors, and other supportive measures should be employed, as needed. ECG monitoring is essential since ventricular fibrillation or cardiac arrest can occur. Gastric lavage, followed by instillation of activated charcoal, may be useful if performed within 4 h of ingestion. In moderately severe cases of salicylate poisoning, cautiously administer sodium bicarbonate IV in sufficient quantity, if possible, to maintain an alkaline diuresis; intermittent peritoneal dialysis may also be helpful. In severe cases, hemodialysis should be seriously considered. Hyperthermia, particularly in children, and dehydration require prompt correction. Hemorrhagic phenomena may necessitate whole-blood transfusions and phytonadione (vitamin K_1). Do not administer barbiturates to treat excitement or convulsions. Dialysis is of little value in propoxyphene poisoning. If possible, determine whether the patient has ingested other agents, such as alcohol, barbiturates, tranquilizers, or other CNS depressants, since these increase CNS depression as well as cause specific toxic effects.

DRUG INTERACTIONS

Other narcotic analgesics; sedative-hypnotics, antianxiety agents, phenothiazines, general anesthetics, muscle relaxants, and other CNS depressants; MAO inhibitors; tricyclic antidepressants	△ CNS depression; use with caution in patients who require concomitant administration of other CNS depressants
Anticoagulants	△ Risk of bleeding
Alcohol	△ Risk of GI ulceration and CNS depression; use with caution in patients who consume excessive amounts of alcohol
Carbamazepine, tricyclic antidepressants, barbiturates, oral anticoagulants	△ Pharmacologic effect of interacting drug
Corticosteroids, phenylbutazone, oxyphenbutazone	△ Risk of GI ulceration

DARVON Compound ■ DEMEROL

Probenecid, sulfinpyrazone	▽ Uricosuric effect
Spironolactone	▽ Diuretic effect
Methotrexate	△ Methotrexate plasma level and risk of toxicity

ALTERED LABORATORY VALUES

Blood/serum values	△ Prothrombin time △ Uric acid (with low doses) ▽ Uric acid (with high doses) ▽ Thyroxine (T₄) ▽ Thyroid-stimulating hormone △ Glucose ▽ Bilirubin
Urinary values	△ Glucose (with Clinitest tablets) △ 5-HIAA (with nitrosonaphthol reagent test)

USE IN CHILDREN

Not recommended for use in children

USE IN PREGNANT AND NURSING WOMEN

Safety for use during pregnancy has not been established in regard to fetal development; neonatal withdrawal symptoms have been reported following propoxyphene usage during pregnancy. Use in pregnant women only if the expected therapeutic benefit outweighs the possible hazards. Although low levels of propoxyphene have been found in human milk, no adverse effects have been noted in nursing infants.

CONTROLLED ANALGESICS

DEMEROL (meperidine hydrochloride) Winthrop-Breon   C-II

Tablets: 50, 100 mg **Syrup (per 5 ml):** 50 mg (16 fl oz) *banana-flavored* **Ampuls:** 50 mg/ml (0.5, 1.0, 1.5, 2.0 ml), 100 mg/ml (1 ml) **Vials:** 50 mg/ml (30 ml), 100 mg/ml (20 ml) **Cartridge-needle units:** 25, 50, 75, 100 mg/ml (1 ml)

INDICATIONS	ORAL DOSAGE	PARENTERAL DOSAGE
Moderate to severe pain	Adult: 50–150 mg q3–4h, as needed Child: 0.5–0.8 mg/lb, up to 150 mg, q3–4h, as needed	Adult: 50–150 mg SC or IM q3–4h, as needed Child: 0.5–0.8 mg/lb, up to 150 mg, SC or IM q3-4h, as needed
Preoperative medication	—	Adult: 50–100 mg SC or IM, given 30–90 min before onset of anesthesia Child: 0.5–1.0 mg/lb, up to 100 mg, SC or IM, given 30–90 min before onset of anesthesia
Anesthesia support		Adult: repeated slow IV injections of fractional doses (eg, 10 mg/ml) or continuous IV infusion of a more dilute solution (eg, 1 mg/ml); titrate dose to individual needs, based on patient response, premedication, type of anesthesia, and nature and duration of operation Child: same as adult
Obstetrical analgesia		Adult: 50–100 mg SC or IM q1–3h, as needed, when pain is regular; repeat injection q1–3h, as needed

CONTRAINDICATIONS

Hypersensitivity to meperidine	MAO inhibitor therapy (see WARNINGS/PRECAUTIONS)

ADMINISTRATION/DOSAGE ADJUSTMENTS

Intravenous administration	Rapid IV injection increases risk of adverse reactions, including severe respiratory depression, apnea, hypotension, peripheral circulatory collapse, and cardiac arrest. If IV route is necessary, inject very slowly, preferably in dilute form, and have a narcotic antagonist and facilities for assisted or controlled respiration on hand. Patient should be lying down. Do not mix with barbiturates; solutions are incompatible.
Combination therapy	Use with caution and reduce dosage in patients who are concurrently receiving other CNS depressants. Respiratory depression, hypotension, and profound sedation or coma may result.

WARNINGS/PRECAUTIONS

MAO inhibitor therapy	Therapeutic doses of meperidine have precipitated unpredictable, severe, and occasionally fatal reactions in patients who have received MAO inhibitors within 14 days of treatment with meperidine
Drug dependence	Psychic and/or physical dependence and tolerance may develop, especially in addiction-prone individuals

DEMEROL

Ambulatory patients	Caution patients that their ability to engage in potentially hazardous activities requiring full mental alertness or physical coordination may be impaired
Patients with head injuries or other intracranial lesions	The respiratory depressant effects of this drug and its capacity to elevate CSF pressure may be markedly exaggerated in such patients; side effects may also interfere with the clinical evaluation of head injuries. Administer with extreme caution and only if use of this drug is deemed essential.
Patients with acute abdominal conditions	Use of this drug may obscure the diagnosis or clinical course of acute abdominal conditions
Patients with asthma or other respiratory conditions	Therapeutic doses may decrease respiratory drive while increasing airway resistance to the point of apnea; use with extreme caution during an acute asthmatic attack and in the presence of chronic obstructive pulmonary disease, cor pulmonale, substantially decreased respiratory reserve, respiratory depression, hypoxia, or hypercapnia
Increased ventricular response rate	May occur due to potential vagolytic action of meperidine; use with caution in patients with atrial flutter and other supraventricular tachycardias
Convulsive disorders	May be aggravated; convulsions may occur in patients with no prior history of seizures if tolerance develops and doses substantially exceeding recommended levels are taken
Other special-risk patients	Reduce initial dosage and use with caution in the elderly or debilitated and patients with hepatic or renal impairment, hypothyroidism, Addison's disease, prostatic hypertrophy, or urethral stricture

ADVERSE REACTIONS[1]

	Frequent reactions (incidence $\geq$ 1%) are printed in *italics*
Central nervous system and neuromuscular	*Light-headedness, dizziness, sedation,* euphoria, dysphoria, weakness, agitation, tremor, transient hallucinations, disorientation, visual disturbances, headache, sensory motor paralysis caused by inadvertent injection too near a nerve trunk, uncoordinated muscle movements
Gastrointestinal	*Nausea, vomiting,* dry mouth, constipation, biliary tract spasm
Dermatological	Pruritus, urticaria, rash, wheal and flare over vein at IV site
Respiratory	Respiratory depression, respiratory arrest
Cardiovascular	Flushed face, tachycardia, bradycardia, palpitations, hypotension, shock, syncope, phlebitis with IV use, cardiac arrest
Genitourinary	Urinary retention
Other	*Sweating,* pain at injection site, local induration and irritation after SC injection, edema

OVERDOSAGE

Signs and symptoms	Respiratory depression, miosis, extreme somnolence progressing to stupor or coma, skeletal-muscle flaccidity, cold and clammy skin, hypotension, bradycardia, and, in severe cases, apnea, circulatory collapse, and cardiac arrest
Treatment	Give primary attention to reestablishing adequate respiratory exchange through provision of an adequate airway and assisted or controlled ventilation; positive-pressure respiration may be desirable if pulmonary edema is present. If respiratory depression is significant, promptly administer naloxone (adult, 0.4 mg; child, 0.01 mg/kg), preferably IV, and repeat at 2- to 3-min intervals until satisfactory breathing is restored. *Do not use analeptic agents.* Oxygen, IV fluids, vasopressors, and other supportive measures should be employed, as needed. Gastric lavage, followed by instillation of activated charcoal, may be useful; dialysis is of little value unless other, dialyzable substances (such as barbiturates) have been simultaneously ingested.

DRUG INTERACTIONS

Other narcotic analgesics; sedative-hypnotics, antianxiety agents, phenothiazines, general anesthetics, and other CNS depressants (including alcohol); MAO inhibitors; tricyclic antidepressants	△ CNS depression; reduce dose of one or both agents if used concomitantly or in close succession
Anticholinergic agents	△ Risk of paralytic ileus

ALTERED LABORATORY VALUES

Blood/serum values	△ Amylase △ Lipase

No clinically significant alterations in urinary values occur at therapeutic dosages

---

USE IN CHILDREN

See INDICATIONS and dosage recommendations

USE IN PREGNANT AND NURSING WOMEN

Safety for use during pregnancy (except during labor) has not been established. Use during labor may result in neonatal respiratory depression, possibly requiring resuscitation. Meperidine is excreted in human milk.

---

[1] Some adverse reactions in ambulatory patients may be alleviated if the patient lies down

DILAUDID

CONTROLLED ANALGESICS

DILAUDID (hydromorphone hydrochloride) Knoll   C-II

Tablets: 1, 2, 3, 4 mg   **Ampuls:** 1, 2, 4 mg/ml (1 ml)   **Vials:** 2 mg/ml (20 ml)   **Suppositories:** 3 mg   **Powder:** 15 gr (for prescription compounding)

INDICATIONS	ORAL DOSAGE	PARENTERAL DOSAGE
Moderate to severe pain	**Adult:** 2 mg q4–6h, as needed; for more severe pain, 4 mg or more q4–6h	**Adult:** 1–2 mg SC or IM q4–6h, as needed, to start

CONTRAINDICATIONS

Intracranial lesion associated with increased intracranial pressure	Depressed ventilatory function	Hypersensitivity to hydromorphone

ADMINISTRATION/DOSAGE ADJUSTMENTS

Rectal use	Suppositories provide long-lasting relief and are particularly useful at night; usual adult dosage: 1 suppository q6–8h
Intravenous administration	Rapid IV injection increases risk of hypotension and respiratory depression; if IV route must be used, inject very slowly, taking at least 2–3 min to administer, and monitor patient closely
Dosage adjustment	A gradual increase in dosage may be necessary if tolerance to narcotic drugs has occurred, tolerance to hydromorphone develops, or pain becomes more severe

WARNINGS/PRECAUTIONS

Drug dependence	Psychic and/or physical dependence and tolerance may develop with prolonged use, especially in addiction-prone patients
Respiratory depression	Characterized by an increase in respiratory rate and/or tidal volume, Cheyne-Stokes respiration, and cyanosis, as well as irregular and periodic breathing, may occur, depending on dose (see OVERDOSAGE)
Ambulatory patients	Caution patients that their ability to engage in potentially hazardous activities requiring full mental alertness or physical coordination may be impaired
Patients with head injuries or other intracranial lesions	The respiratory depressant effects of this drug and its capacity to elevate CSF pressure may be markedly exaggerated in such patients; side effects may also interfere with the clinical evaluation of head injuries
Patients with acute abdominal conditions	Use of this drug may obscure the diagnosis or clinical course of acute abdominal conditions
Cough suppression	May occur; use with caution postoperatively and in patients with pulmonary disease
Other special-risk patients	Use with caution in elderly or debilitated patients and in the presence of hepatic or renal impairment, hypothyroidism, Addison's disease, prostatic hypertrophy, and urethral stricture
Tartrazine sensitivity	Presence of FD&C Yellow No. 5 (tartrazine) in 1-, 2-, and 4-mg tablets may cause allergic-type reactions, including bronchial asthma, in susceptible individuals

ADVERSE REACTIONS

Central nervous system	Sedation, drowsiness, mental clouding, lethargy, impairment of mental and physical performance, anxiety, fear, dysphoria, dizziness, psychic dependence, mood changes
Gastrointestinal	Nausea, vomiting; constipation (with prolonged use)
Cardiovascular	Circulatory depression, peripheral circulatory collapse, and cardiac arrest following rapid IV injection; orthostatic hypotension and fainting upon sudden standing after injection
Genitourinary	Ureteral spasm, vesical sphincter spasm, urinary retention
Respiratory	Depression, irregularities

OVERDOSAGE

Signs and symptoms	Respiratory depression, miosis, extreme somnolence progressing to stupor or coma, skeletal-muscle flaccidity, cold and clammy skin, hypotension, bradycardia, and, in severe cases, apnea, circulatory collapse, and cardiac arrest
Treatment	Maintain patent airway and institute assisted or controlled ventilation, if needed. If drug is not completely absorbed and patient is conscious, induce emesis or use gastric lavage to empty stomach. For significant respiratory depression, administer naloxone (adult, 0.4–0.8 mg) simultaneously with ventilatory assistance. Administer oxygen, IV fluids, vasopressors, and other supportive measures, as needed.

DILAUDID ■ EMPIRIN with Codeine

DRUG INTERACTIONS

Other narcotic analgesics; sedative-hypnotics, antianxiety agents, phenothiazines, general anesthetics, and other CNS depressants (including alcohol); MAO inhibitors; tricyclic antidepressants	⌂ CNS depression; reduce dose of one or both agents if used concomitantly or in close succession
Anticholinergic agents	⌂ Risk of paralytic ileus

ALTERED LABORATORY VALUES

No clinically significant alterations in blood/serum or urinary values occur at therapeutic dosages

USE IN CHILDREN

Safety and effectiveness for use in children have not been established

USE IN PREGNANT AND NURSING WOMEN

Pregnancy Category C: use during pregnancy only if the expected benefit justifies the potential risk to the fetus. Teratogenicity has been reported in hamsters at doses 600 times the normal human dose. Infants born to mothers taking opioids regularly prior to delivery will be physically dependent; those born to mothers taking opioids shortly before delivery may have respiratory depression. It is not known whether hydromorphone is excreted in human milk. Because many drugs are excreted in breast milk and because of the potential for serious adverse reactions, the patient should not nurse if use of this drug is deemed essential.

CONTROLLED ANALGESICS

EMPIRIN with Codeine (aspirin and codeine phosphate) Burroughs Wellcome   C-III

Tablets: 325 mg aspirin and 15 mg (No. 2), 30 mg (No. 3), or 60 mg (No. 4) codeine phosphate

INDICATIONS

Mild, moderate, and moderate to severe pain

ORAL DOSAGE

Adult: 1–2 No. 2 or No. 3 tabs q4h, as needed, or 1 No. 4 tab q4h, as needed; the drug should be taken with food or a full glass of milk or water to lessen gastric irritation

CONTRAINDICATIONS

Hypersensitivity or intolerance to aspirin or codeine	Severe bleeding	Peptic ulcer or other serious gastrointestinal lesions
Anticoagulant therapy	Disorders affecting blood coagulation or primary hemostasis[1]	

WARNINGS/PRECAUTIONS

Aspirin sensitivity	Therapeutic doses of aspirin can cause severe allergic reactions, including anaphylactic shock (see ADVERSE REACTIONS), even in the absence of a history of allergy or prior reaction to aspirin; hypersensitivity is particularly likely in patients with nasal polyps or asthma. Aspirin sensitivity cannot be detected by skin testing or radioimmunoassay procedures.
Bleeding	Significant bleeding may be caused by aspirin therapy in patients with peptic ulcer or other GI lesions, and in those with bleeding disorders; excessive bleeding can also occur following injury or surgery in patients who have taken therapeutic doses of aspirin within the preceding 10 days. A bleeding tendency can be detected by observation of the platelet count, bleeding time, activated partial thromboplastin time, or prothrombin time.
Ambulatory patients	Caution patients not to engage in potentially hazardous activities requiring full mental alertness or physical coordination and to avoid alcohol and other CNS depressants, which may produce additional CNS depression
Patients with head injuries or other intracranial lesions	The respiratory depressant effects of this drug and its capacity to elevate CSF pressure may be markedly exaggerated in such patients; side effects may also interfere with the clinical evaluation of head injuries. Administer with extreme caution and only if use of this drug is deemed essential.
Patients with acute abdominal conditions	Use of this drug may obscure the diagnosis or clinical course of acute abdominal conditions
Patients with hepatic or renal impairment	Use with caution in patients with severe hepatic or renal insufficiency, and monitor the effects of therapy by serial liver and renal function tests

EMPIRIN with Codeine

Other special-risk patients	Use with caution in the elderly or debilitated and in patients with gallbladder disease or gallstones, respiratory impairment, cardiac arrhythmias, inflammatory GI disorders, hypothyroidism, Addison's disease, prostatic hypertrophy, urethral stricture, coagulation disorders, head injuries, or acute abdominal conditions. Hepatotoxicity has occurred with prolonged use of large doses of aspirin in patients with lupus erythematosus, rheumatoid arthritis, and rheumatic disease. Aspirin may cause a mild hemolytic anemia in patients with glucose-6-phosphate dehydrogenase (G6PD) deficiency, and in hyperuricemic patients, it may reduce the effectiveness of uricosuric therapy or precipitate an attack of gout.
Reye's syndrome	Results from pilot epidemiologic studies suggest an association between aspirin and Reye's syndrome; use this product with caution in children, including teenagers, with chicken pox or influenza
Prolonged salicylate therapy	May cause painless erosion of gastric mucosa, occult bleeding, and, rarely, iron-deficiency anemia. Chronic use of large doses of aspirin may result in mild aspirin intoxication (salicylism), manifested by nausea, vomiting, hearing impairment, tinnitus, diminished vision, headache, dizziness, drowsiness, mental confusion, hyperpnea, hyperventilation, tachycardia, sweating, and thirst. Unless specifically indicated, this preparation should not be prescribed for long-term use.
Drug dependence	Codeine may be addictive when used in high doses or over a long period; caution patients not to exceed the dosage, frequency of administration, or duration of therapy prescribed. Dependence may occur at therapeutic doses after 1–2 mo of therapy; withdrawal symptoms are mild. Most patients show no signs of physical dependence on oral codeine upon abrupt withdrawal of long-term therapy.
Carcinogenicity, mutagenicity	Long-term studies in mice and rats have not demonstrated any carcinogenic effects of aspirin, whether given alone or in combination with other drugs. Adequate studies have not been done to determine the carcinogenicity of codeine or the mutagenicity of either aspirin or codeine.

ADVERSE REACTIONS

Central nervous system	Light-headedness, dizziness, drowsiness, euphoria, dysphoria, headache, mental confusion
Gastrointestinal	Nausea, vomiting, constipation, dyspepsia or heartburn (sometimes accompanied by occult bleeding), exacerbation of peptic ulcer symptoms with occasionally extensive bleeding (with high doses)
Dermatological	Pruritus, rash
Otic and ophthalmic	Hearing impairment, tinnitus, diminished vision
Allergic	Skin rash, urticaria, angioedema, rhinorrhea, asthma, abdominal pain, nausea, vomiting, anaphylactic shock
Other	Respiratory depression; hyperpnea; tachycardia; sweating; thirst; bone marrow depression, manifested by weakness, fatigue, or abnormal bruising or bleeding

OVERDOSAGE

Signs and symptoms	*Codeine-related effects:* respiratory depression, miosis, extreme somnolence progressing to stupor or coma, skeletal-muscle flaccidity, cold and clammy skin, bradycardia, hypotension, and, in severe cases, apnea, circulatory collapse, and cardiac arrest; *aspirin-related effects:* hyperpnea, nausea, vomiting, vertigo, tinnitus, flushing, sweating, thirst, headache, drowsiness, diarrhea, and tachycardia, progressing to hyperthermia, hemorrhage, acid-base disturbances, restlessness, confusion, convulsions, vasomotor depression, coma, and respiratory failure
Treatment	Give primary attention to reestablishing adequate respiratory exchange through provision of an adequate airway and assisted or controlled ventilation; positive-pressure respiration may be desirable if pulmonary edema is present. If respiratory depression is significant, promptly administer naloxone (adult, 0.4 mg; child, 0.01 mg/kg), preferably IV, and repeat at 2- to 3-min intervals until satisfactory breathing is restored. *Do not use analeptic agents.* Oxygen, IV fluids, vasopressors, and other supportive measures should be employed, as needed. Gastric lavage, followed by instillation of activated charcoal, may be used if performed within 4 h of ingestion. In moderately severe cases of salicylate poisoning, cautiously administer sodium bicarbonate IV in sufficient quantity, if possible, to maintain an alkaline diuresis; intermittent peritoneal dialysis may also be helpful. In severe cases, hemodialysis should be seriously considered. Hyperthermia, particularly in children, and dehydration require prompt correction. Hemorrhagic phenomena may necessitate whole-blood transfusions and phytonadione (vitamin K$_1$). Do not use barbiturates to treat excitement or convulsions.

DRUG INTERACTIONS

MAO inhibitors	⇧ Pharmacologic effects of MAO inhibitors
Oral anticoagulants	⇧ Hypoprothrombinemia
Oral hypoglycemic agents, insulin	⇧ Hypoglycemia

EMPIRIN with Codeine ■ EMPRACET with Codeine

Mercaptopurine, methotrexate	⇧ Bone marrow toxicity and blood dyscrasias
Penicillins, sulfonamides	⇧ Blood antibiotic levels
Nonsteroidal anti-inflammatory agents	⇧ Risk of peptic ulceration and bleeding
Other narcotic analgesics, alcohol, general anesthetics, tranquilizers (eg, chlordiazepoxide), sedative-hypnotics, other CNS depressants	⇧ CNS depression
Corticosteroids	⇧ Steroid anti-inflammatory effects ⇧ Renal clearance of aspirin, potentially resulting in aspirin intoxication when steroid medication is withdrawn
Para-aminosalicylic acid, furosemide, vitamin C	Accumulation of aspirin and its metabolites to potentially toxic levels
Uricosuric agents (eg, probenecid and sulfinpyrazone)	⇩ Uricosuria

ALTERED LABORATORY VALUES

Blood/serum values	⇧ Amylase ⇧ Lipase ⇧ Prothrombin time ⇧ Uric acid (with low doses) ⇩ Uric acid (with high doses) ⇩ Thyroxine (T$_4$) ⇩ Thyroid-stimulating hormone
Urinary values	⇧ Glucose (with Clinitest tablets)

USE IN CHILDREN

Consult manufacturer

USE IN PREGNANT AND NURSING WOMEN

Pregnancy Category C: use during pregnancy only if clearly needed. Animal reproduction studies have not been conducted with this drug. *Aspirin:* Aspirin has been shown to be teratogenic and embryocidal in mice and rats at 4–6 times the human dose. No teratogenic effects have been observed in women given aspirin, although therapeutic doses in women close to term or prior to delivery may cause bleeding in the mother, fetus, or neonate. Regular use of aspirin in high doses during the last 6 mo of pregnancy has been shown to prolong pregnancy and delivery. *Codeine:* Rats and rabbits given up to 150 times the human dose have shown no evidence of impaired fertility or fetal harm; however, codeine given during labor may depress respiration in the neonate. Both aspirin and codeine are excreted in human breast milk in small amounts; because of the potential for harm to the infant, a decision should be made whether to stop nursing or discontinue use of the drug.

[1] Including hemophilia, hypoprothrombinemia, von Willebrand's disease, the thrombocytopenias, thrombasthenia and other ill-defined hereditary platelet dysfunctions, and associated conditions, such as severe vitamin K deficiency and severe liver damage

---

CONTROLLED ANALGESICS

EMPRACET with Codeine (acetaminophen and codeine phosphate) Burroughs Wellcome C-III

Tablets: 300 mg acetaminophen and 30 mg (No. 3) or 60 mg (No. 4) codeine phosphate

INDICATIONS

Mild to moderate pain

Moderate to moderately severe pain

ORAL DOSAGE

Adult: 1–2 No. 3 tabs q4h, as needed

Adult: 1 No. 4 tab q4h, as needed

CONTRAINDICATIONS

Hypersensitivity to acetaminophen or codeine

WARNINGS/PRECAUTIONS

Drug dependence	Psychic and/or physical dependence and tolerance may develop, especially in addiction-prone individuals
Ambulatory patients	Caution patients that their ability to engage in potentially hazardous activities requiring full mental alertness or physical coordination may be impaired
Patients with head injuries or other intracranial lesions	The respiratory depressant effects of this drug and its capacity to elevate CSF pressure may be markedly exaggerated in such patients; side effects may also interfere with the clinical evaluation of head injuries
Patients with acute abdominal conditions	Use of this drug may obscure the diagnosis or clinical course of acute abdominal conditions

EMPRACET with Codeine ■ EQUAGESIC

Other special-risk patients	Use with caution in the elderly or debilitated and in patients with severe hepatic or renal impairment, hypothyroidism, Addison's disease, prostatic hypertrophy, or urethral stricture

ADVERSE REACTIONS[1]

The most frequent reactions, regardless of incidence, are printed in *italics*

Central nervous system	*Light-headedness, dizziness, sedation,* euphoria, dysphoria
Gastrointestinal	*Nausea, vomiting,* constipation
Other	*Shortness of breath,* pruritus

OVERDOSAGE

Signs and symptoms	*Codeine-related effects:* respiratory depression, miosis, extreme somnolence progressing to stupor or coma, skeletal-muscle flaccidity, cold and clammy skin, bradycardia, hypotension, and, in severe cases, apnea, circulatory collapse, and cardiac arrest; *acetaminophen-related effects:* nausea, anorexia, vomiting, abdominal pain, diarrhea, diaphoresis, malaise; hepatotoxicity may not be evident until after 2–4 days
Treatment	Give primary attention to reestablishing adequate respiratory exchange through provision of an adequate airway and assisted or controlled ventilation; positive-pressure respiration may be desirable if pulmonary edema is present. If respiratory depression is significant, promptly administer naloxone. For adults, give 0.4–2 mg IV (or, if necessary, IM or SC) at 2- to 3-min intervals, as needed; for children, give 0.01 mg/kg IV, followed, if necessary, by 0.1 mg/kg IV (administer IM or SC in divided doses if IV administration is not feasible). Keep the patient under constant surveillance since the duration of action of codeine may exceed that of naloxone; if significant respiratory depression recurs, repeat naloxone dose. *Do not use analeptic agents.* Oxygen, IV fluids, vasopressors, and other supportive measures should be employed, as needed.
	Promptly empty stomach by performing gastric lavage or inducing emesis. Administer oral acetylcysteine as soon as possible (no later than 24 h after ingestion); give a loading dose of 140 mg/kg and then, at 4-h intervals, 17 maintenance doses of 70 mg/kg. (Activated charcoal, if used, should be removed before acetylcysteine is given.) Measure the plasma level of unconjugated acetaminophen as early as possible, but no sooner than 4 h after ingestion. Determine prothrombin time, SGOT and SGPT levels, and serum concentrations of bilirubin, creatinine, BUN, glucose, and electrolytes every 24 h. If the prothrombin time exceeds 1.5 times the control value, give vitamin K_1; if the prothrombin time exceeds 3 times this value, give fresh frozen plasma. Institute appropriate measures to treat hypoglycemia and electrolyte and fluid imbalance. Avoid forced diuresis or use of diuretics when treating an acetaminophen overdose. For additional information on use of acetylcysteine and interpretation of the plasma acetaminophen level, see Mucomyst chart.

DRUG INTERACTIONS

Other narcotic analgesics; sedative-hypnotics, antianxiety agents, phenothiazines, general anesthetics, and other CNS depressants (including alcohol); MAO inhibitors; tricyclic antidepressants	△ CNS depression; reduce dose of one or both agents if used concomitantly or in close succession
Anticholinergic agents	△ Risk of paralytic ileus

ALTERED LABORATORY VALUES

Blood/serum values	△ Amylase △ Lipase ▽ Glucose (with glucose oxidase/peroxidase tests)
Urinary values	△ 5-HIAA (with nitrosonaphthol reagent test)

USE IN CHILDREN
Consult manufacturer

USE IN PREGNANT AND NURSING WOMEN
Safety for use during pregnancy has not been established; use during pregnancy only if the potential benefits outweigh the possible hazards. It is not known whether acetaminophen or codeine is excreted in human milk; use with caution in nursing mothers because many drugs are excreted in human milk.

[1] Some frequent reactions may be alleviated if the patient lies down

---

CONTROLLED ANALGESICS

EQUAGESIC (meprobamate and aspirin) Wyeth

C-IV

Tablets: 200 mg meprobamate and 325 mg aspirin

INDICATIONS

Pain, when it is associated with musculoskeletal disease and accompanied by tension or anxiety[1] (adjunctive therapy)

ORAL DOSAGE

Adult: 1–2 tabs tid or qid, as needed; to avoid oversedation, use the lowest effective dosage, particularly for elderly or debilitated patients

EQUAGESIC

CONTRAINDICATIONS

Acute intermittent porphyria	Allergic or idiosyncratic reaction to aspirin, meprobamate, or related compounds

WARNINGS/PRECAUTIONS

Drug dependence	Psychic and/or physical dependence and tolerance may develop, especially in addiction-prone patients; chronic intoxication is characterized by ataxia, slurred speech, and vertigo. Abrupt withdrawal after prolonged and excessive use may precipitate anxiety, anorexia, insomnia, vomiting, ataxia, tremors, muscle twitching, confusional states, hallucinosis, or, in rare cases, convulsions; to avoid withdrawal reactions when excessive doses have been taken for weeks or months, reduce the dosage of this preparation gradually over a period of 1–2 wk or, alternatively, substitute a short-acting barbiturate and discontinue that drug gradually.
Drowsiness, ataxia, dizziness	Caution patients about driving or engaging in other potentially hazardous activities that require mental alertness or physical coordination
Seizures	This preparation may occasionally cause seizures in epileptic patients; abrupt withdrawal after prolonged and excessive use is more likely to precipitate convulsions in patients with CNS damage or convulsive disorders than in other patients
Patients with renal or hepatic impairment	Use with caution in patients with compromised renal or hepatic function; meprobamate is metabolized in the liver and excreted by the kidney
Potentially suicidal patients	Use with caution in patients with suicidal tendencies; prescribe in small quantities
Other special-risk patients	Use in patients allergic to salicylates is contraindicated because, in rare instances, life-threatening allergic episodes may occur. Use with extreme caution in patients with peptic ulcer, asthma, or coagulation disorders (eg, hypoprothrombinemia, vitamin K deficiency).

ADVERSE REACTIONS

Central nervous system	Drowsiness, ataxia, dizziness, slurred speech, headache, vertigo, weakness, paresthesias, impaired visual accommodation, euphoria, overstimulation, paradoxical excitement, fast EEG activity, tinnitus
Gastrointestinal	Nausea, vomiting, diarrhea, epigastric discomfort
Cardiovascular	Palpitations, arrhythmia (including tachycardia), transient ECG changes, syncope, hypotensive crisis
Allergic or idiosyncratic	Urticaria; itchy, urticarial, or erythematous maculopapular rash; leukopenia; purpura (including acute nonthrombocytopenic purpura); petechiae; ecchymoses; eosinophilia; peripheral edema; adenopathy; fixed drug eruption; fever; hyperpyrexia; chills; angioneurotic edema; bronchospasm; asthma; oliguria; anuria; anaphylaxis; exfoliative dermatitis; stomatitis; proctitis; Stevens-Johnson syndrome; bullous dermatitis
Other	Exacerbation of porphyric symptoms; thrombocytopenic purpura[2]

OVERDOSAGE

Signs and symptoms	*Aspirin-related effects:* hyperpnea, nausea, vomiting, vertigo, tinnitus, flushing, sweating, thirst, headache, drowsiness, diarrhea, and tachycardia, progressing to hyperthermia, dehydration, hemorrhage, acid-base disturbances, restlessness, confusion, convulsions, vasomotor depression, coma, and respiratory failure; *meprobamate-related effects:* drowsiness, lethargy, stupor, ataxia, and light coma (with serum levels of 3–10 mg/dl); deeper coma, shock, and vasomotor and respiratory collapse (with serum levels exceeding 10 mg/dl)
Treatment	If less than 4 h have elapsed since ingestion, induce emesis or perform gastric lavage, followed by activated charcoal, to remove any remaining drug from the stomach. Initial therapy should be directed at reducing hyperthemia by external sponging with tepid water, correcting dehydration by appropriate IV fluid replacement, and maintaining adequate cardiorespiratory and renal function. Use CNS stimulants and vasopressors with caution. In moderately severe cases of salicylate poisoning, cautiously administer sodium bicarbonate IV in sufficient quantity, if possible, to maintain an alkaline diuresis; carefully monitor urinary output and avoid overhydration. Hemodialysis, peritoneal dialysis, and diuretics (including mannitol) may be useful. Potassium should be added to the repair solution to compensate for potassium losses once urine formation is deemed adequate. Glucose may be provided to correct ketosis and hypoglycemia. Plasma transfusion may be beneficial if shock intervenes. Hemorrhagic phenomena may necessitate whole-blood transfusions and phytonadione (vitamin K_1). Do not administer barbiturates to treat excitement or convulsions.

DRUG INTERACTIONS

Anticoagulants	⟁ Risk of bleeding; use with extreme caution in patients receiving anticoagulants
Alcohol	⟁ CNS depression; exercise appropriate caution ⟁ Risk of GI ulceration
Other narcotic analgesics; sedative-hypnotics, antianxiety agents, phenothiazines, general anesthetics, and other CNS depressants; MAO inhibitors; tricyclic antidepressants	⟁ CNS depression; exercise appropriate caution

EQUAGESIC ■ FIORINAL

Probenecid, sulfinpyrazone	⇩ Uricosuria
Sulfonylureas	⇧ Hypoglycemic effect
Methotrexate	⇧ Risk of methotrexate toxicity
Antacids, other urinary alkalinizers, corticosteroids	⇩ Serum level of aspirin component
Ammonium chloride, other urinary acidifiers	⇧ Serum level of aspirin component

ALTERED LABORATORY VALUES

Blood/serum values	⇧ Prothrombin time ⇧ Uric acid (with low doses) ⇩ Uric acid (with high doses) ⇩ Thyroxine (T$_4$) ⇩ Thyroid-stimulating hormone
Urinary values	⇧ Glucose (with Clinitest tablets)

USE IN CHILDREN

This preparation is not recommended for children under 13 yr of age

USE IN PREGNANT AND NURSING WOMEN

Several studies have suggested that meprobamate increases the risk of congenital malformations; use of this preparation during the first trimester of pregnancy should almost always be avoided. The concentration of meprobamate in human milk is 2–4 times the maternal plasma level.

[1] Effectiveness for long-term use (> 4 mo) has not been established
[2] Agranulocytosis and aplastic anemia have been reported; however, a causal relationship has not been established

---

CONTROLLED ANALGESICS

FIORINAL (butalbital, aspirin, and caffeine)   Sandoz Pharmaceuticals   C-III

Capsules: 50 mg butalbital, 325 mg aspirin, and 40 mg caffeine   **Tablets:** 50 mg butalbital, 325 mg aspirin, and 40 mg caffeine

INDICATIONS	ORAL DOSAGE
Tension (muscle contraction) headache	Adult: 1–2 caps or tabs q4h, up to 6 caps or tabs per day

CONTRAINDICATIONS	
Porphyria	Hypersensitivity to aspirin, caffeine, or barbiturates

WARNINGS/PRECAUTIONS	
Drug dependence	Psychic and/or physical dependence and tolerance may develop, especially in addiction-prone individuals
Ambulatory patients	Caution patients that their ability to engage in potentially hazardous activities requiring full mental alertness or physical coordination may be impaired and to avoid alcohol and other CNS depressants, which may produce additional CNS depression

ADVERSE REACTIONS	Frequent reactions (incidence ≥ 1%) are printed in *italics*
Central nervous system	*Drowsiness, dizziness,* light-headedness
Gastrointestinal	Nausea, vomiting, flatulence

OVERDOSAGE	
Signs and symptoms	*Butalbital-related effects:* drowsiness, confusion, coma, respiratory depression, hypotension, shock; *aspirin-related effects:* hyperpnea, nausea, vomiting, vertigo, tinnitus, flushing, sweating, thirst, headache, drowsiness, diarrhea, and tachycardia, progressing to hyperthermia, hemorrhage, acid-base disturbances, restlessness, confusion, convulsions, vasomotor depression, coma, and respiratory failure; *caffeine-related effects:* insomnia, restlessness, and excitement, progressing to mild delirium, dehydration, fever, tachycardia, extrasystoles, tremor, and convulsions
Treatment	Induce emesis if patient is conscious. Gastric lavage may be used if pharyngeal and laryngeal reflexes are intact and less than 4 h have elapsed since ingestion; a cuffed endotracheal tube should be inserted before performing lavage on an unconscious patient or when necessary to provide assisted respiration. Meticulous attention should be given to maintaining adequate pulmonary ventilation. Severe hypotension may require IV use of norepinephrine or phenylephrine for correction. In moderately severe cases of salicylate poisoning, cautiously administer sodium bicarbonate in sufficient quantity, if possible, to maintain an alkaline diuresis; intermittent peritoneal dialysis may also be helpful. In severe cases, hemodialysis should be seriously considered. Hyperthermia, particularly in children, and dehydration require prompt correction. Hemorrhagic phenomena may necessitate whole-blood transfusions and phytonadione (vitamin K$_1$). Do not administer barbiturates to treat excitement or convulsions.

FIORINAL ■ FIORINAL with Codeine

DRUG INTERACTIONS

Other sedative-hypnotics; narcotic analgesics, antianxiety agents, phenothiazines, general anesthetics, and other CNS depressants (including alcohol); MAO inhibitors	△ CNS depression; reduce dose of one or both agents if used concomitantly or in close succession
Alcohol, corticosteroids, phenylbutazone, oxyphenbutazone	△ Risk of GI ulceration
Probenecid, sulfinpyrazone	▽ Uricosuric effect
Spironolactone	▽ Diuretic effect
Methotrexate	△ Methotrexate plasma level and risk of toxicity
Corticosteroids, digitalis, digitoxin, doxycycline, tricyclic antidepressants	▽ Serum half-life and drug effect
Griseofulvin	▽ Absorption of griseofulvin

ALTERED LABORATORY VALUES

Blood/serum values	△ Prothrombin time △ Uric acid (with low doses) ▽ Uric acid (with high doses) ▽ Thyroxine (T_4) ▽ Thyroid-stimulating hormone △ Glucose ▽ Bilirubin
Urinary values	△ Glucose (with Clinitest tablets) △ 5-HIAA (with nitrosonaphthol reagent test)

USE IN CHILDREN

Safety and effectiveness for use in children under 12 yr of age have not been established

---

USE IN PREGNANT AND NURSING WOMEN

Safety for use during pregnancy has not been established; may be administered to pregnant women only when clearly indicated. Aspirin and barbiturates appear in breast milk. Effects on infants are unknown, although serum levels are considered insignificant with therapeutic doses.

CONTROLLED ANALGESICS

FIORINAL with Codeine (butalbital, aspirin, caffeine, and codeine phosphate) Sandoz Pharmaceuticals   C-III

Capsules: 50 mg butalbital, 325 mg aspirin, 40 mg caffeine, and 7.5 mg (No. 1), 15 mg (No. 2), or 30 mg (No. 3) codeine phosphate

INDICATIONS	ORAL DOSAGE
Pain that does not need to be treated with morphine or equipotent analgesics	**Adult:** 1–2 caps, as needed, up to 6 caps/day; give each dose with solid food or a full glass of milk or water

CONTRAINDICATIONS

Hypersensitivity or intolerance to aspirin, caffeine, butalbital, or codeine   Peptic ulcer or other serious GI lesions   Porphyria

WARNINGS/PRECAUTIONS

Hypersensitivity to aspirin	To reduce the risk of hypersensitivity reactions, use with caution in patients with a history of allergies; bear in mind that these reactions are relatively common in patients with asthma and are particularly likely to occur in patients with nasal polyps
Drowsiness, dizziness	Caution patients about driving or engaging in other potentially hazardous activities requiring mental alertness or physical coordination
Drug dependence	Tolerance, psychological dependence, and physical addiction may develop with use at high doses or for long periods; caution patients not to exceed the dose, frequency of administration, and duration of therapy that have been prescribed. To treat butalbital dependence, reduce dosage cautiously and gradually; abrupt cessation after prolonged use of high doses may precipitate withdrawal reactions, including delirium and convulsions.

ADVERSE REACTIONS

Central nervous system	Dizziness, weakness, drowsiness, lethargy
Gastrointestinal	Nausea, vomiting, constipation

OVERDOSAGE

Signs and symptoms	Drowsiness, confusion, restlessness, delirium, convulsions, coma, miosis, respiratory depression, tinnitus, hypotension, shock, hyperpnea, acid-base disturbances (including metabolic acidosis), hypoprothrombinemia, hyperthermia, vomiting, abdominal pain

FIORINAL with Codeine ■ MEPERGAN

Treatment	Induce emesis if patient is conscious. Gastric lavage may be performed when pharyngeal and laryngeal reflexes are intact and less than 4 h have elapsed since ingestion; use a cuffed endotracheal tube for unconscious patients. Give meticulous attention to maintenance of pulmonary function and provide assisted or controlled ventilation when necessary. For reversal of hypotension, administration of norepinephrine or phenylephrine may be required. If respiratory or cardiovascular depression is significant, naloxone may be used; however, bear in mind that respiratory depression may result from both butalbital and codeine and therefore may not be fully reversed by a narcotic antagonist such as naloxone. To enhance urinary output, alkalinize urine, and to correct electrolyte disturbances, use an IV solution such as 1% sodium bicarbonate in 5% dextrose. Treat hypoprothrombinemia with IV vitamin K_1 and methemoglobinemia over 30% with IV methylene blue. For severe toxicity, perform peritoneal dialysis, hemodialysis, or an exchange transfusion.

DRUG INTERACTIONS

Other CNS depressants, including alcohol	△ CNS depression; reduce dose of one or both agents if used concomitantly or in close succession. Instruct patients to avoid consuming alcohol during therapy and to use CNS depressants with this preparation only when so directed.
Oral anticoagulants	△ or ▽ Hematological response (aspirin increases the risk of bleeding, while butalbital reduces the pharmacologic effect of anticoagulants)
Heparin	△ Risk of bleeding
Chloramphenicol	▽ Plasma level of chloramphenicol △ Plasma level of butalbital component
Methotrexate	△ Pharmacologic effect of methotrexate
Oral contraceptives	▽ Pharmacologic effect of oral contraceptives
Methoxyflurane	△ Risk of methoxyflurane-induced nephrotoxicity
Corticosteroids	▽ Pharmacologic effect of corticosteroids ▽ Plasma level of aspirin
Naltrexone	▽ Pharmacologic effect of codeine
Doxycycline, griseofulvin, quinidine, theophylline, metoprolol, propranolol, digitoxin, doxorubicin, metronidazole, tricyclic antidepressants	▽ Plasma level of interacting drug

ALTERED LABORATORY VALUES

Blood/serum values	△ Amylase △ Lipase ▽ Potassium
Urinary values	▽ PSP ▽ VMA (with Pisano method) △ VMA (with other methods) Interference with fluorescent test for 5-HIAA and with Gerhardt test for acetoacetic acid

USE IN CHILDREN

Safety and effectiveness for use in children under 12 yr of age have not been established

USE IN PREGNANT AND NURSING WOMEN

Pregnancy Category C: no adequate, well-controlled studies have been performed to determine whether this preparation can affect fertility or fetal development. Although no adverse effects on fetal development have been reported in over 20 yr of marketing and clinical experience, the possibility of infrequent or subtle damage to the fetus cannot be ruled out. Use during pregnancy only if clearly needed. Salicylates, codeine, caffeine, and barbiturates are excreted in human milk; use with caution in nursing mothers.

CONTROLLED ANALGESICS

MEPERGAN (meperidine hydrochloride and promethazine hydrochloride) Wyeth   C-II

Cartridge-needle units: 25 mg meperidine hydrochloride and 25 mg promethazine hydrochloride per ml (2 ml)   **Vials:** 25 mg meperidine hydrochloride and 25 mg promethazine hydrochloride per ml (10 ml)

INDICATIONS

Preanesthetic medication, when both analgesia and sedation are desired
As an adjunct to local or general anesthesia

PARENTERAL DOSAGE

Adult: 1–2 ml (25–50 mg of each component) IM, repeated q3–4h, as needed
Child: 0.02 ml (0.5 mg of each component)/lb IM, repeated q3–4h, as needed

MEPERGAN

MEPERGAN Fortis (meperidine hydrochloride and promethazine hydrochloride) Wyeth   C-II

Capsules: 50 mg meperidine hydrochloride and 25 mg promethazine hydrochloride

INDICATIONS	ORAL DOSAGE
Moderate pain, when both analgesia and sedation are desired	Adult: 1 cap q4–6h, as needed

CONTRAINDICATIONS

Subcutaneous or intraarterial injection (see WARNINGS/PRECAUTIONS)	MAO inhibitor therapy (see WARNINGS/PRECAUTIONS)	Hypersensitivity to meperidine or promethazine

ADMINISTRATION/DOSAGE ADJUSTMENTS

Intravenous administration	Rapid IV injection increases risk of adverse reactions, including severe respiratory depression, apnea, hypotension, peripheral circulatory collapse, and cardiac arrest. If IV administration is necessary, inject very slowly ($\leq$ 1 ml/min), preferably through the tubing of an IV infusion set that is functioning satisfactorily. Patient should be lying down, and a narcotic antagonist and facilities for assisted or controlled respiration should be on hand. If patient complains of pain, perivascular extravasation or inadvertent intraarterial injection, which can result in gangrene of the affected extremity, may have occurred; stop injection immediately and evaluate cause of pain. Injection into or near peripheral nerves may result in permanent neurological deficit.
Concomitant use of other CNS depressants	Use with great caution and at reduced dosage in patients who are concurrently receiving other CNS depressants (see DRUG INTERACTIONS); respiratory depression, hypotension, and profound sedation or coma may result. Reduce dosage of barbiturates by at least $1/2$ and of other analgesic CNS depressants by $1/4$ to $1/2$. Do not mix barbiturates with Mepergan in the same syringe; solutions are chemically incompatible.
Concomitant use of anticholinergic agents for preoperative medication	If desired, Mepergan may be mixed in the same syringe with 0.3–0.4 mg atropine sulfate, 0.25–0.4 mg scopolamine hydrobromide, or other appropriate atropine-like drugs

WARNINGS/PRECAUTIONS

Subcutaneous or intraarterial injection	Chemical irritation and, rarely, necrotic lesions, may occur with subcutaneous injection, and severe arteriospasm and resultant gangrene may occur with intraarterial injection
MAO inhibitor therapy	Therapeutic doses of meperidine have precipitated unpredictable, severe, and occasionally fatal reactions in patients who have received MAO inhibitors within 14 days of treatment with meperidine
Drug dependence	Psychic and/or physical dependence and tolerance may develop, especially in addiction-prone individuals
Ambulatory patients	Caution patients that their ability to engage in potentially hazardous activities requiring full mental alertness or physical coordination may be impaired
Patients with head injuries or other intracranial lesions	The respiratory depressant effects of this drug and its capacity to elevate CSF pressure may be markedly exaggerated in such patients; side effects may also interfere with the clinical evaluation of head injuries. Administer with extreme caution and only if use of this drug is deemed essential.
Patients with acute abdominal conditions	Use of this drug may obscure the diagnosis or clinical course of acute abdominal conditions
Patients with asthma or other respiratory conditions	Therapeutic doses may decrease respiratory drive while increasing airway resistance to the point of apnea; use with extreme caution during an acute asthmatic attack and in the presence of chronic obstructive pulmonary disease, cor pulmonale, substantially decreased respiratory reserve, respiratory depression, hypoxia, or hypercapnia
Severe hypotension	May occur in postoperative patients or in any patient whose ability to maintain blood pressure is lowered by depleted blood volume or by administration of phenothiazines or certain anesthetics; ambulatory patients may experience orthostatic hypotension
Increased ventricular response rate	May occur due to potential vagolytic action of meperidine; use with caution in patients with atrial flutter and other supraventricular tachycardias
Convulsive disorders	May be aggravated; convulsions may occur in patients with no prior history of seizures if tolerance develops and doses substantially exceeding recommended levels are taken
Antiemetic effect	Use of this drug may mask symptoms of unrecognized disease and interfere with diagnosis
Other special-risk patients	Use with caution and reduce initial dosage in elderly or debilitated patients and in patients with severe hepatic or renal impairment, hypothyroidism, Addison's disease, and prostatic hypertrophy or urethral stricture

MEPERGAN ■ MICRAININ

ADVERSE REACTIONS[1]	Frequent reactions (incidence ≥ 1%) are printed in *italics*
Central nervous system and neuromuscular	*Light-headedness, dizziness, sedation,* euphoria, dysphoria, weakness, headache, agitation, tremor, uncoordinated muscle movements, transient hallucinations, disorientation, visual disturbances; extrapyramidal reactions (rare)
Respiratory	Depression, arrest
Gastrointestinal	*Nausea, vomiting,* dry mouth, constipation, biliary tract spasm
Cardiovascular	Flushing of the face, tachycardia, bradycardia, palpitations, faintness, syncope, mild hypotension or hypertension, venous thrombosis (at injection site), circulatory depression, shock, cardiac arrest
Genitourinary	Urinary retention, antidiuretic effect
Hypersensitivity	Pruritus, urticaria, rash, wheal and flare over vein at IV site; photosensitivity (rare)
Hematological	Leukopenia (rare), agranulocytosis (one case)
Other	*Sweating,* pain at injection site, local induration and irritation following SC injection

OVERDOSAGE

Signs and symptoms	*Meperidine-related effects:* respiratory depression, miosis, extreme somnolence progressing to stupor or coma, skeletal-muscle flaccidity, cold and clammy skin, bradycardia, hypotension, and, in severe cases, apnea, circulatory collapse, and cardiac arrest; *promethazine-related effects:* deep sedation, coma, and (rarely) convulsions and cardiorespiratory symptoms compatible with the depth of sedation present; extrapyramidal reactions
Treatment	Give primary attention to reestablishing adequate respiratory exchange through provision of an adequate airway and assisted or controlled ventilation; positive-pressure respiration may be desirable if pulmonary edema is present. If respiratory depression is significant, promptly administer naloxone (adult, 0.4 mg; child, 0.01 mg/kg), preferably IV, and repeat at 2- to 3-min intervals until satisfactory breathing is restored. *Do not use analeptic agents.* Oxygen, IV fluids, vasopressors, and other supportive measures should be employed, as needed. Treat extrapyramidal reactions with anticholinergic antiparkinson agents or diphenhydramine. Severe hypotension may be treated with norepinephrine or phenylephrine; do not use epinephrine. Gastric lavage, followed by instillation of activated charcoal, may be useful in cases of acute overdose ingestion; dialysis is of little value unless other, dialyzable substances (such as barbiturates) have been simultaneously ingested.

DRUG INTERACTIONS

Other narcotic analgesics and phenothiazines; sedative-hypnotics, antianxiety agents, general anesthetics, and other CNS depressants (including alcohol); MAO inhibitors; tricyclic antidepressants	△ CNS depression; reduce dose of one or both agents if used concomitantly or in close succession
Anticholinergic agents	△ Risk of paralytic ileus
Anticonvulsants	▽ Convulsive threshold; anticonvulsant dosage may need upward adjustment
Epinephrine	Severe hypotension

ALTERED LABORATORY VALUES

Blood/serum values	△ Amylase △ Lipase
Urinary values	False-positive or false-negative pregnancy tests

USE IN CHILDREN

See INDICATIONS and PARENTERAL DOSAGE for Mepergan; consult manufacturer for use of Mepergan Fortis in children

USE IN PREGNANT AND NURSING WOMEN

Safety for use during pregnancy (except during labor) has not been established. Use during labor may result in neonatal respiratory depression, possibly requiring resuscitation. Meperidine is excreted in breast milk.

[1] Some adverse reactions in ambulatory patients may be alleviated if the patient lies down

---

CONTROLLED ANALGESICS

MICRAININ (meprobamate and aspirin) Wallace C-IV

Tablets: 200 mg meprobamate and 325 mg aspirin

INDICATIONS	**ORAL DOSAGE**
Pain accompanied by tension and/or anxiety in patients with musculoskeletal disease (adjunctive therapy)	**Adult:** 1–2 tabs tid or qid, as needed, up to 2,400 mg of meprobamate/day

MICRAININ

CONTRAINDICATIONS

Acute intermittent porphyria	Hypersensitivity or severe intolerance to aspirin, meprobamate, or related compounds

WARNINGS/PRECAUTIONS

Drug dependence	Psychic and/or physical dependence and tolerance may develop; use with caution in addiction-prone individuals and watch for signs of chronic intoxication, such as ataxia, slurred speech, and vertigo
Abrupt discontinuation of therapy after prolonged or excessive use	May precipitate recurrence of preexisting symptoms, such as anxiety, anorexia, or insomnia, or withdrawal symptoms, such as vomiting, ataxia, tremors, muscle twitching, confusion, hallucinations, and rarely, convulsive seizures, especially in patients with CNS damage or preexisting or latent convulsive disorders; to minimize withdrawal symptoms, gradually reduce dosage over a period of 1–2 wk or substitute (and then gradually withdraw) a short-acting barbiturate
Ambulatory patients	Caution patients that their ability to engage in potentially hazardous activities requiring full mental alertness or physical coordination may be impaired by the meprobamate component
Patients with hepatic or renal impairment	Use with caution and monitor patient for signs of excessive drug accumulation (see OVERDOSAGE)
Seizures	May be precipitated occasionally in epileptic patients
Allergic or idiosyncratic reactions	May occur due to meprobamate component (see ADVERSE REACTIONS); cross-sensitivity with metabumate and carbromal may exist. Institute appropriate symptomatic therapy, including, where appropriate, antihistamines, epinephrine, and, in severe cases, corticosteroids. Rarely, use of aspirin in persons allergic to salicylates can result in life-threatening allergic episodes.
Other special-risk patients	Use with extreme caution in patients with peptic ulcer or coagulation abnormalities

ADVERSE REACTIONS

Central nervous system	Drowsiness, ataxia, dizziness, slurred speech, headache, vertigo, weakness, paresthesias, impairment of visual accommodation, euphoria, overstimulation, paradoxical excitement, fast EEG activity
Gastrointestinal	Nausea, vomiting, diarrhea
Cardiovascular	Palpitations, tachycardia, arrhythmias, transient ECG changes, syncope, hypotensive crisis (one fatal case)
Hypersensitivity	Itchy, urticarial, or erythematous maculopapular rash (either generalized or confined to groin); leukopenia; acute nonthrombocytopenic purpura; petechiae, ecchymoses; eosinophilia; peripheral edema; adenopathy; fever; fixed drug eruption; rarely, hyperpyrexia, chills, angioneurotic edema, bronchospasm, oliguria, anuria, anaphylaxis, erythema multiforme, exfoliative dermatitis, stomatitis, proctitis, Stevens-Johnson syndrome, and bullous dermatitis (one fatal case)
Hematological	Thrombocytopenic purpura (rare)[1]
Other	Exacerbation of porphyric symptoms

OVERDOSAGE

Signs and symptoms	*Meprobamate-related effects:* drowsiness, lethargy, stupor, ataxia, coma, shock, vasomotor and respiratory collapse; *aspirin-related effects:* hyperpnea, nausea, vomiting, vertigo, tinnitus, flushing, sweating, thirst, headache, drowsiness, diarrhea, and tachycardia progressing to hyperthermia, hemorrhage, acid-base disturbances, restlessness, confusion, convulsions, vasomotor depression, coma, and respiratory failure
Treatment	Induce emesis or perform gastric lavage, followed by activated charcoal, to remove any remaining drug from stomach. (Incomplete gastric emptying and delayed absorption may lead to fatal relapse.) Institute appropriate supportive measures, including respiratory assistance, and cautious use of pressor agents, as indicated. In moderately severe cases of salicylate poisoning, cautiously administer sodium bicarbonate IV in sufficient quantity, if possible, to maintain an alkaline diuresis; intermittent peritoneal dialysis may also be helpful. In severe cases, hemodialysis should be seriously considered. Hyperthermia, particularly in children, and dehydration require prompt correction. Hemorrhagic phenomena may necessitate whole-blood transfusions and phytonadione (vitamin K_1). Do not administer barbiturates to treat excitement or convulsions.

DRUG INTERACTIONS

Other narcotic analgesics and sedative-hypnotics; antianxiety agents, phenothiazines, general anesthetics, and other CNS depressants (including alcohol); MAO inhibitors; tricyclic antidepressants	↑ CNS depression; reduce dose of one or both agents if used concomitantly or in close succession
Alcohol, corticosteroids phenylbutazone, oxyphenbutazone	↑ Risk of GI ulceration
Probenecid, sulfinpyrazone	↓ Uricosuric effect

MICRAININ ■ Morphine

| Spironolactone | ⇩ Diuretic effect |
| Methotrexate | ⇧ Methotrexate plasma level and/or toxicity |

ALTERED LABORATORY VALUES

| Blood/serum values | ⇧ Prothrombin time   ⇧ Uric acid (with low doses)   ⇩ Uric acid (with high doses)
⇩ Thyroxine (T_4)   ⇩ Thyroid-stimulating hormone |
| Urinary values | ⇧ Glucose (with Clinitest tablets) |

USE IN CHILDREN
Not recommended for use in children under 12 yr of age

USE IN PREGNANT AND NURSING WOMEN
Use of antianxiety agents during pregnancy should almost always be avoided. An increased risk of congenital malformations during the first trimester has been associated with minor tranquilizers, including meprobamate. Aspirin may also have teratogenic effects. Both meprobamate and aspirin cross the placental barrier and have been detected in human milk. Meprobamate appears in breast milk in concentrations 2–4 times that of maternal plasma.

[1] Other reactions for which a causal relationship has not been established include agranulocytosis and aplastic anemia

---

CONTROLLED ANALGESICS

Morphine sulfate injection

C-II

Ampuls: 8, 10, 15 mg (1 ml)   **Vials:** 5, 8, 10 mg/ml (1 ml); 15 mg/ml (1, 20 ml)   **Cartridge-needle units:** 2, 4, 8, 10, 15 mg/ml (1 ml)   **Soluble hypodermic tablets:** 10, 15, 30 mg

INDICATIONS
Severe pain
Preoperative medication

PARENTERAL DOSAGE
Adult: 5–20 mg SC or IM q4h, as needed
Child: 0.1–0.2 mg/kg, up to 15 mg, SC or IM q4h, as needed

CONTRAINDICATIONS
Hypersensitivity to morphine

Prematurity or delivery of a premature infant

ADMINISTRATION/DOSAGE ADJUSTMENTS

| Intravenous administration | If necessary, 4–10 mg, diluted in 4–5 ml of Sterile Water for Injection, may be given IV. Inject the drug very slowly over a period of 4–5 min; rapid IV administration increases the risk of adverse reactions and may cause severe respiratory depression, apnea, hypotension, peripheral circulatory collapse, and cardiac arrest, as well as anaphylactoid reactions. A narcotic antagonist (eg, naloxone) and facilities for resuscitation and assisted or controlled respiration must be immediately available, and the patient should be lying down. |

WARNINGS/PRECAUTIONS

Drug dependence	Psychic and/or physical dependence and tolerance may develop, especially in addiction-prone individuals
Hypotensive effect	Severe hypotension may occur in patients whose ability to maintain blood pressure has been compromised by a depleted blood volume or concurrent administration of phenothiazines or certain anesthetics
Impaired perfusion of injection site	Exercise caution in injecting morphine SC or IM if the area is chilled or if the patient is hypotensive or in shock; repeated administration may result in an excessive amount being suddenly absorbed if normal circulation is reestablished
Ambulatory patients	Caution patients that their ability to engage in potentially hazardous activities requiring full mental alertness or physical coordination may be impaired, that alcohol and other CNS depressants may produce additional CNS depression, and that orthostatic hypotension may occur
Patients with head injuries or other intracranial lesions	The respiratory depressant effects of this drug and its capacity to elevate CSF pressure may be markedly exaggerated in such patients; side effects may also interfere with the clinical evaluation of head injuries. Administer with extreme caution and only if use of this drug is deemed essential.
Patients with asthma or other respiratory conditions	Use with extreme caution during an acute asthmatic attack or in the presence of chronic obstructive pulmonary disease, cor pulmonale, substantially decreased respiratory reserve, or preexisting respiratory depression, hypoxia, or hypercapnia; under such circumstances, even usual therapeutic doses may decrease respiratory drive while increasing airway resistance to the point of apnea. Morphine produces dose-dependent respiratory depression by acting directly on brain-stem respiratory centers; it also affects centers that control respiratory rhythm and may produce irregular and periodic breathing. Indiscriminate use of this drug may precipitate severe respiratory insufficiency due to increased viscosity of bronchial secretions and suppression of the cough reflex.

Morphine

Patients with acute abdominal conditions	Use of this drug may obscure the diagnosis or clinical course of acute abdominal conditions; use with caution and reduce the initial dosage
Patients with convulsive disorders	Use of this drug may aggravate preexisting conditions; use with caution and reduce the initial dosage
Other special-risk patients	Use with caution and reduce the initial dosage in very young or elderly patients, debilitated persons, alcoholics, and patients with severe hepatic or renal impairment, hypothyroidism (myxedema), Addison's disease, ulcerative colitis, prostic hypertrophy, urethral stricture, fever, toxic psychosis, cardiac arrhythmias, or recent GI or urinary tract surgery
Carcinogenicity, mutagenicity	The carcinogenic and mutagenic potential of this drug has not been studied

ADVERSE REACTIONS

The most frequent reactions, regardless of incidence, are printed in *italics*

Central nervous system	*Light-headedness, dizziness, sedation,* euphoria, dysphoria, weakness, headache, agitation, tremor, mental clouding, fear, anxiety, transient hallucinations, disorientation, visual disturbances, uncoordinated muscle movements
Gastrointestinal	*Nausea, vomiting,* constipation, biliary-tract spasm
Cardiovascular	Flushing, tachycardia, bradycardia, palpitations, orthostatic hypotension, faintness, syncope
Genitourinary	Oliguria, urinary retention or hesitancy, antidiuretic effect
Allergic	Pruritus, urticaria, rash; anaphylactoid reactions following IV administration (rare)
Other	*Sweating,* irritation, pain, and induration following repeated SC injection, wheal at injection site

OVERDOSAGE

Signs and symptoms	Respiratory depression (decreased respiratory rate and/or tidal volume, Cheyne-Stokes respiration, cyanosis), miosis, extreme somnolence progressing to stupor or coma, skeletal-muscle flaccidity, cold and clammy skin, bradycardia, hypotension, and, in severe cases, apnea, circulatory collapse, and cardiac arrest
Treatment	Give primary attention to reestablishing adequate respiratory exchange through provision of an adequate airway and assisted or controlled ventilation; positive-pressure respiration may be desirable if pulmonary edema is present. If respiratory depression is significant, promptly administer naloxone (adult, 0.4 mg; child, 0.01 mg/kg), preferably IV, and repeat at 2- to 3-min intervals until satisfactory breathing is restored. *Do not use analeptic agents.* Oxygen, IV fluids, vasopressors, and other supportive measures should be employed, as needed. Gastric lavage, followed by instillation of activated charcoal, may be useful; dialysis is of little value unless other, dialyzable substances (such as barbiturates) have been simultaneously ingested.

DRUG INTERACTIONS

Other narcotic analgesics; sedative-hypnotics, antianxiety agents, phenothiazines, general anesthetics, and other CNS depressants (including alcohol); MAO inhibitors; tricyclic antidepressants	△ CNS depression; reduce dose of one or both agents if used concomitantly or in close succession
Anticholinergic agents	△ Risk of paralytic ileus

ALTERED LABORATORY VALUES

Blood/serum values	△ Amylase △ Lipase ▽ Lactate

No clinically significant alterations in urinary values occur at therapeutic dosages

---

USE IN CHILDREN

See INDICATIONS and PARENTERAL DOSAGE. Administration of this drug in the pediatric age group should be limited to patients with pulmonary stenosis and infundibular spasm, congestive heart failure, severe visceral pain of known origin, intractable pain, severe postoperative pain, and pain associated with terminal illness. If used in infants and small children, exercise great caution and monitor dosage carefully. The safety and effectiveness of morphine in newborns has not been established; use in premature infants is contraindicated.

USE IN PREGNANT AND NURSING WOMEN

Pregnancy Category C: use during pregnancy only if the potential therapeutic benefit justifies the possible risk to the fetus. Morphine is teratogenic in hamsters at several hundred times the human dose; however, no adequate, well-controlled studies have been done in pregnant women. Morphine crosses the placental barrier, and drug dependence has been observed in newborns whose mothers took opioids regularly prior to delivery. This drug also prolongs labor and can produce respiratory depression in the newborn; resuscitation may be necessary if morphine is administered during labor, especially if higher doses are used. It is not known whether morphine is excreted in human milk in clinically significant amounts following administration of therapeutic doses; because of the potential for serious adverse effects in nursing infants, however, breast-feeding may be inadvisable if use of this drug is continued.

CONTROLLED ANALGESICS

NUMORPHAN (oxymorphone hydrochloride) Du Pont   C-II

Ampuls: 1 mg/ml (1 ml), 1.5 mg/ml (1 ml) **Vials:** 1.5 mg/ml (10 ml) **Suppositories:** 5 mg

INDICATIONS	PARENTERAL DOSAGE
Moderate to severe pain **Preoperative medication** **Anesthesia support** **Anxiety** in patients with dyspnea associated with acute left ventricular failure and pulmonary edema	Adult: 1–1.5 mg SC or IM or 0.5 mg IV q4–6h, as needed; in nondebilitated patients, the dose can be cautiously increased until satisfactory pain relief is obtained
Obstetrical analgesia	Adult: 0.5–1 mg IM during labor

CONTRAINDICATIONS

Age < 12 yr

Hypersensitivity to morphine analogs

ADMINISTRATION/DOSAGE ADJUSTMENTS

Rectal use	For moderate to severe pain, insert 1 suppository q4–6h; in nondebilitated patients, the dose can be cautiously increased until satisfactory pain relief is obtained

WARNINGS/PRECAUTIONS

Drug dependence	Psychic and/or physical dependence and tolerance may develop, especially in addiction-prone individuals
Patients with head injuries or other intracranial lesions	The respiratory depressant effects of this drug and its capacity to elevate CSF pressure may be markedly exaggerated in such patients; side effects may also interfere with the clinical evaluation of head injuries
Other special-risk patients	Use with caution in the elderly and debilitated and in patients with cardiovascular, pulmonary, or hepatic disease, hypothyroidism (myxedema), acute alcoholism, delirium tremens, convulsive disorders, bronchial asthma, and kyphoscoliosis; reduce dosage in debilitated and elderly patients and in patients with severe liver disease

ADVERSE REACTIONS

Central nervous system	Drowsiness, miosis, dysphoria, light-headedness, headache
Respiratory	Depression
Gastrointestinal	Nausea, vomiting
Dermatological	Pruritus

OVERDOSAGE

Signs and symptoms	Respiratory depression, miosis, extreme somnolence progressing to stupor or coma, skeletal-muscle flaccidity, cold and clammy skin, bradycardia, hypotension, and, in severe cases, apnea, circulatory collapse, and cardiac arrest
Treatment	Give primary attention to reestablishing adequate respiratory exchange through provision of an adequate airway and assisted or controlled ventilation; positive-pressure respiration may be desirable if pulmonary edema is present. If respiratory depression is significant, promptly administer naloxone (adult, 0.4 mg; child, 0.01 mg/kg), preferably IV, and repeat at 2- to 3-min intervals until satisfactory breathing is restored. *Do not use analeptic agents.* Oxygen, IV fluids, vasopressors, and other supportive measures should be employed, as needed. Gastric lavage, followed by instillation of activated charcoal, may be useful; dialysis is of little value unless other, dialyzable substances (such as barbiturates) have been simultaneously ingested.

DRUG INTERACTIONS

Other narcotic analgesics; sedative-hypnotics, antianxiety agents, phenothiazines, general anesthetics, and other CNS depressants (including alcohol); MAO inhibitors, tricyclic antidepressants	⇧ CNS depression; reduce dose of one or both agents if used concomitantly or in close succession
Anticholinergic agents	⇧ Risk of paralytic ileus

ALTERED LABORATORY VALUES

Blood/serum values — ⇧ Amylase ⇧ Lipase

No clinically significant alterations in urinary values occur at therapeutic dosages

CONTROLLED ANALGESICS

USE IN CHILDREN	USE IN PREGNANT AND NURSING WOMEN
Contraindicated for use in children under 12 yr of age	Safety for use in pregnant or nursing women has not been established

PERCOCET (oxycodone hydrochloride and acetaminophen) Du Pont   C-II

Tablets: 5 mg oxycodone hydrochloride and 325 mg acetaminophen

INDICATIONS	ORAL DOSAGE
Moderate to moderately severe pain	Adult: 1 tab q6h, as needed; dosage may need to be increased in cases of more severe pain or if tolerance to narcotic analgesics has developed

CONTRAINDICATIONS
Hypersensitivity to oxycodone or acetaminophen

WARNINGS/PRECAUTIONS

Drug dependence	Psychic and/or physical dependence and tolerance may develop, especially in addiction-prone individuals
Ambulatory patients	Caution patients that their ability to engage in potentially hazardous activities requiring full mental alertness or physical coordination may be impaired
Patients with head injuries or other intracranial lesions	The respiratory depressant effects of this drug and its capacity to elevate CSF pressure may be markedly exaggerated in such patients; side effects may also interfere with the clinical evaluation of head injuries
Patients with acute abdominal conditions	Use of this drug may obscure the diagnosis or clinical course of acute abdominal conditions
Other special-risk patients	Use with caution in the elderly or debilitated and in patients with severe hepatic or renal impairment, hypothyroidism, Addison's disease, prostatic hypertrophy, or urethral stricture

ADVERSE REACTIONS[1]

The most frequent reactions, regardless of incidence, are printed in *italics*

Central nervous system	*Light-headedness, dizziness, sedation,* euphoria, dysphoria
Gastrointestinal	*Nausea, vomiting,* constipation
Dermatological	Rash, pruritus
Other	Respiratory depression and other opioid side effects (with higher doses)

OVERDOSAGE

Signs and symptoms	*Oxycodone-related effects:* respiratory depression, miosis, extreme somnolence progressing to stupor or coma, skeletal-muscle flaccidity, cold and clammy skin, bradycardia, hypotension, and, in severe cases, apnea, circulatory collapse, and cardiac arrest; *acetaminophen-related effects:* nausea, anorexia, vomiting, abdominal pain, diarrhea, diaphoresis, malaise; hepatotoxicity may not be evident until after 2–4 days
Treatment	Give primary attention to reestablishing adequate respiratory exchange through provision of an adequate airway and assisted or controlled ventilation; positive-pressure respiration may be desirable if pulmonary edema is present. If respiratory depression is significant, promptly administer naloxone. For adults, give 0.4–2 mg IV (or, if necessary, IM or SC) at 2- to 3-min intervals, as needed; for children, give 0.01 mg/kg IV, followed, if necessary, by 0.1 mg/kg IV (administer IM or SC in divided doses if IV administration is not feasible). Keep the patient under constant surveillance since the duration of action of oxycodone may exceed that of naloxone; if significant respiratory depression recurs, repeat naloxone dose. *Do not use analeptic agents.* Oxygen, IV fluids, vasopressors, and other supportive measures should be employed, as needed.
	Promptly empty stomach by performing gastric lavage or inducing emesis. Administer oral acetylcysteine as soon as possible (no later than 24 h after ingestion); give a loading dose of 140 mg/kg and then, at 4-h intervals, 17 maintenance doses of 70 mg/kg. (Activated charcoal, if used, should be removed before acetylcysteine is given.) Measure the plasma level of unconjugated acetaminophen as early as possible, but no sooner than 4 h after ingestion. Determine prothrombin time, SGOT and SGPT levels, and serum concentrations of bilirubin, creatinine, BUN, glucose, and electrolytes every 24 h. If the prothrombin time exceeds 1.5 times the control value, give vitamin K$_1$; if the prothrombin time exceeds 3 times this value, give fresh frozen plasma. Institute appropriate measures to treat hypoglycemia and electrolyte and fluid imbalance. Avoid forced diuresis or use of diuretics when treating an acetaminophen overdose. For additional information on use of acetylcysteine and interpretation of the plasma acetaminophen level, see Mucomyst chart.

PERCOCET ■ PERCODAN

DRUG INTERACTIONS

Other narcotic analgesics; sedative-hypnotics, antianxiety agents, phenothiazines, general anesthetics, and other CNS depressants (including alcohol)	△ CNS depression; reduce dose of one or both agents if used concomitantly or in close succession
Tricyclic antidepressants, MAO inhibitors	△ Pharmacologic effect of the antidepressant or oxycodone
Anticholinergic agents	△ Risk of paralytic ileus

ALTERED LABORATORY VALUES

Blood/serum values	△ Amylase △ Lipase ▽ Glucose (with glucose oxidase/peroxidase tests)
Urinary values	△ 5-HIAA (with nitrosonaphthol reagent test)

USE IN CHILDREN
Safety and effectiveness for use in children have not been established

USE IN PREGNANT AND NURSING WOMEN
Pregnancy Category C: reproduction studies have not been done in animals; it is not known whether this preparation can cause fetal harm or affect reproductive capacity in humans. Use in pregnant women only if the expected therapeutic benefit outweighs the possible hazards. Infants born to mothers taking opioids during pregnancy may be physically dependent; administration of opioids to the mother shortly before delivery may produce some respiratory depression in both the neonate and the mother, especially if higher doses are used. It is not known whether this preparation is excreted in human milk; because many drugs are excreted in human milk, use with caution in nursing mothers.

[1] Some frequent reactions may be alleviated if the patient lies down

---

CONTROLLED ANALGESICS

PERCODAN (oxycodone hydrochloride, oxycodone terephthalate, and aspirin) Du Pont   C-II
Tablets: 4.5 mg oxycodone hydrochloride, 0.38 mg oxycodone terephthalate, and 325 mg aspirin

PERCODAN-Demi (oxycodone hydrochloride, oxycodone terephthalate, and aspirin) Du Pont   C-II
Tablets: 2.25 mg oxycodone hydrochloride, 0.19 mg oxycodone terephthalate, and 325 mg aspirin

INDICATIONS
Moderate to moderately severe pain

ORAL DOSAGE
Adult: 1 Percodan tab or 1–2 Percodan-Demi tabs q6h
Child (6–12 yr): ¼ Percodan-Demi tab q6h
Child (> 12 yr): ½ Percodan-Demi tab q6h

CONTRAINDICATIONS
Hypersensitivity to oxycodone or aspirin

WARNINGS/PRECAUTIONS

Drug dependence	Psychic and/or physical dependence and tolerance may develop, especially in addiction-prone individuals
Ambulatory patients	Caution patients that their ability to engage in potentially hazardous activities requiring full mental alertness or physical coordination may be impaired
Patients with head injuries or other intracranial injuries	The respiratory depressant effects of this drug and its capacity to elevate CSF pressure may be markedly exaggerated in such patients; side effects may also interfere with the clinical evaluation of head injuries
Patients with acute abdominal conditions	Use of this drug may obscure the diagnosis or clinical course of acute abdominal conditions
Other special-risk patients	Use with caution in the elderly or debilitated and in patients with severe hepatic or renal impairment, hypothyroidism, Addison's disease, prostatic hypertrophy, urethral stricture, peptic ulcer, or coagulation abnormalities
Reye's syndrome	Some reports claim that aspirin or salicylates may increase the risk of developing Reye's syndrome, a rare but serious disease that can follow chicken pox or influenza in children and teenagers

ADVERSE REACTIONS
Frequent reactions (incidence ≥ 1%) are printed in *italics*

Central nervous system	*Light-headedness, dizziness, sedation,* euphoria, dysphoria
Gastrointestinal	*Nausea, vomiting,* constipation

PERCODAN ■ PHENAPHEN with Codeine

Dermatological — Pruritus

OVERDOSAGE

Signs and symptoms — *Oxycodone-related effects:* respiratory depression, extreme somnolence progressing to stupor or coma, skeletal-muscle flaccidity, cold and clammy skin, bradycardia, hypotension, and, in severe cases, apnea, circulatory collapse, and cardiac arrest; *aspirin-related effects:* hyperpnea, nausea, vomiting, vertigo, tinnitus, flushing, sweating, thirst, headache, drowsiness, diarrhea, and tachycardia progressing to hyperthermia, hemorrhage, acid-base disturbances, restlessness, confusion, convulsions, vasomotor depression, coma, and respiratory failure

Treatment — Give primary attention to reestablishing adequate respiratory exchange through provision of an adequate airway and assisted or controlled ventilation; positive-pressure respiration may be desirable if pulmonary edema is present. If respiratory depression is significant, promptly administer naloxone. For adults, give 0.4–2 mg IV (or, if necessary, IM or SC) at 2- to 3-min intervals, as needed; for children, give 0.01 mg/kg IV, followed, if necessary, by 0.1 mg/kg IV (administer IM or SC in divided doses if IV administration is not feasible). Keep the patient under constant surveillance since the duration of action of oxycodone may exceed that of naloxone; if significant respiratory depression recurs, repeat naloxone dose. *Do not use analeptic agents.* Oxygen, IV fluids, vasopressors, and other supportive measures should be employed, as needed. Gastric lavage, followed by instillation of activated charcoal, may be useful if performed within 4 h of ingestion. In moderately severe cases of salicylate poisoning, cautiously administer sodium bicarbonate IV in sufficient quantity, if possible, to maintain an alkaline diuresis; intermittent peritoneal dialysis may also be helpful. In severe cases, hemodialysis should be seriously considered. Hyperthermia, particularly in children, and dehydration require prompt correction. Hemorrhagic phenomena may necessitate whole-blood transfusions and phytonadione (vitamin K$_1$). Do not administer barbiturates to treat excitement or convulsions.

DRUG INTERACTIONS

Other narcotic analgesics; sedative-hypnotics, antianxiety agents, phenothiazines, general anesthetics, and other CNS depressants (including alcohol); MAO inhibitors; tricyclic antidepressants — △ CNS depression; reduce dose of one or both agents if used concomitantly or in close succession

Anticholinergic agents — △ Risk of paralytic ileus

Anticoagulants — △ Risk of bleeding

Alcohol, corticosteroids, phenylbutazone, oxyphenbutazone — △ Risk of GI ulceration

Probenecid, sulfinpyrazone — ▽ Uricosuric effect

Spironolactone — ▽ Diuretic effect

Methotrexate — △ Methotrexate plasma level and risk of toxicity

ALTERED LABORATORY VALUES

Blood/serum values — △ Amylase △ Lipase △ Prothrombin time △ Uric acid (with low doses) ▽ Uric acid (with high doses) ▽ Thyroxine (T$_4$) ▽ Thyroid-stimulating hormone

Urinary values — △ Glucose (with Clinitest tablets)

USE IN CHILDREN

Percodan should not be administered to children; Percodan-Demi may be considered in children who are at least 6 yr of age (see INDICATIONS and ORAL DOSAGE)

USE IN PREGNANT AND NURSING WOMEN

Safety for use during pregnancy has not been established. Consult manufacturer for use in nursing mothers.

CONTROLLED ANALGESICS

PHENAPHEN with Codeine (acetaminophen and codeine phosphate) Robins   C-III

Capsules: 325 mg acetaminophen and 15 mg (No. 2), 30 mg (No. 3), or 60 mg (No. 4) codeine phosphate

PHENAPHEN-650 with Codeine (acetaminophen and codeine phosphate) Robins   C-III

Tablets: 650 mg acetaminophen and 30 mg codeine phosphate

INDICATIONS	ORAL DOSAGE
Mild to moderately severe pain	**Adult:** 1 tab, 1 No. 4 cap, or 1–2 No. 2 or No. 3 caps q4h **Child (≥30 kg):** 1 No. 2 cap (0.5 mg/kg codeine) q4h

PHENAPHEN with Codeine

CONTRAINDICATIONS
Hypersensitivity to acetaminophen or codeine

WARNINGS/PRECAUTIONS

Drug dependence	Psychic and/or physical dependence and tolerance may develop with repeated use, especially in addiction-prone individuals; use with the same degree of caution appropriate to the use of other oral narcotic preparations
Ambulatory patients	Caution patients that their ability to engage in potentially hazardous activities requiring full mental alertness or physical coordination may be impaired
Patients with head injuries or other intracranial lesions	The respiratory depressant effects of this drug and its capacity to elevate CSF pressure may be markedly exaggerated in such patients; side effects may also interfere with the clinical evaluation of head injuries
Patients with acute abdominal conditions	Use of this drug may obscure the diagnosis or clinical course of acute abdominal conditions
Other special-risk patients	Use with caution in the elderly or debilitated and in patients with severe renal or hepatic impairment, Addison's disease, prostatic hypertrophy, or urethral stricture
Severe or intractable pain	Do not use this preparation at recommended or higher doses for relief of severe or intractable pain; doses exceeding those recommended above not only fail to provide sufficient analgesia for severe or intractable pain, but also produce an increase in adverse effects
Carcinogenicity, mutagenicity, effect on fertility	No long-term studies have been done with acetaminophen and codeine to determine their carcinogenic potential or their effect on fertility. Acetaminophen and codeine have been found to have no mutagenic activity in the Ames, Basc *Drosophila,* and mouse micronucleus tests.

ADVERSE REACTIONS[1]

The most frequent reactions, regardless of incidence, are printed in *italics*

Central nervous system	*Light-headedness, dizziness, sedation,* euphoria, dysphoria
Gastrointestinal	*Nausea, vomiting,* constipation
Other	*Shortness of breath;* pruritus; morphine-like effects, including respiratory depression (at higher doses)

OVERDOSAGE

Signs and symptoms	*Codeine-related effects:* respiratory depression, miosis, extreme somnolence progressing to stupor or coma, skeletal-muscle flaccidity, cold and clammy skin, bradycardia, hypotension, and, in severe cases, apnea, circulatory collapse, and cardiac arrest; *acetaminophen-related effects:* nausea, anorexia, vomiting, abdominal pain, diarrhea, diaphoresis, malaise; hepatotoxicity may not be evident until after 2–4 days
Treatment	Give primary attention to reestablishing adequate respiratory exchange through provision of an adequate airway and assisted or controlled ventilation; positive-pressure respiration may be desirable if pulmonary edema is present. If respiratory depression is significant, promptly administer naloxone. For adults, give 0.4–2 mg IV (or, if necessary, IM or SC) at 2- to 3-min intervals, as needed; for children, give 0.01 mg/kg IV, followed, if necessary, by 0.1 mg/kg IV (administer IM or SC in divided doses if IV administration is not feasible). Keep the patient under constant surveillance since the duration of action of codeine may exceed that of naloxone; if significant respiratory depression recurs, repeat naloxone dose. *Do not use analeptic agents.* Oxygen, IV fluids, vasopressors, and other supportive measures should be employed, as needed.
	Promptly empty stomach by performing gastric lavage or inducing emesis. Administer oral acetylcysteine as soon as possible (no later than 24 h after ingestion); give a loading dose of 140 mg/kg and then, at 4-h intervals, 17 maintenance doses of 70 mg/kg. (Activated charcoal, if used, should be removed before acetylcysteine is given.) Measure the plasma level of unconjugated acetaminophen as early as possible, but no sooner than 4 h after ingestion. Determine prothrombin time, SGOT and SGPT levels, and serum concentrations of bilirubin, creatinine, BUN, glucose, and electrolytes every 24 h. If the prothrombin time exceeds 1.5 times the control value, give vitamin K_1; if the prothrombin time exceeds 3 times this value, give fresh frozen plasma. Institute appropriate measures to treat hypoglycemia and electrolyte and fluid imbalance. Avoid forced diuresis or use of diuretics when treating an acetaminophen overdose. For additional information on use of acetylcysteine and interpretation of the plasma acetaminophen level, see Mucomyst chart.

DRUG INTERACTIONS

Other narcotic analgesics; sedative-hypnotics, antianxiety agents, phenothiazines, general anesthetics, and other CNS depressants (including alcohol); MAO inhibitors; tricyclic antidepressants	⇧ CNS depression; reduce dose of one or both agents if used concomitantly or in close succession
Anticholinergic agents	⇧ Risk of paralytic ileus

ALTERED LABORATORY VALUES

Blood/serum values — △ Amylase   △ Lipase   ▽ Glucose (with glucose oxidase/peroxidase tests)

Urinary values — △ 5-HIAA (with nitrosonaphthol reagent test)

USE IN CHILDREN

See INDICATIONS and ORAL DOSAGE

USE IN PREGNANT AND NURSING WOMEN

Pregnancy Category C: codeine has caused teratogenic effects in mice when given in doses 17 times the maximum human daily dose; use this preparation during pregnancy only if the expected benefit justifies the potential risk to the fetus. It is not known whether codeine or acetaminophen is excreted in human milk; use with caution in nursing mothers.

---

[1] The frequency of adverse reactions is dose-related.

CONTROLLED ANALGESICS

SUBLIMAZE (fentanyl citrate) Janssen   C-II

Ampuls: 50 μg fentanyl[1] per milliliter (2, 5, 10, 20 ml)

INDICATIONS

Preoperative medication

Adjunct to general anesthesia

Adjunct to regional anesthesia

General anesthesia

Postoperative medication

PARENTERAL DOSAGE

Adult: 50–100 μg IM 30–60 min before surgery

Adult: for minor surgical procedures, 2 μg/kg IV; for more major procedures, 2–20 μg/kg IV, followed by 25–100 μg IV or IM whenever surgical stress or lightening of anesthesia is detected; for procedures requiring attenuation of the stress response (eg, open heart surgery and certain longer and more complicated neurosurgical and orthopedic procedures), 20–50 μg/kg IV, with nitrous oxide and oxygen, followed by doses ranging from 25 μg to one-half the initial loading dose whenever surgical stress or lightening of anesthesia is detected

Adult: 50–100 μg IM or by slow IV injection over a period of 1–2 min

Adult: for procedures requiring attenuation of the stress response (eg, open heart surgery, certain other major procedures, certain complicated neurosurgical and orthopedic procedures), 50–100 μg/kg IV or, if necessary, up to 150 μg/kg IV, with oxygen and a neuromuscular blocker
Child (2–12 yr): for induction and maintenance, as little as 2–3 μg/kg

Adult: for control of pain, tachypnea, and emergence delirium, 50–100 μg IM q1–2h, as needed

CONTRAINDICATIONS

Intolerance to fentanyl

ADMINISTRATION/DOSAGE ADJUSTMENTS

Elderly and debilitated patients — Reduce initial dose; determine subsequent doses on the basis of response

Vital signs — Monitor vital signs routinely (see WARNINGS/PRECAUTIONS)

WARNINGS/PRECAUTIONS

Respiratory depression — Fentanyl frequently reduces the respiratory rate and diminishes sensitivity to carbon dioxide stimulation; both effects may last longer than the analgesic effect and may persist or recur during the postoperative period. Fentanyl can also cause bronchoconstriction. When using this drug, particularly at doses exceeding 10 μg/kg, make sure that facilities for postoperative observation are adequate and that oxygen, an opioid antagonist, resuscitative and intubation equipment, and trained personnel are readily available. Provide assisted or controlled ventilation when anesthetic doses are used. To minimize drug-induced rigidity of muscles affecting ventilation, use a neuromuscular blocker (see warning below). Monitor patient response after surgery, particularly when anesthetic doses have been used; do not discharge patient from recovery area until adequate spontaneous breathing has been established and maintained in the absence of stimulation. Use with caution in patients with chronic obstructive pulmonary disease, decreased respiratory reserve, or potentially compromised respiratory function; when they undergo anesthesia, provide assisted or controlled respiration. For management of respiratory depression, see OVERDOSAGE.

SUBLIMAZE

Neuromuscular effects	Fentanyl can cause rigidity of muscles, particularly those affecting pulmonary function; during induction of anesthesia, the drug can also produce skeletal movements in the extremities, neck, and eye that, in rare cases, may be strong enough to affect management of the patient. The severity of neuromuscular reactions depends on dose and rate of injection. To minimize these effects, give a full paralyzing dose of a nondepolarizing neuromuscular blocker with anesthetic doses of fentanyl or up to 25% of a full paralyzing dose just prior to administration of nonanesthetic doses; during slow IV infusion of anesthetic doses, wait until loss of eyelash reflex occurs before giving the neuromuscular blocker.
Bradycardia	Use with caution in patients with bradyarrhythmias, since this drug can cause bradycardia; the effect may be reversed with atropine
Drug dependence	Fentanyl can produce morphine-type drug dependence
Use with tranquilizers such as droperidol	A decrease in pulmonary artery pressure and hypotension can occur when fentanyl is used with a tranquilizer such as droperidol. When using droperidol with fentanyl, make sure that measures for the management of hypotension are available. Treat hypotension by giving IV fluids and, when conditions permit, reposition the patient for optimal venous return; take care to avoid orthostatic hypotension when handling the patient. If hypotension persists, consider using a vasopressor; however, do not give epinephrine, since it may produce a paradoxical decrease in pressure. Hypertension, chills, shivering, restlessness, hallucinations, mental depression, and extrapyramidal reactions can also occur with combined use of fentanyl and droperidol. Bear in mind that the duration of action for these two drugs differs markedly and that the EEG pattern may return to normal more slowly after surgery when these two drugs are used together.
Use with or after MAO inhibitors	Severe reactions, including hypertension, have occurred with concomitant use of other narcotic analgesics and MAO inhibitors; although this interaction has not been seen with fentanyl, the risk cannot be ruled out. If fentanyl is given to patients who have received MAO inhibitors within the past 14 days, monitor response and make sure that vasodilators and beta blockers are readily available for treatment of hypertension.
Intracranial disorders	Fentanyl can increase CSF pressure; use with caution in patients who may be particularly susceptible to this effect, such as comatose patients who may have head injuries or brain tumors. Bear in mind that the side effects of this drug may interfere with clinical evaluation of head injuries.
Renal or hepatic impairment	Use with caution in patients with renal or hepatic impairment; the drug is metabolized in the liver
Carcinogenicity, mutagenicity	No long-term studies have been done to evaluate the carcinogenic or mutagenic potential of this drug
Impairment of fertility	Studies in rats have shown that fentanyl causes a significant decrease in the pregnancy rate

ADVERSE REACTIONS

The most common reactions are italicized

Respiratory	*Respiratory depression, apnea,* respiratory arrest, laryngospasm, bronchoconstriction
Cardiovascular	*Bradycardia,* circulatory depression, cardiac arrest, hypertension, hypotension
Central nervous system	*Muscular rigidity,* dizziness, euphoria
Ophthalmic	Blurred vision, miosis
Gastrointestinal	Nausea, vomiting
Other	Diaphoresis

OVERDOSAGE

Signs and symptoms	See ADVERSE REACTIONS
Treatment	For hypoventilation or apnea, administer oxygen and assist or control ventilation mechanically. Maintain a patent airway; when necessary, provide an oropharyngeal airway or insert an endotracheal tube. Give a narcotic antagonist, such as naloxone, as needed; bear in mind that the duration of respiratory depression may be longer than the duration of action of the antagonist. Keep the patient under close observation for at least 24 h. If respiratory depression is associated with muscular rigidity, an IV neuromuscular blocker may be required. Use IV fluids to manage severe or persistent hypotension. Maintain body warmth and adequate fluid intake.

DRUG INTERACTIONS

Other CNS depressants	⚠ CNS depression; reduce the dose of fentanyl after administering other CNS depressants and reduce the dose of other CNS depressants after administering fentanyl. The initial dose of narcotic analgesics given postoperatively following administration of fentanyl should be as low as 25–33% of the usual recommended dose.
Diazepam	Cardiovascular depression (with higher or anesthetic doses of fentanyl given with doses of diazepam that may even be relatively small)
Droperidol	Hypotension, other effects (see WARNINGS/PRECAUTIONS)

SUBLIMAZE ■ SYNALGOS-DC

Nitrous oxide	Cardiovascular depression (with higher doses of fentanyl)
Spinal and certain peridural anesthetics	⇧ Respiratory depression

ALTERED LABORATORY VALUES

Blood/serum values	⇧ Amylase ⇧ Lipase

No clinically significant alterations in urinary values occur at therapeutic dosages

---

USE IN CHILDREN

Safety and effectiveness for use in children under 2 yr of age have not been established. In rare cases, clinically significant methemoglobinemia has been seen in premature neonates following combined use of fentanyl, pancuronium, and atropine; a direct causal relationship has not been established.

USE IN PREGNANT AND NURSING WOMEN

Pregnancy Category C: fentanyl produced an embryocidal effect in rats given 0.3 times the maximum human dose for 12 days; use during pregnancy only if the expected benefit justifies the potential risk to the fetus. Use during labor and delivery is not recommended because of insufficient data. It is not known if fentanyl is excreted in human milk; use with caution in nursing mothers.

---

[1] As the citrate salt

CONTROLLED ANALGESICS

SYNALGOS-DC (dihydrocodeine bitartrate, aspirin, and caffeine) Wyeth   C-III

Capsules: 16 mg dihydrocodeine bitartrate, 356.4 mg aspirin, and 30 mg caffeine

INDICATIONS	**ORAL DOSAGE**
Moderate to moderately severe pain	Adult: 2 caps q4h, as needed

CONTRAINDICATIONS

Hypersensitivity to dihydrocodeine or aspirin

WARNINGS/PRECAUTIONS

Drug dependence	Psychic and/or physical dependence and tolerance may develop, especially in addiction-prone individuals
Ambulatory patients	Caution patients that their ability to engage in potentially hazardous activities requiring full mental alertness or physical coordination may be impaired
Special-risk patients	Use with caution in the elderly or debilitated; use with extreme caution in the presence of peptic ulcer or coagulation abnormalities

ADVERSE REACTIONS

Central nervous system	Light-headedness, dizziness, drowsiness, sedation
Gastrointestinal	Nausea, vomiting, constipation
Dermatological	Pruritus, skin reactions

OVERDOSAGE

Signs and symptoms	*Dihydrocodeine-related effects:* respiratory depression, miosis, extreme somnolence progressing to stupor or coma, skeletal-muscle flaccidity, cold and clammy skin, bradycardia, hypotension, and, in severe cases, apnea, circulatory collapse, and cardiac arrest; *aspirin-related effects:* hyperpnea, nausea, vomiting, vertigo, tinnitus, flushing, sweating, thirst, headache, drowsiness, diarrhea, and tachycardia, progressing to hyperthermia, hemorrhage, acid-base disturbances, restlessness, confusion, convulsions, vasomotor depression, coma, and respiratory failure; *caffeine-related effects:* insomnia, restlessness, and excitement progressing to mild delirium, dehydration, fever, tachycardia, extrasystoles, tremor, convulsions
Treatment	Give primary attention to reestablishing adequate respiratory exchange through provision of an adequate airway and assisted or controlled ventilation; positive-pressure respiration may be desirable if pulmonary edema is present. If respiratory depression is significant, promptly administer naloxone (adult, 0.4 mg; child, 0.01 mg/kg), preferably IV, and repeat at 2- to 3-min intervals until satisfactory breathing is restored. *Do not use analeptic agents.* Oxygen, IV fluids, vasopressors, and other supportive measures should be employed, as needed. Gastric lavage, followed by instillation of activated charcoal, may be useful if performed within 4 h of ingestion. In moderately severe cases of salicylate poisoning, cautiously administer sodium bicarbonate IV in sufficient quantity, if possible, to maintain an alkaline diuresis; intermittent peritoneal dialysis may also be helpful. In severe cases, hemodialysis should be seriously considered. Hyperthermia, particularly in children, and dehydration require prompt correction. Hemorrhagic phenomena may necessitate whole-blood transfusions and phytonadione (vitamin K_1). Do not administer barbiturates to treat excitement or convulsions.

DRUG INTERACTIONS

Other narcotic analgesics; sedative-hypnotics, anti-anxiety agents, general anesthetics, and other CNS depressants (including alcohol); MAO inhibitors; tricyclic antidepressants	△ CNS depression; reduce dose of one or both agents if used concomitantly or in close succession
Anticholinergic agents	△ Risk of paralytic ileus
Alcohol, corticosteroids, phenylbutazone, oxyphenbutazone	△ Risk of GI ulceration
Probenecid, sulfinpyrazone	▽ Uricosuric effect
Spironolactone	▽ Diuretic effect
Methotrexate	△ Methotrexate plasma level and risk of toxicity
Anticoagulants	△ Anticoagulant effects

ALTERED LABORATORY VALUES

Blood/serum values	△ Amylase △ Lipase △ Prothrombin time △ Uric acid (with low doses) ▽ Uric acid (with high doses) ▽ Thyroxine (T_4) ▽ Thyroid-stimulating hormone
Urinary values	△ Glucose (with Clinitest tablets) ▽ Bilirubin △ 5-HIAA (with nitrosonaphthol reagent test)

USE IN CHILDREN

Safety and effectiveness for use in children have not been established; use in children 12 yr of age or younger is not recommended

USE IN PREGNANT AND NURSING WOMEN

Safety for use during pregnancy has not been established. Animal reproduction studies have not been done, nor is there any adequate information on whether this drug can affect human fetal development or fertility. Consult manufacturer for use in nursing mothers.

CONTROLLED ANALGESICS

TALACEN (pentazocine hydrochloride and acetaminophen) Winthrop-Breon   C-IV

Tablets: pentazocine hydrochloride, equivalent to 25 mg pentazocine and 650 mg acetaminophen

INDICATIONS	ORAL DOSAGE
Mild to moderate pain	**Adult:** 1 tab q4h, as needed, up to 6 tabs/day

CONTRAINDICATIONS

Hypersensitivity to pentazocine or acetaminophen

WARNINGS/PRECAUTIONS

Drug dependence	Psychic and/or physical dependence and tolerance may develop, especially in addiction-prone patients; abrupt discontinuation after prolonged use may precipitate withdrawal reactions. Patients with a history of drug dependence should be closely supervised. When prescribing this drug for long-term use, precautions should be taken to prevent patients from increasing the dosage.
Patients receiving other narcotics	Administration of pentazocine, a mild narcotic antagonist, may precipitate withdrawal reactions in patients taking methadone or other opioid substances
Ambulatory patients	Caution patients not to drive or engage in other potentially hazardous activities, because sedation, dizziness, and/or euphoria may occur. Patients have experienced transient hallucinations (usually visual), disorientation, and confusion; if such reactions occur, observe patient very closely and monitor vital signs. Since these acute CNS reactions may recur, exercise caution if use of this drug is reinstituted. Also, caution patients about the concomitant use of alcohol or other CNS depressants with this drug (see DRUG INTERACTIONS).
Patients with head injuries or increased intracranial pressure	The respiratory depressant effects of pentazocine and its capacity to elevate CSF pressure may be markedly exaggerated in patients with head injuries, other intracranial lesions, or increased intracranial pressure; side effects may also interfere with the clinical evaluation of head injuries. Administer with extreme caution and only if use of this drug is deemed essential.
Patients with respiratory conditions	Use with caution in patients with respiratory depression, severe bronchial asthma or other obstructive respiratory conditions, severely limited respiratory reserve, or cyanosis, because pentazocine can, in rare instances, depress respiration after oral administration

TALACEN

Patients with myocardial infarction	Use with caution in patients with myocardial infarction who are nauseated or vomiting
Patients with hepatic or renal impairment	Use with caution. Pentazocine and acetaminophen are metabolized by the liver; in patients with extensive hepatic disease, the risk of side effects may be increased.
Patients predisposed to seizures	Use with caution. Seizures have occurred in a few such patients who were given pentazocine; however, a causal relationship has not been established.
Biliary tract surgery	Some evidence suggests that pentazocine, unlike other narcotic drugs, may cause little or no increase in biliary tract pressure
Drug accumulation	Administration every 4 h over an extended period may cause accumulation of pentazocine (mean plasma half-life, 3.6 h; range 1.5–10 h) and, to a lesser extent, accumulation of acetaminophen (mean plasma half-life, 2.8 h; range, 2–4 h)
Carcinogenicity, mutagenicity	Long-term studies in animals given pentazocine have shown no evidence of carcinogenicity; mutagenicity and carcinogenicity studies have not been performed with Talacen
Effect on fertility	Adverse effects on reproductive capacity have not been detected in rabbits and rats given pentazocine orally or parenterally; in addition, no adverse effect on fertility rate was observed in female rats given 4–20 mg/kg/day SC, beginning 14 days before mating and continuing until day 13 of pregnancy. However, animal reproduction studies have not been performed with Talacen, and it is not known whether Talacen can affect reproductive capacity.

ADVERSE REACTIONS[1]

Central nervous system	Dizziness, light-headedness, hallucinations, sedation, euphoria, headache, confusion, disorientation, weakness, disturbed dreams, insomnia, syncope, depression; tremor, irritability, excitement, tinnitus and paresthesia (rare)
Ophthalmic	Visual blurring, focusing difficulty
Gastrointestinal	Nausea, vomiting, constipation; abdominal distress, anorexia, and diarrhea
Cardiovascular	Decreased blood pressure, tachycardia
Hematological	Leukopenia (particularly granulocytopenia; usually reversible) and moderate, transient eosinophilia (rare)
Hypersensitivity	Rash, thrombocytopenic purpura; urticaria, facial edema, hemolytic anemia, and agranulocytosis (rare)
Other	Sweating, flushing; chills, respiratory depression, urinary retention, and toxic epidermal necrolysis (rare)

OVERDOSAGE

Signs and symptoms	*Pentazocine-related effects:* anxiety, nightmares, strange thoughts, hallucinations, dizziness, nausea, vomiting, lethargy, paresthesia; marked respiratory depression associated with increased blood pressure and tachycardia; *acetaminophen-related effects:* nausea, anorexia, vomiting, abdominal pain, diarrhea, diaphoresis, malaise; hepatotoxicity may not be evident until after 2–4 days.
Treatment	Give primary attention to reestablishing adequate respiratory exchange through provision of an adequate airway and assisted or controlled ventilation; positive-pressure respiration may be desirable if pulmonary edema is present. If respiratory depression is significant, promptly administer naloxone. For adults, give 0.4–2 mg IV (or, if necessary, IM or SC) at 2- to 3-min intervals, as needed; for children, give 0.01 mg/kg IV, followed, if necessary, by 0.1 mg/kg IV (administer IM or SC in divided doses if IV administration is not feasible). *Do not use analeptic agents.* Oxygen, IV fluids, vasopressors, and other supportive measures should be employed, as needed.
	Promptly empty stomach by performing gastric lavage or inducing emesis and then giving activated charcoal. Administer oral acetylcysteine as soon as possible (no later than 24 h after ingestion); give a loading dose of 140 mg/kg and then, at 4-h intervals, 17 maintenance doses of 70 mg/kg. (Activated charcoal should be removed before acetylcysteine is given.) Measure the plasma level of unconjugated acetaminophen as early as possible, but no sooner than 4 h after ingestion. Determine prothrombin time, SGOT and SGPT levels, and serum concentrations of bilirubin, creatinine, BUN, glucose, and electrolytes every 24 h. If the prothrombin time exceeds 1.5 times the control value, give vitamin K_1; if the prothrombin time exceeds 3 times this value, give fresh frozen plasma. Institute appropriate measures to treat hypoglycemia and electrolyte and fluid imbalance. Start hemodialysis within 12 h after ingestion if the plasma acetaminophen level 4 h after ingestion exceeds 120 µg/ml. Avoid forced diuresis or use of diuretics when treating an acetaminophen overdose. For additional information on use of acetylcysteine and interpretation of the plasma acetaminophen level, see Mucomyst chart.

DRUG INTERACTIONS

Other narcotic analgesics; sedative-hypnotics, antianxiety agents, phenothiazines, general anesthetics, and other CNS depressants (including alcohol); MAO inhibitors; tricyclic antidepressants	△ CNS depression; reduce dose of one or both agents if used concomitantly or in close succession

TALACEN ■ TALWIN Injection

Anticholinergic agents —— △ Risk of paralytic ileus

ALTERED LABORATORY VALUES

Blood/serum values —— △ Amylase △ Lipase ▽ Glucose (with glucose oxidase/peroxidase tests)
Urinary values —— △ 5-HIAA (with nitrosonaphthol reagent test)

USE IN CHILDREN

Safety and effectiveness for use in children under 12 yr of age have not been established

USE IN PREGNANT AND NURSING WOMEN

Pregnancy Category C: use during pregnancy only if clearly needed; animal reproduction studies have not been performed with Talacen, and it is not known whether this preparation can cause harm to the fetus. Studies of rats and rabbits given pentazocine orally or parenterally have shown no adverse effect on the course of pregnancy nor any evidence of embryotoxicity. There have been rare reports of a possible neonatal withdrawal syndrome occurring after prolonged use of pentazocine during pregnancy. Use of Talacen during labor and delivery has not been studied; patients given pentazocine during labor have experienced only those adverse effects that are associated with commonly used analgesics. Talacen should be used with caution during the delivery of premature infants. It is not known whether Talacen is excreted in human milk; use with caution in nursing mothers, because many drugs are so excreted.

[1] The reactions listed here are primarily reactions associated with oral administration of 50-mg doses of pentazocine hydrochloride (twice the amount in one Talacen tablet); when taken in recommended doses, acetaminophen is relatively free of adverse effects

---

CONTROLLED ANALGESICS

TALWIN Injection (pentazocine lactate) Winthrop-Breon   C-IV

Ampuls: 30 mg/ml (1, 1½, 2 ml)   **Vials:** 30 mg/ml (10 ml)   **Cartridge-needle units:** 30 mg/ml (1, 1½, 2 ml)

INDICATIONS	PARENTERAL DOSAGE
Moderate to severe pain **Preoperative, preanesthetic medication** **As an adjunct to surgical anesthesia**	Adult: 30 mg IV, IM, or SC; may be repeated q3–4h, up to 360 mg/day, not to exceed 30 mg/dose IV or 60 mg/dose IM or SC
Labor	Adult: 30 mg IM or 20 mg IV when contractions become regular; repeat 2 or 3 times q2–3h, as needed

CONTRAINDICATIONS
Hypersensitivity to pentazocine

ADMINISTRATION/DOSAGE ADJUSTMENTS

Parenteral administration —— If frequent injections are needed, give the drug IM and rotate injection sites (eg, upper outer quadrant of the buttocks, midlateral aspect of the thighs, and deltoid area of the shoulders). Because severe tissue damage may occur, the SC route should be avoided, if possible. Do not mix pentazocine in the same syringe with soluble barbiturates, since precipitation will occur.

WARNINGS/PRECAUTIONS

Drug dependence —— Psychic and/or physical dependence may develop, especially in addiction-prone and emotionally unstable patients, who should be supervised if the duration of therapy is more than 4–5 days. Abrupt discontinuation may result in abdominal cramps, fever, rhinorrhea, restlessness, anxiety, and lacrimation. If more than minor difficulty is encountered in withdrawing the drug, reinstitute parenteral administration of pentazocine and then gradually taper the dosage until the drug can be completely withdrawn; do not substitute methadone or other narcotics.

Patients dependent on narcotics —— Administration of pentazocine may precipitate withdrawal symptoms

Ambulatory patients —— Caution patients not to engage in potentially hazardous activities requiring full mental alertness or physical coordination and to avoid alcohol and other CNS depressants, which may produce additional CNS depression

Patients with head injuries or other intracranial lesions —— The respiratory depressant effects of this drug and its capacity to elevate CSF pressure may be markedly exaggerated in such patients; side effects may also interfere with the clinical evaluation of head injuries. Administer with extreme caution and only if use of this drug is deemed essential.

Respiratory depression —— May result or worsen; use cautiously and lower dosage in patients with bronchial asthma, severely limited respiratory reserve, respiratory obstruction, or cyanosis

TALWIN Injection ■ TALWIN Nx

Patients with hepatic or renal impairment	Use with caution; extensive hepatic disease may predispose to increased side effects
Patients with myocardial infarction	IV administration may increase systemic and pulmonary arterial pressure and systemic vascular resistance in cases of acute myocardial infarction accompanied by hypertension or left ventricular failure
Seizures	May occur in predisposed patients
Biliary surgery	Some evidence suggests that pentazocine, unlike other narcotic drugs, may cause little or no increase in biliary tract pressure
Acute CNS manifestations	Transient hallucinations, disorientation, and confusion have occurred and cleared spontaneously after several hours. If CNS reactions occur, closely observe patient and monitor vital signs. Use with caution if drug is reinstated.

ADVERSE REACTIONS

The most frequent reactions, regardless of incidence, are printed in *italics*

Gastrointestinal	*Nausea, vomiting,* constipation, dry mouth; taste alterations, diarrhea, and cramps (rare)
Central nervous system and neuromuscular	*Dizziness, light-headedness, euphoria,* hallucinations, sedation, headache, confusion, disorientation, weakness, disturbed dreams, insomnia, syncope, depression; tremor, irritability, excitement, and tinnitus (rare)
Dermatological	*Soft-tissue induration, nodules, and cutaneous depression at injection site; ulceration and local sclerosis with multiple injection;* sting on injection; flushed skin (including plethora); dermatitis (including pruritus); toxic epidermal necrolysis (rare)
Hypersensitivity	Allergic reactions, including facial edema (rare)
Ophthalmic	Blurred vision, nystagmus, diplopia, and miosis (rare)
Cardiovascular	Circulatory depression, shock, hypertension; tachycardia (rare)
Respiratory	Depression, dyspnea, transient apnea in neonates exposed during labor
Hematological	Depression of WBC count (usually reversible) and moderate transient eosinophilia (rare)
Other	Sweating, urinary retention, irregular uterine contractions; chills (rare)

OVERDOSAGE

Signs and symptoms	See ADVERSE REACTIONS
Treatment	Employ IV fluids, oxygen, vasopressors, and other supportive measures. For respiratory depression, administer naloxone (usual adult dose: 0.4 mg, preferably IV), simultaneously with respiratory resuscitation. Assisted or controlled ventilation may be indicated.

DRUG INTERACTIONS

Other narcotic analgesics; sedative-hypnotics, antianxiety agents, phenothiazines, general anesthetics, and other CNS depressants (including alcohol); MAO inhibitors; tricyclic antidepressants	△ CNS depression; reduce dose of one or both agents if used concomitantly or in close succession. Before anesthesia, ensure that adequate equipment and facilities are available for treatment of emergencies.
Anticholinergic agents	△ Risk of paralytic ileus
Morphine, meperidine	▽ Analgesic effect of morphine or meperidine

ALTERED LABORATORY VALUES

Blood/serum values	△ Amylase △ Lipase

No clinically significant alterations in urinary values occur at therapeutic dosages

---

USE IN CHILDREN

Not recommended for use in children under 12 yr of age

USE IN PREGNANT AND NURSING WOMEN

Safety for use during pregnancy (except during labor) has not been established; use with caution in women delivering premature infants. There are rare reports of a possible abstinence syndrome in newborns following prolonged use of pentazocine during pregnancy. Pentazocine is excreted in human milk.[1]

[1] *United States Pharmacopeia Dispensing Information 1981.* Rockville, Md, United States Pharmacopeial Convention, Inc, 1981

CONTROLLED ANALGESICS

TALWIN Nx (pentazocine hydrochloride and naloxone hydrochloride) Winthrop-Breon C-IV

Tablets: pentazocine hydrochloride equivalent to 50 mg pentazocine and naloxone hydrochloride equivalent to 0.5 mg naloxone; for oral use only (see WARNINGS/PRECAUTIONS)

INDICATIONS	ORAL DOSAGE
Moderate to severe pain	**Adult:** 1 tab q3–4h to start, followed, if necessary, by 2 tabs q3–4h, up to 12 tabs/day

COMPENDIUM OF DRUG THERAPY

TALWIN Nx

CONTRAINDICATIONS

Hypersensitivity to pentazocine or naloxone

WARNINGS/PRECAUTIONS

Drug dependence	Psychic and/or physical dependence and tolerance may develop, especially in addiction-prone patients; abrupt discontinuation after prolonged use may precipitate withdrawal reactions. Patients with a history of drug dependence should be closely supervised. When prescribing this drug for long-term use, precautions should be taken to prevent patients from increasing the dosage.
Hazards of parenteral administration	This preparation is not indicated for parenteral use. The naloxone component is inactive when taken orally, but it acts as a narcotic antagonist when taken parenterally. Injection may have severe and potentially lethal consequences, including pulmonary emboli, ulceration and abscesses, vascular occlusion, and withdrawal reactions, in narcotic-dependent individuals.
Patients receiving other narcotics	Administration of pentazocine, a mild narcotic antagonist, may precipitate withdrawal reactions in patients taking methadone or other opioid substances
Ambulatory patients	Caution patients not to drive or engage in other potentially hazardous activities, because sedation, dizziness, and/or euphoria may occur. Patients have experienced transient hallucinations (usually visual), disorientation, and confusion; if such reactions occur, observe patient very closely and monitor vital signs. Since these acute CNS reactions may recur, exercise caution if use of this drug is reinstituted. Also, caution patients about the concomitant use of alcohol or other CNS depressants with this drug (see DRUG INTERACTIONS).
Patients with head injuries or increased intracranial pressure	The respiratory depressant effects of pentazocine and its capacity to elevate CSF pressure may be markedly exaggerated in patients with head injuries, other intracranial lesions, or increased intracranial pressure; side effects may also interfere with the clinical evaluation of head injuries. Administer with extreme caution and only if use of this drug is deemed essential.
Patients with respiratory conditions	Use with caution in patients with respiratory depression, severe bronchial asthma or other obstructive respiratory conditions, severely limited respiratory reserve, or cyanosis, because pentazocine can, in rare instances, depress respiration after oral administration
Patients with myocardial infarction	Use with caution in patients with myocardial infarction who are nauseated or vomiting
Patients with hepatic or renal impairment	Use with caution. Pentazocine is metabolized by the liver; in patients with extensive hepatic disease, the risk of side effects may be increased.
Patients predisposed to seizures	Use with caution. Seizures have occurred in a few such patients who were given pentazocine; however, a causal relationship has not been established.
Biliary tract surgery	Some evidence suggests that pentazocine, unlike other narcotic drugs, may cause little or no increase in biliary tract pressure
Carcinogenicity	No long-term studies of carcinogenicity have been performed with this preparation in animals

ADVERSE REACTIONS

Central nervous system	Dizziness, light-headedness, hallucinations, sedation, euphoria, headache, confusion, disorientation, weakness, disturbed dreams, insomnia, depression, paresthesia; tremor, irritability, excitement, and tinnitus (rare)
Ophthalmic	Visual blurring, focusing difficulty
Gastrointestinal	Nausea, vomiting, constipation, diarrhea, anorexia; abdominal distress (rare)
Cardiovascular	Hypotension, tachycardia, syncope, flushing
Hematological	Leukopenia (particularly granulocytopenia; usually reversible); moderate, transient eosinophilia
Hypersensitivity	Facial edema, dermatitis (including pruritus), flushing (including plethora), rash; urticaria (rare)
Other	Chills, sweating, urinary retention; respiratory depression (rare)

OVERDOSAGE

Signs and symptoms	See ADVERSE REACTIONS
Treatment	Employ IV fluids, oxygen, vasopressors, and other supportive measures. For respiratory depression, administer naloxone (usual adult dose: 0.4 mg, preferably IV), simultaneously with respiratory resuscitation. Assisted or controlled ventilation may be indicated.

DRUG INTERACTIONS

Other narcotic analgesics; sedative-hypnotics, antianxiety agents, phenothiazines, general anesthetics, and other CNS depressants (including alcohol); MAO inhibitors; tricyclic antidepressants	△ CNS depression; reduce dose of one or both agents if used concomitantly or in close succession

TALWIN Nx ■ TYCOLET

Anticholinergic agents — ⌂ Risk of paralytic ileus

ALTERED LABORATORY VALUES

Blood/serum values — ⌂ Amylase   ⌂ Lipase

No clinically significant alterations in urinary values occur at therapeutic dosages

USE IN CHILDREN

Safety and effectiveness for use in children under 12 yr of age have not been established

USE IN PREGNANT AND NURSING WOMEN

Pregnancy Category C: use during pregnancy only if clearly needed; animal reproduction studies have not been performed with Talwin Nx, and it is not known whether this preparation can cause harm to the fetus or adversely affect reproductive capacity. Studies of animals given pentazocine have shown no evidence of embryotoxicity. There have been rare reports of a possible neonatal withdrawal syndrome occurring after prolonged use of pentazocine during pregnancy. Use of Talwin Nx during labor and delivery has not been studied; patients given pentazocine during labor have experienced only those adverse effects that are associated with commonly used analgesics. Talwin Nx should be used with caution during the delivery of premature infants. It is not known whether Talwin Nx is excreted in human milk; use with caution in nursing mothers, because many drugs are so excreted.

CONTROLLED ANALGESICS

TYCOLET (hydrocodone bitartrate and acetaminophen) McNeil Pharmaceutical   C-III

Caplets: 5 mg hydrocodone bitartrate and 500 mg acetaminophen

INDICATIONS
Moderate to moderately severe pain

ORAL DOSAGE
Adult: 1 caplet q4–6h, as needed; for more severe pain, 2 caplets q6h, up to 8 caplets/24 h

CONTRAINDICATIONS
Hypersensitivity to hydrocodone or acetaminophen

WARNINGS/PRECAUTIONS

Drug dependence	Psychic and/or physical-dependence and tolerance may develop with prolonged use, especially in addiction-prone individuals
Respiratory depression	A decrease in respiratory rate and/or tidal volume, Cheyne-Stokes respiration, and cyanosis, as well as irregular and periodic breathing, may occur in patients who receive high doses of hydrocodone or are sensitive to this preparation (for treatment, see OVERDOSAGE)
Cough suppression	Hydrocodone suppresses the cough reflex; use with caution postoperatively and in patients with pulmonary disease
Gastrointestinal effects	Nausea and vomiting are more likely to occur in ambulatory patients than in recumbent patients. Antiemetic phenothiazines are useful in managing nausea and vomiting; however, some of these drugs seem to reduce the analgesic effect of this preparation, while others increase the effect.
Ambulatory patients	Caution patients that their ability to engage in potentially hazardous activities requiring full mental alertness or physical coordination may be impaired
Patients with head injuries, other intracranial lesions, or increased intracranial pressure	The respiratory depressant effects of hydrocodone and its capacity to elevate CSF pressure may be markedly exaggerated in such patients; side effects may also interfere with the clinical evaluation of head injuries
Patients with acute abdominal conditions	Use of this preparation may obscure the diagnosis or clinical course of acute abdominal conditions
Other special-risk patients	Use with caution in the elderly and debilitated and in patients with severe hepatic or renal impairment, hypothyroidism, Addison's disease, prostatic hypertrophy, or urethral stricture

ADVERSE REACTIONS

Central nervous system	Sedation, drowsiness, mental clouding, lethargy, impairment of mental and physical performance, anxiety, fear, dysphoria, dizziness, psychic dependence, mood changes
Gastrointestinal	Nausea, vomiting; constipation (with prolonged use)
Genitourinary	Ureteral spasm, vesical sphincter spasm, urinary retention
Respiratory	Depression, irregularities

TYCOLET ■ TYLENOL with Codeine

OVERDOSAGE

Signs and symptoms — *Hydrocodone-related effects:* respiratory depression, miosis, extreme somnolence progressing to stupor or coma, skeletal-muscle flaccidity, cold and clammy skin, bradycardia, hypotension, and, in severe cases, apnea, circulatory collapse, and cardiac arrest; *acetaminophen-related effects:* nausea, anorexia, vomiting, abdominal pain, diarrhea, diaphoresis, malaise; hepatotoxicity may not be evident until after 2–4 days

Treatment — Give primary attention to reestablishing adequate respiratory exchange through provision of an adequate airway and assisted or controlled ventilation; positive-pressure respiration may be desirable if pulmonary edema is present. If respiratory depression is significant, promptly administer naloxone. For adults, give 0.4–2 mg IV (or, if necessary, IM or SC) at 2- to 3-min intervals, as needed; for children, give 0.01 mg/kg IV, followed, if necessary, by 0.1 mg/kg IV (administer IM or SC in divided doses if IV administration is not feasible). Keep the patient under constant surveillance since the duration of action of hydrocodone may exceed that of naloxone; if significant respiratory depression recurs, repeat naloxone dose. *Do not use analeptic agents.* Oxygen, IV fluids, vasopressors, and other supportive measures should be employed, as needed.

Promptly empty stomach by performing gastric lavage or inducing emesis. Administer oral acetylcysteine as soon as possible (no later than 24 h after ingestion); give a loading dose of 140 mg/kg and then, at 4-h intervals, 17 maintenance doses of 70 mg/kg. (Activated charcoal, if used, should be removed before acetylcysteine is given.) Measure the plasma level of unconjugated acetaminophen as early as possible, but no sooner than 4 h after ingestion. Determine prothrombin time, SGOT and SGPT levels, and serum concentrations of bilirubin, creatinine, BUN, glucose, and electrolytes every 24 h. If the prothrombin time exceeds 1.5 times the control value, give vitamin K_1; if the prothrombin time exceeds 3 times this value, give fresh frozen plasma. Institute appropriate measures to treat hypoglycemia and electrolyte and fluid imbalance. Avoid forced diuresis or use of diuretics when treating an acetaminophen overdose. For additional information on use of acetylcysteine and interpretation of the plasma acetaminophen level, see Mucomyst chart.

DRUG INTERACTIONS

Other narcotic analgesics; sedative-hypnotics, antianxiety agents, antipsychotic agents, and other CNS depressants (including alcohol); MAO inhibitors; tricyclic antidepressants — △ CNS depression; reduce dose of one or both agents if used concomitantly or in close succession

Anticholinergic agents — △ Risk of paralytic ileus

ALTERED LABORATORY VALUES

Blood/serum values — △ Amylase △ Lipase ▽ Glucose (with glucose oxidase/peroxidase tests)
Urinary values — △ 5-HIAA (with nitrosonaphthol reagent test)

USE IN CHILDREN

Safety and effectiveness for use in children have not been established

---

USE IN PREGNANT AND NURSING WOMEN

Pregnancy Category C: use during pregnancy only if the expected benefit justifies the potential risk to the fetus. Doses 700 times the normal human dose have resulted in teratogenicity in hamsters; no adequate, well-controlled studies have been conducted in pregnant women. Infants born to mothers who have been taking opioids regularly prior to delivery will be physically dependent and will exhibit withdrawal symptoms. Although the best method of managing neonatal withdrawal signs has not been determined, these reactions have been treated by giving 0.7–1 mg/kg of chlorpromazine q6h or 2–4 drops/kg of paregoric q4h initially and then reducing the dosage, as tolerated, over a period of 4–28 days. Use of this preparation shortly before delivery may cause neonatal respiratory depression, especially at higher doses. It is not known whether this preparation is excreted in human milk. Because many drugs are excreted in breast milk and because of the potential for serious adverse reactions, the patient should not nurse if use of this preparation is deemed essential.

CONTROLLED ANALGESICS

TYLENOL with Codeine (acetaminophen and codeine phosphate) **McNeil Pharmaceutical** C-III
Capsules: 300 mg acetaminophen and 30 mg (No. 3) or 60 mg (No. 4) codeine phosphate **Tablets:** 300 mg acetaminophen and 7.5 mg (No. 1), 15 mg (No. 2), 30 mg (No. 3), or 60 mg (No. 4) codeine phosphate

TYLENOL with Codeine Elixir (acetaminophen and codeine phosphate) **McNeil Pharmaceutical** C-V
Elixir (per 5 ml): 120 mg acetaminophen and 12 mg codeine phosphate[1] (5, 15 ml; 1 pt) *cherry flavored*

INDICATIONS
Mild to moderate pain

ORAL DOSAGE
Adult: 15 ml (1 tbsp) of the elixir q4h, as needed
Child (3–6 yr): 5 ml (1 tsp) (0.5 mg of codeine/kg) of the elixir tid or qid
Child (7–12 yr): 10 ml (2 tsp) (0.5 mg of codeine/kg) of the elixir tid or qid

TYLENOL with Codeine

Mild to moderately severe pain	Adult: 1–2 No. 1, No. 2, or No. 3 tabs, 1–2 No. 3 caps, or 1 No. 4 tab or cap q4h, as needed

CONTRAINDICATIONS

Hypersensitivity to acetaminophen or codeine

WARNINGS/PRECAUTIONS

Drug dependence	Psychic and/or physical dependence and tolerance may develop with continued use, especially in addiction-prone individuals
Ambulatory patients	Caution patients that their ability to engage in potentially hazardous activities requiring full mental alertness or physical coordination may be impaired
Patients with head injuries or other intracranial lesions	The respiratory depressant effects of this drug and its capacity to elevate CSF pressure may be markedly exaggerated in such patients; side effects may also interfere with the clinical evaluation of head injuries
Patients with acute abdominal conditions	Use of this drug may obscure the diagnosis or clinical course of acute abdominal conditions
Other special-risk patients	Use with caution in the elderly and debilitated and in patients with severe renal or hepatic impairment, hypothyroidism, Addison's disease, prostatic hypertrophy, or urethral stricture
Carcinogenicity, mutagenicity	No long-term carcinogenicity studies have been performed in animals; the Ames test, the Basc test on *Drosophila* germ cells, and the Micronucleus test on mouse bone marrow have shown no evidence of mutagenicity
Effect on fertility	No long-term studies have been performed in animals
Sulfite sensitivity	Sodium metabisulfite in capsules and tablets may cause urticaria, pruritus, wheezing, anaphylaxis, or other allergic-type reactions in susceptible patients, such as those with asthma or atopy

ADVERSE REACTIONS

The most frequent reactions, regardless of incidence, are printed in *italics*

Central nervous system	*Light-headedness, dizziness, sedation,* euphoria, dysphoria
Gastrointestinal	*Nausea, vomiting,* constipation
Other	*Shortness of breath,* pruritus, allergic reactions

OVERDOSAGE

Signs and symptoms	*Codeine-related effects:* respiratory depression (a decrease in respiratory rate and/or tidal volume, Cheyne-Stokes respiration, cyanosis), miosis, extreme somnolence progressing to stupor or coma, skeletal-muscle flaccidity, cold and clammy skin, bradycardia, hypotension, and, in severe cases, apnea, circulatory collapse, and cardiac arrest; *acetaminophen-related effects:* nausea, anorexia, vomiting, abdominal pain, diarrhea, diaphoresis, malaise; hepatotoxicity may not be evident until after 2–4 days
Treatment	Give primary attention to reestablishing adequate respiratory exchange through provision of an adequate airway and assisted or controlled ventilation; positive-pressure respiration may be desirable if pulmonary edema is present. If respiratory depression is significant, promptly administer naloxone. For adults, give 0.4–2 mg IV (or, if necessary, IM or SC) at 2- to 3-min intervals, as needed; for children, give 0.01 mg/kg IV, followed, if necessary, by 0.1 mg/kg IV (administer IM or SC in divided doses if IV administration is not feasible). Keep the patient under constant surveillance since the duration of action of codeine may exceed that of naloxone; if significant respiratory depression recurs, repeat naloxone dose. *Do not use analeptic agents.* Oxygen, IV fluids, vasopressors, and other supportive measures should be employed, as needed.
	Promptly empty stomach by performing gastric lavage or inducing emesis. Administer oral acetylcysteine as soon as possible (no later than 24 h after ingestion); give a loading dose of 140 mg/kg and then, at 4-h intervals, 17 maintenance doses of 70 mg/kg. (Activated charcoal, if used, should be removed before acetylcysteine is given.) Measure the plasma level of unconjugated acetaminophen as early as possible, but no sooner than 4 h after ingestion. Determine prothrombin time, SGOT and SGPT levels, and serum concentrations of bilirubin, creatinine, BUN, glucose, and electrolytes every 24 h. If the prothrombin time exceeds 1.5 times the control value, give vitamin K$_1$; if the prothrombin time exceeds 3 times this value, give fresh frozen plasma. Institute appropriate measures to treat hypoglycemia and electrolyte and fluid imbalance. Avoid forced diuresis or use of diuretics when treating an acetaminophen overdose. For additional information on use of acetylcysteine and interpretation of the plasma acetaminophen level, see Mucomyst chart and contact the Rocky Mountain Poison Center (800–525–6115).

DRUG INTERACTIONS

Other narcotic analgesics; sedative-hypnotics, antianxiety agents, phenothiazines, general anesthetics, and other CNS depressants (including alcohol); MAO inhibitors; tricyclic antidepressants	⌂ CNS depression; reduce dose of one or both agents if used concomitantly or in close succession

TYLENOL with Codeine ■ TYLOX

| Anticholinergic agents | △ Risk of paralytic ileus |

ALTERED LABORATORY VALUES

| Blood/serum values | △ Amylase △ Lipase ▽ Glucose (with glucose oxidase/peroxidase tests) |
| Urinary values | △ 5-HIAA (with nitrosonaphthol reagent test) |

USE IN CHILDREN
See INDICATIONS and ORAL DOSAGE. Safety of the elixir for use in children under 3 yr of age has not been established; the tablets and capsules should not be given to children under 12 yr of age.

USE IN PREGNANT AND NURSING WOMEN
Pregnancy Category C: codeine has caused teratogenic effects in mice when given in doses 17 times the maximum human daily dose; no adequate, well-controlled studies have been done in pregnant women. Use this preparation during pregnancy only if the expected benefit justifies the potential risk to the fetus. It is not known whether codeine or acetaminophen is excreted in human milk; use with caution in nursing mothers.

[1] Contains 7% alcohol

CONTROLLED ANALGESICS

TYLOX (oxycodone hydrochloride and acetaminophen) McNeil Pharmaceutical   C-II

Capsules: 5 mg oxycodone hydrochloride and 500 mg acetaminophen

INDICATIONS	ORAL DOSAGE
Moderate to moderately severe pain	**Adult:** 1 cap q6h, as needed

CONTRAINDICATIONS
Hypersensitivity to oxycodone or acetaminophen

WARNINGS/PRECAUTIONS

Drug dependence	Psychic and/or physical dependence and tolerance may develop with continued use, especially in addiction-prone individuals
Ambulatory patients	Caution patients that their ability to engage in potentially hazardous activities requiring full mental alertness or physical coordination may be impaired
Patients with head injuries or other intracranial lesions	The respiratory depressant effects of this drug and its capacity to elevate CSF pressure may be markedly exaggerated in such patients; side effects may also interfere with the clinical evaluation of head injuries
Patients with acute abdominal conditions	Use of this drug may obscure the diagnosis or clinical course of acute abdominal conditions
Other special-risk patients	Use with caution in the elderly or debilitated and in patients with severe hypothyroidism, Addison's disease, prostatic hypertrophy, or urethral stricture
Sulfite sensitivity	Sodium metabisulfite in this product may cause urticaria, pruritus, wheezing, anaphylaxis, or other allergic-type reactions in susceptible patients, such as those with asthma or atopy

ADVERSE REACTIONS
The most frequent reactions, regardless of incidence, are printed in *italics*

Central nervous system	*Light-headedness, dizziness, sedation,* euphoria, dysphoria
Gastrointestinal	*Nausea, vomiting,* constipation
Dermatological	Pruritus, rash
Other	Allergic reactions

OVERDOSAGE

| Signs and symptoms | *Oxycodone-related effects:* respiratory depression, extreme somnolence progressing to stupor or coma, skeletal-muscle flaccidity, cold and clammy skin, bradycardia, hypotension, and, in severe cases, apnea, circulatory collapse, and cardiac arrest; *acetaminophen-related effects:* nausea, anorexia, vomiting, abdominal pain, diarrhea, diaphoresis, malaise; hepatotoxicity may not be evident until after 2–4 days |

Treatment

Give primary attention to reestablishing adequate respiratory exchange through provision of an adequate airway and assisted or controlled ventilation; positive-pressure respiration may be desirable if pulmonary edema is present. If respiratory depression is significant, promptly administer naloxone. For adults, give 0.4–2 mg IV (or, if necessary, IM or SC) at 2- to 3-min intervals, as needed; for children, give 0.01 mg/kg IV, followed, if necessary, by 0.1 mg/kg IV (administer IM or SC in divided doses if IV administration is not feasible). Keep the patient under constant surveillance since the duration of action of oxycodone may exceed that of naloxone; if significant respiratory depression recurs, repeat naloxone dose. *Do not use analeptic agents.* Oxygen, IV fluids, vasopressors, and other supportive measures should be employed, as needed.

Promptly empty stomach by performing gastric lavage or inducing emesis. Administer oral acetylcysteine as soon as possible (no later than 24 h after ingestion); give a loading dose of 140 mg/kg and then, at 4-h intervals, 17 maintenance doses of 70 mg/kg. (Activated charcoal, if used, should be removed before acetylcysteine is given.) Measure the plasma level of unconjugated acetaminophen as early as possible, but no sooner than 4 h after ingestion. Determine prothrombin time, SGOT and SGPT levels, and serum concentrations of bilirubin, creatinine, BUN, glucose, and electrolytes every 24 h. If the prothrombin time exceeds 1.5 times the control value, give vitamin K_1; if the prothrombin time exceeds 3 times this value, give fresh frozen plasma. Institute appropriate measures to treat hypoglycemia and electrolyte and fluid imbalance. Avoid forced diuresis or use of diuretics when treating an acetaminophen overdose. For additional information on use of acetylcysteine and interpretation of the plasma acetaminophen level, see Mucomyst chart and contact the Rocky Mountain Poison Center (800–525–6115).

DRUG INTERACTIONS

Other narcotic analgesics; sedative-hypnotics, antianxiety agents, phenothiazines, general anesthetics, and other CNS depressants (including alcohol); MAO inhibitors; tricyclic antidepressants	△ CNS depression; reduce dose of one or both agents if used concomitantly or in close succession
Anticholinergic agents	△ Risk of paralytic ileus

ALTERED LABORATORY VALUES

Blood/serum values	△ Amylase △ Lipase ▽ Glucose (with glucose oxidase/peroxidase tests)
Urinary values	△ 5-HIAA (with nitrosonaphthol reagent test)

USE IN CHILDREN
Not recommended for use in children

USE IN PREGNANT AND NURSING WOMEN
Pregnancy Category C: reproduction studies have not been done with this preparation. However, it is known that infants born to mothers receiving opioids during pregnancy may be physically dependent and that administration of opioids shortly before delivery may produce respiratory depression in neonates and mothers, especially when higher doses are used. Use during pregnancy only if the expected benefit outweighs the possible hazards. It is not known whether the components of this preparation are excreted in human milk; because many drugs are excreted in human milk, use with caution in nursing mothers.

CONTROLLED ANALGESICS

VICODIN (hydrocodone bitartrate and acetaminophen) Knoll   C-III

Tablets: 5 mg hydrocodone bitartrate and 500 mg acetaminophen

INDICATIONS
Moderate to moderately severe pain

ORAL DOSAGE
Adult: 1 tab q4–6h, as needed; for more severe pain, 2 tabs q6h, up to 8 tabs/24 h

CONTRAINDICATIONS
Hypersensitivity to hydrocodone or acetaminophen

WARNINGS/PRECAUTIONS

Drug dependence	Psychic and/or physical dependence and tolerance may develop with prolonged use, especially in addiction-prone individuals

VICODIN

Respiratory depression	A decrease in respiratory rate and/or tidal volume, Cheyne-Stokes respiration, and cyanosis, as well as irregular and periodic breathing, may occur in patients who receive high doses of hydrocodone or are sensitive to this preparation (for treatment, see OVERDOSAGE)
Cough suppression	Hydrocodone suppresses the cough reflex; use with caution postoperatively and in patients with pulmonary disease
Gastrointestinal effects	Nausea and vomiting are more likely to occur in ambulatory patients than in recumbent patients. Antiemetic phenothiazines are useful in managing nausea and vomiting; however, some of these drugs seem to reduce the analgesic effect of this preparation, while others increase the effect.
Ambulatory patients	Caution patients that their ability to engage in potentially hazardous activities requiring full mental alertness or physical coordination may be impaired
Patients with head injuries, other intracranial lesions, or increased intracranial pressure	The respiratory depressant effects of hydrocodone and its capacity to elevate CSF pressure may be markedly exaggerated in such patients; side effects may also interfere with the clinical evaluation of head injuries
Patients with acute abdominal conditions	Use of this preparation may obscure the diagnosis or clinical course of acute abdominal conditions
Other special-risk patients	Use with caution in the elderly and debilitated and in patients with severe hepatic or renal impairment, hypothyroidism, Addison's disease, prostatic hypertrophy, or urethral stricture

ADVERSE REACTIONS

Central nervous system	Sedation, drowsiness, mental clouding, lethargy, impairment of mental and physical performance, anxiety, fear, dysphoria, dizziness, psychic dependence, mood changes
Gastrointestinal	Nausea, vomiting; constipation (with prolonged use)
Genitourinary	Ureteral spasm, vesical sphincter spasm, urinary retention
Respiratory	Depression, irregularities

OVERDOSAGE

Signs and symptoms	*Hydrocodone-related effects:* respiratory depression, miosis, extreme somnolence progressing to stupor or coma, skeletal-muscle flaccidity, cold and clammy skin, bradycardia, hypotension, and, in severe cases, apnea, circulatory collapse, and cardiac arrest; *acetaminophen-related effects:* nausea, anorexia, vomiting, abdominal pain, diarrhea, diaphoresis, malaise; hepatotoxicity may not be evident until after 2–4 days
Treatment	Give primary attention to reestablishing adequate respiratory exchange through provision of an adequate airway and assisted or controlled ventilation; positive-pressure respiration may be desirable if pulmonary edema is present. If respiratory depression is significant, promptly administer naloxone. For adults, give 0.4–2 mg IV (or, if necessary, IM or SC) at 2- to 3-min intervals, as needed; for children, give 0.01 mg/kg IV, followed, if necessary, by 0.1 mg/kg IV (administer IM or SC in divided doses if IV administration is not feasible). Keep the patient under constant surveillance since the duration of action of hydrocodone may exceed that of naloxone; if significant respiratory depression recurs, repeat naloxone dose. *Do not use analeptic agents.* Oxygen, IV fluids, vasopressors, and other supportive measures should be employed, as needed.
	Promptly empty stomach by performing gastric lavage or inducing emesis. Administer oral acetylcysteine as soon as possible (no later than 24 h after ingestion); give a loading dose of 140 mg/kg and then, at 4-h intervals, 17 maintenance doses of 70 mg/kg. (Activated charcoal, if used, should be removed before acetylcysteine is given.) Measure the plasma level of unconjugated acetaminophen as early as possible, but no sooner than 4 h after ingestion. Determine prothrombin time, SGOT and SGPT levels, and serum concentrations of bilirubin, creatinine, BUN, glucose, and electrolytes every 24 h. If the prothrombin time exceeds 1.5 times the control value, give vitamin K_1; if the prothrombin time exceeds 3 times this value, give fresh frozen plasma. Institute appropriate measures to treat hypoglycemia and electrolyte and fluid imbalance. Avoid forced diuresis or use of diuretics when treating an acetaminophen overdose. For additional information on use of acetylcysteine and interpretation of the plasma acetaminophen level, see Mucomyst chart.

DRUG INTERACTIONS

Other narcotic analgesics; sedative-hypnotics, antianxiety agents, antipsychotic agents, and other CNS depressants (including alcohol); MAO inhibitors; tricyclic antidepressants	⚠ CNS depression; reduce dose of one or both agents if used concomitantly or in close succession
Anticholinergic agents	⚠ Risk of paralytic ileus

ALTERED LABORATORY VALUES

Blood/serum values — △ Amylase △ Lipase ▽ Glucose (with glucose oxidase/peroxidase tests)

Urinary values — △ 5-HIAA (with nitrosonaphthol reagent test)

USE IN CHILDREN
Safety and effectiveness for use in children have not been established

USE IN PREGNANT AND NURSING WOMEN
Pregnancy Category C: use during pregnancy only if the expected benefit justifies the potential risk to the fetus. Doses 700 times the normal human dose have resulted in teratogenicity in hamsters; no adequate, well-controlled studies have been conducted in pregnant women. Infants born to mothers who have been taking opioids regularly prior to delivery will be physically dependent and will exhibit withdrawal symptoms. Although the best method of managing neonatal withdrawal signs has not been determined, these reactions have been treated by giving 0.7–1 mg/kg of chlorpromazine q6h or 2–4 drops/kg of paregoric q4h initially and then reducing the dosage, as tolerated, over a period of 4–28 days. Use of this preparation shortly before delivery may cause neonatal respiratory depression, especially at higher doses. It is not known whether this preparation is excreted in human milk. Because many drugs are excreted in breast milk and because of the potential for serious adverse reactions, the patient should not nurse if use of this preparation is deemed essential.

CONTROLLED ANALGESICS

WYGESIC (propoxyphene hydrochloride and acetaminophen) Wyeth C-IV

Tablets: 65 mg propoxyphene hydrochloride and 650 mg acetaminophen

INDICATIONS
Mild to moderate pain alone or accompanied by fever

ORAL DOSAGE
Adult: 1 tab q4h, as needed, up to 6 tabs/24 h

CONTRAINDICATIONS
Suicidal or addiction-prone individuals — Hypersensitivity to propoxyphene or acetaminophen

WARNINGS/PRECAUTIONS

Drug dependence — Psychic dependence and, less often, physical dependence and tolerance may develop when taken in higher-than-recommended doses for prolonged periods, especially in addiction-prone individuals; prescribe with the same degree of caution appropriate to the use of codeine

Overdosage — Excessive doses of propoxyphene, either alone or in combination with other CNS depressants, including alcohol (see DRUG INTERACTIONS), are a major cause of drug-related fatalities; caution patients not to exceed recommended dosage and to limit their intake of alcohol, and that other CNS depressants have an additive depressant effect

Ambulatory patients — Caution patients that their ability to engage in potentially hazardous activities requiring full mental alertness or physical coordination may be impaired and that alcohol and other CNS depressants may produce additional CNS depression

ADVERSE REACTIONS
The most frequent reactions, regardless of incidence, are printed in *italics*

Central nervous system — *Dizziness, sedation,* light-headedness, headache, weakness, euphoria, dysphoria, minor visual disturbances

Gastrointestinal — *Nausea, vomiting,* constipation, abdominal pain, liver dysfunction

Dermatological — Rash

OVERDOSAGE
Signs and symptoms — *Propoxyphene-related effects:* CNS depression, ranging from somnolence (usually) to stupor and coma; respiratory depression, progressing to Cheyne-Stokes respiration, cyanosis, hypoxia, and apnea; pinpoint pupils, becoming dilated as hypoxia increases; fall in blood pressure and deterioration in cardiac performance, culminating in pulmonary edema and circulatory collapse; respiratory and metabolic acidosis; cardiac conduction delay and arrhythmias; convulsions; *acetaminophen-related effects:* nausea, anorexia, vomiting, abdominal pain, diarrhea, diaphoresis, malaise; hepatotoxicity may not be evident until after 2–4 days

Treatment	Give primary attention to reestablishing adequate respiratory exchange through provision of an adequate airway and assisted or controlled ventilation; positive-pressure respiration may be desirable if pulmonary edema is present. If respiratory depression is significant, promptly administer naloxone. For adults, give 0.4–2 mg IV (or, if necessary, IM or SC) at 2- to 3-min intervals, as needed; for children, give 0.01 mg/kg IV, followed, if necessary, by 0.1 mg/kg IV (administer IM or SC in divided doses if IV administration is not feasible). Reevaluate diagnosis if no response is seen after giving 10 mg of naloxone. *Do not use analeptic agents.* Monitor blood gases, pH, and electrolytes, and promptly correct any acid-base or electrolyte abnormalities present (lactic acidosis may require IV sodium bicarbonate for prompt correction). Administer an anticonvulsant in carefully titrated doses if seizures occur. Oxygen, IV fluids, vasopressors, and other supportive measures should be employed, as needed. ECG monitoring is essential since ventricular fibrillation or cardiac arrest can occur.
	Promptly empty stomach by performing gastric lavage or inducing emesis; activated charcoal may also be used to remove propoxyphene. Administer oral acetylcysteine as soon as possible (no later than 24 h after ingestion); give a loading dose of 140 mg/kg and then, at 4-h intervals, 17 maintenance doses of 70 mg/kg. (Activated charcoal, if used, should be removed before acetylcysteine is given.) Measure the plasma level of unconjugated acetaminophen as early as possible, but no sooner than 4 h after ingestion. Determine prothrombin time, SGOT and SGPT levels, and serum concentrations of bilirubin, creatinine, BUN, glucose, and electrolytes every 24 h. If the prothrombin time exceeds 1.5 times the control value, give vitamin K_1; if the prothrombin time exceeds 3 times this value, give fresh frozen plasma. Institute appropriate measures to treat hypoglycemia and electrolyte and fluid imbalance. Avoid forced diuresis or use of diuretics when treating an acetaminophen overdose. For additional information on use of acetylcysteine and interpretation of the plasma acetaminophen level, see Mucomyst chart.

DRUG INTERACTIONS

Other narcotic analgesics; sedative-hypnotics, antianxiety agents, phenothiazines, general anesthetics, and other CNS depressants (including alcohol); MAO inhibitors; tricyclic antidepressants	△ CNS depression

ALTERED LABORATORY VALUES

Blood/serum values	▽ Glucose (with glucose oxidase/peroxidase tests)
Urinary values	△ 5-HIAA (with nitrosonaphthol reagent test)

USE IN CHILDREN
Not recommended for use in children

USE IN PREGNANT AND NURSING WOMEN
Safety for use during pregnancy has not been established in regard to fetal development; neonatal withdrawal symptoms have been reported following propoxyphene usage during pregnancy. Although low levels of propoxyphene have been found in human milk, no adverse effects have been noted in nursing infants.

CONTROLLED ANALGESICS

ZYDONE (hydrocodone bitartrate and acetaminophen) Du Pont   C-III

Capsules: 5 mg hydrocodone bitartrate and 500 mg acetaminophen

INDICATIONS	ORAL DOSAGE
Moderate to moderately severe pain	Adult: 1 cap q4–6h, as needed; for more severe pain, 2 caps q6h, up to 8 caps/24 h

CONTRAINDICATIONS
Hypersensitivity to hydrocodone or acetaminophen

WARNINGS/PRECAUTIONS

Drug dependence	Psychic and/or physical dependence and tolerance may develop with prolonged use, especially in addiction-prone individuals
Respiratory depression	A decrease in respiratory rate and/or tidal volume, Cheyne-Stokes respiration, and cyanosis, as well as irregular and periodic breathing, may occur in patients who receive high doses of hydrocodone or are sensitive to this preparation (for treatment, see OVERDOSAGE)

ZYDONE

Cough suppression	Hydrocodone suppresses the cough reflex; use with caution postoperatively and in patients with pulmonary disease
Gastrointestinal effects	Nausea and vomiting are more likely to occur in ambulatory patients than in recumbent patients. Antiemetic phenothiazines are useful in managing nausea and vomiting; however, some of these drugs seem to reduce the analgesic effect of this preparation, while others increase the effect.
Ambulatory patients	Caution patients that their ability to engage in potentially hazardous activities requiring full mental alertness or physical coordination may be impaired
Patients with head injuries, other intracranial lesions, or increased intracranial pressure	The respiratory depressant effects of hydrocodone and its capacity to elevate CSF pressure may be markedly exaggerated in such patients; side effects may also interfere with the clinical evaluation of head injuries
Patients with acute abdominal conditions	Use of this preparation may obscure the diagnosis or clinical course of acute abdominal conditions
Other special-risk patients	Use with caution in the elderly and debilitated and in patients with severe hepatic or renal impairment, hypothyroidism, Addison's disease, prostatic hypertrophy, or urethral stricture

ADVERSE REACTIONS

Central nervous system	Sedation, drowsiness, mental clouding, lethargy, impairment of mental and physical performance, anxiety, fear, dysphoria, dizziness, psychic dependence, mood changes
Gastrointestinal	Nausea, vomiting; constipation (with prolonged use)
Genitourinary	Ureteral spasm, vesical sphincter spasm, urinary retention
Respiratory	Depression, irregularities

OVERDOSAGE

Signs and symptoms	*Hydrocodone-related effects:* respiratory depression, miosis, extreme somnolence progressing to stupor or coma, skeletal-muscle flaccidity, cold and clammy skin, bradycardia, hypotension, and, in severe cases, apnea, circulatory collapse, and cardiac arrest; *acetaminophen-related effects:* nausea, anorexia, vomiting, abdominal pain, diarrhea, diaphoresis, malaise; hepatotoxicity may not be evident until after 2–4 days
Treatment	Give primary attention to reestablishing adequate respiratory exchange through provision of an adequate airway and assisted or controlled ventilation; positive-pressure respiration may be desirable if pulmonary edema is present. If respiratory depression is significant, promptly administer naloxone. For adults, give 0.4–2 mg IV (or, if necessary, IM or SC) at 2- to 3-min intervals, as needed; for children, give 0.01 mg/kg IV, followed, if necessary, by 0.1 mg/kg IV (administer IM or SC in divided doses if IV administration is not feasible). Keep the patient under constant surveillance since the duration of action of hydrocodone may exceed that of naloxone; if significant respiratory depression recurs, repeat naloxone dose. *Do not use analeptic agents.* Oxygen, IV fluids, vasopressors, and other supportive measures should be employed, as needed.
	Promptly empty stomach by performing gastric lavage or inducing emesis. Administer oral acetylcysteine as soon as possible (no later than 24 h after ingestion); give a loading dose of 140 mg/kg and then, at 4-h intervals, 17 maintenance doses of 70 mg/kg. (Activated charcoal, if used, should be removed before acetylcysteine is given.) Measure the plasma level of unconjugated acetaminophen as early as possible, but no sooner than 4 h after ingestion. Determine prothrombin time, SGOT and SGPT levels, and serum concentrations of bilirubin, creatinine, BUN, glucose, and electrolytes every 24 h. If the prothrombin time exceeds 1.5 times the control value, give vitamin K$_1$; if the prothrombin time exceeds 3 times this value, give fresh frozen plasma. Institute appropriate measures to treat hypoglycemia and electrolyte and fluid imbalance. Avoid forced diuresis or use of diuretics when treating an acetaminophen overdose. For additional information on use of acetylcysteine and interpretation of the plasma acetaminophen level, see Mucomyst chart.

DRUG INTERACTIONS

Other narcotic analgesics; sedative-hypnotics, antianxiety agents, antipsychotic agents, and other CNS depressants (including alcohol); MAO inhibitors; tricyclic antidepressants	△ CNS depression; reduce dose of one or both agents if used concomitantly or in close succession
Anticholinergic agents	△ Risk of paralytic ileus

ALTERED LABORATORY VALUES

Blood/serum values	△ Amylase △ Lipase ▽ Glucose (with glucose oxidase/peroxidase tests)
Urinary values	△ 5-HIAA (with nitrosonaphthol reagent test)

USE IN CHILDREN

Safety and effectiveness for use in children have not been established

USE IN PREGNANT AND NURSING WOMEN

Pregnancy Category C: use during pregnancy only if the expected benefit justifies the potential risk to the fetus. Doses 700 times the normal human dose have resulted in teratogenicity in hamsters; no adequate, well-controlled studies have been conducted in pregnant women. Infants born to mothers who have been taking opioids regularly prior to delivery will be physically dependent and will exhibit withdrawal symptoms. Although the best method of managing neonatal withdrawal signs has not been determined, these reactions have been treated by giving 0.7–1 mg/kg of chlorpromazine q6h or 2–4 drops/kg of paregoric q4h initially and then reducing the dosage, as tolerated, over a period of 4–28 days. Use of this preparation shortly before delivery may cause neonatal respiratory depression, especially at higher doses. It is not known whether this preparation is excreted in human milk. Because many drugs are excreted in breast milk and because of the potential for serious adverse reactions, the patient should not nurse if use of this preparation is deemed essential.

Chapter 8

Nonnarcotic Analgesics/Antipyretics

ADVIL (Whitehall) — 281
Ibuprofen *OTC*

ANACIN (Whitehall) — 281
Aspirin and caffeine *OTC*

Maximum Strength ANACIN (Whitehall) — 282
Aspirin and caffeine *OTC*

Children's ANACIN-3 (Whitehall) — 283
Acetaminophen *OTC*

Maximum Strength ANACIN-3 (Whitehall) — 283
Acetaminophen *OTC*

Regular Strength ANACIN-3 (Whitehall) — 282
Acetaminophen *OTC*

ANAPROX (Syntex) — 284
Naproxen sodium *Rx*

APF ARTHRITIS PAIN FORMULA (Whitehall) — 286
Acetaminophen *OTC*

ARTHRITIS PAIN FORMULA (Whitehall) — 286
Aspirin, aluminum hydroxide, and magnesium hydroxide *OTC*

ARTHROPAN (Purdue Frederick) — 287
Choline salicylate *OTC*

ASCRIPTIN (Rorer) — 288
Aspirin, magnesium hydroxide, and aluminum hydroxide *OTC*

ASCRIPTIN A/D (Rorer) — 288
Aspirin, magnesium hydroxide, and aluminum hydroxide *OTC*

Extra Strength ASCRIPTIN (Rorer) — 289
Aspirin, magnesium hydroxide, and aluminum hydroxide *OTC*

BAYER Aspirin (Glenbrook) — 290
Aspirin *OTC*

Maximum BAYER Aspirin (Glenbrook) — 290
Aspirin *OTC*

BAYER Children's Chewable Aspirin (Glenbrook) — 290
Aspirin *OTC*

8-Hour BAYER Aspirin (Glenbrook) — 290
Aspirin *OTC*

BUFFERIN (Bristol-Myers) — 292
Aspirin, aluminum glycinate, and magnesium carbonate *OTC*

Arthritis Strength BUFFERIN (Bristol-Myers) — 292
Aspirin, aluminum glycinate, and magnesium carbonate *OTC*

Extra Strength BUFFERIN (Bristol-Myers) — 292
Aspirin, aluminum glycinate, and magnesium carbonate *OTC*

Extra Strength DATRIL (Bristol-Myers) — 293
Acetaminophen *OTC*

DOLOBID (Merck Sharp & Dohme) — 294
Diflunisal *Rx*

Maximum Strength ECOTRIN (SmithKline Consumer Products) — 296
Aspirin *OTC*

Regular Strength ECOTRIN (SmithKline Consumer Products) — 296
Aspirin *OTC*

EMPIRIN (Burroughs Wellcome) — 297
Aspirin *OTC*

FIORICET (Sandoz Pharmaceuticals) — 299
Butalbital, acetaminophen, and caffeine *Rx*

GEMNISYN (Kremers-Urban) — 300
Aspirin and acetaminophen *OTC*

HALTRAN (Upjohn) — 301
Ibuprofen *OTC*

LEVOPROME (Lederle) — 302
Methotrimeprazine *Rx*

MAGAN (Adria) — 303
Magnesium salicylate *Rx*

MEDIPREN (McNeil Consumer Products) — 305
Ibuprofen *OTC*

MIDOL 200 (Glenbrook) — 305
Ibuprofen *OTC*

MOTRIN (Upjohn) — 306
Ibuprofen *Rx*

NALFON (Dista) — 308
Fenoprofen calcium *Rx*

NAPROSYN (Syntex) — 310
Naproxen *Rx*

NUBAIN (Du Pont) — 312
Nalbuphine hydrochloride *Rx*

NUPRIN (Bristol-Myers) — 313
Ibuprofen *OTC*

PANADOL (Glenbrook) — 314
Acetaminophen *OTC*

PANADOL Jr. (Glenbrook) — 315
Acetaminophen *OTC*

Children's PANADOL (Glenbrook) — 314
Acetaminophen *OTC*

PERCOGESIC (Richardson-Vicks Health Care Products) — 315
Acetaminophen and phenyltoloxamine citrate *OTC*

PONSTEL (Parke-Davis) — 316
Mefenamic acid *Rx*

RUFEN (Boots) — 318
Ibuprofen *Rx*

ST. JOSEPH Aspirin for Children (Plough) — 320
Aspirin *OTC*

Aspirin-Free ST. JOSEPH (Plough) — 321
Acetaminophen *OTC*

STADOL (Bristol) — 322
Butorphanol tartrate *Rx*

SUPROL (McNeil Pharmaceutical/Ortho) — 323
Suprofen *Rx*

SYNALGOS (Wyeth) — 325
Aspirin and caffeine *OTC*

continued

COMPENDIUM OF DRUG THERAPY

Nonnarcotic Analgesics/Antipyretics continued

TEMPRA (Mead Johnson) 326
Acetaminophen *OTC*

TRENDAR (Whitehall) 327
Ibuprofen *OTC*

Children's TYLENOL (McNeil Consumer Products) 328
Acetaminophen *OTC*

Extra-Strength TYLENOL 328
(McNeil Consumer Products)
Acetaminophen *OTC*

Junior Strength TYLENOL 328
(McNeil Consumer Products)
Acetaminophen *OTC*

Regular Strength TYLENOL 328
(McNeil Consumer Products)
Acetaminophen *OTC*

Other Nonnarcotic Analgesics/ 279
Antipyretics

AXOTAL (Adria) 279
Butalbital and aspirin *Rx*

CAMA (Sandoz Consumer Health Care Group) 279
Aspirin, magnesium oxide, and dried aluminum
hydroxide gel *OTC*

COPE (Mentholatum) 279
Aspirin, caffeine, magnesium hydroxide, and
dried aluminum hydroxide gel *OTC*

DILONE (Richardson-Vicks Health Care Products) 279
Acetaminophen, phenyltoloxamine citrate,
and caffeine *OTC*

DIMENSYN (Advanced Health Care Products) 279
Acetaminophen, pamabrom, and pyrilamine
maleate *OTC*

DORCOL Fever and Pain Reducer 279
(Sandoz Consumer Health Care Group)
Acetaminophen *OTC*

EASPRIN (Parke-Davis) 279
Aspirin *Rx*

ENCAPRIN (Richardson-Vicks Health Care Products) 279
Aspirin *OTC*

ESGIC (Gilbert) 279
Butalbital, caffeine, and acetaminophen *Rx*

EXCEDRIN (Bristol-Myers) 279
Acetaminophen, aspirin, and caffeine *OTC*

EXCEDRIN P.M. (Bristol-Myers) 279
Acetaminophen and diphenhydramine citrate *OTC*

LIQUIPRIN (Norcliff Thayer) 279
Acetaminophen *OTC*

MIDOL (Glenbrook) 279
Aspirin, cinnamedrine hydrochloride, and caffeine
OTC

Maximum Strength MIDOL (Glenbrook) 279
Aspirin, cinnamedrine hydrochloride, and caffeine
OTC

Maximum Strength MIDOL PMS (Glenbrook) 279
Acetaminophen, pamabrom, and pyrilamine
maleate *OTC*

MOMENTUM (Whitehall) 279
Aspirin and phenyltoloxamine citrate *OTC*

PABALATE (Robins) 280
Sodium salicylate and sodium aminobenzoate *OTC*

PABALATE-SF (Robins) 280
Potassium salicylate and potassium
aminobenzoate *Rx*

PHENAPHEN (Robins) 280
Acetaminophen *OTC*

Sodium salicylate *OTC, Rx* 280

Sodium thiosalicylate *Rx* 280

VANQUISH (Glenbrook) 280
Aspirin, acetaminophen, caffeine, dried aluminum
hydroxide gel, and magnesium hydroxide *OTC*

ZORPRIN (Boots) 280
Aspirin *Rx*

OTHER NONNARCOTIC ANALGESICS/ANTIPYRETICS

DRUG	HOW SUPPLIED	USUAL DOSAGE[1]
AXOTAL (Adria) Butalbital and aspirin *Rx*	**Tablets:** 50 mg butalbital and 650 mg aspirin	**Adult:** 1 tab q4h, as needed, with food or 8 fl oz of water or milk
CAMA (Sandoz Consumer Health Care Group) Aspirin, magnesium oxide, and dried aluminum hydroxide gel *OTC*	**Tablets:** 500 mg aspirin, 150 mg magnesium oxide, and 150 mg dried aluminum hydroxide gel	**Adult:** 2 tabs q6h with 8 fl oz of water, as needed
COPE (Mentholatum) Aspirin, caffeine, magnesium hydroxide, and dried aluminum hydroxide gel *OTC*	**Tablets:** 421 mg aspirin, 32 mg caffeine, 50 mg magnesium hydroxide, and 25 mg dried aluminum hydroxide gel	**Adult:** 2 tabs to start, followed by 1 tab q3h, as needed, up to 9 tabs/24 h; each dose should be given with a full glass of water
DILONE (Richardson-Vicks Health Care Products) Acetaminophen, phenyltoloxamine citrate, and caffeine *OTC*	**Tablets:** 325 mg acetaminophen, 30 mg phenyltoloxamine citrate, and 30 mg caffeine	**Adult:** 1–2 tabs q4h, up to 8 tabs/day **Child (6–12 yr):** ½–1 tab q4h, up to 4 tabs/day
DIMENSYN (Advanced Care Products) Acetaminophen, pamabrom, and pyrilamine maleate *OTC*	**Capsules:** 500 mg acetaminophen, 25 mg pamabrom, and 15 mg pyrilamine maleate	**Adult:** 2 caps q3–4h, as needed, up to 8 caps/24 h
DORCOL Children's Fever and Pain Reducer (Sandoz Consumer Health Care Group) Acetaminophen *OTC*	**Elixir (per 5 ml):** 160 mg (4 fl oz)	**Child (2–4 yr; 25–35 lb):** 5 ml (1 tsp) q4h, up to 5 times/24 h **Child (4–6 yr; 36–45 lb):** 7.5 ml (1½ tsp) q4h, up to 5 times/24 h **Child (6 yr; 46–60 lb):** 10 ml (2 tsp) q4h, up to 5 times/24h
EASPRIN (Parke-Davis) Aspirin *Rx*	**Tablets (enteric coated):** 975 mg	**Adult:** 975 mg (1 tab) tid or qid; if long-term qid use is tolerated, bid regimen may be instituted
ENCAPRIN (Richardson-Vicks Health Care Products) Aspirin *OTC*	**Capsules (with enteric-coated granules):** 325, 500 mg	**Adult:** 650–1,000 mg with water q4h, up to 4,000 mg/24 h; dosing may be gradually changed from q4h to bid
ESGIC (Gilbert) Butalbital, caffeine, and acetaminophen *Rx*	**Capsules:** 50 mg butalbital, 40 mg caffeine, and 325 mg acetaminophen **Tablets:** 50 mg butalbital, 40 mg caffeine, and 325 mg acetaminophen	**Adult:** 1–2 caps or tabs q4h, as needed, up to 6 caps or tabs/day
EXCEDRIN (Bristol-Myers) Acetaminophen, aspirin, and caffeine *OTC*	**Caplets:** 250 mg acetaminophen, 250 mg aspirin, and 65 mg caffeine **Tablets:** 250 mg acetaminophen, 250 mg aspirin, and 65 mg caffeine	**Adult:** 2 caplets or tabs q4h, up to 8 caplets or tabs/24 h **Child (≥ 12 yr):** same as adult
EXCEDRIN P.M. (Bristol-Myers) Acetaminophen and diphenhydramine citrate *OTC*	**Tablets:** 500 mg acetaminophen and 38 mg diphenhydramine citrate	**Adult:** 2 tabs at bedtime
LIQUIPRIN (Norcliff Thayer) Acetaminophen *OTC*	**Drops (per 1.66-ml dropperful):** 80 mg (35 ml) *raspberry flavored*	**Child (2–3 yr):** 160 mg (2 dropperful) q4h, up to 5 times/day **Child (4–5 yr):** 240 mg (3 dropperful) q4h, up to 5 times/day
MIDOL (Glenbrook) Aspirin, cinnamedrine hydrochloride, and caffeine *OTC*	**Caplets:** 454 mg aspirin, 14.9 mg cinnamedrine hydrochloride, and 32.4 mg caffeine	**Adult:** 2 caplets with water q4h, as needed, up to 8 caplets/day
Maximum Strength MIDOL (Glenbrook) Aspirin, cinnamedrine hydrochloride, and caffeine *OTC*	**Caplets:** 500 mg aspirin, 14.9 mg cinnamedrine hydrochloride, and 32.4 mg caffeine	**Adult:** 2 caplets with water q4h, as needed, up to 8 caplets/24 h
Maximum Strength MIDOL PMS (Glenbrook) Acetaminophen, pamabrom, and pyrilamine maleate *OTC*	**Caplets:** 500 mg acetaminophen, 25 mg pamabrom, and 15 mg pyrilamine maleate	**Adult:** 2 caplets with water q4h, as needed, up to 8 caplets/day
MOMENTUM (Whitehall) Aspirin and phenyltoloxamine citrate *OTC*	**Tablets:** 500 mg aspirin and 15 mg phenyltoloxamine citrate	**Adult:** 2 tabs upon arising, followed, if needed, by 2 tabs at lunch, dinner, and bedtime, up to 8 tabs/24 h

[1] Where pediatric dosages are not given, consult manufacturer

continued

OTHER NONNARCOTIC ANALGESICS/ANTIPYRETICS continued

DRUG	HOW SUPPLIED	USUAL DOSAGE[1]
PABALATE (Robins) Sodium salicylate and sodium aminobenzoate *OTC*	**Tablets (enteric coated):** 300 mg sodium salicylate and 300 mg sodium aminobenzoate	**Adult:** 2 tabs q4h
PABALATE-SF (Robins) Potassium salicylate and potassium aminobenzoate *Rx*	**Tablets (enteric coated):** 300 mg potassium salicylate and 300 mg potassium aminobenzoate	**Adult:** 2 tabs q4h
PHENAPHEN (Robins) Acetaminophen *OTC*	**Capsules:** 325 mg	**Adult:** 325–650 mg tid or qid **Child (6–12 yr):** 325 mg tid or qid
Sodium salicylate *OTC, Rx*	**Tablets:** 325, 650 mg *OTC* **Ampuls:** 1 g (10 ml) *Rx*	**Adult:** 325–650 mg PO q4–8h; 500 mg/day IV
Sodium thiosalicylate *Rx*	**Vials:** 50 mg/ml (30 ml)	**Adult:** 50–100 mg IM daily or every other day
VANQUISH (Glenbrook) Aspirin, acetaminophen, caffeine, dried aluminum hydroxide gel, and magnesium hydroxide *OTC*	**Tablets:** 227 mg aspirin, 194 mg acetaminophen, 33 mg caffeine, 25 mg dried aluminum hydroxide gel, and 50 mg magnesium hydroxide	**Adult:** 2 tabs with water q4h, as needed
ZORPRIN (Boots) Aspirin *Rx*	**Tablets (controlled release):** 800 mg	**Adult:** 1,600 mg (2 tabs) with at least 8 fl oz of water bid for the 1st week; thereafter, titrate dosage according to patient response **Child (≥ 12 yr):** same as adult

[1] Where pediatric dosages are not given, consult manufacturer

NONNARCOTIC ANALGESICS/ANTIPYRETICS

ADVIL (ibuprofen) Whitehall — OTC

Tablets: 200 mg **Caplets:** 200 mg

INDICATIONS

Headache, toothache, backache, muscle ache, menstrual pain, minor pain of arthritis, and minor ache and pain of colds

Fever

ORAL DOSAGE

Adult: 200–400 mg q4–6h, up to 1,200 mg/24 h, for a period of up to 10 days; initial dosage: 200 mg q4–6h. The package labeling warns patients not to exceed these recommendations unless otherwise directed by a physician.
Child (> 12 yr): same as adult

Adult: 200–400 mg q4–6h, up to 1,200 mg/24 h, for a period of up to 3 days; initial dosage: 200 mg q4–6h. The package labeling warns patients not to exceed these recommendations unless otherwise directed by a physician.
Child (> 12 yr): same as adult

CONTRAINDICATIONS
Consult manufacturer

WARNINGS/PRECAUTIONS

Special-risk patients — The package labeling warns patients not to take this product if they have had a severe allergic reaction to aspirin, such as asthma, swelling, shock, or hives; the labeling also cautions patients to consult a physician before using this product if they have experienced any problems or serious adverse reactions while taking an OTC analgesic, if they are under medical supervision for the treatment of a serious condition, or if they are receiving a prescription drug (see also USE IN CHILDREN and USE IN PREGNANT AND NURSING WOMEN)

Adverse reactions — The package labeling instructs patients to take the tablets with food or milk if occasional, mild heartburn, upset stomach, or stomach pain occurs and to consult a physician if gastric symptoms, pain, or fever becomes persistent or more severe, if other new symptoms develop, or if a painful area becomes red or swollen

Concomitant use of other drugs — The package labeling cautions patients not to combine this product with any other ibuprofen-containing product and to consult a physician before using this product in combination with aspirin or acetaminophen (see also DRUG INTERACTIONS)

ADVERSE REACTIONS
Consult manufacturer

OVERDOSAGE

Signs and symptoms — Apnea, cyanosis, dizziness, nystagmus

Treatment — Following recent ingestion (< 1 h), induce emesis or perform gastric lavage to remove drug from stomach. Activated charcoal may be helpful. If drug is already absorbed, it may be useful to induce diuresis and alkalinize the urine.

DRUG INTERACTIONS

Coumarin anticoagulants — ⇧ Risk of bleeding; use with caution
Aspirin — ⇩ Anti-inflammatory activity (potential)

ALTERED LABORATORY VALUES

Blood/serum values — ⇧ SGOT ⇧ SGPT
No clinically significant alterations in urinary values occur at therapeutic dosages

---

USE IN CHILDREN
The package labeling warns adults to consult a physician before giving this product to children under 12 yr of age

USE IN PREGNANT AND NURSING WOMEN
The package labeling cautions pregnant or nursing women to consult a health professional before using this product and, because ibuprofen may cause premature closure of the ductus arteriosus or complications during delivery, warns patients not to use this product during the last 3 mo of pregnancy unless specifically directed to do so by a physician

---

NONNARCOTIC ANALGESICS/ANTIPYRETICS

ANACIN (aspirin and caffeine) Whitehall — OTC

Caplets: 400 mg aspirin and 32 mg caffeine **Tablets:** 400 mg aspirin and 32 mg caffeine

INDICATIONS

Headache, neuralgia, neuritis, sprains, muscular aches, tooth-extraction pain, toothache, menstrual discomfort, and minor aches and pains of arthritis and rheumatism

Fever and discomfort of colds

ORAL DOSAGE

Adult: 2 caplets or tabs with water q4h, as needed, up to 10 caplets or tabs per day
Child (6–12 yr): 1 caplet or tab with water q4h, as needed, up to 5 caplets or tabs per day

Maximum Strength ANACIN (aspirin and caffeine) Whitehall OTC
Tablets: 500 mg aspirin and 32 mg caffeine

INDICATIONS
Headache, neuralgia, neuritis, sprains, muscular aches, tooth-extraction pain, toothache, menstrual discomfort, and minor aches and pains of arthritis and rheumatism
Fever and discomfort associated with colds

ORAL DOSAGE
Adult and child ($\geq$ 12 yr): 2 tabs with water tid or qid

WARNINGS/PRECAUTIONS
Patient self-medication	Package labels caution patients to consult a physician immediately if pain persists for more than 10 days or redness is present or for arthritic or rheumatic conditions affecting children under 12 yr of age; labels also advise patients who are pregnant or nursing to seek the advice of a health-care professional before using these products
Reye's syndrome	There is evidence suggesting that use of aspirin in children or adolescents with chicken pox or influenza may increase the risk of Reye's syndrome

OVERDOSAGE
Signs and symptoms	*Aspirin-related effects:* hyperpnea, nausea, vomiting, vertigo, tinnitus, flushing, sweating, thirst, headache, drowsiness, diarrhea, and tachycardia, progressing to hyperthermia, hemorrhage, acid-base disturbances, restlessness, confusion, convulsions, vasomotor depression, coma, and respiratory failure; *caffeine-related effects:* insomnia, restlessness, tremors, delirium, tachycardia, extrasystoles, tinnitus, urinary frequency
Treatment	If less than 4 h have elapsed since ingestion, induce emesis or perform gastric lavage, followed by activated charcoal, to remove any remaining drug from the stomach. Initial therapy should be directed at reducing hyperthermia by external sponging with tepid water, correcting dehydration by appropriate IV fluid replacement, and maintaining adequate cardiorespiratory and renal function. In moderately severe cases of salicylate poisoning, cautiously administer sodium bicarbonate IV in sufficient quantity, if possible, to maintain an alkaline diuresis; intermittent peritoneal dialysis may also be helpful. In severe cases, hemodialysis should be seriously considered. Potassium should be added to the repair solution to compensate for potassium losses once urine formation is deemed adequate. Glucose may be provided to correct ketosis and hypoglycemia. Plasma transfusion may be beneficial if shock intervenes. Hemorrhagic phenomena may necessitate whole-blood transfusions and phytonadione (vitamin K_1). Do not administer barbiturates to treat excitement or convulsions.

DRUG INTERACTIONS
Anticoagulants	△ Risk of bleeding
Alcohol, corticosteroids, phenylbutazone, oxyphenbutazone	△ Risk of GI ulceration
Probenecid, sulfinpyrazone	▽ Uricosuria
Spironolactone	▽ Diuretic effect
Methotrexate	△ Methotrexate plasma level and risk of toxicity

ALTERED LABORATORY VALUES
Blood/serum values	△ Prothrombin time △ Uric acid (with low doses) ▽ Uric acid (with high doses) ▽ Thyroxine (T_4) ▽ Thyroid-stimulating hormone
Urinary values	△ Glucose (with Clinitest tablets)

USE IN CHILDREN
Anacin is not recommended for use in children under 6 yr of age; Maximum Strength Anacin is not recommended for use in children under 12 yr of age

USE IN PREGNANT AND NURSING WOMEN
Consult manufacturer for use during pregnancy and in nursing mothers

---

NONNARCOTIC ANALGESICS/ANTIPYRETICS

Regular Strength ANACIN-3 (acetaminophen) Whitehall OTC
Tablets: 325 mg

INDICATIONS
Pain (headache, colds, flu, sinusitis, muscle aches, bursitis, sprains, overexertion, backache, menstrual discomfort, minor arthritic pain, and toothaches)
Fever

ORAL DOSAGE
Adult: 650–975 mg (2–3 tablets) q4h, up to 3,900 mg (12 tablets)/24 h
Child (6–12 yr): 162.5–325 mg (1/2–1 tab) tid or qid

Maximum Strength ANACIN-3 (acetaminophen) Whitehall — OTC

Caplets: 500 mg **Tablets:** 500 mg

INDICATIONS	ORAL DOSAGE
Pain (headache, colds, flu, sinusitis, muscle aches, bursitis, sprains, overexertion, backache, menstrual discomfort, minor arthritic pain, and toothaches) Fever	Adult: 1,000 mg (2 caplets or tablets) tid or qid, up to 4,000 mg (8 caplets or tablets)/24 h

Children's ANACIN-3 (acetaminophen) Whitehall — OTC

Chewable tablets: 80 mg *cherry flavored* **Liquid (per 5 ml):** 160 mg (2, 4 fl oz) *cherry flavored, alcohol free* **Drops (per 0.8-ml dropperful):** 80 mg (0.5 fl oz) *fruit flavored, alcohol free*

INDICATIONS	ORAL DOSAGE
Fever and pain associated with mild upper respiratory infections, headache, myalgia, immunization, tonsillectomy, gastroenteritis, and other conditions requiring reduction of fever and/or relief of pain	Infant (0–3 mo; 6–11 lb): 40 mg (½ dropperful) q4h, up to 5 doses/24 h Infant (4–11 mo; 12–17 lb): 80 mg (1 dropperful or ½ tsp liquid) q4h, up to 5 doses/24 h Child (12–23 mo; 18–23 lb): 120 mg (1½ dropperful, ¾ tsp liquid, or 1½ tablets) q4h, up to 5 doses/24 h Child (2–3 yr; 24–35 lb): 160 mg (2 dropperful, 1 tsp liquid, or 2 tablets) q4h, up to 5 doses/24 h Child (4–5 yr; 36–47 lb): 240 mg (3 dropperful, 1½ tsp liquid, or 3 tablets) q4h, up to 5 doses/24 h Child (6–8 yr; 48–59 lb): 320 mg (2 tsp liquid or 4 tablets) q4h, up to 5 doses/24 h Child (9–10 yr; 60–71 lb): 400 mg (2½ tsp liquid or 5 tablets) q4h, up to 5 doses/24 h Child (11–12 yr; 72–95 lb): 480 mg (3 tsp liquid or 6 tablets) q4h, up to 5 doses/24 h

ADMINISTRATION/DOSAGE ADJUSTMENTS

Use of drops and liquid	The pediatric drops and liquid may be given directly or mixed with milk, formula, or fruit juice

WARNINGS/PRECAUTIONS

Hypersensitivity	On rare occasions, a hypersensitivity reaction may occur; if reaction is seen, discontinue use
Patients with phenylketonuria	The chewable tablets contain phenylalanine; warn patients with phenylketonuria
Patient instructions	Regular and Maximum Strength Anacin-3: patients are cautioned on the package label to consult a physician immediately "if pain persists for more than 10 days, or redness is present, or in arthritic or rheumatic conditions affecting children under 12...." Children's Anacin-3: the label warns parents to consult a physician immediately "if fever persists for more than three days or recurs, or if pain continues for more than five days."

OVERDOSAGE

Signs and symptoms	*Early:* nausea, vomiting, diaphoresis, and general malaise (some patients may be asymptomatic); *late:* clinical and laboratory evidence of hepatotoxicity (vomiting; right upper quadrant tenderness; increased SGOT, SGPT, serum bilirubin, and prothrombin time; and possible hypoglycemia) may not be apparent until 48–72 h after ingestion
Treatment	Promptly empty stomach by performing gastric lavage or inducing emesis with syrup of ipecac (15–30 ml for children, 30–45 ml for adults). Give ipecac with copious quantities of water; if emesis does not occur within 20 min, repeat dose. Activated charcoal may be given if acetaminophen has been ingested with certain other drugs. Administer oral acetylcysteine as soon as possible (no later than 24 h after ingestion); give a loading dose of 140 mg/kg and then, at 4-h intervals, 17 maintenance doses of 70 mg/kg. (Charcoal, if used, should be removed before acetylcysteine is given.) Measure the plasma level of unconjugated acetaminophen as early as possible, but no sooner than 4 h after ingestion. Determine prothrombin time, SGOT and SGPT levels, and serum concentrations of bilirubin, creatinine, BUN, glucose, and electrolytes every 24 h. If the prothrombin time exceeds 1.5 times the control value, give vitamin K_1; if the prothrombin time exceeds 3 times this value, give fresh frozen plasma. Institute appropriate measures to treat hypoglycemia and electrolyte and fluid imbalance. Avoid forced diuresis or use of diuretics when treating an acetaminophen overdose. For additional information on use of acetylcysteine and interpretation of the plasma acetaminophen level, see Mucomyst chart and contact the Rocky Mountain Poison Center (800–525–6115).

ALTERED LABORATORY VALUES

Blood/serum values	▽ Glucose (with glucose oxidase/peroxidase tests)
Urinary values	+ 5-HIAA (with nitrosonaphthol reagent tests)

USE IN CHILDREN	USE IN PREGNANT AND NURSING WOMEN
See INDICATIONS and ORAL DOSAGE	The package label warns patients who are pregnant or nursing to seek the advice of a health professional before using these products

ANAPROX

NONNARCOTIC ANALGESICS/ANTIPYRETICS

ANAPROX (naproxen sodium) Syntex   Rx
Tablets: 275 mg

INDICATIONS	ORAL DOSAGE
Mild to moderate pain **Primary dysmenorrhea** **Acute tendinitis and bursitis**	**Adult:** 550 mg to start, followed by 275 mg q6–8h, as needed, up to 1,375 mg/day
Rheumatoid arthritis, osteoarthritis, and ankylosing spondylitis	**Adult:** 275 mg bid (AM and PM) or 275 mg in the morning and 550 mg at night to start; for long-term administration, adjust dosage as needed, depending on clinical response. Smaller daily doses may suffice for long-term therapy. Dosages exceeding 1,100 mg/day have not been studied.
Acute gout	**Adult:** 825 mg to start, followed by 275 mg q8h until attack has subsided

CONTRAINDICATIONS	
History of allergic reaction to naproxen or naproxen sodium	History of asthma, rhinitis, and nasal polyps precipitated by aspirin or other nonsteroidal, anti-inflammatory/analgesic drugs

ADMINISTRATION/DOSAGE ADJUSTMENTS	
Therapeutic response in arthritis	Should be observed within 2 wk; in some patients, symptomatic improvement may not be seen for up to 4 wk
Combination therapy	Added benefits in arthritis have not been demonstrated with corticosteroids; however, use with gold salts has resulted in greater improvement. Use with salicylates is not recommended. Use with related drug naproxen is not recommended.
Adrenal function tests	Discontinue naproxen sodium therapy 72 h prior to testing

WARNINGS/PRECAUTIONS	
Anaphylactic reactions	Potentially fatal allergic or idiosyncratic anaphylactic reactions may occur. Before beginning therapy, determine whether the patient has experienced reactions such as asthma, nasal polyps, urticaria, or hypotension in association with nonsteroidal anti-inflammatory drugs (see CONTRAINDICATIONS); if such reactions occur during therapy, discontinue use.
Peptic ulcer, perforation, GI bleeding	May occur and can be severe or even fatal; patients with a history of peptic ulcer disease or active gastric or duodenal ulcers should be closely supervised during therapy
Renal toxicity	Proteinuria, acute interstitial nephritis with hematuria, and occasionally the nephrotic syndrome may occur during therapy. In patients with reduced renal blood flow or volume owing to conditions such as heart failure, renal or hepatic impairment, advanced age, or use of diuretics, administration of a nonsteroidal anti-inflammatory agent may cause a critical decrease in the formation of renal prostaglandins and thereby precipitate overt renal failure; reaction is reversible upon discontinuation of the drug. To avoid renal toxicity, monitor serum creatinine level and/or creatinine clearance and exercise great caution if a patient has significant renal impairment.
Drug accumulation	Naproxen is eliminated primarily by the kidneys; exercise caution if creatinine clearance is less than 20 mg/ml since drug accumulation can occur in such a case. Chronic alcoholic liver disease, probably other forms of cirrhosis, and, according to one study, advanced age all produce an increase in the serum level of unbound naproxen; if a cirrhotic or elderly patient requires high doses, exercise caution, and be prepared to adjust dose.
Liver function abnormalities	Borderline elevations may occur in up to 15% of patients; meaningful elevations 3 times the upper limit of normal in SGOT or SGPT levels have been reported in less than 1% of patients. If abnormal liver function tests or other manifestations of liver dysfunction arise during therapy, evaluate the patient for evidence of a more severe hepatic reaction. Although such reactions as jaundice and fatal hepatitis have occurred rarely, discontinue therapy if abnormal liver function test results persist or worsen, signs and symptoms of liver disease develop, or secondary manifestations (eg, eosinophilia, rash) occur.
Ophthalmic changes	Have occurred in animals treated with related drugs; perform an ophthalmologic examination within a reasonable period after starting therapy and periodically thereafter if drug is used for an extended period
Peripheral edema	May occur; use with caution in patients with fluid retention, hypertension, or heart failure. Each tablet contains approximately 25 mg (about 1 mEq) of sodium.
Corticosteroid therapy	If discontinued, reduce dosage gradually to avoid complications of sudden steroid withdrawal and observe patient closely for adverse effects
Mental impairment	Performance of potentially hazardous activities may be impaired; advise patients to exercise caution if they experience drowsiness, dizziness, vertigo, or depression

ANAPROX

Prolonged bleeding time	May occur due to inhibition of platelet aggregation; use with caution in patients with coagulation defects or in those on anticoagulant therapy
Patients with initially low hemoglobin values ($\leq$ 10 g)	Obtain periodic hemoglobin determinations during long-term therapy
Diagnostic interference	Complications of presumably noninfectious, noninflammatory painful conditions may escape detection because of reduction in fever and inflammation
Carcinogenicity	No evidence of carcinogenicity has been found in rats after 2 yr of study

ADVERSE REACTIONS[1]

Frequent reactions (incidence $\geq$ 1%) are printed in *italics*

Gastrointestinal	*Constipation, heartburn, abdominal pain, and nausea (3-9%); dyspepsia, diarrhea, and stomatitis (1-3%);* bleeding and/or perforation, peptic ulcer with bleeding and/or perforation, vomiting, melena, hematemesis
Respiratory	Eosinophilic pneumonitis
Central nervous system and neuromuscular	*Headache, dizziness, and drowsiness (3-9%); light-headedness and vertigo (1-3%);* myalgia, muscle weakness, inability to concentrate, depression, malaise, dream abnormalities, insomnia
Dermatological	*Pruritus, eruption, and ecchymoses (3-9%); sweating and purpura (1-3%);* rash, alopecia, photosensitive dermatitis[2]
Cardiovascular	*Edema and dyspnea (3-9%); palpitations (1-3%);* congestive heart failure
Hepatic	Abnormal liver function tests, jaundice
Renal	Glomerular nephritis, interstitial nephritis, nephrotic syndrome, hematuria, renal disease
Hematological	Thrombocytopenia, leukopenia, granulocytopenia, eosinophilia[2]
Other	*Tinnitus (3-9%); thirst, visual disturbances, and hearing disturbances (1-3%);* hearing impairment, anaphylactoid reactions, menstrual disorders, chills, fever[2]

OVERDOSAGE

Signs and symptoms	Drowsiness, heartburn, indigestion, nausea, vomiting
Treatment	Induce emesis or use gastric lavage to empty stomach, and institute supportive measures. Activated charcoal may be helpful.

DRUG INTERACTIONS

Albumin-bound drugs	Displacement of either drug
Coumarin anticoagulants	△ Prothrombin time
Hydantoins	△ Hydantoin plasma level
Sulfonylureas	△ Sulfonylurea plasma level
Sulfonamides	△ Sulfonamide plasma level
Furosemide	▽ Natriuretic effect of furosemide
Lithium	△ Lithium plasma level
Propranolol, other beta blockers	▽ Antihypertensive effect
Aspirin	△ Excretion of naproxen sodium
Probenecid	△ Naproxen sodium plasma half-life
Methotrexate	△ Methotrexate plasma level (based on animal studies); exercise caution

ALTERED LABORATORY VALUES

Blood/serum values	△ BUN △ Creatinine △ SGOT △ SGPT
Urinary values	△ 17-Ketogenic steroids Interference with 5-HIAA determinations

USE IN CHILDREN

Pediatric dosages have not been established

USE IN PREGNANT AND NURSING WOMEN

Pregnancy Category B: use during pregnancy only if clearly needed; because premature closure of the ductus arteriosus may occur, administration during late pregnancy should be avoided. An increased incidence of dystocia and delayed parturition has been observed in rats. Reproduction studies in rats, rabbits, and mice given up to 6 times the human dose have shown no evidence of teratogenicity or impaired fertility. No adequate, well-controlled studies have been performed in pregnant women. Naproxen anion appears in human breast milk at a concentration of 1% of maternal plasma levels; avoid use in nursing mothers due to potential adverse effects of prostaglandin inhibition.

---

[1] Adverse reactions occurring in patients treated for rheumatoid arthritis or osteoarthritis are listed; in general, these reactions were reported 2-10 times more frequently than they were in patients treated for mild-to-moderate pain or dysmenorrhea

[2] Other reactions for which a causal relationship has not been established include epidermal necrolysis, erythema multiforme, Stevens-Johnson syndrome, urticaria, agranulocytosis, aplastic anemia, hemolytic anemia, cognitive dysfunction, ulcerative stomatitis, vasculitis, angioneurotic edema, hypoglycemia, and hyperglycemia

APF ARTHRITIS PAIN FORMULA ■ ARTHRITIS PAIN FORMULA

NONNARCOTIC ANALGESICS/ANTIPYRETICS

APF ARTHRITIS PAIN FORMULA (acetaminophen) Whitehall   OTC

Caplets: 500 mg

INDICATIONS	**ORAL DOSAGE**
Minor aches and pains of arthritis, rheumatism, headache, low back pain, toothache, and menstrual discomfort Fever	Adult: 1,000 mg (2 caplets) tid or qid; do not exceed 4,000 mg (8 caplets)/24 h

WARNINGS/PRECAUTIONS

Patient instructions — Package label cautions patients to consult a physician in arthritic or rheumatic conditions affecting children under 12 yr of age, if pain persists more than 10 days, or if redness is present

OVERDOSAGE

Signs and symptoms — *Early:* nausea, vomiting, diaphoresis, and general malaise (some patients may be asymptomatic); *late:* clinical and laboratory evidence of hepatotoxicity (vomiting; right upper quadrant tenderness; increased SGOT, SGPT, serum bilirubin, and prothrombin time; and possible hypoglycemia) may not be apparent until 48–72 h after ingestion

Treatment — Promptly empty stomach by performing gastric lavage or inducing emesis with syrup of ipecac (15–30 ml for children, 30–45 ml for adults). Give ipecac with copious quantities of water; if emesis does not occur within 20 min, repeat dose. Activated charcoal may be given if acetaminophen has been ingested with certain other drugs. Administer oral acetylcysteine as soon as possible (no later than 24 h after ingestion); give a loading dose of 140 mg/kg and then, at 4-h intervals, 17 maintenance doses of 70 mg/kg. (Charcoal, if used, should be removed before acetylcysteine is given.) Measure the plasma level of unconjugated acetaminophen as early as possible, but no sooner than 4 h after ingestion. Determine prothrombin time, SGOT and SGPT levels, and serum concentrations of bilirubin, creatinine, BUN, glucose, and electrolytes every 24 h. If the prothrombin time exceeds 1.5 times the control value, give vitamin K_1; if the prothrombin time exceeds 3 times this value, give fresh frozen plasma. Institute appropriate measures to treat hypoglycemia and electrolyte and fluid imbalance. Avoid forced diuresis or use of diuretics when treating an acetaminophen overdose. For additional information on use of acetylcysteine and interpretation of the plasma acetaminophen level, see Mucomyst chart.

ALTERED LABORATORY VALUES

Blood/serum values — ▽ Glucose (with glucose oxidase/peroxidase tests)

Urinary values — + 5-HIAA (with nitrosonaphthol reagent tests)

USE IN CHILDREN	**USE IN PREGNANT AND NURSING WOMEN**
Consult manufacturer	Consult manufacturer

NONNARCOTIC ANALGESICS/ANTIPYRETICS

ARTHRITIS PAIN FORMULA (aspirin, aluminum hydroxide, and magnesium hydroxide) Whitehall   OTC

Tablets: 500 mg aspirin, 33 mg aluminum hydroxide, and 100 mg magnesium hydroxide

INDICATIONS	**ORAL DOSAGE**
Minor aches and pains of arthritis and rheumatism and low back pain Pain, including headache, neuralgia, neuritis, sprains, muscular aches, tooth-extraction pain, toothache, and menstrual discomfort Fever and discomfort of colds	Adult: 2 tabs tid or qid, up to 8 tabs/24 h

WARNINGS/PRECAUTIONS

Patient self-medication — Patient should not use product if pain persists more than 10 days or redness is present or for arthritic or rheumatic conditions in children under 12 yr of age without advice and supervision of physician

Reye's syndrome	There is evidence suggesting that use of aspirin in children or adolescents with chicken pox or influenza may increase the risk of Reye's syndrome

OVERDOSAGE

Signs and symptoms	Hyperpnea, nausea, vomiting, vertigo, tinnitus, flushing, sweating, thirst, headache, drowsiness, diarrhea, and tachycardia, progressing to hyperthermia, hemorrhage, acid-base disturbances, restlessness, confusion, convulsions, vasomotor depression, coma, and respiratory failure
Treatment	If less than 4 h have elapsed since ingestion, induce emesis or perform gastric lavage, followed by activated charcoal, to remove any remaining drug from the stomach. Initial therapy should be directed at reducing hyperthermia by external sponging with tepid water, correcting dehydration by appropriate IV fluid replacement, and maintaining adequate cardiorespiratory and renal function. In moderately severe cases of salicylate poisoning, cautiously administer sodium bicarbonate IV in sufficient quantity, if possible, to maintain an alkaline diuresis; intermittent peritoneal dialysis may also be helpful. In severe cases, hemodialysis should be seriously considered. Potassium should be added to the repair solution to compensate for potassium losses once urine formation is deemed adequate. Glucose may be provided to correct ketosis and hypoglycemia. Plasma transfusion may be beneficial if shock intervenes. Hemorrhagic phenomena may necessitate whole-blood transfusions and phytonadione (vitamin K_1). Do not administer barbiturates to treat excitement or convulsions.

DRUG INTERACTIONS

Anticoagulants	△ Risk of bleeding
Alcohol, corticosteroids, phenylbutazone, oxyphenbutazone	△ Risk of GI ulceration
Probenecid, sulfinpyrazone	▽ Uricosuria
Spironolactone	▽ Diuretic effect
Tetracycline	▽ Absorption of tetracycline
Methotrexate	△ Methotrexate plasma level and risk of toxicity

ALTERED LABORATORY VALUES

Blood/serum values	△ Prothrombin time △ Uric acid (with low doses) ▽ Uric acid (with high doses) ▽ Thyroxine (T_4) ▽ Thyroid-stimulating hormone
Urinary values	△ Glucose (with Clinitest tablets)

USE IN CHILDREN

Use according to medical judgment

USE IN PREGNANT AND NURSING WOMEN

Consult manufacturer for use in pregnant or nursing women

NONNARCOTIC ANALGESICS/ANTIPYRETICS

ARTHROPAN (choline salicylate) Purdue Frederick OTC

Liquid (per 5 ml): choline salicylate equivalent to 650 mg aspirin (8, 16 fl oz) *mint-flavored*

INDICATIONS

Inflammatory conditions, including rheumatoid arthritis, rheumatic fever, and osteoarthritis
Other conditions for which oral salicylates are recommended, particularly when a liquid dosage form is desirable

ORAL DOSAGE

Adult: 5 ml (1 tsp) q3–4h, as necessary, up to 30 ml (6 tsp)/day; for rheumatoid arthritis, 5–10 ml (1–2 tsp) qid to start
Child (> 12 yr): same as adult

CONTRAINDICATIONS

Consult manufacturer

WARNINGS/PRECAUTIONS

Overdosage	May lead to salicylism (see OVERDOSAGE)

ADVERSE REACTIONS

Gastrointestinal	Minimal blood loss and gastric irritation

OVERDOSAGE

Signs and symptoms — Hyperpnea, nausea, vomiting, vertigo, tinnitus, flushing, sweating, thirst, headache, drowsiness, diarrhea, and tachycardia, progressing to hyperthermia, hemorrhage, acid-base disturbances, restlessness, confusion, convulsions, vasomotor depression, coma, and respiratory failure

Treatment — If less than 4 h have elapsed since ingestion, induce emesis or perform gastric lavage, followed by activated charcoal, to remove any remaining drug from the stomach. Initial therapy should be directed at reducing hyperthermia by external sponging with tepid water, correcting dehydration by appropriate IV fluid replacement, and maintaining adequate cardiorespiratory and renal function. In moderately severe cases of salicylate poisoning, cautiously administer sodium bicarbonate IV in sufficient quantity, if possible, to maintain an alkaline diuresis; intermittent peritoneal dialysis may also be helpful. In severe cases, hemodialysis should be seriously considered. Potassium should be added to the repair solution to compensate for potassium losses once urine formation is deemed adequate. Glucose may be provided to correct ketosis and hypoglycemia. Plasma transfusion may be beneficial if shock intervenes. Hemorrhagic phenomena may necessitate whole-blood transfusions and phytonadione (vitamin K_1). Do not administer barbiturates to treat excitement or convulsions.

DRUG INTERACTIONS

Anticoagulants	△ Risk of bleeding
Alcohol, corticosteroids, phenylbutazone, oxyphenbutazone	△ Risk of GI ulceration
Probenecid, sulfinpyrazone	▽ Uricosuria
Spironolactone	▽ Diuretic effect
Methotrexate	△ Methotrexate plasma level and risk of toxicity

ALTERED LABORATORY VALUES

Blood/serum values — △ Prothrombin time △ Uric acid (with low doses) ▽ Uric acid (with high doses)
▽ Thyroxine (T_4) ▽ Thyroid-stimulating hormone

Urinary values — △ Glucose (with Clinitest tablets)

USE IN CHILDREN
Consult manufacturer for use in children under 12 yr of age

USE IN PREGNANT AND NURSING WOMEN
Consult manufacturer for use in pregnant or nursing women

NONNARCOTIC ANALGESICS/ANTIPYRETICS

ASCRIPTIN (aspirin, magnesium hydroxide, and aluminum hydroxide) Rorer — OTC

Tablets: 325 mg aspirin, 75 mg magnesium hydroxide, and 75 mg dried aluminum hydroxide gel

INDICATIONS	ORAL DOSAGE
Headache, neuralgia **Pain** of minor injuries and dysmenorrhea **Pain and fever** of colds and influenza **Pain and inflammation** of arthritis and other rheumatic diseases	**Adult:** 2–3 tabs qid
Reducing the risk of **recurrent transient ischemic attacks or stroke in men** who have had transient ischemia of the brain due to fibrin platelet emboli	**Adult:** 1 tab qid or 2 tabs bid
Reducing the risk of **myocardial infarction and subsequent death** in patients with unstable angina or a prior infarction[1]	**Adult:** 1 tab once daily

ASCRIPTIN A/D (aspirin, magnesium hydroxide, and aluminum hydroxide) Rorer — OTC

Tablets: 325 mg aspirin, 150 mg magnesium hydroxide, and 150 mg dried aluminum hydroxide gel

INDICATIONS	ORAL DOSAGE
Pain, inflammation, and fever associated with rheumatoid arthritis, osteoarthritis, and other arthritic conditions	**Adult:** 2–3 tabs qid

Extra Strength ASCRIPTIN (aspirin, magnesium hydroxide, and aluminum hydroxide) Rorer   OTC

Tablets: 500 mg aspirin, 82.5 mg magnesium hydroxide, and 82.5 mg dried aluminum hydroxide gel

INDICATIONS	ORAL DOSAGE
Headache, neuralgia **Pain** of minor injuries and dysmenorrhea **Discomfort** of colds **Minor aches and pains** associated with arthritis and rheumatism	**Adult:** 2 tabs, with a full glass of water, tid or qid

CONTRAINDICATIONS
Consult manufacturer

WARNINGS/PRECAUTIONS

Evaluation of patients with transient ischemic attacks (TIA's)	Before initiating treatment of patients presenting with signs and symptoms of TIA's, perform a complete medical and neurological evaluation, taking into account other disorders that resemble TIA's. Attention should also be given to risk factors; disorders frequently associated with TIA's, such as hypertension and diabetes, should be evaluated and treatment instituted if appropriate.
Monitoring of prophylactic therapy for myocardial infarction	Check blood pressure, BUN level, and serum uric acid level regularly when using aspirin for long-term prophylaxis of myocardial infarction; small increases in these values have been detected during one clinical trial
Information for patients	Package labels caution patients not to use aspirin without medical supervision if they are undergoing medical treatment, have arthritis or rheumatism, are hypersensitive to aspirin, or have a history of one of the following conditions: asthma, renal or gastric disease, or a hematological disorder; patients are instructed to immediately consult a physician if they experience tinnitus or other symptoms, erythema is seen, or pain persists for more than 10 days. Women who are pregnant or nursing are advised to consult a health professional before using aspirin.
Reye's syndrome	Do not give this preparation to children, including teenagers, with chicken pox or influenza

OVERDOSAGE

Signs and symptoms	Hyperpnea, nausea, vomiting, vertigo, tinnitus, flushing, sweating, thirst, headache, drowsiness, diarrhea, and tachycardia, progressing to hyperthermia, hemorrhage, acid-base disturbances, restlessness, confusion, convulsions, vasomotor depression, coma, and respiratory failure
Treatment	If less than 4 h have elapsed since ingestion, induce emesis or perform gastric lavage, followed by activated charcoal, to remove any remaining drug from the stomach. Initial therapy should be directed at reducing hyperthermia by external sponging with tepid water, correcting dehydration by appropriate IV fluid replacement, and maintaining adequate cardiorespiratory and renal function. In moderately severe cases of salicylate poisoning, cautiously administer sodium bicarbonate IV in sufficient quantity, if possible, to maintain an alkaline diuresis; intermittent peritoneal dialysis may also be helpful. In severe cases, hemodialysis should be seriously considered. Potassium should be added to the repair solution to compensate for potassium losses once urine formation is deemed adequate. Glucose may be provided to correct ketosis and hypoglycemia. Plasma transfusion may be beneficial if shock intervenes. Hemorrhagic phenomena may necessitate whole-blood transfusions and phytonadione (vitamin K_1). Do not administer barbiturates to treat excitement or convulsions.

DRUG INTERACTIONS

Anticoagulants	△ Risk of bleeding
Alcohol, corticosteroids, phenylbutazone, oxyphenbutazone	△ Risk of GI ulceration
Probenecid, sulfinpyrazone	▽ Uricosuria
Spironolactone	▽ Diuretic effect
Methotrexate	△ Methotrexate plasma level and risk of toxicity
Tetracycline	▽ Absorption of tetracycline; do not use concomitantly
Absorbable antacids	△ Clearance of salicylate
Nonabsorbable antacids	▽ Rate of absorption of aspirin ▽ Plasma aspirin/salicylate ratio

ALTERED LABORATORY VALUES

Blood/serum values	△ Prothrombin time △ Uric acid (with low doses) ▽ Uric acid (with high doses) ▽ Thyroxine (T_4) ▽ Thyroid-stimulating hormone
Urinary values	△ Glucose (with Clinitest tablets)

USE IN CHILDREN	USE IN PREGNANT AND NURSING WOMEN
Use according to medical judgment in children under 12 yr of age	Consult manufacturer for use in pregnant or nursing women

[1] *FDA Drug Bulletin* 15(4):34, 1985

BAYER Aspirin

NONNARCOTIC ANALGESICS/ANTIPYRETICS

BAYER Aspirin (aspirin) Glenbrook   OTC

Tablets: 325 mg **Caplets:** 325 mg

INDICATIONS	ORAL DOSAGE
Headache, muscular aches and pains, bursitis, menstrual discomfort, toothache, minor aches and pains of arthritis and rheumatism **Fever and discomfort** of colds and influenza	Adult: 325–650 mg (1–2 tablets or caplets) with water q4h, as needed
Reducing the risk of **recurrent transient ischemic attacks or stroke in men** who have had transient ischemia of the brain due to fibrin platelet emboli[1]	Adult: 325 mg (1 tablet or caplet) qid or 650 mg (2 tablets or caplets) bid, with water
Reducing the risk of **myocardial infarction and subsequent death** in patients with unstable angina or a prior infarction[2]	Adult: 325 mg (1 tablet or caplet) once daily

Maximum BAYER Aspirin (aspirin) Glenbrook   OTC

Tablets: 500 mg **Caplets:** 500 mg

INDICATIONS	ORAL DOSAGE
Headache, muscular aches and pains, bursitis, menstrual discomfort, toothache, minor aches and pains of arthritis and rheumatism **Fever and discomfort** of colds and influenza	Adult: 1,000 mg (2 tablets or caplets) with water or fruit juice q4h, as needed, up to 4,000 mg (8 tablets or caplets)/24 h

8-Hour BAYER Aspirin (aspirin) Glenbrook   OTC

Tablets (timed release): 650 mg

INDICATIONS	ORAL DOSAGE
Backache, bursitis, sprains, headache, sinusitis, minor pain and stiffness of arthritis **Fever and discomfort** of colds and influenza	Adult: 1,300 mg (2 tablets) with water, followed by 650–1,300 mg (1–2 tablets) q8h, as needed, up to 3,900 mg (6 tablets)/day; for prevention of nighttime and early morning stiffness, 1,300 mg (2 tablets) with water at bedtime. Tablets may be broken up (but not ground) between the teeth or gently crumbled in the mouth and swallowed with water without loss of timed-release action.

BAYER Children's Chewable Aspirin (aspirin) Glenbrook   OTC

Chewable tablets: 81.25 mg *orange flavored*

INDICATIONS	ORAL DOSAGE
Headache, sore throat, other minor aches and pains **Fever and discomfort** of colds	Child (3–4 yr; 32–35 lb): 162.5 mg (2 tablets) with water q4h, up to 5 doses/day Child (4–6 yr; 36–45 lb): 243.75 mg (3 tablets) with water q4h, up to 5 doses/day Child (6–9 yr; 46–65 lb): 325 mg (4 tablets) with water q4h, up to 5 doses/day Child (9–11 yr; 66–76 lb): 406.25 mg (5 tablets) with water q4h, up to 5 doses/day Child (11–12 yr; 77–83 lb): 487.5 mg (6 tablets) with water q4h, up to 5 doses/day Child ($\geq$ 12 yr; $\geq$ 84 lb): 650 mg (8 tablets) with water q4h, up to 5 doses/day

CONTRAINDICATIONS

Bleeding ulcer   Hemorrhagic states   Hypersensitivity to salicylates
Hemophilia

ADMINISTRATION/DOSAGE ADJUSTMENTS

Administration of chewable tablets —— Chewable tablets may be swallowed whole with half a glass of water, milk, or fruit juice; chewed or dissolved on the tongue and then ingested with half a glass of one of these liquids; dissolved in a small amount of one of these liquids, which is then drunk; or crushed in a teaspoonful of water and then ingested with part of a glass of water

WARNINGS/PRECAUTIONS

Gastric irritation —— May occur, especially in patients with gastric ulcers, erosive gastritis, or bleeding tendencies; use with caution

Patients with blood-coagulation abnormalities —— Use with caution in patients with preexisting hypoprothrombinemia or vitamin K deficiency

Nasal polyps, asthma, hay fever —— May predispose to salicylate hypersensitivity; use with caution

BAYER Aspirin

Interference with platelet aggregation	Use with caution prior to surgery
Monitoring of prophylactic therapy for myocardial infarction	Check blood pressure, BUN level, and serum uric acid level regularly when using aspirin for long-term prophylaxis of myocardial infarction; small increases in these values have been detected during one clinical trial
Patient instructions	Bayer, Maximum Bayer, and 8-Hour Bayer: the package label advises consultation with a physician if pain persists for more than 10 days, redness is present, or the patient is less than 12 yr of age. Children's Bayer: the package label advises consultation with a physician if nausea, vomiting, headache, high or continued fever, or severe or persistent sore throat occurs. The package labels also advise pregnant or nursing women to consult a health professional before using these products.
Reye's syndrome	There is evidence suggesting that use of aspirin in children or adolescents with chicken pox or influenza may increase the risk of Reye's syndrome

ADVERSE REACTIONS

Gastrointestinal	Nausea, dyspepsia, heartburn, epigastric discomfort, anorexia, diarrhea, occult blood loss, hemorrhage
Central nervous system	Dizziness, tinnitus, headache, deafness
Respiratory	Hyperventilation
Cardiovascular	Increased pulse rate
Dermatological	Skin eruptions
Other	Sweating, thirst, electrolyte and acid-base imbalance

OVERDOSAGE

Signs and symptoms	Hyperpnea, nausea, vomiting, vertigo, tinnitus, flushing, sweating, thirst, headache, drowsiness, diarrhea, and tachycardia, progressing to hyperthermia, hemorrhage, acid-base disturbances, restlessness, confusion, convulsions, vasomotor depression, coma, and respiratory failure
Treatment	If less than 4 h have elapsed since ingestion, induce emesis or perform gastric lavage, followed by activated charcoal, to remove any remaining drug from the stomach. Initial therapy should be directed at reducing hyperthermia by external sponging with tepid water, correcting dehydration by appropriate IV fluid replacement, and maintaining adequate cardiorespiratory and renal function. In moderately severe cases of salicylate poisoning, cautiously administer sodium bicarbonate IV in sufficient quantity, if possible, to maintain an alkaline diuresis; intermittent peritoneal dialysis may also be helpful. In severe cases, hemodialysis should be seriously considered. Potassium should be added to the repair solution to compensate for potassium losses once urine formation is deemed adequate. Glucose may be provided to correct ketosis and hypoglycemia. Plasma transfusion may be beneficial if shock intervenes. Hemorrhagic phenomena may necessitate whole-blood transfusions and phytonadione (vitamin K_1). Do not administer barbiturates to treat excitement or convulsions.

DRUG INTERACTIONS

Anticoagulants	↑ Risk of bleeding; exercise caution during combination therapy
Alcohol, corticosteroids, phenylbutazone, oxyphenbutazone	↑ Risk of GI ulceration
Probenecid, sulfinpyrazone	↓ Uricosuria
Spironolactone	↓ Diuretic effect
Methotrexate	↑ Methotrexate plasma level and risk of toxicity

ALTERED LABORATORY VALUES

Blood/serum values	↑ Prothrombin time ↑ Uric acid (with low doses) ↓ Uric acid (with high doses) ↓ Thyroxine (T_4) ↓ Thyroid-stimulating hormone
Urinary values	↑ Glucose (with Clinitest tablets)

USE IN CHILDREN

See INDICATIONS and ORAL DOSAGE. *Bayer Aspirin and Children's Chewable Aspirin:* use according to medical judgment in children under 2 yr of age; *Maximum Bayer Aspirin and 8-Hour Bayer Aspirin:* use according to medical judgment in children under 12 yr of age.

USE IN PREGNANT AND NURSING WOMEN

Consult manufacturer for use in pregnant or nursing women

---

[1] *FDA Drug Bulletin* 10(1):2, 1980
[2] *FDA Drug Bulletin* 15(4):34, 1985

NONNARCOTIC ANALGESICS/ANTIPYRETICS

BUFFERIN (aspirin, aluminum glycinate, and magnesium carbonate) Bristol-Myers — OTC

Tablets: 324 mg aspirin, 48.6 mg aluminum glycinate, and 97.2 mg magnesium carbonate

INDICATIONS	ORAL DOSAGE
Headache, muscular aches, toothache, menstrual cramps, and minor **pain and inflammation of arthritis and rheumatism** **Pain and fever** of colds and influenza	**Adult:** 2 tabs q4h, as needed **Child (6–12 yr):** 1 tab q4h, as needed
Reducing the risk of **recurrent transient ischemic attacks or stroke in men** who have had transient ischemia of the brain due to fibrin platelet emboli[1]	**Adult:** 1 tab qid or 2 tabs bid
Reducing the risk of **myocardial infarction and subsequent death** in patients with unstable angina or a prior infarction[2]	**Adult:** 1 tab once daily

Arthritis Strength BUFFERIN (aspirin, aluminum glycinate, and magnesium carbonate) Bristol-Myers — OTC

Tablets: 486 mg aspirin, 72.9 mg aluminum glycinate, and 145.8 mg magnesium carbonate

Extra Strength BUFFERIN (aspirin, aluminum glycinate, and magnesium carbonate) Bristol-Myers — OTC

Tablets: 500 mg aspirin, 75 mg aluminum glycinate, and 150 mg magnesium carbonate

INDICATIONS	ORAL DOSAGE
Minor aches and pains, stiffness, swelling, and inflammation of arthritis and rheumatism **Pain and fever** of colds and influenza **Pain,** including that of simple headache, lower backache, sinusitis, neuralgia, neuritis, tooth extraction, muscle strain, athletic soreness, and menstrual distress	**Adult:** 2 tabs q4h, as needed, up to 8 tabs per 24 h

CONTRAINDICATIONS
Hypersensitivity to salicylates

WARNINGS/PRECAUTIONS

Monitoring of prophylactic therapy for myocardial infarction	Check blood pressure, BUN level, and serum uric acid level regularly when using aspirin for long-term prophylaxis of myocardial infarction; small increases in these values have been detected during one clinical trial
Information for patients	Package labels caution patients not to use these products without medical supervision if one of the following conditions exists: (1) chicken pox or influenza in a child or teenager, (2) erythema, (3) arthritis or rheumatism in a child under 12 yr of age, (4) pregnancy, or (5) nursing. Patients are instructed to discontinue administration if they experience dizziness, tinnitus, or hearing impairment and to also consult a physician if overdose or erythema occurs or pain persists for more than 10 days.
Reye's syndrome	There is evidence suggesting that use of aspirin in children or adolescents with chicken pox or influenza may increase the risk of Reye's syndrome

OVERDOSAGE

Signs and symptoms	Hyperpnea, nausea, vomiting, vertigo, tinnitus, flushing, sweating, thirst, headache, drowsiness, diarrhea, restlessness, and tachycardia, progressing to hyperthermia, hemorrhage, acid-base disturbances, restlessness, confusion, convulsions, vasomotor depression, coma, and respiratory failure
Treatment	If less than 4 h have elapsed since ingestion, induce emesis or perform gastric lavage, followed by activated charcoal, to remove any remaining drug from the stomach. Initial therapy should be directed at reducing hyperthermia by external sponging with tepid water, correcting dehydration by appropriate IV fluid replacement, and maintaining adequate cardiorespiratory and renal function. In moderately severe cases of salicylate poisoning, cautiously administer sodium bicarbonate IV in sufficient quantity, if possible, to maintain an alkaline diuresis; intermittent peritoneal dialysis may also be helpful. In severe cases, hemodialysis should be seriously considered. Potassium should be added to the repair solution to compensate for potassium losses once urine formation is deemed adequate. Glucose may be provided to correct ketosis and hypoglycemia. Plasma transfusion may be beneficial if shock intervenes. Hemorrhagic phenomena may necessitate whole-blood transfusions and phytonadione (vitamin K_1). Do not administer barbiturates to treat excitement or convulsions.

DRUG INTERACTIONS

Anticoagulants	⇧ Risk of bleeding
Alcohol, corticosteroids, phenylbutazone, oxyphenbutazone	⇧ Risk of GI ulceration
Probenecid, sulfinpyrazone	⇩ Uricosuria
Spironolactone	⇩ Diuretic effect
Tetracycline	⇩ Absorption of tetracycline
Methotrexate	⇧ Methotrexate plasma level and risk of toxicity

ALTERED LABORATORY VALUES

Blood/serum values	⇧ Prothrombin time ⇧ Uric acid (with low doses) ⇩ Uric acid (with high doses) ⇩ Thyroxine (T$_4$) ⇩ Thyroid-stimulating hormone
Urinary values	⇧ Glucose (with Clinitest tablets)

USE IN CHILDREN

See INDICATIONS and ORAL DOSAGE

USE IN PREGNANT AND NURSING WOMEN

Consult manufacturer for use in pregnant or nursing women

---

[1] *FDA Drug Bulletin* 10(1):2, 1980
[2] *FDA Drug Bulletin* 15(4):34, 1985

NONNARCOTIC ANALGESICS/ANTIPYRETICS

Extra-Strength DATRIL (acetaminophen) Bristol-Myers OTC

Caplets: 500 mg **Tablets:** 500 mg

INDICATIONS Minor aches, pains, headaches, and fever	**ORAL DOSAGE** Adult: 1,000 mg (2 caplets or tabs) q4h, as needed; do not exceed 4,000 mg (8 caplets or tabs)/24 h

CONTRAINDICATIONS

Hypersensitivity to acetaminophen

WARNINGS/PRECAUTIONS

Hypersensitivity	On rare occasions, a hypersensitivity reaction such as rash or glossitis may occur; if a reaction is seen, discontinue use
Patient instructions	Package label advises patients to consult a physician for "severe or recurrent pain or high or continued fever...." Patients are also warned not to use this product for more than 10 days or in children 12 yr of age or younger unless directed to do so by a physician. Women who are pregnant or nursing are advised to consult a health professional before using this product.

OVERDOSAGE

Signs and symptoms	*Early:* nausea, vomiting, diaphoresis, and general malaise (some patients may be asymptomatic); *late:* clinical and laboratory evidence of hepatotoxicity (vomiting, right upper quadrant tenderness; increased SGOT, SGPT, serum bilirubin, and prothrombin time; and possible hypoglycemia) may not be apparent until 48–72 h after ingestion
Treatment	Promptly empty stomach by performing gastric lavage or inducing emesis with syrup of ipecac (15–30 ml for children, 30–45 ml for adults). Give ipecac with copious quantities of water; if emesis does not occur within 20 min, repeat dose. Activated charcoal may be given if acetaminophen has been ingested with certain other drugs. Administer oral acetylcysteine as soon as possible (no later than 24 h after ingestion); give a loading dose of 140 mg/kg and then, at 4-h intervals, 17 maintenance doses of 70 mg/kg. (Charcoal, if used, should be removed before acetylcysteine is given.) Measure the plasma level of unconjugated acetaminophen as early as possible, but no sooner than 4 h after ingestion. Determine prothrombin time, SGOT and SGPT levels, and serum concentrations of bilirubin, creatinine, BUN, glucose, and electrolytes every 24 h. If the prothrombin time exceeds 1.5 times the control value, give vitamin K$_1$; if the prothrombin time exceeds 3 times this value, give fresh frozen plasma. Institute appropriate measures to treat hypoglycemia and electrolyte and fluid imbalance. Avoid forced diuresis or use of diuretics when treating an acetaminophen overdose. For additional information on use of acetylcysteine and interpretation of the plasma acetaminophen level, see Mucomyst chart.

Extra-Strength DATRIL ■ DOLOBID

ALTERED LABORATORY VALUES

Blood/serum values	▽ Glucose (with glucose oxidase/peroxidase tests)
Urinary values	+ 5-HIAA (with nitrosonaphthol reagent test)

USE IN CHILDREN	USE IN PREGNANT AND NURSING WOMEN
Consult manufacturer	Consult manufacturer

NONNARCOTIC ANALGESICS/ANTIPYRETICS

DOLOBID (diflunisal) Merck Sharp & Dohme   Rx

Tablets: 250, 500 mg

INDICATIONS	ORAL DOSAGE
Mild to moderate pain	**Adult:** 1,000 mg to start, followed by 500 mg q12h or, if necessary, q8h; depending on pain severity, patient response, weight, or advanced age, a lower dosage may be appropriate (eg, 500 mg to start, followed by 250 mg q8–12h)
Osteoarthritis Rheumatoid arthritis	**Adult:** 500–1,000 mg/day in two divided doses, adjusted according to patient response; for maintenance, do not exceed 1,500 mg/day

CONTRAINDICATIONS	
Hypersensitivity to diflunisal	History of acute asthmatic attacks, urticaria, or rhinitis precipitated by aspirin or other nonsteroidal anti-inflammatory drugs

ADMINISTRATION/DOSAGE ADJUSTMENTS	
Administration	Diflunisal may be administered with water, milk, or meals; tablets should not be crushed or chewed

WARNINGS/PRECAUTIONS	
Peptic ulceration, GI bleeding	May occur and, in rare instances, can be fatal; patients with a history of upper GI tract disease should be closely supervised during therapy. In patients with active GI bleeding or an active peptic ulcer, benefits of therapy should be weighed against possible hazards; institute an appropriate ulcer regimen and monitor patient's progress carefully.
Interference with platelet function	Monitor closely patients who may be adversely affected by diflunisal's inhibition of platelet function
Visual disturbances	May occur; if eye complaints develop, perform an ophthalmologic examination
Renal toxicity	roteinuria, acute interstitial nephritis with hematuria, and occasionally the nephrotic syndrome may occur during therapy. In patients with reduced renal blood flow or volume owing to conditions such as renal or hepatic dysfunction, advanced age, hypovolemia, congestive heart failure, sepsis, or use of nephrotoxic agents, administration of a nonsteroidal anti-inflammatory agent may cause a critical decrease in the formation of renal prostaglandins and thereby precipitate overt renal failure; this reaction is reversible upon discontinuation of the drug. To avoid renal toxicity, use with caution in patients at risk and monitor renal function periodically in any patient with possible renal impairment.
Drug accumulation	Diflunisal is eliminated primarily by the kidneys; closely monitor patients with significant renal impairment and be prepared to reduce the daily dose
Peripheral edema	May occur; use with caution in patients with compromised cardiac function, hypertension, or other conditions predisposing to fluid retention
Liver function abnormalities	Borderline elevations may occur in up to 15% of patients; meaningful elevations (3 times the upper limit of normal) in SGOT or SGPT levels have been reported in less than 1% of patients. If abnormal liver function tests or other manifestations of liver dysfunction arise during therapy, evaluate the patient for evidence of a more severe hepatic reaction. Although such reactions as jaundice have occurred rarely, discontinue therapy if abnormal liver function test results persist or worsen, signs and symptoms of liver disease develop, or secondary manifestations (eg, eosinophilia, rash) occur, because hepatic reactions can be fatal.
Renal toxicity	Papillary edema has been observed occasionally in rats and dogs receiving high dosages, and papillary necrosis has been seen in mice during long-term studies

DOLOBID

Carcinogenicity, mutagenicity, effect on fertility	An apparent, but not statistically significant, increase in pulmonary and hepatocellular adenomas has been observed in mice (because the results of this study were inconclusive, it is being repeated). A long-term study in the rat has shown no evidence of carcinogenicity, and both in vitro and in vivo studies have failed to demonstrate any mutagenic potential. No evidence of impaired fertility has been found in rats given up to 50 mg/kg/day.

ADVERSE REACTIONS[1]

Frequent reactions (incidence $\geq$ 1%) are printed in *italics*

Gastrointestinal	*Nausea, dyspepsia, gastrointestinal pain, and diarrhea (3–9%); vomiting, constipation, and flatulence (1–3%);* peptic ulcer, gastrointestinal bleeding, anorexia, eructation, gastrointestinal perforation
Otic	*Tinnitus (1–3%)*
Ophthalmic	Transient visual disturbances, including blurred vision
Hepatic	Liver function abnormalities, jaundice (sometimes with fever), cholestasis, hepatitis
Central nervous system	*Dizziness, somnolence, and insomnia (1–3%);* vertigo, nervousness, depression, hallucinations, confusion, disorientation, vertigo, light-headedness, paresthesias
Dermatological	*Rash (3–9%);* erythema multiforme, exfoliative dermatitis, Stevens-Johnson syndrome, toxic epidermal necrolysis, urticaria, pruritus, sweating, dry mucous membranes, stomatitis, photosensitivity
Genitourinary	Dysuria, renal impairment (including renal failure), interstitial nephritis, hematuria, proteinuria
Hypersensitivity	Acute anaphylactic reaction with bronchospasm; potentially fatal syndrome characterized by fever, chills, dermatological reactions (see above), changes in liver function, jaundice, leukopenia, thrombocytopenia, eosinophilia, renal impairment (including renal failure), adenitis, arthralgia, arthritis, malaise, anorexia, and disorientation
Other	*Headache (3–9%); fatigue/tiredness (1–3%);* asthenia, edema, thrombocytopenia

OVERDOSAGE

Signs and symptoms	Drowsiness, vomiting, nausea, diarrhea, hyperventilation, tachycardia, sweating, tinnitus, disorientation, stupor, coma, diminished urine output, cardiorespiratory arrest
Treatment	Empty stomach by inducing emesis or by gastric lavage, and institute symptomatic and supportive measures, as needed. Hemodialysis is not likely to be beneficial in removing the drug from the circulation because of high protein binding.

DRUG INTERACTIONS

Oral anticoagulants	△ Prothrombin time; closely monitor the prothrombin time during concomitant therapy and for several days afterwards, and adjust the anticoagulant dosage as needed
Acetaminophen	△ Plasma level of acetaminophen; exercise caution and carefully monitor patient response during concomitant therapy because of the increased risk of hepatotoxicity[2]
Indomethacin	△ Plasma level of indomethacin; diflunisal and indomethacin should not be administered concomitantly because, in some patients, combined use has been associated with fatal GI hemorrhage
Sulindac	▽ Plasma level of active sulfide metabolite of sulindac
Aspirin	▽ Plasma level of diflunisal
Naproxen	▽ Urinary excretion of naproxen and its glucuronide metabolite; the plasma level of naproxen is not affected
Antacids	▽ Plasma level of diflunisal with continuous use of antacids
Hydrochlorothiazide	△ Plasma level of hydrochlorothiazide ▽ Hyperuricemic effect of hydrochlorothiazide
Furosemide	▽ Hyperuricemic effect of furosemide; the diuretic effect of furosemide is not affected

ALTERED LABORATORY VALUES

Blood/serum values	△ SGOT △ SGPT ▽ Uric acid
Urinary values	△ Uric acid + Protein

USE IN CHILDREN

Safety and effectiveness have not been established; not recommended for use in children under 12 yr of age

USE IN PREGNANT AND NURSING WOMEN

Pregnancy Category C: use during the first two trimesters of pregnancy only if the expected benefit justifies the potential risk to the fetus; because premature closure of the ductus arteriosus may occur, use during the third trimester is not recommended. A dose of 60 mg/kg/day (twice the maximum human dose) was shown to be maternotoxic, embryotoxic, and teratogenic in rabbits. In three other rabbit studies, teratogenicity was observed at doses of 40–50 mg/kg/day. Studies in mice and rats receiving up to 45 mg/kg/day and 100 mg/kg/day, respectively, showed no evidence of fetal harm. Prolonged gestation has been observed in rats receiving 1½ times the maximum human dose; nonsteroidal anti-inflammatory drugs have caused dystocia and delayed parturition in animals. No adequate, well-controlled studies have been performed with diflunisal in pregnant women. This drug is excreted in human milk in concentrations reaching 2–7% of plasma levels. Because of the potential for serious adverse effects in the nursing infant, patient should stop nursing while taking diflunisal.

---

[1] In general, a lower incidence of adverse reactions may be anticipated in patients receiving short-term treatment for mild to moderate pain. Reactions for which a causal relationship has not been established include dyspnea, palpitation, syncope, muscle cramps, and chest pain; the prescriber should also be aware of the adverse reactions associated with the use of other nonsteroidal anti-flammatory agents which may potentially develop in patients treated with diflunisal.

[2] An increase in GI toxicity has been observed in dogs, but not in rats, at dosages of 40–52 mg/kg/day of diflunisal and acetaminophen (approximately twice the maximum human dose of each drug); the clinical significance of this finding is not known

NONNARCOTIC ANALGESICS/ANTIPYRETICS

Regular Strength ECOTRIN (aspirin) SmithKline Consumer Products — OTC

Tablets (enteric coated): 325 mg

INDICATIONS	ORAL DOSAGE
Arthritis and rheumatism	**Adult:** for minor aches and pain, 325–650 mg q4h, as needed; for chronic therapy, up to 650 mg q4h or up to 975 mg q6h without medical supervision (higher doses may be given *with* supervision)
Reducing the risk of **recurrent transient ischemic attacks or stroke in men** who have had transient ischemia of the brain due to fibrin platelet emboli	**Adult:** 325 mg qid or 650 mg bid
Reducing the risk of **myocardial infarction and subsequent death** in patients with unstable angina or a prior infarction[1]	**Adult:** 325 mg once daily

Maximum Strength ECOTRIN (aspirin) SmithKline Consumer Products — OTC

Tablets (enteric coated): 500 mg **Caplets (enteric coated):** 500 mg

INDICATIONS	ORAL DOSAGE
Arthritis and rheumatism	**Adult:** for minor aches and pain, 1 g q6h, as needed; for chronic therapy, up to 1 g q6h without medical supervision (higher doses may be given *with* supervision)

CONTRAINDICATIONS
Consult manufacturer

ADMINISTRATION/DOSAGE ADJUSTMENTS

Administration	Give each dose with water or fruit juice
Chronic therapy	Anti-inflammatory effect is generally associated with a serum salicylate level of 15 mg/dl, attained in healthy men with 3 days of treatment at 5.2 g/day or with 4 days of treatment at 3.9 g/day and attained in healthy women with 2 days at 5.2 g/day or with 3 days at 3.9 g/day. If 3.9-4 g/day is exceeded, monitor serum levels and watch for tinnitus and other clinical manifestations of toxicity; bear in mind that high-frequency hearing loss, which often occurs in the elderly, makes detection of tinnitus difficult and use of tinnitus as an index of toxicity questionable.

WARNINGS/PRECAUTIONS

Information for patients	Package labels caution patients not to use these products without medical supervision if one of the following conditions exists: (1) history of ulcers, (2) erythema, (3) chicken pox or influenza in a child or teenager, (4) arthritis or rheumatism in a child under 12 yr of age, (5) pregnancy, or (6) nursing. Patients are instructed to discontinue administration if they experience dizziness, tinnitus, or hearing impairment and to also consult a physician if persistent or unexplained stomach upset develops, overdose or erythema occurs, or pain persists for more than 10 days.
Evaluation of patients with transient ischemic attacks (TIA's)	Before initiating treatment of patients presenting with signs and symptoms of TIA's, perform a complete medical and neurological evaluation, taking into account other disorders that resemble TIA's. Attention should also be given to risk factors; disorders frequently associated with TIA's, such as hypertension and diabetes, should be evaluated and treatment instituted if appropriate.
Monitoring of prophylactic therapy for myocardial infarction	Check blood pressure, BUN level, and serum uric acid level regularly when using aspirin for long-term prophylaxis of myocardial infarction; small increases in these values have been detected during one clinical trial
Patients with impaired gastric emptying	Tablet accumulation and subsequent formation of a bezoar in the stomach have occurred occasionally in patients with impaired gastric emptying, apparently as a result of outlet obstruction due to peptic ulcer disease alone or in combination with hypotonic gastric peristalsis. Telltale symptoms include early satiety and vague upper abdominal distress. Tablet accumulation may be confirmed roentgenographically or by endoscopy. The bezoar can be removed by gastric lavage, alternating between neutral and slightly basic solutions, or by gastrotomy. Alternatively, in a clinically untested approach, parenteral cimetidine, followed by sips of a slightly basic liquid, may be administered in an attempt to dissolve the bezoar; dissolution can be assessed by monitoring the plasma salicylate level or by watching for the development of tinnitus.
Patients with gastrectomy	The acid-resistant enteric coating of these products may offer no benefit to patients with partial or complete gastrectomy since gastric pH may be elevated in these patients
Reye's syndrome	There is evidence suggesting that use of aspirin in children or adolescents with chicken pox or influenza may increase the risk of Reye's syndrome

OVERDOSAGE

Signs and symptoms — Hyperpnea, nausea, vomiting, vertigo, tinnitus, flushing, sweating, thirst, headache, drowsiness, diarrhea, and tachycardia, progressing to hyperthermia, hemorrhage, acid-base disturbances, restlessness, confusion, convulsions, vasomotor depression, coma, and respiratory failure

Treatment — If less than 4 h have elapsed since ingestion, induce emesis or perform gastric lavage, followed by activated charcoal, to remove any remaining drug from the stomach. Initial therapy should be directed at reducing hyperthermia by external sponging with tepid water, correcting dehydration by appropriate IV fluid replacement, and maintaining adequate cardiorespiratory and renal function. In moderately severe cases of salicylate poisoning, cautiously administer sodium bicarbonate IV in sufficient quantity, if possible, to maintain an alkaline diuresis; intermittent peritoneal dialysis may also be helpful. In severe cases, hemodialysis should be seriously considered. Potassium should be added to the repair solution to compensate for potassium losses once urine formation is deemed adequate. Glucose may be provided to correct ketosis and hypoglycemia. Plasma transfusion may be beneficial if shock intervenes. Hemorrhagic phenomena may necessitate whole-blood transfusions and phytonadione (vitamin K_1). Do not administer barbiturates to treat excitement or convulsions.

DRUG INTERACTIONS

Anticoagulants — △ Risk of bleeding

Alcohol, corticosteroids, phenylbutazone, oxyphenbutazone — △ Risk of GI ulceration

Probenecid, sulfinpyrazone — ▽ Uricosuria

Spironolactone — ▽ Diuretic effect

Methotrexate — △ Methotrexate plasma level and risk of toxicity

ALTERED LABORATORY VALUES

Blood/serum values — △ Prothrombin time △ Uric acid (with low doses) ▽ Uric acid (with high doses)
▽ Thyroxine (T_4) ▽ Thyroid-stimulating hormone

Urinary values — △ Glucose (with Clinitest tablets)

USE IN CHILDREN
Use according to medical judgment in children under 12 yr of age

USE IN PREGNANT AND NURSING WOMEN
Consult manufacturer for use in pregnant or nursing women

---

[1] *FDA Drug Bulletin* 15(4):34, 1985

NONNARCOTIC ANALGESICS/ANTIPYRETICS

EMPIRIN (aspirin) Burroughs Wellcome OTC

Tablets: 325 mg (5 gr)

INDICATIONS

Pain, including headache, muscular aches and pains, and toothache
Fever and discomfort of colds and flu
Pain and discomfort due to sore throat, neuralgia, menstrual pain, arthritis and rheumatism, bursitis, lumbago, and sciatica; **sleeplessness** caused by minor pain and discomfort

Reducing the risk of **recurrent transient ischemic attacks or stroke in men** who have had transient ischemia of the brain due to fibrin platelet emboli[1]

Reducing the risk of **myocardial infarction and subsequent death** in patients with unstable angina or a prior infarction[2]

ORAL DOSAGE

Adult: 325–650 mg (1–2 tabs) with a full glass of water q4h, up to 3,900 mg (12 tabs)/day

Adult: 325 mg (1 tab) qid or 650 mg (2 tabs) bid

Adult: 325 mg once daily

EMPIRIN

CONTRAINDICATIONS

Gastric ulcer and peptic ulcer symptoms	Asthma	Hypersensitivity to aspirin
Anticoagulant therapy		

WARNINGS/PRECAUTIONS

Gastric irritation	May occur, especially in patients with gastric ulcers, erosive gastritis, or bleeding tendencies; use with caution
Patients with blood-coagulation abnormalities	Use with caution in patients with preexisting hypoprothrombinemia or vitamin K deficiency
Nasal polyps, asthma, hay fever	May predispose to salicylate hypersensitivity; use with caution
Interference with platelet aggregation	Use with caution prior to surgery
Monitoring of prophylactic therapy for myocardial infarction	Check blood pressure, BUN level, and serum uric acid level regularly when using aspirin for long-term prophylaxis of myocardial infarction; small increases in these values have been detected during one clinical trial
Patient instructions	The package label advises consultation with a physician if the patient experiences high or continued fever or severe or persistent sore throat, especially when accompanied by fever, headache, nausea, or vomiting; pregnant or nursing women are advised to consult a health professional before using this product
Reye's syndrome	There is evidence suggesting that use of aspirin in children or adolescents with chicken pox or influenza may increase the risk of Reye's syndrome

ADVERSE REACTIONS

Gastrointestinal	Nausea, dyspepsia, heartburn, epigastric discomfort, anorexia, diarrhea, occult blood loss, hemorrhage
Central nervous system	Dizziness, tinnitus, headache, deafness
Respiratory	Hyperventilation
Cardiovascular	Increased pulse rate
Dermatological	Skin eruptions
Other	Sweating, thirst, electrolyte and acid-base imbalance

OVERDOSAGE

Signs and symptoms	Hyperpnea, nausea, vomiting, vertigo, tinnitus, flushing, sweating, thirst, headache, drowsiness, diarrhea, and tachycardia, progressing to hyperthermia, hemorrhage, acid-base disturbances, restlessness, confusion, convulsions, vasomotor depression, coma, and respiratory failure
Treatment	If less than 4 h have elapsed since ingestion, induce emesis or perform gastric lavage, followed by activated charcoal, to remove any remaining drug from the stomach. Initial therapy should be directed at reducing hyperthermia by external sponging with tepid water, correcting dehydration by appropriate IV fluid replacement, and maintaining adequate cardiorespiratory and renal function. In moderately severe cases of salicylate poisoning, cautiously administer sodium bicarbonate IV in sufficient quantity, if possible, to maintain an alkaline diuresis; intermittent peritoneal dialysis may also be helpful. In severe cases, hemodialysis should be seriously considered. Potassium should be added to the repair solution to compensate for potassium losses once urine formation is deemed adequate. Glucose may be provided to correct ketosis and hypoglycemia. Plasma transfusion may be beneficial if shock intervenes. Hemorrhagic phenomena may necessitate whole-blood transfusions and phytonadione (vitamin K_1). Do not administer barbiturates to treat excitement or convulsions.

DRUG INTERACTIONS

Anticoagulants	△ Risk of bleeding
Alcohol, corticosteroids, phenylbutazone, oxyphenbutazone	△ Risk of GI ulceration
Probenecid, sulfinpyrazone	▽ Uricosuria
Spironolactone	▽ Diuretic effect
Methotrexate	△ Methotrexate plasma level and risk of toxicity

ALTERED LABORATORY VALUES

Blood/serum values	△ Prothrombin time △ Uric acid (with low doses) ▽ Uric acid (with high doses) ▽ Thyroxine (T_4) ▽ Thyroid-stimulating hormone
Urinary values	△ Glucose (with Clinitest tablets)

USE IN CHILDREN	USE IN PREGNANT AND NURSING WOMEN
Consult manufacturer	Aspirin has been shown to be teratogenic and embryocidal in rats and mice given 4–6 times the normal human dose. Clinical studies, however, have not shown that aspirin given during the first trimester increases the risk of abnormalities. Use of aspirin close to term may cause bleeding in the mother, fetus, or neonate. Pregnancy and delivery may be prolonged by regular, high-dosage use during the last two trimesters. Use before delivery may also prolong delivery. Aspirin is excreted in breast milk in small amounts; its clinical effect on nursing infants is not known. Because of the potential for serious adverse reactions in nursing infants, a decision should be made not to nurse or to discontinue use of this preparation, taking into account its importance to the mother.

[1] *FDA Drug Bulletin* 10(1):2, 1980
[2] *FDA Drug Bulletin* 15(4):34, 1985

NONNARCOTIC ANALGESICS/ANTIPYRETICS

FIORICET (butalbital, acetaminophen, and caffeine) Sandoz Pharmaceuticals — Rx

Tablets: 50 mg butalbital, 325 mg acetaminophen, and 40 mg caffeine

INDICATIONS	ORAL DOSAGE
Tension (muscle contraction) headache	**Adult:** 1–2 tabs q4h, up to 6 tabs/day

CONTRAINDICATIONS	
Porphyria	Hypersensitivity to acetaminophen, caffeine, or barbiturates

WARNINGS/PRECAUTIONS	
Drug dependence	Psychic and/or physical dependence and tolerance may develop with prolonged use, especially in addiction-prone individuals. Warn patients not to increase the dosage on their own. Use with caution, if at all, in patients with a history of drug abuse.
Ambulatory patients	Caution patients that their ability to drive or engage in other potentially hazardous activities requiring mental alertness or physical coordination may be impaired
Depressed or suicidal patients	Use with caution, if at all, in patients who are mentally depressed or who have suicidal tendencies
Elderly or debilitated patients	Barbiturates may cause marked excitement, depression, or confusion in elderly or debilitated patients
Paradoxical excitement	In some patients, barbiturates repeatedly produce excitement rather than depression

ADVERSE REACTIONS	The most frequent reactions, regardless of incidence, are printed in *italics*
Central nervous system	*Drowsiness, dizziness,* light-headedness, mental confusion, depression
Gastrointestinal	Nausea, vomiting, flatulence

OVERDOSAGE	
Signs and symptoms	*Butalbital-related effects:* drowsiness, confusion, coma, respiratory depression, hypotension, shock; *acetaminophen-related effects:* nausea, anorexia, vomiting, abdominal pain, diarrhea, diaphoresis, malaise; hepatotoxicity may not be evident until after 2–4 days
Treatment	Maintain an adequate airway, assist ventilation, and administer oxygen, as needed. Induce emesis if patient is conscious, taking care to avoid pulmonary aspiration; if emesis is contraindicated, perform gastric lavage with a cuffed endotracheal tube and with the patient in a face-down position. Activated charcoal, followed by a saline cathartic, may be administered after emesis or lavage. Monitor vital signs and fluid balance. Treat shock with fluids and other standard measures. If renal function is normal, forced diuresis may enhance elimination of butalbital. Hemodialysis may be helpful in patients who are anuric, in shock, or severely intoxicated. Administer oral acetylcysteine as soon as possible (no later than 24 h after ingestion); give a loading dose of 140 mg/kg and then, at 4-h intervals, 17 maintenance doses of 70 mg/kg. (Activated charcoal should be removed before acetylcysteine is given.) Measure the plasma level of unconjugated acetaminophen as early as possible, but no sooner than 4 h after ingestion. Determine prothrombin time, SGOT and SGPT levels, and serum concentrations of bilirubin, creatinine, BUN, glucose, and electrolytes every 24 h. If the prothrombin time exceeds 1.5 times the control value, give vitamin K_1; if the prothrombin time exceeds 3 times this value, give fresh frozen plasma. Institute appropriate measures to treat hypoglycemia and electrolyte and fluid imbalance. For additional information on use of acetylcysteine and interpretation of the plasma acetaminophen level, see Mucomyst chart.

FIORICET ■ GEMNISYN

DRUG INTERACTIONS

Alcohol, narcotic analgesics, antipsychotic agents, antianxiety agents, and other CNS depressants	△	CNS depression; instruct patients not to consume alcohol during therapy
Oral anticoagulants	▽	Anticoagulant effect
Tricyclic antidepressants	▽	Serum level of antidepressant

ALTERED LABORATORY VALUES

Blood/serum values	▽	Glucose (with glucose oxidase/peroxidase tests)
Urinary values	+	5-HIAA (with nitrosonaphthol reagent test)

USE IN CHILDREN
Safety and effectiveness for use in children under 12 yr of age have not been established

USE IN PREGNANT AND NURSING WOMEN
No adequate studies have been performed in animals or pregnant women; use during pregnancy only if clearly needed since the risk of harm to the fetus cannot be ruled out. Barbiturates appear in human milk; effects on nursing infants are not known, although serum levels attained in infants at therapeutic dosages are believed to be insignificant.

NONNARCOTIC ANALGESICS/ANTIPYRETICS

GEMNISYN (aspirin and acetaminophen) Kremers-Urban   OTC

Tablets: 325 mg (5 gr) aspirin and 325 mg (5 gr) acetaminophen

INDICATIONS
Pain that cannot be adequately treated with usual doses of mild analgesics

ORAL DOSAGE
Adult: 1–2 tabs q4–6h while pain persists, up to 6 tabs/24 h

CONTRAINDICATIONS
Sensitivity to aspirin or acetaminophen

WARNINGS/PRECAUTIONS

Persistent pain	Advise patient to report if pain persists more than 10 days
Special-risk patients	Use with caution in patients with peptic ulcer, asthma, or liver damage and in patients receiving anticoagulant therapy
Reye's syndrome	Do not use in children or teenagers with chicken pox or influenza

OVERDOSAGE

Signs and symptoms	*Aspirin-related effects:* hyperpnea, nausea, vomiting, vertigo, tinnitus, flushing, sweating, thirst, headache, drowsiness, diarrhea, and tachycardia, progressing to hyperthermia, hemorrhage, acid-base disturbances, restlessness, confusion, convulsions, vasomotor depression, coma, and respiratory failure; *acetaminophen-related effects:* nausea, anorexia, vomiting, abdominal pain, diarrhea, diaphoresis, malaise; hepatotoxicity may not be evident until after 2–4 days
Treatment	Promptly empty stomach by performing gastric lavage or inducing emesis; then instill activated charcoal. Administer oral acetylcysteine as soon as possible (no later than 24 h after ingestion); give a loading dose of 140 mg/kg and then, at 4-h intervals, 17 maintenance doses of 70 mg/kg. (Activated charcoal should be removed before acetylcysteine is given.) Measure the plasma level of unconjugated acetaminophen as early as possible, but no sooner than 4 h after ingestion. For additional information on use of acetylcysteine and interpretation of the plasma acetaminophen level, see Mucomyst chart. To treat hyperthermia, sponge body with tepid water. For hypoglycemia, dehydration, electrolyte deficiencies, and acid-base disturbances, administer appropriate IV replacement solutions. If salicylate poisoning is severe, cautiously alkalinize the urine with IV bicarbonate. In rare cases, it may be necessary to perform hemodialysis or hemoperfusion in an adult or older child and exchange transfusions or peritoneal dialysis in a younger child or infant. Check urinary output hourly during therapy and determine the following values frequently (at least every 24 h): prothrombin time, arterial pH, pCO_2, pO_2, serum bicarbonate level, total CO_2 concentration, SGOT and SGPT levels, and serum levels of sodium, chloride, potassium, bilirubin, creatinine, BUN, and glucose. If the prothrombin time exceeds 1.5 times the control value, give vitamin K_1; if the prothrombin time exceeds 3 times this value, give fresh frozen plasma. For treatment of hemorrhage, vitamin K_1 as well as blood transfusions may be necessary.

GEMNISYN ■ HALTRAN

DRUG INTERACTIONS

Anticoagulants	△ Risk of bleeding
Alcohol, corticosteroids, phenylbutazone, oxyphenbutazone	△ Risk of GI ulceration
Probenecid, sulfinpyrazone	▽ Uricosuria
Spironolactone	▽ Diuretic effect
Methotrexate	△ Methotrexate plasma level and risk of toxicity

ALTERED LABORATORY VALUES

Blood/serum values	△ Prothrombin time △ or ▽ Uric acid ▽ Glucose (with glucose oxidase/peroxidase tests) ▽ Thyroxine (T_4) ▽ TSH
Urinary values	+ Glucose (with Clinitest tablets) + 5-HIAA (with nitrosonaphthol reagent test)

USE IN CHILDREN
Not recommended for use in children under 12 yr of age

USE IN PREGNANT AND NURSING WOMEN
Consult manufacturer

NONNARCOTIC ANALGESICS/ANTIPYRETICS

HALTRAN (ibuprofen) Upjohn   OTC
Tablets: 200 mg

INDICATIONS

Headache, toothache, backache, muscle ache, menstrual pain, minor pain of arthritis, and minor ache and pain of colds

Fever

ORAL DOSAGE

Adult: 200–400 mg q4–6h, up to 1,200 mg/24 h, for a period of up to 10 days; initial dosage: 200 mg q4–6h. The package labeling warns patients not to exceed these recommendations unless otherwise directed by a physician.
Child (> 12 yr): same as adult

Adult: 200–400 mg q4–6h, up to 1,200 mg/24 h, for a period of up to 3 days; initial dosage: 200 mg q4–6h. The package labeling warns patients not to exceed these recommendations unless otherwise directed by a physician.
Child (> 12 yr): same as adult

CONTRAINDICATIONS
Consult manufacturer

WARNINGS/PRECAUTIONS

Special-risk patients	The package labeling warns patients not to take this product if they have had a severe allergic reaction to aspirin, such as asthma, swelling, shock, or hives; the labeling also cautions patients to consult a physician before using this product if they have experienced any problems or serious adverse reactions while taking an OTC analgesic, if they are under medical supervision for the treatment of a serious condition, or if they are receiving a prescription drug (see also USE IN CHILDREN and USE IN PREGNANT AND NURSING WOMEN)
Adverse reactions	The package labeling instructs patients to take the tablets with food or milk if occasional, mild heartburn, upset stomach, or stomach pain occurs and to consult a physician if gastric symptoms, pain, or fever becomes persistent or more severe, if other new symptoms develop, or if a painful area becomes red or swollen
Concomitant use of aspirin or acetaminophen	The package labeling cautions patients to consult a physician before using this product in combination with aspirin or acetaminophen (see also DRUG INTERACTIONS)

ADVERSE REACTIONS
Consult manufacturer

OVERDOSAGE

Signs and symptoms	Apnea, cyanosis, dizziness, nystagmus
Treatment	Following recent ingestion (< 1 h), induce emesis or perform gastric lavage to remove drug from stomach. Activated charcoal may be helpful. If drug is already absorbed, it may be useful to induce diuresis and alkalinize the urine.

DRUG INTERACTIONS

Coumarin anticoagulants	△ Risk of bleeding; use with caution

| Aspirin | ▽ Anti-inflammatory activity (potential) |

ALTERED LABORATORY VALUES

| Blood/serum values | △ SGOT △ SGPT |

No clinically significant alterations in urinary values occur at therapeutic dosages

---

USE IN CHILDREN

The package labeling warns adults to consult a physician before giving this product to children under 12 yr of age

USE IN PREGNANT AND NURSING WOMEN

The package labeling cautions pregnant or nursing women to consult a health professional before using this product and, because ibuprofen may cause premature closure of the ductus arteriosus or complications during delivery, warns patients not to use this product during the last 3 mo of pregnancy unless specifically directed to do so by a physician

---

NONNARCOTIC ANALGESICS/ANTIPYRETICS

LEVOPROME (methotrimeprazine) Lederle   Rx

Vials: 20 mg/ml (10 ml) for IM use only

INDICATIONS / PARENTERAL DOSAGE

Acute or intractable pain	**Adult:** 10–20 mg IM to start, followed by similar or higher or lower doses, as needed, q4–6h
Obstetrical analgesia and sedation	**Adult:** 15–20 mg IM to start, followed by similar or higher or lower doses, as needed
Preanesthetic medication for producing sedation, somnolence, and relief of apprehension and anxiety	**Adult:** 2–20 mg IM, given 45 min to 3 h before surgery
Postoperative analgesia	**Adult:** 2.5–7.5 mg IM to start, followed by similar or higher or lower doses, as needed, q4–6h

CONTRAINDICATIONS

Age < 12 yr	Hypersensitivity to phenothiazines	CNS depressant overdosage
Antihypertensive therapy with MAO inhibitors	Severe myocardial, renal, or hepatic disease	Comatose states
Clinically significant hypotension		

ADMINISTRATION/DOSAGE ADJUSTMENTS

IM administration	Inject deeply into large muscle mass; rotate the injection site when giving multiple injections. Methotrimeprazine may be given in the same syringe with atropine or scopolamine, but it should *not* be mixed in the same syringe with other drugs. Reduce usual dosage of atropine or scopolamine when used concurrently (see WARNINGS/PRECAUTIONS).
Combination therapy	Reduce dosage of both methotrimeprazine and CNS depressant drugs when administered concomitantly or in close succession
Elderly or debilitated patients with heart disease	Initiate therapy at 5–10 mg and adjust subsequent doses according to patient response; check pulse, blood pressure, and general circulatory status frequently until dosage requirements and responses are stabilized
Duration of therapy	Administer for no more than 30 days unless narcotic drugs are contraindicated or illness is terminal (see WARNINGS/PRECAUTIONS)

WARNINGS/PRECAUTIONS

Concomitant use of atropine, scopolamine, and succinylcholine	May cause tachycardia, fall in blood pressure, and undesirable CNS effects, including stimulation, delirium and extrapyramidal symptoms; use methotrimeprazine with caution
Prolonged high-dose therapy	May cause agranulocytosis or jaundice; perform periodic blood counts and liver-function studies when therapy exceeds 30 days
Orthostatic hypotension	May occur after each of the first several injections; patients should remain in bed or be closely supervised for about 6 h after injection until tolerance to this effect is obtained
Effect on fertility	Depressed spermatogenesis has been reported in experimental animals with doses of phenothiazines that greatly exceed the recommended human dose

ADVERSE REACTIONS[1]

Cardiovascular	Orthostatic hypotension, fainting, syncope, weakness
Central nervous system	Disorientation, dizziness, excessive sedation, slurred speech
Gastrointestinal	Abdominal discomfort, nausea, vomiting, dry mouth
Hepatic	Jaundice (with long-term use of high dosages)
Genitourinary	Difficult urination
Hematological	Agranulocytosis (with long-term use of high dosages)
Other	Nasal congestion, chills, pain at IM injection site, local inflammation and swelling; uterine inertia (rare)

OVERDOSAGE

Signs and symptoms	Blood dyscrasias (agranulocytosis, pancytopenia, leukopenia, eosinophilia, thrombocytopenia); hepatoxicity (jaundice, biliary stasis); extrapyramidal symptoms (dyskinesia, tilting stance, dystonia, parkinsonism, opisthotonos, hyperreflexia, especially in patients with previous brain damage); grand mal convulsions; potentiation of CNS depressants (opiates, barbiturates, antihistamines, alcohol, analgesics), atropine, phosphorous insecticides, heat; cerebral edema and altered CSF proteins; reactivation of psychotic processes; catatonia; autonomic reactions (dryness of mouth, constipation); cardiac arrest, tachycardia, hyperpyrexia; endocrine disturbances (menstrual and lactation irregularities); dermatological disorders (photosensitivity, itching, erythema, urticaria, pigmentation, rash, exfoliative dermatitis); ocular changes (lenticular and corneal deposits and pigmentary retinopathy); hypersensitivity reactions (angioneurotic, laryngeal, and peripheral edema; anaphylactoid reactions; and asthma)
Treatment	Discontinue use. Institute supportive measures, as required. Treat hypotension with phenylephrine or methoxamine; reserve levarterenol for hypotension not reversed by other vasopressors. Do not use epinephrine.

DRUG INTERACTIONS

Other narcotic analgesics and sedative-hypnotics; antianxiety agents, phenothiazines, general anesthetics, and other CNS depressants (including alcohol); MAO inhibitors; tricyclic antidepressants	△ CNS depression; reduce dose of one or both agents if used concomitantly or in close succession
Anticonvulsants	▽ Convulsion threshold
Epinephrine	Severe hypotension
Guanethidine	▽ Antihypertensive effect
Antimuscarinics	△ Atropine-like effect (see WARNINGS/PRECAUTIONS)
Amphetamines	▽ Amphetamine effect
Antacids containing aluminum or magnesium ions	▽ Absorption of methotrimeprazine
Levodopa	▽ Antiparkinsonism effect
MAO inhibitors, tricyclic antidepressants	△ Sedation and antimuscarinic effects

ALTERED LABORATORY VALUES

Urinary values	False-positive or false-negative pregnancy tests △ Bilirubin (false elevation)

No clinically significant alterations in blood/serum values occur at therapeutic dosages

---

USE IN CHILDREN

Contraindicated for use in children under 12 yr of age

USE IN PREGNANT AND NURSING WOMEN

Safety for use during early pregnancy has not been established, but there is no evidence of this drug having adverse developmental effects when administered during late pregnancy and labor. Use with caution in nursing mothers, as phenothiazines are probably excreted in human milk.

---

[1] Other adverse reactions to phenothiazines have been reported during use as antipsychotics, but do not necessarily occur with analgesic doses of methotrimeprazine (see OVERDOSAGE)

NONNARCOTIC ANALGESICS/ANTIPYRETICS

MAGAN (magnesium salicylate) Adria   Rx

Tablets: 545 mg

INDICATIONS	ORAL DOSAGE
Rheumatoid arthritis, osteoarthritis, bursitis, and other musculoskeletal disorders	**Adult:** 1,090 mg (2 tabs) tid to start; adjust dosage, if necessary, to meet individual patient needs

CONTRAINDICATIONS

Advanced chronic renal insufficiency	Uricosuric therapy

WARNINGS/PRECAUTIONS

Patients with known salicylate sensitivity, erosive gastritis, or peptic ulcer	Use with caution; discontinue use if a reaction to magnesium salicylate develops
Patients with renal impairment	Use with caution; discontinue other drugs containing magnesium and monitor serum magnesium levels if dosage levels are high
Other special-risk patients	Use with caution, if at all, in patients receiving anticoagulants, those with liver damage, preexisting hypoprothrombinemia, or vitamin K deficiency, and before surgery
Carcinogenicity, mutagenicity	The carcinogenic and mutagenic potential of this drug has not been studied
Impairment of fertility	The effect, if any, that this drug may have on fertility is unknown; however, aspirin causes testicular atrophy and inhibition of spermatogenesis in animals

ADVERSE REACTIONS

Same as aspirin, with the exception of asthmatic reactions and inhibition of platelet aggregation and increased bleeding time with recommended doses

OVERDOSAGE

Signs and symptoms	Hyperpnea, nausea, vomiting, vertigo, tinnitus, flushing, sweating, thirst, headache, drowsiness, diarrhea, and tachycardia, progressing to hyperthermia, hemorrhage, acid-base disturbances, restlessness, confusion, convulsions, vasomotor depression, coma, and respiratory failure
Treatment	If less than 4 h have elapsed since ingestion, induce emesis or perform gastric lavage, followed by activated charcoal, to remove any remaining drug from the stomach. Initial therapy should be directed at reducing hyperthermia by external sponging with tepid water, correcting dehydration by appropriate IV fluid replacement, and maintaining adequate cardiorespiratory and renal function. In moderately severe cases of salicylate poisoning, cautiously administer sodium bicarbonate IV in sufficient quantity, if possible, to maintain an alkaline diuresis; intermittent peritoneal dialysis may also be helpful. In severe cases, hemodialysis should be seriously considered. Potassium should be added to the repair solution to compensate for potassium losses once urine formation is deemed adequate. Glucose may be provided to correct ketosis and hypoglycemia. Plasma transfusion may be beneficial if shock intervenes. Hemorrhagic phenomena may necessitate whole-blood transfusions and phytonadione (vitamin K_1). Do not administer barbiturates to treat excitement or convulsions.

DRUG INTERACTIONS

Oral anticoagulants	⇧ Risk of bleeding; if possible, avoid concomitant use
Alcohol, corticosteroids, phenylbutazone, oxyphenbutazone	⇧ Risk of GI ulceration
Probenecid, sulfinpyrazone	⇩ Uricosuria
Spironolactone	⇩ Diuretic effect
Methotrexate	⇧ Methotrexate plasma level and risk of toxicity
Sulfonylurea hypoglycemic agents	⇧ Hypoglycemic effect
Barbiturates	⇧ Pharmacologic effects of barbiturates
Phenytoin	⇧ Pharmacologic effects of phenytoin
Magnesium-containing antacids and other drugs	⇧ Risk of hypermagnesemia in patients with renal impairment

ALTERED LABORATORY VALUES

Blood/serum values	⇧ Prothrombin time ⇧ Uric acid (with low doses) ⇩ Uric acid (with high doses) ⇩ Thyroxine (T_4) ⇩ Thyroid-stimulating hormone
Urinary values	⇧ Glucose (with Clinitest tablets)

USE IN CHILDREN

Safety and effectiveness for use in children have not been established

USE IN PREGNANT AND NURSING WOMEN

Pregnancy Category C: use during pregnancy only if expected benefit of therapy outweighs potential risk to the fetus. Salicylate have been shown to be teratogenic in animals, and have increased the number of stillbirths and neonatal deaths in women. Pregnant women given chronic high doses of salicylates have shown longer gestation periods, more frequent postmaturity, and prolonged spontaneous labor. There have been no adequate well-controlled studies of magnesium salicylate in pregnant women. Salicylates are excreted in human milk; use with caution in nursing mothers.

NONNARCOTIC ANALGESICS/ANTIPYRETICS

MEDIPREN (ibuprofen) McNeil Consumer Products OTC

Caplets: 200 mg   **Tablets:** 200 mg

INDICATIONS

Headache, toothache, backache, muscle ache, menstrual pain, minor pain of arthritis, and minor ache and pain of colds

Fever

ORAL DOSAGE

Adult: 200–400 mg q4–6h, up to 1,200 mg/24 h, for a period of up to 10 days; initial dosage: 200 mg q4–6h. The package labeling warns patients not to exceed these recommendations unless otherwise directed by a physician.
Child (> 12 yr): same as adult

Adult: 200–400 mg q4–6h, up to 1,200 mg/24 h, for a period of up to 3 days; initial dosage: 200 mg q4–6h. The package labeling warns patients not to exceed these recommendations unless otherwise directed by a physician.
Child (> 12 yr): same as adult

CONTRAINDICATIONS

Consult manufacturer

WARNINGS/PRECAUTIONS

Special-risk patients — The package labeling warns patients not to take this product if they have had a severe allergic reaction to aspirin, such as asthma, swelling, shock, or hives; the labeling also cautions patients to consult a physician before using this product if they have experienced any problems or serious adverse reactions while taking an OTC analgesic, if they are under medical supervision for the treatment of a serious condition, or if they are receiving a prescription drug (see also USE IN CHILDREN and USE IN PREGNANT AND NURSING WOMEN)

Adverse reactions — The package labeling instructs patients to take this product with food or milk if occasional, mild heartburn, upset stomach, or stomach pain occurs and to consult a physician if gastric symptoms, pain, or fever becomes persistent or more severe, if other new symptoms develop, or if a painful area becomes red or swollen

Concomitant use of other drugs — The package labeling cautions patients not to combine this product with any other ibuprofen-containing product and to consult a physician before using this product in combination with aspirin or acetaminophen (see also DRUG INTERACTIONS)

ADVERSE REACTIONS

Consult manufacturer

OVERDOSAGE

Signs and symptoms — Apnea, cyanosis, dizziness, nystagmus

Treatment — Following recent ingestion (< 1 h), induce emesis or perform gastric lavage to remove drug from stomach. Activated charcoal may be helpful. If drug is already absorbed, it may be useful to induce diuresis and alkalinize the urine.

DRUG INTERACTIONS

Coumarin anticoagulants — ⇧ Risk of bleeding; use with caution
Aspirin — ⇩ Anti-inflammatory activity (potential)

ALTERED LABORATORY VALUES

Blood/serum values — ⇧ SGOT ⇧ SGPT

No clinically significant alterations in urinary values occur at therapeutic dosages

---

USE IN CHILDREN

The package labeling warns adults to consult a physician before giving this product to children under 12 yr of age

USE IN PREGNANT AND NURSING WOMEN

The package labeling cautions pregnant or nursing women to consult a health professional before using this product and, because ibuprofen may cause premature closure of the ductus arteriosus or complications during delivery, warns patients not to use this product during the last 3 mo of pregnancy unless specifically directed to do so by a physician

---

NONNARCOTIC ANALGESICS/ANTIPYRETICS

MIDOL 200 (ibuprofen) Glenbrook OTC

Tablets: 200 mg

INDICATIONS

Headache, toothache, backache, muscle ache, menstrual pain, minor pain of arthritis, and minor ache and pain of colds

ORAL DOSAGE

Adult: 200–400 mg q4–6h, up to 1,200 mg/24 h, for a period of up to 10 days; initial dosage: 200 mg q4–6h. The package labeling warns patients not to exceed these recommendations unless otherwise directed by a physician.
Child (> 12 yr): same as adult

MIDOL 200 ■ MOTRIN

Fever — Adult: 200–400 mg q4–6h, up to 1,200 mg/24 h, for a period of up to 3 days; initial dosage: 200 mg q4–6h. The package labeling warns patients not to exceed these recommendations unless otherwise directed by a physician.
Child (> 12 yr): same as adult

CONTRAINDICATIONS
Consult manufacturer

WARNINGS/PRECAUTIONS

Special-risk patients — The package labeling warns patients not to take this product if they have had a severe allergic reaction to aspirin, such as asthma, swelling, shock, or hives; the labeling also cautions patients to consult a physician before using this product if they have experienced any problems or serious adverse reactions while taking an OTC analgesic, if they are under medical supervision for the treatment of a serious condition, or if they are receiving a prescription drug (see also USE IN CHILDREN and USE IN PREGNANT AND NURSING WOMEN)

Adverse reactions — The package labeling instructs patients to take the tablets with food or milk if occasional, mild heartburn, upset stomach, or stomach pain occurs and to consult a physician if gastric symptoms, pain, or fever becomes persistent or more severe, if other new symptoms develop, or if a painful area becomes red or swollen

Concomitant use of aspirin or acetaminophen — The package labeling cautions patients to consult a physician before using this product in combination with aspirin or acetaminophen (see also DRUG INTERACTIONS)

ADVERSE REACTIONS
Consult manufacturer

OVERDOSAGE

Signs and symptoms — Apnea, cyanosis, dizziness, nystagmus

Treatment — Following recent ingestion (< 1 h), induce emesis or perform gastric lavage to remove drug from stomach. Activated charcoal may be helpful. If drug is already absorbed, it may be useful to induce diuresis and alkalinize the urine.

DRUG INTERACTIONS

Coumarin anticoagulants — △ Risk of bleeding; use with caution

Aspirin — ▽ Anti-inflammatory activity (potential)

ALTERED LABORATORY VALUES

Blood/serum values — △ SGOT △ SGPT

No clinically significant alterations in urinary values occur at therapeutic dosages

---

USE IN CHILDREN

The package labeling warns adults to consult a physician before giving this product to children under 12 yr of age

USE IN PREGNANT AND NURSING WOMEN

The package labeling cautions pregnant or nursing women to consult a health professional before using this product and, because ibuprofen may cause premature closure of the ductus arteriosus or complications during delivery, warns patients not to use this product during the last 3 mo of pregnancy unless specifically directed to do so by a physician

---

NONNARCOTIC ANALGESICS/ANTIPYRETICS

MOTRIN (ibuprofen) Upjohn   Rx

Tablets: 300, 400, 600, 800 mg

INDICATIONS	ORAL DOSAGE
Rheumatoid arthritis Osteoarthritis	Adult: 300 mg qid or 400–800 mg tid or qid; once a satisfactory response is obtained (usually by 2 wk), adjust dosage as needed; higher doses may be required for rheumatoid arthritis than for osteoarthritis
Mild to moderate pain	Adult: 400 mg q4–6h, as needed
Primary dysmenorrhea	Adult: 400 mg q4h, as needed

MOTRIN

CONTRAINDICATIONS

Hypersensitivity to ibuprofen	History of nasal polyps, angioedema, and bronchospastic reactivity to aspirin or other nonsteroidal anti-inflammatory drugs

ADMINISTRATION/DOSAGE ADJUSTMENTS

Gastric irritation	May be minimized by administering drug with meals or milk
Arthritis	An increase in dosage from 2,400 to 3,200 mg/day may be beneficial for certain patients, although it should be borne in mind that in well-controlled clinical trials such an increase caused a slight increase in adverse reactions and failed to enhance mean effectiveness
Combination therapy	Additional symptomatic relief has been obtained in combination with gold salts. Neither benefits nor harmful interactions have been demonstrated with corticosteroids; if prolonged corticosteroid therapy is discontinued, reduce dosage gradually to avoid the complications of abrupt withdrawal.

WARNINGS/PRECAUTIONS

Anaphylactoid reactions	May occur in patients who are hypersensitive to other nonsteroidal anti-inflammatory agents (see CONTRAINDICATIONS)
Peptic ulceration, perforation, GI bleeding	May occur and can be severe and even fatal; patients with a history of upper GI tract disease or with an active peptic ulcer should be closely supervised during therapy
Renal toxicity	Proteinuria, acute interstitial nephritis with hematuria, and occasionally the nephrotic syndrome may occur during therapy. In patients with reduced renal blood flow or volume owing to conditions such as heart failure, renal or hepatic impairment, advanced age, or use of diuretics, administration of a nonsteroidal anti-inflammatory agent may cause a dose-dependent decrease in the formation of renal prostaglandins and thereby precipitate overt renal failure; the reaction is reversible upon discontinuation of the drug.
Drug accumulation	Ibuprofen is eliminated primarily by the kidneys; closely monitor patients with significant renal impairment and be prepared to reduce the daily dose. The safety of ibuprofen in patients with chronic renal failure has not been studied.
Ophthalmic changes	May occur (see ADVERSE REACTIONS); if visual complaints develop, discontinue drug and perform an ophthalmologic examination, including testing of central visual fields and color vision
Fluid retention and edema	May occur; use with caution in patients with a history of cardiac decompensation or hypertension
Prolonged bleeding time	May occur due to inhibition of platelet aggregation; use with caution in patients with coagulation defects and in those receiving anticoagulants
Decreased hemoglobin and hematocrit	A slight dose-related reduction in hemoglobin and hemotocrit may occur. The total decrease in hemoglobin, even at 3,200 mg/day, usually does not exceed 1 g; this effect is probably not clinically important if there are no signs of bleeding.
Liver function abnormalities	Borderline elevations may occur in up to 15% of patients; meaningful elevations (3 times the upper limit of normal) in SGOT or SGPT levels have been reported in less than 1% of patients. If abnormal liver function tests or other manifestations of liver dysfunction arise during therapy, evaluate the patient for evidence of a more severe hepatic reaction. Although such reactions as jaundice and fatal hepatitis have occurred rarely, discontinue therapy if abnormal liver function test results persist or worsen, signs and symptoms of liver disease develop, or secondary manifestations (eg, eosinophilia, rash) occur.
Diagnostic interference	Complications of presumably noninfectious, noninflammatory painful conditions may escape detection because of reduction in fever and inflammation

ADVERSE REACTIONS

Frequent reactions (incidence $\geq$ 1%) are printed in *italics*

Gastrointestinal	*Nausea, epigastric pain, and heartburn (3-9%); diarrhea, abdominal distress, nausea and vomiting, indigestion, constipation, abdominal cramps or pain, bloating, and flatulence (1-3%);* gastric or duodenal ulcer with bleeding and/or perforation, GI hemorrhage, melena, gastritis, pancreatitis[1]
Hepatic	Hepatitis, jaundice, abnormal liver function tests
Central nervous system	*Dizziness (3-9%); headache and nervousness (1-3%);* depression, insomnia, confusion, emotional lability, somnolence, aseptic meningitis with fever and coma[1]
Otic	*Tinnitus (1-3%),* hearing loss
Ophthalmic	Amblyopia, characterized by blurred and/or diminished vision, scotomata, and/or changes in color vision[1]
Dermatological	*Rash, including maculopapular rash (3-9%); pruritus (1-3%);* vesiculobullous eruptions, urticaria, erythema multiforme, Stevens-Johnson syndrome, alopecia[1]
Cardiovascular	*Edema and fluid retention (1-3%),* congestive heart failure in patients with marginal cardiac function, elevated blood pressure, palpitations[1]

Hematological	Neutropenia, agranulocytosis, aplastic anemia, hemolytic anemia (occasionally Coombs' positive), thrombocytopenia with or without purpura, eosinophilia, decreased hemoglobin and hematocrit[1]
Metabolic and endocrinological	*Decreased appetite (1–3%)*[1]
Renal	Acute renal failure in patients with preexisting significant renal impairment, decreased creatinine clearance, polyuria, azotemia, cystitis, hematuria[1]
Allergic	Syndrome of abdominal pain, fever, chills, nausea, and vomiting; anaphylaxis; bronchospasm[1]
Other	Dry eyes and mouth, gingival ulcer, rhinitis

OVERDOSAGE

Signs and symptoms	Apnea, cyanosis, dizziness, nystagmus
Treatment	Following recent ingestion (< 1 h), remove drug by induced emesis or gastric lavage. Activated charcoal may be helpful. If drug is already absorbed, it may be useful to induce diuresis and alkalinize the urine.

DRUG INTERACTIONS

Coumarin anticoagulants	△ Risk of bleeding; use with caution
Aspirin	▽ Anti-inflammatory activity (potential)

ALTERED LABORATORY VALUES

Blood/serum values	△ SGOT △ SGPT

No clinically significant alterations in urinary values occur at therapeutic dosages

---

USE IN CHILDREN

Safety and effectiveness for use in children have not been established

USE IN PREGNANT AND NURSING WOMEN

Not recommended for use in pregnant or nursing women. Animal reproduction studies have shown no evidence of developmental abnormalities; however, no adequate, well-controlled studies have been done in pregnant women and, hence, the drug should be used only if clearly needed. Because of the risk of premature closure of the ductus arteriosus, use during late pregnancy should be avoided. An increased incidence of dystocia and delayed parturition has been observed in rats. Limited studies in nursing women have not demonstrated significant excretion of this drug in human milk; however, because this remains a possibility and because of the potential for serious adverse effects in neonates, the patient should not nurse while taking ibuprofen.

---

[1] Other reactions for which a causal relationship has not been established include paresthesias, hallucinations, dream abnormalities, pseudotumor cerebri, conjunctivitis, diplopia, optic neuritis, cataracts, toxic epidermal necrolysis, photoallergic skin reactions, sinus tachycardia, sinus bradycardia, bleeding episodes, gynecomastia, hypoglycemic reaction, acidosis, renal papillary necrosis, serum sickness, lupus erythematosus syndrome, angioedema, and Henoch-Schönlein vasculitis

---

NONNARCOTIC ANALGESICS/ANTIPYRETICS

NALFON (fenoprofen calcium) Dista   Rx

Capsules: 200, 300 mg   **Tablets:** 600 mg

INDICATIONS	ORAL DOSAGE
Rheumatoid arthritis **Osteoarthritis**	Adult: 300–600 mg tid or qid, or up to 3,200 mg/day if needed
Mild to moderate pain	Adult: 200 mg q4–6h, as needed

CONTRAINDICATIONS

Hypersensitivity to fenoprofen	History of asthma, rhinitis, or urticaria precipitated by aspirin or other nonsteroidal anti-inflammatory drugs
Significant renal impairment	

ADMINISTRATION/DOSAGE ADJUSTMENTS

Timing of administration	Since food decreases fenoprofen blood levels, administer 30 min before or 2 h after meals; if gastrointestinal complaints occur, administer with meals or milk
Combination therapy	Neither benefits nor harmful interactions have been demonstrated with gold salts or corticosteroids. Concomitant therapy with salicylates is not recommended; aspirin may increase excretion rate of fenoprofen, and no additional benefit is obtained beyond the effect of aspirin alone.

WARNINGS/PRECAUTIONS

Peptic ulcer, perforation, GI bleeding	May occur and can be severe and even fatal; patients with a history of upper GI tract disease or with an active peptic ulcer should be closely supervised during therapy. Patients with an active peptic ulcer should be placed on a vigorous antiulcer treatment regimen.
Renal toxicity	Acute interstitial nephritis and the nephrotic syndrome may occur during therapy. The nephrotic syndrome associated with fenoprofen may be preceded by fever, rash, arthralgia, oliguria, and azotemia; substantial proteinuria may also occur, and the syndrome may progress to anuria. Patients who have had these reactions to other nonsteroidal anti-inflammatory agents should not be given fenoprofen. Rapid recovery has occurred with early detection and discontinuation of the drug; treatment may also require dialysis and steroids. In patients with reduced renal blood flow or volume owing to conditions such as heart failure, renal or hepatic impairment, advanced age, or use of diuretics, administration of a nonsteroidal anti-inflammatory agent may cause a critical decrease in the formation of renal prostaglandins and thereby precipitate overt renal failure; the reaction is reversible upon discontinuation of the drug. To avoid renal toxicity, perform renal function tests periodically in patients with possible renal impairment.
Drug accumulation	Fenoprofen is eliminated primarily by the kidneys; closely monitor patients with possibly compromised renal function and be prepared to lower the daily dose
Liver function abnormalities	Test periodically for increases in serum liver enzyme levels. Borderline elevations may occur in up to 15% of patients; meaningful increases (3 times the upper limit of normal) in SGOT or SGPT levels have been reported in less than 1% of patients. If abnormal liver function tests or other manifestations of liver dysfunction occur during therapy, evaluate the patient for evidence of a more severe hepatic reaction. Although such reactions as jaundice and fatal hepatitis have occurred rarely, discontinue therapy if abnormal liver function test results persist or worsen, signs and symptoms of liver disease develop, or secondary manifestations (eg, eosinophilia, rash) occur.
Corticosteroid therapy	If discontinued, reduce dosage gradually to avoid complications of sudden steroid withdrawal
Patients with initially low hemoglobin values	Obtain periodic hemoglobin determinations during long-term therapy
Peripheral edema	May occur; use with caution in patients with compromised cardiac function or hypertension
Prolonged bleeding time	May occur due to inhibition of platelet aggregation; closely monitor patients who may be affected
Impaired hearing	Monitor auditory function periodically
Mental impairment	Performance of potentially hazardous activities may be impaired; caution patients accordingly
Visual impairment	Has occurred with some nonsteroidal anti-inflammatory drugs; if eye complaints develop perform an ophthalmologic examination

ADVERSE REACTIONS[1]

Frequent reactions (incidence $\geq$ 1%) are printed in *italics*

Gastrointestinal	*Dyspepsia, constipation, nausea, and vomiting (3–9%); abdominal pain, anorexia, occult blood loss, diarrhea, flatulence, and dry mouth (1–2%)*; gastritis, peptic ulcer with or without perforation and/or GI hemorrhage[2]
Central nervous system	*Headache and somnolence (15%); dizziness, nervousness, and asthenia (3–9%); tremor, confusion, insomnia, fatigue, and malaise (1–2%)*[2]
Ophthalmic	*Blurred vision (1–2%)*[2]
Otic	*Tinnitus and decreased hearing (1–2%)*
Dermatological	*Pruritus (3–9%); rash, increased sweating and urticuria (1–2%)*[2]
Cardiovascular	*Palpitations (3–9%); tachycardia (1–2%)*[2]
Genitourinary	Dysuria, cystitis, hematuria, oliguria, azotemia, anuria, interstitial nephritis, nephrosis, papillary necrosis
Hepatic	Jaundice, cholestatic hepatitis
Hematological	Purpura, bruising, hemorrhage, thrombocytopenia, hemolytic anemia, aplastic anemia, agranulocytosis, pancytopenia[2]
Other	*Dyspnea (1–2%)*, peripheral edema, anaphylaxis; lymphadenopathy, mastodynia, burning tongue[2]

OVERDOSAGE

Signs and symptoms	See ADVERSE REACTIONS
Treatment	Induce emesis or use gastric lavage to empty stomach, followed by activated charcoal. Employ supportive measures, as indicated. Urinary alkalinization and forced diuresis may be helpful. Furosemide does *not* lower blood levels of fenoprofen.

NALFON ■ NAPROSYN

DRUG INTERACTIONS

Albumin-bound drugs	Displacement of either drug
Hydantoins	⇧ Hydantoin plasma level; observe for signs of toxicity
Sulfonamides	⇧ Sulfonamide plasma level; observe for signs of toxicity
Sulfonylureas	⇧ Sulfonylurea plasma level; observe for signs of toxicity
Coumarin anticoagulants	⇧ Prothrombin time; observe patient carefully
Aspirin	⇩ Plasma half-life of fenoprofen; do not use concomitantly
Phenobarbital	⇩ Plasma half-life of fenoprofen; if necessary, adjust fenoprofen dosage

ALTERED LABORATORY VALUES

Blood/serum values	⇧ Alkaline phosphatase ⇧ SGOT ⇧ Lactate dehydrogenase ⇧ BUN

No clinically significant alterations in urinary values occur at therapeutic dosages

---

USE IN CHILDREN	USE IN PREGNANT AND NURSING WOMEN
Safety and effectiveness for use in children have not been established	Not recommended for use in pregnant or nursing women because of lack of sufficient evidence demonstrating safety in these patients

[1] Reactions observed during clinical trials of fenoprofen in the treatment of rheumatoid arthritis and osteoarthritis; when fenoprofen was used for analgesia in short-term studies, the incidence of adverse reactions was markedly lower than that observed during long-term trials
[2] Other adverse reactions for which a causal relationship has not been established include burning tongue, aphthous ulcerations of the buccal mucosa, metallic taste, pancreatitis, depression, disorientation, seizures, trigeminal neuralgia, personality changes, Stevens-Johnson syndrome, angioneurotic edema, exfoliative dermatitis, alopecia, atrial fibrillation, pulmonary edema, ECG changes, supraventricular tachycardia, lymphadenopathy, mastodynia, fever, diplopia, and optic neuritis

---

NONNARCOTIC ANALGESICS/ANTIPYRETICS

NAPROSYN (naproxen) Syntex   Rx

Tablets: 250, 375, 500 mg

INDICATIONS / ORAL DOSAGE

Rheumatoid arthritis, osteoarthritis, and ankylosing spondylitis	**Adult:** 250–375 mg bid (morning and evening; doses do not have to be equal); during long-term therapy, adjust dosage up or down depending upon clinical response of patient (dosages exceeding 1 g/day have not been studied in these indications)
Acute gout	**Adult:** 750 mg to start, followed by 250 mg q8h until attack has subsided
Mild to moderate pain / Primary dysmenorrhea / Acute tendinitis and bursitis	**Adult:** 500 mg to start, followed by 250 mg q6–8h, as needed, up to 1,250 mg/day

CONTRAINDICATIONS

History of allergic reaction to naproxen or naproxen sodium	History of asthma, rhinitis, and nasal polyps precipitated by aspirin or other nonsteroidal anti-inflammatory/analgesic drugs

ADMINISTRATION/DOSAGE ADJUSTMENTS

Onset of clinical response	Should be observed within 2 wk in arthritic patients; in some patients, symptomatic improvement may not be seen for up to 4 wk
Combination therapy	Added benefits in arthritis have not been demonstrated with corticosteroids; however, coadministration with gold salts has resulted in greater improvement. Use with salicylates or related drug naproxen sodium is not recommended.
Adrenal function tests	Discontinue naproxen therapy 72 h prior to testing

WARNINGS/PRECAUTIONS

Anaphylactoid reactions	Potentially fatal allergic or idiosyncratic anaphylactoid reactions may occur. Before beginning therapy, determine whether the patient has experienced reactions such as asthma, nasal polyps, urticaria, or hypotension in association with nonsteroidal anti-inflammatory drugs (see CONTRAINDICATIONS); if such reactions occur during therapy, discontinue use.
Peptic ulcer, perforation, GI bleeding	May occur and can be severe or even fatal; patients with a history of peptic ulcer disease or active gastric or duodenal ulcers should be closely supervised during therapy

NAPROSYN

Renal toxicity	Proteinuria, acute interstitial nephritis with hematuria, and occasionally the nephrotic syndrome may occur during therapy. In patients with reduced renal blood flow or volume owing to conditions such as heart failure, renal or hepatic impairment, advanced age, or use of diuretics, administration of a nonsteroidal anti-inflammatory agent may cause a critical decrease in the formation of renal prostaglandins and thereby precipitate overt renal failure; reaction is reversible upon discontinuation of the drug. To avoid renal toxicity, monitor serum creatinine level and/or creatinine clearance and exercise great caution if a patient has significant renal impairment.
Drug accumulation	Naproxen is eliminated primarily by the kidneys; use with caution if creatinine clearance is less than 20 mg/ml since drug accumulation can occur in such a case. Chronic alcoholic liver disease, probably other forms of cirrhosis, and, according to one study, advanced age all produce an increase in the serum level of unbound naproxen; if a cirrhotic or elderly patient requires high doses, exercise caution, and be prepared to adjust dose.
Liver function abnormalities	Borderline elevations may occur in up to 15% of patients; meaningful elevations (3 times the upper limit of normal) in SGOT or SGPT levels have been reported in less than 1% of patients. If abnormal liver function tests or other manifestations of liver dysfunction arise during therapy, evaluate the patient for evidence of a more severe hepatic reaction. Although such reactions as jaundice and fatal hepatitis have occurred rarely, discontinue therapy if abnormal liver function test results persist or worsen, signs and symptoms of liver disease develop, or secondary manifestations (eg, eosinophilia, rash) occur.
Ophthalmic changes	Have occurred in animals treated with related drugs; perform an ophthalmological examination within a reasonable period after initiating therapy and periodically thereafter if drug is used for an extended period
Peripheral edema	May occur; use with caution in patients with fluid retention, hypertension, or heart failure
Corticosteroid therapy	If discontinued, reduce dosage gradually to avoid complications of sudden steroid withdrawal and observe patient closely for adverse effects
Mental impairment	Performance of potentially hazardous activities may be impaired; advise patients to exercise caution if they experience drowsiness, dizziness, vertigo, or depression
Prolonged bleeding time	May occur due to inhibition of platelet aggregation; use with caution in patients with coagulation defects or in those on anticoagulant therapy
Patients with initially low hemoglobin values (≤ 10 g)	Obtain periodic hemoglobin determinations during long-term therapy
Diagnostic interference	Complications of presumably noninfectious, noninflammatory painful conditions may escape detection because of reduction in fever and inflammation
Carcinogenicity	No evidence of carcinogenicity has been found in rats after 2 yr of study

ADVERSE REACTIONS[1]

	Frequent reactions (incidence ≥ 1%) are printed in *italics*
Gastrointestinal	*Constipation, heartburn, abdominal pain, and nausea (3-9%); dyspepsia, diarrhea, and stomatitis (1-3%);* bleeding and/or perforation, peptic ulcer with bleeding and/or perforation, vomiting, melena, hematemesis
Respiratory	Eosinophilic pneumonitis
Central nervous system and neuromuscular	*Headache, dizziness, and drowsiness (3-9%); light-headedness and vertigo (1-3%);* myalgia, muscle weakness, inability to concentrate, depression, malaise, dream abnormalities, insomnia
Dermatological	*Pruritus, eruption, and ecchymoses (3-9%); sweating and purpura (1-3%);* rash, alopecia, photosensitive dermatitis[2]
Cardiovascular	*Edema and dyspnea (3-9%); palpitations (1-3%);* congestive heart failure
Hepatic	Abnormal liver function tests, jaundice
Renal	Glomerular nephritis, interstitial nephritis, nephrotic syndrome, hematuria, renal disease
Hematological	Thrombocytopenia, leukopenia, granulocytopenia, eosinophilia[2]
Other	*Tinnitus (3-9%); thirst, visual disturbances, and hearing disturbances (1-3%);* hearing impairment, anaphylactoid reactions, menstrual disorders, chills, fever[2]

OVERDOSAGE

Signs and symptoms	Drowsiness, heartburn, indigestion, nausea, vomiting
Treatment	Induce emesis or use gastric lavage to empty stomach, and institute supportive measures, as needed. Activated charcoal may be helpful.

DRUG INTERACTIONS

Albumin-bound drugs	Displacement of either drug
Coumarin anticoagulants	⇧ Prothrombin time

Hydantoins	⇧ Hydantoin plasma level
Sulfonylureas	⇧ Sulfonylurea plasma level
Sulfonamides	⇧ Sulfonamide plasma level
Furosemide	⇩ Natriuretic effect of furosemide
Lithium	⇧ Lithium plasma level
Propranolol, other beta blockers	⇩ Antihypertensive effect
Aspirin	⇧ Excretion of naproxen
Probenecid	⇧ Naproxen plasma half-life
Methotrexate	⇧ Methotrexate plasma level (based on animal studies); exercise caution

ALTERED LABORATORY VALUES

Blood/serum values	⇧ BUN ⇧ Creatinine ⇧ SGOT ⇧ SGPT
Urinary values	⇧ 17-Ketogenic steroids Interference with 5-HIAA determinations

USE IN CHILDREN

Pediatric dosages have not been established

USE IN PREGNANT AND NURSING WOMEN

Pregnancy Category B: use during pregnancy only if clearly needed; because premature closure of the ductus arteriosus may occur, administration during late pregnancy should be avoided. An increased incidence of dystocia and delayed parturition has been observed in rats. Reproduction studies in rats, rabbits, and mice given up to 6 times the human dose have shown no evidence of teratogenicity or impaired fertility. No adequate, well-controlled studies have been performed in pregnant women. Naproxen anion appears in human breast milk at a concentration of 1% of maternal plasma levels; avoid use in nursing mothers due to potential adverse effects of prostaglandin inhibition.

[1] Adverse reactions occurring in patients treated for rheumatoid arthritis or osteoarthritis are listed; in general, these reactions were reported 2–10 times more frequently than they were in patients treated for mild-to-moderate pain or dysmenorrhea
[2] Other reactions for which a causal relationship has not been established incude epidermal necrolysis, erythema multiforme, Stevens-Johnson syndrome, urticaria, agranulocytosis, aplastic anemia, hemolytic anemia, cognitive dysfunction, ulcerative stomatitis, vasculitis, angioneurotic edema, hypoglycemia, and hyperglycemia

---

NONNARCOTIC ANALGESICS/ANTIPYRETICS

NUBAIN (nalbuphine hydrochloride) Du Pont   Rx

Ampuls: 10 mg/ml (1 ml), 20 mg/ml (1 ml)   **Vials:** 10 mg/ml (10 ml), 20 mg/ml (10 ml)   **Prefilled syringes:** 20 mg/ml (1 ml)

INDICATIONS   PARENTERAL DOSAGE

Moderate to severe pain
Preoperative analgesia

Adult: 10 mg/70 kg SC, IM, or IV q3–6h, as needed; for nontolerant patients, do not exceed 20 mg/dose or 160 mg/day

Anesthesia support
Obstetrical analgesia

Adult: 10–20 mg SC, IM, or IV q3–6h, up to a total of 160 mg/day, as needed[1]

CONTRAINDICATIONS

Hypersensitivity to nalbuphine

ADMINISTRATION/DOSAGE ADJUSTMENTS

Patients dependent on morphine, meperidine, codeine, or similar narcotics	Reduce dose to ¼ the usual dose and observe patient for signs of withdrawal; if untoward reactions do not occur, increase dose gradually to optimal level

WARNINGS/PRECAUTIONS

Drug dependence	Psychic and/or physical dependence and tolerance may develop, especially in addiction-prone individuals, although potential for abuse is less than that of controlled analgesics. Abrupt withdrawal following prolonged use may cause abdominal cramps, nausea, vomiting, and other signs of narcotic withdrawal; withdraw drug gradually.
Ambulatory patients	Caution patients not to engage in potentially hazardous activities requiring full mental alertness or physical coordination and to avoid alcohol and other CNS depressants, which may produce additional CNS depression
Patients with head injuries or other intracranial lesions	The respiratory depressant effects of this drug and its capacity to elevate CSF pressure may be markedly exaggerated in such patients; side effects may also interfere with the clinical evaluation of head injuries. Administer with extreme caution and only if use of this drug is deemed essential.

Other special-risk patients	Reduce dosage and administer with caution to patients with impaired respiration or hepatic or renal impairment; use with caution also in patients with myocardial infarction who are nauseous or vomiting and in patients scheduled for biliary tract surgery
Narcotic withdrawal symptoms	May be precipitated in patients dependent on narcotics; unduly troublesome symptoms may be controlled by slow IV administration of morphine in small increments until relief is obtained
Sulfite sensitivity	Sodium metabisulfite in this product may cause urticaria, pruritus, wheezing, anaphylaxis, or other allergic-type reactions in susceptible patients, such as those with asthma or atopy

ADVERSE REACTIONS

Frequent reactions (incidence ≥ 1%) are printed in *italics*

Central nervous system	*Sedation (36%), dizziness/vertigo (5%), headache (3%)*, nervousness, depression, restlessness, crying, euphoria, a "floating" feeling, hostility, unusual dreams, confusion, faintness, hallucinations, dysphoria, a feeling of heaviness, numbness, tingling, distortion of reality
Gastrointestinal	*Nausea/vomiting (6%), dry mouth (4%)*, cramps, dyspepsia, bitter taste
Cardiovascular	Hypertension, hypotension, bradycardia, tachycardia
Respiratory	Depression, dyspnea, asthma
Dermatological	Itching, burning, urticaria
Other	*Sweaty/clammy skin (9%)*, speech difficulty, urinary urgency, blurred vision, flushing and warmth

OVERDOSAGE

Signs and symptoms	Sleepiness, mild dysphoria, respiratory depression
Treatment	Administer naloxone IV immediately as an antidote. Provide oxygen, IV fluids, vasopressors, and other supportive measures, as needed.

DRUG INTERACTIONS

Narcotic analgesics, sedative-hypnotics, tranquilizers, phenothiazine antipsychotics, general anesthetics, and other CNS depressants	⌂ CNS depression; reduce dose of one or both agents if used concomitantly or in close succession

ALTERED LABORATORY VALUES

No clinically significant alterations in blood/serum or urinary values occur at therapeutic dosages

---

USE IN CHILDREN	USE IN PREGNANT AND NURSING WOMEN
Not recommended for use in patients under 18 yr of age	Safety for use during pregnancy has not been established. Use during labor and delivery may result in neonatal respiratory depression; exercise caution if infant is premature. Consult manufacturer for use in nursing mothers.

[1] Beaver WT, Feise GA: *J Pharmacol Exp Ther* 904:487–496, 1978; Elliott HW et al: *J Med* 1:74–89, 1970; *The Medical Letter* 21:81–84, 1979; Nubain (Nalbuphine HCl): A Physician's Monograph, Endo Laboratories, Garden City, N.Y.; Tammisto T, Tigerstedt I: *Acta Anaesth Scand* 91:390–394, 1977

NONNARCOTIC ANALGESICS/ANTIPYRETICS

NUPRIN (ibuprofen) Bristol-Myers OTC

Tablets: 200 mg

INDICATIONS	ORAL DOSAGE
Headache, toothache, backache, muscle ache, menstrual pain, minor pain of arthritis, and minor ache and pain of colds	**Adult:** 200–400 mg q4–6h, up to 1,200 mg/24 h, for a period of up to 10 days; initial dosage: 200 mg q4–6h. The package labeling warns patients not to exceed these recommendations unless otherwise directed by a physician. **Child (> 12 yr):** same as adult
Fever	**Adult:** 200–400 mg q4–6h, up to 1,200 mg/24 h, for a period of up to 3 days; initial dosage: 200 mg q4–6h. The package labeling warns patients not to exceed these recommendations unless otherwise directed by a physician. **Child (> 12 yr):** same as adult

CONTRAINDICATIONS

Consult manufacturer

WARNINGS/PRECAUTIONS

Special-risk patients	The package labeling warns patients not to take this product if they have had a severe allergic reaction to aspirin, such as asthma, swelling, shock, or hives; the labeling also cautions patients to consult a physician before using this product if they have experienced any problems or serious adverse reactions while taking an OTC analgesic, if they are under medical supervision for the treatment of a serious condition, or if they are receiving a prescription drug (see also USE IN CHILDREN and USE IN PREGNANT AND NURSING WOMEN)
Adverse reactions	The package labeling instructs patients to take the tablets with food or milk if occasional, mild heartburn, upset stomach, or stomach pain occurs and to consult a physician if gastric symptoms, pain, or fever becomes persistent or more severe, if other new symptoms develop, or if a painful area becomes red or swollen
Concomitant use of aspirin or acetaminophen	The package labeling cautions patients to consult a physician before using this product in combination with aspirin or acetaminophen (see also DRUG INTERACTIONS)

ADVERSE REACTIONS

Consult manufacturer

OVERDOSAGE

Signs and symptoms	Apnea, cyanosis, dizziness, nystagmus
Treatment	Following recent ingestion (< 1 h), induce emesis or perform gastric lavage to remove drug from stomach. Activated charcoal may be helpful. If drug is already absorbed, it may be useful to induce diuresis and alkalinize the urine.

DRUG INTERACTIONS

Coumarin anticoagulants	↑ Risk of bleeding; use with caution
Aspirin	↓ Anti-inflammatory activity (potential)

ALTERED LABORATORY VALUES

Blood/serum values	↑ SGOT ↑ SGPT

No clinically significant alterations in urinary values occur at therapeutic dosages

---

USE IN CHILDREN

The package labeling warns adults to consult a physician before giving this product to children under 12 yr of age

USE IN PREGNANT AND NURSING WOMEN

The package labeling cautions pregnant or nursing women to consult a health professional before using this product and, because ibuprofen may cause premature closure of the ductus arteriosus or complications during delivery, warns patients not to use this product during the last 3 mo of pregnancy unless specifically directed to do so by a physician

---

NONNARCOTIC ANALGESICS/ANTIPYRETICS

PANADOL (acetaminophen) Glenbrook   OTC

Caplets: 500 mg   **Tablets:** 500 mg

INDICATIONS	ORAL DOSAGE
Pain (headache, colds, flu, sinusitis, backaches, muscle aches, menstrual discomfort, arthritis, and toothaches)	**Adult:** 1,000 mg (2 caplets or tablets) q4h, up to 4,000 mg (8 caplets or tablets)/24 h

Children's PANADOL (acetaminophen) Glenbrook   OTC

Chewable tablets: 80 mg *fruit flavored*   **Liquid (per 5 ml):** 160 mg (2, 4 fl oz) *fruit flavored, alcohol free*   **Drops (per 0.8-ml dropperful):** 80 mg (0.5 fl oz) *fruit flavored, alcohol free*

INDICATIONS	ORAL DOSAGE
Pain and fever associated with colds and flu, earaches, headaches, teething, immunizations, tonsillectomy, and childhood illnesses	**Child (2–3 yr; 24–35 lb):** 160 mg (2 dropperful, 1 tsp liquid, or 2 tablets) q4h, up to 5 doses/24 h **Child (4–5 yr; 36–47 lb):** 240 mg (3 dropperful, 1½ tsp liquid, or 3 tablets) q4h, up to 5 doses/24 h **Child (6–8 yr; 48–59 lb):** 320 mg (4 dropperful, 2 tsp liquid, or 4 tablets) q4h, up to 5 doses/24 h **Child (9–10 yr; 60–71 lb):** 400 mg (2½ tsp liquid or 5 tablets) q4h, up to 5 doses/24 h **Child (11–12 yr; 72–95 lb):** 480 mg (3 tsp liquid or 6 tablets) q4h, up to 5 doses/24 h

PANADOL ■ PERCOGESIC

PANADOL Jr. (acetaminophen) Glenbrook OTC
Caplets: 160 mg

INDICATIONS	**ORAL DOSAGE**
Pain and fever associated with colds and flu, headaches, minor muscular aches, sprains, and menstrual discomfort	Child (6–8 yr; 48–59 lb): 320 mg (2 caplets) q4h, up to 1,600 mg (10 caplets)/24 h Child (9–10 yr; 60–71 lb): 400 mg (2½ caplets) q4h, up to 2,000 mg (12½ caplets)/24 h Child (11–12 yr; 72–95 lb): 480 mg (3 caplets) q4h, up to 2,400 mg (15 caplets)/24 h Child (>12 yr; >96 lb): 640 mg (4 caplets) q4h, up to 3,200 mg (20 caplets)/24 h
CONTRAINDICATIONS	
Hypersensitivity to acetaminophen	
ADMINISTRATION/DOSAGE ADJUSTMENTS	
Use of drops and liquid	The pediatric drops and liquid may be given directly or mixed with milk, formula, fruit juice, cereal, or other foods
WARNINGS/PRECAUTIONS	
Hypersensitivity	On rare occasions, a hypersensitivity reaction may occur; if reaction is seen, discontinue use
Patient instructions	Panadol: the package label cautions patients not to give this drug to children under 12 yr of age or use it for more than 10 days unless directed to do so by a physician; the label also advises patients to consult a physician for conditions associated with severe, recurrent pain or high, continued fever. Children's Panadol and Panadol Jr.: the package labels caution patients not to use these products for more than 5 days and to consult a physician if symptoms persist or new ones occur, if fever persists for more than 3 days or recurs, or if high fever, severe or persistent sore throat, headache, nausea, or vomiting occurs
OVERDOSAGE	
Signs and symptoms	*Early:* nausea, vomiting, diaphoresis, and general malaise (some patients may be asymptomatic); *late:* clinical and laboratory evidence of hepatotoxicity (vomiting; right upper quadrant tenderness; increased SGOT, SGPT, serum bilirubin, and prothrombin time; and possible hypoglycemia) may not be apparent until 48–72 h after ingestion
Treatment	Promptly empty stomach by performing gastric lavage or inducing emesis with syrup of ipecac (15–30 ml for children, 30–45 ml for adults). Give ipecac with copious quantities of water; if emesis does not occur within 20 min, repeat dose. Activated charcoal may be given if acetaminophen has been ingested with certain other drugs. Administer oral acetylcysteine as soon as possible (no later than 24 h after ingestion); give a loading dose of 140 mg/kg and then, at 4-h intervals, 17 maintenance doses of 70 mg/kg. (Charcoal, if used, should be removed before acetylcysteine is given.) Measure the plasma level of unconjugated acetaminophen as early as possible, but no sooner than 4 h after ingestion. Determine prothrombin time, SGOT and SGPT levels, and serum concentrations of bilirubin, creatinine, BUN, glucose, and electrolytes every 24 h. If the prothrombin time exceeds 1.5 times the control value, give vitamin K_1; if the prothrombin time exceeds 3 times this value, give fresh frozen plasma. Institute appropriate measures to treat hypoglycemia and electrolyte and fluid imbalance. Avoid forced diuresis or use of diuretics when treating an acetaminophen overdose. For additional information on use of acetylcysteine and interpretation of the plasma acetaminophen level, see Mucomyst chart.
ALTERED LABORATORY VALUES	
Blood/serum values	▽ Glucose (with glucose oxidase/peroxidase tests)
Urinary values	+ 5-HIAA (with nitrosonaphthol tests)

USE IN CHILDREN	USE IN PREGNANT AND NURSING WOMEN
See INDICATIONS and ORAL DOSAGE	The package labeling cautions pregnant or nursing women to consult a health professional before using these products

---

NONNARCOTIC ANALGESICS/ANTIPYRETICS

PERCOGESIC (acetaminophen and phenyltoloxamine citrate) Richardson-Vicks Health Care Products OTC
Tablets: 325 mg acetaminophen and 30 mg phenyltoloxamine citrate

INDICATIONS	**ORAL DOSAGE**
Pain and discomfort due to headache **Pain** associated with muscle and joint soreness, neuralgia, sinusitis, minor menstrual cramps, the common cold, and toothache **Minor aches and pains** associated with rheumatism and arthritis	Adult and child (≥ 12 yr): 1–2 tabs q4h, up to 8 tabs/24 h Child (6–12 yr): ½–1 tab q4h, up to 4 tabs/24 h

COMPENDIUM OF DRUG THERAPY

WARNINGS/PRECAUTIONS

Patient self-medication — Package label cautions patients not to exceed recommended dosage and to consult a physician in arthritic or rheumatic conditions affecting children under 12 yr of age, if arthritic or rheumatic pain persists for more than 10 days, or if redness or swelling is present; the label also advises that therapy be discontinued after 3 days when used for temporary, symptomatic relief of colds. In addition, the label cautions patients who are pregnant or nursing to seek the opinion of a health-care professional before using this product.

Drowsiness — Caution patients not to drive or engage in other potentially hazardous activities during therapy

OVERDOSAGE

Signs and symptoms — *Antihistaminic effects:* CNS depression ranging from drowsiness to coma; CNS stimulation ranging from excitement to hallucinations and convulsions (with postictal depression); hypotension and cardiovascular collapse; anticholinergic reactions (dry mouth, mydriasis, flushing, fever); toxic effects are seen within 30–120 min after ingestion. In children, excitement, hallucinations, cyanosis, anticholinergic effects, ataxia, incoordination, muscle twitching, athetosis, tremors, hyperreflexia, and tonic-clonic convulsions may occur initially (convulsions can also occur after mild depression); reactions may be followed by postictal depression and cardiorespiratory arrest. *Acetaminophen-related effects:* nausea, anorexia, vomiting, abdominal pain, diarrhea, diaphoresis, malaise; hepatotoxicity may not be evident until after 2–4 days.

Treatment — If patient is conscious, induce vomiting even though it may have occurred spontaneously. If emesis is not possible, perform gastric lavage. Take appropriate precautions against aspiration, especially in children. The airway should be secured with a cuffed endotracheal tube before lavage if the patient is unconscious. After emptying stomach, instill a charcoal slurry or another suitable agent; a saline cathartic such as milk of magnesia may also be helpful. Maintain pulmonary function; if necessary, establish an adequate airway, provide mechanically assisted ventilation, and administer oxygen. For hypotension, give IV fluids; if great caution is exercised, a vasopressor other than epinephrine may also be used. To control convulsions, carefully administer IV diazepam or a short-acting barbiturate, as needed; physostigmine may also be considered if convulsions are centrally mediated. Treat fever with ice packs and cooling sponge baths, not with alcohol. Do not use CNS stimulants. Administer oral acetylcysteine as soon as possible (no later than 24 h after ingestion); give a loading dose of 140 mg/kg and then, at 4-h intervals, 17 maintenance doses of 70 mg/kg. Activated charcoal should be removed before acetylcysteine is given.) Measure the plasma level of unconjugated acetaminophen as early as possible, but no sooner than 4 h after ingestion. Determine prothrombin time, SGOT and SGPT levels, and serum concentrations of bilirubin, creatinine, BUN, glucose, and electrolytes every 24 h. If the prothrombin time exceeds 1.5 times the control value, give vitamin K_1; if the prothrombin time exceeds 3 times this value, give fresh frozen plasma. Institute appropriate measures to treat hypoglycemia and electrolyte and fluid imbalance. Avoid forced diuresis or use of diuretics when treating an acetaminophen overdose. For additional information on use of acetylcysteine and interpretation of the plasma acetaminophen level, see Mucomyst chart.

DRUG INTERACTIONS

Alcohol, tranquilizers, sedative-hypnotics, and other CNS depressants	⇧ CNS depression
MAO inhibitors	⇧ Anticholinergic effects

ALTERED LABORATORY VALUES

Blood/serum values	⇩ Glucose (with glucose oxidase/peroxidase tests)
Urinary values	+ 5-HIAA (with nitrosonaphthol reagent test)

USE IN CHILDREN

Safety and effectiveness for use in children under 6 yr of age has not been established; use according to medical judgment

USE IN PREGNANT AND NURSING WOMEN

Specific guidelines are not available; use according to medical judgment

---

NONNARCOTIC ANALGESICS/ANTIPYRETICS

PONSTEL (mefenamic acid) Parke-Davis   Rx
Capsules: 250 mg

INDICATIONS
Moderate pain

ORAL DOSAGE
Adult: 500 mg to start, followed by 250 mg q6h, as needed, for generally not more than 1 wk

PONSTEL

Primary dysmenorrhea	**Adult:** 500 mg to start, followed by 250 mg q6h, beginning with the onset of menses and continuing for generally not more than 2–3 days

CONTRAINDICATIONS

Hypersensitivity to mefenamic acid	History of bronchospasm, allergic rhinitis, or urticaria precipitated by aspirin or other nonsteroidal anti-inflammatory drugs
Active ulceration or chronic inflammation of the upper or lower GI tract	Preexisting renal disease

ADMINISTRATION/DOSAGE ADJUSTMENTS

Timing of administration	The capsules should preferably be taken with food

WARNINGS/PRECAUTIONS

Special-risk patients	Therapy in patients with a history of ulceration or chronic inflammation of the upper or lower GI tract should be closely supervised (see ADVERSE REACTIONS)
Management of side effects	Diarrhea occurs in approximately 5% of patients; the diarrhea is usually dose-dependent and can be controlled by reducing the dosage or, if necessary, temporarily suspending therapy. Once the diarrhea subsides, the drug may be reintroduced; certain patients, however, may re-experience diarrhea upon subsequent exposure to mefenamic acid. If rash develops, discontinue therapy.
Concomitant anticoagulant therapy	Mefenamic acid may prolong the prothrombin time; monitor the prothrombin time frequently in patients who are taking oral anticoagulants concomitantly
Suspected biliuria	Mefenamic acid may produce a false-positive reaction for urinary bile in the diazo tablet test; if biliuria is suspected, an alternative diagnostic procedure, such as the Harrison spot test, should be performed
Liver function abnormalities	Borderline elevations may occur in some patients; meaningful elevations (3 times the upper limit of normal) in SGOT or SGPT levels have been reported in less than 1% of patients. If abnormal liver function tests or other manifestations of liver dysfunction arise during therapy, evaluate the patient for evidence of a more severe hepatic reaction. Although such reactions as jaundice and fatal hepatitis have occurred rarely, discontinue therapy if abnormal liver function test results persist or worsen, signs and symptoms of liver disease develop, or secondary manifestations (eg, eosinophilia, rash) occur.
Renal toxicity	Proteinuria, acute interstitial nephritis with hematuria, and occasionally the nephrotic syndrome may occur during therapy; renal effects may not be completely reversible. In patients with reduced renal blood flow or volume owing to conditions such as heart failure, renal or hepatic impairment, advanced age, or use of diuretics, administration of a nonsteroidal anti-inflammatory agent may cause a critical decrease in the formation of renal prostaglandins and thereby precipitate overt renal failure; reaction is reversible upon discontinuation of the drug. In elderly patients, renal failure has occurred after 2–6 wk of therapy.
Drug accumulation	Mefenamic acid is eliminated primarily by the kidneys; do not administer to patients with significant renal impairment
Long-term safety	The long-term effects of intermittent therapy of dysmenorrhea with mefenamic acid have not been determined

ADVERSE REACTIONS

Gastrointestinal	Diarrhea, nausea (with or without vomiting), other GI symptoms, abdominal pain, anorexia, pyrosis, flatulence, constipation, ulceration (with or without hemorrhage), mild hepatic toxicity
Hematological	Reversible autoimmune hemolytic anemia (with continuous administration for 1 yr or longer), decreased hematocrit (generally with prolonged therapy), leukopenia, eosinophilia, thrombocytopenic purpura, agranulocytosis, pancytopenia, bone marrow hypoplasia
Central nervous system and special senses	Drowsiness, dizziness, nervousness, headache, blurred vision, insomnia, eye irritation, ear pain; reversible loss of color vision (rare)
Dermatological	Urticaria, rash
Renal	Hematuria, dysuria, renal failure (including papillary necrosis)
Other	Sweating, increased insulin requirements in diabetics, facial edema; palpitation and dyspnea (rare)

OVERDOSAGE

Signs and symptoms	Drowsiness, dizziness, nausea, vomiting, diarrhea, rash, various blood dyscrasias
Treatment	Empty stomach by inducing emesis or by gastric lavage, followed by administration of activated charcoal. Monitor vital signs and institute supportive measures, as needed. Dialysis is of little value because the drug and its metabolites are firmly bound to plasma proteins

DRUG INTERACTIONS

Aspirin and other salicylates, corticosteroids, indomethacin, phenylbutazone, oxyphenbutazone	⇧ Risk of GI ulceration

Oral anticoagulants	△ Prothrombin time
Insulin	▽ Hypoglycemic effect

ALTERED LABORATORY VALUES

Blood/serum values	△ SGOT △ SGPT △ BUN (with prolonged therapy at excessive doses)
Urinary values	+ Bile (with diazo tablet test)

USE IN CHILDREN

Safety and effectiveness for use in children under 14 yr of age have not been established

USE IN PREGNANT AND NURSING WOMEN

Pregnancy Category C: use during pregnancy only if clearly needed. Administration of this drug in late pregnancy is not recommended because of the cardiovascular effects of prostaglandin inhibitors. Decreased fertility, delayed parturition, and a decreased rate of survival to weaning have been observed in rats at 10 times the human dose, and an increase in resorptions has been found in rabbits at 2.5 times the human dose. Fetal anomalies have not occurred in these species, nor in dogs at up to 10 times the human dose. No adequate, well-controlled studies have been done in pregnant women. Because trace amounts of mefenamic acid may be present in breast milk and transmitted to nursing infants, this drug should not be given to women who are breast-feeding.

NONNARCOTIC ANALGESICS/ANTIPYRETICS

RUFEN (ibuprofen) Boots Rx

Tablets: 400, 600, 800 mg

INDICATIONS

	ORAL DOSAGE
Rheumatoid arthritis **Osteoarthritis**	Adult: 300 mg qid or 400–800 mg tid or qid; once a satisfactory response is obtained (usually by 2 wk), adjust dosage as needed; higher doses may be required for rheumatoid arthritis than for osteoarthritis
Mild to moderate pain	Adult: 400 mg q4–6h, as needed
Primary dysmenorrhea	Adult: 400 mg q4h, as needed

CONTRAINDICATIONS

Hypersensitivity to ibuprofen

History of nasal polyps, angioedema, or bronchospasm precipitated by aspirin or other nonsteroidal anti-inflammatory drugs

ADMINISTRATION/DOSAGE ADJUSTMENTS

Gastric irritation	May be minimized by administering drug with meals or milk
Arthritis	An increase in dosage from 2,400 to 3,200 mg/day may be beneficial for certain patients, although it should be borne in mind that in well-controlled studies such an increase caused a slight increase in adverse reactions and failed to enhance mean effectiveness
Combination therapy	Additional symptomatic relief has been obtained in combination with gold salts. Neither benefits nor harmful interactions have been demonstrated with corticosteroids; if prolonged corticosteroid therapy is discontinued, reduce dosage gradually to avoid the complications of abrupt withdrawal

WARNINGS/PRECAUTIONS

Anaphylactoid reactions	May occur in patients hypersensitive to other nonsteroidal anti-inflammatory agents (see CONTRAINDICATIONS)
Peptic ulceration, perforation, GI bleeding	May occur and can be severe and even fatal; patients with a history of upper GI tract disease or with an active peptic ulcer should be closely supervised during therapy
Renal toxicity	Proteinuria, acute interstitial nephritis with hematuria, and occasionally the nephrotic syndrome may occur during therapy. In patients with reduced renal blood flow or volume owing to conditions such as heart failure, renal or hepatic impairment, advanced age, or use of diuretics, administration of a nonsteroidal anti-inflammatory agent may cause a dose-dependent decrease in the formation of renal prostaglandins and thereby precipitate overt renal failure; the reaction is reversible upon discontinuation of the drug.
Drug accumulation	Ibuprofen is eliminated primarily by the kidneys; closely monitor patients with significant renal impairment and be prepared to reduce the daily dose. The safety of ibuprofen in patients with chronic renal failure has not been studied.

RUFEN

Ophthalmic changes	May occur (see ADVERSE REACTIONS); if visual complaints develop, discontinue drug and perform an ophthalmologic examination, including testing of central visual fields and color vision
Fluid retention and edema	May occur; use with caution in patients with a history of cardiac decompensation or hypertension. Fluid retention can generally be reversed by discontinuing the drug.
Prolonged bleeding time	May occur due to inhibition of platelet aggregation; use with caution in patients with coagulation defects or with those on anticoagulant therapy
Decreased hemoglobin and hematocrit	A slight dose-related reduction in hemoglobin and hematocrit may occur. The total decrease in hemoglobin, even at 3,200 mg/day, usually does not exceed 1 g; this effect is probably not clinically important if there are no signs of bleeding.
Liver function abnormalities	Borderline elevations may occur in up to 15% of patients; meaningful elevations (3 times the upper limit of normal) in SGOT or SGPT levels have been reported in less than 1% of patients. If abnormal liver function tests or other manifestations of liver dysfunction arise during therapy, evaluate the patient for evidence of a more severe hepatic reaction. Although such reactions as jaundice and fatal hepatitis have occurred rarely, discontinue therapy if abnormal liver function test results persist or worsen, signs and symptoms of liver disease develop, or secondary manifestations (eg, eosinophilia, rash) occur.
Diagnostic interference	Complications of presumably noninfectious, noninflammatory painful conditions may escape detection because of reduction in fever and inflammation

ADVERSE REACTIONS[1]

Frequent reactions (incidence $\geq$ 1%) are printed in *italics*

Gastrointestinal	*Nausea, epigastric pain, and heartburn (3–9%); diarrhea, abdominal distress, nausea and vomiting, indigestion, constipation, abdominal cramps or pain, bloating, and flatulence ($<$ 3%);* gastric or duodenal-ulcer bleeding and/or perforation, GI hemorrhage, pancreatitis, melena, gastritis, hepatitis, jaundice, abnormal liver function tests
Central nervous system	*Dizziness (3–9%); headache and nervousness ($<$ 3%);* depression, insomnia, confusion, emotional lability, somnolence, aseptic meningitis with fever and coma
Ophthalmic	Blurred and/or diminished vision; scotomata; changes in color vision
Otic	*Tinnitus ($<$ 3%),* hearing loss
Dermatological	*Rash, including maculopapular rash (3–9%), pruritus ($<$ 3%),* vesiculobullous eruptions, urticaria, erythema multiforme, Stevens-Johnson syndrome, alopecia
Metabolic	*Decreased appetite ($<$ 3%)*
Cardiovascular	*Edema and fluid retention ($<$ 3%),* congestive heart failure in patients with marginal cardiac function; elevated blood pressure, palpitations
Hematological	Neutropenia, agranulocytosis, aplastic anemia, hemolytic anemia (occasionally Coombs' positive), thrombocytopenia with or without purpura, eosinophilia, decreased hemoglobin and hematocrit
Renal	Acute renal failure in patients with significant renal impairment; decreased creatinine clearance, polyuria, azotemia, cystitis, hematuria
Allergic	Syndrome of abdominal pain, fever, chills, nausea, and vomiting; anaphylaxis; bronchospasm
Other	Dry eyes and mouth, gingival ulcer, rhinitis

OVERDOSAGE

Signs and symptoms	Apnea, cyanosis, dizziness, nystagmus
Treatment	Following recent ingestion ($<$ 1 h), induce emesis or perform gastric lavage to remove drug from stomach. Activated charcoal may be helpful. If drug is already absorbed, it may be useful to induce diuresis and alkalinize the urine.

DRUG INTERACTIONS

Coumarin anticoagulants	⇧ Risk of bleeding; use with caution
Aspirin	⇩ Anti-inflammatory activity (potential)

ALTERED LABORATORY VALUES

Blood/serum values	⇧ SGOT ⇧ SGPT

No clinically significant alterations in urinary values occur at therapeutic dosages

---

USE IN CHILDREN

Safety and effectiveness for use in children have not been established

USE IN PREGNANT AND NURSING WOMEN

Not recommended for use in pregnant or nursing women. Animal reproduction studies have shown no evidence of developmental abnormalities; however, no adequate, well-controlled studies have been done in pregnant women and, hence, the drug should be used only if clearly needed. Because of the risk of premature closure of the ductus arteriosus, use during late pregnancy should be avoided. An increased incidence of dystocia and delayed parturition has been observed in rats. Limited studies in nursing women have not demonstrated significant excretion of this drug in human milk; however, because this remains a possibility and because of the potential for serious adverse effects in neonates, the patient should not nurse while taking ibuprofen.

---

[1] Reactions for which a causal relationship has not been established include paresthesias, hallucinations, dream abnormalities, pseudotumor cerebri, toxic epidermal necrolysis, photoallergic skin reactions, conjunctivitis, diplopia, optic neuritis, cataracts, bleeding episodes (eg, epistaxis, menorrhagia), serum sickness, lupus erythematosus syndrome, Henoch-Schonlein vasculitis, angioedema, gynecomastia, hypoglycemic reaction, acidosis, sinus tachycardia, sinus bradycardia, and renal papillary necrosis

NONNARCOTIC ANALGESICS/ANTIPYRETICS

ST. JOSEPH Aspirin for Children (aspirin) Plough   OTC

Chewable tablets: 81 mg (1¼ gr) *orange flavored*

INDICATIONS	ORAL DOSAGE
Fever **Aches and pains** caused by colds, inoculations, headaches, and teething **Sore throat** caused by colds	**Child (12–23 mo; 22–26 lb):** 121.5 mg (1½ tabs) q4h, as needed, up to 5 doses/24 h **Child (2–3 yr; 27–35 lb):** 162 mg (2 tabs) q4h, as needed, up to 5 doses/24 h **Child (4–5 yr; 36–45 lb):** 243 mg (3 tabs) q4h, as needed, up to 5 doses/24 h **Child (6–8 yr; 46–65 lb):** 324 mg (4 tabs) q4h, as needed, up to 5 doses/24 h **Child (9–10 yr; 66–76 lb):** 405 mg (5 tabs) q4h, as needed, up to 5 doses/24 h **Child (11 yr; 77–83 lb):** 486 mg (6 tabs) q4h, as needed, up to 5 doses/24 h **Child ($\geq$ 12 yr; $\geq$ 84 lb):** 648 mg (8 tabs) q4h, as needed, up to 5 doses/24 h

CONTRAINDICATIONS[1]

Bleeding ulcer	Hemorrhagic states	Hypersensitivity to salicylates
Hemophilia		

ADMINISTRATION/DOSAGE ADJUSTMENTS

Administration	Tablets may be chewed, dissolved on the tongue, or swallowed whole or, for younger children, crushed or dissolved in a teaspoon of liquid; always follow administration with ½ glass of water, milk, or fruit juice. The tablets may also be powdered for infant use.

WARNINGS/PRECAUTIONS

Reye's syndrome	According to some reports, the risk of Reye's syndrome in children or teenagers with influenza or chicken pox may be increased by the use of aspirin; the package label warns consumers not to use this product in such patients without medical supervision
Other precautions for consumers	Package label cautions against using this product for more than 5 days or, unless specifically directed by a physician, with other medications containing aspirin. The label also advises consumers to consult a physician if indications of potentially serious illness (eg, severe or persistent sore throat, high fever, headache, nausea, or vomiting) are not relieved within 24 h, if symptoms persist or new ones develop, or if fever persists for more than 3 days or recurs. Patients are also warned not to exceed the recommended dosage.

ADVERSE REACTIONS[1,2]

Gastrointestinal	Nausea, dyspepsia, heartburn, epigastric discomfort, anorexia, diarrhea, occult blood loss, hemorrhage
Central nervous system	Dizziness, tinnitus, headache, deafness
Respiratory	Hyperventilation
Cardiovascular	Increased pulse rate
Dermatological	Skin eruptions
Other	Sweating, thirst, electrolyte and acid-base imbalance

OVERDOSAGE

Signs and symptoms	Hyperpnea, nausea, vomiting, vertigo, tinnitus, flushing, sweating, thirst, headache, drowsiness, diarrhea, and tachycardia, progressing to hyperthermia, hemorrhage, acid-base disturbances, restlessness, confusion, convulsions, vasomotor depression, coma, and respiratory failure
Treatment	If less than 4 h have elapsed since ingestion, induce emesis or perform gastric lavage, followed by activated charcoal, to remove any remaining drug from the stomach. Initial therapy should be directed at reducing hyperthermia by external sponging with tepid water, correcting dehydration by appropriate IV fluid replacement, and maintaining adequate cardiorespiratory and renal function. In moderately severe cases of salicylate poisoning, cautiously administer sodium bicarbonate IV in sufficient quantity, if possible, to maintain an alkaline diuresis; intermittent peritoneal dialysis may also be helpful. In severe cases, hemodialysis should be seriously considered. Potassium should be added to the repair solution to compensate for potassium losses once urine formation is deemed adequate. Glucose may be provided to correct ketosis and hypoglycemia. Plasma transfusion may be beneficial if shock intervenes. Hemorrhagic phenomena may necessitate whole-blood transfusions and phytonadione (vitamin K$_1$). Do not administer barbiturates to treat excitement or convulsions.

DRUG INTERACTIONS

Anticoagulants	⇧ Risk of bleeding
Alcohol, corticosteroids, phenylbutazone, oxyphenbutazone	⇧ Risk of GI ulceration
Probenecid, sulfinpyrazone	⇩ Uricosuria

ST. JOSEPH Aspirin for Children ■ ST. JOSEPH Aspirin-Free

Spironolactone	⇩ Diuretic effect
Methotrexate	⇧ Methotrexate plasma level and risk of toxicity

ALTERED LABORATORY VALUES

Blood/serum values	⇧ Prothrombin time ⇧ Uric acid (with low doses) ⇩ Uric acid (with high doses) ⇩ Thyroxine (T$_4$) ⇩ Thyroid-stimulating hormone
Urinary values	⇧ Glucose (with Clinitest tablets)

USE IN CHILDREN

See INDICATIONS and ORAL DOSAGE

USE IN PREGNANT AND NURSING WOMEN

Consult manufacturer for use in pregnant and nursing women

---

[1] Miller RL et al, in Melmon KL, Morelli HF (eds): *Clinical Pharmacology.* New York, Macmillan, 1978, pp 657–708; Moertel CG et al: *N Engl J Med* 286:813–815, 1972; Tainter ML, Ferus AJ: *Aspirin in Modern Therapy: A Review.* New York, Bayer Company, Division of Sterling Drug, Inc, 1969, pp 1–128; *United States Pharmacopeia Dispensing Information 1981.* Rockville, Md, United States Pharmacopeial Convention, Inc, 1981
[2] Adverse reactions are dose-related. Most reactions are associated with intoxication resulting from continued use of large doses.

NONNARCOTIC ANALGESICS/ANTIPYRETICS

Aspirin-Free ST. JOSEPH (acetaminophen) Plough   OTC

Chewable tablets: 80 mg *fruit flavored, sugar-free* **Liquid (per 5 ml):** 160 mg (2, 4 fl oz) *cherry flavored, sugar-free* **Drops (per 0.8-ml dropperful):** 80 mg (½ fl oz) *fruit flavored, sugar-free*

INDICATIONS

Fever
Minor aches and pains associated with colds, influenza, immunizations, and headaches

ORAL DOSAGE

Child (0–3 mo; 7–12 lb): 40 mg (½ dropperful) q4h, up to 5 doses/24 h
Child (4–11 mo; 13–21 lb): 80 mg (1 dropperful or ½ tsp liquid) q4h, up to 5 doses/24 h
Child (12–23 mo; 22–26 lb): 120 mg (1½ dropperfuls, ¾ tsp liquid, or 1½ chewable tabs) q4h, up to 5 doses/24 h
Child (2–3 yr; 27–35 lb): 160 mg (2 dropperfuls, 1 tsp liquid, or 2 chewable tabs) q4h, up to 5 doses/24 h
Child (4–5 yr; 36–45 lb): 240 mg (3 dropperfuls, 1½ tsp liquid, or 3 chewable tabs) q4h, up to 5 doses/24 h
Child (6–8 yr; 46–65 lb): 320 mg (4 dropperfuls, 2 tsp liquid, or 4 chewable tabs) q4h, up to 5 doses/24 h
Child (9–10 yr; 66–76 lb): 400 mg (5 dropperfuls, 2½ tsp liquid, or 5 chewable tabs) q4h, up to 5 doses/24 h
Child (11 yr; 77–83 lb): 480 mg (3 tsp liquid or 6 chewable tabs) q4h, up to 5 doses/24 h
Child ($\geq$ 12 yr; $\geq$ 84 lb): 640 mg (4 tsp liquid or 8 chewable tabs) q4h, up to 5 doses/24 h

ADMINISTRATION/DOSAGE ADJUSTMENTS

Administration	Chewable tablets may also be crushed or dissolved in a teaspoon of liquid for use in younger children or powdered for use in infants; always give one half glass of water, milk, or fruit juice after administration of chewable tablets

WARNINGS/PRECAUTIONS

Patient instructions	The package label cautions against using these products for more than 5 days or, unless specifically directed by a physician, with other medications containing acetaminophen. The label also advises consumers to consult a physician if indications of potentially serious illness (eg, severe or persistent sore throat, high fever, headache, nausea, or vomiting) are not relieved within 24 h, if symptoms persist or new ones develop, or if fever persists for more than 3 days or recurs. Because severe liver damage may occur, patients should be warned not to exceed the recommended dosage.

OVERDOSAGE

Signs and symptoms	*Early:* nausea, vomiting, diaphoresis, and general malaise (some patients may be asymptomatic); *late:* clinical and laboratory evidence of hepatotoxicity (vomiting; right upper quadrant tenderness; increased SGOT, SGPT, serum bilirubin, and prothrombin time; and possible hypoglycemia) may not be apparent until 48–72 h after ingestion

Treatment	Promptly empty stomach by performing gastric lavage or inducing emesis with syrup of ipecac (15–30 ml for children, 30–45 ml for adults). Give ipecac with copious quantities of water; if emesis does not occur within 20 min, repeat dose. Activated charcoal may be given if acetaminophen has been ingested with certain other drugs. Administer oral acetylcysteine as soon as possible (no later than 24 h after ingestion); give a loading dose of 140 mg/kg and then, at 4-h intervals, 17 maintenance doses of 70 mg/kg. (Charcoal, if used, should be removed before acetylcysteine is given.) Measure the plasma level of unconjugated acetaminophen as early as possible, but no sooner than 4 h after ingestion. Determine prothrombin time, SGOT and SGPT levels, and serum concentrations of bilirubin, creatinine, BUN, glucose, and electrolytes every 24 h. If the prothrombin time exceeds 1.5 times the control value, give vitamin K_1; if the prothrombin time exceeds 3 times this value, give fresh frozen plasma. Institute appropriate measures to treat hypoglycemia and electrolyte and fluid imbalance. Avoid forced diuresis or use of diuretics when treating an acetaminophen overdose. For additional information on use of acetylcysteine and interpretation of the plasma acetaminophen level, see Mucomyst chart.

ALTERED LABORATORY VALUES

Blood/serum values	▽ Glucose (with glucose oxidase/peroxidase tests)
Urinary values	+ 5-HIAA (with nitrosonaphthol reagent test)

USE IN CHILDREN
See INDICATIONS and ORAL DOSAGE

USE IN PREGNANT AND NURSING WOMEN
Consult manufacturer

NONNARCOTIC ANALGESICS/ANTIPYRETICS

STADOL (butorphanol tartrate) Bristol   Rx

Prefilled syringes: 2 mg/ml (1 ml)   **Vials:** 1 mg/ml (1 ml), 2 mg/ml (1, 2, 10 ml)

INDICATIONS	PARENTERAL DOSAGE
Moderate to severe pain **Preoperative or preanesthetic medication** As a supplement to **balanced anesthesia** **Prepartum pain**	Adult: 1–4 mg IM or 0.5–2 mg IV q3–4h, as needed; usual dose: 2 mg IM or 1 mg IV

CONTRAINDICATIONS
Hypersensitivity to butorphanol tartrate

ADMINISTRATION/DOSAGE ADJUSTMENTS

Combination therapy	Reduce dosage of butorphanol when administered concomitantly with phenothiazines and other tranquilizers

WARNINGS/PRECAUTIONS

Patients dependent on narcotics	Prior to using butorphanol, detoxify patients physically dependent on narcotics; detoxification should also be considered in patients who have recently received substantial amounts of narcotics
Drug dependence	Patients who are emotionally unstable or have a history of drug misuse should be closely supervised during long-term therapy
Patients with head injuries	The side effects of this drug may interfere with the clinical evaluation of head injuries; administer with extreme caution and only if use of this drug is deemed essential
Patients with cardiovascular disease	Limit use in cases of acute myocardial infarction, ventricular dysfunction, or coronary insufficiency to patients hypersensitive to morphine or meperidine
Patients with pulmonary disease	Use with caution and in low dosage in patients with respiratory depression, severely limited respiratory reserve, bronchial asthma, obstructive respiratory conditions, or cyanosis
Patients with hepatic or renal impairment	Use with caution; extensive hepatic disease may predispose to increased drug activity and side effects
Biliary surgery	Safety for use in this procedure has not been established
Preoperative or preanesthetic use	Slight increases in systolic blood pressure may occur; use with caution in hypertensive patients

STADOL ■ SUPROL

| Balanced anesthesia | Use in combination with pancuronium may increase conjunctival changes |

ADVERSE REACTIONS
Frequent reactions (incidence ≥ 1%) are printed in *italics*

Central nervous system	*Sedation (40%); headache, vertigo, and floating sensation (3%); dizziness and lethargy (2%); confusion and light-headedness (1%)*, nervousness, unusual dreams, agitation, euphoria, hallucinations
Gastrointestinal	*Nausea (6%)*, vomiting
Autonomic nervous system	*Clamminess/sweating (6%)*, flushing, warmth, dry mouth, cold sensitivity
Cardiovascular	Palpitations, blood pressure changes
Respiratory	Slowing of respiration, shallow breathing
Dermatological	Rash, hives
Ophthalmic	Diplopia, blurred vision

OVERDOSAGE

| Signs and symptoms | Respiratory depression, various cardiovascular and CNS effects |
| Treatment | Maintain a patent airway and administer IV naloxone; monitor respiratory and cardiac status and institute appropriate supportive measures, including oxygen, IV fluids, vasopressors, and assisted or controlled respiration, as indicated |

DRUG INTERACTIONS

Methadone and other narcotics	Narcotic withdrawal symptoms
Alcohol, tranquilizers, sedative-hypnotics, and other CNS depressants	⇧ CNS depression
Pancuronium	⇧ Conjunctival changes

ALTERED LABORATORY VALUES
No clinically significant alterations in blood/serum or urinary values occur at therapeutic dosages

---

USE IN CHILDREN

Safety and efficacy for use in children under 18 yr of age have not been established

USE IN PREGNANT AND NURSING WOMEN

Safety for use during pregnancy prior to labor has not been established. Animal reproduction studies have shown no evidence of impaired fertility or fetal damage. Patients receiving butorphanol during labor have experienced no adverse effects other than those observed with commonly used analgesics; exercise caution if infant is premature. Butorphanol should not be given to nursing mothers; however, it has been used safely for labor pain in women who subsequently nursed.

NONNARCOTIC ANALGESICS/ANTIPYRETICS

SUPROL (suprofen) McNeil Pharmaceutical/Ortho   Rx
Capsules: 200 mg

INDICATIONS	ORAL DOSAGE
Mild to moderate pain Primary dysmenorrhea	Adult: 200 mg q4–6h, as needed, up to 800 mg/day

CONTRAINDICATIONS

| Intolerance to suprofen | History of bronchospasm, rhinitis, urticaria, or other allergic reactions precipitated by aspirin or other nonsteroidal anti-inflammatory drugs |

ADMINISTRATION/DOSAGE ADJUSTMENTS

| Food-drug interaction | Absorption (area under the curve) decreases by 10% following administration with milk and 20% following solid food |

WARNINGS/PRECAUTIONS

| Second-line therapy | This drug should not be considered as initial treatment for either of its indications because flank pain with renal dysfunction may occur with its use |
| Gastrointestinal effects | Suprofen can cause GI bleeding and peptic ulcers; patients with a history of upper GI tract disease should be closely supervised |

SUPROL

Renal toxicity	Acute flank pain with renal insufficiency has been seen in patients who have taken as few as 1 or 2 doses of suprofen; abnormal urinary sediment has been detected in some cases. If flank pain occurs during therapy, discontinue this drug and monitor renal function. Proteinuria, acute interstitial nephritis with hematuria, and occasionally the nephrotic syndrome may occur during therapy. In patients with reduced renal blood flow or volume owing to conditions such as heart failure, renal or hepatic impairment, advanced age, or use of diuretics, administration of a nonsteroidal anti-inflammatory agent may cause a critical decrease in the formation of renal prostaglandins and thereby precipitate overt renal failure; the reaction is reversible upon discontinuation of the drug.
Uricosuria	Substantial uricosuria may occur within an hour or more after the first dose of suprofen; all patients, particularly those who are hyperuricemic, should be well-hydrated before the first dose is given and thereafter during therapy
Drug accumulation	Suprofen is eliminated primarily by the kidneys; closely monitor patients with renal impairment and be prepared to reduce the daily dose
Liver function abnormalities	Borderline elevations may occur in up to 15% of patients; meaningful elevations (3 times the upper limit of normal) in SGOT or SGPT levels have been reported in approximately 1% of patients. If abnormal liver function tests or other manifestations of liver dysfunction arise during therapy, evaluate the patient for evidence of a more severe hepatic reaction. Although potentially fatal reactions such as jaundice have occurred rarely, discontinue therapy if abnormal liver function tests persist or worsen, clinical signs and symptoms of liver disease develop, or secondary manifestations (eg, eosinophilia, rash) occur.
Peripheral edema	During long-term therapy, peripheral edema has been observed in 5% of patients; use with caution in patients with fluid retention, heart failure, or hypertension
Ophthalmic effects	Changes in visual acuity have been reported by 3–9% of patients; although ophthalmological examinations have failed to demonstrate any drug-related effects, attenuation of retinal vasculature, retinal degeneration, and cortical opacities have been detected in rats given 25 or 35 mg/kg/day for 24 mo. Therefore, if the patient experiences visual disturbances during therapy, perform an ophthalmologic evaluation.
Anemia	Decreases in hemoglobin level and hematocrit have occurred during long-term therapy; if signs or symptoms of anemia are seen, perform appropriate tests
Long-term therapy	Watch for clinical signs of anemia, gastric irritation, and liver disease during long-term therapy
Carcinogenicity, mutagenicity	An increase in benign hepatic tumors has been detected in female mice given 40 mg/kg/day (approximately 3 times the human dose) and in male mice given 2.5–40 mg/kg/day; however, no evidence of carcinogenicity has been found in rats and mice at dosages of up to 40 mg/kg/day. Suprofen does not appear to be mutagenic on the basis of the Ames, micronucleus, or dominant lethal tests.
Impairment of fertility	Testicular atrophy and hypoplasia have been observed in dogs given 80 mg/kg/day (approximately 6 times the human dose) for 6 mo and in rats given 40 mg/kg/day (approximately 3 times the human dose) for 12 mo

ADVERSE REACTIONS[1]

Frequent reactions (incidence ≥ 1%) are printed in *italics*

Gastrointestinal	*Nausea (15%), dyspepsia (13%), loose stools/diarrhea (10%); GI distress, abdominal pain, constipation, vomiting, and flatulence (3–9%); GI bleeding, other bowel changes, and stomatitis (1–3%)*; peptic ulcers, gastroenteritis
Central nervous system	*Headache, dizziness, sedation, mood changes, sleep disturbances, and pain (3–9%); paresthesias (1–3%)*, appetite changes
Musculoskeletal	*Muscle cramps (3–9%), bursitis and asthenia (1–3%)*
Ophthalmic	*Changes in vision and conjunctivitis (1–3%)*
Cardiovascular	*Edema (3–9%), hypertension and palpitations (1–3%)*, epistaxis
Respiratory	*Upper respiratory tract congestion (3–9%)*
Dermatological	*Dermatitis and pruritus (3–9%); skin irritation (1–3%)*, rash
Hematological	*Purpura and bleeding (1–3%)*; thrombocytopenia, leukopenia, agranulocytosis, aplastic anemia
Genitourinary	*Urinary frequency, dysuria, and pyuria (1–3%)*; acute nephritis, acute flank pain with renal insufficiency
Other	*Tinnitus (1–3%)*; anaphylactoid reactions, characterized by dyspnea and epiglottal and/or laryngeal edema

OVERDOSAGE

Signs and symptoms	See ADVERSE REACTIONS

Treatment	Induce emesis or perform gastric lavage; then instill activated charcoal. Institute supportive measures, as needed.

DRUG INTERACTIONS
Diuretics	⇧ Risk of renal failure
Anticoagulants	⇧ Risk of bleeding; carefully observe patients during combination therapy
Insulin, sulfonylureas	⇧ Risk of hypoglycemia; carefully observe patients during combination therapy

ALTERED LABORATORY VALUES
Blood/serum values	⇧ SGOT ⇧ SGPT ⇧ Bleeding time
Urinary values	⇧ Uric acid

USE IN CHILDREN
Safety and effectiveness for use in children have not been established

USE IN PREGNANT AND NURSING WOMEN
Pregnancy Category B: an increase in stillbirths and a decrease in postnatal survival have been seen in rats given 2.5 mg/kg/day; an increase in fetal resorptions has occurred in rats and rabbits at maternally toxic doses (40 mg/kg/day, approximately 3 times the human dose, in rats and 80 mg/kg/day, approximately 6 times the human dose, in rabbits). Suprofen has also caused an increase in delayed parturition in rats. When given to women during late pregnancy, the drug can precipitate premature closure of the ductus arteriosus. Use during pregnancy only if clearly needed and avoid administration during late pregnancy. A maximum of 0.03–0.06 mg/kg/day is excreted in human milk; use with caution in nursing mothers.

[1] Reactions for which a causal relationship has not been established include jaundice, tachycardia, acute hemolytic anemia, and lime-green urine

---

NONNARCOTIC ANALGESICS/ANTIPYRETICS

SYNALGOS (aspirin and caffeine) Wyeth   OTC
Capsules: 356.4 mg aspirin and 30 mg caffeine

INDICATIONS
Minor aches and pains, including headaches, dental pain, and minor aches and pains of arthritis and rheumatism
Fever

ORAL DOSAGE
Adult: 2 caps, with a full glass of water, q4h, up to 10 caps/day

WARNINGS/PRECAUTIONS
Patient instructions	Patients are cautioned by the package label not to use this product without the advice and supervision of a physician if they are allergic to aspirin, have asthma, stomach distress, ulcers, or bleeding disorders, or are taking anticoagulants or a medication for the treatment of diabetes, gout, or arthritis; the label also warns patients to discontinue use if tinnitus or other symptoms of overdosage occur and to consult a physician immediately if "pain persists for more than ten days or redness is present or in arthritic or rheumatic conditions affecting children under 12 yr of age. . . ."

ADVERSE REACTIONS
Central nervous system	Drowsiness, dizziness, light-headedness, sedation
Gastrointestinal	Nausea, vomiting, constipation
Dermatological	Skin reactions
Cardiovascular	Hypotension (rare)

OVERDOSAGE
Signs and symptoms	*Aspirin-related effects:* hyperpnea, nausea, vomiting, vertigo, tinnitus, flushing, sweating, thirst, headache, drowsiness, diarrhea, and tachycardia, progressing to hyperthermia, hemorrhage, acid-base disturbances, restlessness, confusion, convulsions, vasomotor depression, coma, and respiratory failure; *caffeine-related effects:* insomnia, restlessness, tremors, delirium, tachycardia, extrasystoles, tinnitus, urinary frequency
Treatment	If less than 4 h have elapsed since ingestion, induce emesis or perform gastric lavage, followed by activated charcoal, to remove any remaining drug from the stomach. Initial therapy should be directed at reducing hyperthermia by external sponging with tepid water, correcting dehydration by appropriate IV fluid replacement, and maintaining adequate cardiorespiratory and renal function. In moderately severe cases of salicylate poisoning, cautiously administer sodium bicarbonate IV in sufficient quantity, if possible, to maintain an alkaline diuresis; intermittent peritoneal dialysis may also be helpful. In severe cases, hemodialysis should be seriously considered. Potassium should be added to the repair solution to compensate for potassium losses once urine formation is deemed adequate. Glucose may be provided to correct ketosis and hypoglycemia. Plasma transfusion may be beneficial if shock intervenes. Hemorrhagic phenomena may necessitate whole-blood transfusions and phytonadione (vitamin K_1). Do not administer barbiturates to treat excitement or convulsions.

DRUG INTERACTIONS

Anticoagulants	△ Risk of bleeding
Sulfonylureas	△ Hypoglycemic effect
Alcohol, corticosteroids, phenylbutazone, oxyphenbutazone	△ Risk of GI ulceration
Probenecid, sulfinpyrazone	▽ Uricosuric effect
Spironolactone	▽ Diuretic effect
Methotrexate	△ Methotrexate plasma level and risk of toxicity

ALTERED LABORATORY VALUES

Blood/serum values	△ Prothrombin time △ Uric acid (with low doses) ▽ Uric acid (with high doses) ▽ Thyroxine (T_4) ▽ Thyroid-stimulating hormone
Urinary values	△ Glucose (with Clinitest tablets)

USE IN CHILDREN
Consult manufacturer; the package label states that a physician should be consulted for use in children under 12 yr of age

USE IN PREGNANT AND NURSING WOMEN
Consult manufacturer; the package label instructs pregnant and nursing patients to seek the advice of a health-care professional before they take this preparation

---

NONNARCOTIC ANALGESICS/ANTIPYRETICS

TEMPRA (acetaminophen) Mead Johnson OTC

Chewable tablets: 80 mg *grape flavored, sugar-free* **Syrup (per 5 ml):** 160 mg (4, 16 fl oz) *cherry flavored, alcohol-free* **Drops (per 0.8-ml dropperful):** 80 mg[1] (15 ml) *cherry flavored*

INDICATIONS
Fever, minor aches and pains, and headaches associated with colds, viral infections, and immunizations
Earache, toothache, pain associated with tonsillectomy and adenoidectomy

ORAL DOSAGE
Infant (< 3 mo; < 13 lb): 40 mg (½ dropperful or ¼ tsp syrup) q4h, up to 5 times/day
Infant (3–9 mo; 13–20 lb): 80 mg (1 dropperful or ½ tsp syrup) q4h, up to 5 times/day
Infant and child (10–24 mo; 21–26 lb): 120 mg (1½ dropperful or ¾ tsp syrup) q4h, up to 5 times/day
Child (2–3 yr; 27–35 lb): 160 mg (2 dropperful, 1 tsp syrup, or 2 chewable tabs) q4h, up to 5 times/day
Child (4–5 yr; 36–43 lb): 240 mg (3 dropperful, 1½ tsp syrup, or 3 chewable tabs) q4h, up to 5 times/day
Child (6–8 yr; 44–62 lb): 320 mg (2 tsp syrup or 4 chewable tabs) q4h, up to 5 times/day
Child (9–10 yr; 63–79 lb): 400 mg (2½ tsp syrup or 5 chewable tabs) q4h, up to 5 times/day
Child (11 yr; 80–89 lb): 480 mg (3 tsp syrup or 6 chewable tabs) q4h, up to 5 times/day
Child (> 12 yr; > 90 lb): 480–640 mg (3–4 tsp syrup or 6–8 chewable tabs) q4h, up to 5 times/day

ADMINISTRATION/DOSAGE ADJUSTMENTS

Use of drops	The drops may be given directly or mixed with water or fruit juice
Dosage adjustment	If the child is significantly under- or overweight, adjust dosage accordingly

WARNINGS/PRECAUTIONS

Patients with phenylketonuria	The chewable tablets contain phenylalanine; warn patients with phenylketonuria
Patient instructions	The package labeling advises patients to consult a physician "if fever persists for more than 3 days (72 hours) or if pain continues for more than 5 days...." The labeling also includes the following warning: "As with any drug, if you are pregnant or nursing a baby, seek the advice of a health professional before using this product."

OVERDOSAGE

Signs and symptoms	*Early:* nausea, vomiting, diaphoresis, and general malaise (some patients may be asymptomatic); *late (up to 72 h after ingestion):* clinical and laboratory evidence of hepatotoxicity, characterized by vomiting; right upper quadrant tenderness; increases in SGOT, SGPT, serum bilirubin, and prothrombin time; and possible hypoglycemia

TEMPRA ■ TRENDAR

Treatment	Promptly empty stomach by performing gastric lavage or inducing emesis with syrup of ipecac (15–30 ml for children, 30–45 ml for adults). Give ipecac with copious quantities of water; if emesis does not occur within 20 min, repeat dose. Activated charcoal may be given if acetaminophen has been ingested with certain other drugs. Administer oral acetylcysteine as soon as possible (no later than 24 h after ingestion); give a loading dose of 140 mg/kg and then, at 4-h intervals, 17 maintenance doses of 70 mg/kg. (Charcoal, if used, should be removed before acetylcysteine is given.) Measure the plasma level of unconjugated acetaminophen as early as possible, but no sooner than 4 h after ingestion. Determine prothrombin time, SGOT and SGPT levels, and serum concentrations of bilirubin, creatinine, BUN, glucose, and electrolytes every 24 h. If the prothrombin time exceeds 1.5 times the control value, give vitamin K_1; if the prothrombin time exceeds 3 times this value, give fresh frozen plasma. Institute appropriate measures to treat hypoglycemia and electrolyte and fluid imbalance. Avoid forced diuresis or use of diuretics when treating an acetaminophen overdose. For additional information on use of acetylcysteine and interpretation of the plasma acetaminophen level, see Mucomyst chart.

ALTERED LABORATORY VALUES

Blood/serum values	▽ Glucose (with glucose oxidase/peroxidase tests)
Urinary values	+ 5-HIAA (with nitrosonaphthol test)

USE IN CHILDREN See INDICATIONS and ORAL DOSAGE	**USE IN PREGNANT AND NURSING WOMEN** See "Patient instructions" in WARNINGS/PRECAUTIONS

[1] Contains 10% alcohol

NONNARCOTIC ANALGESICS/ANTIPYRETICS

TRENDAR (ibuprofen) Whitehall   OTC

Tablets: 200 mg

INDICATIONS **Dysmenorrhea** **Headaches, backaches, and muscular aches and pains** associated with premenstrual syndrome	**ORAL DOSAGE** **Adult:** 200–400 mg q4–6h at the onset of symptoms and while pain persists, up to 1,200 mg/24 h, for a period of up to 10 days; initial dosage: 200 mg q4–6h. The package labeling warns patients not to exceed these recommendations unless otherwise directed by a physician. **Child (> 12 yr):** same as adult

CONTRAINDICATIONS Consult manufacturer	

WARNINGS/PRECAUTIONS	
Special-risk patients	The package labeling warns patients not to take this product if they have had a severe allergic reaction to aspirin, such as asthma, swelling, shock, or hives; the labeling also cautions patients to consult a physician before using this product if they have experienced any problems or serious adverse reactions while taking an OTC analgesic, if they are under medical supervision for the treatment of a serious condition, or if they are receiving a prescription drug (see also USE IN CHILDREN and USE IN PREGNANT AND NURSING WOMEN)
Adverse reactions	The package labeling instructs patients to take the tablets with food or milk if occasional, mild heartburn, upset stomach, or stomach pain occurs and to consult a physician if gastric symptoms or pain becomes persistent or more severe or if other new symptoms develop
Concomitant use of other medications	The package labeling cautions patients not to use this product with other ibuprofen preparations and to consult a physician before using this product in combination with aspirin or acetaminophen (see also DRUG INTERACTIONS)

ADVERSE REACTIONS Consult manufacturer	

OVERDOSAGE	
Signs and symptoms	Apnea, cyanosis, dizziness, nystagmus

TRENDAR ■ TYLENOL

| Treatment | Following recent ingestion (< 1 h), induce emesis or perform gastric lavage to remove drug from stomach. Activated charcoal may be helpful. If drug is already absorbed, it may be useful to induce diuresis and alkalinize the urine. |

DRUG INTERACTIONS

| Coumarin anticoagulants | △ Risk of bleeding; use with caution |
| Aspirin | ▽ Anti-inflammatory activity (potential) |

ALTERED LABORATORY VALUES

| Blood/serum values | △ SGOT △ SGPT |

No clinically significant alterations in urinary values occur at therapeutic dosages

---

USE IN CHILDREN

The package labeling warns adults to consult a physician before giving this product to children under 12 yr of age

USE IN PREGNANT AND NURSING WOMEN

The package labeling cautions pregnant or nursing women to consult a health professional before using this product and, because ibuprofen may cause premature closure of the ductus arteriosus or complications during delivery, warns patients not to use this product during the last 3 mo of pregnancy unless specifically directed to do so by a physician

---

NONNARCOTIC ANALGESICS/ANTIPYRETICS

Regular Strength TYLENOL (acetaminophen) McNeil Consumer Products OTC

Caplets: 325 mg   **Tablets:** 325 mg

INDICATIONS

Arthritic and musculoskeletal pain, headache, dysmenorrhea, myalgia, neuralgia, and other painful conditions
Discomfort and fever associated with viral infections and other diseases

ORAL DOSAGE

Adult: 325–650 mg (1–2 caplets or tablets) q4–6h, up to 3,900 mg (12 caplets or tablets)/day
Child (6–12 yr): 162.5–325 mg (1/2–1 tablet) tid or qid

Extra-Strength TYLENOL (acetaminophen) McNeil Consumer Products OTC

Caplets: 500 mg   **Tablets:** 500 mg   **Liquid (per 15 ml):** 500 mg[1] (8 fl oz) mint flavored

INDICATIONS

Pain and fever (caplets, tablets)
Pain and/or fever (liquid)

ORAL DOSAGE

Adult: 1,000 mg (2 caplets or tablets) tid or qid, up to 4,000 mg (8 caplets or tablets) /24 h, or 1,000 mg (30 ml or 2 tbsp) q4–6h, up to 4,000 mg (120 ml or 8 tbsp)/24 h

Children's TYLENOL (acetaminophen) McNeil Consumer Products OTC

Chewable tablets: 80 mg fruit flavored   **Elixir (per 5 ml):** 160 mg (2, 4 fl oz) cherry flavored, alcohol free   **Drops (per 0.8-ml dropperful):** 80 mg (0.5 fl oz) fruit flavored, alcohol free

INDICATIONS

Fever and pain associated with mild upper respiratory infections, headache, myalgia, immunization, tonsillectomy, gastroenteritis, and other conditions requiring reduction of fever and/or relief of pain

ORAL DOSAGE

Infant (6–11 lb): 40 mg (1/2 dropperful) q4h, up to 5 doses/24 h
Infant (12–17 lb): 80 mg (1 dropperful, 1/2 tsp elixir, or 1 tablet) q4h, up to 5 doses/24 h
Child (18–23 lb): 120 mg (1 1/2 dropperful, 3/4 tsp elixir, or 1 1/2 tablets) q4h, up to 5 doses/24 h
Child (24–35 lb): 160 mg (2 dropperful, 1 tsp elixir, or 2 tablets) q4h, up to 5 doses/24 h
Child (36–47 lb): 240 mg (1 1/2 tsp elixir or 3 tablets) q4h, up to 5 doses/24 h
Child (48–59 lb): 320 mg (2 tsp elixir or 4 tablets) q4h, up to 5 doses/24 h
Child (60–71 lb): 400 mg (2 1/2 tsp elixir or 5 tablets) q4h, up to 5 doses/24 h
Child (72–95 lb): 480 mg (3 tsp elixir or 6 tablets) q4h, up to 5 doses/24 h

Junior Strength TYLENOL (acetaminophen) McNeil Consumer Products OTC

Caplets: 160 mg

INDICATIONS

Fever and pain associated with mild upper respiratory infections, headache, myalgia, immunization, tonsillectomy, gastroenteritis, and other conditions requiring reduction of fever and/or relief of pain

ORAL DOSAGE

Child (6–8 yr or 48–59 lb): 320 mg (2 caplets) q4h, up to 1,600 mg (10 caplets)/24 h
Child (9–10 yr or 60–71 lb): 400 mg (2 1/2 caplets) q4h, up to 2,000 mg (12 1/2 caplets)/24 h
Child (11 yr or 72–95 lb): 480 mg (3 caplets) q4h, up to 2,400 mg (15 caplets)/24 h
Child (12–14 yr or >96 lb): 640 mg (4 caplets) q4h, up to 3,200 mg (20 caplets)/24 h

TYLENOL

ADMINISTRATION/DOSAGE ADJUSTMENTS

Use of drops and elixir	The pediatric drops and elixir may be given directly or mixed with milk, formula, fruit juice, apple sauce, or other foods

WARNINGS/PRECAUTIONS

Hypersensitivity	On rare occasions, a hypersensitivity reaction may occur; if reaction is seen, discontinue use
Patients with phenylketonuria	The chewable tablets contain phenylalanine; warn patients with phenylketonuria
Patient instructions	Regular Strength Tylenol: patients are cautioned on the package label to consult a physician immediately "if pain persists for more than 10 days, or redness is present, or in arthritic or rheumatic conditions affecting children under 12. . . ." Extra-Strength Tylenol: the label advises patients to consult a physician for "severe or recurrent pain or high or continued fever." Children's Tylenol: the label warns parents to consult a physician "if fever persists for more than three days or if pain continues for more than five days." Junior Strength Tylenol: the label includes the same warning as Children's Tylenol, but adds that parents should not use the junior strength product in children who have difficulty swallowing tablets. Regular, Extra-, and Junior Strength Tylenol also provide the following warning: "As with any drug, if you are pregnant or nursing a baby, seek the advice of a health professional before using this product."

OVERDOSAGE

Signs and symptoms	*Early:* nausea, vomiting, diaphoresis, and general malaise (some patients may be asymptomatic); *late:* clinical and laboratory evidence of hepatotoxicity (vomiting; right upper quadrant tenderness; increased SGOT, SGPT, serum bilirubin, and prothrombin time; and possible hypoglycemia) may not be apparent until 48–72 h after ingestion
Treatment	Promptly empty stomach by performing gastric lavage or inducing emesis with syrup of ipecac (15–30 ml for children, 30–45 ml for adults). Give ipecac with copious quantities of water; if emesis does not occur within 20 min, repeat dose. Activated charcoal may be given if acetaminophen has been ingested with certain other drugs. Administer oral acetylcysteine as soon as possible (no later than 24 h after ingestion); give a loading dose of 140 mg/kg and then, at 4-h intervals, 17 maintenance doses of 70 mg/kg. (Charcoal, if used, should be removed before acetylcysteine is given.) Measure the plasma level of unconjugated acetaminophen as early as possible, but no sooner than 4 h after ingestion. Determine prothrombin time, SGOT and SGPT levels, and serum concentrations of bilirubin, creatinine, BUN, glucose, and electrolytes every 24 h. If the prothrombin time exceeds 1.5 times the control value, give vitamin K_1; if the prothrombin time exceeds 3 times this value, give fresh frozen plasma. Institute appropriate measures to treat hypoglycemia and electrolyte and fluid imbalance. Avoid forced diuresis or use of diuretics when treating an acetaminophen overdose. For additional information on use of acetylcysteine and interpretation of the plasma acetaminophen level, see Mucomyst chart and contact the Rocky Mountain Poison Center (800–525–6115).

ALTERED LABORATORY VALUES

Blood/serum values	▽ Glucose (with glucose oxidase/peroxidase tests)
Urinary values	+ 5-HIAA (with nitrosonaphthol reagent test)

USE IN CHILDREN

See INDICATIONS and ORAL DOSAGE. Extra-Strength Adult Liquid is not indicated for use in children under 12 yr of age.

USE IN PREGNANT AND NURSING WOMEN

See "Patient instructions" in WARNINGS/PRECAUTIONS

---

[1] Contains 7% alcohol

Chapter 9

Antacids/Antiflatulents/Digestants

Antacids/Antiflatulents — 334

ALGICON (Rorer) — 334
Aluminum hydroxide/magnesium carbonate gel and magnesium carbonate *OTC*

ALKA-SELTZER (Miles Laboratories) — 334
Sodium bicarbonate, citric acid, and potassium bicarbonate *OTC*

ALternaGEL (Stuart) — 334
Aluminum hydroxide *OTC*

BASALJEL (Wyeth) — 335
Aluminum carbonate gel, basic *OTC*

CAMALOX (Rorer) — 336
Magnesium hydroxide, aluminum hydroxide, and calcium carbonate *OTC*

GAVISCON (Marion) — 336
Aluminum hydroxide and magnesium trisilicate *OTC*

GAVISCON Liquid (Marion) — 336
Aluminum hydroxide and magnesium carbonate *OTC*

GAVISCON-2 (Marion) — 336
Aluminum hydroxide and magnesium trisilicate *OTC*

GELUSIL (Warner-Lambert) — 337
Aluminum hydroxide, magnesium hydroxide, and simethicone *OTC*

GELUSIL-II (Warner-Lambert) — 337
Aluminum hydroxide, magnesium hydroxide, and simethicone *OTC*

GELUSIL-M (Warner-Lambert) — 337
Aluminum hydroxide, magnesium hydroxide, and simethicone *OTC*

ILOPAN-CHOLINE (Adria) — 337
Dexpanthenol and choline bitartrate *Rx*

MAALOX (Rorer) — 338
Magnesium hydroxide and aluminum hydroxide *OTC*

MAALOX Plus (Rorer) — 338
Magnesium hydroxide, aluminum hydroxide, and simethicone *OTC*

MAALOX TC (Rorer) — 338
Magnesium hydroxide and aluminum hydroxide *OTC*

MYLANTA (Stuart) — 339
Aluminum hydroxide, magnesium hydroxide, and simethicone *OTC*

MYLANTA-II (Stuart) — 339
Aluminum hydroxide, magnesium hydroxide, and simethicone *OTC*

MYLICON (Stuart) — 340
Simethicone *OTC*

MYLICON-80 (Stuart) — 340
Simethicone *OTC*

PHAZYME (Reed & Carnrick) — 340
Simethicone *OTC*

PHAZYME 95 (Reed & Carnrick) — 340
Simethicone *OTC*

PHAZYME 125 (Reed & Carnrick) — 340
Simethicone *OTC*

PHAZYME-PB (Reed & Carnrick) — 341
Simethicone and phenobarbital *C-IV*

RIOPAN (Ayerst) — 341
Magaldrate *OTC*

RIOPAN PLUS (Ayerst) — 342
Magaldrate and simethicone *OTC*

Extra Strength RIOPAN PLUS (Ayerst) — 342
Magaldrate and simethicone *OTC*

SIMECO (Wyeth) — 342
Aluminum hydroxide gel, magnesium hydroxide, and simethicone *OTC*

TITRALAC (3M) — 343
Calcium carbonate *OTC*

TUMS (Norcliff Thayer) — 343
Calcium carbonate *OTC*

TUMS E-X (Norcliff Thayer) — 343
Calcium carbonate *OTC*

Digestants — 344

COTAZYM (Organon) — 344
Pancrelipase *Rx*

COTAZYM-S (Organon) — 344
Pancrelipase *Rx*

ILOZYME (Adria) — 344
Pancrelipase *Rx*

KANULASE (Sandoz Consumer Health Care Group) — 345
Cellulase, pancreatin, glutamic acid and hydrochloride, ox bile extract, and pepsin *OTC*

PANCREASE (McNeil Pharmaceutical) — 346
Pancrelipase *Rx*

VIOKASE (Robins) — 346
Pancrelipase *Rx*

Other Antacids — 331

ALKA-MINTS (Miles Laboratories) — 331
Calcium carbonate *OTC*

ALKA-SELTZER Pain Reliever and Antacid (Miles Laboratories) — 331
Aspirin, sodium bicarbonate, and citric acid *OTC*

ALKETS (Upjohn) — 331
Calcium carbonate, magnesium carbonate, and magnesium oxide *OTC*

ALU-CAP (Riker) 332
Aluminum hydroxide gel *OTC*

ALUDROX (Wyeth) 332
Aluminum hydroxide gel and magnesium hydroxide *OTC*

ALU-TAB (Riker) 332
Aluminum hydroxide gel *OTC*

AMPHOJEL (Wyeth) 332
Aluminum hydroxide gel *OTC*

CALCITREL (Glenbrook) 332
Calcium carbonate and magnesium hydroxide *OTC*

CREAMALIN (Mentholatum) 332
Aluminum hydroxide and magnesium hydroxide *OTC*

DELCID (Lakeside) 332
Aluminum hydroxide and magnesium hydroxide *OTC*

DICARBOSIL (Norcliff Thayer) 332
Calcium carbonate *OTC*

DI-GEL Liquid (Plough) 332
Simethicone, aluminum hydroxide, and magnesium hydroxide *OTC*

DI-GEL Tablets (Plough) 332
Simethicone and magnesium hydroxide *OTC*

GAS-X (Sandoz Consumer Health Care Group) 332
Simethicone *OTC*

Extra Strength GAS-X (Sandoz Consumer Health Care Group) 332
Simethicone *OTC*

KOLANTYL (Lakeside) 332
Aluminum hydroxide and magnesium hydroxide *OTC*

Milk of magnesia *OTC* 332

REMEGEL (Warner-Lambert) 332
Aluminum hydroxide and magnesium carbonate *OTC*

ROLAIDS (Warner-Lambert) 333
Dihydroxyaluminum sodium carbonate *OTC*

Sodium Free ROLAIDS (Warner-Lambert) 333
Calcium carbonate and magnesium hydroxide *OTC*

SILAIN-GEL (Robins) 333
Aluminum hydroxide, magnesium hydroxide, and simethicone *OTC*

Sodium bicarbonate *OTC* 333

TEMPO (Richardson-Vicks Health Care Products) 333
Calcium carbonate, aluminum hydroxide, magnesium hydroxide, and simethicone *OTC*

WinGel (Winthrop Consumer Products) 333
Aluminum hydroxide and magnesium hydroxide *OTC*

Other Digestants 333

DONNAZYME (Robins) 333
Pancreatin, pepsin, bile salts, hyoscyamine sulfate, atropine sulfate, scopolamine hydrobromide, and phenobarbital *Rx*

ENTOZYME (Robins) 333
Pancreatin, pepsin, and bile salts *Rx*

FESTAL II (Hoechst-Roussel) 333
Pancreatic enzymes *OTC*

FESTALAN (Hoechst-Roussel) 333
Atropine methyl nitrate and pancreatic enzymes *Rx*

LACTAID (LactAid) 333
Lactase *OTC*

LACTRASE (Kremers-Urban) 333
Lactase *OTC*

OTHER ANTACIDS

DRUG	HOW SUPPLIED	USUAL DOSAGE[1]
ALKA-MINTS (Miles Laboratories) Calcium carbonate *OTC*	**Chewable tablets:** 850 mg *spearmint flavored*	**Adult:** 1 tab q2h, up to 9 tabs/24 h
ALKA-SELTZER Pain Reliever and Antacid (Miles Laboratories) Aspirin, sodium bicarbonate, and citric acid *OTC*	**Effervescent tablets:** 324 mg aspirin, 1,916 mg sodium bicarbonate, and 1,000 mg citric acid *regular flavored*; 324 mg aspirin, 1,710 mg sodium bicarbonate, and 1,220 mg citric acid *lemon-lime flavored*	**Adult:** 2 tabs, dissolved in 6 fl oz of water, q4h, as needed, up to 8 tabs/24 h
ALKETS (Upjohn) Calcium carbonate, magnesium carbonate, and magnesium oxide *OTC*	**Chewable tablets:** 780 mg calcium carbonate, 130 mg magnesium carbonate, and 65 mg magnesium oxide	**Adult:** 1–2 tabs 1–3 times/day; may be chewed, swallowed, or allowed to dissolve under the tongue

[1] Where pediatric dosages are not given, consult manufacturer

continued

COMPENDIUM OF DRUG THERAPY

OTHER ANTACIDS continued

DRUG	HOW SUPPLIED	USUAL DOSAGE[1]
ALU-CAP (Riker) Aluminum hydroxide gel *OTC*	**Capsules:** 475 mg	**Adult:** 3 caps tid
ALUDROX (Wyeth) Aluminum hydroxide gel and magnesium hydroxide *OTC*	**Chewable tablets:** 233 mg dried aluminum hydroxide gel and 83 mg magnesium hydroxide **Suspension (per 5 ml):** 307 mg aluminum hydroxide gel and 103 mg magnesium hydroxide (12 fl oz)	**Adult:** 2 tabs or 10 ml (2 tsp) q4h, as needed, not to exceed 16 tabs or 60 ml (12 tsp)/24 h
ALU-TAB (Riker) Aluminum hydroxide gel *OTC*	**Tablets:** 600 mg	**Adult:** 3 tabs tid
AMPHOJEL (Wyeth) Aluminum hydroxide gel *OTC*	**Tablets:** 0.3, 0.6 g **Suspension (per 5 ml):** 320 mg (12 fl oz) *plain and peppermint flavored*	**Adult:** 0.6 g or 10 ml (2 tsp) 5–6 times/day, between meals and at bedtime, up to 3.6 g in tablets or 60 ml (12 tsp)/24 h
CALCITREL (Glenbrook) Calcium carbonate and magnesium hydroxide *OTC*	**Chewable tablets:** 585 mg calcium carbonate and 120 mg magnesium hydroxide **Liquid (per 5 ml):** 585 mg calcium carbonate and 120 mg magnesium hydroxide *berry flavored*	**Adult:** 1–2 tabs or 5–10 ml (1–2 tsp), as needed, up to 12 tabs (12 tsp)/24 h **Child (> 6 yr):** same as adult
CREAMALIN (Mentholatum) Aluminum hydroxide and magnesium hydroxide *OTC*	**Chewable tablets:** 248 mg aluminum hydroxide and 75 mg magnesium hydroxide	**Adult:** 2–4 tabs, as needed, up to 16 tabs/24 h **Child (> 6 yr):** same as adult
DELCID (Lakeside) Aluminum hydroxide and magnesium hydroxide *OTC*	**Liquid (per 5 ml):** 600 mg aluminum hydroxide and 665 mg magnesium hydroxide (8 fl oz)	**Adult:** 5 ml (1 tsp) 1/2–1 h after meals and at bedtime, up to 30 ml (6 tsp)/24 h
DICARBOSIL (Norcliff Thayer) Calcium carbonate *OTC*	**Chewable tablets:** 500 mg *peppermint flavored*	**Adult:** 500–2,000 mg, as needed, chewed or dissolved in mouth, 1 h after meals and at bedtime, up to 16 tabs/24 h
DI-GEL Liquid (Plough) Simethicone, aluminum hydroxide, and magnesium hydroxide *OTC*	**Liquid (per 5 ml):** 20 mg simethicone, aluminum hydroxide equivalent to 200 mg dried aluminum hydroxide gel, and 200 mg magnesium hydroxide (6, 12 fl oz) *mint and lemon/orange flavored*	**Adult:** 10 ml (2 tsp) q2h, up to 100 ml (20 tsp)/24 h
DI-GEL Tablets (Plough) Simethicone, calcium carbonate, and magnesium hydroxide *OTC*	**Tablets:** 20 mg simethicone, 280 mg calcium carbonate, and 128 mg magnesium hydroxide *mint and lemon/orange flavored*	**Adult:** 2 tabs q2h, or after or between meals and at bedtime
GAS-X (Sandoz Consumer Health Care Group) Simethicone *OTC*	**Chewable tablets:** 80 mg *peppermint flavored*	**Adult:** 80–160 mg after meals and at bedtime, as needed, up to 480 mg/24 h
Extra Strength GAS-X (Sandoz Consumer Health Care Group) Simethicone *OTC*	**Chewable tablets:** 125 mg *peppermint flavored*	**Adult:** 125–250 mg after meals and at bedtime, as needed, up to 600 mg/24 h
KOLANTYL (Lakeside) Aluminum hydroxide and magnesium hydroxide *OTC*	**Wafers:** 180 mg aluminum hydroxide and 170 mg magnesium hydroxide *mint flavored* **Gel (per 5 ml):** 150 mg aluminum hydroxide and 150 mg magnesium hydroxide (12 fl oz) *mint flavored*	**Adult:** 1–4 wafers or 5–20 ml (1–4 tsp) 1/2–1 h after meals and at bedtime, up to 12 wafers or 60 ml (12 tsp)/24 h
Milk of magnesia *OTC*	**Tablets:** 325 mg **Liquid (per 30 ml):** 2.27–2.62 g	**Adult and child (> 12 yr):** for hyperacidity, 2–4 tabs or 5–10 ml (1–2 tsp) qid
REMEGEL (Warner-Lambert) Aluminum hydroxide and magnesium carbonate *OTC*	**Chewable pieces:** 476.4 mg aluminum hydroxide-magnesium carbonate co-dried gel	**Adult:** 1–2 pieces, repeated hourly, as needed, up to 12 pieces/24 h

[1] Where pediatric dosages are not given, consult manufacturer

OTHER ANTACIDS continued

DRUG	HOW SUPPLIED	USUAL DOSAGE[1]
ROLAIDS (Warner-Lambert) Dihydroxyaluminum sodium carbonate *OTC*	**Chewable tablets:** 334 mg *regular, spearmint, and wintergreen flavored*	**Adult:** 1–2 tabs/h, as needed, up to 24 tabs/24 h
Sodium Free ROLAIDS (Warner-Lambert) Calcium carbonate and magnesium hydroxide *OTC*	**Tablets:** 317 mg calcium carbonate and 64 mg magnesium hydroxide	**Adult:** 1–2 tabs/h, as needed, up to 18 tabs/24 h
SILAIN-GEL (Robins) Aluminum hydroxide, magnesium hydroxide, and simethicone *OTC*	**Liquid (per 5 ml):** 282 mg aluminum hydroxide, 285 mg magnesium hydroxide, and 25 mg simethicone (12 fl oz) *lemon-orange flavored*	**Adult:** 5–10 ml (1–2 tsp) after or between meals and at bedtime, as needed, up to 100 ml (20 tsp)/24 h
Sodium bicarbonate *OTC*	**Tablets:** 325, 487.5, 520, 650 mg	**Adult:** 0.3–2 g 1–4 times/day, as needed
TEMPO (Richardson-Vicks Health Care Products) Calcium carbonate, aluminum hydroxide, magnesium hydroxide, and simethicone *OTC*	**Chewable drops:** 414 mg calcium carbonate, 133 mg aluminum hydroxide, 81 mg magnesium hydroxide, and 20 mg simethicone	**Adult:** 1 drop, chewed until dissolved, as needed, up to 12 drops/24 h
WinGel (Winthrop Consumer Products) Aluminum hydroxide and magnesium hydroxide *OTC*	**Chewable tablets:** 180 mg aluminum hydroxide and 160 mg magnesium hydroxide *mint flavored* **Liquid (per 5 ml):** 180 mg aluminum hydroxide and 160 mg magnesium hydroxide (6, 12 fl oz) *mint flavored*	**Adult:** 1–2 tabs or 5–10 ml (1–2 tsp) 1–4 times/day, up to 8 tabs or 40 ml (8 tsp)/24 h **Child (> 6 yr):** same as adult

[1] Where pediatric dosages are not given, consult manufacturer

OTHER DIGESTANTS

DRUG	HOW SUPPLIED	USUAL DOSAGE[1]
DONNAZYME (Robins) Pancreatin, pepsin, bile salts, hyoscyamine sulfate, atropine sulfate, scopolamine hydrobromide, and phenobarbital *Rx*	**Tablets:** 300 mg pancreatin, 150 mg pepsin, 150 mg bile salts, 0.0518 mg hyoscyamine sulfate, 0.0097 mg atropine sulfate, 0.0033 mg scopolamine hydrobromide, and 8.1 mg phenobarbital	**Adult:** 2 tabs after meals
ENTOZYME (Robins) Pancreatin, pepsin, and bile salts *Rx*	**Tablets:** 300 mg pancreatin, 250 mg pepsin, and 150 mg bile salts	**Adult:** 2 tabs with meals and 1–2 tabs with snacks
FESTAL II (Hoechst-Roussel) Pancreatic enzymes *OTC*	**Tablets:** 6,000 units lipase, 30,000 units amylase, and 20,000 units protease	**Adult:** 1–2 tabs with meals
FESTALAN (Hoechst-Roussel) Atropine methyl nitrate and pancreatic enzymes *Rx*	**Tablets:** 1 mg atropine methyl nitrate, 6,000 units lipase, 30,000 units amylase, and 20,000 units protease	**Adult:** 1–2 tabs with meals
LACTAID (LactAid) Lactase *OTC*	**Tablets:** not less than 3,300 FCC lactase units of β-D-galactosidase **Liquid (per 5 drops):** not less than 1,000 neutral lactase units of β-D-galactosidase	**Adult and child:** 1 tab with a lactose-containing medication or vitamin, 1–3 tabs just before a lactose-containing food, or 8–10 drops, to start, sprinkled on a dairy food. To break down lactose in milk, add 4–10 drops/qt and refrigerate for 24 h; for severe intolerance, use 12–15 drops/qt and refrigerate for 24 h or use 8–10 drops/qt and refrigerate for 48 h
LACTRASE (Kremers-Urban) Lactase *OTC*	**Capsules:** 125 mg	**Adult:** 125–250 mg, given with, or sprinkled on, milk or dairy products; milk may be pretreated by adding the contents of 1–2 caps to 1 qt of milk and refrigerating for 24 h

[1] Where pediatric dosages are not given, consult manufacturer

COMPENDIUM OF DRUG THERAPY

ANTACIDS/ANTIFLATULENTS

ALGICON (aluminum hydroxide/magnesium carbonate gel and magnesium carbonate) Rorer — OTC

Chewable tablets: 360 mg aluminum hydroxide/magnesium carbonate gel and 320 mg magnesium carbonate *lemon swiss-creme flavored*

INDICATIONS	ORAL DOSAGE
Gastric hyperacidity Gastritis, peptic esophagitis, heartburn, and hiatal hernia associated with hyperacidity	**Adult:** 1–2 tabs after meals and at bedtime; maximum 24-h dose without medical supervision: 8 tabs. Tablets should be well chewed and then followed by 4 fl oz (½ glass) of a liquid. The package labeling advises patients that, unless otherwise directed by a physician, they should follow these dosage recommendations and should not use this product at the maximum dosage for more than 2 wk.

ADMINISTRATION/DOSAGE ADJUSTMENTS	
Acid-neutralizing capacity	17.5 mEq/tab

WARNINGS/PRECAUTIONS	
Sodium content	0.12 mEq/tab
Patients with renal impairment	Use with caution in patients with renal impairment

DRUG INTERACTIONS	
Tetracycline	▽ Absorption of tetracycline; do not use concomitantly

USE IN CHILDREN	USE IN PREGNANT AND NURSING WOMEN
Use according to medical judgment	Consult manufacturer

ANTACIDS/ANTIFLATULENTS

ALKA-SELTZER (sodium bicarbonate, citric acid, and potassium bicarbonate) Miles Laboratories — OTC

Effervescent tablets: 958 mg sodium bicarbonate, 832 mg citric acid, and 312 mg potassium bicarbonate

INDICATIONS	ORAL DOSAGE
Acid indigestion, heartburn, and sour stomach	**Adult:** 1–2 tabs q4h, as needed; maximum dosage without medical supervision: 8 tabs or, if 60 yr of age or older, 7 tabs/24 h. Dissolve tabs in 2–3 fl oz of water before administering. **Child:** ½–1 tab q4h, as needed; maximum dosage without medical supervision: 4 tabs/24 h. Dissolve tabs in 2–3 fl oz of water before administering.

ADMINISTRATION/DOSAGE ADJUSTMENTS	
Acid-neutralizing capacity	10.6 mEq/tab
Instructions for patients	The package labeling advises patients that, unless otherwise directed by a physician, they should follow the dosage recommendations and should not use this product at the maximum dosage for more than 2 wk

WARNINGS/PRECAUTIONS	
Sodium content	311 mg/tab; do not give to patients on a sodium-restricted diet

USE IN CHILDREN	USE IN PREGNANT AND NURSING WOMEN
See INDICATIONS and ORAL DOSAGE	Consult manufacturer

ANTACIDS/ANTIFLATULENTS

ALternaGEL (aluminum hydroxide) Stuart — OTC

Liquid (per 5 ml): 600 mg (5, 12 fl oz)

INDICATIONS	ORAL DOSAGE
Gastric hyperacidity Peptic ulcer, gastritis, peptic esophagitis, hiatal hernia, and heartburn associated with gastric hyperacidity	**Adult:** 5–10 ml (1–2 tsp), as needed, between meals and at bedtime, followed by a sip of water, if desired; maximum 24-h dose without medical supervision: 90 ml (18 tsp). The package labeling advises patients that, unless otherwise directed by a physician, they should follow these dosage recommendations and should not use this product at the maximum dosage for more than 2 wk. **Child:** use according to medical judgment

ALternaGEL ■ BASALJEL

ADMINISTRATION/DOSAGE ADJUSTMENTS

Acid-neutralizing capacity	16 mEq/tsp

WARNINGS/PRECAUTIONS

Sodium content	< 2.5 mg/tsp
Constipation	Use of this product may cause constipation

DRUG INTERACTIONS

Tetracycline	▽ Absorption of tetracycline; do not use concomitantly

---

USE IN CHILDREN
Use according to medical judgment

USE IN PREGNANT AND NURSING WOMEN
Consult manufacturer

ANTACIDS/ANTIFLATULENTS

BASALJEL (aluminum carbonate gel, basic) Wyeth — OTC

Capsules: aluminum carbonate equivalent to 608 mg dried aluminum hydroxide gel or 500 mg aluminum hydroxide **Tablets:** aluminum carbonate equivalent to 608 mg dried aluminum hydroxide gel or 500 mg aluminum hydroxide **Suspension (per 5 ml):** aluminum carbonate equivalent to 400 mg aluminum hydroxide (regular strength) (12 fl oz) or 1,000 mg aluminum hydroxide (extra strength) (12 fl oz)

INDICATIONS / ORAL DOSAGE

INDICATIONS	ORAL DOSAGE
Management of **hyperphosphatemia** Prevention of **phosphate stones**	**Adult:** 2 caps or tabs, 12 ml (2½ tsp) of the regular-strength suspension, or 5 ml (1 tsp) of the extra-strength suspension tid or qid with meals to start, up to 3–4 g/day; to determine the optimal dosage, carefully monitor dietary intake of phosphate (instruct patient to maintain a low phosphate diet) and regularly measure serum phosphorus level
Gastric hyperacidity **Peptic ulcer, gastritis, peptic esophagitis, and hiatal hernia associated with gastric hyperacidity**	**Adult:** 2 caps or tabs, 10 ml (2 tsp) of the regular-strength suspension, or 5 ml (1 tsp) of the extra-strength suspension as often as q2h

ADMINISTRATION/DOSAGE ADJUSTMENTS

Acid-neutralizing capacity	12 mEq/cap; 12.5 mEq/tab; 11.5 mEq/tsp of the regular-strength suspension; 22 mEq/tsp of the extra-strength suspension
Maximum 24-h dose	24 caps or tabs; 120 ml (24 tsp) of the regular-strength suspension; 60 ml (24 tsp) of the extra-strength suspension
Administration of suspension	Dilute suspension in water or fruit juice before administering

WARNINGS/PRECAUTIONS

Sodium content	0.12 mEq/cap or tab; 0.13 mEq/tsp of the regular-strength suspension; 1 mEq/tsp of the extra-strength suspension
Hypophosphatemia	Prolonged use may cause hypophosphatemia if the serum phosphate level is normal at the start of therapy, but intake of phosphate is inadequate during treatment; severe hypophosphatemia can lead to anorexia, malaise, muscle weakness, and osteomalacia
Dialysis encephalopathy syndrome	Prolonged use may contribute to an increase in the tissue level of aluminum and, as a result, possibly enhance the risk of encephalopathy in patients undergoing dialysis
Mild hypercalciuria	May occur during the early weeks of therapy and is usually transient
Constipation	May occur; maintain adequate fluid intake in addition to specific medical or surgical requirements

DRUG INTERACTIONS

Tetracycline	▽ Absorption of tetracycline; do not use concomitantly

---

USE IN CHILDREN
Use according to medical judgment

USE IN PREGNANT AND NURSING WOMEN
The package labeling cautions patients to consult a health professional before using this product

ANTACIDS/ANTIFLATULENTS

CAMALOX (magnesium hydroxide, aluminum hydroxide, and calcium carbonate) Rorer OTC

Chewable tablets: 200 mg magnesium hydroxide, 225 mg aluminum hydroxide, and 250 mg calcium carbonate *vanilla-mint flavored* **Suspension (per 5 ml):** 200 mg magnesium hydroxide, 225 mg aluminum hydroxide, and 250 mg calcium carbonate (12 fl oz) *vanilla-mint flavored*

INDICATIONS	ORAL DOSAGE
Gastric hyperacidity Peptic ulcer, gastritis, peptic esophagitis, heartburn, and hiatal hernia associated with gastric hyperacidity	**Adult:** 2–4 tabs ½–1 h after meals and at bedtime or 10–20 ml (2–4 tsp) qid, ½ h after meals and at bedtime; maximum 24-h dose without medical supervision: 16 tabs or 80 ml (16 tsp). Tablets should be well chewed. The package labeling advises patients that, unless otherwise directed by a physician, they should follow these dosage recommendations and should not use these products at the maximum dosage for more than 2 wk. **Child:** use according to medical judgment

ADMINISTRATION/DOSAGE ADJUSTMENTS

Acid-neutralizing capacity	18.0 mEq/tab or tsp

WARNINGS/PRECAUTIONS

Sodium content	1 mg/tab; 1.2 mg/tsp
Patients with renal impairment	Use with caution in patients with renal impairment

DRUG INTERACTIONS

Tetracycline	⇩ Absorption of tetracycline; do not use concomitantly

ALTERED LABORATORY VALUES

Blood/serum values	⇧ Magnesium (with renal failure)

No clinically significant alterations in urinary values occur at therapeutic dosages

USE IN CHILDREN	USE IN PREGNANT AND NURSING WOMEN
Use according to medical judgment	Consult manufacturer

ANTACIDS/ANTIFLATULENTS

GAVISCON (aluminum hydroxide and magnesium trisilicate) Marion OTC

Chewable tablets: 80 mg aluminum hydroxide and 20 mg magnesium trisilicate

GAVISCON-2 (aluminum hydroxide and magnesium trisilicate) Marion OTC

Chewable tablets: 160 mg aluminum hydroxide and 40 mg magnesium trisilicate

GAVISCON Liquid (aluminum hydroxide and magnesium carbonate) Marion OTC

Liquid (per 15 ml): 95 mg aluminum hydroxide and 412 mg magnesium carbonate (6, 12 fl oz) *spearmint flavored*

INDICATIONS	ORAL DOSAGE
Heartburn, sour stomach, and acid indigestion	**Adult:** 2–4 Gaviscon tabs, 1–2 Gaviscon-2 tabs, or 15–30 ml (1–2 tbsp) qid, after meals and at bedtime (or as needed) followed by ½ glass of water; maximum 24-h dose without medical supervision: 16 Gaviscon tabs, 8 Gaviscon-2 tabs, or 120 ml (8 tbsp). Tablets should be well chewed. The package labeling advises patients that, unless otherwise directed by a physician, they should follow these dosage recommendations and should not use these products at the maximum dosage for more than 2 wk. **Child:** use according to medical judgment

WARNINGS/PRECAUTIONS

Sodium content	Gaviscon: 0.8 mEq/tab; Gaviscon-2: 1.6 mEq/tab; Gaviscon Liquid: 1.7 mEq/tbsp. These products should not be used by patients on a sodium-restricted diet.
Patients with renal impairment	Use tablets with caution in patients with renal impairment; the liquid should not be used in such patients
Laxative effect	Use of the liquid form may cause a laxative effect

GAVISCON ■ ILOPAN-CHOLINE

DRUG INTERACTIONS

Tetracycline — ▽ Absorption of tetracycline; do not use concomitantly

USE IN CHILDREN
Use according to medical judgment

USE IN PREGNANT AND NURSING WOMEN
Consult manufacturer

ANTACIDS/ANTIFLATULENTS

GELUSIL (aluminum hydroxide, magnesium hydroxide, and simethicone) Warner-Lambert   OTC

Chewable tablets: 200 mg aluminum hydroxide, 200 mg magnesium hydroxide, and 25 mg simethicone *peppermint flavored*
Liquid (per 5 ml): 200 mg aluminum hydroxide, 200 mg magnesium hydroxide, and 25 mg simethicone (6, 12 fl oz) *peppermint flavored*

GELUSIL-M (aluminum hydroxide, magnesium hydroxide, and simethicone) Warner-Lambert   OTC

Chewable tablets: 300 mg aluminum hydroxide, 200 mg magnesium hydroxide, and 25 mg simethicone *spearmint flavored*
Liquid (per 5 ml): 300 mg aluminum hydroxide, 200 mg magnesium hydroxide, and 25 mg simethicone (12 fl oz) *spearmint flavored*

GELUSIL-II (aluminum hydroxide, magnesium hydroxide, and simethicone) Warner-Lambert   OTC

Chewable tablets: 400 mg aluminum hydroxide, 400 mg magnesium hydroxide, and 30 mg simethicone *orange flavored* **Liquid (per 5 ml):** 400 mg aluminum hydroxide, 400 mg magnesium hydroxide, and 30 mg simethicone (12 fl oz) *citrus flavored*

INDICATIONS

Heartburn, sour stomach, and acid indigestion, when accompanied by **gas**
Gastric **hyperacidity**
Peptic **ulcer, gastritis, peptic esophagitis, and hiatal hernia associated with gastric hyperacidity**
Gas, postoperative gas pain

ORAL DOSAGE

Adult: 2 tabs or 10 ml (2 tsp), or more, 1 h after meals and at bedtime; maximum 24-h dose without medical supervision: 12 tabs or 60 ml (12 tsp) of Gelusil, 10 tabs or 50 ml (10 tsp) of Gelusil-M, or 8 tabs or 40 ml (8 tsp) of Gelusil-II. Tablets should be chewed. The package labeling advises patients that, unless otherwise directed by a physician, they should follow these dosage recommendations and should not use these products at the maximum dosage for more than 2 wk.
Child: use according to medical judgment

ADMINISTRATION/DOSAGE ADJUSTMENTS

Acid-neutralizing capacity — Gelusil: 11.0 mEq/tab, 12.0 mEq/tsp; Gelusil-M: 12.5 mEq/tab, 15.0 mEq/tsp; Gelusil-II: 21.0 mEq/tab, 24.0 mEq/tsp

WARNINGS/PRECAUTIONS

Sodium content — Gelusil: 0.8 mg/tab, 0.7 mg/tsp; Gelusil-M: 1.3 mg/tab, 1.2 mg/tsp; Gelusil-II: 2.1 mg/tab, 1.3 mg/tsp

Patients with renal impairment — Use with caution in patients with renal impairment

DRUG INTERACTIONS

Tetracycline — ▽ Absorption of tetracycline; do not use concomitantly

USE IN CHILDREN
Use according to medical judgment

USE IN PREGNANT AND NURSING WOMEN
Consult manufacturer

ANTACIDS/ANTIFLATULENTS

ILOPAN-CHOLINE (dexpanthenol and choline bitartrate) Adria   Rx

Tablets: 50 mg dexpanthenol and 25 mg choline bitartrate

INDICATIONS

Gas retention associated with splenic flexure syndrome, cholecystitis, gastritis, gastric hyperacidity, irritable colon, regional ileitis, post-antibiotic and postoperative gas retention, or laxative withdrawal

ORAL DOSAGE

Adult: 2–3 tabs tid

COMPENDIUM OF DRUG THERAPY

ILOPAN-CHOLINE ■ MAALOX

CONTRAINDICATIONS
None known

WARNINGS/PRECAUTIONS
Allergic reactions — Have been reported rarely during concomitant use of dexpanthenol with antibiotics, narcotics, barbiturates and other drugs; if hypersensitivity occurs, discontinue use

ADVERSE REACTIONS
No clearly established reactions to this drug have been documented[1]

OVERDOSAGE
Toxicity has not occurred in clinical use

DRUG INTERACTIONS
Succinylcholine — Prolongation of neuromuscular blockade due to interaction with dexpanthenol; do not administer Ilopan-Choline within 1 h of injecting succinylcholine

ALTERED LABORATORY VALUES
No clinically significant alterations in blood/serum or urinary values occur at therapeutic dosages

USE IN CHILDREN
Safety and effectiveness have not been established for use in children under 12 yr of age

USE IN PREGNANT AND NURSING WOMEN
Pregnancy Category C: use during pregnancy only if clearly needed. Reproductive studies have not been done in animals, nor is it known whether this drug can cause fetal harm when administered to a pregnant woman or can affect reproductive capacity. Excretion of this drug in human milk is unknown; use with caution in nursing mothers.

[1] Reactions for which a causal relationship has not been established include generalized dermatitis in two patients, urticaria in one patient, and a dull headache in one patient

---

ANTACIDS/ANTIFLATULENTS

MAALOX (magnesium hydroxide and aluminum hydroxide) Rorer — OTC
Chewable tablets: 200 mg magnesium hydroxide and 200 mg aluminum hydroxide (Maalox No. 1); 400 mg magnesium hydroxide and 400 mg aluminum hydroxide (Maalox No. 2) *mint flavored* **Suspension (per 5 ml):** 200 mg magnesium hydroxide and 225 mg aluminum hydroxide (5, 12, 26 fl oz) *mint flavored*

MAALOX Plus (magnesium hydroxide, aluminum hydroxide, and simethicone) Rorer — OTC
Chewable tablets: 200 mg magnesium hydroxide, 200 mg aluminum hydroxide, and 25 mg simethicone *lemon swiss-creme flavored* **Suspension (per 5 ml):** 200 mg magnesium hydroxide, 225 mg aluminum hydroxide, and 25 mg simethicone (12 fl oz) *lemon swiss-creme flavored*

INDICATIONS	ORAL DOSAGE
Gastric hyperacidity Peptic ulcer, gastritis, peptic esophagitis, heartburn, and hiatal hernia associated with hyperacidity Gas, postoperative gas pain (Maalox Plus only)	**Adult:** 2–4 Maalox No. 1 or Maalox Plus tabs, or 1–2 Maalox No. 2 tabs, or 10–20 ml (2–4 tsp) qid, 20–60 min after meals and at bedtime; maximum 24-h dose without medical supervision: 16 Maalox No. 1 or Maalox Plus tabs, 8 Maalox No. 2 tabs, or 80 ml (16 tsp). Tablets should be well chewed. **Child:** use according to medical judgment

MAALOX TC (magnesium hydroxide and aluminum hydroxide) Rorer — OTC
Chewable tablets: 300 mg magnesium hydroxide and 600 mg aluminum hydroxide *peppermint lemon-creme flavored*
Suspension (per 5 ml): 300 mg magnesium hydroxide and 600 mg aluminum hydroxide (12 fl oz) *peppermint flavored*

INDICATIONS	ORAL DOSAGE	NASOGASTRIC DOSAGE
Prevention of stress-induced upper GI hemorrhage	**Adult:** 20 ml q2h **Child:** use according to medical judgment	**Adult:** 10 ml to start, followed by a doubling of the dose every hour until the pH equals or exceeds 4 (usual dose: 20 ml; maximum dose: 80 ml); thereafter, administer the titrated dose q2h. Immediately after instillation of each dose, administer 30 ml of water. **Child:** use according to medical judgment
Gastric hyperacidity associated with peptic ulcer and other GI conditions, when a high degree of acid neutralization is required	**Adult:** 1–2 tabs or 5–10 ml (1–2 tsp) 1 h after meals and at bedtime; maximum 24-h dose without medical supervision: 8 tabs or 40 ml (8 tsp). This dose may be exceeded when treating active peptic ulcer disease if direct medical supervision is provided. Tablets should be well chewed. **Child:** use according to medical judgment	

ADMINISTRATION/DOSAGE ADJUSTMENTS

Acid-neutralizing capacity	Maalox No. 1 tabs: 9.7 mEq/tab; Maalox Plus tabs: 11.4 mEq/tab; Maalox No. 2 tabs: 23.4 mEq/tab; Maalox suspension: 13.3 mEq/tsp; Maalox Plus suspension: 13.35 mEq/tsp; Maalox TC tabs: 28 mEq/tab; Maalox TC suspension: 27.2 mEq/tsp
Nasogastric administration	Before starting therapy and then every hour thereafter, aspirate stomach contents and check pH. After instillation of each dose, clamp the tube for 1 h; then, after checking pH, drain or apply intermittent suction for 1 h (if pH equals or exceeds 4) or administer another dose (if pH is less than 4).
Instructions for patient	The package labeling advises patients that, unless otherwise directed by a physician, they should follow the stated dosage recommendations and should not use this product at the maximum dosage for more than 2 wk

WARNINGS/PRECAUTIONS

Sodium content	Maalox No. 1 tabs: 0.7 mg/tab; Maalox Plus tabs: 0.8 mg/tab; Maalox No. 2 tabs: 1.4 mg/tab; Maalox suspension: 1.4 mg/tsp; Maalox Plus suspension: 1.2 mg/tsp; Maalox TC tabs: 0.5 mg/tab; Maalox TC suspension: 0.8 mg/tsp
Patients with renal impairment	Use with caution in patients with renal impairment
Regurgitation, mild diarrhea	When used for prevention of hemorrhage, Maalox TC suspension has occasionally caused regurgitation and mild diarrhea

DRUG INTERACTIONS

Tetracycline	▽ Absorption of tetracycline; do not use concomitantly

USE IN CHILDREN
Use according to medical judgment

USE IN PREGNANT AND NURSING WOMEN
Consult manufacturer

ANTACIDS/ANTIFLATULENTS

MYLANTA (aluminum hydroxide, magnesium hydroxide, and simethicone) Stuart — OTC

Chewable tablets: 200 mg aluminum hydroxide, 200 mg magnesium hydroxide, and 20 mg simethicone **Liquid (per 5 ml):** 200 mg aluminum hydroxide, 200 mg magnesium hydroxide, and 20 mg simethicone (1, 5, 12 fl oz)

MYLANTA-II (aluminum hydroxide, magnesium hydroxide, and simethicone) Stuart — OTC

Chewable tablets: 400 mg aluminum hydroxide, 400 mg magnesium hydroxide, and 40 mg simethicone **Liquid (per 5 ml):** 400 mg aluminum hydroxide, 400 mg magnesium hydroxide, and 40 mg simethicone (1, 2, 5, 12 fl oz)

INDICATIONS

Heartburn and gas
Gastric hyperacidity
Peptic ulcer, gastritis, peptic esophagitis, and hiatal hernia associated with gastric hyperacidity

ORAL DOSAGE

Adult: 1–2 tabs or 5–10 ml (1–2 tsp) of Mylanta q2–4h or 1–2 tabs or 5–10 ml (1–2 tsp) of Mylanta-II; maximum 24-h dose without medical supervision: 24 tabs or 120 ml (24 tsp) of Mylanta or 12 tabs or 60 ml (12 tsp) of Mylanta-II. These preparations should be given between meals and at bedtime, and the tablets should be chewed thoroughly. The package labeling advises patients that, unless otherwise directed by a physician, they should follow these dosage recommendations and should not use these products at the maximum dosage for more than 2 wk.
Child: use according to medical judgment

ADMINISTRATION/DOSAGE ADJUSTMENTS

Acid-neutralizing capacity	Mylanta: 11.5 mEq/tab, 12.7 mEq/tsp; Mylanta-II: 23.0 mEq/tab, 25.4 mEq/tsp
Dosage adjustment	Dosage should be adjusted on the basis of acid output and gastric emptying time (these two factors vary greatly among patients with peptic ulcer)

WARNINGS/PRECAUTIONS

Sodium content	Mylanta: 0.77 mg/tab, 0.68 mg/tsp; Mylanta-II: 1.3 mg/tab, 1.14 mg/tsp
Patients with renal impairment	Use with caution in patients with renal impairment; watch for CNS depression and other symptoms of hypermagnesemia

DRUG INTERACTIONS

Tetracycline	▽ Absorption of tetracycline; do not use concomitantly

ANTACIDS/ANTIFLATULENTS

MYLICON (simethicone) Stuart   OTC
Chewable tablets: 40 mg   Drops: 40 mg/0.6 ml (30 ml)

MYLICON-80 (simethicone) Stuart   OTC
Chewable tablets: 80 mg

INDICATIONS
Painful symptoms of excess gas in the digestive tract caused by postoperative gaseous distention, aerophagia, functional dyspepsia, peptic ulcer, spastic or irritable colon, diverticulitis, and similar conditions

ORAL DOSAGE
Adult: 40–80 mg or 0.6 ml qid, after meals and at bedtime; maximum 24–h dose without medical supervision: 480 mg or 7.5 ml. Tablets should be well chewed.
Child: use according to medical judgment

USE IN CHILDREN	USE IN PREGNANT AND NURSING WOMEN
Use according to medical judgment	Consult manufacturer

ANTACIDS/ANTIFLATULENTS

PHAZYME (simethicone) Reed & Carnrick   OTC
Tablets: 60 mg

INDICATIONS
Gas pain caused by aerophagia, postoperative distention, dyspepsia, or food intolerance

ORAL DOSAGE
Adult: 1 tab with each meal and at bedtime, or as needed

PHAZYME 95 (simethicone) Reed & Carnrick   OTC
Tablets: 95 mg

PHAZYME 125 (simethicone) Reed & Carnrick   OTC
Capsules: 125 mg

INDICATIONS
Acute, severe lower intestinal gas pain caused by aerophagia, postoperative distention, dyspepsia, or food intolerance

ORAL DOSAGE
Adult: 1 tab or cap with each meal and at bedtime, or as needed

CONTRAINDICATIONS
Hypersensitivity to any component

WARNINGS/PRECAUTIONS
Persistent symptoms — Instruct patient to report gas pain that persists despite medication

USE IN CHILDREN	USE IN PREGNANT AND NURSING WOMEN
Consult manufacturer	This product may be used in pregnant and nursing women; the active ingredient is not systemically absorbed

ANTACIDS/ANTIFLATULENTS

PHAZYME-PB (simethicone and phenobarbital) Reed & Carnrick   C-IV

Tablets: 60 mg simethicone and 15 mg phenobarbital

INDICATIONS	ORAL DOSAGE
Gas associated with chronic anxiety	**Adult:** 1 or 2 tabs with meals and at bedtime, or as needed

CONTRAINDICATIONS

Hypersensitivity to any component

WARNINGS/PRECAUTIONS

Drug dependence	Psychic and/or physical dependence and tolerance may develop, especially in addiction-prone individuals
Drowsiness	May occur with excessive use

ADVERSE REACTIONS

None reported by manufacturer

OVERDOSAGE

Signs and symptoms	*Toxic effects attributable to phenobarbital:* respiratory depression, depressed superficial and deep reflexes, miosis or mydriasis, decreased urine formation, hypothermia, coma
Treatment	Empty stomach immediately by gastric lavage, taking care to prevent pulmonary aspiration. Maintain patent airway, assist ventilation, and administer oxygen, as needed. Monitor vital signs and fluid balance. Treat shock with fluids and other standard measures. If renal function is normal, force diuresis and alkalinize urine to help eliminate drug. Dialysis may be helpful.

DRUG INTERACTIONS

Alcohol, tranquilizers, and other CNS depressants	⇧ CNS depression
Coumarin anticoagulants	⇩ Prothrombin time
Digitoxin	⇩ Digitoxin plasma level
Doxycycline	⇩ Doxycycline half-life

ALTERED LABORATORY VALUES

No clinically significant alterations in blood/serum or urinary values occur at therapeutic dosages

USE IN CHILDREN	USE IN PREGNANT AND NURSING WOMEN
Not indicated for use in children	Use according to medical discretion; phenobarbital in high doses has been known to depress fetal respiration

---

ANTACIDS/ANTIFLATULENTS

RIOPAN (magaldrate) Ayerst   OTC

Chewable tablets: 480 mg **Swallowable tablets:** 480 mg **Suspension (per 5 ml):** 540 mg (30 ml, 12 fl oz)

INDICATIONS	ORAL DOSAGE
Heartburn, sour stomach, and acid indigestion **Gastric hyperacidity** **Peptic ulcer, gastritis, peptic esophagitis, and hiatal hernia associated with gastric hyperacidity**	**Adult:** 1–2 tabs (swallowed with water or chewed, depending on formulation) or 5–10 ml (1–2 tsp) between meals and at bedtime; maximum 24-h dose without medical supervision: 20 tabs or 90 ml (18 tsp) **Child:** use according to medical judgment

COMPENDIUM OF DRUG THERAPY

RIOPAN PLUS (magaldrate and simethicone) Ayerst — OTC

Chewable tablets: 480 mg magaldrate and 20 mg simethicone **Suspension (per 5 ml):** 540 mg magaldrate and 20 mg simethicone (30 ml, 12 fl oz)

Extra Strength RIOPAN PLUS (magaldrate and simethicone) Ayerst — OTC

Chewable tablets: 1,080 mg magaldrate and 20 mg simethicone **Suspension (per 5 ml):** 1,080 mg magaldrate and 30 mg simethicone (12 fl oz)

INDICATIONS

Heartburn, sour stomach, and acid indigestion accompanied by gas
Gastric hyperacidity
Peptic ulcer, gastritis, peptic esophagitis, and hiatal hernia associated with gastric hyperacidity
Postoperative gas pain

ORAL DOSAGE

Adult: 1–2 tabs (well chewed) or 5–10 ml (1–2 tsp) between meals and at bedtime; maximum 24-h dose without medical supervision: Riopan Plus, 20 tabs or 90 ml (18 tsp); Extra Strength Riopan Plus, 9 tabs or 45 ml (9 tsp)
Child: use according to medical judgment

ADMINISTRATION/DOSAGE ADJUSTMENTS

Acid-neutralizing capacity	Riopan, Riopan Plus: 13.5 mEq/tab, 15.0 mEq/tsp; Extra Strength Riopan Plus: 30.0 mEq/tab or tsp
Instructions for patient	The package labeling advises patients that, unless otherwise directed by a physician, they should follow the stated dosage recommendations and should not use these products at the maximum dosage for more than 2 wk

WARNINGS/PRECAUTIONS

Sodium content	Riopan, Riopan Plus: $\leq$ 0.1 mg/tab, $\leq$ 0.1 mg/tsp; Extra Strength Riopan Plus: $\leq$ 0.5 mg/tab, $\leq$ 0.3 mg/tsp
Patients with renal impairment	Use with caution in patients with renal impairment

DRUG INTERACTIONS

Tetracycline	▽ Absorption of tetracycline; do not use concomitantly

USE IN CHILDREN
Use according to medical judgment

USE IN PREGNANT AND NURSING WOMEN
Consult manufacturer

ANTACIDS/ANTIFLATULENTS

SIMECO (aluminum hydroxide gel, magnesium hydroxide, and simethicone) Wyeth — OTC

Suspension (per 5 ml): aluminum hydroxide gel equivalent to 365 mg dried gel, 300 mg magnesium hydroxide, and 30 mg simethicone (12 fl oz) *cool mint flavored*

INDICATIONS

Heartburn, upset stomach, sour stomach, and acid indigestion, when accompanied by gas
Gas
Gastric hyperacidity
Peptic ulcer, gastritis, peptic esophagitis, and hiatal hernia associated with hyperacidity

ORAL DOSAGE

Adult: 5–10 ml (1–2 tsp), undiluted or with a small amount of water, tid or qid, between meals and at bedtime; maximum 24-h dose without medical supervision: 40 ml (8 tsp). The package labeling advises patients that, unless otherwise directed by a physician, they should follow these dosage recommendations and should not use this product at the maximum dosage for more than 2 wk.
Child: use according to medical judgment

ADMINISTRATION/DOSAGE ADJUSTMENTS

Acid-neutralizing capacity	22 mEq/tsp

WARNINGS/PRECAUTIONS

Sodium content	0.53 mEq/tsp
Patients with renal impairment	Use with caution in patients with renal impairment

DRUG INTERACTIONS

Tetracycline	▽ Absorption of tetracycline; do not use concomitantly

SIMECO ■ TUMS

USE IN CHILDREN	USE IN PREGNANT AND NURSING WOMEN
Use according to medical judgment	The package labeling cautions pregnant or nursing women to consult a health professional before using this product

---

ANTACIDS/ANTIFLATULENTS

TITRALAC (calcium carbonate) 3M — OTC

Chewable tablets: 0.42 g *spearmint flavored, sugar-free* **Liquid (per 5 ml):** 1 g (12 fl oz) *spearmint flavored, sugar-free*

INDICATIONS	ORAL DOSAGE
Gastric hyperacidity Peptic ulcer, gastritis, peptic esophagitis, and hiatal hernia associated with gastric hyperacidity	**Adult:** 0.84 g (2 tabs) q2–3h, as needed, or 5 ml (1 tsp) between meals and at bedtime; maximum 24-h dose without medical supervision: 19 tabs or 40 ml (8 tsp). Tablets may be chewed, swallowed, or allowed to melt in the mouth. The package labeling advises patients that, unless otherwise directed by a physician, they should follow these dosage recommendations and should not use these products at the maximum dosage for more than 2 wk. **Child:** use according to medical judgment

ADMINISTRATION/DOSAGE ADJUSTMENTS

Acid-neutralizing capacity	7.5 mEq/tab; 19 mEq/tsp

WARNINGS/PRECAUTIONS

Sodium content	$\leq$ 0.3 mg/tab; $\leq$ 11 mg/tsp

DRUG INTERACTIONS

Tetracycline	▽ Absorption of tetracycline

USE IN CHILDREN	USE IN PREGNANT AND NURSING WOMEN
Use according to medical judgment	Consult manufacturer

ANTACIDS/ANTIFLATULENTS

TUMS (calcium carbonate) Norcliff Thayer — OTC

Tablets: 500 mg *peppermint, cherry, lemon, orange, and wintergreen flavored*

TUMS E-X (calcium carbonate) Norcliff Thayer — OTC

Tablets: 750 mg *wintergreen flavored*

INDICATIONS	ORAL DOSAGE
Gastric hyperacidity Peptic ulcer, gastritis, peptic esophagitis, and hiatal hernia associated with gastric hyperacidity	**Adult:** 1–2 tabs, repeated hourly, as needed; maximum 24-h dose without medical supervision: 16 tabs of Tums or 10 tabs of Tums E-X. The package labeling advises patients that, unless otherwise directed by a physician, they should follow these dosage recommendations and should not use these products at the maximum dosage for more than 2 wk. **Child:** use according to medical judgment

ADMINISTRATION/DOSAGE ADJUSTMENTS

Administration of tablets	Tablets may be well chewed or, to prolong the effective relief time, kept between the gum and the cheek and allowed to dissolve gradually by continuous sucking
Acid-neutralizing capacity	Tums: 10 mEq/tab; Tums E-X: 15 mEq/tab

WARNINGS/PRECAUTIONS

Sodium content	Tums: $\leq$ 2 mg/tab; Tums E-X: $\leq$ 2 mg/tab

DRUG INTERACTIONS

Tetracycline ──────────── ▽ Absorption of tetracycline

USE IN CHILDREN	USE IN PREGNANT AND NURSING WOMEN
Use according to medical judgment	Consult manufacturer

DIGESTANTS

COTAZYM (pancrelipase) Organon Rx
Capsules: 8,000 units lipase, 30,000 units protease, and 30,000 units amylase[1] *regular or cherry flavored*

COTAZYM-S (pancrelipase) Organon Rx
Capsules: 5,000 units lipase, 20,000 units protease, and 20,000 units amylase, supplied as enteric-coated spheres

INDICATIONS
Pancreatic enzyme insufficiency resulting in inadequate fat digestion due to chronic pancreatitis, pancreatectomy, cystic fibrosis, steatorrhea, or other causes

ORAL DOSAGE
Adult: 1–3 Cotazym caps immediately before each meal or snack or 1–2 Cotazym-S caps with each meal or snack, or use according to medical judgment; for severe cases, a higher dosage and dietary adjustment may be necessary
Child: same as adult

CONTRAINDICATIONS
Hypersensitivity to pork protein

ADMINISTRATION/DOSAGE ADJUSTMENTS
Administration of Cotazym-S capsules ──── Capsules should be swallowed, not chewed or crushed. If swallowing is difficult, the capsules can be opened, and the contents may be added to a liquid or a soft food that does not require chewing.

WARNINGS/PRECAUTIONS
Opened Cotazym capsules ──── Spilled powder may be irritating to skin or mucous membranes; if capsule is opened for any reason, caution patient not to inhale powder or spill it on hands

ADVERSE REACTIONS
No adverse reactions have been reported; however, extremely high doses of exogenous pancreatic enzymes have been associated with hyperuricosuria and hyperuricemia

OVERDOSAGE
Toxicity has not occurred in clinical use

DRUG INTERACTIONS
No clinically significant drug interactions have been identified

ALTERED LABORATORY VALUES
No clinically significant alterations in blood/serum or urinary values occur at therapeutic dosages

USE IN CHILDREN	USE IN PREGNANT AND NURSING WOMEN
See INDICATIONS and ORAL DOSAGE	No clinically significant problems have resulted from use of this drug during pregnancy. It is not known whether exogenous pancreatic enzymes are excreted in human milk.

[1] Plus 25 mg precipitated calcium carbonate

DIGESTANTS

ILOZYME (pancrelipase) Adria Rx
Tablets: 11,000 units lipase, not less than 30,000 units protease, and not less than 30,000 units amylase

INDICATIONS
Exocrine pancreatic insufficiency due to chronic pancreatitis, pancreatectomy, cystic fibrosis, or obstruction caused by cancer of the pancreas

ORAL DOSAGE
Adult: 1–3 tabs with meals and 1 tab with any food eaten between meals
Child: same as adult

ILOZYME ■ KANULASE

CONTRAINDICATIONS
None known

ADMINISTRATION/DOSAGE ADJUSTMENTS

Severe deficiency	Increase the dose to 8 tablets (with each meal) or the frequency of administration to hourly intervals, provided that nausea, diarrhea, or cramps do not develop at the higher dosage

WARNINGS/PRECAUTIONS

Treatment of primary disorder	Should not be delayed or supplanted by pancreatic exocrine replacement therapy
Hypersensitivity	Use with caution in patients hypersensitive to pork or enzymes; discontinue therapy if symptoms of hypersensitivity appear
Dietary restriction	If patient continues to experience significant steatorrhea and diarrhea, limiting the amount of dietary fat to 30–50 g/day and increasing the amount of protein in the diet may help; additional calories, if needed, may be supplied in the form of medium-chain triglycerides
Carcinogenicity, mutagenicity, and effect on fertility	No studies have been done in animals to evaluate the carcinogenic or mutagenic potential of this product or its effect on reproductive capacity

ADVERSE REACTIONS

Gastrointestinal	Nausea, abdominal cramps, and/or diarrhea (with high doses)

OVERDOSAGE
Toxicity has not occurred in clinical use

DRUG INTERACTIONS

Antacids containing calcium carbonate or magnesium hydroxide	▽ Therapeutic effect of pancrelipase
Iron supplements	▽ Serum iron levels

ALTERED LABORATORY VALUES
No clinically significant alterations in blood/serum or urinary values occur at therapeutic dosages

---

USE IN CHILDREN
See INDICATIONS and ORAL DOSAGE

USE IN PREGNANT AND NURSING WOMEN
Consult manufacturer

DIGESTANTS

KANULASE (cellulase, pancreatin, glutamic acid hydrochloride, ox bile extract, and pepsin) Sandoz Consumer Health Care Group OTC

Tablets: 9 mg cellulase, 1,000 units lipase, 1,000 units amylase, 12,000 units protease, 200 mg glutamic acid hydrochloride, 100 mg ox bile extract, and 150 mg pepsin

INDICATIONS
Belching, bloating, flatulence, and other intestinal gas discomforts

ORAL DOSAGE
Adult: 1 or 2 tabs, swallowed whole, with meals

CONTRAINDICATIONS
Hypersensitivity to any component

WARNINGS/PRECAUTIONS

Loose stools	May occur; reduce dosage
Special-risk patients	Patients with peptic ulcer are not normally given glutamic acid hydrochloride

COMPENDIUM OF DRUG THERAPY

ADVERSE REACTIONS
None reported by manufacturer

OVERDOSAGE
Toxicity has not occurred in clinical use

DRUG INTERACTIONS
No clinically significant drug interactions have been identified

ALTERED LABORATORY VALUES
No clinically significant alterations in blood/serum or urinary values occur at therapeutic dosages

USE IN CHILDREN
Not indicated for use in children

USE IN PREGNANT AND NURSING WOMEN
Safety for use during pregnancy has not been established; use with caution, weighing the possible benefits of therapy against the potential risk to the fetus. It is not known whether this drug is excreted in human milk; use with caution in nursing mothers.

DIGESTANTS

PANCREASE (pancrelipase) McNeil Pharmaceutical — Rx

Capsules: not less than 4,000 units lipase, 20,000 units amylase, and 25,000 units protease, supplied as enteric-coated microspheres

INDICATIONS
Exocrine pancreatic enzyme deficiency associated with cystic fibrosis, chronic pancreatitis, pancreatectomy, gastrointestinal bypass surgery, ductal obstruction from neoplasm (eg, of pancreas or common bile duct), and other disorders

ORAL DOSAGE
Adult: 1 or 2 caps with each meal, or up to 3 caps per meal, if needed, and 1 cap with snacks
Child: same as adult, titrated according to the amount of steatorrhea the child exhibits

CONTRAINDICATIONS
Hypersensitivity to pork protein

ADMINISTRATION/DOSAGE ADJUSTMENTS
Administration — Capsules should be swallowed, not chewed or crushed. If swallowing is difficult, the capsules can be opened, and the contents may be added to a small amount of a soft food (eg, applesauce, gelatin) that does not require chewing and does not have a pH exceeding 5.5.

WARNINGS/PRECAUTIONS
Hypersensitivity — May occur; discontinue use and treat symptomatically

ADVERSE REACTIONS
The most frequent reactions, regardless of incidence, are printed in *italics*
Gastrointestinal — *GI disturbances*
Hypersensitivity — Allergic reactions
Other — Hyperuricosuria and hyperuricemia (with extremely high doses)

OVERDOSAGE
Toxicity has not occurred in clinical use

DRUG INTERACTIONS
No clinically significant drug interactions have been identified

ALTERED LABORATORY VALUES
No clinically significant alterations in blood/serum or urinary values occur at therapeutic dosages

USE IN CHILDREN
See INDICATIONS and ORAL DOSAGE

USE IN PREGNANT AND NURSING WOMEN
Pregnancy Category C: use during pregnancy only when expected benefit outweighs potential risk to the fetus. Diethyl phthalate, an enteric-coating component, is teratogenic in rats at high intraperitoneal doses; however, no evidence of embryotoxicity or teratogenicity has been observed following oral administration of doses 100 times the human dose. No adequate, well-controlled studies have been done in pregnant women. This drug is not absorbed systemically and may safely be used in nursing mothers.

DIGESTANTS

VIOKASE (pancrelipase) Robins — Rx

Tablets: 8,000 units lipase, 30,000 units protease, and 30,000 units amylase[1]   **Powder (per ¼ tsp):** 16,800 units lipase, 70,000 units protease, and 70,000 units amylase[1] (113.5, 227 g)

INDICATIONS
Pancreatic replacement in cystic fibrosis

ORAL DOSAGE
Adult: 1–3 tabs or ¼ tsp (0.7 g) with meals
Child: titrate dosage according to amount of fat in stool

VIOKASE

Exocrine pancreatic deficiency due to chronic pancreatitis	**Adult:** 1–3 tabs with meals or according to medical judgment **Child:** titrate dosage according to amount of fat in stool
Exocrine pancreatic deficiency due to pancreatectomy or obstruction of the pancreatic ducts	**Adult:** 1–2 tabs, given q2h or according to medical judgment **Child:** titrate dosage according to amount of fat in stool

CONTRAINDICATIONS

Hypersensitivity to pork protein

WARNINGS/PRECAUTIONS

Oral irritation	To avoid irritation of the oral mucosa, this preparation should not be held in the mouth
Hypersensitivity	Use with caution in patients allergic to trypsin, pancreatin, or pancrelipase
Respiratory tract irritation, asthma	Inhalation of the powder should be avoided; inhalation will produce irritation of the nasal mucosa and respiratory tract and may precipitate an asthmatic attack, particularly in patients sensitive to pancreatic enzyme concentrates
Hyperuricemia, hyperuricosuria	At extremely high dosages, hyperuricemia and hyperuricosuria may occur
Carcinogenicity	No long-term studies have been done in animals to evaluate the carcinogenic potential of this preparation

ADVERSE REACTIONS

Gastrointestinal	Diarrhea, other transient GI disorders

OVERDOSAGE

Signs and symptoms	Diarrhea, other transient GI disorders
Treatment	Discontinue medication

DRUG INTERACTIONS

No clinically significant drug interactions have been identified

ALTERED LABORATORY VALUES

No clinically significant alterations in blood/serum or urinary values occur at therapeutic dosages

---

USE IN CHILDREN

See INDICATIONS and ORAL DOSAGE

USE IN PREGNANT AND NURSING WOMEN

Pregnancy Category C: reproduction studies have not been performed; use during pregnancy only if clearly needed. It is not known whether this preparation is excreted in human milk; use with caution in nursing mothers.

---

[1] Plus other pancreatic enzymes

Chapter 10

Anthelmintics/Scabicides/Pediculides

Anthelmintics 349

ANTIMINTH (Pfizer) 349
Pyrantel pamoate *Rx*

MINTEZOL (Merck Sharp & Dohme) 349
Thiabendazole *Rx*

NICLOCIDE (Miles Pharmaceuticals) 351
Niclosamide *Rx*

POVAN (Parke-Davis) 352
Pyrvinium pamoate *Rx*

VERMOX (Janssen) 352
Mebendazole *Rx*

Scabicides/Pediculicides 353

KWELL (Reed & Carnrick) 353
Lindane *Rx*

NIX (Burroughs Wellcome) 354
Permethrin *Rx*

R&C SHAMPOO (Reed & Carnrick) 355
Pyrethrins, piperonyl butoxide, and petroleum
distillate *OTC*

RID (Leeming) 356
Pyrethrins, piperonyl butoxide, petroleum distillate,
and benzyl alcohol *OTC*

Other Anthelmintics 348

BILTRICIDE (Miles Pharmaceuticals) 348
Praziquantel *Rx*

VANSIL (Pfizer) 348
Oxamniquine *Rx*

OTHER ANTHELMINTICS

DRUG	HOW SUPPLIED	USUAL DOSAGE
BILTRICIDE (Miles Pharmaceuticals) Praziquantel *Rx*	**Tablets:** 600 mg	**Adult:** for schistosomiasis, 3 doses of 20 mg/kg each, unchewed, given with water or other liquid at 4- to 6-h intervals over a single day **Child ($\geq$ 4 yr):** same as adult
VANSIL (Pfizer) Oxamniquine *Rx*	**Capsules:** 250 mg	**Adult:** for schistosomiasis, 12–15 mg/kg, given in a single dose **Child ($<$ 30 kg):** for schistosomiasis, 20 mg/kg, given in 2 equally divided doses 2–8 h apart **Child ($>$ 30 kg):** same as adult

ANTHELMINTICS

ANTIMINTH (pyrantel pamoate) Pfizer   Rx

Suspension: 50 mg/ml (60 ml) *caramel-flavored*

INDICATIONS	ORAL DOSAGE
Ascariasis (roundworm infection) Enterobiasis (pinworm infection)	**Adult:** 11 mg/kg (1 ml/10 lb), up to 1 g, given in a single dose with milk or fruit juice, if desired **Child (> 2 yr):** same as adult

CONTRAINDICATIONS

None

ADMINISTRATION/DOSAGE ADJUSTMENTS

Timing of administration	May be administered without regard to meal times or time of day
Adjunctive measures	Purging is unnecessary prior to, during, or after therapy

WARNINGS/PRECAUTIONS

Hepatic impairment	Use with caution; drug may cause minor transient elevations of SGOT

ADVERSE REACTIONS

Frequent reactions (incidence ≥ 1%) are printed in *italics*

Gastrointestinal	*Anorexia, nausea, vomiting, gastralgia, abdominal cramps, diarrhea, tenesmus*
Central nervous system	Headache, dizziness, drowsiness, insomnia
Dermatological	Rash

OVERDOSAGE

Signs and symptoms	See ADVERSE REACTIONS
Treatment	Discontinue medication and treat symptomatically

DRUG INTERACTIONS

Piperazine	▽ Anthelmintic effect

ALTERED LABORATORY VALUES

Blood/serum values	△ SGOT (transient)

No clinically significant alterations in urinary values occur at therapeutic dosages

---

USE IN CHILDREN

See INDICATIONS and ORAL DOSAGE; safety for use in children under 2 yr has not been established

USE IN PREGNANT AND NURSING WOMEN

Safety for use in pregnant or nursing women has not been established because no adequate, well-controlled studies have been performed in these populations. No cases of fetal harm or teratogenicity have been reported.

ANTHELMINTICS

MINTEZOL (thiabendazole) Merck Sharp & Dohme   Rx

Chewable tablets: 500 mg   **Suspension (per 5 ml):** 500 mg (120 ml)

INDICATIONS	ORAL DOSAGE
Strongyloidiasis (threadworm infection) **Uncinariasis** (hookworm infection), **trichuriasis** (whipworm infection), and **ascariasis**[1] (large roundworm infection), when more specific treatment cannot be used or a second agent is desired	**Adult:** 10 mg/lb, up to 1.5 g, bid after meals for 2 consecutive days; alternatively, 20 mg/lb, up to 3 g, once daily for 2 consecutive days (side effects are more likely with administration of a single daily dose) **Child (≥ 30 lb):** same as adult
Cutaneous larva migrans (creeping eruption)	**Adult:** 10 mg/lb, up to 1.5 g, bid after meals for 2 consecutive days; if active lesions are still present 2 days after completion of therapy, repeat course **Child:** same as adult
Toxocariasis (visceral larva migrans)	**Adult:** 10 mg/lb, up to 1.5 g, bid after meals for 7 consecutive days (safety and effectiveness of this regimen are based on limited data) **Child:** same as adult

MINTEZOL

Trichinosis during the invasive stage	**Adult:** to reduce eosinophilia and relieve fever and other symptoms, 10 mg/lb, up to 1.5 g, bid after meals for 2–4 consecutive days **Child (≥ 30 lb):** same as adult

CONTRAINDICATIONS

Hypersensitivity to thiabendazole

ADMINISTRATION/DOSAGE ADJUSTMENTS

Administration	Tablets should be chewed before being swallowed
Enterobiasis (pinworm infection)	For most patients, no additional treatment is necessary if any of the indicated infections occurs in combination with enterobiasis

WARNINGS/PRECAUTIONS

Hypersensitivity reactions	Erythema multiforme and other hypersensitivity reactions have occurred during therapy and, in some cases, have resulted in death; discontinue use immediately if hypersensitivity is evident
Drowsiness, dizziness	Caution patients to avoid activities requiring mental alertness; CNS reactions may occur quite frequently
Special-risk patients	Provide supportive therapy for anemic, dehydrated, or malnourished patients before beginning use of thiabendazole; carefully observe patients with hepatic or renal impairment during treatment
Prophylactic therapy	This preparation should not be used for prophylactic treatment
Carcinogenicity, mutagenicity, effect of fertility	No evidence of carcinogenicity has been seen in animals given up to 15 times the human dose, no mutagenic activity has been detected in microbial assays (in vitro and host-mediated) or the micronucleus test, and no adverse effect on fertility has occurred in mice given 2.5 times the human dose or in rats given the equivalent of the human dose

ADVERSE REACTIONS

Gastrointestinal	Anorexia, nausea, vomiting, diarrhea, epigastric distress
Hepatic	Jaundice, cholestasis, parenchymal liver damage
Central nervous system	Dizziness, weariness, drowsiness, giddiness, headache, numbness, hyperirritability, convulsions, collapse, psychic disturbances
Ophthalmic	Abnormal sensation in eyes, blurred vision, xanthopsia, dry eyes
Genitourinary	Hematuria, enuresis, malodorous urine, crystalluria
Hypersensitivity	Pruritus, fever, facial flushing, chills, conjunctival infection, angioedema, anaphylaxis, perianal rash and other skin rashes, erythema multiforme (including Stevens-Johnson syndrome), lymphadenopathy
Other	Tinnitus, hypotension, hyperglycemia, transient leukopenia, appearance of live *Ascaris* in the mouth and nose, drying of mucous membranes

OVERDOSAGE

Signs and symptoms	Visual disturbances, CNS reactions
Treatment	Induce emesis or perform gastric lavage carefully; treat symptomatically, and institute supportive measures

DRUG INTERACTIONS

Theophylline	⇧ Serum theophylline level; monitor serum level and, if necessary, adjust dosage

ALTERED LABORATORY VALUES

Blood/serum values	⇧ Glucose ⇧ SGOT (transient) ⇧ Cephalin flocculation (transient)

No clinically significant alterations in urinary values occur at therapeutic dosages

---

USE IN CHILDREN

See INDICATIONS and ORAL DOSAGE; clinical experience with thiabendazole for treatment of strongyloidiasis, ascariasis, uncinariasis, trichuriasis, and trichinosis in children weighing under 30 lb is limited

USE IN PREGNANT AND NURSING WOMEN

Pregnancy Category C: no evidence of harm to the fetus has been detected in rabbits given up to 15 times the human dose, rats given the equivalent of the human dose, mice given 2.5 times the human dose, and mice given an aqueous suspension containing 10 times the human dose; however, cleft palate and axial skeletal defects have occurred in mice given an olive oil suspension containing 10 times the human dose. No adequate, well-controlled studies have been done in pregnant women. Use during pregnancy only if the expected benefit justifies the potential risk to the fetus. It is not known whether thiabendazole is excreted in human milk; patients should not nurse while taking this drug.

---

[1] For treatment of mixed infections associated with *Ascaris*, thiabendazole is not considered a suitable agent because it may cause the worms to migrate

ANTHELMINTICS

NICLOCIDE (niclosamide) Miles Pharmaceuticals   Rx

Chewable tablets: 500 mg *vanilla-flavored*

INDICATIONS	ORAL DOSAGE
Tapeworm infections caused by *Taenia saginata* (beef tapeworm) or *Diphyllobothrium latum* (fish tapeworm)	**Adult:** 2 g, given in a single dose **Child (11–34 kg):** 1 g, given in a single dose **Child (> 34 kg):** 1.5 g, given in a single dose
Tapeworm infections caused by *Hymenolepsis nana* (dwarf tapeworm)	**Adult:** 2 g/day, given in single daily doses for a period of 7 days **Child (11–34 kg):** 1 g, given in a single dose on the first day, followed by 0.5 g/day, given in single daily doses for the next 6 days **Child (> 34 kg):** 1.5 g, given in a single dose on the first day, followed by 1 g/day, given in single daily doses for the next 6 days

CONTRAINDICATIONS
Hypersensitivity to any component

ADMINISTRATION/DOSAGE ADJUSTMENTS

Oral administration	Tablets must be thoroughly chewed, and then swallowed with a little water, preferably after a light meal (eg, after breakfast); for young children, tablets should be pulverized and then mixed with a small amount of water to form a paste
Evaluation of treatment	It is not always possible to identify the scolex in stools, because after the tapeworm is killed, the scolex and proximal segments may be digested during their passage through the intestine; thus, the sooner the tapeworm is passed and examined after treatment, the better the chance of identifying the scolex. In constipated patients, it may be desirable to use a mild laxative. *T saginata* or *D latum* segments and/or ova may appear in the stool for up to 3 days after therapy; if they are still present 7 days after therapy, the course of treatment may be repeated. Complete cure is indicated by the absence of tapeworm segments and ova in the stool for a minimum of 3 mo.

WARNINGS/PRECAUTIONS

Patients with *H nana* infections	Caution patients to observe strict personal and environmental hygiene to avoid autoinfection
Patients with cysticercosis	Because niclosamide is active only against intestinal cestodes, it is not effective in the treatment of cysticercosis
Carcinogenicity, mutagenicity	Long-term studies in rats and mice of the ethanolamine salt of niclosamide have shown no evidence of carcinogenicity; mutagenicity tests have not been performed

ADVERSE REACTIONS
Frequent reactions (incidence ≥ 1%) are printed in *italics*

Gastrointestinal	*Nausea and vomiting (4.1%); abdominal discomfort, including anorexia (3.4%); diarrhea (1.6%);* constipation
Central nervous system	*Drowsiness, dizziness, and/or headache (1.4%);* irritability
Dermatological	Rash, including pruritus ani (0.3%); alopecia[1]
Other	Oral irritation, fever, rectal bleeding, bad taste in mouth, sweating, palpitations, edema of an arm, backache

OVERDOSAGE

Signs and symptoms	See ADVERSE REACTIONS
Treatment	A fast-acting laxative and enema should be given; *do not induce vomiting*

DRUG INTERACTIONS
No clinically significant drug interactions have been identified

ALTERED LABORATORY VALUES

Blood/serum values	⇧ SGOT (transient; observed in a narcotic addict)

No clinically significant alterations in urinary values occur at therapeutic dosages

---

USE IN CHILDREN

Safety for use in children under 2 yr of age has not been established

USE IN PREGNANT AND NURSING WOMEN

Pregnancy Category B: use during pregnancy only if clearly needed. Reproduction studies in rabbits and rats given 25 times the human dose and in mice given 12 times the human dose have shown no evidence of impaired fertility or harm to the fetus; however, no adequate, well-controlled studies have been done in pregnant women. No studies on the use of this drug in nursing mothers have been reported.

---

[1] Two cases of urticaria possibly due to the tapeworm's breakdown products have been reported

COMPENDIUM OF DRUG THERAPY

ANTHELMINTICS

POVAN (pyrvinium pamoate) Parke-Davis Rx

Tablets: 50 mg

INDICATIONS	ORAL DOSAGE
Enterobiasis (pinworm infection)	**Adult:** 5 mg/kg, up to 350 mg, given in a single dose; if necessary, dose may be repeated in 2 or 3 wk **Child:** same as adult

CONTRAINDICATIONS

None known

ADMINISTRATION/DOSAGE ADJUSTMENTS

Mass treatment of enterobiasis	To ensure complete parasite eradication, consider treatment of all members of family or institution group

WARNINGS/PRECAUTIONS

Red stool and vomitus	Patient (or parent) should be cautioned in advance to expect red discoloration due to pyrvinium pamoate; vomitus will stain most materials
Gastrointestinal reactions	Occur more often in older children and adults who have received large doses

ADVERSE REACTIONS

Gastrointestinal	Nausea, vomiting (especially with suspension), cramping, diarrhea
Hypersensitivity	Photosensitivity, allergic reactions

OVERDOSAGE

Signs and symptoms	See ADVERSE REACTIONS
Treatment	Discontinue medication; treat symptomatically

DRUG INTERACTIONS

No clinically significant drug interactions have been identified

ALTERED LABORATORY VALUES

No clinically significant alterations in blood/serum or urinary values occur at therapeutic dosages

USE IN CHILDREN	USE IN PREGNANT AND NURSING WOMEN
See INDICATIONS and ORAL DOSAGE	Safety for use during pregnancy has not been established. Consult manufacturer for use in nursing mothers.

ANTHELMINTICS

VERMOX (mebendazole) Janssen Rx

Chewable tablets: 100 mg

INDICATIONS	ORAL DOSAGE
Enterobiasis (pinworm infection)	**Adult:** 100 mg, given in a single dose; if patient is not cured 3 wk later, repeat; tablet may be chewed, swallowed whole, or crushed and mixed with food **Child (> 2 yr):** same as adult
Ascariasis (roundworm infection) Trichuriasis (whipworm infection) Uncinariasis (hookworm infection) caused by *Necator americanus* and *Ancylostoma duodenale*	**Adult:** 100 mg bid (AM and PM) for 3 consecutive days; if patient is not cured 3 wk later, repeat; tablet may be chewed, swallowed whole, or crushed and mixed with food **Child (> 2 yr):** same as adult

CONTRAINDICATIONS

Hypersensitivity to mebendazole

ADMINISTRATION/DOSAGE ADJUSTMENTS

Adjunctive measures	Fasting and purging are unnecessary

VERMOX ■ KWELL

WARNINGS/PRECAUTIONS

Pregnancy	Caution patients about the potential risk of use during pregnancy (see USE IN PREGNANT AND NURSING MOTHERS)
Cleanliness	Inform patients that cleanliness is important in preventing transmission of disease and reinfection
Hydatid disease	There is no evidence that mebendazole is effective, even at high doses, in the treatment of hydatid disease
Carcinogenicity, mutagenicity	No evidence of carcinogenicity has been observed in mice or rats given up to 40 mg/kg/day for 2 yr; no mutagenic effects have been demonstrated in the dominant lethal mutation test (in rats given up to 640 mg/kg) or in the spermatocyte, F_1 translocation, and Ames tests
Effect on fertility	No evidence of impaired fertility has been seen in mice after doses of up to 40 mg/kg had been given for a period of 60 days (males) or 14 days (females) before gestation; however, slight maternal toxicity has been detected at this dose level

ADVERSE REACTIONS

Gastrointestinal	Transient abdominal pain and diarrhea in cases of massive infection and expulsion of worms

OVERDOSAGE

Signs and symptoms	Gastrointestinal reactions persisting for up to a few hours may occur
Treatment	Induce vomiting and purging

DRUG INTERACTIONS

No clinically significant drug interactions have been identified

ALTERED LABORATORY VALUES

No clinically significant alterations in blood/serum or urinary values occur at therapeutic dosages

---

USE IN CHILDREN

See INDICATIONS and ORAL DOSAGE; safety for use in children under 2 yr of age has not been established

USE IN PREGNANT AND NURSING WOMEN

Pregnancy Category C: embryotoxic and teratogenic effects have been detected in rats given single oral doses as low as 10 mg/kg; however, a limited post-marketing survey of women who had inadvertently taken this drug during the first trimester of pregnancy showed no increase in the incidence of spontaneous abortion or malformation, and observation of 170 deliveries at term revealed no increase in teratogenic risk. Use during pregnancy, particularly during the first trimester, is not recommended; administer only if the expected benefits justify the potential risk to the fetus. It is now known whether mebendazole is excreted in human milk; use with caution in nursing mothers.

SCABICIDES/PEDICULICIDES

KWELL (lindane) Reed & Carnrick   Rx

Cream: 1% (57, 454 g)   **Lotion:** 1% (59, 472 ml; 3.8 liters)   **Shampoo:** 1% (59, 472 ml; 3.8 liters)

INDICATIONS

Scabies (*Sarcoptes scabiei* and their ova)

Pediculosis capitis (head lice and their ova)
Pediculosis pubis (pubic lice and their ova)

TOPICAL DOSAGE

Adult and child: apply a thin layer of the cream or lotion to dry skin in sufficient quantity (usually 2 oz for an adult) to cover the entire body from the neck down, including the soles of the feet. Thoroughly massage the preparation into all skin surfaces, leave it in place for 8–12 h, and then remove by thorough washing.

Adult and child: apply a sufficient amount of shampoo to dry hair (approximately 30 ml for short, 45 ml for medium, and 60 ml for long hair), work it thoroughly into the hair, and allow it to remain in place for 4 min. Add small quantities of water until a good lather forms, then rinse thoroughly and towel dry briskly. When hair is dry, remove any remaining nits or nit shells with a nit comb or tweezers.

CONTRAINDICATIONS

Prematurity (see USE IN CHILDREN)	Known seizure disorder	Sensitivity to any component

ADMINISTRATION/DOSAGE ADJUSTMENTS

Application	Avoid unnecessary skin contact or use on open cuts or extensive excoriations; those assisting in lindane therapy, especially pregnant or nursing women, should wear rubber gloves

KWELL ■ NIX

Preparation for shampooing	If an oil-based hair dressing has been used, the hair should be shampooed and dried before application of lindane shampoo
Crusted scabies lesions	A tepid bath preceding application may be helpful; allow the skin to dry before applying the cream or lotion
Duration of therapy	One application of cream or lotion for scabies is usually curative; retreatment of lice infestations is usually unnecessary and should be performed only if living lice are demonstrable after 7 days
Treatment of sexual contacts	Sexual contacts of infested patients should be treated simultaneously
Prophylactic use	This preparation has no residual effects and, therefore, should not be used to ward off a possible infestation

WARNINGS/PRECAUTIONS

CNS toxicity	Lindane penetrates human skin and may cause CNS toxicity, particularly in the young; be especially careful not to exceed the recommended dosage when using on infants, pregnant women, or nursing mothers (see also USE IN PREGNANT AND NURSING WOMEN). Seizures have been reported following excessive topical use or oral ingestion (see OVERDOSAGE). Simultaneous application of creams, ointments, or oils should be avoided since it may enhance the percutaneous absorption of lindane.
Contact with eyes	Avoid contact with the eyes; if accidental contact occurs, flush eyes with water immediately
Irritation or sensitization	Discontinue use if irritation or sensitization occurs
Pruritus	Many patients experience persistent pruritus after treatment for scabies; persistent itching is rarely a sign of treatment failure and is not in itself an indication for retreatment, unless living mites can be found
Carcinogenicity, mutagenicity	Long-term studies in mice and rats have shown no evidence of carcinogenicity, except for one unconfirmed report that linked 600 ppm of lindane with an increased incidence of hepatoma. The results of numerous mutagenicity tests have been negative.

ADVERSE REACTIONS

Central nervous system	Stimulation ranging from dizziness to convulsions (usually associated with accidental ingestion or misuse)
Local	Eczematous eruptions due to irritation

OVERDOSAGE

Signs and symptoms	Central nervous system excitation and convulsions
Treatment	Empty stomach immediately by gastric lavage and administer a saline cathartic to dilute bowel contents and hasten evacuation; avoid use of oil laxatives, which may promote lindane absorption. Treat CNS excitation with pentobarbital, phenobarbital, or diazepam. Institute supportive measures, as needed.

DRUG INTERACTIONS

Oil-based hair dressings, creams, and ointments	△ Absorption of lindane; do not use oil-based products with lindane

ALTERED LABORATORY VALUES

No clinically significant alterations in blood/serum or urinary values occur at therapeutic dosages

---

USE IN CHILDREN

See INDICATIONS and TOPICAL DOSAGE; contraindicated for use on premature neonates because their skin may be more permeable than that of full-term infants and their liver enzymes may be insufficiently developed (see also "CNS toxicity," above)

USE IN PREGNANT AND NURSING WOMEN

Pregnancy Category B: reproduction studies performed in mice, rats, rabbits, pigs, and dogs at doses up to 10 times the human dose of lindane have revealed no evidence of impaired fertility or fetal harm. However, no adequate, well-controlled studies have been done in pregnant women. Use with caution in pregnant women, do not exceed the recommended dose in these patients, and treat them no more than twice during a pregnancy (see WARNINGS/PRECAUTIONS). Small amounts of lindane are excreted in human milk; although these amounts are unlikely to cause serious adverse effects, an alternative method of feeding may be used for 2 days following lindane treatment.

VEHICLE/BASE
Cream (scented, water-dispersible): stearic acid, glycerin, lanolin, 2-amino-2-methyl-1-propanol, perfume, and purified water
Lotion (nongreasy): glycerol monostearate, cetyl alcohol, stearic acid, trolamine, 2-amino-2-methyl-1-propanol, methyl *p*-hydroxybenzoate, butyl-*p*-hydroxybenzoate, carrageenan, perfume, and purified water
Shampoo: trolamine lauryl sulfate, polysorbate 60, acetone, and purified water

---

SCABICIDES/PEDICULICIDES

NIX (permethrin) Burroughs Wellcome Rx
Cream rinse: 1% (2 fl oz)

INDICATIONS

Pediculosis capitis (head lice and their ova)

TOPICAL DOSAGE

Adult and child ($\geq$ 2 yr): after scalp hair has been shampooed, rinsed with water, and dried with a towel, apply a sufficient amount of the cream rinse to saturate hair and scalp, wait 10 min, and then rinse hair with water. Nits may be removed with a comb after hair has been dried; combing is not necessary, but it may be done for cosmetic or other reasons.

NIX ■ R & C SHAMPOO

CONTRAINDICATIONS
Hypersensitivity to any component, chrysanthemums, or any synthetic pyrethroid or pyrethrin

ADMINISTRATION/DOSAGE ADJUSTMENTS

Re-treatment	A single application of the cream rinse is usually effective; if living lice are observed 7 or more days after the initial application, the cream rinse may be applied again[1]

WARNINGS/PRECAUTIONS

Irritation	Pruritus, erythema, and edema, which are often associated with head lice infestation, may be temporarily exacerbated by use of this preparation; instruct patient to report persistent irritation
Contact with eyes	Although this drug is not irritating to the eyes, patients should be instructed to avoid contact with eyes during application and to flush their eyes with water immediately following accidental contact
Ingestion of product	To prevent accidental ingestion by children, discard the contents remaining in the bottle after use; if ingestion occurs, perform gastric lavage and institute general supportive measures
Carcinogenicity, mutagenicity	An increase in pulmonary alveolar-cell carcinomas and benign liver adenomas has been observed in female mice fed permethrin at a concentration of 5,000 ppm; no evidence of tumorigenicity has been seen in rats. Results of all mutagenicity assays have been negative.
Effect on fertility	When fed to three generations of rats at a dose of 180 mg/kg/day, permethrin caused no adverse effect on reproductive function

ADVERSE REACTIONS
Frequent reactions (incidence ≥ 1%) are printed in *italics*

Local	*Mild temporary itching (5.9%); mild transient burning/stinging, tingling, numbness, or discomfort (3.4%); mild transient erythema, edema, or rash of the scalp (2.1%)*

USE IN CHILDREN
See INDICATIONS and TOPICAL DOSAGE; safety and effectiveness for use in children under 2 yr of age have not been established

USE IN PREGNANT AND NURSING WOMEN
Pregnancy Category B: reproduction studies in mice, rats, and rabbits fed 200–400 mg/kg/day have shown no evidence of harm to the fetus; however, no adequate, well controlled studies have been performed in pregnant women. Use during pregnancy only if clearly needed. It is not known whether permethrin is excreted in human milk; since animal studies have produced evidence of tumorigenicity and since many drugs are excreted in human milk, it may be advisable to withhold this drug from women who are nursing or to discontinue nursing temporarily while it is being used.

VEHICLE/BASE
Cream rinse: stearalkonium chloride, hydrolyzed animal protein, cetyl alcohol, polyoxyethylene 10 cetyl ether, hydroxyethylcellulose, balsam canada, fragrance, citric acid, propylene glycol, FD&C Yellow No. 6, 20% isopropyl alcohol, methylparaben, propylparaben, and imidazolidinyl urea

[1] In clinical trials, re-treatment was necessary in less than 1% of patients

---

SCABICIDES/PEDICULICIDES

R&C SHAMPOO (pyrethrins, piperonyl butoxide, and petroleum distillate) Reed & Carnrick OTC
Liquid: 0.3% pyrethrins, 3% piperonyl butoxide (technical grade), and 1.2% petroleum distillate (2, 4 fl oz)

INDICATIONS
Pediculosis capitis (head lice and their ova)
Pediculosis corporis (body lice and their ova)
Pediculosis pubis (crab lice and their ova)

TOPICAL DOSAGE
Adult: apply a sufficient quantity of shampoo to thoroughly wet dry hair and skin, paying particular attention to infested and adjacent hairy areas; allow shampoo to remain in place for 10 min, then add small amounts of water, working the shampoo into the hair and skin to form a lather. Rinse thoroughly. If indicated, remove dead lice and eggs with fine-tooth comb. Do not exceed two applications within 24 h.
Child: same as adult

WARNINGS/PRECAUTIONS

Internal consumption	Ingestion or inhalation of this product may be harmful; avoid contamination of feed and foodstuffs
Contact with mucous membranes	Avoid contact with mucous membranes; if accidental contact with the eyes occurs, flush immediately with water
Ragweed sensitivity	This product should not be used by ragweed-sensitized persons
To prevent reinfestation and infesting others	Clothes, linens, and hair tools used by the infested person during the last month should be washed in hot water (130° F) or dry-cleaned; toilet seats should be scrubbed and rugs and upholstery vacuumed frequently. Spray noncleanable items with R & C Spray. All family members should be examined for 3 wk for signs of infestation.

COMPENDIUM OF DRUG THERAPY

Infestation of eyelashes or eyebrows	This product should not be applied to eyelashes or eyebrows; label cautions patient to consult a physician in the event of louse infestation of eyelashes or eyebrows
Skin infection or irritation	Discontinue use in the event of infection or irritation

ADVERSE REACTIONS
None reported by manufacturer

USE IN CHILDREN	USE IN PREGNANT AND NURSING WOMEN
See INDICATIONS and TOPICAL DOSAGE	There are no warnings regarding use of this product in pregnant or nursing women

VEHICLE/BASE
Shampoo: C-13-14 isoparaffin, fragrance, isocetyl alcohol, isopropyl alcohol, lauramine oxide, laureth-4, laureth-23, TEA-lauryl sulfate, and water

---

SCABICIDES/PEDICULICIDES

RID (pyrethrins, piperonyl butoxide, petroleum distillate, and benzyl alcohol) Leeming   OTC

Liquid: 0.3% pyrethrins, 3.00% piperonyl butoxide (technical grade), 1.20% petroleum distillate, and 2.4% benzyl alcohol (2, 4 fl oz)

INDICATIONS
Pediculosis capitis (head lice and their ova)
Pediculosis corporis (body lice and their ova)
Pediculosis pubis (crab lice and their ova)

TOPICAL DOSAGE
Adult: apply liquid undiluted to dry hair and scalp (avoiding eyelashes and eyebrows) or to other infested areas until entirely wet; wait 10 min (but no longer), then wash thoroughly with warm water and soap or shampoo, dry hair, and comb out dead lice and eggs. Do not exceed two applications within 24 h. Treatment should be repeated in 7–10 days in order to kill any newly hatched lice.
Child: same as adult

WARNINGS/PRECAUTIONS

Internal consumption	Ingestion or inhalation of this product may be harmful; avoid contamination of feed and foodstuffs
Contact with mucous membranes	Avoid contact with mucous membranes; if accidental contact with the eyes occurs, flush immediately with water
Ragweed sensitivity	This product should be used with caution by ragweed-sensitized persons
Patient instructions	This product should not be used for infestations of the eyebrows or eyelashes or inhaled; advise patient to discontinue use and seek medical attention if infection or skin irritation occurs; patients should not use on acutely inflamed skin or raw weeping surfaces
Concurrent infestation of other family members	Infested family members should be treated promptly to avoid reinfestation of previously treated patients or spread to uninfested individuals
Contaminated clothing and other apparel (eg, hats)	Should be dry-cleaned, washed in hot (130° F), soapy water, or otherwise decontaminated to avoid reinfestation or spread

ADVERSE REACTIONS

Local	Irritation, urticaria, pruritus, erythema, edema

USE IN CHILDREN	USE IN PREGNANT AND NURSING WOMEN
See INDICATIONS and TOPICAL DOSAGE	Safety for use in pregnant or nursing women has not been established because no adequate, well-controlled studies have been done in these populations; however, no cases of fetal harm or teratogenicity have been reported.

Chapter 11

Antianginal Agents

Beta-Adrenergic Blockers — 358

CORGARD (Princeton) — 358
Nadolol *Rx*

INDERAL (Ayerst) — 359
Propranolol hydrochloride *Rx*

INDERAL LA (Ayerst) — 362
Propranolol hydrochloride *Rx*

LOPRESSOR (Geigy) — 363
Metoprolol tartrate *Rx*

TENORMIN (Stuart) — 366
Atenolol *Rx*

Calcium Antagonists — 368

ADALAT (Miles Pharmaceuticals) — 368
Nifedipine *Rx*

CALAN (Searle) — 370
Verapamil hydrochloride *Rx*

CALAN SR (Searle) — 370
Verapamil hydrochloride *Rx*
370

CALAN SR (Searle) — 370
Verapamil hydrochloride *Rx*

CARDIZEM (Marion) — 372
Diltiazem hydrochloride *Rx*

ISOPTIN (Knoll) — 374
Verapamil hydrochloride *Rx*

ISOPTIN SR (Knoll) — 374
Verapamil hydrochloride *Rx*

PROCARDIA (Pfizer) — 376
Nifedipine *Rx*

Nitrates — 379

CARDILATE (Burroughs Wellcome) — 379
Erythrityl tetranitrate *Rx*

DEPONIT (Wyeth) — 379
Nitroglycerin *Rx*

DILATRATE-SR (Reed & Carnrick) — 380
Isosorbide dinitrate *Rx*

ISORDIL (Wyeth) — 382
Isosorbide dinitrate *Rx*

NITRO-BID (Marion) — 383
Nitroglycerin *Rx*

NITRO-BID Ointment (Marion) — 384
Nitroglycerin *Rx*

NITRO-BID IV (Marion) — 385
Nitroglycerin *Rx*

NITRO-DUR (Key) — 386
Nitroglycerin *Rx*

NITRO-DUR II (Key) — 386
Nitroglycerin *Rx*

NITRODISC (Searle) — 387
Nitroglycerin *Rx*

NITROGARD (Parke-Davis) — 388
Nitroglycerin *Rx*

NITROL Ointment (Rorer) — 390
Nitroglycerin *Rx*

NITROL IV (Rorer) — 391
Nitroglycerin *Rx*

NITROLINGUAL (Rorer) — 393
Nitroglycerin *Rx*

NITROSTAT (Parke-Davis) — 394
Nitroglycerin *Rx*

NITROSTAT Ointment (Parke-Davis) — 394
Nitroglycerin *Rx*

NITROSTAT IV (Parke-Davis) — 395
Nitroglycerin *Rx*

NTS (Bolar) — 397
Nitroglycerin *Rx*

PERITRATE (Parke-Davis) — 398
Pentaerythritol tetranitrate *Rx*

PERITRATE SA (Parke-Davis) — 398
Pentaerythritol tetranitrate *Rx*

SORBITRATE (Stuart) — 399
Isosorbide dinitrate *Rx*

TRANSDERM-Nitro (CIBA) — 400
Nitroglycerin *Rx*

TRIDIL (Du Pont Critical Care) — 402
Nitroglycerin *Rx*

Other Antianginal Agents — 357

Amyl nitrite *Rx* — 357

OTHER ANTIANGINAL AGENTS

DRUG	HOW SUPPLIED	USUAL DOSAGE[1]
Amyl nitrite *Rx*	Ampuls: 0.18, 0.3 ml	Adult: 0.18–0.3 ml by inhalation, as needed

[1] Where pediatric dosages are not given, consult manufacturer

COMPENDIUM OF DRUG THERAPY

CORGARD

BETA-ADRENERGIC BLOCKERS

CORGARD (nadolol) Princeton   Rx
Tablets: 40, 80, 120, 160 mg

INDICATIONS	**ORAL DOSAGE**
Angina pectoris	**Adult:** 40 mg once daily to start, followed by increments of 40–80 mg/day every 3–7 days until optimal response is achieved, pronounced slowing of heart rate occurs, or a maximum dosage of 240 mg/day is reached; usual maintenance dosage: 40–80 mg once daily
Hypertension	**Adult:** 40 mg once daily (alone or with a diuretic) to start, followed by increments of 40–80 mg/day, as needed, up to 320 mg/day; usual maintenance dosage: 40–80 mg once daily

CONTRAINDICATIONS		
Bronchial asthma	Conduction block greater than first degree	Overt cardiac failure (see WARNINGS/PRECAUTIONS)
Sinus bradycardia	Cardiogenic shock	

ADMINISTRATION/DOSAGE ADJUSTMENTS	
Patients with renal impairment	Increase interval between doses as follows: administer q24h when creatinine clearance rate (Ccr) > 50 ml/min; q24–36h when Ccr = 31–50 ml/min; q24–48h when Ccr = 10–30 ml/min; q40–60h when Ccr < 10 ml/min
Combination therapy	May be used at full dosage in combination with other antihypertensive agents, especially thiazide-type diuretics
Discontinuation of therapy	Reduce dosage gradually over 1–2 wk, if possible, and monitor patient closely. Caution patients with angina or hyperthyroidism against interruption or abrupt cessation of therapy (see WARNINGS/PRECAUTIONS).

WARNINGS/PRECAUTIONS	
Cardiac failure	May be precipitated by further or continued depression of myocardial contractility; discontinue use (gradually, if possible) if cardiac failure occurs or persists despite adequate digitalization and diuretic therapy. In cases of well-compensated congestive heart failure, use with caution.
Abrupt discontinuation	May exacerbate angina pectoris and, in some cases, lead to myocardial infarction in patients with ischemic heart disease
Impaired response to reflex adrenergic stimuli	May augment the risks of general anesthesia and surgery, resulting in protracted hypotension or low cardiac output, and, occasionally, difficulty in restarting and maintaining heartbeat. If possible, discontinue use well before surgery takes place. Excessive beta blockade occurring during emergency surgery can be reversed by IV administration of a beta-receptor agonist (eg, isoproterenol, dopamine, dobutamine, or norepinephrine).
Diabetes mellitus	Beta blockade may mask symptoms of hypoglycemia and potentiate insulin-induced hypoglycemia; use with caution, especially in patients with labile diabetes
Thyrotoxicosis	Clinical signs of hyperthyroidism may be masked; abrupt withdrawal may precipitate thyroid storm
Nonallergic bronchospasm	Use with caution in patients with bronchospastic diseases, since bronchodilation produced by beta stimulation may be blocked
Hepatic or renal impairment	Use with caution and monitor for signs of excessive drug accumulation (see OVERDOSAGE)

ADVERSE REACTIONS[1]	Frequent reactions (incidence ≥ 1%) are printed in *italics*
Cardiovascular	*Heart rate < 40 beats/min and/or symptomatic bradycardia, peripheral vascular insufficiency (2%); cardiac failure, hypotension, and rhythm and/or conduction disturbances (1%);* first- and third-degree heart block
Central nervous system	*Dizziness and fatigue (2%);* paresthesias, sedation, changed behavior, headache, slurred speech
Respiratory	Bronchospasm, cough, nasal stuffiness
Gastrointestinal	Nausea, diarrhea, abdominal discomfort, constipation, vomiting, indigestion, anorexia, bloating, flatulence, dry mouth
Dermatological	Rash, pruritus, dry skin, facial swelling, diaphoresis, reversible alopecia
Ophthalmic	Dry eyes, blurred vision
Genitourinary	Impotence or decreased libido
Other	Weight gain, tinnitus

CORGARD ■ INDERAL

OVERDOSAGE

Signs and symptoms	Excessive bradycardia, cardiac failure, hypotension, bronchospasm
Treatment	Empty stomach by gastric lavage. Hemodialysis may be useful. For excessive bradycardia, administer 0.25–1.0 mg atropine; if there is no response to vagal blockade, administer isoproterenol cautiously. For cardiac failure, administer digitalis and a diuretic; IV glucagon may be helpful. For hypotension, administer a vasopressor, such as norepinephrine or (preferably) epinephrine. Treat bronchospasm with a beta$_2$-stimulating agent (eg, isoproterenol) and/or a theophylline derivative.

DRUG INTERACTIONS

Digitalis	▽ AV conduction
Reserpine, *Rauwolfia* alkaloids	△ Risk of vertigo, syncope, or orthostatic hypotension
Insulin, sulfonylureas	Hypo- or hyperglycemic effect; if necessary, adjust antidiabetic dosage
General anesthetics	△ Hypotension (see WARNINGS/PRECAUTIONS)

ALTERED LABORATORY VALUES

No clinically significant alterations in blood/serum or urinary values have yet been reported at therapeutic dosages

USE IN CHILDREN

Safety and effectiveness for use in children have not been established

USE IN PREGNANT AND NURSING WOMEN

Pregnancy Category C: embryotoxicity and fetotoxicity have been shown in rabbits, but not in rats or hamsters, at 5–10 times the maximum human dose; women receiving nadolol at parturition have given birth to neonates manifesting bradycardia, hypoglycemia, and associated symptoms. Use this drug during pregnancy only if the expected benefits justify the potential risks to the fetus. Nadolol is excreted in human milk; patients should not nurse during therapy.

[1] Other reactions associated with beta blocker therapy but not observed with nadolol include intensification of AV block (see CONTRAINDICATIONS); reversible mental depression progressing to catatonia; visual disturbances, hallucinations; an acute reversible syndrome characterized by temporal and spatial disorientation, short-term memory loss, emotional lability, slightly clouded sensorium, and decreased performance on neuropsychometric tests; mesenteric arterial thrombosis, ischemic colitis, elevated liver enzymes, agranulocytosis; thrombocytopenic and nonthrombocytopenic purpura; fever combined with aching and sore throat; laryngospasm; respiratory distress, pemphigoid rash, hypertensive reactions in patients with pheochromocytoma, sleep disturbances, and Peyronie's disease

---

BETA-ADRENERGIC BLOCKERS

INDERAL (propranolol hydrochloride) Ayerst   Rx

Tablets: 10, 20, 40, 60, 80, 90 mg   **Ampuls:** 1 mg/ml (1 ml)

INDICATIONS	ORAL DOSAGE
Hypertension	**Adult:** 40 mg bid (alone or with a diuretic) to start, followed by gradual increments until optimal response is achieved, up to 640 mg/day; usual maintenance dosage: 120–240 mg/day **Child:** 0.5 mg/kg bid to start, followed by gradual increments until optimal response is achieved, up to 16 mg/kg/day; usual maintenance dosage: 1–2 mg/kg bid
Long-term management of **angina pectoris**	**Adult:** 80–320 mg/day, given in 2–4 divided doses
Cardiac arrhythmias, including supraventricular arrhythmias, ventricular tachycardias, digitalis-induced tachyarrhythmias, and resistant tachyarrhythmias due to excessive catecholamine activity during anesthesia	**Adult:** 10–30 mg tid or qid, before meals and at bedtime
Reduction of cardiovascular mortality in clinically stable patients following **acute myocardial infarction**	**Adult:** 180–240 mg/day, given in divided doses bid or tid; patients with angina, hypertension, or other coexisting cardiovascular diseases may require dosages exceeding 240 mg/day. In clinical studies, long-term therapy was started 5–21 days after infarction.
Migraine prophylaxis	**Adult:** 80 mg/day in divided doses to start, followed, if necessary, by gradual increments, up to 240 mg/day; usual dosage: 160–240 mg/day. If satisfactory prophylaxis is not obtained after giving 240 mg/day for 4–6 wk, discontinue use.
Familial or hereditary **essential tremor**	**Adult:** 40 mg bid to start, followed, if necessary, by increases in dosage, up to 320 mg/day; usual maintenance dosage: 120 mg/day
Hypertrophic subaortic stenosis	**Adult:** 20–40 mg tid or qid, before meals and at bedtime

COMPENDIUM OF DRUG THERAPY

INDERAL

As an adjunct to alpha-adrenergic blocking agents in the management of **pheochromocytoma**

Adult: 60 mg/day in divided doses for 3 days prior to surgery, concomitantly with an alpha-adrenergic blocking agent, or 30 mg/day in divided doses for inoperable tumors

CONTRAINDICATIONS

Sinus bradycardia	Cardiogenic shock	Overt congestive heart failure, unless it results from a tachyarrhythmia treatable with propranolol
Heart block greater than first degree	Bronchial asthma	

ADMINISTRATION/DOSAGE ADJUSTMENTS

Intravenous use	For life-threatening arrhythmias or those occurring under anesthesia in adults, give 1–3 mg IV. To minimize risk of hypotension and possibility of cardiac standstill, administer slowly ($\leq$ 1 mg/min) and monitor ECG and CVP continuously. Initial dose may be repeated after 2 min; thereafter, wait at least 4 h before administering additional propranolol.
Inadequate control of hypertension	Twice-daily dosing is usually effective. Some patients, however, experience a modest rise in blood pressure toward the end of the 12-h dosing interval, especially when lower dosages are used. If control is inadequate, a larger dose or tid therapy may be indicated.
Discontinuation of therapy	Reduce dosage gradually over a period of several weeks; caution patients who experience angina or who may have occult coronary artery disease not to interrupt or discontinue therapy on their own
Tremor	Essential tremor is usually limited to the upper limbs; it appears only when a limb moves or is held in a fixed position against gravity. Propranolol reduces the intensity of tremors, but not their frequency; this drug is not indicated for treatment of tremor associated with parkinsonism.

WARNINGS/PRECAUTIONS

Cardiac failure	Beta blockade may cause or exacerbate cardiac failure; discontinue use if this disorder does not stabilize after diuretic therapy and digitalization. If necessary, propranolol may be given to patients with well-compensated congestive heart failure; observe such patients closely.
Thyrotoxicosis	Propranolol may mask certain clinical signs of hyperthyroidism; abrupt withdrawal may exacerbate manifestations of this disorder and precipitate a thyroid storm
Patients with angina	Abrupt withdrawal in such patients may exacerbate angina and, in some cases, lead to myocardial infarction; reinstitute therapy if withdrawal reactions occur (see ADMINISTRATION/DOSAGE ADJUSTMENTS)
Patients with Wolff-Parkinson-White (WPW) syndrome	Severe bradycardia, necessitating use of a demand pacemaker, has occurred in several patients with WPW syndrome following use of propranolol
Patients with diabetes	Propranolol may mask tachycardia associated with hypoglycemia; however, this drug may not significantly affect other manifestations such as dizziness and diaphoresis. Propranolol may delay return of normal plasma glucose levels following insulin-induced hypoglycemia. Use with caution in patients with diabetes.
Patients with bronchospastic disease	In general, such patients should not receive propranolol because it may block catecholamine-induced bronchodilation. Propranolol is specifically contraindicated for use in patients with bronchial asthma; use with caution in patients with nonallergic bronchospasm (eg, chronic bronchitis, emphysema).
Patients with renal or hepatic impairment	Use with caution in such patients
Major surgery	The necessity or desirability of discontinuing use before major surgery is controversial. Beta blockade can increase the risks associated with general anesthesia and surgery (because cardiac responsiveness to reflex beta-adrenergic stimuli is impaired) and may cause protracted severe hypotension and difficulty in restarting and maintaining the heartbeat. However, beta-adrenergic agonists (eg, dobutamine, isoproterenol) can reverse the effects of propranolol.
Fatigue, lethargy, vivid dreams	Daily doses exceeding 160 mg, given in divided doses of more than 80 mg, may increase the risk of fatigue, lethargy, and vivid dreams
Glaucoma testing	Propranolol can reduce intraocular pressure and thereby affect the results of glaucoma screening tests
Carcinogenicity	No evidence of tumorigenicity has been seen in rats or mice given up to 150 mg/kg/day for a period of 18 mo
Effect on fertility	No impairment of fertility has been observed in animals

ADVERSE REACTIONS

Cardiovascular	Bradycardia, congestive heart failure, AV-block intensification, hypotension, paresthesia of the hands, Raynaud-type arterial insufficiency, purpura

INDERAL

Central nervous system	Light-headedness, depression, insomnia, weakness, fatigue, lassitude, catatonia, visual disturbances, hallucinations, vivid dreams; an acute reversible syndrome characterized by spatial and temporal disorientation, short-term memory loss, emotional lability, slightly clouded sensorium, and decreased neuropsychometric performance
Gastrointestinal	Nausea, vomiting, epigastric distress, abdominal cramps, diarrhea, constipation, mesenteric arterial thrombosis, ischemic colitis
Respiratory	Bronchospasm
Allergic	Pharyngitis, agranulocytosis, erythematous rash, fever with aching and sore throat, laryngospasm and respiratory distress
Other	Alopecia, lupus erythematosus-like reactions, psoriasiform rashes, dry eyes, impotence, and Peyronie's disease (rare); systemic lupus erythematosus (extremely rare)

OVERDOSAGE

Signs and symptoms	Severe bradycardia, cardiac failure, hypotension, bronchospasm
Treatment	Empty stomach (avoid pulmonary aspiration). For excessive bradycardia, administer 0.25–1.0 mg atropine IV; if there is no response to vagal blockade, administer isoproterenol cautiously. For cardiac failure, administer digitalis and a diuretic. For hypotension, use norepinephrine or (preferably) epinephrine. Treat bronchospasm with isoproterenol and aminophylline. Significant amounts of propranolol cannot be removed by dialysis.

DRUG INTERACTIONS

Reserpine, other catecholamine-depleting drugs	△ Risk of hypotension, marked bradycardia, vertigo, syncope, or orthostatic hypotension; closely observe patients during concomitant therapy
Calcium channel blockers	▽ AV conduction and myocardial contractility; concomitant IV administration of a beta blocker and verapamil has resulted in serious reactions, particularly in patients with severe cardiomyopathy, cardiac failure, or recent myocardial infarction. When using propranolol with a calcium channel blocker, especially IV verapamil, exercise caution.
Phenytoin, phenobarbital, rifampin	▽ Plasma level of propranolol
Cimetidine	△ Plasma level of propranolol
Chlorpromazine	△ Plasma level of propranolol and chlorpromazine
Theophylline, lidocaine, antipyrine	△ Plasma level of theophylline, lidocaine, and antipyrine
Thyroxine	△ Plasma T_4 level (due to decreased peripheral conversion of T_4 to T_3)
Aluminum hydroxide	▽ Absorption of propranolol
Digitalis	▽ AV conduction
Ephedrine, isoproterenol, other beta-adrenergic bronchodilators	▽ Bronchodilation
Thiazide-type diuretics, other antihypertensive agents	△ Antihypertensive effect
Alcohol	▽ Rate of absorption

ALTERED LABORATORY VALUES

Blood/serum values	△ SGOT △ SGPT △ Alkaline phosphatase △ LDH △ T_4 △ rT_3 ▽ T_3 △ BUN (in patients with severe heart disease)

No clinically significant alterations in urinary values occur at therapeutic dosages

USE IN CHILDREN

See INDICATIONS and ORAL DOSAGE; do not give IV to children. High plasma drug levels have been detected in patients with Down's syndrome, which suggests that bioavailability may be increased in these patients. If echocardiography is used to monitor therapy, bear in mind that the characteristics of a normal echocardiogram vary with age in children.

USE IN PREGNANT AND NURSING WOMEN

Pregnancy Category C: embryotoxic effects have been observed in animals given approximately 10 times the maximum human dose; no adequate, well-controlled studies have been done in pregnant women. Use during pregnancy only if the expected benefit justifies the potential risk to the fetus. Propranolol is excreted in human milk; use with caution in nursing mothers.

BETA-ADRENERGIC BLOCKERS

INDERAL LA (propranolol hydrochloride) Ayerst   Rx

Capsules (long-acting): 80, 120, 160 mg

INDICATIONS	ORAL DOSAGE
Hypertension	**Adult:** 80 mg once daily (alone or with a diuretic) to start, followed, if necessary, by 120 mg or more once daily, up to 640 mg once daily (the full therapeutic effect of a given dosage may not be evident for a few days to several weeks); usual dosage: 120–160 mg/day
Prophylaxis and long-term management of angina pectoris	**Adult:** 80 mg once daily to start, followed, if necessary, by gradual increments every 3–7 days, up to 320 mg once daily; usual dosage: 160 mg/day
Prophylaxis of migraine	**Adult:** 80 mg once daily to start, followed, if necessary, by gradual increments, up to 240 mg once daily; usual dosage: 160–240 mg/day. If satisfactory prophylaxis is not obtained after giving 240 mg/day for 4–6 wk, discontinue use.
Hypertrophic subaortic stenosis	**Adult:** 80–160 mg once daily

CONTRAINDICATIONS

Sinus bradycardia	Cardiogenic shock	Overt congestive heart failure, unless it results from a tachyarrhythmia treatable with immediate-release propranolol
Heart block greater than first degree	Bronchial asthma	

ADMINISTRATION/DOSAGE ADJUSTMENTS

Switching from immediate-release propranolol	To maintain therapeutic effectiveness, especially at the end of a 24-h dosing interval, it may be necessary to increase the dosage, because the long-acting form produces lower serum propranolol levels. However, retitration may not be required if, in the treatment of a disorder (eg, hypertension, angina), there is little correlation between serum level and therapeutic effect.
Discontinuation of therapy	Reduce dosage gradually over a period of several weeks; caution patients who experience angina or who may have occult coronary artery disease not to interrupt or discontinue therapy on their own

WARNINGS/PRECAUTIONS

Cardiac failure	Beta blockade may cause or exacerbate cardiac failure; discontinue use if this disorder does not stabilize after diuretic therapy and digitalization. If necessary, propranolol may be given to patients with well-compensated congestive heart failure; observe such patients closely.
Thyrotoxicosis	Propranolol may mask certain clinical signs of hyperthyroidism; abrupt withdrawal may exacerbate manifestations of this disorder and precipitate a thyroid storm
Patients with angina	Abrupt withdrawal in such patients may exacerbate angina and, in some cases, lead to myocardial infarction; reinstitute therapy if withdrawal reactions occur (see ADMINISTRATION/DOSAGE ADJUSTMENTS)
Patients with Wolff-Parkinson-White (WPW) syndrome	Severe bradycardia, necessitating use of a demand pacemaker, has occurred in several patients with WPW syndrome following use of propranolol
Patients with diabetes	Adjustment of insulin dosage in patients with labile insulin-dependent diabetes may be more difficult, because propranolol may mask certain clinical signs (eg, changes in pulse rate and blood pressure) of acute hypoglycemia
Patients with bronchospastic disease	In general, such patients should not receive propranolol because it may block catecholamine-induced bronchodilation. Propranolol is specifically contraindicated for use in patients with bronchial asthma; use with caution in patients with nonallergic bronchospasm (eg, chronic bronchitis, emphysema).
Patients with renal or hepatic impairment	Use with caution in such patients
Major surgery	The necessity or desirability of discontinuing use before major surgery is controversial. Beta blockade can increase the risks associated with general anesthesia and surgery (because cardiac responsiveness to reflex beta-adrenergic stimuli is impaired) and may cause protracted severe hypotension and difficulty in restarting and maintaining the heartbeat. However, beta-adrenergic agonists (eg, dobutamine, isoproterenol) can reverse the effects of propranolol.
Glaucoma testing	Propranolol can reduce intraocular pressure and thereby affect the results of glaucoma screening tests
Carcinogenicity	No evidence of tumorigenicity has been seen in rats or mice given up to 150 mg/kg/day for a period of 18 mo
Effect on fertility	No impairment of fertility has been observed in animals

INDERAL LA ■ LOPRESSOR

ADVERSE REACTIONS

Cardiovascular	Bradycardia, congestive heart failure, AV-block intensification, hypotension, paresthesia of the hands, Raynaud-type arterial insufficiency, purpura
Central nervous system	Light-headedness, depression, insomnia, weakness, fatigue, lassitude, catatonia, visual disturbances, hallucinations, disorientation, short-term memory loss, emotional lability, slightly clouded sensorium, decreased neuropsychometric performance
Gastrointestinal	Nausea, vomiting, epigastric distress, abdominal cramps, diarrhea, constipation, mesenteric arterial thrombosis, ischemic colitis
Respiratory	Bronchospasm
Allergic	Pharyngitis, agranulocytosis, erythematous rash, fever with aching and sore throat, laryngospasm and respiratory distress
Other	Alopecia, lupus erythematosus-like reactions, psoriasiform rashes, dry eyes, impotence, and Peyronie's disease (rare); systemic lupus erythematosus (extremely rare)

OVERDOSAGE

Signs and symptoms	Severe bradycardia, cardiac failure, hypotension, bronchospasm
Treatment	Empty stomach (avoid pulmonary aspiration). For excessive bradycardia, administer 0.25–1.0 mg atropine IV; if there is no response to vagal blockade, administer isoproterenol cautiously. For cardiac failure, administer digitalis and a diuretic. For hypotension, use norepinephrine or (preferably) epinephrine. Treat bronchospasm with isoproterenol and aminophylline. Significant amounts of propranolol cannot be removed by dialysis.

DRUG INTERACTIONS

Reserpine, other catecholamine-depleting drugs	⇧ Risk of hypotension, marked bradycardia, vertigo, syncope, or orthostatic hypotension; closely observe patients during concomitant therapy
Digitalis	⇩ AV conduction
Ephedrine, isoproterenol, other beta-adrenergic bronchodilators	⇩ Bronchodilation
Thiazide-type diuretics, other antihypertensive agents	⇧ Antihypertensive effect

ALTERED LABORATORY VALUES

Blood/serum values	⇧ SGOT ⇧ SGPT ⇧ Alkaline phosphatase ⇧ Lactate dehydrogenase ⇧ BUN (in patients with severe heart disease)

No clinically significant alterations in urinary values occur at therapeutic dosages

---

USE IN CHILDREN

Safety and effectiveness for use in children have not been established

USE IN PREGNANT AND NURSING WOMEN

Pregnancy Category C: embryotoxic effects have been observed in animals given approximately 10 times the maximum human dose; no adequate, well-controlled studies have been done in pregnant women. Use during pregnancy only if the expected benefit justifies the potential risk to the fetus. Propranolol is excreted in human milk; use with caution in nursing mothers.

BETA-ADRENERGIC BLOCKERS

LOPRESSOR (metoprolol tartrate) Geigy Rx
Tablets: 50, 100 mg   Ampuls: 1 mg/ml (5 ml)   Prefilled syringes: 1 mg/ml (5 ml)

INDICATIONS	ORAL DOSAGE	PARENTERAL DOSAGE
Hypertension	**Adult:** 100 mg/day, given in single or divided doses (alone or with a diuretic), to start, followed by weekly (or less frequent) increases until optimal response is achieved, up to 450 mg/day	—
Long-term management of **angina pectoris**	**Adult:** 100 mg/day, given in two divided doses to start, followed, if necessary, by gradual increases at weekly intervals, up to 400 mg/day, until optimal response is obtained or pronounced slowing of the heart rate occurs	—
Reduction of cardiovascular mortality in clinically stable patients following **acute myocardial infarction**	**Adult:** for early treatment of patients who tolerate the full IV dose, 50 mg q6h, beginning 15 min after the last IV dose and continuing for 48 h (if IV therapy is not well tolerated, give 25 or 50 mg q6h, beginning 15 min after the last IV dose or as soon as the clinical condition permits and continuing for 48 h); for late treatment or maintenance therapy following early treatment, 100 mg bid	**Adult:** for early treatment, 5 mg IV every 2 min for a total of 15 mg, followed by oral therapy

LOPRESSOR

CONTRAINDICATIONS

Hypertension and angina
Sinus bradycardia
Second- or third-degree AV block
Cardiogenic shock
Overt cardiac failure

Myocardial infarction
Bradycardia (heart rate < 45 beats/min)
Significant first-degree AV block (P-R interval ≥ 0.24 s); second- or third-degree AV block
Hypotension (systolic pressure < 100 mm Hg)
Moderate or severe cardiac failure

ADMINISTRATION/DOSAGE ADJUSTMENTS

Hypertension — Once-daily administration of lower doses (especially 100 mg) may be inadequate to maintain a full antihypertensive effect at the end of the 24-h dosing interval; in these cases, larger doses or more frequent dosing may be necessary. The initial daily dose for patients with bronchospastic disease should be given in 3 divided doses.

Myocardial infarction — Immediately after the hemodynamic condition stabilizes, treatment may be started in a coronary care unit (or a similar unit) with injection of 3 IV doses and oral administration q6h (see "early treatment" in dosage section). During IV administration, blood pressure, heart rate, and the ECG should be carefully monitored; if severe intolerance occurs, metoprolol should be discontinued. Therapy should begin 3–10 days after infarction—as soon as the clinical condition permits—if early treatment is contraindicated, undesirable, or not tolerated (see "late treatment"). Metoprolol should be given for at least 3 mo; although effectiveness beyond this period has not been conclusively established, studies with other beta blockers suggest that treatment should be continued for 1–3 yr.

Oral therapy — Tablets should be given with or immediately after meals. Caution patients not to double the dose after a missed dose and not to interrupt or discontinue therapy on their own.

WARNINGS/PRECAUTIONS

Cardiac failure — Beta blockade may cause or exacerbate cardiac failure (see CONTRAINDICATIONS); carefully monitor hemodynamic function during therapy, and use with caution in patients with congestive heart failure controlled by digitalis and diuretics. If cardiac failure occurs or worsens during treatment and does not respond to digitalis and diuretic therapy, discontinue administration of metoprolol.

Thyrotoxicosis — Abrupt withdrawal of beta blockade can precipitate a thyroid storm in patients with hyperthyroidism; discontinue therapy gradually if thyrotoxicosis is suspected. Beta blockade can mask certain signs of hyperthyroidism, such as tachycardia.

Discontinuation of therapy — When discontinuing chronic administration, especially in patients with ischemic heart disease, reduce dosage gradually over a period of 1–2 wk and monitor patient carefully. In patients with ischemic heart disease, abrupt discontinuation of therapy can exacerbate angina and, in some cases, lead to myocardial infarction. If, after discontinuation, angina markedly worsens or acute coronary insufficiency occurs, reinstate use promptly, at least temporarily, and take other appropriate measures for managing unstable angina. Caution patients not to interrupt or discontinue therapy on their own. Therapy should not be discontinued abruptly in patients treated for hypertension, since coronary artery disease is common and may go unrecognized.

Bradycardia, AV block, hypotension — Use of metoprolol following acute myocardial infarction may result in bradycardia, particularly in patients with inferior infarction, and may also produce hypotension and AV block (significant first-degree block [P-R interval ≥ 0.26 s] or second- or third-degree block). To reverse significant bradycardia (heart rate < 40 beats/min), especially when it is associated with decreased cardiac output, or to treat AV block, give 0.25–0.5 mg of atropine IV; if atropine treatment is unsuccessful, cautious administration of isoproterenol or installation of a pacemaker should be considered. To manage hypotension, characterized by a decrease in systolic pressure to 90 mm Hg or less, carefully evaluate hemodynamic condition (invasive monitoring of central venous, pulmonary capillary wedge, and arterial pressures may be necessary), assess extent of myocardial damage, and institute appropriate therapy, such as balloon counterpulsation or administration of IV fluids or positive inotropic agents. Metoprolol should be discontinued if AV block or hypotension occurs or if atropine fails to reverse bradycardia.

Bronchospasm — Instruct patients to report any difficulty in breathing. If bronchospasm unrelated to congestive heart failure occurs during myocardial infarction (MI) therapy, metoprolol should be discontinued. If necessary, theophylline or a $beta_2$ agonist may be given for bronchospasm; this should be done cautiously, however, because serious cardiac arrhythmias may occur.

In general, patients with bronchospastic disease should not receive beta blockers. However, if other antihypertensive treatment is not effective or tolerated, metoprolol may be used with caution in these patients since the drug has a relative selectivity for $beta_1$ receptors; because this selectivity is not absolute and diminishes at higher doses, a $beta_2$ agonist should be given concomitantly, and the lowest possible dose of metoprolol should be used (see ADMINISTRATION/DOSAGE ADJUSTMENTS). Metoprolol may also be used with extreme caution in patients with bronchospastic disease for MI therapy; however, a $beta_2$ agonist, which may exacerbate myocardial ischemia and the extent of infarction, should not be administered prophylactically to these patients.

LOPRESSOR

Surgery	The necessity or desirability of discontinuing use before major surgery is controversial. Beta blockade can increase the risks associated with general anesthesia and surgery (because cardiac responsiveness to reflex beta-adrenergic stimuli is impaired) and may cause protracted severe hypotension and difficulty in restarting and maintaining the heartbeat. However, beta-adrenergic agonists (eg, dobutamine, isoproterenol) can reverse the effects of metoprolol. Instruct patients to inform their physician or dentist that they are taking metoprolol before undergoing any surgical procedure.
Fatigue	Instruct patients to determine how they react to this drug before they drive or engage in other activities requiring alertness
Patients with diabetes	Beta blockade may mask hypoglycemia-induced tachycardia but may not significantly affect the manifestation of other hypoglycemic reactions, such as dizziness or sweating; use with caution in diabetic patients
Patients with hepatic impairment	Use with caution in patients with impaired hepatic function; approximately 90% of an IV dose and more than 95% of an oral dose are converted to inactive metabolites by the liver
Dry eyes, reversible alopecia, agranulocytosis	Rare instances of these reactions have been reported; consider discontinuing therapy if any such reaction cannot be explained by causes other than the drug
Carcinogenicity, mutagenicity	No evidence of carcinogenicity has been detected in rats fed up to 800 mg/kg/day for 2 yr. A 21-mo study has shown an increase in benign lung tumors (small adenomas) in female mice fed 750 mg/kg/day; however, when this study was repeated, no significant results were observed. The results of all mutagenicity tests with metoprolol have been negative.
Effect on fertility	The fertility of rats has not been affected by administration of up to 55.5 times the maximum human dose of metoprolol

ADVERSE REACTIONS

Frequent reactions (incidence $\geq$ 1%) are printed in *italics*

When used to treat hypertension or angina

Central nervous system, neuromuscular	*Tiredness and dizziness (10%), depression (5%),* mental confusion, short-term memory loss, headache, nightmares, insomnia, musculoskeletal pain, blurred vision, tinnitus
Cardiovascular	*Shortness of breath and bradycardia (3%);* cold extremities, arterial insufficiency (usually Raynaud type), palpitations, congestive heart failure peripheral edema, and hypotension (1%)
Respiratory	*Wheezing (bronchospasm) and dyspnea (1%)*
Gastrointestinal	*Diarrhea (5%);* nausea, dry mouth, gastric pain, constipation, flatulence, and heartburn (1%)
Dermatological	*Pruritus and rash (5%),* worsening of psoriasis; reversible alopecia (rare)
Other	Peyronie's disease, agranulocytosis, and dry eyes (rare)

When used to treat myocardial infarction[1]

Central nervous system	*Tiredness (1%)*
Cardiovascular	*Hypotension (27% vs 24% for placebo), bradycardia (16% vs 7% for placebo), first-degree heart block (5% vs 2% for placebo), second- or third-degree heart block (5% vs 5% for placebo), heart failure (28% vs 30% for placebo)*
Respiratory	Dyspnea
Gastrointestinal	Nausea, abdominal pain

OVERDOSAGE

Signs and symptoms	Bradycardia, hypotension, cardiac failure, bronchospasm; cardiovascular instability is generally greater in patients with acute or recent myocardial infarction than in other patients
Treatment	Empty stomach by gastric lavage. For bradycardia, administer atropine IV; if there is no response to vagal blockade, give isoproterenol cautiously. For hypotension, use a vasopressor such as norepinephrine or dopamine. For cardiac failure, administer digitalis and a diuretic; for cardiogenic shock, consider using dobutamine, isoproterenol, or glucagon. Treat bronchospasm with a $beta_2$ agonist and/or theophylline.

DRUG INTERACTIONS

Reserpine, other catecholamine-depleting drugs	△ Risk of hypotension (including orthostatic hypotension), marked bradycardia, vertigo, and syncope
Digitalis	▽ AV conduction
Thiazide-type diuretics, other antihypertensive agents	△ Antihypertensive effect

ALTERED LABORATORY VALUES

Blood/serum values	△ SGOT △ SGPT △ Alkaline phosphatase △ LDH

LOPRESSOR ■ TENORMIN

No clinically significant alterations in urinary values occur at therapeutic dosages

---

USE IN CHILDREN

Safety and effectiveness for use in children have not been established

USE IN PREGNANT AND NURSING WOMEN

Pregnancy Category C: an increase in postimplantation loss and a decrease in neonatal survival have been seen in rats given up to 55.5 times the maximum human dose of metoprolol; no evidence of teratogenicity or impaired fertility has been observed. No adequate, well-controlled studies have been performed in pregnant women. Use during pregnancy only if clearly needed. A very small amount of metoprolol ($<$ 1 mg/liter) is excreted in human milk; use with caution in nursing mothers.

---

[1] Reactions for which a causal relationship has not been established that have occurred in patients being treated for myocardial infarction include headache, sleep disturbances, hallucinations, visual disturbances, dizziness, vertigo, confusion, reduced libido, rash, exacerbation of psoriasis, unstable diabetes, and claudication. Reactions that are associated with use of other beta blockers include intensification of AV block; reversible mental depression progressing to catatonia; an acute reversible syndrome characterized by temporal and spatial disorientation, short-term memory loss, emotional lability, slightly clouded sensorium, and decreased performance on neuropsychometric tests; agranulocytosis; purpura; and fever combined with aching and sore throat, laryngospasm, and respiratory distress.

BETA-ADRENERGIC BLOCKERS

TENORMIN (atenolol) Stuart   Rx

Tablets: 50, 100 mg

INDICATIONS	ORAL DOSAGE
Hypertension	**Adult:** 50 mg/day (alone or with a diuretic) to start, followed in 1–2 wk by 100 mg/day, if needed
Long-term management of **angina pectoris** caused by coronary atherosclerosis	**Adult:** 50 mg once daily to start, followed, if necessary, by 100 mg once daily (the full therapeutic effect may not be seen for 1 wk at a given dosage); maximum dosage: 200 mg given once daily

CONTRAINDICATIONS

Sinus bradycardia	Heart block greater than first degree	Cardiogenic shock
Overt cardiac failure (see WARNINGS/PRECAUTIONS)		

ADMINISTRATION/DOSAGE ADJUSTMENTS

Combination therapy	May be used in combination with other antihypertensive agents, including thiazide-type diuretics, hydralazine, prazosin, and methyldopa
Patients with renal impairment	Administer up to 50 mg/day when creatinine clearance rate (CCr) = 15–35 ml/min and up to 50 mg every other day when CCr $<$ 15 ml/min. Give patients on hemodialysis 50 mg after each dialysis treatment; hospital supervision is needed since marked falls in blood pressure can occur.
Effect on exercise tolerance	The maximum early effect on exercise tolerance occurs with doses of 50–100 mg; at these doses, however, the effect at 24 h is attenuated and averages about 50–75% of that observed with once-daily administration of 200 mg
Cessation of therapy	Withdraw atenolol gradually over a period of 2 wk and observe patient carefully; instruct patient to limit physical activity to a minimum during this time (see WARNINGS/PRECAUTIONS)
Discontinuation of therapy in patients receiving clonidine concomitantly	Discontinue use of atenolol several days before gradually withdrawing clonidine

WARNINGS/PRECAUTIONS

Cardiac failure	May be precipitated by further or continued depression of myocardial contractility; discontinue use if cardiac failure persists despite adequate digitalization and diuretic therapy. In cases of well-compensated congestive heart failure, use with caution.
Patients with angina	Abrupt withdrawal of beta blockers in such patients has exacerbated angina and, in some cases, led to myocardial infarction and ventricular arrhythmias; reinstitute therapy, at least temporarily, if angina worsens or acute coronary insufficiency develops
Bronchospastic disease in patients refractory to or intolerant of other antihypertensive agents	Administer with caution, using the lowest possible dose (50 mg); since beta$_1$ (cardiac) selectivity is not absolute, a beta$_2$-stimulating agent should be made available; if atenolol dosage must be increased, consider divided doses to reduce peak blood levels

TENORMIN

Patients undergoing anesthesia and major surgery	Beta blockade may augment the risks. If atenolol is withdrawn before surgery, allow 48 h to elapse between the last dose and anesthesia; if treatment is continued, anesthetic agents that depress the myocardium (eg, ether, cyclopropane, and trichloroethylene) should be used with caution. Excessive beta blockade during surgery may be reversed by cautious administration of a beta-receptor agonist (eg, dobutamine or isoproterenol). Profound bradycardia and hypotension may be corrected with atropine, 1–2 mg IV.
Diabetes and hypoglycemia	Use with caution in diabetic patients; beta blockade may mask some (eg, tachycardia), but not other (eg, dizziness and sweating), symptoms of hypoglycemia. Insulin-induced hypoglycemia is *not* potentiated, nor is recovery of normal blood glucose levels delayed.
Thyrotoxicosis	Clinical signs of hyperthyroidism (eg, tachycardia) may be masked. Abrupt withdrawal may precipitate thyroid storm; if therapy is discontinued, closely monitor patients suspected of developing thyrotoxicosis.
Patients with renal impairment	Use with caution (see ADMINISTRATION/DOSAGE ADJUSTMENTS)
Skin rash and/or dry eyes	Have been associated with use of other beta blockers; consider discontinuing atenolol therapy if any such reaction cannot be explained otherwise and closely follow patient after drug is withdrawn
Carcinogenicity, mutagenicity	Long-term studies in rats and mice treated with doses as high as 150 times the maximum recommended human dose have shown no evidence of carcinogenicity; results of various mutagenicity studies have also been negative
Impairment of fertility	Administration of atenolol in doses as high as 100 times the maximum recommended human dose has had no effect on fertility of male and female rats

ADVERSE REACTIONS[1]

Cardiovascular	Bradycardia, cold extremities, postural hypotension, leg pain
Central nervous system	Dizziness, vertigo, light-headedness, tiredness, fatigue, lethargy, drowsiness, depression, dreaming
Gastrointestinal	Diarrhea, nausea
Respiratory	Wheeziness, dyspnea
Other	Dry eyes

OVERDOSAGE

Signs and symptoms	Bradycardia, congestive heart failure, hypotension, bronchospasm, and hypoglycemia (based on overdosage experience with other beta blockers)
Treatment	Discontinue medication. Empty stomach by gastric lavage, and initiate hemodialysis to eliminate drug from general circulation. For bradycardia, administer atropine or another anticholinergic drug. For second- or third-degree heart block, administer isoproterenol or use a transvenous cardiac pacemaker. Treat congestive heart failure with digitalis, diuretics, and other conventional measures. For hypotension, epinephrine may be useful in addition to atropine and digitalis. For bronchospasm, administer aminophylline, isoproterenol, or atropine. For hypoglycemia, give IV glucose.

DRUG INTERACTIONS

Digitalis	▽ AV conduction time
Reserpine, other *Rauwolfia* alkaloids	Hypotension and/or marked bradycardia
Thiazide-type diuretics, methyldopa, hydralazine, prazosin	△ Antihypertensive effect

ALTERED LABORATORY VALUES

No clinically significant alterations in blood/serum or urinary values occur at therapeutic dosages

USE IN CHILDREN

Safety and effectiveness for use in children have not been established

USE IN PREGNANT AND NURSING WOMEN

Pregnancy Category C: use during pregnancy only if anticipated benefit outweighs potential fetal risk. Atenolol has been shown to produce a dose-related increase in embryonic and fetal resorptions in rats at doses ≥ 25 times the maximum recommended human dose. No adequate, well-controlled studies have been done in pregnant women. Atenolol is excreted in human milk at a ratio of 1.5:6.8 when compared to the concentration in plasma; use with caution in nursing women.

---

[1] Other reactions associated with beta blocker therapy but not observed with atenolol include intensification of AV block (see CONTRAINDICATIONS); reversible mental depression progressing to catatonia; visual disturbances, hallucinations; an acute reversible syndrome characterized by temporal and spatial disorientation, short-term memory loss, emotional lability, slightly clouded sensorium, and decreased performance on neuropsychometric tests; agranulocytosis; thrombocytopenic and nonthrombocytopenic purpura; erythematous rash; fever combined with aching and sore throat; laryngospasm; respiratory distress; reversible alopecia; Peyronie's disease; and Raynaud's phenomenon

CALCIUM ANTAGONISTS

ADALAT (nifedipine) Miles Pharmaceuticals   Rx
Capsules: 10, 20 mg

INDICATIONS

Vasospastic angina confirmed by (1) a classical pattern of angina at rest accompanied by ST-segment elevation, (2) angina or coronary artery spasm provokable by ergonovine, *or* (3) angiographically demonstrable coronary artery spasm[1]

Chronic stable angina (effort-associated angina) in patients without evidence of vasospasm who (1) remain symptomatic despite adequate doses of beta blockers or organic nitrates *or* (2) cannot tolerate these agents[2]

ORAL DOSAGE

Adult: 10 mg tid to start, followed by gradual increases in dosage (see "frequency of dosage adjustment," below), as needed and tolerated. The usual effective dosage is 10–20 mg tid; however, some patients, especially those with evidence of coronary artery spasm, may require 20–30 mg tid or qid. Dosages above 120 mg/day are rarely necessary, and dosages exceeding 180 mg/day are not recommended.

CONTRAINDICATIONS

Hypersensitivity to nifedipine

ADMINISTRATION/DOSAGE ADJUSTMENTS

Frequency of dosage adjustment — In most cases, 7–14 days should elapse between dosage increases to permit adequate assessment of clinical response and patient tolerance; however, if the patient's level of physical activity, attack frequency, and sublingual nitroglycerin consumption warrant, the dosage may be increased from 10 mg tid to 20 mg tid and then to 30 mg tid over a 3-day period, provided that the patient is frequently evaluated. In hospitalized patients under close observation, the dosage may be increased by 10 mg q4–6h, as needed to control pain and arrhythmias due to ischemia; more than 30 mg should generally not be given as a single dose. No rebound effect has been observed upon discontinuation of therapy; nevertheless, if discontinuation is necessary, dosage should be decreased gradually under close supervision.

Concomitant administration of other antianginal agents — Sublingual nitroglycerin tablets may be taken as needed for acute anginal symptoms, especially during the period of initial dosage titration. Co-administration of nifedipine and beta blockers may be beneficial in patients with chronic stable angina and is usually well tolerated; however, the effects of this combination, particularly in patients with compromised left ventricular function or cardiac conduction abnormalities, cannot be predicted with confidence until more data are obtained. (See warnings, below, concerning hypotension, exacerbation of angina, and congestive heart failure.) Nifedipine may be given safely with organic nitrates, but there have been no controlled studies to evaluate the effectiveness of this combination on angina.

WARNINGS/PRECAUTIONS

Hypotension — Occasional patients may develop excessive or poorly tolerated hypotension, particularly when nifedipine is introduced or when the dosage is subsequently increased; co-administration of beta blockers increases the risk. Blood pressure should be carefully monitored during the period of initial dosage adjustment, especially if the patient is taking drugs that are known to produce hypotension.

Exacerbation of angina and myocardial infarction — An increase in the frequency, duration, or severity of angina or acute myocardial infarction has occurred at the start of therapy and when the dosage has been increased. This rare effect has been seen most commonly in patients with severe obstructive coronary artery disease. Nifedipine may also exacerbate the increase in angina that can develop during or after withdrawal of a beta blocker; discontinue a beta blocker gradually, if possible, when switching to nifedipine.

Congestive heart failure — Has occurred rarely after initiation of nifedipine therapy, usually in patients receiving beta blockers; patients with "tight" aortic stenosis may be at increased risk

Peripheral edema — Approximately 10% of patients develop peripheral edema, primarily in the lower extremities; the edema is typically associated with arterial vasodilation and usually responds to diuretics. Peripheral edema occurring in nifedipine-treated patients with congestive heart failure should be carefully differentiated from the effects of increasing left ventricular dysfunction.

Hematological effects — Limited clinical studies have demonstrated that in some patients nifedipine can moderately decrease platelet aggregation, presumably by inhibiting calcium ion flux across the platelet membrane, and thereby increase bleeding time; it has not been shown that these findings are clinically significant. The use of nifedipine in patients receiving coumarin anticoagulants has been associated, in rare cases, with an increase in prothrombin time; however, a causal relationship has not been established.

Hepatotoxicity — In rare instances, significantly elevated hepatic enzyme levels, cholestasis, cholestatic jaundice, and allergic hepatitis have occurred during therapy

ADALAT

Patients with renal impairment	Rare, reversible elevations in BUN and serum creatinine levels have been seen in patients with chronic renal insufficiency; in at least some cases, the increases were probably due to nifedipine
Surgery with fentanyl	Nifedipine therapy should be interrupted, if possible, at least 36 h before any surgical procedure that requires high doses of fentanyl. Severe hypotension and hypovolemia have occurred in patients who were given high doses of fentanyl during coronary artery bypass surgery; although these reactions were apparently due to the combination of nifedipine and a beta blocker, the possibility that such reactions may also occur in other surgical procedures or with other narcotic analgesics, low doses of fentanyl, or nifedipine alone cannot be ruled out.
Patients receiving digoxin	Measure serum digoxin levels at the beginning and end of nifedipine therapy and whenever the dosage of nifedipine is changed; administration of this drug has been reported to elevate serum digoxin levels. In one study, nifedipine increased serum digoxin levels in 9 of 12 normal subjects by an average of 45%. However, a study in 13 patients with coronary artery disease showed no increase in serum levels, and no evidence of digitalis toxicity was found in an uncontrolled study that involved over 200 patients with congestive heart failure.
Carcinogenicity, mutagenicity	There is no evidence that nifedipine is carcinogenic or mutagenic
Impairment of fertility	Reduced fertility has been observed in rats given approximately 30 times the maximum recommended human dose prior to mating

ADVERSE REACTIONS[3]

	Frequent reactions (incidence $\geq$ 1%) are printed in *italics*
Central nervous system	*Dizziness/light-headedness, headache, and weakness (each ~10%)*; shakiness, nervousness, jitteriness, sleep disturbances, and difficulties in maintaining balance (each $\leq$ 2%); depression and paranoid syndrome (each $<$ 0.5%)
Ophthalmic	Blurred vision ($\leq$ 2%), transient blindness at peak plasma level ($<$ 0.5%)
Cardiovascular	*Peripheral edema and flushing (each ~10%), transient hypotension (~5%), palpitation (2%)*, syncope (~0.5%), ventricular arrhythmias and conduction disturbances (each $<$ 0.5%), increased angina (rare)[4]
Hematological	Thrombocytopenia, anemia, leukopenia, and purpura (each $<$ 0.5%)
Gastrointestinal	*Nausea (~10%)*; diarrhea, constipation, cramps, and flatulence (each $\leq$ 2%); allergic hepatitis ($<$ 0.5%); cholestasis with or without jaundice (rare)
Respiratory	Nasal/chest congestion and shortness of breath (each $\leq$ 2%)
Musculoskeletal	Inflammation, joint stiffness, and muscle cramps (each $\leq$ 2%)
Dermatological	Dermatitis, pruritus, and urticaria (each $\leq$ 2%); erythromelalgia ($<$ 0.5%)
Other	Fever, sweating, chills, and sexual difficulties (each $\leq$ 2%); gingival hyperplasia and arthritis with positive ANA (each $<$ 0.5%)

OVERDOSAGE

Signs and symptoms	Marked and probably prolonged systemic hypotension
Treatment	Empty stomach by inducing emesis or by gastric lavage. Monitor cardiac and respiratory function, elevate the lower extremities, and pay careful attention to the patient's circulating fluid volume and urine output, instituting supportive measures, as needed. A vasoconstrictor (eg, norepinephrine) may be given to help restore vascular tone and blood pressure, unless there is a contraindication to its use. Clearance may be prolonged in patients with liver disease. Dialysis is not likely to be beneficial, since the drug is highly protein bound.

DRUG INTERACTIONS

Beta blockers	⇧ Risk of severe hypotension, congestive heart failure, and exacerbation of angina
Oral anticoagulants	⇧ Anticoagulant effect (see WARNINGS/PRECAUTIONS)
Cimetidine	⇧ Serum nifedipine level; if treatment is initiated in a patient currently receiving cimetidine, cautious titration is advised

ALTERED LABORATORY VALUES

Blood/serum values	⇧ SGOT ⇧ SGPT ⇧ Alkaline phosphatase ⇧ Lactate dehydrogenase ⇧ Creatine phosphokinase + Coombs' test + ANA

No clinically significant alterations in urinary values occur at therapeutic dosages

USE IN CHILDREN

No clinical experience with this drug in children has been reported

USE IN PREGNANT AND NURSING WOMEN

Pregnancy Category C: use during pregnancy only if anticipated benefit of therapy justifies the potential fetal risk. Nifedipine has been shown to be teratogenic in rats at 30 times the maximum recommended human dose and embryotoxic in rats, mice, and rabbits at 3–10 times the maximum recommended human dose. Administration of two-thirds and twice the maximum recommended human dose to pregnant monkeys has resulted in small placentas with underdeveloped chorionic villi. Prolongation of pregnancy has been observed in rats at 3 times the maximum human dose. No adequate, well-controlled studies have been done in pregnant women. It is not known whether nifedipine is excreted in human milk; because many drugs are excreted in human milk, patient should not nurse while taking this drug.

---

[1] Nifedipine may also be used when the clinical presentation suggests a possible vasospastic component but vasospasm has not been confirmed (eg, when pain on exertion has a variable threshold, when ECG findings are compatible with intermittent vasospasm in unstable angina, or when angina is refractory to organic nitrates and/or adequate doses of beta blockers)
[2] The effectiveness and safety of using nifedipine beyond 8 wk in these patients have not been established
[3] Adverse reactions reported in uncontrolled clinical trials of nifedipine in over 2,100 patients in the United States. The pattern and incidence of major adverse effects observed in worldwide controlled studies were as follows: dizziness/light-headedness/giddiness, 27%; flushing/heat sensation, 25%; headache, 23%; weakness, 12%; nausea/heartburn, 11%; muscle cramps/tremor, 8%; peripheral edema, 7%; nervousness/mood changes, 7%; palpitation, 7%; dyspnea/cough/wheezing, 6%; and nasal congestion/sore throat, 6%.
[4] Other reactions for which a causal relationship has not been established include myocardial infarction (reported incidence of 4%) and congestive heart failure/pulmonary edema (2%)

CALCIUM ANTAGONISTS

CALAN (verapamil hydrochloride) Searle   Rx

Tablets: 80, 120 mg

INDICATIONS

Angina at rest, including vasospastic (Prinzmetal's variant) and unstable (crescendo, preinfarction) angina

Chronic stable angina (classic effort-associated angina)

Control of ventricular rate in digitalized patients with chronic atrial flutter and/or atrial fibrillation

Prophylaxis of repetitive paroxysmal supraventricular tachycardia in undigitalized patients

Essential hypertension

ORAL DOSAGE

Adult: 80–120 mg tid, followed by daily or weekly increases in dosage, up to 480 mg/day, as needed, until optimum clinical response is obtained

Adult: 240–320 mg/day, given in divided doses tid or qid

Adult: 240–480 mg/day

Adult: 240 mg/day to start, given in equally divided doses tid

CALAN SR (verapamil hydrochloride) Searle   Rx

Caplets (sustained release): 240 mg

INDICATIONS

Essential hypertension

ORAL DOSAGE

Adult: 240 mg/day, given in a single morning dose; if an adequate response is not obtained, titrate the dosage upward by giving 240 mg each morning to start, followed by 240 mg each morning plus 120 mg each evening, and then 240 mg q12h

CONTRAINDICATIONS

Severe left ventricular dysfunction

Accessory bypass tracts (Wolff-Parkinson-White, Lown-Ganong-Levine syndromes), when associated with atrial fibrillation

Second- or third-degree AV block (except in patients with a functioning artificial ventricular pacemaker)

Hypotension (systolic pressure < 90 mm Hg)

Sick sinus syndrome (except in patients with a functioning artificial ventricular pacemaker)

Cardiogenic shock

ADMINISTRATION/DOSAGE ADJUSTMENTS

Titration of dosage — Starting treatment at 40 mg tid should be considered in anginal and hypertensive patients who may exhibit an increased response to verapamil as a result of hepatic dysfunction, advanced age, small body size, or other conditions. Titrate dosage upward based on therapeutic efficacy and safety, evaluated approximately 8 h after the immediate-release tablets are taken or 24 h after the sustained-release formulation has been taken. Since the half-life of verapamil increases with repeated administration, the maximum response may be delayed during chronic dosing. In general, the maximum antiarrhythmic effect of this drug will be apparent during the first 48 h of administration, whereas the antihypertensive effect should be evident within the first week of therapy.

Timing of administration	The sustained-release formulation should be administered with food; the immediate-release tablets may be taken without regard to meals
Switching formulations	The total daily dose of verapamil may remain the same when switching from the immediate-release to the sustained-release form
Concomitant therapy	Concomitant use of this drug with both short- and long-acting nitrates may be beneficial in patients with angina and is apparently free of harmful drug interactions. Concomitant use of verapamil with beta blockers may also be beneficial in certain patients with chronic stable angina or hypertension, but the combination can adversely affect cardiac function (see WARNINGS/PRECAUTIONS). Monitor vital signs and clinical status closely, and reassess the need for concomitant beta-blocker therapy periodically.

WARNINGS/PRECAUTIONS

Heart failure	Control heart failure with digitalis and/or diuretics before giving verapamil; do not administer to patients with severe left ventricular dysfunction (ejection fraction < 30%), patients with moderate to severe cardiac failure, or those with any degree of ventricular dysfunction who are concomitantly receiving a beta blocker.
Hypotension	Blood pressure may fall in some patients and may result in dizziness or symptomatic hypotension; decreases in blood pressure below normal levels are unusual in hypertensive patients. If severe hypotension occurs, administer isoproterenol, norepinephrine, atropine, or 10% calcium gluconate immediately *(in patients with hypertrophic cardiomyopathy [IHSS], use phenylephrine, metaraminol, or methoxamine, instead of isoproterenol or norepinephrine, to maintain blood pressure)*. If further support is needed, administer dopamine or dobutamine.
Hepatotoxicity	Elevations of SGOT, SGPT, alkaline phosphatase, and bilirubin levels have been reported. In some cases, these increases have been transient. However, in several patients, drug-induced hepatocellular injury has been reported; half of these patients experienced malaise, fever, and/or right quadrant pain as well as elevated hepatic enzyme levels. To reduce the risk of hepatotoxicity, periodically monitor liver function in all patients.
Rapid ventricular response, fibrillation	In some patients with paroxysmal and/or chronic atrial flutter or atrial fibrillation and an accessory AV pathway (eg, Wolff-Parkinson-White or Lown-Ganong-Levine syndrome), IV verapamil may produce a very rapid ventricular response or ventricular fibrillation following increased antegrade conduction; treat with DC cardioversion. While these risks have not been established with oral verapamil, use in this patient group is contraindicated.
Atrioventricular block	The effect of this drug on AV conduction and the SA node may cause asymptomatic first-degree AV block and transient bradycardia, sometimes accompanied by nodal escape rhythms; prolongation of the P-R interval is correlated with plasma concentrations of verapamil, especially during early titration of therapy. If marked first-degree block occurs, reduce dosage or discontinue verapamil administration and institute appropriate therapy (see suggested management of severe hypotension, above).
Impairment of neuromuscular transmission	Verapamil reportedly decreases neuromuscular transmission in patients with Duchenne's muscular dystrophy; the drug may also enhance the effects of neuromuscular blockers and delay reversal of vecuronium-induced blockade. A decrease in dosage may be necessary for patients with attenuated neuromuscular transmission; when verapamil is given in combination with a neuromuscular blocker, it may be necessary to reduce the dosage of one or both of the drugs.
Patients with hypertrophic cardiomyopathy (IHSS)	Serious adverse effects, including pulmonary edema and/or severe hypotension, sinus bradycardia, second-degree AV block, and sinus arrest, may occur in these patients; reduce dosage if adverse effects occur or discontinue therapy, if necessary
Drug accumulation	Use with caution in patients with significant renal or hepatic impairment; administer 30% of the usual dose to patients with hepatic impairment. Carefully monitor patients for abnormal prolongation of the P-R interval or other signs of overdosage (see below).
Carcinogenicity	Studies in rate fed verapamil at doses of 10, 35, and 120 mg/kg/day for 2 yr showed no evidence of carcinogenic potential; verapamil has shown no evidence of tumorigenicity in rats given 6 times the maximum human dose for 18 mo
Mutagenicity	Verapamil has shown no evidence of mutagenicity in the Ames test
Effect on fertility	Studies in female rats fed 5.5 times the recommended human dose of verapamil showed no evidence of impaired fertility; the effect of this drug on male fertility has not been determined

ADVERSE REACTIONS[1]

Frequent reactions (incidence ≥ 1%) are printed in *italics*

Cardiovascular	*Hypotension (2.5%), edema (2.1%), congestive heart failure/pulmonary edema (1.8%), bradycardia (< 50 beats/min) (1.4%), first, second, and third-degree AV block (1.3%),* third-degree AV block alone (0.8%), flushing (0.1%)
Gastrointestinal	*Constipation (8.4%), nausea (2.7%),* elevation of liver enzyme levels
Central nervous system	*Dizziness (3.5%), headache (1.9%), fatigue (1.7%)*

CALAN ■ CARDIZEM

OVERDOSAGE

Signs and symptoms	Abnormal prolongation of P-R interval, severe hypotension, second- or third-degree AV block, asystole
Treatment	Institute standard supportive measures (eg, IV fluids). Administer beta-adrenergic stimulating agents or parenteral calcium solutions to increase calcium ion flux across the slow channel. Treat clinically significant hypotensive reactions or fixed high-degree AV block with vasopressors or cardiac pacing, respectively. Treat asystole with usual measures, including cardiopulmonary resuscitation.

DRUG INTERACTIONS

Beta blockers	↑ Antianginal and antihypertensive effect ↑ Risk of negative inotropic, chronotropic, or dromotropic effects during high-dose beta-blocker therapy; closely monitor patients during concomitant therapy. Avoid concomitant use in patients with AV conduction abnormalities and those with depressed left ventricular function ↓ Clearance of metoprolol
Digitalis	↑ Serum digoxin level and digitalis toxicity; reduce dosage or discontinue use, if necessary
Oral antihypertensive agents (eg, vasodilators, angiotensin-converting enzyme inhibitors, diuretics, beta blockers)	↑ Reduction of blood pressure; monitor patient during concomitant therapy
Prazosin	Excessive hypotension
Disopyramide	↑ Risk of decreased myocardial contractility; do not give disopyramide within 48 h before or 24 h after administration of verapamil
Quinidine	Significant hypotension in patients with hypertrophic cardiomyopathy (IHSS); avoid concomitant use in these patients ↑ Serum levels of quinidine ↓ Pharmacologic effects of quinidine on AV conduction
Cimetidine	↓ Clearance of verapamil
Lithium	↓ Serum levels of lithium; adjust dosage of lithium, if necessary
Carbamazepine	↑ Serum levels of carbamazepine, possibly leading to diplopia, headache, ataxia, or dizziness
Rifampin	↓ Bioavailability of rifampin
Inhalation anesthetics	↓ Cardiovascular activity; titrate dose of each agent carefully
Curare-like and depolarizing neuromuscular blocking agents	↑ Neuromuscular blockade; decrease dosage of one or both agents, if necessary
Nitrates	↑ Antianginal effect

ALTERED LABORATORY VALUES

Blood/serum values	↑ SGOT ↑ SGPT ↑ Alkaline phosphatase ↑ Bilirubin

No clinically significant alterations in urinary values occur at therapeutic dosages

USE IN CHILDREN

Safety and effectiveness for use in children under 18 yr of age have not been established

USE IN PREGNANT AND NURSING WOMEN

Pregnancy Category C: reproductive studies in rabbits and rats at oral doses up to 1.5 and 6 times the oral human dose, respectively, have shown no evidence of teratogenicity; in the rat, however, the drug caused hypotension, was embryocidal, and retarded fetal growth and development. Verapamil crosses the placental barrier and can be detected in umbilical vein blood at delivery; it is not known whether verapamil administration during labor and delivery has any immediate or delayed adverse effect on the fetus, prolongs labor, or increases the need for obstetric intervention. No adequate, well-controlled studies have been performed in pregnant women; use during pregnancy only if clearly needed. Verapamil is excreted in human milk; patients who are taking this drug should not nurse.

[1] Reactions for which a causal relationship is uncertain include angina pectoris, chest pain, claudication, myocardial infarction, palpitations, purpura (vasculitis), syncope, diarrhea, dry mouth, GI distress, gingival hyperplasia, ecchymosis, bruising, confusion, equilibrium disorders, insomnia, muscle cramps, paresthesia, psychotic symptoms, shakiness, somnolence; dyspnea, arthralgia and rash, exanthema, hair loss, hyperkeratosis, macules, sweating, urticaria, blurred vision, gynecomastia, increased urination, spotty menstruation; and impotence (reported only with sustained-release form)

CALCIUM ANTAGONISTS

CARDIZEM (diltiazem hydrochloride) Marion   Rx
Tablets: 30, 60 mg

INDICATIONS

Vasospastic angina, characterized by angina at rest and ST-segment elevation
Chronic stable angina (effort-associated angina) in patients who (1) remain symptomatic despite adequate doses of beta-adrenergic blockers or organic nitrates or (2) cannot tolerate these agents[1]

ORAL DOSAGE

Adult: 30 mg qid, before meals and at bedtime, to start, followed, if necessary, by a gradual dosage increase every 1–2 days; usual maintenance dosage: 180–360 mg/day. A daily dose exceeding 120 mg should be given in 3 or 4 divided doses.

CARDIZEM

CONTRAINDICATIONS

Sick sinus syndrome (unless a functioning ventricular pacemaker is present)	Hypotension (systolic pressure < 90 mm Hg)	Second- or third-degree AV block (unless a functioning pacemaker is present)

ADMINISTRATION/DOSAGE ADJUSTMENTS

Concomitant administration of other antianginal agents	Sublingual nitroglycerin tablets may be taken as needed for acute anginal attacks. Diltiazem may be given safely with organic nitrates, but there have been no controlled studies to evaluate the prophylactic effect of this combination. The safety and effectiveness of concomitant use with digitalis or beta-adrenergic blockers have not been established; although controlled studies suggest that such use is usually well-tolerated, the effects, particularly in patients with left ventricular dysfunction or conduction abnormalities, cannot be predicted because available data are insufficient (see DRUG INTERACTIONS).

WARNINGS/PRECAUTIONS

Prolonged cardiac conduction time	Bradycardia or second- or third-degree AV block may occur because diltiazem prolongs AV-node refractory periods without significantly prolonging sinus-node recovery time, except in patients with sick sinus syndrome; in such patients (see CONTRAINDICATIONS), bradycardia is more likely. A patient with Prinzmetal's angina experienced asymptomatic asystole lasting 2–5 s approximately 5 h after receiving a single 60-mg dose of diltiazem.
Hypotension	Decreases in blood pressure due to diltiazem may occasionally cause symptomatic hypotension
Hepatic injury	In rare cases, diltiazem has caused acute reversible hepatic injury, characterized by mild increases in alkaline phosphatase, SGOT, SGPT, LDH, and CPK levels and appropriate symptoms
Patients with ventricular dysfunction	Use with caution; clinical experience in such patients is very limited. Although a negative inotropic effect occurs in isolated animal tissue preparations, neither consistent negative effects on contractility nor a reduction in cardiac index have been reported in studies in patients with normal ventricular function.
Patients with renal or hepatic impairment	Use with particular caution; no data is available concerning dosage requirements for such patients. Diltiazem undergoes extensive hepatic metabolism, and only 2–4% of the unchanged drug appears in the urine.
Prolonged therapy	Laboratory parameters should be monitored at regular intervals during prolonged therapy
Carcinogenicity, mutagenicity	No evidence of carcinogenicity has been reported in long-term studies of mice or rats; no mutagenic response has been detected in bacterial tests

ADVERSE REACTIONS[2]

Frequent reactions (incidence ≥ 1%) are printed in *italics*

Cardiovascular	*Edema (2.4%)*, angina, arrhythmia, AV block, bradycardia, congestive heart failure, flushing, hypotension, palpitations, syncope
Central nervous system	*Headache (2.1%), dizziness (1.5%), asthenia (1.2%)*, paresthesia, nervousness, somnolence, tremor, insomnia, hallucinations, amnesia, gait abnormality, personality change, tinnitus
Ophthalmic	Amblyopia, eye irritation
Gastrointestinal	*Nausea (1.9%)*, anorexia, dysgeusia, weight increase, constipation, dyspepsia, diarrhea, vomiting; elevation of SGOT, SGPT, alkaline phosphatase, CPK, and LDH levels
Dermatological	*Rash (1.3%)*, pruritus, petechiae, urticaria, photosensitivity
Genitourinary	Polyuria, nocturia, sexual difficulties
Other	Dyspnea, epistaxis, nasal congestion, hyperglycemia, osteoarticular pain

OVERDOSAGE

Signs and symptoms	Bradycardia, high-degree AV block, hypotension, and cardiac failure may be anticipated; actual overdosage has not been reported
Treatment	Empty stomach by gastric lavage, and institute supportive measures. For bradycardia and high-degree AV block, use atropine (0.6–1 mg); if there is no response to vagal blockade, cautiously administer isoproterenol. Fixed high-degree AV block should be treated with cardiac pacing. For hypotension, use vasopressors (eg, dopamine or norepinephrine). For cardiac failure, administer inotropic agents (eg, isoproterenol, dopamine, or dobutamine) and diuretics.

DRUG INTERACTIONS

Beta-adrenergic blockers, digitalis	⇧ AV conduction time ⇧ Serum digoxin level

ALTERED LABORATORY VALUES

Blood/serum values	⇧ SGOT ⇧ SGPT ⇧ Alkaline phosphatase ⇧ LDH ⇧ CPK ⇧ Glucose

CARDIZEM ■ ISOPTIN

No clinically significant alterations in urinary values occur at therapeutic dosages

USE IN CHILDREN

Safety and effectiveness for use in children have not been established

USE IN PREGNANT AND NURSING WOMEN

Pregnancy Category C: use during pregnancy only if the expected benefit justifies the potential risk to the fetus. Administration of 5–10 times the recommended human dose to mice, rats, and rabbits has resulted in skeletal abnormalities and fetal deaths. An increased incidence of stillbirths (at ≥ 20 times the human dose), decreased pup body weights, and decreased survival rates have been reported. An intrinsic effect on fertility has not been observed in rats. No adequate, well-controlled studies have been performed in humans. The concentration of diltiazem in human milk may be equivalent to that of blood; do not use in nursing mothers.

[1] Long-term effectiveness in the management of chronic stable angina has not been established
[2] Reactions for which a causal relationship has not been established include alopecia, gingival hyperplasia, erythema multiforme, and leukopenia

CALCIUM ANTAGONISTS

ISOPTIN (verapamil hydrochloride) Knoll   Rx

Tablets: 80, 120 mg

INDICATIONS	ORAL DOSAGE
Angina at rest, including vasospastic (Prinzmetal's variant) and unstable (crescendo, preinfarction) angina **Chronic stable angina** (classic effort-associated angina)	**Adult:** 80–120 mg tid, followed by daily or weekly increases in dosage, up to 480 mg/day, as needed, until optimum clinical response is obtained
Control of ventricular rate in digitalized patients with chronic atrial flutter and/or atrial fibrillation	**Adult:** 240–320 mg/day, given in divided doses tid or qid
Prophylaxis of repetitive paroxysmal supraventricular tachycardia in undigitalized patients	**Adult:** 240–480 mg/day
Essential hypertension	**Adult:** 240 mg/day to start, given in equally divided doses tid

ISOPTIN SR (verapamil hydrochloride) Knoll   Rx

Tablets (sustained release): 240 mg

INDICATIONS	ORAL DOSAGE
Essential hypertension	**Adult:** 240 mg/day, given in a single morning dose; if an adequate response is not obtained, titrate the dosage upward by giving 240 mg each morning to start, followed by 240 mg each morning plus 120 mg each evening, and then 240 mg q12h

CONTRAINDICATIONS

Severe left ventricular dysfunction Hypotension (systolic pressure < 90 mm Hg)	Second- or third-degree AV block (except in patients with a functioning artificial ventricular pacemaker) Cardiogenic shock	Sick sinus syndrome (except in patients with a functioning artificial ventricular pacemaker)

ADMINISTRATION/DOSAGE ADJUSTMENTS

Titration of dosage	Starting treatment at 40 mg tid should be considered in anginal and hypertensive patients who may exhibit an increased response to verapamil as a result of hepatic dysfunction, advanced age, small body size, or other conditions. Titrate dosage upward based on therapeutic efficacy and safety, evaluated approximately 8 h after the immediate-release tablets are taken or 24 h after the sustained-release formulation has been taken. Since the half-life of verapamil increases with repeated administration, the maximum response may be delayed during chronic dosing. In general, the maximum antiarrhythmic effect of this drug will be apparent during the first 48 h of administration, whereas the antihypertensive effect should be evident within the first week of therapy.
Timing of administration	The sustained-release formulation should be administered with food; the immediate-release tablets may be taken without regard to meals
Switching formulations	The total daily dose of verapamil may remain the same when switching from the immediate-release to the sustained-release form

ISOPTIN

Concomitant therapy — Concomitant use of this drug with both short- and long-acting nitrates may be beneficial in patients with angina and is apparently free of harmful drug interactions. Concomitant use of verapamil with beta blockers may also be beneficial in certain patients with chronic stable angina or hypertension, but the combination can adversely affect cardiac function (see WARNINGS/PRECAUTIONS). Monitor vital signs and clinical status closely, and reassess the need for concomitant beta-blocker therapy periodically.

WARNINGS/PRECAUTIONS

Heart failure — Control heart failure with digitalis and/or diuretics before giving verapamil; do not administer to patients with severe left ventricular dysfunction (ejection fraction < 30%), patients with moderate to severe cardiac failure, or those with significant ventricular dysfunction who are concomitantly receiving a beta blocker.

Hypotension — Blood pressure may fall in some patients and may result in dizziness or symptomatic hypotension; decreases in blood pressure below normal levels are unusual in hypertensive patients (tilt table testing [60°] has not induced orthostatic hypotension). If severe hypotension occurs, administer isoproterenol, norepinephrine, atropine, or 10% calcium gluconate immediately *(in patients with hypertrophic cardiomyopathy [IHSS], use phenylephrine, metaraminol, or methoxamine, instead of isoproterenol or norepinephrine, to maintain blood pressure)*. If further support is needed, administer dopamine or dobutamine.

Hepatotoxicity — Elevations of SGOT, SGPT, alkaline phosphatase, and bilirubin levels have been reported. In some cases, these increases have been transient. However, in several patients, drug-induced hepatocellular injury has been reported; half of these patients experienced malaise, fever, and/or right quadrant pain, as well as elevated hepatic enzyme levels. To reduce the risk of hepatotoxicity, periodically monitor liver function in all patients.

Rapid ventricular response, fibrillation — In patients with paroxysmal and/or chronic atrial flutter or atrial fibrillation and an accessory AV pathway (eg, Wolff-Parkinson-White or Lown-Ganong-Levine syndrome), IV verapamil may produce a very rapid ventricular response or ventricular fibrillation following increased antegrade conduction; treat with DC cardioversion. While these effects have not been reported with oral verapamil, they should be considered during therapy.

Antrioventricular block — The effect of this drug on AV conduction and the SA node may cause asymptomatic first-degree AV block and transient bradycardia, sometimes accompanied by nodal escape rhythms; prolongation of the P-R interval is correlated with plasma concentrations of verapamil, especially during early titration of therapy. If marked first-degree block occurs, reduce dosage or discontinue verapamil administration and institute appropriate therapy (see suggested management of severe hypotension, above).

Patients with hypertrophic cardiomyopathy (IHSS) — Serious adverse effects, including pulmonary edema and/or severe hypotension, sinus bradycardia, second-degree AV block, and sinus arrest, may occur in these patients; reduce dosage if adverse effects occur or discontinue therapy, if necessary

Drug accumulation — Use with caution in patients with significant renal or hepatic impairment; administer 30% of the usual dose to patients with hepatic impairment. Carefully monitor patients for abnormal prolongation of the P-R interval or other signs of overdosage (see below).

Carcinogenicity — Studies in rats fed verapamil at doses of 10, 35, and 120 mg/kg/day for 2 yr showed no evidence of carcinogenic potential; verapamil has shown no evidence of tumorigenicity in rats given 6 times the maximum human dose for 18 mo

Mutagenicity — Verapamil has shown no evidence of mutagenicity in the Ames test

Effect on fertility — Studies in female rats fed 5.5 times the recommended human dose of verapamil showed no evidence of impaired fertility; the effect of this drug on male fertility has not been determined

ADVERSE REACTIONS[1]

Frequent reactions (incidence ≥ 1%) are printed in *italics*

Cardiovascular — *Hypotension (2.5%), edema (2.1%), congestive heart failure/pulmonary edema (1.8%), bradycardia (< 50 beats/min) (1.4%); first, second, and third-degree AV block (1.3%);* third-degree AV block (0.8%), flushing (0.1%)

Gastrointestinal — *Constipation (8.4%), nausea (2.7%),* elevation of liver enzyme levels

Central nervous system — *Dizziness (3.5%), headache (1.9%), fatigue (1.7%)*

OVERDOSAGE

Signs and symptoms — Abnormal prolongation of P-R interval, severe hypotension, second- or third-degree AV block, asystole

Treatment — Institute standard supportive measures (eg, IV fluids). Administer beta-adrenergic stimulating agents or parenteral calcium solutions to increase calcium ion flux across the slow channel. Treat clinically significant hypotensive reactions or high-degree AV block with vasopressors or cardiac pacing, respectively. Treat asystole with usual measures, including cardiopulmonary resuscitation.

ISOPTIN ■ PROCARDIA

DRUG INTERACTIONS

Beta blockers	△ Antianginal and antihypertensive effects △ Risk of negative inotropic and chronotropic effects during high-dose beta-blocker therapy; closely monitor patients during concomitant therapy ▽ Clearance of metoprolol
Digoxin	△ Serum digoxin level and digitalis toxicity; reduce dosage or discontinue use of digoxin, if necessary
Oral antihypertensive agents (eg, vasodilators, angiotensin-converting enzyme inhibitors, diuretics, beta blockers)	△ Reduction of blood pressure; monitor patient during concomitant therapy
Prazosin	Excessive hypotension
Disopyramide	△ Risk of decreased myocardial contractility; do not give disopyramide within 48 h before or 24 h after administration of verapamil
Quinidine	Significant hypotension in patients with hypertrophic cardiomyopathy (IHSS); avoid concomitant use in these patients △ Serum levels of quinidine ▽ Pharmacologic effects of quinidine on AV conduction
Cimetidine	▽ Clearance of verapamil △ Elimination half-life of verapamil
Lithium	▽ Serum levels of lithium; adjust dosage of lithium, if necessary
Carbamazepine	△ Serum levels of carbamazepine
Rifampin	▽ Bioavailability of rifampin
Neuromuscular blocking agents, inhalation anesthetics	△ Pharmacologic activity of neuromuscular blocking agents and inhalation anesthetics
Nitrates	△ Antianginal effect of verapamil and nitrates

ALTERED LABORATORY VALUES

Blood/serum values — △ SGOT △ SGPT △ Alkaline phosphatase △ Bilirubin

No clinically significant alterations in urinary values occur at therapeutic dosages

USE IN CHILDREN

Safety and effectiveness for use in children under 18 yr of age have not been established

USE IN PREGNANT AND NURSING WOMEN

Pregnancy Category C: reproductive studies in rabbits and rats at oral doses up to 1.5 and 6 times the oral human dose, respectively, have shown no evidence of teratogenicity; in the rat, however, the drug caused hypotension, was embryocidal, and retarded fetal growth and development. Verapamil crosses the placental barrier and can be detected in umbilical vein blood at delivery; it is not known whether verapamil administration during labor and delivery has any immediate or delayed adverse effect on the fetus, prolongs labor, or increases the need for obstetric intervention. No adequate, well-controlled studies have been performed in pregnant women; use during pregnancy only if clearly needed. Verapamil is excreted in human milk; patients who are taking this drug should not nurse.

[1] Reactions for which a causal relationship is uncertain include angina pectoris, chest pain, claudication, myocardial infarction, palpitations, purpura (vasculitis), syncope, diarrhea, dry mouth, GI distress, gingival hyperplasia, ecchymosis, bruising, confusion, equilibrium disorders, insomnia, muscle cramps, paresthesia, psychotic symptoms, shakiness, somnolence; dyspnea, arthralgia and rash, exanthema, hair loss, hyperkeratosis, maculae, sweating, urticaria, blurred vision, gynecomastia, increased urination, spotty menstruation; cerebrovascular accident and impotence (reported only with sustained-release form)

CALCIUM ANTAGONISTS

PROCARDIA (nifedipine) Pfizer   Rx

Capsules: 10, 20 mg

INDICATIONS

Vasospastic angina confirmed by (1) a classical pattern of angina at rest accompanied by ST-segment elevation, (2) angina or coronary artery spasm provokable by ergonovine, *or* (3) angiographically demonstrable coronary artery spasm[1]

Chronic stable angina (effort-associated angina) in patients without evidence of vasospasm who (1) remain symptomatic despite adequate doses of beta blockers or organic nitrates *or* (2) cannot tolerate these agents[2]

ORAL DOSAGE

Adult: 10 mg tid to start, followed by gradual increases in dosage (see "frequency of dosage adjustment," below), as needed and tolerated. The usual effective dosage is 10–20 mg tid; however, some patients, especially those with evidence of coronary artery spasm, may require 20–30 mg tid or qid. Dosages above 120 mg/day are rarely necessary, and dosages exceeding 180 mg/day are not recommended.

PROCARDIA

CONTRAINDICATIONS

Hypersensitivity to nifedipine

ADMINISTRATION/DOSAGE ADJUSTMENTS

Frequency of dosage adjustment	In most cases, 7–14 days should elapse between dosage increases to permit adequate assessment of clinical response and patient tolerance; however, if the patient's level of physical activity, attack frequency, and sublingual nitroglycerin consumption warrant, the dosage may be increased from 10 mg tid to 20 mg tid and then to 30 mg tid over a 3-day period, provided that the patient is frequently evaluated. In hospitalized patients under close observation, the dosage may be increased by 10 mg q4–6h, as needed to control pain and arrhythmias due to ischemia; more than 30 mg should generally not be given as a single dose. No rebound effect has been observed upon discontinuation of therapy; nevertheless, if discontinuation is necessary, dosage should be decreased gradually under close supervision.
Concomitant administration of other antianginal agents	Sublingual nitroglycerin tablets may be taken as needed for acute anginal symptoms, especially during the period of initial dosage titration. Co-administration of nifedipine and beta blockers may be beneficial in patients with chronic stable angina and is usually well tolerated; however, the effects of this combination, particularly in patients with compromised left ventricular function or cardiac conduction abnormalities, cannot be predicted with confidence until more data are obtained. (See warnings, below, concerning hypotension, exacerbation of angina, and congestive heart failure.) Nifedipine may be given safely with organic nitrates, but there have been no controlled studies to evaluate the effectiveness of this combination on angina.

WARNINGS/PRECAUTIONS

Hypotension	Occasional patients may develop excessive or poorly tolerated hypotension, particularly when nifedipine is introduced or when the dosage is subsequently increased; co-administration of beta blockers increases the risk. Blood pressure should be carefully monitored during the period of initial dosage adjustment, especially if the patient is taking drugs that are known to produce hypotension.
Exacerbation of angina and myocardial infarction	An increase in the frequency, duration, or severity of angina or acute myocardial infarction has occurred at the start of therapy and when the dosage has been increased. This rare effect has been seen most commonly in patients with severe obstructive coronary artery disease. Nifedipine may also exacerbate the increase in angina that can develop during or after withdrawal of a beta blocker; discontinue a beta blocker gradually, if possible, when switching to nifedipine.
Congestive heart failure	Has occurred rarely after initiation of nifedipine therapy, usually in patients receiving beta blockers; patients with "tight" aortic stenosis may be at increased risk
Peripheral edema	Approximately 10% of patients develop peripheral edema, primarily in the lower extremities; the edema is typically associated with arterial vasodilation and usually responds to diuretics. Peripheral edema occurring in nifedipine-treated patients with congestive heart failure should be carefully differentiated from the effects of increasing left ventricular dysfunction.
Hematological effects	Hemolytic anemia has occurred during therapy. Limited clinical studies have demonstrated that in some patients nifedipine can moderately decrease platelet aggregation, presumably by inhibiting calcium ion flux across the platelet membrane, and thereby increase bleeding time; thrombocytopenia has been reported. The use of nifedipine in patients receiving coumarin anticoagulants has been associated, in rare cases, with an increase in prothrombin time; however, a causal relationship has not been established.
Hepatotoxicity	In rare instances, significantly elevated hepatic enzyme levels, cholestasis, cholestatic jaundice, and allergic hepatitis have occurred during therapy
Patients with renal impairment	Rare, reversible elevations in BUN and serum creatinine levels have been seen in patients with chronic renal insufficiency; in at least some cases, the increases were probably due to nifedipine
Surgery with fentanyl	Nifedipine therapy should be interrupted, if possible, at least 36 h before any surgical procedure that requires high doses of fentanyl. Severe hypotension and hypovolemia have occurred in patients who were given high doses of fentanyl during coronary artery bypass surgery; although these reactions were apparently due to the combination of nifedipine and a beta blocker, the possibility that such reactions may also occur in other surgical procedures or with other narcotic analgesics, low doses of fentanyl, or nifedipine alone cannot be ruled out.
Patients receiving digoxin	Measure serum digoxin levels at the beginning and end of nifedipine therapy and whenever the dosage of nifedipine is changed; administration of this drug has been reported to elevate serum digoxin levels. In one study, nifedipine increased serum digoxin levels in 9 of 12 normal subjects by an average of 45%. However, a study in 13 patients with coronary artery disease showed no increase in serum levels, and no evidence of digitalis toxicity was found in an uncontrolled study that involved over 200 patients with congestive heart failure.
Carcinogenicity, mutagenicity	There is no evidence that nifedipine is carcinogenic or mutagenic

PROCARDIA

Impairment of fertility	Reduced fertility has been observed in rats given approximately 30 times the maximum recommended human dose prior to mating

ADVERSE REACTIONS[3]

Frequent reactions (incidence $\geq$ 1%) are printed in *italics*

Central nervous system	*Dizziness/light-headedness, headache, and weakness (each ~10%)*; shakiness, nervousness, jitteriness, sleep disturbances, and difficulties in maintaining balance (each $\leq$ 2%); depression and paranoid syndrome (each < 0.5%)
Ophthalmic	Blurred vision ($\leq$ 2%), transient blindness at peak plasma level (< 0.5%)
Cardiovascular	*Peripheral edema and flushing (each ~10%), transient hypotension (~5%), myocardial infarction (4%), palpitation and congestive heart failure/pulmonary edema (2%)*, syncope (~0.5%), ventricular arrhythmias and conduction disturbances (each < 0.5%), increased angina (rare)
Hematological	Thrombocytopenia, anemia, leukopenia, and purpura (each < 0.5%)
Gastrointestinal	*Nausea (~10%)*; diarrhea, constipation, cramps, and flatulence (each $\leq$ 2%); allergic hepatitis (< 0.5%); cholestasis with or without jaundice (rare)
Respiratory	Nasal/chest congestion and shortness of breath (each $\leq$ 2%)
Musculoskeletal	Inflammation, joint stiffness, and muscle cramps (each $\leq$ 2%)
Dermatological	Dermatitis, pruritus, and urticaria (each $\leq$ 2%); erythromelalgia (< 0.5%)
Other	Fever, sweating, chills, and sexual difficulties (each $\leq$ 2%); gingival hyperplasia and arthritis with positive ANA (each < 0.5%)

OVERDOSAGE

Signs and symptoms	Marked and probably prolonged systemic hypotension
Treatment	Empty stomach by inducing emesis or by gastric lavage. Monitor cardiac and respiratory function, elevate the lower extremities, and pay careful attention to the patient's circulating fluid volume and urine output, instituting supportive measures, as needed. A vasoconstrictor (eg, norepinephrine) may be given to help restore vascular tone and blood pressure, unless there is a contraindication to its use. Clearance may be prolonged in patients with liver disease. Dialysis is not likely to be beneficial, since the drug is highly protein bound.

DRUG INTERACTIONS

Beta blockers	⇧ Risk of severe hypotension, congestive heart failure, and exacerbation of angina
Oral anticoagulants	⇧ Anticoagulant effect (see WARNINGS/PRECAUTIONS)
Cimetidine	⇧ Serum nifedipine level; if treatment is initiated in a patient currently receiving cimetidine, cautious titration is advised

ALTERED LABORATORY VALUES

Blood/serum values	⇧ SGOT ⇧ SGPT ⇧ Alkaline phosphatase ⇧ LDH ⇧ CPK + Coombs' test + ANA

No clinically significant alterations in urinary values occur at therapeutic dosages

---

USE IN CHILDREN

No clinical experience with this drug in children has been reported

USE IN PREGNANT AND NURSING WOMEN

Pregnancy Category C: use during pregnancy only if anticipated benefit of therapy justifies the potential fetal risk. Nifedipine has been shown to be teratogenic in rats at 30 times the maximum recommended human dose and embryotoxic in rats, mice, and rabbits at 3–10 times the maximum recommended human dose. Administration of two-thirds and twice the maximum recommended human dose to pregnant monkeys has resulted in small placentas with underdeveloped chorionic villi. Prolongation of pregnancy has been observed in rats at 3 times the maximum human dose. No adequate, well-controlled studies have been done in pregnant women. It is not known whether nifedipine is excreted in human milk; because many drugs are excreted in human milk, patient should not nurse while taking this drug.

---

[1] Nifedipine may also be used when the clinical presentation suggests a possible vasospastic component but vasospasm has not been confirmed (eg, when pain on exertion has a variable threshold, when ECG findings are compatible with intermittent vasospasm in unstable angina, or when angina is refractory to organic nitrates and/or adequate doses of beta blockers)
[2] The effectiveness and safety of using nifedipine beyond 8 wk in these patients have not been established
[3] Adverse reactions reported in uncontrolled clinical trials of nifedipine in over 2,100 patients in the United States. The pattern and incidence of major adverse effects observed in worldwide controlled studies were as follows: dizziness/light-headedness/giddiness, 27%; flushing/heat sensation, 25%; headache, 23%; weakness, 12%; nausea/heartburn, 11%; muscle cramps/tremor, 8%; peripheral edema, 7%; nervousness/mood changes, 7%; palpitation, 7%; dyspnea/cough/wheezing, 6%; and nasal congestion/sore throat, 6%.

NITRATES

CARDILATE (erythrityl tetranitrate) Burroughs Wellcome   Rx
Oral/sublingual tablets: 5, 10 mg

INDICATIONS	SUBLINGUAL DOSAGE	ORAL DOSAGE
Prophylaxis and long-term management of **angina pectoris**	**Adult:** 5–10 mg to start prior to anticipated period of stress and at bedtime for patients subject to nocturnal attacks; adjust subsequent dosage as needed, up to 100 mg/day	**Adult:** 10 mg to start before each meal, as well as midmorning, midafternoon (if needed), and at bedtime for patients subject to nocturnal attacks; adjust subsequent dosage as needed, up to 100 mg/day

CONTRAINDICATIONS
Hypersensitivity or idiosyncratic reaction to organic nitrates

ADMINISTRATION/DOSAGE ADJUSTMENTS
Administration	Oral/sublingual tablets may be placed under the tongue or swallowed
Management of headache	If headache occurs, reduce dosage for a few days and, if necessary, give an analgesic

WARNINGS/PRECAUTIONS
Special-risk patients	Administration to patients with acute myocardial infarction or congestive heart failure should be undertaken only in conjunction with close clinical observation or hemodynamic monitoring. Use with caution in patients with severe hepatic or renal disease.
Tolerance	Patients may develop tolerance to this drug and cross-tolerance to other organic nitrates; however, studies in patients with chronic heart failure have shown that nitrates produce beneficial hemodynamic effects even after prolonged use.
Carcinogenicity, mutagenicity, effect on fertility	No long-term studies in animals have been done to evaluate the carcinogenic or mutagenic potential of this drug or its effect on fertility

ADVERSE REACTIONS
The most frequent reaction is italicized

Central nervous system	*Headache;* transient dizziness, weakness, and other signs of cerebral ischemia associated with postural hypotension; restlessness
Cardiovascular	Cutaneous vasodilation with flushing, pallor
Gastrointestinal	Nausea, vomiting
Dermatological	Rash, exfoliative dermatitis
Other	Sweating, collapse

OVERDOSAGE
Signs and symptoms	Severe hypotension, reflex tachycardia
Treatment	Place patient in a supine position and elevate the legs; IV fluids or other measures may be indicated if further treatment of hypotension is necessary

DRUG INTERACTIONS
Alcohol, antihypertensive agents, other vasodilators	⇧ Orthostatic hypotensive effect of erythrityl tetranitrate
Sympathomimetics	⇩ Antianginal effect of erythrityl tetranitrate

ALTERED LABORATORY VALUES
No clinically significant alterations in blood/serum or urinary values occur at therapeutic dosages

---

USE IN CHILDREN

Safety and effectiveness for use in children have not been established

USE IN PREGNANT AND NURSING WOMEN

Pregnancy Category C: use during pregnancy only if clearly needed. Animal reproduction studies have not been done, nor is it known whether this drug can affect human fetal development or reproductive capacity. It is also not known whether this drug is excreted in human milk; use with caution in nursing mothers because many drugs are excreted in human milk.

NITRATES

DEPONIT (nitroglycerin) Wyeth   Rx
Transdermal drug delivery systems: 5 mg/24 h (16 cm^2), 10 mg/24 h (32 cm^2)

INDICATIONS	TRANSCUTANEOUS DOSAGE
Prevention and treatment of **angina pectoris** due to coronary artery disease[1]	**Adult:** to start, firmly apply a 16-cm^2 system q24h to a convenient skin site, other than the distal extremities, that is clean, intact, dry, and hairless (clip hair first, if necessary); preferable sites are the chest, inner side of the upper arm, and shoulders. To minimize irritation, change the site daily.

DEPONIT ■ DILATRATE-SR

CONTRAINDICATIONS

| Intolerance to organic nitrates | Marked anemia |

ADMINISTRATION/DOSAGE ADJUSTMENTS

| Titration of dose | An increase in dose may be necessary for some patients; use a larger system or an appropriate combination of systems. When titrating dosage, monitor clinical response, heart rate, and blood pressure. |
| Discontinuation of therapy | To prevent sudden withdrawal reactions, gradually reduce both the daily dose and the frequency of application over a period of 4–6 wk |

WARNINGS/PRECAUTIONS

Headache	Transient headaches may occur, particularly at higher doses; treat with mild analgesics while continuing therapy. If headaches persist, reduce dosage or discontinue use.
Symptomatic hypotension	Faintness, weakness, or dizziness, particularly upon standing, may indicate overdosage; reduce dosage or discontinue use if such symptoms occur
Other reactions	Nausea, vomiting, flushing, or increased heart rate can occur during therapy; if reaction persists, reduce dose or discontinue use
Abrupt withdrawal of therapy	Sudden withdrawal reactions may occur following abrupt discontinuation of therapy (see ADMINISTRATION/DOSAGE ADJUSTMENTS)
Cardioversion	To avoid electrical arcing during defibrillation or cardioversion, remove the system before performing the procedure
Special-risk patients	Provide for close clinical surveillance and/or hemodynamic monitoring when the patient has acute myocardial infarction or congestive heart failure
Anginal attacks	This preparation is not intended for immediate relief of acute anginal episodes; sublingual nitroglycerin may be needed occasionally to provide prompt relief

ADVERSE REACTIONS

Cardiovascular	Transient headache, hypotension, increased heart rate, faintness, flushing, dizziness
Gastrointestinal	Nausea, vomiting
Dermatological	Dermatitis

OVERDOSAGE

| Signs and symptoms | See ADVERSE REACTIONS |
| Treatment | Reduce dosage or discontinue use |

DRUG INTERACTIONS

| Alcohol, antihypertensive agents, other vasodilators | ⇧ Orthostatic hypotensive effect of nitroglycerin |

ALTERED LABORATORY VALUES

| Blood/serum values | ⇩ Cholesterol (with Zlatkis-Zak color reaction) |
| Urinary values | ⇧ Catecholamines   ⇧ VMA |

USE IN CHILDREN

Safety and effectiveness for use in children have not been established

USE IN PREGNANT AND NURSING WOMEN

Pregnancy Category C: reproduction studies have not been done; it is not known whether nitroglycerin can affect reproductive capacity or cause harm to the fetus. Use during pregnancy only if clearly needed. It is also not known whether nitroglycerin is excreted in human milk; use with caution in nursing mothers.

[1] Conditionally approved

NITRATES

DILATRATE-SR (isosorbide dinitrate) Reed & Carnrick   Rx

Capsules (controlled release): 40 mg

INDICATIONS
Management of chronic stable angina

ORAL DOSAGE
Adult: 40 mg to start, followed by 40–80 mg q8–12h; capsules should not be chewed

CONTRAINDICATIONS
Hypersensitivity or idiosyncratic reaction to nitrates or nitrites

DILATRATE-SR

ADMINISTRATION/DOSAGE ADJUSTMENTS

Titration of dosage	Increase dosage until angina is relieved or adverse reactions limit further titration; if the patient is ambulatory, measure standing blood pressure to determine the magnitude of each dosage increase

WARNINGS/PRECAUTIONS

Acute myocardial infarction	When used during the early days of an acute myocardial infarction, nitrates can cause potentially deleterious hypotension; moreover, it has not been established that use at that time is beneficial. If isosorbide dinitrate is given at the early stage of an infarction, assess clinical response frequently and monitor hemodynamic parameters.
Hypotension	Severe hypotension, particularly with upright posture, may occur even with small doses; however, hypotension is generally dose-related. Transient dizziness and weakness as well as other symptoms of orthostatic hypotension occur in 2–36% of patients. Hypotension may be accompanied by paradoxical bradycardia and exacerbation of angina. Exercise caution if systolic pressure is less than 90 mm Hg or if blood volume may have been depleted by diuretic therapy.
Hypertrophic cardiomyopathy	Nitrates can exacerbate angina associated with hypertrophic cardiomyopathy
Tolerance	Although nitrate tolerance has been demonstrated in clinical trials, isolated-tissue experiments, and studies with industrial workers continuously exposed to nitroglycerin, the relative importance of this effect has not been determined. In one clinical study, the duration of action of oral isosorbide dinitrate decreased from 8 h to 2 h after 1 wk of continuous use; however, several controlled studies have demonstrated a therapeutic effect after 4 wk of use, and, in open trials, an effect seemed detectable even with administration for as long as several months. If tolerance to isosorbide dinitrate develops, cross-tolerance to nitrites and other nitrates may occur.
Physical dependence	Chest pain, acute myocardial infarction, and even sudden death have occurred in workers who were constantly exposed to nitroglycerin and then temporarily withdrawn from such a setting. During clinical trials, there were reports that soon after discontinuation of nitrates, adverse hemodynamic effects recurred and angina was more easily provoked. Although the relative importance of these findings has not been determined, it seems prudent to terminate therapy in a gradual manner, rather than abruptly.
Headache	The most frequent reaction to nitrates, seen in approximately 25% of patients, is headache. Although headache may be severe and persistent, it generally can be relieved by standard headache remedies or a reduction in dosage, and it usually tends to disappear 1–2 wk after the onset of therapy.
Methemoglobinemia	At therapeutic dosages, nitrates can produce methemoglobinemia in patients with hemoglobin abnormalities that favor formation of methemoglobin
Carcinogenicity, effect on fertility	No long-term studies have been done to evaluate the carcinogenic potential of isosorbide dinitrate; a modified two-litter reproduction study in rats fed 25 or 100 mg/kg/day has shown no adverse effect on fertility

ADVERSE REACTIONS

Cardiovascular	Headache, orthostatic hypotension, cutaneous vasodilation with flushing, weakness, pallor, perspiration, circulatory collapse
Gastrointestinal	Nausea, vomiting
Dermatological	Drug rash, exfoliative dermatitis
Other	Restlessness; methemoglobinemia (rare)

OVERDOSAGE

Signs and symptoms	*Cardiovascular:* persistent, throbbing headache; severe hypotension; flushing and diaphoresis followed by cutaneous chilling and cyanosis; dicrotic, intermittent pulse; palpitations, vertigo, syncope, heart block, circulatory collapse; *CNS:* visual disturbances, increased intracranial pressure (with confusion and moderate fever), paralysis and coma followed by clonic convulsions; *GI:* nausea, vomiting, colic, bloody diarrhea; *respiratory:* methemoglobinemia with cyanosis and anoxia, initial hyperpnea, dyspnea, hypopnea
Treatment	Promptly perform gastric lavage. To treat hypotension, place patient in a recumbent (shock) position and keep comfortably warm; passive movements of the extremities may enhance venous return. Do not use epinephrine or related compounds to reverse hypotension. Institute mechanical ventilation and administer oxygen, as needed. For methemoglobinemia, give 1–2 mg/kg of 1% methylene blue IV. It is not known whether isosorbide dinitrate can be removed by dialysis.

DRUG INTERACTIONS

Alcohol, antihypertensive drugs, and other vasodilators	⇧ Risk of hypotension
Calcium-channel blockers	Marked symptomatic orthostatic hypotension; if necessary, adjust dosage of nitrate or calcium-channel blocker

DILATRATE-SR ■ ISORDIL

ALTERED LABORATORY VALUES

Blood/serum values	▽ Cholesterol (with Zlatkis-Zak color reaction)
Urinary values	△ Catecholamines △ VMA

USE IN CHILDREN
Safety and effectiveness for use in children have not been established

USE IN PREGNANT AND NURSING WOMEN
Pregnancy Category C: isosorbide dinitrate has been shown to be embryotoxic in rabbits, causing an increase in mummified pups at oral doses of 35 and 150 times the maximum human daily dose; no adequate, well-controlled studies have been done in pregnant women. Use during pregnancy only if the expected benefit justifies the potential risk to the fetus. It is not known whether isosorbide dinitrate is excreted in human milk; use with caution in nursing mothers.

NITRATES

ISORDIL (isosorbide dinitrate) Wyeth Rx

Sublingual tablets: 2.5, 5, 10 mg **Chewable tablets:** 10 mg **Swallowable tablets:** 5, 10, 20, 30, 40 mg **Capsules (controlled release):** 40 mg **Tablets (controlled release):** 40 mg

INDICATIONS

Management of chronic stable angina

Prevention of acute angina that can be anticipated

Treatment of acute angina in patients intolerant or unresponsive to sublingual nitroglycerin

ORAL DOSAGE

Adult: when using swallowable tablets, 5–20 mg to start, followed by 10–40 mg q6h; when using controlled-release preparations, 40 mg to start, followed by 40–80 mg q8–12h. Swallowable tablets and controlled-release products should not be chewed.

Adult: 5–10 mg to start, using sublingual or chewable tablets; administer a few minutes before a situation likely to provoke an attack. Doses may be given q2–3h to maintain prophylactic effect; however, no adequate, controlled studies have been done to demonstrate the effectiveness of long-term therapy with these dosage forms.

Adult: when using sublingual tablets, 2.5–5 mg to start; when using chewable tablets, 5 mg to start

CONTRAINDICATIONS
Hypersensitivity or idiosyncratic reaction to nitrates or nitrites

ADMINISTRATION/DOSAGE ADJUSTMENTS

Titration of dosage — Increase dosage until angina is relieved or adverse reactions limit further titration; if the patient is ambulatory, measure standing blood pressure to determine the magnitude of each dosage increase

WARNINGS/PRECAUTIONS

Acute myocardial infarction — When used during the early days of an acute myocardial infarction, nitrates can cause potentially deleterious hypotension; moreover, it has not been established that use at that time is beneficial. If isosorbide dinitrate is given at the early stage of an infarction, assess clinical response frequently and monitor hemodynamic parameters.

Hypotension — Severe hypotension, particularly with upright posture, may occur even with small doses; however, hypotension is generally dose-related. Transient dizziness and weakness as well as other symptoms of orthostatic hypotension occur in 2–36% of patients. Hypotension may be accompanied by paradoxical bradycardia and exacerbation of angina. Exercise caution if systolic pressure is less than 90 mm Hg or if blood volume may have been depleted by diuretic therapy.

Hypertrophic cardiomyopathy — Nitrates can exacerbate angina associated with hypertrophic cardiomyopathy

Tolerance — Although nitrate tolerance has been demonstrated in clinical trials, isolated-tissue experiments, and studies with industrial workers continuously exposed to nitroglycerin, the relative importance of this effect has not been determined. In one clinical study, the duration of action of oral isosorbide dinitrate decreased from 8 h to 2 h after 1 wk of continuous use; however, several controlled studies have demonstrated a therapeutic effect after 4 wk of use, and, in open trials, an effect seemed detectable even with administration for as long as several months. If tolerance to isosorbide dinitrate develops, cross-tolerance to nitrites and other nitrates may occur.

Physical dependence — Chest pain, acute myocardial infarction, and even sudden death have occurred in workers who were constantly exposed to nitroglycerin and then temporarily withdrawn from such a setting. During clinical trials, there were reports that soon after discontinuation of nitrates, adverse hemodynamic effects recurred and angina was more easily provoked. Although the relative importance of these findings has not been determined, it seems prudent to terminate therapy in a gradual manner, rather than abruptly.

ISORDIL ■ NITRO-BID

Headache	The most frequent reaction to nitrates, seen in approximately 25% of patients, is headache. Although headache may be severe and persistent, it generally can be relieved by standard headache remedies or a reduction in dosage, and it usually tends to disappear 1–2 wk after the onset of therapy.
Methemoglobinemia	At therapeutic dosages, nitrates can produce methemoglobinemia in patients with hemoglobin abnormalities that favor formation of methemoglobin
Carcinogenicity, effect on fertility	No long-term studies have been done to evaluate the carcinogenic potential of isosorbide dinitrate; a modified two-litter reproduction study in rats fed 25 or 100 mg/kg/day has shown no adverse effect on fertility

ADVERSE REACTIONS

Cardiovascular	Headache, orthostatic hypotension, cutaneous vasodilation with flushing, weakness, pallor, perspiration, circulatory collapse
Gastrointestinal	Nausea, vomiting
Dermatological	Drug rash, exfoliative dermatitis
Other	Restlessness; methemoglobinemia (rare)

OVERDOSAGE

Signs and symptoms	*Cardiovascular:* persistent, throbbing headache; severe hypotension; flushing and diaphoresis followed by cutaneous chilling and cyanosis; dicrotic, intermittent pulse; palpitations, vertigo, syncope, heart block, circulatory collapse; *CNS:* visual disturbances, increased intracranial pressure (with confusion and moderate fever), paralysis and coma followed by clonic convulsions; *GI:* nausea, vomiting, colic, bloody diarrhea; *respiratory:* methemoglobinemia with cyanosis and anoxia, initial hyperpnea, dyspnea, hypopnea
Treatment	Promptly perform gastric lavage. To treat hypotension, place patient in a recumbent (shock) position and keep comfortably warm; passive movements of the extremities may enhance venous return. Do not use epinephrine or related compounds to reverse hypotension. Institute mechanical ventilation and administer oxygen, as needed. For methemoglobinemia, give 1–2 mg/kg of 1% methylene blue IV. It is not known whether isosorbide dinitrate can be removed by dialysis.

DRUG INTERACTIONS

Alcohol, antihypertensive drugs, and other vasodilators	△ Risk of hypotension
Calcium-channel blockers	Marked symptomatic orthostatic hypotension; if necessary, adjust dosage of nitrate or calcium-channel blocker

ALTERED LABORATORY VALUES

Blood/serum values	▽ Cholesterol (with Zlatkis-Zak color reaction)
Urinary values	△ Catecholamines △ VMA

USE IN CHILDREN

Safety and effectiveness for use in children have not been established

USE IN PREGNANT AND NURSING WOMEN

Pregnancy Category C: isosorbide dinitrate has been shown to be embryotoxic in rabbits, causing an increase in mummified pups at oral doses of 35 and 150 times the maximum human daily dose; no adequate, well-controlled studies have been done in pregnant women. Use during pregnancy only if the expected benefit justifies the potential risk to the fetus. It is not known whether isosorbide dinitrate is excreted in human milk; use with caution in nursing mothers.

NITRATES

NITRO-BID (nitroglycerin) Marion   Rx

Capsules (controlled release): 2.5, 6.5, 9 mg

INDICATIONS

Management, prophylaxis, and treatment of **anginal attacks**[1]

ORAL DOSAGE

Adult: administer smallest effective dose bid or tid, at 8- to 12-h intervals; titrate to anginal relief or hemodynamic response (fall in systolic blood pressure)

NITRO-BID Ointment (nitroglycerin) Marion　　Rx

Ointment: 2% (1-g pouch; 20- and 60-g tubes)

INDICATIONS	TOPICAL DOSAGE
Prevention and treatment of **angina pectoris** due to coronary artery disease[2]	**Adult:** 30 mg (2 in.) q8h; some patients may require up to 60–75 mg (4–5 in.) per application and/or application q4h

CONTRAINDICATIONS

For oral use only		For topical use only
Acute or recent myocardial infarction	Severe anemia	Intolerance to organic nitrates
Closed-angle glaucoma	Increased intracranial pressure	
Postural hypotension	Idiosyncratic reaction to nitroglycerin	

ADMINISTRATION/DOSAGE ADJUSTMENTS

Application of ointment	Squeeze the necessary amount of ointment from the tube or pouch onto the dose-measuring applicator supplied with the package; then, using the applicator to prevent absorption through the fingers, spread the ointment onto the skin in a thin, even layer, covering an area of 6 × 6 in. To protect clothing, cover the area with plastic film, which may be held in place with adhesive tape. The 1-g unit dose package contains the equivalent of 1 in. of ointment as squeezed from the tube.
Initial dosage titration for patients using the ointment	Start with 7.5 mg (1/2 in.) q8h and increase the dose by 7.5 mg (1/2 in.) with each successive application until the desired response is obtained. Optimal dosage may be gauged by the greatest reduction in resting blood pressure that is not associated with clinical symptoms of hypotension, especially orthostatic hypotension; to decrease adverse reactions, tailor the dose and frequency of application to individual needs.

WARNINGS/PRECAUTIONS

Anginal attacks	These preparations should not be used for the immediate relief of acute anginal symptoms
Headache	Transient headaches are the most common side effect of topical therapy, especially at higher dosages, and should be treated with mild analgesics; reduce dosage only if the headaches prove untreatable. Oral therapy may cause severe, persistent headaches.
Hypotension	If hypotension occurs, particularly when the patient rises from a recumbent position, reduce the dosage
Special-risk patients	Patients with acute myocardial infarction or congestive heart failure should be kept under careful clinical and/or hemodynamic surveillance during topical therapy (oral therapy is contraindicated in patients with acute or recent myocardial infarction); because oral administration may increase intraocular pressure, patients with glaucoma should be treated with caution
Contact dermatitis	Change the site of application or use topical corticosteroids if contact dermatitis occurs with use of the ointment
Blurred vision, dry mouth	May occur with oral use; discontinue medication
Tolerance	May develop, as well as cross-tolerance to other organic nitrates and nitrites, with oral use

ADVERSE REACTIONS

Central nervous system	Headache, dizziness, weakness (with oral use)
Cardiovascular	Hypotension, tachycardia, faintness, and flushing (with topical use); cutaneous flushing (with oral use)
Gastrointestinal	Nausea, vomiting (with oral use)
Dermatologic	Rash or exfoliative dermatitis (with oral use); contact dermatitis (with continued topical application)

OVERDOSAGE

Signs and symptoms	Hypotension, increased heart rate, faintness, flushing, dizziness, nausea
Treatment	Reduce dosage

DRUG INTERACTIONS

Acetylcholine	▽ Cholinergic receptor stimulation
Norepinephrine	▽ Pressor effect
Histamine	▽ Histamine effect
Alcohol, antihypertensive agents, other vasodilators	△ Orthostatic hypotensive effect of nitroglycerin
Sympathomimetics	▽ Antianginal effect of nitroglycerin

NITRO-BID ■ NITRO-BID IV

ALTERED LABORATORY VALUES

Urinary values — ◊ Catecholamines   ◊ Vanillylmandelic acid (VMA)

No clinically significant alterations in blood/serum values occur at therapeutic dosages

---

USE IN CHILDREN
Safety and effectiveness for use in children have not been established because of insufficient data

USE IN PREGNANT AND NURSING WOMEN
Consult manufacturer

VEHICLE/BASE
Ointment: lanolin and white petrolatum

[1] Possibly effective
[2] Conditionally approved

NITRATES

NITRO-BID IV (nitroglycerin) Marion   Rx

Vials: 5 mg/ml (1, 5, 10 ml) for IV infusion only

INDICATIONS
Angina pectoris unresponsive to recommended doses of organic nitrates and/or beta blockers
Congestive heart failure associated with acute myocardial infarction
Perioperative hypertension[1]
Production of controlled hypotension during surgical procedures

PARENTERAL DOSAGE
Adult: 5 µg/min via IV infusion, using an administration set made of nonabsorbing materials (see WARNINGS/PRECAUTIONS), to start; increase dosage in increments of 5 µg/min at 3- to 5-min intervals until some response is noted (if no response is seen at 20 µg/min, increments of 10 and then 20 µg/min may be used). Once a partial blood pressure response is observed, reduce the size of the dosage increments and lengthen the interval between increases.

CONTRAINDICATIONS
Hypersensitivity to nitroglycerin or idiosyncratic reaction to organic nitrates

Hypotension or uncorrected hypovolemia[2]

Increased intracranial pressure (eg, head trauma or cerebral hemorrhage)

Inadequate cerebral circulation

Constrictive pericarditis

Pericardial tamponade

ADMINISTRATION/DOSAGE ADJUSTMENTS

Dilution — Nitroglycerin must be diluted in 5% dextrose injection USP or 0.9% sodium chloride injection USP prior to infusion; the fluid requirements of the patient, as well as the expected duration of the infusion, should be considered in choosing an appropriate dilution. To obtain a concentration of 50 µg/ml, add 5 mg of nitroglycerin to 100 ml of diluent, 25 mg to 500 ml, or 50 mg to 1 liter; for a concentration of 100 µg/ml, add 5 mg to 50 ml, 25 mg to 250 ml, 50 mg to 500 ml, or 100 mg to 1 liter; for a concentration of 200 µg/ml, add 10 mg to 50 ml, 50 mg to 250 ml, 100 mg to 500 ml, or 200 mg to 1 liter. Do not mix nitroglycerin with other drugs in the same IV bottle.

Dosage titration — Titrate dosage to desired level of hemodynamic function; blood pressure, heart rate, and other appropriate physiologic parameters must be monitored continuously to obtain the correct dose. Adequate systemic blood pressure and coronary perfusion pressure must be maintained. Since a fall in pulmonary capillary wedge pressure precedes the onset of arterial hypotension, wedge pressure can serve as a useful guide to safe titration of this drug. Patients with normal or low left ventricular filling pressures or pulmonary capillary wedge pressures (eg, patients with uncomplicated angina pectoris) may respond fully to doses as small as 5 µg/min and, therefore, require especially careful titration and monitoring.

WARNINGS/PRECAUTIONS

Absorption of nitroglycerin by IV administration sets — Nitroglycerin is readily absorbed by many plastics; use glass IV bottles to dilute and store this drug and avoid filters that absorb nitroglycerin. Common administration sets made of polyvinyl chloride (PVC) tubing can absorb 40–80% of the total amount of nitroglycerin in the final solution. Since the loss is neither constant nor self-limited, it cannot be simply calculated or corrected for. Use of the least absorptive tubing available is recommended to minimize the loss of nitroglycerin. PVC tubing has been utilized exclusively in published studies, and the doses recommended (25 µg/min or more to start) will be too high if administration sets with nonabsorbing materials are used.

COMPENDIUM OF DRUG THERAPY

NITRO-BID IV ■ NITRO-DUR

Patients with hepatic or renal impairment	Use with caution in patients with severe liver or kidney disease
Excessive hypotension	Must be avoided because of possible deleterious effects on vital organs resulting from poor perfusion, especially if the hypotension is prolonged, and the attendant risk of ischemia, thrombosis, and physiologic impairment; paradoxical bradycardia and increased angina pectoris may accompany nitroglycerin-induced hypotension. Patients with normal or low pulmonary capillary wedge pressures are especially sensitive to the hypotensive effects of IV nitroglycerin (see ADMINISTRATION/DOSAGE ADJUSTMENTS).
Carcinogenicity	No long-term studies have been done in animals to evaluate the carcinogenic potential of nitroglycerin

ADVERSE REACTIONS[3]

Frequent reactions (incidence ≥ 1%) are printed in *italics*

Central nervous system and neuromuscular	*Headache (2%)*, apprehension, restlessness, muscle twitching, dizziness
Cardiovascular	Tachycardia, retrosternal discomfort, palpitations
Gastrointestinal	Nausea, vomiting, abdominal pain

OVERDOSAGE

Signs and symptoms	Severe hypotension, reflex tachycardia
Treatment	Elevate the patient's legs and decrease or temporarily discontinue the infusion until the patient's condition stabilizes. The duration of hemodynamic effects of nitroglycerin is short, and additional corrective measures are usually unnecessary; however, if further therapy is needed, concomitant use of an IV alpha-adrenergic agonist (eg, methoxamine or phenylephrine) should be considered.

DRUG INTERACTIONS

Acetylcholine	⇩ Cholinergic receptor stimulation
Norepinephrine	⇩ Pressor effect
Histamine	⇩ Histamine effect
Alcohol, antihypertensive agents, other vasodilators	⇧ Orthostatic hypotensive effect of nitroglycerin
Sympathomimetics	⇩ Antianginal effect of nitroglycerin

ALTERED LABORATORY VALUES

Urinary values	⇧ Catecholamines ⇧ Vanillylmandelic acid (VMA)

No clinically significant alterations in blood/serum values occur at therapeutic dosages

---

USE IN CHILDREN

Safety and effectiveness for use in children have not been established

USE IN PREGNANT AND NURSING WOMEN

Pregnancy Category C: use during pregnancy only if clearly needed. Reproduction studies have not been done in animals. It is also not known whether nitroglycerin can cause fetal harm when administered to pregnant women or can affect reproductive capacity. No information is available on excretion in human milk; use with caution in nursing mothers.

---

[1] Hypertension associated with surgical procedures, especially cardiovascular procedures, eg, hypertension associated with intratracheal intubation, anesthesia, skin incision, sternotomy, cardiac bypass, and the immediate postoperative period
[2] Use in such states could produce severe hypotension or shock
[3] Oral and/or topical use of nitroglycerin has resulted in cutaneous flushing, weakness, and occasional drug rash or exfoliative dermatitis

---

NITRATES

NITRO-DUR (nitroglycerin) Key   Rx

Transdermal drug delivery systems: 2.5 mg/24 h (5 cm²), 5 mg/24 h (10 cm²), 7.5 mg/24 h (15 cm²), 10 mg/24 h (20 cm²)

NITRO-DUR II (nitroglycerin) Key   Rx

Transdermal drug delivery systems: 2.5 mg/24 h (5 cm²), 5 mg/24 h (10 cm²), 7.5 mg/24 h (15 cm²), 10 mg/24 h (20 cm²), 15 mg/24 h (30 cm²)

INDICATIONS	TRANSCUTANEOUS DOSAGE
Prevention and treatment of **angina pectoris** due to coronary artery disease[1]	**Adult:** to start, apply a 10-cm² system firmly to any convenient skin area, other than the distal extremities (area may be shaved, if necessary); keep system in place for up to 24 h to provide continuous prophylactic levels of nitroglycerin

NITRO-DUR ■ NITRODISC

CONTRAINDICATIONS

Marked anemia	Intolerance to organic nitrates

ADMINISTRATION/DOSAGE ADJUSTMENTS

Dosage titration	For optimal effect, dose may be decreased or increased; when titrating dosage, monitor blood pressure, the number of anginal episodes, and the use of sublingual nitroglycerin
Discontinuation of therapy	To prevent sudden withdrawal reactions, gradually reduce both the dose used daily and the frequency of application over a period of 4–6 wk; use the 5-cm^2 system to decrease the dose

WARNINGS/PRECAUTIONS

Transient headaches	May occur, particularly at higher doses; treat with mild analgesics while continuing therapy. If headaches persist, reduce dosage or discontinue use.
Anginal attacks	This preparation is not intended for immediate relief of acute anginal episodes; sublingual nitroglycerin tablets may be needed occasionally to provide prompt relief
Symptomatic hypotension	Faintness, weakness, or dizziness, particularly upon standing, may indicate overdosage; reduce dosage or discontinue use if such symptoms occur
Abrupt withdrawal of therapy	May produce sudden withdrawal reactions (see ADMINISTRATION/DOSAGE ADJUSTMENTS)
Special-risk patients	Provide for close clinical surveillance and/or hemodynamic monitoring when treating patients with acute myocardial infarction or congestive heart failure

ADVERSE REACTIONS

Central nervous system	Transient headache, faintness, dizziness
Cardiovascular	Hypotension, increased heart rate, flushing
Gastrointestinal	Nausea, vomiting
Dermatological	Dermatitis

OVERDOSAGE

Signs and symptoms	See ADVERSE REACTIONS
Treatment	Reduce dosage or discontinue use

DRUG INTERACTIONS

Acetylcholine	▽ Cholinergic receptor stimulation
Norepinephrine	▽ Pressor effect
Histamine	▽ Histamine effect
Alcohol, antihypertensive agents, other vasodilators	△ Orthostatic hypotensive effect of nitroglycerin
Sympathomimetics	▽ Antianginal effect of nitroglycerin

ALTERED LABORATORY VALUES

Urinary values	△ Catecholamines △ Vanillylmandelic acid (VMA)

No clinically significant alterations in blood/serum values occur at therapeutic dosages

---

USE IN CHILDREN

No information on use in children is available

USE IN PREGNANT AND NURSING WOMEN

Pregnancy Category C: reproduction studies have not been done in animals; it is also not known whether nitroglycerin can cause fetal harm when administered to pregnant women or can affect reproductive capacity. Use during pregnancy only if clearly needed. It is not known whether nitroglycerin is excreted in human milk; use with caution in nursing mothers.

---

[1] Conditionally approved

NITRATES

NITRODISC (nitroglycerin) Searle   Rx

Transdermal drug delivery system: 5 mg/24 h (8 cm^2), 7.5 mg/24 h (12 cm^2), 10 mg/24 h (16 cm^2)

INDICATIONS

Prevention and treatment of **angina pectoris** due to coronary artery disease[1]

TRANSCUTANEOUS DOSAGE

Adult: initially apply an 8-cm^2 pad once daily to any suitable site on the skin, other than the distal extremities, that is free of hair (area should be shaved, if necessary) and not subject to excessive movement; replace the pad daily, using a slightly different site each time to avoid excessive skin irritation, or if it becomes loose. If a greater response is desired, use the 12- or 16-cm^2 pad or, if necessary, more than one pad daily.

NITRODISC ■ NITROGARD

CONTRAINDICATIONS
Marked anemia	Intolerance to organic nitrates

ADMINISTRATION/DOSAGE ADJUSTMENTS
Dosage titration	Determine optimal dosage on the basis of clinical response, side effects, and effects of therapy on blood pressure and heart rate
Discontinuation of therapy	To prevent potential withdrawal reactions, gradually reduce both the dose used daily and the frequency of application over a period of 4–6 wk

WARNINGS/PRECAUTIONS
Transient headaches	May occur, particularly at higher doses; treat with mild analgesics while continuing therapy. If headaches persist, reduce dosage or discontinue use.
Anginal attacks	This preparation is not intended for immediate relief of acute anginal episodes; sublingual nitroglycerin tablets may be needed occasionally to provide prompt relief
Symptomatic hypotension	Faintness, weakness, or dizziness, particularly upon standing, may indicate overdosage; reduce dosage or discontinue use if such symptoms occur
Abrupt withdrawal of therapy	May produce sudden withdrawal reactions (see ADMINISTRATION/DOSAGE ADJUSTMENTS)
Special-risk patients	Provide for close clinical surveillance and/or hemodynamic monitoring when treating patients with acute myocardial infarction or congestive heart failure

ADVERSE REACTIONS
Central nervous system	Transient headache, faintness, dizziness
Cardiovascular	Hypotension, increased heart rate, flushing
Gastrointestinal	Nausea, vomiting
Dermatological	Dermatitis

OVERDOSAGE
Signs and symptoms	See ADVERSE REACTIONS
Treatment	Reduce dosage or discontinue use

DRUG INTERACTIONS
Acetylcholine	⇩	Cholinergic receptor stimulation
Norepinephrine	⇩	Pressor effect
Histamine	⇩	Histamine effect
Alcohol, antihypertensive agents, other vasodilators	⇧	Orthostatic hypotensive effect of nitroglycerin
Sympathomimetics	⇩	Antianginal effect of nitroglycerin

ALTERED LABORATORY VALUES
Urinary values	⇧ Catecholamines ⇧ Vanillylmandelic acid (VMA)

No clinically significant alterations in blood/serum values occur at therapeutic dosages

---

USE IN CHILDREN
Safety and effectiveness for use in children have not been established

USE IN PREGNANT AND NURSING WOMEN
Pregnancy Category C: reproduction studies have not been done in animals; it is also not known whether nitroglycerin can cause fetal harm when administered to pregnant women or can affect reproductive capacity. Use during pregnancy only if clearly needed. It is not known whether nitroglycerin is excreted in human milk; use with caution in nursing mothers.

[1] Conditionally approved

NITRATES

NITROGARD (nitroglycerin) Parke-Davis   Rx
Transmucosal tablets (controlled-release): 1, 2, 3 mg

INDICATIONS
Prevention of acute angina pectoris that can be anticipated

TRANSMUCOSAL DOSAGE
Adult: 1 mg placed on the oral mucosa q5h during waking hours. Assess response over the next 4–5 days. If angina occurs while the tablet is in place, increase dosage to the next tablet strength; if angina occurs after the tablet has dissolved, increase the frequency of dosing (eg, to q4h).

NITROGARD

Treatment of acute angina	**Adult:** 1 mg placed on the oral mucosa; titrate dosage incrementally upward until an effective dose is obtained or side effects intervene (if prompt relief is not obtained, sublingual nitroglycerin is recommended)

CONTRAINDICATIONS
Hypersensitivity or idiosyncratic reaction to nitrates or nitrites

ADMINISTRATION/DOSAGE ADJUSTMENTS

Administration	The tablet should be placed on the oral mucosa between the lip and gum, above the upper incisors, or in the buccal pouch between the cheek and gum, whichever is more comfortable. Advise patient that the tablet should be allowed to dissolve slowly over a 3–5 h period and that it should not be placed under the tongue, chewed, or swallowed. Touching the tablet with the tongue or drinking hot liquids increases the rate of tablet dissolution. Patients are able to talk, eat, and drink while using the tablets. Bedtime administration is not recommended because of the risk of aspiration.
Ambulatory patients	The magnitude of incremental doses in ambulatory patients should be guided by measurements of standing blood pressure

WARNINGS/PRECAUTIONS

Hypotension	Although hypotension is generally dose-related, severe hypotension, particularly with upright posture, may occur even with small doses. Hypotension may be accompanied by paradoxical bradycardia and worsening of angina. Exercise caution if systolic pressure is below 90 mm Hg or if blood volume may have been depleted by prior diuretic therapy. Because hypotension may be harmful during the early days of acute myocardial infarction, careful clinical assessment and hemodynamic monitoring are essential if the drug is to be used during this period.
Hypertrophic cardiomyopathy	Nitrates can exacerbate angina associated with hypertrophic cardiomyopathy
Tolerance	Tolerance to the vascular and antianginal effects of nitrates has been demonstrated in vitro, following occupational exposure, and in controlled clinical trials. Patients who develop tolerance to nitroglycerin may exhibit cross-tolerance to other nitrates and also nitrites. Although the relative importance of nitrate tolerance for users of buccal nitroglycerin has not been established, a controlled study of repeated buccal nitroglycerin use over a 2-wk period showed no significant decline in treadmill performance
Physical dependence	Chest pain, acute myocardial infarction, and even sudden death have occurred in industrial workers who were constantly exposed to nitroglycerin and then temporarily withdrawn from such a setting. During clinical trials, there were reports that soon after discontinuation of nitrates, adverse hemodynamic effects recurred and angina was more easily provoked. Although the relative importance of these findings has not been determined, it seems prudent to withdraw patients from buccal nitroglycerin use gradually, rather than abruptly.
Headache	The most common reaction to nitroglycerin, seen in approximately 50% of patients in some studies, is headache; this reaction, which is generally dose-related, may be severe and persistent. Although headaches tend to disappear 1–2 wk after the initiation of therapy, they may be relieved by use of standard remedies or lowering of the dosage.
Methemoglobinemia	At therapeutic dosages, nitrates can produce methemoglobinemia in patients with genetic hemoglobin abnormalities that favor formation of methemoglobin
Carcinogenicity, mutagenicity, effect on fertility	No long-term studies have been done to evaluate the carcinogenic or mutagenic potential of this preparation or its effect on fertility

ADVERSE REACTIONS

Cardiovascular	Headache, orthostatic hypotension and associated transient signs of cerebral ischemia (ie, dizziness, weakness), cutaneous vasodilation with flushing, pallor, perspiration, circulatory collapse
Gastrointestinal	Nausea, vomiting
Dermatological	Drug rash, exfoliative dermatitis
Other	Restlessness; methemoglobinemia (rare)

OVERDOSAGE

Signs and symptoms	*Cardiovascular:* persistent, throbbing headache; severe hypotension; flushing and diaphoresis followed by cutaneous chilling and cyanosis; dicrotic, intermittent pulse; palpitations, vertigo, syncope, heart block, circulatory collapse; *CNS:* visual disturbances, increased intracranial pressure (with confusion and moderate fever), paralysis and coma followed by clonic convulsions; *GI:* nausea, vomiting, colic, bloody diarrhea; *respiratory:* methemoglobinemia with cyanosis and anoxia, initial hyperpnea, dyspnea, hypopnea
Treatment	Remove any residue of the tablet from the oral mucosa and wipe the gum clean at the site of insertion. If the medication has been swallowed recently, gastric lavage may be useful. To treat hypotension, place patient in a recumbent (shock) position and keep comfortably warm; passive movements of the extremities may enhance venous return. Do not use epinephrine or related compounds to reverse hypotension. Institute mechanical ventilation and administer oxygen, as needed. For methemoglobinemia, give 1–2 mg/kg of 1% methylene blue IV.

NITROGARD ■ NITROL

DRUG INTERACTIONS

Alcohol, antihypertensive drugs, and other vasodilators	⌂ Risk of hypotension
Calcium-channel blockers	Marked symptomatic orthostatic hypotension, based on experience with oral controlled-release preparations; if necessary, adjust dosage of nitrate or calcium-channel blocker

ALTERED LABORATORY VALUES

Blood/serum values	▽ Cholesterol (with Zlatkis-Zak color reaction)
Urinary values	⌂ Catecholamines ⌂ VMA

USE IN CHILDREN
Safety and effectiveness for use in children have not been established

USE IN PREGNANT AND NURSING WOMEN
Pregnancy Category C: reproduction studies have not been done in animals; it is not known whether nitroglycerin can cause harm to the fetus or adversely affect reproductive capacity. Use during pregnancy only if clearly needed. It is also not known whether nitroglycerin is excreted in human milk; use with caution in nursing mothers.

NITRATES

NITROL Ointment (nitroglycerin) Rorer Rx
Ointment: 2% (3, 30, 60 g)

INDICATIONS	TOPICAL DOSAGE
Prevention and treatment of **angina pectoris** due to coronary artery disease[1]	**Adult:** 15–30 mg (1–2 in.) q8h; some patients may require up to 60–75 mg (4–5 in.) per application and/or application q4h

CONTRAINDICATIONS
Intolerance to organic nitrates

ADMINISTRATION/DOSAGE ADJUSTMENTS

Application of ointment	Squeeze the necessary amount of ointment onto the regular or adhesive dose-measuring applicator supplied with the tube. Use the regular applicator to spread the ointment in a thin, uniform layer over an area of skin of at least 2¼ × 3½ in.; then, cover the area with plastic film and secure the film with adhesive tape. Alternatively, carefully fold the adhesive applicator to spread the ointment over the area bounded by the adhesive border; then, peel off the backing, place the applicator on the skin, and press the adhesive border firmly to the skin. To ensure proper contact of the ointment with the skin, gently press the entire surface of the applicator against the skin.
Initial dosage titration	Start with 7.5 mg (½ in.) q8h and increase the dose by 7.5 mg (½ in.) with each successive application until the desired response is obtained. Optimal dosage may be gauged by the greatest reduction in resting blood pressure that is not associated with clinical symptoms of hypotension, especially orthostatic hypotension; to decrease adverse reactions, tailor the dose and frequency of application to individual needs.

WARNINGS/PRECAUTIONS

Anginal attacks	This preparation should not be used for the immediate relief of acute anginal symptoms
Headache	Transient headaches are the most common side effect, especially at higher dosages, and should be treated with mild analgesics; reduce dosage only if the headaches prove untreatable
Hypotension	If hypotension occurs, particularly when the patient rises from a recumbent position, reduce the dosage
Contact dermatitis	May occur with continued use; the incidence may be reduced by changing the site of application
Special-risk patients	Patients with acute myocardial infarction or congestive heart failure should be kept under careful clinical and/or hemodynamic surveillance

ADVERSE REACTIONS

Central nervous system	Transient headache, faintness, dizziness
Cardiovascular	Hypotension, increased heart rate, flushing
Gastrointestinal	Nausea
Dermatological	Contact dermatitis

NITROL ■ NITROL IV

OVERDOSAGE

Signs and symptoms	Hypotension, increased heart rate, faintness, flushing, dizziness, nausea
Treatment	If severe hypotension occurs, quickly remove the ointment, place the patient in a recumbent position, and elevate the legs; if hypotension persists, administer 5% dextrose by IV infusion

DRUG INTERACTIONS

Acetylcholine	▽ Cholinergic receptor stimulation
Norepinephrine	▽ Pressor effect
Alcohol, antihypertensive agents, other vasodilators	△ Orthostatic hypotensive effect of nitroglycerin
Sympathomimetics	▽ Antianginal effect of nitroglycerin

ALTERED LABORATORY VALUES

Urinary values	△ Catecholamines △ Vanillylmandelic acid (VMA)

No clinically significant alterations in blood/serum values occur at therapeutic dosages

---

USE IN CHILDREN

This drug has been used safely in children

USE IN PREGNANT AND NURSING WOMEN

Because of the short half-life of nitroglycerin (approximately 3–4 min), it is not known whether this drug crosses the placental barrier or is excreted in breast milk. Consequently, it should not be administered to pregnant or nursing women unless it is absolutely needed.

VEHICLE/BASE
Ointment: lactose, lanolin, white petrolatum

[1] Conditionally approved

NITRATES

NITROL IV (nitroglycerin) Rorer   Rx

Ampuls: 0.8 mg/ml (1, 10, 30 ml)

INDICATIONS

Angina pectoris unresponsive to recommended doses of organic nitrates and/or a beta blocker
Congestive heart failure associated with acute myocardial infarction
Perioperative hypertension[1]
Production of controlled hypotension during surgical procedures

PARENTERAL DOSAGE

Adult: 5 μg/min via IV infusion, using a nonabsorbing administration set (see WARNINGS/PRECAUTIONS), to start; increase dosage in increments of 5 μg/min at 3- to 5-min intervals until some response is noted (if no response is seen at 20 μg/min, increments of 10 and then 20 μg/min may be used). Once a partial blood pressure response is observed, reduce the size of the dosage increments and lengthen the interval between increases.

CONTRAINDICATIONS

Hypersensitivity to nitroglycerin or idiosyncratic reaction to organic nitrates	Increased intracranial pressure (eg, head trauma or cerebral hemorrhage)	Constrictive pericarditis and pericardial tamponade
Hypotension or uncorrected hypovolemia	Inadequate cerebral circulation	

ADMINISTRATION/DOSAGE ADJUSTMENTS

Preparation of solution	Aseptically add the required amount of nitroglycerin to a glass IV bottle containing 5% dextrose injection USP or 0.9% sodium chloride injection USP. To obtain a concentration of approximately 30 μg/ml, dilute the contents of one 0.8-mg ampul in 25 ml of diluent or the contents of one 8-mg ampul in 250 ml of diluent. For a concentration of approximately 60 μg/ml, add the contents of two 8-mg ampuls to 250 ml of diluent; for a concentration of approximately 85 μg/ml, add the contents of three 8-mg ampuls or one 24-mg ampul to 250 ml of diluent. (The patient's fluid requirements and the expected duration of infusion should be considered when choosing an appropriate dilution.) Mix solution well. Do not add nitroglycerin to a bottle containing other drugs. Flush or replace the infusion set whenever the concentration of a solution is changed; otherwise, administration of the new solution may be delayed.

NITROL IV

Dosage titration	Titrate dosage to desired level of hemodynamic function; blood pressure, heart rate, and other appropriate physiologic parameters must be monitored continuously to obtain the correct dose. Adequate systemic blood pressure and coronary perfusion pressure must be maintained. Since a fall in pulmonary capillary wedge pressure precedes the onset of arterial hypotension, wedge pressure can serve as a useful guide to safe titration of this drug. Patients with normal or low left ventricular filling pressures or pulmonary capillary wedge pressures (eg, patients with uncomplicated angina pectoris) may respond fully to doses as small as 5 μg/min and, therefore, require especially careful titration and monitoring.

WARNINGS/PRECAUTIONS

Absorption of nitroglycerin by IV administration sets	Nitroglycerin is readily absorbed by many plastics; use glass IV bottles to dilute and store this drug and avoid filters that absorb nitroglycerin. Common administration sets made of polyvinyl chloride (PVC) tubing can absorb 40–80% of the total amount of nitroglycerin in the final solution. Since the loss is neither constant nor self-limited, it cannot be simply calculated or corrected for. To minimize loss, use an administration set with the least absorptive tubing available; keep in mind that although initial dosages of 25 μg/min or more have been recommended in the literature, these dosages have been derived from studies in which PVC tubing was used and are therefore not appropriate for administration with low-absorbing tubing.
Improper regulation of infusion	When used with some non-PVC infusion sets, certain infusion pumps may fail to properly regulate flow of drug solution at off or low settings: the solution may flow when the pump is turned off and the amount delivered may be excessive when the pump is at a low setting
Hepatic or renal impairment	Use with caution in patients with severe liver or kidney disease
Excessive hypotension	Must be avoided because of possible deleterious effects on vital organs resulting from poor perfusion, especially if the hypotension is prolonged, and the attendant risk of ischemia, thrombosis, and physiologic impairment; paradoxical bradycardia and increased angina pectoris may accompany nitroglycerin-induced hypotension. Use in patients with hypotension or uncorrected hypovolemia is contraindicated. Patients with normal or low pulmonary capillary wedge pressures are especially sensitive to the hypotensive effects of IV nitroglycerin (see ADMINISTRATION/DOSAGE ADJUSTMENTS).
Carcinogenicity	No long-term studies have been done in animals to evaluate the carcinogenic potential of nitroglycerin

ADVERSE REACTIONS[2]

Frequent reactions (incidence ≥ 1%) are printed in *italics*

Central nervous system and neuromuscular	*Headache (2%)*, apprehension, restlessness, muscle twitching, dizziness
Cardiovascular	Tachycardia, retrosternal discomfort, palpitations
Gastrointestinal	Nausea, vomiting, abdominal pain

OVERDOSAGE

Signs and symptoms	Severe hypotension, reflex tachycardia
Treatment	Elevate the patient's legs and decrease or temporarily discontinue the infusion until the patient's condition stabilizes. The duration of hemodynamic effects of nitroglycerin is short, and additional corrective measures are usually unnecessary; however, if further therapy is needed, concomitant use of an IV alpha-adrenergic agonist (eg, methoxamine or phenylephrine) should be considered.

DRUG INTERACTIONS

Alcohol, antihypertensive drugs, and other vasodilators	⇧ Risk of hypotension

ALTERED LABORATORY VALUES

Blood/serum values	⇩ Cholesterol (with Zlatkis-Zak color reaction)
Urinary values	⇧ Catecholamines ⇧ VMA

USE IN CHILDREN

Safety and effectiveness for use in children have not been established

---

USE IN PREGNANT AND NURSING WOMEN

Pregnancy Category C: reproduction studies have not been done; it is not known whether nitroglycerin can cause harm to the fetus or adversely affect reproductive capacity. Use during pregnancy only if clearly needed. It is also not known whether nitroglycerin is excreted in human milk; use with caution in nursing mothers.

---

[1] Hypertension associated with surgical procedures, especially cardiovascular procedures, eg, hypertension associated with intratracheal intubation, anesthesia, skin incision, sternotomy, cardiac bypass, and the immediate postoperative period
[2] Oral and/or topical use of nitroglycerin has resulted in cutaneous flushing, weakness, and occasional drug rash or exfoliative dermatitis, in addition to these reactions

NITRATES

NITROLINGUAL (nitroglycerin) Rorer   Rx

Metered-dose spray: 0.4 mg/spray (13.8 g, equivalent to 200 metered doses)

INDICATIONS	ORAL DOSAGE
Prevention of acute angina that can be anticipated	Adult: 0.4–0.8 mg (1–2 doses), sprayed onto the oral mucosa (preferably the tongue) 5–10 min before an activity that might precipitate an attack
Treatment of acute angina	Adult: 0.4–0.8 mg (1–2 doses), sprayed onto the oral mucosa (preferably the tongue) at the onset of an attack; do not give more than 0.12 mg (3 doses) within a period of 15 min

CONTRAINDICATIONS

Hypersensitivity or idiosyncratic reaction to nitrates or nitrites

ADMINISTRATION/DOSAGE ADJUSTMENTS

Administration	The patient should be sitting (if possible), holding the canister upright and the spray orifice as close to the mouth as possible. The grooved button on top of the canister is then pressed firmly with a forefinger to release the spray onto or under the tongue, and the mouth is closed immediately; the vapor should not be inhaled or swallowed. At night, it may be necessary to determine the position of the spray orifice by touch; to facilitate use at that time, instruct the patient to become familiar with how the grooved button feels when the spray orifice is properly positioned.

WARNINGS/PRECAUTIONS

Acute myocardial infarction	When using this preparation during the early days of an acute myocardial infarction, pay particular attention to hemodynamic and clinical responses
Hypotension	Severe hypotension, particularly with upright posture, may occur even with small doses; however, hypotension is generally dose-related. Transient dizziness and weakness, as well as other symptoms of orthostatic hypotension, occur occasionally. Hypotension may be accompanied by paradoxical bradycardia and exacerbation of angina. Exercise caution if systolic pressure is less than 90 mm Hg or if blood volume may have been depleted by diuretic therapy.
Hypertrophic cardiomyopathy	Nitrates can exacerbate angina associated with hypertrophic cardiomyopathy
Tolerance	Nitrate tolerance has been demonstrated in clinical trials, isolated-tissue experiments, and studies with industrial workers continuously exposed to nitroglycerin; if tolerance develops, cross-tolerance to nitrites and other nitrates may occur
Physical dependence	Chest pain, acute myocardial infarction, and even sudden death have occurred in workers who were constantly exposed to nitroglycerin and then temporarily withdrawn from such a setting. During clinical trials, there were reports that soon after discontinuation of nitrates, adverse hemodynamic effects recurred and angina was more easily provoked. The relative importance of these findings has not been determined.
Headache	The most frequent reaction to nitrates, seen in approximately 50% of patients in some studies, is headache; this reaction, which is generally dose-related, may be severe and persistent
Persistent chest pain	Instruct patients to promptly report persistent chest pain
Methemoglobinemia	At therapeutic dosages, nitrates can produce methemoglobinemia in patients with hemoglobin abnormalities that favor formation of methemoglobin
Carcinogenicity	No long-term studies have been done to evaluate the carcinogenic potential of this preparation

ADVERSE REACTIONS

Cardiovascular	Headache, orthostatic hypotension, cutaneous vasodilation with flushing, weakness, pallor, perspiration, circulatory collapse
Gastrointestinal	Nausea, vomiting
Dermatological	Drug rash, exfoliative dermatitis
Other	Restlessness; methemoglobinemia (rare)

OVERDOSAGE

Signs and symptoms	*Cardiovascular:* persistent, throbbing headache; severe hypotension; flushing and diaphoresis followed by cutaneous chilling and cyanosis; dicrotic, intermittent pulse; palpitations, vertigo, syncope, heart block, circulatory collapse; *CNS:* visual disturbances, increased intracranial pressure (with confusion and moderate fever), paralysis and coma followed by clonic convulsions; *GI:* nausea, vomiting, colic, bloody diarrhea; *respiratory:* methemoglobinemia with cyanosis and anoxia, initial hyperpnea, dyspnea, hypopnea

NITROLINGUAL ■ NITROSTAT

Treatment	If vapor has been swallowed recently, gastric lavage may be useful. To treat hypotension, place patient in a recumbent (shock) position and keep comfortably warm; passive movements of the extremities may enhance venous return. Do not use epinephrine or related compounds to reverse hypotension. Institute mechanical ventilation and administer oxygen, as needed. For methemoglobinemia, give 1–2 mg/kg of 1% methylene blue IV.

DRUG INTERACTIONS

Alcohol, antihypertensive drugs, and other vasodilators	△ Risk of hypotension
Calcium-channel blockers	Marked symptomatic orthostatic hypotension (reported with oral controlled-release preparations, potential effect with spray); if necessary, adjust dosage of nitrate or calcium-channel blocker

ALTERED LABORATORY VALUES

Blood/serum values	▽ Cholesterol (with Zlatkis-Zak color reaction)
Urinary values	△ Catecholamines △ VMA

USE IN CHILDREN
Safety and effectiveness for use in children have not been established

USE IN PREGNANT AND NURSING WOMEN
Pregnancy Category C: reproduction studies have not been done; it is not known whether nitroglycerin can cause harm to the fetus or adversely affect reproductive capacity. Use during pregnancy only if clearly needed. It is also not known whether nitroglycerin is excreted in human milk; use with caution in nursing mothers.

NITRATES

NITROSTAT (nitroglycerin) Parke-Davis Rx
Sublingual tablets: 0.15, 0.3, 0.4, 0.6 mg

INDICATIONS
Prophylaxis, treatment, and management of **angina pectoris**

SUBLINGUAL DOSAGE
Adult: 1 tab (smallest effective dose) dissolved under tongue or in the buccal pouch at the first sign of an attack. The dose may be repeated every 5 min until relief is obtained; angina that persists after a total of 3 tabs have been given in a 15-min period should be reported by the patient.

NITROSTAT Ointment (nitroglycerin) Parke-Davis Rx
Ointment: 2% (30, 60 g)

INDICATIONS
Prevention and treatment of **angina pectoris** due to coronary artery disease[1]

TOPICAL DOSAGE
Adult: 30 mg (2 in.) q8h; some patients may require up to 60–75 mg (4–5 in.) per application and/or application q4h

CONTRAINDICATIONS

For sublingual use only

Early myocardial infarction

Severe anemia

Increased intracranial pressure

Hypersensitivity to nitroglycerin

For topical use only

Intolerance to organic nitrates

ADMINISTRATION/DOSAGE ADJUSTMENTS

Use of sublingual tablets	Caution patients to sit down, if possible, when taking a tablet, because, if they stand, they may become dizzy or light-headed and fall. For prophylaxis, patients may use this preparation 5–10 min before engaging in activities that might precipitate an anginal attack.
Application of ointment	Squeeze the necessary amount of ointment from the tube onto the dose-measuring applicator supplied with the package; then, using the applicator to prevent absorption through the fingers, spread the ointment onto the skin in a thin, even layer, covering an area equal to or greater than the size of the applicator. Cover the area, including the applicator, with plastic film, which may be held in place with adhesive tape.
Initial dosage titration for patients using the ointment	Start with 7.5 mg (½ in.) q8h and increase the dose by 7.5 mg (½ in.) with each successive application until the desired response is obtained. Optimal dosage may be gauged by the greatest reduction in resting blood pressure that is not associated with clinical symptoms of hypotension, especially orthostatic hypotension; to decrease adverse reactions, tailor the dose and frequency of application to individual needs.

NITROSTAT ■ NITROSTAT IV

WARNINGS/PRECAUTIONS

Anginal attacks	Use the sublingual tablets; the ointment should not be used for the immediate relief of acute anginal symptoms
Headache	Transient headaches are the most common side effect of topical therapy, especially at higher dosages, and should be treated with mild analgesics; reduce dosage only if the headaches prove untreatable. Excessive sublingual dosage may produce severe headaches.
Hypotension	If hypotension occurs, particularly when the patient rises from a recumbent position, reduce the dosage
Special-risk patients	Patients with acute myocardial infarction or congestive heart failure should be kept under careful clinical and/or hemodynamic surveillance during topical therapy (use of the sublingual tablets is contraindicated in patients with early myocardial infarction)
Blurred vision, dry mouth	Discontinue use if these reactions occur
Tolerance	Excessive use of the sublingual tablets may lead to the development of tolerance
Carcinogenicity	No long-term studies of carcinogenicity have been performed in animals

ADVERSE REACTIONS

Central nervous system	Transient headache
Cardiovascular	Hypotension (including orthostatic hypotension), increased heart rate, palpitation, flushing, dizziness, vertigo, weakness, faintness; syncope (with sublingual tablets)
Gastrointestinal	Nausea

OVERDOSAGE

Signs and symptoms	See ADVERSE REACTIONS
Treatment	Reduce dosage

DRUG INTERACTIONS

Acetylcholine	▽ Cholinergic receptor stimulation
Norepinephrine	▽ Pressor effect
Histamine	▽ Histamine effect
Alcohol, antihypertensive agents, beta blockers, phenothiazines	△ Orthostatic hypotensive effect of nitroglycerin
Sympathomimetics	▽ Antianginal effect of nitroglycerin

ALTERED LABORATORY VALUES

Blood/serum values	▽ Cholesterol (with Zlatkis-Zak color reaction)
Urinary values	△ Catecholamines △ Vanillylmandelic acid (VMA)

USE IN CHILDREN

Safety and effectiveness for use in children have not been established

---

USE IN PREGNANT AND NURSING WOMEN

Pregnancy Category C: reproduction studies have not been performed in animals or humans. It is not known whether nitroglycerin can cause harm to the fetus or affect reproductive capacity; use during pregnancy only if clearly needed. It is not known whether this drug is excreted in human milk (use IV nitroglycerin with caution in nursing mothers).

VEHICLE/BASE
Ointment: lanolin, lactose, and white petrolatum

[1] Conditionally approved

NITRATES

NITROSTAT IV (nitroglycerin) Parke-Davis   Rx

Ampuls: 0.8, 5 mg/ml (10 ml)[1]

INDICATIONS

Angina pectoris unresponsive to recommended doses of organic nitrates and/or a beta blocker
Congestive heart failure associated with acute myocardial infarction
Perioperative hypertension[2]
Production of controlled hypotension during surgical procedures

PARENTERAL DOSAGE

Adult: 5 μg/min via IV infusion, using a nonabsorbing administration set (see WARNINGS/PRECAUTIONS), to start; increase dosage in increments of 5 μg/min at 3- to 5-min intervals until some response is noted (if no response is seen at 20 μg/min, increments of 10 and then 20 μg/min may be used). Once a partial blood pressure response is observed, reduce the size of the dosage increments and lengthen the interval between increases.

NITROSTAT IV

CONTRAINDICATIONS

- Hypersensitivity to nitroglycerin or idiosyncratic reaction to organic nitrates
- Hypotension or uncorrected hypovolemia
- Increased intracranial pressure (eg, head trauma or cerebral hemorrhage)
- Constrictive pericarditis and pericardial tamponade

ADMINISTRATION/DOSAGE ADJUSTMENTS

Preparation of solution — Aseptically add the required amount of nitroglycerin to a glass IV bottle containing 5% dextrose injection USP or 0.9% sodium chloride injection USP. Dilute the contents of one, two, or three 8-mg ampuls in 250 ml of diluent to obtain a final concentration of approximately 30 µg/ml (with 1 ampul), 60 µg/ml (with 2 ampuls), or 85 µg/ml (with 3 ampuls); dilute the contents of one or two 50-mg ampuls in 500 ml of diluent to obtain a final concentration of approximately 100 µg/ml (with 1 ampul) or 200 µg/ml (with 2 ampuls). (The patients's fluid requirements and the expected duration of infusion should be considered when choosing an appropriate dilution.) Mix solution well. Do not add nitroglycerin to a bottle containing other drugs. Flush or replace the infusion set whenever the concentration of a solution is changed; otherwise, administration of the new solution may be delayed.

Dosage titration — Titrate dosage to desired level of hemodynamic function; blood pressure, heart rate, and other appropriate physiologic parameters must be monitored continuously to obtain the correct dose. Adequate systemic blood pressure and coronary perfusion pressure must be maintained. Since a fall in pulmonary capillary wedge pressure precedes the onset of arterial hypotension, wedge pressure can serve as a useful guide to safe titration of this drug. Patients with normal or low left ventricular filling pressures or pulmonary capillary wedge pressures (eg, patients with uncomplicated angina pectoris) may respond fully to doses as small as 5 µg/min and, therefore, require especially careful titration and monitoring.

WARNINGS/PRECAUTIONS

Absorption of nitroglycerin by IV administration sets — Nitroglycerin is readily absorbed by many plastics; use glass IV bottles to dilute and store this drug and avoid filters that absorb nitroglycerin. Common administration sets made of polyvinyl chloride (PVC) tubing can absorb 40–80% of the total amount of nitroglycerin in the final solution. Since the loss is neither constant nor self-limited, it cannot be simply calculated or corrected for. Use of the disposable IV infusion set supplied with the drug or a similar administration set is recommended to keep the loss of nitroglycerin to a minimum (< 5%). PVC tubing has been utilized in published studies, and the doses recommended (25 µg/min or more to start) will be too high if administration sets with nonabsorbing tubing are used.

Hepatic or renal impairment — Use with caution in patients with severe liver or kidney disease

Excessive hypotension — Must be avoided because of possible deleterious effects on vital organs resulting from poor perfusion, especially if the hypotension is prolonged, and the attendant risk of ischemia, thrombosis, and physiologic impairment; paradoxical bradycardia and increased angina pectoris may accompany nitroglycerin-induced hypotension. Use in patients with hypotension or uncorrected hypovolemia is contraindicated. Patients with normal or low pulmonary capillary wedge pressures are especially sensitive to the hypotensive effects of IV nitroglycerin (see ADMINISTRATION/DOSAGE ADJUSTMENTS).

Intracoronary administration — This preparation contains alcohol; safety of intracoronary injection has not been established

Carcinogenicity — No long-term studies have been done in animals to evaluate the carcinogenic potential of nitroglycerin

ADVERSE REACTIONS[3]

Frequent reactions (incidence ≥ 1%) are printed in *italics*

Central nervous system and neuromuscular — *Headache (2%)*, apprehension, restlessness, muscle twitching, dizziness

Cardiovascular — Tachycardia, retrosternal discomfort, palpitations

Gastrointestinal — Nausea, vomiting, abdominal pain

OVERDOSAGE

Signs and symptoms — Severe hypotension, reflex tachycardia

Treatment — Elevate the patient's legs and decrease or temporarily discontinue the infusion until the patient's condition stabilizes. The duration of hemodynamic effects of nitroglycerin is short, and additional corrective measures are usually unnecessary; however, if further therapy is needed, concomitant use of an IV alpha-adrenergic agonist (eg, methoxamine or phenylephrine) should be considered.

DRUG INTERACTIONS

Acetylcholine	▽ Cholinergic receptor stimulation
Norepinephrine	▽ Pressor effect
Histamine	▽ Histamine effect
Alcohol, antihypertensive agents, other vasodilators	△ Orthostatic hypotensive effect of nitroglycerin

NITROSTAT IV ■ NTS

Sympathomimetics ──────────── ▽ Antianginal effect

ALTERED LABORATORY VALUES

Urinary values ──────────── △ Catecholamines   △ Vanillylmandelic acid (VMA)

No clinically significant alterations in blood/serum values occur at therapeutic dosages

---

USE IN CHILDREN
Safety and effectiveness for use in children have not been established

USE IN PREGNANT AND NURSING WOMEN
Pregnancy Category C: use during pregnancy only if clearly needed. Reproduction studies have not been done in animals. It is also not known whether nitroglycerin can cause fetal harm when administered to pregnant women or can affect reproductive capacity. No information is available on excretion in human milk; use with caution in nursing mothers.

---

[1] Ampuls can be obtained alone or with a disposable, nonabsorbing IV infusion set
[2] Hypertension associated with surgical procedures, especially cardiovascular procedures, eg, hypertension associated with intratracheal intubation, anesthesia, skin incision, sternotomy, cardiac bypass, and the immediate postoperative period
[3] Oral and/or topical use of nitroglycerin has resulted in cutaneous flushing, weakness, and occasional drug rash or exfoliative dermatitis, in addition to these reactions

---

NITRATES

NTS (nitroglycerin) Bolar   Rx

Transdermal drug delivery systems: 5 mg/24 h (10 cm^2), 15 mg/24 h (30 cm^2)

INDICATIONS
Prevention and treatment of **angina pectoris** due to coronary artery disease[1]

TRANSCUTANEOUS DOSAGE
Adult: to start, firmly apply a 10-cm^2 system once daily to any suitable site on the chest or inner side of the upper arm that is free of hair (area should be shaved, if necessary); to provide continuous prophylactic levels of nitroglycerin, keep system in place for up to 24 h

CONTRAINDICATIONS
Intolerance to organic nitrates   Marked anemia

ADMINISTRATION/DOSAGE ADJUSTMENTS

Titration of dose	An increase in dose may be necessary for some patients; when titrating dose, monitor blood pressure, the number of anginal episodes, and the use of sublingual nitroglycerin
Sensitive skin	For patients with sensitive skin, reduce adhesion strength by lightly touching the adhesive with a dry, lint-free cloth; however, avoid excessive removal of adhesive
Discontinuation of therapy	To prevent sudden withdrawal reactions, gradually reduce both the daily dose and the frequency of application over a period of 4–6 wk

WARNINGS/PRECAUTIONS

Headache	Transient headaches may occur, particularly at higher doses; treat with mild analgesics while continuing therapy. If headaches persist, reduce dose or discontinue use
Symptomatic hypotension	Faintness, weakness, or dizziness, particularly upon standing, may indicate overdosage; reduce dose or discontinue use if such symptoms occur
Other reactions	Nausea, vomiting, flushing, or increased heart rate can occur during therapy; if reaction persists, reduce dose or discontinue use
Abrupt withdrawal of therapy	Sudden withdrawal reactions may occur following abrupt discontinuation of therapy (see ADMINISTRATION/DOSAGE ADJUSTMENTS)
Special-risk patients	Provide for close clinical surveillance and/or hemodynamic monitoring when the patient has acute myocardial infarction or congestive heart failure
Anginal attacks	This preparation is not intended for immediate relief of acute anginal episodes; sublingual nitroglycerin may be needed occasionally to provide prompt relief

ADVERSE REACTIONS

Cardiovascular	Transient headache, hypotension, increased heart rate, faintness, flushing, dizziness
Gastrointestinal	Nausea, vomiting
Dermatological	Dermatitis

OVERDOSAGE
Signs and symptoms ──────── See ADVERSE REACTIONS

NTS ■ PERITRATE

Treatment	Reduce dosage or discontinue use

DRUG INTERACTIONS

Alcohol, antihypertensive agents, other vasodilators	⇧ Orthostatic hypotensive effect of nitroglycerin

ALTERED LABORATORY VALUES

Blood/serum values	⇩ Cholesterol (with Zlatkis-Zak color reaction)
Urinary values	⇧ Catecholamines ⇧ VMA

USE IN CHILDREN

Safety and effectiveness for use in children have not been established

USE IN PREGNANT AND NURSING WOMEN

Pregnancy Category C: reproduction studies have not been done; it is not known whether nitroglycerin can affect reproductive capacity or cause harm to the fetus. Use during pregnancy only if clearly needed. It is also not known whether nitroglycerin is excreted in human milk; use with caution in nursing mothers.

[1] Conditionally approved

NITRATES

PERITRATE (pentaerythritol tetranitrate) Parke-Davis   Rx

Tablets: 10, 20, 40 mg

INDICATIONS	ORAL DOSAGE
Prophylaxis and long-term management of **angina pectoris**[1]	**Adult:** 10–20 mg qid to start, followed by up to 40 mg qid, taken 1/2 h before or 1 h after meals and at bedtime

PERITRATE SA (pentaerythritol tetranitrate) Parke-Davis   Rx

Tablets (sustained release): 80 mg

INDICATIONS	ORAL DOSAGE
Same as Peritrate	**Adult:** 80 mg bid, taken immediately upon arising and again 12 h later on an empty stomach

CONTRAINDICATIONS

Hypersensitivity to pentaerythritol tetranitrate

WARNINGS/PRECAUTIONS

Patients with recent acute myocardial infarction	Safety for use during the period when clinical and laboratory findings are still unstable has not been established
Increased intraocular pressure	Administer with caution to patients with glaucoma
Tolerance	May develop, as well as cross-tolerance to other organic nitrates and nitrites

ADVERSE REACTIONS

Frequent reactions (incidence ≥ 1%) are printed in *italics*

Central nervous system	*Headache* (sometimes severe and persistent), dizziness, weakness, and other signs of cerebral ischemia associated with postural hypotension; restlessness
Cardiovascular	Cutaneous vasodilation with flushing, pallor
Gastrointestinal	*Distress*, nausea, vomiting
Dermatological	*Rash*
Other	Sweating, collapse

OVERDOSAGE

Signs and symptoms	See ADVERSE REACTIONS
Treatment	Discontinue use of drug; treat symptomatically

DRUG INTERACTIONS

Acetylcholine	⇩ Cholinergic receptor stimulation
Norepinephrine	⇩ Pressor effect
Histamine	⇩ Histamine effect

PERITRATE ■ SORBITRATE

Alcohol, antihypertensive agents, other vasodilators ——— △ Orthostatic hypotensive effect of pentaerythritol tetranitrate

Sympathomimetics ——————————— ▽ Antianginal effect of pentaerythritol tetranitrate

ALTERED LABORATORY VALUES
No clinically significant alterations in blood/serum or urinary values occur at therapeutic dosages

USE IN CHILDREN	USE IN PREGNANT AND NURSING WOMEN
Consult manufacturer	Consult manufacturer

[1] Possibly effective

NITRATES

SORBITRATE (isosorbide dinitrate) Stuart — Rx

Sublingual tablets: 2.5, 5, 10 mg **Chewable tablets:** 5, 10 mg **Swallowable tablets:** 5, 10, 20, 30, 40 mg **Tablets (controlled release):** 40 mg (Sorbitrate SA)

INDICATIONS

Management of chronic stable angina

ORAL DOSAGE

Adult: when using swallowable tablets, 5–20 mg to start, followed by 10–40 mg q6h; when using controlled-release tablets, 40 mg to start, followed by 40–80 mg q8–12h. Swallowable and controlled-release tablets should not be chewed.

Prevention of acute angina that can be anticipated

Adult: 5–10 mg to start, using sublingual or chewable tablets; administer a few minutes before a situation likely to provoke an attack. Doses may be given q2–3h to maintain prophylactic effect; however, no adequate, controlled studies have been done to demonstrate the effectiveness of long-term therapy with these dosage forms.

Treatment of acute angina in patients intolerant or unresponsive to sublingual nitroglycerin

Adult: when using sublingual tablets, 2.5–5 mg to start; when using chewable tablets, 5 mg to start

CONTRAINDICATIONS
Hypersensitivity or idiosyncratic reaction to nitrates or nitrites

ADMINISTRATION/DOSAGE ADJUSTMENTS

Titration of dosage — Increase dosage until angina is relieved or adverse reactions limit further titration; if the patient is ambulatory, measure standing blood pressure to determine the magnitude of each dosage increase

WARNINGS/PRECAUTIONS

Acute myocardial infarction — When used during the early days of an acute myocardial infarction, nitrates can cause potentially deleterious hypotension; moreover, it has not been established that use at that time is beneficial. If isosorbide dinitrate is given at the early stage of an infarction, assess clinical response frequently and monitor hemodynamic parameters.

Hypotension — Severe hypotension, particularly with upright posture, may occur even with small doses; however, hypotension is generally dose-related. Transient dizziness and weakness as well as other symptoms of orthostatic hypotension occur in 2–36% of patients. Hypotension may be accompanied by paradoxical bradycardia and exacerbation of angina. Exercise caution if systolic pressure is less than 90 mm Hg or if blood volume may have been depleted by diuretic therapy.

Hypertrophic cardiomyopathy — Nitrates can exacerbate angina associated with hypertrophic cardiomyopathy

Tolerance — Although nitrate tolerance has been demonstrated in clinical trials, isolated-tissue experiments, and studies with industrial workers continuously exposed to nitroglycerin, the relative importance of this effect has not been determined. In one clinical study, the duration of action of oral isosorbide dinitrate decreased from 8 h to 2 h after 1 wk of continuous use; however, several controlled studies have demonstrated a therapeutic effect after 4 wk of use, and, in open trials, an effect seemed detectable even with administration for as long as several months. If tolerance to isosorbide dinitrate develops, cross-tolerance to nitrites and other nitrates may occur.

Physical dependence — Chest pain, acute myocardial infarction, and even sudden death have occurred in workers who were constantly exposed to nitroglycerin and then temporarily withdrawn from such a setting. During clinical trials, there were reports that soon after discontinuation of nitrates, adverse hemodynamic effects recurred and angina was more easily provoked. Although the relative importance of these findings has not been determined, it seems prudent to terminate therapy in a gradual manner, rather than abruptly.

COMPENDIUM OF DRUG THERAPY

SORBITRATE ■ TRANSDERM-Nitro

Headache	The most frequent reaction to nitrates, seen in approximately 25% of patients, is headache. Although headache may be severe and persistent, it generally can be relieved by standard headache remedies or a reduction in dosage, and it usually tends to disappear 1–2 wk after the onset of therapy.
Methemoglobinemia	At therapeutic dosages, nitrates can produce methemoglobinemia in patients with hemoglobin abnormalities that favor formation of methemoglobin
Carcinogenicity, effect on fertility	No long-term studies have been done to evaluate the carcinogenic potential of isosorbide dinitrate; a modified two-litter reproduction study in rats fed 25 or 100 mg/kg/day has shown no adverse effect on fertility

ADVERSE REACTIONS

Cardiovascular	Headache, orthostatic hypotension, cutaneous vasodilation with flushing, weakness, pallor, perspiration, circulatory collapse
Gastrointestinal	Nausea, vomiting
Dermatological	Drug rash, exfoliative dermatitis
Other	Restlessness; methemoglobinemia (rare)

OVERDOSAGE

Signs and symptoms	*Cardiovascular:* persistent, throbbing headache; severe hypotension; flushing and diaphoresis followed by cutaneous chilling and cyanosis; dicrotic, intermittent pulse; palpitations, vertigo, syncope, heart block, circulatory collapse; *CNS:* visual disturbances, increased intracranial pressure (with confusion and moderate fever), paralysis and coma followed by clonic convulsions; *GI:* nausea, vomiting, colic, bloody diarrhea; *respiratory:* methemoglobinemia with cyanosis and anoxia, initial hyperpnea, dyspnea, hypopnea
Treatment	Promptly perform gastric lavage. To treat hypotension, place patient in a recumbent (shock) position and keep comfortably warm; passive movements of the extremities may enhance venous return. Do not use epinephrine or related compounds to reverse hypotension. Institute mechanical ventilation and administer oxygen, as needed. For methemoglobinemia, give 1–2 mg/kg of 1% methylene blue IV. It is not known whether isosorbide dinitrate can be removed by dialysis.

DRUG INTERACTIONS

Alcohol, antihypertensive drugs, and other vasodilators	⇧ Risk of hypotension
Calcium-channel blockers	Marked symptomatic orthostatic hypotension; if necessary, adjust dosage of nitrate or calcium-channel blocker

ALTERED LABORATORY VALUES

Blood/serum values	⇩ Cholesterol (with Zlatkis-Zak color reaction)
Urinary values	⇧ Catecholamines ⇧ VMA

USE IN CHILDREN
Safety and effectiveness for use in children have not been established

USE IN PREGNANT AND NURSING WOMEN
Pregnancy Category C: isosorbide dinitrate has been shown to be embryotoxic in rabbits, causing an increase in mummified pups at oral doses of 35 and 150 times the maximum human daily dose; no adequate, well-controlled studies have been done in pregnant women. Use during pregnancy only if the expected benefit justifies the potential risk to the fetus. It is not known whether isosorbide dinitrate is excreted in human milk; use with caution in nursing mothers.

NITRATES

TRANSDERM-Nitro (nitroglycerin) CIBA Rx

Transcutaneous drug delivery system: 2.5 mg/24 h (5 cm²), 5 mg/24 h (10 cm²), 10 mg/24 h (20 cm²), 15 mg/24 h (30 cm²)

INDICATIONS
Prevention and treatment of **angina pectoris** due to coronary artery disease[1]

TRANSCUTANEOUS DOSAGE
Adult: apply required size and number of systems (see "initial dosage titration," below) to any desired skin area, other than the distal extremities, that is dry, free of cuts and irritations, and preferably hairless (clip hair first if adhesion or removal of the system may be interfered with). Replace system(s) q24h, using a different skin area each time; contact with water will not affect a system.

TRANSDERM-Nitro

CONTRAINDICATIONS

Increased intraocular or intracranial pressure	Marked anemia	Intolerance to organic nitrates

ADMINISTRATION/DOSAGE ADJUSTMENTS

Initial dosage titration	Start with a single Transderm-Nitro 5 system (5 mg/24 h); if clinical response is inadequate, advise patient to replace it with either two Transderm-Nitro 5 systems or one Transderm-Nitro 10 system (10 mg/24 h). Additional systems may be added, if indicated by careful monitoring of the clinical response. For some patients, the Transderm-Nitro 2.5 system may be adequate. The optimal dosage is determined by the clinical response, side effects, and effects of therapy on blood pressure; the goal in adjusting dosage is to obtain the greatest reduction in resting blood pressure without producing symptomatic hypotension, especially upon standing.
Discontinuation of therapy	To prevent sudden withdrawal reactions, gradually reduce both the dose used daily and the frequency of application over a period of 4–6 wk; use the Transderm-Nitro 2.5 system to decrease the dose

WARNINGS/PRECAUTIONS

Transient headaches	May occur, particularly at higher doses; treat with mild analgesics while continuing therapy. If headaches persist, reduce dosage or discontinue use.
Anginal attacks	This preparation is not designed for immediate relief of acute anginal episodes; sublingual nitroglycerin tablets may be needed occasionally to provide prompt relief
Symptomatic hypotension	Faintness, weakness, or dizziness, particularly upon standing, may indicate overdosage; reduce dosage or discontinue use if such symptoms occur
Abrupt withdrawal of therapy	May produce sudden withdrawal reactions (see ADMINISTRATION/DOSAGE ADJUSTMENTS)
Cardioversion	To avoid electrical arcing during defibrillation or cardioversion, remove the system before performing the procedure
Special-risk patients	Provide for close clinical surveillance and/or hemodynamic monitoring when treating patients with acute myocardial infarction or congestive heart failure

ADVERSE REACTIONS

Central nervous system	Transient headache, faintness, dizziness
Cardiovascular	Hypotension, increased heart rate, flushing
Gastrointestinal	Nausea, vomiting
Dermatological	Dermatitis

OVERDOSAGE

Signs and symptoms	See ADVERSE REACTIONS
Treatment	Reduce dosage or discontinue use

DRUG INTERACTIONS

Acetylcholine	↓ Cholinergic receptor stimulation
Norepinephrine	↓ Pressor effect
Histamine	↓ Histamine effect
Alcohol, antihypertensive agents, other vasodilators	↑ Orthostatic hypotensive effect of nitroglycerin
Sympathomimetics	↓ Antianginal effect of nitroglycerin

ALTERED LABORATORY VALUES

Urinary values	↑ Catecholamines ↑ Vanillylmandelic acid (VMA)

No clinically significant alterations in blood/serum values occur at therapeutic dosages

---

USE IN CHILDREN
Evaluate potential benefits and risks before using in children

USE IN PREGNANT AND NURSING WOMEN
Evaluate potential benefits and risks before using in pregnant or nursing women

---

[1] Conditionally approved

NITRATES

TRIDIL (nitroglycerin) Du Pont Critical Care   Rx

Ampuls: 0.5 mg/ml (10 ml), 5 mg/ml (5, 10 ml)   **Vials:** 5 mg/ml (5, 10 ml)

INDICATIONS

Angina pectoris in patients who have not responded to organic nitrates and/or beta blockade
Congestive heart failure associated with **acute myocardial infarction**
Perioperative hypertension[1]
Production of **controlled hypotension** during surgical procedures

PARENTERAL DOSAGE

Adult: 5 µg/min via IV infusion, using Tridilset or Tridilset V.I.P. (see WARNINGS/PRECAUTIONS), to start; increase dosage in increments of 5 µg/min at 3- to 5-min intervals until some response is noted (if no response is seen at 20 µg/min, increments of 10 and then 20 µg/min may be used). Once a partial blood pressure response is observed, reduce the size of the dosage increments and lengthen the interval between increases.

CONTRAINDICATIONS

Hypersensitivity to nitroglycerin or idiosyncratic reaction to organic nitrates

Hypotension or uncorrected hypovolemia

Increased intracranial pressure (eg, head trauma or cerebral hemorrhage)

Constrictive pericarditis and pericardial tamponade

ADMINISTRATION/DOSAGE ADJUSTMENTS

Preparation of solution — Transfer the contents of the ampuls or vials to glass bottles containing either 5% dextrose injection USP or 0.9% sodium chloride injection USP; assure uniform dilution by inverting the container several times. For the initial dilution, prepare a solution of 50 or 100 µg/ml: to obtain a concentration of 50 µg/ml, add 5 mg of nitroglycerin to 100 ml of diluent or 25 mg to 500 ml; to obtain a concentration of 100 µg/ml, add 5 mg to 50 ml, 25 mg to 250 ml, or 50 mg to 500 ml. After the dosage has been titrated, a more concentrated solution may be prepared if fluid restriction is necessary: to obtain a solution of 200 µg/ml, add 10 mg to 50 ml, 50 mg to 250 ml, or 100 mg to 500 ml; to obtain a solution of 400 µg/ml, the maximum recommended concentration, add 100 mg to 250 ml or 200 mg to 500 ml. Do not mix nitroglycerin with other drugs in the same bottle. Whenever the concentration of a solution is changed, the infusion set must be flushed; otherwise, administration of the new solution may be delayed.

Dosage titration — Titrate dosage to desired level of hemodynamic function; blood pressure, heart rate, and other appropriate physiologic parameters must be monitored continuously to obtain the correct dose. Adequate systemic blood pressure and coronary perfusion pressure must be maintained. Since a fall in pulmonary capillary wedge pressure precedes the onset of arterial hypotension, wedge pressure can serve as a useful guide to safe titration of this drug. Patients with normal or low left ventricular filling pressures or pulmonary capillary wedge pressures (eg, patients with uncomplicated angina pectoris) may respond fully to doses as small as 5 µg/ml and, therefore, require especially careful titration and monitoring.

Stability — When stored in glass containers, the diluted solution is physically and chemically stable for up to 48 h at room temperature and for up to 7 days under refrigeration

WARNINGS/PRECAUTIONS

Absorption of nitroglycerin by IV administration sets — Nitroglycerin is readily absorbed by many plastics; use glass IV bottles to dilute and store this drug and avoid filters that absorb nitroglycerin. Common administration sets made of polyvinyl chloride (PVC) tubing can absorb 40–80% of the total amount of nitroglycerin in the final solution. Since the loss is neither constant nor self-limited, it cannot be simply calculated or corrected for. To minimize the loss of nitroglycerin, use the Tridilset IV administration set with a peristaltic action infusion pump or the Tridilset V.I.P. connector set with a volumetric infusion pump. PVC tubing has been utilized exclusively in published studies, and the doses recommended (25 µg/min or more to start) will be too high if administration sets with nonabsorbing materials are used.

Hepatic or renal impairment — Use with caution in patients with severe liver or kidney disease

Excessive hypotension — Must be avoided because of possible deleterious effects on vital organs resulting from poor perfusion, especially if the hypotension is prolonged, and the attendant risk of ischemia, thrombosis, and physiologic impairment; paradoxical bradycardia and increased angina pectoris may accompany nitroglycerin-induced hypotension. Use in patients with hypotension or uncorrected hypovolemia is contraindicated. Patients with normal or low pulmonary capillary wedge pressures are especially sensitive to the hypotensive effects of IV nitroglycerin (see ADMINISTRATION/DOSAGE ADJUSTMENTS).

Intracoronary administration — Safety of intracoronary injection has not been established

Carcinogenicity — No long-term studies have been done in animals to evaluate the carcinogenic potential of nitroglycerin

ADVERSE REACTIONS[2]

Frequent reactions (incidence ≥ 1%) are printed in *italics*

Central nervous system and neuromuscular — *Headache (2%)*, apprehension, restlessness, muscle twitching, dizziness

TRIDIL ■ PERSANTINE

Cardiovascular	Tachycardia, retrosternal discomfort, palpitations
Gastrointestinal	Nausea, vomiting, abdominal pain

OVERDOSAGE

Signs and symptoms	Severe hypotension, reflex tachycardia
Treatment	Elevate the patient's legs and decrease or temporarily discontinue the infusion until the patient's condition stabilizes. The duration of hemodynamic effects of nitroglycerin is short, and additional corrective measures are usually unnecessary; however, if further therapy is needed, concomitant use of an IV alpha-adrenergic agonist (eg, methoxamine or phenylephrine) should be considered.

DRUG INTERACTIONS

Acetylcholine	▽ Cholinergic receptor stimulation
Norepinephrine	▽ Pressor effect
Histamine	▽ Histamine effect
Alcohol, antihypertensive agents, other vasodilators	△ Orthostatic hypotensive effect of nitroglycerin
Sympathomimetics	▽ Antianginal effect of nitroglycerin

ALTERED LABORATORY VALUES

Urinary values	△ Catecholamines △ Vanillylmandelic acid (VMA)

No clinically significant alterations in blood/serum values occur at therapeutic dosages

---

USE IN CHILDREN

Safety and effectiveness for use in children have not been established

USE IN PREGNANT AND NURSING WOMEN

Pregnancy Category C: use during pregnancy only if clearly needed. Reproduction studies have not been done in animals. It is also not known whether nitroglycerin can cause fetal harm when administered to pregnant women or can affect reproductive capacity. No information is available on excretion of this drug in human milk; use with caution in nursing mothers.

---

[1] Hypertension associated with surgical procedures, especially cardiovascular procedures, eg, hypertension associated with intratracheal intubation, anesthesia, skin incision, sternotomy, cardiac bypass, and the immediate postoperative period
[2] Oral and/or topical use of nitroglycerin has resulted in cutaneous flushing, weakness, and occasional drug rash or exfoliative dermatitis

Chapter 12

Antianxiety Agents

Benzodiazepines — 405

ATIVAN (Wyeth) — 405
Lorazepam *C-IV*

ATIVAN Injection (Wyeth) — 406
Lorazepam *C-IV*

CENTRAX (Parke-Davis) — 407
Prazepam *C-IV*

LIBRITABS (Roche) — 408
Chlordiazepoxide hydrochloride *C-IV*

LIBRIUM (Roche) — 408
Chlordiazepoxide hydrochloride *C-IV*

PAXIPAM (Schering) — 410
Halazepam *C-IV*

SERAX (Wyeth) — 411
Oxazepam *C-IV*

TRANXENE (Abbott) — 413
Clorazepate dipotassium *C-IV*

TRANXENE-SD (Abbott) — 413
Clorazepate dipotassium *C-IV*

VALIUM (Roche) — 414
Diazepam *C-IV*

VALRELEASE (Roche) — 415
Diazepam *C-IV*

XANAX (Upjohn) — 416
Alprazolam *C-IV*

Nonbenzodiazepines — 417

ATARAX (Roerig) — 417
Hydroxyzine hydrochloride *Rx*

ATARAX 100 (Roerig) — 417
Hydroxyzine hydrochloride *Rx*

BUSPAR (Mead Johnson) — 418
Buspirone hydrochloride *Rx*

EQUANIL (Wyeth) — 420
Meprobamate *C-IV*

INAPSINE (Janssen) — 421
Droperidol *Rx*

MILTOWN (Wallace) — 423
Meprobamate *C-IV*

MILTOWN 600 (Wallace) — 423
Meprobamate *C-IV*

TRANCOPAL (Winthrop-Breon) — 424
Chlormezanone *Rx*

VISTARIL (Pfizer) — 425
Hydroxyzine pamoate *Rx*

VISTARIL Intramuscular Solution (Roerig) — 426
Hydroxyzine hydrochloride *Rx*

Other Antianxiety Agents — 404

MEPROSPAN (Wallace) — 404
Meprobamate *C-IV*

OTHER ANTIANXIETY AGENTS

DRUG	HOW SUPPLIED	USUAL DOSAGE
MEPROSPAN (Wallace) Meprobamate *C-IV*	Capsules (sustained release): 200, 400 mg	**Adult:** 400–800 mg in the morning and at bedtime, or up to 2,400 mg/day, if needed **Child (6–12 yr):** 200 mg in the morning and at bedtime

BENZODIAZEPINES

ATIVAN (lorazepam) Wyeth

Tablets: 0.5, 1, 2 mg

C-IV

INDICATIONS

Anxiety disorders and short-term relief of symptoms of anxiety or of anxiety mixed with depressive symptoms[1]

ORAL DOSAGE

Adult: 2–3 mg bid or tid to start, followed by 1–10 mg/day, as needed, in divided doses, with the largest being taken before bedtime; usual maintenance dosage: 2–6 mg/day, given in divided doses

CONTRAINDICATIONS

Hypersensitivity to benzodiazepines — Acute narrow-angle glaucoma

ADMINISTRATION/DOSAGE ADJUSTMENTS

Insomnia	Administer 2–4 mg in a single daily dose at bedtime
Elderly and debilitated patients	Initiate therapy with 1–2 mg/day in divided doses; adjust dosage as needed
Long-term use (> 4 mo)	Effectiveness for prolonged use as an antianxiety agent has not been tested in systematic clinical studies; reassess need for continued therapy periodically

WARNINGS/PRECAUTIONS

Primary depressive disorder or psychosis	Should not be treated with this drug
Gastrointestinal or cardiovascular disorders associated with anxiety	Lorazepam has not been shown to be of significant benefit in treating GI tract or cardiovascular symptoms
Drug dependence	Psychic and/or physical dependence may develop, especially in addiction-prone individuals
Mental impairment, reflex-slowing	Caution patients not to engage in potentially hazardous activities requiring full mental alertness and that alcohol and other CNS depressants may cause further impairment
Potentially suicidal patients	Should not have access to large quantities of lorazepam; prescribe smallest amount feasible
Abrupt discontinuation of therapy	May produce barbiturate-like withdrawal symptoms or precipitate recurrence of pre-existing symptoms, including anxiety, agitation, irritability, tension, insomnia, and convulsions[2]
Prolonged therapy	Blood counts and liver-function tests should be performed periodically; use with caution in the elderly and monitor frequently for symptoms of upper GI disease
Hepatic or renal impairment	May lead to excessive drug accumulation; monitor patient closely
Ataxia or oversedation	May develop in elderly and/or debilitated patients (see ADMINISTRATION/DOSAGE ADJUSTMENTS)

ADVERSE REACTIONS

Frequent reactions (incidence ≥ 1%) are printed in *italics*

Central nervous system	*Sedation (16%), dizziness (6.9%), weakness (4.2%), unsteadiness (3.4%)*, disorientation, depression, headache, sleep disturbance, agitation, transient amnesia or memory impairment
Cardiovascular	Slight hypotension
Gastrointestinal	Nausea, altered appetite, various disturbances
Other	Dermatological symptoms, visual disturbances, autonomic manifestations

OVERDOSAGE

Signs and symptoms	Somnolence, confusion, coma
Treatment	Empty stomach immediately by inducing emesis or by gastric lavage. Employ general supportive measures, as needed, and monitor vital signs. Combat hypotension with norepinephrine. The benefit of dialysis is unknown.

DRUG INTERACTIONS

Alcohol, tricyclic antidepressants, sedative-hypnotics, MAO inhibitors, and other CNS depressants	⇧ CNS depression

ALTERED LABORATORY VALUES

Blood/serum values — ⇧ Lactate dehydrogenase

No clinically significant alterations in urinary values occur at therapeutic dosages

COMPENDIUM OF DRUG THERAPY

ATIVAN ■ ATIVAN Injection

USE IN CHILDREN	USE IN PREGNANT AND NURSING WOMEN
Safety and effectiveness for use in children under 12 yr of age have not been established	Use of antianxiety agents during early pregnancy should almost always be avoided. Although lorazepam has not been sufficiently studied to determine conclusively its effects during pregnancy, an increased risk of congenital malformations during the first trimester has been associated with minor tranquilizers (chlordiazepoxide, diazepam, meprobamate). It is not known whether lorazepam is excreted in human milk; because many drugs are excreted in human milk, patient should stop nursing if drug is prescribed.

[1] Anxiety or tension associated with the stress of everyday life usually does not require treatment with an antianxiety agent
[2] Withdrawal symptoms have also been observed following abrupt discontinuation of therapeutic levels of benzodiazepines used continuously for several months

BENZODIAZEPINES

ATIVAN Injection (lorazepam) Wyeth   C-IV

Cartridge-needle units: 2, 4 mg/ml (1 ml)   **Vials:** 2, 4 mg/ml (1, 10 ml) for IM or IV injection

INDICATIONS	PARENTERAL DOSAGE
Preanesthetic medication to produce sedation, relieve anxiety, and diminish recall of preoperative and postoperative events	**Adult:** when sedation and relief of anxiety are primary considerations, 0.044 mg/kg (0.02 mg/lb), up to 2 mg, IV to start; when a greater degree of lack of recall is desired, 0.05 mg/kg, up to 4 mg, given IM at least 2 h prior to surgery or IV 15–20 min prior to surgery for optimum effect

CONTRAINDICATIONS	
Hypersensitivity to benzodiazepines or vehicle (polyethylene glycol, propylene glycol, and benzyl alcohol)	Intraarterial injection

ADMINISTRATION/DOSAGE ADJUSTMENTS	
Intramuscular administration	Inject lorazepam undiluted deeply into muscle mass
Intravenous administration	Immediately prior to use, dilute drug with an equal volume of compatible solution (Sterile Water for Injection USP, Sodium Chloride Injection USP, or 5% Dextrose Injection USP). Inject diluted solution directly into vein or into tubing of an existing IV line at a rate not exceeding 2 mg/min. Aspirate repeatedly and exercise caution to avoid inadvertent intra-arterial injection and perivascular extravasation.

WARNINGS/PRECAUTIONS	
Mental impairment, reflex-slowing	Performance of potentially hazardous activities may be impaired for 24–48 h or longer because of age, general condition, stress of surgery, or concomitant use of other drugs; premature ambulation (up to 8 h) following injection may result in falling and injury
Partial airway obstruction	May occur in heavily sedated patients, especially when more than 0.05 mg/kg is given IV or recommended doses are given IV with other drugs used during administration of anesthesia; have on hand equipment necessary to maintain a patent airway and to support ventilation and respiration prior to IV administration
Concomitant use of other CNS depressants	May potentiate and prolong the effects of lorazepam, resulting in excessive sleepiness or drowsiness and, rarely, interference with recall or recognition of events occurring on the day of surgery and the day after. Reduce dosage of other CNS depressants (see DRUG INTERACTIONS) given concomitantly with parenteral lorazepam or within 6–8 h following injection of the drug. Tolerance to alcoholic beverages may also be diminished; caution patient not to consume any form of alcohol for at least 24–48 h after receiving lorazepam
Concomitant use of scopolamine	Provides no additional therapeutic benefit and may result in increased sedation, hallucination, and irrational behavior
Patients with hepatic or renal impairment	Since effect of drug may be prolonged, use the lowest effective dose in patients with mild to moderate hepatic or renal disease; use in patients with hepatic or renal failure is not recommended
Patients in coma or shock or experiencing acute alcohol intoxication	Should not be given parenteral lorazepam, owing to the lack of clinical experience in these situations
Other special-risk patients	Use with extreme care in elderly and/or very ill patients and patients with limited pulmonary reserve, owing to the increased risk of hypoventilation and/or hypoxia and cardiac arrest; resuscitative equipment to support ventilation should be readily available. Patients over 50 yr of age may experience profound, prolonged sedation following IV injection of lorazepam; ordinarily, doses exceeding 2 mg should not be exceeded, unless a greater degree of lack of recall is desired.

ATIVAN Injection ■ CENTRAX

Intravenous use prior to local or regional anesthesia	May produce excessive sedation or drowsiness and possible interference with patient cooperation in determining level of anesthesia, especially when doses exceeding 0.05 mg/kg are given or with concomitant use of narcotic analgesics
Inadvertent intraarterial injection	May produce arteriospasm, resulting in gangrene and possible amputation; inject drug carefully to preclude intraarterial placement or peripheral extravasation
Physical and psychological dependence	Repeated administration over a prolonged period may result in limited dependence, although there are no data on injectable lorazepam in this respect
Endoscopic procedures	Since pharyngeal reflexes are not impaired by lorazepam, adequate topical or regional anesthesia is recommended to minimize reflex activity associated with per-oral endoscopic procedures. Inpatients should be kept under observation in a recovery room following endoscopy; outpatient use of parenteral lorazepam for endoscopic procedures has not been adequately studied.

ADVERSE REACTIONS

Frequent reactions (incidence ≥ 1%) are printed in *italics*

Central nervous system	*Excessive sleepiness or drowsiness (10–20% following IV injection, depending on age); restlessness, confusion, depression, crying, sobbing, and delirium (1.3%); visual hallucinations (1%);* dizziness
Cardiovascular	Increase or decrease in blood pressure
Respiratory	Partial airway obstruction during regional anesthesia, possibly related to excessive sleepiness (rare)
Local	*Pain and burning sensation immediately following IM injection (17%), pain immediately following IV injection (1.6%), redness immediately following IM injection (2%), redness occurring 24 h after IV injection (2.5%)*
Other	Diplopia and/or blurred vision; depressed hearing coincident with peak effect; skin rash, nausea, and vomiting with concomitant use of other drugs during anesthesia and surgery

OVERDOSAGE

Signs and symptoms	*Mild cases:* drowsiness, mental confusion, and lethargy; *more severe cases:* ataxia, hypotonia, hypotension, hypnosis, coma, and, very rarely, death
Treatment	Until drug is eliminated, treatment is largely supportive. Carefully monitor vital signs and fluid balance. Maintain an adequate airway and provide assisted ventilation, if necessary. If renal function is normal, force diuresis with IV fluids and electrolytes to accelerate elimination; osmotic diuretics (eg, mannitol) may be effective adjuncts to parenteral fluid therapy. If situation becomes critical, renal dialysis and exchange transfusions may be indicated. Physostigmine, given IV at a rate of 1 mg/min for a total dose of 0.5–4 mg, may reverse central anticholinergic manifestations (confusion, memory disturbances, visual disturbances, hallucinations, delirium); however, the risk of inducing seizures should be weighed against the possible clinical benefit of using physostigmine.

DRUG INTERACTIONS

Alcohol, barbiturates, narcotic analgesics, phenothiazines, MAO inhibitors and other antidepressants	⇧ CNS depression
Scopolamine	⇧ Risk of sedation, hallucination, and irrational behavior

ALTERED LABORATORY VALUES

No clinically significant alterations in blood/serum or urinary values occur at therapeutic dosages

---

USE IN CHILDREN

Not recommended for use in patients under 18 yr of age because of insufficient data

USE IN PREGNANT AND NURSING WOMEN

Pregnancy Category D: do not use during pregnancy. An increased risk of congenital malformations has been associated with the use of minor tranquilizers (chlordiazepoxide, diazepam, and meprobamate) during the first trimester. Lorazepam and its major metabolite have been detected in human umbilical cord blood, indicating placental transfer. Obstetrical safety has not been established, and, hence, use during labor or delivery, including cesarean section, is not recommended. The drug should not be given to nursing mothers to preclude the possibility of excretion in human milk and sedation of the nursing infant.

BENZODIAZEPINES

CENTRAX (prazepam) Parke-Davis

C-IV

Capsules: 5, 10, 20 mg   **Tablets:** 10 mg

INDICATIONS

Anxiety disorders and short-term relief of **symptoms of anxiety**[1]

ORAL DOSAGE

Adult: 30 mg/day in divided doses to start, followed by 20–60 mg/day in divided doses, as needed; alternative regimen: 20 mg at bedtime, followed several days later by 20–40 mg/day in divided doses, as needed

CENTRAX ■ LIBRITABS/LIBRIUM

CONTRAINDICATIONS

Hypersensitivity to prazepam	Acute narrow-angle glaucoma

ADMINISTRATION/DOSAGE ADJUSTMENTS

Elderly or debilitated patients	Reduce initial dosage to 10–15 mg/day in divided doses
Long-term use (> 4 mo)	Effectiveness for prolonged use as an antianxiety agent has not been tested in systematic clinical studies; reassess need for continued therapy periodically

WARNINGS/PRECAUTIONS

Psychotic reactions and psychiatric disorders in which anxiety is not prominent	Should not be treated with this drug
Drug dependence	Psychic and/or physical dependence may develop, especially in addiction-prone individuals
Mental impairment, reflex-slowing	Caution patients not to engage in potentially hazardous activities requiring full mental alertness and that alcohol and other CNS depressants may cause further impairment
Potentially suicidal patients	Should not have access to large quantities of prazepam; prescribe smallest amount feasible
Barbiturate-like withdrawal symptoms	May result when drug is discontinued abruptly[2]
Prolonged therapy	Blood counts and liver-function tests should be performed periodically
Hepatic or renal impairment	May lead to excessive drug accumulation; monitor patient closely
Ataxia or oversedation	May develop in elderly or debilitated patients (see ADMINISTRATION/DOSAGE ADJUSTMENTS)

ADVERSE REACTIONS

Frequent reactions (incidence ≥ 1%) are printed in *italics*

Central nervous system	*Fatigue (12%), dizziness (8.7%), weakness, (7.7%), drowsiness and light-headedness (6.8%), ataxia (5.0%),* headache, confusion, tremor, vivid dreams, slurred speech, stimulation, blurred vision
Cardiovascular	Palpitations, syncope, slight hypotension
Gastrointestinal	Dry mouth, various other complaints
Dermatological	Diaphoresis, pruritus, skin rash
Hepatic	Altered liver-function tests
Genitourinary	Various complaints
Other	Swelling of feet, joint pains, slight weight gain

OVERDOSAGE

Signs and symptoms	See ADVERSE REACTIONS
Treatment	Induce emesis if vomiting has not occurred spontaneously and use gastric lavage immediately to empty stomach. Monitor vital signs frequently and employ general supportive measures, as needed. Combat hypotension with levarterenol or metaraminol.

DRUG INTERACTIONS

Alcohol, tricyclic antidepressants, sedative-hypnotics, MAO inhibitors, and other CNS depressants	△ CNS depression

ALTERED LABORATORY VALUES

No clinically significant alterations in blood/serum or urinary values occur at therapeutic dosages

---

USE IN CHILDREN

Safety and effectiveness for use in patients under 18 yr of age have not been established

USE IN PREGNANT AND NURSING WOMEN

Use of antianxiety agents during early pregnancy should almost always be avoided. Although prazepam has not been sufficiently studied to determine conclusively its effects during pregnancy, an increased risk of congenital malformations during the first trimester has been associated with minor tranquilizers (chlordiazepoxide, diazepam, meprobamate). Prazepam and its metabolites are probably excreted in human milk; patients should stop nursing if drug is prescribed.

---

[1] Anxiety or tension associated with the stress of everyday life usually does not require treatment with an antianxiety agent
[2] Withdrawal symptoms have also been observed following abrupt discontinuation of therapeutic levels of benzodiazepines used continuously for several months

---

BENZODIAZEPINES

LIBRITABS (chlordiazepoxide hydrochloride) Roche   C-IV
Tablets: 5, 10, 25 mg

LIBRIUM (chlordiazepoxide hydrochloride) Roche   C-IV
Capsules: 5, 10, 25 mg   Ampuls: 100 mg (5 ml)

INDICATIONS	ORAL DOSAGE	PARENTERAL DOSAGE
Mild to moderate anxiety disorders and symptoms of anxiety[1]	**Adult:** 5–10 mg tid or qid **Child (> 6 yr):** 5 mg bid to qid, or up to 10 mg bid or tid, if needed	

LIBRITABS/LIBRIUM

Acute (parenteral only) or severe anxiety and symptoms of anxiety[1]	Adult: 20–25 mg tid or qid Child: same as child's dosage above	Adult: 50–100 mg IM (preferred) or IV to start, followed by 25–50 mg tid or qid, if needed Child ($>$ 12 yr): 25–50 mg IM (preferred) or IV to start, followed by 25–50 mg tid or qid, if needed
Preoperative apprehension and anxiety	Adult: 5–10 mg tid or qid on days before surgery Child: same as child's dosage above	Adult: 50–100 mg IM 1 h before surgery Child ($>$ 12 yr): 25–50 mg IM 1 h before surgery
Withdrawal symptoms of acute alcoholism	Adult: 50–100 mg, repeated as needed, up to 300 mg/day, until agitation is controlled; thereafter, reduce dosage to maintenance levels	Adult: 50–100 mg IM (preferred) or IV, repeated in 2–4 h, if needed Child ($>$ 12 yr): 25–50 mg IM (preferred) or IV, repeated in 2–4 h, if needed

CONTRAINDICATIONS

Hypersensitivity to chloridiazepoxide	Shock or comatose states (for parenteral use only)

ADMINISTRATION/DOSAGE ADJUSTMENTS

Intramuscular administration	Immediately before use, prepare solution by adding 2 ml of special IM diluent (supplied) to contents of 5-ml amber ampul; agitate gently until powder is completely dissolved. Inject slowly and deeply into upper outer quadrant of gluteus muscle. Patient should be kept under observation, preferably in bed, for up to 3 h after injection.
Intravenous administration	Immediately before use, prepare solution by adding 5 ml of physiologic saline or sterile water for injection to contents of 5-ml ampul; agitate gently until powder is completely dissolved. Inject slowly over a period of 1 min. Patient should be kept under observation, preferably in bed, for up to 3 h after injection.
Maximum parenteral dosage	Up to 300 mg may be given IM or IV during a 6-h period, but not more than this amount in any 24-h period
Elderly or debilitated patients	Reduce oral dosage to 5 mg bid to qid and parenteral dosage 25–50 mg IM or IV
Long-term use ($>$ 4 mo)	Effectiveness for prolonged use as an antianxiety agent has not been tested in systematic clinical studies; reassess need for continued therapy periodically

WARNINGS/PRECAUTIONS

Mental impairment, reflex-slowing	Caution patients not to engage in potentially hazardous activities requiring full mental alertness and that alcohol and other CNS depressants may cause further impairment; ambulatory patients should not be permitted to drive after receiving an injection
Drug dependence	Psychic and/or physical dependence may develop, especially in addiction-prone individuals
Abrupt discontinuation of therapy	May precipitate barbiturate-like withdrawal symptoms, including convulsions, in patients receiving excessive doses for extended periods. Milder withdrawal symptoms have also been observed infrequently following abrupt discontinuation of several months of continuous benzodiazepine therapy, generally when higher therapeutic doses have not been used. After prolonged therapy, reduce dosage gradually.
Prolonged therapy	Blood counts and liver-function tests should be performed periodically
Hepatic or renal impairment	May lead to excessive drug accumulation; monitor patient closely
Concomitant psychotropic therapy	Use with extreme caution, if at all, particularly when use of known potentiating compounds (see DRUG INTERACTIONS) is contemplated
Paradoxical reactions	Excitement, stimulation, and acute rage may occur in psychiatric patients and in hyperactive children; monitor such patients closely during therapy
Ataxia or oversedation	May develop in elderly and/or debilitated patients (see ADMINISTRATION/DOSAGE ADJUSTMENTS)
Porphyria	May be exacerbated; use with caution in patients with porphyria

ADVERSE REACTIONS

Central nervous system	Drowsiness, ataxia, confusion, EEG pattern changes, extrapyramidal symptoms, blurred vision (with parenteral use)
Cardiovascular	Syncope, hypotension (with parenteral use), tachycardia (with parenteral use)
Gastrointestinal	Nausea, constipation
Dermatological	Skin eruptions, edema
Hematological	Blood dyscrasias, including agranulocytosis
Hepatic	Jaundice, dysfunction
Genitourinary	Menstrual irregularities, altered libido

OVERDOSAGE

Signs and symptoms	Somnolence, confusion, coma, diminished reflexes, excitation, hypotension
Treatment	Empty stomach immediately by gastric lavage. Employ general supportive measures, as needed. Administer IV fluids and maintain adequate airway. Combat hypotension with levarterenol or metaraminol. If excitation occurs, do not give barbiturates. Dialysis is of limited value.

LIBRITABS/LIBRIUM ■ PAXIPAM

DRUG INTERACTIONS

Alcohol, tricyclic antidepressants, sedative-hypnotics, MAO inhibitors, and other CNS depressants	⇧ CNS depression
Oral anticoagulants	⇧ or ⇩ Anticoagulant effect

ALTERED LABORATORY VALUES

No clinically significant alterations in blood/serum or urinary values occurs at therapeutic dosages

---

USE IN CHILDREN

See INDICATIONS and dosage recommendations. Oral form is not recommended for use in children under 6 yr of age; parenteral form is not recommended for use in children under 12 yr of age.

USE IN PREGNANT AND NURSING WOMEN

Use of antianxiety agents during early pregnancy should almost always be avoided. Although chlordiazepoxide has not been sufficiently studied to determine conclusively its effects during pregnancy, an increased risk of congenital malformations during the first trimester has been associated with minor tranquilizers, including chlordiazepoxide. Chlordiazepoxide is excreted into breast milk in minimal amounts.

---

[1] Anxiety or tension associated with the stress of everyday life usually does not require treatment with an antianxiety agent

---

BENZODIAZEPINES

PAXIPAM (halazepam) Schering   C-IV

Tablets: 20, 40 mg

INDICATIONS	ORAL DOSAGE
Anxiety disorders and short-term relief of **symptoms of anxiety**[1]	Adult: 20–40 mg tid or qid, depending upon patient response and severity of symptoms; usual optimal dosage: 80–160 mg/day

CONTRAINDICATIONS	
Sensitivity to halazepam or other benzodiazepines	Acute narrow-angle glaucoma

ADMINISTRATION/DOSAGE ADJUSTMENTS

Long-term use (> 4 mo)	Effectiveness for long-term use has not been established; reassess need for continued therapy periodically
Elderly (≥ 70 yr) or debilitated patients	Start with 20 mg 1–2 times/day and adjust dosage as needed and tolerated
Higher-than-usual daily dosages	May be required in some patients; in such cases, increase dosage cautiously to avoid side effects. If side effects occur with starting dose, lower the dose.

WARNINGS/PRECAUTIONS

Psychoses and major depressive disorders	Halazepam is not of value in the treatment of psychotic patients and should not be used in place of appropriate treatment for psychosis; halazepam is not recommended as the primary treatment for major depressive disorders
Drowsiness	Caution patients not to engage in potentially hazardous activities requiring full mental alertness and that alcohol and other CNS depressants may cause further impairment
Concomitant psychotropic or anticonvulsant therapy	Consider carefully the pharmacology of the agents to be used, particularly if they might potentiate the action of halazepam (see DRUG INTERACTIONS)
Severely depressed or potentially suicidal patients	Employ the usual precautions with regard to administration of psychotropic drugs and size of prescription
Ataxia or oversedation	May develop in elderly or debilitated patients; administer the smallest effective dose (see ADMINISTRATION/DOSAGE ADJUSTMENTS)
Hepatic or renal impairment	Observe the usual precautions to avoid excessive drug accumulation
Carcinogenicity, mutagenicity	Results of oral oncogenicity studies in rats and mice given 5–50 times the usual human dose (120 mg/day) showed no evidence of carcinogenicity or other significant pathology; mutagenicity studies have not been done
Drug dependence	Psychic and/or physical dependence may develop, especially in addiction-prone individuals, who should be under careful surveillance while receiving this drug

PAXIPAM ■ SERAX

Barbiturate-like withdrawal symptoms	May occur when drug is discontinued abruptly and may range from mild dysphoria and insomnia to major symptoms (including abdominal and muscle cramps, vomiting, sweating, tremor, and convulsions); although withdrawal symptoms are more commonly seen after prolonged use of excessive doses, they have also been observed following abrupt discontinuation of benzodiazepine therapy when therapeutic doses have been used continuously for several months. Taper dosage gradually after prolonged use.
Patients with a history of seizures or epilepsy	Should not be abruptly withdrawn from this drug or any CNS depressant, regardless of their concomitant anticonvulsant drug therapy

ADVERSE REACTIONS[2]

Frequent reactions (incidence $\geq$ 1%) are printed in *italics*

Central nervous system	*Drowsiness (29%); headache, apathy, psychomotor retardation, disorientation, confusion, euphoria, dysarthria, depression, and syncope (9%); dizziness (8%); ataxia (5%); fatigue (4%); visual disturbances and paradoxical reactions (1%);* sleep disturbances, changes in libido, auditory disturbances
Gastrointestinal	*Motion sickness, nausea, constipation, increased salivation, difficulty in swallowing, vomiting, and gastric disorders (9%); dry mouth (3%); change in appetite (1%)*
Hematological	*Clinically insignificant fluctuations in total and differential leukocyte counts (< 5%)*
Cardiovascular	*Tachycardia, bradycardia, hypotension, and other disturbances (2%)*
Musculoskeletal	*Muscular disturbances (2%)*
Other	Allergic manifestations, genitourinary disturbances, paresthesias, respiratory disturbances

OVERDOSAGE

Signs and symptoms	Somnolence, confusion, impaired coordination, diminished reflexes, and coma
Treatment	Empty stomach immediately by gastric lavage. Monitor respiration, pulse, and blood pressure, and employ general supportive measures, as needed. Administer IV fluids and maintain an adequate airway. Combat hypotension with norepinephrine or metaraminol. Dialysis is of limited value.

DRUG INTERACTIONS

Alcohol, sedative-hypnotics, anticonvulsants, antihistamines, and other CNS depressants	↑ CNS depression

ALTERED LABORATORY VALUES

Blood/serum values	↑ Alkaline phosphatase ↑ SGOT ↑ SGPT

No clinically significant alterations in urinary values occur at therapeutic dosages

USE IN CHILDREN

Safety and effectiveness for use in patients under 18 yr of age have not been established

USE IN PREGNANT AND NURSING WOMEN

Pregnancy Category D: use of this drug during the first trimester of pregnancy should almost always be avoided. Based on experience with other benzodiazepines, an increased risk of congenital abnormalities can be assumed if halazepam is taken during the first trimester. If this drug is used during pregnancy, or if the patient becomes pregnant or intends to become pregnant while taking it, she should be apprised of the potential hazard to the fetus. Neonates of mothers who used benzodiazepines during pregnancy may experience withdrawal symptoms; neonatal flaccidity has also been reported. Since halazepam and its major metabolites are excreted in human breast milk and accumulation to toxic levels is possible in neonates, patients should stop nursing if drug is prescribed. Studies performed in rats have shown no evidence of impaired fertility.

[1] Anxiety or tension associated with the stress of everyday life usually does not require treatment with an antianxiety agent
[2] Benzodiazepines have also been reported to cause jaundice, agranulocytosis, edema, slurred speech, minor menstrual irregularities, dystonia, pruritus, incontinence, urinary retention, and diplopia; these reactions have not been seen with halazepam

---

BENZODIAZEPINES

SERAX (oxazepam) Wyeth

C-IV

Capsules: 10, 15, 30 mg   **Tablets:** 15 mg

INDICATIONS

Anxiety disorders and short-term relief of **symptoms of anxiety**[1]

ORAL DOSAGE

Adult: for mild to moderate anxiety associated with tension, irritability, agitation, or related symptoms of functional origin or secondary to organic disease: 10–15 mg tid or qid; for severe anxiety syndromes, agitation, or anxiety mixed with depression: 15–30 mg tid or qid

COMPENDIUM OF DRUG THERAPY

SERAX

Acute inebriation, tremulousness, or anxiety upon withdrawal of alcohol	Adult: 15–30 tid or qid

CONTRAINDICATIONS

Hypersensitivity to oxazepam

ADMINISTRATION/DOSAGE ADJUSTMENTS

Elderly patients with anxiety, tension, irritability, and agitation	Initiate therapy with 10 mg tid; if necessary, increase dosage gradually to 15 mg tid or qid
Long-term use (> 4 mo)	Effectiveness for prolonged use as an antianxiety agent has not been tested in systematic clinical studies; reassess need for continued therapy periodically

WARNINGS/PRECAUTIONS

Psychoses	Should not be treated with this drug
Drug dependence	Psychic and/or physical dependence may develop, especially in addiction-prone individuals
Drowsiness, dizziness	Caution patients not to engage in potentially hazardous activities requiring full mental alertness; alcohol and other CNS depressants may cause further impairment
Abrupt discontinuation of therapy	May cause epileptiform seizures or barbiturate-like withdrawal symptoms[2]; reduce dosage gradually after prolonged therapy
Special-risk patients	Use with caution in patients in whom a drop in blood pressure could lead to cardiac complications, especially the elderly
Potentially suicidal patients	Should not have access to large quantities of oxazepam; prescribe smallest amount feasible
Prolonged therapy	Blood counts and liver-function tests should be performed periodically
Tartrazine sensitivity	Presence of FD&C Yellow No. 5 (tartrazine) in tablets may cause allergic-type reactions, including bronchial asthma, in susceptible individuals

ADVERSE REACTIONS

Central nervous system	Transient mild drowsiness, dizziness, vertigo, headache, paradoxical excitement or stimulation of affect, lethargy, slurred speech, tremor, transient amnesia or memory impairment; syncope and ataxia (rare)
Gastrointestinal	Nausea
Dermatological	Morbilliform, urticarial, or maculopapular rash
Hematological	Leukopenia (rare)
Hepatic	Dysfunction, including jaundice (rare)
Other	Altered libido, edema

OVERDOSAGE

Signs and symptoms	Somnolence, confusion, coma, diminished reflexes, excitation, hypotension
Treatment	Empty stomach immediately by gastric lavage. Employ general supportive measures, as needed. Administer IV fluids and maintain adequate airway. Combat hypotension with levarterenol or metaraminol.

DRUG INTERACTIONS

Alcohol, tricyclic antidepressants, sedative-hypnotics, MAO inhibitors, and other CNS depressants	⇧ CNS depression

ALTERED LABORATORY VALUES

No clinically significant alterations in blood/serum or urinary values occurs at therapeutic dosages

USE IN CHILDREN

Not indicated for use in children under 6 yr of age; optimum dosage for children 6–12 yr of age has not been established

USE IN PREGNANT AND NURSING WOMEN

Use of antianxiety agents should almost always be avoided during early pregnancy. Although oxazepam has not been sufficiently studied to determine conclusively its effects during pregnancy, an increased risk of congenital malformations during the first trimester has been associated with minor tranquilizers (chlordiazepoxide, diazepam, meprobamate). Consult manufacturer for use in nursing mothers.

---

[1] Anxiety or tension associated with the stress of everyday life usually does not require treatment with an antianxiety agent
[2] Withdrawal symptoms have also been observed following abrupt discontinuation of therapeutic levels of benzodiazepines used continuously for several months

TRANXENE

BENZODIAZEPINES

TRANXENE (clorazepate dipotassium) Abbott   C-IV
Tablets: 3.75, 7.5, 15 mg (Tranxene T-Tab)

TRANXENE-SD (clorazepate dipotassium) Abbott   C-IV
Tablets: 11.25 (Tranxene-SD Half Strength), 22.5 mg (Tranxene-SD)

INDICATIONS	ORAL DOSAGE
Anxiety disorders and short-term relief of symptoms of anxiety[1]	**Adult:** 15 mg/day to start, followed by 15–60 mg/day, given in a single daily dose at bedtime or in divided doses; 1 Tranxene-SD Half Strength or Tranxene-SD tab may be given q24h if the titrated daily dose equals 11.25 or 22.5 mg, respectively (Tranxene-SD should not be used to initiate therapy)
Acute alcohol withdrawal symptoms	**Adult:** day 1, 30 mg to start, followed by 30–60 mg, given in divided doses; day 2, 45–90 mg, given in divided doses; day 3, 22.5–45 mg, given in divided doses; day 4, 15–30 mg, given in divided doses; thereafter, gradually reduce dosage to 7.5–15 mg/day and discontinue as soon as patient's condition stabilizes
Partial seizures (adjunctive therapy)	**Adult:** up to 7.5 mg tid to start, followed by weekly increases of not more than 7.5 mg/day, as needed, up to 90 mg/day **Child (9–12 yr):** up to 7.5 mg bid to start, followed by weekly increases of not more than 7.5 mg/day, as needed, up to 60 mg/day

CONTRAINDICATIONS
Hypersensitivity to clorazepate   Acute narrow-angle glaucoma

ADMINISTRATION/DOSAGE ADJUSTMENTS

Elderly or debilitated patients	Initiate treatment with 7.5–15 mg/day; increase dosage gradually, as needed
Long-term use (> 4 mo)	Effectiveness for prolonged use as an antianxiety agent has not been tested in systematic clinical studies; long-term studies in epileptic patients, however, have shown continued therapeutic activity. Reassess need for continued therapy periodically.

WARNINGS/PRECAUTIONS

Psychotic reactions and depressive neuroses	Should not be treated with this drug
Drug dependence	Psychic and/or physical dependence may develop, especially in addiction-prone individuals
Mental impairment, reflex-slowing	Caution patients not to engage in potentially hazardous activities requiring full mental alertness and that alcohol and other CNS depressants may cause further impairment; to minimize drowsiness when clorazepate is used as an adjunct to antiepileptic drugs, do not exceed the recommended initial dosage and dosage increments
Potentially suicidal patients	Should not have access to large quantities of clorazepate; prescribe smallest amount feasible
Barbiturate-like withdrawal symptoms	May result when drug is discontinued abruptly; withdrawal symptoms have also been reported following abrupt discontinuation of benzodiazepines taken continuously at therapeutic levels for several months
Prolonged therapy	Blood counts and liver-function tests should be performed periodically
Hepatic or renal impairment	May lead to excessive drug accumulation (see OVERDOSAGE); monitor patient closely
Ataxia or oversedation	May develop in elderly and/or debilitated patients (see ADMINISTRATION/DOSAGE ADJUSTMENTS)

ADVERSE REACTIONS

Central nervous system	Drowsiness, dizziness, nervousness, headache, fatigue, ataxia, confusion, insomnia, blurred vision, irritability, diplopia, depression, slurred speech
Cardiovascular	Decreased systolic blood pressure
Gastrointestinal	Various complaints, dry mouth
Dermatological	Skin rash, edema
Other	Altered renal and hepatic function tests, decreased hematocrit, genitourinary complaints

OVERDOSAGE

Signs and symptoms	Somnolence, confusion, coma, diminished reflexes, excitation, hypotension
Treatment	Empty stomach immediately by induction of emesis and/or gastric lavage. Employ general supportive measures, as needed. Monitor vital signs frequently and keep patient under close observation. For hypotension, use norepinephrine or metaraminol.

TRANXENE ■ VALIUM/VALRELEASE

DRUG INTERACTIONS

Alcohol, tricyclic antidepressants, sedative-hypnotics, MAO inhibitors, and other CNS depressants	⇧	CNS depression

ALTERED LABORATORY VALUES

No clinically significant alterations in blood/serum or urinary values usually occur at therapeutic dosages

USE IN CHILDREN	USE IN PREGNANT AND NURSING WOMEN
See INDICATIONS and ORAL DOSAGE; not recommended for use in children under 9 yr of age	Use of antianxiety agents during early pregnancy should almost always be avoided. Although clorazepate has not been sufficiently studied to determine conclusively its effects during pregnancy, an increased risk of congenital malformations during the first trimester has been associated with minor tranquilizers (chlordiazepoxide, diazepam, meprobamate). Nordiazepam, the primary metabolite of clorazepate, is excreted in human milk; patient should stop nursing if drug is prescribed.

[1] Anxiety or tension associated with the stress of everyday life usually does not require treatment with an antianxiety agent

---

BENZODIAZEPINES

VALIUM (diazepam) Roche C-IV

Tablets: 2, 5, 10 mg **Ampuls:** 5 mg/ml (2 ml) **Prefilled syringes:** 5 mg/ml (2 ml) **Vials:** 5 mg/ml (10 ml)

INDICATIONS	ORAL DOSAGE	PARENTERAL DOSAGE
Anxiety disorders and short-term relief of **symptoms of anxiety**[1]	Adult: 2–10 mg bid to qid, depending upon severity	Adult: 2–10 mg IM or IV to start; repeat 3–4 h later, if needed
Acute alcohol withdrawal syndrome	Adult: 10 mg tid or qid over initial 24 h; then 5 mg tid or qid, as needed	Adult: 10 mg IM or IV to start, then 5–10 mg 3–4 h later, if needed
Preoperative medication	—	Adult: 10 mg IM (preferred) before surgery
Skeletal muscle spasm due to reflex spasm secondary to muscle or joint inflammation, trauma, or other local pathology (adjunctive therapy)	Adult: 2–10 mg tid or qid Child (> 6 mo): 1–2.5 mg tid or qid to start; increase gradually, as needed	Adult: 5–10 mg IM or IV to start; repeat 3–4 h later, if needed
Spasticity due to upper motor neuron disorders, such as cerebral palsy and paraplegia (adjunctive therapy)		
Athetosis (adjunctive therapy)		
Stiff-man syndrome (adjunctive therapy)		
Tetanus (adjunctive therapy)	—	Adult: same as for muscle spasm, except that larger doses may be needed Child (1 mo to 5 yr): 1–2 mg IM or IV (slowly); repeat q3–4h, as needed Child (> 5 yr): 5–10 mg IM or IV (slowly); repeat q3–4h, as needed
Convulsive disorders (adjunctive therapy)	Adult: 2–10 mg bid to qid Child (> 6 mo): 1–2.5 mg tid or qid to start; increase gradually, as needed	—
Status epilepticus **Severe recurrent convulsive seizures**		Adult: 5–10 mg IM or IV (preferred), slowly, every 10–15 min, up to 30 mg; repeat 2–4 h later, if needed Child (1 mo to 5 yr): 0.2–0.5 mg IM or IV (preferred), slowly, every 2–5 min, up to 5 mg; repeat 2–4 h later, if needed Child (> 5 yr): 1 mg IM or IV (preferred), slowly, every 2–5 min, up to 10 mg; repeat 2–4 h later, if needed
Endoscopic procedures (adjunctive therapy)	—	Adult: 5–10 mg IM 30 min prior to procedure or 10–20 mg, or less, IV (preferred), slowly, just prior to procedure
Cardioversion (adjunctive therapy)		Adult: 5–15 mg IV within 5–10 min before procedure

VALIUM/VALRELEASE

VALRELEASE (diazepam) Roche C-IV

Capsules (slow release): 15 mg

INDICATIONS

Anxiety disorders and short-term relief of **symptoms of anxiety**[1]
Skeletal muscle spasm due to reflex spasm secondary to muscle or joint inflammation, trauma, or other local pathology (adjunctive therapy)
Spasticity due to upper motor neuron disorders, such as cerebral palsy and paraplegia (adjunctive therapy)
Athetosis (adjunctive therapy)
Stiff-man syndrome (adjunctive therapy)
Convulsive disorders (adjunctive therapy)

Acute alcohol withdrawal syndrome

ORAL DOSAGE

Adult: 15–30 mg once daily, depending upon severity
Child (> 6 mo): 15 mg once daily if 5 mg tid is the optimum dosage of the tablet form

Adult: 30 mg for the initial 24 h, followed by 15 mg once daily, as needed

CONTRAINDICATIONS

Hypersensitivity to diazepam	Depression of vital signs in patients undergoing acute alcohol intoxication	Shock or coma (for parenteral use only)
Acute narrow-angle glaucoma		
Open-angle glaucoma (unless patient is receiving appropriate antiglaucoma therapy)		

ADMINISTRATION/DOSAGE ADJUSTMENTS

Elderly and/or debilitated patients	To preclude ataxia or oversedation, start with 2–2.5 mg 1–2 times/day orally and increase the dosage gradually; if the optimum dosage is 5 mg tid, slow-release capsules may be substituted in a dosage of 15 mg once daily. When using the injectable form, start with 2–5 mg and then increase the dosage gradually (see WARNINGS/PRECAUTIONS).
Intravenous use	May result in venous thrombosis, phlebitis, local irritation, swelling, and (rarely) vascular impairment. Administer solution slowly, no faster than 5 mg (1 ml)/min, *into large veins only;* carefully avoid intraarterial administration or extravasation. Do not mix or dilute with other drugs or solutions. If direct IV administration is not possible, slow injection through infusion tubing as close as possible to vein insertion (since diazepam is sparingly soluble) may be substituted.
Concomitant therapy with narcotic analgesics	Reduce narcotic dosage by a least one third and administer in small increments
Long-term use (> 4 mo)	Effectiveness for prolonged use as an antianxiety agent has not been tested in systematic clinical studies; reassess need for continued therapy periodically

WARNINGS/PRECAUTIONS

Psychosis	Diazepam is of no value in psychotic patients
Mental impairment, reflex-slowing	Caution patients not to engage in potentially hazardous activities requiring full mental alertness and that alcohol and other CNS depressants may cause further impairment
Drug dependence	Psychic and/or physical dependence may develop, especially in addiction-prone individuals
Abrupt discontinuation of therapy	May precipitate barbiturate-like withdrawal symptoms, including convulsions, tremor, abdominal and muscle cramps, vomiting, and sweating; milder withdrawal symptoms have also been observed infrequently following abrupt discontinuation of several months of continuous benzodiazepine therapy, generally when higher therapeutic doses have been used. Taper dosage gradually after extended treatment.
Potentially suicidal patients	Should not have access to large quantities of diazepam; prescribe smallest amount feasible
Apnea and/or cardiac arrest	May occur in the elderly or gravely ill or in patients with limited pulmonary reserve when parenteral route (particularly IV) is used; risk of apnea is increased by concomitant use of CNS depressants (see DRUG INTERACTIONS)
Convulsive disorders	May increase frequency and/or severity of grand mal seizures. Dosages of standard anticonvulsants may have to be increased. Abrupt withdrawal may also be associated temporarily with increased seizure activity. The parenteral form should be used with extreme caution in patients with chronic lung disease or unstable cardiovascular status.
Hepatic or renal impairment	Monitor patient closely to avoid excessive drug accumulation (see OVERDOSAGE)
Prolonged therapy	Blood counts and liver-function tests should be performed periodically

ADVERSE REACTIONS

Frequent reactions (incidence ≥ 1%) are printed in *italics*

Central nervous system and neuromuscular	*Drowsiness, fatigue, ataxia,* confusion, depression, dysarthria, headache, hypoactivity, slurred speech, syncope, tremor, vertigo, acute hyperexcitability, anxiety, hallucinations, increased muscle spasticity, insomnia, rage, sleep disturbances, stimulation, EEG changes, muscular weakness (with parenteral use)

Cardiovascular	Bradycardia, cardiovascular collapse, hypotension, cardiac arrest
Gastrointestinal	Constipation, nausea, hiccoughs, salivary changes
Hepatic	Jaundice
Genitourinary	Incontinence, urinary retention
Ophthalmic	Blurred vision, diplopia, nystagmus
Respiratory	Coughing, depressed respiration, dyspnea, hyperventilation, laryngospasm, throat or chest pain (during peroral endoscopy)
Dermatological	Urticaria, skin rash
Hematological	Neutropenia
Other	*Venous thrombosis and phlebitis at injection site*, changes in libido

OVERDOSAGE

Signs and symptoms	Somnolence, confusion, coma, diminished reflexes, hypotension
Treatment	Empty stomach immediately by gastric lavage. Monitor respiration, pulse, and blood pressure. Employ general supportive measures, as needed. Administer IV fluids and maintain adequate airway. Hypotension may be combated with levarterenol or metaraminol. Dialysis is of limited value.

DRUG INTERACTIONS

Alcohol, narcotic analgesics, sedative-hypnotics, and other CNS depressants	⇧ CNS depression ⇧ Hypotension (with parenteral use) ⇧ Muscular weakness (with parenteral use)
MAO inhibitors and other antidepressants	⇧ CNS effects
Cimetidine	⇩ Clearance of diazepam

ALTERED LABORATORY VALUES

No clinically significant alterations in blood/serum or urinary values occur at therapeutic dosages

USE IN CHILDREN

See INDICATIONS and ORAL DOSAGE. When using the injectable form, give not more than 0.25 mg/kg over a 3-min period; the initial dose may be safely repeated after 15–30 min. Oral diazepam is not indicated for use in infants under 6 mo of age. Consult manufacturer for use of the injectable form in newborns (< 30 days of age); prolonged CNS depression has been observed in neonates.

USE IN PREGNANT AND NURSING WOMEN

Use of antianxiety agents during early pregnancy should almost always be avoided. Although diazepam has not been sufficiently studied to determine conclusively its effects during pregnancy, an increased risk of congenital malformations during the first trimester has been associated with minor tranquilizers (meprobamate, diazepam, and chlordiazepoxide). Patient should stop breast-feeding if drug is prescribed; lethargy, weight loss, and hyperbilirubinemia in nursing infants have been reported.[1]

[1] Erkkola R, Kanto J: *Lancet* 1:542, 1972; Patrick MJ, Tilstone WJ; *Lancet* 1:542, 1972; Takyi BE: *J Hosp Pharm* 28:317, 1970

[1] Anxiety or tension associated with the stress of everyday life usually does not require treatment with an antianxiety agent

---

BENZODIAZEPINES

XANAX (alprazolam) Upjohn   C-IV

Tablets: 0.25, 0.5, 1 mg

INDICATIONS

Anxiety disorders and short-term relief of **symptoms of anxiety**[1]
Anxiety associated with depression[1]

ORAL DOSAGE

Adult: 0.25–0.5 mg tid to start, followed by up to 4 mg/day in divided doses, if needed, or, if adverse reactions occur, by a reduction in dosage

CONTRAINDICATIONS

Sensitivity to alprazolam or other benzodiazepines	Acute narrow-angle glaucoma

ADMINISTRATION/DOSAGE ADJUSTMENTS

Long-term use (> 4 mo)	Effectiveness for long-term use has not been established; reassess need for continued therapy periodically. If therapy is protracted, periodic blood counts, urinalyses, and blood chemistry tests should be performed.
Elderly and/or debilitated patients	To avoid ataxia or oversedation, initiate treatment at 0.25 mg bid or tid; increase dosage gradually, as needed and tolerated
Reduction in dosage, termination of therapy	To avoid withdrawal seizures, closely supervise any decrease in dosage and reduce the daily dose by not more than 1 mg every 3 days; treatment of patients with a history of seizures or epilepsy should not be discontinued abruptly, even when anticonvulsants are given concomitantly

WARNINGS/PRECAUTIONS

Withdrawal reactions	Abrupt discontinuation or a rapid decrease in dosage can precipitate withdrawal seizures (see ADMINISTRATION/DOSAGE ADJUSTMENTS). Other barbiturate-like reactions, ranging from mild dysphoria and insomnia to a major syndrome characterized by abdominal and muscle cramps, vomiting, sweating, tremors, and convulsions, have resulted from abrupt withdrawal of benzodiazepine drugs.

XANAX ■ ATARAX

Drowsiness	Caution patients not to engage in potentially hazardous activities requiring full mental alertness and that alcohol and other CNS depressants may cause further mental impairment
Psychoses	Alprazolam is not of value in the treatment of psychotic patients and should not be used in place of appropriate treatment for psychoses
Concomitant psychotropic or anticonvulsant therapy	Consider carefully the pharmacology of the agents to be used, particularly if they might potentiate the action of alprazolam (see DRUG INTERACTIONS)
Severely depressed or potentially suicidal patients	Employ the usual precautions with regard to administration of psychotropic drugs and size of prescription
Patients with hepatic or renal impairment	Observe the usual precautions to avoid excessive drug accumulation
Drug dependence	Psychic and/or physical dependence may develop, especially in addiction-prone individuals, who should be under careful surveillance while receiving this drug
Paradoxical reactions	Discontinue use of alprazolam if stimulation, agitation, increased muscle spasticity, sleep disturbances, hallucinations, or other adverse behavioral effects occur
Carcinogenicity, mutagenicity	Results of oncogenicity studies in rats given up to 375 times the human dose showed no evidence of carcinogenicity; alprazolam was not mutagenic in the rat micronucleus test at doses up to 1,250 times the human dose

ADVERSE REACTIONS[2]

Central nervous system and neuromuscular	Drowsiness, light-headedness, depression, headache, confusion, insomnia, blurred vision, rigidity, nervousness, tremor, syncope, dizziness, akathisia, tiredness/sleepiness
Gastrointestinal	Dry mouth, constipation, diarrhea, nausea/vomiting, increased salivation
Cardiovascular	Tachycardia/palpitations, hypotension
Dermatological	Dermatitis/allergy
Other	Nasal congestion, weight gain, weight loss

OVERDOSAGE

Signs and symptoms	Somnolence, confusion, impaired coordination, diminished reflexes, and coma
Treatment	Empty stomach immediately by gastric lavage. Monitor respiration, pulse, and blood pressure, and employ general supportive measures, as needed. Administer IV fluids and maintain adequate airway. Combat hypotension with norepinephrine or metaraminol. Dialysis is of limited value.

DRUG INTERACTIONS

Alcohol, sedative-hypnotics, anticonvulsants, antihistamines, and other CNS depressants	◇ CNS depression

ALTERED LABORATORY VALUES

No clinically significant alterations in blood/serum or urinary values occur at therapeutic dosages[3]

USE IN CHILDREN

Safety and effectiveness for use in patients under 18 yr of age have not been established

---

USE IN PREGNANT AND NURSING WOMEN

Pregnancy Category D: use of this drug during the first trimester of pregnancy should almost always be avoided. Based on experience with benzodiazepines, an increased risk of congenital abnormalities can be assumed if alprazolam is taken during the first trimester. If this drug is used during pregnancy, or if the patient becomes pregnant or intends to become pregnant while taking it, she should be apprised of the potential hazard to the fetus. Neonates of mothers who used benzodiazepines during pregnancy may experience withdrawal symptoms; neonatal flaccidity has also been reported. Alprazolam has no established use in labor or delivery. Benzodiazepines are excreted in human breast milk, and adverse effects in nursing infants have been observed; as a rule, patient should stop nursing if drug is prescribed. Studies performed in rats at doses up to 62.5 times the human dose have shown no evidence of impaired fertility.

---

[1] Anxiety or tension associated with the stress of everyday life usually does not require treatment with an antianxiety agent
[2] Anxiolytic benzodiazepines have also been reported to cause jaundice, slurred speech, menstrual irregularities, dystonia, pruritus, incontinence, urinary retention, diplopia, irritability, concentration difficulties, anorexia, loss of coordination, fatigue, sedation, musculoskeletal weakness, dysarthria, and changes in libido; these reactions have not been seen with alprazolam
[3] The changes in laboratory values observed in 565 subjects who participated in a 4-wk controlled clinical trial were considered to be of no physiological significance

---

NONBENZODIAZEPINES

ATARAX (hydroxyzine hydrochloride) Roerig   Rx
Tablets: 10, 25, 50 mg   Syrup (per 5 ml): 10 mg[1] (1 pt)

ATARAX 100 (hydroxyzine hydrochloride) Roerig   Rx
Tablets: 100 mg

INDICATIONS
Anxiety and tension associated with psychoneurosis
Anxiety associated with organic disease (adjunctive therapy)

ORAL DOSAGE
Adult: 50–100 mg qid
Child (< 6 yr): 50 mg/day, given in divided doses
Child (> 6 yr): 50–100 mg/day, given in divided doses

Pruritus due to allergic conditions, including chronic urticaria and atopic and contact dermatoses **Histamine-mediated pruritus**	**Adult:** 25 mg tid or qid **Child (< 6 yr):** 50 mg/day, given in divided doses **Child (> 6 yr):** 50–100 mg/day, given in divided doses
Preoperative sedation and following general anesthesia	**Adult:** 50–100 mg **Child:** 0.6 mg/kg

CONTRAINDICATIONS

Early pregnancy	Hypersensitivity to hydroxyzine

ADMINISTRATION/DOSAGE ADJUSTMENTS

Long-term use (> 4 mo)	Effectiveness for prolonged use as an antianxiety agent has not been tested in systematic clinical studies; reassess need for continued therapy periodically

WARNINGS/PRECAUTIONS

Drowsiness	Caution patients not to engage in potentially hazardous activities requiring full mental alertness
Concomitant use of CNS depressants	May potentiate hydroxyzine's effect; reduce dosage of these agents accordingly and caution patients that simultaneous use of alcohol and other CNS depressants may have addictive effects

ADVERSE REACTIONS

Central nervous system	Transient drowsiness; involuntary motor activity, including tremor and convulsions (rare)
Gastrointestinal	Dry mouth

OVERDOSAGE

Signs and symptoms	Excessive sedation, hypotension, CNS depression
Treatment	Induce emesis or use gastric lavage to empty stomach. Monitor respiration, pulse, and blood pressure. Employ general supportive measures, as needed. Hypotension may be combatted with IV fluids and levarterenol or metaraminol. Do not use epinephrine, since hydroxyzine counteracts its pressor action. Dialysis is of limited value, unless other agents, such as barbiturates, have been ingested concomitantly.

DRUG INTERACTIONS

Alcohol, narcotic analgesics, sedative-hypnotics, other CNS depressants, and tricyclic antidepressants	⌂ CNS depression

ALTERED LABORATORY VALUES

Urinary values	⌂ 17-Hydroxycorticosteroids
No clinically significant alterations in blood/serum values occur at therapeutic dosages	

USE IN CHILDREN
See INDICATIONS and ORAL DOSAGE

USE IN PREGNANT AND NURSING WOMEN
Contraindicated during early pregnancy. Fetal abnormalities have been reported in mice, rats, and rabbits at doses well above the maximum human dose. Clinical data are inadequate to establish safety for use in pregnant women during this period. It is not known whether hydroxyzine is excreted in human milk; because many drugs are excreted in human milk, patient should stop nursing if drug is prescribed.

[1] Contains 0.5% alcohol

NONBENZODIAZEPINES

BUSPAR (buspirone hydrochloride) Mead Johnson Pharmaceutical   Rx

Tablets: 5, 10 mg

INDICATIONS	ORAL DOSAGE
Anxiety disorders and short-term relief of **symptoms of anxiety**[1]	**Adult:** 5 mg tid to start, followed by increases of 5 mg/day every 2–3 days, as needed, up to 60 mg/day (usual dosage: 20–30 mg/day, given in divided doses)

BUSPAR

CONTRAINDICATIONS

Hypersensitivity to buspirone

ADMINISTRATION/DOSAGE ADJUSTMENTS

Long-term use (> 3–4 wk)	Effectiveness of prolonged use has not been demonstrated in controlled trials; however, patients have been treated with buspirone for several months with no ill effect. Reassess need for continued therapy periodically.
Elderly patients	No dosage adjustment for age appears to be necessary

WARNINGS/PRECAUTIONS

Psychoses	Buspirone is not of value in the treatment of psychotic patients and should not be used in place of appropriate antipsychotic treatment
CNS effects	Studies have indicated that buspirone is less sedating than other anxiolytics, does not produce significant functional impairment, and does not increase alcohol-induced impairment of motor and mental performance; however, since patient response can vary, caution patients not to engage in potentially hazardous activities requiring full mental alertness until individual response to the drug has been established and to avoid ingestion of alcoholic beverages during therapy
Patients receiving other CNS depressants	Buspirone does not exhibit cross-tolerance with benzodiazepines and other common sedative-hypnotics and, therefore, will not block the withdrawal reactions that may follow cessation of prior sedative-hypnotic or anxiolytic therapy. Rebound or withdrawal symptoms (eg, irritability, anxiety, agitation, insomnia, abdominal cramps, muscle cramps, vomiting, sweating, flu-like symptoms without fever, and, occasionally, even seizures) following withdrawal of such drugs may occur over various time periods, depending on the type of drug that was taken and its effective elimination half-life. Before starting buspirone therapy, gradually withdraw patients from prior CNS depressant drug therapy, especially if it has been used chronically.
Drug dependence	Buspirone has shown no potential for abuse or diversion, tolerance, or either physical or psychological dependence in human and animal studies; however, it is difficult to predict the extent to which a psychoactive drug will be misused, diverted, and/or abused. Carefully evaluate patients for a history of drug abuse and follow such patients closely for evidence of buspirone misuse or abuse (eg, development of tolerance, dose incrementation, or drug-seeking behavior).
Dopamine-receptor binding	Although buspirone can bind to central dopamine receptors, clinical experience in controlled trials have failed to identify any significant neuroleptic-like activity resulting from therapy; however, a syndrome of restlessness, which appears shortly after initiation of treatment, has been reported in a small fraction of patients and may be due to an increase in central noradrenergic activity or a dopaminergic effect (ie, it may represent akathisia)
Patients with impaired renal or hepatic function	Use of buspirone is not recommended in patients with severe renal or hepatic dysfunction, since the drug is metabolized by the liver and excreted by the kidneys
Carcinogenicity	No evidence of carcinogenicity was seen in rats during a 24-mo study at approximately 133 times the maximum recommended human oral dose or in mice during an 18-mo study at approximately 167 times the maximum recommended human oral dose
Mutagenicity	With or without metabolic activation, no point mutations were induced in five strains of *Salmonella typhosa* (Ames test) or mouse lymphoma L5178YTK$^+$ cell cultures, nor was DNA damage observed in Wi-38 human cells. Chromosomal aberrations and abnormalities did not occur in bone marrow cells of mice given 1 or 5 daily doses of buspirone.

ADVERSE REACTIONS[2]

Frequent reactions (incidence ≥ 1%) are printed in *italics*

Cardiovascular	*Tachycardia/palpitations, nonspecific chest pain;* syncope, hypotension, and hypertension (infrequent); cerebrovascular accident, congestive heart failure, myocardial infarction, cardiomyopathy, and bradycardia (rare)
Central nervous system, neuromuscular	*Dizziness (12%), drowsiness (10%), nervousness (5%), insomnia and light-headedness (3%), decreased concentration, excitement, anger/hostility, confusion, depression, and numbness (2%); musculoskeletal aches/pains, paresthesia, incoordination, tremor, dream disturbances;* depersonalization, dysphoria, noise intolerance, euphoria, akathisia, fearfulness, loss of interest, disassociative reaction, hallucinations, suicidal ideation, seizures, involuntary movements, slow reaction time, muscle cramps, muscle spasms, rigid/stiff muscles, and arthralgias (infrequent); muscle weakness, claustrophobia, cold intolerance, stupor, slurred speech, and psychosis (rare)
Ophthalmic	*Blurred vision (2%);* redness and itching of the eyes and conjunctivitis (infrequent); eye pain, photophobia, and pressure on the eyes (rare)
Otic	*Tinnitus;* inner ear abnormality (rare)
Gastrointestinal	*Nausea (8%), dry mouth (3%); abdominal/gastric distress and diarrhea (2%); constipation, vomiting;* flatulence, anorexia, increased appetite, salivation, irritable colon, and rectal bleeding (infrequent); burning of the tongue (rare)
Endocrinological	Galactorrhea and thyroid abnormality (rare)

BUSPAR ■ EQUANIL

Hematological	Eosinophilia, leukopenia, and thrombocytopenia (rare)
Hepatic	Increases in serum transaminase levels (infrequent)
Genitourinary	Urinary frequency, urinary hesitancy, menstrual irregularity and spotting, dysuria, and increased or decreased libido (infrequent); amenorrhea, pelvic inflammatory disease, enuresis, nocturia, delayed ejaculation, and impotence (rare)
Respiratory	Hyperventilation, shortness of breath, and chest congestion (infrequent)
Dermatological	*Rash;* edema, pruritus, flushing, hair loss, dry skin, facial edema, and blisters (infrequent); acne and thinning of nails (rare)
Other	*Headache (6%), fatigue (4%), weakness (2%), sweating/clamminess, sore throat, nasal congestion;* altered taste, altered smell, weight gain, fever, roaring sensation in the head, weight loss, and malaise (infrequent); alcohol abuse, bleeding disturbance, epistaxis, loss of voice, and hiccoughs (rare)

OVERDOSAGE

Signs and symptoms	Nausea, vomiting, dizziness, drowsiness, miosis, gastric distress
Treatment	Institute general symptomatic and supportive measures and perform immediate gastric lavage; monitor respiration, pulse, and blood pressure. No specific antidote to buspirone is known; the dialyzability of buspirone has not been determined.

DRUG INTERACTIONS

Trazodone	⇧ SGPT (unconfirmed)
Digoxin	Displacement of digoxin from serum proteins (clinical effect unknown)

ALTERED LABORATORY VALUES

Blood/serum values	⇧ SGOT ⇧ SGPT
Urinary values	No clinically significant alterations in urinary values have been reported at therapeutic dosages

---

USE IN CHILDREN

Safety and effectiveness for use in children under 18 yr of age have not been established

USE IN PREGNANT AND NURSING WOMEN

Pregnant women: Pregnancy Category B: no impairment of fertility or fetal damage has been observed in reproduction studies performed in rats and rabbits at doses approximately 30 times the maximum recommended human dose; however, no adequate, well-controlled studies have been performed in pregnant women. Use during pregnancy only if clearly needed. **Nursing mothers:** Buspirone and its metabolites are excreted in the milk of rats; however, the extent of excretion in human milk is not known. Avoid administration to nursing women if clinically possible.

---

[1] Anxiety or tension associated with the stress of everyday life usually does not require treatment with an antianxiety agent
[2] Approximately 10% of 2,200 anxious patients in a premarketing clinical efficacy trial lasting 3–4 wk discontinued treatment due to an adverse event; the more common events causing discontinuation included CNS disturbances (3.4%), primarily dizziness, insomnia, nervousness, drowsiness, and light-headedness; GI disturbances (1.2%), primarily nausea; and miscellaneous effects (1.1%), primarily headache and fatigue. In addition, 3.4% of patients had multiple complaints, none of which could be categorized as primary.

NONBENZODIAZEPINES

EQUANIL (meprobamate) Wyeth   C-IV

Tablets: 200, 400 mg   **Tablets (coated):** 400 mg

INDICATIONS	ORAL DOSAGE
Anxiety disorders and short-term relief of **symptoms of anxiety**[1]	**Adult:** 1,200–1,600 mg/day, given in divided doses, or up to 2,400 mg/day, if needed **Child (6–12 yr):** 100–200 mg bid or tid

CONTRAINDICATIONS

Hypersensitivity or idiosyncratic reaction to meprobamate and related compounds	Acute intermittent porphyria

ADMINISTRATION/DOSAGE ADJUSTMENTS

Long-term use (> 4 mo)	Effectiveness for prolonged use as an antianxiety agent has not been tested in systematic clinical studies; reassess need for continued therapy periodically

WARNINGS/PRECAUTIONS

Drug dependence	Psychic and/or physical dependence may develop, especially in addiction-prone individuals

EQUANIL ■ INAPSINE

Mental impairment, reflex-slowing	Caution patients not to engage in potentially hazardous activities requiring full mental alertness and that alcohol and other CNS depressants may cause further impairment
Potentially suicidal patients	Should not have access to large quantities of meprobamate; prescribe smallest amount feasible
Abrupt discontinuation of therapy	May precipitate recurrence of preexisting symptoms, including anxiety, anorexia, or insomnia, or withdrawal reactions, including vomiting, ataxia, tremors, muscle twitching, confusion, hallucinosis, and convulsive seizures (rare). Seizures are more likely to occur in patients with CNS damage or preexisting or latent convulsive disorders. After prolonged high-dose therapy, reduce dosage gradually over a period of 1–2 wk or substitute a short-acting barbiturate.
Hepatic or renal impairment	May lead to excessive drug accumulation (see OVERDOSAGE); monitor patient closely
Ataxia or oversedation	May develop in elderly and/or debilitated patients; administer the lowest effective dose
Seizures	May develop in epileptic patients
Tartrazine sensitivity	Presence of FD&C Yellow No. 5 (tartrazine) in 400-mg coated tablets may cause allergic-type reactions, including bronchial asthma, in susceptible individuals

ADVERSE REACTIONS

Central nervous system	Drowsiness, ataxia, dizziness, slurred speech, headache, vertigo, weakness, paresthesias, impairment of visual accommodation, euphoria, overstimulation, paradoxical excitement, fast EEG activity
Gastrointestinal	Nausea, vomiting, diarrhea
Cardiovascular	Palpitations, tachycardia, arrhythmias, transient ECG changes, syncope, hypotensive crisis
Allergic or idiosyncratic	Pruritic, urticarial, or erythematous maculopapular rash in groin area or generalized; leukopenia, acute nonthrombocytopenic purpura, petechiae, ecchymoses, eosinophilia, peripheral edema, adenopathy, fever, fixed drug eruption with cross-reaction to carisoprodol, cross-sensitivity between meprobamate/mebutamate and meprobamate/carbromal; in severe cases (rare): hyperpyrexia, chills, angioneurotic edema, bronchospasm, oliguri, anuria, anaphylaxis, exfoliative dermatitis, stomatitis, proctitis, Stevens-Johnson syndrome, bullous dermatitis
Hematological	Thrombocytopenic purpura[2]
Other	Exacerbation of porphyric symptoms

OVERDOSAGE

Signs and symptoms	Drowsiness, lethargy, stupor, ataxia, coma, shock, vasomotor and respiratory collapse
Treatment	Empty stomach immediately by gastric lavage. Treat symptomatically. Provide respiratory assistance, CNS stimulants, and pressor agents cautiously, as needed. Diuretics, osmotic (mannitol) diuresis, peritoneal dialysis, and hemodialysis may be helpful. Monitor urinary output and avoid overhydration.

DRUG INTERACTIONS

Alcohol, tricyclic antidepressants, sedative-hypnotics, MAO inhibitors, and other CNS depressants	⇧ CNS depression

ALTERED LABORATORY VALUES

No clinically significant alterations in blood/serum or urinary values occur at therapeutic dosages

---

USE IN CHILDREN

Safety and effectiveness for use in children under 6 yr of age have not been established

USE IN PREGNANT AND NURSING WOMEN

Use of antianxiety agents during early pregnancy should almost always be avoided. Meprobamate crosses the placental barrier and reaches concentrations in umbilical cord blood approximating maternal plasma levels. The drug is also excreted in human milk, reaching concentrations 2- to 4-fold greater than maternal plasma levels, which should be taken into consideration before prescribing meprobamate to nursing mothers.

---

[1] Anxiety or tension associated with the stress of everyday life usually does not require treatment with an antianxiety agent
[2] Other reactions for which a causal relationship has not been established include agranulocytosis and aplastic anemia

---

NONBENZODIAZEPINES

INAPSINE (droperidol) Janssen Rx

Ampuls: 2.5 mg/ml (2, 5 ml)   **Vials:** 2.5 mg/ml (10 ml)

INDICATIONS

Preoperative tranquilization and reduction of nausea and vomiting

PARENTERAL DOSAGE

Adult: 2.5–10 mg IM 30–60 min before surgery
Child (2–12 yr): as low as 1.0–1.5 mg/20–25 lb IM 30–60 min before surgery

INAPSINE

Adjunct to induction and maintenance of general anesthesia	**Adult:** for induction, 2.5 mg/20–25 lb, usually IV; for maintenance, 1.25–2.5 mg, usually IV **Child (2–12 yr):** for induction, as low as 1.0–1.5 mg/20–25 lb, usually IV
Tranquilization and reduction of nausea and vomiting during diagnostic procedures	**Adult:** 2.5–10 mg IM 30–60 min before procedure, followed by doses of 1.25–2.5 mg, usually IV, as needed
Adjunct to regional anesthesia	**Adult:** 2.5–5 mg IV (slowly) or IM

CONTRAINDICATIONS

Hypersensitivity to droperidol

ADMINISTRATION/DOSAGE ADJUSTMENTS

Elderly, debilitated, or other poor-risk patients	Reduce initial dosage

WARNINGS/PRECAUTIONS

Hypertension	Elevated blood pressure, with or without preexisting hypertension, has been reported following combined use of droperidol and fentanyl or other parenteral analgesics
Conduction anesthesia	Certain forms of conduction anesthesia, such as spinal anesthesia and some peridural forms, can alter respiration by blocking intercostal nerves and can cause peripheral vasodilation and hypotension via sympathetic blockade; droperidol can also alter the circulation. If hypotension occurs, institute appropriate IV fluid therapy and reposition the patient for optimal venous return to the heart, taking care to avoid orthostatic hypotension; pressor agents other than epinephrine may be administered if hypotension persists.
Pulmonary arterial pressure	Droperidol may cause a decrease in pulmonary arterial pressure; this should be taken into account when conducting diagnostic or surgical procedures where interpretation of such measurements might influence treatment
Patient monitoring	Monitor vital signs routinely following administration of droperidol; during postoperative EEG monitoring, the EEG pattern may return to normal slowly
Hepatic or renal impairment	Use with caution in patients with hepatic or renal impairment
Carcinogenicity, mutagenicity, effect on fertility	No studies have been performed to determine the carcinogenic potential of droperidol; the micronucleus test in female rats revealed no mutagenic effects of single oral doses as high as 160 mg/kg, and no impairment of fertility was found in either male or female rats fed 2, 9, and 36 times the maximum recommended human IV or IM dose

ADVERSE REACTIONS

Frequent reactions (incidence ≥ 1%) are printed in *italics*

Cardiovascular	*Hypotension; tachycardia;* hypovolemia; blood-pressure elevation, with or without preexisting hypertension[1]
Central nervous system	*Postoperative drowsiness,* dizziness, dystonia, akathisia, oculogryic crisis, restlessness, hyperactivity, anxiety, postoperative hallucinatory episodes sometimes associated with transient mental depression, muscular rigidity[1]
Respiratory	Depression,[1] apnea,[1] arrest,[1] bronchospasm
Other	Chills, shivering, laryngospasm

OVERDOSAGE

Signs and symptoms	See WARNINGS/PRECAUTIONS and ADVERSE REACTIONS
Treatment	For hypoventilation or apnea, administer oxygen and assist respiration. Maintain a patent airway; an oropharyngeal airway or endotracheal tube may be indicated. Maintain body temperature and adequate fluid intake. For hypovolemia, provide appropriate parenteral fluid therapy. Control extrapyramidal symptoms with antiparkinson agents. Observe patient closely for 24 h.

DRUG INTERACTIONS

Opioids, general anesthetics, barbiturates, anxiolytics, and other CNS depressants	⇧ CNS depression; reduce initial dosage if used concomitantly
Epinephrine	⇩ Blood pressure

INAPSINE ■ MILTOWN

ALTERED LABORATORY VALUES

No clinically significant alterations in blood/serum or urinary values occurs at therapeutic dosages

USE IN CHILDREN

See INDICATIONS and PARENTERAL DOSAGE; where child dosages are not given, consult manufacturer. Safety for use in children under 2 yr of age has not been established.

USE IN PREGNANT AND NURSING WOMEN

Pregnant women: Pregnancy Category C: a slight increase in mortality has occurred in newborn rats at IV doses of 4.4 times the upper human dose; at 44 times this dose, neonatal mortality was comparable to that of control animals. Following IM administration of 1.8 times the upper human dose, increased offspring mortality occurred in rats but was attributable to CNS depression in the dams, who neglected to remove the placentae from their offspring. Droperidol has caused no teratogenic effects in animal studies. There are no adequate, well-controlled studies in pregnant women; use during pregnancy only if the expected benefit justifies the potential risk to the fetus. Use during labor and delivery is not recommended. **Nursing mothers:** It is not known whether this drug is excreted in human milk; because many drugs are excreted in human milk, use with caution in nursing mothers.

[1] Reactions observed when droperidol has been combined with a parenteral or narcotic analgesic

---

NONBENZODIAZEPINES

MILTOWN (meprobamate) Wallace   C-IV
Tablets: 200, 400 mg

MILTOWN 600 (meprobamate) Wallace   C-IV
Tablets: 600 mg

INDICATIONS
Anxiety disorders and short-term relief of **symptoms of anxiety**[1]

ORAL DOSAGE
Adult: 1,200–1,600 mg/day, given in 3–4 divided doses, or 1 Miltown 600 tab bid, or up to 2,400 mg/day, if needed
Child (6–12 yr): 100–200 mg bid or tid

CONTRAINDICATIONS

Acute intermittent porphyria	Hypersensitivity or idiosyncratic reaction to meprobamate or related compounds carisoprodol, mebutamate, tybamate, or carbromal

ADMINISTRATION/DOSAGE ADJUSTMENTS

Long-term use (> 4 mo)	Effectiveness for prolonged use as an antianxiety agent has not been tested in systematic clinical studies; reassess need for continued therapy periodically

WARNINGS/PRECAUTIONS

Drug dependence	Psychic and/or physical dependence may develop, especially in addiction-prone individuals
Mental impairment, reflex-slowing	Caution patients about driving or engaging in other potentially hazardous activities requiring mental alertness or physical coordination, and about using alcohol or other CNS depressants (see DRUG INTERACTIONS)
Potentially suicidal patients	Should not have access to large quantities of meprobamate; prescribe smallest amount feasible
Abrupt discontinuation of therapy	May precipitate recurrence of preexisting symptoms, including anxiety, anorexia, or insomnia, or withdrawal reactions, including vomiting, ataxia, tremors, muscle twitching, confusion, hallucinosis, and convulsive seizures (rare). Seizures are more likely to occur in patients with CNS damage or preexisting or latent convulsive disorders. After prolonged high-dose therapy, reduce dosage gradually over a period of 1–2 wk or substitute a short-acting barbiturate.
Hepatic or renal impairment	May lead to excessive drug accumulation (see OVERDOSAGE); monitor patient closely
Ataxia or oversedation	May develop in elderly and/or debilitated patients; administer the lowest effective dose
Seizures	May develop in epileptic patients

ADVERSE REACTIONS

Central nervous system	Drowsiness, ataxia, dizziness, slurred speech, headache, vertigo, weakness, paresthesias, impairment of visual accommodation, euphoria, overstimulation, paradoxical excitement, fast EEG activity
Gastrointestinal	Nausea, vomiting, diarrhea

MILTOWN ■ TRANCOPAL

Cardiovascular	Palpitations, tachycardia, arrhythmias, transient ECG changes, syncope, hypotensive crisis
Allergic or idiosyncratic	Pruritic, urticarial, or erythematous maculopapular rash in groin area or generalized; leukopenia, acute nonthrombocytopenic purpura, petechiae, ecchymoses, eosinophilia, peripheral edema, adenopathy, fever, fixed drug eruption with cross-reaction to carisoprodol, cross-sensitivity between meprobamate/mebutamate and meprobamate/carbromal; in severe cases (rare): hyperpyrexia, chills, angioneurotic edema, bronchospasm, oliguria, anuria, anaphylaxis, erythema multiforme, exfoliative dermatitis, stomatitis, proctitis, Stevens-Johnson syndrome, bullous dermatitis
Hematological	Thrombocytopenic purpura (rare)[2]
Other	Exacerbation of porphyric symptoms

OVERDOSAGE

Signs and symptoms	Drowsiness, lethargy, stupor, ataxia, coma, shock, vasomotor and respiratory collapse
Treatment	Empty stomach immediately by gastric lavage. Treat symptomatically. Provide respiratory assistance, CNS stimulants, and pressor agents cautiously, as needed. Diuretics, osmotic (mannitol) diuresis, peritoneal dialysis, and hemodialysis may be helpful. Monitor urinary output and avoid overhydration.

DRUG INTERACTIONS

Alcohol, tricyclic antidepressants, sedative-hypnotics, MAO inhibitors, and other CNS depressants	⬦ CNS depression

ALTERED LABORATORY VALUES

No clinically significant alterations in blood/serum or urinary values occur at therapeutic dosages

---

USE IN CHILDREN

Safety and effectiveness for use in children under 6 yr of age have not been established. The 600-mg tablet is not intended for use in children.

USE IN PREGNANT AND NURSING WOMEN

Use of antianxiety agents during early pregnancy should almost always be avoided. Meprobamate crosses the placental barrier and reaches concentrations in umbilical cord blood approximating maternal plasma levels. The drug is also excreted in human milk, reaching concentrations 2- to 4-fold greater than maternal plasma levels, which should be taken into consideration before prescribing meprobamate to nursing mothers.

---

[1] Anxiety or tension associated with the stress of everyday life usually does not require treatment with an antianxiety agent
[2] Other reactions for which a causal relationship has not been established include agranulocytosis and aplastic anemia

---

NONBENZODIAZEPINES

TRANCOPAL (chlormezanone) Winthrop-Breon   Rx

Capsules: 100, 200 mg

INDICATIONS	ORAL DOSAGE
Mild anxiety and tension	**Adult:** 100–200 mg tid or qid **Child (5–12 yr):** 50–100 mg tid or qid

CONTRAINDICATIONS

Hypersensitivity to chlormezanone

ADMINISTRATION/DOSAGE ADJUSTMENTS

Drowsiness	May be minimized or avoided by reducing dosage
Long-term use (> 4 mo)	Effectiveness for prolonged use as an antianxiety agent has not been tested in systematic clinical studies; reassess need for continued therapy periodically

WARNINGS/PRECAUTIONS

Mental impairment, reflex-slowing	Caution patients not to engage in potentially hazardous activities requiring full mental alertness and that alcohol and other CNS depressants may cause further impairment

ADVERSE REACTIONS

Central nervous system	Drowsiness, dizziness, depression, weakness, excitement, tremors, confusion, headache
Gastrointestinal	Nausea, cholestatic jaundice (rare and reversible)

TRANCOPAL ■ VISTARIL

Dermatological	Rash
Genitourinary	Difficult micturition
Other	Flushing, edema

OVERDOSAGE

Signs and symptoms	See ADVERSE REACTIONS
Treatment	Treat symptomatically and institute supportive measures, as required

DRUG INTERACTIONS

Alcohol, tricyclic antidepressants, sedative-hypnotics, MAO inhibitors, and other CNS depressants	△ CNS depression

ALTERED LABORATORY VALUES

No clinically significant alterations in blood/serum or urinary values occur at therapeutic dosages

---

USE IN CHILDREN
See INDICATIONS and ORAL DOSAGE

USE IN PREGNANT AND NURSING WOMEN
Safety for use in pregnant or nursing women has not been established; animal reproduction studies have not been done with chlormezanone

---

NONBENZODIAZEPINES

VISTARIL (hydroxyzine pamoate) Pfizer   Rx

Capsules: 25, 50, 100 mg   **Suspension (per 5 ml):** 25 mg

INDICATIONS

Anxiety and tension associated with psychoneurosis
Anxiety associated with organic disease (adjunctive therapy)

Pruritus due to allergic conditions, including chronic urticaria and atopic and contact dermatoses
Histamine-mediated pruritus

Preoperative sedation and following general anesthesia

ORAL DOSAGE

Adult: 50–100 mg qid
Child (< 6 yr): 50 mg/day, given in divided doses
Child (> 6 yr): 50–100 mg/day, given in divided doses

Adult: 25 mg tid or qid
Child (< 6 yr): 50 mg/day, given in divided doses
Child (> 6 yr): 50–100 mg/day, given in divided doses

Adult: 50–100 mg
Child: 0.6 mg/kg

CONTRAINDICATIONS

Early pregnancy	Hypersensitivity to hydroxyzine

ADMINISTRATION/DOSAGE ADJUSTMENTS

Long-term use (> 4 mo)	Effectiveness for prolonged use as an antianxiety agent has not been tested in systematic clinical studies; reassess need for continued therapy periodically

WARNINGS/PRECAUTIONS

Drowsiness	Caution patients not to engage in potentially hazardous activities requiring full mental alertness
Concomitant use of CNS depressants	May potentiate hydroxyzine's effect; reduce dosage of these agents accordingly and caution patients that simultaneous use of alcohol and other CNS depressants may have addictive effects

ADVERSE REACTIONS

Central nervous system	Transient drowsiness; involuntary motor activity, including tremor and convulsions
Gastrointestinal	Dry mouth

OVERDOSAGE

Signs and symptoms	Excessive sedation, hypotension, CNS depression

VISTARIL ■ VISTARIL Intramuscular Solution

Treatment	Induce emesis or use gastric lavage immediately to empty stomach. Monitor respiration, pulse, and blood pressure. Employ general supportive measures, as needed. Hypotension may be combatted with IV fluids and levarterenol or metaraminol. Do not use epinephrine, since hydroxyzine counteracts its pressor action. Caffeine and sodium benzoate may be used to counteract CNS depression. Dialysis is of limited value, unless other agents such as barbiturates have been ingested concomitantly.

DRUG INTERACTIONS

Alcohol, narcotic analgesics, sedative-hypnotics, other CNS depressants, and tricyclic antidepressants	⇧ CNS depression

ALTERED LABORATORY VALUES

Urinary values	⇧ 17-Hydroxycorticosteroids

No clinically significant alterations in blood/serum values occur at therapeutic dosages

USE IN CHILDREN	**USE IN PREGNANT AND NURSING WOMEN**
See INDICATIONS and ORAL DOSAGE	Contraindicated during early pregnancy. Fetal abnormalities have been reported in mice, rats, and rabbits at doses well above the maximum human dose. Clinical data are inadequate to establish safety for use in pregnant women during this period. It is not known whether hydroxyzine is excreted in human milk; because many drugs are excreted in human milk, patient should stop nursing if drug is prescribed.

NONBENZODIAZEPINES

VISTARIL Intramuscular Solution (hydroxyzine hydrochloride) Roerig   Rx

Vials: 25 mg/ml (10 ml), 50 mg/ml (1, 2, 10 ml) for IM injection only

INDICATIONS	**PARENTERAL DOSAGE**
Psychiatric and emotional emergencies, including acute alcoholism	Adult: 50–100 mg IM at once, followed by 50–100 mg IM q4-6h, as needed
Preoperative and postoperative and prepartum and postpartum adjunctive medication to permit reduction in narcotic dosage, allay anxiety, and control emesis	Adult: 25–100 mg IM Child: 0.5 mg/lb IM
Nausea and vomiting, excluding nausea and vomiting of pregnancy (see box below)	

CONTRAINDICATIONS

Early pregnancy	Hypersensitivity to hydroxyzine

ADMINISTRATION/DOSAGE ADJUSTMENTS

Intramuscular administration	To help prevent inadvertent vascular injection, aspirate syringe before administration. Inject deeply into a relatively large muscle, preferably a midlateral thigh muscle for children and either that muscle or the gluteus maximus for adults. To minimize the possibility of sciatic nerve damage, use the periphery of the gluteus maximus for infants and small children only if necessary (eg, for patients with burns). The deltoid area should be used only if it is well developed and only if caution is exercised to avoid radial nerve injury; injections should not be made into the lower or middle third of the upper arm. Avoid SC administration, which may result in significant tissue damage.
Long-term use (> 4 mo)	Effectiveness for prolonged use as an antianxiety agent has not been tested in systematic clinical studies; reassess need for continued therapy periodically

WARNINGS/PRECAUTIONS

Drowsiness	Caution patients not to engage in potentially hazardous activities requiring full mental alertness
Concomitant use of CNS depressants	May potentiate hydroxyzine's effect; reduce the dosage of these agents by up to 50%. The concomitant use of narcotics and barbiturates as preanesthetic medication should be modified on an individual basis; atropine and other belladonna alkaloids are not affected.

VISTARIL Intramuscular Solution

ADVERSE REACTIONS

Central nervous system	Transient drowsiness; involuntary motor activity, including tremor and convulsions (rare)
Gastrointestinal	Dry mouth

OVERDOSAGE

Signs and symptoms	Excessive sedation, hypotension, CNS depression
Treatment	Monitor respiration, pulse, and blood pressure. Employ general supportive measures, as needed. Hypotension may be combatted with IV fluids and levarterenol or metaraminol. Do not use epinephrine, since hydroxyzine counteracts its pressor action. Caffeine and sodium benzoate may be used to counteract CNS depression. Dialysis is of limited value.

DRUG INTERACTIONS

Alcohol, narcotic analgesics, sedative-hypnotics, other CNS depressants, and tricyclic antidepressants	⇧ CNS depression

ALTERED LABORATORY VALUES

Urinary values	⇧ 17-Hydroxycorticosteroids

No clinically significant alterations in blood/serum values occur at therapeutic dosages

---

USE IN CHILDREN

See INDICATIONS and PARENTERAL DOSAGE

USE IN PREGNANT AND NURSING WOMEN

Contraindicated during early pregnancy. Fetal abnormalities have been reported in mice, rats, and rabbits at doses well above the maximum human dose. Clinical data are inadequate to establish safety for use in pregnant women during this period. It is not known whether hydroxyzine is excreted in human milk; because many drugs are excreted in human milk, patient should not nurse if drug is prescribed.

Chapter 13

Antiarrhythmics

BRETYLOL (Du Pont Critical Care) Bretylium tosylate *Rx*	429
CALAN (Searle) Verapamil hydrochloride *Rx*	430
CALAN SR (Searle) Verapamil hydrochloride *Rx*	430
CALAN Injection (Searle) Verapamil hydrochloride *Rx*	432
CORDARONE (Wyeth) Amiodarone *Rx*	434
CRYSTODIGIN (Lilly) Digitoxin *Rx*	437
INDERAL (Ayerst) Propranolol hydrochloride *Rx*	439
ISOPTIN (Knoll) Verapamil hydrochloride *Rx*	442
ISOPTIN SR (Knoll) Verapamil hydrochloride *Rx*	442
ISOPTIN Injection (Knoll) Verapamil hydrochloride *Rx*	444
LANOXICAPS (Burroughs Wellcome) Digoxin *Rx*	446
LANOXIN (Burroughs Wellcome) Digoxin *Rx*	447
MEXITIL (Boehringer Ingelheim) Mexiletine hydrochloride *Rx*	451
NORPACE (Searle) Disopyramide phosphate *Rx*	453
NORPACE CR (Searle) Disopyramide phosphate *Rx*	453
PROCAN SR (Parke-Davis) Procainamide hydrochloride *Rx*	455
PRONESTYL (Princeton) Procainamide hydrochloride *Rx*	457
PRONESTYL Injection (Princeton) Procainamide hydrochloride *Rx*	457
PRONESTYL-SR (Princeton) Procainamide hydrochloride *Rx*	458
QUINAGLUTE (Berlex) Quinidine gluconate *Rx*	460
QUINIDEX (Robins) Quinidine sulfate *Rx*	462
Quinidine sulfate (Warner-Chilcott) *Rx*	463
SECTRAL (Wyeth) Acebutolol hydrochloride *Rx*	465
TAMBOCOR (Riker) Flecainide acetate *Rx*	467
TONOCARD (Merck Sharp & Dohme) Tocainide hydrochloride *Rx*	470
XYLOCAINE for Ventricular Arrhythmias (Astra) Lidocaine hydrochloride *Rx*	472

BRETYLOL

ANTIARRHYTHMICS

BRETYLOL (bretylium tosylate) Du Pont Critical Care Rx
Ampuls: 50 mg/ml (10 ml)   **Prefilled syringes:** 50 mg/ml (10 ml)

INDICATIONS	PARENTERAL DOSAGE
Immediately life-threatening ventricular arrhythmias, such as ventricular fibrillation, refractory to adequate doses of a first-line antiarrhythmic agent, such as lidocaine **Hemodynamically unstable ventricular tachycardia**	Adult: 5 mg/kg IV (rapidly) to start, in conjunction with other cardiopulmonary resuscitative measures; if ventricular fibrillation persists, increase dosage to 10 mg/kg and repeat as necessary
Other ventricular arrhythmias	Adult: 5–10 mg/kg, given IM or diluted and given by slow ($>$ 8 min) IV infusion; if arrhythmia persists, repeat the same dose at 1- to 2-h intervals

CONTRAINDICATIONS
None known

ADMINISTRATION/DOSAGE ADJUSTMENTS

Maintenance therapy	For continuous suppression of life-threatening ventricular arrhythmias or tachycardia, dilute solution (see below) and give via continuous IV infusion at a rate of 1–2 mg/min or intermittently at a dose of 5–10 mg/kg q6h by slow ($>$ 8 min) IV infusion. For other ventricular arrhythmias, give 5–10 mg/kg q6h IM or dilute and give the same dose by slow ($>$ 8 min) IV infusion q6h. If indicated, substitute an oral antiarrhythmic agent as soon as possible.
Intramuscular administration	Do not inject more than 5 ml into any one site; vary injection site if drug is used repeatedly, to avoid atrophy and necrosis of muscle tissue, fibrosis, vascular degeneration, and inflammation
Preparation of solution for intravenous infusion	Dilute contents of one ampul (10 ml containing 500 mg bretylium) with at least 40 ml of Dextrose Injection USP or Sodium Chloride Injection USP. For immediately life-threatening arrhythmias or IM use, bretylium should be injected undiluted.
Patients with renal impairment	Increase dosage interval to avoid excessive accumulation, since drug is eliminated by the kidney

WARNINGS/PRECAUTIONS

Orthostatic hypotension	Occurs frequently, characterized by dizziness, light-headedness, vertigo, or faintness; keep patient supine until tolerance develops
Transient hypertension and increased frequency of arrhythmias	May occur early in treatment due to release of norepinephrine from adrenergic postganglionic nerve terminals
Severe aortic stenosis or pulmonary hypertension	Severe hypotension may result from a fall in peripheral resistance without a compensatory increase in cardiac output; combat with vasoconstrictive catecholamines
Digitalis toxicity	May be enhanced; avoid concomitant administration of digitalis glycosides and bretylium
Nausea, vomiting	May occur in about 3% of patients, generally because of overly rapid IV administration

ADVERSE REACTIONS
Frequent reactions (incidence $\geq$ 1%) are printed in *italics*

Cardiovascular	*Hypotension, postural hypotension,* bradycardia, increased frequency of premature ventricular contractions, transitory hypertension, initial increase in arrhythmias, anginal attacks, substernal pressure
Gastrointestinal	*Nausea, vomiting,* diarrhea, abdominal pain, hiccoughs
Central nervous system	Vertigo, dizziness, lightheadedness, syncope, hyperthermia, confusion, paranoid psychosis, emotional lability, lethargy, anxiety
Genitourinary	Renal dysfunction
Dermatological	Erythematous macular rash
Other	Flushing, generalized tenderness, shortness of breath, diaphoresis, nasal stuffiness, mild conjunctivitis

OVERDOSAGE

Signs and symptoms	Hypotension (supine systolic blood pressure $<$ 75 mm Hg)
Treatment	To raise blood pressure, administer a diluted solution of dopamine or norepinephrine and monitor pressure closely. If indicated, administer blood or plasma to expand blood volume and IV fluids to correct dehydration.

DRUG INTERACTIONS

Digitalis glycosides	⇧ Risk of digitalis toxicity

Catecholamines	△ Pressor effect
Procainamide, quinidine	△ Hypotension
Tricyclic antidepressants	▽ Hypotension

ALTERED LABORATORY VALUES

No clinically significant alterations in blood/serum or urinary values occur at therapeutic dosages

---

USE IN CHILDREN
Safety and effectiveness for use in children have not been established

USE IN PREGNANT AND NURSING WOMEN
Safety for use in pregnant or nursing women has not been established

---

ANTIARRHYTHMICS

CALAN (verapamil hydrochloride) Searle   Rx
Tablets: 80, 120 mg

INDICATIONS

Angina at rest, including vasospastic (Prinzmetal's variant) and unstable (crescendo, preinfarction) angina
Chronic stable angina (classic effort-associated angina)

Control of ventricular rate in digitalized patients with chronic atrial flutter and/or atrial fibrillation

Prophylaxis of repetitive paroxysmal supraventricular tachycardia in undigitalized patients

Essential hypertension

ORAL DOSAGE

Adult: 80–120 mg tid, followed by daily or weekly increases in dosage, up to 480 mg/day, as needed, until optimum clinical response is obtained

Adult: 240–320 mg/day, given in divided doses tid or qid

Adult: 240–480 mg/day

Adult: 240 mg/day to start, given in equally divided doses tid

CALAN SR (verapamil hydrochloride) Searle   Rx
Caplets (sustained release): 240 mg

INDICATIONS
Essential hypertension

ORAL DOSAGE
Adult: 240 mg/day, given in a single morning dose; if an adequate response is not obtained, titrate the dosage upward by giving 240 mg each morning to start, followed by 240 mg each morning plus 120 mg each evening, and then 240 mg q12h

CONTRAINDICATIONS

Severe left ventricular dysfunction

Accessory bypass tracts (Wolff-Parkinson-White, Lown-Ganong-Levine syndromes), when associated with atrial fibrillation

Second- or third-degree AV block (except in patients with a functioning artificial ventricular pacemaker)

Hypotension (systolic pressure < 90 mm Hg)

Sick sinus syndrome (except in patients with a functioning artificial ventricular pacemaker)

Cardiogenic shock

ADMINISTRATION/DOSAGE ADJUSTMENTS

Titration of dosage	Starting treatment at 40 mg tid should be considered in anginal and hypertensive patients who may exhibit an increased response to verapamil as a result of hepatic dysfunction, advanced age, small body size, or other conditions. Titrate dosage upward based on therapeutic efficacy and safety, evaluated approximately 8 h after the immediate-release tablets are taken or 24 h after the sustained-release formulation has been taken. Since the half-life of verapamil increases with repeated administration, the maximum response may be delayed during chronic dosing. In general, the maximum antiarrhythmic effect of this drug will be apparent during the first 48 h of administration, whereas the antihypertensive effect should be evident within the first week of therapy.
Timing of administration	The sustained-release formulation should be administered with food; the immediate-release tablets may be taken without regard to meals
Switching formulations	The total daily dose of verapamil may remain the same when switching from the immediate-release to the sustained-release form

CALAN

Concomitant therapy	Concomitant use of this drug with both short- and long-acting nitrates may be beneficial in patients with angina and is apparently free of harmful drug interactions. Concomitant use of verapamil with beta blockers may also be beneficial in certain patients with chronic stable angina or hypertension, but the combination can adversely affect cardiac function (see WARNINGS/PRECAUTIONS). Monitor vital signs and clinical status closely, and reassess the need for concomitant beta-blocker therapy periodically.

WARNINGS/PRECAUTIONS

Heart failure	Control heart failure with digitalis and/or diuretics before giving verapamil; do not administer to patients with severe left ventricular dysfunction (ejection fraction < 30%), patients with moderate to severe cardiac failure, or those with any degree of ventricular dysfunction who are concomitantly receiving a beta blocker.
Hypotension	Blood pressure may fall in some patients and may result in dizziness or symptomatic hypotension; decreases in blood pressure below normal levels are unusual in hypertensive patients. If severe hypotension occurs, administer isoproterenol, norepinephrine, atropine, or 10% calcium gluconate immediately *(in patients with hypertrophic cardiomyopathy [IHSS], use phenylephrine, metaraminol, or methoxamine, instead of isoproterenol or norepinephrine, to maintain blood pressure)*. If further support is needed, administer dopamine or dobutamine.
Hepatotoxicity	Elevations of SGOT, SGPT, alkaline phosphatase, and bilirubin levels have been reported. In some cases, these increases have been transient. However, in several patients, drug-induced hepatocellular injury has been reported; half of these patients experienced malaise, fever, and/or right quadrant pain as well as elevated hepatic enzyme levels. To reduce the risk of hepatotoxicity, periodically monitor liver function in all patients.
Rapid ventricular response, fibrillation	In some patients with paroxysmal and/or chronic atrial flutter or atrial fibrillation and an accessory AV pathway (eg, Wolff-Parkinson-White or Lown-Ganong-Levine syndrome), IV verapamil may produce a very rapid ventricular response or ventricular fibrillation following increased antegrade conduction; treat with DC cardioversion. While these risks have not been established with oral verapamil, use in this patient group is contraindicated.
Atrioventricular block	The effect of this drug on AV conduction and the SA node may cause asymptomatic first-degree AV block and transient bradycardia, sometimes accompanied by nodal escape rhythms; prolongation of the P-R interval is correlated with plasma concentrations of verapamil, especially during early titration of therapy. If marked first-degree block occurs, reduce dosage or discontinue verapamil administration and institute appropriate therapy (see suggested management of severe hypotension, above).
Impairment of neuromuscular transmission	Verapamil reportedly decreases neuromuscular transmission in patients with Duchenne's muscular dystrophy; the drug may also enhance the effects of neuromuscular blockers and delay reversal of vecuronium-induced blockade. A decrease in dosage may be necessary for patients with attenuated neuromuscular transmission; when verapamil is given in combination with a neuromuscular blocker, it may be necessary to reduce the dosage of one or both of the drugs.
Patients with hypertrophic cardiomyopathy (IHSS)	Serious adverse effects, including pulmonary edema and/or severe hypotension, sinus bradycardia, second-degree AV block, and sinus arrest, may occur in these patients; reduce dosage if adverse effects occur or discontinue therapy, if necessary
Drug accumulation	Use with caution in patients with significant renal or hepatic impairment; administer 30% of the usual dose to patients with hepatic impairment. Carefully monitor patients for abnormal prolongation of the P-R interval or other signs of overdosage (see below).
Carcinogenicity	Studies in rate fed verapamil at doses of 10, 35, and 120 mg/kg/day for 2 yr showed no evidence of carcinogenic potential; verapamil has shown no evidence of tumorigenicity in rats given 6 times the maximum human dose for 18 mo
Mutagenicity	Verapamil has shown no evidence of mutagenicity in the Ames test
Effect on fertility	Studies in female rats fed 5.5 times the recommended human dose of verapamil showed no evidence of impaired fertility; the effect of this drug on male fertility has not been determined

ADVERSE REACTIONS[1]

	Frequent reactions (incidence ≥ 1%) are printed in *italics*
Cardiovascular	*Hypotension (2.5%), edema (2.1%), congestive heart failure/pulmonary edema (1.8%), bradycardia (< 50 beats/min) (1.4%), first, second, and third-degree AV block (1.3%),* third-degree AV block alone (0.8%), flushing (0.1%)
Gastrointestinal	*Constipation (8.4%), nausea (2.7%),* elevation of liver enzyme levels
Central nervous system	*Dizziness (3.5%), headache (1.9%), fatigue (1.7%)*

OVERDOSAGE

Signs and symptoms	Abnormal prolongation of P-R interval, severe hypotension, second- or third-degree AV block, asystole

CALAN ■ CALAN Injection

Treatment	Institute standard supportive measures (eg, IV fluids). Administer beta-adrenergic stimulating agents or parenteral calcium solutions to increase calcium ion flux across the slow channel. Treat clinically significant hypotensive reactions or fixed high-degree AV block with vasopressors or cardiac pacing, respectively. Treat asystole with usual measures, including cardiopulmonary resuscitation.

DRUG INTERACTIONS

Beta blockers	△ Antianginal and antihypertensive effect △ Risk of negative inotropic, chronotropic, or dromotropic effects during high-dose beta-blocker therapy; closely monitor patients during concomitant therapy. Avoid concomitant use in patients with AV conduction abnormalities and those with depressed left ventricular function ▽ Clearance of metoprolol
Digitalis	△ Serum digoxin level and digitalis toxicity; reduce dosage or discontinue use, if necessary
Oral antihypertensive agents (eg, vasodilators, angiotensin-converting enzyme inhibitors, diuretics, beta blockers)	△ Reduction of blood pressure; monitor patient during concomitant therapy
Prazosin	Excessive hypotension
Disopyramide	△ Risk of decreased myocardial contractility; do not give disopyramide within 48 h before or 24 h after administration of verapamil
Quinidine	Significant hypotension in patients with hypertrophic cardiomyopathy (IHSS); avoid concomitant use in these patients △ Serum levels of quinidine ▽ Pharmacologic effects of quinidine on AV conduction
Cimetidine	▽ Clearance of verapamil
Lithium	▽ Serum levels of lithium; adjust dosage of lithium, if necessary
Carbamazepine	△ Serum levels of carbamazepine, possibly leading to diplopia, headache, ataxia, or dizziness
Rifampin	▽ Bioavailability of rifampin
Inhalation anesthetics	▽ Cardiovascular activity; titrate dose of each agent carefully
Curare-like and depolarizing neuromuscular blocking agents	△ Neuromuscular blockade; decrease dosage of one or both agents, if necessary
Nitrates	△ Antianginal effect

ALTERED LABORATORY VALUES

Blood/serum values	△ SGOT △ SGPT △ Alkaline phosphatase △ Bilirubin

No clinically significant alterations in urinary values occur at therapeutic dosages

USE IN CHILDREN

Safety and effectiveness for use in children under 18 yr of age have not been established

USE IN PREGNANT AND NURSING WOMEN

Pregnancy Category C: reproductive studies in rabbits and rats at oral doses up to 1.5 and 6 times the oral human dose, respectively, have shown no evidence of teratogenicity; in the rat, however, the drug caused hypotension, was embryocidal, and retarded fetal growth and development. Verapamil crosses the placental barrier and can be detected in umbilical vein blood at delivery; it is not known whether verapamil administration during labor and delivery has any immediate or delayed adverse effect on the fetus, prolongs labor, or increases the need for obstetric intervention. No adequate, well-controlled studies have been performed in pregnant women; use during pregnancy only if clearly needed. Verapamil is excreted in human milk; patients who are taking this drug should not nurse.

[1] Reactions for which a causal relationship is uncertain include angina pectoris, chest pain, claudication, myocardial infarction, palpitations, purpura (vasculitis), syncope, diarrhea, dry mouth, GI distress, gingival hyperplasia, ecchymosis, bruising, confusion, equilibrium disorders, insomnia, muscle cramps, paresthesia, psychotic symptoms, shakiness, somnolence; dyspnea, arthralgia and rash, exanthema, hair loss, hyperkeratosis, macules, sweating, urticaria, blurred vision, gynecomastia, increased urination, spotty menstruation; and impotence (reported only with sustained-release form).

ANTIARRHYTHMICS

CALAN Injection (verapamil hydrochloride) Searle   Rx

Ampuls: 2.5 mg/ml (2 ml) for IV use only   **Vials:** 2.5 mg/ml (2, 4 ml) for IV use only   **Prefilled syringes:** 2.5 mg/ml (2, 4 ml) for IV use only

INDICATIONS

Rapid conversion to sinus rhythm of **paroxysmal supraventricular tachycardias** (including those associated with accessory bypass tracts)

Temporary control[1] of rapid ventricular rate in **atrial flutter** or **atrial fibrillation** (except when flutter or fibrillation is associated with accessory bypass tracts)

PARENTERAL DOSAGE

Adult: 5–10 mg (0.075–0.15 mg/kg) IV, followed by 10 mg (0.15 mg/kg) IV after 30 min, if needed

Infant (0–1 yr): 0.1–0.2 mg/kg (usually 0.75–2 mg) IV; repeat after 30 min, if needed

Child (1–15 yr): 0.1–0.3 mg/kg (usually 2–5 mg), up to 5 mg, IV; repeat after 30 min, if needed (maximum single dose: 10 mg)

CONTRAINDICATIONS

Severe hypotension

Sick sinus syndrome (except in patients with a functioning artificial ventricular pacemaker)

Accessory bypass tracts (Wolff-Parkinson-White, Lown-Ganong-Levine syndromes), when associated with atrial flutter or fibrillation

Cardiogenic shock

Severe congestive heart failure (unless secondary to a supraventricular tachycardia amenable to verapamil therapy)

Wide-complex ventricular tachycardia (QRS $\geq$ 0.12 s)

Second- or third-degree AV block (except in patients with a functioning artificial ventricular pacemaker)

Recent (within a few hours) IV administration of beta blockers

Hypersensitivity to verapamil

ADMINISTRATION/DOSAGE ADJUSTMENTS

Intravenous injection	Administer each dose over a period of at least 2 min or, if the patient is elderly, over a period of at least 3 min; monitor ECG and blood pressure continuously during administration
Vagal maneuvers	When advisable, try to control paroxysmal supraventricular tachycardia with the Valsalva maneuver or other appropriate vagal maneuvers before using verapamil
Treatment setting	If possible, begin therapy in a setting that has facilities for monitoring, resuscitation, and DC cardioversion, since life-threatening reactions can occur with use of this drug; after the limits of the patient's response have been defined, this drug may be given in an office
Physical incompatibility	Do not mix verapamil with albumin, amphotericin B, hydralazine, trimethoprim-sulfamethoxazole, or solutions with a pH $>$ 6; do not dilute with sodium lactate injection USP in PVC bags

WARNINGS/PRECAUTIONS

Hypotension	Transient, asymptomatic decreases in blood pressure occur often during therapy; symptomatic hypotension has been seen in 1.5% of patients. If treatment is required, place patient in Trendelenburg's position, give IV fluids, and administer norepinephrine, metaraminol, calcium, isoproterenol, or dopamine by the IV route.
Bradycardia, asystole, AV block	Bradycardia and asystole can occur during treatment, particularly in patients with sick sinus syndrome (see CONTRAINDICATIONS); this syndrome is more common in elderly patients. Asystole in patients other than those with sick sinus syndrome usually lasts for no more than a few seconds; if normal rhythm is not seen within a few seconds after asystole, immediately institute appropriate measures. Verapamil can also prolong AV conduction and, in rare cases, has produced second- and third-degree AV block; if bundle branch block or second- or third-degree AV block occurs, reduce subsequent doses or discontinue therapy. Treat bradycardia, asystole, and AV block by using a cardiac pacemaker or administering atropine, calcium chloride, norepinephrine, or isoproterenol by the IV route; for supportive therapy, give fluids by slow IV infusion.
Heart failure	Verapamil reduces afterload and myocardial contractility; it may exacerbate moderately severe to severe cardiac dysfunction (pulmonary wedge pressure $>$ 20 mm Hg and ejection fraction $<$ 30%). If heart failure is not severe or rate-related, control with diuretics and digitalis before beginning therapy; give verapamil to patients with severe cardiac failure only when they have a verapamil-sensitive supraventricular tachycardia (see CONTRAINDICATIONS).
Ventricular fibrillation	In patients with atrial flutter or fibrillation and an accessory bypass tract (Wolf-Parkinson-White syndrome, Lown-Ganong-Levine syndrome) and in patients with wide-complex ventricular tachycardia, verapamil can produce ventricular fibrillation and other severe reactions; use in these patients is contraindicated. When diagnosing arrhythmia, carefully distinguish between the ventricular and supraventricular forms of wide-complex tachycardia. If a ventricular tachyarrhythmia develops in patients with atrial flutter or fibrillation and an accessory bypass tract as a result of antegrade conduction, give fluids by slow IV infusion and either perform DC-cardioversion or give IV procainamide or IV lidocaine.
Drug accumulation	In patients with significant renal or hepatic impairment, pharmacologic effects may be prolonged following a single dose and may be excessive after repeated doses. Administration of multiple doses to these patients should generally be avoided; if repeated injections are essential, reduce amount of second and subsequent doses and closely monitor blood pressure and P-R interval.
Respiratory failure	Verapamil can precipitate respiratory muscle failure in patients with Duchenne's muscular dystrophy; use with caution in these patients.
Increased intracranial pressure	In patients with supratentorial tumors, use of verapamil during induction of anesthesia can produce an increase in intracranial pressure; to reduce this risk, exercise caution and institute appropriate monitoring measures
PVC-like complexes	A few benign, unusual appearing complexes, sometimes similar to PVCs, may be seen after treatment; these complexes seem to have no clinical significance

ADVERSE REACTIONS

Frequent reactions (incidence $\geq$ 1%) are printed in *italics*

Cardiovascular	*Symptomatic hypotension (1.5%), bradycardia (1.2%), severe tachycardia (1%),* AV block, asystole

Central nervous system	*Dizziness and headache (1.2%);* seizures; emotional depression, rotary nystagmus, sleepiness, and vertigo (one case each)
Gastrointestinal	Nausea (0.9%), abdominal discomfort (0.6%)
Hypersensitivity	Bronchospasm/laryngospasm, accompanied by itch and urticaria (rare)
Other	Muscle fatigue and diaphoresis (one case each)

OVERDOSAGE

Signs and symptoms	Hypotension, bradycardia, AV block
Treatment	See WARNINGS/PRECAUTIONS for treatment of cardiovascular reactions; beta-adrenergic agonists and IV calcium chloride have been effective in treating overdose of oral verapamil

DRUG INTERACTIONS

Intravenous beta blockers	▽ Myocardial contractility and AV conduction. Serious reactions have occurred during combination therapy, especially in patients with severe cardiomyopathy, congestive heart failure, or recent myocardial infarction; do not use verapamil and an IV beta blocker within a few hours of each other.
Oral beta blockers	▽ Myocardial contractility and AV conduction; although no serious reactions have been reported during combination therapy, the possibility of such effects should be kept in mind
Disopyramide	▽ Myocardial contractility. Serious reactions have occurred during combination therapy, especially in patients with severe cardiomyopathy, congestive heart failure, or recent myocardial infarction; do not give disopyramide within 48 h before or 24 h after administration of verapamil.
Digitalis	▽ AV conduction; watch for AV block or excessive bradycardia during combination therapy
Quinidine, alpha-adrenergic blockers	Marked hypotension; exercise caution during combination therapy
General anesthetics	△ Risk of cardiovascular depression; titrate anesthetic dose carefully
Neuromuscular blocking agents	△ Risk of neuromuscular blockade; reducing dose of verapamil, the neuromuscular blocking agent, or both drugs may be necessary during combination therapy
Drugs with high protein-binding capacity	△ Plasma level of interacting drug
Intravenous dantrium	Cardiovascular collapse (based on two animal studies)

ALTERED LABORATORY VALUES

No clinically significant alterations in blood/serum or urinary values occur at therapeutic dosages

---

USE IN CHILDREN

See INDICATIONS and PARENTERAL DOSAGE. Use with caution in neonates and infants since, in rare instances, severe hemodynamic effects have occurred in these patients; provide continuous ECG monitoring when giving IV verapamil to infants under 12 mo of age.

USE IN PREGNANT AND NURSING WOMEN

Pregnant women: Pregnancy Category C: embryocidal effects and decreases in fetal growth and development have been seen in rats fed 60 mg/kg/day (6 times the human oral dose); it is likely that these reactions resulted from the drug's effect on the dams since hypotension and a reduction in maternal weight gain were also observed. Use during pregnancy only if clearly needed. **Labor:** In Europe, there is a long history of using IV verapamil to reverse the cardiac effects of beta-adrenergic agonists given for premature labor; no adverse effects on labor or the fetus have been reported following such use. **Nursing mothers:** Verapamil is excreted in human milk; nursing should be discontinued during therapy.

---

[1] A single dose slows the ventricular rate for 30–60 min when conversion to sinus rhythm does not occur

---

ANTIARRHYTHMICS

CORDARONE (amiodarone) Wyeth   Rx

Tablets: 200 mg

INDICATIONS

Life-threatening, recurrent **ventricular fibrillation** and life-threatening, recurrent, hemodynamically unstable **ventricular tachycardia,** when other antiarrhythmic agents have not been effective or tolerated

ORAL DOSAGE

Adult: 800–1,600 mg/day for 1–3 wk (or longer), until arrhythmia has been adequately controlled or adverse effects have become prominent, followed by 600–800 mg/day for 1 mo and then 400 mg/day for maintenance; some patients may require less than 400 mg/day or up to 600 mg/day as a maintenance dosage

CORDARONE

CONTRAINDICATIONS

Marked sinus bradycardia associated with severe sinus dysfunction	Episodes of bradycardia severe enough to cause syncope (unless a pacemaker is used during therapy)	Second- and third-degree AV block

ADMINISTRATION/DOSAGE ADJUSTMENTS

Administration — Give daily doses of less than 1 g in a single dose; however, if GI intolerance occurs, administer the daily dose in 2 divided doses with meals. Give daily doses of 1 g or more bid with meals. Hospitalize patients during the initial phase of therapy (when 800–1,600 mg/day is given); after discharge, make sure that facilities for the treatment of life-threatening arrhythmias are accessible.

Monitoring of therapy — Facilities that permit adequate monitoring of therapeutic response and adverse effects, including those facilities required for continuous ECG monitoring and electrophysiologic techniques, must be accessible throughout therapy. During the initial phase of therapy (when 800–1,600 mg/day is given), closely monitor clinical and electrophysiological responses, particularly until the risk of recurrent arrhythmia has abated.

The maintenance dosage should be based on clinical response, Holter monitoring, and/or programmed electrical stimulation. Determination of the serum amiodarone level may be helpful in evaluating an inadequate or toxic response since serum levels much below 1 mg/liter are often ineffective and those above 2.5 mg/liter generally do not enhance efficacy. At maintenance doses of 100–600 mg/day, an increase in dosage of 100 mg/day elevates the serum amiodarone level by approximately 0.5 mg/liter (this value varies considerably).

Amiodarone undergoes biphasic elimination, with an initial half-life of 2.5–10 days and a terminal half-life of 26–107 days (usually 40–55 days); therefore, after adjusting dosage or discontinuing use, closely monitor patient for an extended period of time and, if necessary, keep patient in the hospital during that period since the consequences, such as loss of arrhythmia control or toxicity, may not be apparent for weeks or months. If the drug is discontinued and an arrhythmia recurs, control can generally be reestablished relatively soon when compared to the initial response, presumably because the drug has not been completely eliminated. Keep in mind the long and variable half-life of amiodarone when substituting another antiarrhythmic drug.

Switching from other antiarrhythmic agents — Several days after amiodarone has been incorporated into the regimen, the dosage of other antiarrhythmic agents should be reduced by 30–50% (decrease procainamide dosage by 33%); if possible, an attempt should be made to gradually discontinue these agents once the effects of amiodarone have been established

Long-term prophylaxis — To predict the effectiveness of amiodarone in long-term prevention of recurrent ventricular tachycardia or fibrillation, many experts recommend ambulatory monitoring, programmed electrical stimulation (PES), or both techniques. A provocative test, using either exercise or PES, is required for patients with a history of cardiac arrest who fail to manifest a hemodynamically unstable arrhythmia during ECG monitoring; although there are reasons to consider a provocative test for patients who manifest the arrhythmia spontaneously, there is no consensus on whether this test is necessary for such patients.

The complete elimination of nonsustained tachycardia during ambulatory monitoring and the detection of less than 1 premature ventricular contraction per 1,000 normal beats have been suggested as signs indicating that amiodarone will be effective for prevention of arrhythmias. When amiodarone can prevent a PES-induced arrhythmia, the prognosis is almost uniformly excellent; the rate of recurrence may also be reduced if amiodarone makes induction by PES more difficult. The absence of severe symptoms during PES-induced ventricular tachycardia has been associated with greater likelihood of survival, but not with a lower rate of recurrence. If amiodarone facilitates induction or causes poorer tolerance of the PES-induced arrhythmia, consider a change in treatment. Keep in mind that in 20–40% of patients who were considered appropriate candidates for long-term therapy, arrhythmias have recurred after treatment for 1 yr or longer.

WARNINGS/PRECAUTIONS

Pulmonary toxicity — Amiodarone can cause potentially fatal interstitial pneumonitis or alveolitis. The risk appears to increase with duration of therapy and daily and cumulative dose; thus, although these effects have generally been seen in 2–7% of patients, it has occurred, according to a preliminary study, in 11–15% of patients given this drug for more than 1 yr. In a much larger proportion of patients, asymptomatic abnormalities in diffusion capacity have been detected. Pulmonary toxicity has been fatal in 10% of cases. To reduce risk of toxicity, examine patient and obtain chest x-rays every 3–6 mo; in addition, perform baseline tests of pulmonary function (including diffusion capacity) before the start of therapy. If cough, dyspnea, or any other pulmonary reaction occurs during therapy, evaluate clinical condition, obtain x-rays, and, if necessary, perform pulmonary function tests and a gallium scan. Do not assume that symptoms are due to cardiac failure. Among pulmonary function tests, the diffusion capacity test appears to be the one most likely to show a pulmonary abnormality. Once evidence of pulmonary toxicity has been seen, reduce dosage or, if possible, discontinue drug; corticosteroids may be necessary for reversal of toxic effects.

CORDARONE

Arrhythmogenicity	Amiodarone can cause new ventricular fibrillation, incessant ventricular tachycardia, increased resistance to cardioversion, torsade de pointes, or significant heart block in 2–5% of patients and produce symptomatic bradycardia or sinus arrest with suppression of escape foci in 2–4% of patients; use of other antiarrhythmic agents increases the risk of these reactions. Arrhythmogenic effects are prolonged. To control bradycardia, reduce dosage and, if necessary, use a pacemaker; to reverse conduction disturbances, discontinue drug.
Hepatotoxicity	Asymptomatic increases in SGOT and SGPT levels are seen frequently during therapy; in rare cases, potentially fatal hepatic failure has occurred. Check liver enzyme levels regularly in patients receiving relatively high maintenance doses. If the serum level exceeds 3 times the normal level or is twice an elevated baseline level or if hepatomegaly occurs, consider reducing dosage or discontinuing use.
Visual disturbances	Corneal microdeposits, discernible only by slit-lamp examination, occur in almost all patients after 6 mo of therapy and produce visual halos or blurred vision in up to 10% of patients. Visual disturbances can be reversed by a reduction in dosage or discontinuation of therapy; if microdeposits are asymptomatic, therapy should not be altered.
Photosensitivity	Photosensitivity, seen in approximately 10% of patients, can be ameliorated by use of sunscreens and protective clothing; it is usually not necessary to discontinue therapy. During long-term use, a blue-gray discoloration may develop on exposed skin; following discontinuation of therapy, discoloration disappears slowly and occasionally is not completely reversed. The risk of discoloration may be related to cumulative dose and duration of therapy and may be increased if the patient has a fair complexion or has had excessive exposure to the sun.
Hyper- and hypothyroidism	Amiodarone has caused hypothyroidism in 2–10% of patients and hyperthyroidism in 1–3% of patients; check thyroid function before therapy and periodically thereafter, especially in any patient with a history of thyroid nodules, goiter, or other thyroid dysfunction. An elevated serum TSH level is probably the best indication of drug-induced hypothyroidism; treat with thyroid hormone. Hyperthyroidism is best identified by a serum T_3 level of more than 200 mg/dl; the presence of this disorder may be sufficient reason to discontinue this drug.
Open-heart surgery	In patients receiving amiodarone, hypotension has occurred during open-heart surgery after discontinuation of cardiopulmonary bypass; a causal relationship has not been established for this rare reaction
Electrolyte disorders	Hypokalemia or hypomagnesemia may render amiodarone ineffective or increase the risk of arrhythmia; correct electrolyte deficiencies before beginning therapy
Neurological effects	Amiodarone produces neurological reactions, including fatigue, malaise, tremor, ataxia, and peripheral neuropathy, in 20–40% of patients; these effects may be alleviated by a reduction in dose
Gastrointestinal effects	Approximately 25% of patients experience GI symptoms, most commonly anorexia, nausea, vomiting, and constipation; effects are dose-related (see guidelines for administration, above)
Effect on mortality	No controlled studies have shown that amiodarone reduces mortality
Carcinogenicity, mutagenicity	An increase in thyroid carcinoma and thyroid follicular adenoma has been seen in rats at one-half the maximum human maintenance dose; no evidence of mutagenicity has been detected in the Ames, micronucleus, and lysogenic tests
Effect on fertility	Amiodarone has caused a reduction in the fertility of male and female rats at 8 times the maximum human maintenance dose

ADVERSE REACTIONS[1]

The most frequent reactions (> 3%) are italicized

Gastrointestinal	*Nausea and vomiting (10–33%); constipation and anorexia (4–9%);* abdominal pain (1–3%)
Central nervous system	*Malaise, fatigue, tremor, abnormal involuntary movements, lack of coordination, abnormal gait, ataxia, dizziness, and paresthesias (4–9%);* decreased libido, insomnia, headache, and sleep disturbances (1–3%)
Ophthalmic	*Visual disturbances, photophobia, and dry eyes (4–9%)*
Respiratory	*Pulmonary inflammation and fibrosis (4–9%)*
Hepatic	*Abnormal liver function tests (4–9%);* nonspecific hepatic disorders (1–3%); hepatitis and cirrhosis (rare)
Dermatological	*Solar dermatitis/photosensitivity (4–9%);* blue-gray discoloration, rash, spontaneous ecchymosis, alopecia
Cardiovascular	Congestive heart failure, cardiac arrhythmias, SA node dysfunction, flushing, and edema (1–3%); hypotension, cardiac conduction disturbances
Other	Hypothyroidism, hyperthyroidism, abnormal taste and smell, abnormal salivation, and coagulation abnormalities (1–3%)

OVERDOSAGE

Signs and symptoms	Cardiovascular disturbances

CORDARONE ■ CRYSTODIGIN

Treatment	Institute supportive measures. Monitor cardiac rhythm and blood pressure. For bradycardia, administer a beta-adrenergic agonist or use a pacemaker; treat hypotension associated with inadequate perfusion by giving a vasopressor or an inotropic agent.

DRUG INTERACTIONS[2]

Quinidine, procainamide, other antiarrhythmic agents	△ Risk of adverse effects, especially conduction disturbances and exacerbation of tachyarrhythmias. When starting amiodarone in patients receiving another antiarrhythmic agent, reduce dosage of that agent (see ADMINISTRATION/DOSAGE ADJUSTMENTS); when using another antiarrhythmic drug in patients receiving amiodarone, reduce the initial dosage of the added drug by 50%. Monitor electrophysiological and clinical responses very carefully during combination therapy.
Phenytoin	△ Risk of phenytoin toxicity
Digoxin, digitoxin	△ Risk of digitalis toxicity; when starting amiodarone in patients receiving digitalis, either reduce dosage of digitalis by 50% or discontinue the drug. If amiodarone and digitalis are given concomitantly, closely monitor serum digitalis level and clinical response
Oral anticoagulants	△ Risk of serious bleeding; when starting amiodarone in patients receiving an oral anticoagulant, reduce dosage of the anticoagulant by 33-50% and closely monitor prothrombin time
Beta blockers, calcium blockers	△ Risk of bradycardia, sinus arrest, and AV block; exercise caution during combination therapy. Use a pacemaker if concomitant therapy is necessary in patients with severe bradycardia or sinus arrest.

ALTERED LABORATORY VALUES

Blood/serum values	△ SGPT △ SGOT △ T_4 ▽ T_3 △ rT_3

No clinically significant alterations in urinary values occur at therapeutic dosages

---

USE IN CHILDREN
Safety and effectiveness for use in children have not been established

USE IN PREGNANT AND NURSING WOMEN
Pregnancy Category C: embryotoxicity, characterized by increased resorption and retardation of growth, has been seen in rats fed 18 times the maximum human maintenance dose; similar findings have been observed in one of two strains of mice given one-half the maximum human maintenance dose, but have not been detected in rabbits given 9 times the maximum human maintenance dose. In rodents, amiodarone has not affected parturition or the duration of gestation. Use during pregnancy only if the expected benefits justify the potential risks. Amiodarone is excreted in human milk; women who require this drug should not nurse because decreases in weight gain and viability have been seen in nursing rats.

---

[1] Reactions are often reversed by a reduction in dosage and almost always disappear following withdrawal of therapy; the frequency of most effects appears to increase when the duration of treatment exceeds 6 mo, but appears to remain relatively constant once the duration exceeds 1 yr
[2] Amiodarone undergoes biphasic elimination, with an initial half-life of 2.5-10 days and a terminal half-life of 26-107 days (usually 40-55 days); drug interactions can therefore occur after amiodarone has been discontinued

---

ANTIARRHYTHMICS

CRYSTODIGIN (digitoxin) Lilly   Rx
Tablets: 0.05, 0.1, 0.15 mg   **Ampuls:** 0.2 mg/ml (1 ml)

INDICATIONS
Heart failure
Atrial fibrillation and flutter
Paroxysmal atrial tachycardia

ORAL DOSAGE
Adult: for slow digitalization, 0.2 mg bid for 4 days, followed by maintenance dosage; for rapid digitalization, preferably 0.6 mg to start, followed by 0.4 mg and then 0.2 mg at 4- to 6-h intervals; for maintenance, 0.05-0.3 mg/day (usual maintenance dosage: 0.15 mg/day)

Infant (2 wk to 1 yr): 0.045 mg/kg in 3 or more divided doses at least 6 h apart; for maintenance, give 10% of digitalizing dose

Child (1-2 yr): 0.04 mg/kg in 3 or more divided doses at least 6 h apart; for maintenance, give 10% of digitalizing dose

Child (> 2 yr): 0.03 mg/kg (0.75 mg/m²) in 3 or more divided doses at least 6 h apart; for maintenance, give 10% of digitalizing dose

PARENTERAL DOSAGE
Adult: 0.6 mg IV (slowly) to start, followed by 0.4 mg 4-6 h later and then 0.2 mg at 4- to 6-h intervals until full therapeutic effect is apparent (average digitalizing dose: 1.2-1.6 mg IV); for maintenance, 0.05-0.3 mg/day IV or switch to oral therapy

Newborn (< 2 wk), premature infant, or infant with renal impairment or myocarditis: 0.022 mg/kg (0.3-0.35 mg/m²) IV (slowly) in 3 or more divided doses at least 6 h apart; for maintenance, give 10% of digitalizing dose

Infant (2 wk to 1 yr): 0.045 mg/kg IV (slowly) in 3 or more divided doses at least 6 h apart; for maintenance, give 10% of digitalizing dose

Child (1-2 yr): 0.04 mg/kg IV (slowly) in 3 or more divided doses at least 6 h apart; for maintenance, give 10% of digitalizing dose

Child (> 2 yr): 0.03 mg/kg (0.75 mg/m²) IV (slowly) in 3 or more divided doses at least 6 h apart; for maintenance, give 10% of digitalizing dose

CRYSTODIGIN

CONTRAINDICATIONS

Toxic response or idiosyncratic reaction to any digitalis preparation	Ventricular tachycardia[1]	Hypersensitive carotid sinus syndrome (some cases)[2]
Hypersensitivity to digitoxin	Beriberi heart disease[2]	

ADMINISTRATION/DOSAGE ADJUSTMENTS

Parenteral administration	Use only when oral therapy is contraindicated. The doses given above are for patients who have not received any digitalis preparation for 3 wk; reduce the dose proportionately for partially digitalized patients.
Duration of oral therapy	For *heart failure,* continue treatment after signs and symptoms have been abolished, unless some precipitating factor has been corrected. For *atrial fibrillation,* continue use of digitoxin in adequate doses to maintain the desired ventricular rate and other clinical effects. For *atrial flutter,* continue treatment if heart failure ensues or atrial flutter recurs frequently. For *paroxysmal atrial tachycardia,* continue treatment if heart failure ensues or paroxysms recur frequently.
Serum digitoxin levels	Must be evaluated in conjunction with clinical observations, ECG findings, and results of laboratory tests. The therapeutic serum level ranges from 10 to 35 ng/ml; however, a "therapeutic" serum level for one patient may be excessive or inadequate for another, with approximately 50% of patients showing toxicity at levels exceeding 35 ng/ml.[3]

WARNINGS/PRECAUTIONS

Arrhythmias	May be caused by underlying heart disease or reflect digitalis intoxication; if the latter cannot be excluded, withhold digitoxin temporarily, provided the clinical situation permits
Anorexia, nausea, vomiting	May accompany heart failure or reflect digitalis intoxication; determine the cause of these symptoms before continuing administration of digitoxin
Acute glomerulonephritis	Administer digitoxin with extreme caution, in conjunction with constant ECG monitoring, to patients with heart disease accompanied by acute glomerulonephritis; divided doses, relatively low total doses, and concomitant treatment with reserpine or other antihypertensive drugs may be necessary. Discontinue use of digitoxin in such patients as soon as possible.
Rheumatic carditis	Patients with rheumatic carditis, especially if severe, are unusually sensitive to digitoxin and prone to rhythm disturbances. Relatively low doses may be tried in these patients if heart failure develops; increase the dosage cautiously until a beneficial effect is obtained. If no improvement occurs, discontinue use of digitoxin.
Idiopathic hypertrophic subaortic stenosis (IHSS)	Must be managed with extreme care, since outflow obstruction may increase; digitoxin probably should not be used in patients with IHSS, unless cardiac failure is severe
Progression of heart block	Incomplete AV block may progress to advanced or complete heart block in digitalized patients; heart failure in these patients can usually be managed by other measures and by increasing the heart rate
Chronic atrial fibrillation	Digitoxin may not normalize the ventricular rate in patients with acute or unstable chronic atrial fibrillation, even at serum levels exceeding usual therapeutic concentrations; although such patients may be less susceptible to digitoxin-induced arrhythmias, do not increase the dosage to potentially toxic levels
Myxedema	Delays the excretion of digitoxin, resulting in significantly higher serum levels than in patients with normal thyroid function; reduce dosage accordingly
Elderly patients	Digitalis toxicity is more likely to occur in older than in younger adults because body mass tends to be small and renal function is frequently impaired; exercise caution in giving digitoxin to elderly patients, particularly if coronary artery disease is present
Hepatic impairment	Digitoxin is completely metabolized by the liver; accordingly, smaller doses may be required in patients with impaired liver function
Renal impairment	Digitoxin is partly metabolized to digoxin. Although elimination of digitoxin is independent of renal function, the elimination of digoxin is primarily renal; accordingly, dosages may need to be reduced in patients with renal insufficiency to avoid toxicity.
Potassium depletion	Sensitizes the myocardium to digitalis, increasing the risk of serious arrhythmias, and also tends to diminish the positive inotropic effect of digitoxin. Hypokalemia may result from malnutrition, old age, long-standing heart failure, concomitant use of other drugs (see DRUG INTERACTIONS), hemodialysis, and other therapy. Serum potassium levels may be maintained by administering a potassium-sparing diuretic (spironolactone, triamterene, or amiloride) concomitantly with kaliuretic diuretics (eg, furosemide or thiazides) or by use of oral potassium supplements.
Hypercalcemia	May produce serious arrhythmias in digitalized patients; do not give calcium IV and exercise great caution in giving digitoxin parenterally to patients with hypercalcemia
Special-risk patients	Patients with acute myocardial infarction, severe pulmonary disease, or greatly advanced heart failure may be prone to digitoxin-induced rhythm disturbances. Exercise caution in giving digitoxin to patients with active heart disease (eg, acute myocardial infarction or acute myocarditis), extensive myocardial damage, or conduction defects, and reduce the dosage when necessary. The parenteral route should be used with great caution in the presence of multiple ventricular extrasystoles, carotid sinus hypersensitivity, Adams-Stokes syndrome, or heart block and when patients are still under the influence of prior digitalis therapy. Patients with chronic constrictive pericarditis are likely to respond unfavorably to digitoxin. In patients at great risk, use of a short-acting, rapidly eliminated cardiac glycoside, such as digoxin, may be advisable.

CRYSTODIGIN ■ INDERAL

Electrical cardioversion	Adjustment of digitoxin dosage may be advisable prior to electrical cardioversion to prevent induction of ventricular arrhythmias

ADVERSE REACTIONS

Cardiovascular	*In adults:* ventricular premature contractions; paroxysmal and nonparoxysmal nodal rhythms; AV dissociation; paroxysmal atrial tachycardia with block; AV block of increasing degree, progressing to complete heart block; *in children:* nodal and atrial systoles; atrial arrhythmias; atrial ectopic rhythms; paroxysmal atrial tachycardia, particularly with AV block; ventricular arrhythmias (rare)
Gastrointestinal	Anorexia, nausea, vomiting, diarrhea, abdominal pain or discomfort
Central nervous system	Headache, weakness, apathy, visual disturbances (blurred or yellow vision), mental depression, confusion, disorientation, delirium
Endocrinological	Gynecomastia

OVERDOSAGE

Signs and symptoms	Anorexia, nausea, vomiting, and CNS disturbances are common signs of toxicity in adults but are rarely conspicuous in infants and children. Excessive slowing of the pulse ($\leq$ 60 beats/min) and almost any kind of arrhythmia may occur, but vary in frequency with age (see ADVERSE REACTIONS). Sinus bradycardia, sinoatrial arrest, and prolongation of the P-R interval are premonitory signs of toxicity in the newborn.
Treatment	Discontinue administration of digitoxin until all signs of toxicity have disappeared. In severe cases, and particularly if hypokalemia is present, administer potassium chloride in divided oral doses totaling 3–6 g (40–80 mEq) for adults and 1–1.5 mEq/kg for children, provided that renal function is normal. If correction of the arrhythmia is urgent and the serum potassium level is low or normal, potassium may be given IV in 5% Dextrose Injection, with careful ECG monitoring. Adults may be given a total of 40–80 mEq (using a concentration of 40 mEq/500 ml) at a rate of up to 20 mEq/h; infants and children may be given approximately 0.5 mEq/kg/h, using a solution dilute enough to avoid local irritation but with care to avoid fluid overload, especially in infants. Additional amounts may be given if the arrhythmia is uncontrolled and the potassium well tolerated. (Potassium should *not* be given, however, to patients with digitalis-induced heart block, unless primarily related to supraventricular tachycardia.) Discontinue the infusion when the desired effect is achieved. Other antiarrhythmic agents that may be tried include lidocaine, procainamide, propranolol, and phenytoin (experimental). Temporary ventricular pacing may be helpful in advanced heart block.

DRUG INTERACTIONS

Potassium-depleting diuretics and corticosteroids, amphotericin B	△ Risk of digitoxin toxicity due to hypokalemia
Calcium, particularly when administered IV; succinylcholine; sympathomimetics	△ Risk of cardiac arrhythmias
Colestipol, cholestyramine	▽ Serum concentration of digitoxin due to impaired absorption
Phenobarbital and other barbiturates, phenytoin, phenylbutazone	▽ Serum concentration of digitoxin due to accelerated hepatic metabolism

ALTERED LABORATORY VALUES

Urinary values	△ 17-Ketogenic steroids (with Zimmerman reaction)
No clinically significant alterations in blood/serum values occur at therapeutic dosages	

USE IN CHILDREN

See INDICATIONS; dosage must be carefully titrated, and ECG monitoring may be necessary to avoid toxicity if the drug is given IV to newborns. Infants under 1 mo of age have a sharply defined tolerance to digitoxin; premature and immature infants are particularly sensitive and generally require lower doses. Renal function must also be considered.

USE IN PREGNANT AND NURSING WOMEN

Pregnancy Category C: use during pregnancy only when clearly needed. No studies have been done with digitoxin in either animals or pregnant women to determine whether it can cause fetal harm or affect reproductive capacity. No data are available on the effects of this drug on labor or delivery. It is not known whether digitoxin is excreted in human milk; since this remains a possibility, exercise caution in giving it to nursing mothers.

---

[1] The drug may be used, however, if heart failure supervenes after a protracted episode of tachycardia and the patient has not already received digitalis
[2] Contraindications listed by the manufacturer for oral administration only
[3] Gilman AG, Goodman LS, Gilman A (eds): *Goodman and Gilman's The Pharmacological Basis of Therapeutics*, ed 6. New York, Macmillan Publishing Co, Inc, 1980

ANTIARRHYTHMICS

INDERAL (propranolol hydrochloride) Ayerst   Rx
Tablets: 10, 20, 40, 60, 80, 90 mg   **Ampuls:** 1 mg/ml (1 ml)

INDICATIONS	ORAL DOSAGE
Hypertension	**Adult:** 40 mg bid (alone or with a diuretic) to start, followed by gradual increments until optimal response is achieved, up to 640 mg/day; usual maintenance dosage: 120–240 mg/day **Child:** 0.5 mg/kg bid to start, followed by gradual increments until optimal response is achieved, up to 16 mg/kg/day; usual maintenance dosage: 1–2 mg/kg bid

INDERAL

Long-term management of **angina pectoris**	**Adult:** 80–320 mg/day, given in 2–4 divided doses
Cardiac arrhythmias, including supraventricular arrhythmias, ventricular tachycardias, digitalis-induced tachyarrhythmias, and resistant tachyarrhythmias due to excessive catecholamine activity during anesthesia	**Adult:** 10–30 mg tid or qid, before meals and at bedtime
Reduction of cardiovascular mortality in clinically stable patients following **acute myocardial infarction**	**Adult:** 180–240 mg/day, given in divided doses bid or tid; patients with angina, hypertension, or other coexisting cardiovascular diseases may require dosages exceeding 240 mg/day. In clinical studies, long-term therapy was started 5–21 days after infarction.
Migraine prophylaxis	**Adult:** 80 mg/day in divided doses to start, followed, if necessary, by gradual increments, up to 240 mg/day; usual dosage: 160–240 mg/day. If satisfactory prophylaxis is not obtained after giving 240 mg/day for 4–6 wk, discontinue use.
Familial or hereditary **essential tremor**	**Adult:** 40 mg bid to start, followed, if necessary, by increases in dosage, up to 320 mg/day; usual maintenance dosage: 120 mg/day
Hypertrophic subaortic stenosis	**Adult:** 20–40 mg tid or qid, before meals and at bedtime
As an adjunct to alpha-adrenergic blocking agents in the management of **pheochromocytoma**	**Adult:** 60 mg/day in divided doses for 3 days prior to surgery, concomitantly with an alpha-adrenergic blocking agent, or 30 mg/day in divided doses for inoperable tumors

CONTRAINDICATIONS

Sinus bradycardia	Cardiogenic shock	Overt congestive heart failure, unless it results from a tachyarrhythmia treatable with propranolol
Heart block greater than first degree	Bronchial asthma	

ADMINISTRATION/DOSAGE ADJUSTMENTS

Intravenous use	For life-threatening arrhythmias or those occurring under anesthesia in adults, give 1–3 mg IV. To minimize risk of hypotension and possibility of cardiac standstill, administer slowly ($\leq$ 1 mg/min) and monitor ECG and CVP continuously. Initial dose may be repeated after 2 min; thereafter, wait at least 4 h before administering additional propranolol.
Inadequate control of hypertension	Twice-daily dosing is usually effective. Some patients, however, experience a modest rise in blood pressure toward the end of the 12-h dosing interval, especially when lower dosages are used. If control is inadequate, a larger dose or tid therapy may be indicated.
Discontinuation of therapy	Reduce dosage gradually over a period of several weeks; caution patients who experience angina or who may have occult coronary artery disease not to interrupt or discontinue therapy on their own
Tremor	Essential tremor is usually limited to the upper limbs; it appears only when a limb moves or is held in a fixed position against gravity. Propranolol reduces the intensity of tremors, but not their frequency; this drug is not indicated for treatment of tremor associated with parkinsonism.

WARNINGS/PRECAUTIONS

Cardiac failure	Beta blockade may cause or exacerbate cardiac failure; discontinue use if this disorder does not stabilize after diuretic therapy and digitalization. If necessary, propranolol may be given to patients with well-compensated congestive heart failure; observe such patients closely.
Thyrotoxicosis	Propranolol may mask certain clinical signs of hyperthyroidism; abrupt withdrawal may exacerbate manifestations of this disorder and precipitate a thyroid storm
Patients with angina	Abrupt withdrawal in such patients may exacerbate angina and, in some cases, lead to myocardial infarction; reinstitute therapy if withdrawal reactions occur (see ADMINISTRATION/DOSAGE ADJUSTMENTS)
Patients with Wolff-Parkinson-White (WPW) syndrome	Severe bradycardia, necessitating use of a demand pacemaker, has occurred in several patients with WPW syndrome following use of propranolol
Patients with diabetes	Propranolol may mask tachycardia associated with hypoglycemia; however, this drug may not significantly affect other manifestations such as dizziness and diaphoresis. Propranolol may delay return of normal plasma glucose levels following insulin-induced hypoglycemia. Use with caution in patients with diabetes.
Patients with bronchospastic disease	In general, such patients should not receive propranolol because it may block catecholamine-induced bronchodilation. Propranolol is specifically contraindicated for use in patients with bronchial asthma; use with caution in patients with nonallergic bronchospasm (eg, chronic bronchitis, emphysema).
Patients with renal or hepatic impairment	Use with caution in such patients

INDERAL

Major surgery	The necessity or desirability of discontinuing use before major surgery is controversial. Beta blockade can increase the risks associated with general anesthesia and surgery (because cardiac responsiveness to reflex beta-adrenergic stimuli is impaired) and may cause protracted severe hypotension and difficulty in restarting and maintaining the heartbeat. However, beta-adrenergic agonists (eg, dobutamine, isoproterenol) can reverse the effects of propranolol.
Fatigue, lethargy, vivid dreams	Daily doses exceeding 160 mg, given in divided doses of more than 80 mg, may increase the risk of fatigue, lethargy, and vivid dreams
Glaucoma testing	Propranolol can reduce intraocular pressure and thereby affect the results of glaucoma screening tests
Carcinogenicity	No evidence of tumorigenicity has been seen in rats or mice given up to 150 mg/kg/day for a period of 18 mo
Effect on fertility	No impairment of fertility has been observed in animals

ADVERSE REACTIONS

Cardiovascular	Bradycardia, congestive heart failure, AV-block intensification, hypotension, paresthesia of the hands, Raynaud-type arterial insufficiency, purpura
Central nervous system	Light-headedness, depression, insomnia, weakness, fatigue, lassitude, catatonia, visual disturbances, hallucinations, vivid dreams; an acute reversible syndrome characterized by spatial and temporal disorientation, short-term memory loss, emotional lability, slightly clouded sensorium, and decreased neuropsychometric performance
Gastrointestinal	Nausea, vomiting, epigastric distress, abdominal cramps, diarrhea, constipation, mesenteric arterial thrombosis, ischemic colitis
Respiratory	Bronchospasm
Allergic	Pharyngitis, agranulocytosis, erythematous rash, fever with aching and sore throat, laryngospasm and respiratory distress
Other	Alopecia, lupus erythematosus-like reactions, psoriasiform rashes, dry eyes, impotence, and Peyronie's disease (rare); systemic lupus erythematosus (extremely rare)

OVERDOSAGE

Signs and symptoms	Severe bradycardia, cardiac failure, hypotension, bronchospasm
Treatment	Empty stomach (avoid pulmonary aspiration). For excessive bradycardia, administer 0.25–1.0 mg atropine IV; if there is no response to vagal blockade, administer isoproterenol cautiously. For cardiac failure, administer digitalis and a diuretic. For hypotension, use norepinephrine or (preferably) epinephrine. Treat bronchospasm with isoproterenol and aminophylline. Significant amounts of propranolol cannot be removed by dialysis.

DRUG INTERACTIONS

Reserpine, other catecholamine-depleting drugs	△ Risk of hypotension, marked bradycardia, vertigo, syncope, or orthostatic hypotension; closely observe patients during concomitant therapy
Calcium channel blockers	▽ AV conduction and myocardial contractility; concomitant IV administration of a beta blocker and verapamil has resulted in serious reactions, particularly in patients with severe cardiomyopathy, cardiac failure, or recent myocardial infarction. When using propranolol with a calcium channel blocker, especially IV verapamil, exercise caution.
Phenytoin, phenobarbital, rifampin	▽ Plasma level of propranolol
Cimetidine	△ Plasma level of propranolol
Chlorpromazine	△ Plasma level of propranolol and chlorpromazine
Theophylline, lidocaine, antipyrine	△ Plasma level of theophylline, lidocaine, and antipyrine
Thyroxine	△ Plasma T_4 level (due to decreased peripheral conversion of T_4 to T_3)
Aluminum hydroxide	▽ Absorption of propranolol
Digitalis	▽ AV conduction
Ephedrine, isoproterenol, other beta-adrenergic bronchodilators	▽ Bronchodilation
Thiazide-type diuretics, other antihypertensive agents	△ Antihypertensive effect
Alcohol	▽ Rate of absorption

ALTERED LABORATORY VALUES

Blood/serum values	△ SGOT △ SGPT △ Alkaline phosphatase △ LDH △ T_4 △ rT_3 ▽ T_3 △ BUN (in patients with severe heart disease)

No clinically significant alterations in urinary values occur at therapeutic dosages

USE IN CHILDREN	USE IN PREGNANT AND NURSING WOMEN
See INDICATIONS and ORAL DOSAGE; do not give IV to children. High plasma drug levels have been detected in patients with Down's syndrome, which suggests that bioavailability may be increased in these patients. If echocardiography is used to monitor therapy, bear in mind that the characteristics of a normal echocardiogram vary with age in children.	Pregnancy Category C: embryotoxic effects have been observed in animals given approximately 10 times the maximum human dose; no adequate, well-controlled studies have been done in pregnant women. Use during pregnancy only if the expected benefit justifies the potential risk to the fetus. Propranolol is excreted in human milk; use with caution in nursing mothers.

ANTIARRHYTHMICS

ISOPTIN (verapamil hydrochloride) Knoll   Rx

Tablets: 80, 120 mg

INDICATIONS

Angina at rest, including vasospastic (Prinzmetal's variant) and unstable (crescendo, preinfarction) angina

Chronic stable angina (classic effort-associated angina)

Control of ventricular rate in digitalized patients with chronic atrial flutter and/or atrial fibrillation

Prophylaxis of repetitive paroxysmal supraventricular tachycardia in undigitalized patients

Essential hypertension

ORAL DOSAGE

Adult: 80–120 mg tid, followed by daily or weekly increases in dosage, up to 480 mg/day, as needed, until optimum clinical response is obtained

Adult: 240–320 mg/day, given in divided doses tid or qid

Adult: 240–480 mg/day

Adult: 240 mg/day to start, given in equally divided doses tid

ISOPTIN SR (verapamil hydrochloride) Knoll   Rx

Tablets (sustained release): 240 mg

INDICATIONS

Essential hypertension

ORAL DOSAGE

Adult: 240 mg/day, given in a single morning dose; if an adequate response is not obtained, titrate the dosage upward by giving 240 mg each morning to start, followed by 240 mg each morning plus 120 mg each evening, and then 240 mg q12h

CONTRAINDICATIONS

Severe left ventricular dysfunction	Second- or third-degree AV block (except in patients with a functioning artificial ventricular pacemaker)	Sick sinus syndrome (except in patients with a functioning artificial ventricular pacemaker)
Hypotension (systolic pressure < 90 mm Hg)	Cardiogenic shock	

ADMINISTRATION/DOSAGE ADJUSTMENTS

Titration of dosage	Starting treatment at 40 mg tid should be considered in anginal and hypertensive patients who may exhibit an increased response to verapamil as a result of hepatic dysfunction, advanced age, small body size, or other conditions. Titrate dosage upward based on therapeutic efficacy and safety, evaluated approximately 8 h after the immediate-release tablets are taken or 24 h after the sustained-release formulation has been taken. Since the half-life of verapamil increases with repeated administration, the maximum response may be delayed during chronic dosing. In general, the maximum antiarrhythmic effect of this drug will be apparent during the first 48 h of administration, whereas the antihypertensive effect should be evident within the first week of therapy.
Timing of administration	The sustained-release formulation should be administered with food; the immediate-release tablets may be taken without regard to meals
Switching formulations	The total daily dose of verapamil may remain the same when switching from the immediate-release to the sustained-release form

ISOPTIN

Concomitant therapy	Concomitant use of this drug with both short- and long-acting nitrates may be beneficial in patients with angina and is apparently free of harmful drug interactions. Concomitant use of verapamil with beta blockers may also be beneficial in certain patients with chronic stable angina or hypertension, but the combination can adversely affect cardiac function (see WARNINGS/PRECAUTIONS). Monitor vital signs and clinical status closely, and reassess the need for concomitant beta-blocker therapy periodically.

WARNINGS/PRECAUTIONS

Heart failure	Control heart failure with digitalis and/or diuretics before giving verapamil; do not administer to patients with severe left ventricular dysfunction (ejection fraction < 30%), patients with moderate to severe cardiac failure, or those with significant ventricular dysfunction who are concomitantly receiving a beta blocker.
Hypotension	Blood pressure may fall in some patients and may result in dizziness or symptomatic hypotension; decreases in blood pressure below normal levels are unusual in hypertensive patients (tilt table testing [60°] has not induced orthostatic hypotension). If severe hypotension occurs, administer isoproterenol, norepinephrine, atropine, or 10% calcium gluconate immediately *(in patients with hypertrophic cardiomyopathy [IHSS], use phenylephrine, metaraminol, or methoxamine, instead of isoproterenol or norepinephrine, to maintain blood pressure)*. If further support is needed, administer dopamine or dobutamine.
Hepatotoxicity	Elevations of SGOT, SGPT, alkaline phosphatase, and bilirubin levels have been reported. In some cases, these increases have been transient. However, in several patients, drug-induced hepatocellular injury has been reported; half of these patients experienced malaise, fever, and/or right quadrant pain, as well as elevated hepatic enzyme levels. To reduce the risk of hepatotoxicity, periodically monitor liver function in all patients.
Rapid ventricular response, fibrillation	In patients with paroxysmal and/or chronic atrial flutter or atrial fibrillation and an accessory AV pathway (eg, Wolff-Parkinson-White or Lown-Ganong-Levine syndrome), IV verapamil may produce a very rapid ventricular response or ventricular fibrillation following increased antegrade conduction; treat with DC cardioversion. While these effects have not been reported with oral verapamil, they should be considered during therapy.
Antrioventricular block	The effect of this drug on AV conduction and the SA node may cause asymptomatic first-degree AV block and transient bradycardia, sometimes accompanied by nodal escape rhythms; prolongation of the P-R interval is correlated with plasma concentrations of verapamil, especially during early titration of therapy. If marked first-degree block occurs, reduce dosage or discontinue verapamil administration and institute appropriate therapy (see suggested management of severe hypotension, above).
Patients with hypertrophic cardiomyopathy (IHSS)	Serious adverse effects, including pulmonary edema and/or severe hypotension, sinus bradycardia, second-degree AV block, and sinus arrest, may occur in these patients; reduce dosage if adverse effects occur or discontinue therapy, if necessary
Drug accumulation	Use with caution in patients with significant renal or hepatic impairment; administer 30% of the usual dose to patients with hepatic impairment. Carefully monitor patients for abnormal prolongation of the P-R interval or other signs of overdosage (see below).
Carcinogenicity	Studies in rats fed verapamil at doses of 10, 35, and 120 mg/kg/day for 2 yr showed no evidence of carcinogenic potential; verapamil has shown no evidence of tumorigenicity in rats given 6 times the maximum human dose for 18 mo
Mutagenicity	Verapamil has shown no evidence of mutagenicity in the Ames test
Effect on fertility	Studies in female rats fed 5.5 times the recommended human dose of verapamil showed no evidence of impaired fertility; the effect of this drug on male fertility has not been determined

ADVERSE REACTIONS[1]

Frequent reactions (incidence ≥ 1%) are printed in *italics*

Cardiovascular	*Hypotension (2.5%), edema (2.1%), congestive heart failure/pulmonary edema (1.8%), bradycardia (< 50 beats/min) (1.4%); first, second, and third-degree AV block (1.3%);* third-degree AV block (0.8%), flushing (0.1%)
Gastrointestinal	*Constipation (8.4%), nausea (2.7%),* elevation of liver enzyme levels
Central nervous system	*Dizziness (3.5%), headache (1.9%), fatigue (1.7%)*

OVERDOSAGE

Signs and symptoms	Abnormal prolongation of P-R interval, severe hypotension, second- or third-degree AV block, asystole
Treatment	Institute standard supportive measures (eg, IV fluids). Administer beta-adrenergic stimulating agents or parenteral calcium solutions to increase calcium ion flux across the slow channel. Treat clinically significant hypotensive reactions or high-degree AV block with vasopressors or cardiac pacing, respectively. Treat asystole with usual measures, including cardiopulmonary resuscitation.

ISOPTIN ■ ISOPTIN Injection

DRUG INTERACTIONS

Beta blockers	△ Antianginal and antihypertensive effects △ Risk of negative inotropic and chronotropic effects during high-dose beta-blocker therapy; closely monitor patients during concomitant therapy ▽ Clearance of metoprolol
Digoxin	△ Serum digoxin level and digitalis toxicity; reduce dosage or discontinue use of digoxin, if necessary
Oral antihypertensive agents (eg, vasodilators, angiotensin-converting enzyme inhibitors, diuretics, beta blockers)	△ Reduction of blood pressure; monitor patient during concomitant therapy
Prazosin	Excessive hypotension
Disopyramide	△ Risk of decreased myocardial contractility; do not give disopyramide within 48 h before or 24 h after administration of verapamil
Quinidine	Significant hypotension in patients with hypertrophic cardiomyopathy (IHSS); avoid concomitant use in these patients △ Serum levels of quinidine ▽ Pharmacologic effects of quinidine on AV conduction
Cimetidine	▽ Clearance of verapamil △ Elimination half-life of verapamil
Lithium	▽ Serum levels of lithium; adjust dosage of lithium, if necessary
Carbamazepine	△ Serum levels of carbamazepine
Rifampin	▽ Bioavailability of rifampin
Neuromuscular blocking agents, inhalation anesthetics	△ Pharmacologic activity of neuromuscular blocking agents and inhalation anesthetics
Nitrates	△ Antianginal effect of verapamil and nitrates

ALTERED LABORATORY VALUES

Blood/serum values — △ SGOT △ SGPT △ Alkaline phosphatase △ Bilirubin

No clinically significant alterations in urinary values occur at therapeutic dosages

USE IN CHILDREN

Safety and effectiveness for use in children under 18 yr of age have not been established

USE IN PREGNANT AND NURSING WOMEN

Pregnancy Category C: reproductive studies in rabbits and rats at oral doses up to 1.5 and 6 times the oral human dose, respectively, have shown no evidence of teratogenicity; in the rat, however, the drug caused hypotension, was embryocidal, and retarded fetal growth and development. Verapamil crosses the placental barrier and can be detected in umbilical vein blood at delivery; it is not known whether verapamil administration during labor and delivery has any immediate or delayed adverse effect on the fetus, prolongs labor, or increases the need for obstetric intervention. No adequate, well-controlled studies have been performed in pregnant women; use during pregnancy only if clearly needed. Verapamil is excreted in human milk; patients who are taking this drug should not nurse.

[1] Reactions for which a causal relationship is uncertain include angina pectoris, chest pain, claudication, myocardial infarction, palpitations, purpura (vasculitis), syncope, diarrhea, dry mouth, GI distress, gingival hyperplasia, ecchymosis, bruising, confusion, equilibrium disorders, insomnia, muscle cramps, paresthesia, psychotic symptoms, shakiness, somnolence; dyspnea, arthralgia and rash, exanthema, hair loss, hyperkeratosis, maculae, sweating, urticaria, blurred vision, gynecomastia, increased urination, spotty menstruation; cerebrovascular accident and impotence (reported only with sustained-release form)

ANTIARRHYTHMICS

ISOPTIN Injection (verapamil hydrochloride) Knoll   Rx

Ampuls: 2.5 mg/ml (2, 4 ml) for IV use only   **Vials:** 2.5 mg/ml (2, 4 ml) for IV use only   **Prefilled syringes:** 2.5 mg/ml (2, 4 ml) for IV use only

INDICATIONS

Rapid conversion to sinus rhythm of **paroxysmal supraventricular tachycardias** (including those associated with accessory bypass tracts)

Temporary control[1] of rapid ventricular rate in **atrial flutter** or **atrial fibrillation** (except when flutter or fibrillation is associated with accessory bypass tracts)

PARENTERAL DOSAGE

Adult: 5–10 mg (0.075–0.15 mg/kg) IV, followed by 10 mg (0.15 mg/kg) IV after 30 min, if needed

Infant (0–1 yr): 0.1–0.2 mg/kg (usually 0.75–2 mg) IV, given under continuous ECG monitoring; repeat after 30 min, if needed

Child (1–15 yr): 0.1–0.3 mg/kg (usually 2–5 mg), up to 5 mg, IV; repeat after 30 min, if needed (maximum single dose: 10 mg)

ISOPTIN Injection

CONTRAINDICATIONS

Severe hypotension

Sick sinus syndrome (except in patients with a functioning artificial ventricular pacemaker)

Accessory bypass tracts (Wolff-Parkinson-White, Lown-Ganong-Levine syndromes), when associated with atrial flutter or fibrillation

Cardiogenic shock

Severe congestive heart failure (unless secondary to a supraventricular tachycardia amenable to verapamil therapy)

Wide-complex ventricular tachycardia (QRS $\geq$ 0.12 s)

Second- or third-degree AV block (except in patients with a functioning artificial ventricular pacemaker)

Recent (within a few hours) IV administration of beta blockers

Hypersensitivity to verapamil

ADMINISTRATION/DOSAGE ADJUSTMENTS

Intravenous injection	Administer each dose over a period of at least 2 min or, if the patient is elderly, over a period of at least 3 min
Vagal maneuvers	When advisable, try to control paroxysmal supraventricular tachycardia with the Valsalva maneuver or other appropriate vagal maneuvers before using verapamil
Treatment setting	If possible, begin therapy in a setting that has facilities for monitoring, resuscitation, and DC cardioversion, since life-threatening reactions can occur with use of this drug; after the limits of the patient's response have been defined, this drug may be given in an office
Physical incompatibility	Do not mix verapamil with albumin, amphotericin B, hydralazine, trimethoprim-sulfamethoxazole, or solutions with a pH $>$ 6

WARNINGS/PRECAUTIONS

Hypotension	Transient, asymptomatic decreases in blood pressure occur often during therapy; symptomatic hypotension has been seen in 1.5% of patients. If treatment is required, place patient in Trendelenburg's position, give IV fluids, and administer norepinephrine, metaraminol, calcium, isoproterenol, or dopamine by the IV route.
Bradycardia, asystole, AV block	Bradycardia and asystole can occur during treatment, particularly in patients with sick sinus syndrome (see CONTRAINDICATIONS); this syndrome is more common in elderly patients. Asystole in patients other than those with sick sinus syndrome usually lasts for no more than a few seconds; if normal rhythm is not seen within a few seconds after asystole, immediately institute appropriate measures. Verapamil can also prolong AV conduction and, in rare cases, has produced second- and third-degree AV block; if bundle branch block or second- or third-degree AV block occurs, reduce subsequent doses or discontinue therapy. Treat bradycardia, asystole, and AV block by using a cardiac pacemaker or administering atropine, calcium chloride, norepinephrine, or isoproterenol by the IV route; for supportive therapy, give fluids by slow IV infusion.
Heart failure	Verapamil reduces afterload and myocardial contractility; it may exacerbate moderately severe to severe cardiac dysfunction (pulmonary wedge pressure $>$ 20 mm Hg and ejection fraction $<$ 30%). If heart failure is not severe or rate-related, control with diuretics and digitalis before beginning therapy; give verapamil to patients with severe cardiac failure only when they have a verapamil-sensitive supraventricular tachycardia (see CONTRAINDICATIONS).
Ventricular fibrillation	In patients with atrial flutter or fibrillation and an accessory bypass tract (Wolf-Parkinson-White syndrome, Lown-Ganong-Levine syndrome) and in patients with wide-complex ventricular tachycardia, verapamil can produce ventricular fibrillation and other severe reactions; use in these patients is contraindicated. When diagnosing arrhythmia, carefully distinguish between the ventricular and supraventricular forms of wide-complex tachycardia. If a ventricular tachyarrhythmia develops in patients with atrial flutter or fibrillation and an accessory bypass tract as a result of antegrade conduction, give fluids by slow IV infusion and either perform DC-cardioversion or give IV procainamide or IV lidocaine.
Drug accumulation	In patients with significant renal or hepatic impairment, pharmacologic effects may be prolonged following a single dose and may be excessive after repeated doses. Administration of multiple doses to these patients should generally be avoided; if repeated injections are essential, reduce amount of second and subsequent doses and closely monitor blood pressure and P-R interval.
Respiratory failure	Verapamil can precipitate respiratory muscle failure in patients with Duchenne's muscular dystrophy; use with caution in these patients
Increased intracranial pressure	In patients with supratentorial tumors, use of verapamil during induction of anesthesia can produce an increase in intracranial pressure; to reduce this risk, exercise caution and institute appropriate monitoring measures
PVC-like complexes	A few benign, unusual appearing complexes, sometimes similar to PVCs, may be seen after treatment; these complexes seem to have no clinical significance

ADVERSE REACTIONS

Frequent reactions (incidence $\geq$ 1%) are printed in *italics*

Cardiovascular	*Symptomatic hypotension (1.5%), bradycardia (1.2%), severe tachycardia (1%),* AV block, asystole

ISOPTIN Injection ■ LANOXICAPS/LANOXIN

Central nervous system	*Dizziness and headache (1.2%);* seizures; emotional depression, rotary nystagmus, sleepiness, and vertigo (one case each)
Gastrointestinal	Nausea (0.9%), abdominal discomfort (0.6%)
Hypersensitivity	Bronchospasm/laryngospasm, accompanied by itch and urticaria (rare)
Other	Muscle fatigue and diaphoresis (one case each)

OVERDOSAGE

Signs and symptoms	Hypotension, bradycardia, AV block
Treatment	See WARNINGS/PRECAUTIONS for treatment of cardiovascular reactions; beta-adrenergic agonists and IV calcium chloride have been effective in treating overdose of oral verapamil

DRUG INTERACTIONS

Intravenous beta blockers	▽ Myocardial contractility and AV conduction. Serious reactions have occurred during combination therapy, especially in patients with severe cardiomyopathy, congestive heart failure, or recent myocardial infarction; do not use verapamil and an IV beta blocker within a few hours of each other.
Oral beta blockers	▽ Myocardial contractility and AV conduction; although no serious reactions have been reported during combination therapy, the possibility of such effects should be kept in mind
Disopyramide	▽ Myocardial contractility. Serious reactions have occurred during combination therapy, especially in patients with severe cardiomyopathy, congestive heart failure, or recent myocardial infarction; do not give disopyramide within 48 h before or 24 h after administration of verapamil.
Digitalis	▽ AV conduction; watch for AV block or excessive bradycardia during combination therapy
Quinidine, alpha-adrenergic blockers	Marked hypotension; exercise caution during combination therapy
General anesthetics	△ Risk of cardiovascular depression; titrate anesthetic dose carefully
Neuromuscular blocking agents	△ Risk of neuromuscular blockade; reducing dose of verapamil, the neuromuscular blocking agent, or both drugs may be necessary during combination therapy
Drugs with high protein-binding capacity	△ Plasma level of interacting drug
Intravenous dantrium	Cardiovascular collapse (based on two animal studies)

ALTERED LABORATORY VALUES

No clinically significant alterations in blood/serum or urinary values occur at therapeutic dosages

---

USE IN CHILDREN

See INDICATIONS and PARENTERAL DOSAGE. Use with caution in neonates and infants since, in rare instances, severe hemodynamic effects have occurred in these patients; provide continuous ECG monitoring when giving IV verapamil to infants under 12 mo of age.

USE IN PREGNANT AND NURSING WOMEN

Pregnant women: Pregnancy Category C: embryocidal effects and decreases in fetal growth and development have been seen in rats fed 60 mg/kg/day (6 times the human oral dose); it is likely that these reactions resulted from the drug's effect on the dams since hypotension and a reduction in maternal weight gain were also observed. Use during pregnancy only if clearly needed. **Labor:** In Europe, there is a long history of using IV verapamil to reverse the cardiac effects of beta-adrenergic agonists given for premature labor; no adverse effects on labor or the fetus have been reported following such use. **Nursing mothers:** Verapamil is excreted in human milk; nursing should be discontinued during therapy.

---

[1] A single dose slows the ventricular rate for 30–60 min

ANTIARRHYTHMICS

LANOXICAPS (digoxin) Burroughs Wellcome   Rx

Capsules: 50, 100, 200 µg

INDICATIONS

Heart failure
Atrial fibrillation and flutter
Paroxysmal atrial tachycardia

ORAL DOSAGE

Adult: for rapid digitalization, 400–600 µg to start, followed by 100–300 µg at 6- to 8-h intervals until clinical response is adequate (usual loading dose for a 70-kg patient: 600–1,000 µg); for maintenance, see "maintenance dosage for adults" below
Child (2–5 yr): for rapid digitalization, 25–35 µg/kg, with roughly half given at once and the remainder in fractional doses at 6- to 8-h intervals; for maintenance, give 25–35% of *oral or IV* loading dose daily
Child (5–10 yr): for rapid digitalization, 15–30 µg/kg, with roughly half given at once and the remainder in fractional doses at 6- to 8-h intervals; for maintenance, give 25–35% of *oral or IV* loading dose daily
Child (> 10 yr): for rapid digitalization, 8–12 µg/kg, with roughly half given at once and the remainder in fractional doses at 6- to 8-h intervals; for maintenance, give 25–35% of *oral or IV* loading dose daily

LANOXIN (digoxin) Burroughs Wellcome Rx

Tablets: 125, 250, 500 µg **Pediatric elixir:** 50 µg/ml[1] (2 fl oz) *lime-flavored* **Ampuls:** 100 µg/ml (Pediatric Injection) (1 ml), 250 µg/ml (2 ml)

INDICATIONS

Heart failure
Atrial fibrillation and flutter
Paroxysmal atrial tachycardia

ORAL DOSAGE

Adult: for rapid digitalization, 500–750 µg to start, followed by 125–375 µg at 6- to 8-h intervals until clinical response is adequate (usual loading dose for a 70-kg patient: 750–1,250 µg); for maintenance, see "maintenance dosage for adults" below

Premature infant: for rapid digitalization, 20–30 µg/kg, with roughly half given at once and the remainder in fractional doses at 6- to 8-h intervals; for maintenance, give 20–30% of *oral* loading dose daily

Full-term infant: for rapid digitalization, 25–35 µg/kg, with roughly half given at once and the remainder in fractional doses at 6- to 8-h intervals; for maintenance, give 25–35% of *oral* loading dose daily

Infant (1–24 mo): for rapid digitalization, 35–60 µg/kg, with roughly half given at once and the remainder in fractional doses at 6- to 8-h intervals; for maintenance, give 25–35% of *oral* loading dose daily

Child (2–5 yr): for rapid digitalization, 30–40 µg/kg, with roughly half given at once and the remainder in fractional doses at 6- to 8-h intervals; for maintenance, give 25–35% of *oral* loading dose daily

Child (5–10 yr): for rapid digitalization, 20–35 µg/kg, with roughly half given at once and the remainder in fractional doses at 6- to 8-h intervals; for maintenance give 25–35% of *oral* loading dose daily

Child (> 10 yr): for rapid digitalization, 10–15 µg/kg, with roughly half given at once and the remainder in fractional doses at 6- to 8-h intervals; for maintenance, give 25–35% of *oral* loading dose daily

PARENTERAL DOSAGE

Adult: for rapid digitalization, 400–600 µg IV to start, followed by 100–300 µg IV at 4- to 8-h intervals until clinical response is adequate (usual IV loading dose for a 70-kg patient: 600–1,000 µg); for maintenance, see "maintenance dosage for adults" below

Premature infant: for rapid digitalization, 15–25 µg/kg IV, with roughly half given at once and the remainder in fractional doses at 4- to 8-h intervals; for maintenance, give 20–30% of *IV* loading dose daily

Full-term infant: for rapid digitalization, 20–30 µg/kg IV, with roughly half given at once and the remainder in fractional doses at 4- to 8-h intervals; for maintenance, give 25–35% of *IV* loading dose daily

Infant (1–24 mo): for rapid digitalization, 30–50 µg/kg IV, with roughly half given at once and the remainder in fractional doses at 4- to 8-h intervals; for maintenance, give 25–35% of *IV* loading dose daily

Child (2–5 yr): for rapid digitalization, 25–35 µg/kg IV, with roughly half given at once and the remainder in fractional doses at 4- to 8-h intervals; for maintenance, give 25–35% of *IV* loading dose daily

Child (5–10 yr): for rapid digitalization, 15–30 µg/kg IV, with roughly half given at once and the remainder in fractional doses at 4- to 8-h intervals; for maintenance, give 25–35% of *IV* loading dose daily

Child (> 10 yr): for rapid digitalization, 8–12 µg/kg IV, with roughly half given at once and the remainder in fractional doses at 4- to 8-h intervals; for maintenance, give 25–35% of *IV* loading dose daily

CONTRAINDICATIONS

Untoward reaction sufficient to require discontinuation of other digitalis preparations	Hypersensitivity to digoxin	Ventricular fibrillation

ADMINISTRATION/DOSAGE ADJUSTMENTS

Dosage requirements — The recommended doses given in this chart are average values and may require substantial modification depending upon individual sensitivity and other factors, including (1) the indication for using digoxin (larger doses are often required for adequate control of ventricular rate in atrial flutter or fibrillation), (2) body weight (calculate doses on the basis of lean, or ideal, body weight), (3) renal status (smaller doses are usually required in patients with diminished renal function), (4) age (infants [other than newborns] and children generally require larger doses than adults on the basis of lean body weight or body surface area), and (5) associated conditions, such as concomitant disease states and use of other drugs (see WARNINGS/PRECAUTIONS and DRUG INTERACTIONS). Oral administration with meals that are high in bran may result in reduced GI absorption. In some patients, colonic bacteria convert oral digoxin to inactive metabolites (in 10% of patients who receive the tablets, 40% or more of a single dose is metabolized); use of the capsules, which are rapidly absorbed in the upper GI tract, minimizes this effect.

Initiation of therapy — Digitalization may be accomplished by either (1) administering a loading dose and then calculating the maintenance dose as a percentage of the loading dose or (2) beginning with an appropriate maintenance dose (see tables below) and allowing digoxin body stores to accumulate slowly. Loading doses should be based upon projected peak body stores and administered in several portions, with roughly half given as the first dose; *carefully assess the patient's response to the drug before giving each additional dose.* If maintenance doses are used to initiate therapy, steady-state serum levels will be achieved in approximately 5 half-lives, ie, 1–3 wk depending upon the patient's renal status.

| | Maintenance dosage for adults |

The daily maintenance dose is based upon the percentage of peak body stores (ie, the loading dose) lost each day through renal elimination and may be calculated from the *actual* loading dose and the corrected creatinine clearance rate (CCr), in ml/min/70 kg or 1.73 m², by use of the following formula: loading dose $\times$ (14 + CCr/5)/100. To determine the appropriate oral maintenance dose for gradual digitalization of patients with heart failure, use the following tables:

LANOXICAPS
Usual daily maintenance dose (μg) for estimated peak body stores of 10 μg/kg

CCr[1]	Lean body weight (kg)						Days[2]
	50	60	70	80	90	100	
0	50	100	100	100	150	150	22
10	100	100	100	150	150	150	19
20	100	100	150	150	150	200	16
30	100	150	150	150	200	200	14
40	100	150	150	200	200	250	13
50	150	150	200	200	250	250	12
60	150	150	200	200	250	300	11
70	150	200	200	250	250	300	10
80	150	200	200	250	300	300	9
90	150	200	250	250	300	350	8
100	200	200	250	300	300	350	7

[1] Corrected creatinine clearance rate (ml/min/70 kg)
[2] Number of days before steady-state concentration is achieved

LANOXIN Tablets
Usual daily maintenance dose (μg) for estimated peak body stores of 10 μg/kg

CCr[1]	Lean body weight (kg)						Days[2]
	50	60	70	80	90	100	
0	63[3]	125	125	125	188[4]	188	22
10	125	125	125	188	188	188	19
20	125	125	188	188	188	250	16
30	125	188	188	188	250	250	14
40	125	188	188	250	250	250	13
50	188	188	250	250	250	250	12
60	188	188	250	250	250	375	11
70	188	250	250	250	250	375	10
80	188	250	250	250	375	375	9
90	188	250	250	250	375	500	8
100	250	250	250	375	375	500	7

[1] Corrected creatinine clearance rate (ml/min/70 kg)
[2] Number of days before steady-state concentration is achieved
[3] One half of a 125-μg tab or 125 μg every other day
[4] One and one-half 125-μg tabs

If necessary, the CCr may be estimated from the serum creatinine concentration in adult males as (140 − age)/[creatinine]; this value should be reduced by 15% for women. Do not use this formula for estimating the CCr in infants or children.

| Frequency of administration of maintenance doses |

Divided daily dosing is recommended for infants and children under 10 yr of age; older children and adults may be given single daily maintenance doses, usually after breakfast. Because the significance of the higher serum levels obtained by once-daily administration of the soft gelatin capsules is not established, divided daily dosing of the capsule form is currently recommended not only for children under 10 yr of age but also for (1) patients requiring 300 μg or more daily, (2) patients with a history of digitalis toxicity or who are likely to become toxic, and (3) patients in whom compliance is not a problem (if it is a problem, single daily dosing may then be appropriate).

| Parenteral administration |

Use only when need for rapid digitalization is urgent or oral therapy is contraindicated. Digoxin should be administered *slowly* by IV injection over a period of 5 min or longer; rapid infusion may cause systemic and arteriolar constriction. IM injection is extremely painful. If IM route must be used, inject the drug deeply into the muscle and massage afterward; do not give more than 2 ml into a single site. If using a tuberculin syringe to measure minute doses, be careful not to overadminister digoxin; never flush the syringe with the parenteral fluid after the contents are expelled into an indwelling catheter.

| Dilution of injectable form |

Both the standard and pediatric injection forms can be given undiluted; if dilution is desired, mix the injection form with a 4-fold or greater volume of Sterile Water for Injection, 0.9% Sodium Choride Injection, or 5% Dextrose Injection (use of smaller volumes may result in precipitation). The diluted solution should be used immediately. Do not mix digoxin with other parenteral drugs in the same container or administer it simultaneously with other drugs in the same IV line.

| Adjustment of dosage when changing preparations |

When switching a patient from an IV loading regimen to oral maintenance therapy, allow for the difference in bioavailability between the different dosage forms; a 100-μg IV dose is approximately equivalent to a 100-μg dose of the capsules but 125 μg of the tablets or elixir

LANOXICAPS/LANOXIN

Duration of therapy	For *heart failure,* continue use of digoxin after acute symptoms have been controlled, unless some known precipitating factor has been corrected; however, if therapy is difficult to regulate or if the patient is at great risk of becoming toxic (eg, because of unstable renal function or fluctuating potassium levels), consider cautiously withdrawing the drug (if the drug is withdrawn, monitor the patient regularly for signs of recurrent heart failure). Long-term administration may be required for children who have been digitalized for acute heart failure, unless the cause is transient, and for children with severe congenital heart disease, even after surgery. For *atrial fibrillation,* continue use of digoxin in adequate doses to maintain the desired ventricular rate. For *atrial flutter,* continue treatment if atrial fibrillation persists. For *paroxysmal atrial tachycardia,* continue treatment if heart failure ensues or paroxysms recur frequently; in infants, continue use of digoxin for 3–6 mo after a single episode to prevent recurrence.
Serum digoxin levels	May be helpful in assessing the degree of digitalization and in evaluating the probability of intoxication. Proper interpretation of serum digoxin concentrations must always take into account the observed clinical response; *never use an isolated serum concentration value alone as a basis for adjusting dosage.* The usual therapeutic range is 0.8–2.0 ng/ml in adults; infants and young children may tolerate slightly higher serum levels. Obtain samples at least 6–8 h after the last dose, regardless of the route or dosage form used or, if sampling for assessment of steady-state serum levels, ideally just before the next dose. Once steady-state conditions are achieved, maintenance doses may be adjusted upward or downward in direct proportion to the ratio of the desired versus measured serum concentration, provided the measurement is correct, renal function remains stable, and the needed adjustment is not the result of lack of compliance.

WARNINGS/PRECAUTIONS

Treatment of obesity	Use of digoxin solely for the treatment of obesity is unwarranted and can be dangerous, since potentially fatal arrhythmias and other adverse effects may occur
Anorexia, nausea, vomiting, arrhythmias	May accompany heart failure or reflect digitalis intoxication; determine cause of symptoms before continuing administration. If digitalis intoxication cannot be excluded, withhold digoxin temporarily, provided the clinical situation permits. Measurement of the serum digoxin level may be helpful.
Renal impairment	Decreases excretion of digoxin, increasing the risk of toxicity and its duration; reduce dosage in patients with moderate to severe renal disease (see "maintenance dosage for adults" above). Because of the prolonged serum half-life of digoxin in such patients, more time is needed to achieve steady-state conditions initially and when the dosage is adjusted. Assess renal function periodically by measurement of BUN and/or serum creatinine.
Acute glomerulonephritis	Administer digoxin with extreme caution, and with careful monitoring, to patients with heart failure accompanied by acute glomerulonephritis; relatively low loading and maintenance doses and concomitant antihypertensive therapy may be necessary. Discontinue use of digoxin in such patients as soon as possible.
Hypokalemia	Sensitizes the myocardium to digoxin, increasing the risk of toxicity, even at normal serum digoxin levels. Hypokalemia may result from malnutrition, diarrhea, prolonged vomiting, old age, long-standing heart failure, concomitant use of other drugs (see DRUG INTERACTIONS), dialysis, or mechanical suction of GI secretions. Maintain normal serum levels of potassium during digoxin administration, and avoid rapid changes in serum electrolyte levels. Reserve IV potassium administration for the treatment of digoxin-induced arrhythmias.
Other electrolyte disturbances	Hypercalcemia increases the risk of toxicity; calcium administration, particularly if IV and rapid, may produce serious arrhythmias. Hypomagnesemia also increases the risk of toxicity; institute replacement therapy if serum magnesium levels are low. Hypocalcemia can nullify the effects of digoxin. Monitor serum electrolyte levels periodically.
Thyroid disease	Atrial arrhythmias associated with hypermetabolic states, such as hyperthyroidism, are particularly resistant to digoxin; care must be taken to avoid toxicity if large doses of digoxin are needed (digoxin should not be used alone to treat these arrhythmias). Hypothyroidism reduces digoxin requirements. Patients with compensated thyroid disease respond normally to digoxin.
Electrical cardioversion	A reduction in digoxin dosage prior to cardioversion may be desirable to avoid induction of ventricular arrhythmias; however, the consequences of a rapid increase in ventricular response to atrial fibrillation if digoxin is withheld for 1–2 days should be considered. Elective cardioversion should be delayed if digoxin toxicity is suspected; if this would not be prudent, select a minimal energy level to start and increase the level carefully.
Special-risk patients	Patients with severe carditis (eg, carditis associated with rheumatic fever or viral myocarditis), acute myocardial infarction, or severe pulmonary disease may be particularly sensitive to digoxin-induced rhythm disturbances. Incomplete AV block may progress to advanced or complete heart block, especially in patients with Stokes-Adams attacks. Sinus bradycardia or sinoatrial block may worsen in patients with sinus node disease (sick sinus syndrome). Extremely rapid ventricular rates, and even ventricular fibrillation, may occur in patients with WPW syndrome and atrial fibrillation. Outflow obstruction may worsen in patients with idiopathic hypertrophic subaortic stenosis (IHSS); digoxin probably should not be used in these patients, unless cardiac failure is severe.

LANOXICAPS/LANOXIN

Other cardiac conditions	Patients with heart failure resulting from amyloid heart disease or constrictive cardiomyopathies respond poorly to digoxin. Patients with chronic constrictive pericarditis may not only fail to respond but may suffer a further reduction in cardiac output due to slowing of the heart rate by digoxin. Digoxin should not be used to treat sinus tachycardia in the absence of heart failure.
Carcinogenicity	No long-term studies have been done in animals to evaluate the carcinogenic potential of digoxin

ADVERSE REACTIONS

Cardiovascular	*In adults:* unifocal or multiform ventricular premature contractions, especially in bigeminal or trigeminal patterns; ventricular tachycardia; false-positive ST-T changes (with exercise testing); AV dissociation; accelerated junctional (nodal) rhythm; atrial tachycardia, with block; AV block (Wenckebach) of increasing degree, progressing to complete heart block; *in children:* conduction disturbances or supraventricular tachyarrhythmias, including AV block (Wenckebach); atrial tachycardia, with or without block; junctional (nodal) tachycardia; ventricular arrhythmias, including ventricular premature contractions; ventricular tachycardia; sinus bradycardia; other arrhythmias and cardiac conduction abnormalities
Gastrointestinal	Anorexia, nausea, vomiting, diarrhea
Central nervous system	Visual disturbances (blurred or yellow vision), headache, weakness, apathy, psychosis
Endocrinological	Gynecomastia

OVERDOSAGE

Signs and symptoms	Anorexia, nausea, vomiting, and CNS disturbances are common signs of toxicity in adults but are rarely conspicuous in infants and children. Excessive slowing of the pulse ($\leq$ 60 beats/min) and almost any kind of arrhythmia may occur, but vary in frequency with age (see ADVERSE REACTIONS). Sinus bradycardia, sinoatrial arrest, and prolongation of the P-R interval are premonitory signs of toxicity in the newborn.
Treatment	Discontinue administration of digoxin until all signs of toxicity have disappeared; treatment may not be necessary if toxic manifestations are not severe and only occur near the time of peak effect. In severe cases, and particularly if hypokalemia is present, administer potassium chloride in divided oral doses totaling 3–6 g (40–80 mEq) for adults and 1–1.5 mEq/kg for children, provided that renal function is normal. If correction of the arrhythmia is urgent and the serum potassium level is low or normal, potassium may be given IV in 5% dextrose injection, with careful ECG monitoring. Adults may be given a total of 40–80 mEq (using a concentration of 40 mEq/500 ml) at a rate of up to 20 mEq/h; infants and children may be given approximately 0.5 mEq/kg/h, using a solution dilute enough to avoid local irritation but with care to avoid fluid overload, especially in infants. Additional amounts may be given if the arrhythmia is uncontrolled and the potassium well tolerated. (Potassium should *not* be given, however, to patients with digitalis-induced heart block, unless primarily related to supraventricular tachycardia.) Discontinue the infusion when the desired effect is achieved. Other antiarrhythmic agents that may be tried include lidocaine, procainamide, propranolol, and phenytoin (experimental). Temporary ventricular pacing may be helpful in managing advanced heart block. An investigational procedure involving the IV administration of ovine, digoxin-specific, Fab antibody fragments has been used to rapidly reverse potentially life-threatening toxicity unresponsive to conventional measures.

DRUG INTERACTIONS

Potassium-depleting diuretics and corticosteroids, amphotericin B, quinidine	⇧ Risk of digoxin toxicity
Beta-adrenergic blockers, calcium channel blockers	⇧ Risk of complete AV block; nevertheless, combination therapy may be useful for control of atrial fibrillation) ⇧ Risk of digoxin toxicity (with verapamil)
Tetracycline, erythromycin	⇧ Risk of digoxin toxicity if, before antibiotic therapy, colonic bacteria generally convert a portion of an oral dose of digoxin to inactive metabolites; use of the capsules, which are rapidly absorbed in the upper GI tract, significantly reduces this risk
Calcium, particularly when administered IV; succinylcholine; sympathomimetics	⇧ Risk of cardiac arrhythmias
Antacids, kaolin-pectin antidiarrheal suspensions, sulfasalazine, neomycin, cholestyramine, cyclophosphamide, vincristine, vinblastine, procarbazine, cytarabine, doxorubicin, bleomycin	⇩ Serum level of oral digoxin
Propantheline, diphenoxylate	⇧ Serum level of oral digoxin
Thyroid preparations	⇧ Dosage requirement for digoxin in hypothyroid patients

ALTERED LABORATORY VALUES

No clinically significant alterations in blood/serum or urinary values occur at therapeutic dosages

USE IN CHILDREN
See INDICATIONS and ADMINISTRATION/DOSAGE ADJUSTMENTS. Newborns vary considerably in their tolerance to digoxin; premature and immature infants are especially sensitive, and dosage must not only be reduced but carefully individualized according to maturity. Beyond the newborn period, children generally require proportionally larger doses, on a mg/kg basis, than adults. The soft gelatin capsules may not be appropriate for young children who require fractional doses and/or frequent dosage adjustment.

USE IN PREGNANT AND NURSING WOMEN
Pregnancy Category C: reproduction studies have not been done; it is not known whether digoxin can cause harm to the fetus or affect reproductive capacity. Use during pregnancy only if clearly needed. Digoxin concentrations in human milk and serum are similar; although the amount present is unlikely to have any pharmacologic effect on the nursing infant, caution should be exercised in giving digoxin to a nursing mother.

[1] Contains 10% alcohol

ANTIARRHYTHMICS

MEXITIL (mexiletine hydrochloride) Boehringer Ingelheim   Rx

Capsules: 150, 200, 250 mg

INDICATIONS
Symptomatic ventricular arrhythmias, including frequent premature ventricular contractions (unifocal or multifocal), couplets, and ventricular tachycardia

ORAL DOSAGE
Adult: for rapid control of arrhythmias, 400 mg to start, followed by 200 mg 8 h later; onset of action is usually seen within 30 min to 2 h. When rapid control is not essential, give 200 mg q8h to start, followed as needed and tolerated, by an increase or decrease in dose of 50 or 100 mg; if response is not satisfactory at 300 mg q8h and drug is well-tolerated at that level, dosage may be increased to the maximum level, 400 mg q8h. Usual dosage is 200–300 mg q8h. Allow at least 2–3 days to elapse between dosage adjustments.

CONTRAINDICATIONS
Cardiogenic shock

Second- or third-degree AV block (if no pacemaker is present)

ADMINISTRATION/DOSAGE ADJUSTMENTS

Administration — Give mexiletine with food or an antacid; bear in mind that a magnesium or aluminum antacid may decrease the rate of absorption of mexiletine and reduce the bioavailability of digoxin

Twice-daily administration — If titrated dosage is 300 mg or less q8h, the total daily dose may be given in 2 divided doses q12h; however, bid dosing will enhance the difference in peak and trough serum levels, increasing the likelihood of adverse reactions at the peak level and the risk of recurrent arrhythmias at the trough level. When switching from tid to bid dosing, carefully monitor therapeutic response.

Patients with hepatic impairment — Mexiletine is metabolized in the liver; when hepatic function is impaired, the drug's elimination half-life is prolonged. Closely monitor response of patients with hepatic impairment (including those with liver dysfunction owing to congestive heart failure); a reduction in dosage may be necessary for these patients.

Switching from other antiarrhythmic drugs — To switch to mexiletine, give the first dose of this drug 3–6 h after the last dose of procainamide, 8–12 h after the last dose of tocainide, or 6–12 h after the last dose of quinidine sulfate or disopyramide. To transfer from lidocaine, stop infusion of the drug and then give the first dose of mexiletine; keep the infusion line open until suppression of the arrhythmia seems to be satisfactorily maintained. Bear in mind that the adverse effects of lidocaine and mexiletine may be additive. If withdrawal of an antiarrhythmic agent is likely to produce life-threatening arrhythmias, hospitalize the patient during the transition from that agent to mexiletine.

Monitoring of therapy — Assess effectiveness and tolerance by clinical and ECG evaluation (Holter monitoring may be necessary)

WARNINGS/PRECAUTIONS

Conduction disturbances — Depression of sinus rhythm and conduction velocity, prolongation of sinus node recovery time, and an increase in the effective refractory period of the intraventricular conduction system have occasionally been observed in patients with conduction disturbances. Use with caution in patients with first-degree AV block, sinus node dysfunction, or intraventricular conduction abnormalities; if response to therapy is continuously monitored and a ventricular pacemaker is used, mexiletine may be given to patients with second- or third-degree AV block.

Arrhythmogenicity — Mexiletine can exacerbate ventricular arrhythmias; this effect is particularly important when the patient has a life-threatening arrhythmia, such as sustained ventricular tachycardia

Hepatotoxicity — Elevated SGOT levels, 3 times the upper limit of normal or higher, have been detected in 1–2% of patients; the increases were often asymptomatic and transient and usually did not necessitate discontinuation of therapy. However, hepatic necrosis and other manifestations of severe liver injury have been observed in foreign marketing experience. If a hepatic function test produces abnormal results or signs and symptoms suggesting liver dysfunction are seen, carefully evaluate the patient; consider discontinuing therapy if elevation of the hepatic enzyme level persists or progresses.

Blood dyscrasias — Thrombocytopenia has been detected in 0.16% of patients; marked leukopenia (neutrophil count $<1,000/mm^3$) and agranulocytosis have occurred in 0.06% of patients. If significant hematological changes are detected during therapy, carefully evaluate the patient and then, if necessary, withdraw mexiletine. Blood counts usually return to normal within 1 mo after termination of therapy.

Convulsions — Approximately 0.2% of patients have experienced convulsions; these effects have occurred not only in patients with a history of seizures, but also in patients without such a history. Use with caution in patients who have a seizure disorder.

Hypotension, congestive heart failure — Small decreases in cardiac output can occur during therapy; use with caution in patients with hypotension or severe congestive heart failure

Changes in urinary pH — Marked acidification of the urine enhances excretion, while marked alkalinization reduces excretion; avoid drugs or dietary regimens that can markedly alter urinary pH

Common GI and CNS effects — Upper GI distress, light-headedness, tremor, and coordination difficulties are the most frequent reactions to mexiletine; these effects can be reversed by a reduction in dosage or withdrawal of the drug

Decreased absorption rate — By causing an increase in gastric emptying time, disorders such as acute myocardial infarction and drugs such as atropine and narcotic analgesics can decrease the rate of absorption of mexiletine

Effect on mortality — Mexiletine has not been shown to prevent sudden death in patients with severe ventricular ectopic activity

Carcinogenicity, mutagenicity, effect on fertility — No evidence of carcinogenicity has been observed in rats given mexiletine for 24 mo or in mice given the drug for 18 mo; no mutagenic activity has been shown in the Ames test. Mexiletine has not caused impaired fertility in rats.

ADVERSE REACTIONS

Frequent reactions (incidence ≥ 1%) are printed in *italics*

Cardiovascular — *Palpitations (4.3%), chest pain (2.6%), angina/angina-like pain (1.7%), increased ventricular arrhythmias/premature ventricular contractions (1%)*, syncope, edema, hot flashes, hypertension, hypotension, bradycardia, AV block/conduction disturbances, atrial arrhythmias, cardiogenic shock

Gastrointestinal — *Nausea/vomiting/heartburn (39.3%), diarrhea (5.2%), constipation (4%), changes in appetite (2.6%), abdominal pain/cramps/discomfort (1.2%)*, dysphagia, peptic ulcer, upper GI tract bleeding, esophageal ulceration

Central nervous system — *Dizziness/light-headedness (18.9%), tremor (13.2%), coordination difficulties (9.7%), changes in sleep habits (7.1%), headache (5.7%), weakness and nervousness (5%), fatigue (3.8%), speech difficulties and confusion/clouded sensorium (2.6%), paresthesias/numbness, tinnitus, and depression (2.4%);* short-term memory loss, loss of consciousness, hallucinations, psychosis, other psychological changes, convulsions/seizures

Ophthalmic — *Blurred vision/visual disturbances (5.7%)*

Hepatic — Abnormal liver function tests

Genitourinary — Urinary hesitancy/retention, impotence/decreased libido

Hematological — Thrombocytopenia, leukopenia (including neutropenia and agranulocytosis), myelofibrosis

Other — *Rash (4.2%), dyspnea/respiratory reactions (3.3%), dry mouth (2.8%), arthralgia (1.7%), fever (1.2%)*, diaphoresis, malaise, pharyngitis, altered taste, salivary changes, hair loss, hiccups, dry skin, changes in oral mucous membranes, laryngeal and pharyngeal changes, positive ANA test, systemic lupus erythematosus

OVERDOSAGE

Signs and symptoms	Neurological reactions, including ataxia and convulsions
Treatment	Institute supportive treatment. Atropine may be administered if hypotension or bradycardia occurs. To enhance excretion of mexiletine, acidify the urine.

DRUG INTERACTIONS

Phenytoin, rifampin, phenobarbital, and other drugs capable of inducing hepatic enzymes	▽ Serum mexiletine level; monitor serum drug level during combination therapy
Urinary acidifiers	▽ Serum mexiletine level; avoid using urinary acidifiers in combination with mexiletine
Cimetidine	△ Serum mexiletine level; watch carefully for adverse effects during combination therapy
Narcotics, atropine, magnesium-aluminum hydroxide	▽ Rate of absorption of mexiletine
Metoclopramide	△ Rate of absorption of mexiletine

ALTERED LABORATORY VALUES

Blood/serum values	△ SGOT

No clinically significant alterations in urinary values occur at therapeutic dosages

USE IN CHILDREN

Safety and effectiveness for use in children have not been established

USE IN PREGNANT AND NURSING WOMEN

Pregnancy Category C: reproduction studies in rats, mice, and rabbits at up to 4 times the maximum human oral dose have shown an increase in fetal resorptions; use during pregnancy only if the expected benefit justifies the potential risk to the fetus. Mexiletine appears in human milk at concentrations similar to plasma levels; women who require this drug should not nurse.

ANTIARRHYTHMICS

NORPACE (disopyramide phosphate) Searle   Rx
Capsules: 100, 150 mg

NORPACE CR (disopyramide phosphate) Searle   Rx
Capsules (controlled release): 100, 150 mg

INDICATIONS

Unifocal, paired, and multifocal **premature ventricular contractions**
Episodes of **ventricular tachycardia**

ORAL DOSAGE

Adult: 400–800 mg/day, given in equally divided doses; usual maintenance dosage: 150 mg q6h if immediate-release capsules are used or 300 mg q12h if controlled-release capsules are used
Infant (< 1 yr): 10–30 mg/kg/day, given in equally divided doses q6h or as needed
Child (1–4 yr): 10–20 mg/kg/day, given in equally divided doses q6h or as needed
Child (4–12 yr): 10–15 mg/kg/day, given in equally divided doses q6h or as needed
Adolescent (12–18 yr): 6–15 mg/kg/day, given in equally divided doses q6h or as needed

CONTRAINDICATIONS

Second- or third-degree AV block (unless a pacemaker is present)
Cardiogenic shock
Congenital prolongation of Q-T interval
Hypersensitivity to disopyramide

ADMINISTRATION/DOSAGE ADJUSTMENTS

Patients weighing under 110 lb (50 kg)	Administer either 100 mg q6h if immediate-release capsules are used or 200 mg q12h if controlled-release capsules are used; if rapid control of ventricular arrhythmias is essential, administer a loading dose of 200 mg, using the immediate-release capsules only (see below)
Patients requiring prompt control of ventricular arrhythmias	Administer a loading dose of 300 mg, using the immediate-release capsules only (Norpace CR should not be used initially when therapeutic disopyramide serum levels must be attained rapidly); the loading dose is then followed by the appropriate maintenance dosage. If there is no response to the loading dose within 6 h and the patient is not showing signs of toxicity, administer 200 mg q6h, using the immediate-release capsules. If there is still no response after 48 h, either discontinue use of the drug or consider hospitalizing the patient for careful monitoring while subsequent doses of 250–300 mg are given q6h, again using the immediate-release capsules only. Some patients with severe, refractory ventricular tachycardia have tolerated up to 400 mg q6h; such dosages may be given only if patients are hospitalized for close observation and continuous monitoring.

NORPACE

Patients with cardiomyopathy or possible cardiac decompensation	Limit the initial dosage to 100 mg q6h, using the immediate-release capsules, and do not give a loading dose; subsequent dosage adjustments should be made gradually, with the patient under close observation for hypotension and/or congestive heart failure
Patients with hepatic or renal impairment	For patients with hepatic insufficiency or *moderate* renal impairment (creatinine clearance rate [CCr] > 40 ml/min), administer 100 mg q6h, using the immediate-release capsules, or 200 mg q12h, using the controlled-release capsules. For patients with *severe* renal impairment, use the immediate-release capsules only and administer 100 mg q8h if CCr = 30–40 ml/min, q12h if CCr = 15–30 ml/min, or q24h if CCr < 15 ml/min; if a loading dose is needed for these patients, give 150 mg.
Transferring patients with normal renal function from procainamide or quinidine to disopyramide	Begin using the ordinary maintenance dosage 3–6 h after the last dose of procainamide was taken or 6–12 h after the last dose of quinidine; do not give a loading dose
Transferring patients from immediate-release to controlled-release capsules	Advise patient to begin taking Norpace CR 6 h after the last Norpace capsule was taken
Concomitant therapy with phenytoin or other hepatic enzyme-inducing drugs	Lower plasma levels of disopyramide may occur, resulting in ineffectual antiarrhythmic therapy; monitor disopyramide plasma level if drugs capable of inducing hepatic enzymes are given concomitantly
Preparation of pediatric suspension	For pediatric dosing, a 1–10 mg/ml liquid suspension may be prepared by adding the entire contents of an immediate-release capsule to the appropriate amount of Cherry Syrup NF; the resulting suspension is stable for 1 mo when refrigerated and should be shaken thoroughly before use. Do not use Norpace CR for this preparation.
Carcinogenicity, mutagenicity	Studies in rats fed up to 30 times the usual human daily dose for 18 mo showed no evidence of carcinogenicity. Results of the Ames test were negative.
Effect on fertility	No adverse effects on fertility have been seen in rats given up to 250 mg/kg/day

WARNINGS/PRECAUTIONS

Congestive heart failure	May be precipitated or worsen; do not use in patients with uncompensated or marginally compensated heart failure, unless failure is due to an arrhythmia. May be used in patients with a history of heart failure, provided that cardiac function is being adequately maintained. If congestive heart failure worsens, discontinue disopyramide therapy and reinstitute at a lower dosage only after cardiac failure has been adequately compensated.
Severe hypotension	May occur, particularly in patients with primary cardiomyopathy or inadequately compensated congestive heart failure; do not use in patients with hypotension, unless hypotension is secondary to cardiac arrhythmia. If hypotension occurs during disopyramide therapy, discontinue use of the drug and, if necessary, reinstitute therapy at a lower dosage.
Heart block	If first-degree heart block develops, reduce dosage; if the block persists despite dosage reduction, the benefits of continuing therapy should be weighed against the risk of higher degrees of heart block. If second- or third-degree AV block or unifascicular, bifascicular, or trifascicular block develops, discontinue use of disopyramide, unless ventricular rate is controlled with an artificial pacemaker.
ECG changes	If the QRS complex widens by more than 25% (an unusual occurrence), administration should be discontinued. Disopyramide can prolong the Q-T interval, exacerbate the arrhythmia, and cause ventricular tachycardia or fibrillation; if the Q-T interval increases by more than 25% and the arrhythmia persists, clinical response should be monitored and termination of disopyramide should be considered. Use with particular caution if an increase in the Q-T interval has occurred following administration of quinidine.
Patients with atrial tachyarrhythmias	Patients with atrial flutter or fibrillation should be digitalized prior to initiating disopyramide therapy to prevent an excessive increase in ventricular rate
Patients with conduction abnormalities	Use with caution in patients with sick sinus syndrome, Wolff-Parkinson-White syndrome, or bundle branch block
Patients with hepatic or renal impairment	Hepatic or renal insufficiency may lead to excessive drug accumulation; reduce dosage (see ADMINISTRATION/DOSAGE ADJUSTMENTS) and monitor ECG for signs of toxicity. Patients with cardiac dysfunction have a higher potential for hepatic impairment; this should be considered before prescribing disopyramide.
Anticholinergic activity	Unless adequate overriding measures have been taken, do not use in patients with glaucoma, myasthenia gravis, or urinary retention. Urinary retention may occur during disopyramide administration, particularly in males with benign prostatic hypertrophy. Before intiating therapy in patients with a family history of glaucoma, measure intraocular pressure to rule out glaucoma. Use with particular caution in patients with myasthenia gravis due to increased risk of myasthenic crisis.
Hypoglycemia	May occur in rare instances; follow blood glucose levels closely in patients with congestive heart failure, chronic malnutrition, hepatic, renal, or other diseases, or who are taking drugs that could compromise normal glucoregulation in the absence of food, such as beta blockers or alcohol.

NORPACE ■ PROCAN SR

Potassium imbalance	Hypokalemia may reduce antiarrhythmic effectiveness, while hyperkalemia may aggravate toxicity; correct any preexisting potassium abnormalities before initiating disopyramide therapy

ADVERSE REACTIONS

Frequent reactions (incidence ≥ 1%) are printed in *italics*

Autonomic nervous system	*Dry mouth (32%); urinary hesitancy (14%); constipation (11%); blurred vision and dry nose, eyes, and throat (3–9%)*
Genitourinary	*Urinary retention or urinary frequency and urgency (3–9%)*, impotence, dysuria
Gastrointestinal	*Nausea, pain, bloating, and flatulence (3–9%); anorexia, diarrhea, and vomiting (1–3%)*
Central nervous system	*Dizziness, fatigue/muscle weakness, headache, malaise, and aches/pains (3–9%); nervousness (1–3%)*; depression, insomnia, numbness/tingling; acute psychoses (rare)
Cardiovascular	*Hypotension, congestive heart failure, cardiac conduction disturbances, edema/weight gain, shortness of breath, syncope, and chest pain (1–3%)*; AV block
Dermatological	*Rash, dermatoses, and itching (1–3%)*
Hepatic	Cholestatic jaundice (rare)
Other	Hypoglycemia; reversible agranulocytosis, thrombocytopenia, and gynecomastia (rare)

OVERDOSAGE

Signs and symptoms	Hypotension, worsening of heart failure, excessive widening of QRS complex and Q-T interval, conduction disturbances, bradycardia, asystole, anticholinergic effects (eg, dry mouth, nose, and throat; blurred vision; urinary hesitancy or retention), apnea, cardiac arrhythmias, loss of consciousness
Treatment	Treat overdosage promptly and vigorously, even when symptoms are not immediately evident. Induce emesis or perform gastric lavage; administer a cathartic and then activated charcoal. To lower serum drug levels, perform hemoperfusion with charcoal (the preferred technique) or hemodialysis. If renal function is impaired, toxicity may be reduced by measures that increase the GFR. Institute supportive measures, as needed, including intra-aortic balloon counterpulsation, mechanically assisted ventilation, digitalization, diuretic therapy, and the administration of IV isoproterenol or dopamine. Provide endocardial pacing if progressive AV block occurs. Consider using neostigmine to reverse anticholinergic reactions. Monitor ECG.

DRUG INTERACTIONS

Other antiarrhythmic drugs	△ Conduction time ▽ Myocardial contractility (use with particular caution in patients with cardiac decompensation [or a history of this disorder])
Phenytoin and other drugs capable of inducing hepatic enzymes	▽ Plasma disopyramide level and possible loss of antiarrhythmic effectiveness

ALTERED LABORATORY VALUES

Blood/serum values	△ SGOT △ SGPT △ BUN △ Creatinine △ Cholesterol △ Triglycerides ▽ Potassium ▽ Glucose ▽ Hemoglobin ▽ Hematocrit

No clinically significant alterations in urinary values occur at therapeutic dosages

---

USE IN CHILDREN

See INDICATIONS and ORAL DOSAGE; child should be hospitalized during initial treatment, and dosage titration should start toward the lower end of the range given for each age group. Monitor plasma disopyramide level and therapeutic response closely.

USE IN PREGNANT AND NURSING WOMEN

Pregnancy Category C: a decrease in the number of implantation sites and a reduction in pup growth and survival have been seen in rats given 250 mg/kg/day (20 or more times the usual human daily dose); at this dosage, food intake and weight gain of the dams were also lowered. An increase in resorption rate has occurred in rabbits given 60 mg/kg/day (5 times the usual human daily dose). According to reports, disopyramide can stimulate uterine contractions. Use during pregnancy only if the expected benefits justify the potential risks to the fetus. Disopyramide is excreted in human milk; because of the potential for serious adverse reactions in nursing infants, women should not nurse during therapy.

ANTIARRHYTHMICS

PROCAN SR (procainamide hydrochloride) Parke-Davis   Rx

Tablets (sustained release): 250, 500, 750, 1,000 mg

INDICATIONS
Premature ventricular contractions
Ventricular tachycardia
Atrial fibrillation
Paroxysmal atrial tachycardia

ORAL DOSAGE
Adult: ¼ the total daily dose of an immediate-release procainamide preparation q6h (usual dosage: 50 mg/kg/day), starting 2–3 h after the last dose of the immediate-release preparation was taken; monitor serum level of procainamide and its active metabolite, N-acetylprocainamide, after substituting Procan SR

CONTRAINDICATIONS

Complete AV block

Hypersensitivity to procainamide

Second- or third-degree AV block (unless a pacemaker is used)

Myasthenia gravis

ADMINISTRATION/DOSAGE ADJUSTMENTS

Administration — To maintain dissolution characteristics, tablets should be swallowed whole, not broken in half, crushed, or chewed. A dose may be taken as late as 1 h after its scheduled time; however, if a dose is missed, the next dose should not be doubled. The tablet-shaped wax matrix containing the drug is not absorbed and, therefore, may be detected by patients in the stool.

Titration of dosage — Use an oral or parenteral immediate-release preparation of procainamide to determine the required total daily dose. For treatment of ventricular arrhythmias with oral procainamide, give 1 g, followed by 50 mg/kg/day in divided doses q3h, to start; then increase the dosage, as needed and tolerated. For treatment of atrial arrhythmias with oral procainamide, give 1.25 g, followed by 0.75 g 1 h later if no ECG changes are seen, and then 0.5–1 g q2h, as needed and tolerated.

Long-term therapy — During prolonged use, occasionally check ECG to determine whether the drug is still needed

WARNINGS/PRECAUTIONS

Cross-sensitivity — Use with caution in patients hypersensitive to procaine or related drugs

Granulocytopenia — Death from sepsis has occurred as a result of procainamide-induced granulocytopenia. This blood dyscrasia seems to occur more frequently with sustained-release tablets than with immediate-release tablets. To reduce the risk, obtain routine blood counts at least every 2 wk during the first 3 mo of therapy and at longer intervals thereafter; instruct patients to promptly report flu-like symptoms such as malaise and ache (which are often associated with granulocytopenia), as well as other possible signs and symptoms, such as rash, unexplained fever, upper respiratory tract infection, unusual bleeding or bruising, and soreness of the mouth, throat, or gums. If signs or symptoms are observed and CBC results indicate granulocyte depression, procainamide should be discontinued immediately and appropriate therapy instituted; the leukocyte count usually returns to normal within a few weeks after discontinuation.

Lupus-like syndrome — Long-term use often induces the formation of antinuclear antibodies and, less frequently, causes a syndrome resembling systemic lupus erythematosus. Common symptoms of the syndrome are polyarthralgia, other arthritic-like symptoms, and pleuritic pain; less frequent signs and symptoms include fever, myalgia, skin lesions, pleural effusion, pericarditis, headache, fatigue, weakness, nausea, and abdominal pain. Thrombocytopenia, Coombs' positive hemolytic anemia, and increases in SGOT, SGPT, and serum amylase levels, which have been reported in rare cases, may also be associated with this syndrome. To reduce the risk, test for systemic lupus erythematosus at regular intervals; instruct patients to report arthritic-like reactions, as well as any other possible signs and symptoms. If ANA test is positive, weigh the potential risks and benefits of continuing therapy; if a rising ANA titer or clinical signs and symptoms are seen, therapy should generally be discontinued. For reactions that persist despite termination of therapy or that develop during treatment of recurrent, life-threatening arrhythmias unresponsive to other antiarrhythmic agents, corticosteroids may be used.

Cardiac reactions — Carefully monitor all patients for evidence of an untoward myocardial response. During treatment of atrial fibrillation or flutter, the decline in atrial rate may be accompanied by a sudden increase in the ventricular rate, particularly in patients with myocardial damage; adequate digitalization reduces, but does not eliminate, this risk. Dislodgement of mural thrombi and embolism may also occur during conversion of atrial fibrillation; however, it has been suggested that when emboli are already being discharged, procainamide is more likely to stop this process rather than aggravate it. Exercise extreme caution when treating ventricular tachycardia during an occlusive coronary episode. Use with caution in patients with marked AV conduction disturbances such as AV block (see CONTRAINDICATIONS), bundle branch block, or severe digitalis toxicity since procainamide may further depress conduction and precipitate ventricular asystole or fibrillation. Bear in mind that complete heart block may not be apparent in patients with severe organic heart disease and ventricular tachycardia; if procainamide produces a significant reduction in the ventricular rate without causing AV conduction to return to normal, treatment should be discontinued and the diagnosis reassessed because of the risk of asystole occurring under these circumstances.

Toxicity — At high serum levels, procainamide can cause severe hypotension, reflex tachycardia, complete AV block, ventricular extrasystoles and fibrillation, and cardiac arrest; ECG findings include widening of the QRS complex and, less frequently, prolongation of the Q-T and P-R intervals and a reduction in the amplitude of the QRS complex and T wave. Toxic reactions are initially seen at serum procainamide levels exceeding 8 μg/ml; frequency remains quite low at serum levels up to 12 μg/ml but progressively increases at higher concentrations. Since drug accumulation may occur in patients with renal or hepatic disease, cardiac failure, or any condition associated with reduced cardiac output, serum levels of procainamide and its active metabolite, N-acetylprocainamide, should be monitored in these patients.

PROCAN SR ■ PRONESTYL

ADVERSE REACTIONS[1]	The most frequent reactions, regardless of incidence, are printed in *italics*
Gastrointestinal	*Anorexia, nausea, vomiting, diarrhea*
Dermatological	*Urticaria, pruritus*
Central nervous system	Convulsions, psychosis with hallucinations, confusion, depression, giddiness, light-headedness, weakness
Hypersensitivity	Angioneurotic edema, maculopapular rash, fever, eosinophilia, hypergammaglobulinemia
Other	Lupus-like syndrome, granulocytopenia, bitter taste; hypotension (rare)

OVERDOSAGE

Signs and symptoms	Severe hypotension, ventricular fibrillation, widening of the QRS complex, junctional tachycardia, intraventricular conduction delay, oliguria, lethargy, confusion, nausea, vomiting
Treatment	Institute symptomatic measures; monitor ECG and blood pressure. A vasopressor such as dopamine, phenylephrine, or norepinephrine can be given, if necessary, after adequate fluid volume replacement; IV infusion of 1/6 M sodium lactate injection has been reported to be effective in reducing cardiotoxic effects. Cardiac pacing has been suggested as a reasonable precautionary measure in light of the potential risk of high-grade AV block. If ingestion is recent, perform gastric lavage or induce emesis. If severe hypotension and renal insufficiency occur, hemodialysis may be necessary.

DRUG INTERACTIONS

Other antiarrhythmic agents	△ Pharmacologic effects of procainamide
Anticholinergic agents	△ Anticholinergic effects; exercise extreme caution when using procainamide in combination with an anticholinergic drug
Anticholinesterase agents	▽ Anticholinesterase effect Myasthenic crisis; it has been suggested that procainamide be contraindicated for patients with myasthenia gravis
Antihypertensive agents	△ Antihypertensive effect; dosage adjustment may be necessary
Histamine H$_2$-receptor antagonists (eg, cimetidine, ranitidine)	△ Serum level of procainamide and its active metabolite, N-acetylprocainamide. Exercise caution when using procainamide in combination with a histamine H$_2$-receptor antagonist, especially when patient is elderly; dosage adjustment may be necessary.
Succinylcholine, gramicidin, bacitracin, polymyxins, aminoglycosides	△ Risk of respiratory depression

ALTERED LABORATORY VALUES

Blood/serum values	+ ANA

No clinically significant alterations in urinary values occur at therapeutic dosages

---

USE IN CHILDREN

Specific guidelines for use of sustained-release procainamide preparations in children are not available

USE IN PREGNANT AND NURSING WOMEN

Pregnancy Category C: reproduction studies have not been done; it is not known whether procainamide can cause harm to the fetus or affect reproductive capacity. Use during pregnancy only if clearly needed. It is also not known whether this drug is excreted in human milk; use with caution in nursing mothers.

---

[1] Fever and chills, nausea, vomiting, abdominal pain, acute hepatomegaly, and an increase in SGOT have occurred in a patient given a single dose of the drug

---

ANTIARRHYTHMICS

PRONESTYL (procainamide hydrochloride) Princeton   Rx
Capsules: 250, 375, 500 mg   **Tablets:** 250, 375, 500 mg

INDICATIONS

Treatment of **premature ventricular contractions**
Prevention of recurrence of **ventricular tachycardia, paroxysmal supraventricular tachycardia, and atrial flutter or fibrillation** following conversion to normal sinus rhythm

ORAL DOSAGE

Adult: for younger patients with normal renal function, up to 50 mg/kg/day, given in 8 divided doses q3h; for older patients and others at risk, see "dosage adjustment," below

PRONESTYL Injection (procainamide hydrochloride) Princeton   Rx
Vials: 100 mg/ml (10 ml), 500 mg/ml (2 ml)

INDICATIONS

Treatment of **premature ventricular contractions and transient ventricular tachycardia**
Prevention of recurrence of **ventricular tachycardia, paroxysmal supraventricular tachycardia, and atrial flutter or fibrillation** following conversion to normal sinus rhythm

PARENTERAL DOSAGE

Adult: for IM use, 50 mg/kg/day, given in 4–8 divided doses q3–6h, to start, followed by an adjustment in dosage, if necessary, after 3 doses have been given. For IV use, 100 mg every 5 min for up to 10 doses or 20 mg/min by continuous infusion for 25–30 min (or, if necessary, for up to 50 min), followed in either case by a maintenance infusion of 2–6 mg/min.

COMPENDIUM OF DRUG THERAPY

| Treatment of arrhythmias associated with **anesthesia or surgery** | **Adult:** 100–500 mg IM |

PRONESTYL-SR (procainamide hydrochloride) Princeton   Rx
Tablets (sustained release): 500 mg

INDICATIONS

Premature ventricular contractions
Ventricular tachycardia

Atrial fibrillation
Paroxysmal atrial tachycardia

ORAL DOSAGE

Adult: 50 mg/kg/day, given in 4 divided doses q6h

Adult: 1 g q6h

CONTRAINDICATIONS

| Complete heart block | Hypersensitivity to procainamide | Systemic lupus erythematosus (with oral forms) |
| Torsades de pointes | | |

ADMINISTRATION/DOSAGE ADJUSTMENTS

Preparation for IV use — For the initial infusion, add 1 g of procainamide to 50 ml of 5% dextrose injection USP (resulting concentration: 20 mg/ml); for the maintenance infusion, add 1 g to 500 ml (resulting concentration: 2 mg/ml) or, if fluid intake must be limited, add 1 g to 250 ml (resulting concentration: 4 mg/ml). Dilute solutions that are to be given by intermittent injection.

Parenteral administration — Before starting parenteral therapy, ensure that facilities for intensive supportive care are available; keep the patient supine during administration. Intermittent IV doses should be injected slowly, either directly into the vein or through IV tubing, at a rate not greater than 50 mg/min; after 5 doses (500 mg) have been given, wait at least 10 min before resuming use.

Monitoring of therapy — During parenteral administration, monitor blood pressure and ECG; during oral therapy, check vital signs and ECG frequently. If blood pressure decreases by 15 mm Hg or more, discontinue use temporarily. Consider the possibility of overdosage if the QRS complex widens by more than 25% or the Q-T interval is markedly prolonged; if the QRS complex widens by 50% or more, interrupt parenteral therapy or reduce oral dosage.

Dosage adjustment — To determine optimal dosage, closely observe clinical response. A reduction in dosage may be necessary for patients who are over 50 yr of age since renal excretion of procainamide and its active metabolite, *N*-acetylprocainamide, decreases by 25% at 50 yr of age and by 50% at 75 yr of age; a reduction may also be required for patients with decreased creatinine clearance, increased BUN or serum creatinine levels, cardiac or hepatic impairment, or a history of renal insufficiency. Measurement of BUN or serum creatinine level may be helpful in evaluating renal status. Serum levels of procainamide and *N*-acetylprocainamide, if available, can facilitate dosage adjustment; however, bear in mind that although therapeutic serum levels have been reported to be 3–10 µg/ml, a higher, potentially toxic level may be necessary for certain patients, such as those with sustained ventricular tachycardia. A maintenance infusion of 50 µg/kg/min in a patient with a normal procainamide half-life of 3 h can be expected to produce a serum level of approximately 6.5 µg/ml. To reduce the dosage when using immediate-release oral preparations, decrease the amount given at each dosing interval or, alternatively, increase the dosing interval from 3 h to 4 or 6 h.

Switching from parenteral to oral therapy — If possible, terminate parenteral therapy as soon as basic cardiac rhythm stabilizes; after giving the last IV dose, wait a period equivalent to the elimination half-life (generally, 3–4 h) before administering the first oral dose

Sustained-release tablets — Do not use the sustained-release tablets for initial therapy; start with an immediate-release preparation and then switch to the tablets for maintenance. Instruct patients not to break or chew the tablets, and warn them that the tablet matrix may appear in the stool.

WARNINGS/PRECAUTIONS

Heart block — Procainamide can exacerbate heart block and precipitate asystole. Exercise caution in patients with first-degree block; use only if an electrical pacemaker is present in patients with second-degree block or hemiblock. Do not administer the drug to patients with complete heart block. (It may be difficult to detect complete heart block in patients with ventricular tachycardia; the diagnosis can be made in these patients if a significant decrease in ventricular rate occurs during therapy without evidence of AV conduction.) If first-degree block occurs during treatment, reduce dosage; if the block persists, weigh the expected benefits of therapy against the risk of more severe block. Discontinue administration if hemiblock or second-degree block occurs, unless the ventricular rate can be controlled by an electrical pacemaker.

Digitalis-induced arrhythmias — Although procainamide can suppress digitalis-induced arrhythmias, the drug can also cause ventricular asystole or fibrillation if the arrhythmias are accompanied by a marked AV conduction disturbance; administration of procainamide should only be considered when the arrhythmias persist after discontinuation of digitalis and fail to respond to potassium, lidocaine, or phenytoin

PRONESTYL

Ventricular tachycardia	Use of procainamide in patients with atrial flutter or fibrillation may produce an intolerable increase in the ventricular rate, since the drug can enhance AV conduction in this circumstance; adequate digitalization reduces, but does not eliminate, this risk. Convert atrial flutter or fibrillation to normal sinus rhythm with vagotonic maneuvers, electric cardioversion, digitalis, or other measures before beginning use of procainamide. Bear in mind that during conversion of atrial fibrillation, dislodgement of mural thrombi can lead to embolization.
Myocardial depression	Procainamide can produce a slight depression in myocardial contractility; use with caution in patients with congestive heart failure, acute ischemic heart disease, or cardiomyopathy, since cardiac output in these patients may be further reduced
Hypotension	Transient hypotension can occur, especially during IV administration; monitor blood pressure during parenteral administration and avoid giving the drug at an overly rapid rate (see PARENTERAL DOSAGE and ADMINISTRATION/DOSAGE ADJUSTMENTS)
Myasthenia gravis	Procainamide can exacerbate myasthenia gravis; in patients with this disorder, adjust anticholinesterase dosage and take other appropriate measures when using procainamide. If myasthenia gravis is suspected, watch closely for muscle weakness immediately after beginning procainamide therapy.
Hypersensitivity	Immediately after beginning treatment, watch closely for possible allergic reactions, especially when hypersensitivity to procaine or other local anesthetics is suspected; discontinue use if acute allergic dermatitis, asthma, or anaphylaxis occurs
Blood dyscrasias	Long-term use can precipitate potentially fatal agranulocytosis; neutropenia, thrombocytopenia, and hemolytic anemia can also occur during prolonged therapy. Obtain a CBC before beginning therapy and periodically thereafter.
Lupus-like syndrome	Long-term use often induces the formation of antinuclear antibodies. After administration for 1–12 mo, a syndrome resembling systemic lupus erythematosus may occur in 20–30% of patients; the presence of a rapid acetylation rate may increase the risk. Common symptoms of the syndrome are pleural, abdominal, and joint pains; less frequent signs and symptoms include arthritis, pleural effusion, pericarditis, fever, chills, myalgia, blood dyscrasias, hepatomegaly, and skin lesions. To reduce the risk of this syndrome, perform an ANA test before therapy and periodically thereafter; a rising titer may precede clinical symptoms. If results of an ANA test are positive or clinical signs and symptoms develop, weigh the risks and benefits of continued use; bear in mind that the dangerous renal pathological changes associated with lupus occur rarely. For reactions that persist despite termination of therapy or that develop during treatment of recurrent, life-threatening arrhythmias unresponsive to other antiarrhythmic agents, corticosteroids may be used.
Reactions to be reported	Instruct patient to report promptly arthralgia, myalgia, fever, chills, rash, easy bruising, sore throat or mouth, infections, dark urine or icterus, wheezing, muscle weakness, chest or abdominal pain, palpitations, nausea, vomiting, anorexia, diarrhea, hallucinations, dizziness, and/or depression
Tartrazine sensitivity	Presence of FD&C Yellow No. 5 (tartrazine) in immediate-release tablets may cause allergic-type reactions, including bronchial asthma, in susceptible patients (eg, patients hypersensitive to aspirin)
Carcinogenicity, mutagenicity, effect on fertility	No long-term studies have been done to evaluate the carcinogenic or mutagenic potential of procainamide or its effect on fertility

ADVERSE REACTIONS

Cardiovascular	Hypotension (especially with IV use), ventricular asystole or fibrillation; second-degree heart block (with oral use)
Hematological	Neutropenia, thrombocytopenia, hemolytic anemia, agranulocytosis
Gastrointestinal	Anorexia, nausea, vomiting, abdominal pain, bitter taste, and diarrhea (frequency with oral use: 3–4%); hepatomegaly with increased SGOT and SGPT levels
Central nervous system	Dizziness, giddiness, weakness, mental depression, psychosis, hallucinations
Dermatological	Angioneurotic edema, urticaria, pruritus, flushing, maculopapular rash
Other	Fever, chills, serositis with effusions, myalgia, lupus erythematosus-like syndrome

OVERDOSAGE

Signs and symptoms	Progressive widening of QRS complex, prolonged Q-T and P-R intervals, lowered R and T waves, increase in ventricular extrasystoles, more severe AV block, ventricular tachycardia or fibrillation; with parenteral, especially IV, use and, in rare cases, with oral use: hypotension, CNS depression, tremor, and respiratory depression
Treatment	Institute general supportive measures, closely observe patient, and monitor vital signs; if necessary, use vasopressors and provide mechanical cardiorespiratory support. Serum levels of procainamide and its active metabolite, N-acetylprocainamide, can be useful. Both procainamide and N-acetylprocainamide can be removed from the blood by hemodialysis.

DRUG INTERACTIONS

Quinidine, disopyramide	Hypotension ▽ Cardiac conduction ▽ Myocardial contractility These reactions are especially likely to occur in patients with cardiac decompensation. Institute combination therapy only when close observation is possible and the arrhythmia is serious and unresponsive to a single drug; a reduction in dosage may be necessary.

PRONESTYL ■ QUINAGLUTE

Other antiarrhythmic drugs	↑ Pharmacologic effects associated with antiarrhythmic agents; a reduction in dosage may be necessary
Anticholinesterase agents	↓ Anticholinesterase effect; adjust anticholinesterase dosage
Anticholinergic agents	↑ Anticholinergic effects
Cimetidine	↑ Serum level of procainamide and its active metabolite, N-acetylprocainamide
Succinylcholine	↑ Risk of respiratory depression; a reduction in succinylcholine dosage may be necessary

ALTERED LABORATORY VALUES

Blood/serum values	+ ANA ↓ Procainamide and N-acetylprocainamide (with fluorometric tests of serum containing these two drugs and excessive levels of lidocaine or meprobamate) ↑ Procainamide and N-acetylprocainamide (with fluorometric tests of serum containing these two drugs and propranolol)

No clinically significant alterations in urinary values occur at therapeutic dosages

---

USE IN CHILDREN
Safety and effectiveness for use in children have not been established

USE IN PREGNANT AND NURSING WOMEN
Pregnancy Category C: no reproduction studies have been done; it is not known whether procainamide can cause harm to the fetus or affect reproductive capacity. Use during pregnancy only if clearly needed. Procainamide and its active metabolite, N-acetylprocainamide, are excreted in human milk; because of the potential for serious adverse reactions in nursing infants, patients should not nurse during therapy.

ANTIARRHYTHMICS

QUINAGLUTE (quinidine gluconate) Berlex   Rx

Tablets (sustained release): 324 mg quinidine gluconate equivalent to 202 mg quinidine

INDICATIONS
Ventricular arrhythmias, including tachycardia (when not associated with complete heart block) and premature contractions
Junctional (nodal) arrhythmias, including premature complexes and paroxysmal tachycardia
Supraventricular (atrial) arrhythmias, including flutter, fibrillation, (chronic and paroxysmal), premature contractions, and paroxysmal tachycardia

ORAL DOSAGE
Adult: for prevention of premature contractions or complexes, 1–2 tabs q8–12h; for maintenance of normal sinus rhythm following conversion of paroxysmal tachycardias, 2 tabs q12h or 1½–2 tabs q8h

CONTRAINDICATIONS

Complete AV block

Digitalis intoxication manifested by AV conduction disorders

Myasthenia gravis

Complete bundle branch block or other severe intraventricular conduction defects, especially those causing a marked widening of the QRS complex

Hypersensitivity or idiosyncratic reaction to quinidine

Aberrant impulses and abnormal rhythms due to escape mechanisms

ADMINISTRATION/DOSAGE ADJUSTMENTS

Maintenance therapy	The dosages recommended for maintenance of normal rhythm may be reduced (eg, to 1 tab q8–12h) or, if indicated by clinical and laboratory findings (including measurement of serum drug levels and, when feasible, serial ECG monitoring), increased by giving larger individual doses or by administering the drug more frequently (eg, q6h). Treatment may be initiated 2–3 days before cardioversion in order to determine whether a patient can tolerate quinidine therapy.
Hospitalization	Hospitalization for close clinical observation, ECG monitoring, and determination of serum quinidine levels is recommended when large dosages are indicated or when the drug is administered to patients at increased risk
Oral administration	Gastrointestinal disturbances may be minimized by administering the drug with food. To facilitate swallowing, patients should stand up and take the tablets with an adequate amount of fluid. Instruct patients not to crush or chew tablets, since sustained-release properties will be lost as a result.

QUINAGLUTE

Idiosyncratic reactions	Idiosyncrasy to quinidine may be determined by administering a preliminary test dose of 1 tab; tinnitus, headache, nausea, visual disturbances and/or other symptoms of cinchonism may appear in sensitive patients after a single dose

WARNINGS/PRECAUTIONS

Treatment of atrial flutter	Reversion to sinus rhythm may be preceded by a progressive reduction in the degree of AV block to a 1:1 ratio, resulting in an extremely rapid ventricular rate; the risk of ventricular tachycardia may be reduced by digitalization prior to administering quinidine
Cardiotoxicity	Excessive prolongation of the Q-T interval, widening of the QRS complex, ventricular tachyarrhythmias, or other signs of quinidine cardiotoxicity require immediate discontinuation of the drug and/or close clinical and ECG monitoring
Hepatotoxicity	Hepatic toxicity, including granulomatous hepatitis, due to hypersensitivity has been observed in a few patients. Monitoring liver function during the first 4–8 wk of therapy should be considered, because elevation of serum hepatic enzyme levels and/or unexplained fever, especially if they occur in this period, may indicate hepatotoxicity; discontinuation of quinidine therapy usually results in disappearance of the toxicity.
Syncope	Occasional syncopal episodes due (usually) to ventricular tachycardia or fibrillation may occur and have sometimes proved fatal; however, most such episodes end spontaneously or in response to treatment
Patients with signs and symptoms of digitalis intoxication	Treatment with quinidine may cause cardiac rhythm abnormalities in digitalized patients (see also DRUG INTERACTIONS); use with caution if digitalis intoxication is known or suspected. The drug is contraindicated in the presence of digitalis-induced AV conduction disorders.
Patients with hepatic, renal, or cardiac insufficiency	Use with caution to avoid accumulation and potential toxicity
Other special-risk patients	Complete heart block and asystole may occur in patients with incomplete AV block; use with extreme caution. Carefully monitor susceptible patients, such as those with marginally compensated cardiovascular disease, since cardiac depression (eg, hypotension, bradycardia, or heart block) may occur.
Carcinogenicity, mutagenicity, effect on fertility	No studies have been performed to determine the carcinogenic or mutagenic potential of this drug or its effect on fertility

ADVERSE REACTIONS

Gastrointestinal	Nausea, vomiting, abdominal pain, diarrhea
Central nervous system	Headache, fever, vertigo, apprehension, excitement, confusion, delirium, syncope
Auditory	Tinnitus, decreased acuity
Ophthalmic	Mydriasis, blurred vision, disturbed color perception, reduced visual field, photophobia, diplopia, night blindness, scotomata, optic neuritis
Cardiovascular	Widening of QRS complex, cardiac asystole, ectopic ventricular beats, idioventricular rhythms (including ventricular tachycardia and fibrillation), paradoxical tachycardia, arterial embolism, hypotension
Hematological	Acute hemolytic anemia, hypoprothrombinemia, thrombocytopenic purpura, agranulocytosis
Dermatological	Rash, cutaneous flushing with intense pruritus, urticaria, photosensitivity
Hypersensitivity	Angioedema, acute asthmatic episodes, vascular collapse, respiratory arrest, hepatotoxicity (including granulomatous hepatitis); lupus erythematosus (rare)

OVERDOSAGE

Signs and symptoms	Hypotension, heart failure, ventricular arrhythmias, widening of QRS complex ($>$ 0.04 s), prolongation of Q-T interval ($>$ 25%), bradycardia, heart block; symptoms of cinchonism (see ADVERSE REACTIONS)
Treatment	Discontinue use of all antiarrhythmic agents. If ingestion is recent, reduce absorption by emesis, gastric lavage, and/or use of activated charcoal. Management of overdosage includes symptomatic treatment, ECG and blood pressure monitoring, acidification of the urine, and, if necessary, cardiac pacing, artificial respiration, and other supportive measures. Cardiotoxic effects may be treated by IV infusion of 1/6 M sodium lactate. Do not use CNS depressants, since marked CNS depression may occur even in the presence of convulsions. If necessary, treat hypotension with metaraminol or norepinephrine after adequate fluid-volume replacement. Hemodialysis is effective, but rarely warranted.

DRUG INTERACTIONS

Other anticholinergic agents	△ Vagolytic effects
Cholinergic agents	▽ Cholinergic effects
Digoxin	△ Serum level of digoxin, possibly resulting in toxicity; carefully monitor patients on concomitant therapy, and reduce digoxin dosage if indicated

QUINAGLUTE ■ QUINIDEX

Carbonic anhydrase inhibitors, sodium bicarbonate, thiazide diuretics	▽ Excretion of quinidine (due to alkalinization of urine)
Coumarin anticoagulants	▽ Clotting factor concentrations, possibly resulting in hemorrhage
Neuromuscular blocking agents (tubocurare, succinylcholine, decamethonium)	△ Neuromuscular blockade
Phenothiazines, reserpine	△ Cardiac depression
Cimetidine	△ Serum level of quinidine
Hepatic-enzyme-inducing agents (phenobarbital, phenytoin, rifampin)	▽ Serum half-life of quinidine

ALTERED LABORATORY VALUES

No clinically significant alterations in blood/serum or urinary values occur at therapeutic dosages

USE IN CHILDREN

Safety and effectiveness for use in children have not been established

USE IN PREGNANT AND NURSING WOMEN

Pregnancy Category C: use during pregnancy only if clearly needed. Animal reproduction studies have not been done, nor are there any adequate, well-controlled studies in pregnant women. Quinidine does have oxytocic effects, but the clinical significance of this is unknown. The drug is excreted in breast milk; use with caution in nursing mothers.

ANTIARRHYTHMICS

QUINIDEX (quinidine sulfate) Robins   Rx

Tablets (sustained release): 300 mg

INDICATIONS

Premature atrial and ventricular contractions
Paroxysmal atrial tachycardia
Paroxysmal AV junctional rhythm
Atrial flutter
Paroxysmal atrial fibrillation
Established atrial fibrillation when therapy is appropriate
Paroxysmal ventricular tachycardia, except when associated with complete heart block
Maintenance of normal sinus rhythm following electrical conversion of atrial fibrillation and/or flutter

ORAL DOSAGE

Adult: 300–600 mg q8–12h

CONTRAINDICATIONS

Intraventricular conduction defects	Atrioventricular block	Aberrant impulses and abnormal rhythms due to escape mechanisms
Hypersensitivity or idiosyncratic reaction to quinidine		

ADMINISTRATION/DOSAGE ADJUSTMENTS

Gastrointestinal disturbances	May be minimized by administering the drug with food

WARNINGS/PRECAUTIONS

Treatment of atrial flutter	Reversion to sinus rhythm may be preceded by a progressive reduction in the degree of AV block to a 1:1 ratio, resulting in an extremely rapid ventricular rate; the risk of ventricular tachycardia may be reduced by digitalization prior to administering quinidine
Cardiotoxicity	Excessive prolongation of the Q-T interval, 50% widening of the QRS complex, frequent ventricular ectopic beats, or other signs of quinidine cardiotoxicity require immediate discontinuation of the drug, followed by close clinical and ECG monitoring
Patients with signs and symptoms of digitalis intoxication	Treatment with quinidine may cause unpredictable cardiac rhythm abnormalities in digitalized patients (see also DRUG INTERACTIONS); use with particular caution if digitalis intoxication is known or suspected
Potassium serum levels	Hypokalemia may reduce antiarrhythmic effectiveness, while hyperkalemia may enhance quinidine toxicity

QUINIDEX ■ Quinidine sulfate

Patients with congestive heart failure or hypotension	Cardiac contractility and arterial blood pressure are depressed; use quinidine only if heart failure or hypotension are due to, or aggravated by, the arrhythmia
Patients with hepatic or renal impairment	Hepatic or renal insufficiency may delay excretion, increase serum levels, and lead to systemic accumulation (see OVERDOSAGE); use with caution
Other special-risk patients	Use with caution in patients with incomplete heart block, bronchial asthma or other respiratory disorders, myasthenia gravis, muscle weakness, acute infection, or hyperthyroidism
Long-term therapy	Perform periodic blood counts and liver and kidney function tests; discontinue use if blood dyscrasias or signs of hepatic or renal impairment occur

ADVERSE REACTIONS

Allergic and idiosyncratic	Fever, skin eruptions, thrombocytopenia (extremely rare)
Central nervous system	Tinnitus, blurred vision, dizziness, light-headedness, tremor
Gastrointestinal	Nausea, vomiting, diarrhea, colic
Cardiovascular	Ventricular extrasystoles, widening of QRS complex, complete AV block, ventricular tachycardia

OVERDOSAGE

Signs and symptoms	Hypotension, heart failure, ventricular arrhythmias, widening of QRS complex ($>$ 0.04 s), prolongation of Q-T interval ($>$ 25%), bradycardia, heart block; symptoms of cinchonism (see ADVERSE REACTIONS)
Treatment	Discontinue use of all antiarrhythmic agents. If ingestion is recent, reduce absorption by emesis, gastric lavage, and/or use of activated charcoal. Management of overdosage includes symptomatic treatment, ECG and blood pressure monitoring, acidification of the urine, and, if necessary, cardiac pacing, artificial respiration, and other supportive measures. Cardiotoxic effects may be treated by IV infusion of 1/6 M sodium lactate. Do not use CNS depressants, since marked CNS depression may occur even in the presence of convulsions. If necessary, treat hypotension with metaraminol or norepinephrine after adequate fluid-volume replacement. Hemodialysis is effective, but rarely warranted.

DRUG INTERACTIONS

Other antiarrhythmic agents	△ Depression of excitability
Oral anticoagulants	△ Hypoprothrombinemia, possibly resulting in hemorrhage
Neuromuscular blocking agents	△ Neuromuscular blockade
Phenobarbital, phenytoin	▽ Serum half-life of quinidine
Digoxin	△ Digoxin serum level, possibly resulting in toxicity

ALTERED LABORATORY VALUES

No clinically significant alterations in blood/serum or urinary values occur at therapeutic dosages

---

USE IN CHILDREN

Not recommended for use in children under 12 yr of age

USE IN PREGNANT AND NURSING WOMEN

Pregnancy Category C: use during pregnancy only if clearly needed. Animal reproduction studies have not been done, nor are there any adequate, well-controlled studies in pregnant women. Quinidine does have oxytocic effects, but the clinical significance of this is unknown. The drug is excreted in breast milk; use with caution in nursing mothers.

ANTIARRHYTHMICS

Quinidine sulfate Warner-Chilcott   Rx

Tablets: 200 mg

INDICATIONS

Atrial arrhythmias characterized by flutter, fibrillation (paroxysmal or established), premature contractions, or paroxysmal tachycardia
Paroxysmal AV junctional rhythm
Ventricular arrhythmias characterized by paroxysmal tachycardia (when not associated with complete heart block) or premature contractions

ORAL DOSAGE

Adult: for premature atrial and ventricular contractions and for maintenance after electrical conversion of atrial flutter or fibrillation, 200–300 mg tid or qid; for paroxysmal supraventricular tachycardias, 400–600 mg q2–3h; for conversion of atrial fibrillation, 200 mg q2–3h for 5–8 doses, followed, as tolerated and needed, by daily increases in dosage, up to a maximum of 3–4 g/day

COMPENDIUM OF DRUG THERAPY

Quinidine sulfate

CONTRAINDICATIONS

Hypersensitivity or idiosyncratic reaction to quinidine

History of thrombocytopenic purpura associated with quinidine

Digitalis toxicity manifested by AV conduction disorders

Complete AV block with an AV nodal or idioventricular pacemaker

Left bundle branch block or other severe intraventricular conduction defects with marked QRS widening

Ectopic impulses and abnormal rhythms due to escape mechanisms

Myasthenia gravis

ADMINISTRATION/DOSAGE ADJUSTMENTS

Test dose — To test for idiosyncrasy to quinidine, give a preliminary dose of 200 mg; look for symptoms of cinchonism, such as tinnitus, headache, nausea, and visual disturbances

High-risk patients — Hospitalize patients who are receiving more than 2 g/day or who have special-risk conditions (see WARNINGS/PRECAUTIONS); close clinical observation, continuous ECG monitoring, and determination of plasma drug levels are recommended for these patients

Monitoring of plasma drug levels — Therapeutic plasma drug levels, based on assays that measured metabolites as well as the intact drug, have been reported to be 2–7 μg/ml; the therapeutic range will be lower when a more specific assay is used. Ask laboratories to indicate in their reports the method of analysis as well as the plasma levels. Since response to therapy varies widely among patients, optimal dosage should be based not only on plasma drug levels, but also on clinical response and ECG results.

Treatment of atrial flutter or fibrillation — During conversion of atrial flutter or fibrillation, the degree of AV block may be progressively reduced to a 1:1 ratio and the ventricular rate may become extremely rapid; to reduce this risk and to control the ventricular rate and congestive heart failure (when present), digitalize before giving quinidine for conversion. For treatment of fibrillation, see ORAL DOSAGE; the dosage for atrial flutter should be individualized.

Maintenance therapy — If the recommended dosage for maintenance therapy appears to be inadequate, the dosage may be increased—but only if clinical and laboratory findings (including the plasma drug level) are carefully evaluated beforehand and serial ECGs are obtained, if possible

Management of GI reactions — To minimize GI disturbances, give this drug with food

WARNINGS/PRECAUTIONS

Cardiotoxicity — If excessive prolongation of the Q–T interval, 50% widening of the QRS complex, or frequent ventricular ectopic beats are detected, discontinue administration immediately and closely monitor ECG. The pharmacologic effects of quinidine are directly related to the plasma potassium level.

Cardiovascular depression — Quinidine depresses cardiac function and arterial blood pressure. Carefully monitor patients with marginally compensated cardiovascular disease, since clinically significant hypotension, bradycardia, or heart block may occur in these patients. To avoid complete heart block or asystole in patients with incomplete AV block, exercise extreme caution. Use in patients with congestive heart failure or hypotension only if these conditions are associated with an arrhythmia and the benefits and risks of therapy have been weighed.

Syncope — Syncope may occur occasionally, usually as a result of ventricular tachycardia or fibrillation, and sometimes may be fatal; this reaction is not related to dose or plasma drug level

Hypersensitivity — The risk of hypersensitivity should always be considered, especially during the first weeks of therapy. Hepatotoxic effects, including granulomatous hepatitis, have occurred in a few patients as a result of hypersensitivity; these effects have usually been reversed by discontinuation of therapy. Consider monitoring hepatic function during the first 4–8 wk of therapy; if unexplained fever or elevation of hepatic enzymes is detected, particularly during the early stages of therapy, consider a diagnosis of quinidine-induced hepatotoxicity.

Drug accumulation — To avoid toxic plasma drug levels, use with caution in patients with renal, hepatic, or cardiac impairment; quinidine is metabolized in the liver and excreted by the kidney

Carcinogenicity, mutagenicity, effect on fertility — No long-term studies have been done to evaluate the carcinogenic effect of quinidine. No evidence of mutagenicity or impairment of fertility has been reported.

ADVERSE REACTIONS[1]

The most frequent reactions, regardless of incidence, are printed in *italics*

Gastrointestinal — *Nausea, vomiting, abdominal pain, diarrhea*

Cardiovasular — Widening of QRS complex, cardiac asystole, ventricular ectopic beats, idioventricular rhythms (including ventricular tachycardia and fibrillation), paradoxical tachycardia, arterial embolism, hypotension

Hematological — Acute hemolytic anemia, hypoprothrombinemia, thrombocytopenic purpura, agranulocytosis

Central nervous system — Headache, fever, vertigo, apprehension, excitement, confusion, delirium, syncope

Quinidine sulfate ■ SECTRAL

Ophthalmic	Mydriasis, blurred vision, disturbed color perception, reduced visual field, photophobia, diplopia, night blindness, scotomata, optic neuritis
Otic	Tinnitus, decreased auditory acuity
Dermatological	Rash, cutaneous flushing with intense pruritus, urticaria, photosensitivity
Hypersensitivity	Angioedema, acute asthmatic episode, vascular collapse, respiratory arrest, hepatotoxicity (including granulomatous hepatitis)

OVERDOSAGE

Signs and symptoms	See ADVERSE REACTIONS
Treatment	Induce emesis and then administer activated charcoal. Give IV fluids for hypotension; norepinephrine may be administered if arrhythmias are not present and ECG is monitored. Maintain respiratory function. Use M/6 sodium lactate injection to increase protein binding of the drug and lower the plasma potassium level. Institute forced diuresis to enhance excretion of the drug.

DRUG INTERACTIONS

Digoxin	△ Risk of digitalis toxicity and arrhythmias; if combination therapy is necessary, reduce dosage of digoxin, monitor the plasma digoxin level, and watch closely for evidence of toxicity
Oral anticoagulants	△ Risk of bleeding; exercise caution during combination therapy
Anticholinergic drugs	△ Vagolytic effect
Cholinergic drugs	▽ Cholinergic effect
Thiazide diuretics, carbonic anhydrase inhibitors, sodium bicarbonate, and other urinary alkalinizers	△ Plasma level of quinidine
Phenobarbital, phenytoin, rifampin, and other drugs capable of inducing hepatic enzymes	▽ Plasma level of quinidine
Tubocurarine, succinylcholine, decamethonium, pancuronium	△ Neuromuscular blockade
Phenothiazines, reserpine	△ Cardiac depression

ALTERED LABORATORY VALUES

No clinically significant alterations in blood/serum or urinary values occur at therapeutic dosages

---

USE IN CHILDREN

No adequate, well-controlled studies have been done in children to establish safety and effectiveness

---

USE IN PREGNANT AND NURSING WOMEN

Pregnant women: Pregnancy Category C: reproduction studies have not been done. It has been reported that quinidine has oxytocic properties; the clinical significance of this finding is not known. Use during pregnancy only if clearly needed. **Nursing mothers:** Quinidine is excreted in human milk; use with caution in nursing mothers.

---

[1] Extremely rare cases of lupus erythematosus have been reported, but a causal relationship has not been established

---

ANTIARRHYTHMICS

SECTRAL (acebutolol hydrochloride) Wyeth   Rx

Capsules: 200, 400 mg

INDICATIONS	ORAL DOSAGE
Hypertension	**Adult:** for uncomplicated mild to moderate hypertension, 400 mg/day, given once daily or, in certain cases, in 2 divided doses, to start; for maintenance, 400–800 mg/day or, in some cases, 200 mg/day. To treat refractory or more severe hypertension, administer another antihypertensive agent (eg, a thiazide diuretic) in combination with acebutolol or, alternatively, give 1,200 mg/day of acebutolol in 2 divided doses.
Premature ventricular contractions, including paired and multiform ectopic beats and R-on-T beats	**Adult:** 200 mg bid to start, followed by a gradual increase in dosage; for maintenance, 600–1,200 mg/day

SECTRAL

CONTRAINDICATIONS

Overt cardiac failure
Cardiogenic shock
Second- and third-degree AV block
Persistently severe bradycardia

ADMINISTRATION/DOSAGE ADJUSTMENTS

Patients with renal impairment	Reduce recommended daily dose by 50% if creatinine clearance (Ccr) is less than 50 ml/min and by 75% if Ccr is less than 25 ml/min
Elderly patients	A lower maintenance dosage may be necessary for elderly patients, since the bioavailability of acebutolol and its major metabolite, diacetolol, is increased approximately two-fold in these patients. Dosage in elderly patients should not exceed 800 mg/day.

WARNINGS/PRECAUTIONS

Cardiac failure	Beta blockade may exacerbate cardiac failure and, in patients with aortic or mitral valve disease or compromised left ventricular function, may precipitate cardiac failure. Nevertheless, acebutolol may be used with caution in patients with well-compensated congestive heart failure; it should be borne in mind that acebutolol as well as digitalis increase AV conduction time. If cardiac failure occurs during treatment and does not respond to digitalization and diuretic therapy, acebutolol should be discontinued.
Angina	Abrupt withdrawal of certain beta blockers can exacerbate angina and, in some cases, precipitate myocardial infarction and death. Caution patients not to interrupt or terminate therapy on their own. To discontinue acebutolol, even if ischemic heart disease is not evident, gradually withdraw the drug over a period of approximately 2 wk and restrict to a minimum the level of physical activity. During this period, carefully observe the patient; if exacerbation of angina occurs, the patient should be hospitalized and acebutolol therapy reinstituted immediately.
Bronchospasm	In general, patients with bronchospastic disease should not receive beta blockers. However, if other antihypertensive treatment is not effective or tolerated, acebutolol may be used with caution in these patients because of its *relative* selectivity for beta$_1$ receptors. For these patients, acebutolol should be given initially at the lowest possible daily dose (preferably in divided doses) since beta$_1$ selectivity diminishes as the dosage is increased; in addition, a bronchodilator (eg, theophylline) or a beta$_2$ agonist should be provided for emergency treatment.
Arterial insufficiency	In patients with peripheral or mesenteric vascular disease, beta blockade may cause or exacerbate symptoms of arterial insufficiency; use with caution in such patients, watching closely for progression of arterial obstruction
Major surgery	The necessity or desirability of discontinuing therapy before major surgery is controversial; beta blockade may prevent arrhythmia during surgery by reducing cardiac responsiveness to reflex stimuli, yet may increase the risk of myocardial depression and cause difficulty in restarting and maintaining the heartbeat. If acebutolol is not withdrawn, use at the lowest possible dosage, and exercise particular care when administering general anesthetics that can depress the myocardium, such as ether, cyclopropane, and trichlorethylene.
Hypoglycemia	Beta blockade may mask certain manifestations of hypoglycemia, such as tachycardia; however, in most cases, symptomatic dizziness and sweating are not significantly affected
Hyperthyroidism	Abrupt withdrawal of beta blockade can precipitate a thyroid storm in patients with hyperthyroidism; since certain clinical signs of this disorder (such as tachycardia) can be masked during therapy, patients should be closely observed during the period of withdrawal, even if thyrotoxicosis is only suspected.
Positive ANA titers	In <1% of patients, positive ANA titers were seen in association with persistent arthralgia or myalgia; these reactions disappeared following discontinuation of therapy
Patients with hepatic impairment	Use with caution in patients with hepatic impairment
Carcinogenicity, mutagenicity, effect on fertility	No evidence of carcinogenicity has been seen in rats and mice fed 15 times the maximum human dose of acebutolol or in rats given up to 1.8 g/kg/day of diacetolol, the major metabolite. Use of acebutolol and diacetolol in the Ames test has resulted in negative findings. No significant effect on reproductive performance or fertility has occurred in rats fed up to 12 times the maximum human dose of acebutolol or given up to 1 g/kg/day of diacetolol.

ADVERSE REACTIONS[1]

Frequent reactions (≥ 2%) are italicized

Cardiovascular	*Chest pain and edema (2%)*, hypotension, bradycardia, heart failure
Respiratory	*Dyspnea (4%), rhinitis (2%)*, cough, pharyngitis, wheezing
Central nervous system	*Fatigue (11%), headache and dizziness (6%), insomnia (3%), depression and abnormal dreams (2%)*, anxiety, hyper- or hypoesthesia, impotence
Ophthalmic	*Abnormal vision (2%)*, conjunctivitis, dry eyes, eye pain
Musculoskeletal	*Arthralgia and myalgia (2%)*, back pain, joint pain

SECTRAL ■ TAMBOCOR

Gastrointestinal	*Constipation, diarrhea, dyspepsia, and nausea (4%), flatulence (3%),* vomiting, abdominal pain
Genitourinary	*Urinary frequency (3%),* dysuria, nocturia
Dermatological	*Rash (2%),* pruritus

OVERDOSAGE

Signs and symptoms	Extreme bradycardia, advanced AV block, intraventricular conduction defects, hypotension, severe congestive heart failure, seizures, and, in susceptible patients, bronchospasm and hypoglycemia
Treatment	Induce emesis or perform gastric lavage; remove acebutolol from the blood by hemodialysis. For excessive bradycardia, give 1–3 mg of atropine in fractional IV doses. If response to vagal blockade is inadequate, administer isoproterenol; exercise caution since unusually large doses may be necessary. For persistent hypotension, give a vasopressor such as epinephrine, norepinephrine, dopamine, or dobutamine; monitor blood pressure and heartbeat frequently. Treat bronchospasm with a theophylline derivative, such as aminophylline, and/or beta$_2$ agonist, such as terbutaline. For cardiac failure, administer digitalis and a diuretic; glucagon may also be helpful.

DRUG INTERACTIONS

Reserpine, other catecholamine-depleting drugs	⇧ Risk of marked bradycardia and hypotension; watch carefully for vertigo, syncope/presyncope, and other manifestations of orthostatic hypotension
Phenylephrine, phenylpropanolamine, other alpha-adrenergic agonists	⇧ Hypertension; warn patients that this reaction can occur with use of certain OTC cold or decongestant preparations
General anesthetics	⇧ Risk of excessive myocardial depression (see warning, above, concerning major surgery)
Insulin	⇧ Hypoglycemic effect

ALTERED LABORATORY VALUES

Blood/serum values	+ ANA

No clinically significant alterations in urinary values occur at therapeutic dosages

USE IN CHILDREN

Safety and effectiveness for use in children have not been established

USE IN PREGNANT AND NURSING WOMEN

Pregnancy Category B: an increase in postimplantation loss (along with a reduction in food consumption and weight gain) has been seen in rabbits given 450 mg/kg/day of acebutolol's major metabolite, diacetolol; no evidence of harm to the fetus has been shown in rats and rabbits at up to 3 times the maximum human dose of acebutolol or in rats at up to 1.8 g/kg/day of diacetolol. Use during pregnancy only if the expected benefit justifies the potential risk to the fetus. In animal studies using acebutolol, no adverse effects on the usual course of labor and delivery have been demonstrated. Acebutolol and diacetolol are excreted in human milk; use by nursing mothers is not recommended.

[1] Reactions associated with the use of other beta blockers include intensification of AV block; reversible mental depression progressing to catatonia; an acute reversible syndrome characterized by temporal and spatial disorientation, short-term memory loss, emotional lability, slightly clouded sensorium, and decreased performance on neuropsychometric tests; erythematous rash; fever with sore throat and aching; laryngospasm; respiratory distress; agranulocytosis; purpura; mesenteric artery thrombosis; ischemic colitis; reversible alopecia; and Peyronie's disease.

ANTIARRHYTHMICS

TAMBOCOR (flecainide acetate) Riker   Rx

Tablets: 100 mg

INDICATIONS

Life-threatening ventricular arrhythmias, such as sustained ventricular tachycardia

Symptomatic nonsustained ventricular tachycardia and frequent premature ventricular complexes

ORAL DOSAGE

Adult: 100 mg q12h to start, followed by increases of 50 mg bid every 4 days until optimal response is achieved; for maintenance dosage, see ADMINISTRATION/DOSAGE ADJUSTMENTS. Do not give a loading dose.

TAMBOCOR

CONTRAINDICATIONS

Preexisting second- or third-degree AV block

Hypersensitivity to flecainide

Right bundle branch block associated with left hemiblock (bifascicular block), unless a pacemaker is present

Cardiogenic shock

ADMINISTRATION/DOSAGE ADJUSTMENTS

Limitations of treatment	The effects of flecainide in patients with supraventricular arrhythmias and in patients with recent acute myocardial infarction have not been adequately studied; flecainide, like other antiarrhythmics, has not been shown to have a favorable effect on mortality or sudden death
Maintenance dosage	Most patients with sustained ventricular tachycardia do not require more than 150 mg q12h, but may be given up to 400 mg/day. Likewise, most patients with symptomatic nonsustained ventricular tachycardia, couplets, or premature ventricular complexes do not require more than 200 mg q12h; should such patients still show symptoms at 400 mg/day, and the plasma level is below 0.6 μg/ml, cautiously increase the dosage up to 600 mg/day. Patients who are not adequately controlled by (or intolerant to) dosing at 12-h intervals may be given the drug q8h.
Hospitalization	Because of the relatively high frequency of arrhythmogenic events in patients with sustained ventricular tachycardia and serious underlying structural heart disease, therapy should be initiated in the hospital to permit close clinical observation and ECG monitoring
Patients with a history of congestive heart failure or myocardial dysfunction	Do not give more than 100 mg q12h initially or exceed 200 mg q12h (400 mg/day) in patients with congestive heart failure or myocardial dysfunction; exacerbation of congestive heart failure may occur at higher doses
Patients with renal impairment	Increase dosage cautiously at longer than 4-day intervals in patients with renal impairment; observe patient closely for signs of adverse cardiac effects or toxicity. Because more than 4 days may be needed to reach a new steady-state plasma level following a change in dosage, plasma level monitoring should guide adjustments of dosage.
Plasma level monitoring	Optimal results have been observed in patients with trough plasma levels of 0.2–1.0 μg/ml. The probability of adverse cardiac effects may increase with higher trough plasma levels, especially at levels exceeding 1.0 μg/ml. Elimination of flecainide may be slower in patients with severe chronic renal failure or severe congestive heart failure; plasma level monitoring may be especially helpful in these patients.
Patients with electronic pacemakers	Determine the pacing threshold prior to starting flecainide therapy; repeat after 1 wk of therapy and at regular intervals thereafter. When threshold changes are within the range of multiprogrammable pacemakers, a doubling of either voltage or pulse width is sufficient to regain capture.
Transferring patients from other antiarrhythmic agents	Allow at least 2–4 plasma half-lives to elapse for the drug being discontinued before starting flecainide therapy; when withdrawal of a previous antiarrhythmic agent may produce life-threatening arrhythmias, consider hospitalization of the patient

WARNINGS/PRECAUTIONS

Heart block	Clinically significant conduction changes, including sinus node dysfunction such as sinus pause, sinus arrest, and symptomatic bradycardia (1.2%), second-degree AV block (0.5%), and third-degree AV block (0.4%), have occurred; manage patients on the lowest effective dosage to minimize these effects. If second- or third-degree AV block or right bundle branch block associated with a left hemiblock occurs, discontinue use of flecainide, unless the ventricular rate is controlled with an artificial pacemaker.
ECG changes	Flecainide can increase the P–R, QRS, and Q–T intervals. The P–R interval increases by an average of 25% (0.04 s), but may increase by as much as 118% in some patients; approximately one-third of patients may develop new first-degree AV heart block (P–R interval $\geq$ 0.20 s). Likewise, the QRS interval increases by an average of 25% (0.02 s), but may increase by as much as 150% (many patients develop QRS complexes $\geq$ 0.12 s). The Q–T interval widens approximately 8%, about 60%–90% resulting from widening of the QRS complex. The J–T interval (Q–T minus QRS) widens an average of 4%; significant J–T prolongation occurs in less than 2% of patients. Increases of the P–R interval to $\geq$ 0.30 s or of the QRS interval to $\geq$ 0.18 s are uncommon; use with caution and consider reducing the dose when such intervals occur.
Arrhythmogenic effects	Flecainide can cause new arrhythmias or worsen existing arrhythmias, including an increased frequency of PVCs and development of more severe and potentially fatal ventricular tachycardia (eg, tachycardia that is more sustained or resistant to conversion to sinus rhythm)
Congestive heart failure (CHF)	Use with caution in patients with a history of congestive heart failure or myocardial dysfunction (see ADMINISTRATION/DOSAGE ADJUSTMENTS). Flecainide may cause or worsen CHF, particularly in patients with cardiomyopathy, preexisting severe heart failure (NYHA functional class III or IV), or low ejection fractions (< 30%); in clinical trials, new or worsened CHF occurred in approximately 5% of patients taking flecainide, and approximately 1% of patients with no previous history developed CHF.

TAMBOCOR

Sick sinus syndrome	Flecainide may cause sinus bradycardia, sinus pause, or sinus arrest in patients with sick sinus syndrome; use with extreme caution in such patients
Patients with electronic pacemakers	Flecainide increases endocardial pacing thresholds and may suppress ventricular escape rhythms; these effects are reversible upon discontinuation of the drug. Use with caution in patients with permanent pacemakers or those with temporary pacing electrodes; do not use in patients with existing poor thresholds or nonprogrammable pacemakers unless suitable pacing rescue is available.
Potassium imbalance	Hypokalemia or hyperkalemia may alter the effects of Class I antiarrhythmic drugs; correct preexisting potassium imbalance before instituting flecainide therapy
Patients with hepatic impairment	Flecainide undergoes extensive biotransformation, most probably in the liver; do not use in patients with significant hepatic impairment unless the expected benefits outweigh the potential risks of therapy. Although hepatic dysfunction has been reported rarely after administration of flecainide, discontinue use in patients developing unexplained jaundice or other signs of hepatic dysfunction.
Blood dyscrasias	Discontinue use if signs of blood dyscrasias develop
Carcinogenicity, mutagenicity, effect on fertility	No evidence of carcinogenicity has been seen in rats and mice fed up to 8 times the usual human dose. No mutagenic activity has been shown in the Ames test, the mouse lymphoma test, or in vivo cytogenetic studies. Oral administration of up to 7 times the usual human dose has not adversely affected fertility in rats.

ADVERSE REACTIONS

Frequent reactions (incidence $\geq$ 1%) are printed in *italics*

Central nervous system	*Dizziness, including lightheadedness, faintness, unsteadiness, and near syncope (18.9%); headache (9.6%), fatigue (7.7%), asthenia (4.9%), tremor (4.7%); hypothesia, paresthesia, paresis, ataxia, flushing, increased sweating, vertigo, syncope, somnolence, tinnitus, anxiety, insomnia, and depression (1–3%);* twitching, weakness, change in taste, dry mouth, convulsions, impotence, speech disorder, stupor, amnesia, confusion, decreased libido, depersonalization, euphoria, morbid dreams, apathy
Cardiovascular	*New or exacerbated ventricular arrhythmias (7%); chest pain (5.4%); new or worsened congestive heart failure (5%); edema (3.5%); sinus bradycardia, sinus pause, or sinus arrest (1.2%);* unresuscitatable ventricular tachycardia or ventricular fibrillation, second- or third-degree AV block, angina pectoris, bradycardia, hypertension, hypotension
Ophthalmic	*Visual disturbance, including blurred vision, difficulty in focusing, and spots before the eyes (15.9%), diplopia (1–3%),* eye pain or irritation, photophobia, nystagmus
Respiratory	*Dyspnea (10.3%),* bronchospasm
Gastrointestinal	*Nausea (8.9%), constipation (4.4%), abdominal pain (3.3%), vomiting, diarrhea, dyspepsia, and anorexia (1–3%),* flatulence
Hematological	Leukopenia, thrombocytopenia; blood dyscrasias (extremely rare)
Genitourinary	Polyuria, urinary retention
Dermatological	*Rash (1–3%),* urticaria, exfoliative dermatitis, pruritus
Hepatic	Hepatic dysfunction, including cholestasis and hepatic failure (rare)
Other	*Malaise and fever (1–3%),* arthralgia, myalgia, swollen lips, tongue, and mouth

OVERDOSAGE

Signs and symptoms	Lengthening of P–R interval, increase in QRS duration, prolongation of Q–T interval, increase in amplitude of T-wave, reduction in myocardial rate and contractility, conduction disturbances, hypotension, death from respiratory failure or asystole
Treatment	Management of overdosage includes symptomatic treatment, administration of inotropic agents or cardiac stimulants such as dopamine, dobutamine, or isoproterenol; mechanically assisted ventilation, and intra-aortic counterpulsation. Institute transvenous pacing for conduction block. Supportive measures may be necessary for extended periods because of the long plasma half-life of flecainide (12–27 h in patients receiving usual doses). Hemodialysis is not effective.

DRUG INTERACTIONS

Digoxin	⇧ Plasma digoxin level
Propranolol	⇧ Plasma propranolol and flecainide levels ⇧ Negative inotropic effect
Calcium-channel blockers, disopyramide	Effects unknown; concomitant administration of nifedipine or diltiazem with flecainide is not recommended and, because of their negative inotropic effect, verapamil and disopyramide should not be given with flecainide unless the expected benefit outweighs the potential risk

ALTERED LABORATORY VALUES

Blood/serum	⇧ Alkaline phosphatase ⇧ SGOT ⇧ SGPT

No clinically significant alterations in urinary values occur at therapeutic dosages

TAMBOCOR ■ TONOCARD

USE IN CHILDREN

Safety and effectiveness for use in children and adolescents under 18 yr of age have not been established

USE IN PREGNANT AND NURSING WOMEN

Pregnancy Category C: reproduction studies in rabbits given 4 times the usual human dose of flecainide have shown teratogenic effects (club paws, sternebrae and vertebrae abnormalities, pale hearts with contracted ventricular septum) and an increase in resorptions in the New Zealand White breed but not in the Dutch Belted breed. No teratogenic effects have been observed in rats or mice; however, delayed sternebral and vertebral ossification was observed in rats given 50 mg/kg/day. No adequate, well-controlled studies have been done in pregnant women. Use during pregnancy only if the expected benefit justifies the potential risk to the fetus. It is not known if flecainide is excreted in human milk; because of the potential for serious adverse effects in nursing infants, patients who require the drug should not nurse.

ANTIARRHYTHMICS

TONOCARD (tocainide hydrochloride) Merck Sharp & Dohme   Rx

Tablets: 400, 600 mg

INDICATIONS

Symptomatic ventricular arrhythmias, including frequent premature ventricular contractions (unifocal or multifocal), couplets, and ventricular tachycardia

ORAL DOSAGE

Adult: 400 mg q8h to start; usual maintenance dosage: 400–600 mg q8h. For patients with renal or hepatic impairment, who may eliminate this drug at a significantly slower rate, and for some other patients, a dosage of less than 1,200 mg/day may be adequate. Use at dosages exceeding 2,400 mg/day has been infrequent. Twice-daily administration, with careful monitoring, may be tried in patients who tolerate the tid regimen.

CONTRAINDICATIONS

Hypersensitivity to tocainide or amide-type local anesthetics

Second- or third-degree AV block (except when an artificial ventricular pacemaker is present)

ADMINISTRATION/DOSAGE ADJUSTMENTS

Monitoring of therapy — Assess effectiveness and tolerance by clinical and ECG evaluation (Holter monitoring may be necessary). If no therapeutic effect is observed, look for evidence of hypokalemia, since antiarrhythmic drugs may be ineffective in patients with below-normal serum potassium levels; correct any underlying potassium deficit and then reassess response. If control of arrhythmias decreases at the end of a dosing interval, increase the dose and/or use a shorter dose interval. Watch for tremor when titrating dosage, since this symptom, when it occurs, may be a useful indication that the maximum dose is being approached. Manage dizziness, paresthesias, nausea, and tremor, which are generally the most frequent reactions, by reducing the dosage, administering with food, or discontinuing therapy. If adverse reactions occur soon after administration of a dose, divide the daily dose into smaller individual doses. Use of tocainide should be reconsidered if a clear response is not evident.

WARNINGS/PRECAUTIONS

Blood dyscrasias — Agranulocytosis, bone marrow depression, leukopenia, neutropenia, hypoplastic anemia, and thrombocytopenia have occurred in 0.18% of patients, usually during the first 12 wk of therapy; these reactions have been fatal (approximately 25% of those with agranulocytosis subsequently died). To reduce the risk, perform a complete blood count (including a white cell, differential, and platelet count) weekly during the first 3 mo of therapy and periodically thereafter. Instruct patients to report immediately the development of bruising or bleeding, or any sign of infection, such as fever, sore throat, chills, or stomatitis. Promptly determine blood counts whenever a sign or symptom of dyscrasia is seen; if any of the hematological disorders cited above is diagnosed, withdraw tocainamide, and, if necessary, institute appropriate treatment (blood counts usually return to normal within 1 mo after termination of therapy). Use tocainamide with caution in patients with preexisting bone marrow failure or any type of cytopenia.

Pulmonary disorders — Tocainide may be associated with the development of pulmonary fibrosis, interstitial pneumonitis, fibrosing alveolitis, pulmonary edema, and pneumonia. Fibrosis has occurred in 0.11% of patients, and the other reactions have been seen in less than 1% of patients; signs and symptoms have usually appeared 3–18 wk after the start of therapy. Instruct patients to report promptly the development of pulmonary symptoms, such as exertional dyspnea, cough, and wheezing; if symptoms occur, take chest x-rays and look for evidence of bilateral infiltration. If any of these pulmonary disorders is diagnosed, therapy should be discontinued.

Arrhythmogenicity — Worsening of arrhythmias can occur in some patients; infrequently, tocainide causes an increase in the ventricular rate in patients with atrial flutter or fibrillation

COMPENDIUM OF DRUG THERAPY

TONOCARD

Myocardial depression	Use with caution in patients with cardiac failure or minimal cardiac reserve, especially when administering a beta blocker concomitantly, because tocainide has a small negative inotropic effect and, therefore, may exacerbate heart failure
AV block	Exercise caution if cardiac conductivity becomes increasingly depressed during therapy (see CONTRAINDICATIONS)
Hepatic impairment	Abnormal liver function tests (particularly in the early stages of therapy) and some cases of hepatitis and jaundice have been reported; consider periodic monitoring of liver function
Prophylactic use	Tocainide has not been shown to prevent sudden death in patients with serious ventricular ectopic activity
Carcinogenicity, mutagenicity, effect of fertility	No evidence of carcinogenicity has been seen in rats fed up to 8 times the usual human dose for 24 mo or in mice fed up to 12 times the usual human dose for 94 wk (male mice) or 102 wk (female mice). No mutagenic activity has been shown in the Ames test, the mouse micronucleus test (with oral doses of up to 7 times the usual human dose), or the mouse lymphoma forward mutation assay. Oral administration of up to 8 times the usual human dose has not adversely affected fertility in rats.

ADVERSE REACTIONS

Frequent reactions (incidence ≥ 1%) are printed in *italics*

Cardiovascular	*Increase in ventricular arrhythmias (including premature ventricular contractions), congestive heart failure, exacerbation of heart failure, tachycardia, hypotension, conduction disturbances, bradycardia, palpitations, chest pain, left ventricular failure,* ventricular fibrillation, extension of acute myocardial infarction, cardiogenic shock, angina, AV block, hypertension, widening of QRS complex, pleurisy/pericarditis, prolonged Q-T interval, right bundle branch block, syncope, vasovagal episodes, cardiomegaly, sinus arrest, claudication, cold extremities, edema, pallor, flush
Gastrointestinal	*Nausea, vomiting, anorexia, diarrhea/loose stools,* hepatitis, jaundice, abnormal liver function tests, stomatitis, abdominal pain/discomfort, constipation, dysphagia, digestive symptoms (including dyspepsia), dry mouth, thirst
Musculoskeletal	*Arthritis/arthralgia, myalgia,* muscle cramps, muscle twitching/spasm, neck pain, pain radiating from neck, pressure on shoulder
Central nervous system	*Dizziness/vertigo, tremor, nervousness, confusion/disorientation/hallucinations, altered mood/awareness, ataxia, paresthesia, headache, tiredness/drowsiness/ fatigue/lethargy/lassitude/sleepiness, incoordination/unsteadiness/walking disturbances, anxiety, hot/cold feelings,* coma, convulsions/seizures, myasthenia gravis, depression, psychosis, psychic disturbances, agitation, decreased mental acuity, dysarthria, impaired memory, increased stuttering/slurred speech, insomnia/sleeping disturbances, local anesthesia, dream abnormalities
Dermatological	*Rash/skin lesion, diaphoresis, lupus,* Stevens-Johnson syndrome, exfoliative dermatitis, erythema multiforme, urticaria, alopecia, pruritus, pallor/flushed face
Ophthalmic	*Blurred vision/visual disturbances, nystagmus,* diplopia
Otic	*Tinnitus/hearing loss,* earache
Hematological	Agranulocytosis, bone marrow depression, hypoplastic anemia, anemia, leukopenia, neutropenia, thrombocytopenia
Pulmonary	Respiratory arrest, pulmonary edema, pulmonary embolism, pulmonary fibrosis, fibrosing alveolitis, pneumonia, interstitial pneumonitis, dyspnea, hiccoughs, yawning
Genitourinary	Urinary retention, polyuria/increased diuresis
Other	Increased ANA titer, fever, cinchonism, asthenia, malaise, taste/smell perversion

OVERDOSAGE

Signs and symptoms	Central nervous system reactions, followed by GI disturbances and other adverse effects
Treatment	If convulsions or respiratory depression occurs, take immediate steps to maintain a patent airway and ensure adequate ventilation; if convulsions persist despite oxygen administration, give an anticonvulsant agent, such as diazepam, thiopental, thiamylal, pentobarbital, or secobarbital, in small IV increments. Renal clearance and clearance by hemodialysis of tocainide are approximately equivalent.

DRUG INTERACTIONS

Metoprolol	⇧ Pulmonary wedge pressure ⇩ Cardiac index (see warning, above, concerning myocardial depression)
Lidocaine	⇧ Risk of CNS adverse reactions, including seizures

ALTERED LABORATORY VALUES

Blood/serum values	⇧ Liver function values + ANA titer

No clinically significant alterations in urinary values occur at therapeutic dosages

USE IN CHILDREN

Safety and effectiveness for use in children have not been established

USE IN PREGNANT AND NURSING WOMEN

Pregnancy Category C: reproduction studies have shown an increase in abortions and stillbirths in rabbits fed 1–4 times the usual human dose, an increase in resorptions in rats fed 12 times the usual human dose, and dystocia, delayed parturition, an increase in stillbirths, and reduced survival of offspring during the first week after birth in rats fed 8 or 12 times the usual human dose; maternal toxicity was evident in all of the studies. No adequate, well-controlled studies have been done in pregnant women. Use during pregnancy only if the expected benefit justifies the potential risk to the fetus. It is not known whether tocainide is excreted in human milk; because of the potential for adverse effects in nursing infants, this drug should not be given to women who elect to breast-feed.

ANTIARRHYTHMICS

XYLOCAINE for Ventricular Arrhythmias (lidocaine hydrochloride) Astra   Rx

Ampuls: 20 mg/ml (5 ml) for direct IV injection; 100 mg/ml (5 ml) for IM injection **Prefilled syringes:** 20 mg/ml (5 ml) for direct IV injection **Additive syringes:** 200 mg/ml (5, 10 ml) for IV infusion **Vials:** 40 mg/ml (25, 50 ml) for IV infusion

INDICATIONS

Ventricular arrhythmias such as those associated with cardiac surgery, other cardiac procedures, and acute myocardial infarction

PARENTERAL DOSAGE

Adult: 50–100 mg (0.7–1.4 mg/kg), given in a single IV dose at a rate of 25–50 mg/min (0.35–0.7 mg/kg/min) and then repeated, if necessary, after 5 min (maximum dosage: 200–300 mg/h); alternatively, 300 mg (~ 4.3 mg/kg), given in a single IM dose and then repeated, if necessary, after 60–90 min. For continuous IV infusion, give 1–4 mg/min (14–57 µg/kg/min) to start after administration of a loading dose; adjust dosage when basic cardiac rhythm stabilizes or if signs of toxicity appear (prolonged infusion is rarely necessary).
Child: 3 µg/kg/min, given by IV infusion after administration of a loading dose of 1 mg/kg

CONTRAINDICATIONS

Stokes-Adams syndrome

Wolff-Parkinson-White syndrome

Severe SA, AV, or intraventricular block (when an artificial pacemaker is not present)

Hypersensitivity to amide-type local anesthetics

ADMINISTRATION/DOSAGE ADJUSTMENTS

Intramuscular administration — Inject solution preferably into the deltoid muscle; administration at this site produces a more rapid onset of action and higher peak serum levels than injection into the gluteus or lateral thigh muscles. To avoid inadvertent intravascular injection, aspirate frequently. After the initial IM dose, switch to IV infusion, if possible.

Intravenous infusion — Immediately before administration, add 1–2 g to 1 liter of 5% dextrose in water (use aseptic technique); a more concentrated solution may be prepared if fluid restriction is necessary. Continuous infusion for more than 24 h may result in a serum half-life of 3 h or more (the usual half-life after direct IV injection is 1.5–2 h).

WARNINGS/PRECAUTIONS

Cardiotoxicity — Constant ECG monitoring during administration is essential; signs of excessive cardiac depression, including sinus node dysfunction, prolongation of the P-R interval and QRS complex, and activation or exacerbation of arrhythmia, necessitate dosage adjustment or prompt discontinuation of use

Respiratory depression — Make sure that oxygen and resuscitative drugs and equipment are immediately available to treat respiratory depression and arrest (see OVERDOSAGE)

Accumulation of lidocaine or its metabolites — Altered liver function and changes in liver blood flow may affect metabolism of lidocaine; use with caution in patients with hypovolemia, congestive heart failure, shock, or severe hepatic impairment (see also DRUG INTERACTIONS). Accumulation of active metabolites may occur in patients with severe renal impairment; exercise caution.

Elderly or debilitated patients — Reduce dosage according to physical status

Patients with atrial flutter or fibrillation — The ventricular rate in such patients may occasionally increase during therapy

Patients with sinus bradycardia or incomplete heart block — Intravenous administration to such patients for the treatment of ectopic ventricular beats may produce more frequent and serious ventricular arrhythmias or complete heart block; to prevent these reactions, increase the heart rate (eg, with atropine, isoproterenol, or electric pacing) before administration. Use with caution in patients with any form of heart block.

XYLOCAINE for Ventricular Arrhythmias

Patients predisposed to malignant hyperthermia	Safety for use in such patients has not been fully assessed; use with caution. Although it is not known whether lidocaine can precipitate malignant hyperthermia, significant serum levels such as those attained by IV infusion of large doses increase the risk of this reaction. During therapy, watch for premonitory signs (tachycardia, tachypnea, labile blood pressure, and metabolic acidosis), and, if hyperthermia occurs, promptly discontinue administration and institute appropriate treatment, including use of oxygen and dantrolene.
Carcinogenicity, mutagenicity, effect on fertility	No long-term studies have been done to evaluate the carcinogenic and mutagenic potential of this drug or its effect on fertility

ADVERSE REACTIONS

Central nervous system	Light-headedness; nervousness; apprehension; euphoria; confusion; dizziness; drowsiness; tinnitus; blurred or double vision; sensation of heat, cold, or numbness; twitching; tremors; convulsions; unconsciousness; respiratory depression and arrest
Cardiovascular	Bradycardia, hypotension, cardiovascular collapse, cardiac arrest
Other	Vomiting; allergic reactions (extremely rare)

OVERDOSAGE

Signs and symptoms	Cardiovascular depression, CNS stimulation and/or depression (see ADVERSE REACTIONS)
Treatment	Institute emergency resuscitative procedures; establish a patent airway, provide adequate ventilatory support, and administer oxygen. If convulsions persist, give small incremental IV doses of a benzodiazepine (eg, diazepam), an ultrashort-acting barbiturate (eg, thiopental or thiamylal), a short-acting barbiturate (eg, pentobarbital or secobarbital), or, if the patient is under general anesthesia, a short-acting muscle relaxant (eg, succinylcholine); longer-acting drugs should be used only for recurrent convulsions. Vasopressors may be given if circulatory depression occurs. Dialysis is of negligible value.

DRUG INTERACTIONS

Beta-adrenergic blockers, cimetidine	△ Serum half-life of lidocaine
Phenytoin	△ Cardiac depression ▽ Serum half-life of lidocaine
Succinylcholine	△ Neuromuscular blockade (with prolonged or repeated use)

ALTERED LABORATORY VALUES

Blood/serum values	△ Creatine phosphokinase (with IM use); isoenzyme separation may be necessary when testing for acute myocardial infarction

No clinically significant alterations in urinary values occur at therapeutic dosages

---

USE IN CHILDREN

The dosage recommended by the American Heart Association (see PARENTERAL DOSAGE) has not been established by controlled clinical studies

USE IN PREGNANT AND NURSING WOMEN

Pregnancy Category B: reproduction studies in rats given up to 6.6 times the maximum human dose have shown no significant evidence of harm to the fetus; however, no adequate well-controlled studies have been performed in pregnant women. The effects of use during labor and delivery are not known. Lidocaine readily crosses the placental barrier. Use during pregnancy only if clearly needed. It is not known whether lidocaine is excreted in human milk; use with caution in nursing mothers.

Chapter 14

Antiarthritic Agents

ANACIN (Whitehall) — 476
Aspirin and caffeine *OTC*

Maximum Strength ANACIN (Whitehall) — 476
Aspirin and caffeine *OTC*

ANAPROX (Syntex) — 477
Naproxen sodium *Rx*

ARTHRITIS PAIN FORMULA (Whitehall) — 479
Aspirin, aluminum hydroxide, and magnesium hydroxide *OTC*

ARTHROPAN (Purdue Frederick) — 479
Choline salicylate *OTC*

ASCRIPTIN (Rorer) — 480
Aspirin, magnesium hydroxide, and aluminum hydroxide *OTC*

ASCRIPTIN A/D (Rorer) — 481
Aspirin, magnesium hydroxide, and aluminum hydroxide *OTC*

Extra Strength ASCRIPTIN (Rorer) — 481
Aspirin, magnesium hydroxide, and aluminum hydroxide *OTC*

BAYER Aspirin (Glenbrook) — 482
Aspirin *OTC*

Maximum BAYER Aspirin (Glenbrook) — 482
Aspirin *OTC*

BAYER Children's Chewable Aspirin (Glenbrook) — 482
Aspirin *OTC*

8-Hour BAYER Aspirin (Glenbrook) — 482
Aspirin *OTC*

BUFFERIN (Bristol-Myers) — 484
Aspirin, aluminum glycinate, and magnesium carbonate *OTC*

Arthritis Strength BUFFERIN (Bristol-Myers) — 484
Aspirin, aluminum glycinate, and magnesium carbonate *OTC*

Extra Strength BUFFERIN (Bristol-Myers) — 484
Aspirin, aluminum glycinate, and magnesium carbonate *OTC*

BUTAZOLIDIN (Geigy) — 485
Phenylbutazone *Rx*

CLINORIL (Merck Sharp & Dohme) — 488
Sulindac *Rx*

CUPRIMINE (Merck Sharp & Dohme) — 490
Penicillamine *Rx*

DEPEN (Wallace) — 492
Penicillamine *Rx*

DISALCID (Riker) — 495
Salsalate *Rx*

DOLOBID (Merck Sharp & Dohme) — 496
Diflunisal *Rx*

Maximum Strength ECOTRIN (SmithKline Consumer Products) — 498
Aspirin *OTC*

Regular Strength ECOTRIN (SmithKline Consumer Products) — 498
Aspirin *OTC*

EMPIRIN (Burroughs Wellcome) — 500
Aspirin *OTC*

FELDENE (Pfizer) — 501
Piroxicam *Rx*

IMURAN (Burroughs Wellcome) — 503
Azathioprine *Rx*

INDOCIN (Merck Sharp & Dohme) — 504
Indomethacin *Rx*

INDOCIN SR (Merck Sharp & Dohme) — 504
Indomethacin *Rx*

MAGAN (Adria) — 507
Magnesium salicylate *Rx*

MECLOMEN (Parke-Davis) — 508
Meclofenamate sodium *Rx*

MOTRIN (Upjohn) — 510
Ibuprofen *Rx*

MYOCHRYSINE (Merck Sharp & Dohme) — 511
Gold sodium thiomalate *Rx*

NALFON (Dista) — 513
Fenoprofen calcium *Rx*

NAPROSYN (Syntex) — 515
Naproxen *Rx*

ORUDIS (Wyeth) — 517
Ketoprofen *Rx*

RIDAURA (Smith Kline & French) — 519
Auranofin *Rx*

RUFEN (Boots) — 520
Ibuprofen *Rx*

SOLGANAL (Schering) — 522
Aurothioglucose *Rx*

SYNALGOS (Wyeth) — 524
Aspirin and caffeine *OTC*

TOLECTIN 200 (McNeil Pharmaceutical) — 525
Tolmetin sodium *Rx*

TOLECTIN DS (McNeil Pharmaceutical) — 525
Tolmetin sodium *Rx*

TRILISATE (Purdue Frederick) — 527
Choline magnesium trisalicylate *Rx*

Other Antiarthritic Agents — 475

AZOLID (Rorer) — 475
Phenylbutazone *Rx*

OTHER ANTIARTHRITIC AGENTS

DRUG	HOW SUPPLIED	USUAL DOSAGE[1]
AZOLID (Rorer) Phenylbutazone *Rx*	**Capsules:** 100 mg **Tablets:** 100 mg	**Adult:** for rheumatoid arthritis, ankylosing spondylitis, and acute degenerative joint disease, 300–600 mg/day, given in 3–4 divided doses, to start, followed, when improvement is noted, by a prompt reduction to minimum effective level for maintenance, as low as 100–200 mg/day or up to 400 mg/day, if needed; for acute gouty arthritis, 400 mg to start, followed by 100 mg q4h for not more than 1 wk; doses should be taken with milk or with meals **Child ($\geq$ 14 yr):** same as adult

[1] Where pediatric dosages are not given, consult manufacturer

COMPENDIUM OF DRUG THERAPY

ANTIARTHRITIC AGENTS

ANACIN (aspirin and caffeine) Whitehall — OTC

Caplets: 400 mg aspirin and 32 mg caffeine **Tablets:** 400 mg aspirin and 32 mg caffeine

INDICATIONS

Headache, neuralgia, neuritis, sprains, muscular aches, tooth-extraction pain, toothache, menstrual discomfort, and minor aches and pains of arthritis and rheumatism

Fever and discomfort of colds

ORAL DOSAGE

Adult: 2 caplets or tabs with water q4h, as needed, up to 10 caplets or tabs per day
Child (6–12 yr): 1 caplet or tab with water q4h, as needed, up to 5 caplets or tabs per day

Maximum Strength ANACIN (aspirin and caffeine) Whitehall — OTC

Tablets: 500 mg aspirin and 32 mg caffeine

INDICATIONS

Headache, neuralgia, neuritis, sprains, muscular aches, tooth-extraction pain, toothache, menstrual discomfort, and minor aches and pains of arthritis and rheumatism

Fever and discomfort associated with colds

ORAL DOSAGE

Adult and child ($\geq$ 12 yr): 2 tabs with water tid or qid

WARNINGS/PRECAUTIONS

Patient self-medication — Package labels caution patients to consult a physician immediately if pain persists for more than 10 days or redness is present or for arthritic or rheumatic conditions affecting children under 12 yr of age; labels also advise patients who are pregnant or nursing to seek the advice of a health-care professional before using these products

Reye's syndrome — There is evidence suggesting that use of aspirin in children or adolescents with chicken pox or influenza may increase the risk of Reye's syndrome

OVERDOSAGE

Signs and symptoms — *Aspirin-related effects:* hyperpnea, nausea, vomiting, vertigo, tinnitus, flushing, sweating, thirst, headache, drowsiness, diarrhea, and tachycardia, progressing to hyperthermia, hemorrhage, acid-base disturbances, restlessness, confusion, convulsions, vasomotor depression, coma, and respiratory failure; *caffeine-related effects:* insomnia, restlessness, tremors, delirium, tachycardia, extrasystoles, tinnitus, urinary frequency

Treatment — If less than 4 h have elapsed since ingestion, induce emesis or perform gastric lavage, followed by activated charcoal, to remove any remaining drug from the stomach. Initial therapy should be directed at reducing hyperthermia by external sponging with tepid water, correcting dehydration by appropriate IV fluid replacement, and maintaining adequate cardiorespiratory and renal function. In moderately severe cases of salicylate poisoning, cautiously administer sodium bicarbonate IV in sufficient quantity, if possible, to maintain an alkaline diuresis; intermittent peritoneal dialysis may also be helpful. In severe cases, hemodialysis should be seriously considered. Potassium should be added to the repair solution to compensate for potassium losses once urine formation is deemed adequate. Glucose may be provided to correct ketosis and hypoglycemia. Plasma transfusion may be beneficial if shock intervenes. Hemorrhagic phenomena may necessitate whole-blood transfusions and phytonadione (vitamin K$_1$). Do not administer barbiturates to treat excitement or convulsions.

DRUG INTERACTIONS

Anticoagulants	△ Risk of bleeding
Alcohol, corticosteroids, phenylbutazone, oxyphenbutazone	△ Risk of GI ulceration
Probenecid, sulfinpyrazone	▽ Uricosuria
Spironolactone	▽ Diuretic effect
Methotrexate	△ Methotrexate plasma level and risk of toxicity

ALTERED LABORATORY VALUES

Blood/serum values — △ Prothrombin time △ Uric acid (with low doses) ▽ Uric acid (with high doses) ▽ Thyroxine (T$_4$) ▽ Thyroid-stimulating hormone

Urinary values — △ Glucose (with Clinitest tablets)

USE IN CHILDREN

Anacin is not recommended for use in children under 6 yr of age; Maximum Strength Anacin is not recommended for use in children under 12 yr of age

USE IN PREGNANT AND NURSING WOMEN

Consult manufacturer for use during pregnancy and in nursing mothers

ANTIARTHRITIC AGENTS

ANAPROX (naproxen sodium) Syntex   Rx

Tablets: 275 mg

INDICATIONS	ORAL DOSAGE
Mild to moderate pain Primary dysmenorrhea Acute tendinitis and bursitis	**Adult:** 550 mg to start, followed by 275 mg q6–8h, as needed, up to 1,375 mg/day
Rheumatoid arthritis, osteoarthritis, and ankylosing spondylitis	**Adult:** 275 mg bid (AM and PM) or 275 mg in the morning and 550 mg at night to start; for long-term administration, adjust dosage as needed, depending on clinical response. Smaller daily doses may suffice for long-term therapy. Dosages exceeding 1,100 mg/day have not been studied.
Acute gout	**Adult:** 825 mg to start, followed by 275 mg q8h until attack has subsided

CONTRAINDICATIONS

History of allergic reaction to naproxen or naproxen sodium	History of asthma, rhinitis, and nasal polyps precipitated by aspirin or other nonsteroidal, anti-inflammatory/analgesic drugs

ADMINISTRATION/DOSAGE ADJUSTMENTS

Therapeutic response in arthritis	Should be observed within 2 wk; in some patients, symptomatic improvement may not be seen for up to 4 wk
Combination therapy	Added benefits in arthritis have not been demonstrated with corticosteroids; however, use with gold salts has resulted in greater improvement. Use with salicylates is not recommended. Use with related drug naproxen is not recommended.
Adrenal function tests	Discontinue naproxen sodium therapy 72 h prior to testing

WARNINGS/PRECAUTIONS

Anaphylactic reactions	Potentially fatal allergic or idiosyncratic anaphylactic reactions may occur. Before beginning therapy, determine whether the patient has experienced reactions such as asthma, nasal polyps, urticaria, or hypotension in association with nonsteroidal anti-inflammatory drugs (see CONTRAINDICATIONS); if such reactions occur during therapy, discontinue use.
Peptic ulcer, perforation, GI bleeding	May occur and can be severe or even fatal; patients with a history of peptic ulcer disease or active gastric or duodenal ulcers should be closely supervised during therapy
Renal toxicity	Proteinuria, acute interstitial nephritis with hematuria, and occasionally the nephrotic syndrome may occur during therapy. In patients with reduced renal blood flow or volume owing to conditions such as heart failure, renal or hepatic impairment, advanced age, or use of diuretics, administration of a nonsteroidal anti-inflammatory agent may cause a critical decrease in the formation of renal prostaglandins and thereby precipitate overt renal failure; reaction is reversible upon discontinuation of the drug. To avoid renal toxicity, monitor serum creatinine level and/or creatinine clearance and exercise great caution if a patient has significant renal impairment.
Drug accumulation	Naproxen is eliminated primarily by the kidneys; exercise caution if creatinine clearance is less than 20 mg/ml since drug accumulation can occur in such a case. Chronic alcoholic liver disease, probably other forms of cirrhosis, and, according to one study, advanced age all produce an increase in the serum level of unbound naproxen; if a cirrhotic or elderly patient requires high doses, exercise caution, and be prepared to adjust dose.
Liver function abnormalities	Borderline elevations may occur in up to 15% of patients; meaningful elevations 3 times the upper limit of normal) in SGOT or SGPT levels have been reported in less than 1% of patients. If abnormal liver function tests or other manifestations of liver dysfunction arise during therapy, evaluate the patient for evidence of a more severe hepatic reaction. Although such reactions as jaundice and fatal hepatitis have occurred rarely, discontinue therapy if abnormal liver function test results persist or worsen, signs and symptoms of liver disease develop, or secondary manifestations (eg, eosinophilia, rash) occur.
Ophthalmic changes	Have occurred in animals treated with related drugs; perform an ophthalmologic examination within a reasonable period after starting therapy and periodically thereafter if drug is used for an extended period
Peripheral edema	May occur; use with caution in patients with fluid retention, hypertension, or heart failure. Each tablet contains approximately 25 mg (about 1 mEq) of sodium.
Corticosteroid therapy	If discontinued, reduce dosage gradually to avoid complications of sudden steroid withdrawal and observe patient closely for adverse effects
Mental impairment	Performance of potentially hazardous activities may be impaired; advise patients to exercise caution if they experience drowsiness, dizziness, vertigo, or depression

ANAPROX

Prolonged bleeding time	May occur due to inhibition of platelet aggregation; use with caution in patients with coagulation defects or in those on anticoagulant therapy
Patients with initially low hemoglobin values (≤ 10 g)	Obtain periodic hemoglobin determinations during long-term therapy
Diagnostic interference	Complications of presumably noninfectious, noninflammatory painful conditions may escape detection because of reduction in fever and inflammation
Carcinogenicity	No evidence of carcinogenicity has been found in rats after 2 yr of study

ADVERSE REACTIONS[1]

Frequent reactions (incidence $\geq 1\%$) are printed in *italics*

Gastrointestinal	*Constipation, heartburn, abdominal pain, and nausea (3–9%); dyspepsia, diarrhea, and stomatitis (1–3%);* bleeding and/or perforation, peptic ulcer with bleeding and/or perforation, vomiting, melena, hematemesis
Respiratory	Eosinophilic pneumonitis
Central nervous system and neuromuscular	*Headache, dizziness, and drowsiness (3–9%); light-headedness and vertigo (1–3%);* myalgia, muscle weakness, inability to concentrate, depression, malaise, dream abnormalities, insomnia
Dermatological	*Pruritus, eruption, and ecchymoses (3–9%); sweating and purpura (1–3%);* rash, alopecia, photosensitive dermatitis[2]
Cardiovascular	*Edema and dyspnea (3–9%); palpitations (1–3%);* congestive heart failure
Hepatic	Abnormal liver function tests, jaundice
Renal	Glomerular nephritis, interstitial nephritis, nephrotic syndrome, hematuria, renal disease
Hematological	Thrombocytopenia, leukopenia, granulocytopenia, eosinophilia[2]
Other	*Tinnitus (3–9%); thirst, visual disturbances, and hearing disturbances (1–3%);* hearing impairment, anaphylactoid reactions, menstrual disorders, chills, fever[2]

OVERDOSAGE

Signs and symptoms	Drowsiness, heartburn, indigestion, nausea, vomiting
Treatment	Induce emesis or use gastric lavage to empty stomach, and institute supportive measures. Activated charcoal may be helpful.

DRUG INTERACTIONS

Albumin-bound drugs	Displacement of either drug
Coumarin anticoagulants	△ Prothrombin time
Hydantoins	△ Hydantoin plasma level
Sulfonylureas	△ Sulfonylurea plasma level
Sulfonamides	△ Sulfonamide plasma level
Furosemide	▽ Natriuretic effect of furosemide
Lithium	△ Lithium plasma level
Propranolol, other beta blockers	▽ Antihypertensive effect
Aspirin	△ Excretion of naproxen sodium
Probenecid	△ Naproxen sodium plasma half-life
Methotrexate	△ Methotrexate plasma level (based on animal studies); exercise caution

ALTERED LABORATORY VALUES

Blood/serum values	△ BUN △ Creatinine △ SGOT △ SGPT
Urinary values	△ 17-Ketogenic steroids Interference with 5-HIAA determinations

---

USE IN CHILDREN

Pediatric dosages have not been established

USE IN PREGNANT AND NURSING WOMEN

Pregnancy Category B: use during pregnancy only if clearly needed; because premature closure of the ductus arteriosus may occur, administration during late pregnancy should be avoided. An increased incidence of dystocia and delayed parturition has been observed in rats. Reproduction studies in rats, rabbits, and mice given up to 6 times the human dose have shown no evidence of teratogenicity or impaired fertility. No adequate, well-controlled studies have been performed in pregnant women. Naproxen anion appears in human breast milk at a concentration of 1% of maternal plasma levels; avoid use in nursing mothers due to potential adverse effects of prostaglandin inhibition.

---

[1] Adverse reactions occurring in patients treated for rheumatoid arthritis or osteoarthritis are listed; in general, these reactions were reported 2–10 times more frequently than they were in patients treated for mild-to-moderate pain or dysmenorrhea

[2] Other reactions for which a causal relationship has not been established include epidermal necrolysis, erythema multiforme, Stevens-Johnson syndrome, urticaria, agranulocytosis, aplastic anemia, hemolytic anemia, cognitive dysfunction, ulcerative stomatitis, vasculitis, angioneurotic edema, hypoglycemia, and hyperglycemia

ANTIARTHRITIC AGENTS

ARTHRITIS PAIN FORMULA (aspirin, aluminum hydroxide, and magnesium hydroxide) Whitehall   OTC

Tablets: 500 mg aspirin, 33 mg aluminum hydroxide, and 100 mg magnesium hydroxide

INDICATIONS	**ORAL DOSAGE**
Minor aches and pains of arthritis and rheumatism and low back pain **Pain,** including headache, neuralgia, neuritis, sprains, muscular aches, tooth-extraction pain, toothache, and menstrual discomfort **Fever and discomfort** of colds	**Adult:** 2 tabs tid or qid, up to 8 tabs/24 h

WARNINGS/PRECAUTIONS

Patient self-medication	Patient should not use product if pain persists more than 10 days or redness is present or for arthritic or rheumatic conditions in children under 12 yr of age without advice and supervision of physician
Reye's syndrome	There is evidence suggesting that use of aspirin in children or adolescents with chicken pox or influenza may increase the risk of Reye's syndrome

OVERDOSAGE

Signs and symptoms	Hyperpnea, nausea, vomiting, vertigo, tinnitus, flushing, sweating, thirst, headache, drowsiness, diarrhea, and tachycardia, progressing to hyperthermia, hemorrhage, acid-base disturbances, restlessness, confusion, convulsions, vasomotor depression, coma, and respiratory failure
Treatment	If less than 4 h have elapsed since ingestion, induce emesis or perform gastric lavage, followed by activated charcoal, to remove any remaining drug from the stomach. Initial therapy should be directed at reducing hyperthermia by external sponging with tepid water, correcting dehydration by appropriate IV fluid replacement, and maintaining adequate cardiorespiratory and renal function. In moderately severe cases of salicylate poisoning, cautiously administer sodium bicarbonate IV in sufficient quantity, if possible, to maintain an alkaline diuresis; intermittent peritoneal dialysis may also be helpful. In severe cases, hemodialysis should be seriously considered. Potassium should be added to the repair solution to compensate for potassium losses once urine formation is deemed adequate. Glucose may be provided to correct ketosis and hypoglycemia. Plasma transfusion may be beneficial if shock intervenes. Hemorrhagic phenomena may necessitate whole-blood transfusions and phytonadione (vitamin K_1). Do not administer barbiturates to treat excitement or convulsions.

DRUG INTERACTIONS

Anticoagulants	⬆ Risk of bleeding
Alcohol, corticosteroids, phenylbutazone, oxyphenbutazone	⬆ Risk of GI ulceration
Probenecid, sulfinpyrazone	⬇ Uricosuria
Spironolactone	⬇ Diuretic effect
Tetracycline	⬇ Absorption of tetracycline
Methotrexate	⬆ Methotrexate plasma level and risk of toxicity

ALTERED LABORATORY VALUES

Blood/serum values	⬆ Prothrombin time ⬆ Uric acid (with low doses) ⬇ Uric acid (with high doses) ⬇ Thyroxine (T_4) ⬇ Thyroid-stimulating hormone
Urinary values	⬆ Glucose (with Clinitest tablets)

USE IN CHILDREN	USE IN PREGNANT AND NURSING WOMEN
Use according to medical judgment	Consult manufacturer for use in pregnant or nursing women

---

ANTIARTHRITIC AGENTS

ARTHROPAN (choline salicylate) Purdue Frederick   OTC

Liquid (per 5 ml): choline salicylate equivalent to 650 mg aspirin (8, 16 fl oz) *mint-flavored*

INDICATIONS	**ORAL DOSAGE**
Inflammatory conditions, including rheumatoid arthritis, rheumatic fever, and osteoarthritis **Other conditions for which oral salicylates are recommended,** particularly when a liquid dosage form is desirable	**Adult:** 5 ml (1 tsp) q3–4h, as necessary, up to 30 ml (6 tsp)/day; for rheumatoid arthritis, 5–10 ml (1–2 tsp) qid to start **Child (> 12 yr):** same as adult

COMPENDIUM OF DRUG THERAPY

ARTHROPAN ■ ASCRIPTIN

CONTRAINDICATIONS
Consult manufacturer

WARNINGS/PRECAUTIONS
Overdosage — May lead to salicylism (see OVERDOSAGE)

ADVERSE REACTIONS
Gastrointestinal — Minimal blood loss and gastric irritation

OVERDOSAGE

Signs and symptoms — Hyperpnea, nausea, vomiting, vertigo, tinnitus, flushing, sweating, thirst, headache, drowsiness, diarrhea, and tachycardia, progressing to hyperthermia, hemorrhage, acid-base disturbances, restlessness, confusion, convulsions, vasomotor depression, coma, and respiratory failure

Treatment — If less than 4 h have elapsed since ingestion, induce emesis or perform gastric lavage, followed by activated charcoal, to remove any remaining drug from the stomach. Initial therapy should be directed at reducing hyperthermia by external sponging with tepid water, correcting dehydration by appropriate IV fluid replacement, and maintaining adequate cardiorespiratory and renal function. In moderately severe cases of salicylate poisoning, cautiously administer sodium bicarbonate IV in sufficient quantity, if possible, to maintain an alkaline diuresis; intermittent peritoneal dialysis may also be helpful. In severe cases, hemodialysis should be seriously considered. Potassium should be added to the repair solution to compensate for potassium losses once urine formation is deemed adequate. Glucose may be provided to correct ketosis and hypoglycemia. Plasma transfusion may be beneficial if shock intervenes. Hemorrhagic phenomena may necessitate whole-blood transfusions and phytonadione (vitamin K$_1$). Do not administer barbiturates to treat excitement or convulsions.

DRUG INTERACTIONS

Anticoagulants	△ Risk of bleeding
Alcohol, corticosteroids, phenylbutazone, oxyphenbutazone	△ Risk of GI ulceration
Probenecid, sulfinpyrazone	▽ Uricosuria
Spironolactone	▽ Diuretic effect
Methotrexate	△ Methotrexate plasma level and risk of toxicity

ALTERED LABORATORY VALUES

Blood/serum values — △ Prothrombin time △ Uric acid (with low doses) ▽ Uric acid (with high doses)
▽ Thyroxine (T$_4$) ▽ Thyroid-stimulating hormone

Urinary values — △ Glucose (with Clinitest tablets)

USE IN CHILDREN
Consult manufacturer for use in children under 12 yr of age

USE IN PREGNANT AND NURSING WOMEN
Consult manufacturer for use in pregnant or nursing women

ANTIARTHRITIC AGENTS

ASCRIPTIN (aspirin, magnesium hydroxide, and aluminum hydroxide) Rorer — OTC
Tablets: 325 mg aspirin, 75 mg magnesium hydroxide, and 75 mg dried aluminum hydroxide gel

INDICATIONS	ORAL DOSAGE
Headache, neuralgia **Pain** of minor injuries and dysmenorrhea **Pain and fever** of colds and influenza **Pain and inflammation** of arthritis and other rheumatic diseases	**Adult:** 2–3 tabs qid
Reducing the risk of **recurrent transient ischemic attacks or stroke in men** who have had transient ischemia of the brain due to fibrin platelet emboli	**Adult:** 1 tab qid or 2 tabs bid
Reducing the risk of **myocardial infarction and subsequent death** in patients with unstable angina or a prior infarction[1]	**Adult:** 1 tab once daily

ASCRIPTIN A/D (aspirin, magnesium hydroxide, and aluminum hydroxide) Rorer — OTC

Tablets: 325 mg aspirin, 150 mg magnesium hydroxide, and 150 mg dried aluminum hydroxide gel

INDICATIONS

Pain, inflammation, and fever associated with rheumatoid arthritis, osteoarthritis, and other arthritic conditions

ORAL DOSAGE

Adult: 2–3 tabs qid

Extra Strength ASCRIPTIN (aspirin, magnesium hydroxide, and aluminum hydroxide) Rorer — OTC

Tablets: 500 mg aspirin, 82.5 mg magnesium hydroxide, and 82.5 mg dried aluminum hydroxide gel

INDICATIONS

Headache, neuralgia
Pain of minor injuries and dysmenorrhea
Discomfort of colds
Minor aches and pains associated with arthritis and rheumatism

ORAL DOSAGE

Adult: 2 tabs, with a full glass of water, tid or qid

CONTRAINDICATIONS

Consult manufacturer

WARNINGS/PRECAUTIONS

Evaluation of patients with transient ischemic attacks (TIA's)	Before initiating treatment of patients presenting with signs and symptoms of TIA's, perform a complete medical and neurological evaluation, taking into account other disorders that resemble TIA's. Attention should also be given to risk factors; disorders frequently associated with TIA's, such as hypertension and diabetes, should be evaluated and treatment instituted if appropriate.
Monitoring of prophylactic therapy for myocardial infarction	Check blood pressure, BUN level, and serum uric acid level regularly when using aspirin for long-term prophylaxis of myocardial infarction; small increases in these values have been detected during one clinical trial
Information for patients	Package labels caution patients not to use aspirin without medical supervision if they are undergoing medical treatment, have arthritis or rheumatism, are hypersensitive to aspirin, or have a history of one of the following conditions: asthma, renal or gastric disease, or a hematological disorder; patients are instructed to immediately consult a physician if they experience tinnitus or other symptoms, erythema is seen, or pain persists for more than 10 days. Women who are pregnant or nursing are advised to consult a health professional before using aspirin.
Reye's syndrome	Do not give this preparation to children, including teenagers, with chicken pox or influenza

OVERDOSAGE

Signs and symptoms	Hyperpnea, nausea, vomiting, vertigo, tinnitus, flushing, sweating, thirst, headache, drowsiness, diarrhea, and tachycardia, progressing to hyperthermia, hemorrhage, acid-base disturbances, restlessness, confusion, convulsions, vasomotor depression, coma, and respiratory failure
Treatment	If less than 4 h have elapsed since ingestion, induce emesis or perform gastric lavage, followed by activated charcoal, to remove any remaining drug from the stomach. Initial therapy should be directed at reducing hyperthermia by external sponging with tepid water, correcting dehydration by appropriate IV fluid replacement, and maintaining adequate cardiorespiratory and renal function. In moderately severe cases of salicylate poisoning, cautiously administer sodium bicarbonate IV in sufficient quantity, if possible, to maintain an alkaline diuresis; intermittent peritoneal dialysis may also be helpful. In severe cases, hemodialysis should be seriously considered. Potassium should be added to the repair solution to compensate for potassium losses once urine formation is deemed adequate. Glucose may be provided to correct ketosis and hypoglycemia. Plasma transfusion may be beneficial if shock intervenes. Hemorrhagic phenomena may necessitate whole-blood transfusions and phytonadione (vitamin K_1). Do not administer barbiturates to treat excitement or convulsions.

DRUG INTERACTIONS

Anticoagulants	⇧ Risk of bleeding
Alcohol, corticosteroids, phenylbutazone, oxyphenbutazone	⇧ Risk of GI ulceration
Probenecid, sulfinpyrazone	⇩ Uricosuria
Spironolactone	⇩ Diuretic effect
Methotrexate	⇧ Methotrexate plasma level and risk of toxicity
Tetracycline	⇩ Absorption of tetracycline; do not use concomitantly
Absorbable antacids	⇧ Clearance of salicylate

ASCRIPTIN ■ BAYER Aspirin

| Nonabsorbable antacids | ▽ Rate of absorption of aspirin | ▽ Plasma aspirin/salicylate ratio |

ALTERED LABORATORY VALUES

Blood/serum values	△ Prothrombin time △ Uric acid (with low doses) ▽ Uric acid (with high doses)
	▽ Thyroxine (T$_4$) ▽ Thyroid-stimulating hormone
Urinary values	△ Glucose (with Clinitest tablets)

USE IN CHILDREN

Use according to medical judgment in children under 12 yr of age

USE IN PREGNANT AND NURSING WOMEN

Consult manufacturer for use in pregnant or nursing women

---

[1] *FDA Drug Bulletin* 15(4):34, 1985

ANTIARTHRITIC AGENTS

BAYER Aspirin (aspirin) Glenbrook   OTC

Tablets: 325 mg   **Caplets:** 325 mg

INDICATIONS	ORAL DOSAGE
Headache, muscular aches and pains, bursitis, menstrual discomfort, toothache, minor aches and pains of arthritis and rheumatism Fever and discomfort of colds and influenza	**Adult:** 325–650 mg (1–2 tablets or caplets) with water q4h, as needed
Reducing the risk of **recurrent transient ischemic attacks or stroke in men** who have had transient ischemia of the brain due to fibrin platelet emboli[1]	**Adult:** 325 mg (1 tablet or caplet) qid or 650 mg (2 tablets or caplets) bid, with water
Reducing the risk of **myocardial infarction and subsequent death** in patients with unstable angina or a prior infarction[2]	**Adult:** 325 mg (1 tablet or caplet) once daily

Maximum BAYER Aspirin (aspirin) Glenbrook   OTC

Tablets: 500 mg   **Caplets:** 500 mg

INDICATIONS	ORAL DOSAGE
Headache, muscular aches and pains, bursitis, menstrual discomfort, toothache, minor aches and pains of arthritis and rheumatism Fever and discomfort of colds and influenza	**Adult:** 1,000 mg (2 tablets or caplets) with water or fruit juice q4h, as needed, up to 4,000 mg (8 tablets or caplets)/24 h

8-Hour BAYER Aspirin (aspirin) Glenbrook   OTC

Tablets (timed release): 650 mg

INDICATIONS	ORAL DOSAGE
Backache, bursitis, sprains, headache, sinusitis, minor pain and stiffness of arthritis Fever and discomfort of colds and influenza	**Adult:** 1,300 mg (2 tablets) with water, followed by 650–1,300 mg (1–2 tablets) q8h, as needed, up to 3,900 mg (6 tablets)/day; for prevention of nighttime and early morning stiffness, 1,300 mg (2 tablets) with water at bedtime. Tablets may be broken up (but not ground) between the teeth or gently crumbled in the mouth and swallowed with water without loss of timed-release action.

BAYER Children's Chewable Aspirin (aspirin) Glenbrook   OTC

Chewable tablets: 81.25 mg *orange flavored*

INDICATIONS	ORAL DOSAGE
Headache, sore throat, other minor aches and pains Fever and discomfort of colds	**Child (3–4 yr; 32–35 lb):** 162.5 mg (2 tablets) with water q4h, up to 5 doses/day **Child (4–6 yr; 36–45 lb):** 243.75 mg (3 tablets) with water q4h, up to 5 doses/day **Child (6–9 yr; 46–65 lb):** 325 mg (4 tablets) with water q4h, up to 5 doses/day **Child (9–11 yr; 66–76 lb):** 406.25 mg (5 tablets) with water q4h, up to 5 doses/day **Child (11–12 yr; 77–83 lb):** 487.5 mg (6 tablets) with water q4h, up to 5 doses/day **Child ($\geq$ 12 yr; $\geq$ 84 lb):** 650 mg (8 tablets) with water q4h, up to 5 doses/day

BAYER Aspirin

CONTRAINDICATIONS

Bleeding ulcer	Hemorrhagic states	Hypersensitivity to salicylates
Hemophilia		

ADMINISTRATION/DOSAGE ADJUSTMENTS

Administration of chewable tablets	Chewable tablets may be swallowed whole with half a glass of water, milk, or fruit juice; chewed or dissolved on the tongue and then ingested with half a glass of one of these liquids; dissolved in a small amount of one of these liquids, which is then drunk; or crushed in a teaspoonful of water and then ingested with part of a glass of water

WARNINGS/PRECAUTIONS

Gastric irritation	May occur, especially in patients with gastric ulcers, erosive gastritis, or bleeding tendencies; use with caution
Patients with blood-coagulation abnormalities	Use with caution in patients with preexisting hypoprothrombinemia or vitamin K deficiency
Nasal polyps, asthma, hay fever	May predispose to salicylate hypersensitivity; use with caution
Interference with platelet aggregation	Use with caution prior to surgery
Monitoring of prophylactic therapy for myocardial infarction	Check blood pressure, BUN level, and serum uric acid level regularly when using aspirin for long-term prophylaxis of myocardial infarction; small increases in these values have been detected during one clinical trial
Patient instructions	Bayer, Maximum Bayer, and 8-Hour Bayer: the package label advises consultation with a physician if pain persists for more than 10 days, redness is present, or the patient is less than 12 yr of age. Children's Bayer: the package label advises consultation with a physician if nausea, vomiting, headache, high or continued fever, or severe or persistent sore throat occurs. The package labels also advise pregnant or nursing women to consult a health professional before using these products.
Reye's syndrome	There is evidence suggesting that use of aspirin in children or adolescents with chicken pox or influenza may increase the risk of Reye's syndrome

ADVERSE REACTIONS

Gastrointestinal	Nausea, dyspepsia, heartburn, epigastric discomfort, anorexia, diarrhea, occult blood loss, hemorrhage
Central nervous system	Dizziness, tinnitus, headache, deafness
Respiratory	Hyperventilation
Cardiovascular	Increased pulse rate
Dermatological	Skin eruptions
Other	Sweating, thirst, electrolyte and acid-base imbalance

OVERDOSAGE

Signs and symptoms	Hyperpnea, nausea, vomiting, vertigo, tinnitus, flushing, sweating, thirst, headache, drowsiness, diarrhea, and tachycardia, progressing to hyperthermia, hemorrhage, acid-base disturbances, restlessness, confusion, convulsions, vasomotor depression, coma, and respiratory failure
Treatment	If less than 4 h have elapsed since ingestion, induce emesis or perform gastric lavage, followed by activated charcoal, to remove any remaining drug from the stomach. Initial therapy should be directed at reducing hyperthermia by external sponging with tepid water, correcting dehydration by appropriate IV fluid replacement, and maintaining adequate cardiorespiratory and renal function. In moderately severe cases of salicylate poisoning, cautiously administer sodium bicarbonate IV in sufficient quantity, if possible, to maintain an alkaline diuresis; intermittent peritoneal dialysis may also be helpful. In severe cases, hemodialysis should be seriously considered. Potassium should be added to the repair solution to compensate for potassium losses once urine formation is deemed adequate. Glucose may be provided to correct ketosis and hypoglycemia. Plasma transfusion may be beneficial if shock intervenes. Hemorrhagic phenomena may necessitate whole-blood transfusions and phytonadione (vitamin K_1). Do not administer barbiturates to treat excitement or convulsions.

DRUG INTERACTIONS

Anticoagulants	⇧ Risk of bleeding; exercise caution during combination therapy
Alcohol, corticosteroids, phenylbutazone, oxyphenbutazone	⇧ Risk of GI ulceration
Probenecid, sulfinpyrazone	⇩ Uricosuria
Spironolactone	⇩ Diuretic effect
Methotrexate	⇧ Methotrexate plasma level and risk of toxicity

ALTERED LABORATORY VALUES

Blood/serum values — ⇧ Prothrombin time   ⇧ Uric acid (with low doses)   ⇩ Uric acid (with high doses)
⇩ Thyroxine (T$_4$)   ⇩ Thyroid-stimulating hormone

Urinary values — ⇧ Glucose (with Clinitest tablets)

USE IN CHILDREN
See INDICATIONS and ORAL DOSAGE. *Bayer Aspirin and Children's Chewable Aspirin:* use according to medical judgment in children under 2 yr of age; *Maximum Bayer Aspirin and 8–Hour Bayer Aspirin:* use according to medical judgment in children under 12 yr of age.

USE IN PREGNANT AND NURSING WOMEN
Consult manufacturer for use in pregnant or nursing women

[1] *FDA Drug Bulletin* 10(1):2, 1980
[2] *FDA Drug Bulletin* 15(4):34, 1985

ANTIARTHRITIC AGENTS

BUFFERIN (aspirin, aluminum glycinate, and magnesium carbonate) Bristol-Myers   OTC

Tablets: 324 mg aspirin, 48.6 mg aluminum glycinate, and 97.2 mg magnesium carbonate

INDICATIONS	ORAL DOSAGE
Headache, muscular aches, toothache, menstrual cramps, and **minor pain and inflammation of arthritis and rheumatism** **Pain and fever** of colds and influenza	**Adult:** 2 tabs q4h, as needed **Child (6–12 yr):** 1 tab q4h, as needed
Reducing the risk of **recurrent transient ischemic attacks or stroke in men** who have had transient ischemia of the brain due to fibrin platelet emboli[1]	**Adult:** 1 tab qid or 2 tabs bid
Reducing the risk of **myocardial infarction and subsequent death** in patients with unstable angina or a prior infarction[2]	**Adult:** 1 tab once daily

Arthritis Strength BUFFERIN (aspirin, aluminum glycinate, and magnesium carbonate) Bristol-Myers   OTC

Tablets: 486 mg aspirin, 72.9 mg aluminum glycinate, and 145.8 mg magnesium carbonate

Extra Strength BUFFERIN (aspirin, aluminum glycinate, and magnesium carbonate) Bristol-Myers   OTC

Tablets: 500 mg aspirin, 75 mg aluminum glycinate, and 150 mg magnesium carbonate

INDICATIONS	ORAL DOSAGE
Minor aches and pains, stiffness, swelling, and **inflammation** of arthritis and rheumatism **Pain and fever** of colds and influenza **Pain,** including that of simple headache, lower backache, sinusitis, neuralgia, neuritis, tooth extraction, muscle strain, athletic soreness, and menstrual distress	**Adult:** 2 tabs q4h, as needed, up to 8 tabs per 24 h

CONTRAINDICATIONS
Hypersensitivity to salicylates

WARNINGS/PRECAUTIONS

Monitoring of prophylactic therapy for myocardial infarction — Check blood pressure, BUN level, and serum uric acid level regularly when using aspirin for long-term prophylaxis of myocardial infarction; small increases in these values have been detected during one clinical trial

BUFFERIN ■ BUTAZOLIDIN

Information for patients	Package labels caution patients not to use these products without medical supervision if one of the following conditions exists: (1) chicken pox or influenza in a child or teenager, (2) erythema, (3) arthritis or rheumatism in a child under 12 yr of age, (4) pregnancy, or (5) nursing. Patients are instructed to discontinue administration if they experience dizziness, tinnitus, or hearing impairment and to also consult a physician if overdose or erythema occurs or pain persists for more than 10 days.
Reye's syndrome	There is evidence suggesting that use of aspirin in children or adolescents with chicken pox or influenza may increase the risk of Reye's syndrome

OVERDOSAGE

Signs and symptoms	Hyperpnea, nausea, vomiting, vertigo, tinnitus, flushing, sweating, thirst, headache, drowsiness, diarrhea, and tachycardia, progressing to hyperthermia, hemorrhage, acid-base disturbances, restlessness, confusion, convulsions, vasomotor depression, coma, and respiratory failure
Treatment	If less than 4 h have elapsed since ingestion, induce emesis or perform gastric lavage, followed by activated charcoal, to remove any remaining drug from the stomach. Initial therapy should be directed at reducing hyperthermia by external sponging with tepid water, correcting dehydration by appropriate IV fluid replacement, and maintaining adequate cardiorespiratory and renal function. In moderately severe cases of salicylate poisoning, cautiously administer sodium bicarbonate IV in sufficient quantity, if possible, to maintain an alkaline diuresis; intermittent peritoneal dialysis may also be helpful. In severe cases, hemodialysis should be seriously considered. Potassium should be added to the repair solution to compensate for potassium losses once urine formation is deemed adequate. Glucose may be provided to correct ketosis and hypoglycemia. Plasma transfusion may be beneficial if shock intervenes. Hemorrhagic phenomena may necessitate whole-blood transfusions and phytonadione (vitamin K$_1$). Do not administer barbiturates to treat excitement or convulsions.

DRUG INTERACTIONS

Anticoagulants	△ Risk of bleeding
Alcohol, corticosteroids, phenylbutazone, oxyphenbutazone	△ Risk of GI ulceration
Probenecid, sulfinpyrazone	▽ Uricosuria
Spironolactone	▽ Diuretic effect
Tetracycline	▽ Absorption of tetracycline
Methotrexate	△ Methotrexate plasma level and risk of toxicity

ALTERED LABORATORY VALUES

Blood/serum values	△ Prothrombin time △ Uric acid (with low doses) ▽ Uric acid (with high doses) ▽ Thyroxine (T$_4$) ▽ Thyroid-stimulating hormone
Urinary values	△ Glucose (with Clinitest tablets)

USE IN CHILDREN See INDICATIONS and ORAL DOSAGE	**USE IN PREGNANT AND NURSING WOMEN** Consult manufacturer for use in pregnant or nursing women

[1] FDA Drug Bulletin 10(1):2, 1980
[2] FDA Drug Bulletin 15(4):34, 1985

ANTIARTHRITIC AGENTS

BUTAZOLIDIN (phenylbutazone) Geigy   Rx

Capsules: 100 mg   **Tablets:** 100 mg

INDICATIONS	ORAL DOSAGE
Active ankylosing spondylitis[1] **Active rheumatoid arthritis**[1] **Acute attacks of degenerative joint disease** of the hips and knees[1]	**Adult:** 300–600 mg/day, given in 3–4 divided doses, for a trial period of up to 1 wk; maximal therapeutic response usually occurs at 400 mg/day. Once improvement is attained, promptly reduce dosage to lowest effective level (100–200 mg/day may be satisfactory); maintenance dosage should not exceed 400 mg/day. If a favorable response is not seen after 1 wk of therapy, the drug should be discontinued.
Acute gouty arthritis[1]	**Adult:** 400 mg to start, followed by 100 mg q4h for up to 1 wk; articular inflammation usually subsides within 4 days

COMPENDIUM OF DRUG THERAPY

BUTAZOLIDIN

CONTRAINDICATIONS

Hypersensitivity to phenylbutazone or oxyphenbutazone	History of bronchospastic reaction to aspirin or other nonsteroidal anti-inflammatory drugs

ADMINISTRATION/DOSAGE ADJUSTMENTS

Administration	Give each dose with milk or meals
Duration of therapy	Discontinue phenylbutazone as soon as possible; if the patient is 60 yr of age or older, terminate administration on, or as soon as possible after, the seventh day of therapy

WARNINGS/PRECAUTIONS

Blood dyscrasias	Phenylbutazone can cause agranulocytosis and aplastic anemia; elderly patients, especially elderly women, and patients undergoing long-term therapy are especially susceptible. This drug can also precipitate other blood dyscrasias, including thrombocytopenia and hemorrhagic diathesis (see ADVERSE REACTIONS). Hematological reactions, which may develop abruptly or gradually, can occur shortly after onset of therapy, following prolonged use, or days or weeks after cessation of therapy. Before beginning treatment, obtain a careful, detailed history, perform a complete physical examination, and obtain a complete laboratory evaluation that includes examination of erythrocytes, leukocytes, and platelets; use with caution in patients with blood dyscrasias. Instruct patients that if they detect fever, sore throat, oral lesions, or unusual bruising or bleeding, they should discontinue use and immediately report these reactions. The physical and laboratory examinations that were done before therapy should be repeated whenever any sign or symptom suggesting a blood dyscrasia appears. If a significant change in the total leukocyte count, a relative decrease in granulocytes, a fall in hematocrit or platelet count, or an immature blood cell form is detected, treatment should be discontinued immediately and a complete hematological investigation initiated.
Gastrointestinal effects	New or reactivated peptic ulcer, perforation, and severe GI bleeding can occur during therapy; use with caution in patients with active ulcers, GI inflammation, or a history of peptic ulcers. Instruct patients that if they experience dyspepsia, epigastric pain, symptoms of anemia, unusual bleeding or bruising, black or tarry stools, or any other manifestation of intestinal ulceration, they should discontinue use and immediately report these reactions.
Renal toxicity	Proteinuria, acute interstitial nephritis with hematuria, and occasionally the nephrotic syndrome may occur during therapy. In patients with reduced renal blood flow or volume owing to conditions such as heart failure, renal or hepatic impairment, advanced age, or use of diuretics, administration of a nonsteroidal anti-inflammatory agent may cause a critical decrease in the formation of renal prostaglandins and thereby precipitate overt renal failure; the reaction is reversible upon discontinuation of the drug.
Drug accumulation	To avoid drug accumulation, closely monitor patients with renal impairment and be prepared to reduce the daily dose
Liver function abnormalities	Borderline elevations may occur in up to 15% of patients; meaningful elevations (3 times the upper limit of normal) in SGOT or SGPT levels have been reported in less than 1% of patients. Use with caution in patients with severe hepatic disease. If abnormal liver function tests or other manifestations of liver dysfunction arise during therapy, evaluate the patient for evidence of a more severe hepatic reaction. Although such reactions as jaundice and fatal hepatitis have occurred rarely, discontinue therapy if abnormal liver function test results persist or worsen, clinical signs and symptoms of liver disease develop, or secondary manifestations (eg, eosinophilia, rash) occur.
Acute asthma	Asthmatic attacks may be precipitated in patients with asthma
Peripheral edema	Phenylbutazone increases sodium retention; use with caution in patients with incipient cardiac failure, severe cardiac or renal disease, or any other condition that can be exacerbated by fluid retention. Instruct all patients that if they detect significant weight gain or edema, they should discontinue use and immediately report these reactions.
Visual disturbances	Ophthalmic reactions, including optic neuritis, retinal hemorrhage, toxic amblyopia, scotomata, retinal detachment, and oculomotor palsy, have been reported; if the patient complains of visual disturbances, discontinue treatment and perform an ophthalmological examination
Rash	Severe dermatological reactions can occur during therapy; instruct patients that if they see a rash they should discontinue use and immediately report the reaction
Stomatitis, parotitis, pancreatitis, temporal arteritis	Phenylbutazone may exacerbate stomatitis, parotitis, pancreatitis, or temporal arteritis; use with caution in patients with any one of these disorders or polymyalgia rheumatica
Age-related toxicity	Beginning at 40 yr of age, the risk of adverse reactions increases with age; use with caution in patients 40 yr of age or older, especially those who are elderly (see recommendations for duration of therapy, above)
Thyroid toxicity	Hyper- and hypothyroidism, thyroid hyperplasia, and goiter have been reported

BUTAZOLIDIN

Carcinogenicity	Leukemia has been reported; however, a causal relationship has not been clearly established. No long-term animal studies have been done to determine the carcinogenic potential of this drug.
Mutagenicity	An increase in chromosomal anomalies has been detected in cultured leukocyte cells taken from patients given therapeutic doses of phenylbutazone; however, results of other similar studies in humans and horses have been inconclusive or negative. Chromosomal aberrations have been induced in Chinese hamster fibroblast cells exposed in vitro to a solution containing 20 times the human plasma level of 43 mg/liter. No evidence of mutagenicity has been seen in bacteria or fungi or, at up to 33 times the maximum daily human dose, in mice, Chinese hamsters, or rats.
Effect on fertility	No adverse effect on fertility has been seen in mice, Chinese hamsters, or rats given up to 33 times the maximum daily human dose

ADVERSE REACTIONS[2]

Frequent reactions (incidence ≥ 1%) are printed in *italics*

Gastrointestinal	*Abdominal discomfort and distress (3–9%), nausea, dyspepsia, indigestion, and heartburn (1–3%),* vomiting, abdominal distention with flatulence, constipation, diarrhea, esophagitis, gastritis, salivary gland enlargement, stomatitis (sometimes with ulceration), ulceration and perforation of the intestinal tract (including acute and reactivated peptic ulcer), anemia from occult GI bleeding, hepatitis
Hematological	Aplastic anemia, agranulocytosis, bone marrow depression, thrombocytopenia, pancytopenia, leukopenia, anemia, hemolytic anemia
Dermatological	*Rash (1–3%),* pruritus, erythema nodosum, erythema multiforme, nonthrombocytopenic purpura
Cardiovascular	*Fluid retention (3–9%), edema (1–3%),* sodium and chloride retention, plasma dilution, congestive heart failure, metabolic acidosis, respiratory alkalosis, hypertension, pericarditis, interstitial myocarditis
Renal	Hematuria, proteinuria, ureteral obstruction with uric acid crystals, anuria, glomerulonephritis, acute tubular necrosis, cortical necrosis, renal stones, nephrotic syndrome, renal impairment and failure, interstitial nephritis
Central nervous system	Headache, drowsiness, agitation, confusion, lethargy, tremors, numbness, weakness
Hypersensitivity	Urticaria, anaphylactic shock, arthralgia, fever, vasculitis, Lyell's syndrome, serum sickness, Stevens-Johnson syndrome, activation of systemic lupus erythematosus, aggravation of temporal arteritis
Other	Hyperglycemia, hearing loss, tinnitus

OVERDOSAGE

Signs and symptoms	*Mild poisoning:* nausea, abdominal pain, drowsiness; *severe poisoning, early manifestations:* upper abdominal pain, nausea, vomiting, hematemesis, diarrhea, restlessness, dizziness, agitation, hallucinations, psychosis, coma, convulsions (more common in children), hyperpyrexia, electrolyte disturbances, hyperventilation, alkalosis or acidosis, respiratory arrest, hypotension, hypertension, cyanosis; *severe poisoning, late manifestations (2–7 days):* acute renal failure, edema, hematuria, oliguria, jaundice, ECG abnormalities, cardiac arrest, anemia, thrombocytopenia, leukopenia, leukocytosis, hypoprothrombinemia
Treatment	If the patient is alert, induce emesis and then perform gastric lavage. If the patient is obtunded, secure the airway with a cuffed endotracheal tube before starting lavage; do not induce emesis. Maintain adequate respiratory exchange; avoid stimulants. Treat shock with appropriate supportive measures. Control seizures with IV diazepam or a short-acting barbiturate. If the prognosis is poor, hemoperfusion can be instituted.

DRUG INTERACTIONS

Other anti-inflammatory agents, oral anticoagulants, sulfonylureas, insulin, sulfonamides, phenytoin, valproic acid, divalproex, methotrexate, lithium	⇧ Risk of toxicity associated with these drugs
Barbiturates, promethazine, chlorpheniramine, rifampin, prednisone	⇩ Serum half-life of phenylbutazone
Methylphenidate	⇧ Serum level of phenylbutazone
Dicumarol, digitoxin, cortisone	⇩ Serum level of these drugs
Cholestyramine	⇩ Absorption of phenylbutazone

ALTERED LABORATORY VALUES

Blood/serum values	⇧ RT$_3$U ⇩ ^{131}I ⇩ Uric acid ⇧ Glucose ⇧ SGOT ⇧ SGPT

No clinically significant alterations in urinary values occur at therapeutic dosages

USE IN CHILDREN

Safety and effectiveness for use in children 14 yr of age or younger have not been established

USE IN PREGNANT AND NURSING WOMEN

Pregnancy Category C: reproduction studies in rats and rabbits fed up to 16 times the maximum daily human dose have shown no evidence of teratogenicity; however, a slight reduction in litter size has been observed in rats and rabbits given oral or SC doses during pregnancy, and an increase in stillbirths along with a drop in the number of surviving offspring has occurred in rats following oral administration at 3.5 times the maximum daily human dose. Use during pregnancy only if the expected benefit justifies the potential risk to the fetus. Small quantities of phenylbutazone are excreted in breast milk; because of the potential for serious adverse reactions in nursing infants, a decision should be made to discontinue either nursing or therapy.

---

[1] This drug should be used only after other therapeutic measures, including other nonsteroidal anti-inflammatory agents, have been found to be unsatisfactory
[2] Reactions for which a causal relationship has not been established include leukemia, blurred vision, optic neuritis, toxic amblyopia, scotomata, retinal detachment, retinal hemorrhage, oculomotor palsy, thyroid hyperplasia, goiters with hyper- and hypothyroidism, and pancreatitis

---

ANTIARTHRITIC AGENTS

CLINORIL (sulindac) Merck Sharp & Dohme   Rx

Tablets: 150, 200 mg

INDICATIONS

Osteoarthritis
Rheumatoid arthritis[1]
Ankylosing spondylitis

Acute painful shoulder
Acute gouty arthritis

ORAL DOSAGE

Adult: 150 mg bid, with food, to start, followed by up to 400 mg/day, as needed; adjust dosage depending upon response. About 50% of patients respond within 1 wk of initiating therapy; others may take longer to respond.

Adult: 200 mg bid, with food, to start; after a satisfactory response is achieved, reduce dosage according to response

CONTRAINDICATIONS

Hypersensitivity to sulindac

History of asthmatic attacks, urticaria, or rhinitis precipitated by aspirin or other nonsteroidal anti-inflammatory drugs

ADMINISTRATION/DOSAGE ADJUSTMENTS

Duration of therapy for acute conditions — Generally 7–14 days for acute painful shoulder, 1 wk for acute gouty arthritis

WARNINGS/PRECAUTIONS

Peptic ulceration, GI bleeding — Potentially fatal peptic ulceration and GI bleeding may occur, particularly in patients at risk, such as the elderly and those with hemorrhagic disorders; patients with a history of upper GI tract disease should be closely supervised during therapy. If treatment is started or continued in patients with active GI bleeding or an active peptic ulcer, institute an appropriate ulcer regimen.

Interference with platelet function — Monitor closely patients who may be adversely affected by sulindac's inhibition of platelet function

Visual disturbances — May occur; if visual complaints develop, perform an ophthalmologic examination

Liver function abnormalities — Borderline elevations may occur in up to 15% of patients; meaningful elevations (3 times the upper limit of normal) in SGOT or SGPT levels have been reported in less than 1% of patients. Hepatic reactions may result from hypersensitivity (see warning, below). If abnormal liver function tests or other manifestations of liver dysfunction arise during therapy, evaluate the patient for evidence of a more severe hepatic reaction. Although such reactions as jaundice and hepatitis (including cholestatic hepatitis) have occurred rarely, discontinue therapy if abnormal liver function test results persist or worsen, signs and symptoms of liver disease develop, or secondary manifestations (eg, eosinophilia, rash) occur. Do not give more than 400 mg/day; administration of 600 mg/day has been associated with an increased incidence of mildly abnormal liver test results.

Hypersensitivity — Potentially fatal hypersensitivity reactions (see ADVERSE REACTIONS) may occur in rare cases; hepatitis, jaundice, or both may occur with or without fever during the first 1–3 mo of therapy. If unexplained fever, rash, or other manifestations of hypersensitivity develop, discontinue use and test liver function.

Pancreatitis — Sulindac can cause pancreatitis; if this condition is suspected, discontinue administration, institute supportive therapy, closely monitor appropriate laboratory values, and determine the cause of the observed disorder

CLINORIL

Renal toxicity	Proteinuria, acute interstitial nephritis with hematuria, and occasionally the nephrotic syndrome may occur during therapy. In patients with reduced renal blood flow or volume owing to conditions such as renal or hepatic dysfunction, advanced age, hypovolemia, congestive heart failure, sepsis, or use of nephrotoxic agents, administration of a nonsteroidal anti-inflammatory agent may cause a critical decrease in the formation of renal prostaglandins and thereby precipitate overt renal failure; this reaction is reversible upon discontinuation of the drug. Although sulindac may affect renal function less than other nonsteroidal anti-inflammatory agents in patients with chronic glomerular kidney disease, it should nevertheless be used with caution in patients at risk.
Drug accumulation	Monitor closely patients with poor liver function or significant renal impairment and, if necessary, reduce the daily dose to avoid excessive drug accumulation
Edema	May occur; use with caution in patients with compromised cardiac function, hypertension, or other conditions predisposing to fluid retention
Corticosteroid therapy	Therapy with sulindac may permit a reduction in corticosteroid dosage or elimination of chronic corticosteroid therapy for rheumatoid arthritis patients; reduce dosage gradually over a period of several months
Aspirin administration	Do not give aspirin concomitantly, as it decreases plasma levels of the active sulfide metabolite of sulindac, has no beneficial effect on the therapeutic response to sulindac, and increases the incidence of GI reactions to treatment
Concomitant oral anticoagulant or hypoglycemic therapy	Although studies have shown no clinically significant drug interactions when sulindac has been given at a dosage of 400 mg/day, patients should be monitored carefully until it is certain that no change in their anticoagulant or hypoglycemic dosage is required, especially if higher than recommended doses are used or metabolic conditions exist that might elevate sulindac blood levels, such as renal insufficiency (see DRUG INTERACTIONS)

ADVERSE REACTIONS[2]

Frequent reactions (incidence ≥ 1%) are printed in *italics*

Gastrointestinal	*Pain (10%); dyspepsia, nausea with or without vomiting, diarrhea and constipation (3–9%); flatulence, anorexia, and cramps (1–3%);* gastritis or gastroenteritis, peptic ulcer, bleeding; perforation (rare)
Dermatological	*Rash (3–9%), pruritus (1–3%),* stomatitis, sore or dry mucous membranes, alopecia, photosensitivity, toxic epidermal necrolysis, erythema multiforme, Stevens-Johnson syndrome, exfoliative dermatitis
Central nervous system	*Dizziness and headache (3–9%); nervousness and tinnitus (1–3%),* decreased hearing, blurred vision, vertigo, insomnia, paresthesia, depression, psychic disturbances (including acute psychosis), convulsions, syncope, aseptic meningitis, metallic or bitter taste
Hepatic and pancreatic	Liver function abnormalities, jaundice, cholestasis, hepatitis, pancreatitis
Genitourinary	Urine discoloration, vaginal bleeding, hematuria, proteinuria, renal impairment (including renal failure), interstitial nephritis, nephrotic syndrome
Hematological	Thrombocytopenia, ecchymosis, purpura, leukopenia, agranulocytosis, neutropenia, bone marrow depression (including aplastic anemia), hemolytic anemia
Cardiovascular	Congestive heart failure (especially in patients with marginal cardiac function), palpitation, hypertension
Hypersensitivity	Anaphylaxis, angioneurotic edema; potentially fatal syndrome characterized by fever, chills, rash or other dermatological reactions (see above), changes in liver function, jaundice, pancreatitis, pneumonitis, leukopenia, eosinophilia, anemia, adenitis, renal impairment (including renal failure), arthralgia, fatigue, and/or chest pain
Other	*Edema (1–3%),* epistaxis

OVERDOSAGE

Signs and symptoms	Stupor, coma, diminished urine output, hypotension
Treatment	Empty stomach by inducing emesis or by gastric lavage. Administration of activated charcoal and alkalinization of the urine may be helpful in eliminating the drug from the circulation, based on animal studies. Observe patient carefully, and institute symptomatic and supportive therapy, as needed.

DRUG INTERACTIONS

Oral anticoagulants	⇧ Prothrombin time
Dimethyl sulfoxide (DMSO)	⇩ Plasma level of active sulfide metabolite of sulindac Peripheral neuropathy; avoid concomitant use
Diflunisal	⇩ Plasma level of active sulfide metabolite of sulindac
Aspirin	⇩ Plasma level of active sulfide metabolite of sulindac ⇧ Incidence of GI reactions
Probenecid	⇧ Plasma levels of sulindac and sulfone metabolite ⇩ Uricosuric effect

Other anti-inflammatory agents, alcohol	⇧ Risk of ulcer

ALTERED LABORATORY VALUES

Blood/serum values	⇧ Alkaline phosphatase ⇧ SGOT ⇧ SGPT
Urinary values	+ Protein

USE IN CHILDREN
Pediatric indications and dosage have not been established

USE IN PREGNANT AND NURSING WOMEN
Not recommended for use during pregnancy because safety has not been established in pregnant women and because administration during the third trimester may induce premature closure of the ductus arteriosus. Prolonged gestation, dystocia, and delayed parturition have been observed in animals. Reproduction studies in rats given 20 or 40 mg/kg/day have shown a decrease in average fetal weight and the number of surviving pups on the first postpartum day. Sulindac is excreted in the milk of rats; it is not known whether it is excreted in human milk. Patient should stop nursing if drug is prescribed.

---

[1] Safety and effectiveness have not been established for rheumatoid arthritis patients designated by the American Rheumatism Association as Functional Class IV (incapacitated; largely or wholly bedridden or confined to a wheelchair; little or no self-care)
[2] Other reactions for which a causal relationship has not been established include hyperglycemia, neuritis, transient visual disturbances, and gynecomastia

---

ANTIARTHRITIC AGENTS

CUPRIMINE (penicillamine) Merck Sharp & Dohme Rx

Capsules: 125, 250 mg

INDICATIONS	ORAL DOSAGE
Severe, active rheumatoid arthritis in patients refractory to conventional therapy	**Adult:** 125–250 mg/day to start, given in a single dose, followed, as needed and tolerated, by increases of 125–250 mg/day every 1–3 mo, up to 500–750 mg/day, and then, if still necessary after 2–3 mo at this level, by further increases of 250 mg/day every 2–3 mo; if, after administration of 1–1.5 g/day for 3–4 mo, patient does not respond, discontinue use; average maintenance dosage: 500–750 mg/day. Total daily doses exceeding 500 mg should be given in divided doses; smaller amounts can be administered once daily.
Wilson's disease	**Adult:** 1 g/day to start, followed, if necessary, by increases in dosage up to 2 g/day **Child:** same as adult
Cystinuria	**Adult:** 250 mg/day at bedtime to start, followed by gradual increases to 1–4 g/day in 4 equally divided doses; usual maintenance dosage: 2 g/day in divided doses **Child:** 30 mg/kg/day in 4 equally divided doses

CONTRAINDICATIONS

History of aplastic anemia or agranulocytosis associated with prior penicillamine therapy	History or evidence of renal insufficiency in patients with rheumatoid arthritis	Pregnancy in patients with rheumatoid arthritis Breast-feeding

ADMINISTRATION/DOSAGE ADJUSTMENTS

Timing of administration	Give each dose at least 1 h before or 2 h after a meal and at least 1 h apart from snacks or other drugs
Rheumatoid arthritis	Clinical response may not be apparent for 2–3 mo after onset of therapy or dosage adjustment. If disease suppression is inadequate after first 6–9 mo, increase maintenance dosage by 125–250 mg/day at 3-mo intervals, up to 1 g/day in divided doses or, if necessary, 1.5 g/day in divided doses. If patient has been in remission for 6 mo or more, attempt to reduce dosage by 125–250 mg/day approximately every 3 mo. If therapy is interrupted, reintroduce drug at a lower dosage and increase dosage slowly.
Management of arthritic exacerbations	Flare-ups of rheumatoid arthritis may be controlled by adding a nonsteroidal anti-inflammatory agent. Do not increase the dosage of penicillamine unless flare persists more than 12 wk. Penicillamine-induced migratory polyarthralgia may closely mimic a disease exacerbation and can be distinguished from it by discontinuing or substantially reducing the dosage of penicillamine for up to several weeks.
Concomitant antiarthritic therapy	Do not use with gold salts, antimalarials, cytotoxic (immunosuppressive) agents, phenylbutazone, or oxyphenbutazone; treatment with salicylates, other nonsteroidal anti-inflammatory agents, or systemic corticosteroids may be continued when penicillamine is started or withdrawn gradually as symptoms permit

CUPRIMINE

Wilson's disease	Clinical improvement may not be apparent for 1–3 mo. During this period, neurologic symptoms may worsen; if necessary, therapy may be interrupted *temporarily,* but not without risk (see WARNINGS/PRECAUTIONS). For patients unable to tolerate 1 g/day to start, therapy may be initiated with 250 mg/day and dosage gradually increased to recommended level. Dosage should be titrated according to urinary copper excretion and therapy monitored every 3 mo by measuring 24-h urinary excretion of copper (optimum therapeutic level with patient on a low-copper diet, 0.5–1 mg/24 h).
Cystinuria	Individualize dosage to limit cystine excretion to 100–200 mg/day in patients with no history of stones and to below 100 mg/day in patients with stones and/or pain. Instruct patient to drink about a pint of fluid at bedtime and another pint once during the night. Fluid intake during the day should be adequate to maintain urine specific gravity below 1.010; in addition, patient should take sufficient alkali to maintain a urinary pH of 7.5–8 and be placed on a diet low in methionine (except growing children and pregnant patients). If doses cannot be divided equally, give the largest at bedtime. Bedtime dose should be retained if daily dosage is lowered due to adverse reactions. An annual x-ray examination for renal stones is advisable.

WARNINGS/PRECAUTIONS

Blood dyscrasias	May occur and can be fatal; monitor hemoglobin, WBC count, differential count, and direct platelet count every 2 wk for at least first 6 mo of therapy and monthly thereafter, and instruct patient to report signs such as fever, sore throat, chills, bruising, or bleeding. If WBC count falls below 3,500/mm^3 discontinue therapy; if platelet count falls below 100,000/mm^3 or either platelet count or WBC count decreases progressively over three successive determinations, suspend therapy temporarily or discontinue treatment.
Renal impairment	May occur; perform a routine urinalysis every 2 wk for at least first 6 mo of therapy and monthly thereafter. Proteinuria and/or hematuria may indicate incipient membranous glomerulopathy; if proteinuria exceeds 1 g/24 h or increases progressively, reduce dosage or discontinue therapy; in rheumatoid arthritis patients, discontinue therapy if unexplained gross hematuria develops or microscopic hematuria persists. Urinary abnormalities may persist for a year or more after drug is discontinued.
Intrahepatic cholestasis and toxic hepatitis	May occur rarely; perform liver-function tests every 6 mo for the duration of therapy
Goodpasture's syndrome	May occur rarely; if urinary findings are abnormal in conjunction with hemoptysis and pulmonary infiltrates on x-ray, discontinue therapy immediately
Myasthenic syndrome	May occur and may progress to myasthenia gravis; discontinue therapy if suggestive signs occur
Pemphigoid-type reactions	May occur; discontinue use of penicillamine and treat with corticosteroids
Interruption of therapy in Wilson's disease or cystinuria	May be followed by sensitivity reactions when drug is restarted, even if interruption is only for a few days
Skin rash	May occur during first few months of therapy or, less often, later. If pruritus and/or rash occurs early, add an antihistamine; if necessary, suspend therapy temporarily and reinstitute drug at a lower dosage level when reaction clears. If rash occurs after first 6 mo of therapy or is accompanied by fever, arthralgia, lymphadenopathy, or other allergic reactions, discontinue therapy.
Drug fever	May occur, sometimes accompanied by macular cutaneous eruptions. In Wilson's disease and cystinuria, suspend therapy temporarily and reinstitute drug at a lower dosage level when reaction has subsided; if reaction recurs, add a systemic corticosteroid. In patients with rheumatoid arthritis, discontinue therapy permanently.
Positive ANA test	May occur and may foreshadow development of lupus erythematosus-like syndrome
Oral ulcerations	May occur and may resemble aphthous stomatitis; reduce dosage or, if necessary, discontinue therapy. Rarely, cheilosis, glossitis, or gingivostomatitis may occur and may be dose related, precluding further dosage increases or requiring withdrawal of therapy.
Obliterative bronchiolitis	May occur rarely; instruct patient to report immediately pulmonary symptoms such as exertional dyspnea, unexplained cough, or wheezing; pulmonary function studies should be considered in suspicious cases
Collagen changes	May occur, resulting in increased skin friability at sites subject to pressure or trauma, extravasation of blood, and development of papules at venipuncture and surgical sites; reduce dosage to 250 mg/day prior to surgery and until wound healing is complete
Special-risk patients	Use with caution in patients who have experienced a major toxic reaction to chrysotherapy, since the risk of a serious adverse reaction to penicillamine may be increased
Dietary supplementation	Pyridoxine (25 mg/day) is necessary in patients with Wilson's disease or cystinuria and in rheumatoid arthritis patients with impaired nutrition; short courses of iron supplements may be necessary, especially in children and menstruating women (allow 2 h to elapse between administration of iron and penicillamine)

CUPRIMINE ■ DEPEN

Carcinogenicity	Leukemia has been associated with penicillamine therapy, but a causal relationship has not been established. Intraperitoneal administration of 400 mg/kg, 5 days/wk, for 6 mo has resulted in lymphocytic leukemia in 5 of 10 autoimmune, disease-prone NZB mice; long-term studies have not been done.

ADVERSE REACTIONS
Frequent reactions (incidence ≥ 1%) are printed in *italics*

Allergic	*Rash (5%)*; generalized pruritus; pemphigoid-type reactions; eruptions accompanied by fever, arthralgia, or lymphadenopathy; urticaria; exfoliative dermatitis; thyroiditis and hypoglycemia associated with anti-insulin antibodies (extremely rare); migratory polyarthralgia, often with objective synovitis; lupus erythematosus-like syndrome
Gastrointestinal	*Anorexia, epigastric pain, nausea, vomiting, and diarrhea (17%); decreased taste perception (12%)*; reactivated peptic ulcer; hepatic dysfunction; pancreatitis; oral ulcerations; cheilosis, glossitis, gingivostomatitis, intrahepatic cholestasis, and toxic hepatitis (rare)
Hematological	*Thrombocytopenia (4%), leukopenia (2%)*, agranulocytosis, aplastic anemia, thrombotic thrombocytopenic purpura, hemolytic anemia, red-cell aplasia, monocytosis, leukocytosis, eosinophilia, thrombocytosis, thrombophlebitis (rare)
Renal	*Proteinuria (6%)* and/or hematuria, progressing to membranous glomerulonephropathy and the nephrotic syndrome; Goodpasture's syndrome and fatal renal vasculitis (rare)
Central nervous system; neuromuscular	Tinnitus; optic neuritis; peripheral sensory and motor neuropathies (including Guillain-Barré syndrome), with or without muscular weakness; myasthenia gravis
Dermatological	Increased skin friability, excessive wrinkling, white papules at venipuncture and surgical sites; lichen planus, elastosis perforans serpiginosa, toxic epidermal necrolysis, and anetoderma (rare)
Other	Bronchial asthma; hyperpyrexia, hair loss, polymyositis, dermatomyositis, and mammary hyperplasia (rare)[1]

OVERDOSAGE

Signs and symptoms	See ADVERSE REACTIONS
Treatment	Treat symptomatically and institute supportive measures, as needed

DRUG INTERACTIONS

Gold salts, antimalarials, cytotoxic drugs, phenylbutazone, oxyphenbutazone	△ Risk of renal or hematological toxicity; do not administer concomitantly
Iron preparations, mineral supplements	▽ Therapeutic effect of penicillamine

ALTERED LABORATORY VALUES

Blood/serum values	△ Alkaline phosphatase △ Lactic dehydrogenase + Cephalin flocculation test + Thymol turbidity test
Urinary values	▽ Cystine △ Copper △ Zinc △ Mercury △ Lead

USE IN CHILDREN
See INDICATIONS and ORAL DOSAGE; the effectiveness of this drug in juvenile rheumatoid arthritis has not been established

USE IN PREGNANT AND NURSING WOMEN
Congenital cutis laxa and other associated birth defects have been reported in infants whose mothers received penicillamine during pregnancy. This drug is contraindicated in pregnant women with rheumatoid arthritis. It has been reported that continued treatment with penicillamine throughout pregnancy protects the mother from relapses of Wilson's disease, and that discontinuation has deleterious effects on the mother. If this drug is given to a pregnant woman with Wilson's disease, limit dosage to 1 g/day, and when cesarean section is planned, limit dosage to 250 mg/day during the last 6 wk of pregnancy and postoperatively (until wound healing is completed). If possible, penicillamine should not be used in pregnant women with cystinuria; if stone formation persists in these patients, the benefit to the mother should be weighed against the risk to the fetus. Penicillamine should not be used in nursing mothers.

[1] In addition, allergic alveolitis, obliterative bronchiolitis, interstitial pneumonitis, and pulmonary fibrosis have been reported in patients with severe rheumatoid arthritis, some of whom were receiving penicillamine. Leukemia has also been reported; however, a causal relationship has not been established.

ANTIARTHRITIC AGENTS

DEPEN (penicillamine) Wallace   Rx
Tablets: 250 mg

INDICATIONS
Severe, active rheumatoid arthritis in patients refractory to conventional therapy

ORAL DOSAGE
Adult: 125–250 mg/day, at least 1 h before eating or 1 h apart from other drugs, food, or milk, followed by increases of 125–250 mg/day every 1–3 mo, up to 500–750 mg/day, and then, if still necessary after 2–3 mo at this level, by further increases of 250 mg/day every 2–3 mo; if, after administration of 1–1.5 g/day for 3–4 mo, patient does not respond, discontinue use; average maintenance dosage: 500–750 mg/day in divided doses

DEPEN

Wilson's disease	**Adult:** 250 mg qid, 1/2–1 h before meals and at bedtime (at least 2 h after evening meal), increased if needed up to 2 g/day in divided doses **Child:** same as adult
Cystinuria	**Adult:** 250 mg/day at bedtime to start, followed by gradual increases to 1–4 g/day in 4 equally divided doses; usual maintenance dosage: 2 g/day in divided doses **Child:** 30 mg/kg/day in 4 equally divided doses

CONTRAINDICATIONS

History of aplastic anemia or agranulocytosis associated with prior penicillamine therapy	History or evidence of renal insufficiency in patients with rheumatoid arthritis	Pregnancy in patients with rheumatoid arthritis

ADMINISTRATION/DOSAGE ADJUSTMENTS

Rheumatoid arthritis	Clinical response may not be apparent for 2–3 mo after onset of therapy or dosage adjustment. If disease suppression is inadequate after first 6–9 mo, increase maintenance dosage by 125–250 mg/day at 3-mo intervals, up to 1 g/day in divided doses or, if necessary, 1.5 g/day in divided doses. If patient has been in remission for 6 mo or more, attempt to reduce dosage by 125–250 mg/day approximately every 3 mo. If therapy is interrupted, reintroduce drug at a lower dosage and increase dosage slowly.
Management of arthritic exacerbations	Flare-ups of rheumatoid arthritis may be controlled by adding a nonsteroidal anti-inflammatory agent. Do not increase the dosage of penicillamine unless flare persists more than 12 wk. Penicillamine-induced migratory polyarthralgia may closely mimic a disease exacerbation and can be distinguished from it by discontinuing or substantially reducing the dosage of penicillamine.
Concomitant antiarthritic therapy	Do not use with gold salts, antimalarials, cytotoxic (immunosuppressive) agents, phenylbutazone, or oxyphenbutazone; treatment with salicylates, other nonsteroidal anti-inflammatory agents, or systemic corticosteroids may be continued when penicillamine is started or withdrawn gradually as symptoms permit
Wilson's disease	Clinical improvement may not be apparent for 1–3 mo. During this period, neurologic symptoms may worsen; if necessary, therapy may be interrupted *temporarily,* but not without risk (see WARNINGS/PRECAUTIONS). For patients unable to tolerate 1 g/day to start, therapy may be initiated with 250 mg/day and dosage gradually increased to recommended level. Dosage should be titrated according to urinary copper excretion and therapy monitored every 3 mo by measuring 24 h urinary excretion of copper (optimum therapeutic level with patient on a low-copper diet, 0.5–1 mg/24 h).
Cystinuria	Individualize dosage to limit cystine excretion to 100–200 mg/day in patients with no history of stones and to below 100 mg/day in patients with stones and/or pain. Instruct patient to drink about a pint of fluid at bedtime and another pint once during the night. Fluid intake during the day should be adequate to maintain urine specific gravity below 1.010; in addition, patient should take sufficient alkali to maintain a urinary pH of 7.5–8 and be placed on a diet low in methionine (except growing children and pregnant patients). If doses cannot be divided equally, give the largest at bedtime. Bedtime dose should be retained if daily dosage is lowered due to adverse reactions. An annual x-ray examination for renal stones is advisable.
Dosage frequency	Up to 500 mg/day may be given in a single daily dose; divide dosages exceeding 500 mg/day

WARNINGS/PRECAUTIONS

Blood dyscrasias	May occur and can be fatal; monitor hemoglobin, WBC count, differential count, and direct platelet count every 2 wk for first 6 mo of therapy and monthly thereafter, and instruct patient to report signs such as fever, sore throat, chills, bruising, or bleeding. If WBC count falls below 3,500/mm^3, discontinue therapy; if platelet count falls below 100,000/mm^3 or either platelet count or WBC count decreases progressively over three successive determinations, suspend therapy temporarily or discontinue treatment.
Renal impairment	May occur; perform a routine urinalysis every 2 wk for first 6 mo of therapy and monthly thereafter. Proteinuria and/or hematuria may indicate incipient membranous glomerulopathy; if proteinuria exceeds 1 g/24 h or increases progressively, reduce dosage or discontinue therapy; in rheumatoid arthritis patients, discontinue therapy if unexplained gross hematuria develops or microscopic hematuria persists. Urinary abnormalities may persist for a year or more after drug is discontinued.
Intrahepatic cholestasis and toxic hepatitis	May occur rarely; perform liver-function tests every 6 mo for the duration of therapy
Goodpasture's syndrome	May occur rarely; if urinary findings are abnormal in conjunction with hemoptysis and pulmonary infiltrates on x-ray, discontinue therapy immediately
Myasthenic syndrome	May occur and may progress to myasthenia gravis; discontinue therapy if suggestive signs occur
Pemphigoid-type reactions	May occur; discontinue use of penicillamine and treat with corticosteroids
Interruption of therapy in Wilson's disease or cystinuria	May be followed by sensitivity reactions when drug is restarted, even if interruption is only for a few days

DEPEN

Skin rash	May occur during first few months of therapy or, less often, later. If pruritus and/or rash occurs early, add an antihistamine; if necessary, suspend therapy temporarily and reinstitute drug at a lower dosage level when reaction clears. If rash occurs after first 6 mo of therapy or is accompanied by fever, arthralgia, lymphadenopathy, or other allergic reactions, discontinue therapy.
Drug fever	May occur, sometimes accompanied by macular cutaneous eruptions. In Wilson's disease and cystinuria, suspend therapy temporarily and reinstitute drug at a lower dosage level when reaction has subsided; if reaction recurs, add a systemic corticosteroid. In patients with rheumatoid arthritis, discontinue therapy permanently.
Positive ANA test	May occur and may foreshadow development of lupus erythematosus-like syndrome
Oral ulcerations	May occur and may resemble aphthous stomatitis; reduce dosage or, if necessary, discontinue therapy. Rarely, cheilosis, glossitis, or gingivostomatitis may occur and may be dose related, precluding further dosage increases or requiring withdrawal of therapy.
Obliterative bronchiolitis	May occur rarely; instruct patient to report immediately pulmonary symptoms such as exertional dyspnea, unexplained cough, or wheezing; pulmonary function studies should be considered in suspicious cases
Collagen changes	May occur, resulting in increased skin friability at sites subject to pressure or trauma, extravasation of blood, and development of papules at venipuncture and surgical sites; reduce dosage to 250 mg/day prior to surgery and until wound healing is complete
Special-risk patients	Use with caution in patients who have experienced a major toxic reaction to chrysotherapy, since the risk of a serious adverse reaction to penicillamine may be increased
Dietary supplementation	Pyridoxine (25 mg/day) is necessary in patients with Wilson's disease or cystinuria and in rheumatoid arthritis patients with impaired nutrition; short courses of iron supplements may be necessary, especially in children and menstruating women (allow 2 h to elapse between administration of iron and penicillamine)
Carcinogenicity	Leukemia has been associated with penicillamine therapy, but a causal relationship has not been established. Intraperitoneal administration of 400 mg/kg, 5 days/wk, for 6 mo has resulted in lymphocytic leukemia in 5 of 10 autoimmune, disease-prone NZB mice; long-term studies have not been done.

ADVERSE REACTIONS

Frequent reactions (incidence $\geq$ 1%) are printed in *italics*

Allergic	*Rash (5%);* generalized pruritus; pemphigoid-type reactions; eruptions accompanied by fever, arthralgia, or lymphadenopathy; urticaria; exfoliative dermatitis; thyroiditis (rare); migratory polyarthralgia, often with objective synovitis; lupus erythematosus-like syndrome
Gastrointestinal	*Anorexia, epigastric pain, nausea, vomiting, and diarrhea (17%); decreased taste perception (12%);* reactivated peptic ulcer; hepatic dysfunction; cholestatic jaundice; pancreatitis; oral ulcerations; cheilosis, glossitis, and gingivostomatitis (rare)
Hematological	*Thrombocytopenia (4%), leukopenia (2%),* agranulocytosis, aplastic anemia, thrombotic thrombocytopenic purpura, hemolytic anemia, red-cell aplasia, monocytosis, leukocytosis, eosinophilia, thrombocytosis, thrombophlebitis (rare)
Renal	*Proteinuria (6%)* and/or hematuria, progressing to membranous glomerulonephropathy and the nephrotic syndrome; Goodpasture's syndrome and fatal renal vasculitis (rare)
Central nervous system	Tinnitus, optic neuritis
Dermatological	Increased skin friability, excessive wrinkling, white papules at venipuncture and surgical sites; elastosis perforans serpiginosa, toxic epidermal necrolysis, and anetoderma (rare)
Other	Hyperpyrexia, hair loss, myasthenia gravis, polymyositis, dermatomyositis, and mammary hyperplasia (rare)[1]

OVERDOSAGE

Signs and symptoms	See ADVERSE REACTIONS
Treatment	Treat symptomatically and institute supportive measures, as needed

DRUG INTERACTIONS

Gold salts, antimalarials, cytotoxic drugs, phenylbutazone, oxyphenbutazone	⇧ Risk of renal or hematological toxicity; do not administer concomitantly
Iron preparations, mineral supplements	⇩ Therapeutic effect of penicillamine

ALTERED LABORATORY VALUES

Blood/serum values	⇧ Alkaline phosphatase ⇧ Lactic dehydrogenase + Cephalin flocculation test + Thymol turbidity test

DEPEN ■ DISALCID

Urinary values — ▽ Cystine △ Copper △ Zinc △ Mercury △ Lead

USE IN CHILDREN	USE IN PREGNANT AND NURSING WOMEN
See INDICATIONS and ORAL DOSAGE; the effectiveness of this drug in juvenile rheumatoid arthritis has not been established	Contraindicated in pregnant women with rheumatoid arthritis. In pregnant women with Wilson's disease, limit dosage to 1 g/day; if cesarean section is planned, limit dosage to 250 mg/day during last 6 wk of pregnancy and postoperatively until wound healing is completed. Not recommended for use in pregnant women with cystinuria. Consult manufacturer for use in nursing mothers.

[1] In addition, allergic alveolitis and obliterative bronchiolitis have been reported in patients with severe rheumatoid arthritis, some of whom were receiving penicillamine. Leukemia has also been reported; however, a causal relationship has not been established.

ANTIARTHRITIC AGENTS

DISALCID (salsalate) Riker   Rx
Capsules: 500 mg **Tablets:** 500, 750 mg

INDICATIONS
Rheumatoid arthritis, osteoarthritis, and related rheumatic disorders

ORAL DOSAGE
Adult: 1 g tid or 1.5 g bid; titrate dosage according to individual response (full benefits of therapy may not be evident for 3–4 days)

CONTRAINDICATIONS
Hypersensitivity to salicylates

WARNINGS/PRECAUTIONS

Reye's syndrome	Salicylates may precipitate Reye's syndrome in patients who have chicken pox, influenza, or influenza-like symptoms; use in such patients is not recommended
Factors influencing plasma salicylic acid levels	Nutritional status, competitive binding of other drugs, and fluctuations in serum protein levels caused by disease (eg, rheumatoid arthritis) can influence the protein binding of salicylic acid and, therefore, the free salicylic acid level. Drugs and food that increase urinary pH increase the urinary excretion of salicylic acid and thus lower plasma levels, whereas acidifying drugs and food decrease urinary excretion and thus increase plasma salicylic acid levels. Regularly monitor urinary pH, as sudden acidification of the urine (eg, from pH 6.5 to 5.5) can double the plasma salicylic acid concentration, resulting in toxicity. To maintain therapeutic serum levels, an increase in dosage may be necessary because induction of hepatic enzymes may occur during therapy. Exercise great caution in prescribing this drug to patients with chronic renal insufficiency.
Long-term therapy	Caution patients on long-term therapy not to take other salicylates in order to avoid potentially toxic plasma salicylate levels. Periodically monitor the plasma salicylic acid concentration to help maintain therapeutic levels (10–30 mg/dl); toxicity is not usually seen until the plasma level exceeds 30 mg/dl.
Carcinogenicity	No long-term studies have been done to evaluate the carcinogenic potential of this drug; however, several such studies in animals have failed to demonstrate any association of aspirin and other salicylates with cancer

ADVERSE REACTIONS

Otic	Tinnitus, temporary hearing loss
Gastrointestinal	Nausea, dyspepsia, heartburn

OVERDOSAGE

Signs and symptoms	Tinnitus, vertigo, headache, confusion, drowsiness, sweating, hyperventilation, vomiting, diarrhea; in severe cases, electrolyte and acid-base disturbances, hyperthermia, and dehydration
Treatment	Administer syrup of ipecac to induce emesis and, if necessary, perform gastric lavage. Correct fluid and electrolyte imbalances with appropriate IV therapy. Maintain adequate renal function. Extreme cases may require hemodialysis or peritoneal dialysis.

DRUG INTERACTIONS

Aspirin and other salicylates	△ Plasma salicylate levels and possible toxicity
Uricosuric agents (eg, probenecid and sulfinpyrazone)	▽ Uricosuric effect
Urinary alkalinizers	△ Urinary excretion of salicylic acid

COMPENDIUM OF DRUG THERAPY

Urinary acidifiers	▽ Urinary excretion of salicylic acid
Oral anticoagulants	△ Risk of bleeding and hemorrhage
Tolbutamide, chlorpropamide, acetohexamide, tolazamide	△ Hypoglycemic effect

ALTERED LABORATORY VALUES

Blood/serum values	▽ Thyroxine (T$_4$)

No clinically significant alterations in urinary values have been reported at therapeutic dosages

USE IN CHILDREN

Safety and effectiveness for use in children have not been established

USE IN PREGNANT AND NURSING WOMEN

Pregnancy Category C: use during pregnancy only if expected benefit justifies the potential risk to the fetus. Salsalate and salicylic acid have been shown to be teratogenic and embryocidal in rats at 4–5 times the usual human dose, but not at twice the human dose. No adequate, well-controlled studies have been done in pregnant women. Although adverse maternal and fetal effects have not been reported when salsalate has been used during labor, it should be used with caution if anti-inflammatory doses are required. Other salicylates have been associated with prolonged gestation and labor, maternal and neonatal bleeding complications, potentiation of narcotic and barbiturate effects, delivery problems, and stillbirth. Salicylic acid is excreted in human milk in concentrations approximating maternal blood levels; use with caution in nursing mothers.

ANTIARTHRITIC AGENTS

DOLOBID (diflunisal) Merck Sharp & Dohme   Rx

Tablets: 250, 500 mg

INDICATIONS	ORAL DOSAGE
Mild to moderate pain	**Adult:** 1,000 mg to start, followed by 500 mg q12h or, if necessary, q8h; depending on pain severity, patient response, weight, or advanced age, a lower dosage may be appropriate (eg, 500 mg to start, followed by 250 mg q8–12h)
Osteoarthritis Rheumatoid arthritis	**Adult:** 500–1,000 mg/day in two divided doses, adjusted according to patient response; for maintenance, do not exceed 1,500 mg/day

CONTRAINDICATIONS	
Hypersensitivity to diflunisal	History of acute asthmatic attacks, urticaria, or rhinitis precipitated by aspirin or other nonsteroidal anti-inflammatory drugs

ADMINISTRATION/DOSAGE ADJUSTMENTS	
Administration	Diflunisal may be administered with water, milk, or meals; tablets should not be crushed or chewed

WARNINGS/PRECAUTIONS	
Peptic ulceration, GI bleeding	May occur and, in rare instances, can be fatal; patients with a history of upper GI tract disease should be closely supervised during therapy. In patients with active GI bleeding or an active peptic ulcer, benefits of therapy should be weighed against possible hazards; institute an appropriate ulcer regimen and monitor patient's progress carefully.
Interference with platelet function	Monitor closely patients who may be adversely affected by diflunisal's inhibition of platelet function
Visual disturbances	May occur; if eye complaints develop, perform an ophthalmologic examination
Renal toxicity	Proteinuria, acute interstitial nephritis with hematuria, and occasionally the nephrotic syndrome may occur during therapy. In patients with reduced renal blood flow or volume owing to conditions such as renal or hepatic dysfunction, advanced age, hypovolemia, congestive heart failure, sepsis, or use of nephrotoxic agents, administration of a nonsteroidal anti-inflammatory agent may cause a critical decrease in the formation of renal prostaglandins and thereby precipitate overt renal failure; this reaction is reversible upon discontinuation of the drug. To avoid renal toxicity, use with caution in patients at risk and monitor renal function periodically in any patient with possible renal impairment.
Drug accumulation	Diflunisal is eliminated primarily by the kidneys; closely monitor patients with significant renal impairment and be prepared to reduce the daily dose

DOLOBID

Peripheral edema	May occur; use with caution in patients with compromised cardiac function, hypertension, or other conditions predisposing to fluid retention
Liver function abnormalities	Borderline elevations may occur in up to 15% of patients; meaningful elevations (3 times the upper limit of normal) in SGOT or SGPT levels have been reported in less than 1% of patients. If abnormal liver function tests or other manifestations of liver dysfunction arise during therapy, evaluate the patient for evidence of a more severe hepatic reaction. Although such reactions as jaundice have occurred rarely, discontinue therapy if abnormal liver function test results persist or worsen, signs and symptoms of liver disease develop, or secondary manifestations (eg, eosinophilia, rash) occur, because hepatic reactions can be fatal.
Renal toxicity	Papillary edema has been observed occasionally in rats and dogs receiving high dosages, and papillary necrosis has been seen in mice during long-term studies
Carcinogenicity, mutagenicity, effect on fertility	An apparent, but not statistically significant, increase in pulmonary and hepatocellular adenomas has been observed in mice (because the results of this study were inconclusive, it is being repeated). A long-term study in the rat has shown no evidence of carcinogenicity, and both in vitro and in vivo studies have failed to demonstrate any mutagenic potential. No evidence of impaired fertility has been found in rats given up to 50 mg/kg/day.

ADVERSE REACTIONS[1]

Frequent reactions (incidence ≥ 1%) are printed in *italics*

Gastrointestinal	*Nausea, dyspepsia, gastrointestinal pain, and diarrhea (3–9%); vomiting, constipation, and flatulence (1–3%);* peptic ulcer, gastrointestinal bleeding, anorexia, eructation, gastrointestinal perforation
Otic	*Tinnitus (1–3%)*
Ophthalmic	Transient visual disturbances, including blurred vision
Hepatic	Liver function abnormalities, jaundice (sometimes with fever), cholestasis, hepatitis
Central nervous system	*Dizziness, somnolence, and insomnia (1–3%);* vertigo, nervousness, depression, hallucinations, confusion, disorientation, vertigo, light-headedness, paresthesias
Dermatological	*Rash (3–9%);* erythema multiforme, exfoliative dermatitis, Stevens-Johnson syndrome, toxic epidermal necrolysis, urticaria, pruritus, sweating, dry mucous membranes, stomatitis, photosensitivity
Genitourinary	Dysuria, renal impairment (including renal failure), interstitial nephritis, hematuria, proteinuria
Hypersensitivity	Acute anaphylactic reaction with bronchospasm; potentially fatal syndrome characterized by fever, chills, dermatological reactions (see above), changes in liver function, jaundice, leukopenia, thrombocytopenia, eosinophilia, renal impairment (including renal failure), adenitis, arthralgia, arthritis, malaise, anorexia, and disorientation
Other	*Headache (3–9%); fatigue/tiredness (1–3%);* asthenia, edema, thrombocytopenia

OVERDOSAGE

Signs and symptoms	Drowsiness, vomiting, nausea, diarrhea, hyperventilation, tachycardia, sweating, tinnitus, disorientation, stupor, coma, diminished urine output, cardiorespiratory arrest
Treatment	Empty stomach by inducing emesis or by gastric lavage, and institute symptomatic and supportive measures, as needed. Hemodialysis is not likely to be beneficial in removing the drug from the circulation because of high protein binding.

DRUG INTERACTIONS

Oral anticoagulants	△ Prothrombin time; closely monitor the prothrombin time during concomitant therapy and for several days afterwards, and adjust the anticoagulant dosage as needed
Acetaminophen	△ Plasma level of acetaminophen; exercise caution and carefully monitor patient response during concomitant therapy because of the increased risk of hepatotoxicity[2]
Indomethacin	△ Plasma level of indomethacin; diflunisal and indomethacin should not be administered concomitantly because, in some patients, combined use has been associated with fatal GI hemorrhage
Sulindac	▽ Plasma level of active sulfide metabolite of sulindac
Aspirin	▽ Plasma level of diflunisal
Naproxen	▽ Urinary excretion of naproxen and its glucuronide metabolite; the plasma level of naproxen is not affected
Antacids	▽ Plasma level of diflunisal with continuous use of antacids
Hydrochlorothiazide	△ Plasma level of hydrochlorothiazide ▽ Hyperuricemic effect of hydrochlorothiazide
Furosemide	▽ Hyperuricemic effect of furosemide; the diuretic effect of furosemide is not affected

ALTERED LABORATORY VALUES

Blood/serum values	△ SGOT △ SGPT ▽ Uric acid

Urinary values — ⇧ Uric acid   + Protein

USE IN CHILDREN

Safety and effectiveness have not been established; not recommended for use in children under 12 yr of age

USE IN PREGNANT AND NURSING WOMEN

Pregnancy Category C: use during the first two trimesters of pregnancy only if the expected benefit justifies the potential risk to the fetus; because premature closure of the ductus arteriosus may occur, use during the third trimester is not recommended. A dose of 60 mg/kg/day (twice the maximum human dose) was shown to be maternotoxic, embryotoxic, and teratogenic in rabbits. In three other rabbit studies, teratogenicity was observed at doses of 40–50 mg/kg/day. Studies in mice and rats receiving up to 45 mg/kg/day and 100 mg/kg/day, respectively, showed no evidence of fetal harm. Prolonged gestation has been observed in rats receiving 1½ times the maximum human dose; nonsteroidal anti-inflammatory drugs have caused dystocia and delayed parturition in animals. No adequate, well-controlled studies have been performed with diflunisal in pregnant women. This drug is excreted in human milk in concentrations reaching 2–7% of plasma levels. Because of the potential for serious adverse effects in the nursing infant, patient should stop nursing while taking diflunisal.

[1] In general, a lower incidence of adverse reactions may be anticipated in patients receiving short-term treatment for mild to moderate pain. Reactions for which a causal relationship has not been established include dyspnea, palpitation, syncope, muscle cramps, and chest pain; the prescriber should also be aware of the adverse reactions associated with the use of other nonsteroidal anti-inflammatory agents which may potentially develop in patients treated with diflunisal.

[2] An increase in GI toxicity has been observed in dogs, but not in rats, at dosages of 40–52 mg/kg/day of diflunisal and acetaminophen (approximately twice the maximum human dose of each drug); the clinical significance of this finding is not known

---

ANTIARTHRITIC AGENTS

Regular Strength ECOTRIN (aspirin) SmithKline Consumer Products   OTC

Tablets (enteric coated): 325 mg

INDICATIONS	ORAL DOSAGE
Arthritis and rheumatism	**Adult:** for minor aches and pain, 325–650 mg q4h, as needed; for chronic therapy, up to 650 mg q4h or up to 975 mg q6h without medical supervision (higher doses may be given *with* supervision)
Reducing the risk of **recurrent transient ischemic attacks or stroke in men** who have had transient ischemia of the brain due to fibrin platelet emboli	**Adult:** 325 mg qid or 650 mg bid
Reducing the risk of **myocardial infarction and subsequent death** in patients with unstable angina or a prior infarction[1]	**Adult:** 325 mg once daily

Maximum Strength ECOTRIN (aspirin) SmithKline Consumer Products   OTC

Tablets (enteric coated): 500 mg   **Caplets (enteric coated):** 500 mg

INDICATIONS	ORAL DOSAGE
Arthritis and rheumatism	**Adult:** for minor aches and pain, 1 g q6h, as needed; for chronic therapy, up to 1 g q6h without medical supervision (higher doses may be given *with* supervision)

CONTRAINDICATIONS

Consult manufacturer

ADMINISTRATION/DOSAGE ADJUSTMENTS

Administration — Give each dose with water or fruit juice

Chronic therapy — Anti-inflammatory effect is generally associated with a serum salicylate level of 15 mg/dl, attained in healthy men with 3 days of treatment at 5.2 g/day or with 4 days of treatment at 3.9 g/day and attained in healthy women with 2 days at 5.2 g/day or with 3 days at 3.9 g/day. If 3.9–4 g/day is exceeded, monitor serum levels and watch for tinnitus and other clinical manifestations of toxicity; bear in mind that high-frequency hearing loss, which often occurs in the elderly, makes detection of tinnitus difficult and use of tinnitus as an index of toxicity questionable.

WARNINGS/PRECAUTIONS

Information for patients	Package labels caution patients not to use these products without medical supervision if one of the following conditions exists: (1) history of ulcers, (2) erythema, (3) chicken pox or influenza in a child or teenager, (4) arthritis or rheumatism in a child under 12 yr of age, (5) pregnancy, or (6) nursing. Patients are instructed to discontinue administration if they experience dizziness, tinnitus, or hearing impairment and to also consult a physician if persistent or unexplained stomach upset develops, overdose or erythema occurs, or pain persists for more than 10 days.
Evaluation of patients with transient ischemic attacks (TIA's)	Before initiating treatment of patients presenting with signs and symptoms of TIA's, perform a complete medical and neurological evaluation, taking into account other disorders that resemble TIA's. Attention should also be given to risk factors; disorders frequently associated with TIA's, such as hypertension and diabetes, should be evaluated and treatment instituted if appropriate.
Monitoring of prophylactic therapy for myocardial infarction	Check blood pressure, BUN level, and serum uric acid level regularly when using aspirin for long-term prophylaxis of myocardial infarction; small increases in these values have been detected during one clinical trial
Patients with impaired gastric emptying	Tablet accumulation and subsequent formation of a bezoar in the stomach have occurred occasionally in patients with impaired gastric emptying, apparently as a result of outlet obstruction due to peptic ulcer disease alone or in combination with hypotonic gastric peristalsis. Telltale symptoms include early satiety and vague upper abdominal distress. Tablet accumulation may be confirmed roentgenographically or by endoscopy. The bezoar can be removed by gastric lavage, alternating between neutral and slightly basic solutions, or by gastrotomy. Alternatively, in a clinically untested approach, parenteral cimetidine, followed by sips of a slightly basic liquid, may be administered in an attempt to dissolve the bezoar; dissolution can be assessed by monitoring the plasma salicylate level or by watching for the development of tinnitus.
Patients with gastrectomy	The acid-resistant enteric coating of these products may offer no benefit to patients with partial or complete gastrectomy since gastric pH may be elevated in these patients
Reye's syndrome	There is evidence suggesting that use of aspirin in children or adolescents with chicken pox or influenza may increase the risk of Reye's syndrome

OVERDOSAGE

Signs and symptoms	Hyperpnea, nausea, vomiting, vertigo, tinnitus, flushing, sweating, thirst, headache, drowsiness, diarrhea, and tachycardia, progressing to hyperthermia, hemorrhage, acid-base disturbances, restlessness, confusion, convulsions, vasomotor depression, coma, and respiratory failure
Treatment	If less than 4 h have elapsed since ingestion, induce emesis or perform gastric lavage, followed by activated charcoal, to remove any remaining drug from the stomach. Initial therapy should be directed at reducing hyperthermia by external sponging with tepid water, correcting dehydration by appropriate IV fluid replacement, and maintaining adequate cardiorespiratory and renal function. In moderately severe cases of salicylate poisoning, cautiously administer sodium bicarbonate IV in sufficient quantity, if possible, to maintain an alkaline diuresis; intermittent peritoneal dialysis may also be helpful. In severe cases, hemodialysis should be seriously considered. Potassium should be added to the repair solution to compensate for potassium losses once urine formation is deemed adequate. Glucose may be provided to correct ketosis and hypoglycemia. Plasma transfusion may be beneficial if shock intervenes. Hemorrhagic phenomena may necessitate whole-blood transfusions and phytonadione (vitamin K_1). Do not administer barbiturates to treat excitement or convulsions.

DRUG INTERACTIONS

Anticoagulants	△ Risk of bleeding
Alcohol, corticosteroids, phenylbutazone, oxyphenbutazone	△ Risk of GI ulceration
Probenecid, sulfinpyrazone	▽ Uricosuria
Spironolactone	▽ Diuretic effect
Methotrexate	△ Methotrexate plasma level and risk of toxicity

ALTERED LABORATORY VALUES

Blood/serum values	△ Prothrombin time △ Uric acid (with low doses) ▽ Uric acid (with high doses) ▽ Thyroxine (T_4) ▽ Thyroid-stimulating hormone
Urinary values	△ Glucose (with Clinitest tablets)

USE IN CHILDREN

Use according to medical judgment in children under 12 yr of age

USE IN PREGNANT AND NURSING WOMEN

Consult manufacturer for use in pregnant or nursing women

---

[1] *FDA Drug Bulletin* 15(4):34, 1985

ANTIARTHRITIC AGENTS

EMPIRIN (aspirin) Burroughs Wellcome OTC
Tablets: 325 mg (5 gr)

INDICATIONS	ORAL DOSAGE
Pain, including headache, muscular aches and pains, and toothache **Fever and discomfort** of colds and flu **Pain and discomfort** due to sore throat, neuralgia, menstrual pain, arthritis and rheumatism, bursitis, lumbago, and sciatica; **sleeplessness** caused by minor pain and discomfort	**Adult:** 325–650 mg (1–2 tabs) with a full glass of water q4h, up to 3,900 mg (12 tabs)/day
Reducing the risk of **recurrent transient ischemic attacks or stroke in men** who have had transient ischemia of the brain due to fibrin platelet emboli[1]	**Adult:** 325 mg (1 tab) qid or 650 mg (2 tabs) bid
Reducing the risk of **myocardial infarction and subsequent death** in patients with unstable angina or a prior infarction[2]	**Adult:** 325 mg once daily

CONTRAINDICATIONS
Gastric ulcer and peptic ulcer symptoms   Asthma   Hypersensitivity to aspirin
Anticoagulant therapy

WARNINGS/PRECAUTIONS

Gastric irritation	May occur, especially in patients with gastric ulcers, erosive gastritis, or bleeding tendencies; use with caution
Patients with blood-coagulation abnormalities	Use with caution in patients with preexisting hypoprothrombinemia or vitamin K deficiency
Nasal polyps, asthma, hay fever	May predispose to salicylate hypersensitivity; use with caution
Interference with platelet aggregation	Use with caution prior to surgery
Monitoring of prophylactic therapy for myocardial infarction	Check blood pressure, BUN level, and serum uric acid level regularly when using aspirin for long-term prophylaxis of myocardial infarction; small increases in these values have been detected during one clinical trial
Patient instructions	The package label advises consultation with a physician if the patient experiences high or continued fever or severe or persistent sore throat, especially when accompanied by fever, headache, nausea, or vomiting; pregnant or nursing women are advised to consult a health professional before using this product
Reye's syndrome	There is evidence suggesting that use of aspirin in children or adolescents with chicken pox or influenza may increase the risk of Reye's syndrome

ADVERSE REACTIONS

Gastrointestinal	Nausea, dyspepsia, heartburn, epigastric discomfort, anorexia, diarrhea, occult blood loss, hemorrhage
Central nervous system	Dizziness, tinnitus, headache, deafness
Respiratory	Hyperventilation
Cardiovascular	Increased pulse rate
Dermatological	Skin eruptions
Other	Sweating, thirst, electrolyte and acid-base imbalance

OVERDOSAGE

Signs and symptoms	Hyperpnea, nausea, vomiting, vertigo, tinnitus, flushing, sweating, thirst, headache, drowsiness, diarrhea, and tachycardia, progressing to hyperthermia, hemorrhage, acid-base disturbances, restlessness, confusion, convulsions, vasomotor depression, coma, and respiratory failure
Treatment	If less than 4 h have elapsed since ingestion, induce emesis or perform gastric lavage, followed by activated charcoal, to remove any remaining drug from the stomach. Initial therapy should be directed at reducing hyperthermia by external sponging with tepid water, correcting dehydration by appropriate IV fluid replacement, and maintaining adequate cardiorespiratory and renal function. In moderately severe cases of salicylate poisoning, cautiously administer sodium bicarbonate IV in sufficient quantity, if possible, to maintain an alkaline diuresis; intermittent peritoneal dialysis may also be helpful. In severe cases, hemodialysis should be seriously considered. Potassium should be added to the repair solution to compensate for potassium losses once urine formation is deemed adequate. Glucose may be provided to correct ketosis and hypoglycemia. Plasma transfusion may be beneficial if shock intervenes. Hemorrhagic phenomena may necessitate whole-blood transfusions and phytonadione (vitamin K$_1$). Do not administer barbiturates to treat excitement or convulsions.

DRUG INTERACTIONS

Anticoagulants	↑ Risk of bleeding
Alcohol, corticosteroids, phenylbutazone, oxyphenbutazone	↑ Risk of GI ulceration
Probenecid, sulfinpyrazone	↓ Uricosuria
Spironolactone	↓ Diuretic effect
Methotrexate	↑ Methotrexate plasma level and risk of toxicity

ALTERED LABORATORY VALUES

Blood/serum values	↑ Prothrombin time ↑ Uric acid (with low doses) ↓ Uric acid (with high doses) ↓ Thyroxine (T_4) ↓ Thyroid-stimulating hormone
Urinary values	↑ Glucose (with Clinitest tablets)

USE IN CHILDREN
Consult manufacturer

USE IN PREGNANT AND NURSING WOMEN
Aspirin has been shown to be teratogenic and embryocidal in rats and mice given 4–6 times the normal human dose. Clinical studies, however, have not shown that aspirin given during the first trimester increases the risk of abnormalities. Use of aspirin close to term may cause bleeding in the mother, fetus, or neonate. Pregnancy and delivery may be prolonged by regular, high-dosage use during the last two trimesters. Use before delivery may also prolong delivery. Aspirin is excreted in breast milk in small amounts; its clinical effect on nursing infants is not known. Because of the potential for serious adverse reactions in nursing infants, a decision should be made not to nurse or to discontinue use of this preparation, taking into account its importance to the mother.

[1] *FDA Drug Bulletin* 10(1):2, 1980
[2] *FDA Drug Bulletin* 15(4):34, 1985

ANTIARTHRITIC AGENTS

FELDENE (piroxicam) Pfizer   Rx
Capsules: 10, 20 mg

INDICATIONS	**ORAL DOSAGE**
Osteoarthritis Rheumatoid arthritis	**Adult:** 20 mg/day, given in a single daily dose or divided; although therapeutic effects are evident early, allow 2 wk before assessing effect of treatment

CONTRAINDICATIONS

Hypersensitivity to piroxicam	History of nasal polyps, angioedema, and bronchospasm precipitated by aspirin or other nonsteroidal anti-inflammatory drugs

WARNINGS/PRECAUTIONS

Peptic ulceration, perforation, GI bleeding	May occur and can be severe and, in rare instances, fatal; patients with a history of upper GI tract disease should be closely supervised during therapy
Renal toxicity	Proteinuria, acute interstitial nephritis with hematuria, and, occasionally, the nephrotic syndrome may occur during therapy. In patients with reduced renal blood flow or volume owing to conditions such as heart failure, renal or hepatic impairment, advanced age, or use of diuretics, administration of a nonsteroidal anti-inflammatory agent may cause a critical decrease in the formation of renal prostaglandins and thereby precipitate overt renal failure; reaction is reversible upon discontinuation of the drug.
Drug accumulation	Patients with renal impairment should be carefully observed and a reduction in their dosage should be considered because of the extensive renal excretion of piroxicam and its metabolites
Visual impairment	May occur; if visual complaints develop, perform an ophthalmologic evaluation
Anemia	Determine hemoglobin and hematocrit values if signs and symptoms of anemia occur
Peripheral edema	May occur; use with caution in patients with congestive heart failure, hypertension, or other conditions predisposing to fluid retention

Liver function abnormalities	Borderline elevations may occur in up to 15% of patients; meaningful elevations (3 times the upper limit of normal) in SGOT or SGPT levels have been reported in less than 1% of patients. If abnormal liver function tests or other manifestations of liver dysfunction arise during therapy, evaluate the patient for evidence of a more severe hepatic reaction. Although such reactions as jaundice and fatal hepatitis have occurred rarely, discontinue therapy if abnormal liver function test results persist or worsen, signs and symptoms of liver disease develop, or secondary manifestations (eg, eosinophilia, rash) occur.
Interference with platelet function	May occur; closely monitor patients who may be affected
Serum sickness	A serum sickness-like syndrome, characterized by arthralgia, fever, fatigue, pruritus, and rash (including vesiculobullous reactions and exfoliative dermatitis), has occurred occasionally

ADVERSE REACTIONS[1]

Frequent reactions (incidence ≥ 1%) are printed in *italics*

Gastrointestinal	*Epigastric distress and nausea (3–9%); stomatitis, anorexia, constipation, abdominal discomfort, flatulence, diarrhea, abdominal pain, and indigestion (1–3%);* pain (colic), liver function abnormalities, jaundice, hepatitis, vomiting, hematemesis, melena, gastrointestinal bleeding, perforation, ulceration, dry mouth
Hematological	*Decreases in hemoglobin and hematocrit (3–9%); anemia, leukopenia, and eosinophilia (1–3%);* thrombocytopenia, petechial rash, ecchymosis, bone marrow depression (including aplastic anemia), epistaxis
Central nervous system	*Dizziness, somnolence, vertigo, headache, and malaise (1–3%);* depression, insomnia, nervousness
Genitourinary	Hematuria, proteinuria, interstitial nephritis, renal failure, hyperkalemia, glomerulitis, papillary necrosis, nephrotic syndrome
Special senses	*Tinnitus (1–3%);* swollen eyes, blurred vision, eye irritation
Cardiovascular	*Edema (2%);* hypertension, exacerbation of congestive heart failure and angina
Dermatological	*Pruritus and rash (1–3%);* sweating, erythema, bruising, desquamation, exfoliative dermatitis, erythema multiforme, toxic epidermal necrolysis, Stevens-Johnson syndrome, vesiculobullous reactions, photoallergic skin reactions
Other	Anaphylaxis, bronchospasm, urticaria/angioedema, vasculitis, serum sickness-like syndrome, fever, hyperglycemia, hypoglycemia, weight gain and loss

OVERDOSAGE

Signs and symptoms	See ADVERSE REACTIONS
Treatment	Induce emesis or use gastric lavage to empty stomach. Observe patient, and give symptomatic and supportive treatment, as needed. Activated charcoal may be effective in reducing absorption and hastening elimination.

DRUG INTERACTIONS

Coumarin-type anticoagulants and other highly protein-bound drugs	Monitor patients closely for a change in dosage requirements
Aspirin	⇩ Plasma levels of piroxicam
Lithium	⇧ Plasma levels of lithium; monitor lithium level when initiating or discontinuing piroxicam therapy or when adjusting the dosage of piroxicam

ALTERED LABORATORY VALUES

Blood/serum values	⇧ BUN ⇧ Creatinine ⇧ SGOT ⇧ SGPT
Urinary values	+ Protein

USE IN CHILDREN

Pediatric indications and dosages have not been established

USE IN PREGNANT AND NURSING WOMEN

Not recommended for use in pregnant or nursing women because of adverse findings in animals and because the safety of using piroxicam during pregnancy or lactation has not been established in humans. An increased incidence of dystocia and delayed parturition has been observed in animals, as well as an increase in gastrointestinal tract toxicity when piroxicam was administered during the third trimester.

---

[1] Other reactions for which a causal relationship has not been established include pancreatitis, onycholysis, loss of hair, akathisia, hallucinations, mood alterations, dream abnormalities, mental confusion, paresthesias, dysuria, weakness, palpitations, dyspnea, and positive ANA test

ANTIARTHRITIC AGENTS

IMURAN (azathioprine) Burroughs Wellcome   Rx

Tablets: 50 mg   **Vials:** 100 mg (20 ml)

INDICATIONS	ORAL DOSAGE	PARENTERAL DOSAGE
Severe, active **rheumatoid arthritis** unresponsive to rest, nonsteroidal anti-inflammatory agents, or gold	**Adult:** 1 mg/kg/day, given in a single dose or divided (bid), to start, followed, if necessary, after a period of 6–8 wk by increments of 0.5 mg/kg/day every 4 wk, up to 2.5 mg/kg/day	—
Renal homotransplantation, as an adjunct for prevention of rejection	**Adult:** 3–5 mg/kg/day to start, beginning on day of transplantation or 1–3 days before; usual maintenance dosage: 1–3 mg/kg/day	**Adult:** 3–5 mg/kg/day IV to start, beginning on day of transplantation or 1–3 days before; switch to oral form after postoperative period, if possible, at the same dose level used IV

CONTRAINDICATIONS

Previous treatment of rheumatoid arthritis patients with alkylating agents (eg, cyclophosphamide, chlorambucil, or melphalan)	Pregnancy in patients with rheumatoid arthritis	Hypersensitivity to azathioprine

ADMINISTRATION/DOSAGE ADJUSTMENTS

Duration of effect	Drug is considered slow acting, and effects may persist after its discontinuation
Threatened transplant rejection	Do not increase dose to toxic levels; discontinuation of therapy may be necessary if severe hematological or other toxicity develops, even if transplant rejection results
Maintenance therapy for rheumatoid arthritis	To obtain lowest effective maintenance dose and reduce risk of toxicity, lower dose by 0.5 mg/kg (approximately 25 mg/day) every 4 wk while keeping other therapy constant and monitoring patient carefully
Therapeutic response time in rheumatoid arthritis	Usually occurs after 6–8 wk of treatment; consider patient refractory if no improvement is observed after 12 wk
Concomitant therapy	Continue rest, physiotherapy, and use of salicylates; reduce dose of corticosteroids if possible; concurrent use of gold, antimalarials, or penicillamine is not recommended
Concomitant allopurinol therapy	Reduce dosage of azathioprine to approximately one-third to one-fourth the usual dosage
Parenteral administration	Add 10 ml of Sterile Water for Injection and swirl until clear solution results; use within 24 h. For IV infusion, dilute further with sterile saline or dextrose; the final volume depends upon the infusion period (usually 30–60 min).
Gastric disturbances	May be reduced in frequency by administering drug in divided doses and/or after meals
Renal impairment	Relatively oliguric patients, especially those with tubular necrosis in the immediate post-cadaveric transplant period, may exhibit delayed clearance of the drug or its metabolites, may be particularly sensitive to the drug, and may require lower doses

WARNINGS/PRECAUTIONS

Risk of neoplasia	May be increased with chronic therapy, particularly in transplant recipients, although acute myelogenous leukemia and solid tumors have been reported in rheumatoid arthritis patients
Mutagenicity	Reversible chromosomal abnormalities have been documented in patients receiving this drug
Hematological toxicity	Severe leukopenia and/or thrombocytopenia, macrocytic anemia, and severe bone marrow depression may occur. These are dose-related and may be more severe in renal transplant patients whose homograft is undergoing rejection; risk is lower for patients with rheumatoid arthritis than for transplant recipients. Delayed hematological suppression may occur. A prompt reduction in dosage or temporary withdrawal of the drug may be necessary if patient shows a rapid fall in or persistently low leukocyte count or other evidence of bone marrow depression.
Serious infections	May occur, especially in homograft recipients, and may be fatal; treat vigorously and consider reducing azathioprine dosage and/or addition of other drugs
Patient monitoring	Perform complete blood counts, including platelet counts, weekly during first month of treatment, twice monthly for second and third months, then monthly or more frequently if dosage alterations or other therapy changes are necessary. Instruct patient to report any unusual bleeding or bruising or signs of infection.
Hepatotoxicity	May occur in homograft recipients but is generally reversible after interruption of therapy; occurrence in rheumatoid arthritis patients is $< 1\%$

IMURAN ■ INDOCIN

ADVERSE REACTIONS	Frequent reactions (incidence ≥ 1%) are printed in *italics*
Hematological	*Leukopenia*, thrombocytopenia, bone marrow suppression, macrocytic anemia and/or bleeding (two cases)
Gastrointestinal	*Nausea and vomiting (~ 12%)*; hypersensitivity pancreatitis (rare); toxic hepatitis with biliary stasis; diarrhea and steatorrhea (< 1%)
Dermatological	*Rash (~ 2%)*, alopecia (< 1%)
Other	Fever, arthralgias, and negative nitrogen balance (< 1%); secondary infection

OVERDOSAGE	
Signs and symptoms	See ADVERSE REACTIONS
Treatment	Discontinue medication; treat symptomatically and institute supportive measures, as required

DRUG INTERACTIONS	
Allopurinol	⇧ Risk of azathioprine toxicity
Alkylating agents (eg, cyclophosphamide, chlorambucil, melphalan)	⇧ Risk of neoplasia (see CONTRAINDICATIONS)
Myelosuppressive drugs	⇧ Effects of both drugs

ALTERED LABORATORY VALUES	
Blood/serum values	⇧ Amylase ⇧ SGOT ⇧ SGPT ⇧ Bilirubin ⇧ Alkaline phosphatase ⇩ Uric acid ⇩ Albumin
Urinary values	⇩ Uric acid

USE IN CHILDREN
See INDICATIONS and ORAL DOSAGE; in children, use only to prevent rejection of renal homotransplants

USE IN PREGNANT AND NURSING WOMEN
Contraindicated for treatment of rheumatoid arthritis in pregnant women. Use in pregnant renal homograft recipients should be avoided unless potential benefits outweigh possible risks to fetus; azathioprine is mutagenic in humans and teratogenic in rodents, crosses the placental barrier, and has been associated with the occurrence of limited immunological and other abnormalities in some infants born to renal homograft recipients. Patients should be advised of the potential risks of using azathioprine during pregnancy and the nursing period.

ANTIARTHRITIC AGENTS

INDOCIN (indomethacin) Merck Sharp & Dohme   Rx

Capsules: 25, 50 mg **Suppositories:** 50 mg **Suspension (per 5 ml):** 25 mg[1] (237 ml) *Pineapple-coconut-mint flavored*

INDICATIONS	ORAL AND RECTAL DOSAGE
Moderate to severe **rheumatoid arthritis**, including acute flares Moderate to severe **ankylosing spondylitis** Moderate to severe **osteoarthritis**	**Adult:** 25 mg bid or tid to start, followed by increases of 25–50 mg/day at weekly intervals, if necessary, up to 150–200 mg/day **Child (> 2 yr):** 2 mg/kg/day, given in divided doses, to start; do not exceed 4 mg/kg/day or 150–200 mg/day, whichever is less
Acute **painful shoulder** (bursitis and/or tendinitis)	**Adult:** 75–150 mg/day in 3 or 4 divided doses until signs and symptoms of inflammation have been controlled for several days (usual course: 7–14 days)
Acute **gouty arthritis**	**Adult:** 50 mg tid, as needed

INDOCIN SR (indomethacin) Merck Sharp & Dohme   Rx

Capsules (sustained release): 75 mg

INDICATIONS	ORAL DOSAGE
Moderate to severe **rheumatoid arthritis**, including acute flares Moderate to severe **ankylosing spondylitis** Moderate to severe **osteoarthritis**	**Adult:** 75 mg once daily in the morning or at bedtime to start, followed, if necessary, by 75 mg bid; watch closely for evidence of intolerance
Acute **painful shoulder** (bursitis and/or tendinitis)	**Adult:** 75 mg 1–2 times/day; watch closely for evidence of intolerance

INDOCIN

CONTRAINDICATIONS

History of acute asthma, urticaria, or rhinitis precipitated by aspirin or other nonsteroidal anti-inflammatory drugs	Recent rectal bleeding or history of proctitis (suppositories only)	Hypersensitivity to indomethacin

ADMINISTRATION/DOSAGE ADJUSTMENTS

Persistent night pain and/or morning stiffness	Up to 100 mg of the total daily dose may be given at bedtime
Acute flare-ups of chronic rheumatoid arthritis	Increase dosage temporarily by 25–50 mg/day until acute phase is under control. If minor adverse reactions occur, reduce dosage rapidly to a tolerable level. If severe adverse reactions occur, discontinue therapy.
Therapeutic response of acute gouty arthritis	Pain is generally relieved within 2–4 h, tenderness and heat usually subside in 24–36 h, and swelling gradually disappears in 3–5 days. Reduce dosage rapidly until drug is withdrawn completely.
Combination therapy	May allow reduction in dosage or elimination of corticosteroids
Gastric irritation	May be minimized by administering capsules or suspension after meals, with food, or with antacids

WARNINGS/PRECAUTIONS

Elderly patients	Are more likely to experience adverse reactions; use with greater care in the aged
High doses (> 150–200 mg/day)	Increase the risk of adverse effects without increasing clinical benefits and are not recommended
Gastrointestinal reactions	Can be severe and even fatal (see ADVERSE REACTIONS); use with extreme caution in patients with a history of recurrent GI lesions or with active GI tract disease and only if such patients can be monitored very closely
Renal toxicity	Proteinuria, acute interstitial nephritis with hematuria, and occasionally the nephrotic syndrome may occur during therapy. In patients with reduced renal blood flow or volume owing to conditions such as congestive heart failure, renal or hepatic impairment, hypovolemia, sepsis, advanced age, or use of nephrotoxic drugs, administration of a nonsteroidal anti-inflammatory agent may cause a critical decrease in the formation of renal prostaglandins and thereby precipitate overt renal failure; the reaction is reversible upon discontinuation of the drug. Use with caution and monitor renal function in any patient who may have diminished renal reserve.
Hyperkalemia	Increases in serum potassium concentrations, including hyperkalemia, have been reported in patients with and without renal impairment; in patients with normal renal function, these effects have been attributed to a hyporeninemic-hypoaldosteronism state
Drug accumulation	Indomethacin is eliminated primarily by the kidneys; closely monitor patients with significant renal impairment and be prepared to reduce the daily dose
Circulatory dysfunction	Indomethacin can cause peripheral edema; use with caution in patients with cardiac dysfunction, hypertension, or other conditions likely to precipitate fluid retention. In patients with severe heart failure and hyponatremia, this drug has produced a significant deterioration in circulatory function.
Ocular effects	Corneal deposits and retinal disturbances (including macular changes) have occurred during prolonged therapy. An ophthalmological examination should be performed whenever vision becomes blurred and, because the ocular changes may be asymptomatic, at periodic intervals during prolonged therapy; if ocular effects are detected, discontinue use.
Psychiatric disturbances, epilepsy, or parkinsonism	May be aggravated; if CNS reactions are severe, discontinue therapy
Drowsiness	Caution patients that their ability to engage in potentially hazardous activities requiring mental alertness or motor coordination may be impaired
Headache	May occur; if headache persists despite a reduction in dosage, discontinue therapy
Infection	Indomethacin may mask the usual signs and symptoms of infection; use with extra care in the presence of a controlled infection
Prolonged bleeding time	May occur due to inhibition of platelet aggregation; use with caution in patients with coagulation defects or in those on anticoagulant therapy
Plasma renin activity	Indomethacin reduces basal plasma renin activity and attenuates the increase in activity associated with hypovolemia, hyponatremia, and loop diuretics
Liver function abnormalities	Borderline elevations may occur in up to 15% of patients; meaningful elevations (3 times the upper limit of normal) in SGOT or SGPT levels have been reported in less than 1% of patients. If abnormal liver function tests or other manifestations of liver dysfunction arise during therapy, evaluate the patient for evidence of a more severe hepatic reaction. Although such reactions as jaundice and fatal hepatitis have occurred rarely, discontinue therapy if abnormal liver function test results persist or worsen, signs and symptoms of liver disease develop, or secondary manifestations (eg, eosinophilia, rash) occur.

INDOCIN

Carcinogenicity, mutagenicity, effect on fertility	No carcinogenic effects have been seen in rats given up to 1 mg/kg/day for 81 wk or in mice and rats given up to 1.5 mg/kg/day throughout their life. No evidence of mutagenicity has been detected in a host-mediated assay or in the Ames, mouse micronucleus, and *Drosophila* tests. Reproduction studies in rats and mice have shown no adverse effect on fertility.

ADVERSE REACTIONS

Frequent reactions (incidence ≥ 1%) are printed in *italics*

Central nervous system and neuromuscular	*Headache (> 10%); dizziness (3–9%); vertigo, somnolence, depression, and fatigue (1–3%);* anxiety, muscle weakness, involuntary muscle activity, insomnia, muzziness, psychic disturbances (including psychosis), mental confusion, drowsiness, light-headedness, syncope, paresthesias, aggravation of epilepsy and parkinsonism, depersonalization, coma, peripheral neuropathy, convulsions
Otic	*Tinnitus (1–2%),* hearing disturbances, deafness
Gastrointestinal	*Nausea (with or without vomiting) and dyspepsia (indigestion, heartburn, epigastric pain) (3–9%); diarrhea, abdominal distress or pain, and constipation (1–3%);* anorexia, bloating, flatulence, peptic ulcer, gastroenteritis, rectal bleeding, proctitis, perforation and hemorrhage of the esophagus, stomach, duodenum, or small and large intestine, intestinal ulceration associated with stenosis and obstruction, bleeding without obvious ulceration, perforation of preexisting sigmoid lesions, ulcerative colitis, regional ileitis, ulcerative stomatitis
Genitourinary	Hematuria, vaginal bleeding, proteinuria, nephrotic syndrome, interstitial nephritis, renal insufficiency (including renal failure)[2]
Cardiovascular	Hypertension, hypotension, tachycardia, chest pain, congestive heart failure, arrhythmia, palpitations
Dermatological	Pruritus, rash, urticaria, petechiae or ecchymosis, exfoliative dermatitis, erythema nodosum, hair loss, Stevens-Johnson syndrome, erythema multiforme, toxic epidermal necrolysis
Hepatic	Toxic hepatitis, jaundice
Ophthalmic	Corneal deposits, retinal disturbances (including macular disturbances), blurred vision
Hematological	Leukopenia, bone-marrow depression anemia secondary to GI bleeding, aplastic or hemolytic anemia, agranulocytosis, thrombocytopenic purpura[1]
Metabolic	Edema, weight gain, fluid retention, flushing or sweating, hyperglycemia, glycosuria, hyperkalemia
Hypersensitivity	Acute respiratory distress, shock-like hypotension, angioedema, dyspnea, asthma, purpura, angiitis, pulmonary edema
Other	Epistaxis, breast enlargement or tenderness, gynecomastia; rectal irritation and tenesmus (with suppositories only)

OVERDOSAGE

Signs and symptoms	Nausea, vomiting, intense headache, dizziness, mental confusion, disorientation, lethargy, paresthesias, numbness, convulsions
Treatment	Empty stomach as soon as possible when overdose is recent. Induce emesis with syrup of ipecac if vomiting has not already occurred; if emesis is not possible, perform gastric lavage. After emptying stomach, instill 25–50 g of activated charcoal. Institute symptomatic and supportive therapy, as needed. Watch patient carefully for several days, with particular attention to possibility of GI ulceration and hemorrhage; administration of antacids may be helpful.

DRUG INTERACTIONS

Diflunisal	Gastrointestinal hemorrhage (may be fatal); indomethacin should not be used in combination with diflunisal
Salicylates	△ Risk of GI reactions; indomethacin should not be used in combination with salicylates
Probenecid	△ Pharmacological effects of indomethacin; titrate dosage carefully and in small increments, bearing in mind that a satisfactory therapeutic response may be attained at a lower than usual dosage
Lithium	△ Risk of lithium toxicity; during combination therapy, carefully watch for signs of lithium toxicity and check the serum drug level more frequently
Loop and thiazide-type diuretics	▽ Diuretic and antihypertensive effects; closely monitor therapeutic response during combination therapy △ Risk of nephrotoxicity
Potassium-sparing diuretics	△ Risk of hyperkalemia and nephrotoxicity Acute renal failure (with triamterene); indomethacin should not be used in combination with triamterene
Beta blockers	▽ Antihypertensive effect; carefully monitor therapeutic response during combination therapy
Captopril	▽ Antihypertensive effect

INDOCIN ■ MAGAN

ALTERED LABORATORY VALUES

Blood/serum values — △ Glucose △ BUN △ Potassium △ SGOT △ SGPT ▽ Renin activity (PRA)

Urinary values — △ Glucose

USE IN CHILDREN

Effectiveness for use in children 14 yr of age or younger has not been established; moreover, during treatment of juvenile rheumatoid arthritis, fatal hepatic reactions have occurred. Give to children who are between 2 and 14 yr of age only when toxicity or ineffectiveness of other agents warrants the risks associated with this drug. For dosing recommendations, see ORAL DOSAGE. During therapy, watch children closely and assess liver function periodically.

USE IN PREGNANT AND NURSING WOMEN

Not recommended for use during pregnancy because safety has not been established in pregnant women and because administration during the third trimester may induce premature closure of the ductus arteriosus. Teratogenic studies in mice and rats have shown no increase in fetal malformations at 0.5–4 mg/kg/day, except for retarded fetal ossification and a decrease in average fetal weight at the highest dosage level. In other studies, administration of 5–15 mg/kg/day has led to maternal toxicity and death and an increase in fetal resorptions and malformations in mice. Decreased maternal weight gain and some maternal and fetal deaths have also been observed in mice and rats receiving 4 mg/kg/day during the last 3 days of gestation; this dosage, but not 2 mg/kg/day, also increased the incidence of neuronal necrosis in the diencephalon in live-born fetuses. Delayed parturition has occurred in rats. Indomethacin is excreted in milk and is not recommended for use in nursing mothers.

VEHICLE/BASE
Suppositories: glycerin, polyethylene glycol 6000, polyethylene glycol 4000, sodium chloride, edetic acid, butylated hydroxyanisole, and butylated hydroxytoluene

[1] Contains 1% alcohol
[2] Other reactions for which a causal relationship has not been established include urinary frequency and leukemia

---

ANTIARTHRITIC AGENTS

MAGAN (magnesium salicylate) Adria   Rx

Tablets: 545 mg

INDICATIONS	ORAL DOSAGE
Rheumatoid arthritis, osteoarthritis, bursitis, and other musculoskeletal disorders	**Adult:** 1,090 mg (2 tabs) tid to start; adjust dosage, if necessary, to meet individual patient needs

CONTRAINDICATIONS	
Advanced chronic renal insufficiency	Uricosuric therapy

WARNINGS/PRECAUTIONS	
Patients with known salicylate sensitivity, erosive gastritis, or peptic ulcer	Use with caution; discontinue use if a reaction to magnesium salicylate develops
Patients with renal impairment	Use with caution; discontinue other drugs containing magnesium and monitor serum magnesium levels if dosage levels are high
Other special-risk patients	Use with caution, if at all, in patients receiving anticoagulants, those with liver damage, preexisting hypoprothrombinemia, or vitamin K deficiency, and before surgery
Carcinogenicity, mutagenicity	The carcinogenic and mutagenic potential of this drug has not been studied
Impairment of fertility	The effect, if any, that this drug may have on fertility is unknown; however, aspirin causes testicular atrophy and inhibition of spermatogenesis in animals

ADVERSE REACTIONS

Same as aspirin, with the exception of asthmatic reactions and inhibition of platelet aggregation and increased bleeding time with recommended doses

OVERDOSAGE

Signs and symptoms	Hyperpnea, nausea, vomiting, vertigo, tinnitus, flushing, sweating, thirst, headache, drowsiness, diarrhea, and tachycardia, progressing to hyperthermia, hemorrhage, acid-base disturbances, restlessness, confusion, convulsions, vasomotor depression, coma, and respiratory failure

Treatment	If less than 4 h have elapsed since ingestion, induce emesis or perform gastric lavage, followed by activated charcoal, to remove any remaining drug from the stomach. Initial therapy should be directed at reducing hyperthermia by external sponging with tepid water, correcting dehydration by appropriate IV fluid replacement, and maintaining adequate cardiorespiratory and renal function. In moderately severe cases of salicylate poisoning, cautiously administer sodium bicarbonate IV in sufficient quantity, if possible, to maintain an alkaline diuresis; intermittent peritoneal dialysis may also be helpful. In severe cases, hemodialysis should be seriously considered. Potassium should be added to the repair solution to compensate for potassium losses once urine formation is deemed adequate. Glucose may be provided to correct ketosis and hypoglycemia. Plasma transfusion may be beneficial if shock intervenes. Hemorrhagic phenomena may necessitate whole-blood transfusions and phytonadione (vitamin K$_1$). Do not administer barbiturates to treat excitement or convulsions.

DRUG INTERACTIONS

Oral anticoagulants	△ Risk of bleeding; if possible, avoid concomitant use
Alcohol, corticosteroids, phenylbutazone, oxyphenbutazone	△ Risk of GI ulceration
Probenecid, sulfinpyrazone	▽ Uricosuria
Spironolactone	▽ Diuretic effect
Methotrexate	△ Methotrexate plasma level and risk of toxicity
Sulfonylurea hypoglycemic agents	△ Hypoglycemic effect
Barbiturates	△ Pharmacologic effects of barbiturates
Phenytoin	△ Pharmacologic effects of phenytoin
Magnesium-containing antacids and other drugs	△ Risk of hypermagnesemia in patients with renal impairment

ALTERED LABORATORY VALUES

Blood/serum values	△ Prothrombin time △ Uric acid (with low doses) ▽ Uric acid (with high doses) ▽ Thyroxine (T$_4$) ▽ Thyroid-stimulating hormone
Urinary values	△ Glucose (with Clinitest tablets)

USE IN CHILDREN	USE IN PREGNANT AND NURSING WOMEN
Safety and effectiveness for use in children have not been established	Pregnancy Category C: use during pregnancy only if expected benefit of therapy outweighs potential risk to the fetus. Salicylate have been shown to be teratogenic in animals, and have increased the number of stillbirths and neonatal deaths in women. Pregnant women given chronic high doses of salicylates have shown longer gestation periods, more frequent postmaturity, and prolonged spontaneous labor. There have been no adequate well-controlled studies of magnesium salicylate in pregnant women. Salicylates are excreted in human milk; use with caution in nursing mothers.

ANTIARTHRITIC AGENTS

MECLOMEN (meclofenamate sodium) Parke-Davis Rx

Capsules: meclofenamate sodium equivalent to 50 or 100 mg meclofenamic acid

INDICATIONS	ORAL DOSAGE
Rheumatoid arthritis[1] Osteoarthritis	**Adult:** 200–400 mg/day, given in 3–4 equally divided doses; optimum therapeutic benefit may not be obtained for 2–3 wk

CONTRAINDICATIONS	
Hypersensitivity to meclofenamate	History of bronchospasm, allergic rhinitis, or urticaria precipitated by aspirin or other nonsteroidal anti-inflammatory drugs

ADMINISTRATION/DOSAGE ADJUSTMENTS

Elderly patients	Because adverse reactions are more common in older patients, reduce the initial dosage for these patients and follow them carefully
Gastrointestinal complaints	Diarrhea, irritation, or abdominal pain may be minimized by administering meclofenamate with meals; concomitant use of an antacid (ie, aluminum or magnesium hydroxide) does not interfere with absorption of the drug

MECLOMEN

WARNINGS/PRECAUTIONS

Peptic ulceration, GI bleeding	May occur and can be severe or even fatal (one case); patients with a history of upper GI tract disease should be closely supervised during therapy
Diarrhea, GI irritation, abdominal pain	May occur (see ADMINISTRATION/DOSAGE ADJUSTMENTS); if intolerance develops, reduce dosage or temporarily discontinue use
Liver function abnormalities	Borderline elevations may occur in up to 15% of patients; meaningful elevations (3 times the upper limit of normal) in SGOT or SGPT levels have been reported in less than 1% of patients. If abnormal liver function tests or other manifestations of liver dysfunction arise during therapy, evaluate the patient for evidence of a more severe hepatic reaction. Although such reactions as jaundice and fatal hepatitis have occurred rarely, discontinue therapy if abnormal liver function test results persist or worsen, signs and symptoms of liver disease develop, or secondary manifestations (eg, eosinophilia, rash) occur.
Renal toxicity	Proteinuria, acute interstitial nephritis with hematuria, and occasionally the nephrotic syndrome may occur during therapy. In patients with reduced renal blood flow or volume owing to conditions such as heart failure, renal or hepatic impairment, advanced age, or use of diuretics, administration of a nonsteroidal anti-inflammatory agent may cause a critical decrease in the formation of renal prostaglandins and thereby precipitate overt renal failure; reaction is reversible upon discontinuation of the drug.
Drug accumulation	Meclofenamate is eliminated primarily by the kidneys; closely monitor patients with significant renal impairment and be prepared to reduce the daily dose
Long-term therapy	Determine hemoglobin and hematocrit values if anemia is suspected
Visual disturbances	Discontinue use if visual disturbances[2] occur, and perform a complete ophthalmologic examination
Corticosteroid therapy	If discontinued, reduce dosage gradually to avoid the possible complications of sudden steroid withdrawal
Leukopenia	May occur (rarely) and is usually transient; persistent blood dyscrasias warrant further clinical evaluation and possible discontinuation of therapy

ADVERSE REACTIONS

Frequent reactions (incidence ≥ 1%) are printed in *italics*

Gastrointestinal	*Diarrhea (10–33%); nausea with or without vomiting (11%); other GI disorders (10%); abdominal pain, pyrosis, and flatulence (3–9%); anorexia, constipation, stomatitis, and peptic ulcer (1–3%);* bleeding and/or perforation, ulcer, colitis, cholestatic jaundice[2]
Cardiovascular	*Edema (1–3%)*[2]
Dermatological	*Rash (3–9%); urticaria and pruritus (1–3%);* erythema multiforme, Stevens-Johnson syndrome, exfoliative dermatitis
Central nervous system	*Headache and dizziness (3–9%); tinnitus (1–3%)*[2]
Hematological	Neutropenia, thrombocytopenic purpura, leukopenia, agranulocytosis, hemolytic anemia, eosinophilia, decrease in hemoglobin and/or hematocrit
Other	Renal failure; lupus-like and serum sickness–like reactions[2]

OVERDOSAGE

Signs and symptoms	CNS stimulation, manifested by irrational behavior, marked agitation, and generalized seizures, followed by renal reactions, including decreased urinary output, increased serum creatinine levels, abnormal cellular elements in the urine, and, in some cases, azotemia with oliguria or anuria
Treatment	Empty stomach by emesis or gastric lavage, followed by administration of activated charcoal. Institute supportive measures, as needed, and carefully monitor vital functions and fluid and electrolyte balance. Dialysis and hemoperfusion may be less effective than charcoal in removing the drug because of plasma protein binding; however, dialysis may be necessary to correct serious azotemia or electrolyte imbalance.

DRUG INTERACTIONS

Warfarin	↑ Anticoagulant effect
Aspirin	↑ Fecal blood loss ↓ Plasma meclofenamate level

ALTERED LABORATORY VALUES

Blood/serum values	↑ SGOT ↑ SGPT ↑ Alkaline phosphatase ↑ BUN ↑ Creatinine

No clinically significant alterations in urinary values occur at therapeutic dosages

---

USE IN CHILDREN

Safety and effectiveness for use in children under 14 yr of age have not been established

USE IN PREGNANT AND NURSING WOMEN

Not recommended for use during pregnancy, particularly the first and third trimesters, because of potential risk to the fetus. Not recommended for use in nursing mothers because of adverse effects on suckling rodents.

---

[1] Safety and effectiveness have not been established for rheumatoid arthritis patients designated by the American Rheumatism Association as Functional Class IV (incapacitated; largely or wholly bedridden or confined to a wheelchair; little or no self-care)

[2] Other reactions for which a causal relationship has not been established include palpitations, malaise, fatigue, paresthesia, insomnia, depression, blurred vision, nocturia, taste disturbances, decreased visual acuity, temporary blindness, reversible loss of color vision, retinal changes (including macular fibrosis and macular and perimacular edema), conjunctivitis, iritis, paralytic ileus, erythema nodosum, and hair loss

ANTIARTHRITIC AGENTS

MOTRIN (ibuprofen) Upjohn Rx
Tablets: 300, 400, 600, 800 mg

INDICATIONS	ORAL DOSAGE
Rheumatoid arthritis **Osteoarthritis**	**Adult:** 300 mg qid or 400–800 mg tid or qid; once a satisfactory response is obtained (usually by 2 wk), adjust dosage as needed; higher doses may be required for rheumatoid arthritis than for osteoarthritis
Mild to moderate pain	**Adult:** 400 mg q4–6h, as needed
Primary dysmenorrhea	**Adult:** 400 mg q4h, as needed

CONTRAINDICATIONS	
Hypersensitivity to ibuprofen	History of nasal polyps, angioedema, and bronchospastic reactivity to aspirin or other nonsteroidal anti-inflammatory drugs

ADMINISTRATION/DOSAGE ADJUSTMENTS	
Gastric irritation	May be minimized by administering drug with meals or milk
Arthritis	An increase in dosage from 2,400 to 3,200 mg/day may be beneficial for certain patients, although it should be borne in mind that in well-controlled clinical trials such an increase caused a slight increase in adverse reactions and failed to enhance mean effectiveness
Combination therapy	Additional symptomatic relief has been obtained in combination with gold salts. Neither benefits nor harmful interactions have been demonstrated with corticosteroids; if prolonged corticosteroid therapy is discontinued, reduce dosage gradually to avoid the complications of abrupt withdrawal.

WARNINGS/PRECAUTIONS	
Anaphylactoid reactions	May occur in patients who are hypersensitive to other nonsteroidal anti-inflammatory agents (see CONTRAINDICATIONS)
Peptic ulceration, perforation, GI bleeding	May occur and can be severe and even fatal; patients with a history of upper GI tract disease or with an active peptic ulcer should be closely supervised during therapy
Renal toxicity	Proteinuria, acute interstitial nephritis with hematuria, and occasionally the nephrotic syndrome may occur during therapy. In patients with reduced renal blood flow or volume owing to conditions such as heart failure, renal or hepatic impairment, advanced age, or use of diuretics, administration of a nonsteroidal anti-inflammatory agent may cause a dose-dependent decrease in the formation of renal prostaglandins and thereby precipitate overt renal failure; the reaction is reversible upon discontinuation of the drug.
Drug accumulation	Ibuprofen is eliminated primarily by the kidneys; closely monitor patients with significant renal impairment and be prepared to reduce the daily dose. The safety of ibuprofen in patients with chronic renal failure has not been studied.
Ophthalmic changes	May occur (see ADVERSE REACTIONS); if visual complaints develop, discontinue drug and perform an ophthalmologic examination, including testing of central visual fields and color vision
Fluid retention and edema	May occur; use with caution in patients with a history of cardiac decompensation or hypertension
Prolonged bleeding time	May occur due to inhibition of platelet aggregation; use with caution in patients with coagulation defects and in those receiving anticoagulants
Decreased hemoglobin and hematocrit	A slight dose-related reduction in hemoglobin and hematocrit may occur. The total decrease in hemoglobin, even at 3,200 mg/day, usually does not exceed 1 g; this effect is probably not clinically important if there are no signs of bleeding.
Liver function abnormalities	Borderline elevations may occur in up to 15% of patients; meaningful elevations (3 times the upper limit of normal) in SGOT or SGPT levels have been reported in less than 1% of patients. If abnormal liver function tests or other manifestations of liver dysfunction arise during therapy, evaluate the patient for evidence of a more severe hepatic reaction. Although such reactions as jaundice and fatal hepatitis have occurred rarely, discontinue therapy if abnormal liver function test results persist or worsen, signs and symptoms of liver disease develop, or secondary manifestations (eg, eosinophilia, rash) occur.
Diagnostic interference	Complications of presumably noninfectious, noninflammatory painful conditions may escape detection because of reduction in fever and inflammation

ADVERSE REACTIONS	Frequent reactions (incidence $\geq$ 1%) are printed in *italics*
Gastrointestinal	*Nausea, epigastric pain, and heartburn (3–9%); diarrhea, abdominal distress, nausea and vomiting, indigestion, constipation, abdominal cramps or pain, bloating, and flatulence (1–3%);* gastric or duodenal ulcer with bleeding and/or perforation, GI hemorrhage, melena, gastritis, pancreatitis[1]
Hepatic	Hepatitis, jaundice, abnormal liver function tests

MOTRIN ■ MYOCHRYSINE

Central nervous system	*Dizziness (3–9%); headache and nervousness (1–3%);* depression, insomnia, confusion, emotional lability, somnolence, aseptic meningitis with fever and coma[1]
Otic	*Tinnitus (1–3%),* hearing loss
Ophthalmic	Amblyopia, characterized by blurred and/or diminished vision, scotomata, and/or changes in color vision[1]
Dermatological	*Rash, including maculopapular rash (3–9%); pruritus (1–3%);* vesiculobullous eruptions, urticaria, erythema multiforme, Stevens-Johnson syndrome, alopecia[1]
Cardiovascular	*Edema and fluid retention (1–3%),* congestive heart failure in patients with marginal cardiac function, elevated blood pressure, palpitations[1]
Hematological	Neutropenia, agranulocytosis, aplastic anemia, hemolytic anemia (occasionally Coombs' positive), thrombocytopenia with or without purpura, eosinophilia, decreased hemoglobin and hematocrit[1]
Metabolic and endocrinological	*Decreased appetite (1–3%)*[1]
Renal	Acute renal failure in patients with preexisting significant renal impairment, decreased creatinine clearance, polyuria, azotemia, cystitis, hematuria[1]
Allergic	Syndrome of abdominal pain, fever, chills, nausea, and vomiting; anaphylaxis; bronchospasm[1]
Other	Dry eyes and mouth, gingival ulcer, rhinitis

OVERDOSAGE

Signs and symptoms	Apnea, cyanosis, dizziness, nystagmus
Treatment	Following recent ingestion (< 1 h), remove drug by induced emesis or gastric lavage. Activated charcoal may be helpful. If drug is already absorbed, it may be useful to induce diuresis and alkalinize the urine.

DRUG INTERACTIONS

Coumarin anticoagulants	⇧ Risk of bleeding; use with caution
Aspirin	⇩ Anti-inflammatory activity (potential)

ALTERED LABORATORY VALUES

Blood/serum values	⇧ SGOT ⇧ SGPT

No clinically significant alterations in urinary values occur at therapeutic dosages

USE IN CHILDREN

Safety and effectiveness for use in children have not been established

USE IN PREGNANT AND NURSING WOMEN

Not recommended for use in pregnant or nursing women. Animal reproduction studies have shown no evidence of developmental abnormalities; however, no adequate, well-controlled studies have been done in pregnant women and, hence, the drug should be used only if clearly needed. Because of the risk of premature closure of the ductus arteriosus, use during late pregnancy should be avoided. An increased incidence of dystocia and delayed parturition has been observed in rats. Limited studies in nursing women have not demonstrated significant excretion of this drug in human milk; however, because this remains a possibility and because of the potential for serious adverse effects in neonates, the patient should not nurse while taking ibuprofen.

[1] Other reactions for which a causal relationship has not been established include paresthesias, hallucinations, dream abnormalities, pseudotumor cerebri, conjunctivitis, diplopia, optic neuritis, cataracts, toxic epidermal necrolysis, photoallergic skin reactions, sinus tachycardia, sinus bradycardia, bleeding episodes, gynecomastia, hypoglycemic reaction, acidosis, renal papillary necrosis, serum sickness, lupus erythematosus syndrome, angioedema, and Henoch-Schönlein vasculitis

ANTIARTHRITIC AGENTS

MYOCHRYSINE (gold sodium thiomalate) Merck Sharp & Dohme   Rx

Ampuls: 10, 25, 50 mg/ml (1 ml) for IM use only   **Vials:** 50 mg/ml (10 ml) for IM use only

INDICATIONS

Active rheumatoid arthritis (adjunctive therapy)

PARENTERAL DOSAGE

Adult: 10 mg IM (preferably intragluteally), followed in 1 wk by 25 mg IM, and subsequently by 25–50 mg/wk IM until major improvement or toxicity occurs or total cumulative dose reaches 1 g; for maintenance: 25–50 mg IM every 2 wk for 2–20 wk, followed by 25–50 mg IM every 3–4 wk
Child: 10 mg IM (preferably intragluteally), followed by 1 mg/kg/wk IM up to 50 mg/dose; other guidelines: same as adult

COMPENDIUM OF DRUG THERAPY

MYOCHRYSINE

CONTRAINDICATIONS

Prior severe toxic reaction to gold or other heavy metals	Severe debilitation	Systemic lupus erythematosus

ADMINISTRATION/DOSAGE ADJUSTMENTS

Position of patient	Patient should be lying down during injection and should remain recumbent for approximately 10 min after solution is injected
Failure of initial therapy	If patient fails to improve after receiving a cumulative dose of 1 g, discontinue therapy, continue giving 25–50 mg/wk for 10 wk more, or increase dose by 10 mg every 1–4 wk, up to 100 mg/injection; if significant improvement occurs, initiate maintenance therapy as described under PARENTERAL DOSAGE
Management of exacerbations	Resume weekly injections until disease activity is suppressed
Resumption of therapy following resolution of mild reactions	Administer an initial test dose of 5 mg IM; if dose is well tolerated, give progressively larger doses, in increments of 5–10 mg, at weekly to monthly intervals until usual maintenance dose of 25–50 mg is reached
Concomitant antiarthritic therapy	Do not use with penicillamine. The safety of coadministration with cytotoxic agents has not been established. Treatment with salicylates, other nonsteroidal anti-inflammatory agents, or systemic corticosteroids may be continued when gold therapy is started or withdrawn gradually as symptoms permit.

WARNINGS/PRECAUTIONS

Hematological, renal, and dermatological toxicity	May occur; obtain baseline hemoglobin, erythrocyte, WBC, differential, and platelet counts and urinalysis; analyze urine for protein and sediment changes prior to each injection and repeat complete blood and platelet counts before every second injection and whenever purpura or ecchymoses develop. If hemoglobin drops rapidly, WBC count falls below 4,000/mm^3, eosinophilia exceeds 5%, platelet count falls below 100,000/mm^3, or albuminuria, hematuria, pruritus, skin eruption, stomatitis, or persistent diarrhea develops, discontinue therapy until another cause of the abnormality can be determined.
Neurological toxicity	Central nervous system and peripheral complications, including hallucinations, seizures, and the Guillain-Barré syndrome, have been reported (see ADVERSE REACTIONS); these effects have usually disappeared upon discontinuation of therapy
Special-risk patients	Use with caution in patients with a history of drug-related blood dyscrasias, allergy, or hypersensitivity; skin rashes; previous kidney or liver disease; marked hypertension; or compromised cerebral or cardiovascular circulation. Diabetes mellitus and congestive heart failure must be under control before instituting gold therapy.
Pruritus	May occur as a warning signal of impending dermatological reaction
Metallic taste	May occur as warning signal or impending oral mucous membrane reactions

ADVERSE REACTIONS

Dermatological	Dermatitis, pruritus, actinic rash, exfoliative dermatitis leading to alopecia and nail shedding, partial or complete hair loss
Mucous membrane	Stomatitis, buccal ulceration, glossitis, gingivitis
Renal	Nephrotic syndrome, glomerulitis with hematuria
Hematological	Granulocytopenia, thrombocytopenia (with or without purpura), hypoplastic and aplastic anemia, and eosinophilia (rare)
Nitritoid and allergic	Flushing, fainting, dizziness, sweating, nausea, vomiting, malaise, weakness, anaphylactic shock, syncope, bradycardia, difficulty in swallowing and breathing, angioneurotic edema
Gastrointestinal	Nausea, vomiting, anorexia, abdominal cramps, diarrhea; ulcerative enterocolitis (rare)
Neurological	Confusion, hallucinations, seizures, peripheral neuropathy with and without fasciculations, sensorimotor effects (including Guillain-Barré syndrome), and elevated CSF protein (rare)
Ophthalmic	Iritis, corneal ulcers, gold deposits in ocular tissues, and conjunctivitis (rare)
Other	Arthralgia (transient), hepatitis, jaundice (including cholestatic jaundice), gold bronchitis, interstitial pneumonitis, pulmonary fibrosis, fever

OVERDOSAGE

Signs and symptoms	See ADVERSE REACTIONS
Treatment	Discontinue treatment immediately. Severe or generalized dermatitis or stomatitis may benefit from systemic corticosteroids (eg, prednisone, 10–40 mg/day in divided doses). Less severe skin and mucous membrane reactions often benefit from topical corticosteroids, oral antihistaminics, or soothing or anesthetic lotions. For serious renal, hematological, pulmonary, and enterocolitic complications, high doses of systemic corticosteroids (eg, prednisone, 40–100 mg/day in divided doses) are recommended. The chelating agent dimercaprol may be given in addition to corticosteroids to enhance gold excretion in patients who do not improve on steroids alone, but careful monitoring is required.

DRUG INTERACTIONS

Penicillamine	⇧ Risk of renal or hematological toxicity; do not administer concomitantly
Other dermatitis-causing drugs	⇧ Risk of severe skin reactions

ALTERED LABORATORY VALUES

Blood/serum values — ⇧ or ⇩ PBI (with chloric acid method)

No clinically significant alterations in urinary values occur at therapeutic dosages

USE IN CHILDREN
See INDICATIONS and PARENTERAL DOSAGE

USE IN PREGNANT AND NURSING WOMEN
Pregnancy Category C: use during pregnancy only when expected benefit outweighs potential hazard to the fetus. No adequate, well-controlled studies have been conducted in pregnant women. Teratogenicity has been demonstrated in rats and rabbits at doses 140 and 175 times the usual human dose. Gold is excreted in the milk of lactating women and has been detected in the serum and red blood cells of a nursing infant. Because of the potential for serious adverse effects in the infant, a decision should be made to discontinue nursing or use of the drug. Significant gold levels may persist after therapy is withdrawn.

ANTIARTHRITIC AGENTS

NALFON (fenoprofen calcium) Dista   Rx

Capsules: 200, 300 mg   **Tablets:** 600 mg

INDICATIONS

Rheumatoid arthritis
Osteoarthritis

Mild to moderate pain

ORAL DOSAGE

Adult: 300–600 mg tid or qid, or up to 3,200 mg/day if needed

Adult: 200 mg q4–6h, as needed

CONTRAINDICATIONS

Hypersensitivity to fenoprofen

Significant renal impairment

History of asthma, rhinitis, or urticaria precipitated by aspirin or other nonsteroidal anti-inflammatory drugs

ADMINISTRATION/DOSAGE ADJUSTMENTS

Timing of administration	Since food decreases fenoprofen blood levels, administer 30 min before or 2 h after meals; if gastrointestinal complaints occur, administer with meals or milk
Combination therapy	Neither benefits nor harmful interactions have been demonstrated with gold salts or corticosteroids. Concomitant therapy with salicylates is not recommended; aspirin may increase excretion rate of fenoprofen, and no additional benefit is obtained beyond the effect of aspirin alone.

WARNINGS/PRECAUTIONS

Peptic ulcer, perforation, GI bleeding	May occur and can be severe and even fatal; patients with a history of upper GI tract disease or with an active peptic ulcer should be closely supervised during therapy. Patients with an active peptic ulcer should be placed on a vigorous antiulcer treatment regimen.
Renal toxicity	Acute interstitial nephritis and the nephrotic syndrome may occur during therapy. The nephrotic syndrome associated with fenoprofen may be preceded by fever, rash, arthralgia, oliguria, and azotemia; substantial proteinuria may also occur, and the syndrome may progress to anuria. Patients who have had these reactions to other nonsteroidal anti-inflammatory agents should not be given fenoprofen. Rapid recovery has occurred with early detection and discontinuation of the drug; treatment may also require dialysis and steroids. In patients with reduced renal blood flow or volume owing to conditions such as heart failure, renal or hepatic impairment, advanced age, or use of diuretics, administration of a nonsteroidal anti-inflammatory agent may cause a critical decrease in the formation of renal prostaglandins and thereby precipitate overt renal failure; the reaction is reversible upon discontinuation of the drug. To avoid renal toxicity, perform renal function tests periodically in patients with possible renal impairment.
Drug accumulation	Fenoprofen is eliminated primarily by the kidneys; closely monitor patients with possibly compromised renal function and be prepared to lower the daily dose

Liver function abnormalities	Test periodically for increases in serum liver enzyme levels. Borderline elevations may occur in up to 15% of patients; meaningful increases (3 times the upper limit of normal) in SGOT or SGPT levels have been reported in less than 1% of patients. If abnormal liver function tests or other manifestations of liver dysfunction occur during therapy, evaluate the patient for evidence of a more severe hepatic reaction. Although such reactions as jaundice and fatal hepatitis have occurred rarely, discontinue therapy if abnormal liver function test results persist or worsen, signs and symptoms of liver disease develop, or secondary manifestations (eg, eosinophilia, rash) occur.
Corticosteroid therapy	If discontinued, reduce dosage gradually to avoid complications of sudden steroid withdrawal
Patients with initially low hemoglobin values	Obtain periodic hemoglobin determinations during long-term therapy
Peripheral edema	May occur; use with caution in patients with compromised cardiac function or hypertension
Prolonged bleeding time	May occur due to inhibition of platelet aggregation; closely monitor patients who may be affected
Impaired hearing	Monitor auditory function periodically
Mental impairment	Performance of potentially hazardous activities may be impaired; caution patients accordingly
Visual impairment	Has occurred with some nonsteroidal anti-inflammatory drugs; if eye complaints develop perform an ophthalmologic examination

ADVERSE REACTIONS[1]

Frequent reactions (incidence $\geq$ 1%) are printed in *italics*

Gastrointestinal	*Dyspepsia, constipation, nausea, and vomiting (3-9%); abdominal pain, anorexia, occult blood loss, diarrhea, flatulence, and dry mouth (1-2%)*; gastritis, peptic ulcer with or without perforation and/or GI hemorrhage[2]
Central nervous system	*Headache and somnolence (15%); dizziness, nervousness, and asthenia (3-9%); tremor, confusion, insomnia, fatigue, and malaise (1-2%)*[2]
Ophthalmic	*Blurred vision (1-2%)*[2]
Otic	*Tinnitus and decreased hearing (1-2%)*
Dermatological	*Pruritus (3-9%); rash, increased sweating and urticuria (1-2%)*[2]
Cardiovascular	*Palpitations (3-9%); tachycardia (1-2%)*[2]
Genitourinary	Dysuria, cystitis, hematuria, oliguria, azotemia, anuria, interstitial nephritis, nephrosis, papillary necrosis
Hepatic	Jaundice, cholestatic hepatitis
Hematological	Purpura, bruising, hemorrhage, thrombocytopenia, hemolytic anemia, aplastic anemia, agranulocytosis, pancytopenia[2]
Other	*Dyspnea (1-2%)*, peripheral edema, anaphylaxis; lymphadenopathy, mastodynia, burning tongue[2]

OVERDOSAGE

Signs and symptoms	See ADVERSE REACTIONS
Treatment	Induce emesis or use gastric lavage to empty stomach, followed by activated charcoal. Employ supportive measures, as indicated. Urinary alkalinization and forced diuresis may be helpful. Furosemide does *not* lower blood levels of fenoprofen.

DRUG INTERACTIONS

Albumin-bound drugs	Displacement of either drug
Hydantoins	△ Hydantoin plasma level; observe for signs of toxicity
Sulfonamides	△ Sulfonamide plasma level; observe for signs of toxicity
Sulfonylureas	△ Sulfonylurea plasma level; observe for signs of toxicity
Coumarin anticoagulants	△ Prothrombin time; observe patient carefully
Aspirin	▽ Plasma half-life of fenoprofen; do not use concomitantly
Phenobarbital	▽ Plasma half-life of fenoprofen; if necessary, adjust fenoprofen dosage

ALTERED LABORATORY VALUES

Blood/serum values	△ Alkaline phosphatase △ SGOT △ Lactate dehydrogenase △ BUN

No clinically significant alterations in urinary values occur at therapeutic dosages

NALFON ■ NAPROSYN

USE IN CHILDREN	USE IN PREGNANT AND NURSING WOMEN
Safety and effectiveness for use in children have not been established	Not recommended for use in pregnant or nursing women because of lack of sufficient evidence demonstrating safety in these patients

[1] Reactions observed during clinical trials of fenoprofen in the treatment of rheumatoid arthritis and osteoarthritis; when fenoprofen was used for analgesia in short-term studies, the incidence of adverse reactions was markedly lower than that observed during long-term trials
[2] Other adverse reactions for which a causal relationship has not been established include burning tongue, aphthous ulcerations of the buccal mucosa, metallic taste, pancreatitis, depression, disorientation, seizures, trigeminal neuralgia, personality changes, Stevens-Johnson syndrome, angioneurotic edema, exfoliative dermatitis, alopecia, atrial fibrillation, pulmonary edema, ECG changes, supraventricular tachycardia, lymphadenopathy, mastodynia, fever, diplopia, and optic neuritis

ANTIARTHRITIC AGENTS

NAPROSYN (naproxen) Syntex   Rx

Tablets: 250, 375, 500 mg

INDICATIONS	ORAL DOSAGE
Rheumatoid arthritis, osteoarthritis, and ankylosing spondylitis	**Adult:** 250–375 mg bid (morning and evening; doses do not have to be equal); during long-term therapy, adjust dosage up or down depending upon clinical response of patient (dosages exceeding 1 g/day have not been studied in these indications)
Acute gout	**Adult:** 750 mg to start, followed by 250 mg q8h until attack has subsided
Mild to moderate pain **Primary dysmenorrhea** **Acute tendinitis and bursitis**	**Adult:** 500 mg to start, followed by 250 mg q6–8h, as needed, up to 1,250 mg/day

CONTRAINDICATIONS	
History of allergic reaction to naproxen or naproxen sodium	History of asthma, rhinitis, and nasal polyps precipitated by aspirin or other nonsteroidal anti-inflammatory/analgesic drugs

ADMINISTRATION/DOSAGE ADJUSTMENTS	
Onset of clinical response	Should be observed within 2 wk in arthritic patients; in some patients, symptomatic improvement may not be seen for up to 4 wk
Combination therapy	Added benefits in arthritis have not been demonstrated with corticosteroids; however, coadministration with gold salts has resulted in greater improvement. Use with salicylates or related drug naproxen sodium is not recommended.
Adrenal function tests	Discontinue naproxen therapy 72 h prior to testing

WARNINGS/PRECAUTIONS	
Anaphylactoid reactions	Potentially fatal allergic or idiosyncratic anaphylactoid reactions may occur. Before beginning therapy, determine whether the patient has experienced reactions such as asthma, nasal polyps, urticaria, or hypotension in association with nonsteroidal anti-inflammatory drugs (see CONTRAINDICATIONS); if such reactions occur during therapy, discontinue use.
Peptic ulcer, perforation, GI bleeding	May occur and can be severe or even fatal; patients with a history of peptic ulcer disease or active gastric or duodenal ulcers should be closely supervised during therapy
Renal toxicity	Proteinuria, acute interstitial nephritis with hematuria, and occasionally the nephrotic syndrome may occur during therapy. In patients with reduced renal blood flow or volume owing to conditions such as heart failure, renal or hepatic impairment, advanced age, or use of diuretics, administration of a nonsteroidal anti-inflammatory agent may cause a critical decrease in the formation of renal prostaglandins and thereby precipitate overt renal failure; reaction is reversible upon discontinuation of the drug. To avoid renal toxicity, monitor serum creatinine level and/or creatinine clearance and exercise great caution if a patient has significant renal impairment.
Drug accumulation	Naproxen is eliminated primarily by the kidneys; use with caution if creatinine clearance is less than 20 mg/ml since drug accumulation can occur in such a case. Chronic alcoholic liver disease, probably other forms of cirrhosis, and, according to one study, advanced age all produce an increase in the serum level of unbound naproxen; if a cirrhotic or elderly patient requires high doses, exercise caution, and be prepared to adjust dose.
Liver function abnormalities	Borderline elevations may occur in up to 15% of patients; meaningful elevations (3 times the upper limit of normal) in SGOT or SGPT levels have been reported in less than 1% of patients. If abnormal liver function tests or other manifestations of liver dysfunction arise during therapy, evaluate the patient for evidence of a more severe hepatic reaction. Although such reactions as jaundice and fatal hepatitis have occurred rarely, discontinue therapy if abnormal liver function test results persist or worsen, signs and symptoms of liver disease develop, or secondary manifestations (eg, eosinophilia, rash) occur.

COMPENDIUM OF DRUG THERAPY

Ophthalmic changes	Have occurred in animals treated with related drugs; perform an ophthalmological examination within a reasonable period after initiating therapy and periodically thereafter if drug is used for an extended period
Peripheral edema	May occur; use with caution in patients with fluid retention, hypertension, or heart failure
Corticosteroid therapy	If discontinued, reduce dosage gradually to avoid complications of sudden steroid withdrawal and observe patient closely for adverse effects
Mental impairment	Performance of potentially hazardous activities may be impaired; advise patients to exercise caution if they experience drowsiness, dizziness, vertigo, or depression
Prolonged bleeding time	May occur due to inhibition of platelet aggregation; use with caution in patients with coagulation defects or in those on anticoagulant therapy
Patients with initially low hemoglobin values ($\leq$ 10 g)	Obtain periodic hemoglobin determinations during long-term therapy
Diagnostic interference	Complications of presumably noninfectious, noninflammatory painful conditions may escape detection because of reduction in fever and inflammation
Carcinogenicity	No evidence of carcinogenicity has been found in rats after 2 yr of study

ADVERSE REACTIONS[1]

	Frequent reactions (incidence $\geq$ 1%) are printed in *italics*
Gastrointestinal	*Constipation, heartburn, abdominal pain, and nausea (3–9%); dyspepsia, diarrhea, and stomatitis (1–3%);* bleeding and/or perforation, peptic ulcer with bleeding and/or perforation, vomiting, melena, hematemesis
Respiratory	Eosinophilic pneumonitis
Central nervous system and neuromuscular	*Headache, dizziness, and drowsiness (3–9%); light-headedness and vertigo (1–3%);* myalgia, muscle weakness, inability to concentrate, depression, malaise, dream abnormalities, insomnia
Dermatological	*Pruritus, eruption, and ecchymoses (3–9%); sweating and purpura (1–3%);* rash, alopecia, photosensitive dermatitis[2]
Cardiovascular	*Edema and dyspnea (3–9%); palpitations (1–3%);* congestive heart failure
Hepatic	Abnormal liver function tests, jaundice
Renal	Glomerular nephritis, interstitial nephritis, nephrotic syndrome, hematuria, renal disease
Hematological	Thrombocytopenia, leukopenia, granulocytopenia, eosinophilia[2]
Other	*Tinnitus (3–9%); thirst, visual disturbances, and hearing disturbances (1–3%);* hearing impairment, anaphylactoid reactions, menstrual disorders, chills, fever[2]

OVERDOSAGE

Signs and symptoms	Drowsiness, heartburn, indigestion, nausea, vomiting
Treatment	Induce emesis or use gastric lavage to empty stomach, and institute supportive measures, as needed. Activated charcoal may be helpful.

DRUG INTERACTIONS

Albumin-bound drugs	Displacement of either drug
Coumarin anticoagulants	△ Prothrombin time
Hydantoins	△ Hydantoin plasma level
Sulfonylureas	△ Sulfonylurea plasma level
Sulfonamides	△ Sulfonamide plasma level
Furosemide	▽ Natriuretic effect of furosemide
Lithium	△ Lithium plasma level
Propranolol, other beta blockers	▽ Antihypertensive effect
Aspirin	△ Excretion of naproxen
Probenecid	△ Naproxen plasma half-life
Methotrexate	△ Methotrexate plasma level (based on animal studies); exercise caution

ALTERED LABORATORY VALUES

Blood/serum values	△ BUN △ Creatinine △ SGOT △ SGPT
Urinary values	△ 17-Ketogenic steroids Interference with 5-HIAA determinations

---

USE IN CHILDREN

Pediatric dosages have not been established

USE IN PREGNANT AND NURSING WOMEN

Pregnancy Category B: use during pregnancy only if clearly needed; because premature closure of the ductus arteriosus may occur, administration during late pregnancy should be avoided. An increased incidence of dystocia and delayed parturition has been observed in rats. Reproduction studies in rats, rabbits, and mice given up to 6 times the human dose have shown no evidence of teratogenicity or impaired fertility. No adequate, well-controlled studies have been performed in pregnant women. Naproxen anion appears in human breast milk at a concentration of 1% of maternal plasma levels; avoid use in nursing mothers due to potential adverse effects of prostaglandin inhibition.

---

[1] Adverse reactions occurring in patients treated for rheumatoid arthritis or osteoarthritis are listed; in general, these reactions were reported 2–10 times more frequently than they were in patients treated for mild-to-moderate pain or dysmenorrhea

[2] Other reactions for which a causal relationship has not been established incude epidermal necrolysis, erythema multiforme, Stevens-Johnson syndrome, urticaria, agranulocytosis, aplastic anemia, hemolytic anemia, cognitive dysfunction, ulcerative stomatitis, vasculitis, angioneurotic edema, hypoglycemia, and hyperglycemia

ANTIARTHRITIC AGENTS

ORUDIS (ketoprofen) Wyeth   Rx
Capsules: 50, 75 mg

INDICATIONS	ORAL DOSAGE
Rheumatoid arthritis Osteoarthritis	**Adult:** 75 mg tid or 50 mg qid to start, followed, if needed and tolerated, by up to 150–300 mg/day, given in 3–4 divided doses (maximum recommended dosage: 300 mg/day)

CONTRAINDICATIONS	
Hypersensitivity to ketoprofen	History of asthma, urticaria, or other allergic-type reactions precipitated by aspirin or other nonsteroidal anti-inflammatory drugs

ADMINISTRATION/DOSAGE ADJUSTMENTS

Dosage titration	Dosage may be increased up to 300 mg/day if needed for optimal effectiveness; patients of relatively small stature may require smaller doses. Individual patients may show a better response to 300 mg/day than to 200 mg/day, although clinical studies of patients taking 300 mg/day have not shown a greater mean effectiveness; these studies did show, however, an increased frequency of upper- and lower-GI distress and headaches at the higher dosage, especially in women. Give 300 mg/day only if the observed clinical benefit justifies the potentially increased risk; if minor side effects occur, they may disappear at a lower therapeutic dose.
Gastric intolerance	Gastric intolerance may be minimized by administration of milk, food, or antacids with ketoprofen; food and milk affect the rate but not the extent of absorption
Patients with impaired renal function, elderly patients, and hypoalbuminemic patients	Reduce initial dosage by 33–50% in patients with impaired renal function and in the elderly; patients with hypoalbuminemia and renal impairment should also be started on lower doses and closely monitored

WARNINGS/PRECAUTIONS

Peptic ulceration, GI bleeding	Ketoprofen may cause peptic ulceration and GI bleeding, with new peptic ulcers appearing in patients on ketoprofen therapy at a rate greater than 1% a year; patients with a history of GI tract disease should be closely supervised during therapy. In patients with GI tract bleeding or an active peptic ulcer, the benefits of therapy should be weighed against the possible hazards; institute an appropriate anti-ulcer regimen and monitor patient's progress carefully.
Renal toxicity	Interstitial nephritis and the nephrotic syndrome may occur during therapy. In patients with reduced renal blood flow or volume owing to conditions such as heart failure, renal or hepatic impairment, advanced age, or use of diuretics, administration of a nonsteroidal anti-inflammatory agent may cause a dose-dependent decrease in renal prostaglandin synthesis, reducing renal blood flow and possibly precipitating overt renal failure; the reaction is reversible upon discontinuation of the drug.
Liver function abnormalities	Borderline elevations in the results of liver function tests may occur in up to 15% of patients; meaningful elevations (3 times the upper limit of normal) in SGOT or SGPT levels have been reported in less than 1% of patients. If abnormal liver function tests or other manifestations of liver dysfunction arise during therapy, evaluate the patient for evidence of a more severe hepatic reaction. Although serious hepatic reactions such as jaundice have occurred rarely, discontinue therapy if abnormal liver function tests persist or worsen, clinical signs and symptoms of liver disease develop, or secondary manifestations (eg, eosinophilia, rash) occur.
Drug accumulation	Ketoprofen is eliminated primarily by the kidneys; closely monitor patients with significant renal impairment and be prepared to reduce the daily dose to avoid accumulation
Peripheral edema	Peripheral edema has been observed in 2% of patients taking ketoprofen; use with caution in patients with fluid retention, heart failure, or hypertension
Anemia	Patients with rheumatoid arthritis commonly develop anemia that may be aggravated by nonsteroidal anti-inflammatory drugs; determine hemoglobin values frequently in patients with initial hemoglobin values of 10 g/dl or less who are on long-term therapy
Prolonged bleeding time	Ketoprofen decreases platelet adhesion and aggregation; bleeding time may be prolonged by approximately 3–4 min from baseline values
Discontinuation of steroid therapy	If steroid dosage is reduced or eliminated during ketoprofen therapy, reduce the dosage slowly and closely observe patient for evidence of adverse effects, including adrenal insufficiency and exacerbation of arthritic symptoms
Concomitant arthritis therapy	The risk of drug interactions increases when single doses exceeding 50 mg or more than 200 mg/day are used concomitantly with drugs that are highly bound to serum proteins
Carcinogenicity, mutagenicity	No evidence of carcinogenicity has been found in rats given up to 32 mg/kg/day (8 times the maximum recommended human dose); no mutagenic potential has been found using the Ames test

ORUDIS

Impairment of fertility	A decrease in the number of implantation sites has been found in female rats fed ketoprofen at doses of 6 or 9 mg/kg/day; no significant effect on reproductive performance or fertility has been detected in male rats fed up to 9 mg/kg/day

ADVERSE REACTIONS[1]

The most frequent reactions, regardless of incidence, are printed in *italics*

Gastrointestinal	*Dyspepsia (11.5%); nausea, abdominal pain, diarrhea, constipation, and flatulence ($>$ 3%); anorexia, vomiting, and stomatitis (1–3%);* appetite increase, dry mouth, eructation, gastritis, rectal hemorrhage, melena, fecal occult blood, salivation, peptic ulcer, gastrointestinal perforation, hematemesis, and intestinal ulceration (rare)
Central nervous system	*Headache and CNS inhibition (including somnolence, malaise, and depression) or excitation (including insomnia, nervousness, and dreams) ($>$ 3%); dizziness (1–3%);* amnesia, confusion, impotence, migraine, paresthesia, and vertigo (rare)
Ophthalmic	*Visual disturbances (1–3%);* conjunctivitis, conjunctivitis sicca, eye pain, retinal hemorrhage and pigmentation change (rare)
Otic	*Tinnitus (1–3%),* hearing impairment (rare)
Dermatological, hypersensitivity	*Rash (1–3%);* alopecia, eczema, pruritus, purpuric rash, sweating, urticaria, bullous rash, exfoliative dermatitis, photosensitivity, skin discoloration, onycholysis, allergic reaction, and anaphylaxis (rare)
Genitourinary	*Impairment of renal function, including edema and increased BUN ($>$ 3%); signs or symptoms of urinary tract irritation (1–3%);* menometrorrhagia, hematuria, renal failure, interstitial nephritis, and nephrotic syndrome (rare)
Cardiovascular	Hypertension, palpitation, tachycardia, congestive heart failure, peripheral vascular disease, and vasodilation (rare)
Hematological	Hypocoagulability, agranulocytosis, anemia, hemolysis, purpura, and thrombocytopenia (rare)
Metabolic	Thirst, weight gain, weight loss, hepatic dysfunction, and hyponatremia (rare)
Musculoskeletal	Myalgia (rare)
Respiratory	Dyspnea, hemoptysis, epistaxis, pharyngitis, rhinitis, bronchospasm, and laryngeal edema (rare)
Other	Chills, facial edema, infection, taste perversion, and pain (rare)

OVERDOSAGE

Signs and symptoms	Vomiting, drowsiness
Treatment	Induce emesis or use gastric lavage to empty stomach, and institute supportive measures, as needed. Hemodialysis may be useful in removing the drug from the circulation and in the event of renal failure.

DRUG INTERACTIONS

Aspirin	▽ Protein binding of ketoprofen △ Plasma clearance of ketoprofen Concomitant use is not recommended
Diuretics	▽ Urinary excretion of potassium and chloride △ Risk of developing renal failure
Warfarin	△ Bleeding time; closely monitor patient for adverse effects on bleeding and platelet function
Probenecid	▽ Protein binding and plasma clearance of ketoprofen; monitor patient closely

ALTERED LABORATORY VALUES

Blood/serum values	△ Bleeding time △ BUN ▽ Sodium △ SGOT △ SGPT

No clinically significant alterations in urinary values occur at therapeutic dosages

---

USE IN CHILDREN

Safety and effectiveness for use in children have not been established

USE IN PREGNANT AND NURSING WOMEN

Pregnancy Category B: maternally toxic doses of ketoprofen administered to rabbits have been associated with embryotoxicity but not teratogenicity; no teratogenic effects have been observed in mice at doses up to 12 mg/kg/day or in rats given up to 9 mg/kg/day. Studies in rats have shown that a dose of 6 mg/kg (approximately the same as the maximum recommended human dose) can prolong pregnancy when given before the onset of labor. No adequate, well-controlled studies have been performed in pregnant women; use during pregnancy only if the expected benefit justifies the potential risk to the fetus. Because of the known effects of prostaglandin-inhibiting drugs on the fetal cardiovascular system (ie, closure of the ductus arteriosus), avoid use during late pregnancy. It is not known whether ketoprofen is excreted in human milk, although it is excreted in dog milk; because many drugs are excreted in human milk, use of ketoprofen by nursing mothers is not recommended.

---

[1] Reactions for which no causal relationship have been established include buccal necrosis, ulcerative colitis, dysphoria, hallucinations, libido disturbance, nightmares, personality disorder, septicemia, shock, arrhythmias, myocardial infarction, aggravated diabetes mellitus, jaundice, acute genitourinary tubulopathy, and gynecomastia

ANTIARTHRITIC AGENTS

RIDAURA (auranofin) Smith Kline & French — Rx
Capsules: 3 mg

INDICATIONS	ORAL DOSAGE
Active classical or definite **rheumatoid arthritis** in patients who respond inadequately to or cannot tolerate nonsteroidal anti-inflammatory drugs	**Adult:** 3 mg bid or 6 mg once daily, followed after 6 mo, if response is inadequate, by 3 mg tid; if administration at 9 mg/day does not produce an adequate response within 3 mo, the drug should be discontinued

CONTRAINDICATIONS
History of severe toxicity to gold, characterized by anaphylaxis, necrotizing enterocolitis, bone marrow aplasia or other severe hematologic disorders, pulmonary fibrosis, exfoliative dermatitis, or other severe effects

ADMINISTRATION/DOSAGE ADJUSTMENTS

Chrysotherapy	Gold is most beneficial when used in the treatment of active synovitis, particularly at the early stage of inflammation; the drug cannot reverse structural damage to the joints. Anyone planning to use auranofin should be experienced with chrysotherapy and aware of the relative risks and benefits. In controlled clinical trials comparing auranofin and parenteral gold, the oral drug was associated with a smaller number of withdrawals owing to adverse reactions, but with a larger number of withdrawals owing to inadequate therapeutic response.
Switching from parenteral gold	Discontinue the injectable drug; administer auranofin as recommended in the ORAL DOSAGE section
Management of GI reactions	Diarrhea or loose stools, which occur in approximately 50% of patients, can generally be managed by a reduction in dosage, eg, from 6 mg/day to 3 mg/day
Concomitant antiarthritic therapy	Auranofin can be given to patients receiving either corticosteroids at low dosages or nonsteroidal anti-inflammatory drugs; safety for concomitant use with parenteral gold, hydroxychloroquine, penicillamine, high doses of corticosteroids, or immunosuppressive agents (such as cyclophosphamide, azathioprine, and methotrexate) has not been established

WARNINGS/PRECAUTIONS

Blood dyscrasias	Auranofin may cause hematological reactions, including thrombocytopenia, leukopenia, and granulocytopenia, that can have serious effects. Thrombocytopenia, usually peripheral in origin, can progress rapidly and result in bleeding. Obtain a CBC plus differential and platelet count before therapy and then at least monthly thereafter. Signs of possible toxicity include fall in hemoglobin, WBC count under 4,000/mm^3, granulocyte count below 1,500/mm^3, and platelet count under 150,000/mm^3. If purpura, ecchymoses, petechiae, or other manifestations of thrombocytopenia are seen or if the platelet count declines precipitously or is less than 100,000/mm^3, therapy should be immediately discontinued; administration may be resumed only if thrombocytopenia is reversed and studies show that the disorder was not caused by the drug.
Renal disease	Gold can cause a nephrotic syndrome and glomerulitis, manifested by proteinuria or hematuria. Renal effects are, in general, relatively mild and fully reversible when they first become evident, but may become severe and chronic with continued treatment. To avoid nephrotoxicity, perform a urinalysis at least monthly and renal function tests at appropriate intervals after baseline values have been established. If proteinuria or hematuria is detected, administration should be promptly discontinued.
Rash	Any dermatological eruption, especially if pruritic, should initially be seen as a sign of possible toxicity; pruritus should be considered a premonitory sign of dermatitis. Exposure to sunlight during therapy may cause a rash or exacerbate dermatitis. Parenteral gold has caused generalized exfoliative dermatitis.
Oral reactions	Stomatitis, glossitis, and gingivitis are signs of possible toxicity; stomatitis is characterized by shallow ulcers on the palate, pharynx, buccal membranes, or borders of the tongue. A metallic taste should be considered a premonitory sign of oral mucous membrane reactions.
Hepatic disorders	Auranofin may produce an increase in hepatic enzyme levels and, in rare cases, cause jaundice; perform liver function tests before therapy and at appropriate intervals thereafter
Ulcerative colitis	Watch for GI bleeding in patients with GI symptoms, since auranofin can cause ulcerative enterocolitis
Other reactions	Peripheral neuropathy, hair loss, and interstitial pneumonitis have been seen in patients receiving auranofin; parenteral gold has caused fibrosis, gold bronchitis, and fever. Watch for these reactions during therapy.
Special-risk patients	Before using auranofin in patients with progressive renal disease, rash, significant hepatocellular disease, inflammatory bowel disease, or a history of bone marrow depression, consider the potential risks of toxicity as well as the difficulty of quickly detecting and diagnosing a reaction to auranofin. Any condition that may mask a sign or symptom of toxicity should be corrected before the start of therapy.

Carcinogenicity, mutagenicity	Increases in malignant renal epithelial tumors, renal adenomas, and renal tubular cell karyomegaly and cytomegaly have been detected in rats fed 8 or 21 times the human dose of auranofin for 24 mo. In a 12-mo study, rats developed renal tubular epithelial tumors when given 192, but not 30, times the recommended human dose. Administration of up to 72 times the human dose to mice produced no increase in tumors over an 18-mo period. When used at high concentrations in the mouse lymphoma forward mutation assay, auranofin induced increases in the mutation rate; however, no mutagenic effects have been observed in other assays.

ADVERSE REACTIONS[1]

Frequent reactions (incidence ≥ 1%) are printed in *italics*

Gastrointestinal	*Loose stools or diarrhea (47%), abdominal pain (14%), nausea, with or without vomiting (10%); anorexia, flatulence, and dyspepsia (3–9%); constipation and dysgeusia (1–3%);* GI bleeding, melena, occult blood in stool; dysphagia and ulcerative enterocolitis (rare)
Dermatological	*Rash (24%), pruritus (17%), hair loss and urticaria (1–3%),* angioedema (rare)
Oral	*Stomatitis (13%), glossitis (1–3%),* gingivitis
Hematological	*Anemia, leukopenia, thrombocytopenia, and eosinophilia (1–3%),* neutropenia; agranulocytosis (rare)
Renal	*Proteinuria (3–9%), hematuria (1–3%)*
Hepatic	*Elevated liver enzyme levels (1–3%),* jaundice (rare)
Ophthalmic	*Conjunctivitis (3–9%)*
Other	Interstitial pneumonitis and peripheral neuropathy (rare)

OVERDOSAGE

Signs and symptoms	Encephalopathy, peripheral neuropathy
Treatment	Immediately induce emesis or perform gastric lavage; institute supportive measures. Use of chelating agents may be considered.

DRUG INTERACTIONS

Phenytoin	⇧ Serum phenytoin level

ALTERED LABORATORY VALUES

Blood/serum values	⇧ Hepatic enzymes
Urinary values	+ Protein

USE IN CHILDREN

Safety and effectiveness for use in children have not been established; use in these patients is not recommended

USE IN PREGNANT AND NURSING WOMEN

Pregnancy Category C: increases in resorptions, abortions, and congenital abnormalities (mainly abdominal defects such as gastroschisis and umbilical hernia) and decreases in food intake and maternal and fetal weight gain have been seen in rabbits given 4.2–50 times the human dose of auranofin. Administration of 42 times the human dose produced maternal toxicity (resulting in an increase in resorptions and reduced litter size and weight) in rats, but had no teratogenic effects in mice. Use of this drug in pregnant women is not recommended. Caution women of childbearing potential about the potential risks of use during pregnancy. Injectable gold has been detected in human milk, and auranofin has been seen in the milk of rats and mice; administration of auranofin to nursing mothers is not recommended.

[1] Reactions reported with parenteral gold, but not with auranofin, include generalized exfoliative dermatitis, pancytopenia, aplastic anemia, and nitritoid (anaphylactoid) reactions

ANTIARTHRITIC AGENTS

RUFEN (ibuprofen) Boots   Rx

Tablets: 400, 600, 800 mg

INDICATIONS	ORAL DOSAGE
Rheumatoid arthritis **Osteoarthritis**	**Adult:** 300 mg qid or 400–800 mg tid or qid; once a satisfactory response is obtained (usually by 2 wk), adjust dosage as needed; higher doses may be required for rheumatoid arthritis than for osteoarthritis
Mild to moderate pain	**Adult:** 400 mg q4–6h, as needed
Primary dysmenorrhea	**Adult:** 400 mg q4h, as needed

CONTRAINDICATIONS

Hypersensitivity to ibuprofen	History of nasal polyps, angioedema, or bronchospasm precipitated by aspirin or other nonsteroidal anti-inflammatory drugs

ADMINISTRATION/DOSAGE ADJUSTMENTS

Gastric irritation	May be minimized by administering drug with meals or milk
Arthritis	An increase in dosage from 2,400 to 3,200 mg/day may be beneficial for certain patients, although it should be borne in mind that in well-controlled studies such an increase caused a slight increase in adverse reactions and failed to enhance mean effectiveness
Combination therapy	Additional symptomatic relief has been obtained in combination with gold salts. Neither benefits nor harmful interactions have been demonstrated with corticosteroids; if prolonged corticosteroid therapy is discontinued, reduce dosage gradually to avoid the complications of abrupt withdrawal

WARNINGS/PRECAUTIONS

Anaphylactoid reactions	May occur in patients hypersensitive to other nonsteroidal anti-inflammatory agents (see CONTRAINDICATIONS)
Peptic ulceration, perforation, GI bleeding	May occur and can be severe and even fatal; patients with a history of upper GI tract disease or with an active peptic ulcer should be closely supervised during therapy
Renal toxicity	Proteinuria, acute interstitial nephritis with hematuria, and occasionally the nephrotic syndrome may occur during therapy. In patients with reduced renal blood flow or volume owing to conditions such as heart failure, renal or hepatic impairment, advanced age, or use of diuretics, administration of a nonsteroidal anti-inflammatory agent may cause a dose-dependent decrease in the formation of renal prostaglandins and thereby precipitate overt renal failure; the reaction is reversible upon discontinuation of the drug.
Drug accumulation	Ibuprofen is eliminated primarily by the kidneys; closely monitor patients with significant renal impairment and be prepared to reduce the daily dose. The safety of ibuprofen in patients with chronic renal failure has not been studied.
Ophthalmic changes	May occur (see ADVERSE REACTIONS); if visual complaints develop, discontinue drug and perform an ophthalmologic examination, including testing of central visual fields and color vision
Fluid retention and edema	May occur; use with caution in patients with a history of cardiac decompensation or hypertension. Fluid retention can generally be reversed by discontinuing the drug.
Prolonged bleeding time	May occur due to inhibition of platelet aggregation; use with caution in patients with coagulation defects or with those on anticoagulant therapy
Decreased hemoglobin and hematocrit	A slight dose-related reduction in hemoglobin and hematocrit may occur. The total decrease in hemoglobin, even at 3,200 mg/day, usually does not exceed 1 g; this effect is probably not clinically important if there are no signs of bleeding.
Liver function abnormalities	Borderline elevations may occur in up to 15% of patients; meaningful elevations (3 times the upper limit of normal) in SGOT or SGPT levels have been reported in less than 1% of patients. If abnormal liver function tests or other manifestations of liver dysfunction arise during therapy, evaluate the patient for evidence of a more severe hepatic reaction. Although such reactions as jaundice and fatal hepatitis have occurred rarely, discontinue therapy if abnormal liver function test results persist or worsen, signs and symptoms of liver disease develop, or secondary manifestations (eg, eosinophilia, rash) occur.
Diagnostic interference	Complications of presumably noninfectious, noninflammatory painful conditions may escape detection because of reduction in fever and inflammation

ADVERSE REACTIONS[1]

Frequent reactions (incidence ≥ 1%) are printed in *italics*

Gastrointestinal	*Nausea, epigastric pain, and heartburn (3–9%); diarrhea, abdominal distress, nausea and vomiting, indigestion, constipation, abdominal cramps or pain, bloating, and flatulence (< 3%);* gastric or duodenal-ulcer bleeding and/or perforation, GI hemorrhage, pancreatitis, melena, gastritis, hepatitis, jaundice, abnormal liver function tests
Central nervous system	*Dizziness (3–9%); headache and nervousness (< 3%);* depression, insomnia, confusion, emotional lability, somnolence, aseptic meningitis with fever and coma
Ophthalmic	Blurred and/or diminished vision; scotomata; changes in color vision
Otic	*Tinnitus (< 3%),* hearing loss
Dermatological	*Rash, including maculopapular rash (3–9%), pruritus (< 3%),* vesiculobullous eruptions, urticaria, erythema multiforme, Stevens-Johnson syndrome, alopecia
Metabolic	*Decreased appetite (< 3%)*
Cardiovascular	*Edema and fluid retention (< 3%),* congestive heart failure in patients with marginal cardiac function; elevated blood pressure, palpitations
Hematological	Neutropenia, agranulocytosis, aplastic anemia, hemolytic anemia (occasionally Coombs' positive), thrombocytopenia with or without purpura, eosinophilia, decreased hemoglobin and hematocrit
Renal	Acute renal failure in patients with significant renal impairment; decreased creatinine clearance, polyuria, azotemia, cystitis, hematuria

Allergic	Syndrome of abdominal pain, fever, chills, nausea, and vomiting; anaphylaxis; bronchospasm
Other	Dry eyes and mouth, gingival ulcer, rhinitis

OVERDOSAGE

Signs and symptoms	Apnea, cyanosis, dizziness, nystagmus
Treatment	Following recent ingestion (< 1 h), induce emesis or perform gastric lavage to remove drug from stomach. Activated charcoal may be helpful. If drug is already absorbed, it may be useful to induce diuresis and alkalinize the urine.

DRUG INTERACTIONS

Coumarin anticoagulants	△ Risk of bleeding; use with caution
Aspirin	▽ Anti-inflammatory activity (potential)

ALTERED LABORATORY VALUES

Blood/serum values	△ SGOT △ SGPT

No clinically significant alterations in urinary values occur at therapeutic dosages

USE IN CHILDREN

Safety and effectiveness for use in children have not been established

USE IN PREGNANT AND NURSING WOMEN

Not recommended for use in pregnant or nursing women. Animal reproduction studies have shown no evidence of developmental abnormalities; however, no adequate, well-controlled studies have been done in pregnant women and, hence, the drug should be used only if clearly needed. Because of the risk of premature closure of the ductus arteriosus, use during late pregnancy should be avoided. An increased incidence of dystocia and delayed parturition has been observed in rats. Limited studies in nursing women have not demonstrated significant excretion of this drug in human milk; however, because this remains a possibility and because of the potential for serious adverse effects in neonates, the patient should not nurse while taking ibuprofen.

[1] Reactions for which a causal relationship has not been established include paresthesias, hallucinations, dream abnormalities, pseudotumor cerebri, toxic epidermal necrolysis, photoallergic skin reactions, conjunctivitis, diplopia, optic neuritis, cataracts, bleeding episodes (eg, epistaxis, menorrhagia), serum sickness, lupus erythematosus syndrome, Henoch-Schonlein vasculitis, angioedema, gynecomastia, hypoglycemic reaction, acidosis, sinus tachycardia, sinus bradycardia, and renal papillary necrosis

ANTIARTHRITIC AGENTS

SOLGANAL (aurothioglucose) Schering   Rx

Vials: 50 mg/ml (10 ml) for IM use only

INDICATIONS

Early, active **rheumatoid arthritis** inadequately controlled by other anti-inflammatory agents and conservative measures (adjunctive therapy)

PARENTERAL DOSAGE

Adult: 10 mg IM (preferably intragluteally), followed 1 and 2 wk later by 25 mg IM, and subsequently by 50 mg/wk IM until total cumulative dose reaches 0.8–1.0 g; for maintenance: 25–50 mg IM every 3–4 wk
Child (6–12 yr): ¼ adult dose, determined by body weight, up to 25 mg/dose

CONTRAINDICATIONS

- Uncontrolled diabetes or congestive heart failure
- Severe debilitation
- Renal disease
- Hepatic dysfunction
- History of infectious hepatitis
- Marked hypertension
- Agranulocytosis, other blood dyscrasias, or hemorrhagic diathesis
- Recent radiotherapy
- Prior severe toxic reaction to gold or other heavy metals
- Hypersensitivity to aurothioglucose or other components
- Urticaria
- Eczema
- Systemic lupus erythematosus
- Colitis
- Pregnancy, unless continued therapy is deemed essential

ADMINISTRATION/DOSAGE ADJUSTMENTS

Preparation of dose and administration	Heat the vial to body temperature by immersing it in warm water. Hold the vial horizontally and shake it thoroughly to suspend all of the active material. Using a dry syringe and 18-gauge, 1½-inch needle (or 2-inch needle if patient is obese), withdraw required dose and inject into the upper outer quadrant of the gluteal region. Patient should be lying down and remain recumbent for approximately 10 min after suspension is injected; keep patient under observation for at least 15 min after injection.

SOLGANAL

Failure of initial therapy	If no clinical improvement is apparent after patient has received a total of 1 g of the drug, reevaluate the need for chrysotherapy
Concomitant antiarthritic therapy	Do not use with penicillamine or antimalarials. The safety of coadministration with cytotoxic (immunosuppressive) agents has not been established. Treatment with salicylates, other nonsteroidal anti-inflammatory agents, or systemic corticosteroids may be continued when gold therapy is started or withdrawn gradually as symptoms permit.

WARNINGS/PRECAUTIONS

Hematological, renal, and dermatological toxicity	May occur; obtain baseline complete blood count, platelet count, and urinalysis; repeat urinalysis prior to each injection, and repeat complete blood count and platelet count every 2 wk and whenever purpura or ecchymoses develop. If hemoglobin drops rapidly, WBC count falls below 4,000/mm^3, eosinophilia exceeds 5%, platelet count falls below 100,000/mm^3, or albuminuria, hematuria, pruritus, dermatitis, stomatitis, jaundice, or petechiae develops, discontinue therapy until another cause of the abnormality can be determined.
Special-risk patients	Use with caution in the elderly, in patients with HLA-D histocompatibility antigens DRw2 and DRw3, and in those with compromised cardiovascular or cerebral circulation; use with extreme caution in patients with skin rash or a history of renal or hepatic disease or hypersensitivity to other drugs
Patient instructions	Instruct patient to minimize exposure to sunlight or artificial UV light, maintain good oral hygiene, and report promptly any unusual signs and symptoms, such as pruritus, rash, sore mouth, ingestion, or metallic taste
Arthralgia	May occur for 1–2 days after injection, but usually subsides after the first few injections; warn patient that he or she may experience increased joint pain for this period until therapy is well established
Pruritus	May occur as a warning signal of impending dermatological reaction
Metallic taste	May occur as a warning signal of impending oral mucous membrane reaction

ADVERSE REACTIONS

Dermatological	Dermatitis, pruritus, erythema, actinic rash, chrysiasis, papular and vesicular eruptions, exfoliative dermatitis leading to alopecia and nail shedding
Mucous membrane	Stomatitis, buccal ulceration, glossitis, gingivitis, upper respiratory tract inflammation, pharyngitis, gastritis, colitis, tracheitis, vaginitis
Renal	Nephrotic syndrome, glomerulitis with hematuria
Hematological	Granulocytopenia, agranulocytosis, thrombocytopenia (with or without purpura), leukopenia, eosinophilia, panmyelopathy, hemorrhagic diathesis, and hypoplastic and aplastic anemia (rare)
Nitritoid and allergic	Flushing, fainting, dizziness, sweating, malaise, weakness, nausea, vomiting, anaphylactic shock, syncope, bradycardia, thickening of the tongue, difficulty in swallowing and breathing, and angioneurotic edema (rare)
Gastrointestinal	Nausea, vomiting, colic, anorexia, abdominal cramps, diarrhea, ulcerative enterocolitis
Ophthalmic	Transient, asymptomatic gold deposits in cornea or conjunctiva; iritis, corneal ulcers, and conjunctivitis (rare)
Hepatic	Intrahepatic cholestasis, hepatitis with jaundice, toxic hepatitis
Central nervous system	Headache (rare), encephalitis, EEG abnormalities
Other	Arthralgia (transient), immunological destruction of the synovia, acute yellow atrophy, peripheral neuritis, gold bronchitis, interstitial pneumonitis, pulmonary fibrosis, fever, partial or complete hair loss

OVERDOSAGE

Signs and symptoms	Renal damage, manifested by hematuria and proteinuria; hematological changes, including thrombocytopenia and granulocytopenia; fever; nausea; vomiting; diarrhea; skin disorders (eg, papulovesicular lesions, urticaria, and exfoliative dermatitis) accompanied by severe pruritus
Treatment	Discontinue treatment immediately. If symptoms are mild, treatment may be reinstituted at lower doses. Treat dermatitis and pruritus with soothing lotions, antipruritics, or topical glucocorticoids. Systemic glucocorticoid treatment may be required for severe or generalized dermatitis or stomatitis; treatment with larger doses for many months may be required for renal, hematological, and most other adverse reactions. Reactions unresponsive to glucocorticoids may require the use of a chelating agent such as dimercaprol. Institute specific supportive measures for renal and hematological effects. Adjunctive use of an anabolic steroid with dimercaprol, penicillamine, or corticosteroids may help restore bone marrow function.

DRUG INTERACTIONS

Antimalarial agents, penicillamine	⇧ Risk of renal and hematological toxicity

ALTERED LABORATORY VALUES

Blood/serum values — ⇧ or ⇩ PBI (with chloric acid method)

No clinically significant alterations in urinary values occur at therapeutic dosages

USE IN CHILDREN

See INDICATIONS and PARENTERAL DOSAGE; safety and effectiveness for use in children under 6 yr of age have not been established

USE IN PREGNANT AND NURSING WOMEN

Pregnancy Category C: use during pregnancy is usually contraindicated unless continued therapy is considered essential, since the potential nephrotoxicity of chrysotherapy can compound the already increased renal burden associated with pregnancy. Patients should be aware of the potential hazards of becoming pregnant while receiving gold therapy; the slow excretion of gold and its persistence in body tissues after therapy is discontinued should be kept in mind if the patient plans to become pregnant. Teratogenic effects probably related to maternal toxicity have been observed in rats and rabbits treated with gold sodium thiomalate at doses 140 and 175 times the usual human dose. No adequate, well-controlled studies have been conducted in pregnant women; however, extensive clinical experience with aurothioglucose has shown no evidence of human teratogenicity. Gold is excreted in the milk of lactating mothers and has been detected in the serum and red blood cells of a nursing infant. Because of the potential for serious adverse effects in the infant, a decision should be made to discontinue nursing or use of the drug. Significant gold levels may persist after therapy is withdrawn.

ANTIARTHRITIC AGENTS

SYNALGOS (aspirin and caffeine) Wyeth   OTC

Capsules: 356.4 mg aspirin and 30 mg caffeine

INDICATIONS

Minor aches and pains, including headaches, dental pain, and minor aches and pains of arthritis and rheumatism
Fever

ORAL DOSAGE

Adult: 2 caps, with a full glass of water, q4h, up to 10 caps/day

WARNINGS/PRECAUTIONS

Patient instructions — Patients are cautioned by the package label not to use this product without the advice and supervision of a physician if they are allergic to aspirin, have asthma, stomach distress, ulcers, or bleeding disorders, or are taking anticoagulants or a medication for the treatment of diabetes, gout, or arthritis; the label also warns patients to discontinue use if tinnitus or other symptoms of overdosage occur and to consult a physician immediately if "pain persists for more than ten days or redness is present or in arthritic or rheumatic conditions affecting children under 12 yr of age. . . ."

ADVERSE REACTIONS

Central nervous system — Drowsiness, dizziness, light-headedness, sedation

Gastrointestinal — Nausea, vomiting, constipation

Dermatological — Skin reactions

Cardiovascular — Hypotension (rare)

OVERDOSAGE

Signs and symptoms — *Aspirin-related effects:* hyperpnea, nausea, vomiting, vertigo, tinnitus, flushing, sweating, thirst, headache, drowsiness, diarrhea, and tachycardia, progressing to hyperthermia, hemorrhage, acid-base disturbances, restlessness, confusion, convulsions, vasomotor depression, coma, and respiratory failure; *caffeine-related effects:* insomnia, restlessness, tremors, delirium, tachycardia, extrasystoles, tinnitus, urinary frequency

Treatment — If less than 4 h have elapsed since ingestion, induce emesis or perform gastric lavage, followed by activated charcoal, to remove any remaining drug from the stomach. Initial therapy should be directed at reducing hyperthermia by external sponging with tepid water, correcting dehydration by appropriate IV fluid replacement, and maintaining adequate cardiorespiratory and renal function. In moderately severe cases of salicylate poisoning, cautiously administer sodium bicarbonate IV in sufficient quantity, if possible, to maintain an alkaline diuresis; intermittent peritoneal dialysis may also be helpful. In severe cases, hemodialysis should be seriously considered. Potassium should be added to the repair solution to compensate for potassium losses once urine formation is deemed adequate. Glucose may be provided to correct ketosis and hypoglycemia. Plasma transfusion may be beneficial if shock intervenes. Hemorrhagic phenomena may necessitate whole-blood transfusions and phytonadione (vitamin K_1). Do not administer barbiturates to treat excitement or convulsions.

DRUG INTERACTIONS

Anticoagulants	⇧ Risk of bleeding
Sulfonylureas	⇧ Hypoglycemic effect
Alcohol, corticosteroids, phenylbutazone, oxyphenbutazone	⇧ Risk of GI ulceration
Probenecid, sulfinpyrazone	⇩ Uricosuric effect
Spironolactone	⇩ Diuretic effect
Methotrexate	⇧ Methotrexate plasma level and risk of toxicity

ALTERED LABORATORY VALUES

Blood/serum values	⇧ Prothrombin time ⇧ Uric acid (with low doses) ⇩ Uric acid (with high doses) ⇩ Thyroxine (T$_4$) ⇩ Thyroid-stimulating hormone
Urinary values	⇧ Glucose (with Clinitest tablets)

USE IN CHILDREN

Consult manufacturer; the package label states that a physician should be consulted for use in children under 12 yr of age

USE IN PREGNANT AND NURSING WOMEN

Consult manufacturer; the package label instructs pregnant and nursing patients to seek the advice of a health-care professional before they take this preparation

---

ANTIARTHRITIC AGENTS

TOLECTIN 200 (tolmetin sodium) McNeil Pharmaceutical Rx

Tablets: tolmetin sodium equivalent to 200 mg tolmetin

TOLECTIN DS (tolmetin sodium) McNeil Pharmaceutical Rx

Capsules: tolmetin sodium equivalent to 400 mg tolmetin

INDICATIONS

	ORAL DOSAGE
Rheumatoid arthritis	**Adult:** 400 mg tid to start, followed by 600–1,800 mg/day in 3–4 divided doses, or up to 2,000 mg/day, if needed
Osteoarthritis	**Adult:** 400 mg tid to start, followed by 600–1,600 mg/day in 3–4 divided doses
Juvenile rheumatoid arthritis	**Child (≥ 2 yr):** 20 mg/kg/day in 3–4 divided doses to start, followed by 15–30 mg/kg/day in divided doses

CONTRAINDICATIONS

Hypersensitivity to tolmetin

History of asthma, rhinitis, urticaria, or other allergic reactions precipitated by aspirin or other nonsteroidal anti-inflammatory drugs

ADMINISTRATION/DOSAGE ADJUSTMENTS

Onset of action	A therapeutic response can be expected to occur in a few days to a week, followed by progressive improvement over the succeeding weeks
Management of GI reactions	If GI symptoms occur, an antacid other than sodium bicarbonate can be given with tolmetin
Food-drug interaction	Administration with milk or immediately after a meal produces a 16% decrease in total bioavailability
Combination therapy	Use of tolmetin in patients receiving gold or a corticosteroid has produced an additional therapeutic effect (this effect is greater with gold than with a steroid). When reducing the dosage of a corticosteroid, be sure to do it in a gradual manner; complications can occur if the drug is suddenly withdrawn.

WARNINGS/PRECAUTIONS

Gastrointestinal effects	Tolmetin can cause severe GI bleeding and peptic ulcers; patients with a history of upper GI tract disease or with an active peptic ulcer should be closely supervised
Anaphylactoid reactions	Institute conventional measures to treat anaphylactoid reactions; eg, administer epinephrine, antihistamines, and/or corticosteroids

Renal toxicity	Proteinuria, acute interstitial nephritis with hematuria, and occasionally the nephrotic syndrome may occur during therapy. In patients with reduced renal blood flow or volume owing to conditions such as heart failure, renal or hepatic impairment, advanced age, or use of diuretics, administration of a nonsteroidal anti-inflammatory agent may cause a critical decrease in the formation of renal prostaglandins and thereby precipitate overt renal failure; reaction is reversible upon discontinuation of the drug.
Drug accumulation	Tolmetin is eliminated primarily by the kidneys; closely monitor patients with renal impairment and be prepared to reduce the daily dose
Liver function abnormalities	Borderline elevations may occur in up to 15% of patients; meaningful elevations (3 times the upper limit of normal) in SGOT or SGPT levels have been reported in less than 1% of patients. If abnormal liver function tests or other manifestations of liver dysfunction arise during therapy, evaluate the patient for evidence of a more severe hepatic reaction. Although severe reactions such as jaundice and fatal hepatitis have occurred rarely, discontinue therapy if abnormal liver function tests persist or worsen, clinical signs and symptoms of liver disease develop, or secondary manifestations (eg, eosinophilia, rash) occur.
Peripheral edema	Use with caution in patients with compromised cardiac function, hypertension, or other conditions that are likely to produce fluid retention since tolmetin may cause peripheral edema in these patients
Ophthalmic effects	Ocular changes have been produced in animals by tolmetin and in humans by other nonsteroidal anti-inflammatory agents; optic neuropathy and macular and retinal changes have been detected in patients given tolmetin, but a causal relationship has not been established. If the patient experiences visual disturbances during therapy, perform an ophthalmologic evaluation.
Prolonged bleeding time	Since tolmetin prolongs bleeding time, patients who may be adversely affected by this effect should be carefully observed (see DRUG INTERACTIONS)
Carcinogenicity, mutagenicity, effect on fertility	No evidence of carcinogenicity has been seen in rats given up to 75 mg/kg/day for 24 mo or in mice given up to 50 mg/kg/day for 18 mo. The Ames test has shown no mutagenic effects. Reproduction studies have failed to demonstrate any adverse effect on fertility.

ADVERSE REACTIONS[1]

Frequent reactions (incidence ≥ 1%) are printed in *italics*

Gastrointestinal	*Nausea (11%); dyspepsia, abdominal pain, GI distress, flatulence, diarrhea, and vomiting (3–9%); constipation, peptic ulcer, and gastritis (1–3%);* GI bleeding, with or without peptic ulcer; stomatitis; glossitis
Hepatic	Hepatitis, liver function abnormalities
Central nervous system	*Headache and dizziness (3–9%); drowsiness, depression, tinnitus, visual disturbance (1–3%)*
Cardiovascular	*Elevated blood pressure and edema (3–9%);* congestive heart failure (in patients with marginal cardiac function)
Dermatological	*Skin irritation (1–3%);* urticaria, purpura, erythema multiforme, toxic epidermal necrolysis
Hematological	*Small, transient decreases in hemoglobin and hematocrit (1–3%);* hemolytic anemia, thrombocytopenia, granulocytopenia, agranulocytosis
Genitourinary	*Urinary tract infection (1–3%);* hematuria, proteinuria, dysuria, renal failure
Other	*Weight gain or loss and asthenia (3–9%), chest pain (1–3%),* fever, anaphylactoid reactions, lymphadenopathy, serum sickness

OVERDOSAGE

Signs and symptoms	See ADVERSE REACTIONS
Treatment	Induce vomiting or use gastric lavage, followed by activated charcoal

DRUG INTERACTIONS

Anticoagulants	⇧ Risk of bleeding; exercise caution during concomitant therapy
Salicylates	⇧ Risk of adverse reactions; salicylates should not be used with tolmetin

ALTERED LABORATORY VALUES

Blood/serum values	⇧ Sodium ⇧ BUN ⇧ SGOT ⇧ SGPT
Urinary values	+ Protein (with sulfosalicylic acid tests)

USE IN CHILDREN

See INDICATIONS and ORAL DOSAGE; safety and effectiveness for use in children under 2 yr of age have not been established

USE IN PREGNANT AND NURSING WOMEN

Pregnancy Category C: reproduction studies in rats and rabbits given up to 50 mg/kg have shown no evidence of teratogenicity or impaired fertility; however, an increased incidence of dystocia and delayed parturition has been observed in animals. Moreover, when given to women during the third trimester, tolmetin may precipitate constriction of the ductus arteriosus and, as a result, cause persistent pulmonary hypertension in the neonate. Use during pregnancy only if the expected benefit justifies the potential risk to the fetus. Tolmetin is excreted in human milk; use in nursing mothers should be avoided.

---

[1] Reactions for which a causal relationship has not been established include optic neuropathy, macular and retinal changes, and epistaxis

ANTIARTHRITIC AGENTS

TRILISATE (choline magnesium trisalicylate) Purdue Frederick   Rx

Tablets: 500, 750, 1,000 mg   **Liquid (per 5 ml):** 500 mg (8 fl oz) *cherry-cordial flavored*

INDICATIONS

Rheumatoid arthritis[1]
Osteoarthritis
The more severe arthritides
Acute painful shoulder

Juvenile rheumatoid arthritis[1]

Mild to moderate pain
Fever

ORAL DOSAGE

Adult: 3,000 mg once daily at bedtime or 1,500 mg bid to start

Child (12–37 kg): 50 mg/kg/day, given in 2 divided doses, to start
Child (> 37 kg): 2,250 mg/day, given in 2 divided doses, to start

Adult: 2,000–3,000 mg/day, given in 2 divided doses, to start
Child (12–37 kg): 50 mg/kg/day, given in 2 divided doses, to start
Child (> 37 kg): 2,250 mg/day, given in 2 divided doses, to start

CONTRAINDICATIONS

Hypersensitivity to nonacetylated salicylates

ADMINISTRATION/DOSAGE ADJUSTMENTS

Onset of action	Some patients may require 2–3 wk of therapy for optimal effect
Dilution of liquid form	If desired, liquid may be mixed with fruit juice immediately before ingestion
Dosage titration	Adjust dosage to achieve appropriate therapeutic effect or therapeutic blood salicylate levels (for analgesic and antipyretic effect, 5–15 mg/dl; for anti-inflammatory effect, 15–30 mg/dl)
Dosage equivalents	Each 500-mg tab or 5 ml (1 tsp) is equivalent in salicylate content to 10 gr of aspirin; each 750-mg tablet is equivalent to 15 gr of aspirin
Alternative dosage schedule	If preferred, recommended daily dose may be given in divided doses tid

WARNINGS/PRECAUTIONS

Special-risk patients	Use with caution in patients with chronic renal insufficiency, active erosive gastritis, or peptic ulcer and in patients requiring oral anticoagulants or heparin
Salicylism and/or salicylate intoxication	May occur if taken in large doses or for a prolonged period; reduce dosage if tinnitus develops (see OVERDOSAGE)

ADVERSE REACTIONS

General	Salicylism (see WARNINGS/PRECAUTIONS)

OVERDOSAGE

Signs and symptoms	Hyperpnea, nausea, vomiting, vertigo, tinnitus, flushing, sweating, thirst, headache, drowsiness, diarrhea, and tachycardia, progressing to hyperthermia, hemorrhage, restlessness, confusion, convulsions, vasomotor depression, coma, and respiratory failure
Treatment	If less than 4 h have elapsed since ingestion, induce emesis or perform gastric lavage, followed by activated charcoal, to remove any remaining drug from the stomach. Initial therapy should be directed at reducing hyperthermia by external sponging with tepid water, correcting dehydration by appropriate IV fluid replacement, and maintaining adequate cardiorespiratory and renal function. In moderately severe cases of salicylate poisoning, cautiously administer sodium bicarbonate IV in sufficient quantity, if possible, to maintain an alkaline diuresis; intermittent peritoneal dialysis may also be helpful. In severe cases, hemodialysis should be seriously considered. Potassium should be added to the repair solution to compensate for potassium losses once urine formation is deemed adequate. Glucose may be provided to correct ketosis and hypoglycemia. Plasma transfusion may be beneficial if shock intervenes. Hemorrhagic phenomena may necessitate whole-blood transfusions and phytonadione (vitamin K). Do not administer barbiturates to treat excitement or convulsions.

DRUG INTERACTIONS

Anticoagulants	△ Anticoagulant effect
Antacids, urinary alkalinizers	▽ Plasma salicylate levels
Urinary acidifiers	△ Plasma salicylate levels
Oral hypoglycemics	△ Hypoglycemic effect
Methotrexate	△ Plasma methotrexate plasma level and risk of toxicity
Probenecid, sulfinpyrazone	▽ Uricosuric effect

TRILISATE

ALTERED LABORATORY VALUES

Blood/serum values — △ or ▽ Uric acid
Urinary values — △ or ▽ VMA

USE IN CHILDREN
See INDICATIONS and ORAL DOSAGE

USE IN PREGNANT AND NURSING WOMEN
Use with caution during pregnancy. Because of possible prostaglandin inhibition with high doses of salicylates, do not administer immediately prior to the onset of labor. Consult manufacturer for use in nursing mothers.

[1] Safety and effectiveness have not been established for rheumatoid arthritis patients designated by the American Rheumatism Association as belonging to Functional Class IV (incapacitated; largely or wholly bedridden or confined to a wheelchair; little or no self-care)

528   COMPENDIUM OF DRUG THERAPY

Chapter 15

Anticoagulants/Thrombolytic Agents/Other Blood Modifiers

Anticoagulants	**530**
CALCIPARINE (Du Pont Critical Care) Heparin calcium Rx	530
COUMADIN (Du Pont) Warfarin sodium, crystalline Rx	532
EMBOLEX (Sandoz Pharmaceuticals) Heparin sodium and dihydroergotamine mesylate Rx	534
Heparin sodium Rx	536
PANWARFIN (Abbott) Warfarin sodium Rx	539
Thrombolytic Agents	**541**
ABBOKINASE (Abbott) Urokinase Rx	541
ABBOKINASE OPEN-CATH (Abbott) Urokinase Rx	541
KABIKINASE (KabiVitrum) Streptokinase Rx	543
STREPTASE (Hoechst-Roussel) Streptokinase Rx	545
Antifibrinolytic Agents	**547**
AMICAR (Lederle) Aminocaproic acid Rx	547
Hemorheologic Agents	**548**
TRENTAL (Hoechst-Roussel) Pentoxifylline Rx	548
Antiplatelet Agents	**549**
ASCRIPTIN (Rorer) Aspirin, magnesium hydroxide, and aluminum hydroxide OTC	549
ASCRIPTIN A/D (Rorer) Aspirin, magnesium hydroxide, and aluminum hydroxide OTC	550
Extra Strength ASCRIPTIN (Rorer) Aspirin, magnesium hydroxide, and aluminum hydroxide OTC	550
BAYER Aspirin (Glenbrook) Aspirin OTC	551
Maximum BAYER Aspirin (Glenbrook) Aspirin OTC	551
BAYER Children's Chewable Aspirin (Glenbrook) Aspirin OTC	551
8-Hour BAYER Aspirin (Glenbrook) Aspirin OTC	551
BUFFERIN (Bristol-Myers) Aspirin, aluminum glycinate, and magnesium carbonate OTC	553
Arthritis Strength BUFFERIN (Bristol-Myers) Aspirin, aluminum glycinate, and magnesium carbonate OTC	553
Extra Strength BUFFERIN (Bristol-Myers) Aspirin, aluminum glycinate, and magnesium carbonate OTC	553
Maximum Strength ECOTRIN (SmithKline Consumer Products) Aspirin OTC	554
Regular Strength ECOTRIN (SmithKline Consumer Products) Aspirin OTC	554
EMPIRIN (Burroughs Wellcome) Aspirin OTC	556
Hemostatic Agents	**558**
AVITENE (Alcon) Microfibrillar collagen hemostat (MCH) Rx	558
THROMBOSTAT (Parke-Davis) Thrombin Rx	559
Other Anticoagulants	**529**
Dicumarol Rx	529

OTHER ANTICOAGULANTS

DRUG	HOW SUPPLIED	USUAL DOSAGE[1]
Dicumarol Rx	Tablets: 25, 50 mg	Adult: 200–300 mg/day to start, followed by 25–200 mg/day, as needed to maintain the prothrombin time at 1.5–2.5 times the normal value

[1] Where pediatric dosages are not given, consult manufacturer

COMPENDIUM OF DRUG THERAPY

CALCIPARINE

ANTICOAGULANTS

CALCIPARINE (heparin calcium) Du Pont Critical Care   Rx

Ampuls: 12,500 units (0.5 ml), 20,000 units (0.8 ml)   **Prefilled syringes:** 5,000 units (0.2 ml)

INDICATIONS[1]

Venous thrombosis, pulmonary embolism, atrial fibrillation with embolization, and peripheral arterial embolism (full-dose therapy)

Prevention of **postoperative deep venous thrombosis and pulmonary embolism** in patients over 40 yr of age who are undergoing major abdominal or thoracic surgery (low-dose therapy)

Prevention of clotting in patients undergoing total body perfusion during **open-heart surgery**

PARENTERAL DOSAGE

Adult (68 kg): for *SC administration*, 10,000–20,000 units SC to start (usually preceded by an IV loading dose of 5,000 units), followed by 8,000–10,000 units SC q8h or 15,000–20,000 units SC q12h; for *intermittent IV administration*, 10,000 units IV to start, followed by 5,000–10,000 units IV q4–6h (initial and maintenance doses may be given undiluted or in 50–100 ml of 0.9% sodium chloride injection USP); for *continuous IV infusion*, 5,000 units by IV injection to start, followed by continuous IV infusion of 20,000–40,000 units in 1 liter of 0.9% sodium chloride injection USP or another compatible diluent/24 h

Child: 50 units/kg by IV infusion to start, followed by either 100 units/kg by IV infusion q4h or 20,000 units/m^2/24 h by continuous IV infusion

Adult: 5,000 units SC 2 h before surgery, followed by 5,000 units SC q8–12h for 7 days or until patient is fully ambulatory, whichever is longer

Adult: not less than 150 units/kg IV to start; as a rule, 300 units/kg IV may be given for procedures lasting less than 60 min and 400 units/kg is given for longer procedures

CONTRAINDICATIONS

Uncontrollable active bleeding, except when caused by disseminated intravascular coagulation

Inability to perform suitable coagulation tests at appropriate intervals (full-dose therapy only)

Severe thrombocytopenia

ADMINISTRATION/DOSAGE ADJUSTMENTS

Formulation — This product is derived from porcine intestinal mucosa; the dosage strengths (and dosage) are given in terms of USP heparin units

Administration — Heparin may be given by IV injection, IV infusion, or deep SC injection. Intramuscular administration is not recommended since it frequently results in hematoma. Inject each SC dose into the abdominal fat layer or into fat tissue above the iliac crest; minimize tissue trauma by using a 25- or 26-gauge needle. To avoid massive hematoma, use a different site for each SC injection. Containers to be used for continuous IV infusion should be inverted at least 6 times before use to ensure adequate mixing and prevent pooling of the drug.

Monitoring of full-dose therapy — To monitor therapeutic response to full doses of heparin, check activated partial thromboplastin time (APTT) or whole blood clotting time (WBCT) frequently; adjust dosage on the basis of coagulation test results. If heparin is given by intermittent IV injection, check the coagulation time before each dose during the early stages and at appropriate intervals thereafter; if the drug is given by continuous IV infusion, check every 4 h during the early stages; if the drug is given SC, check 4–6 h after each dose. Dosage is considered adequate when the APTT is 1.5–2 times the normal value or the WBCT is 2.5–3 times the control value.

Guidelines for prevention of postoperative thromboembolism — Determine coagulation values before beginning prophylactic therapy and just before surgery; these values should be normal or only slightly elevated. Monitoring of coagulation values during low-dose therapy is usually unnecessary. Do not institute prophylactic therapy if the patient has a bleeding disorder, is receiving antiplatelet drugs or oral anticoagulants, or is undergoing spinal anesthesia, potentially sanguineous procedures, or brain, ophthalmic, or spinal cord surgery. The effectiveness of prophylactic therapy for patients undergoing hip surgery has not been established. Low-dose therapy may increase the risk of bleeding during or after surgery (see warning below concerning hemorrhage). If thromboembolism develops during therapy, administer full therapeutic doses (unless contraindicated).

Switching to oral anticoagulants — To switch from heparin to an oral anticoagulant, first give heparin and the oral anticoagulant together; then, after the prothrombin time has remained at the therapeutic level for several days, discontinue heparin. Since heparin affects prothrombin time, blood samples should be drawn during concomitant therapy at least 5 h after the last IV dose of heparin or 24 h after the last SC dose; prothrombin time may usually be measured any time during continuous IV infusion.

Blood transfusions — To prevent clotting in blood transfusions, dissolve 7,500 units of heparin in 100 ml of 0.9% sodium chloride injection USP (or 75,000 units in 1 liter) and then add 6–8 ml of this solution to each 100 ml of whole blood

Blood samples — To prevent clotting of blood samples used for laboratory tests, add 70–150 units of heparin to each 10–20 ml of whole blood. Leukocyte counts should be done within 2 h after addition of the drug. Do not use heparinized blood for isoagglutinin, complement, or erythrocyte fragility tests or for platelet counts.

CALCIPARINE

Extracorporeal dialysis	For use of heparin in extracorporeal dialysis, carefully follow the operating directions of the equipment manufacturer

WARNINGS/PRECAUTIONS

Hemorrhage	The chief risk of this preparation is hemorrhage, which is dose-related and can occur at virtually any site. Overdosage may be manifested initially by petechiae, easy bruising, and prolonged coagulation test results, followed by epistaxis, hematuria, and tarry stools. Use with extreme caution during continuous tube drainage of the stomach and small intestine and during and immediately after a spinal tap, spinal anesthesia, or major surgery (especially eye, brain, or spinal cord surgery); exercise extreme caution in patients who are menstruating or have subacute bacterial endocarditis, severe hypertension, liver disease with impaired hemostasis, hemophilia, certain vascular purpuras, thrombocytopenia, or ulcerative lesions. Use with caution in women over 60 yr of age. Periodically check hematocrit and test for occult blood in the stool; if full doses are given, perform coagulation tests frequently (see ADMINISTRATION/DOSAGE ADJUSTMENTS). If minor bleeding occurs or the clotting time or activated partial thromboplastin time is overly prolonged, discontinue treatment. The possibility of hemorrhage should be seriously considered whenever an unexplained decrease in hematocrit or blood pressure or any other unexplained effect occurs. Bear in mind that adrenal, ovarian, and retroperitoneal hemorrhage may be difficult to detect and that GI or urinary tract bleeding may be a sign of an occult lesion. For more severe bleeding or overdose, give 1% protamine sulfate IV; the dosage of protamine depends on the heparin dose, the organ source of the heparin product, and the amount of time that has elapsed since injection. If signs and symptoms of acute adrenal hemorrhage and insufficiency are seen, discontinue therapy and immediately institute corrective measures; do not wait for laboratory confirmation of the diagnosis, since any delay may be fatal.
Thrombocytopenia	Heparin may produce mild or severe thrombocytopenia in up to 30% of patients. In rare cases, the drug may induce irreversible platelet aggregation and thereby cause a "white clot" syndrome characterized by thrombosis and thrombocytopenia. This syndrome may precipitate severe thromboembolic disorders, including skin necrosis, gangrene of the extremities, myocardial infarction, pulmonary embolism, and stroke. Periodically check the platelet count during therapy. If thrombocytopenia occurs, closely monitor condition; if platelet count drops below 100,000/mm^3 or new thrombi develop, promptly discontinue administration or, when therapy must be continued, cautiously switch to a heparin product derived from a different organ source.
Resistance	Heparin is frequently less effective after surgery and in the presence of fever, thrombosis, thrombophlebitis, infections with a thrombosing tendency, myocardial infarction, and cancer
Hypersensitivity	Patients with documented hypersensitivity should be given heparin only in clearly life-threatening situations
Carcinogenicity, mutagenicity, effect on fertility	No long-term studies have been done in animals to evaluate the carcinogenic or mutagenic potential of heparin or its effect on fertility

ADVERSE REACTIONS

Hematological	Bleeding, hemorrhage, thrombocytopenia; thromboembolic complications of thrombocytopenia, including skin necrosis, gangrene of the extremities, myocardial infarction, pulmonary embolism, and stroke; pain, ischemia, and cyanosis of limbs
Hypersensitivity	Chills, fever, urticaria, asthma, rhinitis, lacrimation, headache, nausea, vomiting, pruritus and burning (especially on the plantar side of the feet); anaphylactoid reactions, including shock
Local	Cutaneous necrosis (with IV or SC use); irritation, erythema, mild pain, hematoma, and ulceration (with SC injection)
Other	Suppression of aldosterone synthesis, delayed transient alopecia, priapism, osteoporosis (with long-term, high-dose therapy), rebound hyperlipidemia following discontinuation of therapy

OVERDOSAGE

For signs and symptoms and treatment of overdosage, see warning, above, concerning hemorrhage

DRUG INTERACTIONS

Aspirin, sulfinpyrazone, oral anticoagulants, thrombolytic agents, dextran, phenylbutazone, ibuprofen, indomethacin, dipyridamole, azlocillin, mezlocillin, piperacillin, ticarcillin, parenteral carbenicillin, valproic acid, divalproex, cefamandole, cefoperazone, moxalactam, plicamycin, methimazole, propylthiouracil, probenecid, hydroxychloroquine, chloroquine	⚠ Risk of bleeding and hemorrhage; exercise caution

CALCIPARINE ■ COUMADIN

Digitalis, tetracyclines, antihistamines, nicotine —— ▽ Anticoagulant effect

ALTERED LABORATORY VALUES

Blood/serum values —— △ SGOT △ SGPT △ Prothrombin time △ Clotting time △ APTT
▽ Triglycerides △ Free fatty acids ▽ Cholesterol (with doses of 15,000–20,000 units) △ T_4 (with competitive protein-binding tests) Interference with BSP test

No clinically significant alterations in urinary values occur at therapeutic dosages

USE IN CHILDREN

See INDICATIONS and PARENTERAL DOSAGE

USE IN PREGNANT AND NURSING WOMEN

Pregnant women: Pregnancy Category C: reproduction studies have not been done. Although heparin does not cross the placental barrier, this drug has caused stillbirths and premature births in 13–22% of pregnant patients and increased the risk of maternal hemorrhage associated with the last trimester and the postpartum period.[2] Use during pregnancy only if clearly needed; bear in mind that prolonged, high-dose therapy can cause osteoporosis. **Nursing mothers:** Heparin is not excreted in human milk; however, it has been reported that use of the drug in nursing women for 2–4 wk can, in rare cases, result in severe osteoporosis and vertebral collapse.[2]

[1] Although heparin is indicated for diagnosis and treatment of disseminated intravascular coagulation, such use is controversial; for appropriate guidelines, consult manufacturer
[2] USP DI, Drug Information for the Health Care Provider. Rockville, MD, The United States Pharmacopeial Convention, Inc., 1986

ANTICOAGULANTS

COUMADIN (warfarin sodium, crystalline) Du Pont   Rx

Tablets: 2, 2.5, 5, 7.5, 10 mg **Vials:** 50 mg (2 ml)

INDICATIONS

Venous thrombosis
Pulmonary embolism
Atrial fibrillation with embolization
Coronary occlusion (adjunctive therapy)

ORAL DOSAGE

Adult: 10–15 mg/day (usually for 2–3 days) or a single dose of 40–60 mg to start; for maintenance, adjust dosage according to prothrombin-time response (usual maintenance dosage: 2–10 mg/day)

PARENTERAL DOSAGE

Adult: 10–15 mg/day IM or IV (usually for 2–3 days) or a single IM or IV dose of 40–60 mg to start; for maintenance, adjust dosage according to prothrombin-time response (usual maintenance dosage: 2–10 mg/day)

CONTRAINDICATIONS

Pregnancy

Active ulceration or bleeding associated with pericarditis, pericardial effusions, subacute bacterial endocarditis, or cerebral or dissecting aortic aneurysm

Active GI, genitourinary, or respiratory tract ulceration or bleeding

Diagnostic or therapeutic procedures (eg, spinal puncture) with a potential for uncontrollable bleeding

Inadequate laboratory facilities

Blood dyscrasias

Recent or anticipated traumatic surgery that has produced or may result in large exposed surfaces

Cerebrovascular hemorrhage

Major regional or lumbar block anesthesia

Lack of supervision of senile, alcoholic, or psychotic patients

Hemorrhagic tendencies

Recent or anticipated CNS or ophthalmic surgery

Preeclampsia, eclampsia, possible abortion

Malignant hypertension

Lack of patient compliance

ADMINISTRATION/DOSAGE ADJUSTMENTS

Induction of hypoprothrombinemia —— A therapeutic prothrombin time is usually attained in 36–72 h. Administration of small daily doses instead of a loading dose will not delay depression of factors II, IX, and X and may reduce the possibility of an excessive increase in prothrombin time. If an elderly or debilitated patient requires a loading dose, administer 20–30 mg rather than 40–60 mg.

Monitoring of therapy —— After giving the initial dose, determine the prothrombin time daily until a therapeutic value of 1.5–2.5 times the normal prothrombin time is reached; then recheck the prothrombin time every 1–4 wk. Additional determinations should be done during the period immediately after discharge from the hospital and whenever other medications are initiated, discontinued, or taken haphazardly. The following factors may reduce the expected prothrombin-time response: edema, hyperlipidemia, hypothyroidism, hereditary resistance to warfarin, and a diet high in vitamin K (see also DRUG INTERACTIONS); other factors may enhance this response (see DRUG INTERACTIONS and "special-risk conditions" in WARNINGS/PRECAUTIONS).

COUMADIN

Concomitant use of heparin	Since the onset of action of warfarin is not immediate, it may be advisable in emergency situations to give heparin as well as warfarin; heparin and parenteral warfarin may be mixed in the same syringe. Since heparin affects prothrombin time, blood samples should be drawn just before the next heparin dose (at least 5 h after the last IV dose of heparin or 24 h after the last SC dose).
Dental or surgical procedures	To minimize the risk of hemorrhage during dental or surgical procedures, keep the operative site sufficiently limited in size so as to permit, when necessary, effective use of local hemostatic procedures, including sutures, pressure dressings, and absorbable hemostatic agents; maintain the prothrombin time at 1.5–2.5 times the normal time
Withdrawal of therapy	To terminate anticoagulant treatment, reduce the dosage of warfarin gradually over a period of 3–4 wk

WARNINGS/PRECAUTIONS

Excessive hypoprothrombinemia and bleeding	An excessive anticoagulant effect can produce bleeding or potentially fatal hemorrhage in any tissue or organ; the risk of hemorrhage is directly related to dosage and duration of treatment. Consider the possibility of hemorrhage when investigating any complaint whose cause is not obvious. If bleeding is seen in a patient with a therapeutic prothrombin time, it may be due to unmasking of a previously unsuspected lesion, such as an ulcer or tumor. During therapy, watch for early signs of excessive hypoprothrombinemia, such as microscopic hematuria, excessive menstrual bleeding, melena, petechiae, and oozing from shaving nicks; bear in mind that bleeding does not always occur when the prothrombin time is excessive. For treatment of excessive hypoprothrombinemia associated with mild or no bleeding, omit one or more doses of warfarin and, if necessary, give 2.5–10 mg of vitamin K_1 orally. If minor bleeding persists or progresses, give 5–25 mg of vitamin K_1 parenterally; consider fresh whole blood transfusions if bleeding is severe or does not respond to vitamin K_1.
Necrosis	Potentially fatal gangrene and necrosis of the skin, breast, penis, or other tissues can occur, usually within a few days after the start of treatment. Necrosis seems to be associated with local thrombosis and is more likely to occur in patients with a personal or family history of protein C deficiency; look for evidence of this deficiency in patients who have a personal or family history of recurrent thromboembolic disorders. According to reports, the risk of necrosis may be minimized if heparin is given for a period of 4–5 days immediately before the start of warfarin therapy. If necrosis occurs during therapy, it should be carefully diagnosed; if warfarin is the suspected cause, discontinue the drug and consider substituting heparin. No treatment of necrosis has been uniformly effective; severe cases have been treated by debridement or amputation of the affected area.
Special-risk conditions	Use with caution if one of the following conditions is present: severe to moderate hepatic or renal impairment, infectious disease, disturbances of intestinal flora (eg, sprue, antibiotic-induced disturbances), severe to moderate hypertension, cardiac failure, indwelling catheter, polycythemia vera, vasculitis, severe diabetes, severe allergic or anaphylactic disorders, nursing, protein C deficiency, or trauma that has produced or may result in internal bleeding or large exposed surfaces. The following factors may enhance the prothrombin-time response: carcinoma, collagen disease, cardiac failure, diarrhea, elevated temperature, infectious hepatitis, jaundice, hyperthyroidism, malnutrition, dietary deficiency, vitamin K deficiency, steatorrhea, or prolonged hot weather (see also DRUG INTERACTIONS). For patients with cardiac failure, it may be necessary to check the prothrombin time more frequently and reduce the dose.

ADVERSE REACTIONS[1]

Hematological	Bleeding, hemorrhage, necrosis, "purple toes" syndrome
Gastrointestinal	Nausea, diarrhea, abdominal cramping
Dermatological	Alopecia, urticaria, dermatitis
Other	Fever, hypersensitivity reactions

OVERDOSAGE

For signs and symptoms and treatment of overdosage, see warning, above, concerning excessive hypoprothrombinemia

DRUG INTERACTIONS

Urokinase, streptokinase	⚠ Risk of bleeding; do not use concomitantly

Allopurinol, aminosalicylic acid, amiodarone, anabolic steroids, antibiotics, bromelains, chloramphenicol, chymotrypsin, cimetidine, cinchophen, clofibrate, dextran, dextrothyroxine, diazoxide, diflunisal, disulfiram, drugs affecting blood elements, ethacrynic acid, fenoprofen, glucagon, hepatotoxic drugs, ibuprofen, indomethacin, influenza virus vaccine, inhalation anesthetics, MAO inhibitors, mefenamic acid, methyldopa, methylphenidate, metronidazole, miconazole, nalidixic acid, naproxen, narcotics (prolonged use), nortriptyline, oxolinic acid, oxyphenbutazone, pentoxifylline, phenylbutazone, phenyramidol, propylthiouracil, quinidine, quinine, salicylates, sulfinpyrazone, sulfonamides (long-acting), sulindac, thyroid drugs, triclofos sodium, trimethoprim-sulfamethoxazole	△ Prothrombin-time response	
Adrenocorticosteroids, antacids, antihistamines, barbiturates, carbamazepine, chlordiazepoxide, cholestyramine, ethchlorvynol, estrogens, glutethimide, griseofulvin, haloperidol, meprobamate, oral contraceptives, paraldehyde, primidone, rifampin, vitamin C, vitamin K	▽ Prothrombin-time response	
Alcohol, chloral hydrate, ranitidine, diuretics	△ or ▽ Prothrombin-time response	
Chlorpropamide, tolbutamide	△ Prothrombin-time response	△ Pharmacological effect of chlorpropamide and tolbutamide
Phenobarbital	▽ Prothrombin-time response	△ Pharmacological effect of phenobarbital
Phenytoin	△ Prothrombin-time response	△ Pharmacological effect of phenytoin

ALTERED LABORATORY VALUES

Blood/serum values — △ Prothrombin time

No clinically significant alterations in urinary values occur at therapeutic dosages

USE IN CHILDREN
Consult manufacturer

USE IN PREGNANT AND NURSING WOMEN
Warfarin can cause malformations and fatal hemorrhage in the fetus; do not use during pregnancy. Women who become pregnant during therapy should be apprised of the potential risks and should consider the possibility of an abortion. Hypoprothrombinemia may occur in nursing infants whose mothers are given warfarin.

[1] Priapism has been reported, but a causal relationship has not been established

ANTICOAGULANTS

EMBOLEX (heparin sodium and dihydroergotamine mesylate) Sandoz Pharmaceuticals   Rx

Ampuls: 2,500 USP units heparin sodium and 0.5 mg dihydroergotamine mesylate[1] (0.5 ml); 5,000 USP units heparin sodium and 0.5 mg dihydroergotamine mesylate[1] (0.7 ml)

INDICATIONS

Prevention of postoperative deep vein thrombosis and pulmonary embolism in patients (generally over 40 yr of age) undergoing major abdominal, thoracic, or pelvic surgery

PARENTERAL DOSAGE

Adult: 5,000 USP units of heparin and 0.5 mg of dihydroergotamine (one 0.7-ml ampul), given by deep SC (intrafat) injection 2 h before surgery and then q12h for a period of 5–7 days

EMBOLEX

CONTRAINDICATIONS

Peripheral vascular disease	Uncontrollable active bleeding	Hepatic or renal impairment
Angina or coronary artery insufficiency	Severe hypertension	Sepsis
Hypersensitivity to heparin, ergot alkaloids, or lidocaine	Oral anticoagulant therapy	Pregnancy
	Severe thrombocytopenia	

ADMINISTRATION/DOSAGE ADJUSTMENTS

Administration — Using a 25- or 26-gauge needle, inject solution into a fold in the anterior abdominal wall above the iliac crest (for abdominal procedures, an alternative site may be used); IM administration substantially increases the risk of local reactions and is not recommended

Special-risk patients — For some elderly patients, as well as for patients with compromised hepatic function, increased partial thromboplastin time, or other disorders, it may be advisable to use a heparin dose of 2,500 USP units in place of the higher amount. When selecting an appropriate dosage strength for these patients, consider such factors as age, duration of procedure, history of deep vein thrombosis or pulmonary embolism, and presence of malignancy, obesity, varicosities, cardiovascular disease, or chronic pulmonary obstructive disease.

WARNINGS/PRECAUTIONS

Bleeding — Hemorrhage is the chief risk of this preparation. Perform appropriate coagulation tests when considering use and then again just before starting surgery; values should be normal or only slightly elevated. Use with extreme caution in patients with subacute bacterial endocarditis, liver disease with impaired hemostasis, or ulcerative GI lesions necessitating continuous drainage; do not give to patients who have bleeding disorders (including certain vascular purpuras) or who are undergoing lumbar puncture, spinal anesthesia, potentially sanguineous procedures, or brain, ophthalmic, or spinal cord surgery (see also CONTRAINDICATIONS). Bear in mind that the risk of bleeding increases during and after surgery and, according to reports, with use in women over 60 yr of age. During therapy, periodically check hematocrit and test for occult blood. An especially prolonged clotting time or minor bleeding complication can usually be managed by discontinuing use of this preparation. For more serious complications, protamine sulfate may be necessary.

Thrombocytopenia — Heparin may produce mild or severe thrombocytopenia. In rare cases, the drug may induce irreversible aggregation of platelets and thereby cause a "white clot" syndrome characterized by thrombosis and thrombocytopenia; this syndrome may precipitate severe thromboembolic disorders, including skin necrosis, gangrene of the extremities, myocardial infarction, pulmonary embolism, and stroke. Check platelet count periodically. If thrombocytopenia occurs, closely monitor condition; if platelet count drops below 100,000/mm^3 or new thrombi develop, administration should be promptly discontinued.

Vasospasm — Dihydroergotamine can cause intense arterial vasoconstriction, manifested by angina, mesenteric ischemia, or signs and symptoms of peripheral vascular ischemia, such as myalgia, numbness, coldness, and pallor of the fingers and toes; persistent vasospasm can result in gangrene or death. In worldwide use, this preparation has caused vasospasm most frequently in patients with severe injuries or severe debilitating conditions (such as sepsis). If signs or symptoms of vasoconstriction are observed during therapy, administration should be immediately discontinued.

Hypertension — Dihydroergotamine can exacerbate hypertension; use with caution in patients with this disorder. Do not give this preparation to patients with severe hypertension.

Inadequate prophylactic response — Increased resistance to heparin has frequently been seen in patients who have undergone surgery or who have thrombosis, thrombophlebitis, infections with thrombosing tendencies, cancer, fever, or myocardial infarction. If evidence of thromboembolism is detected during use of this preparation, administration should be discontinued and, unless contraindicated, therapeutic doses of an anticoagulant should be given.

Hip surgery — The effectiveness of this preparation in patients undergoing hip surgery has not been established

Carcinogenicity, mutagenicity, effect on fertility — No studies have been done to determine the carcinogenic or mutagenic potential of this preparation or its effect on fertility

ADVERSE REACTIONS[2]

Hematological — Excessive postoperative bleeding, decrease in hemoglobin level, wound hematoma, microscopic hematuria

Gastrointestinal — Nausea, vomiting, abdominal discomfort, GI bleeding, mesenteric ischemia, bowel necrosis, other GI reactions

Cardiovascular — Chest pain, hypertension, myocardial infarction, shortness of breath, tachycardia, other cardiovascular reactions

Local — Irritation, mild pain, ecchymosis, hematoma

EMBOLEX ■ Heparin sodium

Other	Pyrexia, CNS reactions; rash and other dermatological reactions

OVERDOSAGE

Signs and symptoms	Epistaxis, hematuria, tarry stools, petechiae, easy bruising, hemorrhage; peripheral manifestations of ergotism
Treatment	To manage peripheral vasospasm and prevent ischemia, apply heat to affected area, take other supportive measures, and administer a vasodilator. For severe bleeding, use 1% protamine sulfate; when calculating the dose, bear in mind that the heparin component of this preparation is derived from porcine intestinal mucosa. It is not known whether dialysis is useful in the treatment of overdosage.

DRUG INTERACTIONS

Oral anticoagulants; antiplatelet agents (eg, aspirin, dextran, phenylbutazone, ibuprofen, indomethacin, hydroxychloroquine, dipyridamole)	Bleeding; heparin should not be given in combination with oral anticoagulants or antiplatelet agents
Erythromycin, troleandomycin	△ Risk of ergot toxicity
Digitalis, tetracycline, nicotine, antihistamines	▽ Anticoagulant effect of heparin

ALTERED LABORATORY VALUES

Blood/serum values	△ SGOT △ SGPT

No clinically significant alterations in urinary values occur at therapeutic dosages

USE IN CHILDREN
Safety and effectiveness for use in children have not been established

USE IN PREGNANT AND NURSING WOMEN
Pregnancy Category X: dihydroergotamine is an oxytocic drug; do not use in pregnant women. Although heparin does not appear in human milk, it is not known whether dihydroergotamine is excreted in human milk; exercise caution when using this preparation in nursing mothers.

[1] This preparation also contains 1% lidocaine hydrochloride
[2] Reactions associated with heparin or dihydroergotamine, but not commonly seen in US clinical trials with this preparation, include numbness and tingling of fingers and toes; myalgia in the extremities; weakness, cramping, or soreness in the legs; precordial distress; bradycardia; local pruritus and edema; headache; thrombocytopenia; severe thromboembolic disorders, such as skin necrosis, gangrene of the extremities, pulmonary embolism, and stroke; and hypersensitivity to heparin, characterized by chills, fever, urticaria, and, more rarely, asthma, rhinitis, lacrimation, headache, nausea, vomiting, pruritus and burning (especially on the plantar side of the feet), and anaphylactoid reactions, including shock

ANTICOAGULANTS

Heparin sodium Rx

Ampuls: 1,000 units/ml (1 ml), 5,000 units/ml (1 ml), 10,000 units/ml (1 ml) **Vials:** 2 units/ml (500, 1,000 ml), 10 units/ml (500 ml), 25 units/ml (1,000 ml), 40 units/ml (500 ml), 50 units/ml (250, 500 ml), 100 units/ml (100, 250 ml), 1,000 units/ml (1, 5, 10, 30 ml), 5,000 units/ml (1, 5, 10 ml), 10,000 units/ml (1, 4, 5, 10 ml), 20,000 units/ml (1, 2, 5, 10 ml), 40,000 units/ml (1, 5 ml) **Cartridge-needle units:** 1,000 units/ml (1 ml), 2,500 units/ml (1 ml), 5,000 units/ml (1 ml), 7,500 units/ml (1 ml), 10,000 units/ml (1 ml), 15,000 units/ml (1 ml), 20,000 units/ml (1 ml) **Plastic containers:** 2 units/ml (500, 1,000 ml), 5 units/ml (1,000 ml), 10 units/ml (500 ml), 40 units/ml (500 ml), 50 units/ml (250, 500 ml), 100 units/ml (250 ml) **Add-Vantage vials:** 2,000 units/ml (5, 10 ml), 2,500 units/ml (5, 10 ml)

INDICATIONS[1]

Venous thrombosis, pulmonary embolism, atrial fibrillation with embolization, and peripheral arterial embolism (full-dose therapy)

Prevention of **postoperative deep venous thrombosis and pulmonary embolism** in patients over 40 yr of age who are undergoing major abdominal or thoracic surgery (low-dose therapy)

PARENTERAL DOSAGE

Adult (68 kg): for *SC administration,* 10,000–20,000 units SC to start (usually preceded by an IV loading dose of 5,000 units), followed by 8,000–10,000 units SC q8h or 15,000–20,000 units SC q12h; for *intermittent IV administration,* 10,000 units IV to start, followed by 5,000–10,000 units IV q4–6h (initial and maintenance doses may be given undiluted or in 50–100 ml of 0.9% sodium chloride injection USP); for *continuous IV infusion,* 5,000 units IV to start, followed by continuous IV infusion of 20,000–40,000 units in 1 liter of 0.9% sodium chloride injection USP or other compatible diluent/24 h
Child: 50 units/kg by IV infusion to start, followed by either 100 units/kg by IV infusion q4h or 20,000 units/m²/24 h by continuous IV infusion

Adult: 5,000 units SC 2 h before surgery, followed by 5,000 units SC q8–12h for 7 days or until patient is fully ambulatory, whichever is longer

Heparin sodium

Prevention of clotting in patients undergoing total body perfusion during **open-heart surgery**	**Adult:** not less than 150 units/kg IV to start; as a rule, 300 units/kg IV may be given for procedures lasting less than 60 min and 400 units/kg for longer procedures

CONTRAINDICATIONS

Uncontrollable active bleeding, except when caused by disseminated intravascular coagulation	Inability to perform suitable coagulation tests at appropriate intervals (full-dose therapy only)	Severe thrombocytopenia

ADMINISTRATION/DOSAGE ADJUSTMENTS

Formulation	Heparin sodium products are derived from porcine intestinal mucosa or bovine lung tissue; the dosage strengths (and dosage) of these products are given in terms of USP heparin units
Administration	Heparin may be given by IV injection, IV infusion, or deep SC injection. Intramuscular administration is not recommended since it frequently results in hematoma. Inject each SC dose into the abdominal fat layer or into fat tissue above the iliac crest; minimize tissue trauma by using a 25- or 26-gauge needle. To avoid massive hematoma, use a different site for each SC injection. Containers to be used for continuous IV infusion should be inverted at least 6 times before use to ensure adequate mixing and prevent pooling of the drug.
Monitoring of full-dose therapy	To monitor therapeutic response to full doses of heparin, check activated partial thromboplastin time (APTT) or whole blood clotting time (WBCT) frequently; adjust dosage on the basis of coagulation test results. If heparin is given by intermittent IV injection, check the coagulation time before each dose during the early stages and at appropriate intervals thereafter; if the drug is given by continuous IV infusion, check every 4 h during the early stages; if the drug is given SC, check 4–6 h after each dose. Dosage is considered adequate when the APTT is 1.5–2 times the normal value or the WBCT is 2.5–3 times the control value.
Guidelines for prevention of postoperative thromboembolism	Determine coagulation values before beginning prophylactic therapy and just before surgery; these values should be normal or only slightly elevated. Monitoring of coagulation values during low-dose therapy is usually unnecessary. Do not institute prophylactic therapy if the patient has a bleeding disorder, is receiving antiplatelet drugs or oral anticoagulants, or is undergoing spinal anesthesia, potentially sanguineous procedures, or brain, ophthalmic, or spinal cord surgery. The effectiveness of prophylactic therapy for patients undergoing hip surgery has not been established. Low-dose therapy may increase the risk of bleeding during or after surgery (see warning, below, concerning hemorrhage). If thromboembolism develops during therapy, administer full therapeutic doses (unless contraindicated).
Switching to oral anticoagulants	To switch from heparin to an oral anticoagulant, first give heparin and the oral anticoagulant together; then, after the prothrombin time has remained at the therapeutic level for several days, discontinue heparin. Since heparin affects prothrombin time, blood samples should be drawn during concomitant therapy at least 5 h after the last IV dose of heparin or 24 h after the last SC dose; prothrombin time may usually be measured any time during continuous IV infusion.
Blood transfusions	To prevent clotting in blood transfusions, dilute 7,500 units of heparin in 100 ml of 0.9% sodium chloride injection USP (or 75,000 units in 1 liter) and then add 6–8 ml of this solution to each 100 ml of whole blood
Blood samples	To prevent clotting of blood samples used for laboratory tests, add 70–150 units of heparin to each 10–20 ml of whole blood. Leukocyte counts should be done within 2 h after addition of the drug. Do not use heparinized blood for isoagglutinin, complement, or erythrocyte fragility tests or for platelet counts.
Extracorporeal dialysis	For use of heparin in extracorporeal dialysis, carefully follow the operating directions of the equipment manufacturer

Heparin sodium

WARNINGS/PRECAUTIONS

Hemorrhage — The chief risk of this preparation is hemorrhage, which is dose-related and can occur at virtually any site. Overdosage may be manifested initially by petechiae, easy bruising, and prolonged coagulation test results, followed by epistaxis, hematuria, and tarry stools. Use with extreme caution during continuous tube drainage of the stomach and small intestine and during and immediately after a spinal tap, spinal anesthesia, or major surgery (especially eye, brain, or spinal cord surgery); exercise extreme caution in patients who are menstruating or have subacute bacterial endocarditis, severe hypertension, liver disease with impaired hemostasis, hemophilia, certain vascular purpuras, thrombocytopenia, or ulcerative lesions. Use with caution in women over 60 yr of age.

Periodically check hematocrit and test for occult blood in the stool; if full doses are given, perform coagulation tests frequently (see ADMINISTRATION/DOSAGE ADJUSTMENTS). If minor bleeding occurs or the clotting time or activated partial thromboplastin time is overly prolonged, discontinue treatment. The possibility of hemorrhage should be seriously considered whenever an unexplained decrease in hematocrit or blood pressure or any other unexplained effect occurs. Bear in mind that adrenal, ovarian, and retroperitoneal hemorrhage may be difficult to detect and that GI or urinary tract bleeding may be a sign of an occult lesion. For more severe bleeding or overdose, give 1% protamine sulfate IV; the dosage of protamine depends on the heparin dose, the organ source of the heparin product, and the amount of time that has elapsed since injection. If signs and symptoms of acute adrenal hemorrhage and insufficiency are seen, discontinue therapy and immediately institute corrective measures; do not wait for laboratory confirmation of the diagnosis, since any delay may be fatal.

Thrombocytopenia — Heparin may produce mild or severe thrombocytopenia in up to 30% of patients. In rare cases, the drug may induce irreversible platelet aggregation and thereby cause a "white clot" syndrome characterized by thrombosis and thrombocytopenia. This syndrome may precipitate severe thromboembolic disorders, including skin necrosis, gangrene of the extremities, myocardial infarction, pulmonary embolism, and stroke. Periodically check the platelet count during therapy. If thrombocytopenia occurs, closely monitor condition; if platelet count drops below 100,000/mm^3 or new thrombi develop, promptly discontinue administration or, when therapy must be continued, cautiously switch to a heparin product derived from a different organ source.

Resistance — Heparin is frequently less effective after surgery and in the presence of fever, thrombosis, thrombophlebitis, infections with a thrombosing tendency, myocardial infarction, and cancer

Hypersensitivity — Patients with documented hypersensitivity should be given heparin only in clearly life-threatening situations

Sensitivity to preservatives — Benzyl alcohol, which is contained in some preparations, may precipitate a potentially fatal gasping syndrome in premature infants; sodium metabisulfite, which is included in some other products, may cause urticaria, pruritus, wheezing, anaphylaxis, or other allergic-type reactions in susceptible patients, such as those with asthma or atopy

Carcinogenicity, mutagenicity, effect on fertility — No long-term studies have been done in animals to evaluate the carcinogenic or mutagenic potential of heparin or its effect on fertility

ADVERSE REACTIONS

Hematological — Bleeding, hemorrhage, thrombocytopenia; thromboembolic complications of thrombocytopenia, including skin necrosis, gangrene of the extremities, myocardial infarction, pulmonary embolism, and stroke; pain, ischemia, and cyanosis of limbs

Hypersensitivity — Chills, fever, urticaria, asthma, rhinitis, lacrimation, headache, nausea, vomiting, pruritus and burning (especially on the plantar side of the feet); anaphylactoid reactions, including shock

Local — Cutaneous necrosis (with IV or SC use); irritation, erythema, mild pain, hematoma, and ulceration (with SC injection)

Other — Suppression of aldosterone synthesis, delayed transient alopecia, priapism, osteoporosis (with long-term, high-dose therapy), rebound hyperlipidemia following discontinuation of therapy

OVERDOSAGE

For signs and symptoms and treatment of overdosage, see warning, above, concerning hemorrhage

DRUG INTERACTIONS

Aspirin, sulfinpyrazone, oral anticoagulants, thrombolytic agents, dextran, phenylbutazone, ibuprofen, indomethacin, dipyridamole, azlocillin, mezlocillin, piperacillin, ticarcillin, parenteral carbenicillin, valproic acid, divalproex, cefamandole, cefoperazone, moxalactam, plicamycin, methimazole, propylthiouracil, probenecid, hydroxychloroquine, chloroquine — △ Risk of bleeding and hemorrhage; exercise caution

Heparin sodium ■ PANWARFIN

Digitalis, tetracyclines, antihistamines, nicotine ——————— ▽ Anticoagulant effect

ALTERED LABORATORY VALUES

Blood/serum values ——————— △ SGOT △ SGPT △ Prothrombin time △ Clotting time △ APTT
▽ Triglycerides △ Free fatty acids ▽ Cholesterol (with doses of 15,000–20,000 units) △ T_4 (with competitive protein-binding tests) Interference with BSP test

No clinically significant alterations in urinary values occur at therapeutic dosages

USE IN CHILDREN

See INDICATIONS and PARENTERAL DOSAGE

USE IN PREGNANT AND NURSING WOMEN

Pregnant women: Pregnancy Category C: reproduction studies have not been done. Although heparin does not cross the placental barrier, this drug has caused stillbirths and premature births in 13–22% of pregnant patients and increased the risk of maternal hemorrhage associated with the last trimester and the postpartum period.[2] Use during pregnancy only if clearly needed; bear in mind that prolonged, high-dose therapy can cause osteoporosis. **Nursing mothers:** Heparin is not excreted in human milk; however, it has been reported that use of the drug in nursing women for 2–4 wk can, in rare cases, result in severe osteoporosis and vertebral collapse.[2]

[1] Although heparin is indicated for diagnosis and treatment of disseminated intravascular coagulation, such use is controversial; for appropriate guidelines, consult manufacturer
[2] *USP DI, Drug Information for the Health Care Provider.* Rockville, MD, The United States Pharmacopeial Convention, Inc., 1986

ANTICOAGULANTS

PANWARFIN (warfarin sodium) Abbott   Rx

Tablets: 2, 2.5, 5, 7.5, 10 mg

INDICATIONS

Venous thrombosis
Atrial fibrillation with embolism
Pulmonary embolism
Coronary occlusion (adjunctive therapy)

ORAL DOSAGE

Adult: 40–60 mg in a single dose to start, followed by 5–10 mg/day, as determined by the prothrombin-time response, for maintenance

CONTRAINDICATIONS

Bleeding	Ulcerations of GI tract	Vitamin K deficiency
Hemorrhagic tendencies	Severe hepatic or renal disease	Recent eye, brain, or spinal-cord surgery
Open wounds	Severe uncontrolled hypertension	
Visceral carcinoma	Subacute bacterial endocarditis	

ADMINISTRATION/DOSAGE ADJUSTMENTS

Elderly or debilitated patients ——————— Reduce starting dose to 20–30 mg

Monitoring of therapy ——————— Determine prothrombin time daily after initiating therapy until the results stabilize in the therapeutic range ($2^{1}/_{2}$–3 times the normal value); subsequent determinations may be made less frequently

Concomitant use of heparin ——————— Draw blood for prothrombin-time determinations just prior to next heparin dose (at least 5 h after last IV injection or 24 h after last SC injection)

Gastric irritation ——————— May be minimized by dividing the daily dose

Cessation of therapy ——————— Taper dosage gradually to avert rebound thromboembolic complications; hypercoagulability may follow rapid reversal of a prolonged prothrombin time

WARNINGS/PRECAUTIONS

Laboratory monitoring ——————— Control dosage by periodic determinations of prothrombin time or by use of other suitable coagulation tests; clotting and bleeding times are not effective measures of prothrombin activity

Patients with congestive heart failure ——— May become more sensitive to warfarin; reduce dosage, if necessary

Other special-risk patients ——————— Use with caution in patients with diverticulitis, colitis, regional and lumbar block anesthesia, mild or moderate uncontrolled hypertension, mild or moderate renal or hepatic disease, drainage tubes in any orifice, active tuberculosis, severe diabetes, a history of ulcerative disease of the GI tract, and during menstruation and the post-partum period

PANWARFIN

Factors that alter anticoagulant activity	An alteration in prothrombin time may result from such factors as a change in the intake of vitamin K, fat, or leafy green vegetables, vitamin K deficiency in the newborn, x-ray therapy, alcoholism, vitamin C deficiency, fever, or diarrhea. Furthermore, an increase or decrease in anticoagulant effect may result from interaction with many drugs (see DRUG INTERACTIONS); carefully monitor prothrombin time whenever adding or withdrawing a drug from the therapeutic regimen.
Careful patient selection	Is desirable to ensure cooperation, particularly from alcoholic, emotionally unstable, psychotic, or senile patients
Bleeding	Does not always correlate with prothrombin time during anticoagulant therapy; significant GI- or urinary-tract bleeding may indicate the presence of an underlying occult lesion
Acute adrenal hemorrhage or insufficiency	Discontinue anticoagulant therapy; measure plasma cortisol levels immediately and promptly institute vigorous IV corticosteroid therapy. Do not delay treatment for laboratory confirmation of diagnosis, as death may intervene.

ADVERSE REACTIONS

Hematological	Bleeding, hemorrhage, leukopenia
Gastrointestinal	Nausea, vomiting, cramps, diarrhea, paralytic ileus and intestinal obstruction (resulting from submucosal or intramural hemorrhage)
Genitourinary	Excessive uterine bleeding, ovarian hemorrhage on ovulation
Dermatological	Dermatitis, urticaria, alopecia, hemorrhagic necrosis (bleeding into the skin and subcutaneous tissue, with necrosis, vasculitis, and thrombosis) of the female breast and other areas
Other	Fever, adrenal hemorrhage (resulting in adrenal insufficiency), priapism

OVERDOSAGE

Signs and symptoms	Excessive prothrombinopenia, with or without bleeding, as manifested by microscopic hematuria, excessive menstrual bleeding, melena, petechiae, and/or oozing from shaving nicks
Treatment	Discontinue anticoagulant therapy temporarily if prothrombin activity falls below 15% of normal or hemorrhage occurs. If the clinical situation warrants, give 1–5 mg vitamin K_1 IV in cases of mild overdosage and 20–40 mg in severe cases. Whole-blood transfusion may be necessary in some situations.

DRUG INTERACTIONS

Allopurinol, aminosalicylic acid, anabolic steroids, antibiotics, bromelains, chloramphenicol, chymotrypsin, cimetidine, cinchophen, clofibrate, dextran, dextrothyroxine, diazoxide, disulfiram, drugs affecting blood elements, ethacrynic acid, glucagon, hepatotoxic drugs, indomethacin, inhalation anesthetics, MAO inhibitors, mefenamic acid, methyldopa, methylphenidate, methylthiouracil, metronidazole, nalidixic acid, narcotics (with prolonged use), nortriptyline, oxolinic acid, oxyphenbutazone, phenylbutazone, phenyramidol, phenytoin, propylthiouracil, quinidine, quinine, salicylates, sulfinpyrazone, sulfonamides (long-acting), sulindac, thyroid drugs, tolbutamide, triclofos sodium, trimethoprim-sulfamethoxazole	△ Prothrombin-time response
Adrenocorticosteroids, antacids, antihistamines, barbiturates, carbamazepine, chlordiazepoxide, cholestyramine, ethchlorvynol, estrogens, glutethimide, griseofulvin, haloperidol, meprobamate, oral contraceptives, paraldehyde, phenytoin, primidone, rifampin, vitamin C, vitamin K	▽ Prothrombin-time response
Alcohol, chloral hydrate, diuretics	△ or ▽ Prothrombin-time response
Alkylating agents, antimetabolites, corticosteroids, dipyridamole, indomethacin, oxyphenbutazone, phenylbutazone, quinidine, salicylates, streptokinase, sulfinpyrazone, urokinase	△ Risk of bleeding
Chlorpropamide, tolbutamide	△ Hypoglycemic effect

PANWARFIN ■ ABBOKINASE

Phenobarbital, phenytoin —————————— ⬆ Anticonvulsant blood level and/or toxicity

ALTERED LABORATORY VALUES

Blood/serum values —————————— ⬆ Prothrombin time

No clinically significant alterations in urinary values occur at therapeutic dosages

---

USE IN CHILDREN

Use of this drug in children has not been studied by the manufacturer, and specific dosage recommendations cannot be made. However, the drug has been used successfully to prevent thromboembolism in 19 children with idiopathic nonobstructive cardiomyopathies or following prosthetic valve insertions; therapeutic prothrombin times of 1½–2½ times the control value were achieved within 36–48 h with a loading dose of 0.5–0.7 mg/kg and maintained with doses ranging from 15% to 25% of the loading dose used.[1]

[1]Carpentieri U et al: *Arch Dis Child* 51:445–448, 1976

USE IN PREGNANT AND NURSING WOMEN

Use during pregnancy may cause congenital malformations or fatal fetal hemorrhage. Warfarin should be used during pregnancy only when the potential benefits outweigh the possible risks. If the drug must be used during pregnancy or if the patient becomes pregnant while taking warfarin, she should be apprised of the potential risks to the fetus. Since warfarin appears in breast milk, the nursing infant should be observed for evidence of unexpected bleeding.

THROMBOLYTIC AGENTS

ABBOKINASE (urokinase) Abbott   Rx
Vials: 250,000 IU

ABBOKINASE OPEN-CATH (urokinase) Abbott   Rx
Vials: 5,000 IU (1 ml) for catheter clearance only

INDICATIONS

Acute **pulmonary embolism,** when it is associated with shock or characterized by obstruction of blood flow to a lobe or multiple segments

Acute **coronary artery thrombosis** associated with evolving transmural myocardial infarction[1]

Clearance of IV catheters, including central venous catheters, obstructed by clotted blood or fibrin

PARENTERAL DOSAGE

Adult: 4,400 IU/kg (15 ml), given by IV infusion over a period of 10 min, followed by 4,400 IU/kg/h (15 ml/h), given by continuous IV infusion for 12 h; total dose: 57,200 IU/kg (195 ml). At the end of the infusion, flush the entire length of the infusion set with 0.9% sodium chloride injection or 5% dextrose injection, using a volume approximating that of the tubing and an infusion rate of 15 ml/h.

Adult: 6,000 IU (4 ml)/min, given by infusion into the occluded artery for up to 2 h; the infusion should be maintained until the artery reaches maximal patency (usually 15–30 min after initial recanalization). Start treatment within 6 h after the onset of infarction symptoms. Before beginning infusion, give 2,500–10,000 units of heparin in a single IV dose (when calculating this dose, consider prior heparin use).

Adult: for each procedure, up to 5,000 IU (1 ml) or, in resistant cases, up to 10,000 IU (2 ml)

CONTRAINDICATIONS[2]

Recent (within past 2 mo) cerebrovascular accident or intracranial or intraspinal surgery

Active internal bleeding

Intracranial neoplasm

ADMINISTRATION/DOSAGE ADJUSTMENTS

Preparation of solution —————————— Immediately before administration, add 5.2 ml of sterile water for injection USP to each 250,000-IU vial, or transfer the diluent in the upper chamber of the 5,000-IU vial to the lower compartment. To minimize the formation of filaments, roll and tilt the vial instead of shaking it. The solution in the 250,000-IU vial may be filtered (a cellulose membrane filter with a pore size of 0.45 μ or less can be used). Do not add any other medication to a vial; discard any solution that is highly colored. Use a solution that has been reconstituted in 250,000-IU vials if IV or intracoronary administration is anticipated. For IV use, dilute the reconstituted solution with 0.9% sodium chloride injection USP or 5% dextrose injection USP to a final volume of 195 ml. For intracoronary use, dilute a 750,000-IU solution with 500 ml of 5% dextrose injection USP. For catheter clearance, combine 9 ml of sterile water for injection USP with 1 ml of a solution that has been reconstituted in a 250,000-IU vial; reconstituted solutions supplied in 5,000-IU vials may be used without further dilution.

COMPENDIUM OF DRUG THERAPY

ABBOKINASE

Monitoring of therapy	Before beginning therapy, determine the hematocrit, platelet count, and either the thrombin time (TT), activated partial thromboplastin time (APTT), or prothrombin time; the TT or APTT should be less than twice the normal control value. During infusion, observe the clinical response frequently, and check vital signs (pulse, temperature, respiratory rate, and blood pressure) at least every 4 h; to avoid dislodgement of possible deep vein thrombi, do not use a lower extremity to determine blood pressure. Tests for coagulation and fibrinolytic activity may be done during therapy, but they will not provide reliable indications of efficacy or risk of bleeding. To monitor thrombolytic response during intracoronary administration, perform angiography every 15 min. Following intracoronary infusion, determine hemostatic parameters.
Use of anticoagulants	Give heparin before intracoronary infusion (see PARENTERAL DOSAGE). Heparin may also be given, if necessary, during intracoronary administration; however, carefully watch for signs of excessive bleeding, even though a clinical study has shown that heparin does not increase the risk of bleeding associated with this particular procedure. Discontinue administration of heparin before beginning IV infusion of urokinase. After intracoronary use, institute or continue heparin therapy; following IV infusion, wait until the thrombin or activated partial thromboplastin time has decreased to less than twice the normal control value, and then give heparin (without a loading dose) by continuous IV infusion. Oral anticoagulants should eventually be given in place of heparin.
Clearance of IV catheters	Disconnect the IV tubing connection at the catheter hub and attach an empty 10-ml syringe to the catheter. (To prevent air from entering a central venous catheter, instruct patient to exhale and hold his or her breath whenever the catheter is not connected to IV tubing or a syringe.) Gently attempt to aspirate blood from the catheter with the 10-ml syringe; avoid vigorous suction, which may cause damage to the vascular wall or collapse of a soft-wall catheter. If aspiration is not possible, remove the 10-ml syringe and attach a 1-ml tuberculin syringe filled with 5,000 IU of urokinase. Slowly and gently inject an amount of urokinase equal to the volume of the catheter; avoid excessive pressure, as such force may rupture the catheter or expel the clot into the circulation. Remove the tuberculin syringe and connect an empty 5-ml syringe to the catheter. After waiting at least 5 min, try to aspirate the drug and residual clot; repeat attempt every 5 min, as needed, until patency is restored. However, if the catheter does not open within 30 min, cap it and wait 30–60 min before trying again. In resistant cases, a second injection of urokinase may be necessary. (Remember that catheters may be occluded by substances other than blood products, such as a drug precipitate; urokinase is not effective in such cases, and its use might force the precipitate into the circulation.) Once patency is restored, aspirate 4–5 ml of blood to assure removal of all drug material and clot residue. Remove the blood-filled syringe and attach a 10-ml syringe filled with 0.9% sodium chloride injection USP. Gently irrigate the catheter, remove the syringe, and reconnect the IV tubing to the catheter hub.

WARNINGS/PRECAUTIONS

Bleeding	To prevent bleeding during therapy, avoid IM injections and unnecessary handling of the patient. Perform venipunctures carefully and as infrequently as possible. If intraarterial puncture (except for intracoronary injection) is necessary, use an upper extremity vessel; following puncture, apply pressure for at least 30 min, put on a pressure dressing, and check the site frequently. If bleeding occurs during therapy and cannot be controlled by application of local pressure, discontinue urokinase immediately, and, if necessary, administer whole blood (preferably fresh), packed red blood cells, and cryoprecipitate or fresh frozen plasma; do not use dextran. For emergency situations, consider using aminocaproic acid.
	Use with particular caution in the presence of (1) recent (within past 10 days) major surgery, obstetrical delivery, organ biopsy, needle puncture of a noncompressable vessel, or serious GI bleeding; (2) recent trauma, including cardiopulmonary resuscitation; (3) severe, uncontrolled hypertension; (4) suspected left heart thrombus (eg, mitral stenosis with atrial fibrillation); (5) subacute bacterial endocarditis; (6) hemostatic defects, including defects due to severe hepatic or renal disease; (7) pregnancy; (8) cerebrovascular disease; (9) diabetic hemorrhagic retinopathy; or (10) any other condition in which bleeding constitutes a significant hazard or would be particularly difficult to control because of its location.
Arrhythmias	Rapid lysis of coronary thrombi has occasionally caused reperfusion atrial or ventricular dysrhythmias requiring immediate treatment; monitor patient carefully for arrhythmias both during and immediately after intracoronary infusion of urokinase
Fever	Approximately 2–3% of patients may experience fever; for symptomatic treatment, use acetaminophen rather than aspirin
Carcinogenicity	Available data do not permit adequate evaluation of this drug's carcinogenic potential

ADVERSE REACTIONS[3]

Hematological	Superficial or surface bleeding (mainly at sites of invasive procedures); GI, genitourinary, IM, retroperitoneal, and cerebral bleeding; cerebral and retroperitoneal hemorrhage (occasionally fatal)
Allergic	Bronchospasm and skin rash (rare)

OVERDOSAGE

Signs and symptoms	Severe bleeding

ABBOKINASE ■ KABIKINASE

Treatment — See WARNINGS/PRECAUTIONS

DRUG INTERACTIONS

Antiplatelet agents (eg, aspirin, indomethacin, phenylbutazone)	⇧ Risk of bleeding; do not use concomitantly
Anticoagulants	⇧ Risk of bleeding (see ADMINISTRATION/DOSAGE ADJUSTMENTS)

ALTERED LABORATORY VALUES

Blood/serum values — ⇧ Thrombin time   ⇧ Activated partial thromboplastin time   ⇧ Prothrombin time

No clinically significant alterations in urinary values occur at therapeutic dosages

USE IN CHILDREN

Safety and effectiveness for use in children have not been established

USE IN PREGNANT AND NURSING WOMEN

Pregnancy Category B: reproduction studies in mice and rats given up to 1,000 times the human dose have shown no evidence of impaired fertility or harm to the fetus; however, no adequate, well-controlled studies have been done in pregnant women. Use during pregnancy only if clearly needed. It is not known whether urokinase is excreted in human milk; use with caution in nursing mothers.

---

[1] It is not known whether the use of urokinase results in reduced damage to myocardial tissue or decreased mortality
[2] No reports suggest that these contraindications should apply to use of urokinase for catheter clearance
[3] Although these reactions have been associated with IV therapy, they may also occur with intracoronary administration and should be considered a possible risk of catheter clearance. Fever has occurred during IV use, but a causal relationship has not been established.

THROMBOLYTIC AGENTS

KABIKINASE (streptokinase) KabiVitrum   Rx

Vials: 250,000, 600,000, 750,000 IU (5 ml)

INDICATIONS

Acute **pulmonary embolism,** when it is associated with shock or characterized by obstruction of blood vessels to a lobe or multiple segments

Acute extensive **deep vein thrombosis**
Acute **arterial thrombosis or embolism**[1]

Acute **coronary artery thrombosis** associated with evolving transmural myocardial infarction[2]

PARENTERAL DOSAGE

Adult: 250,000 IU, given by IV infusion over a period of 30 min to start, followed by 100,000 IU/h, given by continuous IV infusion for 24 h (or up to 72 h if concurrent deep vein thrombosis is suspected)

Adult: 250,000 IU, given by IV infusion over a period of 30 min to start, followed by 100,000 IU/h, given by continuous IV infusion for 72 h

Adult: 20,000 IU, given as a bolus directly into the thrombosed coronary artery, followed by 2,000 IU/min, given by intracoronary infusion. Use the Judkins or Sones technique to insert the catheter; administer the solution within 6 h after the onset of infarction symptoms. To ensure complete thrombolysis, continue the infusion after recanalization has been achieved.

CONTRAINDICATIONS

Recent (within past 2 mo) cerebrovascular accident or intracranial or intraspinal surgery

Active internal bleeding

Intracranial neoplasm

ADMINISTRATION/DOSAGE ADJUSTMENTS

Preparation of solution	To reconstitute the solution, add 5 ml of 0.9% sodium chloride injection USP (the preferred diluent) or 5 ml of 5% dextrose injection USP to the vial. For the IV loading dose, dilute the solution to a total volume of 50–250 ml; for the subsequent IV infusion, dilute to a total volume of 50–500 ml.
Timing of administration	Begin IV therapy as soon as possible after onset of thrombosis, preferably within 7 days. When started within 6 h after onset of symptoms, intracoronary administration has produced recanalization within 1 h in 75% of cases.
Monitoring of therapy	Before beginning therapy, determine the thrombin time (TT), activated partial thromboplastin time (APTT), prothrombin time (PT), hematocrit, and platelet count; the TT or APTT should be less than twice the normal control value. Obtain a second determination of the TT or PT approximately 4 h after starting the IV infusion; if this determination shows no prolongation, discontinue streptokinase. Monitor hemostatic parameters during intracoronary administration since treatment causes certain changes in these parameters, including a marked decrease in the serum fibrinogen level.

KABIKINASE

Use of anticoagulants — Heparin may be given, if necessary, immediately before or after intracoronary administration (or at both times); carefully watch for signs of excessive bleeding, especially at the catheterization site, since both heparin and streptokinase can cause bleeding and, at the dose usually given for angiography, heparin can produce major hematomas at the catheterization site. Discontinue administration of heparin before beginning IV infusion of streptokinase. After intracoronary use, institute or continue heparin therapy. Following IV infusion, wait until the thrombin time (TT) has decreased to less than twice the normal control value (check TT within 3–4 h after infusion); then give heparin (without a loading dose) by continuous IV infusion. Oral anticoagulants should eventually be given in place of heparin.

WARNINGS/PRECAUTIONS

Bleeding — Minor bleeding has often been detected, especially at puncture sites; more severe bleeding, including potentially fatal internal hemorrhaging, has also occurred. To prevent bleeding during therapy, avoid IM injections and unnecessary handling of the patient. Perform venipunctures carefully and as infrequently as possible. If intraarterial puncture is necessary, use an upper extremity vessel; following puncture, apply pressure for at least 30 min, put on a pressure dressing, and check the site frequently. Control minor bleeding with local measures; if treatment is continued, do not reduce the dose. (By increasing the fraction of plasminogen available for conversion to plasmin, a reduction in dose may enhance the risk of more serious bleeding.) If bleeding occurs during therapy and cannot be controlled by application of local pressure, discontinue streptokinase immediately, administer whole blood (preferably fresh), packed red blood cells, and cryoprecipitate or fresh frozen plasma; for emergency situations, consider using aminocaproic acid.

Fever — Approximately one third of patients experience fever; treat symptomatically, and use acetaminophen rather than aspirin

Allergic reactions — For mild or moderate reactions, continue streptokinase therapy and administer corticosteroids and/or antihistamines concomitantly; for severe reactions, discontinue streptokinase immediately and give IV sympathomimetics, antihistamines, or corticosteroids, as needed

Arrhythmias — Rapid lysis of coronary thrombi has occasionally caused reperfusion atrial or ventricular dysrhythmias requiring immediate treatment; monitor patient carefully for arrhythmias both during and immediately after intracoronary infusion of streptokinase

Pulmonary reactions — Noncardiogenic pulmonary edema, a rare reaction, is most likely to occur when patients with large myocardial infarcts undergo intracoronary therapy. Pulmonary emboli occasionally develop or recur during use of streptokinase; if pulmonary emboli are detected during treatment, continue administration in an attempt to lyse both the newly formed emboli and those present before therapy.

Polyneuropathy — In rare cases, polyneuropathy has been temporally related to use of streptokinase

Special-risk patients — Use with particular caution in the following conditions: (1) recent (within past 10 days) major surgery, obstetrical delivery, organ biopsy, needle puncture of a noncompressible vessel, or serious GI bleeding; (2) recent trauma, including cardiopulmonary resuscitation; (3) severe, uncontrolled hypertension or chronic, controlled hypertension; (4) suspected left heart thrombus (eg, mitral stenosis with atrial fibrillation); (5) subacute bacterial endocarditis; (6) hemostatic defects, including defects due to severe hepatic or renal disease; (7) pregnancy; (8) cerebrovascular disease; (9) diabetic hemorrhagic retinopathy; (10) any condition in which bleeding constitutes a significant hazard or would be particularly difficult to control because of its location; (11) prior severe allergic reaction to streptokinase; or (12) septic thrombophlebitis or serious infection at the site of an occluded AV cannula

ADVERSE REACTIONS

The most frequent reactions, regardless of incidence, are printed in *italics*

Hematological — *Minor bleeding (mainly at sites of invasive procedures);* severe gastrointestinal, genitourinary, retroperitoneal, or intracerebral bleeding and hemorrhage (occasionally fatal); pulmonary emboli

Allergic — Minor breathing difficulty, bronchospasm, periorbital swelling, angioneurotic edema, urticaria, itching, flushing, nausea, headache, musculoskeletal pain

Other — *Fever ($\geq 1.5°$ F);* noncardiogenic pulmonary edema and polyneuropathy (rare)

OVERDOSAGE

Signs and symptoms — Severe bleeding

Treatment — See WARNINGS/PRECAUTIONS

DRUG INTERACTIONS

Antiplatelet agents (eg, aspirin, phenylbutazone, dipyridamole) — ⚠ Risk of bleeding; do not use concomitantly

Anticoagulants — ⚠ Risk of bleeding (see ADMINISTRATION/DOSAGE ADJUSTMENTS)

KABIKINASE ■ STREPTASE

ALTERED LABORATORY VALUES

Blood/serum values —————————— ◇ Thrombin time ◇ Activated partial thromboplastin time ◇ Prothrombin time

No clinically significant alterations in urinary values occur at therapeutic dosages

---

USE IN CHILDREN

Safety and effectiveness for use in children have not been established

USE IN PREGNANT AND NURSING WOMEN

Pregnancy Category A: clinical studies have shown that streptokinase does not increase the risk of fetal abnormalities; nevertheless, use during pregnancy only if clearly needed because such studies cannot rule out the possibility of harm. Consult manufacturer for use in nursing mothers.

---

[1] Do not use streptokinase for arterial emboli emanating from the left side of the heart (eg, in mitral stenosis associated with atrial fibrillation) due to the danger of new embolic phenomena

[2] Increasing, though not unequivocal, evidence indicates that if streptokinase produces reperfusion within 6 h after the onset of symptoms, infarct size may be limited, cardiac function improved, and cardiac mortality reduced; in high-risk patients with anterior myocardial infarction, mortality after 1 yr is reduced when reperfusion is complete, but not when it is partial

---

THROMBOLYTIC AGENTS

STREPTASE (streptokinase) Hoechst-Roussel   Rx

Vials: 250,000, 750,000 IU (6.5 ml)

INDICATIONS

Acute **pulmonary embolism,** when it is associated with shock or characterized by obstruction of blood vessels to a lobe or multiple segments

Acute extensive **deep vein thrombosis**
Acute **arterial thrombosis or embolism**[1]

Acute **coronary artery thrombosis** associated with evolving transmural myocardial infarction[2]

PARENTERAL DOSAGE

Adult: 250,000 IU, given by IV infusion over a period of 30 min to start, followed by 100,000 IU/h, given by continuous IV infusion for 24 h (or for up to 72 h if concurrent deep vein thrombosis is suspected)

Adult: 250,000 IU, given by IV infusion over a period of 30 min to start, followed by 100,000 IU/h, given by continuous IV infusion for 72 h (deep vein thrombosis) or 24–72 h (arterial thrombosis or embolism)

Adult: 20,000 IU (10 ml), given as a bolus directly into the thrombosed coronary artery, followed by intracoronary infusion of 2,000 IU (1 ml)/min; use Judkins or Sones technique to insert coronary catheter

---

CONTRAINDICATIONS

Recent (within past 2 mo) cerebrovascular accident or intracranial or intraspinal surgery

Active internal bleeding

Intracranial neoplasm

ADMINISTRATION/DOSAGE ADJUSTMENTS

Reconstitution and dilution for parenteral administration

To minimize flocculation, *slowly* add 5 ml of Sodium Chloride Injection USP or 5% Dextrose Injection USP, directing the stream toward the side of the vial rather than into the powder. Gently roll and tilt the vial to reconstitute; *do not shake.* For intracoronary use, dilute the contents of a 250,000-IU vial to a total volume of 125 ml. For the IV loading dose, use a 250,000-IU or 750,000-IU vial, and prepare a solution with a total volume of 45 ml; for the subsequent IV infusion, use a 750,000-IU vial and prepare a solution with a total volume of 45 ml (or, if necessary, up to 500 ml, in 45-ml increments). Solution may be filtered; solutions containing *large* amounts of flocculation should be discarded. Do not add any other drug to the container. To administer the solution, use a volumetric or syringe infusion pump, rather than a drop-counting infusion device, because streptokinase may change the size of the drop.

Timing of administration

In treating deep vein thrombosis, pulmonary or arterial embolism, or arterial thrombosis, streptokinase therapy should be started as soon as possible after the thrombotic event, preferably within 7 days. In clinical studies where streptokinase was given within 6 h of the onset of symptoms of acute transmural myocardial infarction, 75% of occlusions opened within 1 h of the infusion

Monitoring of therapy

Before beginning therapy, determine the thrombin time (TT), activated partial thromboplastin time (APTT), prothrombin time (PT), hematocrit, and platelet count; the TT or APTT should be less than twice the normal control value. Obtain a second determination of the TT or PT approximately 4 h after starting the IV infusion; if the TT or PT shows no prolongation, discontinue streptokinase. During intracoronary infusion, there is generally little, if any, change in hemostatic parameters, although in some patients a marked decrease in fibrinogen may occur.

STREPTASE

Use of anticoagulants	Heparin may be given, if necessary, during intracoronary administration; however, carefully watch for signs of excessive bleeding, even though clinical studies have shown that heparin does not increase the risk of bleeding associated with this particular procedure. Discontinue administration of heparin before beginning IV infusion of streptokinase. After intracoronary use, institute or continue heparin therapy; following IV infusion, wait until the thrombin time has decreased to less than twice the normal control value, and then give heparin (without a loading dose) by continuous IV infusion. Oral anticoagulants should eventually be given in place of heparin.
Treatment of arteriovenous cannula occlusion	Before using streptokinase, attempt to clear the cannula by careful syringe technique, using heparinized saline solution; if adequate flow is not re-established, streptokinase may be employed: Allow the effect of pretreatment anticoagulants to diminish. Slowly reconstitute 250,000 IU streptokinase with 2 ml Sodium Chloride Injection USP or 5% Dextrose Injection USP and slowly instill solution into each occluded limb of the cannula. After clamping off cannula limb(s) for 2 h, aspirate contents, flush with saline, and reconnect cannula.

WARNINGS/PRECAUTIONS

Minor bleeding	May occur, mainly at invaded or disturbed sites; during therapy, avoid IM injections and unnecessary handling of patient. Perform venipunctures carefully and as infrequently as possible. Control minor bleeding by applying local pressure; if streptokinase therapy is continued, *do not reduce the dose,* as this may increase fibrinolytic activity. If arterial puncture is necessary, upper extremity vessels are preferable; apply pressure for at least 30 min after puncture, then a pressure dressing. Frequently check puncture site for signs of bleeding.
Special-risk patients	Use with particular caution in the presence of (1) recent (within past 10 days) major surgery, obstetrical delivery, organ biopsy, needle puncture of a noncompressible vessel, or serious GI bleeding; (2) recent trauma, including cardiopulmonary resuscitation; (3) severe, uncontrolled hypertension; (4) suspected left heart thrombus (eg, mitral stenosis with atrial fibrillation); (5) subacute bacterial endocarditis; (6) hemostatic defects, including defects due to severe hepatic or renal disease; (7) pregnancy; (8) cerebrovascular disease; (9) diabetic hemorrhagic retinopathy; (10) any condition in which bleeding constitutes a significant hazard or would be particularly difficult to control because of its location; (11) prior severe allergic reaction to streptokinase; or (12) septic thrombophlebitis or serious infection at the site of an occluded AV cannula. If serious bleeding, uncontrollable by local measures, occurs, discontinue infusion of streptokinase immediately and treat as described under OVERDOSAGE.
Allergic reactions	May occur (see ADVERSE REACTIONS); if reaction is mild or moderate, continue streptokinase therapy and treat concomitantly with antihistamines or corticosteroids; if reaction is severe, discontinue infusion and administer sympathomimetics, antihistamines, or corticosteroids IV, as needed
Fever	May occur in about one third of patients; treat symptomatically, preferably with acetaminophen (see DRUG INTERACTIONS)
Atrial or ventricular arrhythmias	Rapid lysis of coronary thrombi has occasionally caused reperfusion atrial or ventricular dysrhythmias requiring immediate treatment; monitor patient carefully for arrhythmias both during and after intracoronary infusion of streptokinase
Pulmonary reactions	Noncardiogenic pulmonary edema, a rare reaction, is most likely to occur when patients with large myocardial infarcts undergo intracoronary therapy. Pulmonary emboli occasionally develop during treatment of deep-vein thrombosis; if the emboli occur during therapy, administration should be continued in an attempt to lyse them as well as the deep-vein thrombi.

ADVERSE REACTIONS

Frequent reactions (incidence $\geq$ 1%) are printed in *italics*

Hematological	*Minor bleeding* (mainly at invaded or disturbed sites); severe gastrointestinal, genitourinary, retroperitoneal, or intracerebral bleeding and hemorrhage (occasionally fatal)
Allergic	Minor breathing difficulty, bronchospasm, periorbital swelling, angioneurotic edema, urticaria, itching, flushing, nausea, headache, musculoskeletal pain
Other	*Fever ($\geq$ 1.5° F);* noncardiogenic pulmonary edema (rare)

OVERDOSAGE

Signs and symptoms	See ADVERSE REACTIONS
Treatment	For uncontrollable bleeding, discontinue streptokinase and administer whole blood (preferably fresh), packed red blood cells, and cryoprecipitate or fresh frozen plasma; consider use of aminocaproic acid in emergency situations

DRUG INTERACTIONS

Antiplatelet agents (eg, aspirin, indomethacin, phenylbutazone)	⚠ Risk of bleeding; do not use concomitantly
Anticoagulants	⚠ Risk of bleeding; concomitant use is not recommended

ALTERED LABORATORY VALUES

Blood/serum values —————————————— ⇧ Thrombin time ⇧ Activated partial thromboplastin time ⇧ Prothrombin time

No clinically significant alterations in urinary values occur at therapeutic dosages

USE IN CHILDREN

Not recommended for use in children, since safety and effectiveness have not been established in pediatric populations

USE IN PREGNANT AND NURSING WOMEN

Not recommended for use during pregnancy, as safety and effectiveness have not been established.

[1] Do not use streptokinase for arterial emboli emanating from left side of heart (eg, in mitral stenosis with atrial fibrillation) due to danger of new embolic phenomena
[2] It is not known whether the use of streptokinase results in reduced damage to myocardial tissue or decreased mortality

---

ANTIFIBRINOLYTIC AGENTS

AMICAR (aminocaproic acid) Lederle   Rx

Tablets: 500 mg   **Syrup:** 250 mg/ml (16 fl oz) *raspberry flavored*   **Vials:** 250 mg/ml (20, 96 ml)

INDICATIONS

Excessive bleeding resulting from elevated fibrinolytic activity or urinary fibrinolysis[1]

ORAL DOSAGE

Adult: 5 g to start, followed in 1 h by 1–1.25 g/h over a period of 8 h or until bleeding is controlled, up to 30 g/24 h

PARENTERAL DOSAGE

Adult: 4–5 g, given by slow IV infusion over a period of 1 h to start, followed by 1 g/h over a period of 8 h or until bleeding is controlled, up to 30 g/24 h

CONTRAINDICATIONS

Presence of an active intravascular clotting process

ADMINISTRATION/DOSAGE ADJUSTMENTS

Intravenous administration —— Give the initial dose (4–5 g) in 250 ml of a compatible diluent (eg, sterile water for injection, isotonic saline, 5% dextrose, or Ringer's solution); administer each subsequent hourly dose (1 g) in 50 ml of diluent. Rapid administration may induce hypotension, bradycardia, and/or arrhythmia; infuse *slowly*. To minimize the possibility of thrombophlebitis, pay strict attention to proper insertion of needle and fixing of its position.

WARNINGS/PRECAUTIONS

Pretreatment evaluation —— Hyperfibrinolysis must be definitely diagnosed or indicated by laboratory findings and differentiated from disseminated intravascular coagulation (DIC); in primary hyperfibrinolysis, the platelet count is normal, precipitation does not occur when protamine is added to citrated blood, and the time required for lysis of a euglobulin clot is less than normal, whereas in DIC, the platelet count is usually decreased, precipitation occurs in the protamine test, and the results of the euglobulin test are normal. Aminocaproic acid may be given to patients with DIC only if heparin is administered concomitantly.

Myopathy —— Skeletal myopathy, including, on rare occasions, rhabdomyolysis with myoglobinuria and renal failure, may occur and may be accompanied by general weakness, fatigue, elevated serum enzymes, and necrosis of muscle fibers. Cardiac (and hepatic) lesions have been reported in one patient; endocardial hemorrhages and myocardial fat degeneration have been seen in animals. If skeletal myopathy is evident, consider the possibility that myocardial damage may have also occurred; use with caution in patients with cardiac disease. Monitor serum CPK level during long-term therapy; if an increase is seen, discontinue administration.

Patients with upper urinary tract bleeding —— Aminocaproic acid has caused clots in the renal pelvis and ureters and glomerular capillary thrombosis in patients with upper urinary tract bleeding; this drug should not be used in the management of hematuria originating in the upper urinary tract unless the possible benefits outweigh the risks

Patients with renal or hepatic diseases —— Use with caution in patients with renal or hepatic diseases; kidney concretions have been detected in animals, and hepatic (and cardiac) lesions have been reported in one patient

Clotting or thrombosis —— May occur (no definite evidence); the few reported cases of intravascular clotting probably resulted from a preexisting condition (eg, disseminated intravascular coagulation). It has been postulated that extravascular clots, unlike normal clots, may not undergo spontaneous lysis.

AMICAR ■ TRENTAL

Neurological reactions	Use of antifibrinolytic agents in the treatment of subarachnoid hemorrhage has been associated with an increased incidence of certain neurological reactions, including hydrocephalus, cerebral vasospasm, and cerebral ischemia; a causal relationship has not been established
Effect on fertility	Some studies in rodents have suggested that aminocaproic acid can adversely affect fertility

ADVERSE REACTIONS

Gastrointestinal	Nausea, cramps, diarrhea
Central nervous system	Dizziness, tinnitus, malaise, headache[2]
Musculoskeletal	Myopathy, general weakness, fatigue; rhabdomyolysis (rare)
Cardiovascular	Hypotension; thrombophlebitis (with IV use)
Genitourinary	Reversible dry ejaculation (observed in hemophiliacs who received this drug after dental surgery)
Dermatological	Rash
Other	Conjunctival suffusion, nasal stuffiness, elevated serum muscle enzymes, myoglobinuria, renal failure

OVERDOSAGE

Signs and symptoms	See ADVERSE REACTIONS
Treatment	Discontinue medication; treat symptomatically and institute supportive measures, as required

DRUG INTERACTIONS

Oral contraceptives, estrogens	△ Potential for blood clotting

ALTERED LABORATORY VALUES

No clinically significant alterations in blood/serum or urinary values occur at therapeutic dosages

---

USE IN CHILDREN
No studies have been done regarding the use of this drug in children

USE IN PREGNANT AND NURSING WOMEN
Safety for use during pregnancy has not been established with regard to fetal development; studies in rats have shown evidence of teratogenicity. Do not use in pregnant women (particularly during early pregnancy) or in women of childbearing age unless the expected therapeutic benefits outweigh the possible hazards. No studies have been done with this drug in nursing mothers.

---

[1] In life-threatening situations, transfusions of fresh whole blood, infusion of fibrinogen, and other emergency measures may be required
[2] Convulsions have occurred in two patients after IV administration; however, a causal relationship has not been established

---

HEMORHEOLOGIC AGENTS

TRENTAL (pentoxifylline) Hoechst-Roussel Rx

Tablets (controlled release): 400 mg

INDICATIONS
Intermittent claudication owing to chronic occlusive arterial disease of the limbs

ORAL DOSAGE
Adult (≥ 18 yr): 400 mg, given tid with meals for at least 8 wk. If digestive or neurological reactions occur, reduce dosage to 400 mg bid; if reactions persist at this lower dosage, discontinue use.

CONTRAINDICATIONS
Intolerance to pentoxifylline or other xanthines

WARNINGS/PRECAUTIONS

Cardiovascular effects	Angina, hypotension, or arrhythmia may occur occasionally; use with caution in patients with coronary artery or cerebrovascular disease
Treatment of peripheral vascular disease	Although this drug can improve vascular function and provide symptomatic relief, it should not be considered a substitute for more definitive modes of therapy, such as removal of the obstructions or surgical bypass.

TRENTAL ■ ASCRIPTIN

Bleeding	Increased prothrombin times and bleeding have been reported with pentoxifylline. Although a causal relationship has not been established, monitor the prothrombin time more frequently when using this drug in patients receiving warfarin, and periodically check for evidence of bleeding, including changes in hematocrit or hemoglobin, when giving it to patients at risk of hemorrhage, such as those who have peptic ulcers or who have recently undergone surgery.
Carcinogenicity	Oral administration of 24 times the maximum human daily dose for 18 mo has produced no carcinogenic effects in mice, but has resulted in an increase in benign mammary fibroadenomas in female rats. No evidence of mutagenicity has been detected in the Ames test.

ADVERSE REACTIONS[1]

Frequent reactions (incidence $\geq$ 1%) are printed in *italics*

Cardiovascular	Angina/chest pain
Gastrointestinal	*Dyspepsia (2.8%), nausea (2.2%), vomiting (1.2%)*, belching, flatulence, bloating
Central nervous system	*Dizziness (1.9%), headache (1.2%), tremor*

OVERDOSAGE

Signs and symptoms	Flushing, hypotension, convulsions, somnolence, coma, fever, agitation
Treatment	Support respiratory function, maintain systemic blood pressure, and control convulsions. To remove the drug, perform gastric lavage; activated charcoal can also be given.

DRUG INTERACTIONS

Antihypertensive agents	⇩ Antihypertensive response; check systemic blood pressure periodically during concomitant therapy and, if necessary, reduce dosage of the antihypertensive agent
Warfarin	⇧ Risk of bleeding (see WARNINGS/PRECAUTIONS)

ALTERED LABORATORY VALUES

No clinically significant alterations in blood/serum or urinary values occur at therapeutic dosages

---

USE IN CHILDREN

Safety and effectiveness for use in children under 18 yr of age have not been established

USE IN PREGNANT AND NURSING WOMEN

Pregnancy Category C: an increase in resorptions has been seen in rats following administration of 25 times the maximum human daily dose; no teratogenic effects have been detected in rabbits give 10 times this dose or in rats given 25 times this dose. Use during pregnancy only if clearly needed. Pentoxifylline and its metabolites are excreted in human milk; patients should not nurse while taking this drug.

---

[1] Other reactions, which have been associated with use of immediate-release capsules containing pentoxifylline, include arrhythmia/palpitation, flushing, abdominal discomfort, diarrhea, agitation/nervousness, drowsiness, insomnia, and blurred vision. Reactions to pentoxifylline for which a causal relationship has not been established include dyspnea, edema, hypotension, tachycardia, decrease in serum fibrinogen, pancytopenia, purpura, thrombocytopenia, leukopenia, anorexia, cholecystitis, constipation, dry mouth/thirst, hepatitis, jaundice, anxiety, confusion, epistaxis, flu-like symptoms, laryngitis, nasal congestion, brittle fingernails, pruritus, rash, urticaria, conjunctivitis, earache, scotoma, bad taste, excessive salivation, malaise, sore throat/swollen neck glands, and weight change.

ANTIPLATELET AGENTS

ASCRIPTIN (aspirin, magnesium hydroxide, and aluminum hydroxide) Rorer   OTC

Tablets: 325 mg aspirin, 75 mg magnesium hydroxide, and 75 mg dried aluminum hydroxide gel

INDICATIONS	ORAL DOSAGE
Headache, neuralgia **Pain** of minor injuries and dysmenorrhea **Pain and fever** of colds and influenza **Pain and inflammation** of arthritis and other rheumatic diseases	**Adult:** 2–3 tabs qid
Reducing the risk of **recurrent transient ischemic attacks or stroke in men** who have had transient ischemia of the brain due to fibrin platelet emboli	**Adult:** 1 tab qid or 2 tabs bid
Reducing the risk of **myocardial infarction and subsequent death** in patients with unstable angina or a prior infarction[1]	**Adult:** 1 tab once daily

COMPENDIUM OF DRUG THERAPY

ASCRIPTIN A/D (aspirin, magnesium hydroxide, and aluminum hydroxide) Rorer — OTC

Tablets: 325 mg aspirin, 150 mg magnesium hydroxide, and 150 mg dried aluminum hydroxide gel

INDICATIONS

Pain, inflammation, and fever associated with rheumatoid arthritis, osteoarthritis, and other arthritic conditions

ORAL DOSAGE

Adult: 2–3 tabs qid

Extra Strength ASCRIPTIN (aspirin, magnesium hydroxide, and aluminum hydroxide) Rorer — OTC

Tablets: 500 mg aspirin, 82.5 mg magnesium hydroxide, and 82.5 mg dried aluminum hydroxide gel

INDICATIONS

Headache, neuralgia
Pain of minor injuries and dysmenorrhea
Discomfort of colds
Minor aches and pains associated with arthritis and rheumatism

ORAL DOSAGE

Adult: 2 tabs, with a full glass of water, tid or qid

CONTRAINDICATIONS

Consult manufacturer

WARNINGS/PRECAUTIONS

Evaluation of patients with transient ischemic attacks (TIA's)	Before initiating treatment of patients presenting with signs and symptoms of TIA's, perform a complete medical and neurological evaluation, taking into account other disorders that resemble TIA's. Attention should also be given to risk factors; disorders frequently associated with TIA's, such as hypertension and diabetes, should be evaluated and treatment instituted if appropriate.
Monitoring of prophylactic therapy for myocardial infarction	Check blood pressure, BUN level, and serum uric acid level regularly when using aspirin for long-term prophylaxis of myocardial infarction; small increases in these values have been detected during one clinical trial
Information for patients	Package labels caution patients not to use aspirin without medical supervision if they are undergoing medical treatment, have arthritis or rheumatism, are hypersensitive to aspirin, or have a history of one of the following conditions: asthma, renal or gastric disease, or a hematological disorder; patients are instructed to immediately consult a physician if they experience tinnitus or other symptoms, erythema is seen, or pain persists for more than 10 days. Women who are pregnant or nursing are advised to consult a health professional before using aspirin.
Reye's syndrome	Do not give this preparation to children, including teenagers, with chicken pox or influenza

OVERDOSAGE

Signs and symptoms	Hyperpnea, nausea, vomiting, vertigo, tinnitus, flushing, sweating, thirst, headache, drowsiness, diarrhea, and tachycardia, progressing to hyperthermia, hemorrhage, acid-base disturbances, restlessness, confusion, convulsions, vasomotor depression, coma, and respiratory failure
Treatment	If less than 4 h have elapsed since ingestion, induce emesis or perform gastric lavage, followed by activated charcoal, to remove any remaining drug from the stomach. Initial therapy should be directed at reducing hyperthermia by external sponging with tepid water, correcting dehydration by appropriate IV fluid replacement, and maintaining adequate cardiorespiratory and renal function. In moderately severe cases of salicylate poisoning, cautiously administer sodium bicarbonate IV in sufficient quantity, if possible, to maintain an alkaline diuresis; intermittent peritoneal dialysis may also be helpful. In severe cases, hemodialysis should be seriously considered. Potassium should be added to the repair solution to compensate for potassium losses once urine formation is deemed adequate. Glucose may be provided to correct ketosis and hypoglycemia. Plasma transfusion may be beneficial if shock intervenes. Hemorrhagic phenomena may necessitate whole-blood transfusions and phytonadione (vitamin K$_1$). Do not administer barbiturates to treat excitement or convulsions.

DRUG INTERACTIONS

Anticoagulants	△ Risk of bleeding
Alcohol, corticosteroids, phenylbutazone, oxyphenbutazone	△ Risk of GI ulceration
Probenecid, sulfinpyrazone	▽ Uricosuria
Spironolactone	▽ Diuretic effect
Methotrexate	△ Methotrexate plasma level and risk of toxicity
Tetracycline	▽ Absorption of tetracycline; do not use concomitantly
Absorbable antacids	△ Clearance of salicylate

ASCRIPTIN ■ BAYER Aspirin

Nonabsorbable antacids	⇩ Rate of absorption of aspirin	⇩ Plasma aspirin/salicylate ratio

ALTERED LABORATORY VALUES

Blood/serum values	⇧ Prothrombin time ⇧ Uric acid (with low doses) ⇩ Uric acid (with high doses)
	⇩ Thyroxine (T₄) ⇩ Thyroid-stimulating hormone
Urinary values	⇧ Glucose (with Clinitest tablets)

USE IN CHILDREN
Use according to medical judgment in children under 12 yr of age

USE IN PREGNANT AND NURSING WOMEN
Consult manufacturer for use in pregnant or nursing women

[1] *FDA Drug Bulletin* 15(4):34, 1985

ANTIPLATELET AGENTS

BAYER Aspirin (aspirin) Glenbrook OTC
Tablets: 325 mg **Caplets:** 325 mg

INDICATIONS	ORAL DOSAGE
Headache, muscular aches and pains, bursitis, menstrual discomfort, toothache, minor aches and pains of arthritis and rheumatism **Fever and discomfort** of colds and influenza	**Adult:** 325–650 mg (1–2 tablets or caplets) with water q4h, as needed
Reducing the risk of **recurrent transient ischemic attacks or stroke in men** who have had transient ischemia of the brain due to fibrin platelet emboli[1]	**Adult:** 325 mg (1 tablet or caplet) qid or 650 mg (2 tablets or caplets) bid, with water
Reducing the risk of **myocardial infarction and subsequent death** in patients with unstable angina or a prior infarction[2]	**Adult:** 325 mg (1 tablet or caplet) once daily

Maximum BAYER Aspirin (aspirin) Glenbrook OTC
Tablets: 500 mg **Caplets:** 500 mg

INDICATIONS	ORAL DOSAGE
Headache, muscular aches and pains, bursitis, menstrual discomfort, toothache, minor aches and pains of arthritis and rheumatism **Fever and discomfort** of colds and influenza	**Adult:** 1,000 mg (2 tablets or caplets) with water or fruit juice q4h, as needed, up to 4,000 mg (8 tablets or caplets)/24 h

8-Hour BAYER Aspirin (aspirin) Glenbrook OTC
Tablets (timed release): 650 mg

INDICATIONS	ORAL DOSAGE
Backache, bursitis, sprains, headache, sinusitis, minor pain and stiffness of arthritis **Fever and discomfort** of colds and influenza	**Adult:** 1,300 mg (2 tablets) with water, followed by 650–1,300 mg (1–2 tablets) q8h, as needed, up to 3,900 mg (6 tablets)/day; for prevention of nighttime and early morning stiffness, 1,300 mg (2 tablets) with water at bedtime. Tablets may be broken up (but not ground) between the teeth or gently crumbled in the mouth and swallowed with water without loss of timed-release action.

BAYER Children's Chewable Aspirin (aspirin) Glenbrook OTC
Chewable tablets: 81.25 mg *orange flavored*

INDICATIONS	ORAL DOSAGE
Headache, sore throat, other minor aches and pains **Fever and discomfort** of colds	**Child (3–4 yr; 32–35 lb):** 162.5 mg (2 tablets) with water q4h, up to 5 doses/day **Child (4–6 yr; 36–45 lb):** 243.75 mg (3 tablets) with water q4h, up to 5 doses/day **Child (6–9 yr; 46–65 lb):** 325 mg (4 tablets) with water q4h, up to 5 doses/day **Child (9–11 yr; 66–76 lb):** 406.25 mg (5 tablets) with water q4h, up to 5 doses/day **Child (11–12 yr; 77–83 lb):** 487.5 mg (6 tablets) with water q4h, up to 5 doses/day **Child (≥ 12 yr; ≥ 84 lb):** 650 mg (8 tablets) with water q4h, up to 5 doses/day

BAYER Aspirin

CONTRAINDICATIONS

Bleeding ulcer	Hemorrhagic states	Hypersensitivity to salicylates
Hemophilia		

ADMINISTRATION/DOSAGE ADJUSTMENTS

Administration of chewable tablets	Chewable tablets may be swallowed whole with half a glass of water, milk, or fruit juice; chewed or dissolved on the tongue and then ingested with half a glass of one of these liquids; dissolved in a small amount of one of these liquids, which is then drunk; or crushed in a teaspoonful of water and then ingested with part of a glass of water

WARNINGS/PRECAUTIONS

Gastric irritation	May occur, especially in patients with gastric ulcers, erosive gastritis, or bleeding tendencies; use with caution
Patients with blood-coagulation abnormalities	Use with caution in patients with preexisting hypoprothrombinemia or vitamin K deficiency
Nasal polyps, asthma, hay fever	May predispose to salicylate hypersensitivity; use with caution
Interference with platelet aggregation	Use with caution prior to surgery
Monitoring of prophylactic therapy for myocardial infarction	Check blood pressure, BUN level, and serum uric acid level regularly when using aspirin for long-term prophylaxis of myocardial infarction; small increases in these values have been detected during one clinical trial
Patient instructions	Bayer, Maximum Bayer, and 8–Hour Bayer: the package label advises consultation with a physician if pain persists for more than 10 days, redness is present, or the patient is less than 12 yr of age. Children's Bayer: the package label advises consultation with a physician if nausea, vomiting, headache, high or continued fever, or severe or persistent sore throat occurs. The package labels also advise pregnant or nursing women to consult a health professional before using these products.
Reye's syndrome	There is evidence suggesting that use of aspirin in children or adolescents with chicken pox or influenza may increase the risk of Reye's syndrome

ADVERSE REACTIONS

Gastrointestinal	Nausea, dyspepsia, heartburn, epigastric discomfort, anorexia, diarrhea, occult blood loss, hemorrhage
Central nervous system	Dizziness, tinnitus, headache, deafness
Respiratory	Hyperventilation
Cardiovascular	Increased pulse rate
Dermatological	Skin eruptions
Other	Sweating, thirst, electrolyte and acid-base imbalance

OVERDOSAGE

Signs and symptoms	Hyperpnea, nausea, vomiting, vertigo, tinnitus, flushing, sweating, thirst, headache, drowsiness, diarrhea, and tachycardia, progressing to hyperthermia, hemorrhage, acid-base disturbances, restlessness, confusion, convulsions, vasomotor depression, coma, and respiratory failure
Treatment	If less than 4 h have elapsed since ingestion, induce emesis or perform gastric lavage, followed by activated charcoal, to remove any remaining drug from the stomach. Initial therapy should be directed at reducing hyperthermia by external sponging with tepid water, correcting dehydration by appropriate IV fluid replacement, and maintaining adequate cardiorespiratory and renal function. In moderately severe cases of salicylate poisoning, cautiously administer sodium bicarbonate IV in sufficient quantity, if possible, to maintain an alkaline diuresis; intermittent peritoneal dialysis may also be helpful. In severe cases, hemodialysis should be seriously considered. Potassium should be added to the repair solution to compensate for potassium losses once urine formation is deemed adequate. Glucose may be provided to correct ketosis and hypoglycemia. Plasma transfusion may be beneficial if shock intervenes. Hemorrhagic phenomena may necessitate whole-blood transfusions and phytonadione (vitamin K_1). Do not administer barbiturates to treat excitement or convulsions.

DRUG INTERACTIONS

Anticoagulants	⇧ Risk of bleeding; exercise caution during combination therapy
Alcohol, corticosteroids, phenylbutazone, oxyphenbutazone	⇧ Risk of GI ulceration
Probenecid, sulfinpyrazone	⇩ Uricosuria
Spironolactone	⇩ Diuretic effect
Methotrexate	⇧ Methotrexate plasma level and risk of toxicity

ALTERED LABORATORY VALUES

Blood/serum values	⇧ Prothrombin time ⇧ Uric acid (with low doses) ⇩ Uric acid (with high doses) ⇩ Thyroxine (T_4) ⇩ Thyroid-stimulating hormone

Urinary values — ⌂ Glucose (with Clinitest tablets)

USE IN CHILDREN	USE IN PREGNANT AND NURSING WOMEN
See INDICATIONS and ORAL DOSAGE. *Bayer Aspirin and Children's Chewable Aspirin:* use according to medical judgment in children under 2 yr of age; *Maximum Bayer Aspirin and 8-Hour Bayer Aspirin:* use according to medical judgment in children under 12 yr of age.	Consult manufacturer for use in pregnant or nursing women

[1] *FDA Drug Bulletin* 10(1):2, 1980
[2] *FDA Drug Bulletin* 15(4):34, 1985

ANTIPLATELET AGENTS

BUFFERIN (aspirin, aluminum glycinate, and magnesium carbonate) Bristol-Myers OTC

Tablets: 324 mg aspirin, 48.6 mg aluminum glycinate, and 97.2 mg magnesium carbonate

INDICATIONS	ORAL DOSAGE
Headache, muscular aches, toothache, menstrual cramps, and minor pain and inflammation of arthritis and rheumatism **Pain and fever** of colds and influenza	**Adult:** 2 tabs q4h, as needed **Child (6–12 yr):** 1 tab q4h, as needed
Reducing the risk of **recurrent transient ischemic attacks or stroke in men** who have had transient ischemia of the brain due to fibrin platelet emboli[1]	**Adult:** 1 tab qid or 2 tabs bid
Reducing the risk of **myocardial infarction and subsequent death** in patients with unstable angina or a prior infarction[2]	**Adult:** 1 tab once daily

Arthritis Strength BUFFERIN (aspirin, aluminum glycinate, and magnesium carbonate) Bristol-Myers OTC

Tablets: 486 mg aspirin, 72.9 mg aluminum glycinate, and 145.8 mg magnesium carbonate

Extra Strength BUFFERIN (aspirin, aluminum glycinate, and magnesium carbonate) Bristol-Myers OTC

Tablets: 500 mg aspirin, 75 mg aluminum glycinate, and 150 mg magnesium carbonate

INDICATIONS	ORAL DOSAGE
Minor aches and pains, stiffness, swelling, and inflammation of arthritis and rheumatism **Pain and fever** of colds and influenza **Pain,** including that of simple headache, lower backache, sinusitis, neuralgia, neuritis, tooth extraction, muscle strain, athletic soreness, and menstrual distress	**Adult:** 2 tabs q4h, as needed, up to 8 tabs per 24 h

CONTRAINDICATIONS

Hypersensitivity to salicylates

WARNINGS/PRECAUTIONS

Monitoring of prophylactic therapy for myocardial infarction	Check blood pressure, BUN level, and serum uric acid level regularly when using aspirin for long-term prophylaxis of myocardial infarction; small increases in these values have been detected during one clinical trial
Information for patients	Package labels caution patients not to use these products without medical supervision if one of the following conditions exists: (1) chicken pox or influenza in a child or teenager, (2) erythema, (3) arthritis or rheumatism in a child under 12 yr of age, (4) pregnancy, or (5) nursing. Patients are instructed to discontinue administration if they experience dizziness, tinnitus, or hearing impairment and to also consult a physician if overdose or erythema occurs or pain persists for more than 10 days.

BUFFERIN ■ ECOTRIN

Reye's syndrome	There is evidence suggesting that use of aspirin in children or adolescents with chicken pox or influenza may increase the risk of Reye's syndrome

OVERDOSAGE

Signs and symptoms	Hyperpnea, nausea, vomiting, vertigo, tinnitus, flushing, sweating, thirst, headache, drowsiness, diarrhea, and tachycardia, progressing to hyperthermia, hemorrhage, acid-base disturbances, restlessness, confusion, convulsions, vasomotor depression, coma, and respiratory failure
Treatment	If less than 4 h have elapsed since ingestion, induce emesis or perform gastric lavage, followed by activated charcoal, to remove any remaining drug from the stomach. Initial therapy should be directed at reducing hyperthermia by external sponging with tepid water, correcting dehydration by appropriate IV fluid replacement, and maintaining adequate cardiorespiratory and renal function. In moderately severe cases of salicylate poisoning, cautiously administer sodium bicarbonate IV in sufficient quantity, if possible, to maintain an alkaline diuresis; intermittent peritoneal dialysis may also be helpful. In severe cases, hemodialysis should be seriously considered. Potassium should be added to the repair solution to compensate for potassium losses once urine formation is deemed adequate. Glucose may be provided to correct ketosis and hypoglycemia. Plasma transfusion may be beneficial if shock intervenes. Hemorrhagic phenomena may necessitate whole-blood transfusions and phytonadione (vitamin K$_1$). Do not administer barbiturates to treat excitement or convulsions.

DRUG INTERACTIONS

Anticoagulants	△ Risk of bleeding
Alcohol, corticosteroids, phenylbutazone, oxyphenbutazone	△ Risk of GI ulceration
Probenecid, sulfinpyrazone	▽ Uricosuria
Spironolactone	▽ Diuretic effect
Tetracycline	▽ Absorption of tetracycline
Methotrexate	△ Methotrexate plasma level and risk of toxicity

ALTERED LABORATORY VALUES

Blood/serum values	△ Prothrombin time △ Uric acid (with low doses) ▽ Uric acid (with high doses) ▽ Thyroxine (T$_4$) ▽ Thyroid-stimulating hormone
Urinary values	△ Glucose (with Clinitest tablets)

USE IN CHILDREN

See INDICATIONS and ORAL DOSAGE

USE IN PREGNANT AND NURSING WOMEN

Consult manufacturer for use in pregnant or nursing women

---

[1] FDA Drug Bulletin 10(1):2, 1980
[2] FDA Drug Bulletin 15(4):34, 1985

ANTIPLATELET AGENTS

Regular Strength ECOTRIN (aspirin)   SmithKline Consumer Products   OTC

Tablets (enteric coated): 325 mg

INDICATIONS	ORAL DOSAGE
Arthritis and rheumatism	**Adult:** for minor aches and pain, 325–650 mg q4h, as needed; for chronic therapy, up to 650 mg q4h or up to 975 mg q6h without medical supervision (higher doses may be given *with* supervision)
Reducing the risk of **recurrent transient ischemic attacks or stroke in men** who have had transient ischemia of the brain due to fibrin platelet emboli	**Adult:** 325 mg qid or 650 mg bid
Reducing the risk of **myocardial infarction and subsequent death** in patients with unstable angina or a prior infarction[1]	**Adult:** 325 mg once daily

Maximum Strength ECOTRIN (aspirin) SmithKline Consumer Products OTC

Tablets (enteric coated): 500 mg **Caplets (enteric coated):** 500 mg

INDICATIONS

Arthritis and rheumatism

ORAL DOSAGE

Adult: for minor aches and pain, 1 g q6h, as needed; for chronic therapy, up to 1 g q6h without medical supervision (higher doses may be given *with* supervision)

CONTRAINDICATIONS

Consult manufacturer

ADMINISTRATION/DOSAGE ADJUSTMENTS

Administration	Give each dose with water or fruit juice
Chronic therapy	Anti-inflammatory effect is generally associated with a serum salicylate level of 15 mg/dl, attained in healthy men with 3 days of treatment at 5.2 g/day or with 4 days of treatment at 3.9 g/day and attained in healthy women with 2 days at 5.2 g/day or with 3 days at 3.9 g/day. If 3.9-4 g/day is exceeded, monitor serum levels and watch for tinnitus and other clinical manifestations of toxicity; bear in mind that high-frequency hearing loss, which often occurs in the elderly, makes detection of tinnitus difficult and use of tinnitus as an index of toxicity questionable.

WARNINGS/PRECAUTIONS

Information for patients	Package labels caution patients not to use these products without medical supervision if one of the following conditions exists: (1) history of ulcers, (2) erythema, (3) chicken pox or influenza in a child or teenager, (4) arthritis or rheumatism in a child under 12 yr of age, (5) pregnancy, or (6) nursing. Patients are instructed to discontinue administration if they experience dizziness, tinnitus, or hearing impairment and to also consult a physician if persistent or unexplained stomach upset develops, overdose or erythema occurs, or pain persists for more than 10 days.
Evaluation of patients with transient ischemic attacks (TIA's)	Before initiating treatment of patients presenting with signs and symptoms of TIA's, perform a complete medical and neurological evaluation, taking into account other disorders that resemble TIA's. Attention should also be given to risk factors; disorders frequently associated with TIA's, such as hypertension and diabetes, should be evaluated and treatment instituted if appropriate.
Monitoring of prophylactic therapy for myocardial infarction	Check blood pressure, BUN level, and serum uric acid level regularly when using aspirin for long-term prophylaxis of myocardial infarction; small increases in these values have been detected during one clinical trial
Patients with impaired gastric emptying	Tablet accumulation and subsequent formation of a bezoar in the stomach have occurred occasionally in patients with impaired gastric emptying, apparently as a result of outlet obstruction due to peptic ulcer disease alone or in combination with hypotonic gastric peristalsis. Telltale symptoms include early satiety and vague upper abdominal distress. Tablet accumulation may be confirmed roentgenographically or by endoscopy. The bezoar can be removed by gastric lavage, alternating between neutral and slightly basic solutions, or by gastrotomy. Alternatively, in a clinically untested approach, parenteral cimetidine, followed by sips of a slightly basic liquid, may be administered in an attempt to dissolve the bezoar; dissolution can be assessed by monitoring the plasma salicylate level or by watching for the development of tinnitus.
Patients with gastrectomy	The acid-resistant enteric coating of these products may offer no benefit to patients with partial or complete gastrectomy since gastric pH may be elevated in these patients
Reye's syndrome	There is evidence suggesting that use of aspirin in children or adolescents with chicken pox or influenza may increase the risk of Reye's syndrome

OVERDOSAGE

Signs and symptoms	Hyperpnea, nausea, vomiting, vertigo, tinnitus, flushing, sweating, thirst, headache, drowsiness, diarrhea, and tachycardia, progressing to hyperthermia, hemorrhage, acid-base disturbances, restlessness, confusion, convulsions, vasomotor depression, coma, and respiratory failure
Treatment	If less than 4 h have elapsed since ingestion, induce emesis or perform gastric lavage, followed by activated charcoal, to remove any remaining drug from the stomach. Initial therapy should be directed at reducing hyperthermia by external sponging with tepid water, correcting dehydration by appropriate IV fluid replacement, and maintaining adequate cardiorespiratory and renal function. In moderately severe cases of salicylate poisoning, cautiously administer sodium bicarbonate IV in sufficient quantity, if possible, to maintain an alkaline diuresis; intermittent peritoneal dialysis may also be helpful. In severe cases, hemodialysis should be seriously considered. Potassium should be added to the repair solution to compensate for potassium losses once urine formation is deemed adequate. Glucose may be provided to correct ketosis and hypoglycemia. Plasma transfusion may be beneficial if shock intervenes. Hemorrhagic phenomena may necessitate whole-blood transfusions and phytonadione (vitamin K_1). Do not administer barbiturates to treat excitement or convulsions.

ECOTRIN ■ EMPIRIN

DRUG INTERACTIONS

Anticoagulants	△ Risk of bleeding
Alcohol, corticosteroids, phenylbutazone, oxyphenbutazone	△ Risk of GI ulceration
Probenecid, sulfinpyrazone	▽ Uricosuria
Spironolactone	▽ Diuretic effect
Methotrexate	△ Methotrexate plasma level and risk of toxicity

ALTERED LABORATORY VALUES

Blood/serum values	△ Prothrombin time △ Uric acid (with low doses) ▽ Uric acid (with high doses) ▽ Thyroxine (T$_4$) ▽ Thyroid-stimulating hormone
Urinary values	△ Glucose (with Clinitest tablets)

USE IN CHILDREN
Use according to medical judgment in children under 12 yr of age

USE IN PREGNANT AND NURSING WOMEN
Consult manufacturer for use in pregnant or nursing women

---

[1] *FDA Drug Bulletin* 15(4):34, 1985

ANTIPLATELET AGENTS

EMPIRIN (aspirin) Burroughs Wellcome   OTC

Tablets: 325 mg (5 gr)

INDICATIONS

Pain, including headache, muscular aches and pains, and toothache
Fever and discomfort of colds and flu
Pain and discomfort due to sore throat, neuralgia, menstrual pain, arthritis and rheumatism, bursitis, lumbago, and sciatica; **sleeplessness** caused by minor pain and discomfort

Reducing the risk of **recurrent transient ischemic attacks or stroke in men** who have had transient ischemia of the brain due to fibrin platelet emboli[1]

Reducing the risk of **myocardial infarction and subsequent death** in patients with unstable angina or a prior infarction[2]

ORAL DOSAGE

Adult: 325–650 mg (1–2 tabs) with a full glass of water q4h, up to 3,900 mg (12 tabs)/day

Adult: 325 mg (1 tab) qid or 650 mg (2 tabs) bid

Adult: 325 mg once daily

CONTRAINDICATIONS

Gastric ulcer and peptic ulcer symptoms	Asthma	Hypersensitivity to aspirin
Anticoagulant therapy		

WARNINGS/PRECAUTIONS

Gastric irritation	May occur, especially in patients with gastric ulcers, erosive gastritis, or bleeding tendencies; use with caution
Patients with blood-coagulation abnormalities	Use with caution in patients with preexisting hypoprothrombinemia or vitamin K deficiency
Nasal polyps, asthma, hay fever	May predispose to salicylate hypersensitivity; use with caution
Interference with platelet aggregation	Use with caution prior to surgery
Monitoring of prophylactic therapy for myocardial infarction	Check blood pressure, BUN level, and serum uric acid level regularly when using aspirin for long-term prophylaxis of myocardial infarction; small increases in these values have been detected during one clinical trial

EMPIRIN

Patient instructions	The package label advises consultation with a physician if the patient experiences high or continued fever or severe or persistent sore throat, especially when accompanied by fever, headache, nausea, or vomiting; pregnant or nursing women are advised to consult a health professional before using this product
Reye's syndrome	There is evidence suggesting that use of aspirin in children or adolescents with chicken pox or influenza may increase the risk of Reye's syndrome

ADVERSE REACTIONS

Gastrointestinal	Nausea, dyspepsia, heartburn, epigastric discomfort, anorexia, diarrhea, occult blood loss, hemorrhage
Central nervous system	Dizziness, tinnitus, headache, deafness
Respiratory	Hyperventilation
Cardiovascular	Increased pulse rate
Dermatological	Skin eruptions
Other	Sweating, thirst, electrolyte and acid-base imbalance

OVERDOSAGE

Signs and symptoms	Hyperpnea, nausea, vomiting, vertigo, tinnitus, flushing, sweating, thirst, headache, drowsiness, diarrhea, and tachycardia, progressing to hyperthermia, hemorrhage, acid-base disturbances, restlessness, confusion, convulsions, vasomotor depression, coma, and respiratory failure
Treatment	If less than 4 h have elapsed since ingestion, induce emesis or perform gastric lavage, followed by activated charcoal, to remove any remaining drug from the stomach. Initial therapy should be directed at reducing hyperthermia by external sponging with tepid water, correcting dehydration by appropriate IV fluid replacement, and maintaining adequate cardiorespiratory and renal function. In moderately severe cases of salicylate poisoning, cautiously administer sodium bicarbonate IV in sufficient quantity, if possible, to maintain an alkaline diuresis; intermittent peritoneal dialysis may also be helpful. In severe cases, hemodialysis should be seriously considered. Potassium should be added to the repair solution to compensate for potassium losses once urine formation is deemed adequate. Glucose may be provided to correct ketosis and hypoglycemia. Plasma transfusion may be beneficial if shock intervenes. Hemorrhagic phenomena may necessitate whole-blood transfusions and phytonadione (vitamin K_1). Do not administer barbiturates to treat excitement or convulsions.

DRUG INTERACTIONS

Anticoagulants	⇧ Risk of bleeding
Alcohol, corticosteroids, phenylbutazone, oxyphenbutazone	⇧ Risk of GI ulceration
Probenecid, sulfinpyrazone	⇩ Uricosuria
Spironolactone	⇩ Diuretic effect
Methotrexate	⇧ Methotrexate plasma level and risk of toxicity

ALTERED LABORATORY VALUES

Blood/serum values	⇧ Prothrombin time ⇧ Uric acid (with low doses) ⇩ Uric acid (with high doses) ⇩ Thyroxine (T_4) ⇩ Thyroid-stimulating hormone
Urinary values	⇧ Glucose (with Clinitest tablets)

USE IN CHILDREN

Consult manufacturer

USE IN PREGNANT AND NURSING WOMEN

Aspirin has been shown to be teratogenic and embryocidal in rats and mice given 4–6 times the normal human dose. Clinical studies, however, have not shown that aspirin given during the first trimester increases the risk of abnormalities. Use of aspirin close to term may cause bleeding in the mother, fetus, or neonate. Pregnancy and delivery may be prolonged by regular, high-dosage use during the last two trimesters. Use before delivery may also prolong delivery. Aspirin is excreted in breast milk in small amounts; its clinical effect on nursing infants is not known. Because of the potential for serious adverse reactions in nursing infants, a decision should be made not to nurse or to discontinue use of this preparation, taking into account its importance to the mother.

---

[1] FDA Drug Bulletin 10(1):2, 1980
[2] FDA Drug Bulletin 15(4):34, 1985

HEMOSTATIC AGENTS

AVITENE (microfibrillar collagen hemostat [MCH]) Alcon   Rx

Fibrous form: 1, 5 g   **Nonwoven web form:** 70 × 35 × 1 mm and 70 × 70 × 1 mm sheets

INDICATIONS

As an aid during surgery for the **production of hemostasis** when bleeding cannot be controlled by ligature or conventional procedures

TOPICAL DOSAGE

Adult: apply, with pressure, directly to source of bleeding in a sufficient amount to produce hemostasis; remove material after several minutes (see ADMINISTRATION/DOSAGE ADJUSTMENTS)

CONTRAINDICATIONS

Closure of skin incisions (may interfere with healing)

Use on bone surfaces to which prosthetic materials are to be attached with methylmethacrylate materials

ADMINISTRATION/DOSAGE ADJUSTMENTS

Application	MCH must be applied dry. Immediately before use, compress surface to be treated with dry sponges. Apply MCH directly to source of bleeding with dry smooth forceps, and exert pressure over the site with a dry sponge *(do not use gloved fingers to apply pressure)* until bleeding is controlled; this may range from 1 min for capillary bleeding (eg, skin-graft donor sites and following dermatological curettage) to 3–5 min or more for brisk bleeding (eg, splenic tears) or high-pressure leaks in major artery suture holes. To control oozing from cancellous bone, firmly pack MCH into spongy bone surface.
Break-through bleeding	If break-through bleeding occurs, apply additional MCH. The amount required depends upon the severity of bleeding: for capillary bleeding, 1 g is usually enough for a 50-cm² area; for more brisk bleeding, apply a thicker amount.
Removal of material after bleeding is controlled	After 5–10 min, remove excess MCH with a blunt forceps; this can be facilitated by wetting with sterile 0.9% saline solution and irrigation
Use of nonwoven web in neurosurgical and other procedures	Apply small squares of the material to bleeding areas and then cover the sites with moist cottonoid "patties." To prevent wetting of the MCH (and to apply needed pressure), hold a suction tip against the cottonoid patty for one to several minutes, depending on the briskness of bleeding. After 5–10 min, excess MCH may be removed by teasing and irrigation.

WARNINGS/PRECAUTIONS

Autoclaving	Will inactivate MCH; do not resterilize. Discard any unused portion.
Concealed hematoma	The possibility of concealment of an underlying hematoma should be considered in suspected cases (eg, penetrating liver wounds), since the material may seal over the exit site of a deeper hemorrhage due to its adhesiveness
Impairment of hemostatic efficacy	Can occur if MCH is moistened or wetted with saline or thrombin; the material should be applied dry
Spillage on nonbleeding surfaces	Should be avoided, especially on abdominal or thoracic organs
Use in contaminated wounds	May enhance infection, as with any foreign substance (see ADVERSE REACTIONS)
Removal of excess material	Bowel adhesion or mechanical pressure sufficient to compromise the ureter may occur if excess MCH is not removed within several minutes after application
Otolaryngological surgery	To prevent aspiration, remove all excess dry material and thoroughly irrigate the pharynx
Patients with systemic coagulation disorders	Institute appropriate therapy to correct the underlying coagulopathy before using MCH
Immunologic response to MCH	MCH contains a low amount of intercalated bovine serum protein that reacts immunologically like beef serum albumin (BSA); increases in anti-BSA titers have been observed after treatment with MCH. Intradermal skin tests have occasionally shown a weak positive reaction to BSA or MCH, but these results have not been correlated with IgG titers to BSA. Tests have failed to elicit clinically significant IgE antibodies to BSA following MCH therapy.
Blood salvage	Fragments of MCH may pass through the filters of blood scavenging systems; avoid reintroducing blood from operative sites treated with MCH. This product should not be used in conjunction with autologous blood salvaging circuits.
Intraocular bleeding	Do not use MCH intraocularly

ADVERSE REACTIONS

Local	Potentiation of infection, including abscess formation, hematoma, wound dehiscence, and mediastinitis

AVITENE ■ THROMBOSTAT

| Other | Adhesions, allergic reactions, foreign body reactions, subgaleal seroma (one case), alveolalgia (following use in dental extraction sockets), transient laryngospasm due to aspiration of dry material (following use in tonsillectomy) |

USE IN CHILDREN
Use according to surgical discretion

USE IN PREGNANT AND NURSING WOMEN
Use during pregnancy only when clearly needed. Although teratology studies in rats and rabbits have shown no evidence of fetal damage, no adequate, well-controlled studies have been done in pregnant women. There are no known contraindications for use of this drug in nursing mothers.

HEMOSTATIC AGENTS

THROMBOSTAT (thrombin) Parke-Davis   Rx
Vials: 1,000, 5,000, 10,000, 20,000 units for topical use only[1]

INDICATIONS
As an aid for the **production of hemostasis** whenever oozing blood from capillaries and small venules is accessible

TOPICAL DOSAGE
Adult: for general use in controlling surgical bleeding (associated with plastic surgery, dental extractions, skin grafting, neurosurgery, etc), 100 units/ml, applied directly to bleeding surface or used in conjunction with absorbable gelatin sponge; for profuse bleeding (eg, hepatic and splenic tears), up to 1,000–2,000 units/ml, applied directly or used with absorbable gelatin sponge (see ADMINISTRATION/DOSAGE ADJUSTMENTS)

CONTRAINDICATIONS
Sensitivity to any component and/or bovine material

ADMINISTRATION/DOSAGE ADJUSTMENTS

Preparation of solution	For 100 units/ml, add 10 ml of sterile distilled water or isotonic saline to the 1,000-unit package; for 1,000–2,000 units/ml, dissolve 5,000 units in, respectively, 5 or 2.5 ml of the diluent. For intermediate strengths, dissolve the contents of the proper strength package in an appropriate volume of diluent. Use solutions within 6 h after preparation if stored at room temperature, within 24 h if refrigerated, and within 48 h if frozen.
Application of solution	Before treatment, sponge surface free of blood *(do not wipe)*. Spray surface with appropriate thrombin solution, or use a sterile syringe and small-gauge needle to flood the surface; efficacy is greatest when thrombin mixes freely with blood as soon as it reaches the surface. Avoid sponging the treated surface so that the clot remains securely in place.
Application of powder	Oozing surfaces may often be effectively treated with thrombin in dry form. Open the vial by removing the metal ring by flipping up the plastic cap and tearing counterclockwise. Break the dried thrombin up into a powder with a sterile glass rod or other suitable sterile instrument and apply directly to oozing surface.
Use in conjunction with absorbable gelatin sponge	Prepare thrombin solution of desired strength. Immerse sponge strips of the desired size in the solution. Knead the sponge strips vigorously with moistened fingers to remove trapped air, thereby facilitating saturation of the sponge. Apply saturated sponge to bleeding area. Hold in place for 10–15 s with a cotton pledget or a small gauze sponge.[2]

WARNINGS/PRECAUTIONS

| Injection of thrombin | Thrombin must not be injected or otherwise allowed to enter large blood vessels; extensive intravascular clotting and even death may result |
| Sensitivity and allergic reactions | Have been reported in animals given thrombin by injection |

ADVERSE REACTIONS

| Hypersensitivity | Anaphylactoid reaction (following use for treatment of epistaxis) |
| Other | Febrile reactions (causal relationship not established) |

USE IN CHILDREN
Safety and effectiveness for use in children have not been established

USE IN PREGNANT AND NURSING WOMEN
Pregnancy Category C: reproduction studies have not been done; it is not known whether topical thrombin can cause harm to the fetus or affect reproductive capacity. Use during pregnancy only if clearly needed. Consult manufacturer for use in nursing mothers.

[1] Each 5,000- and 10,000-unit vial is supplied with 1 vial of isotonic saline; the 20,000-unit vial is supplied in a package with 1 vial of isotonic saline and in a kit with 1 pump sprayer cap and 1 vial of isotonic saline
[2] Consult the absorbable gelatin sponge product labeling for complete use information prior to utilizing this procedure

Chapter 16

Anticonvulsants/Antiparkinson Agents

Barbiturates — 562

AMYTAL (Lilly) — 562
Amobarbital C-II

AMYTAL Sodium (Lilly) — 562
Amobarbital sodium C-II

GEMONIL (Abbott) — 563
Metharbital C-III

MEBARAL (Winthrop-Breon) — 564
Mephobarbital C-IV

NEMBUTAL Elixir (Abbott) — 566
Pentobarbital C-II

NEMBUTAL Sodium Capsules and Solution (Abbott) — 566
Pentobarbital sodium C-II

NEMBUTAL Sodium Suppositories (Abbott) — 567
Pentobarbital sodium C-III

Phenobarbital C-IV — 569

Phenobarbital sodium C-IV — 569

SECONAL Sodium Capsules (Lilly) — 571
Secobarbital sodium C-II

SECONAL Sodium Injection (Lilly) — 571
Secobarbital sodium C-II

SECONAL Sodium Suppositories (Lilly) — 571
Secobarbital sodium C-III

Hydantoins — 573

DILANTIN (Parke-Davis) — 573
Phenytoin Rx

DILANTIN (Parke-Davis) — 573
Phenytoin sodium, extended Rx

DILANTIN Parenteral (Parke-Davis) — 575
Phenytoin sodium Rx

MESANTOIN (Sandoz Pharmaceuticals) — 578
Mephenytoin Rx

PEGANONE (Abbott) — 579
Ethotoin Rx

Succinimides — 580

CELONTIN (Parke-Davis) — 580
Methsuximide Rx

MILONTIN (Parke-Davis) — 581
Phensuximide Rx

ZARONTIN (Parke-Davis) — 582
Ethosuximide Rx

Miscellaneous Anticonvulsants — 583

DEPAKENE (Abbott) — 583
Valproic acid Rx

DEPAKOTE (Abbott) — 583
Divalproex sodium Rx

KLONOPIN (Roche) — 585
Clonazepam C-IV

MYSOLINE (Ayerst) — 587
Primidone Rx

PHENURONE (Abbott) — 588
Phenacemide Rx

TEGRETOL (Geigy) — 589
Carbamazepine Rx

TRANXENE (Abbott) — 592
Clorazepate dipotassium C-IV

TRANXENE-SD (Abbott) — 592
Clorazepate dipotassium C-IV

TRIDIONE (Abbott) — 593
Trimethadione Rx

VALIUM (Roche) — 594
Diazepam C-IV

VALRELEASE (Roche) — 595
Diazepam C-IV

Antiparkinson Agents — 597

AKINETON (Knoll) — 597
Biperiden Rx

ARTANE (Lederle) — 598
Trihexyphenidyl hydrochloride Rx

BENADRYL (Parke-Davis) — 600
Diphenhydramine hydrochloride Rx

BENADRYL 25 (Warner-Lambert) — 599
Diphenhydramine hydrochloride OTC

BENADRYL Elixir (Warner-Lambert) — 599
Diphenhydramine hydrochloride OTC

COGENTIN (Merck Sharp & Dohme) — 601
Benztropine mesylate Rx

DOPAR (Norwich Eaton) — 603
Levodopa Rx

KEMADRIN (Burroughs Wellcome) — 604
Procyclidine hydrochloride Rx

LARODOPA (Roche) — 605
Levodopa Rx

PARLODEL (Sandoz Pharmaceuticals) — 607
Bromocriptine mesylate Rx

SINEMET (Merck Sharp & Dohme) — 610
Carbidopa and levodopa Rx

SYMMETREL (Du Pont) — 612
Amantadine hydrochloride Rx

Other Anticonvulsants

DILANTIN with Phenobarbital (Parke-Davis) — 561
Phenytoin sodium and phenobarbital *Rx*

PARADIONE (Abbott) — 561
Paramethadione *Rx*

Other Antiparkinson Agents

DISIPAL (Riker) — 561
Orphenadrine hydrochloride *Rx*

PARSIDOL (Parke-Davis) — 561
Ethopropazine hydrochloride *Rx*

OTHER ANTICONVULSANTS

DRUG	HOW SUPPLIED	USUAL DOSAGE
DILANTIN with Phenobarbital (Parke-Davis) Phenytoin sodium and phenobarbital *Rx*	**Capsules:** 100 mg phenytoin sodium and 16 mg phenobarbital; 100 mg phenytoin sodium and 32 mg phenobarbital	**Adult:** 3–4 caps/day, followed, if necessary, by up to 6 caps/day **Child:** 5 mg/kg/day of phenytoin and 2–3 mg/kg/day of phenobarbital, given in 2–3 equally divided doses, up to 300 mg to start; maximum daily dose of phenytoin: 300 mg
PARADIONE (Abbott) Paramethadione *Rx*	**Capsules:** 150, 300 mg **Solution:** 300 mg/ml (50 ml)	**Adult:** 900 mg/day, given in 3–4 equally divided doses, to start, followed by weekly increases of 300 mg/day, if needed, up to 2.4 g/day, given in 3–4 divided doses **Child:** 300–900 mg/day, given in 3–4 equally divided doses

OTHER ANTIPARKINSON AGENTS

DRUG	HOW SUPPLIED	USUAL DOSAGE[1]
DISIPAL (Riker) Orphenadrine hydrochloride *Rx*	**Tablets:** 50 mg	**Adult:** 1 tab tid
PARSIDOL (Parke-Davis) Ethopropazine hydrochloride *Rx*	**Tablets:** 10, 50 mg	**Adult:** 50 mg 1–2 times/day to start, followed, if necessary, by a gradual increase in dosage; usual maintenance dosage: 100–400 mg/day for mild to moderate symptoms, 500–600 mg/day or higher for severe symptoms

[1] Where pediatric dosages are not given, consult manufacturer

COMPENDIUM OF DRUG THERAPY

AMYTAL

BARBITURATES

AMYTAL (amobarbital) Lilly   C-II
Tablets: 30, 50, 100 mg

INDICATIONS	ORAL DOSAGE
Daytime sedation	**Adult:** 15–120 mg 2–4 times/day; usual sedative dosage, 30–50 mg bid or tid
Insomnia Preanesthetic sedation	**Adult:** 100–200 mg; higher doses may be given if needed

AMYTAL Sodium (amobarbital sodium) Lilly   C-II
Capsules: 65, 200 mg   Vials: 250, 500 mg

INDICATIONS	ORAL DOSAGE	PARENTERAL DOSAGE
Insomnia	**Adult:** 65–200 mg at bedtime	—
Preanesthetic sedation	**Adult:** 200 mg 1–2 h prior to surgery	—
Labor	**Adult:** 200–400 mg to start, followed by 200–400 mg q1-3h, if needed, up to a total of 1,000 mg	—
Convulsive seizures, including seizures due to chorea, eclampsia, meningitis, tetanus, procaine or cocaine reactions, and strychnine or picrotoxin poisoning **Epileptiform seizures** **Catatonic, negativistic, or manic reactions** **Narcoanalysis** **Narcotherapy** **Diagnosis of schizophrenia**	—	**Adult:** 65–500 mg IM or IV, up to 500 mg IM or 1 g IV, as needed **Child (6–12 yr):** 65–500 mg IM or IV, as needed

CONTRAINDICATIONS

Hypersensitivity to barbiturates	History of manifest or latent porphyria	Severe hepatic impairment
Respiratory disease accompanied by dyspnea or obstruction	Prior addiction to sedative-hypnotics	Acute or chronic pain

ADMINISTRATION/DOSAGE ADJUSTMENTS

Preparation of parenteral solution	Dilute contents of ampul with Sterile Water for Injection; ordinarily, a 10% solution is used for IV administration and a 20% solution for IM injection. Discard solution if drug does not dissolve completely within 5 min of mixing with diluent or if a precipitate forms after the solution clears. Inject within 30 min of opening the ampul. Do not use drug supplied in capsules for injection.
Intramuscular administration	Inject deeply into a large muscle mass, such as the gluteus maximus; to preclude irritation, give no more than 5 ml at any one site
Intravenous administration	Administer slowly ($\leq$ 1 ml/min); overly rapid IV administration may result in apnea and/or hypotension

WARNINGS/PRECAUTIONS

Patients with hepatic impairment	Use with caution to avoid excessive accumulation
Elderly or debilitated patients	May experience marked excitement or CNS depression; use with caution
Patients with borderline hypoadrenal function	Systemic effects of both endogenous and exogenous hydrocortisone may be diminished; use with caution
Mental and/or physical impairment	Caution patients that their ability to drive or perform other potentially hazardous activities may be impaired
Overdosage	Excessive doses, either alone or in combination with other CNS depressants, may result in toxicity and death; warn patients not to exceed recommended dosage and to limit alcohol intake, and that the concomitant use of other CNS depressants can cause additional CNS depression. Use with caution in patients who have a history of emotional disturbances or suicidal ideation.
Drug dependence	Psychic and/or physical dependence and tolerance may develop, especially in addiction-prone individuals; abrupt discontinuation after chronic use of large doses may result in withdrawal reactions, including delirium, convulsions, and death

ADVERSE REACTIONS

Central nervous system	Residual sedation ("hangover"), drowsiness; lethargy and headache (with oral use); idiosyncratic excitement and pain (with parenteral use)
Respiratory	Depression, apnea; laryngospasm (with parenteral use)

AMYTAL ■ GEMONIL

Cardiovascular	Circulatory collapse; vasodilation and hypotension (with rapid IV injection)
Hypersensitivity	Allergic reactions, skin eruptions
Gastrointestinal	Nausea, vomiting
Other	Postoperative atelectasis (with parenteral use)

OVERDOSAGE

Signs and symptoms	Early hypothermia followed by fever, sluggish or absent reflexes, respiratory depression, circulatory collapse, pulmonary edema, and coma
Treatment	Empty stomach by gastric lavage and institute general supportive measures, as needed, including IV fluid replacement and maintenance of blood pressure, body temperature, and adequate respiratory exchange. Dialysis may be helpful. Antibiotics may be required to control pulmonary complications.

DRUG INTERACTIONS

Alcohol, antihistamines, tranquilizers, and other CNS depressants	△ CNS depression
Oral anticoagulants	▽ Prothrombin time
Corticosteroids	▽ Corticosteroid effects
Digitalis, digitoxin	▽ Cardiac glycoside effects
Doxycycline	▽ Anti-infective effect
Tricyclic antidepressants	▽ Antidepressant effect
Griseofulvin	▽ Griseofulvin absorption
MAO inhibitors	△ Antidepressant or barbiturate effects

ALTERED LABORATORY VALUES

Blood/serum values	▽ Bilirubin

No clinically significant alterations in urinary values occur at therapeutic dosages

---

USE IN CHILDREN

See INDICATIONS for use of parenteral form; the safety and effectiveness of oral administration have not been established in children

USE IN PREGNANT AND NURSING WOMEN

Pregnancy Category B: use during pregnancy only if clearly needed. Animal reproduction studies have shown no evidence of impaired fertility or fetal harm; however, no adequate, well-controlled studies have been done in pregnant women. Neonatal depression may occur following use during labor. Administer with caution to nursing mothers.

BARBITURATES

GEMONIL (metharbital) Abbott C-III

Tablets: 100 mg

INDICATIONS	ORAL DOSAGE
Grand mal, petit mal, myoclonic, and mixed-type seizures	**Adult:** 100 mg 1–3 times/day, to start, followed by gradual increases in dosage, if needed and tolerated, up to 600–800 mg/day, until optimal clinical response is achieved **Child:** 50 mg 1–3 times/day, depending upon age and weight, or 5–15 mg/kg/day to start, followed by gradual increases in dosage until optimal clinical response is achieved

CONTRAINDICATIONS

Hypersensitivity to barbiturates	History of manifest or latent porphyria

ADMINISTRATION/DOSAGE ADJUSTMENTS

Combination therapy	May be used concomitantly with trimethadione, paramethadione, phenacemide, ethotoin, phenytoin, or mephenytoin; when adding metharbital to an established anticonvulsant regimen, gradually increase the dosage of metharbital while decreasing the dosage of the other agent

WARNINGS/PRECAUTIONS

Drug dependence	Psychic and/or physical dependence and tolerance may develop, especially in addiction-prone individuals

COMPENDIUM OF DRUG THERAPY

GEMONIL ■ MEBARAL

Patients with hepatic impairment	Use with caution and observe for signs of excessive drug accumulation
Patients with renal impairment	Use with caution; metharbital is converted in the liver to barbital (a long-acting barbiturate), which is excreted unchanged in urine[1]
Abrupt discontinuation of therapy	May precipitate status epilepticus; withdraw drug gradually

ADVERSE REACTIONS

Gastrointestinal	Gastric distress
Central nervous system	Dizziness, increased irritability; drowsiness (with large doses)
Dermatological	Rash

OVERDOSAGE

Signs and symptoms	Drowsiness, irritability, dizziness, and gastric distress, followed in cases of very large ingestions by loss of consciousness and coma
Treatment	Maintain and assist respiration and support circulation with vasopressors and IV fluids, as indicated. Evacuate stomach by gastric lavage, taking care to avoid pulmonary aspiration. Administer an osmotic diuretic and measure intake and output of fluids. Perform dialysis, if indicated. Administer antibiotics to control pulmonary complications, when necessary.

DRUG INTERACTIONS

Alcohol, general anesthetics, CNS depressants, MAO inhibitors	△ CNS depression
Oral anticoagulants	▽ Prothrombin time
Corticosteroids	▽ Corticosteroid effects
Digitalis, digitoxin	▽ Cardiac glycoside effects
Tricyclic antidepressants	▽ Antidepressant effect
Doxycycline	▽ Anti-infective effect
Griseofulvin	▽ Griseofulvin absorption
Phenytoin	△ or ▽ Phenytoin effects, depending on dosage of metharbital

ALTERED LABORATORY VALUES

Blood/serum values	▽ Bilirubin
No clinically significant alterations in urinary values occur at therapeutic dosages	

USE IN CHILDREN

See INDICATIONS and ORAL DOSAGE

USE IN PREGNANT AND NURSING WOMEN

An increased incidence of birth defects may be associated with the use of anticonvulsants during pregnancy. However, discontinuation of therapy may be considered only if removal of the drug does not pose any serious risk, such as the precipitation of status epilepticus with hypoxia in patients with serious convulsive disorders. Maternal ingestion of anticonvulsants may cause neonatal hemorrhage due to a coagulation defect. Administer prophylactic vitamin K_1 to mother 1 mo prior to and during delivery, and to infant intravenously immediately after birth. The safety of metharbital for use in nursing mothers has not been established.

[1] Gilman AG et al (eds): *The Pharmacological Basis of Therapeutics*, ed 6. New York, Macmillan, 1980, p 458.

BARBITURATES

MEBARAL (mephobarbital) Winthrop-Breon C-IV

Tablets: 32, 50, 100 mg

INDICATIONS	ORAL DOSAGE
Sedation for the relief of anxiety, tension, and apprehension	**Adult:** 32–100 mg (optimally, 50 mg) tid or qid **Child:** 16–32 mg tid or qid
Grand mal and petit mal seizures	**Adult:** 400–600 mg/day **Child (< 5 yr):** 16–32 mg tid or qid **Child (> 5 yr):** 32–64 mg tid or qid

MEBARAL

CONTRAINDICATIONS

Hypersensitivity to barbiturates	History of manifest or latent porphyria

ADMINISTRATION/DOSAGE ADJUSTMENTS

Special-risk patients	Reduce dosage in elderly or debilitated patients and patients with hepatic or renal impairment (see WARNINGS/PRECAUTIONS
Initiating anticonvulsant therapy	Start with small doses, and gradually titrate dosage upward over a period of 4–5 days until optimal dosage level is obtained (see ORAL DOSAGE). In patients receiving other anticonvulsants, gradually increase the dosage of mephobarbital while tapering the dosage of other agents.
Maintenance anticonvulsant therapy	Gradually reduce the dosage of mephobarbital over a period of 4–5 days to the lowest effective level
Combination anticonvulsant therapy	Mephobarbital may be alternated with phenobarbital or given concurrently (for adults, give 200–300 mg/day of mephobarbital combined with 50–100 mg/day of phenobarbital); when used in combination with phenytoin in adults, give 600 mg/day of mephobarbital and reduce the dosage of phenytoin to 230 mg/day
Timing of administration in epileptic patients	For nocturnal seizures, dosage should be taken at night; for diurnal seizures, dosage should be taken during the day

WARNINGS/PRECAUTIONS

Drug dependence	Psychic and/or physical dependence and tolerance may develop, especially after prolonged use of high doses. Instruct patients to adhere strictly to the dosage regimen. Use with caution, if at all, in mentally depressed patients and patients with suicidal tendencies or a history of drug abuse.
Excitement	In some patients, barbiturates repeatedly produce excitement rather than depression
Mental and/or physical impairment	Caution patients that their performance of potentially hazardous activities may be impaired while taking barbiturates, and that concurrent use with other CNS depressants (see DRUG INTERACTIONS) may cause increased CNS depression; instruct patients not to consume alcohol while taking this drug
Long-term therapy	Periodic laboratory evaluations, including tests of renal, hepatic, and hematopoietic function, should be performed during prolonged therapy
Elderly or debilitated patients	Reduce dosage, since such patients may be more sensitive to barbiturates, and may respond to usual doses with marked excitement, depression, or confusion
Patients with acute or chronic pain	Use with caution because paradoxical excitement may be induced or important symptoms masked; however, use as a sedative after surgery or as an adjunct to cancer chemotherapy is well established
Patients with hepatic or renal impairment	Reduce initial dosage and use with caution in patients with hepatic damage. Barbiturates should not be given to patients with premonitory signs of hepatic coma.
Abrupt discontinuation of therapy	May produce withdrawal symptoms after chronic use of high doses, resulting in tremors, weakness, insomnia, convulsions, and delirium. In epileptic patients, abrupt cessation of therapeutic doses may precipitate status epilepticus. Dosage should be gradually reduced over a period of 4–5 days.
Vitamin D deficiency	Vitamin D requirements may be increased; rickets and osteomalacia have occurred rarely following prolonged use of barbiturates
Other special-risk patients	Use with caution and adjust dosage carefully in patients with impaired hepatic, renal, cardiac, or respiratory function, and in patients with myasthenia gravis or myxedema
Status epilepticus	May be precipitated if treatment of epilepsy is suddenly discontinued; reduce the dosage of mephobarbital gradually over a period of 4–5 days
Carcinogenicity	Lifetime administration of phenobarbital sodium has caused benign and malignant liver-cell tumors in mice and benign liver-cell tumors in aged rats; phenobarbital is the major metabolite of mephobarbital

ADVERSE REACTIONS[1]

Frequent reactions (incidence ≥ 1%) are printed in *italics*

Central nervous system	*Somnolence (1–3%)*, agitation, confusion, hyperkinesia, ataxia, CNS depression, nightmares, nervousness, psychiatric disturbance, hallucinations, insomnia, anxiety, dizziness, thinking abnormality
Respiratory	Hypoventilation, apnea
Cardiovascular	Bradycardia, hypotension, syncope
Gastrointestinal	Nausea, vomiting, constipation
Other	Headache, injection site reactions, hypersensitivity reactions (angioedema, skin rashes, exfoliative dermatitis), fever, hepatic damage, megaloblastic anemia (following chronic phenobarbital use)

OVERDOSAGE

Signs and symptoms	Respiratory and CNS depression, possibly progressing to Cheyne-Stokes respiration, absent reflexes, slight miosis (in severe cases, paralytic dilation may occur), oliguria, tachycardia, hypotension, hypothermia, coma, and, in severe cases, apnea, circulatory collapse, respiratory arrest, and death
Treatment	Maintain an adequate airway, assist ventilation, and administer oxygen, as needed. Empty stomach by gastric lavage, taking care to avoid pulmonary aspiration. Monitor vital signs and fluid balance. Treat shock with fluids and other standard measures. If renal function is normal, force diuresis and alkalinize urine to help eliminate drug. Dialysis may be helpful in patients who are anuric, in shock, or severely intoxicated. For pulmonary complications, administer antibiotics.

DRUG INTERACTIONS

Alcohol, antihistamines, tranquilizers, and other CNS depressants	⇧ CNS depression
Oral anticoagulants	⇩ Prothrombin time
Corticosteroids	⇩ Corticosteroid effects
Digitalis, digitoxin	⇩ Cardiac glycoside effects
Doxycycline	⇩ Anti-infective effect
Griseofulvin	⇩ Griseofulvin absorption
Tricyclic antidepressants	⇩ Antidepressant effect
MAO inhibitors	⇧ Antidepressant or barbiturate effects

ALTERED LABORATORY VALUES

Blood/serum values	⇩ Bilirubin

No clinically significant alterations in urinary values occur at therapeutic dosages

USE IN CHILDREN

See INDICATIONS and dosage recommendations

USE IN PREGNANT AND NURSING WOMEN

Pregnancy Category D: barbiturates can cause harm to the fetus, and patients who use this drug during pregnancy or who become pregnant while taking it should be apprised of the potential hazards. Barbiturates readily cross the placental barrier and, following parenteral administration, can attain concentrations in fetal blood approaching those in the maternal circulation. They are distributed in all fetal tissues, reaching the highest concentration in the placenta, liver, and brain. Retrospective, case-controlled studies have suggested a connection between maternal barbiturate use and an increased incidence of fetal abnormalities; prenatal exposure to barbiturates has also been linked to an increased risk of brain tumors. Long-term exposure to barbiturates in utero (eg, throughout the last trimester) can result in neonatal dependence on barbiturates and withdrawal reactions, including hyperirritability and seizures, 0–14 days after birth. Although hypnotic doses do not significantly impair uterine activity, full anesthetic doses given during labor decrease the force and frequency of uterine contractions. Administration of barbiturates during labor and delivery, however, may cause respiratory depression in newborns, especially premature infants, and resuscitation equipment should be available. Neonatal coagulation defects, which have been observed in infants following exposure to anticonvulsants in utero, may be prevented by administering vitamin K_1 to the mother before delivery or to the infant at birth. Because small amounts of barbiturates have been detected in human milk, this drug should be used with caution in nursing mothers.

[1] These reactions have been reported in hospitalized patients, who may be less aware than fully ambulatory patients of some of the milder adverse effects of barbiturates; the incidence of such effects, therefore, may be somewhat higher in fully ambulatory patients

---

BARBITURATES

NEMBUTAL Elixir (pentobarbital) Abbott   C-II

Elixir (per 5 ml): pentobarbital equivalent to 20 mg pentobarbital sodium[1] (1 pt, 1 gal)

NEMBUTAL Sodium Capsules and Solution (pentobarbital sodium) Abbott   C-II

Capsules: 50, 100 mg   Ampuls: 50 mg/ml (2 ml)   Vials: 50 mg/ml (20, 50 ml)

INDICATIONS

Daytime sedation
Short-term (up to 2 wk) treatment of **insomnia**
Preanesthetic medication
Control of **acute convulsive episodes,** including those associated with status epilepticus, cholera, eclampsia, meningitis, tetanus, and toxic reactions to strychnine and local anesthetics (parenteral use only)

ORAL DOSAGE

Adult: for use as a sedative, 5 ml (1 tsp) tid or qid; for use as a hypnotic, 25 ml (5 tsp) or 100 mg at bedtime
Child: preoperatively, 2–6 mg/kg/24 h, up to 100 mg/day, depending upon age, weight, and desired degree of sedation; for use as a hypnotic, adjust dosage according to age and weight

PARENTERAL DOSAGE

Adult: 150–200 mg, given in a single IM injection, or 100 mg/70 kg IV to start, followed, if necessary, by additional small IV doses, up to a total of 200–500 mg IV
Child: 2–6 mg/kg, up to 100 mg, given in a single IM injection, or administer IV, using a proportionate reduction of the adult IV dose

NEMBUTAL Sodium Suppositories (pentobarbital sodium) Abbott

Suppositories: 30, 60, 120, 200 mg

INDICATIONS

Daytime sedation
Short-term (up to 2 wk) treatment of **insomnia**

RECTAL DOSAGE

Adult (average to above-average weight): for use as a hypnotic, one 120-mg or one 200-mg suppository; for use as a sedative, reduce dose appropriately
Child (2 mo to 1 yr; 10–20 lb): for use as a hypnotic, one 30-mg suppository
Child (1–4 yr; 20–40 lb): for use as a hypnotic, one 30-mg or one 60-mg suppository
Child (5–12 yr; 40–80 lb): for use as a hypnotic, one 60-mg suppository; for use as a sedative, reduce dose appropriately
Child (12–14 yr; 80–110 lb): for use as a hypnotic, one 60-mg or one 120-mg suppository; for use as a sedative, reduce dose appropriately

CONTRAINDICATIONS

Sensitivity to barbiturates

History of manifest or latent porphyria

ADMINISTRATION/DOSAGE ADJUSTMENTS

Parenteral therapy	Parenteral routes should be used only if oral administration is impossible or impractical. Since parenteral solutions are highly alkaline, exercise extreme caution to avoid extravascular or intraarterial injection. Any complaint of pain warrants stopping the injection.
Intramuscular administration	Intramuscular injection should be made deeply into a large muscle mass; to avoid possible tissue irritation, inject not more than 5 ml into any one site. Monitor vital signs after IM injection of hypnotic doses.
Intravenous administration	Use the IV route when prompt action is essential or when other routes are not feasible because of unconsciousness or patient resistance. Inject slowly ($\leq$ 50 mg/min), using fractional doses; wait at least 1 min after each dose to determine its full effect. Too rapid administration may cause vasodilation and decreased blood pressure, respiratory depression, apnea, and/or laryngospasm. During IV administration, monitor blood pressure, respiration, and cardiac function, and have equipment for resuscitation and artificial ventilation on hand.
Rectal administration	Use the rectal route when oral or parenteral routes are undesirable. Suppositories should not be divided.
Anticonvulsant use	Anesthetic doses are required for controlling seizures in emergencies; to avoid compounding the postictal depression that may occur, use the smallest effective dose. Inject slowly, and allow time for the drug to penetrate the blood-brain barrier and for the anticonvulsant effect to develop before administering a second dose.
Discontinuation of therapy	Reduce hypnotic doses gradually after regular use (eg, decrease the daily dose by one therapeutic dose every 5 or 6 days), since drug-withdrawal insomnia, increased dreaming, and nightmares may accompany abrupt cessation. Gradual discontinuation is essential after prolonged use by patients dependent on barbiturates since withdrawal manifestations (including delirium, convulsions, and possibly death) may otherwise result.

WARNINGS/PRECAUTIONS

Drug dependence	Psychic and/or physical dependence and tolerance may develop, especially after prolonged use of high doses. Instruct patients to adhere strictly to the dosage regimen. Use with caution, if at all, in mentally depressed patients and patients with suicidal tendencies or a history of drug abuse.
Excitement	In some patients, barbiturates repeatedly produce excitement rather than depression
Elderly or debilitated patients	Reduce dosage, since such patients may be more sensitive to barbiturates, and may respond to usual doses with marked excitement, depression, or confusion
Patients with acute or chronic pain	Use with caution because paradoxical excitement may be induced or important symptoms masked; however, use as a sedative after surgery or as an adjunct to cancer chemotherapy is well established
Patients with hepatic or renal impairment	Reduce initial dosage. Use with caution in patients with hepatic damage, since pentobarbital is almost entirely metabolized in the liver before it is excreted. Barbiturates should not be given to patients with premonitory signs of hepatic coma.
Ambulatory patients	Caution patients that their performance of potentially hazardous activities may be impaired while taking barbiturates, and that concurrent use with other CNS depressants (see DRUG INTERACTIONS) may cause increased CNS depression; instruct patients not to consume alcohol while taking this drug
Long-term therapy	Periodic laboratory evaluations, including tests of renal, hepatic, and hematopoietic function, should be performed during prolonged therapy
Tartrazine sensitivity	Presence of FD&C Yellow No. 5 (tartrazine) in the 100-mg capsules may cause allergic-type reactions, including bronchial asthma, in susceptible individuals
Carcinogenicity	Adequate data on the long-term potential for carcinogenicity have not been reported

NEMBUTAL

ADVERSE REACTIONS[2]

Frequent reactions (incidence ≥ 1%) are printed in *italics*

Central nervous system	*Somnolence (1–3%)*, agitation, confusion, hyperkinesia, ataxia, CNS depression, nightmares, nervousness, psychiatric disturbance, hallucinations, insomnia, anxiety, dizziness, thinking abnormality
Respiratory	Hypoventilation, apnea
Cardiovascular	Bradycardia, hypotension, syncope
Gastrointestinal	Nausea, vomiting, constipation
Other	Headache, injection site reactions, hypersensitivity reactions (angioedema, skin rashes, exfoliative dermatitis), fever, hepatic damage

OVERDOSAGE

Signs and symptoms	Respiratory and CNS depression, possibly progressing to Cheyne-Stokes respiration, absent reflexes, slight miosis (in severe cases, paralytic dilation may occur), oliguria, tachycardia, hypotension, hypothermia, coma, and, in severe cases, apnea, circulatory collapse, respiratory arrest, and death
Treatment	Maintain an adequate airway, assist ventilation, and administer oxygen, as needed. If patient is conscious, empty stomach by emesis and administer 30 mg of activated charcoal; if emesis is contraindicated, perform gastric lavage and instill activated charcoal. Take measures to prevent pulmonary aspiration during emesis; use a cuffed endotracheal tube for lavage. Administer a saline cathartic. Monitor vital signs and fluid balance. Treat shock with fluids and other standard measures. If renal function is normal, force diuresis to help eliminate drug. Dialysis may be helpful in patients who are anuric, in shock, or severely intoxicated. For pulmonary complications, administer antibiotics.

DRUG INTERACTIONS

Alcohol, antihistamines, tranquilizers, and other CNS depressants	⇧ CNS depression
Oral anticoagulants	⇩ Prothrombin time
Corticosteroids	⇩ Corticosteroid effects
Digitalis, digitoxin	⇩ Cardiac glycoside effects
Doxycycline	⇩ Anti-infective effect
Griseofulvin	⇩ Griseofulvin absorption
Tricyclic antidepressants	⇩ Antidepressant effect
MAO inhibitors	⇧ Antidepressant or barbiturate effects
Valproic acid	⇧ Barbiturate effects

ALTERED LABORATORY VALUES

Blood/serum values	⇩ Bilirubin

No clinically significant alterations in urinary values occur at therapeutic dosages

USE IN CHILDREN

See INDICATIONS and dosage recommendations

USE IN PREGNANT AND NURSING WOMEN

Pregnancy Category D: barbiturates can cause harm to the fetus, and patients who use this drug during pregnancy or who become pregnant while taking it should be apprised of the potential hazards. Barbiturates readily cross the placental barrier and, following parenteral administration, can attain concentrations in fetal blood approaching those in the maternal circulation. They are distributed in all fetal tissues, reaching the highest concentration in the placenta, liver, and brain. Retrospective, case-controlled studies have suggested a connection between maternal barbiturate use and an increased incidence of fetal abnormalities; prenatal exposure to barbiturates has also been linked to an increased risk of brain tumors. Long-term exposure to barbiturates in utero (eg, throughout the last trimester) can result in neonatal dependence on barbiturates and withdrawal reactions, including hyperirritability and seizures, 0–14 days after birth. Although hypnotic doses do not significantly impair uterine activity, full anesthetic doses given during labor decrease the force and frequency of uterine contractions. Administration of barbiturates during labor and delivery, however, may cause respiratory depression in newborns, especially premature infants, and resuscitation equipment should be available. Because small amounts of barbiturates have been detected in human milk, this drug should be used with caution in nursing mothers.

VEHICLE/BASE
Suppositories: semisynthetic glycerides and other ingredients

[1] Contains 18% alcohol
[2] These reactions have been reported in hospitalized patients, who may be less aware than fully ambulatory patients of some of the milder adverse effects of barbiturates; the incidence of such effects, therefore, may be somewhat higher in fully ambulatory patients

BARBITURATES

Phenobarbital   C-IV
Capsules: 16 mg   **Capsules (sustained release):** 65 mg   **Drops:** 16 mg/ml   **Elixir (per 5 ml):** 20 mg   **Tablets:** 8, 15, 16, 30, 32, 65, 100 mg

Phenobarbital sodium   C-IV
Ampuls: 65 mg/ml (2 ml), 130 mg/ml (1 ml), 163 mg/ml (2 ml)   **Vials:** 65, 120, 130, 325 mg   **Cartridge-needle units:** 30 mg/ml (1 ml)   **Prefilled syringes:** 65 mg/ml (1 ml), 130 mg/ml (1 ml)

INDICATIONS	ORAL DOSAGE	PARENTERAL DOSAGE
Daytime sedation	Adult: 30–120 mg/day, given in 2–3 divided doses; if sustained-release capsules are used, 65 mg bid (AM and PM) Child: 2 mg/kg or 60 mg/m² tid	Adult: 30–120 mg/day IM or IV, given in 2–3 divided doses
Preanesthetic medication	Child: 1–3 mg/kg	Adult: 100–200 mg IM 60–90 min before surgery Child: 16–100 mg or 1–3 mg/kg IM 60–90 min before surgery
Short-term (up to 2 wk) treatment of **insomnia**	Adult: 100–320 mg at bedtime Child: individualize dosage according to age and weight	Adult: 100–320 mg IM or IV at bedtime Child: 3–5 mg/kg IM or IV
Long-term treatment of **generalized tonic-clonic and cortical focal seizures**	Adult: 50–100 mg bid or tid Child: 3–5 mg/kg/day or 125 mg/m²/day given as a single dose at bedtime or divided	—
Control of **acute convulsive episodes**, including those associated with status epilepticus, cholera, eclampsia, meningitis, tetanus, and toxic reactions to strychnine and local anesthetics	—	Adult: for status epilepticus, 200–320 mg IV, repeated after 6 h, if needed Child: for status epilepticus, 15–20 mg/kg IV, given over a period of 10–15 min

CONTRAINDICATIONS
Sensitivity to barbiturates	History of manifest or latent porphyria

ADMINISTRATION/DOSAGE ADJUSTMENTS
Parenteral therapy	Parenteral routes should be used only if oral administration is impossible or impractical. Since parenteral solutions are highly alkaline, exercise extreme caution to avoid extravascular or intraarterial injection. Any complaint of pain warrants stopping the injection.
Intramuscular administration	Intramuscular injection should be made deeply into a large muscle mass; to avoid possible tissue irritation, inject not more than 5 ml into any one site. Monitor vital signs after IM injection of hypnotic doses.
Intravenous administration	Use the IV route when prompt action is essential or when other routes are not feasible because of unconsciousness or patient resistance. Inject slowly ($\leq$ 60 mg/min), using fractional doses (however, in the treatment of status epilepticus, use a full anticonvulsant dose initially). Wait after each dose to determine its full effect; it may take 15 min or longer before peak levels in the brain are attained. Too rapid administration may cause vasodilation and decreased blood pressure, respiratory depression, apnea, and/or laryngospasm. During IV administration, monitor blood pressure, respiration, and cardiac function, and have equipment for resuscitation and artificial ventilation on hand.
Anticonvulsant use	Subhypnotic, oral doses of phenobarbital are effective in long-term anticonvulsant therapy. Adjust dosage to achieve a serum phenobarbital level of 10–25 μg/ml; children may require higher per-kilogram dosages than adults to achieve therapeutic serum levels. For acute convulsant episodes, use the smallest effective dose to avoid compounding the postictal depression that may occur. Inject slowly, and allow time for the drug to penetrate the blood-brain barrier.
Discontinuation of therapy	Reduce hypnotic doses gradually after regular use (eg, decrease the daily dose by one therapeutic dose every 5 or 6 days), since drug-withdrawal insomnia, increased dreaming, and nightmares may accompany abrupt cessation. Gradual discontinuation is essential after prolonged use by patients dependent on barbiturates, since withdrawal manifestations (including delirium, convulsions, and possibly death) may otherwise result.

WARNINGS/PRECAUTIONS
Drug dependence	Psychic and/or physical dependence and tolerance may develop, especially after prolonged use of high doses. Instruct patients to adhere strictly to the dosage regimen. Use with caution, if at all, in mentally depressed patients and patients with suicidal tendencies or a history of drug abuse.
Excitement	In some patients, barbiturates repeatedly produce excitement rather than depression
Elderly or debilitated patients	Reduce dosage, since such patients may be more sensitive to barbiturates, and may respond to usual doses with marked excitement, depression, or confusion
Patients with acute or chronic pain	Use with caution because paradoxical excitement may be induced or important symptoms masked; however, use as a sedative after surgery or as an adjunct to cancer chemotherapy is well established

Phenobarbital

Patients with hepatic or renal impairment	Reduce initial dosage; approximately 25–50% of a phenobarbital dose is excreted unchanged. Use with caution in patients with hepatic damage; barbiturates should not be given to patients with premonitory signs of hepatic coma.
Ambulatory patients	Caution patients that their performance of potentially hazardous activities may be impaired while taking barbiturates, and that concurrent use with other CNS depressants (see DRUG INTERACTIONS) may cause increased CNS depression; instruct patients not to consume alcohol while taking this drug
Long-term therapy	Periodic laboratory evaluations, including tests of renal, hepatic, and hematopoietic function, should be performed during prolonged therapy
Treatment and prophylaxis of febrile seizures	Phenobarbital has been used in the treatment and prophylaxis of febrile seizures; however, it has not been established that prevention of febrile seizures can influence the subsequent development of epilepsy
Carcinogenicity	Lifetime administration of phenobarbital sodium has caused benign and malignant liver-cell tumors in mice and benign liver-cell tumors in rats

ADVERSE REACTIONS[1]

Frequent reactions (incidence ≥ 1%) are printed in *italics*

Central nervous system	*Somnolence (1–3%)*, agitation, confusion, hyperkinesia, ataxia, CNS depression, nightmares, nervousness, psychiatric disturbance, hallucinations, insomnia, anxiety, dizziness, thinking abnormality
Respiratory	Hypoventilation, apnea
Cardiovascular	Bradycardia, hypotension, syncope
Gastrointestinal	Nausea, vomiting, constipation
Other	Headache, injection site reactions, hypersensitivity reactions (angioedema, skin rashes, exfoliative dermatitis), fever, hepatic damage, megaloblastic anemia (following chronic use)

OVERDOSAGE

Signs and symptoms	Respiratory and CNS depression, possibly progressing to Cheyne-Stokes respiration, absent reflexes, slight miosis (in severe cases, paralytic dilation may occur), oliguria, tachycardia, hypotension, hypothermia, coma, and, in severe cases, apnea, circulatory collapse, respiratory arrest, and death
Treatment	Maintain an adequate airway, assist ventilation, and administer oxygen, as needed. Empty stomach by gastric lavage, taking care to avoid pulmonary aspiration. Monitor vital signs and fluid balance. Treat shock with fluids and other standard measures. If renal function is normal, force diuresis and alkalinize urine to help eliminate drug. Dialysis may be helpful in patients who are anuric, in shock, or severely intoxicated. For pulmonary complications, administer antibiotics.

DRUG INTERACTIONS

Alcohol, antihistamines, tranquilizers, and other CNS depressants	△ CNS depression
Oral anticoagulants	▽ Prothrombin time
Corticosteroids	▽ Corticosteroid effects
Digitalis, digitoxin	▽ Cardiac glycoside effects
Doxycycline	▽ Anti-infective effect
Griseofulvin	▽ Griseofulvin absorption
Tricyclic antidepressants	▽ Antidepressant effect
MAO inhibitors	△ Antidepressant or barbiturate effects

ALTERED LABORATORY VALUES

Blood/serum values	▽ Bilirubin

No clinically significant alterations in urinary values occur at therapeutic dosages

USE IN CHILDREN

See INDICATIONS and dosage recommendations

USE IN PREGNANT AND NURSING WOMEN

Pregnancy Category D: barbiturates can cause harm to the fetus, and patients who use this drug during pregnancy or who become pregnant while taking it should be apprised of the potential hazards. Barbiturates readily cross the placental barrier and, following parenteral administration, can attain concentrations in fetal blood approaching those in the maternal circulation. They are distributed in all fetal tissues, reaching the highest concentration in the placenta, liver, and brain. Retrospective, case-controlled studies have suggested a connection between maternal barbiturate use and an increased incidence of fetal abnormalities; prenatal exposure to barbiturates has also been linked to an increased risk of brain tumors. Long-term exposure to barbiturates in utero (eg, throughout the last trimester) can result in neonatal dependence on barbiturates and withdrawal reactions, including hyperirritability and seizures, 0–14 days after birth. Although hypnotic doses do not significantly impair uterine activity, full anesthetic doses given during labor decrease the force and frequency of uterine contractions. Administration of barbiturates during labor and delivery, however, may cause respiratory depression in newborns, especially premature infants, and resuscitation equipment should be available. Because small amounts of barbiturates have been detected in human milk, this drug should be used with caution in nursing mothers.

---

[1] These reactions have been reported in hospitalized patients, who may be less aware than fully ambulatory patients of some of the milder adverse effects of barbiturates; the incidence of such effects, therefore, may be somewhat higher in fully ambulatory patients

BARBITURATES

SECONAL Sodium Capsules (secobarbital sodium) Lilly C-II
Capsules: 50, 100 mg

INDICATIONS	ORAL DOSAGE
Insomnia	**Adult:** 100 mg at bedtime for up to 2 wk
Preanesthetic medication	**Adult:** 200–300 mg 1–2 h before surgery **Child:** 2–6 mg/kg, up to 100 mg, 1–2 h before surgery

SECONAL Sodium Injection (secobarbital sodium) Lilly C-II
Vials: 50 mg/ml (20 ml)

INDICATIONS	PARENTERAL DOSAGE	RECTAL DOSAGE
Preanesthetic medication	**Adult:** for general, spinal, or regional anesthesia or for intubation procedures, up to 250 mg IV (usual dosage for spinal or regional anesthesia: 50–100 mg); if the desired degree of hypnosis is not attained after use of 250 mg, give a small quantity of meperidine. For dental nerve block, administer 100–150 mg IV.	**Child (< 40 kg):** for ear, nose, and throat procedures, 5 mg/kg of a 1–1.5% solution **Child (≥ 40 kg):** for ear, nose, and throat procedures, 4 mg/kg of a 1–1.5% solution
Preoperative sedation	**Adult:** 2.2 mg/kg, up to 100 mg, IM 10–15 min before a dental procedure; for lighter sedation, reduce dose to 1.1–1.6 mg/kg **Child:** same as adult	—
Convulsions associated with tetanus	**Adult:** 5.5 mg/kg IM or IV q3–4h, as needed	—

SECONAL Sodium Suppositories (secobarbital sodium) Lilly C-III
Suppositories: 200 mg

INDICATIONS	RECTAL DOSAGE
Sedative-hypnotic use	**Adult:** 120–200 mg for up to 2 wk

CONTRAINDICATIONS

Hypersensitivity to barbiturates	History of addiction to a sedative-hypnotic	Significant cardiac disease (vials only)
History of manifest or latent porphyria	Marked hepatic impairment	Obstetrical delivery (vials only)
Respiratory disease associated with dyspnea or obstruction	Acute or chronic pain	Renal impairment (vials only)

ADMINISTRATION/DOSAGE ADJUSTMENTS

Use of vials — For IV or IM administration, the solution may be used as supplied or diluted with sterile water for injection, 0.9% sodium chloride injection, or Ringer's injection. The rate of IV injection should not exceed 50 mg/15 s; respiratory depression, apnea, laryngospasm, or vasodilation with hypotension may occur if IV administration is too rapid. If the IM route is used, inject deeply into a large muscle, and do not give more than 5 ml (regardless of dilution) at any one site; after IM injection of large hypnotic doses, observe patient for 20–30 min, since excessive narcosis may occur. For rectal administration to children, the solution should be diluted with lukewarm water to a concentration of 1–1.5% and then given after a cleansing enema; atropine may be administered concomitantly to dry respiratory-tract secretions. After rectal administration, children should be observed for 15–20 min.

WARNINGS/PRECAUTIONS

Drug dependence — Psychic and/or physical dependence and tolerance may develop with continued use. Administration of more than 400 mg/day for 90 days can produce physical dependence; use of 600–800 mg/day for at least 35 days, when followed by abrupt discontinuation, can result in withdrawal seizures. (A barbiturate addict usually takes 1.5 g/day.) Symptoms of dependence are similar to those of chronic alcoholism; withdrawal reactions range in severity from anxiety, muscle twitching, and dizziness to convulsions, delirium, and death. To avoid dependence, limit each prescription to an amount required until the next appointment, warn patients not to increase the dosage on their own, and use with caution, if at all, in patients with a history of drug abuse. To treat dependence, cautiously and gradually reduce the dosage of secobarbital or a substituted drug. The specific method of withdrawal may vary. In one regimen, phenobarbital is given orally 3–4 times/day as a substitute for the total daily dose of secobarbital (30 mg/day of phenobarbital for each 100–200 mg/day of secobarbital). Once the patient is stabilized, the dosage is reduced daily by 10%. In a modification of this regimen, up to 600 mg/day of phenobarbital is substituted; however, if withdrawal reactions occur on the first day of treatment, an additional 200–300 mg of phenobarbital is given IM as a loading dose. Once the patient is stabilized, the dosage is reduced daily by 30 mg.

SECONAL Sodium

Depressed or suicidal patients	Use with caution, if at all, in patients who are mentally depressed or who have suicidal tendencies
Elderly or debilitated patients	Reduce dosage for elderly or debilitated patients, since these patients may be more sensitive to barbiturates and may respond to usual doses with marked excitement, depression, or confusion
Patients with hepatic or renal impairment	Reduce the dosage for patients with decreased hepatic function, and do not use in patients with marked hepatic impairment, since secobarbital is metabolized in the liver. Reduce the dosage of the capsules and suppositories for patients with renal impairment; do not administer the solution contained in the vials to such patients because the polyethylene glycol vehicle may irritate the kidneys.
Patients with borderline hypoadrenal function	Secobarbital may diminish the systemic effects of cortisol and exogenous hydrocortisone; use secobarbital with caution in patients with borderline hypoadrenal function
Drowsiness	Caution patients that their ability to drive or perform other potentially hazardous activities may be impaired. If secobarbital has been used in an office procedure, the patient should be discharged in the company of another person.
Paradoxical response	In some patients, barbiturates repeatedly produce excitement rather than depression
Long-term therapy	Periodic laboratory evaluations, including tests of renal, hepatic, and hematopoietic function, should be performed during prolonged therapy

ADVERSE REACTIONS[1]

The most frequent reaction is italicized

Central nervous system	*Somnolence (1–3%)*, agitation, confusion, hyperkinesia, ataxia, CNS depression, nightmares, nervousness, psychiatric disturbance, hallucinations, insomnia, anxiety, dizziness, thinking abnormality
Respiratory	Hypoventilation, apnea
Cardiovascular	Bradycardia, hypotension, syncope
Gastrointestinal	Nausea, vomiting, constipation
Other	Headache, injection site reactions, hypersensitivity reactions (angioedema, skin rashes, exfoliative dermatitis), fever, hepatic damage

OVERDOSAGE

Signs and symptoms	Respiratory and CNS depression, possibly progressing to Cheyne-Stokes respiration, absent reflexes, slight miosis (in severe cases, paralytic dilation may occur), oliguria, tachycardia, hypotension, hypothermia, coma, and, in severe cases, apnea, circulatory collapse, respiratory arrest, and death. A flat EEG, which may be observed following extreme overdosage, does not indicate death; cessation of electric activity in the brain can be fully reversed if hypoxic damage has not occurred.
Treatment	Maintain an adequate airway, assist ventilation, and administer oxygen, as needed. Induce emesis if patient is conscious, taking care to avoid pulmonary aspiration; if emesis is contraindicated, perform gastric lavage with a cuffed endotracheal tube and with the patient in a face-down position. Activated charcoal, followed by a saline cathartic, may be administered after emesis or lavage. Monitor vital signs and fluid balance. Treat shock with fluids and other standard measures. If renal function is normal, force diuresis to help eliminate drug. Dialysis may be helpful in patients who are anuric, in shock, or severely intoxicated. For pulmonary complications, administer antibiotics. To prevent hypostatic pneumonia, decubiti, aspiration, and other complications, roll patient from side to side every 30 min and take other appropriate measures.

DRUG INTERACTIONS

Alcohol, antihistamines, tranquilizers, and other CNS depressants	△ CNS depression; instruct patients not to consume alcohol during therapy, and warn them about using other CNS depressants in combination with secobarbital
Oral anticoagulants	▽ Prothrombin time; during concomitant therapy, check the prothrombin time more frequently
Corticosteroids	▽ Corticosteroid effects
Digitalis, digitoxin	▽ Cardiac glycoside effects
Doxycycline	▽ Anti-infective effect
Griseofulvin	▽ Griseofulvin absorption
Tricyclic antidepressants	▽ Antidepressant effect
MAO inhibitors	△ Antidepressant or barbiturate effects

ALTERED LABORATORY VALUES

Blood/serum values	▽ Bilirubin

No clinically significant alterations in urinary values occur at therapeutic dosages

USE IN CHILDREN

See INDICATIONS and dosage recommendations

USE IN PREGNANT AND NURSING WOMEN

Pregnancy Category D: barbiturates can cause harm to the fetus, and patients who use this drug during pregnancy or who become pregnant while taking it should be apprised of the potential hazards. Retrospective, case-controlled studies have suggested a connection between maternal barbiturate use and an increased incidence of fetal abnormalities. Exposure to barbiturates in utero throughout the last trimester can result in neonatal dependence and in withdrawal reactions, including hyperirritability and seizures, 0–14 days after birth; phenobarbital may be used to treat dependence (3–10 mg/kg/day is given until withdrawal reactions cease, and then the dosage is decreased gradually over a period of 2 wk). Full anesthetic doses of barbiturates decrease the force and frequency of uterine contractions; however, hypnotic doses do not significantly impair uterine activity. Administration of barbiturates during labor and delivery may cause respiratory depression in newborns, especially premature infants, and resuscitation equipment should be available. Because small amounts of some barbiturates have been detected in human milk, this drug should be used with caution in nursing mothers.

[1] These reactions have been reported in hospitalized patients, who may be less aware than fully ambulatory patients of some of the milder adverse effects of barbiturates; the incidence of such effects, therefore, may be somewhat higher in fully ambulatory patients

---

HYDANTOINS

DILANTIN (phenytoin sodium, extended) Parke-Davis   Rx

Capsules: 30, 100 mg

DILANTIN (phenytoin) Parke-Davis   Rx

Chewable tablets: 50 mg (Dilantin Infatabs)   **Suspension (per 5 ml):** 30 mg[1] (Dilantin-30 Pediatric Suspension), 125 mg[1] (Dilantin-125 Suspension)

INDICATIONS

Control of **generalized tonic-clonic (grand mal) and complex partial (psychomotor, temporal lobe) seizures**
Prevention and treatment of seizures associated with **neurosurgery**

ORAL DOSAGE

Adult: one 100-mg cap, two 50-mg tabs, or 5 ml of Dilantin-125 suspension tid to start, followed, if necessary, by up to 600–625 mg/day; usual maintenance dosage: 300–400 mg/day. For most patients taking the capsules, a maintenance dosage of 100 mg tid or qid is satisfactory; however, if desired, the dosage for a patient requiring 300 mg/day may be changed from 100 mg tid to 300 mg once daily.
Child: 5 mg/kg/day, given in 2–3 equally divided doses, to start, followed, if necessary, by up to 300 mg/day (children over 6 yr of age may require this maximum dosage); usual maintenance dosage: 4–8 mg/kg/day. If the daily dose cannot be divided equally, give the larger dose at bedtime.

CONTRAINDICATIONS

Hypersensitivity to hydantoins

ADMINISTRATION/DOSAGE ADJUSTMENTS

Administration of tablets	Tablets may be chewed thoroughly or swallowed whole
Dosage adjustment	Allow at least 7–10 days to elapse after each change in dosage. To achieve optimal dosage in some patients, determination of the serum level may be necessary; the therapeutic level is usually 10–20 µg/ml.
Loading dose	The capsules can be used in adults for rapid attainment of a steady-state therapeutic serum level when IV administration is undesirable. Give 1 g in 3 divided doses (400 mg, 300 mg, 300 mg), allowing 2 h between each dose; 24 h after the loading dose, begin administration at the normal maintenance dosage (100 mg tid or qid). Closely monitor the serum level during the initial 24-h period (patients should be in a clinic or hospital); determine the serum level frequently once the normal regimen is instituted. A loading dose should not be given to patients with renal or hepatic disease.
Adjusting for differences in bioavailability of phenytoin preparations	Whenever a preparation is changed (eg, from phenytoin sodium to phenytoin or from extended phenytoin sodium to prompt phenytoin sodium), the serum level should be monitored and caution exercised. Careful dosage adjustment and monitoring of serum phenytoin levels may also be necessary when switching from preparations containing the free acid form of the drug (the tablets and suspensions) to those containing the sodium salt (such as the capsules) and vice versa.

DILANTIN

WARNINGS/PRECAUTIONS

General toxicity — The optimal serum phenytoin level generally ranges from 10 to 20 µg/ml, with nystagmus (on lateral gaze) usually occurring at 20 µg/ml, ataxia at 30 µg/ml, and dysarthria and lethargy at over 40 µg/ml; however, in some cases, concentrations as high as 50 µg/ml have been seen without evidence of toxicity. If a toxic serum level is sustained, confusional states (delirium, psychosis, encephalopathy) or, in rare cases, irreversible cerebellar dysfunction may result. Elderly or gravely ill patients, as well as those who have hepatic impairment or who metabolize phenytoin slowly, are particularly likely to manifest toxic effects. At the first sign of acute toxicity in a patient, determine the serum level and, if the value is excessive, reduce the dosage; if symptoms persist, treatment should be discontinued.

Lymphadenopathy — Localized or generalized lymphadenopathy, ranging from pseudolymphoma and benign lymph node hyperplasia to lymphoma and Hodgkin's disease, may occur during therapy; serum sickness-like signs and symptoms, such as fever, rash, and hepatic reactions, may accompany lymph node changes. If lymphadenopathy is seen, the possibility that the condition results from phenytoin should be considered, even though a causal relationship has not been established; every effort should be made to substitute another anticonvulsant, and the patient should be observed for an extended period.

Rash — Dermatological reactions, sometimes accompanied by fever, range in severity from morbilliform rash (the most common reaction) to Stevens-Johnson syndrome. If an exfoliative, purpuric, or bullous rash appears or if lupus erythematosus or Stevens-Johnson syndrome is suspected, administration should be permanently discontinued. If a milder rash (eg, a morbilliform or scarlatiniform rash) is seen, therapy should be halted until the rash completely disappears; if the rash recurs when treatment is resumed, the drug must be permanently withdrawn.

Blood dyscrasias — Severe, potentially fatal hematological reactions, including thrombocytopenia, leukopenia, granulocytopenia, agranulocytosis, and pancytopenia, have been associated with phenytoin; these reactions have occurred with and without bone marrow suppression. Macrocytosis and megaloblastic anemia have also been seen; these disorders usually can be treated with folic acid.

Hyperglycemia — Phenytoin may increase the serum glucose level in diabetic patients and cause hyperglycemia in normal patients

Alcoholic beverages — The serum phenytoin level may be increased by acute intake of alcohol, but may be decreased by chronic use

Osteomalacia — Phenytoin may interfere with the metabolism of vitamin D and cause osteomalacia

Gingival hyperplasia — To minimize the risk of gingival hyperplasia, instruct patients to maintain good dental hygiene

Absence seizures, convulsions owing to metabolic disorders — Phenytoin is not effective in the treatment of absence (petit mal) seizures, but may be used in combination with other drugs if a patient exhibits both tonic-clonic and absence seizures; this drug should not be used for seizures owing to hypoglycemia or other metabolic disorders

Discontinuation of phenytoin — Abrupt withdrawal may precipitate status epilepticus. In general, phenytoin should be discontinued or its dosage reduced in a gradual manner; however, if a hypersensitivity reaction occurs, a nonhydantoin anticonvulsant may be rapidly substituted for phenytoin

ADVERSE REACTIONS

The most frequent reactions, regardless of incidence, are printed in *italics*

Central nervous system — *Nystagmus, ataxia, slurred speech, decreased coordination, confusion,* dizziness, insomnia, transient nervousness, motor twitchings, headaches; neuroleptic-type dyskinesias (rare), including chorea, dystonia, tremor, and asterixis; predominantly sensory peripheral polyneuropathy (with long-term use of phenytoin)

Gastrointestinal — Nausea, vomiting, constipation

Dermatological — Scarlatiniform or morbilliform rash, lupus erythematosus, Stevens-Johnson syndrome; bullous, exfoliative, and purpuric dermatitis

Hematological — Thrombocytopenia, leukopenia, granulocytopenia, agranulocytosis, pancytopenia, macrocytosis, megaloblastic anemia

Hepatic — Toxic hepatitis, liver damage

Oral — Gingival hyperplasia, enlargement of the lips

Other — Lymphadenopathy, coarsening of facial features, hypertrichosis, Peyronie's disease, systemic lupus erythematosus, periarteritis nodosa, immunoglobulin abnormalities

OVERDOSAGE

Signs and symptoms — Nystagmus, ataxia, dysarthria, tremor, hyperreflexia, lethargy, slurred speech, nausea, vomiting, hypotension, coma, respiratory and circulatory depression

Treatment — Monitor respiratory and circulatory function; institute appropriate measures. Hemodialysis may be considered for removal of the drug from the blood; total exchange transfusion has been used for the treatment of severe toxicity in children.

DILANTIN ■ DILANTIN Parenteral

DRUG INTERACTIONS

Acute alcohol ingestion, chloramphenicol, chlordiazepoxide, cimetidine, diazepam, dicumarol, disulfiram, ethosuximide, halothane, isoniazid, methylphenidate, phenothiazines, phenylbutazone, salicylates, sulfonamides, tolbutamide, trazodone	⇧ Serum phenytoin level; monitor serum level and, if necessary, adjust dosage
Calcium-containing antacids, chronic alcohol abuse, carbamazepine, molindone, reserpine	⇩ Serum phenytoin level; monitor serum level and, if necessary, adjust dosage. Separate administration of phenytoin and a calcium-containing antacid if the patient's serum level is low.
Phenobarbital, valproic acid, divalproex sodium	⇧ or ⇩ Serum phenytoin level; monitor serum level and, if necessary, adjust dosage ⇧ or ⇩ Serum level of interacting drug
Corticosteroids, digitoxin, doxycycline, furosemide, oral anticoagulants, quinidine, rifampin, vitamin D	⇩ Pharmacologic effect of interacting drug
Estrogens (including oral contraceptives)	⇧ Serum phenytoin level; monitor serum level and, if necessary, adjust dosage ⇩ Pharmacologic effect of estrogens
Tricyclic antidepressants	⇧ Risk of seizures; monitor serum level and, if necessary, adjust dosage

ALTERED LABORATORY VALUES

Blood/serum values	⇩ PBI ⇧ Glucose ⇧ Alkaline phosphatase ⇧ SGGT
Urinary values	Subnormal increase in 17-OHCS and 17-KS (with dexamethasone and metyrapone tests)

USE IN CHILDREN

See INDICATIONS and PARENTERAL DOSAGE

USE IN PREGNANT AND NURSING WOMEN

In a number of reports, use of phenytoin during pregnancy has been associated with an increase in adverse congenital effects, such as heart malformations, cleft lip and palate, microcephaly, mental deficiency, and impaired prenatal growth; isolated cases of malignancy, including neuroblastomas, have also been seen in children whose mothers received this drug during pregnancy. Nevertheless, prophylactic treatment of major seizures should not be discontinued during pregnancy, since there is a strong possibility that withdrawal may precipitate status epilepticus with attendant hypoxia and threat to life. However, if removal of the drug will not pose a serious risk, discontinuation of phenytoin may be considered, although it should be recognized that even minor seizures may pose some hazard to the embryo or fetus. In a large proportion of women, pregnancy increases the risk of seizures by altering the absorption or metabolism of phenytoin; serum levels should be determined periodically during pregnancy and, if necessary, the dosage should be adjusted. Coagulation defects may occur within the first 24 h postpartum in a neonate whose mother was receiving phenytoin; to reduce this risk, vitamin K should be given to the mother before delivery and to the neonate after birth. Phenytoin is excreted in low concentrations in human milk; woman taking this drug should not nurse.

[1] Contains not more than 0.6% alcohol

HYDANTOINS

DILANTIN Parenteral (phenytoin sodium) Parke-Davis Rx

Ampuls: 50 mg/ml (2, 5 ml)   **Prefilled syringes:** 50 mg/ml

INDICATIONS	PARENTERAL DOSAGE
Control of grand mal **status epilepticus**	**Adult:** 10–15 mg/kg IV, followed by 100 mg IV or orally (using a suitable oral phenytoin preparation) q6–8h; the rate of injection should not exceed 50 mg/min **Child:** 15–20 mg/kg IV; the rate of injection in neonates should not exceed 1–3 mg/kg/min
Prevention of seizures associated with **neurosurgery**	**Adult:** 100–200 mg IM q4h during and after surgery; for patients requiring more than 1 wk of treatment, consider using an alternative route, such as gastric intubation

CONTRAINDICATIONS

Hypersensitivity to hydantoins	Adams-Stokes syndrome	Second- or third-degree AV block
Sinus bradycardia	Sinoatrial block	

DILANTIN Parenteral

ADMINISTRATION/DOSAGE ADJUSTMENTS

Status epilepticus	Using a large-gauge needle or IV catheter, inject the solution directly into a large vein; to prevent local venous irritation, follow with sterile saline through the same needle or catheter. SC or perivascular injection should be avoided. Continuous IV infusion is not advisable because precipitation may occur. IM injection is also not recommended because of delayed absorption. Monitor ECG and blood pressure continuously, watch for signs of respiratory depression, and measure serum phenytoin level (see warning, below, regarding toxicity). For rapid control of seizures, an IV benzodiazepine (eg, diazepam) or an IV short-acting barbiturate will usually be necessary because phenytoin must be injected slowly. If seizures persist despite administration of phenytoin, consider general anesthesia, use of other anticonvulsants, or other appropriate measures.
Adjusting for differences in oral and parenteral bioavailability	To maintain therapeutic serum levels when switching from oral to IM administration, give an IM dose that is 50% greater than the oral dose; when resuming oral therapy, administer one-third the IM dose (one-half the original oral dose) for a period of time equal to the duration of IM administration. Careful dosage adjustment and monitoring of serum phenytoin levels may be necessary when switching from preparations containing the free acid form of the drug (chewable tablets and oral suspensions) to parenteral phenytoin and vice versa.

WARNINGS/PRECAUTIONS

General toxicity	The optimal serum phenytoin level generally ranges from 10 to 20 $\mu g/ml$, with nystagmus (on lateral gaze) usually occurring at 20 $\mu g/ml$, ataxia at 30 $\mu g/ml$, and dysarthria and lethargy at over 40 $\mu g/ml$; however, in some cases, concentrations as high as 50 $\mu g/ml$ have been seen without evidence of toxicity. If a toxic serum level is sustained, confusional states (delirium, psychosis, encephalopathy) or, in rare cases, irreversible cerebellar dysfunction may result. Elderly or gravely ill patients, as well as those who have hepatic impairment or who metabolize phenytoin slowly, are particularly likely to manifest toxic effects. At the first sign of acute toxicity in a patient, determine the serum level and, if the value is excessive, reduce the dosage; if symptoms persist, treatment should be discontinued.
Cardiotoxicity	Rapid IV administration usually causes hypotension. Severe, potentially fatal cardiotoxicity, with depression of atrial and ventricular conduction and ventricular fibrillation, has occurred during therapy, most commonly in elderly or gravely ill patients. Exercise caution in patients with hypotension or severe myocardial insufficiency.
Lymphadenopathy	Localized or generalized lymphadenopathy, ranging from pseudolymphoma and benign lymph node hyperplasia to lymphoma and Hodgkin's disease, may occur during therapy; serum sickness-like signs and symptoms, such as fever, rash, and hepatic reactions, may accompany lymph node changes. If lymphadenopathy is seen, the possibility that the condition results from phenytoin should be considered, even though a causal relationship has not been established; every effort should be made to substitute another anticonvulsant, and the patient should be observed for an extended period.
Rash	Dermatological reactions, sometimes accompanied by fever, range in severity from morbilliform rash (the most common reaction) to Stevens-Johnson syndrome. If an exfoliative, purpuric, or bullous rash appears or if lupus erythematosus or Stevens-Johnson syndrome is suspected, administration should be permanently discontinued. If a milder rash (eg, a morbilliform or scarlatiniform rash) is seen, therapy should be halted until the rash completely disappears; if the rash recurs when treatment is resumed, the drug must be permanently withdrawn.
Blood dyscrasias	Severe, potentially fatal hematological reactions, including thrombocytopenia, leukopenia, granulocytopenia, agranulocytosis, and pancytopenia, have been associated with phenytoin; these reactions have occurred with and without bone marrow suppression. Macrocytosis and megaloblastic anemia have also been seen; these disorders usually can be treated with folic acid.
Hyperglycemia	Phenytoin may increase the serum glucose level in diabetic patients and cause hyperglycemia in normal patients
Alcoholic beverages	The serum phenytoin level may be increased by acute intake of alcohol, but may be decreased by chronic use
Absence seizures, convulsions owing to metabolic disorders	Phenytoin is not effective in the treatment of absence (petit mal) seizures, but may be used in combination with other drugs if a patient exhibits both tonic-clonic and absence seizures; this drug should not be used for seizures owing to hypoglycemia or other metabolic disorders
Local irritation	Soft tissue irritation and inflammation, ranging from slight tenderness to extensive necrosis and sloughing, can occur at the site of IV injection; local reactions are not always associated with extravasation

ADVERSE REACTIONS

The most frequent reactions, regardless of incidence, are printed in *italics*

Cardiovascular	Hypotension, cardiovascular collapse, depression of atrial and ventricular conduction, ventricular fibrillation
Central nervous system	*Nystagmus, ataxia, slurred speech, decreased coordination, confusion,* dizziness, insomnia, transient nervousness, motor twitchings, headaches; neuroleptic-type dyskinesias (rare), including chorea, dystonia, tremor, and asterixis; predominantly sensory peripheral polyneuropathy (with long-term use of phenytoin)

DILANTIN Parenteral

Gastrointestinal	Nausea, vomiting, constipation
Dermatological	Scarlatiniform and morbilliform rash, lupus erythematosus, Stevens-Johnson syndrome; bullous, exfoliative, and purpuric dermatitis
Hematological	Thrombocytopenia, leukopenia, granulocytopenia, agranulocytosis, pancytopenia, macrocytosis, megaloblastic anemia
Hepatic	Toxic hepatitis, liver damage
Oral	Gingival hyperplasia, enlargement of the lips
Local	Irritation, inflammation, tenderness, necrosis, and sloughing (with IV use)
Other	Lymphadenopathy, coarsening of facial features, hypertrichosis, Peyronie's disease, systemic lupus erythematosus, periarteritis nodosa, immunoglobulin abnormalities

OVERDOSAGE

Signs and symptoms	Nystagmus, ataxia, and dysarthria, tremor, hyperflexia, lethargy, slurred speech, nausea, vomiting, hypotension, coma, respiratory and circulatory depression
Treatment	Monitor respiratory and circulatory function; institute appropriate measures. Hemodialysis may be considered for removal of the drug from the blood; total exchange transfusion has been used for the treatment of severe toxicity in children.

DRUG INTERACTIONS

Acute alcohol ingestion, chloramphenicol, chlordiazepoxide, cimetidine, diazepam, dicumarol, disulfiram, ethosuximide, halothane, isoniazid, methylphenidate, phenothiazines, phenylbutazone, salicylates, sulfonamides, tolbutamide, trazodone	△ Serum phenytoin level; monitor serum level and, if necessary, adjust dosage
Calcium-containing antacids, chronic alcohol abuse, carbamazepine, molindone, reserpine	▽ Serum phenytoin level; monitor serum level and, if necessary, adjust dosage. Separate administration of phenytoin and a calcium-containing antacid if the patient's serum level is low.
Phenobarbital, valproic acid, divalproex sodium	△ or ▽ Serum phenytoin level; monitor serum level and, if necessary, adjust dosage △ or ▽ Serum level of interacting drug
Corticosteroids, digitoxin, doxycyline, furosemide, oral anticoagulants, quinidine, rifampin, vitamin D	▽ Pharmacologic effect of interacting drug
Estrogens (including oral contraceptives)	△ Serum phenytoin level; monitor serum level and, if necessary, adjust dosage ▽ Pharmacologic effect of estrogens
Tricyclic antidepressants	△ Risk of seizures; monitor serum level and, if necessary, adjust dosage

ALTERED LABORATORY VALUES

Blood/serum values	▽ PBI △ Glucose △ Alkaline phosphatase △ SGGT
Urinary values	Subnormal increase in 17-OHCS and 17-KS (with dexamethasone and metyrapone tests)

USE IN CHILDREN

See INDICATIONS and PARENTERAL DOSAGE

USE IN PREGNANT AND NURSING WOMEN

In a number or reports, use of phenytoin during pregnancy has been associated with an increase in adverse congenital effects, such as heart malformations, cleft lip and palate, microcephaly, mental deficiency, and impaired prenatal growth; isolated cases of malignancy, including neuroblastomas, have also been seen in children whose mothers received this drug during pregnancy. Nevertheless, prophylactic treatment of major seizures should not be discontinued during pregnancy, since there is a strong possibility that withdrawal may precipitate status epilepticus with attendant hypoxia and threat to life. However, if removal of the drug will not pose a serious risk, discontinuation of phenytoin may be considered, although it should be recognized that even minor seizures may pose some hazard to the embryo or fetus. In a large proportion of women, pregnancy increases the risk of seizures by altering the absorption or metabolism of phenytoin; serum levels should be determined periodically during pregnancy and, if necessary, the dosage should be adjusted. Coagulation defects may occur within the first 24 h postpartum in a neonate whose mother was receiving phenytoin; to reduce this risk, vitamin K should be given to the mother before delivery and to the neonate after birth. Phenytoin is excreted in low concentrations in human milk; women taking this drug should not nurse.

COMPENDIUM OF DRUG THERAPY

HYDANTOINS

MESANTOIN (mephenytoin) Sandoz Pharmaceuticals Rx

Tablets: 100 mg

INDICATIONS
Grand mal, focal, Jacksonian, and psychomotor seizures refractory to less toxic anticonvulsants

ORAL DOSAGE
Adult: 50–100 mg/day to start, followed by weekly increases of 50–100 mg/day, up to 800 mg/day, if needed; usual maintenance dosage: 200–600 mg/day
Child: 50–100 mg/day to start, followed by weekly increases of 50–100 mg/day; usual maintenance dosage: 100–400 mg/day

CONTRAINDICATIONS
Hypersensitivity to hydantoins

ADMINISTRATION/DOSAGE ADJUSTMENTS

Patients receiving other anticonvulsants	Gradually add mephenytoin (see ORAL DOSAGE) while tapering dose of anticonvulsant to be discontinued, over a period of 3–6 wk; thereafter, dosage may be increased by 100 mg/day at weekly intervals, if needed. Phenobarbital may be continued until optimal mephenytoin dosage is achieved, and then gradually withdrawn.
Dosage reduction	Must be gradual to minimize risk of precipitating seizures

WARNINGS/PRECAUTIONS

Medical supervision	Patient must be kept under close supervision at all times due to possibility of serious adverse effects (see ADVERSE REACTIONS)
Patients with hepatic impairment	Use with caution and observe for signs of excessive drug accumulation; pretreatment liver-function tests are recommended
Blood dyscrasias	May occur (see ADVERSE REACTIONS). Instruct patient to discontinue drug and report for examination if sore throat, fever, mucous membrane bleeding, glandular swelling, or cutaneous reactions develop. Obtain total WBC and differential counts before starting treatment, 2 wk after starting therapy, 2 wk after optimal dosage is reached, monthly thereafter for 1 yr, and every 3 mo subsequently. If neutrophil count drops to between 1,600 and 2,500/mm³, obtain counts every 2 wk. If neutrophil count falls below 1,600/mm³, discontinue therapy.
Alcohol intoxication	Acute intoxication may increase anticonvulsant effect of mephenytoin due to decreased catabolism, whereas chronic alcohol abuse may decrease anticonvulsant effect due to enzyme induction; caution patient that alcohol and other CNS depressants may have an additive effect

ADVERSE REACTIONS

Hematological	Leukopenia, neutropenia, agranulocytosis, thrombocytopenia, pancytopenia, eosinophilia, monocytosis, leukocytosis; simple anemia, hemolytic anemia, megaloblastic anemia, and aplastic anemia (rare)
Dermatological	Maculopapular, morbilliform, scarlatiniform, urticarial, purpuric, and nonspecific rashes; pigmentation, rash associated with lupus erythematosus syndrome, alopecia; exfoliative dermatitis, erythema multiforme (Stevens-Johnson syndrome), toxic epidermal necrolysis, and fatal dermatides (rare)
Central nervous system and neuromuscular	Drowsiness (dose-related), ataxia, fatigue, irritability, choreiform movements, depression, tremor, nervousness, sleeplessness, dizziness, dysarthria, polyarthropathy[1]
Ophthalmic	Diplopia, nystagmus, photophobia, conjunctivitis
Gastrointestinal	Nausea, vomiting
Other	Weight gain, gum hyperplasia, edema, pulmonary fibrosis, lymphadenopathy resembling Hodgkin's disease[1]

OVERDOSAGE

Signs and symptoms	See ADVERSE REACTIONS
Treatment	Induce emesis or perform gastric lavage to empty stomach. Treat symptomatically and institute supportive measures, as required.

DRUG INTERACTIONS[2]

Tricyclic antidepressants (high doses), antipsychotics (high doses)	△ Risk of seizures
Oral hypoglycemics	▽ Hypoglycemic effect
Alcohol, CNS depressants	△ CNS depression

ALTERED LABORATORY VALUES

Blood/serum values	△ Glucose △ Alkaline phosphatase ▽ PBI

MESANTOIN ■ PEGANONE

No clinically significant alterations in urinary values occur at therapeutic dosages

---

USE IN CHILDREN
See INDICATIONS and ORAL DOSAGE

USE IN PREGNANT AND NURSING WOMEN
An increased incidence of birth defects may be associated with the use of anticonvulsants during pregnancy. However, discontinuation of therapy may be considered only if removal of the drug does not pose any serious risk, such as the precipitation of status epilepticus with hypoxia in patients with serious convulsive disorders. The effects of mephenytoin on nursing infants are unknown.

---

[1] Other reactions for which a causal relationship has not been established include mental confusion, psychotic disturbances, increased seizures, hepatitis, jaundice, and nephrosis
[2] Other interactions have been reported with hydantoins, but not with mephenytoin

---

HYDANTOINS

PEGANONE (ethotoin) Abbott   Rx
Tablets: 250, 500 mg

INDICATIONS
Grand mal (tonic-clonic) and psychomotor (complex partial) seizures

ORAL DOSAGE
Adult: up to 1,000 mg/day, given in 4–6 divided doses to start, followed by gradual increases over several days until optimal response is achieved; usual maintenance dosage: 2,000–3,000 mg/day, given in 4–6 divided doses
Child: up to 750 mg/day, given in 4–6 divided doses to start, depending upon age and weight, followed by gradual increases, as needed, up to 3,000 mg/day; usual maintenance dosage: 500–1,000 mg/day, given in 4–6 divided doses

CONTRAINDICATIONS
Hepatic abnormalities   Hematological disorders

ADMINISTRATION/DOSAGE ADJUSTMENTS

Timing of administration	Nausea and vomiting may be minimized by instructing patient to take medication after meals
Patients receiving other anticonvulsants	Gradually increase ethotoin dosage while tapering dosage of other agent, until optimal combination dosage is achieved or the other agent is completely withdrawn
Combination therapy	Ethotoin may be combined with metharbital or phenobarbital for grand mal seizures, or with trimethadione or paramethadione as adjunctive therapy for petit mal seizures associated with grand mal seizures. Use with phenacemide is not recommended (see DRUG INTERACTIONS).

WARNINGS/PRECAUTIONS

Blood dyscrasias	May occur; obtain a baseline and monthly CBC and instruct patient to report immediately any signs or symptoms of infection or bleeding tendency (eg, sore throat, fever, malaise, easy bruising, petechiae, or epistaxis). Discontinue therapy if blood count is markedly depressed. Avoid use of other drugs with adverse hematological effects.
Monitoring of hepatic function	Observe patient for clinical signs of hepatic dysfunction; if confirmed by liver function studies, discontinue use of ethotoin
Monitoring of renal function	Perform a urinalysis when therapy is begun and at monthly intervals for several months thereafter
Concomitant anticoagulant therapy	The related anticonvulsant phenytoin has been reported to decrease serum levels of coumarin anticoagulants; conversely, these anticoagulants have been reported to increase the serum level and prolong the half-life of phenytoin. Although a similar interaction has not been observed between ethotoin and coumarin anticoagulants, caution should be exercised.
Megaloblastic anemia	May occur due to interference with folic acid metabolism
Lymphoma-like syndrome	May occur; discontinue therapy until signs and symptoms remit
Carcinogenicity	The long-term carcinogenic potential of this drug has not been evaluated

ADVERSE REACTIONS

Gastrointestinal	Nausea, vomiting, diarrhea; gum hypertrophy (rare)[1]
Central nervous system and neuromuscular	Fatigue, insomnia, dizziness, headache, numbness, fever; ataxia (rare)[1]
Ophthalmic	Diplopia, nystagmus

COMPENDIUM OF DRUG THERAPY

PEGANONE ■ CELONTIN

Dermatological	Rash
Other	Chest pain; lymphadenopathy and systemic lupus erythematosus (rare)

OVERDOSAGE

Signs and symptoms	Drowsiness, visual disturbance, nausea, and ataxia, followed by coma if massive doses have been ingested
Treatment	Induce emesis or perform gastric lavage to empty stomach. Institute general supportive measures. Following recovery, evaluate blood-forming organs.

DRUG INTERACTIONS[2]

Phenacemide	Paranoid symptoms
Antipsychotics (high doses)	⇧ Risk of seizures
Oral hypoglycemics	⇩ Hypoglycemic effect

ALTERED LABORATORY VALUES

Blood/serum values	⇧ Glucose

No clinically significant alterations in urinry values occur at therapeutic dosages

USE IN CHILDREN

See INDICATIONS and ORAL DOSAGE

USE IN PREGNANT AND NURSING WOMEN

Pregnancy Category C: an increased incidence of birth defects may be associated with the use of anticonvulsants during pregnancy. However, discontinuation of therapy may be considered only if removal of the drug does not pose any serious risk, such as the precipitation of status epilepticus in patients with serious convulsive disorders. Maternal ingestion of anticonvulsants may cause neonatal bleeding (usually within 24 h of birth) due to a coagulation defect. Administer prophylactic vitamin K$_1$ to pregnant women 1 mo prior to and during delivery, and to infant IV immediately after birth. If megaloblastic anemia occurs during pregnancy, folic acid therapy should be considered. Ethotoin is excreted in breast milk; because of the potential for serious adverse reactions in nursing infants, a decision should be made to discontinue either nursing or use of this drug.

[1] As a rule, these reactions have occurred only in patients receiving an additional hydantoin derivative
[2] Other interactions have been reported with hydantoins, but not with ethotoin

---

SUCCINIMIDES

CELONTIN (methsuximide) Parke-Davis   Rx

Capsules: 150, 300 mg

INDICATIONS

Absence (petit mal) seizures refractory to other anticonvulsants

ORAL DOSAGE

Adult: 300 mg/day to start, followed by weekly increases of 300 mg/day, up to 1.2 g/day, if needed
Child: same as adult; adjust dosage in small children by 150-mg increments or decrements[1]

CONTRAINDICATIONS

Hypersensitivity to succinimides

ADMINISTRATION/DOSAGE ADJUSTMENTS

Combination therapy	Methsuximide may be combined with other anticonvulsants when other forms of epilepsy coexist with absence (petit mal) seizures

WARNINGS/PRECAUTIONS

Blood dyscrasias	May occur and may be fatal (see ADVERSE REACTIONS); obtain a CBC periodically
Patients with hepatic or renal disease	Use with extreme caution in patients with known hepatic or renal disorders; perform a urinalysis and liver function studies periodically in all patients
Mental and/or physical impairment	Caution patients that this drug may impair their ability to drive or perform other potentially hazardous activities
Abrupt discontinuation of therapy	May precipitate absence (petit mal) status; all dosage adjustments must be gradual
Grand mal seizures	May increase in frequency when methsuximide is used alone to treat mixed types of epilepsy

CELONTIN ■ MILONTIN

Behavioral alterations	May occur, including unusual depression or aggressiveness; withdraw drug gradually

ADVERSE REACTIONS
Frequent reactions (incidence ≥ 1%) are printed in *italics*

Gastrointestinal	*Nausea, vomiting, anorexia, diarrhea, weight loss, epigastric and abdominal pain, constipation*
Hematological	Eosinophilia, leukopenia, monocytosis, pancytopenia
Central nervous system and neuromuscular	*Drowsiness, ataxia, dizziness*, headache, irritability, nervousness, hiccups, insomnia, confusion, instability, mental slowness, depression, hypochondriacal behavior, aggressiveness; psychosis, suicidal behavior, and auditory hallucinations (rare)
Ophthalmic	Blurred vision, photophobia, periorbital edema
Dermatological	Urticaria, Stevens-Johnson syndrome, pruritic erythematous rashes
Other	Hyperemia[2]

OVERDOSAGE

Signs and symptoms	See ADVERSE REACTIONS
Treatment	Induce emesis or perform gastric lavage to empty stomach. Treat symptomatically and institute supportive measures, as required.

DRUG INTERACTIONS

Tricyclic antidepressants (high doses), antipsychotics (high doses)	◇ Risk of seizures

ALTERED LABORATORY VALUES
No clinically significant alterations in blood/serum or urinary values occur at therapeutic dosages

---

USE IN CHILDREN

See INDICATIONS AND ORAL DOSAGE

USE IN PREGNANT AND NURSING WOMEN

An increased incidence of birth defects may be associated with the use of anticonvulsants during pregnancy. However, discontinuation of therapy may be considered only if removal of the drug does not pose any serious risk, such as the precipitation of status epilepticus in patients with serious convulsive disorders. The effects of methsuximide on nursing infants are unknown.

---

[1] *United States Pharmacopeia Dispensing Information 1982*. Rockville, Md, The United States Pharmacopeial Convention, Inc, 1982
[2] Systemic lupus erythematosus has occurred in patients receiving succinimides

---

SUCCINIMIDES

MILONTIN (phensuximide) Parke-Davis   Rx

Capsules: 500 mg

INDICATIONS	ORAL DOSAGE
Absence (petit mal) seizures	**Adult:** 500–1,000 mg bid or tid; usual maintenance dosage: 1,500 mg/day **Child:** same as adult

CONTRAINDICATIONS
Hypersensitivity to succinimides

ADMINISTRATION/DOSAGE ADJUSTMENTS

Combination therapy	Phensuximide may be combined with other anticonvulsants when other forms of epilepsy coexist with absence (petit mal) seizures

WARNINGS/PRECAUTIONS

Blood dyscrasias	May occur and may be fatal (see ADVERSE REACTIONS); obtain a CBC periodically
Patients with hepatic or renal disease	Use with extreme caution in patients with known hepatic or renal disorders; perform a urinalysis and liver function studies periodically in all patients
Mental and/or physical impairment	Caution patients that this drug may impair their ability to drive or perform other potentially hazardous activities
Grand mal seizures	May increase in frequency when phensuximide is used alone to treat mixed types of epilepsy
Abrupt discontinuation of therapy	May precipitate absence (petit mal) status; all dosage adjustments must be gradual

ADVERSE REACTIONS[1]

Frequent reactions (incidence ≥ 1%) are printed in *italics*

Gastrointestinal	*Nausea, vomiting, anorexia*
Central nervous system and neuromuscular	Drowsiness, dizziness, ataxia, headache, dream-like state, lethargy, muscle weakness
Dermatological	Pruritus, skin eruptions, erythema multiforme, erythematous rashes, alopecia
Genitourinary	Urinary frequency, renal damage, hematuria
Hematological	Granulocytopenia, transient leukopenia, pancytopenia

OVERDOSAGE

Signs and symptoms	See ADVERSE REACTIONS
Treatment	Induce emesis or perform gastric lavage to empty stomach. Treat symptomatically and institute supportive measures, as required.

DRUG INTERACTIONS

Tricyclic antidepressants (high doses), antipsychotics (high doses)	⌂ Risk of seizures

ALTERED LABORATORY VALUES

No clinically significant alterations in blood/serum or urinary values occur at therapeutic dosages

---

USE IN CHILDREN

See INDICATIONS and ORAL DOSAGE

USE IN PREGNANT AND NURSING WOMEN

An increased incidence of birth defects may be associated with the use of anticonvulsants during pregnancy. However, discontinuation of therapy may be considered only if removal of the drug does not pose any serious risk, such as the precipitation of status epilepticus in patients with serious convulsive disorders. The effects of phensuximide on nursing infants are unknown.

---

[1] Systemic lupus erythematosus has occurred in patients receiving succinimides

---

SUCCINIMIDES

ZARONTIN (ethosuximide) Parke-Davis   Rx

Capsules: 250 mg   **Syrup (per 5 ml):** 250 mg (16 fl oz) *raspberry-flavored*

INDICATIONS

Absence (petit mal) seizures

ORAL DOSAGE

Adult: 500 mg/day to start, followed by increases of 250 mg/day every 4–7 days until optimal clinical response is achieved; dosages exceeding 1.5 g/day should be divided and administered only under strict medical supervision

Child (3–6 yr): 250 mg/day to start, followed by increases of 250 mg/day every 4–7 days until optimal clinical response is achieved; dosages exceeding 1.5 g/day should be divided and administered only under strict medical supervision (normal optimal dosage: 20 mg/kg/day)

Child (> 6 yr): same as adult

CONTRAINDICATIONS

Hypersensitivity to succinimides

ADMINISTRATION/DOSAGE ADJUSTMENTS

Combination therapy	Ethosuximide may be combined with other anticonvulsants when other forms of epilepsy coexist with absence (petit mal) seizures
Serum level monitoring	Therapeutic serum levels range from 40 to 100 µg/ml, which can be achieved in most children with a dosage of 20 mg/kg/day; use the actual serum level and the patient's response to the drug to determine the subsequent dosage schedule

WARNINGS/PRECAUTIONS

Blood dyscrasias	May occur and may be fatal (see ADVERSE REACTIONS); obtain a CBC periodically
Patients with hepatic or renal impairment	Use with extreme caution to patients with known hepatic or renal disorders; perform a urinalysis and liver function studies periodically in all patients
Mental and/or physical impairment	Caution patients that this drug may impair their ability to drive or perform other potentially hazardous activities

Grand mal seizures	May increase in frequency when ethosuximide is used alone to treat mixed types of epilepsy
Abrupt discontinuation of therapy	May precipitate absence (petit mal) status; all dosage adjustments must be gradual

ADVERSE REACTIONS
Frequent reactions (incidence ≥ 1%) are printed in *italics*

Gastrointestinal	*Anorexia, vague gastric upset, nausea, vomiting, cramps, epigastric and abdominal pain, diarrhea,* swelling of the tongue, gum hypertrophy
Hematological	Leukopenia, agranulocytosis, pancytopenia, aplastic anemia, eosinophilia
Central nervous system	Drowsiness, headache, dizziness, euphoria, hiccups, irritability, hyperactivity, lethargy, fatigue, ataxia, sleep disturbances, night terrors, poor concentration, aggressiveness; paranoid psychosis and depression with overt suicidal tendencies (rare)
Dermatological	Urticaria, Stevens-Johnson syndrome, pruritic erythematous rash, hirsutism
Other	Myopia, vaginal bleeding, systemic lupus erythematosus

OVERDOSAGE

Signs and symptoms	See ADVERSE REACTIONS
Treatment	Induce emesis or perform gastric lavage to empty stomach. Treat symptomatically and institute supportive measures, as required.

DRUG INTERACTIONS

Tricyclic antidepressants (high doses), antipsychotics (high doses)	⇧ Risk of seizures

ALTERED LABORATORY VALUES
No clinically significant alterations in blood/serum or urinary values occur at therapeutic dosages

---

USE IN CHILDREN
See INDICATIONS and ORAL DOSAGE

USE IN PREGNANT AND NURSING WOMEN
An increased incidence of birth defects may be associated with the use of anticonvulsants during pregnancy. However, discontinuation of therapy may be considered only if removal of the drug does not pose any serious risk, such as the precipitation of status epilepticus with hypoxia in patients with serious convulsive disorders. The effects of ethosuximide on nursing infants are unknown.

MISCELLANEOUS ANTICONVULSANTS

DEPAKENE (valproic acid) Abbott   Rx
Capsules: 250 mg **Syrup (per 5 ml):** 250 mg (16 fl oz)

DEPAKOTE (divalproex sodium) Abbott   Rx
Tablets (enteric coated): divalproex sodium equivalent to 125, 250, 500 mg valproic acid

INDICATIONS	ORAL DOSAGE
Simple and complex absence seizures, including petit mal **Multiple seizure types** which include absence seizures (adjunctive therapy)	**Adult:** 15 mg/kg/day to start, followed, as tolerated, by weekly increases of 5–10 mg/kg/day until optimal clinical response is achieved, up to 60 mg/kg/day. Daily doses exceeding 250 mg should be divided. **Child:** same as adult

CONTRAINDICATIONS

Hypersensitivity to valproic acid	Hepatic disease or significant dysfunction

ADMINISTRATION/DOSAGE ADJUSTMENTS

Serum level monitoring	Therapeutic serum levels range from 50 to 100 μg/ml; occasionally, good control may be obtained at levels above or below this range
Gastrointestinal irritation	May be avoided by administering drug with meals, initiating therapy gradually, or using the enteric-coated tablets
Switching from capsules or syrup to enteric-coated tablets	In patients previously receiving the capsules or syrup, therapy with the enteric-coated tablets may be initiated at the same total daily dose and dosing schedule; after stabilization, selected patients may take the tablets bid or tid
Combination therapy	Serum levels of phenytoin and phenobarbital may be affected by valproic acid (see DRUG INTERACTIONS); periodic serum determinations are recommended

DEPAKENE/DEPAKOTE

WARNINGS/PRECAUTIONS

Hepatic failure	Potentially fatal hepatic failure may occur, usually within the first 6 mo of therapy. The risk of fatal hepatotoxicity is considerably increased in children under 2 yr of age, but declines considerably in progressively older patient groups; this risk is enchanced by concomitant use of other anticonvulsants, a history of hepatic disease, and the presence of congenital metabolic disorders, severe seizure disorders accompanied by mental retardation, and organic brain disease. Before using in patients at risk, weigh the benefits and risks. Use alone (ie, with no other anticonvulsants) and with extreme caution in children under 2 yr of age; use with caution in older patients at risk.
	Serious or fatal hepatotoxicity may be preceded by nonspecific signs and symptoms, including loss of seizure control, malaise, weakness, lethargy, facial edema, anorexia, and vomiting; watch closely for these symptoms. Perform liver function tests prior to initiating therapy and at frequent intervals thereafter, especially during the first 6 mo; in addition, obtain a careful interim medical history and examine patient for evidence of hepatic dysfunction, as serum liver enzymes may not always be elevated. Use with caution in children, patients receiving other anticonvulsants, and those with a prior history of hepatic disease, congenital disorders, severe seizure disorders accompanied by mental retardation, or organic brain disease. Discontinue therapy immediately in the presence of suspected or apparent significant hepatic dysfunction and follow patient closely, as hepatic impairment may progress despite discontinuation of the drug.
Thrombocytopenia, coagulation disorders	May occur; perform platelet counts and coagulation tests before initiating therapy and at periodic intervals thereafter, especially prior to planned surgery. Reduce dosage or withdraw drug pending investigation if hemorrhage, bruising, or a hemostasis/coagulation disorder develops.
Mental impairment	Caution patients not to drive or engage in other potentially hazardous activities if they become drowsy after taking this drug
Local irritation of mouth and throat	May occur if capsules are chewed; caution patient to swallow capsules without chewing
Hyperammonemia	May occur, with or without lethargy or coma, and in the absence of abnormal liver function tests; discontinue use if clinically significant hyperammonemia is detected
Concomitant anticonvulsant therapy	Other antiepileptic drugs may interact with valproic acid (see DRUG INTERACTIONS); monitor the serum levels of these drugs periodically during the early phase of therapy
Carcinogenicity	Long-term studies on rats and mice have shown a statistically significant increase in the incidence of subcutaneous fibrosarcomas in male rats receiving high doses of valproic acid and a dose-related trend in the incidence of benign pulmonary adenomas in male mice; the clinical significance of these findings is not known
Mutagenicity	No evidence of mutagenicity has been detected in bacteria or laboratory animals
Effect on fertility	Chronic toxicity studies have demonstrated reduced spermatogenesis and testicular atrophy in rats given over 200 mg/kg/day and in dogs given over 90 mg/kg/day; however, in segment I studies on rats, no effect on fertility has been found following administration of up to 350 mg/kg/day for 60 days. The effect of this drug on testicular development, sperm production, and fertility in humans is unknown.

ADVERSE REACTIONS[1]

	Frequent reactions (incidence $\geq$ 1%) are printed in *italics*
Gastrointestinal	*Nausea, vomiting, indigestion,* diarrhea, abdominal cramps, constipation, anorexia with weight loss, increased appetite with weight gain
Central nervous system and neuromuscular	Sedation (usually with combination therapy), tremor, weakness, emotional upset, depression, psychosis, aggression, hyperactivity, behavioral deterioration; ataxia, headache, asterixis, dysarthria, dizziness, incoordination, and coma (rare)
Dermatological	Alopecia (transient); rash and erythema multiforme (rare)
Ophthalmic	Nystagmus, diplopia, and "spots before eyes" (rare)
Hematological	Thrombocytopenia, altered bleeding time, lymphocytosis, hypofibrinogenemia, anemia, bone marrow suppression, leukopenia, eosinophilia, petechiae, bruising, hematoma formation, frank hemorrhage
Endocrine	Irregular menses, secondary amenorrhea, altered thyroid function tests; breast enlargement and galactorrhea (rare)
Metabolic	Hyperammonemia, hyperglycinemia (one case with fatal outcome in a patient with preexisting nonketotic hyperglycinemia)
Hepatic	*Elevated serum transaminase and LDH levels (dose-related),* other abnormal changes in liver function tests, hepatic failure
Pancreatic	Acute pancreatitis (in rare cases, fatal)
Other	Edema of the extremities

OVERDOSAGE

Signs and symptoms	Deep coma

DRUG INTERACTIONS

Alcohol, CNS depressants	↑ CNS depression
Phenobarbital, other barbiturates	↑ Severe CNS depression; monitor patient for neurotoxicity and reduce barbiturate dosage, if necessary[2]
Phenytoin	↑ or ↓ Serum phenytoin level; adjust phenytoin dosage as clinical situation dictates
Ethosuximide	↑ Serum ethosuximide level; monitor serum level of ethosuximide and valproic acid (or divalproex) during combination therapy
Carbamazepine	↓ Serum level of valproic acid or divalproex ↑ or ↓ Serum level of carbamazepine
Clonazepam	Absence (petit mal) status
Warfarin, dipyridamole, sulfinpyrazone	↑ Bleeding time
Salicylates	↑ Bleeding time ↑ Serum level of valproic acid or divalproex
Dicumarol	↑ Bleeding time Altered serum level of valproic acid or divalproex

ALTERED LABORATORY VALUES

Blood/serum values	↑ Alkaline phosphatase ↑ SGOT ↑ SGPT ↑ Lactate dehydrogenase ↑ Bilirubin Altered thyroid function tests
Urinary values	False-positive ketone tests

USE IN CHILDREN

See INDICATIONS and ORAL DOSAGE; use with great caution in children under 2 yr of age (see WARNINGS/PRECAUTIONS)

USE IN PREGNANT AND NURSING WOMEN

Pregnancy Category D: valproic acid may be teratogenic in humans; use in women of childbearing potential only if clearly essential. It has been estimated that the risk of having a child with spina bifida following exposure to valproic acid during pregnancy is approximately 1–2%; this is similar to the risk for nonepileptic women who have given birth to children with neural tube defects. Skeletal and soft-tissue abnormalities, fetal resorptions, delayed parturition, and adverse effects on postnatal growth and survival have been observed in animal studies. Discontinuation of valproic acid (or divalproex) before or during pregnancy may be considered, provided that removal of the drug does not pose a serious risk to the patient (it is not known whether even minor seizures can have adverse developmental effects). Prophylactic treatment of major seizures should not be discontinued, however, because of the strong possibility of precipitating status epilepticus with attendant hypoxia and threat to life. Valproic acid has been detected in breast milk at concentrations that are 1–10% of serum levels. The effect of such concentrations on nursing infants is not known; use with caution in nursing mothers.

[1] The frequency of adverse reactions, particularly of an elevation in hepatic enzyme levels, may be dose-dependent; consequently, the benefit of improved seizure control that may accompany the use of higher doses should be weighed against the risk of a greater incidence of side effects
[2] Primidone is partially metabolized to phenobarbital and may similarly interact with valproic acid

---

MISCELLANEOUS ANTICONVULSANTS

KLONOPIN (clonazepam) Roche
C-IV

Tablets: 0.5, 1, 2 mg

INDICATIONS

Lennox-Gastaut syndrome (petit mal variant)
Akinetic and myoclonic seizures
Absence (petit mal) seizures refractory to succinimides

ORAL DOSAGE

Adult: up to 1.5 mg/day, given in 3 divided doses to start, followed by increases of 0.5–1.0 mg/day every 3 days until optimal clinical response is achieved, up to 20 mg/day

Infant and child (< 10 yr or < 30 kg): 0.01–0.03 mg/kg/day, or up to 0.05 mg/kg/day, if necessary, given in 2–3 divided doses to start, followed by increases of 0.25–0.5 mg every 3 days, up to 0.1–0.2 mg/kg/day in 3 equally divided doses, until optimal clinical response is achieved

KLONOPIN

CONTRAINDICATIONS

Hypersensitivity to benzodiazepines	Acute narrow angle glaucoma	Significant hepatic disease
Open angle glaucoma (unless patient is receiving appropriate therapy)		

ADMINISTRATION/DOSAGE ADJUSTMENTS

Division of doses	Whenever possible, divide daily dose into 3 equal parts; if doses are divided unequally, give the largest one at bedtime

WARNINGS/PRECAUTIONS

Drug dependence	Psychic and/or physical dependence and tolerance may develop, especially in addiction-prone individuals
Mental and/or physical impairment	Caution patients against driving or engaging in other potentially hazardous activities requiring full mental alertness and that alcohol and other CNS depressants may cause additional CNS depression if taken concomitantly
Abrupt discontinuation of therapy	May precipitate barbiturate-like withdrawal symptoms of status epilepticus, especially with prolonged high-dose therapy; always withdraw drug gradually and, if necessary, administer another anticonvulsant concomitantly
Patients with renal impairment	Use with caution to avoid excessive accumulation of metabolites
Generalized tonic-clonic (grand mal) seizures	May be precipitated in patients with mixed-type seizures; if needed, administer additional appropriate anticonvulsants or increase anticonvulsant dosage
Increased salivation	May occur; use with caution in patients who have difficulty handling secretions
Respiratory depression	May occur; use with caution in patients with chronic respiratory disease
Long-term therapy	Perform a CBC and liver function tests periodically (see ADVERSE REACTIONS)

ADVERSE REACTIONS

Frequent reactions (incidence ≥ 1%) are printed in *italics*

Central nervous system and neuromuscular	*Drowsiness (50%), ataxia (30%), behavioral problems (25%)*, aphonia, choreiform movements, coma, dysarthria, dysdiadochokinesis, headache, hemiparesis, hypotonia, slurred speech, tremor, vertigo, confusion, depression, forgetfulness, hallucinations, hysteria, increased libido, insomnia, psychosis, muscle weakness, pain
Ophthalmic	Abnormal eye movements, diplopia, "glassy-eyed" appearance, nystagmus
Respiratory	Depression, chest congestion, rhinorrhea, shortness of breath, hypersecretion in upper respiratory passages
Cardiovascular	Palpitations
Dermatological	Alopecia, hirsutism, rash, ankle and facial edema
Gastrointestinal	Anorexia or increased appetite, coated tongue, constipation, diarrhea, dry mouth, encopresis, gastritis, hepatomegaly, nausea, sore gums
Genitourinary	Dysuria, enuresis, nocturia, urinary retention
Hematological	Anemia, leukopenia, thrombocytopenia, eosinophilia
Other	Dehydration, general deterioration, lymphadenopathy, fever, weight loss or gain

OVERDOSAGE

Signs and symptoms	Somnolence, confusion, coma, diminished reflexes
Treatment	Empty stomach immediately by gastric lavage. Institute general supportive measures, including IV fluids and airway maintenance, and monitor vital signs. Treat hypotension with norepinephrine or metaraminol. The value of dialysis is unknown.

DRUG INTERACTIONS

Valproic acid	Absence (petit mal) status
Alcohol, narcotic analgesics, barbiturates, sedative-hypnotics, anxiolytics, phenothiazine, thioxanthene and butyrophenone antipsychotics, MAO inhibitors, tricyclic antidepressants, other anticonvulsants	⇧ CNS depression

ALTERED LABORATORY VALUES

Blood/serum values	⇧ SGOT ⇧ SGPT ⇧ Alkaline phosphatase

No clinically significant alterations in urinary values occur at therapeutic dosages

USE IN CHILDREN
See INDICATIONS and ORAL DOSAGE; the long-term effects of this drug on development are unknown

USE IN PREGNANT AND NURSING WOMEN
An increased incidence of birth defects may be associated with the use of anticonvulsants during pregnancy. However, discontinuation of therapy may be considered only if removal of the drug does not pose any serious risk, such as the precipitation of status epilepticus with hypoxia in patients with serious convulsive disorders. Patients taking this drug should not breast feed their infants.

MISCELLANEOUS ANTICONVULSANTS

MYSOLINE (primidone) Ayerst Rx
Tablets: 50, 250 mg Suspension (per 5 ml): 250 mg (8 fl oz)

INDICATIONS
Grand mal, psychomotor, and focal epileptic seizures

ORAL DOSAGE
Adult: days 1–3, 100–125 mg at bedtime; days 4–6, 100–125 mg bid; days 7–9, 100–125 mg tid; day 10, 250 mg tid; thereafter, adjust dosage as needed, up to 500 mg qid if necessary, to maintain good control; usual maintenance dosage: 250 mg tid or qid
Child (< 8 yr): days 1–3, 50 mg at bedtime; days 4–6, 50 mg bid; days 7–9, 100 mg bid; day 10, 125–250 mg tid; thereafter, adjust dosage as needed to maintain good control; usual maintenance dosage: 125–250 mg tid or 10–25 mg/kg/day, given in divided doses
Child (≥ 8 yr): same as adult

CONTRAINDICATIONS
Porphyria	Hypersensitivity to phenobarbital (one of the active metabolites of primidone)

ADMINISTRATION/DOSAGE ADJUSTMENTS
Patients receiving other anticonvulsants	Initiate primidone therapy with 100–125 mg at bedtime and then gradually increase primidone dosage to maintenance levels while decreasing dosage of other agent(s) until optimal combination dosage is achieved. If other medication is to be completely withdrawn, transition should not be completed for at least 2 wk.
Serum level monitoring	May be useful for optimal dosage adjustment; therapeutic range is 5–12 µg/ml

WARNINGS/PRECAUTIONS
Abrupt discontinuation of therapy	May precipitate status epilepticus; withdraw drug gradually
Prolonged therapy	Perform a CBC and sequential multiple analysis-12 (SMA-12) every 6 mo
Megaloblastic anemia	Occurs rarely and may be treated with folic acid without interruption of therapy

ADVERSE REACTIONS
Frequent reactions (incidence ≥ 1%) are printed in *italics*

Central nervous system	*Ataxia, vertigo,* fatigue, hyperirritability, emotional disturbances, drowsiness
Gastrointestinal	Nausea, anorexia, vomiting
Ophthalmic	Diplopia, nystagmus
Hematological	Megaloblastic anemia (see WARNINGS/PRECAUTIONS)
Dermatological	Morbilliform skin eruptions
Genitourinary	Impotence

OVERDOSAGE
Signs and symptoms	See ADVERSE REACTIONS
Treatment	Treat symptomatically. Institute supportive measures, as required.

DRUG INTERACTIONS
Alcohol, general anesthetics, CNS depressants, MAO inhibitors	⇧ Drug effects and/or anticonvulsant toxicity
Oral anticoagulants	⇩ Prothrombin time
Corticosteroids	⇩ Corticosteroid effects
Digitalis, digitoxin	⇩ Cardiac glycoside effects
Doxycycline	⇩ Anti-infective effect
Tricyclic antidepressants	⇩ Antidepressant effect
Griseofulvin	⇩ Griseofulvin absorption

Phenytoin, other anticonvulsants	Change in pattern of epileptiform seizures

ALTERED LABORATORY VALUES

Blood/serum values	▽ Bilirubin

No clinically significant alterations in urinary values occur at therapeutic dosages

USE IN CHILDREN
See INDICATIONS and ORAL DOSAGE

USE IN PREGNANT AND NURSING WOMEN
An increased incidence of birth defects may be associated with the use of anticonvulsants during pregnancy. However, discontinuation of therapy may be considered only if removal of the drug does not pose any serious risk, such as the precipitation of status epilepticus with hypoxia in patients with serious convulsive disorders. Neonatal hemorrhage due to a coagulation deficiency resembling vitamin K deficiency may occur. Administer prophylactic vitamin K_1 to pregnant women 1 mo prior to and during delivery. Primidone appears in breast milk in substantial quantities; patient should stop nursing if undue somnolence and drowsiness occur in the infant.

MISCELLANEOUS ANTICONVULSANTS

PHENURONE (phenacemide) Abbott   Rx

Tablets: 500 mg

INDICATIONS
Severe epilepsy, especially mixed forms of complex partial (psychomotor) seizures refractory to other anticonvulsants

ORAL DOSAGE
Adult: 250–500 mg tid to start, followed, if needed (and if drug is well tolerated), by an additional 500 mg, taken upon arising, after the first week of therapy and 500 mg more at bedtime after the second week, up to 5 g/day in divided doses; usual maintenance dosage: 2–3 g/day, given in divided doses
Child (5–10 yr): one half the adult dose, given at the same time intervals as for adults

CONTRAINDICATIONS
Satisfactory control of seizures with other anticonvulsants (use phenacemide only if other medications are ineffective)

ADMINISTRATION/DOSAGE ADJUSTMENTS

Combination therapy	Phenacemide may be combined with other anticonvulsants; use with extreme caution if toxic effects are similar
Patients receiving other anticonvulsants	Gradually increase phenacemide dosage while tapering dosage of anticonvulsant to be discontinued to maintain seizure control

WARNINGS/PRECAUTIONS

Personality disorders, including severe psychoses and suicide attempts	May occur; use with extreme caution in patients with a history of personality disorders and observe for behavioral changes (eg, apathy, depression, or aggressiveness). Hospitalization during the first week of therapy may be advisable. Withdraw the drug if severe or exacerbated personality changes occur.
Severe hepatic impairment	May occur and may be fatal; use with caution in patients with hepatic dysfunction. Perform liver function tests before and during therapy, and discontinue use if jaundice or other signs of hepatitis appear.
Blood dyscrasias	May occur and may be fatal (see ADVERSE REACTIONS); obtain a baseline and monthly CBC and instruct patient to report immediately any signs or symptoms of a possible developing blood dyscrasia (eg, sore throat, malaise, or fever).[1] For a better indication of possible blood dyscrasia, obtain the number, rather than the percentage, of each formed cellular element. Discontinue therapy if blood count is markedly depressed.
Nephritis	May occur; perform a urinalysis periodically and discontinue therapy if abnormalities develop
Hypersensitivity reactions	Use with caution in patients with a history of allergy, especially to other anticonvulsants, and discontinue therapy at the first sign of a skin rash or other allergic manifestation
Combination anticonvulsant therapy	Use with extreme caution if given in combination with any other anticonvulsant that may cause similar toxic effects; exercise considerable caution if ethotoin is given concomitantly (see DRUG INTERACTIONS)
Carcinogenicity	No data on carcinogenicity in animals or humans have been reported

PHENURONE ■ TEGRETOL

ADVERSE REACTIONS	Frequent reactions (incidence ≥ 1%) are printed in *italics*
Central nervous system	*Psychic changes (17%), drowsiness (4%), headache (2%), insomnia (1%)*, dizziness, paresthesias
Gastrointestinal	*Anorexia (5%), nausea and vomiting (2%)*, abdominal distress, diarrhea
Dermatological	*Rash (5%)*, pruritus
Hematological	*Leukopenia (≤ 4,000/mm³) (1.4%)*; leukocytosis, low platelet count, aplastic anemia, granulocytopenia
Other	*Hepatitis (2%)*, nephritis, fatigue, fever, muscle pain, weight loss, palpitation

OVERDOSAGE

Signs and symptoms	Excitement or mania, followed by drowsiness, dizziness, ataxia, and coma
Treatment	Induce emesis or perform gastric lavage to empty stomach. Institute general supportive measures. Following recovery, carefully evaluate hepatic and renal function, mental state, and blood-forming organs.

DRUG INTERACTIONS

Ethotoin	Paranoid symptoms

ALTERED LABORATORY VALUES

Blood/serum values	⇧ Creatinine
Urinary values	⇧ Creatinine ⇧ Albumin ⇧ Glucose ⇧ Acetone

USE IN CHILDREN

See INDICATIONS and ORAL DOSAGE; the safety and effectiveness of this drug for use in children under 5 yr of age have not been established

USE IN PREGNANT AND NURSING WOMEN

Pregnancy Category D: phenacemide can cause harm to the fetus; use of anticonvulsants during pregnancy increases the probability of birth defects. Patients who are or who may become pregnant while taking this drug should be apprised of the potential hazard to the fetus. Maternal ingestion of anticonvulsants may cause neonatal bleeding (usually within 24 h of birth) owing to a coagulation defect; for prophylactix, vitamin K may be given to the mother 1 mo prior to and during delivery and to the infant IV immediately after birth. It is not known whether phenacemide is excreted in human milk; because many drugs are so excreted and because of the potential for serious adverse reactions in nursing infants, patients should not nurse while taking this drug.

---

¹ The interval between blood counts may be extended if no abnormality occurs for 12 mo

---

MISCELLANEOUS ANTICONVULSANTS

TEGRETOL (carbamazepine) Geigy   Rx

Chewable tablets: 100 mg   **Tablets:** 200 mg

INDICATIONS	ORAL DOSAGE
Epilepsy, including partial seizures with complex symptomatology (eg, psychomotor, temporal lobe), generalized tonic-clonic (grand mal) seizures, and mixed seizure patterns, in patients unmanageable with other anticonvulsants	**Adult:** 200 mg bid to start, followed by gradual increases of 200 mg/day or less, up to 1,200 or (rarely) 1,600 mg/day, given in 3-4 divided doses, until optimal clinical response is obtained; usual maintenance dosage: 800-1,200 mg/day **Child (6-12 yr):** 100 mg bid to start, followed by gradual increases of 100 mg/day, up to 1,000 mg/day, given in 3-4 divided doses, until optimal clinical response is obtained; usual maintenance dosage: 400-800 mg/day **Child (12-15 yr):** same as adult, up to 1,000 mg/day, given in divided doses, if needed
Pain associated with true **trigeminal neuralgia**	**Adult:** 100 mg bid on the first day, followed by increases of 100 mg q12h, up to 1,200 mg/day, given in divided doses, if needed; usual maintenance dosage: 400-800 mg/day

CONTRAINDICATIONS

History of previous bone marrow depression caused by carbamazepine	Hypersensitivity to carbamazepine or any tricyclic compound	MAO inhibitor therapy (see WARNINGS/PRECAUTIONS)

ADMINISTRATION/DOSAGE ADJUSTMENTS

Timing of administration	Tablets should be taken with meals
Combination anticonvulsant therapy	Carbamazepine may be added gradually to an existing anticonvulsant regimen while the dosage of other anticonvulsants is maintained or gradually reduced; however, it may be necessary to increase the dosage of phenytoin (see DRUG INTERACTIONS)

TEGRETOL

Maintenance therapy	Adjust dosage gradually to minimum effective level; for trigeminal neuralgia, reassess dosage at least every 3 mo and discontinue therapy, if possible

WARNINGS/PRECAUTIONS

MAO inhibitor therapy	Wait at least 14 days (or longer if clinically permissible) after discontinuing MAO inhibitors before initiating carbamazepine therapy
Blood dyscrasias	May occur and may be fatal (see ADVERSE REACTIONS). Obtain a CBC prior to treatment, at weekly intervals for the first 3 mo of therapy, and monthly thereafter for at least 2–3 yr. Instruct patient to discontinue drug and report immediately any signs or symptoms of a potential hematological problem (eg, fever, sore throat, mouth ulcers, easy bruising, petechiae, or purpura). Discontinue treatment if evidence of bone marrow depression appears (RBC $< 4.0 \times 10^6/mm^3$, hematocrit $< 32\%$, hemoglobin < 11 g/dl, WBC $< 4,000/mm^3$, platelets $< 100,000/mm^3$, reticulocytes $< 0.3\%$ [$20,000/mm^3$], serum iron > 150 μg/dl); obtain a daily CBC plus platelet and reticulocyte counts, and perform a bone marrow aspiration and trephine biopsy immediately and at sufficiently frequent intervals thereafter to monitor recovery. Patients with a history of hematological reaction to any drug may be especially at risk.
Latent psychoses	May be activated
Elderly patients	May become agitated or confused
Eye changes	Have occurred in patients taking related drugs; perform eye examinations, including a slit-lamp examination, funduscopy, and tonometry, before starting therapy and periodically thereafter
Hepatic damage	May occur; perform liver function studies before starting therapy, especially in patients with hepatic disease, and repeat the tests periodically during therapy. Discontinue use of the drug immediately if hepatic disease is activated or hepatic insufficiency is aggravated.
Renal dysfunction	May occur; perform a complete urinalysis and obtain a BUN determination before starting therapy and at periodic intervals during therapy
Dizziness, drowsiness	Caution patients about driving or engaging in other potentially hazardous activities after taking this drug
Dermatological reactions	Although extremely rare, severe and potentially fatal dermatological reactions, including toxic epidermal necrolysis (Lyell's syndrome) and Stevens-Johnson syndrome, have been reported
Patients with mixed seizure disorders	Use with caution in patients with a mixed seizure disorder that includes atypical absence seizures, since an increased incidence of generalized convulsions has occurred in such patients during carbamazepine therapy
Other special-risk patients	Use with caution in patients with cardiac, hepatic, or renal damage, increased intraocular pressure, or a history of drug-induced hematological reactions, and in those who have had interrupted courses of carbamazepine therapy
Abrupt discontinuation of therapy	May precipitate seizures or status epilepticus
Carcinogenicity, mutagenicity	Carbamazepine is carcinogenic in Sprague-Dawley rats; bacterial and mammalian studies have shown no evidence of mutagenicity
Impairment of fertility	Rats given carbamazepine orally for 4–52 wk at dose levels of 50–400 mg/kg/day showed testicular atrophy, and both aspermatogenesis and testicular atrophy have been observed in rats given 25, 75, and 250 mg/kg/day for 2 yr; the relevance of these findings to clinical use of this drug is unknown
Drug dependence	No evidence of abuse potential has been associated with carbamazepine, nor is there any evidence of psychological or physical dependence in humans
Unwarranted uses	Carbamazepine should not be used for absence (petit mal) seizures or seizures that are responsive to other anticonvulsants (eg, phenytoin, phenobarbital, or primidone)

ADVERSE REACTIONS

The most frequent reactions, regardless of incidence, are printed in *italics*

Central nervous system and neuromuscular	*Dizziness, drowsiness, unsteadiness,* incoordination, confusion, headache, fatigue, speech disturbances, abnormal involuntary movements, peripheral neuritis, paresthesias, depression with agitation, talkativeness, tinnitus, hyperacusis, aching joints and muscles, leg cramps
Gastrointestinal	*Nausea, vomiting,* gastric distress, abdominal pain, diarrhea, constipation, anorexia, dry mouth and pharynx, glossitis, stomatitis
Hepatic	Abnormal liver function tests, cholestatic and hepatocellular jaundice, hepatitis
Respiratory	Pulmonary hypersensitivity characterized by fever, dyspnea, pneumonitis, or pneumonia
Hematological	Aplastic anemia, leukopenia, agranulocytosis, eosinophilia, leukocytosis, thrombocytopenia
Genitourinary	Urinary frequency, acute urinary retention, oliguria with elevated blood pressure, renal failure, azotemia, impotence

TEGRETOL

Ophthalmic	Blurred vision, visual hallucinations, transient diplopia, oculomotor disturbances, nystagmus[1]
Dermatological	Pruritic and erythematous rashes, urticaria, toxic epidermal necrolysis (Lyell's syndrome), Stevens-Johnson syndrome, photosensitivity, altered pigmentation, exfoliative dermatitis, alopecia, erythema multiforme and nodosum, purpura, aggravation of disseminated lupus erythematosus
Cardiovascular	Congestive heart failure, aggravation of hypertension, hypotension, syncope and collapse, edema, primary thrombophlebitis, recurrence of thrombophlebitis, aggravation of coronary artery disease, adenopathy or lymphadenopathy, arrhythmias, AV block[1]
Other	Diaphoresis, fever, chills, inappropriate secretion of antidiuretic hormone syndrome; altered thyroid function (with combination anticonvulsant therapy)

OVERDOSAGE

Signs and symptoms	*Respiratory:* irregular breathing, respiratory depression. *Cardiovascular:* tachycardia, hypotension or hypertension, shock, conduction disorders. *Central nervous system and neuromuscular:* impairment of consciousness ranging up to deep coma; convulsions (especially in small children), motor restlessness, muscular twitching, tremor, athetoid movements, opisthotonus, ataxia, drowsiness, mydriasis, nystagmus, adiadochokinesis, ballism, psychomotor disturbances, dysmetria, hyperreflexia followed by hyporeflexia. *Gastrointestinal:* nausea, vomiting. *Genitourinary:* anuria or oliguria, urinary retention. *Laboratory findings:* leukocytosis, reduced WBC count, glycosuria, acetonuria, ECG abnormalities (dysrhythmias).
Treatment	Induce vomiting and irrigate the stomach repeatedly by lavage, especially if the patient has also consumed alcohol (gastric lavage should be performed even if more than 4 h have elapsed since the drug was ingested). Administer activated charcoal and a cathartic, and force diuresis; dialysis is indicated only in severe cases associated with renal failure (small children who have been severely poisoned should receive replacement transfusions). Maintain a patent airway and, if necessary, resort to endotracheal intubation, artificial ventilation, and oxygen administration to treat respiratory depression. If hypotension or shock intervenes, elevate the patient's legs and administer a plasma volume expander; if these measures fail to raise the blood pressure, a vasopressor should be considered. Diazepam or barbiturates may be used to treat convulsions; however, these drugs may aggravate respiratory depression (especially in children), hypotension, and coma. (If the patient has taken an MAO inhibitor within the past week, do *not* give barbiturates.) Monitor respiration, cardiac function (ECG), blood pressure, body temperature, pupillary reflexes, and kidney and bladder function for several days until the patient has fully recovered.

DRUG INTERACTIONS

Oral contraceptives	Breakthrough bleeding
MAO inhibitors	Hyperpyrexia, excitability, seizures
Phenobarbital, primidone	▽ Carbamazepine serum level
Phenytoin	▽ Phenytoin and carbamazepine serum levels; dosage of phenytoin may have to be increased
Theophylline, warfarin, doxycycline, haloperidol	▽ Serum levels of these drugs, possibly requiring an increase in dosage
Erythromycin, cimetidine, propoxyphene, isoniazid, calcium channel blockers	△ Carbamazepine plasma level, with potential toxicity
Lithium	△ Risk of neurotoxicity

ALTERED LABORATORY VALUES

Blood/serum values	△ BUN ▽ Thyroid function values Abnormal liver function tests
Urinary values	△ Albumin △ Glucose

USE IN CHILDREN

See INDICATIONS and ORAL DOSAGE; the safety and effectiveness of this drug in children under 6 yr of age have not been established

USE IN PREGNANT AND NURSING WOMEN

Pregnancy Category C: use during pregnancy only if the anticipated therapeutic benefit justifies the potential risk to the fetus. Teratogenicity, including kinked ribs, cleft palate, and other anomalies, has been demonstrated in rats. However, no adequate, well-controlled studies have been done in pregnant women. Discontinuation of therapy may be considered only if removal of the drug does not pose any serious risk, such as the precipitation of status epilepticus with hypoxia in patients with serious convulsive disorders. The effect, if any, of carbamazepine on human labor and delivery is unknown. The concentration of carbamazepine in human milk is approximately 60% of the maternal plasma concentration; because of the potential for serious adverse effects in nursing infants, a decision should be made to either discontinue use of the drug or stop nursing, taking into consideration the importance of the drug to the mother.

---

[1] Other reactions for which a causal relationship has not been established include scattered, punctate cortical lens opacities, conjunctivitis, and cerebral arterial insufficiency with paralysis; in addition, myocardial infarction has been associated with other tricyclic compounds

TRANXENE

MISCELLANEOUS ANTICONVULSANTS

TRANXENE (clorazepate dipotassium) Abbott   C-IV
Tablets: 3.75, 7.5, 15 mg (Tranxene T-Tab)

TRANXENE-SD (clorazepate dipotassium) Abbott   C-IV
Tablets: 11.25 (Tranxene-SD Half Strength), 22.5 mg (Tranxene-SD)

INDICATIONS	ORAL DOSAGE
Anxiety disorders and short-term relief of symptoms of anxiety[1]	Adult: 15 mg/day to start, followed by 15–60 mg/day, given in a single daily dose at bedtime or in divided doses; 1 Tranxene-SD Half Strength or Tranxene-SD tab may be given q24h if the titrated daily dose equals 11.25 or 22.5 mg, respectively (Tranxene-SD should not be used to initiate therapy)
Acute alcohol withdrawal symptoms	Adult: day 1, 30 mg to start, followed by 30–60 mg, given in divided doses; day 2, 45–90 mg, given in divided doses; day 3, 22.5–45 mg, given in divided doses; day 4, 15–30 mg, given in divided doses; thereafter, gradually reduce dosage to 7.5–15 mg/day and discontinue as soon as patient's condition stabilizes
Partial seizures (adjunctive therapy)	Adult: up to 7.5 mg tid to start, followed by weekly increases of not more than 7.5 mg/day, as needed, up to 90 mg/day
Child (9–12 yr): up to 7.5 mg bid to start, followed by weekly increases of not more than 7.5 mg/day, as needed, up to 60 mg/day

CONTRAINDICATIONS	
Hypersensitivity to clorazepate	Acute narrow-angle glaucoma

ADMINISTRATION/DOSAGE ADJUSTMENTS	
Elderly or debilitated patients	Initiate treatment with 7.5–15 mg/day; increase dosage gradually, as needed
Long-term use (> 4 mo)	Effectiveness for prolonged use as an antianxiety agent has not been tested in systematic clinical studies; long-term studies in epileptic patients, however, have shown continued therapeutic activity. Reassess need for continued therapy periodically.

WARNINGS/PRECAUTIONS	
Psychotic reactions and depressive neuroses	Should not be treated with this drug
Drug dependence	Psychic and/or physical dependence may develop, especially in addiction-prone individuals
Mental impairment, reflex-slowing	Caution patients not to engage in potentially hazardous activities requiring full mental alertness and that alcohol and other CNS depressants may cause further impairment; to minimize drowsiness when clorazepate is used as an adjunct to antiepileptic drugs, do not exceed the recommended initial dosage and dosage increments
Potentially suicidal patients	Should not have access to large quantities of clorazepate; prescribe smallest amount feasible
Barbiturate-like withdrawal symptoms	May result when drug is discontinued abruptly; withdrawal symptoms have also been reported following abrupt discontinuation of benzodiazepines taken continuously at therapeutic levels for several months
Prolonged therapy	Blood counts and liver-function tests should be performed periodically
Hepatic or renal impairment	May lead to excessive drug accumulation (see OVERDOSAGE); monitor patient closely
Ataxia or oversedation	May develop in elderly and/or debilitated patients (see ADMINISTRATION/DOSAGE ADJUSTMENTS)

ADVERSE REACTIONS	
Central nervous system	Drowsiness, dizziness, nervousness, headache, fatigue, ataxia, confusion, insomnia, blurred vision, irritability, diplopia, depression, slurred speech
Cardiovascular	Decreased systolic blood pressure
Gastrointestinal	Various complaints, dry mouth
Dermatological	Skin rash, edema
Other	Altered renal and hepatic function tests, decreased hematocrit, genitourinary complaints

OVERDOSAGE	
Signs and symptoms	Somnolence, confusion, coma, diminished reflexes, excitation, hypotension
Treatment	Empty stomach immediately by induction of emesis and/or gastric lavage. Employ general supportive measures, as needed. Monitor vital signs frequently and keep patient under close observation. For hypotension, use norepinephrine or metaraminol.

DRUG INTERACTIONS	
Alcohol, tricyclic antidepressants, sedative-hypnotics, MAO inhibitors, and other CNS depressants	△ CNS depression

ALTERED LABORATORY VALUES

No clinically significant alterations in blood/serum or urinary values usually occur at therapeutic dosages

USE IN CHILDREN

See INDICATIONS and ORAL DOSAGE; not recommended for use in children under 9 yr of age

USE IN PREGNANT AND NURSING WOMEN

Use of antianxiety agents during early pregnancy should almost always be avoided. Although clorazepate has not been sufficiently studied to determine conclusively its effects during pregnancy, an increased risk of congenital malformations during the first trimester has been associated with minor tranquilizers (chlordiazepoxide, diazepam, meprobamate). Nordiazepam, the primary metabolite of clorazepate, is excreted in human milk; patient should stop nursing if drug is prescribed.

[1] Anxiety or tension associated with the stress of everyday life usually does not require treatment with an antianxiety agent

---

MISCELLANEOUS ANTICONVULSANTS

TRIDIONE (trimethadione) Abbott Rx

Capsules: 300 mg **Chewable tablets:** 150 mg **Solution (per 5 ml):** 200 mg (1 pt)

INDICATIONS

Absence (petit mal) seizures refractory to less toxic anticonvulsants

ORAL DOSAGE

Adult: 900 mg/day to start, followed by weekly increases of 300 mg/day, if needed and tolerated, until optimal clinical response is achieved; usual maintenance dosage: 300–600 mg tid or qid
Child: 300–900 mg/day, given in 3–4 equally divided doses

CONTRAINDICATIONS

Hypersensitivity to trimethadione

WARNINGS/PRECAUTIONS

Medical supervision	Patient must be carefully supervised, especially during the first year of therapy, because of possibility of serious side effects
Exfoliative dermatitis, severe erythema multiforme	May develop; discontinue therapy at the first sign of even mild skin rash and reinstitute therapy (cautiously) only after the rash has cleared completely
Blood dyscrasias	May occur and may be fatal (see ADVERSE REACTIONS); obtain a baseline and monthly CBC and instruct patient to report immediately any signs or symptoms of infection or bleeding tendency (eg, sore throat, fever, malaise, bruises, petechiae, or epistaxis).[1] Discontinue therapy if blood count is markedly depressed or neutrophil count drops to 2,500/mm^3 or less. Do not use ordinarily in patients with severe blood dyscrasias.
Hepatic impairment	May occur; perform liver function studies before starting therapy and at monthly intervals thereafter. Discontinue use if jaundice or other signs of hepatic dysfunction occur. Do not use ordinarily in patients with severe hepatic impairment.
Nephrosis	May occur and may be fatal; perform a urinalysis prior to initiating therapy and at monthly intervals thereafter. Discontinue use of the drug if persistent or increasing albuminuria or other significant renal abnormality occurs. Do not use ordinarily in patients with severe renal dysfunction.
Drowsiness	May occur but usually subsides with continued therapy; if drowsiness persists, reduce dosage
Visual disturbances	May occur; use with caution in patients with diseases of the retina or optic nerve. Hemeralopia may be reversed by dosage reduction. Discontinue use of the drug if scotomata occur.
Systemic lupus erythematosus	May occur; discontinue therapy if lupus-like manifestations occur
Lymphadenopathies	May occur, simulating malignant lymphoma; discontinue therapy if lymph-node enlargement occurs
Myasthenia gravis-like syndrome	May occur with chronic use; discontinue therapy if suggestive symptoms occur
Concomitant drug therapy	Drugs with similar side effects should be avoided or used with extreme caution during therapy
Abrupt discontinuation of therapy	May precipitate petit mal status; if abrupt withdrawal is required (eg, because of serious effects), substitute another anticonvulsant

TRIDIONE ■ VALIUM/VALRELEASE

ADVERSE REACTIONS

Gastrointestinal	Nausea, vomiting, abdominal pain, gastric distress, anorexia, weight loss; hepatitis (rare)
Central nervous system and neuromuscular	Drowsiness, fatigue, malaise, insomnia, vertigo, headache, paresthesias, grand mal seizures, increased irritability, personality changes
Hematological	Neutropenia, leukopenia, eosinophilia, thrombocytopenia, pancytopenia, agranulocytosis, hypoplastic anemia, fatal aplastic anemia, bleeding gums, epistaxis, petechial hemorrhage, vaginal bleeding
Dermatological	Acneform or morbilliform rash progressing to exfoliative dermatitis or severe erythema multiforme; alopecia
Ophthalmic	Hemeralopia, photophobia, diplopia, retinal hemorrhage
Hypersensitivity	Pruritus associated with lymphadenopathy and hepatosplenomegaly
Other	Hiccups, blood-pressure changes, fatal nephrosis, lupus erythematosus, lymphadenopathies simulating malignant lymphoma, myasthenia gravis-like syndrome

OVERDOSAGE

Signs and symptoms	Drowsiness, nausea, dizziness, ataxia, and visual disturbances, followed by coma in cases of massive ingestion
Treatment	Induce emesis or perform gastric lavage to empty stomach. Institute general supportive measures and monitor vital signs. Alkalinization of the urine may increase metabolite excretion. Following recovery, obtain a CBC and evaluate hepatic and renal function.

DRUG INTERACTIONS

Tricyclic antidepressants (high doses), antipsychotics (high doses)	⇧ Risk of seizures

ALTERED LABORATORY VALUES

Urinary values	⇧ Albumin

No clinically significant alterations in blood/serum values occur at therapeutic dosges

USE IN CHILDREN
See INDICATIONS and ORAL DOSAGE

USE IN PREGNANT AND NURSING WOMEN
An increased incidence of birth defects may be associated with the use of trimethadione during pregnancy. Administer to women of childbearing potential only if essential to management of seizures; effective contraception should be used and, if patient becomes pregnant, termination of pregnancy should be considered. Maternal ingestion of anticonvulsants may cause neonatal hemorrhage (usually within 24 h of birth) due to a coagulation defect. Administer prophylactic vitamin K_1 to mother 1 mo prior to and during delivery, and to infant IV immediately after birth. The safety of trimethadione for use in nursing mothers has not been established.

[1] The interval between blood counts may be extended if no abnormality occurs for 12 mo

---

MISCELLANEOUS ANTICONVULSANTS

VALIUM (diazepam) Roche

C-IV

Tablets: 2, 5, 10 mg   **Ampuls:** 5 mg/ml (2 ml)   **Prefilled syringes:** 5 mg/ml (2 ml)   **Vials:** 5 mg/ml (10 ml)

INDICATIONS	ORAL DOSAGE	PARENTERAL DOSAGE
Anxiety disorders and short-term relief of **symptoms of anxiety**[1]	Adult: 2–10 mg bid to qid, depending upon severity	Adult: 2–10 mg IM or IV to start; repeat 3–4 h later, if needed
Acute alcohol withdrawal syndrome	Adult: 10 mg tid or qid over initial 24 h; then 5 mg tid or qid, as needed	Adult: 10 mg IM or IV to start, then 5–10 mg 3–4 h later, if needed
Preoperative medication		Adult: 10 mg IM (preferred) before surgery
Skeletal muscle spasm due to reflex spasm secondary to muscle or joint inflammation, trauma, or other local pathology (adjunctive therapy) **Spasticity** due to upper motor neuron disorders, such as cerebral palsy and paraplegia (adjunctive therapy) **Athetosis** (adjunctive therapy) **Stiff-man syndrome** (adjunctive therapy)	Adult: 2–10 mg tid or qid Child (> 6 mo): 1–2.5 mg tid or qid to start; increase gradually, as needed	Adult: 5–10 mg IM or IV to start; repeat 3–4 h later, if needed

VALIUM/VALRELEASE

Indication	Adult Dosage	Child Dosage
Tetanus (adjunctive therapy)	Adult: same as for muscle spasm, except that larger doses may be needed	Child (1 mo to 5 yr): 1–2 mg IM or IV (slowly); repeat q3–4h, as needed Child (> 5 yr): 5–10 mg IM or IV (slowly); repeat q3–4h, as needed
Convulsive disorders (adjunctive therapy)	Adult: 2–10 mg bid to qid	Child (> 6 mo): 1–2.5 mg tid or qid to start; increase gradually, as needed
Status epilepticus Severe recurrent convulsive seizures	Adult: 5–10 mg IM or IV (preferred), slowly, every 10–15 min, up to 30 mg; repeat 2–4 h later, if needed	Child (1 mo to 5 yr): 0.2–0.5 mg IM or IV (preferred), slowly, every 2–5 min, up to 5 mg; repeat 2–4 h later, if needed Child (> 5 yr): 1 mg IM or IV (preferred), slowly, every 2–5 min, up to 10 mg; repeat 2–4 h later, if needed
Endoscopic procedures (adjunctive therapy)	Adult: 5–10 mg IM 30 min prior to procedure or 10–20 mg, or less, IV (preferred), slowly, just prior to procedure	
Cardioversion (adjunctive therapy)	Adult: 5–15 mg IV within 5–10 min before procedure	

VALRELEASE (diazepam) Roche   C-IV

Capsules (slow release): 15 mg

INDICATIONS

Anxiety disorders and short-term relief of **symptoms of anxiety**[1]
Skeletal muscle spasm due to reflex spasm secondary to muscle or joint inflammation, trauma, or other local pathology (adjunctive therapy)
Spasticity due to upper motor neuron disorders, such as cerebral palsy and paraplegia (adjunctive therapy)
Athetosis (adjunctive therapy)
Stiff-man syndrome (adjunctive therapy)
Convulsive disorders (adjunctive therapy)

Acute alcohol withdrawal syndrome

ORAL DOSAGE

Adult: 15–30 mg once daily, depending upon severity
Child (> 6 mo): 15 mg once daily if 5 mg tid is the optimum dosage of the tablet form

Adult: 30 mg for the initial 24 h, followed by 15 mg once daily, as needed

CONTRAINDICATIONS

Hypersensitivity to diazepam	Depression of vital signs in patients undergoing acute alcohol intoxication	Shock or coma (for parenteral use only)
Acute narrow-angle glaucoma		
Open-angle glaucoma (unless patient is receiving appropriate antiglaucoma therapy)		

ADMINISTRATION/DOSAGE ADJUSTMENTS

Elderly and/or debilitated patients	To preclude ataxia or oversedation, start with 2–2.5 mg 1–2 times/day orally and increase the dosage gradually; if the optimum dosage is 5 mg tid, slow-release capsules may be substituted in a dosage of 15 mg once daily. When using the injectable form, start with 2–5 mg and then increase the dosage gradually (see WARNINGS/PRECAUTIONS).
Intravenous use	May result in venous thrombosis, phlebitis, local irritation, swelling, and (rarely) vascular impairment. Administer solution slowly, no faster than 5 mg (1 ml)/min, *into large veins only;* carefully avoid intraarterial administration or extravasation. Do not mix or dilute with other drugs or solutions. If direct IV administration is not possible, slow injection through infusion tubing as close as possible to vein insertion (since diazepam is sparingly soluble) may be substituted.
Concomitant therapy with narcotic analgesics	Reduce narcotic dosage by a least one third and administer in small increments
Long-term use (> 4 mo)	Effectiveness for prolonged use as an antianxiety agent has not been tested in systematic clinical studies; reassess need for continued therapy periodically

WARNINGS/PRECAUTIONS

Psychosis	Diazepam is of no value in psychotic patients
Mental impairment, reflex-slowing	Caution patients not to engage in potentially hazardous activities requiring full mental alertness and that alcohol and other CNS depressants may cause further impairment
Drug dependence	Psychic and/or physical dependence may develop, especially in addiction-prone individuals

VALIUM/VALRELEASE

Abrupt discontinuation of therapy	May precipitate barbiturate-like withdrawal symptoms, including convulsions, tremor, abdominal and muscle cramps, vomiting, and sweating; milder withdrawal symptoms have also been observed infrequently following abrupt discontinuation of several months of continuous benzodiazepine therapy, generally when higher therapeutic doses have been used. Taper dosage gradually after extended treatment.
Potentially suicidal patients	Should not have access to large quantities of diazepam; prescribe smallest amount feasible
Apnea and/or cardiac arrest	May occur in the elderly or gravely ill or in patients with limited pulmonary reserve when parenteral route (particularly IV) is used; risk of apnea is increased by concomitant use of CNS depressants (see DRUG INTERACTIONS)
Convulsive disorders	May increase frequency and/or severity of grand mal seizures. Dosages of standard anticonvulsants may have to be increased. Abrupt withdrawal may also be associated temporarily with increased seizure activity. The parenteral form should be used with extreme caution in patients with chronic lung disease or unstable cardiovascular status.
Hepatic or renal impairment	Monitor patient closely to avoid excessive drug accumulation (see OVERDOSAGE)
Prolonged therapy	Blood counts and liver-function tests should be performed periodically

ADVERSE REACTIONS

Frequent reactions (incidence ≥ 1%) are printed in *italics*

Central nervous system and neuromuscular	*Drowsiness, fatigue, ataxia,* confusion, depression, dysarthria, headache, hypoactivity, slurred speech, syncope, tremor, vertigo, acute hyperexcitability, anxiety, hallucinations, increased muscle spasticity, insomnia, rage, sleep disturbances, stimulation, EEG changes, muscular weakness (with parenteral use)
Cardiovascular	Bradycardia, cardiovascular collapse, hypotension, cardiac arrest
Gastrointestinal	Constipation, nausea, hiccoughs, salivary changes
Hepatic	Jaundice
Genitourinary	Incontinence, urinary retention
Ophthalmic	Blurred vision, diplopia, nystagmus
Respiratory	Coughing, depressed respiration, dyspnea, hyperventilation, laryngospasm, throat or chest pain (during peroral endoscopy)
Dermatological	Urticaria, skin rash
Hematological	Neutropenia
Other	*Venous thrombosis and phlebitis at injection site,* changes in libido

OVERDOSAGE

Signs and symptoms	Somnolence, confusion, coma, diminished reflexes, hypotension
Treatment	Empty stomach immediately by gastric lavage. Monitor respiration, pulse, and blood pressure. Employ general supportive measures, as needed. Administer IV fluids and maintain adequate airway. Hypotension may be combated with levarterenol or metaraminol. Dialysis is of limited value.

DRUG INTERACTIONS

Alcohol, narcotic analgesics, sedative-hypnotics, and other CNS depressants	⇧ CNS depression ⇧ Hypotension (with parenteral use) ⇧ Muscular weakness (with parenteral use)
MAO inhibitors and other antidepressants	⇧ CNS effects
Cimetidine	⇩ Clearance of diazepam

ALTERED LABORATORY VALUES
No clinically significant alterations in blood/serum or urinary values occur at therapeutic dosages

USE IN CHILDREN
See INDICATIONS and ORAL DOSAGE. When using the injectable form, give not more than 0.25 mg/kg over a 3-min period; the initial dose may be safely repeated after 15–30 min. Oral diazepam is not indicated for use in infants under 6 mo of age. Consult manufacturer for use of the injectable form in newborns (< 30 days of age); prolonged CNS depression has been observed in neonates.

USE IN PREGNANT AND NURSING WOMEN
Use of antianxiety agents during early pregnancy should almost always be avoided. Although diazepam has not been sufficiently studied to determine conclusively its effects during pregnancy, an increased risk of congenital malformations during the first trimester has been associated with minor tranquilizers (meprobamate, diazepam, and chlordiazepoxide). Patient should stop breast-feeding if drug is prescribed; lethargy, weight loss, and hyperbilirubinemia in nursing infants have been reported.[1]

[1] Erkkola R, Kanto J: *Lancet* 1:542, 1972; Patrick MJ, Tilstone WJ: *Lancet* 1:542, 1972; Takyi BE: *J Hosp Pharm* 28:317, 1970

[1] Anxiety or tension associated with the stress of everyday life usually does not require treatment with an antianxiety agent

---

ANTIPARKINSON AGENTS

AKINETON (biperiden) Knoll Rx
Tablets: 2 mg biperiden hydrochloride   **Ampuls:** 5 mg biperiden lactate/ml (1 ml)

INDICATIONS	ORAL DOSAGE	PARENTERAL DOSAGE
Parkinsonism, including postencephalitic, arteriosclerotic, and idiopathic forms (adjunctive therapy)	Adult: 2 mg tid or qid to start, followed, as needed, by up to 16 mg/24 h	
Drug-induced extrapyramidal disturbances	Adult: 2 mg 1–3 times/day	Adult: 2 mg IM or IV q½h, as needed, up to 4 doses/24 h

CONTRAINDICATIONS
Hypersensitivity to biperiden	Narrow angle glaucoma	Bowel obstruction
Megacolon		

ADMINISTRATION/DOSAGE ADJUSTMENTS
Gastric irritation	May be avoided with oral form by administering drug during or after meals
Parenteral side effects	May be minimized or avoided by slow IV administration

WARNINGS/PRECAUTIONS
Special-risk patients	Use with caution in patients with glaucoma, prostatism, or cardiac arrythmias
Drowsiness	Caution patients who drive or engage in other potentially hazardous activities that drowsiness may occasionally occur

ADVERSE REACTIONS
Central nervous system	Mental confusion, euphoria, agitation, disturbed behavior, disorientation, drowsiness
Gastrointestinal	Gastric irritation (with oral use), constipation
Cardiovascular	Mild, transient postural hypotension
Other	Dry mouth, blurred vision, urinary retention

OVERDOSAGE
Signs and symptoms	Warm, dry skin, dilated and sluggish pupils, facial flushing, decreased secretions of the mouth, pharynx, nose, and bronchi, foul-smelling breath, hyperthermia, tachycardia, decreased bowel sounds, urinary retention, delirium, disorientation, anxiety, hallucinations, illusions, confusion, incoherence, agitation, hyperactivity, ataxia, loss of memory, paranoia, combativeness, seizures, stupor, coma, paralysis, respiratory and cardiac arrest
Treatment	If drug was ingested, perform gastric lavage or other measures to limit absorption. Respiratory support, artificial ventilation, and/or vasopressors may be required. Hyperthermia must be reversed, fluid volume replaced, and acid-base balance maintained. Urinary catheterization may be necessary. For CNS excitation, administer a small dose of diazepam or a short-acting barbiturate. Do not give phenothiazines, as coma may ensue. To treat anticholinergic symptoms, physostigmine may be administered, but its routine use is controversial; delirium, hallucinations, coma, and supraventricular tachycardia (not ventricular tachycardias or conduction defects) seem to respond. If indicated, give 1 mg of physostigmine salicylate (halve the dose for children and elderly patients), administered IM or by slow IV infusion. If there is no response after 20 min, repeat the dose until toxic effects are reversed, excessive cholinergic signs are seen, or a total of 4 mg has been given. Additional injections may be required q1–2h to maintain control. Observe patient closely for 8–12 h after last episode for relapse.

DRUG INTERACTIONS

Alcohol and other CNS depressants	△ Sedative effects; instruct patients to avoid alcohol and other CNS depressants during therapy
Amantadine, antihistamines, antimuscarinics, haloperidol, MAO inhibitors, tricyclic antidepressants, phenothiazines, procainamide, quinidine	△ Atropine-like effects
Antacids, antidiarrheals	▽ Absorption of biperiden; allow 1–2 h between doses of different medications

ALTERED LABORATORY VALUES

No clinically significant alterations in blood/serum or urinary values occur at therapeutic dosages

USE IN CHILDREN

Safety and effectiveness for use in children have not been established

USE IN PREGNANT AND NURSING WOMEN

Pregnancy Category C: possibility of fetal harm and effect, if any, on reproductive capacity are unknown. Use only when clearly indicated in pregnant women. Administer with caution to nursing mothers, since it is not known whether this drug is excreted in human milk.

ANTIPARKINSON AGENTS

ARTANE (trihexyphenidyl hydrochloride) Lederle Rx

Tablets: 2, 5 mg   **Capsules (sustained release):** 5 mg   **Elixir (per 5 ml):** 2 mg[1] *lime-mint flavored*

INDICATIONS

Parkinsonism, including postencephalitic, arteriosclerotic, and idiopathic forms (adjunctive therapy)

Drug-induced extrapyramidal disturbances

ORAL DOSAGE

Adult: 1 mg/day to start, followed, if needed, by increases of 2 mg/day at 3- to 5-day intervals, up to 6–10 mg/day, given in 3 divided doses at mealtimes
Child: use according to medical judgment

Adult: 1 mg to start, followed by increases, if needed, after several hours, up to 15 mg/day; usual dosage range: 5–15 mg/day
Child: use according to medical judgment

CONTRAINDICATIONS

None known

ADMINISTRATION/DOSAGE ADJUSTMENTS

High doses (> 10 mg/day)	May be divided into 4 parts, with 3 doses given at mealtimes and the 4th at bedtime
Neuroleptic-induced extrapyramidal reactions	Satisfactory control occasionally may be achieved more rapidly by temporarily reducing the antipsychotic dosage upon starting treatment with trihexyphenidyl and then adjusting the dosage of both drugs until desired ataractic effect is retained without extrapyramidal symptoms. Once the reactions have been controlled for several days, it may be possible to lower the dosage of trihexyphenidyl or even eliminate the drug.
Patients with arteriosclerosis or idiosyncratic reactions to other drugs	Initiate therapy with small doses and increase dosage gradually to avoid untoward effects (see ADVERSE REACTIONS); if severe reactions occur, discontinue therapy for several days and resume at a lower dosage
Postencephalitic patients	May require 12–15 mg/day; excessive salivation may be reduced by administration after meals or by concomitant use of small amounts of atropine
Excessive dryness of the mouth, thirst	May be allayed by taking the drug prior to meals, by drinking water, or by using mints or chewing gum
Combination therapy	Administer 3–6 mg/day when used with levodopa; when used with another parasympathetic agent, gradually increase trihexyphenidyl dosage while decreasing the dosage of the other agent
Sustained-release capsules	May be used for maintenance therapy after patient has been stabilized on conventional dosage forms; administer daily dose as a single dose after breakfast, or as 2 divided doses q12h. Do not use for initial therapy.

WARNINGS/PRECAUTIONS

Increased intraocular pressure	May develop; perform gonioscope evaluation prior to therapy and closely monitor intraocular pressure at regular intervals thereafter. Incipient glaucoma may be precipitated.
Special-risk patients	Use with caution in patients with cardiac, hepatic, or renal disorders, hypertension, glaucoma, or obstructive gastrointestinal or genitourinary tract disease and in elderly males with possible prostatic hypertrophy

Elderly patients	Exhibit increased sensitivity to drug; strict dosage regulation is necessary
Prolonged therapy	Observe patient carefully for allergic or other untoward reactions
Tardive dyskinesia	Antiparkinson drugs do not alleviate the symptoms of tardive dyskinesia, and, in some instances, may aggravate them; do not use this drug in patients with tardive dyskinesia

ADVERSE REACTIONS[2]

Frequent reactions (incidence $\geq$ 1%) are printed in *italics*

Central nervous system	*Dizziness and nervousness (30–50%);* mental confusion, agitation, and disturbed behavior (in patients with arteriosclerosis or idiosyncratic reactions to other drugs); drowsiness; weakness; headache; psychiatric disturbances (with indiscriminate use to sustain continued euphoria); delusions, hallucinations, and paranoia (rare)
Gastrointestinal	*Dry mouth and mild nausea (30–50%);* vomiting; constipation; colonic dilatation, paralytic ileus, and suppurative parotitis (rare)
Dermatological	Rash (rare)
Cardiovascular	Tachycardia
Ophthalmic	*Blurred vision (30–50%);* mydriasis; increased intraocular tension; narrow-angle glaucoma (with prolonged use)
Genitourinary	Urinary hesitancy, urinary retention

OVERDOSAGE

Signs and symptoms	May range from CNS stimulation (confusion, excitement, hyperpyrexia, agitation, disorientation, delirium, hallucinations) to CNS depression (drowsiness, sedation, coma); atropine-like effects (see ADVERSE REACTIONS)
Treatment	If patient is neither precomatose nor convulsive, empty stomach by emesis or gastric lavage. Support respiration with artificial respiration or mechanical assistance, if needed. For CNS excitation, administer a short-acting barbiturate *carefully,* since excitation may precede depression. Treat circulatory collapse with vasopressors. Control hyperthermia with tepid bathing.

DRUG INTERACTIONS

Alcohol and other CNS depressants	⇧	Sedative effect
Amantadine, antihistamines, antimuscarinics, haloperidol, MAO inhibitors, phenothiazines, procainamide, quinidine, tricyclic antidepressants	⇧	Atropine-like effects
Antacids, antidiarrheals	⇩	Absorption of trihexyphenidyl; allow 1–2 h between doses of different medications

ALTERED LABORATORY VALUES

No clinically significant alterations in blood/serum or urinary values occur at therapeutic dosages

---

USE IN CHILDREN

Use according to medical judgment

USE IN PREGNANT AND NURSING WOMEN

Safety for use during pregnancy has not been established; use with caution. It is not known whether trihexyphenidyl is excreted in human milk; because many drugs are excreted in breast milk, use with caution in nursing mothers.

---

[1] Contains 5% alcohol
[2] Includes reactions common to atropine-like drugs in general

---

ANTIPARKINSON AGENTS

BENADRYL 25 (diphenhydramine hydrochloride) Warner-Lambert — OTC

Capsules: 25 mg

BENADRYL Elixir (diphenhydramine hydrochloride) Warner-Lambert — OTC

Elixir (per 5 ml): 12.5 mg[1] (4 fl oz)

INDICATIONS	ORAL DOSAGE
Runny nose, sneezing, itchy nose and throat, and itchy, watery eyes associated with **hay fever** or other upper respiratory tract allergies Runny nose and sneezing associated with the **common cold**	**Adult:** 25–50 mg or 10–20 ml (2–4 tsp) q4–6h **Child (6–12 yr):** 25 mg or 5–10 ml (1–2 tsp) q4–6h

BENADRYL (diphenhydramine hydrochloride) Parke-Davis Rx

Capsules: 25, 50 mg **Elixir (per 5 ml):** 12.5 mg[1] (5 ml, 4 fl oz, 1 pt, 1 gal) **Ampuls:** 50 mg/ml (1 ml) **Vials:** 10 mg/ml (10, 30 ml), 50 mg/ml (10 ml) **Prefilled syringes:** 50 mg/ml (1 ml)

INDICATIONS	ORAL DOSAGE	PARENTERAL DOSAGE
Allergic conjunctivitis due to foods Mild, uncomplicated **urticaria** and **angioedema** **Dermatographism** **Allergic reactions to blood or plasma** **Anaphylactic reactions,** as an adjunct to epinephrine and other standard measures after acute symptoms have been controlled **Motion sickness** **Parkinsonism** (including drug-induced symptoms), for use in elderly patients unable to tolerate more potent agents, for mild cases in other age groups, and for more severe cases when combined with centrally acting anticholinergic agents	**Adult:** 25–50 mg or 10–20 ml (2–4 tsp) tid or qid **Child (> 20 lb):** 12.5–25 mg or 5–10 ml (1–2 tsp) tid or qid, or 5 mg/kg/24 h (150 mg/m²/24 h), up to 300 mg/day, given in 3–4 divided doses	**Adult:** 10–50 mg (or up to 100 mg, if needed) IM (deeply) or IV, up to 400 mg/day **Child:** 5 mg/kg/24 h (150 mg/m²/24 h), up to 300 mg/day, given in 4 divided doses IM (deeply) or IV
Insomnia	**Adult:** 50 mg or 20 ml (4 tsp) at bedtime	—

CONTRAINDICATIONS

Hypersensitivity to diphenhydramine or structurally related antihistamines	Breast-feeding	Full-term or premature neonates

ADMINISTRATION/DOSAGE ADJUSTMENTS

Parenteral administration	The injectable forms may be used when oral therapy is impractical for active treatment of motion sickness, amelioration of allergic reactions to blood or plasma, or adjunctive therapy of anaphylactic reactions, and when oral therapy is contraindicated or impossible in cases of parkinsonism or other uncomplicated, immediate-type allergic reactions
Treatment of motion sickness	The full oral dosage is recommended for prophylactic use; the first dose should be given 30 min before the patient is exposed to motion, followed by similar doses before meals and upon retiring for the duration of the exposure

WARNINGS/PRECAUTIONS

Drowsiness	Caution patients about driving or engaging in other activities requiring mental alertness, and about using alcohol or other CNS depressants (see DRUG INTERACTIONS)
Elderly patients	Dizziness, sedation, and hypotension occur more frequently in patients over 60 yr of age
Special-risk patients	Use with considerable caution in patients with narrow-angle glaucoma, stenosing peptic ulcer, pyloroduodenal obstruction, symptomatic prostatic hypertrophy, or bladder-neck obstruction and with caution in patients with increased intraocular pressure, hyperthyroidism, cardiovascular disease, hypertension, or a history of asthma or other lower respiratory tract diseases
Carcinogenicity, mutagenicity	No studies have been done to evaluate the carcinogenic or mutagenic potential of this drug

ADVERSE REACTIONS

The most frequent reactions, regardless of incidence, are printed in *italics*

Cardiovascular	Hypotension, headache, palpitations, tachycardia, extrasystoles
Hematological	Hemolytic anemia, thrombocytopenia, agranulocytosis
Central nervous system	*Sedation, sleepiness, dizziness, disturbed coordination,* fatigue, confusion, restlessness, excitation, nervousness, tremor, irritability, insomnia, euphoria, paresthesias, vertigo, tinnitus, acute labyrinthitis, neuritis, convulsions
Ophthalmic	Blurred vision, diplopia
Gastrointestinal	*Epigastric distress,* anorexia, nausea, vomiting, diarrhea, constipation
Genitourinary	Urinary frequency, difficult urination, urinary retention, early menses
Respiratory	*Thickening of bronchial secretions,* tightness in the chest and wheezing, nasal stuffiness
Dermatological	Urticaria, drug rash, photosensitivity
Hypersensitivity	Anaphylactic shock
Other	Dry mouth, nose, and throat; chills, excessive perspiration

OVERDOSAGE

Signs and symptoms	Varies from CNS depression (drowsiness, sedation, diminished mental alertness, apnea, cardiovascular collapse) to CNS stimulation (insomnia, excitement, hallucinations, ataxia, incoordination, athetosis, tremors, convulsions) and may include dizziness, tinnitus, blurred vision, and hypotension; CNS stimulation, followed by postictal depression, and atropine-like symptoms (dry mouth; fixed, dilated pupils; fever, flushing, GI disturbances) are particularly likely in children

BENADRYL ■ COGENTIN

Treatment	If patient is conscious, induce emesis with syrup of ipecac, even though vomiting may have occurred spontaneously. If vomiting is unsuccessful or contraindicated, perform gastric lavage with isotonic or 1/2 isotonic saline solution. Remove any remaining drug in the stomach by instillation of activated charcoal. Administer a saline cathartic to rapidly dilute bowel content. Treatment is symptomatic and supportive. If breathing is significantly impaired, maintain an adequate airway and provide mechanically assisted ventilation; *do not use analeptics*. Vasopressors (eg, norepinephrine) may be used for significant hypotension. Treat hyperpyrexia by sponging with tepid water or use of ice packs or a hypothermal blanket. For seizures, administer a short-acting barbiturate, diazepam, or paraldehyde.

DRUG INTERACTIONS

Alcohol, tranquilizers, sedative-hypnotics, and other CNS depressants	↕ CNS depression
MAO inhibitors	↕ Anticholinergic effects

ALTERED LABORATORY VALUES

No clinically significant alterations in blood/serum or urinary values occur at therapeutic dosages

---

USE IN CHILDREN

See INDICATIONS and dosage recommendations; contraindicated for use in full-term or premature neonates. Antihistamines may produce excitation in young children.

USE IN PREGNANT AND NURSING WOMEN

Pregnancy Category B: reproduction studies in rats and rabbits given up to 5 times the human dose have shown no evidence of impaired fertility or harm to the fetus; use during pregnancy only if clearly needed. Contraindicated for use in nursing mothers due to the increased risk of antihistaminic side effects in newborns and infants.

---

[1] Contains 5% alcohol
[2] Contains 14% alcohol

ANTIPARKINSON AGENTS

COGENTIN (benztropine mesylate) Merck Sharp & Dohme — Rx

Tablets: 0.5, 1, 2 mg **Ampuls:** 1 mg/ml[1] (2 ml)

INDICATIONS	ORAL DOSAGE	PARENTERAL DOSAGE
Idiopathic parkinsonism (adjunctive therapy)	**Adult:** 0.5–1 mg, given in a single daily dose at bedtime, to start, followed by up to 4–6 mg/day, if needed; usual dosage: 1–2 mg/day	**Adult:** 0.5–1 mg IM, given in a single daily dose at bedtime, to start, followed by up to 4–6 mg/day, if needed; usual dosage: 1–2 mg/day
Postencephalitic parkinsonism (adjunctive therapy)	**Adult:** 2 mg/day to start, followed by up to 6 mg/day, if needed; usual dosage: 1–2 mg/day	**Adult:** 2 mg/day IM to start, followed by up to 6 mg/day, if needed; usual dosage: 1–2 mg/day IM
Drug-induced extrapyramidal disorders	**Adult:** 1–4 mg 1–2 times/day	**Adult:** 1–4 mg IM 1–2 times/day
Drug-induced acute dystonic reactions	—	**Adult:** 1–2 mg IM, followed by 1–2 mg orally bid to prevent recurrence
Prophylaxis of recurrent or transient drug-induced extrapyramidal disorders	**Adult:** 1–2 mg bid or tid, as needed; reassess need for continued therapy after 1–2 wk by withdrawing drug temporarily	—

CONTRAINDICATIONS

Age < 3 yr	Hypersensitivity to benztropine mesylate or any component of injectable form

ADMINISTRATION/DOSAGE ADJUSTMENTS

Initiating therapy and frequency of dosage adjustments	Begin with a low dose and increase dosage gradually in increments of 0.5 mg every 5–6 days until optimal results are achieved without excessive adverse reactions; for highly sensitive patients with postencephalitic parkinsonism, initiate therapy with 0.5 mg at bedtime and increase dosage as necessary
Frequency of administration	Daily dose may be given as a single dose, preferably at bedtime, or divided into 2–4 parts
Intravenous use	As there is no significant difference in the onset of effect after IM or IV administration, the IV route is rarely needed

COMPENDIUM OF DRUG THERAPY

COGENTIN

Patients receiving other anti-parkinson agents	Reduce or discontinue dosage of other agents gradually when adding benztropine mesylate
Combination therapy	May be used with levodopa/carbidopa or with levodopa alone; periodic dosage adjustments may be needed to maintain optimum response
Atropine-like effects	May be minimized by careful adjustment of daily dosage or time of administration; if dry mouth causes anorexia, weight loss, or difficulty in swallowing or speaking, reduce dosage or temporarily discontinue drug
Nausea, vomiting	Reduce dosage slightly to control nausea; if vomiting occurs, temporarily discontinue drug and reinstitute therapy at a lower dosage. Nausea unaccompanied by vomiting can usually be disregarded.

WARNINGS/PRECAUTIONS

Medical supervision	Continued supervision is recommended due to cumulative action
Mental and/or physical impairment	Caution patients that their performance of potentially hazardous activities may be impaired
Paralytic ileus	May occur in patients who are also receiving phenothiazines or tricyclic antidepressants, and can be fatal; advise patient to report GI disturbances promptly
Anhidrosis	Possibly leading to fatal hyperthermia, may occur. Use with caution during hot weather and in patients with sweating disorders. Concomitant administration of other atropine-like drugs to patients with chronic diseases, CNS disease, or alcoholism or to patients who perform manual labor in a hot environment increases risk. Monitor patient for early signs and reduce dosage accordingly.
Muscle weakness, inability to move particular muscle groups	May occur with large dosages; reduce dosage accordingly
Mental confusion, excitement	May occur with large doses or in susceptible individuals
Intensification of preexisting mental disorders	May occur during treatment of neuroleptic-induced extrapyramidal disorders; toxic psychosis may be precipitated if dosage is increased. Monitor such patients carefully when therapy is started or dosage is increased.
Hypersensitivity	Allergic reactions, including rash, may occur occasionally; if an allergic reaction is seen and it cannot be controlled by a reduction in dosage, therapy should be discontinued
Patients with glaucoma	Therapy is inadvisable in patients with angle-closure glaucoma; simple glaucoma is not affected by the drug
Other special-risk patients	Closely supervise therapy in patients with a tendency toward tachycardia or with prostatic hypertrophy; dysuria may occur but is rarely problematic
Tardive dyskinesia	Antiparkinson agents do not alleviate and may exacerbate symptoms of phenothiazine-induced tardive dyskinesia

ADVERSE REACTIONS

Cardiovascular	Tachycardia
Gastrointestinal	Constipation, dry mouth, nausea, vomiting
Central nervous system	Toxic psychosis, including confusion, disorientation, memory impairment, and visual hallucinations; exacerbation of psychotic symptoms; nervousness, depression, listlessness, numbness of fingers
Ophthalmic	Blurred vision, dilated pupils
Genitourinary	Urinary retention, dysuria
Hypersensitivity	Allergic reactions, including rash

OVERDOSAGE

Signs and symptoms	CNS depression, preceded or followed by stimulation, confusion, nervousness, listlessness, intensification of mental symptoms, toxic psychoses, visual hallucinations, dizziness, muscle weakness, ataxia, dry mouth, mydriasis, blurred vision, palpitations, tachycardia, nausea, vomiting, dysuria, numbness of fingers, dysphagia, allergic reactions, including skin rash; headache, hot, dry, flushed skin; delirium, coma, shock, convulsions, respiratory arrest, anhidrosis, hyperthermia, glaucoma, constipation
Treatment	Empty stomach by emesis or gastric lavage, except in precomatose, convulsive, or psychotic states. Maintain respiration. For anticholinergic intoxication, give 1–2 mg physostigmine SC or IV; repeat after 2 h, if needed. CNS excitement may be treated with a short-acting barbiturate; exercise caution, however, to avoid subsequent depression. Do not use convulsant stimulants for depression. Treat mydriasis and cycloplegia with a local miotic. Use ice bags or other cold applications and alcohol sponges for hyperpyrexia. Vasopressors and fluids may be required for circulatory collapse. Darken room for photophobia.

DRUG INTERACTIONS

Alcohol and other CNS depressants	⇧ Sedative effects

Amantadine, antihistamines, antimuscarinics, haloperidol, MAO inhibitors, tricyclic antidepressants, procainamide, quinidine	⇧ Atropine-like effects
Antacids, antidiarrheals	⇩ Absorption of benztropine; allow 1–2 h between doses of different medications

ALTERED LABORATORY VALUES
No clinically significant alterations in blood/serum or urinary values occur at therapeutic dosages

USE IN CHILDREN
Contraindicated for use in children under 3 yr of age; use with caution in older children (dosage not established)

USE IN PREGNANT AND NURSING WOMEN
Safety for use during pregnancy has not been established. There are no data available regarding use of this drug in nursing women; because most drugs are excreted in human milk, caution should be exercised when this drug is administered to a nursing woman.

[1] Contains 9.0 mg sodium chloride/ml

ANTIPARKINSON AGENTS

DOPAR (levodopa) Norwich Eaton Rx
Capsules: 100, 250, 500 mg

INDICATIONS
Idiopathic Parkinson's disease (paralysis agitans)
Postencephalitic parkinsonism
Symptomatic parkinsonism caused by carbon monoxide or manganese intoxication
Parkinsonism in the elderly associated with cerebral arteriosclerosis

ORAL DOSAGE
Adult: 0.5–1 g/day, given in 2 or more divided doses, with food, to start, followed by increases of up to 0.75 g/day, as tolerated, every 3–7 days, up to a total of 8 g/day, until desired therapeutic response is achieved. An exceptional patient may require higher doses; administer doses exceeding 8 g/day with caution.

CONTRAINDICATIONS
Hypersensitivity to levodopa	Suspicious, undiagnosed skin lesions or history of melanoma	MAO inhibitor therapy (see WARNINGS/PRECAUTIONS)
Narrow-angle glaucoma		

ADMINISTRATION/DOSAGE ADJUSTMENTS
Duration of therapy	Up to 6 mo of treatment may be required in some patients to obtain a significant therapeutic response; during prolonged therapy, perform periodic evaluations of hepatic, hematopoietic, cardiovascular, and renal function
Concomitant use with general anesthetics	Levodopa may be continued as long as the patient is able to take fluids and medication by mouth; if therapy is interrupted, give the usual daily dose as soon as the patient is able to take oral medication
Reinstitution of therapy after prolonged interruptions	Adjust dosage gradually, although in many cases the dosage can be rapidly titrated to the previous therapeutic level

WARNINGS/PRECAUTIONS
MAO inhibitor therapy	Wait at least 14 days after discontinuing MAO inhibitors before initiating levodopa therapy
Postural hypotension	May occur; use with caution in patients receiving antihypertensive agents. Dosage adjustment of antihypertensive agents may be necessary.
Patients with a history of myocardial infarction and residual arrhythmias	If levodopa is essential, administer with caution in a facility with a coronary or intensive care unit
Gastrointestinal hemorrhage	May occur in patients with a history of active peptic ulcer disease
Depression with suicidal tendencies	May develop; observe patient carefully. Administer with caution to psychotics.
Patients with chronic wide-angle glaucoma	Use with caution, provided intraocular pressure is well controlled; observe for changes in intraocular pressure
Other special-risk patients	Use with caution in patients with severe cardiovascular or pulmonary disease, bronchial asthma, or renal, hepatic, or endocrine disease
Leukopenia	May occur, requiring at least temporary cessation of therapy

COMPENDIUM OF DRUG THERAPY

DOPAR ■ KEMADRIN

Tartrazine sensitivity	Presence of FD&C Yellow No. 5 (tartrazine) in capsules may cause allergic-type reactions, including bronchial asthma, in susceptible individuals

ADVERSE REACTIONS

Frequent reactions (incidence ≥ 1%) are printed in *italics*

Musculoskeletal	*Adventitious movements (eg, choreiform movements, dystonia), ataxia, increased hand tremor,* muscle twitching, blepharospasm, trismus
Cardiovascular	Orthostatic hypotension, cardiac irregularities, palpitations; hypertension and phlebitis (rare)
Central nervous system	*Headache, dizziness, numbness, weakness, faintness, bruxism, confusion, insomnia, nightmares, hallucinations, delusions, agitation, anxiety, malaise, fatigue, euphoria,* mental changes (eg, paranoid ideation and psychotic episodes), bradykinetic episodes, depression with or without suicidal tendencies, dementia[1]
Gastrointestinal	*Anorexia, nausea, and vomiting with or without abdominal pain and distress; dry mouth, dysphagia, sialorrhea,* diarrhea, constipation, flatulence; hiccoughs, bleeding, and duodenal ulcer (rare)
Hematological	Reduced WBC count, hemoglobin, and hematocrit, leukopenia; hemolytic anemia and agranulocytosis (rare)
Dermatological	Rash, flushing; alopecia (rare)
Respiratory	Bizarre breathing patterns
Genitourinary	Urinary retention, urinary incontinence, dark urine; priapism (rare)
Ophthalmic	Diplopia, blurred vision, dilated pupils; oculogyric crisis and activation of latent Horner's syndrome (rare)
Other	Burning sensation of the tongue, bitter taste, diaphoresis, hot flashes, weight gain or loss, dark sweat; edema and hoarseness (rare)

OVERDOSAGE

Signs and symptoms	See ADVERSE REACTIONS
Treatment	Empty stomach immediately by gastric lavage. Institute general supportive measures as needed, including maintenance of an adequate airway and administration of IV fluids. Institute ECG monitoring and observe patient carefully for possible arrhythmias; give appropriate antiarrhythmic agents, if required. Value of pyridoxine hydrochloride (vitamin B_6) in reversing the effects of levodopa has not been established. Value of dialysis is unknown. Consider the possibility of multiple-drug ingestion.

DRUG INTERACTIONS

Pyridoxine hydrochloride (vitamin B_6)	Antagonism of levodopa
Antihypertensive agents	⇧ Hypotensive effect
Methyldopa	⇩ Antiparkinson effect ⇧ Hypotensive effect
Butyrophenones (haloperidol), papaverine, phenothiazines, phenytoin, reserpine	⇩ Antiparkinson effect
MAO inhibitors	⇧ Risk of hypertensive crisis
Sympathomimetics	⇧ Risk of cardiac arrhythmias

ALTERED LABORATORY VALUES

Blood/serum values	⇧ BUN ⇧ SGOT ⇧ SGPT ⇧ Lactic dehydrogenase ⇧ Bilirubin ⇧ Alkaline phosphatase ⇧ PBI + Coombs' test (with prolonged therapy)
Urinary values	⇧ Uric acid (with colorimetric method)

USE IN CHILDREN

Safety for use in children under 12 yr of age has not been established

USE IN PREGNANT AND NURSING WOMEN

Safety for use during pregnancy or in women who may become pregnant has not been established; levodopa adversely affects fetal and postnatal growth and viability in rodents. Do not use in nursing mothers.

---

[1] Stimulation and convulsions have been reported rarely, but a causal relationship has not been established

---

ANTIPARKINSON AGENTS

KEMADRIN (procyclidine hydrochloride) Burroughs Wellcome Rx

Tablets: 5 mg

INDICATIONS

Mild to moderate **postencephalitic, arteriosclerotic, and idiopathic parkinsonism; severe parkinsonism** (adjunctive therapy)

ORAL DOSAGE

Adult: 2.5 mg tid, after meals, to start, followed by a gradual increase in dosage to 5 mg tid plus an additional dose of 5 mg at bedtime, if needed

KEMADRIN ■ LARODOPA

Drug-induced extrapyramidal disorders, including sialorrhea — Adult: 2.5 mg tid, after meals, to start, followed by increases of 2.5 mg/day until symptoms are relieved; usual dosage: 10–20 mg/day

CONTRAINDICATIONS
Narrow-angle glaucoma

ADMINISTRATION/DOSAGE ADJUSTMENTS

Bedtime dose	If dose is not well tolerated, divide total daily requirement into 3 equal daytime doses
Patients receiving other antiparkinson agents	Gradually substitute all or part of original drug with procyclidine, starting with 2.5 mg tid, after meals, and then increasing the dosage, as needed, while omitting or tapering the dosage of the other drug until complete replacement is achieved; thereafter, adjust total daily dose of procyclidine to optimal level
Elderly or arteriosclerotic patients	Lower dosage may be required
Atropine-like effects, mydriasis	May be minimized by careful dosage adjustment

WARNINGS/PRECAUTIONS

Special-risk patients	Use with caution in patients with hypotension or conditions in which inhibition of parasympathetic nervous system is undesirable, such as tachycardia or urinary retention
Mental confusion, disorientation	May occur, particularly in the elderly, with development of agitation, hallucinations, and psychotic-like symptoms
Psychotic episodes	May be precipitated in patients with mental disorders when dosage is increased in the treatment of drug-induced extrapyramidal disorders

ADVERSE REACTIONS

Central nervous system	Giddiness, light-headedness
Gastrointestinal	Nausea, vomiting, epigastric distress, constipation, dry mouth, acute suppurative parotitis
Other	Skin rash, muscular weakness, blurred vision, mydriasis

OVERDOSAGE

Signs and symptoms	May range from CNS stimulation (confusion, excitement, hyperpyrexia, agitation, disorientation, delirium, hallucinations) to CNS depression (drowsiness, sedation, coma); atropine-like effects (see ADVERSE REACTIONS)
Treatment	If patient is neither precomatose nor convulsive, empty stomach by emesis or gastric lavage. Support respiration with artificial respiration or mechanical assistance, if needed. For CNS excitation, administer a short-acting barbiturate *carefully,* since excitation may precede depression. Treat circulatory collapse with vasopressors. Control hyperthermia with tepid bathing.

DRUG INTERACTIONS

Alcohol and other CNS depressants	⇧ Sedative effect
Antihistamines, antimuscarinics, haloperidol, MAO inhibitors, tricyclic antidepressants, phenothiazines, procainamide, quinidine, amantadine	⇧ Atropine-like effects
Antacids, antidiarrheals	⇩ Absorption of procyclidine; allow 1–2 h between doses of different medications

ALTERED LABORATORY VALUES
No clinically significant alterations in blood/serum or urinary values occur at therapeutic dosages

---

USE IN CHILDREN

Safety and efficacy has not been established for use in children

USE IN PREGNANT AND NURSING WOMEN

Safety for use in pregnant or nursing women has not been established

---

ANTIPARKINSON AGENTS

LARODOPA (levodopa) Roche   Rx
Capsules: 100, 250, 500 mg   **Tablets:** 100, 250, 500 mg

INDICATIONS
Idiopathic Parkinson's disease (paralysis agitans)
Postencephalitic parkinsonism
Symptomatic parkinsonism caused by carbon monoxide or manganese intoxication
Parkinsonism in the elderly associated with cerebral arteriosclerosis

ORAL DOSAGE
Adult: 0.5–1 g/day, given in 2 or more divided doses, with food, to start, followed by increases of up to 0.75 g/day, as tolerated, every 3–7 days, up to a total of 8 g/day, until desired therapeutic response is achieved. An exceptional patient may require higher doses; administer doses exceeding 8 g/day with caution.

COMPENDIUM OF DRUG THERAPY

LARODOPA

CONTRAINDICATIONS

Hypersensitivity to levodopa	Suspicious, undiagnosed skin lesions or history of melanoma	MAO inhibitor therapy (see WARNINGS/PRECAUTIONS)
Narrow-angle glaucoma		

ADMINISTRATION/DOSAGE ADJUSTMENTS

Duration of therapy	Up to 6 mo of treatment may be required in some patients to obtain a significant therapeutic response; during prolonged therapy, perform periodic evaluations of hepatic, hematopoietic, cardiovascular, and renal function
Concomitant use with general anesthetics	Levodopa may be continued as long as the patient is able to take fluids and medication by mouth; if therapy is interrupted, give the usual daily dose as soon as the patient is able to take oral medication
Reinstitution of therapy after prolonged interruptions	Adjust dosage gradually, although in many cases the dosage can be rapidly titrated to the previous therapeutic level

WARNINGS/PRECAUTIONS

MAO inhibitor therapy	Wait at least 14 days after discontinuing MAO inhibitors before initiating levodopa therapy
Postural hypotension	May occur; use with caution in patients receiving antihypertensive agents. Dosage adjustment of antihypertensive agents may be necessary.
Patients with a history of myocardial infarction and residual arrhythmias	If levodopa is essential, administer with caution in a facility with a coronary or intensive care unit
Gastrointestinal hemorrhage	May occur in patients with a history of active peptic ulcer disease
Depression with suicidal tendencies	May develop; observe patient carefully. Administer with caution to psychotics.
Patients with chronic wide-angle glaucoma	Use with caution, provided intraocular pressure is well controlled; observe for changes in intraocular pressure
Other special-risk patients	Use with caution in patients with severe cardiovascular or pulmonary disease, bronchial asthma, or renal, hepatic, or endocrine disease
Leukopenia	May occur, requiring at least temporary cessation of therapy

ADVERSE REACTIONS

Frequent reactions (incidence ≥ 1%) are printed in *italics*

Musculoskeletal	*Adventitious movements (eg, choreiform movements, dystonia), ataxia, increased hand tremor,* muscle twitching, blepharospasm, trismus
Cardiovascular	Orthostatic hypotension, cardiac irregularities, palpitations; hypertension and phlebitis (rare)
Central nervous system	*Headache, dizziness, numbness, weakness, faintness, bruxism, confusion, insomnia, nightmares, hallucinations, delusions, agitation, anxiety, malaise, fatigue, euphoria, mental changes (eg, paranoid ideation and psychotic episodes), bradykinetic episodes, depression with or without suicidal tendencies, dementia*[1]
Gastrointestinal	*Anorexia, nausea, and vomiting with or without abdominal pain and distress; dry mouth, dysphagia, sialorrhea,* diarrhea, constipation, flatulence; hiccoughs, bleeding, and duodenal ulcer (rare)
Hematological	Reduced WBC count, hemoglobin, and hematocrit, leukopenia; hemolytic anemia and agranulocytosis (rare)
Dermatological	Rash, flushing; alopecia (rare)
Respiratory	Bizarre breathing patterns
Genitourinary	Urinary retention, urinary incontinence, dark urine; priapism (rare)
Ophthalmic	Diplopia, blurred vision, dilated pupils; oculogyric crisis and activation of latent Horner's syndrome (rare)
Other	Burning sensation of the tongue, bitter taste, diaphoresis, hot flashes, weight gain or loss, dark sweat; edema and hoarseness (rare)

OVERDOSAGE

Signs and symptoms	See ADVERSE REACTIONS
Treatment	Empty stomach immediately by gastric lavage. Institute general supportive measures as needed, including maintenance of an adequate airway and administration of IV fluids. Institute ECG monitoring and observe patient carefully for possible arrhythmias; give appropriate antiarrhythmic agents, if required. Value of pyridoxine hydrochloride (vitamin B_6) in reversing the effects of levodopa has not been established. Value of dialysis is unknown. Consider the possibility of multiple-drug ingestion.

DRUG INTERACTIONS

Pyridoxine hydrochloride (vitamin B_6)	Antagonism of levodopa
Antihypertensive agents	⇧ Hypotensive effect
Methyldopa	⇩ Antiparkinson effect ⇧ Hypotensive effect

Butyrophenones (haloperidol), papaverine, phenothiazines, phenytoin, reserpine	⇩ Antiparkinson effect
MAO inhibitors	⇧ Risk of hypertensive crisis
Sympathomimetics	⇧ Risk of cardiac arrhythmias

ALTERED LABORATORY VALUES

Blood/serum values	⇧ BUN ⇧ SGOT ⇧ SGPT ⇧ Lactic dehydrogenase ⇧ Bilirubin ⇧ Alkaline phosphatase ⇧ PBI + Coombs' test (with prolonged therapy)
Urinary values	⇧ Uric acid (with colorimetric method)

USE IN CHILDREN

Safety for use in children under 12 yr of age has not been established

USE IN PREGNANT AND NURSING WOMEN

Safety for use during pregnancy or in women who may become pregnant has not been established; levodopa adversely affects fetal and postnatal growth and viability in rodents. Do not use in nursing mothers.

---

[1] Stimulation and convulsions have been reported rarely, but a causal relationship has not been established

---

ANTIPARKINSON AGENTS

PARLODEL (bromocriptine mesylate) Sandoz Pharmaceuticals   Rx

Capsules: 5 mg   **Tablets:** 2.5 mg

INDICATIONS	ORAL DOSAGE
Hyperprolactinemic disorders, including amenorrhea, galactorrhea, hypogonadism (infertility), and prolactin-secreting adenomas	**Adult:** 1.25–2.5 mg/day to start, followed, as tolerated, by an increase in dosage of 2.5 mg/day every 3–7 days, until an optimal response is achieved; therapeutic dosage is usually 5–7.5 mg/day, but may range from 2.5–15 mg/day. To manage adverse reactions, temporarily reduce dosage to 1.25 mg bid or tid.
Prevention of physiological lactation after parturition, stillbirth, or abortion	**Adult:** 2.5 mg bid for 14 days or, if necessary, up to 21 days (dosage range: 2.5–7.5 mg/day); begin administration after vital signs have stabilized, but not sooner than 4 h after delivery
Acromegaly	**Adult:** 1.25–2.5 mg/day, given at bedtime with food for 3 days, followed, as tolerated, by an increase in dosage of 1.25–2.5 mg/day every 3–7 days until optimal response or a maximum of 100 mg/day is achieved; usual dosage: 20–30 mg/day
Idiopathic or postencephalitic Parkinson's disease, as an adjunct to levodopa (alone or with a peripheral decarboxylase inhibitor, such as carbidopa)	**Adult:** 1.25 mg bid to start, followed, as needed, by an increase in dosage of 2.5 mg/day every 14–28 days until optimal response or a maximum of 100 mg/day is achieved. If possible, maintain dosage of levodopa while titrating dosage of bromocriptine; if dosage of levodopa is subsequently reduced, retitrate dosage of bromocriptine.

CONTRAINDICATIONS

Sensitivity to ergot alkaloids

ADMINISTRATION/DOSAGE ADJUSTMENTS

Administration	Give each dose with food
Use of contraceptives and pregnancy tests	Bromocriptine can restore fertility, which may not only be undesirable, but may also pose the following two risks: (1) the drug may subsequently affect fetal development if pregnancy is not detected at the time of conception (see USE IN PREGNANT AND NURSING WOMEN) and (2) the hormonal changes during pregnancy may cause optic nerve compression if the woman has a prolactin-secreting macroadenoma (see WARNINGS/PRECAUTIONS). Instruct women who do not wish to become pregnant to use a contraceptive, other than an oral contraceptive, as long as they are undergoing treatment. To avoid prolonged in utero exposure in the event of an unsuspected pregnancy, instruct women seeking to become pregnant to use such a contraceptive during the period of amenorrhea. Test for pregnancy in all patients at least every 4 wk during the period of amenorrhea and, after a normal ovulatory cycle has been restored, whenever menstruation does not occur within 3 days of the expected date. Discontinue therapy any time pregnancy is suspected.
Amenorrhea, galactorrhea	In patients with amenorrhea, menses is usually seen after 6–8 wk of therapy; however, response may vary from a few days to up to 8 mo. Control of galactorrhea depends on the degree of mammary stimulation prior to therapy. A reduction in secretion of at least 75% usually occurs after 8–12 wk of therapy; however, galactorrhea may fail to respond even after 12 mo of treatment.

PARLODEL

Prolactinomas	Bromocriptine may be given alone to treat prolactin-secreting adenomas or, alternatively, may be used to reduce the size of macroadenomas prior to adenectomy. It is not known whether drug therapy or surgery is the more effective treatment for patients experiencing loss of visual field; if loss progresses rapidly, the appropriate form of therapy should be decided after a neurosurgeon has examined the patient. Caution patients that discontinuation of drug therapy usually results in rapid regrowth of macroadenomas and recurrence of symptoms.
Acromegaly	When used alone or in conjunction with surgery or radiotherapy, bromocriptine reduces the serum growth hormone level by at least 50% in approximately one-half of patients; however, a normal serum level is usually not attained. After each adjustment in dosage, reevaluate diagnosis and then evaluate clinical response and check serum level; if no significant reduction in the serum level occurs after a brief trial, either continue to titrate dosage or terminate administration. Once a maintenance dosage has been established, monitor clinical response and serum level monthly and then at periodic intervals. If a patient has undergone radiotherapy, use of the drug should be interrupted annually for a period of 4–8 wk to assess the relative effects of radiation and drug treatment, since the full therapeutic effect of radiotherapy may not occur until after several years; if signs or symptoms recur or the serum level increases, consider resuming therapy.
Parkinson's disease	Bromocriptine can enhance therapeutic response in patients receiving levodopa and may also permit a reduction in the maintenance dose when these patients experience adverse effects such as dyskinesia and "on-off" phenomenon; bear in mind that safety and effectiveness of bromocriptine for use as an antiparkinson agent for more than 2 yr have not been established. When titrating dosage of bromocriptine, assess therapeutic response every 2 wk. During chronic therapy, check renal, hepatic, cardiovascular, and hematopoietic functions periodically.

WARNINGS/PRECAUTIONS

Dizziness, drowsiness, syncope	Caution all patients that their ability to drive, operate machinery, or engage in other activities requiring rapid and precise response may be impaired during therapy
Renal, hepatic disease	Safety and effectiveness for use in patients with renal or hepatic disease have not been established
Compression of the optic nerve	Hormonal changes during pregnancy can cause expansion of prolactin-secreting adenomas and result in compression of the optic or other cranial nerves. Although compression usually disappears after delivery, emergency surgery may be necessary in some cases. Bromocriptine has reportedly caused improvement of visual field symptoms owing to nerve compression; however, safety for use during pregnancy has not been established. To reduce the risk of nerve compression, carefully assess the pituitary gland and look for evidence of a prolactin-secreting adenoma before beginning treatment of hyperprolactinemic disorders such as hypogonadism and amenorrhea since these disorders may be due to a pituitary adenoma. Avoid pregnancy, when possible (see ADMINISTRATION/DOSAGE ADJUSTMENTS). If or when the patient becomes pregnant, watch closely for signs and symptoms that may indicate enlargement of a known or previously undetected adenoma.
CSF rhinorrhea	In rare instances, bromocriptine may cause CSF rhinorrhea in patients who have macroadenomas that extend into the sphenoid sinus or who have undergone transsphenoidal surgery or pituitary radiotherapy; caution these patients to report any persistent watery nasal discharge
Effects on blood pressure	Bromocriptine can cause symptomatic hypotension, particularly when given postpartum; in 28% of patients who received this drug for prevention of lactation, systolic pressure decreased by more than 20 mm Hg and diastolic pressure declined by more than 10 mm Hg. In rare instances, postpartum use may precipitate hypertension in patients who have toxemia or are receiving other drugs, including other ergot alkaloids, that can increase blood pressure. Do not begin postpartum administration until vital signs have stabilized (wait at least 4 h after delivery); exercise particular caution if a patient has toxemia or has received within the preceding 24-h period a drug that can affect blood pressure. Monitor blood pressure periodically, especially during the first few days of therapy, and exercise caution if patient is taking other medications that are known to lower blood pressure.
Rebound lactation	Discontinuing bromocriptine following use for prevention of lactation results in mild to moderate breast engorgement, congestion, or secretion in 18–40% of patients
Digital vasospasm	In some acromegalic patients receiving bromocriptine, digital vasospasm may occur following exposure to the cold; reaction can be prevented by keeping the fingers warm and reversed by lowering the dosage
Peptic ulcers	In acromegalic patients, severe GI bleeding, sometimes followed by death, has occurred as a result of peptic ulcers; however, no evidence has shown that bromocriptine affects the incidence of peptic ulcers. Nevertheless, during therapy, thoroughly investigate any sign or symptom suggestive of peptic ulcer.
Tumor expansion	Possible expansion of growth hormone secreting tumors has been seen in a few acromegalic patients; since the natural course of these tumors is not known, any acromegalic patient should be carefully observed and, if evidence of tumor expansion is detected, therapy should be discontinued

PARLODEL

Confusion and mental disturbances	May occur in Parkinson's disease patients receiving high doses; since these patients may manifest mild degrees of dementia, use bromocriptine with caution
Pulmonary reactions	In a few patients receiving 20–100 mg/day for 6–36 mo, bromocriptine has produced pulmonary infiltrates, pleural effusion, and thickening of the pleura; these effects were slowly reversed following discontinuation of therapy
Hallucinations, confusion	Bromocriptine has caused visual hallucinations in patients with acromegaly and visual and auditory hallucinations in patients with Parkinson's disease; in rare instances, hallucinations have persisted for several weeks after discontinuation of high-dose antiparkinson therapy. If hallucinations occur, reduce dosage or, if necessary, discontinue bromocriptine. High doses of bromocriptine can produce confusion and other CNS disturbances; exercise caution during antiparkinson therapy.
Arrhythmia	During antiparkinson therapy, exercise caution if the patient has a history of myocardial infarction and a residual arrhythmia

ADVERSE REACTIONS

Frequent reactions (incidence ≥ 1%) are printed in *italics*

When used to treat hyperprolactinemic disorders

Gastrointestinal	*Nausea (49%), vomiting (5%), abdominal cramps (4%), constipation and diarrhea (3%)*
Central nervous system	*Headache (19%), dizziness (17%), fatigue (7%), light-headedness (5%), drowsiness (3%)*, CSF rhinorrhea (rare)
Other	*Nasal congestion (3%)*, slight hypotension

When used to prevent physiological lactation

Gastrointestinal	*Nausea (7%), vomiting (3%)*, abdominal cramps and diarrhea (0.4%)
Central nervous system	*Headache (10%), dizziness (8%), fatigue (1%)*
Cardiovascular	*Hypotension (28%)*, syncope (0.7%); hypertension, cerebrovascular accident, and seizures (rare)

When used to treat acromegaly

Gastrointestinal	*Nausea (18%), constipation (14%), anorexia and dyspepsia (4%), vomiting (2%)*, GI bleeding (< 2%)
Central nervous system	*Drowsiness/tiredness (3%), dizziness and headache (< 2%)*, alcohol potentiation, faintness, light-headedness, decreased sleep requirement, visual hallucinations, lassitude, vertigo, paresthesia, sluggishness, delusional psychosis, paranoia, insomnia, heavy headedness
Cardiovascular	*Orthostatic hypotension (6%), digital vasospasm (3%), syncope and exacerbation of Raynaud's syndrome (< 2%)*, vasovagal attack, arrhythmia, ventricular tachycardia, bradycardia, reduced tolerance to cold, tingling of ears, facial pallor, muscle cramps
Other	*Dry mouth/nasal congestion (4%)*, hair loss, shortness of breath

When used as an adjunct to levodopa in Parkinson's disease

Gastrointestinal	*Nausea, vomiting, abdominal discomfort, constipation*, anorexia, dry mouth, dysphagia
Central nervous system	*Abnormal involuntary movements, hallucinations, confusion, "on-off" phenomenon, dizziness, drowsiness, faintness/fainting, asthenia, visual disturbance, ataxia, insomnia, depression, vertigo*, anxiety, blepharospasm, epileptiform seizure, fatigue, headache, lethargy, nervousness, nightmares, paresthesia
Cardiovascular	*Hypotension, pedal and ankle edema, erythromelalgia*, signs and symptoms of ergotism (eg, tingling of the fingers, cold feet, numbness, muscle cramps of the feet and legs, exacerbation of Raynaud's syndrome; rare)
Dermatological	Mottling, rash
Genitourinary	Urinary frequency, incontinence, or retention
Other	*Shortness of breath*, nasal congestion

OVERDOSAGE

Signs and symptoms	See ADVERSE REACTIONS
Treatment	Discontinue medication; treat symptomatically and institute supportive measures, as required

DRUG INTERACTIONS

Diuretics, antihypertensive agents	⇧ Risk of hypotension; exercise caution
Dopamine antagonists (eg, phenothiazines, haloperidol)	⇩ Therapeutic effect of bromocriptine, especially in patients undergoing treatment of macroadenomas
Estrogens, progestins (including oral contraceptives)	⇩ Antiamenorrheic effect of bromocriptine

PARLODEL ■ SINEMET

ALTERED LABORATORY VALUES

Blood/serum values — ⇧ Prolactin ⇧ Growth hormone ⇧ BUN ⇧ SGOT ⇧ SGPT ⇧ GGPT
⇧ Creatine phosphokinase ⇧ Alkaline phosphatase ⇧ Uric acid

No clinically significant alterations in urinary values occur at therapeutic dosages

USE IN CHILDREN

Safety and effectiveness for use in children under 15 yr of age have not been established

USE IN PREGNANT AND NURSING WOMEN

Pregnant women: Congenital malformations have been seen in 3.3% of infants born to women who received this drug during pregnancy; spontaneous abortions have occurred in 11% of pregnancies during which this drug was used. Although these frequencies do not exceed those generally reported for the population at large, safety for use during pregnancy has not been established. Women who wish to become pregnant should use a contraceptive, other than an oral contraceptive, during the period of amenorrhea (see ADMINISTRATION/DOSAGE ADJUSTMENTS). Bromocriptine has been used during pregnancy to treat optic nerve compression and visual field defects associated with macroadenomas (see WARNINGS/PRECAUTIONS). **Nursing mothers:** Since bromocriptine inhibits lactation, it should not be administered to women who elect to breast-feed.

ANTIPARKINSON AGENTS

SINEMET (carbidopa and levodopa) Merck Sharp & Dohme   Rx

Tablets: 10 mg carbidopa and 100 mg levodopa (Sinemet 10–100); 25 mg carbidopa and 100 mg levodopa (Sinemet 25–100); 25 mg carbidopa and 250 mg levodopa (Sinemet 25–250)

INDICATIONS

Idiopathic Parkinson's disease (paralysis agitans)
Postencephalitic parkinsonism
Symptomatic parkinsonism due to carbon monoxide or manganese intoxication

ORAL DOSAGE

Adult: initiate therapy with 1 Sinemet 25–100 tab tid, followed, if needed, by increases of 1 tab daily or every other day, up to 6 tabs/day; if Sinemet 10–100 is used, start with 1 tab tid or qid, followed, if needed, by increases of 1 tab daily or every other day, up to 8 tabs/day (2 tabs qid)

CONTRAINDICATIONS

Hypersensitivity to carbidopa or levodopa	Suspicious, undiagnosed skin lesions or history of melanoma	MAO inhibitor therapy (see WARNINGS/PRECAUTIONS)
Narrow-angle glaucoma	Breast-feeding	

ADMINISTRATION/DOSAGE ADJUSTMENTS

Transferring patients from levodopa — Discontinue levodopa at least 8 h before initiating Sinemet therapy. For most patients who received more than 1,500 mg levodopa/day, the suggested starting dosage is 1 Sinemet 25–250 tab tid or qid; for patients who required less than 1,500 mg levodopa/day, start with 1 Sinemet 25–100 tab tid or qid. Choose a daily dosage that will provide ~ 25% of the previous levodopa dosage.

Combination therapy — May be used with other antiparkinson agents; adjust dosages accordingly

Maintenance — Therapy should be individualized and adjusted according to desired therapeutic response. If a greater proportion of carbidopa is required, substitute 1 Sinemet 25–100 tab for each Sinemet 10–100 tab; if more levodopa is required, substitute 1 Sinemet 25–250 tab tid or qid. Dosage may be increased, as needed, by ½–1 tab daily or every other day, up to 8 tabs/day. Monitor patients closely during the dose adjustment period, as both therapeutic and adverse responses occur more rapidly with this combination drug than with levodopa alone. The occurrence of involuntary movements may require dosage reduction. In some patients, blepharospasm may be a useful early sign of excess dosage.

Patients requiring general anesthesia — Therapy may be continued as long as the patient is able to take fluids and medication by mouth; if therapy is interrupted, give the usual daily dose as soon as the patient is able to take oral medication

WARNINGS/PRECAUTIONS

MAO inhibitor therapy — Discontinue use of MAO inhibitors at least 14 days prior to Sinemet therapy

Depression with suicidal tendencies — May develop; observe patient carefully

Dyskinesias — May occur at lower dosages than with levodopa alone; adjust dosage accordingly. Blepharospasm is an early sign of excess dosage.

SINEMET

Patients with a history of myocardial infarction and residual arrhythmias	Monitor cardiac function during initial dosage adjustment in a facility with provisions for intensive cardiac care
Gastrointestinal hemorrhage	May occur in patients with a history of peptic ulcer
NMS-like syndrome	A symptom complex resembling the neuroleptic malignant syndrome, characterized by muscular rigidity, elevated temperature, mental changes, and increased serum CPK levels, has occurred following abrupt withdrawal of antiparkinson agents; carefully observe patients, especially those receiving neuroleptics, when dosage is abruptly reduced or drug is discontinued
Other special-risk patients	Use with caution in patients with recurrent or past psychoses, severe cardiovascular or pulmonary disease, bronchial asthma, or renal, hepatic, or endocrine disease
Prolonged therapy	Monitor hepatic, hematopoietic, cardiovascular, and renal function periodically
Chronic wide-angle glaucoma	Use with caution, provided intraocular pressure is well controlled; observe for changes in intraocular pressure

ADVERSE REACTIONS[1]

Frequent reactions (incidence $\geq$ 1%) are printed in *italics*

Musculoskeletal	*Choreiform, dystonic, and other involuntary movements;* ataxia, increased hand tremor, muscle twitching, blepharospasm, trismus
Central nervous system	Mental changes (eg, paranoid ideation and psychotic episodes), bradykinetic episodes, depression with or without suicidal tendencies, dementia, dizziness, headache, numbness, weakness, faintness, confusion, bruxism, sleepiness, insomnia, nightmares, hallucinations, delusions, agitation, anxiety, stimulation, malaise, fatigue, euphoria[2]
Gastrointestinal	*Nausea,* anorexia, vomiting, abdominal pain and distress, dry mouth, dysphagia, hiccoughs, sialorrhea, diarrhea, constipation, flatulence; rarely, bleeding and duodenal ulcer
Cardiovascular	Cardiac irregularities and/or palpitations, orthostatic hypotension; rarely, hypertension and phlebitis
Hematological	Hemolytic and nonhemolytic anemia, thrombocytopenia, leukopenia, and agranulocytosis (rare)
Dermatological	Flushing, rash, alopecia
Respiratory	Bizarre breathing patterns
Genitourinary	Urinary retention, urinary incontinence, dark urine, priapism
Ophthalmic	Diplopia, blurred vision, mydriasis, oculogyric crises, activation of latent Horner's syndrome
Other	Burning sensation of the tongue, bitter taste, diaphoresis, hot flashes, weight gain or loss, dark sweat, edema, hoarseness, neuroleptic malignant syndrome

OVERDOSAGE

Signs and symptoms	See ADVERSE REACTIONS
Treatment	Empty stomach immediately by gastric lavage. Institute general supportive measures as needed, including maintenance of an adequate airway and administration of IV fluids. Institute ECG monitoring and observe patient carefully for possible arrhythmias; give appropriate antiarrhythmic agents, if required. Pyridoxine hydrochloride (vitamin B_6) will not reverse the effects of Sinemet. Value of dialysis is unknown. Consider the possibility of multiple-drug ingestion.

DRUG INTERACTIONS

Antihypertensive agents	Postural hypotension; dosage adjustment of antihypertensive agent may be necessary
Methyldopa	▽ Antiparkinson effect △ Hypotensive effect
Butyrophenones (haloperidol), papaverine, phenothiazines, phenytoin, reserpine	▽ Antiparkinson effect
Tricyclic antidepressants	Hypertension and dyskinesia (rare)
MAO inhibitors	△ Risk of hypertensive crisis
Sympathomimetics	△ Risk of cardiac arrhythmias

ALTERED LABORATORY VALUES

Blood/serum values	△ BUN △ SGOT △ SGPT △ Alkaline phosphatase △ Lactic dehydrogenase △ Bilirubin △ PBI + Coombs' test
Urinary values	△ Uric acid (with colorimetric method) + Ketones (with nitroprusside method) + Glucose (with copper reduction method) − Glucose (with glucose oxidase method)

SINEMET ■ SYMMETREL

USE IN CHILDREN	USE IN PREGNANT AND NURSING WOMEN
Safety for use in children under 18 yr of age has not been established	Safety for use during pregnancy has not been established; levodopa alone and in combination with carbidopa has caused skeletal and visceral malformations in rabbits. This drug is contraindicated for use in nursing mothers.

[1] Includes reactions associated with levodopa alone; see also ALTERED LABORATORY VALUES
[2] Convulsions have been reported, but a causal relationship has not been established

---

ANTIPARKINSON AGENTS

SYMMETREL (amantadine hydrochloride) Du Pont   Rx

Capsules: 100 mg   **Syrup (per 5 ml):** 50 mg

INDICATIONS	ORAL DOSAGE
Idiopathic and postencephalitic parkinsonism **Symptomatic parkinsonism** caused by carbon monoxide intoxication **Parkinsonism** associated with cerebral arteriosclerosis in the elderly	**Adult:** 100 mg bid to start, followed, if necessary, by up to 400 mg/day, given in divided doses under close medical supervision
Drug-induced extrapyramidal reactions	**Adult:** 100 mg bid to start, followed, if necessary, by up to 300 mg/day in divided doses
Prophylaxis and symptomatic treatment of **respiratory tract illness** caused by influenza A virus strains	**Adult:** 200 mg/day, given in a single daily dose or 2 divided doses **Child (1–9 yr):** 2–4 mg/lb/day, up to 150 mg/day, given in 2–3 equally divided doses **Child (9–12 yr):** same as adult

CONTRAINDICATIONS

Hypersensitivity to amantadine

ADMINISTRATION/DOSAGE ADJUSTMENTS

Concomitant therapy	Reduce dosage of amantadine hydrochloride or concomitant anticholinergics if atropine-like effects occur; use cautiously with CNS stimulants
Combination therapy with levodopa	When adding levodopa, maintain a constant amantadine dosage of 100 mg 1–2 times/day, while gradually increasing levodopa dosage to optimal level
Prolonged therapy	Effectiveness may decrease after several months; increase dosage to 300 mg/day or temporarily discontinue therapy for several weeks
Seriously ill patients or those receiving other antiparkinson agents in high doses	Initiate therapy with 100 mg/day, followed by 100 mg bid, if necessary, after one to several weeks
CNS disturbances	May be alleviated by twice-daily administration
Duration of therapy for influenza A virus respiratory illness	For prophylaxis, continue treatment at least 10 days following known exposure. When used chemoprophylactically with inactivated influenza A virus vaccine, administer for 2–3 wk after vaccine has been given. When vaccine is unavailable or contraindicated, administer amantadine for up to 90 days. Symptomatic treatment should be started as soon as possible after the onset of symptoms and continued for 24–48 h after symptoms disappear.

WARNINGS/PRECAUTIONS

Congestive heart failure	May occur; closely supervise therapy in patients with a history of congestive heart failure or peripheral edema
Patients with convulsive disorders	Closely monitor patients with a history of epilepsy or other seizure disorders for possible increased seizure activity
Other special-risk patients	Adjust dosage carefully in patients with renal impairment, congestive heart failure, peripheral edema, or orthostatic hypotension; use with caution in patients with hepatic disease, a history of recurrent eczematoid rash, or psychosis or severe psychoneurosis not controlled by drugs
Mental impairment, blurred vision	Caution patients to avoid driving or other potentially hazardous activities if they experience CNS effects or blurred vision
Resumption of normal activities	Caution patients with Parkinson's disease whose symptoms improve to resume their normal activities gradually and with caution
Abrupt discontinuation of therapy	May precipitate parkinsonian crisis in patients with Parkinson's disease

SYMMETREL

Carcinogenicity, mutagenicity	The carcinogenic and mutagenic potential of this drug have not been investigated

ADVERSE REACTIONS

Frequent reactions (incidence ≥ 1%) are printed in *italics*

Central nervous system	*Depression, psychosis,* hallucinations, confusion, anxiety, irritability, dizziness, lightheadedness, headache, fatigue, insomnia, weakness, slurred speech, ataxia; convulsions (rare)
Cardiovascular	*Congestive heart failure, orthostatic hypotension,* peripheral edema
Hematological	Leukopenia and neutropenia (rare)
Gastrointestinal	Anorexia, nausea, constipation, vomiting, dry mouth
Dermatological	Skin rash, livedo reticularis; eczematoid dermatitis (rare)
Ophthalmic	Visual disturbances; oculogyric episodes (rare)
Other	Urinary retention, dyspnea

OVERDOSAGE

Signs and symptoms	Urinary retention, hyperactivity, convulsions, arrhythmias, hypotension, acid-base disturbances, and acute toxic psychosis manifested by disorientation, confusion, visual hallucinations, and aggressive behavior
Treatment	Empty stomach by gastric lavage or emesis and institute supportive measures, including forced or IV fluids, if necessary. Acidification of the urine may speed elimination of the drug. For CNS effects, slowly administer physostigmine (1-2 mg IV q1-2h in adults and 0.5 mg IV at 5- to 10-min intervals, up to 2 mg/h, in children). Monitor vital signs, serum electrolytes, urine pH, and urinary output. Catheterization should be done if patient has not recently voided. Employ appropriate anticonvulsant, antiarrhythmic, and vasopressor therapy, as needed.

DRUG INTERACTIONS

Anticholinergic agents	⇧ Atropine-like effects

ALTERED LABORATORY VALUES

No clinically significant alterations in blood/serum or urinary values occur at therapeutic dosages

---

USE IN CHILDREN

See INDICATIONS and ORAL DOSAGE; safety and effectiveness for use in newborns and infants under 1 yr of age have not been established

USE IN PREGNANT AND NURSING WOMEN

Pregnancy Category C: use during pregnancy only if the expected benefit of therapy outweighs the potential risk to the embryo or fetus. Amantadine has been shown to be embryotoxic and teratogenic in rats at 12 times the recommended human dose but not in rabbits receiving up to 25 times the human dose. No adequate, well-controlled studies have been done in pregnant women. Amantadine is excreted in human milk; use with caution in nursing women.

Chapter 17

Antidepressants

Antidepressants	**615**
ADAPIN (Pennwalt) Doxepin hydrochloride *Rx*	615
ASENDIN (Lederle) Amoxapine *Rx*	616
DESYREL (Mead Johnson) Trazodone hydrochloride *Rx*	618
ELAVIL (Merck Sharp & Dohme) Amitriptyline hydrochloride *Rx*	620
ENDEP (Roche) Amitriptyline hydrochloride *Rx*	622
LUDIOMIL (CIBA) Maprotiline hydrochloride *Rx*	624
MARPLAN (Roche) Isocarboxazid *Rx*	626
NARDIL (Parke-Davis) Phenelzine sulfate *Rx*	627
NORPRAMIN (Merrell Dow) Desipramine hydrochloride *Rx*	629
PAMELOR (Sandoz Pharmaceuticals) Nortriptyline hydrochloride *Rx*	631
PARNATE (Smith Kline & French) Tranylcypromine sulfate *Rx*	633
SINEQUAN (Roerig) Doxepin hydrochloride *Rx*	635
SURMONTIL (Wyeth) Trimipramine maleate *Rx*	636
TOFRANIL (Geigy) Imipramine hydrochloride *Rx*	638
TOFRANIL-PM (Geigy) Imipramine pamoate *Rx*	640
VIVACTIL (Merck Sharp & Dohme) Protriptyline hydrochloride *Rx*	642
Antidepressant Combinations	**644**
ETRAFON (Schering) Perphenazine and amitriptyline hydrochloride *Rx*	644
LIMBITROL (Roche) Chlordiazepoxide and amitriptyline hydrochloride *C-IV*	647
LIMBITROL DS (Roche) Chlordiazepoxide and amitriptyline hydrochloride *C-IV*	647
TRIAVIL (Merck Sharp & Dohme) Perphenazine and amitriptyline hydrochloride *Rx*	649
Other Antidepressants	**614**
DEPROL (Wallace) Meprobamate and benactyzine hydrochloride *C-IV*	614
PERTOFRANE (Rorer) Desipramine hydrochloride *Rx*	614

OTHER ANTIDEPRESSANTS

DRUG	HOW SUPPLIED	USUAL DOSAGE[1]
DEPROL (Wallace) Meprobamate and benactyzine hydrochloride *C-IV*	**Tablets:** 400 mg meprobamate and 1 mg benactyzine hydrochloride	**Adult:** 1 tab tid or qid to start, followed by up to 6 tabs/day, if needed; reduce dosage gradually to maintenance level when relief is obtained
PERTOFRANE (Rorer) Desipramine hydrochloride *Rx*	**Capsules:** 25, 50 mg	**Adult:** 75–150 mg/day, given in single or divided daily doses, to start, followed by up to 200 mg/day, given in divided doses, if needed; for elderly and adolescent patients, 25–50 mg/day, given in single or divided daily doses, to start, followed, if needed, by up to 100 mg/day, given in single or divided daily doses

[1] Where pediatric dosages are not given, consult manufacturer

ANTIDEPRESSANTS

ADAPIN (doxepin hydrochloride) Pennwalt   Rx

Capsules: 10, 25, 50, 75, 100 mg

INDICATIONS

Psychoneurotic anxiety and/or depressive reactions
Mixed symptoms of anxiety and depression
Anxiety and/or depression associated with alcoholism
Anxiety associated with organic disease
Psychotic depressive disorders, including involutional depression and manic-depression

ORAL DOSAGE

Adult: for mild to moderate symptoms, 25 mg tid to start, followed by an increase or decrease in dosage at appropriate intervals according to individual response (usual optimum dosage, 75–150 mg/day; mild symptoms or emotional symptoms accompanying organic disease may be adequately controlled in some patients with as little as 25–50 mg/day); for more severe symptoms, 50 mg tid to start, followed by a gradual increase in dosage up to 300 mg/day, if needed

CONTRAINDICATIONS

| Hypersensitivity to doxepin | Glaucoma | Urinary retention |

ADMINISTRATION/DOSAGE ADJUSTMENTS

| Alternative once-a-day regimen | If desired, the entire daily dose, but not more than 150 mg, may be given at bedtime |

WARNINGS/PRECAUTIONS

MAO inhibitor therapy	Wait at least 14 days after discontinuing use of an MAO inhibitor before initiating therapy with this drug; start treatment cautiously
Mental and/or physical impairment	Caution patients not to drive or engage in other potentially hazardous activities while taking this drug because they may become drowsy, and that their response to alcohol may be enhanced
Alcohol usage	Because the effects of alcohol are potentiated, its ingestion may increase the danger inherent in any suicide attempt or accidental overdose; this is especially important in patients who may use alcohol excessively
Latent psychotic symptoms	May be activated or unmasked, despite the anxiolytic activity of this drug
Potentially suicidal patients	Should be closely supervised during the early phases of therapy
Withdrawal reactions	Nausea, headache, and malaise may result from abrupt withdrawal following prolonged use

ADVERSE REACTIONS

Cardiovascular	Hypotension, tachycardia
Central nervous system and neuromuscular	Drowsiness, weakness, dizziness, fatigue, paresthesias, extrapyramidal symptoms, tinnitus
Autonomic nervous system	Dry mouth, blurred vision, constipation
Endocrinological	Decreased libido, inappropriate ADH secretion syndrome
Allergic	Rash, edema, photophobia, pruritus
Other	Weight gain, GI disturbances, diaphoresis, flushing, chills, photophobia, edema

OVERDOSAGE

Signs and symptoms	Excessive sedation, anticholinergic effects, such as dry mouth and blurred vision; pronounced tachycardia; hypotension, extrapyramidal symptoms (see also ADVERSE REACTIONS)
Treatment	Institute standard supportive measures. Empty stomach by gastric lavage and activated charcoal. Obtain ECG and begin close monitoring of cardiac function if abnormalities appear. Maintain an open airway and adequate fluid intake. Regulate body temperature. Cardiac function should be closely monitored for at least 5 days under these circumstances. Dialysis is of no value because of low plasma drug concentrations and because of extensive tissue distribution of drug.

DRUG INTERACTIONS

Alcohol, anticonvulsants, sedative-hypnotics, and other CNS depressants	△ CNS depression
MAO inhibitors	Hyperpyrexia, excitability, severe convulsions, coma, death
Anticholinergic agents	Acute glaucoma, urinary retention, paralytic ileus
Ethchlorvynol	Transient delirium
Guanethidine	▽ Antihypertensive effect (at dosages of 300 mg/day or higher)
Sympathomimetic agents	Severe hypertension, hyperpyrexia

| Cimetidine | ⇧ Serum doxepin level; close supervision and careful adjustment of dosage are necessary during combination therapy |

ALTERED LABORATORY VALUES

| Blood/serum values | ⇧ or ⇩ Glucose |

No clinically significant alterations in urinary values occur at therapeutic dosages

USE IN CHILDREN

Not recommended for use in children under 12 yr of age because conditions for the safe use of this drug in children have not been established

USE IN PREGNANT AND NURSING WOMEN

Use during pregnancy only if this drug is considered essential to the welfare of the mother. Animal reproduction studies have shown no evidence of teratogenicity or adverse effects on the number of live births or litter size. However, no studies have been done in pregnant women. Doxepin is excreted in human milk; respiratory depression has been reported in an 8-wk-old nursing infant. Because of the potential for adverse effects in infants, mothers should not nurse during therapy.

ANTIDEPRESSANTS

ASENDIN (amoxapine) Lederle Rx

Tablets: 25, 50, 100, 150 mg

INDICATIONS

Neurotic or reactive depression
Endogenous depression
Psychotic depression
Depression accompanied by anxiety or agitation

ORAL DOSAGE

Adult: 50 mg 2–3 times/day to start, followed, if tolerated, by 100 mg 2–3 times/day at the end of the first week of therapy; usual maintenance dosage: 200–300 mg/day, given in a single bedtime dose. An initial dosage of 300 mg/day may be given; however, during the first few days, some patients may experience notable sedation.

CONTRAINDICATIONS

| MAO inhibitor therapy (see WARNINGS/PRECAUTIONS) | During the acute recovery phase following myocardial infarction | Hypersensitivity to dibenzoxazepines |

ADMINISTRATION/DOSAGE ADJUSTMENTS

Dosage adjustment	If no response is seen at 300 mg/day during a trial period of at least 2 wk, dosage may be increased, if tolerated, up to 400 mg/day in divided doses. Amoxapine has a more rapid onset of action than amitriptyline or imipramine; initial clinical effect may occur within 4–7 days and generally within 2 wk of initiating therapy.
Refractory patients	Hospitalized patients who have no history of convulsive seizures may be given up to 600 mg/day in divided doses, with caution
Elderly patients	Give 25 mg 2–3 times/day to start, followed, if tolerated, by 50 mg 2–3 times/day at the end of the first week of therapy; if necessary, dosage may be carefully increased up to 300 mg/day
Maintenance therapy	Use the lowest dose that will control symptoms; if symptoms reappear, increase dosage to earlier level until they are controlled

WARNINGS/PRECAUTIONS

| Tardive dyskinesia | Neuroleptic drugs can cause tardive dyskinesia, a potentially irreversible syndrome characterized by involuntary choreoathetoid movements of the tongue, face, mouth, lips, jaw, trunk, and/or extremities. Protrusion of the tongue, puffing of the cheeks, puckering of the mouth, chewing movements, and other manifestations may become evident during treatment, upon dosage reduction, or after the drug is discontinued. The likelihood that tardive dyskinesia will develop or become irreversible increases with duration of treatment and total cumulative dose; however, even relatively brief use of low doses can cause it. Although this reaction appears to occur most often in the elderly, especially among older women, it is impossible to use this information to predict, before therapy is started, which patients are likely to develop the syndrome.

In general, reserve chronic therapy for patients who respond to neuroleptics and who cannot undergo another, equally effective form of treatment that is potentially less harmful. Use the lowest effective dosage, keep the duration of therapy as short as possible, and periodically reassess the need for the drug. Watch carefully for manifestations of tardive dyskinesia since neuroleptic therapy can itself mask the signs and symptoms of tardive dyskinesia. If evidence of the syndrome is seen, consider terminating use of the drug, bearing in mind that some patients may require continued neuroleptic treatment despite the development of dyskinesia. There is no known treatment for tardive dyskinesia; however, after discontinuation, some or all manifestations of this syndrome may disappear spontaneously. |

ASENDIN

MAO inhibitor therapy	Wait at least 14 days after discontinuing use of an MAO inhibitor before initiating therapy with this drug; start treatment cautiously with gradual increases in dosage until optimum response is achieved
Atropine-like action	Use with caution in patients with a history of urinary retention, narrow-angle glaucoma, or increased intraocular pressure; even average doses may precipitate an attack in patients with narrow-angle glaucoma
Cardiovascular disease	May worsen; use with caution and keep patient under close supervision. Tricyclic antidepressants, especially in high doses, may produce arrhythmias, sinus tachycardia, and prolongation of conduction time; myocardial infarction and stroke have followed use of these agents.
Mental and/or physical impairment	Caution patients that their ability to drive or perform other potentially hazardous activities may be impaired by drowsiness, and that their response to alcohol, barbiturates, and other CNS depressants may be enhanced
Psychotic symptoms	May increase in schizophrenic patients; paranoia may worsen, and manic-depressive patients may shift to manic phase. Reduce dosage of amoxapine or add a major tranquilizing agent, as indicated.
Seizures	Amoxapine may cause seizures; use with extreme caution in patients with seizure disorders or a history of convulsions
Allergic reactions	Discontinue use if skin rash or drug fever occur; these reactions are more likely to occur during the first few days of therapy and, in rare cases, may be severe
Potentially suicidal patients	Should not have access to large quantities of amoxapine; prescribe the smallest feasible amount
Electroconvulsive therapy	Hazard may be increased
Carcinogenicity	Pancreatic islet cell hyperplasia has occurred in rats at doses 5–10 times the human dose
Impairment of fertility	Male rats treated with 5–10 times the human dose have shown a slight decrease in fertile matings; female rats treated with therapeutic doses display a reversible increase in estrous cycle length

ADVERSE REACTIONS[1]

Frequent reactions (incidence $\geq$ 1%) are printed in *italics*

Central nervous system and neuromuscular	*Drowsiness (14%), anxiety, insomnia, restlessness, nervousness, tremors, confusion, excitement, nightmares, ataxia, EEG changes, dizziness, headache, fatigue, weakness, excessive appetite,* tingling, paresthesias of extremities, tinnitus, disorientation, extrapyramidal symptoms (including, rarely, tardive dyskinesia), seizures, hypomania, numbness, incoordination, hyperthermia, disturbed concentration, neuroleptic malignant syndrome
Autonomic nervous system	*Dry mouth (14%), constipation (12%), blurred vision (7%),* disturbances of accommodation, mydriasis, delayed micturition, nasal stuffiness, urinary retention
Cardiovascular	*Palpitations,* hypotension, hypertension, syncope, tachycardia
Allergic	*Skin rash, edema,* drug fever, photosensitization, pruritus; vasculitis (rare)
Gastrointestinal	*Nausea,* excessive appetite, epigastric distress, vomiting, flatulence, abdominal pain, peculiar taste, weight gain or loss, diarrhea
Hematological	Leukopenia, agranulocytosis
Endocrinological	*Hyperprolactinemia,* increased or decreased libido, impotence, menstrual irregularity, breast enlargement and galactorrhea (in females), inappropriate ADH secretion syndrome
Other	Increased perspiration, lacrimation, altered liver function

OVERDOSAGE

Signs and symptoms	Grand mal convulsions, status epilepticus, coma, and acidosis; acute tubular necrosis with rhabdomyolysis and myoglobinuria may occur 2–5 days after overdosage, especially in patients who had multiple seizures
Treatment	Empty stomach as soon as possible; if the patient is conscious, induce vomiting and then perform gastric lavage. Give an initial dose of activated charcoal to reduce absorption and subsequent doses to facilitate elimination. Maintain pulmonary function; if the patient is comatose, establish an open airway and, if necessary, institute mechanical ventilation. Convulsions usually begin within 12 h after ingestion and may occur even in an asymptomatic patient; prophylactic use of anticonvulsants during this 12-h period may be considered. To control seizures, use standard anticonvulsants such as IV diazepam and/or IV phenytoin; treat status epilepticus vigorously.

DRUG INTERACTIONS

Alcohol, sedative-hypnotics, and other CNS depressants	⇧ CNS depression
MAO inhibitors	Hyperpyrexia, excitability, severe convulsions, coma, death
Anticholinergic agents	Acute glaucoma, urinary retention, paralytic ileus

ASENDIN ■ DESYREL

Epinephrine	⇧ Pressor response, arrhythmias
Ethchlorvynol	Transient delirium
Guanethidine	⇩ Antihypertensive effect
Sympathomimetic agents	Severe hypertension, hyperpyrexia
Thyroid preparations	⇧ Antidepressant effect and possible risk of arrhythmias
Cimetidine	⇧ Serum level of amoxapine

ALTERED LABORATORY VALUES

No clinically significant alterations in blood/serum or urinary values occur at therapeutic dosages

USE IN CHILDREN

Safety and effectiveness for use in children under 16 yr of age have not been established

USE IN PREGNANT AND NURSING WOMEN

Pregnancy Category C: use during pregnancy only if the expected therapeutic benefit outweighs the possible hazards. Animal reproduction studies have shown no evidence of teratogenicity; however, embryotoxicity has been reported in rats and rabbits at oral doses approximating the human oral dose, and fetotoxicity, as well as decreased postnatal survival, has been observed at higher doses. No adequate, well-controlled studies have been done in pregnant women. Amoxapine is excreted in human milk; use with caution in nursing mothers because the effects of this drug on nursing infants are unknown.

[1] Reactions for which a causal relationship has not been established and which are very rare include paralytic ileus, atrial arrhythmias (including fibrillation), myocardial infarction, stroke, heart block, hallucinations, thrombocytopenia, eosinophilia, purpura, petechiae, parotid swelling, change in serum glucose level, pancreatitis, hepatitis, jaundice, urinary frequency, testicular swelling, anorexia, and alopecia; reactions reported with other tricyclic antidepressants include sublingual adenitis, dilation of the urinary tract, delusions, stomatitis, black tongue, and gynecomastia

ANTIDEPRESSANTS

DESYREL (trazodone hydrochloride) Mead Johnson   Rx

Tablets: 50, 100, 150 mg

INDICATIONS

Depression, with or without prominent anxiety

ORAL DOSAGE

Adult: 150 mg/day, in divided doses, to start, followed by an increase of 50 mg/day every 3–4 days, as needed and tolerated, up to 400 mg/day, in divided doses, for most outpatients or 600 mg/day, in divided doses, for inpatients or more severely depressed patients; once the response is adequate, reduce the dosage gradually to the lowest effective level

CONTRAINDICATIONS

Hypersensitivity to trazodone

ADMINISTRATION/DOSAGE ADJUSTMENTS

Onset of action	Symptomatic improvement may be seen within the 1st wk of administration and optimum improvement, within the 2d wk; 25% of those who eventually respond may require up to 4 wk of continuous therapy for significant improvement to occur
Timing of administration	The tablets should be taken shortly after a meal or light snack, since up to 20% more of the drug may be absorbed than when the tablets are taken on an empty stomach, and the patient is less likely to become dizzy or light-headed
Drowsiness	If necessary, administer a major portion of the daily dose at bedtime or reduce the dosage
MAO inhibitor therapy	Clinical experience with concomitant administration is lacking; if MAO inhibitors are discontinued shortly before trazodone is started or given concomitantly, initiate trazodone therapy with caution and gradually increase the dosage until an optimum response is achieved

WARNINGS/PRECAUTIONS

Priapism	Surgical treatment has been necessary in approximately one-third of men with trazodone-induced priapism; permanent impairment of erectile function or impotence has occurred in a portion of those who underwent surgery. Caution male patients that they should immediately discontinue use if they experience prolonged or inappropriate penile erection.
Mental and/or physical impairment	Caution patients that their ability to drive or perform other potentially hazardous activities may be impaired, and that their response to alcohol, barbiturates, and other CNS depressants may be enhanced

DESYREL

Cardiac effects	Arrythmias have been observed, generally in patients with cardiac disease; ventricular couplets, short episodes of ventricular tachycardia (two cases), and isolated premature ventricular contractions have been detected in such patients during clinical studies. Patients with preexisting cardiac disease should be closely monitored during therapy, particularly for arrhythmias. Trazodone should not be used during the initial recovery phase following acute myocardial infarction.
Suicidal tendencies	May persist until significant remission occurs and should be kept in mind when treating severely depressed patients; prescribe the smallest number of tablets possible consistent with good patient management
Blood counts	Obtain a total and differential WBC count if fever, sore throat, or other signs of infection develop; discontinue therapy if the WBC count or absolute neutrophil count falls below normal
Elective surgery	Discontinue therapy for as long as clinically feasible prior to elective surgery, as extent of interaction with general anesthetics is little known
Electroconvulsive therapy	Should be avoided during treatment with trazodone because of the lack of clinical experience in this area
Carcinogenicity	Studies in rats receiving trazodone in oral dosages of up to 300 mg/kg/day for 18 mo have shown no evidence of carcinogenesis

ADVERSE REACTIONS

Autonomic nervous system	Dry mouth, blurred vision, constipation, urinary hesitancy
Central nervous system and neuromuscular	Drowsiness, dizziness/light-headedness, headache, nervousness, agitation, insomnia, fatigue, weakness, confusion, musculoskeletal aches/pains, tremors, excitement, nightmares/vivid dreams, incoordination, anger/hostility, decreased concentration, disorientation, impaired memory, paresthesia, akathisia, hallucinations/delusions, hypomania, impaired speech, muscle twitches, grand mal seizures, numbness
Cardiovascular	Hypotension (including orthostatic hypotension and syncope), hypertension, shortness of breath, chest pain, palpitations, arrhythmia, bradycardia, ventricular ectopic activity, tachycardia, atrial fibrillation, myocardial infarction, cardiac arrest
Gastrointestinal	Nausea/vomiting, abdominal/gastric disorder, diarrhea, decreased appetite, bad taste in mouth, flatulence, increased salivation, increased appetite
Hematological	Anemia (including hemolytic anemia), methemoglobinemia
Respiratory	Apnea, nasal/sinus congestion
Genitourinary	Decreased libido, early or missed menses, impotence, priapism, increased libido, increased urinary frequency, delayed urine flow, retrograde ejaculation, hematuria
Other	Skin condition/edema; rash; weight loss; weight gain; sweating/clamminess; red, tired, or itching eyes; "full" or "heavy" head; malaise; tinnitus; diplopia; allergic reactions

OVERDOSAGE

Signs and symptoms	Vomiting and drowsiness are the most frequent manifestations; other signs and symptoms (see ADVERSE REACTIONS), including priapism, respiratory arrest, seizures, and ECG changes, have been reported
Treatment	Empty stomach by gastric lavage and institute symptomatic and supportive therapy for hypotension or excessive sedation. Forced diuresis may facilitate elimination of the drug.

DRUG INTERACTIONS

Antihypertensive agents	↕ Risk of hypotension; reduce dosage of antihypertensive drug, if necessary
Alcohol, barbiturates, and other CNS depressants	↕ CNS depression
Digoxin, phenytoin	↕ Serum levels of digoxin and phenytoin

ALTERED LABORATORY VALUES

Blood/serum values	Changes in liver enzyme activity

No clinically significant alterations in urinary values occur at therapeutic dosages

---

USE IN CHILDREN

Safety and effectiveness for use in children and adolescents under 18 yr of age have not been established

USE IN PREGNANT AND NURSING WOMEN

Pregnancy Category C: use during pregnancy only if the anticipated benefit of therapy justifies the potential risk to the fetus. Increased fetal resorption and other adverse fetal effects have been observed in rats at doses 30–50 times the maximum human dose. An increase in congenital anomalies has also been seen in one of three studies in the rabbit at doses 15–50 times the maximum human dose. No adequate, well-controlled studies have been done in pregnant women. The drug may be excreted in human milk, based on findings in the rat; use with caution in nursing mothers.

ELAVIL

ANTIDEPRESSANTS

ELAVIL (amitriptyline hydrochloride) Merck Sharp & Dohme   Rx

Tablets: 10, 25, 50, 75, 100, 150 mg   **Vials:** 10 mg/ml (10 ml) for IM use only

INDICATIONS	ORAL DOSAGE	PARENTERAL DOSAGE
Depression, especially endogenous depression	**Adult:** 75 mg/day, given in divided doses, to start, followed by an increase in the late-afternoon or bedtime dose, up to a total of 150 mg/day in divided doses, if needed; alternatively, give 50–100 mg at bedtime to start, followed by increases of 25–50 mg in the bedtime dose, up to a total of 150 mg/day, if needed	**Adult:** 20–30 mg IM qid to start; replace with oral therapy as soon as possible

CONTRAINDICATIONS

MAO inhibitor therapy (see WARNINGS/PRECAUTIONS)	During the acute recovery phase following myocardial infarction	Hypersensitivity to amitriptyline

ADMINISTRATION/DOSAGE ADJUSTMENTS

Hospitalized patients	May require 100 mg/day to start, followed by a gradual increase up to a total of 200 or, occasionally, 300 mg/day, if necessary
Adolescent and elderly patients	Reduce dosage to 10 mg tid, with 20 mg given at bedtime, if higher dosages are not tolerated
Maintenance regimen	Usually, 50–100 mg/day, given in a single dose preferably at bedtime; some patients may require only 40 mg/day. To lessen the possibility of relapse, maintenance therapy should be continued for 3 mo or longer
Plasma-level determinations	May be useful in identifying patients with apparent toxic effects due to excessive plasma levels or when lack of absorption or noncompliance is suspected; however, dosage adjustments should be based on clinical response and not plasma levels

WARNINGS/PRECAUTIONS

MAO inhibitor therapy	Wait at least 14 days after discontinuing use of an MAO inhibitor before initiating therapy with this drug; start treatment cautiously with gradual increases in dosage until optimum response is achieved
Atropine-like action	Use with caution in patients with a history of urinary retention, narrow-angle glaucoma, or increased intraocular pressure; even average doses may precipitate an attack in patients with narrow-angle glaucoma
Cardiovascular disease	May worsen; use with caution and keep patient under close supervision. Tricyclic antidepressants, especially in high doses, may produce arrhythmias, sinus tachycardia, and prolongation of conduction time; myocardial infarction and stroke have followed use of these agents
Mental and/or physical impairment	Caution patients that their ability to drive or perform other potentially hazardous activities may be impaired, and that their response to alcohol, barbiturates, and other CNS depressants may be enhanced
Alcohol usage	Because the effects of alcohol are potentiated, its ingestion may increase the danger inherent in any suicide attempt or accidental overdose; this is especially important in patients who may use alcohol excessively
Psychotic symptoms	May increase in schizophrenic patients; paranoia may worsen, and depressed patients (particularly those with manic-depressive illness) may become manic or hypomanic. Reduce dosage of amitriptyline or add an antipsychotic agent, such as perphenazine.
Potentially suicidal patients	Should not have access to large quantities of amitriptyline; prescribe the smallest feasible amount
Discontinuation of prolonged therapy	Abrupt withdrawal may produce nausea, headache, and malaise; transient symptoms, including irritability, restlessness, and dream and sleep disturbances, may occur within the first 2 wk of gradual dosage reduction. These symptoms are not indicative of addiction. Hypomania or mania occurring within 2–7 days of stopping chronic tricyclic antidepressant therapy has been reported rarely.
Elective surgery	If possible, discontinue medication several days prior to surgery
Electroconvulsive therapy (ECT)	Hazard may be increased; use ECT only when essential
Special-risk patients	Use with caution in patients with hepatic impairment, hyperthyroidism, or a history of seizures and in those taking thyroid medication, anticholinergic agents, or sympathomimetics (see DRUG INTERACTIONS)

ADVERSE REACTIONS[1]

Cardiovascular	Hypotension (particularly orthostatic hypotension), hypertension, tachycardia, palpitations, myocardial infarction, arrhythmias, heart block, stroke

ELAVIL

Central nervous system and neuromuscular	Confusion, disturbed concentration, disorientation, delusions, hallucinations, excitement, anxiety, restlessness, insomnia, nightmares, numbness, tingling, and paresthesias of the extremities; peripheral neuropathy, incoordination, ataxia, tremors, seizures, alteration in EEG patterns, extrapyramidal symptoms, tinnitus, dizziness, weakness, headache, fatigue, inappropriate antidiuretic hormone secretion syndrome
Autonomic nervous system	Dry mouth, blurred vision, disturbance of accommodation, increased intraocular pressure, constipation, paralytic ileus, urinary retention, dilatation of urinary tract
Hematological	Bone marrow depression, including agranulocytosis, leukopenia, eosinophilia, purpura, and thrombocytopenia
Gastrointestinal	Nausea, epigastric distress, vomiting, anorexia, stomatitis, peculiar taste, diarrhea, parotid swelling, black tongue; hepatitis, including altered liver function and jaundice (rare)
Endocrinological	Testicular swelling and gynecomastia (in males), breast enlargement and galactorrhea (in females), increased or decreased libido
Allergic	Skin rash, urticaria, photosensitization, edema of face and tongue
Other	Weight gain or loss, edema, diaphoresis, urinary frequency, mydriasis, drowsiness, alopecia

OVERDOSAGE

Signs and symptoms	Drowsiness, hypothermia, tachycardia and other arrhythmias, ECG evidence of impaired conduction, congestive heart failure, mydriasis, convulsions, severe hypotension, stupor, coma, agitation, hyperactive reflexes, muscle rigidity, vomiting, hyperpyrexia (see also ADVERSE REACTIONS)
Treatment	Admit patient to hospital. Empty stomach by inducing emesis, followed by gastric lavage and activated charcoal (20–30 g q4–6h during initial 24–48 h). Obtain ECG and begin close monitoring of cardiac function if abnormalities appear. Maintain an open airway and adequate fluid intake. Regulate body temperature. Administer 1–3 mg physostigmine salicylate IV and repeat as needed, especially if life-threatening signs recur or persist. (Physostigmine should not be used routinely, however, as it may itself be toxic.) For circulatory shock and metabolic acidosis, institute standard supportive measures. Treat cardiac arrhythmias with neostigmine, pyridostigmine, or propranolol. If cardiac failure occurs, consider digitalization. (Cardiac function should be closely monitored for at least 5 days under these circumstances.) To control convulsions, use diazepam, paraldehyde, or an inhalation anesthetic; *do not use barbiturates*. Dialysis is of no value because of low plasma drug concentrations and because of extensive tissue distribution of drug.

DRUG INTERACTIONS

Alcohol, sedative-hypnotics, and other CNS depressants	↑ CNS depression
MAO inhibitors	Hyperpyrexia, excitability, severe convulsions, coma, death
Anticholinergic agents	Acute glaucoma, urinary retention, paralytic ileus
Epinephrine	↑ Pressor response, arrhythmias
Ethchlorvynol, disulfiram	Delirium
Guanethidine	↓ Antihypertensive effect
Sympathomimetic agents	Severe hypertension, hyperpyrexia
Thyroid preparations	↑ Antidepressant effect and possible risk of arrhythmias
Cimetidine	↑ Pharmacologic effects of amitriptyline

ALTERED LABORATORY VALUES

Blood/serum values	↑ or ↓ Glucose

No clinically significant alterations in urinary values occur at therapeutic dosages

USE IN CHILDREN

Not recommended for use in children under 12 yr of age because of insufficient clinical experience

USE IN PREGNANT AND NURSING WOMEN

Safety for use in pregnant or nursing women has not been established. Animal reproduction studies have been inconclusive, and clinical experience with this drug in pregnant women has been limited.

[1] Included are some tricyclic antidepressant adverse reactions not reported with this drug, but which must be considered before and during therapy

ANTIDEPRESSANTS

ENDEP (amitriptyline hydrochloride) Roche   Rx

Tablets: 10, 25, 50, 75, 100, 150 mg

INDICATIONS	**ORAL DOSAGE**
Depression, especially endogenous depression	**Adult:** 25 mg tid to start, followed by increases in late-afternoon and/or bedtime dose, up to a total of 150 mg/day, if needed; alternatively, give 50–100 mg at bedtime to start, followed by increases of 25–50 mg in the bedtime dose, up to a total of 150 mg/day, if needed

CONTRAINDICATIONS

MAO inhibitor therapy (see WARNINGS/PRECAUTIONS)	During the acute recovery phase following myocardial infarction	Hypersensitivity to amitriptyline[1]

ADMINISTRATION/DOSAGE ADJUSTMENTS

Hospitalized patients	May require 100 mg/day to start, followed by gradual increases up to a total of 200 mg/day or, occasionally, 300 mg/day, if necessary
Adolescent and elderly patients	Reduce dosage to 10 mg tid with 20 mg at bedtime if higher dosages are not tolerated
Maintenance regimen	The usual maintenance dosage is 50–100 mg/day, although some patients may require only 40 mg/day; for maintenance therapy, the entire daily dose may be given as a single dose, preferably at bedtime. Once symptoms are controlled satisfactorily, reduce the dosage to the lowest effective amount; to lessen the possibility of relapse, maintenance therapy should be continued for at least 3 mo.

WARNINGS/PRECAUTIONS

MAO inhibitor therapy	Wait at least 14 days after discontinuing use of an MAO inhibitor before initiating therapy with this drug; start treatment cautiously with gradual decreases in dosage until optimum response is achieved
Atropine-like action	Use with caution in patients with a history of urinary retention, narrow-angle glaucoma, or increased intraocular pressure; even average doses may precipitate an attack in patients with narrow-angle glaucoma
Cardiovascular disease	May worsen; use with caution and keep patient under close supervision. Tricyclic antidepressants, especially in high doses, may produce arrhythmias, sinus tachycardia, and prolongation of conduction time; myocardial infarction and stroke have followed use of these agents.
Mental and/or physical impairment	Caution patients that their ability to drive or perform other potentially hazardous activities may be impaired, and that their response to alcohol, barbiturates, and other CNS depressants may be enhanced
Alcohol usage	Because the effects of alcohol are potentiated, its ingestion may increase the danger inherent in any suicide attempt or accidental overdose; this is especially important in patients who may use alcohol excessively
Psychotic symptoms	May increase in schizophrenic patients; paranoia may worsen and manic-depressive patients may shift to manic phase. Reduce dosage of amitriptyline or add an antipsychotic agent.
Potentially suicidal patients	Should not have access to large quantities of amitriptyline; prescribe the smallest feasible amount
Abrupt discontinuation of therapy	May produce nausea, headache, and malaise after prolonged administration; symptoms are not indicative of addiction
Elective surgery	If possible, discontinue medication several days prior to surgery
Electroconvulsive therapy (ECT)	Hazard may be increased; use ECT only when essential
Special-risk patients	Use with caution in patients with impaired hepatic function, hyperthyroidism or a history of seizures and in those taking thyroid medication, anticholinergic agents, or sympathomimetics (see DRUG INTERACTIONS)
Carcinogenicity	Adequate studies have not been done in animals to evaluate the carcinogenic potential of this drug; however, no increase in the incidence of any tumor has been found in relatively small numbers of rats that received amitriptyline in their diet at dosages up to 100 mg/kg/day for 78 wk
Mutagenicity	No evidence of mutagenicity has been observed in vitro (Ames test)

ADVERSE REACTIONS[2]

Cardiovascular	Hypotension, hypertension, tachycardia, palpitations, myocardial infarction, arrhythmias, heart block, stroke

ENDEP

Central nervous system and neuromuscular	Confusion, disturbed concentration, disorientation, delusions, hallucinations, excitement, anxiety, restlessness, insomnia, nightmares, numbness, tingling and paresthesias of the extremities; peripheral neuropathy, incoordination, ataxia, tremors, seizures, alteration in EEG patterns, extrapyramidal symptoms, tinnitus, dizziness, weakness, fatigue, headache, drowsiness, inappropriate antidiuretic hormone secretion syndrome
Autonomic nervous system	Dry mouth, blurred vision, disturbance of accommodation, constipation, paralytic ileus, urinary retention, dilatation of urinary tract
Hematological	Bone marrow depression, including agranulocytosis, eosinophilia, purpura, and thrombocytopenia
Gastrointestinal	Nausea, epigastric distress, vomiting, anorexia, stomatitis, peculiar taste, diarrhea, parotid swelling, black tongue; hepatitis, including altered liver function and jaundice (rare)
Endocrinological	Testicular swelling and gynecomastia (in males), breast enlargement and galactorrhea (in females), increased or decreased libido, inappropriate ADH secretion syndrome
Allergic	Skin rash, urticaria, photosensitization, edema of face and tongue
Other	Weight gain or loss, diaphoresis, urinary frequency, mydriasis, alopecia

OVERDOSAGE

Signs and symptoms	Drowsiness, hypothermia, tachycardia and other arrhythmias, ECG evidence of impaired conduction, congestive heart failure, mydriasis, convulsions, severe hypotension, stupor, coma, agitation, hyperactive reflexes, muscle rigidity, vomiting, hyperpyrexia (see also ADVERSE REACTIONS)
Treatment	Admit patient to hospital. Empty stomach by inducing emesis, followed by gastric lavage and activated charcoal (20–30 g q4–6h during initial 24–48 h). Obtain ECG and begin close monitoring of cardiac function if abnormalities appear. Maintain an open airway and adequate fluid intake. Regulate body temperature. Administer 1–3 mg physostigmine salicylate IV and repeat as needed, especially if life-threatening signs recur or persist. (Physostigmine should not be used routinely, however, as it may itself be toxic.) For circulatory shock and metabolic acidosis, institute standard supportive measures. Treat cardiac arrhythmias with neostigmine, pyridostigmine, or propranolol. If cardiac failure occurs, consider digitalization. (Cardiac function should be closely monitored for at least 5 days under these circumstances.) To control convulsions, use diazepam, paraldehyde, or an inhalation anesthetic; *do not use barbiturates.* Dialysis is of no value because of low plasma drug concentrations and because of extensive tissue distribution of drug.

DRUG INTERACTIONS

Alcohol, sedative-hypnotics, and other CNS depressants	△ CNS depression
MAO inhibitors	Hyperpyrexia, excitability, severe convulsions, coma, death
Anticholinergic agents	Acute glaucoma, urinary retention, paralytic ileus
Epinephrine	△ Pressor response, arrhythmias
Ethchlorvynol	Transient delirium
Guanethidine	▽ Antihypertensive effect
Sympathomimetic agents	Severe hypertension, hyperpyrexia
Thyroid preparations	△ Antidepressant effect and possible risk of arrhythmias

ALTERED LABORATORY VALUES

Blood/serum values	△ or ▽ Glucose

No clinically significant alterations in urinary values occur at therapeutic dosages

USE IN CHILDREN

Not recommended for use in children under 12 yr of age because of insufficient clinical experience

USE IN PREGNANT AND NURSING WOMEN

Pregnancy Category C: use during pregnancy only if the expected therapeutic benefit justifies the potential risk to the infant. Animal reproduction studies have been inconclusive. Dosages of up to 20 mg/kg/day have caused stunting and decreased neonatal survival in rabbits but no significant adverse effects on peri- or postnatal growth and development of rat pups or teratogenic effects in either species. Teratogenic effects in animals have been seen, however, at dosages 10.5–70 times the maximum recommended adult maintenance dosage and 3.5–23 times the maximum recommended initial dosage for hospitalized patients (300 mg/day). No adequate, well-controlled studies have been done in pregnant women, and clinical experience is limited. Amitriptyline and its active metabolite, nortriptyline, are excreted in breast milk; because of the potential for serious adverse effects in nursing infants, a decision should be made to either discontinue use of the drug or stop nursing.

---

[1] Cross-sensitivity to other tricyclic antidepressants should also be considered
[2] Included are some tricyclic antidepressant adverse reactions not reported with this drug, but which must be considered before and during therapy

ANTIDEPRESSANTS

LUDIOMIL (maprotiline hydrochloride) CIBA Rx

Tablets: 25, 50, 75 mg

INDICATIONS

Depressive neurosis (dysthymic disorder)
Manic-depressive illness, depressed type (major depressive disorder)
Anxiety associated with depression

ORAL DOSAGE

Adult: for outpatients with mild-to-moderate depression, 75 mg/day, given in single or divided daily doses for 2 wk to start (some patients, particularly the elderly, may require only 25 mg/day to start), followed, if needed and tolerated, by a gradual increase in dosage, in 25-mg increments, until response is satisfactory (maximum dosage for most outpatients: 150 mg/day; this dosage should not be exceeded except for the most severely depressed outpatients, who may be given up to 225 mg/day when necessary); for more severely depressed, hospitalized patients, 100–150 mg/day, given in single or divided daily doses, to start, followed, if needed and tolerated, by a gradual increase in dosage until response is satisfactory (most hospitalized patients with moderate-to-severe depression respond to 150 mg/day, but some may require as much as 225 mg/day, the maximum recommended dosage)

CONTRAINDICATIONS

MAO inhibitor therapy (see WARNINGS/PRECAUTIONS)	During the acute recovery phase following myocardial infarction	Hypersensitivity to maprotiline
Known or suspected seizure disorders		

ADMINISTRATION/DOSAGE ADJUSTMENTS

Maintenance therapy	Reduce dosage to 75–150 mg/day; therapeutic response should guide subsequent dosage adjustments
Elderly patients	Use lower dosages for patients over 60 yr of age; for maintenance, give 50–75 mg/day to elderly patients who do not tolerate higher amounts

WARNINGS/PRECAUTIONS

MAO inhibitor therapy	Wait at least 14 days after discontinuing use of an MAO inhibitor before initiating therapy with this drug; start treatment with patient under observation and increase dosage gradually until optimum response is achieved
Cardiovascular effects	Conduction defects, arrhythmias, myocardial infarction, stroke, and tachycardia may occur in patients with a history of myocardial infarction or when a history of or active cardiovascular disease is present; use with extreme caution
Mental and/or physical impairment	Caution patients that their ability to drive or perform other potentially hazardous activities may be impaired, and that their response to alcohol, barbiturates, and other CNS depressants may be enhanced
Alcohol usage	Because the effects of alcohol are potentiated, its ingestion may increase the danger inherent in any suicide attempt or accidental overdose; this is especially important in patients who may use alcohol excessively
Seizures	Have occurred in less than 0.1% of patients, mainly in those without a history of seizure disorders; seizures are more likely to occur with rapid escalation of dosage, use of excessive dosages, concomitant administration of a phenothiazine, or rapid tapering of the dosage of a benzodiazepine given with maprotiline. Although a causal relationship has not been established, the risk may be minimized by starting therapy at a low dosage for a period of 2 wk before gradually increasing the dosage to the required level (see ORAL DOSAGE) and by keeping the dosage at the minimum effective level during maintenance therapy.
Hypomanic or manic episodes	May occur, especially in patients with manic-depressive illness, although incidence is rare
Elective surgery	Discontinue medication for as long as clinically feasible prior to surgery
Anticholinergic effect	Use with caution in patients with increased intraocular pressure or a history of urinary retention or narrow-angle glaucoma
Fever and sore throat	May occur; discontinue therapy if leukocyte and differential counts show evidence of pathologic neutrophil depression
Potentially suicidal patients	Should not have access to large quantities of maprotiline; prescribe the smallest feasible amount
Electroconvulsive therapy (ECT)	Should be avoided because of lack of experience in this area
Hyperthyroid patients	The potential for cardiovascular toxicity is enhanced in hyperthyroid patients and in those receiving thyroid medication; use with caution
Carcinogenicity, mutagenicity	Studies in rats receiving up to 60 mg/kg/day for 18 mo and in dogs receiving up to 30 mg/kg/day for 1 yr have shown no evidence of carcinogenic potential; no evidence of mutagenicity has been found in the offspring of female mice mated with males that had been treated with up to 60 times the recommended maximum human daily dose

LUDIOMIL

ADVERSE REACTIONS[1]

Frequent reactions (incidence ≥ 1%) are printed in *italics*

Central nervous system and neuromuscular	*Drowsiness (16%); dizziness (8%); nervousness (6%); weakness/fatigue and headache (4%); anxiety and tremor (3%); insomnia and agitation (2%);* numbness, tingling, motor hyperactivity, akathisia, seizures, EEG alterations, tinnitus, confusional states (especially in the elderly), hallucinations, disorientation, delusions, restlessness, nightmares, hypomania, mania, exacerbation of psychosis, decrease in memory, and feelings of unreality (rare)
Cardiovascular	Hypotension, hypertension, tachycardia, palpitation, arrhythmia, heart block, and syncope (rare)
Autonomic nervous system	*Dry mouth (22%), constipation (6%), blurred vision (4%);* accommodation disturbances, mydriasis, urinary retention, and delayed micturition (rare)
Allergic	Skin rash, petechiae, pruritus, photosensitization, edema, and drug fever (rare)
Gastrointestinal	*Nausea (2%);* vomiting, epigastric distress, diarrhea, bitter taste, abdominal cramps, dysphagia, altered liver function, and jaundice (rare)
Endocrinological	Increased or decreased libido, impotence, and hyper- or hypoglycemia (rare)
Other	Weight loss or gain, diaphoresis, flushing, urinary frequency, increased salivation, and nasal congestion (rare)

OVERDOSAGE

Signs and symptoms	Based on limited clinical experience, signs and symptoms may include drowsiness, tachycardia, ataxia, vomiting, cyanosis, hypotension, shock, restlessness, agitation, hyperpyrexia, muscle rigidity, athetoid movements, mydriasis, cardiac arrhythmias, impaired cardiac condition, and, in severe cases, loss of consciousness and generalized convulsions; congestive heart failure, a manifestation of tricyclic antidepressant overdosage, may also occur.
Treatment	Empty stomach contents by emesis or gastric lavage; to help promote more rapid elimination of the drug, leave the tube in the stomach for irrigation and continual aspiration of stomach contents. To reduce the tendency to convulsions, darken the room, allowing only minimal external stimulation. Physostigmine is not recommended since it may increase the risk of seizures. *Do not use barbiturates.* Paraldehyde may be used effectively in some children to counteract muscular hypertonus and convulsions with less likelihood of causing respiratory depression. Treat shock (circulatory collapse) with supportive measures, such as IV fluids, oxygen, and corticosteroids. Control hyperpyrexia by whatever means available, including ice packs. Employ rapid digitalization for congestive heart failure. Dialysis is of little value.

DRUG INTERACTIONS

Alcohol, sedative-hypnotics, and other CNS depressants	△ CNS depression
MAO inhibitors	Hyperpyrexia, excitability, severe convulsions, coma, death
Benzodiazepines (with rapid decrease in dosage), phenothiazines	△ Risk of seizures
Anticholinergic agents	Acute glaucoma, urinary retention, paralytic ileus
Guanethidine and similar agents	▽ Antihypertensive effect
Sympathomimetic agents	Severe hypertension, hyperpyrexia
Thyroid preparations	△ Antidepressant effect and possible risk of arrhythmias
Cimetidine	△ Pharmacologic effect of maprotiline; dosage adjustment may be necessary

ALTERED LABORATORY VALUES

Blood/serum values	△ or ▽ Glucose

No clinically significant alterations in urinary values occur at therapeutic dosages

---

USE IN CHILDREN

Safety and effectiveness for use in children under 18 yr of age have not been established

USE IN PREGNANT AND NURSING WOMEN

Pregnancy Category B: use during pregnancy only if clearly needed. Reproduction studies in rabbits, mice, and rats at doses up to 1.3, 7, and 9 times the recommended maximum human dose, respectively, have shown no evidence of impaired fertility or harm to the fetus. Maprotiline is excreted in human milk in concentrations approximating those in whole blood; use with caution in nursing mothers.

---

[1] Although the following adverse reactions have not been reported with maprotiline, its pharmacologic similarity to tricyclic antidepressants requires that each reaction be considered when administering this drug: bone marrow depression, including agranulocytosis, eosinophilia, purpura, and thrombocytopenia; myocardial infarction; stroke; peripheral neuropathy, sublingual adenitis; black tongue; stomatitis; paralytic ileus; gynecomastia in the male; breast enlargement and galactorrhea in the female; and testicular swelling

MARPLAN

ANTIDEPRESSANTS

MARPLAN (isocarboxazid) Roche   Rx
Tablets: 10 mg

INDICATIONS

Depression in patients who are refractory to tricyclic antidepressants or electroconvulsive therapy, or in whom tricyclic antidepressants are contraindicated[1]

ORAL DOSAGE

Adult: 30 mg/day, given in single or divided doses, to start; as soon as clinical improvement is observed, reduce dosage to 10–20 mg/day or less, for maintenance. If no response is obtained after 3–4 wk, further administration is unlikely to be beneficial.

CONTRAINDICATIONS

Hypersensitivity to isocarboxazid

Severe hepatic or renal impairment

Congestive heart failure

Pheochromocytoma

Sympathomimetic agents, other MAO inhibitors, tricyclic antidepressants, narcotic drugs, alcohol, and certain foods (see DRUG INTERACTIONS)

Elective surgery requiring general anesthesia (see DRUG INTERACTIONS)

WARNINGS/PRECAUTIONS

Hypertensive crisis	May occur within hours of ingestion of contraindicated substances; crises are characterized by headache, palpitation, neck stiffness or soreness, nausea, vomiting, sweating (sometimes with fever or cold, clammy skin), photophobia, tachycardia or bradycardia, constricting chest pain, and dilated pupils, and may lead to potentially fatal intracranial bleeding or circulatory collapse. Monitor blood pressure frequently, and caution patients to report promptly the occurrence of headache or any other unusual symptoms. Therapy should be discontinued immediately if palpitations or frequent headaches are observed. To treat, administer phentolamine, 5 mg IV (slowly); manage fever by external cooling.
Use of other psychotropic agents	Concomitant use of other psychotropic agents with isocarboxazid is not recommended because of possible potentiation of their individual effects and a reduced margin of safety, especially if the patient is likely to attempt suicide by overdosage. Allow at least 10 days to elapse after discontinuing this drug before initiating therapy with another psychotropic agent.
Special-risk patients	Because the most serious reactions to this drug relate to changes in blood pressure, use of isocarboxazid is not recommended in elderly or debilitated patients and in the presence of hypertension or cardiovascular or cerebrovascular disease. Because headaches may be the first symptom of a hypertensive reaction to isocarboxazid, patients with frequent or severe headaches should not be considered as candidates for therapy.
Suicidal patients	Should be under strict medical supervision, and preferably hospitalized, as reliance on drug therapy (or any other single therapeutic measure) to prevent suicide attempts is unwarranted
Manic-depressive states	If a swing from a depressive to a manic phase occurs, discontinue use of isocarboxazid briefly and resume therapy at a lower dosage
Epileptic patients	May experience a decrease or increase in seizures
Altered liver function, hepatocellular jaundice	May occur in rare cases; obtain liver function studies periodically and discontinue use at the first sign of hepatic dysfunction or jaundice
Excessive stimulation	May occur in hyperactive, agitated, or schizophrenic patients; use with caution
Orthostatic hypotension	May occur; if necessary, reduce dosage or discontinue therapy
Patients with renal impairment	Use with caution to avoid drug accumulation
Diabetic patients	There is conflicting evidence as to whether MAO inhibitors affect glucose metabolism or potentiate hypoglycemic agents

ADVERSE REACTIONS

Cardiovascular	Orthostatic hypotension, disturbances in cardiac rate and rhythm
Central nervous system	Dizziness, vertigo, headache, overactivity, hyperreflexia, tremors, muscle twitching, mania, hypomania, jitteriness, confusion, memory impairment, insomnia, fatigue, weakness, akathisia, ataxia, coma, euphoria, neuritis; hallucinations (rare)
Genitourinary	Dysuria, incontinence, urinary retention; impaired water excretion (associated with inappropriate ADH secretion syndrome)
Gastrointestinal	Constipation, dry mouth, anorexia, other disturbances
Dermatological	Rash, spider telangiectases
Ophthalmic	Blurred vision, photosensitivity[2]

MARPLAN ■ NARDIL

Other — Peripheral edema, hyperhidrosis, black tongue, weight changes, hematological changes, sexual disturbances

OVERDOSAGE

Signs and symptoms — Tachycardia, hypotension, coma, convulsions, respiratory depression, sluggish reflexes, pyrexia, diaphoresis

Treatment — Empty stomach by gastric lavage or emesis. Maintain an open airway and supply oxygen, if necessary. Employ general supportive measures. For hypotension, plasma may be of value; pressor amines, such as norepinephrine, may be of limited value. Perform liver-function tests and follow liver function for 4–6 wk after recovery.

DRUG INTERACTIONS

Sympathomimetic agents (including levodopa, dopamine, cocaine, tryptophan, tyramine, and caffeine) — Hypertensive crisis; do not give a sympathomimetic agent in combination with isocarboxazid. Caution patients to moderate their use of caffeine, to avoid taking OTC cold, hay fever, and weight-reducing preparations, and to refrain from consuming foods with a high concentration of tryptophan or tyramine, such as broad bean pods (fava beans), cheese, beer, wine, pickled herring, chicken livers, and yeast extract.

Other MAO inhibitors, tricyclic antidepressants — Hypertensive crisis, fever, marked sweating, excitation, delirium, tremor, twitching, convulsions, coma, and circulatory collapse. Do not give isocarboxazid and either a tricyclic antidepressant or another MAO inhibitor concomitantly or in rapid succession; when switching to a tricyclic antidepressant or switching to or from another MAO inhibitor, allow a drug-free interval of at least 10 days to elapse.

Meperidine and other narcotic drugs, alcohol — △ CNS depression (with alcohol or narcotic drugs); circulatory collapse, severe hyperpyrexia, and death (with meperidine). Caution patients not to consume alcohol during antidepressant therapy, and do not give a narcotic drug in combination with isocarboxazid.

General anesthetics — △ CNS depression; isocarboxazid should be discontinued at least 10 days before performance of elective surgery requiring general anesthesia

Spinal anesthetics — Hypotension; give a spinal anesthetic in combination with isocarboxazid only if such use is essential

Barbiturates — △ CNS depression; reduce dosage of barbiturates given in combination with isocarboxazid

Methyldopa, guanethidine, rauwolfia alkaloids, and other antihypertensive drugs — Hypertensive crisis (with methyldopa); do not give methyldopa in combination with isocarboxazid

Hypertension (with guanethidine or rauwolfia alkaloids); hypotension (with other antihypertensive drugs). Exercise caution if an antihypertensive drug other than methyldopa is given in combination with isocarboxazid.

ALTERED LABORATORY VALUES

Blood/serum values — ▽ Glucose
Urinary values — ▽ 5-HIAA ▽ VMA

USE IN CHILDREN

Not recommended for use in children under 16 yr of age because there are no controlled studies of safety or effectiveness in this age group

USE IN PREGNANT AND NURSING WOMEN

Safety for use in pregnant or nursing women has not been established; before giving this drug to such patients or to women of childbearing age, weigh the expected benefits against the possible hazards to mother and child. No evidence of teratogenic effects nor significant differences in litter size have been detected in reproduction studies on rats receiving 0.5 and 5 mg/kg/day in their diet through two mating cycles.

[1] Probably effective
[2] Toxic amblyopia has also been reported (once), but a causal relationship could not be established

---

ANTIDEPRESSANTS

NARDIL (phenelzine sulfate) Parke-Davis Rx

Tablets: 15 mg

INDICATIONS

Atypical, nonendogenous, or neurotic depression, generally in patients who fail to respond to other antidepressant therapy

ORAL DOSAGE

Adult: 15 mg tid to start, followed by a rapid increase in dosage to 60–90 mg/day until maximum benefit is achieved; thereafter, reduce dosage slowly over several weeks to as low as 15 mg daily or every other day. Clinical response may not be apparent until 60 mg/day has been given for 4 wk or more.

NARDIL

CONTRAINDICATIONS

Hypersensitivity to phenelzine	Elective surgery requiring general anesthesia (see DRUG INTERACTIONS)	Sympathomimetic agents, other MAO inhibitors, narcotic drugs, alcohol, guanethidine, and certain foods (see DRUG INTERACTIONS)
Pheochromocytoma	History of liver disease	
Congestive heart failure	Abnormal liver function tests	

WARNINGS/PRECAUTIONS

Hypertensive crisis	May occur within hours of ingestion of contraindicated substances; crises are characterized by headache, palpitation, neck stiffness or soreness, nausea, vomiting, sweating (sometimes with fever or cold, clammy skin), photophobia, tachycardia or bradycardia, constricting chest pain, and dilated pupils, may lead to intracranial bleeding, and can be fatal. Monitor blood pressure frequently and caution patients to report promptly the occurrence of headache or any other unusual symptoms. Therapy should be discontinued immediately if palpitations or frequent headaches are observed. To treat, administer phentolamine, 5 mg IV (slowly); manage fever by external cooling.
Suicidal patients	Should be kept under careful observation until depression is controlled; if necessary, institute additional measures (electroconvulsive therapy, hospitalization, etc) to prevent suicide attempts
Epileptic patients	May experience a decrease or increase in seizures; take adequate precautions
Orthostatic hypotension	May occur in hypertensive, as well as normotensive and hypotensive, patients; if necessary, reduce the dosage of phenelzine or discontinue therapy
Diabetic patients	There is conflicting evidence as to whether MAO inhibitors affect glucose metabolism or potentiate hypoglycemic agents
Hypomania or increased agitation	May occur if hyperkinetic symptoms coexist with depression or agitation is present or, less frequently, if higher than recommended doses are used or following long-term therapy; schizophrenic patients may show excessive stimulation. In manic-depressive states, a swing from a depressive phase to a manic phase may occur.
Withdrawal	Abrupt withdrawal may infrequently precipitate symptoms ranging from vivid nightmares and agitation to frank psychosis; these reactions are usually first seen 24–72 h after discontinuation of the drug. If such symptoms occur, reinstitute therapy with a low dose of phenelzine and then cautiously reduce the dosage before discontinuing therapy.
Carcinogenicity	Induction of pulmonary and vascular tumors has been observed in an uncontrolled, life-time study in mice

ADVERSE REACTIONS

Frequent reactions (incidence $\geq$ 1%) are printed in *italics*

Cardiovascular	*Orthostatic hypotension,* transient depression following electroconvulsive therapy
Hepatic	Jaundice; fatal progressive necrotizing hepatocellular damage (rare)
Respiratory	Transient depression following electroconvulsive therapy
Central nervous system	*Dizziness, drowsiness, weakness, fatigue, tremors, muscle twitching, hyperreflexia,* mania, hypomania, jitteriness, euphoria, palilalia, ataxia, coma, toxic delirium, convulsions, acute anxiety reaction, precipitation of schizophrenia
Genitourinary	Anorgasmia, ejaculatory disturbances, urinary retention
Gastrointestinal	*Constipation, dry mouth, other disturbances*
Dermatological	Rash, diaphoresis
Ophthalmic	Blurred vision, glaucoma, nystagmus
Hematological	Leukopenia
Other	*Edema,* weight gain, hypernatremia, glottal edema

OVERDOSAGE

Signs and symptoms	Drowsiness, dizziness, faintness, irritability, hyperactivity, agitation, severe headache, hallucinations, trismus, opisthotonus, convulsions, coma, rapid and irregular pulse, hypertension, hypotension, vascular collapse, precordial pain, respiratory depression and failure, hyperpyrexia, diaphoresis, cool and clammy skin
Treatment	Admit patient to hospital immediately. Empty stomach by gastric lavage or induction of emesis and by instillation of activated charcoal (avoid aspiration). Maintain an open airway; if necessary, assist ventilation and give oxygen. Regulate body temperature and maintain fluid and electrolyte balance. For CNS stimulation, including convulsions, slowly administer IV diazepam; avoid phenothiazines and CNS stimulants. Combat hypotension and vascular collapse with IV fluids; administer a dilute vasopressor solution by IV infusion if necessary (titrate dosage carefully; adrenergic agents may produce a marked increase in blood pressure). In cases of massive overdosage, hemodialysis, peritoneal dialysis, and charcoal hemoperfusion may be useful.

DRUG INTERACTIONS

Sympathomimetic agents (including phenylalanine, tyrosine, levodopa, dopamine, tyramine, tryptophan, cocaine, amphetamines, methylphenidate, and caffeine)	Hypertensive crisis; do not use sympathomimetic drugs during therapy or for 2 wk after discontinuation of treatment. Caution patients that during this period they should moderate their use of caffeine and chocolate, avoid taking OTC respiratory tract, weight-reducing, or tryptophan-containing preparations, and refrain from consuming foods with a high tryptophan or tyramine content such as liver, broad bean pods (fava beans), yeast extracts, beer, wine, and protein-rich foods that have spoiled or that have undergone aging, fermentation, pickling, or smoking (eg, pickled herring, dry sausage, cheeses other than cottage and cream cheese, and yogurt)
Other MAO inhibitors	Hypertensive crisis, convulsive seizures, fever, marked sweating, excitation, delirium, tremor, coma, and circulatory collapse; do not give phenelzine and another MAO inhibitor concomitantly or in rapid succession
Meperidine and other narcotic drugs, alcohol	Excitation, seizures, delirium, hyperpyrexia, circulatory collapse, coma, and death (with meperidine) △ CNS depression (with alcohol or narcotic drugs)
	Alcohol and certain narcotic drugs should not be used in combination with phenelzine
General anesthetics	△ CNS depression; phenelzine should be discontinued at least 10 days before performance of elective surgery requiring general anesthesia
Spinal anesthetics	Hypotension; exercise caution
Barbiturates	△ CNS depression; reduce dosage of barbiturates given in combination with phenelzine
Methyldopa, guanethidine, rauwolfia alkaloids, and other antihypertensive drugs	CNS excitation, hypertension (with methyldopa); hypertension (with guanethidine); do not give methyldopa or guanethidine in combination with phenelzine
	Hypertension (with rauwolfia alkaloids); hypotension (with other antihypertensive drugs); exercise caution if an antihypertensive drug other than methyldopa or guanethidine is given in combination with phenelzine
Tricyclic compounds (including maprotiline, cyclobenzapine, and carbamazepine)	Possible adverse reactions; although a significant incidence of serious side effects has not occurred with concomitant use of phenelzine and tricyclic antidepressants, patients should be warned that adverse reactions may result from combination therapy or from administration of phenelzine within less than 10 days after discontinuation of a tricyclic antidepressant

ALTERED LABORATORY VALUES

Blood/serum values	▽ Glucose
Urinary values	▽ 5-HIAA ▽ VMA

USE IN CHILDREN

Not recommended for use in children under 16 yr of age because there are no controlled studies of safety or effectiveness in this age group

USE IN PREGNANT AND NURSING WOMEN

Safety for use in pregnant or nursing women has not been established. A significant decrease in the number of surviving mice per litter has been observed at doses well above the recommended maximum human dose, and growth retardation has been seen in young dogs and rats at doses exceeding the recommended maximum human dose.

ANTIDEPRESSANTS

NORPRAMIN (desipramine hydrochloride) Merrell Dow   Rx

Tablets: 10, 25, 50, 75, 100, 150 mg

INDICATIONS

Depression, especially endogenous depression

ORAL DOSAGE

Adult: 100–200 mg/day, given in one or more doses; for more severe depression, dosage may be further increased gradually, up to 300 mg/day. Begin therapy with lower dosages and increase level as needed and tolerated.

CONTRAINDICATIONS

MAO inhibitor therapy (see WARNINGS/PRECAUTIONS)   During the acute recovery phase following myocardial infarction   Hypersensitivity to desipramine[1]

ADMINISTRATION/DOSAGE ADJUSTMENTS

Adolescent and geriatric patients — Administer 25–100 mg/day (begin at a lower level); for more severe depression, dosage may be further increased, up to 150 mg/day

NORPRAMIN

Patients requiring high doses	Treatment of patients requiring doses approaching 300 mg should be initiated in the hospital, where close supervision is available and frequent ECG monitoring can be accomplished

WARNINGS/PRECAUTIONS

MAO inhibitor therapy	Wait at least 14 days after discontinuing use of an MAO inhibitor before initiating therapy with this drug; start treatment cautiously and increase dosage gradually
Atropine-like action	Use with extreme caution in patients with a history of urinary retention or narrow-angle glaucoma
Cardiovascular disease	Use with extreme caution; conduction defects, arrhythmias, tachycardias, stroke, and acute myocardial infarction may occur
Mental and/or physical impairment	Caution patients that their ability to drive or perform other potentially hazardous activities may be impaired, and that their response to alcohol may be enhanced
Alcohol usage	Because the effects of alcohol are potentiated, its ingestion may increase the danger inherent in any suicide attempt or accidental overdose; this is especially important in patients who may use alcohol excessively
Psychotic symptoms	May increase in schizophrenic patients; paranoia may worsen and manic-depressive patients may shift to manic phase; reduce dosage of desipramine or add an antipsychotic agent
Potentially suicidal patients	Should not have access to large quantities of desipramine; prescribe the smallest feasible amount
Abrupt discontinuation of therapy	May produce nausea, headache, and malaise after prolonged administration; symptoms are not indicative of addiction
Elective surgery	If possible, discontinue medication several days prior to surgery
Electroconvulsive therapy (ECT)	Hazard may be increased; use ECT only when essential
Special-risk patients	Use with extreme caution in patients with thyroid disease or a history of seizures, and in those taking thyroid medication, anticholinergic agents, or sympathomimetics (see DRUG INTERACTIONS)
Fever and sore throat developing during therapy	Discontinue therapy if leukocyte and differential counts show evidence of pathologic neutrophil depression
Tartrazine sensitivity	Presence of FD&C Yellow No. 5 (tartrazine) in all tablets except 10-mg and 150-mg strengths may cause allergic-type reactions, including bronchial asthma, in susceptible individuals

ADVERSE REACTIONS[2]

Cardiovascular	Hypotension, hypertension, tachycardia, palpitations, myocardial infarction, arrhythmias, heart block, stroke
Central nervous system and neuromuscular	Confusion, hallucinations, disorientation, delusions, anxiety, restlessness, agitation, insomnia, nightmares, hypomania, exacerbated psychosis, numbness, tingling, paresthesias of the extremities, incoordination, ataxia, tremors, peripheral neuropathy, extrapyramidal symptoms, seizures, alteration in EEG patterns, tinnitus, drowsiness, dizziness, weakness, fatigue, headache
Autonomic nervous system	Dry mouth (associated rarely with sublingual adenitis), blurred vision, disturbance of accommodation, increased intraocular pressure, mydriasis, constipation, paralytic ileus, urinary retention, dilatation of urinary tract
Hematological	Bone marrow depression, including agranulocytosis, eosinophilia, purpura, and thrombocytopenia
Gastrointestinal	Anorexia, nausea, vomiting, epigastric distress, stomatitis, peculiar taste, abdominal cramps, diarrhea, parotid swelling, black tongue, altered liver function, jaundice
Endocrinological	Testicular swelling and gynecomastia (in males), breast enlargement and galactorrhea (in females), increased or decreased libido, impotence, inappropriate ADH secretion syndrome
Allergic	Skin rash, petechiae, urticaria, itching, photosensitization, edema of face and tongue or generalized, drug fever
Other	Weight gain or loss, diaphoresis, flushing, urinary frequency, nocturia, alopecia

OVERDOSAGE

Signs and symptoms	Tachycardia and other arrhythmias, cardiac output disturbances, ECG evidence of impaired conduction, congestive heart failure, mydriasis, grand mal seizures, severe hypotension, stupor, coma, agitation, hyperactive reflexes, muscle rigidity, vomiting, hyperpyrexia, shock, renal shutdown (see also ADVERSE REACTIONS)
Treatment	Admit patient to hospital. Empty stomach by gastric lavage. Obtain ECG and begin close monitoring of cardiac function for at least 72 h if abnormalities appear. Maintain an open airway and adequate fluid intake. Regulate body temperature. For cardiac arrhythmias, circulatory shock, and metabolic acidosis, institute standard supportive measures. If cardiac failure occurs, consider digitalization. (Cardiac function should be closely monitored for at least 5 days under these circumstances.) Dialysis is of no value because of low plasma drug concentrations and because of extensive tissue distribution of drug.

NORPRAMIN ■ PAMELOR

DRUG INTERACTIONS

Alcohol, sedative-hypnotics, and other CNS depressants	△ CNS depression
MAO inhibitors	Hyperpyrexia, excitability, severe convulsions, coma, death
Anticholinergic agents	Acute glaucoma, urinary retention, paralytic ileus
Ethchlorvynol	Transient delirium
Clonidine, guanethidine	▽ Antihypertensive effect
Sympathomimetic agents	Severe hypertension, hyperpyrexia
Thyroid preparations	△ Antidepressant effect and possible risk of arrhythmias
Cimetidine	△ Pharmacologic effects of desipramine

ALTERED LABORATORY VALUES

Blood/serum values —————— △ or ▽ Glucose

No clinically significant alterations in urinary values occur at therapeutic dosages

USE IN CHILDREN
Not recommended for use in children because safety and effectiveness have not been established in the pediatric age group

USE IN PREGNANT AND NURSING WOMEN
Safety for use in pregnant or nursing women has not been established. Animal reproduction studies have been inconclusive.

[1] Cross-sensitivity to other dibenzazepines should also be considered
[2] Included are some tricyclic antidepressant adverse reactions not reported with this drug, but which must be considered before and during therapy

---

ANTIDEPRESSANTS

PAMELOR (nortriptyline hydrochloride) Sandoz Pharmaceuticals   Rx

Capsules: 10, 25, 50, 75 mg   **Solution (per 5 ml):** 10 mg[1] (16 fl oz)

INDICATIONS	ORAL DOSAGE
Depression, especially endogenous depression	**Adult:** initiate therapy with low doses and increase dosage gradually as needed, according to clinical response and tolerance; usual dosage, 25 mg tid or qid or 75–100 mg/day, given in a single daily dose; once remission has occurred, reduce dosage to lowest effective level for maintenance

CONTRAINDICATIONS

MAO inhibitor therapy (see WARNINGS/PRECAUTIONS)	During the acute recovery phase following myocardial infarction	Hypersensitivity to nortriptyline[2]

ADMINISTRATION/DOSAGE ADJUSTMENTS

Dosages > 100 mg/day	If dosages greater than 100 mg/day are required, monitor nortriptyline plasma level and adjust dosage to maintain an optimum level of 50–150 ng/ml; dosages exceeding 150 mg/day are not recommended
Adolescent or elderly patients	Reduce dosage to 30–50 mg/day, given in a single daily dose or divided

WARNINGS/PRECAUTIONS

MAO inhibitor therapy	Wait at least 14 days after discontinuing use of an MAO inhibitor before initiating therapy with this drug
Atropine-like action	Use with great caution in patients with a history of urinary retention or narrow-angle glaucoma
Cardiovascular disease	May worsen; use with caution, keep patient under close supervision. Tricyclic antidepressants, especially in high doses, may produce arrhythmias, sinus tachycardia, and prolongation of conduction time; myocardial infarction and stroke have followed use of these agents.
Mental and/or physical impairment	Caution patients that their ability to drive or perform other potentially hazardous activities may be impaired, and that their response to alcohol may be enhanced
Alcohol usage	Because the effects of alcohol are potentiated, its ingestion may increase the danger inherent in any suicide attempt or accidental overdose; this is especially important in patients who may use alcohol excessively
Psychotic symptoms	May increase in schizophrenic patients; hostility may be aroused, latent symptoms may be unmasked, and manic-depressive patients may shift to manic phase

PAMELOR

Potentially suicidal patients	Should not have access to large quantities of nortriptyline; prescribe the smallest feasible amount
Abrupt discontinuation of therapy	May produce nausea, headache, and malaise after prolonged administration; symptoms are not indicative of addiction
Elective surgery	If possible, discontinue medication several days prior to surgery
Electroconvulsive therapy (ECT)	May increase hazard; use ECT only when essential
Special-risk patients	Use with caution in patients with hyperthyroidism or a history of seizures and in those taking thyroid medications, anticholinergic agents, or sympathomimetics (see DRUG INTERACTIONS)

ADVERSE REACTIONS[3]

Cardiovascular	Hypotension, hypertension, tachycardia, palpitations, myocardial infarction, arrhythmias, heart block, stroke
Central nervous system and neuromuscular	Confusion, disorientation, delusions, hallucinations, excitement, anxiety, restlessness, agitation, insomnia, panic, nightmares, hypomania, exacerbation of psychosis, numbness, tingling, paresthesias of the extremities, peripheral neuropathy, incoordination, ataxia, tremors, seizures, alteration in EEG patterns, extrapyramidal symptoms, tinnitus, drowsiness, dizziness, weakness, fatigue, headache
Autonomic nervous system	Dry mouth (associated rarely with sublingual adenitis), blurred vision, disturbance of accommodation, increased intraocular pressure, mydriasis, constipation, paralytic ileus, urinary retention, dilatation of urinary tract, delayed micturition
Hematological	Bone marrow depression, including agranulocytosis, eosinophilia, purpura, and thrombocytopenia
Gastrointestinal	Nausea, epigastric distress, vomiting, anorexia, stomatitis, peculiar taste, abdominal cramps, diarrhea, parotid swelling, black tongue, altered liver function, jaundice
Endocrinological	Testicular swelling, gynecomastia, and impotence (in males), breast enlargement and galactorrhea (in females), increased or decreased libido, inappropriate ADH secretion syndrome
Allergic	Skin rash, urticaria, photosensitization, edema of face and tongue or generalized, petechiae, itching, drug fever
Other	Weight gain or loss, diaphoresis, flushing, urinary frequency, nocturia, alopecia

OVERDOSAGE

Signs and symptoms	Confusion, restlessness, agitation, vomiting, hyperpyrexia, muscle rigidity, hyperactive reflexes, tachycardia, ECG evidence of impaired conduction, shock, congestive heart failure, convulsions, stupor, coma, respiratory depression, death (see also ADVERSE REACTIONS)
Treatment	Admit patient to hospital. Empty stomach by gastric lavage. Employ general supportive measures. Maintain an open airway and adequate fluid intake. To control convulsions, use diazepam or paraldehyde; *do not use barbiturates*. The value of dialysis has not been established.

DRUG INTERACTIONS

Alcohol, sedative-hypnotics, and other CNS depressants	△ CNS depression
MAO inhibitors	Hyperpyrexia, excitability, severe convulsions, coma, death
Anticholinergic agents	Acute glaucoma, urinary retention, paralytic ileus
Ethchlorvynol	Transient delirium
Reserpine	Stimulation ▽ Antihypertensive effect
Guanethidine	▽ Antihypertensive effect
Sympathomimetic agents	Severe hypertension, hyperpyrexia
Thyroid preparations	△ Antidepressant effect and possible risk of arrhythmias
Cimetidine	△ Serum nortriptyline level

ALTERED LABORATORY VALUES

Blood/serum values	△ or ▽ Glucose

No clinically significant alterations in urinary values occur at therapeutic dosages

USE IN CHILDREN

Not recommended for use in children because safety and effectiveness have not been established in the pediatric age group

USE IN PREGNANT AND NURSING WOMEN

Safety for use in pregnant or nursing women has not been established. Animal reproduction studies have been inconclusive.

---

[1] Contains 4% alcohol
[2] Cross-sensitivity to other dibenzazepines should also be considered
[3] Included are some tricyclic antidepressant adverse reactions not reported with this drug, but which must be considered before and during therapy

ANTIDEPRESSANTS

PARNATE (tranylcypromine sulfate) Smith Kline & French Rx

Tablets: 10 mg

INDICATIONS

Major depressive episode *without* melancholia[1] in patients who can be closely supervised and who have not responded to other, more commonly used antidepressants

ORAL DOSAGE

Adult: 30 mg/day in divided doses; if improvement is not seen within 2 wk, increase dosage in increments of 10 mg/day at intervals of 1–3 wk, up to a maximum of 60 mg/day

CONTRAINDICATIONS

Hypersensitivity to tranylcypromine	Elective surgery requiring general anesthesia (see DRUG INTERACTIONS)	Sympathomimetic agents, other MAO inhibitors, tricyclic compounds, antihypertensive drugs, narcotic drugs, alcohol, and certain foods (see DRUG INTERACTIONS)
Age > 60 yr	History of liver disease	
Confirmed or suspected cerebrovascular defect	Abnormal liver function tests	
Cardiovascular disease or hypertension		
Pheochromocytoma		

ADMINISTRATION/DOSAGE ADJUSTMENTS

Discontinuation of therapy	Withdrawal of the drug should be gradual

WARNINGS/PRECAUTIONS

Hypertensive crisis	May occur within hours of ingestion of contraindicated substances; crises are characterized by headache, palpitation, neck stiffness or soreness, nausea, vomiting, sweating (sometimes with fever or cold, clammy skin), photophobia, tachycardia or bradycardia, constricting chest pain, and dilated pupils, and may lead to potentially fatal intracranial bleeding. Monitor blood pressure frequently, and caution patients to report promptly the occurrence of headache or any other unusual symptoms. Therapy should be discontinued immediately if palpitations or frequent headaches are observed. To treat, administer phentolamine, 5 mg IV (slowly); *do not use parenteral reserpine*. Manage fever by external cooling.
Orthostatic hypotension	May occur, most commonly in patients with preexisting hypertension; at dosages above 30 mg/day, orthostatic hypotension is a major side effect and may result in syncope. Increase dosage more gradually in patients prone to hypotension at the beginning of therapy. When tranylcypromine is combined with phenothiazine derivatives or other compounds known to cause hypotension, the possibility of additive hypotensive effects should be considered.
Concomitant antiparkinson therapy	Use with caution, as severe antimuscarinic reactions may occur
Suicidal patients	Should be kept under close supervision, as reliance on drug therapy alone to prevent suicide attempts is unwarranted
Convulsive threshold	May be raised or lowered; use with caution in epileptic patients
Hypoglycemia	May occur in diabetic patients receiving insulin or oral hypoglycemics; use with caution
Anginal pain	May be suppressed, resulting in the masking of myocardial ischemia
Patients with renal impairment	Use with caution to avoid drug accumulation
Hyperthyroid patients	May show increased sensitivity to pressor amines; use with caution
Concomitant use of disulfiram	Use with caution; conflicting results have been obtained in animal studies
Excessive stimulation	May occur, including increased anxiety, agitation, and manic symptoms; reduce dosage or administer a phenothiazine antipsychotic agent concomitantly
Drug dependence	Has been observed in patients using doses significantly above the therapeutic range; some of these patients had a history of prior substance abuse. Withdrawal of the drug from patients physically dependent on it reportedly may cause restlessness, anxiety, depression, confusion, hallucinations, headache, weakness, and diarrhea.

ADVERSE REACTIONS[2]

Central nervous system	Overstimulation (including anxiety, agitation, and manic symptoms), restlessness, insomnia, weakness, drowsiness, dizziness, headache (without hypertension)
Gastrointestinal	Dry mouth, nausea, diarrhea, abdominal pain, constipation, anorexia; hepatitis (rare)
Cardiovascular	Orthostatic hypotension, tachycardia, edema, palpitation
Ophthalmic	Blurred vision
Dermatological	Rash (rare)
Other	Impotence, inappropriate secretion of antidiuretic hormone (ADH) syndrome

PARNATE

OVERDOSAGE

Signs and symptoms	See WARNINGS/PRECAUTIONS and ADVERSE REACTIONS; insomnia, restlessness, and anxiety, progressing to agitation, mental confusion, and incoherence; or hypotension, dizziness, weakness, and drowsiness progressing to extreme dizziness or shock; or hypertension with severe headache, in rare cases accompanied by twitching or myoclonic fibrillation of skeletal muscles with hyperpyrexia progressing to generalized rigidity and coma
Treatment	Empty stomach by gastric lavage. Employ general supportive measures. For hyperpyrexia, provide external cooling. Administer barbiturates with caution to control myoclonic reactions. For hypotension, use standard measures for managing circulatory shock. If pressor agents are used, regulate rate of infusion carefully to preclude an excessive rise in blood pressure. Continue to observe patient closely for 1 wk.

DRUG INTERACTIONS

Sympathomimetic agents (including levodopa, dopamine, cocaine, tryptophan, tyramine, and caffeine)	Hypertensive crisis; also disorientation and impairment of memory (with tryptophan). Do not use a sympathomimetic drug in combination with tranylcypromine. Caution patients to moderate their use of caffeine, to avoid taking OTC cold, hay fever, or weight-reducing preparations that contain vasoconstrictors, and to refrain from consuming foods with a high tyramine content (usually owing to protein degradation), such as cheese (especially if strong or aged), sour cream, Chianti wine, sherry, beer, pickled herring, liver, canned figs, raisins, bananas and avocados (especially if overripe), chocolate, soy sauce, broad bean pods (fava beans), yeast extracts, and tenderized meat.
Other MAO inhibitors (including furazolidone and procarbazine), tricyclic compounds (including maprotiline, cyclobenzaprine, and carbamazepine)	Hypertensive crisis, severe convulsive seizures; when switching to or from a tricyclic compound or another MAO inhibitor, allow a drug-free interval of at least 1 wk to elapse. During at least the first week of tranylcypromine therapy, patients who have been switched from a tricyclic compound or another MAO inhibitor should be given 10 mg/day (one half the usual starting dosage).
Meperidine and other narcotic drugs, alcohol	Coma, severe hypertension or hypotension, severe respiratory depression, convulsions, malignant hyperpyrexia, excitation, peripheral vascular collapse, and death (with meperidine); do not give meperidine in combination with tranylcypromine or within 2–3 wk after discontinuation of tranylcypromine therapy
	△ CNS depression (with alcohol or narcotic drugs); caution patients not to consume alcohol during antidepressant therapy, and do not give a narcotic drug in combination with tranylcypromine
General anesthetics	△ CNS depression; tranylcypromine should be discontinued at least 10 days before performance of elective surgery requiring general anesthesia
Spinal anesthetics	Hypotension; exercise caution
Methyldopa, guanethidine, rauwolfia alkaloids, and other antihypertensive drugs	Hypertensive crisis (with methyldopa); hypertension (with guanethidine or rauwolfia alkaloids); hypotension (with other antihypertensive drugs). Do not use an antihypertensive drug in combination with tranylcypromine.
Metrizamide	Seizures; discontinue use of tranylcypromine at least 48 h before administration of metrizamide for myelography, and wait at least 24 h after performance of the procedure before resuming therapy

ALTERED LABORATORY VALUES

Blood/serum values	▽ Glucose
Urinary values	▽ 5-HIAA ▽ VMA

USE IN CHILDREN

Consult manufacturer for use in children

USE IN PREGNANT AND NURSING WOMEN

Safety for use in pregnant or nursing women has not been established. Tranylcypromine crosses the placental barrier in the rat and has been detected in the milk of lactating dogs.

---

[1] A major depressive episode without melancholia is described in the American Psychiatric Association's Diagnostic and Statistic Manual III as a prominent depressed or dysphoric mood that occurs nearly every day for at least 2 wk, usually interferes with daily functioning, and includes at least 4 of the following 8 symptoms: change in appetite, change in sleep, psychomotor agitation or retardation, loss of interest in usual activities or decrease in sexual drive, increased fatigue, feelings of guilt or worthlessness, slowed thinking or impaired concentration, and suicidal ideation or attempts. The effectiveness of tranylcypromine for treatment of a major depressive episode with melancholia has not been established.

[2] Reactions for which a causal relationship has not been established include tinnitus, muscle spasm and tremors, paresthesia, and urinary retention

ANTIDEPRESSANTS

SINEQUAN (doxepin hydrochloride) Roerig   Rx
Capsules: 10, 25, 50, 75, 100, 150 mg   **Concentrate:** 10 mg/ml (120 ml)

INDICATIONS	ORAL DOSAGE
Depression and/or anxiety in psychoneurotic patients Depression and/or anxiety associated with alcoholism Depression and/or anxiety associated with organic disease Psychotic depressive disorders associated with anxiety, including involutional depression and manic-depressive disorders	**Adult:** for mild to moderate symptoms, 25 mg tid to start, followed by an increase or decrease in dosage at appropriate intervals according to individual response (usual optimum dosage, 75–150 mg/day; very mild symptoms or emotional symptoms accompanying organic disease may be adequately controlled in some patients with as little as 25–50 mg/day); for more severe symptoms, higher doses may be needed initially, followed by a gradual increase in dosage up to 300 mg/day, if necessary. Oral concentrate should be diluted, just prior to administration, with 120 ml of water, milk, or fruit juice *(do not use carbonated beverages)*.

CONTRAINDICATIONS

Hypersensitivity to doxepin[1]	Glaucoma	Urinary retention

ADMINISTRATION/DOSAGE ADJUSTMENTS

Alternative once-a-day regimen	If desired, the entire daily dose, but not more than 150 mg, may given at bedtime (the 150-mg capsule is intended for maintenance therapy only and should not be used to initiate treatment with this drug); adjust the dosage carefully in elderly patients and in patients with intercurrent illness or taking other medications, particularly drugs with anticholinergic effects
Patients on methadone maintenance programs	The oral concentrate and methadone syrup can be mixed together with Gatorade, lemonade, orange juice, sugar water, Tang, or plain water (but not with grape juice) for patients requiring antidepressant therapy

WARNINGS/PRECAUTIONS

MAO inhibitor therapy	Wait at least 14 days after discontinuing use of an MAO inhibitor before initiating therapy with this drug; start treatment cautiously
Mental and/or physical impairment	Caution patients not to drive or engage in other potentially hazardous activities while taking this drug because they may become drowsy, and that their response to alcohol may be enhanced
Alcohol usage	Because the effects of alcohol are potentiated, its ingestion may increase the danger inherent in any suicide attempt or accidental overdose; this is especially important in patients who may use alcohol excessively
Psychotic symptoms	May increase; manic-depressive patients may shift to manic phase; reduce dosage of doxepin or add an antipsychotic agent
Potentially suicidal patients	Should be closely supervised during the early phases of therapy and should not have access to large quantities of doxepin; prescribe the smallest feasible amount
Withdrawal reactions	Abrupt discontinuation following prolonged use may result in withdrawal reactions

ADVERSE REACTIONS[2]

Cardiovascular	Hypotension, tachycardia
Central nervous system and neuromuscular	Drowsiness, confusion, disorientation, hallucinations, numbness, paresthesias, ataxia, seizures, extrapyramidal symptoms, tinnitus, dizziness, weakness, fatigue, headache
Autonomic nervous system	Dry mouth, blurred vision, constipation, urinary retention
Hematological	Bone marrow depression, including agranulocytosis, leukopenia, eosinophilia, purpura, and thrombocytopenia
Gastrointestinal	Nausea, vomiting, indigestion, anorexia, stomatitis, peculiar taste, diarrhea, jaundice
Endocrinological	Testicular swelling and gynecomastia (in males), breast enlargement and galactorrhea (in females), increased or decreased libido, inappropriate ADH secretion syndrome
Allergic	Skin rash, edema, photosensitization, pruritus
Other	Weight gain, diaphoresis, alopecia, chills, flushing

OVERDOSAGE

Signs and symptoms	Drowsiness, stupor, blurred vision, dry mouth, respiratory depression, hypotension, coma, tachycardia and other arrhythmias, hypothermia, hyperthermia, urinary retention, paralytic ileus, convulsions, hypertension, mydriasis, hyperactive reflexes
Treatment	Institute standard supportive measures. If patient is conscious, empty stomach by gastric lavage with saline, followed by activated charcoal. Obtain ECG and begin close monitoring of cardiac function if abnormalities appear. Maintain an open airway and adequate fluid intake; assist ventilation, if necessary. Regulate body temperature. Treat arrhythmias with an appropriate antiarrhythmic agent. Slow IV administration of physostigmine salicylate (1–3 mg for adults) may reverse many of the cardiovascular and CNS signs and symptoms. Control convulsions with standard anticonvulsant therapy; however, barbiturates potentiate respiratory depression. Dialysis is of no value because of high tissue and protein binding.

SINEQUAN ■ SURMONTIL

DRUG INTERACTIONS

Alcohol, sedative-hypnotics, and other CNS depressants	△ CNS depression
Cimetidine	△ Pharmacologic effect of doxepin
Anticonvulsants	△ CNS depression
MAO inhibitors	Hyperpyrexia, excitability, severe convulsions, coma, death
Anticholinergic agents	Acute glaucoma, urinary retention, paralytic ileus
Ethchlorvynol	Transient delirium
Guanethidine	▽ Antihypertensive effect (at dosages above 150 mg/day)
Sympathomimetic agents	Severe hypertension, hyperpyrexia

ALTERED LABORATORY VALUES

Blood/serum	△ or ▽ Glucose

No clinically significant alterations in urinary values occur at therapeutic dosages

USE IN CHILDREN

Not recommended for use in children under 12 yr of age because conditions for the safe use of this drug in children have not been established

USE IN PREGNANT AND NURSING WOMEN

Safety for use during pregnancy has not been established. Reproduction studies in rats, rabbits, monkeys, and dogs have shown no evidence of harm to the animal fetus; however, the relevance of these findings to humans is unknown. There has been no clinical experience with this drug in pregnant women. It is not known whether doxepin is excreted in human milk or can affect nursing infants.

[1] Cross-sensitivity to other dibenzoxepines should also be considered
[2] Included are some tricyclic antidepressant adverse reactions not reported with this drug, but which must be considered before and during therapy

---

ANTIDEPRESSANTS

SURMONTIL (trimipramine maleate) Wyeth   Rx

Capsules: 25, 50, 100 mg

INDICATIONS

Depression, especially endogenous depression

ORAL DOSAGE

Adult: 75 mg/day, given in divided doses, to start, followed by gradual increases in dosage up to 200 mg/day, if needed; usual maintenance dosage, 50–150 mg/day, given in a single daily dose at bedtime for approximately 3 mo

CONTRAINDICATIONS

MAO inhibitor therapy (see WARNINGS/PRECAUTIONS)	During the acute recovery phase following myocardial infarction	Hypersensitivity to trimipramine[1]

ADMINISTRATION/DOSAGE ADJUSTMENTS

Adolescent and elderly patients	Reduce initial dosage to 50 mg/day, followed by gradual increases in dosage up to 100 mg/day, depending on patient response and tolerance
Hospitalized patients	Give 100 mg/day in divided doses, to start, followed in a few days by gradual increases in dosage up to 200 mg/day. If improvement does not occur in 2–3 wk, increase dosage to 250–300 mg/day. If dosage exceeds 2.5 mg/kg/day, monitor ECG when initiating therapy and at appropriate intervals during dosage stabilization phase.

WARNINGS/PRECAUTIONS

MAO inhibitor therapy	Wait at least 14 days after discontinuing use of an MAO inhibitor before initiating therapy with this drug; start treatment with a low dose, and increase dosage gradually with caution and careful observation of the patient
Atropine-like action	Use with caution in patients with increased intraocular pressure, a history of urinary retention, or a history of narrow-angle glaucoma
Mental and/or physical impairment	Caution patients that their ability to drive or perform other potentially hazardous activities may be impaired, and that their response to alcohol may be enhanced
Cardiovascular disease	Use with extreme caution; conduction defects, arrhythmias, myocardial infarction, stroke, and tachycardia may occur
Cardiovascular toxicity	May be precipitated in patients with hyperthyroidism or those on thyroid medication; use with caution
Lowered seizure threshold	Use with caution in patients with a history of seizure disorder

Fever and sore throat developing during therapy	Discontinue therapy if leukocyte and differential counts show evidence of pathologic neutrophil depression
Psychotic symptoms	May increase in schizophrenic patients; reduce dosage of trimipramine or add an antipsychotic agent
Manic or hypomanic episodes	May occur; if necessary, discontinue use of the drug until episode is relieved and then reinstitute therapy at a lower dosage
Potentially suicidal patients	Should not have access to large quantities of trimipramine; prescribe the smallest feasible amount
Abrupt discontinuation of therapy	May produce nausea, headache, and malaise after prolonged administration; symptoms are not indicative of addiction
Elective surgery	If possible, discontinue medication several days prior to surgery
Electroconvulsive therapy (ECT)	Hazard may be increased; use ECT only when essential
Special-risk patients	Use with caution in patients with hepatic impairment and in those taking atropine or other anticholinergic agents, sympathomimetics, local decongestants, epinephrine-containing local anesthetics, clonidine, or guanethidine

ADVERSE REACTIONS[2]

Cardiovascular	Hypotension, hypertension, tachycardia, palpitations, myocardial infarction, arrhythmias, heart block, stroke
Central nervous system and neuromuscular	Confusion, hallucinations, disorientation, delusions, anxiety, restlessness, agitation, insomnia, nightmares, hypomania, exacerbated psychosis, numbness, tingling, paresthesias of the extremities, incoordination, ataxia, tremors, peripheral neuropathy, extrapyramidal symptoms, seizures, altered EEG patterns, tinnitus, drowsiness, dizziness, weakness, fatigue, headache
Autonomic nervous system	Dry mouth (associated rarely with sublingual adenitis), blurred vision, disturbance of accommodation, mydriasis, constipation, paralytic ileus, urinary retention, delayed micturition, dilatation of urinary tract
Hematological	Bone marrow depression, including agranulocytosis, eosinophilia, purpura, and thrombocytopenia
Gastrointestinal	Nausea, vomiting, anorexia, epigastric distress, diarrhea, peculiar taste, stomatitis, abdominal cramps, black tongue, jaundice, altered liver function, parotid swelling
Endocrinological	Gynecomastia (in males), breast enlargement and galactorrhea (in females); increased or decreased libido; impotence; testicular swelling
Allergic	Skin rash, petechiae, urticaria, itching, photosensitization, edema of face and tongue
Other	Weight gain or loss, diaphoresis, flushing, urinary frequency, alopecia

OVERDOSAGE

Signs and symptoms	Drowsiness, stupor, coma, ataxia, restlessness, agitation, hyperactive reflexes, muscle rigidity, athetoid and choreiform movements, convulsions, tachycardia and other arrhythmias, ECG evidence of impaired conduction, congestive heart failure, respiratory depression, cyanosis, hypotension, vomiting, hyperpyrexia, mydriasis, diaphoresis, shock
Treatment	Admit patient to hospital. If patient is alert, empty stomach by induction of emesis, followed by gastric lavage. (In the obtunded patient, secure airway with a cuffed endotracheal tube before beginning lavage; do not induce emesis.) Administration of activated charcoal may be helpful. Obtain ECG and begin continuous monitoring of cardiac function for a minimum of 72 h if abnormalities appear. Maintain an open airway and adequate fluid intake. Regulate body temperature with ice packs and cooling sponge baths, if necessary. For cardiac arrhythmias and circulatory shock, institute standard supportive measures. If cardiac failure occurs, rapid digitalization may be necessary; use with extreme care. Minimize external stimulation to reduce convulsive tendency. If anticonvulsants are needed, use diazepam, short-acting barbiturates, paraldehyde, or methocarbamol. Dialysis, exchange transfusions, and forced diuresis are generally ineffective.

DRUG INTERACTIONS

Alcohol, sedative-hypnotics, and other CNS depressants	△ CNS depression
MAO inhibitors	Hyperpyrexia, excitability, severe convulsions, coma, death
Anticholinergic agents	Acute glaucoma, urinary retention, paralytic ileus
Guanethidine, clonidine	▽ Antihypertensive effect
Sympathomimetic agents	Severe hypertension, hyperpyrexia
Thyroid preparations	△ Antidepressant effect and possible risk of arrhythmias
Cimetidine	△ Serum level of trimipramine; adjustment of trimipramine dosage may be needed

ALTERED LABORATORY VALUES

Blood/serum values —————————— △ or ▽ Glucose

No clinically significant alterations in urinary values occur at therapeutic dosages

USE IN CHILDREN

Not recommended for use in children because safety and effectiveness have not been established in the pediatric age group

USE IN PREGNANT AND NURSING WOMEN

Pregnancy Category C: use during pregnancy only if the expected therapeutic benefits justify the potential risk to the fetus. Embryotoxicity and/or an increased incidence of major anomalies has been observed in rats or rabbits at doses 20 times the human dose. No adequate, well-controlled studies have been done in pregnant women. It is not known whether trimipramine is excreted in human milk; use with caution in nursing mothers because many drugs are excreted in human milk.

[1] Cross-sensitivity to other dibenzazepines should also be considered
[2] Included are some tricyclic antidepressant adverse reactions not reported with this drug, but which must be considered before and during therapy.

ANTIDEPRESSANTS

TOFRANIL (imipramine hydrochloride) Geigy   Rx

Tablets: 10, 25, 50 mg **Ampuls:** 12.5 mg/ml (2 ml) for IM use only

INDICATIONS

Depression, especially endogenous depression

Childhood enuresis (temporary, adjunctive therapy)

ORAL DOSAGE

Adult: for outpatients, 75 mg/day to start, followed, as needed, by 150 mg/day and then 200 mg/day; usual maintenance dosage: 50–150 mg/day. For hospitalized patients, give 100 mg/day in divided doses to start, followed, as needed, by a gradual increase in dosage; if no response is achieved after 2 wk at 200 mg/day, increase dosage to 250–300 mg/day.

Child ($\geq$ 6 yr): 25 mg/day 1 h before bedtime to start; if a satisfactory response is not attained after 1 wk, increase dosage to 50 mg/day in children under 12 or up to 75 mg/day in children over 12 (do not give more than 2.5 mg/kg/day). For enuresis early in the night, administer in divided doses (eg, give 25 mg in the midafternoon and then again at bedtime).

PARENTERAL DOSAGE

Adult: up to 100 mg/day IM in divided doses to start; switch to oral therapy as soon as possible

CONTRAINDICATIONS

MAO inhibitor therapy (see WARNINGS/PRECAUTIONS)

During the acute recovery phase following myocardial infarction

Hypersensitivity to imipramine[1]

ADMINISTRATION/DOSAGE ADJUSTMENTS

Adolescent and elderly patients ——— Administer 30–40 mg/day to start, followed by up to 100 mg/day

Onset of action ——————————— Optimal response may not occur until after 1–3 wk of treatment

Treatment of enuresis ——————— Consider discontinuing administration once enuresis has been controlled since the effectiveness of treatment may decrease with continued use; to reduce the possibility of relapse, decrease the dosage gradually. If a child relapses after the drug has been discontinued, a second course of treatment will not always be effective.

WARNINGS/PRECAUTIONS

MAO inhibitor therapy ——————— Wait at least 14 days after discontinuing use of an MAO inhibitor before initiating therapy with this drug; start treatment with a low dose and increase dosage gradually and cautiously

Atropine-like action ———————— Use with extreme caution in patients with a history of urinary retention, narrow-angle glaucoma, or increased intraocular pressure

Cardiovascular disease ——————— Use with extreme caution; conduction defects, congestive heart failure, arrhythmias, tachycardia, myocardial infarction, and stroke may occur, especially in the elderly and in patients with a history of cardiac disease

TOFRANIL

Mental and/or physical impairment	Caution patients that their ability to drive or perform other potentially hazardous activities may be impaired, and that their response to alcohol may be enhanced
Alcohol usage	Because the effects of alcohol are potentiated, its ingestion may increase the danger inherent in any suicide attempt or accidental overdose; this is especially important in patients who may use alcohol excessively
Psychotic symptoms	May increase in schizophrenic patients; manic-depressive patients may shift to manic phase. Reduce dosage of imipramine or add a tranquilizing agent, or phenothiazine, as indicated.
Potentially suicidal patients	Should not have access to large quantities of imipramine; prescribe smallest amount feasible
Abrupt discontinuation of therapy	May produce nausea, headache, and malaise after prolonged administration; symptoms are not indicative of addiction
Elective surgery	If possible, discontinue medication several days prior to surgery
Electroconvulsive therapy (ECT)	Hazard may be increased; use ECT only when essential
Special-risk patients	Use with caution in patients with renal or hepatic impairment, hyperthyroidism, or a history of seizures and in those taking thyroid medication, anticholinergic agents, decongestants, guanethidine, clonidine, methylphenidate, or sympathomimetics (see DRUG INTERACTIONS)
Fever and sore throat developing during therapy	Discontinue therapy if leukocyte and differential counts show evidence of pathologic neutrophil depression

ADVERSE REACTIONS[2]

Cardiovascular	Orthostatic hypotension, hypertension, tachycardia, palpitations, myocardial infarction, arrhythmias, heart block, ECG changes, congestive heart failure, stroke
Central nervous system and neuromuscular	Confusion, disorientation, delusions, agitation, hallucinations, anxiety, restlessness, insomnia, nightmares, numbness, tingling and paresthesias of the extremities, peripheral neuropathy, incoordination, ataxia, tremors, seizures, alteration in EEG patterns, extrapyramidal symptoms, tinnitus, drowsiness, dizziness, weakness, fatigue, headache, hypomania, exacerbated psychosis
Autonomic nervous system	Dry mouth (associated rarely with sublingual adenitis), blurred vision, disturbance of accommodation, constipation, paralytic ileus, urinary retention, dilatation of urinary tract, mydriasis, delayed micturition
Hematological	Bone marrow depression (including agranulocytosis), eosinophilia, purpura, thrombocytopenia
Gastrointestinal	Nausea, epigastric distress, vomiting, anorexia, stomatitis, peculiar taste, diarrhea, parotid swelling, black tongue, altered liver function, jaundice, abdominal cramps
Endocrinological	Testicular swelling and gynecomastia (in males), breast enlargement and galactorrhea (in females), increased or decreased libido, impotence, inappropriate ADH secretion syndrome
Allergic	Skin rash, petechiae, urticaria, photosensitization, edema, itching, drug fever, cross-sensitivity with desipramine
Other	Weight gain or loss, diaphoresis, urinary frequency, alopecia, flushing, proneness to falling

OVERDOSAGE

Signs and symptoms	Drowsiness, tachycardia and other arrhythmias, ECG evidence of impaired conduction, congestive heart failure, mydriasis, convulsions, severe hypotension, stupor, coma, agitation, hyperactive reflexes, muscle rigidity, vomiting, hyperpyrexia, ataxia, restlessness, athetoid and choreiform movements, respiratory depression, cyanosis, shock, diaphoresis (see also ADVERSE REACTIONS)
Treatment	Admit patient to hospital. If patient is alert, empty stomach by inducing emesis, followed by gastric lavage and activated charcoal. (In the obtunded patient, secure airway with a cuffed endotracheal tube before beginning lavage; do not induce emesis.) Continue lavage for 24 h or longer. Obtain ECG and begin close monitoring of cardiac function for at least 72 h if abnormalities appear. Maintain an open airway and adequate fluid intake. Regulate body temperature with ice packs and cooling sponge baths, if necessary. For circulatory shock, institute standard supportive measures. If cardiac failure occurs, rapid digitalization may be necessary; use with extreme care. Minimize external stimulation to reduce convulsive tendency. To control convulsions, use diazepam, paraldehyde, or methocarbamol; *do not use barbiturates.* Dialysis, exchange transfusions, and forced diuresis are generally ineffective because of low plasma drug concentrations and because of extensive tissue distribution of drug.

DRUG INTERACTIONS

Alcohol, sedative-hypnotics, and other CNS depressants	⇧ CNS depression
MAO inhibitors	Hyperpyrexia, excitability, severe convulsions, coma, death

TOFRANIL ■ TOFRANIL-PM

Anticholinergic agents	Acute glaucoma, urinary retention, paralytic ileus
Epinephrine	⇧ Pressor response, arrhythmias
Ethchlorvynol	Transient delirium
Clonidine, guanethidine	⇩ Antihypertensive effect
Methylphenidate	⇧ Imipramine side effects
Sympathomimetic agents	Severe hypertension, hyperpyrexia
Thyroid preparations	⇧ Antidepressant effect and possible risk of arrhythmias
Cimetidine	⇧ Serum imipramine level; adjustment of imipramine dosage may be necessary when cimetidine therapy is initiated or discontinued

ALTERED LABORATORY VALUES

Blood/serum values	⇧ or ⇩ Glucose

No clinically significant alterations in urinary values occur at therapeutic dosages

USE IN CHILDREN

See INDICATIONS and ORAL DOSAGE; not recommended for use in children under 6 yr of age. Rule out genitourinary disease before instituting therapy for enuresis. Safety of long-term chronic use has not been established. In enuretic children, the most common adverse reactions are nervousness, sleep disorders, tiredness, and mild GI disturbances; these reactions usually disappear when administration is continued or dosage is reduced. Constipation, convulsions, anxiety, emotional instability, syncope, and collapse, as well as reactions reported with adults, may also occur during enuresis therapy.

USE IN PREGNANT AND NURSING WOMEN

Safety for use during pregnancy has not been established; use in women who are or who may become pregnant only if the clinical condition clearly justifies the potential risk to the fetus. Animal reproduction studies have been inconclusive, and no adequate, well-controlled studies have been done in pregnant women. However, there have been clinical reports of congenital malformations associated with the use of imipramine during pregnancy; although a causal relationship could not be established, the possibility of harm to the fetus cannot be excluded. Limited data suggest that imipramine is excreted in human milk; since the possibility exists that the drug may be harmful to the infant if it is excreted in breast milk, nursing is inadvisable.

[1] Cross-sensitivity to other dibenzazepines should also be considered
[2] Included are some tricyclic antidepressant adverse reactions not reported with this drug, but which must be considered before and during therapy

---

ANTIDEPRESSANTS

TOFRANIL-PM (imipramine pamoate) Geigy   Rx

Capsules: 75, 100, 125, 150 mg

INDICATIONS

Depression, especially endogenous depression

ORAL DOSAGE

Adult: for outpatients, 75 mg/day to start, followed, as needed, by 150 mg/day and then 200 mg/day; usual maintenance dosage: 75–150 mg/day. For hospitalized patients, give 100–150 mg/day to start, followed, as needed, by 200 mg/day and then, if no response is achieved after 2 wk, by 250–300 mg/day.

CONTRAINDICATIONS

MAO inhibitor therapy (see WARNINGS/PRECAUTIONS)	During the acute recovery phase following myocardial infarction	Hypersensitivity to imipramine[1]

ADMINISTRATION/DOSAGE ADJUSTMENTS

Adolescent and elderly patients	Initiate imipramine therapy with 25–50 mg/day of imipramine hydrochloride and increase the dosage as needed and tolerated, up to 100 mg/day; if the total established dosage is 75 or 100 mg/day, imipramine pamoate may be substituted
Frequency of administration	The initial dosage may be given as a single daily bedtime dose. A higher dosage may also be administered once daily if it has been determined by titration to be optimal. However, a divided-dose schedule may be necessary for some patients.
Onset of action	Optimal response may not occur until after 1–3 wk of treatment

TOFRANIL-PM

WARNINGS/PRECAUTIONS

MAO inhibitor therapy	Wait at least 14 days after discontinuing use of an MAO inhibitor before initiating therapy with this drug; start treatment with a low dose and increase dosage gradually and cautiously
Atropine-like action	Use with extreme caution in patients with a history of urinary retention, narrow-angle glaucoma, or increased intraocular pressure
Cardiovascular disease	Use with extreme caution; conduction defects, congestive heart failure, arrhythmias, tachycardia, myocardial infarction, and stroke may occur, especially in the elderly and in patients with a history of cardiac disease
Mental and/or physical impairment	Caution patients that their ability to drive or perform other potentially hazardous activities may be impaired, and that their response to alcohol may be enhanced
Alcohol usage	Because the effects of alcohol are potentiated, its ingestion may increase the danger inherent in any suicide attempt or accidental overdose; this is especially important in patients who may use alcohol excessively
Psychotic symptoms	May increase in schizophrenic patients; manic-depressive patients may shift to manic phase. Reduce dosage of imipramine or add a tranquilizing agent or phenothiazine, as indicated
Potentially suicidal patients	Should not have access to large quantities of imipramine; prescribe smallest amount feasible
Abrupt discontinuation of therapy	May produce nausea, headache, and malaise after prolonged administration; symptoms are not indicative of addiction
Elective surgery	Discontinue medication several days prior to surgery, if possible
Electroconvulsive therapy (ECT)	May increase hazard; use ECT only when necessary
Special-risk patients	Use with caution in patients with renal or hepatic impairment, hyperthyroidism, or a history of seizures and in those taking thyroid medication, anticholinergic agents, decongestants, guanethidine, clonidine, methylphenidate, or sympathomimetics (see DRUG INTERACTIONS)
Fever and sore throat developing during therapy	Discontinue therapy if leukocyte and differential counts show evidence of pathologic neutrophil depression
Tartrazine sensitivity	Presence of FD&C Yellow No. 5 (tartrazine) in 100- and 125-mg capsules may cause allergic-type reactions, including bronchial asthma, in susceptible individuals

ADVERSE REACTIONS[2]

Cardiovascular	Orthostatic hypotension, hypertension, tachycardia, palpitations, myocardial infarction, arrhythmias, heart block, ECG changes, congestive heart failure, stroke
Central nervous system, neuromuscular	Confusion, disorientation, delusions, agitation, hallucinations, anxiety, restlessness, insomnia, nightmares, numbness, tingling and paresthesias of the extremities; peripheral neuropathy, incoordination, ataxia, tremors, seizures, alteration in EEG patterns, extrapyramidal symptoms, tinnitus, dizziness, weakness, fatigue, headache, hypomania, exacerbated psychosis
Autonomic nervous system	Dry mouth (associated rarely with sublingual adenitis), blurred vision, disturbance of accommodation, constipation, paralytic ileus, urinary retention, dilatation of urinary tract, mydriasis, delayed micturition
Hematological	Bone marrow depression (including agranulocytosis), eosinophilia, purpura, thrombocytopenia
Gastrointestinal	Nausea, epigastric distress, vomiting, anorexia, stomatitis, peculiar taste, diarrhea, parotid swelling, black tongue, altered liver function, jaundice, abdominal cramps
Endocrinological	Testicular swelling and gynecomastia (in males), breast enlargement and galactorrhea (in females), increased or decreased libido, impotence, inappropriate ADH secretion syndrome
Allergic	Skin rash, petechiae, photosensitization, edema, itching, drug fever, cross-sensitivity with desipramine
Other	Weight gain or loss, diaphoresis, urinary frequency, alopecia, flushing, proneness to falling

OVERDOSAGE

Signs and symptoms	Drowsiness, tachycardia and other arrhythmias, ECG evidence of impaired conduction, congestive heart failure, mydriasis, convulsions, severe hypotension, stupor, coma, agitation, hyperactive reflexes, muscle rigidity, vomiting, hyperpyrexia, ataxia, restlessness, athetoid and choreiform movements, respiratory depression, cyanosis, shock, diaphoresis (see also ADVERSE REACTIONS)
Treatment	Admit patient to hospital. If patient is alert, empty stomach by inducing emesis, followed by gastric lavage and activated charcoal. (In the obtunded patient, secure airway with a cuffed endotracheal tube before beginning lavage; do not induce emesis.) Continue lavage for 24 h or longer. Obtain ECG and begin close monitoring of cardiac function for at least 72 h if abnormalities appear. Maintain an open airway and adequate fluid intake. Regulate body temperature with ice packs and cooling sponge baths, if necessary. For circulatory shock, institute standard supportive measures. If cardiac failure occurs, rapid digitalization may be necessary; use with extreme care. Minimize external stimulation to reduce convulsive tendency. To control convulsions, use diazepam, paraldehyde, or methocarbamol; *do not use barbiturates*. Dialysis, exchange transfusions, and forced diuresis are generally ineffective because of low plasma drug concentrations and because of extensive tissue distribution of drug.

TOFRANIL-PM ■ VIVACTIL

DRUG INTERACTIONS

Alcohol, sedative-hypnotics, and other CNS depressants	△ CNS depression
MAO inhibitors	Hyperpyrexia, excitability, severe convulsions, coma, death
Anticholinergic agents	Acute glaucoma, urinary retention, paralytic ileus
Epinephrine	△ Pressor response, arrhythmias
Ethchlorvynol	Transient delirium
Clonidine, guanethidine	▽ Antihypertensive effect
Methylphenidate	△ Imipramine side effects
Sympathomimetic agents	Severe hypertension, hyperpyrexia
Thyroid preparations	△ Antidepressant effect and possible risk of arrhythmias
Cimetidine	△ Serum imipramine level; adjustment of imipramine dosage may be necessary when cimetidine therapy is initiated or discontinued

ALTERED LABORATORY VALUES

Blood/serum values — △ or ▽ Glucose

No clinically significant alterations in urinary values occur at therapeutic dosages

USE IN CHILDREN

Not recommended for use in children of any age because of the increased potential of acute overdosage due to the large amount of imipramine contained in each capsule

USE IN PREGNANT AND NURSING WOMEN

Safety for use during pregnancy has not been established; use in women who are or who may become pregnant only if the clinical condition clearly justifies the potential risk to the fetus. Animal reproduction studies have been inconclusive, and no adequate, well-controlled studies have been done in pregnant women. However, there have been clinical reports of congenital malformations associated with the use of imipramine during pregnancy; although a causal relationship could not be established, the possibility of harm to the fetus cannot be excluded. Limited data suggest that imipramine is excreted in human milk; since the possibility exists that the drug may be harmful to the infant if it is excreted in breast milk, nursing is inadvisable.

[1] Cross-sensitivity to other dibenzazepines should also be considered
[2] Included are some tricyclic antidepressant adverse reactions not reported with this drug, but which must be considered before and during therapy

---

ANTIDEPRESSANTS

VIVACTIL (protriptyline hydrochloride) Merck Sharp & Dohme   Rx

Tablets: 5, 10 mg

INDICATIONS

Depression, especially in withdrawn and anergic patients

ORAL DOSAGE

Adult: 15–40 mg/day, given in 3–4 divided doses, to start, followed by up to 60 mg/day, if necessary

CONTRAINDICATIONS

MAO inhibitor therapy (see WARNINGS/PRECAUTIONS)	During the acute recovery phase following myocardial infarction	Hypersensitivity to protriptyline

ADMINISTRATION/DOSAGE ADJUSTMENTS

Dosage increases	If needed, should be made in morning dose
Elderly or adolescent patients	Give 5 mg tid to start, followed by a gradual increase in dosage, if necessary; monitor cardiovascular status in elderly patients if dosage exceeds 20 mg/day

WARNINGS/PRECAUTIONS

MAO inhibitor therapy	Wait at least 14 days after discontinuing use of an MAO inhibitor before initiating therapy with this drug; start treatment cautiously with gradual increases in dosage until optimum response is achieved
Atropine-like action	Use with caution in patients with a history of urinary retention or increased intraocular pressure

VIVACTIL

Cardiovascular disease	May worsen; use with caution and keep patient under close supervision. Tricyclic antidepressants may produce arrhythmias, tachycardia, and prolongation of conduction time; myocardial infarction and stroke have followed use of these agents. Tachycardia and postural hypotension may occur more frequently with protriptyline than with other tricyclic antidepressants.
Mental and/or physical impairment	Caution patients that their ability to drive or perform other potentially hazardous activities may be impaired, and that their response to alcohol, barbiturates, and other CNS depressants may be enhanced
Alcohol usage	Because the effects of alcohol are potentiated, its ingestion may increase the danger inherent in any suicide attempt or accidental overdose; this is especially important in patients who may use alcohol excessively
Psychotic symptoms	May increase in schizophrenic patients; paranoia may worsen and manic-depressive patients may shift to manic phase. Reduce dosage of protriptyline or add an antipsychotic agent.
Potentially suicidal patients	Should not have access to large quantities of protriptyline; prescribe smallest amount feasible
Abrupt discontinuation of therapy	May produce nausea, headache, and malaise after prolonged administration; symptoms are not indicative of addiction
Elective surgery	If possible, discontinue medication several days prior to surgery
Electroconvulsive therapy (ECT)	Hazard may be increased; use ECT only when essential
Special-risk patients	Use with caution in patients with hyperthyroidism or a history of seizures and in those taking thyroid medications, anticholinergic agents, or sympathomimetics (see DRUG INTERACTIONS)
Anxiety or agitation	May be aggravated in overactive or agitated patients

ADVERSE REACTIONS[1]

Cardiovascular	Hypotension (particularly orthostatic hypotension), hypertension, tachycardia, palpitations, myocardial infarction, arrhythmias, heart block, stroke
Central nervous system and neuromuscular	Confusion, disturbed concentration, disorientation, delusions, hallucinations, excitement, anxiety, restlessness, insomnia, panic, hypomania, exacerbation of psychosis, nightmares, numbness, tingling and paresthesias of the extremities, peripheral neuropathy, incoordination, ataxia, tremors, seizures, alteration in EEG patterns, extrapyramidal symptoms, tinnitus, dizziness, weakness, fatigue, headache, drowsiness
Autonomic nervous system	Dry mouth (associated rarely with sublingual adenitis), blurred vision, disturbance of accommodation, mydriasis, constipation, paralytic ileus, urinary retention, dilation of urinary tract, delayed micturition
Hematological	Bone marrow depression, agranulocytosis, leukopenia, eosinophilia, purpura, thrombocytopenia
Gastrointestinal	Nausea, epigastric distress, vomiting, anorexia, stomatitis, peculiar taste, diarrhea, abdominal cramps, black tongue, parotid swelling, altered liver function, jaundice
Endocrinological	Testicular swelling and gynecomastia (in males), breast enlargement and galactorrhea (in females), increased or decreased libido, impotence, inappropriate ADH secretion syndrome
Allergic	Skin rash, petechiae, itching, urticaria, photosensitization, edema of face and tongue, drug fever
Other	Weight gain or loss, edema, diaphoresis, flushing, urinary frequency, nocturia, alopecia

OVERDOSAGE

Signs and symptoms	Drowsiness, hypothermia, tachycardia and other arrhythmias, ECG evidence of impaired conduction, congestive heart failure, mydriasis, convulsions, severe hypotension, stupor, coma, agitation, hyperactive reflexes, muscle rigidity, vomiting, hyperpyrexia (see also ADVERSE REACTIONS)
Treatment	Admit patient to hospital. Empty stomach by inducing emesis, followed by gastric lavage and activated charcoal (20–30 g q4–6h during initial 24–48 h). Obtain ECG and begin close monitoring of cardiac function if abnormalities appear. Maintain an open airway and adequate fluid intake. Regulate body temperature. Administer 1–3 mg physostigmine salicylate IV and repeat as needed, especially if life-threatening signs recur or persist. (Physostigmine should not be used routinely, however, as it may itself be toxic.) For circulatory shock and metabolic acidosis, institute standard supportive measures. Treat cardiac arrhythmias with neostigmine, pyridostigmine, or propranolol. If cardiac failure occurs, consider digitalization. (Cardiac function should be closely monitored for at least 5 days under these circumstances.) Control convulsions with anticonvulsants. Dialysis is of no value because of low plasma drug concentrations and because of extensive tissue distribution of drug.

VIVACTIL ■ ETRAFON

DRUG INTERACTIONS

Alcohol and other CNS depressants	△ CNS depression
Anticonvulsants	△ CNS depression ▽ Anticonvulsant effect
MAO inhibitors	Hyperpyrexia, excitability, severe convulsions, coma, death
Anticholinergic agents	Acute glaucoma, urinary retention, paralytic ileus
Epinephrine	△ Pressor response, arrhythmias
Estrogens	▽ Antidepressant effect
Clonidine, guanethidine	▽ Antihypertensive effect
Sympathomimetic agents	Severe hypertension, hyperpyrexia
Thyroid preparations	Possible risk of arrhythmias
Cimetidine	△ Pharmacologic effects of protriptyline

ALTERED LABORATORY VALUES

Blood/serum values —— △ or ▽ Glucose

No clinically significant alterations in urinary values occur at therapeutic dosages

USE IN CHILDREN

Not recommended for use in children because safety and effectiveness have not been established in the pediatric age group

USE IN PREGNANT AND NURSING WOMEN

Safety for use in pregnant or nursing women has not been established. Reproduction studies in mice, rats, and rabbits at doses approximately 10 times the recommended human dose have shown no adverse effects.

[1] Included are some tricyclic antidepressant adverse reactions not reported with this drug, but which must be considered before and during therapy

ANTIDEPRESSANT COMBINATIONS

ETRAFON (perphenazine and amitriptyline hydrochloride) Schering   Rx

Tablets: 2 mg perphenazine and 10 mg amitriptyline hydrochloride (Etrafon 2-10); 2 mg perphenazine and 25 mg amitriptyline hydrochloride (Etrafon 2-25 [Etrafon]); 4 mg perphenazine and 10 mg amitriptyline hydrochloride (Etrafon 4-10 [Etrafon-A]); 4 mg perphenazine and 25 mg amitriptyline hydrochloride (Etrafon 4-25 [Etrafon-Forte])

INDICATIONS

Moderate to severe anxiety and/or agitation and depression or depressed mood

Anxiety and depression associated with chronic physical disease

Cases in which **depression and anxiety** cannot be clearly differentiated

Depressive symptoms in schizophrenic patients

ORAL DOSAGE

Adult: 1 Etrafon 2-25 or 4-25 tab tid or qid to start; for more severely ill patients with schizophrenia, 2 Etrafon 4-25 tabs tid or, if necessary, qid to start (give the fourth dose at bedtime); for adolescents and elderly patients, 1 Etrafon 4-10 tab tid or qid to start. Total daily dose should not exceed 8 tabs of any dosage strength. For maintenance, reduce dosage to the lowest effective level; a useful maintenance dosage: 1 Etrafon 2-25 or 4-25 tab 2-4 times/day.

CONTRAINDICATIONS

MAO inhibitor therapy (see WARNINGS/PRECAUTIONS)

Suspected or known subcortical brain damage, with or without hypothalamic brain damage (see WARNINGS/PRECAUTIONS)

CNS depression induced by large doses of CNS depressants (see DRUG INTERACTIONS)

Comatose or greatly obtunded patients

Blood dyscrasia

Bone marrow depression

Liver damage

During the acute recovery phase following myocardial infarction

Hypersensitivity to perphenazine, amitriptyline, or related compounds

ETRAFON

WARNINGS/PRECAUTIONS

Tardive dyskinesia — Neuroleptic drugs can cause tardive dyskinesia, a potentially irreversible syndrome characterized by involuntary choreoathetoid movements of the tongue, face, mouth, lips, jaw, trunk, and/or extremities. Protrusion of the tongue, puffing of the cheeks, puckering of the mouth, chewing movements, and other manifestations may become evident during treatment, upon dosage reduction, or after the drug is discontinued. The likelihood that tardive dyskinesia will develop or become irreversible increases with duration of treatment and total cumulative dose; however, even relatively brief use of low doses can cause it. Although this reaction appears to occur most often in the elderly, especially among older women, it is impossible to use this information to predict, before therapy is started, which patients are likely to develop the syndrome.

In general, reserve chronic therapy for patients who respond to neuroleptics and who cannot undergo another, equally effective form of treatment that is potentially less harmful. Use the lowest effective dosage, keep the duration of therapy as short as possible, and periodically reassess the need for the drug. Watch carefully for manifestations of tardive dyskinesia; fine vermicular movements of the tongue reportedly may be an early sign. However, do not forget that neuroleptic therapy can itself mask the signs and symptoms of tardive dyskinesia. If evidence of the syndrome is seen, consider terminating use of the drug, bearing in mind that some patients may require continued neuroleptic treatment despite the development of dyskinesia. There is no known treatment for tardive dyskinesia; however, after discontinuation, some or all manifestations of this syndrome may disappear spontaneously.

Other extrapyramidal effects — Extrapyramidal reactions other than tardive dyskinesia can usually be controlled by a reduction in dosage, use of an antiparkinson agent such as benztropine, or a combination of both approaches

MAO inhibitor therapy — Wait at least 14 days after discontinuing use of an MAO inhibitor before initiating therapy with this drug; start treatment cautiously, increasing the dosage gradually until a satisfactory response is obtained

Suspected or known subcortical brain damage, with or without hypothalamic damage — A hyperthermic reaction (temperature > 104° F) may occur up to 14–16 h after administration; if reaction occurs, pack body in ice and administer antipyretics

Atropine-like action — Use with caution in patients with a history of urinary retention, narrow-angle glaucoma, or increased intraocular pressure; even average doses may precipitate an attack in patients with narrow-angle glaucoma

Cardiovascular disease — May worsen; use with caution and keep patient under close supervision. Tricyclic antidepressants, especially in high doses, may produce arrhythmias, sinus tachycardia, and prolongation of conduction time; myocardial infarction and stroke have followed use of these agents.

Mental and/or physical impairment — Caution patients that their ability to drive or perform other potentially hazardous activities may be impaired, and that their response to alcohol, barbiturates, and other CNS depressants may be enhanced. If drowsiness proves troublesome, reduce the dosage of Etrafon.

Psychotic symptoms — Paranoia may worsen, and manic-depressive patients may shift to manic phase; perphenazine component minimizes the occurrences of these effects

Potentially suicidal patients — Should not have access to large quantities of this drug; prescribe smallest amount feasible

Electroconvulsive therapy (ECT) — May increase hazard; use ECT only when essential

Antiemetic effect — May mask signs of toxicity due to overdosage of other drugs or render more difficult the diagnosis of such disorders as brain tumors or intestinal obstruction

Unexplained rise in temperature — May suggest intolerance to perphenazine component; discontinue use if a significant rise occurs

Severe acute hypotension — May occur, especially in patients with mitral insufficiency or pheochromocytoma; the latter may experience rebound hypertension

Adynamic ileus — May occur occasionally and, if severe, can lead to complications and death; psychiatric patients should be closely supervised, as they may fail to seek treatment

Bone marrow depression — May occur; observe patient closely, especially during the 4th to 10th weeks of therapy (when most cases of agranulocytosis have occurred), for the sudden appearance of sore throat or infection. Monitor WBC count and differential; if count is significantly depressed, discontinue use of drug and institute appropriate therapy.

Reduction in convulsion threshold — May occur in susceptible patients (eg, patients with EEG abnormalities or a history of seizures). Use with caution in patients with convulsive disorders or alcohol withdrawal syndrome; dosage of concomitantly used anticonvulsants may need to be increased.

Jaundice — May occur as a hypersensitivity reaction to perphenazine, usually between 2nd and 4th weeks of therapy; reaction resembles infectious hepatitis clinically, but with laboratory features of obstructive jaundice. Discontinue use of drug if abnormalities in hepatic-function tests occur.

ETRAFON

Photosensitivity	May occur; advise patient to avoid undue exposure to the sun
Effects of long-term therapy	Blood dyscrasias, hepatic or renal damage, corneal and lenticular deposits, and irreversible dyskinesias may occur; blood counts and hepatic and renal function should be monitored periodically. If signs of blood dyscrasias or abnormal renal or hepatic function develop, discontinue therapy.
Surgical candidates	Patients receiving large doses of phenothiazines may develop hypotension during surgery. Reduce dosage of anesthetic agents and/or CNS depressants, if necessary. If possible, discontinue use of Etrafon several days prior to surgery.
Abrupt discontinuation of therapy	May produce nausea, headache, and malaise after prolonged use and gastritis, nausea, vomiting, dizziness, and tremulousness when high doses have been taken; symptoms may be reduced by administering antiparkinson agents for several weeks after Etrafon is withdrawn
Patients with renal impairment	Use with caution in patients with diminished renal function; discontinue therapy if BUN level rises
Patients with respiratory impairment	Use with caution in patients with impaired respiratory function due to acute pulmonary infection or chronic respiratory disorders, such as severe asthma and emphysema
Patients with previously detected breast cancer	Use with caution, as perphenazine component may cause a persistent elevation of serum prolactin levels, which may be of importance in patients with prolactin-dependent breast cancers. Although endocrine disturbances have been reported, no association between chronic neuroleptic administration and mammary tumorigenesis has been demonstrated; the available evidence is considered too limited to be conclusive at this time.
Other special-risk patients	Closely supervise therapy in hyperthyroid patients, as well as patients receiving thyroid preparations, atropine or other anticholinergic drugs, or sympathomimetics, including epinephrine-containing local anesthetic solutions (see DRUG INTERACTIONS); use with caution in patients who have experienced severe adverse reactions to other phenothiazines and in those who may be exposed to extreme heat or organophosphorous insecticides

ADVERSE REACTIONS[1]

Central nervous system and neuromuscular	Extrapyramidal reactions (opisthotonus; trismus; torticollis; retrocollis; aching and numbness of the limbs; motor restlessness; oculogyric crisis; hyperreflexia; dystonia, including protrusion, discoloration, aching, and rounding of the tongue; tonic spasm of the masticatory muscles; tightness in the throat; slurred speech; dysphagia; akathisia; dyskinesia; parkinsonism; ataxia; persistent tardive dyskinesia;) numbness, tingling, and paresthesias of the extremities; peripheral neuropathy; incoordination; tremors; altered EEG patterns; convulsive seizures; cerebral edema; abnormal CSF proteins; headache; drowsiness; dizziness; tinnitus; paradoxical exacerbation of psychotic symptoms; catatonic-like states; paranoid reactions; weakness; fatigue; lethargy; muscle weakness; paradoxical excitement; restlessness; hyperactivity; confusion; disturbed concentration; disorientation; delusions; hallucinations; jitteriness; anxiety; insomnia; bizarre dreams; nightmares; activation of latent schizophrenia; epileptiform seizures in chronic schizophrenics (rare)
Autonomic nervous system	Dry mouth or salivation; nausea; vomiting; diarrhea; anorexia; constipation; obstipation; fecal impaction; urinary retention, frequency, or incontinence; dilatation of urinary tract; polyuria; bladder paralysis; nasal congestion; pallor; adynamic or paralytic ileus; miosis or mydriasis; blurred vision; accommodation disturbances; glaucoma; diaphoresis; altered pulse rate; hypotension or hypertension
Cardiovascular	Postural hypotension, faintness, dizziness, hypertension, tachycardia, bradycardia, shock-like syndrome, palpitations, arrhythmias, nonspecific quinidine-like ECG changes, myocardial infarction, stroke, heart block, cardiac arrest
Hematological	Bone marrow depression, including agranulocytosis, eosinophilia, leukopenia, hemolytic anemia, thrombocytopenia, thrombocytopenic purpura, and pancytopenia
Gastrointestinal	Nausea, epigastric distress, heartburn, vomiting, anorexia, stomatitis, peculiar taste, diarrhea, biliary stasis, jaundice, parotid swelling; hepatitis (rare)
Endocrinological	Lactation, galactorrhea, and breast enlargement (in females); testicular swelling and gynecomastia (in males); menstrual cycle disturbances; amenorrhea; inhibition of ejaculation; altered libido; hyperglycemia; hypoglycemia; glycosuria; inappropriate antidiuretic hormone secretion syndrome
Ophthalmic	Deposition of fine particulate matter in cornea and lens, progressing in more severe cases to stellate lenticular opacities; epithelial keratopathies; pigmentary retinopathy; photophobia
Allergic	Rash; pruritus; erythema; eczema; exfoliative dermatitis; photosensitivity; asthma; fever; anaphylactoid reactions; edema of face, tongue, and larynx; contact dermatitis (in nursing personnel handling the drug); jaundice; cerebral edema, circulatory collapse, and death (extremely rare)
Other	Peripheral edema, weight changes, reversed epinephrine effect, increased PBI, hyperpyrexia, alopecia, increased appetite, SLE-like syndrome, polyphagia; neuroleptic malignant syndrome, a potentially fatal reaction characterized by hyperthermia, autonomic disturbances, and severe extrapyramidal dysfunction (muscular rigidity followed by stupor or coma)[2]

OVERDOSAGE

Signs and symptoms — Drowsiness, hypothermia, tachycardia and other arrhythmias, ECG evidence of impaired conduction, congestive heart failure, mydriasis, oculomotor paresis, convulsions, severe hypotension, stupor, coma, agitation, hyperactive reflexes, muscle rigidity, vomiting, hyperpyrexia (see also ADVERSE REACTIONS)

Treatment — Admit patient to hospital immediately. Induce emesis with syrup of ipecac, along with 8–12 fl oz of water, even if vomiting has occurred spontaneously. If necessary, repeat dose of ipecac in 15 min. Following emesis, administer a slurry of activated charcoal with water. If emesis is unsuccessful or contraindicated, perform gastric lavage, preferably with isotonic or ½ isotonic saline. To rapidly dilute bowel contents, administer a saline cathartic (eg, milk of magnesia). Obtain an ECG and begin monitoring cardiac function closely if abnormalities appear. Maintain an open airway and adequate fluid intake. If CNS depression occurs, do not use stimulants that may cause convulsions (eg, picrotoxin or pentylenetetrazol). Signs of arousal may not occur for 48 h. Regulate body temperature; hypothermia is expected, but if hyperthermia occurs, treat vigorously by packing body in ice and administering antipyretics. To treat central anticholinergic effects, administer 1–3 mg physostigmine salicylate IV and repeat, as needed, especially if life-threatening signs recur or persist. For cardiac arrhythmias, circulatory shock, and metabolic acidosis, institute standard supportive measures. Treat cardiac arrhythmias with neostigmine, pyridostigmine, or propranolol. If cardiac failure occurs, consider digitalization. (Cardiac function should be closely monitored for at least 5 days under these circumstances.) To control convulsions, use diazepam, paraldehyde, or an inhalation anesthetic; *do not use barbiturates*. Combat hypotension with norepinephrine, not epinephrine. Administer benztropine mesylate or diphenhydramine for acute parkinsonian symptoms. Dialysis is of no value because of low plasma drug concentrations and because of extensive tissue distribution of the drug.

DRUG INTERACTIONS

Alcohol	△ CNS depression and risk of hypotension; avoid using concomitantly
Opiates, analgesics, antihistamines, barbiturates, and other CNS depressants	△ CNS depression; use with caution and at lower than usual doses
MAO inhibitors	Hyperpyrexia, excitability, severe convulsions, coma, death
Anticholinergic agents	Acute glaucoma, urinary retention, paralytic ileus
Epinephrine	Severe hypotension
Ethchlorvynol	Transient delirium
Clonidine, guanethidine, and related antihypertensive agents	▽ Antihypertensive effect; do not give concomitantly with Etrafon
Sympathomimetic agents	Severe hypertension, hyperpyrexia
Thyroid preparations	△ Antidepressant effect and possible risk of arrhythmias
Anticonvulsants	▽ Anticonvulsant effect; increase anticonvulsant dosage, if necessary
Cimetidine	△ Pharmacologic effect of amitriptyline component

ALTERED LABORATORY VALUES

Blood/serum values	△ or ▽ Glucose △ Prolactin
Urinary values	△ Glucose False-positive pregnancy tests

USE IN CHILDREN
Not recommended for use in children because a dosage has not been established

USE IN PREGNANT AND NURSING WOMEN
Safety for use in pregnant or nursing women has not been established; hyperreflexia in the newborn has been reported following use of a phenothiazine during pregnancy

[1] Includes reactions common to phenothiazines and tricyclic antidepressants in general which should be considered because of pharmacological similarities to this specific drug

[2] Sudden death has occasionally been reported in patients receiving phenothiazines, in some cases due to cardiac arrest and in others to asphyxia caused by failure of the cough reflex; in still other patients the cause could not be determined, nor could a causal relationship to use of the drug be established

---

ANTIDEPRESSANT COMBINATIONS

LIMBITROL (chlordiazepoxide and amitriptyline hydrochloride) Roche   C-IV
Tablets: 5 mg chlordiazepoxide and 12.5 mg amitriptyline hydrochloride

LIMBITROL DS (chlordiazepoxide and amitriptyline hydrochloride) Roche   C-IV
Tablets: 10 mg chlordiazepoxide and 25 mg amitriptyline hydrochloride

INDICATIONS
Moderate to severe depression associated with moderate to severe anxiety

ORAL DOSAGE
Adult: 3–4 Limbitrol DS tabs/day, given in divided doses, to start, followed by 2–6 tabs/day, as required

LIMBITROL

CONTRAINDICATIONS

MAO inhibitor therapy (see WARNINGS/PRECAUTIONS)	During the acute recovery phase following myocardial infarction	Hypersensitivity to benzodiazepines or tricyclic antidepressants

ADMINISTRATION/DOSAGE ADJUSTMENTS

Patients who cannot tolerate higher doses	Administer 3–4 Limbitrol tabs/day in divided doses to start; reduce dosage to the smallest amount needed to maintain remission
Timing of administration	The larger portion or, in some cases, all of the daily dose may be given at bedtime

WARNINGS/PRECAUTIONS

MAO inhibitor therapy	Wait at least 14 days after discontinuing use of an MAO inhibitor before initiating therapy with this drug; start treatment cautiously, with a gradual increase in dosage until optimum response is achieved
Atropine-like action	Use with great caution in patients with a history of urinary retention or narrow-angle glaucoma; even average doses may precipitate an attack in patients with narrow-angle glaucoma
Cardiovascular disease	May worsen; use with caution and keep patient under close supervision. Tricyclic antidepressants, especially in high doses, may produce arrhythmias, sinus tachycardia, and prolongation of conduction time; myocardial infarction and stoke have followed use of these agents.
Drug dependence	Psychic and/or physical dependence may develop, especially in addiction-prone individuals
Mental and/or physical impairment	Caution patients that their ability to drive or perform other potentially hazardous activities may be impaired, and that use of alcohol, barbiturates, and other CNS depressants may produce a harmful degree of sedation and CNS depression
Potentially suicidal patients	Should not have access to large quantities of this preparation; prescribe the smallest feasible amount
Concomitant psychotropic therapy	Use with extreme caution, if at all, particularly when use of known potentiating compounds is contemplated (see DRUG INTERACTIONS)
Prolonged therapy	Blood counts and liver-function tests should be performed periodically
Abrupt discontinuation of therapy	May produce nausea, headache, malaise, and barbiturate-like withdrawal symptoms after prolonged administration
Elective surgery	If possible, discontinue medication several days prior to surgery
Electroconvulsive therapy (ECT)	Hazard may be increased; use ECT only when essential
Elderly or debilitated patients	Ataxia, oversedation, confusion, or anticholinergic effects may develop in elderly or debilitated patients; limit dosage to smallest effective amount
Other special-risk patients	Use with caution in patients with renal or hepatic impairment, hyperthyroidism, or a history of seizures and in those taking thyroid medication, anticholinergic agents, or sympathomimetics (see DRUG INTERACTIONS)

ADVERSE REACTIONS[1]

The most frequent reactions, regardless of incidence, are printed in *italics*

Cardiovascular	Hypotension, hypertension, tachycardia, palpitations, myocardial infarction, arrhythmias, heart block, stroke
Central nervous system and neuromuscular	*Drowsiness, dizziness,* vivid dreams, tremor, confusion, euphoria, apprehension, poor concentration, delusions, hallucinations, hypomania, excitement, numbness, tingling, and paresthesias of the extremities, incoordination, ataxia, alteration in EEG patterns, extrapyramidal symptoms, syncope, headache, fatigue, weakness, restlessness, lethargy
Autonomic nervous system	*Dry mouth, blurred vision, constipation,* nasal congestion, disturbance of accommodation, paralytic ileus, urinary retention, dilatation of urinary tract
Hematological	Bone marrow depression (including agranulocytosis), eosinophilia, purpura, thrombocytopenia; granulocytopenia (rare)
Gastrointestinal	*Bloated feeling,* nausea, epigastric distress, vomiting, anorexia, stomatitis, peculiar taste, parotid swelling, diarrhea, black tongue; jaundice and hepatic dysfunction (rare)
Endocrinological	Impotence, testicular swelling and gynecomastia (in males), breast enlargement, galactorrhea, menstrual irregularities (in females), increased or decreased libido, inappropriate ADH secretion syndrome
Allergic	Skin rash, urticaria, photosensitization, edema of face and tongue, pruritus
Other	Headache, weight gain or loss, diaphoresis, urinary frequency, mydriasis, alopecia

OVERDOSAGE

Signs and symptoms	*Toxicity primarily attributable to amitriptyline component:* hypothermia, tachycardia and other arrhythmias, ECG evidence of impaired conduction, congestive heart failure, mydriasis, convulsions, severe hypotension, stupor, coma, agitation, hyperactive reflexes, muscle rigidity, vomiting, hyperpyrexia (see also ADVERSE REACTIONS)

LIMBITROL ▪ TRIAVIL

Treatment	Admit patient to hospital. Empty stomach by inducing emesis or by gastric lavage, followed by activated charcoal. (If patient is comatose, secure airway with a cuffed endotracheal tube before beginning lavage.) Obtain ECG and begin close monitoring of cardiac function if abnormalities appear. Maintain an open airway and adequate fluid intake. Regulate body temperature. Administer 1–3 mg physostigmine salicylate IV and repeat as needed, especially if life-threatening signs recur or persist. (Physostigmine should not be used routinely, however, as it may itself be toxic.) For circulatory shock, institute standard supportive measures. If cardiac failure occurs, consider digitalization. (Cardiac function should be closely monitored for at least 5 days under these circumstances.) Treat arrhythmias with appropriate antiarrhythmic agents. To control convulsions, use an inhalation anesthetic; *do not use barbiturates.* Dialysis is of no value because of low plasma drug concentrations, but may be useful in cases of multiple drug ingestions.

DRUG INTERACTIONS

Alcohol, sedative-hypnotics, and other CNS depressants	△ CNS depression
MAO inhibitors	Hyperpyrexia, excitability, severe convulsions, coma, death
Anticholinergic agents	Acute glaucoma, urinary retention, severe constipation, paralytic ileus
Ethchlorvynol	Transient delirium
Guanethidine	▽ Antihypertensive effect
Sympathomimetic agents	△ Sympathomimetic effects
Thyroid preparations	△ Antidepressant effect and possible risk of arrhythmias
Oral anticoagulants	△ Anticoagulant effect
Cimetidine	△ Pharmacologic effects of amitriptyline component

ALTERED LABORATORY VALUES

Blood/serum values	△ or ▽ Glucose

No clinically significant alterations in urinary values occur at therapeutic dosages

USE IN CHILDREN

Safety and effectiveness for use in children under 12 yr of age have not been established

USE IN PREGNANT AND NURSING WOMEN

Antianxiety agents should almost always be avoided during early pregnancy; an increased risk of congenital malformations during the first trimester has been associated with minor tranquilizers, including chlordiazepoxide. It is not known whether the components of this preparation are excreted in human milk; because many drugs are excreted in human milk, nursing is generally inadvisable during therapy.

[1] Included are some benzodiazepine and tricyclic antidepressant adverse reactions not reported with this drug, but which must be considered before and during therapy

ANTIDEPRESSANT COMBINATIONS

TRIAVIL (perphenazine and amitriptyline hydrochloride) Merck Sharp & Dohme   Rx

Tablets: 2 mg perphenazine and 25 mg amitriptyline hydrochloride (Triavil 2-25); 4 mg perphenazine and 25 mg amitriptyline hydrochloride (Triavil 4-25); 4 mg perphenazine and 50 mg amitriptyline hydrochloride (Triavil 4-50); 2 mg perphenazine and 10 mg amitriptyline hydrochloride (Triavil 2-10); 4 mg perphenazine and 10 mg amitriptyline hydrochloride (Triavil 4-10)

INDICATIONS

Moderate to severe anxiety and/or agitation and depression or depressed mood
Anxiety and depression associated with chronic physical disease
Depressive symptoms in schizophrenic patients

ORAL DOSAGE

Adult: 1 Triavil 2-25 or 4-25 tab tid or qid or 1 Triavil 4-50 tab bid to start; for more severely ill patients with schizophrenia, 2 Triavil 4–25 tabs tid or, if necessary, qid to start (give the fourth dose at bedtime); for adolescents, elderly patients, and patients with anxiety as the predominant symptom, 1 Triavil 4–10 tab tid or qid to start. Total daily dose should not exceed 4 Triavil 4-50 tabs or 8 tabs of any other dosage strength. For maintenance, reduce dosage to the lowest effective level; maintenance dosage: 1 Triavil 2–25 or 4–25 tab 2–4 times/day or 1 Triavil 4–50 tab bid.

CONTRAINDICATIONS

MAO inhibitor therapy (see WARNINGS/PRECAUTIONS)

Drug-induced CNS depression

During the acute recovery phase following myocardial infarction

Hypersensitivity to phenothiazines or amitriptyline

WARNINGS/PRECAUTIONS

Tardive dyskinesia — Neuroleptic drugs can cause tardive dyskinesia, a potentially irreversible syndrome characterized by involuntary choreoathetoid movements of the tongue, face, mouth, lips, jaw, trunk, and/or extremities. Protrusion of the tongue, puffing of the cheeks, puckering of the mouth, chewing movements, and other manifestations may become evident during treatment, upon dosage reduction, or after the drug is discontinued. The likelihood that tardive dyskinesia will develop or become irreversible increases with duration of treatment and total cumulative dose; however, even relatively brief use of low doses can cause it. Although this reaction appears to occur most often in the elderly, especially among older women, it is impossible to use this information to predict, before therapy is started, which patients are likely to develop the syndrome.

In general, reserve chronic therapy for patients who respond to neuroleptics and who cannot undergo another, equally effective form of treatment that is potentially less harmful. Use the lowest effective dosage, keep the duration of therapy as short as possible, and periodically reassess the need for the drug. Watch for evidence of tardive dyskinesia; fine vermicular movements of the tongue reportedly may be an early sign. Since neuroleptic therapy can mask the signs of tardive dyskinesia, periodically reduce the dosage (if clinically feasible) and observe patient. If signs of dyskinesia appear, consider terminating use of the drug, bearing in mind that some patients may require continued neuroleptic treatment despite the development of dyskinesia. There is no known treatment for tardive dyskinesia; however, after discontinuation, some or all manifestations of this syndrome may disappear spontaneously.

Other extrapyramidal reactions — Dystonia may manifest as torticollis, opisthotonos, carpopedal spasm, trismus, dysphagia, dyspnea, oculogyric crisis, or protrusion of the tongue; treat by administering parenterally either diphenhydramine or an anticholinergic antiparkinson drug. If akathisia occurs, dosage may be reduced until the reaction subsides; the effectiveness of anticholinergic therapy has not be established. For pseudoparkinsonism, reduce dosage and, if necessary, give benztropine, biperiden, procyclidine, trihexphenidyl, or amantadine; antiparkinson therapy, if instituted, should be periodically reevaluated. The value of prophylactic antiparkinson treatment has not been demonstrated.

MAO inhibitor therapy — Wait at least 14 days after discontinuing use of an MAO inhibitor before initiating therapy with this drug; start treatment cautiously, with gradual increases in dosage until optimum response is achieved

Atropine-like action — Use with caution in patients with a history of urinary retention, narrow-angle glaucoma, or increased intraocular pressure; even average doses may precipitate an attack in patients with narrow-angle glaucoma

Cardiovascular disease — May worsen; use with caution and keep patient under close supervision. Tricyclic antidepressants, especially in high doses, may produce arrhythmias, sinus tachycardia, and prolongation of conduction time; myocardial infarction and stroke have followed use of these agents.

Mental and/or physical impairment — Caution patients that their ability to drive or perform other potentially hazardous activities may be impaired, and that their response to alcohol, barbiturates, and other CNS depressants may be enhanced

Alcohol usage — Because the effects of alcohol are potentiated, its ingestion may increase the danger inherent in any suicide attempt or accidental overdose; this is especially important in patients who may use alcohol excessively

Psychotic symptoms — Paranoia may worsen, and depressed patients (particularly those with manic-depressive illness) may become manic or hypomanic; the tranquilizing effect of this preparation seems to reduce the likelihood of these effects

Potentially suicidal patients — Should not have access to large quantities of this drug; prescribe smallest amount feasible

Discontinuation of prolonged therapy — Abrupt withdrawal may produce nausea, headache, and malaise; transient symptoms, including irritability, restlessness, and dream and sleep disturbances, may occur within the first 2 wk of gradual dosage reduction. These symptoms are not indicative of addiction. Hypomania or mania occurring within 2–7 days of stopping chronic antidepressant therapy has been reported rarely.

Elective surgery — If possible, discontinue medication several days prior to surgery

Electroconvulsive therapy (ECT) — Hazard may be increased; use ECT only when essential

Antiemetic effect — May mask signs of toxicity due to overdosage of other drugs or render more difficult the diagnosis of such disorders as brain tumors or intestinal obstruction

Unexplained fever — May suggest intolerance to perphenazine component; discontinue use if a significant rise occurs

Patients with previously detected breast cancer — Use with caution, as perphenazine component may cause persistent elevation of serum prolactin levels, which may be of importance in patients with prolactin-dependent breast cancers. Although endocrine disturbances have been reported, no association between chronic neuroleptic administration and mammary tumorigenesis has been demonstrated; the available evidence is considered too limited to be conclusive at this time.

TRIAVIL

Other special-risk patients	Use with caution in patients with hepatic impairment, convulsive disorders, hyperthyroidism, or a history of adverse reaction to phenothiazines or amitriptyline; patients exposed to heat or phosphorous insecticides; and those taking thyroid medication, anticholinergic agents, or sympathomimetics (see DRUG INTERACTIONS)

ADVERSE REACTIONS[1]

Central nervous system and neuromuscular	Dystonia, akathisia, pseudoparkinsonism, acute dyskinesia, tardive dyskinesia, hyperreflexia, ataxia, reactivation of psychosis, catatonic-like states, muscle weakness, insomnia, hypnotic effects, fatigue, drowsiness, lassitude, weakness, headache, altered CSF proteins, confusion, dizziness, disturbed concentration, disorientation, delusions, hallucinations, excitement, anxiety, restlessness, nightmares, numbness, tingling, paresthesias of the extremities, peripheral neuropathy, incoordination, tremors, seizures, grand mal convulsions, altered EEG patterns, cerebral edema
Ophthalmic	Pigmentation of the cornea and lens, pigmentary retinopathy, blurred vision, accommodation disturbances, mydriasis, increased intraocular pressure
Cardiovascular	Hypotension, orthostatic hypotension, hypertension, tachycardia, palpitations, peripheral edema, occasional change in pulse rate, quinidine-like ECG abnormalities, myocardial infarction, arrhythmias, heart block, stroke, edema
Gastrointestinal	Obstipation, vomiting, nausea, constipation, anorexia, epigastric distress, diarrhea, paralytic ileus, polyphagia
Oral	Dry mouth, salivation, peculiar taste, parotid swelling, black tongue, stomatitis
Hepatic	Jaundice, biliary stasis, hepatitis, altered liver function
Hematological	Pancytopenia, agranulocytosis, leukopenia, purpura, thrombocytopenia, thrombocytopenic purpura, eosinophilia
Genitourinary	Urinary frequency, incontinence, urinary retention, dilatation of urinary tract, change in libido, ejaculation failure
Endocrinological	Lactation, galactorrhea, breast enlargement, gynecomastia, menstrual irregularities, testicular swelling, hyperglycemia, decrease in serum glucose level, inappropriate ADH secretion syndrome
Dermatological	Eczema, exfoliative dermatitis, urticaria, erythema, pruritus, photosensitivity, photophobia, pigmentation, alopecia
Hypersensitivity	Anaphylactoid reactions, laryngeal edema, asthma, angioneurotic edema, rash, urticaria, photosensitivity, edema of face and tongue
Other	Nasal congestion, increased perspiration, change in weight, tinnitus

OVERDOSAGE

Signs and symptoms	Drowsiness, hypothermia, tachycardia and other arrhythmias, ECG evidence of impaired conduction, congestive heart failure, mydriasis, convulsions, severe hypotension, stupor, coma, agitation, hyperactive reflexes, muscle rigidity, vomiting, hyperpyrexia (see also ADVERSE REACTIONS)
Treatment	Admit patient to hospital. Empty stomach by inducing emesis, followed by gastric lavage and activated charcoal (20–30 g q4–6h during initial 24–48 h). Obtain ECG and begin close monitoring of cardiac function if abnormalities appear. Maintain an open airway and adequate fluid intake. Regulate body temperature. Administer 1–3 mg physostigmine salicylate IV and repeat as needed, especially if life-threatening signs recur or persist. (Physostigmine should not be used routinely, however, as it may itself be toxic.) For cardiac arrhythmias, circulatory shock, and metabolic acidosis, institute standard supportive measures. Treat cardiac arrhythmias with neostigmine, pyridostigmine, or propranolol. If cardiac failure occurs, consider digitalization. (Cardiac function should be closely monitored for at least 5 days under these circumstances.) To control convulsions, use diazepam, paraldehyde, or an inhalation anesthetic; *do not use barbiturates*. Combat hypotension with norepinephrine, not epinephrine. Administer benztropine mesylate or diphenhydramine for acute parkinsonian symptoms. Dialysis is of no value because of low plasma drug concentrations and because of extensive tissue distribution of the drug.

DRUG INTERACTIONS

Alcohol, sedative-hypnotics, and other CNS depressants	↑ CNS depression
MAO inhibitors	Hyperpyrexia, excitability, severe convulsions, coma, death
Anticholinergic agents	Acute glaucoma, urinary retention, paralytic ileus
Epinephrine	↑ Severe hypotension
Ethchlorvynol, disulfiram	Delirium
Guanethidine	↓ Antihypertensive effect
Sympathomimetic agents	Severe hypertension, hyperpyrexia
Thyroid preparations	↑ Antidepressant effect and possible risk of arrhythmias

TRIAVIL

Cimetidine	⇧ Pharmacologic effects of amitriptyline
Anticonvulsants	⇩ Convulsion threshold ⇧ CNS depression

ALTERED LABORATORY VALUES

Blood/serum values	⇧ or ⇩ Glucose
Urinary values	False-positive pregnancy tests

USE IN CHILDREN

Not recommended for use in children because a dosage for children has not been established

USE IN PREGNANT AND NURSING WOMEN

Not recommended for use in pregnant women or nursing mothers. Reproduction studies in rats have shown no evidence of fetal abnormalities; however, clinical experience and follow-up have been limited, and the possibility remains that this drug may adversely affect human fetal development.

[1] Included are some phenothiazine and tricyclic antidepressant adverse reactions not reported with this drug, but which must be considered before and during therapy

652

COMPENDIUM OF DRUG THERAPY

Chapter 18

Antidiarrheal Agents/Oral Electrolyte Solutions

Antidiarrheal Agents — 654

DIASORB (Key) — 654
Attapulgite *OTC*

DONNAGEL (Robins) — 654
Kaolin, pectin, hyoscyamine sulfate, atropine sulfate, and scopolamine hydrobromide *OTC*

DONNAGEL-PG (Robins) — 655
Opium, kaolin, pectin, hyoscyamine sulfate, atropine sulfate, and scopolamine hydrobromide *OTC*

IMODIUM (Janssen) — 656
Loperamide hydrochloride *Rx*

KAOPECTATE (Upjohn) — 658
Kaolin and pectin *OTC*

KAOPECTATE Concentrate (Upjohn) — 658
Kaolin and pectin *OTC*

KAOPECTATE Tablets (Upjohn) — 658
Attapulgite *OTC*

LACTINEX (Hynson, Westcott & Dunning) — 659
Lactobacillus acidophilus and *L bulgaricus* cultures *OTC*

LOMOTIL (Searle) — 659
Diphenoxylate hydrochloride and atropine sulfate *C-V*

MITROLAN (Robins) — 661
Calcium polycarbophil *OTC*

Paregoric (Lilly) — 661
Camphorated tincture of opium *C-III*

PAREPECTOLIN (Rorer) — 663
Paregoric, pectin, and kaolin *C-V*

PEPTO-BISMOL (Procter & Gamble) — 663
Bismuth subsalicylate *OTC*

RHEABAN (Leeming) — 664
Attapulgite *OTC*

Oral Electrolyte Solutions — 665

GASTROLYTE (Rorer) *OTC* — 665
INFALYTE (Pennwalt) *OTC* — 665
LYTREN (Mead Johnson) *OTC* — 666
PEDIALYTE (Ross) *OTC* — 666
PEDIALYTE RS (Ross) *OTC* — 667

Other Antidiarrheal Agents — 653

BACID (Fisons) — 653
Lactobacillus acidophilus and sodium carboxymethylcellulose *OTC*

FUROXONE (Norwich Eaton) — 653
Furazolidone *Rx*

OTHER ANTIDIARRHEAL AGENTS

DRUG	HOW SUPPLIED	USUAL DOSAGE
BACID (Fisons) *Lactobacillus acidophilus* and sodium carboxymethylcellulose *OTC*	**Capsules:** not less than 5×10^8 *Lactobacillus acidophilus* and 100 mg sodium carboxymethylcellulose	**Adult and child ($\geq$ 3 yr):** 2 caps bid to qid, given preferably with milk
FUROXONE (Norwich Eaton) Furazolidone *Rx*	**Tablets:** 100 mg **Liquid (per 15 ml):** 50 mg (60, 473 ml) *sugar-free*	**Adult:** 1 tab or 30 ml (2 tbsp) qid for 2–5 days **Infant (1 mo to 1 yr):** 2.5–5 ml (1/2–1 tsp) qid for 2–5 days **Child (1–4 yr):** 5–7.5 ml (1–1 1/2 tsp) qid for 2–5 days **Child ($\geq$ 5 yr):** 7.5–15 ml (1/2–1 tbsp) or 1/4–1/2 tab qid for 2–5 days

COMPENDIUM OF DRUG THERAPY

ANTIDIARRHEAL AGENTS

DIASORB (attapulgite) Key   OTC

Tablets: 750 mg   **Liquid (per 5 ml):** 750 mg (4 fl oz) *cola flavored*

INDICATIONS
Diarrhea

ORAL DOSAGE
Adult and child (> 12 yr): 3,000 mg (4 tsp or tabs) to start, repeated after each bowel movement or q2h, as needed, up to 9,000 mg (12 tsp or tabs)/24 h
Infant and child (< 3 yr): use according to medical judgment
Child (3–6 yr): 750 mg (1 tsp or tab) to start, repeated after each bowel movement or q2h, as needed, up to 2,250 mg (3 tsp or tabs)/24 h
Child (6–12 yr): 1,500 mg (2 tsp or tabs) to start, repeated after each bowel movement or q2h, as needed, up to 4,500 mg (6 tsp or tabs)/24 h

CONTRAINDICATIONS
None known

WARNINGS/PRECAUTIONS
Consult manufacturer

ADVERSE REACTIONS

Gastrointestinal	Constipation, diarrhea, vomiting
Other	Miscellaneous effects, refusal

DRUG INTERACTIONS

Rifampin	↓ Absorption of rifampin; administer 1 h before or 2 h after administering attapulgite
Tetracycline	↓ Absorption of tetracycline; administer 1 h before or 2 h after administering attapulgite
Trimethoprim	↓ Absorption of trimethoprim; administer 1 h before or 2 h after administering attapulgite

ALTERED LABORATORY VALUES
No clinically significant alterations in blood/serum or urinary values occur at therapeutic dosages

---

USE IN CHILDREN
See INDICATIONS and ORAL DOSAGE

USE IN PREGNANT AND NURSING WOMEN
Consult manufacturer

ANTIDIARRHEAL AGENTS

DONNAGEL (kaolin, pectin, hyoscyamine sulfate, atropine sulfate, and scopolamine hydrobromide) Robins   OTC

Suspension (per 30 ml): 6 g kaolin, 142.8 mg pectin, 0.1037 mg hyoscyamine sulfate, 0.0194 mg atropine sulfate, and 0.0065 mg scopolamine hydrobromide[1] (4, 16 fl oz) *mint flavored*

INDICATIONS
Diarrhea

ORAL DOSAGE
Adult: 30 ml (2 tbsp) to start, followed by 15 ml (1 tbsp) q3h, up to 4 doses/24 h
Child (6–12 yr): 10 ml (2 tsp) to start, followed by 5–10 ml (1–2 tsp) q3h, up to 4 doses/24 h
Child (> 12 yr): same as adult

WARNINGS/PRECAUTIONS

Patient instructions	Patients with glaucoma, excessive intraocular pressure, under 6 yr of age, or of advanced age are cautioned not to use this preparation unless otherwise directed by a physician. Patients are instructed not to use this preparation for more than 2 days, in the presence of high fever, or to exceed the recommended dosage. A decrease in dosage is advised if dryness of the mouth occurs. Patients are warned to discontinue use if blurred vision, rapid pulse, or dizziness occurs and, in addition, to consult a physician immediately if they experience eye pain.

DONNAGEL ■ DONNAGEL-PG

OVERDOSAGE

Signs and symptoms — *Central nervous system:* confusion, disorientation, delusions, paranoia, disturbed speech, anxiety, agitation, excitement, hyperactivity, restlessness, headache, dizziness, ataxia, lack of coordination, delirium, hallucinations, convulsions, CNS depression (usually follows CNS stimulation); in severe cases, coma; *ophthalmic:* mydriasis, blurred vision; *dermatological:* hot and dry skin, flushing, rash; *digestive:* dry mouth and throat, difficulty in swallowing, foul breath, nausea, vomiting, abdominal distention; *urinary:* retention of urine; *cardiovascular:* tachycardia, other arrhythmias, hypertension; in severe cases, hypotension and circulatory collapse; *respiratory:* increased respiratory rate, hoarseness, dry nose; in severe cases, respiratory paralysis; *other:* fever

Treatment — Monitor cardiovascular and respiratory responses and institute standard measures, as needed. Give diazepam to control excitement and convulsions; however, avoid large doses since the action of diazepam may coincide with the onset of CNS depression owing to the overdose. Do not treat psychotic symptoms with phenothiazines; these drugs have anticholinergic effects. Use a miotic to reverse mydriasis. For relief of fever, cool body with tepid water, ice packs, or mechanical cooling devices. To avoid urinary retention in comatose patients, perform urethral catheterization. Physostigmine has been given for certain severe conditions, such as delirium, hallucinations, arrhythmias, severe hypertension, and coma; routine use has been controversial since the drug has produced serious adverse reactions. For adults, give 2 mg IV; for children, titrate the dose as follows: give 0.02 mg/kg IV to start and then, if signs persist and no cholinergic signs are seen, repeat dose every 5–10 min until a therapeutic effect has been obtained or a total of 2 mg has been given. Administer each dose by slow IV injection; rate should not exceed 1 mg/min for adults or 0.5 mg/min for children. The duration of action of physostigmine is only 45–60 min; therefore, monitor clinical response and ECG and repeat dose (2 mg for adults, titrated dose for children), as needed. To remove this preparation from the body, induce emesis or, if the patient is unconscious or experiencing seizures, perform gastric lavage; then instill activated charcoal.

DRUG INTERACTIONS

Chloroquine	▽ Absorption of chloroquine
Digoxin	▽ Absorption of digoxin
Lincomycin	▽ Absorption of lincomycin

USE IN CHILDREN

See INDICATIONS and ORAL DOSAGE

USE IN PREGNANT AND NURSING WOMEN

Use with caution in pregnant or nursing women; atropine is excreted in breast milk[1]

[1] Speika N: *J Obstet Gynaecol Br Commonw* 54:426, 1947; Knowles JA: *J Pediatr* 66:1068, 1965; Takyi BE: *J Hosp Pharm* 28:317, 1970

---

[1] Contains 3.8% alcohol

ANTIDIARRHEAL AGENTS

DONNAGEL-PG (opium, kaolin, pectin, hyoscyamine sulfate, atropine sulfate, and scopolamine hydrobromide) Robins   C-V

Suspension (per 30 ml): 24 mg opium, 6 g kaolin, 142.8 mg pectin, 0.1037 mg hyoscyamine sulfate, 0.0194 mg atropine sulfate, and 0.0065 mg scopolamine hydrobromide[1] (6, 16 fl oz) *banana-flavored*

INDICATIONS
Acute nonspecific diarrhea

ORAL DOSAGE
Adult: 30 ml (2 tbsp) to start, followed by 15 ml (1 tbsp) q3h, up to 4 doses/24 h
Child (6–12 yr): 10 ml (2 tsp) to start, followed by 5–10 ml (1–2 tsp) q3h, up to 4 doses/24 h
Child (> 12 yr): same as adult

WARNINGS/PRECAUTIONS

Patient instructions — Patients with glaucoma, excessive intraocular pressure, under 6 yr of age, or of advanced age are cautioned not to use this preparation unless otherwise directed by a physician. Patients are instructed not to use this preparation for more than 2 days, in the presence of high fever, or to exceed the recommended dosage. A decrease in dosage is advised if dryness of the mouth occurs. Patients are warned to discontinue use if blurred vision, rapid pulse, or dizziness occurs and, in addition, to consult a physician immediately if they experience eye pain.

Drug dependence	Psychic and/or physical dependence and tolerance may develop, especially in addiction-prone individuals

OVERDOSAGE

Signs and symptoms	*Central nervous system:* extreme somnolence progressing to stupor or coma, skeletal-muscle flaccidity, confusion, disorientation, delusions, paranoia, disturbed speech, anxiety, agitation, excitement, hyperactivity, restlessness, headache, dizziness, ataxia, lack of coordination, delirium, hallucinations, convulsions; *ophthalmic:* miosis, mydriasis, blurred vision; *dermatological:* cold and clammy skin, hot and dry skin, flushing, rash; *digestive:* dry mouth and throat, difficulty in swallowing, foul breath, nausea, vomiting, abdominal distention; *urinary:* retention of urine; *cardiovascular:* bradycardia, tachycardia, other arrhythmias, hypertension, hypotension, shock, cardiac arrest; *respiratory:* increased respiratory rate, hoarseness, dry nose, respiratory depression, apnea; *other:* fever
Treatment	Monitor cardiovascular and respiratory responses. Give primary attention to reestablishing adequate respiratory exchange through provision of an adequate airway and through assisted or controlled ventilation; if pulmonary edema is present, positive-pressure respiration may be desirable. If respiratory depression is significant, promptly administer naloxone, preferably IV. For adults, give 0.4–2 mg at intervals of 2–3 min, as needed; for children, give 0.01 mg/kg and then, if dose is not adequate, 0.1 mg/kg. Reevaluate diagnosis if no response is seen after a total of 10 mg has been given. Keep the patient under constant surveillance since the duration of action of opium may exceed that of naloxone. *Do not administer analeptic agents to reverse CNS depression.* Use diazepam to control excitement and convulsions; however, avoid large doses since the action of diazepam may coincide with the onset of CNS depression owing to the overdose. Do not treat psychotic symptoms with phenothiazines; these drugs have anticholinergic effects. Use a miotic to reverse mydriasis. For relief of fever, cool body with tepid water, ice packs, or mechanical cooling devices. To avoid urinary retention in comatose patients, perform urethral catheterization. Physostigmine has been given for certain severe conditions associated with anticholinergic overdose, such as delirium, hallucinations, arrhythmias, severe hypertension, and coma; routine use has been controversial since the drug has produced serious adverse reactions. For adults, give 2 mg IV; for children, titrate the dose as follows: give 0.02 mg/kg IV to start and then, if signs persist and no cholinergic signs are seen, repeat dose every 5–10 min until a therapeutic effect has been obtained or a total of 2 mg has been given. Administer each dose by slow IV injection; rate should not exceed 1 mg/min for adults or 0.5 mg/min for children. The duration of action of physostigmine is only 45–60 min; therefore, monitor clinical response and ECG and repeat dose (2 mg for adults, titrated dose for children), as needed. To remove this preparation from the body, induce emesis or, if the patient is unconscious or experiencing seizures, perform gastric lavage; then instill activated charcoal.

DRUG INTERACTIONS

Chloroquine	▽ Absorption of chloroquine
Digoxin	▽ Absorption of digoxin
Lincomycin	▽ Absorption of lincomycin

USE IN CHILDREN
See INDICATIONS and ORAL DOSAGE

USE IN PREGNANT AND NURSING WOMEN
Use with caution in pregnant or nursing women; atropine is excreted in breast milk[1]

[1]Speika N: *J Obstet Gynaecol Br Commonw* 54:426, 1947; Knowles JA: *J Pediatr* 66:1068, 1965; Takyi BE: *J Hosp Pharm* 28:317, 1970

[1] Contains 5.0% alcohol

ANTIDIARRHEAL AGENTS

IMODIUM (loperamide hydrochloride) Janssen   Rx
Capsules: 2 mg   **Liquid (per 5 ml):** 1 mg (4 fl oz)

INDICATIONS[1]
Acute nonspecific diarrhea

ORAL DOSAGE
Adult: 4 mg or 20 ml (4 tsp) to start, followed by 2 mg or 10 ml (2 tsp) after each unformed stool, up to 16 mg or 80 ml (16 tsp) per day
Child (2–5 yr; 13–20 kg): 5 ml (1 tsp) tid on the first day, followed by 5 ml (1 tsp)/10 kg after each unformed stool, up to 15 ml (3 tsp)/day
Child (5–8 yr; 20–30 kg): 2 mg or 10 ml (2 tsp) bid on the first day, followed by 1 mg or 5 ml (1 tsp) per 10 kg after each unformed stool, up to 4 mg or 20 ml (4 tsp) per day
Child (8–12 yr; > 30 kg): 2 mg or 10 ml (2 tsp) tid on the first day, followed by 1 mg or 5 ml (1 tsp) per 10 kg after each unformed stool, up to 6 mg or 30 ml (6 tsp) per day

IMODIUM

Chronic diarrhea due to inflammatory bowel disease	Adult: 4 mg or 20 ml (4 tsp) to start, followed by 2 mg or 10 ml (2 tsp) after each unformed stool, up to 16 mg or 80 ml (16 tsp)/day, until diarrhea is controlled; thereafter, reduce dosage to meet individual requirements (the optimum daily dose may be given as a single dose or divided; average maintenance dosage: 4–8 mg/day). It is unlikely that loperamide will control diarrhea if no clinical improvement has occurred after 16 mg/day has been given for at least 10 days; nevertheless, administration may be continued if other measures (diet, specific treatment) are not adequate alternatives.

CONTRAINDICATIONS

Hypersensitivity to loperamide — Conditions in which constipation must be avoided

ADMINISTRATION/DOSAGE ADJUSTMENTS

Refractory acute diarrhea	Discontinue administration if clinical improvement of acute diarrhea is not observed within 48 h after the onset of therapy

WARNINGS/PRECAUTIONS

Toxic megacolon	Use of agents that inhibit intestinal motility or delay intestinal transit time has reportedly caused toxic megacolon in patients with antibiotic-induced pseudomembranous colitis and in some patients with acute ulcerative colitis; discontinue therapy promptly if abdominal distention occurs or if other untoward symptoms develop in patients with acute ulcerative colitis
Acute dysentery	Loperamide should not be used for acute dysentery that is characterized by bloody stools and fever; instruct patient to report any fever developing during therapy
Patients with hepatic impairment	Closely watch patients with hepatic impairment for signs of CNS depression, because the metabolism of loperamide is likely to be inhibited in these patients
Patients with fluid and electrolyte depletion	Use of this drug does not preclude the need for appropriate replacement therapy when fluid and electrolyte depletion has occurred
Drug dependence	Loperamide, when given at doses exceeding those recommended for humans, prevents withdrawal reactions in morphine-dependent monkeys; however, physical dependence has not been seen in humans, and when the naloxone challenge pupil test has been performed in humans after administration of a single high dose of loperamide or after more than 2 yr of therapeutic use, no opiate-like effects have been detected
Carcinogenicity, mutagenicity	No evidence of carcinogenicity has been seen in rats given up to 133 times the maximum human dose for 18 mo; mutagenicity tests have not been done
Impairment of fertility	Administration of 150–200 times the human dose to rats has resulted in marked female infertility and reduced male fertility

ADVERSE REACTIONS

Gastrointestinal	Abdominal pain, distention, discomfort, constipation, nausea, vomiting
Central nervous system	Drowsiness, dizziness, fatigue
Other	Hypersensitivity reactions, including rash; dry mouth

OVERDOSAGE

Signs and symptoms	Constipation, CNS depression, GI irritation, nausea, vomiting
Treatment	If vomiting has occurred spontaneously, administer a slurry of 100 g of activated charcoal as soon as patient is able to retain fluids. If vomiting has not occurred, perform gastric lavage, followed by administration of 100 g of activated charcoal through the gastric tube. Watch for CNS depression, especially in children, for at least 24 h; if CNS depression is observed, administer naloxone as needed (repeated use may be required), and then, after the last dose of naloxone, monitor vital signs for at least 24 h. Forced diuresis is unlikely to be beneficial, since little of the drug is excreted in urine.

DRUG INTERACTIONS

No clinically significant drug interactions have been identified

ALTERED LABORATORY VALUES

No clinically significant alterations in blood/serum or urinary values occur at therapeutic dosages

USE IN CHILDREN

See INDICATIONS and ORAL DOSAGE; loperamide is not recommended for children under 2 yr of age. The liquid form should be prescribed for children under 6 yr of age. Loperamide has been used in a limited number of children with chronic diarrhea, but a therapeutic dosage has not been established. Exercise special caution when treating young children, particularly if they are dehydrated, because the response to loperamide may be more variable.

USE IN PREGNANT AND NURSING WOMEN

Pregnancy Category B: reproduction studies in rats and rabbits given up to 30 times the human dose have shown no evidence of harm to the fetus; however, no adequate, well-controlled studies have been done in pregnant women. Use during pregnancy only if clearly needed. It is not known whether this drug is excreted in human milk; use with caution in nursing mothers.

[1] Loperamide can also be used to reduce the volume of discharge in patients who have undergone an ileostomy; consult manufacturer for the appropriate dosage

ANTIDIARRHEAL AGENTS

KAOPECTATE (kaolin and pectin) Upjohn — OTC

Liquid (per 30 ml): 90 gr kaolin and 2 gr pectin (3, 8, 12, 16 fl oz; 1 gal)

INDICATIONS
Diarrhea

ORAL DOSAGE
Adult: 60–120 ml (4–8 tbsp) after each bowel movement or as needed
Child (< 3 yr): use according to medical judgment
Child (3–6 yr): 15–30 ml (1–2 tbsp) after each bowel movement or as needed
Child (6–12 yr): 30–60 ml (2–4 tbsp) after each bowel movement or as needed
Child (> 12 yr): 60 ml (4 tbsp) after each bowel movement or as needed

KAOPECTATE Concentrate (kaolin and pectin) Upjohn — OTC

Liquid (per 30 ml): 135 gr kaolin and 3 gr pectin (3, 8, 12 fl oz) *peppermint flavored*

INDICATIONS
Diarrhea

ORAL DOSAGE
Adult: 45–90 ml (3–6 tbsp) after each bowel movement or as needed
Child (< 3 yr): use according to medical judgment
Child (3–6 yr): 15 ml (1 tbsp) after each bowel movement or as needed
Child (6–12 yr): 30 ml (2 tbsp) after each bowel movement or as needed
Child (> 12 yr): 45 ml (3 tbsp) after each bowel movement or as needed

KAOPECTATE Tablets (attapulgite) Upjohn — OTC

Tablets: 600 mg

INDICATIONS
Diarrhea and associated cramps and pain

ORAL DOSAGE
Adult: 1,200 mg (2 tabs) after each bowel movement, up to 14 tabs/24 h; swallow tablets whole with a full glass of water
Child (6–12 yr): 600 mg (1 tab) after each bowel movement, up to 7 tabs/24 h; swallow tablets whole with a full glass of water

CONTRAINDICATIONS
Consult manufacturer

WARNINGS/PRECAUTIONS

Patient instructions — Patients are cautioned on the package label to consult a physician if diarrhea continues for more than 2 days or is accompanied by high fever

OVERDOSAGE

Signs and symptoms — Constipation

Treatment — Stop medication

KAOPECTATE ■ LOMOTIL

DRUG INTERACTIONS

| Digoxin | ⇓ Digoxin absorption |
| Lincomycin | ⇓ Lincomycin absorption |

ALTERED LABORATORY VALUES
No clinically significant alterations in blood/serum or urinary values occur at therapeutic dosages

---

USE IN CHILDREN
See INDICATIONS and ORAL DOSAGE; do not use tablets in children under 6 yr of age

USE IN PREGNANT AND NURSING WOMEN
Consult manufacturer

ANTIDIARRHEAL AGENTS

LACTINEX (*Lactobacillus acidophilus* and *L bulgaricus* cultures) Hynson, Westcott & Dunning   OTC

Chewable tablets: 2.5 million *Lactobacillus acidophilus* and 2.5 million *L bulgaricus*   **Granules:** 10 million *Lactobacillus acidophilus* and 10 million *L bulgaricus* per 1-g packet

INDICATIONS
Uncomplicated diarrhea

ORAL DOSAGE
Adult and child: 4 tabs or 1 packet of granules, added to or taken with cereal, food, milk, fruit juice, or water, tid or qid

CONTRAINDICATIONS
Hypersensitivity to milk products or lactose intolerance

WARNINGS/PRECAUTIONS
Must be kept refrigerated

ADVERSE REACTIONS
None reported

OVERDOSAGE
Toxicity of *Lactobacillus* cultures in man has not been reported

DRUG INTERACTIONS
No clinically significant drug interactions have been identified

ALTERED LABORATORY VALUES
No clinically significant alterations in blood/serum or urinary values occur at therapeutic dosages

---

USE IN CHILDREN
See INDICATIONS and ORAL DOSAGE

USE IN PREGNANT AND NURSING WOMEN
There is no basis for contraindicating use of these products by pregnant or nursing women; however, no studies have been conducted in appropriate populations

---

ANTIDIARRHEAL AGENTS

LOMOTIL (diphenoxylate hydrochloride and atropine sulfate) Searle   C-V

Tablets: 2.5 mg diphenoxylate hydrochloride and 0.025 mg atropine sulfate   **Liquid (per 5 ml):** 2.5 mg diphenoxylate hydrochloride and 0.025 mg atropine sulfate (2 fl oz)

INDICATIONS
Diarrhea (adjunctive therapy)

ORAL DOSAGE
Adult: 2 tabs or 10 ml (2 tsp) qid, until the diarrhea is controlled, followed by as little as 2 tabs or 10 ml (2 tsp)/day for maintenance. It is unlikely that diphenoxylate will control chronic diarrhea if no clinical improvement has occurred after 20 mg of the drug has been given daily for 10 days.

Child ($\geq$ 2 yr): 0.3–0.4 mg/kg/day, given in 4 divided doses, until the diarrhea is controlled; use liquid, not tablets. Consider the nutritional status and degree of dehydration of the child when determining the dosage; do not exceed the recommended level. For maintenance, the initial dosage may be reduced by as much as 75%. If no clinical response has occurred after 48 h, it is unlikely that diphenoxylate will control the diarrhea.

LOMOTIL

CONTRAINDICATIONS

Hypersensitivity to diphenoxylate or atropine	Pseudomembranous enterocolitis	Obstructive jaundice

WARNINGS/PRECAUTIONS

Risk of overdosage	Severe respiratory depression and coma, followed by permanent brain damage or death, may result from acute overdosage; caution patients not to exceed the recommended dosage, and instruct them to use a child-resistant container, which they should keep out of the reach of children
Fluid and electrolyte therapy	Institute appropriate fluid and electrolyte therapy, as needed. If dehydration or electrolyte imbalance is severe, give this preparation only after suitable corrective therapy has been started; drug-induced inhibition of peristalsis may cause fluid retention in the intestine and thereby exacerbate dehydration or electrolyte imbalance.
Diarrhea owing to drugs or toxigenic bacteria	If diarrhea is associated with antibiotic-induced pseudomembranous colitis or with infections owing to toxigenic *E coli*, *Salmonella*, *Shigella*, or other organisms that penetrate the intestinal mucosa, this preparation should not be given because such use may exacerbate these conditions
Drowsiness, dizziness	Caution patients about driving or engaging in other potentially hazardous activities requiring mental alertness
Patients with acute ulcerative colitis	Use of agents that inhibit intestinal motility or delay intestinal transit time has been associated with toxic megacolon in some patients with acute ulcerative colitis; keep such patients under close observation during therapy, and discontinue use of this drug if abdominal distention or other untoward symptoms develop
Hepatic coma	May be precipitated in patients with advanced hepatorenal disease or abnormal liver-function tests; use with extreme caution
Drug dependence	Psychic and/or physical dependence may develop at high dosages; however, diphenoxylate has not produced addiction at dosages used for the treatment of diarrhea
Carcinogenicity	No long-term studies have been done to evaluate the carcinogenic potential of this preparation
Effect on fertility	A decrease in fertility has been seen in rats fed 50 times the human dose of diphenoxylate

ADVERSE REACTIONS

Gastrointestinal	Anorexia, nausea, vomiting, abdominal discomfort, paralytic ileus, toxic megacolon
Central nervous system	Dizziness, drowsiness/sedation, headache, malaise/lethargy, confusion, restlessness, euphoria, depression, numbness in the extremities
Cardiovascular	Flushing, tachycardia
Allergic	Pruritus, swelling of the gums, urticaria, angioneurotic edema, anaphylaxis
Other	Hyperthermia, urinary retention, dryness of the skin and mucous membranes

OVERDOSAGE

Signs and symptoms	Dryness of skin and mucous membranes, mydriasis, restlessness, flushing, hyperthermia, and tachycardia followed by lethargy or coma, hypotonic reflexes, nystagmus, pinpoint pupils, and respiratory depression
Treatment	Maintain pulmonary function; if necessary, establish a patent airway and institute mechanical ventilation. For control of respiratory depression, administer naloxone (0.4 mg IV in adults, 0.01 mg/kg IV in children) every 2–3 min, as needed. Maintain medical observation, preferably with continuous hospital care, for at least 48 h; respiratory depression can start as late as 30 h after ingestion and, because of naloxone's relatively short duration of action, may recur after pulmonary function has been restored. To remove the drug from the GI tract, induce emesis or perform gastric lavage, and then, if patient is conscious, give 100 g of activated charcoal.

DRUG INTERACTIONS

MAO inhibitors	May precipitate hypertensive crisis
Antimuscarinics	△ Risk of paralytic ileus
Barbiturates, alcohol, tranquilizers, and other CNS depressants	△ CNS depression; caution patients accordingly

ALTERED LABORATORY VALUES

Blood/serum values	△ Amylase

No clinically significant alterations in urinary values occur at therapeutic dosages

LOMOTIL ■ Paregoric

USE IN CHILDREN
See INDICATIONS and ORAL DOSAGE; use in children under 2 yr of age is not recommended. Do not give the tablets to children under 13 yr of age. Signs of atropinism may occur at the recommended dosage in children, especially in those with Down's syndrome. Exercise particular caution when treating young children because their response may be more variable, and the risk of delayed toxicity is greater in these patients.

USE IN PREGNANT AND NURSING WOMEN
Pregnancy Category C: a study of general reproductive function has shown decreases in litter size and maternal weight gain in rats fed 10 times the human dose of diphenoxylate; no adequate studies have been done in animals to specifically evaluate the teratogenic potential of this drug. Use during pregnancy only if the expected benefit justifies the potential risk to the fetus. Atropine is known, and diphenoxylic acid (the major metabolite) is likely, to be present in breast milk; use with caution in nursing mothers.

ANTIDIARRHEAL AGENTS

MITROLAN (calcium polycarbophil) Robins   OTC
Chewable tablets: calcium polycarbophil equivalent to 500 mg polycarbophil *citrus-vanilla flavored*

INDICATIONS
Constipation or diarrhea

ORAL DOSAGE
Adult: 2 tabs qid or as needed, up to 12 tabs/24 h, to be chewed before swallowing
Child (3–5 yr): 1 tab bid or as needed, up to 3 tabs/24 h, to be chewed before swallowing
Child (6–11 yr): 1 tab tid or as needed, up to 6 tabs/24 h, to be chewed before swallowing

CONTRAINDICATIONS
Gastrointestinal obstruction

ADMINISTRATION/DOSAGE ADJUSTMENTS

Acute diarrhea	If necessary, repeat dose every 1/2 h, without exceeding maximum daily dosage
Laxative use	Each dose should be taken with 8 fl oz of liquid
Avoidance of abdominal fullness	Give smaller doses at more frequent, equally spaced intervals

WARNINGS/PRECAUTIONS

Self-medication for constipation	Package label cautions patients to consult a physician before using this product if there has been a sudden change in bowel habits that has persisted over a period of 2 wk, to discontinue use and seek medical attention if taking this product has had no effect after 1 wk, and not to use it, unless directed by a physician, if abdominal pain, nausea, or vomiting is present
Self-medication for diarrhea	Package label cautions patients against using this product for more than 2 days, in the presence of a high fever, or in children under 3 yr of age, unless directed by a physician; patients are also advised to seek medical attention if diarrhea is accompanied by a high fever

ADVERSE REACTIONS

Gastrointestinal	Abdominal fullness (see ADMINISTRATION/DOSAGE ADJUSTMENTS)

OVERDOSAGE
Product is not absorbed; no toxic effects have been observed in clinical use

DRUG INTERACTIONS

Tetracycline	▽ Absorption of tetracycline; do not use concomitantly

ALTERED LABORATORY VALUES
No clinically significant alterations in blood/serum or urinary values occur at therapeutic dosages

USE IN CHILDREN
See INDICATIONS and ORAL DOSAGE

USE IN PREGNANT AND NURSING WOMEN
The package labeling cautions pregnant or nursing women to consult a health professional before using this product

---

ANTIDIARRHEAL AGENTS

Paregoric (camphorated tincture of opium) Lilly   C-III
Liquid (per 5 ml): camphorated tincture of opium (16 fl oz, 1 gal) equivalent to 2 mg anhydrous morphine[1]

INDICATIONS
Diarrhea

ORAL DOSAGE
Adult: 5–10 ml (1–2 tsp) 1–4 times/day
Child: 0.25–0.5 ml/kg 1–4 times/day

COMPENDIUM OF DRUG THERAPY

Paregoric

CONTRAINDICATIONS

Convulsive states (eg, status epilepticus, tetanus, or strychnine poisoning)	Diarrhea caused by poisoning (until toxic material is eliminated from GI tract)	Hypersensitivity to morphine

WARNINGS/PRECAUTIONS

Drug dependence	Psychic and/or physical dependence and tolerance may develop, especially in addiction-prone individuals. Patients receiving therapeutic dosage regimens of 10 mg q4h for 1–2 wk have experienced mild withdrawal symptoms; severe symptoms may require use of a replacement narcotic.
Patients with head injuries or other intracranial lesions	The respiratory depressant effects of this drug and its capacity to elevate CSF pressure may be markedly exaggerated in such patients; side effects may also interfere with the clinical evaluation of head injuries
Patients with acute abdominal conditions	Use of this drug may obscure the diagnosis or clinical course of acute abdominal conditions
Hypoxia	Use with extreme caution in patients with disorders characterized by hypoxia, since even usual therapeutic doses may decrease respiratory drive to the point of apnea, while simultaneously increasing airway resistance
Patients with supraventricular tachycardias	Use with caution in patients with atrial flutter or other supraventricular tachycardias; a vagolytic action is possible, which may cause a significant increase in the ventricular response rate
Severe hypotension	May occur in the postoperative patient or in any patient whose ability to maintain blood pressure has been compromised by a depleted blood volume or use of such drugs as phenothiazines or certain anesthetics
Convulsions	May occur in individuals without a history of convulsive disorders, if dosage is increased substantially above recommended levels because of tolerance development; preexisting convulsions may be aggravated in patients with convulsive disorders (see CONTRAINDICATIONS)
Other special-risk patients	Use with caution in elderly or debilitated patients and in those with severe hepatic or renal impairment, hypothyroidism, Addison's disease, prostatic hypertrophy, or urethral stricture
Mental and/or physical impairment	Caution patients that their abilities to engage in potentially hazardous activities may be impaired and that alcohol and other CNS depressants may cause further impairment
Carcinogenicity, mutagenicity	No long-term studies have been performed in animals to evaluate the carcinogenic or mutagenic potential of morphine

ADVERSE REACTIONS

Frequent reactions (incidence ≥ 1%) are printed in *italics*

Central nervous system	*Light-headedness, dizziness, sedation,* euphoria, dysphoria
Gastrointestinal	*Nausea, vomiting,* constipation
Dermatological	Pruritus

OVERDOSAGE

Signs and symptoms	Respiratory depression, extreme somnolence progressing to stupor and coma, skeletal-muscle flaccidity, cold and clammy skin, bradycardia, hypotension, and, in severe cases, apnea, circulatory collapse, cardiac arrest, and death
Treatment	Give primary attention to reestablishing adequate respiratory exchange through provision of an adequate airway and assisted or controlled ventilation; positive-pressure respiration may be desirable if pulmonary edema is present. If respiratory depression is significant, promptly administer naloxone (adult, 0.4 mg; child, 0.01 mg/kg), preferably IV, and repeat at 2- to 3-min intervals until satisfactory breathing is restored. *Do not use analeptic agents.* Oxygen, IV fluids, vasopressors, and other supportive measures should be employed, as needed. Gastric lavage, followed by instillation of activated charcoal, may be useful; dialysis is of little value unless other, dialyzable substances (such as barbiturates) have been simultaneously ingested.

DRUG INTERACTIONS

Other narcotics; sedative-hypnotics, antianxiety agents, phenothiazines, general anesthetics, and other CNS depressants (including alcohol); MAO inhibitors; tricyclic antidepressants	⌂ CNS depression; reduce dose of one or both agents if used concomitantly or in close succession
Phenothiazines, certain anesthetics	⌂ Risk of hypotension

ALTERED LABORATORY VALUES
No clinically significant alterations in blood/serum or urinary values occur at therapeutic dosages

USE IN CHILDREN	USE IN PREGNANT AND NURSING WOMEN
See INDICATIONS and ORAL DOSAGE	Pregnancy Category C: use during pregnancy only when clearly needed. Animal reproduction studies have not been done, nor is it known what effect, if any, this drug may have on human fetal development or reproductive capacity. Morphine is excreted in human milk; use with caution in nursing mothers.

[1] Contains 45% alcohol

ANTIDIARRHEAL AGENTS

PAREPECTOLIN (paregoric, pectin, and kaolin) Rorer   C-V
Suspension (per 30 ml): 3.7 ml paregoric, 162 mg pectin, and 5.5 g kaolin[1] (4, 8 fl oz)

INDICATIONS	ORAL DOSAGE
Nonspecific diarrhea	**Adult:** 15–30 ml (1–2 tbsp) after each loose bowel movement, up to 4 doses/12 h **Child (1 yr):** 2.5 ml ($1/2$ tsp) after each loose bowel movement, up to 4 doses/12 h **Child (3 yr):** 7.5 ml ($1 1/2$ tsp) after each loose bowel movement, up to 4 doses/12 h **Child (6 yr):** 10 ml (2 tsp) after each loose bowel movement, up to 4 doses/12 h

CONTRAINDICATIONS
None reported by manufacturer

WARNINGS/PRECAUTIONS

Drug dependence	Psychic and/or physical dependence and tolerance may develop, especially in addiction-prone individuals
Patient instructions	Package label advises patients not to use this product for more than 2 days, in the presence of high fever, or in infants or children under 3 yr of age without medical supervision; the label also cautions pregnant or nursing women to seek the advice of a health professional before using this product

ADVERSE REACTIONS
None reported by manufacturer

OVERDOSAGE

Signs and symptoms	Constipation, CNS depression
Treatment	Maintain a patent airway; institute artificial respiration, if indicated. If patient is conscious, induce emesis or perform gastric lavage to empty stomach, and give activated charcoal. For respiratory depression, administer naloxone (0.4 mg IV in adults, 0.01 mg/kg IV in children); repeat dose, as needed, at 2- to 3-min intervals. Observe patient for recurrence of drug overdose symptoms for at least 48 h after the last dose of naloxone.

DRUG INTERACTIONS

Digoxin	▽ Absorption of digoxin
Lincomycin	▽ Absorption of lincomycin

ALTERED LABORATORY VALUES
No clinically significant alterations in blood/serum or urinary values occur at therapeutic dosages

USE IN CHILDREN	USE IN PREGNANT AND NURSING WOMEN
See INDICATIONS and ORAL DOSAGE	Consult manufacturer

[1] Contains 0.69% alcohol

ANTIDIARRHEAL AGENTS

PEPTO-BISMOL (bismuth subsalicylate) Procter & Gamble   OTC
Chewable tablets: 262 mg[1] *sugar-free*   **Liquid (per 5 ml):** 87.3 mg[1] (4, 8, 12, 16 fl oz) *sugar-free*

INDICATIONS	ORAL DOSAGE
Diarrhea, indigestion, heartburn, nausea, and upset stomach	**Adult:** 524 mg (2 tabs or 30 ml [2 tbsp]) q$1/2$–1h, as needed, up to a maximum of 4,192 mg (8 doses)/24 h **Child (3–6 yr):** 87.3 mg ($1/3$ tab or 5 ml [1 tsp]) q$1/2$–1h, as needed, up to a maximum of approximately 698 mg (8 doses)/24 h **Child (6–9 yr):** 174.6 mg ($2/3$ tab or 10 ml [2 tsp]) q$1/2$–1h, as needed, up to a maximum of approximately 1,397 mg (8 doses)/24 h **Child (9–12 yr):** 262 mg (1 tab or 15 ml [1 tbsp]) q$1/2$–1h, as needed, up to a maximum of 2,096 mg (8 doses)/24 h

COMPENDIUM OF DRUG THERAPY

CONTRAINDICATIONS

Hypersensitivity to salicylates

ADMINISTRATION/DOSAGE ADJUSTMENTS

Administration of tablets	Tablets may be chewed or dissolved in the mouth

WARNINGS/PRECAUTIONS

Reye's syndrome	Package label warns patients to consult a physician before they give this product to a child or teen-ager during or after recovery from chicken pox or influenza
Persistent diarrhea, fever	Package label cautions patients to consult a physician if diarrhea continues for more than 2 days or is accompanied by high fever
Sodium content	< 2 mg/tab; for sodium content of liquid, consult manufacturer
Concomitant therapy	If tinnitus occurs after concomitant use with aspirin, discontinue use of bismuth subsalicylate; use with caution in patients requiring oral anticoagulant, antidiabetic, or antigout medication (see DRUG INTERACTIONS)

ADVERSE REACTIONS

Gastrointestinal	Temporary darkening of stool and tongue (reaction is harmless)

OVERDOSAGE

No toxic effects have been observed in clinical use

DRUG INTERACTIONS

Oral anticoagulants	△ Risk of bleeding
Insulin, oral hypoglycemics	△ Risk of hypoglycemia
Probenecid, sulfinpyrazone	▽ Uricosuric effect

ALTERED LABORATORY VALUES

Blood/serum values	△ Uric acid

No clinically significant alterations in urinary values occur at therapeutic dosages

---

USE IN CHILDREN
See INDICATIONS and ORAL DOSAGE

USE IN PREGNANT AND NURSING WOMEN
Consult manufacturer

---

[1] Salicylate content: 102 mg per tab or tbsp

ANTIDIARRHEAL AGENTS

RHEABAN (attapulgite) Leeming   OTC
Tablets: 750 mg

INDICATIONS
Diarrhea

ORAL DOSAGE
Adult: 2 tabs after initial bowel movement, followed by 2 tabs after each subsequent bowel movement
Child (6–12 yr): 1 tab after initial bowel movement, followed by 1 tab after each subsequent bowel movement

ADMINISTRATION/DOSAGE ADJUSTMENTS

Administration	Tablets should be swallowed with water; they should not be chewed
Maximum dosage	12 tabs/24 h
Duration of therapy	Labeling instructs patients not to use product for more than 2 days except under medical supervision

WARNINGS/PRECAUTIONS

Fever	Labeling cautions patients not to use product in the presence of high fever except under medical supervision

---

USE IN CHILDREN
See INDICATIONS and ORAL DOSAGE; labeling instructs parents not to use in children under 6 yr of age except under medical supervision

USE IN PREGNANT AND NURSING WOMEN
Consult manufacturer

ORAL ELECTROLYTE SOLUTIONS

GASTROLYTE Rorer
Concentrate

OTC
Calories: 16 kcal/packet

INGREDIENT	AMOUNT/packet	INGREDIENT	AMOUNT/packet
Carbohydrate (glucose)	4 g	Chloride (sodium chloride)	16 mEq
Sodium (sodium citrate, sodium chloride)	18 mEq	Citrate (sodium citrate)	6 mEq
Potassium (potassium citrate)	4 mEq		

INDICATIONS

For **maintenance of water and electrolyte levels and replacement of mild to moderate fluid losses**, particularly in mild to moderate diarrhea

ORAL DOSAGE

For children 2–12 yr of age, give up to 2 fl oz/lb/day; for adults, give 7 fl oz after each loose bowel movement. For children 2 yr of age and younger, use according to medical judgment.

CONTRAINDICATIONS

Consult manufacturer

ADMINISTRATION/DOSAGE ADJUSTMENTS

Preparation of solution — Immediately before use, dissolve contents of 1 packet in 7 fl oz (200 ml) of drinking water. The solution may be stored for up to 24 h, if refrigerated.

Patient instructions — The package labeling instructs patients to consult a physician if vomiting or fever is present or if diarrhea continues beyond 48 h

---

ORAL ELECTROLYTE SOLUTIONS

INFALYTE Pennwalt
Solution, prepared from powder

OTC
Calories: 18 kcal/8 fl oz

INGREDIENT	AMOUNT/8 fl oz	INGREDIENT	AMOUNT/8 fl oz
Carbohydrate (dextrose)	4.8 g	Chloride (sodium and potassium chloride)	9.5 mEq
Sodium (sodium chloride, sodium bicarbonate)	11.8 mEq	Bicarbonate (sodium bicarbonate)	7.1 mEq
Potassium (potassium chloride)	4.7 mEq		

INDICATIONS

For **maintenance and replacement of water and electrolytes** in mild to moderate diarrhea; in severe diarrhea, for maintenance and replacement of water and electrolyte losses following corrective parenteral therapy

ORAL DOSAGE

Administer solution at frequent intervals during the day; discontinue use once diarrhea has ceased. For infants and young children, use the table below; infants receiving breast milk will require lesser amounts. For children 4–12 yr of age, administer 1–2 qt/day for maintenance or 2–3 qt/day for replacement; for older children and adults, administer 2–3 qt/day for maintenance or 3–4 qt/day for replacement.

Weight		Daily amount of Infalyte (fl oz)[1]		Weight		Daily amount of Infalyte (fl oz)[1]	
lb	kg	For maintenance	For replacement	lb	kg	For maintenance	For replacement
5	2.3	8	14	25	11.4	27	44
10	4.5	14	22	30	13.6	31	50
15	6.8	19	30	35	15.9	35	56
20	9.1	23	37	40	18.2	38	61

ADMINISTRATION/DOSAGE ADJUSTMENTS

Preparation of solution — Dissolve contents of 24-g packet in 1 qt of water or contents of 6-g packet in 8 fl oz of water; use solution within 24 h. Store covered in refrigerator.

INFALYTE ■ PEDIALYTE

Concomitant administration of food	During the first 8 h of treatment, do not administer liquids or solid food; however, breast-feeding may be continued. Lactose-free products, such as soy-based formula (diluted 1:1 with water), rice cereal (mixed with water), pureed fruit, or other age-appropriate foods, may be given after the first 8 h, even if diarrhea has not ceased; cow's milk or lactose-containing products prepared from cow's milk should not be given until 24 h after cessation of diarrhea.
Patients who have been severely dehydrated	Infalyte may be given once dehydration has been reduced to 5–8% and blood pressure and pulse rate have stabilized

WARNINGS/PRECAUTIONS

Special-risk patients	Use with caution in patients with renal insufficiency or diabetes, as well as in those taking digitalis, diuretics, or potassium supplements

[1] Daily amount in the table is for infants who are not breast-feeding; if the infant will receive breast milk during therapy, use a smaller amount

---

ORAL ELECTROLYTE SOLUTIONS

LYTREN Mead Johnson   OTC
Solution, ready to use   Calories: 24 kcal/8 fl oz

INGREDIENT	AMOUNT/ 8 fl oz	INGREDIENT	AMOUNT/ 8 fl oz
Carbohydrate (glucose, corn syrup solids)	6 g	Chloride (sodium chloride)	11 mEq
Sodium (sodium citrate, sodium chloride)	12 mEq	Citrate (sodium and potassium citrate, citric acid)	7 mEq
Potassium (potassium citrate)	6 mEq		

INDICATIONS
For **maintenance of water and electrolyte levels and replacement of mild to moderate fluid losses,** particularly in mild to moderate diarrhea, for prevention of dehydration, and after surgery

ORAL DOSAGE
Begin administration of Lytren as soon as usual foods and liquids are discontinued. Intake should approximate patient's calculated daily water requirements for maintenance and replacement of losses, and may be given in divided doses, as desired or appropriate. For infants and young children, give 50 fl oz/m^2/day for maintenance and 80 fl oz/m^2/day for maintenance and replacement to start or, alternatively, administer an initial dosage based on body weight (see following table).

Weight lb.	kg	Daily amount of Lytren (fl oz) For maintenance	For maintenance and replacement	Weight lb.	kg	Daily amount of Lytren (fl oz) For maintenance	For maintenance and replacement
6–7	3	10	16	26	12	28	44
11	5	15	23	33	15	32	51
15	7	19	30	40	18	38	61
22	10	25	40				

Adjust intake according to individual needs and clinical conditions. For children 5–10 yr of age, give 1–2 qt daily; for older children and adults, give 2 qt or more daily. Do not mix Lytren with, or give concomitantly with, other electrolyte-containing liquids, such as milk or fruit juice; intake of Lytren should be discontinued upon reintroduction of other electrolyte-containing foods into the patient's diet.

CONTRAINDICATIONS

Severe, continuing diarrhea or other critical fluid losses requiring parenteral fluid therapy	Intractable vomiting, adynamic ileus, intestinal obstruction, or perforated bowel	Depressed renal function or impaired homeostatic mechanisms

ADMINISTRATION/DOSAGE ADJUSTMENTS

Additional liquids	Water or other non-electrolyte-containing liquids should be given to satisfy thirst
Concomitant parenteral therapy	Lytren may be given simultaneously to supplement parenteral fluid therapy in emergency cases; however, do not exceed total water and electrolyte requirements. Lytren alone may be used after emergency needs have been met.

ORAL ELECTROLYTE SOLUTIONS

PEDIALYTE Ross   OTC
Ready to use solution   Calories: 24 kcal/8 fl oz

INGREDIENT[1]	AMOUNT/ 8 fl oz	INGREDIENT[1]	AMOUNT/ 8 fl oz
Carbohydrate (dextrose)	5.9 g	Potassium (potassium citrate)	4.7 mEq
Sodium (sodium chloride, sodium citrate)	10.6 mEq	Citrate (sodium citrate, potassium citrate)	7.1 mEq
Chloride (sodium chloride)	8.3 mEq		

INDICATIONS
For **maintenance of water and electrolytes** in infants and children either during mild to moderate diarrhea or following corrective parenteral treatment of severe diarrhea

PEDIALYTE

ORAL DOSAGE

Divide daily intake into frequent feedings, adjusting dosage to meet individual needs based on thirst and patient response. For infants and children 1 wk to 4 yr of age, use the table below. Ongoing stool loss is not considered in this table; therefore, to determine the appropriate dosage, add the amount of fluid lost daily in loose stools to the daily amount recommended in this table.

Age	Weight (kg)	Daily amount of Pedialyte (fl oz)	Age	Weight (kg)	Daily amount of Pedialyte (fl oz)
2 wk	3.2	13–16	2 yr	12.6	48–53
3 mo	6.0	28–32	2½ yr	13.6	51–56
6 mo	7.8	34–40	3 yr	14.6	54–58
9 mo	9.2	38–44	3½ yr	16.0	56–60
1 yr	10.2	41–46	4 yr	17.0	57–62
1½ yr	11.4	45–50			

For children over 4 yr of age, give 2 qt or more daily

PEDIALYTE RS Ross

OTC

Ready to use solution Calories: 24 kcal/8 fl oz

INGREDIENT	AMOUNT/ 8 fl oz	INGREDIENT	AMOUNT/ 8 fl oz
Carbohydrate (dextrose)	5.9 g	Potassium (potassium citrate)	4.7 mEq
Sodium (sodium chloride, sodium citrate)	17.7 mEq	Citrate (sodium citrate, potassium citrate)	7.1 mEq
Chloride (sodium chloride)	15.4 mEq		

INDICATIONS

For **replacement of water and electrolytes** during moderate to severe diarrhea

ORAL DOSAGE

Divide daily intake into frequent feedings, adjusting dosage to meet individual needs based on thirst and patient response. For infants and children 1 wk to 4 yr of age, use the table below. Ongoing stool loss is not considered in this table; therefore, to determine the appropriate dosage, add the amount of fluid lost daily in loose stools to the daily amount recommended in this table.

Age	Weight (kg)	Daily amount of Pedialyte RS (fl oz) For 5% dehydration	For 10% dehydration	Age	Weight (kg)	Daily amount of Pedialyte RS (fl oz) For 5% dehydration	For 10% dehydration
2 wk	3.2	18–21	23–26	2 yr	12.6	69–74	90–95
3 mo	6.0	38–42	48–52	2½ yr	13.6	74–79	97–102
6 mo	7.8	47–53	60–66	3 yr	14.6	78–82	102–106
9 mo	9.2	53–59	68–74	3½ yr	16.0	83–87	110–114
1 yr	10.2	58–63	75–80	4 yr	17.0	85–90	113–118
1½ yr	11.4	64–69	83–88				

For children over 4 yr of age, give 2 qt or more daily

[1] Composition of unflavored Pedialyte; fruit-flavored solution is similar in composition and nutrient values (see package label for specific information)

Chapter 19

Antifungal/Antitrichomonal/Antiviral Agents/Other Topicals

Topical Preparations — 673

GARAMYCIN Cream (Schering) — 673
Gentamicin sulfate *Rx*

GARAMYCIN Ointment (Schering) — 673
Gentamicin sulfate *Rx*

HALOTEX (Westwood) — 674
Haloprogin *Rx*

LOPROX (Hoechst-Roussel) — 674
Ciclopirox olamine *Rx*

LOTRIMIN (Schering) — 675
Clotrimazole *Rx*

LOTRISONE (Schering) — 676
Clotrimazole and betamethasone dipropionate *Rx*

MONISTAT-DERM (Ortho) — 677
Miconazole nitrate *Rx*

MYCELEX (Miles Pharmaceuticals) — 677
Clotrimazole *Rx*

MYCELEX Troche (Miles Pharmaceuticals) — 678
Clotrimazole *Rx*

MYCOLOG-II (Squibb) — 679
Nystatin and triamcinolone acetonide *Rx*

MYCOSTATIN Cream, Ointment, and Powder (Squibb) — 680
Nystatin *Rx*

NEOSPORIN Cream (Burroughs Wellcome) — 680
Polymyxin B sulfate and neomycin sulfate *OTC*

NEOSPORIN Ointment (Burroughs Wellcome) — 680
Polymyxin B sulfate, bacitracin zinc, and neomycin sulfate *OTC*

NIZORAL Cream (Janssen) — 681
Ketoconazole *Rx*

POLYSPORIN (Burroughs Wellcome) — 682
Polymyxin B sulfate and bacitracin zinc *OTC*

SILVADENE (Marion) — 682
Silver sulfadiazine *Rx*

SPECTAZOLE (Ortho) — 683
Econazole nitrate *Rx*

TINACTIN (Schering) — 684
Tolnaftate *OTC*

ZOVIRAX Ointment (Burroughs Wellcome) — 685
Acyclovir *Rx*

Vaginal Preparations — 685

AVC (Merrell Dow) — 685
Sulfanilamide, aminacrine hydrochloride, and allantoin *Rx*

FEMSTAT (Syntex) — 686
Butoconazole nitrate *Rx*

GYNE-LOTRIMIN (Schering) — 687
Clotrimazole *Rx*

MONISTAT 3 (Ortho) — 687
Miconazole nitrate *Rx*

MONISTAT 7 (Ortho) — 687
Miconazole nitrate *Rx*

MONISTAT DUAL-PAK (Ortho) — 687
Miconazole nitrate *Rx*

MYCELEX-G (Miles Pharmaceuticals) — 688
Clotrimazole *Rx*

MYCELEX TWIN PACK (Miles Pharmaceuticals) — 688
Clotrimazole *Rx*

MYCOSTATIN Vaginal Tablets (Squibb) — 689
Nystatin *Rx*

SULTRIN (Ortho) — 690
Sulfathiazole, sulfacetamide, and sulfabenzamide (triple sulfa) *Rx*

VAGISEC (Schmid) — 691
Polyoxyethylene nonyl phenol, sodium edetate, and sodium dioctyl sulfosuccinate *OTC*

VAGISEC PLUS (Schmid) — 691
9-Aminoacridine hydrochloride, polyoxyethylene nonyl phenol, sodium edetate, and sodium dioctyl sulfosuccinate *Rx*

VAGITROL (Lemmon) — 692
Sulfanilamide *Rx*

Systemic Agents — 692

ANCOBON (Roche) — 692
Flucytosine *Rx*

FLAGYL (Searle) — 693
Metronidazole *Rx*

FULVICIN P/G 165 and 330 (Schering) — 695
Griseofulvin, ultramicrosize *Rx*

FULVICIN-U/F (Schering) — 695
Griseofulvin, microsize *Rx*

FUNGIZONE (Squibb) — 696
Amphotericin B *Rx*

MONISTAT i.v. (Janssen) — 698
Miconazole *Rx*

MYCOSTATIN (Squibb) — 700
Nystatin *Rx*

NIZORAL (Janssen) — 700
Ketoconazole *Rx*

PROTOSTAT (Ortho) — 702
Metronidazole *Rx*

SYMMETREL (Du Pont) — 704
Amantadine hydrochloride *Rx*

VIRA-A (Parke-Davis) — 705
Vidarabine monohydrate *Rx*

VIRAZOLE (ICN Pharmaceuticals) — 707
Ribavirin *Rx*

ZOVIRAX Capsules (Burroughs Wellcome) — 708
Acyclovir *Rx*

ZOVIRAX Sterile Powder (Burroughs Wellcome) — 709
Acyclovir sodium *Rx*

Debriding Agents	**711**
BIOZYME-C (Armour) Collagenase Rx	711
ELASE (Parke-Davis) Fibrinolysin and desoxyribonuclease, combined (bovine) Rx	712
ELASE-CHLOROMYCETIN (Parke-Davis) Fibrinolysin and desoxyribonuclease, combined (bovine), and chloramphenicol Rx	712
SANTYL (Knoll) Collagenase Rx	713
TRAVASE (Flint) Sutilains Rx	714

Other Antifungal Agents	**669**
AFTATE (Plough) Tolnaftate OTC	669
DESENEX (Pharmacraft) Undecylenate OTC	670
GRIFULVIN V (Ortho) Griseofulvin microsize Rx	670
GRISACTIN (Ayerst) Griseofulvin microsize Rx	670
GRISACTIN Ultra (Ayerst) Griseofulvin ultramicrosize Rx	670
Gris-PEG (Herbert) Griseofulvin ultramicrosize Rx	670
MICATIN (Advanced Care Products) Miconazole nitrate OTC	670
NILSTAT (Lederle) Nystatin Rx	670
VIOFORM (CIBA) Clioquinol OTC	670

Other Topical Anti-Infectives	**671**
ACHROMYCIN Ointment (Lederle) Tetracycline hydrochloride OTC	671
AUREOMYCIN Ointment (Lederle) Chlortetracycline hydrochloride OTC	671
BACIGUENT Ointment (Upjohn) Bacitracin OTC	671
BETADINE (Purdue Frederick) Povidone-iodine OTC	671
CHLOROMYCETIN Cream (Parke-Davis) Chloramphenicol Rx	672
FLINT SSD (Travenol) Silver sulfadiazine Rx	672
FURACIN (Norwich Eaton) Nitrofurazone Rx	672
HIBICLENS Antiseptic Antimicrobial Skin Cleanser (Stuart) Chlorhexidine gluconate OTC	672
HIBISTAT Germicidal Hand Rinse (Stuart) Chlorhexidine gluconate OTC	672
MYCIGUENT Ointment (Upjohn) Neomycin sulfate OTC	672
MYCITRACIN (Upjohn) Bacitracin, neomycin sulfate, and polymyxin B sulfate OTC	672
NEO-POLYCIN (Lakeside) Neomycin sulfate, polymyxin B sulfate, and bacitracin zinc OTC	672

OTHER ANTIFUNGAL AGENTS

DRUG	HOW SUPPLIED	USUAL DOSAGE[1]
AFTATE (Plough) Tolnaftate OTC	Gel: 1% (0.5 fl oz) Spray liquid: 1% (4 fl oz) Powder: 1% (1.5, 2.25 oz) Spray powder: 1% (3.5 oz)	Adult: apply liberally over affected area bid; wash and dry area before each application. After symptoms disappear, continue use for 2 wk; to help prevent recurrence, apply powder or spray powder daily.

[1] Where pediatric dosages are not given, consult manufacturer

OTHER ANTIFUNGAL AGENTS continued

DRUG	HOW SUPPLIED	USUAL DOSAGE[1]
DESENEX (Pharmacraft) Undecylenate *OTC*	**Cream:** 20% (0.5, 1 oz) **Ointment:** 22% (0.9, 1.8 oz) **Powder:** 19% (1.5, 3 oz) **Spray powder:** 19% (2.7, 5.5 oz) **Liquid:** 10% undecylenic acid (1.5 fl oz) **Foam:** 10% undecylenic acid (1.5 oz)	Adult and child (2–12 yr): apply over affected area bid (morning and night); pay special attention to the space between the toes. Wash and dry area before each application. For persistent cases, use cream or ointment at night and powder or spray powder during the day. To prevent recurrence, use powder or spray powder daily.
GRIFULVIN V (Ortho) Griseofulvin microsize *Rx*	**Tablets:** 250, 500 mg **Suspension (per 5 ml):** 125 mg (4 fl oz)	**Adult:** 500 mg/day, or 1 g/day in severe cases **Child (30–50 lb):** 125–250 mg/day **Child (> 50 lb):** 250–500 mg/day
GRISACTIN (Ayerst) Griseofulvin microsize *Rx*	**Capsules:** 125, 250 mg **Tablets:** 500 mg	**Adult:** 500 mg/day, given in a single dose or 2–4 divided doses; some patients may require less or more, up to 1 g/day, depending on severity of infection **Child (30–50 lb):** 125–250 mg/day **Child (> 50 lb):** 250–500 mg/day, given in divided doses
GRISACTIN Ultra (Ayerst) Griseofulvin ultramicrosize *Rx*	**Tablets:** 125, 250, 330 mg	**Adult:** for tinea corporis, cruris, or capitis, 330 mg/day, given in a single dose or divided doses; for tinea pedis or unguium, 660 mg/day, given in divided doses **Child (35–50 lb):** 125–165 mg/day **Child (50–75 lb):** 165–250 mg/day **Child (≥ 75 lb):** 250–330 mg/day
Gris-PEG (Herbert) Griseofulvin ultramicrosize *Rx*	**Tablets:** 125, 250 mg	**Adult:** for tinea corporis, cruris, or capitis, 375 mg/day, given in a single dose or divided doses; for tinea pedis or unguium, 750 mg/day, given in divided doses **Child (> 2 yr and ≥ 35 lb):** 3.3 mg/lb/day, not to exceed 375 mg/day; for tinea capitis, give in a single daily dose
MICATIN (Advanced Care Products) Miconazole nitrate *OTC*	**Cream:** 2% (0.5, 1 oz) **Powder:** 2% (1.5 oz) **Spray liquid:** 2% (3.5 oz) **Spray powder:** 2% (3 oz)	Adult and child (2–12 yr): apply a thin layer of cream, powder, or liquid over affected area bid (morning and evening)
NILSTAT (Lederle) Nystatin *Rx*	**Oral tablets:** 500,000 units **Powder:** 500,000 units per 1/8 tsp (0.15, 1, 2 billion units) **Suspension:** 100,000 units/ml (2, 16 fl oz) **Vaginal tablets:** 100,000 units	**Adult:** 500,000–1,000,000 units tid **Adult and older child:** 500,000 units, mixed in 4–8 fl oz of water, qid; rinse mouth thoroughly with each dose and retain as long as possible **Adult and child:** 400,000–600,000 units (2–3 ml in each side of mouth) qid **Infant:** 200,000 units (1 ml in each side of mouth) qid; for premature and low-birth-weight infants, 100,000 units qid may be effective **Adult:** 100,000 units (1 tab)/day for 14 days
VIOFORM (CIBA) Clioquinol *OTC*	**Cream:** 3% (1 oz) **Ointment:** 3% (1 oz)	**Adult:** apply to affected area bid or tid

[1] Where pediatric dosages are not given, consult manufacturer

OTHER TOPICAL ANTI-INFECTIVES

DRUG	HOW SUPPLIED	USUAL DOSAGE[1]
ACHROMYCIN Ointment (Lederle) Tetracycline hydrochloride *OTC*	Ointment: 3% (28.4 g)	**Adult and child:** after cleansing, apply to affected area 1–2 times/day
AUREOMYCIN Ointment (Lederle) Chlortetracycline hydrochloride *OTC*	Ointment: 3% (1/2, 1 oz)	**Adult:** apply to affected area 1 or more times/day, preferably on sterile gauze; for severe local infection, supplement treatment with appropriate oral antibiotic
BACIGUENT Ointment (Upjohn) Bacitracin *OTC*	Ointment (per gram): 500 units (0.5, 1, 4 oz)	**Adult and child:** apply liberally to affected area 1–2 times/day and cover with sterile gauze
BETADINE (Purdue Frederick) Povidone-iodine *OTC*	**Aerosol Spray:** 5% povidone-iodine (0.5% available iodine) (3 fl oz)	**Adult:** spray affected area thoroughly, as needed
	Douche: 10% povidone-iodine (1% available iodine) (0.5-fl oz packet; 1-, 8-fl oz bottle)	**Adult:** for vaginitis, 0.5 fl oz (1 tbsp) in 1 qt of lukewarm water once daily, preferably before bedtime, for the entire menstrual cycle; for minor irritation and pruritus, 0.5 fl oz in 1 qt of lukewarm water once daily for 5 days; for cleansing, 0.5 fl oz in 1 qt of lukewarm water once or twice weekly
	Douche kit: 10% povidone-iodine (8 fl oz)	**Adult:** for vaginitis, 2 douches (each containing 0.5 fl oz [1 tbsp] in ~ 14 fl oz of lukewarm water) once daily, preferably before bedtime, for the entire menstrual cycle; for minor irritation and pruritus, 0.5 fl oz in ~ 14 fl oz of lukewarm water once daily for 5 days; for cleansing, 0.5 fl oz in ~ 14 fl oz of lukewarm water once or twice weekly
	Gauze pad: 10% povidone-iodine (1% available iodine)	**Adult:** apply directly to affected area
	Helafoam solution: 10% povidone-iodine (1% available iodine) (9 fl oz)	**Adult:** apply liberally to affected area, as needed
	Medicated douche: 0.25% povidone-iodine (0.18-fl oz packet with 6 fl oz sanitized water)	**Adult:** for minor irritation and pruritus, 0.18 fl oz in 6 fl oz of water once daily for 5 days; for cleansing, 0.18 fl oz in 6 fl oz of water once or twice weekly
	Microbicidal bath concentrate: 10% povidone-iodine (1 pt)	**Adult:** for routine disinfection, add 2½ fl oz to 50 gal (1 tubful) of water and stir
	Mouthwash/gargle: 0.5% povidone-iodine (0.05% available iodine) in 8% alcohol (6, 12 fl oz)	**Adult:** dilute with 2 parts water or use full strength
	Ointment: 10% povidone-iodine (1% available iodine) (1/32, 1/8, 1 oz; 1, 5 lb)	**Adult:** apply directly to affected area, as needed
	Perineal wash: 10% povidone-iodine (8 fl oz)	**Adult:** fill dispenser bottle to bottom line with concentrate, add water to top line, and irrigate area until bottle empties; repeat, as needed
	Skin cleanser: 7.5% povidone-iodine (0.75% available iodine) (1, 4 fl oz)	**Adult:** apply to wetted skin, lather, and allow to remain for 3 min; repeat bid, tid, or as needed
	Skin Cleanser Foam: 10% povidone-iodine (6 oz)	**Adult:** apply to wetted skin, rub to develop lather, and rinse
	Solution: 10% povidone-iodine (1% available iodine) (0.5, 4, 8, 16, 32, 128 fl oz)	**Adult:** apply full strength to affected area, as needed
	Sponge brush: 7.5% povidone-iodine	**Adult:** for preoperative hand scrubbing, rub on wetted hands and arms to develop lather, and rinse
	Surgical scrub: 7.5% povidone-iodine (0.75% available iodine) (0.5, 16, 32, 128 fl oz)	**Adult:** for microbicidal washing and scrubbing of hands and forearms, rub 1 tsp over wetted areas for 5 min, add water to develop suds, rinse, and repeat; for preoperative preparation of patient, lather and scrub 1 ml/20–30 in² over shaved, wetted area for 5 min and rinse

[1] Where pediatric dosages are not given, consult manufacturer

continued

OTHER TOPICAL ANTI-INFECTIVES continued

DRUG	HOW SUPPLIED	USUAL DOSAGE[1]
BETADINE (Purdue Frederick) Povidone-iodine *OTC*	**Swab aid:** 10% povidone-iodine	**Adult:** swab affected areas thoroughly, as needed
	Swabsticks: 10% povidone-iodine	**Adult:** apply directly to affected area, as needed
	Vaginal gel: 10% povidone-iodine (1% available iodine) (18 g, 3 oz)	**Adult:** 1 applicatorful at night for 7 days
	Vaginal suppositories: 10% povidone-iodine	**Adult:** 1 suppository at night for 7 days
	Viscous formula gauze pad: 10% povidone-iodine (1% available iodine)	**Adult:** apply directly to affected area, as needed
	Whirlpool concentrate: 10% povidone-iodine (1% available iodine) (1 gal)	**Adult:** for routine disinfection, add 1 fl oz to each 20 gal of water
CHLOROMYCETIN Cream (Parke-Davis) Chloramphenicol *Rx*	**Cream:** 1% (1 oz)	**Adult:** after cleansing, apply to affected area tid or qid
FLINT SSD (Travenol) Silver sulfadiazine *Rx*	**Cream:** 1% (50, 400 g)	**Adult:** apply a layer at least 1/16 in. thick to selected burn areas, using sterile gloves, 1-2 times/day; reapply cream immediately after hydrotherapy and promptly if removed by patient movement; continue treatment until spontaneous healing or grafting of the wound is achieved
FURACIN (Norwich Eaton) Nitrofurazone *Rx*	**Cream:** 0.2% (14, 28, 368 g) **Soluble dressing:** 0.2% (28, 56, 135, 454 g)	**Adult:** for burns, apply directly to lesion or first place on gauze; reapply once daily or less often, depending on preferred dressing technique
HIBICLENS Antiseptic Antimicrobial Skin Cleanser (Stuart) Chlorhexidine gluconate *OTC*	**Skin cleanser:** 4% (1/2, 4, 8, 16, 32 fl oz; 1 gal)	**Adult:** for skin wounds and general skin cleansing, rinse area thoroughly with water, apply liberally to involved area, wash gently, and rinse again thoroughly; for preoperative skin preparation, swab surgical site for 2 min, dry with a sterile towel, and repeat once; for use as a surgical hand scrub, wet hands and forearms, scrub for 3 min with about 5 ml and wet brush, rinse thoroughly, repeat once, and dry; for hand washing, wet hands, scrub vigorously for 15 s with about 5 ml, rinse, and dry thoroughly
	Sponge/brush: 4% (22 ml of solution)	**Adult:** for preoperative hand scrubbing, rub wetted sponge side on wet hands and forearms to develop lather, scrub fngers and nails with brush for 3 min, and rinse; repeat scrubbing for 3 min with sponge side only, rinse thoroughly, and dry
HIBISTAT Germicidal Hand Rinse (Stuart) Chlorhexidine gluconate *OTC*	**Liquid:** 0.5% chlorhexidine gluconate, 70% isopropyl alcohol, and emollients (4, 8 fl oz) **Towelettes:** 0.5% chlorhexidine gluconate, 70% isopropyl alcohol, and emollients (5 ml)	**Adult:** dispense about 5 ml of liquid into cupped hands or use towelette and rub vigorously until dry (about 15 s), paying particular attention to nails and interdigital spaces
MYCIGUENT Ointment (Upjohn) Neomycin sulfate *OTC*	**Ointment (per gram):** 5 mg neomycin sulfate equivalent to 3.5 mg neomycin (0.5, 1, 4 oz)	**Adult and child:** apply liberally to affected area 1-2 times/day; cover with sterile gauze
MYCITRACIN (Upjohn) Bacitracin, neomycin sulfate, and polymyxin B sulfate *OTC*	**Ointment (per gram):** 500 units bacitracin, neomycin sulfate equivalent to 3.5 mg neomycin, and 5,000 units polymyxin B sulfate (1/32, 1/2, 1 oz)	**Adult:** apply liberally to affected area 1-2 times/day **Child:** same as adult
NEO-POLYCIN (Lakeside) Neomycin sulfate, polymyxin B sulfate, and bacitracin zinc *OTC*	**Ointment (per gram):** neomycin sulfate equivalent to 3.5 mg neomycin, 5,000 units polymyxin B sulfate, and 400 units bacitracin zinc (1/2 oz)	**Adult and child:** apply a thin film to affected area 1-2 times/day

[1] Where pediatric dosages are not given, consult manufacturer

TOPICAL PREPARATIONS

GARAMYCIN Cream (gentamicin sulfate) Schering   Rx
Cream: 0.1% (15 g)

GARAMYCIN Ointment (gentamicin sulfate) Schering   Rx
Ointment: 0.1% (15 g)

INDICATIONS

Primary skin infections,[1] including impetigo contagiosa, superficial folliculitis, ecthyma, furunculosis, sycosis barbae, and pyoderma gangrenosum
Secondary skin infections,[1] including infectious eczematoid dermatitis, pustular acne, pustular psoriasis, infected contact dermatitis (including poison ivy), infected excoriations, and bacterial superinfections of fungal or viral infections
Infected skin cysts and other skin abscesses, when preceded by incision and drainage; **infected stasis and other skin ulcers; infected superficial burns; paronychia; infected insect bites and stings; infected lacerations and abrasions; infected wounds from minor surgery**

TOPICAL DOSAGE

Adult: apply a small amount of cream or ointment to the lesion tid or qid; cover area with gauze dressing, if desired
Infant ($>$ 1 yr) and child: same as adult

CONTRAINDICATIONS
Hypersensitivity to any of the components

ADMINISTRATION/DOSAGE ADJUSTMENTS

Impetigo contagiosa	Crusts should be removed before application to permit maximum contact between the antibiotic and the infecting bacteria
Infected stasis ulcers	Have responded well to topical gentamicin therapy under gelatin packing
Choice of dosage form	Ointment aids in retaining moisture and is useful on dry eczematous or psoriatic skin; cream is recommended for wet, oozing primary infections and greasy secondary infections, such as pustular acne or infected seborrheic dermatitis, or when a water-washable preparation is desired

WARNINGS/PRECAUTIONS

Overgrowth of nonsusceptible organisms	Nonsusceptible organisms, including fungi, may proliferate during treatment; discontinue use and institute appropriate therapy
Irritation, sensitization, or superinfection	May occur; discontinue treatment and institute appropriate measures
Patients sensitive to topical antibiotics	Topical gentamicin can be used in patients sensitive to neomycin, with periodic observation

ADVERSE REACTIONS

Local	Erythema, pruritus[2]

USE IN CHILDREN
Same as adult indications and dosage; safety and effectiveness have not been established for use in infants under 1 yr of age

USE IN PREGNANT AND NURSING WOMEN
Safety for use during pregnancy has not been established; use only if clearly needed. Aminoglycosides cross the placental barrier. Total irreversible bilateral congenital deafness has been reported in children whose mothers received streptomycin during pregnancy. However, serious side effects have not been reported in pregnant women given other aminoglycosides. Trace amounts of gentamicin are excreted in human milk; use with caution in nursing mothers. No adverse effect was observed in animal pups nursed by dams receiving gentamicin.

VEHICLE/BASE
Cream (bland, emulsion type): stearic acid, propylene glycol monostearate, isopropyl myristate, propylene glycol, polysorbate 40, sorbitol solution, and purified water, with methylparaben and butylparaben as preservatives
Ointment (bland, unctuous): petrolatum, with methylparaben and propylparaben as preservatives

[1] Not effective against viruses or fungi in skin infections
[2] Photosensitization has also been reported, but a causal relationship has not been established

TOPICAL PREPARATIONS

HALOTEX (haloprogin) Westwood Rx
Cream: 1% (15, 30 g) **Solution:** 1% (10, 30 ml)

INDICATIONS	
Tinea pedis, tinea cruris, tinea corporis, and tinea manuum caused by *Trichophyton rubrum, T tonsurans, T mentagrophytes, Microsporum canis,* and *Epidermophyton floccosum* **Tinea versicolor** caused by *Malassezia furfur*	**TOPICAL DOSAGE** **Adult:** apply cream or solution liberally to affected areas bid for 2–3 wk or, if lesion is intertriginous, for up to 4 wk

CONTRAINDICATIONS
Hypersensitivity to haloprogin or other components

WARNINGS/PRECAUTIONS

KOH tests	To confirm the diagnosis, obtain KOH smears and/or cultures before starting therapy; to monitor therapeutic response, repeat the test every 2 wk during therapy and then 2–4 wk after treatment. Reassess the diagnosis if no improvement is evident after 4 wk of use.
Mixed infections	Other antibiotics may be necessary in mixed infections where bacteria or nonsusceptible fungi are also present
Irritation	If irritation occurs, patch testing with the components of these products may be useful to verify the reaction and identify its cause; if sensitization is observed or irritation persists, discontinue use. Caution patients to avoid contact with the eyes.
Carcinogenicity, mutagenicity	No studies have been done to evaluate the carcinogenic potential of this drug; mutagenic effects have not been detected with the Ames test

ADVERSE REACTIONS
The most frequent reactions, regardless of incidence, are printed in *italics*

Local	*Burning and/or irritation (0.8% with cream, 1.7% with solution);* pruritus and vesiculation (with solution); erythema, scaling, pruritus, and folliculitis (with cream)

USE IN CHILDREN
Safety and effectiveness for use in children have not been established

USE IN PREGNANT AND NURSING WOMEN
Pregnancy Cagegory B: no evidence of impaired fertility or harm to the fetus has been detected following topical use on rats and rabbits; the animals were given over a period of 10 days 3 times the estimated total human dose required for a 30-day course of therapy. No adequate, well-controlled studies have been done in pregnant women. Use during pregnancy only if clearly needed. It is not known whether haloprogin is excreted in human milk; caution should be exercised when these preparations are used by nursing mothers.

VEHICLE/BASE
Cream (water-dispersible): polyethylene glycol 400, polyethylene glycol 4000, diethyl sebacate, and polyvinylpyrrolidone
Solution (colorless): diethyl sebacate and 75% alcohol

TOPICAL PREPARATIONS

LOPROX (ciclopirox olamine) Hoechst-Roussel Rx
Cream: 1% (15, 30, 90 g)

INDICATIONS	**TOPICAL DOSAGE**
Tinea pedis, tinea cruris, and tinea corporis caused by *Trichophyton rubrum, T mentagrophytes, Epidermophyton floccosum,* and *Microsporum canis* **Candidiasis** caused by *Candida albicans* **Tinea versicolor** caused by *Malassezia furfur*	**Adult:** gently massage cream into affected and surrounding skin areas bid (morning and evening) **Child ($\geq$ 10 yr):** same as adult

CONTRAINDICATIONS
Hypersensitivity to any component

WARNINGS/PRECAUTIONS

Lack of response	Pruritus and other symptoms will usually improve within the first week of treatment; tinea versicolor usually responds in 2 wk. If no clinical improvement is evident after 4 wk of continued use, the diagnosis should be reconsidered.

Sensitivity or chemical irritation	Discontinue use of this medication and institute appropriate therapy if erythema, pruritus, burning, blistering, edema, or other reactions suggesting sensitivity or irritation occur
Occlusive dressings	Caution patient not to use occlusive wrappings or dressings
Carcinogenicity, mutagenicity	Topical administration of ciclopirox for 50 wk produced no evidence of carcinogenicity in female mice; several tests have shown no indication of mutagenicity

ADVERSE REACTIONS

Local	Pruritus, burning sensation, clinical worsening of underlying lesion

---

USE IN CHILDREN

See INDICATIONS and TOPICAL DOSAGE; safety and effectiveness for use in children under 10 yr of age have not been established

USE IN PREGNANT AND NURSING WOMEN

Pregnancy Category B: reproduction studies in mice, rats, rabbits, and monkeys at doses 10 or more times greater than the recommended human dose have shown no significant evidence of impaired fertility or harm to the fetus; however, no adequate, well-controlled studies have been done in pregnant women. Use during pregnancy only if clearly needed. It is not known whether ciclopirox is excreted in human milk; use with caution in nursing mothers.

VEHICLE/BASE
Cream (water miscible): 2-octyldodecanol, mineral oil, stearyl alcohol, cetyl alcohol, polysorbate 60, myristyl alcohol, cocamide DEA, sorbitan monostearate, lactic acid, purified water, and 1% benzyl alcohol

---

TOPICAL PREPARATIONS

LOTRIMIN (clotrimazole) Schering   Rx

Cream: 1% (15, 30, 45, 90 g)   **Lotion:** 1% (30 ml)   **Solution:** 1% (10, 30 ml)

INDICATIONS

Tinea pedis, tinea cruris, and tinea corporis caused by *Trichophyton rubrum, T mentagrophytes, Epidermophyton floccosum,* and *Microsporum canis*
Candidiasis caused by *Candida albicans*
Tinea versicolor caused by *Malassezia furfur*

TOPICAL DOSAGE

Adult: gently massage cream, lotion, or solution into affected and surrounding areas bid (AM and PM)
Child: same as adult

CONTRAINDICATIONS

Hypersensitivity to clotrimazole or other components

WARNINGS/PRECAUTIONS

Irritation or sensitivity	Discontinue therapy and institute appropriate treatment; avoid contact with eyes
Lack of response	Pruritus and other symptoms usually improve within the first week of treatment; if no clinical improvement is evident after 4 wk of continual use, the diagnosis should be reconsidered and appropriate microbiological studies repeated. A second course of therapy may be administered if the diagnosis is confirmed and other pathogens are ruled out
Carcinogenicity, mutagenicity	Oral administration of clotrimazole for 18 mo has produced no evidence of carcinogenicity in rats; no mutagenic effects have been detected in Chinese hamsters following administration of 5 oral doses of 100 mg/kg each

ADVERSE REACTIONS

Local	Erythema, stinging, blistering, peeling, edema, pruritus, urticaria, burning, irritation

---

USE IN CHILDREN

See INDICATIONS and TOPICAL DOSAGE

USE IN PREGNANT AND NURSING WOMEN

Pregnancy Category B: no evidence of harm to the fetus has been detected in rats given up to 100 mg/kg intravaginally; reproduction studies have demonstrated embryotoxicity (possibly due to maternal toxicity), impairment of mating, and decreases in litter size, number of viable young, and pup survival in mice and rats given oral doses of 50–120 mg/kg, but have shown no evidence of teratogenicity in mice fed up to 200 mg/kg, rats (100 mg/kg), or rabbits (180 mg/kg). In humans, clotrimazole is very poorly absorbed following topical administration; however, no adequate, well-controlled studies have evaluated the safety of topical use during the first trimester. Administer during the first trimester only if clearly needed. In clinical studies, intravaginal administration during the second and third trimesters has not adversely affected fetal development. It is not known whether clotrimazole is excreted in human milk; use with caution in nursing mothers.

VEHICLE/BASE
Cream (vanishing): sorbitan monostearate, polysorbate 60, cetyl esters wax, cetearyl alcohol, 2-octyldodecanol, and purified water, with 1% benzyl alcohol as a preservative
Lotion: sorbitan monostearate, polysorbate 60, cetyl esters wax, cetearyl alcohol, 2-octyldodecanol, 1% benzyl alcohol, sodium phosphate dibasic, sodium biphosphate, and purified water
Solution (nonaqueous): polyethylene glycol 400

LOTRISONE

TOPICAL PREPARATIONS

LOTRISONE (clotrimazole and betamethasone dipropionate) Schering   Rx

Cream: 1% clotrimazole and 0.05% betamethasone (15, 45 g)

INDICATIONS

Tinea pedis, tinea cruris, and tinea corporis caused by *Trichophyton rubrum, T mentagrophytes, Epidermophyton floccosum,* and *Microsporum canis*

TOPICAL DOSAGE

Adult: gently massage cream into affected and surrounding areas bid (morning and evening); use for 4 wk when treating tinea pedis and for 2 wk when treating tinea cruris or tinea corporis

Child: same as adult (see USE IN CHILDREN)

CONTRAINDICATIONS

Hypersensitivity to any component, other imidazoles, or other corticosteroids

WARNINGS/PRECAUTIONS

Occlusive dressings — Do not use this preparation under occlusive dressings; caution patients not to bandage or otherwise cover the treated area and not to use tight-fitting diapers or plastic pants on a child if the preparation is applied to the diaper area

Systemic absorption — Reversible hypothalamic-pituitary-adrenal (HPA) axis suppression, Cushing's syndrome, hyperglycemia, and glucosuria may result from systemic absorption of the steroidal component, particularly in children (see USE IN CHILDREN). Use over extensive areas, for prolonged periods, or under occlusive dressings increases percutaneous absorption. Periodically evaluate HPA axis function (by ACTH stimulation or measurement of urinary free cortisol) when large doses are being applied over extensive areas. If HPA axis suppression occurs, discontinue use of this preparation, reduce the frequency of application, or substitute a less potent steroid. Infrequently, systemic corticosteroids may be needed to treat manifestations of topical steroid withdrawal.

Irritation — Instruct patients to report any signs of a local reaction; if a hypersensitivity reaction or other irritation is observed, discontinue use. Caution patients not to let this preparation come into contact with their eyes.

Lack of response — Therapeutic response, with relief of pruritus and erythema, is usually evident after 3–5 days of treatment. If no clinical improvement occurs after treating tinea pedis for 2 wk or after treating tinea cruris or tinea corporis for 1 wk, reconsider the diagnosis and repeat the appropriate microbiological studies. If no improvement is seen after one course of therapy has been completed, a second course may be instituted, provided the diagnosis is once again confirmed and other pathogens are ruled out.

Carcinogenicity, mutagenicity — Oral administration of clotrimazole for 18 mo has produced no evidence of carcinogenicity in rats; no mutagenic effects have been detected in Chinese hamsters following administration of 5 oral doses of 100 mg/kg each

ADVERSE REACTIONS[1]

Local — Paresthesias, maculopapular rash, edema, secondary infection, erythema, stinging, blistering, peeling, pruritus, urticaria, irritation, burning, itching, dryness, folliculitis, hypertrichosis, acneform eruptions, hypopigmentation, perioral dermatitis, allergic contact dermatitis, maceration of the skin, skin atrophy, striae, miliaria

---

USE IN CHILDREN

Safety and effectiveness for use in children under 12 yr of age have been established for betamethasone and clotrimazole, but not for the combination of the two drugs. When using this preparation, apply the smallest amount necessary for effective treatment; children may be more susceptible than adults to HPA axis suppression and Cushing's syndrome because of the larger ratio of surface area to body weight. Intracranial hypertension has also been seen in children receiving topical corticosteroids. Chronic corticosteroid therapy may interfere with growth and development.

USE IN PREGNANT AND NURSING WOMEN

Pregnancy Category C: systemic administration of corticosteroids at relatively low dosages, as well as topical application of the more potent corticosteroids, is generally teratogenic in laboratory animals. Reproduction studies with high oral doses of clotrimazole have demonstrated embryotoxicity (possibly due to maternal toxicity), impairment of mating, and decreases in litter size, number of viable young, and pup survival in mice and rats, but have shown no evidence of teratogenicity in these animals or in rabbits; no evidence of harm to the fetus has been detected in rats given up to 100 mg/kg intravaginally. Use this preparation during pregnancy only if the expected benefit justifies the potential risks to the fetus; do not apply over an extensive area, in a large amount, or for a prolonged period if a patient is pregnant and requires this preparation. It is not known whether components of this preparation are excreted in human milk; caution should be exercised when this preparation is used by nursing mothers.

VEHICLE/BASE

Cream (hydrophilic, emollient): mineral oil, white petrolatum, cetearyl alcohol, ceteareth-30, propylene glycol, sodium phosphate monobasic, phosphoric acid, benzyl alcohol, and purified water

[1] Reactions other than paresthesias, maculopapular rash, edema, and secondary infection have not been reported following use of this preparation, but have occurred when either clotrimazole or a topical corticosteroid was used alone

TOPICAL PREPARATIONS

MONISTAT-DERM (miconazole nitrate) Ortho   Rx

Cream: 2% (15 g; 1, 3 oz; Monistat Dual-Pak[1])   **Lotion:** 2% (30, 60 ml)

INDICATIONS	TOPICAL DOSAGE
Tinea pedis, tinea cruris, and **tinea corporis** caused by *Trichophyton rubrum, T mentagrophytes,* and *Epidermophyton floccosum* **Cutaneous candidiasis**	**Adult:** apply cream or lotion to affected areas bid (AM and PM) for 2 wk (for candidiasis, tinea cruris, and tinea corporis) or 1 mo (for tinea pedis)
Tinea versicolor	**Adult:** apply cream or lotion to affected areas once daily

CONTRAINDICATIONS
None known

ADMINISTRATION/DOSAGE ADJUSTMENTS

Intertriginous areas	Use lotion form; if cream is used, apply sparingly and smooth in well

WARNINGS/PRECAUTIONS

Irritation or sensitivity	Discontinue use immediately; avoid contact with eyes
Lack of response after 4 wk	Re-evaluate diagnosis

ADVERSE REACTIONS

Local	Irritation, burning, maceration, allergic contact dermatitis

USE IN CHILDREN	USE IN PREGNANT AND NURSING WOMEN
Consult manufacturer	Consult manufacturer

VEHICLE/BASE
Cream and lotion (water-miscible): pegoxol 7 stearate, peglicol 5 oleate, mineral oil, benzoic acid, and butylated hydroxyanisole

[1] Combination package of 2% dermatological cream with three 200-mg Monistat 3 (miconazole nitrate) vaginal suppositories; see Monistat 3/Monistat 7 chart for additional prescribing information

---

TOPICAL PREPARATIONS

MYCELEX (clotrimazole) Miles Pharmaceuticals   Rx

Cream: 1% (15, 30, 45, 90 g; Mycelex Twin Pack[1])   **Solution:** 1% (10, 30 ml)

INDICATIONS	TOPICAL DOSAGE
Tinea pedis, tinea cruris, and **tinea corporis** caused by *Trichophyton rubrum, T mentagrophytes, Epidermophyton floccosum* and *Microsporum canis* **Candidiasis** caused by *Candida albicans* **Tinea versicolor** caused by *Malassezia furfur*	**Adult:** massage gently into affected and surrounding areas bid (AM and PM) **Child:** same as adult

CONTRAINDICATIONS
Hypersensitivity to any component

WARNINGS/PRECAUTIONS

Irritation or sensitivity	Discontinue therapy and institute appropriate treatment; avoid contact with eyes
Lack of response	Pruritus and other symptoms usually improve within the first week of treatment; if no clinical improvement is evident after 4 wk of continual use, the diagnosis should be reconsidered and appropriate microbiological studies repeated. A second course of therapy may be administered if the diagnosis is confirmed and other pathogens are ruled out
Occlusive dressings	Caution patients not to use occlusive wrappings or dressings
Carcinogenicity, mutagenicity	Oral administration of clotrimazole for 18 mo has produced no evidence of carcinogenicity in rats; no mutagenic effects have been detected in Chinese hamsters following administration of 5 oral doses of 100 mg/kg each

ADVERSE REACTIONS

Local — Erythema, stinging, blistering, peeling, edema, pruritus, urticaria, burning, irritation

USE IN CHILDREN

See INDICATIONS and TOPICAL DOSAGE

USE IN PREGNANT AND NURSING WOMEN

Pregnancy Category B: no evidence of harm to the fetus has been detected in rats given up to 100 mg/kg intravaginally; reproduction studies have demonstrated embryotoxicity (possibly due to maternal toxicity), impairment of mating, and decreases in litter size, number of viable young, and pup survival in mice and rats given oral doses of 50–120 mg/kg, but have shown no evidence of teratogenicity in mice fed up to 200 mg/kg, rats (100 mg/kg), or rabbits (180 mg/kg). In humans, clotrimazole is very poorly absorbed following topical administration; however, no adequate, well-controlled studies have evaluated the safety of topical use during the first trimester. Administer during the first trimester only if clearly needed. In clinical studies, intravaginal administration during the second and third trimesters has not adversely affected fetal development. It is not known whether clotrimazole is excreted in human milk; use with caution in nursing mothers.

VEHICLE/BASE
Cream (vanishing): sorbitan monostearate, polysorbate 60, cetyl esters wax, cetostearyl alcohol, 2-octyldodecanol, and purified water, with 1% benzyl alcohol as a preservative
Solution (nonaqueous): polyethylene glycol 400

[1] Combination package of 1% dermatological cream with one 500-mg Mycelex-G (clotrimazole) vaginal tablet; see Mycelex-G chart for additional prescribing information

---

TOPICAL PREPARATIONS

MYCELEX Troche (clotrimazole) Miles Pharmaceuticals   Rx

Tablets: 10 mg

INDICATIONS

Oropharyngeal candidiasis

ORAL DOSAGE

Adult: 10 mg, given 5 times/day at 3-h intervals for 14 consecutive days; administer as a lozenge, which must be dissolved slowly in the mouth

CONTRAINDICATIONS

Hypersensitivity to any component

WARNINGS/PRECAUTIONS

Diagnostic confirmation	Obtain KOH smears and/or cultures before beginning therapy
Liver function abnormalities	Elevated SGOT levels have been detected in approximately 15% of patients; in many cases, it has not been possible to determine whether these increases, which were usually minimal, resulted from therapy or the underlying disease. Periodically assess hepatic function, particularly in patients with hepatic impairment.
Systemic mycoses	This preparation is not indicated for the treatment of systemic mycoses
Carcinogenicity	No evidence of carcinogenicity has been observed in an 18-mo study in rats

ADVERSE REACTIONS

Frequent reactions (incidence ≥ 1%) are printed in *italics*

Hepatic	*Abnormal liver function tests* (see WARNINGS/PRECAUTIONS)
Gastrointestinal	*Nausea and vomiting (5%)*

USE IN CHILDREN

Safety and effectiveness for use in children under 3 yr of age have not been established; use in such patients is not recommended

USE IN PREGNANT AND NURSING WOMEN

Pregnancy Category C: embryotoxic effects have been observed in rats and mice given 100 times the adult human dose; no evidence of teratogenicity has been detected in mice, rabbits, and rats given up to 200, 180, and 100 times the human dose. Reproduction studies, beginning 9 wk before mating and continuing through the period of weaning, have demonstrated impairment of mating in mice, a slight decrease in litter size in rats, and a decrease in pup viability in mice and rats; mice were fed 120 times the human dose, and rats were fed 50 times the human dose (no effects occurred in mice fed 60 times the human dose). No adequate, well-controlled studies have been done in pregnant women; use during pregnancy only if the expected benefit justifies the potential risk to the fetus.

MYCOLOG-II

TOPICAL PREPARATIONS

MYCOLOG-II (nystatin and triamcinolone acetonide) Squibb Rx

Cream (per gram): 100,000 units nystatin and 1 mg triamcinolone acetonide (15, 30, 60, 120 g) **Ointment (per gram):** 100,000 units nystatin and 1 mg triamcinolone acetonide (15, 30, 60, 120 g)

INDICATIONS	TOPICAL DOSAGE
Cutaneous candidiasis	Adult and child ($\geq$ 2 mo): apply cream or a thin film of ointment to affected area bid, in the morning and evening; the cream should be gently and thoroughly massaged into the skin

CONTRAINDICATIONS

Hypersensitivity to any component

WARNINGS/PRECAUTIONS

Occlusive dressings	Do not use under occlusive dressings
Patient instructions	Caution patients not to bandage or otherwise cover the treated area so that it becomes occluded; thus tight-fitting diapers or plastic pants should not be used on children being treated in the diaper area, and patients who are undergoing treatment in the inguinal area should apply the preparation sparingly and wear loose-fitting clothing. Warn patients not to let the preparation come into contact with their eyes. Patients should be advised to report any signs of adverse reactions and to take measures to avoid reinfection.
Irritation, other hypersensitivity reactions	Discontinue use and institute appropriate therapy
Lack of response	If signs or symptoms persist after 25 days of treatment, discontinue use; before beginning a second course, repeat appropriate microbiological studies (eg, KOH smears and/or cultures) in order to confirm diagnosis and rule out other pathogens
Systemic absorption	Reversible hypothalamic-pituitary-adrenal (HPA) axis suppression, Cushing's syndrome, hyperglycemia, and glucosuria may result from systemic absorption after topical application, particularly in children (see USE IN CHILDREN). Use over extensive areas, for prolonged periods, or of occlusive dressings increases percutaneous absorption. If large doses are applied over extensive areas, periodically evaluate thermal homeostasis and HPA axis function; ACTH stimulation test and measurement of urinary free cortisol facilitate diagnosis of HPA axis suppression. If pyrexia or HPA axis suppression occurs, discontinue use of this drug, reduce the frequency of application, or administer a less potent steroid. Infrequently, systemic corticosteroids may be needed to treat manifestations of topical steroid withdrawal.
Carcinogenicity, mutagenicity, effect on fertility	No studies have been done to evaluate the carcinogenic or mutagenic potential of this preparation or its effect on fertility

ADVERSE REACTIONS[1]

Local	Acneform eruptions, irritation, burning, itching, dryness, folliculitis, hypertrichosis, hypopigmentation, perioral dermatitis, allergic contact dermatitis, maceration of the skin, secondary infection, skin atrophy, striae, miliaria

USE IN CHILDREN

Use smallest amount necessary for effective treatment. Children may be more susceptible than adults to HPA axis suppression and Cushing's syndrome because of the larger ratio of surface area to body weight; intracranial hypertension has also been reported in children receiving topical corticosteroids. Chronic therapy may interfere with growth and development.

USE IN PREGNANT AND NURSING WOMEN

Pregnancy Category C: in animal studies, systemic corticosteroids have generally been teratogenic at relatively low doses; the more potent corticosteroids have also been shown to be teratogenic when applied to animal skin. Use during pregnancy only if the expected benefit justifies the potential risk to the fetus. Do not use over extensive areas, in large amounts, or for prolonged periods. It is not known whether triamcinolone or nystatin is excreted in human milk; use with caution in nursing mothers.

VEHICLE/BASE
Cream (aqueous, perfumed, vanishing): aluminum hydroxide concentrated wet gel, titanium dioxide, glyceryl monostearate, polyethylene glycol monostearate, simethicone, sorbic acid, propylene glycol, white petrolatum, cetearyl alcohol (and) ceteareth-20, and sorbitol solution
Ointment (gel): mineral oil and polyethylene

[1] Acneform eruptions occurred in 1 of 100 patients during clinical trials; nystatin-induced irritation has been seen in rare cases. Other reactions listed here have been associated with use of topical corticosteroids in general.

TOPICAL PREPARATIONS

MYCOSTATIN Cream, Ointment, and Powder (nystatin) Squibb Rx

Cream: 100,000 units/g (15, 30 g)   **Ointment:** 100,000 units/g (15, 30 g)   **Powder:** 100,000 units/g in talc (15 g)

INDICATIONS
Cutaneous or mucocutaneous candidiasis

TOPICAL DOSAGE
Adult: apply cream or ointment liberally to affected areas bid or as needed until healing is complete; if powder is used, apply to candidal lesions bid or tid until lesions have healed

CONTRAINDICATIONS
Hypersensitivity to nystatin or other components

ADMINISTRATION/DOSAGE ADJUSTMENTS

Choice of topical preparation	The cream is usually preferred to the ointment for treating candidiasis involving intertriginous areas; very moist lesions, however, are best treated with the topical dusting powder
Candidal infections of the feet	Powder should be dusted freely on feet, shoes, and socks

WARNINGS/PRECAUTIONS

Local sensitization or irritation	Caution patients to report promptly the occurrence of sensitization or irritation; discontinue use if these reactions to therapy develop

ADVERSE REACTIONS

Local	Irritation, sensitization

OVERDOSAGE

Signs and symptoms	See ADVERSE REACTIONS
Treatment	Discontinue medication; treat symptomatically

DRUG INTERACTIONS
No clinically significant drug interactions have been identified

ALTERED LABORATORY VALUES
No clinically significant alterations in blood/serum or urinary values occur at therapeutic dosages

---

USE IN CHILDREN
See INDICATIONS and dosage recommendations. The topical preparations are well tolerated by all age groups, including debilitated infants

USE IN PREGNANT AND NURSING WOMEN
Consult manufacturer

VEHICLE/BASE
Cream (aqueous, perfumed, vanishing): aluminum hydroxide gel, titanium dioxide, propylene glycol, cetearyl alcohol, ceteareth-20, white petrolatum, sorbitol solution, glyceryl monostearate, polyethylene glycol monostearate, sorbic acid, and simethicone
Ointment (gel): mineral oil, polyethylene glycol 300, polyethylene glycol 400, polyethylene glycol 1540, and polyethylene glycol 6000 distearate, with butylated hydroxytoluene as a preservative
Powder: talc

TOPICAL PREPARATIONS

NEOSPORIN Cream (polymyxin B sulfate and neomycin sulfate) Burroughs Wellcome OTC
Cream (per gram): 10,000 units polymyxin B sulfate and neomycin sulfate equivalent to 3.5 mg neomycin (15 g)

NEOSPORIN Ointment (polymyxin B sulfate, bacitracin zinc, and neomycin sulfate) OTC
Burroughs Wellcome

Ointment (per gram): 5,000 units polymyxin B sulfate, 400 units bacitracin zinc, and neomycin sulfate equivalent to 3.5 mg neomycin (14.2, 28.4 g)

INDICATIONS
To help prevent infection of **minor cuts, scrapes, and burns**

TOPICAL DOSAGE
Adult and child: apply ointment or a small amount of cream to the affected area; if necessary, cover with a sterile dressing. Use cream 1–3 times/day or ointment 2–5 times/day.

NEOSPORIN ■ NIZORAL Cream

ADMINISTRATION/DOSAGE ADJUSTMENTS

Cleansing of wound	Instruct patients to remove all debris and thoroughly cleanse wound with soap and water before application

WARNINGS/PRECAUTIONS

Toxicity	Do not apply over large areas of the body or use for more than 1 wk
Information for patients	Caution patients not to apply to the eyes. Package labels warn patients to consult a physician in the following circumstances: (1) if the cut is deep or a puncture wound or is due to an animal bite, (2) if the burn is serious, or (3) if the bleeding does not stop; patients are instructed to discontinue use and consult a physician if an infection occurs, the wound does not heal, or reactions such as erythema, irritation, swelling, and pain persist or become more severe.

USE IN CHILDREN	USE IN PREGNANT AND NURSING WOMEN
See INDICATIONS and TOPICAL DOSAGE	Consult manufacturer

VEHICLE/BASE
Cream: white petrolatum, emulsifying wax, mineral oil, polyoxyethylene polyoxypropylene compound, propylene glycol, 0.25% methylparaben, and purified water
Ointment: white petrolatum

TOPICAL PREPARATIONS

NIZORAL Cream (ketoconazole) Janssen — Rx

Cream: 2% (15, 30 g)

INDICATIONS	TOPICAL DOSAGE
Tinea corporis and tinea cruris caused by *Trichophyton rubrum*, *T mentagrophytes*, and *Epidermophyton floccosum* **Tinea versicolor** caused by *Malassezia furfur*	**Adult:** apply cream to affected and surrounding skin areas once daily; patients with more resistant cases may be treated bid, according to response

CONTRAINDICATIONS

Hypersensitivity to any component

WARNINGS/PRECAUTIONS

Lack of response	Although the majority of patients experience symptomatic relief shortly after initiation of therapy, tinea corporis and tinea cruris should be treated for 2 wk to reduce the possibility of recurrence; patients with tinea versicolor will exhibit improvement after 2 wk of therapy. If no clinical improvement occurs within the treatment period, reconsider the diagnosis and repeat microbiological studies.
Irritation or sensitivity	Discontinue therapy and institute appropriate treatment if sensitivity or chemical irritation occurs; avoid contact with the eyes
Carcinogenicity, mutagenicity	A long-term study in Swiss albino mice and Wistar rats receiving oral ketoconazole produced no evidence of carcinogenicity; no mutagenic effects have been seen in the Ames *Salmonella* microsomal activator assay or in a dominant lethal mutation test in male and female mice fed single doses as high as 80 mg/kg/day

ADVERSE REACTIONS

Local	Severe irritation, pruritus, stinging; painful allergic reaction (one case)

USE IN CHILDREN	USE IN PREGNANT AND NURSING WOMEN
Safety and effectiveness for use in children have not been established	Pregnancy Category C: syndactylia and oligodactylia have occurred in the offspring of rats fed 80 mg/kg/day (10 times the maximum recommended human dose) of ketoconazole; however, these effects may have resulted from maternal toxicity, which has been observed at this and higher dose levels. No adequate, well controlled studies have been performed in pregnant women; use during pregnancy only if the expected benefit justifies the potential risk to the fetus. It is not known whether topical ketoconazole is excreted in human milk; use with caution in nursing mothers.

VEHICLE/BASE
Cream: propylene glycol, stearyl and cetyl alcohols, sorbitan monostearate, polysorbate 60, isopropyl myristate, sodium sulfite anhydrous, polysorbate 80, and water

TOPICAL PREPARATIONS

POLYSPORIN (polymyxin B sulfate and bacitracin zinc) Burroughs Wellcome — OTC

Ointment (per gram): 10,000 units polymyxin B sulfate and 500 units bacitracin zinc (0.44, 14.2, 28.4 g) **Powder (per gram):** 10,000 units polymyxin B sulfate and 500 units bacitracin zinc (10 g) **Spray (per 90 g):** 200,000 units polymyxin B sulfate and 10,000 units bacitracin zinc (90 g)

INDICATIONS	TOPICAL DOSAGE
To prevent infection of **minor cuts, scrapes, and burns**	**Adult and child:** apply ointment or lightly dust powder on affected area; alternatively, spray a small amount in 1-s bursts from a distance of approximately 8 in. (avoid prolonged spraying). Affected area may be covered with a sterile dressing. Use ointment 2-5 times/day or spray or powder 1-3 times/day.

ADMINISTRATION/DOSAGE ADJUSTMENTS

Cleansing of wound	Instruct patients to remove all debris and thoroughly cleanse wound with soap and water before application

WARNINGS/PRECAUTIONS

Toxicity	Do not apply over large areas of the body or use for more than 1 wk
Information for patients	Caution patients not to apply to the eyes. Package labels warn patients to consult a physician in the following circumstances: (1) if the cut is deep or a puncture wound or is due to an animal bite or (2) if the burn is serious; patients are instructed to discontinue use and consult a physician if the condition persists or deteriorates.

USE IN CHILDREN	USE IN PREGNANT AND NURSING WOMEN
See INDICATIONS and TOPICAL DOSAGE	Consult manufacturer

VEHICLE/BASE
Ointment: white petrolatum
Powder: lactose
Spray: dichlorodifluoromethane and trichloromonofluoromethane

---

TOPICAL PREPARATIONS

SILVADENE (silver sulfadiazine) Marion — Rx

Cream: 1% (20, 50, 400, 1,000 g)

INDICATIONS	TOPICAL DOSAGE
Prevention and treatment of **wound infections resulting from second- or third-degree burns** (adjunctive therapy)	**Adult:** after burn wounds have been cleaned and debrided, apply a layer approximately 1/16 in. thick, using a sterile, gloved hand, once or twice daily; reapply as needed to any area from which the cream has been removed by patient movement (burn areas should be covered with cream at all times) **Infant (> 1 mo) and child:** same as adult

CONTRAINDICATIONS

Pregnancy at term	Administration to premature infants or during the first month of life

ADMINISTRATION/DOSAGE ADJUSTMENTS

Duration of treatment	Continue treatment until satisfactory healing has occurred or until the burn site is ready for grafting; unless a significant adverse reaction occurs, do not discontinue use of this preparation while the possibility of infection remains
Bathing	When feasible, the patient should be bathed daily, preferably in a whirlpool bath, as an aid in debridement
Dressings	Wound dressings are unnecessary but may be used when indicated
Escharotomy	In some cases escharotomy may be necessary to prevent contracture if separation is delayed because of the reduction in bacterial colonization

WARNINGS/PRECAUTIONS

Hypersensitivity	Use with great caution on patients with a history of hypersensitivity to this preparation; if an allergic reaction to it occurs during therapy, consideration must be given to discontinuing further use. It is not known whether cross-sensitivity to other sulfonamides exists.

Fungal colonization	Bacterial growth inhibition may lead to fungal colonization in and below the eschar; fungal dissemination, however, is rare
Patients with extensive burns	Application of this preparation over extensive areas of the body may result in serum sulfonamide levels approaching adult therapeutic levels (8–12 mg/dl); when treating such patients, monitor serum sulfonamide levels and renal function, and examine the urine for sulfa crystals
Patients with G6PD deficiency	Administration of this drug to patients deficient in glucose-6-phosphate dehydrogenase (G6PD) may result in hemolysis
Patients with hepatic or renal impairment	Impairment of hepatic or renal function may lead to drug accumulation as elimination decreases, necessitating reappraisal of the benefit-risk involved by continuing therapy
Concomitant use of proteolytic enzymes	The presence of silver in this preparation may inactivate topical proteolytic enzymes

ADVERSE REACTIONS

Local	Burning sensation, rash, itching
Systemic	Interstitial nephritis[1]

USE IN CHILDREN

See INDICATIONS and TOPICAL DOSAGE; contraindicated for premature infants and newborns under 1 mo of age because of the risk of kernicterus

USE IN PREGNANT AND NURSING WOMEN

Safety has not been established during pregnancy; use of this preparation on women of childbearing potential is not recommended unless the burned area covers more than 20% of the total body surface area or the expected therapeutic benefit from it exceeds the potential risk to the fetus. Administration at term is contraindicated because of the risk of kernicterus. Consult manufacturer if patient is breast feeding.

VEHICLE/BASE
Cream (water miscible): white petrolatum, stearyl alcohol, isopropyl myristate, sorbitan monooleate, polyoxyl 40 stearate, propylene glycol, and water, with 0.3% methylparaben as a preservative

[1] Because significant quantities of silver sulfadiazine are absorbed, any of the adverse reactions that have been attributed to sulfonamide therapy hypothetically may occur

TOPICAL PREPARATIONS

SPECTAZOLE (econazole nitrate) Ortho Rx

Cream: 1% (15, 30, 85 g)

INDICATIONS

Tinea pedis, tinea cruris, and tinea corporis caused by *Trichophyton rubrum, T mentagrophytes, T tonsurans, Microsporum audouni, M gypseum,* and *Epidermophyton floccosum*
Candidiasis caused by *Candida albicans*

Tinea versicolor caused by *Malassezia furfur*

TOPICAL DOSAGE

Adult: apply a sufficient amount to cover affected areas bid (morning and evening)

Adult: apply a sufficient amount to cover affected areas once daily

CONTRAINDICATIONS

Hypersensitivity to any component

ADMINISTRATION/DOSAGE ADJUSTMENTS

Duration of treatment	Although symptomatic relief and clinical improvement may occur fairly early, treatment of candidal infections, tinea cruris, and tinea corporis should be continued for 2 wk and of tinea pedis for 1 mo to lessen the possibility of relapse; tinea versicolor usually responds after 2 wk of regular use

WARNINGS/PRECAUTIONS

Lack of response	If no clinical improvement is evident after 2 wk of regular use in candidiasis or tinea cruris, corporis, or versicolor or after 4 wk in tinea pedis, the diagnosis should be reconsidered
Sensitivity or chemical irritation	Discontinue use of this medication if burning, itching, stinging, redness, or other reactions suggesting sensitivity or irritation occur
Potential for hepatotoxicity	Although hepatic effects have not been documented in clinical trials, several cases of hepatocellular dysfunction have occurred during systemic use of a different imidazole

Carcinogenicity	No long-term studies have been done in animals to determine the carcinogenic potential of this drug
Effect on fertility	Intravaginal administration of econazole has had no adverse effects on reproduction in women

ADVERSE REACTIONS

Local	Burning sensation, itching, stinging, erythema

USE IN CHILDREN
Consult manufacturer

USE IN PREGNANT AND NURSING WOMEN
Pregnancy Category C: reproduction studies in mice, rats, and rabbits have shown no evidence of teratogenicity; oral administration of 10–80 times the human topical dose has produced embryotoxicity and fetotoxicity in these species. Use during the first trimester of pregnancy only when considered essential to the welfare of the patient. During the second and third trimesters, use only if clearly needed. It is not known whether econazole is excreted in human milk. The drug has been detected in the milk of lactating rats and in nursing pups; administration of large doses to lactating rats has resulted in a reduction in postpartum viability of nursing pups and survival to weaning, possibly as a result of maternal toxicity. Administer with caution to nursing women.

VEHICLE/BASE
Cream (water miscible): pegoxol 7 stearate, peglicol 5 oleate, mineral oil, benzoic acid, butylated hydroxyanisole, and purified water

TOPICAL PREPARATIONS

TINACTIN (tolnaftate) Schering OTC

Cream (water-washable): 1% (Tinactin Jock Itch Cream) (15 g) **Cream (nonaqeous):** 1% (Tinactin Cream) (15, 30 g) **Solution:** 1% (Tinactin Solution) (10 ml) **Liquid aerosol:** 1% (Tinactin Liquid Aerosol) (113 g) **Powder:** 1% (Tinactin Powder) (45, 90 g) **Powder aerosol:** 1% (Tinactin Jock Itch Spray Powder; Tinactin Powder aerosol) (100 g)

INDICATIONS
Tinea pedis
Tinea cruris
Tinea corporis (solution only)

TOPICAL DOSAGE
Adult and child (> 2 yr): after washing and drying affected area, spray liquid, sprinkle or spray powder liberally, gently rub in 1/2 in. of cream, or gently massage in 2–3 drops of the solution; administer preparation bid (morning and evening). Sprinkle powder in shoes or socks as well as on affected area when using for tinea pedis. Spray aerosols from a distance of 6–10 in. Duration of therapy is usually 2 wk for tinea cruris and 4 wk for tinea pedis and tinea corporis. After signs and symptoms have disappeared, continue treatment for 2 wk. To help prevent tinea pedis, instruct patient to bathe daily, dry carefully, and sprinkle or spray powder.

ADMINISTRATION/DOSAGE ADJUSTMENTS

Use of powder	The drying action of the powder and power aerosol may be useful when treating infections in naturally moist areas
Onset of action	Preparations begin to relieve burning, itching, and soreness within 24 h

WARNINGS/PRECAUTIONS

Care of eyes	Keep these preparations out of the eyes
Irritation, lack of response	Discontinue use if irritation occurs or symptoms do not improve within 10 days
Nail and scalp infections	Tolnaftate is not effective in the treatment of nail or scalp infections

USE IN CHILDREN
See INDICATIONS and TOPICAL DOSAGE; administration by children under 12 yr of age should be supervised. Use with caution in children under 2 yr of age.

USE IN PREGNANT AND NURSING WOMEN
No problems with use in women who are pregnant or nursing have been reported

VEHICLE/BASE
Cream (water-washable): white petrolatum, propylene glycol, cetearyl alcohol, mineral oil, ceteareth-30, sodium phosphate monobasic monohydrate, chlorocresol, phosphoric acid, and sodium hydroxide
Cream (nonaqueous): polyethylene glycol-400, propylene glycol, carboxypolymethylene, monoamylamine, titanium dioxide, and butylated hydroxytoluene
Solution (nonaqueous): butylated hydroxytoluene and polyethylene glycol-400
Liquid aerosol: butylated hydroxytoluene, polyethylene-polypropylene glycol monobutyl ether, 36% denatured alcohol, and isobutane
Powder: corn starch and talc
Powder aerosol: butylated hydroxytoluene, talc, polyethylene-polypropylene glycol monobutyl ether, 14% denatured alcohol, and isobutane

TOPICAL PREPARATIONS

ZOVIRAX Ointment (acyclovir) Burroughs Wellcome — Rx
Ointment: 5% (15 g)

INDICATIONS	**TOPICAL DOSAGE**
Initial herpes genitalis Limited, non-life-threatening, mucocutaneous **herpes simplex virus infections** in immunocompromised patients	**Adult:** apply enough ointment (approximately 1/2 in. per 4 sq in. of surface area) to adequately cover all lesions q3h, 6 times/day, for 7 consecutive days; therapy should be started as early as possible following the onset of signs and symptoms **Child:** same as adult
CONTRAINDICATIONS	
Hypersensitivity or chemical intolerance	Ophthalmic or prophylactic use (see WARNINGS/PRECAUTIONS)
WARNINGS/PRECAUTIONS	
Recurrence and transmission of infection	There are no data showing that use of this drug will prevent recurrent herpesvirus infections in the absence of signs and symptoms, nor prevent transmission of infection to other individuals (see "patient instructions," below)
Viral resistance	Although clinically significant viral resistance has not been associated with use of this drug, this possibility still exists
Carcinogenicity	No evidence of carcinogenicity has been observed in lifetime bioassays in rats and mice given 50, 150, and 450 mg/kg/day by gavage; conflicting results have been found in two in vitro assays
Mutagenicity	Parenteral doses of 100 mg/kg have not caused chromosomal damage in rats or Chinese hamsters; however, higher doses (500 and 1,000 mg/kg) are clastogenic in Chinese hamsters. A dominant lethal study in mice has shown no evidence of mutagenicity. In 2 of 11 microbial and mammalian cell assays, evidence of mutagenicity and chromosomal damage has been found, but only at concentrations at least 1,000 times those achieved in human plasma following topical application.
Patient instructions	Advise patient not to exceed the recommended dosage, frequency of application, or length of treatment and to wear a finger cot or rubber glove when applying the ointment to prevent autoinoculation of other body sites and transmission of the infection to other persons

ADVERSE REACTIONS
Some patients may experience discomfort upon application due to the characteristic sensitivity and tenderness of ulcerated genital lesions. No significant difference in the rate or type of adverse reactions—mild pain (including transient burning or stinging), pruritus, rash, and vulvitis—has been observed between drug- and placebo-treated patients.

OVERDOSAGE
Overdosage by topical application is unlikely because of limited percutaneous absorption

DRUG INTERACTIONS
No clinically significant drug interactions have been identified

ALTERED LABORATORY VALUES
No clinically significant alterations in blood/serum or urinary values occur at therapeutic dosages

USE IN CHILDREN	USE IN PREGNANT AND NURSING WOMEN
Same as adult indications and dosage	Pregnancy Category C: use during pregnancy only if the expected benefit outweighs the potential risk to the fetus. Acyclovir does not impair either fertility or reproduction in mice at oral doses up to 450 mg/kg/day or in rats at subcutaneous doses up to 25 mg/kg/day. Rabbits given 50 mg/kg/day subcutaneously have shown a statistically significant decrease in implantation efficiency. Teratogenic effects have not been detected in animals; however, there are no adequate, well-controlled studies in pregnant women. It is not known whether this drug is excreted in human milk; use with caution in nursing mothers.

VEHICLE/BASE
Ointment: polyethylene glycol

VAGINAL PREPARATIONS

AVC (sulfanilamide, aminacrine hydrochloride, and allantoin) Merrell Dow — Rx
Vaginal cream: 15% sulfanilamide, 0.2% aminacrine hydrochloride, and 2% allantoin (1/4, 4 oz) **Vaginal suppositories:** 1.05 g sulfanilamide, 0.014 g aminacrine hydrochloride, and 0.14 g allantoin

INDICATIONS	**INTRAVAGINAL DOSAGE**
Vulvovaginitis, when isolation of the causative organism is not possible[1] **Trichomoniasis, vulvovaginal candidiasis, and vaginitis** caused by *Hemophilus vaginalis* or other susceptible bacteria[2]	**Adult:** 1 applicatorful or suppository 1–2 times/day through one complete menstrual cycle, unless specific therapy is initiated

COMPENDIUM OF DRUG THERAPY

AVC ■ FEMSTAT

CONTRAINDICATIONS	
Sensitivity to sulfonamides	

WARNINGS/PRECAUTIONS	
Local or systemic toxicity or sensitivity	May occur; discontinue therapy if manifestations (eg, skin rash) appear
Tartrazine sensitivity	Presence of FD&C Yellow No. 5 (tartrazine) in the suppository may cause allergic-type reactions, including bronchial asthma, in susceptible individuals

ADVERSE REACTIONS	
Local	Increased discomfort, burning

USE IN CHILDREN	USE IN PREGNANT AND NURSING WOMEN
Consult manufacturer	Consult manufacturer

VEHICLE/BASE
Cream (water-miscible): lactose, propylene glycol, stearic acid, diglycol stearate, and trolamine, buffered with lactic acid to an acid pH
Suppository: lactose, polyethylene glycol 400, polysorbate 80, polyethylene glycol 4000, and glycerin, buffered with lactic acid to an acid pH; inert covering contains gelatin, glycerin, water, methylparaben, and propylparaben

[1] Probably effective
[2] Possibly effective

VAGINAL PREPARATIONS

FEMSTAT (butoconazole nitrate) Syntex — Rx
Vaginal cream: 2% (28 g)

INDICATIONS	INTRAVAGINAL DOSAGE
Vulvovaginal candidiasis	Adult: 1 applicatorful at bedtime for 3 days or, if necessary, for 6 days; for use during the second or third trimester of pregnancy, 1 applicatorful at bedtime for 6 days (do not administer during the first trimester; see USE IN PREGNANT AND NURSING WOMEN)

CONTRAINDICATIONS	
Hypersensitivity to any component	

WARNINGS/PRECAUTIONS	
Diagnostic confirmation	Obtain KOH smears and/or cultures; rule out other pathogens commonly associated with vulvovaginitis by appropriate laboratory methods
Lack of response	If clinical symptoms persist after a course of treatment, repeat appropriate microbiological studies to confirm diagnosis and rule out other pathogens
Hypersensitivity, irritation	If sensitization or irritation occurs, discontinue treatment
Premature termination of therapy	Caution patients not to discontinue drug prematurely because of menses or symptomatic relief
Carcinogenicity, mutagenicity, effect on fertility	No long-term studies have been performed to determine the carcinogenic potential of butoconazole. Microbial tests have shown no evidence of mutagenicity. No impairment of fertility has been observed in rabbits fed up to 30 mg/kg/day or in rats fed up to 100 mg/kg/day.

ADVERSE REACTIONS	
Local	Vulvar/vaginal burning (2.3%), vulvar itching (0.9%), discharge, soreness, swelling, and itching of the fingers (0.2%)

USE IN CHILDREN	USE IN PREGNANT AND NURSING WOMEN
Safety and effectiveness for use in children have not been established	Pregnancy Category C: in rats, intravaginal administration of 6 mg/kg/day (3–7 times the human dose) during organogenesis has caused an increase in the resorption rate and a decrease in litter size; oral administration throughout this period has produced cleft palate and abdominal wall defects at maternally stressful dosages of 100–750 mg/kg/day, but no apparent adverse reaction at up to 50 mg/kg/day. Adverse effects have not been seen in rabbits, even at the maternally stressful dosage of 150 mg/kg/day. No adequate, well-controlled studies have been done in pregnant women during the first trimester. Use of butoconazole from organogenesis through parturition has caused dystocia in rats; however, this effect has not been observed in rabbits given up to 100 mg/kg/day orally. In clinical studies with pregnant women, use of the 2% cream during the second or third trimester for 3 or 6 days had no adverse effect on the fetus or the course of pregnancy. Butoconazole should be used in pregnant women only during the second or third trimester. It is not known whether butoconazole is excreted in human milk; use with caution in nursing mothers.

VEHICLE/BASE
Cream (water-washable, emollient): stearyl alcohol, propylene glycol, cetyl alcohol, sorbitan monostearate, glyceryl stearate (and) PEG-100 stearate, mineral oil, polysorbate 60, methylparaben, propylparaben, and purified water

VAGINAL PREPARATIONS

GYNE-LOTRIMIN (clotrimazole) Schering   Rx

Vaginal cream: 1% (45 g)   **Vaginal tablets:** 100, 500 mg

INDICATIONS	**INTRAVAGINAL DOSAGE**
Vulvovaginal candidiasis	**Adult:** for single-dose therapy, one 500-mg tab, given preferably at bedtime; alternatively, administer one 100-mg tab or one applicatorful daily, preferably at bedtime, for 7 consecutive days (100-mg tab) or 7–14 days (cream) or, if patient is not pregnant, two 100-mg tabs/day for 3 consecutive days **Child:** same as adult

CONTRAINDICATIONS
Hypersensitivity to any component

ADMINISTRATION/DOSAGE ADJUSTMENTS
Severe infection	To treat severe vulvovaginitis, use a preparation such as the cream or 100-mg tablets that requires administration for more than one day; do not use the 500-mg tablets

WARNINGS/PRECAUTIONS
Diagnostic confirmation	Obtain KOH smears and/or cultures; rule out other pathogens commonly associated with vulvovaginitis (*Trichomonas* and *Gardnerella vaginalis*) by appropriate laboratory methods
Lack of response	If signs or symptoms of vaginitis persist after a course of treatment with the cream or 100-mg tablets, or 5 days after the 500-mg dose, repeat appropriate microbiological studies to confirm diagnosis and rule out other pathogens before instituting another course of antimycotic therapy
Carcinogenicity	No indication of carcinogenicity has been observed in a long-term study in Wistar rats given oral doses of the clotrimazole; long-term studies have not been performed in animals with intravaginal doses

ADVERSE REACTIONS
With cream
Local	Burning, erythema, irritation
Genitourinary	Intercurrent cystitis

With tablets
Local	Burning, rash, pruritus, and vulval irritation (with either strength); vaginal irritation, dyspareunia, and vaginal soreness with coitus (with 500-mg strength only)
Genitourinary	Slight cramping and slight urinary frequency (with either strength)
Gastrointestinal	Lower abdominal cramps and bloating (with either strength); vomiting (with 500-mg strength only)
Other	Burning or irritation in sexual partner (with either strength)

USE IN CHILDREN
See INDICATIONS and INTRAVAGINAL DOSAGE

USE IN PREGNANT AND NURSING WOMEN
Pregnancy Category B: no evidence of harm to the fetus has been detected in rats given up to 100 mg/kg/day intravaginally; reproduction studies have demonstrated embryotoxicity (possibly due to maternal toxicity), impairment of mating, and decreases in litter size, number of viable young, and pup survival in mice and rats given oral doses of 50–120 mg/kg, but have shown no evidence of teratogenicity in mice fed up to 200 mg/kg, rats fed up to 100 mg/kg, or rabbits fed up to 180 mg/kg. In humans, clotrimazole is poorly absorbed following topical administration; however, no adequate, well-controlled studies have evaluated the safety of topical use during the first trimester. Administer during the first trimester only if clearly needed. Use of cream and 100-mg tablets during the second and third trimesters has not adversely affected fetal development. Consult manufacturer for use in nursing mothers.

VEHICLE/BASE
Cream: sorbitan monostearate, polysorbate 60, cetyl esters wax, cetostearyl alcohol, 2-octyldodecanol, and purified water, with 1% benzyl alcohol as a preservative
Tablets (500 mg): lactose, microcrystalline cellulose, lactic acid, corn starch, crospovidone, calcium lactate, magnesium stearate, silicon dioxide, and hydroxypropylmethyl cellulose

---

VAGINAL PREPARATIONS

MONISTAT DUAL-PAK (miconazole nitrate) Ortho   Rx
Vaginal suppositories and cream: three 200-mg suppositories and 2% Monistat-Derm dermatological cream[1]

MONISTAT 3 (miconazole nitrate) Ortho   Rx
Vaginal suppositories: 200 mg

MONISTAT 7 (miconazole nitrate) Ortho   Rx
Vaginal cream: 2% (45 g)   **Vaginal suppositories:** 100 mg

INDICATIONS	**INTRAVAGINAL DOSAGE**
Vulvovaginal candidiasis (moniliasis)	**Adult:** one applicatorful of vaginal cream or one 100-mg suppository at bedtime for 7 days or, alternatively, one 200-mg suppository at bedtime for 3 days; if necessary, repeat course

MONISTAT ■ MYCELEX-G

CONTRAINDICATIONS

Hypersensitivity to miconazole

WARNINGS/PRECAUTIONS

Diagnostic confirmation	Obtain KOH smears and/or cultures; rule out other pathogens commonly associated with vulvovaginitis (*Trichomonas* and *Gardnerella vaginalis*) by appropriate laboratory methods
Diabetic patients	Effectiveness of the 200-mg suppositories for use in diabetic patients has not been established
Lack of response	Repeat appropriate microbiological studies to confirm the diagnosis and rule out other pathogens before instituting another course of antimycotic therapy
Irritation or sensitivity	Discontinue use
Concomitant use of a diaphragm	The suppository and certain latex products, such as vaginal diaphragms, should not be used concomitantly; the suppository base may interact with the latex in these products
Carcinogenicity	No long-term carcinogenicity studies have been performed in animals

ADVERSE REACTIONS

Local	*Cream:* vulvovaginal burning, itching, or irritation (6.6%), vaginal burning ($<$ 0.2%); *suppositories:* vulvovaginal burning, itching, or irritation (2% with 200-mg strength, 0.5% with 100-mg strength)
Other	*Cream:* skin rash, hives, pelvic cramps, and headaches ($<$ 0.2%); *suppositories:* skin rash ($<$ 0.5% with 200-mg strength, 0.2% with 100-mg strength), hives ($<$ 0.5% with 200-mg strength), pelvic cramps (2% with 200-mg strength), headaches (1.3% with 200-mg strength)

USE IN CHILDREN
Consult manufacturer

USE IN PREGNANT AND NURSING WOMEN
Oral doses of 80 mg/kg or more have caused dystocia in rats and embryo- and fetotoxic effects in both rats and rabbits; oral administration has also resulted in prolonged gestation in rats, but not in rabbits. These effects have not been observed in rats after intravaginal administration, and no adverse reactions have occurred in infants whose mothers used the cream or suppositories for up to 14 days during clinical studies. Nevertheless, since small amounts of miconazole are absorbed from the vagina, this drug should be administered intravaginally during the first trimester only if such use is deemed essential. Effectiveness of the suppositories for use during pregnancy has not been established. It is not known whether this drug is excreted in human milk; use with caution in nursing mothers.

VEHICLE/BASE
Cream (white, water-miscible): pegoxol 7 stearate, peglicol 5 oleate, mineral oil, benzoic acid, and butylated hydroxyanisole
Suppositories (white to off-white, water-miscible): hydrogenated vegetable oil

[1] See Monistat-Derm chart for additional prescribing information

---

VAGINAL PREPARATIONS

MYCELEX-G (clotrimazole) Miles Pharmaceuticals   Rx
Vaginal cream: 1% (45, 90 g)   Vaginal tablets: 100, 500 mg

MYCELEX TWIN PACK (clotrimazole) Miles Pharmaceuticals   Rx
Vaginal tablets and cream: one 500-mg vaginal tablet with 1% dermatological cream[1]

INDICATIONS
Vulvovaginal candidiasis

INTRAVAGINAL DOSAGE
Adult: for single-dose therapy, one 500-mg tab, given preferably at bedtime; alternatively, administer one 100-mg tab or one applicatorful daily, preferably at bedtime, for 7 consecutive days (100-mg tab) or 7–14 days (vaginal cream) or, if patient is not pregnant, two 100-mg tabs/day for 3 consecutive days
Child: same as adult

CONTRAINDICATIONS
Hypersensitivity to any component

MYCELEX-G ■ MYCOSTATIN Vaginal Tablets

ADMINISTRATION/DOSAGE ADJUSTMENTS

Severe infection	To treat severe vulvovaginitis, use a preparation such as the cream or 100-mg tablets that requires administration for more than one day; do not use the 500-mg tablets

WARNINGS/PRECAUTIONS

Diagnostic confirmation	Obtain KOH smears and/or cultures; rule out other pathogens commonly associated with vulvovaginitis (*Trichomonas* and *Gardnerella vaginalis*) by appropriate laboratory methods
Lack of response	If signs or symptoms of vaginitis persist after a course of treatment with the cream or 100-mg tablets, or 5 days after the 500-mg dose, repeat appropriate microbiological studies to confirm diagnosis and rule out other pathogens before instituting another course of antimycotic therapy
Carcinogenicity	No indication of carcinogenicity has been observed in a long-term study in Wistar rats given oral doses of the clotrimazole; long-term studies have not been performed in animals with intravaginal doses

ADVERSE REACTIONS

With cream

Local	Burning, erythema, irritation
Genitourinary	Intercurrent cystitis

With tablets

Local	Burning, rash, pruritus, and vulval irritation (with either strength); vaginal irritation, dyspareunia, and vaginal soreness with coitus (with 500-mg strength only)
Genitourinary	Slight cramping and slight urinary frequency (with either strength)
Gastrointestinal	Lower abdominal cramps and bloating (with either strength); vomiting (with 500-mg strength only)
Other	Burning or irritation in sexual partner (with either strength)

USE IN CHILDREN
See INDICATIONS and INTRAVAGINAL DOSAGE

USE IN PREGNANT AND NURSING WOMEN
Pregnancy Category B: no evidence of harm to the fetus has been detected in rats given up to 100 mg/kg/day intravaginally; reproduction studies have demonstrated embryotoxicity (possibly due to maternal toxicity), impairment of mating, and decreases in litter size, number of viable young, and pup survival in mice and rats given oral doses of 50-120 mg/kg, but have shown no evidence of teratogenicity in mice fed up to 200 mg/kg, rats fed up to 100 mg/kg, or rabbits fed up to 180 mg/kg. In humans, clotrimazole is poorly absorbed following topical administration; however, no adequate, well-controlled studies have evaluated the safety of topical use during the first trimester. Administer during the first trimester only if clearly needed. Use of cream and 100-mg tablets during the second and third trimesters has not adversely affected fetal development. Consult manufacturer for use in nursing mothers.

VEHICLE/BASE
Cream: sorbitan monostearate, polysorbate 60, cetyl esters wax, cetostearyl alcohol, 2-octyldodecanol, purified water, and 1% benzyl alcohol

[1] See Mycelex chart for additional prescribing information

VAGINAL PREPARATIONS

MYCOSTATIN Vaginal Tablets (nystatin) Squibb   Rx

Vaginal tablets: 100,000 units

INDICATIONS	TOPICAL DOSAGE
Vulvovaginal candidiasis	**Adult:** 100,000 units (1 vaginal tablet) once daily for 2 wk

CONTRAINDICATIONS

Hypersensitivity to nystatin or other components

COMPENDIUM OF DRUG THERAPY

MYCOSTATIN Vaginal Tablets ■ SULTRIN

WARNINGS/PRECAUTIONS

Pretreatment evaluation of vulvovaginitis	Confirm diagnosis prior to therapy by obtaining KOH smears and/or cultures; since other pathogens commonly associated with vulvovaginitis (*Trichomonas* and *Hemophilus vaginalis*) are not affected by nystatin, they should be ruled out by appropriate laboratory methods. If the condition does not respond, repeat appropriate microbiological studies to reconfirm the diagnosis and rule out nonsusceptible pathogens before instituting a second course of antimycotic therapy.
Patient instructions	Caution patients being treated for vulvovaginitis to continue taking the medication for the entire treatment course, even during their menstrual period and even though symptomatic improvement may occur within a few days of starting therapy; they should also be advised that adjunctive measures, such as therapeutic douches, are unnecessary and sometimes unwise (however, cleansing douches may be used for esthetic reasons if the patient is not pregnant)
Local sensitization or irritation	Caution patients to report promptly the occurrence of sensitization or irritation; discontinue use if these reactions to therapy develop

ADVERSE REACTIONS

Local	Irritation, sensitization

OVERDOSAGE

Signs and symptoms	See ADVERSE REACTIONS
Treatment	Discontinue medication; treat symptomatically

DRUG INTERACTIONS

No clinically significant drug interactions have been identified

ALTERED LABORATORY VALUES

No clinically significant alterations in blood/serum or urinary values occur at therapeutic dosages

USE IN CHILDREN

Safety and effectiveness for use in children have not been established

USE IN PREGNANT AND NURSING WOMEN

Pregnancy Category A: use during pregnancy only if essential to the patient's welfare. Animal reproduction studies have not been done; however, there have been no reports that use of this product by pregnant women increases the risk of fetal abnormalities or affects the subsequent growth, development, and functional maturation of the child. Consult manufacturer for information pertaining to the use of nystatin by nursing women.

VEHICLE/BASE
Vaginal tablets: lactose, ethyl cellulose, stearic acid, and starch

---

VAGINAL PREPARATIONS

SULTRIN (sulfathiazole, sulfacetamide, and sulfabenzamide [triple sulfa]) Ortho   Rx

Cream: 3.42% sulfathiazole, 2.86% sulfacetamide, and 3.7% sulfabenzamide (2.75 oz)   **Vaginal tablets:** 172.5 mg sulfathiazole, 143.75 mg sulfacetamide, and 184.0 mg sulfabenzamide

INDICATIONS

Hemophilus (Gardnerella) vaginalis vaginitis

INTRAVAGINAL DOSAGE

Adult: one applicatorful of cream intravaginally bid for 4–6 days, followed by $1/2$ to $1/4$ the dosage, if needed, or 1 tab intravaginally upon retiring and again in the morning for 10 days; repeat, if necessary
Child: use according to medical judgment

CONTRAINDICATIONS

Hypersensitivity to sulfonamides   Kidney disease

WARNINGS/PRECAUTIONS

Consult manufacturer

ADVERSE REACTIONS

Consult manufacturer

SULTRIN ■ VAGISEC

USE IN CHILDREN	USE IN PREGNANT AND NURSING WOMEN
Indications and dosage for use in children have not been established; use according to medical judgment	Use according to medical judgment during pregnancy. It is not known whether this drug is excreted in human milk; use with caution in nursing women.

VEHICLE/BASE
Cream: 0.64% urea, glyceryl monostearate, 2% cetyl alcohol, stearic acid, cholesterol, lanolin, lecithin, peanut oil, propylparaben, propylene glycol, diethylaminoethyl stearamide, phosphoric acid, methylparaben, and water
Vaginal tablets: urea, lactose, guar gum, starch, and magnesium stearate

---

VAGINAL PREPARATIONS

VAGISEC (polyoxyethylene nonyl phenol, sodium edetate, and sodium dioctyl sulfosuccinate) Schmid   OTC

Vaginal liquid: exact amounts not specified by manufacturer (4 fl oz)

VAGISEC PLUS (9-aminoacridine hydrochloride, polyoxyethylene nonyl phenol, sodium edetate, and sodium dioctyl sulfosuccinate) Schmid   Rx

Vaginal suppositories: 6 mg 9-aminoacridine hydrochloride, 5.25 mg polyoxyethylene nonyl phenol, 0.66 mg sodium edetate, and 0.07 mg sodium dioctyl sulfosuccinate

INDICATIONS
Vaginitis caused by *Trichomonas vaginalis*
Vaginal infection caused by bacteria and *Trichomonas vaginalis*

INTRAVAGINAL DOSAGE
Adult: in the office, scrub the vagina with a 1:100 dilution of the liquid and then insert 1 suppository; perform this procedure 3 times during the first week of therapy and twice during the second week. Patient should continue treatment at home for a period of 14 days; she should insert 1 suppository every morning after douching with a quart of solution containing 1 tsp of the liquid and insert 1 suppository every evening at bedtime. Products should not be used in the evening and morning before an office visit.

CONTRAINDICATIONS
Pregnancy	Attempting to conceive (products are spermicidal)

ADMINISTRATION/DOSAGE ADJUSTMENTS
Chronic or stubborn cases	Repeat regimen, continuing treatment through two menstrual periods; after home treatment has been discontinued for 3 days, reexamine patient
Demonstration of cure	Vaginal smears or cultures, obtained once monthly for 3 mo after treatment, should show normal bacterial flora and no evidence of trichomonads
Use during menstruation	To guard against potential flare-ups, continue treatment during menstruation; blood enhances the growth of trichomonads
Preventive therapy	To maintain vaginal cleanliness and prevent flare-ups after completion of treatment, patient should douche with liquid up to twice weekly

WARNINGS/PRECAUTIONS
Sexual intercourse	During treatment, the patient should refrain from intercourse or ask her partner to use a prophylactic
Minor irritation	Discontinue use of liquid for 24 h if minor irritation occurs
Overdose	Use copious amounts of water to treat overdose; the liquid, when diluted, is not toxic
Recurrent vaginitis	Extravaginal foci or infection (eg, in cervical, vestibular, or urethral glands) or reinfection by a sexual partner are frequent causes of recurrent vaginitis

USE IN CHILDREN	USE IN PREGNANT AND NURSING WOMEN
Not indicated	Douching during pregnancy is not recommended

VEHICLE/BASE
Suppositories: polyethylene glycol, glycerin, and citric acid
Liquid: 5% alcohol

VAGINAL PREPARATIONS

VAGITROL (sulfanilamide) Lemmon   Rx
Cream: 15% (4 oz)

INDICATIONS
Vulvovaginitis caused by *Candida albicans*

INTRAVAGINAL DOSAGE
Adult: 1 applicatorful 1–2 times/day for one complete menstrual cycle (approximately 30 days)

CONTRAINDICATIONS
Hypersensitivity to sulfonamides

ADMINISTRATION/DOSAGE ADJUSTMENTS
Intravaginal administration	After removing cap from tube and puncturing opening with point of cap, screw applicator onto tube and tighten. Pull plunger out as far as it will go, squeeze tube from the bottom, and fill applicator completely with cream. Detach applicator from tube, hold applicator by the cylinder, and gently insert into vagina as far as it will go comfortably; then push plunger down until contact is made with cylinder. Withdraw applicator with plunger still fully pushed in.
Douching	For hygienic purposes, douching may be performed before insertion
Protection of underclothing	A sanitary pad may be used to protect underclothing

WARNINGS/PRECAUTIONS
Systemic absorption	Oral sulfonamides have caused severe, potentially fatal reactions, including blood dyscrasias such as agranulocytosis and aplastic anemia as well as serious hypersensitivity reactions; in rare cases, goiter, diuresis, and hypoglycemia have developed. These systemic effects can also occur with intravaginal use since sulfonamides are absorbed from the vaginal mucosa. Therefore, watch for rash or any other systemic reaction; discontinue use if a systemic effect is seen.
Cross-sensitivity	Patients allergic to acetazolamide, thiazide-type diuretics, sulfonylureas, or certain goitrogens may also be hypersensitive to this preparation
Local reactions	Discontinue use if a local reaction occurs
Carcinogenicity	In rats, an animal especially susceptible to the goitrogenic effect of sulfonamides, long-term use of these drugs has produced thyroid malignancies

ADVERSE REACTIONS
Local	Increased discomfort, burning sensation

USE IN CHILDREN
Consult manufacturer

USE IN PREGNANT AND NURSING WOMEN
Safety for use during pregnancy has not been established. Sulfonamides cross the placental barrier, producing a fetal serum level 50–90% of the maternal level; if the fetal concentration reaches a sufficiently high level, toxic effects can occur. A significant increase in the incidence of cleft palate and other bony abnormalities has been detected when rats and mice were fed certain sulfonamides in large amounts (7–25 times the human therapeutic dose); however, the teratogenic potential of most sulfonamides has not been thoroughly studied in animals or humans. Sulfonamides are excreted in human milk and may cause kernicterus; patient should stop nursing if drug is prescribed.

VEHICLE/BASE
Cream (water-miscible): lactose, stearic acid, cetyl alcohol, trolamine, sodium lauryl sulfate, glycerin, methylparaben, propylparaben, and lactic acid (pH ~4.5)

SYSTEMIC AGENTS

ANCOBON (flucytosine) Roche   Rx
Capsules: 250, 500 mg

INDICATIONS
Serious mycotic infections caused by susceptible strains of *Candida* (septicemia; endocarditis; pulmonary and urinary tract infections) and/or *Cryptococcus* (meningitis; septicemia; pulmonary and urinary tract infections)

ORAL DOSAGE
Adult: 50–150 mg/kg/day, given in divided doses q6h

CONTRAINDICATIONS

Hypersensitivity to flucytosine

ADMINISTRATION/DOSAGE ADJUSTMENTS

Gastrointestinal disturbances	Nausea or vomiting may be reduced or eliminated by administering the capsules a few at a time over a 15-min period
Patients with renal impairment	Initiate therapy at 50 mg/kg/day if the BUN or serum creatinine level is elevated or other signs of renal impairment exist

WARNINGS/PRECAUTIONS

Patient monitoring	Close monitoring of hepatic, renal, and hematopoietic function is essential; determine the patient's renal and hematological status prior to using flucytosine and monitor liver enzyme (alkaline phosphatase, SGOT, and SGPT) levels and hematopoietic function at frequent intervals during therapy, as indicated
Renal impairment	May lead to drug accumulation; use with extreme caution in patients with impaired renal function and assay the blood level of flucytosine periodically to determine the adequacy of renal excretion of the drug
Bone marrow suppression	Use with extreme caution in patients with evidence of hematological disease and in patients who are now being treated or have a history of treatment with myelosuppressive drugs or radiation

ADVERSE REACTIONS

Gastrointestinal	Nausea, vomiting, diarrhea
Hematological	Anemia, leukopenia, thrombocytopenia
Central nervous system	Confusion, hallucinations, headache, sedation, vertigo
Dermatological	Rash

OVERDOSAGE

Signs and symptoms	See ADVERSE REACTIONS
Treatment	Discontinue medication; treat symptomatically and institute supportive measures, as required

DRUG INTERACTIONS

Myelosuppressive agents	⇧ Risk of hematological toxicity
Amphotericin B	⇧ Antifungal activity and toxicity

ALTERED LABORATORY VALUES

Blood/serum values	⇧ Alkaline phosphatase ⇧ Lactate dehydrogenase ⇧ SGOT ⇧ SGPT ⇧ BUN ⇧ Creatinine

No clinically significant alterations in urinary values occur at therapeutic dosages

---

USE IN CHILDREN
Consult manufacturer

USE IN PREGNANT AND NURSING WOMEN
Safety has not been established for use in pregnant or nursing women

---

SYSTEMIC AGENTS

FLAGYL (metronidazole) Searle   Rx

Tablets: 250, 500 mg

INDICATIONS

Symptomatic trichomoniasis, when the presence of trichomonads has been confirmed by appropriate laboratory procedures
Asymptomatic trichomoniasis associated with endocervicitis, cervicitis, or cervical erosion
Treatment of **asymptomatic partners** of treated patients

Acute intestinal amebiasis (acute amebic dysentery)

ORAL DOSAGE

Adult: 250 mg tid for 7 days or, if patient is not pregnant, 2 g given in a single dose or 2 divided doses of 1 g each on the same day. Repeated courses may be given at 4- to 6-wk intervals, upon laboratory confirmation that trichomonads are still present; obtain total and differential leukocyte counts before and after retreatment.

Adult: 750 mg tid for 5–10 days
Child: 35–50 mg/kg/24 h, given in 3 divided doses for 10 days

FLAGYL

Amebic liver abscess

Adult: 500–750 mg tid for 5–10 days
Child: same as child's dosage above

Intraabdominal infections, including peritonitis, intraabdominal abscess, and liver abscess, caused by susceptible strains of *Bacteroides* (including the *B fragilis* group), *Clostridium, Eubacterium, Peptococcus,* and *Peptostreptococcus*
Skin and skin structure infections caused by susceptible strains of *Bacteroides* (including the *B fragilis* group), *Clostridium, Peptococcus, Peptostreptococcus,* and *Fusobacterium*
Gynecologic infections, including endometritis, endomyometritis, tubo-ovarian abscess, and postsurgical vaginal cuff infection, caused by susceptible strains of *Bacteroides* (including the *B fragilis* group), *Clostridium, Peptococcus,* and *Peptostreptococcus*
Bacterial septicemia caused by susceptible strains of *Bacteroides* (including the *B fragilis* group) and *Clostridium*
Bone and joint infections caused by susceptible strains of *Bacteroides* (including the *B fragilis* group) (adjunctive therapy)
Central nervous system infections, including meningitis and brain abscess, caused by susceptible strains of *Bacteroides* (including the *B fragilis* group)
Lower respiratory tract infections including pneumonia, empyema, and lung abscess, caused by susceptible strains of *Bacteroides* (including the *B fragilis* group)
Endocarditis caused by susceptible strains of *Bacteroides* (including the *B fragilis* group)

Adult: 7.5 mg/kg q6h, up to 4.0 g/24 h

CONTRAINDICATIONS

First trimester of pregnancy, when used to treat trichomoniasis	Hypersensitivity to metronidazole or other nitroimidazole derivatives

ADMINISTRATION/DOSAGE ADJUSTMENTS

Duration of therapy for anaerobic infections	Usual duration is 7–10 days; bone and joint infections, lower respiratory tract infections, and endocarditis may require longer treatment
Serious anaerobic infections	Are usually treated first with intravenous metronidazole (Flagyl I.V.)

WARNINGS/PRECAUTIONS

Convulsive seizures and peripheral neuropathy	May occur; warn patient to discontinue use immediately if abnormal neurologic signs appear. Use with caution in patients with CNS diseases.
Tumorigenicity, mutagenicity	Carcinogenic activity has been observed following chronic oral administration to mice and rats; similar studies in hamsters gave negative results. Mutagenic activity has been reported in a number of in vitro assays, but studies in mammals have failed to demonstrate a potential for genetic damage.
Patients with severe hepatic disease	Accumulation of metronidazole and its metabolites may occur. Reduce dosage and use with caution; closely monitor plasma metronidazole levels and observe patient for signs of toxicity.
Anuric patients	Accumulated metabolites may be rapidly removed by dialysis; do not reduce dosage
Known or previously unrecognized candidiasis	May present more prominent symptoms during therapy; treat with a candicidal agent
Mild leukopenia	May occur; use with caution in patients with evidence or a history of blood dyscrasias. Obtain total and differential leukocyte counts before and after therapy.
Amebic liver abscess	Therapy does not obviate need to aspirate pus

ADVERSE REACTIONS

Frequent reactions (incidence ≥ 1%) are printed in *italics*

Gastrointestinal	*Nausea (12%); anorexia; vomiting; diarrhea; epigastric distress; abdominal cramping;* constipation; sharp, metallic, unpleasant taste; furry tongue; glossitis; stomatitis
Central nervous system and neurological	Headache, dizziness, vertigo, incoordination, ataxia, convulsive seizures, confusion, irritability, depression, weakness, insomnia, peripheral neuropathy (numbness, paresthesia of extremities)
Hematological	Leukopenia (reversible)
Hypersensitivity	Urticaria, erythematous rash, flushing, nasal congestion, dry mouth, dryness of the vagina or vulva, fever
Genitourinary	Dysuria, cystitis, dyspareunia, polyuria, incontinence, decreased libido, dark urine, pelvic pressure, proliferation of *Candida* in the vagina
Other	Joint pain (resembling serum sickness), proctitis, flattening of T-wave on ECG

OVERDOSAGE

Signs and symptoms	See ADVERSE REACTIONS; nausea, vomiting, and ataxia have occurred following accidental overdoses and in suicide attempts. Neurotoxic effects, including seizures and peripheral neuropathy, have been reported after 5–7 days of ingestion of 6–10.4 g every other day.

Treatment	Treat symptomatically and institute supportive measures, as needed

DRUG INTERACTIONS

Alcohol	Abdominal cramps, nausea, vomiting, headache, or flushing; alcoholic beverages should be avoided during therapy and for at least 1 day afterward
Oral anticoagulants	↑ Prothrombin time
Cimetidine and other drugs capable of reducing hepatic enzyme activity	↑ Serum metronidazole level
Phenytoin, phenobarbital, and other drugs capable of inducing hepatic enzymes	↓ Serum metronidazole level

ALTERED LABORATORY VALUES

Blood/serum values	↓ SGOT, SGPT, LDH, triglycerides, and hexokinase glucose (with tests based on oxidation-reduction of NAD)

No clinically significant alterations in urinary values occur at therapeutic dosages

USE IN CHILDREN

See INDICATIONS and ORAL DOSAGE; safety and efficacy have not been established for use in children except for the treatment of amebiasis

USE IN PREGNANT AND NURSING WOMEN

Pregnancy Category B: fetotoxicity is caused in mice by intraperitoneal administration, but not by oral administration, of a dose approximating the human dose; reproduction studies in rats given up to 5 times the human dose have shown no evidence of impaired fertility or harm to the fetus. Use during pregnancy only if clearly needed because no adequate, well-controlled studies have been performed in pregnant women and because metronidazole is carcinogenic in mice and rats. Antitrichomonal therapy with metronidazole is contraindicated during the first trimester and, during the second and third trimesters, should be restricted to patients in whom local palliative treatment has been inadequate. Metronidazole crosses the placental barrier and enters the fetal circulation rapidly. It is also excreted in breast milk; patient should stop nursing if drug is prescribed.

SYSTEMIC AGENTS

FULVICIN P/G 165 and 330 (griseofulvin, ultramicrosize) Schering   Rx

Tablets: 165, 330 mg

INDICATIONS

Tinea corporis, tinea pedis, tinea cruris, tinea barbae, tinea capitis, and tinea unguium (onychomycosis) caused by *Trichophyton rubrum, T tonsurans, T mentagrophytes, T interdigitalis, T verrucosum, T megninii, T gallinae, T crateriform, T sulphureum, T schoenleinii, Microsporum audouini, M canis, M gypseum,* and *Epidermophyton floccosum* unresponsive or likely to be unresponsive to topical therapy alone

ORAL DOSAGE

Adult: for tinea corporis, cruris, or capitis, 330 mg/day, given in single or divided daily doses until infecting organism is completely eradicated; for tinea pedis, tinea unguium, and other more resistant infections, 660 mg/day, given in divided daily doses until infecting organism is completely eradicated (see "duration of treatment," below)
Child (30–50 lb): 82.5–165 mg/day (see "duration of treatment," below)
Child (> 50 lb): 165–330 mg/day (see "duration of treatment," below)

FULVICIN-U/F (griseofulvin, microsize) Schering   Rx

Tablets: 250, 500 mg

INDICATIONS

Same as for Fulvicin P/G

ORAL DOSAGE

Adult: for tinea corporis, cruris, or capitis, 500 mg/day, given in single or divided daily doses until infecting organism is completely eradicated; for tinea pedis, tinea unguium, and other more resistant infections, 1,000 mg/day, given in divided daily doses until infecting organism is completely eradicated (see "duration of treatment," below)
Child (30–50 lb): 125–250 mg/day (see "duration of treatment," below)
Child (> 50 lb): 250–500 mg/day (see "duration of treatment," below)

CONTRAINDICATIONS

History of hypersensitivity to griseofulvin	Porphyria	Hepatocellular failure

FULVICIN ■ FUNGIZONE

ADMINISTRATION/DOSAGE ADJUSTMENTS

Pretreatment evaluation	The type of fungi responsible for the infection should be identified before initiating therapy; identification may be made by direct microscopic examination or culture
Duration of treatment	Therapy must be continued until infecting organism is completely eradicated. Representative treatment periods are for tinea corporis, 2–4 wk; tinea capitis, 4–6 wk; tinea pedis, 4–8 wk; tinea unguium, depending on rate of nail growth, at least 4 mo for fingernails and at least 6 mo for toenails (see WARNINGS/PRECAUTIONS)
Concomitant antifungal therapy	Concomitant use of topical agents is usually necessary, particularly in the treatment of tinea pedis (athlete's foot); general hygienic measures should be observed to control sources of infection or reinfection

WARNINGS/PRECAUTIONS

Unwarranted uses	Griseofulvin should not be used for bacterial infections, candidiasis (moniliasis), histoplasmosis, actinomycosis, sporotrichosis, chromoblastomycosis, coccidioidomycosis, North American blastomycosis, cryptococcosis (torulosis), tinea versicolor, and nocardiosis, or for minor or trivial infections that will respond to topical agents alone
Antifungal prophylaxis	Safety and efficacy of griseofulvin for prophylaxis of fungal infections have not been established
Prolonged therapy	Periodically monitor organ system functions, including renal, hepatic, and hematopoietic function, of patients on long-term therapy
Penicillin-allergic patients	May be treated without difficulty, despite theoretical possibility of cross-sensitivity with penicillin
Photosensitivity	May occur; caution patients against undue exposure to artificial or natural sunlight
Hypersensitivity reactions	May occur (see ADVERSE REACTIONS); therapy may need to be withdrawn and appropriate countermeasures instituted
Granulocytopenia	May occur; discontinue medication
Toxicity	Hepatocellular necrosis has been reported in mice, and disturbances in porphyrin metabolism have been observed in laboratory animals
Carcinogenicity	Hepatomas have been observed in mice, and thyroid tumors, mostly adenomas, have been reported in rats. In laboratory animals, griseofulvin has been reported to have a colchicine-like effect on mitosis and act as a cocarcinogen with methylcholanthrene in inducing cutaneous tumors

ADVERSE REACTIONS

Hypersensitivity	Skin rash, urticaria; angioneurotic edema (rare)
Central nervous system	Headache, fatigue, dizziness, insomnia, mental confusion, impaired performance of routine activities; paresthesias of hands and feet (rare)
Gastrointestinal	Nausea, vomiting, epigastric distress, diarrhea
Hematological	Leukopenia and granulocytopenia (rare)
Other	Oral thrush, photosensitivity, lupus erythematosus or lupus-like syndrome; proteinuria (rare)

OVERDOSAGE

Signs and symptoms	See ADVERSE REACTIONS
Treatment	Discontinue medication; treat symptomatically

DRUG INTERACTIONS

Oral anticoagulants	▽ Anticoagulant effect
Barbiturates	▽ Antifungal effect
Alcohol	Tachycardia, flushing

ALTERED LABORATORY VALUES

No clinically significant alterations in blood/serum or urinary values occur at therapeutic dosages

---

USE IN CHILDREN

See INDICATIONS and ORAL DOSAGE; dosage has not been established for children under 2 yr of age. A single daily dose is effective in the treatment of tinea capitis.

USE IN PREGNANT AND NURSING WOMEN

Safety for use during pregnancy has not been established; embryotoxicity and teratogenic effects have been reported in the rat and dog but have not yet been confirmed in other animal species or man. Because of the potential for serious adverse reactions in the nursing infant, the patient should not nurse if use of the drug is deemed essential.

SYSTEMIC AGENTS

FUNGIZONE (amphotericin B) Squibb   Rx
Cream: 3% (20 g)   Lotion: 3% (30 ml)   Ointment: 3% (20 g)   Vials: 50 mg (10 ml)

INDICATIONS	TOPICAL DOSAGE	PARENTERAL DOSAGE
Cutaneous and mucocutaneous candidiasis	**Adult:** apply liberally to candidal lesion 2–4 times/day **Child:** same as adult	

FUNGIZONE

Cryptococcosis
North American blastomycosis
Coccidioidomycosis
Invasive phycomycosis caused by *Mucor, Rhizopus, Absidia, Entomophthora,* and *Basidiobolus*
Invasive aspergillosis
Disseminated sporotrichosis, histoplasmosis, and candidiasis

Adult: 0.25 mg/kg/day IV (slowly) to start, followed by gradual increases, as needed and tolerated, up to 1 mg/kg daily or 1.5 mg/kg every other day, usually for several months
Child: same as adult

CONTRAINDICATIONS

Hypersensitivity to amphotericin B, unless condition is life-threatening and amenable only to amphotericin B therapy

ADMINISTRATION/DOSAGE ADJUSTMENTS

Selection of patients for intravenous therapy	Use only in hospitalized patients, or in those under close clinical observation; use should be restricted to patients with diagnosis of progressive, potentially fatal forms of susceptible mycotic infections that have been firmly established, preferably by culture or histologically
Rate of intravenous infusion	Administer slowly over a period of 6 h; recommended concentration, 0.1 mg/ml (1 mg/10 ml)
Supplemental medication	Adverse reactions resulting from IV therapy may be partially alleviated by giving aspirin, antihistamines, and antiemetics. Alternate-day therapy may decrease anorexia and phlebitis. IV administration of adrenal corticosteroids just prior to, or during, infusion of amphotericin B may decrease febrile reactions. (Dosage and duration of corticosteroid treatment should be kept to a minimum.) Adding small amounts of heparin to the infusion may decrease incidence of thrombophlebitis.
Interruption of intravenous therapy	If lapse is longer than 7 days, reinstitute therapy at lowest dosage level and increase dosage gradually
Clinical response of mycotic skin infections	Intertriginous lesions usually respond within a few days, and treatment may be completed within 1–3 wk. Candidiasis in other than interdigital areas usually resolves within 1–2 wk, whereas interdigital lesions and paronychias may require 2–4 wk of intensive treatment. Onychomycotic infections that respond may require several months or more of treatment.

WARNINGS/PRECAUTIONS[1]

Renal impairment	Determine BUN and serum creatinine levels (or endogenous creatinine clearance) at least weekly; if BUN > 40 mg/dl or serum creatinine > 3.0 mg/dl, discontinue therapy or reduce dosage markedly until renal function improves. Some permanent impairment often occurs, especially with cumulative doses > 5 g. Supplemental alkalinization of the urine may reduce renal tubular acidosis complications
Hepatic impairment	Obtain weekly liver-function studies; if sulfobromophthalein retention, serum alkaline phosphatase concentration, and/or bilirubin level rise, therapy may have to be discontinued
Hematopoietic abnormalities	May occur (see ADVERSE REACTIONS); obtain weekly hemograms
Hypokalemia	Occurs frequently and may be potentiated by concomitant corticosteroid therapy; determine serum potassium level at least weekly during therapy
Hypersensitivity reactions	Discontinue therapy and institute appropriate treatment
Concomitant therapy	Other nephrotoxic antibiotics should be used with great caution, if at all, in combination with amphotericin B; concomitant treatment with antineoplastic agents (eg, nitrogen mustard) also should be avoided, if possible
Rhinocerebral phycomycosis	Generally occurs in association with diabetic ketoacidosis; diabetic control must be restored before successful antifungal treatment can be accomplished
Oleaginous ointment	May be irritating to moist intertriginous areas

ADVERSE REACTIONS[1]

Frequent reactions (incidence ≥ 1%) are printed in *italics*

Central nervous system	*Headache, malaise,* convulsions
Otic	Hearing loss, tinnitus, transient vertigo
Ophthalmic	Blurred vision or diplopia
Gastrointestinal	*Anorexia, nausea, vomiting, dyspepsia, diarrhea, cramping epigastric pain,* melena or hemorrhagic gastroenteritis, acute liver failure
Hematological	*Normochromic, normocytic anemia;* coagulation defects, thrombocytopenia, leukopenia, agranulocytosis, eosinophilia, leukocytosis
Renal	*Hypokalemia, azotemia, hyposthenuria, renal tubular acidosis, nephrocalcinosis,* anuria, oliguria
Cardiovascular	Arrhythmias, ventricular fibrillation, cardiac arrest, hypertension, hypotension
Dermatological	Slight sensitization (with topical preparations); erythema, pruritus, or burning sensation (with cream); pruritus, with or without other signs of local irritation (with lotion and IV form); maculopapular rash (with IV form)

FUNGIZONE ■ MONISTAT i.v.

Other	Fever, sometimes with shaking chills; weight loss; generalized pain, including muscle and joint pain; pain and irritation at injection site, with phlebitis and thrombophlebitis; peripheral neuropathy, anaphylactoid reactions, flushing

OVERDOSAGE

Signs and symptoms	See ADVERSE REACTIONS
Treatment	Discontinue medication; institute supportive measures, as required

DRUG INTERACTIONS

Digitalis	△ Risk of digitalis toxicity
Corticosteroids	△ Risk of hypokalemia
Flucytosine	△ Toxicity of flucytosine
Nephrotoxic antibiotics	△ Risk of renal toxicity

ALTERED LABORATORY VALUES

Blood/serum values	△ BUN △ Creatinine △ Sulfobromophthalein retention △ Alkaline phosphatase △ Bilirubin ▽ Potassium ▽ Magnesium ▽ Sodium ▽ Calcium

No clinically significant alterations in urinary values occur at therapeutic dosages

---

USE IN CHILDREN
See INDICATIONS and dosage recommendations

USE IN PREGNANT AND NURSING WOMEN
Safety of parenteral administration during pregnancy has not been established. Consult manufacturer for use in nursing mothers.

VEHICLE/BASE
Cream (aqueous, tinted): titanium dioxide, thimerosal, propylene glycol, cetearyl alcohol (and) ceteareth-20, white petrolatum, sorbitol solution, glyceryl monostearate, polyethylene glycol monostearate, simethicone, sorbic acid, methylparaben, and propylparaben
Lotion (aqueous, tinted, scented): titanium dioxide, thimerosal, guar gum, propylene glycol, cetyl alcohol, stearyl alcohol, sorbitan monopalmitate, polysorbate 20, glyceryl monostearate, polyethylene glycol monostearate, simethicone, sorbic acid, methylparaben, and propylparaben
Ointment (tinted; gel): titanium dioxide, mineral oil, polyethylene glycol 300, polyethylene glycol 400, polyethylene glycol 1540, and polyethylene glycol 6000 distearate, with butylated hydroxytoluene as a preservative

[1] The topical preparations have no evident systemic toxicity or side effects

---

SYSTEMIC AGENTS

MONISTAT i.v. (miconazole) Janssen   Rx
Ampuls: 10 mg/ml[1] (20 ml)

INDICATIONS	PARENTERAL DOSAGE
Coccidioidomycosis	**Adult:** 1,800–3,600 mg/day, given by IV infusion (30–60 min) in a single daily dose or in 3 divided doses for 3–20 wk or longer; for relapse or reinfection, repeat course **Child:** 20–40 mg/kg/day, given by IV infusion (30–60 min) in divided doses of up to 15 mg/kg
Cryptococcosis	**Adult:** 1,200–2,400 mg/day, given by IV infusion (30–60 min) in a single daily dose or in 3 divided doses for 3–12 wk or longer; for relapse or reinfection, repeat course **Child:** 20–40 mg/kg/day, given by IV infusion (30–60 min) in divided doses of up to 15 mg/kg
Candidiasis Chronic mucocutaneous candidiasis	**Adult:** 600–1,800 mg/day, given by IV infusion (30–60 min) in a single daily dose or in 3 divided doses for 1–20 wk or longer; for relapse or reinfection, repeat course **Child:** 20–40 mg/kg/day, given by IV infusion (30–60 min) in divided doses of up to 15 mg/kg
Petriellidiosis (allescheriosis)	**Adult:** 600–3,000 mg/day, given by IV infusion (30–60 min) in a single dose or in 3 divided doses for 5–20 wk or longer; for relapse or reinfection, repeat course **Child:** 20–40 mg/kg/day, given by IV infusion (30–60 min) in divided doses of up to 15 mg/kg
Paracoccidioidomycosis	**Adult:** 200–1,200 mg/day, given by IV infusion (30–60 min) in a single daily dose or in 3 divided doses for 2–16 wk or longer; for relapse or reinfection, repeat course **Child:** 20–40 mg/kg/day, given by IV infusion (30–60 min) in divided doses of up to 15 mg/kg
Fungal meningitis (adjunctive therapy)	**Adult:** 20 mg (undiluted), given intrathecally every 3–7 days by alternate lumbar, cervical, and cisternal punctures

MONISTAT i.v.

Urinary bladder mycoses (adjunctive therapy)   **Adult:** 200 mg by bladder instillation

CONTRAINDICATIONS

Hypersensitivity to miconazole

ADMINISTRATION/DOSAGE ADJUSTMENTS

Preparation of IV infusion	Dilute contents of each ampul in at least 200 ml of 0.9% sodium chloride or 5% dextrose
Initial therapy	Give 200 mg to start with the physician in attendance and under stringent hospital conditions
Nausea and vomiting	May be mitigated by giving antihistaminic or antiemetic drugs before miconazole infusion or by reducing the dose, slowing the rate of infusion, or avoiding administration at mealtime

WARNINGS/PRECAUTIONS

Transient tachycardia or arrhythmia	May occur with rapid injection of undiluted miconazole
Petriellidiosis	Obtain cultures if petriellidiosis is suspected because of the difficulty in distinguishing *Petriellidium boydii* from *Aspergillus* histologically
Patient monitoring	Obtain hemoglobin, hematocrit, electrolyte, and lipid determinations
Ambulatory patients	Closely monitor suitable patients
Unwarranted use	Trivial forms of fungal diseases should not be treated with IV miconazole
Systemic fungal mycoses	May be complications of chronic underlying disease; take appropriate diagnostic and therapeutic measures, if indicated
Severe pruritus and skin rashes	May occur; discontinue medication

ADVERSE REACTIONS

Frequent reactions (incidence ≥ 1%) are printed in *italics*

Dermatological	*Pruritus (21%), rash (9%)*
Gastrointestinal	*Nausea (18%), vomiting (7%),* diarrhea, anorexia
Central nervous system	Drowsiness
Hematological	Decreased hematocrit, thrombocytopenia, RBC aggregation or rouleau formation on blood smears
Other	*Phlebitis (29%), fever and chills (10%),* hyperlipemia (due to vehicle), flushes

OVERDOSAGE

Signs and symptoms	See WARNINGS/PRECAUTIONS and ADVERSE REACTIONS
Treatment	Discontinue medication; treat symptomatically and institute supportive measures, as required

DRUG INTERACTIONS

Oral anticoagulants	⇧ Anticoagulant effect; monitor anticoagulant response and, if necessary, reduce dosage of the anticoagulant
Sulfonylureas	Severe hypoglycemia
Rifampin	⇩ Serum miconazole level; avoid concomitant use
Cyclosporine	⇧ Serum cyclosporine level; monitor serum level during concomitant use
Phenytoin	⇧ or ⇩ Serum level of phenytoin and miconazole; consider monitoring serum levels of both drugs during concomitant use

ALTERED LABORATORY VALUES

Blood/serum values	⇩ Sodium Abnormal lipoprotein electrophoresis (due to vehicle)

No clinically significant alterations in urinary values occur at therapeutic dosages

---

USE IN CHILDREN

Safety has not been established for use in children under 1 yr of age

USE IN PREGNANT AND NURSING WOMEN

Safety for use during pregnancy has not been established. Reproduction studies in rats and rabbits have shown no evidence of impaired fertility or harm to the fetus; however, no studies have been performed in pregnant women. Information on use in nursing mothers is not available.

---

[1] Contains PEG 40 castor oil (Cremophor EL), which may cause hyperlipidemia and affect lipoprotein electrophoresis

SYSTEMIC AGENTS

MYCOSTATIN (nystatin) Squibb   Rx

Suspension: 100,000 units/ml (5, 60, 473 ml)   **Tablets:** 500,000 units

INDICATIONS	ORAL DOSAGE
Candidiasis of the oral cavity	Adult and child: 400,000–600,000 units (2–3 ml in each side of mouth) qid Infant: 200,000 units (1 ml in each side of mouth) qid
Intestinal candidiasis	Adult: 500,000–1,000,000 units (1–2 tabs) tid

CONTRAINDICATIONS

Hypersensitivity to nystatin or other components

ADMINISTRATION/DOSAGE ADJUSTMENTS

Premature or low-birth-weight infants	For treatment of oral candidiasis, 100,000 units (1 ml) qid may be effective
Duration of therapy	Continue treatment of candidiasis of the oral cavity for at least 48 h after perioral symptoms have cleared and cultures have returned to normal; to prevent relapse, treatment of intestinal candidiasis should be continued for at least 48 h after clinical cure has been achieved

ADVERSE REACTIONS

Gastrointestinal	Diarrhea, distress, nausea, and vomiting

OVERDOSAGE

Signs and symptoms	See ADVERSE REACTIONS
Treatment	Discontinue medication; treat symptomatically

DRUG INTERACTIONS

No clinically significant drug interactions have been identified

ALTERED LABORATORY VALUES

No clinically significant alterations in blood/serum or urinary values occur at therapeutic dosages

---

USE IN CHILDREN

See INDICATIONS and dosage recommendations. The oral preparations are well tolerated by all age groups, including debilitated infants.

USE IN PREGNANT AND NURSING WOMEN

No adverse effects or complications in infants have been attributed to oral administration of nystatin during pregnancy. Consult manufacturer for information pertaining to the use of nystatin by nursing women.

SYSTEMIC AGENTS

NIZORAL (ketoconazole) Janssen   Rx

Tablets: 200 mg   **Suspension (per 5 ml):** 100 mg (4 fl oz) *cherry flavored*

INDICATIONS	ORAL DOSAGE
Candidiasis[1] Chronic mucocutaneous candidiasis Oral thrush Candiduria Blastomycosis Coccidioidomycosis[1] Histoplasmosis Chromomycosis Paracoccidioidomycosis[1] **Severe, recalcitrant cutaneous dermatophytoses** in patients who have not responded to topical therapy or oral griseofulvin or who are unable to take griseofulvin	Adult: 200 mg/day to start; if clinical response is inadequate within expected period or if infection is very severe, increase dosage to 400 mg once daily Child (> 2 yr): 3.3–6.6 mg/kg once daily

CONTRAINDICATIONS

Hypersensitivity to ketoconazole

ADMINISTRATION/DOSAGE ADJUSTMENTS

Duration of therapy — Perform clinical and laboratory testing prior to initiating ketoconazole therapy, and continue treatment until all tests indicate subsidence of active infection. Candidiasis requires a minimum of 1–2 wk of treatment; patients with chronic mucocutaneous candidiasis usually require maintenance therapy. Treat other systemic mycoses for at least 6 mo. Patients with recalcitrant dermatophyte infections should be treated for a minimum of 4 wk in cases involving glabrous skin; palmar and plantar infections may respond more slowly. In some cases, the infection may recur after discontinuation of therapy.

Concomitant use of drugs that reduce gastric acidity — Wait at least 2 h after administering ketoconazole before giving antacids, anticholinergics, or H_2-blockers (see DRUG INTERACTIONS). In cases of achlorhydria, instruct patient to dissolve each tablet in 4 ml of 0.2N hydrochloric acid and to sip the resulting mixture through a glass or plastic straw to avoid contact with the teeth; follow with a cup of tap water.

WARNINGS/PRECAUTIONS

Hepatic toxicity — Hepatic dysfunction has occurred and has been fatal in rare instances, mainly as a result of hepatocellular toxicity; symptomatic hepatotoxicity has developed in patients treated with ketoconazole for a median duration of 28 days, although it has occurred after 3 days, and mostly in patients treated for onychomycosis and, less commonly, chronic recalcitrant dermatophytoses. Several cases of hepatitis have been seen in children. The disorders have usually, but not always, been reversible. Instruct patient to report any signs or symptoms of liver dysfunction, such as unusual fatigue, anorexia, nausea, vomiting, jaundice, dark urine, and pale stools; determine hepatic enzyme and bilirubin levels frequently. Use of ketoconazole in combination with other potentially hepatotoxic drugs should be carefully monitored, particularly if therapy is prolonged or if the patient has a history of liver disease. Minor elevations of hepatic enzyme levels may return to normal with continued treatment; however, if abnormal enzyme levels persist, continue to rise, or are accompanied by symptoms of possible hepatic injury, use of ketoconazole should be discontinued.

Hypersensitivity — Anaphylaxis has occurred in rare cases, and other allergic reactions, including urticaria, have been seen in several instances

Increased fragility of long bones, occasional fractures — Have occurred in female rats receiving 80 mg/kg or more for 3–6 mo; no effect was seen with doses $\leq$ 20 mg/kg (2.5 times the maximum recommended human dose). Limited studies in dogs have failed to demonstrate a similar effect on the metacarpals and ribs. Clinical significance is unknown.

Hormonal fluctuations — Ketoconazole may reversibly lower serum testosterone levels, beginning at a dosage of 800 mg/day; testosterone secretion is abolished at a dosage of 1,600 mg/day. ACTH-induced corticosteroid secretion is also reduced at similar dosages and may have contributed to the death of 11 patients with metastatic prostatic cancer who were treated with 1,200 mg/day of ketoconazole, although it was not possible to establish a causal relationship in these cases. Follow the recommended dosages closely.

Carcinogenicity, mutagenicity — No evidence of carcinogenicity has been found in the Ames test or in a long-term study in mice and rats; a dominant lethal mutation study in mice given up to 80 mg/kg (10 times the maximum human dose) in single oral doses has shown no evidence of mutagenicity

ADVERSE REACTIONS

Frequent reactions (incidence $\geq$ 1%) are printed in *italics*

Gastrointestinal — *Nausea, with or without vomiting (3%); abdominal pain (1.2%);* diarrhea; hepatic dysfunction (rare)

Dermatological — *Pruritus (1.5%)*

Central nervous system — Headache, dizziness, somnolence

Endocrinological — Gynecomastia, impotence; oligospermia (at dosages exceeding 400 mg/day)

Hypersensitivity — Urticaria and other allergic reactions; anaphylaxis (rare)

Other — Fever, chills, photophobia, thrombocytopenia, leukopenia, hemolytic anemia, bulging fontanelles

OVERDOSAGE

Signs and symptoms — See ADVERSE REACTIONS

Treatment — Discontinue medication; treat symptomatically and institute supportive measures, including gastric lavage with sodium bicarbonate, as needed

DRUG INTERACTIONS

Antacids, anticholinergic agents, H_2-blockers — ▽ Dissolution and absorption of ketoconazole (see ADMINISTRATION/DOSAGE ADJUSTMENTS)

Oral anticoagulants — △ Anticoagulant effect; monitor anticoagulant response and, if necessary, reduce dosage of the anticoagulant

Sulfonylureas — Severe hypoglycemia

NIZORAL ■ PROTOSTAT

Rifampin, isoniazid — ⇩ Serum ketoconazole level; avoid concomitant use

Cyclosporine — ⇧ Serum cyclosporine level; monitor serum level during concomitant use

Phenytoin — ⇧ or ⇩ Serum level of phenytoin and ketoconazole; consider monitoring serum levels of both drugs during concomitant use

ALTERED LABORATORY VALUES

Blood/serum values — ⇧ Liver enzymes ⇩ Testosterone ⇩ Corticosteroids

No clinically significant alterations in urinary values occur at therapeutic dosages

USE IN CHILDREN
See INDICATIONS and ORAL DOSAGE. Safety and effectiveness for use in children under 2 yr of age have not been established; use in children only if expected benefit justifies the potential risk.

USE IN PREGNANT AND NURSING WOMEN
Pregnancy Category C: use during pregnancy only if the expected benefits justify the potential risk to the fetus. Teratogenicity (possibly related to maternal toxicity) and embryotoxicity have been demonstrated in rats fed approximately 10 times the maximum recommended human dose; difficult labor has been noted in rats that had received doses exceeding 1.25 times the maximum human dose during the third trimester. No adequate, well-controlled studies have been performed in pregnant women. Patient should stop nursing if drug is prescribed, since ketoconazole is probably excreted in human breast milk.

[1] Because of poor penetration into CSF, ketoconazole should not be used for fungal meningitis

---

SYSTEMIC AGENTS

PROTOSTAT (metronidazole) Ortho   Rx
Tablets: 250, 500 mg

INDICATIONS

Symptomatic trichomoniasis, when the presence of trichomonads has been confirmed by appropriate laboratory procedures
Asymptomatic trichomoniasis associated with endocervicitis, cervicitis, or cervical erosion
Treatment of **asymptomatic partners** of treated patients

ORAL DOSAGE

Adult: 250 mg tid for 7 days or, if patient is not pregnant, 2 g given in a single dose or 2 divided doses of 1 g each on the same day. Repeated courses may be given at 4- to 6-wk intervals, upon laboratory confirmation that trichomonads are still present; obtain total and differential leukocyte counts before and after retreatment.

Acute intestinal amebiasis (acute amebic dysentery)

Adult: 750 mg tid for 5–10 days
Child: 35–50 mg/kg/24 h, given in 3 divided doses for 10 days

Amebic liver abscess

Adult: 500–750 mg tid for 5–10 days
Child: same as child's dosage above

Intraabdominal infections, including peritonitis, intraabdominal abscess, and liver abscess, caused by susceptible strains of *Bacteroides* (including the *B fragilis* group), *Clostridium, Eubacterium, Peptococcus,* and *Peptostreptococcus*
Skin and skin structure infections caused by susceptible strains of *Bacteroides* (including the *B fragilis* group), *Clostridium, Peptococcus, Peptostreptococcus,* and *Fusobacterium*
Gynecologic infections, including endometritis, endomyometritis, tubo-ovarian abscess, and postsurgical vaginal cuff infection, caused by susceptible strains of *Bacteroides* (including the *B fragilis* group), *Clostridium, Peptococcus,* and *Peptostreptococcus*
Bacterial septicemia caused by susceptible strains of *Bacteroides* (including the *B fragilis* group) and *Clostridium*
Bone and joint infections caused by susceptible strains of *Bacteroides* (including the *B fragilis* group) (adjunctive therapy)
Central nervous system infections, including meningitis and brain abscess, caused by susceptible strains of *Bacteroides* (including the *B fragilis* group)
Lower respiratory tract infections, including pneumonia, empyema, and lung abscess, caused by susceptible strains of *Bacteroides* (including the *B fragilis* group)
Endocarditis caused by susceptible strains of *Bacteroides* (including the *B fragilis* group)

Adult: 7.5 mg/kg q6h, up to 4.0 g/24 h

PROTOSTAT

CONTRAINDICATIONS

First trimester of pregnancy, when used to treat trichomoniasis	Hypersensitivity to metronidazole or other nitroimidazole derivatives

ADMINISTRATION/DOSAGE ADJUSTMENTS

Duration of therapy for anaerobic infections	Usual duration is 7–10 days; bone and joint infections, lower respiratory tract infections, and endocarditis may require longer treatment
Serious anaerobic infections	Are usually treated first with intravenous metronidazole

WARNINGS/PRECAUTIONS

Convulsive seizures and peripheral neuropathy	May occur; warn patient to discontinue use immediately if abnormal neurologic signs appear. Use with caution in patients with CNS diseases.
Tumorigenicity, mutagenicity	Carcinogenic activity has been observed following chronic oral administration to mice and rats; similar studies in hamsters gave negative results. Mutagenic activity has been reported in a number of in vitro assays, but studies in mammals have failed to demonstrate a potential for genetic damage.
Patients with severe hepatic disease	Accumulation of metronidazole and its metabolites may occur. Reduce dosage and use with caution; closely monitor plasma metronidazole levels and observe patient for signs of toxicity.
Anuric patients	Accumulated metabolites may be rapidly removed by dialysis; do not reduce dosage
Known or previously unrecognized candidiasis	May present more prominent symptoms during therapy; treat with a candicidal agent
Mild leukopenia	May occur; use with caution in patients with evidence or a history of blood dyscrasias. Obtain total and differential leukocyte counts before and after therapy.
Amebic liver abscess	Therapy does not obviate need to aspirate pus
Alcohol ingestion	Should be avoided (see DRUG INTERACTIONS); patient may also find that the taste of alcoholic beverages is altered

ADVERSE REACTIONS

Frequent reactions (incidence $\geq$ 1%) are printed in *italics*

Gastrointestinal	*Nausea; anorexia; vomiting; diarrhea; epigastric distress; abdominal cramping;* constipation; sharp, metallic, unpleasant taste, furry tongue, glossitis, and stomatitis possibly associated with a sudden proliferation of *Candida* in the mouth
Central nervous system and neurological	Headache, dizziness, vertigo, incoordination, ataxia, convulsive seizures, confusion, irritability, depression, weakness, insomnia, peripheral neuropathy (numbness, paresthesia of extremities)
Hematological	Leukopenia (reversible)
Hypersensitivity	Urticaria, erythematous rash, flushing, nasal congestion, dry mouth, dryness of the vagina or vulva, fever
Genitourinary	Dysuria, cystitis, dyspareunia, polyuria, incontinence, decreased libido, dark urine, pelvic pressure, proliferation of *Candida* in the vagina
Other	Joint pain (resembling serum sickness), proctitis, flattening of T-wave on ECG

OVERDOSAGE

Signs and symptoms	See ADVERSE REACTIONS; nausea, vomiting, and ataxia have occurred following accidental overdoses and in suicide attempts. Neurotoxic effects, including seizures and peripheral neuropathy, have been reported after 5–7 days of ingestion of 6–10.4 g every other day.
Treatment	Treat symptomatically and institute supportive measures, as needed

DRUG INTERACTIONS

Alcohol	Abdominal cramps, nausea, vomiting, headache, or flushing
Oral anticoagulants	⇧ Prothrombin time
Phenytoin, phenobarbital, other drugs capable of inducing hepatic enzymes	⇩ Serum metronidazole level

ALTERED LABORATORY VALUES

Blood/serum values	⇩ SGOT (test interference)

No clinically significant alterations in urinary values occur at therapeutic dosages

---

USE IN CHILDREN

See INDICATIONS and ORAL DOSAGE; safety and efficacy have not been established for use in children except for the treatment of amebiasis

USE IN PREGNANT AND NURSING WOMEN

Pregnancy Category B: reproduction studies in rabbits and rats given up to 5 times the human dose have shown no evidence of impaired fertility or harm to the fetus. Nevertheless, use during pregnancy only if clearly needed because no adequate, well-controlled studies have been performed in pregnant women and because metronidazole is carcinogenic in mice and rats. Antitrichomonal therapy with metronidazole is contraindicated during the first trimester and, during the second and third trimesters, should be restricted to patients in whom local palliative treatment has been inadequate. Metronidazole crosses the placental barrier and enters the fetal circulation rapidly. It is also excreted in breast milk; patient should stop nursing if drug is prescribed.

SYSTEMIC AGENTS

SYMMETREL (amantadine hydrochloride) Du Pont Rx

Capsules: 100 mg **Syrup (per 5 ml):** 50 mg

INDICATIONS	ORAL DOSAGE
Idiopathic and postencephalitic parkinsonism **Symptomatic parkinsonism** caused by carbon monoxide intoxication **Parkinsonism** associated with cerebral arteriosclerosis in the elderly	**Adult:** 100 mg bid to start, followed, if necessary, by up to 400 mg/day, given in divided doses under close medical supervision
Drug-induced extrapyramidal reactions	**Adult:** 100 mg bid to start, followed, if necessary, by up to 300 mg/day in divided doses
Prophylaxis and symptomatic treatment of **respiratory tract illness** caused by influenza A virus strains	**Adult:** 200 mg/day, given in a single daily dose or 2 divided doses **Child (1–9 yr):** 2–4 mg/lb/day, up to 150 mg/day, given in 2–3 equally divided doses **Child (9–12 yr):** same as adult

CONTRAINDICATIONS

Hypersensitivity to amantadine

ADMINISTRATION/DOSAGE ADJUSTMENTS

Concomitant therapy	Reduce dosage of amantadine hydrochloride or concomitant anticholinergics if atropine-like effects occur; use cautiously with CNS stimulants
Combination therapy with levodopa	When adding levodopa, maintain a constant amantadine dosage of 100 mg 1–2 times/day, while gradually increasing levodopa dosage to optimal level
Prolonged therapy	Effectiveness may decrease after several months; increase dosage to 300 mg/day or temporarily discontinue therapy for several weeks
Seriously ill patients or those receiving other antiparkinson agents in high doses	Initiate therapy with 100 mg/day, followed by 100 mg bid, if necessary, after one to several weeks
CNS disturbances	May be alleviated by twice-daily administration
Duration of therapy for influenza A virus respiratory illness	For prophylaxis, continue treatment at least 10 days following known exposure. When used chemoprophylactically with inactivated influenza A virus vaccine, administer for 2–3 wk after vaccine has been given. When vaccine is unavailable or contraindicated, administer amantadine for up to 90 days. Symptomatic treatment should be started as soon as possible after the onset of symptoms and continued for 24–48 h after symptoms disappear.

WARNINGS/PRECAUTIONS

Congestive heart failure	May occur; closely supervise therapy in patients with a history of congestive heart failure or peripheral edema
Patients with convulsive disorders	Closely monitor patients with a history of epilepsy or other seizure disorders for possible increased seizure activity
Other special-risk patients	Adjust dosage carefully in patients with renal impairment, congestive heart failure, peripheral edema, or orthostatic hypotension; use with caution in patients with hepatic disease, a history of recurrent eczematoid rash, or psychosis or severe psychoneurosis not controlled by drugs
Mental impairment, blurred vision	Caution patients to avoid driving or other potentially hazardous activities if they experience CNS effects or blurred vision
Resumption of normal activities	Caution patients with Parkinson's disease whose symptoms improve to resume their normal activities gradually and with caution
Abrupt discontinuation of therapy	May precipitate parkinsonian crisis in patients with Parkinson's disease
Carcinogenicity, mutagenicity	The carcinogenic and mutagenic potential of this drug have not been investigated

ADVERSE REACTIONS

Frequent reactions (incidence $\geq$ 1%) are printed in *italics*

Central nervous system	*Depression, psychosis,* hallucinations, confusion, anxiety, irritability, dizziness, lightheadedness, headache, fatigue, insomnia, weakness, slurred speech, ataxia; convulsions (rare)
Cardiovascular	*Congestive heart failure, orthostatic hypotension,* peripheral edema
Hematological	Leukopenia and neutropenia (rare)
Gastrointestinal	Anorexia, nausea, constipation, vomiting, dry mouth
Dermatological	Skin rash, livedo reticularis; eczematoid dermatitis (rare)
Ophthalmic	Visual disturbances; oculogyric episodes (rare)
Other	Urinary retention, dyspnea

OVERDOSAGE

Signs and symptoms	Urinary retention, hyperactivity, convulsions, arrhythmias, hypotension, acid-base disturbances, and acute toxic psychosis manifested by disorientation, confusion, visual hallucinations, and aggressive behavior
Treatment	Empty stomach by gastric lavage or emesis and institute supportive measures, including forced or IV fluids, if necessary. Acidification of the urine may speed elimination of the drug. For CNS effects, slowly administer physostigmine (1–2 mg IV q1–2h in adults and 0.5 mg IV at 5- to 10-min intervals, up to 2 mg/h, in children). Monitor vital signs, serum electrolytes, urine pH, and urinary output. Catheterization should be done if patient has not recently voided. Employ appropriate anticonvulsant, antiarrhythmic, and vasopressor therapy, as needed.

DRUG INTERACTIONS

Anticholinergic agents	⇧	Atropine-like effects

ALTERED LABORATORY VALUES

No clinically significant alterations in blood/serum or urinary values occur at therapeutic dosages

---

USE IN CHILDREN
See INDICATIONS and ORAL DOSAGE; safety and effectiveness for use in newborns and infants under 1 yr of age have not been established

USE IN PREGNANT AND NURSING WOMEN
Pregnancy Category C: use during pregnancy only if the expected benefit of therapy outweighs the potential risk to the embryo or fetus. Amantadine has been shown to be embryotoxic and teratogenic in rats at 12 times the recommended human dose but not in rabbits receiving up to 25 times the human dose. No adequate, well-controlled studies have been done in pregnant women. Amantadine is excreted in human milk; use with caution in nursing women.

SYSTEMIC AGENTS

VIRA-A (vidarabine monohydrate) Parke-Davis   Rx

Vials: 200 mg/ml (5 ml) for IV infusion only

INDICATIONS	PARENTERAL DOSAGE
Herpes simplex virus encephalitis	**Adult:** 15 mg/kg/day, given by IV infusion for a period of 10 days
Herpes zoster in immunosuppressed patients	**Adult:** 10 mg/kg/day, given by IV infusion for a period of 5 days

CONTRAINDICATIONS
Hypersensitivity to vidarabine

ADMINISTRATION/DOSAGE ADJUSTMENTS

Herpes simplex virus encephalitis	Vidarabine does not alter morbidity or the resulting serious neurological sequelae in comatose patients; thus, early diagnosis and treatment are essential. Encephalitis due to herpes simplex virus should be suspected in patients with a history of acute febrile encephalopathy associated with disordered mentation, an altered level of consciousness, and focal cerebral signs, particularly after CSF examination and localization of an intracerebral lesion by brain scan, CAT scan, or EEG. Brain biopsy, following viral isolation in cell cultures or by use of specific fluorescent antibody techniques, is necessary to confirm the diagnosis; discontinue use of vidarabine if cell culture results are negative. Detection of *Herpesvirus*-like particles by electron microscopy or intranuclear inclusion by histopathological techniques provides only a presumptive diagnosis.
Herpes zoster	Skin eruptions occur along a sensory nerve network as vesicles and develop into pustules and then scabs; begin treatment as early as possible—within 72 h after the appearance of vesicular lesions. Fever, local pain, and erythema may precede formation of vesicles. Varicella-zoster virus can be detected by isolation from lesions or by immunofluorescent techniques.
Preparation of infusion	Shake the vial well to obtain a homogeneous suspension, and then aseptically transfer the proper dose to an appropriate prewarmed (35–40° C) IV infusion fluid; do not use biological or colloidal fluids (eg, blood products and protein solutions) as diluents. Each milligram of vidarabine monohydrate requires 2.22 ml of IV infusion fluid for complete solubilization (ie, 1 liter for every 450 mg). Thoroughly agitate admixture until it is *completely* clear; after solubilization, subsequent agitation is unnecessary. Use an in-line membrane filter (pore size $\leq 45\ \mu m$) for final filtration. Prepare dilution immediately before administration, and use within 48 h; do not refrigerate.

VIRA-A

Parenteral administration	Using aseptic technique, slowly infuse the total daily dose at a constant rate over a period of 12–24 h; avoid rapid or bolus injection. Because of its low solubility and poor absorption, this drug should not be administered IM or SC.

WARNINGS/PRECAUTIONS

Efficacy	Vidarabine is effective only if some degree of immunocompetence is present. This drug is not effective against bacterial or fungal infections or those caused by adenoviruses or RNA viruses, nor is there any evidence that vidarabine would be effective in treating infections due to cytomegalovirus, vaccinia virus, or smallpox virus or encephalitis due to varicella-zoster virus.
Patients undergoing allopurinol therapy	Use with caution in patients receiving allopurinol because, according to laboratory studies, allopurinol may interfere with vidarabine metabolism (however, clear evidence of adverse effects in humans has not been reported)
Patients with hepatic impairment	Observe patients with impaired liver function for possible adverse effects
Other special-risk patients	Use with special care in patients susceptible to fluid overload or cerebral edema (eg, patients with CNS infection or renal impairment). Since this drug is principally eliminated by the kidneys, carefully monitor patients with renal impairment (eg, postoperative renal transplant recipients) and, if necessary, adjust dosage.
Carcinogenicity	Chronic IM administration to mice and rats has resulted in a significantly increased incidence of thyroid adenomas in rats, kidney neoplasia in male mice, liver tumors in female mice, and hepatic megalocytosis in mice and rats; an increase in transformed foci in vitro has been observed in the Balb/3T3 assay
Mutagenicity	In vitro studies have shown that vidarabine can be incorporated into mammalian DNA and that it can cause mutagenic effects in mouse cells and *Salmonella* (with the Ames test) and chromosomal aberrations in human leukocytes and Chinese hamster ovary cells; although the results of in vivo studies have not been as conclusive, the evidence obtained from the dominant lethal assay in mice indicates that vidarabine may be able to produce mutagenic changes in male germ cells.

ADVERSE REACTIONS

The most frequent reactions, regardless of incidence, are printed in *italics*

Gastrointestinal	*Anorexia, nausea, vomiting, diarrhea,* hematemesis
Central nervous system	Tremor, dizziness, hallucinations, confusion, psychosis, ataxia, headache, encephalopathy, malaise
Hematological	Decreased hemoglobin or hematocrit; decreased WBC, reticulocyte, and platelet counts
Dermatological	Pruritus, rash
Other	Weight loss, pain at injection site

OVERDOSAGE

Signs and symptoms	Acute massive overdosage without serious adverse effects has been reported; however, dosages exceeding 20 mg/kg/day can cause bone marrow depression with concomitant thrombocytopenia and leukopenia. Acute water overloading could occur with overdosage (due to vidarabine's low solubility) and would pose a greater risk than excessive amounts of the drug itself.
Treatment	Carefully monitor hematological, hepatic, and renal function and institute supportive measures, as indicated

DRUG INTERACTIONS

Allopurinol	Interference with vidarabine metabolism (theoretical); use with caution

ALTERED LABORATORY VALUES

Blood/serum values	⇧ SGOT ⇧ Bilirubin

No clinically significant alterations in urinary values occur at therapeutic dosages

---

USE IN CHILDREN

Consult manufacturer for use in children

USE IN PREGNANT AND NURSING WOMEN

Pregnancy Category C: use during pregnancy only if the expected therapeutic benefit justifies the potential risk to the fetus. Vidarabine is teratogenic in rats at doses of 150–250 mg/kg and in rabbits at doses of 5 mg/kg or higher. No adequate, well-controlled studies have been performed in pregnant women. It is not known whether vidarabine is excreted in human milk. Because many drugs are excreted in human milk and because of this drug's tumorigenic potential, a decision should be made to either discontinue nursing or not use this drug.

SYSTEMIC AGENTS

VIRAZOLE (ribavirin) ICN Pharmaceuticals   Rx

Vials: 6 g

INDICATIONS
Severe lower respiratory tract infections due to respiratory syncytial virus (RSV) in selected hospitalized infants and young children

INHALANT DOSAGE
Infant and child: 190 μg/liter of air, delivered for 12–18 h per day over a period of 3–7 days (see ADMINISTRATION/DOSAGE ADJUSTMENTS)

CONTRAINDICATIONS
Pregnancy

ADMINISTRATION/DOSAGE ADJUSTMENTS

Preparation of aerosol solution	Reconstitute the contents of the vial with 100 ml of sterile water for injection or sterile water for inhalation (no preservatives added). Transfer the reconstituted solution to a clean, sterilized 500-mg wide-mouth Erlenmeyer flask (SPAG-2 reservoir) and further dilute with sterile water for injection or inhalation, USP, to a final volume of 300 ml (final concentration: 20 mg/ml). Do not use a diluent that contains any antimicrobial agent or other added substance.
Delivery	Ribavirin is normally delivered to an infant oxygen hood from a small-particle aerosol generator (Viratek SPAG-2); do not use with any other aerosol-generating device or together with other aerosol medications. If necessary, a face mask or oxygen tent may be used; however, the distribution volume and condensation area of an oxygen tent are larger, and the efficacy of delivering the drug by means of a tent has been evaluated in only a small number of patients.
Duration of treatment	Treatment is effective when initiated within the first 3 days of RSV lower respiratory tract infection; early treatment in the course of severe infections may be necessary for maximum efficacy. Continue treatment 12–18 h/day for 3–7 days in conjunction with standard supportive fluid and respiratory measures.

WARNINGS/PRECAUTIONS

Selection of patients for therapy	Document RSV infections by a rapid diagnostic method (eg, immunofluorescence or ELISA) prior to administration or during the first 24 h of therapy; discontinue treatment if RSV infection cannot be documented. Use only in patients with severe RSV lower respiratory tract infections; many children with mild lower respiratory tract infections require shorter hospitalization than the 3–7 days necessary for a course of ribavirin. In general, the decision whether to use ribavirin should be based on the severity of the RSV infection. The presence of underlying conditions, including prematurity and cardiopulmonary disease, may increase the severity of RSV infection; high-risk infants and young children with such conditions may benefit from ribavirin treatment.
Patients requiring assisted ventilation	Precipitation of ribavirin in the ventilatory apparatus (including the endotracheal tube), resulting in increased positive end expiratory pressure, increased positive inspiratory pressure, and accumulation of fluid in the tubing, may jeopardize adequate ventilation and gas exchange in infants
↑Toxicity in animals	Aerosol administration of ribavirin has produced cardiac lesions in mice and rats given 30 and 36 mg/kg, respectively, for 4 wk; oral administration to monkeys has produced similar effects. Inflammatory and possibly emphysematous pulmonary and proliferative changes have occurred in developing ferrets after treatment with ribavirin aerosol; however, the significance of these findings to human treatment is unknown.
Pulmonary function	Pulmonary function has deteriorated in infants, and also in adults with chronic obstructive lung disease or asthma, following ribavirin therapy; several serious adverse events have occurred in severely ill infants with life-threatening underlying diseases; however, the role of ribavirin in these events has not been determined. Monitor respiratory function carefully during treatment. If initiation of treatment produces a sudden deterioration of respiratory function, stop treatment immediately; reinstitute therapy with extreme caution and continuous monitoring.
Carcinogenicity, mutagenicity	Chronic oral administration of ribavirin at doses of 16–60 mg/kg has produced benign mammary, pancreatic, pituitary, and adrenal tumors in rats; the drug has also induced cell transformation in vitro. Ribavirin is mutagenic to mammalian cells in culture; however, there has been no evidence of mutagenicity in microbial assays or the dominant mouse lethal assay in mice.
Effect on fertility	Testicular changes (tubular atrophy) have occurred in adult rats fed 16 mg/kg/day; the effect of ribavirin on fertility in animals has not been adequately studied

ADVERSE REACTIONS[1]

Pulmonary	Worsening of respiratory status (see WARNINGS/PRECAUTIONS), bacterial pneumonia, pneumothorax, apnea, and ventilator dependence
Cardiovascular	Cardiac arrest, hypotension, digitalis toxicity

COMPENDIUM OF DRUG THERAPY

VIRAZOLE ■ ZOVIRAX Capsules

Hematological	Anemia, reticulocytosis
Hypersensitivity	Rash, conjunctivitis

OVERDOSAGE

Signs and symptoms	Hypoactivity and GI symptoms
Treatment	Reduce dosage and/or frequency of administration

DRUG INTERACTIONS

No clinically significant drug interactions have been identified

ALTERED LABORATORY VALUES

No clinically significant alterations in blood/serum or urinary values have occurred at therapeutic dosages

---

USE IN CHILDREN

See INDICATIONS and INHALANT DOSAGE

USE IN PREGNANT AND NURSING WOMEN

Pregnancy Category X: ribavirin may cause fetal harm in pregnant women; this drug has proven teratogenic and/or embryolethal in nearly all species that have been tested. Malformations of the skull, palate, eye, jaw, skeleton, and GI tract were found in hamsters fed single doses of 2.5 mg/kg and rats fed 10 mg/kg; fetal and offspring survival were also reduced. Embryolethality was observed in rabbits at daily oral doses as low as 1 mg/kg. Although no adequate, well-controlled studies have been performed in pregnant women, this drug should not be used during pregnancy. It is not known whether ribavirin is excreted in human milk; however, because it is toxic to lactating animals and their offspring, ribavirin should not be used by nursing mothers.

---

[1] Seven deaths have occurred during or shortly after treatment with ribavirin aerosol; however, no causal relationship has been established

---

SYSTEMIC AGENTS

ZOVIRAX Capsules (acyclovir) Burroughs Wellcome   Rx

Capsules: 200 mg

INDICATIONS	ORAL DOSAGE
Initial episodes of **genital herpes**	**Adult:** 200 mg 5 times/day at 4-h intervals for a period of 10 consecutive days
Recurrent episodes of **genital herpes**	**Adult:** for treatment of a recurrent episode, 200 mg 5 times/day at 4-h intervals for a period of 5 consecutive days; for prevention of recurrent episodes, 200 mg 3–5 times/day for up to 6 mo

CONTRAINDICATIONS

Hypersensitivity or intolerance to acyclovir

ADMINISTRATION/DOSAGE ADJUSTMENTS

Treatment of an initial episode	This preparation has been shown to reduce the duration of acute infection, the time required for healing of lesions, and, in some cases, the duration of pain and the incidence of new lesion formation. The effectiveness of therapy may depend on how promptly treatment is started and whether the patient has been previously exposed to the herpes simplex virus. Patients with mild disease may benefit less from therapy than those with more severe signs and symptoms. For extremely severe episodes that necessitate hospitalization and more aggressive management, IV therapy may be advisable.
Management of recurrent episodes	In patients who have experienced six or more episodes annually, use for 4–6 mo has been shown to prevent recurrences or reduce their frequency or severity. However, some animal studies have produced evidence that acyclovir may cause chromosomal damage and decreased spermatogenesis (see WARNINGS/PRECAUTIONS); furthermore, the first episode that occurs after cessation of chronic therapy may, in some cases, be more severe than previous episodes. Therefore, the benefits and risks should be weighed before instituting long-term treatment. Chronic therapy should be limited to a period of 6 mo and should not be instituted in patients with mild disease. For patients with infrequent recurrences, intermittent short-term treatment may be more appropriate than a chronic regimen. Each course should be started at the earliest sign or symptom of recurrence. For immunocompromised patients, acyclovir can be given either intermittently or chronically (see warning, below, concerning resistance).
Patients with renal impairment	For patients whose creatinine clearance equals or is less than 10 ml/min, give 200 mg q12h

ZOVIRAX Capsules ■ ZOVIRAX Sterile Powder

WARNINGS/PRECAUTIONS

Resistance	Treatment may result in the emergence of less sensitive viruses. All patients should be advised to take particular care whenever active lesions develop during therapy to avoid the potential transmission of a virus. In severely immunocompromised patients, clinically significant resistance may occur with repeated or prolonged use.
Carcinogenicity	No evidence of carcinogenicity has been observed in lifetime bioassays in rats and mice given 50, 150, and 450 mg/kg/day by gavage; conflicting results have been found in two in vitro assays
Mutagenicity	Acute studies in Chinese hamsters given 500 or 1,000 mg/kg have demonstrated clastrogenic effects; in vitro cell assays with human lymphocytes and mouse lymphoma cells have shown evidence of mutagenicity and chromosomal damage at concentrations that were at least 400 times those achieved in human plasma with oral administration
Impairment of male fertility	Testicular atrophy has been observed in rats given intraperitoneally 80 mg/kg/day for 6 mo or 320 mg/kg/day for 1 mo; atrophy persisted during the drug-free 4-wk period that followed administration of the higher dose, although some evidence of recovery of sperm production was seen 30 days after the last dose. Administration of 100 or 200 mg/kg/day IV for 31 days has caused aspermatogenesis in dogs. Preliminary analysis of the results of a 6-mo clinical study with 400 or 1,000 mg/day has shown no evidence of decreased spermatogenesis.

ADVERSE REACTIONS

Frequent reactions (incidence ≥ 1%) are printed in *italics*

With short-term use

Gastrointestinal	*Nausea and/or vomiting (2.7%)*, diarrhea, anorexia
Central nervous system	Headache, dizziness, fatigue
Other	Edema, rash, leg pain, inguinal adenopathy, medication taste, sore throat

With long-term use

Gastrointestinal	*Diarrhea (8.8%), nausea and/or vomiting (8%)*
Central nervous system	*Headache (13.1%), vertigo (3.6%), fatigue (2.8%), insomnia (1.6%)*, irritability, depression
Musculoskeletal	*Arthralgia (3.6%)*, muscle cramps
Dermatological	*Rash (2.8%), acne (1.2%)*
Other	*Fever (1.6%), menstrual abnormality (1.6%)*, sore throat, lymphadenopathy, superficial thrombophlebitis, pars planitis, accelerated hair loss, palpitations

OVERDOSAGE

Signs and symptoms	No untoward effects have occurred with a dosage as high as 800 mg 6 times/day for 5 days; acute massive overdosage has not been reported. Precipitation of acyclovir in the renal tubules can occur if the intratubular concentration exceeds 2.5 mg/ml; elevation of BUN and serum creatinine levels, followed by renal failure, has been seen with IV overdosage.
Treatment	Hemodialysis may be used to remove the drug from the blood; a single 6-h dialysis treatment results in a 60% decrease in the serum acyclovir level. Hemodialysis may also be helpful as a supportive measure when acute renal failure and anuria occur.

DRUG INTERACTIONS

Probenecid	⇧ Serum half-life of acyclovir

ALTERED LABORATORY VALUES

No clinically significant alterations in blood/serum or urinary values occur at therapeutic dosages

USE IN CHILDREN

Safety and effectiveness for use in children have not been established

USE IN PREGNANT AND NURSING WOMEN

Pregnancy Category C: no teratogenic effects have been seen in mice, rats, or rabbits; however, administration of 50 mg/kg/day SC has caused an increase in postimplantation loss in rats, a decrease in implantation efficiency in rabbits (not seen with IV administration at this dosage), and, in a peri- and postnatal study in rats, a decrease in the number of corpora lutea, total implantation sites, and live fetuses. Reduction in litter size has been seen in rabbits at a dosage (100 mg/kg/day IV) associated with obstructive nephropathy. Use acyclovir during pregnancy only if the expected benefits justify the potential risk to the fetus; bear in mind the mutagenic as well as embryotoxic potential of this drug. It is not known whether acyclovir is excreted in human milk; use with caution in nursing mothers. Consideration should be given to either discontinuing breast-feeding or not using this drug.

SYSTEMIC AGENTS

ZOVIRAX Sterile Powder (acyclovir sodium) Burroughs Wellcome   Rx

Vials: acyclovir sodium equivalent to 500 mg acyclovir (10 ml) for IV infusion only

INDICATIONS

Initial and recurrent episodes of mucocutaneous **herpes simplex virus (HSV-1 and HSV-2) infections** in immunocompromised patients

PARENTERAL DOSAGE

Adult: 5 mg/kg, given at a constant rate over a period of 1 h by IV infusion q8h for 7 days

Child (< 12 yr): 250 mg/m², given at a constant rate over a period of 1 h by IV infusion q8h for 7 days

ZOVIRAX Sterile Powder

Severe initial episodes of **herpes genitalis** in nonimmunocompromised patients	**Adult:** 5 mg/kg, given at a constant rate over a period of 1 h by IV infusion q8h for 5 days **Child (< 12 yr):** 250 mg/m^2, given at a constant rate over a period of 1 h by IV infusion q8h for 5 days

CONTRAINDICATIONS

Hypersensitivity to acyclovir

ADMINISTRATION/DOSAGE ADJUSTMENTS

Preparation of solution	To reconstitute solution, add 10 ml of sterile water for injection or bacteriostatic water for injection with benzyl alcohol to the 500-mg vial and then shake well; to avoid precipitation of the solution, do not use paraben-containing bacteriostatic water for injection. For infusion, withdraw the calculated dose from the vial and dilute to a final concentration of ~ 7 mg/ml or less. (If higher concentrations are used, phlebitis or inflammation at the injection site may occur upon inadvertent extravasation.) Use any standard electrolyte or glucose solution as a diluent; biological or colloidal fluids (eg, blood products, protein solutions, etc) are not recommended. Reconstituted solutions (50 mg/ml) should be used within 12 h, diluted solutions within 24 h.
Administration	Administer by IV infusion only; do not inject SC or IM. To prevent renal impairment (see WARNINGS/PRECAUTIONS), maintain adequate hydration, particularly during the first 2 h after each infusion, and avoid rapid or bolus injection.
Patients with renal impairment	The half-life of acyclovir is dependent on renal function. Administer 5 mg/kg q12h if creatinine clearance (Ccr) equals 25–50 ml/min or q24h if Ccr equals 10–25 ml/min; administer 2.5 mg/kg q24h if Ccr equals 0–10 ml/min. No dosage change is necessary if Ccr exceeds 50 ml/min. For patients undergoing hemodialysis, adjust dosing schedules so that a dose can be given after each dialysis treatment.

WARNINGS/PRECAUTIONS

Renal impairment	If the maximum solubility of free acyclovir (2.5 mg/ml at 37°C in water) is exceeded in the renal tubules, precipitation of crystals can occur, causing an increase in serum creatinine and BUN, a decrease in creatinine clearance, and, in some cases, acute renal failure. Bolus injection, dehydration, preexisting renal disease, and the concomitant use of other nephrotoxic drugs increase the risk of renal impairment due to acyclovir. In most cases, the renal dysfunction has been transient or has resolved following improvement in water and electrolyte balance, dosage adjustment, or discontinuation of acyclovir administration (see ADMINISTRATION/DOSAGE ADJUSTMENTS).
Special-risk patients	Encephalopathic changes (see ADVERSE REACTIONS) have been observed in ~ 1% of patients; use with caution in patients with neurological disorders, serious renal, hepatic, or electrolyte disorders, or significant hypoxia, and in patients who have had neurological reactions to cytotoxic drugs or who are currently receiving intrathecal methotrexate therapy or interferon
Severely immunocompromised patients	Intravenous administration of acyclovir to patients with combined severe congenital immunodeficiencies and to bone marrow transplant recipients has resulted in the emergence of less sensitive herpes simplex viruses; these less sensitive viruses have not, however, been associated with a worsening of illness, and, in some cases, have disappeared spontaneously
Carcinogenicity	No evidence of carcinogenicity has been observed in lifetime bioassays in rats and mice given 50, 150, and 450 mg/kg/day by gavage; conflicting results have been found in two in vitro assays
Mutagenicity	Parenteral doses of 100 mg/kg have not caused chromosomal damage in rats or Chinese hamsters; however, higher doses (500 and 1,000 mg/kg) were clastogenic in Chinese hamsters. A dominant lethal study in mice has shown no evidence of mutagenicity. In 2 of 11 microbial and mammalian cell assays, evidence of mutagenicity and chromosomal damage has been found, but only at concentrations at least 25 times those achieved in human plasma following IV administration.

ADVERSE REACTIONS

The most frequent reactions, regardless of incidence, are printed in *italics*

Central nervous system	Encephalopathic changes, characterized by lethargy, obtundation, tremors, confusion, hallucinations, agitation, seizures, or coma[1]; headache, jitters
Renal	*Increased serum creatinine levels*
Dermatological	*Rash,*[2] hives
Other	*Inflammation or phlebitis at injection site*[2] *(after extravasation)*, diaphoresis, hematuria,[2] hypotension, nausea,[2] thrombocytosis

OVERDOSAGE

Signs and symptoms	Elevation of BUN and serum creatinine levels, followed by renal failure (see warning, above, concerning renal impairment)

ZOVIRAX Sterile Powder ■ BIOZYME-C

Treatment	Hemodialysis may be used to remove the drug from the blood; a single 6-h dialysis treatment results in a 60% decrease in the serum acyclovir level. Hemodialysis may also be helpful as a supportive measure when acute renal failure and anuria occur.

DRUG INTERACTIONS

Probenecid	△ Serum half-life of acyclovir

ALTERED LABORATORY VALUES

Blood/serum values	△ Creatinine △ BUN
Urinary values	▽ Creatinine

USE IN CHILDREN
See INDICATIONS and PARENTERAL DOSAGE

USE IN PREGNANT AND NURSING WOMEN
Pregnancy Category C: use during pregnancy only if the expected benefit justifies the potential risk to the fetus. Acyclovir crosses the placental barrier in laboratory animals. Evidence of teratogenicity or impaired fertility has not been observed in mice given orally up to 450 mg/kg/day; teratogenic effects have not been detected in rabbits and rats receiving 50 mg/kg/day SC. A decrease in implantation efficiency, but not in litter size, has been shown in rabbits given 50 mg/kg/day SC after mating. Adequate, well-controlled studies have not been performed in pregnant women. It is not known whether acyclovir is excreted in human milk; use with caution in nursing mothers because many drugs are excreted in human milk.

[1] A bone marrow transplant recipient with pneumonitis experienced seizures, cerebral edema, and coma, and then died, apparently because of cerebral anoxia; another immunocompromised patient exhibited coarse tremor and clonus
[2] This reaction was also reported by placebo recipients during controlled clinical trials

---

DEBRIDING AGENTS

BIOZYME-C (collagenase) Armour   Rx

Ointment (per gram): 250 units

INDICATIONS
Debridement of chronic dermal ulcers and severely burned areas

TOPICAL DOSAGE
Adult: apply once daily or more frequently if the dressing becomes soiled (see ADMINISTRATION/DOSAGE ADJUSTMENTS)

CONTRAINDICATIONS
Hypersensitivity to collagenase

ADMINISTRATION/DOSAGE ADJUSTMENTS

Use of ointment	Gently cleanse debris and digested material from the lesion using a gauze pad saturated with hydrogen peroxide or Dakin's solution, followed by sterile normal saline. If infection is present, apply an appropriate compatible topical antibiotic before using the ointment; if the infection fails to respond, discontinue the enzyme treatment until the infection remits. For shallow lesions, place the ointment on a sterile gauze pad and secure it to the wound; for deep lesions, apply the ointment directly from the tube. Cross-hatch any thick eschar with a #10 scalpel blade to allow the enzyme more surface contact with necrotic debris; remove as much loosened detritus as possible with forceps and scissors. Remove excess ointment each time a dressing is changed; terminate treatment when debridement of the necrotic tissue is complete and granulation tissue is well established.

WARNINGS/PRECAUTIONS

Effect of pH	The optimal pH range for collagenase is 6–8; take precautions to keep the pH within this range, since higher or lower pH conditions decrease enzymatic activity
Compatibility with other agents	Detergents, hexachlorophene, and/or antiseptics or soaks containing heavy metal ions (eg, mercury, silver) adversely affect the enzymatic activity of collagenase; if prior use of such agents is suspected, carefully and repeatedly wash the site with normal saline before applying the ointment. Burow's solution, which has a low pH (3.6–4.4) and contains aluminum ions, should be avoided.
Debilitated patients	There is a theoretical risk that debriding enzymes may increase the risk of bacteremia in debilitated patients; closely monitor such patients for systemic bacterial infections
Erythema	Slight, transient erythema has occurred occasionally, especially when application of the ointment was not confined to the lesion; use care when applying this preparation

BIOZYME-C ■ ELASE

ADVERSE REACTIONS

No allergic or toxic reactions to collagenase have been observed, except for one report of a systemic hypersensitivity reaction in a patient using collagenase with cortisone for more than a year

OVERDOSAGE

Signs and symptoms	Pain, burning sensation, erythema
Treatment	If necessary, apply Burow's solution to the lesion and surrounding area to stop the action of the enzyme

USE IN CHILDREN	USE IN PREGNANT AND NURSING WOMEN
Consult manufacturer	Consult manufacturer

VEHICLE/BASE
Ointment: white petrolatum

DEBRIDING AGENTS

ELASE (fibrinolysin and desoxyribonuclease, combined [bovine]) Parke-Davis Rx

Vials: 25 units fibrinolysin and 15,000 units desoxyribonuclease (30 ml) **Ointment (per gram):** 1 unit fibrinolysin and 666 units desoxyribonuclease (10, 30 g)

INDICATIONS

Debridement of inflamed and infected lesions, including general surgical wounds, ulcerative lesions (trophic, decubitus, stasis, arteriosclerotic), second- and third-degree burns, circumcisions, and episiotomies

Cervicitis (benign, postpartum, and postconization) **and vaginitis**

TOPICAL DOSAGE

Adult: use solution as directed under ADMINISTRATION/DOSAGE ADJUSTMENTS or apply a thin layer of ointment at least once daily and, preferably, bid or tid (see "Use of ointment," below)

Adult: for mild to moderate cases, deposit 5 ml of the ointment deep into the vagina at bedtime for 5 consecutive nights or until an entire 30-g tube is depleted. For severe cases, instill 10 ml of the solution (see ADMINISTRATION/DOSAGE ADJUSTMENTS) intravaginally; wait 1–2 min for the enzyme to disperse, and insert a cotton tampon. Remove the tampon the next day and continue treatment with the ointment.

ELASE-CHLOROMYCETIN (fibrinolysin and desoxyribonuclease, combined [bovine], and chloramphenicol) Parke-Davis Rx

Ointment (per gram): 1 unit fibrinolysin, 666 units desoxyribonuclease, and 10 mg chloramphenicol (10, 30 g)

INDICATIONS

Debridement and topical antibiotic treatment of infected lesions, including infected burns, ulcers, and wounds

TOPICAL DOSAGE

Adult: apply a thin layer of ointment at least once daily and, preferably, bid or tid (see ADMINISTRATION/DOSAGE ADJUSTMENTS)

CONTRAINDICATIONS

Hypersensitivity to any component	Parenteral use

ADMINISTRATION/DOSAGE ADJUSTMENTS

Preparation of solution	Reconstitute contents of each vial with 10 ml of normal saline; the amount of diluent may be varied to prepare higher or lower concentrations, if desired. Use freshly prepared solutions. Refrigeration retards loss of enzyme activity; however, do not use solution more than 24 h after reconstitution, even if refrigerated.
Use of solution	The solution may be applied as a liquid, spray (using a conventional atomizer), or wet dressing as follows: Prepare a solution with 10–50 ml of normal saline (as above) and saturate strips of fine-mesh gauze or an unfolded sterile gauze sponge with the solution. Pack the ulcerated area with the gauze, making sure it remains in contact with the necrotic substrate for about 6–8 h (any heavy eschar covering the lesion should be surgically removed before debridement). As the gauze dries in place, the necrotic tissue sloughs off and becomes enmeshed in the gauze. Remove the dried gauze. Repeat tid or qid, since frequent dressing changes enhance healing. In 2–4 days the area will become clean and start to fill in with granulation tissue.

ELASE ■ SANTYL

Use of ointment	Cleanse the wound with water, hydrogen peroxide, or normal saline, and dry gently. If any dry eschar is present, remove it surgically before using the ointment. Apply a thin layer of ointment, and cover the site with petrolatum gauze or other nonadhering dressing. Change the dressing at least once daily, and preferably 2–3 times (frequency of application is more important than the amount of preparation used because the enzyme action of the ointment is rapidly and progressively exhausted within 24 h). Flush away the necrotic debris and fibrinous exudate with normal saline, hydrogen peroxide, or warm water to allow the freshly applied ointment to remain in direct contact with the substrate.
Use as an irrigating agent	The prepared solution may be used as an irrigating agent in the treatment of abscesses, empyema cavities, fistulae, sinus tracts, otorhinolaryngologic wounds, or subcutaneous hematomas (except those adjacent to or within adipose tissue). After irrigating the wound, drain off the solution and replace it at 6- to 10-h intervals to reduce the amount of by-product accumulation and minimize the loss of enzyme activity. Traces of blood in the discharge usually indicate active filling in of the cavity.
Wound dressing	Careful aseptic wound-dressing techniques are mandatory. Surgically remove any dense, dry eschar before attempting debridement, and periodically remove accumulated necrotic debris. Make sure that the enzyme remains in constant contact with the substrate, and replenish it at least once daily. As soon as possible after optimal debridement has been attained, secondary closure or skin grafting must be performed.
Systemic antibiotic treatment	If clinically indicated, administer an appropriate systemic antibiotic concomitantly; the chloramphenicol-containing ointment should be used alone only for very superficial infections.

WARNINGS/PRECAUTIONS

Systemic absorption	Bone marrow hypoplasia, including aplastic anemia and death, has been reported following local application of chloramphenicol. Blood dyscrasias have also been associated with the use of chloramphenicol.
Superinfection	Overgrowth of nonsusceptible organisms, including fungi, may occur with prolonged use of topical antibiotics; if secondary infection occurs during therapy, discontinue the chloramphenicol-containing ointment and institute appropriate therapeutic measures
Hypersensitivity	Observe the usual precautions against allergic reactions, especially in patients hypersensitive to products of bovine origin or to mercury compounds (these products contain thimerosal as a preservative). A number of side effects have been reported in patients sensitive to chloramphenicol or other materials in topical preparations (see ADVERSE/REACTIONS); should such reactions occur, discontinue use.

ADVERSE REACTIONS

Local	Hyperemia (with higher than recommended concentrations of all preparations); irritation, itching, burning, angioneurotic edema, urticaria, and vesicular and maculopapular dermatitis (with use of chloramphenicol)

USE IN CHILDREN	USE IN PREGNANT AND NURSING WOMEN
Consult manufacturer	Consult manufacturer

VEHICLE/BASE
Ointment: 0.0004% thimerosal, liquid petrolatum, and polyethylene

DEBRIDING AGENTS

SANTYL (collagenase) Knoll   Rx

Ointment (per gram): 250 units

INDICATIONS

Debridement of chronic dermal ulcers and severely burned areas

TOPICAL DOSAGE

Adult: apply once daily or more frequently if the dressing becomes soiled (see ADMINISTRATION/DOSAGE ADJUSTMENTS)

CONTRAINDICATIONS

Hypersensitivity to collagenase

ADMINISTRATION/DOSAGE ADJUSTMENTS

Use of ointment — Gently cleanse debris and digested material from the lesion using a gauze pad saturated with hydrogen peroxide or Dakin's solution, followed by sterile normal saline. If infection is present, apply an appropriate compatible topical antibiotic before using the ointment; if the infection fails to respond, discontinue the enzyme treatment until the infection remits. For shallow lesions, place the ointment on a sterile gauze pad and secure it to the wound; use a wooden tongue depressor or spatula to apply the ointment directly to deep lesions. Cross-hatch any thick eschar with a #10 scalpel blade to allow the enzyme more surface contact with necrotic debris; remove as much loosened detritus as possible with forceps and scissors. Remove excess ointment each time a dressing is changed; terminate treatment when debridement of the necrotic tissue is complete and granulation tissue is well established.

WARNINGS/PRECAUTIONS

Effect of pH — The optimal pH range for collagenase is 6–8; take precautions to keep the pH within this range, since higher or lower pH conditions decrease enzymatic activity

Compatibility with other agents — Detergents, hexachlorophene, and/or antiseptics or soaks containing heavy metal ions (eg, mercury, silver) adversely affect the enzymatic activity of collagenase; if prior use of such agents is suspected, carefully and repeatedly wash the site with normal saline before applying the ointment. Burow's solution, which has a low pH (3.6–4.4) and contains aluminum ions, should be avoided.

Debilitated patients — There is a theoretical risk that debriding enzymes may increase the risk of bacteremia in debilitated patients; closely monitor such patients for systemic bacterial infections

Erythema — Slight, transient erythema has occurred occasionally, especially when application of the ointment was not confined to the lesion; use care when applying this preparation

ADVERSE REACTIONS

No allergic or toxic reactions to collagenase have been observed, except for one report of a systemic hypersensitivity reaction in a patient using collagenase with cortisone for more than a year

OVERDOSAGE

Signs and symptoms — Pain, burning sensation, erythema

Treatment — If necessary, apply Burow's solution to the lesion and surrounding area to stop the action of the enzyme

---

USE IN CHILDREN
Consult manufacturer

USE IN PREGNANT AND NURSING WOMEN
Consult manufacturer

VEHICLE/BASE
Ointment: white petrolatum

DEBRIDING AGENTS

TRAVASE (sutilains) Flint   Rx

Ointment (per gram): sutilains equivalent to 82,000 casein units of proteolytic activity (14.2 g)

INDICATIONS

Debridement of second- and third-degree burns; incisional, traumatic, and pyogenic wounds; decubitus ulcers; and ulcers due to peripheral vascular disease

TOPICAL DOSAGE

Adult: apply a thin layer of ointment at least once daily and, preferably, tid or qid (see ADMINISTRATION/DOSAGE ADJUSTMENTS)

CONTRAINDICATIONS

Wounds communicating with major body cavities

Fungating neoplastic ulcers

Wounds containing exposed major nerves or nervous tissue

Wounds in women of child-bearing potential

TRAVASE

ADMINISTRATION/DOSAGE ADJUSTMENTS

Use of ointment — Thoroughly cleanse and irrigate the wound with normal saline or water to remove any detergents or antiseptics that may impair enzyme activity (see "Compatibility with other agents," below). Moisten the wound area thoroughly by bathing, showering, or water or saline soaks. Apply a thin layer of ointment; ensure that it is in close contact with the necrotic debris and completely covers the wound, extending 1/4–1/2 in. beyond the area to be debrided. Apply loose, moist dressings (a moist environment is essential for optimal enzyme activity). For best results, repeat the entire procedure tid or qid.

WARNINGS/PRECAUTIONS

Compatibility with other agents — Certain detergents (eg, hexachlorophene, benzalkonium chloride), antiseptics (eg, nitrofurazone, iodine), and antibacterial agents containing heavy metal ions (eg, silver nitrate) have been shown in vitro to impair enzyme activity by either denaturing the enzyme or altering the substrate characteristics. Neomycin, sulfamylon, streptomycin, and penicillin do not interfere with enzyme activity, whereas thimerosal causes a slight decrease in enzyme activity. In instances where the ointment has been used concomitantly with other topical agents and no dissolution or slough occurs 24–48 h after its application, it is likely that these adjuncts have interfered with the enzyme activity of sutilains, and further use of the ointment would probably be of no value.

Existing or threatened invasive infection — Institute appropriate concomitant systemic antibiotic therapy in patients with an existing or threatened invasive infection

Hypersensitivity and/or other reactions — Studies in humans have shown that there may be an antibody response to absorbed enzyme material; however, there have been no reports of systemic allergic reactions or toxicity. Occasionally, side effects severe enough to warrant discontinuation of therapy have occurred (see ADVERSE REACTIONS); terminate therapy if bleeding or dermatitis occurs as a result of ointment application. Any pain experienced can usually be controlled with mild analgesics.

Contact with eyes — Do not allow the ointment to come in contact with the eyes; should this occur inadvertently during treatment of head or neck burns or lesions, flush the eyes with copious amounts of water, preferably sterile

ADVERSE REACTIONS

Local — Mild transient pain, paresthesias, bleeding, transient dermatitis

USE IN CHILDREN
Consult manufacturer

USE IN PREGNANT AND NURSING WOMEN
The effects of this preparation on fetal development have not been evaluated; use is contraindicated in women who are pregnant or who may become pregnant. Consult manufacturer for use in nursing mothers.

VEHICLE/BASE
Ointment: 95% white petrolatum and 5% polyethylene

Chapter 20

Antigout Agents

ANTURANE (CIBA)   717
Sulfinpyrazone *Rx*

BENEMID (Merck Sharp & Dohme)   717
Probenecid *Rx*

ColBENEMID (Merck Sharp & Dohme)   719
Probenecid and colchicine *Rx*

Colchicine *Rx*   721

LOPURIN (Boots)   722
Allopurinol *Rx*

ZYLOPRIM (Burroughs Wellcome)   724
Allopurinol *Rx*

ANTIGOUT AGENTS

ANTURANE (sulfinpyrazone) CIBA Rx
Capsules: 200 mg **Tablets:** 100 mg

INDICATIONS	**ORAL DOSAGE**
Chronic or intermittent gouty arthritis	Adult: 200–400 mg/day, given in 2 divided doses with milk or meals, followed by 400 mg/day in 2 divided doses

CONTRAINDICATIONS
Active peptic ulcer	Hypersensitivity to phenylbutazone or other pyrazole compounds	History or evidence of blood dyscrasias
Gastrointestinal inflammation or ulceration		

ADMINISTRATION/DOSAGE ADJUSTMENTS
Initiating therapy	Increase initial dosage gradually within 1 wk up to maintenance dosage; use full maintenance dosage when transferring patients previously controlled by other uricosuric agents
Maintenance	Dosage may be increased to 800 mg/day, if needed; after blood urate level has been controlled, dosages as low as 200 mg/day may be adequate
Gastric irritation	May be minimized by administering drug with food, milk, or antacids

WARNINGS/PRECAUTIONS
Acute gouty attacks	May be precipitated in initial stages of therapy; treat with colchicine or phenylbutazone while therapy continues
Renal colic, urolithiasis	May result, especially in initial stages of therapy; maintain an adequate fluid intake and alkaline urine
Renal impairment	Requires periodic assessment; renal failure has been reported, but a causal relationship has not been established
Past peptic ulcer	May be reactivated; use with caution in patients with healed ulcers
Blood counts	Monitor periodically (see ADVERSE REACTIONS)

ADVERSE REACTIONS[1]
Gastrointestinal	Various upper GI tract disturbances
Dermatological	Rash

OVERDOSAGE
Signs and symptoms	Nausea, vomiting, diarrhea, epigastric pain, ataxia, labored respiration, convulsions, coma (also anemia, jaundice, ulceration[2])
Treatment	No specific antidote. Induce emesis or use gastric lavage to empty stomach. Treat symptomatically and institute supportive measures, as needed.

DRUG INTERACTIONS
Salicylates	▽ Uricosuric effect
Sulfonamides	△ Sulfonamide effect
Insulin, oral hypoglycemic agents	△ Risk of hypoglycemia
Coumarin anticoagulants	△ Prothrombin time

ALTERED LABORATORY VALUES
No clinically significant alterations in blood/serum or urinary values occur at therapeutic dosages

USE IN CHILDREN	**USE IN PREGNANT AND NURSING WOMEN**
Safety and effectiveness for use in children have not been established	Use with caution in pregnant women, weighing the potential risks against the possible benefits. Teratogenic studies in animals have yielded inconclusive results; there have been no clinical reports of teratogenicity associated with the use of sulfinpyrazone. It is not known whether this drug is excreted in human milk. Because many drugs are excreted in human milk and because of the potential for serious adverse reactions in nursing infants, the patient should not nurse if use of the drug is deemed essential.

[1] Other reactions for which a causal relationship has not been established include anemia, leukopenia, agranulocytosis, thrombocytopenia, aplastic anemia, and leukemia (two cases)
[2] Possible symptoms, seen after overdosage with other pyrazolone derivatives

---

ANTIGOUT AGENTS

BENEMID (probenecid) Merck Sharp & Dohme Rx
Tablets: 0.5 g

INDICATIONS	**ORAL DOSAGE**
Hyperuricemia associated with gout and gouty arthritis	Adult: 0.25 g bid for 1 wk, followed by 0.5 g bid

BENEMID

Adjuvant to **penicillin therapy**	**Adult:** 2 g/day, given in divided doses **Child (2–14 yr and ≤ 50 kg):** 25 mg/kg or 0.7 g/m² to start, followed by 40 mg/kg/day or 1.2 g/m²/day, given in 4 divided doses **Child (2–14 yr and > 50 kg):** same as adult
Adjuvant to antibiotic treatment of **sexually transmitted diseases**	**Adult:** for uncomplicated urethral, endocervical, or rectal gonorrhea (treatment or prevention); disseminated gonococcal infections; acute pelvic inflammatory disease in ambulatory patients; and acute sexually transmitted epididymo-orchitis, 1 g with the appropriate antibiotic[1]; for neurosyphilis, 0.5 g qid for 10 days with 2.4 million units of penicillin G procaine once daily[1] **Child (< 45 kg):** for uncomplicated gonococcal vulvovaginitis and urethritis, 25 mg/kg, up to 1 g, with 50 mg/kg of amoxicillin[1] **Child (≥ 45 kg):** for gonococcal infections, same as adult[1]

CONTRAINDICATIONS

Blood dyscrasias	Hypersensitivity to probenecid	Age < 2 yr
Uric acid kidney stones	Acute gouty attack	

ADMINISTRATION/DOSAGE ADJUSTMENTS

Treatment of hyperuricemia	Wait until an acute gouty attack subsides before beginning probenecid therapy. If, at 1 g/day, symptoms of gout still occur in patients with some renal impairment or uric acid excretion in these patients does not exceed 700 mg/24 h, the dosage may be further increased, as needed and tolerated, by 0.5 g/day every 4 wk; dosage generally should not exceed 2 g/day. Probenecid may not be effective in patients with chronic renal insufficiency, particularly when the GFR is 30 ml/min or less. To prevent urinary complications such as hematuria, renal colic, costovertebral pain, and uric acid stones, encourage all patients to drink plenty of fluids and alkalinize urine with 7.5 g/day of potassium citrate or 3–7.5 g/day of sodium bicarbonate; monitor acid-base balance during therapy. When the serum uric acid level is normal and tophaceous deposits disappear, alkalinization of urine and the usual restrictions on consumption of purine-containing food may be somewhat relaxed. When acute attacks have been absent for at least 6 mo and the serum uric acid level has remained normal during that period, the dosage may be reduced by 0.5 g/day every 6 mo; monitor serum uric acid level after each decrease in dosage.
Adjuvant therapy	Reduce the dosage of probenecid when using it as a adjuvant in elderly patients who may have renal impairment; do not use this drug as an adjuvant in patients who are known to have renal impairment. A PSP excretion test may be done to gauge the effectiveness of adjuvant therapy; when the renal clearance of PSP is reduced to approximately 20% the normal rate, the dosage of probenecid can be considered adequate.

WARNINGS/PRECAUTIONS

Acute attack of gout	Probenecid can exacerbate gout. If an acute attack occurs during therapy, give full therapeutic doses of colchicine or take other appropriate measures; probenecid therapy may be continued, with the dosage unchanged.
Hypersensitivity	Severe allergic reactions, including anaphylaxis, have been seen in rare instances, most frequently within several hours after administration to patients who had previously received the drug; if an allergic reaction occurs during therapy, discontinue use
Gastric intolerance	A reduction in dosage may eliminate gastric complaints
Peptic ulcer	Use with caution in patients with a history of peptic ulcer
Hemolytic anemia	Instances of hemolytic anemia seen during therapy may be related to G6PD deficiency

ADVERSE REACTIONS

Central nervous system	Headache, dizziness
Digestive	Hepatic necrosis, vomiting, nausea, anorexia, sore gums
Genitourinary	Nephrotic syndrome, uric acid stones, hematuria, renal colic, costovertebral pain, urinary frequency
Hematological	Aplastic anemia, leukopenia, hemolytic anemia, anemia
Dermatological	Dermatitis, alopecia, flushing, urticaria, pruritus
Hypersensitivity	Anaphylaxis, fever, urticaria, pruritus
Other	Precipitation of acute gouty arthritis

OVERDOSAGE

Signs and symptoms	Vomiting, tonic-clonic convulsions, stupor, coma
Treatment	Institute appropriate symptomatic and supportive measures

BENEMID ■ ColBENEMID

DRUG INTERACTIONS

Methotrexate	△ Serum level of methotrexate; if probenecid and methotrexate are given concomitantly, reduce dosage of methotrexate and monitor its serum level
Salicylates	▽ Uricosuric effect of probenecid; do not use salicylates during probenecid therapy
Penicillin, cephalosporins (except ceftazidime and ceforanide), other beta-lactam antibiotics	△ Serum level of beta-lactam antibiotics △ Risk of psychic disturbances and other reactions associated with antibiotic toxicity
Sulfonamides	△ Serum level of sulfonamides; periodically check serum sulfonamide level during prolonged combination therapy
Sulfonylureas	△ Risk of hypoglycemia
General anesthetics	▽ Induction dose of thiopental △ Duration of thiopental-induced anesthesia △ Duration of ketamine-induced anesthesia (based on studies in rats)
Indomethacin	△ Serum level of indomethacin; titrate dosage of indomethacin cautiously and in small increments
Pyrazinamide, diazoxide, mecamylamine, diuretics, alcohol	▽ Uricosuric effect of probenecid
Clofibrate, dyphylline, dapsone, nitrofurantoin, heparin, acyclovir, p-aminosalicylic acid, rifampin	△ Serum level of interacting drug
Iodohippurate	▽ Renal uptake of iodohippurate

ALTERED LABORATORY VALUES

Blood/serum values	△ Theophylline (with Schack and Wexler method) ▽ Uric acid
Urinary values	+ Glucose (with copper reduction tests) ▽ 17-KS ▽ PSP ▽ BSP ▽ PAH △ Uric acid

USE IN CHILDREN

Probenecid may be used in children as an adjuvant to antibiotic therapy; see ORAL DOSAGE. Do not give this drug to children under 2 yr of age.

USE IN PREGNANT AND NURSING WOMEN

Probenecid appears in cord blood; before using this drug in women of childbearing potential, weigh expected benefit against potential hazards. Consult manufacturer for use in nursing mothers.

[1] Dosage is based on the current recommendations of the Centers for Disease Control (CDC); for complete information on dosage, see CDC guidelines (*MMWR* 34[suppl 4S], 1985)

ANTIGOUT AGENTS

ColBENEMID (probenecid and colchicine) Merck Sharp & Dohme   Rx

Tablets: 0.5 g probenecid and 0.5 mg colchicine

INDICATIONS	ORAL DOSAGE
Chronic gouty arthritis complicated by frequent, recurrent gouty attacks	**Adult:** 1 tab/day for 1 wk, followed by 1 tab bid

CONTRAINDICATIONS

Hypersensitivity to probenecid or colchicine, alone or in combination	Uric acid kidney stones	Age < 2 yr
	Blood dyscrasias	Pregnancy
Acute gouty attacks		

ADMINISTRATION/DOSAGE ADJUSTMENTS

Initiating therapy	Wait until acute attack subsides; acute attacks arising during therapy may be controlled with additional colchicine while drug is continued
Maintenance	Maintain a liberal fluid intake and alkaline urine until serum uric-acid levels are normal and tophaceous deposits disappear. Reduce daily dosage by 1 tab every 6 mo if attacks have subsided for at least 6 mo and serum uric-acid levels have normalized.
Patients with renal impairment	Increase daily dosage by 1 tab every 4 wk, as needed (especially if 24-h urate excretion < 700 mg) and tolerated, up to generally no more than 4 tabs/day. This preparation may not be effective in patients with chronic renal impairment, particularly when the glomerular filtration rate is 30 ml/min or less.

ColBENEMID

Management of side effects	Decrease dosage or discontinue therapy

WARNINGS/PRECAUTIONS

Exacerbation of gout	May occur; increase colchicine dosage or institute other appropriate therapy
Hypersensitivity reactions	Severe allergic reactions and anaphylaxis have occurred in rare cases, usually within several hours after therapy has been reinstituted; discontinue drug if hypersensitivity reactions appear
Genitourinary complaints	Hematuria, renal colic, costovertebral pain, and uric acid stone formation may be prevented by alkalinization of the urine and a liberal fluid intake; monitor acid-base balance periodically
Toxicity	Generalized vascular damage, gastric intolerance (including severe diarrhea), and renal impairment with hematuria and oliguria may occur at toxic doses; gastric intolerance may be reversed by a decrease in dosage
Special-risk patients	Use with caution in patients with a history of peptic ulcer or active peptic ulcer disease, spastic colon, hepatic dysfunction, or glucose-6-phosphate dehydrogenase (G6PD) deficiency
Carcinogenicity	Colchicine, an established mutagen, may be carcinogenic; adequate studies have not been conducted to determine the carcinogenic potential of probenecid or the combination of probenecid and colchicine. Weigh the risks and benefits before long-term use.
Impaired spermatogenesis	May occur; reversible azoospermia has been reported in one patient

ADVERSE REACTIONS

Gastrointestinal	Hepatic necrosis, nausea, vomiting, abdominal pain, diarrhea, anorexia, sore gums
Central nervous system and neuromuscular	Headache, dizziness, peripheral neuritis, muscular weakness
Genitourinary	Nephrotic syndrome, uric acid stones with or without hematuria, renal colic, costovertebral pain, urinary frequency
Dermatological	Dermatitis, alopecia, flushing, purpura
Hematological	Aplastic anemia, agranulocytosis, leukopenia, hemolytic anemia (possibly owing to G6PD deficiency), anemia
Hypersensitivity	Anaphylaxis, fever, urticaria, pruritus
Other	Precipitation of acute gouty arthritis

OVERDOSAGE

Signs and symptoms	See ADVERSE REACTIONS
Treatment	Induce emesis or perform gastric lavage; institute appropriate symptomatic and supportive measures

DRUG INTERACTIONS

Penicillin and other beta-lactam antibiotics	△ Antibiotic plasma level Psychic disturbances
Pyrazinamide, salicylates	▽ Uricosuric effect; do not use salicylates with this preparation
Sulfonamides	△ Conjugated sulfonamide plasma level; periodically measure plasma level during prolonged combination therapy
Oral sulfonylureas	△ Risk of hypoglycemia
Thiopental, ketamine	△ Anesthetic effect of thiopental; patients receiving probenecid reportedly need a lower dose of thiopental for induction of anesthesia △ Duration of thiopental and ketamine anesthesia (in rats)
Indomethacin	△ Indomethacin plasma level; titrate dosage of indomethacin cautiously and in small increments when patients are receiving probenecid, since a lower than usual dosage may be sufficient
Rifampin	△ Rifampin plasma level
Methotrexate	△ Methotrexate plasma level and risk of toxicity; reduce dosage of methotrexate and, if necessary, monitor plasma level during combination therapy
Para-aminohippuric acid (PAH)	▽ Excretion of PAH
Para-aminosalicylic acid (PAS)	▽ Excretion of PAS
Sodium iodomethamate	▽ Excretion of sodium iodomethamate
Pantothenic acid	▽ Excretion of pantothenic acid
Phenolsulfonphthalein	▽ Excretion of phenolsulfonphthalein

ColBENEMID ■ Colchicine

ALTERED LABORATORY VALUES

Blood/serum values — ▽ Uric acid △ Theophylline (with Schack and Wexler method)

Urinary values — △ Glucose (with Benedict's solution) △ Uric acid ▽ 17-Ketosteroids

---

USE IN CHILDREN

Contraindicated for use in children under 2 yr of age. Consult manufacturer for dosage recommendations for older children.

USE IN PREGNANT AND NURSING WOMEN

Contraindicated during pregnancy. Probenecid crosses placental barrier and appears in cord blood. Colchicine can arrest cell division and has proved teratogenic in certain animals under certain conditions. Consult manufacturer for use in nursing mothers.

ANTIGOUT AGENTS

Colchicine   Rx

Tablets: 0.432, 0.5, 0.6 mg   **Granules:** 0.5 mg   **Ampuls:** 0.5 mg/ml (2 ml) for IV use only

INDICATIONS	ORAL DOSAGE	PARENTERAL DOSAGE
Acute gouty arthritis	**Adult:** 0.5–1.2 mg to start, followed by 0.5–0.6 mg q1–2h or 1–1.2 mg q2h until pain ceases or nausea, vomiting, or diarrhea develops	**Adult:** 2 mg IV to start, followed by 0.5 mg IV q6h, as needed, up to 4 mg for the first 24 h (do not give more than 4 mg over one course of treatment); alternative regimens: 3 mg in a single IV dose or 1 mg IV to start, followed by 0.5 mg IV 1–2 times/day, as needed

CONTRAINDICATIONS		
Serious gastrointestinal, renal, or cardiac disease	Hypersensitivity to colchicine	Blood dyscrasias

ADMINISTRATION/DOSAGE ADJUSTMENTS

Initiating therapy	Begin treatment at first sign of attack; if second course is required, wait 3 days
Parenteral administration	Administer IV only; IM or SC injection can cause severe local irritation. To avoid extravasation and the considerable irritation that may result, properly position the needle in the vein; inject slowly, over a period of 2–5 min. If extravasation occurs, use of analgesics and local application of heat or cold may relieve the irritation. If solution must be diluted, use only 0.9% Sodium Chloride Injection, which does not contain a bacteriostatic agent (do not use 5% dextrose in water). Discard any solutions that become turbid.
Prophylaxis (interval therapy)	Oral route is preferred, in conjunction with a uricosuric agent. For mild to moderate gout, give 0.5–0.6 mg orally 1–4 times/wk; for severe gout, give 0.5–0.6 mg 1–2 times/day. If IV route is used, give 0.5–1 mg 1–2 times/day.

WARNINGS/PRECAUTIONS

Special-risk patients	Use with great caution in elderly or debilitated patients, especially if renal, gastrointestinal, or heart disease is present; reduce dosage if weakness, anorexia, nausea, vomiting, or diarrhea occurs
Diarrhea	May be severe, even with IV route; administer paregoric concomitantly or as needed

ADVERSE REACTIONS

Frequent reactions (incidence ≥ 1%) are printed in *italics*

Gastrointestinal	*Abdominal pain, nausea, vomiting, diarrhea*
Dermatological	Hair loss
Neuromuscular	Peripheral neuritis
Hematological	Bone marrow depression (including agranulocytosis, thrombocytopenia, and aplastic anemia) with prolonged use; thrombophlebitis at injection site (rare)

OVERDOSAGE

Signs and symptoms	Onset is usually delayed, regardless of route. Signs and symptoms include nausea, vomiting, abdominal pain, diarrhea (possibly severe and bloody), burning sensations in the throat, stomach, and skin, vascular damage, hematuria, oliguria, severe dehydration, hypotension, shock, marked muscular weakness, ascending paralysis, delirium, convulsions, and death due to respiratory depression.

COMPENDIUM OF DRUG THERAPY

Colchicine ■ LOPURIN

Treatment	Remove drug by gastric lavage, combined with hemodialysis or peritoneal dialysis. Establish a patent airway and provide respiratory assistance, if needed. Observe for signs of shock and provide appropriate supportive measures. Atropine or morphine may relieve abdominal pain.

DRUG INTERACTIONS

Vitamin B$_{12}$ (cyanocobalamin)	▽ Absorption of vitamin B$_{12}$

ALTERED LABORATORY VALUES

No clinically significant alterations in blood/serum or urinary values occur at therapeutic dosages

USE IN CHILDREN
Safety and effectiveness for use in children have not been established

USE IN PREGNANT AND NURSING WOMEN
Pregnancy Category B: may cause fetal harm if used during pregnancy. If drug is used or if patient conceives while taking it, she should be apprised of the potential hazard to the fetus. It is not known whether colchicine is excreted in human milk; use with caution in nursing mothers.

ANTIGOUT AGENTS

LOPURIN (allopurinol) Boots   Rx
Tablets: 100, 300 mg

INDICATIONS

Treatment of primary and secondary **gout**	**Adult:** 100 mg/day to start, followed by weekly increases in dosage of 100 mg/day, until serum uric acid level falls to 6 mg/dl (or less) or until a maximum of 800 mg/day is reached; usual dosage: 200–300 mg/day for mild gout, 400–600 mg/day for moderately severe tophaceous gout
Prevention of uric acid nephropathy associated with vigorous **antineoplastic therapy**	**Adult:** 600–800 mg/day for 2–3 days **Child (< 6 yr):** 150 mg/day to start; assess response after 48 h and, if necessary, adjust dosage **Child (6–10 yr):** 300 mg/day to start; assess response after 48 h and, if necessary, adjust dosage
Management of **recurrent calcium oxalate stones** in women whose uric acid excretion exceeds 750 mg/day and in men whose uric acid excretion exceeds 800 mg/day	**Adult:** 200–300 mg/day to start; adjust dosage, as needed, on the basis of uric acid content in 24-h urine samples

ORAL DOSAGE

CONTRAINDICATIONS
Severe reaction to allopurinol

ADMINISTRATION/DOSAGE ADJUSTMENTS

Administration	A daily dose of 300 mg or less may be given as a single dose or divided; higher daily doses should be divided. Gastric irritation can be minimized by administering the drug after meals. If a dose is missed, it is not necessary to double the next dose. Maintain a neutral or, preferably, slightly alkaline urine during therapy, and instruct patients to drink an amount of fluid sufficient to yield an urinary output of at least 2 liters/day; these measures reduce the risk of xanthine calculi and, during concomitant uricosuric therapy, help prevent uric acid stones. A high fluid intake is especially important when allopurinol is given for prevention of uric acid nephropathy associated with antineoplastic therapy.
Determination of serum uric acid level	Do not rely heavily on a single determination of the serum uric acid level since, for technical reasons, estimation of uric acid may be difficult
Patients with renal impairment	Do not exceed 200 mg/day if creatinine clearance (Ccr) is 10–20 ml/min or 100 mg/day if Ccr is less than 10 ml/min. A dosing interval of more than 24 h may be necessary if Ccr is less than 3 ml/min; in some cases, administration twice weekly may be sufficient
Anti-inflammatory drugs	During the early stages of allopurinol therapy, when an increase in attacks of gout may occur, colchicine should generally be given prophylactically and other anti-inflammatory drugs, if used immediately prior to therapy, should also be administered; anti-inflammatory drugs, including colchicine, can be discontinued when the serum uric level becomes normal and freedom from attacks of gout has been achieved for a period of several months

LOPURIN

Uricosuric drugs	To transfer a patient from a uricosuric drug to allopurinol, gradually reduce the dosage of the uricosuric agent over a period of several weeks and, at the same time, gradually increase the dosage of allopurinol. Bear in mind that, in certain cases, use of a uricosuric agent in combination with allopurinol may be necessary for attaining a normal serum uric acid level.
Recurrent calcium oxalate stones	Treatment with allopurinol of recurrent calcium oxalate stones should be carefully evaluated initially and then reassessed periodically, with benefits and risks weighed each time

WARNINGS/PRECAUTIONS

Hypersensitivity	In some cases, a rash may be followed by severe, potentially fatal hypersensitivity reactions (eg, Stevens-Johnson syndrome, generalized vasculitis, toxic epidermal necrolysis); these reactions may be accompanied by fever, chills, arthralgia, mild leukocytosis or leukopenia, eosinophilia, cholestatic jaundice, or, in rare cases, renal failure. If rash or any other sign suggesting hypersensitivity is seen, administration of allopurinol should be discontinued immediately; patients with renal impairment may be more likely than others to develop a rash.
Hepatotoxicity	Hepatic reactions range from asymptomatic increases in transaminase and alkaline phosphatase levels to hepatitis and cholestatic jaundice; these reactions may occur in conjunction with allergic skin reactions (see warning, above, concerning hypersensitivity). If anorexia, weight loss, or pruritus is detected during treatment, hepatic function should be assessed. During the early stages of therapy, perform liver function tests periodically in patients with hepatic disease.
Acute gout	An increase in attacks of gout may occur during the early stages of therapy, even after the serum uric acid level has fallen to a normal or subnormal level; drug-induced mobilization of urates from tissue deposits may be the cause of this reaction. Administer colchicine as a prophylactic measure (see discussion of anti-flammatory drugs in ADMINISTRATION/DOSAGE ADJUSTMENTS). In some cases, therapeutic doses of colchicine or another anti-inflammatory drug may be necessary to treat an attack of gout. After several months of allopurinol therapy, attacks usually become shorter and less severe and eventually are controlled.
Renal impairment	Renal failure has been seen in patients with hyperuricemia owing to neoplastic disease. Precipitation of oxypurines, intermediate products of purine metabolism, should be borne in mind as a possible risk, even though xanthine crystalluria has been detected in only three patients (two with Lesch-Nyhan syndrome and a third with severe hyperuricemia owing to chemotherapy). Caution all patients to report the incidence of hematuria and dysuria.
	An increase in BUN level has occurred in some patients with renal disease or poor urate clearance, and exacerbation of renal impairment has been seen in patients with disorders such as multiple myeloma and congestive heart failure. Patients who have either renal impairment or a nephropathic disorder such as hypertension or diabetes should be closely observed during the early stages of therapy, and the renal function values for these patients, especially their BUN level and creatinine clearance (estimated or measured), should be determined periodically throughout treatment. If a persistent increase in a renal function abnormality is detected, the dosage should be decreased or the drug withdrawn.
Bone marrow depression	Allopurinol can, in rare cases, cause bone marrow depression; reactions can occur 6 wk to 6 yr after the start of therapy. In patients with neoplastic disorders other than leukemia, myelosuppression caused by cytotoxic drugs has reportedly been enhanced by allopurinol; however, a well-controlled study has shown in patients with lymphoma that allopurinol does not increase the bone marrow toxicity associated with cyclophosphamide, doxorubicin, bleomycin, procarbazine, or mechlorethamine.
Drowsiness	Instruct patients to take due precaution when they engage in activities requiring mental alertness
Ophthalmic and oral reactions	Caution patients to report irritation of the eyes (conjunctivitis, iritis) and swelling of the mouth or lips (stomatitis, edema of the tongue, swelling of salivary glands); these reactions have been seen during therapy, but a causal relationship has not yet been established
Asymptomatic hyperuricemia	Do not use allopurinol for asymptomatic hyperuricemia

ADVERSE REACTIONS[1]

The most frequent reactions, regardless of incidence, are printed in *italics*

Dermatological	*Rash (usually maculopapular rash);* Stevens-Johnson syndrome, toxic epidermal necrolysis (Lyell's syndrome), hypersensitivity vasculitis, purpura, vesicular bullous dermatitis, exfoliative dermatitis, eczematoid dermatitis, pruritus, urticaria, alopecia, onycholysis, lichen planus, ecchymosis
Gastrointestinal	*Diarrhea, nausea, increased SGOT, SGPT, and alkaline phosphatase levels,* hepatic necrosis, granulomatous hepatitis, hepatomegaly, hyperbilirubinemia, cholestatic jaundice, vomiting, intermittent abdominal pain, gastritis, dyspepsia
Hematological	Thrombocytopenia, eosinophilia, leukocytosis, leukopenia
Renal	Renal failure, uremia

LOPURIN ■ ZYLOPRIM

Central nervous system	Peripheral neuropathy, neuritis, paresthesia, somnolence, taste loss/change, headache
Musculoskeletal	Myopathy, arthralgias
Cardiovascular	Necrotizing angiitis, vasculitis
Other	*Attacks of gout,* fever, epistaxis

OVERDOSAGE

Signs and symptoms	Acute overdose has not been reported; see ADVERSE REACTIONS for possible effects
Treatment	Allopurinol and its active metabolite, oxipurinol, can be removed from the blood by dialysis; however, it is not known whether this technique is useful in the management of acute overdose

DRUG INTERACTIONS

Mercaptopurine, azathioprine	△ Pharmacologic effect of mercaptopurine and azathioprine; if a patient is receiving 300–600 mg/day of allopurinol, reduce the usual dosage of mercaptopurine or azathioprine by 67–75% to start and then adjust the dosage, as needed and tolerated
Thiazide-type diuretics	△ Risk of hypersensitivity reactions to allopurinol in patients with renal impairment. Monitor renal function, even if normal, during combination therapy. Closely observe patients and adjust dosage with particular care if renal impairment either develops during therapy or is already present at the outset.
Dicumarol	△ Pharmacologic effect of dicumarol; periodically check prothrombin time during combination therapy
Ampicillin, amoxicillin	△ Risk of rash
Cyclophosphamide	△ Risk of bone marrow depression (see warning, above, concerning this effect)
Probenecid	△ Hypouricemic effect
Chlorpropamide	△ Risk of hypoglycemia in patients with renal impairment
Tolbutamide	▽ Metabolism of tolbutamide (based on animal studies)

ALTERED LABORATORY VALUES

Blood/serum values	△ SGPT △ SGOT △ Alkaline phosphatase ▽ Uric acid
Urinary values	▽ Uric acid

USE IN CHILDREN

See INDICATIONS and ORAL DOSAGE; use in children is generally limited to correction of certain congenital defects of purine metabolism and to treatment of hyperuricemia caused by malignancy

USE IN PREGNANT AND NURSING WOMEN

Pregnancy Category C: intraperitoneal administration to mice has resulted in fetotoxicity (at 20 times the usual human dose) and external and skeletal malformations (at 10 and 20 times this dose); however, no evidence of impaired fertility or harm to the fetus has been seen rats or rabbits given up to 20 times the usual human dose, and women have reportedly given birth to normal children after receiving allopurinol during pregnancy. Use this drug in pregnant women only if clearly needed. Allopurinol and its active metabolite, oxipurinol, are excreted in human milk; use with caution in nursing mothers.

[1] The incidence of these reactions, including the most frequent ones, is less than 1%. Reactions for which a causal relationship has not been established include malaise, pericarditis, peripheral vascular disease, thrombophlebitis, bradycardia, vasodilation, male infertility, hypercalcemia, gynecomastia, hemorrhagic pancreatitis, GI bleeding, stomatitis, salivary gland swelling, hyperlipidemia, tongue edema, anorexia, aplastic anemia, agranulocytosis, eosinophilic fibrohistiocytic lesion of bone marrow, pancytopenia, prothrombin decrease, anemia, hemolytic anemia, reticulocytosis, lymphadenopathy, lymphocytosis, myalgia, optic neuritis, confusion, dizziness, vertigo, foot drop, decrease in libido, depression, amnesia, tinnitus, asthenia, insomnia, bronchospasm, asthma, pharyngitis, rhinitis, furunculosis, facial edema, sweating, skin edema, cataracts, macular retinitis, iritis, conjunctivitis, amblyopia, nephritis, impotence, primary hematuria, and albuminuria

---

ANTIGOUT AGENTS

ZYLOPRIM (allopurinol) Burroughs Wellcome   Rx

Tablets: 100, 300 mg

INDICATIONS

Treatment of primary and secondary **gout**

Prevention of uric acid nephropathy associated with vigorous **antineoplastic therapy**

ORAL DOSAGE

Adult: 100 mg/day to start, followed by weekly increases in dosage of 100 mg/day, until serum uric acid level falls to 6 mg/dl (or less) or until a maximum of 800 mg/day is reached; usual dosage: 200–300 mg/day for mild gout, 400–600 mg/day for moderately severe tophaceous gout

Adult: 600–800 mg/day for 2–3 days
Child (< 6 yr): 150 mg/day to start; assess response after 48 h and, if necessary, adjust dosage
Child (6–10 yr): 300 mg/day to start; assess response after 48 h and, if necessary, adjust dosage

ZYLOPRIM

Management of **recurrent calcium oxalate stones** in women whose uric acid excretion exceeds 750 mg/day and in men whose uric acid excretion exceeds 800 mg/day	**Adult:** 200–300 mg/day to start; adjust dosage, as needed, on the basis of uric acid content in 24-h urine samples

CONTRAINDICATIONS
Severe reaction to allopurinol

ADMINISTRATION/DOSAGE ADJUSTMENTS

Administration	A daily dose of 300 mg or less may be given as a single dose or divided; higher daily doses should be divided. Gastric irritation can be minimized by administering the drug after meals. If a dose is missed, it is not necessary to double the next dose. Maintain a neutral or, preferably, slightly alkaline urine during therapy, and instruct patients to drink an amount of fluid sufficient to yield an urinary output of at least 2 liters/day; these measures reduce the risk of xanthine calculi and, during concomitant uricosuric therapy, help prevent uric acid stones. A high fluid intake is especially important when allopurinol is given for prevention of uric acid nephropathy associated with antineoplastic therapy.
Determination of serum uric acid level	Do not rely heavily on a single determination of the serum uric acid level since, for technical reasons, estimation of uric acid may be difficult
Patients with renal impairment	Do not exceed 200 mg/day if creatinine clearance (Ccr) is 10–20 ml/min or 100 mg/day if Ccr is less than 10 ml/min. A dosing interval of more than 24 h may be necessary if Ccr is less than 3 ml/min; in some cases, administration twice weekly may be sufficient
Anti-inflammatory drugs	During the early stages of allopurinol therapy, when an increase in attacks of gout may occur, colchicine should generally be given prophylactically and other anti-inflammatory drugs, if used immediately prior to therapy, should also be administered; anti-inflammatory drugs, including colchicine, can be discontinued when the serum uric level becomes normal and freedom from attacks of gout has been achieved for a period of several months
Uricosuric drugs	To transfer a patient from a uricosuric drug to allopurinol, gradually reduce the dosage of the uricosuric agent over a period of several weeks and, at the same time, gradually increase the dosage of allopurinol. Bear in mind that in certain cases use of a uricosuric agent in combination with allopurinol may be necessary for attaining a normal serum uric acid level.
Recurrent calcium oxalate stones	Treatment with allopurinol of recurrent calcium oxalate stones should be carefully evaluated initially and then reassessed periodically, with benefits and risks weighed each time

WARNINGS/PRECAUTIONS

Hypersensitivity	In some cases, a rash may be followed by severe, potentially fatal hypersensitivity reactions (eg, Stevens-Johnson syndrome, generalized vasculitis, toxic epidermal necrolysis); these reactions may be accompanied by fever, chills, arthralgia, mild leukocytosis or leukopenia, eosinophilia, cholestatic jaundice, or, in rare cases, renal failure. If rash or any other sign suggesting hypersensitivity is seen, administration of allopurinol should be discontinued immediately; patients with renal impairment may be more likely than others to develop a rash.
Hepatotoxicity	Hepatic reactions range from asymptomatic increases in transaminase and alkaline phosphatase levels to hepatitis and cholestatic jaundice; these reactions may occur in conjunction with allergic skin reactions (see warning, above, concerning hypersensitivity). If anorexia, weight loss, or pruritus is detected during treatment, hepatic function should be assessed. During the early stages of therapy, perform liver function tests periodically in patients with hepatic disease.
Acute gout	An increase in attacks of gout may occur during the early stages of therapy, even after the serum uric acid level has fallen to a normal or subnormal level; drug-induced mobilization of urates from tissue deposits may be the cause of this reaction. Administer colchicine as a prophylactic measure (see discussion of anti-flammatory drugs in ADMINISTRATION/DOSAGE ADJUSTMENTS). In some cases, therapeutic doses of colchicine or another anti-inflammatory drug may be necessary to treat an attack of gout. After several months of allopurinol therapy, attacks usually become shorter and less severe and eventually are controlled.
Renal impairment	Renal failure has been seen in patients with hyperuricemia owing to neoplastic disease. Precipitation of oxypurines, intermediate products of purine metabolism, should be borne in mind as a possible risk, even though xanthine crystalluria has been detected in only three patients (two with Lesch-Nyhan syndrome and a third with severe hyperuricemia owing to chemotherapy). Caution all patients to report the incidence of hematuria and dysuria.
	An increase in BUN level has occurred in some patients with renal disease or poor urate clearance, and exacerbation of renal impairment has been seen in patients with disorders such as multiple myeloma and congestive heart failure. Patients who have either renal impairment or a nephropathic disorder such as hypertension or diabetes should be closely observed during the early stages of therapy, and the renal function values for these patients, especially their BUN level and creatinine clearance (estimated or measured), should be determined periodically throughout treatment. If a persistent increase in a renal function abnormality is detected, the dosage should be decreased or the drug withdrawn.

ZYLOPRIM

Bone marrow depression	Allopurinol can, in rare cases, cause bone marrow depression; reactions can occur 6 wk to 6 yr after the start of therapy. In patients with neoplastic disorders other than leukemia, myelosuppression caused by cytotoxic drugs has reportedly been enhanced by allopurinol; however, a well-controlled study has shown in patients with lymphoma that allopurinol does not increase the bone marrow toxicity associated with cyclophosphamide, doxorubicin, bleomycin, procarbazine, or mechlorethamine.
Drowsiness	Instruct patients to take due precaution when they engage in activities requiring mental alertness
Ophthalmic and oral reactions	Caution patients to report irritation of the eyes (conjunctivitis, iritis) and swelling of the mouth or lips (stomatitis, edema of the tongue, swelling of salivary glands); these reactions have been seen during therapy, but a causal relationship has not yet been established
Asymptomatic hyperuricemia	Do not use allopurinol for asymptomatic hyperuricemia

ADVERSE REACTIONS[1]

The most frequent reactions, regardless of incidence, are printed in *italics*

Dermatological	*Rash (especially maculopapular rash),* Stevens-Johnson syndrome, toxic epidermal necrolysis (Lyell's syndrome), hypersensitivity vasculitis, purpura, vesicular bullous dermatitis, exfoliative dermatitis, eczematoid dermatitis, pruritus, urticaria, alopecia, onycholysis, lichen planus, ecchymosis
Gastrointestinal	*Diarrhea, nausea, increased SGOT, SGPT, and alkaline phosphatase levels,* hepatic necrosis, granulomatous hepatitis, hepatomegaly, hyperbilirubinemia, cholestatic jaundice, vomiting, intermittent abdominal pain, gastritis, dyspepsia
Hematological	Thrombocytopenia, eosinophilia, leukocytosis, leukopenia
Renal	Renal failure, uremia
Central nervous system	Peripheral neuropathy, neuritis, paresthesia, somnolence, taste loss/change, headache
Musculoskeletal	Myopathy, arthralgias
Cardiovascular	Necrotizing angiitis, vasculitis
Other	*Attacks of gout,* fever, epistaxis

OVERDOSAGE

Signs and symptoms	Acute overdose has not been reported; see ADVERSE REACTIONS for possible effects
Treatment	Allopurinol and its active metabolite, oxipurinol, can be removed from the blood by dialysis; however, it is not known whether this technique is useful in the management of acute overdose

DRUG INTERACTIONS

Mercaptopurine, azathioprine	△ Pharmacologic effect of mercaptopurine and azathioprine; if a patient is receiving 300–600 mg/day of allopurinol, reduce the usual dosage of mercaptopurine or azathioprine by 67–75% to start and then adjust the dosage, as needed and tolerated
Thiazide-type diuretics	△ Risk of hypersensitivity reactions to allopurinol in patients with renal impairment. Monitor renal function, even if normal, during combination therapy. Closely observe patients and adjust dosage with particular care if renal impairment either develops during therapy or is already present at the outset.
Dicumarol	△ Pharmacologic effect of dicumarol; periodically check prothrombin time during combination therapy
Ampicillin, amoxicillin	△ Risk of rash
Cyclophosphamide	△ Risk of bone marrow depression (see warning, above, concerning this effect)
Probenecid	△ Hypouricemic effect
Chlorpropamide	△ Risk of hypoglycemia in patients with renal impairment
Tolbutamide	▽ Metabolism of tolbutamide (based on animal studies)

ALTERED LABORATORY VALUES

Blood/serum values	△ SGPT △ SGOT △ Alkaline phosphatase ▽ Uric acid
Urinary values	▽ Uric acid

USE IN CHILDREN

See INDICATIONS and ORAL DOSAGE; use in children is generally limited to correction of certain congenital defects of purine metabolism and to treatment of hyperuricemia caused by malignancy

USE IN PREGNANT AND NURSING WOMEN

Pregnancy Category C: intraperitoneal administration to mice has resulted in fetotoxicity (at 20 times the usual human dose) and external and skeletal malformations (at 10 and 20 times this dose); however, no evidence of impaired fertility or harm to the fetus has been seen in rats or rabbits given up to 20 times the usual human dose, and women have reportedly given birth to normal children after receiving allopurinol during pregnancy. Use this drug in pregnant women only if clearly needed. Allopurinol and its active metabolite, oxipurinol, are excreted in human milk; use with caution in nursing mothers.

---

[1] The incidence of these reactions, including the most frequent ones, is less than 1%. Reactions for which a causal relationship has not been established include malaise, pericarditis, peripheral vascular disease, thrombophlebitis, bradycardia, vasodilation, male infertility, hypercalcemia, gynecomastia, hemorrhagic pancreatitis, GI bleeding, stomatitis, salivary gland swelling, hyperlipidemia, tongue edema, anorexia, aplastic anemia, agranulocytosis, eosinophilic fibrohistiocytic lesion of bone marrow, pancytopenia, prothrombin decrease, anemia, hemolytic anemia, reticulocytosis, lymphadenopathy, lymphocytosis, myalgia, optic neuritis, confusion, dizziness, vertigo, foot drop, decrease in libido, depression, amnesia, tinnitus, asthenia, insomnia, bronchospasm, asthma, pharyngitis, rhinitis, furunculosis, facial edema, sweating, skin edema, cataracts, macular retinitis, iritis, conjunctivitis, amblyopia, nephritis, impotence, primary hematuria, and albuminuria

Chapter 21

Antihistamines/Antipruritics/Mast-Cell Stabilizers

Anthistamines/Antipruritics — 729

ATARAX (Roerig) — 729
Hydroxyzine hydrochloride *Rx*

ATARAX 100 (Roerig) — 729
Hydroxyzine hydrochloride *Rx*

BENADRYL (Parke-Davis) — 730
Diphenhydramine hydrochloride *Rx*

BENADRYL 25 (Warner-Lambert) — 730
Diphenydramine hydrochloride *OTC*

BENADRYL Elixir (Warner-Lambert) — 730
Diphenhydramine hydrochloride *OTC*

CHLOR-TRIMETON (Schering) — 731
Chlorpheniramine maleate *OTC*

CHLOR-TRIMETON Injection (Schering) — 732
Chlorpheniramine maleate *Rx*

DIMETANE (Robins) — 733
Brompheniramine maleate *OTC*

DIMETANE-TEN (Robins) — 733
Brompheniramine maleate *Rx*

OPTIMINE (Schering) — 735
Azatadine maleate *Rx*

PBZ (Geigy) — 736
Tripelennamine *Rx*

PBZ-SR (Geigy) — 736
Tripelennamine hydrochloride *Rx*

PERIACTIN (Merck Sharp & Dohme) — 737
Cyproheptadine hydrochloride *Rx*

PHENERGAN (Wyeth) — 739
Promethazine hydrochloride *Rx*

PHENERGAN Injection (Wyeth) — 740
Promethazine hydrochloride *Rx*

POLARAMINE (Schering) — 742
Dexchlorpheniramine maleate *Rx*

SELDANE (Merrell Dow) — 743
Terfenadine *Rx*

TAVIST (Sandoz Pharmaceuticals) — 744
Clemastine fumarate *Rx*

TAVIST Syrup (Sandoz Pharmaceuticals) — 745
Clemastine fumarate *Rx*

TAVIST-1 (Sandoz Pharmaceuticals) — 745
Clemastine fumarate *Rx*

TELDRIN (SmithKline Consumer Products) — 746
Chlorpheniramine maleate *OTC*

TEMARIL (Herbert) — 747
Trimeprazine tartrate *Rx*

VISTARIL (Pfizer) — 749
Hydroxyzine pamoate *Rx*

Mast-Cell Stabilizers — 749

INTAL Capsules (Fisons) — 749
Cromolyn sodium *Rx*

INTAL Inhaler (Fisons) — 750
Cromolyn sodium *Rx*

INTAL Nebulizer Solution (Fisons) — 750
Cromolyn sodium *Rx*

NASALCROM (Fisons) — 752
Cromolyn sodium *Rx*

OPTICROM 4% Ophthalmic Solution (Fisons) — 752
Cromolyn sodium *Rx*

Other Anthistamines/Antipruritics — 728

ACTIDIL (Burroughs Wellcome) — 728
Triprolidine hydrochloride *OTC*

BENADRYL Cream (Warner-Lambert) — 728
Diphenhydramine hydrochloride *OTC*

CALADRYL (Warner-Lambert) — 728
Calamine and diphenhydramine hydrochloride *OTC*

CLISTIN (McNeil Pharmaceutical) — 728
Carbinoxamine maleate *Rx*

HISPRIL (Smith Kline & French) — 728
Diphenylpyraline hydrochloride *Rx*

NOLAHIST (Carnrick) — 728
Phenindamine tartrate *OTC*

TACARYL (Westwood) — 728
Methdilazine hydrochloride *Rx*

continued

COMPENDIUM OF DRUG THERAPY

OTHER ANTIHISTAMINES/ANTIPRURITICS

DRUG	HOW SUPPLIED	USUAL DOSAGE[1]
ACTIDIL (Burroughs Wellcome) Triprolidine hydrochloride *OTC*	Tablets: 2.5 mg Syrup (per 5 ml): 1.25 mg (1 pt)	**Adult:** 2.5 mg or 10 ml (2 tsp) q4–6h, up to 10 mg or 40 ml (8 tsp)/24 h **Child (6–12 yr):** 1.25 mg or 5 ml (1 tsp) q4–6h, up to 5 mg or 20 ml (4 tsp)/24 h
BENADRYL Cream (Warner-Lambert) Diphenhydramine hydrochloride *OTC*	Cream: 2% (1, 2 oz)	**Adult and child (> 2 yr):** apply to affected area up to tid or qid
CALADRYL (Warner-Lambert) Calamine and diphenhydramine hydrochloride *OTC*	Cream: calamine, 1% diphenhydramine hydrochloride, and camphor (1½ oz) Lotion: calamine, 1% diphenhydramine hydrochloride, and camphor (2½, 6 fl oz)	**Adult:** apply to affected area tid or qid; wash skin with soap and water and dry before each application
CLISTIN (McNeil Pharmaceutical) Carbinoxamine maleate *Rx*	Tablets: 4 mg	**Adult:** 4–8 mg tid or qid **Child (1–3 yr):** 2 mg tid or qid **Child (3–6 yr):** 2–4 mg tid or qid **Child (> 6 yr):** 4–6 mg tid or qid
HISPRIL (Smith Kline & French) Diphenylpyraline hydrochloride *Rx*	Capsules (sustained release): 5 mg	**Adult:** 5 mg q12h **Child (6–12 yr):** 5 mg once daily
NOLAHIST (Carnrick) Phenindamine tartrate *OTC*	Tablets: 25 mg	**Adult:** 25 mg q4–6h **Child (6–12 yr):** 12.5 mg q4–6h
TACARYL (Westwood) Methdilazine hydrochloride *Rx*	Tablets: 8 mg Chewable tablets: 3.6 mg methdilazine (equivalent to 4 mg methdilazine hydrochloride) Syrup (per 5 ml): 4 mg (16 fl oz)	**Adult:** 8 mg, 10 ml (2 tsp), or 2 chewable tablets bid to qid **Child (> 3 yr):** 4 mg, 5 ml (1 tsp), or 1 chewable tablet bid to qid

[1] Where pediatric dosages are not given, consult manufacturer

ANTIHISTAMINES/ANTIPRURITICS

ATARAX (hydroxyzine hydrochloride) Roerig — Rx
Tablets: 10, 25, 50 mg Syrup (per 5 ml): 10 mg[1] (1 pt)

ATARAX 100 (hydroxyzine hydrochloride) Roerig — Rx
Tablets: 100 mg

INDICATIONS	ORAL DOSAGE
Anxiety and tension associated with psychoneurosis **Anxiety** associated with organic disease (adjunctive therapy)	Adult: 50–100 mg qid Child ($<$ 6 yr): 50 mg/day, given in divided doses Child ($>$ 6 yr): 50–100 mg/day, given in divided doses
Pruritus due to allergic conditions, including chronic urticaria and atopic and contact dermatoses **Histamine-mediated pruritus**	Adult: 25 mg tid or qid Child ($<$ 6 yr): 50 mg/day, given in divided doses Child ($>$ 6 yr): 50–100 mg/day, given in divided doses
Preoperative sedation and following general anesthesia	Adult: 50–100 mg Child: 0.6 mg/kg

CONTRAINDICATIONS	
Early pregnancy	Hypersensitivity to hydroxyzine

ADMINISTRATION/DOSAGE ADJUSTMENTS	
Long-term use ($>$ 4 mo)	Effectiveness for prolonged use as an antianxiety agent has not been tested in systematic clinical studies; reassess need for continued therapy periodically

WARNINGS/PRECAUTIONS	
Drowsiness	Caution patients not to engage in potentially hazardous activities requiring full mental alertness
Concomitant use of CNS depressants	May potentiate hydroxyzine's effect; reduce dosage of these agents accordingly and caution patients that simultaneous use of alcohol and other CNS depressants may have addictive effects

ADVERSE REACTIONS	
Central nervous system	Transient drowsiness; involuntary motor activity, including tremor and convulsions (rare)
Gastrointestinal	Dry mouth

OVERDOSAGE	
Signs and symptoms	Excessive sedation, hypotension, CNS depression
Treatment	Induce emesis or use gastric lavage to empty stomach. Monitor respiration, pulse, and blood pressure. Employ general supportive measures, as needed. Hypotension may be combatted with IV fluids and levarterenol or metaraminol. Do not use epinephrine, since hydroxyzine counteracts its pressor action. Dialysis is of limited value, unless other agents, such as barbiturates, have been ingested concomitantly.

DRUG INTERACTIONS	
Alcohol, narcotic analgesics, sedative-hypnotics, other CNS depressants, and tricyclic antidepressants	△ CNS depression

ALTERED LABORATORY VALUES	
Urinary values	△ 17-Hydroxycorticosteroids

No clinically significant alterations in blood/serum values occur at therapeutic dosages

---

USE IN CHILDREN

See INDICATIONS and ORAL DOSAGE

USE IN PREGNANT AND NURSING WOMEN

Contraindicated during early pregnancy. Fetal abnormalities have been reported in mice, rats, and rabbits at doses well above the maximum human dose. Clinical data are inadequate to establish safety for use in pregnant women during this period. It is not known whether hydroxyzine is excreted in human milk; because many drugs are excreted in human milk, patient should stop nursing if drug is prescribed.

---

[1] Contains 0.5% alcohol

BENADRYL

ANTIHISTAMINES/ANTIPRURITICS

BENADRYL 25 (diphenhydramine hydrochloride) Warner-Lambert — OTC
Capsules: 25 mg

BENADRYL Elixir (diphenhydramine hydrochloride) Warner-Lambert — OTC
Elixir (per 5 ml): 12.5 mg[1] (4 fl oz)

INDICATIONS	ORAL DOSAGE
Runny nose, sneezing, itchy nose and throat, and itchy, watery eyes associated with **hay fever** or other upper respiratory tract allergies Runny nose and sneezing associated with the **common cold**	**Adult:** 25–50 mg or 10–20 ml (2–4 tsp) q4–6h **Child (6–12 yr):** 25 mg or 5–10 ml (1–2 tsp) q4–6h

BENADRYL (diphenhydramine hydrochloride) Parke-Davis — Rx
Capsules: 25, 50 mg **Elixir (per 5 ml):** 12.5 mg[1] (5 ml, 4 fl oz, 1 pt, 1 gal) **Ampuls:** 50 mg/ml (1 ml) **Vials:** 10 mg/ml (10, 30 ml), 50 mg/ml (10 ml) **Prefilled syringes:** 50 mg/ml (1 ml)

INDICATIONS	ORAL DOSAGE	PARENTERAL DOSAGE
Allergic conjunctivitis due to foods Mild, uncomplicated **urticaria** and **angioedema** **Dermatographism** **Allergic reactions to blood or plasma** **Anaphylactic reactions,** as an adjunct to epinephrine and other standard measures after acute symptoms have been controlled **Motion sickness** **Parkinsonism** (including drug-induced symptoms), for use in elderly patients unable to tolerate more potent agents, for mild cases in other age groups, and for more severe cases when combined with centrally acting anticholinergic agents	**Adult:** 25–50 mg or 10–20 ml (2–4 tsp) tid or qid **Child (> 20 lb):** 12.5–25 mg or 5–10 ml (1–2 tsp) tid or qid, or 5 mg/kg/24 h (150 mg/m²/24 h), up to 300 mg/day, given in 3–4 divided doses	**Adult:** 10–50 mg (or up to 100 mg, if needed) IM (deeply) or IV, up to 400 mg/day **Child:** 5 mg/kg/24 h (150 mg/m²/24 h), up to 300 mg/day, given in 4 divided doses IM (deeply) or IV
Insomnia	**Adult:** 50 mg or 20 ml (4 tsp) at bedtime	

CONTRAINDICATIONS		
Hypersensitivity to diphenhydramine or structurally related antihistamines	Breast-feeding	Full-term or premature neonates

ADMINISTRATION/DOSAGE ADJUSTMENTS

Parenteral administration	The injectable forms may be used when oral therapy is impractical for active treatment of motion sickness, amelioration of allergic reactions to blood or plasma, or adjunctive therapy of anaphylactic reactions, and when oral therapy is contraindicated or impossible in cases of parkinsonism or other uncomplicated, immediate-type allergic reactions
Treatment of motion sickness	The full oral dosage is recommended for prophylactic use; the first dose should be given 30 min before the patient is exposed to motion, followed by similar doses before meals and upon retiring for the duration of the exposure

WARNINGS/PRECAUTIONS

Drowsiness	Caution patients about driving or engaging in other activities requiring mental alertness, and about using alcohol or other CNS depressants (see DRUG INTERACTIONS)
Elderly patients	Dizziness, sedation, and hypotension occur more frequently in patients over 60 yr of age
Special-risk patients	Use with considerable caution in patients with narrow-angle glaucoma, stenosing peptic ulcer, pyloroduodenal obstruction, symptomatic prostatic hypertrophy, or bladder-neck obstruction and with caution in patients with increased intraocular pressure, hyperthyroidism, cardiovascular disease, hypertension, or a history of asthma or other lower respiratory tract diseases
Carcinogenicity, mutagenicity	No studies have been done to evaluate the carcinogenic or mutagenic potential of this drug

ADVERSE REACTIONS
The most frequent reactions, regardless of incidence, are printed in *italics*

Cardiovascular	Hypotension, headache, palpitations, tachycardia, extrasystoles
Hematological	Hemolytic anemia, thrombocytopenia, agranulocytosis

BENADRYL ■ CHLOR-TRIMETON

Central nervous system	*Sedation, sleepiness, dizziness, disturbed coordination,* fatigue, confusion, restlessness, excitation, nervousness, tremor, irritability, insomnia, euphoria, paresthesias, vertigo, tinnitus, acute labyrinthitis, neuritis, convulsions
Ophthalmic	Blurred vision, diplopia
Gastrointestinal	*Epigastric distress,* anorexia, nausea, vomiting, diarrhea, constipation
Genitourinary	Urinary frequency, difficult urination, urinary retention, early menses
Respiratory	*Thickening of bronchial secretions,* tightness in the chest and wheezing, nasal stuffiness
Dermatological	Urticaria, drug rash, photosensitivity
Hypersensitivity	Anaphylactic shock
Other	Dry mouth, nose, and throat; chills, excessive perspiration

OVERDOSAGE

Signs and symptoms	Varies from CNS depression (drowsiness, sedation, diminished mental alertness, apnea, cardiovascular collapse) to CNS stimulation (insomnia, excitement, hallucinations, ataxia, incoordination, athetosis, tremors, convulsions) and may include dizziness, tinnitus, blurred vision, and hypotension; CNS stimulation, followed by postictal depression, and atropine-like symptoms (dry mouth; fixed, dilated pupils; fever, flushing, GI disturbances) are particularly likely in children
Treatment	If patient is conscious, induce emesis with syrup of ipecac, even though vomiting may have occurred spontaneously. If vomiting is unsuccessful or contraindicated, perform gastric lavage with isotonic or $^1/_2$ isotonic saline solution. Remove any remaining drug in the stomach by instillation of activated charcoal. Administer a saline cathartic to rapidly dilute bowel content. Treatment is symptomatic and supportive. If breathing is significantly impaired, maintain an adequate airway and provide mechanically assisted ventilation; *do not use analeptics.* Vasopressors (eg, norepinephrine) may be used for significant hypotension. Treat hyperpyrexia by sponging with tepid water or use of ice packs or a hypothermal blanket. For seizures, administer a short-acting barbiturate, diazepam, or paraldehyde.

DRUG INTERACTIONS

Alcohol, tranquilizers, sedative-hypnotics, and other CNS depressants	⇧ CNS depression
MAO inhibitors	⇧ Anticholinergic effects

ALTERED LABORATORY VALUES

No clinically significant alterations in blood/serum or urinary values occur at therapeutic dosages

---

USE IN CHILDREN

See INDICATIONS and dosage recommendations; contraindicated for use in full-term or premature neonates. Antihistamines may produce excitation in young children.

USE IN PREGNANT AND NURSING WOMEN

Pregnancy Category B: reproduction studies in rats and rabbits given up to 5 times the human dose have shown no evidence of impaired fertility or harm to the fetus; use during pregnancy only if clearly needed. Contraindicated for use in nursing mothers due to the increased risk of antihistaminic side effects in newborns and infants.

---

[1] Contains 5% alcohol
[2] Contains 14% alcohol

ANTIHISTAMINES/ANTIPRURITICS

CHLOR-TRIMETON (chlorpheniramine maleate) Schering   OTC

Tablets: 4 mg   **Tablets (sustained release):** 8, 12 mg   **Syrup (per 5 ml):** 2 mg[1] (4 fl oz)

INDICATIONS

Hay fever symptoms, including sneezing, running or itchy nose, watery, itchy eyes, and itchy throat

ORAL DOSAGE

Adult: 4 mg or 10 ml (2 tsp) q4–6h; if sustained-release tablets are used, 8 mg q8–12h or 12 mg q12h
Child (2–5 yr): 1 mg or 2.5 ml ($^1/_2$ tsp) q4–6h
Child (6–11 yr): 2 mg or 5 ml (1 tsp) q4–6h; if sustained-release tablets are used, 8 mg at bedtime or during the day
Child ($\geq$ 12 yr): same as adult

CHLOR-TRIMETON Injection (chlorpheniramine maleate) Schering   Rx

Ampuls: 10 mg/ml (1 ml)

INDICATIONS

Seasonal and perennial **allergic rhinitis**
Vasomotor rhinitis
Allergic conjunctivitis due to inhalant allergens and foods
Mild, uncomplicated **urticaria** and **angioedema**
Dermatographism

Allergic reactions to blood or plasma

Anaphylactic reactions as an adjunct to epinephrine and other standard measures after acute symptoms have been controlled

PARENTERAL DOSAGE

Adult and child ($\geq$ 12 yr): 5–20 mg SC, IM, or IV

Adult and child ($\geq$ 12 yr): 10–20 mg SC, IM, or IV; maximum 24-h dose: 40 mg

Adult and child ($\geq$ 12 yr): 10–20 mg IV

CONTRAINDICATIONS

Hypersensitivity to chlorpheniramine or structurally related antihistamines

ADMINISTRATION/DOSAGE ADJUSTMENTS

Use of parenteral solution	Do not mix parenteral solution with other drugs

WARNINGS/PRECAUTIONS

Drowsiness	Caution patients about driving or engaging in other activities requiring mental alertness, and about using alcohol or other CNS depressants (see DRUG INTERACTIONS)
Elderly patients	Dizziness, sedation, and hypotension occur more frequently in patients over 60 yr of age
Special-risk patients	Use with caution in patients with narrow-angle glaucoma, stenosing peptic ulcer, pyloroduodenal obstruction, urinary bladder obstruction (owing to symptomatic prostatic hypertrophy or narrowing of the bladder neck), increased intraocular pressure, hyperthyroidism, cardiovascular disease, hypertension, or a history of bronchial asthma
Interference with skin tests	Antihistamines may prevent or diminish otherwise positive reactions to allergens used in skin tests; discontinue chlorpheniramine about 4 days before a skin test
Patients receiving anticoagulants	Chlorpheniramine should not be used in combination with oral anticoagulants since it may reduce their effectiveness
Carcinogenicity, mutagenicity	Long-term studies in rats fed chlorpheniramine have shown no evidence of carcinogenicity; no signs of mutagenicity due to chlorpheniramine or its nitrosation metabolite have been seen in the Ames test
Effect on fertility	No adverse effects on fertility have been detected in rats fed up to 67 times the human dose

ADVERSE REACTIONS[2]

	Frequent reactions (incidence $\geq$ 1%) are printed in *italics*
Cardiovascular	Hypotension, headache, palpitations, tachycardia, extrasystoles
Hematological	Hemolytic anemia, hypoplastic anemia, thrombocytopenia, agranulocytosis
Central nervous system	*Drowsiness, sedation, dizziness, disturbed coordination,* fatigue, confusion, restlessness, excitation, nervousness, tremor, irritability, insomnia, euphoria, paresthesias, vertigo, tinnitus, acute labyrinthitis, hysteria, neuritis, convulsions
Ophthalmic	Blurred vision, diplopia
Gastrointestinal	*Epigastric distress,* anorexia, nausea, vomiting, diarrhea, constipation
Genitourinary	Urinary frequency, difficult urination, urinary retention, early menses
Respiratory	*Thickening bronchial secretions,* tightness in the chest and wheezing, nasal stuffiness
Dermatological	Urticaria, drug rash, photosensitivity
Other	Anaphylactic shock, excessive perspiration, chills; dry mouth, nose, and throat

OVERDOSAGE

Signs and symptoms	Varies from CNS depression (sedation, apnea, diminished mental alertness, cyanosis, hyperreflexia, cardiovascular collapse) to CNS stimulation (insomnia, hallucinations, tremors, convulsions) and may also include dizziness, tinnitus, ataxia, blurred vision, and hypotension; excitation, hallucinations, athetosis, tonic-clonic convulsions with postictal depression, and atropine-like symptoms (dry mouth; fixed, dilated pupils; flushing; fever; GI disturbances) are particularly likely to occur in children

CHLOR-TRIMETON ■ DIMETANE

Treatment — If the patient is conscious, induce emesis with syrup of ipecac, even though vomiting may have occurred spontaneously; the action of ipecac is facilitated by physical–activity and the ingestion of 8-12 fl oz of water. If emesis does not occur within 15 min, the dose of ipecac should be repeated. Take precautions to avoid aspiration, particularly in infants and children. If vomiting is unsuccessful or contraindicated, perform gastric lavage; isotonic saline solution should be used, particularly with children (tap water, although not preferred, can be used with adults). Remove any drug remaining in the stomach by instillation of a slurry containing activated charcoal. Administer a saline cathartic to rapidly dilute bowel content. Dialysis is of little value. Treatment is symptomatic and supportive. If breathing is significantly impaired, maintain an adequate airway and provide mechanically assisted ventilation; *do not use analeptics.* Vasopressors (eg, norepinephrine) may be used for significant hypotension. Treat hyperpyrexia by sponging with tepid water or using a hypothermal blanket. For seizures, administer a short-acting barbiturate, diazepam, or paraldehyde.

DRUG INTERACTIONS

Alcohol, tranquilizers, barbiturates, sedative-hypnotics, and other CNS depressants — ◇ CNS depression

MAO inhibitors — ◇ Anticholinergic effects

ALTERED LABORATORY VALUES

No clinically significant alterations in blood/serum or urinary values occur at therapeutic dosages

---

USE IN CHILDREN

See INDICATIONS and dosage recommendations. The parenteral solution and 12-mg sustained-release tablets are not recommended for use in children under 12 yr of age; the 8-mg sustained-release tablets are not indicated for use in children under 6 yr of age. Antihistamines may produce excitation in young children.

USE IN PREGNANT AND NURSING WOMEN

Pregnancy Category B: reproduction studies in rats given up to 50 times the human dose and in rabbits given up to 30 times the human dose have shown no evidence of impaired fertility or harm to the fetus. Use during the first two trimesters of pregnancy only if clearly needed; do not use in the third trimester because of the risk of severe reactions, such as convulsions, in neonates. It is not known whether chlorpheniramine is excreted in human milk; however, low concentrations of other antihistamines have been detected in human milk. Because of the increased risk of antihistaminic side effects in infants, particularly in neonates, patients should not nurse while taking this drug.

---

[1] Contains approximately 7% alcohol
[2] Includes reactions common to antihistamines in general

ANTIHISTAMINES/ANTIPRURITICS

DIMETANE (brompheniramine maleate) Robins OTC

Tablets: 4 mg   **Elixir (per 5 ml):** 2 mg[1] (4 fl oz, 1 pt, 1 gal)   **Tablets (sustained release):** 8, 12 mg

INDICATIONS

Hay fever symptoms, including sneezing, itchy or running nose, watery, itchy eyes, and itchy throat

ORAL DOSAGE

Adult: 4 mg or 10 ml (2 tsp) q4–6h; if sustained-release tablets are used, 8 mg q8–12h or 12 mg q12h
Child (6–12 yr): 2 mg or 5 ml (1 tsp) q4–6h
Child (≥ 12 yr): same as adult

DIMETANE-TEN (brompheniramine maleate) Robins Rx

Ampuls: 10 mg/ml (1 ml)

INDICATIONS

Seasonal and perennial **allergic rhinitis**
Vasomotor rhinitis
Allergic conjunctivitis due to inhalant allergens and foods
Mild, uncomplicated **urticaria** and **angioedema**
Dermatographism
Allergic reactions to blood or plasma
Anaphylactic reactions, as an adjunct to epinephrine and other standard measures after acute symptoms have been controlled

PARENTERAL DOSAGE

Adult: 5–20 mg SC, IM, or IV (slowly) bid, up to 40 mg/24 h; usual dosage: 10 mg bid
Child (< 12 yr): 0.5 mg/kg/24 h or 15 mg/m^2/24 h SC, IM, or IV (slowly), divided into 3–4 doses

DIMETANE

CONTRAINDICATIONS

Lower respiratory tract conditions, including asthma	Full-term or premature neonates	MAO inhibitor therapy (see DRUG INTERACTIONS)
Hypersensitivity to brompheniramine		

ADMINISTRATION/DOSAGE ADJUSTMENTS

Intravenous administration	The solution may be given undiluted or, before injection, may be diluted 1:10 with sterile saline for injection. Administer slowly, preferably with the patient lying down.

WARNINGS/PRECAUTIONS

Drowsiness	Caution patients that they should not drive or engage in any other potentially hazardous activity until their response to this drug has been established
Elderly patients	Dizziness, sedation, and hypotension occur more frequently in patients over 60 yr of age
Special-risk patients	Use with caution in patients with narrow-angle glaucoma, gastrointestinal obstruction, prostatic hypertrophy, or a history of bronchial asthma
Carcinogenicity, mutagenicity	No studies have been done to evaluate the carcinogenic or mutagenic potential of this drug

ADVERSE REACTIONS

The most frequent reactions, regardless of incidence, are printed in *italics*

Cardiovascular	Hypotension, headache, palpitations, tachycardia, extrasystoles
Hematological	Hemolytic anemia, thrombocytopenia, agranulocytosis
Central nervous system	*Sedation, sleepiness, dizziness, disturbed coordination,* fatigue, confusion, restlessness, excitation, nervousness, tremor, irritability, insomnia, euphoria, paresthesias, vertigo, tinnitus, acute labyrinthitis, hysteria, neuritis, convulsions
Ophthalmic	Blurred vision, diplopia
Gastrointestinal	*Epigastric distress,* anorexia, nausea, vomiting, diarrhea, constipation
Genitourinary	Urinary frequency, difficult urination, urinary retention, early menses
Respiratory	*Thickening of bronchial secretions,* tightness in the chest and wheezing, nasal stuffiness
Dermatological	Urticaria, drug rash, photosensitivity
Hypersensitivity	Anaphylactic shock
Other	Dry mouth, nose, and throat, chills, excessive perspiration

OVERDOSAGE

Signs and symptoms	*CNS:* depressant effects, including drowsiness, lethargy, fatigue, hypnosis, and coma; stimulative effects (particularly in children), including tremors, anxiety, insomnia, excitement, hallucinations, delirium, toxic psychosis, and convulsions; vertigo, ataxia, tinnitus, blurred vision; *cardiovascular:* tachycardia, hypotension, cardiovascular collapse; *other:* hyperpyrexia (in children), respiratory arrest
Treatment	Maintain pulmonary function; if necessary, provide mechanically assisted ventilation, and administer oxygen. For control of seizures, a short-acting depressant such as thiopental is preferable, but IV diazepam may also be considered. Vasopressors may be used for hypotension, and physostigmine can be given to reverse anticholinergic effects. Do not administer analeptic drugs. To remove the drug from the GI tract, induce emesis or, if vomiting is not possible, perform gastric lavage; saline cathartics can also be used.

DRUG INTERACTIONS

Alcohol, tranquilizers, sedative-hypnotics, and other CNS depressants	⬆ CNS depression
MAO inhibitors	⬆ Anticholinergic effects

ALTERED LABORATORY VALUES

No clinically significant alterations in blood/serum or urinary values occur at therapeutic dosages

---

USE IN CHILDREN

See INDICATIONS and dosage recommendations; contraindicated for use in full-term or premature neonates. Use of the elixir in children 2–6 yr of age and the sustained-release tablets in children 6–12 yr of age should be determined by medical judgment. Antihistamines may produce excitation in young children.

USE IN PREGNANT AND NURSING WOMEN

Pregnancy Category B: reproduction studies in rats and mice given up to 16 times the maximum human dose have shown no evidence of impaired fertility or harm to the fetus; however, no adequate, well-controlled studies have been performed in pregnant women. Use during pregnancy only if clearly needed. It is not known whether this drug is excreted in human milk; use with caution in nursing mothers.

---

[1] Contains 3% alcohol

ANTIHISTAMINES/ANTIPRURITICS

OPTIMINE (azatadine maleate) Schering   Rx
Tablets: 1 mg

INDICATIONS	**ORAL DOSAGE**	
Seasonal and perennial **allergic rhinitis** Chronic urticaria	Adult: 1–2 mg bid	
CONTRAINDICATIONS		
Lower respiratory tract conditions, including asthma	MAO inhibitor therapy (see DRUG INTERACTIONS)	Hypersensitivity to azatadine or structurally related antihistamines

WARNINGS/PRECAUTIONS

Drowsiness	Caution patients that they should not drive or engage in other activities requiring mental alertness only until their response to azatadine has been determined; also warn patients about using alcohol or other CNS depressants in combination with azatadine (see DRUG INTERACTIONS)
MAO inhibitors, oral anticoagulants	Caution patients that they should not use azatadine if they are taking an MAO inhibitor or an oral anticoagulant (see DRUG INTERACTIONS)
Elderly patients	Dizziness, sedation, and hypotension occur more frequently in patients over 60 yr of age
Special-risk patients	Use with caution in patients with narrow-angle glaucoma, stenosing peptic ulcer, pyloroduodenal obstruction, urinary bladder obstruction owing to symptomatic prostatic hypertrophy and narrowing of the bladder neck, increased intraocular pressure, hyperthyroidism, cardiovascular disease, hypertension, or a history of bronchial asthma
Laboratory testing	Use of azatadine should be discontinued approximately 4 days before performing skin tests (antihistamines can prevent or diminish otherwise positive reactions)
Carcinogenicity, mutagenicity	No evidence of carcinogenicity has been observed in long-term studies of rats and mice given oral doses; a dominant lethal assay study in mice given oral and intraperitoneal doses showed no mutagenic effect
Effect on fertility	No impairment of fertility occurred in rats fed more than 150 times the recommended human daily dose
Drug dependence	Abuse and dependence have not been reported

ADVERSE REACTIONS
The most frequent reactions, regardless of incidence, are printed in *italics*

Cardiovascular	Hypotension, headache, palpitations, tachycardia, extrasystoles
Hematological	Hemolytic anemia, hypoplastic anemia, thrombocytopenia, agranulocytosis
Central nervous system	*Drowsiness, sedation, sleepiness, dizziness, disturbed coordination,* fatigue, confusion, restlessness, excitation, nervousness, tremor, irritability, insomnia, euphoria, paresthesias, vertigo, tinnitus, acute labyrinthitis, hysteria, neuritis, convulsions
Ophthalmic	Blurred vision, diplopia
Gastrointestinal	*Epigastric distress,* anorexia, nausea, vomiting, diarrhea, constipation
Genitourinary	Urinary frequency, difficult urination, urinary retention, early menses
Respiratory	*Thickening of bronchial secretions,* tightness in the chest and wheezing, nasal stuffiness
Dermatological	Urticaria, drug rash, photosensitivity
Hypersensitivity	Anaphylactic shock
Other	Dry mouth, nose, and throat, chills, excessive perspiration

OVERDOSAGE

Signs and symptoms	Varies from CNS depression (drowsiness, sedation, diminished mental alertness, apnea, cardiovascular collapse) to CNS stimulation (insomnia, excitement, hallucinations, ataxia, incoordination, athetosis, tremors, convulsions) and may include dizziness, tinnitus, blurred vision, and hypotension; CNS stimulation, followed by postictal depression, and atropine-like symptoms (dry mouth; fixed, dilated pupils; fever; flushing; GI disturbances) are particularly likely in children
Treatment	If patient is conscious, induce emesis with syrup of ipecac, even though vomiting may have occurred spontaneously; the action of ipecac is facilitated by physical activity and by the ingestion of 8–12 fl oz of water. If emesis does not occur within 15 min, the dose of ipecac should be repeated. Take precautions to avoid aspiration, particularly in infants and children. If vomiting is unsuccessful or contraindicated, perform gastric lavage; isotonic saline solution should be used, particularly in children (tap water, although not preferred, can be used with adults). Remove any remaining drug in the stomach by instillation of activated charcoal. Administer a saline cathartic to rapidly dilute bowel content. Treatment is symptomatic and supportive; dialysis is of little value. If breathing is significantly impaired, maintain an adequate airway and provide mechanically assisted ventilation; *do not use analeptics.* Vasopressors (eg, norepinephrine) may be used for significant hypotension. Treat hyperpyrexia by sponging with tepid water or using a hypothermal blanket. For seizures, administer a short-acting barbiturate, diazepam, or paraldehyde.

DRUG INTERACTIONS

Alcohol, tricyclic antidepressants, tranquilizers, sedative-hypnotics, and other CNS depressants	△ CNS depression
MAO inhibitors	△ Anticholinergic and sedative effects
Oral anticoagulants	▽ Anticoagulant effect

ALTERED LABORATORY VALUES

No clinically significant alterations in blood/serum or urinary values occur at therapeutic dosages

USE IN CHILDREN

Caution patients that azatadine should not be given to children under 12 yr of age; safety and effectiveness for use in such children have not been established

USE IN PREGNANT AND NURSING WOMEN

Pregnancy Category B: use during the first two trimesters of pregnancy only if clearly needed. Reproduction studies in rats given up to 188 times the human dose and in rabbits given up to 38 times the human dose have shown no evidence of harm to the fetus; however, no adequate, well-controlled studies have been performed in pregnant women. Azatadine should not be used during the third trimester because of the risk of severe reactions, such as convulsions, in premature infants and newborns. It is not known whether azatadine is excreted in human milk; however, low concentrations of certain other antihistamines have been detected in human milk. Because of the increased risk of antihistaminic side effects in infants, particularly in premature infants and neonates, patients should not nurse while taking this drug.

ANTIHISTAMINES/ANTIPRURITICS

PBZ (tripelennamine) Geigy Rx

Tablets: 25, 50 mg tripelennamine hydrochloride **Elixir (per 5 ml):** tripelennamine citrate equivalent to 25 mg tripelennamine hydrochloride[1] (473 ml) *cinnamon flavored*

PBZ-SR (tripelennamine hydrochloride) Geigy Rx

Tablets (sustained release): 100 mg

INDICATIONS

Seasonal and perennial **allergic rhinitis**
Vasomotor rhinitis
Allergic conjunctivitis due to inhalant allergens and foods
Mild, uncomplicated **urticaria** and **angioedema**
Allergic reactions to blood or plasma
Dermatographism
Anaphylactic reactions, as an adjunct to epinephrine and other standard measures after acute symptoms have been controlled

ORAL DOSAGE

Adult: 25–50 mg q4–6h, up to 600 mg/day, or, alternatively, one 100-mg tab bid (morning and evening) or, if necessary, q8h; sustained-release tablets must be swallowed whole, not chewed or crushed
Infant and child: 5 mg/kg/24 h or 150 mg/m^2/24 h, up to 300 mg/24 h, given in 4–6 divided doses; do not use sustained-release tablets in children

CONTRAINDICATIONS

Stenosing peptic ulcer
Pyloroduodenal obstruction
Symptomatic prostatic hypertrophy
Bladder-neck obstruction

Narrow-angle glaucoma
Hypersensitivity to tripelennamine or related compounds
MAO inhibitor therapy (see DRUG INTERACTIONS)

Full-term or premature neonates
Breast-feeding
Lower respiratory tract conditions, including asthma

WARNINGS/PRECAUTIONS

Drowsiness	Caution patients about driving or engaging in other activities requiring mental alertness, and about using alcohol or other CNS depressants (see DRUG INTERACTIONS)
Elderly patients	Dizziness, sedation, and hypotension occur more frequently in patients over 60 yr of age
Special-risk patients	Use with caution in patients with increased intraocular pressure, hyperthyroidism, cardiovascular disease, hypertension, or a history of bronchial asthma

ADVERSE REACTIONS[2]

The most frequent reactions, regardless of incidence, are printed in *italics*

Cardiovascular	Hypotension, palpitations, tachycardia, extrasystoles

PBZ ■ PERIACTIN

Hematological	Leukopenia, hemolytic anemia, thrombocytopenia, agranulocytosis, aplastic anemia
Central nervous system	*Sedation, sleepiness, dizziness, disturbed coordination,* fatigue, confusion, restlessness, excitation, hysteria, nervousness, irritability, insomnia, euphoria, vertigo, tinnitus, convulsions, headache, tremor, paresthesias, acute labyrinthitis, neuritis
Ophthalmic	Blurred vision, diplopia
Gastrointestinal	*Epigastric distress,* anorexia, nausea, vomiting, diarrhea, constipation
Genitourinary	Urinary frequency, difficult urination, urinary retention, early menses
Respiratory	*Thickening of bronchial secretions,* tightness in the chest and wheezing, nasal stuffiness
Dermatological	Urticaria, rash, photosensitivity
Hypersensitivity	Anaphylactic shock
Other	*Dry mouth, nose, and throat;* chills, excessive perspiration

OVERDOSAGE

Signs and symptoms	Varies from CNS depression (drowsiness, sedation, diminished mental alertness, apnea, cardiovascular collapse) to CNS stimulation (insomnia, excitement, hallucinations, ataxia, incoordination, athetosis, tremors, convulsions) and may include dizziness, tinnitus, blurred vision, and hypotension; CNS stimulation, followed by postictal depression, and atropine-like symptoms (dry mouth; fixed, dilated pupils; fever; flushing; GI disturbances) are particularly likely in children
Treatment	If patient is conscious, induce emesis with syrup of ipecac, even though vomiting may have occurred spontaneously. If vomiting is unsuccessful or contraindicated, perform gastric lavage with isotonic or 1/2 isotonic saline solution. Remove any remaining drug in the stomach by instillation of activated charcoal. Administer a saline cathartic to rapidly dilute bowel content. Treatment is symptomatic and supportive. If breathing is significantly impaired, maintain an adequate airway and provide mechanically assisted ventilation; *do not use analeptics.* Vasopressors (eg, norepinephrine) may be used for significant hypotension. Treat hyperpyrexia by sponging with tepid water or use of ice packs or a hypothermal blanket. For seizures, administer a short-acting barbiturate, diazepam, or paraldehyde.

DRUG INTERACTIONS

Alcohol, tranquilizers, sedative-hypnotics, and other CNS depressants	⇧ CNS depression
MAO inhibitors	⇧ Anticholinergic effects

ALTERED LABORATORY VALUES

No clinically significant alterations in blood/serum or urinary values occur at therapeutic dosages

USE IN CHILDREN

See INDICATIONS and ORAL DOSAGE; contraindicated for use in full-term or premature neonates. The 100-mg tablets are not indicated for use in children. Antihistamines may produce excitation in children.

USE IN PREGNANT AND NURSING WOMEN

Use during pregnancy only if the expected therapeutic benefit outweighs the potential risks. Safety for use during pregnancy has not been established; however, limited reproduction studies in animals have not demonstrated teratogenic or other adverse effects on the fetus. Use of tripelennamine in nursing mothers is contraindicated.

[1] Contains 12% alcohol
[2] Includes reactions common to antihistamines in general

ANTIHISTAMINES/ANTIPRURITICS

PERIACTIN (cyproheptadine hydrochloride) Merck Sharp & Dohme Rx

Tablets: 4 mg **Syrup (per 5 ml):** 2 mg[1] (473 ml)

INDICATIONS

Perennial and seasonal **allergic rhinitis**
Vasomotor rhinitis
Allergic conjunctivitis due to inhalant allergens and foods
Mild, uncomplicated **urticaria** and **angioedema**
Cold urticaria
Dematographism
Allergic reactions to blood or plasma
Anaphylactic reactions, as an adjunct to epinephrine and other standard measures after acute symptoms have been controlled

ORAL DOSAGE

Adult: 4 mg tid to start; adjust dosage according to response, up to 0.5 mg/kg/day; usual dosage range: 4–20 mg/day
Child (2–6 yr): 2 mg bid or tid, or 0.25 mg/kg/day, or 8 mg/m²/day to start; adjust dosage according to response, up to 12 mg/day
Child (7–14 yr): 4 mg bid or tid, or 0.25 mg/kg/day, or 8 mg/m²/day to start; adjust dosage according to response, up to 16 mg/day

PERIACTIN

CONTRAINDICATIONS

Elderly, debilitated patients	Stenosing peptic ulcer	Hypersensitivity to cyproheptadine or structurally related compounds
Full-term or premature neonates	Pyloroduodenal obstruction	MAO inhibitor therapy (see DRUG INTERACTIONS)
Breast-feeding	Symptomatic prostatic hypertrophy	
Narrow-angle glaucoma	Bladder-neck obstruction	

WARNINGS/PRECAUTIONS

Drowsiness, disturbed coordination	Caution patients about driving or engaging in other activities requiring mental alertness and physical coordination, and about using alcohol or other CNS depressants
Elderly patients	Dizziness, sedation, and hypotension occur more frequently in patients over 60 yr of age
Special-risk patients	Use with caution in patients with increased intraocular pressure, hyperthyroidism, cardiovascular disease, hypertension, or a history of bronchial asthma
Carcinogenicity, mutagenicity	Long-term studies of carcinogenicity have not been performed; no evidence of mutagenicity has been seen in the Ames test or in cultured human lymphocytes and fibroblasts
Effect on fertility	No effect on fertility has been detected in rats or mice given approximately 10 times the human dose

ADVERSE REACTIONS[2]

Cardiovascular	Faintness, hypotension, palpitations, tachycardia, extrasystoles
Hematological	Hemolytic anemia, leukopenia, thrombocytopenia, agranulocytosis
Central nervous system	Sedation and sleepiness (often transient); dizziness, disturbed coordination, fatigue, confusion, restlessness, excitation, nervousness, tremor, irritability, insomnia, euphoria, paresthesias, vertigo, tinnitus, acute labyrinthitis, hysteria, neuritis, convulsions, hallucinations, headache
Ophthalmic	Blurred vision, diplopia
Gastrointestinal	Epigastric distress, anorexia, nausea, vomiting, diarrhea, constipation, jaundice
Genitourinary	Urinary frequency, difficult urination, urinary retention, early menses
Respiratory	Thickening of bronchial secretions, tightness in the chest and wheezing, nasal stuffiness
Dermatological	Urticaria, rash, photosensitivity
Hypersensitivity	Anaphylactic shock
Other	Dry mouth, nose, and throat; chills, excessive perspiration, edema

OVERDOSAGE

Signs and symptoms	Varies from CNS depression (drowsiness, sedation, diminished mental alertness, apnea, cardiovascular collapse) to CNS stimulation (insomnia, excitement, hallucinations, ataxia, incoordination, athetosis, tremors, convulsions) and may include dizziness, tinnitus, blurred vision, and hypotension; CNS stimulation, followed by postictal depression, and atropine-like symptoms (dry mouth; fixed, dilated pupils; fever; flushing; GI disturbances) are particularly likely in children
Treatment	If patient is conscious, induce emesis with syrup of ipecac if vomiting has not occurred spontaneously. If vomiting is contraindicated or not possible, perform gastric lavage with isotonic or 1/2 isotonic saline solution. Take measures to prevent aspiration, especially in infants and children. Remove any remaining drug in the stomach by instillation of activated charcoal. Administer a saline cathartic to rapidly dilute bowel content. Treatment is symptomatic and supportive. If breathing is significantly impaired, maintain an adequate airway and provide mechanically assisted ventilation; *do not use analeptics.* Vasopressors (eg, norepinephrine) may be used for significant hypotension. Treat hyperpyrexia by sponging with tepid water or use of ice packs or a hypothermal blanket. For seizures, administer a short-acting barbiturate, diazepam, or paraldehyde. If life-threatening CNS reactions occur, IV physostigmine may be considered.

DRUG INTERACTIONS

Alcohol, tranquilizers, sedative-hypnotics, and other CNS depressants	△ CNS depression
MAO inhibitors	△ Anticholinergic effects

ALTERED LABORATORY VALUES

No clinically significant alterations in blood/serum or urinary values occur at therapeutic dosages

USE IN CHILDREN
See INDICATIONS and ORAL DOSAGE; contraindicated for use in full-term or premature neonates. Safety and effectiveness for use in children under 2 yr of age have not been established. Antihistamines may produce excitation in young children.

USE IN PREGNANT AND NURSING WOMEN
Pregnancy Category B: reproduction studies in rabbits, mice, and rats given up to 32 times the human dose have shown no evidence of harm to the fetus; however, no adequate, well-controlled studies have been performed in pregnant women. Use during pregnancy only if clearly needed. It is not known whether cyproheptadine is excreted in human milk; because serious adverse reactions may occur if this drug is ingested by nursing infants, use in nursing mothers is contraindicated.

[1] Contains 5% alcohol
[2] Includes reactions common to antihistamines in general

ANTIHISTAMINES/ANTIPRURITICS

PHENERGAN (promethazine hydrochloride) Wyeth — Rx

Tablets: 12.5, 25, 50 mg **Syrup (per 5 ml):** 6.25 mg (Syrup Plain—4, 6, 8 fl oz; 1 pt; 1 gal) *fruit flavored,* 25 mg (Syrup Fortis—1 pt) **Rectal suppositories:** 12.5, 25, 50 mg

INDICATIONS

Seasonal and perennial **allergic rhinitis**
Vasomotor rhinitis
Allergic conjunctivitis owing to inhalant allergens and foods
Mild, uncomplicated, allergic manifestations of **urticaria and angioedema**
Allergic reactions to blood or plasma
Dermatographism
Anaphylactic reactions (adjunctive therapy)

ORAL AND RECTAL DOSAGE

Adult: for minor reactions to blood or plasma, 25 mg; for other allergic reactions, oral doses of 25 mg, given at bedtime, to start or, if necessary, oral doses of 12.5 mg, given before meals and at bedtime, to start, or, alternatively, when oral administration is not feasible, a rectal dose of 25 mg, repeated, if necessary, within 2 h after the first dose. Treat anaphylactic reactions after the acute manifestations have been controlled; use promethazine in conjunction with epinephrine and other standard measures.
Child (> 2 yr): for minor reactions to blood or plasma, 25 mg; for other allergic reactions, oral doses of 25 mg, given at bedtime, to start or, if necessary, oral doses of 6.25–12.5 mg, given tid, to start, or, alternatively, when oral administration is not feasible, a rectal dose of 25 mg, repeated, if necessary, within 2 h after the first dose. Treat anaphylactic reactions after the acute manifestations have been controlled; use promethazine in conjunction with epinephrine and other standard measures.

Motion sickness

Adult: 25 mg, given 30–60 min before departure, 8–12 h later, and then, on each subsequent day of travel, at the time of arising and before the evening meal
Child (> 2 yr): 12.5–25 mg, given 30–60 min before departure, 8–12 h later, and then, on each subsequent day of travel, at the time of arising and before the evening meal

Nausea and vomiting associated with anesthesia and surgery

Adult: for prophylaxis, 25 mg q4–6h; for treatment, 25 mg to start, followed, if necessary, by 12.5–25 mg q4–6h
Child (> 2 yr): for treatment, 0.5 mg/lb q4–6h

Sedation

Adult: for *nighttime sedation,* 25–50 mg or, before surgery, 50 mg, given in either case at bedtime; for use as a *preoperative medication,* 50 mg, given with 50 mg of meperidine and the appropriate dose of a belladonna alkaloid; for *obstetric sedation,* 25–50 mg, given alone or with a narcotic analgesic; for *postoperative pain* (adjunctive therapy), 25–50 mg, given with meperidine or another analgesic
Child (> 2 yr): for *nighttime sedation* before surgery or at other times, 12.5–25 mg, given at bedtime; for use as a *preoperative medication,* an oral dose of 0.5 mg/lb or a rectal dose of either 25 mg (for children under 3 yr of age) or 50 mg (for children over 3 yr of age), given with an equal dose of meperidine and the appropriate dose of an atropine-like drug; for *postoperative pain* (adjunctive therapy), 12.5–25 mg, given with meperidine or another analgesic

CONTRAINDICATIONS

Asthma or other lower respiratory tract conditions

Hypersensitivity or idiosyncratic reaction to promethazine or other phenothiazines

WARNINGS/PRECAUTIONS

Drowsiness, dizziness — Caution patients that they may drive or engage in other potentially hazardous activities requiring mental alertness or physical coordination only after it has been established that this preparation does not make them drowsy or dizzy (see also USE IN CHILDREN)

Photosensitivity, extrapyramidal reactions — Photosensitivity and extrapyramidal reactions such as oculogyric crisis, torticollis, and tongue protrusion have occurred in rare instances; the extrapyramidal reactions have usually resulted from excessive dosage. Instruct patients to report any involuntary muscle movements or unusual sensitivity to sunlight.

PHENERGAN ■ PHENERGAN Injection

Patients with a history of sleep apnea	Avoid use in patients with a history of sleep apnea
Patients with GI or GU conditions	Use with caution in patients with hepatic impairment, stenosing peptic ulcer, pyloroduodenal obstruction, symptomatic prostatic hypertrophy, or bladder neck obstruction
Other special-risk patients	Use with caution in patients with convulsive disorders, cardiovascular disease, or narrow angle glaucoma
Carcinogenicity, mutagenicity, effect on fertility	No long-term studies have been performed in animals to evaluate the carcinogenic potential of promethazine. Use in the Ames test has produced no evidence of mutagenicity. The effect of promethazine on fertility has not been assessed.

ADVERSE REACTIONS

Central nervous system	Sedation, sleepiness, blurred vision, dizziness, disorientation, confusion, and extrapyramidal reactions (rare)
Cardiovascular	Hypertension, hypotension
Gastrointestinal	Nausea, vomiting, cholestatic jaundice
Hematological	Leukopenia and thrombocytopenia (rare), agranulocytosis (one case)
Dermatological	Rash; photosensitivity (rare)
Other	Dry mouth

OVERDOSAGE

Signs and symptoms	*CNS:* extreme somnolence, stupor, coma, hyperexcitability, nightmares, convulsions (CNS stimulation is especially likely to occur in children and the elderly); *respiratory:* decrease in respiratory rate and/or tidal volume; *cardiovascular:* flushing, hypotension; *other:* mydriasis, dry mouth, GI reactions
Treatment	To maintain pulmonary function, establish a patent airway, and provide assisted or controlled ventilation. Correct acidosis and electrolyte losses. To treat severe hypotension, use norepinephrine or phenylephrine, not epinephrine. Diazepam may be given to control convulsions. Do not give analeptic drugs for CNS depression. Monitor vital signs only in cases of extreme overdosage or individual sensitivity. To remove this preparation from the body, administer activated charcoal or use sodium or magnesium sulfate as a cathartic; limited experience indicates that dialysis is not helpful.

DRUG INTERACTIONS

Alcohol, narcotic drugs, sedative-hypnotics (eg, barbiturates), tranquilizers, local anesthetics, and other CNS depressants	⌂ CNS depression; instruct patients requiring this preparation that other CNS depressants should be avoided or used at a lower dosage (for concomitant use with this preparation, reduce the dosage of a narcotic analgesic by 25–50% and the dosage of a barbiturate by at least 50% ⌂ Risk of convulsions (with concomitant use of narcotic drugs or local anesthetics)

ALTERED LABORATORY VALUES

Blood/serum values	⌂ Glucose
Urinary values	False-positive and false-negative pregnancy test

---

USE IN CHILDREN

See INDICATIONS and ORAL DOSAGE; do not give to children under 2 yr of age because safety for use in such patients has not been established. Children undergoing treatment should be supervised whenever they ride a bicycle or engage in other potentially hazardous activities requiring mental alertness or physical coordination.

USE IN PREGNANT AND NURSING WOMEN

Pregnancy Category C: promethazine has been shown to be fetotoxic in rodents; no evidence of teratogenicity has been observed in rats fed 6.25 or 12.5 mg/kg/day. Inhibition of platelet aggregation may occur in a neonate if this preparation is taken within 2 wk before delivery. This medication should be used during pregnancy only if the expected benefit justifies the potential risk to the fetus or neonate. It is not known whether promethazine is excreted in human milk; use with caution in nursing mothers.

VEHICLE/BASE
Suppository: ascorbyl palmitate, silicon dioxide, white wax, and cocoa butter
Syrup Fortis: 1.5% alcohol
Syrup Plain: 7% alcohol

ANTIHISTAMINES/ANTIPRURITICS

PHENERGAN Injection (promethazine hydrochloride) Wyeth Rx

Ampuls: 25, 50 mg/ml (1 ml) **Cartridge-needle units:** 25, 50 mg/ml (1 ml)

INDICATIONS

Uncomplicated **immediate-type allergic reactions,** when oral therapy is impossible or contraindicated
Allergic reactions to blood or plasma
Anaphylactic reactions, as an adjunct to epinephrine and other standard measures after acute symptoms have been controlled

PARENTERAL DOSAGE

Adult: 25 mg IM (deeply) or IV, repeated within 2 h, if needed
Child: up to 12.5 mg IM (deeply) or IV, repeated within 2 h, if needed

PHENERGAN Injection

Motion sickness **Nausea and vomiting** associated with anesthesia and surgery	**Adult:** 12.5–25 mg IM (deeply) or IV, repeated not more often than q4h, as needed **Child:** up to 6.25–12.5 mg IM (deeply) or IV, repeated not more often than q4h, as needed (see warning concerning pediatric use)
Nighttime sedation in hospitalized patients	**Adult:** 25–50 mg IM (deeply) or IV **Child:** up to 12.5–25 mg IM (deeply) or IV
As an adjunct to **preoperative or postoperative medication**	**Adult:** 25–50 mg IM (deeply) or IV; reduce dosage of analgesics, hypnotics, and atropine-like drugs accordingly **Child:** 0.5 mg/lb IM (deeply) or IV, with an equal dose of a narcotic analgesic or barbiturate and the appropriate amount of atropine-like drug
As an adjunct to **analgesia and anesthesia** in special surgical situations, including repeated bronchoscopy, ophthalmic surgery, and poor-risk patients	**Adult:** 25–50 mg IV; reduce dosage of narcotic analgesics accordingly **Child:** up to 12.5–25 mg IV; reduce dosage of narcotic analgesics accordingly
Obstetric sedation	**Adult:** for sedation and relief of apprehension in early stages of labor, 50 mg IM (deeply) or IV; when labor is definitely established, 25–75 mg IM (deeply) or IV, repeated once or twice q4h up to 100 mg/24 h; reduce dosage of narcotic analgesics accordingly

CONTRAINDICATIONS

Hypersensitivity or idiosyncratic reaction to promethazine	Drug-induced CNS depression Comatose states	Intraarterial or SC injection (see ADMINISTRATION/DOSAGE ADJUSTMENTS)

ADMINISTRATION/DOSAGE ADJUSTMENTS

Route of administration	Preferred route is by deep IM injection. Extreme care should be taken when using IV route that intraarterial injection or perivascular extravasation does not occur (see WARNINGS/PRECAUTIONS); IV concentration should not exceed 25 mg/ml, nor rate of administration exceed 25 mg/min. The SC route is contraindicated; necrotic lesions (on rare occasions) and chemical irritation have occurred after SC injection.
Elderly patients	Reduce dosage in patients over 60 yr of age
Concomitant therapy	Reduce the usual dose of barbiturates by at least one half and of narcotic analgesics by one fourth to one half

WARNINGS/PRECAUTIONS

Inadvertent intraarterial injection, perivascular extravasation	Pain, severe chemical irritation, severe spasm of distal vessels, and resultant gangrene requiring amputation may occur. Although there is no proven successful management, sympathetic block and heparinization are commonly used. Aspiration of dark blood does not preclude intraarterial needle placement, since blood is discolored upon contact with promethazine.
Drowsiness, disturbed coordination	Caution ambulatory patients about driving or engaging in other potentially hazardous activities requiring mental alertness and/or physical coordination, and about using alcohol or other CNS depressants (see DRUG INTERACTIONS)
Infants and children	Not recommended for treatment of uncomplicated vomiting; use only for prolonged vomiting of known etiology. Extrapyramidal symptoms secondary to use of promethazine may be confused with CNS signs of undiagnosed primary disease; avoid use when signs and symptoms suggest the presence of Reye's syndrome or other hepatic diseases. Excessively large doses may cause hallucinations, convulsions, and sudden death. Paradoxical hyperexcitability and abnormal movements may occur following a single dose, which may indicate relative overdosage; discontinue drug. Acutely ill, dehydrated children may be susceptible to dystonias.
Patients with pain	Excessive amounts of promethazine relative to narcotic analgesic dose may cause restlessness and motor hyperactivity
Patients with bone-marrow depression	Use with caution; leukopenia and agranulocytosis have been reported, usually when promethazine has been used with other known toxic agents
Special-risk patients	Use with caution in patients with cardiovascular disease, impaired liver function, asthmatic attacks, narrow-angle glaucoma, stenosing peptic ulcer, pyroloduodenal obstruction, prostatic hypertrophy, or bladder-neck obstruction
Diagnostic interference	Antiemetic effects may mask signs and symptoms of unrecognized disease

ADVERSE REACTIONS

Central nervous system	Drowsiness, extrapyramidal effects, dizziness, lassitude, tinnitus, incoordination, fatigue, euphoria, nervousness, insomnia, tremors, convulsive seizures, oculogyric crises, excitation, catatonic-like states, hysteria
Ophthalmic	Blurred vision, diplopia
Cardiovascular	Tachycardia, bradycardia, faintness, dizziness, hypotension or hypertension, venous thrombosis at injection site
Gastrointestinal	Nausea, vomiting, dry mouth, obstructive jaundice
Hypersensitivity	Urticaria, dermatitis, asthma, photosensitivity, angioneurotic edema
Hematological	Leukopenia, agranulocytosis, thrombocytopenic purpura

PHENERGAN Injection ■ POLARAMINE

| Other | Nasal stuffiness; tissue necrosis following SC injection |

OVERDOSAGE

Signs and symptoms	Range from mild CNS and cardiovascular depression to profound hypotension, respiratory depression, and unconsciousness. Stimulation may be present, especially in children and in geriatric patients. Atropine-like signs and symptoms (eg, dry mouth; fixed, dilated pupils; flushing) and GI disturbances may occur
Treatment	Generally supportive and symptomatic; *do not use stimulants* for CNS depression. Treat severe hypotension with norepinephrine or phenylephrine; *do not use epinephrine*. Treat extrapyramidal reactions with anticholinergic antiparkinsonism agents, diphenhydramine, or barbiturates. Additional measures include administration of oxygen and IV fluids. Dialysis does not seem to be helpful.

DRUG INTERACTIONS

Alcohol, tranquilizers, sedative-hypnotics (including barbiturates), general anesthetics, narcotic preparations, and other CNS depressants	⇧ CNS depression
MAO inhibitors	⇧ Risk of extrapyramidal side effects[1]

ALTERED LABORATORY VALUES

Blood/serum values	⇧ Glucose tolerance
Urinary values	False-negative and false-positive pregnancy tests

USE IN CHILDREN

See INDICATIONS, dosage recommendations, and WARNINGS/PRECAUTIONS

USE IN PREGNANT AND NURSING WOMEN

Pregnancy Category C: use during pregnancy only if the expected therapeutic benefit justifies the potential risk to the fetus. Reproduction studies have been done in animals (consult manufacturer for information); however, no adequate, well-controlled studies have been performed in pregnant women. It is not known whether this drug is excreted in human milk.

[1] Although such a reaction has not been reported with promethazine, it has occurred when other phenothiazines and some MAO inhibitors have been used concomitantly

---

ANTIHISTAMINES/ANTIPRURITICS

POLARAMINE (dexchlorpheniramine maleate) Schering   Rx

Tablets: 2 mg   **Tablets (sustained release):** 4, 6 mg   **Syrup (per 5 ml):** 2 mg[1] (473 ml) *orange-flavored*

INDICATIONS	ORAL DOSAGE
Seasonal and perennial **allergic rhinitis** **Vasomotor rhinitis** **Allergic conjunctivitis** Mild, uncomplicated **urticaria** and **angioedema** **Dermatographism** **Allergic reactions to blood or plasma** **Anaphylactic reactions,** as an adjunct to epinephrine and other standard measures after acute symptoms have been controlled	**Adult:** 2 mg or 5 ml (1 tsp) q4–6h; if sustained-release tablets are used, 4 or 6 mg at bedtime or q8–10h during the day **Child (2–5 yr):** 0.5 mg or 1.25 ml (¼ tsp) q4–6h **Child (6–12 yr):** 1 mg or 2.5 ml (½ tsp) q4–6h; if sustained-release tablets are used, 4 mg/day, preferably at bedtime

CONTRAINDICATIONS

| Full-term or premature neonates
Lower respiratory tract conditions | Hypersensitivity to dexchlorpheniramine or structurally related antihistamines | MAO inhibitor therapy (see DRUG INTERACTIONS) |

WARNINGS/PRECAUTIONS

Drowsiness	Caution patients not to drive or engage in other activities requiring mental alertness, and that the use of alcohol or other CNS depressants (see DRUG INTERACTIONS) may enhance antihistamine-induced drowsiness
Elderly patients	Dizziness, sedation, and hypotension occur more frequently in patients over 60 yr of age
Special-risk patients	Use with caution in patients with narrow-angle glaucoma, stenosing peptic ulcer, pyroduodenal obstruction, symptomatic prostatic hypertrophy, bladder-neck obstruction, increased intraocular pressure, hyperthyroidism, cardiovascular disease, hypertension, or a history of bronchial asthma

POLARAMINE ■ SELDANE

Carcinogenicity, mutagenicity	Although there have been no oncogenic or mutagenic studies of dexchlorpheniramine, a 103-wk study in rats given chlorpheniramine (the racemic mixture) showed no increase in tumor incidence; results of an Ames mutagenicity test of chlorpheniramine and its nitrosation products were also negative

ADVERSE REACTIONS[2]

The most frequent reactions, regardless of incidence, are printed in *italics*

Cardiovascular	Headache, palpitations, tachycardia, extrasystoles, hypotension
Hematological	Hemolytic or hypoplastic anemia, thrombocytopenia, agranulocytosis
Central nervous system	*Drowsiness (slight to moderate)*, sedation, dizziness, disturbed coordination, fatigue, confusion, restlessness, excitation, nervousness, tremor, irritability, insomnia, euphoria, paresthesias, vertigo, tinnitus, acute labyrinthitis, hysteria, neuritis, convulsions
Ophthalmic	Blurred vision
Gastrointestinal	Epigastric distress, anorexia, nausea, vomiting, diarrhea, constipation
Genitourinary	Urinary frequency, difficult urination, urinary retention, early menses
Respiratory	Thickening of bronchial secretions, tightness in the chest and wheezing, nasal stuffiness
Dermatological and hypersensitivity	Urticaria, rash, photosensitivity, anaphylactic shock
Other	Excessive perspiration, chills; dry mouth, nose, and throat

OVERDOSAGE

Signs and symptoms	Varies from CNS depression (drowsiness, sedation, diminished mental alertness, apnea, cardiovascular collapse) to CNS stimulation (insomnia, hallucinations, tremors, convulsions) and may include dizziness, tinnitus, ataxia, blurred vision, and hypotension. CNS stimulation and atropine-like signs and symptoms (dry mouth; fixed, dilated pupils; hyperthermia; flushing; GI disturbances) are particularly likely in children.
Treatment	If patient is conscious, induce emesis with syrup of ipecac, even though vomiting may have occurred spontaneously. If emesis does not occur within 15 min, repeat the dose of ipecac. If vomiting is unsuccessful or contraindicated, perform gastric lavage with isotonic or 1/2 isotonic saline solution. Remove any remaining drug in the stomach by instillation of activated charcoal. Administer a saline cathartic to rapidly dilute bowel content. Dialysis is of little value. Treatment is symptomatic and supportive. If breathing is significantly impaired, maintain an adequate airway and provide mechanically assisted ventilation; *do not use analeptics.* Vasopressors (eg, norepinephrine) may be used for hypotension. Treat hyperpyrexia by sponging with tepid water or use of a hypothermal blanket. For seizures, administer a short-acting barbiturate, diazepam, or paraldehyde.

DRUG INTERACTIONS

Alcohol, tranquilizers, sedative-hypnotics, and other CNS depressants	⇧ CNS depression
MAO inhibitors	Risk of severe hypotension
Oral anticoagulants	⇩ Anticoagulant effect

ALTERED LABORATORY VALUES

No clinically significant alterations in blood/serum or urinary values occur at therapeutic dosages

---

USE IN CHILDREN

See INDICATIONS and ORAL DOSAGE; contraindicated for use in full-term or premature neonates, due to possible severe reactions (including convulsions). Overdosage may cause hallucinations, convulsions, or death. Safety and efficacy have not been established for use of the syrup or the immediate-release tablet in children under 2 yr of age; the 4-mg sustained-release tablet in children under 6 yr of age; or the 6-mg sustained-release tablet in children under 12 yr of age.

USE IN PREGNANT AND NURSING WOMEN

Pregnancy Category B: use during the first two trimesters of pregnancy only if clearly needed. This drug should not be used during the third trimester, due to the risk of severe reactions in premature and full-term infants. Studies in rabbits and rats (at doses up to 50 and 85 times the human dose, respectively) have shown no evidence of fetal harm or reduction in fertility due to chlorpheniramine maleate, the racemic mixture; however, studies in rats have found a decrease in the postnatal survival rate of pups of animals given 33 and 67 times the human dose. No adequate, well-controlled studies have been done in pregnant women. Since dexchlorpheniramine is contraindicated in newborns and it is not known whether it is excreted in human milk, it should be used with caution in nursing mothers.

---

[1] Contains 6% alcohol
[2] Includes reactions common to antihistamines in general

ANTIHISTAMINES/ANTIPRURITICS

SELDANE (terfenadine) Merrell Dow   Rx

Tablets: 60 mg

INDICATIONS	ORAL DOSAGE
Sneezing, rhinorrhea, pruritus, lacrimation and other symptoms of seasonal allergic rhinitis	Adult: 60 mg bid Child ($\geq$ 12 yr): same as adult

COMPENDIUM OF DRUG THERAPY

SELDANE ■ TAVIST

CONTRAINDICATIONS
Hypersensitivity to any component

WARNINGS/PRECAUTIONS

Special-risk patients	In considering use of this drug for patients with asthma or other lower respiratory tract diseases, bear in mind that anticholinergic (drying) reactions may occur; administration to pregnant or nursing women may adversely affect fetal growth and development (see discussion, below)
Carcinogenicity, mutagenicity, effect on fertility	No evidence of tumorigenicity has been seen in rats and mice following long-term oral administration of 63 times the human daily dose. Microbial and micronucleus test assays have shown no signs of mutagenicity. No effect on fertility has been demonstrated in rats given up to 21 times the human daily dose.

ADVERSE REACTIONS[1]

Frequent reactions (incidence $\geq$ 1%) are printed in *italics*

Central nervous system	*Drowsiness (9%), headache (6.3%), fatigue (2.9%), dizziness (1.4%)*, nervousness, weakness, increase in appetite, depression, insomnia, musculoskeletal pain, nightmares, tremor, paresthesias
Gastrointestinal	*Gastrointestinal distress, characterized by nausea, vomiting, abdominal distress, or a change in bowel habits (4.6%)*
Respiratory	*Dry mouth/nose/throat (2.3%)*, cough, sore throat, bronchospasm
Dermatological	*Eruption or itching (1%)*, alopecia, angioedema
Cardiovascular	Palpitations, tachycardia
Other	Anaphylaxis, galactorrhea, menstrual disorders (including dysmenorrhea), sweating, urinary frequency, visual disturbances

OVERDOSAGE

Signs and symptoms	See ADVERSE REACTIONS (in the only reported case of acute overdosage, blood pressure decreased from 110/90 to 90/50 mm Hg)
Treatment	Induce emesis; if vomiting is contraindicated or cannot be induced (eg, when patient is unconscious), perform gastric lavage with normal saline. After emesis or lavage, administer activated charcoal. Saline cathartics may also be helpful. It is not known whether terfenadine can be removed from the blood by dialysis.

DRUG INTERACTIONS
No clinically significant drug interactions have been identified

ALTERED LABORATORY VALUES
No clinically significant alterations in blood/serum or urinary values occur at therapeutic dosages[1]

USE IN CHILDREN
Safety and effectiveness for use in children under 12 yr of age have not been established

USE IN PREGNANT AND NURSING WOMEN
Pregnancy Category C: reproduction studies in rats given 63 and 125 times the human daily dose have shown decreases in the number of implants, pup weight gain, and pup survival; an increase in postimplantation loss, caused by maternal toxicity, has also occurred at the higher dose. Use during pregnancy only if the expected benefit justifies the potential risk to the fetus. Studies limited to the period of lactation have not been done in animals; however, because the decreases in weight gain and survival that were seen in rats resulted from administration throughout pregnancy and lactation, this drug should not be used by nursing mothers.

VEHICLE/BASE
Tablets: corn starch, gelatin, lactose, magnesium stearate, and sodium bicarbonate

[1] Jaundice, hepatitis (including cholestatic hepatitis), and increases in SGOT and SGPT levels have been reported; however, a causal relationship has not been established

---

ANTIHISTAMINES/ANTIPRURITICS

TAVIST (clemastine fumarate) Sandoz Pharmaceuticals Rx
Tablets: 2 mg clemastine[1]

INDICATIONS	ORAL DOSAGE
Allergic rhinitis Mild, uncomplicated **urticaria and angioedema**	**Adult:** 2 mg 1–3 times/day, as needed

TAVIST Syrup (clemastine fumarate) Sandoz Pharmaceuticals Rx

Syrup (per 5 ml): 0.5 mg clemastine[2] (4 fl oz) *citrus flavored*

INDICATIONS	ORAL DOSAGE
Allergic rhinitis	**Adult:** 10 ml (2 tsp) bid to start; maximum dosage: 60 ml (12 tsp)/day **Child (6–12 yr):** 5 ml (1 tsp) bid to start; maximum dosage: 30 ml (6 tsp)/day **Child ($\geq$ 12 yr):** same as adult
Mild, uncomplicated **urticaria and angio-edema**	**Adult:** 20 ml (4 tsp) bid to start; maximum dosage: 60 ml (12 tsp)/day **Child (6–12 yr):** 10 ml (2 tsp) bid to start; maximum dosage: 30 ml (6 tsp)/day **Child ($\geq$ 12 yr):** same as adult

TAVIST-1 (clemastine fumarate) Sandoz Pharmaceuticals Rx

Tablets: 1 mg clemastine[1]

INDICATIONS	ORAL DOSAGE	
Allergic rhinitis	**Adult:** 1 mg bid to start; maximum dosage: 6 mg/day	

CONTRAINDICATIONS

Breast-feeding	Hypersensitivity to clemastine or structurally related antihistamines	MAO inhibitors (see DRUG INTERACTIONS)
Premature or full-term neonates		

WARNINGS/PRECAUTIONS

Drowsiness	Caution patients not to drive or engage in any other potentially hazardous activity requiring mental alertness until after they have assessed the effects of this drug
Elderly patients	Dizziness, sedation, and hypotension occur more frequently in patients 60 yr of age or older
Other special-risk patients	Use with considerable caution in patients with narrow angle glaucoma, stenosing peptic ulcer, pyloroduodenal obstruction, symptomatic prostatic hypertrophy, or bladder neck obstruction and with caution in patients with increased intraocular pressure, hyperthyroidism, cardiovascular disease (including hypertension), or a history of bronchial asthma
Carcinogenicity, mutagenicity	No evidence of carcinogenicity has been seen in a 2-yr study in which rats were fed approximately 500 times the adult human dose and mice were fed about 1,300 times this dose; no mutagenicity tests have been done
Impairment of fertility	Clemastine produced a decrease in the mating ability of male rats at 312 times the adult human dose, but not at 156 times this dose

ADVERSE REACTIONS

The most frequent reactions, regardless of incidence, are printed in *italics*

Central nervous system	*Sedation, sleepiness, dizziness, disturbed coordination,* fatigue, confusion, restlessness, excitation, nervousness, tremor, irritability, insomnia, euphoria, paresthesias, vertigo, hysteria, neuritis, convulsions
Ophthalmic	Blurred vision, diplopia
Otic	Tinnitus, acute labyrinthitis
Gastrointestinal	*Epigastric distress,* anorexia, nausea, vomiting, diarrhea, constipation
Respiratory	*Thickening of bronchial secretions,* tightness in the chest and wheezing, nasal congestion
Cardiovascular	Hypotension, headache, palpitations, tachycardia, extrasystoles
Hematological	Hemolytic anemia, thrombocytopenia, agranulocytosis
Genitourinary	Urinary frequency, difficult urination, urinary retention, early menses
Dermatological	Urticaria, drug rash, photosensitivity
Other	Anaphylactic shock, chills, excessive perspiration; dry mouth, nose, and throat

OVERDOSAGE

Signs and symptoms	CNS depression ranging from drowsiness to coma, CNS stimulation, hypotension, cardiovascular collapse, anticholinergic reactions (dry mouth, mydriasis, flushing, fever); toxic effects are seen within 30–120 min after ingestion. In children, excitement, hallucinations, cyanosis, anticholinergic effects, ataxia, incoordination, muscle twitching, athetosis, tremors, hyperreflexia, and tonic-clonic convulsions may occur initially (convulsions can also occur after mild depression); reactions may be followed by postictal depression and cardiorespiratory arrest.
Treatment	If patient is conscious, induce vomiting even though it may have occurred spontaneously. If emesis is not possible, perform gastric lavage. Take appropriate precautions against aspiration, especially in children. The airway should be secured with a cuffed endotracheal tube before lavage if the patient is unconscious. After emptying stomach, instill a charcoal slurry or another suitable agent; a saline cathartic such as milk of magnesia may also be helpful. If breathing is significantly impaired, establish an adequate airway and provide mechanically assisted ventilation. Treat hypotension vigorously; a vasopressor may be necessary. To control convulsions, carefully administer IV diazepam or a short-acting barbiturate, as needed; physostigmine may also be considered if convulsions are centrally mediated. Treat fever with ice packs and cooling sponge baths, not with alcohol. Do not use CNS stimulants.

DRUG INTERACTIONS

Alcohol, barbiturates, tranquilizers, and other CNS depressants	◊ CNS depression; caution patients not to use alcohol or other CNS depressants in combination with clemastine
MAO inhibitors	◊ Anticholinergic effects

ALTERED LABORATORY VALUES

No clinically significant alterations in blood/serum or urinary values occur at therapeutic dosages

USE IN CHILDREN	USE IN PREGNANT AND NURSING WOMEN
See INDICATIONS and ORAL DOSAGE	Pregnancy Category B: reproduction studies in rats given up to 312 times the adult human dose and in rabbits given up to 188 times the adult human dose have shown no evidence of teratogenicity; use during pregnancy only if clearly needed. Although it is not known whether clemastine is excreted in human milk, other antihistamines have been detected in human milk; because of the potential for adverse reactions in infants, use of clemastine in nursing mothers is contraindicated.

[1] As the fumarate salt
[2] As the fumarate salt; the syrup also contains 5.5% alcohol

---

ANTIHISTAMINES/ANTIPRURITICS

TELDRIN (chlorpheniramine maleate) SmithKline Consumer Products   OTC

Tablets: 4 mg   **Capsules (sustained release):** 12 mg (Maximum Strength)

INDICATIONS

Allergic rhinitis and other **upper respiratory tract allergies**

ORAL DOSAGE

Adult: 4 mg q4–6h, up to 24 mg/24 h; if sustained-release capsules are used, 12 mg bid (morning and evening)
Child (> 12 yr): same as adult

CONTRAINDICATIONS

Consult manufacturer

WARNINGS/PRECAUTIONS

Drowsiness	Caution patients not to drive or engage in other activities requiring mental alertness, and to avoid using alcohol or other CNS depressants (see DRUG INTERACTIONS)
Special-risk patients	Should not be used by patients with asthma, glaucoma, or difficulty in urination due to prostatic enlargement, except under medical supervision

ADVERSE REACTIONS

Central nervous system	Drowsiness

OVERDOSAGE

Signs and symptoms	Varies from CNS depression (drowsiness, sedation, diminished mental alertness, apnea, cardiovascular collapse) to CNS stimulation (insomnia, excitement, hallucinations, ataxia, incoordination, athetosis, tremors, convulsions) and may include dizziness, tinnitus, blurred vision, and hypotension; CNS stimulation, followed by postictal depression and atropine-like symptoms (dry mouth; fixed, dilated pupils; fever; flushing; GI disturbances) are particularly likely in children
Treatment	If patient is conscious, induce emesis with syrup of ipecac, even though vomiting may have occurred spontaneously. If vomiting is unsuccessful or contraindicated, perform gastric lavage with isotonic or 1/2 isotonic saline solution. Remove any remaining drug in the stomach by instillation of activated charcoal. Administer a saline cathartic to rapidly dilute bowel content. Treatment is symptomatic and supportive. If breathing is significantly impaired, maintain an adequate airway and provide mechanically assisted ventilation; *do not use analeptics.* Vasopressors (eg, norepinephrine) may be used for significant hypotension. Treat hyperpyrexia by sponging with tepid water or use of ice packs or a hypothermal blanket. For seizures, administer a short-acting barbiturate, diazepam, or paraldehyde.

DRUG INTERACTIONS

Alcohol, tranquilizers, sedative-hypnotics, and other CNS depressants	◊ CNS depression
MAO inhibitors	◊ Anticholinergic effects

ALTERED LABORATORY VALUES

No clinically significant alterations in blood/serum or urinary values occur at therapeutic dosages

---

USE IN CHILDREN
Not recommended for use in children under 12 yr of age, except under medical supervision. May produce excitability in children.

USE IN PREGNANT AND NURSING WOMEN
No teratogenic effects have been reported. Use with caution in nursing mothers.

ANTIHISTAMINES/ANTIPRURITICS

TEMARIL (trimeprazine tartrate) Herbert   Rx

Capsules (sustained release): trimeprazine tartrate equivalent to 5 mg trimeprazine **Tablets:** trimeprazine tartrate equivalent to 2.5 mg trimeprazine **Syrup (per 5 ml):** trimeprazine tartrate equivalent to 2.5 mg trimeprazine[1] (4 fl oz)

INDICATIONS

Pruritus associated with urticaria
Pruritus associated with other allergic and nonallergic conditions, including atopic dermatitis, neurodermatitis, contact dermatitis, pityriasis rosea, poison ivy dermatitis, eczematous dermatitis, pruritus ani and vulvae, and drug rash

ORAL DOSAGE

Adult: 2.5 mg or 5 ml (1 tsp) qid; if sustained-release capsules are used, 5 mg q12h
Child (6 mo to 3 yr): 2.5 ml (1/2 tsp) at bedtime or, if necessary, tid
Child (3–6 yr): 2.5 mg or 5 ml (1 tsp) at bedtime or, if necessary, tid
Child (> 6 yr): 2.5 mg or 5 ml (1 tsp) at bedtime or, if necessary, tid; if sustained-release capsules are used, 5 mg/day

CONTRAINDICATIONS

Breast-feeding	Hypersensitivity or idiosyncratic reaction to trimeprazine or other phenothiazines	Bone marrow depression
Full-term or premature neonates		Drug-induced CNS depression
Acutely ill or dehydrated children	Comatose states	

ADMINISTRATION/DOSAGE ADJUSTMENTS

Concomitant therapy	Reduce the usual dose of narcotics or barbiturates by one half to three fourths

WARNINGS/PRECAUTIONS

Drowsiness, disturbed coordination	Caution patients about driving or engaging in other potentially hazardous activities requiring mental alertness and/or physical coordination, and about using alcohol or other CNS depressants (see DRUG INTERACTIONS)
Antiemetic action	May mask signs and symptoms of overdosage of other drugs or such conditions as intestinal obstruction or brain tumor
MAO inhibitor therapy	Use with extreme caution in patients taking MAO inhibitors (see DRUG INTERACTIONS)
Patients with respiratory impairment	Use with caution in patients with acute or chronic respiratory impairment, especially children, since cough reflex may be suppressed
Elderly patients	Hypotension, syncope, toxic confusional states, extrapyramidal symptoms (especially parkinsonism), and excessive sedation occur more frequently in patients over 60 yr of age
Special-risk patients	Use with caution in patients with cardiovascular disease, hepatic impairment, or a history of ulcer disease, and with extreme caution in patients with asthmatic attacks, narrow-angle glaucoma, prostatic hypertrophy, stenosing peptic ulcer, pyloroduodenal obstruction, or bladder-neck obstruction
Myelography with metrizamide	Discontinue use of trimeprazine at least 48 h before administration of metrizamide for myelography; wait at least 24 h after performance of procedure before resuming therapy. Trimeprazine is not indicated for control of nausea and vomiting.
Patients with previously detected breast cancer	Use with caution, as chronic therapy may cause a persistent elevation of serum prolactin levels, which may be of importance in patients with prolactin-dependent breast cancers. Although endocrine disturbances have been reported, no association between chronic neuroleptic administration and mammary tumorigenesis has been demonstrated; the available evidence is considered too limited to be conclusive at this time.

TEMARIL

ADVERSE REACTIONS[2]	The most frequent reactions, regardless of incidence, are printed in *italics*
Central nervous system	*Drowsiness*, extrapyramidal reactions (including opisthotonos, dystonia, akathisia, dyskinesia, and parkinsonism), dizziness, headache, lassitude, tinnitus, incoordination, fatigue, euphoria, nervousness, insomnia, tremors, grand mal seizures, excitation, catatonic-like states, neuritis, hysteria, disturbing dreams/nightmares, pseudoschizophrenia
Cardiovascular	*Postural hypotension*, reflex tachycardia, bradycardia, syncope, cardiac arrest, ECG changes (including blunting of T waves and prolongation of Q-T interval)
Gastrointestinal	Anorexia, nausea, vomiting, epigastric distress, diarrhea, constipation, dry mouth
Endocrinological	Early menses, induced lactation, gynecomastia, decreased libido
Genitourinary	Urinary frequency, urinary retention, dysuria, inhibition of ejaculation
Respiratory	Thickening of bronchial secretions, tightness in the chest, wheezing, nasal stuffiness
Allergic	Urticaria, dermatitis, asthma, laryngeal edema, angioneurotic edema, photosensitivity, lupus erythematosus-like syndrome, anaphylactoid reactions
Hematological	Leukopenia, agranulocytosis, pancytopenia, hemolytic anemia, thrombocytopenic purpura
Dermatological	Erythema; pigmentation of skin, especially exposed skin (with prolonged high-dose therapy)
Ophthalmic	Diplopia; blurred vision; oculogyric crises; lenticular and corneal opacities, epithelial keratopathies, pigmentary retinopathy, and impaired vision (with prolonged high-dose therapy)
Other	Obstructive jaundice, increased appetite, weight gain, peripheral edema, stomatitis, high or prolonged glucose tolerance curves, elevated spinal-fluid proteins; neuroleptic malignant syndrome, a potentially fatal reaction characterized by hyperthermia, altered consciousness, muscular rigidity, and autonomic dysfunction (rare)
OVERDOSAGE	
Signs and symptoms	CNS depression, cardiovascular depression, severe hypotension, respiratory depression, unconsciousness; dry mouth, fixed dilated pupils, flushing, GI disturbances; stimulation, especially in children (eg, hallucinations, convulsions, sudden death) and the elderly
Treatment	Early gastric lavage may be useful; *do not induce emesis*. Treat extrapyramidal symptoms with antiparkinsonism drugs, barbiturates, or diphenhydramine. Avoid analeptics. Severe hypotension may be treated with norepinephrine or phenylephrine; do not administer epinephrine. Institute additional symptomatic and supportive measures, including the use of oxygen and IV fluids, as indicated. Saline cathartics are useful for hastening evacuation of sustained-release pellets.
DRUG INTERACTIONS	
Narcotics	△ CNS depression and analgesia Restlessness and motor hyperactivity with excessive amounts of trimeprazine
Alcohol, barbiturates, anesthetics, and other CNS depressants	△ CNS depression
Epinephrine	▽ Vasopressor effect Hypotension
Atropine, thiazide diuretics	△ Anticholinergic effects
MAO inhibitors	△ Anticholinergic effects Hypertension, extrapyramidal reactions
Oral contraceptives, progesterone, reserpine, nylidrin hydrochloride	△ Phenothiazine activity
ALTERED LABORATORY VALUES	
Blood/serum values	△ Cholesterol △ Serum prolactin
Urinary values	△ Glucose False-positive tests for bilirubin and pregnancy

USE IN CHILDREN

See INDICATIONS and ORAL DOSAGE; contraindicated for use in full-term or premature neonates, as well as acutely ill or dehydrated children, due to increased susceptibility to dystonias. Use with caution in children with a history of sleep apnea or a family history of sudden infant death syndrome; use with caution in young children, since this drug may cause excitation. Sustained-release capsules are not recommended for use in children under 6 yr of age.

USE IN PREGNANT AND NURSING WOMEN

Trimeprazine should not be used in women of childbearing potential; safety for use during pregnancy has not been established. It is not known whether this drug can adversely affect fetal development. Jaundice, hyperreflexia, and prolonged extrapyramidal symptoms have occurred in infants born to mothers who received phenothiazines during pregnancy. Contraindicated for use in nursing mothers.

[1] Contains 5.7% alcohol
[2] Includes reactions common to phenothiazines in general

ANTIHISTAMINES/ANTIPRURITICS

VISTARIL (hydroxyzine pamoate) Pfizer   Rx
Capsules: 25, 50, 100 mg   **Suspension (per 5 ml):** 25 mg

INDICATIONS

Anxiety and tension associated with psychoneurosis

Anxiety associated with organic disease (adjunctive therapy)

Pruritus due to allergic conditions, including chronic urticaria and atopic and contact dermatoses

Histamine-mediated pruritus

Preoperative sedation and following general anesthesia

ORAL DOSAGE

Adult: 50–100 mg qid
Child (< 6 yr): 50 mg/day, given in divided doses
Child (> 6 yr): 50–100 mg/day, given in divided doses

Adult: 25 mg tid or qid
Child (< 6 yr): 50 mg/day, given in divided doses
Child (> 6 yr): 50–100 mg/day, given in divided doses

Adult: 50–100 mg
Child: 0.6 mg/kg

CONTRAINDICATIONS

Early pregnancy

Hypersensitivity to hydroxyzine

ADMINISTRATION/DOSAGE ADJUSTMENTS

Long-term use (> 4 mo) — Effectiveness for prolonged use as an antianxiety agent has not been tested in systematic clinical studies; reassess need for continued therapy periodically

WARNINGS/PRECAUTIONS

Drowsiness — Caution patients not to engage in potentially hazardous activities requiring full mental alertness

Concomitant use of CNS depressants — May potentiate hydroxyzine's effect; reduce dosage of these agents accordingly and caution patients that simultaneous use of alcohol and other CNS depressants may have addictive effects

ADVERSE REACTIONS

Central nervous system — Transient drowsiness; involuntary motor activity, including tremor and convulsions

Gastrointestinal — Dry mouth

OVERDOSAGE

Signs and symptoms — Excessive sedation, hypotension, CNS depression

Treatment — Induce emesis or use gastric lavage immediately to empty stomach. Monitor respiration, pulse, and blood pressure. Employ general supportive measures, as needed. Hypotension may be combatted with IV fluids and levarterenol or metaraminol. Do not use epinephrine, since hydroxyzine counteracts its pressor action. Caffeine and sodium benzoate may be used to counteract CNS depression. Dialysis is of limited value, unless other agents such as barbiturates have been ingested concomitantly.

DRUG INTERACTIONS

Alcohol, narcotic analgesics, sedative-hypnotics, other CNS depressants, and tricyclic antidepressants — ⌂ CNS depression

ALTERED LABORATORY VALUES

Urinary values — ⌂ 17-Hydroxycorticosteroids

No clinically significant alterations in blood/serum values occur at therapeutic dosages

---

USE IN CHILDREN

See INDICATIONS and ORAL DOSAGE

USE IN PREGNANT AND NURSING WOMEN

Contraindicated during early pregnancy. Fetal abnormalities have been reported in mice, rats, and rabbits at doses well above the maximum human dose. Clinical data are inadequate to establish safety for use in pregnant women during this period. It is not known whether hydroxyzine is excreted in human milk; because many drugs are excreted in human milk, patient should stop nursing if drug is prescribed.

MAST-CELL STABILIZERS

INTAL Capsules (cromolyn sodium) Fisons   Rx
Capsules: 20 mg,[1] for inhalation only

INDICATIONS

Management of **bronchial asthma**

INHALANT DOSAGE

Adult and child (≥ 2 yr): 20 mg qid at regular intervals to start, using a Spinhaler turbo-inhaler for administration

INTAL

Prevention of **acute bronchospasm** owing to exercise, aspirin, cold dry air, environmental agents (eg, toluene diisocyanate, pollutants, animal dander), or other causes	Adult and child ($\geq$ 2 yr): 20 mg shortly before the precipitating activity or exposure to the precipitating factor, using a Spinhaler turbo-inhaler for administration

INTAL Nebulizer Solution (cromolyn sodium) Fisons   Rx

Ampuls: 20 mg (2 ml), for inhalation only

INDICATIONS	INHALANT DOSAGE
Management of **bronchial asthma**	Adult and child ($\geq$ 2 yr): 20 mg qid at regular intervals, using a power-operated nebulizer for administration
Prevention of **exercise-induced bronchospasm**	Adult and child ($\geq$ 2 yr): 20 mg within 1 h before exercise, using a power-operated nebulizer for administration

INTAL Inhaler (cromolyn sodium) Fisons   Rx

Metered-dose oral inhaler: 800 µg per inhalation (8.1, 14.2 g)

INDICATIONS	INHALANT DOSAGE
Management of **bronchial asthma**	Adult and child ($\geq$ 5 yr): 2 inhalations qid, given at regular intervals (see ADMINISTRATION/DOSAGE ADJUSTMENTS)
Prevention of **acute bronchospasm** owing to exercise, cold dry air, environmental agents (eg, toluene diisocyanate, pollutants, animal dander), or other causes	Adult and child ($\geq$ 5 yr): 2 inhalations within 10–15 min, but not more than 60 min, before exposure to precipitating factor

CONTRAINDICATIONS

Hypersensitivity to cromolyn or other components	Hypersensitivity to lactose (capsules only)

ADMINISTRATION/DOSAGE ADJUSTMENTS

Administration of nebulizer solution and capsules	The solution should be administered by a means of a power-operated nebulizer that has an adequate flow rate and a suitable face mask; a hand-operated nebulizer should not be used. To empty the contents of the capsule, several deep inhalations may be necessary; it is normal for a light dusting of powder to remain. If the patient experiences difficulty in emptying the capsule, determine whether directions for use of the Spinhaler have been carefully followed. At least once every week, the Spinhaler should be washed in warm water and then dried thoroughly.
Patients with renal or hepatic impairment	Decrease dosage in patients with renal or hepatic impairment
Starting treatment of chronic asthma	When the acute episode has been controlled, the airway has been cleared, and the patient is able to inhale adequately, cromolyn may be given; clinical effect is usually evident within 2–4 wk
Patients receiving nonsteroidal antiasthmatic agents	Maintain use of other nonsteroidal antiasthmatic agents when beginning treatment of chronic asthma with cromolyn; if a clinical response to cromolyn is seen and asthma is well-controlled, dosage of the other agents may be gradually reduced
Patients receiving corticosteroids	Maintain steroidal antiasthmatic regimen when beginning treatment with cromolyn. If symptoms improve, try to reduce the dosage of the corticosteroid. If improvement is not seen, a reduction may nonetheless be possible and an attempt to decrease the dosage may be made. To avoid exacerbation of asthma, reduce dosage of the corticosteroid slowly and monitor clinical response carefully. Prolonged corticosteroid therapy frequently causes HPA-axis suppression, which may persist even after gradual discontinuation. If a significant stress (eg, severe asthmatic attack, surgery, trauma, severe illness) occurs during concomitant therapy, consider increasing the dosage of the corticosteroid; if such a stress occurs within 1–2 yr after termination of steroid therapy, consider resuming use. A temporary increase in steroid dosage may also be necessary during concomitant therapy if respiratory function becomes impaired (eg, if severe exacerbation of asthma occurs). Exercise great care and provide continued close supervision when discontinuing cromolyn after the drug has permitted termination or a reduced dosage of the corticosteroid; severe asthma may suddenly recur and necessitate not only immediate treatment, but also reintroduction or increased dosage of the corticosteroid.
Reduction in dosage	If asthma has been controlled and other agents are required only occasionally or have been eliminated, the frequency of administration may be reduced from qid to tid or bid. To avoid exacerbation of asthma, reduce dosage gradually. If asthmatic condition deteriorates in a patient receiving less than 4 doses/day, an increase in dosage and introduction or more frequent use of symptomatic medications may be necessary.

WARNINGS/PRECAUTIONS

Status asthmaticus	Do not use cromolyn for treatment of status asthmaticus

INTAL

Bronchospasm	Cromolyn can cause bronchospasm, which, on rare occasions, may be very severe; if bronchospasm cannot be controlled by prior administration of bronchodilators, discontinue use
Cough, wheezing	The powder in the capsules causes transient cough in 20% of patients and mild wheezing in 4% of patients; the solution produces cough occasionally. In some cases, cough and irritation of the throat can be prevented if mouth is rinsed or water is drunk immediately before and/or after use of the Spinhaler.
Anaphylaxis	Severe anaphylactic reactions may occur following administration of cromolyn sodium
Eosinophilic pneumonia	If the patient develops eosinophilic pneumonia or pulmonary infiltrates with eosinophilia, discontinue use of the metered-dose inhaler
Patients with exercise-induced bronchospasm	Use of the metered-dose inhaler may be effective in relieving bronchospasm in some, but not all, of these patients
Use in patients with impaired renal or hepatic function	Because cromolyn is excreted via the biliary and renal routes, decrease the dosage or discontinue use in patients with renal or hepatic dysfunction
Special-risk patients	Use the metered-dose inhaler with caution in patients with coronary artery disease or a history of cardiac arrhythmias because of the type of propellants contained in this preparation
Carcinogenicity, mutagenicity, effect on fertility	No cromolyn-induced neoplastic effects have been detected in rats following SC administration for 18 mo or in mice and hamsters following intraperitoneal administration for 12 mo. No evidence of chromosomal damage or cytotoxicity has been found in mutagenicity tests. Reproduction studies in animals have shown no evidence of impaired fertility.

ADVERSE REACTIONS[2]

The most frequent reactions, regardless of incidence, are printed in *italics*

With use of capsules and solution

Respiratory	*Bronchospasm, wheezing, cough, nasal congestion; laryngeal edema* (rare)
Central nervous system	Dizziness, headache
Dermatological	Rash, urticaria, angioedema
Genitourinary	Dysuria, urinary frequency
Gastrointestinal	Nausea
Other	Joint swelling and pain, lacrimation, swollen parotid glands; inhalation of gelatin particles, mouthpiece, or propeller (with use of capsules and Spinhaler)

With use of inhaler

Gastrointestinal	*Bad taste, nausea*
Respiratory	*Throat irritation or dryness, cough, wheeze;* pulmonary infiltrates with eosinophilia
Hypersensitivity	Anaphylaxis, angioedema, rash, urticaria
Central nervous system	Dizziness, headache
Genitourinary	Dysuria, urinary frequency
Other	Joint swelling and pain, lacrimation, swollen parotid glands, substernal burning, myopathy

OVERDOSAGE

No clinical signs or symptoms have been seen with overdosage; in studies with mammals, it has not been possible to attain an inhalant dose comparable to the toxic parenteral or oral dose

DRUG INTERACTIONS

See USE IN PREGNANT AND NURSING WOMEN

ALTERED LABORATORY VALUES

No clinically significant alterations in blood/serum or urinary values occur at therapeutic dosages

USE IN CHILDREN

See INDICATIONS and INHALANT DOSAGE; safety and effectiveness of capsules and nebulizer solution have not been established for use in children under 2 yr of age. Safety and effectiveness of the metered-dose inhaler have not been established for use in children under 5 yr of age; for younger children unable to use the Spinhaler or metered-dose inhaler, use the nebulizer solution. Cromolyn may cause adverse effects that could become apparent only after many years; use over a prolonged period in children only if the expected benefit outweighs the potential risk to the child.

USE IN PREGNANT AND NURSING WOMEN

Pregnancy Category B: reproduction studies in mice, rats, and rabbits injected with up to 338 times the human dose have shown no evidence of fetal malformations; an increase in resorptions and a decrease in fetal weight have been seen only at dosages that produced maternal toxicity. In mice, the frequency of resorptions and major fetal malformations associated with SC injection of isoproterenol (at 90 times the human dose) has been increased by the simultaneous SC administration of cromolyn (at 338 times the human dose). No adequate, well-controlled studies have been done in pregnant women; use during pregnancy only if clearly needed. It is not known whether cromolyn is excreted in human milk; use with caution in nursing mothers.

---

[1] Capsules also contain 20 mg of lactose (see CONTRAINDICATIONS)

[2] Reactions associated with use of the capsules or solution for which a causal relationship has not been established include anaphylaxis, nephrosis, periarteritic vasculitis, pericarditis, peripheral neuritis, pulmonary infiltrates with eosinophilia, polymyositis, exfoliative dermatitis, hemoptysis, anemia, myalgia, hoarseness, photodermatitis, and vertigo; reactions associated with use of the metered-dose inhaler for which a causal relationship has not been established include anemia, exfoliative dermatitis, hemoptysis, hoarseness, myalgia, nephrosis, periarteritic vasculitis, pericarditis, peripheral neuritis, photodermatitis, sneezing, drowsiness, nasal itching, nasal bleeding, nasal burning, serum sickness, stomachache, polymyositis, vertigo, and liver disease

NASALCROM ■ OPTICROM 4%

MAST-CELL STABILIZERS

NASALCROM (cromolyn sodium) Fisons   Rx
Solution: 40 mg/ml (13 ml, sufficient for a minimum of 100 inhalations)

INDICATIONS	INTRANASAL DOSAGE
Allergic rhinitis	Adult: 1 spray (5.2 mg) in each nostril tid or qid at regular intervals to start; if necessary, this dosage may be increased to 1 spray in each nostril 6 times/day Child ($\geq$ 6 yr): same as adult

CONTRAINDICATIONS
Hypersensitivity to any component[1]

ADMINISTRATION/DOSAGE ADJUSTMENTS

Intranasal administration	Nasalcrom is supplied in a spray bottle together with a refillable metered spray pump; refills are available separately. Instruct patients to clear their nasal passages before actuating the device and to inhale through the nose during administration.
Seasonal rhinitis	For patients with allergic rhinitis caused by pollen or other specific inhalant allergens, preferably begin treatment prior to expected contact and continue use until the pollen season or exposure to the offending allergen has ended
Perennial rhinitis	A therapeutic benefit in perennial allergic rhinitis may not be apparent until after 2–4 wk of regular use; during this initial period, concomitant administration of an antihistamine or a nasal decongestant, or both, may be necessary

WARNINGS/PRECAUTIONS

Patients with renal or hepatic impairment	Reduction in dosage and discontinuation of use should be considered as possible courses of action, since cromolyn is excreted in the urine and bile
Nasal stinging, sneezing	If these reactions occur, it may be necessary, in rare instances, to discontinue use
Carcinogenicity, mutagenicity, effect on fertility	Long-term SC or intraperitoneal administration of cromolyn had no effect on the incidence of neoplasia in mice, hamsters, and rats. No evidence of chromosomal damage or cytotoxicity has been found in mutagenicity tests. Reproduction studies in animals have shown no evidence of impaired fertility.

ADVERSE REACTIONS[2]
Frequent reactions (incidence $\geq$ 1%) are printed in *italics*

Respiratory	*Sneezing (10%); nasal stinging (5%); burning (4%), and irritation (2.5%);* epistaxis, postnasal drip
Other	*Headache and bad taste (2%);* rash; anaphylaxis (one case)

OVERDOSAGE

Signs and symptoms	See ADVERSE REACTIONS
Treatment	Discontinue medication; treat symptomatically and institute supportive measures, as required

DRUG INTERACTIONS
See USE IN PREGNANT AND NURSING WOMEN, below, concerning concomitant use of isoproterenol

ALTERED LABORATORY VALUES
No clinically significant alterations in blood/serum or urinary values occur at therapeutic dosages

USE IN CHILDREN	USE IN PREGNANT AND NURSING WOMEN
Safety and effectiveness for use in children under 6 yr of age have not been established	Pregnancy Category B: reproduction studies in mice, rats, and rabbits injected with up to 338 times the human dose have shown no evidence of fetal malformations; an increase in resorptions and a decrease in fetal weight have been observed only at dosages that produced maternal toxicity. In mice, simultaneous SC administration of cromolyn (at 338 times the human dose) increased the incidence of resorptions and fetal malformations related to SC injection of isoproterenol (at 90 times the human dose) alone. No adequate, well-controlled studies have been performed in pregnant women; use during pregnancy only if clearly needed. It is not known whether cromolyn is excreted in human milk; use with caution in nursing mothers.

[1] The solution also contains 0.01% benzalkonium chloride and 0.01% EDTA
[2] Reactions reported with the use of other dosage forms include angioedema, joint pain and swelling, urticaria, coughing, wheezing, and, in rare cases, serum sickness, periarteritic vasculitis, polymyositis, pericarditis, photodermatitis, exfoliative dermatitis, peripheral neuritis, and nephrosis

---

MAST-CELL STABILIZERS

OPTICROM 4% Ophthalmic Solution (cromolyn sodium) Fisons   Rx
Solution: 4% (10 ml)

INDICATIONS	TOPICAL DOSAGE
Vernal keratoconjunctivitis, vernal conjunctivitis, giant papillary conjunctivitis, vernal keratitis, and allergic keratoconjunctivitis	Adult and child ($\geq$ 4 yr): 1–2 drops instilled into each eye 4–6 times/day at regular intervals

OPTICROM 4%

CONTRAINDICATIONS

Hypersensitivity to cromolyn sodium or any other component	Wearing of soft contact lenses (due to benzalkonium chloride preservative)

ADMINISTRATION/DOSAGE ADJUSTMENTS

Duration of therapy	Symptomatic response (decreased itching, tearing, redness, and discharge) usually occurs within a few days; however, therapy for up to 6 wk is sometimes needed. Once symptomatic improvement has been established, continue therapy for as long as is needed to sustain improvement.
Concomitant therapy	If needed, corticosteroids may be given concomitantly

WARNINGS/PRECAUTIONS

Soft contact lenses	As with all preparations containing benzalkonium chloride, this solution should not be used while soft contact lenses are worn; patient can resume wearing soft lenses a few hours after the drug is discontinued
Transient stinging or burning	Following application, some transient stinging or burning may be experienced
Carcinogenicity, mutagenicity, effect on fertility	Long-term SC or intraperitoneal administration of cromolyn had no effect on the incidence of neoplasia in mice, hamsters, and rats. No evidence of chromosomal damage or cytotoxicity has been found in mutagenicity tests. Reproduction studies in animals have shown no evidence of impaired fertility.
Patient instructions	To avoid contamination, advise patient to discard the bottle and any remaining contents 4 wk after the blister pack is opened

ADVERSE REACTIONS

The most frequent reaction is italicized

Ophthalmic	*Transient stinging or burning,* conjunctival injection, watery or itchy eyes, dryness around the eye, puffiness, irritation, styes

OVERDOSAGE

Cromolyn is poorly absorbed; in normal volunteers, approximately 0.03% of a dose is absorbed systematically after ophthalmic administration

DRUG INTERACTIONS

No clinically significant drug interactions have been identified

---

USE IN CHILDREN

See INDICATIONS and TOPICAL DOSAGE; safety and effectiveness have not been established in children under 4 yr of age

USE IN PREGNANT AND NURSING WOMEN

Pregnancy Category B: reproduction studies in mice, rats, and rabbits injected with up to 338 times the human dose have shown no evidence of fetal malformations; an increase in resorptions and a decrease in fetal weight have been observed only at dosages that produced maternal toxicity. No adequate, well-controlled studies have been performed in pregnant women; use during pregnancy only if clearly needed. It is not known whether cromolyn is excreted in human milk; use with caution in nursing mothers.

VEHICLE/BASE
Solution: 0.4% phenylethyl alcohol, 0.01% benzalkonium chloride, 0.01% EDTA, and purified water

Chapter 22

Anthihypertensive Agents

Alpha- and Beta-Adrenergic Blockers — 758
NORMODYNE (Schering) — 758
Labetalol hydrochoride *Rx*

TRANDATE (Glaxo) — 760
Labetalol hydrochloride *Rx*

Angiotensin-Converting Enzyme Inhibitors — 763
CAPOTEN (Squibb) — 763
Captopril *Rx*

VASOTEC (Merck Sharp & Dohme) — 765
Enalapril maleate *Rx*

Beta-Adrenergic Blockers — 767
BLOCADREN (Merck Sharp & Dohme) — 767
Timolol maleate *Rx*

CORGARD (Princeton) — 769
Nadolol *Rx*

INDERAL (Ayerst) — 771
Propranolol hydrochloride *Rx*

INDERAL LA (Ayerst) — 773
Propranolol hydrochloride *Rx*

LOPRESSOR (Geigy) — 775
Metoprolol tartrate *Rx*

SECTRAL (Wyeth) — 778
Acebutolol hydrochloride *Rx*

TENORMIN (Stuart) — 779
Atenolol *Rx*

VISKEN (Sandoz Pharmaceuticals) — 781
Pindolol *Rx*

Calcium Antagonists — 783
CALAN (Searle) — 783
Verapamil hydrochloride *Rx*

CALAN SR (Searle) — 783
Verapamil hydrochloride *Rx*

ISOPTIN (Knoll) — 785
Verapamil hydrochloride *Rx*

ISOPTIN SR (Knoll) — 786
Verapamil hydrochloride *Rx*

Central Alpha$_2$-Adrenergic Agonists — 788
ALDOMET (Merck Sharp & Dohme) — 788
Methyldopa *Rx*

CATAPRES (Boehringer Ingelheim) — 789
Clonidine hydrochloride *Rx*

CATAPRES-TTS (Boehringer Ingelheim) — 791
Clonidine *Rx*

WYTENSIN (Wyeth) — 792
Guanabenz acetate *Rx*

Indolines — 794
LOZOL (Rorer) — 794
Indapamide *Rx*

Peripheral Vasodilators — 795
APRESOLINE (CIBA) — 795
Hydralazine hydrochloride *Rx*

HYPERSTAT I.V. (Schering) — 797
Diazoxide *Rx*

LONITEN (Upjohn) — 799
Minoxidil *Rx*

MINIPRESS (Pfizer) — 800
Prazosin hydrochloride *Rx*

NIPRIDE (Roche) — 802
Sodium nitroprusside *Rx*

REGITINE (CIBA) — 803
Phentolamine mesylate *Rx*

Sympatholytics — 805
ARFONAD (Roche) — 805
Trimethaphan camsylate *Rx*

HYLOREL (Pennwalt) — 806
Guanadrel sulfate *Rx*

ISMELIN (CIBA) — 807
Guanethidine monosulfate *Rx*

SERPASIL (CIBA) — 809
Reserpine *Rx*

Antihypertensives with Diuretics — 811
ALDOCLOR (Merck Sharp & Dohme) — 811
Methyldopa and chlorothiazide *Rx*

ALDORIL (Merck Sharp & Dohme) — 813
Methyldopa and hydrochlorothiazide *Rx*

APRESAZIDE (CIBA) — 815
Hydralazine hydrochloride and hydrochlorothiazide *Rx*

CAPOZIDE (Squibb) — 818
Captopril and hydrochlorothiazide *Rx*

COMBIPRES (Boehringer Ingelheim) — 821
Clonidine hydrochloride and chlorthalidone *Rx*

CORZIDE (Princeton) — 823
Nadolol and bendroflumethiazide *Rx*

Demi-REGROTON (Rorer) — 845
Chlorthalidone and reserpine *Rx*

DIUPRES (Merck Sharp & Dohme) — 825
Chlorothiazide and reserpine *Rx*

ENDURONYL (Abbott) — 827
Methyclothiazide and deserpidine *Rx*

ENDURONYL Forte (Abbott) — 827
Methyclothiazide and deserpidine *Rx*

ESIMIL (CIBA) Guanethidine monosulfate and hydrochlorothiazide *Rx*	829
HYDROPRES (Merck Sharp & Dohme) Hydrochlorothiazide and reserpine *Rx*	832
INDERIDE (Ayerst) Propranolol hydrochloride and hydrochlorothiazide *Rx*	834
INDERIDE LA (Ayerst) Propranolol hydrochloride and hydrochlorothiazide *Rx*	836
LOPRESSOR HCT (Geigy) Metoprolol tartrate and hydrochlorothiazide *Rx*	839
MINIZIDE (Pfizer) Prazosin hydrochloride and polythiazide *Rx*	841
RAUZIDE (Princeton) *Rauwolfia serpentina* and bendroflumethiazide *Rx*	843
REGROTON (Rorer) Chlorthalidone and reserpine *Rx*	845
SALUTENSIN (Bristol) Hydroflumethiazide and reserpine *Rx*	847
SALUTENSIN-Demi (Bristol) Hydroflumethiazide and reserpine *Rx*	847
SER-AP-ES (CIBA) Reserpine, hydralazine hydrochloride, and hydrochlorothiazide *Rx*	850
TENORETIC (Stuart) Atenolol and chlorthalidone *Rx*	853
TIMOLIDE (Merck Sharp & Dohme) Timolol maleate and hydrochlorothiazide *Rx*	855
VASERETIC (Merck Sharp & Dohme) Enalapril maleate and hydrochlorothiazide *Rx*	858

Other Antihypertensive Agents 756

ARFONAD (Roche) Trimethaphan camsylate *Rx*	756
DIBENZYLINE (Smith Kline & French) Phenoxybenzamine hydrochloride *Rx*	756
EUTONYL (Abbott) Pargyline hydrochloride *Rx*	756
HARMONYL (Abbott) Deserpidine *Rx*	756
MODERIL (Pfizer) Rescinnamine *Rx*	756
NITROPRESS (Abbott) Sodium nitroprusside *Rx*	756
RAUDIXIN (Princeton) *Rauwolfia serpentina*, whole root *Rx*	756
RAUWILOID (Riker) Alseroxylon *Rx*	756
REGITINE (CIBA) Phentolamine mesylate *Rx*	756

Other Antihypertensives with Diuretics 756

APRESOLINE-ESIDRIX (CIBA) Hydralazine hydrochloride and hydrochlorothiazide *Rx*	756
DIUTENSEN (Wallace) Cryptenamine tannate and methyclothiazide *Rx*	756
DIUTENSEN-R (Wallace) Methyclothiazide and reserpine *Rx*	756
EUTRON (Abbott) Pargyline hydrochloride and methyclothiazide *Rx*	756
HYDROMOX R (Lederle) Quinethazone and reserpine *Rx*	756
METATENSIN (Merrell Dow) Trichlormethiazide and reserpine *Rx*	757
NAQUIVAL (Schering) Trichlormethiazide and reserpine *Rx*	757
ORETICYL (Abbott) Hydrochlorothiazide and deserpidine *Rx*	757
RAUTRAX (Princeton) *Rauwolfia serpentina*, flumethiazide, and potassium chloride *Rx*	757
RENESE-R (Pfizer) Polythiazide and reserpine *Rx*	757
SERPASIL-APRESOLINE (CIBA) Reserpine and hydralazine hydrochloride *Rx*	757
SERPASIL-ESIDRIX (CIBA) Reserpine and hydrochlorothiazide *Rx*	757

continued

COMPENDIUM OF DRUG THERAPY

OTHER ANTIHYPERTENSIVE AGENTS

DRUG	HOW SUPPLIED	USUAL DOSAGE[1]
ARFONAD (Roche) Trimethaphan camsylate *Rx*	**Ampuls:** 50 mg/ml (10 ml)	**Adult:** 3–4 mg (3–4 ml)/min, given by IV infusion, to start; thereafter, adjust rate of administration to maintain desired level of hypotension
DIBENZYLINE (Smith Kline & French) Phenoxybenzamine hydrochloride *Rx*	**Capsules:** 10 mg	**Adult:** 10 mg bid to start; increase daily dose every other day, usually to 20–40 mg bid or tid, until optimum dosage is reached
EUTONYL (Abbott) Pargyline hydrochloride *Rx*	**Tablets:** 10, 25 mg	**Adult:** 25 mg/day to start, given in a single daily dose; increase daily dose at weekly intervals by 10 mg until desired response is achieved, up to 200 mg/day; for elderly or postsympathectomy patients, 10–25 mg/day to start; usual daily dosage: 25–50 mg/day
HARMONYL (Abbott) Deserpidine *Rx*	**Tablets:** 0.25 mg	**Adult:** for mild essential hypertension, 0.75–1 mg/day to start; adjust dosage to clinical response after 10–14 days for maintenance
MODERIL (Pfizer) Rescinnamine *Rx*	**Tablets:** 0.25, 0.5 mg	**Adult:** 0.5 mg bid to start; for maintenance, 0.25–0.5 mg/day
NITROPRESS (Abbott) Sodium nitroprusside *Rx*	**Vials:** 50 mg (2 ml)	**Adult:** 0.5–10 μg/kg/min, given by IV infusion (average dosage: 3 μg/kg/min)
RAUDIXIN (Princeton) *Rauwolfia serpentina* (whole root) *Rx*	**Tablets:** 50, 100 mg	**Adult:** 200–400 mg/day, given in 2 divided doses (AM and PM) to start; for maintenance, 50–300 mg/day, given in a single daily dose or 2 divided doses; for the elderly and severely debilitated, reduce dosage
RAUWILOID (Riker) Alseroxylon *Rx*	**Tablets:** 2 mg	**Adult:** 2–4 mg/day to start; for maintenance, 2 mg/day
REGITINE (CIBA) Phentolamine mesylate *Rx*	**Vials:** 5 mg	**Adult:** 5 mg IM or IV 1–2 h before surgery **Child:** 1 mg IM or IV 1–2 h before surgery

[1] Where pediatric dosages are not given, consult manufacturer

OTHER ANTIHYPERTENSIVES WITH DIURETICS

DRUG	HOW SUPPLIED	USUAL DOSAGE[1]
APRESOLINE-ESIDRIX (CIBA) Hydralazine hydrochloride and hydrochlorothiazide *Rx*	**Tablets:** 25 mg hydralazine hydrochloride and 15 mg hydrochlorothiazide	**Adult:** determine dosage by titration of individual components; usual dosage, 1 tab tid; adjust dosage as needed for maintenance, up to 2 tabs tid
DIUTENSEN (Wallace) Cryptenamine tannate and methyclothiazide *Rx*	**Tablets:** 2 mg cryptenamine tannate and 2.5 mg methyclothiazide	**Adult:** determine dosage by titration of individual components; usual dosage, 1–4 tabs/day
DIUTENSEN-R (Wallace) Methyclothiazide and reserpine *Rx*	**Tablets:** 2.5 mg methyclothiazide and 0.1 mg reserpine	**Adult:** determine dosage by titration of individual components; usual dosage, 1–4 tabs/day
EUTRON (Abbott) Pargyline hydrochloride and methyclothiazide *Rx*	**Tablets:** 25 mg pargyline hydrochloride and 5 mg methyclothiazide	**Adult:** determine dosage by titration of individual components; usual dosage, 1 tab/day; adjust dosage as needed for maintenance, up to 2 tabs/day
HYDROMOX R (Lederle) Quinethazone and reserpine *Rx*	**Tablets:** 50 mg quinethazone and 0.125 mg reserpine	**Adult:** determine dosage by titration of individual components; if necessary, give 3–4 tabs once daily for up to 2 wk to start; for maintenance, 1–2 tabs once daily

OTHER ANTIHYPERTENSIVES WITH DIURETICS continued

DRUG	HOW SUPPLIED	USUAL DOSAGE[1]
METATENSIN (Merrell Dow) Trichlormethiazide and reserpine Rx	**Tablets:** 2 or 4 mg trichlormethiazide and 0.1 mg reserpine	**Adult:** determine dosage by titration of individual components; administer up to 4–8 mg of trichlormethiazide, as needed, once daily in AM
NAQUIVAL (Schering) Trichlormethiazide and reserpine Rx	**Tablets:** 4 mg trichlormethiazide and 0.1 mg reserpine	**Adult:** determine dosage by titration of individual components; 1 tab bid may be given to start; reduce dosage according to clinical response for maintenance
ORETICYL (Abbott) Hydrochlorothiazide and deserpidine Rx	**Tablets:** 25 mg hydrochlorothiazide and 0.125 mg deserpidine (Oreticyl 25); 50 mg hydrochlorothiazide and 0.125 mg deserpidine (Oreticyl 50); 25 mg hydrochlorothiazide and 0.25 mg deserpidine (Oreticyl Forte)	**Adult:** determine dosage by titration of each component; usual dosage, 1 Oreticyl 50 tab bid
RAUTRAX (Princeton) Rauwolfia serpentina, flumethiazide, and potassium chloride Rx	**Tablets:** 50 mg powdered Rauwolfia serpentina, 400 mg flumethiazide, and 400 mg potassium chloride	**Adult:** 2–6 tabs/day to start, given in divided doses and preferably at mealtimes; for maintenance, 1–6 tabs/day, given in divided doses (usual dose: 2 tabs/day)
RENESE-R (Pfizer) Polythiazide and reserpine Rx	**Tablets:** 2 mg polythiazide and 0.25 mg reserpine	**Adult:** determine dosage by titration of each component to start, followed by 1/2–2 tabs/day for maintenance
SERPASIL-APRESOLINE (CIBA) Reserpine and hydralazine hydrochloride Rx	**Tablets:** 0.1 mg reserpine and 25 mg hydralazine hydrochloride (No. 1); 0.2 mg reserpine and 50 mg hydralazine hydrochloride (No. 2)	**Adult:** determine dosage by titration of individual components; if reserpine alone (0.5 mg/day) does not adequately control hypertension, administer 1 No. 2 tab qid to start, followed by a gradual reduction in dosage to 1 No. 1 tab qid for maintenance
SERPASIL-ESIDRIX (CIBA) Reserpine and hydrochlorothiazide Rx	**Tablets:** 0.1 mg reserpine and 25 mg hydrochlorothiazide (No. 1); 0.1 mg reserpine and 50 mg hydrochlorothiazide (No. 2)	**Adult:** determine dosage by titration of individual components; usual dosage, 2 No. 1 or No. 2 tabs/day, given in a single daily dose or divided; reduce dosage to lowest effective level for maintenance

[1] Where pediatric dosages are not given, consult manufacturer

COMPENDIUM OF DRUG THERAPY

ALPHA- AND BETA-ADRENERGIC BLOCKERS

NORMODYNE (labetalol hydrochloride) Schering   Rx

Tablets: 100 mg (scored), 200 mg (scored), 300 mg **Vials:** 5 mg/ml (20, 60 ml)

INDICATIONS

Hypertension

ORAL DOSAGE

Adult: 100 mg bid (alone or with a diuretic) to start, followed, as needed, by increases of 100 mg bid every 2–3 days; usual dosage: 200–400 mg bid. For patients with severe hypertension, who may require 600–1,200 mg bid, the dosage may be increased in increments of up to 200 mg bid. For hospitalized patients who have received labetalol IV, give 200 mg to start, followed by 200 or 400 mg 6–12 h later, 200 mg bid on day 2, and then, as needed, 400 mg bid on day 3, 800 mg bid on day 4, and 1,200 mg bid on day 5.

PARENTERAL DOSAGE

Adult: for severe hypertension in hospitalized patients, 20 mg, given by IV injection over a period of 2 min, followed, if necessary, by 40- or 80-mg doses at 10-min intervals, up to a total of 300 mg; alternatively, 50–300 mg, given by continuous IV infusion at an initial rate of 2 mg/min

CONTRAINDICATIONS

Bronchial asthma	Cardiogenic shock	Second- or third-degree AV block
Overt cardiac failure	Severe bradycardia	

ADMINISTRATION/DOSAGE ADJUSTMENTS

Preparation for IV infusion — Dilute 200 mg (40 ml) of labetalol in either 160 ml of diluent (final concentration: 2 mg/2 ml) or 250 ml of diluent (final concentration: approximately 2 mg/3 ml). Use as a diluent Ringer's or lactated Ringer's injection USP, 5% dextrose injection USP, 0.9% sodium chloride injection USP, 5% dextrose and Ringer's or 5% lactated Ringer's injection, 5% dextrose and 0.2%, 0.33%, or 0.9% sodium chloride injection USP, or 2.5% dextrose and 0.45% sodium chloride injection USP; do not use 5% sodium bicarbonate injection USP.

Intravenous administration — Reduce blood pressure slowly, taking as much time as possible and avoiding any rapid or excessive decreases; angina, ischemic changes in the ECG, and cerebral and optic nerve infarction have occurred when other antihypertensive drugs have been used for as long as 1–2 days to reduce extremely high blood pressure. Maintain patients in a supine position during and immediately after administration; allow patients to walk only after it is established that they can tolerate a standing position because a change in position within 3 h after IV use is especially likely to precipitate orthostatic hypotension.

Monitoring of therapy — To evaluate response to oral therapy, measure standing blood pressure 1–3 h after administration when therapy is started or the dosage is changed and immediately before the next dose when the same dose has been given repeatedly. To monitor response to IV therapy, check supine blood pressure immediately before and 5 and 10 min after each injection (maximum effect usually occurs within 5 min), or measure supine pressure during and after infusion. Discontinue IV administration when a satisfactory response is achieved; once it is established that the supine diastolic blood pressure has begun to rise, switch to oral therapy.

Management of adverse effects — If reactions such as nausea and dizziness occur during oral therapy, the total daily dose may be given in 3 divided doses

WARNINGS/PRECAUTIONS

Cardiac failure — Beta blockade may exacerbate cardiac failure and, in patients with latent cardiac insufficiency, may cause cardiac failure. If necessary, however, labetalol may be used with caution in patients with well-compensated congestive heart failure. If cardiac failure occurs during treatment and does not respond to digitalization and diuretic therapy, discontinue administration of labetalol (withdraw the drug gradually, if possible).

Angina — Abrupt withdrawal of certain beta blockers can exacerbate angina and, in some cases, precipitate myocardial infarction. After chronic use, labetalol should generally be discontinued over a period of 1–2 wk, even if coronary artery disease is not evident. During the period of withdrawal, carefully observe the patient and restrict physical activity; if acute coronary artery insufficiency develops or angina markedly worsens, promptly reinstitute use of labetalol and take measures appropriate for the management of unstable angina. Caution patients not to interrupt or discontinue labetalol therapy on their own.

Bronchospasm — In general, patients with nonallergic bronchospastic diseases such as emphysema and chronic bronchitis should not receive beta blockers; oral labetalol may be used with caution in these patients if other antihypertensive agents are not effective or tolerated

Jaundice — On rare occasions, jaundice has occurred; discontinue use immediately if jaundice or laboratory evidence of hepatic injury is detected

NORMODYNE

Major surgery	The necessity or desirability of discontinuing therapy before major surgery is controversial and has not been fully assessed; severe protracted hypotension and difficulty in restarting or maintaining the heartbeat have occurred with use of beta blockers during surgery (see also DRUG INTERACTIONS)
Pheochromocytoma	Use with caution in patients with pheochromocytoma because paradoxical hypertensive responses have occasionally occurred. For IV treatment of pheochromocytoma-related hypertension, unusually high doses may be necessary.
Hypoglycemia	Beta blockade may mask tachycardia and other premonitory signs and symptoms of acute hypoglycemia; this effect is of particular importance when treating patients with labile diabetes
Drug metabolism	Use with caution in patients with hepatic impairment since labetalol metabolism may be reduced in these patients
Laboratory testing	During prolonged treatment, laboratory parameters should be checked regularly; to monitor renal impairment or other concomitant disorders, appropriate tests should be done during therapy
Carcinogenicity, mutagenicity	No evidence of carcinogenicity has been seen in mice or rats following long-term oral administration; mutagenic effects have not been detected in the Ames test or in dominant lethal assays using rats and mice

ADVERSE REACTIONS[1]

Frequent reactions (incidence $\geq$ 1%) are printed in *italics*

Oral therapy

Central nervous system	*Dizziness (11%), fatigue (5%), headache and vertigo (2%), asthenia (1%)*, drowsiness, paresthesias (especially tingling of the scalp), drowsiness
Ophthalmic	*Vision abnormality (1%)*, dry eyes
Cardiovascular	*Edema and orthostatic hypotension (1%)*; syncope (rare)
Gastrointestinal	*Nausea (6%), dyspepsia (3%), distortion of taste (1%)*, vomiting, diarrhea, cholestasis (with or without jaundice)
Genitourinary	*Ejaculation failure (2%), impotence (1%)*, urinary retention, difficult urination
Respiratory	*Nasal congestion (3%), dyspnea (2%)*, bronchospasm
Dermatological	*Rash, including urticaria, facial erythema, bullous lichen planus, and lichenoid, psoriasiform, and generalized maculopapular rash (1%)*, Peyronie's disease, alopecia
Other	Diaphoresis, systemic lupus erythematosus, muscle cramps, toxic myopathy

Intravenous therapy

Central nervous system	*Dizziness (9%), tingling of the scalp or skin (7%), somnolence/yawning (3%), numbness and vertigo (1%)*
Cardiovascular	*Orthostatic hypotension (58%), ventricular arrhythmias, flushing, and hypotension (1%)*
Gastrointestinal	*Nausea (13%), vomiting (4%), dyspepsia and distortion of taste (1%)*
Respiratory	*Wheezing (1%)*
Dermatological	*Pruritis (1%)*
Other	*Diaphoresis (4%)*

OVERDOSAGE

Signs and symptoms	Hypotension, excessive bradycardia, cardiac failure, bronchospasm
Treatment	If orthostatic hypotension occurs, lay patient down and, if necessary, raise the patient's legs. Administer atropine or epinephrine for excessive bradycardia and a vasopressor such as norepinephrine for hypotension. Alternatively, reverse bradycardia or hypotension with glucagon, giving 5–10 mg over a period of 30 s and then 5 mg/h by continuous infusion (infusion rate may be reduced as patient improves). For cardiac failure, administer digitalis and a diuretic; dopamine or dobutamine may also be useful. Treat bronchospasm with epinephrine and/or an aerosolized beta$_2$ agonist. Control seizures with diazepam. To empty stomach shortly after ingestion, induce emesis with syrup of ipecac or perform gastric lavage. Neither peritoneal dialysis nor hemodialysis removes a significant amount of labetalol from the blood.

DRUG INTERACTIONS

Diuretics	△ Antihypertensive effect; if necessary, reduce labetalol dosage
Insulin, sulfonylureas	▽ Hypoglycemic effect; if necessary, increase antidiabetic dosage
Halothane	△ Antihypertensive effect, with possible increase in central venous pressure and decrease in cardiac output; halothane concentrations of 3% or higher should not be used concomitantly
Cimetidine	△ Bioavailability of oral labetalol; exercise special care when titrating dosage of labetalol

NORMODYNE ■ TRANDATE

Ephedrine, isoproterenol, other beta-adrenergic bronchodilators	▽ Bronchodilation; if necessary, increase bronchodilator dosage
Nitroglycerin	△ Antihypertensive effect
Tricyclic antidepressants	Tremors

ALTERED LABORATORY VALUES

Blood/serum values	With oral therapy: △ BUN △ SGPT △ SGOT + ANA titer + Antimitochondrial antibodies
	With IV therapy: △ BUN △ Creatinine
Urinary values	△ Catecholamines (with nonspecific trihydroxyindole reaction); to avoid falsely elevated results, use specific radioenzymatic assay or high performance liquid chromatography

USE IN CHILDREN

Safety and effectiveness for use in children have not been established

USE IN PREGNANT AND NURSING WOMEN

Pregnancy Category C: an increase in resorptions has been seen in rats and rabbits fed the maximum human dose, and an decrease in neonatal survival has been observed when rats have been fed 2–4 times this dose from late gestation to the time of weaning; no fetal malformations have been detected in rats at 6 times this dose or in rabbits at 4 times this dose. Administration of labetalol to pregnant women has not caused any apparent reactions in infants; however, no adequate, well-controlled, clinical studies have been done. Use during pregnancy only if the expected benefit justifies the potential risk to the fetus. Labetalol does not appear to affect the usual course of labor and delivery. Small amounts of this drug are excreted in human milk; use with caution in nursing mothers.

[1] Reactions associated with use of other beta blockers include intensification of AV block; reversible mental depression progressing to catatonia; an acute reversible syndrome characterized by temporal and spatial disorientation, short-term memory loss, emotional lability, slightly clouded sensorium, and decreased performance on neuropsychometric tests; agranulocytosis; purpura; mesenteric artery thrombosis; ischemic colitis; fever with sore throat and aching; laryngospasm; and respiratory distress

---

ALPHA- AND BETA-ADRENERGIC BLOCKERS

TRANDATE (labetalol hydrochloride) Glaxo   Rx

Tablets: 100 mg (scored), 200 mg (scored), 300 mg (scored)   **Vials:** 5 mg/ml (20, 40 ml)

INDICATIONS	ORAL DOSAGE	PARENTERAL DOSAGE
Hypertension	**Adult:** 100 mg bid (alone or with a diuretic) to start, followed, as needed, by increases of 100 mg bid every 2–3 days; usual dosage: 200–400 mg bid. For patients with severe hypertension, who may require 600–1,200 mg bid, the dosage may be increased in increments of up to 200 mg bid. For hospitalized patients who have received labetalol IV, give 200 mg to start, followed by 200 or 400 mg 6–12 h later, 200 mg bid on day 2, and then, as needed, 400 mg bid on day 3, 800 mg bid on day 4, and 1,200 mg bid on day 5.	**Adult:** for severe hypertension in hospitalized patients, 20 mg, given by IV injection over a period of 2 min, followed, if necessary, by 40- or 80-mg doses at 10-min intervals, up to a total of 300 mg; alternatively, 50–300 mg, given by continuous IV infusion at an initial rate of 2 mg/min

CONTRAINDICATIONS

Bronchial asthma	Cardiogenic shock	Second- or third-degree AV block
Overt cardiac failure	Severe bradycardia	

ADMINISTRATION/DOSAGE ADJUSTMENTS

Preparation for IV infusion	Dilute 200 mg (40 ml) of labetalol in either 160 ml of diluent (final concentration: 2 mg/2 ml) or 250 ml of diluent (final concentration: approximately 2 mg/3 ml). Use as a diluent Ringer's or lactated Ringer's injection USP, 5% dextrose injection USP, 0.9% sodium chloride injection USP, 5% dextrose and Ringer's or 5% lactated Ringer's injection, 5% dextrose and 0.2%, 0.33%, or 0.9% sodium chloride injection USP, or 2.5% dextrose and 0.45% sodium chloride injection USP; do not use 5% sodium bicarbonate injection USP.

TRANDATE

Intravenous administration	Reduce blood pressure slowly, taking as much time as possible and avoiding any rapid or excessive decreases; angina, ischemic changes in the ECG, and cerebral and optic nerve infarction have occurred when other antihypertensive drugs have been used for as long as 1–2 days to reduce extremely high blood pressure. Maintain patients in a supine position during and immediately after administration; allow patients to walk only after it is established that they can tolerate a standing position, because a change in position within 3 h after IV use is especially likely to precipitate orthostatic hypotension.
Monitoring of therapy	To evaluate response to oral therapy, measure standing blood pressure 1–3 h after administration when therapy is started or the dosage is changed and immediately before the next dose when the same dose has been given repeatedly. To monitor response to IV therapy, check supine blood pressure immediately before and 5 and 10 min after each injection (maximum effect usually occurs within 5 min), or measure supine pressure during and after infusion. Discontinue IV administration when a satisfactory response is achieved; once it is established that the supine diastolic blood pressure has begun to rise, switch to oral therapy.
Management of adverse effects	If reactions such as nausea and dizziness occur during oral therapy, the total daily dose may be given in 3 divided doses

WARNINGS/PRECAUTIONS

Cardiac failure	Beta blockade may exacerbate cardiac failure and, in patients with latent cardiac insufficiency, may cause cardiac failure. If necessary, however, labetalol may be used with caution in patients with well-compensated congestive heart failure. If cardiac failure occurs during treatment and does not respond to digitalization and diuretic therapy, discontinue administration of labetalol (withdraw the drug gradually, if possible).
Angina	Abrupt withdrawal of certain beta blockers can exacerbate angina and, in some cases, precipitate myocardial infarction. After chronic use, labetalol should generally be discontinued over a period of 1–2 wk, even if coronary artery disease is not evident. During the period of withdrawal, carefully observe the patient and restrict physical activity; if acute coronary artery insufficiency develops or angina markedly worsens, promptly reinstitute use of labetalol and take measures appropriate for the management of unstable angina. Caution patients not to interrupt or discontinue labetalol therapy on their own.
Bronchospasm	In general, patients with nonallergic bronchospastic diseases, such as emphysema and chronic bronchitis, should not receive beta blockers; oral labetalol may be used with caution in these patients if other antihypertensive agents are not effective or tolerated
Jaundice	On rare occasions, jaundice has occurred; discontinue use immediately if jaundice or laboratory evidence of hepatic injury is detected
Major surgery	The necessity or desirability of discontinuing therapy before major surgery is controversial and has not been fully assessed; severe protracted hypotension and difficulty in restarting or maintaining the heartbeat have occurred with use of beta blockers during surgery (see also DRUG INTERACTIONS)
Pheochromocytoma	Use with caution in patients with pheochromocytoma because paradoxical hypertensive responses have occasionally occurred. For IV treatment of pheochromocytoma-related hypertension, unusually high doses may be necessary.
Hypoglycemia	Beta blockade may mask tachycardia and other premonitory signs and symptoms of acute hypoglycemia; this effect is of particular importance when treating patients with labile diabetes
Drug metabolism	Use with caution in patients with hepatic impairment, since labetalol metabolism may be reduced in these patients
Laboratory testing	During prolonged treatment, laboratory parameters should be checked regularly; to monitor renal impairment or other concomitant disorders, appropriate tests should be done during therapy
Carcinogenicity, mutagenicity	No evidence of carcinogenicity has been seen in mice or rats following long-term oral administration; mutagenic effects have not been detected in the Ames test or in dominant lethal assays using rats and mice

ADVERSE REACTIONS[1]

Frequent reactions (incidence ≥ 1%) are printed in *italics*

Oral therapy

Central nervous system	*Dizziness (11%), fatigue (5%), headache and vertigo (2%), asthenia (1%),* drowsiness, paresthesias (especially tingling of the scalp), drowsiness
Ophthalmic	*Vision abnormality (1%),* dry eyes
Cardiovascular	*Edema and orthostatic hypotension (1%),* syncope (rare)
Gastrointestinal	*Nausea (6%), dyspepsia (3%), distortion of taste (1%),* vomiting, diarrhea, cholestasis (with or without jaundice)
Genitourinary	*Ejaculation failure (2%), impotence (1%),* urinary retention, difficult urination

TRANDATE

Respiratory	Nasal congestion (3%), dyspnea (2%), bronchospasm
Dermatological	Rash, including urticaria, facial erythema, bullous lichen planus, and lichenoid, psoriasiform, and generalized maculopapular rash (1%); Peyronie's disease, alopecia
Other	Diaphoresis, systemic lupus erythematosus, muscle cramps, toxic myopathy

Intravenous therapy

Central nervous system	Dizziness (9%), tingling of the scalp or skin (7%), somnolence/yawning (3%), numbness and vertigo (1%)
Cardiovascular	Orthostatic hypotension (58%), ventricular arrhythmias, flushing, and hypotension (1%)
Gastrointestinal	Nausea (13%), vomiting (4%), dyspepsia and distortion of taste (1%)
Respiratory	Wheezing (1%)
Dermatological	Pruritus (1%)
Other	Diaphoresis (4%)

OVERDOSAGE

Signs and symptoms	Hypotension, excessive bradycardia, cardiac failure, bronchospasm
Treatment	If orthostatic hypotension occurs, lay patient down and, if necessary, raise the patient's legs. Administer atropine or epinephrine for excessive bradycardia and a vasopressor such as norepinephrine for hypotension. Alternatively, reverse bradycardia or hypotension with glucagon, giving 5–10 mg over a period of 30 s and then 5 mg/h by continuous infusion (infusion rate may be reduced as patient improves). For cardiac failure, administer digitalis and a diuretic; dopamine or dobutamine may also be useful. Treat bronchospasm with epinephrine and/or an aerosolized beta$_2$ agonist. Control seizures with diazepam. To empty stomach shortly after ingestion, induce emesis with syrup of ipecac or perform gastric lavage. Neither peritoneal dialysis nor hemodialysis removes a significant amount of labetalol from the blood.

DRUG INTERACTIONS

Diuretics	△ Antihypertensive effect; if necessary, reduce labetalol dosage
Insulin, sulfonylureas	▽ Hypoglycemic effect; if necessary, increase antidiabetic dosage
Halothane	△ Antihypertensive effect, with possible increase in central venous pressure and decrease in cardiac output; halothane concentrations of 3% or higher should not be used concomitantly
Cimetidine	△ Bioavailability of oral labetalol; exercise special care when titrating dosage of labetalol
Ephedrine, isoproterenol, other beta-adrenergic bronchodilators	▽ Bronchodilation; if necessary, increase bronchodilator dosage
Nitroglycerin	△ Antihypertensive effect
Tricyclic antidepressants	Tremors

ALTERED LABORATORY VALUES

Blood/serum values	With oral therapy: △ BUN △ SGPT △ SGOT + ANA titer + Antimitochondrial antibodies With IV therapy: △ BUN △ Creatinine
Urinary values	△ Catecholamines (with nonspecific trihydroxyindole reaction); to avoid falsely elevated results, use specific radioenzymatic assay or high-performance liquid chromatography

---

USE IN CHILDREN

Safety and effectiveness for use in children have not been established

USE IN PREGNANT AND NURSING WOMEN

Pregnancy Category C: an increase in resorptions has been seen in rats and rabbits fed the maximum human dose, and a decrease in neonatal survival has been observed when rats have been fed 2–4 times this dose from late gestation to the time of weaning; no fetal malformations have been detected in rats at 6 times this dose or in rabbits at 4 times this dose. Administration of labetalol to pregnant women has not caused any apparent reactions in infants; however, no adequate, well-controlled, clinical studies have been done. Use during pregnancy only if the expected benefit justifies the potential risk to the fetus. Labetalol does not appear to affect the usual course of labor and delivery. Small amounts of this drug are excreted in human milk; use with caution in nursing mothers.

---

[1] Reactions associated with use of other beta blockers include intensification of AV block; reversible mental depression progressing to catatonia; an acute reversible syndrome characterized by temporal and spatial disorientation, short-term memory loss, emotional lability, slightly clouded sensorium, and decreased performance on neuropsychometric tests; agranulocytosis; purpura; mesenteric artery thrombosis; ischemic colitis; fever with sore throat and aching; laryngospasm; and respiratory distress

ANGIOTENSIN-CONVERTING ENZYME INHIBITORS

CAPOTEN (captopril) Squibb   Rx
Tablets: 12.5, 25, 37.5, 50, 100 mg

INDICATIONS
Hypertension in patients with normal renal function

Hypertension in patients with renal impairment who have experienced unacceptable side effects with other antihypertensive drugs or have failed to respond satisfactorily to a combination of other antihypertensive drugs

Heart failure inadequately controlled by conventional diuretic and digitalis therapy

ORAL DOSAGE
Adult: 25 mg bid or tid, administered 1 h before meals, to start; if necessary, increase dosage to 50 mg bid or tid after 1–2 wk. If blood pressure is not satisfactorily controlled after another 1–2 wk, add a thiazide diuretic, beginning with a modest dose (eg, 25 mg/day of hydrochlorothiazide). Increase the dose of the diuretic, as needed, at intervals of 1–2 wk until its maximum antihypertensive dosage is reached. If blood pressure is still not satisfactorily controlled, increase captopril dosage to 100 mg bid or tid and then, if necessary, to 150 mg bid or tid, while continuing the diuretic. Do not exceed 450 mg/day.

Adult: 25 mg tid, administered 1 h before meals, to start, in addition to the usual diuretic and digitalis regimen; if necessary, increase the dosage to 50 mg tid. If heart failure is still not satisfactorily controlled after at least 2 wk, increase the dosage to 100 mg tid or, if necessary, 150 mg tid; usual therapeutic dosage: 50–100 mg tid.

CONTRAINDICATIONS
None known

ADMINISTRATION/DOSAGE ADJUSTMENTS

Initiating therapy for hypertension — Captopril may be used to initiate treatment of hypertension in patients with normal renal function. When planning to give this drug to patients who are currently receiving other antihypertensive agents, discontinue the existing antihypertensive drug regimen (including diuretics) 1 wk before starting captopril, if possible. When captopril is given alone, sodium restriction may be helpful. To avoid excessive hypotension in patients who must continue diuretic therapy, increase salt intake approximately 1 wk before starting captopril, begin with a small dose (6.25 or 12.5 mg), or observe patient for at least 1 h after administering the first dose. Transient hypotension is not a contraindication to further use since this effect should not recur once hypovolemia disappears and blood pressure increases. To begin treatment in patients who require prompt reduction in blood pressure and in patients with severe hypertension (eg, accelerated or malignant hypertension) who cannot interrupt their antihypertensive regimen, discontinue all antihypertensive drugs except diuretics and, under close supervision, promptly substitute captopril; administer the usual starting dosage (25 mg bid or tid) and then, if necessary, increase the daily dose q24h or more frequently, under continuous medical supervision, until a satisfactory response is obtained or the maximum dosage of 450 mg/day is reached. To achieve a satisfactory response, a more potent diuretic, such as furosemide, may be necessary.

Initiating therapy for heart failure — To minimize the risk of hypotension, observe patients closely during the first 2 wk of treatment and whenever the dosage of captopril or the diuretic is increased. For patients who have undergone vigorous diuretic therapy, start with 6.25 or 12.5 mg tid; increase dosage over the next several days, as tolerated, to the usual initial dosage of 25 mg tid.

Patients with significant renal impairment — Reduce initial daily dose; increase dosage in small increments every 1–2 wk, as needed and tolerated. After desired therapeutic effect has been attained, reduce dosage to the minimum effective level. When concomitant diuretic therapy is necessary in a patient with severe renal impairment, use a loop diuretic rather than a thiazide.

WARNINGS/PRECAUTIONS

Neutropenia, agranulocytosis — Captopril has caused myeloid hypoplasia, neutropenia, and agranulocytosis within 3 mo after the start of therapy; oral and systemic infections or other manifestations of agranulocytosis have developed in approximately 50% of patients with neutropenia. On bone marrow examination, erythroid hypoplasia and a decreased number of megakaryocytes have frequently been seen in conjunction with myeloid hypoplasia; in some cases, neutropenia has been accompanied by anemia and thrombocytopenia. Neutropenia has occurred in approximately 0.012% of patients with normal renal function (serum creatinine level <1.6 mg/dl), about 0.2% of patients with renal impairment (serum creatinine level >1.6 mg/dl), and 3.7% of patients with a combination of renal impairment and collagen vascular disease (eg, systemic lupus erythematosus, scleroderma). In over 75% of cases seen during treatment of heart failure, procainamide was given in combination with captopril. Thirteen percent of patients who developed neutropenia while receiving captopril have died; however, almost all of the deaths were associated with one or more of the following complicating factors: serious illness, collagen vascular disease, renal or heart failure, or immunosuppressant therapy.

To reduce the risk of agranulocytosis, instruct all patients to report any sign of infection, such as sore throat or fever. Promptly obtain a WBC count whenever an infection is suspected. If a neutrophil count of less than 1,000/mm^3 is detected, discontinue captopril and closely watch patient; neutropenia generally reverses within 2 wk after termination of therapy. Always assess renal function before beginning therapy. If renal impairment is seen, obtain WBC and differential counts before therapy, every 2 wk during the initial 3-mo period, and then periodically thereafter. In patients who have collagen vascular disease or who are receiving other drugs known to affect leukocytes or the immune response, use with caution and only after weighing benefits and risks, particularly when these patients also have renal impairment.

CAPOTEN

Proteinuria, nephrotic syndrome	Urinary protein exceeding 1 g/day has been seen in approximately 0.7% of patients; the nephrotic syndrome has developed in about 20% of those with proteinuria. Creatinine and BUN levels were seldom affected. In most cases, proteinuria occurred within 8 mo after the start of therapy and, regardless of whether or not therapy was continued, subsided or disappeared within 6 mo after detection. Instruct patients to report any sign of progressive edema that may indicate proteinuria or the nephrotic syndrome. Patients who had a history of renal disease or who received more than 150 mg/day have accounted for 90% of the cases of proteinuria. If captopril is to be used in these patients, obtain estimates of urinary protein before therapy (or before giving 150 mg/day) and then periodically thereafter; use first morning urine samples for these determinations.
Increases in BUN and creatinine	In some patients with hypertension and renal disease, especially those with severe renal artery stenosis, BUN and serum creatinine levels may increase; if necessary, reduce the dosage of captopril and/or discontinue diuretic therapy since it may not be possible to simultaneously maintain both normal blood pressure and adequate renal perfusion. Although stable increases in BUN and serum creatinine levels of about 20% above normal or baseline may develop in about 20% of patients with heart failure, progressive increases may occur in up to 5% of these patients, generally those with severe renal disease, and necessitate discontinuation of treatment. Transient elevations have also been seen, especially in association with hypovolemia, renovascular hypertension, and rapid control of severe or prolonged hypertension.
Hypotension	Although hypotension rarely occurs during antihypertensive therapy, transient decreases in blood pressure of more than 20% occur in about 50% of patients with heart failure; these episodes, which may occur after the first of several doses, are usually well tolerated, producing either no symptoms or brief, mild light-headedness, but in rare instances may result in arrhythmias or conduction defects; the effects lessen in severity after 1–2 wk and generally disappear within 2 mo. During treatment of heart failure *or* hypertension, excessive hypotension may occur in patients with severe hyponatremia or hypovolemia, such as those who undergo diuretic therapy (especially if vigorous or instituted recently), have dialysis treatments, or severely restrict their intake of salt; this effect usually occurs within 1 h after the initial dose. If hypotension occurs during therapy, place patient in a supine position and, if necessary, give normal saline by IV infusion. Caution patients that dehydration owing to excessive perspiration, vomiting, or diarrhea may precipitate hypotension. To avoid excessive hypotension, start treatment of heart failure under very close medical supervision. If possible, discontinue diuretic therapy before beginning antihypertensive therapy with captopril; if a diuretic must be used concomitantly, provide close medical supervision when starting treatment. For other appropriate measures, see ADMINISTRATION/DOSAGE ADJUSTMENTS.
Surgery	In patients undergoing major surgery or receiving anesthetics that can cause hypotension, captopril will block a compensatory increase in angiotensin II; if captopril-induced hypotension occurs, correct by volume expansion
Aortic stenosis	Theoretically, patients with aortic stenosis may be at particular risk of decreased coronary perfusion during therapy because of a smaller reduction in afterload
Physical activity	Caution patients with heart failure against rapid increases in physical activity
Rash	Maculopapular or, in rare cases, urticarial rash has been seen in 4–7% of patients, usually during the first 4 wk of therapy; it occurs frequently with pruritus, sometimes with fever and arthralgia, and, in 7–10% of cases, with eosinophilia or a positive ANA test. Rash is usually mild and generally disappears within a few days after reduction of dosage, short-term use of an antihistamine, or termination of therapy.
Impairment of taste	Dysgeusia, seen in 2–4% of patients, is usually reversible even with continued use and generally disappears within 2–3 mo. Weight loss may occur along with dysgeusia.
Concomitant use of other vasodilators	No information is available on the effects of combining captopril with nitroglycerin or other vasodilators in patients with heart failure. If possible, discontinue use of any drug with vasodilator activity before starting captopril; if use of such drugs is resumed, administer them with caution and perhaps at a lower dosage.
Carcinogenicity, effect on fertility	No evidence of carcinogenicity has been seen in mice and rats given 50–1,350 mg/kg/day for 2 yr; studies in rats have shown no adverse effect on fertility

ADVERSE REACTIONS[1]

Frequent reactions (incidence ≥ 1%) are printed in *italics*

Cardiovascular	*Hypotension; tachycardia, chest pain, and palpitations (1%);* angina, myocardial infarction, Raynaud's syndrome, congestive heart failure, flushing, pallor
Hematological	Neutropenia, agranulocytosis, anemia, thrombocytopenia, pancytopenia
Dermatological	*Rash (4–7%), pruritus (2%),* pemphigoid-like lesions, photosensitivity; angioedema of the face, mouth, or extremities; laryngeal edema (one case)
Renal	Proteinuria, nephrotic syndrome
Hepatic	Hepatocellular injury and cholestatic jaundice (rare)
Other	*Diminution or loss of taste (2–4%),* weight loss

OVERDOSAGE

Signs and symptoms	Excessive hypotension

CAPOTEN ■ VASOTEC

| Treatment | To restore blood pressure, administer normal saline by IV infusion; captopril may be removed from the blood by hemodialysis |

DRUG INTERACTIONS

Diuretics	⇧ Antihypertensive effect; the combined effect of captopril and thiazide diuretics is additive ⇧ Risk of hypotension (see ADMINISTRATION/DOSAGE ADJUSTMENTS)
Adrenergic blockers, ganglionic blockers	⇧ Antihypertensive effect; the combined effect of captopril and beta blockers is less than additive ⇧ Risk of hypotension; exercise caution during concomitant therapy
Potassium-sparing diuretics (see also diuretics interaction, above), potassium supplements, potassium-containing salt substitutes	⇧ Serum potassium level; use potassium supplements or potassium-sparing diuretics with caution and only for documented hypokalemia. Use salt substitutes with caution.
Indomethacin, possibly other nonsteroidal anti-inflammatory agents	⇩ Antihypertensive effect, especially in patients with low renin hypertension

ALTERED LABORATORY VALUES

| Blood/serum values | ⇧ BUN ⇧ Creatinine ⇧ Potassium, especially in patients with renal impairment |
| Urinary values | False-positive for acetone |

USE IN CHILDREN

Although safety and effectiveness for use in children have not been established, captopril may be given to such patients if other antihypertensive measures have not been effective; in limited experience, captopril has been given at a weight-adjusted adult dosage to children 2 mo to 15 yr of age who had secondary hypertension and varying degrees of renal insufficiency

USE IN PREGNANT AND NURSING WOMEN

Pregnancy Category C: captopril has been shown to be embryocidal in rabbits at 2–70 times the maximum human dose (probably as a result of severe hypotension) and has caused a reduction in neonatal survival in rats at 400 times the recommended human dose; no teratogenic effects have been seen in hamsters, rats, or rabbits following administration of large doses. Captopril crosses the human placenta. Use during pregnancy only if the expected benefit justifies the potential risk to the fetus. The concentration of captopril in human milk is approximately 1% of the maternal serum level. Patients should generally not nurse during therapy; if a patient does nurse, exercise caution.

[1] Reactions for which a causal relationship has not been established include renal insufficiency and failure, polyuria, oliguria, urinary frequency, gastric irritation, abdominal pain, nausea, vomiting, diarrhea, anorexia, constipation, aphthous ulcers, peptic ulcers, dizziness, headache, malaise, fatigue, insomnia, dry mouth, dyspnea, cough, alopecia, and paresthesias

---

ANGIOTENSIN-CONVERTING ENZYME INHIBITORS

VASOTEC (enalapril maleate) Merck Sharp & Dohme Rx

Tablets: 5, 10, 20 mg

INDICATIONS

Hypertension

ORAL DOSAGE

Adult: 5 mg once daily to start for patients not on diuretics; if necessary, increase dosage to 10–40 mg/day, given in a single dose or 2 divided doses. In patients unresponsive to a once-daily regimen, consider an increase in dosage or twice-daily administration and, if necessary, addition of a diuretic.

CONTRAINDICATIONS

Hypersensitivity to enalapril

ADMINISTRATION/DOSAGE ADJUSTMENTS

| Initiating therapy for hypertension | When planning to give enalapril to patients who are currently receiving other antihypertensive agents, discontinue the existing antihypertensive drug regimen (including diuretics) 2–3 days before starting enalapril, if possible. To avoid excessive hypotension in patients who must continue diuretic therapy, increase salt intake approximately 1 wk before starting enalapril and begin with a small dose (2.5 mg) to determine whether excessive hypotension will occur. |
| Patients with significant renal impairment | If creatinine clearance (Ccr) ≤ 30 ml/min, use an initial dosage of 2.5 mg once daily; titrate the dosage upward until blood pressure is controlled or a maximum dosage of 40 mg/day is reached. For patients undergoing dialysis, give 2.5 mg on the day of dialysis, and adjust dosage for nondialysis days according to blood pressure response. |

VASOTEC

WARNINGS/PRECAUTIONS

Hypotension — Excessive hypotension has occurred in patients with congestive heart failure and may be associated with oliguria and/or progressive azotemia and, rarely, acute renal failure and/or death. During treatment of hypertension, excessive hypotension has also occurred rarely in patients with severe hyponatremia or hypovolemia, such as those undergoing vigorous diuretic therapy or patients on dialysis. Because of the risk of excessive hypotension in these patients, initiate therapy under very close medical supervision; monitor such patients closely for the first 2 wk of enalapril therapy and whenever the dosage of enalapril or the diuretic is increased.

Caution patient that light-headedness may occur, especially during the first days of treatment; discontinue therapy if actual syncope occurs. If hypotension occurs, place the patient in a supine position and, if necessary, give normal saline by IV infusion. Caution patients that dehydration owing to excessive perspiration, vomiting, or diarrhea may precipitate hypotension. To avoid excessive hypotension, discontinue diuretic therapy 2–3 days before beginning antihypertensive therapy with enalapril. For other appropriate measures, see ADMINISTRATION/DOSAGE ADJUSTMENTS.

Angioedema — Following the first dose of enalapril, angioedema, including potentially fatal laryngeal edema and/or shock, may occur; immediately discontinue therapy if swelling of the face, eyes, lips, or tongue or difficulty in breathing occurs, and institute appropriate supportive therapy

Neutropenia, agranulocytosis — Bone marrow depression and agranulocytosis have occurred rarely in patients taking captopril (another angiotensin converting enzyme inhibitor), primarily in patients with renal impairment and/or collagen vascular disease. Available clinical data are insufficient to show that enalapril does not cause agranulocytosis at a rate similar to that of captopril. Instruct all patients to report any sign of infection, such as sore throat or fever. Monitor WBC count periodically in patients with collagen vascular disease and renal disease.

Increases in BUN and creatinine — In some patients with hypertension and renal disease, especially those with unilateral or bilateral renal artery stenosis, BUN and serum creatinine levels have increased. Some patients with no apparent preexisting renal vascular disease have developed reversible increases in BUN and serum creatinine levels, especially when enalapril was given concomitantly with a diuretic; however, this reaction is more likely to occur in patients with preexisting renal impairment. If necessary, reduce the dosage of enalapril and/or discontinue diuretic therapy, since it may not be possible to simultaneously maintain both normal blood pressure and adequate renal perfusion. Patients with renal artery stenosis should be monitored for changes in renal function during the first few weeks of therapy.

Hyperkalemia — Elevated serum potassium levels ($>$ 5.7 mEq/liter) have been observed in approximately 1% of patients and in some cases have warranted discontinuation of therapy. Patients at highest risk of hyperkalemia include those with renal insufficiency or diabetes mellitus and those using potassium supplements, potassium salt substitutes, or potassium-sparing agents; advise patients not to use potassium supplements or salt substitutes.

Surgery, anesthesia — In patients undergoing major surgery or receiving anesthetics that can cause hypotension, enalapril can block a compensatory increase in angiotensin II; if enalapril-induced hypotension occurs, correct by volume expansion

Carcinogenicity, mutagenicity, effect on fertility — No evidence of carcinogenicity has been seen in rats and male mice given up to 90 mg/kg/day or in female mice given up to 180 mg/kg/day for 2 yr; these dosages represent 150 and 300 times the maximum recommended daily dose for humans. No mutagenic effects have been observed in various studies with enalapril, both in vitro and in vivo. Studies in male and female rats have shown no adverse effect on reproductive performance at dosages ranging from 10 to 90 mg/kg/day.

ADVERSE EFFECTS[1]

Frequent reactions (incidence $\geq$ 1%) are printed in *italics*

Central nervous system — *Headache (4.8%), dizziness (4.6%), fatigue (2.8%),* insomnia, nervousness, paresthesia, somnolence

Gastrointestinal — *Diarrhea (1.6%), nausea (1.3%),* abdominal pain, vomiting, dyspepsia

Cardiovascular — *Hypotension (1.4%), orthostatic effects (1.3%),* syncope, orthostatic hypotension, palpitations, chest pain

Hypersensitivity — *Rash (1.5%),* pruritus, angioedema

Respiratory — *Cough (1.3%),* dyspnea

Other — Decreased hemoglobin and hematocrit, muscle cramps, hyperhidrosis, impotence, asthenia

OVERDOSAGE

Signs and symptoms — Excessive hypotension

Treatment — To restore blood pressure, administer normal saline by IV infusion; enalapril may be removed from the blood by hemodialysis

VASOTEC ■ BLOCADREN

DRUG INTERACTIONS

Diuretics	Excessive hypotension (see "hypotension," above, and ADMINISTRATION/DOSAGE ADJUSTMENTS)
Potassium-sparing diuretics, potassium supplements, potassium-containing salt substitutes	⇧ Serum potassium level; exercise caution and monitor serum potassium frequently

ALTERED LABORATORY VALUES

Blood/serum values — ⇧ BUN ⇧ Creatinine ⇧ Potassium, especially in patients with renal impairment

No clinically significant alterations in urinary values have occurred at therapeutic dosages

USE IN CHILDREN

Safety and effectiveness for use in children have not been established

USE IN PREGNANT AND NURSING WOMEN

Pregnancy Category C: no teratogenic effects have been seen in rats or rabbits. Enalapril caused a decrease in average fetal weight in rats given 1,200 mg/kg/day, but this reaction did not occur when these animals were supplemented with saline. Although maternal and fetal toxicity occurred in rabbits at doses of 1 mg/kg/day or more, saline supplementation prevented these effects at doses of 3 and 10 mg/kg/day, but not at 30 mg/kg/day. No adequate, well-controlled studies have been done in pregnant women. Use during pregnancy only if the expected benefit outweighs the potential risk to the fetus. It is not known whether this drug is excreted in human milk; because many drugs are excreted in human milk, use with caution in nursing mothers.

[1] Reactions for which no causal relationship has been established include elevations of liver enzymes and/or serum bilirubin; rare cases of neutropenia, thrombocytopenia, and bone marrow depression have been reported in overseas marketing studies

---

BETA-ADRENERGIC BLOCKERS

BLOCADREN (timolol maleate) Merck Sharp & Dohme   Rx

Tablets: 5, 10, 20 mg

INDICATIONS	ORAL DOSAGE
Hypertension	**Adult:** 10 mg bid (alone or with a diuretic) to start, followed by up to 60 mg/day, if needed, in 2 divided doses; usual maintenance dosage: 20–40 mg/day
Long-term prophylaxis following acute myocardial infarction, to reduce cardiovascular mortality and the risk of reinfarction in clinically stable patients	**Adult:** 10 mg bid; in the clinical trial, therapy was started 1–4 wk after infarction

CONTRAINDICATIONS

Bronchial asthma or a history of bronchial asthma

Severe chronic obstructive pulmonary disease

Sinus bradycardia

Second- or third-degree AV block

Overt cardiac failure (see WARNINGS/PRECAUTIONS)

Cardiogenic shock

Hypersensitivity to timolol

ADMINISTRATION/DOSAGE ADJUSTMENTS

Frequency of dosage adjustments for hypertension	Do not increase dosage more frequently than once every 7 days; dosage adjustment may require several weeks to obtain optimal antihypertensive effect, as determined by reduction in heart rate and/or blood pressure response
Combination antihypertensive therapy	Timolol may be used alone or in combination with other antihypertensive agents, especially thiazide-type diuretics; observe patient closely when initiating concomitant therapy
Patients with hepatic or renal impairment	May require a reduction in dosage; use with particular caution in patients with marked renal failure who undergo dialysis, since such patients have experienced marked hypotension subsequent to treatment with 20-mg doses

WARNINGS/PRECAUTIONS

Cardiac failure	May be precipitated by further or continued depression of myocardial contractility; discontinue use if cardiac failure persists despite adequate digitalization and diuretic therapy. In cases of well-compensated congestive heart failure, use with caution.

BLOCADREN

Abrupt discontinuation of therapy	May exacerbate angina and in some cases lead to myocardial infarction in patients with ischemic heart disease; caution patients accordingly. When discontinuing chronic administration of timolol, reduce dosage gradually over 1–2 wk and monitor patient carefully. If angina worsens markedly or acute coronary artery insufficiency develops, reinstate timolol promptly and take other appropriate therapeutic measures.
Pulmonary disease	Since timolol can block catecholamine-dependent bronchodilation, it is contraindicated for use in patients with bronchial asthma, a history of bronchial asthma, or severe nonasthmatic chronic obstructive pulmonary disease (COPD) and it is to be used with caution and only if necessary in patients with nonasthmatic bronchospastic disease, a history of such a disorder, or mild-to-moderate nonasthmatic COPD
Patients undergoing anesthesia and major surgery	Beta blockade may augment the risks; gradual withdrawal of beta blockers prior to elective surgery is recommended by some authorities. If necessary, the effects of beta blockade may be reversed during surgery by sufficient doses of such beta-adrenergic agonists as isoproterenol, dobutamine, or norepinephrine.
Diabetes and hypoglycemia	Use with caution in patients subject to spontaneous hypoglycemia and in diabetic patients (especially labile diabetics) who are taking insulin or oral hypoglycemic agents; beta blockade may mask the signs and symptoms of acute hypoglycemia
Thyrotoxicosis	Clinical signs of hyperthyroidism (eg, tachycardia) may be masked; manage patients suspected of developing thyrotoxicosis carefully to avoid abrupt withdrawal of beta blockade, which might precipitate a thyroid storm
Muscle weakness	Beta blockade can cause certain myasthenic signs and symptoms (eg, diplopia, ptosis, generalized weakness) and, in rare cases, may exacerbate myasthenia
Cerebrovascular insufficiency	Since beta blockers affect blood pressure and heart rate, they should be used with caution in patients with cerebrovascular insufficiency; if signs or symptoms suggesting reduced cerebral blood flow are noted, consider discontinuing timolol
Carcinogenicity, mutagenicity	A 2-yr study in male rats showed a statistically significant increase in adrenal pheochromocytomas at 300 times the maximum recommended human dose (1 mg/kg/day), and a lifetime study in female mice showed a statistically significant increase in the overall incidence of neoplasms (including benign and malignant pulmonary tumors, benign uterine polyps, and mammary adenocarcinomas associated with increased serum prolactin levels) at 500 mg/kg/day. Results of various mutagenicity studies were negative.
Impairment of fertility	Administration of timolol at doses up to 150 times the maximum recommended human dose had no adverse effect on the fertility of male or female rats

ADVERSE REACTIONS[1]

Frequent reactions (incidence ≥ 1%) are printed in *italics*

Cardiovascular	*Bradycardia (9.1% [heart rate < 40 beats/min, 5%]), nonfatal cardiac failure [8%], cold hands and feet [8%], claudication [3%], hypotension [3%], arrhythmia (1.1%)*, second- or third-degree AV block [< 1%], sinoatrial block [< 1%], syncope (0.6%), edema (0.6%), chest pain (0.6%), decreased exercise tolerance, cardiac arrest, worsening of angina pectoris, extremity pain, worsening of arterial insufficiency, Raynaud's phenomenon, palpitations, vasodilation, cerebral vascular accident
Central nervous system and neuromuscular	*Fatigue/tiredness (3.4% [fatigue or asthenia, 5%]), dizziness (2.3% [6%]), headache (1.7%)*; asthenia, vertigo, paresthesia, decreased libido, and tinnitus (0.6%); local weakness, exacerbation of myasthenia gravis, arthralgia, depression, nightmares, somnolence, insomnia, nervousness, diminished concentration, hallucinations
Ophthalmic	*Eye irritation (1.1%)*, visual disturbances, diplopia, ptosis, dry eyes
Gastrointestinal	Nausea (0.6% [nausea or digestive disturbances, 8%]), dyspepsia (0.6%), pain, hepatomegaly, vomiting, diarrhea
Respiratory	*Bronchial obstruction [2%], nonfatal pulmonary edema [2%], dyspnea (1.7%)*; bronchial spasm and rales (0.6%); cough
Dermatological	*Pruritus (1.1%)*, rash, skin irritation, increased pigmentation, sweating
Endocrine	Hyperglycemia, hypoglycemia
Genitourinary	Impotence, urination difficulties[2]
Other	Weight loss, decreased hemoglobin and hematocrit (slight), nonthrombocytopenic purpura

OVERDOSAGE

Signs and symptoms	Symptomatic bradycardia, hypotension, bronchospasm, and acute cardiac failure, based on the anticipated effects of excessive beta blockade
Treatment	Discontinue medication. Empty stomach by gastric lavage. For symptomatic bradycardia, administer atropine sulfate (0.25–2 mg IV) to induce vagal blockade; if bradycardia persists, give IV isoproterenol cautiously and, in refractory cases, consider using a transvenous cardiac pacemaker. For hypotension, administer a sympathomimetic amine (eg, dopamine, dobutamine, or norepinephrine); in refractory cases, try glucagon HCl. For bronchospasm, give isoproterenol and possibly also aminophylline. For acute cardiac failure, institute treatment with digitalis, diuretics, and oxygen immediately; in refractory cases, try IV aminophylline, followed, if necessary, by glucagon HCl. For second- or third-degree heart block, use isoproterenol or a transvenous cardiac pacemaker. Hemodialysis may or may not be helpful in removing the drug from the circulation.

BLOCADREN ■ CORGARD

DRUG INTERACTIONS

Calcium antagonists	Hypotension (with oral antagonists, especially nifedipine), left ventricular failure (with oral antagonists, especially verapamil and diltiazem), AV conduction disturbance (with oral or IV antagonists, especially verapamil and diltiazem). Although timolol can be given with an oral calcium antagonist if heart function is normal, this combination should be avoided if heart function is impaired. Exercise caution when administering an IV antagonist with timolol.
Reserpine, other catecholamine-depleting drugs	Hypotension and/or marked bradycardia
Thiazide-type diuretics, other antihypertensive agents	⇧ Antihypertensive effect
Nonsteroidal anti-inflammatory agents	⇩ Antihypertensive effect

ALTERED LABORATORY VALUES

Blood/serum values	⇧ BUN ⇧ Potassium ⇧ Uric acid ⇧ or ⇩ Glucose

No clinically significant alterations in urinary values occur at therapeutic dosages

---

USE IN CHILDREN

Safety and effectiveness for use in children have not been established

USE IN PREGNANT AND NURSING WOMEN

Pregnancy Category C: use during pregnancy only if the anticipated benefit of treatment exceeds the potential fetal risk. An increase in fetal resorption has been observed in mice and rabbits at 1,000 and 100 times the maximum recommended human dose, respectively. While teratogenic effects have not been seen in rodents at doses up to 50 times the maximum recommended human dose, no adequate, well-controlled studies have been done in pregnant women. Because of the potential for serious adverse effects in nursing infants, a decision should be made to either discontinue nursing or discontinue use of this drug, taking into account its importance to the mother.

---

[1] Figures in parentheses are representative of the incidence of adverse reactions that may be expected in a properly selected hypertensive patient population, while those given in brackets represent the reported frequency of reactions among 941 timolol-treated patients with coronary artery disease who were enrolled in a Norwegian multicenter trial to evaluate the cardioprotective effect of timolol following acute myocardial infarction; these reactions, however, can also occur in patients treated for hypertension and *vice versa*. Other reactions associated with beta blocker therapy but not observed with timolol include intensification of AV block (see CONTRAINDICATIONS); reversible mental depression, progressing to catatonia; hallucinations; an acute reversible syndrome characterized by temporal and spatial disorientation, short-term memory loss, emotional lability, slightly cloudy sensorium, and decreased performance on neuropsychometric tests; mesenteric arterial thrombosis; ischemic colitis; agranulocytosis; thrombocytopenic and nonthrombocytopenic purpura; erythematous rash; fever combined with aching and sore throat; laryngospasm; respiratory distress; reversible alopecia; and Peyronie's disease.
[2] Retroperitoneal fibrosis has been reported, but a causal relationship has not been established

---

BETA-ADRENERGIC BLOCKERS

CORGARD (nadolol) Princeton   Rx

Tablets: 40, 80, 120, 160 mg

INDICATIONS

Angina pectoris

ORAL DOSAGE

Adult: 40 mg once daily to start, followed by increments of 40–80 mg/day every 3–7 days until optimal response is achieved, pronounced slowing of heart rate occurs, or a maximum dosage of 240 mg/day is reached; usual maintenance dosage: 40–80 mg once daily

Hypertension

Adult: 40 mg once daily (alone or with a diuretic) to start, followed by increments of 40–80 mg/day, as needed, up to 320 mg/day; usual maintenance dosage: 40–80 mg once daily

CONTRAINDICATIONS

Bronchial asthma	Conduction block greater than first degree	Overt cardiac failure (see WARNINGS/PRECAUTIONS)
Sinus bradycardia	Cardiogenic shock	

ADMINISTRATION/DOSAGE ADJUSTMENTS

Patients with renal impairment	Increase interval between doses as follows: administer q24h when creatinine clearance rate (Ccr) > 50 ml/min; q24–36h when Ccr = 31–50 ml/min; q24–48h when Ccr = 10–30 ml/min; q40–60h when Ccr < 10 ml/min
Combination therapy	May be used at full dosage in combination with other antihypertensive agents, especially thiazide-type diuretics

CORGARD

Discontinuation of therapy	Reduce dosage gradually over 1–2 wk, if possible, and monitor patient closely. Caution patients with angina or hyperthyroidism against interruption or abrupt cessation of therapy (see WARNINGS/PRECAUTIONS).

WARNINGS/PRECAUTIONS

Cardiac failure	May be precipitated by further or continued depression of myocardial contractility; discontinue use (gradually, if possible) if cardiac failure occurs or persists despite adequate digitalization and diuretic therapy. In cases of well-compensated congestive heart failure, use with caution.
Abrupt discontinuation	May exacerbate angina pectoris and, in some cases, lead to myocardial infarction in patients with ischemic heart disease
Impaired response to reflex adrenergic stimuli	May augment the risks of general anesthesia and surgery, resulting in protracted hypotension or low cardiac output, and, occasionally, difficulty in restarting and maintaining heartbeat. If possible, discontinue use well before surgery takes place. Excessive beta blockade occurring during emergency surgery can be reversed by IV administration of a beta-receptor agonist (eg, isoproterenol, dopamine, dobutamine, or norepinephrine).
Diabetes mellitus	Beta blockade may mask symptoms of hypoglycemia and potentiate insulin-induced hypoglycemia; use with caution, especially in patients with labile diabetes
Thyrotoxicosis	Clinical signs of hyperthyroidism may be masked; abrupt withdrawal may precipitate thyroid storm
Nonallergic bronchospasm	Use with caution in patients with bronchospastic diseases, since bronchodilation produced by beta stimulation may be blocked
Hepatic or renal impairment	Use with caution and monitor for signs of excessive drug accumulation (see OVERDOSAGE)

ADVERSE REACTIONS[1]

Frequent reactions (incidence ≥ 1%) are printed in *italics*

Cardiovascular	*Heart rate < 40 beats/min and/or symptomatic bradycardia, peripheral vascular insufficiency (2%); cardiac failure, hypotension, and rhythm and/or conduction disturbances (1%);* first- and third-degree heart block
Central nervous system	*Dizziness and fatigue (2%);* paresthesias, sedation, changed behavior, headache, slurred speech
Respiratory	Bronchospasm, cough, nasal stuffiness
Gastrointestinal	Nausea, diarrhea, abdominal discomfort, constipation, vomiting, indigestion, anorexia, bloating, flatulence, dry mouth
Dermatological	Rash, pruritus, dry skin, facial swelling, diaphoresis, reversible alopecia
Ophthalmic	Dry eyes, blurred vision
Genitourinary	Impotence or decreased libido
Other	Weight gain, tinnitus

OVERDOSAGE

Signs and symptoms	Excessive bradycardia, cardiac failure, hypotension, bronchospasm
Treatment	Empty stomach by gastric lavage. Hemodialysis may be useful. For excessive bradycardia, administer 0.25–1.0 mg atropine; if there is no response to vagal blockade, administer isoproterenol cautiously. For cardiac failure, administer digitalis and a diuretic; IV glucagon may be helpful. For hypotension, administer a vasopressor, such as norepinephrine or (preferably) epinephrine. Treat bronchospasm with a beta$_2$-stimulating agent (eg, isoproterenol) and/or a theophylline derivative.

DRUG INTERACTIONS

Digitalis	⇩ AV conduction
Reserpine, *Rauwolfia* alkaloids	⇧ Risk of vertigo, syncope, or orthostatic hypotension
Insulin, sulfonylureas	Hypo- or hyperglycemic effect; if necessary, adjust antidiabetic dosage
General anesthetics	⇧ Hypotension (see WARNINGS/PRECAUTIONS)

ALTERED LABORATORY VALUES

No clinically significant alterations in blood/serum or urinary values have yet been reported at therapeutic dosages

USE IN CHILDREN

Safety and effectiveness for use in children have not been established

USE IN PREGNANT AND NURSING WOMEN

Pregnancy Category C: embryotoxicity and fetotoxicity have been shown in rabbits, but not in rats or hamsters, at 5–10 times the maximum human dose; women receiving nadolol at parturition have given birth to neonates manifesting bradycardia, hypoglycemia, and associated symptoms. Use this drug during pregnancy only if the expected benefits justify the potential risks to the fetus. Nadolol is excreted in human milk; patients should not nurse during therapy.

[1] Other reactions associated with beta blocker therapy but not observed with nadolol include intensification of AV block (see CONTRAINDICATIONS); reversible mental depression progressing to catatonia; visual disturbances, hallucinations; an acute reversible syndrome characterized by temporal and spatial disorientation, short-term memory loss, emotional lability, slightly clouded sensorium, and decreased performance on neuropsychometric tests; mesenteric arterial thrombosis, ischemic colitis, elevated liver enzymes, agranulocytosis; thrombocytopenic and nonthrombocytopenic purpura; fever combined with aching and sore throat; laryngospasm; respiratory distress, pemphigoid rash, hypertensive reactions in patients with pheochromocytoma, sleep disturbances, and Peyronie's disease

---

BETA-ADRENERGIC BLOCKERS

INDERAL (propranolol hydrochloride) Ayerst   Rx

Tablets: 10, 20, 40, 60, 80, 90 mg **Ampuls:** 1 mg/ml (1 ml)

INDICATIONS	ORAL DOSAGE
Hypertension	**Adult:** 40 mg bid (alone or with a diuretic) to start, followed by gradual increments until optimal response is achieved, up to 640 mg/day; usual maintenance dosage: 120–240 mg/day **Child:** 0.5 mg/kg bid to start, followed by gradual increments until optimal response is achieved, up to 16 mg/kg/day; usual maintenance dosage: 1–2 mg/kg bid
Long-term management of **angina pectoris**	**Adult:** 80–320 mg/day, given in 2–4 divided doses
Cardiac arrhythmias, including supraventricular arrhythmias, ventricular tachycardias, digitalis-induced tachyarrhythmias, and resistant tachyarrhythmias due to excessive catecholamine activity during anesthesia	**Adult:** 10–30 mg tid or qid, before meals and at bedtime
Reduction of cardiovascular mortality in clinically stable patients following **acute myocardial infarction**	**Adult:** 180–240 mg/day, given in divided doses bid or tid; patients with angina, hypertension, or other coexisting cardiovascular diseases may require dosages exceeding 240 mg/day. In clinical studies, long-term therapy was started 5–21 days after infarction.
Migraine prophylaxis	**Adult:** 80 mg/day in divided doses to start, followed, if necessary, by gradual increments, up to 240 mg/day; usual dosage: 160–240 mg/day. If satisfactory prophylaxis is not obtained after giving 240 mg/day for 4–6 wk, discontinue use.
Familial or hereditary **essential tremor**	**Adult:** 40 mg bid to start, followed, if necessary, by increases in dosage, up to 320 mg/day; usual maintenance dosage: 120 mg/day
Hypertrophic subaortic stenosis	**Adult:** 20–40 mg tid or qid, before meals and at bedtime
As an adjunct to alpha-adrenergic blocking agents in the management of **pheochromocytoma**	**Adult:** 60 mg/day in divided doses for 3 days prior to surgery, concomitantly with an alpha-adrenergic blocking agent, or 30 mg/day in divided doses for inoperable tumors

CONTRAINDICATIONS

Sinus bradycardia	Cardiogenic shock	Overt congestive heart failure, unless it results from a tachyarrhythmia treatable with propranolol
Heart block greater than first degree	Bronchial asthma	

ADMINISTRATION/DOSAGE ADJUSTMENTS

Intravenous use — For life-threatening arrhythmias or those occurring under anesthesia in adults, give 1–3 mg IV. To minimize risk of hypotension and possibility of cardiac standstill, administer slowly ($\leq$ 1 mg/min) and monitor ECG and CVP continuously. Initial dose may be repeated after 2 min; thereafter, wait at least 4 h before administering additional propranolol.

INDERAL

Inadequate control of hypertension	Twice-daily dosing is usually effective. Some patients, however, experience a modest rise in blood pressure toward the end of the 12-h dosing interval, especially when lower dosages are used. If control is inadequate, a larger dose or tid therapy may be indicated.
Discontinuation of therapy	Reduce dosage gradually over a period of several weeks; caution patients who experience angina or who may have occult coronary artery disease not to interrupt or discontinue therapy on their own
Tremor	Essential tremor is usually limited to the upper limbs; it appears only when a limb moves or is held in a fixed position against gravity. Propranolol reduces the intensity of tremors, but not their frequency; this drug is not indicated for treatment of tremor associated with parkinsonism.

WARNINGS/PRECAUTIONS

Cardiac failure	Beta blockade may cause or exacerbate cardiac failure; discontinue use if this disorder does not stabilize after diuretic therapy and digitalization. If necessary, propranolol may be given to patients with well-compensated congestive heart failure; observe such patients closely.
Thyrotoxicosis	Propranolol may mask certain clinical signs of hyperthyroidism; abrupt withdrawal may exacerbate manifestations of this disorder and precipitate a thyroid storm
Patients with angina	Abrupt withdrawal in such patients may exacerbate angina and, in some cases, lead to myocardial infarction; reinstitute therapy if withdrawal reactions occur (see ADMINISTRATION/DOSAGE ADJUSTMENTS)
Patients with Wolff-Parkinson-White (WPW) syndrome	Severe bradycardia, necessitating use of a demand pacemaker, has occurred in several patients with WPW syndrome following use of propranolol
Patients with diabetes	Propranolol may mask tachycardia associated with hypoglycemia; however, this drug may not significantly affect other manifestations such as dizziness and diaphoresis. Propranolol may delay return of normal plasma glucose levels following insulin-induced hypoglycemia. Use with caution in patients with diabetes.
Patients with bronchospastic disease	In general, such patients should not receive propranolol because it may block catecholamine-induced bronchodilation. Propranolol is specifically contraindicated for use in patients with bronchial asthma; use with caution in patients with nonallergic bronchospasm (eg, chronic bronchitis, emphysema).
Patients with renal or hepatic impairment	Use with caution in such patients
Major surgery	The necessity or desirability of discontinuing use before major surgery is controversial. Beta blockade can increase the risks associated with general anesthesia and surgery (because cardiac responsiveness to reflex beta-adrenergic stimuli is impaired) and may cause protracted severe hypotension and difficulty in restarting and maintaining the heartbeat. However, beta-adrenergic agonists (eg, dobutamine, isoproterenol) can reverse the effects of propranolol.
Fatigue, lethargy, vivid dreams	Daily doses exceeding 160 mg, given in divided doses of more than 80 mg, may increase the risk of fatigue, lethargy, and vivid dreams
Glaucoma testing	Propranolol can reduce intraocular pressure and thereby affect the results of glaucoma screening tests
Carcinogenicity	No evidence of tumorigenicity has been seen in rats or mice given up to 150 mg/kg/day for a period of 18 mo
Effect on fertility	No impairment of fertility has been observed in animals

ADVERSE REACTIONS

Cardiovascular	Bradycardia, congestive heart failure, AV-block intensification, hypotension, paresthesia of the hands, Raynaud-type arterial insufficiency, purpura
Central nervous system	Light-headedness, depression, insomnia, weakness, fatigue, lassitude, catatonia, visual disturbances, hallucinations, vivid dreams; an acute reversible syndrome characterized by spatial and temporal disorientation, short-term memory loss, emotional lability, slightly clouded sensorium, and decreased neuropsychometric performance
Gastrointestinal	Nausea, vomiting, epigastric distress, abdominal cramps, diarrhea, constipation, mesenteric arterial thrombosis, ischemic colitis
Respiratory	Bronchospasm
Allergic	Pharyngitis, agranulocytosis, erythematous rash, fever with aching and sore throat, laryngospasm and respiratory distress
Other	Alopecia, lupus erythematosus-like reactions, psoriasiform rashes, dry eyes, impotence, and Peyronie's disease (rare); systemic lupus erythematosus (extremely rare)

OVERDOSAGE

Signs and symptoms	Severe bradycardia, cardiac failure, hypotension, bronchospasm

INDERAL ■ INDERAL LA

Treatment	Empty stomach (avoid pulmonary aspiration). For excessive bradycardia, administer 0.25–1.0 mg atropine IV; if there is no response to vagal blockade, administer isoproterenol cautiously. For cardiac failure, administer digitalis and a diuretic. For hypotension, use norepinephrine or (preferably) epinephrine. Treat bronchospasm with isoproterenol and aminophylline. Significant amounts of propranolol cannot be removed by dialysis.

DRUG INTERACTIONS

Reserpine, other catecholamine-depleting drugs	△ Risk of hypotension, marked bradycardia, vertigo, syncope, or orthostatic hypotension; closely observe patients during concomitant therapy
Calcium channel blockers	▽ AV conduction and myocardial contractility; concomitant IV administration of a beta blocker and verapamil has resulted in serious reactions, particularly in patients with severe cardiomyopathy, cardiac failure, or recent myocardial infarction. When using propranolol with a calcium channel blocker, especially IV verapamil, exercise caution.
Phenytoin, phenobarbital, rifampin	▽ Plasma level of propranolol
Cimetidine	△ Plasma level of propranolol
Chlorpromazine	△ Plasma level of propranolol and chlorpromazine
Theophylline, lidocaine, antipyrine	△ Plasma level of theophylline, lidocaine, and antipyrine
Thyroxine	△ Plasma T_4 level (due to decreased peripheral conversion of T_4 to T_3)
Aluminum hydroxide	▽ Absorption of propranolol
Digitalis	▽ AV conduction
Ephedrine, isoproterenol, other beta-adrenergic bronchodilators	▽ Bronchodilation
Thiazide-type diuretics, other antihypertensive agents	△ Antihypertensive effect
Alcohol	▽ Rate of absorption

ALTERED LABORATORY VALUES

Blood/serum values	△ SGOT △ SGPT △ Alkaline phosphatase △ LDH △ T_4 △ rT_3 ▽ T_3 △ BUN (in patients with severe heart disease)

No clinically significant alterations in urinary values occur at therapeutic dosages

---

USE IN CHILDREN

See INDICATIONS and ORAL DOSAGE; do not give IV to children. High plasma drug levels have been detected in patients with Down's syndrome, which suggests that bioavailability may be increased in these patients. If echocardiography is used to monitor therapy, bear in mind that the characteristics of a normal echocardiogram vary with age in children.

USE IN PREGNANT AND NURSING WOMEN

Pregnancy Category C: embryotoxic effects have been observed in animals given approximately 10 times the maximum human dose; no adequate, well-controlled studies have been done in pregnant women. Use during pregnancy only if the expected benefit justifies the potential risk to the fetus. Propranolol is excreted in human milk; use with caution in nursing mothers.

BETA-ADRENERGIC BLOCKERS

INDERAL LA (propranolol hydrochloride) Ayerst Rx

Capsules (long-acting): 80, 120, 160 mg

INDICATIONS	ORAL DOSAGE
Hypertension	**Adult:** 80 mg once daily (alone or with a diuretic) to start, followed, if necessary, by 120 mg or more once daily, up to 640 mg once daily (the full therapeutic effect of a given dosage may not be evident for a few days to several weeks); usual dosage: 120–160 mg/day
Prophylaxis and long-term management of **angina pectoris**	**Adult:** 80 mg once daily to start, followed, if necessary, by gradual increments every 3–7 days, up to 320 mg once daily; usual dosage: 160 mg/day
Prophylaxis of **migraine**	**Adult:** 80 mg once daily to start, followed, if necessary, by gradual increments, up to 240 mg once daily; usual dosage: 160–240 mg/day. If satisfactory prophylaxis is not obtained after giving 240 mg/day for 4–6 wk, discontinue use.

COMPENDIUM OF DRUG THERAPY

INDERAL LA

| Hypertrophic subaortic stenosis | Adult: 80–160 mg once daily |

CONTRAINDICATIONS

| Sinus bradycardia | Cardiogenic shock | Overt congestive heart failure, unless it results from a tachyarrhythmia treatable with immediate-release propranolol |
| Heart block greater than first degree | Bronchial asthma | |

ADMINISTRATION/DOSAGE ADJUSTMENTS

| Switching from immediate-release propranolol | To maintain therapeutic effectiveness, especially at the end of a 24-h dosing interval, it may be necessary to increase the dosage, because the long-acting form produces lower serum propranolol levels. However, retitration may not be required if, in the treatment of a disorder (eg, hypertension, angina), there is little correlation between serum level and therapeutic effect. |
| Discontinuation of therapy | Reduce dosage gradually over a period of several weeks; caution patients who experience angina or who may have occult coronary artery disease not to interrupt or discontinue therapy on their own |

WARNINGS/PRECAUTIONS

Cardiac failure	Beta blockade may cause or exacerbate cardiac failure; discontinue use if this disorder does not stabilize after diuretic therapy and digitalization. If necessary, propranolol may be given to patients with well-compensated congestive heart failure; observe such patients closely.
Thyrotoxicosis	Propranolol may mask certain clinical signs of hyperthyroidism; abrupt withdrawal may exacerbate manifestations of this disorder and precipitate a thyroid storm
Patients with angina	Abrupt withdrawal in such patients may exacerbate angina and, in some cases, lead to myocardial infarction; reinstitute therapy if withdrawal reactions occur (see ADMINISTRATION/DOSAGE ADJUSTMENTS)
Patients with Wolff-Parkinson-White (WPW) syndrome	Severe bradycardia, necessitating use of a demand pacemaker, has occurred in several patients with WPW syndrome following use of propranolol
Patients with diabetes	Adjustment of insulin dosage in patients with labile insulin-dependent diabetes may be more difficult, because propranolol may mask certain clinical signs (eg, changes in pulse rate and blood pressure) of acute hypoglycemia
Patients with bronchospastic disease	In general, such patients should not receive propranolol because it may block catecholamine-induced bronchodilation. Propranolol is specifically contraindicated for use in patients with bronchial asthma; use with caution in patients with nonallergic bronchospasm (eg, chronic bronchitis, emphysema).
Patients with renal or hepatic impairment	Use with caution in such patients
Major surgery	The necessity or desirability of discontinuing use before major surgery is controversial. Beta blockade can increase the risks associated with general anesthesia and surgery (because cardiac responsiveness to reflex beta-adrenergic stimuli is impaired) and may cause protracted severe hypotension and difficulty in restarting and maintaining the heartbeat. However, beta-adrenergic agonists (eg, dobutamine, isoproterenol) can reverse the effects of propranolol.
Glaucoma testing	Propranolol can reduce intraocular pressure and thereby affect the results of glaucoma screening tests
Carcinogenicity	No evidence of tumorigenicity has been seen in rats or mice given up to 150 mg/kg/day for a period of 18 mo
Effect on fertility	No impairment of fertility has been observed in animals

ADVERSE REACTIONS

Cardiovascular	Bradycardia, congestive heart failure, AV-block intensification, hypotension, paresthesia of the hands, Raynaud-type arterial insufficiency, purpura
Central nervous system	Light-headedness, depression, insomnia, weakness, fatigue, lassitude, catatonia, visual disturbances, hallucinations, disorientation, short-term memory loss, emotional lability, slightly clouded sensorium, decreased neuropsychometric performance
Gastrointestinal	Nausea, vomiting, epigastric distress, abdominal cramps, diarrhea, constipation, mesenteric arterial thrombosis, ischemic colitis
Respiratory	Bronchospasm
Allergic	Pharyngitis, agranulocytosis, erythematous rash, fever with aching and sore throat, laryngospasm and respiratory distress
Other	Alopecia, lupus erythematosus-like reactions, psoriasiform rashes, dry eyes, impotence, and Peyronie's disease (rare); systemic lupus erythematosus (extremely rare)

OVERDOSAGE

| Signs and symptoms | Severe bradycardia, cardiac failure, hypotension, bronchospasm |

INDERAL LA ■ LOPRESSOR

Treatment	Empty stomach (avoid pulmonary aspiration). For excessive bradycardia, administer 0.25–1.0 mg atropine IV; if there is no response to vagal blockade, administer isoproterenol cautiously. For cardiac failure, administer digitalis and a diuretic. For hypotension, use norepinephrine or (preferably) epinephrine. Treat bronchospasm with isoproterenol and aminophylline. Significant amounts of propranolol cannot be removed by dialysis.

DRUG INTERACTIONS

Reserpine, other catecholamine-depleting drugs	△ Risk of hypotension, marked bradycardia, vertigo, syncope, or orthostatic hypotension; closely observe patients during concomitant therapy
Digitalis	▽ AV conduction
Ephedrine, isoproterenol, other beta-adrenergic bronchodilators	▽ Bronchodilation
Thiazide-type diuretics, other antihypertensive agents	△ Antihypertensive effect

ALTERED LABORATORY VALUES

Blood/serum values	△ SGOT △ SGPT △ Alkaline phosphatase △ Lactate dehydrogenase △ BUN (in patients with severe heart disease)

No clinically significant alterations in urinary values occur at therapeutic dosages

---

USE IN CHILDREN
Safety and effectiveness for use in children have not been established

USE IN PREGNANT AND NURSING WOMEN
Pregnancy Category C: embryotoxic effects have been observed in animals given approximately 10 times the maximum human dose; no adequate, well-controlled studies have been done in pregnant women. Use during pregnancy only if the expected benefit justifies the potential risk to the fetus. Propranolol is excreted in human milk; use with caution in nursing mothers.

BETA-ADRENERGIC BLOCKERS

LOPRESSOR (metoprolol tartrate) Geigy Rx

Tablets: 50, 100 mg   **Ampuls:** 1 mg/ml (5 ml)   **Prefilled syringes:** 1 mg/ml (5 ml)

INDICATIONS	ORAL DOSAGE	PARENTERAL DOSAGE
Hypertension	**Adult:** 100 mg/day, given in single or divided doses (alone or with a diuretic), to start, followed by weekly (or less frequent) increases until optimal response is achieved, up to 450 mg/day	—
Long-term management of **angina pectoris**	**Adult:** 100 mg/day, given in two divided doses to start, followed, if necessary, by gradual increases at weekly intervals, up to 400 mg/day, until optimal response is obtained or pronounced slowing of the heart rate occurs	—
Reduction of cardiovascular mortality in clinically stable patients following **acute myocardial infarction**	**Adult:** for early treatment of patients who tolerate the full IV dose, 50 mg q6h, beginning 15 min after the last IV dose and continuing for 48 h (if IV therapy is not well tolerated, give 25 or 50 mg q6h, beginning 15 min after the last IV dose or as soon as the clinical condition permits and continuing for 48 h); for late treatment or maintenance therapy following early treatment, 100 mg bid	**Adult:** for early treatment, 5 mg IV every 2 min for a total of 15 mg, followed by oral therapy

CONTRAINDICATIONS

Hypertension and angina	Myocardial infarction	
Sinus bradycardia	Bradycardia (heart rate < 45 beats/min)	Hypotension (systolic pressure < 100 mm Hg)
Second- or third-degree AV block	Significant first-degree AV block (P-R interval ≥ 0.24 s); second- or third-degree AV block	Moderate or severe cardiac failure
Cardiogenic shock		
Overt cardiac failure		

COMPENDIUM OF DRUG THERAPY

LOPRESSOR

ADMINISTRATION/DOSAGE ADJUSTMENTS

Hypertension — Once-daily administration of lower doses (especially 100 mg) may be inadequate to maintain a full antihypertensive effect at the end of the 24-h dosing interval; in these cases, larger doses or more frequent dosing may be necessary. The initial daily dose for patients with bronchospastic disease should be given in 3 divided doses.

Myocardial infarction — Immediately after the hemodynamic condition stabilizes, treatment may be started in a coronary care unit (or a similar unit) with injection of 3 IV doses and oral administration q6h (see "early treatment" in dosage section). During IV administration, blood pressure, heart rate, and the ECG should be carefully monitored; if severe intolerance occurs, metoprolol should be discontinued. Therapy should begin 3–10 days after infarction—as soon as the clinical condition permits—if early treatment is contraindicated, undesirable, or not tolerated (see "late treatment"). Metoprolol should be given for at least 3 mo; although effectiveness beyond this period has not been conclusively established, studies with other beta blockers suggest that treatment should be continued for 1–3 yr.

Oral therapy — Tablets should be given with or immediately after meals. Caution patients not to double the dose after a missed dose and not to interrupt or discontinue therapy on their own.

WARNINGS/PRECAUTIONS

Cardiac failure — Beta blockade may cause or exacerbate cardiac failure (see CONTRAINDICATIONS); carefully monitor hemodynamic function during therapy, and use with caution in patients with congestive heart failure controlled by digitalis and diuretics. If cardiac failure occurs or worsens during treatment and does not respond to digitalis and diuretic therapy, discontinue administration of metoprolol.

Thyrotoxicosis — Abrupt withdrawal of beta blockade can precipitate a thyroid storm in patients with hyperthyroidism; discontinue therapy gradually if thyrotoxicosis is suspected. Beta blockade can mask certain signs of hyperthyroidism, such as tachycardia.

Discontinuation of therapy — When discontinuing chronic administration, especially in patients with ischemic heart disease, reduce dosage gradually over a period of 1–2 wk and monitor patient carefully. In patients with ischemic heart disease, abrupt discontinuation of therapy can exacerbate angina and, in some cases, lead to myocardial infarction. If, after discontinuation, angina markedly worsens or acute coronary insufficiency occurs, reinstate use promptly, at least temporarily, and take other appropriate measures for managing unstable angina. Caution patients not to interrupt or discontinue therapy on their own. Therapy should not be discontinued abruptly in patients treated for hypertension, since coronary artery disease is common and may go unrecognized.

Bradycardia, AV block, hypotension — Use of metoprolol following acute myocardial infarction may result in bradycardia, particularly in patients with inferior infarction, and may also produce hypotension and AV block (significant first-degree block [P-R interval ≥ 0.26 s] or second- or third-degree block). To reverse significant bradycardia (heart rate < 40 beats/min), especially when it is associated with decreased cardiac output, or to treat AV block, give 0.25–0.5 mg of atropine IV; if atropine treatment is unsuccessful, cautious administration of isoproterenol or installation of a pacemaker should be considered. To manage hypotension, characterized by a decrease in systolic pressure to 90 mm Hg or less, carefully evaluate hemodynamic condition (invasive monitoring of central venous, pulmonary capillary wedge, and arterial pressures may be necessary), assess extent of myocardial damage, and institute appropriate therapy, such as balloon counterpulsation or administration of IV fluids or positive inotropic agents. Metoprolol should be discontinued if AV block or hypotension occurs or if atropine fails to reverse bradycardia.

Bronchospasm — Instruct patients to report any difficulty in breathing. If bronchospasm unrelated to congestive heart failure occurs during myocardial infarction (MI) therapy, metoprolol should be discontinued. If necessary, theophylline or a beta$_2$ agonist may be given for bronchospasm; this should be done cautiously, however, because serious cardiac arrhythmias may occur.

In general, patients with bronchospastic disease should not receive beta blockers. However, if other antihypertensive treatment is not effective or tolerated, metoprolol may be used with caution in these patients since the drug has a relative selectivity for beta$_1$ receptors; because this selectivity is not absolute and diminishes at higher doses, a beta$_2$ agonist should be given concomitantly, and the lowest possible dose of metoprolol should be used (see ADMINISTRATION/DOSAGE ADJUSTMENTS). Metoprolol may also be used with extreme caution in patients with bronchospastic disease for MI therapy; however, a beta$_2$ agonist, which may exacerbate myocardial ischemia and the extent of infarction, should not be administered prophylactically to these patients.

Surgery — The necessity or desirability of discontinuing use before major surgery is controversial. Beta blockade can increase the risks associated with general anesthesia and surgery (because cardiac responsiveness to reflex beta-adrenergic stimuli is impaired) and may cause protracted severe hypotension and difficulty in restarting and maintaining the heartbeat. However, beta-adrenergic agonists (eg, dobutamine, isoproterenol) can reverse the effects of metoprolol. Instruct patients to inform their physician or dentist that they are taking metoprolol before undergoing any surgical procedure.

Fatigue — Instruct patients to determine how they react to this drug before they drive or engage in other activities requiring alertness

LOPRESSOR

Patients with diabetes	Beta blockade may mask hypoglycemia-induced tachycardia but may not significantly affect the manifestation of other hypoglycemic reactions, such as dizziness or sweating; use with caution in diabetic patients
Patients with hepatic impairment	Use with caution in patients with impaired hepatic function; approximately 90% of an IV dose and more than 95% of an oral dose are converted to inactive metabolites by the liver
Dry eyes, reversible alopecia, agranulocytosis	Rare instances of these reactions have been reported; consider discontinuing therapy if any such reaction cannot be explained by causes other than the drug
Carcinogenicity, mutagenicity	No evidence of carcinogenicity has been detected in rats fed up to 800 mg/kg/day for 2 yr. A 21-mo study has shown an increase in benign lung tumors (small adenomas) in female mice fed 750 mg/kg/day; however, when this study was repeated, no significant results were observed. The results of all mutagenicity tests with metoprolol have been negative.
Effect on fertility	The fertility of rats has not been affected by administration of up to 55.5 times the maximum human dose of metoprolol

ADVERSE REACTIONS

Frequent reactions (incidence $\geq$ 1%) are printed in *italics*

When used to treat hypertension or angina

Central nervous system, neuromuscular	*Tiredness and dizziness (10%), depression (5%)*, mental confusion, short-term memory loss, headache, nightmares, insomnia, musculoskeletal pain, blurred vision, tinnitus
Cardiovascular	*Shortness of breath and bradycardia (3%)*; cold extremities, arterial insufficiency (usually Raynaud type), palpitations, congestive heart failure peripheral edema, and *hypotension (1%)*
Respiratory	*Wheezing (bronchospasm) and dyspnea (1%)*
Gastrointestinal	*Diarrhea (5%)*; *nausea, dry mouth, gastric pain, constipation, flatulence, and heartburn (1%)*
Dermatological	*Pruritus and rash (5%)*, worsening of psoriasis; reversible alopecia (rare)
Other	Peyronie's disease, agranulocytosis, and dry eyes (rare)

When used to treat myocardial infarction[1]

Central nervous system	*Tiredness (1%)*
Cardiovascular	*Hypotension (27% vs 24% for placebo), bradycardia (16% vs 7% for placebo), first-degree heart block (5% vs 2% for placebo), second- or third-degree heart block (5% vs 5% for placebo), heart failure (28% vs 30% for placebo)*
Respiratory	Dyspnea
Gastrointestinal	Nausea, abdominal pain

OVERDOSAGE

Signs and symptoms	Bradycardia, hypotension, cardiac failure, bronchospasm; cardiovascular instability is generally greater in patients with acute or recent myocardial infarction than in other patients
Treatment	Empty stomach by gastric lavage. For bradycardia, administer atropine IV; if there is no response to vagal blockade, give isoproterenol cautiously. For hypotension, use a vasopressor such as norepinephrine or dopamine. For cardiac failure, administer digitalis and a diuretic; for cardiogenic shock, consider using dobutamine, isoproterenol, or glucagon. Treat bronchospasm with a beta$_2$ agonist and/or theophylline.

DRUG INTERACTIONS

Reserpine, other catecholamine-depleting drugs	⇧ Risk of hypotension (including orthostatic hypotension), marked bradycardia, vertigo, and syncope
Digitalis	⇩ AV conduction
Thiazide-type diuretics, other antihypertensive agents	⇧ Antihypertensive effect

ALTERED LABORATORY VALUES

Blood/serum values	⇧ SGOT ⇧ SGPT ⇧ Alkaline phosphatase ⇧ LDH

No clinically significant alterations in urinary values occur at therapeutic dosages

---

USE IN CHILDREN

Safety and effectiveness for use in children have not been established

USE IN PREGNANT AND NURSING WOMEN

Pregnancy Category C: an increase in postimplantation loss and a decrease in neonatal survival have been seen in rats given up to 55.5 times the maximum human dose of metoprolol; no evidence of teratogenicity or impaired fertility has been observed. No adequate, well-controlled studies have been performed in pregnant women. Use during pregnancy only if clearly needed. A very small amount of metoprolol ($<$ 1 mg/liter) is excreted in human milk; use with caution in nursing mothers.

---

[1] Reactions for which a causal relationship has not been established that have occurred in patients being treated for myocardial infarction include headache, sleep disturbances, hallucinations, visual disturbances, dizziness, vertigo, confusion, reduced libido, rash, exacerbation of psoriasis, unstable diabetes, and claudication. Reactions that are associated with use of other beta blockers include intensification of AV block; reversible mental depression progressing to catatonia; an acute reversible syndrome characterized by temporal and spatial disorientation, short-term memory loss, emotional lability, slightly clouded sensorium, and decreased performance on neuropsychometric tests; agranulocytosis; purpura; and fever combined with aching and sore throat, laryngospasm, and respiratory distress.

BETA-ADRENERGIC BLOCKERS

SECTRAL (acebutolol hydrochloride) Wyeth   Rx
Capsules: 200, 400 mg

INDICATIONS	ORAL DOSAGE
Hypertension	**Adult:** for uncomplicated mild to moderate hypertension, 400 mg/day, given once daily or, in certain cases, in 2 divided doses, to start; for maintenance, 400–800 mg/day or, in some cases, 200 mg/day. To treat refractory or more severe hypertension, administer another antihypertensive agent (eg, a thiazide diuretic) in combination with acebutolol or, alternatively, give 1,200 mg/day of acebutolol in 2 divided doses.
Premature ventricular contractions, including paired and multiform ectopic beats and R-on-T beats	**Adult:** 200 mg bid to start, followed by a gradual increase in dosage; for maintenance, 600–1,200 mg/day

CONTRAINDICATIONS
Overt cardiac failure
Cardiogenic shock
Second- and third-degree AV block
Persistently severe bradycardia

ADMINISTRATION/DOSAGE ADJUSTMENTS

Patients with renal impairment	Reduce recommended daily dose by 50% if creatinine clearance (Ccr) is less than 50 ml/min and by 75% if Ccr is less than 25 ml/min
Elderly patients	A lower maintenance dosage may be necessary for elderly patients, since the bioavailability of acebutolol and its major metabolite, diacetolol, is increased approximately two-fold in these patients. Dosage in elderly patients should not exceed 800 mg/day.

WARNINGS/PRECAUTIONS

Cardiac failure	Beta blockade may exacerbate cardiac failure and, in patients with aortic or mitral valve disease or compromised left ventricular function, may precipitate cardiac failure. Nevertheless, acebutolol may be used with caution in patients with well-compensated congestive heart failure; it should be borne in mind that acebutolol as well as digitalis increase AV conduction time. If cardiac failure occurs during treatment and does not respond to digitalization and diuretic therapy, acebutolol should be discontinued.
Angina	Abrupt withdrawal of certain beta blockers can exacerbate angina and, in some cases, precipitate myocardial infarction and death. Caution patients not to interrupt or terminate therapy on their own. To discontinue acebutolol, even if ischemic heart disease is not evident, gradually withdraw the drug over a period of approximately 2 wk and restrict to a minimum level of physical activity. During this period, carefully observe the patient; if exacerbation of angina occurs, the patient should be hospitalized and acebutolol therapy reinstituted immediately.
Bronchospasm	In general, patients with bronchospastic disease should not receive beta blockers. However, if other antihypertensive treatment is not effective or tolerated, acebutolol may be used with caution in these patients because of its *relative* selectivity for beta$_1$ receptors. For these patients, acebutolol should be given initially at the lowest possible daily dose (preferably in divided doses) since beta$_1$ selectivity diminishes as the dosage is increased; in addition, a bronchodilator (eg, theophylline) or a beta$_2$ agonist should be provided for emergency treatment.
Arterial insufficiency	In patients with peripheral or mesenteric vascular disease, beta blockade may cause or exacerbate symptoms of arterial insufficiency; use with caution in such patients, watching closely for progression of arterial obstruction
Major surgery	The necessity or desirability of discontinuing therapy before major surgery is controversial; beta blockade may prevent arrhythmia during surgery by reducing cardiac responsiveness to reflex stimuli, yet may increase the risk of myocardial depression and cause difficulty in restarting and maintaining the heartbeat. If acebutolol is not withdrawn, use at the lowest possible dosage, and exercise particular care when administering general anesthetics that can depress the myocardium, such as ether, cyclopropane, and trichlorethylene.
Hypoglycemia	Beta blockade may mask certain manifestations of hypoglycemia, such as tachycardia; however, in most cases, symptomatic dizziness and sweating are not significantly affected
Hyperthyroidism	Abrupt withdrawal of beta blockade can precipitate a thyroid storm in patients with hyperthyroidism; since certain clinical signs of this disorder (such as tachycardia) can be masked during therapy, patients should be closely observed during the period of withdrawal, even if thyrotoxicosis is only suspected.
Positive ANA titers	In <1% of patients, positive ANA titers were seen in association with persistent arthralgia or myalgia; these reactions disappeared following discontinuation of therapy
Patients with hepatic impairment	Use with caution in patients with hepatic impairment
Carcinogenicity, mutagenicity, effect on fertility	No evidence of carcinogenicity has been seen in rats and mice fed 15 times the maximum human dose of acebutolol or in rats given up to 1.8 g/kg/day of diacetolol, the major metabolite. Use of acebutolol and diacetolol in the Ames test has resulted in negative findings. No significant effect on reproductive performance or fertility has occurred in rats fed up to 12 times the maximum human dose of acebutolol or given up to 1 g/kg/day of diacetolol.

SECTRAL ■ TENORMIN

ADVERSE REACTIONS[1]	Frequent reactions (≥ 2%) are italicized
Cardiovascular	*Chest pain and edema (2%)*, hypotension, bradycardia, heart failure
Respiratory	*Dyspnea (4%), rhinitis (2%)*, cough, pharyngitis, wheezing
Central nervous system	*Fatigue (11%), headache and dizziness (6%), insomnia (3%), depression and abnormal dreams (2%)*, anxiety, hyper- or hypoesthesia, impotence
Ophthalmic	*Abnormal vision (2%)*, conjunctivitis, dry eyes, eye pain
Musculoskeletal	*Arthralgia and myalgia (2%)*, back pain, joint pain
Gastrointestinal	*Constipation, diarrhea, dyspepsia, and nausea (4%), flatulence (3%)*, vomiting, abdominal pain
Genitourinary	*Urinary frequency (3%)*, dysuria, nocturia
Dermatological	*Rash (2%)*, pruritus

OVERDOSAGE

Signs and symptoms	Extreme bradycardia, advanced AV block, intraventricular conduction defects, hypotension, severe congestive heart failure, seizures, and, in susceptible patients, bronchospasm and hypoglycemia
Treatment	Induce emesis or perform gastric lavage; remove acebutolol from the blood by hemodialysis. For excessive bradycardia, give 1–3 mg of atropine in fractional IV doses. If response to vagal blockade is inadequate, administer isoproterenol; exercise caution since unusually large doses may be necessary. For persistent hypotension, give a vasopressor such as epinephrine, norepinephrine, dopamine, or dobutamine; monitor blood pressure and heartbeat frequently. Treat bronchospasm with a theophylline derivative, such as aminophylline, and/or beta$_2$ agonist, such as terbutaline. For cardiac failure, administer digitalis and a diuretic; glucagon may also be helpful.

DRUG INTERACTIONS

Reserpine, other catecholamine-depleting drugs	⇧ Risk of marked bradycardia and hypotension; watch carefully for vertigo, syncope/presyncope, and other manifestations of orthostatic hypotension
Phenylephrine, phenylpropanolamine, other alpha-adrenergic agonists	⇧ Hypertension; warn patients that this reaction can occur with use of certain OTC cold or decongestant preparations
General anesthetics	⇧ Risk of excessive myocardial depression (see warning, above, concerning major surgery)
Insulin	⇧ Hypoglycemic effect

ALTERED LABORATORY VALUES

Blood/serum values	+ ANA

No clinically significant alterations in urinary values occur at therapeutic dosages

---

USE IN CHILDREN

Safety and effectiveness for use in children have not been established

USE IN PREGNANT AND NURSING WOMEN

Pregnancy Category B: an increase in postimplantation loss (along with a reduction in food consumption and weight gain) has been seen in rabbits given 450 mg/kg/day of acebutolol's major metabolite, diacetolol; no evidence of harm to the fetus has been shown in rats and rabbits at up to 3 times the maximum human dose of acebutolol or in rats at up to 1.8 g/kg/day of diacetolol. Use during pregnancy only if the expected benefit justifies the potential risk to the fetus. In animal studies using acebutolol, no adverse effects on the usual course of labor and delivery have been demonstrated. Acebutolol and diacetolol are excreted in human milk; use by nursing mothers is not recommended.

---

[1] Reactions associated with the use of other beta blockers include intensification of AV block; reversible mental depression progressing to catatonia; an acute reversible syndrome characterized by temporal and spatial disorientation, short-term memory loss, emotional lability, slightly clouded sensorium, and decreased performance on neuropsychometric tests; erythematous rash; fever with sore throat and aching; laryngospasm; respiratory distress; agranulocytosis; purpura; mesenteric artery thrombosis; ischemic colitis; reversible alopecia; and Peyronie's disease.

BETA-ADRENERGIC BLOCKERS

TENORMIN (atenolol) Stuart   Rx

Tablets: 50, 100 mg

INDICATIONS	ORAL DOSAGE
Hypertension	**Adult:** 50 mg/day (alone or with a diuretic) to start, followed in 1–2 wk by 100 mg/day, if needed

COMPENDIUM OF DRUG THERAPY

TENORMIN

Long-term management of **angina pectoris** caused by coronary atherosclerosis — **Adult:** 50 mg once daily to start, followed, if necessary, by 100 mg once daily (the full therapeutic effect may not be seen for 1 wk at a given dosage); maximum dosage: 200 mg given once daily

CONTRAINDICATIONS

- Sinus bradycardia
- Heart block greater than first degree
- Cardiogenic shock
- Overt cardiac failure (see WARNINGS/PRECAUTIONS)

ADMINISTRATION/DOSAGE ADJUSTMENTS

Combination therapy	May be used in combination with other antihypertensive agents, including thiazide-type diuretics, hydralazine, prazosin, and methyldopa
Patients with renal impairment	Administer up to 50 mg/day when creatinine clearance rate (CCr) = 15–35 ml/min and up to 50 mg every other day when CCr < 15 ml/min. Give patients on hemodialysis 50 mg after each dialysis treatment; hospital supervision is needed since marked falls in blood pressure can occur.
Effect on exercise tolerance	The maximum early effect on exercise tolerance occurs with doses of 50–100 mg; at these doses, however, the effect at 24 h is attenuated and averages about 50–75% of that observed with once-daily administration of 200 mg
Cessation of therapy	Withdraw atenolol gradually over a period of 2 wk and observe patient carefully; instruct patient to limit physical activity to a minimum during this time (see WARNINGS/PRECAUTIONS)
Discontinuation of therapy in patients receiving clonidine concomitantly	Discontinue use of atenolol several days before gradually withdrawing clonidine

WARNINGS/PRECAUTIONS

Cardiac failure	May be precipitated by further or continued depression of myocardial contractility; discontinue use if cardiac failure persists despite adequate digitalization and diuretic therapy. In cases of well-compensated congestive heart failure, use with caution.
Patients with angina	Abrupt withdrawal of beta blockers in such patients has exacerbated angina and, in some cases, led to myocardial infarction and ventricular arrhythmias; reinstitute therapy, at least temporarily, if angina worsens or acute coronary insufficiency develops
Bronchospastic disease in patients refractory to or intolerant of other antihypertensive agents	Administer with caution, using the lowest possible dose (50 mg); since $beta_1$ (cardiac) selectivity is not absolute, a $beta_2$-stimulating agent should be made available; if atenolol dosage must be increased, consider divided doses to reduce peak blood levels
Patients undergoing anesthesia and major surgery	Beta blockade may augment the risks. If atenolol is withdrawn before surgery, allow 48 h to elapse between the last dose and anesthesia; if treatment is continued, anesthetic agents that depress the myocardium (eg, ether, cyclopropane, and trichloroethylene) should be used with caution. Excessive beta blockade during surgery may be reversed by cautious administration of a beta-receptor agonist (eg, dobutamine or isoproterenol). Profound bradycardia and hypotension may be corrected with atropine, 1–2 mg IV.
Diabetes and hypoglycemia	Use with caution in diabetic patients; beta blockade may mask some (eg, tachycardia), but not other (eg, dizziness and sweating), symptoms of hypoglycemia. Insulin-induced hypoglycemia is *not* potentiated, nor is recovery of normal blood glucose levels delayed.
Thyrotoxicosis	Clinical signs of hyperthyroidism (eg, tachycardia) may be masked. Abrupt withdrawal may precipitate thyroid storm; if therapy is discontinued, closely monitor patients suspected of developing thyrotoxicosis.
Patients with renal impairment	Use with caution (see ADMINISTRATION/DOSAGE ADJUSTMENTS)
Skin rash and/or dry eyes	Have been associated with use of other beta blockers; consider discontinuing atenolol therapy if any such reaction cannot be explained otherwise and closely follow patient after drug is withdrawn
Carcinogenicity, mutagenicity	Long-term studies in rats and mice treated with doses as high as 150 times the maximum recommended human dose have shown no evidence of carcinogenicity; results of various mutagenicity studies have also been negative
Impairment of fertility	Administration of atenolol in doses as high as 100 times the maximum recommended human dose has had no effect on fertility of male and female rats

ADVERSE REACTIONS[1]

Cardiovascular	Bradycardia, cold extremities, postural hypotension, leg pain
Central nervous system	Dizziness, vertigo, light-headedness, tiredness, fatigue, lethargy, drowsiness, depression, dreaming
Gastrointestinal	Diarrhea, nausea
Respiratory	Wheeziness, dyspnea
Other	Dry eyes

OVERDOSAGE

Signs and symptoms	Bradycardia, congestive heart failure, hypotension, bronchospasm, and hypoglycemia (based on overdosage experience with other beta blockers)
Treatment	Discontinue medication. Empty stomach by gastric lavage, and initiate hemodialysis to eliminate drug from general circulation. For bradycardia, administer atropine or another anticholinergic drug. For second- or third-degree heart block, administer isoproterenol or use a transvenous cardiac pacemaker. Treat congestive heart failure with digitalis, diuretics, and other conventional measures. For hypotension, epinephrine may be useful in addition to atropine and digitalis. For bronchospasm, administer aminophylline, isoproterenol, or atropine. For hypoglycemia, give IV glucose.

DRUG INTERACTIONS

Digitalis	▽ AV conduction time
Reserpine, other *Rauwolfia* alkaloids	Hypotension and/or marked bradycardia
Thiazide-type diuretics, methyldopa, hydralazine, prazosin	△ Antihypertensive effect

ALTERED LABORATORY VALUES

No clinically significant alterations in blood/serum or urinary values occur at therapeutic dosages

USE IN CHILDREN

Safety and effectiveness for use in children have not been established

USE IN PREGNANT AND NURSING WOMEN

Pregnancy Category C: use during pregnancy only if anticipated benefit outweighs potential fetal risk. Atenolol has been shown to produce a dose-related increase in embryonic and fetal resorptions in rats at doses $\geq$ 25 times the maximum recommended human dose. No adequate, well-controlled studies have been done in pregnant women. Atenolol is excreted in human milk at a ratio of 1.5:6.8 when compared to the concentration in plasma; use with caution in nursing women.

[1] Other reactions associated with beta blocker therapy but not observed with atenolol include intensification of AV block (see CONTRAINDICATIONS); reversible mental depression progressing to catatonia; visual disturbances, hallucinations; an acute reversible syndrome characterized by temporal and spatial disorientation, short-term memory loss, emotional lability, slightly clouded sensorium, and decreased performance on neuropsychometric tests; agranulocytosis; thrombocytopenic and nonthrombocytopenic purpura; erythematous rash; fever combined with aching and sore throat; laryngospasm; respiratory distress; reversible alopecia; Peyronie's disease; and Raynaud's phenomenon

---

BETA-ADRENERGIC BLOCKERS

VISKEN (pindolol) Sandoz Pharmaceuticals   Rx

Tablets: 5, 10 mg

INDICATIONS	ORAL DOSAGE
Hypertension	**Adult:** 5 mg bid (alone or combined with other antihypertensives) to start, followed, if necessary, by a dosage increase of 10 mg/day every 3–4 wk, up to 60 mg/day

CONTRAINDICATIONS

Bronchial asthma (see WARNINGS/PRECAUTIONS)	Cardiogenic shock	Overt cardiac failure (see WARNINGS/PRECAUTIONS)
Second- and third-degree heart block	Severe bradycardia	

ADMINISTRATION/DOSAGE ADJUSTMENTS

Combination therapy	Pindolol may be used in combination with other antihypertensive agents, especially with thiazide-type diuretics

WARNINGS/PRECAUTIONS

Cardiac failure	Beta blockade may precipitate cardiac failure in patients with latent cardiac insufficiency and more severe failure in patients with congestive heart failure. Caution patients to report signs or symptoms of impending cardiac failure. If failure persists despite adequate digitalization and diuretic therapy, discontinue use gradually. Use in patients with overt failure is contraindicated; however, if necessary, pindolol can be used with caution in cases of well-compensated congestive heart failure (pindolol does not inhibit the inotropic action of digitalis).
Thyrotoxicosis	Clinical signs of hyperthyroidism (eg, tachycardia) may be masked; manage patients suspected of developing thyrotoxicosis carefully to avoid abrupt withdrawal of beta blockade, which might precipitate a thyroid crisis

VISKEN

Discontinuation of therapy	When discontinuing chronic administration, reduce dosage gradually over a period of 1–2 wk and monitor patient carefully. In patients with ischemic heart disease, abrupt discontinuation can exacerbate angina and, in some cases, lead to myocardial infarction (see also warning, above, concerning thyrotoxicosis). If, after discontinuation, angina markedly worsens or acute coronary artery disease occurs, reinstate use promptly and take other appropriate measures for managing unstable angina. Caution patients not to interrupt or discontinue therapy on their own.
Anesthesia and major surgery	Beta blockade can increase the risks of general anesthesia and surgery, and cause protracted hypotension, low cardiac output, or difficulty in restarting or maintaining the heart beat; beta-adrenergic agonists (eg, isoproterenol, dopamine, dobutamine, or norepinephrine) can reverse these effects. If possible, pindolol therapy should be discontinued *well* before the time of surgery, because increased sensitivity to catecholamines has been observed in patients recently withdrawn from beta-blocker therapy. If emergency surgery is necessary, the anesthesiologist should be informed that the patient is receiving a beta-adrenergic blocker.
Patients with bronchospastic diseases	In general, such patients should not receive pindolol, because it can block catecholamine-induced bronchodilation. Pindolol is specifically contraindicated for use in patients with bronchial asthma; use with caution in patients with nonallergic bronchospasm (eg, chronic bronchitis, emphysema).
Patients with diabetes or hypoglycemia	Beta blockade may mask premonitory signs and symptoms (eg, tachycardia, blood pressure changes) of acute hypoglycemia; this effect is especially important to bear in mind when labile diabetics are being treated with pindolol. Because beta blockade also inhibits the release of insulin in response to hyperglycemia, antidiabetic drug dosage may require adjustment.
Patients with renal or hepatic impairment	Use with caution; renal impairment has only minor effects on pindolol clearance, but hepatic impairment may cause blood levels to increase substantially
Carcinogenicity	No pathological lesions were detected in rats and mice fed up to 59 and 124 mg/kg/day (50 and 100 times the maximum human dose), respectively, for 2 yr
Effect on fertility	Testicular atrophy and decreased spermatogenesis have been observed in rats given 30 mg/kg/day; however, it is not clear that such reactions are drug-related

ADVERSE REACTIONS[1]

Frequent reactions (> 2%) are italicized

Central nervous system	*Insomnia (19%), dizziness (17%), fatigue (15%), nervousness (11%), bizarre or many dreams (8%), weakness (7%), anxiety (4%), lethargy (3%),* hallucinations (1%)
Autonomic nervous system	*Paresthesia (5%), visual disturbances (4%),* hyperhidrosis
Cardiovascular	*Edema (11%), weight gain (3%), palpitations and heart failure (2%),* bradycardia, claudication, cold extremities, heart block, hypotension, syncope, tachycardia
Respiratory	*Dyspnea (9%),* wheezing
Musculoskeletal	*Muscle pain (12%), joint pain (11%), muscle cramps (8%), chest pain (5%)*
Gastrointestinal	*Abdominal discomfort and nausea (7%),* diarrhea, vomiting
Dermatological	Pruritus and rash (2%)
Genitourinary	Impotence, pollakiuria
Other	Discomfort or burning of the eyes

OVERDOSAGE

Signs and symptoms	Excessive bradycardia, cardiac failure, hypotension, bronchospasm; increased blood pressure and heart rate ($\geq$ 80 beats/min) occurred in one case after intake of 500 mg (recovery was uneventful)
Treatment	Discontinue medication and empty stomach by gastric lavage. For excessive bradycardia, use atropine; if there is no response to vagal blockade, cautiously administer isoproterenol. For cardiac failure, digitalize patient and/or use a diuretic (glucagon may also be helpful). For hypotension, use a vasopressor such as norepinephrine or (preferably) epinephrine, with serial monitoring of blood pressure. For bronchospasm, use a beta$_2$-adrenergic agonist (eg, isoproterenol) and/or a theophylline derivative.

DRUG INTERACTIONS

Digitalis	Excessive bradycardia, with possible heart block
Reserpine, other catecholamine-depleting drugs	Hypotension and/or marked bradycardia
Thiazide-type diuretics, other antihypertensive agents	⇧ Antihypertensive effect

ALTERED LABORATORY VALUES

Blood/serum values	⇧ SGOT ⇧ SGPT ⇧ Alkaline phosphatase (rare) ⇧ Lactate dehydrogenase (rare) ⇧ Uric acid (rare)

VISKEN ■ CALAN

No clinically significant alterations in urinary values occur at therapeutic dosages

USE IN CHILDREN

Safety and effectiveness for use in children have not been established

USE IN PREGNANT AND NURSING WOMEN

Pregnancy Category B: use during pregnancy only if the expected benefit justifies the potential risk to the fetus. Reproduction studies in rats and rabbits given more than 100 times the maximum recommended human dose have shown no evidence of embryotoxicity or teratogenicity. Increased mortality of offspring in rats has been reported following administration of 30 and 100 mg/kg/day prior to mating through day 21 of lactation; although increased prenatal mortality has been reported at 10 mg/kg/day, a clear dose-response relationship has not been established. No adequate, well-controlled studies have been performed in pregnant women. Pindolol is excreted in human milk; women receiving this drug should not nurse.

[1] Other reactions attributed to beta-blocker therapy but that have not been observed specifically with pindolol include: reversible mental depression, progressing to catatonia; an acute reversible syndrome characterized by temporal and spatial disorientation, short-term memory loss, emotional lability, slightly cloudy sensorium, and decreased performance on neuropsychometric tests; intensification of AV block (see CONTRAINDICATIONS); mesenteric arterial thrombosis; ischemic colitis; agranulocytosis; thrombocytopenic and nonthrombocytopenic purpura; erythematous rash; fever combined with aching and sore throat; laryngospasm; respiratory distress; reversible alopecia; and Peyronie's disease

---

CALCIUM ANTAGONISTS

CALAN (verapamil hydrochloride) Searle   Rx

Tablets: 80, 120 mg

INDICATIONS	ORAL DOSAGE
Angina at rest, including vasospastic (Prinzmetal's variant) and unstable (crescendo, preinfarction) angina **Chronic stable angina** (classic effort-associated angina)	**Adult:** 80–120 mg tid, followed by daily or weekly increases in dosage, up to 480 mg/day, as needed, until optimum clinical response is obtained
Control of ventricular rate in digitalized patients with chronic atrial flutter and/or atrial fibrillation	**Adult:** 240–320 mg/day, given in divided doses tid or qid
Prophylaxis of repetitive paroxysmal supraventricular tachycardia in undigitalized patients	**Adult:** 240–480 mg/day
Essential hypertension	**Adult:** 240 mg/day to start, given in equally divided doses tid

CALAN SR (verapamil hydrochloride) Searle   Rx

Caplets (sustained release): 240 mg

INDICATIONS	ORAL DOSAGE
Essential hypertension	**Adult:** 240 mg/day, given in a single morning dose; if an adequate response is not obtained, titrate the dosage upward by giving 240 mg each morning to start, followed by 240 mg each morning plus 120 mg each evening, and then 240 mg q12h

CONTRAINDICATIONS

Severe left ventricular dysfunction	Second- or third-degree AV block (except in patients with a functioning artificial ventricular pacemaker)	Sick sinus syndrome (except in patients with a functioning artificial ventricular pacemaker)
Accessory bypass tracts (Wolff-Parkinson-White, Lown-Ganong-Levine syndromes), when associated with atrial fibrillation	Hypotension (systolic pressure < 90 mm Hg)	Cardiogenic shock

ADMINISTRATION/DOSAGE ADJUSTMENTS

Titration of dosage	Starting treatment at 40 mg tid should be considered in anginal and hypertensive patients who may exhibit an increased response to verapamil as a result of hepatic dysfunction, advanced age, small body size, or other conditions. Titrate dosage upward based on therapeutic efficacy and safety, evaluated approximately 8 h after the immediate-release tablets are taken or 24 h after the sustained-release formulation has been taken. Since the half-life of verapamil increases with repeated administration, the maximum response may be delayed during chronic dosing. In general, the maximum antiarrhythmic effect of this drug will be apparent during the first 48 h of administration, whereas the antihypertensive effect should be evident within the first week of therapy.
Timing of administration	The sustained-release formulation should be administered with food; the immediate-release tablets may be taken without regard to meals

COMPENDIUM OF DRUG THERAPY

Switching formulations	The total daily dose of verapamil may remain the same when switching from the immediate-release to the sustained-release form
Concomitant therapy	Concomitant use of this drug with both short- and long-acting nitrates may be beneficial in patients with angina and is apparently free of harmful drug interactions. Concomitant use of verapamil with beta blockers may also be beneficial in certain patients with chronic stable angina or hypertension, but the combination can adversely affect cardiac function (see WARNINGS/PRECAUTIONS). Monitor vital signs and clinical status closely, and reassess the need for concomitant beta-blocker therapy periodically.

WARNINGS/PRECAUTIONS

Heart failure	Control heart failure with digitalis and/or diuretics before giving verapamil; do not administer to patients with severe left ventricular dysfunction (ejection fraction < 30%), patients with moderate to severe cardiac failure, or those with any degree of ventricular dysfunction who are concomitantly receiving a beta blocker.
Hypotension	Blood pressure may fall in some patients and may result in dizziness or symptomatic hypotension; decreases in blood pressure below normal levels are unusual in hypertensive patients. If severe hypotension occurs, administer isoproterenol, norepinephrine, atropine, or 10% calcium gluconate immediately *(in patients with hypertrophic cardiomyopathy [IHSS], use phenylephrine, metaraminol, or methoxamine, instead of isoproterenol or norepinephrine, to maintain blood pressure)*. If further support is needed, administer dopamine or dobutamine.
Hepatotoxicity	Elevations of SGOT, SGPT, alkaline phosphatase, and bilirubin levels have been reported. In some cases, these increases have been transient. However, in several patients, drug-induced hepatocellular injury has been reported; half of these patients experienced malaise, fever, and/or right quadrant pain as well as elevated hepatic enzyme levels. To reduce the risk of hepatotoxicity, periodically monitor liver function in all patients.
Rapid ventricular response, fibrillation	In some patients with paroxysmal and/or chronic atrial flutter or atrial fibrillation and an accessory AV pathway (eg, Wolff-Parkinson-White or Lown-Ganong-Levine syndrome), IV verapamil may produce a very rapid ventricular response or ventricular fibrillation following increased antegrade conduction; treat with DC cardioversion. While these risks have not been established with oral verapamil, use in this patient group is contraindicated.
Atrioventricular block	The effect of this drug on AV conduction and the SA node may cause asymptomatic first-degree AV block and transient bradycardia, sometimes accompanied by nodal escape rhythms; prolongation of the P-R interval is correlated with plasma concentrations of verapamil, especially during early titration of therapy. If marked first-degree block occurs, reduce dosage or discontinue verapamil administration and institute appropriate therapy (see suggested management of severe hypotension, above).
Impairment of neuromuscular transmission	Verapamil reportedly decreases neuromuscular transmission in patients with Duchenne's muscular dystrophy; the drug may also enhance the effects of neuromuscular blockers and delay reversal of vecuronium-induced blockade. A decrease in dosage may be necessary for patients with attenuated neuromuscular transmission; when verapamil is given in combination with a neuromuscular blocker, it may be necessary to reduce the dosage of one or both of the drugs.
Patients with hypertrophic cardiomyopathy (IHSS)	Serious adverse effects, including pulmonary edema and/or severe hypotension, sinus bradycardia, second-degree AV block, and sinus arrest, may occur in these patients; reduce dosage if adverse effects occur or discontinue therapy, if necessary
Drug accumulation	Use with caution in patients with significant renal or hepatic impairment; administer 30% of the usual dose to patients with hepatic impairment. Carefully monitor patients for abnormal prolongation of the P-R interval or other signs of overdosage (see below).
Carcinogenicity	Studies in rate fed verapamil at doses of 10, 35, and 120 mg/kg/day for 2 yr showed no evidence of carcinogenic potential; verapamil has shown no evidence of tumorigenicity in rats given 6 times the maximum human dose for 18 mo
Mutagenicity	Verapamil has shown no evidence of mutagenicity in the Ames test
Effect on fertility	Studies in female rats fed 5.5 times the recommended human dose of verapamil showed no evidence of impaired fertility; the effect of this drug on male fertility has not been determined

ADVERSE REACTIONS[1]

Frequent reactions (incidence ≥ 1%) are printed in *italics*

Cardiovascular	*Hypotension (2.5%), edema (2.1%), congestive heart failure/pulmonary edema (1.8%), bradycardia (< 50 beats/min) (1.4%), first, second, and third-degree AV block (1.3%),* third-degree AV block alone (0.8%), flushing (0.1%)
Gastrointestinal	*Constipation (8.4%), nausea (2.7%),* elevation of liver enzyme levels
Central nervous system	*Dizziness (3.5%), headache (1.9%), fatigue (1.7%)*

CALAN ■ ISOPTIN

OVERDOSAGE

Signs and symptoms	Abnormal prolongation of P-R interval, severe hypotension, second- or third-degree AV block, asystole
Treatment	Institute standard supportive measures (eg, IV fluids). Administer beta-adrenergic stimulating agents or parenteral calcium solutions to increase calcium ion flux across the slow channel. Treat clinically significant hypotensive reactions or fixed high-degree AV block with vasopressors or cardiac pacing, respectively. Treat asystole with usual measures, including cardiopulmonary resuscitation.

DRUG INTERACTIONS

Beta blockers	△ Antianginal and antihypertensive effect △ Risk of negative inotropic, chronotropic, or dromotropic effects during high-dose beta-blocker therapy; closely monitor patients during concomitant therapy. Avoid concomitant use in patients with AV conduction abnormalities and those with depressed left ventricular function ▽ Clearance of metoprolol
Digitalis	△ Serum digoxin level and digitalis toxicity; reduce dosage or discontinue use, if necessary
Oral antihypertensive agents (eg, vasodilators, angiotensin-converting enzyme inhibitors, diuretics, beta blockers)	△ Reduction of blood pressure; monitor patient during concomitant therapy
Prazosin	Excessive hypotension
Disopyramide	△ Risk of decreased myocardial contractility; do not give disopyramide within 48 h before or 24 h after administration of verapamil
Quinidine	Significant hypotension in patients with hypertrophic cardiomyopathy (IHSS); avoid concomitant use in these patients △ Serum levels of quinidine ▽ Pharmacologic effects of quinidine on AV conduction
Cimetidine	▽ Clearance of verapamil
Lithium	▽ Serum levels of lithium; adjust dosage of lithium, if necessary
Carbamazepine	△ Serum levels of carbamazepine, possibly leading to diplopia, headache, ataxia, or dizziness
Rifampin	▽ Bioavailability of rifampin
Inhalation anesthetics	▽ Cardiovascular activity; titrate dose of each agent carefully
Curare-like and depolarizing neuromuscular blocking agents	△ Neuromuscular blockade; decrease dosage of one or both agents, if necessary
Nitrates	△ Antianginal effect

ALTERED LABORATORY VALUES

Blood/serum values	△ SGOT △ SGPT △ Alkaline phosphatase △ Bilirubin

No clinically significant alterations in urinary values occur at therapeutic dosages

USE IN CHILDREN

Safety and effectiveness for use in children under 18 yr of age have not been established

USE IN PREGNANT AND NURSING WOMEN

Pregnancy Category C: reproductive studies in rabbits and rats at oral doses up to 1.5 and 6 times the oral human dose, respectively, have shown no evidence of teratogenicity; in the rat, however, the drug caused hypotension, was embryocidal, and retarded fetal growth and development. Verapamil crosses the placental barrier and can be detected in umbilical vein blood at delivery; it is not known whether verapamil administration during labor and delivery has any immediate or delayed adverse effect on the fetus, prolongs labor, or increases the need for obstetric intervention. No adequate, well-controlled studies have been performed in pregnant women; use during pregnancy only if clearly needed. Verapamil is excreted in human milk; patients who are taking this drug should not nurse.

[1] Reactions for which a causal relationship is uncertain include angina pectoris, chest pain, claudication, myocardial infarction, palpitations, purpura (vasculitis), syncope, diarrhea, dry mouth, GI distress, gingival hyperplasia, ecchymosis, bruising, confusion, equilibrium disorders, insomnia, muscle cramps, paresthesia, psychotic symptoms, shakiness, somnolence; dyspnea, arthralgia and rash, exanthema, hair loss, hyperkeratosis, macules, sweating, urticaria, blurred vision, gynecomastia, increased urination, spotty menstruation; and impotence (reported only with sustained-release form)

CALCIUM ANTAGONISTS

ISOPTIN (verapamil hydrochloride) Knoll   Rx

Tablets: 80, 120 mg

INDICATIONS

Angina at rest, including vasospastic (Prinzmetal's variant) and unstable (crescendo, preinfarction) angina
Chronic stable angina (classic effort-associated angina)

ORAL DOSAGE

Adult: 80–120 mg tid, followed by daily or weekly increases in dosage, up to 480 mg/day, as needed, until optimum clinical response is obtained

ISOPTIN

Control of ventricular rate in digitalized patients with chronic atrial flutter and/or atrial fibrillation	Adult: 240–320 mg/day, given in divided doses tid or qid
Prophylaxis of repetitive paroxysmal supraventricular tachycardia in undigitalized patients	Adult: 240–480 mg/day
Essential hypertension	Adult: 240 mg/day to start, given in equally divided doses tid

ISOPTIN SR (verapamil hydrochloride) Knoll   Rx
Tablets (sustained release): 240 mg

INDICATIONS
Essential hypertension

ORAL DOSAGE
Adult: 240 mg/day, given in a single morning dose; if an adequate response is not obtained, titrate the dosage upward by giving 240 mg each morning to start, followed by 240 mg each morning plus 120 mg each evening, and then 240 mg q12h

CONTRAINDICATIONS

Severe left ventricular dysfunction	Second- or third-degree AV block (except in patients with a functioning artificial ventricular pacemaker)	Sick sinus syndrome (except in patients with a functioning artificial ventricular pacemaker)
Hypotension (systolic pressure < 90 mm Hg)	Cardiogenic shock	

ADMINISTRATION/DOSAGE ADJUSTMENTS

Titration of dosage	Starting treatment at 40 mg tid should be considered in anginal and hypertensive patients who may exhibit an increased response to verapamil as a result of hepatic dysfunction, advanced age, small body size, or other conditions. Titrate dosage upward based on therapeutic efficacy and safety, evaluated approximately 8 h after the immediate-release tablets are taken or 24 h after the sustained-release formulation has been taken. Since the half-life of verapamil increases with repeated administration, the maximum response may be delayed during chronic dosing. In general, the maximum antiarrhythmic effect of this drug will be apparent during the first 48 h of administration, whereas the antihypertensive effect should be evident within the first week of therapy.
Timing of administration	The sustained-release formulation should be administered with food; the immediate-release tablets may be taken without regard to meals
Switching formulations	The total daily dose of verapamil may remain the same when switching from the immediate-release to the sustained-release form
Concomitant therapy	Concomitant use of this drug with both short- and long-acting nitrates may be beneficial in patients with angina and is apparently free of harmful drug interactions. Concomitant use of verapamil with beta blockers may also be beneficial in certain patients with chronic stable angina or hypertension, but the combination can adversely affect cardiac function (see WARNINGS/PRECAUTIONS). Monitor vital signs and clinical status closely, and reassess the need for concomitant beta-blocker therapy periodically.

WARNINGS/PRECAUTIONS

Heart failure	Control heart failure with digitalis and/or diuretics before giving verapamil; do not administer to patients with severe left ventricular dysfunction (ejection fraction < 30%), patients with moderate to severe cardiac failure, or those with significant ventricular dysfunction who are concomitantly receiving a beta blocker.
Hypotension	Blood pressure may fall in some patients and may result in dizziness or symptomatic hypotension; decreases in blood pressure below normal levels are unusual in hypertensive patients (tilt table testing [60°] has not induced orthostatic hypotension). If severe hypotension occurs, administer isoproterenol, norepinephrine, atropine, or 10% calcium gluconate immediately *(in patients with hypertrophic cardiomyopathy [IHSS], use phenylephrine, metaraminol, or methoxamine, instead of isoproterenol or norepinephrine, to maintain blood pressure)*. If further support is needed, administer dopamine or dobutamine.
Hepatotoxicity	Elevations of SGOT, SGPT, alkaline phosphatase, and bilirubin levels have been reported. In some cases, these increases have been transient. However, in several patients, drug-induced hepatocellular injury has been reported; half of these patients experienced malaise, fever, and/or right quadrant pain, as well as elevated hepatic enzyme levels. To reduce the risk of hepatotoxicity, periodically monitor liver function in all patients.
Rapid ventricular response, fibrillation	In patients with paroxysmal and/or chronic atrial flutter or atrial fibrillation and an accessory AV pathway (eg, Wolff-Parkinson-White or Lown-Ganong-Levine syndrome), IV verapamil may produce a very rapid ventricular response or ventricular fibrillation following increased antegrade conduction; treat with DC cardioversion. While these effects have not been reported with oral verapamil, they should be considered during therapy.
Antrioventricular block	The effect of this drug on AV conduction and the SA node may cause asymptomatic first-degree AV block and transient bradycardia, sometimes accompanied by nodal escape rhythms; prolongation of the P-R interval is correlated with plasma concentrations of verapamil, especially during early titration of therapy. If marked first-degree block occurs, reduce dosage or discontinue verapamil administration and institute appropriate therapy (see suggested management of severe hypotension, above).

ISOPTIN

Patients with hypertrophic cardiomyopathy (IHSS)	Serious adverse effects, including pulmonary edema and/or severe hypotension, sinus bradycardia, second-degree AV block, and sinus arrest, may occur in these patients; reduce dosage if adverse effects occur or discontinue therapy, if necessary
Drug accumulation	Use with caution in patients with significant renal or hepatic impairment; administer 30% of the usual dose to patients with hepatic impairment. Carefully monitor patients for abnormal prolongation of the P-R interval or other signs of overdosage (see below).
Carcinogenicity	Studies in rats fed verapamil at doses of 10, 35, and 120 mg/kg/day for 2 yr showed no evidence of carcinogenic potential; verapamil has shown no evidence of tumorigenicity in rats given 6 times the maximum human dose for 18 mo
Mutagenicity	Verapamil has shown no evidence of mutagenicity in the Ames test
Effect on fertility	Studies in female rats fed 5.5 times the recommended human dose of verapamil showed no evidence of impaired fertility; the effect of this drug on male fertility has not been determined

ADVERSE REACTIONS[1]

Frequent reactions (incidence ≥ 1%) are printed in *italics*

Cardiovascular	*Hypotension (2.5%), edema (2.1%), congestive heart failure/pulmonary edema (1.8%), bradycardia (< 50 beats/min) (1.4%); first, second, and third-degree AV block (1.3%);* third-degree AV block (0.8%), flushing (0.1%)
Gastrointestinal	*Constipation (8.4%), nausea (2.7%),* elevation of liver enzyme levels
Central nervous system	*Dizziness (3.5%), headache (1.9%), fatigue (1.7%)*

OVERDOSAGE

Signs and symptoms	Abnormal prolongation of P-R interval, severe hypotension, second- or third-degree AV block, asystole
Treatment	Institute standard supportive measures (eg, IV fluids). Administer beta-adrenergic stimulating agents or parenteral calcium solutions to increase calcium ion flux across the slow channel. Treat clinically significant hypotensive reactions or high-degree AV block with vasopressors or cardiac pacing, respectively. Treat asystole with usual measures, including cardiopulmonary resuscitation.

DRUG INTERACTIONS

Beta blockers	△ Antianginal and antihypertensive effects △ Risk of negative inotropic and chronotropic effects during high-dose beta-blocker therapy; closely monitor patients during concomitant therapy ▽ Clearance of metoprolol
Digoxin	△ Serum digoxin level and digitalis toxicity; reduce dosage or discontinue use of digoxin, if necessary
Oral antihypertensive agents (eg, vasodilators, angiotensin-converting enzyme inhibitors, diuretics, beta blockers)	△ Reduction of blood pressure; monitor patient during concomitant therapy
Prazosin	Excessive hypotension
Disopyramide	△ Risk of decreased myocardial contractility; do not give disopyramide within 48 h before or 24 h after administration of verapamil
Quinidine	Significant hypotension in patients with hypertrophic cardiomyopathy (IHSS); avoid concomitant use in these patients △ Serum levels of quinidine ▽ Pharmacologic effects of quinidine on AV conduction
Cimetidine	▽ Clearance of verapamil △ Elimination half-life of verapamil
Lithium	▽ Serum levels of lithium; adjust dosage of lithium, if necessary
Carbamazepine	△ Serum levels of carbamazepine
Rifampin	▽ Bioavailability of rifampin
Neuromuscular blocking agents, inhalation anesthetics	△ Pharmacologic activity of neuromuscular blocking agents and inhalation anesthetics
Nitrates	△ Antianginal effect of verapamil and nitrates

ALTERED LABORATORY VALUES

Blood/serum values	△ SGOT △ SGPT △ Alkaline phosphatase △ Bilirubin

No clinically significant alterations in urinary values occur at therapeutic dosages

USE IN CHILDREN

Safety and effectiveness for use in children under 18 yr of age have not been established

USE IN PREGNANT AND NURSING WOMEN

Pregnancy Category C: reproductive studies in rabbits and rats at oral doses up to 1.5 and 6 times the oral human dose, respectively, have shown no evidence of teratogenicity; in the rat, however, the drug caused hypotension, was embryocidal, and retarded fetal growth and development. Verapamil crosses the placental barrier and can be detected in umbilical vein blood at delivery; it is not known whether verapamil administration during labor and delivery has any immediate or delayed adverse effect on the fetus, prolongs labor, or increases the need for obstetric intervention. No adequate, well-controlled studies have been performed in pregnant women; use during pregnancy only if clearly needed. Verapamil is excreted in human milk; patients who are taking this drug should not nurse.

[1] Reactions for which a causal relationship is uncertain include angina pectoris, chest pain, claudication, myocardial infarction, palpitations, purpura (vasculitis), syncope, diarrhea, dry mouth, GI distress, gingival hyperplasia, ecchymosis, bruising, confusion, equilibrium disorders, insomnia, muscle cramps, paresthesia, psychotic symptoms, shakiness, somnolence; dyspnea, arthralgia and rash, exanthema, hair loss, hyperkeratosis, maculae, sweating, urticaria, blurred vision, gynecomastia, increased urination, spotty menstruation; cerebrovascular accident and impotence (reported only with sustained-release form)

ALDOMET

CENTRAL ALPHA$_2$-ADRENERGIC AGONISTS

ALDOMET (methyldopa) Merck Sharp & Dohme Rx

Tablets: 125, 250, 500 mg **Suspension (per 5 ml):** 250 mg[1] (473 ml) *citric orange-pineapple flavored* **Vials (per 5 ml):** 250 mg methyldopate hydrochloride (5 ml)

INDICATIONS	ORAL DOSAGE	PARENTERAL DOSAGE
Hypertension	**Adult:** 250 mg bid or tid to start, followed by up to 3 g/day in 2–4 divided doses; usual maintenance dosage: 500 mg to 2 g/day **Child:** 10 mg/kg/day in 2–4 divided doses to start, followed by divided doses totalling up to 65 mg/kg/day or 3 g/day, whichever is less	**Adult:** 250–500 mg IV q6h, as needed, up to 1 g q6h **Child:** 20–40 mg/kg/day IV, given in divided doses q6h, as needed, up to 65 mg/kg/day or 3 g/day, whichever is less
Hypertensive crisis	—	**Adult:** same as adult's dosage above **Child:** same as child's dosage above

CONTRAINDICATIONS		
Active hepatic disease, including acute hepatitis and active cirrhosis	Liver disorders associated with prior methyldopa therapy	Hypersensitivity to any component (see WARNINGS/PRECAUTIONS)

ADMINISTRATION/DOSAGE ADJUSTMENTS

Initiating therapy	Allow at least 48 h between dosage adjustments. Increase or decrease dosage until optimal blood pressure response is obtained; to minimize sedation, increase dosage in the evening.
Intravenous administration	Add the desired dose to 100 ml of 5% Dextrose Injection USP (or, if preferred, the drug may be diluted with 5% dextrose in water to a concentration of 100 mg/10 ml) and give by slow IV infusion over a period of 30–60 min; decline in blood pressure generally begins in 4–6 h and may last 10–16 h after injection
Combination therapy	Thiazide dosages do not need to be altered; when adding methyldopa to other antihypertensive regimens, limit initial dosage to 500 mg/day
Tolerance	May develop occasionally, usually between 2nd and 3rd mo of therapy; to restore control, add a diuretic or increase dosage of methyldopa
Refractory patients	Add a thiazide diuretic if therapy has not been started with a diuretic or if blood pressure cannot be controlled with 2 g/day of methyldopa
Elderly patients	To prevent syncope, which may be related to increased sensitivity and advanced arteriosclerosis, use lower dosages

WARNINGS/PRECAUTIONS

Coombs'-positive hemolytic anemia	May occur in less than 4% of patients, with potentially fatal complications. Obtain a blood count and Coombs' test before initiating therapy and at 6 and 12 mo after inception. With prolonged use of methyldopa, 10–20% of patients develop a positive direct Coombs' test; while this is not a contraindication to further use of the drug, therapy should be discontinued immediately if hemolytic anemia also develops in such patients. Usually, the anemia remits promptly. If it is related to methyldopa use, however, do not reinstitute the drug.
Drug-induced hepatitis	May occur at any time during therapy. Obtain liver-function studies (eg, SGOT, bilirubin) periodically, especially during first 2–3 mo of therapy or if unexplained fever or rash occurs. If drug-related, abnormalities will revert to normal after drug is stopped; do not reinstitute therapy.
Orthostatic hypotension	May occur; reduce dosage
Edema and weight gain	May occur and can usually be relieved with a diuretic; discontinue therapy if edema progresses or signs of heart failure appear
Reversible leukopenia	May occur rarely, manifested primarily by a reduction in granulocytes; discontinue therapy
Circulatory instability during anesthesia	May occur; if necessary, reduce anesthetic dosage. If hypotension does occur, use a vasopressor.
Paradoxical pressor response	May occur with parenteral administration
Involuntary choreoathetotic movements	May occur rarely in patients with severe bilateral cerebrovascular disease; discontinue therapy
Special-risk patients	Use with caution in patients with previous liver disease or dysfunction or in those with severe renal impairment; the latter may respond adequately to lower doses
Suspected pheochromocytoma	Urinary catecholamine level may appear to be elevated due to fluorescence of methyldopa; measurement of vanillylmandelic acid (VMA) by methods that convert VMA to vanillin is not affected
Dialysis patients	Blood pressure may be difficult to control, since methyldopa is removed by dialysis
Sulfite hypersensitivity	Presence of sulfites in vials and suspension may cause severe allergic reactions in certain susceptible patients, such as those with asthma; use of vials or suspension for patients hypersensitive to sulfites is contraindicated

ALDOMET ■ CATAPRES

ADVERSE REACTIONS

Central nervous system and neuromuscular	Sedation, headache, asthenia, weakness, dizziness, light-headedness, symptoms of cerebrovascular insufficiency, paresthesias, parkinsonism, Bell's palsy, decreased mental acuity, involuntary choreoathetotic movements, psychic disturbances (including nightmares and reversible mild psychoses or depression)
Cardiovascular	Bradycardia, prolonged carotid sinus hypersensitivity, aggravation of angina pectoris, orthostatic hypotension, edema (and weight gain); paradoxical pressor response (with IV use)
Digestive	Nausea, vomiting, distention, constipation, flatus, diarrhea, colitis, mild dryness of the mouth, sore or black tongue, pancreatitis, sialadenitis
Hepatic	Abnormal liver function tests, jaundice, liver disorders
Metabolic and endocrinological	Breast enlargement, gynecomastia, lactation, hyperprolactinemia, amenorrhea, impotence, decreased libido
Hematological	Hemolytic anemia, bone marrow depression, leukopenia, granulocytopenia, thrombocytopenia
Dermatological	Eczema-like rash or lichenoid eruption, toxic epidermal necrosis
Hypersensitivity	Drug-related fever, lupus-like syndrome, myocarditis, pericarditis
Other	Nasal stuffiness, mild arthralgia (with or without joint swelling), myalgia

OVERDOSAGE

Signs and symptoms	Sedation, hypotension
Treatment	Institute supportive measures, as indicated. Treat hypotension by elevating feet and by volume expansion, if possible.

DRUG INTERACTIONS

Other antihypertensive agents	⇧ Antihypertensive effect

ALTERED LABORATORY VALUES

Blood/serum values	⇧ Alkaline phosphatase ⇧ SGOT ⇧ SGPT ⇧ Bilirubin ⇧ Creatinine (with alkaline picrate method) ⇧ BUN ⇩ Plasma renin activity + Coombs' test + LE cell reaction + Rheumatoid factor + ANA
Urinary values	⇧ Uric acid (with phosphotungstate method) ⇧ Catecholamines (with fluorescence methods)

USE IN CHILDREN

See INDICATIONS and dosage recommendations

USE IN PREGNANT AND NURSING WOMEN

Use with caution if drug is essential. Methyldopa crosses the placental barrier and appears in cord blood and breast milk. No unusual adverse effects have been reported during pregnancy, nor is there any evidence of teratogenicity. However, the possibility of injury to the fetus or nursing infant cannot be excluded.

---

1 Contains 1% alcohol

CENTRAL ALPHA₂-ADRENERGIC AGONISTS

CATAPRES (clonidine hydrochloride) Boehringer Ingelheim   Rx

Tablets: 0.1, 0.2, 0.3 mg

INDICATIONS	ORAL DOSAGE
Hypertension	**Adult:** 0.1 mg bid to start, followed by increments of 0.1 or 0.2 mg/day, up to 2.4 mg/day, until desired response is achieved; usual maintenance dosage: 0.2–0.8 mg/day, given in divided doses

CONTRAINDICATIONS

None known

ADMINISTRATION/DOSAGE ADJUSTMENTS

Discontinuation of therapy	Reduce dosage gradually over 2–4 days to avoid withdrawal symptoms (see WARNINGS/PRECAUTIONS)

COMPENDIUM OF DRUG THERAPY

CATAPRES

WARNINGS/PRECAUTIONS

Withdrawal syndrome	Nervousness, agitation, headache, elevated serum catecholamine levels, a rapid increase in blood pressure, and, in rare cases, hypertensive encephalopathy and death, have been seen following abrupt cessation of clonidine; reactions have usually occurred after use at dosages exceeding 1.2 mg/day or when beta blockade has been instituted or maintained at the time of cessation. Rebound hypertension can be reversed by reinstitution of oral clonidine therapy or use of IV phentolamine. Caution patients not to terminate therapy on their own. To discontinue clonidine in patients receiving both this drug and a beta blocker, first withdraw the beta blocker and then, several days later, discontinue clonidine.
Visual impairment	Periodic eye examinations (every 6–12 mo) are recommended during prolonged therapy, based on evidence of retinal degeneration in rats[1]
Drowsiness, sedation	Patients who engage in potentially hazardous activities should be cautioned about the sedative effect of clonidine and that it may enhance the CNS depressant effects of alcohol, barbiturates, and other sedatives
Special-risk patients	Use with caution in patients with severe coronary insufficiency, recent myocardial infarction, cerebrovascular disease, or chronic renal failure
Hypersensitivity	If allergic contact sensitization occurs with transdermal clonidine, substitution of this product may produce a generalized rash; if systemic allergic reactions such as angioedema, urticaria, or generalized rash develop with transdermal clonidine, they may recur following substitution of this product.
Tolerance	Some patients may develop tolerance to clonidine; if tolerance occurs, reevaluate therapy

ADVERSE REACTIONS

Frequent reactions (incidence ≥ 1%) are printed in *italics*

Gastrointestinal	*Dry mouth (~ 40%),* constipation, anorexia, malaise, nausea, vomiting, parotid pain, mild transient abnormalities in liver function tests, drug-induced hepatitis without icterus or hyperbilirubinemia (one case)
Metabolic and endocrinological	Weight gain, gynecomastia
Cardiovascular	Congestive heart failure, Raynaud's phenomenon, ECG abnormalities manifested as Wenckebach's period or ventricular trigeminy; sinus bradycardia and AV block (rare)
Central nervous system	*Drowsiness (~ 35%), sedation (~ 8%),* dizziness, headache, fatigue, vivid dreams or nightmares, insomnia, other behavioral changes, nervousness, restlessness, anxiety, mental depression
Dermatological	Rash, angioneurotic edema, hives, urticaria, thinning of hair, pruritus not associated with rash
Genitourinary	Impotence, urinary retention
Other	Increased sensitivity to alcohol; dryness, itching, or burning of the eyes; dryness of the nasal mucosa; pallor; weakly positive Coombs' test

OVERDOSAGE

Signs and symptoms	Profound hypotension, weakness, somnolence, diminished or absent reflexes, vomiting
Treatment	Perform gastric lavage to empty stomach. Administer an analeptic and a vasopressor or, alternatively, 10 mg tolazoline IV every 30 min. Institute supportive measures, as needed.

DRUG INTERACTIONS

Alcohol, tranquilizers, sedative-hypnotics, and other CNS depressants	△ CNS depression
Beta blockers	Rebound hypertension following withdrawal of clonidine (see WARNINGS/PRECAUTIONS)
Diuretics	△ Antihypertensive effect of clonidine
Tricyclic antidepressants[1]	▽ Antihypertensive effect; increase clonidine dosage, if necessary

ALTERED LABORATORY VALUES

Blood/serum values	△ Glucose (transient) △ Creatine phosphokinase ▽ Plasma renin activity
Urinary values	△ Aldosterone △ Catecholamines

USE IN CHILDREN

Safety and effectiveness for use in children have not been established

USE IN PREGNANT AND NURSING WOMEN

Embryotoxic effects have been seen in animals at doses as low as one-third the maximum human dose; use in women who are or may become pregnant is not recommended, unless the expected benefit outweighs the potential risk to the mother and infant. Clonidine is excreted in human milk; use with caution in nursing mothers.

---

[1] Several studies have shown that clonidine produces a dose-dependent increase in the incidence and severity of spontaneous retinal degeneration in albino rats treated for 6 mo or longer; rats treated concurrently with clonidine and amitriptyline have developed corneal lesions within 5 days. Except for dry eyes, however, no adverse ophthalmologic effects have been observed in patients receiving clonidine, some of whom have been examined periodically for 24 mo or longer.

CATAPRES-TTS

CENTRAL ALPHA$_2$-ADRENERGIC AGONISTS

CATAPRES-TTS (clonidine) Boehringer Ingelheim   Rx

Transdermal drug delivery systems: 0.1 mg/day (3.5 cm^2) (Catapres-TTS-1), 0.2 mg/day (7 cm^2) (Catapres-TTS-2), 0.3 mg/day (10.5 cm^2) (Catapres-TTS-3)

INDICATIONS	**TRANSCUTANEOUS DOSAGE**
Hypertension	**Adult:** apply product once every 7 days. Use one Catapres-TTS-1 system to start; if desired reduction in blood pressure is not achieved after 1 or 2 wk, apply two Catapres-TTS-1 systems or a larger system. Use of more than two Catapres-TTS-3 systems usually does not produce an increase in effectiveness.

CONTRAINDICATIONS	
Hypersensitivity to any component	

ADMINISTRATION/DOSAGE ADJUSTMENTS	
Administration	Apply the system to a hairless area of intact skin on the upper arm or torso; use a new site each time. If the system begins to loosen during the week, apply the supplied adhesive overlay directly over the system.
Switching from other antihypertensive drugs	Reduce dosage of other antihypertensive agents gradually when switching to transdermal clonidine because this drug may not produce a therapeutic effect until 2-3 days after initial application
Combination antihypertensive therapy	Concomitant use of other antihypertensive agents may be necessary, particularly for patients with more severe forms of hypertension

WARNINGS/PRECAUTIONS	
Withdrawal syndrome	Nervousness, agitation, headache, elevated serum catecholamine levels, a rapid increase in blood pressure, and, in rare cases, hypertensive encephalopathy and death, have been seen following abrupt cessation of clonidine; reactions have usually occurred after high oral doses have been used or when beta blockade has been instituted or maintained at the time of cessation. Rebound hypertension can be reversed by use of oral clonidine or IV phentolamine. Caution patients not to terminate therapy on their own. To discontinue transdermal clonidine in patients receiving both this drug and a beta blocker, first withdraw the beta blocker and then, several days later, discontinue clonidine.
Surgery	Do not interrupt therapy because of surgery; however, carefully monitor blood pressure during surgery and make sure that emergency measures for control of hypotension are available. When starting the drug during the perioperative period, keep in mind that therapeutic serum levels are not achieved until 2-3 days after initial application.
Drowsiness	Caution patients about driving or engaging in other potentially hazardous activities
Dermatological effects	Instruct patients to promptly report moderate or severe erythema, local vesiculation, and generalized skin rashes. When local irritation occurs, the system can be removed and a new one applied to a different site. Pruritus and erythema occur more frequently when the adhesive overlay is used throughout the 7-day period of application. If allergic contact sensitization occurs with this product, substitution of oral clonidine may produce a generalized rash; if systemic allergic reactions such as angioedema, urticaria, or generalized rash develop with this product, they may recur following substitution of oral clonidine.
Special-risk patients	Use with caution in patients with severe coronary insufficiency, recent myocardial infarction, cerebrovascular disease, or chronic renal failure
Cardioversion	To avoid electrical arcing during defibrillation or cardioversion, remove the transdermal system before performing the procedure
Tolerance	Some patients may develop tolerance to clonidine; if tolerance occurs, reevaluate therapy
Carcinogenicity, mutagenicity	No evidence of carcinogenicity has been seen in rats fed 111-160 times the maximum recommended daily human dose of clonidine for 132 wk; no mutagenicity has been shown in the Ames test
Impairment of fertility	Doses of 35-140 times the maximum recommended daily human dose of clonidine appear to affect fertility in female rats; no impairment of fertility has been shown in male or female rats given up to 10.5 times the maximum recommended daily human dose

ADVERSE REACTIONS[1,2]	The most frequent reactions, regardless of incidence, are printed in *italics*
Central nervous system	*Drowsiness (12%)*, fatigue (6%), headache (5%), lethargy (3%), sedation (3%), insomnia (2%), dizziness (2%), nervousness (1%)
Dermatological	*Pruritus (51%), local erythema (25%), contact dermatitis (5-16%)*, local vesiculization (7%), hyperpigmentation (5%), edema (3%), excoriation (3%), burning (3%), papules (1%), throbbing (1%), blanching (1%), generalized macular rash (1%)

CATAPRES-TTS ■ WYTENSIN

Gastrointestinal	Constipation (1%), nausea (1%), change in taste (1%)
Genitourinary	Impotence/sexual dysfunction (2%)
Other	*Dry mouth (25%)*, dry throat (2%)

OVERDOSAGE

Signs and symptoms	Hypotension, bradycardia, lethargy, irritability, weakness, somnolence, diminished or absent reflexes, miosis, vomiting, hypoventilation, and, with a large overdose, cardiac conduction disturbances or arrhythmias, apnea, seizures, and transient hypertension
Treatment	Immediately remove all transdermal systems. Reverse bradycardia with IV atropine; correct hypotension with IV fluids and, if necessary, dopamine. For hypertension associated with overdosage, use IV furosemide, diazoxide, or an alpha-adrenergic blocker such as phentolamine. If these or other efforts fail to reverse effects of clonidine, give 10 mg of tolazoline IV every 30 min. Routine hemodialysis is of limited value.

DRUG INTERACTIONS

Tricyclic antidepressants[2]	▽ Antihypertensive effect; increase clonidine dosage, if necessary
Alcohol, barbiturates, other sedatives	△ CNS depression
Beta blockers	Rebound hypertension following withdrawal of clonidine (see WARNINGS/PRECAUTIONS)

ALTERED LABORATORY VALUES

Blood/serum values	▽ PRA (plasma renin activity)
Urinary values	▽ Catecholamines ▽ VMA ▽ Aldosterone

USE IN CHILDREN

Safety and effectiveness for use in children under 12 yr of age have not been established

---

USE IN PREGNANT AND NURSING WOMEN

Pregnancy Category C: an increase in resorptions has been observed in female rats given as low as 1.2 times the maximum recommended daily human dose (MRDHD) of clonidine for a period beginning 2 mo before mating and extending through pregnancy; however, no resorptions have been seen in rats given up to 10.5 times the MRDHD on days 6–15 of gestation. An increase in resorptions has also been seen in mice and rats following administration of 140 times the MRDHD during days 1–14 of gestation. In rabbits, no teratogenic or embryotoxic effects have been detected at up to 10.5 times the MRDHD. Use during pregnancy only if clearly needed. Clonidine is excreted in human milk; use with caution in nursing mothers.

---

[1] Reactions for which a causal relationship has not been established include maculopapular rash, urticaria, and angioedema of the face and/or tongue; reactions associated with oral clonidine include dry mouth, drowsiness, sedation, nausea, vomiting, anorexia, malaise, mild transient abnormalities in liver function tests, parotitis, weight gain, gynecomastia, transient elevation of blood glucose or serum CPK, nervousness, agitation, mental depression, insomnia, vivid dreams, nightmares, other behavioral changes, restlessness, anxiety, visual and auditory hallucinations, delirium, orthostatic symptoms, palpitations and tachycardia, bradycardia, Raynaud's phenomenon, congestive heart failure, conduction disturbances, arrhythmias, sinus bradycardia, AV block, rash, pruritus, hives, angioneurotic edema, urticaria, alopecia, decreased sexual activity, impotence, loss of libido, nocturia, difficulty in micturition, urinary retention, weakness, fatigue, headache, withdrawal syndrome, muscle or joint pain, cramps of lower limbs, dryness or burning of the eyes, dryness of the nasal mucosa, pallor, weakly positive Coombs' test, increased sensitivity to alcohol, and fever

[2] Several studies have shown that oral clonidine produces a dose-dependent increase in the incidence and severity of spontaneous retinal degeneration in albino rats treated for 6 mo or longer; rats treated concurrently with oral clonidine and amitriptyline have developed corneal lesions within 5 days. Except for dry eyes, however, no adverse ophthalmologic effects have been observed in patients receiving oral clonidine, some of whom have been examined periodically for 24 mo or longer.

CENTRAL ALPHA$_2$-ADRENERGIC AGONISTS

WYTENSIN (guanabenz acetate) Wyeth   Rx

Tablets: 4, 8, 16 mg

INDICATIONS	**ORAL DOSAGE**
Hypertension	**Adult:** 4 mg bid (alone or with a thiazide diuretic) to start, followed, if necessary, by a dosage increase of 4–8 mg/day every 1–2 wk, up to 32 mg bid

CONTRAINDICATIONS

Sensitivity to guanabenz

WARNINGS/PRECAUTIONS

Discontinuation of therapy	Caution patients against discontinuing therapy abruptly; rebound hypertension (rare), increased serum catecholamine levels, and various symptoms can occur after sudden cessation

WYTENSIN

Mental impairment	Caution patients to be careful driving or engaging in other activities requiring mental alertness until it is determined that they do not become drowsy or dizzy while taking this drug; patients should also be warned that their tolerance of alcohol or other CNS depressants may be diminished (see DRUG INTERACTIONS)
Special-risk patients	Use with caution in patients with severe hepatic or renal failure, severe coronary insufficiency, recent myocardial infarction, or cerebrovascular disease
Carcinogenicity, mutagenicity	No evidence of carcinogenicity has been observed in rats fed up to 9.6 mg/kg/day (~10 times the maximum human dose) for 2 yr. In the Ames test, guanabenz caused dose-related mutagenic effects in one of five *Salmonella typhimurium* strains. However, guanabenz was not mutagenic at dose levels up to those that inhibited the growth of the eukaryote organism *Schizosaccharomyces pombe* or that were lethal in vitro to Chinese hamster ovary cells, and it had no activity in an assay measuring induction of repairable DNA damage in *Saccharomyces cerevisiae*.
Effect on fertility	A decreased pregnancy rate has been reported in rats given high oral doses (9.6 mg/kg)
Drug dependence and tolerance	Dependence or abuse has not been associated with use of this drug, nor is there any evidence that patients develop tolerance to its antihypertensive effect

ADVERSE REACTIONS

Frequent reactions (incidence $\geq$ 1%) are printed in *italics*

Central nervous system	*Drowsiness or sedation (20–39%), dizziness (12–17%), weakness (10%), headache (5%)*, anxiety, ataxia, depression, sleep disturbances, blurring of vision
Cardiovascular	Chest pain, edema, arrhythmias, palpitations
Respiratory	Dyspnea, nasal congestion
Gastrointestinal	Nausea, epigastric pain, diarrhea, vomiting, constipation, abdominal discomfort
Musculoskeletal	Aches in extremities, muscle aches
Dermatological	Rash, pruritus
Genitourinary	Urinary frequency, disturbances of sexual function
Other	*Dry mouth (28–38%)*, taste disorders, gynecomastia

OVERDOSAGE

Signs and symptoms	Hypotension, somnolence, lethargy, irritability, miosis, and bradycardia were reported in two children who were 1 and 3 yr old
Treatment	Empty stomach by gastric lavage, and administer activated charcoal. Carefully monitor vital signs and fluid balance; maintain adequate respiratory exchange through provision of an adequate airway and, if necessary, use of assisted or controlled ventilation. Institute other supportive measures, including vasopressors and fluids, as needed.

DRUG INTERACTIONS

Alcohol, tranquilizers, sedative-hypnotics, and other CNS depressants	⇧ CNS depression
Hydrochlorothiazide	⇧ Antihypertensive effect

ALTERED LABORATORY VALUES

Blood/serum values	⇩ Cholesterol ⇩ Triglycerides (however, HDL fraction is not affected) ⇩ Norepinephrine ⇩ Dopamine beta-hydroxylase ⇩ Renin ⇧ Hepatic enzymes (rare)

No clinically significant alterations in urinary values occur at therapeutic dosages

---

USE IN CHILDREN

Safety and effectiveness for use in children under 12 yr of age have not been established; use in this age group is not recommended

USE IN PREGNANT AND NURSING WOMEN

Pregnancy Category C: use during pregnancy only if the expected benefit justifies the potential risk to the fetus. A possible increase in skeletal abnormalities has been detected in mice fed 3–6 times the maximum human dose of 1 mg/kg. Increased fetal loss has been observed in rabbits (20 mg/kg orally) and rats (14 mg/kg orally). Slightly decreased live-birth indices, decreased fetal survival rate, and decreased pup body weight have also been reported in rats (6.4 and 9.6 mg/kg orally). No adequate, well-controlled studies have been performed in pregnant women. It is not known whether guanabenz is excreted in human milk; this drug should not be given to nursing mothers.

INDOLINES

LOZOL (indapamide) Rorer Rx
Tablets: 2.5 mg

INDICATIONS	ORAL DOSAGE
Hypertension	**Adult:** 2.5 mg once daily in the morning to start, followed, if necessary after 4 wk, by 5 mg once daily.[1] When another antihypertensive agent is given in combination with indapamide, the usual dosage of that agent should be halved initially; during combination therapy, blood pressure should be carefully monitored and dosage should be adjusted when necessary.
Edema associated with congestive heart failure	**Adult:** 2.5 mg once daily in the morning to start, followed, if necessary after 1 wk, by 5 mg once daily[1]

CONTRAINDICATIONS	
Anuria	Hypersensitivity to indapamide or other sulfonamide derivatives

WARNINGS/PRECAUTIONS	
Electrolyte disorders	Hypokalemia may occur, especially when larger doses are used, diuresis is brisk, severe cirrhosis is present, ACTH or corticosteroids are given concomitantly, or oral intake of electrolytes is inadequate; potassium supplements or potassium-rich foods may be given to avoid or treat hypokalemia. Dilutional hyponatremia may occur in edematous patients when the weather is hot; restrict the intake of water, and administer salt only if hyponatremia is life-threatening or actual salt depletion occurs. For hypochloremia, specific treatment is usually unnecessary, except for certain patients (eg, those with hepatic or renal disease). To prevent electrolyte imbalance, measure serum and urinary electrolyte levels periodically in all patients; these determinations are especially important if excessive vomiting occurs, parenteral fluids are being given, salt is restricted in the diet, or patients have disorders that increase the risk of electrolyte imbalance (eg, heart failure, renal impairment, cirrhosis) or diseases that are exacerbated by electrolyte imbalance (eg, arrhythmia, hepatic impairment). Watch for premonitory signs and symptoms of hypokalemia, hyponatremia, and hypochloremic alkalosis, such as dry mouth, thirst, weakness, lethargy, drowsiness, restlessness, muscle pain or cramps, muscular fatigue, hypotension, oliguria, tachycardia, and GI disturbances (eg, nausea, vomiting).
Hyperuricemia, gout	An increase of 1 mg/dl in the serum uric acid level is usually seen during therapy; overt gout may occur in certain patients. Monitor serum uric acid levels periodically.
Parathyroid dysfunction	Indapamide causes slight increases in serum calcium levels. Hypercalcemia and hypophosphatemia, precipitated by physiological changes in parathyroid function, have been associated in rare instances with prolonged use of pharmacologically related drugs; however, even in these cases, the common complications of hyperparathyroidism (eg, renal lithiasis, bone resorption, peptic ulcer) have not been seen. Discontinue use of indapamide before performing parathyroid function tests.
Patients with renal impairment	Indapamide may precipitate or exacerbate azotemia in patients with severe renal disease; use with caution in such patients. Perform renal function tests periodically during therapy; if renal impairment progresses, consider interrupting or discontinuing therapy.
Patients with hepatic disease	Minor changes in fluid and electrolyte balance may precipitate hepatic coma in patients with hepatic impairment or progressive liver disease; use with caution in such patients
Patients with diabetes	Indapamide may activate latent diabetes or affect insulin requirements; monitor serum glucose levels routinely
Patients who have undergone sympathectomy	The antihypertensive effect of indapamide may be enhanced in such patients
Systemic lupus erythematosus	Indapamide may activate or exacerbate systemic lupus erythematosus
Carcinogenicity	No evidence of carcinogenicity has been seen in mice or rats

ADVERSE REACTIONS	The most frequent reactions (≥5%) are italicized
Central nervous system and neuromuscular	*Headache, dizziness, fatigue, weakness, loss of energy, lethargy, tiredness, malaise, muscle cramps or spasm, numbness of the extremities, nervousness, tension, anxiety, irritability, agitation,* light-headedness, drowsiness, vertigo, insomnia, depression, blurred vision, tingling of the extremities
Gastrointestinal	Constipation, nausea, vomiting, diarrhea, gastric irritation, abdominal pain or cramps, anorexia
Cardiovascular	Orthostatic hypotension, arrhythmias (including premature ventricular contractions), palpitations, flushing
Genitourinary	Frequent urination, nocturia, polyuria, reduced libido, impotence
Dermatological/hypersensitivity	Rash, hives, pruritus, vasculitis

LOZOL ■ APRESOLINE

Other	Rhinorrhea, dry mouth, weight loss, hyperuricemia, hyperglycemia, glycosuria, hypokalemia, hyponatremia, hypochloremia

OVERDOSAGE[2]

Signs and symptoms	Diuresis, dehydration, changes in serum electrolyte levels, transient increase in BUN levels, GI irritation and hypermotility, CNS depression; lethargy progressing to coma, possibly accompanied by minimal cardiorespiratory depression and no changes in electrolyte and fluid balance
Treatment	Empty stomach by gastric lavage, taking care to avoid aspiration. Monitor serum electrolyte levels and renal function, and institute supportive measures, as required, to maintain hydration, electrolyte balance, respiration, and cardiovascular and renal function. Treat GI effects symptomatically.

DRUG INTERACTIONS

Other antihypertensive agents	⇧ Antihypertensive effect
Lithium	⇧ Risk of lithium toxicity; diuretics generally should not be given to patients receiving lithium
Digitalis, other cardiac glycosides	⇧ Risk of digitalis toxicity (due to possible indapamide-induced hypokalemia); monitor electrolyte levels
Corticosteroids, ACTH	⇧ Risk of hypokalemia
Insulin, oral hypoglycemic agents	⇧ Hypoglycemic effect
Norepinephrine, other vasopressors	⇩ Vasopressor effect; nevertheless, this interaction does not preclude therapeutic use of vasopressors
Alcohol, barbiturates, narcotic analgesics	⇧ Risk of orthostatic hypotension
Tubocurarine, other nondepolarizing skeletal muscle relaxants	⇧ Skeletal muscle relaxation

ALTERED LABORATORY VALUES

Blood/serum values	⇩ Sodium ⇩ Potassium ⇧ Calcium ⇩ Magnesium ⇩ Chloride ⇩ Phosphate ⇧ Uric acid ⇩ PBI ⇧ Glucose ⇧ Amylase ⇧ BUN ⇧ Creatinine
Urinary values	⇧ Sodium ⇧ Potassium ⇩ Calcium ⇧ Magnesium ⇧ Chloride ⇧ Bicarbonate ⇩ Uric acid ⇧ Glucose

USE IN CHILDREN

Consult manufacturer

USE IN PREGNANT AND NURSING WOMEN

Pregnancy Category B: reproduction studies at up to 6,250 times the human dose have shown no evidence of impaired fertility or harm to the fetus in rats, mice, and rabbits and no effect on postnatal development in rats and mice. However, diuretics cross the placental barrier and may cause fetal or neonatal jaundice, thrombocytopenia, and other possible reactions. No adequate, well-controlled studies have been performed in pregnant women. Use indapamide during pregnancy for the treatment of hypertension or pathological edema only if clearly needed; this drug may also be given in a short course if edema associated with hypervolemia occurs during pregnancy and produces extreme discomfort that cannot be relieved by rest. Do not use for toxemia of pregnancy or for dependent edema resulting from restriction of venous return by uterine expansion. It is not known whether indapamide is excreted in human milk; patients should not nurse while taking this drug.

[1] In general, doses of 5 mg and larger appear to have no additional therapeutic benefit in either hypertension or edema, but do increase the degree of hypokalemia
[2] The information in this section is based on reports of thiazide overdosage; for specific guidelines concerning diagnosis and treatment of indapamide overdosage, consult manufacturer

---

PERIPHERAL VASODILATORS

APRESOLINE (hydralazine hydrochloride) CIBA   Rx

Tablets: 10, 25, 50, 100 mg   **Ampuls:** 20 mg/ml (1 ml)

INDICATIONS	ORAL DOSAGE	PARENTERAL DOSAGE
Hypertension	**Adult:** 10 mg qid for the first 2–4 days, followed by 25 mg qid for the balance of the first week and then 50 mg qid thereafter **Child:** 0.75 mg/kg/day, given in 4 divided doses, to start, followed by a gradual increase in dosage over the next 3–4 wk, up to a maximum of 200 mg/day or 7.5 mg/kg/day	**Adult:** for severe hypertension, 20–40 mg by IM or rapid IV injection, as needed; certain patients, especially those with marked renal impairment, may require a lower dose **Child:** for severe hypertension, 1.7–3.5 mg/kg/day, given by IM or rapid IV injection in 4–6 divided doses

APRESOLINE

CONTRAINDICATIONS

| Coronary artery disease | Rheumatic mitral valve disease | Hypersensitivity to hydralazine |

ADMINISTRATION/DOSAGE ADJUSTMENTS

Food-drug interactions	Administration of oral hydralazine with food results in higher serum levels
Monitoring of parenteral therapy	Check blood pressure frequently after injection. Blood pressure may begin to fall within a few minutes; maximum decrease is usually reached within 10–80 min.
High dosage requirements	Toxic reactions, especially the lupus-like syndrome, are particularly likely to occur at high oral dosages; for patients who require 200–300 mg/day, consider using hydralazine at a lower dosage in combination with a thiazide-type diuretic and either reserpine or a beta blocker
Acetylation rate	Serum levels are generally higher in patients with a slow acetylation rate; these patients usually require lower doses than patients with a rapid rate of acetylation
Management of adverse reactions	Adverse effects are usually reversed by a reduction in dosage; however, in some cases, termination of therapy may be necessary (see WARNINGS/PRECAUTIONS)

WARNINGS/PRECAUTIONS

Lupus-like syndrome	A syndrome resembling systemic lupus erythematosus, with glomerulonephritis and other lupus-like reactions, can occur during therapy; although this syndrome is usually reversible, manifestations can persist and necessitate long-term corticosteroid treatment. To reduce the risk of this syndrome, perform an ANA test before therapy, periodically during prolonged treatment, and whenever arthralgia, fever, chest pain, continued malaise, or any other unexplained reaction occurs. If results of an ANA test are positive or clinical signs and symptoms develop, carefully weigh risks and benefits of continued use.
Angina, myocardial infarction	The myocardial stimulation due to hydralazine may precipitate angina, myocardial ischemia, and myocardial infarction; use with caution in patients with known or suspected coronary artery disease
Postural hypotension, cerebral ischemia	Hydralazine can cause postural hypotension. When given parenterally to patients with increased intracranial pressure, this drug may enhance cerebral ischemia. Exercise caution when using this drug in patients with cerebrovascular accidents.
Renal impairment	Use with caution in patients with advanced renal disease
Peripheral neuritis	Hydralazine may cause peripheral neuritis, characterized by paresthesias, numbness, and tingling; if symptoms develop, administer pyridoxine concomitantly
Blood dyscrasias	Watch for evidence of blood dyscrasias; obtain a CBC before therapy, periodically during prolonged treatment, and whenever symptoms develop. If leukopenia, agranulocytosis, purpura, or a reduction in hemoglobin and erythrocytes is detected, this drug should be discontinued.
Tartrazine sensitivity	Presence of FD&C Yellow No. 5 (tartrazine) in 100-mg tablets may cause allergic-type reactions, including bronchial asthma, in susceptible individuals such as those hypersensitive to aspirin
Carcinogenicity	An increase in adenomas and adenocarcinomas of the lung has occurred in mice fed throughout their lives 80 times the maximum human dose of hydralazine; increases in benign hepatic neoplastic nodules and benign testicular interstitial cell tumors have been observed in rats. Long-term clinical observation has not suggested an association between hydralazine and cancer; however, no adequate epidemiological studies have been done.
Mutagenicity	Hydralazine has been shown to be mutagenic in the Ames test and has elicited DNA repair, a sign of mutagenicity, in *E coli* and cultured rat hepatocytes. In tests with rabbit hepatocytes having either a slow or rapid acetylation rate, the drug has elicited DNA repair only in those hepatocytes with a slow rate; these results suggest that patients with a rapid acetylation rate may be less susceptible to the potentially mutagenic effects of this drug. No evidence of mutagenicity has been seen in the mouse lymphoma assay, host-mediated assay, nucleus anomaly test, or dominant lethal test.

ADVERSE REACTIONS

Frequent reactions (incidence ≥ 1%) are printed in *italics*

Central nervous system	*Headache*, peripheral neuritis, dizziness, tremors, muscle cramps; psychotic reactions characterized by depression, disorientation, or anxiety
Gastrointestinal	*Anorexia, nausea, vomiting, diarrhea,* constipation, paralytic ileus
Cardiovascular	*Palpitations, tachycardia, angina pectoris,* hypotension, paradoxical hypertension, edema
Hematological	Reduction in hemoglobin, erythropenia, leukopenia, agranulocytosis, purpura, lymphadenopathy, splenomegaly
Respiratory	Dyspnea, nasal congestion
Ophthalmic	Lacrimation, conjunctivitis
Hypersensitivity	Rash, urticaria, pruritus, fever, chills, arthralgia, eosinophilia; hepatitis (rare)
Other	Flushing, difficult micturition

OVERDOSAGE

Signs and symptoms	Hypotension, tachycardia, headache, generalized skin flushing, myocardial ischemia and infarction, arrhythmia, severe shock
Treatment	Give primary attention to cardiovascular status. Treat shock with plasma expanders; use vasopressors only if they are necessary and precautions are taken to avoid precipitating or exacerbating an arrhythmia. For tachycardia, give a beta blocker. Digitalization may be necessary for reversal of cardiovascular disorders. Monitor renal function and institute supportive measures as needed. To remove the drug from the GI tract, empty stomach and then, if conditions permit, instill activated charcoal; bear in mind that since these measures can precipitate arrhythmia or enhance shock, it may be necessary to either skip them or wait until cardiovascular function has been restored before doing them.

DRUG INTERACTIONS

Diazoxide	Severe hypotension; after giving diazoxide to patients receiving hydralazine, monitor blood pressure continuously for several hours
MAO inhibitors	△ Risk of hypotension; exercise caution during combination therapy
Propranolol, metoprolol	△ Serum level of propranolol and metoprolol
Epinephrine	▽ Vasopressor effect

ALTERED LABORATORY VALUES

Blood/serum values	+ ANA + Direct Coombs' test △ PRA (plasma renin activity)

No clinically significant alterations in urinary values occur at therapeutic dosages

---

USE IN CHILDREN

Although safety and effectiveness for use in children have not been established in controlled clinical trials, the drug has been used in these patients; see INDICATIONS and dosage recommendations

USE IN PREGNANT AND NURSING WOMEN

Pregnancy Category C: hydralazine has caused cleft palate and malformations of facial and cranial bones in mice at 20–30 times the maximum daily human dose and may be teratogenic in rabbits at 10–15 times the maximum daily human dose. Use during pregnancy only if the expected benefit justifies the potential risk to the fetus. It is not known whether this drug is excreted in human milk; use with caution in nursing mothers.

PERIPHERAL VASODILATORS

HYPERSTAT I.V. (diazoxide) Schering   Rx

Ampuls: 15 mg/ml (20 ml)

INDICATIONS

Severe, nonmalignant or malignant hypertension in hospitalized adults[1]
Acute, severe hypertension in hospitalized children

PARENTERAL DOSAGE

Adult and child: 1–3 mg/kg, up to 150 mg, by rapid IV injection, repeated at intervals of 5–15 min until a satisfactory reduction in blood pressure (diastolic pressure < 100 mm Hg) is achieved; thereafter, repeat at intervals of 4–24 h to control blood pressure until an oral antihypertensive regimen can be instituted

CONTRAINDICATIONS

Compensatory hypertension (eg, hypertension associated with an arteriovenous shunt or coarctation of the aorta)

Hypersensitivity to diazoxide, other thiazides, or other sulfonamide derivatives

ADMINISTRATION/DOSAGE ADJUSTMENTS

IV administration	Inject only into a peripheral vein; avoid extravascular injection into subcutaneous tissues. Do not administer IM, SC, or into body cavities. Inject within 30 s after insertion into the vein for maximal antihypertensive effect; slower injection may fail to reduce blood pressure or produce a very brief response. Adjust the interval between injections by the duration of response; treatment can usually be discontinued after 4–5 days. Do not give IV diazoxide for more than 10 days.
Monitoring of therapy	Both during and following treatment, monitor ECG; hematocrit; hemoglobin; WBC and platelet counts; serum glucose, uric acid, total protein, albumin, sodium, potassium, and creatinine; urinary protein, and osmolality. Because hypotension requiring sympathomimetic treatment may occur, diazoxide should be administered only in a hospital setting or where facilities exist to treat untoward responses. Monitor blood pressure closely until it stabilizes; afterward, take measurements hourly during the balance of the effect. A further decrease in blood pressure 30 min or more after injection should be investigated. The patient should remain supine for at least 1 h after injection; in ambulatory patients, measure blood pressure with patient standing before ending surveillance.

HYPERSTAT I.V.

WARNINGS/PRECAUTIONS

Bolus injection — Intravenous administration of diazoxide in a bolus of 300 mg has resulted in cerebral and myocardial infarction, angina, and permanent blindness secondary to optic-nerve infarction; use only the recommended dosage, and, assuming the patient's condition permits, extend the period of blood-pressure reduction over at least several hours or, preferably, 1–2 days. Hypotension severe enough to require therapy will usually respond to the Trendelenberg maneuver; if necessary, administer a sympathomimetic, such as dopamine or norepinephrine.

Myocardial lesions — Intravenous administration of diazoxide has induced subendocardial and papillary muscle necrosis in dogs; presumably, the lesions are related to anoxia resulting from a combination of reflex tachycardia and decreased perfusion

Sodium and water retention — Repeated administration of diazoxide may cause sodium and water retention; administration of a diuretic may be necessary for maximal reduction of blood pressure and avoidance of congestive heart failure

Special-risk patients — Use with caution in patients with impaired cerebral or cardiac circulation (ie, those in whom mild tachycardia or decreased blood perfusion may be deleterious), diabetes mellitus, and in those in whom retention of salt and water may present serious problems; in patients with preexisting renal failure, avoid prolonged hypotension

Carcinogenicity, mutagenicity, effect on fertility — No long-term studies have been performed in laboratory animals to determine the carcinogenic or mutagenic potential of this drug or its effect on fertility

ADVERSE REACTIONS[2]

The most frequent reactions, regardless of incidence, are printed in *italics*

Cardiovascular — *Hypotension (7%)*, sodium and water retention after repeated injections (especially in patients with impaired cardiac reserve), hypotension to shock levels, transient myocardial ischemia (manifested by angina, atrial and ventricular arrhythmias, and marked ECG changes, but occasionally leading to myocardial infarction), supraventricular tachycardia and palpitation, bradycardia, chest discomfort or nonanginal "tightness in the chest"

Ophthalmic — Optic-nerve infarction (following a too-rapid decrease in severely elevated blood pressure), blurred vision; transient cataracts (one case), papilledema secondary to plasma volume expansion (one case)

Central nervous system — *Dizziness and weakness (7%)*, transient cerebral ischemia, occasionally leading to infarction (manifested by unconsciousness, convulsions, paralysis, confusion, or focal neurological deficit, such as numbness of the hands); vasodilative phenomena (eg, orthostatic hypotension, sweating, flushing, and generalized or localized sensations of warmth), headache (sometimes throbbing), light-headedness, sleepiness (lethargy, somnolence, drowsiness), euphoria or "funny feeling," ringing in the ears and momentary hearing loss, weakness of short duration, apprehension or anxiety

Gastrointestinal — *Nausea and vomiting (4%)*, abdominal discomfort, anorexia, alteration in taste, parotid swelling, salivation, dry mouth, lacrimation, ileus, constipation, diarrhea; acute pancreatitis (rare)

Respiratory — Dyspnea, cough, choking sensation

Hypersensitivity — Rash, leukopenia, fever

Other — Hyperglycemia (in diabetic patients after repeated use), hyperosmolar coma (in infants), transient hyperglycemia (in nondiabetic patients), transient retention of nitrogenous wastes, warmth or pain along injected vein, cellulitis without sloughing and/or phlebitis at the injection site, back pain and increased nocturia, malaise, hirsutism, decreased libido

OVERDOSAGE

Signs and symptoms — Excessive hypotension, excessive hyperglycemia

Treatment — Hypotension can usually be controlled with the Trendelenberg maneuver and, if necessary, sympathomimetics (eg, dopamine or norepinephrine). For hyperglycemia, restore fluid and electrolyte balance and treat with insulin.

DRUG INTERACTIONS

Thiazide diuretics — △ Hyperglycemic, hyperuricemic, and antihypertensive effects ▽ Risk of diazoxide-induced edema

Hydralazine, reserpine, alphaprodine, methyldopa, beta blockers, prazosin, minoxidil, nitrites, papaverine-like compounds — △ Hypotensive effect; do not use diazoxide within 6 h of administering these drugs

Phenytoin — ▽ Serum phenytoin level

Oral anticoagulants — △ Anticoagulant effect

ALTERED LABORATORY VALUES

Blood/serum values — ▽ BUN △ Creatinine △ SGOT △ Alkaline phosphatase △ Free fatty acids ▽ Hematocrit ▽ Hemoglobin ▽ IgG △ Renin △ Cortisol △ Glucose △ Sodium △ Uric acid ▽ Insulin — Insulin response (with glucagon test)

HYPERSTAT I.V. ■ LONITEN

Urinary values ——————————————— ▽ Sodium   ▽ Potassium   ▽ Chloride   ▽ Bicarbonate   ▽ Uric acid   + Glucose

USE IN CHILDREN

See INDICATIONS and PARENTERAL DOSAGE

USE IN PREGNANT AND NURSING WOMEN

Pregnancy Category C: diazoxide has caused reduced fetal and/or pup survival and reduced fetal growth in rats, rabbits, and dogs at daily doses of 30, 21, and 10 mg/kg, respectively; this drug has also caused prolonged parturition in rats treated at term with 10 mg/kg and above. IV administration of diazoxide during labor may cause cessation of uterine contractions, requiring use of an oxytocic agent. One episode of maternal hypotension and fetal bradycardia occurred during labor in a patient who received both reserpine and hydralazine prior to administration of diazoxide; neonatal hyperglycemia following intrapartum administration of diazoxide has also been reported. No adequate, well-controlled studies have been done in pregnant women. Safety for use in pregnant women has not been established. It is not known whether diazoxide is excreted in human milk; because of the potential for adverse effects in nursing infants, patients who require diazoxide should not nurse.

[1] Diazoxide is ineffective against pheochromocytoma-induced hypertension
[2] The reactions reported in this section have all occurred following bolus administration of 300-mg doses; reactions similar in character but with less frequency and severity may be expected to ensue from the currently recommended "minibolus" dosing regimen

---

PERIPHERAL VASODILATORS

LONITEN (minoxidil) Upjohn   Rx

Tablets: 2.5, 10 mg

INDICATIONS

Hypertension that is symptomatic or associated with target-organ damage and that is not manageable with maximum therapeutic doses of a diuretic plus two other antihypertensive agents

ORAL DOSAGE

Adult: 5 mg once daily to start, followed by increases to 10, 20, and then 40 mg/day, in single or divided doses, as needed for optimal control, up to 100 mg/day; usual maintenance dosage: 10–40 mg/day
Child (< 12 yr): 0.2 mg/kg once daily to start, followed by increases in 50–100% increments, as needed for optimal control, up to 50 mg/day; usual maintenance dosage: 0.25–1.0 mg/kg/day

CONTRAINDICATIONS

Pheochromocytoma (catecholamine secretion from tumor may be stimulated)

ADMINISTRATION/DOSAGE ADJUSTMENTS

Frequency of administration	If supine diastolic pressure has been reduced < 30 mm Hg, administer only once daily; if reduced > 30 mm Hg, divide the daily dose into two equal parts
Frequency of dosage adjustments	Titrate dosage according to patient response. Allow at least 3 days between dosage adjustments. When rapid control of hypertension is required, dose adjustments can be made every 6 h, with careful monitoring.
Mandatory concomitant therapy	Administer (1) the equivalent of 80–160 mg/day of propranolol in divided doses or, if beta blockers are contraindicated, 250–750 mg of methyldopa bid (given at least 24 h before beginning minoxidil therapy) or possibly 0.1–0.2 mg of clonidine bid and (2) the equivalent of 50 mg of hydrochlorothiazide bid, 50–100 mg of chlorthalidone once daily, or 40 mg of furosemide bid

WARNINGS/PRECAUTIONS

Salt and water retention, congestive heart failure	Must be prevented by concomitant diuretic therapy; a high-ceiling (loop) diuretic is almost always required. If excessive salt and water retention results in a weight gain > 5 lb on a thiazide-type diuretic, switch to furosemide. If the patient is already taking furosemide and is experiencing edema, increase the dosage. Rarely, refractory fluid retention may require discontinuing minoxidil therapy. Refractory salt retention may resolve by discontinuing minoxidil for 1 or 2 days and then reinstituting treatment in conjunction with vigorous diuretic therapy.
Tachycardia, anginal symptoms	Can be partly or entirely prevented by concomitant administration of a beta-adrenergic blocker or other sympatholytic agent, such as methyldopa (see ADMINISTRATION/DOSAGE ADJUSTMENTS)
Pericardial effusion with or without tamponade	May occur in ~ 3% of patients not on dialysis; more vigorous diuretic therapy, dialysis, pericardiocentesis, or surgery may be required. If the effusion persists, consider withdrawal of minoxidil.

COMPENDIUM OF DRUG THERAPY

LONITEN ■ MINIPRESS

Rapid blood pressure control	Syncope, cerebrovascular accidents, myocardial infarction, and a decrease or loss of vision or hearing (due to local ischemia) may occur in patients with very severe hypertension and ischemic episodes may occur in patients with compromised circulation or cryoglobulinemia if blood pressure is reduced too rapidly (these reactions have not been unequivocally associated with minoxidil). Treatment of patients with malignant hypertension should be initiated in a hospital setting.
Patients with recent myocardial infarction	Use of minoxidil within 1 mo of myocardial infarction may further limit blood flow to the myocardium
Hypersensitivity	May be manifested as a skin rash in < 1% of patients
Patients with renal failure or on dialysis	May require smaller doses and should be closely supervised medically to prevent exacerbation of renal failure or precipitation of cardiac failure
Hypertrichosis	Elongation, thickening, and increased pigmentation of fine body hair may occur in ∼ 80% of patients 3–6 wk after starting therapy; after therapy is discontinued, new hair growth stops, but 1–6 mo may elapse before normal appearance is restored
Laboratory testing	Laboratory values that are abnormal at the onset of therapy should be monitored; perform tests every 1-3 mo initially, and then, as values stabilize, every 6–12 mo
Promotion of hair growth	Use of this product, in any formulation, to promote hair growth is not an approved indication; efficacy, dosage, duration of treatment, and actual side effects for this use are not known and are currently being determined in clinical trials. All risks associated with oral use should be considered if an extemporaneous preparation is applied topically since systemic absorption (as well as skin intolerance) may occur.
Carcinogenicity, mutagenicity	No evidence of tumorigenicity has been seen in rats given 15 times the human dose for 22 mo; no mutagenic effects have been observed in the Ames test

ADVERSE REACTIONS

Frequent reactions (incidence ≥ 1%) are printed in *italics*

Cardiovascular	*ECG (T-wave) changes (∼ 60%), transient edema (7%),* tachycardia, angina, pericardial effusion and tamponade
Hematological	Transient decrease in hematocrit, hemoglobin, and RBC count; leukopenia (WBC < 3,000/mm^3) and thrombocytopenia (rare)
Hypersensitivity	Rash (< 1%)
Other	*Hypertrichosis (∼ 80%),* breast tenderness (< 1%)

OVERDOSAGE

Signs and symptoms	Exaggerated hypotension; in general, a serum level substantially above 2,000 ng/ml should be regarded as evidence of overdosage, unless it is known that the patient has not exceeded the maximum dose
Treatment	To help maintain blood pressure and promote urine formation, administer normal saline IV. Avoid sympathomimetic drugs, such as norepinephrine or epinephrine. If underperfusion of a vital organ is present, administer phenylephrine, angiotensin II (investigational), vasopressin (investigational), or dopamine.

DRUG INTERACTIONS

Guanethidine	Profound orthostatic hypotension

ALTERED LABORATORY VALUES

Blood/serum values	⇧ Alkaline phosphatase ⇧ Creatinine ⇧ BUN

No clinically significant alterations in urinary values occur at therapeutic dosages

---

USE IN CHILDREN

See INDICATIONS and ORAL DOSAGE. Dosage recommendations should be considered only as a rough guide; careful titration is essential, particularly in infants.

USE IN PREGNANT AND NURSING WOMEN

Pregnancy Category C: use during pregnancy only if expected benefit justifies the potential risk to the fetus. Minoxidil has been shown to reduce the conception rate in rats and increase fetal resorptions in rabbits at 5 times the human dose; there has been no evidence of teratogenicity in either species. The effects of this drug on labor and delivery are not known. No adequate, well-controlled studies have been done in pregnant women. It is not known whether minoxidil is excreted in human milk; as a rule, patient should stop nursing if drug is prescribed.

PERIPHERAL VASODILATORS

MINIPRESS (prazosin hydrochloride) Pfizer   Rx

Capsules: 1, 2, 5 mg

INDICATIONS	ORAL DOSAGE
Hypertension	**Adult:** 1 mg bid or tid, followed by up to 20 mg/day in divided doses; usual maintenance dosage: 6–15 mg/day, given in divided doses

MINIPRESS

CONTRAINDICATIONS

None known

ADMINISTRATION/DOSAGE ADJUSTMENTS

Frequency of administration	After initial titration, some patients can be maintained adequately on a bid schedule
Combination therapy	When adding a diuretic or other antihypertensive agent, reduce prazosin dosage to 1 or 2 mg tid, then retitrate
Refractory patients	May benefit from additional increases in dosage up to 40 mg/day in divided doses

WARNINGS/PRECAUTIONS

Syncope	Prazosin may cause syncope, usually within 30–90 min after the first dose and occasionally following a rapid increase in dosage or introduction of another antihypertensive agent while at a high dosage; syncope is usually attributed to excessive orthostatic hypotension, although occasionally this effect has been preceded by severe tachycardia (heart rate, 120–160 beats/min). In most cases, syncope does not recur during therapy. To minimize this risk, limit the initial dose to 1 mg, increase dosage slowly, and exercise caution when introducing additional antihypertensive agents. Instruct patients to limit their alcohol consumption, rise slowly from a sitting or lying position, and exercise special care during hot weather and when standing for long periods or exercising. Caution patients not to drive or engage in other potentially hazardous activities during the first 24 h of therapy and whenever the dosage is increased. If syncope occurs during therapy, place the patient in a recumbent position and take appropriate supportive measures.
Carcinogenicity, mutagenicity	No evidence of carcinogenicity has been demonstrated in rats given more than 225 times the maximum human dose for 18 mo; the results of in vivo genetic toxicology studies have been negative
Effect on fertility	Testicular atrophy and necrosis has been observed in rats and dogs given 75 times the maximum human dose for 1 yr or longer; decreased fertility has been seen in male and female rats at 225 times the maximum human dose. However, no changes in sperm morphology have been observed in 27 male patients who received prazosin for up to 51 mo, and no changes in excretion of 17-ketosteroids have been reported with long-term use in 105 patients.

ADVERSE REACTIONS

Frequent reactions (incidence ≥ 1%) are printed in *italics*

Central nervous system	*Dizziness (10.3%), headache (7.8%), drowsiness (7.6%), lack of energy (6.9%), weakness (6.5%), vertigo, depression, and nervousness (1–4%)*, paresthesias, hallucinations
Cardiovascular	*Palpitations (5.3%), edema, orthostatic hypotension, dyspnea, and syncope (1–4%)*, tachycardia
Gastrointestinal	*Nausea (4.9%), vomiting, diarrhea, and constipation (1–4%)*, abdominal discomfort and/or pain, liver function abnormalities, pancreatitis
Ophthalmic[1]	*Blurred vision and reddened sclera (1–4%)*, cataracts; pigmentary mottling and serious retinopathy (one case each)
Dermatological	*Rash (1–4%)*, pruritus, alopecia, lichen planus
Genitourinary	*Urinary frequency (1–4%)*, incontinence, impotence, priapism
Other	*Epistaxis, nasal congestion, and dry mouth (1–4%)*, tinnitus, diaphoresis, fever, positive ANA titer, arthralgia

OVERDOSAGE

Signs and symptoms	Drowsiness, depressed reflexes, hypotension, shock
Treatment	Support cardiovascular system if hypotension occurs. Keep patient in supine position to restore blood pressure and normalize heart rate. Volume expanders should be used first to treat shock; then, if necessary, use a vasopressor. Monitor renal function, and institute supportive measures, as needed. Dialysis is not beneficial, since drug is protein-bound.

DRUG INTERACTIONS

Beta blockers	⇧ Risk of hypotension
Other antihypertensive agents	⇧ Antihypertensive effect and risk of syncope

ALTERED LABORATORY VALUES

Blood/serum values	+ ANA titer
Urinary values	⇧ Normetanephrine ⇧ VMA; if an elevated VMA level is detected when testing for pheochromocytoma, prazosin should be discontinued and the test repeated 1 mo later

MINIPRESS ■ NIPRIDE

<table>
<tr><td>

USE IN CHILDREN

Safety and effectiveness for use in children have not been established

</td><td>

USE IN PREGNANT AND NURSING WOMEN

Pregnant women: Pregnancy Category C: administration of more than 225 times the maximum human dose has caused a decrease in litter size in rats; however, no fetal abnormalities have been reported with use in pregnant women. Adequate, well-controlled studies have not been done in pregnant women; therefore, use during pregnancy only if the expected benefit outweighs the potential risk to mother and fetus.
Nursing mothers: Small amounts of prazosin are excreted in human milk; use with caution in nursing mothers.

</td></tr>
</table>

[1] Although cataracts, pigmentary mottling, and serious retinopathy have been reported, an exact causal relationship could not be established because the baseline observations were frequently inadequate; slit-lamp and fundoscopic studies, with adequate baseline examinations, have shown no drug-related abnormal ophthalmological findings

---

PERIPHERAL VASODILATORS

NIPRIDE (sodium nitroprusside) Roche   Rx

Vials: 50 mg (5 ml)

INDICATIONS	**PARENTERAL DOSAGE**
Immediate reduction of blood pressure in patients in hypertensive crises **Production of controlled hypotension during anesthesia** to control bleeding	**Adult and child:** 0.5–10 μg/kg/min by IV infusion (see ADMINISTRATION/DOSAGE ADJUSTMENTS); average dosage: 3 μg/kg/min

CONTRAINDICATIONS		
Compensatory hypertension (eg, hypertension associated with an arteriovenous shunt or coarctation of the aorta)	Emergency surgery in moribund patients	Inadequate cerebral circulation

ADMINISTRATION/DOSAGE ADJUSTMENTS	
Preparation of infusion fluid	Dissolve contents of vial in 2–3 ml of dextrose-in-water *(do not use other diluents)*. Dilute the prepared stock solution in 250–1,000 ml of 5% dextrose-in-water. Wrap in foil to protect from light. Prepare freshly for each use, and discard any unused portion. Once prepared, do not keep or use the solution longer than 24 h, and protect from light. Freshly prepared infusion fluids should have a very faint brownish tint; discard blue, green, or dark-red solutions. Do not administer any other drugs simultaneously in the nitroprusside infusion solution.
Administration	Administer infusion solution by infusion pump, micro-drop regulator, or similar device that will allow a precise flow rate. Avoid extravasation. Adjust rate of administration to maintain the desired antihypertensive or hypotensive effect, as determined by frequent blood-pressure measurement. Do not allow blood pressure to drop at too rapid a rate or systolic pressure to fall below 60 mm Hg. The maximum infusion rate should rarely exceed 10 μg/kg/min; if adequate reduction of blood pressure is not obtained within 10 min at this rate, discontinue administration.
Concomitant antihypertensive therapy	Give smaller doses to hypertensive patients receiving concomitant antihypertensive therapy
Elderly patients	Use with caution in the elderly; initiate therapy with low doses
Young, vigorous male patients	Larger-than-ordinary doses may be necessary to initiate hypotensive anesthesia in these patients; however, do not exceed an infusion rate of 10 μg/kg/min. Deepening of anesthesia may permit satisfactory conditions to exist within the dosage guidelines.

WARNINGS/PRECAUTIONS	
Preexisting conditions	Tolerance to anemia, blood loss, and hypovolemia may be diminished; if possible, correct preexisting anemia and hypovolemia before producing controlled hypotension
Pulmonary reactions	The pulmonary ventilation perfusion ratio may be altered by hypotensive anesthetic techniques; patients intolerant of additional dead air space at ordinary oxygen partial pressure may benefit from a higher oxygen partial pressure
Patient monitoring	Have adequate facilities, equipment, and personnel available for frequent, vigilant monitoring of blood pressure
Special-risk patients	Use with extreme caution in patients who are especially poor surgical risks (American Surgical Association Class 4 and 4E) and with caution in patients with hepatic insufficiency, hypothyroidism, or severe renal impairment, and in the elderly

NIPRIDE ■ REGITINE

Toxicity	Thiocyanate toxicity may occur following excessive doses of nitroprusside, causing tinnitus, blurred vision, mental confusion, psychotic behavior, convulsions, delirium, lactic acidosis, bone marrow depression, and hypothyroidism; with gross overdosage, cyanide intoxication is possible (see OVERDOSAGE). Plasma thiocyanate levels should not exceed 10 mg/dl. Metabolic acidosis is the earliest and most reliable evidence of cyanide toxicity; determine blood pH and acid base balance frequently, particularly if increased tolerance occurs. Although plasma thiocyanate concentrations do not reflect cyanide toxicity, they should be monitored daily in any patient receiving nitroprusside for longer than 48 h, especially in those with renal or hepatic impairment.
Tolerance	Failure to respond to sodium nitroprusside may be associated with an increase in free cyanide; should increased tolerance occur, discontinue use and promptly institute appropriate therapy
Carcinogenicity, mutagenicity, effect on fertility	No long-term, adequate studies have been performed in laboratory animals to determine the carcinogenic or mutagenic potential of this drug or its effect on fertility

ADVERSE EFFECTS

Gastrointestinal	Nausea, retching, abdominal pain
Cardiovascular	Retrosternal discomfort, palpitations, flushing, bradycardia, ECG changes, tachycardia
Central nervous system	Apprehension, headache, restlessness, muscle twitching, dizziness, increased intracranial pressure
Other	Diaphoresis, rash, methemoglobinemia, venous streaking, irritation at infusion site, hypothyroidism (one case following long-term use)

OVERDOSAGE

Signs and symptoms	*Early signs:* profound hypotension, metabolic acidosis, dyspnea, headache, vomiting, dizziness, ataxia, loss of consciousness; *late signs:* cyanide intoxication (coma, imperceptible pulse, absent reflexes, widely dilated pupils, pink color, distant heart sounds, hypotension, very shallow breathing)
Treatment	Immediately discontinue use of nitroprusside. For cyanide toxicity, administer amyl nitrate inhalations for 15–30 s/min. Prepare a 3% sodium nitrite solution for IV use and inject at a rate not to exceed 2.5–5.0 ml/min, up to a total dose of 10–15 ml, and carefully monitor blood pressure. Follow with IV sodium thiosulfate, 12.5 g in 50 ml of 5% dextrose-in-water over a 10-min period. Repeat sodium nitrite and thiosulfate injections at 50% of the preceding doses if symptoms of overdosage reappear. If blood pressure drops, correct with vasopressor agents.

DRUG INTERACTIONS

Other antihypertensive agents, ganglionic blocking agents, halothane, enflurane, and other circulatory depressants	△ Hypotensive effect

ALTERED LABORATORY VALUES

Blood/serum values	△ Creatinine ▽ PBI

No clinically significant alterations in urinary values occur at therapeutic dosages

---

USE IN CHILDREN
See INDICATIONS and PARENTERAL DOSAGE

USE IN PREGNANT AND NURSING WOMEN
Pregnancy Category C: studies in pregnant ewes have shown that nitroprusside crosses the placental barrier. Fetal cyanide levels are dose-related to maternal nitroprusside levels; infusion of 25 μg/kg/min for 1 h in pregnant ewes resulted in the deaths of all fetuses, whereas infusion of 1 μg/kg/min for 1 h resulted in the birth of normal lambs. There are no adequate, well-controlled studies in laboratory animals or pregnant women; use during pregnancy only if clearly needed. It is not known whether this drug is excreted in human milk; because many drugs are excreted in human milk, patients who require nitroprusside should not nurse.

PERIPHERAL VASODILATORS

REGITINE (phentolamine mesylate) CIBA Rx
Vials: 5 mg

INDICATIONS
Prevention or control of **hypertensive episodes** that may occur in a patient with pheochromocytoma as a result of stress or manipulation before or during surgery

PARENTERAL DOSAGE
Adult: 5 mg IV or IM 1–2 h before surgery, repeated, if necessary; during surgery, 5 mg IV to control effects of epinephrine intoxication
Child: 1 mg as above

REGITINE

Dermal necrosis and sloughing associated with the intravenous administration or extravasation of norepinephrine	**Adult:** for prevention, add 10 mg to each liter of solution containing norepinephrine; for treatment, inject 5–10 mg in 10 ml saline into area of extravasation within 12 h
Diagnosis of pheochromocytoma by blocking test	**Adult:** 5 mg IV (rapidly) or IM **Child:** 1 mg IV (rapidly) or 3 mg IM (see ADMINISTRATION/DOSAGE ADJUSTMENTS and WARNINGS/PRECAUTIONS)

CONTRAINDICATIONS

Past or present myocardial infarction	Hypersensitivity to phentolamine or related compounds	Angina or other evidence of coronary artery disease
Coronary insufficiency		

ADMINISTRATION/DOSAGE ADJUSTMENTS

Use of phentolamine blocking test	*Preparation:* Sedatives, analgesics, and all other medications except those such as digitalis and insulin that are deemed essential should be withheld for at least 24 h (preferably 48–72 h) before the test. Withhold antihypertensives until blood pressure returns to the untreated, hypertensive level. Do *not* perform test on a normotensive patient. *Procedure:* Keep patient in supine position throughout the test, preferably in a quiet, darkened room. Obtain blood-pressure readings every 10 min for at least ½ h until pressure stabilizes. Dissolve 5 mg phentolamine in 1 ml sterile water. Inject appropriate dose (see INDICATIONS) by IV or IM route; delay IV injection after insertion of syringe needle into vein until pressor response to venipuncture subsides. For IV test, record blood pressure immediately after injection, at 30-s intervals for the first 3 min, and at 60-s intervals for the next 7 min. For IM test, record blood pressure every 5 min for 30–45 min following injection. *Test results:* Positive response is indicated by a drop in blood pressure of more than 35 mm Hg systolic and 25 mm Hg diastolic within 2 min after IV injection or within 20 min after IM injection. Negative response is indicated when the blood pressure is unchanged, elevated, or reduced less than 35 mm Hg systolic and 25 mm Hg diastolic after injection.

WARNINGS/PRECAUTIONS

Myocardial infarction, cerebrovascular spasm, and cerebrovascular occlusion	May occur, usually in association with marked hypotensive episodes
Limitations of phentolamine blocking test	This test is not the procedure of choice for screening patients with hypertension for pheochromocytoma; reserve for cases requiring additional confirmatory evidence once urinary and other biochemical assays for catecholamines have been performed, and consider the relative risks of this procedure. A negative response to this test does not exclude the diagnosis of pheochromocytoma, especially in patients with paroxysmal hypertension. False-positive test results may occur in patients with hypertension without pheochromocytoma.
Tachycardia and cardiac arrhythmias	May occur; if possible, defer use of cardiac glycosides until cardiac rhythm returns to normal
Carcinogenicity, mutagenicity, effect on fertility	No studies have been done to evaluate the carcinogenic or mutagenic potential of phentolamine or its effect on fertility

ADVERSE REACTIONS

Cardiovascular	Acute and prolonged hypotensive episodes, orthostatic hypotension, tachycardia, arrhythmias
Gastrointestinal	Nausea, vomiting, diarrhea
Other	Weakness, dizziness, flushing, nasal stuffiness

OVERDOSAGE

Signs and symptoms	Arrythmias, tachycardia, hypotension, shock, excitation, headache, sweating, pupillary contraction, visual disturbances, nausea, vomiting, diarrhea, hypoglycemia
Treatment	Institute supportive measures immediately. Raise patient's legs and administer a plasma expander. If necessary, administer norepinephrine by IV infusion; titrate to maintain normotensive blood pressure levels. Do *not* use epinephrine.

DRUG INTERACTIONS

Epinephrine	▽ Blood pressure
Sedatives, narcotics, antihypertensive agents	△ Risk of false-positive response to phentolamine blocking test

REGITINE ■ ARFONAD

ALTERED LABORATORY VALUES

No clinically significant alterations in blood/serum or urinary values occur at therapeutic dosages

USE IN CHILDREN
See INDICATIONS and PARENTERAL DOSAGE

USE IN PREGNANT AND NURSING WOMEN
Pregnancy Category C: reproduction studies in rats and mice fed 24-30 times the usual daily human dose have shown a slight decrease in fetal growth, as well as slight increases in partially ossified sternebrae, incomplete or unossified calcanei, and phalangeal nuclei of the hind limb; in rats fed 60 times the usual daily human dose, there was a slightly lower implantation rate. Phentolamine should be used during pregnancy only if the expected benefit outweighs the potential risk to the fetus. It is not known whether phentolamine is excreted in human milk; because of the potential for serious adverse reactions in the nursing infant, a decision should be made to either discontinue nursing or drug therapy.

SYMPATHOLYTICS

ARFONAD (trimethaphan camsylate) Roche Rx
Ampuls: 50 mg/ml (10 ml)

INDICATIONS
Production of controlled hypotension during surgery
Short-term control of blood pressure in hypertensive emergencies
Emergency treatment of **pulmonary edema** in patients with pulmonary hypertension associated with systemic hypertension

PARENTERAL DOSAGE
Adult: 3-4 mg (3-4 ml after dilution)/min, given by IV infusion, to start; thereafter, adjust the rate of administration to maintain the desired level of hypotension (see ADMINISTRATION/DOSAGE ADJUSTMENTS) or antihypertensive effect. In surgical patients, discontinue use prior to wound closure to permit blood pressure to return to normal.

CONTRAINDICATIONS
Inability to replace blood or fluids for technical reasons

Conditions where hypotension may subject the patient to undue risk, including uncorrected anemia, hypovolemia, shock, asphyxia, and uncorrected respiratory insufficiency

ADMINISTRATION/DOSAGE ADJUSTMENTS

Preparing infusion fluid — Dilute contents of one ampul in 500 ml of 5% Dextrose Injection USP (*do not use other diluents*) to a final concentration of 1 mg/ml. Use only freshly prepared solutions; discard all unused portions. Do not employ the infusion fluid used to give trimethaphan as a vehicle for simultaneous administration of any other drugs.

Maintaining hypotension — Rates of administration can vary from 0.3 ml (0.3 mg)/min to > 6 ml (6 mg)/min owing to marked variation of patient response; obtain frequent blood-pressure determinations to maintain proper control. Position the patient so as to avoid cerebral anoxia, and during surgery establish adequate anesthesia.

WARNINGS/PRECAUTIONS

Vigilant monitoring of the circulation — Is essential, as trimethaphan is an extremely potent hypotensive; adequate facilities, equipment, and personnel must be available for this purpose

Adequate oxygenation — Must be assured throughout treatment, especially in regard to coronary and cerebral circulation

Pupillary dilation — May occur but does not necessarily indicate anoxia or depth of anesthesia

Special-risk patients — Use with extreme caution in elderly or debilitated patients; in those with arteriosclerosis, cardiac, hepatic, or renal disease, degenerative disease of the central nervous system, Addison's disease, or diabetes; and in those receiving steroids

Respiratory arrest — Rare cases have been reported (causal relationship not established); monitor respiratory status closely, especially if large doses are given

Histamine-type reaction — May occur; use with caution in patients with allergies

ADVERSE REACTIONS
Consult manufacturer

OVERDOSAGE
Signs and symptoms — Excessive hypotension, apnea, respiratory arrest

COMPENDIUM OF DRUG THERAPY

Treatment	Tilt the patient to the head-down position or elevate the lower extremities. To correct undesirable hypotension during surgery, or to achieve normotensive levels more rapidly, give phenylephrine hydrochloride or mephentermine sulfate. Reserve norepinephrine for refractory cases.

DRUG INTERACTIONS

Diuretics, antihypertensive agents, anesthetics (especially spinal anesthetics), procainamide	⇧ Hypotensive effect
Tubocurarine, succinylcholine	⇧ Neuromuscular blocking effect

ALTERED LABORATORY VALUES

Blood/serum values	⇧ Potassium ⇩ Glucose

No clinically significant alterations in urinary values occur at therapeutic dosages

---

USE IN CHILDREN
Consult manufacturer for dosage recommendations; use with great caution

USE IN PREGNANT AND NURSING WOMEN
Induced hypotension may have serious consequences on the fetus; consult manufacturer for use in nursing mothers

---

SYMPATHOLYTICS

HYLOREL (guanadrel sulfate) Pennwalt   Rx

Tablets: 10, 25 mg

INDICATIONS
Hypertension inadequately controlled by thiazide diuretics (step 2 therapy)

ORAL DOSAGE
Adult: 5 mg bid (with a thiazide diuretic) to start, followed, as needed, by a weekly or monthly adjustment in dosage until blood pressure is controlled; usual therapeutic dosage: 20–75 mg/day, given in 2 divided doses (larger daily doses may need to be given in 3 or 4 divided doses)

CONTRAINDICATIONS

Pheochromocytoma	MAO inhibitor therapy (see DRUG INTERACTIONS)	Hypersensitivity to guanadrel
Overt cardiac failure		

WARNINGS/PRECAUTIONS

Orthostatic hypotension	Warn patients that symptoms of orthostatic hypotension (such as dizziness or weakness) occur frequently during therapy, particularly in the morning, and that alcohol, fever, hot weather, prolonged standing, and exercise increase the risk and intensity of these symptoms. To assess the orthostatic response, especially when starting therapy or changing the dosage, measure the standing blood pressure as well as the supine pressure. Caution patients that whenever they begin to feel dizzy or weak during therapy, they should sit or lie down immediately. Do not give this drug to patients with cerebrovascular or coronary insufficiency unless other drugs with a lower risk of orthostatic hypotension are not effective or tolerated; when using guanadrel in these patients, avoid hypotensive episodes, even if such an effort precludes complete control of blood pressure.
Asthma	The catecholamine depletion produced by guanadrel may exacerbate bronchial asthma, and sympathomimetic agents used to treat asthma may reduce the effectiveness of this drug; use guanadrel with caution in patients with bronchial asthma
Peripheral edema	Salt and fluid retention may occur, especially when a diuretic is not given concomitantly
Cardiac failure	Guanadrel could cause decompensation in patients with a history of cardiac failure; use in such patients has not been studied
Peptic ulcer	Guanadrel may cause peptic ulcer in patients with a history of this disorder; use with caution in such patients
Renal failure	Use in patients with renal failure has not been studied
Tolerance	An increase in dosage may be necessary during long-term therapy because of tolerance
Carcinogenicity, mutagenicity	Endometrial fibromatous polyps have been seen in rats given 100 mg/kg/day for 22 mo; no evidence of carcinogenicity has been observed in mice after administration for 2 yr. The Ames test has shown no evidence of mutagenicity.

ADVERSE REACTIONS

Cardiovascular	Orthostatic hypotension, nonorthostatic faintness, palpitations, chest pain; syncope (rare)
Central nervous system	Fatigue, headache, drowsiness, visual disturbances, paresthesias, confusion, psychological problems, sleep disorders, depression
Musculoskeletal	Aching limbs, leg cramps, joint pain and inflammation, backache, neckache
Respiratory	Shortness of breath, coughing
Gastrointestinal	Gas pain, increase in bowel movements, indigestion, constipation, anorexia, nausea, vomiting, abdominal distress and pain
Genitourinary	Nocturia, urinary urgency and frequency, peripheral edema, ejaculation disturbances, impotence, hematuria; urinary retention (rare)
Other	Weight gain and loss, glossitis, dry mouth and throat

OVERDOSAGE

Signs and symptoms	Marked dizziness, blurred vision, syncope
Treatment	Instruct patient to lie down. For severe persistent hypotension, a vasopressor such as phenylephrine may be given; however, the vasopressor must be used with great caution because patients may be particularly sensitive to its actions (see DRUG INTERACTIONS)

DRUG INTERACTIONS

MAO inhibitors	Severe hypertension (when an MAO inhibitor has been given alone prior to concomitant use); discontinue an MAO inhibitor at least 1 wk before beginning guanadrel
Anesthetics	Vascular collapse; discontinue guanadrel 48–72 h before elective surgery, and cautiously administer preanesthetic and anesthetic agents at a reduced dosage before emergency surgery
Norepinephrine and other direct-acting sympathomimetic agents	Severe hypertension and arrhythmia; exercise caution during concomitant therapy
Ephedrine, phenylpropanolamine, and other indirect-acting sympathomimetic agents	▽ Antihypertensive effect; warn patients not use OTC cold, allergy, asthma, or diet medications on their own
Tricyclic antidepressants, phenothiazines	▽ Antihypertensive effect
Thiazide diuretics	△ Antihypertensive effect; see INDICATIONS and ORAL DOSAGE
Reserpine, adrenergic blockers	△ Pharmacologic effects of guanadrel; although bradycardia and enhanced orthostatic hypotension would be expected to occur, a clinical study with propranolol has failed to show any significant adverse effects, and no studies have been done with other adrenergic blockers or reserpine
Vasodilators	△ Orthostatic hypotension; concomitant use is generally not recommended
Alcohol	△ Orthostatic hypotension

ALTERED LABORATORY VALUES

No clinically significant alterations in blood/serum or urinary values occur at therapeutic dosages

---

USE IN CHILDREN

Safety and effectiveness for use in children have not been established

USE IN PREGNANT AND NURSING WOMEN

Pregnancy Category B: reproduction studies in rats and rabbits given up to 12 times the maximum human dose have shown no evidence of impaired fertility or harm to the fetus; no adequate, well-controlled studies have been done in pregnant women. Use during pregnancy only if the expected benefit justifies the potential risk to the fetus. It is not known whether guanadrel is excreted in human milk; patients should not nurse while taking this drug.

SYMPATHOLYTICS

ISMELIN (guanethidine monosulfate) CIBA   Rx

Tablets: 10, 25 mg

INDICATIONS

Moderate to severe essential hypertension

Renal hypertension, including hypertension secondary to pyelonephritis, renal amyloidosis, and renal artery stenosis

ORAL DOSAGE

Adult (ambulatory): 10 mg once daily to start; blood pressure must be taken at 5- to 7-day intervals to determine if there is a need for an increase in dosage (see ADMINISTRATION/DOSAGE ADJUSTMENTS); if needed on 2nd visit, increase dosage to 20 mg once daily; if needed on 3rd visit, increase dosage to 30 or 37.5 mg once daily; if needed on 4th visit, increase dosage to 50 mg once daily; if needed on 5th or subsequent visits, increase daily dose by 12.5 or 25 mg; usual maintenance dosage: 25–50 mg once daily

Adult (hospitalized): 25–50 mg to start, followed by increases of 25 or 50 mg once daily or every other day, as needed

ISMELIN

CONTRAINDICATIONS

Hypersensitivity to guanethidine	Frank congestive heart failure not due to hypertension	Use of MAO inhibitors (see WARNINGS/PRECAUTIONS)
Pheochromocytoma, either known or suspected		

ADMINISTRATION/DOSAGE ADJUSTMENTS

Initial titration of dosage	Take blood pressure with patient in supine position, after he or she has been standing for 10 min, and immediately after exercise, if feasible. Increase dosage only if there is no decrease in standing blood pressure from previous levels. Reduce dosage if pressure is normal in the supine position or if patient evidences either an excessive orthostatic fall in pressure or severe diarrhea.
Combination therapy	Add guanethidine gradually to thiazides or hydralazine. When thiazide diuretics are added, it is usually necessary to reduce the guanethidine dosage.
Patients with fever	Dosage requirements may be reduced
Transferring patients from ganglionic blockers	Withdraw blocker gradually to prevent a spiking blood pressure response during period of transition

WARNINGS/PRECAUTIONS

Inhibition of ejaculation	Inhibition of ejaculation resulting from sympathetic blockade has been reported in animals and humans; normal ejaculatory function is restored after the drug has been discontinued for several weeks. Guanethidine does not cause parasympathetic blockade, and erectile potency is usually retained during treatment. Keep the possibility of ejaculatory inhibition in mind when treating men of reproductive age, and caution them accordingly.
Orthostatic hypertension	Warn patients that symptoms of orthostatic hypotension occur frequently during therapy, particularly in the morning, and are accentuated by alcohol, fever, hot weather, sudden or prolonged standing, and exercise. Fainting spells may occur unless patients are forewarned to sit or lie down if they begin to feel dizzy or weak.
Cardiovascular instability during surgery	If possible, withdraw therapy 2 wk prior to elective surgery to minimize the risk of vascular collapse and cardiac arrest during anesthesia. For emergency surgery, administer preanesthetic and anesthetic agents with caution and lower the dosage. Oxygen, atropine, vasopressors, and adequate solutions for volume replacement should be available for immediate use; administer vasopressors with extreme caution, since guanethidine can augment their effect (see DRUG INTERACTIONS).
Patients with bronchial asthma	The catecholamine depletion produced by guanethidine may exacerbate bronchial asthma; use with caution
Patients with incipient cardiac decompensation	Monitor patients with incipient cardiac decompensation for weight gain or edema; fluid retention may be averted by concomitant administration of a thiazide diuretic
Patients with severe cardiac failure	Use with extreme caution in patients with severe cardiac failure, since guanethidine may interfere with the compensatory role of the adrenergic system in producing circulatory adjustment
Patients with peptic ulcer disease	Use with caution in patients with a history of peptic ulcer or other chronic disorders that may be aggravated by relative increases in parasympathetic tone
Other special-risk patients	Use very cautiously in hypertensive patients with renal disease coupled with nitrogen retention or rising BUN levels; coronary insufficiency or recent myocardial infarction; or cerebrovascular disease, especially with encephalopathy
Diarrhea	Severe diarrhea may occur and necessitate a reduction in dosage or discontinuation of therapy
Long-term therapy	The effects of guanethidine are cumulative; give small initial doses, and increase dosage gradually in small increments
Carcinogenicity	No long-term studies have been performed to evaluate the carcinogenic potential of this drug
Impairment of fertility	Inhibition of sperm passage and accumulation of sperm debris have been reported in rats and rabbits given 5 or 10 mg/kg/day of guanethidine SC or IP for several weeks; however, recovery of ejaculatory function and fertility has been shown in rats following IM administration of 25 mg/kg/day of the drug IM for 8 wk. Reversible inhibition of ejaculation has also occurred in men (see "Inhibition of ejaculation," above).

ADVERSE REACTIONS[1]

Gastrointestinal	Diarrhea, vomiting, nausea, increased bowel movements, dry mouth, parotid tenderness
Cardiovascular	Chest pains (angina), bradycardia, fluid retention and edema with occasional development of congestive heart failure
Respiratory	Dyspnea, asthma (in susceptible patients), nasal congestion
Central nervous system, neuromuscular	Syncope resulting from postural or exertional hypotension, dizziness, blurred vision, muscle tremor, ptosis, mental depression, chest paresthesias, weakness, lassitude, fatigue, myalgia

ISMELIN ■ SERPASIL

Genitourinary	Rise in BUN level, urinary incontinence, inhibition of ejaculation, nocturia
Hypersensitivity	Dermatitis, scalp hair loss
Other	Weight gain

OVERDOSAGE

Signs and symptoms	Postural hypotension with dizziness, blurred vision, and possible syncope when standing; shock, bradycardia; diarrhea, nausea, vomiting, and, rarely, unconsciousness
Treatment	Evacuate stomach contents by gastric lavage, instill a slurry of activated charcoal, and give laxatives, if conditions permit. Support vital functions and control cardiac irregularities, if present. Treat hypotension by keeping patient's feet up and, if necessary, by replacing lost fluid and electrolytes. For sinus bradycardia, administer atropine. For previously normotensive patients, restore blood pressure and heart rate by keeping patient in a supine position (normal homeostatic control gradually returns within 72 h). For previously hypertensive patients, particularly those with impaired cardiac reserve or other cardiovascular-renal disease, intensive treatment may be needed; maintain patient in a supine position, and, if vasopressors are required, they should be used with extreme caution. Treat severe or persistent diarrhea with anticholinergic agents; maintain hydration and electrolyte balance. Monitor cardiovascular and renal function for several days, until drug is completely eliminated.

DRUG INTERACTIONS

MAO inhibitors	△ Hypertension to crisis proportions
Digitalis	▽ Heart rate
Amphetamine-like compounds, ephedrine, methylphenidate, and other stimulants; tricyclic antidepressants; phenothiazines; other psychotropic agents; oral contraceptives	▽ Antihypertensive effect
Rauwolfia derivatives	Excessive postural hypotension, bradycardia, mental depression
Norepinephrine and other vasopressors	△ Pressor effect and risk of cardiac arrhythmias

ALTERED LABORATORY VALUES

Blood/serum values	△ BUN △ Creatinine △ Plasma renin activity
Urinary values	△ Catecholamines (initially) ▽ Catecholamines (subsequently) ▽ VMA

USE IN CHILDREN

Safety and effectiveness for use in children have not been established

USE IN PREGNANT AND NURSING WOMEN

Pregnancy Category C: reproduction studies have not been performed; use during pregnancy only if clearly needed. Small quantities of guanethidine are excreted in human milk; use with caution in nursing mothers.

---

[1] A few instances of blood dyscrasias (anemia, thrombocytopenia, and leukopenia), priapism, and impotence have been reported, but no causal relationship has been established

---

SYMPATHOLYTICS

SERPASIL (reserpine) CIBA   Rx

Tablets: 100, 250 μg

INDICATIONS	ORAL DOSAGE
Hypertension	**Adult:** for mild hypertension, 500 μg/day for 1–2 wk, followed by 100–250 μg/day for maintenance **Child:** 20 μg/kg/day to start; do not exceed 250 μg/day
Agitated **psychotic states** (eg, schizophrenia)	**Adult:** 100–1,000 μg/day to start; usual initial dosage: 500 μg/day

CONTRAINDICATIONS

Mental depression, especially with suicidal tendencies	Active peptic ulcer	Hypersensitivity to reserpine
Electroconvulsive therapy	Ulcerative colitis	

SERPASIL

ADMINISTRATION/DOSAGE ADJUSTMENTS

Treatment of hypertension	Reserpine can be used alone for mild hypertension or with other drugs for more severe forms; carefully titrate dosage during combination therapy. Exercise caution when giving adult patients with mild or more severe hypertension more than 500 μg/day to start or more than 250 μg/day for maintenance since the frequency of adverse reactions may increase considerably at these higher dosages.
Treatment of psychosis	Reserpine should be used as an antipsychotic primarily in patients who either cannot tolerate phenothiazines or also require antihypertensive medication

WARNINGS/PRECAUTIONS

Mental depression	Reserpine-induced depression is dose-related, may persist for several months after drug withdrawal, and can result in suicide. Use with extreme caution in patients with a history of mental depression; discontinue drug at first sign of despondency, early morning insomnia, loss of appetite, impotence, or self-deprecation.
Gastrointestinal effects	Reserpine can increase GI motility and secretion; use with caution in patients with a history of peptic ulcer or ulcerative colitis. Biliary colic can occur in patients with a history of gallstones; exercise caution when using drug in these patients.
Renal impairment	Reserpine-induced decrease in blood pressure may exacerbate renal insufficiency; use with caution in patients with renal impairment
Surgery	Bradycardia and hypotension can occur during surgery, even if reserpine is withdrawn before the procedure; inform the anesthesiologist before surgery that the patient has received this drug. If cardiovascular reactions occur during surgery, use anticholinergic drugs and direct-acting sympathomimetic agents (eg, norepinephrine, metaraminol) as needed.
Carcinogenicity	Long-term (2-yr) studies in rodents fed 100–300 times the usual human dose of reserpine have shown an increased frequency of mammary fibroadenomas in female mice, malignant tumors of the seminal vesicles in male mice, and malignant adrenal medullary tumors in male rats. No definite conclusion about whether this drug increases the risk of breast cancer in humans has emerged from epidemiological studies or long-term clinical observation; nevertheless, it should be used with caution in patients with previously detected breast cancer because of its prolactin-elevating effect. No studies have been done to determine whether reserpine increases the risks of pheochromocytoma and tumors of the seminal vesicles in humans.

ADVERSE REACTIONS

Gastrointestinal	Vomiting, diarrhea, nausea, anorexia, hypersecretion
Cardiovascular	Arrhythmias, syncope, angina, bradycardia, edema
Respiratory	Dyspnea, epistaxis, nasal congestion
Central nervous system	Extrapyramidal reactions (including parkinsonism), dizziness, headache, paradoxical anxiety, depression, nervousness, nightmares, dull sensorium, drowsiness, muscular aches
Ophthalmic	Optic atrophy, glaucoma, uveitis, conjunctival injection
Genitourinary	Impotence, dysuria, decreased libido
Hypersensitivity	Purpura, rash, pruritus
Other	Deafness, dry mouth, weight gain, pseudolactation, breast engorgement, gynecomastia

OVERDOSAGE

Signs and symptoms	Drowsiness, flushing, conjunctival injection, miosis, hypotension, hypothermia, respiratory depression, bradycardia, increases in gastric and salivary secretion, diarrhea, coma
Treatment	Empty stomach, taking adequate precautions against aspiration, and then instill activated charcoal. Institute symptomatic treatment as needed. If a vasopressor is required, use a direct-acting agent such as phenylephrine, norepinephrine, or metaraminol. When treating marked bradycardia, consider using an anticholinergic drug. Keep patient under careful observation for at least 72 h since reserpine is a long-acting drug.

DRUG INTERACTIONS

MAO inhibitors	Hypertension; institute combination therapy with extreme caution, if at all
Digitalis, quinidine	⇧ Risk of cardiac arrhythmias; exercise caution during combination therapy

ALTERED LABORATORY VALUES

Blood/serum values	⇧ Prolactin
Urinary values	⇩ Catecholamines ⇩ VMA ⇩ 17-OHCS (with modified Glenn-Nelson technique) ⇩ 17-KS (with Holtorff-Koch modification of the Zimmerman reaction)

USE IN CHILDREN

Reserpine is not generally recommended for children because safety and effectiveness for use in these patients have not been established in controlled studies and because adverse effects such as mental depression, emotional lability, sedation, and nasal congestion can occur during therapy; nevertheless, the drug has been used in children (see ORAL DOSAGE).

USE IN PREGNANT AND NURSING WOMEN

Pregnancy Category C: when given parenterally, reserpine has been shown to be teratogenic in rats at up to 2 mg/kg and to be embryocidal in guinea pigs at 0.5 mg/day. In humans, the drug crosses the placental barrier and appears in breast milk; use by pregnant or nursing women can result in anorexia, cyanosis, an increase in respiratory tract secretions, and nasal congestion in neonates. Give this drug during pregnancy only if the expected benefits justify the potential risks; instruct women not to nurse during therapy.

ANTIHYPERTENSIVES WITH DIURETICS

ALDOCLOR (methyldopa and chlorothiazide) Merck Sharp & Dohme Rx

Tablets: 250 mg methyldopa and 150 mg chlorothiazide (Aldoclor 150); 250 mg methyldopa and 250 mg chlorothiazide (Aldoclor 250)

INDICATIONS
Hypertension

ORAL DOSAGE
Adult: 1 tab bid or tid to start, followed by up to 3 g/day of methyldopa and 1–2 g/day of chlorothiazide, as needed (see WARNINGS/PRECAUTIONS)

CONTRAINDICATIONS

Anuria	Active hepatic disease, including acute hepatitis and active cirrhosis	Liver disorders associated with prior methyldopa therapy
Hypersensitivity to chlorothiazide, other sulfonamide derivatives, or methyldopa		

ADMINISTRATION/DOSAGE ADJUSTMENTS

Initiating therapy	Allow at least 48 h between dosage adjustments. Increase or decrease dosage until optimal blood pressure response is obtained; to minimize sedation, increase dosage in the evening.
Combination therapy	Dosage of other antihypertensive agents may need to be adjusted to effect a smooth transition when initiating therapy; limit initial methyldopa dosage to 500 mg/day when adding combination to antihypertensives other than thiazides
Tolerance	May develop occasionally, usually between 2nd and 3rd mo of therapy; to restore control, increase dosage of methyldopa and/or chlorothiazide
Refractory patients	If blood pressure is not adequately controlled with maximal doses of Aldoclor, give additional methyldopa separately
Elderly patients	To prevent syncope, which may be related to increased sensitivity and advanced arteriosclerosis, use lower dosages

WARNINGS/PRECAUTIONS

Fixed combination	Not indicated for initial therapy of hypertension; dosages of component drugs must be individually titrated and then periodically reviewed, as conditions warrant
Coombs'-positive hemolytic anemia	May occur in less than 4% of patients, with potentially fatal complications. Obtain a blood count and Coombs' test before initiating therapy and at 6 and 12 mo after starting. With prolonged use of methyldopa, 10–20% of patients develop a positive direct Coombs' test; while this is not a contraindication to further use of the drug, therapy should be discontinued immediately if hemolytic anemia also develops in such patients. Usually, the anemia remits promptly. If it is related to methyldopa, do not reinstitute the drug.
Drug-induced hepatitis	May occur at any time during therapy. Obtain liver-function studies (eg, SGOT, bilirubin) periodically, especially during first 2–3 mo of therapy, or if unexplained fever or rash occurs. If drug-related, abnormalities will revert to normal after methyldopa is stopped; do not reinstitute therapy.
Hepatic coma	May be precipitated by minor changes in fluid and electrolyte balance in patients with hepatic impairment or progressive liver disease
Special-risk patients	Use with caution in patients with previous liver disease or dysfunction or in those with severe renal impairment; the latter may respond adequately to lower doses
Azotemia	May be precipitated in patients with renal disease

ALDOCLOR

Lithium therapy	Renal clearance is reduced, increasing risk of lithium toxicity; coadministration generally should be avoided unless adequate precautions are taken
Circulatory instability during anesthesia	May occur; if necessary, reduce anesthetic dosage. If hypotension does occur, use a vasopressor.
Orthostatic hypotension	May occur; reduce dosage
Edema and weight gain	May occur; discontinue use of methyldopa if edema progresses or signs of heart failure appear
Suspected pheochromocytoma	Urinary catecholamine level may appear to be elevated due to fluorescence of methyldopa; measurement of vanillylmandelic acid (VMA) by methods that convert VMA to vanillin is not affected
Reversible leukopenia	May occur rarely, manifested primarily by a reduction in granulocytes; discontinue therapy
Involuntary choreoathetotic movements	May occur rarely in patients with severe bilateral cerebrovascular disease; discontinue therapy
Sensitivity reactions	May occur in patients with or without a history of allergy or bronchial asthma
Systemic lupus erythematosus	May be activated or exacerbated
Electrolyte imbalances	Measure serum and urine electrolytes periodically, especially if patient is vomiting excessively or receiving parenteral fluids. Watch for dry mouth, thirst, weakness, lethargy, drowsiness, restlessness, muscle pains or cramps, muscular fatigue, hypotension, oliguria, tachycardia, and GI disturbances.
Hypokalemia	May develop, especially with brisk diuresis, concomitant corticosteroid or ACTH therapy, interference with adequate oral intake of electrolytes, or in the presence of severe cirrhosis; may be minimized by including potassium-rich foods in diet or, if necessary, with potassium supplements
Dilutional hyponatremia	May occur in edematous patients when weather is hot; restrict water and use salt replacement only for life-threatening hyponatremia
Hypomagnesemia	May occur
Hyperuricemia or overt gout	May occur or be precipitated in certain patients
Insulin requirements	May increase, decrease, or remain unchanged; latent diabetes may become active
Dialysis patients	Blood pressure may be difficult to control, since methyldopa is removed by dialysis
Postsympathectomy patients	Antihypertensive effect may be enhanced
Parathyroid function tests	Discontinue drug before testing

ADVERSE REACTIONS

Central nervous system and neuromuscular	Sedation, headache, asthenia, weakness, dizziness, light-headedness, symptoms of cerebrovascular insufficiency, paresthesias, parkinsonism, Bell's palsy, decreased mental acuity, involuntary choreoathetotic movements, psychic disturbances (including nightmares and reversible mild psychoses or depression), vertigo, restlessness, muscle spasm
Ophthalmic	Transient blurred vision, xanthopsia
Cardiovascular	Bradycardia, prolonged carotid sinus hypersensitivity, aggravation of angina pectoris, orthostatic hypotension, edema (and weight gain)
Digestive	Nausea, vomiting, distention, constipation, flatus, diarrhea, colitis, mild dryness of the mouth, sore or "black" tongue, anorexia, gastric irritation, cramping, pancreatitis, sialadenitis
Hepatic	Abnormal liver function tests, jaundice, liver disorders, intrahepatic cholestatic jaundice
Metabolic and endocrinological	Hyperglycemia, glycosuria, hyperuricemia, electrolyte imbalance; breast enlargement, gynecomastia, lactation, impotence, decreased libido, hyperprolactinemia, amenorrhea
Hematological	Bone marrow depression, leukopenia, agranulocytosis, granulocytopenia, thrombocytopenia, aplastic anemia, hemolytic anemia
Dermatological	Eczema-like rash or lichenoid eruption, toxic epidermal necrolysis
Hypersensitivity	Fever, lupus-like syndrome, myocarditis, pericarditis, purpura, photosensitivity, rash, urticaria, necrotizing angiitis, respiratory distress (including pneumonitis and pulmonary edema), anaphylactic reactions
Other	Nasal stuffiness, mild arthralgia (with or without joint swelling), myalgia

OVERDOSAGE

Signs and symptoms	*Methyldopa-related effects:* sedation, hypotension; *chlorothiazide-related effects:* diuresis, lethargy progressing to coma with minimal cardiorespiratory depression, GI irritation, hypermotility, elevated BUN, serum electrolyte changes

ALDOCLOR ■ ALDORIL

Treatment	Monitor serum electrolyte levels and renal function, and institute supportive measures, as required. Treat hypotension by elevating feet and by volume expansion alone, if possible. Treat GI effects symptomatically.

DRUG INTERACTIONS

Beta-adrenergic blockers	▽ Antihypertensive effect (rare)
Other antihypertensive agents	△ Antihypertensive effect
Tubocurarine	△ Skeletal muscle relaxation
Nonsteroidal anti-inflammatory agents	▽ Diuretic, natriuretic, and antihypertensive effects of chlorothiazide component; observe patient closely during concomitant therapy to ensure that desired therapeutic effect is obtained
Norepinephrine	▽ Vasopressor effect
Steroids, ACTH	△ Risk of hypokalemia
Lithium	▽ Lithium clearance
Alcohol, barbiturates, narcotic analgesics	△ Risk of orthostatic hypotension

ALTERED LABORATORY VALUES

Blood/serum values	△ Alkaline phosphatase △ SGOT △ SGPT △ Bilirubin △ Creatinine (with alkaline picrate method) △ BUN △ Uric acid △ Calcium ▽ Magnesium ▽ Sodium ▽ Potassium ▽ Chloride ▽ Bicarbonate ▽ Phosphate ▽ PBI △ or ▽ Glucose ▽ Plasma renin activity + Coombs' test + LE-cell reaction + Rheumatoid factor + ANA titer
Urinary values	△ Sodium △ Potassium △ Chloride △ Bicarbonate △ Uric acid △ Catecholamines (with fluorescence methods) ▽ Calcium △ Magnesium

---

USE IN CHILDREN

Consult manufacturer

USE IN PREGNANT AND NURSING WOMEN

Safety for use during pregnancy has not been established. Both methyldopa and thiazides cross the placental barrier and appear in cord blood and breast milk. No unusual adverse effects of methyldopa have been reported during pregnancy, nor is there any evidence of teratogenicity. The possibility of fetal injury cannot be excluded, however. Thiazides may cause fetal or neonatal jaundice, thrombocytopenia, and other possible reactions. Patient should stop nursing if drug is prescribed.

ANTIHYPERTENSIVES WITH DIURETICS

ALDORIL (methyldopa and hydrochlorothiazide)   Merck Sharp & Dohme   Rx

Tablets: 250 mg methyldopa and 15 mg hydrochlorothiazide (Aldoril 15); 250 mg methyldopa and 25 mg hydrochlorothiazide (Aldoril 25); 500 mg methyldopa and 30 mg hydrochlorothiazide (Aldoril D30); 500 mg methyldopa and 50 mg hydrochlorothiazide (Aldoril D50)

INDICATIONS	ORAL DOSAGE
Hypertension	**Adult:** 1 tab bid or tid to start, followed by up to 3 g/day of methyldopa and 100–200 mg/day of hydrochlorothiazide, as needed (see WARNINGS/PRECAUTIONS)

CONTRAINDICATIONS

Anuria	Active hepatic disease, including acute hepatitis and active cirrhosis	Liver disorders associated with prior methyldopa therapy
Hypersensitivity to hydrochlorothiazide, other sulfonamide derivatives, or methyldopa		

ADMINISTRATION/DOSAGE ADJUSTMENTS

Initiating therapy	Allow at least 48 h between dosage adjustments. Increase or decrease dosage until optimal blood pressure response is obtained; to minimize sedation, increase dosage in the evening.
Combination therapy	Dosage of other antihypertensive agents may need to be adjusted to effect a smooth transition when initiating therapy; limit initial methyldopa dosage to 500 mg/day when adding combination to antihypertensives other than thiazides
Tolerance	May develop occasionally, usually between 2nd and 3rd mo of therapy; to restore control, increase dosage of methyldopa and/or hydrochlorothiazide

ALDORIL

Refractory patients	If blood pressure is not adequately controlled with maximal doses of Aldoril, give additional methyldopa separately
Elderly patients	To prevent syncope, which may be related to increased sensitivity and advanced arteriosclerosis, use lower dosages

WARNINGS/PRECAUTIONS

Fixed combination	Not indicated for initial therapy of hypertension; dosages of component drugs must be individually titrated and then periodically reviewed, as conditions warrant
Coombs'-positive hemolytic anemia	May occur in less than 4% of patients, with potentially fatal complications. Obtain a blood count and Coombs' test before initiating therapy and at 6 and 12 mo after starting. With prolonged use of methyldopa, 10–20% of patients develop a positive direct Coombs' test; while this is not a contraindication to further use of the drug, therapy should be discontinued immediately if hemolytic anemia also develops in such patients. Usually, the anemia remits promptly. If it is related to methyldopa, do not reinstitute the drug.
Drug-induced hepatitis	May occur at any time during therapy. Obtain liver function studies (eg, SGOT, bilirubin) periodically, especially during first 2–3 mo of therapy, or if unexplained fever or rash occurs. If drug-related, abnormalities will revert to normal after methyldopa is stopped; do not reinstitute therapy.
Hepatic coma	May be precipitated by minor changes in fluid and electrolyte balance in patients with hepatic impairment or progressive liver disease
Special-risk patients	Use with caution in patients with previous liver disease or dysfunction or in those with severe renal impairment; the latter may respond adequately to lower doses
Azotemia	May be precipitated in patients with renal disease
Lithium therapy	Renal clearance is reduced, increasing risk of lithium toxicity; coadministration generally should be avoided unless adequate precautions are taken
Circulatory instability during anesthesia	May occur; if necessary, reduce anesthetic dosage. If hypotension does occur, use a vasopressor.
Orthostatic hypotension	May occur; reduce dosage
Edema and weight gain	May occur; discontinue use of methyldopa if edema progresses or signs of heart failure appear
Suspected pheochromocytoma	Urinary catecholamine level may appear to be elevated due to fluorescence of methyldopa; measurement of vanillylmandelic acid (VMA) by methods that convert VMA to vanillin is not affected
Reversible leukopenia	May occur rarely, manifested primarily by a reduction in granulocytes; discontinue therapy
Involuntary choreoathetotic movements	May occur rarely in patients with severe bilateral cerebrovascular disease; discontinue therapy
Sensitivity reactions	May occur in patients with or without a history of allergy or bronchial asthma
Systemic lupus erythematosus	May be activated or exacerbated
Electrolyte imbalances	Measure serum and urine electrolytes periodically, especially if patient is vomiting excessively or receiving parenteral fluids. Watch for dry mouth, thirst, weakness, lethargy, drowsiness, restlessness, muscle pains or cramps, muscular fatigue, hypotension, oliguria, tachycardia, and GI disturbances.
Hypokalemia	May develop, especially with brisk diuresis, concomitant corticosteroid or ACTH therapy, interference with adequate oral intake of electrolytes, or in the presence of severe cirrhosis; may be minimized by including potassium-rich foods in diet or, if necessary, with potassium supplements
Dilutional hyponatremia	May occur in edematous patients when weather is hot; restrict water and use salt replacement only for life-threatening hyponatremia
Hypomagnesemia	May occur
Hyperuricemia or overt gout	May occur or be precipitated in certain patients
Insulin requirements	May increase, decrease, or remain unchanged; latent diabetes may become active
Dialysis patients	Blood pressure may be difficult to control, since methyldopa is removed by dialysis
Postsympathectomy patients	Antihypertensive effect may be enhanced
Parathyroid function tests	Discontinue drug before testing

ADVERSE REACTIONS

Central nervous system and neuromuscular	Sedation, headache, asthenia, weakness, dizziness, light-headedness, symptoms of cerebrovascular insufficiency, paresthesias, parkinsonism, Bell's palsy, decreased mental acuity, involuntary choreoathetotic movements, psychic disturbances (including nightmares and reversible mild psychoses or depression), vertigo, restlessness, muscle spasm

ALDORIL ■ APRESAZIDE

Ophthalmic	Transient blurred vision, xanthopsia
Cardiovascular	Bradycardia, prolonged carotid sinus hypersensitivity, aggravation of angina pectoris, orthostatic hypotension, edema (and weight gain)
Gastrointestinal	Nausea, vomiting, distention, constipation, flatus, diarrhea, colitis, mild dryness of the mouth, sore or "black" tongue, anorexia, gastric irritation, cramping, pancreatitis, sialadenitis
Hepatic	Abnormal liver function tests, jaundice, liver disorders, intrahepatic cholestatic jaundice
Metabolic and endocrinological	Hyperglycemia, glycosuria, hyperuricemia, electrolyte imbalance; breast enlargement, gynecomastia, lactation, impotence, decreased libido, hyperprolactinemia, amenorrhea
Hematological	Bone marrow depression, leukopenia, agranulocytosis, granulocytopenia, thrombocytopenia, aplastic anemia, hemolytic anemia
Dermatological	Eczema-like rash or lichenoid eruption, toxic epidermal necrolysis
Hypersensitivity	Fever, lupus-like syndrome, myocarditis, pericarditis, purpura, photosensitivity, rash, urticaria, necrotizing angiitis, respiratory distress (including pneumonitis and pulmonary edema), anaphylactic reactions
Other	Nasal stuffiness, mild arthralgia (with or without joint swelling), myalgia

OVERDOSAGE

Signs and symptoms	*Methyldopa-related effects:* sedation, hypotension; *hydrochlorothiazide-related effects:* diuresis, lethargy progressing to coma with minimal cardiorespiratory depression, GI irritation, hypermotility, elevated BUN, serum electrolyte changes
Treatment	Monitor serum electrolyte levels and renal function, and institute supportive measures, as required. Treat hypotension by elevating feet and by volume expansion alone, if possible. Treat GI effects symptomatically.

DRUG INTERACTIONS

Beta-adrenergic blockers	▽ Antihypertensive effect (rare)
Other antihypertensive agents	△ Antihypertensive effect
Tubocurarine	△ Skeletal muscle relaxation
Nonsteroidal anti-inflammatory agents	▽ Diuretic, natriuretic, and antihypertensive effects of hydrochlorothiazide component; observe patient closely during concomitant therapy to ensure that desired therapeutic effect is obtained
Norepinephrine	▽ Vasopressor effect
Steroids, ACTH	△ Risk of hypokalemia
Lithium	▽ Lithium clearance
Alcohol, barbiturates, narcotic analgesics	△ Risk of orthostatic hypotension

ALTERED LABORATORY VALUES

Blood/serum values	△ Alkaline phosphatase △ SGOT △ SGPT △ Bilirubin △ Creatinine (with alkaline picrate method) △ Uric acid △ Calcium ▽ Magnesium ▽ Sodium ▽ Potassium ▽ Chloride ▽ Bicarbonate ▽ Phosphate ▽ PBI △ or ▽ Glucose ▽ Plasma renin activity + Coombs' test + LE-cell reaction + Rheumatoid factor + ANA titer
Urinary values	△ Sodium △ Potassium △ Chloride △ Bicarbonate △ Uric acid △ Catecholamines (with fluorescence methods) ▽ Calcium △ Magnesium

---

USE IN CHILDREN
Consult manufacturer

USE IN PREGNANT AND NURSING WOMEN
Safety for use during pregnancy has not been established. Both methyldopa and thiazides cross the placental barrier and appear in cord blood and breast milk. No unusual adverse effects of methyldopa have been reported during pregnancy, nor is there any evidence of teratogenicity. However, the possibility of fetal injury cannot be excluded. Thiazides may cause fetal or neonatal jaundice, thrombocytopenia, and other possible reactions. Patient should stop nursing if drug is prescribed.

ANTIHYPERTENSIVES WITH DIURETICS

APRESAZIDE (hydralazine hydrochloride and hydrochlorothiazide) CIBA   Rx

Capsules: 25 mg hydralazine hydrochloride and 25 mg hydrochlorothiazide (Apresazide 25/25); 50 hydralazine hydrochloride and 50 mg hydrochlorothiazide (Apresazide 50/50); 100 mg hydralazine hydrochloride and 50 mg hydrochlorothiazide (Apresazide 100/50)

INDICATIONS	ORAL DOSAGE
Hypertension	**Adult:** 1 cap bid

APRESAZIDE

CONTRAINDICATIONS

Coronary artery disease	Hypersensitivity to hydrochlorothiazide, other sulfonamide derivatives, or hydralazine	Rheumatic mitral valve disease
Anuria		

ADMINISTRATION/DOSAGE ADJUSTMENTS

Food-drug interactions	Administration of hydralazine with food results in higher serum drug levels; food also enhances absorption of hydrochlorothiazide
Acetylation rate	Serum levels of hydralazine are generally higher in patients who acetylate the drug at a slow rate; these patients usually require lower doses of hydralazine than patients with a rapid rate of acetylation
Combination therapy	Other antihypertensive agents, such as sympatholytics, may be added gradually at a reduced dosage; carefully monitor clinical response

WARNINGS/PRECAUTIONS

Fixed combination	This preparation is not indicated for initial therapy of hypertension; dosages of the component drugs must be individually titrated to the patient's needs before instituting treatment with this combination
Lupus erythematosus	A syndrome resembling systemic lupus erythematosus, with glomerulonephritis and other lupus-like reactions, can occur with use of hydralazine; although this syndrome is usually reversible, manifestations can persist and necessitate long-term corticosteroid treatment. Thiazides can activate or exacerbate systemic lupus erythematosus. To reduce the risk of this syndrome, perform an ANA test before therapy, periodically during prolonged treatment, and whenever arthralgia, fever, chest pain, continued malaise, or any other unexplained reaction occurs. If results of an ANA test are positive or clinical signs and symptoms develop, carefully weigh risks and benefits of continued use.
Angina, myocardial infarction	The myocardial stimulation due to hydralazine may precipitate angina, myocardial ischemia, and myocardial infarction; use with caution in patients with known or suspected coronary artery disease
Postural hypotension	Hydralazine can cause postural hypotension; use with caution in patients with cerebrovascular accidents
Peripheral neuritis	Hydralazine may cause peripheral neuritis, characterized by paresthesias, numbness, and tingling; if symptoms develop, administer pyridoxine concomitantly
Blood dyscrasias	Watch for evidence of blood dyscrasias; obtain a CBC before therapy, periodically during prolonged treatment, and whenever symptoms develop. If leukopenia, agranulocytosis, purpura, or a reduction in hemoglobin and erythrocytes is detected, this preparation should be discontinued.
Drug accumulation, renal dysfunction	Thiazides can accumulate or precipitate azotemia in patients with renal impairment; hydralazine may exacerbate advanced renal disease. Use this preparation with caution in patients with severe or advanced renal disease; if renal impairment progresses, consider interrupting or terminating therapy.
Hepatic coma	Minor changes in fluid and electrolyte balance may precipitate hepatic coma in patients with hepatic impairment or progressive liver disease; use with caution in such patients
Electrolyte disorders	Hypokalemia may occur, especially when diuresis is brisk, severe cirrhosis is present, ACTH or corticosteroids are given concomitantly, or oral intake of electrolytes is inadequate; potassium supplements or potassium-rich foods may be given to avoid or treat hypokalemia. Dilutional hyponatremia may occur in edematous patients when the weather is hot. Treat by restricting the intake of water; administer salt only if hyponatremia is life-threatening or actual salt depletion occurs. For hypochloremia, specific treatment is usually unnecessary, except for certain patients (eg, those with hepatic or renal disease). To prevent electrolyte imbalance, measure serum and urinary electrolyte levels periodically in all patients (these determinations are especially important if excessive vomiting occurs or parenteral fluids are being given); watch for premonitory signs and symptoms of hypokalemia, hyponatremia, and hypochloremic alkalosis, such as dry mouth, thirst, weakness, lethargy, drowsiness, restlessness, muscle pain or cramps, muscular fatigue, hypotension, oliguria, tachycardia, and GI disturbances (eg, nausea and vomiting).
Diabetes	Thiazides can activate latent diabetes or alter insulin requirements
Parathyroid dysfunction	Thiazides decrease calcium excretion. Discontinue use before performing parathyroid function tests. Pathological changes in the parathyroid gland, accompanied by hypercalcemia and hypophosphatemia, have occurred in a few patients after prolonged thiazide therapy; however, the common complications of hyperparathyroidism have not been seen.
Other thiazide-related reactions	Thiazides can cause hyperuricemia or overt gout, precipitate hypersensitivity reactions (especially in patients with a history of allergy or bronchial asthma), and, in postsympathectomy patients, produce an enhanced antihypertensive effect
Carcinogenicity	An increase in adenomas and adenocarcinomas of the lung has occurred in mice fed throughout their lives 80 times the maximum human dose of hydralazine; increases in benign hepatic neoplastic nodules and benign testicular interstitial cell tumors have been observed in rats given hydralazine. Long-term clinical observation has not suggested an association between hydralazine and cancer; however, no adequate epidemiological studies have been done. No long-term studies have been done to evaluate the carcinogenic potential of hydrochlorothiazide.

APRESAZIDE

Mutagenicity	Hydralazine has been shown to be mutagenic in the Ames test and has elicited DNA repair, a sign of mutagenicity, in *E coli* and cultured rat hepatocytes. In tests with rabbit hepatocytes having either a slow or rapid acetylation rate, the drug has elicited DNA repair only in those hepatocytes with a slow rate; these results suggest that patients with a rapid acetylation rate may be less susceptible to the potentially mutagenic effects of this drug. No evidence of mutagenicity has been seen in the mouse lymphoma assay, host-mediated assay, nucleus anomaly test, or dominant lethal test.

ADVERSE REACTIONS

Central nervous system	Headache, paresthesias, peripheral neuritis, dizziness, vertigo, tremors, muscle cramps or spasm, weakness, restlessness; psychotic reactions characterized by depression, disorientation, or anxiety
Ophthalmic	Lacrimation, conjunctivitis, xanthopsia, transient blurred vision
Gastrointestinal	Anorexia, nausea, vomiting, diarrhea, gastric irritation, cramping, constipation, paralytic ileus, intrahepatic cholestatic jaundice, pancreatitis
Cardiovascular	Palpitations, tachycardia, angina, hypotension (including orthostatic hypotension), paradoxical hypertension, edema
Hematological	Reduction in hemoglobin, erythropenia, leukopenia, agranulocytosis, thrombocytopenia, purpura, aplastic anemia, lymphadenopathy, splenomegaly
Respiratory	Dyspnea, nasal congestion
Hypersensitivity	Rash, urticaria, pruritus, fever, chills, arthralgia, eosinophilia, purpura, photosensitivity, necrotizing angiitis, Stevens-Johnson syndrome; hepatitis (rare)
Other	Flushing, difficult urination, sialadenitis, hyperglycemia, glycosuria, hyperuricemia

OVERDOSAGE

Signs and symptoms	Hypotension, shock, tachycardia, headache, generalized skin flushing, myocardial ischemia and infarction, arrhythmia, hypokalemia, hyponatremia, hypochloremia, alkalosis, increased BUN level (especially in patients with renal impairment); anuria, oliguria, or polyuria; nausea, vomiting, thirst, weakness, confusion, dizziness, fatigue, impairment of consciousness, cramped calf muscles, paresthesia
Treatment	Give primary attention to cardiovascular status. To treat shock, raise patient's legs, replace fluids and electrolytes (potassium and sodium), and administer plasma expanders; use vasopressors only if they are necessary and precautions are taken to avoid precipitating or exacerbating an arrhythmia. For tachycardia, give a beta blocker. Digitalization may be necessary for reversal of cardiovascular disorders. Monitor renal function and institute supportive measures as needed. To remove the drug from the GI tract, empty stomach and then, if conditions permit, instill activated charcoal; bear in mind that since these measures can precipitate arrhythmia or enhance shock, it may be necessary to either skip them or wait until cardiovascular function has been restored before doing them.

DRUG INTERACTIONS

Diazoxide	Severe hypotension; after giving diazoxide to patients receiving this preparation, monitor blood pressure continuously for several hours
Other antihypertensive agents	△ Antihypertensive effect
Digitalis	△ Risk of digitalis toxicity owing to thiazide-induced hypokalemia
MAO inhibitors	△ Risk of hypotension; exercise caution during combination therapy
Lithium	△ Risk of lithium toxicity
Norepinephrine, other vasopressors	▽ Vasopressor effect; nevertheless, this interaction does not preclude therapeutic use of vasopressors
Corticosteroids, ACTH	△ Risk of hypokalemia
Tubocurarine, other nondepolarizing skeletal muscle relaxants	△ Skeletal muscle relaxation
Propranolol, metoprolol	△ Serum level of propranolol and metoprolol
Alcohol, barbiturates, narcotic analgesics	△ Risk of orthostatic hypotension

ALTERED LABORATORY VALUES

Blood/serum values	+ ANA + Direct Coombs' test △ PRA (plasma renin activity) ▽ Sodium ▽ Potassium △ Calcium ▽ Magnesium ▽ Chloride ▽ Phosphate △ Uric acid ▽ PBI △ Glucose
Urinary values	△ Sodium △ Potassium ▽ Calcium △ Magnesium △ Chloride △ Bicarbonate ▽ Uric acid △ Glucose

APRESAZIDE ■ CAPOZIDE

USE IN CHILDREN
Safety and effectiveness for use in children have not been established

USE IN PREGNANT AND NURSING WOMEN
Pregnancy Category C: hydralazine has caused cleft palate and malformations of facial and cranial bones in mice at 20–30 times the maximum daily human dose and may be teratogenic in rabbits at 10–15 times the maximum daily human dose. Administration of a thiazide during pregnancy can produce adverse reactions, including jaundice and thrombocytopenia, in a neonate or fetus. Use this preparation during pregnancy only if the expected benefit justifies the potential risks. It is not known whether hydralazine is excreted in human milk; however, thiazides are found in human milk. Instruct women not to nurse during therapy.

ANTIHYPERTENSIVES WITH DIURETICS

CAPOZIDE (captopril and hydrochlorothiazide) Squibb   Rx
Tablets: 25 mg captopril and 15 mg hydrochlorothiazide (Capozide 25/15), 25 mg captopril and 25 mg hydrochlorothiazide (Capozide 25/25), 50 mg captopril and 15 mg hydrochlorothiazide (Capozide 50/15), 50 mg captopril and 25 mg hydrochlorothiazide (Capozide 50/25)

INDICATIONS
Hypertension in patients with normal renal function
Hypertension in patients with renal impairment who have experienced unacceptable side effects with other antihypertensive drugs or have failed to respond satisfactorily to a combination of other antihypertensive drugs

ORAL DOSAGE
Adult: 1 tab bid or tid; if administration of 1 Capozide 50/15 tab tid will not provide sufficient control, add another antihypertensive agent to the regimen. Do not give more than 450 mg/day of captopril.

CONTRAINDICATIONS
Anuria   Hypersensitivity to hydrochlorothiazide or other sulfonamide derivatives

ADMINISTRATION/DOSAGE ADJUSTMENTS
Timing of administration	Give this preparation 1 h before meals
Renal impairment	A reduction in dosage may be necessary for patients with renal impairment since both components of this preparation are excreted primarily by the kidney. Use in patients with severe renal impairment is generally not recommended because when these patients require use of a diuretic in combination with captopril, it is preferable to give them a loop diuretic rather than a thiazide.
Severe hypertension	Dosage can be titrated at intervals of less than 2 wk if the patient has severe hypertension (eg, accelerated or malignant hypertension) and is kept under continuous medical supervision
Combination therapy	To avoid hypotension, reduce the usual starting dosage of the new agent by 50% and increase the dosage gradually. Bear in mind that although beta blockers enhance antihypertensive response, the effect is less than additive.

WARNINGS/PRECAUTIONS
Fixed combination	This preparation is not indicated for initial therapy of hypertension; dosages of the component drugs must be individually titrated to the patient's needs before instituting treatment with this combination
Neutropenia, agranulocytosis	Captopril has caused myeloid hypoplasia, neutropenia, and agranulocytosis within 3 mo after the start of therapy; oral and systemic infections or other manifestations of agranulocytosis have developed in approximately 50% of patients with neutropenia. On bone marrow examination, erythroid hypoplasia and a decreased number of megakaryocytes have frequently been seen with myeloid hypoplasia; in some cases, neutropenia has been accompanied by anemia and thrombocytopenia. Neutropenia has occurred in approximately 0.012% of patients with normal renal function (serum creatinine level < 1.6 mg/dl), about 0.2% of patients with renal impairment (serum creatinine level > 1.6 mg/dl), and 3.7% of patients with a combination of renal impairment and collagen vascular disease (eg, systemic lupus erythematosus, scleroderma). In over 75% of cases seen during treatment of heart failure, procainamide was given in combination with captopril. Thirteen percent of patients who developed neutropenia while receiving captopril have died; however, almost all of the deaths were associated with one or more of the following complicating factors: serious illness, collagen vascular disease, renal or heart failure, or immunosuppressant therapy.

To reduce the risk of agranulocytosis, instruct all patients to report any sign of infection, such as sore throat or fever. Promptly obtain a WBC count whenever an infection is suspected. If a neutrophil count of less than 1,000/mm³ is detected, discontinue captopril and closely watch patient; neutropenia generally reverses within 2 wk after termination of therapy. Always assess renal function before beginning therapy. If renal impairment is seen, obtain WBC and differential counts before therapy, every 2 wk during the initial 3-mo period, and then periodically thereafter. In patients who have collagen vascular disease or who are receiving other drugs known to affect leukocytes or the immune response, use with caution and only after weighing benefits and risks, particularly when these patients also have renal impairment.

Proteinuria, nephrotic syndrome	Urinary protein exceeding 1 g/day has been seen in approximately 0.7% of patients given captopril; the nephrotic syndrome has developed in about 20% of those with proteinuria. Creatinine and BUN levels were seldom affected. In most cases, proteinuria occurred within 8 mo after the start of therapy and, regardless of whether or not therapy was continued, subsided or disappeared within 6 mo after detection. Patients who had a history of renal disease or who received more than 150 mg/day have accounted for 90% of the cases of proteinuria. If captopril is to be used in these patients, obtain estimates of urinary protein before therapy (or before giving 150 mg/day) and then periodically thereafter; use first morning urine samples for these determinations. Instruct all patients to report any sign of progressive edema that may indicate proteinuria or the nephrotic syndrome.
Increases in BUN and creatinine, azotemia	Transient elevations in BUN and serum creatinine levels can occur, especially in association with hypovolemia, renovascular hypertension, or rapid control of severe or prolonged hypertension. In some patients with renal disease, especially those with severe renal artery stenosis, increases in BUN and serum creatinine levels may persist; if necessary, reduce the dosage of captopril and/or discontinue diuretic therapy since it may not be possible to simultaneously maintain both normal blood pressure and adequate renal perfusion. Thiazides may precipitate azotemia in patients with renal impairment; use this preparation with caution in patients with severe renal disease and, if renal impairment progresses, consider interrupting or terminating therapy.
Hepatic coma	Minor changes in fluid and electrolyte balance may precipitate hepatic coma in patients with hepatic impairment or progressive liver disease; use with caution in such patients
Electrolyte disorders	Thiazides can cause hypokalemia, especially when diuresis is brisk, severe cirrhosis is present, ACTH or corticosteroids are given concomitantly, or oral intake of electrolytes is inadequate; however, captopril reduces this risk and, in some cases, may even eliminate the need for prophylactic therapy with potassium supplements or potassium-rich foods. Dilutional hyponatremia may occur in edematous patients when the weather is hot. Treat by restricting the intake of water; administer salt only if hyponatremia is life-threatening or actual salt depletion occurs. For hypochloremia, specific treatment is usually unnecessary, except for certain patients (eg, those with hepatic or renal disease). To prevent electrolyte imbalance, measure serum and urinary electrolyte levels periodically in all patients (these determinations are especially important if excessive vomiting occurs or parenteral fluids are being given); watch for premonitory signs and symptoms of hypokalemia, hyponatremia, and hypochloremic alkalosis, such as dry mouth, thirst, weakness, lethargy, drowsiness, restlessness, muscle pain or cramps, muscular fatigue, hypotension, oliguria, tachycardia, and GI disturbances (eg, nausea and vomiting).
Hypotension	Captopril can precipitate excessive hypotension in patients with severe hyponatremia or hypovolemia, which can result from dialysis, severe congestive heart failure, diuretic therapy (especially if vigorous or instituted recently), or severe salt restriction; hypotension most frequently occurs within 1 h after the initial dose. To avoid excessive hypotension, discontinue diuretic therapy or increase salt intake approximately 1 wk before starting captopril therapy, begin with a small dose (6.25 or 12.5 mg), or observe patient for at least 1 h after administering the first dose. Transient hypotension is not a contraindication to further use since this effect should not recur once hypovolemia disappears and blood pressure increases. If hypotension occurs during therapy, place patient in a supine position and, if necessary, give normal saline by IV infusion. Caution patients that dehydration owing to excessive perspiration, vomiting, or diarrhea may precipitate hypotension.
Surgery	In patients undergoing major surgery or receiving anesthetics that can cause hypotension, captopril will block a compensatory increase in angiotensin II; if captopril-induced hypotension occurs, correct by volume expansion
Rash	Captopril causes rash, usually characterized by maculopapules, in 4–7% of patients; frequency depends on dose and renal status. Rash most frequently occurs during the first 4 wk of therapy; it is often seen with pruritus, sometimes with fever and arthralgia, and, in 7–10% of cases, with eosinophilia or a positive ANA test. Rashes are usually mild and can generally be reversed within a few days by a reduction of dosage, short-term use of an antihistamine, or termination of therapy; reactions may also disappear spontaneously during therapy.
Physical activity	Caution patients with heart failure against rapid increases in physical activity
Impairment of taste	Dysgeusia occurs in 2–4% of patients given captopril; frequency depends on dose and renal status. The reaction is usually reversible even with continued use and generally disappears within 2–3 mo. Weight loss may occur along with dysgeusia.
Concomitant use of other vasodilators	No information is available on the effects of combining captopril with nitroglycerin or other vasodilators in patients with heart failure. If possible, discontinue use of any drug with vasodilator activity before starting captopril; if use of such drugs is resumed, administer them with caution and perhaps at a lower dosage.
Parathyroid dysfunction	Thiazides decrease calcium excretion. Discontinue use before performing parathyroid function tests. Pathological changes in the parathyroid gland, accompanied by hypercalcemia and hypophosphatemia, have occurred in a few patients after prolonged thiazide therapy; however, the common complications of hyperparathyroidism have not been seen.

CAPOZIDE

Other thiazide-related reactions	Thiazides may activate or exacerbate systemic lupus erythematosus, precipitate hypersensitivity reactions, activate latent diabetes, cause hyperuricemia or overt gout, or, in postsympathectomy patients, produce an enhanced antihypertensive response
Carcinogenicity, effect on fertility	No evidence of carcinogenicity has been seen in mice and rats given 50–1,350 mg/kg/day of captopril for 2 yr; studies in rats have shown no adverse effect on fertility. No studies have been done to evaluate the carcinogenic or mutagenic potential of hydrochlorothiazide or its effect on fertility.

ADVERSE REACTIONS[1]

Cardiovascular	Hypotension (including orthostatic hypotension), tachycardia, chest pain, palpitations, angina, myocardial infarction, Raynaud's syndrome, congestive heart failure, flushing, pallor
Hematological	Neutropenia, agranulocytosis, anemia, thrombocytopenia, pancytopenia, leukopenia, aplastic anemia, hemolytic anemia, eosinophilia
Central nervous system	Dizziness, vertigo, paresthesias, headache, weakness, restlessness
Ophthalmic	Xanthopsia, transient blurred vision
Gastrointestinal	Weight loss, anorexia, gastric irritation, nausea, vomiting, cramping, diarrhea, constipation, hepatocellular injury, cholestatic jaundice, pancreatitis
Renal	Proteinuria, nephrotic syndrome
Hypersensitivity	Rash, urticaria, pruritus, pemphigoid-like lesions, photosensitivity, purpura, necrotizing angiitis, fever, respiratory distress, pneumonitis, anaphylactic reactions; angioedema of the face, mouth, or extremities; laryngeal edema (one case)
Other	Diminution or loss of taste, sialadenitis, arthralgia, positive ANA test, muscle spasm, hyperglycemia, glycosuria, hyperuricemia

OVERDOSAGE

Signs and symptoms	Hypotension, diuresis, lethargy, coma, GI irritation and hypermotility, transitory increase in BUN level, serum electrolyte changes
Treatment	To reverse hypotension, administer normal saline by IV infusion. Treat GI effects symptomatically; institute supportive therapy for stupor and coma. Take appropriate measures to restore fluid and electrolyte balance and to maintain renal and cardiorespiratory functions. Empty stomach by performing gastric lavage. Captopril can be removed from the blood by hemodialysis; the extent to which hydrochlorothiazide can be removed has not been clearly established.

DRUG INTERACTIONS

Other diuretics	△ Risk of hypotension (see WARNINGS/PRECAUTIONS)
Adrenergic blockers, ganglionic blockers	△ Risk of hypotension; exercise caution during concomitant therapy
Potassium-sparing diuretics (see also diuretics interaction, above), potassium supplements, potassium-containing salt substitutes	△ Serum potassium level; use potassium supplements or potassium-sparing diuretics with caution and only for documented hypokalemia. Use salt substitutes with caution.
Indomethacin, possibly other nonsteroidal anti-inflammatory agents	△ Antihypertensive effect, especially in patients with low renin hypertension
Lithium	△ Risk of lithium toxicity; lithium should generally not be given with this preparation
Digitalis	△ Risk of digitalis toxicity
Norepinephrine, other vasopressors	▽ Vasopressor effect; nevertheless, this interaction does not preclude therapeutic use of vasopressors
Corticosteroids, ACTH	△ Risk of hypokalemia
Insulin, sulfonylureas	△ Risk of hyperglycemia; adjustment of antidiabetic dosage may be necessary
Tubocurarine, other nondepolarizing skeletal muscle relaxants	△ Skeletal muscle relaxation
Preanesthetic and anesthetic agents	△ Pharmacologic effect of these agents; adjust dosage of these drugs accordingly
Alcohol, barbiturates, narcotic analgesics	△ Risk of orthostatic hypotension

ALTERED LABORATORY VALUES

Blood/serum values	△ BUN △ Creatinine + ANA ▽ Sodium ▽ Potassium △ Calcium ▽ Magnesium ▽ Chloride ▽ Phosphate △ Uric acid ▽ PBI △ Glucose
Urinary values	False positive for acetone △ Sodium △ Potassium △ Calcium △ Magnesium △ Chloride △ Bicarbonate ▽ Uric acid △ Glucose

CAPOZIDE ■ COMBIPRES

USE IN CHILDREN

Use this preparation in children only if other measures to control hypertension have not been effective. Safety and effectiveness of captopril for use in children have not been established; however, in limited experience, captopril has been given at a weight-adjusted adult dosage to children 2 mo to 15 yr of age who had secondary hypertension and varying degrees of renal insufficiency.

USE IN PREGNANT AND NURSING WOMEN

Pregnancy Category C: captopril has been shown to be embryocidal and teratogenic in rabbits at 2–70 times the maximum human dose (probably as a result of severe hypotension) and has caused a reduction in neonatal survival in rats at 400 times the recommended human dose; no teratogenic effects have been seen in hamsters or rats following administration of large doses. Administration of a thiazide during pregnancy can produce adverse reactions, including jaundice and thrombocytopenia, in a fetus or neonate. Use this preparation during pregnancy only if the expected benefit justifies the potential risks. Both captopril and hydrochlorothiazide are excreted in human milk; instruct women not to nurse during therapy.

[1] Reactions for which a causal relationship have not been established include renal insufficiency and failure, polyuria, oliguria, urinary frequency, abdominal pain, aphthous ulcers, peptic ulcers, malaise, fatigue, insomnia, dry mouth, dyspnea, cough, and alopecia

---

ANTIHYPERTENSIVES WITH DIURETICS

COMBIPRES (clonidine hydrochloride and chlorthalidone) Boehringer Ingelheim   Rx

Tablets: 0.1 mg clonidine hydrochloride and 15 mg chlorthalidone (Combipres 0.1); 0.2 mg clonidine hydrochloride and 15 mg chlorthalidone (Combipres 0.2); 0.3 mg clonidine hydrochloride and 15 mg chlorthalidone (Combipres 0.3)

INDICATIONS	ORAL DOSAGE
Hypertension	**Adult:** determine patient dose by individual titration of separate components (see Catapres and Hygroton)

CONTRAINDICATIONS	
Hypersensitivity to chlorthalidone	Severe renal or hepatic disease

ADMINISTRATION/DOSAGE ADJUSTMENTS	
Discontinuation of therapy	Reduce dosage of clonidine gradually over 2–4 days to avoid withdrawal symptoms (see WARNINGS/PRECAUTIONS)

WARNINGS/PRECAUTIONS	
Fixed combination	Not indicated for initial therapy of hypertension; dosages of component drugs must be individually titrated and then periodically reviewed, as conditions warrant
Withdrawal syndrome	Nervousness, agitation, headache, elevated serum catecholamine levels, a rapid increase in blood pressure, and, in rare cases, hypertensive encephalopathy and death, have been seen following abrupt cessation of clonidine; reactions have usually occurred after use of clonidine at dosages exceeding 1.2 mg/day or when beta blockade has been instituted or maintained at the time of cessation. Rebound hypertension can be reversed by reinstitution of oral clonidine therapy or use of IV phentolamine. Caution patients not to terminate therapy on their own. To discontinue clonidine in patients receiving both this drug and a beta blocker, first withdraw the beta blocker and then, several days later, discontinue clonidine.
Drowsiness, sedation	Patients who engage in potentially hazardous activities should be cautioned about the sedative effect of clonidine and that it may enhance the CNS depressant effects of alcohol, barbiturates, and other sedatives
Special-risk patients	Use with caution in patients with severe coronary insufficiency, recent myocardial infarction, cerebrovascular disease, or chronic renal failure
Visual impairment	Periodic eye examinations are recommended during prolonged therapy, based on evidence of retinal degeneration in rats[1]
Decreased glucose tolerance	May occur; periodically test patients predisposed toward or affected by diabetes
Renal failure	Determine BUN periodically; if rise in BUN is significant, stop therapy
Sodium and/or potassium depletion	May occur, resulting in muscular weakness, muscle cramps, anorexia, nausea, vomiting, constipation, lethargy, or mental confusion; severe dietary salt restriction is not recommended
Potassium deficiency, hypokalemia	May develop, often preceded by hypochloremic acidosis. Patients taking corticosteroids, ACTH, or digitalis concomitantly must be closely monitored. Risk of potassium deficiency may be minimized by including potassium-rich foods in diet or, if necessary, with oral potassium supplements supplying 3.0–4.5 g/day of KCl.
Hyperuricemia or acute gout	May occur or be precipitated by chlorthalidone; for significant or prolonged hyperuricemia, administer a uricosuric agent while continuing Combipres therapy

COMBIPRES

Hypersensitivity	If allergic contact sensitization occurs with transdermal clonidine, substitution of this product may produce a generalized rash; if systemic allergic reactions such as angioedema, urticaria, or generalized rash develop with transdermal clonidine, they may recur following substitution of this product.
Tolerance	Some patients may develop tolerance to clonidine; if tolerance occurs, reevaluate therapy

ADVERSE REACTIONS

Frequent reactions (incidence $\geq$ 1%) are printed in *italics*

Gastrointestinal	*Dry mouth ($\sim$ 40%)*, anorexia, malaise, nausea, vomiting, parotid pain, mild transient abnormalities in liver function tests, gastric irritation, constipation, cramping, pancreatitis, jaundice, drug-induced hepatitis without icterus or hyperbilirubinemia (one case)
Metabolic and endocrinological	Weight gain, gynecomastia, hyperglycemia, glycosuria, hypokalemia, gout, hyperuricemia
Cardiovascular	Congestive heart failure, Raynaud's phenomenon, ECG abnormalities manifested as Wenckebach's period or ventricular trigeminy, orthostatic hypotension; sinus bradycardia and AV block (rare)
Central nervous system and neuromuscular	*Drowsiness ($\sim$ 35%), sedation ($\sim$ 8%)*, dizziness, headache, vivid dreams or nightmares, insomnia, other behavioral changes, nervousness, restlessness, anxiety, mental depression, paresthesias, fatigue, weakness
Ophthalmic	Dry, itching, or burning eyes, xanthopsia
Dermatological	Rash, angioneurotic edema, hives, urticaria, thinning of hair, pruritis not associated with a rash, purpura, photosensitization
Genitourinary	Impotence, urinary retention, dysuria
Hematological (idiosyncratic)	Aplastic anemia, thrombocytopenia, leukopenia, agranulocytosis, necrotizing angiitis
Other	Increased sensitivity to alcohol, dryness of the nasal mucosa, pallor, weakly positive Coombs' test

OVERDOSAGE

Signs and symptoms	*Clonidine-related effects:* profound hypotension, weakness, somnolence, diminished or absent reflexes, vomiting; *chlorthalidone-related effects:* nausea, weakness, dizziness, electrolyte balance disturbances
Treatment	Use gastric lavage to empty stomach. Administer an analeptic and vasopressor or, alternatively, 10 mg tolazoline every 30 min. Treat chlorthalidone-related effects supportively, including, when necessary, IV dextrose and saline with potassium, administered with caution.

DRUG INTERACTIONS

Alcohol, barbiturates, narcotic analgesics	△ CNS depression △ Risk of orthostatic hypotension
Tricyclic antidepressants[1]	▽ Antihypertensive effect of clonidine; increase dosage, if necessary
Beta blockers	Rebound hypertension following withdrawal of clonidine (see WARNINGS/PRECAUTIONS)
Tubocurarine	△ Skeletal muscle relaxation
Norepinephrine	▽ Vasopressor effect
Steroids, ACTH	△ Risk of hypokalemia
Lithium	▽ Lithium clearance

ALTERED LABORATORY VALUES

Blood/serum values	△ Glucose (transient) △ Creatine phosphokinase △ Uric acid ▽ Sodium ▽ Potassium ▽ Chloride ▽ Plasma renin activity
Urinary values	△ Aldosterone △ Catecholamines △ Sodium △ Potassium △ Chloride △ Uric acid

---

USE IN CHILDREN

Safety and effectiveness for use in children have not been established

USE IN PREGNANT AND NURSING WOMEN

Embryotoxic effects have been observed in animals given clonidine at doses as low as one-third the maximum dose; use of this preparation in women who are or may become pregnant is not recommended, unless the expected benefit outweighs the potential risk to the mother and infant. Clonidine is excreted in human milk; use with caution in nursing mothers.

---

[1] Several studies have shown that clonidine produces a dose-dependent increase in the incidence and severity of spontaneous retinal degeneration in albino rats treated for 6 mo or longer; rats treated concurrently with clonidine and amitriptyline have developed corneal lesions within 5 days. Except for dry eyes, however, no adverse ophthalmologic effects have been observed in patients receiving clonidine, some of whom have been examined periodically for 24 mo or longer.

ANTIHYPERTENSIVES WITH DIURETICS

CORZIDE (nadolol and bendroflumethiazide) Squibb   Rx

Tablets: 40 mg nadolol and 5 mg bendroflumethiazide (Corzide 40/5); 80 mg nadolol and 5 mg bendroflumethiazide (Corzide 80/5)

INDICATIONS

Hypertension

ORAL DOSAGE

Adult: 1 Corzide 40/5 tab once daily to start, followed, if necessary, by 1 Corzide 80/5 tab once daily

CONTRAINDICATIONS

Cardiogenic shock

Bronchial asthma

Anuria

Conduction block greater than first degree

Overt cardiac failure (see WARNINGS/PRECAUTIONS)

Sinus bradycardia

Hypersensitivity to bendroflumethiazide or other sulfonamide derivatives

ADMINISTRATION/DOSAGE ADJUSTMENTS

Patients with renal impairment	Use with caution; renal insufficiency may lead to excessive drug accumulation. Adjust the interval between doses as follows: administer q24h if creatinine clearance (Ccr) > 50 ml/min; q24–36h if Ccr = 31–50 ml/min; q24–48h if Ccr = 10–30 ml/min; or q40–60h if Ccr < 10 ml/min.
Switching from Naturetin (bendroflumethiazide)	Substitution of Corzide for 5 mg of Naturetin represents a 30% increase in bendroflumethiazide dosage because of the difference in bioavailability
Adding other antihypertensive agents	To avoid an excessive fall in blood pressure, begin with half dosage and increase the dosage gradually
Discontinuation of therapy	Reduce dosage gradually over a period of 1–2 wk and monitor patient carefully. Caution patients, especially those with coronary artery disease, not to interrupt or discontinue therapy on their own.

WARNINGS/PRECAUTIONS

Fixed combination	This preparation is not indicated for initial therapy of hypertension; dosages of the component drugs must be individually titrated to the patient's needs before instituting treatment with this combination
Cardiac failure	Beta blockade may cause or exacerbate cardiac failure; discontinue use if this disorder does not stabilize after diuretic therapy and digitalization. If necessary, nadolol may be given to patients with well-compensated congestive heart failure; observe such patients closely.
Patients with coronary artery disease	Abrupt withdrawal of therapy can exacerbate angina and, in some cases, cause myocardial infarction; reduce dosage gradually. If angina markedly worsens or acute coronary insufficiency develops after the drug is withdrawn, reinstitute therapy promptly and take other appropriate measures.
Patients with hyperthyroidism	Beta blockade can mask certain clinical signs (eg, tachycardia) of hyperthyroidism. Abrupt withdrawal of therapy can precipitate thyroid storm in susceptible patients; reduce dosage gradually.
Patients with diabetes	Adjustment of antidiabetic drug dosage may be necessary because bendroflumethiazide may cause hyperglycemia and nadolol may inhibit the release of insulin induced by hyperglycemia. Beta blockade may also mask the premonitory signs (eg, tachycardia, blood pressure changes) of acute hypoglycemia, which should be kept in mind when treating patients with labile diabetes.
Patients with bronchospastic disease	In general, such patients should not receive beta blockers because both endogenous and exogenous sympathetic stimulation of bronchial beta$_2$ receptors may be blocked. Nadolol is specifically contraindicated for use in patients with bronchial asthma; it may be used with caution in patients with *nonallergic* bronchospastic disease (eg, chronic bronchitis or emphysema).
Major surgery	Beta blockade can increase the risks of general anesthesia and surgery, and cause protracted hypotension, low cardiac output, or difficulty in restarting or maintaining the heartbeat; beta-adrenergic agonists (eg, isoproterenol, dopamine, dobutamine, or norepinephrine) can reverse these effects. If possible, nadolol therapy should be discontinued *well* before the time of surgery, because increased sensitivity to catecholamines has been observed in patients recently withdrawn from beta-blocker therapy. If emergency surgery is necessary, the anesthesiologist should be informed that the patient is receiving a beta blocker.
Postsympathectomy patients	The antihypertensive effects of the thiazide component may be enhanced in sympathectomized patients
Azotemia	Thiazides can precipitate azotemia in patients with renal disease; if renal impairment progresses, as indicated by rising BUN or NPN levels, consider interrupting or discontinuing therapy

CORZIDE

Hepatic coma	Minor changes in fluid and electrolyte balance may precipitate hepatic coma in patients with hepatic impairment or progressive liver disease; use with caution in such patients
Electrolyte disorders	Hypokalemia may occur, especially with brisk diuresis, when severe cirrhosis is present, ACTH or corticosteroids are given concomitantly, or oral intake of electrolytes is inadequate; potassium supplements or potassium-rich foods may be given to avoid or treat hypokalemia. Dilutional hyponatremia may occur in edematous patients when the weather is hot; restrict the intake of water, and administer salt only if hyponatremia is life-threatening or actual salt depletion occurs. For hypochloremia, specific treatment is usually unnecessary, except for certain patients (eg, those with hepatic or renal disease). To prevent electrolyte imbalance, measure serum and urinary electrolyte levels periodically in all patients (these determinations are especially important if excessive vomiting occurs or parenteral fluids are being given); watch for premonitory signs and symptoms of hypokalemia, hyponatremia, and hypochloremic alkalosis, such as dry mouth, thirst, weakness, lethargy, drowsiness, restlessness, muscle pain or cramps, muscular fatigue, hypotension, oliguria, tachycardia, and GI disturbances (eg, nausea and vomiting).
Parathyroid dysfunction	Pathological changes in the parathyroid gland, accompanied by hypercalcemia and hypophosphatemia, have occurred in a few patients after prolonged thiazide therapy; however, the common complications of hyperparathyroidism have not been seen. Discontinue use before performing parathyroid function tests.
Other thiazide-related reactions	Thiazides may activate or exacerbate systemic lupus erythematosus, precipitate hypersensitivity reactions in patients with a history of allergy or bronchial asthma, activate latent diabetes, or cause hyperuricemia or overt gout in certain patients
Carcinogenicity	No evidence of carcinogenicity has been found in mice and rats that were fed nadolol for 2 yr; long-term studies in animals have not been done with bendroflumethiazide
Effect on fertility	No adverse effects on fertility have been observed in rats given nadolol; studies with bendroflumethiazide have not been done

ADVERSE REACTIONS[1]

Cardiovascular	Heart rate < 40 beats/min and/or symptomatic bradycardia, peripheral vascular insufficiency, cardiac failure, hypotension, rhythm and/or conduction disturbances, first- and third-degree heart block, orthostatic hypotension
Central nervous system and neuromuscular	Dizziness, fatigue, paresthesias, sedation, changed behavior, headache, slurred speech, vertigo, muscle spasm, weakness, restlessness
Ophthalmic	Dry eyes, blurred vision, xanthopsia
Respiratory	Bronchospasm, cough, nasal stuffiness
Gastrointestinal	Nausea, diarrhea, abdominal discomfort, constipation, vomiting, indigestion, anorexia, bloating, flatulence, gastric irritation, cramps, intrahepatic cholestatic jaundice, pancreatitis
Genitourinary	Impotence or decreased libido
Hematological	Leukopenia, agranulocytosis, thrombocytopenia, aplastic anemia
Dermatological	Rash, pruritus, dry skin, facial swelling, diaphoresis
Hypersensitivity	Purpura, photosensitivity, rash, urticaria, necrotizing angiitis, allergic glomerulonephritis
Other	Weight gain, tinnitus, dry mouth, hyperglycemia, glycosuria, metabolic acidosis (in diabetic patients), hyperuricemia, hypokalemia, hypochloremia, hyponatremia, reversible alopecia

OVERDOSAGE

Signs and symptoms	*Nadolol-related effects:* excessive bradycardia, cardiac failure, hypotension, bronchospasm; *bendroflumethiazide-related effects:* diuresis, dehydration, changes in serum electrolyte levels, transient increase in BUN levels, GI irritation and hypermotility, CNS depression; lethargy progressing to coma, possibly accompanied by minimal cardiorespiratory depression and no changes in electrolyte and fluid balance
Treatment	Empty stomach by gastric lavage. Hemodialysis may be useful. For excessive bradycardia, administer 0.25–1.0 mg atropine; if there is no response to vagal blockade, administer isoproterenol cautiously. For cardiac failure, administer digitalis and a diuretic; IV glucagon may be helpful. For hypotension, administer a vasopressor, such as norepinephrine or (preferably) epinephrine. Treat bronchospasm with a beta$_2$-stimulating agent (eg, isoproterenol) and/or a theophylline derivative. Monitor serum electrolyte levels and renal function, and institute supportive measures, as required, to maintain hydration, electrolyte balance, respiration, and cardiovascular and renal function. Treat GI effects symptomatically.

DRUG INTERACTIONS

Other antihypertensive agents	⇧ Antihypertensive effect
Other adrenergic blockers	⇧ Adrenergic blockade

CORZIDE ■ DIUPRES

Digitalis	⇧ Risk of digitalis toxicity (due to possible thiazide-induced hypokalemia)
Reserpine, other catecholamine-depleting agents	⇧ Risk of hypotension and/or excessive bradycardia; watch for vertigo, syncope, and orthostatic hypotension
Anesthetics, preanesthetics	⇧ Anesthetic or preanesthetic effect ⇧ Risk of hypotension or reduced cardiac output (with general anesthetics)
Alcohol, barbiturates, narcotic analgesics	⇧ Risk of orthostatic hypotension
Ephedrine, other beta-adrenergic bronchodilators	⇩ Bronchodilation
Insulin, oral hypoglycemic agents	⇧ Hypoglycemic effect
Norepinephrine, other vasopressors	⇩ Vasopressor effect; nevertheless, this interaction does not preclude therapeutic use of vasopressors
Corticosteroids, ACTH	⇧ Risk of hypokalemia
Tubocurarine, other nondepolarizing skeletal muscle relaxants	⇧ Skeletal muscle relaxation

ALTERED LABORATORY VALUES

Blood/serum values	⇩ Sodium ⇩ Potassium ⇧ Calcium ⇩ Magnesium ⇩ Chloride ⇩ Phosphate ⇧ Uric acid ⇩ PBI, ⇧ Glucose ⇧ Amylase
Urinary values	⇧ Sodium ⇧ Potassium ⇩ Calcium ⇧ Magnesium ⇧ Chloride ⇧ Bicarbonate ⇩ Uric acid ⇧ Glucose

USE IN CHILDREN

Safety and effectiveness for use in children have not been established

USE IN PREGNANT AND NURSING WOMEN

Pregnancy Category C: reproduction studies with 5–10 times the maximum human dose of nadolol have shown evidence of embryo- and fetotoxicity in rabbits, but not in rats and hamsters; no teratogenic effects have been detected in these studies. Neonates whose mothers received nadolol at parturition have exhibited bradycardia and hypoglycemia. Thiazides cross the placental barrier and may cause fetal or neonatal jaundice, thrombocytopenia, and other possible reactions; reproduction studies with bendroflumethiazide have not been done. No adequate, well-controlled studies have been performed in pregnant women; use Corzide during pregnancy only if the expected benefit justifies the potential risk to the embryo or fetus. Nadolol and bendroflumethiazide are excreted in human milk; because of the potential for serious adverse reactions in nursing infants, patients should not nurse while taking this preparation.

[1] Reactions for which no causal relationship has been established include intensification of AV block (see CONTRAINDICATIONS); reversible mental depression progressing to catatonia; visual disturbances; hallucinations; an acute reversible syndrome characterized by temporal and spatial disorientation, short-term memory loss, emotional lability, slightly clouded sensorium, and decreased performance on neuropsychometric tests; mesenteric arterial thrombosis; ischemic colitis; elevated liver enzymes; agranulocytosis; thrombocytopenic or nonthrombocytopenic purpura; fever combined with aching and sore throat; laryngospasm; respiratory distress; pemphigoid rash; hypertensive reaction in patients with pheochromocytoma; sleep disturbances; and Peyronie's disease

---

ANTIHYPERTENSIVES WITH DIURETICS

DIUPRES (chlorothiazide and reserpine) Merck Sharp & Dohme   Rx

Tablets: 250 mg chlorothiazide and 0.125 mg reserpine (Diupres 250); 500 mg chlorothiazide and 0.125 mg reserpine (Diupres 500)

INDICATIONS

Hypertension

ORAL DOSAGE

Adult: 1–2 Diupres 250 tabs or 1 Diupres 500 tab 1–2 times/day (see WARNINGS/PRECAUTIONS)

CONTRAINDICATIONS

Hypersensitivity to chlorothiazide, other sulfonamide derivatives, or reserpine

Mental depression, especially in patients with suicidal tendencies

Active peptic ulcer

Ulcerative colitis

Anuria

Electroconvulsive therapy

WARNINGS/PRECAUTIONS

Fixed combination	Not indicated for initial therapy of hypertension; dosages of component drugs must be individually titrated and then periodically reviewed, as conditions warrant

DIUPRES

Patients with renal impairment	Use with caution and monitor for signs of excessive drug accumulation (see OVERDOSAGE); patient may adjust poorly to lowered blood pressure
Azotemia	May be precipitated in patients with renal disease
Hepatic coma	May be precipitated by minor changes in fluid and electrolyte balance in patients with hepatic impairment or progressive liver disease
Sensitivity reactions	May occur in patients with or without a history of allergy or bronchial asthma
Postsympathectomy patients	Antihypertensive effect may be enhanced
Systemic lupus erythematosus	May be activated or exacerbated
Electrolyte imbalances	Measure serum and urine electrolytes periodically, especially if patient is vomiting excessively or receiving parenteral fluids. Watch for dry mouth, thirst, weakness, lethargy, drowsiness, restlessness, muscle pains or cramps, muscular fatigue, hypotension, oliguria, tachycardia, and GI disturbances.
Hypokalemia	May develop, especially with brisk diuresis, concomitant corticosteroid or ACTH therapy, interference with adequate oral intake of electrolytes, or in the presence of severe cirrhosis; may be minimized by including potassium-rich foods in diet or, if necessary, with potassium supplements
Dilutional hyponatremia	May occur in edematous patients when weather is hot; restrict water and use salt replacement only for life-threatening hyponatremia
Hypomagnesemia	May occur
Hyperuricemia or overt gout	May occur or be precipitated in certain patients
Insulin requirements	May increase, decrease, or remain unchanged; latent diabetes may become active
Patients with a history of mental depression	Use with extreme caution; discontinue therapy at the first sign of despondency, early morning insomnia, loss of appetite, impotence, or self-deprecation. Mental depression is unusual with reserpine doses of 0.25 mg/day or less.
Patients undergoing electroconvulsive therapy	Discontinue drug at least 7 days before giving electroshock treatments; severe and even fatal reactions have occurred
Increased gastric secretion and motility	Use with caution in patients with history of peptic ulcer, ulcerative colitis, or other GI disorders
Biliary colic	May be precipitated in patients with gallstones
Bronchial asthma	May be precipitated in susceptible patients
Lithium therapy	Renal clearance is reduced, increasing risk of lithium toxicity; coadministration generally should be avoided unless adequate precautions are taken
Circulatory disturbances	May develop during surgical anesthesia; vagal blocking agents may be needed to prevent or reverse hypotension and/or bradycardia
Parathyroid function tests	Discontinue drug before testing
Carcinogenicity	Long-term (2-yr) studies in rodents fed 100–300 times the usual human dose of reserpine have shown an increased incidence of mammary fibroadenomas in female mice, malignant tumors of the seminal vesicles in male mice, and malignant adrenal medullary tumors in male rats. No definite conclusion about whether this drug increases the risk of breast cancer in humans has emerged from epidemiological studies or long-term clinical observation. Nevertheless, it should be used with caution in patients with previously detected breast cancer because of reserpine's prolactin-elevating effect. The risk of pheochromocytoma or tumors of the seminal vesicles in humans who have used reserpine has not been studied.

ADVERSE REACTIONS

Digestive	Anorexia, gastric irritation, hypersecretion and increased motility, nausea, vomiting, cramps, diarrhea, constipation, dry mouth, increased salivation, intrahepatic cholestatic jaundice, pancreatitis, sialadenitis
Central nervous system and neuromuscular	Dizziness, syncope, nervousness, vertigo, paresthesias, headache, excessive sedation, mental depression, nightmares, paradoxical anxiety, dulled sensorium, deafness, muscle spasm, weakness, restlessness, muscle aches, parkinsonism (usually reversible)
Ophthalmic	Transient blurred vision, glaucoma, uveitis, optic atrophy, xanthopsia
Cardiovascular	Orthostatic hypotension, bradycardia, angina pectoris, arrhythmia, premature ventricular contractions, fluid retention, congestive heart failure
Hematological	Leukopenia, agranulocytosis, thrombocytopenia, aplastic anemia, hemolytic anemia, excessive bleeding following prostatic surgery, thrombocytopenic purpura, epistaxis
Genitourinary	Dysuria, impotence, decreased libido
Metabolic	Hyperglycemia, glycosuria, hyperuricemia, electrolyte imbalance, weight gain
Hypersensitivity	Purpura, photosensitivity, pruritus, rash, urticaria, flushing, necrotizing angiitis, fever, respiratory distress (including pneumonitis and pulmonary edema), anaphylactic reactions

DIUPRES ■ ENDURONYL

Other	Nasal congestion, dyspnea, increased susceptibility to colds, nonpuerperal lactation

OVERDOSAGE

Signs and symptoms	*Chlorothiazide-related effects:* diuresis, lethargy progressing to coma with minimal cardiorespiratory depression, GI irritation, hypermotility, elevated BUN, serum electrolyte changes; *reserpine-related effects:* impairment of consciousness ranging from drowsiness to coma, flushing, conjunctival injection, miosis, hypotension, hypothermia, respiratory depression, bradycardia, diarrhea
Treatment	Induce emesis or use gastric lavage, followed by activated charcoal, to empty stomach. Treat hypotension by elevating feet and by volume expansion, if possible. If a vasopressor is needed, use phenylephrine, levarterenol, or metaraminol. Treat significant bradycardia with vagal blocking agents, along with other appropriate measures. Monitor serum electrolytes and renal function, and institute supportive measures, as required. Treat GI effects symptomatically. Observe patient for at least 72 h, administering treatment as needed.

DRUG INTERACTIONS

Other antihypertensive agents	⇧ Antihypertensive effect
Digitalis	⇧ Risk of cardiac arrhythmias, bradycardia, heart block
Quinidine	⇧ Risk of cardiac arrhythmias
MAO inhibitors	Severe hypertension
Tubocurarine	⇧ Skeletal muscle relaxation
Nonsteroidal anti-inflammatory agents	⇩ Diuretic, natriuretic, and antihypertensive effects of chlorothiazide component; observe patient closely during concomitant therapy to ensure that desired therapeutic effect is obtained
Norepinephrine	⇩ Vasopressor effect
Steroids, ACTH	⇧ Risk of hypokalemia
Lithium	⇩ Lithium clearance
Alcohol, barbiturates, narcotic analgesics	⇧ Risk of orthostatic hypotension

ALTERED LABORATORY VALUES

Blood/serum values	Carbohydrate intolerance ⇧ Uric acid ⇧ Calcium ⇩ Magnesium ⇩ Sodium ⇩ Potassium ⇩ Chloride ⇩ Bicarbonate ⇩ Phosphate ⇩ PBI ⇩ Thyroxine (T$_4$) ⇩ Plasma renin activity
Urinary values	⇧ Sodium ⇧ Potassium ⇧ Chloride ⇧ Bicarbonate ⇧ Uric acid ⇧ 5-HIAA ⇩ Calcium ⇧ Magnesium ⇩ 17-Ketosteroids

USE IN CHILDREN
Consult manufacturer

USE IN PREGNANT AND NURSING WOMEN
Safety for use during pregnancy has not been established. Thiazides cross the placental barrier, appear in cord blood, and may cause fetal or neonatal jaundice, thrombocytopenia, and other possible reactions. Reserpine crosses the placental barrier, appears in cord blood, and may cause nasal congestion, lethargy, depressed Moro reflex, and bradycardia in newborns. Both drugs are also excreted in breast milk; patient should stop nursing if this product is prescribed.

ANTIHYPERTENSIVES WITH DIURETICS

ENDURONYL (methyclothiazide and deserpidine) Abbott   Rx
Tablets: 5 mg methyclothiazide and 0.25 mg deserpidine

ENDURONYL Forte (methyclothiazide and deserpidine) Abbott   Rx
Tablets: 5 mg methyclothiazide and 0.5 mg deserpidine

INDICATIONS	ORAL DOSAGE
Mild to moderately severe hypertension	**Adult:** 1/2–2 tabs/day (see WARNINGS/PRECAUTIONS); usual dosage: 1 Enduronyl tab/day

ENDURONYL

CONTRAINDICATIONS

Hypersensitivity to methyclothiazide, other sulfonamide derivatives, or deserpidine	Active peptic ulcer	Renal decompensation
	Electroconvulsive therapy	Ulcerative colitis
Mental depression, especially in patients with suicidal tendencies		

ADMINISTRATION/DOSAGE ADJUSTMENTS

Frequency of dosage adjustments	Titrate dosage to individual needs; allow at least 10 days to 2 wk between dosage adjustments for full drug effects to become evident
Combination therapy	Addition of other antihypertensive drugs should be gradual; ganglionic blocking agents should be given at only ½ the usual dose, since their effect is potentiated

WARNINGS/PRECAUTIONS

Fixed combination	Not indicated for initial therapy of hypertension; dosages of component drugs must be individually titrated and then periodically reviewed, as conditions warrant
Renal impairment	Use with caution and monitor for signs of excessive drug accumulation (see OVERDOSAGE); patient may adjust poorly to lowered blood pressure
Azotemia	May be precipitated in patients with renal disease
Hepatic coma	May be precipitated by minor changes in fluid and electrolyte balance in patients with hepatic impairment or progressive liver disease
Sensitivity reactions	May occur in patients with a history of allergy or bronchial asthma
Systemic lupus erythematosus	May be activated or exacerbated
Electrolyte imbalances	Measure serum and urine electrolytes periodically, especially if patient is vomiting excessively or receiving parenteral fluids. Watch for dry mouth, thirst, weakness, lethargy, drowsiness, restlessness, muscle pains or cramps, muscular fatigue, hypotension, oliguria, tachycardia, and GI disturbances.
Hypokalemia	May develop, especially with brisk diuresis, concomitant corticosteroid or ACTH therapy, interference with adequate oral intake of electrolytes, or in the presence of severe cirrhosis; may be minimized by including potassium-rich foods in diet or, if necessary, with potassium supplements
Dilutional hyponatremia	May occur in edematous patients when weather is hot; restrict water and use salt replacement only for life-threatening hyponatremia
Hyperuricemia or overt gout	May occur or be precipitated in certain patients
Insulin requirements	May increase, decrease, or remain unchanged; latent diabetes may become active
Postsympathectomy patients	Antihypertensive effect may be enhanced
Patients with a history of mental depression	Use with extreme caution; discontinue treatment at the first sign of despondency, early morning insomnia, loss of appetite, impotence, or self-deprecation
Persistence of drug effects	Drug-induced depression may persist for several months after withdrawal and may be severe enough to result in suicide; cardiac effects may also persist
Increased GI motility and secretion	Use with caution in patients with a history of peptic ulcer or ulcerative colitis
Biliary colic	May be precipitated in patients with gallstones
Circulatory instability and hypotension	May occur during anesthesia; anticholinergic and/or adrenergic agents (metaraminol, norepinephrine) may be needed to correct adverse vagocirculatory effects
Carcinogenicity	Although no studies have shown that deserpidine is tumorigenic in animals, it is structurally related to reserpine and, like reserpine, can stimulate the release of prolactin. Long-term (2-yr) studies in rodents fed 100–300 times the usual human dose of reserpine have shown an increased incidence of mammary fibroadenomas in female mice, malignant tumors of the seminal vesicles in male mice, and malignant adrenal medullary tumors in male rats. No definite conclusion about whether reserpine increases the risk of breast cancer in humans has emerged from epidemiological studies or long-term clinical observation. Nevertheless, because of its prolactin-elevating effect, it has been suggested that reserpine should be used with caution in patients with previously detected breast cancer. The risk of pheochromocytoma or tumors of the seminal vesicles in humans who have used reserpine has not been studied.

ADVERSE REACTIONS

Gastrointestinal	Anorexia, gastric irritation, nausea, vomiting, cramping, diarrhea, constipation, intrahepatic cholestatic jaundice, pancreatitis, hypersecretion
Central nervous system and neuromuscular	Dizziness, vertigo, paresthesias, headache, drowsiness, depression, nervousness, paradoxical anxiety, nightmares, extrapyramidal tract symptoms, dulled sensorium, deafness, muscle spasm, muscular aches, weakness, restlessness
Ophthalmic	Glaucoma, uveitis, optic atrophy, conjunctival injection, xanthopsia
Cardiovascular	Orthostatic hypotension, angina-like symptoms, arrhythmias, bradycardia

ENDURONYL ■ ESIMIL

Hematological	Leukopenia, agranulocytosis, thrombocytopenia, aplastic anemia, thrombocytopenic purpura
Hypersensitivity	Purpura, photosensitivity, rash, urticaria, necrotizing angiitis, pruritus; asthma (in asthmatic patients)
Other	Nasal congestion, weight gain, impotence or decreased libido, dysuria, dyspnea

OVERDOSAGE

Signs and symptoms	*Methyclothiazide-related effects:* electrolyte imbalance, confusion, dizziness, muscular weakness, GI disturbances; *deserpidine-related effects:* flushing, conjunctival injection, pupillary constriction, sedation ranging from drowsiness to coma; in severe cases: hypotension, hypothermia, central respiratory depression, bradycardia
Treatment	Carefully evacuate stomach contents. Treat CNS depression symptomatically. For severe hypotension, use a direct-acting vasopressor, such as norepinephrine. Monitor serum electrolytes and renal function, and replace fluids and electrolytes, as needed.

DRUG INTERACTIONS

Other antihypertensive agents	↑ Antihypertensive effect
Tubocurarine	↑ Skeletal muscle relaxation
Norepinephrine	↓ Vasopressor effect
Steroids, ACTH	↑ Risk of hypokalemia
Lithium	↓ Lithium clearance
Digitalis	↑ Risk of cardiac arrhythmias and heart block
Quinidine	↑ Risk of cardiac arrhythmias
Alcohol, barbiturates, narcotic analgesics	↑ Risk of orthostatic hypotension

ALTERED LABORATORY VALUES

Blood/serum values	↑ Uric acid ↑ Calcium ↓ Sodium ↓ Potassium ↓ Chloride ↓ Bicarbonate ↓ Phosphate ↓ PBI ↑ or ↓ Glucose
Urinary values	↑ Sodium ↑ Potassium ↑ Chloride ↑ Bicarbonate ↑ Uric acid ↓ Calcium

---

USE IN CHILDREN

Safety and effectiveness for use in children have not been established

USE IN PREGNANT AND NURSING WOMEN

Safety for use during pregnancy has not been established. Thiazides cross the placental barrier, appear in cord blood, and may cause fetal or neonatal jaundice, thrombocytopenia, and other possible reactions. *Rauwolfia* alkaloids such as deserpidine also cross the placental barrier, appear in cord blood, and have caused increased respiratory secretions, nasal congestion, cyanosis, and anorexia in neonates. Both drugs are excreted in breast milk; patient should stop nursing if drug is prescribed.

ANTIHYPERTENSIVES WITH DIURETICS

ESIMIL (guanethidine monosulfate and hydrochlorothiazide) CIBA   Rx

Tablets: 10 mg guanethidine monosulfate and 25 mg hydrochlorothiazide

INDICATIONS	ORAL DOSAGE
Hypertension	**Adult:** 1 tab/day to start, followed by increases of 1 tab/day at weekly intervals, up to 4 tabs/day, as needed; usual maintenance dosage: 2 tabs/day (see WARNINGS/PRECAUTIONS)

CONTRAINDICATIONS

Anuria	Pheochromocytoma, either known or suspected	Use of MAO inhibitors (see WARNINGS/PRECAUTIONS)
Hypersensitivity to hydrochlorothiazide, other sulfonamide derivatives, or guanethidine	Overt congestive heart failure not due to hypertension	

ADMINISTRATION/DOSAGE ADJUSTMENTS

Initial titration of dosage	Take blood pressure with patient in supine position and again after patient has been standing for 10 min. Increase dosage only if there is no decrease in standing blood pressure from previous levels.

ESIMIL

Transferring patients from other antihypertensive agents	Begin with 1 tab/day of Esimil and ½ the usual dose of the antihypertensive agent to be substituted. One week later, increase Esimil dosage to 2 tabs/day and give ¼ the usual dose of the previous agent. The following week, discontinue the previous drug and begin titrating Esimil dosage at weekly intervals.
Refractory patients	If blood pressure is not adequately controlled at maximum dosage (4 tabs/day), add guanethidine alone
Patients with fever	Dosage requirements may be reduced

WARNINGS/PRECAUTIONS

Fixed combination	This preparation is not indicated for initial therapy of hypertension; dosages of the component drugs must be individually titrated to the patient's needs before instituting treatment with this combination
Inhibition of ejaculation	Inhibition of ejaculation resulting from sympathetic blockade has been reported in animals and humans; normal ejaculatory function is restored after the drug has been discontinued for several weeks. Guanethidine does not cause parasympathetic blockade, and erectile potency is usually retained during treatment. Keep the possibility of ejaculatory inhibition in mind when treating men of reproductive age, and caution them accordingly.
Orthostatic hypertension	Warn patients that symptoms of orthostatic hypotension occur frequently during therapy, particularly in the morning, and are accentuated by alcohol, fever, hot weather, sudden or prolonged standing, and exercise. Fainting spells may occur unless patients are forewarned to sit or lie down if they begin to feel dizzy or weak.
Cardiovascular instability during surgery	If possible, withdraw therapy 2 wk prior to elective surgery to minimize the risk of vascular collapse and cardiac arrest during anesthesia. For emergency surgery, administer preanesthetic and anesthetic agents with caution and lower the dosage. Oxygen, atropine, vasopressors, and adequate solutions for volume replacement should be available for immediate use; administer vasopressors with extreme caution, since guanethidine can augment their effect (see DRUG INTERACTIONS).
Patients with bronchial asthma	The catecholamine depletion produced by guanethidine may exacerbate bronchial asthma; use with caution
Patients with incipient cardiac decompensation	Monitor patients with incipient cardiac decompensation for weight gain or edema
Patients with severe cardiac failure	Use with extreme caution in patients with severe cardiac failure; guanethidine may interfere with the compensatory role of the adrenergic system in producing circulatory adjustment
Patients with peptic ulcer disease	Use with caution in patients with a history of peptic ulcer or other chronic disorders that may be aggravated by relative increases in parasympathetic tone
Other special-risk patients	Use very cautiously in hypertensive patients with renal disease coupled with nitrogen retention or rising BUN levels; coronary insufficiency or recent myocardial infarction; or cerebrovascular disease, especially with encephalopathy
Patients with diabetes	Thiazides may activate latent diabetes or affect the insulin requirements of diabetic patients; exercise caution during therapy
Patients with renal disease	In patients with renal impairment, thiazides may accumulate or they may precipitate azotemia; use with caution in patients with severe renal disease. If renal impairment progresses, consider interrupting or discontinuing therapy.
Patients with liver disease	Minor changes in fluid and electrolyte balance caused by thiazides may precipitate hepatic coma in patients with hepatic impairment or progressive liver disease; exercise caution when using this preparation in patients with hepatic impairment
Electrolyte disorders	Hypokalemia may occur, especially when diuresis is brisk, severe cirrhosis is present, ACTH or corticosteroids are given concomitantly, or oral intake of electrolytes is inadequate; potassium supplements or potassium-rich foods may be given to avoid or treat hypokalemia. Dilutional hyponatremia may occur in edematous patients when the weather is hot; restrict the intake of water, and administer salt only if hyponatremia is life-threatening or actual salt depletion occurs. For hypochloremia, specific treatment is usually unnecessary, except for certain patients (eg, those with hepatic or renal disease). To minimize the risk of electrolyte imbalance, measure serum electrolyte levels periodically in all patients (urinary as well as serum determinations are especially important if excessive vomiting occurs or parenteral fluids are being given), and watch for premonitory signs and symptoms of hypokalemia, hyponatremia, and hypochloremic alkalosis: dry mouth, thirst, weakness, lethargy, drowsiness, restlessness, muscle pain or cramps, muscular fatigue, hypotension, oliguria, tachycardia, and GI disturbances (eg, nausea, vomiting).
Parathyroid dysfunction	Thiazides decrease calcium excretion. Discontinue therapy before performing parathyroid function tests. Pathological changes in the parathyroid gland, accompanied by hypercalcemia and hypophosphatemia, have occurred in a few patients after prolonged thiazide therapy; however, the common complications of hyperparathyroidism have not been seen.
Hypersensitivity	Allergic reactions to thiazides are more likely to occur in patients with a history of allergy or bronchial asthma

ESIMIL

Other thiazide-related effects	Thiazides may activate or exacerbate systemic lupus erythematosus, cause hyperuricemia or overt gout, or produce an enhanced antihypertensive effect following sympathectomy
Diarrhea	Severe diarrhea may occur and necessitate a reduction in dosage or discontinuation of therapy
Long-term therapy	The effects of guanethidine are cumulative; give small initial doses, and increase dosage gradually in small increments
Carcinogenicity	No long-term studies have been performed to evaluate the carcinogenic potential of this preparation
Impairment of fertility	Inhibition of sperm passage and accumulation of sperm debris have been reported in rats and rabbits given 5 or 10 mg/kg/day of guanethidine SC or IP for several weeks; however, recovery of ejaculatory function and fertility has been shown in rats following IM administration of 25 mg/kg/day of the drug for 8 wk. Reversible inhibition of ejaculation has also occurred in men (see "Inhibition of ejaculation," above).

ADVERSE REACTIONS[1]

Gastrointestinal	Diarrhea, vomiting, nausea, increased bowel movements, dry mouth, parotid tenderness, pancreatitis, intrahepatic cholestatic jaundice, sialadenitis, cramping, gastric irritation, constipation, anorexia
Cardiovascular	Chest pains (angina), bradycardia, fluid retention and edema with occasional development of congestive heart failure, orthostatic hypotension
Respiratory	Dyspnea, asthma (in susceptible patients), nasal congestion
Central nervous system, neuromuscular	Syncope resulting from postural or exertional hypotension, dizziness, blurred vision, muscle tremor, ptosis, mental depression, paresthesias, weakness, lassitude, fatigue, myalgia, vertigo, headache, xanthopsia, restlessness
Genitourinary	Rise in BUN level, urinary incontinence, inhibition of ejaculation, nocturia
Hematological	Aplastic anemia, agranulocytosis, leukopenia, thrombocytopenia
Hypersensitivity	Dermatitis, scalp hair loss, necrotizing angiitis, Stevens-Johnson syndrome, purpura, urticaria, rash, photosensitivity
Other	Weight gain, hyperglycemia, glycosuria, hyperuricemia

OVERDOSAGE

Signs and symptoms	*Guanethidine-related effects:* postural hypotension with dizziness, blurred vision, and possible syncope when standing; shock, bradycardia; diarrhea, nausea, vomiting, and, rarely, unconsciousness; *hydrochlorothiazide-related effects:* acute loss of fluid and electrolytes, tachycardia, hypotension, shock, weakness, confusion, dizziness, cramps of the calf muscles, paresthesia, fatigue, impairment of consciousness, nausea, vomiting, thirst, polyuria, oliguria, or anuria; hypokalemia, hyponatremia, hypochloremia, alkalosis, increased BUN (especially in patients with renal insufficiency)
Treatment	Evacuate stomach contents by gastric lavage, instill a slurry of activated charcoal, and give laxatives, if conditions permit. Support vital functions and control cardiac irregularities, if present. Treat hypotension by keeping patient's feet up and, if necessary, by replacing lost fluid and electrolytes. For sinus bradycardia, administer atropine. For previously normotensive patients, restore blood pressure and heart rate by keeping patient in a supine position (normal homeostatic control gradually returns within 72 h). For previously hypertensive patients, particularly those with impaired cardiac reserve or other cardiovascular-renal disease, intensive treatment may be needed; maintain patient in a supine position, and, if vasopressors are required, they should be used with extreme caution. Treat severe or persistent diarrhea with anticholinergic agents; maintain hydration and electrolyte balance. Monitor cardiovascular and renal function for several days, until drug is completely eliminated.

DRUG INTERACTIONS

MAO inhibitors	⇧ Hypertension to crisis proportions
Digitalis	⇩ Heart rate
Amphetamine-like compounds, ephedrine, methylphenidate, and other stimulants; tricyclic antidepressants, phenothiazines, and other psychotropic agents	⇩ Antihypertensive effect
Oral contraceptives	⇩ Antihypertensive effect
Rauwolfia derivatives	Excessive postural hypotension, bradycardia, mental depression
Norepinephrine and other vasopressors	⇧ Pressor effect ⇧ Risk of cardiac arrhythmias
Tubocurarine	⇧ Skeletal muscle relaxation
Steroids, ACTH	⇧ Risk of hypokalemia

ESIMIL ■ HYDROPRES

Lithium	⇓ Lithium clearance
Alcohol, barbiturates, narcotic analgesics	⇑ Risk of orthostatic hypotension

ALTERED LABORATORY VALUES

Blood/serum values	⇑ BUN ⇑ Creatinine ⇑ Uric acid ⇑ Calcium ⇑ Plasma renin activity ⇓ Sodium ⇓ Potassium ⇓ Chloride ⇓ Bicarbonate ⇓ Phosphate ⇓ PBI ⇑ or ⇓ Glucose
Urinary values	⇑ Sodium ⇑ Potassium ⇑ Chloride ⇑ Bicarbonate ⇑ Uric acid ⇑ Catecholamines (initially) ⇓ Catecholamines (subsequently) ⇓ VMA ⇓ Calcium

USE IN CHILDREN
Safety and effectiveness for use in children have not been established

USE IN PREGNANT AND NURSING WOMEN
Pregnancy Category B: no evidence of impaired fertility or fetal harm was found in a study performed in rats receiving at least 150 times the average human dose of this formulation. Thiazides cross the placental barrier, appear in cord blood, and may cause fetal or neonatal jaundice, thrombocytopenia, and possibly other reactions. No adequate, well controlled studies have been performed in pregnant women; use during pregnancy only if clearly needed. Thiazides and small quantities of guanethidine are excreted in human milk; if use of this preparation is deemed essential, the patient should not nurse.

[1] A few instances of blood dyscrasias (anemia, thrombocytopenia, and leukopenia), priapism, and impotence have been reported in patients receiving guanethidine, but no causal relationship has been established

---

ANTIHYPERTENSIVES WITH DIURETICS

HYDROPRES (hydrochlorothiazide and reserpine) Merck Sharp & Dohme   Rx

Tablets: 25 mg hydrochlorothiazide and 0.125 mg reserpine (Hydropres 25); 50 mg hydrochlorothiazide and 0.125 mg reserpine (Hydropres 50)

INDICATIONS	ORAL DOSAGE
Hypertension	**Adult:** 1–2 Hydropres 25 tabs or 1 Hydropres 50 tab 1–2 times/day, as needed (see WARNINGS/PRECAUTIONS)

CONTRAINDICATIONS

Hypersensitivity to hydrochlorothiazide, other sulfonamide derivatives, or reserpine	Active peptic ulcer	Electroconvulsive therapy
	Ulcerative colitis	
Mental depression, especially in patients with suicidal tendencies	Anuria	

WARNINGS/PRECAUTIONS

Fixed combination	Not indicated for initial therapy of hypertension; dosages of component drugs must be individually titrated and then periodically reviewed, as conditions warrant
Patients with renal impairment	Use with caution and monitor for signs of excessive drug accumulation (see OVERDOSAGE); patient may adjust poorly to lowered blood pressure
Azotemia	May be precipitated in patients with renal disease
Hepatic coma	May be precipitated by minor changes in fluid and electrolyte balance in patients with hepatic impairment or progressive liver disease; use with caution
Sensitivity reactions	May occur in patients with or without a history of allergy or bronchial asthma
Postsympathectomy patients	Antihypertensive effect may be enhanced
Systemic lupus erythematosus	May be activated or exacerbated
Electrolyte imbalances	Measure serum and urine electrolytes periodically, especially if patient is vomiting excessively or receiving parenteral fluids. Watch for dry mouth, thirst, weakness, lethargy, drowsiness, restlessness, muscle pains or cramps, muscular fatigue, hypotension, oliguria, tachycardia, and GI disturbances.
Hypokalemia	May develop, especially with brisk diuresis, concomitant corticosteroid or ACTH therapy, interference with adequate oral intake of electrolytes, or in the presence of severe cirrhosis; may be minimized by including potassium-rich foods in diet or, if necessary, with potassium supplements

HYDROPRES

Dilutional hyponatremia	May occur in edematous patients when weather is hot; restrict water and use salt replacement only for life-threatening hyponatremia
Hypomagnesemia	May occur
Hyperuricemia or overt gout	May occur or be precipitated in certain patients
Insulin requirements	May increase, decrease, or remain unchanged; latent diabetes may become active
Patients with a history of mental depression	Use with extreme caution; discontinue therapy at the first sign of despondency, early morning insomnia, loss of appetite, impotence, or self-deprecation. Mental depression is unusual with reserpine doses of 0.25 mg/day or less.
Patients undergoing electroconvulsive therapy	Discontinue drug at least 7 days before giving electroshock treatments; severe and even fatal reactions have occurred
Increased gastric secretion and motility	Use with caution in patients with a history of peptic ulcer, ulcerative colitis, or other GI disorders
Biliary colic	May be precipitated in patients with gallstones
Bronchial asthma	May be precipitated in susceptible patients
Lithium therapy	Renal clearance is reduced, increasing risk of lithium toxicity; coadministration generally should be avoided unless adequate precautions are taken
Circulatory disturbances	May develop during surgical anesthesia; vagal blocking agents may be needed to prevent or reverse hypotension and/or bradycardia
Parathyroid function tests	Discontinue drug before testing
Carcinogenicity	Long-term (2-yr) studies in rodents fed 100–300 times the usual human dose of reserpine have shown an increased incidence of mammary fibroadenomas in female mice, malignant tumors of the seminal vesicles in male mice, and malignant adrenal medullary tumors in male rats. No definite conclusion about whether this drug increases the risk of breast cancer in humans has emerged from epidemiological studies or long-term clinical observation. Nevertheless, it should be used with caution in patients with previously detected breast cancer because of reserpine's prolactin-elevating effect. The risk of pheochromocytoma or tumors of the seminal vesicles in humans who have used reserpine has not been studied.

ADVERSE REACTIONS

Digestive	Anorexia, gastric irritation, hypersecretion and increased motility, nausea, vomiting, cramps, diarrhea, constipation, dry mouth, increased salivation, intrahepatic cholestatic jaundice, pancreatitis, sialadenitis
Central nervous system and neuromuscular	Dizziness, syncope, nervousness, vertigo, paresthesias, headache, excessive sedation, mental depression, nightmares, paradoxical anxiety, dulled sensorium, deafness, muscle spasm, weakness, restlessness, muscle aches, parkinsonism (usually reversible)
Ophthalmic	Transient blurred vision, glaucoma, uveitis, optic atrophy, xanthopsia
Cardiovascular	Orthostatic hypotension, bradycardia, angina pectoris, arrhythmia, premature ventricular contractions, fluid retention, congestive heart failure
Hematological	Leukopenia, agranulocytosis, thrombocytopenia, aplastic anemia, hemolytic anemia, excessive bleeding following prostatic surgery, thrombocytopenic purpura, epistaxis
Genitourinary	Dysuria, impotence, decreased libido
Metabolic	Hyperglycemia, glycosuria, hyperuricemia, electrolyte imbalance, weight gain
Hypersensitivity	Purpura, photosensitivity, pruritus, rash, urticaria, flushing, necrotizing angiitis, fever, respiratory distress (including pneumonitis and pulmonary edema), anaphylactic reactions
Other	Nasal congestion, dyspnea, increased susceptibility to colds, nonpuerperal lactation

OVERDOSAGE

Signs and symptoms	*Hydrochlorothiazide-related effects:* diuresis, lethargy progressing to coma with minimal cardiorespiratory depression, GI irritation, hypermotility, elevated BUN, serum electrolyte changes; *reserpine-related effects:* impairment of consciousness ranging from drowsiness to coma, flushing, conjunctival injection, miosis, hypotension, hypothermia, respiratory depression, bradycardia, diarrhea
Treatment	Induce emesis or use gastric lavage, followed by activated charcoal, to empty stomach. Treat hypotension by elevating feet and by volume expansion, if possible. If a vasopressor is needed, use phenylephrine, levarterenol, or metaraminol. Treat significant bradycardia with vagal blocking agents, along with other appropriate measures. Monitor serum electrolytes and renal function, and institute supportive measures, as required. Treat GI effects symptomatically. Observe patient for at least 72 h, administering treatment as needed.

DRUG INTERACTIONS

Other antihypertensive agents	⇧ Antihypertensive effect

HYDROPRES ■ INDERIDE

Digitalis	⇧ Risk of cardiac arrhythmias, bradycardia, heart block
Quinidine	⇧ Risk of cardiac arrhythmias
MAO inhibitors	Severe hypertension
Tubocurarine	⇧ Skeletal muscle relaxation
Nonsteroidal anti-inflammatory agents	⇩ Diuretic, natriuretic, and antihypertensive effects of hydrochlorothiazide component; observe patient closely during concomitant therapy to ensure that desired therapeutic effect is obtained
Norepinephrine	⇩ Vasopressor effect
Steroids, ACTH	⇧ Risk of hypokalemia
Lithium	⇩ Lithium clearance
Alcohol, barbiturates, narcotic analgesics	⇧ Risk of orthostatic hypotension

ALTERED LABORATORY VALUES

Blood/serum values	Carbohydrate intolerance ⇧ Uric acid ⇧ Calcium ⇩ Magnesium ⇩ Sodium ⇩ Potassium ⇩ Chloride ⇩ Bicarbonate ⇩ Phosphate ⇩ PBI ⇩ Thyroxine (T_4) ⇩ Plasma renin activity
Urinary values	⇧ Sodium ⇧ Potassium ⇧ Chloride ⇧ Bicarbonate ⇧ Uric acid ⇧ 5-HIAA ⇩ Calcium ⇧ Magnesium ⇩ 17-Ketosteroids

---

USE IN CHILDREN
Consult manufacturer

USE IN PREGNANT AND NURSING WOMEN
Safety for use during pregnancy has not been established. Thiazides cross the placental barrier, appear in cord blood, and may cause fetal or neonatal jaundice, thrombocytopenia, and other possible reactions. Reserpine crosses the placental barrier, appears in cord blood, and may cause nasal congestion, lethargy, depressed Moro reflex, and bradycardia in newborns. Both drugs are also excreted in breast milk; patient should stop nursing if this product is prescribed.

ANTIHYPERTENSIVES WITH DIURETICS

INDERIDE (propranolol hydrochloride and hydrochlorothiazide) Ayerst Rx

Tablets: 40 mg propranolol hydrochloride and 25 mg hydrochlorothiazide (Inderide-40/25); 80 mg propranolol hydrochloride and 25 mg hydrochlorothiazide (Inderide-80/25)

INDICATIONS	ORAL DOSAGE
Hypertension	**Adult:** 1–2 tabs bid (see WARNINGS/PRECAUTIONS)

CONTRAINDICATIONS

Sinus bradycardia	Hypersensitivity to hydrochlorothiazide or other sulfonamide derivatives	Anuria
Greater than first-degree heart block		Bronchial asthma
Cardiogenic shock	Treatment with adrenergic-augmenting psychotropic agents, including MAO inhibitors, within the preceding 2 wk of initiating Inderide therapy	Allergic rhinitis during the pollen season
Right ventricular failure secondary to pulmonary hypertension		
Congestive heart failure not resulting from propranolol-treatable tachyarrhythmias		

ADMINISTRATION/DOSAGE ADJUSTMENTS

Combination therapy	Reduce usual recommended starting dosage of other antihypertensive agents by ½ to avoid an excessive fall in blood pressure
Discontinuation of therapy	Reduce dosage gradually and monitor patient closely. Caution patients with angina or hyperthyroidism against interruption or abrupt cessation of therapy (see WARNINGS/PRECAUTIONS).

WARNINGS/PRECAUTIONS

Fixed combination	Not indicated for initial therapy of hypertension; dosages of component drugs must be individually titrated and then periodically reviewed, as conditions warrant

INDERIDE

Cardiac failure	May be precipitated by further or continued depression of myocardial contractility; discontinue use if cardiac failure persists despite adequate digitalization and diuretic therapy
Abrupt discontinuation of therapy	May exacerbate angina pectoris, lead to myocardial infarction in patients with coronary artery disease, or precipitate thyrotoxicosis in hyperthyroid patients
Thyrotoxicosis	Clinical signs of hyperthyroidism may be masked
Wolff-Parkinson-White syndrome	Tachycardia may be replaced by severe bradycardia requiring a demand pacemaker
Impaired response to reflex adrenergic stimuli	Withdraw drug 48 h prior to surgery, unless surgery is for pheochromocytoma. Patients undergoing emergency surgery may experience protracted severe hypotension and, occasionally, difficulty in restarting and maintaining heartbeat. Excessive beta blockade may be reversed during surgery by IV administration of a beta-receptor agonist (eg, isoproterenol or norepinephrine).
Nonallergic bronchospasm	Use with caution, since bronchodilation produced by beta stimulation may be blocked
Diabetes, hypoglycemia	Beta blockade may prevent appearance of premonitory signs and symptoms of acute hypoglycemia, especially in patients with labile diabetes
Patients with hepatic or renal impairment	Use with caution and monitor patient for signs of excessive drug accumulation (see OVERDOSAGE)
Azotemia	May be precipitated in patients with renal disease
Hepatic coma	May be precipitated by minor changes in fluid and electrolyte balance in patients with hepatic impairment or progressive liver disease
Sensitivity reactions	May occur in patients with a history of allergy or bronchial asthma
Systemic lupus erythematosus	May be activated or exacerbated
Electrolyte imbalances	Measure serum and urine electrolytes periodically, especially if patient is vomiting excessively or receiving parenteral fluids. Watch for dry mouth, thirst, weakness, lethargy, drowsiness, restlessness, muscle pains or cramps, muscular fatigue, hypotension, oliguria, tachycardia, and GI disturbances.
Hypokalemia	May develop, especially with brisk diuresis, concomitant corticosteroid or ACTH therapy, interference with adequate oral intake of electrolytes, or in the presence of severe cirrhosis; may be minimized by including potassium-rich foods in diet or, if necessary, with potassium supplements
Dilutional hyponatremia	May occur in edematous patients when weather is hot; restrict water and use salt replacement only for life-threatening hyponatremia
Hyperuricemia or overt gout	May occur or be precipitated in certain patients
Insulin requirements	May increase, decrease, or remain unchanged; latent diabetes may become active
Postsympathectomy patients	Antihypertensive effect may be enhanced
Parathyroid function tests	Discontinue drug before testing

ADVERSE REACTIONS

Cardiovascular	Bradycardia, congestive heart failure, intensified AV block, hypotension, Raynaud-type arterial insufficiency, orthostatic hypotension
Central nervous system and neuromuscular	Light-headedness, insomnia, lassitude, weakness, fatigue, reversible mental depression progressing to catatonia, visual disturbances, hallucinations, acute reversible syndrome of disorientation, short-term memory loss, emotional lability, clouded sensorium, decreased neuropsychometric performance, dizziness, vertigo, paresthesias, headache, restlessness, muscle spasm
Ophthalmic	Transient blurred vision, xanthopsia
Gastrointestinal	Nausea, vomiting, epigastric distress, abdominal cramping, diarrhea, constipation, mesenteric arterial thrombosis, ischemic colitis, anorexia, gastric irritation, intrahepatic cholestatic jaundice, pancreatitis, sialadenitis
Allergic or hypersensitivity	Pharyngitis, agranulocytosis, erythematous rash, purpura, photosensitivity, urticaria, necrotizing angiitis, fever, aching, sore throat, laryngospasm, respiratory distress (including pneumonitis), anaphylactic reactions
Respiratory	Bronchospasm
Hematological	Agranulocytosis, nonthrombocytopenic purpura, thrombocytopenic purpura, leukopenia, thrombocytopenia, aplastic anemia
Other	Reversible alopecia

OVERDOSAGE

Signs and symptoms	*Propranolol-related effects:* severe bradycardia, congestive heart failure, hypotension, bronchospasm; *hydrochlorothiazide-related effects:* diuresis, lethargy progressing to coma with minimal cardiorespiratory depression, GI irritation, hypermotility, temporarily elevated BUN, serum electrolyte changes

INDERIDE ■ INDERIDE LA

Treatment	Empty stomach, taking care to prevent pulmonary aspiration. For bradycardia, administer 0.25–1.0 mg atropine IV; if there is no response to vagal blockade, administer isoproterenol cautiously. For cardiac failure, administer digitalis and a diuretic. For hypotension, use norepinephrine or (preferably) epinephrine. Treat bronchospasm with isoproterenol and aminophylline. For stupor or coma, employ supportive measures. Treat GI effects symptomatically. Monitor serum electrolyte levels and renal function, and institute supportive measures, as required.

DRUG INTERACTIONS

Other antihypertensive agents	⇧ Antihypertensive effect
MAO inhibitors	Severe hypertension
Alcohol, barbiturates, narcotic analgesics	⇧ Risk of orthostatic hypotension
Digitalis	⇩ AV conduction
Ephedrine, isoproterenol, and other beta-adrenergic bronchodilating agents	⇩ Bronchodilation
Reserpine, *Rauwolfia* alkaloids	⇧ Risk of vertigo, syncope, or orthostatic hypotension
Tubocurarine	⇧ Skeletal muscle relaxation
Norepinephrine	⇩ Vasopressor effect
Steroids, ACTH	⇧ Risk of hypokalemia
Lithium	⇩ Lithium clearance

ALTERED LABORATORY VALUES

Blood/serum values	⇧ BUN ⇧ Alkaline phosphatase ⇧ Lactate dehydrogenase ⇧ SGOT ⇧ SGPT ⇧ Uric acid ⇧ Calcium ⇩ Sodium ⇩ Potassium ⇩ Chloride ⇩ Bicarbonate ⇩ Phosphate ⇩ PBI ⇧ or ⇩ Glucose
Urinary values	⇧ Sodium ⇧ Potassium ⇧ Chloride ⇧ Bicarbonate ⇧ Uric acid ⇩ Calcium

USE IN CHILDREN
Consult manufacturer

USE IN PREGNANT AND NURSING WOMEN
Safety for use during pregnancy has not been established. In animal studies, propranolol has demonstrated embryotoxicity at doses ~ 10 times greater than the maximum recommended human dose. Thiazides cross the placental barrier, appear in cord blood, and may cause fetal or neonatal jaundice, thrombocytopenia, and other possible reactions. Both drugs are excreted in breast milk; patient should stop nursing if this product is prescribed.

ANTIHYPERTENSIVES WITH DIURETICS

INDERIDE LA (propranolol hydrochloride and hydrochlorothiazide) Ayerst Rx

Capsules (long-acting¹): 80 mg propranolol hydrochloride and 50 mg hydrochlorothiazide (Inderide LA 80/50); 120 mg propranolol hydrochloride and 50 mg hydrochlorothiazide (Inderide LA 120/50); 160 mg propranolol hydrochloride and 50 mg hydrochlorothiazide (Inderide LA 160/50)

INDICATIONS	ORAL DOSAGE
Hypertension	**Adult:** 1 cap once daily

CONTRAINDICATIONS

Sinus bradycardia	Overt cardiac failure, when it is not associated with a propranolol-responsive tachyarrhythmia	Hypersensitivity to hydrochlorothiazide or other sulfonamide derivatives
Heart block greater than first degree		Anuria
Cardiogenic shock	Bronchial asthma	

ADMINISTRATION/DOSAGE ADJUSTMENTS

Dosage adjustment	When this product is substituted without a change in the daily dose for a similar combination product (eg, Inderide) or for a regimen in which immediate-release propranolol and hydrochlorothiazide are given separately, therapeutic effects may diminish, especially at the end of a 24-h dosing interval, because of the resulting decreases in the serum propranolol level and 24-h area under the curve; after switching to this product, monitor therapeutic response and, if necessary, increase dosage

INDERIDE LA

Combination therapy	When necessary, add another antihypertensive agent; to avoid hypotensive effects, begin use of the new agent at 50% of its usual starting dose and increase dosage gradually

WARNINGS/PRECAUTIONS

Fixed combination	This preparation is not indicated for initial therapy of hypertension; dosages of the component drugs must be individually titrated to the patient's needs before instituting treatment with this combination
Cardiac failure	Beta blockade may cause or exacerbate cardiac failure. Propranolol should generally not be given to patients with overt cardiac failure; however, the drug may be used when heart failure is well-compensated, provided treatment is necessary and the patient is kept under close observation. If cardiac failure occurs or progresses during therapy and does not respond to digitalis and diuretics, propranolol should be discontinued (gradually, if possible).
Angina	Abrupt withdrawal can exacerbate angina and, in some cases, precipitate myocardial infarction. When discontinuing therapy in patients with angina or suspected occult atherosclerotic heart disease, reduce dosage gradually and monitor clinical response carefully. If exacerbation of angina occurs during withdrawal, reinstitute therapeutic regimen and take other appropriate measures. Caution patients not to interrupt or discontinue treatment on their own.
Bronchospastic disease	Propranolol should generally not be given to patients with bronchospastic disease because it can block catecholamine-induced bronchodilation. The drug is specifically contraindicated for use in patients with bronchial asthma. Exercise caution when using in patients with nonallergic bronchospasm (eg, emphysema or chronic bronchitis).
Thyrotoxicosis	Beta blockade may mask clinical signs of hyperthyroidism; abrupt withdrawal can exacerbate this disorder and precipitate a thyroid storm
Wolff-Parkinson-White syndrome	Severe bradycardia, necessitating use of a demand pacemaker, has occurred in several patients with the Wolff-Parkinson-White syndrome following use of propranolol
Diabetes	When used in patients with labile, insulin-dependent diabetes during a hypoglycemic episode, propranolol can mask certain signs such as tachycardia and cause a precipitous increase in blood pressure. Thiazides can alter insulin requirements or activate latent diabetes.
Major surgery	The necessity or desirability of discontinuing use before major surgery is controversial. By impairing cardiac responsiveness to reflex beta-adrenergic stimuli, beta blockade may increase the risks associated with general anesthesia and surgery.
Glaucoma testing	By reducing intraocular pressure, propranolol can interfere with glaucoma screening tests
Renal impairment, drug accumulation	In patients with renal impairment, thiazides can precipitate azotemia or accumulate; these patients may be more likely to experience adverse effects of propranolol. Use this preparation with caution in patients with renal disorders; if renal impairment progresses, consider interrupting or terminating therapy.
Hepatic impairment	Propranolol undergoes extensive hepatic metabolism. In patients with hepatic impairment or progressive liver disease, thiazides can produce minor changes in fluid and electrolyte balance that may precipitate hepatic coma. Use this preparation with caution in patients with hepatic impairment.
Electrolyte disorders	Hypokalemia may occur, especially when diuresis is brisk, severe cirrhosis is present, ACTH or corticosteroids are given concomitantly, or oral intake of electrolytes is inadequate; potassium supplements or potassium-rich foods may be given to avoid or treat hypokalemia. Dilutional hyponatremia may occur in edematous patients when the weather is hot. Treat by restricting the intake of water; administer salt only if hyponatremia is life-threatening or actual salt depletion occurs. For hypochloremia, specific treatment is usually unnecessary, except for certain patients (eg, those with hepatic or renal disease). To prevent electrolyte imbalance, measure serum and urinary electrolyte levels periodically in all patients (these determinations are especially important if excessive vomiting occurs or parenteral fluids are being given); watch for premonitory signs and symptoms of hypokalemia, hyponatremia, and hypochloremic alkalosis, such as dry mouth, thirst, weakness, lethargy, drowsiness, restlessness, muscle pain or cramps, muscular fatigue, hypotension, oliguria, tachycardia, and GI disturbances (eg, nausea and vomiting).
Parathyroid dysfunction	Thiazides decrease calcium excretion. Discontinue use before performing parathyroid function tests. Pathological changes in the parathyroid gland, accompanied by hypercalcemia and hypophosphatemia, have occurred in a few patients after prolonged thiazide therapy; however, the common complications of hyperparathyroidism have not been seen.
Other thiazide-related reactions	Thiazides may activate or exacerbate systemic lupus erythematosus, cause hyperuricemia or overt gout, precipitate hypersensitivity reactions (especially in patients with a history of allergy or bronchial asthma), or, in postsympathectomy patients, produce an enhanced antihypertensive effect
Carcinogenicity	No evidence of tumorigenicity has been seen in mice and rats given up to 150 mg/kg/day of propranolol for a period of 18 mo

INDERIDE LA

Effect on fertility	No evidence of impaired fertility has been observed in animals given propranolol

ADVERSE REACTIONS

Cardiovascular	Bradycardia, congestive heart failure, intensification of AV block, hypotension (including orthostatic hypotension), Raynaud-type arterial insufficiency
Central nervous system	Light-headedness, insomnia, lassitude, weakness, fatigue, depression, catatonia, hallucinations, dizziness, vertigo, paresthesias, headache, restlessness, muscle spasm; an acute reversible syndrome characterized by spatial and temporal disorientation, short-term memory loss, emotional lability, slightly clouded sensorium, and decreased neuropsychometric performance
Ophthalmic	Transient blurred vision, visual disturbances, xanthopsia, dry eyes
Gastrointestinal	Nausea, vomiting, epigastric distress, abdominal cramping, diarrhea, constipation, mesenteric arterial thrombosis, ischemic colitis, anorexia, gastric irritation, intrahepatic cholestatic jaundice, pancreatitis
Hematological	Agranulocytosis, leukopenia, thrombocytopenia, nonthrombocytopenic and thrombocytopenic purpura, aplastic anemia
Hypersensitivity	Pharyngitis, agranulocytosis, erythematous rash, purpura, rash, photosensitivity, urticaria, necrotizing angiitis, fever (alone or with aching and sore throat), laryngospasm, respiratory distress, pneumonitis, anaphlactic reactions
Other	Bronchospasm, alopecia, lupus erythematosus-like reactions, systemic lupus erythematosus, sialadenitis, psoriasiform rash, impotence, Peyronie's disease, hyperuricemia, hyperglycemia, glycosuria

OVERDOSAGE

Signs and symptoms	Bradycardia, cardiac failure, hypotension, bronchospasm, diuresis, lethargy, coma, GI irritation and hypermotility, transitory increase in BUN level, serum electrolyte changes
Treatment	Empty stomach, taking care to prevent pulmonary aspiration. For bradycardia, administer 0.25–1 mg of atropine IV; if there is no response to vagal blockade, cautiously give isoproterenol. Administer a digitalis preparation and a diuretic for cardiac failure. Correct hypotension with a vasopressor such as norepinephrine or epinephrine. To reverse bronchospasm, use isoproterenol and aminophylline. Treat GI effects symptomatically; institute supportive therapy for stupor and coma. Monitor renal function and serum electrolyte levels and institute supportive measures as needed.

DRUG INTERACTIONS

Other antihypertensive agents	△ Antihypertensive effect
Reserpine, other catecholamine-depleting drugs	△ Risk of hypotension, marked bradycardia, vertigo, syncope, or orthostatic hypotension; closely observe patients during concomitant therapy
Digitalis	△ Risk of digitalis toxicity
Lithium	△ Risk of lithium toxicity
Norepinephrine, other vasopressors	▽ Vasopressor effect; nevertheless, this interaction does not preclude therapeutic use of vasopressors
Corticosteroids, ACTH	△ Risk of hypokalemia
Tubocurarine, other nondepolarizing skeletal muscle relaxants	△ Skeletal muscle relaxation
Alcohol, barbiturates, narcotic analgesics	△ Risk of orthostatic hypotension
Ephedrine, isoproterenol, other beta-adrenergic bronchodilators	▽ Bronchodilation

ALTERED LABORATORY VALUES

Blood/serum values	△ SGOT △ SGPT △ Alkaline phosphatase △ LDH △ BUN (in patients with severe heart disease) ▽ Sodium ▽ Potassium △ Calcium ▽ Magnesium ▽ Chloride ▽ Phosphate △ Uric acid ▽ PBI △ Glucose
Urinary values	△ Sodium △ Potassium ▽ Calcium △ Magnesium ▽ Chloride △ Bicarbonate △ Uric acid △ Glucose

---

USE IN CHILDREN

Safety and effectiveness for use in children have not been established

USE IN PREGNANT AND NURSING WOMEN

Pregnancy Category C: embryotoxic effects have been observed in animals given approximately 10 times the maximum human dose of propranolol. Administration of a thiazide during pregnancy can produce adverse reactions, including jaundice and thrombocytopenia, in a neonate or fetus. Use this preparation during pregnancy only if the expected benefit justifies the potential risk to the fetus or neonate. Propranolol and hydrochlorothiazide are excreted in human milk; instruct patients not to nurse during therapy.

---

[1] Capsules contain a long-acting form of propranolol and a conventional, immediate-release form of hydrochlorothiazide

ANTIHYPERTENSIVES WITH DIURETICS

LOPRESSOR HCT (metoprolol tartrate and hydrochlorothiazide) Geigy   Rx

Tablets: 50 mg metoprolol tartrate and 25 mg hydrochlorothiazide (Lopressor HCT 50/25); 100 mg metoprolol tartrate and 25 mg hydrochlorothiazide (Lopressor HCT 100/25); 100 mg metoprolol tartrate and 50 mg hydrochlorothiazide (Lopressor HCT 100/50)

INDICATIONS

Hypertension

ORAL DOSAGE

Adult: two 50/25 tabs, one to two 100/25 tabs, or one 100/50 tab, given daily in single or divided doses; dosage of hydrochlorothiazide should not exceed 50 mg/day

CONTRAINDICATIONS

Cardiogenic shock	Sinus bradycardia	Hypersensitivity to hydrochlorothiazide or other sulfonamide derivatives
Second- or third-degree AV block	Anuria	
Overt cardiac failure		

ADMINISTRATION/DOSAGE ADJUSTMENTS

Administration	Tablets should be given with or immediately after meals. Caution patients not to double the dose after a missed dose and not to interrupt or discontinue therapy on their own.
Dosage adjustment	Once-daily administration of lower doses of metoprolol (especially 100 mg) may be inadequate to maintain a full antihypertensive effect at the end of the 24-h dosing interval; in these cases, larger doses or more frequent dosing may be necessary. The initial daily dose for patients with bronchospastic disease should be given in 3 divided doses.
Addition of another antihypertensive agent	To avoid an excessive fall in blood pressure, give half the usual dose of the new agent to start, and then gradually increase the dose

WARNINGS/PRECAUTIONS

Fixed combination	This preparation is not indicated for initial therapy of hypertension; dosages of the component drugs must be individually titrated to the patient's needs before instituting treatment with this combination
Cardiac failure	Beta blockade may cause or exacerbate cardiac failure. Use with caution in patients with well-compensated congestive heart failure. If cardiac failure occurs during treatment and does not respond to digitalization and diuretic therapy, administration should be discontinued.
Angina	Abrupt withdrawal of certain beta blockers can exacerbate angina and, in some cases, precipitate myocardial infarction. Discontinue metoprolol gradually, even when overt angina is not evident.
Hyperthyroidism	Abrupt withdrawal of beta blockade can precipitate a thyroid storm in patients with hyperthyroidism; since certain clinical signs of this disorder (such as tachycardia) can be masked during therapy, patients should be closely observed during the period of withdrawal, even if thyrotoxicosis is only suspected.
Diabetes	Beta blockade may mask tachycardia associated with hypoglycemia, but may not significantly affect other manifestations, such as dizziness and sweating. Thiazides may activate latent diabetes or affect the insulin requirements of diabetic patients. Exercise caution during therapy.
Bronchospasm	In general, patients with bronchospastic disease should not receive beta blockers. However, if other antihypertensive treatment is not effective or tolerated, metoprolol may be used with caution in these patients since the drug has a relative selectivity for beta$_1$ receptors; because this selectivity is not absolute and diminishes at higher doses, a beta$_2$ agonist should be given concomitantly, and the lowest possible dose of metoprolol should be used (see ADMINISTRATION/DOSAGE ADJUSTMENTS). Instruct patients to report any difficulty in breathing.
Surgery	The necessity or desirability of discontinuing use before major surgery is controversial. Beta blockade can increase the risks associated with general anesthesia and surgery (because cardiac responsiveness to reflex beta-adrenergic stimuli is impaired) and may cause protracted severe hypotension and difficulty in restarting and maintaining the heartbeat. However, beta-adrenergic agonists (eg, dobutamine, isoproterenol) can reverse the effects of metoprolol. Instruct patients to inform their physician or dentist that they are taking metoprolol whenever they undergo any surgical procedure.
Fatigue	Instruct patients to determine how they react to this preparation before they drive or engage in other activities requiring alertness
Azotemia, drug accumulation	In patients with renal impairment, thiazides may accumulate or they may precipitate azotemia; use with caution in patients with severe renal disease. If renal impairment progresses, consider interrupting or discontinuing therapy.
Hepatic coma, drug metabolism	Minor changes in fluid and electrolyte balance caused by thiazides may precipitate hepatic coma in patients with hepatic impairment or progressive liver disease. More than 95% of an oral dose of metoprolol undergoes hepatic metabolism. Exercise caution when using this preparation in patients with hepatic impairment.

LOPRESSOR HCT

Electrolyte disorders	Hypokalemia may occur, especially when diuresis is brisk, severe cirrhosis is present, ACTH or corticosteroids are given concomitantly, or oral intake of electrolytes is inadequate; potassium supplements or potassium-rich foods may be given to avoid or treat hypokalemia. Dilutional hyponatremia may occur in edematous patients when the weather is hot; restrict the intake of water, and administer salt only if hyponatremia is life-threatening or actual salt depletion occurs. For hypochloremia, specific treatment is usually unnecessary, except for certain patients (eg, those with hepatic or renal disease). To prevent electrolyte imbalance, measure serum and urinary electrolyte levels periodically in all patients (these determinations are especially important if excessive vomiting occurs or parenteral fluids are being given); watch for premonitory signs and symptoms of hypokalemia, hyponatremia, and hypochloremic alkalosis, such as dry mouth, thirst, weakness, lethargy, drowsiness, restlessness, muscle pain or cramps, muscular fatigue, hypotension, oliguria, tachycardia, and GI disturbances (eg, nausea and vomiting).
Parathyroid dysfunction	Thiazides decrease calcium excretion. Discontinue therapy before performing parathyroid function tests. Pathological changes in the parathyroid gland, accompanied by hypercalcemia and hypophosphatemia, have occurred in a few patients after prolonged thiazide therapy; however, the common complications of hyperparathyroidism have not been seen.
Other thiazide-related effects	Thiazides may activate or exacerbate systemic lupus erythematosus, cause hyperuricemia or overt gout, precipitate hypersensitivity reactions (even in patients without a history of allergy), or, in postsympathectomy patients, produce an enhanced antihypertensive effect
Carcinogenicity, mutagenicity	A 21-mo study has shown an increase in benign lung tumors (small adenomas) in female Swiss Albino mice fed 750 mg/kg/day of metoprolol; however, when this study was repeated in CD-1 mice, no significant results were observed. The results of all mutagenicity tests with metoprolol have been negative.
Effect on fertility	The fertility of rats has not been affected by administration of up to 55.5 times the maximum human dose of metoprolol

ADVERSE REACTIONS[1]

Frequent reactions (> 1%) are italicized

Central nervous system	*Dizziness, vertigo, drowsiness, somnolence, fatigue, lethargy, and headache (10%)*; nightmares and myalgia (1%)
Cardiovascular	*Bradycardia (6%)*, edema and decreased exercise tolerance (1%)
Gastrointestinal	Diarrhea, digestive disorders, nausea, vomiting, constipation, and anorexia (1%)
Ophthalmic	Blurred vision (1%)
Otic	Tinnitus and earache (1%)
Other	*Influenza-like syndrome (10%), hypokalemia (< 10%)*, dyspnea, purpura, gout, impotence, dry mouth, and sweating (1%)

OVERDOSAGE

Signs and symptoms	Hypotension, shock, cardiac failure, bradycardia or tachycardia, bronchospasm, hypokalemia, hyponatremia, hypochloremia, alkalosis, increased BUN level (especially in patients with renal impairment); polyuria, oliguria, or anuria; nausea, vomiting, thirst, weakness, confusion, dizziness, cramped calf muscles, paresthesia, fatigue, impairment of consciousness; signs or symptoms may be affected by concomitant intake of other antihypertensive drugs, barbiturates, curare, digitalis, corticosteroids, narcotics, or alcohol
Treatment	Monitor fluid and electrolyte balance (especially serum potassium level) as well as renal function. To treat hypotension, elevate patient's legs, replace fluids and electrolytes, and administer a vasopressor such as norepinephrine or dopamine. For bradycardia, administer atropine IV; if there is no response to vagal blockade, give isoproterenol cautiously. For cardiac failure, administer digitalis and a diuretic; for cardiogenic shock, consider using dobutamine, isoproterenol, or glucagon. Treat bronchospasm with a beta$_2$ agonist and/or theophylline. To remove this preparation from the GI tract, induce vomiting, perform gastric lavage, and administer activated charcoal.

DRUG INTERACTIONS

Other antihypertensive agents	⇧ Antihypertensive effect
Other adrenergic blockers	⇧ Adrenergic blockade
Digitalis	⇧ Risk of digitalis toxicity owing to thiazide-induced hypokalemia
Reserpine, other catecholamine-depleting agents	⇧ Risk of hypotension and bradycardia; watch for vertigo, syncope, and other signs of orthostatic hypotension
Anesthetics	⇧ Risk of hypotension and bradycardia (see warning, above, concerning use during surgery)
Lithium	⇧ Risk of lithium toxicity
Norepinephrine, other vasopressors	⇩ Vasopressor effect; nevertheless, this interaction does not preclude therapeutic use of vasopressors

LOPRESSOR HCT ■ MINIZIDE

Corticosteroids, ACTH	△ Risk of hypokalemia
Tubocurarine, other nondepolarizing skeletal muscle relaxants	△ Skeletal muscle relaxation
Alcohol, barbiturates, narcotic analgesics	△ Risk of orthostatic hypotension

ALTERED LABORATORY VALUES

Blood/serum values	△ SGOT △ SGPT △ Alkaline phosphatase △ LDH ▽ Sodium ▽ Potassium △ Calcium ▽ Magnesium ▽ Chloride ▽ Phosphate △ Uric acid ▽ PBI △ Glucose △ Amylase
Urinary values	△ Sodium △ Potassium ▽ Calcium △ Magnesium △ Chloride △ Bicarbonate ▽ Uric acid △ Glucose

USE IN CHILDREN

Safety and effectiveness for use in children have not been established

USE IN PREGNANT AND NURSING WOMEN

Pregnancy Category C: an increase in postimplantation loss and a decrease in neonatal survival have been seen in rats given up to 55.5 times the maximum human dose of metoprolol; adverse reactions, including jaundice and thrombocytopenia, can occur in a neonate or fetus following administration of thiazides during pregnancy. Use this preparation in pregnant women only if clearly needed. Thiazides, as well as a very small amount of metoprolol (<1 mg/liter), are excreted in human milk; patients should not nurse while taking this preparation.

[1] Reactions associated with metoprolol or hydrochlorothiazide, but not seen in clinical trials with this preparation, include depression, confusion, short-term memory loss, insomnia, weakness, restlessness, paresthesia, muscle spasm, xanthopsia, shortness of breath, bronchospasm, cold extremities, arterial insufficiency (usually Raynaud-type), palpitations, orthostatic hypotension, cardiac failure, gastric pain, flatulence, heartburn, gastric irritation, cramping, cholestatic jaundice, pancreatitis, sialadenitis, leukopenia, agranulocytosis, thrombocytopenia, aplastic anemia, pruritus, photosensitivity, rash, urticaria, necrotizing angiitis, Stevens-Johnson syndrome, Peyronie's disease, alopecia, hyperglycemia, glycosuria, and hyperuricemia; reactions that have not been seen with metoprolol (or hydrochlorothiazide) but have been reported following use of other beta blockers include intensification of AV block; reversible mental depression progressing to catatonia; visual disturbances; hallucinations; an acute reversible syndrome characterized by temporal and spatial disorientation, short-term memory loss, emotional lability, slightly clouded sensorium, and decreased performance on neuropsychometric tests; fever combined with sore throat and aching; laryngospasm; and respiratory distress

ANTIHYPERTENSIVES WITH DIURETICS

MINIZIDE (prazosin hydrochloride and polythiazide) Pfizer   Rx

Capsules: 1 mg prazosin hydrochloride and 0.5 mg polythiazide (Minizide 1); 2 mg prazosin hydrochloride and 0.5 mg polythiazide (Minizide 2); 5 mg prazosin hydrochloride and 0.5 mg polythiazide (Minizide 5)

INDICATIONS	ORAL DOSAGE
Hypertension	**Adult:** determine patient dose by individual titration of separate components; usual dosage: 1 cap bid or tid (see WARNINGS/PRECAUTIONS)

CONTRAINDICATIONS

Anuria	Hypersensitivity to thiazides or other sulfonamide derivatives

WARNINGS/PRECAUTIONS

Fixed combination	Not indicated for initial therapy of hypertension; dosages of component drugs must be individually titrated and then periodically reviewed, as conditions warrant
Syncope, accompanied by dizziness, light-headedness, or sudden loss of consciousness	May occur due to prazosin component, usually within 30–90 min of initial administration and occasionally in association with rapid dose increases or when other antihypertensive agents are added to prazosin. Severe tachycardia (heart rate, 120–160 beats/min) may precede a syncopal episode. Reaction may be minimized by limiting initial dose to 1 mg of prazosin, by increasing dosage slowly, and by using caution when other antihypertensive agents are introduced.
Patients with renal impairment	Observe patient for signs of excessive drug accumulation (see OVERDOSAGE); use with caution in patients with severe renal disease. If renal impairment progresses, consider withholding or discontinuing diuretic therapy.
Azotemia	May be precipitated in patients with renal disease
Hepatic coma	May be precipitated by minor changes in fluid and electrolyte balance in patients with hepatic impairment or progressive liver disease; use with caution
Postsympathectomy patients	Antihypertensive effect may be enhanced
Systemic lupus erythematosus	May be activated or exacerbated
Insulin requirements	May increase, decrease, or remain unchanged; latent diabetes may become active

COMPENDIUM OF DRUG THERAPY

MINIZIDE

Electrolyte imbalances	Measure serum and urine electrolytes periodically, especially if patient is vomiting excessively or receiving parenteral fluids or digitalis. Watch for dry mouth, thirst, weakness, lethargy, drowsiness, restlessness, muscle pains or cramps, muscular fatigue, hypotension, oliguria, tachycardia, and GI disturbances (nausea, vomiting, diarrhea).
Hypokalemia	May develop, especially with brisk diuresis, concomitant corticosteroid or ACTH therapy, interference with adequate oral intake of electrolytes, or in the presence of severe cirrhosis; hypokalemia may result in digitalis cardiotoxicity
Dilutional hyponatremia	May occur in edematous patients in hot weather; replace salt only for actual salt depletion or when hyponatremia is life-threatening
Sensitivity reactions	May occur in patients with a history of bronchial asthma or allergy
Hyperuricemia or overt gout	May occur or be precipitated in certain patients due to thiazide component

ADVERSE REACTIONS

Frequent reactions (incidence ≥ 1%) are printed in *italics*

Central nervous system	*Dizziness (10.3%)*, *headache (7.8%)*, *drowsiness (7.6%)*, *lack of energy (6.9%)*, *weakness (6.5%)*, nervousness, vertigo, depression, paresthesia, hallucinations, restlessness
Gastrointestinal	*Nausea (4.9%)*, vomiting, diarrhea, constipation, abdominal discomfort and/or pain, dry mouth, anorexia, gastric irritation, cramping, liver function abnormalities, intrahepatic cholestatic jaundice, pancreatitis
Cardiovascular	*Palpitations (5.3%)*, edema, dyspnea, syncope, tachycardia, orthostatic hypotension
Dermatological	Rash, pruritus, purpura, photosensitivity, urticaria, necrotizing angiitis, alopecia, lichen planus
Genitourinary	Urinary frequency, incontinence, impotence, priapism
Ophthalmic	Blurred vision, reddened sclera, xanthopsia, pigmentary mottling and serous retinopathy (rare)
Hematological	Leukopenia, agranulocytosis, thrombocytopenia, aplastic anemia
Other	Epistaxis, tinnitus, nasal congestion, diaphoresis, fever, muscle spasm

OVERDOSAGE

Signs and symptoms	*Prazosin-related effects:* profound drowsiness, depressed reflexes, hypotension, shock; *polythiazide-related effects:* electrolyte imbalance; lethargy progressing to coma, with minimal cardiorespiratory depression and with or without significant serum electrolyte changes or dehydration; GI irritation; hypermotility; transient elevation in BUN level
Treatment	Empty stomach by gastric lavage. Support cardiovascular system if hypotension occurs. Keep patient supine to restore blood pressure and normalize heart rate. Treat shock with volume expanders and, if necessary, vasopressors. Institute supportive measures, as needed, to maintain hydration, electrolyte balance, respiration, and cardiovascular and renal function. Treat GI effects symptomatically. Dialysis is not beneficial for the removal of prazosin, since it is protein-bound.

DRUG INTERACTIONS

Beta blockers	△ Risk of hypotension
Other antihypertensive agents	△ Antihypertensive effect and risk of syncope
Steroids, ACTH	△ Risk of hypokalemia
Digitalis	△ Risk of digitalis toxicity associated with hypokalemia
Tubocurarine	△ Skeletal muscle relaxation
Norepinephrine	▽ Vasopressor effect; however, interaction does not preclude therapeutic use of norepinephrine
Alcohol, barbiturates, narcotic analgesics	△ Risk of orthostatic hypotension
Lithium	△ Risk of lithium toxicity due to reduced renal clearance

ALTERED LABORATORY VALUES

Blood/serum values	△ Glucose △ Uric acid ▽ Sodium ▽ Potassium ▽ Chloride △ Calcium △ Bicarbonate ▽ Phosphate ▽ PBI
Urinary values	△ Glucose △ Sodium △ Potassium △ Chloride △ Bicarbonate △ Uric acid ▽ Calcium △ VMA △ Normetanephrine
	If an elevated VMA level is detected when testing for pheochromocytoma, prazosin should be discontinued and the test repeated 1 mo later

USE IN CHILDREN

Safety and effectiveness for use in children have not been established

USE IN PREGNANT AND NURSING WOMEN

Pregnancy Category C: use during pregnancy only if the expected benefit justifies the potential risk to the fetus. In rats, the combination of polythiazide at 40 times the usual maximum human dose and prazosin at 8 times the usual maximum human dose increased the number of stillbirths, prolonged gestation, and decreased survival before weaning. No teratogenic effects have been observed in rats or rabbits at oral doses more than 100 times the usual maximum human dose. No adequate, well-controlled studies have been done in pregnant women. Thiazides are excreted in breast milk; patient should stop nursing if drug is prescribed.

ANTIHYPERTENSIVES WITH DIURETICS

RAUZIDE (*Rauwolfia serpentina* and bendroflumethiazide) Princeton   Rx

Tablets: 50 mg *Rauwolfia serpentina* and 4 mg bendroflumethiazide

INDICATIONS	ORAL DOSAGE
Hypertension	**Adult:** 1–4 tabs/day (see WARNINGS/PRECAUTIONS)

CONTRAINDICATIONS

- Hypersensitivity to thiazides, other sulfonamide derivatives, or *Rauwolfia*
- Mental depression, especially in patients with suicidal tendencies
- Active peptic ulcer
- Ulcerative colitis
- Anuria
- Electroconvulsive therapy

WARNINGS/PRECAUTIONS

Fixed combination — This preparation is not indicated for initial therapy of hypertension; dosages of the component drugs must be individually titrated to the patient's needs before instituting treatment with this combination

Mental depression — Reserpine may cause mental depression, which may be masked by somatic complaints; drug-induced depression may persist for several months following discontinuation of therapy and may be severe enough to result in suicide. This preparation should be discontinued when despondency, early morning insomnia, anorexia, impotence, self-deprecation, or other signs of depression are first seen.

Mental and/or physical impairment — Caution patients that their ability to drive or engage in other potentially hazardous activities may be impaired

Increased GI motility and secretion — Use with caution in patients with a history of peptic ulcer, which may be reactivated by high dosages, or in those with ulcerative colitis

Biliary colic — Use with caution in patients with gallstones; biliary colic may be precipitated

Patients with renal impairment — Use with caution in patients with impaired renal function since they tend to adjust poorly to lowered blood pressure levels. Thiazides can precipitate azotemia in patients with renal disease; if impairment progresses, as indicated by a rising NPN or BUN level, consider withholding or discontinuing treatment.

Major surgery — Circulatory instability and hypotension may occur during surgical anesthesia, even if treatment is withdrawn preoperatively; use anticholinergic and/or adrenergic agents (eg, metaraminol or norepinephrine) to treat adverse vagocirculatory effects. If possible, discontinue use of bendroflumethiazide 1 wk prior to surgery. Apprise anesthesiologist of patient's drug intake.

Postsympathectomy patients — The antihypertensive effects of the thiazide component may be enhanced in sympathectomized patients

Hepatic coma — Minor changes in fluid and electrolyte balance may precipitate hepatic coma in patients with hepatic impairment or progressive liver disease; use with caution in such patients

Electrolyte disorders — Hypokalemia may occur, especially with brisk diuresis, after prolonged thiazide therapy, when severe cirrhosis is present, ACTH, digitalis, or corticosteroids are given concomitantly, or oral intake of electrolytes is inadequate; potassium supplements or potassium-rich foods may be given to avoid or treat hypokalemia. Dilutional hyponatremia may occur in edematous patients when the weather is hot; restrict the intake of water, and administer salt only if hyponatremia is life-threatening or actual salt depletion occurs. For hypochloremia, specific treatment is usually unnecessary, except for certain patients (eg, those with hepatic or renal disease). To prevent electrolyte imbalance, measure serum and urinary electrolyte levels periodically in all patients (these determinations are especially important if excessive vomiting occurs or parenteral fluids are being given); watch for premonitory signs and symptoms of hypokalemia, hyponatremia, and hypochloremic alkalosis, such as dry mouth, thirst, weakness, lethargy, drowsiness, restlessness, muscle pain or cramps, muscular fatigue, hypotension, oliguria, tachycardia, and GI disturbances (nausea, vomiting).

RAUZIDE

Parathyroid dysfunction	Pathological changes in the parathyroid gland, accompanied by hypercalcemia and hypophosphatemia, have occurred in a few patients after prolonged thiazide therapy; however, the common complications of hyperparathyroidism have not been seen. Discontinue use before performing parathyroid function tests.
Other thiazide-related reactions	Thiazides may activate or exacerbate systemic lupus erythematosus, precipitate hypersensitivity reactions in patients with or without a history of allergy or bronchial asthma, activate latent diabetes, or cause hyperuricemia or frank gout in certain patients
Tartrazine sensitivity	Presence of FD&C Yellow No. 5 (tartrazine) in tablets may cause allergic-type reactions, including bronchial asthma, in susceptible individuals
Carcinogenicity	Long-term (2-yr) studies in rodents fed 100–300 times the usual human dose of reserpine have shown an increased incidence of mammary fibroadenomas in female mice, malignant tumors of the seminal vesicles in male mice, and malignant adrenal medullary tumors in male rats. No definite conclusion about whether this drug increases or decreases the risk of breast cancer in humans has emerged form epidemiological studies or long-term clinical observation. Nevertheless, it should be used with caution in patients with previously detected breast cancer because of reserpine's prolactin-elevating effect. The risk of pheochromocytoma or tumors of the seminal vesicles in humans who have used reserpine has not been studied. No long-term animal studies have been performed to evaluate the carcinogenic potential of bendroflumethiazide.

ADVERSE REACTIONS

Gastrointestinal	Anorexia, nausea, vomiting, diarrhea; GI bleeding, hypersecretion, increased intestinal motility, dryness of the mouth; gastric irritation, abdominal cramps or bloating, constipation, pancreatitis, sialadenitis
Central nervous system, neuromuscular	Headache, dizziness; deafness, dull sensorium, extrapyramidal tract symptoms, depression, paradoxical anxiety, nightmares, nervousness, drowsiness, muscular aches; vertigo, paresthesias, lightheadedness, muscle spasm or cramps, weakness, restlessness; parkinsonian disease (rare)
Ophthalmic	Optic atrophy, glaucoma, uveitis, conjunctival injection; xanthopsia, transient blurred vision
Hypersensitivity	Purpura, pruritus, rash; ecchymosis, skin photosensitivity, exfoliative dermatitis, urticaria, necrotizing angiitis, vasculitis, cutaneous vasculitis, fever, anaphylactic reactions
Respiratory	Dyspnea, epistaxis, nasal congestion; respiratory distress, including pneumonitis
Cardiovascular	Bradycardia, arrhythmias, angina-like symptoms; orthostatic hypotension
Hematological	Leukopenia, agranulocytopenia, agranulocytosis, thrombocytopenia, aplastic anemia, hemolytic anemia; hyperglycemia, hyperuricemia
Hepatic	Cholestatic jaundice
Renal and genitourinary	Dysuria; allergic glomerulonephritis, glycosuria, occasional metabolic acidosis (in diabetic patients), impotence or decreased libido, gynecomastia
Other	Weight gain, breast engorgement, pseudolactation

OVERDOSAGE

Signs and symptoms	*Rauwolfia-related effects:* impairment of consciousness ranging from drowsiness to coma, flushing, bradycardia, hypotension, conjunctival congestion, pupillary constriction, hypothermia, central respiratory depression, mental depression, diarrhea, vomiting, ptosis, miosis, and extrapyramidal signs such as stiffness, leg pain, and tremors; *bendroflumethiazide-related effects:* diuresis, lethargy progressing to coma with minimal cardiorespiratory depression, gastrointestinal irritation and hypermotility, transient increase in BUN; serum electrolyte changes, especially in patients with impaired renal function
Treatment	Induce emesis or use gastric lavage, followed by a slurry of activated charcoal, to empty stomach. Treat hypotension by elevating feet and by volume expansion, if possible. For severe hypotension, administer a vasopressor having direct action upon vascular smooth muscle or a direct-acting sympathomimetic. Avoid rapid infusion of IV solutions and use of cathartics. Treat significant bradycardia and parasympathomimetic effects with appropriate anticholinergic agents, along with other appropriate measures. Monitor serum electrolytes and renal function, maintain hydration, and institute supportive measures, as required. Treat GI effects symptomatically. Observe patient for at least 72 h, administering treatment as needed.

DRUG INTERACTIONS

Alcohol, barbiturates, narcotics, other CNS depressants	Orthostatic hypotension △ CNS depression; do not use concomitantly
Other antihypertensives or diuretics	△ Antihypertensive effect; adjust dosage accordingly
Digitalis glycosides, quinidine	Cardiac arrhythmias
Levodopa	▽ Pharmacologic effect of levodopa
Methotrimeprazine	△ Orthostatic hypotension

RAUZIDE ■ REGROTON

MAO inhibitors	⇧ Excitation, hypertension, and sympathetic response	⇧ Hypotensive effect; adjust dosage accordingly
Sympathomimetics	Prolonged sympathomimetic effect (direct-acting sympathomimetics); inhibition of action (indirect-acting sympathomimetics)	
Tricyclic antidepressants	⇩ Antidepressant effect ⇩ Antihypertensive effect	
Amphotericin B, corticosteroids, or ACTH	Intensified electrolyte imbalance (particularly hypokalemia)	
Oral anticoagulants	⇩ Anticoagulant effect; adjust dosage accordingly	
Antigout agents	⇧ Hyperuricemia; adjust dosage accordingly	
Oral antidiabetic agents, insulin	⇧ Hyperglycemic effect; adjust dosage accordingly	
Calcium	⇧ Serum calcium levels	
Cardiac glycosides	⇧ Risk of digitalis toxicity due to hypokalemia	
Cholestyramine resin, colestipol hydrochloride	⇩ or Delayed absorption of bendroflumethiazide; give sulfonamide diuretics at least 1 h before or 4-6 h after these medications	
Diazoxide	⇧ Risk of hyperglycemia, hyperuricemia, and hypertensive effects	
Lithium	⇧ Risk of lithium toxicity	
Nondepolarizing muscle relaxants, preanesthetic medications, surgical anesthetics (eg, tubocurarine chloride and gallamide triethiodide)	⇩ Responsiveness to muscle relaxants	
Pressor amines, norepinephrine	⇩ Arterial responsiveness to pressor amines	
Methenamine	⇩ Effectiveness of methenamine	
Probenecid, sulfinpyrazone	⇧ Hyperuricemic effects; increased dosage may be necessary	

ALTERED LABORATORY VALUES

Blood/serum values	⇧ Uric acid ⇧ Calcium ⇩ Sodium ⇩ Potassium ⇩ Chloride ⇩ Bicarbonate ⇩ Phosphate ⇩ PBI ⇩ Thyroxine (T_4) ⇩ Plasma renin activity
Urinary values	⇧ Sodium ⇧ Potassium ⇧ Chloride ⇧ Bicarbonate ⇧ Uric acid ⇧ 5-HIAA ⇩ Calcium ⇩ 17-Ketosteroids False-negative results on phentolamine and tyramine tests Interference with PSP testing ⇩ Steroid colorimetric determination (with modified Glenn-Nelson technique or Holtorff-Koch modification of the Zimmerman reaction)

USE IN CHILDREN

Safety and effectiveness for use in children have not been established

USE IN PREGNANT AND NURSING WOMEN

Pregnancy Category C: *Rauwolfia* preparations cross the placental barrier, appear in cord blood, and have caused increased respiratory secretions, nasal congestion, cyanosis, hypothermia, and anorexia in newborns. Thiazides also cross the placental barrier, appear in cord blood, and may cause fetal or neonatal jaundice, thrombocytopenia, and other possible reactions. Use during pregnancy only if the expected benefit justifies the potential risk to the fetus. Both drugs are also excreted in breast milk; the patient should stop nursing if this product is prescribed.

ANTIHYPERTENSIVES WITH DIURETICS

REGROTON (chlorthalidone and reserpine) Rorer   Rx

Tablets: 50 mg chlorthalidone and 0.25 mg reserpine

Demi-REGROTON (chlorthalidone and reserpine) Rorer   Rx

Tablets: 25 mg chlorthalidone and 0.125 mg reserpine

INDICATIONS	ORAL DOSAGE
Hypertension	**Adult:** 1–2 tabs once daily given in the morning with food (see WARNINGS/PRECAUTIONS) **Child:** one-half the adult dosage (use Demi-Regroton)

REGROTON

CONTRAINDICATIONS

Hypersensitivity to chlorthalidone or reserpine	Most cases of severe renal or hepatic disease	Electroconvulsive therapy
Mental depression or history of depression		

ADMINISTRATION/DOSAGE ADJUSTMENTS

Initial titration of dosage	Optimal effect on blood pressure may require 2 wk or more to appear, because of slow onset of action of reserpine component; wait at least this long before adjusting dosage
Combination therapy	In more severe cases, other antihypertensive agents may be added gradually at dosages at least 50% lower than customary; monitor patient closely. When used concomitantly, reduce dosage of ganglionic blocking agents, other potent antihypertensive agents, and curare by at least 50% and provide close supervision.

WARNINGS/PRECAUTIONS

Fixed combination	Not indicated for initial therapy of hypertension; dosages of component drugs must be individually titrated and then periodically reviewed, as conditions warrant
Patients with renal impairment	Use with caution in patients with severe renal disease; monitor for signs of excessive drug accumulation
Azotemia	May be precipitated in patients with severe renal disease
Hepatic coma	May be precipitated by minor changes in fluid and electrolyte balance in patients with hepatic impairment or progressive liver disease; discontinue therapy if liver function abnormalities increase
Sensitivity reactions	May occur in patients with a history of allergy or bronchial asthma
Mental depression	May occur; discontinue therapy at the first sign of despondency, early morning insomnia, loss of appetite, impotence, self-deprecation, or other symptoms of depression
Patients undergoing electroconvulsive therapy	Discontinue drug at least 7 days before giving electroshock treatments; severe and even fatal reactions have occurred
Peptic ulcer	May be precipitated or aggravated in susceptible patients; discontinue therapy
Postsympathectomy patients	Antihypertensive effect may be enhanced; use with caution
Electrolyte imbalances	Measure serum and urine electrolytes periodically, especially if patient is vomiting excessively or receiving parenteral fluids. Watch for dry mouth, thirst, weakness, lethargy, drowsiness, restlessness, muscle pains or cramps, muscular fatigue, hypotension, oliguria, tachycardia, and GI disturbances.
Hypokalemia	May develop, especially with brisk diuresis, concomitant corticosteroid or ACTH therapy, interference with adequate oral intake of electrolytes, or in the presence of severe cirrhosis; may be minimized by including potassium-rich foods in diet or, if necessary, with potassium supplements
Dilutional hyponatremia	May occur in edematous patients when weather is hot; restrict water and use salt replacement only for life-threatening hyponatremia
Hyperuricemia or overt gout	May occur or be precipitated in certain patients; combat with a uricosuric agent if serious
Insulin requirements	May increase, decrease, or remain unchanged; latent diabetes may become active
Decreased glucose tolerance	May occur, evidenced by hyperglycemia and glycosuria; discontinue therapy. Monitor diabetics and other susceptible patients closely.
Increased GI motility and secretion	Use with caution in patients with ulcerative colitis
Biliary colic	May be precipitated in patients with gallstones
Hypotension during surgery	May occur; discontinue therapy at least 2 wk before elective surgery. For emergency surgery, use anticholinergic and/or adrenergic agents (eg, metaraminol or norepinephrine) to prevent vagocirculatory responses; other supportive measures may also be indicated.
Progressive renal damage	May occur; perform kidney function tests periodically. Discontinue therapy if BUN rises.
Bronchial asthma	May occur in susceptible patients
Carcinogenicity	Long-term (2-yr) studies in rodents fed 100–300 times the usual human dose of reserpine have shown an increased incidence of mammary fibroadenomas in female mice, malignant tumors of the seminal vesicles in male mice, and malignant adrenal medullary tumors in male rats. No definite conclusion about whether this drug increases the risk of breast cancer in humans has emerged from epidemiological studies or long-term clinical observation. Nevertheless, it should be used with caution in patients with previously detected breast cancer because of reserpine's prolactin-elevating effect. The risk of pheochromocytoma or tumors of the seminal vesicles in humans who have used reserpine has not been studied.

REGROTON ■ SALUTENSIN

ADVERSE REACTIONS	Frequent reactions (incidence ≥ 1%) are printed in *italics*
Gastrointestinal	*Anorexia, gastric irritation, nausea, vomiting, diarrhea, constipation,* dry mouth, pancreatitis (rare)
Central nervous system and neuromuscular	*Muscle cramps, dizziness, weakness, headache, drowsiness, mental depression* (rare at recommended dosages), restlessness, lassitude, paradoxical anxiety, nightmares, dulled sensorium, muscle aches, paralysis agitans-like syndrome (reversible), deafness
Ophthalmic	Transient myopia, blurred vision, conjunctival injection, uveitis, optic atrophy, glaucoma
Dermatological	Skin rash, urticaria, pruritus, eruptions, flushing, ecchymosis (one case)
Cardiovascular	Orthostatic hypotension, bradycardia, ectopic cardiac rhythms, angina pectoris
Genitourinary	Decreased libido, impotence, dysuria
Idiosyncratic	Aplastic anemia, purpura, thrombocytopenia, leukopenia, agranulocytosis, necrotizing angiitis, Lyell's syndrome (toxic epidermal necrolysis)
Other	*Nasal congestion,* increased susceptibility to colds, dyspnea, weight gain
OVERDOSAGE	
Signs and symptoms	Nausea, weakness, dizziness, syncope, electrolyte-balance disturbances, marked hypotension
Treatment	Use gastric lavage, followed by activated charcoal, to empty stomach. Institute supportive measures, as required. Intravenous dextrose-saline with potassium chloride may be given. Vasopressors may be used for marked hypotension.
DRUG INTERACTIONS	
Other antihypertensive agents	△ Antihypertensive effect
Digitalis	△ Risk of cardiac arrhythmias, bradycardia, heart block
Quinidine	△ Risk of cardiac arrhythmias
MAO inhibitors	Severe hypertension
Tubocurarine	△ Skeletal muscle relaxation
Norepinephrine	▽ Vasopressor effect
Steroids, ACTH	△ Risk of hypokalemia
Lithium	▽ Lithium clearance
Alcohol, barbiturates, narcotic analgesics	△ Risk of orthostatic hypotension
ALTERED LABORATORY VALUES	
Blood/serum values	Carbohydrate intolerance △ Uric acid △ Calcium ▽ Sodium ▽ Potassium ▽ Chloride ▽ Bicarbonate ▽ Phosphate ▽ PBI ▽ Thyroxine (T$_4$) ▽ Plasma renin activity
Urinary values	△ Sodium △ Potassium △ Chloride △ Bicarbonate △ Uric acid △ 5-HIAA ▽ Calcium ▽ 17-Ketosteroids

---

USE IN CHILDREN

See INDICATIONS and ORAL DOSAGE

USE IN PREGNANT AND NURSING WOMEN

Safety for use during pregnancy has not been established. Reserpine crosses the placental barrier, appears in cord blood, and has caused increased respiratory secretions, nasal congestion, cyanosis, and anorexia in newborns. Although chlorthalidone has not demonstrated teratogenicity in animal reproduction studies, thiazides—to which it is related—do cross the placental barrier and appear in cord blood. Both drugs are also excreted in breast milk; patient should stop nursing if this product is prescribed.

ANTIHYPERTENSIVES WITH DIURETICS

SALUTENSIN (hydroflumethiazide and reserpine) Bristol   Rx

Tablets: 50 mg hydroflumethiazide and 0.125 mg reserpine

SALUTENSIN-Demi (hydroflumethiazide and reserpine) Bristol   Rx

Tablets: 25 mg hydroflumethiazide and 0.125 mg reserpine

INDICATIONS	ORAL DOSAGE
Hypertension	Adult: 1 tab 1–2 times/day (see WARNINGS/PRECAUTIONS)

COMPENDIUM OF DRUG THERAPY

SALUTENSIN

CONTRAINDICATIONS

Hypersensitivity to hydroflumethiazide, reserpine, or any other component	Active peptic ulcer	Severe depression
Anuria or oliguria	Ulcerative colitis	Electroconvulsive therapy (see WARNINGS/PRECAUTIONS)

ADMINISTRATION/DOSAGE ADJUSTMENTS

Refractory patients	Up to 3–4 tabs/day in divided doses may be given cautiously in refractory cases. Closely monitor serum uric acid, fasting blood sugar, BUN/NPN, and serum electrolytes. Reduce dosage to minimum effective level after desired blood pressure reduction is achieved.
Combination therapy	Reduce dosage of other antihypertensives, especially ganglionic blockers, by at least 50% to avoid an excessive drop in blood pressure. Further dosage reduction or discontinuance of therapy may be necessary.

WARNINGS/PRECAUTIONS

Fixed combination	This preparation is not indicated for initial therapy of hypertension; dosages of the component drugs must be individually titrated to the patient's needs before instituting treatment with this combination
Electroconvulsive therapy	Discontinue use at least 7 days prior to administration of electroconvulsive therapy
Patients with gallstones	Use with caution in patients with gallstones; biliary colic may be precipitated
Patients with renal impairment	Use with caution in patients with impaired renal function since they tend to adjust poorly to lowered blood pressure levels. Thiazides can precipitate or increase azotemia in patients with renal disease; if impairment progresses, as indicated by a rising NPN or BUN level, consider withholding or discontinuing treatment.
Patients with liver disease	Minor changes in fluid and electrolyte balance may precipitate hepatic coma in patients with hepatic impairment or progressive liver disease; use with caution in such patients
Patients with GI disorders	Use with caution in patients with a history of peptic ulcer, ulcerative colitis, or other GI disorders which may be exacerbated by an increase in GI motility or secretion
Major surgery	Thiazides may increase responsiveness to tubocurarine and decrease arterial responsiveness to norepinephrine. Reserpine may cause significant hypotension and bradycardia during surgical anesthesia. If possible, the use of reserpine should be discontinued 2 wk before giving anesthesia; thiazides should be discontinued 48 h before elective surgery. For emergency procedures, parenteral vagal blocking agents may be necessary to prevent or reverse hypotension and/or bradycardia.
Postsympathectomy patients	The antihypertensive effects of the thiazide component may be enhanced in sympathectomized patients
Electrolyte disorders	Hypokalemia may occur, especially with brisk diuresis, after prolonged thiazide therapy, when severe cirrhosis is present, ACTH, digitalis, or corticosteroids are given concomitantly, or intake of electrolytes is inadequate; potassium supplements or potassium-rich foods may be given to avoid or treat hypokalemia. Dilutional hyponatremia may occur in severely edematous patients with congestive heart failure or renal disease when the weather is hot; restrict the intake of water, and administer salt only if hyponatremia is life-threatening or actual salt depletion occurs. For hypochloremia, specific treatment is unnecessary, except for certain patients (eg, those with hepatic or renal disease); chloride deficit may be corrected with use of ammonium chloride (except in patients with hepatic disease) and prevented with a near normal salt intake. To prevent electrolyte imbalance, measure serum and urinary electrolyte levels periodically in all patients (these determinations are especially important if excessive vomiting occurs or parenteral fluids are being given); watch for premonitory signs and symptoms of hypokalemia, hyponatremia, and hypochloremic alkalosis, such as dry mouth, thirst, weakness, lethargy, drowsiness, restlessness, muscle pain or cramps, muscular fatigue, hypotension, oliguria, tachycardia, and GI disturbances (nausea, vomiting).
Parathyroid dysfunction	Pathological changes in the parathyroid gland, accompanied by hypercalcemia and hypophosphatemia, have occurred in a few patients after prolonged thiazide therapy; however, the common complications of hyperparathyroidism have not been seen. Although parathyroidectomy has resulted in subjective clinical improvement in most patients, no effect on hypertension has been documented; following surgery, thiazide therapy may be resumed. Discontinue use before performing parathyroid function tests.
Diabetes	Insulin requirements in diabetic patients may be increased, decreased, or unchanged; thiazides may cause hyperglycemia and glycosuria in latent diabetics
Other thiazide-related effects	Thiazides may activate or exacerbate systemic lupus erythematosus, precipitate hypersensitivity reactions in patients with a history of allergy or bronchial asthma, or cause gout in patients with hyperuricemia or a history of gout
Psychic effects, depression	Anxiety or depression, as well as psychosis, may develop during therapy; existing depression may be aggravated with use of reserpine. Although mental depression is unusual with reserpine doses of 0.25 mg/day or less, use with extreme caution in patients with a history of depression because of the possibility of suicide; discontinue use at the first sign of depression.

SALUTENSIN

Carcinogenicity	Long-term (2-yr) studies in rodents fed 100–300 times the usual human dose of reserpine have shown an increased incidence of mammary fibroadenomas in female mice, malignant tumors of the seminal vesicles in male mice, and malignant adrenal medullary tumors in male rats. No definite conclusion about whether this drug increases the risk of breast cancer in humans has emerged from epidemiological studies or long-term clinical observation. Nevertheless, it should be used with caution in patients with previously detected breast cancer because of reserpine's prolactin-elevating effect. The risk of pheochromocytoma or tumors of the seminal vesicles in humans who have used reserpine has not been studied.

ADVERSE REACTIONS

Gastrointestinal	Anorexia, gastric irritation, nausea, vomiting, cramping, diarrhea, constipation, intrahepatic cholestatic jaundice, pancreatitis, increased intestinal motility, dry mouth, increased salivation
Central nervous system, neuromuscular	Dizziness, vertigo, paresthesias, headache, muscle spasm, weakness, restlessness, excessive sedation, nightmares, impotence or decreased libido, mental depression, nervousness, paradoxical anxiety, dull sensorium, deafness, parkinsonian-like syndrome, muscular aches
Ophthalmic	Xanthopsia, conjunctival injection, blurred vision, syncope, glaucoma, uveitis, optic atrophy
Hematological	Leukopenia, thrombocytopenia, agranulocytosis, aplastic anemia, epistaxis, thrombocytopenic purpura
Dermatological, hypersensitivity	Purpura, photosensitivity, rash, urticaria, necrotizing angiitis, flushing of the skin, pruritus
Cardiovascular	Orthostatic hypotension, bradycardia, angina pectoris, and other direct cardiac effects (including premature ventricular contractions, fluid retention, and congestive heart failure)
Respiratory	Respiratory distress (including pneumonitis, pulmonary edema, and anaphylactic reactions), nasal congestion, dyspnea
Other	Fever, weight gain, increased susceptibility to colds, dysuria, nonpuerperal lactation, hyperglycemia, glycosuria

OVERDOSAGE

Signs and symptoms	*Hydroflumethiazide-related effects:* diuresis, lethargy progressing to coma with minimal cardiorespiratory depression, GI irritation, hypermotility, elevated BUN, serum electrolyte changes; *reserpine-related effects:* impairment of consciousness ranging from drowsiness to coma, flushing, conjunctival injection, miosis, hypotension, hypothermia, respiratory depression, bradycardia, diarrhea
Treatment	Induce emesis or use gastric lavage, followed by activated charcoal, to empty stomach. Treat hypotension by volume expansion, if possible. If a vasopressor is needed, use phenylephrine, norepinephrine, or metaraminol. Treat significant bradycardia with vagal blocking agents, along with other appropriate measures. Monitor serum electrolytes and renal function and institute supportive measures, as required. Treat GI effects symptomatically. Observe patient for at least 72 h, administering treatment as needed.

DRUG INTERACTIONS

Preanesthetic and anesthetic agents, nondepolarizing skeletal muscle relaxants	⇧ Pharmacologic effects of these agents; adjust dosage accordingly, if necessary
Other antihypertensive agents, diuretics	⇧ Antihypertensive effect; adjust dosage accordingly, if necessary
Amphotericin B, corticosteroids, corticotropin	Intensified electrolyte imbalance (especially hypokalemia)
Cardiac glycosides	⇧ Risk of digitalis toxicity associated with hypokalemia
Colestipol	⇩ GI absorption of thiazides; administer 1 h before or 4 h after colestipol
Hypoglycemic agents	⇧ Hyperglycemic effect; adjust dosage accordingly
Lithium	⇧ Risk of lithium toxicity; concurrent use is not recommended
Methenamine	⇩ Pharmacologic effect of methenamine
Alcohol, barbiturates, narcotics, CNS depressants	Orthostatic hypotension ⇧ CNS depression; do not use concomitantly
Beta-blocking agents	⇧ Beta-adrenergic blockade; observe patient closely
Digitalis glycosides, quinidine	Cardiac arrhythmias (controversial); use with caution
Levodopa	⇧ Risk of dopamine depletion and parkinsonism; do not use concomitantly
Methotrimeprazine	⇧ Risk of orthostatic hypotension
MAO inhibitors	Moderate to sudden, severe hypertension and hyperpyrexia, possibly to crisis levels

SALUTENSIN ■ SER-AP-ES

Sympathomimetics	Prolonged sympathomimetic effect (direct-acting sympathomimetics), inhibition of sympathomimetic action (indirect-acting sympathomimetics); use with caution and under close supervision
Tricyclic antidepressants	▽ Antihypertensive effect Interference with antidepressant effect

ALTERED LABORATORY VALUES

Blood/serum values	△ Glucose △ Calcium △ Bilirubin △ Uric acid △ or ▽ Magnesium ▽ Potassium ▽ Sodium ▽ PBI △ Prolactin ▽ Chloride ▽ Thyroxine (T$_4$)
Urinary values	△ Sodium △ Potassium △ Chloride △ Bicarbonate △ Uric acid △ 5-HIAA ▽ Calcium ▽ 17-Ketosteroids △ Glucose ▽ Steroid colorimetric determination (with modified Glenn-Nelson technique or Holtorff-Koch modification of the Zimmerman reaction) ▽ Catecholamine excretion ▽ VMA

USE IN CHILDREN
Safety and effectiveness for use in children have not been established

USE IN PREGNANT AND NURSING WOMEN
Pregnancy Category C: *Rauwolfia* preparations cross the placental barrier, appear in cord blood, and have caused nasal congestion, lethargy, depressed Moro reflex, and bradycardia in newborns. Thiazides also cross the placental barrier, appear in cord blood, and may cause fetal or neonatal jaundice, thrombocytopenia, and other possible reactions. Use during pregnancy only if the expected benefit justifies the potential risk to the fetus. Both drugs are excreted in human milk; the patient should stop nursing if use of this preparation is considered essential.

ANTIHYPERTENSIVES WITH DIURETICS

SER-AP-ES (reserpine, hydralazine hydrochloride, and hydrochlorothiazide) CIBA Rx
Tablets: 0.1 mg reserpine, 25 mg hydralazine hydrochloride, and 15 mg hydrochlorothiazide

INDICATIONS	ORAL DOSAGE
Hypertension	**Adult:** 1–2 tabs tid

CONTRAINDICATIONS
Mental depression, especially with suicidal tendencies	Coronary artery disease	Hypersensitivity to hydrochlorothiazide, other sulfonamide derivatives, reserpine, or hydralazine
Electroconvulsive therapy	Rheumatic mitral valve disease	
Active peptic ulcer	Ulcerative colitis	Anuria

ADMINISTRATION/DOSAGE ADJUSTMENTS

Food-drug interactions	Administration of hydralazine with food results in higher serum drug levels; food also enhances absorption of hydrochlorothiazide
Peak therapeutic effect	Maximal reduction in blood pressure may not occur at a particular dosage until after 2 wk
Acetylation rate	Serum levels of hydralazine are generally higher in patients who acetylate the drug at a slow rate; these patients usually require lower doses of hydralazine than patients with a rapid rate of acetylation
Combination therapy	When necessary, more potent antihypertensive agents may be added gradually at a dosage at least 50% lower than customary; carefully monitor clinical response

WARNINGS/PRECAUTIONS

Fixed combination	This preparation is not indicated for initial therapy of hypertension; dosages of the component drugs must be individually titrated to the patient's needs before instituting treatment with this combination
Mental depression	Reserpine-induced depression is dose-related, may persist for several months after drug withdrawal, and can result in suicide. Use with extreme caution in patients with a history of mental depression; discontinue drug at first sign of despondency, early morning insomnia, loss of appetite, impotence, or self-deprecation.
Gastrointestinal effects	Reserpine can increase GI motility and secretion; use with caution in patients with a history of peptic ulcer or ulcerative colitis. Biliary colic can occur in patients with a history of gallstones; exercise caution when using this drug in these patients.

Surgery	Bradycardia and hypotension can occur during surgery in patients who are receiving reserpine or who have recently discontinued the drug; inform the anesthesiologist before surgery that the patient has received this drug. If cardiovascular reactions occur during surgery, use anticholinergic drugs and direct-acting sympathomimetic agents (eg, norepinephrine, metaraminol), as needed.
Lupus erythematosus	A syndrome resembling systemic lupus erythematosus, with glomerulonephritis and other lupus-like reactions, can occur with use of hydralazine; although this syndrome is usually reversible, manifestations can persist and necessitate long-term corticosteroid treatment. Thiazides can activate or exacerbate systemic lupus erythematosus. To reduce the risk of this syndrome, perform an ANA test before therapy, periodically during prolonged treatment, and whenever arthralgia, fever, chest pain, continued malaise, or any other unexplained reaction occurs. If results of an ANA test are positive or clinical signs and symptoms develop, carefully weigh risks and benefits of continued use.
Angina, myocardial infarction	The myocardial stimulation due to hydralazine may precipitate angina, myocardial ischemia, and myocardial infarction; use with caution in patients with known or suspected coronary artery disease
Postural hypotension	Hydralazine can cause postural hypotension; use with caution in patients with cerebrovascular accidents
Peripheral neuritis	Hydralazine may cause peripheral neuritis, characterized by paresthesias, numbness, and tingling; if symptoms develop, administer pyridoxine concomitantly
Blood dyscrasias	Watch for evidence of blood dyscrasias; obtain a CBC before therapy, periodically during prolonged treatment, and whenever symptoms develop. If leukopenia, agranulocytosis, purpura, or a reduction in hemoglobin and erythrocytes is detected, this preparation should be discontinued.
Renal dysfunction, drug accumulation	Thiazides can accumulate or precipitate azotemia in patients with renal impairment; reserpine may exacerbate renal dysfunction, and hydralazine can aggravate advance renal disease. Use this preparation with caution in patients with renal disorders; if renal impairment progresses, consider interrupting or terminating therapy.
Hepatic coma	Minor changes in fluid and electrolyte balance may precipitate hepatic coma in patients with hepatic impairment or progressive liver disease; use with caution in such patients
Electrolyte disorders	Hypokalemia may occur, especially when diuresis is brisk, severe cirrhosis is present, ACTH or corticosteroids are given concomitantly, or oral intake of electrolytes is inadequate; potassium supplements or potassium-rich foods may be given to avoid or treat hypokalemia. Dilutional hyponatremia may occur in edematous patients when the weather is hot. Treat by restricting the intake of water; administer salt only if the hyponatremia is life-threatening or actual salt depletion occurs. For hypochloremia, specific treatment is usually unnecessary, except for certain patients (eg, those with hepatic or renal disease). To prevent electrolyte imbalance, measure serum and urinary electrolyte levels periodically in all patients (these determinations are especially important if excessive vomiting occurs or parenteral fluids are being given); watch for premonitory signs and symptoms of hypokalemia, hyponatremia, and hypochloremic alkalosis, such as dry mouth, thirst, weakness, lethargy, drowsiness, restlessness, muscle pain or cramps, muscular fatigue, hypotension, oliguria, tachycardia, and GI disturbances (eg, nausea and vomiting).
Diabetes	Thiazides can activate latent diabetes or alter insulin requirements
Parathyroid dysfunction	Thiazides decrease calcium excretion. Discontinue use before performing parathyroid function tests. Pathological changes in the parathyroid gland, accompanied by hypercalcemia and hypophosphatemia, have occurred in a few patients after prolonged thiazide therapy; however, the common complications of hyperparathyroidism have not been seen.
Other thiazide-related reactions	Thiazides may cause hyperuricemia or overt gout, precipitate hypersensitivity reactions (especially in patients with a history of allergy or bronchial asthma), and, in postsympathectomy patients, produce an enhanced antihypertensive effect
Carcinogenicity	An increase in adenomas and adenocarcinomas of the lung has occurred in mice fed throughout their lives 80 times the maximum human dose of hydralazine; increases in benign hepatic neoplastic nodules and benign testicular interstitial cell tumors have been observed in rats given hydralazine. Long-term clinical observation has not suggested an association between hydralazine and cancer; however, no adequate epidemiological studies have been done. Long-term (2-yr) studies in rodents fed 100–300 times the usual human dose of reserpine have shown an increased frequency of mammary fibroadenomas in female mice, malignant tumors of the seminal vesicles in male mice, and malignant adrenal medullary tumors in male rats. No definite conclusion about whether reserpine increases the risk of breast cancer in humans has emerged from epidemiological studies or long-term clinical observation; nevertheless, it should be used with caution in patients with previously detected breast cancer because of its prolactin-elevating effect. No studies have been done to determine whether reserpine increases the risks of pheochromocytoma and tumors of the seminal vesicles in humans.

SER-AP-ES

Mutagenicity	Hydralazine has been shown to be mutagenic in the Ames test and has elicited DNA repair, a sign of mutagenicity, in *E coli* and cultured rat hepatocytes. In tests with rabbit hepatocytes having either a slow or rapid acetylation rate, the drug has elicited DNA repair only in those hepatocytes with a slow rate; these results suggest that patients with a rapid acetylation rate may be less susceptible to the potentially mutagenic effects of this drug. No evidence of mutagenicity has been seen in the mouse lymphoma assay, host-mediated assay, nucleus anomaly test, or dominant lethal test.

ADVERSE REACTIONS

Central nervous system	Headache, paresthesias, peripheral neuritis, dizziness, vertigo, tremors, weakness, restlessness, extrapyramidal reactions (including parkinsonism), paradoxical anxiety, depression, nervousness, nightmares, dull sensorium, drowsiness; psychotic reactions characterized by depression, disorientation, or anxiety; muscle cramps, spasm, and aches; arthralgia
Ophthalmic	Optic atrophy, glaucoma, uveitis, conjunctival injection, lacrimation, conjunctivitis, xanthopsia, transient blurred vision
Gastrointestinal	Anorexia, nausea, vomiting, diarrhea, gastric irritation, hypersecretion, cramping, constipation, paralytic ileus, hepatitis, intrahepatic cholestatic jaundice, pancreatitis
Cardiovascular	Palpitations, tachycardia, bradycardia, arrhythmias, angina, hypotension (including orthostatic hypotension), syncope, paradoxical hypertension, edema, flushing
Hematological	Reduction in hemoglobin, erythropenia, leukopenia, agranulocytosis, thrombocytopenia, aplastic anemia, eosinophilia, lymphadenopathy, splenomegaly
Respiratory	Dyspnea, nasal congestion, epistaxis
Genitourinary	Impotence, decreased libido, dysuria, difficult urination
Hypersensitivity	Rash, urticaria, pruritus, fever, chills, purpura, photosensitivity, necrotizing angiitis, Stevens-Johnson syndrome
Other	Deafness, dry mouth, sialadenitis, weight gain, pseudolactation, breast engorgement, gynecomastia, hyperglycemia, glycosuria, hyperuricemia

OVERDOSAGE

Signs and symptoms	Hypotension, shock, tachycardia, bradycardia, headache, generalized skin flushing, myocardial ischemia and infarction, arrhythmia, hypokalemia, hyponatremia, hypochloremia, alkalosis, increased BUN level (especially in patients with renal impairment); anuria, oliguria, or polyuria; nausea, vomiting, diarrhea, thirst, increases in gastric and salivary secretions, weakness, confusion, dizziness, fatigue, drowsiness, cramped calf muscles, paresthesia, conjunctival injection, miosis, hypothermia, respiratory depression, coma
Treatment	Give primary attention to cardiovascular status. To treat hypotension or shock, raise patient's legs and replace fluids and electrolytes (potassium and sodium). Use vasopressors only if they are necessary and precautions are taken to avoid precipitating or exacerbating an arrhythmia; administer a direct-acting agent such as phenylephrine, norepinephrine, or metaraminol. For tachycardia, give a beta blocker. Digitalization may be necessary for reversal of cardiovascular disorders. To remove this preparation from the GI tract, empty stomach and then, if conditions permit, instill activated charcoal; bear in mind that since these measures can precipitate arrhythmia or enhance shock, it may be necessary to either skip them or wait until cardiovascular function has been restored before doing them. Monitor renal function and fluid and electrolyte balance (especially the serum potassium level) until conditions return to normal. Since reserpine is a long-acting drug, the patient should be kept under careful observation for at least 72 h.

DRUG INTERACTIONS

Diazoxide	Severe hypotension; after giving diazoxide to patients receiving this preparation, monitor blood pressure continuously for several hours
Other antihypertensive agents	△ Antihypertensive effect
Digitalis	△ Risk of digitalis toxicity and arrhythmias; exercise caution during combination therapy
Quinidine	△ Risk of arrhythmias; exercise caution during combination therapy
MAO inhibitors	△ Risk of hypotension or hypertension; institute combination therapy with extreme caution, if at all
Lithium	△ Risk of lithium toxicity
Norepinephrine, other vasopressors	▽ Vasopressor effect (this interaction does not preclude therapeutic use of vasopressors)
Corticosteroids, ACTH	△ Risk of hypokalemia
Tubocurarine, other nondepolarizing skeletal muscle relaxants	△ Skeletal muscle relaxation
Propranolol, metoprolol	△ Serum level of propranolol and metoprolol

Alcohol, barbiturates, narcotic analgesics — ⇧ Risk of orthostatic hypotension

ALTERED LABORATORY VALUES

Blood/serum values — + ANA + Direct Coombs' test ⇧ PRA (plasma renin activity) ⇩ Sodium ⇩ Potassium ⇩ Calcium ⇩ Magnesium ⇩ Chloride ⇩ Phosphate ⇧ Uric acid ⇩ PBI ⇧ Glucose ⇧ Prolactin

Urinary values — ⇧ Sodium ⇧ Potassium ⇩ Calcium ⇧ Magnesium ⇧ Chloride ⇧ Bicarbonate ⇩ Uric acid ⇧ Glucose ⇩ Catecholamines ⇩ VMA ⇩ 17-OHCS (with modified Glenn-Nelson technique) ⇩ 17-KS (with Holtorff-Koch modification of the Zimmerman reaction)

USE IN CHILDREN

Safety and effectiveness for use in children have not been established

USE IN PREGNANT AND NURSING WOMEN

Pregnancy Category C: hydralazine has caused cleft palate and malformations of facial and cranial bones in mice at 20–30 times the maximum daily human dose and may be teratogenic in rabbits at 10–15 times the maximum daily human dose. Administration of a thiazide during pregnancy can produce adverse reactions, including jaundice and thrombocytopenia, in a neonate or fetus; thiazides are excreted in human milk. When given parenterally, reserpine has been shown to be teratogenic in rats at up to 2 mg/kg and to be embryocidal in guinea pigs at 0.5 mg/day; use by pregnant or nursing women has resulted in anorexia, cyanosis, an increase in respiratory tract secretions, and nasal congestion in neonates. Give this preparation during pregnancy only if the expected benefits justify the potential risks; instruct women not to nurse during therapy.

ANTIHYPERTENSIVES WITH DIURETICS

TENORETIC (atenolol and chlorthalidone) Stuart   Rx

Tablets: 50 mg atenolol and 25 mg chlorthalidone (Tenoretic 50); 100 mg atenolol and 25 mg chlorthalidone (Tenoretic 100)

INDICATIONS
Hypertension

ORAL DOSAGE
Adult: 1 Tenoretic 50 tab once daily to start, followed, if necessary, by 1 Tenoretic 100 tab once daily

CONTRAINDICATIONS

Cardiogenic shock

Second- or third-degree AV block

Overt cardiac failure

Sinus bradycardia

Anuria

Hypersensitivity to atenolol, chlorthalidone or other sulfonamide derivatives

ADMINISTRATION/DOSAGE ADJUSTMENTS

Patients with severe renal impairment — Administer 1 Tenoretic 50 tab q24h or less frequently if creatinine clearance (Ccr) = 15–35 ml/min, or q48h or less frequently if Ccr < 15 ml/min; do not use Tenoretic 100 tabs

Addition of another antihypertensive agent — To avoid an excessive fall in blood pressure, give half the usual dose of the new agent to start, and then gradually increase the dose

WARNINGS/PRECAUTIONS[1]

Fixed combination — This preparation is not indicated for initial therapy of hypertension; dosages of the component drugs must be individually titrated to the patient's needs before instituting treatment with this combination

Cardiac failure — Beta blockade may cause or exacerbate cardiac failure. Use with caution in patients with well-compensated congestive heart failure. If cardiac failure occurs during treatment and does not respond to digitalization and diuretic therapy, administration should be discontinued.

Angina — Abrupt withdrawal of certain beta blockers can exacerbate angina and, in some cases, precipitate myocardial infarction. When discontinuing therapy, carefully observe the patient and restrict physical activity, even if overt angina is not evident; if withdrawal symptoms occur, reinstitute use of this preparation. Caution patients not to interrupt or discontinue therapy on their own.

Hyperthyroidism — Abrupt withdrawal of beta blockade can precipitate a thyroid storm in patients with hyperthyroidism; since certain clinical signs of this disorder (such as tachycardia) can be masked during therapy, patients should be closely observed during the period of withdrawal, even if thyrotoxicosis is only suspected.

TENORETIC

Diabetes	Beta blockade may mask tachycardia associated with hypoglycemia, but may not significantly affect other manifestations, such as dizziness and sweating. Thiazides may activate latent diabetes or affect the insulin requirements of diabetic patients. Exercise caution during therapy.
Bronchospasm	In general, patients with bronchospastic disease should not receive beta blockers. However, if other antihypertensive treatment is not effective or tolerated, this preparation may be used with caution in these patients since atenolol has a relative selectivity for beta$_1$ receptors; because this selectivity is not absolute, a beta$_2$ agonist should be available during therapy, and the lowest possible dose of atenolol should be used. If an increase in dosage is necessary, consider dividing the daily dose.
Major surgery	Bradycardia and hypotension may result from beta blockade during surgery, but can be reversed by atropine and beta-adrenergic agonists. To avoid these reactions, use anesthetic agents with caution or, alternatively, discontinue beta blockade at least 48 h before surgery.
Rash, dry eyes	Beta-blocker therapy has been associated with skin rash and dry eyes, which have usually cleared when therapy was stopped. If these reactions occur and cannot be attributed to any cause other than use of this preparation, consider discontinuing therapy. After cessation, monitor patient closely.
Azotemia	Thiazides can precipitate azotemia in patients with renal disease; if renal impairment progresses, therapy should be discontinued
Hepatic coma	Minor changes in fluid and electrolyte balance may precipitate hepatic coma in patients with hepatic impairment or progressive liver disease; use with caution in such patients
Electrolyte disorders	Hypokalemia may occur, especially with brisk diuresis, when severe cirrhosis is present, ACTH or corticosteroids are given concomitantly, or oral intake of electrolytes is inadequate; potassium supplements or potassium-rich foods may be given to avoid or treat hypokalemia. Dilutional hyponatremia may occur in edematous patients when the weather is hot; restrict the intake of water, and administer salt only if hyponatremia is life-threatening or actual salt depletion occurs. For hypochloremia, specific treatment is usually unnecessary, except for certain patients (eg, those with hepatic or renal disease). To prevent electrolyte imbalance, measure serum and urinary electrolyte levels periodically in all patients (these determinations are especially important if excessive vomiting occurs or parenteral fluids are being given); watch for premonitory signs and symptoms of hypokalemia, hyponatremia, and hypochloremic alkalosis, such as dry mouth, thirst, weakness, lethargy, drowsiness, restlessness, muscle pain or cramps, muscular fatigue, hypotension, oliguria, tachycardia, and GI disturbances (eg, nausea and vomiting).
Parathyroid dysfunction	Thiazides decrease calcium excretion. Discontinue therapy before performing parathyroid function tests. Pathological changes in the parathyroid gland, accompanied by hypercalcemia and hypophosphatemia, have occurred in a few patients after prolonged thiazide therapy; however, the common complications of hyperparathyroidism have not been seen.
Other thiazide-related effects	Thiazides may activate or exacerbate systemic lupus erythematosus, cause hyperuricemia or overt gout, precipitate hypersensitivity reactions (even in patients without a history of allergy), or, in postsympathectomy patients, produce an enhanced antihypertensive effect
Carcinogenicity	Long-term studies in mice and rats given up to 150 times the maximum human dose of atenolol have shown no evidence of carcinogenicity; there has also been no evidence of atenolol mutagenicity in the Ames test, mouse dominant lethal assay, or the Chinese hamster in vivo cytogenetic test
Effect on fertility	The fertility of rats has not been affected by administration of up to 100 times the maximum human dose of atenolol

ADVERSE REACTIONS[2]

Cardiovascular	Bradycardia, cold extremities, postural hypotension, leg pain
Central nervous system	Dizziness, vertigo, light-headedness, tiredness, fatigue, lethargy, drowsiness, depression, dreaming, weakness, restlessness, paresthesias
Ophthalmic	Xanthopsia, dry eyes
Gastrointestinal	Diarrhea, nausea, anorexia, gastric irritation, vomiting, cramping, constipation, intrahepatic cholestatic jaundice, pancreatitis
Respiratory	Wheezing, dyspnea
Hematological	Leukopenia, agranulocytosis, thrombocytopenia, aplastic anemia
Hypersensitivity	Purpura, photosensitivity, rash, urticaria, necrotizing angiitis, toxic epidermal necrolysis
Other	Hyperglycemia, hyperuricemia, muscle spasm

TENORETIC ■ TIMOLIDE

OVERDOSAGE

Signs and symptoms	Bradycardia, cardiac failure, hypotension, bronchospasm, hypoglycemia, electrolyte imbalance, nausea, weakness, dizziness
Treatment	Induce emesis or perform gastric lavage. To remove atenolol from the general circulation, use hemodialysis. Correct dehydration and electrolyte imbalance; if necessary, cautiously administer IV dextrose-saline with potassium. For bradycardia, give atropine or another anticholinergic drug. For second- or third-degree AV block, use isoproterenol or a transvenous cardiac pacemaker. Treat cardiac failure with digitalis and diuretics. Epinephrine, in addition to atropine and digitalis, may be useful in reversing hypotension. For bronchospasm, administer aminophylline, isoproterenol, or atropine. For hypoglycemia, give IV glucose.

DRUG INTERACTIONS

Digitalis	⇧ Risk of digitalis toxicity
Reserpine, other catecholamine-depleting agents	⇧ Risk of hypotension and bradycardia; watch for vertigo, syncope, and other signs of orthostatic hypotension
Anesthetics	⇧ Risk of hypotension and bradycardia (see warning, above, concerning use during surgery)
Lithium	⇧ Risk of lithium toxicity; lithium generally should not be given with this preparation
Clonidine	⇧ Rebound hypertension (when clonidine is abruptly discontinued during beta blockade); to terminate use of both atenolol and clonidine, discontinue the beta blocker several days before starting gradual withdrawal of clonidine
Norepinephrine, other vasopressors	⇩ Vasopressor effect; nevertheless, this interaction does not preclude therapeutic use of vasopressors
Corticosteroids, ACTH	⇧ Risk of hypokalemia
Tubocurarine, other nondepolarizing skeletal muscle relaxants	⇧ Skeletal muscle relaxation

ALTERED LABORATORY VALUES

Blood/serum values	⇩ Sodium ⇩ Potassium ⇧ Calcium ⇩ Magnesium ⇩ Chloride ⇩ Phosphate ⇧ Uric acid ⇩ PBI ⇧ Glucose ⇧ Amylase
Urinary values	⇧ Sodium ⇧ Potassium ⇩ Calcium ⇧ Magnesium ⇧ Chloride ⇧ Bicarbonate ⇩ Uric acid ⇧ Glucose

---

USE IN CHILDREN

Safety and effectiveness for use in children have not been established

USE IN PREGNANT AND NURSING WOMEN

Pregnancy Category C: an increase in resorptions has been shown in rats at 25 times the maximum human dose of atenolol and in rabbits at 50 times, but not at 12.5 times, this dose; adverse reactions, including jaundice and thrombocytopenia, can occur in a neonate or fetus following administration of thiazides during pregnancy. Use this preparation in pregnant women only if the expected benefit justifies the potential risk to the fetus. The concentration of atenolol and chlorthalidone in human milk is not known; patients should not nurse while taking this preparation.

---

[1] Chlorthalidone differs chemically, but is similar pharmacologically, to thiazide diuretics
[2] Other reactions associated with beta blockers include intensification of AV block; reversible mental depression progressing to catatonia; hallucinations; an acute reversible syndrome characterized by temporal and spatial disorientation, short-term memory loss, emotional lability, slightly clouded sensorium, and decreased performance on neuropsychometric tests; mesenteric arterial thrombosis; ischemic colitis; fever combined with sore throat and aching; laryngospasm; respiratory distress; reversible alopecia; and Peyronie's disease

---

ANTIHYPERTENSIVES WITH DIURETICS

TIMOLIDE (timolol maleate and hydrochlorothiazide) Merck Sharp & Dohme   Rx

Tablets: 10 mg timolol maleate and 25 mg hydrochlorothiazide

INDICATIONS
Hypertension

ORAL DOSAGE
Adult: 1 tab bid (if response is unsatisfactory, another antihypertensive agent may be added)

CONTRAINDICATIONS

Bronchial asthma or a history of bronchial asthma	Second- or third-degree AV block	Cardiogenic shock
Severe chronic obstructive pulmonary disease	Overt cardiac failure (see WARNINGS/PRECAUTIONS)	Hypersensitivity to this product or sulfonamide derivatives
Sinus bradycardia		

COMPENDIUM OF DRUG THERAPY

TIMOLIDE

WARNINGS/PRECAUTIONS

Fixed combination	Not indicated for initial therapy of hypertension; dosages of component drugs must be individually titrated to patient's needs before instituting treatment with this product
Cardiac failure	May be precipitated by further or continued depression of myocardial contractility; discontinue use if cardiac failure persists despite adequate digitalization and diuretic therapy. In cases of well-compensated congestive heart failure, use with caution.
Abrupt discontinuation of therapy	May exacerbate angina and in some cases lead to myocardial infarction in patients with ischemic heart disease; caution patients accordingly. When discontinuing chronic administration of this product, reduce dosage gradually over 1–2 wk and monitor patient carefully. If angina worsens markedly or acute coronary artery insufficiency develops, reinstitute use of timolol promptly and take other appropriate therapeutic measures.
Patients with obstructive pulmonary disease	This preparation is specifically contraindicated for use in patients with bronchial asthma or a history of bronchial asthma; because this product may block catecholamine-induced bronchodilation, it should be used with caution and only if necessary in patients with nonasthmatic bronchospastic disease, a history of such a disorder, or nonasthmatic, mild to moderate, chronic obstructive pulmonary disease (eg, chronic bronchitis, emphysema)
Patients undergoing anesthesia and major surgery	Beta blockade may augment the risks; gradual withdrawal of beta blockers prior to elective surgery is recommended by some authorities. If necessary, the effects of beta blockade may be reversed during surgery by sufficient doses of such beta-adrenergic agonists as isoproterenol, dobutamine, or norepinephrine.
Diabetes and hypoglycemia	Use with caution in patients subject to spontaneous hypoglycemia and in diabetic patients (especially labile diabetics) who are taking insulin or oral hypoglycemic agents; beta blockade may mask the signs and symptoms of acute hypoglycemia
Thyrotoxicosis	Clinical signs of hyperthyroidism (eg, tachycardia) may be masked; manage patients suspected of developing thyrotoxicosis carefully to avoid abrupt withdrawal of beta blockade, which might precipitate a thyroid storm
Muscle weakness	Beta blockade can cause certain myasthenic signs and symptoms (eg, diplopia, ptosis, generalized weakness) and, in rare instances, may exacerbate myasthenia gravis or myasthenic symptoms
Cerebrovascular insufficiency	Since beta blockers affect blood pressure and heart rate, they should be used with caution in patients with cerebrovascular insufficiency; if signs or symptoms suggesting reduced cerebral blood flow are noted, consider discontinuing this preparation
Patients with renal impairment	Renal insufficiency may result in excessive drug accumulation (see OVERDOSAGE); if renal impairment progresses, consider withholding or discontinuing diuretic therapy
Azotemia	May be precipitated in patients with renal disease
Electrolyte imbalance	Measure serum and urine electrolytes periodically, especially if patient is vomiting excessively or receiving parenteral fluids. Watch for dry mouth, thirst, weakness, lethargy, drowsiness, restlessness, muscle pain or cramps, muscular fatigue, hypotension, oliguria, tachycardia, and GI disturbances.
Hypokalemia	May develop, especially with brisk diuresis, concomitant corticosteroid or ACTH therapy, interference with adequate oral intake of electrolytes, or in the presence of severe cirrhosis; may be minimized by including potassium-rich foods in diet or, if necessary, with potassium supplements. Hypokalemia may result in digitalis toxicity.
Dilutional hyponatremia	May occur in edematous patients when weather is hot; restrict intake of water. Replace salt only for actual salt depletion or when hyponatremia is life-threatening.
Hypomagnesemia	May occur
Hepatic coma	May be precipitated by minor changes in fluid and electrolyte balance in patients with hepatic impairment or progressive liver disease; use with caution
Hyperuricemia or overt gout	May occur in certain patients
Sensitivity reactions	May occur in patients with or without a history of allergy or bronchial asthma
Insulin requirements	May increase, decrease, or remain unchanged; latent diabetes may become active
Lithium therapy	Renal clearance is reduced, increasing risk of lithium toxicity; coadministration generally should be avoided unless adequate precautions are taken
Systemic lupus erythematosus	May be activated or exacerbated
Postsympathectomy patients	Antihypertensive effect may be enhanced
Diagnostic interference	Hydrochlorothiazide may decrease serum PBI levels without signs of thyroid disturbance; because calcium excretion is decreased by thiazides, discontinue use of this product before testing parathyroid function
Carcinogenicity, mutagenicity	A 2-yr study of timolol in male rats showed a statistically significant increase in adrenal pheochromocytomas at 300 times the maximum recommended human dose (1 mg/kg/day), and a lifetime study in female mice showed a statistically significant increase in the overall incidence of neoplasms (including benign and malignant pulmonary tumors, benign uterine polyps, and mammary adenocarcinomas associated with increased serum prolactin levels) at 500 mg/kg/day. Results of various mutagenicity studies were negative.

TIMOLIDE

Impairment of fertility	Administration of timolol at doses up to 150 times the maximum recommended human dose had no adverse effect on the fertility of male or female rats

ADVERSE REACTIONS[1]

Frequent reactions (incidence ≥ 1%) are printed in *italics*

Cardiovascular	*Hypotension (1.6%), bradycardia (1.2%),* arrhythmia, syncope, cardiac failure, cerebrovascular accident
Gastrointestinal	Diarrhea, dyspepsia, nausea, pain, constipation
Dermatological	Rash, increased pigmentation, dry mucous membranes
Central nervous system	*Dizziness (1.2%),* insomnia, decreased libido, nervousness, confusion, difficulty concentrating, somnolence, cerebral ischemia, oculogyric crisis
Musculoskeletal	Myalgia, gout, muscle cramps
Respiratory	*Bronchial spasm (1.6%), dyspnea (1.2%),* rales, worsening of chronic obstructive pulmonary disease
Genitourinary	Renal colic, impotence
Other	*Fatigue/tiredness and asthenia (1.9%),* chest pain, headache, earache

OVERDOSAGE

Signs and symptoms	*Timolol-related effects:* symptomatic bradycardia, hypotension, bronchospasm, and acute cardiac failure, based on the anticipated effects of excessive beta blockade (overdosage in humans has not been observed); *hydrochlorothiazide-related effects:* diuresis; lethargy progressing to coma, with minimal cardiorespiratory depression and with or without significant serum electrolyte changes or dehydration; GI irritation; hypermotility; transient elevation in BUN level
Treatment	Discontinue medication. Empty stomach by gastric lavage. For symptomatic bradycardia, administer atropine sulfate (0.25–2 mg IV) to induce vagal blockade; if bradycardia persists, give IV isoproterenol cautiously and, in refractory cases, consider using a transvenous cardiac pacemaker. For hypotension, administer a sympathomimetic amine (eg, dopamine, dobutamine, or norepinephrine); in refractory cases, try glucagon HCl. For bronchospasm, give isoproterenol and possibly also aminophylline. For acute cardiac failure, institute treatment with digitalis, diuretics, and oxygen immediately; in refractory cases, try IV aminophylline, followed, if necessary, by glucagon HCl. For second- or third-degree heart block, use isoproterenol or a transvenous cardiac pacemaker. Monitor serum electrolyte levels and renal function, and institute supportive measures, as required, to maintain hydration, electrolyte balance, respiration, and cardiovascular and renal function. Treat GI effects symptomatically. Hemodialysis may or may not be helpful in removing the drug from the circulation; although timolol can be readily dialyzed from human plasma or whole blood in vitro, a study in patients with renal failure showed that the drug did not readily dialyze.

DRUG INTERACTIONS

Calcium antagonists	Hypotension (with oral antagonists, especially nifedipine), left ventricular failure (with oral antagonists, especially verapamil and diltiazem), AV conduction disturbances (with oral or IV antagonists, especially verapamil and diltiazem). Although timolol can be given with an oral calcium antagonist if heart function is normal, concomitant use should be avoided if heart function is impaired. Exercise caution when administering an IV antagonist with timolol.
Reserpine, other catecholamine-depleting drugs	Hypotension and/or marked bradycardia
Nonsteroidal anti-inflammatory agents	▽ Diuretic, natriuretic, and antihypertensive effects of hydrochlorothiazide component; observe patient closely during concomitant therapy to ensure that desired therapeutic effect is obtained
Tubocurarine	△ Skeletal-muscle relaxation
Norepinephrine	▽ Vasopressor effect
Steroids, ACTH	△ Risk of hypokalemia
Lithium	▽ Lithium clearance
Alcohol, barbiturates, narcotic analgesics	△ Risk of orthostatic hypotension

ALTERED LABORATORY VALUES

Blood/serum values	△ BUN △ Uric acid △ Calcium ▽ Magnesium ▽ Sodium △ or ▽ Potassium ▽ Chloride ▽ Bicarbonate ▽ Phosphate ▽ PBI △ or ▽ Glucose △ Triglycerides
Urinary values	△ Sodium △ Potassium △ Chloride △ Bicarbonate △ Uric acid ▽ Calcium △ Magnesium

USE IN CHILDREN	USE IN PREGNANT AND NURSING WOMEN
Safety and effectiveness for use in children have not been established	Pregnancy Category C: use during pregnancy only if the anticipated benefit of therapy exceeds the potential risk to the fetus. Studies of this combination in mice and rabbits have shown no evidence of teratogenicity, embryotoxicity, fetotoxicity, or maternotoxicity. However, an increase in fetal resorption has been observed in mice and rabbits given respectively 1,000 and 100 times the maximum recommended human dose of timolol. No adequate, well-controlled studies have been done with timolol in pregnant women. Thiazides cross the placental barrier and may cause fetal or neonatal jaundice, thrombocytopenia, and other possible reactions. Because of the potential for serious adverse effects in nursing infants, a decision should be made to either discontinue nursing or discontinue use of this preparation, taking into account its importance to the mother.

[1] Other reactions have been attributed to the individual components of this drug. These reactions include: for timolol, extremity pain, decreased exercise tolerance, weight loss, cardiac arrest, worsening of angina pectoris, sinoatrial block, AV block, worsening of arterial insufficiency, Raynaud's phenomenon, claudication, palpitations, vasodilatation, cold hands and feet, edema, hepatomegaly, vomiting, nonthrombocytopenic purpura, hyperglycemia, hypoglycemia, skin irritation, pruritus, sweating, arthralgia, local weakness, vertigo, paresthesia, exacerbation of myasthenia gravis, depression, nightmares, hallucinations, cough, visual disturbances, diplopia, ptosis, eye irritation, dry eyes, tinnitus, urination difficulties; for hydrochlorothiazide, anorexia, gastric irritation, vomiting, cramping, jaundice (intrahepatic cholestatic jaundice), pancreatitis, sialadenitis, vertigo, paresthesias, xanthopsia, leukopenia, agranulocytosis, thrombocytopenia, aplastic anemia, hemolytic anemia, orthostatic hypotension (may be aggravated by alcohol, barbiturates, or narcotics), purpura, photosensitivity, urticaria, necrotizing angiitis (vasculitis, cutaneous vasculitis), fever, respiratory distress including pneumonitis and pulmonary edema, anaphylactic reactions, hyperglycemia, glycosuria, hyperuricemia, electrolyte imbalance, muscle spasm, weakness, restlessness, transient blurred vision. Retroperitoneal fibrosis has occurred during timolol therapy, but a causal relationship has not been established. In addition, beta blockers other than timolide have been reported to cause reversible mental depression, progressing to catatonia, an acute reversible syndrome characterized by temporal and spatial disorientation, short-term memory loss, emotional lability, slightly cloudy sensorium, and decreased performance on neuropsychometric tests, intensification of AV block (see CONTRAINDICATIONS), mesenteric arterial thrombosis, ischemic colitis, agranulocytosis, thrombocytopenic purpura, erythematous rash, fever combined with aching and sore throat, laryngospasm, respiratory distress, reversible alopecia, and Peyronie's disease.

ANTIHYPERTENSIVES WITH DIURETICS

VASERETIC (enalapril maleate and hydrochlorothiazide)   Merck Sharp & Dohme   Rx

Tablets: 10 mg enalapril maleate and 25 mg hydrochlorothiazide (Vaseretic 10-25)

INDICATIONS	ORAL DOSAGE
Hypertension	**Adult:** 1–2 tabs, given once daily

CONTRAINDICATIONS
Hypersensitivity to hydrochlorothiazide, other sulfonamide derivatives, or enalapril

ADMINISTRATION/DOSAGE ADJUSTMENTS

Initiating therapy	When planning to give enalapril to patients who are currently receiving other antihypertensive agents, discontinue the existing antihypertensive drug regimen (including any diuretics) 2–3 days before starting enalapril, if possible. The initial dose of enalapril for patients not currently receiving diuretics is 5 mg, given once daily; adjust dosage according to patient response (usual range: 10–40 mg/day, given in a single dose or 2 divided doses). To avoid excessive hypotension in patients who must continue diuretic therapy, begin with a small dose of enalapril (2.5 mg) and keep the patient under medical supervision for at least 1 h to determine whether excessive hypotension will occur. Do not exceed 2 tabs/day, since dosages beyond 50 mg/day of hydrochlorothiazide are usually not required; additional doses of enalapril or other nondiuretic antihypertensive agents may be considered if further blood pressure control is indicated.
Adjustment of dosage interval	During initial titration, patients treated once daily with enalapril may experience diminished antihypertensive effects toward the end of the day; an increase in dosage of enalapril or twice-daily administration should be considered in these patients
Patients with renal impairment	No dosage adjustment is required for patients with a creatinine clearance (Ccr) > 30 ml/min; this combination is not recommended for use in patients with severe renal dysfunction

WARNINGS/PRECAUTIONS

Fixed combination	This preparation is not indicated for initial therapy of hypertension; patients receiving a diuretic when enalapril therapy is initiated, or given a diuretic and enalapril simultaneously, can develop symptomatic hypotension. The fixed-dose combination may be substituted for the individual components if the titrated doses are the same as those in the combination.

VASERETIC

Hypotension — Excessive hypotension has occurred in patients with congestive heart failure and may be associated with oliguria and/or progressive azotemia and, rarely, acute renal failure and/or death. During treatment of hypertension, excessive hypotension has also occurred rarely in patients with severe hyponatremia or hypovolemia, such as those undergoing vigorous diuretic therapy or patients on dialysis. Because of the risk of excessive hypotension in these patients, initiate therapy under very close medical supervision; monitor such patients closely for the first 2 wk of enalapril therapy and whenever the dosage of enalapril or the diuretic is increased.

Caution patient that light-headedness may occur, especially during the first days of treatment; however, since syncope has been reported in fewer patients receiving enalapril alone than in those taking this combination, the overall incidence of syncope may be reduced by proper titration of the individual components. If hypotension occurs, place the patient in a supine position and, if necessary, give normal saline by IV infusion. Caution patients that dehydration owing to excessive perspiration, vomiting, or diarrhea may precipitate hypotension. To avoid excessive hypotension, discontinue diuretic therapy 2–3 days before beginning antihypertensive therapy with enalapril. For other appropriate measures, see ADMINISTRATION/DOSAGE ADJUSTMENTS.

Angioedema — Angioedema of the face, extremities, lips, tongue, and glottis, and/or potentially fatal angioedema of the larynx has been reported in patients treated with enalapril and other angiotensin-converting enzyme inhibitors; advise patient to report any swelling immediately. Discontinue use and monitor patient carefully if angioedema occurs; swelling confined to the face and lips usually resolves without treatment, although antihistamines have been useful in relieving symptoms. For involvement of the tongue, glottis, or larynx likely to cause airway obstruction, give 0.3–0.5 ml of epinephrine 1:1000 SC immediately.

Neutropenia, agranulocytosis — Bone marrow depression and agranulocytosis have occurred rarely in patients taking captopril (another angiotensin converting enzyme inhibitor), primarily in patients with renal impairment and/or collagen vascular disease. Available clinical data are insufficient to show that enalapril does not cause agranulocytosis at a rate similar to that of captopril. Instruct all patients to report any sign of infection, such as sore throat or fever. Monitor WBC count periodically in patients with collagen vascular disease and renal disease.

Increases in BUN and creatinine — In some patients with hypertension and renal disease, especially those with unilateral or bilateral renal artery stenosis, BUN and serum creatinine levels have increased. Some patients with no apparent preexisting renal vascular disease have developed reversible increases in BUN and serum creatinine levels, especially when enalapril was given concomitantly with a diuretic; however, this reaction is more likely to occur in patients with preexisting renal impairment. If necessary, reduce the dosage of enalapril and/or discontinue diuretic therapy, since it may not be possible to simultaneously maintain both normal blood pressure and adequate renal perfusion. Patients with renal artery stenosis should be monitored for changes in renal function during the first few weeks of therapy.

Hyperkalemia — Elevated serum potassium levels ($>$ 5.7 mEq/liter) have been observed in approximately 1% of patients treated with enalapril alone and in some cases has warranted discontinuation of therapy; the incidence of hyperkalemia is less in patients who have been treated with this combination. Patients at highest risk of hyperkalemia include those with renal insufficiency or diabetes mellitus and those using potassium supplements, potassium salt substitutes, or potassium-sparing agents; advise patients not to use potassium supplements or salt substitutes.

Surgery, anesthesia — In patients undergoing major surgery or receiving anesthetics that can cause hypotension, enalapril can block a compensatory increase in angiotensin II; if enalapril-induced hypotension occurs, correct by volume expansion

Drug accumulation, renal dysfunction — Thiazides can accumulate or precipitate azotemia in patients with renal impairment. Use this preparation with caution in patients with severe or advanced renal disease; if renal impairment progresses, consider interrupting or terminating therapy.

Hepatic coma — Minor changes in fluid and electrolyte balance may precipitate hepatic coma in patients with hepatic impairment or progressive liver disease; use with caution in such patients

Electrolyte disorders — Hypokalemia may occur, especially when diuresis is brisk, severe cirrhosis is present, ACTH or corticosteroids are given concomitantly, oral intake of electrolytes is inadequate, or therapy is prolonged; potassium supplements or potassium-rich foods may be given to avoid or treat hypokalemia. Dilutional hyponatremia may occur in edematous patients when the weather is hot. Treat by restricting the intake of water; administer salt only if hyponatremia is life-threatening or actual salt depletion occurs. For hypochloremia, specific treatment is usually unnecessary, except for certain patients (eg, those with hepatic or renal disease). Hypomagnesemia may also occur. To prevent electrolyte imbalance, measure serum and urinary electrolyte levels periodically in all patients (these determinations are especially important if excessive vomiting occurs or parenteral fluids are being given); watch for premonitory signs and symptoms of hypokalemia, hyponatremia, and hypochloremic alkalosis, such as dry mouth, thirst, weakness, lethargy, drowsiness, restlessness, muscle pain or cramps, muscular fatigue, hypotension, oliguria, tachycardia, and GI disturbances (eg, nausea and vomiting); chloride replacement may be needed to treat metabolic alkalosis.

VASERETIC

Diabetes	Thiazides can activate latent diabetes or alter insulin requirements
Parathyroid dysfunction	Thiazides may decrease calcium excretion and may cause intermittent and slight hypercalcemia in the absence of known calcium metabolism disorders. Marked hypercalcemia may be a sign of hidden hyperparathyroidism; discontinue use before performing parathyroid function tests.
Other thiazide-related reactions	Thiazides can cause hyperuricemia or overt gout, precipitate hypersensitivity reactions (especially in patients with a history of allergy or bronchial asthma), and, in postsympathectomized patients, produce an enhanced antihypertensive effect
Carcinogenicity	No evidence of carcinogenicity has been seen in rats and male mice given enalapril at doses of up to 90 mg/kg/day or in female mice given up to 180 mg/kg/day for 2 yr; these dosages represent 150 and 300 times the maximum recommended daily dose for humans. No long-term studies have been done to evaluate the carcinogenic potential of hydrochlorothiazide.
Mutagenicity	No mutagenic effects have been observed in various studies with enalapril, both in vitro and in vivo. Hydrochlorothiazide has caused nondisjunction in studies using *Aspergillus nidulans*. This formulation has shown no mutagenic activity in the Ames microbial mutagen test with or without metabolic activation, nor has it produced DNA single-strand breaks in vitro or in vivo.
Effect on fertility	Studies in male and female rats have shown no adverse effect on reproductive performance at dosages ranging from 10 to 90 mg/kg/day of enalapril; hydrochlorothiazide has shown no effect on fertility.

ADVERSE REACTIONS[1]

Frequent reactions (incidence ≥ 1%) are printed in *italics*

Central nervous system, neuromuscular	*Dizziness (8.6%), headache (5.5%), fatigue (3.9%), muscle cramps (2.7%),* insomnia, nervousness, paresthesia, somnolence, vertigo, back pain, arthralgia
Gastrointestinal	*Nausea (2.5%), diarrhea (2.1%),* abdominal pain, vomiting, dyspepsia, constipation, flatulence, dry mouth
Cardiovascular	*Orthostatic effects (2.3%), orthostatic hypotension (1.5%), syncope (1.3%),* palpitations, chest pain, tachycardia
Respiratory	*Cough (3.5%),* dyspnea
Hypersensitivity	Pruritus, rash, angioedema
Other	*Asthenia (2.4%), impotence (2.2%),* gout, hyperhidrosis, decreased libido, tinnitus, urinary tract infection, decreased hemoglobin and hematocrit

OVERDOSAGE

Signs and symptoms	*Enalapril-related effects:* hypotension; *hydrochlorothiazide-related effects:* effects resulting from electrolyte depletion (eg, hypokalemia, hypochloremia, hyponatremia) and dehydration; cardiac arrhythmias resulting from hypokalemia (with concomitant digitalis therapy)
Treatment	Induce emesis and/or perform gastric lavage to evacuate stomach. Institute appropriate supportive measures to correct dehydration and electrolyte imbalances. For hypotension, administer normal saline by IV infusion. Enalapril may be removed from the blood by hemodialysis.

DRUG INTERACTIONS

Diuretics	Excessive hypotension (see "hypotension," above, and ADMINISTRATION/DOSAGE ADJUSTMENTS)
Potassium-sparing diuretics, potassium supplements, potassium-containing salt substitutes	⇧ Serum potassium level; exercise caution and monitor serum potassium frequently
Other antihypertensive agents causing renin release	⇧ Antihypertensive effect
Digitalis	⇧ Risk of digitalis toxicity owing to thiazide-induced hypokalemia
Lithium	⇧ Risk of lithium toxicity
Norepinephrine, other vasopressors	⇩ Vasopressor effect; nevertheless, this interaction does not preclude therapeutic use of vasopressors
Corticosteroids, ACTH	⇧ Risk of electrolyte depletion, particularly hypokalemia
Tubocurarine, other nondepolarizing skeletal muscle relaxants	⇧ Skeletal muscle relaxation
Insulin, oral hypoglycemic agents	⇧ Hypoglycemic effect; adjust dosage, if necessary
Alcohol, barbiturates, narcotic analgesics	⇧ Risk of orthostatic hypotension
Nonsteroidal anti-inflammatory agents	⇩ Antihypertensive effect of hydrochlorothiazide; monitor patient closely

VASERETIC

ALTERED LABORATORY VALUES

Blood/serum values — ⇧ BUN ⇧ Creatinine ⇧ PRA (plasma renin activity) ⇩ Sodium ⇧ or ⇩ Potassium ⇧ Calcium ⇩ Magnesium ⇩ Chloride ⇩ Phosphate ⇧ Uric acid ⇧ Glucose

Urinary values — ⇩ Sodium ⇧ or ⇩ Potassium ⇧ Calcium ⇧ Magnesium ⇩ Chloride ⇧ Uric acid ⇧ Glucose

USE IN CHILDREN

Safety and effectiveness for use in children have not been established

USE IN PREGNANT AND NURSING WOMEN

Pregnancy Category C: no teratogenic effects have been seen in rats or rabbits. Enalapril caused a decrease in average fetal weight in rats given 1,200 mg/kg/day, but this reaction did not occur when these animals were supplemented with saline. Although maternal and fetal toxicity occurred in rabbits at doses of 1 mg/kg/day or more, saline supplementation prevented these effects at doses of 3 and 10 mg/kg/day, but not at 30 mg/kg/day. Administration of a thiazide during pregnancy can produce adverse reactions, including jaundice and thrombocytopenia, in a neonate or fetus. No evidence teratogenicity or fetotoxicity has been found following use of the combination in rats and rabbits, except for a decrease in fetal weight in both species. Use this preparation during pregnancy only if the expected benefit justifies the potential risks. It is not known whether enalapril is excreted in human milk; however, thiazides are found in human milk. Instruct women not to nurse during therapy.

[1] Reactions for which no causal relationship has been established include rare elevations of liber enzymes and/or serum bilirubin. Reactions associated with use of enalapril or hydrochlorothiazide, but not seen in clinical trials with this specific combination, include renal dysfunction, renal failure, oliguria; rare cases of neutropenia, thrombocytopenia, and bone marrow depression; weakness, anorexia, gastric irritation, cramping, jaundice (intrahepatic cholestatic jaundice); pancreatitis, sialadenitis, leukopenia, agranulocytosis, thrombocytopenia, aplastic anemia, hemolytic anemia, muscle spasm, restlessness, transient blurred vision, xanthopsia, purpura, photosensitivity, urticaria, necrotizing angiitis (vasculitis and cutaneous vasculitis), fever, respiratory distress (including pneumonitis and pulmonary edema), and anaphylactic reactions.

Chapter 23

Anti-Infectives: Aminoglycosides, Sulfonamides, and Miscellaneous

Aminoglycosides — 867

AMIKIN (Bristol) — 867
Amikacin sulfate *Rx*

GARAMYCIN (Schering) — 869
Gentamicin sulfate *Rx*

KANTREX (Apothecon) — 871
Kanamycin sulfate *Rx*

MYCIFRADIN (Upjohn) — 873
Neomycin sulfate *Rx*

NEBCIN (Dista) — 875
Tobramycin sulfate *Rx*

NETROMYCIN (Schering) — 877
Netilmicin sulfate *Rx*

Sulfonamides — 880

AZULFIDINE (Pharmacia) — 880
Sulfasalazine *Rx*

GANTANOL (Roche) — 882
Sulfamethoxazole *Rx*

GANTANOL DS (Roche) — 882
Sulfamethoxazole *Rx*

GANTRISIN (Roche) — 884
Sulfisoxazole *Rx*

RENOQUID (Glenwood) — 885
Sulfacytine *Rx*

THIOSULFIL (Ayerst) — 886
Sulfamethizole *Rx*

THIOSULFIL Forte (Ayerst) — 886
Sulfamethizole *Rx*

Miscellaneous Anti-Infective Agents — 888

BACTRIM (Roche) — 888
Trimethoprim and sulfamethoxazole *Rx*

BACTRIM DS (Roche) — 888
Trimethoprim and sulfamethoxazole *Rx*

BACTRIM I.V. Infusion (Roche) — 890
Trimethoprim and sulfamethoxazole *Rx*

CHLOROMYCETIN (Parke-Davis) — 892
Chloramphenicol *Rx*

CHLOROMYCETIN Palmitate (Parke-Davis) — 892
Chloramphenicol palmitate *Rx*

CHLOROMYCETIN Sodium Succinate (Parke-Davis) — 892
Chloramphenicol sodium succinate *Rx*

CLEOCIN HCl (Upjohn) — 894
Clindamycin hydrochloride *Rx*

CLEOCIN PEDIATRIC (Upjohn) — 894
Clindamycin palmitate hydrochloride *Rx*

CLEOCIN PHOSPHATE (Upjohn) — 894
Clindamycin phosphate *Rx*

COLY-MYCIN M (Parke-Davis) — 896
Colistimethate sodium *Rx*

COLY-MYCIN S (Parke-Davis) — 897
Colistin sulfate *Rx*

FLAGYL (Searle) — 897
Metronidazole *Rx*

FLAGYL I.V. (Searle) — 899
Metronidazole hydrochloride *Rx*

FLAGYL I.V. RTU (Searle) — 899
Metronidazole *Rx*

PEDIAZOLE (Ross) — 901
Erythromycin ethylsuccinate and sulfisoxazole acetyl *Rx*

PRIMAXIN (Merck Sharp & Dohme) — 903
Imipenem and cilastatin sodium *Rx*

PROTOSTAT (Ortho) — 905
Metronidazole *Rx*

SEPTRA (Burroughs Wellcome) — 907
Trimethoprim and sulfamethoxazole *Rx*

SEPTRA DS (Burroughs Wellcome) — 907
Trimethoprim and sulfamethoxazole *Rx*

SEPTRA I.V. Infusion (Burroughs Wellcome) — 909
Trimethoprim and sulfamethoxazole *Rx*

VANOCIN HCl (Lilly) — 911
Vancomycin hydrochloride *Rx*

VANCOCIN HCl IntraVenous (Lilly) — 911
Vancomycin hydrochloride *Rx*

Other Aminoglycosides — 863

HUMATIN (Parke-Davis) — 863
Paromomycin sulfate *Rx*

Streptomycin sulfate (Roerig) *Rx* — 863

Other Sulfonamides — 864

Sulfadiazine *Rx* — 864

Sulfapyridine *Rx* — 864

TERFONYL (Squibb) — 864
Sulfadiazine, sulfamerazine, and sulfamethazine *Rx*

Triple sulfa — 864
Sulfadiazine, sulfamerazine, and sulfamethazine *Rx*

Other Miscellaneous Anti-Infectives — 864

AEROSPORIN (Burroughs Wellcome) — 864
Polymyxin B sulfate *Rx*

LINOCIN (Upjohn) — 865
Lincomycin hydrochloride *Rx*

PENTAM 300 (LyphoMed) — 865
Pentamidine isethionate *Rx*

Polymyxin B sulfate (Roerig) *Rx* — 865

RIFADIN (Merrell Dow) Rifampin *Rx*		865
RIMACTANE (CIBA) Rifampin *Rx*		866
TAO (Roerig) Troleandomycin *Rx*		866
TROBICIN (Upjohn) Spectinomycin hydrochloride *Rx*		866

OTHER AMINOGLYCOSIDES

DRUG	HOW SUPPLIED	USUAL DOSAGE
HUMATIN (Parke-Davis) Paromomycin sulfate *Rx*	**Capsules:** 250 mg	**Adult:** for intestinal amebiasis, 25–35 mg/kg/day, given in 3 divided doses, with meals, for 5–10 days; for hepatic coma, 4 g/day, given in divided doses, for 5–6 days **Child:** for intestinal amebiasis, same as adult
Streptomycin sulfate (Roerig) *Rx*	**Vials:** streptomycin sulfate equivalent to 1 or 5 g of streptomycin (sterile powder for reconstitution)	**Adult:** for tuberculosis, 1 g/day IM along with other antitubercular drugs, followed by 1 g 2–3 times/wk for at least 1 yr; for tularemia, 1–2 g/day IM, given in divided doses, for 7–10 days, until the patient is afebrile for 5–7 days; for plague, 2–4 g/day IM, given in divided doses, until the patient is afebrile for 3 days; for alpha-hemolytic and nonhemolytic streptococcal endocarditis, 1 g IM bid for 1 wk, followed by 0.5 g IM bid for 1 wk, along with penicillin; for enterococcal endocarditis, 1 g IM bid for 2 wk, followed by 0.5 g IM bid for 4 wk, along with penicillin; in combination with other anti-infective agents for meningitis, gram-negative bacillary bacteremia, pneumonia, brucellosis, granuloma inguinale, chancroid, and urinary tract infections, 2–4 g/day IM, given in divided doses q6–12h, if infection is severe and fulminating, or 1–2 g/day IM if infection is less severe and organism is highly susceptible **Child:** for meningitis, gram-negative bacillary bacteremia, pneumonia, brucellosis, granuloma inguinale, chancroid, and urinary tract infections, 20–40 mg/kg/day IM, given in divided doses q6–12h, along with other anti-infective agents

continued

OTHER SULFONAMIDES

DRUG	HOW SUPPLIED	USUAL DOSAGE[1]
Sulfadiazine Rx	**Tablets:** 500 mg	**Adult:** 2–4 g to start, followed by 2–4 g/24 h, given in 3–6 divided doses **Child (> 2 mo):** 75 mg/kg to start, followed by 150 mg/kg/24 h (up to 6 g/24 h) in 4–6 divided doses
Sulfapyridine Rx	**Tablets:** 500 mg	**Adult:** 500 mg qid until improvement is noted, then reduce daily dosage by 500 mg/day at 3-day intervals until patient is asymptomatic
TERFONYL (Squibb) Sulfadiazine, sulfamerazine, and sulfamethazine Rx	**Tablets:** 167 mg sulfadiazine, 167 mg sulfamerazine, and 167 mg sulfamethazine **Suspension (per 5 ml):** 167 mg sulfadiazine, 167 mg sulfamerazine, and 167 mg sulfamethazine	**Adult:** 2–4 g to start, followed by 2–4 g/24 h, given in 3–6 divided doses **Child (> 2 mo):** 75 mg/kg/24 h to start, followed by 150 mg/kg/24 h (up to 6 g/24 h), given in 4–6 divided doses
Triple sulfa Sulfadiazine, sulfamerazine, and sulfamethazine Rx	**Tablets:** 167 mg sulfadiazine, 167 mg sulfamerazine, and 167 mg sulfamethazine **Suspension (per 5 ml):** 167 mg sulfadiazine, 167 mg sulfamerazine, and 167 mg sulfamethazine (pt, gal) *banana/vanilla flavored*	**Adult:** 2–4 g to start, followed by 2–4 g/24 h, given in 3–6 divided doses **Child (> 2 mo):** 75 mg/kg to start, followed by 150 mg/kg/24 h (up to 6 g/24 h), given in 4–6 divided doses

[1] Where pediatric dosages are not given, consult manufacturer

OTHER MISCELLANEOUS ANTI-INFECTIVES

DRUG	HOW SUPPLIED	USUAL DOSAGE
AEROSPORIN (Burroughs Wellcome) Polymyxin B sulfate Rx	**Vials:** 500,000 units	**Adult:** for acute infections, 15,000–25,000 units/kg/day IV, given in a single IV infusion or in divided doses q12h, or 25,000–30,000 units/kg/day IM, given in divided doses q4–6h; for *Pseudomonas aeruginosa* meningitis, 50,000 units once a day intrathecally for 3–4 days, followed by 50,000 units on alternate days for at least 2 wk after negative CSF culture and normalization of sugar content; for *P aeruginosa* infections of the eye, 1–3 drops (of 0.1–0.25% solution) every hour, increasing the intervals as response indicates; for *P aeruginosa* infections of the cornea and conjunctiva, up to 10,000 units/day, given by subconjunctival injection **Infant:** up to 40,000 units/kg/day IV or IM **Child (< 2 yr):** use adult IV and IM dosages; for *Pseudomonas aeruginosa* meningitis, 20,000 units once a day intrathecally for 3–4 days or 25,000 units on alternate days, followed by 25,000 units on alternate days for at least 2 wk after negative CSF culture and normalization of sugar content **Child (≥ 2 yr):** same as adult

OTHER MISCELLANEOUS ANTI-INFECTIVES continued

DRUG	HOW SUPPLIED	USUAL DOSAGE
LINCOCIN (Upjohn) Lincomycin hydrochloride *Rx*	**Capsules:** lincomycin hydrochloride equivalent to 500 mg lincomycin **Pediatric capsules:** lincomycin hydrochloride equivalent to 250 mg lincomycin **Vials:** lincomycin hydrochloride equivalent to 300 mg/ml of lincomycin (2, 10 ml) **Prefilled syringes:** lincomycin hydrochloride equivalent to 300 mg/ml of lincomycin (2 ml)	**Adult:** for serious infections, 500 mg PO tid or 600 mg IM q24h; for more severe infections, 500 mg or more PO qid, 600 mg IM q12h or more often, if needed, or 600 mg to 1 g IV q8–12h, depending on severity of infection; for life-threatening infections, up to 8 g/day IV; for ocular infections, 75 mg, given by subconjunctival injection **Child (> 1 mo):** for serious infections, 30 mg/kg/day PO, given in 3–4 equally divided doses, or 10 mg/kg/day IM, given in a single dose; for more severe infections, 60 mg/kg/day PO, given in 3–4 equally divided doses, or 10 mg/kg IM q12h or more often, if needed, or 10–20 mg/kg/day IV, depending on severity of infection
PENTAM 300 (LyphoMed) Pentamidine isethionate *Rx*	**Vials:** 300 mg	**Adult and child:** 4 mg/kg/day IM or IV, given in a single dose, for 14 days
Polymyxin B sulfate (Roerig) *Rx*	**Vials:** 25,000 units/ml (20 ml)	**Adult:** 15,000–25,000 units/kg/day, given by IV infusion q12h *or*, if necessary, 25,000–30,000 units/kg/day IM, given in divided doses q4–6h; for meningitis due to *Pseudomonas aeruginosa*, 50,000 units, given in a single intrathecal dose daily for 3–4 days and then every other day until at least 2 wk after CSF cultures are negative and sugar level has returned to normal **Infant:** up to 40,000 units/kg/day, given by IV infusion *or*, if necessary, IM; for meningitis due to *Pseudomonas aeruginosa* in children under 2 yr of age, 25,000 units, given in a single intrathecal dose every other day, to start or after administering 20,000 units in a single intrathecal dose daily for 3–4 days (continue treatment until at least 2 wk after CSF cultures are negative and sugar level has returned to normal) **Child:** for IV or IM use, same as adult; for intrathecal use in children over 2 yr of age, same as adult
RIFADIN (Merrell Dow) Rifampin *Rx*	**Capsules:** 150, 300 mg	**Adult:** for pulmonary tuberculosis, 600 mg/day, given in a single dose in conjunction with other antituberculous agent(s), until bacterial conversion and maximal improvement occur; for meningococcal carriers, 600 mg/day, given in a single dose, for 4 consecutive days **Child (≥ 5 yr):** for pulmonary tuberculosis, 10–20 mg/kg/day, given in a single dose, up to 600 mg/day, in conjunction with other antituberculous agent(s), until bacterial conversion and maximal improvement occur; for meningococcal carriers, 10–20 mg/kg/day, given in a single dose, up to 600 mg/day, for 4 consecutive days

continued

OTHER MISCELLANEOUS ANTI-INFECTIVES continued

DRUG	HOW SUPPLIED	USUAL DOSAGE[1]
RIMACTANE (CIBA) Rifampin *Rx*	**Capsules:** 300 mg	**Adult:** for pulmonary tuberculosis, 600 mg/day, given in a single dose in conjunction with other antituberculous agent(s), until bacterial conversion and maximal improvement occur; for meningococcal carriers, 600 mg/day, given in a single dose, for 4 consecutive days **Child ($\geq$ 5 yr):** for pulmonary tuberculosis, 10–20 mg/kg/day, given in a single dose, up to 600 mg/day, in conjunction with other antituberculous agent(s), until bacterial conversion and maximal improvement occur; for meningococcal carriers, 10–20 mg/kg/day, given in a single dose, up to 600 mg/day, for 4 consecutive days
TAO (Roerig) Troleandomycin *Rx*	**Capsules:** troleandomycin equivalent to 250 mg oleandomycin	**Adult:** 250–500 mg qid **Child:** 125–250 mg (6.6–11 mg/kg) q6h
TROBICIN (Upjohn) Spectinomycin hydrochloride *Rx*	**Vials:** spectinomycin hydrochloride equivalent to 2 or 4 g spectinomycin	**Adult:** 2 g IM (deeply); where antibiotic resistance is prevalent, initiate treatment with 4 g IM

[1] Where pediatric dosages are not given, consult manufacturer

AMINOGLYCOSIDES

AMIKIN (amikacin sulfate) Bristol Rx

Vials: 50 mg/ml (2 ml), 250 mg/ml (2, 4 ml) **Prefilled syringes:** 250 mg/ml (2 ml)

INDICATIONS

Serious infections of the **respiratory tract, bones, joints, skin, soft tissue, and central nervous system** (including meningitis); serious complicated and recurrent **urinary tract infections; bacteremia** (including neonatal sepsis); **intraabdominal infections** (including peritonitis); **burn infections; and postoperative infections** (including infections following vascular surgery), when caused by susceptible strains of gram-negative bacteria, including *Pseudomonas, Escherichia coli, Proteus, Providencia, Klebsiella-Enterobacter-Serratia,* and *Acinetobacter,* or when caused by susceptible strains of staphylococci (see "Usage" in ADMINISTRATION/DOSAGE ADJUSTMENTS)

PARENTERAL DOSAGE

Adult, child, and older infant: for uncomplicated urinary tract infections, 250 mg bid IM or IV; for other infections, 7.5 mg/kg q12h or 5 mg/kg q8h IM or IV. Do not exceed 1.5 g/day.
Neonate: 10 mg/kg IM or IV to start, followed by 7.5 mg/kg q12h IM or IV

CONTRAINDICATIONS

Hypersensitivity to amikacin

ADMINISTRATION/DOSAGE ADJUSTMENTS

Usage — Amikacin is indicated for the treatment of serious gram-negative infections and may be given as initial therapy (ie, before the results of susceptibility tests are known) for these infections. This drug is effective against gram-negative infections caused by tobramycin- or gentamicin-resistant strains (especially *Proteus rettgeri, Providencia stuartii, Serratia marcescens,* and *Pseudomonas aeruginosa*). Use for initial episodes of uncomplicated urinary tract infections only when other, less potentially toxic anti-infectives are contraindicated or ineffective. Although amikacin is also effective against staphylococcal infections, such use should be considered only under certain circumstances, eg, when the patient is allergic to other antibiotics, the suspected pathogen is a gram-negative organism or *Staphylococcus,* or the infection is due to both gram-negative pathogens and staphylococci. Concomitant use of penicillin may be necessary for the treatment of certain infections, such as neonatal sepsis, that may also be caused by streptococci or other nonstaphylococcal gram-positive organisms.

Intravenous administration — To prepare solution for IV administration, add the contents of a 500-mg vial to 100 or 200 ml of 0.9% sodium chloride injection USP, 5% dextrose injection USP, lactated Ringer's injection USP, 5% dextrose and 0.2% or 0.45% sodium chloride injection USP, or 5% dextrose and Normosol M or R or Plasma-Lyte 56 or 148; do not mix the solution with penicillins, cephalosporins, or any other drugs. Administer the required dose by IV infusion over a period of 1–2 h for infants or over a period of 30–60 min for other patients.

Patients with renal impairment — Give patients with stable renal impairment an initial loading dose of 7.5 mg/kg and then either administer subsequent 7.5-mg/kg doses at an interval of more than 12 h or give a dose of less than 7.5 mg/kg q12h. To calculate the appropriate dose or dosing interval, use data obtained from measurement of the serum amikacin level. If determination of the serum level and creatinine clearance (Ccr) are not feasible, calculate the dosing interval (in hours) by multiplying the patient's serum creatinine level (in mg/dl) by 9; according to this formula, a patient with a serum creatinine level of 2 mg/dl should receive 7.5 mg/kg q18h. To calculate the appropriate maintenance dose for administration q12h when serum drug levels cannot be obtained, divide the observed Ccr (in ml/min) by the normal Ccr (in ml/min) and then multiply the quotient by the initial loading dose (in mg); for a rough estimate, divide the normally recommended dose by the serum creatinine level. The formulas above for adjustment of dose or dosing interval should not be used for patients who are undergoing dialysis.

Use of serum drug levels — When feasible, peak and trough serum drug levels should be measured intermittently during therapy. For peak levels, take blood samples 30–90 min after IM injection or at the end of an IV infusion; for trough levels, measure just before the next dose. Trough levels exceeding 10 μg/ml and peak levels exceeding 35 μg/ml should be avoided. Concomitant use of penicillin in patients with severe renal impairment can cause significant inactivation of amikacin in body fluids; samples obtained from these patients during combination therapy should be promptly assayed, frozen, or treated with beta-lactamase since inactivation may continue after these fluids are drawn.

Duration of therapy — Keep the duration of treatment as short as possible. Amikacin is usually given for 7–10 days; safety of use for a period longer than 14 days has not been established. Before continuing treatment beyond 10 days, reevaluate therapy; if administration is continued, be sure to monitor serum drug level and renal, auditory, and vestibular functions.

AMIKIN

Lack of response	Uncomplicated infections should respond to treatment in 24–48 h; if a definite clinical response does not occur within 3–5 days, therapy should be stopped and susceptibility of the pathogen retested. Lack of response may be due to resistance or the presence of septic foci that need to be drained.

WARNINGS/PRECAUTIONS

Ototoxicity and nephrotoxicity	Amikin can cause ototoxic and nephrotoxic reactions, especially when patients are elderly or dehydrated, renal function is impaired, the recommended dosage or serum level is exceeded, treatment continues for more than 14 days, or other potentially nephrotoxic or neurotoxic drugs are administered concomitantly. Ototoxic effects are usually irreversible; they are generally characterized by impairment of auditory function, but may also include vestibular injury. The first sign of auditory impairment is usually high frequency deafness, which can only be detected by audiometric tests; subsequent premonitory clinical symptoms can fail to develop during therapy, and partial or total bilateral deafness may be the first clinical manifestation of cochlear damage. Nephrotoxic effects are usually reversible; the risk is low when patients are well-hydrated, renal function is normal, and the recommended dosage and duration of therapy are not exceeded. To prevent ototoxicity and nephrotoxicity, closely monitor renal and eighth-nerve function, especially in patients with renal impairment, and ensure that patients are well-hydrated. Serial audiograms should be obtained when feasible, particularly for high-risk patients. Renal function should be assessed before therapy and daily thereafter. Check for presence of cells, casts, or albumin in urine, measure urinary specific gravity, and either determine creatinine clearance or measure serum creatinine level; for elderly patients, creatinine clearance may be more useful than the serum creatinine level because renal impairment in these patients may escape detection when the serum creatinine level is used to evaluate renal function. If feasible, measure peak and trough serum levels of amikacin intermittently during therapy (see ADMINISTRATION/DOSAGE ADJUSTMENTS). Avoid concomitant or serial use of other potentially nephrotoxic or ototoxic drugs (see DRUG INTERACTIONS). If casts, cells, or albumin are detected in the urine, increase water intake. If any of these urinary changes is accompanied by other evidence of renal impairment, such as oliguria, a decrease in creatinine clearance or urinary specific gravity, or an increase in BUN or serum creatinine level, it may be desirable to reduce dosage. Discontinue treatment if azotemia increases or urinary output continues to decrease. If the patient experiences signs of ototoxicity (dizziness, vertigo, tinnitus, roaring in the ears, hearing loss), adjust dosage or discontinue the drug.
Neuromuscular effects	Acute muscular paralysis or apnea may occur as a result of neuromuscular blockade, particularly in patients who have received anesthetics, neuromuscular blocking agents (eg, succinylcholine, tubocurarine, decamethonium), or massive transfusions of citrate-anticoagulated blood; if neuromuscular blockade occurs, use IV calcium salts and, if necessary, institute mechanical ventilation. Use with caution in patients with neuromuscular disorders, such as myasthenia gravis and parkinsonism.
Cross-sensitivity	Use of amikacin in patients with a history of serious toxic reaction or hypersensitivity to another aminoglycoside may be contraindicated because of aminoglycoside cross-sensitivity
Superinfection	Overgrowth of nonsusceptible organisms may occur
Local irrigation	Aminoglycosides are quickly and almost completely absorbed from body surfaces (except the urinary bladder) after topical application during surgery; local irrigation has caused irreversible deafness, renal failure, and death
Carcinogenicity, mutagenicity, effect on fertility	No studies have been done in humans to determine the carcinogenic or mutagenic potential of aminoglycosides or their effect on fertility

ADVERSE REACTIONS

Central nervous system and neuromuscular	Hearing loss, loss of balance, acute muscular paralysis, apnea, numbness, paresthesia, tremor, convulsions, arthralgia, headache
Renal	Elevated serum creatinine level, albuminuria, red and white blood cells in the urine, cylindruria, azotemia, oliguria
Gastrointestinal	Nausea, vomiting
Hematological	Eosinophilia, anemia
Other	Drug fever, rash, hypotension

OVERDOSAGE

Signs and symptoms	Hearing loss, vertigo, renal dysfunction, neuromuscular blockade, respiratory paralysis
Treatment	To remove the drug from the blood, institute hemodialysis or peritoneal dialysis; for neonates, exchange transfusion may also be considered

DRUG INTERACTIONS

Other aminoglycosides	△ Risk of ototoxicity, nephrotoxicity, and neuromuscular blockade; avoid concomitant or sequential use
Wide-spectrum penicillins (ticarcillin, carbenicillin, piperacillin, mezlocillin, azlocillin)	▽ Serum level or half-life of amikacin in patients with severe renal impairment
Loop diuretics	△ Risk of ototoxicity; avoid concomitant or sequential use
Cephalothin, bacitracin, amphotericin B	△ Risk of nephrotoxicity; avoid concomitant or sequential use
Polymyxins	△ Risk of nephrotoxicity and neuromuscular blockade; avoid concomitant or sequential use
Cisplatin, vancomycin, capreomycin	△ Risk of ototoxicity and nephrotoxicity; avoid concomitant or sequential use
General anesthetics, neuromuscular blockers, massive transfusions of citrated blood	△ Risk of neuromuscular blockade
Anticholinesterase agents	▽ Antimyasthenic effect
Antivertigo agents (eg, diphenhydramine)	Masking of ototoxic symptoms

ALTERED LABORATORY VALUES

Blood/serum values	△ Creatinine[1] △ BUN
Urinary values	+ Protein ▽ Specific gravity

USE IN CHILDREN
See INDICATIONS and PARENTERAL DOSAGE. Use with caution in premature and full-term neonates; the serum half-life of amikacin is prolonged in such patients because of renal immaturity.

USE IN PREGNANT AND NURSING WOMEN
Pregnancy Category D: several cases of total irreversible bilateral congenital deafness have been observed in children whose mothers received streptomycin during pregnancy; although serious adverse effects have not been seen with the use of other aminoglycosides and reproduction studies with amikacin in rats and mice have shown no evidence of harm to the fetus or impaired fertility, it is nevertheless possible that amikacin may adversely affect fetal development or reproductive capacity. Women who are or who become pregnant during therapy should be apprised of the potential hazard to the fetus. It is not known whether this drug is excreted in human milk; women should not nurse during therapy.

[1] Creatinine levels may be spuriously elevated if cephalosporins are used concomitantly; however, serum levels are actually increased if nephrotoxic effects occur

---

AMINOGLYCOSIDES

GARAMYCIN (gentamicin sulfate) Schering   Rx

Vials: 10 mg/ml (2 ml, for pediatric use), 40 mg/ml (2, 20 ml)   **Prefilled syringes:** 40 mg/ml (1.5, 2 ml)   **Ampuls:** 2 mg/ml (2 ml) for intrathecal administration   **Piggyback units:** 1 mg/ml (60, 80 ml) for IV infusion only

INDICATIONS
Neonatal sepsis, septicemia, serious central nervous system infections (meningitis), **complicated urinary tract infections, respiratory tract infections, gastrointestinal tract infections** (including peritonitis), and **skin, bone, and soft tissue infections** (including burn infections) caused by susceptible strains of *Pseudonomas aeruginosa, Proteus, Escherichia coli, Klebsiella-Enterobacter-Serratia, Citrobacter,* and *Staphylococcus*

PARENTERAL DOSAGE[1]
Adult: 3 mg/kg/day IM or IV in 3 equally divided doses q8h; for life-threatening infections, give up to 5 mg/kg/day IM or IV in 3 or 4 equally divided doses, followed by 3 mg/kg/day as soon as clinically indicated
Premature infant and full-term neonate (≤ 1 wk): 2.5 mg/kg q12h
Infant (> 1 wk): 2.5 mg/kg q8h
Child: 2.0–2.5 mg/kg q8h

CONTRAINDICATIONS
Hypersensitivity to gentamicin (absolute contraindication)

Hypersensitivity or toxic reaction to other aminoglycosides (relative contraindication)

ADMINISTRATION/DOSAGE ADJUSTMENTS

Usage — Gentamicin may be given as initial therapy (ie, before the results of susceptibility tests are known) for serious gram-negative infections; when susceptibility test results indicate its use and other, less potentially toxic anti-infectives are ineffective or contraindicated, this drug may also be considered for serious staphylococcal infections and for uncomplicated initial episodes of urinary tract infections. If the causative organism is unknown, gentamicin may be administered in combination with a penicillin or cephalosporin as initial therapy; if an anaerobic organism is suspected, gentamicin should be given in combination with other appropriate anti-infectives. Concomitant use of gentamicin and penicillin is usually indicated for the treatment of suspected sepsis or staphylococcal pneumonia in neonates. Gentamicin, in combination with carbenicillin, is effective in the treatment of life-threatening infections caused by *Pseudomonas aeruginosa* and, in combination with a penicillin, is effective in the treatment of endocarditis caused by Group D streptococci.

GARAMYCIN

Intermittent intravenous infusion	A single dose may be diluted in 50–200 ml (less for infants and children) of isotonic saline or 5% dextrose in water and infused over a period of 30 min to 2 h; gentamicin should not be added to solutions of other drugs. The piggyback units are ready-to-use forms intended for IV infusion only; use the contents promptly after the seal is broken, and discard any unused portion (these units do not contain preservatives).
Intrathecal administration	For serious CNS infections (meningitis, ventriculitis) caused by susceptible strains of *Pseudomonas* in adults, administer 4–8 mg qd intrathecally (for infants > 3 mo of age and children, reduce dosage to 1–2 mg qd) as an adjunct to systemic gentamicin therapy. Draw required dose into a 5- or 10-ml syringe. After lumbar puncture and removal of fluid for laboratory analysis, insert syringe into hub of spinal needle. Allow a small amount of CSF (~ 10% of estimated total CSF volume) to flow into syringe and mix with gentamicin; then inject resultant fluid over a period of 3–5 min, with bevel of needle directed upward. If CSF is grossly purulent or unobtainable, dilute gentamicin with normal saline. The solution may also be injected directly into the subdural space or intraventricularly.
Use of serum drug levels	If feasible, periodically measure both peak and trough serum concentrations of gentamicin; dosage should be adjusted so that prolonged peak levels above 12 μg/ml or trough levels (measured just prior to the next dose) above 2 μg/ml are avoided
Patients with renal impairment	Dosage must be adjusted either by increasing the interval between administration of normal doses (multiply the serum creatinine level [mg/dl] by 8 to determine the dosage interval in hours) or by administering the drug more frequently (q8h) at reduced doses (after the normal initial dose, divide the normally recommended dose by the serum creatinine level); renal function should be carefully monitored, since it may change over the course of the infectious process
Patients undergoing hemodialysis	For adults, 1–1.7 mg/kg should be administered at the end of each dialysis period; for children, 2 mg/kg may be administered

WARNINGS/PRECAUTIONS

Nephrotoxicity and neurotoxicity	Nephrotoxic and neurotoxic reactions may occur, especially if patients are elderly or dehydrated, renal function is impaired, therapy is prolonged, the recommended dosage is exceeded, or other potentially nephrotoxic or neurotoxic drugs have been administered; in rare cases, these reactions may not become evident until soon after completion of therapy. A Fanconi-like syndrome, with aminoaciduria and metabolic acidosis, has been seen in some adults and infants. The risk of toxic reactions in patients with normal renal function is low, provided that the recommended dosage and usual duration of therapy are not exceeded. Nephrotoxic effects are usually mild and reversible, but permanent impairment can occur. Neurotoxic effects include ototoxicity (dizziness, vertigo, tinnitus, hearing loss), numbness, skin tingling, muscle twitching, and convulsions; ototoxic effects are usually irreversible. Cochlear damage is usually manifested initially by small changes in audiometric test results at higher frequencies and may not be associated with perceptible hearing loss. If nephrotoxic or ototoxic reactions occur, reduce dosage or discontinue use.
Prevention of toxic reactions	Patients should be well-hydrated during therapy. The concurrent or sequential use of other potentially nephrotoxic or neurotoxic drugs (see DRUG INTERACTIONS) and the concomitant use of potent diuretics should be avoided. (Some diuretics are directly ototoxic; diuretics can also enhance the risk of aminoglycoside toxicity when given IV by altering the serum and tissue concentrations of the aminoglycoside.) Patients should be closely observed during therapy, and serum drug levels should be measured whenever feasible. If possible, serial audiometric tests should also be performed, particularly in high-risk patients. Urine should be examined periodically for increased excretion of protein, the presence of cells and casts, and decreased specific gravity. Periodically throughout therapy (including the onset and end), obtain serum creatinine levels, or, for a more precise analysis, determine the creatinine clearance by careful measurement or estimation; BUN levels may be measured, although they are generally a much less reliable indication of renal function. More frequent testing should be done if renal function changes.
Neuromuscular effects	Aminoglycosides can exacerbate muscle weakness; use with caution in patients with neuromuscular disorders such as myasthenia gravis (see also DRUG INTERACTIONS). During or after therapy, tetany and muscle weakness have been observed in infants, and paresthesias, tetany, confusion, and positive Chvostek and Trousseau signs have been seen in adults; these clinical effects were accompanied by hypocalcemia, hypomagnesemia, and hypokalemia and were treated by administration of the appropriate electrolytes.
Superinfection	Overgrowth of nonsusceptible organisms may occur
Long-term therapy	Usual duration of therapy is 7–10 days; if a longer course is necessary, renal, auditory, and vestibular functions should be monitored, since the risk of toxicity is increased after 10 days. Dosage should be reduced if clinically indicated.
Elderly patients	Monitoring of renal function in such patients is particularly important. Creatinine clearance should be measured or estimated; renal impairment may not be detected if routine screening tests (eg, measurement of BUN or serum creatinine levels) are given.
Patients with extensive burns	The half-life may be significantly decreased in such patients, and the serum concentrations resulting from a particular dose may be lower than expected; use of serum drug levels as a basis for dosage adjustment is particularly important in this patient group

ADVERSE REACTIONS

Renal	Casts, cells, or protein in the urine; oliguria

GARAMYCIN ■ KANTREX

Hepatic	Transient hepatomegaly, splenomegaly
Gastrointestinal	Nausea, vomiting, increased salivation, stomatitis
Central nervous system and neuromuscular	Peripheral neuropathy or encephalopathy, including numbness, tingling sensation, muscle twitching, convulsions, and a myasthenia gravis-like syndrome; dizziness, vertigo, numbness, tingling sensation, muscle twitching, convulsions, lethargy, confusion, depression, visual disturbances, pseudotumor cerebri, acute organic brain syndrome, joint pain; arachnoiditis or burning at injection site (with intrathecal use)
Otic	Tinnitus, roaring in the ears, hearing loss
Hematological	Anemia, granulocytopenia, leukopenia, transient agranulocytopenia, eosinophilia, increased or decreased reticulocyte count, thrombocytopenia, purpura
Cardiovascular	Hypotension, hypertension
Respiratory	Depression, pulmonary fibrosis
Dermatological and hypersensitivity	Rash, pruritus, urticaria, generalized burning sensation, laryngeal edema, anaphylactoid reactions, fever, headache; subcutaneous atrophy and fat necrosis at injection site (rare)
Other	Decreased appetite, weight loss, alopecia, pain at injection site

OVERDOSAGE

Signs and symptoms	Hearing loss, vertigo, renal dysfunction, neuromuscular blockade, respiratory paralysis
Treatment	Institute appropriate supportive and symptomatic measures. Hemodialysis may be helpful in removing the drug from the blood; it is particularly important when renal function is impaired. For overdosage in neonates, consider exchange transfusions as well as hemodialysis.

DRUG INTERACTIONS

Other aminoglycoside antibiotics	△ Risk of ototoxicity, nephrotoxicity, and neuromuscular blockade
Cephaloridine, cephalothin	△ Risk of nephrotoxicity
Polymyxin antibiotics	△ Risk of nephrotoxicity and neuromuscular blockade
Potent diuretics (eg, ethacrynic acid, furosemide), cisplatin, vancomycin, viomycin, capreomycin	△ Risk of ototoxicity and nephrotoxicity
Anesthetics, neuromuscular blocking agents, massive transfusions of citrate-anticoagulated blood	△ Risk of neuromuscular blockade and respiratory paralysis (reversible with calcium)
Carbenicillin	▽ Gentamicin serum half-life in patients with severe renal impairment

ALTERED LABORATORY VALUES

Blood/serum values	△ BUN △ NPN △ Creatinine △ SGOT △ SGPT △ Lactate dehydrogenase △ Bilirubin ▽ Calcium ▽ Magnesium ▽ Sodium ▽ Potassium
Urinary values	△ Protein ▽ Specific gravity

USE IN CHILDREN
See INDICATIONS; adjust dosage according to body weight and severity of infection

USE IN PREGNANT AND NURSING WOMEN
Several cases of total irreversible bilateral congenital deafness have been observed in children whose mothers received streptomycin during pregnancy; although serious adverse effects have not been seen with the use of other aminoglycosides in pregnant women and reproduction studies with gentamicin in rats and rabbits have shown no evidence of harm to the fetus or impaired fertility, it is nevertheless possible that gentamicin may adversely affect fetal development or reproductive capacity. Women who are or who may become pregnant during therapy should be apprised of the potential hazard to the fetus. Consult manufacturer for use in nursing mothers.

[1] Calculate dosage on the basis of lean body mass

AMINOGLYCOSIDES

KANTREX (kanamycin sulfate) Apothecon   Rx

Capsules: kanamycin sulfate equivalent to 500 mg kanamycin   **Prefilled syringes:** 500 mg (2 ml)   **Vials:** 75 mg (2 ml, for pediatric use), 500 mg (2 ml), 1 g (3 ml)

INDICATIONS
Serious infections caused by susceptible strains of *Escherichia coli, Proteus, Enterobacter aerogenes, Klebsiella pneumoniae, Serratia marcescens,* and *Acinetobacter*
Staphylococcal infections caused by susceptible strains of *Staphylococcus aureus* and *S epidermidis* in patients allergic to other antibiotics, **mixed staphylococcal** and **Gram-negative bacterial infections,** and **severe infections** thought to be caused by either a Gram-negative bacterium or *Staphylococcus*

ORAL DOSAGE

PARENTERAL DOSAGE
Adult: 7.5 mg/kg IM q12h or up to 15 mg/kg/day IM or IV (slowly) in 2 or 3 equally divided doses; to achieve continuously high blood levels, give 15 mg/kg/day IM in equally divided doses q6–8h, not to exceed 1.5 g/day
Child: same as adult

KANTREX

| Suppression of intestinal bacteria (short-term adjunctive therapy) | **Adult:** 1 g q4h, followed by 1 g q6h for 36–72 h | |
| Hepatic coma (adjunctive therapy)[1] | **Adult:** 8–12 g/day, given in divided doses | |

CONTRAINDICATIONS

| Hypersensitivity or toxic reaction to kanamycin or other aminoglycosides (relative contraindication) | Intestinal obstruction (with oral form) | Long-term parenteral use |

ADMINISTRATION/DOSAGE ADJUSTMENTS

Duration of treatment	Usual duration of parenteral therapy is 7–10 days; when used orally as an adjunct to mechanical cleansing of the large bowel, the duration will depend on the patient's condition, whether catharsis or enemas are used and to what degree, and the customary medical routine for bowel preparation before surgery
Patients with renal impairment	Renal dysfunction may necessitate reduced frequency of administration; dosing interval in hours may be calculated by multiplying patient's serum creatinine level (mg/dl) by 9. Since renal function may alter appreciably during therapy, serum creatinine level should be checked frequently.
Intramuscular injection	Inject calculated dose deeply into the upper outer quadrant of gluteus muscle
Intravenous infusion	Dilute contents of 500-mg vial with 100–200 ml of normal saline or 5% dextrose (or contents of 1-g vial with 200–400 ml) and administer over a period of 30–60 min; for children, use sufficient diluent to infuse calculated pediatric dose over a similar period
Intraperitoneal use following exploration for established peritonitis or peritoneal contamination due to fecal spillage during surgery	Dilute contents of 500-mg vial in 20 ml of sterile distilled water and instill via a catheter sutured into the wound at closure; if possible, postpone instillation until effects of anesthesia and muscle-relaxing drugs have dissipated
Aerosol treatment	Dilute 250 mg in 3 ml of normal saline, place in a nebulizer, and administer solution bid to qid
Irrigating solution	Concentrations of 2.5 mg/ml may be used to irrigate abscess cavities, pleural space, and peritoneal and ventricular cavities

WARNINGS/PRECAUTIONS

Lack of response	Discontinue therapy and recheck antibiotic sensitivity if no definite clinical response occurs within 3–5 days; treatment failure may indicate bacterial resistance or the presence of septic foci requiring surgical drainage
Ototoxicity, nephrotoxicity, neurotoxicity	May occur, especially at higher doses or for administration periods longer than recommended; risk is greater in patients with renal damage. Concurrent or serial use of other ototoxic or nephrotoxic agents or diuretics should be avoided (see DRUG INTERACTIONS). Elderly patients, patients with pre-existing tinnitus, vertigo, or known subclinical deafness, patients who have received ototoxic drugs in the past, and patients receiving a total dose of 15 g or more of kanamycin should be carefully observed for signs of eighth-nerve damage; hearing loss may occur in such patients even with normal renal function.
Patients with renal impairment	Closely monitor renal and eighth-nerve function in patients with known or suspected renal impairment or in those who develop renal insufficiency during therapy. Reduce dosage or stop treatment if azotemia increases or urinary output decreases progressively. Audiograms should be taken before initiating treatment and again periodically. Discontinue therapy if patient develops significant loss of high-frequency perception, tinnitus, or subjective hearing loss.
Renal irritation	May be minimized by adequate hydration; increase hydration or reduce dosage if signs of irritation (eg, casts, WBC, RBC, albumin) appear
Intestinal absorption	Although absorption of oral kanamycin is usually negligible, the presence of ulcerated or denuded areas may increase absorption from the intestine
Superinfection	Overgrowth of nonsusceptible organisms, including fungi, may occur
Malabsorption syndrome	Characterized by increased fecal fat and by decreased serum carotene and xylose absorption, may occur with prolonged oral therapy
Neuromuscular blockade and respiratory paralysis	May occur in patients receiving anesthetics, neuromuscular blocking agents, or massive transfusion of citrate-anticoagulated blood; calcium salts or neostigmine may reverse blockade if it occurs
Muscle weakness	May worsen in patients with myasthenia gravis because of curare-like effect of drug on neuromuscular junction
Cross-allergenicity	Use with caution in patients demonstrating sensitivity to other aminoglycosides

ADVERSE REACTIONS[2]

| Renal | Albuminuria, red and white blood cells or granular casts in urine, azotemia, oliguria |

KANTREX ■ MYCIFRADIN

Gastrointestinal	Nausea, vomiting, and diarrhea (with oral use)
Central nervous system and neuromuscular	Headache, paresthesias
Otic	Tinnitus, vertigo, partial to irreversible hearing loss
Hypersensitivity	Skin rash, drug fever
Other	Local irritation or pain following IM injection

OVERDOSAGE

Signs and symptoms	Deafness, vertigo, renal dysfunction, neuromuscular blockade, respiratory paralysis
Treatment	Reduce dosage or discontinue medication; institute supportive measures. Peritoneal dialysis or hemodialysis may be used to eliminate drug from bloodstream. Newborns may, in addition, benefit from exchange transfusion.

DRUG INTERACTIONS

Other aminoglycoside antibiotics	△ Risk of ototoxicity, nephrotoxicity, and neuromuscular blockade
Cephaloridine, cephalothin	△ Risk of nephrotoxicity
Polymyxin antibiotics	△ Risk of nephrotoxicity and neuromuscular blockade
Potent diuretics (eg, ethacrynic acid, furosemide, mannitol, mercaptomerin), cisplatin, vancomycin, viomycin, capreomycin	△ Risk of ototoxicity and nephrotoxicity
Anesthetics, neuromuscular blocking agents	△ Risk of neuromuscular blockade and respiratory paralysis (reversible with calcium or neostigmine)

ALTERED LABORATORY VALUES

Blood/serum values	△ BUN △ Creatinine
Urinary values	△ Protein ▽ Specific gravity

USE IN CHILDREN

See INDICATIONS and PARENTERAL DOSAGE; infants and children generally tolerate the parenteral form well

USE IN PREGNANT AND NURSING WOMEN

Safety for use during pregnancy has not been established. Trace amounts of kanamycin are excreted in breast milk.

---

[1] To lower blood ammonia by suppressing ammonia-forming bacteria in the intestinal tract
[2] Side effects of oral therapy are mainly gastrointestinal; however, prolonged, high-dose oral administration in hepatic coma may result in nephrotoxicity and ototoxicity

---

AMINOGLYCOSIDES

MYCIFRADIN (neomycin sulfate) Upjohn   Rx

Tablets: 0.5 g   **Solution (per 5 ml):** 125 mg (1 pt)

INDICATIONS / ORAL DOSAGE

Bowel preparation prior to elective colorectal surgery (adjunctive therapy)	**Adult:** 1 g, given with 1 g of enteric-coated erythromycin base tablets, 19, 18, and 9 h before surgery
Hepatic encephalopathy (adjunctive therapy)	**Adult:** for hepatic coma, 4–12 g/day, given in divided doses for 5 or 6 days; for chronic hepatic insufficiency when other, less potentially toxic drugs cannot be used, up to 4 g/day for a period of up to 3 wk

CONTRAINDICATIONS

Hypersensitivity to neomycin	Intestinal obstruction

WARNINGS/PRECAUTIONS

Cross-sensitivity	Patients with a history of hypersensitivity or serious toxic reaction to other aminoglycosides may be hypersensitive to neomycin (see CONTRAINDICATIONS)
Nephrotoxocity and neurotoxicity	Nephrotoxic and neurotoxic reactions may occur, especially if patient is elderly or dehydrated, therapy is prolonged, renal function is impaired, higher dosages are used, or other potentially nephrotoxic or neurotoxic drugs (see DRUG INTERACTIONS) are given serially or concomitantly, even though only 3% of a dose is absorbed from the intact intestinal mucosa (if areas are ulcerated or denuded, however, absorption may be enhanced). Neurotoxicity may be manifested by vestibular and auditory disturbances (including partial or total irreversible bilateral deafness), numbness, skin tingling, muscle twitching, and convulsions; ototoxic effects may first appear or become more serious *after* therapy had been discontinued. Caution patients or members of their families about the risks of eighth-nerve damage.

MYCIFRADIN

Prevention of toxicity	To avoid toxic reactions, which may occur even at the recommended dosage, closely monitor clinical response. Extending treatment beyond 3 wk may increase the risk of toxicity; use the smallest possible dose for the shortest period of time necessary to control the patient's condition. Serial audiometric and vestibular tests should be performed; urine should be examined periodically for casts, cells, increased protein, and decreased specific gravity; and the BUN level, serum creatinine level, or creatinine clearance should be checked at regular intervals. To assess renal function in elderly patients, it may be more helpful to determine creatinine clearance, because routine screening of the BUN or serum creatinine level may fail to detect evidence of dysfunction. Exercise particular care when the risks of toxicity are enhanced. Adjust the dosage for patients with renal impairment. Avoid the concomitant or serial use of other potentially nephrotoxic or neurotoxic drugs (see DRUG INTERACTIONS). Monitor serum levels of neomycin and frequently check clinical response during treatment of chronic hepatic insufficiency since the risk of toxicity progressively increases during prolonged therapy. If renal impairment occurs during therapy, reduce dosage or discontinue use.
Neuromuscular effects	Respiratory depression or paralysis may occur, particularly if other drugs that can cause neuromuscular blockade (see DRUG INTERACTIONS) are given; IV calcium and, if necessary, a respirator may reverse the blockade. Aminoglycosides should be used with caution in patients with neuromuscular disorders (eg, myasthenia gravis or parkinsonism).
Superinfection	Overgrowth of nonsusceptible organisms, particularly fungi, may occur
Local irrigation or application	Neomycin is quickly and almost completely absorbed from body surfaces (except the urinary bladder) after local irrigation and after topical application during surgery; irreversible deafness, renal failure, respiratory paralysis, and death have resulted from irrigation with minute quantities of this drug
Carcinogenicity, mutagenicity, effect on fertility	No long-term studies have been done to evaluate the carcinogenic and mutagenic potential of neomycin or its effect on fertility

ADVERSE REACTIONS

The most frequent reactions, regardless of incidence, are printed in *italics*

Neurological	Auditory and vestibular disorders, including partial or total irreversible bilateral deafness; neuromuscular blockade and respiratory depression; numbness, tingling of the skin, muscle twitching, convulsions
Renal	Renal impairment
Gastrointestinal	*Nausea, vomiting, diarrhea;* decrease in absorption of lipids, cholesterol, carotene, protein, glucose, xylose, lactose, sodium, calcium, iron, and vitamin B_{12} (with prolonged therapy or administration of 12 mg/day); increase in fecal bile acid excretion; decrease in intestinal lactase activity

OVERDOSAGE

Signs and symptoms	Neurotoxicity and nephrotoxicity (see WARNINGS/PRECAUTIONS); because oral neomycin is poorly absorbed, toxicity is unlikely to occur following an acute overdose
Treatment	Reduce dosage or discontinue medication; to remove neomycin from the blood, use hemodialysis

DRUG INTERACTIONS

Other aminoglycosides	△ Risk of ototoxicity, nephrotoxicity, and respiratory depression or paralysis
Loop diuretics	△ Risk of ototoxicity
Cephalothin, bacitracin, amphotericin B	△ Risk of nephrotoxicity
Polymyxins	△ Risk of nephrotoxicity and respiratory depression
Capreomycin, cisplatin, vancomycin	△ Risk of ototoxicity and nephrotoxicity
Inhalation anesthetics, neuromuscular blockers, massive transfusions of citrated blood	△ Risk of respiratory depression or paralysis
Anticholinesterase agents	▽ Antimyasthenic effect
Oral digoxin	▽ Absorption of digoxin; monitor serum digoxin level
Oral methotrexate, penicillin V, oral vitamin B_{12}	▽ Serum levels of methotrexate, penicillin V, and vitamin B_{12}
Oral anticoagulants	△ Prothrombin time
Antivertigo agents	Masking of ototoxic symptoms

ALTERED LABORATORY VALUES

Blood/serum values	△ Creatinine △ BUN
Urinary values	△ Protein ▽ Specific gravity

USE IN CHILDREN

If treatment of patients under 18 yr of age is necessary, exercise caution and do not administer for more than 3 wk; safety and effectiveness for use in such patients have not been established

USE IN PREGNANT AND NURSING WOMEN

Pregnancy Category D: aminoglycosides cross the placental barrier and can cause harm to the human fetus. Several cases of total irreversible bilateral congenital deafness have been observed in children whose mothers received streptomycin during pregnancy; although serious side effects to fetus or neonate have not been reported with the use of other aminoglycosides during pregnancy, the possibility that such use may cause harm cannot be ruled out. Reproduction studies with neomycin have not been done. If a patient is or becomes pregnant while taking this drug, she should be apprised of the potential hazard to the fetus. It is not known whether neomycin is excreted in human milk; however, studies have demonstrated the presence of neomycin (given IM) in cow's milk and other aminoglycosides in human milk. Because of the potential for serious adverse reactions in nursing infants, patients should not nurse while taking neomycin.

AMINOGLYCOSIDES

NEBCIN (tobramycin sulfate) Dista   Rx

Prefilled syringes: tobramycin sulfate equivalent to 40 mg/ml tobramycin (1.5, 2 ml) **Vials:** tobramycin sulfate equivalent to 40 mg/ml tobramycin (2 ml, for general use) and 10 mg/ml tobramycin (2 ml, for pediatric use) **Pharmacy bulk package:** tobramycin sulfate equivalent to 40 mg/ml tobramycin (30 ml) for IV use only

INDICATIONS

Septicemia caused by susceptible strains of *Pseudomonas aeruginosa, Escherichia coli,* and *Klebsiella*
Lower respiratory tract infections caused by susceptible strains of *Pseudomonas aeruginosa, Klebsiella, Enterobacter, Serratia, Escherichia coli,* and *Staphylococcus aureus*[1]
Serious central nervous system infections (meningitis) caused by susceptible organisms
Intraabdominal infections, including peritonitis, caused by susceptible strains of *Escherichia coli, Klebsiella,* and *Enterobacter*
Skin, skin structure, and bone infections caused by susceptible strains of *Pseudomonas aeruginosa, Proteus, Escherichia coli, Klebsiella, Enterobacter,* and *Staphylococcus aureus*[1]
Complicated and recurrent urinary tract infections[2] caused by susceptible strains of *Pseudomonas aeruginosa, Proteus, Escherichia coli, Klebsiella, Enterobacter, Serratia, Staphylococcus aureus,*[1] *Providencia,* and *Citrobacter*

PARENTERAL DOSAGE

Adult: 3 mg/kg/day IM or IV, given in 3 equally divided doses q8h; for life-threatening infections, up to 5 mg/kg/day IM or IV, given in 3 or 4 equally divided doses (reduce dosage to 3 mg/kg/day as soon as clinically indicated); do not give more than 5 mg/kg/day unless serum levels are monitored
Premature or full-term newborn ($\leq$ 1 wk): up to 4 mg/kg/day IM or IV, given in 2 equally divided doses q12h
Child: 6–7.5 mg/kg/day IM or IV, given in 3 or 4 equally divided doses (2–2.5 mg/kg q8h or 1.5–1.89 mg/kg q6h)

CONTRAINDICATIONS

Hypersensitivity to any aminoglycoside (absolute contraindication)

History of hypersensitivity or serious toxic reaction to prior aminoglycoside therapy (relative contraindication)

ADMINISTRATION/DOSAGE ADJUSTMENTS

Duration of treatment	Usual duration of treatment is 7–10 days; if a longer course of therapy is required, renal, auditory, and vestibular function should be monitored because neurotoxicity is more likely to occur if treatment is extended beyond 10 days
Intramuscular administration	Withdraw the appropriate dose directly from a vial or use a prefilled disposable syringe
Intravenous administration	Dilute the required amount of tobramycin with 50–100 ml of 0.9% Sodium Chloride Injection or 5% Dextrose Injection for adults and a proportionately smaller volume for children; do not mix tobramycin with other drugs in the same container. Administer IV over a period of 20–60 min; infusion over a shorter period may result in serum levels exceeding 12 μg/ml (see below).
Use of serum drug levels	Measure peak and trough serum levels periodically, especially in patients with renal impairment or when dosages exceeding 5 mg/kg/day are used. Serum levels should be monitored after the first 2 or 3 doses and then every 3 or 4 days until the drug is discontinued; if renal function changes, monitor more often. To measure peak drug levels, draw blood about 30 min following IV infusion or 1 h after IM injection; for trough levels, obtain blood samples 8 h after the previous dose or just before the next dose is given. Rising trough levels ($>$ 2 μg/ml) may indicate tissue accumulation. Prolonged serum levels $>$ 12 μg/ml should be avoided.

NEBCIN

Patients with renal impairment (creatinine clearance rate ≤ 70 ml/min)	Administer 1 mg/kg IM or IV to start, followed by smaller doses administered at 8-h intervals (divide usual dose by patient's serum creatinine level) or normal doses given at prolonged intervals (multiply patient's serum creatinine level by 6 to determine dosage interval in hours); neither method of calculating the appropriate dosage should be used if the patient is undergoing dialysis
Obese patients	Calculate the appropriate dose by using the patient's estimated lean body weight and adding 40% of the excess

WARNINGS/PRECAUTIONS

Nephrotoxicity and neurotoxicity	May occur, especially in elderly or dehydrated patients or when renal damage is present, therapy is prolonged, or higher than recommended doses have been given. Neurotoxicity may manifest itself by bilateral, partial or complete, irreversible hearing loss, vestibular dysfunction (see ADVERSE REACTIONS), numbness, skin tingling, muscle twitching, and/or convulsions. Patients who develop cochlear damage may not have warning symptoms of eighth-nerve toxicity. Ototoxicity may continue to progress after the drug is discontinued, and, rarely, nephrotoxicity may not become evident until the first few days after therapy is stopped. Concomitant use of potent diuretics and concurrent or sequential use of other neurotoxic and/or nephrotoxic drugs (see DRUG INTERACTIONS) should be avoided.
Patients with renal impairment	Closely monitor renal and eighth-nerve function in patients with known or suspected renal impairment and in those who develop renal insufficiency during therapy. Measure serum calcium, magnesium, sodium, and creatinine concentrations, BUN, and creatinine clearance periodically, as well as serum drug levels if renal impairment is known. Examine urine for decreased specific gravity and increased excretion of protein, cells, and casts. When feasible, obtain serial audiograms in any patient old enough to be tested. Reduce dosage or discontinue therapy if renal, vestibular, or auditory function becomes impaired.
Prolonged or secondary apnea	May occur in anesthetized patients who are given neuromuscular blocking agents and in patients receiving massive transfusions of citrated blood; if neuromuscular blockade occurs, administer IV calcium
Cross-allergenicity	Patients who are hypersensitive to other aminoglycosides may also be allergic to tobramycin (see CONTRAINDICATIONS)
Patients with extensive burns	Altered pharmacokinetics may result in reduced serum drug levels; determine proper dosage on the basis of serum level measurements
Elderly patients	Routine screening tests (eg, BUN, serum creatinine) may not detect renal insufficiency in aged patients; measure creatinine clearance to determine renal function in the elderly
Patients with muscular disorders	Muscle weakness may be aggravated in patients with myasthenia gravis, parkinsonism, or other muscular disorders due to drug's curare-like effect on neuromuscular function; use with caution
Local irrigation or application	May result in significant percutaneous absorption of tobramycin and potential neurotoxicity and nephrotoxicity
Superinfection	Overgrowth of nonsusceptible organisms may occur

ADVERSE REACTIONS

Central nervous system and neuromuscular	Dizziness, vertigo, tinnitus, roaring sound in the ears, hearing loss, headache, lethargy, mental confusion, disorientation
Renal	Oliguria, cylinduria, increased proteinuria
Hematological	Anemia, granulocytopenia, thrombocytopenia, leukopenia, leukocytosis, eosinophilia
Gastrointestinal	Nausea, vomiting
Other	Fever, rash, itching, urticaria, pain at injection site

OVERDOSAGE

Signs and symptoms	Hearing loss, vertigo, renal dysfunction, neuromuscular blockade, respiratory paralysis
Treatment	Reduce dosage or discontinue medication; institute supportive measures, as needed. Peritoneal dialysis or (preferably) hemodialysis may be used to eliminate the drug from the bloodstream.

DRUG INTERACTIONS

Other aminoglycoside antibiotics	⚠ Risk of otoxicity, nephrotoxicity, and neuromuscular blockade
Cephalosporin antibiotics	⚠ Risk of nephrotoxicity
Polymyxin antibiotics	⚠ Risk of nephrotoxicity and neuromuscular blockade

NEBCIN ■ NETROMYCIN

Potent diuretics (eg, loop diuretics), cisplatin, vancomycin, viomycin, capreomycin	↑ Risk of ototoxicity and nephrotoxicity
Neuromuscular blocking agents	Prolonged or secondary apnea in anesthetized patients
Beta-lactam antibiotics (penicillins and cephalosporins)	Inactivation of tobramycin in patients with severe renal impairment

ALTERED LABORATORY VALUES

Blood/serum values	↑ BUN ↑ NPN ↑ Creatinine ↑ SGOT ↑ SGPT ↑ Lactate dehydrogenase ↑ Bilirubin ↓ Calcium ↓ Magnesium ↓ Sodium ↓ Potassium
Urinary values	↑ Protein ↓ Specific gravity

USE IN CHILDREN

See INDICATIONS and PARENTERAL DOSAGE; use with caution in premature infants and neonates due to renal immaturity

USE IN PREGNANT AND NURSING WOMEN

Pregnancy Category D: aminoglycosides cross the placental barrier and can cause fetal harm when administered during pregnancy. If therapy is initiated in a pregnant woman or patient becomes pregnant while taking this drug, she should be apprised of the potential hazard to the fetus. Several cases of total irreversible bilateral congenital deafness have been reported where streptomycin was taken during pregnancy; however, no serious side effects to the mother, fetus, or newborn have been associated with the administration of other aminoglycosides to pregnant women. Trace amounts of tobramycin are excreted in human milk.[1]

[1] Takase Z et al: *Chemotherapy* 23:1402, 1975

---

[1] Tobramycin may be considered in serious staphylococcal infections when penicillin or other potentially less toxic drugs are contraindicated and bacterial susceptibility and clinical judgment indicate its use
[2] Aminoglycosides are not indicated in uncomplicated initial episodes of urinary tract infections unless the causative organisms are not susceptible to other, less potentially toxic antibiotics

---

AMINOGLYCOSIDES

NETROMYCIN (netilmicin sulfate) Schering   Rx

Ampuls: netilmicin sulfate equivalent to 10 mg/ml netilmicin (2 ml) for neonatal use   **Vials:** netilmicin sulfate equivalent to 25 mg/ml netilmicin (2 ml) for pediatric use and 100 mg/ml netilmicin (1.5, 15 ml) for general use   **Prefilled syringes:** netilmicin sulfate equivalent to 100 mg/ml netilmicin (1.5 ml) for general use

INDICATIONS

Complicated urinary tract infections[2] caused by susceptible strains of *Escherichia coli, Klebsiella pneumoniae, Pseudomonas aeruginosa, Enterobacter, Proteus mirabilis*, indole-positive *Proteus, Serratia, Citrobacter*, and *Staphylococcus aureus*

Septicemia caused by susceptible strains of *Escherichia coli, Klebsiella pneumoniae, Pseudomonas aeruginosa, Enterobacter, Serratia*, and *Proteus mirabilis*
Intraabdominal infections, including peritonitis and abscesses, caused by susceptible strains of *Escherichia coli, Klebsiella pneumoniae, Pseudomonas aeruginosa, Enterobacter, Proteus mirabilis*, indole-positive *Proteus*, and *Staphylococcus aureus*
Skin, skin structure, and lower respiratory tract infections caused by susceptible strains of *Escherichia coli, Klebsiella pneumoniae, Pseudomonas aeruginosa, Enterobacter, Serratia, Proteus mirabilis*, indole-positive *Proteus*, and *Staphylococcus aureus*

PARENTERAL DOSAGE[1]

Adult: 1.5–2 mg/kg IM or IV q12h
Neonate (< 6 wk): 2–3.25 mg/kg IM or IV q12h
Infant and child (6 wk to 12 yr): 1.8–2.7 mg/kg IM or IV q8h or 2.7–4 mg/kg IM or IV q12h

Adult: 1.3–2.2 mg/kg IM or IV q8h or 2–3.25 mg/kg IM or IV q12h
Neonate (< 6 wk): 2–3.25 mg/kg IM or IV q12h
Infant and child (6 wk to 12 yr): 1.8–2.7 mg/kg IM or IV q8h or 2.7–4 mg/kg IM or IV q12h

CONTRAINDICATIONS

Hypersensitivity to netilmicin or any other component

ADMINISTRATION/DOSAGE ADJUSTMENTS

Usage	Netilmicin is indicated for the treatment of serious or life-threatening infections and should be used only when other, less potentially toxic anti-infectives are contraindicated or ineffective. This drug may be given as initial therapy (ie, before the results of susceptibility tests are known) for gram-negative infections and may be considered for staphylococcal infections when susceptibility test results and clinical judgment indicate its use. If the causative organism is unknown, netilmicin may be administered in combination with a penicillin or cephalosporin as initial therapy; if an anaerobic organism is suspected, netilmicin should be given in combination with other appropriate anti-infectives. Concomitant use of netilmicin and penicillin is usually indicated for the treatment of suspected sepsis in neonates. Netilmicin, in combination with carbenicillin or ticarcillin, is effective in the treatment of life-threatening infections caused by *Pseudomonas aeruginosa* and, in combination with carbenicillin, azlocillin, mezlocillin, cefamandole, cefotaxime, or moxalactam, inhibits many, but not all, strains of *Serratia*.

NETROMYCIN

Duration of therapy	Usual duration of therapy is 7–14 days; if a longer course of therapy is required (eg, for the treatment of complicated infections), renal, auditory, and vestibular function should be carefully monitored, and, if necessary, dosage should be adjusted
Intravenous administration	Dilute the calculated single dose in 50–200 ml of 0.9% sodium chloride injection (alone or with 5% dextrose), 5% or 10% dextrose injection, Ringer's injection, lactated Ringer's injection (alone or with 5% dextrose), or other appropriate diluent (see package insert) and give by infusion over a period of 30–120 min; use a smaller volume of diluent for infants and children, in accordance with their fluid requirements. (Netilmicin may also be given by direct IV injection; serum drug levels observed after rapid injection may be transiently 2–3 times higher than those detected after a 60-min infusion.) Large-volume solutions of 2.1–3 mg/ml are stable for up to 72 h at room or refrigerator temperature.
Use of serum drug levels	Peak and trough serum drug levels should be measured periodically during therapy. For peak levels, take blood samples 30–60 min after IM injection or at the end of an IV infusion; for trough levels, measure just before the next dose. After IM injection or 60-min IV infusion in adults, the peak level (given in $\mu g/ml$) is usually 3–3.5 times the strength (given in mg/kg) of a single dose; thus, a peak level of $\sim$ 7 $\mu g/ml$ can be expected from a single dose of 2 mg/kg. Dosage should be adjusted to maintain, in general, peak levels of 6–10 $\mu g/ml$ and trough levels of 0.5–2 $\mu g/ml$; trough levels exceeding 4 $\mu g/ml$ and prolonged peak levels exceeding 16 $\mu g/ml$ should be avoided. Pharmacokinetic data based on measurements of serum drug levels can be used to individualize dosage. To avoid obtaining spuriously low serum levels, samples taken from patients who are also receiving beta-lactam anti-infectives (see DRUG INTERACTIONS) should be assayed promptly or frozen, or beta-lactamase should be added.
Patients with renal impairment	As an initial dose, give the usual dose, ie, the same dose that would be given to patients with normal renal function (see PARENTERAL DOSAGE); however, patients with renal impairment generally should not be given more than 3.25 mg/kg in a single dose. For subsequent dosage adjustments, use serum drug levels. If such data cannot be obtained and renal function is stable, use serum creatinine levels (divide the usual dose by the patient's serum creatinine level) or creatinine clearance (Ccr) values (either divide the patient's Ccr by the normal Ccr and multiply the quotient by the usual dose or use the table, below). The Ccr can be estimated from serum creatinine levels; for adult men, use the following formula: $(140 - \text{age [yr]})(\text{weight [kg]})/(72)(\text{serum creatinine level [mg/dl]})$, for adult women multiply this quotient by 0.85. If renal function is deteriorating, a greater reduction in dosage may be necessary.

Dosage adjustment for patients with stable renal impairment[1]

Ccr[2]	Adjustment	Ccr[2]	Adjustment	Ccr[2]	Adustment
70	0.70	38	0.40	18	0.20
62	0.65	32	0.35	12	0.15
50	0.55	28	0.30	8	0.10
42	0.50	22	0.25	5	0.05

[1] To obtain the appropriate dosage, multiply the usual dose by the adjustment factor
[2] Creatinine clearance (ml/min/1.73 m^2)

Administer the adjusted daily dose in 3 equally divided doses q8h, 2 equally divided doses q12h, or as a single dose q24h. The amount of drug removed during dialysis in adults may vary, depending on the equipment and methods that are used; administer 2 mg/kg to adults at the end of each dialysis period until serum drug levels have been determined. Information on hemodialysis in children is not available.

WARNINGS/PRECAUTIONS

Nephrotoxicity and neurotoxicity	Nephrotoxic and neurotoxic reactions may occur, especially if patients are elderly or dehydrated, renal function is impaired, therapy is prolonged, the recommended dosage is exceeded, or other potentially nephrotoxic or neurotoxic drugs have been administered; in rare cases, these reactions may not become evident until soon after completion of therapy. The risk of toxic reactions in patients with normal renal function is low, provided that the recommended dosage and usual duration of therapy are not exceeded. Nephrotoxic effects are usually mild and reversible, but permanent impairment can occur. Neurotoxic effects include auditory ototoxic reactions (audiometric changes, hearing loss, tinnitus), vestibular ototoxic reactions (nystagmus, vertigo, nausea, vomiting, acute Meniere's syndrome), numbness, skin tingling, muscle twitching, and convulsions; ototoxic effects are usually irreversible. Cochlear damage is usually manifested initially by small changes in audiometric test results at higher frequencies and may not be associated with perceptible hearing loss. If nephrotoxic reactions occur, adjust dosage; if ototoxic reactions occur, reduce dosage or discontinue use.

NETROMYCIN

Prevention of toxic reactions	Patients should be well-hydrated during therapy. The concurrent or sequential use of other potentially nephrotoxic or neurotoxic drugs (see DRUG INTERACTIONS) and the concomitant use of potent diuretics should be avoided. (Some diuretics are directly ototoxic; diuretics can also enhance the risk of aminoglycoside toxicity when given IV by altering the serum and tissue concentrations of the aminoglycoside.) Patients should be closely observed during therapy, and serum drug levels should be measured whenever feasible. If possible, serial audiometric tests should also be performed, particularly in high-risk patients. Urine should be examined periodically for increased excretion of protein, the presence of cells and casts, and decreased specific gravity. Periodically throughout therapy (including the onset and end), obtain serum creatinine levels, or, for a more precise analysis, determine the creatinine clearance by careful measurement or estimation; BUN levels may be measured, although they are generally a much less reliable indication of renal function. More frequent testing should be done if renal function changes.
Neuromuscular effects	Acute muscular paralysis or apnea may occur as a result of neuromuscular blockade, particularly in patients given neuromuscular blocking agents (eg, succinylcholine, tubocurarine, decamethonium) and in patients who received massive transfusions of citrate-anticoagulated blood; if neuromuscular blockade occurs, use IV calcium and, if necessary, a respirator. Use with caution in patients with neuromuscular disorders (eg, myasthenia gravis, parkinsonism, infant botulism).
Cross-sensitivity	Use very cautiously, if at all, in patients with a history of serious toxic reaction or hypersensitivity to another aminoglycoside, because cross-sensitivity has been reported
Superinfection	Overgrowth of nonsusceptible organisms may occur
Elderly patients	Monitoring of renal function in such patients is particularly important. Creatinine clearance should be measured or estimated; renal impairment may not be detected if routine screening tests (eg, measurement of BUN or serum creatinine levels) are given.
Patients with extensive burns	The half-life may be significantly decreased in such patients, and the serum concentrations resulting from a particular dose may be lower than expected; use of serum drug levels as a basis for dosage adjustment is particularly important in this patient group
Local irrigation or application	Netilmicin may be almost completely absorbed from body surfaces (except the urinary bladder) after local irrigation and after topical application during surgery; the potentially toxic effects of such use should be considered
Carcinogenicity, mutagenicity	No drug-related tumors have been detected in mice or rats that underwent lifetime carcinogenicity studies; the results of mutagenicity tests have been negative
Effect on fertility	No impairment of fertility has been observed in rats injected with 13–15 times the highest adult human dose

ADVERSE REACTIONS

	Frequent reactions (incidence $\geq$ 1%) are printed in *italics*
Central nervous system and neuromuscular	*Audiometric changes (4%)*, vertigo, tinnitus, nystagmus, hearing loss, acute Meniere's syndrome, headache, disorientation, blurred vision, paresthesias, acute muscular paralysis
Renal	*Renal impairment (7%)*, characterized by increased serum creatinine or BUN levels, decreased creatinine clearance, proteinuria, presence of cells in the urine, cylindruria, or oliguria
Gastrointestinal	Nausea, vomiting, diarrhea
Hematological	Eosinophilia, thrombocytosis, prolonged prothrombin time, anemia, leukopenia, thrombocytopenia, leukemoid reactions, immature circulating white blood cells
Cardiovascular	Palpitations, hypotension
Dermatological	Rash, itching
Other	Fever; hyperkalemia; apnea; hematoma, induration, and/or severe pain at administration site

OVERDOSAGE

Signs and symptoms	Hearing loss, vertigo, renal dysfunction, neuromuscular blockade, respiratory paralysis
Treatment	Reduce dosage or discontinue medication; institute supportive measures, as needed. Peritoneal dialysis or (preferably) hemodialysis may be used to eliminate the drug from the bloodstream.

DRUG INTERACTIONS

Other aminoglycosides	△ Risk of neurotoxicity, nephrotoxicity, and neuromuscular blockade
Cephalothin, bacitracin	△ Risk of nephrotoxicity
Polymyxins, amphotericin B	△ Risk of nephrotoxicity and neuromuscular blockade

NETROMYCIN ■ AZULFIDINE

Potent diuretics (eg, loop diuretics), cisplatin, vancomycin, viomycin, capreomycin	△ Risk of neurotoxicity and nephrotoxicity
Neuromuscular blocking agents	Acute muscular paralysis, apnea
Beta-lactam anti-infectives (penicillins and cephalosporins)	Inactivation of netilmicin (usually clinically significant only in patients with severe renal impairment)

ALTERED LABORATORY VALUES

Blood/serum values	△ Creatinine[3] △ BUN △ SGOT △ SGPT △ Alkaline phosphatase △ Bilirubin △ Potassium
Urinary values	△ Protein ▽ Specific gravity

USE IN CHILDREN

See INDICATIONS and PARENTERAL DOSAGE. Use with caution in premature and full-term neonates; the serum half-life of netilmicin is prolonged in such patients because of renal immaturity. During the first week of life, the half-life is ~ 8 h in neonates weighing 1.5–2 kg and ~ 4.5 h in neonates weighing 3–4 kg (by comparison, the half-life in adults is 2–3 h).

USE IN PREGNANT AND NURSING WOMEN

Pregnancy Category D: aminoglycosides cross the placental barrier and can cause harm to the fetus. If the patient is or becomes pregnant while taking netilmicin, she should be apprised of the potential hazard to the fetus. Several cases of total irreversible bilateral congenital deafness have been observed in children whose mothers received streptomycin during pregnancy. Serious side effects to neonate or fetus have not been reported with the use of other aminoglycosides during pregnancy; nevertheless, the possibility that such use may cause harm should not be ruled out. Reproduction studies conducted in rats and rabbits given IM or SC 13–15 times the maximum adult human dose of netilmicin have shown no evidence of harm to the fetus; ototoxic effects have not been detected in the offspring of rats given SC doses during pregnancy and lactation. Small amounts of netilmicin are excreted in human milk; because of the potential for serious adverse reactions in nursing infants, patients should not nurse while taking this drug.

[1] Calculate dosage on the basis of estimated lean body mass
[2] Aminoglycosides are not indicated for the treatment of uncomplicated, initial episodes of urinary tract infections, unless the causative organisms are not susceptible to other, less potentially toxic anti-infectives
[3] Creatinine levels may be spuriously elevated if cephalosporins are used concomitantly; however, serum levels are actually increased if nephrotoxic effects occur

---

SULFONAMIDES

AZULFIDINE (sulfasalazine) Pharmacia Rx

Tablets: 500 mg **Tablets (enteric-coated):** 500 mg **Suspension (per 5 ml):** 250 mg (1 pt)

INDICATIONS	ORAL DOSAGE
Treatment of **mild to moderate ulcerative colitis** Adjunctive therapy for **severe ulcerative colitis**	**Adult:** 3-4 g/day, given in evenly divided doses **Child (>2 yr):** 40-60 mg/kg/day, given in 4-6 evenly divided doses
Prolongation of **remission** following acute ulcerative colitis	**Adult:** 2 g/day, given in evenly divided doses **Child (>2 yr):** 30 mg/kg/day, given in 4 evenly divided doses

CONTRAINDICATIONS

Hypersensitivity to sulfasalazine, sulfapyridine, or other sulfonamides, or to 5-aminosalicylic acid or other salicylates	Intestinal or urinary obstruction Age < 2 yr	Porphyria

ADMINISTRATION/DOSAGE ADJUSTMENTS

Timing of administration	The interval between nighttime doses should not exceed 8 h; when feasible, administer drug after meals
Monitoring of therapeutic response	An endoscopic examination should be done periodically to assess therapeutic response and determine whether dosage should be adjusted. Dosage should be reduced to a maintenance level after clinical signs, including diarrhea, have been controlled and endoscopic findings confirm satisfactory improvement. If diarrhea recurs during maintenance therapy, dosage should be increased to previously effective therapeutic level.
Gastric intolerance	Anorexia, nausea, vomiting, and other gastric reactions occurring after the first few doses of the suspension or regular tablets are usually due to mucosal irritation; they may be alleviated by distributing the daily dose more evenly or by switching to enteric-coated tablets. Gastric reactions that occur after the first few doses of the enteric-coated tablets or after the first few days of treatment with the suspension or regular tablets are probably due to sulfapyridine toxicity and may be alleviated by halving the daily dose and then gradually increasing it over several days; if the reactions persist despite the reduction in dosage, discontinue administration for 5-7 days and then resume giving the drug at a lower dosage. To reduce the likelihood of gastric intolerance, susceptible adults can initially be given 1-2 g/day rather than 3-4 g/day.

AZULFIDINE

Desensitization	To reinstitute therapy in patients who have experienced sensitivity reactions, give 50-250 mg/day to start and then double the dosage every 4-7 days until a satisfactory clinical response is obtained (use the suspension for administering small doses). If a sensitivity reaction recurs, discontinue administration of sulfasalazine. A desensitization-like regimen should not be started until 2 wk after sulfasalazine has been discontinued and symptoms have disappeared; it should not be attempted at all in any patient who has experienced an anaphylactoid reaction to this drug or has a history of agranulocytosis.

WARNINGS/PRECAUTIONS

Toxicity	Drug-induced hypersensitivity reactions, blood dyscrasias, neuromuscular and CNS reactions, hepatotoxicity, nephrotoxicity, or fibrosing alveolitis may result in death. Only after critical appraisal should sulfasalazine be given to a patient with a blood dyscrasia or hepatic or renal impairment. Exercise caution when treating a patient with a severe allergy or bronchial asthma. In general, watch for clinical signs suggesting a serious blood dyscrasia, such as sore throat, fever, pallor, purpura, and jaundice; obtain a CBC frequently. Closely observe patients with glucose-6-phosphate dehydrogenase deficiency for signs of hemolytic anemia. To prevent crystalluria and lithiasis, perform a urinalysis, including a careful microscopic examination, frequently during therapy and instruct patients to maintain an adequate fluid intake. Monitoring of serum sulfapyridine levels may be useful, since concentrations exceeding 50 μg/ml appear to be associated with an increased incidence of adverse reactions. Patients receiving 4 g/day or more are at increased risk of toxicity and therefore should be carefully observed. If a toxic or hypersensitivity reaction occurs during therapy, discontinue administration immediately.
Cross-sensitivity	Patients hypersensitive to acetazolamide, thiazide-type diuretics, or sulfonylureas may be allergic to sulfasalazine
Carcinogenicity	Long-term administration of sulfonamides to rats, a species particularly susceptible to the goitrogenic effects of these drugs, has resulted in thyroid malignancies
Impairment of fertility	Oligospermia and infertility have been seen in men given sulfasalazine; withdrawal of the drug appears to reverse these effects. No evidence of impaired fertility has been seen in female rats or rabbits given up to 6 times the human dose of sulfasalazine.
Skin and urine discoloration	Caution patients that their skin or urine may turn orange-yellow during therapy
Sugar content	Caution diabetic patients being treated with the suspension that it contains sucrose

ADVERSE REACTIONS

The most frequent reactions, regardless of incidence, are printed in *italics*

Gastrointestinal	*Anorexia, nausea, vomiting, and gastric distress (33%)*; hepatitis, pancreatitis, diarrhea (including bloody diarrhea), stomatitis, abdominal pains
Central nervous system	*Headache (33%)*, transverse myelitis, convulsions, transient lesions of the posterior spinal column, peripheral neuropathy, mental depression, vertigo, hearing loss, insomnia, ataxia, hallucinations, tinnitus, drowsiness
Genitourinary	*Oligospermia (33%)*, infertility
Hematological	*Heinz body anemia and hemolytic anemia (3.3%)*; aplastic anemia, agranulocytosis, leukopenia, megaloblastic (macrocytic) anemia, purpura, thrombocytopenia, hypoprothrombinemia, methemoglobinemia
Renal	Toxic nephrosis with oliguria and anuria, nephrotic syndrome, hematuria, crystalluria, and proteinuria; discoloration of urine
Hypersensitivity	*Rash, pruritus, and urticaria (3.3%)*; erythema multiforme (Stevens-Johnson syndrome), exfoliative dermatitis, epidermal necrolysis (Lyell's syndrome) with corneal damage, anaphylaxis, serum sickness syndrome, transient pulmonary changes with eosinophilia and decreased pulmonary function, allergic myocarditis, polyarteritis nodosa, lupus erythematosus, hepatitis with immune complexes, parapsoriasis varioliformis acuta (Mucha-Haberman syndrome), photosensitization, arthralgia, periorbital edema, conjunctival and scleral injection, alopecia
Other	*Cyanosis and fever (3.3%)*; goiter, diuresis, hypoglycemia, discoloration of skin

OVERDOSAGE

Signs and symptoms	Nausea, vomiting, gastric distress, abdominal pains, drowsiness, convulsions
Treatment	Induce emesis or perform gastric lavage; then administer a cathartic, alkalinize urine, and, if renal function is normal, force fluids. Sulfasalazine and its metabolites can be removed from the blood by dialysis. Monitor serum levels. Restrict salt and fluids if anuria occurs; catheterization of the ureter may be necessary to treat complete renal blockage caused by crystals. Hospitalize patients with agranulocytosis. To control hypersensitivity reactions, use antihistamines and, if necessary, systemic corticosteroids.

DRUG INTERACTIONS

Digoxin, folic acid	▽ Absorption of digoxin and folic acid

ALTERED LABORATORY VALUES

Urinary values	△ Protein

AZULFIDINE ■ GANTANOL

No clinically significant alterations in blood/serum values occur at therapeutic dosages

USE IN CHILDREN
See INDICATIONS and ORAL DOSAGE; use in children under 2 yr of age is contraindicated

USE IN PREGNANT AND NURSING WOMEN
Pregnancy Category B: both a study in pregnant women who received sulfasalazine or other sulfonamides and a survey of pregnant women who received sulfasalazine alone or with corticosteroids have shown no evidence of harm to the fetus; similar results have been observed in rats and rabbits given up to 6 times the human dose of sulfasalazine. Nevertheless, bear in mind that no adequate, well-controlled studies have been performed in pregnant women. Sulfapyridine, a major metabolite, crosses the placental barrier and appears in human milk; the metabolite has a poor, but nonetheless significant, capacity to displace bilirubin from plasma proteins and therefore, if present in a pregnant or nursing woman, may cause kernicterus in a neonate. Use sulfasalazine during pregnancy only if clearly needed, and exercise caution if the woman is nursing.

SULFONAMIDES

GANTANOL (sulfamethoxazole) Roche   Rx
Tablets: 0.5 g **Suspension (per 5 ml):** 0.5 g (16 fl oz) *cherry-flavored*

GANTANOL DS (sulfamethoxazole) Roche   Rx
Tablets: 1 g

INDICATIONS
Acute, recurrent, or chronic urinary tract infections caused by susceptible strains of *Escherichia coli*, *Klebsiella-Enterobacter*, staphylococci, *Proteus mirabilis*, and *P vulgaris* in the absence of obstructive uropathy and foreign bodies
Prophylaxis of meningococcal meningitis caused by sulfonamide-sensitive Group A strains
Acute otitis media caused by *Hemophilus influenzae* when used concomitantly with penicillin
Trachoma
Inclusion conjunctivitis
Nocardiosis
Chancroid
Toxoplasmosis (adjunctive therapy with pyrimethamine)
Malaria caused by chloroquine-resistant strains of *Plasmodium falciparum* (adjunctive therapy)

ORAL DOSAGE
Adult: 2 g or 20 ml (4 tsp) to start, followed by 1 g or 10 ml (2 tsp) bid (mild to moderate infections) or tid (severe infections)
Infant (≥ 2 mo) and child: 50–60 mg/kg to start, followed by 25–30 mg/kg bid (up to 75 mg/kg/24 h), as follows:
Infant (20 lb): 0.5 g or 5 ml (1 tsp) to start, followed by 0.25 g or 2.5 ml (½ tsp) bid
Child (40 lb): 1 g or 10 ml (2 tsp) to start, followed by 0.5 g or 5 ml (1 tsp) bid
Child (60 lb): 1.5 g or 15 ml (3 tsp) to start, followed by 0.75 g or 7.5 ml (1½ tsp) bid
Child (80 lb): 2 g or 20 ml (4 tsp) to start, followed by 1 g or 10 ml (2 tsp) bid

CONTRAINDICATIONS
Pregnancy at term

Breast-feeding

Age < 2 mo (see USE IN CHILDREN)   Hypersensitivity to sulfonamides

ADMINISTRATION/DOSAGE ADJUSTMENTS

Susceptibility — In vitro susceptibility tests are not always reliable; carefully coordinate test results with bacteriological and clinical response. Bear in mind that resistance to sulfonamides is becoming more common, especially in the treatment of chronic and recurrent urinary tract infections. When performing follow-up cultures during therapy, add aminobenzoic acid to the culture media.

Patients with renal impairment — Reduce dosage if creatinine clearance is less than 20–30 ml/min (see WARNINGS/PRECAUTIONS)

Therapeutic blood levels — For most infections, 5–15 mg/dl; for serious infections, 12–15 mg/dl; blood levels > 20 mg/dl increase the probability of adverse reactions. Blood levels should be measured in patients with serious infections.

WARNINGS/PRECAUTIONS

Group A beta-hemolytic streptococcal infections — Sulfonamides have no place in the treatment of such infections since they will neither eradicate the causative organism nor prevent complications

GANTANOL

Life-threatening infections	Severe, potentially fatal reactions, including hepatocellular necrosis, hypersensitivity reactions, and serious blood dyscrasias (eg, agranulocytosis, aplastic anemia), have occurred in patients receiving sulfonamides. These drugs have caused hemolytic anemia in patients with G6PD deficiency. When using this product, obtain a CBC frequently and watch for early clinical signs such as sore throat, fever, pallor, purpura, and jaundice; if the count of a formed blood element falls significantly, administration should be discontinued.
Bone marrow depression	High doses or prolonged use may cause bone marrow depression and, as a result, produce thrombocytopenia, leukopenia, and/or megaloblastic anemia; if signs of bone marrow depression appear, give 3–6 mg/day of leucovorin IM until normal hematopoiesis is restored (usual duration of treatment: 3 days)
Cross-sensitivity	Patients allergic to acetazolamide, thiazide-type diuretics, sulfonylureas, or certain goitrogens may also be hypersensitive to sulfamethoxazole
Renal effects	Crystalluria, urolithiasis, and other renal complications have occurred in patients taking sulfonamides; the frequency is considerably lower with a more soluble sulfonamide such as sulfamethoxazole. Caution patients to maintain an adequate fluid intake; renal function tests and urinalyses, including careful microscopic examination, should be performed during therapy, particularly when a patient has renal impairment.
Special-risk patients	Use with caution in patients with renal or hepatic impairment, severe allergy, bronchial asthma, or G6PD deficiency
Carcinogenicity, mutagenicity, effect on fertility	No adequate studies have been done to determine the carcinogenic potential of sulfamethoxazole; chromosomal abnormalities have not been detected in cultured human leukocytes. In rats, oral administration at up to 350 mg/kg/day has produced no adverse effects on fertility.

ADVERSE REACTIONS[1]

Hematological	Agranulocytosis, aplastic anemia, thrombocytopenia, leukopenia, hemolytic anemia, purpura, hypoprothrombinemia, methemoglobinemia, neutropenia, eosinophilia
Dermatological	Stevens-Johnson syndrome, epidermal necrolysis, erythema multiforme, exfoliative dermatitis, photosensitivity, pruritus, urticaria, rash, generalized skin eruptions
Gastrointestinal	Hepatitis, hepatocellular necrosis, pseudomembranous enterocolitis, pancreatitis, stomatitis, glossitis, nausea, emesis, abdominal pain, diarrhea, anorexia
Genitourinary	Elevated serum creatinine level, toxic nephrosis with oliguria and anuria
Central nervous system	Convulsions, peripheral neuritis, ataxia, vertigo, tinnitus, headache, hallucinations, depression, apathy, weakness, fatigue, insomnia
Endocrinological	Diuresis and hypoglycemia (rare)
Musculoskeletal	Arthralgia, myalgia
Hypersensitivity	Anaphylaxis, allergic myocarditis, serum sickness, conjunctival and scleral injection, generalized allergic reactions, periarteritis nodosa, systemic lupus erythematosus
Other	Edema (including periorbital edema), pyrexia, chills

OVERDOSAGE

Signs and symptoms	Anorexia, colic, nausea, vomiting, dizziness, headache, drowsiness, unconsciousness, pyrexia, hematuria, crystalluria, blood dyscrasias, jaundice
Treatment	Induce emesis or perform gastric lavage. To enhance renal elimination, acidify urine and institute forced diuresis; if urine output is low and renal function is normal, administer IV fluids. Monitor blood count and electrolyte balance. Institute appropriate therapy if jaundice or a significant blood dyscrasia occurs. Peritoneal dialysis is not useful and hemodialysis is only moderately effective in removing sulfonamides.

DRUG INTERACTIONS

Diuretics (especially thiazides)	△ Risk of thrombocytopenic purpura in elderly patients
Warfarin	△ Prothrombin time; if sulfamethoxazole is given during warfarin therapy, recheck prothrombin time
Phenytoin	△ Serum half-life of phenytoin; watch for evidence of phenytoin toxicity during combination therapy
Methotrexate	△ Serum level of methotrexate

ALTERED LABORATORY VALUES

Blood/serum values	△ Creatinine (especially with Jaffé test)

No clinically significant alterations in urinary values occur at therapeutic dosages

---

USE IN CHILDREN

See INDICATIONS and ORAL DOSAGE; use in infants under 2 mo of age for disorders other than congenital toxoplasmosis is contraindicated. Prolonged or intermittent treatment of chronic renal disease in children under 6 yr of age has not been adequately studied.

USE IN PREGNANT AND NURSING WOMEN

Pregnancy Category C: in rats, oral doses of 533 mg/kg have produced teratogenic effects characterized mainly by cleft palate; use during pregnancy (except at term) only if the expected benefit justifies the potential risks to the fetus. Administration at term or while the patient is nursing is contraindicated because, after crossing the placenta or being excreted in human milk, sulfonamides can cause kernicterus.

---

[1] Includes reactions common to sulfonamides in general

SULFONAMIDES

GANTRISIN (sulfisoxazole) Roche   Rx

Tablets: 0.5 g sulfisoxazole   **Pediatric suspension (per 5 ml):** acetyl sulfisoxazole equivalent to 0.5 g sulfisoxazole (4, 16 fl oz) *raspberry-flavored*   **Syrup (per 5 ml):** acetyl sulfisoxazole equivalent to 0.5 g sulfisoxazole (16 fl oz) *chocolate-flavored*

INDICATIONS

Acute, recurrent, or chronic urinary tract infections caused by susceptible strains of *Escherichia coli*, *Klebsiella-Enterobacter*, staphylococci, *Proteus mirabilis*, and *P vulgaris* in the absence of obstructive uropathy and foreign bodies
Meningococcal meningitis caused by sulfonamide-sensitive strains
Hemophilus influenzae **meningitis** (as an adjunct to parenteral streptomycin therapy)
Prophylaxis of meningococcal meningitis caused by sulfonamide-sensitive Group A strains
Acute otitis media caused by *Hemophilus influenzae* when used concomitantly with penicillin or erythromycin
Trachoma
Inclusion conjunctivitis
Nocardiosis
Chancroid
Toxoplasmosis (adjunctive therapy with pyrimethamine)
Malaria caused by chloroquine-resistant strains of *Plasmodium falciparum* (adjunctive therapy)

ORAL DOSAGE

Adult: 2–4 g to start, followed by 4–8 g/24 h in 4–6 divided doses
Infant ($\geq$ 2 mo) and child: 75 mg/kg (2 g/m^2) to start, followed by 150 mg/kg/24 h (4 g/m^2/24 h) in 4–6 divided doses, up to 6 g/24 h

CONTRAINDICATIONS

Pregnancy at term   Age < 2 mo (see USE IN CHILDREN)   Hypersensitivity to sulfonamides
Breast-feeding

ADMINISTRATION/DOSAGE ADJUSTMENTS

Susceptibility	In vitro susceptibility tests are not always reliable; carefully coordinate test results with bacteriological and clinical response. Bear in mind that resistance to sulfonamides is becoming more common, especially in the treatment of chronic and recurrent urinary tract infections. When performing follow-up cultures during therapy, add aminobenzoic acid to the culture media.
Therapeutic blood levels	For most infections, 5–15 mg/dl; for serious infections, 12–15 mg/dl; blood levels > 20 mg/dl increase the probability of adverse reactions. Blood levels should be measured in patients with serious infections.

WARNINGS/PRECAUTIONS

Group A beta-hemolytic streptococcal infections	Sulfonamides have no place in the treatment of such infections since they will neither eradicate the causative organism nor prevent complications
Life-threatening infections	Severe, potentially fatal reactions, including hepatocellular necrosis, hypersensitivity reactions, and serious blood dyscrasias (eg, agranulocytosis, aplastic anemia), have occurred in patients receiving sulfonamides. These drugs have caused hemolytic anemia in patients with G6PD deficiency. When using this product, obtain a CBC frequently and watch for early clinical signs such as sore throat, fever, pallor, purpura, and jaundice; if the count of a formed blood element falls significantly, administration should be discontinued.
Cross-sensitivity	Patients allergic to acetazolamide, thiazide-type diuretics, sulfonylureas, or certain goitrogens may also be hypersensitive to sulfisoxazole
Renal effects	Crystalluria, urolithiasis, and other renal complications have occurred in patients taking sulfonamides; the frequency is considerably lower with a more soluble sulfonamide such as sulfisoxazole. Caution patients to maintain an adequate fluid intake; renal function tests and urinalyses, including careful microscopic examination, should be performed during therapy, particularly when a patient has renal impairment.
Special-risk patients	Use with caution in patients with renal or hepatic impairment, severe allergy, bronchial asthma, or G6PD deficiency
Carcinogenicity, mutagenicity, effect of fertility	No evidence of carcinogenicity has been seen after 103 wk in rats given 400 mg/kg/day or in mice given up to 2 g/kg/day. Sulfisoxazole has been shown to be nonmutagenic in *E coli* Sd-4-73. No adverse effects on fertility have been seen in rats given 800 mg/kg/day.

ADVERSE REACTIONS[1]

Hematological	Agranulocytosis, aplastic anemia, thrombocytopenia, leukopenia, hemolytic anemia, purpura, hypoprothrombinemia, methemoglobinemia, eosinophilia
Dermatological	Stevens-Johnson syndrome, epidermal necrolysis, erythema multiforme, exfoliative dermatitis, photosensitivity, pruritus, urticaria, rash, generalized skin eruptions
Gastrointestinal	Hepatitis, hepatocellular necrosis, pseudomembranous enterocolitis, pancreatitis, stomatitis, glossitis, nausea, emesis, abdominal pain, diarrhea, anorexia

GANTRISIN ■ RENOQUID

Genitourinary	Elevated serum creatinine level, toxic nephrosis with oliguria and anuria
Central nervous system	Convulsions, peripheral neuritis, ataxia, vertigo, tinnitus, headache, hallucinations, depression, apathy, weakness, fatigue, insomnia
Endocrinological	Diuresis and hypoglycemia (rare)
Musculoskeletal	Arthralgia, myalgia
Hypersensitivity	Anaphylaxis, allergic myocarditis, serum sickness, conjunctival and scleral injection, generalized allergic reactions, periarteritis nodosa, systemic lupus erythematosus
Other	Edema (including periorbital edema), pyrexia, chills

OVERDOSAGE

Signs and symptoms	Anorexia, colic, nausea, vomiting, dizziness, headache, drowsiness, unconsciousness, pyrexia, hematuria, crystalluria, blood dyscrasias, jaundice
Treatment	Induce emesis or perform gastric lavage. To enhance renal elimination, acidify urine and institute forced diuresis; if urine output is low and renal function is normal, administer IV fluids. Monitor blood count and electrolyte balance. Institute appropriate therapy if jaundice or a significant blood dyscrasia occurs. Peritoneal dialysis is not useful and hemodialysis is only moderately effective in removing sulfonamides.

DRUG INTERACTIONS

Warfarin	⇧ Prothrombin time; if sulfisoxazole is given during warfarin therapy, recheck prothrombin time
Thiopental	⇧ Pharmacological effect of thiopental; a smaller anesthetic dose of thiopental may be required if the patient is receiving sulfisoxazole
Methotrexate	⇧ Serum level of methotrexate
Sulfonylureas	⇧ Hypoglycemic effect of sulfonylureas

ALTERED LABORATORY VALUES

Blood/serum values	⇧ Creatinine

No clinically significant alterations in urinary values occur at therapeutic dosages

---

USE IN CHILDREN

See INDICATIONS and ORAL DOSAGE; use in infants under 2 mo of age for disorders other than congenital toxoplasmosis is contraindicated

USE IN PREGNANT AND NURSING WOMEN

Pregnancy Category C: administration of 1 g/kg/day (9–18 times the usual adult dosage) has produced skeletal defects in rats and cleft palate in both rats and mice; use during pregnancy (except at term) only if the expected benefit justifies the potential risks to the fetus. Administration at term or while the patient is nursing is contraindicated because, after crossing the placenta or being excreted in human milk, sulfonamides can cause kernicterus.

---

[1] Includes reactions common to sulfonamides in general

SULFONAMIDES

RENOQUID (sulfacytine) Glenwood   Rx

Tablets: 250 mg

INDICATIONS

Acute urinary tract infections caused by susceptible strains of *Escherichia coli*, *Klebsiella-Enterobacter*, *Staphylococcus aureus*, *Proteus mirabilis*, and *P vulgaris* in the absence of obstructive uropathy and foreign bodies

ORAL DOSAGE

Adult: 500 mg to start, followed by 250 mg qid for 10 days

CONTRAINDICATIONS

Pregnancy at term	Age < 2 mo	Hypersensitivity to sulfonamides
Breast-feeding		

WARNINGS/PRECAUTIONS

In vitro sulfonamide sensitivity tests	May not be reliable; coordinate test results with bacteriological and clinical response
Blood dyscrasias	May occur and can be fatal (see ADVERSE REACTIONS); obtain CBC frequently and watch for early signs (eg, sore throat, fever, pallor, purpura, jaundice) of serious blood disorders

RENOQUID ■ THIOSULFIL

Hypersensitivity reactions	May occur and can be fatal (see ADVERSE REACTIONS); use with caution in patients allergic to some goitrogens, diuretics, and oral hypoglycemic agents
Renal effects	Crystalluria, urolithiasis, and other renal complications have occurred in patients taking sulfonamides; caution patients to maintain an adequate fluid intake, and perform a urinalysis, including a careful microscopic examination, frequently during therapy
Special-risk patients	Use with caution in patients with impaired renal or hepatic function, severe allergy, bronchial asthma, or G6PD deficiency

ADVERSE REACTIONS[1]

Hematological	Agranulocytosis, aplastic anemia, thrombocytopenia, leukopenia, hemolytic anemia, purpura, hypoprothrombinemia, methemoglobinemia
Allergic	Erythema multiforme (including Stevens-Johnson syndrome), generalized skin eruptions, epidermal necrolysis, urticaria, serum sickness, pruritus, exfoliative dermatitis, anaphylactoid reactions, periorbital edema, conjunctival and scleral injection, photosensitization, arthralgia, allergic myocarditis
Gastrointestinal	Nausea, vomiting, abdominal pain, hepatitis, diarrhea, anorexia, pancreatitis, stomatitis
Central nervous system	Headache, peripheral neuritis, mental depression, convulsions, ataxia, hallucinations, tinnitus, vertigo, insomnia
Renal	Toxic nephrosis with oliguria and anuria, crystalluria, urinary calculi; diuresis (rare)
Endocrinological	Goiter and hypoglycemia (rare)
Other	Drug fever, chills, periarteritis nodosa, lupus erythematosus phenomena

OVERDOSAGE

Signs and symptoms	See ADVERSE REACTIONS
Treatment	Discontinue use of drug; treat symptomatically

DRUG INTERACTIONS

Para-aminobenzoic acid (PABA)	▽ Bacteriostatic effect of sulfacytine
Oral anticoagulants, oral hypoglycemics, methotrexate, phenytoin, thiopental	Pharmacologic effects increased or prolonged △ Risk of toxicity
Methenamine	△ Risk of crystalluria

ALTERED LABORATORY VALUES

Blood-serum values	▽ PBI ▽ ^{131}I thyroid uptake
Urinary values	△ Glucose (with Clinitest tablets)

USE IN CHILDREN

See INDICATIONS; contraindicated for use in infants under 2 mo of age; not recommended for use in children under 14 yr of age

USE IN PREGNANT AND NURSING WOMEN

Safe use has not been established during pregnancy; contraindicated at term and in nursing mothers. Sulfonamides cross the placental barrier, are excreted in breast milk, and may cause kernicterus.

[1] Includes reactions common to sulfonamides in general

SULFONAMIDES

THIOSULFIL (sulfamethizole) Ayerst Rx
Tablets: 0.25 g

THIOSULFIL Forte (sulfamethizole) Ayerst Rx
Tablets: 0.5 g   THIOSULFIL Duo-Pak[1]

INDICATIONS
Urinary tract infections caused by susceptible strains of *Escherichia coli, Klebsiella-Enterobacter, Staphylococcus aureus, Proteus mirabilis,* and *P vulgaris* in the absence of obstructive uropathy and foreign bodies

ORAL DOSAGE
Adult: 0.5–1.0 g tid or qid
Infant (> 2 mo) and child: 30–45 mg/kg/day in 4 divided doses

THIOSULFIL

CONTRAINDICATIONS

Pregnancy at term	Age < 2 mo	Hypersensitivity to sulfonamides
Breast-feeding		

ADMINISTRATION/DOSAGE ADJUSTMENTS

Therapeutic blood levels	For most infections, 5–15 mg/dl; for serious infections, 12–15 mg/dl. Blood levels > 20 mg/dl increase the probability of adverse reactions. Blood levels should be measured in patients with serious infections.

WARNINGS/PRECAUTIONS

Group A beta-hemolytic streptococcal infections	Sulfonamides have no place in the treatment of such infections, as they will neither eradicate the causative organism nor prevent complications
In vitro sulfonamide sensitivity tests	May not be reliable; coordinate test results with bacteriological and clinical response
Blood dyscrasias	May occur and can be fatal (see ADVERSE REACTIONS); obtain frequent blood counts and watch for early signs (eg, sore throat, fever, pallor, purpura, jaundice) of serious blood disorders
Hypersensitivity reactions	May occur and can be fatal (see ADVERSE REACTIONS); use with caution in patients allergic to some goitrogens, diuretics, and oral hypoglycemic agents
Renal effects	Crystalluria, urolithiasis, and other renal complications have occurred in patients taking sulfonamides; caution patients to maintain an adequate fluid intake, conduct renal function tests frequently (especially during prolonged therapy), and perform a urinalysis, including a microscopic examination, once a week if treatment extends beyond 2 wk
Special-risk patients	Use with caution in patients with severe renal or hepatic impairment, severe allergy, bronchial asthma, or G6PD deficiency (hemolysis may occur)
Carcinogenicity	Long-term administration of sulfonamides has been associated with thyroid malignancies in rats

ADVERSE REACTIONS

Hematological	Agranulocytosis, aplastic anemia, thrombocytopenia, leukopenia, hemolytic anemia, purpura, hypoprothrombinemia, methemoglobinemia
Allergic	Erythema multiforme (Stevens-Johnson syndrome), generalized skin eruptions, epidermal necrolysis, urticaria, serum sickness, pruritus, exfoliative dermatitis, anaphylactoid reactions, periorbital edema, conjunctival and scleral injection, photosensitization, arthralgia, allergic myocarditis
Gastrointestinal	Nausea, vomiting, abdominal pain, hepatitis, diarrhea, anorexia, pancreatitis, stomatitis
Central nervous system	Headache, peripheral neuritis, mental depression, convulsions, ataxia, hallucinations, tinnitus, vertigo, insomnia
Renal	Toxic nephrosis with oliguria and anuria; diuresis (rare)
Endocrinological	Goiter and hypoglycemia (rare)
Other	Drug fever, chills, periarteritis nodosa, lupus erythematosus phenomena

OVERDOSAGE

Signs and symptoms	See ADVERSE REACTIONS
Treatment	Discontinue use of drug; treat symptomatically

DRUG INTERACTIONS

Para-aminobenzoic acid (PABA)	▽ Bacteriostatic effect of sulfamethizole
Oral anticoagulants, oral hypoglycemics, methotrexate, phenytoin, thiopental	△ Serum half-life of these drugs
Methenamine	△ Risk of crystalluria

ALTERED LABORATORY VALUES

Blood/serum values	▽ PBI ▽ ^{131}I thyroid uptake
Urinary values	△ Glucose (with Clinitest tablets)

THIOSULFIL ■ BACTRIM

USE IN CHILDREN
See INDICATIONS; contraindicated for use in infants under 2 mo of age

USE IN PREGNANT AND NURSING WOMEN
Safety for use during pregnancy has not been established (sulfonamides cross the placental barrier); administration at term is contraindicated. A significant increase in the incidence of cleft palate and other bony abnormalities has been detected in the offspring of rats and mice fed certain sulfonamides in large amounts (7–25 times the human therapeutic dose); however, the teratogenic potential of most sulfonamides has not been thoroughly studied in animals or humans. Use in nursing mothers is contraindicated; sulfonamides are excreted in breast milk and may cause kernicterus.

[1] Combination of Thiosulfil Forte tablets and Thiosulfil-A Forte (sulfamethizole and phenazopyridine) tablets; see Thiosulfil-A chart for dosage information

---

MISCELLANEOUS ANTI-INFECTIVE AGENTS

BACTRIM (trimethoprim and sulfamethoxazole) Roche — Rx

Tablets: 80 mg trimethoprim and 400 mg sulfamethoxazole **Suspension (per 5 ml):** 40 mg trimethoprim and 200 mg sulfamethoxazole[1] (16 fl oz) *fruit/licorice-flavored* **Pediatric suspension (per 5 ml):** 40 mg trimethoprim and 200 mg sulfamethoxazole[1] (100 ml, 16 fl oz) *cherry-flavored*

BACTRIM DS (trimethoprim and sulfamethoxazole) Roche — Rx

Tablets: 160 mg trimethoprim and 800 mg sulfamethoxazole

INDICATIONS / ORAL DOSAGE

Urinary tract infections caused by susceptible strains of *Escherichia coli*, *Klebsiella*, *Enterobacter*, *Morganella morganii*, *Proteus mirabilis*, and *P vulgaris* [2]

Adult: 2 Bactrim tabs, 1 Bactrim DS tab, or 20 ml (4 tsp) q12h for 10–14 days
Child (≥ 2 mo): 4 mg/kg trimethoprim and 20 mg/kg sulfamethoxazole q12h for 10 days, as follows:
Child (10 kg): 5 ml (1 tsp) q12h for 10 days
Child (20 kg): 1 Bactrim tab or 10 ml (2 tsp) q12h for 10 days
Child (30 kg): 1½ Bactrim tabs or 15 ml (3 tsp) q12h for 10 days
Child (40 kg): 2 Bactrim tabs, 1 Bactrim DS tab, or 20 ml (4 tsp) q12h for 10 days

Acute otitis media caused by susceptible strains of *Hemophilus influenzae* or *Streptococcus pneumoniae*[3]

Child (≥ 2 mo): same as pediatric dosages above

Acute exacerbations of chronic bronchitis caused by susceptible strains of *Hemophilus influenzae* or *Streptococcus pneumoniae*[4]

Adult: same as adult dosage above for 14 days

Enteritis caused by susceptible strains of *Shigella flexneri* and *S sonnei*

Adult: same as adult dosage above for 5 days
Child (≥ 2 mo): same as pediatric dosages above for 5 days

Pneumocystis carinii pneumonitis

Adult: 5 mg/kg trimethoprim and 25 mg/kg sulfamethoxazole q6h for 14 days
Child (≥ 2 mo): same as adult, as follows:
Child (8 kg): 5 ml (1 tsp) q6h for 14 days
Child (16 kg): 1 Bactrim tab or 10 ml (2 tsp) q6h for 14 days
Child (24 kg): 1½ Bactrim tabs or 15 ml (3 tsp) q6h for 14 days
Child (32 kg): 2 Bactrim tabs, 1 Bactrim DS tab, or 20 ml (4 tsp) q6h for 14 days

CONTRAINDICATIONS

Pregnancy at term
Breast-feeding
Age < 2 mo
Hypersensitivity to trimethoprim or sulfonamides
Megaloblastic anemia due to folate deficiency

ADMINISTRATION/DOSAGE ADJUSTMENTS

Patients with renal impairment — Follow the usual dosage regimen if creatinine clearance (Ccr) > 30 ml/min. Administer half the usual dosage if Ccr = 15–30 ml/min. Use is not recommended if Ccr < 15 ml/min.

WARNINGS/PRECAUTIONS

Group A beta-hemolytic streptococcal pharyngitis — Sulfonamides have no place in the treatment of such infections, as they will neither eradicate the causative organism from the tonsillopharyngeal area nor prevent complications

BACTRIM

Life-threatening reactions	Severe, potentially fatal reactions, including Stevens-Johnson syndrome, toxic epidermal necrolysis, fulminant hepatic necrosis, and serious blood dyscrasias (eg, agranulocytosis, aplastic anemia) have occurred on rare occasions in patients receiving sulfonamides. These drugs have caused hemolytic anemia in patients with G6PD deficiency. The risk of severe adverse reactions may be increased in elderly patients, particularly when these patients are receiving other drugs (see DRUG INTERACTIONS) or they have renal or hepatic impairment or another complicating condition; the most frequent serious adverse effects seen in elderly patients are severe skin reactions, generalized bone marrow depression, and thrombocytopenia. When using this preparation, obtain a CBC frequently and watch for early clinical signs such as rash, sore throat, fever, pallor, purpura, and jaundice; *discontinue administration at the first sign of skin rash or any adverse reaction.*
Bone marrow depression	High doses or prolonged use may cause bone marrow depression and, as a result, produce thrombocytopenia, leukopenia, and/or megaloplastic anemia; if signs of bone marrow depression appear, give 5-15 mg/day of leucovorin until normal hematopoiesis is restored
Cross-sensitivity	Patients allergic to acetazolamide, thiazide-type diuretics, sulfonylureas, or certain goitrogens may also be hypersensitive to this preparation
Renal effects	Crystalluria, urolithiasis, and other renal complications have occurred in patients taking sulfonamides. Caution patients to maintain an adequate fluid intake; urinalysis, including careful microscopic examination, and renal function tests should be performed during therapy, particularly when a patient has renal impairment.
Special-risk patients	Use with caution in elderly patients and those with renal or hepatic impairment, possible folate deficiency, severe allergies, bronchial asthma, or G6PD deficiency. Among the conditions that may be associated with folate deficiency are malnutrition, malabsorption syndrome, chronic alcoholism, advanced age, and anticonvulsant therapy.
AIDS	Patients with AIDS may not tolerate or respond to this preparation in the same manner as other patients; the frequency of adverse effects, particularly rash, fever, and leukopenia, has been reported to be greatly increased in AIDS patients who were undergoing treatment of *Pneumocystis carinii* pneumonia
Carcinogenicity	No long-term studies have been done in animals to evaluate the oncogenic potential of this drug
Mutagenicity	Although bacterial mutagenicity studies have not been done with this preparation, trimethoprim alone has shown no mutagenic potential in the Ames assay, and no chromosomal abnormalities have been detected in human leukocytes cultured in vitro with either component alone or in combination or in leukocytes from treated patients
Effect on fertility	No adverse effects on fertility or general reproductive performance have been observed in rats given oral dosages as high as 70 mg/kg/day of trimethoprim plus 350 mg/kg/day of sulfamethoxazole

ADVERSE REACTIONS

Hematological	Agranulocytosis, aplastic anemia, thrombocytopenia, leukopenia, neutropenia, hemolytic anemia, megaloblastic anemia, hypoprothrombinemia, methemoglobinemia, eosinophilia
Gastrointestinal	Hepatitis (including cholestatic jaundice and fulminant hepatic necrosis), elevation of serum transaminase and bilirubin levels, pseudomembranous enterocolitis, pancreatitis, stomatitis, glossitis, nausea, vomiting, abdominal pain, diarrhea, anorexia
Genitourinary	Renal failure, interstitial nephritis, elevation of BUN and serum creatinine levels, toxic nephrosis with oliguria and anuria, crystalluria
Central nervous system	Aseptic meningitis, convulsions, peripheral neuritis, ataxia, vertigo, tinnitus, headache, hallucinations, depression, apathy, nervousness, weakness, fatigue, insomnia
Endocrinological	Diuresis, hypoglycemia
Musculoskeletal	Arthralgia, myalgia
Hypersensitivity	Stevens-Johnson syndrome, toxic epidermal necrolysis, anaphylaxis, allergic myocarditis, erythema multiforme, exfoliative dermatitis, angioedema, drug fever, chills, Henoch-Schoenlein purpura, serum sickness–like syndrome, generalized allergic reactions, generalized skin eruptions, photosensitivity, conjunctival and scleral injection, pruritus, urticaria, rash, periarteritis nodosa, systemic lupus erythematosus

OVERDOSAGE

Signs and symptoms	Anorexia, colic, nausea, vomiting, dizziness, headache, drowsiness, mental depression, confusion, unconsciousness, pyrexia, hematuria, crystalluria, bone marrow depression, other blood dyscrasias, jaundice
Treatment	Induce emesis or perform gastric lavage. To enhance renal elimination, acidify urine and institute forced diuresis; if urine output is low and renal function is normal, administer IV fluids. Monitor blood counts and electrolyte balance. Institute specific therapy if jaundice or a significant blood dyscrasia occurs. Peritoneal dialysis is not useful, and hemodialysis only moderately effective, in removing the components of this preparation.

BACTRIM ■ BACTRIM I.V. Infusion

DRUG INTERACTIONS

Diuretics (especially thiazides)	△ Risk of thrombocytopenic purpura in elderly patients
Warfarin	△ Prothrombin time; if this preparation is given during warfarin therapy, recheck prothrombin time
Phenytoin	△ Serum half-life of phenytoin; watch for evidence of phenytoin toxicity during combination therapy
Methotrexate	△ Serum level of methotrexate

ALTERED LABORATORY VALUES

Blood/serum values	△ Methotrexate (with competitive binding protein assay using dihydrofolate reductase) △ BUN △ Creatinine (especially with Jaffé test) △ Bilirubin △ SGOT △ SGPT ▽ PBI ▽ [131]I thyroid uptake

No clinically significant alterations in urinary values occur at therapeutic dosages

---

USE IN CHILDREN

See INDICATIONS and ORAL DOSAGE. Data on the safety of repeated use in children under 2 yr of age are limited; contraindicated for infants under 2 mo of age.

USE IN PREGNANT AND NURSING WOMEN

Pregnancy Category C: use during pregnancy only if expected benefit justifies the potential fetal risk, since the drug may interfere with folic acid metabolism. Teratogenic effects (mainly cleft palate) have been observed in rats and increased fetal loss has been observed in rats and rabbits at doses several times the recommended human dose. Although no large, well-controlled studies have been done in pregnant women, two limited studies have shown no increase in congenital abnormalities. The drug is contraindicated at term and for use in nursing mothers because sulfonamides cross the placental barrier, are excreted in human milk, and may cause kernicterus.

---

[1] Contains 0.3% alcohol
[2] Initial episodes of uncomplicated infections should be treated with a single, effective antibacterial agent, rather than a combination
[3] Not indicated for prophylaxis or prolonged administration
[4] When in the physician's judgment this preparation offers some advantage over the use of a single antimicrobial agent

---

MISCELLANEOUS ANTI-INFECTIVE AGENTS

BACTRIM I.V. Infusion (trimethoprim and sulfamethoxazole) Roche   Rx

Ampuls (per 5 ml): 80 mg trimethoprim and 400 mg sulfamethoxazole (5 ml) for IV infusion only **Vials (per 5 ml):** 80 mg trimethoprim and 400 mg sulfamethoxazole (5, 10, 30 ml) for IV infusion only

INDICATIONS

PARENTERAL DOSAGE[1]

Pneumocystis carinii pneumonitis

Adult: 15–20 mg/kg/day, given in 3 or 4 equally divided doses via IV infusion q6–8h
Child: same as adult

Severe or complicated **urinary tract infections** caused by susceptible strains of *Escherichia coli, Klebsiella, Enterobacter, Morganella morganii,* and *Proteus,* when oral administration is not feasible or when the organism is not susceptible to single urinary anti-infectives alone
Enteritis caused by susceptible strains of *Shigella flexneri* and *S sonnei*

Adult: 8–10 mg/kg/day, up to 960 mg/day, given in 2–4 equally divided doses via IV infusion q6–12h
Child: same as adult

CONTRAINDICATIONS

Pregnancy at term	Hypersensitivity to trimethoprim or sulfonamides	Documented megaloblastic anemia due to folate deficiency
Breast-feeding	Age < 2 mo	

ADMINISTRATION/DOSAGE ADJUSTMENTS

Preparation of infusion	Dilute each 5 ml of the preparation in 125 ml of 5% dextrose-in-water and use within 6 h; do not refrigerate. If fluid restriction is desired, dilute in 100 ml and use within 4 h or dilute in 75 ml and use within 2 h. Do not mix with other drugs or solutions in the same container. The contents of the 30 ml vial must be used within 48 h after withdrawal of the initial dose.
Intravenous administration	Administer slowly by IV drip over a period of 60–90 min; avoid rapid infusion or bolus injection
Local irritation and inflammation	May occur, due to extravascular infiltration of the infusion; discontinue infusion and restart at another site

BACTRIM I.V. Infusion

Susceptibility tests	Cultures and appropriate microbiological tests should be performed to determine susceptibility; therapy may be started, however, before the results of these tests are available
Duration of therapy	Pneumonitis due to *Pneumocystis carinii* and severe urinary tract infections should be treated for up to 14 days and shigellosis for up to 5 days
Patients with renal impairment	Follow the usual dosage regimen if creatinine clearance (Ccr) > 30 ml/min. Administer half the usual dosage if Ccr = 15–30 ml/min; use is not recommended if Ccr < 15 ml/min.

WARNINGS/PRECAUTIONS

Streptococcal pharyngitis	Should not be treated with this drug, as it may fail to eliminate group A beta-hemolytic streptococci from the tonsillopharyngeal area
Life-threatening reactions	Severe, potentially fatal reactions, including Stevens-Johnson syndrome, toxic epidermal necrolysis, fulminant hepatic necrosis, and serious blood dyscrasias (eg, agranulocytosis, aplastic anemia) have occurred on rare occasions in patients receiving sulfonamides. These drugs have caused hemolytic anemia in patients with G6PD deficiency. The risk of severe adverse reactions may be increased in elderly patients, particularly when these patients are receiving other drugs (see DRUG INTERACTIONS) or they have renal or hepatic impairment or another complicating condition; the most frequent serious adverse effects seen in elderly patients are severe skin reactions, generalized bone marrow depression, and thrombocytopenia. When using this preparation, obtain a CBC frequently and watch for early clinical signs such as rash, sore throat, fever, pallor, purpura, and jaundice; *discontinue administration at the first sign of skin rash or any adverse reaction.*
Bone marrow depression	High doses or prolonged use may cause bone marrow depression and, as a result, produce thrombocytopenia, leukopenia, and/or megaloblastic anemia; if signs of bone marrow depression appear, give 5-15 mg/day of leucovorin until normal hematopoiesis is restored
Cross-sensitivity	Patients allergic to acetazolamide, thiazide-type diuretics, sulfonylureas, or certain goitrogens may also be hypersensitive to this preparation
Renal effects	Crystalluria, urolithiasis, and other renal complications have occurred in patients taking sulfonamides. Caution patients to maintain an adequate fluid intake; urinalysis, including careful microscopic examination, and renal function tests should be performed during therapy, particularly when a patient has renal impairment.
Special-risk patients	Use with caution in elderly patients and those with renal or hepatic impairment, possible folate deficiency, severe allergies, bronchial asthma, or G6PD deficiency. Among the conditions that may be associated with folate deficiency are malnutrition, malabsorption syndrome, chronic alcoholism, advanced age, and anticonvulsant therapy.
AIDS	Patients with AIDS may not tolerate or respond to this preparation in the same manner as other patients; the frequency of adverse effects, particularly rash, fever, and leukopenia, has been reported to be greatly increased in AIDS patients who were undergoing treatment of *Pneumocystis carinii* pneumonia
Sulfite sensitivity	Sodium metabisulfite in this product may cause urticaria, pruritus, wheezing, anaphylaxis, or other allergic-type reactions in susceptible patients, such as those with asthma or atopy
Carcinogenicity	No long-term studies have been done in animals to evaluate the oncogenic potential of this drug
Mutagenicity	Although bacterial mutagenicity studies have not been done with this preparation, trimethoprim alone has shown no mutagenic potential in the Ames assay, and no chromosomal abnormalities have been detected in human leukocytes cultured in vitro with either component alone or in combination or in leukocytes from treated patients
Effect on fertility	No adverse effects on fertility or general reproductive performance have been observed in rats given oral dosages as high as 70 mg/kg/day of trimethoprim plus 350 mg/kg/day of sulfamethoxazole

ADVERSE REACTIONS

Hematological	Agranulocytosis, aplastic anemia, thrombocytopenia, leukopenia, neutropenia, hemolytic anemia, megaloblastic anemia, hypoprothrombinemia, methemoglobinemia, eosinophilia
Gastrointestinal	Hepatitis (including cholestatic jaundice and fulminant hepatic necrosis), elevation of serum transaminase and bilirubin levels, pseudomembranous enterocolitis, pancreatitis, stomatitis, glossitis, nausea, vomiting, abdominal pain, diarrhea, anorexia
Genitourinary	Renal failure, interstitial nephritis, elevation of BUN and serum creatinine levels, toxic nephrosis with oliguria and anuria, crystalluria
Central nervous system	Aseptic meningitis, convulsions, peripheral neuritis, ataxia, vertigo, tinnitus, headache, hallucinations, depression, apathy, nervousness, weakness, fatigue, insomnia
Endocrinological	Diuresis, hypoglycemia

BACTRIM I.V. Infusion ■ CHLOROMYCETIN

Musculoskeletal	Arthralgia, myalgia
Hypersensitivity	Stevens-Johnson syndrome, toxic epidermal necrolysis, anaphylaxis, allergic myocarditis, erythema multiforme, exfoliative dermatitis, angioedema, drug fever, chills, Henoch-Schoenlein purpura, serum sickness-like syndrome, generalized allergic reactions, generalized skin eruptions, photosensitivity, conjunctival and scleral injection, pruritus, urticaria, rash, periarteritis nodosa, systemic lupus erythematosus

OVERDOSAGE

Signs and symptoms	Anorexia, colic, nausea, vomiting, dizziness, headache, drowsiness, mental depression, confusion, unconsciousness, pyrexia, hematuria, crystalluria, bone marrow depression, other blood dyscrasias, jaundice
Treatment	To enhance renal elimination, acidify the urine and institute forced diuresis; if output is low and renal function is normal, administer IV fluids. Monitor blood counts and electrolyte balance. Institute specific therapy if jaundice or a significant blood dyscrasia occurs. Peritoneal dialysis is not useful and hemodialysis is only moderately effective in removing the components of this preparation.

DRUG INTERACTIONS

Diuretics (especially thiazides)	△ Risk of thrombocytopenic purpura in elderly patients
Warfarin	△ Prothrombin time; if this preparation is given during warfarin therapy, recheck prothrombin time
Phenytoin	△ Serum half-life of phenytoin; watch for evidence of phenytoin toxicity during combination therapy
Methotrexate	△ Serum level of methotrexate

ALTERED LABORATORY VALUES

Blood/serum values	△ Methotrexate (with competitive binding protein assay using dihydrofolate reductase) △ BUN △ Creatinine (especially with Jaffé test) △ Bilirubin △ SGOT △ SGPT

No clinically significant alterations in urinary values occur at therapeutic dosages

USE IN CHILDREN
Same as adult indications and dosage; contraindicated for use in infants under 2 mo of age

USE IN PREGNANT AND NURSING WOMEN
Pregnancy Category C: use during pregnancy only if expected benefit justifies the potential fetal risk, since the drug may interfere with folic acid metabolism. Teratogenic effects (mainly cleft palate) have been observed in rats and increased fetal loss has been observed in rats and rabbits at doses several times the recommended human dose. Although no large, well-controlled studies have been done in pregnant women, two limited studies have shown no increase in congenital abnormalities. The drug is contraindicated at term and for use in nursing mothers because sulfonamides cross the placental barrier, are excreted in human milk, and may cause kernicterus.

[1] Dosage is based on trimethoprim component

MISCELLANEOUS ANTI-INFECTIVE AGENTS

CHLOROMYCETIN (chloramphenicol) Parke-Davis Rx
Capsules: 250 mg

CHLOROMYCETIN Palmitate (chloramphenicol palmitate) Parke-Davis Rx
Suspension: chloramphenicol palmitate equivalent to 150 mg chloramphenicol/5 ml

CHLOROMYCETIN Sodium Succinate (chloramphenicol sodium succinate) Parke-Davis Rx
Vials: 100 mg/ml when reconstituted (for IV use only)

INDICATIONS
Acute infections caused by susceptible strains of *Salmonella typhi*[1]
Serious infections caused by susceptible strains of *Salmonella, Hemophilus influenzae* (meningeal infections), rickettsia, lymphogranuloma-psittacosis group, and various Gram-negative bacteria, as well as other susceptible organisms resistant to all other appropriate antibiotics[2]
Cystic fibrosis (adjunctive therapy)

ORAL DOSAGE
Adult: 50 mg/kg/day in divided doses q6h; for infections caused by moderately resistant organisms, up to 100 mg/kg/day to start, followed by lower dosages as soon as possible
Newborn (< 2 wk): 25 mg/kg/day in divided doses q6h
Full-term infant (> 2 wk): up to 50 mg/kg/day in divided doses q6h
Child: same as adult

PARENTERAL DOSAGE
Adult: 50 mg/kg/day IV in divided doses q6h
Newborn (< 2 wk): 25 mg/kg/day IV in divided doses q6h
Full-term infant (> 2 wk): up to 50 mg/kg/day IV in divided doses q6h
Child: same as adult

CHLOROMYCETIN

CONTRAINDICATIONS

Hypersensitivity or (for systemic use) prior toxic reaction to chloramphenicol

ADMINISTRATION/DOSAGE ADJUSTMENTS

Infants and children with impaired metabolic processes	Reduce oral and IV dosage to 25 mg/kg/day and follow blood chloramphenicol levels by microtechniques; therapeutic level ranges from 5 to 20 µg/ml
Intravenous administration	Dilute powder supplied with 10 ml of aqueous diluent to a concentration of 100 mg/ml and inject over at least a 1-min period; replace with oral therapy as soon as possible

WARNINGS/PRECAUTIONS

Blood dyscrasias	May occur after short- or long-term oral or parenteral therapy and may be severe or even fatal (see ADVERSE REACTIONS). Obtain blood studies before starting therapy and approximately every 2 days during treatment. Discontinue use upon first sign of abnormality attributable to chloramphenicol (bone-marrow depression may not be evident prior to development of aplastic anemia).
Prolonged or repeated use	Should be avoided; treatment should not be continued longer than required to effect a cure with little or no risk of relapse
Inappropriate indications	Chloramphenicol should not be used in trivial bacterial infections, where not indicated (eg, viral infections), for prophylaxis, or when other, less potentially dangerous drugs would be effective
Hepatic or renal impairment	May result in excessive blood levels; adjust dosage accordingly or (preferably) monitor blood level at appropriate intervals
Superinfection	Overgrowth of nonsusceptible organisms, including fungi, may occur. If overgrowth occurs during topical therapy, discontinue use of chloramphenicol and institute appropriate therapeutic measures.

ADVERSE REACTIONS

Hematological	Pancytopenia; aplastic anemia; hypoplastic anemia; thrombocytopenia; granulocytopenia; reversible bone-marrow depression characterized by vacuolization of erythroid cells, reduction in reticulocyte count, and leukopenia; paroxysmal nocturnal hemoglobinuria
Gastrointestinal	Nausea, vomiting, glossitis, stomatitis, diarrhea, enterocolitis
Central nervous system	Headache, mild depression, mental confusion, delirium, optic and peripheral neuritis (usually following long-term therapy)
Hypersensitivity	Fever, macular and vesicular rashes, angioedema, urticaria, anaphylaxis, Herxheimer reactions (during therapy for typhoid fever)
Other	"Gray syndrome" in premature and newborn infants

OVERDOSAGE

Signs and symptoms	See ADVERSE REACTIONS
Treatment	Discontinue medication; treat symptomatically and institute supportive methods, as required

DRUG INTERACTIONS

Oral anticoagulants	⇧ Prothrombin time
Myelosuppressive agents	⇧ Risk of bone-marrow depression; do not use concomitantly
Chlorpropamide, tolbutamide	⇧ Risk of hypoglycemia
Phenytoin	⇧ Phenytoin blood level and/or toxicity

ALTERED LABORATORY VALUES

Urinary values	⇧ Glucose (with Clinitest tablets)

No clinically significant alterations in blood/serum values occur at therapeutic dosages

---

USE IN CHILDREN

See INDICATIONS; blood levels of drug should be carefully followed by microtechniques in young infants and other children with known or suspected immature metabolic processes. Toxic reactions, including fatalities, have occurred in premature and newborn infants; follow dosage recommendations closely.

USE IN PREGNANT AND NURSING WOMEN

Safe use not established during pregnancy. Chloramphenicol readily crosses the placental barrier; use with particular caution at term or during labor because of potential toxic effects on the fetus ("gray syndrome"). The drug also appears in breast milk and should be used with caution in nursing mothers.

---

[1] Do not use for routine treatment of the carrier state
[2] When used for initial therapy, perform in vitro sensitivity tests to determine if infecting organism is susceptible to other, potentially less hazardous agents

MISCELLANEOUS ANTI-INFECTIVE AGENTS

CLEOCIN HCl (clindamycin hydrochloride) Upjohn Rx
Capsules: clindamycin hydrochloride equivalent to 75 or 150 mg of clindamycin

CLEOCIN PEDIATRIC (clindamycin palmitate hydrochloride) Upjohn Rx
Granules for oral solution (per 5 ml): clindamycin palmitate hydrochloride equivalent to 75 mg clindamycin when reconstituted (100 ml)

CLEOCIN PHOSPHATE (clindamycin phosphate) Upjohn Rx
Ampuls (per milliliter): clindamycin phosphate equivalent to 150 mg clindamycin (2, 4 ml) **Vials (per milliliter):** clindamycin phosphate equivalent to 150 mg clindamycin (2, 4, 6 ml)

INDICATIONS[1]

Serious infections caused by susceptible anaerobic bacteria, including serious respiratory tract infections (eg, empyema, anaerobic pneumonitis, and lung abscesses); serious skin and soft tissue infections; septicemia; intra-abdominal infections (eg, peritonitis, intraabdominal abscesses); infections of the female pelvis and genital tract (eg, endometritis, nongonococcal tubo-ovarian abscesses, pelvic cellulitis, and postsurgical vaginal cuff infection)

Serious respiratory tract infections and serious skin and soft tissue infections caused by susceptible strains of streptococci and staphylococci in penicillin-allergic patients

Serious respiratory tract infections caused by susceptible strains of *Streptococcus pneumoniae* in penicillin-allergic patients

As an adjunct to surgical treatment of **chronic bone and joint infections** caused by susceptible bacteria

ORAL DOSAGE

Adult: 150–300 mg q6h; for more severe infections, 300–450 mg q6h

Child: 8–16 mg/kg/day in 3–4 equally divided doses; for more severe infections, 16–20 mg/kg/day in 3–4 equally divided doses; **pediatric solution:** 8–12 mg/kg/day in 3–4 equally divided doses; for severe infections, 13–16 mg/kg/day in 3–4 equally divided doses; for more severe infections, 17–25 mg/kg/day in 3–4 equally divided doses. Give at least 2.5 ml (37.5 mg) tid to children weighing 10 kg or less

PARENTERAL DOSAGE

Adult: for infections caused by aerobic and more sensitive anaerobic bacteria, 600–1,200 mg/day IM or IV, given in 2–4 equally divided doses; for infections caused by less sensitive anaerobic bacteria (*Bacteroides fragilis, Peptococcus,* and clostridia other than *Clostridium perfringens*) and for more severe infections caused by aerobic and more sensitive anaerobic bacteria, 1,200–2,700 mg/day IM or IV, given in 2–4 equally divided doses; for more serious or life-threatening infections, dosage may be increased (up to 4,800 mg/day has been given IV)

Neonate (< 1 mo): 15–20 mg/kg/day IM or IV, given in 3–4 equally divided doses; for small, premature neonates, 15 mg/kg/day may suffice

Infant (> 1 mo) and child: 20–40 mg/kg/day or 350–450 mg/m²/day IM or IV, given in 3–4 equally divided doses

Adult: same as above
Neonate, infant, and child: same as above

CONTRAINDICATIONS
Hypersensitivity to clindamycin or lincomycin

ADMINISTRATION/DOSAGE ADJUSTMENTS

Parenteral administration	Clindamycin may be administered by continuous or intermittent IV infusion or by deep IM injection. Dilute solution to a concentration of 12 mg/ml or less before IV administration. For intermittent IV infusion, dilute 300 or 600 mg in 50 ml of diluent or 900 or 1,200 mg in 100 ml of diluent. Administer at a rate of 30 mg/min. (Do not exceed this rate, since cardiovascular reactions may occur if infusion is too rapid.) Do not give more than 1,200 mg in a single 1-h infusion. For continuous IV infusion, administer 10–20 mg/min for the first 30 min and thereafter 0.75–1.25 mg/min. Avoid prolonged use of indwelling IV catheters. Single IM doses should not exceed 600 mg.
Esophageal irritation	May be avoided by administering capsules with a full glass of water
Adjunctive therapy	Perform indicated surgical procedures in conjunction with antibiotic therapy; obtain bacteriological studies to determine the causative organisms and their susceptibility to clindamycin
Beta-hemolytic streptococcal infections	Continue treatment for at least 10 days to prevent rheumatic fever and glomerulonephritis
Anaerobic infections	Although serious anaerobic infections are usually treated by injection, treatment may be initiated or continued with oral therapy

WARNINGS/PRECAUTIONS

Inappropriate indications	Clindamycin should not be used in patients with nonbacterial infections (eg, most upper respiratory tract infections) or in the treatment of meningitis, since adequate diffusion into the CSF does not occur
Superinfection	May result in the overgrowth of nonsusceptible organisms, particularly yeasts

CLEOCIN

Severe, potentially fatal colitis	May occur due to enterotoxin-producing strains of *Clostridium* (particularly *C difficile*). May be characterized by severe persistent diarrhea and abdominal cramps, and may be associated with the passage of blood and mucus; endoscopic examination may reveal pseudomembranous colitis. Onset of signs and symptoms may occur during therapy or up to several weeks after cessation of use. When significant diarrhea occurs, discontinue medication or, if necessary, continue only with close observation; large bowel endoscopy is recommended. Antiperistaltic agents (eg, opiates and diphenyloxylate with atropine) may prolong and/or worsen the condition. Mild cases of colitis may respond to withdrawal of the drug alone. Moderate to severe cases should be managed by fluid and electrolyte replacement and protein supplementation. The use of systemic corticosteroids and steroid retention enemas may help relieve the colitis. For pseudomembranous colitis produced by *Clostridium difficile,* administer vancomycin, 0.5–2 g/day, given orally in 3–4 divided doses for 7–10 days. If cholestyramine or colestipol are administered to bind the toxin, they should not be given at the same time as vancomycin, as vancomycin may also be bound to the resin. Rule out other possible causes.
Hypersensitivity	On rare occasions, anaphylaxis or other serious allergic reactions may occur during therapy; ensure that epinephrine, corticosteroids, and antihistamines are available for emergency treatment. Generalized mild to moderate morbilliform-like rash is the adverse reaction seen most frequently with clindamycin. If a hypersensitivity reaction occurs during therapy, discontinue drug and take appropriate measures.
Special-risk patients	Use with caution in the elderly and in patients with a history of GI disease (particularly colitis), atopic individuals, or patients with very severe renal or hepatic disease accompanied by severe metabolic aberrations. Monitor serum levels during high-dose therapy; severely ill older patients should be closely followed for changes in bowel frequency.
Prolonged therapy	Perform periodic liver- and kidney-function tests and blood counts
Tartrazine sensitivity	Presence of FD&C Yellow No. 5 (tartrazine) in capsules may cause allergic-type reactions, including bronchial asthma, in susceptible individuals

ADVERSE REACTIONS[2]

Gastrointestinal	Abdominal pain, esophagitis, nausea, vomiting, diarrhea, colitis (including pseudomembranous colitis), jaundice, abnormal liver-function tests
Musculoskeletal	Polyarthritis (rare)
Cardiovascular	Thrombophlebitis following IV infusion; cardiopulmonary arrest and hypotension following too rapid infusion (rare)
Hypersensitivity	Maculopapular rash, urticaria, generalized mild to moderate morbilliform-like skin rashes; erythema multiforme (sometimes resembling Stevens-Johnson syndrome) and anaphylactoid reactions (rare)
Other	Pain, induration, and sterile abscess (with IM use)

OVERDOSAGE

Signs and symptoms	See ADVERSE REACTIONS
Treatment	Discontinue medication; treat symptomatically

DRUG INTERACTIONS

General anesthetics, neuromuscular-blocking agents	⇧ Neuromuscular blockade, resulting in skeletal muscle weakness, respiratory depression, or paralysis
Antiperistaltic antidiarrheal agents	⇧ Risk and severity of diarrhea
Chloramphenicol, erythromycin	⇩ Antibacterial effect of clindamycin; do not use concomitantly
Kaolin	⇩ Absorption of clindamycin
Ampicillin, phenytoin sodium, barbiturates, aminophylline, calcium gluconate, magnesium sulfate	Physical incompatibility when mixed in IV solutions

ALTERED LABORATORY VALUES

Blood/serum values	Abnormal liver function values

No clinically significant alterations in urinary values occur at therapeutic dosages

---

USE IN CHILDREN

See INDICATIONS; monitor organ system function when treating newborns and infants

USE IN PREGNANT AND NURSING WOMEN

Safe use during pregnancy not established; clindamycin appears in breast milk at levels approximating maternal blood levels (0.7–3.8 µg/ml)

---

[1] In vitro susceptibility to clindamycin has been shown with anaerobic bacteria, including strains of *Bacteroides, Fusobacterium, Propionibacterium, Eubacterium, Actinomyces, Peptococcus, Peptostreptococcus,* and *Clostridium* and with other bacteria, including strains of *Staphylococcus aureus* and *S epidermidis* and strains of *Streptococcus pneumoniae,* microaerophilic streptococci, and other streptococci (except *Streptococcus fecalis*)
[2] Reactions for which a causal relationship has not been established include azotemia, oliguria, proteinuria, transient neutropenia (leukopenia), eosinophilia, agranulocytosis, and thrombocytopenia

MISCELLANEOUS ANTI-INFECTIVE AGENTS

COLY-MYCIN M (colistimethate sodium) Parke-Davis   Rx

Vials: colistimethate sodium equivalent to 150 mg colistin

INDICATIONS

Acute or chronic infections caused by susceptible strains of *Enterobacter aerogenes, Escherichia coli, Klebsiella pneumoniae,* and *Pseudomonas aeruginosa*

PARENTERAL DOSAGE

Adult: 2.5–5 mg/kg/day IM or IV, given in 2–4 divided doses; do not exceed the maximum dosage
Child: same as adult

CONTRAINDICATIONS

Hypersensitivity to colistimethate

ADMINISTRATION/DOSAGE ADJUSTMENTS

Preparation of parenteral solution	Reconstitute the contents of the vial with 2 ml of Sterile Water for Injection USP; swirl gently to avoid frothing. For infusion, add the required amount of the reconstituted drug to one of the following: 0.9% sodium chloride, 5% dextrose in water or 0.225–0.9% sodium chloride, lactated Ringer's solution, or 10% invert sugar solution (the choice and volume of solution to be used depends on the patient's fluid and electrolyte requirements). Any infusion solution containing colistimethate should be freshly prepared and used within 24 h.
Intermittent intravenous administration	Administer one half the daily dose slowly (over 3–5 min) q12h
Continuous intravenous infusion	Slowly inject one half the daily dose over a period of 3–5 min and administer the remaining half as a slow infusion (5–6 mg/h) 1–2 h after the initial dose
Patients with renal impairment	Modify dosage schedule as follows: 75–115 mg bid when plasma creatinine concentration = 1.3–1.5 mg/dl; 66–150 mg bid or once daily when plasma creatinine concentration = 1.6–2.5 mg/dl; 100–150 mg q36h when plasma creatinine concentration = 2.6–4 mg/dl

WARNINGS/PRECAUTIONS

Neurological disturbances	Transient neurological disturbances may occur, including slurred speech, vertigo, dizziness, circumoral paresthesias or numbness, tingling or formication of the extremities, and generalized pruritus; caution ambulatory patients not to drive or engage in other potentially hazardous activities. If such reactions occur, reduce the dosage and keep the patient under careful observation.
Renal impairment	Use with caution, especially in elderly patients (see ADMINISTRATION/DOSAGE ADJUSTMENTS). Further impairment, acute renal insufficiency, renal shutdown, and further concentration to toxic levels can occur. Interference of nerve transmission at neuromuscular junctions may then occur and result in muscle weakness and apnea. The drug should be discontinued at the first sign of decreased urine output or rising BUN and serum creatinine concentration. In life-threatening situations, therapy may be reinstated at a lower dosage after blood levels have fallen.
Concomitant therapy	Other antibiotics with a Gram-negative antimicrobial spectrum and curariform muscle relaxants should be given only with extreme caution (see DRUG INTERACTIONS)

ADVERSE REACTIONS

Respiratory	Respiratory arrest, apnea
Neurological	Paresthesias, tingling of extremities and/or tongue, neuromuscular blockade, vertigo, slurred speech
Renal	Nephrotoxicity, decreased urine output
Gastrointestinal	Upset
Hypersensitivity	Generalized itching, urticaria, drug fever

OVERDOSAGE

Signs and symptoms	Renal insufficiency, muscular weakness, apnea, neuromuscular blockade
Treatment	Discontinue medication; institute supportive measures, including assisted ventilation, oxygen therapy, and IV calcium chloride, as needed

DRUG INTERACTIONS

Kanamycin, streptomycin, polymyxin B, neomycin	⇧ Risk of neurotoxicity
Cephalothin	⇧ Risk of nephrotoxicity
Curariform muscle relaxants	⇧ Neuromuscular blockade

ALTERED LABORATORY VALUES

Blood/serum values	⇧ BUN ⇧ Creatinine

Urinary values ——————————— ⬆ Protein

USE IN CHILDREN	USE IN PREGNANT AND NURSING WOMEN
Same as adult indications and dosage	Safety for use during pregnancy has not been established; colistimethate crosses the placental barrier. Consult manufacturer for use in nursing mothers.

MISCELLANEOUS ANTI-INFECTIVE AGENTS

COLY-MYCIN S (colistin sulfate) Parke-Davis   Rx
Suspension (per 5 ml): 25 mg after reconstitution (300 mg) *chocolate-flavored*

INDICATIONS	ORAL DOSAGE
Diarrhea caused by susceptible strains of enteropathogenic *Escherichia coli* **Gastroenteritis** due to *Shigella*	**Infant and child:** 5–15 mg/kg/day, given in 3 divided doses; some patients may require higher dosages

CONTRAINDICATIONS
Hypersensitivity to colistin sulfate

ADMINISTRATION/DOSAGE ADJUSTMENTS

Preparation of oral suspension	Reconstitute with 37 ml of distilled water: Slowly add half the diluent to the bottle, replace the cap, and shake well; then add the remaining diluent and shake again. Volume after reconstitution is 60 ml. The reconstituted suspension is stable for 2 wk when stored below 15° C (59° F).

WARNINGS/PRECAUTIONS

Renal toxicity	May occur in the presence of azotemia or if dosages exceeding the recommended level are used; assess renal function prior to initiating therapy
Prolonged therapy	May result in suppression of the intestinal flora with consequent overgrowth of such organisms as *Proteus;* initiate appropriate therapy immediately if bacterial overgrowth occurs

ADVERSE REACTIONS
None at recommended dosage

OVERDOSAGE

Signs and symptoms	Renal insufficiency, muscular weakness, apnea, neuromuscular blockade
Treatment	Empty stomach by inducing emesis or by gastric lavage. Institute symptomatic and supportive measures, as needed, including assisted respiration and administration of oxygen and IV calcium chloride.

DRUG INTERACTIONS
No clinically significant drug interactions have been identified

ALTERED LABORATORY VALUES
No clinically significant alterations in blood/serum or urinary values occur at therapeutic dosages

USE IN CHILDREN	USE IN PREGNANT AND NURSING WOMEN
See INDICATIONS and ORAL DOSAGE	Not indicated for use in pregnant or nursing women

---

MISCELLANEOUS ANTI-INFECTIVE AGENTS

FLAGYL (metronidazole) Searle   Rx
Tablets: 250, 500 mg

INDICATIONS	ORAL DOSAGE
Symptomatic trichomoniasis, when the presence of trichomonads has been confirmed by appropriate laboratory procedures **Asymptomatic trichomoniasis** associated with endocervicitis, cervicitis, or cervical erosion Treatment of **asymptomatic partners** of treated patients	**Adult:** 250 mg tid for 7 days or, if patient is not pregnant, 2 g given in a single dose or 2 divided doses of 1 g each on the same day. Repeated courses may be given at 4- to 6-wk intervals, upon laboratory confirmation that trichomonads are still present; obtain total and differential leukocyte counts before and after retreatment.

FLAGYL

Acute intestinal amebiasis (acute amebic dysentery)	**Adult:** 750 mg tid for 5–10 days **Child:** 35–50 mg/kg/24 h, given in 3 divided doses for 10 days
Amebic liver abscess	**Adult:** 500–750 mg tid for 5–10 days **Child:** same as child's dosage above
Intraabdominal infections, including peritonitis, intraabdominal abscess, and liver abscess, caused by susceptible strains of *Bacteroides* (including the *B fragilis* group), *Clostridium, Eubacterium, Peptococcus,* and *Peptostreptococcus*	**Adult:** 7.5 mg/kg q6h, up to 4.0 g/24 h
Skin and skin structure infections caused by susceptible strains of *Bacteroides* (including the *B fragilis* group), *Clostridium, Peptococcus, Peptostreptococcus,* and *Fusobacterium*	
Gynecologic infections, including endometritis, endomyometritis, tubo-ovarian abscess, and postsurgical vaginal cuff infection, caused by susceptible strains of *Bacteroides* (including the *B fragilis* group), *Clostridium, Peptococcus,* and *Peptostreptococcus*	
Bacterial septicemia caused by susceptible strains of *Bacteroides* (including the *B fragilis* group) and *Clostridium*	
Bone and joint infections caused by susceptible strains of *Bacteroides* (including the *B fragilis* group) (adjunctive therapy)	
Central nervous system infections, including meningitis and brain abscess, caused by susceptible strains of *Bacteroides* (including the *B fragilis* group)	
Lower respiratory tract infections including pneumonia, empyema, and lung abscess, caused by susceptible strains of *Bacteroides* (including the *B fragilis* group)	
Endocarditis caused by susceptible strains of *Bacteroides* (including the *B fragilis* group)	

CONTRAINDICATIONS

First trimester of pregnancy, when used to treat trichomoniasis	Hypersensitivity to metronidazole or other nitroimidazole derivatives

ADMINISTRATION/DOSAGE ADJUSTMENTS

Duration of therapy for anaerobic infections	Usual duration is 7–10 days; bone and joint infections, lower respiratory tract infections, and endocarditis may require longer treatment
Serious anaerobic infections	Are usually treated first with intravenous metronidazole (Flagyl I.V.)

WARNINGS/PRECAUTIONS

Convulsive seizures and peripheral neuropathy	May occur; warn patient to discontinue use immediately if abnormal neurologic signs appear. Use with caution in patients with CNS diseases.
Tumorigenicity, mutagenicity	Carcinogenic activity has been observed following chronic oral administration to mice and rats; similar studies in hamsters gave negative results. Mutagenic activity has been reported in a number of in vitro assays, but studies in mammals have failed to demonstrate a potential for genetic damage.
Patients with severe hepatic disease	Accumulation of metronidazole and its metabolites may occur. Reduce dosage and use with caution; closely monitor plasma metronidazole levels and observe patient for signs of toxicity.
Anuric patients	Accumulated metabolites may be rapidly removed by dialysis; do not reduce dosage
Known or previously unrecognized candidiasis	May present more prominent symptoms during therapy; treat with a candicidal agent
Mild leukopenia	May occur; use with caution in patients with evidence or a history of blood dyscrasias. Obtain total and differential leukocyte counts before and after therapy.
Amebic liver abscess	Therapy does not obviate need to aspirate pus

ADVERSE REACTIONS

Frequent reactions (incidence ≥ 1%) are printed in *italics*

Gastrointestinal	*Nausea (12%); anorexia; vomiting; diarrhea; epigastric distress; abdominal cramping;* constipation; sharp, metallic, unpleasant taste; furry tongue; glossitis; stomatitis
Central nervous system and neurological	Headache, dizziness, vertigo, incoordination, ataxia, convulsive seizures, confusion, irritability, depression, weakness, insomnia, peripheral neuropathy (numbness, paresthesia of extremities)
Hematological	Leukopenia (reversible)
Hypersensitivity	Urticaria, erythematous rash, flushing, nasal congestion, dry mouth, dryness of the vagina or vulva, fever
Genitourinary	Dysuria, cystitis, dyspareunia, polyuria, incontinence, decreased libido, dark urine, pelvic pressure, proliferation of *Candida* in the vagina
Other	Joint pain (resembling serum sickness), proctitis, flattening of T-wave on ECG

FLAGYL ■ FLAGYL I.V.

OVERDOSAGE

Signs and symptoms	See ADVERSE REACTIONS; nausea, vomiting, and ataxia have occurred following accidental overdoses and in suicide attempts. Neurotoxic effects, including seizures and peripheral neuropathy, have been reported after 5–7 days of ingestion of 6–10.4 g every other day.
Treatment	Treat symptomatically and institute supportive measures, as needed

DRUG INTERACTIONS

Alcohol	Abdominal cramps, nausea, vomiting, headache, or flushing; alcoholic beverages should be avoided during therapy and for at least 1 day afterward
Oral anticoagulants	⇧ Prothrombin time
Cimetidine and other drugs capable of reducing hepatic enzyme activity	⇧ Serum metronidazole level
Phenytoin, phenobarbital, and other drugs capable of inducing hepatic enzymes	⇩ Serum metronidazole level

ALTERED LABORATORY VALUES

Blood/serum values	⇩ SGOT, SGPT, LDH, triglycerides, and hexokinase glucose (with tests based on oxidation-reduction of NAD)

No clinically significant alterations in urinary values occur at therapeutic dosages

USE IN CHILDREN

See INDICATIONS and ORAL DOSAGE; safety and efficacy have not been established for use in children except for the treatment of amebiasis

USE IN PREGNANT AND NURSING WOMEN

Pregnancy Category B: fetotoxicity is caused in mice by intraperitoneal administration, but not by oral administration, of a dose approximating the human dose; reproduction studies in rats given up to 5 times the human dose have shown no evidence of impaired fertility or harm to the fetus. Use during pregnancy only if clearly needed because no adequate, well-controlled studies have been performed in pregnant women and because metronidazole is carcinogenic in mice and rats. Antitrichomonal therapy with metronidazole is contraindicated during the first trimester and, during the second and third trimesters, should be restricted to patients in whom local palliative treatment has been inadequate. Metronidazole crosses the placental barrier and enters the fetal circulation rapidly. It is also excreted in breast milk; patient should stop nursing if drug is prescribed.

MISCELLANEOUS ANTI-INFECTIVE AGENTS

FLAGYL I.V. (metronidazole hydrochloride) Searle   Rx

Vials: metronidazole hydrochloride equivalent to 500 mg metronidazole (for IV infusion only)

FLAGYL I.V. RTU (metronidazole) Searle   Rx

Vials: 5 mg/ml (100 ml) for IV infusion only **Plastic containers:** 5 mg/ml (100 ml) for IV infusion only

INDICATIONS

Intraabdominal infections, including peritonitis, intraabdominal abscess, and liver abscess, caused by susceptible strains of *Bacteroides* (including the *B fragilis* group), *Clostridium, Eubacterium, Peptococcus,* and *Peptostreptococcus*
Skin and skin structure infections caused by susceptible strains of *Bacteroides* (including the *B fragilis* group), *Clostridium, Peptococcus, Peptostreptococcus,* and *Fusobacterium*
Gynecologic infections, including endometritis, endomyometritis, tuboovarian abscess, and postsurgical vaginal cuff infection, caused by susceptible strains of *Bacteroides* (including the *B fragilis* group), *Clostridium, Peptococcus,* and *Peptostreptococcus*
Bacterial septicemia caused by susceptible strains of *Bacteroides* (including the *B fragilis* group) and *Clostridium*
Bone and joint infections caused by susceptible strains of Bacteroides (including the *B fragilis* group) (adjunctive therapy)
Central nervous system infections, including meningitis and brain abscess, caused by susceptible strains of *Bacteroides* (including the *B fragilis* group)
Lower respiratory tract infections including pneumonia, empyema, and lung abscess, caused by susceptible strains of *Bacteroides* (including the *B fragilis* group)
Endocarditis caused by susceptible strains of *Bacteroides* (including the *B fragilis* group)

PARENTERAL DOSAGE

Adult: 15 mg/kg IV, infused over a period of 1 h, to start, followed q6h by 7.5 mg/kg IV, infused over a period of 1 h; do not give more than 4 g in a 24-h period

FLAGYL I.V.

Prevention of postoperative infection in patients undergoing elective colorectal surgery that may be classified as contaminated or potentially contaminated	**Adult:** 15 mg/kg IV, infused over a period of 30–60 min, with administration completed approximately 1 h before surgery, and then, 6 and 12 h after the initial dose, 7.5 mg/kg IV, infused over a period of 30–60 min

CONTRAINDICATIONS

Hypersensitivity to metronidazole or other nitroimidazole derivatives

ADMINISTRATION/DOSAGE ADJUSTMENTS

Parenteral administration	Administer by slow IV drip infusion only, either as a continuous or intermittent infusion; avoid IV admixtures containing metronidazole and other drugs. If used with a primary IV fluid system, discontinue infusion of the primary solution during metronidazole administration. *Do not administer by direct IV injection or use equipment containing aluminum (eg, needles, cannulae) that can come in contact with the drug solution.*
Preparation of infusion fluid	Flagyl I.V. RTU is a ready-to-use isotonic solution requiring no dilution or buffering; do not refrigerate. Flagyl I.V. solutions must be reconstituted, further diluted, and then neutralized. To prepare Flagyl I.V. for infusion, proceed as follows: *Step 1:* Reconstitute lyophilized powder by adding 4.4 ml of Sterile Water for Injection USP, Bacteriostatic Water for Injection USP, 0.9% Sodium Chloride Injection USP, or Bacteriostatic 0.9% Sodium Chloride Injection USP to contents of vial (approximate concentration, 100 mg/ml; pH 0.5–2.0). Mix thoroughly. *Step 2:* Dilute reconstituted metronidazole solution in 0.9% Sodium Chloride Injection USP, 5% Dextrose Injection USP, or Lactated Ringer's Injection USP. To avoid precipitation, do not exceed a concentration of 8 mg/ml. *Step 3:* Neutralize the IV solution with approximately 5 mEq of sodium bicarbonate injection for each 500 mg of metronidazole used; mix thoroughly (the pH of the neutralized solution will range from approximately 6.0 to 7.0). CO_2 gas will be generated with neutralization; if necessary, relieve gas pressure within the container. Use diluted, neutralized solutions within 24 h; to avoid precipitate, do not refrigerate.
Use of plastic containers	After removing overwrap, check for minute leaks in container by squeezing it firmly; if leaks are found, discard solution. Do not connect containers in series; residual air (~ 15 ml), drawn from the primary container before administration of the fluid from the secondary container is complete, could cause air embolism.
Duration of therapy	Usual duration is 7–10 days; bone and joint infections, lower respiratory tract infections, and endocarditis may require longer treatment. When conditions warrant, switch to oral metronidazole therapy (usual adult dosage: 7.5 mg/kg q6h).
Mixed aerobic and anaerobic infections	Administer an antibiotic appropriate for the treatment of aerobic infections concomitantly with metronidazole

WARNINGS/PRECAUTIONS

Convulsive seizures and peripheral neuropathy	May occur; if abnormal neurologic signs appear, the benefits of therapy must be weighed against the risks of continued administration
Tumorigenicity, mutagenicity	Reserve use of metronidazole for serious anaerobic infections where expected benefit outweighs the possible risk suggested by reports of carcinogenic activity following chronic oral administration to mice and rats; similar studies in hamsters gave negative results. Mutagenic activity has been reported in a number of in vitro assays, but studies in mammals have failed to demonstrate a potential for genetic damage.
Patients with severe hepatic disease	Accumulation of metronidazole and its metabolites may occur. Reduce dosage and use with caution; closely monitor plasma metronidazole levels and observe patient for signs of toxicity.
Anuric patients	Accumulated metabolites may be rapidly removed by dialysis; do not reduce dosage
Known or previously unrecognized candidiasis	May present more prominent symptoms during therapy; treat with a candicidal agent
Mild leukopenia	May occur; use with caution in patients with evidence of or a history of blood dyscrasias. Obtain total and differential leukocyte counts before and after therapy.
Sodium retention	Administer Flagyl I.V. RTU with caution to patients receiving corticosteroids or those predisposed to edema (sodium content of ready-to-use solution is 14 mEq/100 ml)
Aspiration of the drug	Metronidazole appears in gastric secretions; continuous nasogastric aspiration of these secretions may result in a decrease in the serum drug level

ADVERSE REACTIONS[1]

Central nervous system	Convulsive seizures, peripheral neuropathy (numbness, paresthesia of an extremity), headache, dizziness, syncope, ataxia, confusion
Gastrointestinal	Nausea, vomiting, abdominal discomfort, diarrhea, unpleasant metallic taste
Hematological	Reversible neutropenia (leukopenia)
Dermatological	Erythematous rash, pruritus

FLAGYL I.V. ■ PEDIAZOLE

Local	Thrombophlebitis
Other	Fever, darkened urine (probably of no clinical significance)

OVERDOSAGE

Signs and symptoms	See ADVERSE REACTIONS; nausea, vomiting, and ataxia have occurred following accidental oral overdoses and in suicide attempts
Treatment	Treat symptomatically and institute supportive measures, as required

DRUG INTERACTIONS

Oral anticoagulants	⇧ Prothrombin time
Alcohol	Abdominal cramps, nausea, vomiting, headache, flushing
Cimetidine and other drugs capable of reducing hepatic enzyme activity	⇧ Serum metronidazole level
Phenytoin, phenobarbital, and other drugs capable of inducing hepatic enzymes	⇩ Serum metronidazole level

ALTERED LABORATORY VALUES

Blood/serum values	⇩ SGOT, SGPT, LDH, triglycerides, and hexokinase glucose (with tests based on oxidation-reduction of NAD)

No clinically significant alterations in urinary values occur at therapeutic dosages

USE IN CHILDREN
Safety and effectiveness have not been established for use in children

USE IN PREGNANT AND NURSING WOMEN
Pregnancy Category B: fetotoxicity is caused in mice by intraperitoneal administration, but not by oral administration, of a dose approximating the human dose; reproduction studies in rats given up to 5 times the human dose have shown no evidence of impaired fertility or harm to the fetus. Use during pregnancy only if clearly needed because no adequate, well-controlled studies have been performed in pregnant women and because metronidazole is carcinogenic in mice and rats. Metronidazole crosses the placental barrier and enters the fetal circulation rapidly. It is also excreted in breast milk; patient should stop nursing if drug is prescribed.

[1] Additional reactions have been reported with oral metronidazole

---

MISCELLANEOUS ANTI-INFECTIVE AGENTS

PEDIAZOLE (erythromycin ethylsuccinate and sulfisoxazole acetyl) Ross   Rx

Suspension (per 5 ml): erythromycin ethylsuccinate equivalent to 200 mg erythromycin and sulfisoxazole acetyl equivalent to 600 mg sulfisoxazole after reconstitution (100, 150, 200 ml) *strawberry/banana flavored*

INDICATIONS
Acute otitis media caused by susceptible strains of *Hemophilus influenzae* in infants and children ≥ 2 mo of age

ORAL DOSAGE
Infant (< 8 kg): 50 mg/kg/day erythromycin and 150 mg/kg/day sulfisoxazole, given without regard to meals in 4 equally divided doses q6h for 10 days
Infant (8 kg): 2.5 ml (1/2 tsp) q6h, without regard to meals, for 10 days
Child (16 kg): 5 ml (1 tsp) q6h, without regard to meals, for 10 days
Child (24 kg): 7.5 ml (1 1/2 tsp) q6h, without regard to meals, for 10 days
Child (> 45 kg): 10 ml (2 tsp) q6h, without regard to meals, for 10 days

CONTRAINDICATIONS

Pregnancy at term	Age < 2 mo	Hypersensitivity to either erythromycin or sulfonamides
Breast-feeding		

WARNINGS/PRECAUTIONS

Life-threatening reactions	Severe, potentially fatal reactions, including Stevens-Johnson syndrome, toxic epidermal necrolysis, fulminant hepatic necrosis, and serious blood dyscrasias (eg, agranulocytosis, aplastic anemia), have occurred rarely in patients taking sulfonamides. Watch for early clinical signs of serious reactions, and obtain a CBC frequently. Exercise caution if patient is hypersensitive to acetazolamide, thiazides, sulfonylureas, or certain goitrogens. If rash, sore throat, fever, pallor, purpura, jaundice, or any other adverse reaction occurs, discontinue use.
Concomitant theophylline therapy	May produce elevated serum theophylline levels or theophylline toxicity; reduce theophylline dosage accordingly

COMPENDIUM OF DRUG THERAPY

PEDIAZOLE

Renal effects	Crystalluria, urolithiasis, and other renal complications have occurred in patients taking sulfonamides; caution patients to maintain an adequate fluid intake, and perform a urinalysis, including a careful microscopic examination, frequently during therapy
Ototoxicity	Reversible hearing loss has occurred, primarily in patients who had renal impairment or received high doses of erythromycin
Superinfection	Prolonged or repeated use may cause overgrowth of nonsusceptible bacteria or fungi; if superinfection occurs, discontinue use
Special-risk patients	Use with caution in patients with impaired renal or hepatic function, severe allergy, bronchial asthma, G6PD deficiency (hemolysis can occur), or porphyria[1]
Carcinogenicity	Long-term administration of sulfonamides has been associated with thyroid malignancies in rats

ADVERSE REACTIONS

Hematological	Agranulocytosis, aplastic anemia, thrombocytopenia, leukopenia, hemolytic anemia, purpura, hypoprothrombinemia, methemoglobinemia
Allergic	Erythema multiforme (Stevens-Johnson syndrome), generalized skin eruptions, epidermal necrolysis, urticaria, serum sickness, pruritus, exfoliative dermatitis, anaphylactoid reactions, periorbital edema, conjunctival and scleral injection, photosensitization, arthralgia, allergic myocarditis, anaphylaxis
Gastrointestinal	Hepatic dysfunction (including jaundice and hepatitis), nausea, vomiting, diarrhea, anorexia, pancreatitis, stomatitis; abdominal pain, cramps, and discomfort
Central nervous system	Headache, peripheral neuritis, mental depression, convulsions, ataxia, hallucinations, tinnitus, vertigo, insomnia
Renal	Toxic nephrosis with oliguria and anuria, crystalluria, urinary calculi; diuresis (rare)
Endocrinological	Goiter and hypoglycemia (rare)
Other	Drug fever, chills, periarteritis nodosa, lupus erythematosus phenomena; reversible hearing loss (see WARNINGS/PRECAUTIONS)

OVERDOSAGE

Signs and symptoms	See ADVERSE REACTIONS
Treatment	Discontinue use of drug; treat symptomatically

DRUG INTERACTIONS

Aminophylline, oxtriphylline, theophylline	△ Serum theophylline level and risk of toxicity
Oral anticoagulants, oral hypoglycemics, methotrexate, phenytoin, thiopental	Pharmacologic effects increased or prolonged △ Risk of toxicity

ALTERED LABORATORY VALUES

Blood/serum values	△ Alkaline phosphatse △ Bilirubin △ SGOT △ SGPT ▽ PBI ▽ ^{131}I thyroid uptake ▽ Glucose (rare)
Urinary values	△ Catecholamines (with Hingerty fluorometric method) △ Glucose (with Clinitest tablets) △ Protein (with sulfosalicylic acid method)

USE IN CHILDREN

See INDICATIONS and ORAL DOSAGE; contraindicated for use in infants under 2 mo of age.

USE IN PREGNANT AND NURSING WOMEN

Safety for use during pregnancy has not been established (sulfonamides cross the placental barrier); administration at term is contraindicated. A significant increase in the incidence of cleft palate and other bony abnormalities has been detected in the offspring of rats and mice fed certain sulfonamides in large amounts (7–25 times the human therapeutic dose); however, the teratogenic potential of most sulfonamides has not been thoroughly studied in animals or humans. Use in nursing mothers is contraindicated; sulfonamides are excreted in breast milk and may cause kernicterus.

[1] *1983 USP Dispensing Information*, Rockville, Md., United States Pharmacopeial Convention, Inc, 1982, vol 1

MISCELLANEOUS ANTI-INFECTIVE AGENTS

PRIMAXIN (imipenem and cilastatin sodium) Merck Sharp & Dohme — Rx

Vials: 250 mg imipenem and 250 mg cilastatin[1] (13 ml); 500 mg imipenem and 500 mg cilastatin[1] (13 ml) **Infusion bottles:** 250 mg imipenem and 250 mg cilastatin[1] (120 ml); 500 mg imipenem and 500 mg cilastatin[1] (120 ml)

INDICATIONS

Serious **lower respiratory tract infections** caused by susceptible strains of *Escherichia coli*, penicillinase-producing *Staphylococcus aureus*, *Klebsiella*, *Enterobacter*, *Hemophilus influenzae*, *H parainfluenzae*, *Acinetobacter*, and *Serratia marcescens*

Serious **intraabdominal infections** caused by susceptible strains of Group D streptococci, penicillinase-producing *Staphylococcus aureus*, *S epidermidis*, *Escherichia coli*, *Klebsiella*, *Enterobacter*, *Proteus*, *Morganella morganii*, *Pseudomonas aeruginosa*, *Citrobacter*, *Clostridium*, *Peptococcus*, *Peptostreptococcus*, *Eubacterium*, *Propionibacterium*, *Bifidobacterium*, *Bacteroides* (including *B fragilis*), and *Fusobacterium*

Serious **gynecological infections** caused by susceptible strains of Group B and D streptococci, penicillinase-producing *Staphylococcus aureus*, *S epidermidis*, *Escherichia coli*, *Klebsiella*, *Proteus*, *Enterobacter*, *Peptococcus*, *Peptostreptococcus*, *Propionibacterium*, *Bifidobacterium*, *Bacteroides* (including *B fragilis*), and *Gardnerella vaginalis*

Serious **bacterial septicemia** caused by susceptible strains of Group D streptococci, penicillinase-producing *Straphylococcus aureus*, *Escherichia coli*, *Klebsiella*, *Pseudomonas aeruginosa*, *Serratia*, *Enterobacter*, and *Bacteroides* (including *B fragilis*)

Serious **bone and joint infections** caused by susceptible strains of Group D streptococci, penicillinase-producing *Staphylococcus aureus*, *S epidermidis*, *Enterobacter*, and *Pseudomonas aeruginosa*

Serious **skin and skin structure infections** caused by susceptible strains of Group D streptococci, penicillinase-producing *Staphylococcus aureus*, *S epidermidis*, *Escherichia coli*, *Klebsiella*, *Enterobacter*, *Proteus vulgaris*, *Providencia rettgeri*, *Morganella morganii*, *Pseudomonas aeruginosa*, *Serratia*, *Citrobacter*, *Acinetobacter*, *Peptococcus*, *Peptostreptococcus*, *Bacteroides* (including *B fragilis*), and *Fusobacterium*

Serious **endocarditis** caused by susceptible strains of penicillinase-producing *Staphylococcus aureus*

Serious **urinary tract infections** caused by susceptible strains of Group D streptococci, penicillinase-producing *Staphylococcus aureus*, *Escherichia coli*, *Klebsiella*, *Enterobacter*, *Proteus vulgaris*, *Providencia rettgeri*, *Morganella morganii*, and *Pseudomonas aeruginosa*

PARENTERAL DOSAGE[2]

Adult: for infections owing to anaerobic, gram-positive, or highly susceptible gram-negative organisms, 250 mg IV q6h if infection is mild, 500 mg IV q6–8h if infection is moderate, or 500 mg IV q6h if infection is severe or life-threatening; for infections owing to other gram-negative organisms, 500 mg IV q6h if infection is mild, 500 mg IV q6h or 1 g IV q8h if infection is moderate, or 1 g q6–8h if infection is severe or life-threatening. Daily dose should not exceed 50 mg/kg/day or 4 g/day, whichever is less.

Adult: for uncomplicated infections, 250 mg IV q6h; for complicated infections, 500 mg IV q6h. Daily dose should not exceed 50 mg/kg/day.

CONTRAINDICATIONS

Hypersensitivity to any component

ADMINISTRATION/DOSAGE ADJUSTMENTS

Preparation	Add 10 ml of an appropriate diluent to the vial, shake well, and then transfer solution to a container holding 100 ml of diluent. To ensure complete transfer of vial contents, add another 10 ml of diluent to the vial and repeat procedure. Agitate final solution until it is clear. To prepare the solution in an infusion bottle, add 100 ml of an appropriate diluent and shake until solution is clear. The following diluents can be used for reconstitution and dilution: 0.9% sodium chloride injection, 5% or 10% dextrose injection, Normosol-M in D5-W, 2.5%, 5%, or 10% mannitol, or 5% dextrose injection in combination with either 0.02% sodium bicarbonate solution, 0.15% potassium chloride solution, or 0.9%, 0.45%, or 0.225% sodium chloride injection. Do not mix imipenem with other antibiotics.
Administration	Give drug by IV infusion. Administer each 250- or 500-mg dose over a period of 20–30 min, each 1-g dose over a period of 40–60 min; if nausea occurs, the rate of infusion may be reduced.
Polymicrobial infections	Although infections caused solely by *Streptococcus pneumoniae*, Group A beta-hemolytic streptococci, or nonpenicillinase-producing *Staphylococcus aureus* should be treated with an antibiotic (eg, penicillin G) having a narrower spectrum than imipenem, infections owing to the combination of one of these organisms and one or more of the organisms listed in INDICATIONS can be effectively treated with imipenem
Pseudomonal infections	Some strains of *Pseudomonas aeruginosa* may develop resistance fairly rapidly during treatment; perform susceptibility tests periodically. In patients with cystic fibrosis or chronic pulmonary disease, imipenem may produce clinical improvement of lower respiratory tract infections caused by *Pseudomonas aeruginosa* but fail to eradicate the organism.
Resistant organisms	When treating infections owing to Group D streptococci or penicillinase-producing staphylococci, bear in mind that imipenem is not effective against *Streptococcus faecium* and many strains of methicillin-resistant staphylococci

PRIMAXIN

Patients with renal impairment	For life-threatening infections,[2] give 500 mg q6h if creatinine clearance (Ccr) = 30–70 ml/min, 500 mg q8h if Ccr = 20–30 ml/min, or 500 mg q12h if Ccr = 0–20 ml/min; for infections that are less severe or caused by highly susceptible organisms,[2] give 500 mg q8h if Ccr = 30–70 ml/min, 500 mg q12h if Ccr = 20–30 ml/min, or 250 mg q12h if Ccr = 0–20 ml/min. These dosages are based on a body weight of 70 kg; they should be reduced proportionately for patients weighing less than this amount. The Ccr of patients with stable renal function can be estimated from serum creatinine levels if a measured value cannot be obtained; for adult men, use the following formula: (weight [kg])(140 − age [yr])/(72)(serum creatinine level [mg/dl]), for adult women, multiply this quotient by 0.85. Patients who have undergone hemodialysis should be given a supplemental dose after the procedure unless the next dose is scheduled within 4 h.
Use of probenecid	Concomitant use of probenecid is not recommended since the drug has little effect on the serum level or half-life of imipenem

WARNINGS/PRECAUTIONS

Hypersensitivity	Serious acute hypersensitivity reactions, necessitating epinephrine and other emergency measures, may occur during therapy; use with caution in patients with a history of allergy, especially if they are hypersensitive to other beta-lactam antibiotics or more than one allergen. If an allergic reaction occurs during therapy, discontinue use.
Pseudomembranous colitis	May occur due to alteration of the intestinal flora and should be considered in any patient who develops diarrhea during or after therapy. Mild cases may respond to withdrawal of the drug alone. More severe cases can be managed, as needed, by sigmoidoscopy, appropriate bacteriological studies, fluid and electrolyte replacement, protein supplementation, and use of oral vancomycin. Isolation of the patient may be advisable. Other possible causes of colitis should also be considered.
Convulsions	Myoclonic activity, confusional states, and seizures have occurred, most commonly in patients with renal impairment and either CNS disorders (eg, brain lesions) or a history of seizures; however, in rare cases, these reactions have been seen in patients with no apparent CNS disorder. To reduce risks of CNS reactions, adhere closely to recommended dosage schedules, especially when using in patients predisposed to seizures; in addition, carefully observe patients undergoing hemodialysis and maintain anticonvulsant therapy for patients with seizure disorders. If focal tremors, myoclonus, or seizures occur, institute anticonvulsant treatment; if reactions persist, reduce imipenem dosage or discontinue drug.
Superinfection	Overgrowth of nonsusceptible organisms may occur with prolonged use; repeated clinical observation is essential
Chronic toxicity	Assess organ system function periodically during prolonged therapy
Mutagenicity	No evidence of mutagenicity has been seen in bacterial or mammalian tests

ADVERSE REACTIONS

The most frequent reactions (≥ 0.2%) are italicized

Gastrointestinal	*Nausea (2%), diarrhea (1.8%), vomiting (1.5%),* pseudomembranous colitis, hemorrhagic colitis, gastroenteritis, abdominal pain, glossitis, tongue papillar hypertrophy, heartburn, pharyngeal pain, increased salivation
Central nervous system	*Seizures (0.4%), dizziness (0.3%), somnolence (0.2%),* encephalopathy, confusion, myoclonus, paresthesia, vertigo, headache
Otic	Transient hearing loss (in patients with hearing impairment), tinnitus
Respiratory	Chest discomfort, dyspnea, hyperventilation, thoracic spine pain
Cardiovascular	*Hypotension (0.4%),* palpitations, tachycardia
Renal	Oliguria/anuria, polyuria
Dermatological	*Rash (0.9%), pruritus (0.3%), urticaria (0.2%),* erythema multiforme, facial edema, flushing, cyanosis, hyperhidrosis, skin texture changes, candidiasis, pruritus vulvae
Local	*Phlebitis/thrombophlebitis (3.1%), pain at injection site (0.7%), erythema at injection site (0.4%), vein induration (0.2%),* infused vein infection
Other	*Fever (0.5%),* polyarthralgia, asthenia/weakness

OVERDOSAGE

No information on overdosage in humans is available

DRUG INTERACTIONS

Aminoglycosides	Physical incompatibility; do not mix together

ALTERED LABORATORY VALUES

Changes in laboratory values have been reported (see footnote 3)

USE IN CHILDREN

Safety and effectiveness for use in children under 12 yr of age have not yet been established

USE IN PREGNANT AND NURSING WOMEN

Pregnancy Category C: an apparent intolerance to this preparation, manifested by emesis, anorexia, diarrhea, weight loss, and death, has been suggested by preliminary studies in pregnant rabbits and cynomolgus monkeys given doses equivalent to the usual human dose; this preparation has been well-tolerated by pregnant rats and mice when given at doses up to 11 times the usual human dose. In rats, administration of 8 times the usual human dose has produced a slight decrease in fetal weight. No evidence of teratogenicity has been detected in mice and rats given up to 11 times the usual human dose during the period of major organogenesis. Use during pregnancy only if the expected benefit justifies the potential risks. It is not known whether this drug is excreted in human milk; use with caution in nursing mothers.

[1] As the sodium salt
[2] Dosage is based on the imipenem component
[3] Laboratory findings reported during clinical trials without regard to drug relationship include increases in SGPT, SGOT, alkaline phosphatase, bilirubin, LDH, BUN, creatinine, potassium, and chloride levels; decreases in serum sodium level; increases in platelet, leukocyte, eosinophil, basophil, monocyte, and lymphocyte counts; decreases in leukocyte and neutrophil counts; decreases in hemoglobin level and hematocrit; positive Coombs' test; abnormal prothrombin time; and presence of protein, erythrocytes, leukocytes, casts, bilirubin, and urobilinogen in the urine

---

MISCELLANEOUS ANTI-INFECTIVE AGENTS

PROTOSTAT (metronidazole) Ortho   Rx

Tablets: 250, 500 mg

INDICATIONS

Symptomatic trichomoniasis, when the presence of trichomonads has been confirmed by appropriate laboratory procedures
Asymptomatic trichomoniasis associated with endocervicitis, cervicitis, or cervical erosion
Treatment of **asymptomatic partners** of treated patients

Acute intestinal amebiasis (acute amebic dysentery)

Amebic liver abscess

Intraabdominal infections, including peritonitis, intraabdominal abscess, and liver abscess, caused by susceptible strains of *Bacteroides* (including the *B fragilis* group), *Clostridium, Eubacterium, Peptococcus,* and *Peptostreptococcus*
Skin and skin structure infections caused by susceptible strains of *Bacteroides* (including the *B fragilis* group), *Clostridium, Peptococcus, Peptostreptococcus,* and *Fusobacterium*
Gynecologic infections, including endometritis, endomyometritis, tubo-ovarian abscess, and postsurgical vaginal cuff infection, caused by susceptible strains of *Bacteroides* (including the *B fragilis* group), *Clostridium, Peptococcus,* and *Peptostreptococcus*
Bacterial septicemia caused by susceptible strains of *Bacteroides* (including the *B fragilis* group) and *Clostridium*
Bone and joint infections caused by susceptible strains of *Bacteroides* (including the *B fragilis* group) (adjunctive therapy)
Central nervous system infections, including meningitis and brain abscess, caused by susceptible strains of *Bacteroides* (including the *B fragilis* group)
Lower respiratory tract infections, including pneumonia, empyema, and lung abscess, caused by susceptible strains of *Bacteroides* (including the *B fragilis* group)
Endocarditis caused by susceptible strains of *Bacteroides* (including the *B fragilis* group)

ORAL DOSAGE

Adult: 250 mg tid for 7 days or, if patient is not pregnant, 2 g given in a single dose or 2 divided doses of 1 g each on the same day. Repeated courses may be given at 4- to 6-wk intervals, upon laboratory confirmation that trichomonads are still present; obtain total and differential leukocyte counts before and after retreatment.

Adult: 750 mg tid for 5–10 days
Child: 35–50 mg/kg/24 h, given in 3 divided doses for 10 days

Adult: 500–750 mg tid for 5–10 days
Child: same as child's dosage above

Adult: 7.5 mg/kg q6h, up to 4.0 g/24 h

CONTRAINDICATIONS

First trimester of pregnancy, when used to treat trichomoniasis   Hypersensitivity to metronidazole or other nitroimidazole derivatives

PROTOSTAT

ADMINISTRATION/DOSAGE ADJUSTMENTS

Duration of therapy for anaerobic infections	Usual duration is 7–10 days; bone and joint infections, lower respiratory tract infections, and endocarditis may require longer treatment
Serious anaerobic infections	Are usually treated first with intravenous metronidazole

WARNINGS/PRECAUTIONS

Convulsive seizures and peripheral neuropathy	May occur; warn patient to discontinue use immediately if abnormal neurologic signs appear. Use with caution in patients with CNS diseases.
Tumorigenicity, mutagenicity	Carcinogenic activity has been observed following chronic oral administration to mice and rats; similar studies in hamsters gave negative results. Mutagenic activity has been reported in a number of in vitro assays, but studies in mammals have failed to demonstrate a potential for genetic damage.
Patients with severe hepatic disease	Accumulation of metronidazole and its metabolites may occur. Reduce dosage and use with caution; closely monitor plasma metronidazole levels and observe patient for signs of toxicity.
Anuric patients	Accumulated metabolites may be rapidly removed by dialysis; do not reduce dosage
Known or previously unrecognized candidiasis	May present more prominent symptoms during therapy; treat with a candicidal agent
Mild leukopenia	May occur; use with caution in patients with evidence or a history of blood dyscrasias. Obtain total and differential leukocyte counts before and after therapy.
Amebic liver abscess	Therapy does not obviate need to aspirate pus
Alcohol ingestion	Should be avoided (see DRUG INTERACTIONS); patient may also find that the taste of alcoholic beverages is altered

ADVERSE REACTIONS

Frequent reactions (incidence ≥ 1%) are printed in *italics*

Gastrointestinal	*Nausea; anorexia; vomiting; diarrhea; epigastric distress; abdominal cramping;* constipation; sharp, metallic, unpleasant taste, furry tongue, glossitis, and stomatitis possibly associated with a sudden proliferation of Candida in the mouth
Central nervous system and neurological	Headache, dizziness, vertigo, incoordination, ataxia, convulsive seizures, confusion, irritability, depression, weakness, insomnia, peripheral neuropathy (numbness, paresthesia of extremities)
Hematological	Leukopenia (reversible)
Hypersensitivity	Urticaria, erythematous rash, flushing, nasal congestion, dry mouth, dryness of the vagina or vulva, fever
Genitourinary	Dysuria, cystitis, dyspareunia, polyuria, incontinence, decreased libido, dark urine, pelvic pressure, proliferation of Candida in the vagina
Other	Joint pain (resembling serum sickness), proctitis, flattening of T-wave on ECG

OVERDOSAGE

Signs and symptoms	See ADVERSE REACTIONS; nausea, vomiting, and ataxia have occurred following accidental overdoses and in suicide attempts. Neurotoxic effects, including seizures and peripheral neuropathy, have been reported after 5–7 days of ingestion of 6–10.4 g every other day.
Treatment	Treat symptomatically and institute supportive measures, as needed

DRUG INTERACTIONS

Alcohol	Abdominal cramps, nausea, vomiting, headache, or flushing
Oral anticoagulants	△ Prothrombin time
Phenytoin, phenobarbital, other drugs capable of inducing hepatic enzymes	▽ Serum metronidazole level

ALTERED LABORATORY VALUES

Blood/serum values	▽ SGOT (test interference)

No clinically significant alterations in urinary values occur at therapeutic dosages

---

USE IN CHILDREN

See INDICATIONS and ORAL DOSAGE; safety and efficacy have not been established for use in children except for the treatment of amebiasis

USE IN PREGNANT AND NURSING WOMEN

Pregnancy Category B: reproduction studies in rabbits and rats given up to 5 times the human dose have shown no evidence of impaired fertility or harm to the fetus. Nevertheless, use during pregnancy only if clearly needed because no adequate, well-controlled studies have been performed in pregnant women and because metronidazole is carcinogenic in mice and rats. Antitrichomonal therapy with metronidazole is contraindicated during the first trimester and, during the second and third trimesters, should be restricted to patients in whom local palliative treatment has been inadequate. Metronidazole crosses the placental barrier and enters the fetal circulation rapidly. It is also excreted in breast milk; patient should stop nursing if drug is prescribed.

MISCELLANEOUS ANTI-INFECTIVE AGENTS

SEPTRA (trimethoprim and sulfamethoxazole) Burroughs Wellcome — Rx
Tablets: 80 mg trimethoprim and 400 mg sulfamethoxazole Suspension (per 5 ml): 40 mg trimethoprim and 200 mg sulfamethoxazole[1] (100, 473 ml) cherry-flavored

SEPTRA DS (trimethoprim and sulfamethoxazole) Burroughs Wellcome — Rx
Tablets: 160 mg trimethoprim and 800 mg sulfamethoxazole

INDICATIONS

Urinary tract infections caused by susceptible strains of *Escherichia coli*, *Klebsiella*, *Enterobacter*, *Morganella morganii*, *Proteus mirabilis*, and *P vulgaris*[2]

Acute otitis media caused by susceptible strains of *Hemophilus influenzae* or *Streptococcus pneumoniae*[3]

Acute exacerbations of chronic bronchitis caused by susceptible strains of *Hemophilus influenzae* or *Streptococcus pneumoniae*[4]

Enteritis caused by susceptible strains of *Shigella flexneri* and *S sonnei*

***Pneumocystis carinii* pneumonitis**

ORAL DOSAGE

Adult: 2 Septra tabs, 1 Septra DS tab, or 20 ml (4 tsp) q12h for 10–14 days
Child ($\geq$ 2 mo): 4 mg/kg trimethoprim and 20 mg/kg sulfamethoxazole q12h for 10 days, as follows:
Child (10 kg): 5 ml (1 tsp) q12h for 10 days
Child (20 kg): 1 Septra tab or 10 ml (2 tsp) q12h for 10 days
Child (30 kg): 1½ Septra tabs or 15 ml (3 tsp) q12h for 10 days
Child ($\geq$ 40 kg): 2 Septra tabs, 1 Septra DS tab, or 20 ml (4 tsp) q12h for 10 days

Child ($\geq$ 2 mo): same as pediatric dosages above

Adult: same as adult dosage above for 14 days

Adult: same as above for 5 days
Child ($\geq$ 2 mo): same as above for 5 days

Adult: 5 mg/kg trimethoprim and 25 mg/kg sulfamethoxazole q6h for 14 days
Child ($\geq$ 2 mo): same as adult, as follows:
Child (8 kg): 5 ml (1 tsp) q6h for 14 days
Child (16 kg): 1 Septra tab or 10 ml (2 tsp) q6h for 14 days
Child (24 kg): 1½ Septra tabs or 15 ml (3 tsp) q6h for 14 days
Child ($\geq$ 32 kg): 2 Septra tabs, 1 Septra DS tab, or 20 ml (4 tsp) q6h for 14 days

CONTRAINDICATIONS

Pregnancy at term

Age < 2 mo

Breast-feeding

Hypersensitivity to trimethoprim or sulfonamides

Megaloblastic anemia due to folate deficiency

ADMINISTRATION/DOSAGE ADJUSTMENTS

Patients with renal impairment — Follow the usual dosage regimen if creatinine clearance (Ccr) > 30 ml/min. Administer half the usual dosage if Ccr = 15–30 ml/min. Use is not recommended if Ccr < 15 ml/min.

WARNINGS/PRECAUTIONS

Group A beta-hemolytic streptococcal pharyngitis — Sulfonamides have no place in the treatment of such infections, as they will neither eradicate the causative organism from the tonsillopharyngeal area nor prevent complications

Life-threatening reactions — Severe, potentially fatal reactions, including Stevens-Johnson syndrome, toxic epidermal necrolysis, fulminant hepatic necrosis, and serious blood dyscrasias (eg, agranulocytosis, aplastic anemia) have occurred on rare occasions in patients receiving sulfonamides. These drugs have caused hemolytic anemia in patients with G6PD deficiency. The risk of severe adverse reactions may be increased in elderly patients, particularly when these patients are receiving other drugs (see DRUG INTERACTIONS) or they have renal or hepatic impairment or another complicating condition; the most frequent serious adverse effects seen in elderly patients are severe skin reactions, generalized bone marrow depression, and thrombocytopenia.

When using this preparation, obtain a CBC frequently and watch for early clinical signs such as rash, sore throat, fever, pallor, purpura, and jaundice; *discontinue administration at the first sign of skin rash or any adverse reaction*

Bone marrow depression — High doses or prolonged use may cause bone marrow depression and, as a result, produce thrombocytopenia, leukopenia, and/or megaloplastic anemia; if signs of bone marrow depression appear, give 5–15 mg/day of leucovorin until normal hematopoiesis is restored

Cross-sensitivity — Patients allergic to acetazolamide, thiazide-type diuretics, sulfonylureas, or certain goitrogens may also be hypersensitive to this preparation

Renal effects — Crystalluria, urolithiasis, and other renal complications have occurred in patients taking sulfonamides. Caution patients to maintain an adequate fluid intake; urinalysis, including careful microscopic examination, and renal function tests should be performed during therapy, particularly when a patient has renal impairment

Special-risk patients — Use with caution in elderly patients and those with renal or hepatic impairment, possible folate deficiency, severe allergies, bronchial asthma, or G6PD deficiency. Among the conditions that may be associated with folate deficiency are malnutrition, malabsorption syndrome, chronic alcoholism, advanced age, and anticonvulsant therapy.

SEPTRA

AIDS	Patients with AIDS may not tolerate or respond to this preparation in the same manner as other patients; the frequency of adverse effects, particularly rash, fever, and leukopenia, has been reported to be greatly increased in AIDS patients who were undergoing treatment of *Pneumocystis carinii* pneumonia
Carcinogenicity	No long-term studies have been done in animals to evaluate the oncogenic potential of this drug
Mutagenicity	Although bacterial mutagenicity studies have not been done with this preparation, trimethoprim alone has shown no mutagenic potential in the Ames assay, and no chromosomal abnormalities have been detected in human leukocytes cultured in vitro with either component alone or in combination or in leukocytes from treated patients
Effect on fertility	No adverse effects on fertility or general reproductive performance have been observed in rats given oral dosages as high as 70 mg/kg/day of trimethoprim plus 350 mg/kg/day of sulfamethoxazole

ADVERSE REACTIONS

Hematological	Agranulocytosis, aplastic anemia, thrombocytopenia, leukopenia, neutropenia, hemolytic anemia, megaloblastic anemia, hypoprothrombinemia, methemoglobinemia, eosinophilia
Gastrointestinal	Hepatitis (including cholestatic jaundice and fulminant hepatic necrosis), elevation of serum transaminase and bilirubin levels, pseudomembranous enterocolitis, pancreatitis, stomatitis, glossitis, nausea, vomiting, abdominal pain, diarrhea, anorexia
Genitourinary	Renal failure, interstitial nephritis, elevation of BUN and serum creatinine levels, toxic nephrosis with oliguria and anuria, crystalluria
Central nervous system	Aseptic meningitis, convulsions, peripheral neuritis, ataxia, vertigo, tinnitus, headache, hallucinations, depression, apathy, nervousness, weakness, fatigue, insomnia
Endocrinological	Diuresis, hypoglycemia
Musculoskeletal	Arthralgia, myalgia
Hypersensitivity	Stevens-Johnson syndrome, toxic epidermal necrolysis, anaphylaxis, allergic myocarditis, erythema multiforme, exfoliative dermatitis, angioedema, drug fever, chills, Henoch-Schoenlein purpura, serum sickness-like syndrome, generalized allergic reactions, generalized skin eruptions, photosensitivity, conjunctival and scleral injection, pruritus, urticaria, rash, periarteritis nodosa, systemic lupus erythematosus

OVERDOSAGE

Signs and symptoms	Anorexia, colic, nausea, vomiting, dizziness, headache, drowsiness, mental depression, confusion, unconsciousness, pyrexia, hematuria, crystalluria, bone marrow depression, other blood dyscrasias, jaundice
Treatment	Induce emesis or perform gastric lavage. To enhance renal elimination, acidify urine and institute forced diuresis; if urine output is low and renal function is normal, administer IV fluids. Monitor blood counts and electrolyte balance. Institute specific therapy if jaundice or a significant blood dyscrasia occurs. Peritoneal dialysis is not useful and hemodialysis is only moderately effective in removing the components of this preparation.

DRUG INTERACTIONS

Diuretics (especially thiazides)	△ Risk of thrombocytopenic purpura in elderly patients
Warfarin	△ Prothrombin time; if this preparation is given during warfarin therapy, recheck prothrombin time
Phenytoin	△ Serum half-life of phenytoin; watch for evidence of phenytoin toxicity during combination therapy
Methotrexate	△ Serum level of methotrexate

ALTERED LABORATORY VALUES

Blood/serum values	△ Methotrexate (with competitive binding protein assay using dihydrofolate reductase) △ BUN △ Creatinine (especially with Jaffé test) △ Bilirubin △ SGOT △ SGPT ▽ PBI ▽ [131]I thyroid uptake

No clinically significant alterations in urinary values occur at therapeutic dosages

---

USE IN CHILDREN

See INDICATIONS and ORAL DOSAGE. Data on the safety of repeated use in children under 2 yr of age are limited; contraindicated for infants under 2 mo of age.

USE IN PREGNANT AND NURSING WOMEN

Pregnancy Category C: use during pregnancy only if expected benefit justifies the potential fetal risk, since the drug may interfere with folic acid metabolism. Teratogenic effects (mainly cleft palate) have been observed in rats and increased fetal loss has been observed in rats and rabbits at doses several times the recommended human dose. Although no large, well-controlled studies have been done in pregnant women, two limited studies have shown no increase in congenital abnormalities. The drug is contraindicated at term and for use in nursing mothers because sulfonamides cross the placental barrier, are excreted in human milk, and may cause kernicterus.

---

[1] Contains 0.26% alcohol
[2] Initial episodes of uncomplicated infections should be treated with a single, effective antibacterial agent, rather than a combination
[3] Not indicated for prophylaxis or prolonged administration
[4] When in the physician's judgment this preparation offers some advantage over the use of a single antimicrobial agent

MISCELLANEOUS ANTI-INFECTIVE AGENTS

SEPTRA I.V. Infusion (trimethoprim and sulfamethoxazole) Burroughs Wellcome   Rx

Ampuls (per 5 ml): 80 mg trimethoprim and 400 mg sulfamethoxazole (5 ml) for IV infusion only   **Vials (per 5 ml):** 80 mg trimethoprim and 400 mg sulfamethoxazole (5, 10, 20 ml) for IV infusion only

INDICATIONS

Pneumocystis carinii pneumonitis

Severe or complicated **urinary tract infections** caused by susceptible strains of *Escherichia coli, Klebsiella, Enterobacter, Morganella morganii,* and *Proteus* when oral administration is not feasible or when the organism is not susceptible to single urinary anti-infectives alone

Enteritis caused by susceptible strains of *Shigella flexneri* and *S sonnei*

PARENTERAL DOSAGE[1]

Adult: 15–20 mg/kg/day, given in 3–4 equally divided doses via IV infusion q6–8h
Child: same as adult

Adult: 8–10 mg/kg/day, up to 960 mg/day, given in 2–4 equally divided doses via IV infusion q6–12h
Child: same as adult

CONTRAINDICATIONS

Pregnancy at term

Breast-feeding

Age < 2 mo

Hypersensitivity to trimethoprim or sulfonamides

Documented megaloblastic anemia due to folate deficiency

ADMINISTRATION/DOSAGE ADJUSTMENTS

Preparation of infusion	Dilute each 5 ml of the preparation in 125 ml of 5% dextrose-in-water and use within 6 h; do not refrigerate. If fluid restriction is desired, dilute in 100 ml and use within 4 h or dilute in 75 ml and use within 2 h. Do not mix with other drugs or solutions in the same container. The contents of the 20-ml vial must be used within 48 h after withdrawal of the initial dose.
Intravenous administration	Administer slowly by IV drip over a period of 60–90 min; avoid rapid infusion or bolus injection
Local irritation and inflammation	May occur, due to extravascular infiltration of the infusion; discontinue infusion and restart at another site
Susceptibility tests	Cultures and appropriate microbiological tests should be performed to determine susceptibility; therapy may be initiated, however, before the results of these tests are available
Duration of therapy	Pneumonitis due to *Pneumocystis carinii* and severe urinary tract infections should be treated for up to 14 days and shigellosis for up to 5 days
Patients with renal impairment	Follow the usual dosage regimen if creatinine clearance (Ccr) > 30 ml/min. Administer half the usual dosage if Ccr = 15–30 ml/min; use is not recommended if Ccr < 15 ml/min.

WARNINGS/PRECAUTIONS

Streptococcal pharyngitis	Should not be treated with this drug, as it may fail to eliminate group A beta-hemolytic streptococci from the tonsillopharyngeal area
Life-threatening reactions	Severe, potentially fatal reactions, including Stevens-Johnson syndrome, toxic epidermal necrolysis, fulminant hepatic necrosis, and serious blood dyscrasias (eg, agranulocytosis, aplastic anemia) have occurred on rare occasions in patients receiving sulfonamides. These drugs have caused hemolytic anemia in patients with G6PD deficiency. The risk of severe adverse reactions may be increased in elderly patients, particularly when these patients are receiving other drugs (see DRUG INTERACTIONS) or they have renal or hepatic impairment or another complicating condition; the most frequent serious adverse effects seen in elderly patients are severe skin reactions, generalized bone marrow depression, and thrombocytopenia.
	When using this preparation, obtain a CBC frequently and watch for early clinical signs such as rash, sore throat, fever, pallor, purpura, and jaundice; *discontinue administration at the first sign of skin rash or any adverse reaction*
Bone marrow depression	High doses or prolonged use may cause bone marrow depression and, as a result, produce thrombocytopenia, leukopenia, and/or megaloblastic anemia; if signs of bone marrow depression appear, give 5–15 mg/day of leucovorin until normal hematopoiesis is restored.
Cross-sensitivity	Patients allergic to acetazolamide, thiazide-type diuretics, sulfonylureas, or certain goitrogens may also be hypersensitive to this preparation
Renal effects	Crystalluria, urolithiasis, and other renal complications have occurred in patients taking sulfonamides. Caution patients to maintain an adequate fluid intake; urinalysis, including careful microscopic examination, and renal function tests should be performed during therapy, particularly when a patient has renal impairment.
Special-risk patients	Use with caution in elderly patients and those with renal or hepatic impairment, possible folate deficiency, severe allergies, bronchial asthma, or G6PD deficiency. Among the conditions that may be associated with folate deficiency are malnutrition, malabsorption syndrome, chronic alcoholism, advanced age, and anticonvulsant therapy.

SEPTRA I.V. Infusion

AIDS	Patients with AIDS may not tolerate or respond to this preparation in the same manner as other patients; the frequency of adverse effects, particularly rash, fever, and leukopenia, has been reported to be greatly increased in AIDS patients who were undergoing treatment of *Pneumocystis carinii* pneumonia
Sulfite sensitivity	Sodium metabisulfite in this product may cause urticaria, pruritus, wheezing, anaphylaxis, or other allergic-type reactions in susceptible patients, such as those with asthma or atopy
Carcinogenicity	No long-term studies have been done in animals to evaluate the oncogenic potential of this drug
Mutagenicity	Although bacterial mutagenicity studies have not been done with this preparation, trimethoprim alone has shown no mutagenic potential in the Ames assay, and no chromosomal abnormalities have been detected in human leukocytes cultured in vitro with either component alone or in combination or in leukocytes from treated patients
Effect on fertility	No adverse effects on fertility or general reproductive performance have been observed in rats given oral dosages as high as 70 mg/kg/day of trimethoprim plus 350 mg/kg/day of sulfamethoxazole

ADVERSE REACTIONS

Hematological	Agranulocytosis, aplastic anemia, thrombocytopenia, leukopenia, neutropenia, hemolytic anemia, megaloblastic anemia, hypoprothrombinemia, methemoglobinemia, eosinophilia
Gastrointestinal	Hepatitis (including cholestatic jaundice and fulminant hepatic necrosis), elevation of serum transaminase and bilirubin levels, pseudomembranous enterocolitis, pancreatitis, stomatitis, glossitis, nausea, vomiting, abdominal pain, diarrhea, anorexia
Genitourinary	Renal failure, interstitial nephritis, elevation of BUN and serum creatinine levels, toxic nephrosis with oliguria and anuria, crystalluria
Central nervous system	Aseptic meningitis, convulsions, peripheral neuritis, ataxia, vertigo, tinnitus, headache, hallucinations, depression, apathy, nervousness, weakness, fatigue, insomnia
Endocrinological	Diuresis, hypoglycemia
Musculoskeletal	Arthralgia, myalgia
Hypersensitivity	Stevens-Johnson syndrome, toxic epidermal necrolysis, anaphylaxis, allergic myocarditis, erythema multiform, exfoliative dermatitis, angiodema, drug fever, chills, Henoch-Schoenlein purpura, serum sickness-like syndrome, generalized allergic reactions, generalized skin eruptions, photosensitivity, conjunctival and scleral injection, pruritus, urticaria, rash, periarteritis nodosa, systemic lupus erythematosus

OVERDOSAGE

Signs and symptoms	Anorexia, colic, nausea, vomiting, dizziness, headache, drowsiness, mental depression, confusion, unconsciousness, pyrexia, hematuria, crystalluria, bone marrow depression, other blood dyscrasias, jaundice
Treatment	To enhance renal elimination, acidify urine and institute forced diuresis; if urine output is low and renal function is normal, administer IV fluids. Monitor blood counts and electrolyte balance. Institute specific therapy if jaundice or a significant blood dyscrasia occurs. Peritoneal dialysis is not useful and hemodialysis is only moderately effective in removing the components of this preparation.

DRUG INTERACTIONS

Diuretics (especially thiazides)	△ Risk of thrombocytopenic purpura in elderly patients
Warfarin	△ Prothrombin time; if this preparation is given during warfarin therapy, recheck prothrombin time
Phenytoin	△ Serum half-life of phenytoin; watch for evidence of phenytoin toxicity during combination therapy
Methotrexate	△ Serum level of methotrexate

ALTERED LABORATORY VALUES

Blood/serum values	△ Methotrexate (with competitive binding protein assay using dihydrofolate reductase) △ BUN △ Creatinine (especially with Jaffé test) △ Bilirubin △ SGOT △ SGPT ▽ PBI ▽ ^{131}I thyroid uptake ▽ Glucose (rare)

No clinically significant alterations in urinary values occur at therapeutic dosages

---

USE IN CHILDREN

Same as adult indications and dosage; contraindicated for use in infants under 2 mo of age

USE IN PREGNANT AND NURSING WOMEN

Pregnancy Category C: use during pregnancy only if expected benefit justifies the potential fetal risk, since the drug may interfere with the folic acid metabolism. Teratogenic effects (mainly cleft palate) have been observed in rats and increased fetal loss has been observed in rats and rabbits at doses several times the recommended human dose. Although no large, well-controlled studies have been done in pregnant women, two limited studies have shown no increase in congenital abnormalities. The drug is contraindicated at term and for use in nursing mothers because sulfonamides cross the placental barrier, are excreted in human milk, and may cause kernicterus.

---

[1] Dosage is based on the trimethoprim component

MISCELLANEOUS ANTI-INFECTIVE AGENTS

VANCOCIN HCl (vancomycin hydrochloride) Lilly — Rx
Capsules: 125, 250 mg   Solution: 250 mg/5 ml, 500 mg/6 ml after reconstitution

INDICATIONS	ORAL DOSAGE
Enterocolitis caused by staphylococci **Antibiotic-associated pseudomembranous colitis (AAPC)** caused by *Clostridium difficile*	Adult: 0.5–2 g/day, given in 3–4 divided doses; for AAPC, administer drug for 7–10 days Child: 40 mg/kg/day, up to 2 g/day, given in 4 divided doses; for AAPC, administer drug for 7–10 days

VANCOCIN HCl IntraVenous (vancomycin hydrochloride) Lilly — Rx
Vials: 500 mg (10 ml), 1 g (20 ml)

INDICATIONS[1]	PARENTERAL DOSAGE
Serious or severe infections caused by susceptible strains of **methicillin-resistant staphylococci** **Serious or severe infections** caused by susceptible strains of **other staphylococci** when other anti-infectives, including penicillins and cephalosporins, are ineffective or contraindicated	Adult: 500 mg IV q6h or 1 g IV q12h Neonate (0–7 days): 15 mg/kg IV to start, followed by 10 mg/kg IV q12h Neonate (8 days to 1 mo): 15 mg/kg IV to start, followed by 10 mg/kg IV q8h Infant (> 1 mo) and child: 40 mg/kg/day, given IV in divided doses
Prevention of bacterial endocarditis in penicillin-allergic patients who have prosthetic heart valves or other particularly high-risk conditions and are undergoing **dental procedures or upper respiratory tract surgery or instrumentation**[2]	Adult: 1 g IV over a period of 1 h, beginning 1 h before the procedure Child: 20 mg/kg, up to 1 g, IV over a period of 1 h, beginning 1 h before the procedure
Prevention of bacterial endocarditis in penicillin-allergic patients at risk who are undergoing **GI or genitourinary tract surgery or instrumentation**[2]	Adult: 1 g IV over a period of 1 h, beginning 1 h before the procedure, plus 1.5 mg/kg gentamicin IM or IV 1 h before the procedure; these doses may be repeated once 8–12 h after the initial dose Child: 20 mg/kg, up to 1 g, IV over a period of 1 h, beginning 1 h before the procedure, plus 2 mg/kg gentamicin IM or IV 1 h before the procedure; these doses may be repeated once 8–12 h after the initial dose

CONTRAINDICATIONS
Hypersensitivity to vancomycin

ADMINISTRATION/DOSAGE ADJUSTMENTS
When used orally

Preparation of oral solution — The solution may be prepared in 1- or 10-g screw-cap bottles manufactured for oral use or, alternatively, in 0.5- or 1-g vials manufactured mainly for IV use. To reconstitute the solution in a screw-cap bottle, add 20 ml of distilled or deionized water to the 1-g bottle (resulting concentration: 250 mg/5 ml) or 115 ml to the 10-g bottle (resulting concentration: 500 mg/6 ml). To reconstitute the solution in a parenteral vial, add 1 fl oz of water to the vial. Solutions prepared in the parenteral vials may be given orally (with common flavoring syrups) or via a nasogastric tube.

When used parenterally

Staphylococcal infections — Vancomycin has been shown to be an effective antistaphylococcal agent in the treatment of endocarditis, septicemia, and infections of the bone, skin, skin structure, and lower respiratory tract. This drug may be given for *initial* therapy when methicillin-resistant staphylococci are suspected.

Nonstaphylococcal endocarditis — Vancomycin has been reported to be effective in the treatment of endocarditis caused by diphtheroids, enterococci such as *Streptococcus faecalis* (when used in combination with an aminoglycoside), viridans streptococci, and *Streptococcus bovis*; this drug has been used successfully in combination with rifampin, an aminoglycoside, or both agents to treat early-onset prosthetic valve endocarditis caused by *Streptococcus epidermidis* or diphtheroids

Preparation of IV solution — Add 10 ml of sterile water for injection to the 500-mg vial or 20 ml to the 1-g vial. Dilute solution reconstituted in the 500-mg vial with at least 100 ml of a compatible diluent and dilute solution reconstituted in the 1-g vial with at least 200 ml. The following diluents are compatible with vancomycin: 5% dextrose injection USP, 0.9% sodium chloride injection USP, 5% dextrose injection and 0.9% sodium chloride injection USP, Isolyte E, lactated Ringer's injection USP, acetated Ringer's injection, and 5% dextrose injection with either lactated Ringer's injection or Normosol-M.

Intravenous administration — Adverse effects, including exaggerated hypotension, wheezing, dyspnea, urticaria, pruritus, flushing of the upper body ("red neck"), pain and spasm of the chest and back, and, in rare cases, cardiac arrest, can occur during or soon after IV infusion, particularly when the rate of administration is rapid; these effects usually disappear within 20 min after cessation of infusion, but they may persist for several hours. To minimize the risk of these reactions, administer each dose by slow IV infusion over a period of at least 60 min. Since concomitant administration of anesthetics reportedly increases this risk, infusion of vancomycin should be completed before induction of anesthesia. Inadvertent extravasation or IM injection may produce pain, tenderness, and necrosis; therefore, make sure that IV route is secure. To avoid thrombophlebitis, dilute solution (see "Preparation of solution") and rotate sites of infusion.

VANCOCIN

Obese patients	Adjustment of usual dosage may be necessary for patients who are obese
Elderly patients	A dosage adjustment will be necessary for elderly patients since GFR and renal function decrease with age; see recommendations for patients with renal impairment, below
Patients with renal impairment	If renal function is impaired, give an initial IV dose of at least 15 mg/kg. For maintenance of therapeutic plasma levels when the creatinine clearance is 10–100 ml/min, use the table below. For functionally anephric patients, a maintenance dose may be given every several days; the dose should be the equivalent of 1.9 mg/kg/24 h. If the patient is anuric, give 1 g every 7–10 days. Measurement of the plasma drug level can be helpful in determining the optimal dosage, especially when renal function is changing. Creatinine clearance can be estimated if the serum creatinine level is known and renal function is stable. For adult men, use the following formula: (weight [kg]) (140 − age [yr])/(72) (serum creatinine level [mg/dl]); for adult women, multiply this quotient by 0.85. This formula should *not* be used if one of the following conditions is present: (1) shock, severe heart failure, oliguria, or other disorders associated with a progressive decline in renal function or (2) obesity, liver disease, edema, ascites, debilitation, malnutrition, inactivity, or other conditions in which the normal relationship between muscle mass and total body weight is distorted.

Creatinine clearance (ml/min)	Dosage (mg/24 h)	Creatinine clearance (ml/min)	Dosage (mg/24 h)
10	155	60	925
20	310	70	1,080
30	465	80	1,235
40	620	90	1,390
50	770	100	1,545

Measurement of plasma drug level	Microbiologic assay, RIA, HPLC, fluorescence immunoassay, or fluorescence polarization immunoassay may be used to measure the plasma level of vancomycin
Intrathecal administration	Safety and effectiveness of intralumbar or intraventricular administration have not been established

WARNINGS/PRECAUTIONS

When used orally

Risks of oral therapy	In general, vancomycin is poorly absorbed after oral administration; however, in some patients, the plasma drug level may be clinically significant and the systemic reactions seen with IV administration may develop. Renal function should be monitored serially in patients who are elderly, receiving aminoglycosides, or have renal impairment; serial tests of auditory function may be helpful in minimizing the risk of ototoxicity.

When used parenterally

Ototoxicity	Transient or permanent ototoxicity may occur, particularly in patients who are elderly, receiving excessive doses or ototoxic drugs, or have renal impairment or an underlying hearing loss; serial tests of auditory function may be helpful in minimizing the risk of ototoxicity
Nephrotoxicity	Azotemia, characterized by increases in BUN or serum creatinine level, may occur, particularly in patients who are elderly, receiving aminoglycosides, or have renal impairment; azotemia is usually reversed by discontinuation of therapy. To minimize the risk of nephrotoxicity, monitor renal function serially in patients who are elderly, receiving aminoglycosides, or have renal impairment and carefully adhere to dosing schedules recommended for patients with renal dysfunction (see ADMINISTRATION/DOSAGE ADJUSTMENTS).
Neutropenia	Reversible neutropenia may develop, usually after a cumulative dose of 25 g has been given or after at least 1 wk of therapy has elapsed; periodically monitor WBC count in patients undergoing prolonged therapy or receiving other drugs associated with neutropenia

ADVERSE REACTIONS

When used orally

Hypersensitivity	Anaphylaxis, urticaria, drug fever, macular rash
Other	Chills, nausea

When used parenterally

Otic	Hearing loss, vertigo, dizziness, tinnitus
Renal	Azotemia
Hematological	Neutropenia, thrombocytopenia
Cardiovascular	Hypotension, flushing of the upper body, cardiac arrest
Respiratory	Wheezing, dyspnea
Musculoskeletal	Pain and muscle spasm of the chest and back

VANCOCIN

Other	Anaphylaxis, drug fever, chills, rash, urticaria, pruritus, thrombophlebitis at injection site

OVERDOSAGE

Signs and symptoms	See reactions associated with IV therapy
Treatment	Maintain renal function; institute other supportive measures. Hemoperfusion with Amberlite XAD-4 resin may be of limited benefit in removing vancomycin from the blood; the drug is poorly removed by dialysis.

DRUG INTERACTIONS

Aminoglycosides, amphotericin B, bacitracin, polymyxin B, colistin, viomycin, cisplatin	⌂ Risk of ototoxicity or nephrotoxicity; carefully monitor clinical response and appropriate parameters when vancomycin and any of these drugs is given sequentially or concomitantly
Anesthetics	⌂ Risk of adverse effects associated with IV infusion (see "Intravenous administration")

ALTERED LABORATORY VALUES

Blood/serum values	⌂ BUN ⌂ Creatinine

No clinically significant alterations in urinary values occur at therapeutic dosages

USE IN CHILDREN

See INDICATIONS and dosage recommendations; closely monitor plasma drug level in neonates and young infants given IV doses

USE IN PREGNANT AND NURSING WOMEN

Pregnancy Category C: reproduction studies have not been done; it is not known whether vancomycin can cause harm to the fetus or affect reproductive capacity. Use during pregnancy only if clearly needed. It is not known whether this drug is excreted in human milk; use with caution in nursing mothers. Bear in mind that even if this drug were to appear in human milk, it is unlikely that a nursing infant with a normal GI tract would absorb a significant amount.

---

[1] A solution may be prepared in the vials for oral or nasogastric administration and used to treat antibiotic-associated pseudomembranous colitis caused by *Clostridium difficile*; see recommendations that pertain to oral therapy

[2] Dosage is based on recommendations of the American Heart Association (*Circulation* 70:1123A–1127A, 1984)

Chapter 24

Anti-Infectives: Cephalosporins and Penicillins

Cephalosporins	920
ANCEF (Smith Kline & French) Cefazolin sodium *Rx*	920
ANSPOR (Smith Kline & French) Cephradine *Rx*	921
CECLOR (Lilly) Cefaclor *Rx*	923
CEFADYL (Apothecon) Cephapirin sodium *Rx*	924
CEFIZOX (Smith Kline & French) Ceftizoxime sodium *Rx*	926
CEFOBID (Roerig) Cefoperazone sodium *Rx*	927
CEFOTAN (Stuart) Cefotetan disodium *Rx*	929
CLAFORAN (Hoechst-Roussel) Cefotaxime sodium *Rx*	931
DURICEF (Mead Johnson) Cefadroxil *Rx*	933
FORTAZ (Glaxo) Ceftazidime *Rx*	934
KEFLEX (Dista) Cephalexin *Rx*	936
KEFLIN (Lilly) Cephalothin sodium *Rx*	938
KEFUROX (Lilly) Cefuroxime sodium *Rx*	940
KEFZOL (Lilly) Cefazolin sodium *Rx*	942
MANDOL (Lilly) Cefamandole nafate *Rx*	944
MEFOXIN (Merck Sharp & Dohme) Cefoxitin sodium *Rx*	946
MONOCID (Smith Kline & French) Cefonicid sodium *Rx*	948
MOXAM (Lilly) Moxalactam disodium *Rx*	950
PRECEF (Apothecon) Ceforanide *Rx*	952
ROCEPHIN (Roche) Ceftriaxone sodium *Rx*	954
TAZICEF (Smith Kline & French) Ceftazidime *Rx*	956
TAZIDIME (Lilly) Ceftazidime *Rx*	958
ULTRACEF (Bristol) Cefadroxil *Rx*	960
VELOSEF (Squibb) Cephradine *Rx*	961
ZINACEF (Glaxo) Cefuroxime sodium *Rx*	964

Penicillins	966
AMCILL (Parke-Davis) Ampicillin *Rx*	966
AMOXIL (Beecham) Amoxicillin *Rx*	967
AUGMENTIN (Beecham) Amoxicillin and clavulanate potassium *Rx*	968
AZLIN (Miles Pharmaceuticals) Azlocillin sodium *Rx*	970
BICILLIN C-R (Wyeth) Penicillin G benzathine and penicillin G procaine *Rx*	971
BICILLIN C-R 900/300 (Wyeth) Penicillin G benzathine and penicillin G procaine *Rx*	971
BICILLIN L-A (Wyeth) Penicillin G benzathine *Rx*	972
COACTIN (Roche) Amdinocillin *Rx*	974
CYCLAPEN-W (Wyeth) Cyclacillin *Rx*	975
GEOCILLIN (Roerig) Carbenicillin indanyl sodium *Rx*	976
GEOPEN (Roerig) Carbenicillin disodium *Rx*	977
LAROTID (Beecham) Amoxicillin *Rx*	979
LEDERCILLIN VK (Lederle) Penicillin V potassium *Rx*	980
MEZLIN (Miles Pharmaceuticals) Mezlocillin sodium *Rx*	981
OMNIPEN (Wyeth) Ampicillin *Rx*	983
OMNIPEN-N (Wyeth) Ampicillin sodium *Rx*	983
PENTIDS (Squibb) Penicillin G potassium *Rx*	985
PEN·VEE K (Wyeth) Penicillin V potassium *Rx*	986
PERMAPEN (Roerig) Penicillin G benzathine *Rx*	988
PFIZERPEN-AS (Roerig) Penicillin G procaine *Rx*	989
PIPRACIL (Lederle) Piperacillin sodium *Rx*	991
POLYCILLIN (Apothecon) Ampicillin *Rx*	993
POLYCILLIN-N (Apothecon) Ampicillin sodium *Rx*	993
POLYMOX (Apothecon) Amoxicillin *Rx*	995

PRINCIPEN (Squibb) Ampicillin *Rx*	996
PROSTAPHLIN (Apothecon) Oxacillin sodium *Rx*	997
PYOPEN (Beecham) Carbenicillin disodium *Rx*	999
SK-AMPICILLIN (Smith Kline & French) Ampicillin *Rx*	1001
SPECTROBID (Roerig) Bacampicillin hydrochloride *Rx*	1002
TEGOPEN (Apothecon) Cloxacillin sodium *Rx*	1004
TICAR (Beecham) Ticarcillin disodium *Rx*	1005
TIMENTIN (Beecham) Ticarcillin disodium and clavulanate potassium *Rx*	1007
TOTACILLIN (Beecham) Ampicillin *Rx*	1009
TOTACILLIN-N (Beecham) Ampicillin sodium *Rx*	1009
TRIMOX (Squibb) Ampicillin *Rx*	1010
UNIPEN (Wyeth) Nafcillin sodium *Rx*	1011
V-CILLIN K (Lilly) Penicillin V potassium *Rx*	1012

Other Penicillins	**915**
BETAPEN-VK (Apothecon) Penicillin V potassium *Rx*	915
DYNAPEN (Apothecon) Dicloxacillin sodium *Rx*	916
NAFCIL (Apothecon) Nafcillin sodium *Rx*	916
PFIZERPEN (Roerig) Penicillin G potassium *Rx*	916
PRINCIPEN with Probenecid (Squibb) Ampicillin and probenecid *Rx*	916
ROBICILLIN VK (Robins) Penicillin V potassium *Rx*	917
STAPHCILLIN (Apothecon) Methicillin sodium *Rx*	917
UTICILLIN VK (Upjohn) Penicillin V potassium *Rx*	917
VEETIDS (Squibb) Penicillin V potassium *Rx*	917
WYCILLIN (Wyeth) Penicillin G procaine *Rx*	918
WYMOX (Wyeth) Amoxicillin trihydrate *Rx*	918
Other Cephalosporins	**919**
SEFFIN (Glaxo) Cephalothin sodium *Rx*	919

OTHER PENICILLINS

DRUG	HOW SUPPLIED	USUAL DOSAGE
BETAPEN-VK (Apothecon) Penicillin V potassium *Rx*	**Tablets:** penicillin V potassium equivalent to 250 or 500 mg penicillin V **Solution (per 5 ml):** penicillin V potassium equivalent to 125 or 250 mg penicillin V after reconstitution	**Adult:** for streptococcal infections, 125–250 mg q6–8h for 10 days; for pneumococcal infections, 250 mg q6h until patient is afebrile for at least 2 days; for staphylococcal infections or fusospirochetosis (Vincent's infection), 250 mg q6–8h; to prevent recurrence of rheumatic fever and/or chorea, 125 mg bid; to prevent bacterial endocarditis, 2 g (or 1 million units IM aqueous crystalline penicillin G mixed with 600,000 units procaine penicillin G) ½–1 h prior to surgery or instrumentation, followed by 500 mg q6h for 8 doses **Child (< 60 lb):** to prevent bacterial endocarditis, 1 g (or 30,000 units/kg IM aqueous crystalline penicillin G mixed with 600,000 units procaine penicillin G) ½–1 h prior to surgery or instrumentation, followed by 250 mg q6h for 8 doses **Child (≥ 60 lb):** to prevent bacterial endocarditis, same as adult

continued

OTHER PENICILLINS continued

DRUG	HOW SUPPLIED	USUAL DOSAGE
DYNAPEN (Apothecon) Dicloxacillin sodium *Rx*	**Capsules:** dicloxacillin sodium equivalent to 125, 250, or 500 mg dicloxacillin **Suspension (per 5 ml):** 62.5 mg (80, 100, 200 ml)	**Adult:** for mild to moderate infections, 125 mg q6h; for more severe infections, 250 mg q6h **Child (< 40 kg):** for mild to moderate infections, 12.5 mg/kg/day, given in equally divided doses q6h; for more severe infections, 25 mg/kg/day, given in equally divided doses q6h
NAFCIL (Apothecon) Nafcillin sodium *Rx*	**Vials:** nafcillin sodium equivalent to 500 mg, 1 or 2 g nafcillin **Piggyback units:** nafcillin sodium equivalent to 1 or 2 g nafcillin **Hospital bulk package:** 10 g	**Adult:** 500 mg IV (or 1 g IV for severe infections) q4h for 24–48 h or 500 mg IM q6h (or q4h for severe infections) **Neonate:** 10 mg/kg IM bid **Infant or child:** 25 mg/kg IM bid
PFIZERPEN (Roerig) Penicillin G potassium *Rx*	**Vials:** 1 or 5 million units, for reconstitution and administration by injection (IM, intrathecal) or infusion (intrapleural, other local routes, continuous IV); 20 million units, for reconstitution and administration by continuous IV infusion only **Pharmacy bulk package:** 20 million units, for reconstitution and administration by continuous IV infusion only	**Adult:** for gonorrheal endocarditis, anthrax, and severe infections due to susceptible streptococci, pneumococci, and staphylococci, at least 5 million units/day (for anthrax, use divided doses); for meningococcic meningitis, 1–2 million units IM q2h or 20–30 million units/day by continuous IV infusion; for cervico-facial actinomycosis, 1–6 million units/day; for thoracic and abdominal actinomycosis, 10–20 million units/day; for clostridial infections (adjunctive therapy with antitoxin), 20 million units/day; for severe fusospirochetosis, 5–10 million units/day; for rat-bite infections due to *Spirillum minus* or *Streptobacillus moniliformis*, 12–15 million units/day for 3–4 wk; for meningitis or endocarditis due to *Listeria monocytogenes*, 15–20 million units/day for 2 wk (meningitis) or 4 wk (endocarditis); for bacteremia and meningitis due to *Pasteurella multocida*, 4–6 million units/day for 2 wk; for erysipeloid endocarditis, 2–20 million units/day for 4–6 wk; for gram-negative bacillary bacteremia, 20–80 million units/day; for diphtheria carrier state, 300,000–400,000 units/day, given in divided doses for 10–12 days; for syphilis, determine dosage according to stage of disease and age; for prevention of bacterial endocarditis in patients with congenital heart disease or rheumatic or other acquired valvular heart disease who are undergoing dental procedures or upper respiratory tract surgery, 1 million units aqueous crystalline penicillin G mixed with 600,000 units penicillin G procaine, given IM ½–1 h before procedure or surgery, followed by 500 mg oral penicillin V q6h for 8 doses **Neonate:** for infections due to *Listeria monocytogenes*, 0.5–1 million units/day **Child:** for prevention of bacterial endocarditis (see adult indication), 30,000 units/kg aqueous crystalline penicillin G mixed with 600,000 units penicillin G procaine, given IM ½–1 h before procedure or surgery, followed by 250 mg oral penicillin V (500 mg for child ≥ 60 lb) q6h for 8 doses
PRINCIPEN with Probenecid (Squibb) Ampicillin and probenecid *Rx*	**Capsules:** ampicillin trihydrate equivalent to 389 mg ampicillin and 111 mg probenecid	**Adult:** for gonorrhea, 9 caps given in a single dose

OTHER PENICILLINS continued

DRUG	HOW SUPPLIED	USUAL DOSAGE
ROBICILLIN VK (Robins) Penicillin V potassium *Rx*	**Tablets:** 250, 500 mg	**Adult:** for mild streptococcal infections, 125 mg q6–8h for 10 days; for moderately severe streptococcal infections, 250–500 mg q8h for 10 days; for pneumococcal infections, 250–500 mg q6h until patient is afebrile for at least 2 days; for staphylococcal infections, 250–500 mg q6–8h; for fusospirochetosis (Vincent's infection), 250 mg q6–8h; to prevent recurrence of rheumatic fever and/or chorea, 125 mg bid; to prevent bacterial endocarditis, give 2 g (or 1 million units IM aqueous crystalline penicillin G mixed with 600,000 units procaine penicillin G) $1/2$–1 h before dental or surgical procedure, followed by 500 mg oral penicillin V q6h for 8 doses **Infant or small child:** 15.6–56 mg/kg/day, given in 3–6 divided doses **Child (< 12 yr):** calculate dosage according to body weight; to prevent bacterial endocarditis in children < 60 lb, 1 g (or 30,000 units/kg IM aqueous crystalline penicillin G mixed with 600,000 units procaine penicillin G) $1/2$–1 h before dental or surgical procedure, followed by 250 mg q6h for 8 doses (for children > 60 lb, see adult dosage, above)
STAPHCILLIN (Apothecon) Methicillin sodium *Rx*	**Vials:** 1, 4, 6 g **Piggyback units:** 1, 4 g **Hospital bulk package:** 10 g	**Adult:** 1 g IM q4–6h or 1 g IV q6h **Infant and child (< 40 kg):** 25 mg/kg IM q6h
UTICILLIN VK (Upjohn) Penicillin V potassium *Rx*	**Tablets:** penicillin V potassium equivalent to 250 or 500 mg penicillin V	**Adult:** for streptococcal infections 125–250 mg q6–8h for 10 days; for pneumococcal infections, 250 mg q6h until patient is afebrile for at least 2 days; for staphylococcal infections or fusospirochetosis (Vincent's infection), 250 mg q6–8h; to prevent recurrence of rheumatic fever, 125 mg bid; to prevent bacterial endocarditis, 2 g (or 1 million units IM aqueous crystalline penicillin G mixed with 600,000 units procaine penicillin G) $1/2$–1 h prior to dental or surgical procedure, followed by 500 mg q6h for 8 doses after procedure **Infant or small child:** 15.6–62.5 mg/kg/day, given in 3–6 divided doses **Child (< 12 yr):** calculate dosage according to body weight; to prevent bacterial endocarditis in children < 60 lb, 1 g (or 30,000 units/kg IM aqueous crystalline penicillin G mixed with 600,000 units procaine penicillin G) $1/2$–1 h before dental or surgical procedure, followed by 250 mg q6h for 8 doses (for children > 60 lb, see adult dosage, above)
VEETIDS (Squibb) Penicillin V potassium *Rx*	**Tablets:** penicillin V potassium equivalent to 250 or 500 mg penicillin V **Solution (per 5 ml):** penicillin V potassium equivalent to 125 or 250 mg penicillin V after reconstitution (100, 200 ml)	**Adult:** for mild streptococcal infections, 125 mg tid or qid for 10 days; for moderately severe streptococcal infections, 250 mg tid for 10 days (alternative regimen for streptococcal pharyngitis: 500 mg bid); for pneumococcal infections, 250–500 mg qid until patient is afebrile for at least 2 days; for staphylococcal infections or fusospirochetosis (Vincent's infection), 250 mg tid or qid, or 500 mg tid; to prevent recurrence of rheumatic fever and/or chorea, 125 mg bid; to prevent bacterial endocarditis, 2 g of penicillin V 1 h before dental or

continued

COMPENDIUM OF DRUG THERAPY

OTHER PENICILLINS continued

DRUG	HOW SUPPLIED	USUAL DOSAGE
VEETIDS continued		surgical procedure, followed by 1 g 6 h later; alternatively, 1–2 g of ampicillin IM or IV with 1.5 mg/kg of gentamicin IM or IV 30 min before procedure and then repeat 8 h later *or* give 1 g of penicillin V 6 h later **Infant or small child:** 15–56 mg/kg/day, given in 3–6 divided doses **Child (< 60 kg):** to prevent bacterial endocarditis, 1 g penicillin V 1 h before dental or surgical procedure, followed by 500 mg 6 h later; alternatively, 50 mg/kg of ampicillin IM or IV with 2 mg/kg of gentamicin IM or IV 30 min before procedure and then repeat 8 h later *or* give 500 mg of penicillin V 6 h later (children's dosages should not exceed adult recommendations for a single dose or for a 24-h period) **Child (> 60 kg):** same as adult
WYCILLIN (Wyeth) Penicillin G procaine *Rx*	**Cartridge-needle units:** 600,000 units/ml (1, 2 ml) **Prefilled syringes:** 2,400,000 units (4 ml)	**Adult:** for uncomplicated pneumococcal pneumonia, 600,000–1,000,000 units/day IM; for Group A streptococcal infections, 600,000–1,000,000 units/day IM for 10 days; for staphylococcal infections, 600,000–1,000,000 units/day IM; for bacterial endocarditis (extremely sensitive Group A streptococcal infections only), anthrax, fusospirochetosis (Vincent's infection), erysipeloid, and rat-bite fever, 600,000–1,000,000 units/day IM; to prevent bacterial endocarditis, 1 million units IM aqueous crystalline penicillin G mixed with 600,000 units procaine penicillin G ½–1 h before dental or surgical procedure, followed by 500 mg oral penicillin V q6h for 8 doses; for syphilis, yaws, bejel, or pinta, 600,000 units/day for 8–15 days, depending on disease stage; for uncomplicated gonorrhea, 4.8 million units IM, divided and injected into different sites at one visit, along with 1 g of probenecid PO **Child (< 60 lb):** for pneumococcal, Group A streptococcal, or staphylococcal infections, 300,000 units/day IM; to prevent bacterial endocarditis, 30,000 units/kg IM aqueous crystalline penicillin G mixed with 600,000 units procaine penicillin G ½–1 h before dental or surgical procedure, followed by 250 mg of oral penicillin V q6h for 8 doses **Child (< 70 lb):** for congenital syphilis, 10,000 units/kg/day IM for 10 days
WYMOX (Wyeth) Amoxicillin trihydrate *Rx*	**Capsules:** 250, 500 mg **Suspension (per 5 ml):** amoxicillin trihydrate equivalent to 125 or 250 mg amoxicillin after reconstitution (80, 100, 150 ml)	**Adult:** for ear, nose, throat, genitourinary tract, skin, and soft-tissue infections, 250 mg q8h; for lower respiratory tract infections, severe infections, and infections caused by less-susceptible organisms, 500 mg q8h; for gonorrhea, 3 g, given in a single dose **Child (< 20 kg):** for ear, nose, throat, genitourinary tract, skin, and soft-tissue infections, 20 mg/kg/day, given in divided doses q8h; for lower respiratory tract infections, severe infections, and infections caused by less-susceptible organisms, 40 mg/kg/day, given in divided doses q8h **Child (≥ 20 kg):** same as adult

OTHER CEPHALOSPORINS

DRUG	HOW SUPPLIED	USUAL DOSAGE
SEFFIN (Glaxo) Cephalothin sodium *Rx*	**Vials:** 1, 2 g **Infusion bottles:** 1, 2 g (100 ml) **Pharmacy bulk packages:** 10 g (100 ml)	**Adult:** for treatment, 0.5–1 g IM or IV q4–6h; for life-threatening infections 2 g IM or IV q4h; for prophylactic use, 1–2 g, given IV 30–60 min before surgery, then IM or IV during surgery, and finally IM or IV q6h after surgery for 24 h **Infant and child:** for treatment, 80–160 mg/kg/day, given in divided doses; for prophylactic use, 20–30 mg/kg, given according to the adult schedule

CEPHALOSPORINS

ANCEF (cefazolin sodium) Smith Kline & French   Rx

Vials: 250, 500 mg; 1 g   **Piggyback vials:** 500 mg; 1 g   **Pharmacy bulk vials:** 5, 10 g   **Plastic containers:** 10, 20 mg/ml (50 ml)

INDICATIONS

Respiratory tract infections caused by susceptible strains of *Streptococcus pneumoniae, Klebsiella, Hemophilus influenzae, Staphylococcus aureus,* and Group A beta-hemolytic streptococci

Urinary tract infections caused by susceptible strains of *Escherichia coli, Proteus mirabilis, Klebsiella, Enterobacter,* and enterococci

Skin and skin structure infections caused by susceptible strains of *Staphylococcus aureus,* Group A beta-hemolytic streptococci, and other streptococci

Biliary tract infections caused by susceptible strains of *Escherichia coli,* streptococci, *Proteus mirabilis, Klebsiella,* and *Staphylococcus aureus*

Bone and joint infections caused by susceptible strains of *Staphylococcus aureus*

Septicemia caused by susceptible strains of *Streptococcus pneumoniae, Staphylococcus aureus, Proteus mirabilis, Escherichia coli,* and *Klebsiella*

Endocarditis caused by susceptible strains of *Staphylococcus aureus,* and Group A beta-hemolytic streptococci

Genital infections caused by susceptible strains of *Escherichia coli, Proteus mirabilis, Klebsiella,* and enterococci

Prevention of postoperative infection in patients undergoing contaminated or potentially contaminated procedures or when infection at the operative site would present a serious risk

PARENTERAL DOSAGE

Adult: for mild infections caused by susceptible Gram-positive cocci, 250–500 mg IM of IV q8h; for moderate to severe infections, 500 mg to 1 g IM or IV q6–8h; for acute uncomplicated urinary tract infections, 1 g IM or IV q12h; for pneumococcal pneumonia, 500 mg IM or IV q12h; for life threatening infections, such as endocarditis and septicemia, 1–1.5 g IM or IV q6h or, if necessary, up to 12 g/day

Infant ($\geq$ 1 mo) and child: for mild to moderately severe infections, 25–50 mg/kg/day in 3 or 4 equally divided doses; for severe infections, up to 100 mg/kg/day in 3 or 4 equally divided doses

Adult: 1 g IM or IV $^{1}/_{2}$–1 h prior to surgery, followed by 0.5–1 g IM or IV during lengthy (2 h or more) procedures and then q6–8h for 24 h postoperatively; in cases where postoperative infection would be particularly devastating (eg, open-heart surgery and prosthetic arthroplasty), prophylactic administration may be continued for 3–5 days

CONTRAINDICATIONS

Hypersensitivity to cephalosporins

ADMINISTRATION/DOSAGE ADJUSTMENTS

Intramuscular administration — Add 2 ml of sterile water for injection to the 250- or 500-mg vial or 2.5 ml to the 1-g vial; inject into a large muscle mass

Preparation for IV use — To reconstitute the solution in a regular vial, add 2 ml of sterile water for injection if the vial contains 250 or 500 mg, 2.5 ml if the vial contains 1 g. For IV injection, dilute the reconstituted solution with an additional 5 ml of sterile water for injection; for intermittent or continuous infusion, dilute the solution in 50–100 ml of an appropriate diluent. To reconstitute the solution in a piggyback vial, use 50–100 ml of an appropriate diluent; when adding the diluent, pump the syringe or use a small vent needle in order to allow air to escape. For reconstituting the solution in a piggyback vial or diluting the solution in a regular or bulk vial for IV infusion, use one of the following preparations: 5% dextrose injection (alone, with lactated Ringer's injection, or with 0.2%, 0.45%, or 0.9% sodium chloride injection), 10% dextrose injection, Ringer's or lactated Ringer's injection, 5% or 10% invert sugar in sterile water for injection, or 5% sodium bicarbonate in sterile water for injection. For reconstitution in pharmacy bulk vials, use sterile or bacteriostatic water for injection or sodium chloride injection; add 23 ml to the 5-g vial or 45 ml to the 10-g vial to obtain a concentration of approximately 200 mg/ml, 48 ml to the 5-g vial or 96 ml to the 10-g vial to obtain a concentration of approximately 100 mg/ml. To use a plastic container, thaw contents at room temperature. Check for minute leaks by squeezing the bag firmly; discard it if leaks are found or seal is not intact. Do not put additives into the container.

Intravenous administration — Cefazolin can be given by direct injection or by intermittent or continuous infusion. For bolus administration, slowly inject dose over a period of 3–5 min either directly into a vein or through IV tubing. At least once every 48 h, replace the administration set used with plastic containers. Do not connect these containers in series because residual air in the primary container, withdrawn before administration of the fluid in the secondary container is complete, could produce air embolism.

Adults with renal impairment	Determine the initial dose according to the severity of the infection. Calculate subsequent doses and the dosing interval as follows: If creatinine clearance (Ccr) = 35–54 ml/min or serum creatinine level (Scr) = 1.6–3 mg/dl, maintain dose, but administer at intervals of at least 8 h. If Ccr = 11–34 ml/min or Scr = 3.1–4.5 mg/dl, reduce dose by 50% and give q12h. If Ccr = $\leq$ 10 ml/min or Scr = $\geq$ 4.6 mg/dl, reduce dose by 50% and give q18–24h. For use in patients undergoing peritoneal dialysis, see package insert.
Children with renal impairment	Determine the initial dose according to the severity of the infection. Calculate subsequent doses and the dosing interval as follows: If creatinine clearance (Ccr) = 40–70 ml/min, give 60% of the normal daily dose in 2 equally divided doses q12h. If Ccr = 20–40 ml/min, give 25% of the normal daily dose in 2 equally divided doses q12h. If Ccr = 5–20 ml/min, give 10% of the normal daily dose q24h.

WARNINGS/PRECAUTIONS

Cross-allergenicity	Use with caution in penicillin-allergic patients
Hypersensitivity reactions	Serious acute hypersensitivity reactions may occur, most likely in patients with a history of allergy, particularly to drugs; anaphylactic reactions may require administration of epinephrine and other emergency measures
Pseudomembranous colitis	May occur due to alteration of the normal intestinal flora and should be considered in any patient who develops diarrhea during or after therapy; use with caution in patients with a history of GI disease, particularly colitis. Mild cases may respond to withdrawal of the drug alone. Moderate to severe cases should be managed by fluid and electrolyte replacement and protein supplementation, as needed. Oral vancomycin is the treatment of choice for severe or refractory colitis associated with the overgrowth of *Clostridium difficile;* however, other possible causes should also be considered.
Superinfection	Overgrowth of nonsusceptible organisms may occur with prolonged use; careful clinical observation is essential
Carcinogenicity, mutagenicity	No studies have been done to determine the carcinogenic or mutagenic potential of this drug

ADVERSE REACTIONS

Gastrointestinal	Anorexia, stomach cramps, diarrhea, oral candidiasis, pseudomembranous colitis; nausea and vomiting (rare)
Hypersensitivity	Drug fever, skin rash, pruritus, eosinophilia, anaphylaxis
Genitourinary	Genital and anal pruritus, genital moniliasis, vaginitis
Hematological	Neutropenia, leukopenia, thrombocytosis
Other	Pain on IM injection, sometimes with induration; phlebitis at injection site

OVERDOSAGE

Signs and symptoms	See ADVERSE REACTIONS
Treatment	Discontinue medication; treat symptomatically and institute supportive measures, as required

DRUG INTERACTIONS

Probenecid	⇧ Cefazolin blood level and/or toxicity

ALTERED LABORATORY VALUES

Blood/serum values	⇧ Alkaline phosphatase ⇧ SGOT ⇧ SGPT ⇧ BUN + Coombs' test
Urinary values	+ Glucose (with Benedict's solution, Fehling's solution, and Clinitest tablets)

USE IN CHILDREN

See INDICATIONS; adjust dosage according to body weight and severity of infection. Safety and effectiveness have not been established for use in premature infants or in infants under 1 mo of age.

USE IN PREGNANT AND NURSING WOMEN

Pregnancy Category B: use during pregnancy only if clearly needed. Reproduction studies in rats, mice, and rabbits at doses up to 25 times the human dose have shown no evidence of impaired fertility or harm to the fetus; however, no adequate, well-controlled studies have been done in pregnant women. Positive Coombs' tests have been reported in newborns of mothers who received cephalosporins before delivery. When administered prior to cesarean section, the drug appears to have no adverse effect on the fetus, despite its presence in cord blood. Very low concentrations of cefazolin are excreted in human milk; use with caution in nursing mothers.

CEPHALOSPORINS

ANSPOR (cephradine)   Smith Kline & French   Rx

Capsules: 250, 500 mg   **Suspension (per 5 ml):** 125 mg, 250 mg after reconstitution (100 ml) *fruit-flavored*

INDICATIONS

Respiratory tract infections caused by susceptible strains of Group A beta-hemolytic streptococci and *Streptococcus pneumoniae*

Skin and skin structure infections caused by susceptible strains of staphylococci and beta-hemolytic streptococci

ORAL DOSAGE

Adult: 250 mg q6h or 500 mg q12h; for severe or chronic infections, up to 1 g qid may be given

Infant ($\geq$ 9 mo) and child: 25–50 mg/kg/day in equally divided doses q6h or q12h; for severe or chronic infections, up to 1 g qid may be given

ANSPOR

Urinary tract infections, including prostatis, caused by susceptible strains of *Escherichia coli*, *Proteus mirabilis*, and *Klebsiella*

Adult: 500 mg q6h or 1 g q12h; for severe or chronic infections, up to 1 g qid may be given

Lobar pneumonia caused by susceptible strains of *Streptococcus pneumoniae*

Otitis media caused by susceptible strains of Group A beta-hemolytic streptococci, *Streptococcus pneumoniae*, *Hemophilus influenzae*, and staphylococci

Infant ($\geq$ 9 mo) and child: 75–100 mg/kg/day in equally divided doses q6h or q12h; for severe or chronic infections, up to 1 g qid may be given

CONTRAINDICATIONS

Hypersensitivity to cephalosporins

ADMINISTRATION/DOSAGE ADJUSTMENTS

Timing of administration	Cephradine may be given without regard to meals, unless GI irritation occurs
Patients with renal impairment	For patients not undergoing dialysis, start with 500 mg q6h when creatinine clearance rate (CCr) > 20 ml/min; 250 mg q6h when CCr = 5–20 ml/min; or 250 mg q12h when CCr < 5 ml/min; for patients receiving chronic intermittent hemodialysis, administer 250 mg to start, followed by 250 mg 12 h later and 250 mg 36–48 h after initial dose
Duration of therapy	Continue therapy for a minimum of 48–72 h after patient becomes asymptomatic or evidence of bacterial eradication has been obtained. Infections caused by Group A beta-hemolytic streptococci should be treated for at least 10 days to guard against the risk of rheumatic fever or glomerulonephritis.

WARNINGS/PRECAUTIONS

Cross-allergenicity	Use with caution in penicillin-allergic patients
Hypersensitivity	Serious acute hypersensitivity reactions may occur (most likely in patients with a history of allergy, asthma, hay fever, or urticaria); anaphylactic reactions may require administration of epinephrine, pressor amines, antihistamines, or corticosteroids
Special-risk patients	Patients with markedly impaired renal function should be carefully monitored during therapy, since cephradine accumulates in the serum and tissues (see ADMINISTRATION/DOSAGE ADJUSTMENTS); use with caution in patients with a history of GI disease, particularly colitis
Superinfection	Overgrowth of nonsusceptible organisms may occur with prolonged use
Pseudomembranous colitis	May occur due to alteration of the normal intestinal flora and should be considered in any patient who develops diarrhea during or after therapy. Mild cases may respond to withdrawal of the drug alone. Moderate to severe cases should be managed by fluid and electrolyte replacement and protein supplementation, as needed. Oral vancomycin is the treatment of choice for severe or refractory colitis associated with the overgrowth of *Clostridium difficile;* however, other possible causes should also be considered.
Chronic urinary tract infections	Frequent bacteriological and clinical appraisal is necessary during therapy and may be required for several months afterward; prolonged, intensive therapy is recommended for prostatis
Diabetic patients	Caution diabetics not to independently change their diet or antidiabetic medication dosage, since a false-positive reaction for glucose in the urine may occur if Benedict's solution, Fehling's solution, or Clinitest tablets are used; enzyme-based tests (eg, Clinistix or Tes-Tape) are not affected by cephradine therapy
Carcinogenicity, mutagenicity	The carcinogenic and mutagenic potential of this drug has not been evaluated

ADVERSE REACTIONS

Gastrointestinal	Glossitis, diarrhea or loose stools, abdominal pain, heartburn, pseudomembranous colitis; nausea and vomiting (rare)
Hypersensitivity	Mild urticaria, skin rash, pruritus, joint pains, anaphylaxis (see WARNINGS/PRECAUTIONS)
Hematological	Mild, transient eosinophilia, leukopenia, and neutropenia
Other	Dizziness, tightness in the chest, candidal vaginitis

OVERDOSAGE

Signs and symptoms	See ADVERSE REACTIONS
Treatment	Discontinue medication; treat symptomatically and institute supportive measures, as required

DRUG INTERACTIONS

Probenecid	⇧ Cephradine blood level and/or toxicity

ALTERED LABORATORY VALUES

Blood/serum values	⇧ Alkaline phosphatase ⇧ Bilirubin ⇧ SGOT ⇧ SGPT ⇧ BUN + Coombs' test

| Urinary values | ⇧ Glucose (with Clinitest tablets) |

USE IN CHILDREN
See INDICATIONS; adjust dosage according to body weight and severity of infection. Safety and effectiveness have not been established for use in infants under 9 mo of age.

USE IN PREGNANT AND NURSING WOMEN
Pregnancy Category B: use during pregnancy only if clearly needed. Reproduction studies in mice and rats at doses up to 4 times the maximum human dose have shown no evidence of impaired fertility or harm to the fetus; however, no adequate, well-controlled studies have been done in pregnant women. Cephradine is excreted in human milk in very low concentrations; use with caution in nursing mothers.

CEPHALOSPORINS

CECLOR (cefaclor) Lilly   Rx

Capsules: 250, 500 mg **Suspension (per 5 ml):** 125 mg after reconstitution (75, 150 ml) *strawberry flavored*, 250 mg after reconstitution (75, 150 ml) *strawberry flavored*

INDICATIONS
Otitis media caused by susceptible strains of *Streptococcus pneumoniae, S pyogenes, Hemophilus influenzae,* and staphylococci

Lower respiratory tract infections caused by susceptible strains of *Streptococcus pneumoniae, S pyogenes,* and *Hemophilus influenzae*

Upper respiratory tract infections, including pharyngitis and tonsillitis, caused by susceptible strains of *Streptococcus pyogenes*

Urinary tract infections, including pyelonephritis and cystitis, caused by susceptible strains of *Escherichia coli, Proteus mirabilis, Klebsiella,* and coagulase-negative staphylococci

Skin and skin structure infections caused by *Staphylococcus aureus* and *Streptococcus pyogenes*

ORAL DOSAGE
Adult: 250 mg q8h; for more severe infections or those caused by less susceptible organisms, dosage may be doubled. The daily dose may be given in 2 divided doses q12h for the treatment of otitis media and pharyngitis.

Infant ($\geq$ 1 mo) and child: 20 mg/kg/day in divided doses q8h; for more serious infections, otitis media, or infections caused by less susceptible organisms, 40 mg/kg/day, up to 1 g/day. The daily dose may be given in 2 divided doses q12h for the treatment of otitis media and pharyngitis.

CONTRAINDICATIONS
Hypersensitivity to cephalosporins

ADMINISTRATION/DOSAGE ADJUSTMENTS
| Duration of treatment for streptococcal infections | Infections caused by beta-hemolytic streptococci should be treated for at least 10 days |

WARNINGS/PRECAUTIONS

Hypersensitivity	If allergic reactions occur (see ADVERSE REACTIONS), discontinue use and, if necessary, treat with pressor amines, antihistamines, and/or corticosteroids. Use with caution in patients with a history of allergy, especially if they are hypersensitive to penicillin or other drugs. Reactions other than anaphylaxis usually develop a few days after beginning a second course of therapy and subside within a few days after therapy is discontinued; such reactions occur more frequently in children than in adults.
Pseudomembranous colitis	May occur due to alteration of the normal intestinal flora and should be considered in any patient who develops diarrhea during or after therapy; use with caution in patients with a history of GI disease, particularly colitis. Mild cases may respond to withdrawal of the drug alone. Moderate to severe cases should be managed by sigmoidoscopy, appropriate bacteriological studies, fluid and electrolyte replacement, and protein supplementation, as needed. Oral vancomycin is the treatment of choice for severe or refractory colitis associated with the overgrowth of *Clostridium difficile;* however, other possible causes should also be considered.
Superinfection	Overgrowth of nonsusceptible organisms may occur with prolonged use; careful clinical observation is essential
Patients with renal impairment	Clinical experience with patients having moderate or severe renal impairment is limited; although a dosage adjustment is usually unnecessary, these patients should be carefully observed, and their laboratory values should be monitored

ADVERSE REACTIONS[1]

Frequent reactions (incidence ≥ 1%) are printed in *italics*

Gastrointestinal	*Diarrhea (1.4%)*, pseudomembranous colitis; nausea and vomiting (rare)
Hepatic	Transient hepatitis and cholestatic jaundice (rare)
Hypersensitivity	*Morbilliform eruptions (1.0%)*, pruritus, urticaria; serum sickness-like reactions, including arthralgia, arthritis, fever, erythema multiforme, and Stevens-Johnson syndrome; anaphylaxis
Other	*Eosinophilia (2.0%)*, genital pruritus, vaginitis; thrombocytopenia (rare)

OVERDOSAGE

Signs and symptoms	See ADVERSE REACTIONS
Treatment	Discontinue medication; treat symptomatically and institute supportive measures, as required

DRUG INTERACTIONS

Probenecid	⇧ Cefaclor blood level and/or toxicity

ALTERED LABORATORY VALUES

Blood/serum values	⇧ Alkaline phosphatase ⇧ SGOT ⇧ SGPT ⇧ BUN ⇧ Creatinine + Coombs' test
Urinary values	⇧ Glucose (with Clinitest tablets)

USE IN CHILDREN

See INDICATIONS; adjust dosage according to body weight and severity of infection. Safety and effectiveness have not been established for use in infants under 1 mo of age.

USE IN PREGNANT AND NURSING WOMEN

Pregnancy Category B: use during pregnancy only if clearly needed. Reproduction studies in mice and rats at doses up to 12 times the human dose and in ferrets given 3 times the maximum human dose have shown no evidence of impaired fertility or harm to the fetus; however, no adequate, well-controlled studies have been done in pregnant women. Positive Coombs' tests have been reported in newborns of mothers who received cephalosporins prior to delivery. Cefaclor is excreted in human milk in small amounts; since the effect on nursing infants is unknown, use with caution in nursing mothers.

[1] Reactions for which a causal relationship has not been established include reversible hyperactivity, nervousness, insomnia, confusion, hypertonia, dizziness, somnolence, transient fluctuations in WBC counts (mainly lymphocytosis in infants and young children), abnormal urinalysis, and slight increases in plasma levels of SGOT, SGPT, alkaline phosphatase, BUN, and creatinine

---

CEPHALOSPORINS

CEFADYL (cephapirin sodium) Apothecon   Rx

Vials: cephapirin sodium equivalent to 500 mg, 1 g, and 2 g cephapirin[1] **Piggyback vials:** cephapirin sodium equivalent to 1, 2, and 4 g cephapirin[1] **Hospital bulk package:** cephapirin sodium equivalent to 20 g cephapirin[1]

INDICATIONS

Respiratory tract infections caused by susceptible strains of *Streptococcus pneumoniae, Staphylococcus aureus, Klebsiella, Hemophilus influenzae,* and Group A beta-hemolytic streptococci

Skin and skin structure infections caused by susceptible strains of *Staphylococcus aureus, S epidermidis, Escherichia coli, Proteus mirabilis, Klebsiella,* and Group A beta-hemolytic streptococci

Urinary tract infections caused by susceptible strains of *Staphylococcus aureus, Escherichia coli, Proteus mirabilis,* and *Klebsiella*

Septicemia caused by susceptible strains of *Staphylococcus aureus, viridans*-type streptococci, *Escherichia coli, Klebsiella,* and Group A beta-hemolytic streptococci

Endocarditis caused by susceptible strains of *viridans*-type streptococci and *Staphylococcus aureus*

Osteomyelitis caused by susceptible strains of *Staphylococcus aureus, Klebsiella, Proteus mirabilis,* and Group A beta-hemolytic streptococci

PARENTERAL DOSAGE

Adult: 500 mg to 1 g IM or IV q4–6h; very serious or life-threatening infections may require up to 12 g/day, preferably IV if high doses are indicated. The IV route may also be preferable for patients with bacteremia, septicemia, or other severe or life-threatening infections who may be poor risks because of lowered resistance resulting, eg, from malnutrition, trauma, surgery, diabetes, heart failure, or malignancy, particularly if shock is present or imminent.

Infant (≥ 3 mo) and child: 40–80 mg/kg/day IM or IV in 4 equally divided doses

CEFADYL

Prevention of postoperative infection in patients undergoing contaminated or potentially contaminated procedures or when infection at the operative site would present a serious risk	**Adult:** 1–2 g IM or IV ½–1 h prior to surgery, followed by 1–2 g IM or IV during the procedure, depending on its length, and then 1–2 g IM or IV q6h postoperatively for 24 h; in cases where postoperative infection would be particularly devastating (eg, open-heart surgery and prosthetic arthroplasty), prophylactic administration may be continued for 3–5 days

CONTRAINDICATIONS

Hypersensitivity to cephalosporins

ADMINISTRATION/DOSAGE ADJUSTMENTS

Intramuscular administration	Dilute contents of 500-mg or 1-g vial in 1 or 2 ml, respectively, of Sterile (or Bacteriostatic) Water for Injection USP and inject required dose deeply into the muscle mass
Intermittent intravenous infusion	For intermittent use, dilute contents of 500-mg, 1-g, or 2-g vial in 10 ml or more of diluent and inject required dose slowly over a period of 3–5 min; when administering cephapirin through a Y-type administration set, temporarily discontinue infusion of bulk IV solution
Duration of treatment for streptococcal infections	Treatment of infections caused by beta-hemolytic streptococci should be continued for at least 10 days
Patients with renal impairment	Administer 7.5–15 mg/kg IM or IV q12h when serum creatinine level > 5 mg/dl or moderately severe oliguria is present; patients with severe renal impairment who are to be dialyzed should receive the same dose immediately prior to dialysis and q12h thereafter

WARNINGS/PRECAUTIONS

Cross-allergenicity	Use with great caution in penicillin-allergic patients
Hypersensitivity	Serious anaphylactoid reactions may occur (most likely in patients with a history of allergy, particularly to drugs), necessitating immediate emergency treatment with epinephrine, oxygen, intravenous steroids, and airway management including intubation
Superinfection	Overgrowth of nonsusceptible organisms may occur with prolonged use
Patients with renal impairment	Patients with impaired renal function should be carefully monitored during therapy (see ADMINISTRATION/DOSAGE ADJUSTMENTS)

ADVERSE REACTIONS

Hypersensitivity	Maculopapular rash, urticaria, serum-sickness-like reactions, drug fever, eosinophilia, anaphylaxis (see WARNINGS/PRECAUTIONS)
Hematological	Neutropenia, leukopenia, anemia

OVERDOSAGE

Signs and symptoms	See ADVERSE REACTIONS
Treatment	Discontinue medication; treat symptomatically and institute supportive measures, as required

DRUG INTERACTIONS

Aminoglycoside antibiotics	⌂ Risk of nephrotoxicity
Probenecid	⌂ Cephapirin blood level and/or toxicity

ALTERED LABORATORY VALUES

Blood/serum values	⌂ BUN ⌂ SGOT ⌂ SGPT + Coombs' test
Urinary values	⌂ Glucose (with Clinitest tablets)

USE IN CHILDREN

See INDICATIONS; adjust dosage according to body weight and severity of infection. Safety for use in children under 3 mo of age has not been established.

USE IN PREGNANT AND NURSING WOMEN

Pregnancy Category B: use during pregnancy only if clearly needed. Reproduction studies in mice and rats have shown no evidence of impaired fertility or harm to the fetus; however, no adequate, well-controlled studies have been done in pregnant women. Cephapirin may be present in human milk in small amounts; use with caution in nursing mothers.

---

[1] Each 500 mg of cephapirin sodium contains 1.18 mEq sodium

CEPHALOSPORINS

CEFIZOX (ceftizoxime sodium) Smith Kline & French   Rx

Vials: 1, 2 g   **Piggyback vials:** 1, 2 g   **Plastic containers:** 20, 40 mg/ml (50 ml)

INDICATIONS

Lower respiratory tract infections caused by susceptible strains of *Streptococcus pneumoniae* and other streptococci (except enterococci), *Klebsiella, Proteus mirabilis, Escherichia coli, Hemophilus influenzae* (including ampicillin-resistant strains), *Staphylococcus aureus, Serratia, Enterobacter,* and *Bacteroides*
Urinary tract infections caused by susceptible strains of *Staphylococcus aureus, Escherichia coli, Pseudomonas* (including *P aeruginosa*), *Proteus mirabilis, P vulgaris, Providencia rettgeri, Morganella morganii, Klebsiella, Serratia* (including *S marcescens*), and *Enterobacter*
Intraabdominal infections caused by susceptible strains of *Escherichia coli, Staphylococcus epidermidis, Streptococcus* (except enterococci), *Enterobacter, Klebsiella, Bacteroides* (including *B fragilis*), and anaerobic cocci (including *Peptococcus* and *Peptostreptococcus*)
Septicemia caused by susceptible strains of *Streptococcus pneumoniae* and other streptococci (except enterococci), *Staphylococcus aureus, Escherichia coli, Bacteroides* (including *B fragilis*), *Klebsiella,* and *Serratia*
Skin and skin structure infections caused by susceptible strains of *Staphylococcus aureus, S epidermidis, Escherichia coli, Klebsiella, Streptococcus pyogenes* and other streptococci (except enterococci), *Proteus mirabilis, Serratia, Enterobacter, Bacteroides* (including *B fragilis*), and anaerobic cocci (including *Peptococcus* and *Peptostreptococcus*)
Bone and joint infections caused by susceptible strains of *Staphylococcus aureus, Streptococcus* (except enterococci), *Proteus mirabilis, Bacteroides,* and anaerobic cocci (including *Peptococcus* and *Peptostreptococcus*)
Meningitis caused by susceptible strains of *Hemophilus influenzae* and *Streptococcus pneumoniae*

Uncomplicated cervical and urethral **gonorrhea**

PARENTERAL DOSAGE

Adult: 1 g IM or IV q8–12h; for severe or refractory infections, 1 g IM or IV q8h or 2 g IM or IV q8–12h; for life-threatening infections, 3–4 g IV q8h or up to 2 g IV q4h. For uncomplicated urinary tract infections, give 500 mg IM or IV q12h; use a higher dosage if the infection is caused by *Pseudomonas,* because many strains are only moderately susceptible to ceftizoxime and because such an infection can be serious. The IV route may be preferable for patients with bacterial septicemia, localized parenchymal abscesses, peritonitis, or other severe or life-threatening infections; for conditions such as bacterial septicemia, administer 6–12 g/day IV for several days, and then gradually reduce the dosage.
Child (≥6 mo): 50 mg/kg IM or IV q6–8h; do not exceed the maximum adult dosage for serious infection

Adult: 1 g, given in a single IM dose

CONTRAINDICATIONS

Hypersensitivity to ceftizoxime

ADMINISTRATION/DOSAGE ADJUSTMENTS

Intramuscular administration	Add 3 ml of sterile water for injection to each gram of ceftizoxime; shake well. Aspirate before administration to avoid inadvertent intravascular injection; then inject solution well within the body of a relatively large muscle. A 2-g dose should be divided between different muscle masses.
Intravenous administration	Add 10 ml of sterile water for injection to each gram of ceftizoxime; shake well. Slowly inject solution over a period of 3–5 min. For intermittent or continuous infusion, thaw the contents of a plastic container at room temperature, or add to a reconstituted solution or piggyback vial 50–100 ml of sodium chloride injection, 5% or 10% dextrose injection, 5% dextrose and 0.9%, 0.45%, or 0.2% sodium chloride injection, 10% invert sugar or 5% sodium bicarbonate in sterile water for injection, or Ringer's or lactated Ringer's injection; 5% dextrose in lactated Ringer's injection may be used as a diluent if the ceftizoxime solution has been reconstituted with 4% sodium bicarbonate injection. After thawing the contents of a plastic container, check for minute leaks by squeezing the container firmly; discard if leaks are found. When plastic containers are used, replace the administration set at least once every 48 h; do not connect the containers in series because residual air, drawn from the primary container before administration of the fluid from the secondary container is complete, could cause air embolism.
Patients with renal impairment	Administer an initial loading dose of 0.5–1 g IM or IV; then, for life-threatening infections, give 0.75–1.5 g q8h if creatinine clearance (Ccr) equals 50–79 ml/min, 0.5–1 g q12h if Ccr equals 5–49 ml/min, or 0.5–1 g q48h or 0.5 g q24h if Ccr equals 0–4 ml/min, or, for less severe infections, 0.5 g q8h if Ccr equals 50–79 ml/min, 0.25–0.5 g q12h if Ccr equals 5–49 ml/min, or 0.5 g q48h or 0.25 g q24h if Ccr equals 0–4 ml/min. The Ccr of patients with stable renal function can be estimated from serum creatinine levels if a measured value cannot be obtained; for adult men, use the following formula: (weight [kg])(140 − age [yr])/(72)(serum creatinine level [mg/dl]), for adult women, multiply this quotient by 0.85. Although no additional doses are necessary in patients undergoing hemodialysis, the timing of administration should be arranged so that a dose is given at the end of each dialysis period.

WARNINGS/PRECAUTIONS

Cross-allergenicity	Use with caution in penicillin-sensitive patients
Hypersensitivity	Serious, acute hypersensitivity reactions may occur, especially in patients with a history of allergy (particularly to drugs), and may necessitate emergency measures, including use of epinephrine

Superinfection	Overgrowth of nonsusceptible organisms may occur with prolonged use; careful clinical observation is essential
Pseudomembranous colitis	May occur due to alteration of the normal intestinal flora and should be considered in any patient who develops diarrhea during or after therapy; use with caution in patients with a history of GI disease, particularly colitis. Mild cases may respond to withdrawal of the drug alone. Moderate to severe cases should be managed by fluid and electrolyte replacement and protein supplementation, as needed. Oral vancomycin is the treatment of choice for severe or refractory colitis associated with the overgrowth of *Clostridium difficile;* however, other possible causes should also be considered.
Renal function	Although impairment has not been reported, renal function should be monitored, especially in patients who are receiving the maximum dosage (12 g/day)

ADVERSE REACTIONS

Frequent reactions (incidence ≥ 1%) are printed in *italics*

Gastrointestinal	Diarrhea, nausea, vomiting, pseudomembranous colitis
Hematological	*Thrombocytosis and transient eosinophilia (1-5%);* anemia, neutropenia, leukopenia, and thrombocytopenia (rare)
Genitourinary	Vaginitis (rare)
Hypersensitivity	*Rash, pruritus, and fever (1-5%);* numbness (rare)
Other	*Burning, cellulitis, phlebitis (with IV use), pain, induration, tenderness, and paresthesia at injection site (1-5%)*

OVERDOSAGE

Signs and symptoms	See ADVERSE REACTIONS
Treatment	Discontinue use of drug; treat symptomatically and institute supportive measures, as required

DRUG INTERACTIONS

Aminoglycosides	⇧ Risk of nephrotoxicity
Probenecid	⇧ Ceftizoxime blood level and/or toxicity

ALTERED LABORATORY VALUES

Blood/serum values	⇧ Alkaline phosphatase ⇧ SGOT ⇧ SGPT ⇧ BUN ⇧ Creatinine ⇧ Bilirubin + Coombs' test
Urinary values	⇧ Glucose (with Clinitest tablets)

USE IN CHILDREN

See INDICATIONS and PARENTERAL DOSAGE; safety and effectiveness for use in children under 6 mo of age have not been established. Elevation of the CPK level has been seen in children and may be due to IM administration.

USE IN PREGNANT AND NURSING WOMEN

Pregnancy Category B: reproduction studies in rats and rabbits have shown no evidence of impaired fertility or harm to the fetus; however, no adequate, well-controlled studies have been performed in pregnant women. Use during pregnancy only if clearly needed. Safety for use during labor and delivery has not been established. Ceftizoxime is excreted in human milk in low concentrations; use with caution in nursing mothers.

CEPHALOSPORINS

CEFOBID (cefoperazone sodium) Roerig   Rx

Vials: 1, 2 g   **Piggyback vials:** 1, 2 g   **Plastic containers:** 40 mg/ml (50 ml)

INDICATIONS

Respiratory tract infections caused by susceptible strains of *Streptococcus pneumoniae, Hemophilus influenzae, Staphylococcus aureus, Streptococcus pyogenes, Pseudomonas aeruginosa, Klebsiella pneumoniae, Escherichia coli, Proteus,* and *Enterobacter*
Intraabdominal infections, including peritonitis, caused by susceptible strains of *Escherichia coli, Pseudomonas aeruginosa,* enterococci, anaerobic gram-positive cocci, and anaerobic bacilli (including *Bacteroides fragilis*)
Bacterial septicemia caused by susceptible strains of *Streptococcus pneumoniae, S pyogenes, S agalactiae, Staphylococcus aureus,* enterococci, *Hemophilus influenzae, Pseudomonas aeruginosa, Escherichia coli, Klebsiella, Proteus, Clostridium,* and anaerobic gram-positive cocci
Skin and skin structure infections caused by susceptible strains of *Staphylococcus aureus, Streptococcus pyogenes,* and *Pseudomonas aeruginosa*
Gynecologic infections, including pelvic inflammatory disease and endometritis, caused by susceptible strains of *Neisseria gonorrhoeae, Staphylococcus aureus, S epidermidis, Streptococcus agalactiae, Escherichia coli, Clostridium, Bacteroides* (including *B fragilis*), and anaerobic gram-positive cocci
Urinary tract infections caused by susceptible strains of *Enterococcus, Escherichia coli,* and *Pseudomonas aeruginosa*

PARENTERAL DOSAGE

Adult: 2-4 g/day, by IM injection or IV infusion in 2 divided doses q12h. For infections that are severe or caused by less sensitive organisms, dosage may be increased; administration of 6-12 g/day in 2-4 divided doses of 1.5-4 g/dose has been effective. (In a pharmacokinetic study, 16 g/day has been given by continuous IV infusion to severely immunocompromised patients without producing complications.) Treatment of infections caused by *Streptococcus pyogenes* should be continued for at least 10 days.

CEFOBID

CONTRAINDICATIONS
Hypersensitivity to cephalosporins

ADMINISTRATION/DOSAGE ADJUSTMENTS

Preparation for IM injection	To obtain a concentration of 250 mg/ml, dissolve 1 g of cefoperazone with 2.8 ml of sterile water for injection or 2 g with 5.4 ml and then add 1 ml of 2% lidocaine hydrochloride injection USP to the 1-g solution or 1.8 ml to the 2-g solution. To obtain a concentration of 333 mg/ml, dissolve 1 g of cefoperazone with 2 ml of sterile water for injection or 2 g with 3.8 ml and then add 0.6 ml of 2% lidocaine hydrochloride injection USP to the 1-g solution or 1.2 ml to the 2-g solution. For preparation of solutions containing less than 250 mg/ml, use sterile water for injection, bacteriostatic water for injection USP, or any diluent that can be used to *reconstitute* a solution for IV administration.
Preparation for IV infusion	When the vehicle for infusion is to be 5% or 10% dextrose injection USP, 0.9% sodium chloride injection USP, 5% dextrose and 0.2% or 0.9% sodium chloride injection USP, Normosol R, or Normosol M and 5% dextrose injection, reconstitute solution by adding 2.8–5 ml of diluent to each gram of cefoperazone in a regular vial or 20–40 ml to each gram in a piggyback vial. For intermittent infusion, use the solution reconstituted in the piggyback vial or, alternatively, dilute the solution reconstituted in the regular vial, adding 20–40 ml of diluent for each gram of cefoperazone. For continuous infusion, dilute the solution reconstituted in a regular or piggyback vial to a final concentration of 2–25 mg/ml. When the vehicle for infusion is to be lactated Ringer's injection USP (alone or with 5% dextrose), use one of the diluents listed above to reconstitute the solution, adding 2.8–5 ml to each gram of cefoperazone in a regular or piggyback vial. Then, for intermittent infusion using either a regular or piggyback vial, dilute the reconstituted solution with the lactated Ringer's preparation, adding 20–40 ml for each gram of cefoperazone. For continuous infusion with either vial, take the lactated Ringer's preparation and dilute the reconstituted solution to a final concentration of 2–25 mg/ml. To use a plastic container, thaw contents at room temperature. Check for minute leaks by squeezing the bag firmly; discard if leaks are found or seal is not intact. Additives should not be introduced to the solution. Do not connect plastic containers in series because residual air in the primary container, withdrawn before administration of the fluid in the secondary container is complete, could produce air embolism.
Intermittent IV infusion	Administer each dose over a period of 15–30 min if the drug is to be given intermittently by IV infusion
Solubilization	After reconstitution, allow any foaming in the solution to dissipate; then determine whether the powder is completely solubilized. Vigorous and prolonged agitation may be necessary for concentrations exceeding 333 mg/ml (maximum solubility: 475 mg/ml).
Concomitant use of aminoglycosides	Although a synergistic effect on infections caused by many gram-negative bacilli has been shown, such enhanced activity is not predictable; therefore, susceptibility tests should be performed to determine the effectiveness of concomitant use. Because of physical incompatability, cefoperazone should not be mixed directly with an aminoglycoside. If combination therapy is indicated, give cefoperazone and then the aminoglycoside sequentially by intermittent IV infusion; use separate secondary tubing for each drug and irrigate the primary tubing with an appropriate diluent before giving the aminoglycoside. Renal function should be carefully monitored, as concomitant use has caused nephrotoxicity.
Patients undergoing hemodialysis	Cefoperazone should be administered after hemodialysis, because the serum half-life is slightly reduced by hemodialysis

WARNINGS/PRECAUTIONS

Cross-allergenicity	Use with caution in penicillin-sensitive patients
Hypersensitivity	Serious, acute hypersensitivity reactions may occur, especially in patients with a history of allergy (particularly to drugs), and may necessitate emergency measures, including use of epinephrine
Superinfection	Overgrowth of nonsusceptible organisms may occur with prolonged use; careful clinical observation is essential
Pseudomembranous colitis	May occur due to alteration of the normal intestinal flora and should be considered in any patient who develops diarrhea during or after therapy; use with caution in patients with a history of GI disease, particularly colitis. Mild cases may respond to withdrawal of the drug alone. Moderate to severe cases should be managed by fluid and electrolyte replacement and protein supplementation, as needed. Oral vancomycin is the treatment of choice for severe or refractory colitis associated with the overgrowth of *Clostridium difficile;* however, other possible causes should also be considered.
Vitamin K deficiency	Prothrombin time should be monitored in patients with poor nutritional status, malabsorption states (eg, due to cystic fibrosis), or alcoholism, and in patients undergoing prolonged hyperalimentation; if necessary, vitamin K should be administered. Suppression of the intestinal flora that synthesize vitamin K most probably causes the deficiency.
Disulfiram-like reaction	Caution patients about using alcohol; a disulfiram-like reaction characterized by flushing, sweating, headache, and tachycardia has been reported in patients who ingested alcohol within 72 h after administration of cefoperazone

CEFOBID ■ CEFOTAN

Patients with hepatic or renal impairment	Serum concentrations should be monitored if dosages above 4 g/day are given to patients with hepatic disease and/or biliary obstruction; such high dosages generally should not be necessary, however, because the serum half-life is increased 2- to 4-fold in such patients (cefoperazone is excreted mainly in the bile). Serum levels should also be monitored if high dosages are given to patients with renal failure, and, if necessary, the dosage should be reduced; dosage adjustments are not necessary, however, if usual doses are administered to such patients. Serum concentrations should be monitored closely if dosages exceeding 1–2 g/day are given to patients with both hepatic dysfunction and significant renal disease.
Carcinogenicity, mutagenicity	No long-term studies have been done in animals to evaluate the carcinogenic potential of cefoperazone; genetic toxicology studies have shown no evidence of mutagenicity
Impairment of fertility	Cefoperazone has caused adverse effects on the testes of prepubertal rats; SC administration has resulted in a minor decrease in spermatocytes at approximately 1.6 times the average adult human dose and in reduced testicular weight, arrested spermatogenesis, reduced germinal cell population, and vacuolation of Sertoli cell cytoplasm at 16 times the average adult human dose. Adverse effects on fertility have not been seen in studies with adult rats.

ADVERSE REACTIONS[1]

Frequent reactions (incidence ≥ 1%) are printed in *italics*

Gastrointestinal	*Diarrhea or loose stools (3.3%);* pseudomembranous colitis; nausea and vomiting (rare)
Hematological	*Transient eosinophilia (10%), decreased hemoglobin level or hematocrit (5%), slight decrease in neutrophil count (2%)*
Hypersensitivity	*Skin reactions (2.2%),* drug fever (0.4%)
Other	Phlebitis at infusion site (0.8%), transient pain at IM injection site (0.7%), vitamin K deficiency (rare)

OVERDOSAGE

Signs and symptoms	See ADVERSE REACTIONS
Treatment	Discontinue use of drug; treat symptomatically and institute supportive measures, as required

DRUG INTERACTIONS

Aminoglycoside antibiotics	⇧ Risk of nephrotoxicity
Alcohol	Disulfiram-like reaction (see WARNINGS/PRECAUTIONS)
Probenecid	⇧ Cefoperazone blood level and/or toxicity

ALTERED LABORATORY VALUES

Blood/serum values	⇧ Alkaline phosphatase ⇧ BUN ⇧ Creatinine ⇧ SGOT ⇧ SGPT + Coombs' test
Urinary values	+ Glucose (with Benedict's or Fehling's solution)

USE IN CHILDREN

Safety and effectiveness for use in children have not been established; bacteriostatic water for injection USP (with *benzyl alcohol*) should not be used in neonates

USE IN PREGNANT AND NURSING WOMEN

Pregnancy Category B: use during pregnancy only if clearly needed. Reproduction studies performed in mice, rats, and monkeys given up to 10 times the human dose and in rats given up to 500–1,000 mg/kg/day SC (10–20 times the usual human dose) have shown no evidence of harm to the fetus. No adequate, well-controlled studies have been done in pregnant women. Low concentrations of cefoperazone are excreted in human milk; use with caution in nursing mothers.

---

[1] Significantly elevated hepatic enzyme levels, accompanied by nonspecific hepatitis, have been observed in a patient with a history of liver disease (disorders were reversible)

CEPHALOSPORINS

CEFOTAN (cefotetan disodium) Stuart   Rx

Vials: 1 g[1] (10 ml), 2 g[1] (20 ml)   **Infusion vials:** 1, 2 g[1] (100 ml)

INDICATIONS

Lower respiratory tract infections caused by susceptible strains of *Streptococcus pneumoniae, Staphylococcus aureus, Hemophilus influenzae, Klebsiella,* and *Escherichia coli*

Skin and skin structure infections caused by susceptible strains of *Staphylococcus aureus, S epidermidis, Streptococcus* (except enterococci), and *Escherichia coli*

Gynecological infections caused by susceptible strains of *Staphylococcus aureus, S epidermidis, Streptococcus* (except enterococci), *Escherichia coli, Proteus mirabilis, Neisseria gonorrhoeae, Bacteroides* (except *B distasonis, B ovatus,* and *B thetaiotaomicron*), *Fusobacterium,* and gram-positive anaerobic cocci (including *Peptococcus* and *Peptostreptococcus*)

Intraabdominal infections caused by susceptible strains of *Escherichia coli, Klebsiella, Streptococcus* (except enterococci), and *Bacteroides* (except *B distasonis, B ovatus,* and *B thetaiotaomicron*)

Bone and joint infections caused by susceptible strains of *Staphylococcus aureus*

PARENTERAL DOSAGE

Adult: 1–2 g IM or IV q12h for 5–10 days; for severe infections, 2 g IV q12h for 5–10 days; for life-threatening infections, 3 g IV q12h for 5–10 days

Urinary tract infections caused by susceptible strains of *Escherichia coli, Klebsiella, Proteus mirabilis, P vulgaris, Providencia rettgeri,* and *Morganella morganii*	**Adult:** 500 mg q12h, 1–2 g q24h, or 1–2 g q12h, given IM or IV for 5–10 days
Prevention of certain postoperative infections in patients undergoing surgical procedures (eg, cesarean section, abdominal or vaginal hysterectomy, transurethral surgery, biliary tract surgery, and GI tract surgery) that are classified as contaminated or potentially contaminated	**Adult:** 1–2 g, given IV 30–60 min before surgery; for cesarean section, 1–2 g, given IV as soon as the umbilical cord is clamped

CONTRAINDICATIONS

Hypersensitivity to cephalosporins

ADMINISTRATION/DOSAGE ADJUSTMENTS

Intramuscular administration	To reconstitute solution, use normal saline USP, sterile or bacteriostatic water for injection, or 0.5% or 1% lidocaine hydrochloride; add 2 ml of diluent to the 1-g vial or 3 ml to the 2-g vial. Inject required dose well within the body of a relatively large muscle such as the gluteus maximus; to avoid inadvertent intravascular injection, aspirate before injection.
Preparation for IV use	For injection, add 10 ml of sterile water for injection to the 1-g vial or 10–20 ml to the 2-g vial; for infusion, add 50–100 ml of 5% dextrose solution or 0.9% sodium chloride solution to the 1- or 2-g infusion vial
Intravenous administration	The IV route is preferable for patients with bacteremia, bacterial septicemia, or other severe or life-threatening infections and for patients who may be poor risks because of lowered resistance resulting from malnutrition, trauma, surgery, diabetes, heart failure, malignancy, or other debilitating conditions, particularly if shock is present or imminent. Solutions containing 1–2 g of cefotetan may be injected directly into a suitable vein over a period of 3–5 min or may be given over a longer period by intermittent infusion through the IV tubing; during infusion of cefotetan, temporarily discontinue administration of other solutions at the same IV site. Use butterfly or scalp vein-type needles for infusion. Do not mix cefotetan with solutions containing an aminoglycoside.
Patients with renal impairment	If creatinine clearance (Ccr) > 30 ml/min, give the usual dose q12h; if Ccr $= 10–30$ ml/min, give the usual dose q24h or, alternatively, give 50% of the usual dose q12h; if Ccr < 10 ml/min, give the usual dose q48h or, alternatively, give 25% of the usual dose q12h. The Ccr of patients with stable renal function can be estimated from serum creatinine levels if a measured value cannot be obtained; for adult men, use the following formula: (weight [kg])(140 $-$ age [yr])/(72)(serum creatinine level [mg/dl]), for adult women, multiply this quotient by 0.9. Cefotetan is dialyzable; therefore, for patients undergoing intermittent dialysis, give 25% of the usual dose q24h on days between dialysis and 50% of the usual dose on the day of dialysis.

WARNINGS/PRECAUTIONS

Hypersensitivity	Serious hypersensitivity reactions necessitating emergency measures (such as use of epinephrine) may occur during therapy; use with caution in patients with a history of allergy, especially if they are hypersensitive to penicillin or other drugs. If an allergic reaction occurs, discontinue administration.
Pseudomembranous colitis	May occur due to alteration of the normal intestinal flora and should be considered in any patient who develops diarrhea during or after therapy; use with caution in patients with a history of GI disease, particularly colitis. Mild cases may respond to withdrawal of the drug alone. Moderate to severe cases should be managed by fluid and electrolyte replacement and protein supplementation, as needed. Oral vancomycin is the treatment of choice for severe or refractory colitis associated with the overgrowth of *Clostridium difficile;* however, other possible causes should be considered.
Superinfection	Overgrowth of nonsusceptible organisms may occur with prolonged use; careful observation of patient's condition is essential
Vitamin K deficiency	Cefotetan can cause a decrease in prothrombin activity. Monitor prothrombin time in patients with poor nutritional status and in those with renal or hepatic impairment; administer vitamin K as needed.
Disulfiram-like reaction	A disulfiram-like reaction characterized by flushing, sweating, headache, and tachycardia has been reported in patients who consumed alcohol within 72 h after administration of cefotetan; caution patients about this risk
Carcinogenicity, mutagenicity	No studies have been done to evaluate the carcinogenic potential of cefotetan; standard laboratory tests have shown no evidence of mutagenicity
Impairment of fertility	Degeneration of seminiferous tubules and reduction in testicular weight have been shown in prepubertal rats given SC 120–500 mg/kg/day (2–16 times the usual adult human dose) on days 6–35 of life; the drug affected spermatogonia and spermatocytes, but not Sertoli and Leydig cells. The frequency and severity of lesions were dose-dependent: At 120 mg/kg/day (2–4 times the usual adult human dose), effects were seen in 1 of 10 animals and degeneration was mild; at 500 mg/kg/day (8–16 times the usual adult human dose), lesions were seen in all 10 animals given the drug. No testicular effects have been observed in rats given SC up to 1 g/kg/day for 5 wk, beginning at 7 wk of age; these effects have also not been seen in dogs given IV up to 300 mg/kg/day for 5 wk, beginning at 3 wk of age.

ADVERSE REACTIONS

The most frequent reaction is italicized

Gastrointestinal	*Diarrhea (1.2%)*, nausea
Hepatic	Increases in SGPT, SGOT, alkaline phosphatase, and LDH levels
Hematological	Eosinophilia, thrombocytosis, positive direct Coombs' test
Hypersensitivity	Rash, pruritus
Local	Phlebitis at injection site, discomfort

OVERDOSAGE

Signs and symptoms	See ADVERSE REACTIONS
Treatment	Discontinue medication; treat symptomatically and institute supportive measures, as required

DRUG INTERACTIONS

Aminoglycosides	↑ Risk of nephrotoxicity; carefully monitor renal function during combination therapy, especially when treatment is prolonged or higher aminoglycoside dosages are used
Alcohol	Disulfiram-like reaction (see WARNINGS/PRECAUTIONS)

ALTERED LABORATORY VALUES

Blood/serum values	↑ SGPT ↑ SGOT ↑ Alkaline phosphatase ↑ LDH ↑ Creatinine (with Jaffe reaction) + Coombs' test
Urinary values	+ Glucose (with Benedict's and Fehling's solution) ↑ Creatinine (with Jaffe reaction)

USE IN CHILDREN

Safety and effectiveness for use in children have not been established

USE IN PREGNANT AND NURSING WOMEN

Pregnancy Category B: reproduction studies in rats and monkeys at up to 20 times the usual human dose have shown no evidence of impaired fertility or harm to the fetus; however, no adequate, well-controlled studies have been done in pregnant women. Use during pregnancy only if clearly needed. Cefotetan is excreted in human milk in very low concentrations; use with caution in nursing mothers.

---

[1] As the disodium salt

CEPHALOSPORINS

CLAFORAN (cefotaxime sodium) Hoechst-Roussel   Rx

Vials: 1, 2 g   **Infusion bottles:** 1, 2 g   **Pharmacy bulk bottles:** 10 g   **Plastic containers:** 20, 40 mg/ml (50 ml)

INDICATIONS

Lower respiratory tract infections, including pneumonia, caused by susceptible strains of *Streptococcus pneumoniae, S pyogenes,* and other streptococci (excluding enterococci), *Staphylococcus aureus, Escherichia coli, Klebsiella, Hemophilus influenzae, Proteus mirabilis, Serratia marcescens,* and *Enterobacter*
Urinary tract infections caused by susceptible strains of *Enterococcus, Staphylococcus epidermidis, S aureus, Citrobacter, Enterobacter, Escherichia coli, Klebsiella, Proteus mirabilis, P vulgaris, Morganella morganii, Providencia rettgeri,* and *Serratia marcescens*
Gynecologic infections, including pelvic inflammatory disease, endometritis, and pelvic cellulitis, caused by susceptible strains of *Staphylococcus epidermidis,* streptococci, *Enterococcus, Escherichia coli, Proteus mirabilis, Bacteroides* (including *B fragilis), Clostridium,* and anaerobic cocci (including *Peptococcus* and *Peptostreptococcus*)
Bacteremia/septicemia caused by susceptible strains of *Escherichia coli, Klebsiella,* and *Serratia marcescens*
Skin and skin structure infections caused by susceptible strains of *Staphylococcus aureus, S epidermidis, Streptococcus pyogenes* and other streptococci, *Enterococcus, Escherichia coli, Enterobacter, Klebsiella, Proteus mirabilis, P vulgaris, Morganella morganii, Providencia rettgeri, Pseudomonas, Serratia marcescens, Bacteroides,* and anaerobic cocci (including *Peptococcus* and *Peptostreptococcus*)
Intraabdominal infections, including peritonitis, caused by susceptible strains of *Escherichia coli, Klebsiella, Bacteroides,* and anaerobic cocci (including *Peptococcus* and *Peptostreptococcus*)
Bone and/or joint infections caused by susceptible strains of *Staphylococcus aureus*
Central nervous system infections, including meningitis and ventriculitis, caused by susceptible strains of *Neisseria meningitidis, Hemophilus influenzae, Streptococcus pneumoniae, Klebsiella pneumoniae,* and *Escherichia coli*

PARENTERAL DOSAGE

Adult: for uncomplicated infections, 1 g IM or IV q12h; for moderate to severe infections, 1–2 g IM or IV q8h; for septicemia and similar infections that normally require higher doses of antibiotics, 2 g IV q6-8h; for life-threatening infections, 2 g IV q4h, up to 12 g/day. The IV route is preferable for patients with bacteremia, bacterial septicemia, peritonitis, meningitis, or other severe or life-threatening infections and for patients who may be poor risks because of lowered resistance resulting from malnutrition, trauma, surgery, diabetes, heart failure, malignancy, or other debilitating conditions, particularly if shock is present or imminent.
Neonate (0–1 wk): 50 mg/kg IV q12h
Neonate (1–4 wk): 50 mg/kg IV q8h
Infant and child (1 mo to 12 yr and < 50 kg): 50–180 mg/kg/day, given IM or IV in 4–6 equally divided doses; higher dosages should be used for more severe or serious infections (eg, meningitis)
Infant and child (1 mo to 12 yr and ≥ 50 kg): same as adult

CLAFORAN

Uncomplicated gonorrhea caused by *Neisseria gonorrhoeae*, including penicillinase-producing strains, at single or multiple sites	**Adult:** 1 g, given in a single IM dose
Prevention of infection in patients undergoing elective surgical procedures (eg, abdominal or vaginal hysterectomy, cesarean section, other genitourinary tract surgery, GI tract surgery) that may be classified as contaminated or potentially contaminated	**Adult:** 1 g, given IM or IV 30–90 min before surgery; for cesarean section, 1 g, given IV as soon as the umbilical cord is clamped, followed by 1 g IM or IV 6 and 12 h after the first dose

CONTRAINDICATIONS

Hypersensitivity to cefotaxime sodium or other cephalosporins

ADMINISTRATION/DOSAGE ADJUSTMENTS

Duration of therapy	Continue treatment for at least 48–72 h after fever has subsided or bacteria have been eradicated. Infections caused by Group A beta-hemolytic streptococci should be treated for at least 10 days to guard against the risk of rheumatic fever or glomerulonephritis. Persistent infections may require treatment for several weeks; do not use doses smaller than those indicated above.
Intramuscular administration	Add 3 ml of sterile water for injection or bacteriostatic water for injection to 1-g vial or 5 ml to 2-g vial and shake to dissolve; inject well within the body of a relatively large muscle (eg, the gluteus maximus); individual IM doses of 2 g may be given if dose is divided and administered at different IM sites
Preparation for IV use	To reconstitute solution, add 50–100 ml of a compatible diluent to an infusion bottle, at least 10 ml of sterile water for injection to a vial, or either 47 or 97 ml of a compatible diluent to a pharmacy bulk bottle; solution may be diluted to a final volume of up to 1 liter. Cefotaxime is compatible with the following diluents: 5% or 10% dextrose injection, 0.9% sodium chloride injection (alone or with 5% dextrose), 0.2% or 0.45% sodium chloride injection with 5% dextrose, lactated Ringer's solution, sodium lactate injection (M/6), 10% invert sugar injection, or Freamine II injection. Do not mix solutions of cefotaxime with aminoglycoside solutions or alkaline diluents. To use a plastic container, thaw contents at room temperature. Check for minute leaks by squeezing the bag firmly; discard if leaks are found or seal is not intact. Do not put additives in the container.
Intravenous administration	Cefotaxime can be given by direct injection or by intermittent or continuous infusion. For IV injection, a 10-ml solution prepared in a vial may be used; inject slowly over a period of 3–5 min. When a Y-type set is used for intermittent infusion, administration of the primary solution should be suspended for the duration of the infusion. Do not connect plastic containers in series because residual air in the primary container, withdrawn before administration of the fluid in the secondary container is complete, could produce air embolism.
Patients with renal impairment	Administer half the recommended dose if creatinine clearance rate (Ccr) < 20 ml/min/1.73 m². If necessary, creatinine clearance may be calculated from the serum creatinine concentration by use of the following formula: Ccr (in males) = [patient's weight (*kg*) × (140 − patient's age)]/[72 × creatinine concentration (*ml/dl*)]; for females, multiply the value obtained by this formula by 0.85.
Patients undergoing GI tract surgery	For preoperative bowel preparation in such patients, mechanical cleansing should be performed, and a nonabsorbable antibiotic (eg, neomycin) should be given

WARNINGS/PRECAUTIONS

Cross-allergenicity	Use with caution in penicillin-allergic patients
Hypersensitivity	Serious hypersensitivity reactions may occur, most likely in patients with a history of allergy, particularly to drugs, necessitating epinephrine administration and/or other emergency measures. Discontinue use of drug if hypersensitivity occurs.
Superinfection	Overgrowth of nonsusceptible organisms may occur
Concomitant administration of aminoglycosides	Cefotaxime, unlike some other beta-lactam anti-infectives, is not nephrotoxic when given alone; however, it may potentiate the nephrotoxicity of aminoglycosides if these drugs are given concomitantly. Renal function should be carefully monitored during concomitant therapy, especially if therapy is prolonged or higher dosages are used. Aminoglycosides are also potentially ototoxic.
Pseudomembranous colitis	May occur due to alteration of the normal intestinal flora and should be considered in any patient who develops diarrhea during or after therapy. Mild cases may respond to withdrawal of the drug alone. Moderate to severe cases should be managed by fluid and electrolyte replacement and protein supplementation, as needed. Oral vancomycin is the treatment of choice for severe or refractory colitis associated with the overgrowth of *Clostridium difficile*; however, other possible causes should also be considered.
Special-risk patients	Reduce total daily dose in patients with impaired renal function, since usual dosage can produce high, prolonged serum concentrations in such individuals (see ADMINISTRATION/DOSAGE ADJUSTMENTS). Use with caution in patients with a history of gastrointestinal disease, particularly colitis.

ADVERSE REACTIONS

The most frequent reactions, regardless of incidence, are printed in *italics*

Gastrointestinal	Colitis, diarrhea, pseudomembranous colitis; nausea and vomiting (rare)

CLAFORAN ■ DURICEF

Hematological	Granulocytopenia, transient leukopenia, eosinophilia, neutropenia, thrombocytopenia
Genitourinary	Moniliasis, vaginitis
Hypersensitivity	Rash, pruritus, fever
Other	Inflammation at site of IV injection; pain, induration, and tenderness on IM injection; headache

OVERDOSAGE

Signs and symptoms	See ADVERSE REACTIONS
Treatment	Discontinue medication; treat symptomatically and institute supportive measures, as required

DRUG INTERACTIONS

Aminoglycoside antibiotics	↑ Risk of nephrotoxicity

ALTERED LABORATORY VALUES

Blood/serum values	↑ Alkaline phosphatase (transient) ↑ SGOT (transient) ↑ SGPT (transient) ↑ Lactate dehydrogenase (transient) ↑ BUN (transient) + Coombs' test

No clinically significant alterations in urinary values occur at therapeutic dosages

---

USE IN CHILDREN

See INDICATIONS and PARENTERAL DOSAGE

USE IN PREGNANT AND NURSING WOMEN

Pregnancy Category B: use during pregnancy only if clearly needed. Reproduction studies in mice and rats at doses up to 30 times the usual human dose have shown no evidence of impaired fertility or harm to the fetus; however, no adequate, well-controlled studies have been done in pregnant women. Cefotaxime is excreted in human milk in low concentrations; use with caution in nursing mothers.

CEPHALOSPORINS

DURICEF (cefadroxil) Mead Johnson   Rx

Capsules: 500 mg **Tablets:** 1 g **Suspension (per 5 ml):** 125 mg (50, 100 ml), 250 mg (50, 100 ml), 500 mg (100 ml) after reconstitution *orange/pineapple-flavored*

INDICATIONS

Urinary tract infections caused by susceptible strains of *Escherichia coli*, *Proteus mirabilis*, and *Klebsiella*

Skin and skin structure infections caused by susceptible strains of staphylococci and/or streptococci

Pharyngitis and tonsillitis caused by Group A beta-hemolytic streptococci

ORAL DOSAGE

Adult: for uncomplicated lower urinary tract infections (cystitis), 1–2 g/day in a single daily dose or divided (bid); for all other urinary tract infections: 1 g bid
Infant and child: 30 mg/kg/day in divided doses q12h

Adult: 1 g/day in a single daily dose or divided (bid)
Infant and child: 30 mg/kg/day in divided doses q12h

Adult: 1 g/day in a single daily dose or divided (bid) for 10 days
Infant and child: 30 mg/kg/day in a single daily dose or divided (bid) for 10 days

CONTRAINDICATIONS

Hypersensitivity to cephalosporins

ADMINISTRATION/DOSAGE ADJUSTMENTS

Culture and susceptibility tests	Should be initiated prior to and during therapy
Timing of administration	Cefadroxil may be administered without regard to meals; however, administration with food may help diminish possible GI complaints
Patients with renal impairment	Administer 1 g to start, followed by 500 mg q12h when creatinine clearance rate (CCr) = 25–50 ml/min; 500 mg q24h when CCr = 10–25 ml/min; or 500 mg q36h when CCr = 0–10 ml/min

WARNINGS/PRECAUTIONS

Cross-allergenicity	Use with caution in penicillin-allergic patients
Hypersensitivity	Serious anaphylactic reactions may occur, most likely in patients with a history of allergy, necessitating administration of epinephrine or pressor amines, antihistamines, or corticosteroids

Pseudomembranous colitis	May occur due to alteration of the normal intestinal flora and should be considered in any patient who develops diarrhea during or after therapy. Mild cases may respond to withdrawal of the drug alone. Moderate to severe cases should be managed by fluid and electrolyte replacement and protein supplementation, as needed. Oral vancomycin is the treatment of choice for severe or refractory colitis associated with the overgrowth of *Clostridium difficile;* however, other possible causes should also be considered.
Superinfection	Overgrowth of nonsusceptible organisms may occur with prolonged use; careful clinical observation is essential
Special-risk patients	Patients with markedly impaired renal function (CCr < 50 ml/min) should be carefully monitored prior to and during therapy (see ADMINISTRATION/DOSAGE ADJUSTMENTS); use with caution in patients with a history of GI disease, particularly colitis

ADVERSE REACTIONS

Gastrointestinal	Pseudomembranous colitis; nausea and vomiting (rare)
Hypersensitivity	Rash, urticaria, angioedema
Genitourinary	Genital pruritus, genital moniliasis, vaginitis
Other	Moderate transient neutropenia

OVERDOSAGE

Signs and symptoms	See ADVERSE REACTIONS
Treatment	Discontinue medication; treat symptomatically; institute supportive measures, as required

DRUG INTERACTIONS

Probenecid	△ Cefadroxil blood level and/or toxicity

ALTERED LABORATORY VALUES

Blood/serum values	△ Alkaline phosphatase △ SGOT △ SGPT + Coombs' test
Urinary values	△ Glucose (with Clinitest tablets)

USE IN CHILDREN

See INDICATIONS; adjust dosage according to body weight

USE IN PREGNANT AND NURSING WOMEN

Pregnancy Category B: use during pregnancy only if clearly needed. Reproduction studies in rats and mice at doses up to 11 times the human dose have shown no evidence of impaired fertility or harm to the fetus; however, no adequate, well-controlled studies have been done in pregnant women. Positive Coombs' tests have been reported in newborns of mothers who received cephalosporins prior to delivery. Use with caution in nursing mothers.

CEPHALOSPORINS

FORTAZ (ceftazidime) Glaxo   Rx

Vials: 0.5, 1, 2 g   **Piggyback vials:** 1, 2 g   **Pharmacy bulk vials:** 6 g

INDICATIONS

Lower respiratory tract infections, including pneumonia, caused by susceptible strains of *Pseudomonas* (including *P aeruginosa*), *Hemophilus influenzae, Klebsiella, Enterobacter, Proteus mirabilis, Escherichia coli, Serratia, Citrobacter, Streptococcus pneumoniae,* and methicillin-susceptible *Staphylococcus aureus*

Skin and skin structure infections caused by susceptible strains of *Pseudomonas aeruginosa, Klebsiella, Escherichia coli, Proteus* (including *P mirabilis*), *Enterobacter, Serratia,* methicillin-susceptible *Staphylococcus aureus,* and *Streptococcus pyogenes*

Urinary tract infections caused by susceptible strains of *Pseudomonas aeruginosa, Enterobacter, Proteus* (including *P mirabilis*), *Klebsiella,* and *Escherichia coli*

Septicemia caused by susceptible strains of *Pseudomonas aeruginosa, Klebsiella, Hemophilus influenzae, Escherichia coli, Serratia, Streptococcus pneumoniae,* and methicillin-susceptible *Staphylococcus aureus*

Bone and joint infections caused by susceptible strains of *Pseudomonas aeruginosa, Klebsiella, Enterobacter,* and methicillin-susceptible *Staphylococcus aureus*

Gynecological infections, including endometritis and pelvic cellulitis, caused by susceptible strains of *Escherichia coli*

Intraabdominal infections, including peritonitis, caused by susceptible strains of *Escherichia coli, Klebsiella,* methicillin-susceptible *Staphylococcus aureus,* and *Bacteroides*

Central nervous system infections, including meningitis, caused by susceptible strains of *Hemophilus influenzae, Neisseria meningitidis, Pseudomonas aeruginosa,* and *Streptococcus pneumoniae*

PARENTERAL DOSAGE

Adult: generally, 1 g IV or IM q8–12h; for uncomplicated urinary tract infections, 250 mg IV or IM q12h; for complicated urinary tract infections, 500 mg IV or IM q8–12h; for uncomplicated pneumonia and mild skin and skin structure infections, 0.5–1 g IV or IM q8h; for bone and joint infections, 2 g IV q12h; for meningitis, serious gynecological and intraabdominal infections, and very severe life-threatening infections (especially in immunocompromised patients), 2 g IV q8h; for pseudomonal lung infections in patients with cystic fibrosis, 30–50 mg/kg IV q8h, up to 6 g/day

Neonate (0–4 wk): 30 mg/kg IV q12h

Infant and child (1 mo to 12 yr): 30–50 mg/kg IV q8h, up to 6 g/day; the higher dose should be reserved for children who have meningitis, cystic fibrosis, or an immunocompromised condition

FORTAZ

CONTRAINDICATIONS

Hypersensitivity to ceftazidime or other cephalosporins

ADMINISTRATION/DOSAGE ADJUSTMENTS

Preparation of solution	All containers are supplied, under reduced pressure, with 118 mg of sodium carbonate per gram of ceftazidime; when the drug is dissolved, carbon dioxide is released and pressure in the container increases. To reconstitute the solution in a piggyback vial, add 10 ml of a compatible diluent to the vial and shake well; after product has dissolved, insert a vent needle to release pressure, add 90 ml of diluent, and then remove the vent and syringe needles. To reconstitute solution in a pharmacy bulk vial, add 26 ml of a compatible diluent (for a concentration of approximately 200 mg/ml) and then gently agitate vial; after the product has dissolved, insert a vent needle for 1–2 min to allow gas to escape. Immediately before administering solutions prepared in piggyback or pharmacy vials, vent gas from the vials, especially when the solutions have been stored. To prepare a solution from a regular vial for IV infusion, add 5 ml of sterile water for injection to a 500-mg vial or 10 ml to a 1- or 2-g vial and then withdraw an appropriate quantity of the solution and dilute in a compatible diluent. For IV injection, add 5 ml of sterile water for injection to a regular 500-mg vial or 10 ml to a regular 1- or 2-g vial; for IM injection, reconstitute with sterile or bacteriostatic water for injection or 0.5% or 1% lidocaine hydrochloride injection, adding 1.5 ml to the 500-mg vial or 3 ml to the 1-g vial. Immediately before IM or IV injection, express any accumulated gas from the syringe. Ceftazidime is compatible with the following IV diluents: sterile water for injection, 0.9% sodium chloride injection, M/6 sodium lactate injection, Ringer's and lactated Ringer's injection USP, 5% and 10% dextrose injection, 5% dextrose in 0.225%, 0.45%, and 0.9% sodium chloride injection, 10% invert sugar in water for injection, and Normosol-M in 5% dextrose injection; do not mix ceftazidime with aminoglycoside solutions or sodium bicarbonate injection.
Intramuscular administration	Inject solution into a large muscle mass such as the upper outer quadrant of the gluteus maximus or the lateral part of the thigh
Intravenous administration	The IV route is preferable for treating severe or life-threatening infections such as septicemia, meningitis, and peritonitis as well as for treating less severe infections in patients at increased risk because of debilitating conditions such as malnutrition, trauma, surgery, diabetes, heart failure, or malignancy (especially when shock is present or impending). For direct IV administration, inject the dose into a vein over a period of 3–5 min or, alternatively, give through the tubing of an administration set while a compatible primary IV fluid is being administered. For IV infusion, use a piggyback vial or a solution prepared from a regular vial. During intermittent infusion with a Y-type set, administration of the primary solution should be discontinued.
Patients with renal impairment	For patients whose creatinine clearance (Ccr) is 50 ml/min or less, but who are not undergoing dialysis, give an initial loading dose of 1 g and then either 1 g q12h if Ccr = 31–50 ml/min, 1 g q24h if Ccr = 16–30 ml/min, 0.5 g q24h if Ccr = 6–15 ml/min, or 0.5 g q48h if Ccr < 5 ml/min; to treat a severe infection that under normal circumstances would necessitate 6 g/day, the maintenance dose can be increased by 50% or the dosing interval can be reduced to an appropriate length of time. When determined on the basis of a urine sample and serum creatinine level, the Ccr should be adjusted for body surface area or lean body mass. If a urine sample cannot be obtained, the Ccr can be estimated from the serum creatinine level, provided renal function is stable. For adult men, use the following formula: (weight [kg]) (140 − age [yr])/(72)(serum creatinine level [mg/dl]); for adult women, multiply this quotient by 0.85. To treat infections in patients undergoing peritoneal dialysis, administer 1 g to start and then 500 mg q24h; the drug can be added to the dialysis fluid at a concentration of 125 mg/liter. For patients undergoing hemodialysis, give 1 g at the start of therapy and repeat after each dialysis treatment.
Pseudomonal lung infections	In patients with chronic respiratory disease and cystic fibrosis, treatment of pseudomonal lung infections produces clinical improvement, but cannot be expected to result in a bacteriological cure
Duration of therapy	Treatment generally should be continued for 2 days after signs and symptoms have disappeared; if an infection is complicated, longer treatment may be necessary
Concomitant therapy	For patients with severe or life-threatening infections or immunocompromised conditions, ceftazidime can be given in combination with other antibiotics such as vancomycin, clindamycin, or aminoglycosides (see also DRUG INTERACTIONS)

WARNINGS/PRECAUTIONS

Hypersensitivity	Serious acute hypersensitivity reactions necessitating emergency measures (such as the use of epinephrine) may occur during therapy; use with caution in patients with a history of allergy, especially if they are hypersensitive to penicillin or other drugs. If an allergic reaction occurs, discontinue administration.
Pseudomembranous colitis	May occur due to alteration of the normal intestinal flora and should be considered in any patient who develops diarrhea during or after therapy; use with caution in patients with a history of GI disease, particularly colitis. Mild cases may respond to withdrawal of the drug alone. Moderate to severe cases should be managed by fluid and electrolyte replacement and protein supplementation, as needed. Oral vancomycin is the treatment of choice for severe or refractory colitis associated with the overgrowth of *Clostridium difficile;* however, other possible causes should also be considered.

Superinfection	Overgrowth of nonsusceptible organisms may occur with prolonged use; repeated evaluation of patient's condition is essential
Carcinogenicity, mutagenicity	Long-term animal studies to evaluate the carcinogenic potential of ceftazidime have not been done; no evidence of mutagenicity has been seen in the Ames test or the mouse micronucleus assay

ADVERSE REACTIONS

Frequent reactions (incidence ≥ 1%) are printed in *italics*

Gastrointestinal	*Diarrhea (1.3%)*, nausea, vomiting, abdominal pain
Hematological	*Eosinophilia (7.7%), positive Coombs' test (4.3%), thrombocytosis (2.2%)*; leukopenia, neutropenia, thrombocytopenia, and lymphocytosis (very rare)
Hepatic	*Slight increase in SGOT (6.2%), SGPT (6.6%), LDH (5.5%), SGGT (5.3%), and alkaline phosphatase (4.3%)*
Renal	Increase in BUN, serum urea, and serum creatinine
Central nervous system	Headache, dizziness, paresthesia
Hypersensitivity	*Pruritus, rash, and fever (2%)*, immediate-type hypersensitivity
Local	*Phlebitis and inflammation at injection site (1.4%)*
Other	Candidiasis, vaginitis

OVERDOSAGE

Signs and symptoms	See ADVERSE REACTIONS
Treatment	Treat symptomatically and institute supportive measures, as needed

DRUG INTERACTIONS

Aminoglycosides, potent diuretics (eg, furosemide)	⇧ Risk of nephrotoxicity; carefully monitor renal function when an aminoglycoside is given in combination with ceftazidime, especially when therapy is prolonged or a higher dosage of an aminoglycoside is used
Aminoglycosides	Physical incompatibility; do not mix together

ALTERED LABORATORY VALUES

Blood/serum values	⇧ SGOT ⇧ SGPT ⇧ LDH ⇧ SGGT ⇧ Alkaline phosphatase ⇧ BUN ⇧ Urea ⇧ Creatinine + Coombs' test

No clinically significant alterations in urinary values occur at therapeutic dosages

---

USE IN CHILDREN
See INDICATIONS and PARENTERAL DOSAGE

USE IN PREGNANT AND NURSING WOMEN
Pregnancy Category B: reproduction studies in mice and rats given up to 40 times the human dose have shown no evidence of impaired fertility or harm to the fetus; however, no adequate, well-controlled studies have been done in pregnant women. Use during pregnancy only if clearly needed. Ceftazidime is excreted in human milk; the resulting concentration is low. Use with caution in nursing mothers.

CEPHALOSPORINS

KEFLEX (cephalexin) Dista Rx

Capsules: 250, 500 mg **Tablets:** 1 g **Suspension (per 5 ml):** 125 mg after reconstitution (5, 60, 100, 200 ml), 250 mg after reconstitution (5, 100, 200 ml) **Pediatric drops:** 100 mg/ml after reconstitution (10 ml)

INDICATIONS

Respiratory tract infections caused by susceptible strains of *Streptococcus pneumoniae* and Group A beta-hemolytic streptococci

Bone infections caused by susceptible strains of staphylococci and/or *Proteus mirabilis*

Genitourinary tract infections caused by susceptible strains of *Escherichia coli*, *Proteus mirabilis*, and *Klebsiella*

Skin and skin structure infections caused by susceptible strains of staphylococci and/or streptococci

Otitis media caused by susceptible strains of *Streptococcus pneumoniae*, *Hemophilus influenzae*, staphylococci, streptococci, and *Neisseria catarrhalis*

ORAL DOSAGE

Adult: for streptococcal pharyngitis, uncomplicated cystitis in patients over 15 yr of age, and skin and skin-structure infections, 500 mg q12h; for other infections, 250 mg q6h. Dosages of up to 4 g/day may be necessary for infections that are more severe or are caused by less susceptible organisms; if a dosage exceeding 4 g/day is required, parenteral cephalosporin therapy should be considered.

Infant and child: 25–50 mg/kg/day, given in 2 divided doses q12h (for streptoccocal pharyngitis in patients over 1 yr of age and for skin and skin-structure infections) or given in 4 divided doses (for other infections); dosage may be doubled for severe infections

Infant and child: 75–100 mg/kg/day, given in 4 divided doses

KEFLEX

CONTRAINDICATIONS
Hypersensitivity to cephalosporins

ADMINISTRATION/DOSAGE ADJUSTMENTS

Duration of treatment	Cystitis should be treated for 7–14 days and infections caused by beta-hemolytic streptococci for at least 10 days

WARNINGS/PRECAUTIONS

Cross-allergenicity	Use with caution in penicillin-allergic patients
Hypersensitivity	Serious anaphylactic reactions may occur, most likely in patients with a history of allergy, necessitating administration of epinephrine, pressor amines, antihistamines, or corticosteroids
Pseudomembranous colitis	May occur due to alteration of the normal intestinal flora and should be considered in any patient who develops diarrhea during or after therapy. Mild cases may respond to withdrawal of the drug alone. Moderate to severe cases should be managed by sigmoidoscopy, appropriate bacteriological studies, fluid and electrolyte replacement, and protein supplementation, as needed. Oral vancomycin is the treatment of choice for severe or refractory colitis associated with the overgrowth of *Clostridium difficile*; however, other possible causes should also be considered.
Superinfection	Overgrowth of nonsusceptible organisms may occur with prolonged use; careful clinical observation is essential
Special-risk patients	Patients with markedly impaired renal function should be carefully monitored during therapy, as lower than usual dosage may be required; use with caution in patients with a history of GI disease, particularly colitis

ADVERSE REACTIONS

Frequent reactions (incidence ≥ 1%) are printed in *italics*

Gastrointestinal	*Diarrhea*, dyspepsia, abdominal pain, pseudomembranous colitis; nausea and vomiting (rare)
Hepatic	Slight increase in SGOT and SGPT levels; transient hepatitis and cholestatic jaundice (rare)
Hypersensitivity	Rash, urticaria, angioedema, anaphylaxis
Genitourinary	Genital and anal pruritus, genital moniliasis, vaginitis, vaginal discharge
Central nervous system	Dizziness, fatigue, headache
Hematological	Eosinophilia, neutropenia, thrombocytopenia

OVERDOSAGE

Signs and symptoms	See ADVERSE REACTIONS
Treatment	Discontinue medication; treat symptomatically and institute supportive measures, as required

DRUG INTERACTIONS

Probenecid	⇧ Cephalexin blood level and/or toxicity

ALTERED LABORATORY VALUES

Blood/serum values	⇧ Alkaline phosphatase ⇧ SGOT ⇧ SGPT + Coombs' test
Urinary values	⇧ Glucose (with Clinitest tablets)

USE IN CHILDREN
See INDICATIONS; adjust dosage according to body weight and severity of infection

USE IN PREGNANT AND NURSING WOMEN
Pregnancy Category B: use during pregnancy only if clearly needed. Reproduction studies in mice and rats have shown no adverse effects on fertility, fetal viability, fetal weight, or litter size; however, the safety of cephalexin has not been established in pregnant women. Although enhanced toxicity has not been observed in newborn or weanling rats, clinical studies have not ruled out the possibility of harm. Positive Coombs' tests have been reported in newborns of mothers who received cephalosporins prior to delivery. Cephalexin is excreted in human milk; use with caution in nursing mothers.

CEPHALOSPORINS

KEFLIN (cephalothin sodium) Lilly   Rx

Vials: 1 g (10, 100 ml), 2 g (20, 100 ml), 4 g (50 ml), 20 g (200 ml)   **Add-Vantage vials:** 1, 2 g   **Flexible plastic bags:** 1, 2 g

INDICATIONS

Respiratory tract infections caused by susceptible strains of *Streptococcus pneumoniae,* staphylococci, Group A beta-hemolytic streptococci, *Klebsiella,* and *Hemophilus influenzae*

Skin and soft tissue infections, including peritonitis, caused by susceptible strains of staphylococci, Group A beta-hemolytic streptococci, *Escherichia coli, Proteus mirabilis,* and *Klebsiella*

Genitourinary tract infections caused by susceptible strains of *Escherichia coli, Proteus mirabilis,* and *Klebsiella*

Septicemia, including endocarditis, caused by susceptible strains of *Streptococcus pneumoniae,* staphylococci, Group A beta-hemolytic streptococci, *viridans*-type streptococci, *Escherichia coli, Proteus mirabilis,* and *Klebsiella*

Gastrointestinal infections caused by susceptible strains of *Salmonella* and *Shigella*

Bone and joint infections caused by susceptible strains of staphylococci

Meningitis caused by susceptible strains of *Streptococcus pneumoniae,* Group A beta-hemolytic streptococci, and staphylococci[1]

PARENTERAL DOSAGE

Adult: 500 mg to 1 g IM or IV q4–6h; for uncomplicated pneumonia, furunculosis with cellulitis, and most urinary tract infections, 500 mg q6h; in life-threatening infections, up to 2 g IM or IV q4h may be required. The IV route may be preferable for patients with bacteremia, septicemia, or other severe or life-threatening infections who may be poor risks because of lowered resistance resulting, eg, from malnutrition, trauma, surgery, diabetes, heart failure, or malignancy, particularly if shock is present or imminent.

Infant and child: 80–160 mg/kg/day, given in divided doses IM or IV

Prevention of postoperative infection in patients undergoing contaminated or potentially contaminated procedures or when infection at the operative site would present a serious risk

Adult: 1–2 g IV 1/2–1 h prior to initial incision; repeat dose during surgery and q6h postoperatively for 24 h
Child: 20–30 mg/kg IV, following the same schedule as in adults

CONTRAINDICATIONS

Hypersensitivity to cephalosporins

ADMINISTRATION/DOSAGE ADJUSTMENTS

Patients with renal impairment	Administer 1–2 g IV to start, followed by up to 2 g q6h when creatinine clearance rate (CCr) = 50–80 ml/min; 1.5 g q6h when CCr = 25–50 ml/min; 1 g q6h when CCr = 10–25 ml/min; 0.5 g q6h when CCr = 2–10 ml/min; 0.5 g q8h when CCr < 2 ml/min
Intraperitoneal procedures	During peritoneal dialysis, up to 6 mg cephalothin per 100 ml of dialysis fluid may be instilled into the peritoneal space for 16–30 h; intraperitoneal administration of 0.1–4.0% cephalothin in saline may be used to treat peritonitis or a contaminated peritoneal cavity (the amount given should be considered in the total daily dose)
Streptococcal infections	All infections caused by beta-hemolytic streptococci should be treated for at least 10 days
Intramuscular administration	Dilute 1 g of cephalothin with 4 ml of Sterile Water for Injection and inject required dose into a large muscle mass, eg, the gluteus or lateral aspect of the thigh
Intermittent intravenous infusion	For intermittent use, dilute 1 g of cephalothin in 10 ml of diluent and slowly inject required dose directly into vein over a period of 3–5 min or administer through IV tubing; when administering cephalothin through a Y-type administration set, temporarily discontinue infusion of bulk IV solution
Continuous intravenous infusion	Dilute 1 or 2 g of cephalothin with 10 ml or more of Sterile Water for Injection and add to IV bottle containing compatible solution
Add-Vantage vials	To prepare solutions in the Add-Vantage vials, use Add-Vantage bags containing 50 or 100 ml of 0.9% sodium chloride injection USP or 50 or 100 ml of 5% dextrose injection USP

WARNINGS/PRECAUTIONS

Cross-allergenicity	Use with caution in penicillin-allergic patients
Hypersensitivity	Serious anaphylactic reactions may occur, most likely in patients with a history of allergy, particularly to drugs, necessitating administration of epinephrine or pressor amines, antihistamines, or corticosteroids

KEFLIN

Pseudomembranous colitis	May occur due to alteration of the normal intestinal flora and should be considered in any patient who develops diarrhea during or after therapy. Mild cases may respond to withdrawal of the drug alone. Moderate to severe cases should be managed by sigmoidoscopy, appropriate bacteriological studies, fluid and electrolyte replacement, and protein supplementation, as needed. Oral vancomycin is the treatment of choice for severe or refractory colitis associated with the overgrowth of *Clostridium difficile*; however, other possible causes should also be considered.
Superinfection	Overgrowth of nonsusceptible organisms may occur with prolonged use; constant observation is essential
Special-risk patients	Patients with impaired renal function should be carefully monitored during therapy; usual doses in such patients can result in excessive serum concentrations (see ADMINISTRATION/DOSAGE ADJUSTMENTS); use with caution in patients with a history of GI disease, particularly colitis
Thrombophlebitis	May occur, particularly when IV doses > 6 g/day are given by infusion for periods of more than 3 days; small IV needles and larger veins should be used, and the veins may need to be alternated. The addition of 10–25 mg hydrocortisone to IV solutions of 4–6 g of cephalothin may reduce the incidence of thrombophlebitis.

ADVERSE REACTIONS

Gastrointestinal	Pseudomembranous colitis; nausea and vomiting (rare)
Hypersensitivity	Maculopapular rash, urticaria, serum-sickness-like reactions, anaphylaxis, drug fever, eosinophilia
Hematological	Neutropenia, thrombocytopenia, hemolytic anemia
Other	Pain, induration, tenderness, and elevated temperature with repeated IM injection; thrombophlebitis (see WARNINGS/PRECAUTIONS)

OVERDOSAGE

Signs and symptoms	See ADVERSE REACTIONS
Treatment	Discontinue medication; treat symptomatically and institute supportive measures, as required

DRUG INTERACTIONS

Aminoglycosides, ethacrynic acid, furosemide, polymyxin antibiotics	△ Risk of nephrotoxicity
Probenecid	△ Cephalothin blood level and/or toxicity

ALTERED LABORATORY VALUES

Blood/serum values	△ Alkaline phosphatase △ BUN △ SGOT △ SGPT + Coombs' test
Urinary values	△ Glucose (with Clinitest tablets) ▽ Creatinine clearance

---

USE IN CHILDREN

See INDICATIONS; adjust dosage according to age, weight, and severity of infection

USE IN PREGNANT AND NURSING WOMEN

Pregnancy Category B: use during pregnancy only if clearly needed. Reproduction studies in rabbits at doses of 200 mg/kg have shown no evidence of impaired fertility or harm to the fetus; however, no adequate, well-controlled studies have been done in pregnant women. Use with caution in nursing mothers.

---

[1] Because only low levels of cephalothin appear in cerebrospinal fluid, the drug is not reliable in the treatment of meningitis and may be considered only for unusual circumstances in which more reliable antibiotics cannot be used

CEPHALOSPORINS

KEFUROX (cefuroxime sodium) Lilly Rx

Vials: 750 mg (10 ml), 1.5 g (20 ml) **Infusion bottles:** 750 mg, 1.5 g (100 ml)

INDICATIONS

Lower respiratory tract infections caused by susceptible strains of *Streptococcus pneumoniae, Hemophilus influenzae, Klebsiella, Staphylococcus aureus, Streptococcus pyogenes,* and *Escherichia coli*

Urinary tract infections caused by susceptible strains of *Escherichia coli* and *Klebsiella*

Disseminated gonococcal infections caused by *Neisseria gonorrhoeae*

Skin and skin structure infections caused by susceptible strains of *Staphylococcus aureus, Streptococcus pyogenes, Escherichia coli, Klebsiella,* and *Enterobacter*

Septicemia caused by susceptible strains of *Staphylococcus aureus, Streptococcus pneumoniae, Escherichia coli, Hemophilus influenzae,* and *Klebsiella*

Meningitis caused by susceptible strains of *Streptococcus pneumoniae, Hemophilus influenzae, Neisseria meningitidis,* and *Staphylococcus aureus*

Uncomplicated **gonorrhea** caused by *Neisseria gonorrhoeae*, including penicillinase-producing strains

Prevention of postoperative infection in patients undergoing clean-contaminated or potentially contaminated surgical procedures, or during open heart surgery

PARENTERAL DOSAGE

Adult: for uncomplicated pneumonia and urinary tract infections, disseminated gonococcal infections, and skin and skin structure infections, 750 mg IM or IV q8h; for severe or complicated infections, 1.5 g IM or IV q8h; for life-threatening infections and infections caused by less susceptible organisms, 1.5 g IM or IV q6h; for bacterial meningitis, up to 3 g IV q8h. The IV route may be preferable for patients with bacterial septicemia or other severe or life-threatening infections or for patients who may be poor risks because of lowered resistance, especially if shock is present or impending.

Infant (> 3 mo) and child: 50–100 mg/kg/day IM or IV, given in equally divided doses q6–8h (the higher dosage of 100 mg/kg/day should be given for more severe or serious infections); for bacterial meningitis, 200–240 mg/kg/day IV, given in divided doses q6–8h to start

Adult: 1.5 g, given in a single IM dose (in two different sites) together with 1 g of oral probenecid

Adult: for clean-contaminated or potentially contaminated surgical procedures, 1.5 g IV ½–1 h prior to initial incision, followed by 750 mg IV or IM q8h during prolonged procedures; for open heart surgery, 1.5 g IV at induction of anesthesia, followed by 1.5 g q12h, for a total of 6 g

CONTRAINDICATIONS
Hypersensitivity to cephalosporins

ADMINISTRATION/DOSAGE ADJUSTMENTS

Duration of therapy	Continue administration for at least 48–72 h after the patient has become asymptomatic or evidence of bacterial eradication has been obtained. *Streptococcus pyogenes* infections should be treated for at least 10 days; persistent infections may require several weeks of therapy. Doses lower than those indicated above should not be used.
Patients with renal impairment	Administer 750–1,500 mg q8h when creatinine clearance rate (Ccr) > 20 ml/min, 750 mg q12h when Ccr = 10–20 ml/min, and 750 mg q24h when Ccr < 10 ml/min.[1] Creatinine clearance may be calculated from the serum creatinine concentration by use of the following formula: Ccr (in males) = [patient's weight *(kg)* × (140 − patient's age)]/[72 × creatinine concentration *(mg/dl)*]; for females, multiply the value obtained by this formula by 0.85.
Intramuscular administration	Reconstitute the contents of a 750-mg vial with 3.6 ml of sterile water for injection and withdraw 3.6 ml of the resulting suspension for injection. Inject the drug deeply into a large muscle mass, such as the gluteus or the lateral part of the thigh; to avoid inadvertent injection into a blood vessel, aspirate the syringe prior to injection.
Preparation of solutions for intravenous administration	Reconstitute the contents of each 750-mg vial with 9 ml of sterile water for injection and withdraw 8 ml of the resulting solution for injection; for each 1.5-g vial, use 16 ml of sterile water for injection and withdraw the entire amount of solution for injection. For infusion, add 50–100 ml of one of the following parenteral solutions: sterile water for injection, 5% dextrose injection, 0.9% sodium chloride injection, M/6 sodium lactate injection, Ringer's injection USP, lactated Ringer's injection USP, 5% dextrose and 0.9% sodium chloride injection, 5% dextrose and 0.45% sodium chloride injection, 5% dextrose and 0.225% sodium chloride injection, 10% dextrose injection, or 10% invert sugar in water for injection; if sterile water for injection is used, reconstitute with approximately 20 ml/g to avoid hypotonicity. The solution should be used within 24 h if kept at room temperature and within 48 h if refrigerated.
Intravenous injection	After reconstitution, inject the solution slowly into a vein over a period of 3–5 min, or give it through a tubing system which may already be in place
Intravenous infusion	When a Y-type administration set is used for intermittent infusion, administration of the bulk IV solution should be discontinued for the duration of each infusion. For continuous infusion, a solution of cefuroxime may be added to an IV bottle containing one of the following fluids: 0.9% sodium chloride injection, 5% or 10% dextrose injection, 5% dextrose and 0.9% sodium chloride injection, 5% dextrose and 0.45% sodium chloride injection, or M/6 sodium lactate injection. Do not add cefuroxime to solutions of aminoglycosides because of potential interaction (see DRUG INTERACTIONS); however, these antibiotics may be administered separately.

KEFUROX

WARNINGS/PRECAUTIONS

Cross-allergenicity	Use with caution in penicillin-allergic patients
Hypersensitivity	Serious acute hypersensitivity reactions may occur, most likely in patients with a history of allergy, particularly to drugs; anaphylactic reactions may require administration of epinephrine and other emergency measures
Pseudomembranous colitis	May occur due to alteration of the normal intestinal flora and should be considered in any patient who develops diarrhea during or after therapy. Mild cases may respond to withdrawal of the drug alone. Moderate to severe cases should be managed by fluid and electrolyte replacement and protein supplementation, as needed. Oral vancomycin is the treatment of choice for severe or refractory colitis associated with the overgrowth of *Clostridium difficile;* however, other possible causes should also be considered.
Superinfection	Overgrowth of nonsusceptible organisms may occur with prolonged use; careful observation is essential
Renal impairment	Renal status should be monitored during therapy, especially in seriously ill patients receiving maximum doses. Use this drug with caution in patients who are concomitantly receiving potent diuretics, as these regimens are suspected of adversely affecting renal function. In patients with renal insufficiency, the total daily dose of cefuroxime should be reduced (see ADMINISTRATION/DOSAGE ADJUSTMENTS).
Special-risk patients	Use with caution in patients with known hypersensitivity to penicillin and in patients with a history of gastrointestinal disease, particularly colitis
Carcinogenicity, mutagenicity	Long-term studies have not been done in animals to evaluate the carcinogenic potential of this drug; standard laboratory studies have shown no evidence of mutagenicity

ADVERSE REACTIONS

Frequent reactions (incidence ≥ 1%) are printed in *italics*

Local	*Thrombophlebitis following IV administration (1.7%)*
Gastrointestinal	Diarrhea, nausea, pseudomembranous colitis
Hematological	*Decrease in hemoglobin and hematocrit (10%), transient eosinophilia (7.1%)*, transient neutropenia and leukopenia
Hypersensitivity	Rash, pruritus, urticaria, positive Coombs' test

OVERDOSAGE

Signs and symptoms	See ADVERSE REACTIONS
Treatment	Discontinue medication; treat symptomatically and institute supportive measures, as required

DRUG INTERACTIONS

Aminoglycoside antibiotics	⇧ Risk of nephrotoxicity
Probenecid	⇧ Serum level of cefuroxime

ALTERED LABORATORY VALUES

Blood/serum values	⇧ BUN ⇧ Creatinine ⇧ SGOT ⇧ SGPT ⇧ LDH ⇧ Alkaline phosphatase ⇧ Bilirubin + Coombs' test − Glucose (with ferricyanide test)
Urinary values	⇩ Creatinine clearance + Glucose (with Clinitest tablets or Benedict's or Fehling's solution)

USE IN CHILDREN

See INDICATIONS and PARENTERAL DOSAGE; in calculating dosages by weight, do not exceed the maximum adult dose. Safety and effectiveness for use in infants under 3 mo of age have not been established. Accumulation of cephalosporin drugs in newborn infants has been reported.

USE IN PREGNANT AND NURSING WOMEN

Pregnancy Category B: use during pregnancy only if clearly needed. Reproduction studies in mice and rabbits at doses up to 60 times the human dose have revealed no evidence of impaired fertility or fetal harm; however, no adequate, well-controlled studies have been performed in pregnant women. Cefuroxime is excreted in human milk; use with caution in nursing women.

---

[1] Since cefuroxime sodium is dialyzable, patients on hemodialysis should be given a further dose at the end of the dialysis

CEPHALOSPORINS

KEFZOL (cefazolin sodium) Lilly   Rx

Vials: 250 mg (10 ml), 500 mg (10, 100 ml), 1 g (10, 100 ml), 10 g (100 ml) **Dual-compartment vials:** 500 mg (10 ml), 1 g (10 ml)
Add-Vantage vials: 500 mg, 1 g **Flexible plastic bags:** 500 mg, 1 g

INDICATIONS

Respiratory tract infections caused by susceptible strains of *Streptococcus pneumoniae, Klebsiella, Hemophilus influenzae, Staphylococcus aureus,* and Group A beta-hemolytic streptococci
Genitourinary tract infections caused by susceptible strains of *Escherichia coli, Proteus mirabilis, Klebsiella, Enterobacter,* and enterococci
Skin and soft tissue infections caused by susceptible strains of *Staphylococcus aureus,* Group A beta-hemolytic streptococci, and other streptococci
Biliary tract infections caused by susceptible strains of *Escherichia coli,* streptococci, *Proteus mirabilis, Klebsiella,* and *Staphylococcus aureus*
Bone and joint infections caused by susceptible strains of *Staphylococcus aureus*
Septicemia caused by susceptible strains of *Streptococcus pneumoniae, Staphylococcus aureus, Proteus mirabilis, Escherichia coli,* and *Klebsiella*
Endocarditis caused by susceptible strains of *Staphylococcus aureus* and Group A beta-hemolytic streptococci

Prevention of postoperative infection in patients undergoing contaminated or potentially contaminated procedures or when infection at the operative site would present a serious risk

PARENTERAL DOSAGE

Adult: for mild infections caused by susceptible Gram-positive cocci, 250–500 mg IM or IV q8h; for moderate to severe infections, 500 mg to 1 g IM or IV q6–8h; for acute uncomplicated urinary tract infections, 1 g IM or IV q12h; for pneumococcal pneumonia, 500 mg IM or IV q12h; for life-threatening infections, such as endocarditis and septicemia, 1–1.5 g IM or IV q6h or, if necessary, up to 12 g/day
Infant (≥ 1 mo) and child: for mild to moderately severe infections, 25–50 mg/kg/day IM or IV in 3–4 equally divided doses; for severe infections, up to 100 mg/kg/day IM or IV in 3–4 equally divided doses

Adult: 1 g IM or IV 1/2–1 h prior to surgery, followed by 0.5–1 g IM or IV during lengthy (2 h or more) procedures and then q6–8h for 24 h postoperatively; in cases where postoperative infection would be particularly devastating (eg, open-heart surgery and prosthetic arthroplasty), prophylactic administration may be continued for 3–5 days

CONTRAINDICATIONS
Hypersensitivity to cephalosporins

ADMINISTRATION/DOSAGE ADJUSTMENTS

Intramuscular administration	Add 2 ml of diluent to the 250- or 500-mg vial or 2.5 ml to the 1-g vial; use sterile or bacteriostatic water for injection to reconstitute the 1-g solution, either of these diluents or 0.9% sodium chloride injection to reconstitute the 250- and 500-mg solutions. Inject dose into a large muscle mass.
Preparation for IV use	For IV injection, take a 500-mg or 1-g solution reconstituted in a regular or dual-compartment vial and dilute with at least 10 ml of sterile water for injection. For intermittent infusion, take a 500-mg or 1-g solution reconstituted in a regular or dual-compartment vial and dilute in 50–100 ml of one of the following diluents: 0.9% sodium chloride injection, 5% or 10% dextrose injection, Ringer's or lactated Ringer's injection, 5% or 10% invert sugar in sterile water for injection, Normosol-M in D5-W, or 5% dextrose with Plasma-Lyte, Ionosol B, lactated Ringer's injection, or 0.2%, 0.45%, or 0.9% sodium chloride injection; administer solution in the primary IV fluid or use a separate secondary bottle. To prepare solutions in the Add-Vantage vials, use Add-Vantage bags containing 50 or 100 ml of 0.9% sodium chloride injection USP or 50 or 100 ml of 5% dextrose injection USP.
Intravenous administration	Drug can be given by direct injection or by intermittent or continuous infusion. For bolus administration, slowly inject the dose over a period of 3–5 min either directly into a vein or through IV tubing.
Adults with renal impairment	Determine the initial dose according to the severity of the infection. Calculate subsequent doses and the dosing interval as follows: If creatinine clearance (Ccr) = 35–54 ml/min or serum creatinine level (Scr) = 1.6–3 mg/dl, maintain dose, but administer at intervals of at least 8 h. If Ccr = 11–34 ml/min or Scr = 3.1–4.5 mg/dl, reduce dose by 50% and give q12h. If Ccr = ≤ 10 ml/min or Scr = ≥ 4.6 mg/dl, reduce dose by 50% and give q18–24h. For use in patients undergoing peritoneal dialysis, see package insert.
Children with renal impairment	Determine the initial dose according to the severity of the infection. Calculate subsequent doses and the dosing interval as follows: If creatinine clearance (Ccr) = 40–70 ml/min, give 60% of the normal daily dose in 2 divided doses q12h. If Ccr = 20–40 ml/min, give 25% of the normal daily dose in 2 divided doses q12h. If Ccr = 5–20 ml/min, give 10% of the normal daily dose q24h.

WARNINGS/PRECAUTIONS

Cross-allergenicity	Use with caution in penicillin-allergic patients
Hypersensitivity reactions	Serious acute hypersensitivity reactions may occur, most likely in patients with allergy; anaphylactic reactions may require administration of epinephrine or other pressor amines, antihistamines, or corticosteroids
Pseudomembranous colitis	May occur due to alteration of the normal intestinal flora and should be considered in any patient who develops diarrhea during or after therapy; use with caution in patients with a history of GI disease, particularly colitis. Mild cases may respond to withdrawal of the drug alone. Moderate to severe cases should be managed by sigmoidoscopy, appropriate bacteriological studies, fluid and electrolyte replacement, and protein supplementation, as needed. Oral vancomycin is the treatment of choice for severe or refractory colitis associated with the overgrowth of *Clostridium difficile;* however, other possible causes should also be considered.
Superinfection	Overgrowth of nonsusceptible organisms may occur with prolonged use; careful clinical observation is essential
Carcinogenicity, mutagenicity	No studies have been done to determine the carcinogenic or mutagenic potential of this drug

ADVERSE REACTIONS

Gastrointestinal	Anorexia, diarrhea, oral candidiasis, pseudomembranous colitis; nausea and vomiting (rare)
Renal	Transient increase in BUN level (without clinical evidence of renal impairment)
Hepatic	Transient increase in SGOT, SGPT, and alkaline phosphatase levels (rare); transient hepatitis and cholestatic jaundice (rare)
Hypersensitivity	Drug fever, skin rash, vulvar pruritus, eosinophilia
Genitourinary	Genital and anal pruritus, genital moniliasis, vaginitis
Hematological	Neutropenia, leukopenia, thrombocytopenia
Other	Pain on IM injection, sometimes with induration; phlebitis at injection site

OVERDOSAGE

Signs and symptoms	See ADVERSE REACTIONS
Treatment	Discontinue medication; treat symptomatically and institute supportive measures, as required

DRUG INTERACTIONS

Probenecid	⇧ Cefazolin blood level and/or toxicity

ALTERED LABORATORY VALUES

Blood/serum values	⇧ Alkaline phosphatase ⇧ BUN ⇧ SGOT ⇧ SGPT + Coombs' test
Urinary values	+ Glucose (with Benedict's solution, Fehling's solution, and Clinitest tablets)

USE IN CHILDREN

See INDICATIONS; adjust dosage according to body weight and severity of infection. Safety for use in premature infants and newborns under 1 mo of age has not been established; use in these patients is not recommended.

USE IN PREGNANT AND NURSING WOMEN

Pregnancy Category B: use during pregnancy only if clearly needed. Reproduction studies in rats at doses of 500 or 1,000 mg/kg have shown no evidence of impaired fertility or harm to the fetus; however, no adequate, well-controlled studies have been done in pregnant women. Positive Coombs' tests have been reported for neonates whose mothers received a cephalosporin before delivery. However, when given prior to cesarean section, cefazolin appears to have no adverse effect on the fetus, despite its presence in cord blood. Very low concentrations of cefazolin have been detected in human milk; use with caution in nursing mothers.

CEPHALOSPORINS

MANDOL (cefamandole nafate) Lilly   Rx
Vials: 500 mg (10 ml), 1 g (10, 100 ml), 2 g (20, 100 ml), 10 g (100 ml)   Add-Vantage vials: 1, 2 g   Flexible plastic bags: 1, 2 g

INDICATIONS

Lower respiratory tract infections caused by susceptible strains of *Streptococcus pneumoniae, Hemophilus influenzae, Klebsiella, Staphylococcus aureus,* beta-hemolytic streptococci, and *Proteus mirabilis*

Peritonitis caused by susceptible strains of *Escherichia coli* and *Enterobacter*

Septicemia caused by susceptible strains of *Escherichia coli, Staphylococcus aureus, Streptococcus pneumoniae, Streptococcus pyogenes, Hemophilus influenzae,* and *Klebsiella*

Skin and skin structure infections caused by susceptible strains of *Staphylococcus aureus, Streptococcus pyogenes, Hemophilus influenzae, Escherichia coli, Enterobacter,* and *Proteus mirabilis*

Bone and joint infections caused by susceptible strains of *Staphylococcus aureus*

Urinary tract infections caused by susceptible strains of *Escherichia coli, Proteus, Enterobacter, Klebsiella,* Group D streptococci, and *Streptococcus epidermidis*

Prevention of postoperative infection in patients undergoing contaminated or potentially contaminated procedures or when infection at the operative site would present a serious risk

PARENTERAL DOSAGE

Adult: for skin structure infections and uncomplicated pneumonia, 500 mg IM or IV q6h; for other or more serious infections, 500 mg to 1 g IM or IV q4–8h; for severe infections, 1 g IM or IV q4–6h; for life-threatening or resistant infections caused by less susceptible organisms, up to 2 g IM or IV q4h may be needed. The IV route may be preferable for patients with septicemia, localized parenchymal abscesses (eg, intraabdominal abscess), peritonitis, or other severe or life-threatening infections who may be poor risks because of lowered resistance.

Infant (≥ 6 mo) and child: 50–100 mg/kg/day IM or IV in equally divided doses q4–8h; for severe infections, up to 150 mg/kg/day IM or IV in equally divided doses q4–8h may be needed

Adult: for uncomplicated infections, 500 mg IM or IV q8h; for more serious infections, 1 g IM or IV q8h

Infant (≥ 6 mo) and child: same as pediatric dosages above

Adult: 1–2 g IM or IV 1/2–1 h prior to surgery, followed by 1–2 g IM or IV q6h for 24 h; in cases where postoperative infection would be particularly devastating (eg, open-heart surgery and prosthetic arthroplasty), prophylactic administration may be continued for 72 h

Infant (> 3 mo) and child: 50–100 mg/kg/day IM or IV, given in equally divided doses as above

CONTRAINDICATIONS
Hypersensitivity to cephalosporins

ADMINISTRATION/DOSAGE ADJUSTMENTS

Duration of therapy — Treatment should be continued for at least 48–72 h after patient has become asymptomatic or bacteria have been eradicated. Infections caused by beta-hemolytic streptococci should be treated for at least 10 days to guard against the risk of rheumatic fever or glomerulonephritis. Persistent infections may require treatment for several weeks.

Intramuscular injection — Dilute 1 g of cefamandole with 3 ml of sterile (or bacteriostatic) water for injection, 0.9% sodium chloride, or bacteriostatic sodium chloride injection and inject required dose deeply into a large muscle mass (eg, the gluteus or lateral aspect of the thigh) to minimize pain

Intermittent intravenous infusion — For intermittent use, dilute 1 g of cefamandole with 10 ml of sterile water for injection, 0.9% sodium chloride, or 5% dextrose and slowly inject required dose directly into a vein or administer through IV tubing; when administering cefamandole through a Y–type administration set, temporarily discontinue infusion of bulk IV solution

Continuous intravenous infusion — Dilute 1 g of cefamandole with 10 ml of sterile water for injection and add to IV bottle containing compatible solution; do not mix an aminoglycoside with cefamandole in the same container

Add-Vantage vials — To prepare solutions in the Add-Vantage vials, use Add-Vantage bags containing 50 or 100 ml of 0.9% sodium chloride injection USP or 50 or 100 ml of 5% dextrose injection USP

Patients with renal impairment and life-threatening infections — Administer 1–2 g IM or IV to start, followed by 2 g q4h when creatinine clearance rate (Ccr) > 80 ml/min; 1.5 g q4h or 2 g q6h when Ccr = 50–80 ml/min; 1.5 g q6h or 2 g q8h when Ccr = 25–50 ml/min; 1 g q6h or 1.25 g q8h when Ccr = 10–25 ml/min; 0.67 g q8h or 1 g q12h when Ccr = 2–10 ml/min; or 0.5 g q8h or 0.75 g q12h when Ccr < 2 ml/min. Creatinine clearance may be calculated from the serum creatinine concentration by use of the following formula: Ccr (in males) = [patient's weight *(kg)* × (140 − patient's age)]/[72 × creatinine concentration *(mg/dl)*]; for females, multiply the value obtained by this formula by 0.9.

Patients with renal impairment and less severe infections — Administer 1–2 g IM or IV to start, followed by 1–2 g q6h when creatinine clearance rate (Ccr) > 80 ml/min; 0.75–1.5 g q6h when Ccr = 50–80 ml/min; 0.75–1.5 g q8h when Ccr = 25–50 ml/min; 0.5–1 g q8h when Ccr = 10–25 ml/min; 0.5–0.75 g q12h when Ccr = 2–10 ml/min; or 0.25–0.5 g q12h when Ccr < 2 ml/min. Creatinine clearance may be calculated from the serum creatinine concentration by use of the formula given above.

Prophylactic use following cesarean section	Administer the first dose just prior to surgery or as soon as the umbilical cord is clamped
Chronic urinary tract infections	Frequent bacteriological and clinical appraisal is necessary during therapy and may be required for several weeks afterward

WARNINGS/PRECAUTIONS

Cross-allergenicity	Use with caution in penicillin-allergic patients
Hypersensitivity	Serious acute hypersensitivity reactions may occur, especially in patients with a history of allergy (particularly to drugs), and may necessitate use of epinephrine and other emergency measures
Pseudomembranous colitis	May occur due to alteration of the normal intestinal flora and should be considered in any patient who develops diarrhea during or after therapy. Mild cases may respond to withdrawal of the drug alone. Moderate to severe cases should be managed by sigmoidoscopy, appropriate bacteriological studies, fluid and electrolyte replacement, and protein supplementation, as needed. Oral vancomycin is the treatment of choice for severe or refractory colitis associated with the overgrowth of *Clostridium difficile*; however, other possible causes should also be considered.
Superinfection	Overgrowth of nonsusceptible organisms may occur with prolonged use; careful clinical observation is essential
Special-risk patients	Patients with impaired renal function should be carefully monitored during therapy and should receive a reduced dosage determined by degree of impairment, severity of infection, and susceptibility of organism (see ADMINISTRATION/DOSAGE ADJUSTMENTS); use with caution in patients with a history of GI disease, particularly colitis
Hypoprothrombinemia	May occur rarely, with or without bleeding, particularly in the elderly, debilitated, or otherwise compromised patients with vitamin K deficiencies; may be reversed by administration of vitamin K. Prophylactic administration of vitamin K may be indicated in such patients, especially prior to bowel preparation and/or surgery.
Concomitant ingestion of alcohol	Has produced nausea, vomiting, and vasomotor instability with hypotension and peripheral vasodilation in a few patients; in laboratory animals, cefamandole inhibits the enzyme acetaldehyde dehydrogenase, which causes accumulation of acetaldehyde when alcohol is given concomitantly
Impairment of fertility	Delayed maturity of testicular germinal epithelium, decreased testicular weight, and a reduced number of germinal cells in the leading waves of spermatogenic development have been seen in rats given daily approximately 5 times the maximum human dose during the period of initial spermatogenic development (6–36 days of age); some of the animals were found to be infertile after reaching sexual maturity. Administration of cefamandole in utero, at 0–4 days of age, or for up to 6 mo beginning after 36 days of age has produced no adverse effects on testicular development. The clinical significance of these findings is not known.

ADVERSE REACTIONS

Gastrointestinal	Pseudomembranous colitis; nausea and vomiting (rare)
Hepatic	Transient hepatitis and cholestatic jaundice (rare)
Hypersensitivity	Anaphylaxis, maculopapular rash, urticaria, eosinophilia, drug fever
Hematological	Neutropenia (especially with prolonged use); thrombocytopenia (rare)
Other	Pain on IM injection; thrombophlebitis (rare)

OVERDOSAGE

Signs and symptoms	See ADVERSE REACTIONS
Treatment	Discontinue use of drug; treat symptomatically and institute supportive measures, as required

DRUG INTERACTIONS

Aminoglycoside antibiotics	△ Risk of nephrotoxicity
Alcohol	Nausea, vomiting, and vasomotor instability
Probenecid	△ Cefamandole blood level and/or toxicity

ALTERED LABORATORY VALUES

Blood/serum values	△ Alkaline phosphatase △ BUN △ Creatinine △ SGOT △ SGPT + Coombs' test
Urinary values	△ Glucose (with Clinitest tablets) ▽ Creatinine clearance + Protein (with acid and denaturization-precipitation tests)

USE IN CHILDREN

See INDICATIONS; adjust dosage according to body weight and severity of infection. Cefamandole has been used effectively in infants; however, all laboratory parameters have not been thoroughly studied in 1- to 6-mo-old infants, and safety for use in younger infants and premature newborns has not been established. Thus, in treating infants the potential benefits of the drug should be weighed against the possible risks involved in each situation.

USE IN PREGNANT AND NURSING WOMEN

Pregnancy Category B: use during pregnancy only if clearly needed. Reproduction studies in rats at doses of 500 or 1,000 mg/kg have shown no evidence of impaired fertility or harm to the fetus; however, no adequate, well-controlled studies have been done in pregnant women. Trace amounts of cefamandole are excreted in human milk[1]; use with caution in nursing mothers.

[1] Data on file, Lilly Research Laboratories

CEPHALOSPORINS

MEFOXIN (cefoxitin sodium) Merck Sharp & Dohme   Rx

Vials: 1, 2 g **Infusion bottles:** 1, 2 g **Pharmacy bulk bottles:** 10 g **Plastic containers:** 20, 40 mg/ml (50 ml)

INDICATIONS

Lower respiratory tract infections, including pneumonia and lung abscess, caused by susceptible strains of *Streptococcus pneumoniae,* other streptococci (excluding enterococci), *Staphylococcus aureus, Escherichia coli, Klebsiella, Hemophilus influenzae,* and *Bacteroides*

Urinary tract infections caused by susceptible strains of *Escherichia coli, Klebsiella, Proteus mirabilis,* indole-positive *Proteus,* and *Providencia*

Intraabdominal infections, including peritonitis and intraabdominal abscess, caused by susceptible strains of *Escherichia coli, Klebsiella, Bacteroides* (including the *B fragilis* group[1]), and *Clostridium*

Gynecological infections, including endometritis, pelvic cellulitis, and pelvic inflammatory disease, caused by susceptible strains of *Escherichia coli, Neisseria gonorrhoeae, Bacteroides* (including the *B fragilis* group[1]), *Clostridium, Peptococcus, Peptostreptococcus,* and Group B streptococci

Septicemia caused by susceptible strains of *Streptococcus pneumoniae, Staphylococcus aureus, Escherichia coli, Klebsiella,* and *Bacteroides* (including the *B fragilis* group[1])

Bone and joint infections caused by susceptible strains of *Staphylococcus aureus*

Skin and skin structure infections caused by susceptible strains of *Staphylococcus aureus, S epidermidis,* streptococci (excluding enterococci), *Escherichia coli, Proteus mirabilis, Klebsiella, Bacteroides* (including the *B fragilis* group[1]), *Clostridium, Peptococcus,* and *Peptostreptococcus*

Uncomplicated gonorrhea caused by *Neisseria gonorrhoeae*

Prevention of postoperative infection in patients undergoing contaminated or potentially contaminated procedures or when infection at the operative site would present a serious risk

PARENTERAL DOSAGE

Adult: for uncomplicated infections in which bacteremia is absent or unlikely, 1 g IM or IV q6–8h; for moderately severe to severe infections, 1 g IV q4h or 2 g IV q6–8h; for infections commonly requiring high-dose antibiotic therapy, 2 g IV q4h or 3 g IV q6h. The IV route is preferable for patients with bacteremia, bacterial septicemia, or other severe or life-threatening infections and for patients who may be poor risks because of lowered resistance resulting, eg, from malnutrition, trauma, surgery, diabetes, heart failure, or malignancy, particularly if shock is present or imminent.

Infant (> 3 mo) and child: 80–160 mg/kg/day, up to 12 g/day, IM or IV in 4–6 equally divided doses

Adult: 2 g IM (with 1 g probenecid orally 0–30 min before injection)

Adult: 2 g IM or IV 1/2–1 h prior to surgery, repeated q6h for up to 24 h (or up to 72 h after prosthetic arthroplasty). For prevention of infection associated with cesarean section, administer 2 g IV as soon as the umbilical cord is clamped and then 2 g IV or IM 4 and 8 h later; subsequent doses may be given q6h for up to 24 h. For prevention of infection associated with transurethral prostatectomy, administer 1 g just before surgery and then repeat q8h for up to 5 days.

Infant (≥ 3 mo) and child: 30–40 mg/kg IM or IV 1/2–1 h prior to surgery, repeated q6h for up to 24 h

MEFOXIN

CONTRAINDICATIONS

Hypersensitivity to cefoxitin or other cephalosporins

ADMINISTRATION/DOSAGE ADJUSTMENTS

Intramuscular administration	Add 2 ml of sterile water for injection or 0.5% lidocaine hydrochloride (without epinephrine) to the 1-g standard vial or 4 ml to the 2-g standard vial; following aspiration, inject dose well within the body of a relatively large muscle such as the gluteus maximus
Preparation for IV use	To reconstitute solution, add at least 10 ml of sterile water for injection to the standard 1-g vial, 10 or 20 ml of this diluent to the standard 2-g vial, or 50 or 100 ml of a compatible diluent (see package insert) to the infusion or pharmacy bulk bottle. For IV infusion, dilute solutions prepared in the vials or pharmacy bulk bottles with 50–1,000 ml of a compatible diluent or, alternatively, use the infusion bottles. To use a plastic container, thaw contents at room temperature. Then, check for minute leaks by squeezing the bag firmly; discard it if leaks are found or seal is not intact. Do not put additives into the container. Cefoxitin should not be mixed with solutions containing an aminoglycoside since these drugs are physically incompatible with each other.
Intravenous administration	Cefoxitin can be given by direct injection or by intermittent or continuous infusion. For intermittent administration, a solution containing 1–2 g in 10 ml of sterile water for injection can be injected directly into a vein over a period of 3–5 min; alternatively, this solution can be given through IV tubing over a longer period of time. For continuous infusion, use butterfly or scalp vein-type needles. During intermittent or continuous infusion, no other solution should be administered at the same site. At least once every 48 h, replace the administration set used with plastic containers. Do not connect these containers in series because residual air in the primary container, withdrawn before administration of the fluid in the secondary container is complete, could produce air embolism. Administer cefoxitin and an aminoglycoside at separate sites if concomitant therapy is indicated.
Streptococcal infections	Infections caused by Group A beta-hemolytic streptococci should be treated for at least 10 days to guard against the risk of rheumatic fever or glomerulonephritis
Patients with renal impairment	Administer an initial loading dose of 1–2 g, followed by 1–2 g q8–12h when creatinine clearance rate (CCr) = 30–50 ml/min; 1–2 g q12–24h when CCr = 10–29 ml/min; 0.5–1 g q12–24h when CCr = 5–9 ml/min; 0.5–1 g q24–48h when CCr < 5 ml/min. Creatinine clearance may be calculated from the serum creatinine concentration by use of the following formula: CCr (in males) = [patient's weight (kg) × (140 − patient's age)]/[72 × creatinine concentration (mg/dl)]; for females, multiply the value obtained by this formula by 0.85.
Patients undergoing hemodialysis	Administer 1–2 g after each dialysis treatment and adjust maintenance dosage according to renal impairment schedule

WARNINGS/PRECAUTIONS

Cross-allergenicity	Use with caution in penicillin-allergic patients
Hypersensitivity	Serious hypersensitivity reactions may occur, especially in patients with a history of allergy (particularly to drugs), and may require the use of epinephrine and/or other emergency measures
Pseudomembranous colitis	May occur due to alteration of the normal intestinal flora and should be considered in any patient who develops diarrhea during or after therapy; use with caution in patients with a history of GI disease, particularly colitis. Mild cases may respond to withdrawal of the drug alone. Moderate to severe cases should be managed by sigmoidoscopy, appropriate bacteriological studies, fluid and electrolyte replacement, and protein supplementation, as needed. Isolation of the patient may be advisable. Oral vancomycin is the treatment of choice for severe or refractory colitis associated with the overgrowth of *Clostridium difficile;* however, other possible causes should also be considered.
Superinfection	Overgrowth of nonsusceptible organisms may occur with prolonged use; repeated clinical evaluation is essential
Carcinogenicity, mutagenicity, effect on fertility	No studies have been done to determine the carcinogenic or mutagenic potential of this drug; studies in rats given approximately 3 times the maximum human dose IV have shown no adverse effects on fertility or mating ability

ADVERSE REACTIONS

Hypersensitivity	Rash (including exfoliative dermatitis), pruritus, eosinophilia, fever, other reactions
Gastrointestinal	Diarrhea, pseudomembranous colitis; nausea and vomiting (rare)
Cardiovascular	Hypotension
Hematological	Eosinophilia, leukopenia, granulocytopenia, neutropenia, anemia (including hemolytic anemia), thrombocytopenia, bone marrow depression
Other	Pain, induration, and tenderness at site of IM injection; thrombophlebitis with IV administration; acute renal failure (rare)

MEFOXIN ■ MONOCID

OVERDOSAGE

Signs and symptoms	See ADVERSE REACTIONS
Treatment	Discontinue medication; treat symptomatically and institute supportive measures, as required

DRUG INTERACTIONS

Aminoglycoside antibiotics	△ Risk of nephrotoxicity
Probenecid	△ Cefoxitin blood level and/or toxicity

ALTERED LABORATORY VALUES

Blood/serum values	△ Alkaline phosphatase △ SGOT △ SGPT △ Lactate dehydrogenase △ BUN △ Creatinine + Coombs' test (especially in azotemic patients)
Urinary values	△ Creatinine (with Jaffe reaction) + Glucose (with Clinitest tablets) △ 17-OHCS (with Porter-Silber reaction)

USE IN CHILDREN

See INDICATIONS; adjust dosage according to body weight and severity of infection. Safety and efficacy have not been established in infants from birth to 3 mo of age. In children 3 mo of age and older, doses higher than those recommended are associated with an increased incidence of eosinophilia and elevation in SGOT. Diluents containing benzyl alcohol should not be used in infants; the preservative causes toxic effects in neonates and thus may also produce these reactions in small infants who are over 3 mo of age.

USE IN PREGNANT AND NURSING WOMEN

Pregnancy Category B: reproduction studies in rats and mice given parenterally about 1–7.5 times the maximum human dose have shown a slight decrease in fetal weight, but no evidence of teratogenicity or fetotoxicity. Although a high frequency of abortion and maternal death has been seen in rabbits, these effects have been considered to be the expected results of this species' unusual sensitivity to antibiotic-induced changes in the intestinal flora and therefore have not been viewed as teratogenic reactions. Use cefoxitin during pregnancy only if clearly needed. This drug is excreted in low concentrations in human milk; use with caution in nursing mothers.

[1] B fragilis, B distasonis, B ovatus, B thetaiotaomicron, and B vulgatus

---

CEPHALOSPORINS

MONOCID (cefonicid sodium) Smith Kline & French   Rx

Vials: 0.5, 1 g   **Piggyback vials:** 1 g   **Pharmacy bulk vials:** 10 g

INDICATIONS

Lower respiratory tract infections caused by susceptible strains of *Streptococcus pneumoniae, Klebsiella pneumoniae, Escherichia coli,* and *Hemophilus influenzae*
Urinary tract infections caused by susceptible strains of *Escherichia coli, Proteus mirabilis,* and *Klebsiella pneumoniae*
Skin and skin structure infections caused by susceptible strains of *Staphylococcus aureus, Staphylococcus epidermidis, Streptococcus pyogenes,* and *Streptococcus agalactiae*
Septicemia caused by susceptible strains of *Streptococcus pneumoniae* and *Escherichia coli*
Bone and joint infections caused by susceptible strains of *Staphylococcus aureus*

Prevention of postoperative infection: (1) following contaminated or potentially contaminated procedures such as colorectal surgery, vaginal hysterectomy, cholecystectomy (in high-risk patients), and cesarean section or (2) following procedures such as prosthetic arthroplasty and open-heart surgery in which the occurrence of infection would pose a serious risk

PARENTERAL DOSAGE

Adult: for uncomplicated urinary tract infections, 0.5 g IM or IV q24h; for mild to moderate infections, 1 g IM or IV q24h; for severe or life-threatening infections, 2 g IM or IV q24h

Adult: 1 g IM or IV; administer dose 1 h before surgery or, for prophylaxis following cesarean section, after the umbilical cord has been clamped. For prophylaxis following prosthetic arthoplasty or open-heart surgery, dose may be repeated q24h for 2 days.

CONTRAINDICATIONS

Hypersensitivity to cephalosporins

MONOCID

ADMINISTRATION/DOSAGE ADJUSTMENTS

Preparation of solution — Add 2 ml of sterile water for injection to the 500-mg vial (resulting concentration: 220 mg/ml) or 2.5 ml to the 1-g vial (resulting concentration: 325 mg/ml); shake well. Use sterile or bacteriostatic water for injection or sodium chloride injection to reconstitute the solution in a pharmacy bulk vial; add 25 ml to yield a concentration of 333 mg/ml or 45 ml to yield a concentration of 200 mg/ml. For IV infusion, either reconstitute the contents of a piggyback vial or dilute a solution prepared in a standard or pharmacy bulk vial; use 50–100 ml of 0.9% sodium chloride injection USP, 5% or 10% dextrose injection USP, 5% dextrose and 0.2%, 0.45%, or 0.9% sodium chloride injection USP, Ringer's or lactated Ringer's injection USP, sodium lactate injection USP, 5% dextrose and lactated Ringer's or 0.15% potassium chloride injection, or 10% invert sugar in sterile water for injection.

Administration — Aspirate before IM administration to avoid inadvertent intravascular injection; then inject solution well within the body of a relatively large muscle. A 2-g dose should be divided between different muscle masses. For IV bolus injection, administer the dose over a period of 3–5 min either directly or through IV tubing.

Patients with renal impairment — Administer an initial loading dose of 7.5 mg/kg IM or IV; then adjust dosage according to creatinine clearance and severity of infection (see table). Monitor serum cefonicid level during therapy and, if necessary, change dosage. It is not necessary to give an additional dose after dialysis.

Creatinine clearance (ml/min)	Dosage for mild to moderate infections	Dosage for severe infections
60–79	10 mg/kg q24h	25 mg/kg q24h
40–59	8 mg/kg q24h	20 mg/kg q24h
20–39	4 mg/kg q24h	15 mg/kg q24h
10–19	4 mg/kg q48h	15 mg/kg q48h
5–9	4 mg/kg every 3–5 days	15 mg/kg every 3–5 days
< 5	3 mg/kg every 3–5 days	4 mg/kg every 3–5 days

WARNINGS/PRECAUTIONS

Hypersensitivity — Serious, acute hypersensitivity reactions, necessitating emergency measures such as the use of epinephrine, may occur during therapy; use with caution in patients with a history of allergy, especially if they are hypersensitive to penicillin or other drugs

Pseudomembranous colitis — May occur due to alteration of the normal intestinal flora and should be considered in any patient who develops diarrhea during or after therapy. Mild cases may respond to withdrawal of the drug alone. Moderate to severe cases should be managed by fluid and electrolyte replacement and protein supplementation, as needed. Oral vancomycin is the treatment of choice for severe or refractory colitis associated with the overgrowth of *Clostridium difficile*; however, other possible causes should also be considered.

Superinfection — Overgrowth of nonsusceptible organisms may occur with prolonged use; careful clinical observation is essential

ADVERSE REACTIONS

Frequent reactions (incidence ≥ 1%) are printed in *italics*

Gastrointestinal — Diarrhea

Hepatic — *Increases in liver function values (1.6%)*

Hematological — *Eosinophilia (2.9%), increase in platelet count (1.7%)*, leukopenia, neutropenia, thrombocytopenia, positive Coombs' test

Hypersensitivity — Fever, rash, pruritus, erythema, myalgia, anaphylactoid reactions

Other — *Local pain and discomfort and, with IV use, local burning and phlebitis (5.7%)*

OVERDOSAGE

Signs and symptoms — See ADVERSE REACTIONS

Treatment — Discontinue use of drug; treat symptomatically and institute supportive measures, as required

DRUG INTERACTIONS

Aminoglycosides — ↑ Risk of nephrotoxicity; carefully monitor renal function during concomitant therapy

Probenecid — ↑ Cefonicid blood level and/or toxicity

ALTERED LABORATORY VALUES

Blood/serum levels — ↑ Alkaline phosphatase ↑ SGOT ↑ SGPT ↑ GGTP ↑ LDH + Coombs' test

No clinically significant alterations in urinary values occur at therapeutic dosages

USE IN CHILDREN	USE IN PREGNANT AND NURSING WOMEN
Safety and effectiveness for use in children have not been established	Pregnancy Category B: reproduction studies in mice, rabbits, and rats given up to 40 times the usual human dose have shown no evidence of impaired fertility or harm to the fetus; however, no adequate, well-controlled studies have been done in pregnant women. Use during pregnancy only if clearly needed. Cefonicid can be given during cesarean section to prevent certain postoperative infections (see PARENTERAL DOSAGE). This drug is excreted in human milk in low concentrations; use with caution in nursing mothers.

CEPHALOSPORINS

MOXAM (moxalactam disodium) Lilly   Rx

Vials: 1 g (10 ml), 2 g (20 ml), 10 g (100 ml)

INDICATIONS

Lower respiratory tract infections, including pneumonia, caused by susceptible strains of *Streptococcus pneumoniae, Hemophilus influenzae, Klebsiella, Enterobacter, Staphylococcus aureus, Escherichia coli,* and *Proteus mirabilis*

Intraabdominal infections, including peritonitis, endometritis, and pelvic cellulitis, caused by susceptible strains of *Escherichia coli, Peptostreptococcus, Bacteroides* (including *B fragilis*), and mixed aerobic and anaerobic organisms, including *Klebsiella pneumoniae, Streptococcus agalactiae* (Group B streptococci), *Proteus mirabilis, Enterobacter, Pseudomonas aeruginosa, Peptococcus, Clostridium, Fusobacterium,* and *Eubacterium*

Bacterial septicemia caused by susceptible strains of *Staphylococcus aureus, Escherichia coli, Streptococcus pneumoniae, Klebsiella, Serratia, Pseudomonas,* and *Bacteroides fragilis*

Central nervous system infections, including meningitis and ventriculitis, caused by susceptible strains of *Escherichia coli, Klebsiella, Hemophilus influenzae,* and other Enterobacteriaceae

Skin and skin structure infections caused by susceptible strains of *Staphylococcus aureus, Streptococcus pyogenes* (Group A beta-hemolytic streptococci), *Escherichia coli, Serratia,* and mixed aerobic and anaerobic organisms, including *Proteus, Klebsiella, Enterobacter, Peptococcus, Peptostreptococcus, Bacteroides,* and *Clostridium*

Bone and joint infections caused by susceptible strains of *Staphylococcus aureus, Pseudomonas aeruginosa,* and *Serratia*

Urinary tract infections caused by susceptible strains of *Escherichia coli, Klebsiella, Enterobacter, Proteus,* and *Serratia*

PARENTERAL DOSAGE

Adult: for mild skin and skin structure infections and uncomplicated pneumonia, 500 mg IM or IV q8h; for most other mild to moderate infections, 500 mg to 2 g IM or IV q12h; for other, more serious infections, 2–4 g/day IM or IV, given in divided doses q8–12h for 5–10 days or up to 14 days; for life-threatening infections or those due to less susceptible organisms (eg, *Pseudomonas aeruginosa*), up to 4 g IM or IV q8h. The IV route may be preferable for patients with bacterial septicemia, localized parenchymal abscesses (eg, intraabdominal abscess), peritonitis, meningitis, or other severe or life-threatening infections; in such cases, 3–12 g/day may be given IV if renal function is normal. For conditions such as septicemia, 6–12 g/day may be given IV for several days, followed by a gradual reduction in dosage as clinical and laboratory findings improve.

Neonate (0–1 wk): 50 mg/kg IM or IV q12h; for serious infections, up to 200 mg/kg/day IM or IV

Neonate (1–4 wk): 50 mg/kg IM or IV q8h; for serious infections, up to 200 mg/kg/day IM or IV

Infant: 50 mg/kg IM or IV q6h; for serious infections, up to 200 mg/kg/day IM or IV

Child: 50 mg/kg IM or IV q6–8h; for serious infections, up to 200 mg/kg/day IM or IV

Adult: for mild, uncomplicated infections, 250 mg IM or IV q12h; for more difficult to treat infections, 500 mg IM or IV q12h; for serious infections, 500 mg IM or IV q8h

Neonate, infant, and child: same as pediatric dosages above

CONTRAINDICATIONS
Hypersensitivity to moxalactam

ADMINISTRATION/DOSAGE ADJUSTMENTS

Intramuscular administration ——— Dilute 1 g of moxalactam with 3 ml of Sterile Water for Injection, Bacteriostatic Water for Injection, 0.9% Sodium Chloride Injection, Bacteriostatic Sodium Chloride Injection, or 0.5% or 1% Lidocaine Hydrochloride Injection; shake well until drug is dissolved. Inject deeply into a large muscle mass, such as the upper outer quadrant of the gluteus maximus or the lateral aspect of the thigh. Do not administer doses of 2 g or more at any one site.

Intermittent intravenous administration	Dilute each gram of moxalactam with 10 ml of Sterile Water for Injection, 5% Dextrose Injection, or 0.9% Sodium Chloride Injection. Slowly inject solution directly into vein over a period of 3–5 min or administer through the tubing of an IV administration set while the patient is receiving a compatible IV solution. Alternatively, add 20 ml of Sterile Water for Injection or 50–100 ml of another compatible IV diluent to the 1- or 2-g piggyback (100-ml) vial, and infuse the resulting solution by means of a Y-type administration or volume control set after discontinuing infusion of the other solution; during administration, pay careful attention to the volume of the moxalactam solution to ensure that the proper dose is infused. Avoid solutions containing alcohol.
Continuous intravenous infusion	Dilute each gram of moxalactam with 10 ml of Sterile Water for Injection and add an appropriate amount of the resulting solution to an IV bottle of a compatible solution; avoid IV solutions containing alcohol
Prophylaxis of bleeding abnormalities	To prevent bleeding associated with hypoprothrombinemia, administer vitamin K (10 mg/wk) during therapy. To avoid bleeding related to platelet dysfunction, limit dosage to 4 g/day (if possible). Monitor bleeding time if dosage exceeds 4 g/day for more than 3 days or patient has significant renal impairment, and discontinue use if bleeding time becomes unduly prolonged.
Concomitant use of aminoglycosides	Moxalactam may be used concomitantly with an aminoglycoside antibiotic in cases of confirmed or suspected sepsis or when the causative organism of a serious infection has not been identified. Dosage is dependent upon the severity of the infection and the patient's condition. To avoid inactivating the aminoglycoside, do not mix the solution of moxalactam directly with the aminoglycoside solution; however, the two solutions may be given sequentially by intermittent IV infusion if the tubing is flushed with a compatible diluent before administration of the second solution. Monitor renal function carefully, especially if higher aminoglycoside dosages are used or therapy is prolonged.
Patients with renal impairment and life-threatening infections	Administer 1–2 g IM or IV to start, followed by up to 4 g q8h if creatinine clearance rate (CCr) > 80 ml/min, up to 3 g q8h if CCr = 50–80 ml/min, up to 2 g q8h or 3 g q12h if CCr = 25–50 ml/min, up to 1 g q8h or 1.25 g q12h if CCr = 2–25 ml/min, or up to 1 g q24h if CCr < 2 ml/min. If necessary, the CCr for males may be calculated from the serum creatinine concentration by use of the following formula: CCr = [weight (kg) × (140 − age)]/[72 × creatinine concentration]; for female patients, multiply the value obtained by 0.9.
Patients with renal impairment and less severe infections	Administer 1–2 g IM or IV to start, followed by 0.5–2 g q8–12h if creatinine clearance rate (CCr) > 80 ml/min, 0.5–1 g q8h if CCr = 50–80 ml/min, 0.25–1 g q12h if CCr = 25–50 ml/min, 0.25–0.5 g q8h if CCr = 2–25 ml/min, or 0.25–0.5 g q12h if CCr < 2 ml/min; if necessary, the CCr may be calculated from the serum creatinine concentration by use of the formula given above
Dialysis patients	The serum half-life of moxalactam during dialysis is 2–5 h; maintenance doses should be repeated following regular hemodialysis
Gram-negative meningitis in children	Administer an initial loading dose of 100 mg/kg IM or (preferably) IV prior to utilization of the dosage schedule given under PARENTERAL DOSAGE, above
Bacteriologic cultures and susceptibility tests	Obtain specimens to isolate and identify the causative organism(s); therapy may be initiated before the results of susceptibility tests become available, provided that it is adjusted, if necessary, once the results are known
Impairment of fertility	Delayed maturity of the testicular germinal epithelium, decreased testicular weight, and a reduced number of germinal cells in the leading waves of spermatogenic development have been seen in rats given daily approximately 5 times the maximum human dose during the period of initial spermatogenic development (6–40 days of age); administration in utero or for up to 6 mo at a later stage (ie, when the rats were more than 40 days of age) has produced no adverse effect on testicular development. The clinical significance of these findings is not known.

WARNINGS/PRECAUTIONS

Bleeding abnormalities	Moxalactam may cause hypoprothrombinemia, inhibition of platelet function, or, in very rare cases, immune-mediated thrombocytopenia; bleeding may result, especially in patients with hepatic or renal impairment, poor oral alimentation, or thrombocytopenia and in patients receiving heparin (> 20,000 units/day), oral anticoagulants, or other drugs that affect hemostasis (eg, aspirin). Bleeding during therapy may be related to complications of an underlying disorder; laboratory tests should be performed to rule out disseminated intravascular coagulation, which frequently occurs in patients with sepsis, malignancy, or hepatic disease. If bleeding occurs and the prothrombin time is prolonged, administer vitamin K and, if necessary, fresh frozen plasma, packed erythrocytes, and platelet concentrates; if bleeding is due to platelet dysfunction, discontinue use. For appropriate prophylactic measures, see ADMINISTRATION/DOSAGE ADJUSTMENTS.
Hypersensitivity	Prior to initiating therapy, determine whether patient has a history of hypersensitivity to moxalactam, cephalosporins, penicillins, or other drugs. Use with caution in patients with type I hypersensitivity reactions to penicillin or with other allergies, particularly to drugs. If an allergic reaction occurs, discontinue therapy; serious reactions may require use of epinephrine and other emergency measures.

Ingestion of alcohol	May result in a disulfiram-like reaction (see DRUG INTERACTIONS) due to inhibition of acetaldehyde dehydrogenase and resultant accumulation of acetaldehyde; the reaction occurs only when alcohol is ingested following administration of moxalactam and may be observed as late as 48 h after the last dose of the antibiotic
Prolonged therapy	May result in the overgrowth of nonsusceptible organisms (eg, enterococci); observe patient carefully for signs of superinfection and take appropriate measures, if indicated
Pseudomembranous colitis	May occur due to alteration of the normal intestinal flora and should be considered in any patient who develops diarrhea during or after therapy. Mild cases may respond to withdrawal of the drug alone. Moderate to severe cases should be managed by sigmoidoscopy, appropriate bacteriological studies, fluid and electrolyte replacement, and protein supplementation, as needed. Oral vancomycin is the treatment of choice for severe or refractory colitis associated with the overgrowth of *Clostridium difficile;* however, other possible causes should also be considered.
Special-risk patients	Use with caution in patients with a history of GI disease, particularly colitis

ADVERSE REACTIONS[1]
Frequent reactions (incidence ≥ 1%) are printed in *italics*

Hematological	*Bleeding associated with hypoprothrombinemia, decreased platelet function, or immune-mediated thrombocytopenia (2%;* see WARNINGS/PRECAUTIONS); *reversible neutropenia in children ≤ 3 yr of age (4.3%); eosinophilia (2.9%);* reversible leukopenia (0.7%).
Allergic	*Morbilliform eruptions (1.7%),* fever (0.6%), anaphylaxis (one case)
Gastrointestinal	*Diarrhea (1.7%),* pseudomembranous colitis; nausea and vomiting (rare)
Local	*Phlebitis (2.0%), pain at injection site (1.4%)*

OVERDOSAGE
Signs and symptoms	See ADVERSE REACTIONS
Treatment	Discontinue use; treat symptomatically and institute supportive measures, as required. Treat coagulation abnormalities promptly with vitamin K.

DRUG INTERACTIONS
Aminoglycoside antibiotics	△ Risk of nephrotoxicity
Alcohol	Nausea, vomiting, and vasomotor instability (hypotension, peripheral vasodilatation)

ALTERED LABORATORY VALUES[2]
Blood/serum values	△ BUN △ Creatinine △ SGOT △ SGPT △ Alkaline phosphatase + Coombs' test

No clinically significant alterations in urinary values occur at therapeutic dosages

---

USE IN CHILDREN

See INDICATIONS; in treating serious infections, do not exceed the recommended maximum adult dose

USE IN PREGNANT AND NURSING WOMEN

Pregnancy Category C: use during pregnancy only if the anticipated benefit of therapy justifies the potential fetal risk. Studies in mice and rats at doses up to 20 times the usual human dose have shown no evidence of impaired fertility or teratogenicity. An increased incidence of birth defects and embryotoxicity has been observed in ferrets at 10–20 times the usual human dose, but the significance of these findings is uncertain. No adequate, well-controlled studies have been done in pregnant women. It is not known whether moxalactam is excreted in human milk; use with caution in nursing mothers.

---

[1] Other reactions for which a causal relationship has not been established include pyuria and hematuria (0.4% each)
[2] Hepatic enzyme elevations have occurred in 4% of patients; a causal relationship to moxalactam was established in 10% of these cases. The changes in renal function tests were of unknown etiology.

CEPHALOSPORINS

PRECEF (ceforanide) Apothecon   Rx

Vials: 0.5, 1 g   **Piggyback vials:** 0.5, 1 g   **Pharmacy bulk vials:** 10 g

INDICATIONS

Bone and joint infections caused by susceptible strains of *Staphylococcus aureus*
Endocarditis caused by susceptible strains of *Staphylococcus aureus*
Lower respiratory tract infections caused by susceptible strains of *Staphylococcus aureus, Streptococcus pneumoniae,[1] Klebsiella pneumoniae,* and *Hemophilus influenzae*
Septicemia caused by susceptible strains of *Staphylococcus aureus, Streptococcus pneumoniae,[1]* and *Escherichia coli*
Skin and skin structure infections caused by susceptible strains of *Staphylococcus aureus, S epidermidis,* Group A and B streptococci,[1] *Escherichia coli, Proteus mirabilis,* and *Klebsiella pneumoniae*
Urinary tract infections caused by susceptible strains of *Escherichia coli, Proteus mirabilis,* and *Klebsiella pneumoniae*

PARENTERAL DOSAGE

Adult: 0.5–1 g IM or IV q12h
Child (≥ 1 yr): 20–40 mg/kg/day, given IM or IV in 2 equally divided doses q12h

PRECEF

Prevention of postoperative infection: (1) following contaminated or potentially contaminated procedures such as vaginal hysterectomy or (2) following procedures such as prosthetic arthoplasty and open-heart surgery in which the occurrence of infection would pose a serious risk

Adult: 0.5–1 g IM or IV 1 h before surgery; for prophylaxis when infection would pose a serious risk, dose may be repeated q12h for 2 days

CONTRAINDICATIONS

Hypersensitivity to cephalosporins

ADMINISTRATION/DOSAGE ADJUSTMENTS

Intramuscular administration	Add 1.7 ml of sterile or bacteriostatic water for injection, 0.9% sodium chloride injection, or bacteriostatic sodium chloride injection to a 500-mg vial or 3.2 ml to a 1-g vial (resulting concentration: 250 mg/ml); inject the solution well within the body of the muscle
Intravenous administration	The IV route may be preferable for patients with septicemia or other severe or life-threatening infections. For IV injection, add at least 5 ml of the specified diluent to a 500-mg vial or at least 10 ml to a 1-g vial; slowly administer the dose over a period of 3–5 min. For IV infusion with a regular or piggyback vial, prepare a solution with a final concentration of not less than 10 mg/ml; use one of the following as a diluent: sterile water for injection USP, 5% or 10% dextrose injection USP, 0.9% sodium chloride injection USP, lactated Ringer's injection USP, 5% dextrose injection and lactated Ringer's injection, or 5% dextrose injection and 0.2% or 0.45% sodium chloride injection USP.
Patients with renal impairment	Administer each dose q24h if creatinine clearance (Ccr) = 20–59 ml/min or q48h if Ccr = 5–19 ml/min; if Ccr < 5 ml/min, give each dose q48–72h and monitor serum ceforanide level. The Ccr of patients with stable renal function can be estimated from serum creatinine levels if a measured value cannot be obtained; for adult men, use the following formula: (weight [kg]) (140 − age [yr])/(72) (serum creatinine level [mg/dl]); for adult women, multiply this quotient by 0.85.
Duration of therapy	After symptoms have disappeared or evidence of bacterial eradication has been obtained, continue treatment for at least 48–72 h; to avoid rheumatic fever and glomerulonephritis, treat Group A beta-hemolytic streptococcal infections for at least 10 days

WARNINGS/PRECAUTIONS

Hypersensitivity	Serious, acute hypersensitivity reactions, necessitating emergency measures such as the use of epinephrine, may occur during therapy. Use with caution in patients with a history of allergy, especially if they are hypersensitive to penicillin or other drugs; discontinue administration if an allergic reaction to ceforanide occurs.
Pseudomembranous colitis	May occur due to alteration of the normal intestinal flora and should be considered in any patient who develops diarrhea during or after therapy; use with caution in patients with a history of GI disease, particularly colitis. Mild cases may respond to withdrawal of the drug alone. Moderate to severe cases should be managed by fluid and electrolyte replacement and protein supplementation, as needed. Oral vancomycin is the treatment of choice for severe or refractory colitis associated with the overgrowth of *Clostridium difficile;* however, other possible causes should also be considered.
Renal function abnormalities	Transient elevations of serum creatinine levels have been seen in approximately 11% of patients and of BUN levels in 2% of patients; monitor renal function, especially when using this drug in seriously ill patients at the maximum dosage (2 g/day)
Superinfection	Overgrowth of nonsusceptible organisms may occur with prolonged use; repeated evaluation of the patient's condition is essential
Effect on fertility	No evidence of impaired fertility or reproductive performance has been seen in rats given 50 times the usual human dose

ADVERSE REACTIONS

Frequent reactions (incidence ≥ 1%) are printed in *italics*

Gastrointestinal	Diarrhea, nausea, vomiting, pseudomembranous colitis
Hepatic	*Increase in level of SGPT (11.1%), SGOT (6.3%), and alkaline phosphatase (3.7%)*
Renal	*Increase in level of serum creatinine (11.1%) and BUN (2%)*
Central nervous system	Lethargy, confusion, headache
Hematological	*Thrombocytosis (20%), positive Coombs' test (2.5%)*
Hypersensitivity	*Eosinophilia (8.3%), rash (2.2%),* pruritus
Other	*Increase in CPK level following IM use (33%),* local pain and swelling, phlebitis following IV use, hypotension

OVERDOSAGE

Signs and symptoms	See ADVERSE REACTIONS
Treatment	Discontinue use of drug; treat symptomatically and institute supportive measures, as needed

PRECEF ■ ROCEPHIN

DRUG INTERACTIONS

Potent diuretics, aminoglycosides —— △ Risk of nephrotoxicity; exercise caution if ceforanide and a potent diuretic are used concomitantly

ALTERED LABORATORY VALUES

Blood/serum values —— △ Alkaline phosphatase   △ SGOT   △ SGPT   △ Creatinine   △ BUN   △ CPK (with IM use)   + Coombs' test

No clinically significant alterations in urinary values occur at therapeutic dosages

USE IN CHILDREN

See INDICATIONS and PARENTERAL DOSAGE. Safety and effectiveness for use in infants under 1 yr of age have not been established; evaluate risks and benefits before administering this drug to such patients

USE IN PREGNANT AND NURSING WOMEN

Pregnancy Category B: reproduction studies in mice and rats given up to 25 times the human dose have shown no evidence of teratogenicity. An increase in resorptions and a decrease in the number of viable young have been seen in rats given ceforanide SC up to 50 times the usual human dose perinatally; both reactions may have resulted from drug-induced effects in the mother. No adequate, well-controlled studies have been done in pregnant women. Use during pregnancy only if clearly needed. Safety and effectiveness for use during labor and delivery have not been established. It is not known whether ceforanide is excreted in human milk; use with caution in nursing mothers.

[1] Penicillin G is considered to be the drug of choice for streptococcal infections

---

CEPHALOSPORINS

ROCEPHIN (ceftriaxone sodium) Roche   Rx

Vials: 0.25, 0.5, 1, 2 g   **Piggyback bottles:** 1, 2 g   **Pharmacy bulk containers:** 10 g

INDICATIONS

Lower respiratory tract infections caused by susceptible strains of *Streptococcus pneumoniae* and other streptococci (except enterococci), *Staphylococcus aureus*, *Hemophilus influenzae*, *H parainfluenzae*, *Klebsiella* (including *K pneumoniae*), *Escherichia coli*, *Enterobacter aerogenes*, *Proteus mirabilis*, and *Serratia marcescens*
Skin and skin structure infections caused by susceptible strains of *Staphylococcus aureus*, *S epidermidis*, *Streptococcus* (except enterococci), *Enterobacter cloacae*, *Klebsiella* (including *K pneumoniae*), *Proteus mirabilis*, and *Pseudomonas aeruginosa*
Urinary tract infections caused by susceptible strains of *Escherichia coli*, *Proteus mirabilis*, *P vulgaris*, *Morganella morganii*, and *Klebsiella* (including *K pneumoniae*)
Pelvic inflammatory disease and uncomplicated gonorrhea caused by susceptible strains of *Neisseria gonorrhoeae*
Septicemia caused by susceptible strains of *Staphylococcus aureus*, *Streptococcus pneumoniae*, *Escherichia coli*, *Hemophilus influenzae*, and *Klebsiella pneumoniae*
Bone and joint infections caused by susceptible strains of *Staphylococcus aureus*, *Streptococcus pneumoniae* and other streptococci (except enterococci), *Escherichia coli*, *Proteus mirabilis*, *Klebsiella pneumoniae*, and *Enterobacter*
Intra-abdominal infections caused by susceptible strains of *Escherichia coli* and *Klebsiella pneumoniae*
Meningitis caused by susceptible strains of *Hemophilus influenzae*, *Neisseria meningitidis*, and *Streptococcus pneumoniae*[1]

Prevention of postoperative infection in patients undergoing coronary artery bypass surgery

PARENTERAL DOSAGE

Adult: for meningitis, 100 mg/kg/day, up to 4 g/day, given IM or IV in 2 divided doses q12h (with or without a loading dose of 75 mg/kg); for gonorrhea, 250 mg, given in a single IM dose; for all other infections, 1–4 g/day, given IM or IV either once daily or in 2 equally divided doses (usual dosage: 1–2 g/day)
Neonate, infant, and child: for meningitis, same as adult; for other serious infections, 50–75 mg/kg/day, up to 2 g/day, given IM or IV in 2 divided doses q12h

Adult: 1 g, given in a single IM or IV dose ½ to 2 h before surgery

CONTRAINDICATIONS

Hypersensitivity to cephalosporins

ADMINISTRATION/DOSAGE ADJUSTMENTS

Intramuscular administration —— Reconstitute solution with sterile water for injection, 0.9% sodium chloride injection, 5% dextrose injection, 1% lidocaine injection (without epinephrine), or bacteriostatic water for injection with 0.9% benzyl alcohol; combine diluent and powder in ratio of 0.9 ml/0.25 g. If necessary, the reconstituted solution can be diluted with one of the above preparations. Before IM administration, aspirate in order to avoid inadvertent intravascular injection. The solution should be injected well within the body of a relatively large muscle.

ROCEPHIN

Intravenous administration	Use as a diluent sterile water for injection, 0.9% sodium chloride injection, 5% or 10% dextrose injection, or 5% dextrose and 0.45% or 0.9% sodium chloride injection. If a vial is used, combine diluent and powder in a ratio of 2.4 ml/0.25 g, then dilute the solution to a final concentration of 10–40 mg/ml (if desired, a lower concentration may be used). If a piggyback bottle is used, combine in a ratio of 10 ml/g, then dilute to a final volume of 50 or 100 ml. If a pharmacy bulk container is used, reconstitute with 95 ml of diluent, then withdraw the required dose and dilute to the desired concentration. Do not mix ceftriaxone with solutions containing other antibiotics or combine with diluents other than those listed above. Administer IV solutions by intermittent infusion.
Duration of therapy	Treatment should generally be continued for at least 2 days after signs and symptoms of infection have disappeared; duration of therapy is usually 4–14 days, but may be longer if the infection is complicated. Infections caused by Group A beta-hemolytic streptococci should be treated for at least 10 days.
Patients with renal impairment	No dosage adjustment is generally required for patients with renal impairment; nevertheless, periodically check the serum drug level, particularly in patients with severe renal impairment, and, if necessary, reduce dosage. *Closely* monitor the serum level if the patient has both hepatic and significant renal impairment and is given more than 2 g/day.

WARNINGS/PRECAUTIONS

Hypersensitivity	Serious, acute hypersensitivity reactions, necessitating emergency measures such as the use of epinephrine, may occur during therapy; use with caution in patients with a history of allergy, especially if they are hypersensitive to penicillin or other drugs
Pseudomembranous colitis	May occur due to alteration of the normal intestinal flora and should be considered in any patient who develops diarrhea during or after therapy; use with caution in patients with a history of GI disease, particularly colitis. Mild cases may respond to withdrawal of the drug alone. Moderate to severe cases should be managed by fluid and electrolyte replacement and protein supplementation, as needed. Oral vancomycin is the treatment of choice for severe or refractory colitis associated with the overgrowth of *Clostridium difficile;* however, other possible causes should also be considered.
Renal function abnormalities	Transient elevations of BUN and serum creatinine levels have occurred at the recommended dosage
Vitamin K deficiency	Ceftriaxone may precipitate vitamin K deficiency in susceptible patients, such as those with chronic hepatic disease or malnutrition. It may be necessary to monitor prothrombin time in these patients and, if this time is prolonged, to administer 10 mg of vitamin K weekly.
Superinfection	Overgrowth of nonsusceptible organisms may occur with prolonged use; careful observation is essential
Mutagenicity	No evidence of mutagenicity has been shown in human lymphocyte cultures or the Ames and micronucleus tests
Effect on fertility	No impairment of fertility has been seen in rats given up to 586 mg/kg/day IV

ADVERSE REACTIONS

Frequent reactions (incidence ≥ 1%) are printed in *italics*

Gastrointestinal	*Diarrhea (2.7%)*, nausea, vomiting, dysgeusia; abdominal pain, colitis, flatulence, and dyspepsia (rare)
Hepatic	*Increase in SGPT level (3.3%) and SGOT level (3.1%)*, elevated serum alkaline phosphatase and bilirubin levels; jaundice (rare)
Renal	*Elevated BUN level (1.2%)*, elevated serum creatinine level, cylindruria
Hematological	*Eosinophilia (6%), thrombocytosis (5.1%), leukopenia (2.1%)*, anemia, neutropenia, lymphopenia, thrombocytopenia, increased prothrombin time; leukocytosis, lymphocytosis, monocytosis, basophilia, and decreased prothrombin time (rare)
Central nervous system	Headache, dizziness
Genitourinary	Moniliasis, vaginitis; hematuria (rare)
Hypersensitivity	*Rash (1.7%)*, pruritus, fever, chills; serum sickness (rare)
Other	*Pain, induration, and tenderness at injection site (1%)*, phlebitis (with IV use), diaphoresis, flushing; glycosuria, bronchospasm, palpitations, and epistaxis (rare)

OVERDOSAGE

Signs and symptoms	See ADVERSE REACTIONS
Treatment	Treat symptomatically and institute supportive measures, as needed

DRUG INTERACTIONS

No clinically significant drug interactions have been identified

ALTERED LABORATORY VALUES

Blood/serum values	⇧ BUN ⇧ Creatinine ⇧ SGPT ⇧ SGOT ⇧ Alkaline phosphatase ⇧ Bilirubin

No clinically significant alterations in urinary values generally occur at therapeutic dosages

USE IN CHILDREN

See INDICATIONS and PARENTERAL DOSAGE

USE IN PREGNANT AND NURSING WOMEN

Pregnancy Category B: no evidence of embryotoxicity or teratogenicity has been seen in rats and mice given up to 20 times the usual human dose or in primates given 3 times the human dose; administration of up to 586 mg/kg/day to rats during pregnancy and nursing has not resulted in any adverse effects in their offspring. No adequate, well-controlled studies have been done in pregnant women; therefore, use during pregnancy only if clearly needed. Low concentrations of ceftriaxone are excreted in human milk; use with caution in nursing mothers.

[1] In a limited number of cases, ceftriaxone has been effective in the treatment of meningitis and shunt infections caused by susceptible strains of *Staphylococcus epidermidis* and *Escherichia coli*

CEPHALOSPORINS

TAZICEF (ceftazidime) Smith Kline & French   Rx

Vials: 1, 2 g   **Piggyback vials:** 1, 2 g

INDICATIONS

Lower respiratory tract infections, including pneumonia, caused by susceptible strains of *Pseudomonas* (including *P aeruginosa*), *Hemophilus influenzae*, *Klebsiella*, *Enterobacter*, *Proteus mirabilis*, *Escherichia coli*, *Serratia*, *Citrobacter*, *Streptococcus pneumoniae*, and methicillin-susceptible *Staphylococcus aureus*
Skin and skin structure infections caused by susceptible strains of *Pseudomonas aeruginosa*, *Klebsiella*, *Escherichia coli*, *Proteus* (including *P mirabilis*), *Enterobacter*, *Serratia*, methicillin-susceptible *Staphylococcus aureus*, and *Streptococcus pyogenes*
Urinary tract infections caused by susceptible strains of *Pseudomonas aeruginosa*, *Enterobacter*, *Proteus* (including *P mirabilis*), *Klebsiella*, and *Escherichia coli*
Septicemia caused by susceptible strains of *Pseudomonas aeruginosa*, *Klebsiella*, *Hemophilus influenzae*, *Escherichia coli*, *Serratia*, *Streptococcus pneumoniae*, and methicillin-susceptible *Staphylococcus aureus*
Bone and joint infections caused by susceptible strains of *Pseudomonas aeruginosa*, *Klebsiella*, *Enterobacter*, and methicillin-susceptible *Staphylococcus aureus*
Gynecological infections, including endometritis and pelvic cellulitis, caused by susceptible strains of *Escherichia coli*
Intraabdominal infections, including peritonitis, caused by susceptible strains of *Escherichia coli*, *Klebsiella*, methicillin-susceptible *Staphylococcus aureus*, and *Bacteroides*
Central nervous system infections, including meningitis, caused by susceptible strains of *Hemophilus influenzae*, *Neisseria meningitidis*, *Pseudomonas aeruginosa*, and *Streptococcus pneumoniae*

PARENTERAL DOSAGE

Adult: generally, 1 g IV or IM q8h or q12h; for uncomplicated urinary tract infections, 250 mg IV or IM q12h; for complicated urinary tract infections, 500 mg IV or IM q8–12h; for uncomplicated pneumonia and mild skin and skin structure infections, 0.5–1 g IV or IM q8h; for bone and joint infections, 2 g IV q12h; for meningitis, serious gynecological and intraabdominal infections, and very severe life-threatening infections (especially in immunocompromised patients), 2 g IV q8h; for pseudomonal lung infections in patients with cystic fibrosis, 30–50 mg/kg IV q8h, up to 6 g/day
Neonate (0–4 wk): 30 mg/kg IV q12h
Infant and child (1 mo to 12 yr): 30–50 mg/kg IV q8h, up to 6 g/day; the higher dose should be reserved for children who have meningitis, cystic fibrosis, or an immunocompromised condition

CONTRAINDICATIONS

Hypersensitivity to ceftazidime or other cephalosporins

ADMINISTRATION/DOSAGE ADJUSTMENTS

Preparation of solution — All containers are supplied, under reduced pressure, with 118 mg of sodium carbonate per gram of ceftazidime; when the drug is dissolved, carbon dioxide is released and pressure in the container increases. To reconstitute the solution in a piggyback vial, add 10 ml of sodium chloride injection to the vial and shake well; after product has dissolved, insert a vent needle to release pressure, add 90 ml of sodium chloride injection, and then remove the needle and shake well. To prepare a solution from a regular vial for IV infusion, add 10 ml of sterile water for injection to a regular 1- or 2-g vial, shake well, and then dilute resulting solution in 50–100 ml of a compatible diluent (see below). For IM or IV injection, add 3 ml of sterile water for injection to a regular 1-g vial and shake well; immediately before injection, express any accumulated gas from the syringe. Ceftazidime is compatible with the following diluents: sterile water for injection, 0.9% sodium chloride injection, Ringer's and lactated Ringer's injection USP, 5% and 10% dextrose injection, and 5% dextrose in 0.225%, 0.45%, and 0.9% sodium chloride injection; do not mix ceftazidime with aminoglycoside solutions or sodium bicarbonate injection.

Intramuscular administration — Inject solution into a large muscle mass such as the upper outer quadrant of the gluteus maximus or the lateral part of the thigh

TAZICEF

Intravenous administration	The IV route is preferable for treating severe or life-threatening infections such as septicemia, meningitis, and peritonitis as well as for treating less severe infections in patients at increased risk because of debilitating conditions such as malnutrition, trauma, surgery, diabetes, heart failure, or malignancy (especially when shock is present or impending). For direct IV administration, inject the dose into a vein over a period of 3–5 min or, alternatively, give through the tubing of an administration set while a compatible primary IV fluid is being administered. For IV infusion, use a piggyback vial or a solution prepared from a regular vial. During intermittent infusion with a Y-type set, administration of the primary solution should be discontinued.
Parents with renal impairment	For patients whose creatinine clearance (Ccr) is 50 ml/min or less, but who are not undergoing dialysis, give an initial loading dose of 1 g and then either 1 g q12h if Ccr = 31–50 ml/min, 1 g q24h if Ccr = 16–30 ml/min, 0.5 g q24 h if Ccr = 6–15 ml/min, or 0.5 g q48h if Ccr < 5 ml/min; to treat a severe infection that under normal circumstances would necessitate 6 g/day, the maintenance dose can be increased by 50% or the dosing interval can be reduced to an appropriate length of time. When determined on the basis of a urine sample and serum creatinine level, the Ccr should be adjusted for body surface area or lean body mass. If a urine sample cannot be obtained, the Ccr can be estimated from the serum creatinine level, provided renal function is stable. For adult men, use the following formula: (weight [kg]) (140−age [yr])/(72)(serum creatinine level [mg/dl]); for adult women, multiply this quotient by 0.85. To treat infections in patients undergoing peritoneal dialysis, administer 1 g to start and then 500 mg q24h; the drug can be added to the dialysis fluid at a concentration of 125 mg/liter. For patients undergoing hemodialysis, give 1 g at the start of therapy and repeat after each dialysis treatment.
Pseudomonal lung infections	In patients with chronic respiratory disease and cystic fibrosis, treatment of pseudomonal lung infections produces clinical improvement, but cannot be expected to result in a bacteriological cure
Duration of therapy	Treatment generally should be continued for 2 days after signs and symptoms have disappeared; if an infection is complicated, longer treatment may be necessary
Concomitant therapy	For patients with severe or life-threatening infections or immunocompromised conditions, ceftazidime can be given in combination with other antibiotics such as vancomycin, clindamycin, or aminoglycosides (see also DRUG INTERACTIONS)

WARNINGS/PRECAUTIONS

Hypersensitivity	Serious acute hypersensitivity reactions necessitating emergency measures (such as the use of epinephrine) may occur during therapy; use with caution in patients with a history of allergy, especially if they are hypersensitive to penicillin or other drugs. If an allergic reaction occurs, discontinue administration.
Pseudomembranous colitis	May occur due to alteration of the normal intestinal flora and should be considered in any patient who develops diarrhea during or after therapy; use with caution in patients with a history of GI disease, particularly colitis. Mild cases may respond to withdrawal of the drug alone. Moderate to severe cases should be managed by fluid and electrolyte replacement and protein supplementation, as needed. Oral vancomycin is the treatment of choice for severe or refractory colitis associated with the overgrowth of *Clostridium difficile;* however, other possible causes should also be considered.
Superinfection	Overgrowth of nonsusceptible organisms may occur with prolonged use; repeated evaluation of patient's condition is essential
Carcinogenicity, mutagenicity	Long-term animal studies to evaluate the carcinogenic potential of ceftazidime have not been done; no evidence of mutagenicity has been seen in the Ames test or the mouse micronucleus assay

ADVERSE REACTIONS

Frequent reactions (incidence ≥ 1%) are printed in *italics*

Gastrointestinal	*Diarrhea (1.3%),* nausea, vomiting, abdominal pain
Hematological	*Eosinophilia (7.7%), positive Coombs' test (4.3%), thrombocytosis (2.2%);* leukopenia, neutropenia, thrombocytopenia, and lymphocytosis (very rare)
Hepatic	*Slight increase in SGOT (6.2%), SGPT (6.6%), LDH (5.5%), and alkaline phosphatase (4.3%)*
Renal	Increase in BUN, serum urea, and serum creatinine
Central nervous system	Headache, dizziness, paresthesia
Hypersensitivity	*Pruritus, rash, and fever (2%),* immediate-type hypersensitivity
Local	*Phlebitis and inflammation at injection site (1.4%)*
Other	Candidiasis, vaginitis

OVERDOSAGE

Signs and symptoms	See ADVERSE REACTIONS
Treatment	Treat symptomatically and institute supportive measures, as needed

DRUG INTERACTIONS

Aminoglycosides, potent diuretics (eg, furosemide)	⇧ Risk of nephrotoxicity; carefully monitor renal function when an aminoglycoside is given in combination with ceftazidime, especially when therapy is prolonged or a higher dosage of an aminoglycoside is used

| Aminoglycosides | Physical incompatibility; do not mix together |

ALTERED LABORATORY VALUES

Blood/serum values — ⇧ SGOT ⇧ SGPT ⇧ LDH ⇧ Alkaline phosphatase ⇧ BUN ⇧ Urea ⇧ Creatinine + Coombs' test

No clinically significant alterations in urinary values occur at therapeutic dosages

USE IN CHILDREN

See INDICATIONS and PARENTERAL DOSAGE

USE IN PREGNANT AND NURSING WOMEN

Pregnancy Category B: reproduction studies in mice and rats given up to 40 times the human dose have shown no evidence of impaired fertility or harm to the fetus; however, no adequate, well-controlled studies have been done in pregnant women. Use during pregnancy only if clearly needed. Ceftazidime is excreted in human milk; the resulting concentration is low. Use with caution in nursing mothers.

CEPHALOSPORINS

TAZIDIME (ceftazidime) Lilly   Rx

Vials: 0.5 g (10 ml), 1 g (20 ml), 2 g (50 ml) **Piggyback vials:** 1, 2 g (100 ml) **Pharmacy bulk vials:** 6 g (100 ml) **Plastic containers:** 1, 2 g **Add-Vantage vials:** 1, 2 g

INDICATIONS

Lower respiratory tract infections, including pneumonia, caused by susceptible strains of *Pseudomonas* (including *P aeruginosa*), *Hemophilus influenzae, Klebsiella, Enterobacter, Proteus mirabilis, Escherichia coli, Serratia, Citrobacter, Streptococcus pneumoniae,* and methicillin-susceptible *Staphylococcus aureus*

Skin and skin structure infections caused by susceptible strains of *Pseudomonas aeruginosa, Klebsiella, Escherichia coli, Proteus* (including *P mirabilis*), *Enterobacter, Serratia,* methicillin-susceptible *Staphylococcus aureus,* and *Streptococcus pyogenes*

Urinary tract infections caused by susceptible strains of *Pseudomonas aeruginosa, Enterobacter, Proteus* (including *P mirabilis*), *Klebsiella,* and *Escherichia coli*

Septicemia caused by susceptible strains of *Pseudomonas aeruginosa, Klebsiella, Hemophilus influenzae, Escherichia coli, Serratia, Streptococcus pneumoniae,* and methicillin-susceptible *Staphylococcus aureus*

Bone and joint infections caused by susceptible strains of *Pseudomonas aeruginosa, Klebsiella, Enterobacter,* and methicillin-susceptible *Staphylococcus aureus*

Gynecological infections, including endometritis and pelvic cellulitis, caused by susceptible strains of *Escherichia coli*

Intraabdominal infections, including peritonitis, caused by susceptible strains of *Escherichia coli, Klebsiella,* methicillin-susceptible *Staphylococcus aureus,* and *Bacteroides*

Central nervous system infections, including meningitis, caused by susceptible strains of *Hemophilus influenzae, Neisseria meningitidis, Pseudomonas aeruginosa,* and *Streptococcus pneumoniae*

PARENTERAL DOSAGE

Adult: generally, 1 g IV or IM q8h or q12h; for uncomplicated urinary tract infections, 250 mg IV or IM q12h; for complicated urinary tract infections, 500 mg IV or IM q8–12h; for uncomplicated pneumonia and mild skin and skin structure infections, 0.5–1 g IV or IM q8h; for bone and joint infections, 2 g IV q12h; for meningitis, serious gynecological and intraabdominal infections, and very severe life-threatening infections (especially in immunocompromised patients), 2 g IV q8h; for pseudomonal lung infections in patients with cystic fibrosis, 30–50 mg/kg IV q8h, up to 6 g/day

Neonate (0–4 wk): 30 mg/kg IV q12h

Infant and child (1 mo to 12 yr): 30–50 mg/kg IV q8h, up to 6 g/day; the higher dose should be reserved for children who have meningitis, cystic fibrosis, or an immunocompromised condition

CONTRAINDICATIONS

Hypersensitivity to ceftazidime or other cephalosporins

ADMINISTRATION/DOSAGE ADJUSTMENTS

Preparation of solution — All containers are supplied, under reduced pressure, with 118 mg of sodium carbonate per gram of ceftazidime; when the drug is dissolved, carbon dioxide is released and pressure in the container increases. To reconstitute the solution in a piggyback vial, add 10 ml of a compatible diluent to the vial and shake well; after product has dissolved, insert a vent needle to release pressure, add 40 or 90 ml of diluent, and then remove the vent and syringe needles. To reconstitute solution in a pharmacy bulk vial, add 26 ml of a compatible diluent (for a concentration of approximately 200 mg/ml) or 56 ml of diluent (for a concentration of approximately 100 mg/ml) and then gently agitate vial; after the product has dissolved, insert a vent needle for 1–2 min to allow gas to escape. Immediately before administering solutions prepared in piggyback or pharmacy vials, vent gas from the vials, especially when the solutions have been stored. To prepare a solution from a regular vial for IV infusion, add 5 ml of sterile water for injection to a 500-mg vial, 5 or 10 ml to a 1-g vial, or 10 ml to a 2-g vial and then withdraw an appropriate quantity of the solution and dilute in a compatible diluent. When preparing solutions in the Add-Vantage vials, use Add-Vantage bags containing 0.9% sodium chloride injection or 5% dextrose injection. For IV injection, add 5 ml of sterile water for injection to a regular 500-mg vial, 5 or 10 ml to a regular 1-g vial, or 10 ml to a regular 2-g vial; for IM injection, reconstitute with sterile or bacteriostatic water for injection or 0.5% or 1% lidocaine hydrochloride injection, adding 1.5 ml to the 500-mg vial or 3 ml to the 1-g vial. Before IM or IV injection, express any accumulated gas from the syringe. Ceftazidime is compatible with the following IV diluents: sterile water for injection, 0.9% sodium chloride injection, M/6 sodium lactate injection, Ringer's and lactated Ringer's injection USP, 5% and 10% dextrose injection, 5% dextrose in 0.225%, 0.45%, and 0.9% sodium chloride injection, 10% invert sugar in water for injection, and Normosol-M in 5% dextrose injection; do not mix ceftazidime with aminoglycoside solutions or sodium bicarbonate injection.

TAZIDIME

Intramuscular administration	Inject solution into a large muscle mass such as the upper outer quadrant of the gluteus maximus or the lateral part of the thigh
Intravenous administration	The IV route is preferable for treating severe or life-threatening infections such as septicemia, meningitis, and peritonitis as well as for treating less severe infections in patients at increased risk because of debilitating conditions such as malnutrition, trauma, surgery, diabetes, heart failure, or malignancy (especially when shock is present or impending). For direct IV administration, inject the dose into a vein over a period of 3–5 min or, alternatively, give through the tubing of an administration set while a compatible primary IV fluid is being administered. For IV infusion, use a plastic container, a piggyback or Add-Vantage vial, or a solution prepared from a regular vial. During intermittent infusion with a Y-type set, administration of the primary solution should be discontinued.
Patients with renal impairment	For patients whose creatinine clearance (Ccr) is 50 ml/min or less, but who are not undergoing dialysis, give an initial loading dose of 1 g and then either 1 g q12h if Ccr = 31–50 ml/min, 1 g q24h if Ccr = 16–30 ml/min, 0.5 g q24h if Ccr = 6–15 ml/min, or 0.5 g q48h if Ccr < 5 ml/min; to treat a severe infection that under normal circumstances would necessitate 6 g/day, the maintenance dose can be increased by 50% or the dosing interval can be reduced to an appropriate length of time. When determined on the basis of a urine sample and serum creatinine level, the Ccr should be adjusted for body surface area or lean body mass. If a urine sample cannot be obtained, the Ccr can be estimated from the serum creatinine level, provided renal function is stable. For adult men, use the following formula: (weight [kg])(140 − age [yr])/(72)(serum creatinine level [mg/dl]); for adult women, multiply this quotient by 0.85. To treat infections in patients undergoing peritoneal dialysis, administer 1 g to start and then 500 mg q24h; the drug can be added to the dialysis fluid at a concentration of 125 mg/liter. For patients undergoing hemodialysis, give 1 g at the start of therapy and repeat after each dialysis treatment.
Pseudomonal lung infections	In patients with chronic respiratory disease and cystic fibrosis, treatment of pseudomonal lung infections produces clinical improvement, but cannot be expected to result in a bacteriological cure
Duration of therapy	Treatment generally should be continued for 2 days after signs and symptoms have disappeared; if an infection is complicated, longer treatment may be necessary
Concomitant therapy	For patients with severe or life-threatening infections or immunocompromised conditions, ceftazidime can be given in combination with other antibiotics such as vancomycin, clindamycin, or aminoglycosides (see also DRUG INTERACTIONS)

WARNINGS/PRECAUTIONS

Hypersensitivity	Serious acute hypersensitivity reactions necessitating emergency measures (such as the use of epinephrine) may occur during therapy; use with caution in patients with a history of allergy, especially if they are hypersensitive to penicillin or other drugs. If an allergic reaction occurs, discontinue administration.
Pseudomembranous colitis	May occur due to alteration of the normal intestinal flora and should be considered in any patient who develops diarrhea during or after therapy; use with caution in patients with a history of GI disease, particularly colitis. Mild cases may respond to withdrawal of the drug alone. Moderate to severe cases should be managed by fluid and electrolyte replacement and protein supplementation, as needed. Oral vancomycin is the treatment of choice for severe or refractory colitis associated with the overgrowth of *Clostridium difficile*; however, other possible causes should be ruled out.
Seizures	Administration of inappropriately large doses may cause seizures, especially in patients with renal impairment. Reduce dosage when renal function is impaired (see ADMINISTRATION/DOSAGE ADJUSTMENTS). If seizures occur during therapy, promptly discontinue use and, if necessary, administer anticonvulsants.
Superinfection	Overgrowth of nonsusceptible organisms may occur with prolonged use; repeated evaluation of patient's condition is essential
Carcinogenicity, mutagenicity	Long-term animal studies to evaluate the carcinogenic potential of ceftazidime have not been done; no evidence of mutagenicity has been seen in the Ames test or the mouse micronucleus assay

ADVERSE REACTIONS

	Frequent reactions (incidence ≥ 1%) are printed in *italics*
Gastrointestinal	*Diarrhea (1.3%)*, nausea, vomiting, abdominal pain
Hematological	*Eosinophilia (7.7%), positive Coombs' test (4.3%), thrombocytosis (2.2%)*; leukopenia, neutropenia, thrombocytopenia, and lymphocytosis (very rare)
Hepatic	*Slight increase in SGOT (6.2%), SGPT (6.6%), LDH (5.5%), and alkaline phosphatase (4.3%)*
Renal	Increase in BUN, serum urea, and serum creatinine
Central nervous system	Headache, dizziness, paresthesia
Hypersensitivity	*Pruritus, rash, and fever (2%)*, immediate-type hypersensitivity
Local	*Phlebitis and inflammation at injection site (1.4%)*

TAZIDIME ■ ULTRACEF

Other —— Candidiasis, vaginitis

OVERDOSAGE

Signs and symptoms	Seizures
Treatment	Promptly discontinue use; administer anticonvulsants if necessary. For an overwhelming overdose, hemodialysis may be considered.

DRUG INTERACTIONS

Aminoglycosides, potent diuretics (eg, furosemide)	⌂ Risk of nephrotoxicity; carefully monitor renal function when an aminoglycoside is given in combination with ceftazidime, especially when therapy is prolonged or a higher dosage of an aminoglycoside is used
Aminoglycosides	Physical incompatibility; do not mix together

ALTERED LABORATORY VALUES

Blood/serum values	⌂ SGOT ⌂ SGPT ⌂ LDH ⌂ Alkaline phosphatase ⌂ BUN ⌂ Urea ⌂ Creatinine + Coombs' test

No clinically significant alterations in urinary values occur at therapeutic dosages

USE IN CHILDREN
See INDICATIONS and PARENTERAL DOSAGE

USE IN PREGNANT AND NURSING WOMEN
Pregnancy Category B: reproduction studies in mice and rats given up to 40 times the human dose have shown no evidence of impaired fertility or harm to the fetus; however, no adequate, well-controlled studies have been done in pregnant women. Use during pregnancy only if clearly needed. Ceftazidime is excreted in human milk; the resulting concentration is low. Use with caution in nursing mothers.

CEPHALOSPORINS

ULTRACEF (cefadroxil) Bristol   Rx

Capsules: cefadroxil monohydrate equivalent to 500 mg cefadroxil   **Tablets:** cefadroxil monohydrate equivalent to 1 g cefadroxil
Suspension (per 5 ml): cefadroxil monohydrate equivalent to 125 or 250 mg cefadroxil after reconstitution

INDICATIONS / ORAL DOSAGE

Urinary tract infections caused by susceptible strains of *Escherichia coli, Proteus mirabilis,* and *Klebsiella*	**Adult:** for uncomplicated lower urinary tract infections (cystitis), 1–2 g/day in a single daily dose or divided (bid); for all other urinary tract infections: 1 g bid **Infant and child:** 30 mg/kg/day in divided doses q12h
Skin and skin structure infections caused by susceptible strains of staphylococci and/or streptococci	**Adult:** 1 g/day in a single daily dose or divided (bid) **Infant and child:** 30 mg/kg/day in divided doses q12h
Pharyngitis and tonsillitis caused by Group A beta-hemolytic streptococci	**Adult:** 1 g/day in a single daily dose or divided (bid) for 10 days **Infant and child:** 30 mg/kg/day in a single daily dose or divided (bid) for 10 days

CONTRAINDICATIONS

Hypersensitivity to cephalosporins

ADMINISTRATION/DOSAGE ADJUSTMENTS

Timing of administration	Cefadroxil may be administered without regard to meals; however, administration with food may help diminish possible GI complaints
Culture and susceptibility tests	Should be initiated prior to and during therapy
Patients with renal impairment	Administer 1 g to start, followed by 500 mg q12h when creatinine clearance rate (CCr) = 25–50 ml/min; 500 mg q24h when CCr = 10–25 ml/min; or 500 mg q36h when CCr = 0–10 ml/min

WARNINGS/PRECAUTIONS

Cross-allergenicity	Use with caution in penicillin-allergic patients
Hypersensitivity	Serious anaphylactic reactions may occur, most likely in patients with a history of allergy, necessitating administration of epinephrine or pressor amines, antihistamines, or corticosteroids

ULTRACEF ■ VELOSEF

Pseudomembranous colitis	May occur due to alteration of the normal intestinal flora and should be considered in any patient who develops diarrhea during or after therapy. Mild cases may respond to withdrawal of the drug alone. Moderate to severe cases should be managed by fluid and electrolyte replacement and protein supplementation, as needed. Oral vancomycin is the treatment of choice for severe or refractory colitis associated with the overgrowth of *Clostridium difficile;* however, other possible causes should also be considered.
Superinfection	Overgrowth of nonsusceptible organisms may occur with prolonged use; careful clinical observation is essential
Special-risk patients	Patients with markedly impaired renal function (CCr < 50 ml/min) should be carefully monitored prior to and during therapy (see ADMINISTRATION/DOSAGE ADJUSTMENTS); use with caution in patients with a history of GI disease, particularly colitis

ADVERSE REACTIONS

Gastrointestinal	Diarrhea, pseudomembranous colitis; nausea and vomiting (rare)
Hypersensitivity	Rash, urticaria, angioedema
Genitourinary	Dysuria, genital pruritus, genital moniliasis, vaginitis
Other	Moderate transient neutropenia

OVERDOSAGE

Signs and symptoms	See ADVERSE REACTIONS
Treatment	Discontinue medication; treat symptomatically; institute supportive measures, as required

DRUG INTERACTIONS

Probenecid	⇧ Cefadroxil blood level and/or toxicity

ALTERED LABORATORY VALUES

Blood/serum values	⇧ Alkaline phosphatase ⇧ SGOT ⇧ SGPT + Coombs' test
Urinary values	⇧ Glucose (with Clinitest tablets)

USE IN CHILDREN
See INDICATIONS; adjust dosage according to body weight

USE IN PREGNANT AND NURSING WOMEN
Pregnancy Category B: use during pregnancy only if clearly needed. Reproduction studies in rats and mice at doses up to 11 times the human dose have shown no evidence of impaired fertility or harm to the fetus; however, no adequate, well-controlled studies have been done in pregnant women. Use with caution in nursing mothers.

CEPHALOSPORINS

VELOSEF (cephradine) Squibb   Rx

Capsules: 250, 500 mg   **Suspension (per 5 ml):** 125 and 250 mg after reconstitution (5, 100, 200 ml) *fruit-flavored*   **Vials:** 250, 500 mg; 1 g   **Infusion bottles:** 2 g (100 ml), 4 g (100 ml)

INDICATIONS

Respiratory tract infections caused by susceptible strains of *Streptococcus pneumoniae, Klebsiella, Hemophilus influenzae, Staphylococcus aureus,* and Group A beta-hemolytic streptococci
Skin and skin structure infections caused by susceptible strains of staphylococci and Group A beta-hemolytic streptococci

Lobar pneumonia
Urinary tract infections caused by susceptible strains of *Escherichia coli, Proteus mirabilis, Klebsiella,* and enterococci

ORAL DOSAGE

Adult: 250 mg q6h or 500 mg q12h; for severe or chronic infections, give up to 1 g qid
Infant (≥ 9 mo) and child: 25–50 mg/kg/day in equally divided doses q6h or q12h; for severe or chronic infections, give up to 1 g qid

Adult: 500 mg q6h or 1 g q12h; for severe or chronic infections, give up to 1 g qid

PARENTERAL DOSAGE

Adult: 2–4 g/day IM or IV, given in equally divided doses qid; for severe infections, increase dosage up to 8 g/day or inject q4h
Infant and child: 50–100 mg/kg/day IM or IV, given in equally divided doses qid

Adult: same as adult's dosage above
Infant and child: same as pediatric dosage above

VELOSEF

Otitis media caused by susceptible strains of Group A beta-hemolytic streptococci, *Streptococcus pneumoniae*, *Hemophilus influenzae*, and staphylococci	**Infant (≥ 9 mo) and child:** 25–50 mg/kg/day (or 75–100 mg/kg/day for *H influenzae* infections) in divided doses q6h or q12h; for severe or chronic infections, give up to 1 g qid	
Septicemia caused by susceptible strains of *Streptococcus pneumoniae*, *Staphylococcus aureus*, *Proteus mirabilis*, and *Escherichia coli*	—	**Adult:** same as adult's dosage above **Infant and child:** same as pediatric dosage above
Bone infections caused by susceptible strains of *Staphylococcus aureus*	—	**Adult:** 4 g/day IV, given in equally divided doses
Prevention of postoperative infection in patients undergoing contaminated or potentially contaminated procedures (injection form only)	—	**Adult:** 1 g IM or IV 30–90 min prior to surgery, repeated q4–6h for 1 or 2 doses or up to 24 h postoperatively

CONTRAINDICATIONS

Hypersensitivity to cephalosporins

ADMINISTRATION/DOSAGE ADJUSTMENTS

Duration of treatment	Treatment should be continued for at least 48–72 h after patient has become asymptomatic or bacteria have been eradicated. Infections caused by Group A beta-hemolytic streptococci should be treated for at least 10 days to guard against the risk of rheumatic fever or glomerulonephritis. Persistent infections may require treatment for several weeks; following clinical improvement with parenteral therapy, oral cephradine may be used to continue treatment of persistent or severe conditions. Prolonged intensive therapy is recommended for prostatis.
Timing of oral administration	The presence of food in the GI tract delays absorption but does not affect the total amount of cephradine absorbed; this drug may be taken with food or milk to minimize the possibility of GI complaints
Intramuscular administration	Dilute contents of 250-mg, 500-mg, or 1-g vial in, respectively, 1.2, 2, or 4 ml of Sterile (or Bacteriostatic) Water for Injection and inject deeply into a large muscle mass (eg, the gluteus or lateral aspect of the thigh) to minimize pain and induration
Intravenous injection	Using an appropriate diluent (*do not use lactated Ringer's solution*), prepare a 1 g/10 ml solution of cephradine and slowly inject required dose directly into a vein over a period of 3–5 min; cephradine may also be administered by continuous or intermittent IV infusion. To reduce the risk of phlebitis during long-term therapy, rotate injection site. During prolonged infusions, use a new solution every 10 h.
Patients with renal impairment	For patients not undergoing dialysis, start with 500 mg q6h when creatinine clearance rate (Ccr) > 20 ml/min; 250 mg q6h when Ccr = 5–20 ml/min; or 250 mg q12h when Ccr < 5 ml/min; for patients receiving chronic intermittent hemodialysis, administer 250 mg to start, followed by 250 mg 12 h later and 250 mg 36–48 h after initial dose
Prophylactic use following cesarean section	Administer 1 g IM or IV as soon as the umbilical cord is clamped, followed by 1 g IM or IV 6 and 12 h after the first dose
Chronic urinary tract infections	Frequent bacteriological and clinical appraisal is necessary during therapy, and may be required for several months afterward

WARNINGS/PRECAUTIONS

Cross-allergenicity	Use with caution in penicillin-allergic patients
Hypersensitivity	Serious, potentially fatal anaphylactoid reactions may occur, especially with parenteral use and in patients with a history of allergy (particularly to drugs), necessitating emergency treatment with epinephrine, oxygen, IV steroids, and airway management, including intubation
Pseudomembranous colitis	May occur due to alteration of the normal intestinal flora and should be considered in any patient who develops diarrhea during or after therapy. Mild cases may respond to withdrawal of the drug alone. Moderate to severe cases should be managed by fluid and electrolyte replacement and protein supplementation, as needed. Oral vancomycin is the treatment of choice for severe or refractory colitis associated with the overgrowth of *Clostridium difficile;* however, other possible causes should also be considered.
Special-risk patients	Patients with markedly impaired renal function should be carefully monitored during therapy, since cephradine accumulates in the serum and tissues (see ADMINISTRATION/DOSAGE ADJUSTMENTS); use with caution in patients with a history of GI disease, particularly colitis
Superinfection	Overgrowth of nonsusceptible organisms may occur with prolonged use
Diabetic patients	Caution diabetics that a false-positive reaction for glucose in the urine may occur if Benedict's solution, Fehling's solution, or Clinitest tablets are used; enzyme-based tests (eg, Clinistix or Tes-Tape) are not affected by cephradine therapy

VELOSEF

Concomitant drug therapy	Patients should report the current use of any other medications, and should be cautioned not to take other drugs without the knowledge and approval of their physician (see DRUG INTERACTIONS)
Carcinogenicity, mutagenicity	The carcinogenic and mutagenic potential of this drug has not been evaluated

ADVERSE REACTIONS

Gastrointestinal	Pseudomembranous colitis; nausea and vomiting (rare)
Dermatological and hypersensitivity	Mild urticaria; skin rash; pruritus; joint pains; drug fever, edema, and erythema (with parenteral use)
Hematological	Mild, transient eosinophilia; leukopenia; neutropenia
Other	Headache (with parenteral use), dizziness, dyspnea (with parenteral use), tightness in the chest (with oral use), paresthesias (with parenteral use), candidal overgrowth (with parenteral use), vaginitis, hepatomegaly (with parenteral use), thrombophlebitis at injection site (with parenteral use), pain at injection site (with IM use)

OVERDOSAGE

Signs and symptoms	See ADVERSE REACTIONS
Treatment	Discontinue medication; treat symptomatically and institute supportive measures, as required

DRUG INTERACTIONS

Aminoglycosides, colistin, polymyxins, vancomycin, loop diuretics (ethacrynic acid, furosemide)	⌂ Risk of nephrotoxicity
Bacteriostatic agents	Interference with bactericidal action of cephradine in acute infection
Probenecid	⌂ Cephradine blood level, increasing the risk of nephrotoxicity

ALTERED LABORATORY VALUES

Blood/serum values	⌂ Alkaline phosphatase ⌂ Bilirubin ⌂ SGOT ⌂ SGPT ⌂ Lactate dehydrogenase ⌂ BUN ⌂ Prothrombin time + Coombs' test
Urinary values	⌂ Glucose (with Clinitest tablets) + Protein (with sulfosalicylic acid method) ⌂ 17-Ketosteroids

USE IN CHILDREN

See INDICATIONS; adjust dosage according to body weight and severity of infection. Adequate information is not available on the efficacy of oral bid regimens in infants under 9 mo of age. Parenteral cephradine has been used effectively in infants; however, all laboratory parameters have not been thoroughly studied in 1- to 12-mo-old infants, and safety for use in younger infants and premature newborns has not been established. Thus, in treating infants the potential benefits of the drug should be weighed against the possible risks involved in each situation. Doses for older children should not exceed recommended adult dose.

USE IN PREGNANT AND NURSING WOMEN

Pregnancy Category B: use during pregnancy only if clearly needed. Reproduction studies in mice and rats at doses up to 4 times the maximum recommended human dose have shown no evidence of impaired fertility or harm to the fetus; however, no adequate, well-controlled studies have been done in pregnant women. Positive Coombs' tests have been reported in newborns of mothers who received cephalosporins prior to delivery. Cephradine is excreted in human milk; use with caution in nursing mothers.

CEPHALOSPORINS

ZINACEF (cefuroxime sodium) Glaxo Rx

Vials: 750 mg, 1.5 g   **Infusion bottles:** 750 mg, 1.5 g   **Pharmacy bulk vial:** 7.5 g

INDICATIONS

Lower respiratory tract infections caused by susceptible strains of *Streptococcus pneumoniae, Hemophilus influenzae, Klebsiella, Staphylococcus aureus, Streptococcus pyogenes,* and *Escherichia coli*

Urinary tract infections caused by susceptible strains of *Escherichia coli* and *Klebsiella*

Disseminated gonococcal infections caused by *Neisseria gonorrhoeae*

Skin and skin structure infections caused by susceptible strains of *Staphylococcus aureus, Streptococcus pyogenes, Escherichia coli, Klebsiella,* and *Enterobacter*

Septicemia caused by susceptible strains of *Staphylococcus aureus, Streptococcus pneumoniae, Escherichia coli, Hemophilus influenzae,* and *Klebsiella*

Meningitis caused by susceptible strains of *Streptococcus pneumoniae, Hemophilus influenzae, Neisseria meningitidis,* and *Staphylococcus aureus*

Bone and joint infections caused by susceptible strains of *Staphylococcus aureus*

Uncomplicated gonorrhea caused by *Neisseria gonorrhoeae,* including penicillinase-producing strains

Prevention of postoperative infection in patients undergoing clean-contaminated or potentially contaminated surgical procedures, or during open heart surgery

PARENTERAL DOSAGE

Adult: for uncomplicated pneumonia and urinary tract infections, disseminated gonococcal infections, and skin and skin structure infections, 750 mg IM or IV q8h; for severe or complicated infections, 1.5 g IM or IV q8h; for life-threatening infections and infections caused by less susceptible organisms, 1.5 g IM or IV q6h; for bacterial meningitis, up to 3 g IV q8h. The IV route may be preferable for patients with bacterial septicemia or other severe or life-threatening infections or for patients who may be poor risks because of lowered resistance, especially if shock is present or impending.

Infant ($>$ 3 mo) and child: 50–100 mg/kg/day IM or IV, given in equally divided doses q6–8h (the higher dosage of 100 mg/kg/day should be given for more severe or serious infections); for bacterial meningitis, 200–240 mg/kg/day IV, given in divided doses q6–8h to start

Adult: 1.5 g IM or IV q8h, followed, when appropriate, by a course of oral antibiotics; perform surgery, when indicated, as an adjunctive measure

Infant ($>$ 3 mo) and child: 50 mg/kg, up to 1.5 g, IM or IV q8h, followed by a course of oral antibiotics

Adult: 1.5 g, given in a single IM dose (in two different sites) together with 1 g of oral probenecid

Adult: for clean-contaminated or potentially contaminated surgical procedures, 1.5 g IV ½–1 h prior to initial incision, followed by 750 mg IV or IM q8h during prolonged procedures; for open heart surgery, 1.5 g IV at induction of anesthesia, followed by 1.5 g q12h, for a total of 6 g

CONTRAINDICATIONS

Hypersensitivity to cephalosporins

ADMINISTRATION/DOSAGE ADJUSTMENTS

Duration of therapy — Continue administration for at least 48–72 h after the patient has become asymptomatic or evidence of bacterial eradication has been obtained. *Streptococcus pyogenes* infections should be treated for at least 10 days; persistent infections may require several weeks of therapy. Doses lower than those indicated above should not be used.

Patients with renal impairment — Administer 750–1,500 mg q8h when creatinine clearance rate (Ccr) $>$ 20 ml/min, 750 mg q12h when Ccr = 10–20 ml/min, and 750 mg q24h when Ccr $<$ 10 ml/min.[1] Creatinine clearance may be calculated from the serum creatinine concentration by use of the following formula: Ccr (in males) = [patient's weight *(kg)* $\times$ (140 − patient's age)]/(72 $\times$ creatinine concentration *(mg/dl)*]; for females, multiply the value obtained by this formula by 0.85.

Intramuscular administration — Reconstitute the contents of a 750-mg vial with 3.6 ml of sterile water for injection and withdraw 3.6 ml of the resulting suspension for injection. Inject the drug deeply into a large muscle mass, such as the gluteus or the lateral part of the thigh; to avoid inadvertent injection into a blood vessel, aspirate the syringe prior to injection.

ZINACEF

Preparation of solutions for intravenous administration	Reconstitute the contents of each 750-mg vial with 9 ml of sterile water for injection and withdraw 8 ml of the resulting solution for injection; for each 1.5-g vial, use 16 ml of sterile water for injection and withdraw the entire amount of solution for injection. The approximate drug concentrations after reconstitution are 94 mg/ml for the 750-mg vial and 90 mg/ml for the 1.5-g vial. To reconstitute the contents of an infusion bottle, add 100 ml of one of the following parenteral solutions: sterile water for injection, 5% dextrose injection, 0.9% sodium chloride injection, M/6 sodium lactate injection, Ringer's injection USP, lactated Ringer's injection USP, 5% dextrose and 0.9% sodium chloride injection, 5% dextrose and 0.45% sodium chloride injection, 5% dextrose and 0.225% sodium chloride injection, 10% dextrose injection, or 10% invert sugar in water for injection; the resulting concentration is approximately 15 mg/ml in the 1.5-g bottle and approximately 7.5 mg/ml in the 750-mg bottle. Prepare the solution in the pharmacy bulk vial under a laminar flow hood. Using a sterile dispensing device (not a syringe and needle), reconstitute the contents of the vial with 77 ml of sterile water for injection (resulting concentration: 750 mg/8 ml) and withdraw the required dose; for infusion, dilute this dose to a final concentration of 1–30 mg/ml. All solutions, including those prepared in infusion bottles and vials, should be used within 24 h if they are kept at room temperature; solutions with a concentration of 90 mg/ml or more should be used within 48 h if they are refrigerated, while solutions with a concentration of 1–30 mg/ml should be used within 7 days if they are refrigerated.
Intravenous injection	After reconstitution, inject the solution slowly into a vein over a period of 3–5 min, or give it through a tubing system which may already be in place
Intravenous infusion	When a Y-type administration set is used for intermittent infusion, administration of the bulk IV solution should be discontinued for the duration of each infusion. For continuous infusion, a solution of cefuroxime may be added to an IV bottle containing one of the following fluids: 0.9% sodium chloride injection, 5% or 10% dextrose injection, 5% dextrose and 0.9% sodium chloride injection, 5% dextrose and 0.45% sodium chloride injection, or M/6 sodium lactate injection. Do not add cefuroxime to solutions of aminoglycosides because of potential interaction (see WARNINGS/PRECAUTIONS); however, these antibiotics may be administered separately.

WARNINGS/PRECAUTIONS

Cross-allergenicity	Use with caution in penicillin-allergic patients
Hypersensitivity	Serious acute hypersensitivity reactions may occur, most likely in patients with a history of allergy, particularly to drugs; anaphylactic reactions may require administration of epinephrine and other emergency measures
Pseudomembranous colitis	May occur due to alteration of the normal intestinal flora and should be considered in any patient who develops diarrhea during or after therapy. Mild cases may respond to withdrawal of the drug alone. Moderate to severe cases should be managed by fluid and electrolyte replacement and protein supplementation, as needed. Oral vancomycin is the treatment of choice for severe or refractory colitis associated with the overgrowth of *Clostridium difficile;* however, other possible causes should also be considered.
Superinfection	Overgrowth of nonsusceptible organisms may occur
Renal impairment	Renal status should be monitored during therapy, especially in seriously ill patients receiving maximum doses. Use this drug with caution in patients who are concomitantly receiving potent diuretics, as these regimens are suspected of adversely affecting renal function. In patients with renal insufficiency, the total daily dose of cefuroxime should be reduced (see ADMINISTRATION/DOSAGE ADJUSTMENTS).
Concomitant administration of aminoglycosides	May result in nephrotoxicity and should be avoided
Special-risk patients	Use with caution in patients with known hypersensitivity to penicillin and in patients with a history of gastrointestinal disease, particularly colitis
Carcinogenicity, mutagenicity	Long-term studies have not been done in animals to evaluate the carcinogenic potential of this drug; standard laboratory studies have shown no evidence of mutagenicity

ADVERSE REACTIONS

Frequent reactions (incidence $\geq$ 1%) are printed in *italics*

Local	*Thrombophlebitis following IV administration (1.7%)*
Gastrointestinal	Diarrhea, nausea, pseudomembranous colitis
Hematological	*Decrease in hemoglobin and hematocrit (10%), transient eosinophilia (7.1%),* transient neutropenia and leukopenia
Hypersensitivity	Rash, pruritus, urticaria, positive Coombs' test; anaphylaxis, erythema multiforme, and Stevens-Johnson syndrome (rare)

OVERDOSAGE

Signs and symptoms	See ADVERSE REACTIONS
Treatment	Discontinue medication; treat symptomatically and institute supportive measures, as required

DRUG INTERACTIONS

Aminoglycoside antibiotics	⌂ Risk of nephrotoxicity
Probenecid	⌂ Serum level of cefuroxime

ALTERED LABORATORY VALUES

Blood/serum values	⌂ BUN ⌂ Creatinine ⌂ SGOT ⌂ SGPT ⌂ Lactate dehydrogenase ⌂ Alkaline phosphatase ⌂ Bilirubin + Coombs' test − Glucose (with ferricyanide test)[2]
Urinary values	⌂ Creatinine clearance + Glucose (with Clinitest tablets)

USE IN CHILDREN
See INDICATIONS and PARENTERAL DOSAGE; in calculating dosages by weight, do not exceed the maximum adult dose. Safety and effectiveness for use in infants under 3 mo of age have not been established. Accumulation of cephalosporin drugs in newborn infants has been reported.

USE IN PREGNANT AND NURSING WOMEN
Pregnancy Category B: use during pregnancy only if clearly needed. Reproduction studies in mice and rabbits at doses up to 60 times the human dose have revealed no evidence of impaired fertility or fetal harm; however, no adequate, well-controlled studies have been performed in pregnant women. Cefuroxime is excreted in human milk; use with caution in nursing women.

[1] Since cefuroxime sodium is dialyzable, patients on hemodialysis should be given a further dose at the end of the dialysis
[2] Glucose oxidase or hexokinase methods are recommended for determining serum glucose levels

PENICILLINS

AMCILL (ampicillin) Parke-Davis   Rx

Capsules: 250, 500 mg **Suspension (per 5 ml):** 125, 250 mg after reconstitution

INDICATIONS | ORAL DOSAGE

Upper and lower respiratory tract and soft tissue infections caused by susceptible strains of *Hemophilus influenzae*, penicillin G-sensitive staphylococci, streptococci, and *Streptococcus pneumoniae*

Adult: 250 mg q6h
Child (< 20 kg): 50 mg/kg/day, given in equally divided doses q6–8h
Child (≥ 20 kg): same as adult

Gastrointestinal and genitourinary tract infections caused by susceptible strains of *Shigella*, *Salmonella* (including *S typhosa*), *Escherichia coli*, *Proteus mirabilis*, and enterococci

Adult: 500 mg q6h; for stubborn or severe infections, higher doses may be needed, possibly for several weeks
Child (< 20 kg): 100 mg/kg/day, given in equally divided doses q6–8h; for stubborn or severe infections, higher doses may be needed, possibly for several weeks
Child (≥ 20 kg): same as adult

Urethritis caused by *Neisseria gonorrhoeae*

Adult: 3.5 g, given simultaneously with 1 g probenecid

CONTRAINDICATIONS
Hypersensitivity to penicillins

ADMINISTRATION/DOSAGE ADJUSTMENTS

Duration of treatment	Continue treatment for at least 48–72 h after patient has become asymptomatic or bacteria have been eradicated; beta-hemolytic streptococcal infections should be treated for at least 10 days to prevent rheumatic fever and glomerulonephritis

WARNINGS/PRECAUTIONS

Hypersensitivity	Serious and occasionally fatal anaphylactic reactions may occur, most likely in patients with a history of sensitivity to multiple allergens. Urticaria, other skin rashes, and serum sickness-like reactions may be controlled with antihistamines and, if necessary, systemic corticosteroids. Drug should be discontinued unless infection is life-threatening and amenable only to ampicillin. Severe reactions may necessitate emergency measures, such as immediate use of epinephrine, oxygen, IV corticosteroids, and airway management, including intubation; use with caution in patients who have experienced allergic reactions to cephalosporins.
Long-term therapy	Perform blood, renal, and hepatic studies periodically
Superinfection	Overgrowth of nonsusceptible organisms, including fungi, may occur

AMCILL ■ AMOXIL

Suspected syphilitic lesions	If syphilis is suspected, perform dark-field examination before instituting therapy and perform serology testing monthly for at least 4 mo
Chronic urinary tract and intestinal infections	Require bacteriological and clinical appraisal during therapy, and possibly for several months afterward
Complications of gonorrheal urethritis	Prolonged and intensive therapy is recommended
Inappropriate indications	Ampicillin should not be used for the treatment of infectious mononucleosis; a high percentage of patients with mononucleosis develop a skin rash after receiving ampicillin

ADVERSE REACTIONS

Frequent reactions (incidence ≥ 1%) are printed in *italics*

Gastrointestinal	Glossitis, stomatitis, black hairy tongue, nausea, vomiting, enterocolitis, pseudomembranous colitis, *diarrhea*
Hypersensitivity	*Erythematous maculopapular rash*, urticaria, erythema multiforme, exfoliative dermatitis, anaphylaxis (see WARNINGS/PRECAUTIONS)
Hematological	Anemia, thrombocytopenia, thrombocytopenic purpura, eosinophilia, leukopenia, agranulocytosis

OVERDOSAGE

Signs and symptoms	See ADVERSE REACTIONS
Treatment	Discontinue medication; treat symptomatically

DRUG INTERACTIONS

Probenecid	↑ Ampicillin blood level and/or toxicity

ALTERED LABORATORY VALUES

Blood/serum values	↑ SGOT (especially in infants)

No clinically significant alterations in urinary values occur at therapeutic dosages

---

USE IN CHILDREN

See INDICATIONS and ORAL DOSAGE

USE IN PREGNANT AND NURSING WOMEN

Safety for use during pregnancy has not been established. Consult manufacturer for use in nursing mothers.

PENICILLINS

AMOXIL (amoxicillin) Beecham Rx

Capsules: 250, 500 mg   **Chewable tablets:** 125, 250 mg   **Suspension (per 5 ml):** 125, 250 mg after reconstitution (5, 80, 100, 150 ml)   **Pediatric drops:** 50 mg/ml after reconstitution (15, 30 ml)

INDICATIONS

Ear, nose, and throat infections caused by susceptible strains of streptococci, *Streptococcus pneumoniae*, nonpenicillinase-producing staphylococci, and *Hemophilus influenzae*

Genitourinary tract infections caused by susceptible strains of *Escherichia coli*, *Proteus mirabilis*, and *Streptococcus fecalis*

Skin and soft tissue infections caused by susceptible strains of streptococci, staphylococci, and *Escherichia coli*

Lower respiratory tract infections caused by susceptible strains of streptococci, *Streptococcus pneumoniae*, non-penicillinase-producing staphylococci, and *Hemophilus influenzae*

Gonorrhea, acute uncomplicated anogenital and urethral infections caused by *Neisseria gonorrhoeae*

ORAL DOSAGE

Adult: 250 mg q8h; for infections that are severe or are caused by less susceptible organisms, 500 mg q8h
Infant (< 6 kg): 37.5 mg (0.75 ml of the drops) q8h
Infant (6-7 kg): 50 mg (1 ml of the drops) q8h
Infant (8 kg): 62.5 mg (1.25 ml of the drops) q8h
Infant and child (8-20 kg): 20 mg/kg/day, given in 3 divided doses q8h; for infections that are severe or are caused by less susceptible organisms, 40 mg/kg/day, given in 3 divided doses q8h
Child (≥ 20 kg): same as adult

Adult: 500 mg q8h
Infant (< 6 kg): 62.5 mg (1.25 ml of the drops) q8h
Infant (6-7 kg): 87.5 mg (1.75 ml of the drops) q8h
Infant (8 kg): 112.5 mg (2.25 ml of the drops) q8h
Infant and child (8-20 kg): 40 mg/kg/day, given in 3 divided doses q8h
Child (≥ 20 kg): same as adult

Adult: 3 g, given in a single dose
Prepuberal child (≥ 2 yr): 50 mg/kg, given in a single dose with 25 mg/kg of probenicid

COMPENDIUM OF DRUG THERAPY

CONTRAINDICATIONS
Hypersensitivity to penicillins

ADMINISTRATION/DOSAGE ADJUSTMENTS

Duration of treatment	Continue treatment for at least 48–72 h after patient has become asymptomatic or bacteria have been eradicated; beta-hemolytic streptococcal infections should be treated for at least 10 days to prevent rheumatic fever and glomerulonephritis
Use of oral suspension in children	After reconstitution, place required dose directly on child's tongue for swallowing or add to formula, milk, fruit juice, water, ginger ale, or cold drinks; infants weighing 8 kg (18 lb) or less should be given pediatric drops

WARNINGS/PRECAUTIONS

Hypersensitivity	Serious and occasionally fatal anaphylactoid reactions may occur, most likely in patients with a history of sensitivity to multiple allergens. Urticaria, other skin rashes, and serum sickness-like reactions may be controlled with antihistamines and, if necessary, systemic corticosteroids. Drug should be discontinued unless infection is life-threatening and amenable only to amoxicillin. Severe reactions may require emergency measures, such as immediate use of epinephrine, oxygen, IV corticosteroids, and airway management, including intubation; use with caution in patients who have experienced allergic reactions to cephalosporins
Long-term therapy	Perform blood, renal, and hepatic studies periodically
Superinfection	Overgrowth of nonsusceptible organisms, including fungi, may occur
Suspected syphilitic lesions	If syphilis is suspected, perform dark-field examination before instituting therapy and perform serology testing monthly for at least 4 mo
Chronic urinary tract infection	Requires frequent bacteriological and clinical appraisal during therapy, and possibly for several months afterward; do not use doses smaller than those recommended above

ADVERSE REACTIONS

Gastrointestinal	Nausea, vomiting, diarrhea
Hypersensitivity	Erythematous maculopapular rash, urticaria
Hematological	Anemia, thrombocytopenia, thrombocytopenic purpura, eosinophilia, leukopenia, agranulocytosis

OVERDOSAGE

Signs and symptoms	See ADVERSE REACTIONS
Treatment	Discontinue medication; treat symptomatically

DRUG INTERACTIONS

Probenecid	↑ Amoxicillin blood level and/or toxicity

ALTERED LABORATORY VALUES

Blood/serum values	↑ SGOT

No clinically significant alterations in urinary values occur at therapeutic dosages

---

USE IN CHILDREN
See INDICATIONS and ORAL DOSAGE; do not exceed adult dose

USE IN PREGNANT AND NURSING WOMEN
Safety for use during pregnancy has not been established. Amoxicillin is excreted in human milk (level is unknown); use with caution in nursing mothers.

PENICILLINS

AUGMENTIN (amoxicillin and clavulanate potassium) Beecham — Rx

Tablets: 250 mg amoxicillin and 125 mg clavulanic acid[1] (Augmentin 250); 500 mg amoxicillin and 125 mg clavulanic acid[1] (Augmentin 500) **Chewable tablets:** 125 mg amoxicillin and 31.25 mg clavulanic acid[1] (Augmentin 125); 250 mg amoxicillin and 62.5 mg clavulanic acid[1] (Augmentin 250) **Suspension (per 5 ml):** 125 mg amoxicillin and 31.25 mg clavulanic acid,[1] after reconstitution (Augmentin 125) (75, 150 ml) *banana flavored;* 250 mg amoxicillin and 62.5 mg clavulanic acid,[1] after reconstitution (Augmentin 250) (75, 150 ml) *orange flavored*

INDICATIONS

Lower respiratory tract infections caused by susceptible, beta-lactamase-producing strains of *Hemophilus influenzae*

Otitis media and sinusitis caused by susceptible, beta-lactamase-producing strains of *Hemophilus influenzae* and *Branhamella catarrhalis*

Skin and skin structure infections caused by susceptible, beta-lactamase-producing strains of *Staphylococcus aureus, Escherichia coli,* and *Klebsiella*

Urinary tract infections caused by susceptible, beta-lactamase-producing strains of *Escherichia coli, Klebsiella,* and *Enterobacter*

ORAL DOSAGE

Adult: for respiratory tract infections, 1 Augmentin 500 tab q8h; for other infections, 1 Augmentin 250 tab q8h or, if the infection is severe, 1 Augmentin 500 tab q8h. Do not substitute 2 Augmentin 250 tabs for 1 Augmentin 500 tab because the clavulanic acid content would not be equivalent.

Child (< 40 kg): for otitis media, sinusitis, and lower respiratory tract infections, 40 mg/kg/day, based on the amoxicillin component; for other infections, 20 mg/kg/day, based on the amoxicillin component, or, if the infection is severe, 40 mg/kg/day, based on the amoxicillin component. Administer total daily dose in 3 divided doses q8h.

Child (≥ 40 kg): same as adult

CONTRAINDICATIONS

Hypersensitivity to penicillins

ADMINISTRATION/DOSAGE ADJUSTMENTS

Mixed infections	If an infection is caused by a beta-lactamase-producing organism as well as an ampicillin-susceptible organism, an additional drug should not be necessary, since microorganisms susceptible to ampicillin are also susceptible to amoxicillin

WARNINGS/PRECAUTIONS

Hypersensitivity	Serious, occasionally fatal anaphylactic reactions have occurred in patients receiving oral penicillins; use with caution in patients with a history of allergy, particularly if they have demonstrated hypersensitivity to a number of substances. If an allergic reaction occurs, this preparation should be discontinued. For the treatment of serious anaphylactoid reactions, give epinephrine, oxygen, and IV corticosteroids and take appropriate measures (eg, intubation) to ensure adequate pulmonary function. Dermatological reactions can be controlled with antihistamines and, if necessary, systemic corticosteroids.
Mononucleosis	Aminopenicillins are likely to cause rash in patients with mononucleosis and therefore should not be given to such patients
Superinfection	Bear in mind that superinfection, usually with *Pseudomonas* or *Candida*, may occur; if superinfection occurs, discontinue use and/or institute appropriate therapy
Prolonged therapy	Evaluate hematopoietic, renal, and hepatic function periodically during long-term therapy
Concomitant use of disulfiram	This preparation should not be used with disulfiram
Carcinogenicity, mutagenicity	No studies have been done to evaluate the carcinogenic or mutagenic potential of this preparation

ADVERSE REACTIONS[2]

Frequent reactions (incidence $\geq$ 1%) are printed in *italics*

Gastrointestinal	*Diarrhea/loose stools (9%), nausea (3%), vomiting (1%),* abdominal discomfort, flatulence
Hypersensitivity	*Rash and urticaria (3%)*
Other	*Vaginitis (1%),* headache, increases in SGOT and SGPT levels, thrombocytosis

OVERDOSAGE

Signs and symptoms	See ADVERSE REACTIONS
Treatment	Institute supportive measures and treat symptomatically; amoxicillin and clavulanic acid can be removed from the blood by hemodialysis

DRUG INTERACTIONS

Probenecid	△ Serum amoxicillin level
Allopurinol	△ Risk of rash[3]

ALTERED LABORATORY VALUES

Blood/serum values	△ SGOT △ SGPT
Urinary values	+ Glucose (with Clinitest, Benedict's solution, and Fehling's solution); use enzyme-based tests such as Clinistix or Testape △ Total conjugated estriol △ Estriol-glucuronide △ Conjugated estrone △ Estradiol

---

USE IN CHILDREN

See INDICATIONS and ORAL DOSAGE

USE IN PREGNANT AND NURSING WOMEN

Pregnancy Category B: no evidence of impaired fertility or harm to the fetus has been seen in mice and rats given up to 10 times the human dose of this preparation; however, no adequate, well-controlled studies have been done in pregnant women. Use during pregnancy only if clearly needed. Studies in guinea pigs have shown that IV administration of ampicillin decreases uterine tone as well as the frequency, height, and duration of uterine contractions; it is not known whether these reactions can occur with the use of oral amoxicillin during labor and delivery (oral aminopenicillins are generally not well absorbed during labor). Aminopenicillins are excreted in human milk; use with caution in nursing mothers.

---

[1] As the potassium salt
[2] Reactions associated with the use of other aminopenicillins include gastritis, stomatitis, glossitis, black "hairy" tongue, enterocolitis, pseudomembranous colitis, erythema multiforme, exfoliative dermatitis, anemia, thrombocytopenia, thrombocytopenic purpura, eosinophilia, leukopenia, and agranulocytosis
[3] Use of ampicillin in patients receiving allopurinol has caused an increase in rashes; it is not known whether this effect is due to allopurinol or to the patients' hyperuricemic condition. Concomitant use of amoxicillin has not been studied.

PENICILLINS

AZLIN (azlocillin sodium) Miles Pharmaceuticals Rx

Vials: 2, 3, 4 g **Infusion bottles:** 2, 3, 4 g

INDICATIONS

Lower respiratory tract infections, including pneumonia and lung abscess, caused by susceptible strains of *Pseudomonas aeruginosa, Escherichia coli,* and *Hemophilus influenzae*

Skin and skin structure infections, including ulcers, abscesses, burns, and severe external otitis, caused by susceptible strains of *Pseudomonas aeruginosa, Escherichia coli, Proteus mirabilis,* and *Streptococcus fecalis*

Bone and joint infections, including osteomyelitis, caused by susceptible strains of *Pseudomonas aeruginosa*

Bacterial septicemia, caused by susceptible strains of *Pseudomonas aeruginosa* and *Escherichia coli*

Upper and lower **urinary tract infections** caused by susceptible strains of *Pseudomonas aeruginosa, Escherichia coli, Proteus mirabilis,* and *Streptococcus fecalis*

PARENTERAL DOSAGE

Adult: 3 g IV q4h or 4 g IV q6h (225–300 mg/kg/day); for life-threatening infections, up to 4 g IV q4h (350 mg/kg/day or 24 g/day)

Adult: for uncomplicated infections, 2 g IV q6h (100–125 mg/kg/day); for complicated infections, 3 g IV q6h (150–200 mg/kg/day)

CONTRAINDICATIONS

Hypersensitivity to penicillins

ADMINISTRATION/DOSAGE ADJUSTMENTS

Duration of therapy	Depends upon the severity of the infection, but therapy should usually continue for at least 2 days after the signs and symptoms of infection disappear (usual duration: 10–14 days); in difficult, complicated infections, such as osteomyelitis, more prolonged therapy may be needed
Considerations for individualizing dosage	Include the site and severity of infection, the susceptibility of the causative organisms, and the status of the patient's host defense mechanisms
Deep-seated infections with abscess formation	Appropriate surgical drainage should be performed in conjunction with antimicrobial therapy
Patients with renal impairment	If creatinine clearance rate (CCr) $>$ 30 ml/min, administer the usual recommended dosage; if CCr = 10–30 ml/min, administer 1.5 g q12h for uncomplicated urinary tract infections, 1.5 g q8h for complicated urinary tract infections, or 2 g q8h for serious systemic infections; if CCr $<$ 10 ml/min, administer 1.5 g q12h for uncomplicated urinary tract infections, 2 g q12h for complicated urinary tract infections, or 3 g q12h for serious systemic infections. For patients undergoing hemodialysis for renal failure, administer 3 g after each dialysis treatment and then q12h. For patients with renal failure, especially with hepatic insufficiency, measure azlocillin levels for additional guidance in adjusting dosage.
Intravenous infusion	Reconstitute each gram of azlocillin by shaking vigorously with at least 10 ml of Sterile Water for Injection, 5% Dextrose Injection, or 0.9% Sodium Chloride Injection; dilute further to desired volume with an appropriate IV solution. Inject the solution slowly over a period of 30 min by either direct infusion or through a Y-type infusion set which may already be in place. Discontinue the administration of any other solutions while infusing azlocillin if using this or the "piggy-back" method.
Intermittent intravenous injection	The reconstituted solution (see above) may be injected slowly into a vein or IV tubing over a period of 5 min or longer[1]; to minimize venous irritation, the concentration of the drug should not exceed 10%
Concomitant use of other anti-infectives	Azlocillin has been used effectively in combination with an aminoglycoside antibiotic for the treatment of life-threatening infections; if such combination therapy is indicated, give each drug separately in their full recommended dosages and using the customary route of administration for each drug
Cultures and susceptibility tests	Should be performed prior to treatment to identify the causative organism and determine its susceptibility to azlocillin and then periodically during treatment to monitor for effectiveness and for possible development of bacterial resistance. Therapy can be initiated before test results are known; in certain severe infections, where the causative organisms are unknown and *Pseudomonas aeruginosa* is suspected, azlocillin may be given in combination with an aminoglycoside or a cephalosporin antibiotic as initial therapy and adjusted when test results become available.
Febrile episodes in immunosuppressed patients with granulocytopenia	Azlocillin should be combined with an aminoglycoside or a cephalosporin antibiotic (see "concomitant use of other anti-infectives," above)
Acute pulmonary exacerbations in patients with cystic fibrosis	Azlocillin has been used effectively in combination with an aminoglycoside antibiotic to treat such complications; for children, give 75 mg/kg IV q4h (450 mg/kg/day), not to exceed 24 g/day[2] (see "concomitant use of other anti-infectives," above)

WARNINGS/PRECAUTIONS

Hypersensitivity	Serious and occasionally fatal anaphylactoid reactions may occur, most likely in patients with a history of sensitivity to multiple allergens, and require immediate emergency treatment with epinephrine, oxygen, and IV corticosteroids, and airway management, including intubation; use with caution in patients who have experienced some form of allergy, especially to cephalosporins or other drugs. If an allergic reaction occurs during azlocillin therapy, discontinue use.
Long-term therapy	Perform blood, renal, and hepatic studies periodically during prolonged therapy
Bleeding abnormalities	May occur (rarely), particularly in patients with severe renal impairment receiving maximum doses, and have been associated with abnormalities of coagulation tests, such as clotting time, platelet aggregation, and prothrombin time
Hypokalemia	May occur (rarely), particularly in patients with fluid and electrolyte imbalances; monitor serum potassium level periodically during prolonged therapy
Sodium content	Each gram of azlocillin contains 49.8 mg (2.17 mEq) of sodium; this should be considered when treating patients on salt-restricted diets
Superinfection	Overgrowth of nonsusceptible organisms may occur

ADVERSE REACTIONS

Hypersensitivity	Skin rash, pruritus, urticaria, arthralgia, myalgia, drug fever, chills, chest discomfort, anaphalyactic reactions
Central nervous system	Headache, giddiness, neuromuscular hyperirritability, convulsive seizures
Gastrointestinal	Disturbances of taste and smell, stomatitis, flatulence, nausea, vomiting, diarrhea, epigastric pain
Hematological	Thrombocytopenia, leukopenia, neutropenia, eosinophilia, reduction of hemoglobin or hematocrit, prolongation of prothrombin time and bleeding time
Local	Pain and thrombophlebitis following IV administration

OVERDOSAGE

Signs and symptoms	Neuromuscular hyperirritability, convulsive seizures
Treatment	Hemodialysis (if necessary) will help remove azlocillin from the circulation

DRUG INTERACTIONS

Probenecid	△ Azlocillin serum level and half-life

ALTERED LABORATORY VALUES

Blood/serum values	▽ Uric acid △ SGOT △ SGPT △ Alkaline phosphatase △ Lactate dehydrogenase △ Bilirubin △ Creatinine △ BUN △ Sodium ▽ Potassium
Urinary values	+ Protein (with sulfosalicylic acid and boiling test, acetic acid test, biuret reaction, and nitric acid test)

USE IN CHILDREN

See INDICATIONS and PARENTERAL DOSAGE; until further experience has been gained, do not use this drug in neonates

USE IN PREGNANT AND NURSING WOMEN

Pregnancy Category B: use during pregnancy only if clearly needed. Reproduction studies in rats and mice at doses up to twice the human dose have shown no evidence of impaired fertility or fetal harm; however, no adequate, well-controlled studies have been done in pregnant women. Azlocillin crosses the placenta and is found in cord blood, amniotic fluid, and human milk; use with caution in nursing mothers.

[1] Rapid IV administration of azlocillin has been associated with transient chest discomfort
[2] Only limited data are available on the safety and effectiveness of azlocillin in the treatment of infants with serious infections

---

PENICILLINS

BICILLIN C-R (penicillin G benzathine and penicillin G procaine) Wyeth   Rx

Vials: 300,000 units, 50% penicillin G benzathine and 50% penicillin G procaine, per ml (10 ml) **Cartridge-needle units:** 600,000 units, 50% penicillin G benzathine and 50% penicillin G procaine, per ml (1, 2 ml) **Prefilled syringes:** 600,000 units, 50% penicillin G benzathine and 50% penicillin G procaine, per ml (4 ml)

BICILLIN C-R 900/300 (penicillin G benzathine and penicillin G procaine) Wyeth   Rx

Cartridge-needle units: 1.2 million units, 75% penicillin G benzathine and 25% penicillin G procaine (2 ml)

INDICATIONS

Moderately severe to severe nonbacteremic **upper respiratory tract infections, skin and soft tissue infections, scarlet fever, and erysipelas** caused by penicillin G-sensitive Group A streptococci

Moderately severe **pneumonia and otitis media** caused by penicillin G-sensitive strains of *Streptococcus pneumoniae*

PARENTERAL DOSAGE

Adult: 2.4 million units of Bicillin C-R IM, given at one time (using multiple sites, if necessary) or given half on day 1 and half on day 3

Infant and child: 600,000 units (if infant weighs under 30 lb) or 0.9–1.2 million units (if child weighs 30–60 lb) of Bicillin C-R IM, given at one time (using multiple sites, if necessary) or given half on day 1 and half on day 3; alternatively, 1.2 million units of Bicillin C-R 900/300, given in a single IM dose

Adult: 1.2 million units of Bicillin C-R IM, given every 2–3 days until temperature is normal for 48 h

Child: 600,000 units of Bicillin C-R or 1.2 million units of Bicillin C-R 900/300 IM, given every 2–3 days until temperature is normal for 48 h

BICILLIN C-R ■ BICILLIN L-A

CONTRAINDICATIONS

Hypersensitivity to penicillins or procaine	Injection into or near an artery or nerve

ADMINISTRATION/DOSAGE ADJUSTMENTS

Alternative regimen for streptococcal infections	To ensure adequate serum levels over a 10-day period, administer half the total dose on day 1 and the other half on day 3, provided the patient's cooperation can be assured
Duration of treatment for streptococcal infections	Therapy must be sufficient to eliminate the organism and prevent sequelae of streptococcal disease; cultures should be performed at completion of treatment
Intramuscular injection	Inject deeply into the upper outer quadrant of the buttock (adults) or midlateral aspect of the thigh (infants and small children). Care should be taken to avoid IV or intraarterial administration or injection into or near major peripheral nerves or blood vessels; if blood or any discoloration appears upon aspiration, withdraw the needle and discard the syringe or cartridge.

WARNINGS/PRECAUTIONS

Hypersensitivity	Serious and occasionally fatal anaphylactoid reactions may occur, most likely in patients with a history of sensitivity to multiple allergens. Urticaria, other skin rashes, and serum-sickness-like reactions may be controlled with antihistamines, pressor amines, and, if necessary, systemic corticosteroids. Drug should be discontinued unless infection is life-threatening and amenable only to penicillin. Severe reactions may necessitate emergency measures, such as immediate use of epinephrine, aminophylline, oxygen, and IV corticosteroids; use with caution in patients who have experienced allergic reactions to cephalosporins.
Injection complications	Repeated intramuscular injection into the anterolateral aspect of the thigh may cause quadriceps femoris fibrosis and atrophy. Inadvertent injection into or near a nerve may result in permanent neurological damage. Severe complications have followed inadvertent intravascular administration or injection immediately adjacent to arteries. These complications, which have occurred mainly in infants and small children, have included severe neurovascular damage (eg, transverse myelitis with permanent paralysis, gangrene requiring amputation, and necrosis and sloughing at the injection site), immediate pallor, mottling or cyanosis followed by bleb formation, and severe edema requiring fasciotomy. Discontinue delivery of the dose if patient complains of severe immediate pain at injection site, or if in infants and young children symptoms or signs of severe pain occur. If any compromise of the blood supply occurs at, proximal to, or distal to the site of injection, consult an appropriate specialist promptly.
Superinfection	Overgrowth of nonsusceptible organisms, including fungi, may occur
Procaine reactions	May occur in a small percentage of patients. If there is a history of sensitivity, inject 0.1 ml of 1–2% procaine; subsequent development of an erythema, wheal, flare, or eruption contraindicates the use of procaine penicillin. Treat procaine reactions with barbiturates and possibly antihistamines.
Prolonged therapy	Evaluate renal and hematopoietic function periodically, particularly when using high doses

ADVERSE REACTIONS

Hypersensitivity	Skin rashes, ranging from maculopapular eruptions to exfoliative dermatitis; urticaria; serum-sickness-like reactions, including chills, fever, edema, arthralgia, and prostration; anaphylaxis

OVERDOSAGE

Signs and symptoms	See ADVERSE REACTIONS
Treatment	Discontinue medication; treat symptomatically

DRUG INTERACTIONS

Probenecid	⇧ Penicillin blood level and/or toxicity

ALTERED LABORATORY VALUES

No clinically significant alterations in blood/serum or urinary values occur at therapeutic dosages

---

USE IN CHILDREN

See INDICATIONS and PARENTERAL DOSAGE

USE IN PREGNANT AND NURSING WOMEN

Use during pregnancy only if essential; no teratogenic effects have been documented. Use in nursing women only if essential.

PENICILLINS

BICILLIN L-A (penicillin G benzathine) Wyeth Rx

Vials: 300,000 units/ml (10 ml) **Cartridge-needle units:** 600,000 units/ml (1, 2 ml) **Prefilled syringes:** 600,000 units/ml (4 ml)

INDICATIONS

Mild to moderate nonbacteremic upper respiratory tract infections caused by Group A streptococci

PARENTERAL DOSAGE

Adult: 1.2 million units, given in a single IM dose
Infant: 300,000–600,000 units, given in a single IM dose
Child (< 60 lb): 300,000–600,000 units, given in a single IM dose
Child (> 60 lb): 900,000 units, given in a single IM dose

BICILLIN L-A

Primary, secondary, and latent syphilis	Adult: 2.4 million units, given in a single IM dose
Tertiary syphilis and neurosyphilis	Adult: 2.4 million units, given in a single IM dose at 7-day intervals for 3 doses
Congenital syphilis	Infant ($<$ 2 yr): 50,000 units/kg IM Child (2–12 yr): adjust dosage according to adult schedule
Yaws, bejel, and pinta	Adult: 1.2 million units, given in a single IM dose
Prophylaxis for rheumatic fever, chorea, rheumatic heart disease, and acute glomerulonephritis	Adult: 1.2 million units, given in a single IM dose once a month, or 600,000 units IM every 2 wk following an acute attack Child: same as adult

CONTRAINDICATIONS

Hypersensitivity to penicillins	Injection into or near an artery or nerve

ADMINISTRATION/DOSAGE ADJUSTMENTS

Duration of treatment for streptococcal infections	Therapy must be sufficient to eliminate the organism and prevent sequelae of streptococcal disease; cultures should be performed at completion of treatment
Intramuscular injection	Inject deeply into the upper outer quadrant of the buttock (adults) or midlateral aspect of the thigh (infants and small children). Rate of administration should be slow and steady; otherwise, the needle may be blocked by material suspended in the solution. Rotate injection sites. Care should be taken to avoid IV or intraarterial administration or injection into or near major peripheral nerves or blood vessels; if blood or any discoloration appears upon aspiration, withdraw the needle and discard the syringe or cartridge.

WARNINGS/PRECAUTIONS

Hypersensitivity	Serious and occasionally fatal anaphylactoid reactions may occur, most likely in patients with a history of sensitivity to multiple allergens; use with caution in patients who have experienced allergic reactions to cephalosporins. If an allergic reaction occurs, discontinue medication and employ pressor amines, antihistamines, and corticosteroids, as needed.
Injection complications	Repeated intramuscular injection into the anterolateral aspect of the thigh may cause quadriceps femoris fibrosis and atrophy. Inadvertent injection into or near a nerve may result in permanent neurological damage. Severe complications have followed inadvertent intravascular administration or injection immediately adjacent to arteries. These complications, which have occurred mainly in infants and small children, have included severe neurovascular damage (eg, transverse myelitis with permanent paralysis, gangrene requiring amputation, and necrosis and sloughing at the injection site), immediate pallor, mottling or cyanosis followed by bleb formation, and severe edema requiring fasciotomy. Discontinue delivery of the dose if patient complains of severe immediate pain at injection site, or if in infants and young children symptoms or signs of severe pain occur. If any compromise of the blood supply occurs at, proximal to, or distal to the site of injection, consult an appropriate specialist promptly.
Superinfection	Overgrowth of nonsusceptible organisms, including fungi, may occur with prolonged use

ADVERSE REACTIONS

Hypersensitivity	Skin eruptions ranging from maculopapular rash to exfoliative dermatitis, urticaria, and other serum sickness-like reactions; fever; eosinophilia; laryngeal edema; anaphylaxis (see WARNINGS/PRECAUTIONS)
Hematological	Hemolytic anemia, leukopenia, and thrombocytopenia (with high parenteral doses)
Other	Jarisch-Herxheimer reaction (with syphilis treatment); neuropathy and nephropathy (with high parenteral doses)

OVERDOSAGE

Signs and symptoms	See ADVERSE REACTIONS
Treatment	Discontinue medication; treat symptomatically

DRUG INTERACTIONS

Probenecid	⇧ Penicillin blood level and/or toxicity

ALTERED LABORATORY VALUES

No clinically significant alterations in blood/serum or urinary values occur at therapeutic dosages

---

USE IN CHILDREN
See INDICATIONS and PARENTERAL DOSAGE

USE IN PREGNANT AND NURSING WOMEN
Use during pregnancy only if essential; no teratogenic effects have been documented. Use in nursing women only if essential.

PENICILLINS

COACTIN (amdinocillin) Roche   Rx

Vials: 0.5, 1 g

INDICATIONS

Urinary tract infections caused by susceptible strains of *Escherichia coli*, *Klebsiella* (including *K pneumoniae*), and *Enterobacter*

Bacteremia associated with severe urinary tract infections caused by susceptible strains of *Escherichia coli*

PARENTERAL DOSAGE

Adult: for serious infections, 10 mg/kg, given IV either q4h if used alone or q6h if used in combination with another beta-lactam antibiotic; for less serious infections, drug can also be given by IM injection

CONTRAINDICATIONS

Hypersensitivity to penicillins

ADMINISTRATION/DOSAGE ADJUSTMENTS

Intramuscular administration — To reconstitute solution, add 2.2 ml of sterile water for injection USP or 0.9% sodium chloride injection USP to the 500-mg vial or 4.4 ml to the 1-g vial and then shake well. Before administration, aspirate to help prevent inadvertent intravascular injection. The solution should be injected well within the body of a relatively large muscle, such as the gluteus maximus.

Intravenous administration — To prepare the solution, add 4.8 ml of sterile water for injection USP to the 500-mg vial or 9.6 ml to the 1-g vial; then shake well, withdraw the contents of the vial, and dilute with 5% dextrose injection USP to a final volume of 50 ml. The reconstituted solution can also be diluted with other appropriate solutions (see package insert), and the final concentration can vary from 5 to 100 mg/ml. Administer each dose over a period of 15–30 min by infusion; when using a Y-type set or piggyback arrangement, temporarily discontinue administration of any other solution (amdinocillin should not be mixed with other drugs).

Duration of therapy — Administration should generally be continued for at least 2 days after signs and symptoms of infection have disappeared; duration of therapy is usually 7–10 days, but may be longer if the infection is complicated

Combination therapy — For the treatment of more severe urinary tract infections, the synergistic combination of amdinocillin and another beta-lactam antibiotic may be considered

Patients with renal impairment — If the creatinine clearance is less than 30 ml/min, the dosage should be limited to 10 mg/kg tid or qid

WARNINGS/PRECAUTIONS

Hypersensitivity — Serious, occasionally fatal anaphylactic reactions have occurred in patients receiving penicillin; use with caution in patients with a history of allergy, particularly if they have demonstrated hypersensitivity to a number of substances. If an allergic reaction occurs, amdinocillin should be discontinued; for the treatment of serious reactions, give epinephrine, oxygen, and IV corticosteroids and take appropriate measures (eg, intubation) to ensure adequate pulmonary function.

Prolonged therapy — Evaluate hematopoietic, renal, and hepatic function periodically during long-term therapy; bear in mind that superinfection may occur with prolonged use

Effect on fertility — No evidence of impaired fertility has been seen in rats given daily up to 7.5 times the recommended human dose

ADVERSE REACTIONS

Frequent reactions (incidence ≥ 1%) are printed in *italics*

Hematological — *Eosinophilia and thrombocytosis (5%); anemia, neutropenia, and leukopenia (1%);* thrombocytopenia

Hepatic — *Elevated SGOT and serum alkaline phosphatase levels (5%),* elevated SGPT and serum bilirubin levels

Gastrointestinal	*Diarrhea and nausea (1%)*, vomiting
Central nervous system	*Dizziness (1%)*, drowsiness, lethargy
Dermatological	*Allergic rash (1%)*, pruritus, urticaria
Other	*Thrombophlebitis (1%)*, tenderness and/or pain at injection site, elevated blood pressure, vaginitis

OVERDOSAGE

Signs and symptoms	Neuromuscular hypersensitivity, convulsive seizures
Treatment	If it is necessary to enhance removal of the drug from the blood, hemodialysis can be performed

DRUG INTERACTIONS

Other beta-lactam antibiotics	△ Bactericidal effect
Probenecid	△ Serum amdinocillin level

ALTERED LABORATORY VALUES

Blood/serum values	△ SGOT △ Alkaline phosphatase

No clinically significant alterations in urinary values occur at therapeutic dosages

---

USE IN CHILDREN

Safety and effectiveness for use in children under 12 yr of age have not been established

USE IN PREGNANT AND NURSING WOMEN

Pregnancy Category B: reproduction studies in rats and mice given up to 7.5 times the recommended human dose have shown no evidence of harm to the fetus; however, no adequate, well-controlled studies have been done in pregnant women. Low concentrations of amdinocillin are found in cord blood and amniotic fluid. Use during pregnancy only if clearly needed. In limited, single-dose studies, amdinocillin has not been detected in human milk; use with caution in nursing mothers.

PENICILLINS

CYCLAPEN-W (cyclacillin) Wyeth   Rx

Tablets: 250, 500 mg **Suspension (per 5 ml):** 125, 250 mg (100, 150, 200 ml)

INDICATIONS

Tonsillitis and pharyngitis caused by susceptible strains of Group A beta-hemolytic streptococci

Mild or moderate bronchitis and pneumonia caused by susceptible strains of *Streptococcus pneumoniae*

Otitis media caused by susceptible strains of *Streptococcus pneumoniae, Hemophilus influenzae,* and Group A beta-hemolytic streptococci

Skin and skin structure infections caused by susceptible strains of Group A beta-hemolytic streptococci and non-penicillinase-producing staphylococci

Chronic bronchitis and pneumonia caused by susceptible strains of *Streptococcus pneumoniae*
Acute exacerbations of chronic bronchitis caused by susceptible strains of *Hemophilus influenzae*

Urinary tract infections caused by susceptible strains of *Escherichia coli* and *Proteus mirabilis*

ORAL DOSAGE

Adult: 250 mg qid, given in equally spaced doses
Child (< 20 kg): 125 mg tid, given in equally spaced doses
Child (> 20 kg): 250 mg tid, given in equally spaced doses

Adult: 250 mg qid, given in equally spaced doses
Child: 50 mg/kg/day, given in 4 equally spaced doses

Adult: 250–500 mg, depending on severity, qid, given in equally spaced doses
Child: 50–100 mg/kg/day, depending on severity, given in equally spaced doses

Adult: 250–500 mg, depending on severity, qid, given in equally spaced doses
Child: 50–100 mg/kg/day, depending on severity, given in 3 equally spaced doses

Adult: 500 mg qid, given in equally spaced doses
Child: 100 mg/kg/day, given in 4 equally spaced doses

Adult: 500 mg qid, given in equally spaced doses
Child: 100 mg/kg/day, given in equally spaced doses

CONTRAINDICATIONS

Hypersensitivity to penicillins

COMPENDIUM OF DRUG THERAPY

ADMINISTRATION/DOSAGE ADJUSTMENTS

Cultures and susceptibility tests	Should be initiated prior to therapy and performed periodically during treatment to monitor its effectiveness and bacterial susceptibility
Duration of treatment	Continue treatment for at least 48–72 h after patient has become asymptomatic or bacteria have been eradicated; beta-hemolytic streptococcal infections should be treated for at least 10 days to prevent rheumatic fever and glomerulonephritis
Patients with renal impairment	Administer full doses q12h when creatinine clearance rate (CCr) = 30–50 ml/min, q18h when CCr = 15–30 ml/min, or q24h when CCr = 10–15 ml/min; if CCr $\leq$ 10 ml/min or serum creatinine level $\geq$ 10 mg/dl, determine dosage and frequency by serum drug levels

WARNINGS/PRECAUTIONS

Hypersensitivity	Serious and occasionally fatal anaphylactoid reactions may occur, most likely in patients with a history of sensitivity to multiple allergens, necessitating immediate emergency treatment with epinephrine, oxygen, IV corticosteroids, and airway management, including intubation; use with caution in patients who have experienced allergic reactions to cephalosporins
Superinfection	Overgrowth of nonsusceptible organisms may occur
Chronic urinary tract infection	Requires frequent bacteriological and clinical appraisal during therapy, and possibly for several months afterward

ADVERSE REACTIONS

Frequent reactions (incidence $\geq$ 1%) are printed in *italics*

Gastrointestinal	*Diarrhea (5%), nausea and vomiting (2%)*, abdominal pain
Hypersensitivity	*Skin rash (1.7%)*, urticaria
Hematological	Anemia, thrombocytopenia, thrombocytopenic purpura, leukopenia, neutropenia, eosinophilia
Central nervous system	Headache, dizziness
Other	Vaginitis

OVERDOSAGE

Signs and symptoms	See ADVERSE REACTIONS
Treatment	Discontinue medication; treat symptomatically

DRUG INTERACTIONS

No clinically significant drug interactions have been observed

ALTERED LABORATORY VALUES

Blood/serum values	⇧ SGOT

No clinically significant alterations in urinary values occur at therapeutic dosages

---

USE IN CHILDREN
See INDICATIONS AND ORAL DOSAGE; do not exceed adult dose or use in children under 2 mo of age

USE IN PREGNANT AND NURSING WOMEN
Pregnancy Category B: safety for use during pregnancy not established. Cyclacillin may or may not be excreted in breast milk; use with caution in nursing mothers.

PENICILLINS

GEOCILLIN (carbenicillin indanyl sodium) Roerig　　Rx

Tablets: carbenicillin indanyl sodium equivalent to 382 mg carbenicillin

INDICATIONS

Urinary tract infections and asymptomatic bacteriuria caused by susceptible strains of *Escherichia coli, Proteus mirabilis, P morgani, P rettgeri, P vulgaris,* and *Enterobacter*

Urinary tract infections caused by susceptible strains of *Pseudomonas* and *Streptococcus fecalis*

Prostatitis caused by susceptible strains of *Escherichia coli, Proteus mirabilis, Enterobacter,* and *Streptococcus fecalis*

ORAL DOSAGE

Adult: 1–2 tabs qid

Adult: 2 tabs qid

GEOCILLIN ■ GEOPEN

CONTRAINDICATIONS

Hypersensitivity to penicillins

WARNINGS/PRECAUTIONS

Hypersensitivity	Serious and occasionally fatal anaphylactoid reactions may occur, most likely in patients with a history of sensitivity to multiple allergens, and may necessitate immediate emergency treatment with epinephrine, oxygen, IV corticosteroids, and airway management, including intubation; use with caution in patients who have experienced allergic reactions to cephalosporins
Long-term therapy	Perform blood, renal, and hepatic studies periodically
Superinfection	Overgrowth of nonsusceptible organisms may occur
Patients with renal impairment	Patients with severe renal insufficiency (creatinine clearance < 10 ml/min) will not achieve therapeutic urine levels of carbenicillin

ADVERSE REACTIONS

Gastrointestinal	Nausea, vomiting, diarrhea, flatulence, dry mouth, furry tongue, abdominal cramps
Hypersensitivity	Skin rash, urticaria, pruritus
Hematological	Anemia, thrombocytopenia, leukopenia, neutropenia, eosinophilia
Other	Vaginitis

OVERDOSAGE

Signs and symptoms	See ADVERSE REACTIONS
Treatment	Discontinue medication; treat symptomatically

DRUG INTERACTIONS

Probenecid	△ Carbenicillin blood level and/or toxicity ▽ Urine level

ALTERED LABORATORY VALUES

Blood/serum values	△ SGOT △ SGPT

No clinically significant alterations in urinary values occur at therapeutic dosages

---

USE IN CHILDREN	USE IN PREGNANT AND NURSING WOMEN
Safety for use in children has not been established	Safety for use during pregnancy has not been established. Carbenicillin is excreted in human milk; use with caution in nursing mothers.

PENICILLINS

GEOPEN (carbenicillin disodium) Roerig   Rx

Vials: 1, 2, 5, g   **Piggyback units:** 2, 5, 10 g   **Bulk pharmacy package:** 30 g

INDICATIONS	PARENTERAL DOSAGE
Urinary tract infections caused by susceptible strains of *Pseudomonas aeruginosa, Enterobacter,* and *Streptococcus fecalis*	**Adult:** for uncomplicated infections, 1–2 g IM or IV q6h; for serious infections, 200 mg/kg/day by IV drip **Child:** 50–200 mg/kg/day IM or IV, given in divided doses q4–6h
Urinary tract infections caused by susceptible strains of *Proteus* and *Escherichia coli*	**Adult:** same as above **Child:** 50–100 mg/kg/day IM or IV, given in divided doses q4–6h
Severe systemic infections, septicemia, and **respiratory and soft tissue infections** caused by susceptible strains of *Pseudomonas aeruginosa* and anaerobic bacteria	**Adult:** 400–500 mg/kg/day IV, given in divided doses or by continuous infusion **Child:** same as adult
Severe systemic infections, septicemia, and **respiratory and soft tissue infections** caused by susceptible strains of *Proteus* and *Escherichia coli*	**Adult:** 300–400 mg/kg/day IV, given in divided doses or by continuous infusion **Child:** 300–400 mg/kg/day IM or IV, given in divided doses
Meningitis caused by susceptible strains of *Hemophilus influenzae* and *Streptococcus penumoniae*	**Adult:** 400–500 mg/kg/day IV, given in divided doses or by continuous infusion **Child:** same as adult

COMPENDIUM OF DRUG THERAPY

GEOPEN

Gonorrhea, acute uncomplicated anogenital and urethral infections caused by susceptible strains of *Neisseria gonorrhoeae*	**Adult:** 4 g in a single IM injection divided between two sites (with 1 g probenecid orally 30 min prior to injection)
Neonatal sepsis caused by susceptible strains of *Pseudomonas aeruginosa, Proteus, Escherichia coli, Hemophilus influenzae,* and *Streptococcus pneumoniae*	**Infant (< 2 kg):** 100 mg/kg IM or IV to start, followed by 75 mg/kg IM or IV q8h during 1st wk of life and 100 mg/kg IM or IV q6h thereafter[1] **Infant (> 2 kg):** 100 mg/kg IM or IV to start, followed by 75 mg/kg IM or IV q6h during first 3 days of life and 100 mg/kg IM or IV q6h thereafter[1]

CONTRAINDICATIONS

Hypersensitivity to penicillins

ADMINISTRATION/DOSAGE ADJUSTMENTS

Intravenous infusion	Administer as slowly as possible to avoid vein irritation; to reduce irritation further, dilute to approximately 1 g/20 ml or more
Intramuscular administration	Inject not more than 2 g at once, well within the body of a relatively large muscle
Serious urinary tract and systemic infections	Intravenous therapy in higher doses (up to 40 g/day) may be required
Patients with renal impairment	Administer 2 g IV q8–12h to adults with a creatinine clearance rate < 5 ml/min
Dialysis patients	Administer 2 g IV q6h to adults during peritoneal dialysis or 2 g IV q4h to adults receiving hemodialysis

WARNINGS/PRECAUTIONS

Hypersensitivity	Serious and occasionally fatal anaphylactoid reactions may occur, most likely in patients with a history of sensitivity to multiple allergens; use with caution in patients who have experienced allergic reactions to cephalosporins. If an allergic reaction occurs, institute appropriate therapy and consider discontinuing carbenicillin. Serious reactions may require emergency treatment with epinephrine, oxygen, and IV corticosteroids.
Long-term therapy	Perform blood, renal, and hepatic studies periodically
Superinfection	May result from emergence of resistant organisms, such as *Klebsiella* and *Serratia*
Bleeding abnormalities	May occur in patients with renal impairment; discontinue use of carbenicillin and institute appropriate therapy
Sodium overload	May occur (each gram contains 4.7 mEq of sodium); monitor electrolytes and cardiac status periodically in patients who require sodium restriction (eg, cardiac patients)
Hypokalemia	May occur with high doses; monitor serum potassium level periodically, and institute appropriate corrective measures, as needed
Suspected syphilitic lesions	If syphilis is suspected, perform dark-field examination before instituting therapy, and perform serology testing monthly for at least 4 mo

ADVERSE REACTIONS

Hypersensitivity	Skin rash, pruritus, urticaria, drug fever, anaphylaxis (see WARNINGS/PRECAUTIONS)
Gastrointestinal	Nausea
Hematological	Anemia, thrombocytopenia, leukopenia, neutropenia, eosinophilia
Central nervous system	Convulsions or neuromuscular irritability (with excessively high serum levels)
Other	Pain and (rarely) induration at injection site after IM and IV administration; vein irritation and phlebitis

OVERDOSAGE

Signs and symptoms	See ADVERSE REACTIONS
Treatment	Discontinue medication; treat symptomatically

DRUG INTERACTIONS

Probenecid	△ Carbenicillin blood level and/or toxicity ▽ Urine level

ALTERED LABORATORY VALUES

Blood/serum values	△ SGOT △ SGPT

No clinically significant alterations in urinary values occur at therapeutic dosages

USE IN CHILDREN	USE IN PREGNANT AND NURSING WOMEN
See INDICATIONS and PARENTERAL DOSAGE	Safety for use during pregnancy has not been established. Carbenicillin is excreted in human milk; use with caution in nursing mothers.

[1] Neonatal doses may be given IM or by 15-min IV infusion

PENICILLINS

LAROTID (amoxicillin) Beecham — Rx

Capsules: 250, 500 mg **Suspension (per 5 ml):** 125, 250 mg after reconstitution (5, 80, 100, 150 ml) **Pediatric drops:** 50 mg/ml after reconstitution (15 ml)

INDICATIONS	ORAL DOSAGE
Ear, nose, and throat infections caused by susceptible strains of streptococci, *Streptococcus pneumoniae,* nonpenicillinase-producing staphylococci, and *Hemophilus influenzae* **Genitourinary tract infections** caused by susceptible strains of *Escherichia coli, Proteus mirabilis,* and *Streptococcus fecalis* **Skin and soft tissue infections** caused by susceptible strains of streptococci, staphylococci, and *Escherichia coli*	**Adult:** 250 mg q8h; for infections that are severe or are caused by less susceptible organisms, 500 mg q8h **Infant (< 6 kg):** 37.5 mg (0.75 ml of the drops) q8h **Infant (6–7 kg):** 50 mg (1 ml of the drops) q8h **Infant (8 kg):** 62.5 mg (1.25 ml of the drops) q8h **Infant and child (8–20 kg):** 20 mg/kg/day, given in 3 divided doses q8h; for infections that are severe or are caused by less susceptible organisms, 40 mg/kg/day, given in 3 divided doses q8h **Child (≥ 20 kg):** same as adult
Lower respiratory tract infections caused by susceptible strains of streptococci, *Streptococcus pneumoniae,* nonpenicillinase-producing staphylococci, and *Hemophilus influenzae*	**Adult:** 500 mg q8h **Infant (< 6 kg):** 62.5 mg (1.25 ml of the drops) q8h **Infant (6–7 kg):** 87.5 mg (1.75 ml of the drops) q8h **Infant (8 kg):** 112.5 mg (2.25 ml of the drops) q8h **Infant and child (8–20 kg):** 40 mg/kg/day, given in 3 divided doses q8h **Child (≥ 20 kg):** same as adult
Gonorrhea, acute uncomplicated anogenital and urethral infections caused by *Neisseria gonorrhoeae*	**Adult:** 3 g, given in a single dose **Prepuberal child (≥ 2 yr):** 50 mg/kg, given in a single dose with 25 mg/kg of probenecid

CONTRAINDICATIONS

Hypersensitivity to penicillins

ADMINISTRATION/DOSAGE ADJUSTMENTS

Duration of treatment	Continue treatment for at least 48–72 h after patient becomes asymptomatic or bacteria have been eradicated; beta-hemolytic streptococcal infections should be treated for at least 10 days to prevent rheumatic fever and glomerulonephritis
Use of oral suspension in children	After reconstitution, place required dose directly on child's tongue for swallowing or add to formula, milk, fruit juice, water, ginger ale, or cold drinks; infants weighing 8 kg (18 lb) or less should be given pediatric drops

WARNINGS/PRECAUTIONS

Hypersensitivity	Serious and occasionally fatal anaphylactoid reactions may occur, most likely in patients with a history of sensitivity to multiple allergens. Urticaria, other skin rashes, and serum sickness-like reactions may be controlled with antihistamines and, if necessary, systemic corticosteroids. Drug should be discontinued unless infection is life-threatening and amenable only to amoxicillin. Severe reactions may necessitate emergency measures, such as immediate use of epinephrine, oxygen, IV corticosteroids, and airway management, including intubation; use with caution in patients who have experienced allergic reactions to cephalosporins.
Long-term therapy	Perform blood, renal, and hepatic studies periodically
Superinfection	Overgrowth of nonsusceptible organisms, including fungi, may occur
Suspected syphilitic lesions	If syphilis is suspected, perform dark-field examination before instituting therapy, and perform serology testing monthly for at least 4 mo
Chronic urinary tract infection	Requires frequent bacteriological and clinical appraisal during therapy, and possibly for several months afterward; do not use doses smaller than those recommended above

ADVERSE REACTIONS

Gastrointestinal	Nausea, vomiting, diarrhea
Hypersensitivity	Erythematous maculopapular rash, urticaria, and other serum sickness-like reactions; anaphylaxis (see WARNINGS/PRECAUTIONS)
Hematological	Anemia, thrombocytopenia, thrombocytopenic purpura, eosinophilia, leukopenia, agranulocytosis

OVERDOSAGE

Signs and symptoms	See ADVERSE REACTIONS
Treatment	Discontinue medication; treat symptomatically

DRUG INTERACTIONS

Probenecid	△ Amoxicillin blood level and/or toxicity

ALTERED LABORATORY VALUES

Blood/serum values	△ SGOT

No clinically significant alterations in urinary values occur at therapeutic dosages

---

USE IN CHILDREN

See INDICATIONS and ORAL DOSAGE; do not exceed adult dose

USE IN PREGNANT AND NURSING WOMEN

Safety for use during pregnancy has not been established. No clinical problems have been documented in nursing mothers.

PENICILLINS

LEDERCILLIN VK (penicillin V potassium) Lederle   Rx

Tablets: 250, 500 mg (400,000, 800,000 units)   **Solution (per 5 ml):** 125, 250 mg (200,000, 400,000 units) after reconstitution (100, 150, 200 ml)

INDICATIONS

Mild to moderately severe upper respiratory tract infections, scarlet fever, and mild erysipelas caused by penicillin G-sensitive streptococci (particularly those in groups A, C, H, G, L, and M) in the absence of bacteremia

Otitis media and other mild to moderately severe respiratory tract infections caused by *Streptococcus pneumoniae*

Mild skin and soft tissue infections caused by penicillin G-sensitive staphylococci

Mild to moderately severe fusospirochetosis (Vincent's gingivitis and pharyngitis)

Continuous prophylaxis of rheumatic fever and/or chorea

Prevention of bacterial endocarditis in patients with congenital heart disease or rheumatic or other acquired valvular heart disease who are undergoing dental procedures or upper respiratory tract surgery

ORAL DOSAGE

Adult: 200,000–500,000 units q6–8h for 10 days
Child (< 12 yr): 25,000–90,000 units/kg/day, given in 3–6 divided doses
Child (≥ 12 yr): same as adult

Adult: 400,000–500,000 units q6h until patient has been afebrile for at least 2 days
Child (< 12 yr): 25,000–90,000 units/kg/day, given in 3–6 divided doses
Child (≥ 12 yr): same as adult

Adult: 400,000–500,000 units q6–8h
Child (< 12 yr): 25,000–90,000 units/kg/day, given in 3–6 divided doses
Child (≥ 12 yr): same as adult

Adult: 200,000–250,000 units bid
Child: 25,000–90,000 units/kg/day, given in 3–6 divided doses

Adult and child (> 60 lb): 3,200,000 units (2 g) ½–1 h prior to dental procedure or upper respiratory tract surgery, followed by 800,000 units (500 mg) q6h for 8 doses, *or* combined regimen of 1 million units IM aqueous crystalline penicillin G mixed with 600,000 units procaine penicillin G ½–1 h prior to procedure, followed by 800,000 units (500 mg) oral penicillin V q6h for 8 doses
Child (< 60 lb): 1,600,000 units (1 g) ½–1 h prior to dental procedure or upper respiratory tract surgery, followed by 400,000 units (250 mg) q6h for 8 doses, *or* combined regimen of 30,000 units/kg IM aqueous crystalline penicillin G mixed with 600,000 units procaine penicillin G ½–1 h prior to procedure, followed by 400,000 units (250 mg) q6h for 8 doses

CONTRAINDICATIONS

Hypersensitivity to penicillins

LEDERCILLIN VK ■ MEZLIN

ADMINISTRATION/DOSAGE ADJUSTMENTS

Duration of treatment for streptococcal infections	Therapy should be continued for a minimum of 10 days to prevent sequelae of streptococcal disease; cultures should be taken on completion of therapy to determine whether streptococci have been eradicated
Patients receiving continuous penicillin prophylaxis to prevent recurrence of rheumatic fever	May harbor alpha-hemolytic streptococci that are relatively resistant to penicillin; prophylactic antibiotics other than penicillin may be given to these patients (in addition to their continuous rheumatic fever prophylactic regimen) prior to dental or surgical procedures

WARNINGS/PRECAUTIONS

Hypersensitivity	Serious and occasionally fatal anaphylactoid reactions may occur, most likely in patients with a history of sensitivity to multiple allergens; use with caution in patients who have a history of significant allergies and/or asthma or have experienced allergic reactions to cephalosporins. If an allergic reaction occurs, discontinue medication and employ other agents, eg, epinephrine, antihistamines, and/or corticosteroids, as needed.
Superinfection	Overgrowth of nonsusceptible microorganisms, including fungi, may occur with prolonged use
Impaired absorption	Oral administration should not be relied on in patients with severe illness, nausea, vomiting, gastric dilatation, cardiospasm, or intestinal hypermotility
Inappropriate uses	Oral penicillin V should not be used for treatment during the acute stages of severe pneumonia, empyema, bacteremia, pericarditis, meningitis, or septic arthritis, or for prophylaxis preceding genitourinary instrumentation or surgery, lower-intestinal-tract surgery, sigmoidoscopy, or childbirth

ADVERSE REACTIONS

The most frequent reactions, regardless of incidence, are printed in *italics*

Gastrointestinal	*Nausea, vomiting, epigastric distress, diarrhea, black hairy tongue*
Hypersensitivity	*Skin eruptions, ranging from maculopapular rash to exfoliative dermatitis, urticaria, and other serum sickness-like reactions; fever; eosinophilia; laryngeal edema; anaphylaxis* (see WARNINGS/PRECAUTIONS)
Hematological	Hemolytic anemia, leukopenia, thrombocytopenia (usually only with high parenteral doses)
Other	Neuropathy and nephropathy (usually only with high parenteral doses)

OVERDOSAGE

Signs and symptoms	See ADVERSE REACTIONS
Treatment	Discontinue medication; treat symptomatically

DRUG INTERACTIONS

Probenecid	⇧ penicillin blood level and/or toxicity

ALTERED LABORATORY VALUES

No clinically significant alterations in blood/serum or urinary values occur at therapeutic dosages

---

USE IN CHILDREN
See INDICATIONS and ORAL DOSAGE

USE IN PREGNANT AND NURSING WOMEN
While no teratogenic effects have been reported with this drug, the benefit/risk ratio should be taken into consideration before prescribing for pregnant women. No clinical problems have been documented in nursing mothers.

PENICILLINS

MEZLIN (mezlocillin sodium) Miles Pharmaceuticals Rx

Vials: 1, 2, 3, 4 g **Infusion bottles:** 2, 3, 4 g

INDICATIONS

Lower respiratory tract infections, including pneumonia and lung abscess, caused by susceptible strains of *Hemophilus influenzae, Klebsiella* (including *K pneumoniae*), *Proteus mirabilis, Pseudomonas* (including *P aeruginosa*), *Escherichia coli,* and *Bacteroides* (including *B fragilis*)

Intraabdominal infections, including acute cholecystitis, cholangitis, peritonitis, hepatic abscess, and intraabdominal abscess, caused by susceptible strains of *Escherichia coli, Proteus mirabilis, Klebsiella, Pseudomonas, Streptococcus fecalis, Bacteroides, Peptococcus,* and *Peptostreptococcus*

Gynecological infections, including endometritis, pelvic cellulitis, and pelvic inflammatory disease, associated with susceptible strains of *Neisseria gonorrhoeae, Peptococcus, Peptostreptococcus, Bacteroides, Escherichia coli, Proteus mirabilis, Klebsiella,* and *Enterobacter*

Skin and skin structure infections caused by susceptible strains of *Streptococcus fecalis, Escherichia coli, Proteus mirabilis,* indole-positive *Proteus, Proteus vulgaris, Providencia rettgeri, Klebsiella, Enterobacter, Pseudomonas, Peptococcus,* and *Bacteroides*

Septicemia, including bacteremia, caused by susceptible strains of *Escherichia coli, Klebsiella, Enterobacter, Pseudomonas, Peptococcus,* and *Bacteroides*

PARENTERAL DOSAGE

Adult: 225–300 mg/kg/day IV, given in equally divided doses q4–6h (usual dosage: 4 g q6h or 3 g q4h)

Newborn (≤ 7 days): 75 mg/kg IM or IV, infused over a period of 30 min, q12h

Newborn (8 days to 1 mo): 75 mg/kg IM or IV, infused over a period of 30 min, q8h if body weight ≤ 2 kg or q6h if body weight > 2 kg

Infant (> 1 mo) and child (< 12 yr): 50 mg/kg IM or IV, infused over a period of 30 min, q4h

Urinary tract infections caused by susceptible strains of *Escherichia coli*, *Proteus mirabilis*, indole-positive *Proteus*, *Morganella morganii*, *Klebsiella*, *Enterobacter*, *Serratia*, *Pseudomonas*, and *Streptococcus fecalis*

Adult: for uncomplicated infections, 100–125 mg/kg/day IM or IV, given in 4 equally divided doses q6h (usual dosage: 1.5–2 g q6h); for complicated infections, 150–200 mg/kg/day IV, given in 4 equally divided doses q6h (usual dosage: 3 g q6h)

Newborn, infant, and child: same as pediatric dosages above

CONTRAINDICATIONS

Hypersensitivity to penicillins

ADMINISTRATION/DOSAGE ADJUSTMENTS

Intramuscular administration	Reconstitute each gram of mezlocillin by shaking vigorously with 3–4 ml of Sterile Water for Injection or 0.5% or 1% lidocaine without epinephrine. Inject not more than 2 g well within the body of a relatively large muscle, such as the gluteus maximus, over a period of 12–15 s to minimize patient discomfort.
Intravenous administration	Reconstitute each gram of mezlocillin by shaking vigorously with at least 10 ml of Sterile Water for Injection, 5% Dextrose Injection, or 0.9% Sodium Chloride Injection; dilute further to desired volume (50–100 ml) with an appropriate IV solution. Inject the reconstituted solution over a 30-min period by either direct infusion or through a Y-type infusion set which may already be in place; discontinue administration of any other solutions during the infusion if using a Y-type set or the "piggy-back" method. The reconstituted solution may also be injected directly into a vein or into intravenous tubing over a period of 3–5 min; to minimize venous irritation, the concentration of the drug should not exceed 10%.
Life-threatening infections	May be treated with up to 4 g IV q4h or 350 mg/kg/day IV, but the total daily dose should usually not exceed 24 g; mezlocillin has been used effectively in combination with an aminoglycoside antibiotic for the treatment of life-threatening infections caused by *Pseudomonas aeruginosa*
Duration of therapy	Depends upon the severity of the infection, but therapy should usually continue for at least 2 days after the signs and symptoms of infection disappear (usual duration: 7–10 days); in difficult, complicated infections, more prolonged therapy may be needed
Streptococcal infections (including those caused by Group A beta-hemolytic streptococci and *Streptococcus pneumoniae*)	Although mezlocillin has been shown to be effective for the treatment of these infections, they are usually treated with narrower-spectrum penicillins; antibiotic therapy for Group A beta-hemolytic streptococcal infections should be continued for at least 10 days to reduce the risk of rheumatic fever or glomerulonephritis
Deep-seated infections with abscess formation	Appropriate surgical drainage should be performed in conjunction with antimicrobial therapy
Acute, uncomplicated gonococcal urethritis	Is usually treated with a single IM or IV dose of 1–2 g; 1 g of probenecid may be given orally at the time of dosing or up to 1/2 h before
Patients with impaired renal function	If creatinine clearance rate (CCr) > 30 ml/min, administer the usual recommended dosage; if CCr = 10–30 ml/min, administer 1.5 g q8h for uncomplicated urinary tract infections, 1.5 g q6h for complicated urinary tract infections, 3 g q8h for serious systemic infections, or 3 g q6h for life-threatening infections; if CCr < 10 ml/min, administer 1.5 g q8h for uncomplicated or complicated urinary tract infections, 2 g q8h for serious systemic infections, or 2 g q6h for life-threatening infections. For patients with serious systemic infections undergoing hemodialysis for renal failure, administer 3–4 g after each dialysis treatment and then q12h; for patients undergoing peritoneal dialysis, administer 3 g q12h. For patients with renal failure and hepatic insufficiency, measure mezlocillin serum levels for additional guidance in adjusting dosage.
Cultures and susceptibility tests	Should be performed prior to treatment to identify the causative organism and determine its susceptibility to mezlocillin and then periodically during treatment to monitor for effectiveness and for possible development of bacterial resistance. Therapy can be initiated before test results are known; in certain severe infections, mezlocillin may be given in combination with an aminoglycoside or a cephalosporin antibiotic as initial therapy and adjusted when test results become available.
Febrile episodes in immunosuppressed patients with granulocytopenia	Mezlocillin should be combined with an aminoglycoside or a cephalosporin antibiotic

WARNINGS/PRECAUTIONS

Hypersensitivity	Serious and occasionally fatal anaphylactoid reactions may occur, most likely in patients with a history of sensitivity to multiple allergens, and require immediate emergency treatment with epinephrine, oxygen, and IV corticosteroids, and airway management, including intubation; use with caution in patients who have experienced some form of allergy, especially to cephalosporins or other drugs. If an allergic reaction occurs during mezlocillin therapy, discontinue use.
Long-term therapy	Perform blood, renal, and hepatic studies periodically during prolonged therapy
Acute interstitial nephritis	May occur (rarely)
Bleeding abnormalities	May occur (rarely), particularly in patients with severe renal impairment receiving maximum doses, and have been associated with abnormalities of coagulation tests, such as clotting time, platelet aggregation, and prothrombin time

MEZLIN ■ OMNIPEN

Hypokalemia	May occur (rarely), particularly in patients with fluid and electrolyte imbalances; monitor serum potassium level periodically during prolonged therapy
Sodium content	Each gram of mezlocillin contains 42.6 mg (1.85 mEq) of sodium; this should be considered when treating patients on salt-restricted diets
Superinfection	Overgrowth of nonsusceptible organisms may occur with prolonged use
Patients with venereal disease	Patients with gonorrhea should also be examined for syphilis prior to treatment, since antimicrobial therapy for gonorrhea may mask or delay the symptoms of incubating syphilis. Obtain specimens for dark-field examination from any suspected primary syphilitic lesion and perform other serologic tests before treatment, as well as follow-up tests 3 mo after treatment.

ADVERSE REACTIONS

Hypersensitivity	Skin rash, pruritus, urticaria, drug fever, anaphylactic reactions, acute interstitial nephritis
Gastrointestinal	Abnormal taste sensation, nausea, vomiting, diarrhea
Hematological	Thrombocytopenia, leukopenia, neutropenia, eosinophilia, reduction of hemoglobin or hematocrit
Central nervous system and neuromuscular	Convulsive seizures, neuromuscular hyperirritability
Local	Thrombophlebitis (with IV use), pain (with IM use)

OVERDOSAGE

Signs and symptoms	Neuromuscular hyperirritability, convulsive seizures
Treatment	Hemodialysis (if necessary) will help remove mezlocillin from the circulation

DRUG INTERACTIONS

Probenecid	△ Mezlocillin serum level and half-life

ALTERED LABORATORY VALUES

Blood/serum values	△ SGOT △ SGPT △ Alkaline phosphatase △ Bilirubin △ Creatinine and/or BUN ▽ Potassium
Urinary values	+ Protein (with sulfosalicylic acid and boiling test, acetic acid test, biuret reaction, and nitric acid test)

USE IN CHILDREN
See INDICATIONS and PARENTERAL DOSAGE; data on safety and effectiveness for infants and children with documented serious infection are limited

USE IN PREGNANT AND NURSING WOMEN
Pregnancy Category B: use during pregnancy only if clearly needed. Reproductive studies in rats and mice at doses up to twice the human dose have shown no evidence of impaired fertility or fetal harm; no adequate, well-controlled studies have been done in pregnant women. Mezlocillin is found in low concentrations in cord blood, amniotic fluid, and human milk; use with caution in nursing mothers.

PENICILLINS

OMNIPEN (ampicillin) Wyeth   Rx

Capsules: 250, 500 mg **Suspension (per 5 ml):** 125, 250 mg after reconstitution **Pediatric drops:** 100 mg/ml after reconstitution

OMNIPEN-N (ampicillin sodium) Wyeth   Rx

Vials: 125, 250, 500 mg; 1, 2 g **Piggyback vials:** 500 mg; 1, 2 g **Pharmacy bulk package:** 10 g

INDICATIONS	ORAL DOSAGE[1]	PARENTERAL DOSAGE[1]
Ear, nose, throat, and lower respiratory tract infections caused by susceptible strains of streptococci, *Streptococcus pneumoniae*, and *nonpenicillinase*-producing staphylococci **Upper and lower respiratory tract infections** caused by susceptible strains of *Hemophilus influenzae*	**Adult and child (> 20 kg):** 250 mg q6h **Child (< 20 kg):** 50 mg/kg/day, given in equally divided doses q6h (for capsules and drops) or q6–8h (for suspension)	**Adult and child (> 40 kg):** 250–500 mg IM or IV q6h **Child (< 40 kg):** 25–50 mg/kg/day IM or IV, given in equally divided doses q6h

COMPENDIUM OF DRUG THERAPY

OMNIPEN

Indication	Oral	Parenteral
Gastrointestinal and genitourinary tract infections caused by susceptible strains of *Shigella, Salmonella* (including *S typhosa*), *Escherichia coli, Proteus mirabilis,* and enterococci	**Adult and child ($>$ 20 kg):** 500 mg q6h **Child ($<$ 20 kg):** 100 mg/kg/day, given in equally divided doses q6h (for capsules and drops) or q6–8h (for suspension)	**Adult and child ($>$ 40 kg):** 500 mg IM or IV q6h **Child ($<$ 40 kg):** 50 mg/kg/day IM or IV, given in equally divided doses q6h
Urethral, cervical, rectal, and pharyngeal infections caused by *Neisseria gonorrhoeae*	**Adult:** 3.5 g, given in a single dose simultaneously with 1 g probenecid	—
Urethritis in males caused by *Neisseria gonorrhoeae*	**Adult:** 3.5 g, given in a single dose simultaneously with 1 g probenecid	**Adult:** 500 mg IM bid for 1 day
Meningitis caused by *Neisseria meningitidis* and *Hemophilus influenzae*	—	**Adult:** 8–14 g/day by IV drip to start, followed by IM injection q3–4h **Child:** 100–200 mg/kg/day by IV drip to start, followed by IM injection q3–4h
Prevention of bacterial endocarditis in patients who have prosthetic heart valves or other particularly high risk conditions and are undergoing dental procedures or upper respiratory tract surgery[2]	—	**Adult and child ($>$ 40 kg):** 1–2 g IM or IV with 1.5 mg/kg of gentamicin IM or IV 30 min before the procedure; repeat 8 h later or give 1 g of oral penicillin V 6 h later **Child ($<$ 27 kg):** 50 mg/kg IM or IV with 2 mg/kg of gentamicin IM or IV 30 min before the procedure; repeat 8 h later or give 500 mg of oral penicillin V 6 h later **Child (27–40 kg):** 50 mg/kg IM or IV with 2 mg/kg of gentamicin IM or IV 30 min before the procedure; repeat 8 h later or give 1 g of oral penicillin V 6 h later
Prevention of bacterial endocarditis in patients at risk who are undergoing GI or genitourinary tract surgery or instrumentation[2]	—	**Adult and child ($>$ 40 kg):** 2 g IM or IV with 1.5 mg/kg of gentamicin IM or IV 30 min before the procedure; doses may be repeated 8 h later **Child ($<$ 40 kg):** 50 mg/kg IM or IV with 2 mg/kg of gentamicin 30 min before the procedure; doses may be repeated 8 h later

CONTRAINDICATIONS

Hypersensitivity to penicillins

ADMINISTRATION/DOSAGE ADJUSTMENTS

Use of pediatric drops	Drop administration is especially suitable for newborns (premature and full-term) and small infants; older children and adults are preferably given Omnipen capsules or oral suspension (see ORAL DOSAGE, above). For respiratory tract infections, give 50 mg/kg/24 h in 4 equally divided doses q6h; for gastrointestinal or genitourinary tract infections, give 100 mg/kg/24 h in 4 equally divided doses q6h.
Duration of treatment	Continue treatment for at least 48–72 h after patient has become asymptomatic or bacteria have been eradicated; beta-hemolytic streptococcal infections should be treated for at least 10 days to prevent rheumatic fever and glomerulonephritis. In cases of gonorrhea, perform follow-up cultures within 4–7 days after treating males and 7–14 days after treating females.

WARNINGS/PRECAUTIONS

Hypersensitivity	Serious and occasionally fatal anaphylactoid reactions may occur, most likely in patients with a history of sensitivity to multiple allergens. Urticaria, other skin rashes, and serum sickness-like reactions may be controlled with antihistamines and, if necessary, systemic corticosteroids. Drug should be discontinued unless infection is life-threatening and amenable only to ampicillin. Severe reactions may require emergency measures, such as immediate use of epinephrine, oxygen, IV corticosteroids, and airway management, including intubation; use with caution in patients who have experienced allergic reactions to cephalosporins.
Long-term therapy	Perform blood, renal, and hepatic studies periodically
Superinfection	Overgrowth of nonsusceptible organisms, including fungi, may occur
Suspected syphilitic lesions	If syphilis is suspected, perform dark-field examination before instituting therapy and perform serology testing for at least 4 mo
Chronic urinary tract and intestinal infections	Require frequent bacteriological and clinical appraisal during therapy, and possibly for several months afterward; do not use doses smaller than those recommended above
Complications of gonorrheal urethritis, such as prostatitis and epididymitis	Prolonged and intensive therapy is recommended

OMNIPEN ■ PENTIDS

ADVERSE REACTIONS	Frequent reactions (incidence ≥ 1%) are printed in *italics*
Gastrointestinal	Glossitis, stomatitis, nausea, vomiting, enterocolitis, pseudomembranous colitis, diarrhea
Hypersensitivity	*Erythematous maculopapular rash*, urticaria, erythema multiforme, exfoliative dermatitis, anaphylaxis (see WARNINGS/PRECAUTIONS)
Hematological	Anemia, thrombocytopenia, thrombocytopenic purpura, eosinophilia, leukopenia, agranulocytosis

OVERDOSAGE	
Signs and symptoms	See ADVERSE REACTIONS
Treatment	Discontinue medication; treat symptomatically

DRUG INTERACTIONS	
Probenecid	⇧ Ampicillin blood level and/or toxicity

ALTERED LABORATORY VALUES	
Blood/serum values	⇧ SGOT (especially in infants)

No clinically significant alterations in urinary values occur at therapeutic dosages

---

USE IN CHILDREN

See INDICATIONS; adjust dosage according to body weight and severity of infection

USE IN PREGNANT AND NURSING WOMEN

Safety for use during pregnancy has not been established. Use according to medical judgment in nursing mothers.

---

[1] Larger doses may be needed for stubborn or severe infections
[2] Dosage based on recommendations of the American Heart Association (*Circulation* 70:1123A–1127A, 1984)

PENICILLINS

PENTIDS (penicillin G potassium) Squibb   Rx

Tablets: 125 mg (Pentids), 250 mg (Pentids 400), 500 mg (Pentids 800) **Syrup (per 5 ml):** 125 mg after reconstitution (Pentids) *fruit flavored* (100 ml), 250 mg after reconstitution (Pentids 400) *fruit flavored* (100, 200 ml)

INDICATIONS	ORAL DOSAGE
Mild to moderately severe upper respiratory tract infections, skin and soft tissue infections, scarlet fever, and erysipelas caused by penicillin G-sensitive streptococci in the absence of bacteremia	**Adult:** for mild infections, 125 mg tid or qid for 10 days; for moderately severe infections, 250 mg tid or 500 mg bid for 10 days **Child (< 12 yr):** 15–56 mg/kg/day, given in 3–6 divided doses
Otitis media and other mild to moderately severe upper respiratory tract infections caused by penicillin G-sensitive *Streptococcus pneumoniae*	**Adult:** 250 mg qid until patient has been afebrile for at least 2 days **Child (< 12 yr):** 15–56 mg/kg/day, given in 3–6 divided doses
Mild skin and soft tissue infections caused by penicillin G-sensitive staphylococci	**Adult:** 125–250 mg tid or qid until infection is cured **Child (< 12 yr):** 15–56 mg/kg/day, given in 3–6 divided doses
Fusospirochetosis (Vincent's gingivitis and pharyngitis)	**Adult:** 250 mg tid or qid **Child (< 12 yr):** 15–56 mg/kg/day, given in 3–6 divided doses
Continuous prophylaxis of rheumatic fever and/or chorea	**Adult:** 125 mg bid **Child:** same as adult
Short-term prophylaxis to prevent bacteremia following tooth extraction	Consult manufacturer

CONTRAINDICATIONS
Hypersensitivity to penicillins

ADMINISTRATION/DOSAGE ADJUSTMENTS	
Timing of administration	Administer ½ h before or at least 2 h after meals to assure maximum absorption

PENTIDS ■ PEN·VEE K

Duration of treatment for streptococcal infections	Therapy should be continued for a minimum of 10 days to prevent sequelae of streptococcal disease; cultures should be taken on completion of therapy to determine whether streptococci have been eradicated
Patients receiving prophylactic penicillin	May harbor increased numbers of penicillin-resistant organisms; if penicillin will be used at the time of surgery, interrupt regular program 1 wk before procedure

WARNINGS/PRECAUTIONS

Hypersensitivity	Serious and occasionally fatal anaphylactoid reactions may occur, most likely in patients with a history of sensitivity to multiple allergens. Urticaria, other skin rashes, and serum sickness-like reactions may be controlled with antihistamines and, if necessary, systemic corticosteroids. Drug should be discontinued unless infection is life-threatening and amenable only to penicillin. Severe reactions may necessitate emergency measures, such as immediate use of epinephrine, aminophylline, oxygen, and IV corticosteroids; use with caution in patients who have experienced allergic reactions to cephalosporins.
Long-term therapy	Perform blood, renal, and hepatic studies periodically, particularly with high-dosage schedules
Superinfection	Overgrowth of nonsusceptible organisms, including fungi, may occur
Impaired absorption	Oral administration should not be relied on in patients with severe illness, nausea, vomiting, gastric dilatation, cardiospasm, or intestinal hypermotility (see also ADMINISTRATION/DOSAGE ADJUSTMENTS)
Tartrazine sensitivity	Presence of FD&C Yellow No. 5 (tartrazine) in 500-mg tablets and both syrup formulations may cause allergic-type reactions, including bronchial asthma, in susceptible individuals
Inappropriate indications	Oral penicillin G should not be used for treatment during the acute stages of severe pneumonia, empyema, bacteremia, pericarditis, meningitis, or septic arthritis; for prophylaxis preceding genitourinary instrumentation or surgery, lower intestinal tract surgery, sigmoidoscopy, or childbirth; or for short-term prevention of bacterial endocarditis in patients with valvular heart disease undergoing dental or surgical procedures

ADVERSE REACTIONS

Frequent reactions (incidence ≥ 1%) are printed in *italics*

Gastrointestinal	*Nausea, vomiting, epigastric distress, diarrhea, black hairy tongue,* sore mouth or tongue
Hypersensitivity	Skin rashes ranging from maculopapular rashes to exfoliative dermatitis, urticaria, serum sickness-like reactions (including chills, fever, edema, arthralgia, and prostration), eosinophilia, laryngeal edema, anaphylaxis (see WARNINGS/PRECAUTIONS)
Hematological	Hemolytic anemia, leukopenia, thrombocytopenia
Other	Neuropathy and nephropathy (usually only with high-dosage parenteral therapy)

OVERDOSAGE

Signs and symptoms	See ADVERSE REACTIONS
Treatment	Discontinue medication; treat symptomatically

DRUG INTERACTIONS

Probenecid	⇧ Penicillin blood level and/or toxicity

ALTERED LABORATORY VALUES

No clinically significant alterations in blood/serum or urinary values occur at therapeutic dosages

---

USE IN CHILDREN

See INDICATIONS; adjust dosage according to body weight and severity of infection

USE IN PREGNANT AND NURSING WOMEN

Consult manufacturer for use in pregnant women. Penicillins are excreted in human milk and may increase the risk of allergic sensitization in nursing infants.[1]

[1] Knowles JA: *J Pediatr* 66:1068–1082, 1965; *Med Lett Drugs Ther* 16:25–27, 1974

PENICILLINS

PEN·VEE K (penicillin V potassium) Wyeth   Rx

Tablets: 250, 500 mg **Solution (per 5 ml):** 125 mg after reconstitution (100, 200 ml), 250 mg after reconstitution (100, 150, 200 ml)

INDICATIONS

Mild to moderately severe upper respiratory tract infections, scarlet fever, and erysipelas caused by penicillin G-sensitive streptococci in the absence of bacteremia

ORAL DOSAGE

Adult: 125–250 mg q6–8h for 10 days
Child (≥ 12 yr): same as adult

PEN·VEE K

Otitis media and other mild to moderately severe respiratory tract infections caused by penicillin G-sensitive *Streptococcus pneumoniae*	**Adult:** 250–500 mg q6h until patient has been afebrile for at least 2 days **Child ($\geq$ 12 yr):** same as adult
Mild skin and soft tissue infections caused by penicillin G-sensitive staphylococci	**Adult:** 250–500 mg q6–8h **Child ($\geq$ 12 yr):** same as adult
Fusospirochetosis (Vincent's gingivitis and pharyngitis)	
Continuous prophylaxis of rheumatic fever and/or chorea	**Adult:** 125–250 mg bid **Child ($\geq$ 12 yr):** same as adult
Prevention of bacterial endocarditis in patients with congenital heart disease or rheumatic or other acquired valvular heart disease who are undergoing dental procedures or upper respiratory tract surgery	**Adult and child ($>$ 60 lb):** 2 g 1 h before the procedure, followed by 1 g 6 h later **Child ($<$ 60 lb):** 1 g 1 h before the procedure, followed by 500 mg 6 h later

CONTRAINDICATIONS
Hypersensitivity to penicillins

ADMINISTRATION/DOSAGE ADJUSTMENTS

Duration of treatment for streptococcal infections	Therapy should be continued for a minimum of 10 days to prevent sequelae of streptococcal disease; cultures should be taken on completion of therapy to determine whether streptococci have been eradicated
Prevention of bacterial endocarditis	If the patient has been receiving penicillin for long-term prophylaxis of rheumatic fever or chorea, a drug other than penicillin may be considered for prevention of bacterial endocarditis, since the patient may harbor alpha-hemolytic streptococci that are relatively resistant to penicillin. Penicillin V should not be used for prevention of bacterial endocarditis in a patient who is at particularly high risk (eg, a patient with a prosthetic heart valve or surgically constructed systemic-pulmonary shunt).

WARNINGS/PRECAUTIONS

Hypersensitivity	Serious and occasionally fatal anaphylactoid reactions may occur, most likely in patients with a history of sensitivity to multiple allergens; use with caution in patients who have a history of significant allergies and/or asthma or have experienced allergic reactions to cephalosporins. If an allergic reaction occurs, discontinue medication and employ other agents, eg, epinephrine, antihistamines, and/or corticosteroids, as needed.
Superinfection	Overgrowth of nonsusceptible microorganisms, including fungi, may occur with prolonged use
Impaired absorption	Oral administration should not be relied on in patients with severe illness, nausea, vomiting, gastric dilatation, cardiospasm, or intestinal hypermotility
Inappropriate indications	Oral penicillin V should not be used for treatment during the acute stages of severe pneumonia, empyema, bacteremia, pericarditis, meningitis, or septic arthritis, or for prophylaxis preceding genitourinary instrumentation or surgery, lower intestinal tract surgery, sigmoidoscopy, or childbirth

ADVERSE REACTIONS
The most frequent reactions, regardless of incidence, are printed in *italics*

Gastrointestinal	*Nausea, vomiting, epigastric distress, diarrhea, black hairy tongue*
Hypersensitivity	Skin eruptions ranging from maculopapular rash to exfoliative dermatitis, urticaria, and other serum sickness-like reactions; fever; eosinophilia; laryngeal edema; anaphylaxis (see WARNINGS/PRECAUTIONS)
Hematological	Hemolytic anemia, leukopenia, thrombocytopenia (usually only with high-dose parenteral therapy)
Other	Neuropathy and nephropathy (usually only with high-dosage parenteral therapy)

OVERDOSAGE

Signs and symptoms	See ADVERSE REACTIONS
Treatment	Discontinue medication; treat symptomatically

DRUG INTERACTIONS

Probenecid	⇧ Penicillin blood level and/or toxicity

ALTERED LABORATORY VALUES

No clinically significant alterations in blood/serum or urinary values occur at therapeutic dosages

USE IN CHILDREN	USE IN PREGNANT AND NURSING WOMEN
See INDICATIONS and ORAL DOSAGE	Use during pregnancy only if essential; no teratogenic effects have been documented. Use in nursing women only if essential.

PENICILLINS

PERMAPEN (penicillin G benzathine) Roerig   Rx

Prefilled syringes: 600,000 units/ml (1, 2 ml) for IM use only

INDICATIONS / PARENTERAL DOSAGE

Mild to moderate nonbacteremic upper respiratory tract infections caused by Group A streptococci
- Adult: 1.2 million units, given in a single IM dose
- Child: for older children, 900,000 units, given in a single IM dose

Primary, secondary, and latent syphilis
- Adult: 2.4 million units, given in a single IM dose

Tertiary syphilis and neurosyphilis
- Adult: 3 million units, given in a single IM dose every 7 days, for a total of 6–9 million units

Congenital syphilis
- Infant (< 2 yr): 50,000 units/kg IM
- Child (2–12 yr): adjust dosage according to adult schedule

Yaws, bejel, and pinta
- Adult: 1.2 million units, given in a single IM dose

Prophylaxis for rheumatic fever, chorea, rheumatic heart disease, and acute glomerulonephritis
- Adult: following an acute attack, 1.2 million units every month or 600,000 units every 2 wk, given in a single IM dose

CONTRAINDICATIONS

Hypersensitivity to penicillins

ADMINISTRATION/DOSAGE ADJUSTMENTS

Duration of treatment for streptococcal infections — Therapy must be sufficient to eliminate the organism and prevent sequelae of streptococcal disease; cultures should be performed at completion of treatment

Intramuscular administration — Inject deeply into the mid-lateral muscles of the thigh or, with adults, the upper outer quadrant of the gluteus maximus. The periphery of this quadrant should be used in infants and small children only when necessary (eg, in burn patients) in order to minimize the possibility of sciatic nerve damage. The deltoid area should be used only if it is well-developed (eg, in certain adults and older children), and only if caution is exercised to avoid radial nerve injury; the lower or midthird of the upper arm should not be used. Aspiration is necessary to help prevent inadvertent IV or intraarterial injection. Fat-layer and SC injections should be avoided, because they can cause pain and induration; if these effects occur, an ice pack may be applied.

WARNINGS/PRECAUTIONS

Hypersensitivity — Serious and occasionally fatal anaphylactoid reactions may occur, most likely in patients with a history of sensitivity to multiple allergens; use with caution in patients with a history of asthma or other significant allergies, including allergic reactions to cephalosporins. If an allergic reaction occurs, discontinue medication and employ pressor amines, antihistamines, and corticosteroids, as needed.

Superinfection — Overgrowth of nonsusceptible organisms, including fungi, may occur

ADVERSE REACTIONS

Hypersensitivity — Skin eruptions ranging from maculopapular rash to exfoliative dermatitis; urticaria, and other serum sickness-like reactions; fever; eosinophilia; laryngeal edema; anaphylaxis (see WARNINGS/PRECAUTIONS)

Hematological — Hemolytic anemia, leukopenia, and thrombocytopenia (with high doses)

Other — Irritation at injection site; neuropathy and nephropathy (with high doses)

OVERDOSAGE

Signs and symptoms — See ADVERSE REACTIONS

Treatment — Discontinue medication; treat symptomatically

PERMAPEN ■ PFIZERPEN-AS

DRUG INTERACTIONS

Probenecid ———————————————— ⇧ Penicillin blood level and/or toxicity

ALTERED LABORATORY VALUES

No clinically significant alterations in blood/serum or urinary values occur at therapeutic dosages

USE IN CHILDREN	USE IN PREGNANT AND NURSING WOMEN
See INDICATIONS and PARENTERAL DOSAGE; in children under 12 yr of age, adjust dosage according to age, weight, and severity of infection. In children under 2 yr of age, divide the dose between both buttocks, if necessary.	Consult manufacturer

---

PENICILLINS

PFIZERPEN-AS (penicillin G procaine) Roerig   Rx

Vials: 300,000 units/ml (10 ml) for IM use only

INDICATIONS[1]

Moderately severe to severe nonbacteremic upper respiratory tract infections (including otitis media and tonsillitis), skin and soft tissue infections, scarlet fever, and erysipelas caused by penicillin G-sensitive Group A streptococci

Uncomplicated **pneumonia, otitis media,** and other respiratory tract infections caused by *Streptococcus pneumoniae*

Moderately severe to severe skin and soft tissue infections caused by penicillin G-sensitive staphylococci

Fusospirochetosis (Vincent's gingivitis and pharyngitis)

Cutaneous **anthrax**

Rat-bite fever caused by *Streptobacillus moniliformis* or *Spirillum minus*

Erysipeloid

Subacute **bacterial endocarditis** caused by Group A streptococci extremely sensitive to penicillin G

Primary and secondary syphilis, and latent syphilis with negative spinal fluid examination

Tertiary syphilis, neurosyphilis, and latent syphilis with positive or no spinal fluid examination

Congenital syphilis (early and late)

Yaws, bejel, and pinta

Uncomplicated nonbacteremic **gonorrhea**

Diphtheria (adjunctive therapy with antitoxin)

Prevention of **diphtheria carrier state** (adjunctive therapy with antitoxin)

Prevention of bacterial endocarditis in patients with congenital heart disease or rheumatic or other acquired valvular heart disease who are undergoing dental procedures or upper respiratory tract surgery

PARENTERAL DOSAGE

Adult: 600,000–1,000,000 units/day IM for at least 10 days

Adult: 600,000–1,000,000 units/day IM

Adult: 600,000 units/day IM for 8 days
Child (> 12 yr): same as adult

Adult: 600,000 units/day IM for 10–15 days

Child (< 70 lb): 50,000 units/kg/day IM for 10 days

Adult: treat as with syphilis, according to the corresponding stage of the disease

Adult: 4,800,000 units, given in at least 2 divided IM doses (at different sites), with 1 g oral probenecid, preferably given at least 30 min before injection of penicillin G

Adult: 300,000–600,000 units/day IM

Adult: 300,000 units/day IM for 10 days

Adult: 600,000 units IM mixed with 1 million units aqueous crystalline penicillin G 1/2–1 h prior to procedure, followed by 500 mg oral penicillin V potassium q6h for 8 doses

Child (< 60 lb): 600,000 units IM mixed with 30,000 units/kg aqueous crystalline penicillin G 1/2–1 h prior to procedure, followed by 250 mg oral penicillin V potassium q6h for 8 doses

---

CONTRAINDICATIONS

Hypersensitivity to penicillin or procaine

ADMINISTRATION/DOSAGE ADJUSTMENTS

Intramuscular administration	Inject deeply into the mid-lateral muscles of the thigh or, with adults, the upper outer quadrant of the gluteus maximus. The periphery of this quadrant should be used in infants and small children only when necessary (eg, in burn patients) in order to minimize the possibility of sciatic nerve damage. The deltoid area should be used only if it is well-developed (eg, in certain adults and older children), and only if caution is exercised to avoid radial nerve injury; the lower or midthird of the upper arm should not be used. Aspiration is necessary to help prevent inadvertent IV or intraarterial injection. Fat-layer and SC injections should be avoided, because they can cause pain and induration; if necessary, an ice pack may be applied.
Patients receiving continuous penicillin prophylaxis to prevent recurrence of rheumatic fever	May harbor alpha-hemolytic streptococci that are relatively resistant to penicillin; prophylactic antibiotics other than penicillin may be given to these patients (in addition to their continuous rheumatic fever prophylactic regimen) prior to dental or surgical procedures

WARNINGS/PRECAUTIONS

Hypersensitivity	Serious and occasionally fatal anaphylactoid reactions to penicillin have occurred, especially in patients with a history of hypersensitivity to multiple allergens; patients hypersensitive to penicillin have experienced severe allergic reactions when given cephalosporins. Before initiating therapy, determine whether the patient is hypersensitive to penicillins, cephalosporins, or other allergens; use with caution in patients with a history of asthma or other significant allergies. If allergic reactions occur (see ADVERSE REACTIONS), use of this drug should be discontinued unless the infection is life-threatening and amenable only to penicillin, and vasopressors, antihistamines, corticosteroids, or other similar agents should be administered. Hypersensitive reactions to procaine have not been reported with use of penicillin G procaine.
Sensitivity to procaine	Immediate toxic reactions to procaine (see OVERDOSAGE) may occur, particularly in patients undergoing treatment of gonorrhea. In controlled studies, approximately 0.2% of such patients experienced transient (15–30 min) toxic reactions. Test patients with a history of procaine sensitivity by injecting intradermally 0.1 ml of 1–2% procaine; if erythema, wheal, flare, or eruption occurs, penicillin G procaine should not be used. Sensitivity reactions should be treated with barbiturates or other agents; antihistamines may be helpful.
Superinfection	Overgrowth of nonsusceptible organisms, including fungi, may occur; constant observation is essential
Suspected staphylococcal infections	Culture and sensitivity studies should be performed, because an increasing number of penicillin G-resistant staphylococcal strains have been reported
Suspected syphilitic infections	If primary or secondary syphilis is suspected in patients with gonorrhea, proper diagnostic procedures, including monthly serological tests (for at least 4 mo) and dark-field examinations, should be performed
Prolonged therapy	Evaluate renal and hematopoietic function periodically, particularly when using high doses

ADVERSE REACTIONS

Hypersensitivity	Skin rashes, ranging from maculopapular eruptions to exfoliative dermatitis; urticaria; serum sickness-like reactions, including chills, fever, edema, arthralgia, and prostration; anaphylaxis (see WARNINGS/PRECAUTIONS)
Other	Jarisch-Herxheimer reaction

OVERDOSAGE

Signs and symptoms	*Procaine-related effects:* anxiety, confusion, agitation, depression, weakness, seizures, hallucinations, combativeness, fear of impending death; *penicillin-related effects:* see ADVERSE REACTIONS
Treatment	Discontinue medication; treat symptomatically (see WARNINGS/PRECAUTIONS)

DRUG INTERACTIONS

Probenecid	△ Penicillin blood level and/or toxicity

ALTERED LABORATORY VALUES

No clinically significant alterations in blood/serum or urinary values occur at therapeutic dosages

USE IN CHILDREN
See INDICATIONS and PARENTERAL DOSAGE; in children under 12 yr of age, adjust dosage according to age, weight, and severity of infection. In children under 2 yr of age, divide the dose between both buttocks, if necessary. The absorption of aqueous penicillin G in infants under 3 mo of age produces such high, sustained levels that use of penicillin G procaine in such infants is usually unnecessary.

USE IN PREGNANT AND NURSING WOMEN
Consult manufacturer

[1] Indicated for treatment of moderately severe infections, unless otherwise stated

---

PENICILLINS

PIPRACIL (piperacillin sodium) Lederle　　Rx

Vials: equivalent to 2, 3, and 4 g piperacillin　**Infusion bottles:** equivalent to 2, 3, and 4 g piperacillin　**Pharmacy bulk vials:** equivalent to 40 g piperacillin

INDICATIONS

Intraabdominal infections, including hepatobiliary and surgical infections, caused by susceptible strains of *Escherichia coli, Pseudomonas aeruginosa, Streptococcus fecalis, Clostridium,* anaerobic cocci, and *Bacteroides* (including *B fragilis*)

Gynecologic infections, including endometritis, pelvic inflammatory disease, and pelvic cellulitis, caused by susceptible strains of *Bacteroides* (including *B fragilis*), anaerobic cocci, *Neisseria gonorrhoeae,* and *Streptococcus fecalis*

Septicemia, including bacteremia, caused by susceptible strains of *Escherichia coli, Klebsiella, Enterobacter, Serratia, Proteus mirabilis, Streptococcus pneumoniae, S fecalis, Pseudomonas aeruginosa, Bacteroides,* and anaerobic cocci

Lower respiratory tract infections caused by susceptible strains of *Escherichia coli, Klebsiella, Enterobacter, Pseudomonas aeruginosa, Serratia, Hemophilus influenzae, Bacteroides,* and anaerobic cocci

Skin and skin structure infections caused by susceptible strains of *Escherichia coli, Klebsiella, Serratia, Acinetobacter, Enterobacter, Pseudomonas aeruginosa,* indole-positive *Proteus, Proteus mirabilis, Bacteroides* (including *B fragilis*), anaerobic cocci, and *Streptococcus fecalis*

Bone and joint infections caused by susceptible strains of *Pseudomonas aeruginosa, Streptococcus fecalis, Bacteroides,* and anaerobic cocci

PARENTERAL DOSAGE

Adult: for serious infections, including hospital-acquired pneumonias, 12–18 g/day IV, given in divided doses q4–6h; for most community-acquired pneumonias, 6–8 g/day IM or IV, given in divided doses q6–12h. The maximum daily dose should generally not exceed 24 g, although higher doses have been used.

Urinary tract infections caused by susceptible strains of *Escherichia coli, Klebsiella, Pseudomonas aeruginosa, Proteus* (including *P mirabilis*), and *Streptococcus fecalis*

Adult: for uncomplicated infections, 6–8 g/day IM or IV, given in divided doses q6–12h; for complicated infections, 8–16 g/day IV, given in divided doses q6–8h. The maximum daily dose should generally not exceed 24 g, although higher doses have been used.

Uncomplicated gonococcal urethritis

Adult: 2 g IM, given in a single dose 30 min after oral administration of 1 g probenecid

Gastrointestinal and biliary tract surgery (prophylactic use)

Adults: 2 g IV, given 30–60 min before surgery, again during surgery, and then q6h for up to 24 h after surgery

Abdominal hysterectomy (prophylactic use)

Adult: 2 g IV, given 30–60 min before surgery, upon return to the recovery room, and finally 6 h later

Vaginal hysterectomy (prophylactic use)

Adult: 2 g IV, given 30–60 min before surgery and then 6 and 12 h later

Cesarean section (prophylactic use)

Adult: 2 g IV, given after the umbilical cord is clamped and then 4 and 8 h later

PIPRACIL

CONTRAINDICATIONS

Hypersensitivity to penicillins and/or cephalosporins

ADMINISTRATION/DOSAGE ADJUSTMENTS

Intramuscular administration	When indicated, 6–8 g/day may be given in divided IM doses to initiate therapy; the IM route may also be used for maintenance therapy after clinical and bacteriologic improvement has been obtained via IV administration. Reconstitute the drug with sterile water for injection, bacteriostatic water for injection, sodium chloride injection, bacteriostatic sodium chloride injection, 5% dextrose in water, 5% dextrose and 0.9% sodium chloride, or 0.5–1.0% lidocaine HCl injection (without epinephrine), using at least 2 ml for each gram of piperacillin; shake the vial immediately after adding the diluent. Inject the solution preferably into the upper outer quadrant of the buttock (the deltoid area may be used only if it is well developed, and only with caution to avoid radial nerve damage). *Do not give more than 2 g into any one injection site.*
Intravenous administration	The IV route should be used for serious infections. Reconstitute the drug with sterile water for injection, bacteriostatic water for injection, sodium chloride injection, or bacteriostatic sodium chloride injection, 5% dextrose in water, or 5% dextrose and 0.9% sodium chloride, using at least 5 ml for each gram of piperacillin; shake well until drug is dissolved. Inject the solution slowly over a 3- to 5-min period. Alternatively, dilute the solution, using a compatible diluent, to an appropriate final volume (eg, 50–100 ml) and administer by infusion over a period of approximately 30 min; infusion of the primary solution should be discontinued while piperacillin is being given.
Duration of treatment	For most acute infections, therapy should be continued for at least 48–72 h after the patient becomes asymptomatic; the average duration is 7–10 days, except in gynecologic infections (3–10 days). Treatment of Group A beta-hemolytic streptococcal infections should be continued for at least 10 days to reduce the risk of rheumatic fever and glomerulonephritis (however, narrower-spectrum penicillins are generally more appropriate for streptococcal infections).
Patients with renal impairment	No dosage adjustment is necessary if the creatinine clearance rate (CCr) $>$ 40 ml/min. For uncomplicated urinary tract infections, give the usual dosage if CCr = 20–40 ml/min or 3 g q12h if CCr $<$ 20 ml/min. For complicated urinary tract infections, give 3 g q8h if CCr = 20–40 ml/min or q12h if CCr $<$ 20 ml/min. For serious systemic infections, give 4 g q8h if CCr = 20–40 ml/min or q12h if CCr $<$ 20 ml/min. For patients undergoing hemodialysis, give up to 2 g q8h; after each dialysis treatment, administer an additional 1 g, because 30–50% of piperacillin is removed in 4 h during hemodialysis. Obtain serum piperacillin levels for additional guidance in adjusting dosage for patients with renal failure and hepatic insufficiency.
Empiric therapy	Piperacillin is particularly useful for mixed infections and may be given before the causative organisms are identified; obtain specimens for appropriate cultures and susceptibility testing prior to initiating therapy and adjust the regimen, if necessary, once the results are known
Concomitant use of other anti-infectives	Piperacillin has been used successfully with aminoglycosides, especially in immunodeficient patients; both drugs should be administered in full therapeutic doses. To avoid inactivation of the aminoglycoside, do not mix the two drugs in the same syringe or infusion bottle.
Patients with cystic fibrosis	Piperacillin ameliorates the signs and symptoms of lower respiratory tract infection in patients with cystic fibrosis, but may not completely eradicate the pathogen

WARNINGS/PRECAUTIONS

Hypersensitivity	Serious and occasionally fatal anaphylactic reactions to penicillins have occurred, especially in patients with a history of sensitivity to multiple allergens. Prior to initiating therapy, determine whether patient is allergic to penicillins, cephalosporins, and other allergens (see CONTRAINDICATIONS). If an allergic reaction occurs, discontinue therapy; serious reactions may require immediate use of epinephrine, oxygen, and IV corticosteroids and possible intubation to maintain an open airway.
Prolonged therapy	Assess renal, hepatic, and hematopoietic functions periodically. The possibility of emergence of resistant organisms should be kept in mind, particularly when treatment is prolonged; if superinfection occurs, take appropriate measures. Reversible leukopenia (neutropenia) is also more apt to occur with prolonged administration of high dosages.
Bleeding manifestations	May occur, especially in patients with renal failure, and may be associated with an abnormal clotting or prothrombin time or abnormal platelet aggregation test result; discontinue therapy and institute appropriate corrective measures
Neuromuscular hyperexcitability or convulsions	May occur if higher than recommended doses are given IV
Sodium content	Piperacillin contains 1.85 mEq (42.5 mg) Na^+/g, which should be considered in treating patients who require a restricted salt intake
Hypokalemia	Has occurred rarely in patients with liver disease and in individuals receiving cytotoxic drugs or diuretics concurrently; measure serum electrolyte levels periodically in patients with low or potentially low potassium reserves

PIPRACIL ■ POLYCILLIN

Suspected syphilitic lesions	Patients with gonorrhea should be evaluated for syphilis prior to treatment, since symptoms may be masked or delayed by antimicrobial therapy. Obtain specimens for dark-field examination and perform serological tests if primary syphilis is suspected; repeat the tests monthly for at least 4 mo.
Fever and rash	Patients with cystic fibrosis tend to be more susceptible than others to developing fever or rash during therapy

ADVERSE REACTIONS

Frequent reactions (incidence ≥ 1%) are printed in *italics*

Gastrointestinal	*Diarrhea and loose stools (2%)*, nausea, vomiting, increases in liver enzyme (SGOT, SGPT, and LDH) levels, hyperbilirubinemia, cholestatic hepatitis, bloody diarrhea; pseudomembranous colitis (rare)
Hematological	Reversible leukopenia, neutropenia, thrombocytopenia, eosinophilia, hemorrhagic manifestations
Renal	Increases in BUN and serum creatinine levels; interstitial nephritis (rare)
Central nervous system and neuromuscular	Headache, dizziness, fatigue; prolonged muscle relaxation (rare)
Hypersensitivity	*Rash (1%)*, anaphylactoid reactions, pruritus, vesicular eruptions
Local	*Thrombophlebitis (4%)*; *pain, erythema, and/or induration at the injection site (2%)*; ecchymosis, deep-vein thrombosis, hematoma
Other	Superinfection, including candidiasis

OVERDOSAGE

Signs and symptoms	See ADVERSE REACTIONS
Treatment	Discontinue medication; treat symptomatically and institute supportive measures, as required

DRUG INTERACTIONS

Aminoglycosides	Inactivation of the aminoglycoside when combined *in vitro*
Probenecid	△ Antimicrobial activity in acute gonococcal infections

ALTERED LABORATORY VALUES

Blood/serum values	△ BUN △ Creatinine △ SGOT △ SGPT △ LDH ▽ Potassium (in patients with liver disease or during concomitant cytotoxic or diuretic therapy) + Coombs' test

No clinically significant alterations in urinary values occur at therapeutic dosages

---

USE IN CHILDREN

Dosages for children under 12 yr of age have not been established. Renal tubule dilatation and peritubular hyalinization have been observed in canine neonates; the safety of piperacillin in human neonates is unknown.

USE IN PREGNANT AND NURSING WOMEN

Pregnancy Category B: use during pregnancy only if clearly needed. Reproductive studies in mice and rats at up to 4 times the human dose have shown no evidence of impaired fertility or fetal harm; however, no adequate, well-controlled studies have been done in pregnant women. Piperacillin crosses the placental barrier in rats and is excreted in low concentrations in milk; use with caution in nursing mothers.

PENICILLINS

POLYCILLIN (ampicillin) Apothecon   Rx

Capsules: 250, 500 mg   **Suspension (per 5 ml):** 125 mg, 250 mg, 500 mg after reconstitution   **Pediatric drops:** 100 mg/ml

POLYCILLIN-N (ampicillin sodium) Apothecon   Rx

Vials: 125, 250, 500 mg; 1, 2 g   **Piggyback units:** 500 mg; 1, 2 g   **Hospital bulk package:** 10 g

INDICATIONS

Respiratory tract and soft tissue infections caused by susceptible strains of *Hemophilus influenzae*, penicillin G-sensitive staphylococci, streptococci, and *Streptococcus pneumoniae*

ORAL DOSAGE

Adult: 250 mg q6h
Child (< 20 kg): 50 mg/kg/day, given in equally divided doses q6–8h
Child (≥ 20 kg): same as adult

PARENTERAL DOSAGE

Adult: 250–500 mg IM or IV q6h
Child (< 40 kg): 25–50 mg/kg/day IM or IV, given in equally divided doses q6–8h
Child (≥ 40 kg): same as adult

POLYCILLIN

Gastrointestinal and genitourinary tract infections caused by susceptible strains of *Shigella*, *Salmonella* (including *S typhosa*), *Escherichia coli*, *Proteus mirabilis*, enterococci, and *Neisseria gonorrhoeae* (in females)	**Adult:** 500 mg q6h[1] **Child (< 20 kg):** 100 mg/kg/day, given in equally divided doses q6–8h[1] **Child (≥ 20 kg):** same as adult	**Adult:** 500 mg IM or IV q6h[1] **Child (< 40 kg):** 50 mg/kg/day IM or IV q6–8h[1] **Child (≥ 40 kg):** same as adult
Urethritis caused by *Neisseria gonorrhoeae*	**Adult:** 3.5 g, given simultaneously with 1 g probenecid	—
Urethritis in males caused by *Neisseria gonorrhoeae*	—	**Adult:** 500 mg IM or IV q8–12h for 2 doses; may be repeated or extended, if necessary
Bacterial meningitis caused by susceptible strains of *Neisseria meningitidis* and *Hemophilus influenzae* Septicemia caused by susceptible strains of Gram-positive and Gram-negative bacteria	—	**Adult:** 150–200 mg/kg/day, given in equally divided doses q3–4h, beginning by slow IV infusion (for a minimum of 3 days in treating septicemia) and followed by IM injection q3–4h **Child:** same as adult

CONTRAINDICATIONS

Hypersensitivity to penicillins

ADMINISTRATION/DOSAGE ADJUSTMENTS

Duration of treatment	Continue treatment for at least 48–72 h after patient becomes asymptomatic or bacteria have been eradicated; treatment for several weeks may be necessary for stubborn GI and urinary tract infections. Beta-hemolytic streptococcal infections should be treated for at least 10 days to prevent rheumatic fever and glomerulonephritis

WARNINGS/PRECAUTIONS

Hypersensitivity	Serious and occasionally fatal anaphylactoid reactions may occur, most likely in patients with a history of sensitivity to multiple allergens. Urticaria, other skin rashes, and serum sickness-like reactions may be controlled with antihistamines and, if necessary, systemic corticosteroids. Drug should be discontinued unless infection is life-threatening and amenable only to ampicillin. Severe reactions may necessitate emergency measures, such as immediate use of epinephrine, oxygen, IV corticosteroids, and airway management, including intubation; use with caution in patients who have experienced allergic reactions to cephalosporins.
Long-term therapy	Perform blood, renal, and hepatic studies periodically
Superinfection	Overgrowth of nonsusceptible organisms, including fungi, may occur
Suspected syphilitic lesions	If syphilis is suspected, perform dark-field examination before instituting therapy, and perform serology testing monthly for at least 4 mo
Chronic urinary tract and intestinal infections	Require frequent bacteriological and clinical appraisal during therapy and possibly for several months afterward
Complications of gonorrheal urethritis, such as prostatitis and epididymitis	Prolonged and intensive therapy is recommended
Inappropriate indications	Ampicillin should not be used for the treatment of infectious mononucleosis; a high percentage of patients with mononucleosis develop a skin rash after receiving ampicillin

ADVERSE REACTIONS

Frequent reactions (incidence ≥ 1%) are printed in *italics*

Gastrointestinal	Glossitis, stomatitis, black hairy tongue, nausea, vomiting, enterocolitis, pseudomembranous colitis, diarrhea
Hypersensitivity	*Skin rash*, *urticaria*, exfoliative dermatitis, erythema multiforme, anaphylaxis (see WARNINGS/PRECAUTIONS)
Hematological	Anemia, thrombocytopenia, thrombocytopenic purpura, eosinophilia, leukopenia, agranulocytosis

OVERDOSAGE

Signs and symptoms	See ADVERSE REACTIONS
Treatment	Discontinue medication; treat symptomatically

DRUG INTERACTIONS

Probenecid	⇧ Ampicillin blood level and/or toxicity

ALTERED LABORATORY VALUES

Blood/serum values	⇧ SGOT (especially in infants)
Urinary values	⇧ Glucose (with Clinitest tablets)

USE IN CHILDREN	USE IN PREGNANT AND NURSING WOMEN
See INDICATIONS; adjust dosage according to body weight and severity of infection	Safety for use during pregnancy has not been established. Ampicillin is excreted in human milk in very small amounts.

[1] Higher doses may be needed for stubborn or severe infections

PENICILLINS

POLYMOX (amoxicillin) Apothecon Rx

Capsules: 250, 500 mg **Suspension (per 5 ml):** 125 mg, 250 mg after reconstitution **Pediatric drops:** 50 mg/ml after reconstitution

INDICATIONS

Ear, nose, and throat infections caused by susceptible strains of streptococci, *Streptococcus pneumoniae,* nonpenicillinase-producing staphylococci, and *Hemophilus influenzae*

Genitourinary tract infections caused by susceptible strains of *Escherichia coli, Proteus mirabilis,* and *Streptococcus fecalis*

Skin and soft tissue infections caused by susceptible strains of streptococci, staphylococci, and *Escherichia coli*

Lower respiratory tract infections caused by susceptible strains of streptococci, *Streptococcus pneumoniae,* nonpenicillinase-producing staphylococci, and *Hemophilus influenzae*

Gonorrhea, acute uncomplicated anogenital and urethral infections caused by *Neisseria gonorrhoeae*

ORAL DOSAGE

Adult: 250 mg q8h; for severe infections, 500 mg q8h
Infant ($<$ 6 kg): 25 mg (0.5 ml) q8h
Infant (6–8 kg): 50 mg (1 ml) q8h
Child ($<$ 20 kg): 20 mg/kg/day in divided doses q8h; for severe infections, 40 mg/kg/day in divided doses q8h
Child ($\geq$ 20 kg): same as adult

Adult: 500 mg q8h
Infant ($<$ 6 kg): 50 mg (1 ml) q8h
Infant (6–8 kg): 100 mg (2 ml) q8h
Child ($<$ 20 kg): 40 mg/kg/day in divided doses q8h
Child ($\geq$ 20 kg): same as adult

Adult: 3 g in a single dose

CONTRAINDICATIONS

Hypersensitivity to penicillins

ADMINISTRATION/DOSAGE ADJUSTMENTS

Duration of treatment	Continue treatment for at least 48–72 h after patient becomes asymptomatic or bacteria have been eradicated; beta-hemolytic streptococcal infections should be treated for at least 10 days to prevent rheumatic fever and glomerulonephritis
Use of oral suspension in children	After reconstitution, place required dose directly on child's tongue for swallowing or add to formula, milk, fruit juice, water, ginger ale, or cold drinks; infants weighing 8 kg (18 lb) or less should be given pediatric drops

WARNINGS/PRECAUTIONS

Hypersensitivity	Serious and occasionally fatal anaphylactoid reactions may occur, most likely in patients with a history of sensitivity to multiple allergens. Urticaria, other skin rashes, and serum sickness-like reactions may be controlled with antihistamines and, if necessary, systemic corticosteroids. Drug should be discontinued unless infection is life-threatening and amenable only to amoxicillin. Severe reactions may necessitate emergency measures, such as immediate use of epinephrine, oxygen, IV corticosteroids, and airway management, including intubation; use with caution in patients who have experienced allergic reactions to cephalosporins.
Long-term therapy	Perform blood, renal, and hepatic studies periodically
Superinfection	Overgrowth of nonsusceptible organisms, including fungi, may occur
Suspected syphilitic lesions	If syphilis is suspected, perform dark-field examination before instituting therapy and perform serology testing monthly for at least 4 mo
Chronic urinary tract infections	Require frequent bacteriological and clinical appraisal during therapy and possibly for several months afterward; do not use doses smaller than those recommended above

ADVERSE REACTIONS

Gastrointestinal	Glossitis, stomatitis, black hairy tongue, nausea, vomiting, diarrhea

POLYMOX ■ PRINCIPEN

Hypersensitivity	Skin rash, urticaria, exfoliative dermatitis, anaphylaxis (see WARNINGS/PRECAUTIONS)
Hematological	Anemia, thrombocytopenia, thrombocytopenic purpura, eosinophilia, leukopenia, agranulocytosis

OVERDOSAGE

Signs and symptoms	See ADVERSE REACTIONS
Treatment	Discontinue medication; treat symptomatically

DRUG INTERACTIONS

Probenecid	⇧ Amoxicillin blood level and/or toxicity

ALTERED LABORATORY VALUES

Blood/serum values	⇧ SGOT

Clinically significant alterations in urinary values occur at therapeutic dosages

---

USE IN CHILDREN
See INDICATIONS; do not exceed adult dose

USE IN PREGNANT AND NURSING WOMEN
Safe use not established during pregnancy. Amoxicillin is excreted in human milk in very small amounts.

PENICILLINS

PRINCIPEN (ampicillin) Squibb   Rx

Capsules: 250 mg (Principen 250), 500 mg (Principen 500) **Suspension (per 5 ml):** 125 mg (Principen 125), 250 mg (Principen 250)

INDICATIONS — ORAL DOSAGE[1]

Upper and lower respiratory tract infections caused by susceptible strains of *Hemophilus influenzae*, penicillin G-sensitive staphylococci, streptococci, and *Streptococcus pneumoniae*	**Adult:** 250 mg q6h **Child (≤ 20 kg):** 50 mg/kg/day, given in equally divided doses q6–8h **Child (> 20 kg):** same as adult
Gastrointestinal and genitourinary tract infections caused by susceptible strains of *Shigella*, *Salmonella* (including *S typhosa*), *Escherichia coli*, *Proteus mirabilis*, and enterococci	**Adult:** 500 mg q6h **Child (≤ 20 kg):** 100 mg/kg/day, given in equally divided doses q6h **Child (> 20 kg):** same as adult
Gonorrhea	**Adult:** 3.5 g, given simultaneously with 1 g probenecid

CONTRAINDICATIONS

Infections caused by penicillinase-producing organisms	Hypersensitivity to penicillins

ADMINISTRATION/DOSAGE ADJUSTMENTS

Timing of oral administration	Administer ½ h before or at least 2 h after meals to assure maximum absorption
Duration of treatment	Continue treatment for at least 48–72 h after patient has become asymptomatic or bacteria have been eradicated; beta-hemolytic streptococcal infections should be treated for at least 10 days to prevent rheumatic fever and glomerulonephritis

WARNINGS/PRECAUTIONS

Hypersensitivity	Serious and occasionally fatal anaphylactoid reactions may occur, most likely in patients with a history of sensitivity to multiple allergens. Urticaria, other skin rashes, and serum sickness-like reactions may be controlled with antihistamines and, if necessary, systemic corticosteroids. Drug should be discontinued unless infection is life-threatening and amenable only to ampicillin. Severe reactions may necessitate emergency measures, such as immediate use of epinephrine, oxygen, IV corticosteroids, and airway management, including intubation; use with caution in patients who have experienced allergic reactions to cephalosporins.
Long-term therapy	Perform blood, renal, and hepatic studies periodically, particularly with high-dosage schedules
Superinfection	Overgrowth of nonsusceptible organisms, including fungi, may occur

ADVERSE REACTIONS

Frequent reactions (incidence ≥ 1%) are printed in *italics*

Gastrointestinal	Glossitis, stomatitis, nausea, vomiting, enterocolitis, pseudomembranous colitis, diarrhea
Hypersensitivity	*Erythematous maculopapular rash,* pruritus, urticaria, erythema multiforme, exfoliative dermatitis, anaphylaxis (see WARNINGS/PRECAUTIONS)
Hematological	Anemia, thrombocytopenia, thrombocytopenic purpura, eosinophilia, leukopenia, agranulocytosis
Other	Laryngeal stridor, high fever, sore mouth or tongue

Suspected syphilitic lesions — If syphilis is suspected, perform dark-field examination before instituting therapy and perform serology testing monthly for at least 4 mo

Chronic urinary tract and intestinal infections — Require frequent bacteriological and clinical appraisal during therapy and possibly for several months afterward; do not use doses smaller than those recommended above

OVERDOSAGE

Signs and symptoms	See ADVERSE REACTIONS
Treatment	Discontinue medication; treat symptomatically

DRUG INTERACTIONS

Probenecid	△ Ampicillin blood level and/or toxicity

ALTERED LABORATORY VALUES

Blood/serum values	△ SGOT

No clinically significant alterations in urinary values occur at therapeutic dosages

---

USE IN CHILDREN

See INDICATIONS; adjust dosage according to body weight and severity of infection

---

USE IN PREGNANT AND NURSING WOMEN

Safety for use during pregnancy has not been established. Penicillins are excreted in human milk and may increase the risk of allergic sensitization in nursing infants.[1]

[1] Knowles JA: *J Pediatr* 66:1068–1082, 1965; *Med Lett Drugs Ther* 16:25–27, 1974

---

[1] Higher doses may be needed for severe or chronic infections

---

PENICILLINS

PROSTAPHLIN (oxacillin sodium) Apothecon   Rx

Capsules: 250, 500 mg oxacillin[1] **Solution (per 5 ml):** 250 mg oxacillin[1] after reconstitution **Vials:** 0.25, 0.5, 1, 2, 4 g oxacillin[1]
Piggyback vials: 1, 2 g oxacillin[1] **Pharmacy bulk vials:** 10 g oxacillin[1]

INDICATIONS

Staphylococcal infections caused by susceptible penicillin G-resistant strains

ORAL DOSAGE

Adult: for mild to moderate infections, 500 mg q4–6h; for severe infections, 1 g q4–6h

Child (< 40 kg): for mild to moderate infections, 50 mg/kg/day, given in equally divided doses q6h; for severe infections, 100 mg/kg/day, given in equally divided doses q4–6h

Child (≥ 40 kg): same as adult

PARENTERAL DOSAGE

Adult: for mild to moderate infections, 250–500 mg IM or IV q4–6h; for severe infections, 1 g IM or IV q4–6h

Premature and full-term neonates: 25 mg/kg/day IM or IV

Infant and child (< 40 kg): for mild to moderate infections, 50 mg/kg/day, given IM or IV in equally divided doses q6h; for severe infections, 100 mg/kg/day, given IM or IV in equally divided doses q4–6h

Child (≥ 40 kg): same as adult

CONTRAINDICATIONS

History of anaphylactic reaction to any penicillin

ADMINISTRATION/DOSAGE ADJUSTMENTS

Timing of oral administration	To avoid delayed absorption, administer at least 1 h before meals or at least 2 h after meals
Intramuscular administration	To prepare the solution, add 1.4 ml of sterile water for injection USP to the 250-mg vial, 2.7 ml to the 500-mg vial, 5.7 ml to the 1-g vial, 11.5 ml to the 2-g vial, or 23 ml to the 4-g vial. Avoid sciatic nerve injury during gluteal injection.

PROSTAPHLIN

Intravenous administration	To reconstitute solution, add 5 ml of sterile water for injection USP or sodium chloride injection USP to the 250- or 500-mg vials, 10 ml to the 1-g vial, 20 ml to the 2-g vial, or 40 ml to the 4-g vial. For direct injection, withdraw entire contents and administer slowly over a period of approximately 10 min. For IV infusion, dilute the reconstituted solution to a final concentration of 0.5–2 mg/ml, using 5% dextrose in normal saline, 10% D-fructose in water or normal saline, lactated potassic saline injection, 10% invert sugar in normal saline, 10% invert sugar and 0.3% potassium chloride in water, or Travert 10% Electrolyte #1, #2, or #3. Take care to avoid thrombophlebitis, particularly in elderly patients. If another agent is to be used with oxacillin, do not physically mix with solution, but administer separately.
Impaired absorption	To ensure therapeutic serum levels in patients with nausea, vomiting, gastric dilation, cardiospasm, or intestinal hypermotility, administer IV or IM
Severe infections	If infection is severe, administer initial doses IM or IV; when conditions permit, switch to oral therapy
Duration of therapy	Treatment should be continued for at least 48 h after fever and other symptoms have disappeared and laboratory evidence of bacterial eradication has been obtained; treat severe infections for at least 14 days.
Susceptibility testing	Use a disk containing methicillin, a penicillinase-resistant penicillin, to determine susceptibility to oxacillin; to ensure that methicillin-resistant strains do not escape detection, it may be necessary to incubate a large inocula for 48 h
Suspected staphylococcal infections	Oxacillin may be used to treat suspected penicillin G-resistant staphylococcal infections before the results of cultures and susceptibility tests have been obtained; however, if the laboratory studies indicate that the infection is not due to a susceptible penicillin G-resistant strain, use should be discontinued and a more appropriate antibiotic substituted

WARNINGS/PRECAUTIONS

Hypersensitivity	Severe, potentially fatal anaphylactic reactions have been seen in up to 0.04% of penicillin-treated patients, usually within 20 min after administration. Immediate-type reactions, ranging in severity from urticaria, pruritus, and fever to laryngeal edema, laryngospasm, and hypotension, may also occur within 20 min to 48 h after administration. Still other allergic reactions, such as serum sickness and certain rashes, may manifest themselves not less than 48 h, and sometimes as late as 2–4 wk, after treatment is started. Although immediate-type reactions have usually been seen in patients sensitized during a previous course of penicillin therapy, these reactions have also occurred in patients who have never undergone treatment with the drug, but who are presumed to have been sensitized by exposure to trace amounts of penicillin in milk or vaccines. Whenever an allergic reaction occurs, therapy should generally be discontinued unless the infection is life-threatening and amenable only to penicillin. Anaphylactic reactions should be treated by appropriate supportive measures, including mechanical ventilation and administration of pressor amines, antihistamines, and corticosteroids. To reduce the risk of allergic reactions, avoid, in general, administration to a patient with a history of asthma or other significant allergy; patients who have experienced a penicillin-related anaphylactic reaction should be instructed to wear a medical identification tag or bracelet during therapy (use in such patients is generally contraindicated).
Pseuromembranous colitis	May occur due to alteration of the normal intestinal flora and should be considered in any patient who develops diarrhea during or after therapy. Mild cases may respond to withdrawal of the drug alone. Moderate to severe cases should be managed by fluid and electrolyte replacement and protein supplementation, as needed. Oral vancomycin is the treatment of choice for severe or refractory colitis associated with the overgrowth of Clostridium difficile; however, other possible causes should also be considered.
Detection of septicemia	Perform blood cultures at least weekly during therapy
Superinfection	If overgrowth of nonsusceptible organisms occurs, discontinue use and institute appropriate therapy
Hepatotoxicity	Oxacillin may cause hepatotoxicity, characterized by fever, nausea, vomiting, and abnormal liver function values (mainly increased SGOT levels); periodically measure SGOT and SGPT levels during therapy
Blood dyscrasias	To detect hematological reactions, perform WBC and differential cell counts at least weekly during therapy
Nephrotoxicity	Damage to renal tubules and interstitial nephritis can occur during therapy; possible signs include rash, fever, eosinophilia, hematuria, proteinuria, and renal insufficiency. Periodically measure the BUN level, determine creatinine clearance or serum creatinine level, and perform a urinalysis; if abnormal findings are seen, consider reducing the dosage.
Neurotoxicity	Large IV doses, especially in patients with renal impairment, may produce penicillin G-like neurotoxicity; if renal impairment is known or suspected, monitor the serum oxacillin level and consider reducing the dosage
Carcinogenicity	No long-term studies have been done to evaluate carcinogenic potential of this drug

PROSTAPHLIN ■ PYOPEN

ADVERSE REACTIONS

Gastrointestinal	Nausea, vomiting, diarrhea, GI irritation, increase in liver function values, pseudomembranous colitis
Hematological	Agranulocytosis, neutropenia, bone marrow depression
Renal	Renal tubular damage and interstitial nephritis (infrequent)
Hypersensitivity	Urticaria, pruritus, angioneurotic edema, fever, laryngospasm, laryngeal edema, bronchospasm, hypotension, vascular collapse; serum sickness, characterized by fever, malaise, urticaria, myalgia, arthralgia, and abdominal pain
Other	Penicillin G-like neurotoxicity (see WARNINGS/PRECAUTIONS), stomatitis, black or hairy tongue

OVERDOSAGE

Signs and symptoms	See ADVERSE REACTIONS
Treatment	Treat symptomatically

DRUG INTERACTIONS

Probenecid	↑ Serum oxacillin level; use probenecid in combination with oxacillin only when very high serum levels are necessary
Tetracycline	↓ Anti-infective effect of oxacillin; avoid concomitant use

ALTERED LABORATORY VALUES

Blood/serum values	↑ SGOT

No clinically significant alterations in urinary values occur at therapeutic dosages

---

USE IN CHILDREN

See INDICATIONS and ORAL DOSAGE; when administering this drug to neonates, check serum level frequently and watch closely for evidence of toxicity

USE IN PREGNANT AND NURSING WOMEN

Pregnancy Category B: no evidence of impaired fertility or harm to the fetus has been seen in mice, rats, or rabbits given penicillinase-resistant penicillins, and no adverse effects on a human fetus have been reported following use of these penicillins during pregnancy; however, no adequate, well-controlled studies have been done in pregnant women. Use during pregnancy only if clearly needed. Penicillins are excreted in human milk; use with caution in nursing mothers.

[1] As the sodium salt

PENICILLINS

PYOPEN (carbenicillin disodium) Beecham   Rx

Vials: carbenicillin disodium equivalent to 1, 2, or 5 g carbenicillin   **Piggyback units:** carbenicillin disodium equivalent to 2 or 5 g carbenicillin   **Bulk pharmacy package:** carbenicillin disodium equivalent to 10 or 20 g carbenicillin

INDICATIONS

Urinary tract infections caused by susceptible strains of *Pseudomonas aeruginosa*, *Enterobacter* sp, and *Streptococcus fecalis*

Urinary tract infections caused by susceptible strains of *Proteus* and *Escherichia coli*

Severe systemic infections, septicemia, and respiratory and soft tissue infections caused by susceptible strains of *Pseudomonas aeruginosa* and anaerobic bacteria

Severe systemic infections, septicemia, respiratory and soft tissue infections caused by susceptible strains of *Proteus* and *Escherichia coli*

Meningitis caused by susceptible strains of *Hemophilus influenzae*

PARENTERAL DOSAGE

Adult: for uncomplicated infections, 1–2 g IM or IV q6h; for serious infections, 200 mg/kg/day, given by IV drip
Child: 50–200 mg/kg/day IM or IV, given in divided doses q4–6h

Adult: same as above
Child: 50–100 mg/kg/day IM or IV, given in divided doses q4–6h

Adult: 400–500 mg/kg/day IV, given in divided doses or by continuous infusion
Child: same as adult

Adult: 250–400 mg/kg/day IV, given in divided doses or by continuous infusion
Child: 250–400 mg/kg/day IM or IV, given in divided doses or by continuous infusion

Adult: 400–500 mg/kg/day IV, given in divided doses or by continuous infusion
Child: same as adult

PYOPEN

Gonorrhea; acute uncomplicated anogenital and urethral infections caused by susceptible strains of *Neisseria gonorrhoeae*	**Adult:** 4 g total, given in a single IM injection divided between 2 sites (with 1 g probenecid orally 30 min prior to injection)
Neonatal sepsis caused by susceptible strains of *Pseudomonas aeruginosa*, *Proteus*, *Escherichia coli*, and *Hemophilus influenzae*	**Infant (< 2 kg):** 100 mg/kg IM or IV to start, followed by 75 mg/kg IM or IV q8h during 1st wk of life and 100 mg/kg IM or IV q6h thereafter[1] **Infant (> 2 kg):** 100 mg/kg IM or IV to start, followed by 75 mg/kg IM or IV q6h during first 3 days of life and 100 mg/kg IM or IV q6h thereafter[1]

CONTRAINDICATIONS

Hypersensitivity to penicillins

ADMINISTRATION/DOSAGE ADJUSTMENTS

Intramuscular administration	To reconstitute the solution, add 2–3.6 ml of sterile water for injection USP or 0.5% lidocaine hydrochloride (without epinephrine) to the 1-g vial, 4–6.6 ml to the 2-g vial, or 9.5–17 ml to the 5-g vial. Inject single doses of not more than 2 g well within the body of a relatively large muscle.
Intravenous administration	To reconstitute the solution, use at least the following amount of sterile water for injection USP: 4 ml for the 1-g vial, 8 ml for the 2-g vial, 20 ml for the 5-g vial or 2-g piggyback bottle, 50 ml for the 5-g piggyback bottle, and 95 ml for the 10-g bulk pharmacy bottle; add 85 ml of sterile water for injection USP, sodium chloride injection USP, or 5% dextrose in water injection USP to the 20-g bulk pharmacy bottle. For IV injection, dilute solution to a final concentration of 50 mg/ml or less and administer as slowly as possible in order to avoid irritation of the vein. For continuous or intermittent infusion, dilute solution to a final concentration of 10-50 mg/ml; administer each intermittent dose over a period of 30 min to 2 h.
Serious urinary tract and systemic infections	IV therapy in higher doses up to 40 g/day may be required
Concomitant therapy	Gentamicin may be used concomitantly with carbenicillin for initial therapy until results of cultures and susceptibility tests are known; however, the two antibiotics should not be mixed together in the same IV solution
Patients with renal impairment	For infections caused by *Pseudomonas aeruginosa*, *Proteus*, or *Escherichia coli*, administer 2 g IV q8h to adults with a creatinine clearance rate < 5 ml/min
Dialysis patients	For infections caused by *Pseudomonas aeruginosa*, *Proteus*, or *Escherichia coli*, administer 2 g IV q6h to adults during peritoneal dialysis or 2 g IV q4h to adults receiving hemodialysis

WARNINGS/PRECAUTIONS

Hypersensitivity	Serious and occasionally fatal anaphylactoid reactions may occur, most likely in patients with a history of sensitivity to multiple allergens. If a reaction occurs, drug should be discontinued unless infection is life-threatening and amenable only to carbenicillin. Severe reactions may necessitate immediate emergency treatment with epinephrine, oxygen, IV corticosteroids, and airway management, including intubation; use with caution in patients who have experienced allergic reactions to cephalosporins.
Long-term therapy	Perform blood, renal, and hepatic studies periodically
Superinfection	May result from emergence of resistant organisms, such as *Klebsiella* and *Serratia*
Abnormal bleeding	Hemorrhagic manifestations associated with abnormalities of coagulation tests, such as bleeding time and platelet aggregation, may develop, particularly in uremic patients receiving high doses (eg, 24 g/day); discontinue use of drug and institute appropriate therapy
Patients with renal impairment	Convulsions or neuromuscular excitability may occur when large doses are used
Sodium overload	May occur (each vial contains up to 6.5 mEq sodium/g of carbenicillin); monitor electrolyte and cardiac status carefully
Hypokalemia	May occur; monitor serum potassium level periodically and institute appropriate corrective measures, as needed
Suspected syphilitic lesions	If syphilis is suspected, perform a dark-field examination before instituting therapy and monthly serology tests for at least 4 mo afterward

ADVERSE REACTIONS

Hypersensitivity	Skin rash, eosinophilia, urticaria, pruritus, drug fever, anaphylaxis (see WARNINGS/PRECAUTIONS)
Gastrointestinal	Nausea, unpleasant taste
Hematological	Leukopenia, neutropenia, thrombocytopenia, hemolytic anemia
Central nervous system	Convulsions and neuromuscular excitability, especially with large doses in patients with renal impairment

PYOPEN ■ SK-AMPICILLIN

| Other | Pain and induration at IM injection site, vein irritation and phlebitis |

OVERDOSAGE

| Signs and symptoms | See ADVERSE REACTIONS |
| Treatment | Discontinue medication; treat symptomatically |

DRUG INTERACTIONS

| Probenecid | △ Carbenicillin blood level and/or toxicity   ▽ Urine level |

ALTERED LABORATORY VALUES

| Blood/serum values | △ SGOT   △ SGPT |

No clinically significant alterations in urinary values occur at therapeutic dosages

---

USE IN CHILDREN

See INDICATIONS and PARENTERAL DOSAGE

USE IN PREGNANT AND NURSING WOMEN

Safety for use during pregnancy has not been established. Carbenicillin appears in human milk (level is unknown); use with caution in nursing mothers.

---

[1] Neonatal doses may be given IM or by 15-min IV infusion

PENICILLINS

SK-AMPICILLIN (ampicillin) Smith Kline & French   Rx

Capsules: 250, 500 mg   **Suspension (per 5 ml):** 125 mg (100, 150, 200 ml), 250 mg (100, 150, 200 ml), or 500 mg (20 ml) after reconstitution

INDICATIONS

Upper and lower respiratory tract and soft tissue infections caused by susceptible strains of *Hemophilus influenzae*, penicillin G-sensitive staphylococci, streptococci, and *Streptococcus pneumoniae*

ORAL DOSAGE

Adult: 250 mg q6h
Child (< 20 kg): 50 mg/kg/day, given in equally divided doses q6–8h
Child (≥ 20 kg): same as adult

Gastrointestinal and genitourinary tract infections caused by susceptible strains of *Shigella*, *Salmonella* (including *S typhosa*), *Escherichia coli*, *Proteus mirabilis*, and enterococci

Adult: 500 mg q6h; for stubborn or severe infections, higher doses may be needed, possibly for several weeks
Child (< 20 kg): 100 mg/kg/day, given in equally divided doses q6–8h; for stubborn or severe infections, higher doses may be needed, possibly for several weeks
Child (≥ 20 kg): same as adult

Urethritis caused by *Neisseria gonorrhoeae*

Adult: 3.5 g, given simultaneously with 1 g probenecid

CONTRAINDICATIONS

Hypersensitivity to penicillins

ADMINISTRATION/DOSAGE ADJUSTMENTS

| Duration of treatment | Continue treatment for at least 48–72 h after patient has become asymptomatic or bacteria have been eradicated; beta-hemolytic streptococcal infections should be treated for at least 10 days to prevent rheumatic fever and glomerulonephritis |

WARNINGS/PRECAUTIONS

Hypersensitivity	Serious and occasionally fatal anaphylactic reactions may occur, most likely in patients with a history of sensitivity to multiple allergens. Urticaria, other skin rashes, and serum sickness-like reactions may be controlled with antihistamines and, if necessary, systemic corticosteroids. Drug should be discontinued unless infection is life-threatening and amenable only to ampicillin. Severe reactions may necessitate emergency measures, such as immediate use of epinephrine, oxygen, IV corticosteroids, and airway management, including intubation; use with caution in patients who have experienced allergic reactions to cephalosporins
Long-term therapy	Perform blood, renal, and hepatic studies periodically
Superinfection	Overgrowth of nonsusceptible organisms, including fungi, may occur
Suspected syphilitic lesions	If syphilis is suspected, perform a dark-field examination before instituting therapy and monthly serology tests for at least 4 mo afterward

SK-AMPICILLIN ■ SPECTROBID

Chronic urinary tract and intestinal infections	Require bacteriological and clinical appraisal during therapy, and possibly for several months afterward; do not use doses smaller than those recommended above
Complications of gonorrheal urethritis, (eg, prostatitis and epididymitis)	Prolonged and intensive therapy is recommended
Patients with infectious mononucleosis	Ampicillin should not be used for the treatment of infectious mononucleosis; a high percentage of patients with mononucleosis develop a skin rash after receiving ampicillin

ADVERSE REACTIONS

Frequent reactions (incidence ≥ 1%) are printed in *italics*

Gastrointestinal	Glossitis, stomatitis, black hairy tongue, nausea, vomiting, enterocolitis, pseudomembranous colitis, *diarrhea*
Hypersensitivity	*Skin rash, urticaria,* exfoliative dermatitis, erythema multiforme, anaphylaxis (usually associated with parenteral therapy)
Hematological	Anemia, thrombocytopenia, thrombocytopenic purpura, eosinophilia, leukopenia, agranulocytosis

OVERDOSAGE

Signs and symptoms	See ADVERSE REACTIONS
Treatment	Discontinue medication; treat symptomatically

DRUG INTERACTIONS

Probenecid	△ Ampicillin blood level and/or toxicity

ALTERED LABORATORY VALUES

Blood/serum values	△ SGOT (especially in infants)

No clinically significant alterations in urinary values occur at therapeutic dosages

---

USE IN CHILDREN

See INDICATIONS and ORAL DOSAGE

USE IN PREGNANT AND NURSING WOMEN

Safety for use during pregnancy has not been established. Ampicillin is excreted in human milk in very small amounts; use with caution in nursing mothers.

PENICILLINS

SPECTROBID (bacampicillin hydrochloride) Roerig   Rx

Tablets: 400 mg **Suspension (per 5 ml):** 125 mg after reconstitution (70, 100, 140, 200 ml)

INDICATIONS	ORAL DOSAGE
Upper respiratory tract infections caused by susceptible strains of streptococci, pneumococci, nonpenicillinase-producing staphylococci, and *Hemophilus influenzae* **Urinary tract infections** caused by susceptible strains of *Escherichia coli, Proteus mirabilis,* and *Streptococcus fecalis* (enterococci) **Skin and skin structure infections** caused by susceptible strains of streptococci and staphylococci	Adult: 400 mg q12h; for severe infections or those caused by less susceptible organisms, 800 mg q12h Child: 25 mg/kg/day, given in 2 equally divided doses q12h; for severe infections or those caused by less susceptible organisms, 50 mg/kg/day, given in 2 equally divided doses q12h (for patients weighing ≥ 25 kg, use adult dosage)
Lower respiratory tract infections caused by susceptible strains of streptococci, pneumococci, nonpenicillinase-producing staphylococci, and *Hemophilus influenzae*	Adult: 800 mg q12h Child: 50 mg/kg/day, given in 2 equally divided doses q12h (for patients weighing ≥ 25 kg, use adult dosage)
Acute uncomplicated **urogenital infections** caused by *Neisseria gonorrhoeae*	Adult: 1.6 g, given simultaneously with 1 g probenecid

CONTRAINDICATIONS

Hypersensitivity to penicillins or cephalosporins	Disulfiram therapy (see DRUG INTERACTIONS)

COMPENDIUM OF DRUG THERAPY

SPECTROBID

ADMINISTRATION/DOSAGE ADJUSTMENTS

Timing of administration	Oral suspension should be given to fasting patients; the tablets, which are intended for adults and children weighing 25 kg or more, may be administered without regard to meals
Duration of treatment	Continue treatment for at least 48–72 h after patient has become asymptomatic or bacteria have been eradicated; hemolytic streptococcal infections should be treated for at least 10 days to prevent acute rheumatic fever and glomerulonephritis

WARNINGS/PRECAUTIONS

Hypersensitivity	Serious and occasionally fatal anaphylactic reactions may occur, most likely in patients with a history of penicillin hypersensitivity and/or hypersensitivity to multiple allergens. Urticaria and other skin rashes may be controlled with antihistamines and, if necessary, systemic corticosteroids. Drug should be discontinued unless the opinion of the physician dictates otherwise. Serious anaphylactoid reactions may necessitate emergency measures, such as immediate use of epinephrine, oxygen, IV corticosteroids, and airway management, including intubation; use with caution in patients who have experienced allergic reactions to cephalosporins.
Long-term therapy	Perform blood, renal, and hepatic studies periodically, particularly in premature infants, neonates, and patients with hepatic or renal impairment
Superinfection	Overgrowth of nonsusceptible organisms, including fungi, may occur
Suspected syphilitic lesions	If syphilis is suspected, perform a dark-field examination before instituting therapy and monthly serology tests for at least 4 mo afterward
Chronic urinary tract and intestinal infections	Require bacteriological and clinical appraisal during therapy, and possibly for several months afterward
Complications of gonorrheal urethritis, such as prostatitis and epididymitis	Prolonged and intensive therapy is recommended
Patients with infectious mononucleosis	Ampicillin-class antibiotics should not be used for the treatment of infectious mononucleosis; infectious mononucleosis is viral in origin, and a high percentage of patients who receive ampicillin develop a skin rash

ADVERSE REACTIONS[1]

Frequent reactions (incidence ≥ 1%) are printed in *italics*

Gastrointestinal	*Diarrhea and epigastric upset (2%);* gastritis, stomatitis, nausea, vomiting, glossitis, black hairy tongue, enterocolitis, pseudomembranous colitis
Hypersensitivity	Rash, urticaria, erythema multiforme, exfoliative dermatitis, anaphylaxis (see WARNINGS/PRECAUTIONS)
Hematological	Anemia, thrombocytopenia, thrombocytopenic purpura, eosinophilia, leukopenia, agranulocytosis

OVERDOSAGE

Signs and symptoms	See ADVERSE REACTIONS
Treatment	Discontinue medication; treat symptomatically

DRUG INTERACTIONS[2]

Disulfiram	Risk of disulfiram-like reaction
Probenecid	△ Ampicillin blood level and/or toxicity

ALTERED LABORATORY VALUES

Blood/serum values	△ SGOT ▽ Estrogen (in pregnant women; transient)
Urinary values	△ Glucose (with Clinitest tablets)

USE IN CHILDREN

See INDICATIONS and ORAL DOSAGE

USE IN PREGNANT AND NURSING WOMEN

Pregnancy Category B: use during pregnancy only if clearly needed. Reproduction studies in mice and rats at doses exceeding 25 times the human dose have shown no evidence of impaired fertility or harm to the fetus; however, no adequate, well-controlled studies have been done in pregnant women. Ampicillin-class antibiotics are excreted in breast milk; use with caution in nursing mothers.

---

[1] Includes reactions reported with ampicillin
[2] Co-administration of allopurinol and ampicillin increases substantially the incidence of rashes in patients receiving both drugs as compared to patients receiving ampicillin alone. Whether this potentiation of ampicillin rashes is due to allopurinol or the hyperuricemia present is unknown. No data are available on the incidence of rash in patients treated concurrently with bacampicillin and allopurinol.

PENICILLINS

TEGOPEN (cloxacillin sodium) Apothecon   Rx

Capsules: 250, 500 mg   **Solution (per 5 ml):** 125 mg after reconstitution

INDICATIONS	**ORAL DOSAGE**
Staphylococcal infections caused by susceptible penicillin G-resistant strains	**Adult:** for mild to moderate infections, 250 mg q6h; for severe infections, 500 mg or more q6h **Child (< 20 kg):** for mild to moderate infections, 50 mg/kg/day, given in 4 equally divided doses q6h; for severe infections, 100 mg/kg/day or more, given in 4 equally divided doses q6h **Child (≥ 20 kg):** same as adult

CONTRAINDICATIONS

History of anaphylactic reaction to any penicillin

ADMINISTRATION/DOSAGE ADJUSTMENTS

Timing of administration	To avoid delayed absorption, administer at least 1 h before meals or at least 2 h after meals
Serious infections	To treat serious, life-threatening infections, start with a parenteral agent and then, when conditions permit, switch to cloxacillin
Duration of therapy	Treatment should be continued for at least 48 h after fever and other symptoms have disappeared and laboratory evidence of bacterial eradication has been obtained; treat severe infections for at least 14 days
Susceptibility testing	Use a disk containing methicillin, a penicillinase-resistant penicillin, to determine susceptibility to cloxacillin; to ensure that methicillin-resistant strains do not escape detection, it may be necessary to incubate a large inocula for 48 h
Suspected staphylococcal infections	Cloxacillin may be used to treat suspected penicillin G-resistant staphylococcal infections before the results of cultures and susceptibility tests have been obtained; however, if the laboratory studies indicate that the infection is not due to a susceptible penicillin G-resistant strain, use should be discontinued and a more appropriate antibiotic substituted

WARNINGS/PRECAUTIONS

Hypersensitivity	Severe, potentially fatal anaphylactic reactions have been seen in up to 0.04% of penicillin-treated patients, usually within 20 min after administration. Immediate-type reactions, ranging in severity from urticaria, pruritus, and fever to laryngeal edema, laryngospasm, and hypotension, may also occur within 20 min to 48 h after administration. Still other allergic reactions, such as serum sickness and certain rashes, may manifest themselves not less than 48 h, and sometimes as late as 2–4 wk after, treatment is started. Although immediate-type reactions have usually been seen in patients sensitized during a previous course of penicillin therapy, these reactions have also occurred in patients who have never undergone treatment with the drug, but who are presumed to have been sensitized by exposure to trace amounts of penicillin in milk or vaccines. Whenever an allergic reaction occurs, therapy should generally be discontinued unless the infection is life-threatening and amenable only to penicillin. Anaphylactic reactions should be treated by appropriate supportive measures, including mechanical ventilation and administration of pressor amines, antihistamines, and corticosteroids. To reduce the risk of allergic reactions, avoid, in general, administration to a patient with a history of hypersensitivity to any penicillin, and exercise caution if a patient has a history of asthma or other significant allergy; patients who have experienced a penicillin-related anaphylactic reaction should be instructed to wear a medical identification tag or bracelet during therapy (use in such patients is generally contraindicated).
Impaired absorption	Administer a parenteral form of penicillin to patients with nausea, vomiting, gastric dilation, cardiospasm, or intestinal hypermotility
Detection of septicemia	Perform blood cultures at least weekly during therapy
Superinfection	If overgrowth of nonsusceptible organisms occurs, discontinue use and institute appropriate therapy
Hepatotoxicity	Cloxacillin may cause hepatotoxicity, characterized by fever, nausea, vomiting, and abnormal liver function values (mainly increased SGOT levels); periodically measure SGOT and SGPT levels during therapy
Blood dyscrasias	To detect hematological reactions, perform WBC and differential cell counts at least weekly during therapy
Renal impairment	Perform a urinalysis, measure the BUN level, and determine creatinine clearance or serum creatinine level periodically; if renal impairment is suspected at the outset or becomes apparent during the course of therapy, monitor the serum cloxacillin level and consider reducing the dosage

TEGOPEN ■ TICAR

Carcinogenicity	No studies have been done to evaluate the carcinogenic potential of this drug

ADVERSE REACTIONS

Gastrointestinal	Nausea, vomiting, diarrhea, GI irritation, increase in liver function values
Hematological	Agranulocytosis, neutropenia, bone marrow depression
Hypersensitivity	Urticaria, pruritus, angioneurotic edema, fever, laryngospasm, laryngeal edema, bronchospasm, hypotension, vascular collapse; serum sickness, characterized by fever, malaise, urticaria, myalgia, arthralgia, and abdominal pain
Other	Stomatitis, black or hairy tongue

OVERDOSAGE

Signs and symptoms	See ADVERSE REACTIONS
Treatment	Treat symptomatically

DRUG INTERACTIONS

Probenecid	△ Serum cloxacillin level; use probenecid in combination with cloxacillin only when very high serum levels are necessary
Tetracycline	▽ Anti-infective effect of cloxacillin; avoid concomitant use

ALTERED LABORATORY VALUES

Blood/serum values	△ SGOT

No clinically significant alterations in urinary values occur at therapeutic dosages

---

USE IN CHILDREN

See INDICATIONS and ORAL DOSAGE; when administering this drug to neonates, check serum level frequently and watch closely for evidence of toxicity

USE IN PREGNANT AND NURSING WOMEN

Pregnancy Category B: no evidence of impaired fertility or harm to the fetus has been seen in mice, rats, or rabbits given penicillinase-resistant penicillins, and no adverse effects on a human fetus have been reported following use of these penicillins during pregnancy; however, no adequate, well-controlled studies have been done in pregnant women. Use during pregnancy only if clearly needed. Penicillins are excreted in human milk; use with caution in nursing mothers.

PENICILLINS

TICAR (ticarcillin disodium) Beecham   Rx

Vials: 1, 3, 6 g **Piggyback units:** 3 g **Bulk pharmacy package:** 20, 30 g

INDICATIONS

Bacterial septicemia, skin and soft tissue infections, and acute and chronic respiratory tract infections caused by susceptible strains of *Pseudomonas aeruginosa, Proteus, Escherichia coli,* and anaerobic bacteria

Lower respiratory tract infections, including empyema, anaerobic pneumonitis, and lung abscess, caused by susceptible anaerobic bacteria

Intraabdominal infections, including peritonitis and intraabdominal abscess, caused by susceptible anaerobic bacteria

Female pelvic and genital tract infections, including endometritis, pelvic inflammatory disease, pelvic abscess, and salpingitis, caused by susceptible anaerobic bacteria

Genitourinary tract infections caused by susceptible strains of *Pseudomonas aeruginosa, Proteus, Escherichia coli, Enterobacter,* and *Streptococcus fecalis*

PARENTERAL DOSAGE

Adult: 200–300 mg/kg/day, given by IV infusion in divided doses q4–6h; usual dosage: 3 g q4h or 4 g q6h, depending on weight and the severity of the infection
Child (< 40 kg): 200–300 mg/kg/day, given by IV infusion in divided doses q4–6h
Child (≥ 40 kg): same as adult

Adult: for uncomplicated infections, 1 g IM or by IV injection q6h; for complicated infections, 150–200 mg/kg/day, given by IV infusion in divided doses q4–6h
Child (< 40 kg): for uncomplicated infections, 50–100 mg/kg/day, given IM or by IV injection in divided doses q6–8h; for complicated infections, 150–200 mg/kg/day, given by IV infusion in divided doses q4–6h
Child (≥ 40 kg): same as adult

COMPENDIUM OF DRUG THERAPY

TICAR

Neonatal sepsis caused by susceptible strains of *Pseudomonas*, *Proteus*, and *Escherichia coli*

Infant (< 2 kg): 75 mg/kg, given q12h if 0–7 days of age or q8h if over 7 days of age; administer IM or by 10- to 20-min IV infusion
Infant (> 2 kg): 75 mg/kg q8h if 0–7 days of age or 100 mg/kg q8h if over 7 days of age; administer IM or by 10- to 20-min IV infusion

CONTRAINDICATIONS

Hypersensitivity to penicillins

ADMINISTRATION/DOSAGE ADJUSTMENTS

Intramuscular administration	To reconstitute solution, add 2 ml of sterile water for injection, sodium chloride injection, or 1% lidocaine hydrochloride (without epinephrine) to each gram of ticarcillin. Promptly after reconstitution, inject single doses of not more than 2 g well within the body of a relatively large muscle.
Intravenous administration	To reconstitute solution, add 4 ml of sodium chloride injection, 5% dextrose injection, or lactated Ringer's injection to the 1-g vial, 8 ml to the 2-g vial, 12 ml to the 3-g vial, a minimum of 30 ml to the 3-g piggyback bottle, 85 ml to the 20-g bulk pharmacy package, or 75 ml to the 30-g bulk pharmacy package. For IV injection, dilute solution to a final concentration of 50 mg/ml or less and administer as slowly as possible in order to avoid irritation of the vein. For continuous or intermittent infusion, dilute solution to a final concentration of 10–50 mg/ml; administer each intermittent dose over a period of 30 min to 2 h. Do not mix ticarcillin with gentamicin, tobramycin, or amikacin in the same IV solution.
Serious urinary tract and systemic infections	Intravenous therapy in higher doses may be required
Patients with renal impairment	For children weighing over 40 kg and adults, administer an initial loading dose of 3 g IV, followed by 3 g IV q4h when creatinine clearance rate (CCr) > 60 ml/min, 2 g IV q4h when CCr = 30–60 ml/min, 2 g IV q8h when CCr = 10–30 ml/min, 2 g IV q12h or 1 g IM q6h when CCr < 10 ml/min, or 2 g IV q24h or 1 g IM q12h when CCr < 10 ml/min and hepatic insufficiency exists. CCr may be calculated for men from the serum creatinine (SCr) value using the following formula: CCr = (140 − age) (wt in kg)/72 × SCr (mg/dl); for women, multiply the value obtained by this formula by 0.85.
Dialysis patients	For children weighing over 40 kg and adults, administer 3 g IV q12h if they are on peritoneal dialysis or 2 g q12h IV plus 3 g IV after each dialysis treatment if they are receiving hemodialysis

WARNINGS/PRECAUTIONS

Hypersensitivity	Serious and occasionally fatal anaphylactoid reactions may occur, most likely in patients with a history of sensitivity to multiple allergens. If a reaction occurs, drug should be discontinued unless infection is life-threatening and amenable only to ticarcillin. Severe reactions may necessitate immediate emergency treatment with epinephrine, oxygen, IV corticosteroids, and airway management, including intubation; use with caution in patients who have experienced allergic reactions to cephalosporins.
Long-term therapy	Perform blood, renal, and hepatic studies periodically
Superinfection	Overgrowth of nonsusceptible organisms, including fungi, may occur
Abnormal bleeding	Hemorrhagic manifestations associated with abnormalities of coagulation tests, such as bleeding time and platelet aggregation, may develop, particularly in patients receiving high doses or in those with renal impairment; discontinue use of drug and institute appropriate therapy
Sodium overload	May occur (each vial contains up to 6.5 mEq sodium/g of ticarcillin); monitor electrolyte and cardiac status periodically
Hypokalemia	May occur; monitor serum potassium level periodically and institute appropriate corrective measures, as needed

ADVERSE REACTIONS

Gastrointestinal	Nausea, vomiting
Hypersensitivity	Skin rash, pruritus, urticaria, drug fever
Hematological	Anemia, thrombocytopenia, leukopenia, neutropenia, eosinophilia
Central nervous system	Convulsions and neuromuscular excitability (especially with high doses in patients with renal impairment)
Other	Pain and (rarely) induration at injection site, vein irritation, phlebitis

OVERDOSAGE

Signs and symptoms	See ADVERSE REACTIONS
Treatment	Discontinue medication; treat symptomatically

DRUG INTERACTIONS

Probenecid	⇧ Ticarcillin blood level and/or toxicity

TICAR ■ TIMENTIN

| Gentamicin, tobramycin, amikacin | ↑ Bactericidal activity against certain strains of *Pseudomonas aeruginosa* in vitro (do not mix in same IV bottle) |

ALTERED LABORATORY VALUES

| Blood/serum values | ↑ SGOT ↑ SGPT |

No clinically significant alterations in urinary values occur at therapeutic dosages

USE IN CHILDREN
See INDICATIONS and PARENTERAL DOSAGE

USE IN PREGNANT AND NURSING WOMEN
Safety for use during pregnancy has not been established. Ticarcillin is excreted in human milk (level is unknown); use with caution in nursing mothers.

PENICILLINS

TIMENTIN (ticarcillin disodium and clavulanate potassium) Beecham — Rx

Vials: ticarcillin disodium equivalent to 3 g ticarcillin and clavulanate potassium equivalent to 100 mg clavulanic acid **Piggyback bottles:** ticarcillin disodium equivalent to 3 g ticarcillin and clavulanate potassium equivalent to 100 mg clavulanic acid

INDICATIONS

Septicemia caused by susceptible, beta-lactamase-producing strains of *Klebsiella, Escherichia coli, Staphylococcus aureus,* and *Pseudomonas* (including *P aeruginosa*)
Lower respiratory tract infections caused by susceptible, beta-lactamase-producing strains of *Staphylococcus aureus, Hemophilus influenzae,* and *Klebsiella*
Bone and joint infections caused by susceptible, beta-lactamase-producing strains of *Staphylococcus aureus*
Skin and skin structure infections caused by susceptible, beta-lactamase-producing strains of *Staphylococcus aureus, Klebsiella,* and *Escherichia coli*
Urinary tract infections caused by susceptible, beta-lactamase-producing strains of *Escherichia coli, Klebsiella, Pseudomonas* (including *P aeruginosa*), *Citrobacter, Enterobacter cloacae, Serratia marcescens,* and *Staphylococcus aureus*

PARENTERAL DOSAGE[1]

Adult (60 kg): 3 g, given by intermittent IV infusion q4–6h
Adult (< 60 kg): 200–300 mg/kg/day, given by intermittent IV infusion q4–6h

CONTRAINDICATIONS

Hypersensitivity to penicillins

ADMINISTRATION/DOSAGE ADJUSTMENTS

Preparation and administration	To reconstitute solution, add approximately 13 ml of sterile water for injection USP or sodium chloride injection USP to the vial (resulting concentration of ticarcillin: 200 mg/ml). For IV infusion, dilute solution with sodium chloride injection USP, 5% dextrose injection USP, or lactated Ringer's injection USP to a final concentration of 10–100 mg/ml. Administer each dose, either directly or through a Y-type set, over a period of 30 min. Do not mix this preparation with aminoglycosides, other antimicrobial drugs, or sodium bicarbonate; when a Y-type infusion set is used, administration of the primary IV solution should be discontinued for the duration of the infusion.
Patients with renal impairment	Give 3 g as an initial loading dose[1]; then administer 3 g q4h if creatinine clearance (Ccr) > 60 ml/min, 2 g q4h if Ccr = 30–60 ml/min, 2 g q8h if Ccr = 10–30 ml/min, 2 g q12h if Ccr < 10 ml/min, 2 g q24h if Ccr < 10 ml/min and hepatic function is impaired, or 3 g q12h if the patient is undergoing peritoneal dialysis.[1] For a patient undergoing hemodialysis, give 2 g q12h following the loading dose and an additional 3 g after each dialysis treatment. The Ccr can be estimated from the serum creatinine level if a measured value cannot be obtained. For adult men, use the following formula: (weight [kg]) (140 − age [yr])/(72) (serum creatinine level [mg/dl]); for adult women, multiply this quotient by 0.85.
Pseudomonal infections	On the basis of in vitro synergism, this preparation has been used effectively with aminoglycosides, particularly in immunocompromised patients, for the treatment of infections caused by certain strains of *Pseudomonas aeruginosa*
Chronic urinary tract infections	Frequent evaluation of bacteriological and clinical response is necessary during treatment of chronic urinary tract infections and may be required for several months after therapy
Duration of therapy	After signs and symptoms have disappeared, therapy should generally be continued for at least 2 days. Although treatment usually lasts 10–14 days, a longer period may be required if the infection is difficult and complicated; several weeks may be necessary for the treatment of persistent urinary tract infections.

TIMENTIN

WARNINGS/PRECAUTIONS

Hypersensitivity	Serious, occasionally fatal anaphylactic reactions have occurred in patients receiving penicillin; use with caution in patients with a history of allergy, particularly if they have demonstrated hypersensitivity to a number of substances. If an allergic reaction occurs, this preparation should be discontinued. For the treatment of serious anaphylactoid reactions, give epinephrine, oxygen, and IV corticosteroids and take appropriate measures (eg, intubation) to ensure adequate pulmonary function.
Bleeding	In some patients receiving beta-lactam antibiotics (especially those with renal impairment), bleeding has occurred in association with abnormal clotting test values, such as prolonged bleeding and prothrombin times; if bleeding is seen during therapy, this preparation should be discontinued and appropriate measures taken
Superinfection	Bear in mind that overgrowth of fungi or bacteria may occur, particularly during prolonged therapy; if superinfection is detected, appropriate measures should be taken
Hypokalemia	In rare cases, ticarcillin can cause hypokalemia; keep in mind this risk, particularly if a patient has a fluid or electrolyte imbalance. During prolonged therapy, periodic measurement of the serum potassium level may be advisable.
Salt-restricted diets	The sodium content of this preparation, 4.75 mEq (109 mg)/g, should be considered if salt intake must be restricted
Toxicity	To avoid toxicity, evaluate hematopoietic, renal, and hepatic function periodically during long-term therapy
Carcinogenicity, mutagenicity	No studies have been done to evaluate the carcinogenic or mutagenic potential of this preparation

ADVERSE REACTIONS

Central nervous system	Headache, giddiness, neuromuscular irritability, convulsive seizures
Gastrointestinal	Flatulence, nausea, vomiting, diarrhea, epigastric pain
Hematological	Thrombocytopenia, leukopenia, neutropenia, eosinophilia, reduction of hemoglobin and hematocrit, prolongation of prothrombin and bleeding times
Hepatic	Increases in SGOT and SGPT levels and in serum levels of alkaline phosphatase, bilirubin, and LDH
Renal	Increases in BUN and serum creatinine levels, hypernatremia, hypokalemia, decrease in serum uric acid level
Hypersensitivity	Rash, pruritus, urticaria, arthralgia, myalgia, drug fever, chills, chest discomfort, anaphylaxis
Local	Pain, burning, swelling, induration, thrombophlebitis
Other	Stomatitis, disturbances of taste and smell

OVERDOSAGE

Signs and symptoms	Neuromuscular hyperirritability, convulsive seizures
Treatment	Institute supportive measures and treat symptomatically; ticarcillin and clavulanic acid can be removed from the blood by hemodialysis

DRUG INTERACTIONS

Probenecid	△ Serum ticarcillin level
Aminoglycosides	△ Antibiotic activity against certain pseudomonal strains Physical incompatibility

ALTERED LABORATORY VALUES

Blood/serum values	False-positive Coombs' test + Protein (with biuret reaction and with nitric acid, acetic acid, and sulfosalicylic acid tests) △ SGPT △ SGOT △ Alkaline phosphatase △ LDH △ Bilirubin △ Creatinine △ BUN △ Sodium ▽ Potassium ▽ Uric acid

No clinically significant alterations in urinary values occur at therapeutic dosages

---

USE IN CHILDREN

Safety and effectiveness for use in children under 12 yr of age have not been established

USE IN PREGNANT AND NURSING WOMEN

Pregnancy Category B: reproduction studies in rats given up to 1,050 mg/kg/day of this preparation have shown no evidence of impaired fertility or harm to the fetus; however, no adequate, well-controlled studies have been done in pregnant women. Use this preparation during pregnancy only if clearly needed. Exercise caution when administering to nursing mothers.

---

[1] Dosage based on ticarcillin content

PENICILLINS

TOTACILLIN (ampicillin) Beecham   Rx

Capsules: 250, 500 mg   **Suspension (per 5 ml):** 125, 250 mg after reconstitution (100, 200 ml)

TOTACILLIN-N (ampicillin sodium) Beecham   Rx

Vials: 125, 250, 500 mg; 1, 2 g   **Piggyback units:** 500 mg; 1, 2 g   **Bulk pharmacy package:** 10 g

INDICATIONS	ORAL DOSAGE[1]	PARENTERAL DOSAGE[1]
Ear, nose, throat, and lower respiratory tract infections caused by susceptible strains of streptococci, *Streptococcus pneumoniae*, and nonpenicillinase-producing staphylococci **Upper and lower respiratory tract infections** caused by susceptible strains of *Hemophilus influenzae*	Adult: 250 mg q6h Child ($\leq$ 20 kg): 50 mg/kg/day, given in divided doses q6–8h Child ($>$ 20 kg): same as adult	Adult: 250–500 mg IM or IV (slowly) q6h Child ($\leq$ 20 kg): 12.5 mg/kg IM or IV (slowly) q6h Child ($>$ 20 kg): same as adult
Gastrointestinal and genitourinary tract infections caused by susceptible strains of *Shigella*, *Salmonella* (including *S typhosa*), *Escherichia coli*, *Proteus mirabilis*, and enterococci	Adult: 500 mg q6h Child ($\leq$ 20 kg): 100 mg/kg/day, given in divided doses q6h Child ($>$ 20 kg): same as adult	Adult: 500 mg IM or IV (slowly) q6h Child ($\leq$ 20 kg): 12.5 mg/kg IM or IV (slowly) q6h Child ($>$ 20 kg): same as adult
Uncomplicated urethritis caused by *Neisseria gonorrhoeae*	Adult: 3.5 g, given in a single dose simultaneously with 1 g probenecid	—
Urethritis in males caused by *Neisseria gonorrhoeae*	—	Adult: 500 mg IM q12h for 2 doses
Bacterial meningitis caused by susceptible strains of *Neisseria meningitidis* and *Hemophilus influenzae* **Septicemia** caused by susceptible gram-positive and gram-negative bacteria	—	Adult: 8–14 g/day, beginning by slow IV infusion for a minimum of 3 days and followed by IM injection q3–4h Child: 150–200 mg/kg/day, beginning by slow IV infusion for a minimum of 3 days and followed by IM injection q3–4h

CONTRAINDICATIONS

Hypersensitivity to penicillins

ADMINISTRATION/DOSAGE ADJUSTMENTS

Duration of treament	Continue treatment for at least 48–72 h after patient has become asymptomatic or bacteria have been eradicated; beta-hemolytic streptococcal infections should be treated for at least 10 days to prevent rheumatic fever and glomerulonephritis

WARNINGS/PRECAUTIONS

Hypersensitivity	Serious and occasionally fatal anaphylactoid reactions may occur, most likely in patients with a history of sensitivity to multiple allergens. Urticaria, other skin rashes, and serum sickness-like reactions may be controlled with antihistamines and, if necessary, systemic corticosteroids. Drug should be discontinued unless infection is life-threatening and amenable only to ampicillin. Severe reactions may necessitate emergency measures, such as immediate use of epinephrine, oxygen, IV corticosteroids, and airway management, including intubation; use with caution in patients who have experienced allergic reactions to cephalosporins.
Long-term therapy	Perform blood, renal, and hepatic studies periodically, particularly in premature infants, neonates, and other infants
Superinfection	Overgrowth of nonsusceptible organisms, including fungi, may occur
Suspected syphilitic lesions	If syphilis is suspected, perform a dark-field examination before instituting therapy, and perform serology testing monthly for at least 4 mo
Chronic urinary tract and intestinal infections	Require frequent bacteriological and clinical appraisals during therapy, and possibly for several months afterward; do not use doses smaller than those recommended above

ADVERSE REACTIONS

Frequent reactions (incidence $\geq$ 1%) are printed in *italics*

Gastrointestinal	Glossitis, stomatitis, black hairy tongue, nausea, vomiting, enterocolitis, pseudomembranous colitis, diarrhea
Hypersensitivity	*Erythematous maculopapular rash*, urticaria, erythema multiforme, exfoliative dermatitis, serum sickness-like reactions, anaphylaxis (see WARNINGS/PRECAUTIONS)
Hematological	Anemia, thrombocytopenia, thrombocytopenic purpura, eosinophilia, leukopenia, agranulocytosis

TOTACILLIN ■ TRIMOX

OVERDOSAGE

Signs and symptoms	See ADVERSE REACTIONS
Treatment	Discontinue medication; treat symptomatically

DRUG INTERACTIONS

Probenecid	◊ Ampicillin blood level and/or toxicity

ALTERED LABORATORY VALUES

Blood/serum values	◊ SGOT

No clinically significant alterations in urinary values occur at therapeutic dosages

---

USE IN CHILDREN

See INDICATIONS and dosage recommendations; adjust dosage according to body weight and severity of infection

USE IN PREGNANT AND NURSING WOMEN

Safety for use during pregnancy has not been established. Ampicillin is excreted in human milk; use with caution if given to nursing mothers.

---

[1] Higher doses may be needed for stubborn or severe infections

---

PENICILLINS

TRIMOX (amoxicillin) Squibb   Rx

Capsules: amoxicillin trihydrate equivalent to 250 or 500 mg amoxicillin   **Suspension (per 5 ml):** amoxicillin trihydrate equivalent to 125 or 250 mg amoxicillin after reconstitution

INDICATIONS

Ear, nose, and throat infections caused by susceptible strains of streptococci, *Streptococcus pneumoniae*, nonpenicillinase-producing staphylococci, and *Hemophilus influenzae*

Genitourinary tract infections caused by susceptible strains of *Escherichia coli*, *Proteus mirabilis*, and *Streptococcus fecalis*

Skin and soft tissue infections caused by susceptible strains of streptococci, staphylococci, and *Escherichia coli*

Lower respiratory tract infections caused by susceptible strains of streptococci, *Streptococcus pneumoniae*, non-penicillinase-producing staphylococci, and *Hemophilus influenzae*

Gonorrhea; acute uncomplicated anogenital and urethral infections caused by *Neisseria gonorrhoeae*

ORAL DOSAGE

Adult: 250 mg q8h; for severe infections or those caused by less susceptible organisms, 500 mg q8h
Child (< 20 kg): 20 mg/kg/day, given in divided doses q8h; for severe infections, 40 mg/kg/day, given in divided doses q8h
Child (≥ 20 kg): same as adult

Adult: 500 mg q8h
Child (< 20 kg): 40 mg/kg/day, given in divided doses q8h
Child (≥ 20 kg): same as adult

Adult: 3 g, given in a single dose

CONTRAINDICATIONS

Hypersensitivity to penicillins

ADMINISTRATION/DOSAGE ADJUSTMENTS

Duration of treatment	Continue treatment for at least 48–72 h after patient has become asymptomatic or bacteria have been eradicated; beta-hemolytic streptococcal infections should be treated for at least 10 days to prevent rheumatic fever and glomerulonephritis

WARNINGS/PRECAUTIONS

Hypersensitivity	Serious and occasionally fatal anaphylactoid reactions may occur, most likely in patients with a history of sensitivity to multiple allergens. Urticaria, other skin rashes, and serum sickness-like reactions may be controlled with antihistamines and, if necessary, systemic corticosteroids. Drug should be discontinued unless infection is life-threatening and amenable only to amoxicillin. Severe reactions may necessitate immediate emergency measures, such as immediate use of epinephrine, oxygen, IV corticosteroids, and airway management, including intubation; use with caution in patients who have experienced allergic reactions to cephalosporins.
Long-term therapy	Perform blood, renal, and hepatic studies periodically

TRIMOX ■ UNIPEN

Superinfection	Overgrowth of nonsusceptible organisms, including fungi, may occur
Suspected syphilitic lesions	If syphilis is suspected, perform a dark-field examination before instituting therapy and monthly serology tests for at least 4 mo afterward
Chronic urinary tract infections	Requires frequent bacteriological and clinical appraisal during therapy, and possibly for several months afterward; do not use doses smaller than those recommended above

ADVERSE REACTIONS

Gastrointestinal	Glossitis, stomatitis, black hairy tongue, nausea, vomiting, diarrhea
Hypersensitivity	Erythematous maculopapular rash, urticaria, exfoliative dermatitis, erythema multiforme, serum sickness-like reactions, anaphylaxis (see WARNINGS/PRECAUTIONS)
Hematological	Anemia, thrombocytopenia, thrombocytopenic purpura, eosinophilia, leukopenia, agranulocytosis

OVERDOSAGE

Signs and symptoms	See ADVERSE REACTIONS
Treatment	Discontinue medication; treat symptomatically

DRUG INTERACTIONS

Probenecid	⇧ Amoxicillin blood level and/or toxicity

ALTERED LABORATORY VALUES

Blood/serum values	⇧ SGOT

No clinically significant alterations in urinary values occur at therapeutic dosages

---

USE IN CHILDREN
See INDICATIONS and ORAL DOSAGE

USE IN PREGNANT AND NURSING WOMEN
Safety for use during pregnancy has not been established. Penicillins are excreted in human milk and may increase the risk of allergic sensitization in nursing infants.[1]

[1] Knowles JA: *J Pediatr* 66:1068–1082, 1965; *Med Lett Drugs Ther* 16:25–27, 1974

PENICILLINS

UNIPEN (nafcillin sodium) Wyeth   Rx

Capsules: nafcillin sodium equivalent to 250 mg nafcillin   **Tablets:** nafcillin sodium equivalent to 500 mg nafcillin   **Solution (per 5 ml):** nafcillin sodium equivalent to 250 mg nafcillin after reconstitution (100 ml)   **Vials:** 500 mg; 1, 2 g (equivalent to 250 mg/ml nafcillin after reconstitution)   **Piggyback units:** nafcillin sodium equivalent to 1, 1.5, 2, or 4 g nafcillin   **Bulk pharmacy package:** nafcillin sodium equivalent to 10 g nafcillin

INDICATIONS
Penicillin G-resistant staphylococcal infections[1]

ORAL DOSAGE
Adult: for mild to moderate infections, 250–500 mg q4–6h; for severe infections, 1 g q4–6h
Neonate: 10 mg/kg tid or qid
Infant and child: 50 mg/kg/day, given in 4 divided doses

PARENTERAL DOSAGE
Adult: 500 mg IM q4–6h, depending upon severity, or 500 mg to 1 g IV q4h, depending upon severity
Neonate: 10 mg/kg IM bid
Infant and child: 25 mg/kg IM bid

CONTRAINDICATIONS
Hypersensitivity to penicillins

ADMINISTRATION/DOSAGE ADJUSTMENTS

Streptococcal pharyngitis in children	Administer 250 mg tid orally; treat beta-hemolytic streptococcal infections for at least 10 days to prevent rheumatic fever and glomerulonephritis
Scarlet fever and pneumonia in infants and children	Administer 25 mg/kg/day in 4 divided oral doses; if this is inadequate, switch to parenteral form
Intramuscular administration	Reconstitute contents of vial with Sterile Water for Injection USP, Sodium Chloride Injection USP, or Bacteriostatic Water for Injection USP and inject required dose immediately into the gluteal area

UNIPEN ■ V-CILLIN K

Intravenous administration	Dilute the required amount of drug in 15–30 ml of Sterile Water for Injection USP or Sodium Chloride Injection USP and inject solution slowly over a 5- to 10-min period; this may be accomplished through the tubing of an IV infusion set, if desired. Alternatively, add drug to an IV solution and administer very slowly, over a period of at least 30–60 min, to avoid vein irritation; IV therapy should generally not exceed 24–48 h because of the risk of thrombophlebitis, especially in elderly patients. Take precautions during IV administration to avoid perivascular extravasation, since this could cause severe irritation.

WARNINGS/PRECAUTIONS

Hypersensitivity	Serious and occasionally fatal anaphylactoid reactions may occur, most likely in patients with a history of sensitivity to multiple allergens; use with caution in patients who have experienced severe allergic reactions to cephalosporins. If an allergic reaction occurs, consider discontinuing nafcillin therapy and employ antihistamines, pressor amines, and/or corticosteroids, as needed.
Long-term therapy	Perform blood, renal, and hepatic studies periodically during prolonged therapy
Superinfection	Overgrowth of nonsusceptible organisms, including fungi, may occur
Impaired absorption	Oral administration should not be relied on in patients with severe illness, nausea, vomiting, gastric dilatation, cardiospasm, or intestinal hypermotility
Methicillin resistance	Methicillin-resistant strains of staphylococci should be considered resistant to nafcillin as well

ADVERSE REACTIONS

Hematological	Transient leukopenia, neutropenia with granulocytopenia or thrombocytopenia
Gastrointestinal	Nausea, vomiting, and diarrhea (with oral use)
Hypersensitivity	Skin rash (with IM use), urticaria (with oral use), pruritus (with oral or IM use), drug fever (possible with IM use), serum sickness-like reactions, anaphylactic reactions
Other	Thrombophlebitis (with IV use)

OVERDOSAGE

Signs and symptoms	See ADVERSE REACTIONS
Treatment	Discontinue medication; treat symptomatically

DRUG INTERACTIONS

Probenecid	△ Nafcillin blood level and/or toxicity

ALTERED LABORATORY VALUES

No clinically significant alterations in blood/serum or urinary values occur at therapeutic dosages

---

USE IN CHILDREN
See INDICATIONS and dosage recommendations

USE IN PREGNANT AND NURSING WOMEN
Safety for use during pregnancy has not been established. Nafcillin is excreted in breast milk; use with caution in nursing mothers.

---

[1] Nafcillin should not be used to treat infections caused by organisms susceptible to penicillin G; when necessary, however, it may be used to initiate therapy of suspected penicillin G-resistant staphylococcal infections before definitive culture results are known. If subsequent laboratory studies indicate that the infection is due to an organism other than a penicillinase-producing staphylococcus susceptible to nafcillin, therapy should be continued with a more appropriate antibiotic.

PENICILLINS

V-CILLIN K (penicillin V potassium) Lilly Rx

Tablets: 125, 250, 500 mg (200,000, 400,000, 800,000 units)   **Solution (per 5 ml):** 125, 250 mg (200,000, 400,000 units)

INDICATIONS	ORAL DOSAGE
Mild to moderately severe upper respiratory tract infections, scarlet fever, and mild erysipelas caused by penicillin G-sensitive streptococci in the absence of bacteremia	**Adult:** 200,000–500,000 units q6–8h for 10 days **Infant and small child:** 25,000–90,000 units/kg/day, given in 3–6 divided doses
Otitis media and other mild to moderately severe respiratory tract infections caused by penicillin G-sensitive strains of *Streptococcus pneumoniae*	**Adult:** 400,000–500,000 units q6h until patient has been afebrile for at least 2 days **Infant and small child:** 25,000–90,000 units/kg/day, given in 3–6 divided doses

V-CILLIN K

Mild skin and soft tissue infections caused by susceptible strains of staphylococci **Fusospirochetosis** (Vincent's gingivitis and pharyngitis)	**Adult:** 400,000–500,000 units q6-8h **Infant and small child:** 25,000–90,000 units/kg/day, given in 3–6 divided doses
Long-term prophylaxis of rheumatic fever and/or chorea	**Adult:** 200,000–250,000 units bid **Infant and small child:** 25,000–90,000 units/kg/day, given in 3–6 divided doses
Prevention of bacterial endocarditis in patients with congenital heart disease or rheumatic or other acquired valvular heart disease who are undergoing dental procedures or upper respiratory tract surgery	**Adult and child (> 30 kg):** 3,200,000 units (2 g) ½–1 h prior to dental procedure or upper respiratory tract surgery, followed by 800,000 units (500 mg) q6h for 8 doses, *or* combined regimen of 1 million units IM aqueous crystalline penicillin G mixed with 600,000 units procaine penicillin G ½–1 h prior to procedure, followed by 800,000 units (500 mg) oral penicillin V q6h for 8 doses **Child (< 30 kg):** 1,600,000 units (1 g) ½–1 h prior to dental procedure or upper respiratory tract surgery, followed by 400,000 units (250 mg) q6h for 8 doses, *or* combined regimen of 30,000 units/kg IM aqueous crystalline penicillin G mixed with 600,000 units procaine penicillin G ½–1 h prior to procedure, followed by 400,000 units (250 mg) q6h for 8 doses

CONTRAINDICATIONS

Hypersensitivity to penicillins

ADMINISTRATION/DOSAGE ADJUSTMENTS

Duration of treatment for streptococcal infections	Therapy should be continued for a minimum of 10 days to prevent sequelae of streptococcal disease; cultures should be taken on completion of therapy to determine whether streptococci have been eradicated
Patients receiving continuous penicillin prophylaxis to prevent recurrence of rheumatic fever	May harbor alpha-hemolytic streptococci that are relatively resistant to penicillin; prophylactic antibiotics other than penicillin may be given to these patients (in addition to their continuous rheumatic fever prophylactic regimen) prior to dental or surgical procedures

WARNINGS/PRECAUTIONS

Hypersensitivity	Serious and occasionally fatal anaphylactoid reactions may occur, most likely in patients with a history of sensitivity to multiple allergens; use with caution in patients who have a history of significant allergies and/or asthma or have experienced allergic reactions to cephalosporins. If an allergic reaction occurs, discontinue medication and employ other agents, eg, epinephrine, antihistamines, and/or corticosteroids, as needed.
Superinfection	Overgrowth of nonsusceptible microorganisms, including fungi, may occur with prolonged use
Impaired absorption	Oral administration should not be relied on in patients with severe illness, nausea, vomiting, gastric dilatation, cardiospasm, or intestinal hypermotility
Inappropriate indications	Oral penicillin V should not be used for treatment during the acute stages of severe pneumonia, empyema, bacteremia, pericarditis, meningitis, or septic arthritis, or for prophylaxis preceding genitourinary instrumentation or surgery, lower gastrointestinal tract surgery, sigmoidoscopy, or childbirth

ADVERSE REACTIONS

The most frequent reactions, regardless of incidence, are printed in *italics*

Gastrointestinal	*Nausea, vomiting, epigastric distress, diarrhea, black hairy tongue*
Hypersensitivity	Skin eruptions, ranging from maculopapular rash to exfoliative dermatitis, urticaria, serum sickness-like reactions (including chills, fever, edema, arthralgia, and prostration), laryngeal edema, anaphylaxis (see WARNINGS/PRECAUTIONS)
Hematological	Hemolytic anemia, leukopenia, thrombocytopenia, eosinophilia (usually only with high-dosage parenteral therapy)
Other	Neuropathy and nephropathy (usually only with high-dosage parenteral therapy)

OVERDOSAGE

Signs and symptoms	See ADVERSE REACTIONS
Treatment	Discontinue medication; treat symptomatically

DRUG INTERACTIONS

Probenecid	⇧ Penicillin blood level and/or toxicity

ALTERED LABORATORY VALUES

No clinically significant alterations in blood/serum or urinary values occur at therapeutic dosages

---

USE IN CHILDREN

See INDICATIONS and ORAL DOSAGE

USE IN PREGNANT AND NURSING WOMEN

Safety for use during pregnancy has not been established. Penicillins are excreted in human milk and may increase the risk of allergic sensitization in nursing infants.[1]

[1] Knowles JA: *J Pediatr* 66:1068–1082, 1965; *Med Lett Drugs Ther* 16:25–27, 1974

Chapter 25

Anti-Infectives: Erythromycins and Tetracyclines

Erythromycins — 1016

E.E.S. (Abbott) — 1016
Erythromycin ethylsuccinate *Rx*

E-MYCIN (Boots) — 1017
Erythromycin *Rx*

E-MYCIN E (Boots) — 1017
Erythromycin ethylsuccinate *Rx*

ERYC (Parke-Davis) — 1019
Erythromycin *Rx*

ERYC 125 (Parke-Davis) — 1019
Erythromycin *Rx*

EryPed (Abbott) — 1021
Erythromycin ethylsuccinate *Rx*

ERY-TAB (Abbott) — 1023
Erythromycin *Rx*

ERYTHROCIN Lactobionate-I.V. (Abbott) — 1024
Erythromycin lactobionate *Rx*

ERYTHROCIN Piggyback (Abbott) — 1024
Erythromycin lactobionate *Rx*

ERYTHROCIN Stearate (Abbott) — 1024
Erythromycin stearate *Rx*

ILOSONE (Dista) — 1026
Erythromycin estolate *Rx*

PCE (Abbott) — 1028
Erythromycin *Rx*

PEDIAMYCIN (Ross) — 1030
Erythromycin ethylsuccinate *Rx*

WYAMYCIN E (Wyeth) — 1032
Erythromycin ethylsuccinate *Rx*

WYAMYCIN S (Wyeth) — 1032
Erythromycin stearate *Rx*

Tetracyclines — 1034

ACHROMYCIN (Lederle) — 1034
Tetracycline hydrochloride *Rx*

ACHROMYCIN V (Lederle) — 1034
Tetracycline hydrochloride *Rx*

DECLOMYCIN (Lederle) — 1036
Demeclocycline hydrochloride *Rx*

DORYX (Parke-Davis) — 1037
Doxycycline hyclate *Rx*

MINOCIN (Lederle) — 1039
Minocycline hydrochloride *Rx*

MYSTECLIN-F (Squibb) — 1040
Tetracycline and amphotericin B *Rx*

SUMYCIN (Squibb) — 1042
Tetracycline hydrochloride *Rx*

TERRAMYCIN (Pfizer) — 1044
Oxytetracycline hydrochloride *Rx*

TERRAMYCIN Intramuscular Solution (Roerig) — 1044
Oxytetracycline *Rx*

TERRAMYCIN Intravenous (Roerig) — 1044
Oxytetracycline hydrochloride *Rx*

VIBRAMYCIN (Pfizer) — 1046
Doxycycline *Rx*

VIBRAMYCIN Intravenous (Roerig) — 1046
Doxycycline hyclate *Rx*

VIBRA-TABS (Pfizer) — 1046
Doxycycline hyclate *Rx*

Other Tetracyclines — 1015

PANMYCIN (Upjohn) — 1015
Tetracycline hydrochloride *Rx*

ROBITET (Robins) — 1015
Tetracycline hydrochloride *Rx*

RONDOMYCIN (Wallace) — 1015
Methacycline hydrochloride *Rx*

VIVOX (Squibb) — 1015
Doxycycline hyclate *Rx*

OTHER TETRACYCLINES

DRUG	HOW SUPPLIED	USUAL DOSAGE
PANMYCIN (Upjohn) Tetracycline hydrochloride *Rx*	**Capsules:** 250 mg	**Adult:** 1–2 g/day, given in 2 or 4 equally divided doses; for brucellosis, 500 mg qid for 3 wk with 1 g streptomycin IM bid the first week and once daily the second week; for syphilis, 30–40 g, given in equally divided doses over 10–15 days; for uncomplicated gonorrhea, 0.5 g q6h for a total dosage of 10 g in 5 days; for uncomplicated urethral, endocervical, or rectal infections caused by *Chlamydia trachomatis*, 500 mg qid for at least 7 days **Child (> 8 yr):** 25–50 mg/kg/day, given in 4 equally divided doses
ROBITET (Robins) Tetracycline hydrochloride *Rx*	**Capsules:** 250, 500 mg	**Adult:** 1–2 g/day, given in 2 or 4 equally divided doses; for brucellosis, 500 mg qid for 3 wk with 1 g streptomycin IM bid the first week and once daily the second week; for syphilis, 30–40 g, given in equally divided doses over 10–15 days; for uncomplicated gonorrhea, 1.5 g to start, followed by 500 mg qid for a total of 9 g; for uncomplicated urethral, endocervical, or rectal infections caused by *Chlamydia trachomatis*, 500 mg qid for at least 7 days **Child (> 8 yr):** 25–50 mg/kg/day, given in 4 equally divided doses
RONDOMYCIN (Wallace) Methacycline hydrochloride *Rx*	**Capsules:** 150, 300 mg	**Adult:** 600 mg/day, given in 2–4 equally divided doses; for more severe infections, 300 mg to start, followed by 150 mg q6h or 300 mg q12h; for gonorrhea, 900 mg to start, followed by 300 mg qid for a total of 5.4 g; for syphilis, 18–24 g, given in equally divided doses over a period of 10–15 days; for Eaton Agent pneumonia, 900 mg/day for 6 days **Child (> 8 yr):** 3–6 mg/lb/day, given in 2–4 equally spaced doses
VIVOX (Squibb) Doxycycline hyclate *Rx*	**Capsules:** doxycycline hyclate equivalent to 50 and 100 mg doxycycline **Tablets:** doxycycline hyclate equivalent to 100 mg doxycycline	**Adult:** 100 mg q12h on the first day, followed by 100 mg q24h or 50 mg q12h; for more severe infections (especially chronic urinary tract infections), maintain initial dosage of 100 mg q12h; for acute gonococcal infections, 200 mg to start, followed by 100 mg at bedtime and then 100 mg bid over the next 3 days (alternatively, two 300-mg doses separated by a period of 1 h); for primary and secondary syphilis, 300 mg/day, given in divided doses, for at least 10 days; for uncomplicated urethral, endocervical, and rectal infections caused by *Chlamydia trachomatis*, 100 mg bid for at least 7 days **Child (> 8 yr and ≤ 100 lb):** 2 mg/lb given in 2 divided doses, to start, followed by 1–2 mg/lb, depending on severity, given in a single dose or 2 divided doses **Child (> 8 yr and > 100 lb):** same as adult

COMPENDIUM OF DRUG THERAPY

ERYTHROMYCINS

E.E.S. (erythromycin ethylsuccinate) Abbott Rx

Tablets: 400 mg **Chewable tablets:** 200 mg *cherry flavored* **Suspension (per 5 ml):** 200 mg (E.E.S. 200) (100 ml, 16 fl oz) *fruit flavored*, 400 mg (E.E.S. 400) (100 ml, 16 fl oz) *fruit flavored* **Suspension granules (per 5 ml):** 200 mg after reconstitution (5, 60, 100, 200 ml) *cherry flavored* **Drops (per 2.5 ml):** 100 mg after reconstitution (50 ml) *cherry flavored*

INDICATIONS

Acute mild to moderate **skin and soft tissue infections** caused by susceptible strains of *Staphylococcus aureus*[1]

Mild to moderate **upper and lower respiratory tract, skin, and soft tissue infections** caused by *Streptococcus pyogenes*

Mild to moderate **upper and lower respiratory tract infections** caused by *Streptococcus pneumoniae* and *Mycoplasma pneumoniae*

Mild to moderate **upper respiratory tract infections** caused by susceptible strains of *Hemophilus influenzae* (with appropriate sulfonamide therapy)

As an adjunct to antitoxin for **prevention and/or elimination of the carrier state** in individuals exposed to *Corynebacterium diphtheriae*

Infections caused by *Listeria monocytogenes*

Erythrasma caused by *Corynebacterium minutissimum*

Continuous prophylaxis of rheumatic fever

Prevention of bacterial endocarditis in penicillin-allergic patients with congenital heart disease or rheumatic or other acquired valvular heart disease who are undergoing dental procedures or upper respiratory tract surgery[2]

Urethritis caused by *Chlamydia trachomatis* and *Ureaplasma urealyticum*

Primary syphilis in penicillin-allergic patients

Intestinal amebiasis caused by *Entamoeba histolytica*

Legionnaires' disease

Nasopharyngeal carriage of *Bordetella pertussis*

ORAL DOSAGE

Adult: 400 mg q6h; for severe infections, up to 4 g/day in divided doses
Infant (< 10 lb): 30–50 mg/kg/day in equally divided doses
Infant (10–15 lb): 200 mg/day in equally divided doses
Infant and child (16–25 lb): 400 mg/day in equally divided doses
Child (26–50 lb): 800 mg/day in equally divided doses
Child (51–100 lb): 1,200 mg/day in equally divided doses
Child (> 100 lb): 1,600 mg/day in equally divided doses

Adult: 400 mg bid
Child: same as adult

Adult: 1.6 g 1½–2 h prior to dental procedure or upper respiratory tract surgery, followed by 800 mg q6h for 8 doses
Child: 20 mg/kg 1½–2 h prior to dental procedure or upper respiratory tract surgery, followed by 10 mg/kg q6h for 8 doses

Male adult: 800 mg tid for 7 days

Adult: 48–64 g total, given in divided doses over a period of 10–15 days

Adult: 400 mg qid for 10–14 days
Child: 30–50 mg/kg/day in divided doses for 10–14 days

Adult: 1.6–4 g/day in divided doses

Adult: 40–50 mg/kg/day in divided doses for 5–14 days

CONTRAINDICATIONS

Hypersensitivity to erythromycin

ADMINISTRATION/DOSAGE ADJUSTMENTS

Timing of administration	May be given without regard to meals
Alternative dosing schedule	Half the total daily dose may be given q12h, or, if desired, one third may be given q8h
Duration of treatment for streptococcal infections	Infections caused by Group A beta-hemolytic streptococci should be treated for a minimum of 10 days
Severe infections in children	Dosage given above may be doubled, if necessary
Chewable tablets	Must be chewed thoroughly

WARNINGS/PRECAUTIONS

Hepatic dysfunction	May occur, with or without jaundice, in patients receiving oral erythromycin
Patients with hepatic impairment	Use with caution and watch for signs of excessive accumulation, since drug is excreted primarily by the liver
Concomitant theophylline therapy	May produce elevated serum theophylline levels or theophylline toxicity; reduce theophylline dosage accordingly
Primary syphilis	Spinal-fluid examinations should be performed before treatment and as part of follow-up therapy

E.E.S. ■ E-MYCIN

Localized infections	May require surgical drainage, in addition to antibiotic therapy
Ototoxicity	Reversible hearing loss has occurred, primarily in patients who had renal impairment or received high doses
Superinfection	Prolonged or repeated use may cause overgrowth of nonsusceptible bacteria or fungi; if superinfection occurs, discontinue use

ADVERSE REACTIONS

Gastrointestinal	Nausea, vomiting, abdominal cramping and discomfort, diarrhea
Hypersensitivity	Urticaria, skin rashes, anaphylaxis
Other	Reversible hearing loss (see WARNINGS/PRECAUTIONS)

OVERDOSAGE

Signs and symptoms	See ADVERSE REACTIONS
Treatment	Discontinue medication; treat symptomatically

DRUG INTERACTIONS

Lincomycin	▽ Bactericidal action of lincomycin
Aminophylline, oxtriphylline, theophylline	△ Serum theophylline level

ALTERED LABORATORY VALUES

Blood/serum values	△ Alkaline phosphatase △ Bilirubin △ SGOT △ SGPT
Urinary values	△ Catecholamines (with Hingerty fluorometric method)

USE IN CHILDREN

Age, weight, and severity of infection are important factors in determining the proper dosage; see INDICATIONS

USE IN PREGNANT AND NURSING WOMEN

Safety for use during pregnancy has not been established because no controlled studies or retrospective analyses have been done in pregnant women; erythromycin crosses the placental barrier, but fetal plasma levels are low. Erythromycin is excreted in breast milk.

---

[1] Resistance may develop during treatment
[2] Unsuitable for prevention of bacterial endocarditis in patients undergoing genitourinary or gastrointestinal tract surgery

ERYTHROMYCINS

E-MYCIN (erythromycin) Boots Rx
Tablets (enteric coated): 250, 333 mg

E-MYCIN E (erythromycin ethylsuccinate) Boots Rx
Suspension (per 5 ml): 200 mg, 400 mg (500 ml)

INDICATIONS

Acute mild to moderate **skin and soft tissue infections** caused by susceptible strains of *Staphylococcus aureus*[1]
Mild to moderate **upper and lower respiratory tract, skin, and soft tissue infections** caused by *Streptococcus pyogenes*
Mild to moderate **upper and lower respiratory tract infections** caused by *Streptococcus pneumoniae* and *Mycoplasma pneumoniae*
Mild to moderate **upper respiratory tract infections** caused by susceptible strains of *Hemophilus influenzae* (with appropriate sulfonamide therapy)
As an adjunct to antitoxin for **prevention and/or elimination of the carrier state** in individuals exposed to *Corynebacterium diphtheriae*
Infections caused by *Listeria monocytogenes*
Erythrasma caused by *Corynebacterium minutissimum*

ORAL DOSAGE

Adult: 1 g/day of erythromycin (250 mg qid or 333 mg q8h) or 400 mg of erythromycin ethylsuccinate q6h; for severe infections, up to 4 g/day of erythromycin ethylsuccinate or 4 g/day or more of erythromycin, given in divided doses
Child: 30–50 mg/kg/day in divided doses

E-MYCIN

Acute pelvic inflammatory disease caused by *Neisseria gonorrhoeae* in penicillin-allergic patients	**Adult:** initiate treatment with erythromycin lactobionate (500 mg IV q6h for 3 days), followed by oral erythromycin (250 mg q6h or 333 mg q8h) for 7 days
Continuous prophylaxis of rheumatic fever	**Adult:** 250 mg of erythromycin or 400 mg of erythromycin ethylsuccinate bid **Child:** same as adult
Prevention of bacterial endocarditis in penicillin-allergic patients with congenital heart disease or rheumatic or other acquired valvular heart disease who are undergoing dental procedures or upper respiratory tract surgery[2]	**Adult:** 1 g 1½–2 h prior to dental procedure or upper respiratory tract surgery, followed by 500 mg q6h for 8 doses **Child:** 20 mg/kg 1½–2 h prior to dental procedure or upper respiratory tract surgery, followed by 10 mg/kg q6h for 8 doses
Primary syphilis in penicillin-allergic patients	**Adult:** 30–40 g of erythromycin, given in divided doses over a period of 10–15 days, or 48–64 g of erythromycin ethylsuccinate, given in divided doses over a period of 10–14 days
Intestinal amebiasis caused by *Entamoeba histolytica*	**Adult:** 1 g/day of erythromycin (250 mg qid or 333 mg q8h) or 400 mg of erythromycin ethylsuccinate q6h for 10–14 days **Child:** 30–50 mg/kg/day in divided doses for 10–14 days
Legionnaires' disease	**Adult:** 1–4 g/day in divided doses
Nasopharyngeal carriage of *Bordetella pertussis*	**Adult:** 40–50 mg/kg/day in divided doses for 5–14 days
Conjunctivitis caused by *Chlamydia trachomatis*	**Neonate:** 50 mg/kg/day of erythromycin ethylsuccinate, given in 4 divided doses for at least 2 wk
Pneumonia caused by *Chlamydia trachomatis*	**Infant:** 50 mg/kg/day of erythromycin ethylsuccinate, given in 4 divided doses for at least 3 wk
Uncomplicated urethral, endocervical, and rectal infections caused by *Chlamydia trachomatis,* when tetracycline is contraindicated or cannot be tolerated **Urogenital infections** in pregnant women caused by *Chlamydia trachomatis*	**Adult:** 2 g/day of erythromycin (500 mg qid or 666 mg q8h) or 800 mg of erythromycin ethylsuccinate qid for at least 7 days; pregnant women who cannot tolerate this dosage should be given 1 g/day of erythromycin (250 mg qid or 333 mg q8h) or 400 mg of erythromycin ethylsuccinate qid for at least 14 days

CONTRAINDICATIONS

Hypersensitivity to erythromycin

ADMINISTRATION/DOSAGE ADJUSTMENTS

Timing of administration	May be given without regard to meals
Alternative dosing schedule	Half of the total daily dose may be given q12h; twice-a-day dosing is not recommended when daily doses exceed 1 g
Duration of treatment for streptococcal infections	Infections caused by Group A beta-hemolytic streptococci should be treated for a minimum of 10 days
Severe infections in children	Dosage given above may be doubled, if necessary

WARNINGS/PRECAUTIONS

Hepatic dysfunction	May occur, with or without jaundice, in patients receiving oral erythromycin
Patients with hepatic impairment	Use with caution and watch for signs of excessive accumulation, since drug is excreted primarily by the liver
Concomitant theophylline therapy	May produce elevated serum theophylline levels or theophylline toxicity; reduce theophylline dosage accordingly
Suspected syphilitic lesions	If syphilis is suspected, perform a dark-field examination before instituting therapy and monthly serology tests for at least 4 mo thereafter
Primary syphilis	Spinal fluid examinations should be done before treatment and as part of follow-up therapy
Hypersensitivity	Serious allergic reactions, including anaphylaxis, have been reported; administer epinephrine, corticosteroids, and antihistamines, as indicated
Ototoxicity	Reversible hearing loss has occurred, primarily in patients who had renal impairment or received high doses
Superinfection	Prolonged or repeated use may cause overgrowth of nonsusceptible bacteria or fungi; if superinfection occurs, discontinue use

ADVERSE REACTIONS

Gastrointestinal	Nausea, vomiting, abdominal cramping and discomfort, diarrhea
Hypersensitivity	Urticaria, skin rashes, anaphylaxis
Other	Reversible hearing loss (see WARNINGS/PRECAUTIONS)

OVERDOSAGE

Signs and symptoms	See ADVERSE REACTIONS

E-MYCIN ■ ERYC

| Treatment | Institute supportive measures; remove drug. Treat allergic reactions with epinephrine, corticosteroids, and antihistamines, as needed. |

DRUG INTERACTIONS

Lincomycin	⇓ Bactericidal action of lincomycin
Aminophylline, oxtriphylline, theophylline	⇑ Serum theophylline level
Carbamazepine	⇑ Risk of carbamazepine toxicity (in children)
Warfarin	⇑ Pharmacologic effects of warfarin
Triazolam	⇑ Pharmacologic effect of triazolam

ALTERED LABORATORY VALUES

| Blood/serum values | ⇑ Alkaline phosphatase   ⇑ Bilirubin   ⇑ SGOT   ⇑ SGPT |
| Urinary values | ⇑ Catecholamines (with Hingerty fluorometric method) |

USE IN CHILDREN

Age, weight, and severity of infection are important factors in determining proper dosage; see INDICATIONS

USE IN PREGNANT AND NURSING WOMEN

Safe use not established; erythromycin crosses the placental barrier, but fetal plasma levels are low. Consult manufacturer for use in nursing mothers.

---

[1] Resistance may develop during treatment
[2] Unsuitable for prevention of bacterial endocarditis in patients undergoing genitourinary or gastrointestinal tract surgery

---

ERYTHROMYCINS

ERYC (erythromycin) Parke-Davis   Rx
Capsules (with enteric-coated pellets): 250 mg

ERYC 125 (erythromycin) Parke-Davis   Rx
Capsules (with enteric-coated pellets): 125 mg

INDICATIONS

Mild to moderate **skin and skin structure infections** caused by susceptible strains of *Staphylococcus aureus*[1]

Mild to moderate **upper and lower respiratory tract, skin, and skin structure infections** caused by *Streptococcus pyogenes*

Mild to moderate **upper and lower respiratory tract infections** caused by *Streptococcus pneumoniae* and *Mycoplasma pneumoniae*

Mild to moderate **upper respiratory tract infections** caused by susceptible strains of *Hemophilus influenzae* (with appropriate sulfonamide therapy)

As an adjunct to antitoxin for **prevention and/or elimination of the carrier state** in individuals exposed to *Corynebacterium diphtheriae*

Infections caused by *Listeria monocytogenes*

Erythrasma caused by *Corynebacterium minutissimum*

Continuous prophylaxis of rheumatic fever in patients allergic to penicillins or sulfonamides

Prevention of bacterial endocarditis in susceptible patients[2] who are allergic to penicillin and are about to undergo dental procedures or upper respiratory tract surgery

ORAL DOSAGE

Adult: 250 mg q6h, taken 1 h before meals; for severe infections, up to 4 g/day in divided doses
Child: 30–50 mg/kg/day in divided doses; for severe infections, up to 60–100 mg/kg/day in divided doses

Adult: 250 mg bid
Child: same as adult

Adult: 1 g 1 h prior to dental procedure or upper respiratory tract surgery, followed by 500 mg 6 h later
Child: 20 mg/kg 1 h prior to dental procedure or upper respiratory tract surgery, followed by 10 mg/kg 6 h later

Primary syphilis in penicillin-allergic patients	**Adult:** 30–40 g total, given in divided doses over a period of 10–15 days
Intestinal amebiasis caused by *Entamoeba histolytica*	**Adult:** 250 mg qid for 10–14 days **Child:** 30–50 mg/kg/day in divided doses for 10–14 days
Legionnaires' disease	**Adult:** 1–4 g/day in divided doses
Conjunctivitis caused by *Chlamydia trachomatis*	**Neonate:** 50 mg/kg/day of erythromycin suspension, given in 4 divided doses for at least 2 wk
Pneumonia caused by *Chlamydia trachomatis*	**Infant:** 50 mg/kg/day of erythromycin suspension, given in 4 divided doses for at least 3 wk
Uncomplicated urethral, endocervical, and rectal infections caused by *Chlamydia trachomatis*, and **urethritis** caused by *Ureaplasma urealyticum*, when tetracycline is contraindicated or cannot be tolerated **Urogenital infections** in pregnant women caused by *Chlamydia trachomatis*	**Adult:** 500 mg qid for at least 7 days; pregnant women who cannot tolerate this dosage should be given 250 mg qid for at least 14 days
Nasopharyngeal carriage of *Bordetella pertussis*	**Adult:** 40–50 mg/kg/day in divided doses for 5–14 days

CONTRAINDICATIONS

Hypersensitivity to erythromycin

ADMINISTRATION/DOSAGE ADJUSTMENTS

Timing of administration	Give the 125-mg capsules at least 1 h before meals; administer the 250-mg capsules at least 30 min or, preferably, at least 2 h before or after meals
Administration of 125-mg capsules	The capsules may be swallowed whole or opened and the entire contents sprinkled on a small amount (eg, a spoonful) of applesauce and then swallowed immediately, followed by a small amount of water to ensure that all the pellets are taken. The contents of the capsules should not be subdivided, crushed, or chewed.
Alternative dosing schedule	Half the total daily dose may be given q12h; twice-a-day dosing is not recommended when daily doses exceed 1 g
Duration of treatment for streptococcal infections	Infections caused by Group A beta-hemolytic streptococci should be treated for a minimum of 10 days

WARNINGS/PRECAUTIONS

Hepatic dysfunction	May occur, with or without jaundice, in patients receiving oral erythromycin
Patients with hepatic impairment	Use with caution and watch for signs of excessive accumulation, since drug is excreted primarily by the liver
Concomitant theophylline therapy	May produce elevated serum theophylline levels or theophylline toxicity; reduce theophylline dosage accordingly
Primary syphilis	Spinal fluid examinations should be done before treatment and as part of follow-up therapy; use of erythromycin for treatment of syphilis in utero is not recommended
Ototoxicity	Reversible hearing loss has occurred, primarily in patients who had renal impairment or received high doses
Superinfection	Prolonged or repeated use may cause overgrowth of nonsusceptible bacteria or fungi; if superinfection occurs, discontinue use

ADVERSE REACTIONS

Gastrointestinal	Nausea, vomiting, abdominal pain, diarrhea, anorexia, hepatic dysfunction and/or abnormal liver-function test results
Hypersensitivity	Skin rash, with or without pruritus; urticaria; bullous fixed eruptions; eczema; anaphylaxis
Other	Reversible hearing loss (see WARNINGS/PRECAUTIONS)

OVERDOSAGE

Signs and symptoms	See gastrointestinal ADVERSE REACTIONS
Treatment	Discontinue medication; treat symptomatically

DRUG INTERACTIONS

Lincomycin	▽ Bactericidal action of lincomycin
Aminophylline, oxtriphylline, theophylline	△ Serum theophylline level

ERYC ■ EryPed

| Carbamazepine | ⇧ Risk of carbamazepine toxicity |

ALTERED LABORATORY VALUES

| Blood/serum values | ⇧ Alkaline phosphatase   ⇧ Bilirubin   ⇧ SGOT   ⇧ SGPT |
| Urinary values | ⇧ Catecholamines (with Hingerty fluorometric method) |

USE IN CHILDREN

Age, weight, and severity of infection are important factors in determining proper dosage; see INDICATIONS

USE IN PREGNANT AND NURSING WOMEN

Pregnancy Category B: use during pregnancy only when clearly needed. Animal reproduction studies performed in rats, mice, and rabbits at doses several times the usual human dose have shown no evidence of impaired fertility or fetal harm; however, no adequate, well-controlled studies have been done in pregnant women. Erythromycin is excreted in human milk.

---

[1] Resistance may develop during treatment
[2] Susceptible patients are those with prosthetic cardiac valves, certain congenital heart malformations, systemic-pulmonary shunts, rheumatic or other acquired valvular dysfunction, idiopathic hypertrophic subaortic stenosis, mitral valve prolapse with insufficiency, or a history of bacterial endocarditis

---

ERYTHROMYCINS

EryPed (erythromycin ethylsuccinate) Abbott   Rx

Suspension (per 5 ml): 400 mg after reconstitution (5, 60, 100, 200 ml) *banana flavored*

INDICATIONS	ORAL DOSAGE
Acute mild to moderate **skin and soft tissue infections** caused by susceptible strains of *Staphylococcus aureus*[1] Mild to moderate **upper and lower respiratory tract, skin, and soft tissue infections** caused by *Streptococcus pyogenes* Mild to moderate **upper and lower respiratory tract infections** caused by *Streptococcus pneumoniae* and *Mycoplasma pneumoniae* Mild to moderate **upper respiratory tract infections** caused by susceptible strains of *Hemophilus influenzae* (with appropriate sulfonamide therapy) As an adjunct to antitoxin for **prevention and/or elimination of the carrier state** in individuals exposed to *Corynebacterium diphtheriae* **Infections** caused by *Listeria monocytogenes* **Erythrasma** caused by *Corynebacterium minutissimum*	**Adult:** 400 mg q6h; for severe infections, up to 4 g/day in divided doses **Infant (< 10 lb):** 30–50 mg/kg/day in equally divided doses **Infant (10–15 lb):** 200 mg/day in equally divided doses **Infant and child (16–25 lb):** 400 mg/day in equally divided doses **Child (26–50 lb):** 800 mg/day in equally divided doses **Child (51–100 lb):** 1,200 mg/day in equally divided doses **Child (> 100 lb):** 1,600 mg/day in equally divided doses
Continuous prophylaxis of rheumatic fever	**Adult:** 400 mg bid **Child:** same as adult
Prevention of bacterial endocarditis in penicillin-allergic patients with congenital heart disease or rheumatic or other acquired valvular heart disease who are undergoing dental procedures or upper respiratory tract surgery[2]	**Adult:** 1.6 g 1½–2 h prior to dental procedure or upper respiratory tract surgery, followed by 800 mg q6h for 8 doses **Child:** 20 mg/kg 1½–2 h prior to dental procedure or upper respiratory tract surgery, followed by 10 mg/kg q6h for 8 doses
Urethritis caused by *Chlamydia trachomatis* and *Ureaplasma urealyticum*	**Male adult:** 800 mg tid for 7 days
Primary syphilis in penicillin-allergic patients	**Adult:** 48–64 g total, given in divided doses over a period of 10–15 days
Intestinal amebiasis caused by *Entamoeba histolytica*	**Adult:** 400 mg qid for 10–14 days **Child:** 30–50 mg/kg/day in divided doses for 10–14 days
Legionnaires' disease	**Adult:** 1.6–4 g/day in divided doses
Nasopharyngeal carriage of *Bordetella pertussis*	**Adult:** 40–50 mg/kg/day in divided doses for 5–14 days

COMPENDIUM OF DRUG THERAPY

EryPed

CONTRAINDICATIONS
Hypersensitivity to erythromycin

ADMINISTRATION/DOSAGE ADJUSTMENTS

Timing of administration	May be given without regard to meals
Alternative dosing schedules	Half the total daily dose may be given q12h, or, if desired, one third may be given q8h
Duration of treatment for streptococcal infections	Infections caused by Group A beta-hemolytic streptococci should be treated for a minimum of 10 days
Severe infections in children	Dosage given above may be doubled, if necessary

WARNINGS/PRECAUTIONS

Hepatic dysfunction	May occur, with or without jaundice, in patients receiving oral erythromycin
Patients with hepatic impairment	Use with caution and watch for signs of excessive accumulation, since drug is excreted primarily by the liver
Concomitant theophylline therapy	May produce elevated serum theophylline levels or theophylline toxicity; reduce theophylline dosage accordingly
Primary syphilis	Spinal fluid examinations should be done before treatment and as part of follow-up therapy
Ototoxicity	Reversible hearing loss has occurred, primarily in patients who had renal impairment or received high doses
Superinfection	Prolonged or repeated use may cause overgrowth of nonsusceptible bacteria or fungi; if superinfection occurs, discontinue use

ADVERSE REACTIONS

Gastrointestinal	Nausea, vomiting, abdominal cramping and discomfort, diarrhea
Hypersensitivity	Urticaria, mild skin eruptions, anaphylaxis
Other	Reversible hearing loss (see WARNINGS/PRECAUTIONS)

OVERDOSAGE

Signs and symptoms	See gastrointestinal ADVERSE REACTIONS
Treatment	Discontinue medication; treat symptomatically

DRUG INTERACTIONS

Lincomycin	▽ Bactericidal action of lincomycin
Aminophylline, oxtriphylline, theophylline	△ Serum theophylline level

ALTERED LABORATORY VALUES

Blood/serum values	△ Alkaline phosphatase △ Bilirubin △ SGOT △ SGPT
Urinary values	△ Catecholamines (with Hingerty fluorometric method)

USE IN CHILDREN

Age, weight, and severity of infection are important factors in determining the proper dosage; see INDICATIONS

USE IN PREGNANT AND NURSING WOMEN

Safety for use during pregnancy has not been established because no controlled studies or retrospective analyses have been done in pregnant women; erythromycin crosses the placental barrier, but fetal plasma levels are low. Erythromycin is excreted in breast milk.

---

[1] Resistance may develop during treatment
[2] Unsuitable for prevention of bacterial endocarditis in patients undergoing genitourinary or gastrointestinal tract surgery

ERYTHROMYCINS

ERY-TAB (erythromycin) Abbott Rx
Tablets (enteric coated): 250, 333, 500 mg

INDICATIONS

Acute mild to moderate **skin and soft tissue infections** caused by susceptible strains of *Staphylococcus aureus*[1]

Mild to moderate **upper and lower respiratory tract, skin, and soft tissue infections** caused by *Streptococcus pyogenes*

Mild to moderate **upper and lower respiratory tract infections** caused by *Streptococcus pneumoniae* and *Mycoplasma pneumoniae*

Mild to moderate **upper respiratory tract infections** caused by susceptible strains of *Hemophilus influenzae* (with appropriate sulfonamide therapy)

As an adjunct to antitoxin for **prevention and/or elimination of the carrier state** in individuals exposed to *Corynebacterium diphtheriae*

Infections caused by *Listeria monocytogenes*

Erythrasma caused by *Corynebacterium minutissimum*

Acute pelvic inflammatory disease caused by *Neisseria gonorrhoeae* in penicillin-allergic patients

Continuous prophylaxis of rheumatic fever

Prevention of bacterial endocarditis in penicillin-allergic patients with congenital heart disease or rheumatic or other acquired valvular heart disease who are undergoing dental procedures or upper respiratory tract surgery[2]

Primary syphilis in penicillin-allergic patients

Intestinal amebiasis caused by *Entamoeba histolytica*

Legionnaires' disease

Nasopharyngeal carriage of *Bordetella pertussis*

Conjunctivitis caused by *Chlamydia trachomatis*

Pneumonia caused by *Chlamydia trachomatis*

Uncomplicated **urethral, endocervical, and rectal infections** caused by *Chlamydia trachomatis*, when tetracycline is contraindicated or cannot be tolerated

Urogenital infections in pregnant women caused by *Chlamydia trachomatis*

ORAL DOSAGE

Adult: 250 mg qid, 333 mg q8h, or 500 mg q12h; for severe infections, up to 4 g/day or more, in divided doses
Child: 30–50 mg/kg/day in divided doses; for severe infections, up to 60–100 mg/kg/day in divided doses

Adult: initiate treatment with erythromycin lactobionate (500 mg IV q6h for 3 days), followed by 250 mg of erythromycin orally q6h for 7 days

Adult: 250 mg bid
Child: same as adult

Adult: 1 g 1½–2 h prior to dental procedure or upper respiratory tract surgery, followed by 500 mg q6h for 8 doses
Child: 20 mg/kg 1½–2 h prior to dental procedure or upper respiratory tract surgery, followed by 10 mg/kg q6h for 8 doses

Adult: 30–40 g total, given in divided doses over a period of 10–15 days

Adult: 250 mg qid for 10–14 days
Child: 30–50 mg/kg/day in divided doses for 10–14 days

Adult: 1–4 g/day in divided doses

Adult: 40–50 mg/kg/day in divided doses for 5–14 days

Neonate: 50 mg/kg/day of erythromycin suspension, given in 4 divided doses for at least 2 wk

Infant: 50 mg/kg/day of erythromycin suspension, given in 4 divided doses for at least 3 wk

Adult: 500 mg qid for at least 7 days; pregnant women who cannot tolerate this dosage should be given 250 mg qid for at least 14 days

CONTRAINDICATIONS

Hypersensitivity to erythromycin

ADMINISTRATION/DOSAGE ADJUSTMENTS

Timing of administration	May be given without regard to meals; twice-a-day dosing is not recommended when daily doses exceed 1 g
Duration of treatment for streptococcal infections	Infections caused by Group A beta-hemolytic streptococci should be treated for a minimum of 10 days

WARNINGS/PRECAUTIONS

Hepatic dysfunction	May occur, with or without jaundice, in patients receiving oral erythromycin
Patients with hepatic impairment	Use with caution and watch for signs of excessive accumulation, since drug is excreted primarily by the liver

COMPENDIUM OF DRUG THERAPY

ERY-TAB ■ ERYTHROCIN

Concomitant theophylline therapy	May produce elevated serum theophylline levels or theophylline toxicity; reduce theophylline dosage accordingly
Suspected syphilitic lesions	If syphilis is suspected, perform a dark-field examination before instituting therapy and monthly serology tests for at least 4 mo thereafter
Primary syphilis	Spinal fluid examinations should be done before treatment and as part of follow-up therapy
Hypersensitivity	Serious allergic reactions, including anaphylaxis, have been reported; eliminate unabsorbed drug promptly, and administer epinephrine, corticosteroids, and antihistamines, as indicated
Ototoxicity	Reversible hearing loss has occurred, primarily in patients who had renal impairment or received high doses
Superinfection	Prolonged or repeated use may cause overgrowth of nonsusceptible bacteria or fungi; if superinfection occurs, discontinue use

ADVERSE REACTIONS

Gastrointestinal	Nausea, vomiting, abdominal cramping and discomfort, diarrhea
Hypersensitivity	Urticaria, skin rashes, anaphylaxis
Other	Reversible hearing loss (see WARNINGS/PRECAUTIONS)

OVERDOSAGE

Signs and symptoms	See gastrointestinal ADVERSE REACTIONS
Treatment	Discontinue medication; treat symptomatically

DRUG INTERACTIONS

Lincomycin	▽ Bactericidal action of lincomycin
Aminophylline, oxtriphylline, theophylline	△ Serum theophylline level

ALTERED LABORATORY VALUES

Blood/serum values	△ Alkaline phosphatase △ Bilirubin △ SGOT △ SGPT
Urinary values	Catecholamines (with Hingerty fluorometric method)

USE IN CHILDREN

Age, weight, and severity of infection are important factors in determining proper dosage; see INDICATIONS

USE IN PREGNANT AND NURSING WOMEN

Safety for use during pregnancy has not been established because no controlled studies or retrospective analyses have been done in pregnant women; erythromycin crosses the placental barrier, but fetal plasma levels are low. Erythromycin is excreted in breast milk.

---

[1] Resistance may develop during treatment
[2] Unsuitable for prevention of bacterial endocarditis in patients undergoing genitourinary or gastrointestinal tract surgery

ERYTHROMYCINS

ERYTHROCIN Lactobionate-I.V. (erythromycin lactobionate) Abbott — Rx
Vials: erythromycin lactobionate equivalent to 500 mg or 1 g erythromycin (for IV use only)

ERYTHROCIN Piggyback (erythromycin lactobionate) Abbott — Rx
Piggyback vials: erythromycin lactobionate equivalent to 500 mg erythromycin (for intermittent IV use only)

ERYTHROCIN Stearate (erythromycin stearate) Abbott — Rx
Tablets: 250, 500 mg

INDICATIONS
Acute mild to moderate **skin and soft tissue infections** caused by susceptible strains of *Staphylococcus aureus*[1]
Mild to moderate **upper and lower respiratory tract, skin, and soft tissue infections** caused by *Streptococcus pyogenes*
Mild to moderate **upper and lower respiratory tract infections** caused by *Streptococcus pneumoniae* and *Mycoplasma pneumoniae*
Mild to moderate **upper respiratory tract infections** caused by susceptible strains of *Hemophilus influenzae* (with appropriate sulfonamide therapy)
As an adjunct to antitoxin for **prevention and/or elimination of the carrier state** in individuals exposed to *Corynebacterium diphtheriae*
Infections caused by *Listeria monocytogenes*
Erythrasma caused by *Corynebacterium minutissimum*

ORAL DOSAGE
Adult: 250 mg q6h or 500 mg q12h; for severe infections, up to 4 g/day in divided doses
Child: 30–50 mg/kg/day in 2–4 divided doses; for severe infections, up to 60–100 mg/kg/day in 2–4 divided doses

PARENTERAL DOSAGE
Adult: for severe infections, 15–20 mg/kg/day IV; for very severe infections, up to 4 g/day IV
Child: same as adult

COMPENDIUM OF DRUG THERAPY

ERYTHROCIN

Acute pelvic inflammatory disease caused by *Neisseria gonorrhoeae* in penicillin-allergic patients	**Adult:** 500 mg IV q6h for 3 days, followed by 250 mg q6h orally for 7 days	**Adult:** 500 mg IV q6h for 3 days, followed by 250 mg q6h orally for 7 days
Continuous prophylaxis of rheumatic fever	**Adult:** 250 mg bid **Child:** same as adult	—
Prevention of bacterial endocarditis in penicillin-allergic patients with congenital heart disease or rheumatic or other acquired valvular heart disease who are undergoing dental procedures or upper respiratory tract surgery[2]	**Adult:** 1 g 1½–2 h prior to dental procedure or upper respiratory tract surgery, followed by 500 mg q6h for 8 doses **Child:** 20 mg/kg 1½–2 h prior to dental procedure or upper respiratory tract surgery, followed by 10 mg/kg q6h for 8 doses	—
Conjunctivitis caused by *Chlamydia trachomatis*	**Neonate:** 50 mg/kg/day, given in 4 divided doses for at least 2 wk	—
Pneumonia caused by *Chlamydia trachomatis*	**Infant:** 50 mg/kg/day, given in 4 divided doses for at least 3 wk	—
Uncomplicated urethral, endocervical, and rectal infections caused by *Chlamydia trachomatis,* when tetracycline is contraindicated or cannot be tolerated Urogenital infections in pregnant women caused by *Chlamydia trachomatis*	**Adult:** 500 mg qid for at least 7 days; pregnant women who cannot tolerate this dosage should be given 250 mg qid for at least 14 days	—
Primary syphilis in penicillin-allergic patients	**Adult:** 30–40 g total, given in divided doses over a period of 10–15 days	—
Intestinal amebiasis caused by *Entamoeba histolytica*	**Adult:** 250 mg qid for 10–14 days **Child:** 30–50 mg/kg/day in divided doses for 10–14 days	—
Legionnaires' disease	**Adult:** 1–4 g/day in divided doses	**Adult:** 1–4 g/day IV in divided doses
Nasopharyngeal carriage of *Bordetella pertussis*	**Adult:** 40–50 mg/kg/day in divided doses for 5–14 days	—

CONTRAINDICATIONS

Hypersensitivity to erythromycin

ADMINISTRATION/DOSAGE ADJUSTMENTS

Duration of treatment for streptococcal infections	Infections caused by Group A beta-hemolytic streptococci should be treated for a minimum of 10 days
Preparation of IV solutions	To reconstitute Lactobionate-I.V. solution, add 10 ml of sterile water for injection USP to the 500-mg vial or 20 ml to the 1-g vial *(do not use other diluents);* this solution is stable for 24 h at room temperature and for 2 wk if refrigerated. Using a suitable preparation (see below), dilute this reconstituted solution to a final concentration of 1 mg/ml for continuous infusion or 1–5 mg/ml for intermittent infusion (minimum final volume: 100 ml). To reconstitute the Piggyback solution, add 100 ml of a suitable diluent (see below) to the vial, and then immediately shake well; the drug may be administered directly from the vial. Suitable diluents include: 0.9% sodium chloride injection USP, lactated Ringer's injection USP, Normosol-R, or, after 4% sodium bicarbonate (Neut) has been added (1 ml/100 ml of solution), 5% dextrose injection USP, 5% dextrose injection with Normosol-R or -M (for Piggyback solutions), or 5% dextrose injection with 0.9% sodium chloride injection USP or lactated Ringer's injection. The effect on a solution's stability should be determined before adding any preparation not recommended above.
Intravenous administration	Administer Piggyback solution by intermittent IV infusion and Lactobionate-I.V. solution preferably by slow, continuous IV infusion. For intermittent infusion of either solution, give one fourth of the total daily dose over a period of 20–60 min at intervals not greater than q6h and, to minimize pain along the vein, at a sufficiently slow rate. Use Piggyback solution within 8 h if it was stored at room temperature or within 24 h if it was refrigerated; complete administration of Lactobionate-I.V. solution within 8 h after final dilution.
Timing of oral administration	Optimal serum levels are obtained when tablets are given during the fasting state or immediately before meals

WARNINGS/PRECAUTIONS

Hepatic dysfunction	May occur, with or without jaundice, in patients receiving oral erythromycin
Patients with existing hepatic impairment	Use with caution and watch for signs of excessive accumulation, since drug is excreted by the liver
Ototoxicity	Reversible hearing loss has occurred with oral use, primarily in patients who had renal impairment or received high doses, and, on rare occasions, with IV infusion of 4 g/day or more

Concomitant theophylline therapy	May produce elevated serum theophylline levels or theophylline toxicity; reduce theophylline dosage accordingly
Suspected syphilitic lesions	If syphilis is suspected, perform a dark-field examination before instituting therapy and monthly serology tests for at least 4 mo thereafter
Primary syphilis	Spinal-fluid examinations should be performed before treatment and as part of follow-up therapy
Localized infections	May require surgical drainage, in addition to antibiotic therapy
Superinfection	Prolonged or repeated use may cause overgrowth of nonsusceptible bacteria or fungi; if superinfection occurs, discontinue use

ADVERSE REACTIONS

Gastrointestinal	Abdominal cramping, discomfort, nausea, vomiting, and diarrhea (with oral use)
Hypersensitivity	Urticaria, skin rashes, anaphylaxis
Other	Reversible hearing loss (see WARNINGS/PRECAUTIONS), venous irritation with IV use (rare)

OVERDOSAGE

Signs and symptoms	See ADVERSE REACTIONS
Treatment	Discontinue medication; treat symptomatically

DRUG INTERACTIONS

Lincomycin	▽ Bactericidal action of lincomycin
Aminophylline, oxtriphylline, theophylline	△ Serum theophylline level

ALTERED LABORATORY VALUES

Blood/serum values	△ Alkaline phosphatase △ Bilirubin △ SGOT △ SGPT
Urinary values	△ Catecholamines (with Hingerty fluorometric method)

USE IN CHILDREN

Age, weight, and severity of infection are important factors in determining the proper dosage; see INDICATIONS

USE IN PREGNANT AND NURSING WOMEN

Safety for use during pregnancy has not been established because no controlled studies or retrospective analyses have been done in pregnant women; erythromycin crosses the placental barrier, but fetal plasma levels are low. Erythromycin is excreted in breast milk.

---

[1] Resistance may develop during treatment
[2] Unsuitable for prevention of bacterial endocarditis in patients undergoing genitourinary or gastrointestinal tract surgery

---

ERYTHROMYCINS

ILOSONE (erythromycin estolate) Dista   Rx

Capsules: 250 mg **Tablets:** 500 mg **Chewable tablets:** 125, 250 mg **Drops:** 5 mg/drop (10 ml) **Suspension (per 5 ml):** 125 mg (100 ml, 16 fl oz) *orange flavored*, 250 mg (100 ml, 16 fl oz) *cherry flavored*

INDICATIONS

Acute mild to moderate **skin and soft tissue infections** caused by susceptible strains of *Staphylococcus aureus*[1]

Mild to moderate **upper and lower respiratory tract, skin, and soft tissue infections** caused by *Streptococcus pyogenes*

Mild to moderate **upper and lower respiratory tract infections** caused by *Streptococcus pneumoniae* and *Mycoplasma pneumoniae*

Mild to moderate **upper respiratory tract infections** caused by susceptible strains of *Hemophilus influenzae* (with appropriate sulfonamide therapy)

As an adjunct to antitoxin for **prevention and/or elimination of the carrier state** in individuals exposed to *Corynebacterium diphtheriae*

Infections caused by *Listeria monocytogenes*

Erythrasma caused by *Corynebacterium minutissimum*

ORAL DOSAGE

Adult: 250 mg q6h; for severe infections, up to 4 g/day or more, in divided doses
Child: 30–50 mg/kg/day in divided doses; for severe infections, up to 60–100 mg/kg/day in divided doses

ILOSONE

Streptococcal pharyngitis and tonsillitis	**Adult:** 1,000 mg/day in divided doses **Infant and child (< 25 lb):** 250 mg/day in divided doses **Child (25–40 lb):** 375 mg/day in divided doses **Child (40–55 lb):** 500 mg/day in divided doses **Child (55–80 lb):** 750 mg/day in divided doses **Child (> 80 lb):** same as adult
Continuous prophylaxis of rheumatic fever	**Adult:** 250 mg bid **Child:** same as adult
Prevention of bacterial endocarditis in penicillin-allergic patients with congenital heart disease or rheumatic or other acquired valvular heart disease who are undergoing dental procedures or upper respiratory tract surgery[2]	**Adult:** 1 g 1 h prior to dental procedure or upper respiratory tract surgery, followed by 500 mg 6 h later **Child:** 20 mg/kg 1 h prior to dental procedure or upper respiratory tract surgery, followed by 10 mg/kg 6 h later
Primary syphilis in penicillin-allergic patients	**Adult:** 20 g total, given in divided doses over a period of 10 days
Intestinal amebiasis caused by *Entamoeba histolytica*	**Adult:** 250 mg qid for 10–14 days **Child:** 30–50 mg/kg/day in divided doses for 10–14 days
Nasopharyngeal carriage of *Bordetella pertussis*	**Adult:** 40–50 mg/kg/day in divided doses for 5–14 days
Legionnaires' disease	**Adult:** 1–4 g/day in divided doses
Conjunctivitis caused by *Chlamydia trachomatis*	**Neonate:** 50 mg/kg/day of erythromycin suspension, given in 4 divided doses for at least 2 wk
Pneumonia caused by *Chlamydia trachomatis*	**Infant:** 50 mg/kg/day of erythromycin suspension, given in 4 divided doses for at least 3 wk
Uncomplicated **urethral, endocervical, and rectal infections** caused by *Chlamydia trachomatis*, when tetracycline is contraindicated or cannot be tolerated **Urogenital infections** in pregnant women caused by *Chlamydia trachomatis*	**Adult:** 500 mg qid for at least 7 days; pregnant women who cannot tolerate this dosage should be given 250 mg qid for at least 14 days

CONTRAINDICATIONS

Hypersensitivity to erythromycin	Preexisting liver disease

ADMINISTRATION/DOSAGE ADJUSTMENTS

Timing of administration	May be given without regard to meals
Alternative dosing schedule	If the total daily dose does not exceed 1 g, half of the dose may be given q12h
Duration of treatment for streptococcal infections	Infections caused by Group A beta-hemolytic streptococci should be treated for a minimum of 10 days

WARNINGS/PRECAUTIONS

Reversible hepatic dysfunction, cholestatic hepatitis	May occur, with or without jaundice, generally following 1–2 wk of continuous therapy. Observe patient for malaise, nausea, vomiting, abdominal cramps, and fever; severe abdominal pain simulating an abdominal surgical emergency may also occur. Laboratory findings include abnormal liver-function tests, peripheral eosinophilia, and leukocytosis. Discontinue medication promptly.
Patients with hepatic impairment	Use with caution and watch for signs of excessive accumulation, since drug is excreted primarily by the liver
Primary syphilis	Spinal fluid examinations should be performed before treatment and as part of follow-up therapy
Ototoxicity	Reversible hearing loss has occurred, primarily in patients who had renal impairment or received high doses
Pseudomembranous colitis	May occur due to alteration of the normal intestinal flora and should be considered in any patient who develops diarrhea during or after therapy. Mild cases may respond to withdrawal of the drug alone. Moderate to severe cases should be managed by sigmoidoscopy, appropriate bacteriological studies, fluid and electrolyte replacement, and protein supplementation, as needed. Oral vancomycin is the treatment of choice for severe or refractory colitis associated with the overgrowth of *Clostridium difficile*; however, other possible causes should also be considered.
Superinfection	Prolonged or repeated use may cause overgrowth of nonsusceptible bacteria or fungi; if superinfection occurs, discontinue use

ADVERSE REACTIONS

Gastrointestinal	Nausea, vomiting, abdominal cramping and discomfort, diarrhea
Hypersensitivity	Urticaria, skin rashes, anaphylaxis

COMPENDIUM OF DRUG THERAPY

ILOSONE ■ PCE

| Other | Reversible hearing loss (see WARNINGS/PRECAUTIONS) |

OVERDOSAGE

| Signs and symptoms | See ADVERSE REACTIONS |
| Treatment | Discontinue medication; treat symptomatically |

DRUG INTERACTIONS

Lincomycin	▽ Bactericidal action of lincomycin
Aminophylline, oxtriphylline, theophylline	△ Serum theophylline level; reduce dosage of theophylline if serum level increases or toxicity occurs during combination therapy
Warfarin	△ Risk of bleeding; when erythromycin is given during long-term warfarin therapy, the prothrombin time should be closely monitored, especially in the elderly, and, if necessary, the dosage of warfarin should be reduced

ALTERED LABORATORY VALUES

| Blood/serum values | △ Alkaline phosphatase △ Bilirubin △ SGOT △ SGPT |
| Urinary values | △ Catecholamines (with Hingerty fluorometric method) |

USE IN CHILDREN

Age, weight, and severity of infection are important factors in determining the proper dosage; see INDICATIONS

USE IN PREGNANT AND NURSING WOMEN

Safety for use during pregnancy has not been established; carefully consider the risks and benefits of such use. Trace amounts of erythromycin have been detected in human milk.

---

[1] Resistance may develop during treatment
[2] Unsuitable for prevention of bacterial endocarditis in patients undergoing genitourinary or gastrointestinal tract surgery

---

ERYTHROMYCINS

PCE (erythromycin) Abbott   Rx

Tablets (with polymer-coated particles): 333 mg

INDICATIONS

Mild to moderate **skin and skin structure infections** caused by susceptible strains of *Staphylococcus aureus*[1]

Mild to moderate **upper and lower respiratory tract, skin, and skin structure infections** caused by *Streptococcus pyogenes*

Mild to moderate **upper and lower respiratory tract infections** caused by *Streptococcus pneumoniae* and *Mycoplasma pneumoniae*

Mild to moderate **upper respiratory tract infections** caused by susceptible strains of *Hemophilus influenzae* (with appropriate sulfonamide therapy)

As an adjunct to antitoxin for **prevention and/or elimination of the carrier state** in individuals exposed to *Corynebacterium diphtheriae*

Erythrasma caused by *Corynebacterium minutissimum*

Acute pelvic inflammatory disease caused by *Neisseria gonorrhoeae* in penicillin-allergic patients

Continuous prophylaxis of rheumatic fever in patients allergic to penicillins or sulfonamides

Prevention of bacterial endocarditis in susceptible patients[2] who are allergic to penicillin and are about to undergo dental procedures or upper respiratory tract surgery

ORAL DOSAGE

Adult: 333 mg q8h; for severe infections, up to 4 g/day in divided doses
Child: 30–50 mg/kg/day in equally divided doses; for severe infections, 60–100 mg/kg/day in equally divided doses, up to 4 g/day

Adult: initiate treatment with erythromycin lactobionate (500 mg IV q6h for 3 days), followed by 333 mg of erythromycin orally q8h for 7 days

Adult: 250 mg bid
Child: same as adult

Adult: 1 g 1 h prior to dental procedure or upper respiratory tract surgery, followed by 500 mg 6 h later

Primary syphilis in penicillin-allergic patients	**Adult:** 30–40 g total, given in divided doses over a period of 10–15 days
Intestinal amebiasis caused by *Entamoeba histolytica*	**Adult:** 333 mg q8h or 250 mg q6h for 10–14 days **Child:** 30–50 mg/kg/day in divided doses for 10–14 days
Legionnaires' disease	**Adult:** 1–4 g/day in divided doses
Conjunctivitis caused by *Chlamydia trachomatis*	**Neonate:** 50 mg/kg/day of erythromycin suspension, given in 4 divided doses for at least 2 wk
Pneumonia caused by *Chlamydia trachomatis*	**Infant:** 50 mg/kg/day of erythromycin suspension, given in 4 divided doses for at least 3 wk
Uncomplicated urethral, endocervical, and rectal infections caused by *Chlamydia trachomatis*, and **urethritis** caused by *Ureaplasma urealyticum*, when tetracycline is contraindicated or cannot be tolerated **Urogenital infections** in pregnant women caused by *Chlamydia trachomatis*	**Adult:** 500 mg qid for at least 7 days; pregnant women who cannot tolerate this dosage should be given 250 mg qid for at least 14 days
Nasopharyngeal carriage of *Bordetella pertussis*	**Adult:** 40–50 mg/kg/day in divided doses for 5–14 days

CONTRAINDICATIONS

Hypersensitivity to erythromycin

ADMINISTRATION/DOSAGE ADJUSTMENTS

Timing of administration	Tablets may be given without regard to meals; however, optimal blood levels are obtained when drug is given at least 30 min or, preferably, at least 2 h before meals
Duration of treatment for streptococcal infections	Infections caused by Group A beta-hemolytic streptococci should be treated for a minimum of 10 days

WARNINGS/PRECAUTIONS

Hepatic dysfunction	May occur, with or without jaundice, in patients receiving oral erythromycin
Patients with hepatic impairment	Use with caution and watch for signs of excessive accumulation, since drug is excreted primarily by the liver
Concomitant theophylline therapy	May produce elevated serum theophylline levels or theophylline toxicity; reduce theophylline dosage accordingly
Primary syphilis	Spinal fluid examinations should be done before treatment and as part of follow-up therapy; use of erythromycin for treatment of syphilis in utero is not recommended
Ototoxicity	Reversible hearing loss has occurred, primarily in patients who had renal impairment or received high doses
Superinfection	Prolonged or repeated use may cause overgrowth of nonsusceptible bacteria or fungi; if superinfection occurs, discontinue use
Localized infections	Incision and drainage or surgical procedures should be performed, when indicated, in conjunction with antibiotic therapy
Carcinogenicity, mutagenicity, effect on fertility	No evidence of carcinogenicity has been found in rats fed erythromycin base for 2 yr; no studies have been conducted to evaluate the mutagenic potential of this drug. No effect on male or female fertility has been found in rats fed erythromycin base at levels up to 0.25% of their diet.

ADVERSE REACTIONS

Gastrointestinal	Nausea, vomiting, abdominal pain, diarrhea, anorexia, hepatic dysfunction and/or abnormal liver-function test results; pseudomembranous colitis (rare)
Hypersensitivity	Allergic reactions ranging from urticaria and mild skin eruptions to anaphylaxis
Other	Reversible hearing loss (see WARNINGS/PRECAUTIONS)

OVERDOSAGE

Signs and symptoms	See gastrointestinal ADVERSE REACTIONS
Treatment	Discontinue medication and treat symptomatically; erythromycin is not removed by peritoneal dialysis or hemodialysis

DRUG INTERACTIONS

Lincomycin	▽ Bactericidal action of lincomycin
Aminophylline, oxtriphylline, theophylline	△ Serum theophylline level
Carbamazepine	△ Risk of carbamazepine toxicity

PCE ■ PEDIAMYCIN

Digoxin	△ Serum level of digoxin
Oral anticoagulants	△ Hypoprothrombinemic effect of oral anticoagulants

ALTERED LABORATORY VALUES

Blood/serum values	△ Alkaline phosphatase △ Bilirubin △ SGOT △ SGPT
Urinary values	△ Catecholamines (with Hingerty fluorometric method)

USE IN CHILDREN
Age, weight, and severity of infection are important factors in determining proper dosage; see INDICATIONS

USE IN PREGNANT AND NURSING WOMEN
Pregnancy Category B: reproduction studies in female rats fed erythromycin base at levels up to 0.25% of their diet prior to and during mating, during gestation, and through weaning of two successive litters have shown no teratogenic or other adverse effect on reproduction. No adequate, well-controlled studies have been performed in pregnant women; erythromycin crosses the placental barrier, but fetal plasma levels are generally low. Use during pregnancy only if clearly needed. Erythromycin is excreted in human milk; use with caution in nursing mothers.

[1] Resistance may develop during treatment
[2] Susceptible patients are those with prosthetic cardiac valves, most congenital cardiac malformations, surgically constructed systemic pulmonary shunts, rheumatic or other acquired valvular dysfunction, idiopathic hypertrophic subaortic stenosis, a previous history of bacterial endocarditis, or mitral valve prolapse with insufficiency

---

ERYTHROMYCINS

PEDIAMYCIN (erythromycin ethylsuccinate) Ross   Rx

Oral suspension (per 5 ml): 200 mg[1] (Pediamycin Liquid) (16 fl oz) *cherry flavored*, 400 mg[1] (Pediamycin 400) (16 fl oz) *cherry flavored*, 200 mg after reconstitution (100, 150 ml) *cherry flavored*   **Drops (per 5 ml):** 100 mg (50 ml) *cherry flavored*

INDICATIONS

Acute mild to moderate **skin and soft tissue infections** caused by *Staphylococcus aureus*[3]

Mild to moderate **upper and lower respiratory tract, skin, and soft tissue infections** caused by *Streptococcus pyogenes*

Mild to moderate **upper and lower respiratory tract infections** caused by *Streptococcus pneumoniae* and *Mycoplasma pneumoniae*

Mild to moderate **upper respiratory tract infections** caused by *Hemophilus influenzae* (with appropriate sulfonamide therapy)

As an adjunct to antitoxin for **prevention and/or elimination of the carrier state** in individuals exposed to *Corynebacterium diphtheriae*

Infections caused by *Listeria monocytogenes*

Erythrasma caused by *Corynebacterium minutissimum*

Continuous prophylaxis of rheumatic fever

Prevention of bacterial endocarditis in penicillin-allergic patients with congenital heart disease or rheumatic or other acquired valvular heart disease who are undergoing dental procedures or upper respiratory tract surgery[4]

Urethritis caused by *Chlamydia trachomatis* or *Ureaplasma urealyticum*

Primary syphilis in penicillin-allergic patients

Intestinal amebiasis caused by *Entamoeba histolytica*

Legionnaires' disease

ORAL DOSAGE[2]

Adult: 400 mg q6h; for severe infections, up to 4 g/day in divided doses
Infant (< 10 lb): 40 mg/kg/day in equally divided doses
Infant (10–15 lb): 200 mg/day in 2 or 4 equally divided doses
Infant and child (15–25 lb): 400 mg/day in 2 or 4 equally divided doses
Child (25–50 lb): 800 mg/day in 2 or 4 equally divided doses
Child (50–100 lb): 1,200 mg/day in 2 or 4 equally divided doses
Child (> 100 lb): 1,600 mg/day in 2 or 4 equally divided doses

Adult: 400 mg bid
Child: same as adult

Adult: 1.6 g 1½–2 h prior to dental procedure or respiratory tract surgery, followed by 800 mg q6h for 8 doses
Child: 20 mg/kg 1½–2 h prior to dental procedure or upper respiratory tract surgery, followed by 10 mg/kg for 8 doses

Male adult: 800 mg tid for 7 days

Adult: 48–64 g total, given in divided doses over a period of 10–15 days

Adult: 400 mg qid for 10–14 days
Child: 30–50 mg/kg/day in divided doses for 10–14 days

Adult: 1.6–4 g/day in divided doses

PEDIAMYCIN

Nasopharyngeal carriage of *Bordetella pertussis* — **Adult:** 40–50 mg/kg/day in divided doses for 5–14 days

CONTRAINDICATIONS

Hypersensitivity to erythromycin

ADMINISTRATION/DOSAGE ADJUSTMENTS

Timing of administration	May be given without regard to meals
Alternative dosing schedule	Half the total daily dose may be given q12h, or, if desired, one third may be given q8h
Duration of treatment for streptococcal infections	Infections caused by Group A beta-hemolytic streptococci should be treated for a minimum of 10 days
Severe infections in children	Dosage given above may be doubled, if necessary

WARNINGS/PRECAUTIONS

Hepatic dysfunction	May occur, with or without jaundice, in patients receiving oral erythromycin
Patients with hepatic impairment	Use with caution and watch for signs of excessive accumulation, since drug is excreted primarily by the liver
Concomitant theophylline therapy	May produce elevated serum theophylline levels or theophylline toxicity; reduce theophylline dosage accordingly
Primary syphilis	Spinal fluid examinations should be performed before treatment and as part of follow-up therapy
Ototoxicity	Reversible hearing loss has occurred, primarily in patients who had renal impairment or received high doses
Superinfection	Prolonged or repeated use may cause overgrowth of nonsusceptible bacteria or fungi; if superinfection occurs, discontinue use
Carcinogenicity, mutagenicity	Long-term studies in dogs and rats at doses of 12.5 and 250 times the usual human dose, respectively, have shown no evidence of tumorigenicity; mutagenicity studies have not been done

ADVERSE REACTIONS

Gastrointestinal	Nausea, vomiting, abdominal cramping and discomfort, diarrhea
Hepatic	Hepatic dysfunction, with or without jaundice
Hypersensitivity	Urticaria, mild skin eruptions, anaphylaxis
Other	Reversible hearing loss (see WARNINGS/PRECAUTIONS)

OVERDOSAGE

Signs and symptoms	See ADVERSE REACTIONS
Treatment	Discontinue medication; treat symptomatically

DRUG INTERACTIONS

Chloramphenicol, clindamycin, lincomycin, troleandomycin	▽ Bactericidal activity
Aminophylline, oxtriphylline, theophylline	△ Serum theophylline level

ALTERED LABORATORY VALUES

Blood/serum values	△ Alkaline phosphatase △ Bilirubin △ SGOT △ SGPT
Urinary values	△ Catecholamines (with Hingerty fluorometric method)

USE IN CHILDREN

Age, weight, and severity of infection are important factors in determining the proper dosage; see INDICATIONS and ORAL DOSAGE

USE IN PREGNANT AND NURSING WOMEN

Pregnancy Category B: safety for use during pregnancy has not been established. Reproduction studies in rats at doses of up to 50 mg/kg have shown no adverse effect on reproductive performance, implantation, gestation, parturition, fetal development, lactation, or perinatal and postnatal survival and development; however, a slight increase in fetal resorption was found at the highest dose level. A separate study in rabbits treated with the same doses also showed no evidence of teratogenicity. Although erythromycin reportedly crosses the placental barrier in humans, fetal plasma levels of the drug are generally low. Erythromycin is excreted in breast milk; use with caution in nursing women.

---

[1] Contains <0.1% alcohol
[2] In calculating adult dosages, bear in mind that 400 mg of this drug is equivalent to 250 mg of erythromycin estolate, stearate, or base
[3] Resistance may develop during treatment
[4] Unsuitable for prevention of bacterial endocarditis in patients undergoing genitourinary or gastrointestinal tract surgery

WYAMYCIN

ERYTHROMYCINS

WYAMYCIN E (erythromycin ethylsuccinate) Wyeth   Rx
Suspension (per 5 ml): 200 mg (Wyamycin E 200) (16 fl oz) *fruit-flavored*, 400 mg (Wyamycin E 400) (16 fl oz) *fruit-flavored*

WYAMYCIN S (erythromycin stearate) Wyeth   Rx
Tablets: 250, 500 mg

INDICATIONS	ORAL DOSAGE
Acute mild to moderate **skin and soft tissue infections** caused by susceptible strains of *Staphylococcus aureus*[1] Mild to moderate **upper and lower respiratory tract, skin, and soft tissue infections** caused by *Streptococcus pyogenes* Mild to moderate **upper and lower respiratory tract infections** caused by *Streptococcus pneumoniae* and *Mycoplasma pneumoniae* Mild to moderate **upper respiratory tract infections** caused by susceptible strains of *Hemophilus influenzae* (with appropriate sulfonamide therapy) As an adjunct to antitoxin for **prevention and/or elimination of the carrier state** in individuals exposed to *Corynebacterium diphtheriae* **Infections** caused by *Listeria monocytogenes* **Erythrasma** caused by *Corynebacterium minutissimum*	**Adult:** 250 mg of erythromycin stearate or 400 mg of erythromycin ethylsuccinate q6h; for severe infections, up to 4 g/day or more in divided doses **Child:** 30–50 mg/kg/day in divided doses
Acute pelvic inflammatory disease caused by *Neisseria gonorrhoeae* in penicillin-allergic patients	**Adult:** initiate treatment with erythromycin lactobionate (500 mg IV q6h for 3 days), followed by 250 mg of erythromycin stearate orally q6h for 7 days
Continuous prophylaxis of rheumatic fever	**Adult:** 250 mg of erythromycin stearate or 400 mg of erythromycin ethylsuccinate bid **Child:** same as adult
Prevention of bacterial endocarditis in penicillin-allergic patients with congenital heart disease or rheumatic or other acquired valvular heart disease who are undergoing dental procedures or upper respiratory tract surgery[2]	**Adult:** 1 g 1 h prior to dental procedure or upper respiratory tract surgery, followed by 500 mg 6 h later **Child:** 20 mg/kg 1 h prior to dental procedure or upper respiratory tract surgery, followed by 10 mg/kg 6 h later
Primary syphilis in penicillin-allergic patients	**Adult:** 30–40 g of erythromycin stearate or 48–64 g of erythromycin ethylsuccinate, given in divided doses over a period of 10–15 days
Intestinal amebiasis caused by *Entamoeba histolytica*	**Adult:** 250 mg of erythromycin stearate or 400 mg of erythromycin ethylsuccinate qid for 10–14 days **Child:** 30–50 mg/kg/day in divided doses for 10–14 days
Legionnaires' disease	**Adult:** 1–4 g/day of erythromycin stearate or 1.6–4 g/day of erythromycin ethylsuccinate, given in divided doses
Conjunctivitis caused by *Chlamydia trachomatis*	**Neonate:** 50 mg/kg/day of erythromycin ethylsuccinate, given in 4 divided doses for at least 2 wk
Pneumonia caused by *Chlamydia trachomatis*	**Infant:** 50 mg/kg/day of erythromycin ethylsuccinate, given in 4 divided doses for at least 3 wk
Uncomplicated urethral, endocervical, and rectal infections caused by *Chlamydia trachomatis*, when tetracycline is contraindicated or cannot be tolerated **Urogenital infections** in pregnant women caused by *Chlamydia trachomatis*	**Adult:** 500 mg of erythromycin stearate or 800 mg of erythromycin ethylsuccinate qid for at least 7 days; pregnant women who cannot tolerate this dosage should be given 250 mg of erythromycin stearate or 400 mg of erythromycin ethylsuccinate qid for at least 14 days

CONTRAINDICATIONS
Hypersensitivity to erythromycin

ADMINISTRATION/DOSAGE ADJUSTMENTS

Timing of administration	Suspension form may be given without regard to meals; administer tablets in the fasting state or immediately before meals to obtain optimum serum levels
Alternative dosing schedule	Half the total daily dose may be given q12h, with the tablet given 1 h before meals
Duration of treatment for streptococcal infections	Infections caused by Group A beta-hemolytic streptococci should be treated for a minimum of 10 days

COMPENDIUM OF DRUG THERAPY

WYAMYCIN

Severe infections in children	Dosage given above may be doubled, if necessary

WARNINGS/PRECAUTIONS

Hepatic dysfunction	May occur, with or without jaundice, in patients receiving oral erythromycin
Patients with hepatic impairment	Use with caution and watch for signs of excessive accumulation, since drug is excreted primarily by the liver
Concomitant theophylline therapy	May produce elevated serum theophylline levels or theophylline toxicity; reduce theophylline dosage accordingly
Suspected syphilitic lesions	If syphilis is suspected, perform a dark-field examination before instituting erythromycin stearate therapy and monthly serology tests for at least 4 mo thereafter. Spinal fluid examinations should be done before treatment and as part of follow-up therapy.
Ototoxicity	Reversible hearing loss has occurred, primarily in patients who had renal impairment or received high doses
Superinfection	Prolonged or repeated use may cause overgrowth of nonsusceptible bacteria or fungi; if superinfection occurs, discontinue use

ADVERSE REACTIONS

Gastrointestinal	Nausea, vomiting, abdominal cramping and discomfort, diarrhea
Hypersensitivity	Urticaria, skin rashes, anaphylaxis
Other	Reversible hearing loss (see WARNINGS/PRECAUTIONS)

OVERDOSAGE

Signs and symptoms	See gastrointestinal ADVERSE REACTIONS
Treatment	Discontinue medication; treat symptomatically

DRUG INTERACTIONS

Lincomycin	▽ Bactericidal action of lincomycin
Aminophylline, oxtriphylline, theophylline	△ Serum theophylline level

ALTERED LABORATORY VALUES

Blood/serum values	△ Alkaline phosphatase △ Bilirubin △ SGOT △ SGPT
Urinary values	△ Catecholamines (with Hingerty fluorometric method)

USE IN CHILDREN

Age, weight, and severity of infection are important factors in determining proper dosage; see INDICATIONS

USE IN PREGNANT AND NURSING WOMEN

Safety for use during pregnancy has not been established; erythromycin crosses the placental barrier, but fetal plasma levels are low. Trace amounts of erythromycin have been observed in human milk.

---

[1] Resistance may develop during treatment
[2] Unsuitable for prevention of bacterial endocarditis in patients undergoing genitourinary or gastrointestinal tract surgery

TETRACYCLINES

ACHROMYCIN (tetracycline hydrochloride) Lederle — Rx
Vials: 100, 250 mg (for IM use); 250, 500 mg (for IV use)

ACHROMYCIN V (tetracycline hydrochloride) Lederle — Rx
Capsules: 250, 500 mg Suspension (per 5 ml): 125 mg (2, 16 fl oz) *cherry flavored*

INDICATIONS

Gram-negative bacterial infections caused by *Hemophilus ducreyi* (chancroid), *Calymmatobacterium granulomatis* (granuloma inguinale), *Yersinia pestis* (plague), *Francisella tularensis* (tularemia), *Bartonella bacilliformis* (bartonellosis), *Bacteroides*, *Vibrio cholerae* (cholera), and *Campylobacter fetus* (vibriosis), as well as susceptible strains of *Escherichia coli*, *Enterobacter aerogenes*, *Shigella*, *Acinetobacter*, *Hemophilus influenzae* (respiratory tract infections only), and *Klebsiella* (respiratory and urinary tract infections only)

Mycoplasmal pneumonia (primary atypical pneumonia)

Streptococcal infections caused by susceptible strains[1]

Skin and soft tissue infections caused by susceptible strains of *Staphylococcus aureus*[2]

Rickettsial infections

Psittacosis (ornithosis)

Lymphogranuloma venereum, trachoma, and (when given orally) **inclusion conjunctivitis** and uncomplicated adult **urethral, endocervical, and rectal infections** caused by *Chlamydia trachomatis*

Relapsing fever

As an adjunct to amebicides for **acute intestinal amebiasis**

As an alternative to penicillin for **gonococcal and clostridial infections, listeriosis, yaws, anthrax, Vincent's infection, actinomycosis,** and (when given IV) **meningococcal infections**

Severe acne (oral therapy only)

Syphilis in cases where penicillin is contraindicated

Brucellosis

ORAL DOSAGE

Adult: 1–2 g/day, given in 2 or 4 equally divided doses, depending on the severity of the infection; for acute gonococcal infections, 1.5 g to start, followed by 500 mg q6h for 4 days, for a total of 9 g; for chlamydial urethral, endocervical, and rectal infections, 500 mg qid for at least 7 days

Child (> 8 yr): 25–50 mg/kg/day, given in 2 or 4 equally divided doses

Adult: 30–40 g total, given in equally divided doses over a period of 10–15 days

Adult: 500 mg qid for 3 wk (with 1 g streptomycin IM bid 1st wk and once daily 2nd wk)

PARENTERAL DOSAGE

Adult: 250 mg, given in a single IM dose q24h, or 300 mg/day, given in 2 or 3 divided IM doses q8–12h; if rapid, high blood levels are needed, give 250–500 mg IV q12h, or up to 500 mg IV q6h if necessary

Child (> 8 yr): 15–25 mg/kg/day, up to 250 mg/day, given in a single daily IM dose or 2 or 3 divided IM doses q8–12h; if rapid, high blood levels are needed, give 10–20 mg/kg/day IV, depending on the severity of the infection (usual dosage: 6 mg/kg bid)

CONTRAINDICATIONS
Hypersensitivity to tetracyclines

ADMINISTRATION/DOSAGE ADJUSTMENTS

Duration of treatment	Unless otherwise indicated, continue treatment for at least 24–48 h after symptoms and fever have subsided; infections caused by Group A beta-hemolytic streptococci should be treated for at least 10 days. If patient is started on parenteral therapy, institute oral therapy as soon as possible.
Intramuscular administration	Reserve for situations in which oral therapy is not feasible. Add 2 ml of sterile water for injection or sodium chloride injection to 100- or 250-mg vial, withdraw required dose, and inject deeply into a large muscle mass, such as the gluteus. Use the reconstituted solution within 24 h. IM administration produces lower blood levels than oral administration at recommended dosages.
Intravenous administration	Use only when rapidly attained, high blood levels are needed and oral therapy is not adequate or tolerated. To reconstitute the solution, add 5 ml of sterile water for injection to the 250-mg vial or 10 ml to the 500-mg vial; use within 12 h. Immediately before administration, dilute the solution to a final volume of 100–1,000 ml with 5% dextrose injection USP, sodium chloride injection USP (alone or with 5% dextrose), or 5% protein hydrolysate (low sodium) injection USP (alone, with 5% dextrose, or with 10% invert sugar). Solutions containing calcium generally should be avoided, unless necessary, as they tend to precipitate tetracycline; Ringer's and lactated Ringer's injection USP may be used with caution, however, because their calcium ion content does not normally precipitate tetracycline at acid pH. Prolonged IV administration may cause thrombophlebitis. Avoid rapid administration.

ACHROMYCIN

Timing of oral administration	Food and some dairy products interfere with absorption; give oral forms 1 h before or 2 h after meals

WARNINGS/PRECAUTIONS

Patients with renal impairment	Usual doses may lead to excessive drug accumulation and possible hepatic toxicity. If impairment is significant, azotemia, hyperphosphatemia, and acidosis may occur due to antianabolic action of drug. Reduce dosage by lowering individual doses and/or lengthening interval between doses, monitor kidney and liver function both before and during therapy, and follow serum tetracycline levels periodically (particularly if therapy is prolonged).
Pregnant and postpartum patients with pyelonephritis	Potentially fatal hepatic failure may occur with parenteral administration; do not allow serum level to exceed 15 μg/ml, monitor liver function frequently, and avoid concomitant use of other potentially hepatotoxic drugs
Superinfection	Overgrowth of nonsusceptible organisms, including fungi, may occur
Suspected syphilitic lesions	If syphilis is suspected, perform a dark-field examination before instituting therapy and monthly serology tests for at least 4 mo thereafter
Long-term therapy	Perform hemapoietic, renal, and hepatic studies periodically
Photosensitivity (exaggerated sunburn)	May occur; caution patients likely to be exposed to direct sunlight or UV light and discontinue use of tetracycline at first sign of skin erythema

ADVERSE REACTIONS

Gastrointestinal	Anorexia, nausea, vomiting, diarrhea, glossitis, dysphagia, enterocolitis, inflammatory lesions (with monilial overgrowth) in the anogenital region
Dermatological	Maculopapular and erythematous rashes, exfoliative dermatitis (rare), photosensitivity
Hypersensitivity	Urticaria, angioneurotic edema, anaphylaxis, anaphylactoid purpura, pericarditis, exacerbation of systemic lupus erythematosus
Hematological	Hemolytic anemia, thrombocytopenia, neutropenia, eosinophilia
Other	Microscopic discoloration of thyroid glands, bulging fontanels in infants, local irritation after IM injection

OVERDOSAGE

Signs and symptoms	See ADVERSE REACTIONS
Treatment	Discontinue medication, treat symptomatically, and institute supportive measures, as required

DRUG INTERACTIONS

Oral anticoagulants	△ Prothrombin time
Penicillin	▽ Bactericidal activity of penicillin; avoid concomitant use
Antacids, sodium bicarbonate, iron supplements	▽ Absorption of oral tetracycline; antacids containing aluminum, calcium, or magnesium should not be administered concomitantly
Methoxyflurane	△ Risk of nephrotoxicity

ALTERED LABORATORY VALUES

Blood/serum values	△ Alkaline phosphatase △ BUN △ Amylase △ Bilirubin △ SGOT △ SGPT ▽ Prothrombin activity
Urinary values	△ Catecholamines (with Hingerty fluorometric method)

USE IN CHILDREN

Not recommended for use during infancy through 8 yr of age unless other drugs are not likely to be effective or are contraindicated; use in this age group may cause permanent discoloration of teeth or enamel hypoplasia. A reversible decrease in fibula growth rate has been observed in premature infants given oral tetracycline (100 mg/kg/day).

USE IN PREGNANT AND NURSING WOMEN

Use during latter half of pregnancy (fetal tooth development) may cause permanent discoloration of teeth or enamel hypoplasia. Animal studies indicate that tetracyclines cross the placental barrier, are found in fetal tissues, and can cause both embryotoxicity and fetal toxicity, including retardation of skeletal development. Tetracyclines are excreted in breast milk; if drug is essential, patient should not nurse.

---

[1] Tetracyclines should not be used for streptococcal disease unless bacterial susceptibility has been demonstrated
[2] Tetracyclines are not the drug of choice for treating any staphylococcal infection

TETRACYCLINES

DECLOMYCIN (demeclocycline hydrochloride) Lederle   Rx

Capsules: 150 mg **Tablets:** 150, 300 mg

INDICATIONS

Gram-negative bacterial infections caused by *Hemophilus ducreyi* (chancroid), *Calymmatobacterium granulomatis* (granuloma inguinale), *Yersinia pestis* (plague), *Francisella tularensis* (tularemia), *Bartonella bacilliformis* (bartonellosis), *Bacteroides*, *Brucella* (when combined with streptomycin), *Vibrio cholerae* (cholera), and *Campylobacter fetus* (vibriosis), as well as susceptible strains of *Escherichia coli*, *Enterobacter aerogenes*, *Shigella*, *Acinetobacter*, *Hemophilus influenzae* (respiratory tract infections only), and *Klebsiella* (respiratory and urinary tract infections only)
Mycoplasmal pneumonia (primary atypical pneumonia)
Streptococcal infections caused by susceptible strains[1]
Skin and soft tissue infections caused by susceptible strains of *Staphylococcus aureus*[2]
Rickettsial infections
Psittacosis (ornithosis)
Lymphogranuloma venereum, trachoma, and inclusion conjunctivitis
Relapsing fever
As an adjunct to amebicides for **acute intestinal amebiasis**
As an alternative to penicillin for **gonococcal and clostridial infections, syphilis, yaws, listeriosis, anthrax, Vincent's infection, and actinomycosis**

ORAL DOSAGE

Adult: 150 mg qid or 300 mg bid; for acute gonococcal infections, 600 mg to start, followed by 300 mg q12h for 4 days, for a total of 3 g
Child (> 8 yr): 3–6 mg/lb/day, depending on the severity of the disease, given in 2 or 4 divided doses

CONTRAINDICATIONS

Hypersensitivity to tetracyclines

ADMINISTRATION/DOSAGE ADJUSTMENTS

Duration of treatment	Unless otherwise indicated, continue treatment for at least 24–48 h after symptoms and fever have subsided; infections caused by Group A beta-hemolytic streptococci should be treated for at least 10 days
Timing of oral administration	Food and some dairy products interfere with absorption; give 1 h before or 2 h after meal

WARNINGS/PRECAUTIONS

Patients with renal impairment	Usual doses may lead to excessive drug accumulation and possible hepatic toxicity. If impairment is significant, azotemia, hyperphosphatemia, and acidosis may occur due to antianabolic action of drug. Reduce dosage by lowering individual doses and/or lengthening interval between doses and follow serum tetracycline levels periodically (particularly if therapy is prolonged).
Superinfection	Overgrowth of nonsusceptible organisms, including fungi, may occur
Suspected syphilitic lesions	If syphilis is suspected, perform a dark-field examination before instituting therapy and monthly serology tests for at least 4 mo thereafter
Long-term therapy	Perform hemopoietic, renal, and hepatic studies periodically
Photosensitivity (exaggerated sunburn)	May occur; caution patients likely to be exposed to direct sunlight or UV light and discontinue use of demeclocycline at first sign of skin erythema
Nephrogenic diabetes insipidus	May occur with long-term use, especially with high doses; discontinue therapy if polyuria, polydipsia, and/or unexplained weakness develop
Bacteriologic studies	May be interfered with by persistent inhibitory levels of the drug in both serum and urine following a course of therapy

ADVERSE REACTIONS

Gastrointestinal	Anorexia, nausea, vomiting, diarrhea, glossitis, black hairy tongue, dysphagia, enterocolitis, inflammatory lesions (with monilial overgrowth) in the anogenital region; hepatotoxicity (rare)
Dermatological	Maculopapular and erythematous rashes, exfoliative dermatitis (rare), photosensitivity
Hypersensitivity	Urticaria, angioneurotic edema, anaphylaxis, anaphylactoid purpura, pericarditis, exacerbation of systemic lupus erythematosus
Hematological	Hemolytic anemia, thrombocytopenia, neutropenia, eosinophilia
Renal	Nephrogenic diabetes insipidus (with long-term use)
Other	Microscopic discoloration of thyroid glands, bulging fontanels in infants

OVERDOSAGE

Signs and symptoms	See ADVERSE REACTIONS

DECLOMYCIN ■ DORYX

| Treatment | Discontinue medication; treat symptomatically and institute supportive measures, as required |

DRUG INTERACTIONS

Oral anticoagulants	△ Prothrombin time
Penicillin	▽ Bactericidal activity of penicillin; avoid concomitant use
Antacids, sodium bicarbonate, iron supplements	▽ Absorption of demeclocycline; antacids containing aluminum, calcium, or magnesium should not be administered concomitantly
Methoxyflurane	△ Risk of nephrotoxicity

ALTERED LABORATORY VALUES

| Blood/serum values | △ Alkaline phosphatase △ BUN (dose related) △ Amylase △ Bilirubin △ SGOT △ SGPT ▽ Prothrombin activity |
| Urinary values | △ Catecholamines (with Hingerty fluorometric method) |

USE IN CHILDREN

Not recommended for use during infancy through 8 yr of age unless other drugs are not likely to be effective or are contraindicated; use in this age group may cause permanent discoloration of teeth or enamel hypoplasia. A reversible decrease in fibula growth rate has been observed in premature infants given oral tetracycline (100 mg/kg/day)

USE IN PREGNANT AND NURSING WOMEN

Use during latter half of pregnancy (fetal tooth development) may cause permanent discoloration of teeth or enamel hypoplasia. Animal studies indicate that tetracyclines cross the placental barrier, are found in fetal tissues, and can cause both embryotoxicity and fetal toxicity, including retardation of skeletal development. Tetracyclines are excreted in breast milk; if drug is essential, patient should not nurse.

[1] Tetracyclines should not be used for streptococcal disease unless bacterial susceptibility has been demonstrated
[2] Tetracyclines are not the drug of choice for treating any staphylococcal infection

---

TETRACYCLINES

DORYX (doxycycline hyclate) Parke-Davis   Rx

Capsules: doxycycline hyclate equivalent to 100 mg doxycycline[1]

INDICATIONS

Gram-negative bacterial infections caused by *Hemophilus ducreyi* (chancroid), *Calymmatobacterium granulomatis* (granuloma inguinale), *Yersinia pestis* (plague), *Francisella tularensis* (tularemia), *Bartonella bacilliformis* (bartonellosis), *Bacteroides*, *Brucella* (when combined with streptomycin), *Vibrio cholerae* (cholera), and *Campylobacter fetus* (vibriosis), as well as susceptible strains of *Escherichia coli*, *Enterobacter aerogenes*, *Shigella*, *Acinetobacter*, *Hemophilus influenzae* (respiratory tract infections only), and *Klebsiella* (respiratory and urinary tract infections only)
Mycoplasmal pneumonia (primary atypical pneumonia)
Streptococcal infections caused by susceptible strains[2]
Respiratory, skin, and soft tissue infections caused by susceptible strains of *Staphylococcus aureus*[3]
Rickettsial infections
Psittacosis (ornithosis)
Acute epididymo-orchitis and uncomplicated **gonorrhea** in adults (except for anorectal infection in men), caused by *Neisseria gonorrhoeae*
Lymphogranuloma venereum, trachoma, inclusion conjunctivitis, acute epididymo-orchitis, and uncomplicated adult **urethral, endocervical, and rectal infections** caused by *Chlamydia trachomatis*
Nongonococcal urethritis caused by *Ureaplasma urealyticum*
Relapsing fever
As an adjunct to amebicides for **acute intestinal amebiasis**
As an alternative to penicillin for **clostridial infections, listeriosis, yaws, anthrax, Vincent's infection,** and **actinomycosis**
Severe acne (adjunctive therapy)

Primary and secondary syphilis when penicillin is contraindicated

ORAL DOSAGE

Adult: 200 mg to start, given in 2 divided doses 12 h apart, followed by 100 mg once daily or 50 mg q12h (for more severe infections, especially chronic urinary tract infections, give 100 mg q12h); for uncomplicated gonococcal infections, 100 mg bid for 7 days (or give 2 doses of 300 mg each 1 h apart); for acute epididymo-orchitis, 100 mg bid for at least 10 days; for nongonococcal urethritis and for chlamydial urethral, endocervical, and rectal infections, 100 mg bid for at least 7 days

Child (> 8 yr and ≤ 100 lb): 2 mg/lb to start, given in 2 divided doses 12 h apart, followed by 1-2 mg/lb/day, depending on severity, given in single or 2 divided daily doses

Child (> 8 yr and > 100 lb): same as adult

Adult: 300 mg/day, given in divided doses for at least 10 days

CONTRAINDICATIONS

Hypersensitivity to tetracyclines

COMPENDIUM OF DRUG THERAPY

DORYX

ADMINISTRATION/DOSAGE ADJUSTMENTS

Duration of treatment	Unless otherwise indicated, continue treatment for at least 24–48 h after symptoms and fever have subsided; infections caused by Group A beta-hemolytic streptococci should be treated for at least 10 days
Oral administration	Caution patient to take adequate amounts of fluid with each dose to minimize risk of esophageal irritation or ulceration. If gastric irritation occurs, administer with milk or solid food.

WARNINGS/PRECAUTIONS

Superinfection	Overgrowth of nonsusceptible organisms, including fungi, may occur; if superinfection occurs, discontinue drug
Suspected syphilitic lesions	If syphilis is suspected, perform a dark-field examination before instituting therapy and monthly serology tests for at least 4 mo thereafter
Long-term therapy	Perform hemopoietic, renal, and hepatic studies periodically
Photosensitivity (exaggerated sunburn)	May occur; caution patients likely to be exposed to direct sunlight or UV light and discontinue use of doxycycline at first sign of skin erythema
Elevated BUN level	Although tetracyclines in general can increase BUN, this effect has not been observed in studies to date in patients with renal impairment who received doxycycline
Mutagenicity	Assays with mouse lymphoma cells and Chinese hamster lung cells have shown tetracyclines to be mutagenic; no clinical evidence of this effect has been reported

ADVERSE REACTIONS

Gastrointestinal	Anorexia, nausea, vomiting, diarrhea, glossitis, dysphagia, enterocolitis, inflammatory lesions (with monilial overgrowth) in the anogenital region; esophagitis and esophageal ulceration (rare)
Dermatological	Maculopapular and erythematous rashes, photosensitivity; exfoliative dermatitis (rare)
Hypersensitivity	Urticaria, angioneurotic edema, anaphylaxis, anaphylactoid purpura, pericarditis, exacerbation of systemic lupus erythematosus
Hematological	Hemolytic anemia, thrombocytopenia, neutropenia, eosinophilia
Other	Microscopic discoloration of thyroid glands (with prolonged use), bulging fontanels in infants, benign intracranial hypertension

OVERDOSAGE

Signs and symptoms	See ADVERSE REACTIONS
Treatment	Discontinue medication, treat symptomatically, and institute supportive measures, as required

DRUG INTERACTIONS

Oral anticoagulants	△ Prothrombin time
Penicillin	▽ Bactericidal activity of penicillin; avoid concomitant use
Antacids, sodium bicarbonate, iron supplements	▽ Absorption of oral doxycycline; do not give concomitantly

ALTERED LABORATORY VALUES

Blood/serum values	▽ Prothrombin activity
Urinary values	△ Catecholamines (with Hingerty fluorometric method)

USE IN CHILDREN

Not recommended for use during infancy through 8 yr of age unless other drugs are not likely to be effective or are contraindicated; use in this age group may cause permanent discoloration of teeth or enamel hypoplasia. A reversible decrease in fibula growth rate has been observed in premature infants given oral tetracycline (100 mg/kg/day).

USE IN PREGNANT AND NURSING WOMEN

Pregnant women: Pregnancy Category D: use during latter half of pregnancy (fetal tooth development) may cause permanent discoloration of teeth or enamel hypoplasia. Animal studies indicate that tetracyclines can cause both embryotoxicity and fetal toxicity, including retardation of skeletal development. **Nursing mothers:** Tetracyclines are excreted in human milk; if drug is essential, patient should not nurse.

---

[1] Capsules contain specially coated pellets
[2] Tetracyclines should not be used for streptococcal disease unless bacterial susceptibility has been demonstrated
[3] Tetracyclines are not the drug of choice for treating any staphylococcal infection

TETRACYCLINES

MINOCIN (minocycline hydrochloride) Lederle Rx

Capsules: minocycline hydrochloride equivalent to 50 and 100 mg minocycline **Tablets:** minocycline hydrochloride equivalent to 50 and 100 mg minocycline **Suspension (per 5 ml):** minocycline hydrochloride equivalent to 50 mg minocycline[1] (2 fl oz) custard-flavored **Vials:** 100 mg

INDICATIONS

Gram-negative bacterial infections caused by *Hemophilus ducreyi* (chancroid), *Calymmatobacterium granulomatis* (granuloma inguinale), *Yersinia pestis* (plague), *Francisella tularensis* (tularemia), *Bartonella bacilliformis* (bartonellosis), *Bacteroides*, *Brucella* (when combined with streptomycin), *Vibrio cholerae* (cholera), and *Campylobacter fetus* (vibriosis), as well as susceptible strains of *Escherichia coli*, *Enterobacter aerogenes*, *Shigella*, *Acinetobacter*, *Hemophilus influenzae* (respiratory tract infections only), and *Klebsiella* (respiratory and urinary tract infections only)

Mycoplasmal pneumonia (primary atypical pneumonia)

Streptococcal infections caused by susceptible strains[2]

Skin and soft tissue infections caused by susceptible strains of *Staphylococcus aureus*[3]

Rickettsial infections

Psittacosis (ornithosis)

Lymphogranuloma venereum, trachoma, and (when given orally) **inclusion conjunctivitis** and uncomplicated adult **urethral, endocervical, and rectal infections** caused by *Chlamydia trachomatis* or *Ureaplasma urealyticum*

Relapsing fever

As an adjunct to amebicides for **acute intestinal ambebiasis**

As an alternative to penicillin for **gonococcal and clostridial infections, listeriosis, syphilis, yaws, anthrax, Vincent's infection, actinomycosis,** and (when given IV) **meningococcal infections**

Severe acne (oral therapy only)

Mycobacterium marinum infections

Eradication of **meningococcal carrier state**

ORAL DOSAGE

Adult: 200 mg to start, followed by 100 mg q12h, or 100–200 mg to start, followed by 50 mg qid; for gonorrhea, 200 mg to start, followed by 100 mg q12h for at least 4 days; for gonococcal urethritis in men, 100 mg bid for 5 days; for nongonococcal urethritis in men and women and endocervical and rectal infections caused by *Chlamydia trachomatis* or *Ureaplasma urealyticum*, 100 mg bid for at least 7 days

Child (> 8 yr): 4 mg/kg to start, followed by 2 mg/kg q12h

Adult: 100 mg bid for 6–8 wk

Adult: 100 mg q12h for 5 days

PARENTERAL DOSAGE

Adult: 200 mg IV to start, followed by 100 mg IV q12h, or up to 400 mg/24 h if needed

Child (> 8 yr): 4 mg/kg IV to start, followed by 2 mg/kg IV q12h

CONTRAINDICATIONS

Hypersensitivity to tetracyclines

ADMINISTRATION/DOSAGE ADJUSTMENTS

Duration of treatment	Unless otherwise indicated, continue treatment for at least 24–48 h after symptoms and fever have subsided; infections caused by Group A beta-hemolytic streptococci should be treated for at least 10 days, and syphilis for 10–15 days. If patient is started on parenteral therapy, institute oral therapy as soon as possible.
Intravenous administration	Use only when rapidly attained, high blood levels are needed and oral therapy is not adequate or tolerated. To reconstitute the solution, dissolve the powder and then, just before administration, further dilute the solution to a final volume of 500–1,000 ml with 5% dextrose injection USP or 5% sodium chloride injection USP (with or without 5% dextrose); Ringer's and lactated Ringer's injection USP may also be used, but other diluents containing calcium should not in order to avoid formation of a precipitate. Use the reconstituted solution within 24 h. Prolonged IV administration may cause thrombophlebitis. Avoid rapid administration.
Timing of oral administration	May be administered with food or milk, if desired

WARNINGS/PRECAUTIONS

Patients with renal impairment	Usual doses may lead to excessive drug accumulation and possible hepatic toxicity. If impairment is significant, azotemia, hyperphosphatemia, and acidosis may occur due to antianabolic action of drug. Reduce dosage by lowering individual doses and/or lengthening interval between doses, monitor kidney and liver function both before and during therapy, and follow serum tetracycline levels periodically (particularly if therapy is prolonged).

MINOCIN ■ MYSTECLIN-F

Pregnant and postpartum patients with pyelonephritis	Potentially fatal hepatic failure may occur with parenteral administration; do not allow serum level to exceed 15 μg/ml, monitor liver function frequently, and avoid concomitant use of other potentially hepatotoxic drugs
Superinfection	Overgrowth of nonsusceptible organisms, including fungi, may occur
Suspected syphilitic lesions	If syphilis is suspected, perform a dark-field examination before instituting therapy and monthly serology tests for at least 4 mo therafter
Long-term therapy	Perform hemapoietic, renal, and hepatic studies periodically
Photosensitivity (exaggerated sunburn)	May occur; caution patients likely to be exposed to direct sunlight or UV light and discontinue use of minocycline at first sign of skin erythema
Light-headedness, dizziness, and/or vertigo	May occur; caution patients about driving or engaging in other potentially hazardous activities requiring mental alertness or physical coordination. CNS symptoms may disappear during treatment and usually disappear rapidly upon discontinuation of therapy.
Thrombophlebitis	May result from prolonged IV administration; switch to oral form as soon as possible

ADVERSE REACTIONS

Gastrointestinal	Anorexia, nausea, vomiting, diarrhea, glossitis, dysphagia, enterocolitis, inflammatory lesions (with monilial overgrowth) in the anogenital region, increase in liver enzyme levels; hepatitis (rare)
Dermatological	Maculopapular and erythematous rashes, exfoliative dermatitis (rare), photosensitivity (rare), pigmentation of skin and mucous membranes
Hypersensitivity	Urticaria, angioneurotic edema, anaphylaxis, anaphylactoid purpura, pericarditis, exacerbation of systemic lupus erythematosus; pulmonary infiltrates with eosinophilia (rare)
Hematological	Hemolytic anemia, thrombocytopenia, neutropenia, eosinophilia
Central nervous system	Light-headedness, dizziness, vertigo; pseudotumor cerebri (rare)
Other	Microscopic discoloration of thyroid glands, bulging fontanels in infants

OVERDOSAGE

Signs and symptoms	See ADVERSE REACTIONS
Treatment	Discontinue medication; treat symptomatically and institute supportive measures, as required

DRUG INTERACTIONS

Oral anticoagulants	△ Prothrombin time
Penicillin	▽ Bactericidal activity of penicillin; avoid concomitant use
Antacids, sodium bicarbonate, iron supplements	▽ Absorption of minocycline; antacids containing aluminum, calcium, or magnesium should not be administered concomitantly
Methoxyflurane	△ Risk of nephrotoxicity

ALTERED LABORATORY VALUES

Blood/serum values	△ Alkaline phosphatase △ BUN △ Amylase △ Bilirubin △ SGOT △ SGPT ▽ Prothrombin activity
Urinary values	△ Catecholamines (with Hingerty fluorometric method)

USE IN CHILDREN

Not recommended for use during infancy through 8 yr of age unless other drugs are not likely to be effective or are contraindicated; use in this age group may cause permanent discoloration of teeth or enamel hypoplasia. A reversible decrease in fibula growth rate has been observed in premature infants given oral tetracycline (100 mg/kg/day).

USE IN PREGNANT AND NURSING WOMEN

Use during latter half of pregnancy (fetal tooth development) may cause permanent discoloration of teeth or enamel hypoplasia. Animal studies indicate that tetracyclines cross the placental barrier, are found in fetal tissues, and can cause both embryotoxicity and fetal toxicity, including retardation of skeletal development. Tetracyclines are excreted in breast milk; if drug is essential, patient should not nurse.

---

[1] Contains 5% alcohol
[2] Tetracyclines should not be used for streptococcal disease unless bacterial susceptibility has been demonstrated
[3] Tetracyclines are not the drug of choice for treating any staphylococcal infection

---

TETRACYCLINES

MYSTECLIN-F (tetracycline and amphotericin B) Squibb   Rx

Capsules: tetracycline equivalent to 250 mg tetracycline hydrochloride and 50 mg amphotericin B   **Syrup (per 5 ml):** tetracycline equivalent to 125 mg tetracycline hydrochloride and 25 mg amphotericin B (240 ml) *fruit-flavored*

INDICATIONS

Infections caused by susceptible Gram-positive and Gram-negative bacteria, spirochetes, lympho-granuloma-psittacosis-trachoma viruses, rickettsiae, and *Entamoeba histolytica* in patients susceptible to candidal overgrowth[2]

ORAL DOSAGE[1]

Adult: 250 mg qid; for severe infections, 500 mg qid
Child (> 8 yr): 10–20 mg/lb/day, given in divided doses, or 2.5 ml (½ tsp)/20 lb (up to 80 lb) qid

MYSTECLIN-F

Acne vulgaris (adjunctive therapy)[2]	**Adult:** 1 g/day, given in divided doses, to start, followed by 125–500 mg/day after 1 wk; alternate-day or intermittent therapy may be adequate in some patients for maintenance

CONTRAINDICATIONS

Hypersensitivity to tetracyclines or amphotericin B

ADMINISTRATION/DOSAGE ADJUSTMENTS

Duration of treatment	Continue treatment of most common infections for 24–48 h after symptoms and fever subside; streptococcal infections should be treated for a full 10 days to prevent rheumatic fever and glomerulonephritis. Staphylococcal infections may require prolonged high-dose therapy.
Timing of oral administration	Food and some dairy products interfere with absorption; give 1 h before or 2 h after meals. In treating infants, administer syrup 1 h before feeding; do not add to milk formulas or other food containing calcium.

WARNINGS/PRECAUTIONS

Renal impairment	Usual doses may lead to excessive accumulation and possible liver toxicity; reduce dosage and follow serum tetracycline levels periodically (particularly if therapy is prolonged)
Superinfection	Overgrowth of nonsusceptible organisms, including fungi, may occur
Long-term therapy	Perform hemopoietic, renal, and hepatic studies periodically
Photosensitivity (exaggerated sunburn)	May occur; caution patients with a history of photosensitivity and discontinue use of the drug at first sign of skin discomfort
Sensitivity reactions	Are more likely to occur in patients with a history of allergy, asthma, hay fever, or urticaria; use with caution and discontinue use of drug if an allergic or idiosyncratic reaction occurs. Cross-sensitivity among tetracyclines is common.
Suspected syphilitic lesions	If syphilis is suspected, perform a dark-field examination before instituting therapy and perform monthly serology tests for at least 3 mo thereafter

ADVERSE REACTIONS

Gastrointestinal	Anorexia, epigastric distress, nausea, vomiting, diarrhea, bulky loose stools, glossitis, stomatitis, dysphagia, enterocolitis, proctitis, pruritus ani, peptic ulcer, bleeding, hepatic cholestasis, black hairy tongue
Dermatological	Maculopapular and erythematous rashes, exfoliative dermatitis (rare), photosensitivity (rare), onycholysis, nail discoloration
Hypersensitivity	Urticaria, serum sickness-like reactions (fever, rash, arthralgia), angioneurotic edema, anaphylactoid shock
Hematological	Hemolytic anemia, thrombocytopenic purpura, neutropenia, eosinophilia
Other	Sore throat, hoarseness, increased intracranial pressure with bulging fontanels (in infants)

OVERDOSAGE

Signs and symptoms	See ADVERSE REACTIONS
Treatment	Discontinue medication, treat symptomatically, and institute supportive measures, as required

DRUG INTERACTIONS

Oral anticoagulants	⇧ Prothrombin time
Penicillin	⇩ Bactericidal activity of penicillin
Antacids, sodium bicarbonate, iron supplements	⇩ Absorption of tetracycline component
Methoxyflurane	⇧ Risk of nephrotoxicity
Digitalis	⇧ Digitalis toxicity secondary to hypokalemia
Urinary alkalizers	⇧ Excretion of amphotericin B component

ALTERED LABORATORY VALUES

Blood/serum values	⇧ Alkaline phosphatase ⇧ BUN ⇧ Amylase ⇧ Bilirubin ⇧ SGOT ⇧ SGPT ⇩ Prothrombin activity
Urinary values	⇧ Catecholamines (with Hingerty fluorometric method) ⇧ Nitrogen ⇧ Sodium

USE IN CHILDREN

Not recommended for use during infancy through 8 yr of age unless other drugs are not likely to be effective or are contraindicated; use in this age group may cause permanent discoloration of teeth or enamel hypoplasia

USE IN PREGNANT AND NURSING WOMEN

Use during latter half of pregnancy (fetal tooth development) may cause permanent discoloration of teeth or enamel hypoplasia. Consult manufacturer for use in nursing mothers.

[1] Dosage based on tetracycline content of capsules or syrup
[2] Ineffective as a fixed combination

TETRACYCLINES

SUMYCIN (tetracycline hydrochloride) Squibb   Rx

Capsules: 250, 500 mg **Tablets:** 250, 500 mg **Syrup (per 5 ml):** 125 mg (2, 16 fl oz) *fruit-flavored*

INDICATIONS

Gram-negative bacterial infections caused by *Hemophilus ducreyi* (chancroid), *Calymmatobacterium granulomatis* (granuloma inguinale), *Yersinia pestis* (plague), *Francisella tularensis* (tularemia), *Bartonella bacilliformis* (bartonellosis), *Bacteroides*, *Vibrio cholerae* (cholera), and *Campylobacter fetus* (vibriosis), as well as susceptible strains of *Escherichia coli*, *Enterobacter aerogenes*, *Shigella*, *Acinetobacter*, *Hemophilus influenzae* (respiratory tract infections only), and *Klebsiella* (respiratory and urinary tract infections only)
Mycoplasmal pneumonia (primary atypical pneumonia)
Streptococcal infections caused by susceptible strains[1]
Skin and soft tissue infections caused by susceptible strains of *Staphylococcus aureus*[2]
Rickettsial infections
Psittacosis (ornithosis)
Lymphogranuloma venereum, trachoma, inclusion conjunctivitis, and uncomplicated adult **urethral, endocervical,** and **rectal infections** caused by *Chlamydia trachomatis*
Relapsing fever
As an adjunct to amebicides for **acute intestinal amebiasis**
As an alternative to penicillin for **gonococcal** and **clostridial infections, listeriosis, yaws, anthrax, Vincent's infection,** and **actinomycosis**

Syphilis in cases where penicillin is contraindicated

Brucellosis

Severe acne (adjunctive therapy)

ORAL DOSAGE

Adult: for mild to moderate infections, 500 mg bid or 250 mg qid; for severe infections, higher dosages (eg, 500 mg qid) may be needed; for acute gonococcal infections, 1.5 g to start, followed by 500 mg qid, for a total of 9 g; for chlamydial urethral, endocervical, and rectal infections, 500 mg qid for at least 7 days
Child (> 8 yr): 25–50 mg/kg/day, given in 4 equally divided doses

Adult: 30–40 g total, given in equally divided doses over a period of 10–15 days

Adult: 500 mg qid for 3 wk (with 1 g streptomycin IM bid 1st wk and once daily 2nd wk)

Adult: 1 g/day, given in divided doses, to start, followed, when improvement is noted, by 125–500 mg/day; in some cases, alternate-day or intermittent therapy may be possible for maintenance

CONTRAINDICATIONS

Hypersensitivity to tetracyclines

ADMINISTRATION/DOSAGE ADJUSTMENTS

Duration of treatment — Unless otherwise indicated, continue treatment for at least 24–48 h after symptoms and fever have subsided; infections caused by Group A beta-hemolytic streptococci should be treated for at least 10 days

SUMYCIN

Timing of oral administration	Food and some dairy products interfere with absorption; give 1 h before or 2 h after meals. In treating infants, administer syrup 1 h before feeding; do not add to milk formulas

WARNINGS/PRECAUTIONS

Patients with renal impairment	Usual doses may lead to excessive drug accumulation and possible hepatic toxicity. If impairment is significant, azotemia, hyperphosphatemia, and acidosis may occur due to antianabolic action of drug. Reduce dosage by lowering individual doses and/or lengthening interval between doses and follow serum tetracycline levels periodically (particularly if therapy is prolonged).
Superinfection	Overgrowth of nonsusceptible organisms, including fungi, may occur
Suspected syphilitic lesions	If syphilis is suspected, perform a dark-field examination before instituting therapy and monthly serology tests for at least 4 mo thereafter
Long-term therapy	Perform hemapoietic, renal, and hepatic studies periodically
Photosensitivity (exaggerated sunburn)	May occur; caution patients likely to be exposed to direct sunlight or UV light and discontinue use of tetracycline at first sign of skin erythema
Sensitivity reactions	Are more likely to occur in patients with a history of allergy, asthma, hay fever, or urticaria; use with caution

ADVERSE REACTIONS

Gastrointestinal	Anorexia, nausea, vomiting, diarrhea, glossitis, black hairy tongue, dysphagia, enterocolitis, inflammatory lesions (with candidal overgrowth) in the anogenital region, epigastric distress, bulky loose stools, stomatitis, sore throat, hoarseness, hepatic cholestasis
Dermatological	Maculopapular and erythematous rashes, exfoliative dermatitis (rare), photosensitivity, onycholysis and nail discoloration (rare)
Hypersensitivity	Urticaria, angioneurotic edema, anaphylaxis, anaphylactoid purpura, pericarditis, exacerbation of systemic lupus erythematosus, serum sickness-like reactions (fever, rash, arthralgia)
Hematological	Hemolytic anemia, thrombocytopenia, neutropenia, eosinophilia, anemia, thrombocytopenic purpura
Central nervous system	Dizziness, headache
Other	Microscopic discoloration of thyroid glands, bulging fontanels in infants

OVERDOSAGE

Signs and symptoms	See ADVERSE REACTIONS
Treatment	Discontinue medication; treat symptomatically and institute supportive measures, as required

DRUG INTERACTIONS

Oral anticoagulants	△ Prothrombin time
Penicillin	▽ Bactericidal activity of penicillin; avoid concomitant use
Antacids, sodium bicarbonate, iron supplements	▽ Absorption of tetracycline; antacids containing aluminum, calcium, or magnesium should not be administered concomitantly
Methoxyflurane	△ Risk of nephrotoxicity

ALTERED LABORATORY VALUES

Blood/serum values	△ Alkaline phosphatase △ BUN △ Amylase △ Bilirubin △ SGOT △ SGPT ▽ Prothrombin activity
Urinary values	△ Catecholamines (with Hingerty fluorometric method)

USE IN CHILDREN

Not recommended for use during infancy through 8 yr of age unless other drugs are not likely to be effective or are contraindicated; use in this age group may cause permanent discoloration of teeth or enamel hypoplasia. A reversible decrease in fibula growth rate has been observed in premature infants given oral tetracycline (100 mg/kg/day)

USE IN PREGNANT AND NURSING WOMEN

Use during latter half of pregnancy (fetal tooth development) may cause permanent discoloration of teeth or enamel hypoplasia. Animal studies indicate that tetracyclines cross the placental barrier, are found in fetal tissues, and can cause both embryotoxicity and fetal toxicity, including retardation of skeletal development. Tetracyclines are excreted in breast milk; if drug is essential, patient should not nurse.

---

[1] Tetracyclines should not be used for streptococcal disease unless bacterial susceptibility has been demonstrated
[2] Tetracyclines are not the drug of choice for treating any staphylococcal infection

TERRAMYCIN

TETRACYCLINES

TERRAMYCIN (oxytetracycline hydrochloride) Pfizer Rx
Capsules: 250 mg

TERRAMYCIN Intramuscular Solution (oxytetracycline) Roerig Rx
Ampuls: 50, 125 mg/ml (2 ml) **Vials:** 50 mg/ml (2 ml)

TERRAMYCIN Intravenous (oxytetracycline hydrochloride) Roerig Rx
Vials: 500 mg

INDICATIONS

Gram-negative bacterial infections caused by *Hemophilus ducreyi* (chancroid), *Calymmatobacterium granulomatis* (granuloma inguinale), *Yersinia pestis* (plague), *Francisella tularensis* (tularemia), *Bartonella bacilliformis* (bartonellosis), *Bacteroides*, *Vibrio cholerae* (cholera), and *Campylobacter fetus* (vibriosis), as well as susceptible strains of *Escherichia coli*, *Enterobacter aerogenes*, *Shigella*, *Acinetobacter*, *Hemophilus influenzae* (respiratory tract infections only), and *Klebsiella* (respiratory and urinary tract infections only)

Mycoplasmal pneumonia (primary atypical pneumonia)

Streptococcal infections caused by susceptible strains[1]

Skin and soft tissue infections caused by susceptible strains of *Staphylococcus aureus*[2]

Rickettsial infections

Psittacosis (ornithosis)

Lymphogranuloma venereum, trachoma, and (when given orally) **inclusion conjunctivitis**

Relapsing fever

As an adjunct to amebicides for **acute intestinal amebiasis**

As an alternative to penicillin for **gonococcal and clostridial infections, listeriosis, yaws, anthrax, Vincent's infection,** and **actinomycosis**

Severe acne (oral therapy only)

Syphilis in cases where penicillin is contraindicated

Brucellosis

ORAL DOSAGE

Adult: 1–2 g/day, depending on severity, given in 4 equally divided doses; for uncomplicated gonorrhea, 1.5 g to start, followed by 500 mg qid, for a total of 9 g

Child (> 8 yr): 25–50 mg/kg/day, given in 4 equally divided doses

Adult: 30–40 g total, given in equally divided doses over a period of 10–15 days

Adult: 500 mg qid for 3 wk (with 1 g streptomycin IM bid 1st wk and once daily 2nd wk)

PARENTERAL DOSAGE

Adult: for IM use, 250 mg once daily, 150 mg q12h, or 100 mg q8h; for IV use, 250–500 mg q12h or, if necessary, up to 500 mg q6h

Child (> 8 yr): for IM use, 15–25 mg/kg/day, up to 250 mg/day, given once daily or in 2–3 divided doses; for IV use, 10–20 mg/kg/day, given in 2 divided doses (usual dosage: 12 mg/kg/day)

CONTRAINDICATIONS
Hypersensitivity to tetracyclines

ADMINISTRATION/DOSAGE ADJUSTMENTS

Duration of treatment	Unless otherwise indicated, continue treatment for at least 24–48 h after symptoms and fever have subsided; infections caused by Group A beta-hemolytic streptococci should be treated for at least 10 days. If patient is started on parenteral therapy, institute oral therapy as soon as possible.
Intravenous administration	Reconstitute solution with 10 ml of sterile water for injection USP or 5% dextrose injection USP; dilute solution to a final volume of at least 100 ml using 5% dextrose injection USP, 0.9% sodium chloride injection, or Ringer's injection. Inject each dose directly into the vein; avoid rapid or extravascular injection. Bear in mind that prolonged IV therapy may result in thrombophlebitis.
Intramuscular administration	Reserve for situations in which oral therapy is not feasible; IM administration produces lower blood levels than oral administration at recommended dosages. To help avoid inadvertent vascular injection, aspirate syringe before administration. Inject deeply into a relatively large muscle, preferably a midlateral thigh muscle for children and either that muscle or the gluteus maximus for adults. To minimize the possibility of sciatic nerve damage, use the periphery of the gluteus maximus for infants and small children only if necessary (eg, for patients with burns). The deltoid area should be used only if is well developed and only if caution is exercised to avoid radial nerve injury; injections should not be made into the lower or middle third of the upper arm.

TERRAMYCIN

Timing of oral administration	Food and some dairy products interfere with absorption; give capsules 1 h before or 2 h after meals
Fluid intake	Caution patient to take adequate amounts of fluid with capsules to minimize risk of esophageal irritation and ulceration

WARNINGS/PRECAUTIONS

Hepatotoxicity	Oxytetracycline may accumulate as a result of renal dysfunction or intensive IV therapy and potentially lead to liver damage. When using in patients with renal impairment, reduce the dose or increase the dosing interval; if therapy is prolonged in these patients, monitoring of the serum drug level may be advisable. The risk of hepatotoxicity becomes particularly significant when this drug is given parenterally to women who have pyelonephritis during pregnancy or after birth. If this drug is administered parenterally to these women, test liver function frequently, monitor serum drug level, and reduce dosage; make sure that the serum drug level does not exceed 15 μg/ml. High-dose IV therapy can also cause hepatotoxicity, particularly in pregnant women and patients with renal or hepatic impairment; IV administration of more than 2 g/day has caused fatal liver failure in patients with renal impairment, especially during pregnancy. Before and during intensive IV therapy, monitor the serum drug level and perform renal and liver function texts. Avoid concomitant use of other potentially hepatotoxic drugs during intensive IV therapy and when renal function is impaired.
Renal effects	Tetracyclines can produce an increase in the BUN level; in patients with significant renal impairment, they can precipitate azotemia, hyperphosphatemia, and acidosis at higher serum drug levels
Superinfection	Overgrowth of nonsusceptible organisms, including fungi, may occur
Suspected syphilitic lesions	If syphilis is suspected, perform a dark-field examination before instituting therapy and monthly serology tests for at least 4 mo thereafter
Long-term therapy	Perform hemapoietic, renal, and hepatic studies periodically
Photosensitivity (exaggerated sunburn)	May occur; caution patients likely to be exposed to direct sunlight or UV light and discontinue use of oxytetracycline at first sign of skin erythema

ADVERSE REACTIONS

Gastrointestinal	Anorexia, nausea, vomiting, diarrhea, glossitis, dysphagia, enterocolitis, inflammatory lesions (with monilial overgrowth) in the anogenital region, esophageal irritation or ulceration (capsule form only; rare)
Dermatological	Maculopapular and erythematous rashes, exfoliative dermatitis (rare), photosensitivity
Hypersensitivity	Urticaria, angioneurotic edema, anaphylaxis, anaphylactoid purpura, pericarditis, exacerbation of systemic lupus erythematosus
Hematological	Hemolytic anemia, thrombocytopenia, neutropenia, eosinophilia
Other	Microscopic discoloration of thyroid glands, bulging fontanels in infants, benign intracranial hypertension in adults, local irritation after IM injection

OVERDOSAGE

Signs and symptoms	See ADVERSE REACTIONS
Treatment	Discontinue medication; treat symptomatically and institute supportive measures, as required

DRUG INTERACTIONS

Oral anticoagulants	△ Prothrombin time
Penicillin	▽ Bactericidal activity of penicillin; avoid concomitant use
Antacids, sodium bicarbonate, iron supplements	▽ Absorption of oral oxytetracycline; antacids containing aluminum, calcium, or magnesium should not be administered concomitantly
Methoxyflurane	△ Risk of nephrotoxicity

ALTERED LABORATORY VALUES

Blood/serum values	△ Alkaline phosphatase △ BUN △ Amylase △ Bilirubin △ SGOT △ SGPT ▽ Prothrombin activity
Urinary values	△ Catecholamines (with Hingerty fluorometric method)

USE IN CHILDREN

Not recommended for use during infancy through 8 yr of age unless other drugs are not likely to be effective or are contraindicated; use in this age group may cause permanent discoloration of teeth enamel hypoplasia. A reversible decrease in fibula growth rate has been observed in premature infants given oral tetracycline (100 mg/kg/day).

USE IN PREGNANT AND NURSING WOMEN

Use during latter half of pregnancy (fetal tooth development) may cause permanent discoloration of teeth or enamel hypoplasia. Animal studies indicate that tetracyclines cross the placental barrier, are found in fetal tissues, and can cause both embryotoxicity and fetal toxicity, including retardation of skeletal development. Tetracyclines are excreted in breast milk; if drug is essential, patient should not nurse.

---

[1] Tetracyclines should not be used for streptococcal disease unless bacterial susceptibility has been demonstrated
[2] Tetracyclines are not the drug of choice for treating any staphylococcal infection

COMPENDIUM OF DRUG THERAPY

VIBRAMYCIN/VIBRA-TABS

TETRACYCLINES

VIBRAMYCIN (doxycycline) Pfizer — Rx

Capsules: doxycycline hyclate equivalent to 50 and 100 mg doxycycline **Syrup (per 5 ml):** doxycycline calcium equivalent to 50 mg doxycycline (1, 16 fl oz) *raspberry/apple flavored* **Suspension (per 5 ml):** doxycycline monohydrate equivalent to 25 mg doxycycline after reconstitution (2 fl oz) *raspberry flavored*

VIBRAMYCIN Intravenous (doxycycline hyclate) Roerig — Rx

Vials: doxycycline hyclate equivalent to 100 and 200 mg doxycycline (for IV use only)

VIBRA-TABS (doxycycline hyclate) Pfizer — Rx

Tablets: doxycycline hyclate equivalent to 100 mg doxycycline

INDICATIONS

Gram-negative bacterial infections caused by *Hemophilus ducreyi* (chancroid), *Calymmatobacterium granulomatis* (granuloma inguinale), *Yersinia pestis* (plague), *Francisella tularensis* (tularemia), *Bartonella bacilliformis* (bartonellosis), *Bacteroides*, *Brucella* (when combined with streptomycin), *Vibrio cholerae* (cholera), and *Campylobacter fetus* (vibriosis), as well as susceptible strains of *Escherichia coli*, *Enterobacter aerogenes*, *Shigella*, *Acinetobacter*, *Hemophilus influenzae* (respiratory tract infections only), and *Klebsiella* (respiratory and urinary tract infections only)
Mycoplasmal pneumonia (primary atypical pneumonia)
Streptococcal infections caused by susceptible strains[1]
Respiratory, skin, and soft tissue infections caused by susceptible strains of *Staphylococcus aureus*[2]
Rickettsial infections
Psittacosis (ornithosis)
Acute epididymo-orchitis and uncomplicated **gonorrhea** in adults (except for anorectal infection in men) caused by *Neisseria gonorrhoeae* (oral therapy only)
Lymphogranuloma venereum, **trachoma**, and (when given orally) **inclusion conjunctivitis**, acute **epididymo-orchitis**, and uncomplicated adult **urethral, endocervical, and rectal infections** caused by *Chlamydia trachomatis* **Nongonococcal urethritis** caused by *Ureaplasma urealyticum* (oral therapy only)
Relapsing fever
As an adjunct to amebicides for **acute intestinal amebiasis**
As an alternative to penicillin for **clostridial infections, listeriosis, yaws, anthrax, Vincent's infection, actinomycosis,** and (when given IV) **meningococcal and gonococcal infections**
Severe acne (oral therapy only)

Primary and secondary syphilis when penicillin is contraindicated

ORAL DOSAGE

Adult: 200 mg to start, given in 2 divided doses 12 h apart, followed by 100 mg once daily or 50 mg q12h (for more severe infections, especially chronic urinary tract infections, give 100 mg q12h); for uncomplicated gonococcal infections, 100 mg bid for 7 days (or give 2 doses of 300 mg each 1 h apart); for acute epididymo-orchitis, 100 mg bid for at least 10 days; for nongonococcal urethritis and for chlamydial urethral, endocervical, and rectal infections, 100 mg bid for at least 7 days

Child (> 8 yr and ≤ 100 lb): 2 mg/lb to start, given in 2 divided doses 12 h apart, followed by 1–2 mg/lb/day, depending on severity, given in single or 2 divided daily doses

Child (> 8 yr and > 100 lb): same as adult

Adult: 300 mg/day, given in divided doses for at least 10 days

PARENTERAL DOSAGE

Adult: 200 mg IV the first day, given in 1 or 2 infusions, followed by 100–200 mg/day, depending on severity, with dosages of 200 mg/day given in 1 or 2 infusions

Child (> 8 yr and ≤ 100 lb): 2 mg/lb IV to start, given in 1 or 2 infusions the first day, followed by 1–2 mg/lb/day, depending on severity and given in 1 or 2 infusions

Child (> 8 yr and > 100 lb): same as adult

Adult: 300 mg/day IV for at least 10 days

CONTRAINDICATIONS

Hypersensitivity to tetracyclines

ADMINISTRATION/DOSAGE ADJUSTMENTS

Duration of treatment — Unless otherwise indicated, continue treatment for at least 24–48 h after symptoms and fever have subsided; infections caused by Group A beta-hemolytic streptococci should be treated for at least 10 days. If patient is started on parenteral therapy, institute oral therapy as soon as possible.

VIBRAMYCIN/VIBRA-TABS

Preparation of IV solution	Reconstitute solution with sterile water for injection or other suitable diluents (see below); add 10 ml to the 100-mg vial or 20 ml to the 200-mg vial. Then, withdraw the entire solution from the vial and dilute with sodium chloride injection USP, 5% dextrose injection USP, 10% invert sugar in water, Ringer's injection USP, lactated Ringer's injection USP, 5% dextrose in lactated Ringer's injection, Normosol-M or -R in D5-W, or Plasma-Lyte 56 or 148 in 5% dextrose; add 100–1,000 ml to the 100-mg solution and 200–2,000 ml to the 200-mg solution (recommended final concentration range: 0.1–1 mg/ml). After reconstitution, use solutions containing lactated Ringer's injection within 6 h, solutions containing sodium chloride injection USP or 5% dextrose injection USP within 48 h, and other solutions within 12 h. Solutions with diluents other than lactated Ringer's injection can be refrigerated, if protected from light, for up to 72 h; these preparations must be used within 12 h after refrigeration.
Intravenous administration	Reserve for situations in which oral therapy is not feasible. Prolonged IV administration may cause thrombophlebitis. Avoid rapid administration and inadvertent extravascular injection; the usual duration of infusion varies from 1 to 4 h. Protect solution from direct sunlight during infusion.
Oral administration	If gastric irritation occurs, administer with milk or solid food. Caution patient to take adequate amounts of fluid with capsules or tablets to minimize risk of esophageal irritation or ulceration.

WARNINGS/PRECAUTIONS

Superinfection	Overgrowth of nonsusceptible organisms, including fungi, may occur; if superinfection occurs, discontinue drug
Suspected syphilitic lesions	If syphilis is suspected, perform a dark-field examination before instituting therapy and monthly serology tests for at least 4 mo thereafter
Long-term therapy	Perform hemapoietic, renal, and hepatic studies periodically
Photosensitivity (exaggerated sunburn)	May occur; caution patients likely to be exposed to direct sunlight or UV light and discontinue use of doxycycline at first sign of skin erythema
Elevated BUN level	Although tetracyclines in general can cause an increase in the BUN level, this effect has not been detected in studies to date in patients with renal impairment who received doxycycline

ADVERSE REACTIONS

Gastrointestinal	Anorexia, nausea, vomiting, diarrhea, glossitis, dysphagia, enterocolitis, inflammatory lesions (with monilial overgrowth) in the anogenital region; esophagitis and esophageal ulceration (with capsule and tablet forms; rare)
Dermatological	Maculopapular and erythematous rashes, exfoliative dermatitis (rare), photosensitivity
Hypersensitivity	Urticaria, angioneurotic edema, anaphylaxis, anaphylactoid purpura, pericarditis, exacerbation of systemic lupus erythematosus
Hematological	Hemolytic anemia, thrombocytopenia, neutropenia, eosinophilia
Other	Microscopic discoloration of thyroid glands (with prolonged use), bulging fontanels in infants, benign intracranial hypertension

OVERDOSAGE

Signs and symptoms	See ADVERSE REACTIONS
Treatment	Discontinue medication, treat symptomatically, and institute supportive measures, as required

DRUG INTERACTIONS

Oral anticoagulants	△ Prothrombin time
Penicillin	▽ Bactericidal activity of penicillin; avoid concomitant use
Antacids, sodium bicarbonate, iron supplements	▽ Absorption of oral doxycycline; do not give concomitantly

ALTERED LABORATORY VALUES

Blood/serum values	▽ Prothrombin activity
Urinary values	△ Catecholamines (with Hingerty fluorometric method)

USE IN CHILDREN

Not recommended for use during infancy through 8 yr of age unless other drugs are not likely to be effective or are contraindicated; use in this age group may cause permanent discoloration of teeth or enamel hypoplasia. A reversible decrease in fibula growth rate has been observed in premature infants given oral tetracycline (100 mg/kg/day).

USE IN PREGNANT AND NURSING WOMEN

Use during latter half of pregnancy (fetal tooth development) may cause permanent discoloration of teeth or enamel hypoplasia. Animal studies indicate that tetracyclines cross the placental barrier, are found in fetal tissues, and can cause both embryotoxicity and fetal toxicity, including retardation of skeletal development. Tetracyclines are excreted in breast milk; if drug is essential, patient should not nurse.

---

[1] Tetracyclines should not be used for streptococcal disease unless bacterial susceptibility has been demonstrated
[2] Tetracyclines are not the drug of choice for treating any staphylococcal infection

Chapter 26

Antimigraine Agents

CAFERGOT (Sandoz Pharmaceuticals) 1049
Ergotamine tartrate and caffeine Rx

CAFERGOT P-B (Sandoz Pharmaceuticals) 1049
Ergotamine tartrate, caffeine, belladonna alkaloids,
and pentobarbital Rx

INDERAL (Ayerst) 1050
Propranolol hydrochloride Rx

INDERAL LA (Ayerst) 1053
Propranolol hydrochloride Rx

MIDRIN (Carnrick) 1054
Isometheptene mucate, dichloralphenazone, and
acetaminophen Rx

SANSERT (Sandoz Pharmaceuticals) 1055
Methysergide maleate Rx

WIGRAINE (Organon) 1056
Ergotamine tartrate and caffeine Rx

Other Antimigraine Agents 1048

D.H.E. 45 (Sandoz Pharmaceuticals) 1048
Dihydroergotamine mesylate Rx

ERGOSTAT (Parke-Davis) 1048
Ergotamine tartrate Rx

MEDIHALER ERGOTAMINE (Riker) 1048
Ergotamine tartrate Rx

OTHER ANTIMIGRAINE AGENTS

DRUG	HOW SUPPLIED	USUAL DOSAGE[1]
D.H.E. 45 (Sandoz Pharmaceuticals) Dihydroergotamine mesylate Rx	**Ampuls:** 1 mg/ml (1 ml)	Adult: 1 mg IM or IV at first sign of attack, followed by 1 mg qh, up to 3 mg IM or 2 mg IV, if needed; do not exceed 6 mg/wk
ERGOSTAT (Parke-Davis) Ergotamine tartrate Rx	**Sublingual tablets:** 2 mg	Adult: 2 mg at first sign of attack or as soon as possible thereafter, followed by 2 mg at 30-min intervals, up to a total of 6 mg, if needed; do not exceed 6 mg/24 h or 10 mg/wk
MEDIHALER ERGOTAMINE (Riker) Ergotamine tartrate Rx	**Metered-dose oral inhaler:** 0.36 mg/inhalation (2.5 ml)	Adult: 1 inhalation at first sign of attack, repeated, if necessary, after 5 min; maximum dose: 6 inhalations/24 h or 15 inhalations/wk (allow at least 5 min between inhalations)

[1] Where pediatric dosages are not given, consult manufacturer

ANTIMIGRAINE AGENTS

CAFERGOT (ergotamine tartrate and caffeine) Sandoz Pharmaceuticals Rx

Tablets: 1 mg ergotamine tartrate and 100 mg caffeine **Suppositories:** 2 mg ergotamine tartrate and 100 mg caffeine

INDICATIONS
Vascular headache, including migraine, migraine variants, and histaminic cephalalgia

ORAL DOSAGE
Adult: 2 tabs at once, followed by 1 tab q^1/$_2$h, if needed, up to 6 tabs per attack or 10 per week

RECTAL DOSAGE
Adult: 1 suppository at once, followed by a second suppository 1 h later, if needed, up to 2 suppositories per attack or 5 per week

CONTRAINDICATIONS

Pregnancy	Hypertension	Hypersensitivity to ergotamine tartrate or caffeine
Peripheral vascular disease	Impaired hepatic or renal function	
Coronary heart disease	Sepsis	

ADMINISTRATION/DOSAGE ADJUSTMENTS

Excessive nausea, vomiting	If oral medication is not tolerated, use suppositories
Short-term prevention	Administer at bedtime, within recommended dosage limits; only for carefully selected patients

WARNINGS/PRECAUTIONS

Ergotism	Although rare, signs and symptoms of ergotism may develop, especially with long-term use at relatively high doses; caution patient not to exceed recommended dosage limits

ADVERSE REACTIONS

Cardiovascular	Vasoconstrictive complications (eg, loss of pulse, weakness, muscle pains and paresthesias of the extremities, and precordial distress and pain), transient tachycardia or bradycardia
Gastrointestinal	Nausea, vomiting
Dermatological	Pruritus
Other	Localized edema

OVERDOSAGE

Signs and symptoms	*Ergotamine-related effects:* vomiting, numbness, tingling, pain and cyanosis of extremities with diminished or absent peripheral pulses, hypertension or hypotension, drowsiness, stupor, coma, convulsions, shock; *caffeine-related effects:* insomnia, restlessness, tremors, delirium, tachycardia, extrasystoles
Treatment	Induce emesis or perform gastric lavage to empty stomach, and administer a cathartic. Maintain adequate pulmonary ventilation, correct hypotension, and control convulsions. Treat peripheral vasospasm with warmth *(not heat),* and protect ischemic limbs from cold. Use vasodilators cautiously.

DRUG INTERACTIONS
No clinically significant drug interactions have been observed

ALTERED LABORATORY VALUES
No clinically significant alterations in blood/serum or urinary values occur at therapeutic dosages

---

USE IN CHILDREN
Safety for use in children has not been established

USE IN PREGNANT AND NURSING WOMEN
Contraindicated during pregnancy. Not recommended for use in nursing mothers; ergotamine tartrate may cause adverse reactions in nursing infants, including vomiting, diarrhea, weak pulse, and unstable blood pressure.[1]

[1] Illingworth RS: *Practitioner* 171:533, 1953; Knowles JA: *J Pediatr* 66:1068, 1965; Arena JM: *Clin Pediatr* 5:472, 1966; Katz CS, Giacoia GP: *Symp Pediatr Pharmacol* 19:151, 1972

VEHICLE/BASE
Suppositories: tartaric acid and cocoa butter

ANTIMIGRAINE AGENTS

CAFERGOT P-B (ergotamine tartrate, caffeine, belladonna alkaloids, and pentobarbital) Rx
Sandoz Pharmaceuticals

Tablets: 1 mg ergotamine tartrate, 100 mg caffeine, 0.125 mg belladonna alkaloids, and 30 mg sodium pentobarbital
Suppositories: 2 mg ergotamine tartrate, 100 mg caffeine, 0.25 mg belladonna alkaloids, and 60 mg pentobarbital

INDICATIONS
Vascular headache complicated by tension and GI disturbances

ORAL DOSAGE
Adult: 2 tabs at once, followed by 1 tab q^1/$_2$h, if needed, up to 6 tabs per attack or 10 per week

RECTAL DOSAGE
Adult: 1 suppository at once, followed by a second suppository 1 h later, if needed, up to 2 suppositories per attack or 5 per week

CAFERGOT P-B ■ INDERAL

CONTRAINDICATIONS

Pregnancy	Hypertension	Hypersensitivity to ergotamine, caffeine, belladonna alkaloids, or pentobarbital
Peripheral vascular disease	Impaired hepatic or renal function	
Coronary heart disease	Sepsis	

ADMINISTRATION/DOSAGE ADJUSTMENTS

Excessive nausea, vomiting	If oral medication is not tolerated, use suppositories
Short-term prevention	Administer at bedtime, within recommended dosage limits; only for carefully selected patients

WARNINGS/PRECAUTIONS

Ergotism	Although rare, signs and symptoms of ergotism may develop, especially with long-term use at relatively high doses; caution patient not to exceed recommended dosage limits
Drug dependence	Psychic and/or physical dependence and tolerance may develop, especially in addiction-prone individuals

ADVERSE REACTIONS

Cardiovascular	Vasoconstrictive complications (eg, loss of pulse, weakness, muscle pains and paresthesias of the extremities, and precordial distress and pain), transient tachycardia or bradycardia
Gastrointestinal	Nausea, vomiting
Central nervous system	Drowsiness
Dermatological	Pruritus
Other	Localized edema

OVERDOSAGE

Signs and symptoms	*Ergotamine-related effects:* vomiting, numbness, tingling, pain and cyanosis of extremities with diminished or absent peripheral pulses, hypertension or hypotension, drowsiness, stupor, coma, convulsions, shock; *caffeine-related effects:* insomnia, restlessness, tremors, delirium, tachycardia, extrasystoles; *pentobarbital-related effects:* drowsiness, confusion, coma, respiratory depression, hypotension, shock; *belladonna alkaloid-related effects:* dry mouth and throat, blurred vision, urinary retention, CNS excitation, restlessness, confusion, delirium, convulsions, stupor, and coma, leading to death
Treatment	Induce emesis or perform gastric lavage to empty stomach, and administer a cathartic. Maintain adequate pulmonary ventilation, correct hypotension, and control convulsions. Treat peripheral vasospasm with warmth *(not heat)* and protect ischemic limbs from cold. Use vasodilators cautiously.

DRUG INTERACTIONS

Alcohol, tranquilizers, sedative-hypnotics, and other CNS depressants	△ CNS depression
Oral anticoagulants	▽ Prothrombin time
Corticosteroids	▽ Corticosteroid effects
Digitalis, digitoxin	▽ Cardiac glycoside effects
Doxycycline	▽ Anti-infective effect
Griseofulvin	▽ Griseofulvin absorption
Tricyclic antidepressants	▽ Antidepressant effect
MAO inhibitors	△ Antidepressant or barbiturate effects

ALTERED LABORATORY VALUES
No clinically significant alterations in blood/serum or urinary values occur at therapeutic dosages

---

USE IN CHILDREN

Safety for use in children has not been established

USE IN PREGNANT AND NURSING WOMEN

Contraindicated during pregnancy; not recommended for use in nursing mothers; ergotamine tartrate may cause adverse reactions in nursing infants, including vomiting, diarrhea, weak pulse, and unstable blood pressure.[1]

[1] Illingworth RS: *Practitioner* 171:533, 1953; Knowles JA: *J Pediatr* 66:1068, 1965; Arena JM: *Clin Pediatr* 5:472, 1966; Katz CS, Giacoia GP: *Symp Pediatr Pharmacol* 19:151, 1972

VEHICLE/BASE
Suppositories: tartaric acid, malic acid, lactose, and cocoa butter

---

ANTIMIGRAINE AGENTS

INDERAL (propranolol hydrochloride) Ayerst Rx
Tablets: 10, 20, 40, 60, 80, 90 mg Ampuls: 1 mg/ml (1 ml)

INDICATIONS	ORAL DOSAGE
Hypertension	**Adult:** 40 mg bid (alone or with a diuretic) to start, followed by gradual increments until optimal response is achieved, up to 640 mg/day; usual maintenance dosage: 120–240 mg/day
	Child: 0.5 mg/kg bid to start, followed by gradual increments until optimal response is achieved, up to 16 mg/kg/day; usual maintenance dosage: 1–2 mg/kg bid

INDERAL

Long-term management of **angina pectoris**	**Adult:** 80–320 mg/day, given in 2–4 divided doses
Cardiac arrhythmias, including supraventricular arrhythmias, ventricular tachycardias, digitalis-induced tachyarrhythmias, and resistant tachyarrhythmias due to excessive catecholamine activity during anesthesia	**Adult:** 10–30 mg tid or qid, before meals and at bedtime
Reduction of cardiovascular mortality in clinically stable patients following **acute myocardial infarction**	**Adult:** 180–240 mg/day, given in divided doses bid or tid; patients with angina, hypertension, or other coexisting cardiovascular diseases may require dosages exceeding 240 mg/day. In clinical studies, long-term therapy was started 5–21 days after infarction.
Migraine prophylaxis	**Adult:** 80 mg/day in divided doses to start, followed, if necessary, by gradual increments, up to 240 mg/day; usual dosage: 160–240 mg/day. If satisfactory prophylaxis is not obtained after giving 240 mg/day for 4–6 wk, discontinue use.
Familial or hereditary **essential tremor**	**Adult:** 40 mg bid to start, followed, if necessary, by increases in dosage, up to 320 mg/day; usual maintenance dosage: 120 mg/day
Hypertrophic subaortic stenosis	**Adult:** 20–40 mg tid or qid, before meals and at bedtime
As an adjunct to alpha-adrenergic blocking agents in the management of **pheochromocytoma**	**Adult:** 60 mg/day in divided doses for 3 days prior to surgery, concomitantly with an alpha-adrenergic blocking agent, or 30 mg/day in divided doses for inoperable tumors

CONTRAINDICATIONS

Sinus bradycardia	Cardiogenic shock	Overt congestive heart failure, unless it results from a tachyarrhythmia treatable with propranolol
Heart block greater than first degree	Bronchial asthma	

ADMINISTRATION/DOSAGE ADJUSTMENTS

Intravenous use	For life-threatening arrhythmias or those occurring under anesthesia in adults, give 1–3 mg IV. To minimize risk of hypotension and possibility of cardiac standstill, administer slowly ($\leq$ 1 mg/min) and monitor ECG and CVP continuously. Initial dose may be repeated after 2 min; thereafter, wait at least 4 h before administering additional propranolol.
Inadequate control of hypertension	Twice-daily dosing is usually effective. Some patients, however, experience a modest rise in blood pressure toward the end of the 12-h dosing interval, especially when lower dosages are used. If control is inadequate, a larger dose or tid therapy may be indicated.
Discontinuation of therapy	Reduce dosage gradually over a period of several weeks; caution patients who experience angina or who may have occult coronary artery disease not to interrupt or discontinue therapy on their own
Tremor	Essential tremor is usually limited to the upper limbs; it appears only when a limb moves or is held in a fixed position against gravity. Propranolol reduces the intensity of tremors, but not their frequency; this drug is not indicated for treatment of tremor associated with parkinsonism.

WARNINGS/PRECAUTIONS

Cardiac failure	Beta blockade may cause or exacerbate cardiac failure; discontinue use if this disorder does not stabilize after diuretic therapy and digitalization. If necessary, propranolol may be given to patients with well-compensated congestive heart failure; observe such patients closely.
Thyrotoxicosis	Propranolol may mask certain clinical signs of hyperthyroidism; abrupt withdrawal may exacerbate manifestations of this disorder and precipitate a thyroid storm
Patients with angina	Abrupt withdrawal in such patients may exacerbate angina and, in some cases, lead to myocardial infarction; reinstitute therapy if withdrawal reactions occur (see ADMINISTRATION/DOSAGE ADJUSTMENTS)
Patients with Wolff-Parkinson-White (WPW) syndrome	Severe bradycardia, necessitating use of a demand pacemaker, has occurred in several patients with WPW syndrome following use of propranolol
Patients with diabetes	Propranolol may mask tachycardia associated with hypoglycemia; however, this drug may not significantly affect other manifestations such as dizziness and diaphoresis. Propranolol may delay return of normal plasma glucose levels following insulin-induced hypoglycemia. Use with caution in patients with diabetes.
Patients with bronchospastic disease	In general, such patients should not receive propranolol because it may block catecholamine-induced bronchodilation. Propranolol is specifically contraindicated for use in patients with bronchial asthma; use with caution in patients with nonallergic bronchospasm (eg, chronic bronchitis, emphysema).
Patients with renal or hepatic impairment	Use with caution in such patients
Major surgery	The necessity or desirability of discontinuing use before major surgery is controversial. Beta blockade can increase the risks associated with general anesthesia and surgery (because cardiac responsiveness to reflex beta-adrenergic stimuli is impaired) and may cause protracted severe hypotension and difficulty in restarting and maintaining the heartbeat. However, beta-adrenergic agonists (eg, dobutamine, isoproterenol) can reverse the effects of propranolol.

INDERAL

Fatigue, lethargy, vivid dreams	Daily doses exceeding 160 mg, given in divided doses of more than 80 mg, may increase the risk of fatigue, lethargy, and vivid dreams
Glaucoma testing	Propranolol can reduce intraocular pressure and thereby affect the results of glaucoma screening tests
Carcinogenicity	No evidence of tumorigenicity has been seen in rats or mice given up to 150 mg/kg/day for a period of 18 mo
Effect on fertility	No impairment of fertility has been observed in animals

ADVERSE REACTIONS

Cardiovascular	Bradycardia, congestive heart failure, AV-block intensification, hypotension, paresthesia of the hands, Raynaud-type arterial insufficiency, purpura
Central nervous system	Light-headedness, depression, insomnia, weakness, fatigue, lassitude, catatonia, visual disturbances, hallucinations, vivid dreams; an acute reversible syndrome characterized by spatial and temporal disorientation, short-term memory loss, emotional lability, slightly clouded sensorium, and decreased neuropsychometric performance
Gastrointestinal	Nausea, vomiting, epigastric distress, abdominal cramps, diarrhea, constipation, mesenteric arterial thrombosis, ischemic colitis
Respiratory	Bronchospasm
Allergic	Pharyngitis, agranulocytosis, erythematous rash, fever with aching and sore throat, laryngospasm and respiratory distress
Other	Alopecia, lupus erythematosus-like reactions, psoriasiform rashes, dry eyes, impotence, and Peyronie's disease (rare); systemic lupus erythematosus (extremely rare)

OVERDOSAGE

Signs and symptoms	Severe bradycardia, cardiac failure, hypotension, bronchospasm
Treatment	Empty stomach (avoid pulmonary aspiration). For excessive bradycardia, administer 0.25–1.0 mg atropine IV; if there is no response to vagal blockade, administer isoproterenol cautiously. For cardiac failure, administer digitalis and a diuretic. For hypotension, use norepinephrine or (preferably) epinephrine. Treat bronchospasm with isoproterenol and aminophylline. Significant amounts of propranolol cannot be removed by dialysis.

DRUG INTERACTIONS

Reserpine, other catecholamine-depleting drugs	△ Risk of hypotension, marked bradycardia, vertigo, syncope, or orthostatic hypotension; closely observe patients during concomitant therapy
Calcium channel blockers	▽ AV conduction and myocardial contractility; concomitant IV administration of a beta blocker and verapamil has resulted in serious reactions, particularly in patients with severe cardiomyopathy, cardiac failure, or recent myocardial infarction. When using propranolol with a calcium channel blocker, especially IV verapamil, exercise caution.
Phenytoin, phenobarbital, rifampin	▽ Plasma level of propranolol
Cimetidine	△ Plasma level of propranolol
Chlorpromazine	△ Plasma level of propranolol and chlorpromazine
Theophylline, lidocaine, antipyrine	△ Plasma level of theophylline, lidocaine, and antipyrine
Thyroxine	△ Plasma T_4 level (due to decreased peripheral conversion of T_4 to T_3)
Aluminum hydroxide	▽ Absorption of propranolol
Digitalis	▽ AV conduction
Ephedrine, isoproterenol, other beta-adrenergic bronchodilators	▽ Bronchodilation
Thiazide-type diuretics, other antihypertensive agents	△ Antihypertensive effect
Alcohol	▽ Rate of absorption

ALTERED LABORATORY VALUES

Blood/serum values	△ SGOT △ SGPT △ Alkaline phosphatase △ LDH △ T_4 △ rT_3 ▽ T_3 △ BUN (in patients with severe heart disease)

No clinically significant alterations in urinary values occur at therapeutic dosages

---

USE IN CHILDREN

See INDICATIONS and ORAL DOSAGE; do not give IV to children. High plasma drug levels have been detected in patients with Down's syndrome, which suggests that bioavailability may be increased in these patients. If echocardiography is used to monitor therapy, bear in mind that the characteristics of a normal echocardiogram vary with age in children.

USE IN PREGNANT AND NURSING WOMEN

Pregnancy Category C: embryotoxic effects have been observed in animals given approximately 10 times the maximum human dose; no adequate, well-controlled studies have been done in pregnant women. Use during pregnancy only if the expected benefit justifies the potential risk to the fetus. Propranolol is excreted in human milk; use with caution in nursing mothers.

ANTIMIGRAINE AGENTS

INDERAL LA (propranolol hydrochloride) Ayerst   Rx

Capsules (long-acting): 80, 120, 160 mg

INDICATIONS	ORAL DOSAGE
Hypertension	**Adult:** 80 mg once daily (alone or with a diuretic) to start, followed, if necessary, by 120 mg or more once daily, up to 640 mg once daily (the full therapeutic effect of a given dosage may not be evident for a few days to several weeks); usual dosage: 120–160 mg/day
Prophylaxis and long-term management of **angina pectoris**	**Adult:** 80 mg once daily to start, followed, if necessary, by gradual increments every 3–7 days, up to 320 mg once daily; usual dosage: 160 mg/day
Prophylaxis of **migraine**	**Adult:** 80 mg once daily to start, followed, if necessary, by gradual increments, up to 240 mg once daily; usual dosage: 160–240 mg/day. If satisfactory prophylaxis is not obtained after giving 240 mg/day for 4–6 wk, discontinue use.
Hypertrophic subaortic stenosis	**Adult:** 80–160 mg once daily

CONTRAINDICATIONS

Sinus bradycardia	Cardiogenic shock	Overt congestive heart failure, unless it results from a tachyarrhythmia treatable with immediate-release propranolol
Heart block greater than first degree	Bronchial asthma	

ADMINISTRATION/DOSAGE ADJUSTMENTS

Switching from immediate-release propranolol	To maintain therapeutic effectiveness, especially at the end of a 24-h dosing interval, it may be necessary to increase the dosage, because the long-acting form produces lower serum propranolol levels. However, retitration may not be required if, in the treatment of a disorder (eg, hypertension, angina), there is little correlation between serum level and therapeutic effect.
Discontinuation of therapy	Reduce dosage gradually over a period of several weeks; caution patients who experience angina or who may have occult coronary artery disease not to interrupt or discontinue therapy on their own

WARNINGS/PRECAUTIONS

Cardiac failure	Beta blockade may cause or exacerbate cardiac failure; discontinue use if this disorder does not stabilize after diuretic therapy and digitalization. If necessary, propranolol may be given to patients with well-compensated congestive heart failure; observe such patients closely.
Thyrotoxicosis	Propranolol may mask certain clinical signs of hyperthyroidism; abrupt withdrawal may exacerbate manifestations of this disorder and precipitate a thyroid storm
Patients with angina	Abrupt withdrawal in such patients may exacerbate angina and, in some cases, lead to myocardial infarction; reinstitute therapy if withdrawal reactions occur (see ADMINISTRATION/DOSAGE ADJUSTMENTS)
Patients with Wolff-Parkinson-White (WPW) syndrome	Severe bradycardia, necessitating use of a demand pacemaker, has occurred in several patients with WPW syndrome following use of propranolol
Patients with diabetes	Adjustment of insulin dosage in patients with labile insulin-dependent diabetes may be more difficult, because propranolol may mask certain clinical signs (eg, changes in pulse rate and blood pressure) of acute hypoglycemia
Patients with bronchospastic disease	In general, such patients should not receive propranolol because it may block catecholamine-induced bronchodilation. Propranolol is specifically contraindicated for use in patients with bronchial asthma; use with caution in patients with nonallergic bronchospasm (eg, chronic bronchitis, emphysema).
Patients with renal or hepatic impairment	Use with caution in such patients
Major surgery	The necessity or desirability of discontinuing use before major surgery is controversial. Beta blockade can increase the risks associated with general anesthesia and surgery (because cardiac responsiveness to reflex beta-adrenergic stimuli is impaired) and may cause protracted severe hypotension and difficulty in restarting and maintaining the heartbeat. However, beta-adrenergic agonists (eg, dobutamine, isoproterenol) can reverse the effects of propranolol.
Glaucoma testing	Propranolol can reduce intraocular pressure and thereby affect the results of glaucoma screening tests
Carcinogenicity	No evidence of tumorigenicity has been seen in rats or mice given up to 150 mg/kg/day for a period of 18 mo
Effect on fertility	No impairment of fertility has been observed in animals

ADVERSE REACTIONS

Cardiovascular	Bradycardia, congestive heart failure, AV-block intensification, hypotension, paresthesia of the hands, Raynaud-type arterial insufficiency, purpura

INDERAL LA ■ MIDRIN

Central nervous system	Light-headedness, depression, insomnia, weakness, fatigue, lassitude, catatonia, visual disturbances, hallucinations, disorientation, short-term memory loss, emotional lability, slightly clouded sensorium, decreased neuropsychometric performance
Gastrointestinal	Nausea, vomiting, epigastric distress, abdominal cramps, diarrhea, constipation, mesenteric arterial thrombosis, ischemic colitis
Respiratory	Bronchospasm
Allergic	Pharyngitis, agranulocytosis, erythematous rash, fever with aching and sore throat, laryngospasm and respiratory distress
Other	Alopecia, lupus erythematosus-like reactions, psoriasiform rashes, dry eyes, impotence, and Peyronie's disease (rare); systemic lupus erythematosus (extremely rare)

OVERDOSAGE

Signs and symptoms	Severe bradycardia, cardiac failure, hypotension, bronchospasm
Treatment	Empty stomach (avoid pulmonary aspiration). For excessive bradycardia, administer 0.25–1.0 mg atropine IV; if there is no response to vagal blockade, administer isoproterenol cautiously. For cardiac failure, administer digitalis and a diuretic. For hypotension, use norepinephrine or (preferably) epinephrine. Treat bronchospasm with isoproterenol and aminophylline. Significant amounts of propranolol cannot be removed by dialysis.

DRUG INTERACTIONS

Reserpine, other catecholamine-depleting drugs	△ Risk of hypotension, marked bradycardia, vertigo, syncope, or orthostatic hypotension; closely observe patients during concomitant therapy
Digitalis	▽ AV conduction
Ephedrine, isoproterenol, other beta-adrenergic bronchodilators	▽ Bronchodilation
Thiazide-type diuretics, other antihypertensive agents	△ Antihypertensive effect

ALTERED LABORATORY VALUES

Blood/serum values	△ SGOT △ SGPT △ Alkaline phosphatase △ Lactate dehydrogenase △ BUN (in patients with severe heart disease)

No clinically significant alterations in urinary values occur at therapeutic dosages

---

USE IN CHILDREN
Safety and effectiveness for use in children have not been established

USE IN PREGNANT AND NURSING WOMEN
Pregnancy Category C: embryotoxic effects have been observed in animals given approximately 10 times the maximum human dose; no adequate, well-controlled studies have been done in pregnant women. Use during pregnancy only if the expected benefit justifies the potential risk to the fetus. Propranolol is excreted in human milk; use with caution in nursing mothers.

ANTIMIGRAINE AGENTS

MIDRIN (isometheptene mucate, dichloralphenazone, and acetaminophen) Carnrick   Rx

Capsules: 65 mg isometheptene mucate, 100 mg dichloralphenazone, and 325 mg acetaminophen

INDICATIONS	ORAL DOSAGE
Migraine headache[1]	**Adult:** 2 caps at once, followed by 1 cap every hour, as needed, up to 5 caps/12 h
Tension headache	**Adult:** 1–2 caps q4h, up to 8 caps/day

CONTRAINDICATIONS

Severe renal or hepatic disease, hypertension, or organic heart disease	Glaucoma	MAO inhibitor therapy

WARNINGS/PRECAUTIONS

Special-risk patients	Use with caution in patients with hypertension or peripheral vascular disease or after a recent myocardial infarction

ADVERSE REACTIONS

Central nervous system	Transient dizziness

Dermatological	Rash

OVERDOSAGE

Signs and symptoms	*Early:* nausea, vomiting, diaphoresis, and general malaise (some patients may be asymptomatic); *late:* clinical and laboratory evidence of hepatotoxicity (vomiting; right upper quadrant tenderness; increased SGOT, SGPT, serum bilirubin, and prothrombin time; and possible hypoglycemia) may not be apparent until 48–72 h after ingestion
Treatment	Promptly empty stomach by performing gastric lavage or inducing emesis with syrup of ipecac (15-30 ml for children, 30-45 ml for adults). Give ipecac with copious quantities of water; if emesis does not occur within 20 min, repeat dose. Activated charcoal may be given if acetaminophen has been ingested with certain other drugs. Administer oral acetylcysteine as soon as possible (no later than 24 h after ingestion); give a loading dose of 140 mg/kg and then, at 4-h intervals, 17 maintenance doses of 70 mg/kg. (Charcoal, if used, should be removed before acetylcysteine is given.) Measure the plasma level of unconjugated acetaminophen as early as possible, but no sooner than 4 h after ingestion. Determine prothrombin time, SGOT and SGPT levels, and serum concentrations of bilirubin, creatinine, BUN, glucose, and electrolytes every 24 h. If the prothrombin time exceeds 1.5 times the control value, give vitamin K_1; if the prothrombin time exceeds 3 times this value, give fresh frozen plasma. Institute appropriate measures to treat hypoglycemia and electrolyte and fluid imbalance. Avoid forced diuresis or use of diuretics when treating an acetaminophen overdose. For additional information on use of acetylcysteine and interpretation of the plasma acetaminophen level, see Mucomyst chart.

ALTERED LABORATORY VALUES

Blood/serum values	Glucose (with glucose oxidase/peroxidase tests)
Urinary values	+ 5-HIAA (with nitrosonaphthol reagent tests)

USE IN CHILDREN	USE IN PREGNANT AND NURSING WOMEN
Consult manufacturer	Consult manufacturer

[1] Possibly effective

ANTIMIGRAINE AGENTS

SANSERT (methysergide maleate) Sandoz Pharmaceuticals   Rx

Tablets: 2 mg

INDICATIONS	ORAL DOSAGE
Prophylaxis of frequent and/or severe uncontrollable **vascular headaches**	**Adult:** 4–8 mg/day, with meals, for not more than 6 mo without interruption (see "duration of therapy," below)

CONTRAINDICATIONS

Pregnancy	Coronary artery disease	Serious infections
Peripheral vascular disease	Hepatic or renal impairment	Phlebitis or cellulitis of the lower limbs
Severe arteriosclerosis	Valvular heart disease	Pulmonary disease
Severe hypertension	Debilitated states	Collagen diseases or fibrotic processes

ADMINISTRATION/DOSAGE ADJUSTMENTS

Selection of patients	Reserve for patients suffering from (1) one or more severe vascular headaches per week or (2) vascular headaches that are uncontrollable or so severe that prophylaxis is indicated regardless of their frequency; methysergide has no place in the management of acute headache attacks
Duration of therapy	Do not administer continuously for more than 6 mo; follow each 6-mo course of treatment with a drug-free interval of 3–4 wk. During last 2–3 wk of each treatment course, reduce dosage gradually to avoid "headache rebound."
Initial trial period	If efficacy has not been demonstrated after a 3-wk trial period, longer administration is unlikely to be of benefit
Prevention of GI symptoms	Introduce drug gradually and administer with meals to avert nausea, vomiting, diarrhea, heartburn, and abdominal pain

SANSERT ■ WIGRAINE

WARNINGS/PRECAUTIONS

Fibrotic complications	Retroperitoneal fibrosis, pleuropulmonary fibrosis, and cardiovascular disorders with murmurs or vascular bruits may occur with long-term use; warn patients to report immediately any associated symptoms (see ADVERSE REACTIONS), and discontinue use of the drug if such symptoms develop. There is a high incidence of regression of manifestations once drug is withdrawn, although cardiac murmurs, which may indicate endocardial fibrosis, may persist in some cases.
Patient monitoring	Constant medical supervision is essential. Examine patients regularly for development of fibrotic or vascular complications; an IVP and chest x-ray film should be obtained in suspected cases of retroperitoneal fibrosis and pleuropulmonary fibrosis, respectively
Dependent edema	May occur; correct with lowered doses, salt restriction, or diuretics
Weight gain	May occur; caution patients regarding their caloric intake
Tartrazine sensitivity	Presence of FD&C Yellow No. 5 (tartrazine) in tablets may cause allergic-type reactions, including bronchial asthma, in susceptible individuals

ADVERSE REACTIONS

Fibrotic	Retroperitoneal fibrosis, presenting with general malaise, fatigue, weight loss, backache, low-grade fever (elevated sedimentation rate), urinary obstruction (girdle or flank pain, dysuria, polyuria, oliguria, elevated BUN), and/or vascular insufficiency of the lower limbs (eg, pain, Leriche syndrome, leg edema, thrombophlebitis); pleuropulmonary fibrosis, presenting with dyspnea, chest pain and tightness, pleural friction rubs, and pleural effusion; nonrheumatic fibrotic thickening of the aortic root and of the aortic and mitral valves, presenting with cardiac murmurs and dyspnea; fibrotic plaques simulating Peyronie's disease
Cardiovascular	Vascular insufficiency of the lower limbs (see above); intrinsic arterial vasoconstriction, presenting with chest pain, abdominal pain, or cold, numb, painful extremities, with or without paresthesias and diminished or absent pulses, and rarely progressing to ischemic tissue damage; postural hypotension; tachycardia
Gastrointestinal	Nausea, vomiting, diarrhea, heartburn, abdominal pain, constipation, increased gastric acidity
Central nervous system	Insomnia, drowsiness, mild euphoria, dizziness, ataxia, light-headedness, hyperesthesia, and unworldly feelings (dissociation, hallucination, etc)[1]
Dermatological	Facial flushing, telangiectasia, and rashes (rare); increased hair loss[2]
Hematological	Neutropenia, eosinophilia
Other	Peripheral edema and (more rarely) localized brawny edema; weight gain, weakness, arthralgia, myalgia

OVERDOSAGE

Signs and symptoms	See ADVERSE REACTIONS
Treatment	Discontinue medication; treat symptomatically and institute supportive measures, as required

DRUG INTERACTIONS

Ergotamine	⇧ Vasoconstriction

ALTERED LABORATORY VALUES

Blood/serum values	⇧ BUN

No clinically significant alterations in urinary values occur at therapeutic dosages

---

USE IN CHILDREN
Not recommended for use in children

USE IN PREGNANT AND NURSING WOMEN
Contraindicated for use during pregnancy. Safety for use in nursing women has not been established.

---

[1] Some of these symptoms may be associated with vascular headaches per se and may, therefore, be unrelated to the drug
[2] May abate despite continued therapy

ANTIMIGRAINE AGENTS

WIGRAINE (ergotamine tartrate and caffeine) Organon Rx

Tablets: 1 mg ergotamine tartrate and 100 mg caffeine   Suppositories: 2 mg ergotamine tartrate and 100 mg caffeine

INDICATIONS	ORAL DOSAGE	RECTAL DOSAGE
Vascular headaches, including migraine, migraine variants, and histamine cephalalgia	Adult: 2 tabs at the first sign of attack, followed, if necessary, by 1 tab every 30 min, up to 6 tabs/attack and 10 tabs/wk	Adult: 1 suppository at start of attack, followed, if necessary, by a second suppository 1 h later; maximum dosage: 2 suppositories/attack, 5 suppositories/wk

WIGRAINE

CONTRAINDICATIONS

Pregnancy	Hypertension	Sepsis
Peripheral vascular disease	Hepatic impairment	Hypersensitivity to any component
Coronary artery disease	Renal impairment	

ADMINISTRATION/DOSAGE ADJUSTMENTS

Prophylactic therapy — These preparations may be given at bedtime to carefully selected patients for short-term prophylaxis; the maximum dosage should not be exceeded

WARNINGS/PRECAUTIONS

Ergotism — To prevent ergotism, caution patients not to exceed the dosage limits; manifestations of ergotism rarely occur at recommended dosages, even after long-term intermittent use

ADVERSE REACTIONS

Cardiovascular — Pulselessness, weakness, muscle pains, paresthesia of the extremities, precordial distress and pain, transient tachycardia or bradycardia, localized edema

Gastrointestinal — Vomiting, nausea

Other — Itching

OVERDOSAGE

Signs and symptoms — Vomiting, numbness, tingling, pain and cyanosis of the extremities with diminished or absent peripheral pulses; hypertension or hypotension, drowsiness, stupor, coma, convulsions, shock; bilateral papillitis with ring scotomata

Treatment — Remove drug by induced emesis, gastric lavage, and catharsis. Maintain adequate pulmonary ventilation, correct hypotension, and control convulsions. Treat peripheral vasospasm with warmth *(not heat)* and protect ischemic limbs from cold. Use vasodilators cautiously.

DRUG INTERACTIONS

No clinically significant drug interactions have been identified

ALTERED LABORATORY VALUES

No clinically significant alterations in blood/serum or urinary values occur at therapeutic dosages

---

USE IN CHILDREN

Safety and effectiveness for use in children have not been established

USE IN PREGNANT AND NURSING WOMEN

Pregnancy Category X: these preparations can produce prolonged uterine contractions and thereby cause abortion in pregnant women; use in women who are or may become pregnant is contraindicated. Pregnant patients who are receiving these preparations should be apprised of the potential hazard to the fetus. Although it is not known whether ergotamine tartrate is excreted in human milk, other ergot alkaloids have been detected in human milk and have caused manifestations of ergotism in nursing infants; patients should not nurse while taking these preparations.

VEHICLE/BASE
Suppositories: cocoa butter and 21.5 mg tartaric acid

Chapter 27

Antinauseants/Antiemetics

ANTIVERT (Roerig) Meclizine hydrochloride *Rx*	1060
COMPAZINE (Smith Kline & French) Prochlorperazine *Rx*	1060
DRAMAMINE (Richardson-Vicks Health Care Products) Dimenhydrinate *OTC*	1064
DRAMAMINE Injection (Searle) Dimenhydrinate *Rx*	1064
EMETE-CON (Roerig) Benzquinamide hydrochloride *Rx*	1065
EMETROL (Rorer) Dextrose, levulose, and phosphoric acid *OTC*	1066
MARINOL (Roxane) Dronabinol *C-II*	1067
PEPTO-BISMOL (Procter & Gamble) Bismuth subsalicylate *OTC*	1068
PHENERGAN (Wyeth) Promethazine hydrochloride *Rx*	1069
PHENERGAN Injection (Wyeth) Promethazine hydrochloride *Rx*	1071
REGLAN (Robins) Metoclopramide hydrochloride *Rx*	1073
THORAZINE (Smith Kline & French) Chlorpromazine hydrochloride *Rx*	1075
TIGAN (Beecham) Trimethobenzamide hydrochloride *Rx*	1080
TORECAN (Boehringer Ingelheim) Thiethylperazine maleate *Rx*	1081
TRANSDERM SCŌP (CIBA) Scopolamine *Rx*	1082
VISTARIL Intramuscular Solution (Roerig) Hydroxyzine hydrochloride *Rx*	1083

Other Antinauseants/Antiemetics   1058

BENADRYL (Parke-Davis) Diphenhydramine hydrochloride *Rx*	1058
BONINE (Leeming) Meclizine hydrochloride *Rx*	1058
BUCLADIN-S (Stuart) Buclizine hydrochloride *Rx*	1058
MAREZINE (Burroughs Wellcome) Cyclizine *OTC, Rx*	1059
RU-VERT-M (Reid-Rowell) Meclizine hydrochloride *Rx*	1059
TRILAFON (Schering) Perphenazine *Rx*	1059
VESPRIN (Squibb) Triflupromazine hydrochloride *Rx*	1059
VONTROL (Smith Kline & French) Diphenidol *Rx*	1059

OTHER ANTINAUSEANTS/ANTIEMETICS

DRUG	HOW SUPPLIED	USUAL DOSAGE[1]
BENADRYL (Parke-Davis) Diphenhydramine hydrochloride *Rx*	**Capsules:** 25, 50 mg **Elixir (per 5 ml):** 12.5 mg (5 ml, 4 fl oz, 1 pt, 1 gal) **Ampuls:** 50 mg/ml (1 ml) **Prefilled syringes:** 50 mg/ml (1 ml) **Vials:** 10 mg/ml (10, 30 ml), 50 mg/ml (10 ml)	**Adult:** for motion sickness, 25–50 mg PO tid or qid, or 10–50 mg, up to 400 mg/day, IM (deeply) or IV; give 30 min before exposure to motion and, thereafter, before meals and at bedtime **Child:** for motion sickness, 12.5–25 mg PO tid or qid (in child > 20 lb) or 5 mg/kg/24 h (150 mg/m2/24 h), up to 300 mg/day, PO (in child > 20 lb), IM (deeply), or IV, given in 3–4 (PO) or 4 (IM or IV) divided doses; give 30 min before exposure to motion, and thereafter, before meals and at bedtime
BONINE (Leeming) Meclizine hydrochloride *OTC*	**Chewable tablets:** 25 mg	**Adult:** 25–50 mg 1 h before journey, followed by 25–50 mg q24h, as needed
BUCLADIN-S (Stuart) Buclizine hydrochloride *Rx*	**Tablets:** 50 mg	**Adult:** for nausea, 50–150 mg/day, as needed (usual maintenance dose: 50 mg bid); for motion sickness, 50 mg given 30 min before journey, followed, if needed, by 50 mg 4–6 h later

[1] Where pediatric dosages are not given, consult manufacturer

OTHER ANTINAUSEANTS/ANTIEMETICS continued

DRUG	HOW SUPPLIED	USUAL DOSAGE[1]
MAREZINE (Burroughs Wellcome) Cyclizine *OTC and Rx*	**Tablets:** 50 mg cyclizine hydrochloride (*OTC*) **Ampuls:** 50 mg cyclizine lactate/ml (1 ml) (*Rx*)	**Adult:** 50 mg PO ½ h before journey, followed by 50 mg PO q4–6h, as needed, up to 200 mg/day PO; or 50 mg IM q4–6h, as needed **Child (6–12 yr):** 25 mg PO 1–3 times/day
RU-VERT-M (Reid-Rowell) Meclizine hydrochloride *Rx*	**Tablets:** 25 mg	**Adult:** for vertigo, 25–100 mg/day, given in divided doses; for motion sickness, 25–50 mg 1 h before journey, followed by 25–50 mg q24h, as needed **Child (≥ 12 yr):** same as adult
TRILAFON (Schering) Perphenazine *Rx*	**Tablets:** 2, 4, 8, 16 mg **Tablets (sustained release):** 8 mg **Concentrate (per 5 ml):** 16 mg (4 fl oz) **Ampuls:** 5 mg/ml (1 ml)	**Adult:** for severe nausea and vomiting, 8–16 mg/day PO, given in divided doses, or up to 24 mg/day, if necessary; if sustained-release tablets are used, 8–16 mg bid; alternatively, 5–10 mg IM (deeply) or up to 5 mg IV (slowly)
VESPRIN (Squibb) Triflupromazine hydrochloride *Rx*	**Tablets:** 10, 25, 50 mg **Vials:** 10, 20 mg/ml	**Adult:** 20–30 mg/day PO, 1–3 mg/day IV, or 5–15 mg IM q4h, up to 60 mg/day **Child (> 2½ yr):** 0.2 mg/kg, up to 10 mg/day, PO, given in 3 divided doses, or 0.2–0.25 mg/kg IM up to 10 mg/day
VONTROL (Smith Kline & French) Diphenidol *Rx*	**Tablets:** 25 mg	**Adult:** for vertigo or nausea and vomiting, 25 mg q4h, as needed; some patients may require 50 mg q4h **Child (≥ 50 lb):** for nausea and vomiting, 0.4 mg/lb repeated, if needed, in 1 h, then q4h, as needed, up to 2.5 mg/lb/24 h (the dose for children 50–100 lb is 1 tab)

[1] Where pediatric dosages are not given, consult manufacturer

COMPENDIUM OF DRUG THERAPY

ANTINAUSEANTS/ANTIEMETICS

ANTIVERT (meclizine hydrochloride) Roerig   Rx

Tablets: 12.5 mg (Antivert), 25 mg (Antivert/25), 50 mg (Antivert/50)   **Chewable tablets:** 25 mg (Antivert/25 Chewable Tablets)

INDICATIONS	ORAL DOSAGE
Motion sickness	**Adult:** 25–50 mg 1 h before anticipated exposure to motion, repeated q24h, as needed
Vertigo associated with diseases affecting the vestibular system[1]	**Adult:** 25–100 mg/day, given in divided doses

CONTRAINDICATIONS

Hypersensitivity to meclizine

WARNINGS/PRECAUTIONS

Drowsiness	Caution patients not to drive or engage in other activities requiring alertness, and to avoid alcoholic beverages (see DRUG INTERACTIONS)
Special-risk patients	Use with caution in patients with asthma, glaucoma, or prostate gland enlargement, due to potential anticholinergic action of meclizine

ADVERSE REACTIONS

Central nervous system	Drowsiness
Other	Dry mouth, blurred vision

OVERDOSAGE

Signs and symptoms	Sedation, possible anticholinergic effects (eg, dry mouth, blurred vision, others)
Treatment	Treat symptomatically

DRUG INTERACTIONS

Alcohol, tranquilizers, sedative-hypnotics, and other CNS depressants	⇧ CNS depression

ALTERED LABORATORY VALUES

No clinically significant alterations in blood/serum or urinary values occur at therapeutic dosages

---

USE IN CHILDREN

Not recommended for use in children under 12 yr of age; the safety and effectiveness of this drug have not been established in pediatric patients

USE IN PREGNANT AND NURSING WOMEN

Pregnancy Category B: use during pregnancy only if clearly needed. Although reproduction studies in rats have shown cleft palates at 25–50 times the human dose, epidemiologic studies in pregnant women have detected no increased risk of congenital abnormalities. Consult manufacturer for use in nursing mothers.

[1] Possibly effective

ANTINAUSEANTS/ANTIEMETICS

COMPAZINE (prochlorperazine) Smith Kline & French   Rx

Capsules (sustained release): 10, 15, 30 mg   **Tablets:** 5, 10, 25 mg   **Syrup (per 5 ml):** 5 mg (4 fl oz) *fruit flavored*   **Ampuls:** 5 mg/ml (2 ml)   **Vials:** 5 mg/ml (10 ml)   **Prefilled syringes:** 5 mg/ml (2 ml)   **Rectal suppositories:** 2.5, 5, 25 mg

INDICATIONS	ORAL DOSAGE	PARENTERAL DOSAGE
Severe nausea and vomiting	**Adult:** 5–10 mg tid or qid or, if sustained-release capsules are used, 15 mg on arising or 10 mg q12h **Child (20–29 lb):** 2.5 mg 1–2 times/day, up to 7.5 mg/day **Child (30–39 lb):** 2.5 mg bid or tid, up to 10 mg/day **Child (40–85 lb):** 2.5 mg tid or 5 mg bid, up to 15 mg/day	**Adult:** 5–10 mg IM to start, repeated q3–4h, as needed, up to 40 mg/day. For preoperative use, give 5–10 mg IM 1–2 h before induction of anesthesia (if necessary, dose may be repeated after 30 min); alternatively, give either 5–10 mg by IV injection or 20 mg by IV infusion 15–30 min before induction of anesthesia. To control acute reactions during or after surgery, administer 5–10 mg by IM or IV injection (if necessary, dose may be repeated once). **Child:** 0.06 mg/lb IM

COMPAZINE

Manifestations of **psychotic disorders**	**Adult:** for office patients and outpatients, 5–10 mg tid or qid; for hospitalized or otherwise closely supervised patients, 10 mg tid or qid to start, followed, if necessary, by small increases in dosage every 2–3 days, up to 50–75 mg/day or, in more severe cases, up to 100–150 mg/day **Child (2–12 yr):** 2.5 mg bid or tid, up to 10 mg on 1st day, followed by increases in dosage up to 20 mg/day (2–5 yr) or 25 mg/day (6–12 yr), as needed	**Adult:** for severe cases, 10–20 mg IM to start, repeated q2–4h (in resistant cases, every hour) as needed; for prolonged therapy, 10–20 mg IM q4–6h **Child (< 12 yr):** 0.06 mg/lb IM
Generalized **nonpsychotic anxiety**[1]	**Adult:** 5 mg tid or qid or, if sustained-release capsules are used, 15 mg on arising or 10 mg q12h; do not exceed 20 mg/day or administer for more than 12 wk	—

CONTRAINDICATIONS

Age < 2 yr or weight < 20 lb	Presence of large amounts of CNS depressants	Coma
Use in pediatric surgery		

ADMINISTRATION/DOSAGE ADJUSTMENTS

Initial dosage titration	Adjust dosage according to individual response and severity of the condition; begin with the lowest recommended dose
Parenteral administration	Administer IM by injecting solution deeply into the upper outer quadrant of the buttock; because of local irritation, SC administration is inadvisable. For IV injection, dilute dose in an isotonic solution or give undiluted; rate of administration should not exceed 5 mg/min (do not give as a bolus). For IV infusion, dilute 20 mg in at least 1 liter of isotonic solution and then add to the primary IV solution. Do not mix prochlorperazine with other drugs; do not dilute the contents of the ampuls with any solution that contains parabens.
Rectal dosage	For severe nausea and vomiting in adults, give 25 mg bid. For children, rectal dosages are the same as oral dosages.
Elderly, emaciated, or debilitated patients	Increase dosage more gradually if the patient is elderly, emaciated, or debilitated; for most elderly patients, a dosage in the lower range is sufficient. Carefully monitor clinical response of elderly patients since they appear to be more susceptible to hypotension and extrapyramidal reactions; elderly patients with brain damage are especially susceptible to extrapyramidal effects.
Monitoring of long-term therapy	Periodically evaluate patients with a history of long-term neuroleptic treatment in order to determine whether the maintenance dosage can be reduced or therapy discontinued; watch for tardive dyskinesia, ocular changes, and skin pigmentation during prolonged use

WARNINGS/PRECAUTIONS

Tardive dyskinesia	Neuroleptic drugs can cause tardive dyskinesia, a potentially irreversible syndrome characterized by involuntary choreoathetoid movements of the tongue, face, mouth, lips, jaw, trunk, and/or extremities. Protrusion of the tongue, puffing of the cheeks, puckering of the mouth, chewing movements, and other manifestations may become evident during treatment, upon dosage reduction, or after the drug is discontinued. The likelihood that tardive dyskinesia will develop or become irreversible increases with duration of treatment and total cumulative dose; however, even relatively brief use of low doses can cause it. Although this reaction appears to occur most often in the elderly, especially among older women, it is impossible to use this information to predict, before therapy is started, which patients are likely to develop the syndrome. In general, reserve chronic therapy for patients who respond to neuroleptics and who cannot undergo another, equally effective form of treatment that is potentially less harmful. Use the lowest effective dosage, keep the duration of therapy as short as possible, and periodically reassess the need for the drug. Watch carefully for manifestations of tardive dyskinesia; fine vermicular movements of the tongue reportedly may be an early sign. However, do not forget that neuroleptic therapy can itself mask the signs and symptoms of tardive dyskinesia. If evidence of the syndrome is seen, consider terminating use of the drug, bearing in mind that some patients may require continued neuroleptic treatment despite the development of dyskinesia. There is no known treatment for tardive dyskinesia; however, after discontinuation, some or all manifestations of this syndrome may disappear spontaneously.
Dystonias	To control dystonias, discontinue neuroleptic therapy and take the following measures: for mild cases, provide reassurance or give a barbiturate; for moderate cases, use a barbiturate; for more severe cases, administer an antiparkinson agent other than levodopa; for children, provide reassurance and give either a barbiturate or parenteral diphenhydramine. If antiparkinson agents or diphenhydramine fail to reverse signs and symptoms, reevaluate diagnosis. Appropriate supportive measures, such as those needed to maintain adequate hydration and a patent airway, should be instituted as required. Dystonias usually subside within a few hours and almost always within 24–48 h after the drug has been discontinued. If treatment is resumed, administer at a lower dosage.

COMPAZINE

Akathisia	Symptoms of akathisia often disappear spontaneously; if they become too troublesome, reduce dosage or give a barbiturate. Wait until effects subside before increasing dosage. At times, drug-induced symptoms of akathisia may resemble psychotic or neurotic manifestations seen before therapy.
Pseudoparkinsonism	In most cases, pseudoparkinsonism can be controlled by concomitant use of an antiparkinson agent other than levodopa; occasionally, it is necessary to reduce the dosage of prochlorperazine or discontinue the drug. Administration of antiparkinson drugs for a period ranging from a few weeks to 2–3 mo is generally sufficient; clinical response should be evaluated before continuing therapy for a longer period. Reassurance and sedation are also important in the treatment of pseudoparkinsonism.
Convulsions	Phenothiazines can precipitate petit or grand mal convulsions, particularly in patients with EEG abnormalities or a history of such disorders
Cross-sensitivity	Do not use prochlorperazine in patients with a history of hypersensitivity to a phenothiazine unless potential benefits outweigh possible risks; see also warnings below concerning hepatotoxicity and blood dyscrasias
Hepatotoxicity	Cholestatic jaundice has occurred. If fever with grippe-like symptoms occurs, perform appropriate liver tests; if an abnormality is detected, stop treatment. Do not give prochlorperazine to patients with a history of phenothiazine-induced jaundice unless the potential benefits outweigh the possible risks. Since this drug is potentially hepatotoxic, use in children or adolescents with signs or symptoms suggesting Reye's syndrome should be avoided. Fatty changes have been detected in the livers of patients who died during treatment; however, no causal relationship has been established.
Blood dyscrasias	Agranulocytosis and leukopenia can occur during therapy. Caution patients to report the sudden appearance of sore throat or other signs or symptoms of infection; if signs of infection are seen and WBC and differential counts are depressed, stop therapy and institute appropriate measures. Do not give prochlorperazine to patients with bone marrow depression or a history of phenothiazine-induced blood dyscrasias unless the potential benefits outweigh the possible risks.
Hypotension	Prochlorperazine can cause hypotension. In patients with mitral insufficiency or pheochromocytoma, certain phenothiazines have produced severe hypotension. To minimize risk of hypotension, keep all patients lying down and under observation for at least 30 min after the initial injection. Exercise caution when giving prochlorperazine parenterally or in large doses to patients with cardiovascular dysfunction. If hypotension occurs, place patient in a head-low position with the legs raised; if a vasopressor is needed, use norepinephrine or phenylephrine, not epinephrine.
Masking of nonpsychotic conditions	Extrapyramidal symptoms associated with prochlorperazine may be confused with the neurological manifestations of an undiagnosed primary disease such as Reye's syndrome or another encephalopathy; antiemetic effect may mask nausea and vomiting associated with intestinal obstruction, brain tumor, Reye's syndrome, or toxicity of antineoplastic agents or other drugs
Drowsiness	Caution patients about driving and engaging in other activities requiring mental alertness; drowsiness may occur, especially during the first few days of therapy
Sedation, coma	Deep sleep and coma have occurred, usually as a result of overdosage
Contact dermatitis	To prevent contact dermatitis, avoid getting injectable solution on hands or clothing
Glaucoma	Prochlorperazine may exacerbate glaucoma; use with caution in patients with glaucoma
Extreme heat	Phenothiazines may affect thermal homeostasis; use with caution in patients who will be exposed to extreme heat
Aspiration of vomitus	During postsurgical recovery, aspiration of vomitus has occurred in a few patients given prochlorperazine; bear in mind this risk even though no causal relationship has been established
Sudden death	Patients taking phenothiazines have occasionally died suddenly; in some cases, death appeared to result from cardiac arrest or from asphyxia due to failure of the cough reflex
Abrupt withdrawal	Nausea, vomiting, dizziness, and tremulousness may occur following abrupt discontinuation of high-dose therapy
Carcinogenicity	Chronic use of neuroleptic drugs causes a persistent elevation of the serum prolactin level, an effect that may be of potential importance if the patient has prolactin-dependent breast cancer. Chronic administration has produced an increase in mammary neoplasia in rodents, and endocrine disturbances have been seen in humans; although no clinical or epidemiological studies have shown an association between chronic neuroleptic therapy and mammary tumorigenesis, the available evidence is considered too limited to be conclusive at this time.

ADVERSE REACTIONS[2]

Central nervous system	Drowsiness, dystonias (spasm of neck muscles, torticollis, extensor rigidity of back muscles, opisthotonos, carpopedal spasm, trismus, swallowing difficulty, oculogyric crisis, protrusion of the tongue), akathisia (agitation, jitteriness, insomnia), pseudoparkinsonism (mask-like facies, drooling, tremors, pill-rolling motion, cogwheel rigidity, shuffling gait), tardive dyskinesia, tardive dystonia, hyperreflexia, dyskinesia, reactivation of psychosis, catatonic-like states, grand mal and petit mal seizures, cerebral edema, CSF protein abnormalities, coma

COMPAZINE

Ophthalmic	Blurred vision, miosis, mydriasis, pigmentary retinopathy; corneal and lenticular deposits and epithelial keratopathy (with prolonged use of substantial doses)
Cardiovascular	Hypotension, dizziness, headache, ECG changes (especially distortions of Q and T waves), cardiac arrest, peripheral edema
Hematological	Agranulocytosis, eosinophilia, leukopenia, hemolytic anemia, aplastic anemia, thrombocytopenic purpura, pancytopenia
Gastrointestinal	Jaundice, biliary stasis, nausea, constipation, obstipation, adynamic ileus, atonic colon
Genitourinary	Priapism, ejaculatory disorders/impotence, urinary retention
Endocrinological	Hyperglycemia, hypoglycemia, glucosuria, lactation, galactorrhea, amenorrhea, menstrual irregularities, gynecomastia
Dermatological	Hypersensitivity reactions (see below); skin pigmentation (with prolonged use of substantial doses)
Hypersensitivity	Jaundice, blood dyscrasias, asthma, laryngeal edema, angioneurotic edema, anaphylactoid reactions, urticaria, pruritus, erythema, eczema, photosensitivity, contact dermatitis, exfoliative dermatitis
Other	Dry mouth, nasal congestion, mild fever (with large IM doses), hyperthermia (especially with exposure to extreme heat), hyperpyrexia, increased appetite, weight gain, systemic lupus erythematosus-like syndrome, enhanced effect of organophosphorous insecticides; neuroleptic malignant syndrome, a potentially fatal reaction characterized by hyperthermia, altered consciousness, muscular rigidity, and autonomic dysfunction

OVERDOSAGE

Signs and symptoms	Extrapyramidal effects (see ADVERSE REACTIONS), CNS depression, deep sleep, coma, agitation, restlessness, convulsions, fever, hypotension, dry mouth, ileus
Treatment	Empty stomach by gastric lavage, repeated several times. *Do not induce emesis.* For respiratory depression, administer oxygen and, if needed, perform a tracheostomy, and assist ventilation. For extrapyramidal reactions, keep patient under observation and maintain open airway. Treat extrapyramidal symptoms with antiparkinson drugs (except levodopa), barbiturates, or diphenhydramine. For hypotension, employ standard measures. If a vasoconstrictor is indicated, use norepinephrine or phenylephrine; other pressor agents may lower blood pressure further. Use saline cathartics to hasten evacuation of pellets that have not already released medication. Continue supportive therapy as long as overdosage symptoms remain.

DRUG INTERACTIONS

Other CNS depressants, including alcohol	△ CNS depression
Anticonvulsants	△ Risk of convulsions; adjustment of anticonvulsant dosage may be necessary △ Pharmacologic effect of phenytoin
Metrizamide	△ Risk of convulsions; discontinue use of prochlorperazine at least 48 h before administration of metrizamide for myelography and wait at least 24 h after the procedure before resuming use. Do not use prochlorperazine before or after myelography for control of nausea and vomiting.
Anticholinergic drugs	△ Anticholinergic effects ▽ Antipsychotic effect
Epinephrine	Severe hypotension
Guanethidine	▽ Antihypertensive effect
Thiazide diuretics	△ Orthostatic hypotensive effect
Propranolol	△ Pharmacologic effects of propranolol and prochlorperazine
Amphetamines	▽ Antipsychotic effect ▽ Anorectic effect
Phenmetrazine	▽ Anorectic effect
Lithium	△ Risk of acute encephalopathy and extrapyramidal reactions ▽ Serum prochlorperazine level △ Renal clearance of lithium
Tricyclic antidepressants	△ Serum level of tricyclic antidepressants and prochlorperazine ▽ Antipsychotic effect
Oral anticoagulants	▽ Anticoagulant effect

ALTERED LABORATORY VALUES

Blood/serum values	△ SGOT △ SGPT △ LDH △ Alkaline phosphatase △ Bilirubin △ Prolactin △ or ▽ Glucose
Urinary values	▽ VMA + Glucose + PKU + Pregnancy (with immunologic pregnancy tests) + Bilirubin (with reagent test strips) △ Urobilinogen (with Ehrlich's reagent test) ▽ 5-HIAA (with nitrosonaphthol reagent test) Interference with determination of catecholamines (with Pisano method), 17-KS (with Haltorff-Koch modification of Zimmerman reaction), and 17-OHCS (with modified Glenn-Nelson technique)

COMPAZINE ■ DRAMAMINE

> **USE IN CHILDREN**
>
> See INDICATIONS and dosage recommendations; contraindicated for use in pediatric surgery or children under 2 yr of age. Drug should not be used for conditions in which pediatric dosages have not been established. In children, an IM dose may be effective for up to 12 h. Children appear to be more susceptible to extrapyramidal reactions than adults, even at moderate doses; children who are dehydrated or who have an acute illness such as chicken pox, CNS infection, measles, or gastroenteritis are especially susceptible to these reactions, particularly to dystonias, and therefore must be closely supervised during therapy. If a child experiences an extrapyramidal reaction, discontinue use and do not reinstitute treatment at a later time. Avoid use in children or adolescents with signs or symptoms suggesting Reye's syndrome.

> **USE IN PREGNANT AND NURSING WOMEN**
>
> Jaundice, prolonged extrapyramidal signs, and hyper- and hyporeflexia have been seen in neonates born to mothers who received phenothiazines during pregnancy. Safety for use during pregnancy has not been established; use during pregnancy is not recommended except in serious and intractable cases of severe nausea and vomiting when the potential benefits outweigh possible hazards. If neuromuscular (extrapyramidal) reactions occur in pregnant patients, discontinue therapy and do not reinstitute treatment with prochlorperazine. Phenothiazines are excreted in human milk.

[1] For most patients, prochlorperazine is not the initial treatment of choice because certain risks associated with its use are not shared by common alternatives, such as benzodiazepines. It has not been established that this drug is effective in the treatment of anxiety or anxiety-like signs associated with nonpsychotic conditions (eg, physical illness, organic mental conditions, agitated depression, character pathology) other than generalized anxiety disorder.

ANTINAUSEANTS/ANTIEMETICS

DRAMAMINE (dimenhydrinate) Procter & Gamble — OTC
Tablets: 50 mg **Liquid (per 4 ml):** 12.5 mg[1] (3, 16 fl oz) *cherry flavored*

DRAMAMINE Injection (dimenhydrinate) Searle — Rx
Ampuls: 50 mg/ml (1 ml) **Vials:** 50 mg/ml (5 ml)

INDICATIONS	ORAL DOSAGE	PARENTERAL DOSAGE
Motion sickness	**Adult:** 50–100 mg q4–6h, up to 400 mg/24 h, or 16–32 ml (4–8 tsp) q4–6h, up to 128 ml (32 tsp)/24 h **Child (2–6 yr):** up to 25 mg q6–8h, not to exceed 75 mg/24 h, or 4–8 ml (1–2 tsp) q6–8h, not to exceed 24 ml (6 tsp)/24 h **Child (6–12 yr):** 25–50 mg q6–8h, up to 150 mg/24 h, or 8–16 ml (2–4 tsp) q6–8h, up to 48 ml (12 tsp)/24 h	**Adult:** 50–100 mg q4h IM or IV; for IV use, each milliliter (50 mg) must be diluted in 10 ml of 0.9% sodium chloride injection USP and injected over a 2-min period **Child:** 1.25 mg/kg or 37.5 mg/m² IM qid, up to 300 mg/day

CONTRAINDICATIONS	
Neonates	Hypersensitivity to dimenhydrinate or to diphenhydramine or 8-chlorotheophylline (the two components of dimenhydrinate)

ADMINISTRATION/DOSAGE ADJUSTMENTS	
Use of tablets or liquid for prophylaxis	The first dose should be taken 30–60 min before departure

WARNINGS/PRECAUTIONS	
Masking of ototoxicity	Exercise caution when using this drug with potentially ototoxic preparations because signs and symptoms of ototoxicity may be masked
Drowsiness	Caution patients not to drive or engage in other potentially hazardous activities requiring mental alertness or physical coordination
Special-risk patients	Use with caution in patients with prostatic hypertrophy, stenosing peptic ulcer, pyloroduodenal obstruction, bladder neck obstruction, narrow angle glaucoma, bronchial asthma, or cardiac arrhythmias
Intraarterial administration	Do not give this drug by intraarterial injection
Carcinogenicity, mutagenicity, effect on fertility	No evidence of carcinogenicity or impairment of fertility has been found in humans; mutagenic effects have been detected in bacteria, but not in mammals

ADVERSE REACTIONS

The most frequent reaction is italicized

Central nervous system	*Drowsiness,* dizziness, lassitude, headache, nervousness, restlessness, insomnia, excitation
Gastrointestinal	Anorexia, epigastric distress, nausea
Other	Blurred vision, difficult or painful urination, rash, tachycardia, thickening of bronchial secretions; dry mouth, nose, and throat

OVERDOSAGE

Signs and symptoms	Drowsiness and, in severe cases, convulsions, coma, and respiratory depression; children may also experience hallucinations following severe overdosage
Treatment	Maintain a patent airway; for respiratory depression, give oxygen and provide mechanically assisted ventilation. To treat convulsions in adults, IV diazepam should be used; for children, 5–6 mg/kg of phenobarbital may be given.

DRUG INTERACTIONS

Alcohol, tranquilizers, sedative-hypnotics, and other CNS depressants	⌂ CNS depression; patients should be instructed to avoid alcohol during therapy and cautioned about using other CNS depressants with dimenhydrinate

ALTERED LABORATORY VALUES

No clinically significant alterations in blood/serum or urinary values occur at therapeutic dosages

---

USE IN CHILDREN

See INDICATIONS, CONTRAINDICATIONS, and dosage recommendations; CNS stimulation, including excitation, restlessness, and insomnia, is more likely to occur in young children than in other patients

USE IN PREGNANT AND NURSING WOMEN

Pregnancy Category B: reproduction studies in rats given up to 20 times the human dose and in rabbits given up to 25 times the human dose have shown no evidence of harm to the fetus or impaired fertility, and studies in pregnant women have not demonstrated an increased risk of abnormalities. However, no adequate, well-controlled clinical studies have been done. Use during pregnancy only if clearly needed. Small amounts of dimenhydrinate are excreted in breast milk; because of the potential for adverse reactions in nursing infants, patients should not nurse while taking this drug.

---

[1] Contains 5% alcohol

ANTINAUSEANTS/ANTIEMETICS

EMETE-CON (benzquinamide hydrochloride) Roerig   Rx

Vials: benzquinamide hydrochloride equivalent to 25 mg/ml of benzquinamide after reconstitution (2 ml)

INDICATIONS

Nausea and vomiting associated with anesthesia and surgery

PARENTERAL DOSAGE

Adult: 50 mg (or 0.5–1.0 mg/kg) IM, repeated in 1 h and then q3–4h, as needed, or 25 mg (or 0.2–0.4 mg/kg) IV (slowly), with subsequent doses given IM

CONTRAINDICATIONS

Hypersensitivity to benzquinamide

ADMINISTRATION/DOSAGE ADJUSTMENTS

Reconstitution	Reconstitute contents of vial with 2.2 ml of Sterile Water for Injection or Bacteriostatic Water for Injection
Intramuscular administration	Inject deeply into a large muscle mass; the deltoid area may be used only if it is well developed. To prevent nausea and vomiting during surgery, inject the drug 15 min prior to induction of anesthesia.
Intravenous administration	Administer slowly (1–2 ml/min). If this route must be used for elderly or debilitated patients, limit the dose to 0.2 mg/kg and administer with caution.
Patients receiving epinephrine or other vasopressors	Reduce dosage of benzquinamide and monitor blood pressure during administration

WARNINGS/PRECAUTIONS

Sudden hypertension and transient arrhythmias	May occur following IV administration, making the IM route preferable for most patients; do not use the IV route in the presence of cardiovascular disease or in patients receiving preanesthetic or cardiovascular medications

EMETE-CON ■ EMETROL

Diagnostic interference	The antiemetic action of benzquinamide may mask signs of drug overdosage or obscure diagnosis of such conditions as intestinal obstruction or a brain tumor

ADVERSE REACTIONS

Autonomic nervous system	Dry mouth, shivering, sweating, hiccoughs, flushing, salivation, blurred vision
Central nervous system and neuromuscular	Drowsiness, insomnia, restlessness, headache, excitement, nervousness, twitching, shaking, tremors, weakness, fatigue
Cardiovascular	Hypertension, hypotension, dizziness, atrial fibrillation, premature auricular and ventricular contractions
Gastrointestinal	Anorexia, nausea
Dermatological	Urticaria, rash
Allergic	Fever and urticaria (one case)
Other	Chills, increased temperature

OVERDOSAGE

Signs and symptoms	CNS stimulation or depression may be anticipated, based upon animal toxicology studies
Treatment	Institute general supportive measures, as required. Atropine may be helpful in controlling autonomic signs. Dialysis is not likely to be of value, owing to extensive plasma protein binding of the drug.

DRUG INTERACTIONS

Epinephrine and other vasopressors	⇧ Hypertensive effect of benzquinamide

ALTERED LABORATORY VALUES

No clinically significant alterations in blood/serum or urinary values occur at therapeutic dosages

---

USE IN CHILDREN

Not recommended for use in children because of inadequate clinical experience

USE IN PREGNANT AND NURSING WOMEN

Safety for use during pregnancy has not been established; administration to pregnant women is not recommended, despite the lack of evidence of teratogenicity in chick embryos, mice, rats, and rabbits. Consult manufacturer for use in nursing mothers.

ANTINAUSEANTS/ANTIEMETICS

EMETROL (dextrose, levulose, and phosphoric acid) Rorer   OTC

Solution (per 5 ml): 1.87 g dextrose, 1.87 g levulose, and 21.5 mg phosphoric acid (3, 16 fl oz) *mint-flavored*

INDICATIONS	**ORAL DOSAGE**
Nausea and vomiting due to functional causes, drug therapy, or inhalation anesthesia; **motion sickness**	**Adult:** 15–30 ml (1–2 tbsp) at 15-min intervals until vomiting ceases; if first dose is rejected, resume dosage schedule in 5 min **Infant and child:** 5–10 ml (1–2 tsp) at 15-min intervals until vomiting ceases; if first dose is rejected, resume dosage schedule in 5 min
Regurgitation in infants	**Infant:** 5–10 ml (1–2 tsp) 10–15 min before feeding; for difficult cases; 10–15 ml (2–3 tsp) ½ h before feeding
"Morning sickness"	**Adult:** 15–30 ml (1–2 tbsp) on arising, repeated q3h or whenever nausea threatens

CONTRAINDICATIONS

None known

ADMINISTRATION/DOSAGE ADJUSTMENTS

Administer undiluted	Do not dilute solution or permit oral fluids immediately before or for at least 15 min after dose
Motion sickness	Administer the first dose before starting travel and repeat at convenient intervals during trip

WARNINGS/PRECAUTIONS

Persistent or frequent nausea	This preparation should not be taken without medical consultation for more than 1 h (5 doses) or if nausea continues or recurs frequently

EMETROL ■ MARINOL

ADVERSE REACTIONS
None reported by manufacturer

OVERDOSAGE
No toxicity has occurred in clinical use

DRUG INTERACTIONS
No clinically significant drug interactions have been identified

ALTERED LABORATORY VALUES
No clinically significant alterations in blood/serum or urinary values occur at therapeutic dosages

USE IN CHILDREN	USE IN PREGNANT AND NURSING WOMEN
See INDICATIONS and ORAL DOSAGE	Indicated for treatment of morning sickness. Consult manufacturer for use in nursing mothers.

ANTINAUSEANTS/ANTIEMETICS

MARINOL (dronabinol) Roxane   C-II
Capsules: 2.5, 5, 10 mg

INDICATIONS
Nausea and vomiting associated with cancer chemotherapy in patients who have not responded adequately to conventional antiemetic therapy

ORAL DOSAGE
Adult: 5 mg/m^2 to start, given 1–3 h prior to administration of chemotherapy; repeat q2–4h after chemotherapy, for a total of 4–6 doses/day. If necessary, dosage may be increased by increments of 2.5 mg/m^2; maximum dose: 15 mg/m^2

CONTRAINDICATIONS
Nausea and vomiting due to causes other than cancer chemotherapy

Hypersensitivity to dronabinol or sesame oil

ADMINISTRATION/DOSAGE ADJUSTMENTS
Duration of therapy — Prescribe only the amount necessary for a single cycle of chemotherapy (ie, a few days)

WARNINGS/PRECAUTIONS

Mental impairment — Caution patients about driving or engaging in other potentially hazardous activities requiring sound judgment and unimpaired coordination; the effects of dronabinol may persist for a variable, unpredictable period of time following administration

Patient monitoring — Patients receiving dronabinol should remain under close observation of a responsible adult, if possible within an inpatient setting, for as long as seems clinically warranted. Although close supervision is especially important for patients who are naive about the effects of cannabis, even patients who are experienced users of this drug (or cannabis) may suffer serious, unpredictable reactions.

Special-risk patients — Use with caution in patients with hypertension or heart disease and in manic, depressive, or schizophrenic patients whose symptoms may be unmasked following use of this drug; use with caution in patients receiving other psychoactive agents

Psychoses, mood changes — Advise patient of possible mood changes and other behavioral effects resulting from use of this drug to avoid any panic should such manifestations occur. Closely observe any patient who has a psychotic experience with this drug, and withhold therapy until the patient's mental state returns to normal; counsel the patient about the experience, and allow the patient to share in any decision regarding further use of this drug. If deemed necessary, dronabinol may be reinstituted at a lower dose and under very close medical supervision.

Withdrawal syndrome — A withdrawal syndrome consisting of irritability, insomnia, and restlessness has been observed in some patients within 12 h of abrupt discontinuation of therapy; this syndrome reached peak intensity after 24 h, when patients experienced "hot flashes," sweating, rhinorrhea, loose stools, hiccoughs, and anorexia, and was essentially complete within 96 h

Cardiovascular changes — An initial drug-induced tachycardia successively replaced by normal sinus rhythm and then bradycardia has been observed at high doses (210 mg/day). A fall in supine blood pressure, made worse by standing, has also been observed initially; these effects disappeared within days, however, indicating tolerance development.

MARINOL ■ PEPTO-BISMOL

EEG changes	Following discontinuation of dronabinol use, EEG changes have been consistent with a withdrawal syndrome (see above). Dronabinol has produced a decrease in REM sleep in patients during therapy, followed by a marked rebound of REM sleep after termination of therapy. An impression of disturbed sleep, lasting several weeks after high-dose therapy was discontinued, was reported by several subjects.
Carcinogenicity	No studies have been performed to determine the carcinogenic potential of this drug
Impairment of fertility	A decrease in pregnancy rate has been observed in rats and mice at 8–32 times the human dose and 32–400 times the human dose, respectively. A long-term study in rats fed 3–17 times the human dose of dronabinol revealed reduced ventral prostate, seminal vesicle, and epididymal weights and decreases in seminal fluid volume, spermatogenesis, number of developing germ cells, and number of Leydig cells in the testis; however, sperm count, mating success, and testosterone levels were not affected. The significance of these findings in humans is unknown.

ADVERSE REACTIONS

Frequent reactions (incidence ≥ 1%) are printed in *italics*

Central nervous system	*Drowsiness (48%), dizziness (21%), anxiety (16%), muddled thinking (12%), perceptual difficulties (11%), coordination impairment (9%), irritability/weird feeling and depression (7%), weakness, sluggishness, and headache (6%), hallucinations and memory lapse (5%), unsteadiness and ataxia (4%), paranoia and depersonalization (2%), disorientation and confusion (1%);* tinnitus and nightmares (rare)
Ophthalmic	*Visual distortions (3%)*
Cardiovascular	*Tachycardia and postural hypotension (1%);* syncope (rare)
Musculoskeletal	*Paresthesia (3%);* muscular pains (rare)
Gastrointestinal	Diarrhea and fecal incontinence (rare)
Other	*Dry mouth (3%);* speech difficulty, facial flushing, and perspiring (rare)

OVERDOSAGE

Signs and symptoms	See ADVERSE REACTIONS; physiologic and psychotomimetic reactions may vary widely
Treatment	Observe patient closely in a quiet environment and institute supportive measures, including reassurance; in clinical trials, disturbing reactions have spontaneously disappeared within 24 h without specific medical therapy. Monitor vital signs closely, and observe patient for tachycardia and hyper- or hypotension; treat such symptoms with appropriate measures. Withhold treatment until patient returns to baseline; then, if clinically indicated, therapy may be resumed at a lower dosage.

DRUG INTERACTIONS

Alcohol	⇧ CNS depression; do not use concomitantly ⇩ Absorption of alcohol - ⇧ or ⇩ Metabolism of alcohol
Sedatives, hypnotics, other psychotomimetic substances	⇧ CNS depression; do not use concomitantly

ALTERED LABORATORY VALUES

No clinically significant changes in blood/serum or urinary values occur at therapeutic dosages

---

USE IN CHILDREN

Consult manufacturer

USE IN PREGNANT AND NURSING WOMEN

Pregnancy Category B: substantial reductions in maternal weight gain, decreases in the number of viable pups, and increases in fetal mortality and early resorptions have occurred in mice and rats fed 400 and 32 times the human dose of dronabinol, respectively. These effects were dose-dependent; at lower doses, the effects were less apparent, and less maternal toxicity was produced. No adequate, well-controlled studies have been performed in pregnant women; use during pregnancy only if clearly needed. Dronabinol is excreted in human milk; do not use in nursing mothers.

ANTINAUSEANTS/ANTIEMETICS

PEPTO-BISMOL (bismuth subsalicylate) Procter & Gamble   OTC

Chewable tablets: 262 mg[1] *sugar-free*   **Liquid (per 5 ml):** 87.3 mg[1] (4, 8, 12, 16 fl oz) *sugar-free*

INDICATIONS	ORAL DOSAGE
Diarrhea, indigestion, heartburn, nausea, and upset stomach	**Adult:** 524 mg (2 tabs or 30 ml [2 tbsp]) q1/2–1h, as needed, up to a maximum of 4,192 mg (8 doses)/24 h **Child (3–6 yr):** 87.3 mg (1/3 tab or 5 ml [1 tsp]) q1/2–1h, as needed, up to a maximum of approximately 698 mg (8 doses)/24 h **Child (6–9 yr):** 174.6 mg (2/3 tab or 10 ml [2 tsp]) q1/2–1h, as needed, up to a maximum of approximately 1,397 mg (8 doses)/24 h **Child (9–12 yr):** 262 mg (1 tab or 15 ml [1 tbsp]) q1/2–1h, as needed, up to a maximum of 2,096 mg (8 doses)/24 h

PEPTO-BISMOL ■ PHENERGAN

CONTRAINDICATIONS

Hypersensitivity to salicylates

ADMINISTRATION/DOSAGE ADJUSTMENTS

Administration of tablets	Tablets may be chewed or dissolved in the mouth

WARNINGS/PRECAUTIONS

Reye's syndrome	Package label warns patients to consult a physician before they give this product to a child or teen-ager during or after recovery from chicken pox or influenza
Persistent diarrhea, fever	Package label cautions patients to consult a physician if diarrhea continues for more than 2 days or is accompanied by high fever
Sodium content	< 2 mg/tab; for sodium content of liquid, consult manufacturer
Concomitant therapy	If tinnitus occurs after concomitant use with aspirin, discontinue use of bismuth subsalicylate; use with caution in patients requiring oral anticoagulant, antidiabetic, or antigout medication (see DRUG INTERACTIONS)

ADVERSE REACTIONS

Gastrointestinal	Temporary darkening of stool and tongue (reaction is harmless)

OVERDOSAGE

No toxic effects have been observed in clinical use

DRUG INTERACTIONS

Oral anticoagulants	⇧ Risk of bleeding
Insulin, oral hypoglycemics	⇧ Risk of hypoglycemia
Probenecid, sulfinpyrazone	⇩ Uricosuric effect

ALTERED LABORATORY VALUES

Blood/serum values	⇧ Uric acid

No clinically significant alterations in urinary values occur at therapeutic dosages

---

USE IN CHILDREN
See INDICATIONS and ORAL DOSAGE

USE IN PREGNANT AND NURSING WOMEN
Consult manufacturer

---

[1] Salicylate content: 102 mg per tab or tbsp

ANTINAUSEANTS/ANTIEMETICS

PHENERGAN (promethazine hydrochloride) Wyeth   Rx

Tablets: 12.5, 25, 50 mg   **Syrup (per 5 ml):** 6.25 mg (Syrup Plain—4, 6, 8 fl oz; 1 pt; 1 gal) *fruit flavored*, 25 mg (Syrup Fortis—1 pt)   **Rectal suppositories:** 12.5, 25, 50 mg

INDICATIONS

Seasonal and perennial **allergic rhinitis**
Vasomotor rhinitis
Allergic conjunctivitis owing to inhalant allergens and foods
Mild, uncomplicated, allergic manifestations of **urticaria and angioedema**
Allergic reactions to blood or plasma
Dermatographism
Anaphylactic reactions (adjunctive therapy)

Motion sickness

ORAL AND RECTAL DOSAGE

Adult: for minor reactions to blood or plasma, 25 mg; for other allergic reactions, oral doses of 25 mg, given at bedtime, to start or, if necessary, oral doses of 12.5 mg, given before meals and at bedtime, to start, or, alternatively, when oral administration is not feasible, a rectal dose of 25 mg, repeated, if necessary, within 2 h after the first dose. Treat anaphylactic reactions after the acute manifestations have been controlled; use promethazine in conjunction with epinephrine and other standard measures.
Child (> 2 yr): for minor reactions to blood or plasma, 25 mg; for other allergic reactions, oral doses of 25 mg, given at bedtime, to start or, if necessary, oral doses of 6.25–12.5 mg, given tid, to start, or, alternatively, when oral administration is not feasible, a rectal dose of 25 mg, repeated, if necessary, within 2 h after the first dose. Treat anaphylactic reactions after the acute manifestations have been controlled; use promethazine in conjunction with epinephrine and other standard measures.

Adult: 25 mg, given 30–60 min before departure, 8–12 h later, and then, on each subsequent day of travel, at the time of arising and before the evening meal
Child (> 2 yr): 12.5–25 mg, given 30–60 min before departure, 8–12 h later, and then, on each subsequent day of travel, at the time of arising and before the evening meal

PHENERGAN

Nausea and vomiting associated with anesthesia and surgery	**Adult:** for prophylaxis, 25 mg q4–6h; for treatment, 25 mg to start, followed, if necessary, by 12.5–25 mg q4–6h **Child (> 2 yr):** for treatment, 0.5 mg/lb q4–6h
Sedation	**Adult:** for *nighttime sedation*, 25–50 mg or, before surgery, 50 mg, given in either case at bedtime; for use as a *preoperative medication*, 50 mg, given with 50 mg of meperidine and the appropriate dose of a belladonna alkaloid; for *obstetric sedation*, 25–50 mg, given alone or with a narcotic analgesic; for *postoperative pain* (adjunctive therapy), 25–50 mg, given with meperidine or another analgesic **Child (> 2 yr):** for *nighttime sedation* before surgery or at other times, 12.5–25 mg, given at bedtime; for use as a *preoperative medication*, an oral dose of 0.5 mg/lb or a rectal dose of either 25 mg (for children under 3 yr of age) or 50 mg (for children over 3 yr of age), given with an equal dose of meperidine and the appropriate dose of an atropine-like drug; for *postoperative pain* (adjunctive therapy), 12.5–25 mg, given with meperidine or another analgesic

CONTRAINDICATIONS

Asthma or other lower respiratory tract conditions	Hypersensitivity or idiosyncratic reaction to promethazine or other phenothiazines

WARNINGS/PRECAUTIONS

Drowsiness, dizziness	Caution patients that they may drive or engage in other potentially hazardous activities requiring mental alertness or physical coordination only after it has been established that this preparation does not make them drowsy or dizzy (see also USE IN CHILDREN)
Photosensitivity, extrapyramidal reactions	Photosensitivity and extrapyramidal reactions such as oculogyric crisis, torticollis, and tongue protrusion have occurred in rare instances; the extrapyramidal reactions have usually resulted from excessive dosage. Instruct patients to report any involuntary muscle movements or unusual sensitivity to sunlight.
Patients with a history of sleep apnea	Avoid use in patients with a history of sleep apnea
Patients with GI or GU conditions	Use with caution in patients with hepatic impairment, stenosing peptic ulcer, pyloro-duodenal obstruction, symptomatic prostatic hypertrophy, or bladder neck obstruction
Other special-risk patients	Use with caution in patients with convulsive disorders, cardiovascular disease, or narrow angle glaucoma
Carcinogenicity, mutagenicity, effect on fertility	No long-term studies have been performed in animals to evaluate the carcinogenic potential of promethazine. Use in the Ames test has produced no evidence of mutagenicity. The effect of promethazine on fertility has not been assessed.

ADVERSE REACTIONS

Central nervous system	Sedation, sleepiness, blurred vision, dizziness, disorientation, confusion, and extrapyramidal reactions (rare)
Cardiovascular	Hypertension, hypotension
Gastrointestinal	Nausea, vomiting, cholestatic jaundice
Hematological	Leukopenia and thrombocytopenia (rare), agranulocytosis (one case)
Dermatological	Rash; photosensitivity (rare)
Other	Dry mouth

OVERDOSAGE

Signs and symptoms	*CNS:* extreme somnolence, stupor, coma, hyperexcitability, nightmares, convulsions (CNS stimulation is especially likely to occur in children and the elderly); *respiratory:* decrease in respiratory rate and/or tidal volume; *cardiovascular:* flushing, hypotension; *other:* mydriasis, dry mouth, GI reactions
Treatment	To maintain pulmonary function, establish a patent airway, and provide assisted or controlled ventilation. Correct acidosis and electrolyte losses. To treat severe hypotension, use norepinephrine or phenylephrine, not epinephrine. Diazepam may be given to control convulsions. Do not give analeptic drugs for CNS depression. Monitor vital signs only in cases of extreme overdosage or individual sensitivity. To remove this preparation from the body, administer activated charcoal or use sodium or magnesium sulfate as a cathartic; limited experience indicates that dialysis is not helpful.

DRUG INTERACTIONS

Alcohol, narcotic drugs, sedative-hypnotics (eg, barbiturates), tranquilizers, local anesthetics, and other CNS depressants	⇧ CNS depression; instruct patients requiring this preparation that other CNS depressants should be avoided or used at a lower dosage (for concomitant use with this preparation, reduce the dosage of a narcotic analgesic by 25–50% and the dosage of a barbiturate by at least 50% ⇧ Risk of convulsions (with concomitant use of narcotic drugs or local anesthetics)

ALTERED LABORATORY VALUES

Blood/serum values	⇧ Glucose

PHENERGAN ■ PHENERGAN Injection

Urinary values —— False-positive and false-negative pregnancy test

USE IN CHILDREN
See INDICATIONS and ORAL DOSAGE; do not give to children under 2 yr of age because safety for use in such patients has not been established. Children undergoing treatment should be supervised whenever they ride a bicycle or engage in other potentially hazardous activities requiring mental alertness or physical coordination.

USE IN PREGNANT AND NURSING WOMEN
Pregnancy Category C: promethazine has been shown to be fetotoxic in rodents; no evidence of teratogenicity has been observed in rats fed 6.25 or 12.5 mg/kg/day. Inhibition of platelet aggregation may occur in a neonate if this preparation is taken within 2 wk before delivery. This medication should be used during pregnancy only if the expected benefit justifies the potential risk to the fetus or neonate. It is not known whether promethazine is excreted in human milk; use with caution in nursing mothers.

VEHICLE/BASE
Suppository: ascorbyl palmitate, silicon dioxide, white wax, and cocoa butter
Syrup Fortis: 1.5% alcohol
Syrup Plain: 7% alcohol

ANTINAUSEANTS/ANTIEMETICS

PHENERGAN Injection (promethazine hydrochloride) Wyeth Rx
Ampuls: 25, 50 mg/ml (1 ml) **Cartridge-needle units:** 25, 50 mg/ml (1 ml)

INDICATIONS	PARENTERAL DOSAGE
Uncomplicated **immediate-type allergic reactions,** when oral therapy is impossible or contraindicated **Allergic reactions to blood or plasma** **Anaphylactic reactions,** as an adjunct to epinephrine and other standard measures after acute symptoms have been controlled	**Adult:** 25 mg IM (deeply) or IV, repeated within 2 h, if needed **Child:** up to 12.5 mg IM (deeply) or IV, repeated within 2 h, if needed
Motion sickness **Nausea and vomiting** associated with anesthesia and surgery	**Adult:** 12.5–25 mg IM (deeply) or IV, repeated not more often than q4h, as needed **Child:** up to 6.25–12.5 mg IM (deeply) or IV, repeated not more often than q4h, as needed (see warning concerning pediatric use)
Nighttime sedation in hospitalized patients	**Adult:** 25–50 mg IM (deeply) or IV **Child:** up to 12.5–25 mg IM (deeply) or IV
As an adjunct to **preoperative or postoperative medication**	**Adult:** 25–50 mg IM (deeply) or IV; reduce dosage of analgesics, hypnotics, and atropine-like drugs accordingly **Child:** 0.5 mg/lb IM (deeply) or IV, with an equal dose of a narcotic analgesic or barbiturate and the appropriate amount of atropine-like drug
As an adjunct to **analgesia and anesthesia** in special surgical situations, including repeated bronchoscopy, ophthalmic surgery, and poor-risk patients	**Adult:** 25–50 mg IV; reduce dosage of narcotic analgesics accordingly **Child:** up to 12.5–25 mg IV; reduce dosage of narcotic analgesics accordingly
Obstetric sedation	**Adult:** for sedation and relief of apprehension in early stages of labor, 50 mg IM (deeply) or IV; when labor is definitely established, 25–75 mg IM (deeply) or IV, repeated once or twice q4h up to 100 mg/24 h; reduce dosage of narcotic analgesics accordingly

CONTRAINDICATIONS
Hypersensitivity or idiosyncratic reaction to promethazine
Drug-induced CNS depression
Comatose states
Intraarterial or SC injection (see ADMINISTRATION/DOSAGE ADJUSTMENTS)

ADMINISTRATION/DOSAGE ADJUSTMENTS
Route of administration —— Preferred route is by deep IM injection. Extreme care should be taken when using IV route that intraarterial injection or perivascular extravasation does not occur (see WARNINGS/PRECAUTIONS); IV concentration should not exceed 25 mg/ml, nor rate of administration exceed 25 mg/min. The SC route is contraindicated; necrotic lesions (on rare occasions) and chemical irritation have occurred after SC injection.

Elderly patients —— Reduce dosage in patients over 60 yr of age

Concomitant therapy —— Reduce the usual dose of barbiturates by at least one half and of narcotic analgesics by one fourth to one half

PHENERGAN Injection

WARNINGS/PRECAUTIONS

Inadvertent intraarterial injection, perivascular extravasation	Pain, severe chemical irritation, severe spasm of distal vessels, and resultant gangrene requiring amputation may occur. Although there is no proven successful management, sympathetic block and heparinization are commonly used. Aspiration of dark blood does not preclude intraarterial needle placement, since blood is discolored upon contact with promethazine.
Drowsiness, disturbed coordination	Caution ambulatory patients about driving or engaging in other potentially hazardous activities requiring mental alertness and/or physical coordination, and about using alcohol or other CNS depressants (see DRUG INTERACTIONS)
Infants and children	Not recommended for treatment of uncomplicated vomiting; use only for prolonged vomiting of known etiology. Extrapyramidal symptoms secondary to use of promethazine may be confused with CNS signs of undiagnosed primary disease; avoid use when signs and symptoms suggest the presence of Reye's syndrome or other hepatic diseases. Excessively large doses may cause hallucinations, convulsions, and sudden death. Paradoxical hyperexcitability and abnormal movements may occur following a single dose, which may indicate relative overdosage; discontinue drug. Acutely ill, dehydrated children may be susceptible to dystonias.
Patients with pain	Excessive amounts of promethazine relative to narcotic analgesic dose may cause restlessness and motor hyperactivity
Patients with bone-marrow depression	Use with caution; leukopenia and agranulocytosis have been reported, usually when promethazine has been used with other known toxic agents
Special-risk patients	Use with caution in patients with cardiovascular disease, impaired liver function, asthmatic attacks, narrow-angle glaucoma, stenosing peptic ulcer, pyloroduodenal obstruction, prostatic hypertrophy, or bladder-neck obstruction
Diagnostic interference	Antiemetic effects may mask signs and symptoms of unrecognized disease

ADVERSE REACTIONS

Central nervous system	Drowsiness, extrapyramidal effects, dizziness, lassitude, tinnitus, incoordination, fatigue, euphoria, nervousness, insomnia, tremors, convulsive seizures, oculogyric crises, excitation, catatonic-like states, hysteria
Ophthalmic	Blurred vision, diplopia
Cardiovascular	Tachycardia, bradycardia, faintness, dizziness, hypotension or hypertension, venous thrombosis at injection site
Gastrointestinal	Nausea, vomiting, dry mouth, obstructive jaundice
Hypersensitivity	Urticaria, dermatitis, asthma, photosensitivity, angioneurotic edema
Hematological	Leukopenia, agranulocytosis, thrombocytopenic purpura
Other	Nasal stuffiness; tissue necrosis following SC injection

OVERDOSAGE

Signs and symptoms	Range from mild CNS and cardiovascular depression to profound hypotension, respiratory depression, and unconsciousness. Stimulation may be present, especially in children and in geriatric patients. Atropine-like signs and symptoms (eg, dry mouth; fixed, dilated pupils; flushing) and GI disturbances may occur
Treatment	Generally supportive and symptomatic; *do not use stimulants* for CNS depression. Treat severe hypotension with norepinephrine or phenylephrine; *do not use epinephrine*. Treat extrapyramidal reactions with anticholinergic antiparkinsonism agents, diphenhydramine, or barbiturates. Additional measures include administration of oxygen and IV fluids. Dialysis does not seem to be helpful.

DRUG INTERACTIONS

Alcohol, tranquilizers, sedative-hypnotics (including barbiturates), general anesthetics, narcotic preparations, and other CNS depressants	△ CNS depression
MAO inhibitors	△ Risk of extrapyramidal side effects[1]

ALTERED LABORATORY VALUES

Blood/serum values	△ Glucose tolerance
Urinary values	False-negative and false-positive pregnancy tests

---

USE IN CHILDREN

See INDICATIONS, dosage recommendations, and WARNINGS/PRECAUTIONS

USE IN PREGNANT AND NURSING WOMEN

Pregnancy Category C: use during pregnancy only if the expected therapeutic benefit justifies the potential risk to the fetus. Reproduction studies have been done in animals (consult manufacturer for information); however, no adequate, well-controlled studies have been performed in pregnant women. It is not known whether this drug is excreted in human milk.

---

[1] Although such a reaction has not been reported with promethazine, it has occurred when other phenothiazines and some MAO inhibitors have been used concomitantly

ANTINAUSEANTS/ANTIEMETICS

REGLAN (metoclopramide hydrochloride) Robins Rx

Tablets: 10 mg **Syrup (per 5 ml):** 5 mg (10 ml; 1 pt) *sugar-free* **Ampuls:** 5 mg/ml (2, 10 ml) **Vials:** 5 mg/ml (2, 10, 30 ml)

INDICATIONS	ORAL DOSAGE	PARENTERAL DOSAGE
Gastroesophageal reflux, when conventional therapy is ineffective	**Adult:** for symptomatic relief, 10–15 mg qid, 30 min before each meal and at bedtime, for 4–12 wk; if symptoms only occur at certain times of the day (eg, after the evening meal), consider giving a single dose of up to 20 mg only before each of those times rather than using the drug throughout the day. For treatment of esophageal lesions, give 15 mg qid for up to 12 wk; monitor therapy endoscopically.	—
Symptomatic relief of acute and recurrent **diabetic gastroparesis (diabetic gastric stasis)**	**Adult:** 10 mg 30 min before each meal and at bedtime for 2–8 wk, as needed; reinstitute therapy at earliest sign of recurrence	**Adult:** for severe symptoms, 10 mg IM or IV 30 min before each meal and at bedtime for up to 10 days; switch to oral therapy when symptoms subside
Prevention of nausea and vomiting associated with emetogenic cancer chemotherapy	—	**Adult:** 1 mg/kg, given by slow IV infusion 30 min before administering the antineoplastic agent, then q2h for 2 doses, and finally q3h for 3 doses; if highly emetogenic drugs such as cisplatin and dacarbazine are used, increase the first 2 doses to 2 mg/kg
Facilitation of small bowel intubation if tube has not passed the pylorus with conventional maneuvers in 10 min **Facilitation of radiological examination** of stomach and/or small intestine in cases where delayed gastric emptying interferes with examination		**Adult:** 10 mg IV **Child (< 6 yr):** 0.1 mg/kg IV **Child (6–14 yr):** 2.5–5 mg IV

CONTRAINDICATIONS		
Conditions in which stimulation of GI motility may be hazardous (eg, GI hemorrhage and mechanical obstruction or perforation)	Epilepsy Use of drugs likely to cause extrapyramidal reactions	Pheochromocytoma Hypersensitivity or intolerance to metoclopramide

ADMINISTRATION/DOSAGE ADJUSTMENTS	
Treatment of gastroesophageal reflux	The principal effect of metoclopramide is on symptoms of postprandial and daytime heartburn, with less observed effect on nocturnal symptoms
Symptomatic relief of gastroparesis	The usual manifestations of delayed gastric emptying may respond to therapy within different time intervals: relief of nausea occurs early and continues to improve over a 3-wk period; relief of vomiting and anorexia may precede relief of abdominal fullness by 1 wk or more
Intravenous administration	Inject doses of 10 mg or less, undiluted, over a period of 1–2 min; avoid rapid administration, which may evoke intense anxiety and restlessness initially and then cause drowsiness. To administer doses exceeding 10 mg, dilute the drug in 50 ml of a parenteral solution, preferably 0.9% sodium chloride injection, and then give by infusion over a period of at least 15 min. Ringer's injection, lactated Ringer's injection, and 5% dextrose in water or in 0.45% sodium chloride can be used as alternative diluents; do not freeze preparations diluted with 5% dextrose in water. Prepared solutions exposed to light should be used within 24 h. For information on compatibility, see DRUG INTERACTIONS and package insert.
Patients with renal impairment	If creatinine clearance is less than 40 ml/min, begin treatment at 50% of the usual dosage; since only a small amount of the drug is removed by hemodialysis and continuous peritoneal dialysis, a dosage adjustment to compensate for losses due to dialysis is unlikely to be necessary

REGLAN

WARNINGS/PRECAUTIONS

Tardive dyskinesia — Metoclopramide can cause tardive dyskinesia, a potentially irreversible syndrome characterized by involuntary choreoathetoid movements of the tongue, face, mouth, lips, jaw, trunk, and/or extremities. Protrusion of the tongue, puffing of the cheeks, puckering of the mouth, chewing movements, and other manifestations may become evident during treatment, upon dosage reduction, or after the drug is discontinued. The likelihood that tardive dyskinesia will develop or become irreversible increases with duration of treatment and total cumulative dose; however, even relatively brief use of low doses can cause it. Although this reaction appears to occur most often in the elderly, especially among older women, it is impossible to use this information to predict, before therapy is started, which patients are likely to develop the syndrome. Bear in mind that metoclopramide can itself mask signs of the disorder. There is no known treatment for tardive dyskinesia; however, after discontinuation, some or all manifestations may disappear spontaneously. Although metoclopramide can suppress these manifestations, the drug should not be used for this purpose since the effects of suppression on the long-term course of the disorder are not known.

Dystonia — At a dosage of 30–40 mg/day, acute dystonic reactions occur in approximately 0.2% of patients, with effects more commonly seen in children and young adults than in others; at doses of 1–2 mg/kg, the frequency is 2% among patients over 30–35 yr of age and 25% or higher among younger adults and children. Dystonic reactions are usually seen within 24–48 h after starting treatment; they are characterized by involuntary movements of the limbs, facial grimacing, torticollis, oculogyric crisis, rhythmic protrusion of the tongue, bulbar type of speech, trismus, opisthotonus (tetanus-like reactions), or, in rare cases, stridor or dyspnea. To control symptoms, inject 50 mg of diphenhydramine or 1–2 mg of benztropine IM.

Pseudoparkinsonism, akathisia — Parkinsonian-like symptoms, including bradykinesia, tremor, cogwheel rigidity, and mask-like facies, can first occur within 6 mo after starting treatment or, occasionally, after a longer period; effects generally subside within 2–3 mo after discontinuation of therapy. Akathisia, characterized by anxiety, agitation, jitteriness, insomnia, pacing, foot tapping, and inability to sit still, can also result from therapy; reaction may disappear spontaneously or upon reduction in dosage.

Drowsiness, dizziness — Caution ambulatory patients about driving or engaging in other potentially hazardous activities requiring mental alertness or physical coordination; drowsiness occurs in approximately 10% of patients given 10 mg qid and in approximately 70% of patients given doses of 1–2 mg/kg

Hypertensive crisis — A clinical study has shown that IV administration precipitates the release of catecholamines in patients with hypertension; use metoclopramide with caution in these patients

Depression — A temporal association between metoclopramide and depression has been reported

Diabetic patients — Metoclopramide influences the delivery of food to the intestines and, hence, the rate of absorption; patients dependent upon insulin may require an adjustment in insulin dosage or timing of administration

Carcinogenicity — Metoclopramide causes an increase in serum prolactin levels which persists during chronic administration and may be important in patients with previously detected breast cancer. Although endocrine disturbances have been reported with prolactin-elevating drugs, no association has been shown between chronic administration of these drugs and mammary tumorigenesis; the available evidence is considered too limited to be conclusive at this time.

Mutagenicity — No evidence of mutagenicity has been detected in the Ames test

ADVERSE REACTIONS

Central nervous system — Restlessness, drowsiness, fatigue, lassitude, insomnia, headache, confusion, dizziness, depression; extrapyramidal reactions (dystonia, pseudoparkinsonism, akathisia, tardive dyskinesia), convulsive seizures[1]; hallucinations (rare)

Gastrointestinal — Nausea; diarrhea and other intestinal disturbances

Cardiovascular — Hypotension, hypertension; transient flushing of face and upper body (with high IV doses); supraventricular tachycardia (one case)

Endocrinological — Galactorrhea, amenorrhea, gynecomastia, impotence, fluid retention

Renal — Urinary frequency, incontinence

Hematological — Neutropenia,[1] leukopenia,[1] agranulocytosis[1]

Hypersensitivity — Rash, urticaria, and bronchospasm (especially in patients with a history of asthma); angioneurotic edema, including glossal and laryngeal edema (rare)

Other — Visual disturbances, porphyria; neuroleptic malignant syndrome, a potentially fatal syndrome characterized by hyperthermia, altered consciousness, muscular rigidity, and autonomic dysfunction (rare)

OVERDOSAGE

Signs and symptoms — Drowsiness, disorientation, extrapyramidal reactions; methemoglobinemia (in neonates given 1–2 mg/kg/day IM for 3 days or longer)

REGLAN ■ THORAZINE

Treatment — Discontinue medication. Administer anticholinergic or antiparkinson drugs or antihistamines with anticholinergic properties to control extrapyramidal reactions, if needed. Symptoms are self-limited and usually disappear within 24 h. To reverse methemoglobinemia, administer methylene blue IV. Dialysis is unlikely to be effective, since neither hemodialysis nor peritoneal dialysis removes a significant amount of the drug.

DRUG INTERACTIONS

Phenothiazines, other drugs likely to cause extrapyramidal reactions	△ Extrapyramidal effects; do not use metoclopramide with other drugs likely to produce extrapyramidal effects
MAO inhibitors	Hypertensive crisis; use metoclopramide with caution, if at all, in patients receiving MAO inhibitors
Anticholinergic agents	▽ GI motility
Narcotic analgesics	▽ GI motility △ CNS depression
Alcohol, sedative-hypnotics, tranquilizers	△ CNS depression
Apomorphine	▽ Central and peripheral effects of apomorphine
Drugs absorbed from stomach (eg, digoxin)	▽ Absorption
Drugs absorbed from small intestine (eg, acetaminophen, tetracycline, levodopa, ethanol)	△ Absorption
Cephalolithin, chloramphenicol, sodium bicarbonate	Physical incompatibility in solution; do not mix with metoclopramide

ALTERED LABORATORY VALUES

Blood/serum values — △ Prolactin △ Aldosterone (transient)

No clinically significant alterations in urinary values occur at therapeutic dosages

USE IN CHILDREN

Metoclopramide can be used in children to facilitate small bowel intubation or radiological examination; for dosage recommendations, see PARENTERAL DOSAGE. Extrapyramidal reactions occur more frequently in children; see warning, above, concerning these reactions.

USE IN PREGNANT AND NURSING WOMEN

Pregnancy Category B: use during pregnancy only if clearly needed. Reproductive studies in rats, mice, and rabbits at doses ranging up to 12–250 times the human dose have shown no evidence of impaired fertility or significant fetal harm. No adequate, well-controlled studies have been done in pregnant women. Metoclopramide is excreted in human milk; use with caution in nursing mothers.

[1] No clearcut causal relationship has been established

ANTINAUSEANTS/ANTIEMETICS

THORAZINE (chlorpromazine hydrochloride) Smith Kline & French Rx

Capsules (sustained release): 30, 75, 150, 200, 300 mg **Tablets:** 10, 25, 50, 100, 200 mg **Concentrate:** 30 mg/ml (4 fl oz, 1 gal), 100 mg/ml (8 fl oz) **Syrup (per 5 ml):** 10 mg (4 fl oz) **Ampuls:** 25 mg/ml (1, 2 ml) **Vials:** 25 mg/ml (10 ml) **Rectal suppositories:** 25, 100 mg

INDICATIONS

Manifestations of **psychotic disorders**
Manic episodes of manic-depressive illness
Nonpsychotic anxiety[1]

ORAL DOSAGE

Adult: for excessive anxiety, tension, and agitation, 30–75 mg/day (10 mg, tid or qid, or 25 mg, bid or tid); for more severe symptoms in outpatients and office patients, 25 mg tid for 1–2 days, followed, as needed, by semiweekly increases in dosage of 20–50 mg/day (usual effective dosage: 200–800 mg/day); for more severe symptoms in hospitalized patients, 25 mg tid to start, followed by a gradual increase in dosage (usual effective dosage: 400 mg/day). When treating nonpsychotic anxiety, do not exceed 100 mg/day or administer for more than 12 wk.

PARENTERAL DOSAGE

Adult: for severe symptoms in outpatients and office patients, 25 mg IM for 1 or, if necessary, 2 doses (with 1 h between doses), followed by 25–50 mg orally tid; for acute agitation, mania, or disturbance in hospitalized patients, 25 mg IM, followed, if necessary, by 25–50 mg IM 1 h later, a subsequent gradual increase in the IM dose over a period of several days (up to 400 mg q4–6h in exceptionally severe cases), and then, when the patient becomes quiet and cooperative, further titration of dosage with oral preparations

COMPENDIUM OF DRUG THERAPY

THORAZINE

Manifestations of psychotic disorders Disproportionately severe **explosive hyperexcitability or combativeness** **Conduct disorders,** associated with **hyperactivity** and characterized by impulsiveness, inattention, aggressiveness, mood lability, or poor frustration tolerance (short-term use only)	**Child:** 0.25 mg/lb q4–6h; for severe behavioral disorders or psychoses, younger hospitalized patients may need 50–100 mg/day and older hospitalized patients may require 200 mg/day or more. There is little evidence that dosages exceeding 500 mg/day further improve the behavior of severely disturbed, mentally retarded patients.	**Child:** ($< $ 5 yr or $\leq$ 50 lb): 0.25 mg/lb IM q6–8h, up to 40 mg/day **Child (5–12 yr or 50–100 lb):** 0.25 mg/lb IM q6–8h, up to 75 mg/day, except in unmanageable cases
Preoperative restlessness and apprehension	**Adult:** 25–50 mg 2–3 h before surgery **Child:** 0.25 mg/lb 2–3 h before surgery	**Adult:** 12.5–25 mg IM 1–2 h before surgery **Child:** 0.25 mg/lb IM 1–2 h before surgery
Postoperative medication	**Adult:** 10–25 mg q4–6h, as needed **Child:** 0.25 mg/lb q4–6h, as needed	**Adult:** 12.5–25 mg IM; repeat in 1 h, if needed and if no hypotension occurs **Child:** 0.25 mg/lb IM; repeat in 1 h, if needed and if no hypotension occurs
Nausea and vomiting	**Adult:** 10–25 mg q4–6h, as needed; increase dosage, if necessary **Child:** 0.25 mg/lb q4–6h	**Adult:** 25 mg IM to start; if no hypotension occurs, 25–50 mg q3–4h, as needed, until vomiting ceases; follow with oral regimen **Child ($<$ 5 yr or $<$ 50 lb):** 0.25 mg/lb IM q6–8h, up to 40 mg/day, if needed **Child (5–12 yr or 50–100 lb):** 0.25 mg/lb IM q6–8h, up to 75 mg/day, except in severe cases
Nausea and vomiting during surgery	—	**Adult:** 12.5 mg IM; repeat in ½ h, if needed and if no hypotension occurs; alternative regimen: 2 mg/fractional IV injection every 2 min, up to 25 mg; dilute to 1 mg/ml for IV administration **Child:** 0.125 mg/lb IM; repeat in ½ h if needed and if no hypotension occurs; alternative regimen: 1 mg/fractional IV injection every 2 min, up to 0.125 mg/lb; dilute to 1 mg/ml for IV administration
Intractable hiccups	**Adult:** 25–50 mg tid or qid; if symptoms persist for 2–3 days, switch to IM use	**Adult:** 25–50 mg IM, followed, if necessary, by 25–50 mg, given by slow IV infusion in 500–1,000 ml of saline while patient is lying in bed (closely monitor blood pressure)
Acute intermittent porphyria	**Adult:** 25–50 mg tid or qid	**Adult:** 25 mg IM tid or qid until patient can take oral therapy
Tetanus (adjunctive therapy)	—	**Adult:** 25–50 mg IM tid or qid; alternative regimen: 25–50 mg IV (1 mg/min); dilute to at least 1 mg/ml for IV administration **Child:** 0.25 mg/lb IM or IV (0.5 mg/min) q6–8h, up to 40 mg/day (for children $\leq$ 50 lb) or 75 mg/day (for children 50–100 lb), except in severe cases; dilute to at least 1 mg/ml for IV administration

CONTRAINDICATIONS

Coma	Presence of large amounts of CNS depressants

ADMINISTRATION/DOSAGE ADJUSTMENTS

Parenteral administration	Reserve for bedfast patients and acute ambulatory cases; keep patient lying down for at least ½ h after injection to minimize hypotensive effects. Preferred route is IM; however, IV route may be used during surgery and for tetanus and intractable hiccups. SC administration is not recommended. Intramuscular injections should be given slowly and deeply in upper outer quadrant of buttock. If irritation is a problem, dilute solution with saline or 2% procaine; do not mix with other agents in the syringe.
Rectal use	For nausea and vomiting in adults, insert one 100-mg suppository q6–8h, as needed; in some patients, dosage may be halved. For nausea and vomiting and manifestations of psychiatric disorders in children, administer 0.5 mg/lb q6–8h, as needed (eg, if child is 20–30 lb, use half a 25-mg suppository).
Dilution and storage of concentrate	Immediately prior to use, dilute desired dose of concentrate with 60 ml (2 fl oz) or more of fruit or tomato juice, milk, coffee, tea, water, carbonated beverage, simple syrup, orange syrup, or semisolid food (eg, soup, pudding). Protect concentrate from light and dispense in amber bottles; refrigeration is unnecessary.
Psychiatric regimens	Increase dosage gradually until symptoms are controlled; maximum improvement may take weeks or even months. Continue optimum dosage for 2 wk, then gradually reduce to lowest effective level for maintenance. Therapeutic response is usually not enhanced by exceeding 1 g/day for extended periods.

THORAZINE

Elderly, emaciated, or debilitated patients	Increase dosage more gradually if the patient is elderly, emaciated, or debilitated; for most elderly patients, a dosage in the lower range is sufficient. Carefully monitor clinical response of elderly patients since they appear to be more susceptible to hypotension and extrapyramidal reactions
Monitoring of long-term therapy	Periodically evaluate patients with a history of long-term neuroleptic treatment in order to determine whether the maintenance dosage can be reduced or therapy discontinued; watch for tardive dyskinesia, ocular changes, and skin pigmentation during prolonged use (see warnings below)

WARNINGS/PRECAUTIONS

Tardive dyskinesia	Neuroleptic drugs can cause tardive dyskinesia, a potentially irreversible syndrome characterized by involuntary choreoathetoid movements of the tongue, face, mouth, lips, jaw, trunk, and/or extremities. Protrusion of the tongue, puffing of the cheeks, puckering of the mouth, chewing movements, and other manifestations may become evident during treatment, upon dosage reduction, or after the drug is discontinued. The likelihood that tardive dyskinesia will develop or become irreversible increases with duration of treatment and total cumulative dose; however, even relatively brief use of low doses can cause it. Although this reaction appears to occur most often in the elderly, especially among older women, it is impossible to use this information to predict, before therapy is started, which patients are likely to develop the syndrome.

In general, reserve chronic therapy for patients who respond to neuroleptics and who cannot undergo another, equally effective form of treatment that is potentially less harmful. Use the lowest effective dosage, keep the duration of therapy as short as possible, and periodically reassess the need for the drug. Watch carefully for manifestations of tardive dyskinesia; fine vermicular movements of the tongue reportedly may be an early sign. However, do not forget that neuroleptic therapy can itself mask the signs and symptoms of tardive dyskinesia. If evidence of the syndrome is seen, consider terminating use of the drug, bearing in mind that some patients may require continued neuroleptic treatment despite the development of dyskinesia. There is no known treatment for tardive dyskinesia; however, after discontinuation, some or all manifestations of this syndrome may disappear spontaneously. |
Dystonias	To control dystonias, discontinue neuroleptic therapy and take the following measures: for mild cases, provide reassurance or give a barbiturate; for moderate cases, use a barbiturate; for more severe cases, administer an antiparkinson agent other than levodopa; for children, provide reassurance and give either a barbiturate or parenteral diphenhydramine. If antiparkinson agents or diphenhydramine fail to reverse signs and symptoms, reevaluate diagnosis. Appropriate supportive measures, such as those needed to maintain adequate hydration and a patent airway, should be instituted as required. Dystonias usually subside within a few hours and almost always within 24–48 h after the drug has been discontinued. If treatment is resumed, administer at a lower dosage.
Akathisia	Symptoms of akathisia often disappear spontaneously; if they become too troublesome, reduce dosage or give a barbiturate. Wait until effects subside before increasing dosage. At times, drug-induced symptoms of akathisia may resemble psychotic or neurotic manifestations seen before therapy.
Pseudoparkinsonism	In most cases, pseudoparkinsonism can be controlled by concomitant use of an antiparkinson agent other than levodopa; occasionally, it is necessary to reduce the dosage of chlorpromazine or discontinue the drug. Administration of antiparkinson drugs for a period ranging from a few weeks to 2–3 mo is generally sufficient; clinical response should be evaluated before continuing therapy for a longer period.
Cross-sensitivity	Do not use chlorpromazine in patients with a history of hypersensitivity to a phenothiazine unless potential benefits outweigh possible risks; see also warnings below concerning hepatotoxicity and blood dyscrasias
Hepatotoxicity	Drug-induced jaundice, a hypersensitivity reaction with clinical characteristics of infectious hepatitis and laboratory features of obstructive jaundice, has been seen in most cases between the second and fourth weeks of therapy; the reaction is generally reversible, but may be chronic. Do not give chlorpromazine to patients with a history of phenothiazine-induced jaundice unless the potential benefits outweigh the possible risks. Although there is no conclusive evidence that patients with hepatic disease are particularly susceptible to jaundice, use with caution in such patients. If fever with grippe-like symptoms occurs, perform appropriate liver tests; if an abnormality is detected, stop treatment. Since this drug is potentially hepatotoxic, use in children or adolescents with signs or symptoms suggesting Reye's syndrome should be avoided. Abnormal values associated with extrahepatic obstruction may be similar to those seen with drug-induced jaundice; confirm diagnosis of extrahepatic obstruction before performing exploratory laparotomy.
Blood dyscrasias	Agranulocytosis and other hematological reactions can occur during therapy; caution patients to report the sudden appearance of sore throat or other signs or symptoms of infection. Watch closely for evidence of agranulocytosis between the fourth and tenth week of therapy since the disease is most likely to occur at that time; if signs of infection are seen and WBC and differential counts are depressed, stop therapy and institute appropriate measures. Do not give chlorpromazine to patients with bone marrow depression or a history of phenothiazine-induced blood dyscrasias unless the potential benefits outweigh the possible risks.

THORAZINE

Hypotension	The first parenteral dose may produce orthostatic hypotension, simple tachycardia, momentary faintness, and dizziness; these effects occasionally occur after subsequent injections and, in rare cases, following the first oral dose. Hypotensive effects usually disappear within 30–120 min, but occasionally may be severe and prolonged, causing a shock-like condition. Severe hypotension has occurred in patients with pheochromocytoma or mitral insufficiency. To minimize the risk of hypotension, keep all patients recumbent and under observation for at least 30 min after the initial injection. Exercise caution when giving this drug to patients with cardiovascular disease. If hypotension occurs, place patient in a head-low position with the legs raised; if a vasopressor is needed, use norepinephrine or phenylephrine, not epinephrine (see DRUG INTERACTIONS).
Ocular effects, skin pigmentation	Use of substantial doses for a prolonged period may cause ocular changes and skin pigmentation. Administration of 300 mg or more daily for 2 yr or longer has caused deposition of fine particulate matter in the lens and cornea and, in more severe cases, star-shaped lenticular opacities and visual impairment; epithelial keratopathy and pigmentary retinopathy have also been detected. Changes in skin pigment, seen primarily in women given 500–1,500 mg/day for 3 yr or longer, range from an almost imperceptible darkening to a slate-gray color (sometimes with a violet hue). Following discontinuation of the drug, skin pigmentation may fade and eye lesions may regress. Although the cause of the ophthalmic and dermatological effects is not clear, dosage, duration of use, and exposure to sunlight appear to be the most significant factors. During long-term therapy at moderate-to-high dosage levels, perform ophthalmological examinations periodically. If ocular changes or skin pigmentation is observed during treatment, weigh benefits of continued use against possible risks and then determine whether or not to maintain the current regimen, reduce the dosage, or discontinue the drug.
Masking of nonpsychotic conditions	Extrapyramidal symptoms associated with chlorpromazine may be confused with the neurological manifestations of an undiagnosed primary disease such as Reye's syndrome or another encephalopathy; antiemetic effect may mask nausea and vomiting associated with intestinal obstruction, brain tumor, Reye's syndrome, or toxicity of antineoplastic agents or other drugs
Drowsiness	Caution patients about driving and engaging in other activities requiring mental alertness. Drowsiness may occur, especially during the first or second week of therapy, but usually disappears after this period; if drowsiness is troublesome, reduce dosage.
Cerebral dysfunction	In patients with a history of cirrhotic encephalopathy, chlorpromazine can cause abnormal slowing of the EEG and impairment of cerebral function
Convulsions	Petit mal and grand mal seizures have occurred, especially in patients with EEG abnormalities or a history of such disorders
Respiratory impairment	Use with caution in patients (especially children) with chronic respiratory disorders, such as emphysema, severe asthma, and acute respiratory infections, since this drug is a CNS depressant
Photosensitivity	Instruct patients to avoid undue exposure to the sun
Contact dermatitis	To prevent contact dermatitis, use rubber gloves when handling liquid dosage forms and avoid getting solution on clothing
Swelling of breasts, lactation	Moderate breast engorgement and lactation may occur in women with use of large doses; if reaction persists, reduce dosage or discontinue drug
Hyperthermia, glaucoma	Chlorpromazine may cause hyperthermia or exacerbate glaucoma; use with caution in patients who are exposed to extreme heat or who have glaucoma
Insecticides	Use with caution in patients exposed to organophosphorous insecticides
Aspiration of vomitus	Chlorpromazine suppresses the cough reflex and thus may increase the risk that vomitus will be aspirated
Abrupt withdrawal	Gastritis, nausea, vomiting, dizziness, and tremulousness may occur following abrupt discontinuation of high-dose therapy; to minimize risk, reduce dosage gradually or continue antiparkinson therapy for several weeks after withdrawal
Carcinogenicity	Chronic use of neuroleptic drugs causes a persistent elevation of the serum prolactin level, an effect that may be of potential importance if the patient has prolactin-dependent breast cancer. Chronic administration has produced an increase in mammary neoplasia in rodents, and endocrine disturbances have been seen in humans; although no clinical or epidemiological studies have shown an association between chronic neuroleptic therapy and mammary tumorigenesis, the available evidence is considered too limited to be conclusive at this time.
Tartrazine sensitivity	Presence of FD&C Yellow No. 5 (tartrazine) in tablets may cause allergic-type reactions, including bronchial asthma, in certain susceptible individuals, such as those hypersensitive to aspirin

ADVERSE REACTIONS[2]

Central nervous system	Drowsiness, dystonias (spasm of neck muscles, acute reversible torticollis, extensor rigidity of back muscles, opisthotonos, carpopedal spasm, trismus, swallowing difficulty, oculogyric crisis, protrusion of the tongue), akathisia (agitation, jitteriness, insomnia), pseudoparkinsonism (mask-like facies, drooling, tremors, pill-rolling motion, cogwheel rigidity, shuffling gait), tardive dyskinesia, tardive dystonia, psychotic symptoms, catatonic-like states, convulsive seizures, cerebral edema, CSF protein abnormalities

THORAZINE

Ophthalmic	Miosis, mydriasis, corneal and lenticular changes, visual impairment, epithelial keratopathy, pigmentary retinopathy
Cardiovascular	Orthostatic hypotension, tachycardia, dizziness, syncope, shock, ECG changes (especially distortions of Q and T waves), peripheral edema
Hematological	Agranulocytosis, eosinophilia, leukopenia, hemolytic anemia, aplastic anemia, thrombocytopenic purpura, pancytopenia
Gastrointestinal	Jaundice, nausea, obstipation, constipation, adynamic ileus, atonic colon
Genitourinary	Priapism, urinary retention, ejaculatory disorders/impotence
Endocrinological	Lactation, breast engorgement (in women), amenorrhea, gynecomastia, hyperglycemia, hypoglycemia, glycosuria
Dermatological	Skin pigmentation, hypersensitivity reactions (see below)
Hypersensitivity	Jaundice, blood dyscrasias, urticaria, photosensitivity, exfoliative dermatitis, contact dermatitis, asthma, laryngeal edema, angioneurotic edema, anaphylactoid reactions
Other	Dry mouth, nasal congestion, mild fever (with large IM doses), hyperpyrexia, increased appetite, weight gain, systemic lupus erythematosus–like syndrome; neuroleptic malignant syndrome, a potentially fatal reaction characterized by hyperthermia, altered consciousness, muscular rigidity, and autonomic dysfunction

OVERDOSAGE

Signs and symptoms	CNS depression, somnolence, coma, hypotension, extrapyramidal symptoms, agitation, restlessness, convulsions, fever, dry mouth, ileus, ECG changes, cardiac arrhythmias
Treatment	Empty stomach by gastric lavage. Maintain a patent airway. *Do not induce emesis.* Treat extrapyramidal symptoms with antiparkinson drugs (except levodopa), barbiturates, or diphenhydramine; exercise caution to avoid increasing respiratory depression. Avoid use of convulsion-inducing stimulants (eg, picrotoxin or pentylenetetrazol). Employ standard measures for circulatory shock. If a vasoconstrictor is needed, use norepinephrine or phenylephrine; *do not use epinephrine.* Dialysis is not helpful. Use saline cathartics to hasten the evacuation of sustained-release pellets.

DRUG INTERACTIONS

Other CNS depressants, including alcohol	⇧ CNS depression; before starting chlorpromazine, discontinue other CNS depressants unless this drug is being used to permit a reduction in their dosage. Use of other CNS depressants may be resumed at a later time, with dosage initially at a low level and then increased as needed. The dosage requirement of CNS depressants used in combination with chlorpromazine is 50–75% less than their usual level. Do not give large amounts of CNS depressants in combination with chlorpromazine; avoid concomitant use of alcohol.
Anticonvulsants	⇧ Risk of convulsions; when patients are receiving anticonvulsants, dosage of chlorpromazine should be kept low initially and then increased as needed. Adjustment of anticonvulsant dosage may also be necessary. ⇧ Pharmacologic effect of phenytoin
Metrizamide	⇧ Risk of convulsions; discontinue use of chlorpromazine at least 48 h before administration of metrizamide for myelography and wait at least 24 h after the procedure before resuming use. Do not use chlorpromazine before or after myelography for control of nausea and vomiting.
Anticholinergic drugs	⇧ Anticholinergic effects; exercise caution during combination therapy ⇩ Antipsychotic effect
Epinephrine	Severe hypotension
Guanethidine	⇩ Antihypertensive effect
Propranolol	⇧ Pharmacologic effects of propranolol and chlorpromazine
Amphetamines	⇩ Antipsychotic effect ⇩ Anorectic effect
Phenmetrazine	⇩ Anorectic effect
Lithium	⇧ Risk of acute encephalopathy and extrapyramidal reactions ⇩ Serum chlorpromazine level ⇧ Renal clearance of lithium
Tricyclic antidepressants	⇧ Serum level of tricyclic antidepressants and chlorpromazine ⇩ Antipsychotic effect
Oral anticoagulants	⇩ Anticoagulant effect
Thiazide-type diuretics	⇧ Risk of orthostatic hypotension

ALTERED LABORATORY VALUES

Blood/serum values	⇧ SGOT ⇧ SGPT ⇧ LDH ⇧ Alkaline phosphatase ⇧ Bilirubin ⇧ Prolactin ⇧ or ⇩ Glucose

THORAZINE ■ TIGAN

Urinary values	△ Glucose ▽ VMA + Pregnancy (with immunologic pregnancy tests) + PKU + Bilirubin (with reagent test strips) △ Urobilinogen (with Ehrlich's reagent test) ▽ 5-HIAA (with nitrosonaphthol reagent test) Interference with determination of catecholamines (with Pisano method), 17-KS (with Haltorff-Koch modification of Zimmerman reaction), and 17-OHCS (with modified Glenn-Nelson technique)

USE IN CHILDREN

See INDICATIONS and dosage recommendations; not generally recommended for use in children under 6 mo of age or for conditions in which children's dosages have not been established. After IM administration, the duration of activity may last up to 12 h. If a child experiences dystonia, discontinue use and do not reinstitute treatment at a later time. Avoid use in children or adolescents with signs or symptoms suggesting Reye's syndrome.

USE IN PREGNANT AND NURSING WOMEN

Safety for use during pregnancy has not been established; prolonged jaundice, extrapyramidal signs, and hyperreflexia have occurred in neonates born to mothers who received phenothiazines, and embryotoxicity, increased neonatal mortality, and evidence of possible neurological damage have been seen in reproduction studies with rodents. Use during pregnancy only if essential and only if potential benefits clearly outweigh possible hazards. If a pregnant women experiences dystonia, discontinue use and do not reinstitute treatment at a later time. Chlorpromazine is excreted in human milk.

[1] Possibly effective; for most patients, chlorpromazine is not the initial treatment of choice because certain risks associated with its use are not shared by common alternatives, such as benzodiazepines
[2] Sudden death has occasionally occurred in patients taking phenothiazines; in some cases, death appeared to result from cardiac arrest or from asphyxia due to failure of the cough reflex

---

ANTINAUSEANTS/ANTIEMETICS

TIGAN (trimethobenzamide hydrochloride) Beecham   Rx

Capsules: 100, 250 mg   **Ampuls:** 100 mg/ml (2 ml)   **Vials:** 100 mg/ml (20 ml)   **Prefilled syringes:** 100 mg/ml (2 ml)   **Rectal suppositories:** 200 mg trimethobenzamide and 2% benzocaine   **Pediatric rectal suppositories:** 100 mg trimethobenzamide and 2% benzocaine

INDICATIONS	ORAL DOSAGE	RECTAL DOSAGE
Nausea and vomiting	**Adult:** 250 mg tid or qid **Child (30–90 lb):** 100–200 mg tid or qid	**Adult:** 200 mg (1 regular suppository) tid or qid **Child (< 30 lb):** 100 mg (½ regular suppository or 1 pediatric suppository) tid or qid **Child (30–90 lb):** 100–200 mg (½–1 regular suppository or 1–2 pediatric suppositories) tid or qid

CONTRAINDICATIONS		
Hypersensitivity to trimethobenzamide or, if suppositories are used, benzocaine	Age < 12 yr if injectable form is used	Premature or full-term newborns if rectal form is used

ADMINISTRATION/DOSAGE ADJUSTMENTS

Parenteral use	Usual adult dosage, 200 mg IM tid or qid; IM injection may cause pain, stinging, burning, redness, and swelling at injection site; effects may be minimized by deep injection into upper outer quadrant of gluteal region and by avoiding escape of solution along route

WARNINGS/PRECAUTIONS

Drowsiness	Caution patients not to drive or operate other potentially dangerous machinery until their response can be determined
Reye's syndrome	Centrally acting antiemetics may, in the presence of viral infections, cause or contribute to development of syndrome
Drug-induced extrapyramidal symptoms and other CNS reactions	May mask signs of undiagnosed primary diseases with CNS manifestations
Special-risk patients	Use with caution in patients with acute febrile illness, encephalitis, gastroenteritis, dehydration, and electrolyte imbalances (especially in children, the elderly, or debilitated patients); direct primary attention to restoring body fluids and electrolyte balance, relieving fever, and correction of underlying disease process
Diagnostic interference	Antiemetic effect may mask signs of overdosage of other drugs

ADVERSE REACTIONS

Central nervous system	Parkinsonian-like symptoms, coma, convulsions, mood depression, disorientation, dizziness, drowsiness, headache, opisthotonos
Ophthalmic	Blurred vision
Cardiovascular	Hypotension
Hematological	Blood dyscrasias
Gastrointestinal	Diarrhea
Hypersensitivity	Allergic-type skin reactions
Other	Jaundice, muscle cramps

OVERDOSAGE

Signs and symptoms	See ADVERSE REACTIONS
Treatment	Discontinue use of drug; treat symptomatically

DRUG INTERACTIONS

Alcohol	⇧ CNS depression

ALTERED LABORATORY VALUES

No clinically significant alterations in blood/serum or urinary values occur at therapeutic dosages

---

USE IN CHILDREN

See INDICATIONS and dosage recommendations; limit use to prolonged vomiting of known etiology. Injectable form is contraindicated for use in children. Suppositories are contraindicated for use in premature or newborn infants.

USE IN PREGNANT AND NURSING WOMEN

Safety for use in pregnant or nursing women has not been established. Reproduction studies in rats and rabbits have shown no evidence of teratogenicity. No adequate studies have been done in pregnant women.

ANTINAUSEANTS/ANTIEMETICS

TORECAN (thiethylperazine maleate) Boehringer Ingelheim   Rx

Tablets: 10 mg   **Ampuls:** 10 mg/2 ml (2 ml) for IM use only   **Rectal suppositories:** 10 mg

INDICATIONS	ORAL DOSAGE	PARENTERAL DOSAGE
Nausea and vomiting	**Adult:** 10 mg 1–3 times/day	**Adult:** 10 mg IM 1–3 times/day

CONTRAINDICATIONS

Pregnancy	Severe CNS depression	Comatose states
Hypersensitivity to phenothiazines		

ADMINISTRATION/DOSAGE ADJUSTMENTS

Postoperative nausea and vomiting	Administer drug by deep IM injection, at or shortly before termination of anesthesia
Rectal use	For adults, administer 1 suppository 1–3 times/day

WARNINGS/PRECAUTIONS

Postoperative use	Possible complications due to phenothiazine effects must be considered (see ADVERSE REACTIONS). Restlessness and CNS depression may occur during anesthesia recovery. Use following intracardiac or intracranial surgery not studied.
Postural hypotension	May occur, especially after initial parenteral dose. If vasoconstrictors are required, use norepinephrine or phenylephrine; do not use epinephrine. Intravenous use may result in severe hypotension and, therefore, is contraindicated.
Mental and/or physical impairment	Caution patients that their ability to drive or perform other potentially hazardous activities may be impaired
Extrapyramidal symptoms	May occur, especially in young adults and children, requiring a reduction in dosage or discontinuation of the drug (see ADVERSE REACTIONS)
Tartrazine sensitivity	Presence of FD&C Yellow No. 5 (tartrazine) in tablets may cause allergic-type reactions, including bronchial asthma, in susceptible individuals

TORECAN ■ TRANSDERM SCŌP

ADVERSE REACTIONS[1]

Central nervous system	Convulsions, extrapyramidal reactions (including dystonia, torticollis, oculogyric crises, akathisia, gait disturbances, agitation, motor restlessness, dystonic reactions, trismus, opisthotonos, tremor, muscle rigidity, and akinesia), dizziness, headache, restlessness, drowsiness, excitement, bizarre dreams, aggravation of psychoses, toxic confusional states
Autonomic nervous system	Dry mouth and nose, blurred vision, tinnitus, sialorrhea, altered sense of taste, miosis, obstipation, anorexia, paralytic ileus
Endocrinological	Peripheral edema of the arms, hands, and face; menstrual irregularities; altered libido; gynecomastia; weight gain
Hematological	Agranulocytosis, leukopenia, thrombocytopenia, aplastic anemia, pancytopenia, eosinophilia, leukocytosis
Dermatological	Erythema, exfoliative dermatitis, contact dermatitis
Hepatic	Cholestatic jaundice, biliary stasis, jaundice
Cardiovascular	Hypotension, rarely leading to cardiac arrest; ECG changes
Hypersensitivity	Fever, laryngeal edema, angioneurotic edema, asthma
Other	Cerebral vascular spasm, trigeminal neuralgia, urinary retention or incontinence, hyperpyrexia, progressive pigmentation of skin or conjunctiva accompanied by discoloration or exposed sclera and cornea, irregular or stellate opacities of anterior lens and cornea

OVERDOSAGE

Signs and symptoms	See ADVERSE REACTIONS
Treatment	Discontinue medication; treat symptomatically and institute supportive measures, as required

DRUG INTERACTIONS

Alcohol, opiates, anesthetics, and other CNS depressants	⇩ CNS depression
Atropine	⇧ Antimuscarinic effects
Epinephrine	Severe hypotension

ALTERED LABORATORY VALUES

No clinically significant alterations in blood/serum or urinary values occur at therapeutic dosages

---

USE IN CHILDREN

The safety and effectiveness of this drug for use in children under 12 yr of age have not been established

USE IN PREGNANT AND NURSING WOMEN

Contraindicated for use during pregnancy. It is not known whether thiethylperazine is excreted in human milk; because many drugs are excreted in human milk, nursing is inadvisable.

---

[1] Includes reactions common to phenothiazines in general

ANTINAUSEANTS/ANTIEMETICS

TRANSDERM SCŌP (scopolamine) CIBA Rx

Transcutaneous drug delivery system: 0.5 mg/3 days (2.5 cm²)

INDICATIONS	TRANSCUTANEOUS DOSAGE
Nausea and vomiting associated with motion sickness	Adult: apply to postauricular skin at least 4 h before antiemetic effect is required and leave in place for up to 72 h, if needed; do not use more than one disk at any one time

CONTRAINDICATIONS

Glaucoma	Hypersensitivity to scopolamine or components of adhesive matrix (mineral oil and polyisobutylene)

TRANSDERM SCŌP ■ VISTARIL Intramuscular Solution

ADMINISTRATION/DOSAGE ADJUSTMENTS

Handling of disk	Peel the package open, remove the clear plastic protective backing from the disk, and firmly attach the adhesive surface to a dry, hairless area of skin behind the ear. After 3 days, remove the disk and discard it; wash application site to remove any traces of scopolamine. Immediately after application or removal of the disk, wash hands thoroughly with soap and water and dry them, because scopolamine can cause temporary mydriasis and blurred vision if it comes in contact with the eyes.
Continuation of therapy	If disk is displaced, or if continued therapy beyond 72 h is required, remove the first disk and replace it with a new disk behind the other ear.

WARNINGS/PRECAUTIONS

Drowsiness, disorientation, confusion	Caution patients not to drive or engage in other activities requiring mental alertness
Idiosyncratic reactions	May occur with ordinary therapeutic doses and may be alarming
Withdrawal reactions	Dizziness, nausea, vomiting, headache, and equilibrium disturbances have occurred in a few patients following withdrawal, most frequently after use for more than 3 days
Special-risk patients	Use with caution in patients with pyloric, urinary bladder neck, or intestinal obstruction; use with particular caution in the elderly and patients with impaired renal or hepatic function or metabolic dysfunction because CNS reactions are more likely to occur in such patients
Carcinogenicity	No long-term studies have been performed in animals to determine the carcinogenic potential of this drug

ADVERSE REACTIONS

Frequent reactions (incidence $\geq$ 1%) are printed in *italics*

Central nervous system	*Drowsiness ($<$ 17%)*, disorientation, memory disturbances, restlessness, dizziness, hallucinations, confusion
Autonomic nervous system	*Dry mouth (67%)*, transient impairment of ocular accommodation, acute narrow-angle glaucoma, difficulty urinating
Other	Rash, erythema; dry, itchy, or red eyes

OVERDOSAGE

Signs and symptoms	Disorientation, memory disturbances, restlessness, dizziness, hallucinations, confusion
Treatment	Remove system immediately from skin; if symptoms are severe, initiate appropriate parasympathomimetic therapy (eg, physostigmine)

DRUG INTERACTIONS

Alcohol, tranquilizers, sedative-hypnotics, and other CNS depressants	⇧ CNS depression
Other belladonna alkaloids, antihistamines (including meclizine), antidepressants, and other anticholinergic agents	⇧ Anticholinergic effects

ALTERED LABORATORY VALUES

No clinically significant alterations in blood/serum or urinary values occur at therapeutic dosages

---

USE IN CHILDREN

Children are particularly susceptible to the side effects of belladonna alkaloids; this system should not be used in children because of the unknown potential for serious adverse reactions

USE IN PREGNANT AND NURSING WOMEN

Pregnancy Category C: use during pregnancy only if the expected benefit justifies the potential risk to the fetus. Reproduction studies in female rats have shown no evidence of impaired fertility or fetal harm; however, reduced maternal body weights were observed at plasma drug levels approximately 500 times the human therapeutic level. A marginal embryotoxic effect was detected in rabbits at plasma drug levels approximately 100 times the human therapeutic level, but not at lower plasma drug levels. It is not known whether scopolamine is excreted in human milk; use with caution in nursing mothers.

ANTINAUSEANTS/ANTIEMETICS

VISTARIL Intramuscular Solution (hydroxyzine hydrochloride) Roerig   Rx

Vials: 25 mg/ml (10 ml), 50 mg/ml (1, 2, 10 ml) for IM injection only

INDICATIONS	PARENTERAL DOSAGE
Psychiatric and emotional emergencies, including acute alcoholism	**Adult:** 50–100 mg IM at once, followed by 50–100 mg IM q4-6h, as needed

COMPENDIUM OF DRUG THERAPY

VISTARIL Intramuscular Solution

Preoperative and postoperative and prepartum and postpartum adjunctive medication to permit reduction in narcotic dosage, allay anxiety, and control emesis

Nausea and vomiting, excluding nausea and vomiting of pregnancy (see box below)

Adult: 25–100 mg IM
Child: 0.5 mg/lb IM

CONTRAINDICATIONS

Early pregnancy	Hypersensitivity to hydroxyzine

ADMINISTRATION/DOSAGE ADJUSTMENTS

Intramuscular administration	To help prevent inadvertent vascular injection, aspirate syringe before administration. Inject deeply into a relatively large muscle, preferably a midlateral thigh muscle for children and either that muscle or the gluteus maximus for adults. To minimize the possibility of sciatic nerve damage, use the periphery of the gluteus maximus for infants and small children only if necessary (eg, for patients with burns). The deltoid area should be used only if it is well developed and only if caution is exercised to avoid radial nerve injury; injections should not be made into the lower or middle third of the upper arm. Avoid SC administration, which may result in significant tissue damage.
Long-term use (> 4 mo)	Effectiveness for prolonged use as an antianxiety agent has not been tested in systematic clinical studies; reassess need for continued therapy periodically

WARNINGS/PRECAUTIONS

Drowsiness	Caution patients not to engage in potentially hazardous activities requiring full mental alertness
Concomitant use of CNS depressants	May potentiate hydroxyzine's effect; reduce the dosage of these agents by up to 50%. The concomitant use of narcotics and barbiturates as preanesthetic medication should be modified on an individual basis; atropine and other belladonna alkaloids are not affected.

ADVERSE REACTIONS

Central nervous system	Transient drowsiness; involuntary motor activity, including tremor and convulsions (rare)
Gastrointestinal	Dry mouth

OVERDOSAGE

Signs and symptoms	Excessive sedation, hypotension, CNS depression
Treatment	Monitor respiration, pulse, and blood pressure. Employ general supportive measures, as needed. Hypotension may be combatted with IV fluids and levarterenol or metaraminol. Do not use epinephrine, since hydroxyzine counteracts its pressor action. Caffeine and sodium benzoate may be used to counteract CNS depression. Dialysis is of limited value.

DRUG INTERACTIONS

Alcohol, narcotic analgesics, sedative-hypnotics, other CNS depressants, and tricyclic antidepressants	△ CNS depression

ALTERED LABORATORY VALUES

Urinary values	△ 17-Hydroxycorticosteroids

No clinically significant alterations in blood/serum values occur at therapeutic dosages

---

USE IN CHILDREN

See INDICATIONS and PARENTERAL DOSAGE

USE IN PREGNANT AND NURSING WOMEN

Contraindicated during early pregnancy. Fetal abnormalities have been reported in mice, rats, and rabbits at doses well above the maximum human dose. Clinical data are inadequate to establish safety for use in pregnant women during this period. It is not known whether hydroxyzine is excreted in human milk; because many drugs are excreted in human milk, patient should not nurse if drug is prescribed.

Chapter 28

Antineoplastic Agents

Alkylating Agents — 1088
ALKERAN (Burroughs Wellcome) — 1088
Melphalan *Rx*

BiCNU (Bristol-Myers Oncology) — 1089
Carmustine (BCNU) *Rx*

CeeNU (Bristol-Myers Oncology) — 1090
Lomustine (CCNU) *Rx*

CYTOXAN (Bristol-Myers Oncology) — 1091
Cyclophosphamide *Rx*

DTIC-Dome (Miles Pharmaceuticals) — 1093
Dacarbazine *Rx*

LEUKERAN (Burroughs Wellcome) — 1094
Chlorambucil *Rx*

Thiotepa (Lederle) *Rx* — 1095

ZANOSAR (Upjohn) — 1096
Streptozocin *Rx*

Antimetabolites — 1098
CYTOSAR-U (Upjohn) — 1098
Cytarabine (ara-C) *Rx*

EFUDEX (Roche) — 1099
Fluorouracil *Rx*

Fluorouracil (Roche) *Rx* — 1100

Methotrexate *Rx* — 1101

Antineoplastic Antibiotics — 1103
ADRIAMYCIN (Adria) — 1103
Doxorubicin hydrochloride *Rx*

BLENOXANE (Bristol-Myers Oncology) — 1105
Bleomycin sulfate *Rx*

CERUBIDINE (Wyeth) — 1106
Daunorubicin hydrochloride *Rx*

MITHRACIN (Miles Pharmaceuticals) — 1108
Plicamycin *Rx*

MUTAMYCIN (Bristol-Myers Oncology) — 1109
Mitomycin *Rx*

Hormones — 1111
LUPRON (TAP) — 1111
Leuprolide acetate *Rx*

MEGACE (Bristol-Myers Oncology) — 1112
Megestrol acetate *Rx*

NOLVADEX (Stuart) — 1112
Tamoxifen citrate *Rx*

TESLAC (Squibb) — 1114
Testolactone *Rx*

Interferons — 1114
INTRON-A (Schering) — 1114
Interferon alfa-2b, recombinant *Rx*

ROFERON-A (Roche) — 1116
Interferon alfa-2a, recombinant *Rx*

Miscellaneous Antineoplastic Agents — 1118
EMCYT (Roche) — 1118
Estramustine phosphate sodium *Rx*

HYDREA (Squibb) — 1120
Hydroxyurea *Rx*

ONCOVIN (Lilly) — 1121
Vincristine sulfate *Rx*

PLATINOL (Bristol-Myers Oncology) — 1123
Cisplatin *Rx*

VEPESID (Bristol-Myers Oncology) — 1125
Etoposide *Rx*

Other Antineoplastic Agents — 1086
COSMEGEN (Merck Sharp & Dohme) — 1086
Dactinomycin *Rx*

ELSPAR (Merck Sharp & Dohme) — 1086
Asparaginase *Rx*

FUDR (Roche) — 1086
Floxuridine *Rx*

LYSODREN (Bristol-Myers Oncology) — 1086
Mitotane *Rx*

MATULANE (Roche) — 1086
Procarbazine hydrochloride *Rx*

MEXATE (Bristol-Myers Oncology) — 1086
Methotrexate sodium *Rx*

MEXATE-AQ (Bristol-Myers Oncology) — 1087
Methotrexate sodium *Rx*

MUSTARGEN (Merck Sharp & Dohme) — 1087
Mechlorethamine hydrochloride *Rx*

MYLERAN (Burroughs Wellcome) — 1087
Busulfan *Rx*

PURINETHOL (Burroughs Wellcome) — 1087
Mercaptopurine *Rx*

Thioguanine (Burroughs Wellcome) *Rx* — 1087

VELBAN (Lilly) — 1087
Vinblastine sulfate *Rx*

WELLCOVORIN (Burroughs Wellcome) — 1087
Leucovorin calcium *Rx*

continued

OTHER ANTINEOPLASTIC AGENTS

DRUG	HOW SUPPLIED	USUAL DOSAGE[1]
COSMEGEN (Merck Sharp & Dohme) Dactinomycin *Rx*	**Vials:** 0.5 mg (500 µg/ml after reconstitution)	**Adult:** 500 µg/day IV (not to exceed 15 µg/kg/day or 400–600 µg/m² /day) for up to 5 days; a second course may be given after 3 wk, provided that all signs of toxicity have disappeared **Child:** 15 µg/kg/day IV for up to 5 days or a total of 2.5 mg/m² IV, given in divided doses over a period of 1 wk; a second course may be given after 3 wk, provided that all signs of toxicity have disappeared
ELSPAR (Merck Sharp & Dohme) Asparaginase *Rx*	**Vials:** 10,000 IU (10 ml)	**Adult:** 200 IU/kg/day IV for 28 days when used as the sole agent for induction of remission; for use in combination regimens, consult package literature **Child:** same as adult
FUDR (Roche) Floxuridine *Rx*	**Vials:** 500 mg (5 ml)	**Adult:** 0.1–0.6 mg/kg/day, given by continuous intraarterial infusion; dosage at the upper end of the range (0.4–0.6 mg/kg/day) is generally used for hepatic artery infusion
LYSODREN (Bristol-Myers Oncology) Mitotane *Rx*	**Tablets:** 500 mg	**Adult:** 9–10 g/day, given tid or qid, to start; maximum tolerated dose: usually 9–10 g/day, but may range from 2 to 16 g/day
MATULANE (Roche) Procarbazine hydrochloride *Rx*	**Capsules:** procarbazine hydrochloride equivalent to 50 mg procarbazine	**Adult:** 2–4 mg/kg/day given in single or divided daily doses, for 1 wk, followed by 4–6 mg/kg/day until WBC count falls below 4,000/mm³, platelet count falls below 100,000/mm³, or maximum response is obtained; for maintenance, 1–2 mg/kg/day **Child:** 50 mg/m² /day for 1 wk, followed by 100 mg/m² /day until leukopenia or thrombocytopenia occurs or until maximum response is obtained; for maintenance, 50 mg/m² /day
MEXATE (Bristol-Myers Oncology) Methotrexate sodium *Rx*	**Vials:** 20, 50, 100, 250 mg	**Adult:** for gestational choriocarcinoma and hydatidiform mole, 15–30 mg/day IM, given for 5 consecutive days and repeated 3–5 times at intervals of 1 or more weeks, as needed; for maintenance therapy of acute lymphatic (lymphoblastic) leukemia, 30 mg/m² IM twice weekly or 2.5 mg/kg IV every 14 days; for malignant lymphomas (stage III), 0.625–2.5 mg/kg/day; for meningeal leukemia, 12 mg/m² or 15 mg intrathecally, given every 2–5 days until CSF count returns to normal and followed by one additional dose; for advanced mycosis fungoides, 50 mg IM once weekly or 25 mg IM twice weekly **Child:** for maintenance therapy of acute lymphatic (lymphoblastic) leukemia, 30 mg/m² IM, given twice weekly, or 2.5 mg/kg IV, given every 14 days

[1] Where pediatric dosages are not given, consult manufacturer

OTHER ANTINEOPLASTIC AGENTS continued

DRUG	HOW SUPPLIED	USUAL DOSAGE[1]
MEXATE-AQ (Bristol-Myers Oncology) Methotrexate sodium *Rx*	**Vials:** 25 mg/ml (2, 4, 10 ml)	**Adult:** for gestational choriocarcinoma and hydatidiform mole, 15–30 mg/day IM, given for 5 consecutive days and repeated 3–5 times at intervals of 1 or more weeks, as needed; for induction of remission in leukemia, 3.3 mg/m² with 60 mg/m² prednisone, given once daily and, when remission is achieved, 30 mg/m² IM, given twice weekly, or 2.5 mg/kg IV, given every 14 days; for malignant lymphomas (stage III), 0.625–2.5 mg/kg/day; for meningeal leukemia, 12 mg/m² or 15 mg intrathecally, given every 2–5 days until CSF count returns to normal and followed by one additional dose; for advanced mycosis fungoides, 50 mg IM once weekly or 25 mg IM twice weekly **Child:** for induction of remission in leukemia, 3.3 mg/m² with 60 mg/m² prednisone, given once daily; when remission is achieved, 30 mg/m² IM, given twice weekly, or 2.5 mg/kg IV, given every 14 days
MUSTARGEN (Merck Sharp & Dohme) Mechlorethamine hydrochloride *Rx*	**Vials:** 10 mg (1 mg/ml after reconstitution)	**Adult:** 0.4 mg/kg IV, given in a single dose or 2–4 divided doses
MYLERAN (Burroughs Wellcome) Busulfan *Rx*	**Tablets:** 2 mg	**Adult:** 4–8 mg/day (depending on total leukocyte count and disease severity), or 60 μg/kg/day or 1.8 mg/m²/day, until WBC count falls to 15,000/μl; resume treatment when WBC count reaches ~ 50,000/μl; if remission lasts less than 3 mo, give 1–3 mg/day **Child:** 60 μg/kg/day or 1.8 mg/m²/day, until WBC count falls to 15,000/μl; resume treatment when WBC count is ~ 50,000/μl; if remission lasts less than 3 mo, give 1–3 mg/day
PURINETHOL (Burroughs Wellcome) Mercaptopurine *Rx*	**Tablets:** 50 mg	**Adult:** 2.5 mg/kg/day; if no response is obtained after 4 wk, increase dosage to 5 mg/kg/day; for maintenance, 1.5–2.5 mg/kg/day, given in a single dose **Child:** same as adult
Thioguanine (Burroughs Wellcome) *Rx*	**Tablets:** 40 mg	**Adult and child:** when used alone, 2 mg/kg/day, given in a single dose, to start; if no improvement and no WBC or platelet depression is seen after 4 wk, cautiously increase dosage to 3 mg/kg/day
VELBAN (Lilly) Vinblastine sulfate *Rx*	**Vials:** 10 mg (1 mg/ml after reconstitution) (10 ml)	**Adult:** 3.7 mg/m² IV, given in a single dose, to start, followed by increments of 1.8–1.9 mg/m²/dose at weekly intervals (up to 18.5 mg/m²) until WBC count is reduced to 3,000/mm³; for maintenance, 1.8–1.9 mg/m² less than the dose producing desired degree of leukopenia at weekly intervals (provided the WBC count has returned to at least 4,000/mm³) **Child:** same as adult, but reduce initial dose to 2.5 mg/m² and increase dose in increments of 1.25 mg/m² at weekly intervals (up to 12.5 mg/m²)
WELLCOVORIN (Burroughs Wellcome) Leucovorin calcium *Rx*	**Tablets:** 5, 25 mg **Ampuls:** 5 mg/ml (1, 5 ml)	**Adult:** for rescue with methotrexate, 10 mg/m² PO, IM, or IV, followed by 10 mg/m² PO q6h for 72 h; begin rescue within 24 h after start of methotrexate therapy

[1] Where pediatric dosages are not given, consult manufacturer

ALKERAN

ALKYLATING AGENTS

ALKERAN (melphalan) Burroughs Wellcome Rx
Tablets: 2 mg

INDICATIONS	ORAL DOSAGE
Palliative treatment of **multiple myeloma**	Adult: 6 mg/day, given in a single daily dose for 2–3 wk to start, followed by a rest period of up to 4 wk and then 2 mg/day for maintenance; for alternative regimens, consult manufacturer
Palliative treatment of **nonresectable epithelial ovarian carcinoma**	Adult: 0.2 mg/kg day for 5 consecutive days; repeat at intervals of 4–5 wk, depending upon hematological tolerance

CONTRAINDICATIONS
Prior resistance or hypersensitivity to melphalan

ADMINISTRATION/DOSAGE ADJUSTMENTS

Onset of clinical response	May be very gradual and occur over many months; maximum benefit may be missed if treatment is abandoned too soon
Patients with multiple myeloma	Blood counts should be performed at weekly intervals and dosage adjusted accordingly. During drug-free period (see ORAL DOSAGE), follow blood count carefully; when WBC and platelet counts are rising, institute maintenance dosage. To ensure therapeutic plasma levels, increase the dosage cautiously until some myelosuppression is observed.
Patients with impaired renal function	Although currently available data does not justify a recommendation for dosage reduction, initial use of a reduced dose may be necessary for patients with moderate to severe renal impairment
Combination therapy	Use of melphalan in combination with prednisone may significantly increase the likelihood of response to treatment of multiple myeloma; it is not known whether the addition of other cytotoxic agents to a regimen of melphalan and prednisone increases either the response rate or the duration of survival

WARNINGS/PRECAUTIONS

Myelosuppressive effects	Bone marrow depression can result from excessive dosage. Obtain frequent blood counts to determine optimal dosage and to avoid toxicity; discontinue therapy if WBC count falls below 3,000/mm^3 or platelet count falls below 100,000/mm^3. Use with extreme caution if bone marrow reserve may have been compromised by prior irradiation or chemotherapy or if bone marrow function is recovering from prior cytotoxic therapy.
Azotemic patients	Observe patient closely and reduce dosage, if needed, at the earliest possible moment
Carcinogenicity	Acute nonlymphatic leukemia has reportedly developed in many patients with multiple myeloma following treatment with melphalan and other alkylating agents; similarly, the incidence of acute nonlymphatic leukemia is greatly increased following melphalan treatment in women with ovarian cancer. Melphalan is carcinogenic in animals and must be presumed to be so in humans. Although the potential benefits of therapy are generally considered to far exceed the possible risk of induction of a second neoplasm, the decision to continue treatment must be made on an individual basis.
Mutagenicity	Mutagenic and teratogenic effects may occur, although the extent of risk is unknown; melphalan has produced chromosomal aberrations in human cells, both in vitro and in vivo
Effect on fertility	Melphalan causes suppression of ovarian function in premenopausal women, resulting in amenorrhea in a significant number of women

ADVERSE REACTIONS

Gastrointestinal	Nausea, vomiting, diarrhea, oral ulceration
Hematological	Anemia, neutropenia, thrombocytopenia, hemolytic anemia
Respiratory	Pulmonary fibrosis and interstitial pneumonitis
Other	Skin hypersensitivity, vasculitis, alopecia, allergic reaction

OVERDOSAGE

Signs and symptoms	Bone marrow depression (anemia, neutropenia, thrombocytopenia), vomiting, ulceration of the mouth, diarrhea, GI hemorrhage
Treatment	Closely monitor blood findings for 3–6 wk; institute general supportive measure, including appropriate blood transfusions and administration of antibiotics, if necessary. Hemodialysis does not remove melphalan from the plasma to any significant degree.

DRUG INTERACTIONS

Antigout agents	⇧ Serum uric acid level

Other myelosuppressive agents, radiotherapy	↑ Antineoplastic effect

ALTERED LABORATORY VALUES

Blood/serum values	↑ Uric acid
Urinary values	↑ Uric acid ↑ 5-HIAA

USE IN CHILDREN

Safety and effectiveness for use in children have not been established

USE IN PREGNANT AND NURSING WOMEN

Pregnancy Category D: melphalan may cause fetal harm if administered to a pregnant woman. Animal reproduction studies have not been performed, and no adequate, well controlled studies have been done in pregnant women. If this drug is used during pregnancy, or if a patient becomes pregnant during melphalan therapy, apprise the patient of the potential risk to the fetus. Women of childbearing potential should be advised to avoid becoming pregnant during therapy. It is not known whether melphalan is excreted in human milk. Because many drugs are excreted in breast milk and because of the potential for serious adverse reactions in nursing infants, patient should not nurse if use of this drug is deemed essential.

ALKYLATING AGENTS

BiCNU (carmustine [BCNU]) Bristol-Myers Oncology Rx

Vials: 100 mg (3.3 mg/ml after reconstitution) for IV use only

INDICATIONS

Palliative treatment of **brain tumors,** including glioblastoma, brain-stem glioma, medullablastoma, astrocytoma, ependymoma, and metastatic brain tumors, **multiple myeloma** (in combination with prednisone), **Hodgkin's disease** (secondary adjunctive therapy), and **non-Hodgkin's lymphomas** (secondary adjunctive therapy)

PARENTERAL DOSAGE

Adult: 200 mg/m^2, given in a single IV dose or divided over several days every 6 wk. Adjust dosage as needed to maintain adequate bone marrow function; do not administer until WBC count > 4,000/mm^3 and platelet count > 100,000/mm^3.

CONTRAINDICATIONS

Hypersensitivity to carmustine	Platelet, leukocyte, or erythrocyte depression

ADMINISTRATION/DOSAGE ADJUSTMENTS

Intravenous administration	Reconstitute contents of 100-mg vial with 3 m of absolute alcohol (supplied) plus 27 ml of Sterile Water for Injection USP; if desired, reconstituted solution may be further diluted with Sodium Chloride Injection USP or 5% Dextrose Injection USP. Administer the required dose by IV drip over a period of 1–2 h.
Hematological response to prior dose	If nadir of WBC count following previous dose is 2,000–2,999/mm^3 and/or nadir of platelet count is 25,000–74,999/mm^3, give 70% of prior dose during next course of therapy; if nadir of WBC count is < 2,000/mm^3 and/or nadir of platelet count is < 25,000/mm^3, give 50% of prior dose during next course. Concomitant use of other myelosuppressive agents may require further dosage adjustment.

WARNINGS/PRECAUTIONS

Delayed bone marrow toxicity	Obtain frequent blood counts, as well as liver function studies, for at least 6 wk after administration. Do not repeat dose more often than once every 6 wk. Bone marrow toxicity is cumulative; adjust dosage on the basis of lowest blood counts.
Nausea and/or vomiting	May occur within 2 h of dosing; may be minimized or sometimes prevented by prior antiemetic therapy.

ADVERSE REACTIONS

Gastrointestinal	Nausea, vomiting
Hematological	Delayed thrombocytopenia, leukopenia, anemia
Hepatic	Reversible toxicity
Respiratory	Pulmonary infiltrates and/or fibrosis
Renal	Kidney damage with prolonged therapy and large cumulative doses and occasionally with lower total doses

Other	Burning at injection site, thrombosis (rare), intense flushing of skin and suffusion of conjunctiva with too rapid IV administration

OVERDOSAGE

Signs and symptoms	See ADVERSE REACTIONS
Treatment	Discontinue medication; institute supportive measures, as required

DRUG INTERACTIONS

Hepatotoxic agents	⌂ Hepatotoxicity
Nephrotoxic agents	⌂ Nephrotoxicity
Other myelosuppressive agents, radiotherapy	⌂ Antineoplastic effect

ALTERED LABORATORY VALUES

Blood/serum values	⌂ Alkaline phosphates ⌂ Bilirubin ⌂ SGOT ⌂ SGPT ⌂ BUN

No clinically significant alterations in urinary values occur at therapeutic dosages

USE IN CHILDREN
Consult manufacturer

USE IN PREGNANT AND NURSING WOMEN
Safety for use during pregnancy has not been established; carmustine is embryotoxic and teratogenic in rats and embryotoxic in rabbits at dose levels equivalent to human doses. It is not known whether carmustine is excreted in human milk. Because many drugs are excreted in breast milk and because of the potential for serious adverse reactions in nursing infants, patient should not nurse if use of this drug is deemed essential.

ALKYLATING AGENTS

CeeNU (lomustine [CCNU]) Bristol-Myers Oncology Rx

Capsules: 10, 40, 100 mg

INDICATIONS
Palliative treatment of **primary and metastatic brain tumors** (postoperative and/or postirradiation adjunctive therapy) and **Hodgkin's disease** (secondary adjunctive therapy)

ORAL DOSAGE
Adult: 130 mg/m^2 every 6 wk. Adjust dosage as needed to maintain adequate bone marrow function; do not administer until WBC count > 4,000/mm^3 and platelet count > 100,000/mm^3.
Child: same as adult

CONTRAINDICATIONS
Hypersensitivity to lomustine

ADMINISTRATION/DOSAGE ADJUSTMENTS

Hematological response to prior dose	If nadir of WBC count following previous dose is 2,000–2,999/mm^3, and/or nadir of platelet count is 25,000–74,999/mm^3, give 70% of prior dose during next course of therapy; if nadir of WBC count is < 2,000/mm^3 and/or nadir of platelet count is < 25,000/mm^3, give 50% of prior dose during next course. Concomitant use of other myelosuppressive agents may require further dosage adjustment.
Patients with compromised bone marrow function	Reduce dosage to 100 mg/m^2 every 6 wk

WARNINGS/PRECAUTIONS

Delayed bone marrow toxicity	Use with caution in patients with decreased numbers of circulating platelets, leukocytes, or erythrocytes. Obtain frequent blood counts, as well as liver function studies, for at least 6 wk after administration. Do not repeat dose more often than once every 6 wk. Bone marrow toxicity is cumulative; adjust dosage on the basis of lowest blood counts.
Pulmonary toxicity	Pulmonary infiltrates and/or fibrosis has occurred 6 mo or more after the onset of therapy in three patients given cumulative doses of 600–1,040 mg
Renal toxicity	Decreased kidney size, progressive azotemia, and renal failure have been reported following prolonged administration of lomustine and related nitrosureas; kidney damage has also occurred occasionally in patients who received lower cumulative doses

CeeNU ■ CYTOXAN

Carcinogenicity	Acute leukemia and bone marrow dysplasias have been reported in patients who received nitrosureas

ADVERSE REACTIONS

Gastrointestinal	Nausea, vomiting, stomatitis
Hematological	Delayed thrombocytopenia, leukopenia, anemia
Pulmonary	Infiltrates, fibrosis
Hepatic	Reversible toxicity, manifested by transient increase in liver function test results
Central nervous system and neuromuscular	Disorientation, lethargy, ataxia, dysarthria
Renal	Decreased kidney size, progressive azotemia, renal failure
Other	Alopecia

OVERDOSAGE

Signs and symptoms	See ADVERSE REACTIONS
Treatment	Discontinue medication; institute supportive measures, as required

DRUG INTERACTIONS

Other myelosuppressive agents, radiotherapy	⇧ Antineoplastic effect

ALTERED LABORATORY VALUES

Blood/serum values	⇧ Alkaline phosphatase ⇧ Bilirubin ⇧ SGOT ⇧ SGPT

No clinically significant alterations in urinary values occur at therapeutic dosages

---

USE IN CHILDREN

See INDICATIONS and ORAL DOSAGE

USE IN PREGNANT AND NURSING WOMEN

Safety for use during pregnancy has not been established. It is not known whether lomustine is excreted in human milk. Because many drugs are excreted in breast milk and because of the potential for serious adverse reactions in nursing infants, patient should not nurse if use of this drug is deemed essential.

ALKYLATING AGENTS

CYTOXAN (cyclophosphamide) Bristol-Myers Oncology　　　　　　　　　　　　　　　　Rx

Tablets: 25, 50 mg **Vials:** 0.1, 0.2, 0.5, 1, 2 g[1]

INDICATIONS

Malignant lymphomas (stages III and IV), including Hodgkin's disease, lymphocytic lymphoma, mixed cell lymphoma, histiocytic lymphoma, and Burkitt's lymphoma
Multiple myeloma
Leukemias, including chronic lymphocytic leukemia, chronic granulocytic leukemia, acute myelogenous and monocytic leukemia, and acute lymphoblastic leukemia in children
Advanced mycosis fungoides, neuroblastoma, ovarian adenocarcinoma, retinoblastoma, and breast carcinoma

ORAL DOSAGE

Adult: for induction or maintenance, 1-5 mg/kg/day, depending upon the patient's tolerance

PARENTERAL DOSAGE

Adult: 40-50 mg/kg IV, given in divided doses over a period of 2–5 days to start, followed by 10-15 mg/kg IV every 7–10 days or 3–5 mg/kg IV twice weekly

CONTRAINDICATIONS

None known

ADMINISTRATION/DOSAGE ADJUSTMENTS

Parenteral administration	To reconstitute solution, use bacteriostatic water for injection USP (with parabens) or sterile water for injection USP. Prepare solution from lyophilized powder by adding 5 ml of diluent to the 100-mg vial, 10 ml to the 200-mg vial, 20–25 ml to the 500-mg vial, 50 ml to the 1-g vial, or 80–100 ml to the 2-g vial; prepare solution from nonlyophilized powder by adding 5 ml to the 100-mg vial, 10 ml to the 200-mg vial, 25 ml to the 500-mg vial, 50 ml to the 1-g vial, or 100 ml to the 2-g vial. A solution may be injected IV, IM, intraperitoneally, or intrapleurally or may be infused IV in 5% dextrose injection USP, 0.45% sodium chloride injection USP, 1/6 M sodium lactate injection USP, lactated Ringer's injection USP, 5% dextrose and 0.9% sodium chloride injection USP, or 5% dextrose and Ringer's injection. Solutions prepared with sterile water should be used promptly, preferably within 6 h; solutions prepared with bacteriostatic water should be used within 24 h if stored at room temperature or within 6 days if refrigerated.

CYTOXAN

Preparation of oral solution	A liquid for oral use may be prepared by dissolving the lyophilized or nonlyophilized powder in aromatic elixir NF; refrigerate any unused solution and use within 14 days
Patients with compromised bone marrow function	Previous x-ray or cytotoxic drug treatment or tumor infiltration of the bone marrow may require reduction of the initial loading dose by 33–50%
Adrenalectomized patients	May require dosage adjustment of both replacement steroids and cyclophosphamide
Maintenance therapy	Unless the disease is unusually sensitive to cyclophosphamide, give the largest maintenance dose that can be reasonably tolerated, using the WBC count as a guide (ordinarily a leukopenia of 3,000–4,000 cells/mm^3 can be maintained without undue risk of serious infection or other complications)

WARNINGS/PRECAUTIONS

Cardiac toxicity	Cardiotoxic effects have been observed in some patients who were given a high dose (120–270 mg/kg) over a period of a few days, and severe or fatal congestive heart failure owing primarily to hemorrhagic myocarditis has occurred in a few of these patients within days after the first dose; no residual cardiac abnormalities have been found in surviving patients. Cardiac dysfunction has occurred in a few patients following use of recommended doses; however, no causal relationship has been established. Cyclophosphamide can potentiate the cardiotoxicity of doxorubicin (see DRUG INTERACTIONS).
Concurrent phenobarbital therapy	Chronic high-dose phenobarbital therapy increases the metabolic and leukopenic activity of cyclophosphamide
Normal wound healing	May be impaired
Prevention of cystitis	Ample fluid intake and subsequent frequent voiding may help prevent cystitis; if cystitis occurs, suspend the use of cyclophosphamide
Special-risk patients	Use with caution in patients with hepatic or renal impairment, leukopenia, thrombocytopenia, tumor cell infiltration of bone marrow, or previous x-ray or cytotoxic drug therapy
Immunosuppression	May occur; interruption or modification of dosage should be considered in patients who develop bacterial, fungal, or viral infections, especially in those receiving, or with a recent history of, steroid therapy. Varicella-zoster infections are particularly dangerous under these circumstances and can lead to death.
Carcinogenicity	Secondary malignancies (most frequently urinary bladder and myelo- and lymphoproliferative malignancies) have developed in patients treated with cyclophosphamide alone or in combination with other antineoplastic therapies; occasionally, the secondary malignancy was detected several years after cyclophosphamide was discontinued. Although no causal relationship has been established, the possibility of inducing a secondary malignancy should be considered.
Mutagenicity	Cyclophosphamide is potentially mutagenic; advise both male and female patients to employ adequate contraceptive measures
Tartrazine sensitivity	Presence of FD&C Yellow No. 5 (tartrazine) in tablets may cause allergic-type reactions, including bronchial asthma, in susceptible individuals

ADVERSE REACTIONS

Frequent reactions (incidence ≥ 1%) are printed in *italics*

Hematological	*Leukopenia,* thrombocytopenia, anemia
Gastrointestinal	*Anorexia, nausea, vomiting,* hemorrhagic colitis, oral mucosal ulceration, jaundice
Genitourinary	Severe or fatal hemorrhagic cystitis; nonhemorrhagic cystitis and/or fibrosis of the bladder; nephrotoxicity (including hemorrhage and clot formation in the renal pelvis)
Endocrinological	Gonadal suppression leading to amenorrhea or azoospermia, ovarian fibrosis
Dermatological	*Alopecia,* hyperpigmentation of skin and fingernails, dermatitis
Pulmonary	Interstitial fibrosis (following prolonged use of high doses)

OVERDOSAGE

Signs and symptoms	See ADVERSE REACTIONS
Treatment	Dicontinue medication; institute supportive measures, as required

DRUG INTERACTIONS

Phenobarbital	⇧ Cytotoxic and leukopenic activity
Doxorubicin, daunorubicin	⇧ Risk of hemorrhagic cystitis and cardiotoxicity
Allopurinol, chloramphenicol	⇧ Risk of bone marrow toxicity
Antigout agents	⇧ Blood uric acid levels
Other myelosuppressive agents, radiotherapy	⇧ Antineoplastic effect
Succinylcholine	⇧ Risk of prolonged apnea

ALTERED LABORATORY VALUES

Blood/serum values	⇧ Uric acid ⇧ Pseudocholinesterase

CYTOXAN ■ DTIC-Dome

Urinary values ——————————— ⬆ Uric acid

USE IN CHILDREN	USE IN PREGNANT AND NURSING WOMEN
Consult manufacturer	Cyclophosphamide should not be given during pregnancy, particularly early pregnancy, unless the anticipated benefits of therapy outweigh the possible risk to the fetus. Teratogenicity and increased fetal resorption have been observed in animals. The drug is also excreted in breast milk; patient should stop nursing prior to starting therapy.

[1] All strengths are available as lyophilized and as nonlyophilized powders; solutions prepared from the lyophilized powder are slightly hypotonic (172 mOsm/liter at a concentration of 25 mg/ml, 219 mOsm/liter at a concentration of 20 mg/ml), whereas solutions prepared from the nonlyophilized powder are slightly hypertonic (352 mOsm/liter)

ALKYLATING AGENTS

DTIC-Dome (dacarbazine) Miles Pharmaceuticals Rx

Vials: 100, 200 mg (10 mg/ml after reconstitution) for IV use only

INDICATIONS	PARENTERAL DOSAGE
Metastatic malignant melanoma	**Adult and child:** 2–4.5 mg/kg/day IV, given for 10 consecutive days every 4 wk, or 250 mg/m^2/day IV, given for 5 consecutive days every 3 wk
Hodgkin's disease, when combined with other effective drugs	**Adult and child:** 150 mg/m^2/day IV, given for 5 consecutive days in combination with other effective drugs every 4 wk, or 375 mg/m^2 IV, given on day 1 (ie, once) every 15 days in combination with other effective drugs

CONTRAINDICATIONS	
Hypersensitivity to dacarbazine	

ADMINISTRATION/DOSAGE ADJUSTMENTS	
Preparation of parenteral solution and IV administration	Reconstitute with sterile water for injection USP, using 9.9 ml for the 100-mg vial or 19.7 ml for the 200-mg vial; withdraw required dose into a syringe and inject directly into a vein or, if desired, further dilute reconstituted solution with 5% dextrose injection USP or sodium chloride injection USP and administer as an IV infusion. Use extreme care to avoid extravasation, as subcutaneous infiltration of the drug may cause tissue damage and severe pain.

WARNINGS/PRECAUTIONS	
Myelosuppressive effects	Bone marrow depression may occur and can be fatal; monitor WBC, RBC, and platelet counts carefully. Hematopoietic toxicity may require temporary suspension or cessation of therapy.
Nausea and vomiting	May be minimized by coadministering phenobarbital and/or prochlorperazine; restricting oral intake of food for 4–6 h before treatment may lessen the incidence of these reactions
Hepatotoxicity	Hepatic toxicity accompanied by hepatic vein thrombosis and hepatocellular necrosis have been observed in approximately 0.01% of patients treated with decarbazine alone or, usually, in combination with other antineoplastic agents
Carcinogenicity	Dacarbazine has been shown to induce proliferative endocardial lesions, including fibrosarcomas and sarcomas, in rats and splenic angiosarcomas in mice

ADVERSE REACTIONS	Frequent reactions (incidence ≥ 1%) are printed in *italics*
Gastrointestinal	*Anorexia, nausea, vomiting,* diarrhea (rare), hepatotoxicity and liver necrosis (extremely rare)
Hematological	Leukopenia, thrombocytoenia, anemia
Dermatological	Alopecia, erythematous and urticarial rashes, photosensitivity (rare)
Other	Facial flushing, facial paresthesia, influenza-like syndrome (fever, myalgias, and malaise), renal function test abnormalities, anaphylaxis

OVERDOSAGE	
Signs and symptoms	See ADVERSE REACTIONS
Treatment	Discontinue medication; monitor blood counts and institute supportive measures, as required

DTIC-Dome ■ LEUKERAN

DRUG INTERACTIONS

Allopurinol	⇧ Uricosuric effect of allopurinol
Other myelosuppressive agents, radiotherapy	⇧ Antineoplastic effect

USE IN CHILDREN
See INDICATIONS and PARENTERAL DOSAGE

USE IN PREGNANT AND NURSING WOMEN
Pregnancy Category C: use during pregnancy only if the expected benefit justifies the potential risk to the fetus. Teratogenic effects have been observed in rats and rabbits at 20 and 7 times the human daily dose, respectively. An increased incidence of resorptions has been seen in female rats that were mated to males receiving 10 times the human daily dose twice a week. There are no adequate, well-controlled studies in pregnant women. It is not known whether dacarbazine is excreted in human milk; because many drugs are excreted in breast milk and because of the potential for tumorigenicity, patient should not nurse if use of this drug is deemed essential.

ALKYLATING AGENTS

LEUKERAN (chlorambucil) Burroughs Wellcome   Rx
Tablets: 2 mg

INDICATIONS Palliative treatment of **chronic lymphatic (lymphocytic) leukemia and malignant lymphomas,** including lymphosarcoma, giant follicular lymphoma, and Hodgkin's disease	**ORAL DOSAGE** **Adult:** 0.1–0.2 mg/kg (average dosage: 4–10 mg/day), given in a single daily dose for 3–6 wk, as needed, or 0.4 mg/kg, given in a single dose to start, repeated biweekly or monthly and increased by 0.1 mg/kg until control of lymphocytosis or toxicity occurs; subsequent doses are modified to produce mild hematological toxicity

CONTRAINDICATIONS
Prior resistance or hypersensitivity to chlorambucil[1]

ADMINISTRATION/DOSAGE ADJUSTMENTS

Maintenance therapy	Short courses of treatment, as described under ORAL DOSAGE, are generally considered safer than continuous maintenance therapy. If maintenance therapy is desired, up to 0.1 mg/kg/day may be given (typically 2–4 mg/day, or less, depending upon blood count); in some patients, dosage as low as 0.03 mg/kg/day may be adequate for maintenance. Once maximal control of lymphocytosis is achieved, it may be advisable to withdraw the drug, since intermittent therapy reinstituted at the time of relapse may be as effective as continuous treatment.
Patients with compromised bone marrow function	Reduce initial dose if WBC or platelet count is depressed from bone marrow disease prior to therapy or within 4 wk of a full course of chemotherapy or radiotherapy (full dosage may be used, however, if radiotherapy consisted of only small palliative doses over isolated foci remote from the bone marrow)

WARNINGS/PRECAUTIONS

Myelosuppressive effects	Bone marrow damage can result and may become irreversible as the total dose approaches 6.5 mg/kg (about 450 mg for a typical patient). Hemoglobin levels, total and differential WBC counts, and quantitative platelet counts should be obtained weekly. In addition, during the first 3–6 mo of therapy, obtain a WBC count 3–4 days after each complete blood count. Lymphopenia may slowly progress during treatment but usually rapidly returns to normal upon completion of therapy. Neutropenia generally develops after the 3rd wk of therapy and may continue for 10 days after the last dose, whereupon it usually rapidly returns to normal. Reduce dosage if WBC or platelet count falls below normal and discontinue therapy if more severe depression occurs. Persistent low neutrophil and platelet counts or peripheral lymphocytosis suggests bone marrow infiltration; if confirmed by bone marrow examination, do not administer more than 0.1 mg/kg/day.
Gastrointestinal effects	Single oral doses ≥ 20 mg may produce nausea and vomiting
Carcinogenicity	Acute leukemia has reportedly developed in many patients following treatment with chlorambucil and other alkylating agents. The risk appears to be increased with prolonged therapy and large cumulative doses; however, neither the degree of risk nor unsafe cumulative dose has been adequately defined. The potential benefits of continued therapy must therefore be weighed individually against the possible risk of inducing a second malignancy.
Mutagenicity	Chlorambucil has caused chromatid and chromosomal damage in man

LEUKERAN ■ Thiotepa

Effect on fertility	Both reversible and permanent sterility have occurred in males and females receiving chlorambucil therapy; a high incidence of sterility has been observed in prepubertal and pubertal males receiving the drug, and prolonged or permanent azoospermia has been observed in adults. Induction of amenorrhea in females has occurred with use of alkylating agents, and may occur with chlorambucil use.

ADVERSE REACTIONS

Hematological	Lymphopenia, neutropenia, thrombocytopenia; leukemia
Gastrointestinal	Nausea, vomiting, diarrhea, oral ulceration
Hypersensitivity	Fever, skin hypersensitivity
Respiratory	Pulmonary fibrosis, interstitial pneumonia
Genitourinary	Sterile cystitis, infertility
Other	Secondary malignancy, hepatotoxicity with jaundice, seizures (in children with nephrotic syndrome), peripheral neuropathy, focal fits

OVERDOSAGE

Signs and symptoms	Reversible pancytopenia is the main finding of overdosage; neurological toxicity, ranging from agitated behavior and ataxia to grand mal seizures have also occurred
Treatment	Closely monitor blood findings and institute general supportive measures with, if necessary, blood transfusions; chlorambucil is not dialyzable

DRUG INTERACTIONS

Antigout agents	⇧ Serum uric acid level
Other myelosuppressive agents, radiotherapy	⇧ Antineoplastic effect

ALTERED LABORATORY VALUES

Blood/serum values	⇧ Uric acid
Urinary values	⇧ Uric acid

USE IN CHILDREN

Safety and effectiveness for use in children have not been established

USE IN PREGNANT AND NURSING WOMEN

Pregnancy Category D: unilateral renal agenesis has occurred in two infants whose mothers received chlorambucil during the first trimester; urogenital malformations, including absence of a kidney, were found in fetuses of rats given chlorambucil. However, no adequate, well-controlled studies have been done in pregnant women. If chlorambucil is to be used during pregnancy, or if a patient becomes pregnant during therapy, the patient should be apprised of the potential hazard to the fetus; women of childbearing potential should avoid becoming pregnant during treatment with the drug. It is not known whether chlorambucil is excreted in human milk. Because many drugs are excreted in breast milk and because of the potential for serious adverse reactions in nursing infants, patient should not nurse if use of this drug is deemed essential.

[1] Cross-sensitivity, manifested by skin rash, may occur between chlorambucil and other alkylating agents

---

ALKYLATING AGENTS

Thiotepa Lederle Rx

Vials: 15 mg (10 mg/ml after reconstitution)

INDICATIONS	PARENTERAL DOSAGE
Palliative treatment of **adenocarcinoma of the breast or ovary**	**Adult:** 0.3–0.4 mg/kg, given by rapid IV administration at intervals of 1–4 wk, or 0.6–0.8 mg/kg, injected directly into the tumor, to start, followed by 0.07–0.8 mg/kg at intervals of 1–4 wk, depending upon the patient's condition
Intracavitary effusions secondary to diffuse or localized neoplastic disease of various serosal cavities	**Adult:** 0.6–0.8 mg/kg, injected directly into the cavity
Superficial papillary carcinoma of the urinary bladder	**Adult:** 60 mg dissolved in 30–60 ml of sterile water for injection instilled into the bladder by catheter and retained for 2 h, once a week for 4 wk. If necessary, a second or third course may be given; however, exercise caution since bone marrow depression may be increased.

COMPENDIUM OF DRUG THERAPY

Thiotepa ■ ZANOSAR

CONTRAINDICATIONS

Hepatic, renal, or bone marrow damage[1] | Hypersensitivity to thiotepa

ADMINISTRATION/DOSAGE ADJUSTMENTS

Parenteral administration	Reconstitute with 1.5 ml of sterile water for injection; the reconstituted solution may then be injected directly and rapidly into a suitable vein, injected directly into the tumor mass (see below), or, if desired, added to larger volumes of other diluents for intracavitary administration, continuous IV infusion, or perfusion therapy
Intratumor administration	First inject a small amount of local anesthetic through a 22-gauge needle, remove the syringe, and inject drug through the same needle
Intracavitary administration	Drug may be administered through same tubing used to remove fluid from involved cavity
Intravesical administration	Patient must be dehydrated for 8–12 prior to treatment
Local injection	Drug may be mixed with 2% procaine hydrochloride or 1:1000 epinephrine hydrochloride, or both
Maintenance dose	Adjust weekly on the basis of pretreatment control and subsequent blood counts

WARNINGS/PRECAUTIONS

Myelosuppressive effects	Leukopenia, thrombocytopenia, and anemia may occur, possibly leading to death from septicemia and hemorrhage. Obtain weekly blood and platelet counts during therapy and for at least 3 wk afterward; discontinue therapy if WBC count falls to 3,000/mm^3 or less or if the platelet count falls to 150,000/mm^3. Do not use other myelosuppressive agents concomitantly.
Mutagenicity	Chromosomal aberrations have been shown in vitro, with frequency increasing with increasing patient age
Carcinogenicity	Thiotepa is carcinogenic in animals, and strong circumstantial evidence of human carcinogenicity exists
Concomitant antineoplastic therapy	Do not use other alkylating agents or radiotherapy concomitantly or in close succession with thiotepa; ensure complete hematologic recovery from first agent before instituting therapy with the second agent

ADVERSE REACTIONS

Frequent reactions (incidence $\geq$ 1%) are printed in *italics*

Hematological	*Bone marrow depression, including thrombocytopenia, leukopenia, and anemia*
Gastrointestinal	*Nausea, vomiting, anorexia*
Central nervous system	Dizziness, headache
Endocrinological	*Amenorrhea, interference with spermatogenesis*
Dermatological and hypersensitivity	Hives, rash, alopecia (one case), weeping from subcutaneous lesions (due to breakdown of tumor tissue)
Other	*Pain at injection site*, fever (due to breakdown of tumor tissue)

OVERDOSAGE

Signs and symptoms	Bone marrow depression, including leukopenia, thrombocytopenia, and anemia
Treatment	Discontinue therapy; administer transfusions of whole blood, platelets, or leukocytes, as needed.

DRUG INTERACTIONS

Other myelosuppressive agents, radiotherapy	⇧ Myelosuppression
Succinylcholine	⇧ Risk of prolonged apnea

ALTERED LABORATORY VALUES

No clinically significant alterations in blood/serum or urinary values occur at therapeutic dosages

---

USE IN CHILDREN

Safety for use in children has not been established

USE IN PREGNANT AND NURSING WOMEN

Not recommended for use during pregnancy, unless expected benefit outweighs teratogenic risk. Do not use in nursing mothers.

---

[1] If the need for therapy outweighs risks, drug may be used in low dosage with adequate monitoring of hepatic, renal, and hematopoietic function

---

ALKYLATING AGENTS

ZANOSAR (streptozocin) Upjohn   Rx

Vials: 1 g for IV use only

INDICATIONS

Symptomatic or progressive **metastatic pancreatic islet-cell carcinoma**

PARENTERAL DOSAGE

Adult: 500 mg/m^2 IV for 5 consecutive days every 6 wk, until maximum benefit or treatment-limiting toxicity is observed (dosage escalation on this schedule is not recommended) or start with 1,000 mg/m^2 IV once a week for the first 2 wk; if this dose does not produce a therapeutic response or significant toxicity, it may be increased up to 1,500 mg/m^2, but not any higher

ZANOSAR

CONTRAINDICATIONS
See "renal toxicity" below, under WARNINGS/PRECAUTIONS

ADMINISTRATION/DOSAGE ADJUSTMENTS

Parenteral administration	Streptozocin is administered IV; intraarterial administration is not recommended, pending further investigation of the possibility that adverse renal effects may be evoked more rapidly
Measurement of therapeutic response	For patients with functional tumors, biochemical response may be determined by serial monitoring of fasting insulin levels; for patients with either functional or nonfunctional tumors, therapeutic response may be determined by measurable reductions of tumor size (reduction of organomegaly, masses, or lymph nodes). When streptozocin is administered on a weekly schedule, the median time to onset of therapeutic response is about 17 days (median total dose $\sim$ 2,000 mg/m^2) and to maximum response, about 35 days ($\sim$ 4,000 mg/m^2).
Preparation of solution	Reconstitute the contents of the vial with 9.5 ml of Dextrose Injection USP or 0.9% Sodium Chloride Injection USP to form a 100 mg/ml solution of streptozocin (plus 22 mg/ml citric acid); if desired, the above vehicles may be used to further dilute the solution for IV infusion. Use within 12 h.
Handling of streptozocin	Contact of the powder or solution with the skin or mucosae should be avoided; careful handling and the use of gloves is recommended. If contact occurs, immediately wash affected area with soap and water.

WARNINGS/PRECAUTIONS

Renal toxicity	May occur, and may be evidenced by azotemia, anuria, hypophosphatemia, glycosuria, and renal tubular acidosis. The toxicity is dose-related and cumulative, and may be severe or fatal. Mild proteinuria is one of the first signs of renal toxicity and may herald further deterioration of kidney function; monitor renal function before, during, and after each course of therapy. In patients with preexisting renal disease, the decision to use streptozocin should be made by weighing the possible benefit against the known risk of serious renal damage. Do not use this drug in combination or concomitantly with other potential nephrotoxins. If significant renal toxicity occurs, reduce the dose or discontinue streptozocin therapy.
Carcinogenicity, mutagenicity	Rats exposed to streptozocin on their skin developed benign tumors at the site of application; this drug may therefore pose a carcinogenic hazard following topical exposure if not properly handled (see ADMINISTRATION/DOSAGE ADJUSTMENTS). Streptozocin is mutagenic in bacteria, plants, and mammalian cells, and has been shown to induce tumors in rats, hamsters, and mice following oral and parenteral administration.
Laboratory monitoring during therapy	Monitor patients closely, particularly for evidence of renal, hepatic, and hematopoietic toxicity. A serial urinalysis and measurement of BUN, plasma creatinine, creatinine clearance, and serum electrolytes should be obtained prior to therapy, at least weekly during treatment, and for at least 4 wk afterward (if proteinuria is detected, quantitate the urinalysis by obtaining a 24-h collection). In addition, complete blood counts and liver function tests should be performed at least weekly. If indicated, adjust dosage or discontinue therapy, depending upon the degree of toxicity observed.

ADVERSE REACTIONS

Gastrointestinal	Severe nausea and vomiting, diarrhea, liver dysfunction
Hematological	Mild decrease in hematocrit; significant leukopenia and reduction in platelet count (occasionally fatal)
Endocrinological and metabolic	Mild to moderate abnormalities of glucose tolerance (generally reversible), insulin shock with hypoglycemia

OVERDOSAGE
No specific antidote for streptozocin is known

DRUG INTERACTIONS

Other potentially nephrotoxic drugs	△ Risk of renal toxicity; do not use concomitantly or in combination with streptozocin

ALTERED LABORATORY VALUES

Blood/serum values	△ SGOT △ Lactate dehydrogenase ▽ Albumin

No clinically significant alterations in urinary values occur at therapeutic dosages

USE IN CHILDREN
Consult manufacturer

USE IN PREGNANT AND NURSING WOMEN
Pregnancy Category C: use during pregnancy only if the expected benefit justifies the potential risk to the fetus. Streptozocin is teratogenic in rats and an abortifacient in rabbits; no studies have been done in pregnant women. It is not known whether streptozocin is excreted in human milk. Because many drugs are excreted in human milk, and because of the potential for serious adverse effects in nursing infants, nursing should be discontinued in patients receiving this drug.

ANTIMETABOLITES

CYTOSAR-U (cytarabine [ara-C]) Upjohn   Rx

Vials: 100 mg (20 mg/ml after reconstitution) and 500 mg (50 mg/ml after reconstitution)

INDICATIONS
Acute myelocytic leukemia[1]

PARENTERAL DOSAGE
Adult: for induction of remission, 200 mg/m²/day, given by continuous IV infusion for 5 consecutive days and repeated approximately every 2 wk, as needed. Alternatively, give 100 mg/m²/day in combination with other antineoplastic agents, as follows: cytarabine by continuous IV infusion on days 1–10 plus doxorubicin (30 mg/m²/day) by IV infusion over 30 min on days 1–3; cytarabine by continuous IV infusion on days 1–7 plus (1) daunorubicin (45 mg/m²/day), IV push, on days 1–3 or (2) doxorubicin (30 mg/m²/day) by IV infusion on days 1–3, vincristine (1.5 mg/m²/day) by IV infusion on days 1 and 5, and prednisolone (40 mg/m²/day) by IV infusion q12h on days 1–5; cytarabine by IV infusion over 30 min q12h on days 1–7 plus (1) thioguanine (100 mg/m²) PO q12h on days 1–7 and daunorubicin (60 mg/m²/day) by IV infusion on days 5–7 or (2) daunorubicin (70 mg/m²/day) by IV infusion on days 1–3, thioguanine (100 mg/m²) PO q12h on days 1–7, prednisone (40 mg/m²/day) PO on days 1–7, and vincristine (1 mg/m²/day) by IV infusion on days 1 and 7. Administer additional complete or modified courses every 2–4 wk, as needed. For maintenance of remission, most programs provide a dosage schedule similar to that used for induction, but with a longer interval between courses.
Child: same as adult

CONTRAINDICATIONS
Hypersensitivity to cytarabine

ADMINISTRATION/DOSAGE ADJUSTMENTS

Preparation of parenteral solutions	Reconstitute with bacteriostatic water for injection and 0.945% benzyl alcohol (supplied), using 5 ml for the 100-mg vial or 10 ml for the 500-mg vial; for intrathecal use, substitute preservative-free 0.9% sodium chloride injection and use immediately. Do not use the supplied diluent or any other solution containing benzyl alcohol for intrathecal administration or for experimental high-dose therapy.
Intrathecal use	For acute meningeal leukemia, doses of 5–75 mg/m² have been given intrathecally; the frequency of administration has varied from once daily (for 4 days) to once every 4 days. The most common dosage is 30 mg/m² every 4 days, with one additional dose given after CSF findings have returned to normal. After treatment of an acute meningeal episode, it may be useful as prophylactic therapy to administer cytarabine in combination with hydrocortisone sodium succinate and methotrexate (consult manufacturer). Cytarabine may not be as effective as radiotherapy in the treatment of focal leukemic involvement of the central nervous system.

WARNINGS/PRECAUTIONS

Myelosuppressive effects	Severe bone marrow depression (possibly fatal) may occur; monitor patients carefully and frequently, with frequent bone marrow examinations and daily platelet and WBC counts, and have facilities available to manage secondary infection and hemorrhage. Suspend or modify use if platelet count falls below 50,000/mm³ or polymorphonuclear leukocyte (granulocyte) count falls below 1,000/mm³ and do not restart therapy until counts return to these levels and signs of recovery appear. Use with caution in patients with preexisting drug-induced bone marrow suppression.
Severe nausea and vomiting	May result from rapid administration of large IV doses; effects are less severe with infusion
Acute pancreatitis	Acute pancreatitis has occurred during cytarabine therapy in patients who have had prior treatment with L-asparaginase
Gasping syndrome	Benzyl alcohol, which is contained in the solution used for reconstitution, has been associated with a fatal gasping syndrome in premature infants
Cytarabine syndrome	Some patients may experience a syndrome characterized by fever, myalgia, bone pain, occasional chest pain, maculopapular rash, conjunctivitis, and malaise and occurring usually within 6–12 h of administration; corticosteroids are beneficial in treating or preventing this syndrome. Cytarabine therapy may be continued in those patients whose symptoms are considered treatable with steroids and/or other measures.
Hyperuricemia	May occur; monitor blood uric acid level and institute supportive and pharmacologic measures, as required
Hepatic and renal function	Tests of hepatic and renal function should be performed periodically; reduce dosage and use with caution in patients with poor liver function
Experimental regimens	Use of this drug in some experimental regimens has resulted in severe, potentially fatal CNS, GI, and pulmonary reactions[2]; these effects differ from those seen with conventional regimens

ADVERSE REACTIONS[2]
The most frequent reactions, regardless of incidence, are printed in *italics*

Hematological	*Anemia, leukopenia, thrombocytopenia, megaloblastosis, reduced reticulocyte count, changes in bone marrow cell morphology*

CYTOSAR-U ■ EFUDEX

Gastrointestinal	*Anorexia, nausea, vomiting, diarrhea, oral and anal inflammation or ulceration, hepatic dysfunction,* sore throat, esophagitis, esophageal ulceration, abdominal pain, jaundice
Genitourinary	Urinary retention, renal dysfunction
Dermatological	*Rash,* freckling, ulceration, alopecia, pruritus, urticaria
Other	*Thrombophlebitis, bleeding (all sites), fever,* sepsis, pneumonia, cellulitis at injection site, neuritis, neurotoxicity, chest pain, dizziness, conjunctivitis, anaphylaxis, allergic edema, shortness of breath, headache

OVERDOSAGE

Signs and symptoms	Cerebral and cerebellar dysfunction, including personality changes, somnolence, and coma
Treatment	Discontinue medication; institute supportive measures, as required

DRUG INTERACTIONS

Antigout agents	△ Blood uric acid level
Other myelosuppressive agents, radiotherapy	△ Antineoplastic effect
Methotrexate	Possible synergistic effect

ALTERED LABORATORY VALUES

Blood/serum values	△ SGOT △ Uric acid
Urinary values	△ Uric acid

USE IN CHILDREN

See INDICATIONS and PARENTERAL DOSAGE; numerous studies have shown that children with acute myelocytic leukemia have higher response rates than adults

USE IN PREGNANT AND NURSING WOMEN

Pregnancy Category C: this drug should not be administered to women who are or who may become pregnant without due consideration of the potential therapeutic benefit and the possible hazard to both the mother and fetus. Cytarabine is teratogenic in some animal species. Of 32 cases where this drug was given to pregnant women, 18 normal infants were born; 2 infants were born with congenital anomalies, and 7 others had various problems in the neonatal period. Five of the cases ended in therapeutic abortion; four of the abortuses were grossly normal, but one had an enlarged spleen and another had a trisomy C chromosome abnormality in the chorionic tissue. Because of the potential for abnormalities, particularly during the first trimester, patients who are or who may become pregnant during therapy should be apprised of the risk involved and the advisability of continuing the pregnancy. Although normal infants have been born to mothers who were treated in all three trimesters, follow-up of such infants is advisable. Consult manufacturer for use in nursing mothers.

[1] Cytarabine, alone and in combination with other antineoplastic agents, has also been found useful in the treatment of other leukemias, including acute lymphocytic leukemia, chronic myelocytic leukemia (blast phase), and erythroleukemia. In general, few patients with solid tumors have benefited from cytarabine; however, the drug has been used effectively in combination with other agents for the treatment of non-Hodgkin's lymphoma in children. Consult manufacturer or package literature for applicable references.
[2] Reactions observed in studies where experimental doses were used include cardiomyopathy, pulmonary edema, subacute pulmonary failure, reversible corneal toxicity, hemorrhagic conjunctivitis, cerebral and cerebellar dysfunction (including personality changes, somnolence and coma), severe GI ulceration (including pneumatosis cystoides intestinalis leading to peritonitis), sepsis and liver abscess, liver damage with increased hyperbilirubinemia, bowel necrosis, necrotizing colitis, severe skin rash leading to desquamation, and complete alopecia. Nausea, vomiting, and fever are the most common adverse reactions that occur after intrathecal administration; other reactions include neurotoxicity, paraplegia, necrotizing leukoencephalopathy (in five children who underwent CNS irradiation and were also given intrathecal methotrexate and hydrocortisone), and blindness (in two patients who underwent CNS irradiation and received combination systemic therapy).

ANTIMETABOLITES

EFUDEX (fluorouracil) Roche   Rx

Cream: 5% (25 g)   **Solution:** 2%, 5% (10 ml)

INDICATIONS	TOPICAL DOSAGE
Multiple actinic or solar keratoses	**Adult:** apply cream or solution in an amount sufficient to cover lesions bid for 2–4 wk until inflammatory response (characterized by erythema and vesiculation) progresses to erosion, ulceration, and necrosis
Superficial basal-cell carcinomas, when conventional methods are impractical (eg, multiple lesions or difficult treatment sites)	**Adult:** apply 5% cream or solution in an amount sufficient to cover lesions bid for at least 3–6 wk (up to 10–12 wk, if necessary) until lesions are obliterated

COMPENDIUM OF DRUG THERAPY

EFUDEX ■ Fluorouracil

CONTRAINDICATIONS
Hypersensitivity to any of the components

WARNINGS/PRECAUTIONS

Application	Apply with caution near eyes, nose, and mouth; wash hands immediately afterward
Occlusive dressings	May increase incidence of inflammatory reactions in adjacent normal skin; porous gauze dressings may be applied for cosmetic reasons without increase in reaction
Ultraviolet rays	Prolonged exposure to sunlight or other UV radiation should be avoided during therapy because intensity of reaction may be increased
Unsightly appearance	Forewarn patients that treated areas may be unsightly during and, in some cases, for several weeks after therapy; healing of keratotic lesions may not be complete for 1–2 mo following cessation of therapy
Unresponsive solar keratoses	Perform biopsy to confirm diagnosis
Follow-up	Patients with superficial basal cell carcinoma should be followed and biopsies performed to determine whether cure has been achieved

ADVERSE REACTIONS[1]
The most frequent reactions, regardless of incidence, are printed in *italics*

Local	*Pain, pruritus, hyperpigmentation, burning,* allergic contact dermatitis, scarring, soreness, tenderness, suppuration, scaling, swelling
Hematological	Leukocytosis, thrombocytopenia, toxic granulation, eosinophilia

---

USE IN CHILDREN
Consult manufacturer

USE IN PREGNANT AND NURSING WOMEN
Safety for use during pregnancy has not been established; consult manufacturer for use in nursing mothers

---

VEHICLE/BASE
Cream: white petrolatum, stearyl alcohol, propylene glycol, polysorbate 60, and parabens
Solution: propylene glycol, tris, hydroxypropyl cellulose, parabens, and EDTA

[1] Other reactions for which a causal relationship has not been established include alopecia, insomnia, stomatitis, irritability, medicinal taste, photosensitivity, lacrimation, telangiectasia, and urticaria

---

ANTIMETABOLITES

Fluorouracil Roche   Rx

Ampuls: 50 mg/ml (10 ml) for IV use only   **Vials:** 50 mg/ml (10 ml) for IV use only

INDICATIONS
Palliative treatment of **carcinoma of the colon, rectum, breast, stomach, and pancreas** in patients who are considered incurable by surgery or other means

PARENTERAL DOSAGE
Adult: 12 mg/kg, up to 800 mg/day, given in a single daily IV dose for 4 consecutive days to start, followed by 6 mg/kg IV on the 6th, 8th, 10th, and 12th day, unless toxicity occurs; patient should be hospitalized during the initial course of therapy

CONTRAINDICATIONS

Hypersensitivity to fluorouracil	Depressed bone marrow function	Potentially serious infections
Poor nutritional state		

ADMINISTRATION/DOSAGE ADJUSTMENTS

Calculation of dosage	Base dosage on patient's actual weight; use estimated lean body mass if patient is obese or has gained weight due to edema, ascites, or other causes of abnormal fluid retention
High-risk patients	Administer 6 mg/kg/day, up to 400 mg/day, IV for 3 consecutive days, to start, followed by 3 mg/kg IV on the 5th, 7th, and 9th day unless toxicity occurs
Maintenance therapy	If toxicity does not develop, or if it subsides after treatment, repeat dosage of first course, beginning 30 days after the last day of previous treatment, or administer 10–15 mg/kg/wk; do not give more than 1 g/wk

WARNINGS/PRECAUTIONS

Special-risk patients	Use with caution in patients with a history of high-dose pelvic irradiation, prior use of alkylating agents, widespread involvement of bone marrow by metastatic tumors, or impaired hepatic or renal function

Fluorouracil ■ Methotrexate

Combination therapy	Increase toxicity if it causes additional stress to the patient, interferes with nutrition, or depresses bone marrow function
Patient monitoring and instructions	Therapeutic response is unlikely to occur without some evidence of toxicity; obtain WBC count and differential count before giving each dose and inform patient of expected side effects, particularly oral manifestations (see ADVERSE REACTIONS)
Severe hematological toxicity, GI hemorrhage, and death	May result despite meticulous patient selection and careful dosage adjustment
Conditions necessitating prompt withdrawal of therapy	Discontinue medication if any of the following toxic signs appear: stomatitis, esophagopharyngitis, leukopenia (WBC count $< 3,500/mm^3$), rapidly falling WBC count, intractable vomiting, diarrhea, GI ulceration and bleeding, thrombocytopenia (platelet count $< 100,000/mm^3$), or hemorrhage

ADVERSE REACTIONS

Central nervous system	Euphoria, disorientation, confusion
Gastrointestinal	Stomatitis, esophagopharyngitis, sloughing, ulceration, diarrhea, anorexia, nausea, vomiting
Hematological	Leukopenia, thrombocytopenia, pancytopenia, agranulocytosis, anemia
Dermatological	Alopecia, dermatitis (pruritic maculopapular rash), dry skin, fissuring, photosensitivity, nail changes and possible loss of nails
Ophthalmic	Photophobia, visual changes, lacrimation, lacrimal duct stenosis
Cardiovascular	Myocardial ischemia
Hypersensitivity	Anaphylaxis, bronchospasm, urticaria, pruritus
Other	Epistaxis, acute cerebellar syndrome, thrombophlebitis

OVERDOSAGE

Signs and symptoms	See ADVERSE REACTIONS
Treatment	Discontinue medication; institute supportive measures, as required

DRUG INTERACTIONS

Other myelosuppressive agents, radiotherapy	△ Antineoplastic effect

ALTERED LABORATORY VALUES

Blood/serum values	▽ Albumin
Urinary values	△ 5-HIAA

USE IN CHILDREN

Consult manufacturer

USE IN PREGNANT AND NURSING WOMEN

Safety for use during pregnancy has not been established; consult manufacturer for use in nursing mothers

---

ANTIMETABOLITES

Methotrexate   Rx

Tablets: 2.5 mg   Vials (preserved): 2.5 mg/ml (2 ml), 25 mg/ml (2 ml)   Vials (preservative-free, single use): 25 mg/ml (2, 4, 8 ml)   Vials (cryodessicated powder, preservative-free, single use): 20, 50, 100 mg

INDICATIONS	ORAL DOSAGE	PARENTERAL DOSAGE
Gestational choriocarcinoma **Chorioadenoma destruens** **Hydatidiform mole**	Adult: 15–30 mg/day, given for 5 consecutive days; repeat 3–5 times, at intervals of 1 or more weeks, as required	Adult: 15–30 mg/day IM, given for 5 consecutive days; repeat 3–5 times, at intervals of 1 or more weeks, as required
Palliative treatment of **acute lymphocytic (lymphoblastic) leukemia**	Adult: for induction, 3.3 mg/m²/day, given with 60 mg/m²/day of prednisone for 4–6 wk; for maintenance, 30 mg/m² twice weekly	Adult: for maintenance, 30 mg/m² IM twice weekly or 2.5 mg/kg IV every 14 days
Burkitt's lymphoma (stages I–II)	Adult: 10–25 mg/day, given for 4–8 consecutive days; repeat several times at 7- to 10-day intervals	—
Lymphosarcoma (stage III)	Adult: 0.625–2.5 mg/kg/day	—

COMPENDIUM OF DRUG THERAPY

Methotrexate

Meningeal leukemia	—	**Adult:** 12 mg/m² or 15 mg, given intrathecally every 2–5 days until CSF cell count returns to normal, followed by one additional dose
Advanced mycosis fungoides	**Adult:** 2.5–10 mg/day	**Adult:** 50 mg IM once weekly or 25 mg IM twice weekly
Severe, recalcitrant, disabling **psoriasis** that does not respond to other forms of therapy	**Adult:** 10–25 mg, given in a single weekly dose, up to 50 mg/wk; 2.5 mg q12h for 3 doses or q8h for 4 doses weekly, up to 30 mg/wk; or 2.5 mg/day for 5 days, up to 6.25 mg/day, followed by a drug-free interval of 2 or more days until optimal clinical response is achieved.	**Adult:** 10–25 mg, given in a single weekly IM or IV dose, up to 50 mg/wk, until optimal clinical response is achieved.
Breast cancer; epidermoid cancer of the head and neck; **lung cancer,** particularly squamous cell and small cell types; advanced **lymphosarcoma (stage IV)**	Consult manufacturer	Consult manufacturer

CONTRAINDICATIONS

Pregnancy, severe renal or hepatic disorders, or preexisting blood dyscrasias in patients with psoriasis	Renal impairment (see WARNINGS/PRECAUTION)

ADMINISTRATION/DOSAGE ADJUSTMENTS

Preparation of parenteral solutions	For IM or IV injection, reconstitute solution, not exceeding a concentration of 25 mg/ml, or use supplied solution in diluted or undiluted form; to reconstitute or dilute the solution, immediately before administration add an appropriate, sterile, preservative-free diluent such as sodium chloride injection USP (for IM injection) or 5% dextrose injection USP (for IV injection). For intrathecal injection, reconstitute or dilute solution to a concentration of 1 mg/ml, using sodium chloride injection USP or another appropriate, sterile, preservative-free diluent.

WARNINGS/PRECAUTIONS

Patient monitoring	Fatal or severe toxic reactions may occur; inform patient of the risks involved and monitor carefully. Obtain the following studies periodically: complete hemogram, hematocrit, urinalysis, renal and liver function tests, and chest x-ray. If high doses are used or therapy is prolonged, obtain a liver biopsy or bone marrow aspiration study.
Hepatotoxicity	May occur, particularly at high dosages or with prolonged therapy. Determine hepatic function prior to use and monitor regularly throughout therapy; avoid concomitant use of other hepatotoxic drugs, including alcohol.
Patients with impaired renal function	Toxic accumulation or additional renal damage may occur. Determine patient's renal status prior to and during therapy and use with caution if significant impairment is disclosed; reduce dosage or discontinue medication until renal function improves or is restored.
Other special-risk patients	Use with caution, if at all, in patients with preexisting bone marrow aplasia, anemia, leukopenia, thrombocytopenia, or bleeding; in patients with infection, peptic ulcer, ulcerative colitis, or debility; and in very young or elderly patients
Treatment of psoriasis	Fatalities have occurred following use of this drug in psoriasis; Restrict therapy to severe, recalcitrant, disabling psoriasis that fails to respond to other treatment modalities. The diagnosis must be confirmed by biopsy and/or dermatological examination before starting treatment. Advise patient to take appropriate measures to prevent conception both during therapy and for at least 8 wk after methotrexate is discontinued. Use of the 5-day administration schedule may increase the risk of serious hepatic disease.
Intestinal perforation	May result in hemorrhagic enteritis and death; discontinue use if diarrhea and ulcerative stomatitis develop
Concurrent therapy	Toxicity may be increased by salicylates, sulfonamides, phenytoin, phenylbutazone, and some antibacterial compounds; in addition, Vitamin preparations containing folic acid or folate derivatives may alter the response to methotrexate
Bacterial infection	May follow profound drug-induced leukopenia; discontinue use and institute appropriate antimicrobial therapy (transfusion may also be necessary)
Immunosuppressive effects	Must be considered in evaluating use where immune responses are important or essential

ADVERSE REACTIONS

Gastrointestinal	Nausea, abdominal distress, gingivitis, pharyngitis, stomatitis, anorexia, vomiting, diarrhea, ulcerative stomatitis, hematemesis, melena, ulceration, bleeding, enteritis
Hematological	Leukopenia, bone marrow depression, thrombocytopenia, anemia, hypogamma-globulinemia, hemorrhage

Methotrexate ■ ADRIAMYCIN

Dermatological	Erythematous rashes, pruritus, urticaria, photosensitivity, depigmentation, alopecia, ecchymosis, telangiectasia, acne, furunculosis
Hepatic	Acute atrophy, necrosis, fatty metamorphosis, periportal fibrosis, cirrhosis
Genitourinary	Renal failure, azotemia, cystitis, hematuria, defective oogenesis or spermatogenesis, transient oligospermia, menstrual dysfunction, infertility, abortion, fetal defects, severe nephropathy
Central nervous system	Headaches, drowsiness, blurred vision, aphasia, hemiparesis, paresis, convulsions; leukoencephalopathy (with IV use); arachnoiditis (with intrathecal use)
Other	Malaise, undue fatigue, chills, fever, dizziness, decreased resistance to infection, pneumonitis, septicemia, metabolic changes precipitating diabetes, osteoporotic effects, abnormal tissue cell changes, sudden death

OVERDOSAGE

Signs and symptoms	See ADVERSE REACTIONS
Treatment	Discontinue medication; institute supportive measures, as required. Leucovorin (citrovorum factor) neutralizes the immediate toxic effects on the hematopoietic system. Within 12 h of giving large doses or an inadvertent overdose, administer leucovorin by IV infusion in doses of up to 75 mg, following by 12 mg M q6h for 4 doses. When average doses produce adverse effects, administer 6–12 mg leucovorin IM q6h for 4 doses.

DRUG INTERACTIONS

Alcohol, other hepatotoxic agents	△ Risk of hepatotoxicity
Antigout agents	△ Blood uric acid level
Asparaginase	▽ Antineoplastic effect
Other myelosuppressive agents, radiotherapy	△ Antineoplastic effect
Phenylbutazone, salicylates, sulfonamides, phenytoin, probenecid, tetracycline, chloramphenicol, pyrimethamine, para-aminobenzoic acid	△ Methotrexate toxicity

ALTERED LABORATORY VALUES

Blood/serum values	△ Isocitric acid dehydrogenase (ICD) △ Uric acid
Urinary values	△ Uric acid

USE IN CHILDREN
Only clinicians experienced in antimetabolite therapy and following a rigid, established therapeutic protocol should administer methotrexate to children. Indications in children include palliation of acute lymphoblastic (stem-cell) leukemias and treatment of the advanced stages (III and IV) of lymphosarcoma.

USE IN PREGNANT AND NURSING WOMEN
Not recommended for women of childbearing potential; fetal death and congenital anomalies have occurred. Contraindicated for pregnant psoriatic patients. Methotrexate is excreted in human milk; do not use in nursing mothers (institute an alternative form of infant feeding).

ANTINEOPLASTIC ANTIBIOTICS

ADRIAMYCIN (doxorubicin hydrochloride) Adria   Rx

Vials: 10, 20, 50 mg (2 mg/ml after reconstitution) for IV use only

INDICATIONS
Disseminated neoplastic conditions, including acute lymphoblastic leukemia, acute myeloblastic leukemia, Wilms' tumor, neuroblastoma, soft tissue and bone sarcomas, breast carcinoma, ovarian carcinoma, transitional cell bladder carcinoma, thyroid carcinoma, Hodgkin's disease, non-Hodgkin's lymphomas, and bronchogenic carcinoma (small cells most responsive)

PARENTERAL DOSAGE
Adult: 60–75 mg/m² IV every 21 days (the lower dose should be given to patients with inadequate bone marrow reserves due to old age, prior therapy, or neoplastic infiltration); alternatively, give 20 mg/m² IV once weekly (this regimen reportedly produces a lower incidence of congestive heart failure) or 30 mg/m²/day for 3 consecutive days every 4 wk (this regimen reportedly increases the incidence and severity of mucositis); for combination regimens, consult manufacturer
Child: same as adult

ADRIAMYCIN

CONTRAINDICATIONS

Marked myelosuppression induced by previous treatment with other antitumor agents or by radiotherapy

Previous treatment with complete cumulative doses of doxorubicin and/or daunorubicin

Preexisting heart disease

ADMINISTRATION/DOSAGE ADJUSTMENTS

Preparation of IV solution for injection	Reconstitute with 09% Sodium Chloride Injection USP or Sterile Water for Injection USP (*do not use bacteriostatic diluents*), using 5 ml for the 10-mg vial, 10 ml for the 20-mg vial, and 25 ml for the 50-mg vial. If Sterile Water for Injection USP is used, add 2–3 times the volume of 0.9% Sodium Chloride Injection USP to bring the aqueous solution toward isotonicity before injection. Remove some of the air from the vial to prevent pressure buildup, and shake the vial to dissolve the contents. To avoid precipitation, do not mix the reconstituted solution with other drugs, especially heparin and fluorouracil. The reconstituted solution may be stored for 24 h at room temperature or for 48 h under refrigeration; protect the solution from sunlight and discard any unused portion.
Intravenous administration	Administer the required dose into the tubing of a freely running IV infusion of 0.9% Sodium Chloride Injection USP or 5% Dextrose Injection USP. The tubing should be attached to a scalp-vein needle that has been inserted preferably into a large vein; if possible, avoid veins over joints or in extremities with compromised venous or lymphatic drainage. Inject slowly, over a period of not less than 3–5 min; if facial flushing or erythematous streaking along the vein occurs, injection may be too rapid. Perivascular infiltration may occur painlessly or manifest itself by a burning or stinging sensation (see WARNINGS/PRECAUTIONS).
Patients with elevated serum bilirubin levels	If serum bilirubin level = 1.2–3.0 mg/dl, give ½ the normal dose; if > 3 mg/dl, give ¼ the normal dose

WARNINGS/PRECAUTIONS

Extravasation	Severe cellulitis, vesication, and local tissue necrosis may result if extravasation occurs during IV administration; if signs or symptoms of perivascular infiltration develop, immediately terminate infusion and restart in another vein (extravasation may occur painlessly). Flood the area with normal saline and inject a corticosteroid into the site. If reaction progresses, consult a plastic surgeon; early, wide excision of the site may be necessary if ulceration occurs.
Cardiac effects	Myocardial toxicity with delayed congestive heart failure and/or myopthy may be encountered as the total dose approaches 550 mg/m^2 and is often unresponsive to any cardiac supportive therapy. Myocardial toxicity may occur at lower doses (400 mg/m^2) in patients with prior mediastinal irradiation or patients receiving other potentially cardiotoxic drugs (eg, cyclophosphamide) concurrently. Perform a baseline ECG and repeat prior to each dose or course after a cumulative dose of 300 mg/m^2 has been given. A persistent decrease in QRS voltage, prolongation of systole, and reduction of the ejection fraction (as determined by echocardiography or radionuclide angiography) may indicate that the maximum tolerable dose has been reached, and the benefits of continued therapy should then be carefully weighed against the risk of producing irreversible cardiac damage. Acute, life-threatening arrhythmias have occurred during or within a few hours of administration.
Myelosuppressive effects	Bone marrow depression (primarily leukopenia) may occur and requires careful hematologic monitoring; hematological toxicity may require dose reduction or suspension or delay of therapy. Severe myelosuppression may result in superinfection and hemorrhage.
Mucositis	Stomatitis and esophagitis may occur 5–10 days after administration; in severe cases, ulceration and serious infections may result
Impaired hepatic function	Enhances toxicity; prior to individual dosing, evaluate hepatic function by conventional clinical laboratory tests (eg. SGOT, SGPT, alkaline phosphatase, and bilirubin)
Concurrent antineoplastic therapy	Doxorubicin may potentiate the toxic effects of other anticancer therapies (see DRUG INTERACTIONS); necrotizing colitis manifested by typhlitis (cecal inflammation), bloody stools, and severe, occasionally fatal infections has been reported in patients with acute nonlymphocytic leukemia who were treated with a combination of doxorubicin and cytarabine
Carcinogenicity, mutagenicity	Carcinogenic and mutagenic properties have been observed in experimental models
Patient monitoring	Initial therapy requires close observation of the patient and extensive laboratory monitoring; hospitalize patients during the initial phase of treatment
Hyperuricemia	May occur secondary to rapid lysis of neoplastic cells; monitor blood uric acid level and be prepared to use appropriate supportive and pharmacological measures
Urine discoloration	Urine may turn red for 1–2 days after administration; warn patients to expect this
Skin reactions	May result from accidental contact with powder or solution; wear gloves and handle drug carefully during preparation. If contact with skin or mucosa occurs, wash exposed surface thoroughly with soap and water.

ADVERSE REACTIONS

Hematological	Myelosuppression

ADRIAMYCIN ■ BLENOXANE

Cardiovascular	Cardiotoxicity, arrhythmias, phlebosclerosis, facial flushing
Dermatological	Reversible complete alopecia; hyperpigmentation of nailbeds and dermal creases (primarily in children); recalled skin reaction due to prior radiotherapy; severe cellulitis, vesication, and tissue necrosis; erythematous streaking along the vein proximal to the injection site
Gastrointestinal	Acute nausea and vomiting, mucositis (stomatitis, esophagitis), ulceration and necrosis of the colon (see WARNINGS/PRECAUTIONS), anorexia, diarrhea
Hypersensitivity	Fever, chills, urticaria, anaphylaxis, cross-sensitivity to lincomycin
Other	Conjunctivitis; lacrimation (rare)

OVERDOSAGE

Signs and symptoms	Mucositis, leukopenia, thrombopenia, cardiomyopathy, congestive heart failure
Treatment	Severely myelosuppressed patients should be hospitalized and given antibiotics and platelet and granulocyte infusions, as indicated; treat mucositis symptomatically. Congestive heart failure resulting from chronic overdosage should receive vigorous treatment with digitalis preparations and diuretics; use of peripheral vasodilators is recommended.

DRUG INTERACTIONS

Cyclophosphamide	⇧ Risk of hemorrhage cystitis and cardiotoxicity
Mercaptopurine	⇧ Risk of hepatotoxicity
Radiotherapy	⇧ Risk of cardiac, mucosal skin, and liver toxicity ⇧ Antineoplastic effect
Antigout agents	⇧ Serum uric acid levels
Mitomycin	⇧ Risk of cardiotoxicity
Other myelosuppressive agents	⇧ Antineoplastic effect

ALTERED LABORATORY VALUES

Blood/serum values	⇧ Uric acid
Urinary values	⇧ Uric acid

USE IN CHILDREN
See INDICATIONS and PARENTERAL DOSAGE

USE IN PREGNANT AND NURSING WOMEN
Safety for use during pregnancy has not been established; doxorubicin is embryotoxic and teratogenic in rats and embryotoxic and an abortifacient in rabbits. It is not known whether doxorubicin is excreted in human milk. Use in nursing mothers is not recommended because many drugs are excreted in human milk.

ANTINEOPLASTIC ANTIBIOTICS

BLENOXANE (bleomycin sulfate)   Bristol-Myers Oncology   Rx

Vials: 15 units

INDICATIONS

Palliative treatment of **squamous cell carcinoma** of the mouth, tongue, tonsil, nasopharynx, oropharynx, sinus, palate, lip, buccal mucosa, gingiva, epiglottis, larynx, skin, penis, cervix, or vulva and of **testicular carcinoma**, including embryonal cell carcinoma, choriocarcinoma, and teratocarcinoma

Palliative treatment of **lymphomas**, including Hodgkin's disease, reticulum cell sarcoma, and lymphosarcoma

PARENTERAL DOSAGE

Adult: 0.25–0.50 units/kg SC, IM, or IV weekly or twice weekly

Adult: 2 units or less for first 2 doses, then 0.25–0.50 units/kg SC, IM, or IV weekly or twice weekly; for maintenance of Hodgkin's disease patients, administer 1 unit/day or 5 units/wk IV or IM after achieving a 50% response with initial dosage schedule

CONTRAINDICATIONS

Hypersensitivity or idiosyncratic reaction to bleomycin

COMPENDIUM OF DRUG THERAPY

BLENOXANE ■ CERUBIDINE

ADMINISTRATION/DOSAGE ADJUSTMENTS

Subcutaneous or intramuscular administration	Dissolve contents of vial in 1–5 ml of Sterile Water for Injection USP, Sodium Chloride for Injection USP, 5% Dextrose Injection USP, or Bacteriostatic Water for Injection USP before administration
Intravenous administration	Dissolve contents of vial in 5 ml or more of suitable IV solution (eg, normal saline or glucose) and administer slowly over a period of 10 min
Onset of clinical response	If no improvement in Hodgkin's disease or testicular tumors is seen within 2 wk, improvement is unlikely; squamous cell cancers may take as long as 3 wk to respond

WARNINGS/PRECAUTIONS

Patient monitoring	Monitor patients carefully and frequently for adverse reactions
Pulmonary toxicity	Nonspecific pneumonitis progressing to pulmonary fibrosis may be fatal, especially in elderly patients and those receiving a total dose exceeding 400 units. The pulmonary diffusion capacity for carbon monoxide (DL_{CO}) should be checked monthly, and roentgenograms should be taken every 1–2 wk. If the DL_{CO} falls below 30–35% of the pretreatment value, discontinue use; if radiographic changes are detected, discontinue treatment until it can be determined that they are drug-related. To prevent toxic effects in patients undergoing surgery, maintain the inhaled oxygen fraction at approximately 25% during surgery and the postoperative period because lung damage can occur at higher oxygen levels that, in the absence of bleomycin use, would usually be considered safe; in addition, carefully monitor fluid replacement, and preferably use colloids rather than crystalloids. Total doses over 400 units should be given with great caution because the risk of pulmonary toxicity increases strikingly when this amount is exceeded; toxic effects may occur at lower doses when bleomycin is given in combination with other antineoplastic drugs.
Special-risk patients	Use with extreme caution in patients with significant renal impairment or compromised pulmonary function
Renal or hepatic toxicity	Begins as a deterioration in renal or liver function tests; occurs infrequently
Idiosyncratic reactions	A severe idiosyncratic reaction, consisting of hypotension, mental confusion, fever, chills, and wheezing, may occur in 1% of lymphoma patients after the 1st or 2nd dose; monitor patient carefully

ADVERSE REACTIONS

Pulmonary	Pneumonitis, fibrosis leading to death
Dermatological	Erythema, rash, striae, vesication, hyperpigmentation, tender skin, hyperkeratosis, nail changes, alopecia, pruritus
Gastrointestinal	Stomatitis, vomiting, anorexia
Other	Fever, chills, weight loss, pain at tumor site, phlebitis[1]

OVERDOSAGE

Signs and symptoms	See ADVERSE REACTIONS
Treatment	Discontinue medication; institute supportive measures, as required

DRUG INTERACTIONS

Other antineoplastic agents, radiotherapy	◇ Risk of toxicity, including bone marrow depression

ALTERED LABORATORY VALUES

No clinically significant alterations in blood/serum or urinary values occur at therapeutic dosages

USE IN CHILDREN
Consult manufacturer

USE IN PREGNANT AND NURSING WOMEN
Safety for use during pregnancy has not been established. It is not known whether bleomycin is excreted in human milk. Because many drugs are excreted in breast milk and because of the potential for serious adverse reactions in nursing infants, patient should not nurse if use of this drug is deemed essential.

[1] Isolated cases of Raynaud's phenomenon have been reported in patients with testicular carcinomas who were given bleomycin in combination with vinblastine; a causal relationship has not been established.

ANTINEOPLASTIC ANTIBIOTICS

CERUBIDINE (daunorubicin hydrochloride) Wyeth Rx
Vials: 20 mg (5 mg/ml after reconstitution) for IV use only

INDICATIONS
Induction of remission in **acute non-lymphocytic (myelogenic, monocytic, erythroid) leukemia**

PARENTERAL DOSAGE
Adult: 60 mg/m²/day, given IV for 3 consecutive days every 3–4 wk; alternatively, give 45 mg/m²/day of daunorubicin IV for 3 consecutive days during the first course and 2 consecutive days during subsequent courses, plus 100 mg/kg of cytosine arabinoside by IV infusion daily for 7 days during the first course and 5 days during subsequent courses (up to three courses may be required for remission)

CERUBIDINE

Induction of remission in **acute lymphocytic leukemia**[1] — Child: 25 mg/m² , given IV once a week in combination with vincristine, 1.5 mg/m² IV, and oral prednisone, 40 mg/m²/day; for children under 2 yr of age or whose body surface area is less than 0.5 m², calculate dosage on the basis of body weight. The usual duration of therapy is 4 wk; however, treatment may be continued for an additional 1–2 wk if partial remission is obtained after 4 wk.

CONTRAINDICATIONS

None known

ADMINISTRATION/DOSAGE ADJUSTMENTS

Intravenous administration — Dilute contents of vial with 4 ml of Sterile Water for Injection USP; withdraw desired dose into a syringe containing 10-15 ml of normal saline and inject into tubing or sidearm of a rapidly flowing IV infusion of 5% dextrose or normal saline. Do not administer or mix with other drugs or heparin. Use extreme care to avoid extravasation, as severe local tissue necrosis may occur.

Patients with hepatic or renal impairment — If serum bilirubin = 1.2–3.0 mg/dl, give ¾ the normal dose; if serum bilirubin > 3 mg/dl or serum creatinine > 3 mg/dl, give ½ the normal dose

WARNINGS/PRECAUTIONS

Cardiac effects — Myocardial toxicity, manifested by acute, and possibly fatal, congestive heart failure may occur; there appears to be little risk, however, until the total cumulative dose exceeds 550 mg/m² in adults, 300 mg/m² in children over 2 yr of age, or 10 mg/kg in children under 2 yr of age or with a body surface area of less than 0.5 m². Cardiac effects may occur during therapy or may be delayed for several months. Use with caution in children, patients with preexisting heart disease, patients who have received or are now receiving other potentially cardiotoxic agents or related antineoplastic compounds, such as doxorubicin, and patients who have undergone radiotherapy encompassing the heart. Monitor ECG and/or determine systolic ejection fraction prior to each course of therapy. A decrease equal to or greater than 30% in limb lead QRS voltage or a decline in the systolic ejection fraction may be indicative of a significant risk of drug-induced cardiomyopathy.

Myelosuppressive effects — Severe myelosuppression occurs in all patients at therapeutic doses; do not use in patients with preexisting drug-induced bone marrow suppression unless benefits outweigh risks.

Hepatic or renal impairment — Enhances toxicity; hepatic and renal function should be evaluated prior to therapy, using conventional clinical laboratory tests. Dosage should be reduced accordingly (see ADMINISTRATION/DOSAGE ADJUSTMENTS).

Hyperuricemia — May occur secondary to rapid lysis of leukemic cells; monitor blood uric acid levels and initiate appropriate therapy where needed

Urine discoloration — Urine may turn red temporarily following administration; warn patient to expect this

Systemic infection — Must be controlled with appropriate measures prior to therapy

Patient monitoring — Because of the potential for severe toxicity, therapy requires close patient observation; use only when facilities for extensive laboratory monitoring and immediate supportive resources are available for responding to severe hemorrhagic complications and/or overwhelming infection

ADVERSE REACTIONS

Hematological — Myelosuppression

Cardiovascular — Congestive heart failure; pericarditis-myocarditis (rare)

Dermatological — Reversible alopecia

Gastrointestinal — Acute nausea and vomiting (antiemetic therapy may be helpful), mucositis, diarrhea

Hypersensitivity — Fever, chills, skin rash

OVERDOSAGE

Signs and symptoms — Myelosuppression, cardiotoxicity

Treatment — Discontinue medication and institute supportive measures, as needed; treat congestive heart failure with digitalis, diuretics, sodium restriction, and bed rest

DRUG INTERACTIONS

No clinically significant drug interactions have been identified

ALTERED LABORATORY VALUES

Blood/serum values — △ Uric acid

Urinary values — Discoloration (may interfere with certain colorimetric methods)

USE IN CHILDREN	USE IN PREGNANT AND NURSING WOMEN
See INDICATIONS and PARENTERAL DOSAGE	Pregnancy Category D: may produce teratogenic effects. Pregnant patients who receive daunorubicin should be apprised of the potential hazard to fetus. It is not known whether daunorubicin is excreted in human milk; because many drugs are excreted in breast milk, use with caution in nursing mothers.

[1] Daunorubicin prolongs the duration of complete remission in children who receive only CNS prophylaxis and maintenance therapy after induction; there is no evidence that this effect occurs when the treatment program includes a consolidation (intensification) phase

---

ANTINEOPLASTIC ANTIBIOTICS

MITHRACIN (plicamycin) Miles Pharmaceuticals   Rx

Vials: 2.5 mg (500 µg/ml after reconstitution) for IV use only

INDICATIONS

Malignant testicular tumors, when successful treatment by surgery and/or irradiation is impossible

Hypercalcemia and hypercalciuria associated with advanced malignancy in patients unresponsive to conventional treatment

PARENTERAL DOSAGE[1]

Adult: 25–30 µg/kg/day, given by slow infusion over a period of 4–6 h for 8–10 days unless significant adverse effects or toxicity occurs; maximum daily dosage: 30 µg/kg. Do not give any course of therapy consisting of more than 10 daily doses (see ADMINISTRATION/DOSAGE ADJUSTMENTS)

Adult: 25 µg/kg/day, given by slow IV infusion over a period of 4–6 h for 3–4 days; repeat at intervals of 1 wk or more if desired response is not achieved with initial course. Normal calcium balance may be obtained with single weekly doses or with a schedule of 2–3 doses/wk.

CONTRAINDICATIONS

Thrombocytopenia, thrombocytopathy, coagulation disorder, or increased susceptibility to bleeding	Impaired bone marrow function	Pregnancy

ADMINISTRATION/DOSAGE ADJUSTMENTS

Duration of treatment for tumor therapy	Some degree of tumor regression is usually seen in patients with responsive tumors within 3–4 wk of the initial course; if tumor masses remain unchanged following the initial course, additional courses may be given at monthly intervals. When significant tumor regression is obtained, give additional courses at monthly intervals until complete regression is obtained or definite tumor progression or new tumor masses appear.
Preparation of parenteral solution	Reconstitute by adding 4.9 ml of sterile water for injection to vial contents; shake to dissolve. Dilute the appropriate daily dose with 1 liter of 5% dextrose injection USP or sodium chloride injection USP. Prepare fresh solution for each dose; discard any unused solution.
Administration	Administer by slow IV infusion over a period of 4–6 h; avoid rapid direct IV injection and extravasation (see WARNINGS/PRECAUTIONS). Administer only in a hospital setting where appropriate laboratory facilities are available.

WARNINGS/PRECAUTIONS

Electrolyte balance	Preexisting electrolyte imbalance, especially hypocalcemia, hypokalemia, and hypophosphatemia, should be corrected prior to initiation of plicamycin therapy
Thrombocytopenia, bleeding syndrome	Severe thrombocytopenia, a hemorrhagic tendency, and even death may result from administration of plicamycin; although severe toxicity is most likely to occur in patients with far-advanced disease or who are otherwise severely compromised, serious toxicity may also occur occasionally in patients who are in relatively good physical condition. This bleeding syndrome usually begins with an episode of epistaxis and may consist of a single or several episodes of epistaxis with no further progression; however, this syndrome may also begin with an episode of hematemesis and progress to more widely spread hemorrhaging in the GI tract or to a more generalized bleeding tendency. Determine the platelet count, prothrombin time, and bleeding time frequently during therapy and for several days after the last dose, since thrombocytopenia may appear rapidly and may occur at any time during this period. If thrombocytopenia or significant prolongation of the prothrombin time or bleeding time occurs, discontinue use; infusion of platelet concentrates of platelet-rich plasma may be helpful in elevating the platelet count.
Renal and hepatic function	Abnormalities in renal and hepatic function tests (see ALTERED LABORATORY VALUES) have been observed. Use with extreme caution in patients with significant renal or hepatic impairment. Carefully monitor renal function before, during, and after treatment of hypercalcemia and hypercalciuria.

MITHRACIN ■ MUTAMYCIN

Cross-resistance	No significant cross-resistance between plicamycin and other chemotherapeutic agents has been established; prior radiation therapy or chemotherapy has not altered the response rate with plicamycin
Extravasation	Local irritation and cellulitis at the injection site may result from extravasation of plicamycin solutions; should thrombophlebitis or perivascular cellulitis occur, terminate infusion, reinstitute infusion at another site, and apply moderate heat to the site of extravasation to disperse the compound and minimize discomfort and local tissue irritation
Nausea, vomiting	Avoid rapid direct IV injection, since it may increase the incidence and severity of GI effects; administration of antiemetics prior to and during plicamycin therapy may help relieve nausea and vomiting
Carcinogenicity	No long-term animal studies have been performed to determine the carcinogenic potential of this drug
Impairment of fertility	Histologic evidence of inhibited spermatogenesis has been observed in male rats receiving doses of 0.6 mg/kg/day and above

ADVERSE REACTIONS
The most frequent reactions, regardless of incidence, are printed in *italics*

Hematological	Thrombocytopenia, leukopenia, bleeding syndrome (see WARNINGS/PRECAUTIONS), depression of hemoglobin level and prothrombin time; elevation of clotting time and bleeding time, abnormal clot retraction
Central nervous system	Drowsiness, weakness, lethargy, headache, depression
Gastrointestinal	*Anorexia, nausea, vomiting, diarrhea, stomatitis*
Other	Malaise, fever, phlebitis, facial flushing, rash

OVERDOSAGE

Signs and symptoms	Exaggeration of adverse effects (see ADVERSE REACTIONS)
Treatment	Institute general supportive measures; no specific antidote for plicamycin is known. Closely monitor hematological function (including clotting factors), hepatic and renal function, and serum electolytes.

DRUG INTERACTIONS

Heparin, thrombolytic agents, oral anticoagulants, dextran, dipyrimadole, valproic acid	△ Risk of bleeding and hemorrhage
Salicylates, sulfinpyrazone	△ Risk of hemorrhage and GI ulceration or hemorrhage
Hepatotoxic and nephrotoxic agents, myelosuppressants	△ Risk of plicamycin toxicity
Live virus vaccines	△ Risk of generalized viral infection

ALTERED LABORATORY VALUES

Blood/serum values	△ SGOT △ SGPT △ LDH △ Alkaline phosphatase △ Bilirubin △ Ornithine carbamyl transferase △ Isocitric dehydrogenase △ Bromsulfalein retention △ BUN △ Creatinine ▽ Calcium ▽ Phosphorus ▽ Potassium
Urinary values	△ Protein ▽ Calcium

USE IN CHILDREN

No information is available concerning use in children

USE IN PREGNANT AND NURSING WOMEN

Pregnancy Category X: plicamycin may cause fetal harm and is contraindicated in women who are or who may become pregnant. If this drug is used in a pregnant patient, or if the patient becomes pregnant during therapy, she should be apprised of the potential risk to the fetus. It is not known whether plicamycin is excreted in human milk; because many drugs are excreted in human milk, a decision should be made whether to discontinue nursing or therapy.

---

1 Based on patient's body weight; if the patient has a condition resulting in abnormal fluid retention (eg, edema, hydrothorax, or ascites), base the dosage on the patient's ideal weight, rather than actual body weight

---

ANTINEOPLASTIC ANTIBIOTICS

MUTAMYCIN (mitomycin) Bristol-Myers Oncology   Rx

Vials: 5, 20 mg (0.5 mg/ml after reconstitution) for IV use only

INDICATIONS

Disseminated adenocarcinoma of the stomach or pancreas when used in combination with other chemotherapeutic agents and as palliative treatment when other modalities have failed

PARENTERAL DOSAGE

Adult: 20 mg/m² IV, given in a single dose via IV catheter at intervals of 6–8 wk

MUTAMYCIN

CONTRAINDICATIONS

Hypersensitivity or idiosyncratic reaction to mitomycin	Thrombocytopenia	Coagulation disorders
Increased bleeding tendency	Serum creatinine level > 1.7 mg/dl	

ADMINISTRATION/DOSAGE ADJUSTMENTS

Intravenous administration — Reconstitute with Sterile Water for Injection USP, using 10 ml for the 5-mg vial or 40 ml for the 20-mg vial, and administer via a functioning IV catheter or, if desired, reconstituted solution may be further diluted in various IV solutions to a concentration of 20–40 µg/ml (may be mixed with heparin) before administration. Use extreme care to avoid extravasation and resulting possible cellulitis, ulceration, and sloughing; extravasation, with or without burning and stinging, may occur even if an adequate amount of blood returns upon aspiration.

Dosage adjustment — If nadir of WBC count following previous dose is 2,000–2,999/mm³ and/or nadir of platelet count is 25,000–74,999/mm³, give 70% of prior dose during next course of therapy; if nadir of WBC count is < 2,000/mm³ and/or nadir of platelet count is < 25,000/mm³, give 50% of prior dose during next course. Concomitant use of other myelosuppressive agents may require further dosage adjustment.

Duration of therapy — If disease continues to progress after two courses of therapy, discontinue medication

WARNINGS/PRECAUTIONS

Myelosuppressive effects — Bone marrow suppression occurs frequently; inform patient of the risks involved and obtain the following studies during therapy and for at least 8 wk afterward: platelet count, WBC count, differential count, and hemoglobin. Interrupt therapy if platelet count falls below 150,000/mm³ or WBC count falls below 4,000/mm³ or either declines progressively. Do not reinstitute until WBC count returns to 3,000/mm³ and platelet count to 75,000/mm³.

Renal toxicity — May occur; monitor patient for rise in BUN and serum creatinine level (see CONTRAINDICATIONS)

Pulmonary toxicity — Discontinue therapy if pulmonary reactions are observed (see ADVERSE REACTIONS) and causes other than use of this drug are ruled out

Hemolytic uremic syndrome — A serious, often fatal, syndrome characterized by microangiopathic hemolytic anemia, thrombocytopenia, renal failure, and hypertension has been reported. Most of the patients with this syndrome had been given mitomycin in combination with fluorouracil for 6–12 mo; however, some of the patients had received mitomycin for less than 6 mo or, in combination with other drugs.

Carcinogenicity — Mitomycin, when given at the recommended human dose, has been shown to be carcinogenic in rats and mice

ADVERSE REACTIONS[1]

Frequent reactions (incidence ≥ 1%) are printed in *italics*

Hematological — *Myelosuppression, including thrombocytopenia and/or leukopenia (64%)*

Dermatological — *Integument and mucous membrane toxicity (4%), including cellulitis, ulceration, and sloughing at injection site, delayed erythema and/or ulceration, stomatitis, and alopecia;* rash (rare)

Renal — *Functional impairment, characterized by an elevated serum creatinine level (2%)*

Pulmonary — *Dyspnea, nonproductive cough, radiographic evidence of pulmonary infiltrates*

Gastrointestinal — *Anorexia, nausea, vomiting*

Other — *Fever;* hemolytic uremic syndrome

OVERDOSAGE

Signs and symptoms — See ADVERSE REACTIONS

Treatment — Reduce dosage or, if necessary, discontinue therapy; steroids have been employed for pulmonary toxicity, but their therapeutic value has not been determined

DRUG INTERACTIONS

Other myelosuppressive agents — △ Antineoplastic effect and myelosuppression

ALTERED LABORATORY VALUES

Blood/serum values — △ BUN △ Creatinine

No clinically significant alterations in urinary values occur at therapeutic dosages

---

USE IN CHILDREN

Consult manufacturer

USE IN PREGNANT AND NURSING WOMEN

Safety for use during pregnancy has not been established; teratogenic effects have been observed in laboratory animals. It is not known whether mitomycin is excreted in human milk. Because many drugs are excreted in breast milk and because of the potential for serious adverse reactions in nursing infants, patients should not nurse if use of this drug is deemed essential.

---

[1] Reactions for which a causal relationship has not been established include diarrhea, hematemesis, headache, confusion, drowsiness, syncope, fatigue, pain, blurring of vision, thrombophlebitis, and edema

HORMONES

LUPRON (leuprolide acetate) TAP Rx

Vials: 5 mg/ml (2.8 ml)

INDICATIONS	PARENTERAL DOSAGE
Palliative treatment of **advanced prostatic cancer** when orchiectomy or estrogen administration is either not indicated or unacceptable to the patient	**Adult:** 1 mg/day, given in a single SC dose; injection site should be changed periodically during therapy

CONTRAINDICATIONS
None known

WARNINGS/PRECAUTIONS

Exacerbation and complications of prostatic cancer	The transient increase in testosterone level that commonly occurs during the first few weeks of therapy has occasionally been accompanied by temporary exacerbation of the signs and symptoms of prostatic cancer; bone pain is the reaction that has usually been aggravated, but, in a few cases, urinary tract obstruction and hematuria have been affected. Use of another gonadotropin-releasing hormone analog has resulted in exacerbation of signs and symptoms that, in two cases, may have contributed to a rapid death. Administration during the first few weeks has also been associated, in a few cases, with the temporary development of weakness and paresthesias in the lower limbs. Because use by patients with urinary tract obstruction may lead to increased obstruction and use by patients with vertebral metastases may result in neurological complications, these patients should be closely observed during the first few weeks of therapy.
Laboratory testing	Monitor serum levels of testosterone and acid phosphatase. The testosterone level usually increases above baseline during the first week of therapy, declines to or below baseline by the end of the second week, reaches castrate levels within 2–4 wk, and remains at these levels for the duration of therapy. The acid phosphatase level sometimes increases early in treatment, but then usually decreases to values at or near baseline by the fourth week.
Hypersensitivity to benzyl alcohol	Local erythema and induration may occur in patients allergic to benzyl alcohol, the preservative that has been added to the solution
Carcinogenicity, mutagenicity	An increase in benign pituitary hyperplasia and adenomas has been detected in rats given 0.6–4 mg/kg/day SC for 2 yr; however, no pituitary abnormalities have been seen in patients given up to 10 mg/day for 3 yr or up to 20 mg/day for 2 yr. No evidence of mutagenicity has been seen in tests with bacterial and mammalian systems.
Effect on fertility	Although no studies have been done with leuprolide to determine whether suppression of fertility can be reversed, it has been shown that discontinuation of analogs similar to leuprolide after use for up to 20 wk results in complete reversal of infertility

ADVERSE REACTIONS
Frequent reactions (≥ 3%) are italicized

Endocrinological	*Hot flashes (51%), gynecomastia/breast tenderness (3%)*
Central nervous system	*Dizziness (6%), pain and headache (5%), paresthesia (3%), bone pain (3%),* blurred vision, lethargy, insomnia, memory disorder, sour taste, numbness, myalgia
Cardiovascular	*Peripheral edema (8%),* congestive heart failure, thrombophlebitis, phlebitis, pulmonary emboli, arrhythmias, myocardial infarction
Gastrointestinal	*Nausea/vomiting (5%), constipation (3%),* anorexia, GI bleeding
Genitourinary	Hematuria, decrease in testes size, impotence
Respiratory	Dyspnea, pleural rub, worsening of pulmonary fibrosis
Dermatological	Erythema and ecchymosis at injection site, rash, alopecia, pruritus
Other	Asthenia, fatigue, fever, facial swelling, increases in BUN and creatinine levels, decreases in hematocrit and hemoglobin

OVERDOSAGE

Signs and symptoms	See ADVERSE REACTIONS; no unique reactions have been seen with use of up to 20 mg/day for 2 yr. Although SC administration of 250–500 times the recommended human dose has produced dyspnea, decreased activity, and local irritation in rats, there is no evidence that these reactions are especially likely to occur in humans following acute overdosage.

DRUG INTERACTIONS
No clinically significant drug interactions have been identified

ALTERED LABORATORY VALUES

Blood/serum values	⇧ BUN ⇧ Creatinine

LUPRON ■ NOLVADEX

No clinically significant alterations in urinary values occur at therapeutic dosages

USE IN CHILDREN	USE IN PREGNANT AND NURSING WOMEN
Leuprolide is not indicated for use in children	Leuprolide is not indicated for use in women

VEHICLE/BASE
Vials: benzyl alcohol (9 mg/ml) and sodium chloride, plus sodium hydroxide and/or acetic acid

HORMONES

MEGACE (megestrol acetate) Bristol-Myers Oncology   Rx
Tablets: 20, 40 mg

INDICATIONS	ORAL DOSAGE
Palliative treatment of **recurrent, inoperable, or metastatic breast cancer**	Adult: 40 mg qid; at least 2 mo of continuous treatment is considered adequate to determine efficacy
Palliative treatment of **recurrent, inoperable, or metastatic endometrial carcinoma**	Adult: 40–320 mg/day (usual dosage: 160–320 mg/day), given in divided doses; at least 2 mo of continuous treatment is considered adequate to determine efficacy

CONTRAINDICATIONS
Administration as a diagnostic test for pregnancy

WARNINGS/PRECAUTIONS

Monitoring of therapy	Close, customary surveillance is recommended during treatment of recurrent or metastatic cancer; use with caution in patients with a history of thromboembolism
Carcinogenicity	An increased incidence of both benign and malignant breast tumors has been observed in female dogs treated with megestrol for up to 7 yr; the relevance of this finding to humans is unknown but should be kept in mind when assessing benefit-risk and surveilling patients during therapy. Comparable studies in rats and ongoing studies in monkeys have shown no increase in the incidence of tumors.

ADVERSE REACTIONS

Miscellaneous	Carpal tunnel syndrome, deep vein thrombophlebitis, alopecia

OVERDOSAGE
No serious side effects have resulted with dosages as high as 800 mg/day for up to 6 yr

DRUG INTERACTIONS
No clinically significant drug interactions have been identified

ALTERED LABORATORY VALUES
No clinically significant alterations in blood/serum or urinary values occur at therapeutic dosages

USE IN CHILDREN	USE IN PREGNANT AND NURSING WOMEN
Safety and effectiveness have not been established for use in children	Not recommended for use during the first 4 mo of pregnancy, as intrauterine exposure to exogenous sex hormones, even for very brief periods, may increase the risk of congenital anomalies, including congenital heart defects and limb reduction defects. Patients who have taken this drug during the first 4 mo of pregnancy or who become pregnant while taking it should be apprised of the potential risk to the fetus. Because of the potential for adverse effects on the newborn, nursing should be discontinued if megestrol is prescribed.

HORMONES

NOLVADEX (tamoxifen citrate) Stuart   Rx
Tablets: 10 mg

INDICATIONS	ORAL DOSAGE
Treatment of metastatic breast cancer in postmenopausal women	Adult: 10–20 mg bid (AM and PM)
Delaying recurrence of breast cancer in postmenopausal women after total mastectomy and axillary dissection	

NOLVADEX

CONTRAINDICATIONS
None known

ADMINISTRATION/DOSAGE ADJUSTMENTS

Treatment of metastatic breast cancer	Available evidence indicates that estrogen-receptor-positive tumors are more likely to respond to tamoxifen
Adjuvant therapy	Tamoxifen is indicated for use as an adjuvant in women with primary tumors of any size (T1–3), positive axillary nodes that are not fixed (N1), and no distant metastases (M0); it is most commonly given as an adjuvant to women with stage II, node-positive cancer. In some studies, adjuvant therapy has been most beneficial to date in women with four or more positive axillary nodes. Estrogen- and progesterone-receptor values may help to predict whether therapy is likely to be beneficial. The optimal duration of adjuvant therapy is not known; in clinical trails, the drug was given for 2 yr.

WARNINGS/PRECAUTIONS

Ocular pathology	Retinopathy, corneal changes, and decreased visual acuity have been reported in a few patients who were taking at least 4 times the maximum recommended dosage for more than 1 yr
Hypercalcemia	Has occurred in patients with bone metastases within a few weeks after the start of therapy; if hypercalcemia develops, take appropriate measures and, if severe, discontinue medication
Patients with leukopenia or thrombocytopenia	Use with caution; obtain a CBC, including platelet count, periodically
Thromboembolic effects	During tamoxifen therapy, thromboembolic reactions have been seen; however, a causal relationship to the drug remains conjectural since these effects may be due to the cancer. An increase in thromboembolic reactions has occurred when tamoxifen has been combined with cytotoxic drugs.
Carcinogenicity	Granulosa-cell ovarian tumors and interstitial-cell testicular tumors have been detected in mice given tamoxifen for 13 mo
Mutagenicity	No evidence of mutagenicity has been seen in tests with prokaryotic and eukaryotic tissues or organisms
Impairment of fertility	In separate studies with male and female rats given doses lower than the human dose, tamoxifen has adversely affected fertility, causing a decrease in the number of implantations

ADVERSE REACTIONS

The most frequent reactions, regardless of incidence, are printed in *italics*

Endocrinological	*Hot flashes,* vaginal bleeding or discharge, menstrual irregularities
Gastrointestinal	*Nausea, vomiting,* anorexia
Dermatological	Rash, pruritus vulvae
Central nervous system	Depression, dizziness, light-headedness, headache
Other	Increased bone and tumor pain, local disease flare, increased size of preexisting soft tissue lesions accompanied by marked erythema and/or new lesions, peripheral edema, hypercalcemia

OVERDOSAGE

Signs and symptoms	Respiratory difficulties and convulsions have been observed in animals; there have been no reports of acute overdosage in humans
Treatment	Reduce dosage or discontinue medication; treat symptomatically

DRUG INTERACTIONS
No clinically significant drug interactions have been identified

ALTERED LABORATORY VALUES

Blood/serum values	△ Calcium

No clinically significant alterations in urinary values occur at therapeutic dosages

---

USE IN CHILDREN
Not indicated for use in children

USE IN PREGNANT AND NURSING WOMEN
Pregnancy Category D: tamoxifen may cause harm to the human fetus; spontaneous abortions, birth defects, fetal death, and vaginal bleeding have been reported, and reproduction studies in rats and rabbits at doses lower than the human dose have shown a drug-related increase in fetal death. Instruct patients of childbearing age to avoid becoming pregnant during therapy; women who are or do become pregnant should be apprised of the potential hazards to the fetus. It is not known whether tamoxifen is excreted in human milk; patients should not nurse while taking this drug.

HORMONES

TESLAC (testolactone) Squibb Rx
Tablets: 50 mg

INDICATIONS
Palliative treatment of **advanced or disseminated breast cancer** in postmenopausal women (adjunctive therapy)[1]

ORAL DOSAGE
Adult: 250 mg qid

CONTRAINDICATIONS
Treatment of breast cancer in men

ADMINISTRATION/DOSAGE ADJUSTMENTS
Measurement of therapeutic response — Before evaluating patient response, continue therapy for at least 3 mo, unless there is active progression of the disease

WARNINGS/PRECAUTIONS
Hypercalcemia — Plasma calcium levels should be determined routinely, especially during periods of active remission of bony metastases; if hypercalcemia occurs, institute appropriate therapy

ADVERSE REACTIONS[2]
Gastrointestinal — Glossitis, anorexia, nausea, vomiting
Dermatological — Maculopapular erythema; alopecia with and without disturbance of nail growth (rare)
Other — Aching and edema of the extremities, paresthesias, increased blood pressure

OVERDOSAGE
Acute toxicity has not been reported

DRUG INTERACTIONS
No clinically significant drug interactions have been identified

ALTERED LABORATORY VALUES
Blood/serum values — ⌂ Calcium
Urinary values — ⌂ Creatinine ⌂ 17-Ketosteroids

USE IN CHILDREN
Not indicated for use in children

USE IN PREGNANT AND NURSING WOMEN
This drug is intended for use only in postmenopausal women; for this reason, and because safe use has not been established with respect to adverse effects on fetal development, it should not be administered to a pregnant woman. Testolactone is not indicated for women who are nursing.

---

[1] This drug may also be used in premenopausal women with disseminated breast carcinoma if ovarian function has been terminated
[2] Causal relationship not established

INTERFERONS

INTRON A (interferon alfa-2b, recombinant) Schering Rx
Vials: 3 million, 5 million, 10 million, 25 million IU

INDICATIONS
Hairy cell leukemia in both splenectomized and nonsplenectomized patients

PARENTERAL DOSAGE
Adult ($\geq$ **18 yr**): 2 million IU/m², given SC or IM 3 times/wk

CONTRAINDICATIONS
Hypersensitivity to interferon alfa or any other component

ADMINISTRATION/DOSAGE ADJUSTMENTS
Preparation of solution — Add 1 ml of supplied bacteriostatic water for injection to the 3 million-IU or 5 million-IU vial, 2 ml to the 10 million-IU vial, or 5 ml to the 25 million-IU vial; do not aim the stream of liquid directly at the lyophilized powder. Swirl the vial gently until the contents have completely dissolved.

Administration — If platelet count is less than 50,000/mm³, administer the drug SC, not IM. Injection site should be checked 2 h after administration for signs of inflammation. Rotate injection sites in a regular pattern. Influenza-like reactions may be minimized by administration at bedtime.

INTRON A

Monitoring of hematological response	Before beginning therapy and periodically thereafter, quantitate peripheral blood hemoglobin, platelets, and granulocytes and both bone marrow and peripheral hairy cells. If a positive response to treatment occurs, continue administration until no further improvement is seen and hematological values have been stable for approximately 3 mo; whether treatment beyond this time is beneficial is not known. If the patient does not respond within 6 mo, this drug should be discontinued. In clinical trials, values for peripheral blood erythrocytes, leukocytes, and platelets decreased during the first 1–2 mo of therapy and then subsequently improved; normal median values were seen at the following times: for platelet counts, after 2 mo of therapy; for hemoglobin levels, after 4 mo; and for granulocyte counts, after 5 mo. Bear in mind that these are median values; thus a period of 6 mo or more may be necessary for improvement of all three values. The percentage of patients with a hairy cell index (a measure of bone marrow infiltration) of 50% or more declined from 87% at the start of therapy to 25% after 6 mo and 14% after 1 yr; these results indicate that even after normal peripheral blood values have been achieved, prolonged treatment may be necessary for attainment of a maximal reduction in hairy cell infiltrates.
Management of severe reactions	If severe reactions occur, reduce dosage by 50% or temporarily discontinue therapy until the effects abate; take appropriate corrective measures as needed. If intolerance persists or recurs following adjustment of dosage or if the disease progresses, discontinue treatment. The minimum effective dose of this drug has not been established.
Use of other interferon products	Caution patients not to switch brands of interferon without medical consultation, as a change in dosage may result

WARNINGS/PRECAUTIONS

Patients with cardiac disorders	Cardiovascular effects, including significant hypotension, supraventricular arrhythmias, and a heart rate of 150 beats/min or more, have been seen at doses higher than those recommended for hairy cell leukemia. Hypotension may occur during administration or up to 2 days afterward. Tachycardia has usually been seen in conjunction with high fever. Supraventricular arrhythmias appear to be associated with preexisting conditions and prior use of cardiotoxic drugs. Closely monitor patients with prior or current arrhythmias and those with a recent history of myocardial infarction. Obtain an ECG before therapy and at appropriate intervals thereafter for patients with cardiac abnormalities and/or an advanced stage of cancer. Fever and chills, which occur in almost all patients given this drug, can exacerbate cardiovascular disease; use with caution in patients with a history of unstable angina, uncontrolled congestive heart failure, or other cardiovascular disease. For management of severe reactions, see ADMINISTRATION/DOSAGE ADJUSTMENTS.
Patients with other debilitating medical conditions	Fever and chills, which occur in almost all patients given this drug, can exacerbate debilitating medical conditions such as chronic obstructive pulmonary disease, diabetes associated with episodes of ketoacidosis, and cardiovascular disease (see warning above); use with caution. For management of severe reactions, see ADMINISTRATION/DOSAGE ADJUSTMENTS.
Influenza-like reactions	Almost all patients experience influenza-like reactions, primarily fever, chills, and fatigue; the severity of these effects appears to diminish with continued treatment. Some of these effects may be minimized by administration at bedtime. Acetaminophen may be given to prevent or partially alleviate fever and headache.
Neurological effects	Depression, confusion, and other alterations of mental status have been observed in approximately 2% of patients with hairy cell leukemia. Administration of doses higher than those recommended for hairy cell leukemia has caused more significant obtundation and coma in some, usually elderly, patients. If CNS effects occur, it may be necessary to discontinue therapy; see "Management of severe reactions" in ADMINISTRATION/DOSAGE ADJUSTMENTS. Although CNS effects have usually reversed rapidly, in a few severe cases complete resolution of symptoms has taken up to 3 wk. Patients who experience CNS reactions should be closely observed until these reactions disappear.
Liver function abnormalities	Elevated SGPT levels have been seen in 13% of patients undergoing treatment of hairy cell leukemia; elevated SGOT levels have been detected in 4% of these patients. Liver function abnormalities are usually mild to moderate and transient; severe abnormalities generally disappear rapidly following a reduction in dosage or cessation of therapy. To monitor hepatic response, perform liver function tests before therapy and then periodically thereafter. For management of severe reactions, see ADMINISTRATION/DOSAGE ADJUSTMENTS.
Hematological abnormalities	Thrombocytopenia and granulocytopenia are common during therapy; prolongation of prothrombin and partial thromboplastin times has also been observed. Reductions in platelet and granulocyte counts are usually mild to moderate and transient; when these abnormalities are severe, they generally disappear rapidly following a reduction in dosage or cessation of therapy. For monitoring of hematological response and management of severe reactions, see ADMINISTRATION/DOSAGE ADJUSTMENTS. Use with caution in patients with severe myelosuppression or with coagulation disorders, such as thrombophlebitis or pulmonary embolism.
Electrolyte changes	Determine serum electrolyte levels before therapy and then periodically thereafter
Dehydration	Instruct patients to keep well-hydrated, especially during the initial stages of treatment

INTRON A ■ ROFERON-A

Hypersensitivity reactions	Transient cutaneous rashes have occurred in some patients following injection of the solution, but have not necessitated interruption of treatment. Serious, acute hypersensitivity reactions, such as urticaria, angioedema, bronchoconstriction, and anaphylaxis, have not been reported; should such reactions occur, discontinue use immediately and institute appropriate treatment.
Carcinogenicity, mutagenicity	No studies have been performed to evaluate the carcinogenic potential of this drug. Mutagenicity studies have revealed no adverse effects.
Impairment of fertility	Interferon may impair fertility. Primates treated with interferon alfa-2a have developed menstrual-cycle abnormalities; no studies have been done with interferon alfa-2b. Use with caution in fertile men and women.

ADVERSE REACTIONS
Frequent reactions (> 5%) are italicized

Cardiovascular	*Mild hypotension, hypertension, and tachycardia (> 5%)*; supraventricular arrhythmias and syncope (1–5%)
Gastrointestinal	*Change in taste, anorexia, weight loss, nausea, vomiting, and mild diarrhea (> 5%)*; constipation, stomatitis, paralytic ileus, and pharyngitis (1–5%); dyspepsia, flatulence, increased saliva, and ulcerative stomatitis (< 1%)
Hematological	*Mild thrombocytopenia and transient granulocytopenia (> 5%)*; increases in prothrombin and partial thromboplastin times (1–5%)
Central nervous system	*Headache, myalgia, arthralgia, fatigue, somnolence, confusion, dizziness, ataxia, paresthesia, anxiety, depression, and nervousness (> 5%)*; leg cramps, insomnia, tremor, and emotional lability (1–5%)
Dermatological	*Mild pruritus, mild alopecia, and transient mild rashes (> 5%)*; urticaria (1–5%), purpura (< 1%)
Hepatic	*Increase in SGPT level (13%)*; increase in SGOT level (4%); increases in LDH and alkaline phosphatase levels[1]
Respiratory	Dyspnea, sneezing, and nasal congestion (< 1%)
Ophthalmic	Abnormal vision and syncope (1–5%); oculomotor paralysis (< 1%)
Other	*Fever and chills (> 5%)*; herpetic eruptions, nonherpetic cold sores, dehydration, hot flashes, epistaxis, and chest pain (1–5%); hyperglycemia (< 1%), increase in serum creatinine level[1]

OVERDOSAGE

Signs and symptoms	See ADVERSE REACTIONS
Treatment	See "Management of severe reactions" in ADMINISTRATION/DOSAGE ADJUSTMENTS

DRUG INTERACTIONS

Narcotics, hypnotics, sedatives	△ Risk of CNS depression; use with caution

ALTERED LABORATORY VALUES

Blood/serum values	△ SGOT △ SGPT △ LDH △ Alkaline phosphatase △ Creatinine

No clinically significant alterations in urinary values occur at therapeutic dosages

---

USE IN CHILDREN
Safety and effectiveness for use in children under 18 yr of age have not been established

USE IN PREGNANT AND NURSING WOMEN
Pregnant women: Pregnancy Category C: an increased frequency of spontaneous abortions has been observed in rhesus monkeys given 20–500 times the human dose of interferon alfa-2a; it is not known whether interferon alfa-2b can affect reproductive capacity or cause harm to the human fetus since no studies have been done with this drug. Use during pregnancy only if the expected benefit justifies the potential risk to the fetus. **Nursing mothers:** It is not known whether this drug is excreted in human milk; however, mouse interferons are excreted in mouse milk. Because of the potential for serious adverse effects in nursing infants, this drug should not be given to women who are nursing.

[1] Frequency has not been reported by manufacturer in the package insert

---

INTERFERONS

ROFERON-A (interferon alfa-2a, recombinant) Roche   Rx

Vials: 3 million IU/ml (1 ml), 6 million IU/ml (3 ml)

INDICATIONS
Hairy cell leukemia in both splenectomized and nonsplenectomized patients

PARENTERAL DOSAGE
Adult (>18 yr): for induction, 3 million IU, given SC or IM once daily for 16–24 wk; for maintenance, 3 million IU, given SC or IM 3 times/wk

CONTRAINDICATIONS

Hypersensitivity to alfa interferon, mouse immunoglobulin, or any component of this product

ADMINISTRATION/DOSAGE ADJUSTMENTS

Administration	For patients who are at risk of bleeding or who have a platelet count of less than 50,000/mm³, SC administration is particularly advisable
Monitoring of hematological response	Before beginning therapy and periodically (eg, monthly) thereafter, quantitate peripheral blood hemoglobin, platelets, and granulocytes and both bone marrow and peripheral hairy cells. Therapeutic response is usually not seen until after 1–3 mo. If a positive response to treatment occurs, continue administration until no further improvement is seen and hematological values have been stable for approximately 3 mo; whether treatment beyond this time is beneficial is not known. If no response occurs within 6 mo, this drug should be discontinued. During the initial phase of treatment, watch very carefully for evidence of severe depression of blood counts (see WARNINGS/PRECAUTIONS).
Management of severe reactions	If severe reactions occur, reduce dosage by 50% or temporarily discontinue therapy until the effects abate. The need for dosage reduction should take into account that prior radio- or chemotherapy may have compromised bone marrow reserve. Exercise caution when therapy is reinstituted, as toxicity may recur. The minimum effective dose of this drug has not been established.
Use of other interferon products	Caution patients not to switch brands of interferon without medical consultation, as a change in dosage may result

WARNINGS/PRECAUTIONS

Patients with cardiac disorders	Fever and chills, which are common side effects of therapy, may exacerbate preexisting cardiac disorders. In rare cases, myocardial infarction has occurred in patients receiving this drug. Use with caution in patients with cardiac disease or a history of cardiac illness. Obtain an ECG before therapy and at appropriate intervals thereafter when patients have cardiac abnormalities and/or an advanced stage of cancer.
Myelosuppression	Leukopenia, thrombocytopenia, and other indications of myelosuppression are common during therapy, especially in the first 1–2 mo (see "Monitoring of hematological response" in ADMINISTRATION/DOSAGE ADJUSTMENTS); significant myelosuppressive toxicity has been seen in rare cases. Use with caution in patients with myelosuppression.
Neurological effects	Interferon has caused dizziness, obtundation, CNS stimulation, and, in rare cases, coma. Most CNS reactions have been mild and have disappeared within a few days to 3 wk after a reduction in dose or discontinuation of therapy. Careful evaluation of neuropsychiatric function should be done periodically during therapy. Use with caution in patients with seizure disorders or compromised CNS function.
Hepatotoxicity	An increase in hepatic serum enzyme levels is common during therapy; however, significant hepatotoxicity has occurred only rarely. Perform liver function tests before therapy and then periodically thereafter. Use with caution in patients with severe hepatic disease.
Nephrotoxicity	Proteinuria and increased cells in the urinary sediment have been seen infrequently with this drug; however, significant nephrotoxicity has occurred only rarely. Use with caution in patients with severe renal disease.
Dehydration	Patients should be well-hydrated during therapy, especially during the initial stages
Neutralizing antibodies	Neutralizing antibodies to interferon alfa-2a have been detected in approximately 27% of all patients given this drug and in 3.4% of patients who received this drug for hairy cell leukemia; the clinical significance of this effect is not known. Certain conditions (eg, cancer, systemic lupus erythematosus, herpes zoster) have been associated with the spontaneous development of antibodies to human leukocyte interferon.
Carcinogenicity	No studies have been performed to evaluate the carcinogenic potential of this drug
Mutagenicity	A chromosomal defect has been reported following the addition of human leukocyte interferon to lymphocyte cultures taken from a patient with a lymphoproliferative disorder; the defect has not been detected in interferon-treated cultures obtained from healthy volunteers. No evidence of mutagenicity has been seen in various Ames tests or human leukocyte cultures in which interferon alfa-2a has been used. It has also been shown that human leukocyte interferon protects primary chick embryo fibroblasts against chromosomal aberrations caused by gamma rays.
Impairment of fertility	Rhesus monkeys given 5 and 25 million IU/kg/day of interferon alfa-2a have developed irregular menstrual cycles associated with anovulation; menstrual rhythm returned to normal following discontinuation of the drug. No significant adverse effects on male fertility have been seen to date.

ADVERSE REACTIONS[1]

Frequent reactions (> 3%) are italicized

Central nervous system	*Fatigue (89%), myalgias (73%), headache (71%), dizziness (21%), paresthesias and numbness (6%), arthralgias (5%);* decreased mental status, depression, sleep disturbances, and nervousness (< 3%)

ROFERON-A ■ EMCYT

Hematological	*Leukopenia (59%), decrease in hematocrit (43%), thrombocytopenia (42%), neutropenia (39%), decrease in hemoglobin level (36%)*
Hepatic	*Increases in levels of SGOT (47%), alkaline phosphatase (18%), and LDH (12%); increase in bilirubin level (1.6%)*
Gastrointestinal	*Anorexia (46%), nausea (32%), diarrhea (29%), emesis (10%)*
Dermatological	*Rash (18%), dry skin or pruritus (13%), partial alopecia (8%); petechiae, ecchymosis, and urticaria (< 3%)*
Genitourinary	*Proteinuria (10%), reactivation of herpes labialis (8%), transient impotence and increase in uric acid level (6%); increases in levels of serum creatinine (3%) and BUN (2%)*
Cardiovascular	*Hypertension, chest pain, arrhythmias, and palpitations (< 3%)*
Ophthalmic	*Visual disturbances and conjunctivitis (< 3%)*
Local	*Inflammation at injection site (< 3%)*
Other	*Fever (98%), chills (64%), increase in serum glucose level (33%), dryness or inflammation of the oropharynx (16%), weight loss (14%), change in taste (13%), hypocalcemia (10%), diaphoresis (8%); epistaxis, bleeding gums, and night sweats (< 3%), increase in serum phosphorus level (2%)*

OVERDOSAGE

Signs and symptoms	See ADVERSE REACTIONS
Treatment	If serious reactions occur, reduce dosage by 50% or temporarily discontinue therapy until reactions subside

DRUG INTERACTIONS

No clinically significant drug interactions have been identified

ALTERED LABORATORY VALUES

Blood/serum values	△ SGOT △ Alkaline phosphatase △ LDH △ Bilirubin △ BUN △ Creatinine △ Uric acid ▽ Calcium △ Phosphorus △ Glucose
Urinary values	+ Protein △ Uric acid

USE IN CHILDREN

Safety and effectiveness for use in children under 18 yr of age have not been established

USE IN PREGNANT AND NURSING WOMEN

Pregnant women: Pregnancy Category C: an increased frequency of spontaneous abortions has been observed in rhesus monkeys given 20–500 times the human dose during the period of early to middle fetal development (days 22–70 of gestation); a study (in progress) of treatment of these animals during late pregnancy (days 79–100) has failed so far to show any abortifacient effect. No teratogenic activity has been seen in this species. Use during pregnancy only if the expected benefits justify the potential risks to the fetus. Before giving this product to fertile, nonpregnant women, make sure that they are using effective contraception. **Nursing mothers:** It is not known whether this drug is excreted in human milk; because of the potential for serious adverse effects in nursing infants, this drug should not be given to women who are nursing.

[1] Use of interferon alfa-2a at higher doses for treatment of cancers other than hairy cell leukemia has been associated with all of the effects listed in ADVERSE REACTIONS plus the following: confusion, hypotension, lethargy, edema, abdominal fullness, hypermotility, hepatitis, gait disturbance, poor coordination, hallucinations, syncope, seizures, encephalopathy, psychomotor retardation, coma, stroke, transient ischemic attacks, aphasia, aphonia, dysarthria, dysphasia, forgetfulness, amnesia, sedation, apathy, anxiety, emotional lability, irritability, hyperactivity, involuntary movements, claustrophobia, loss of libido, muscle contractions, congestive heart failure, pulmonary edema, myocardial infarction, Raynaud's phenomenon, hot flashes, bronchospasm, tachypnea, excessive salivation, and flushing of the skin

---

MISCELLANEOUS ANTINEOPLASTIC AGENTS

EMCYT (estramustine phosphate sodium) Roche   Rx

Capsules: estramustine phosphate sodium equivalent to 140 mg estramustine phosphate

INDICATIONS	ORAL DOSAGE
Palliative treatment of **metastatic and/or progressive prostatic carcinoma**	Adult: 14 mg/kg/day (1 cap/10 kg or 22 lb of body weight), given in 3 or 4 divided doses (usual dosage: 10–16 mg/kg/day)

CONTRAINDICATIONS

Hypersensitivity to either estradiol or mechlorethamine (nitrogen mustard)	Active thrombophlebitis or thromboembolic disorders[1]

EMCYT

ADMINISTRATION/DOSAGE ADJUSTMENTS

Duration of therapy	Patient should be treated for 30–90 days before a determination of the possible benefits of continued therapy is made. Continue therapy as long as there is a favorable response; some patients have been maintained on dosages of 10–16 mg/kg/day for more than 3 yr

WARNINGS/PRECAUTIONS

Thrombosis	Men receiving estrogens for prostatic cancer have demonstrated an increased risk of thrombosis, including nonfatal myocardial infarction; use with caution in patients with a history of thrombophlebitis, thrombosis, or thromboembolic disorders, particularly if they were associated with estrogen therapy, and in those with cerebrovascular or coronary artery disease
Diabetic patients	Glucose tolerance may be decreased; observe diabetic patients carefully
Elevated blood pressure	Hypertension may occur; monitor blood pressure periodically
Fluid retention	Exacerbation of preexisting or incipient peripheral edema or congestive heart disease has been observed in patients receiving estramustine phosphate; monitor carefully patients with other conditions which might be affected by fluid retention, such as epilepsy, migraine, or renal dysfunction
Patients with impaired liver function	Use with caution, since drug may be poorly metabolized
Calcium and phosphorous metabolism	May be affected; use with caution in patients with metabolic bone diseases associated with hypercalcemia or if renal function is impaired
Hepatic abnormalities	Increases in bilirubin and hepatic enzyme levels have occurred in some patients, but have seldom been severe enough to require discontinuation of therapy; hepatic function tests should be performed at appropriate intervals during therapy and repeated after the drug has been withdrawn for 2 mo
Carcinogenicity, mutagenicity	Long-term continuous administration of estrogens increases the incidence of breast and liver carcinomas. Compounds structurally related to this drug are carcinogenic in mice. No carcinogenicity studies have been done in human subjects. Although mutagenicity has not been demonstrated in the Ames test, both estradiol and mechlorethamine (nitrogen mustard) are mutagenic; consequently, patients should be advised to use contraceptive measures while receiving this drug.

ADVERSE REACTIONS

Cardiovascular, respiratory	Edema, dyspnea, leg cramps, myocardial infarction, thrombophlebitis, congestive heart failure, cerebrovascular accident, pulmonary emboli, upper respiratory discharge, hoarseness
Gastrointestinal	Nausea, diarrhea, minor gastrointestinal upset, anorexia, flatulence, vomiting, gastrointestinal bleeding, burning throat, thirst
Central nervous system	Lethargy, insomnia, emotional lability, headache, anxiety
Endocrinological	Breast tenderness and/or enlargement
Dermatological	Easy bruising, pruritus, dry skin, rash, flushing, thinning of the hair, peeling of the skin (on fingertips)
Hematological	Leukopenia, thrombopenia
Hepatic	Increased bilirubin and liver enzyme levels
Other	Chest pain, lacrimation

OVERDOSAGE

Signs and symptoms	See ADVERSE REACTIONS
Treatment	Empty stomach by gastric lavage and initiate symptomatic therapy; hematological and hepatic parameters should be monitored at least 6 wk after an overdosage episode

DRUG INTERACTIONS

Milk	▽ Absorption of estramustine; consider giving estramustine at least 1 h before or 2 h after ingestion of milk or other dairy products

ALTERED LABORATORY VALUES

Blood/serum values	△ Lactate dehydrogenase △ SGOT △ Bilirubin

No clinically significant alterations in urinary values occur at therapeutic dosages

---

USE IN CHILDREN

Not applicable

USE IN PREGNANT AND NURSING WOMEN

Not applicable

---

[1] Except in those cases where the actual tumor mass is the cause of the thromboembolic phenomenon and the benefits of therapy may outweigh the risks

MISCELLANEOUS ANTINEOPLASTIC AGENTS

HYDREA (hydroxyurea) Squibb   Rx

Capsules: 500 mg

INDICATIONS	ORAL DOSAGE[1]
Melanoma Recurrent, metastatic, or inoperable **carcinoma of the ovary**	**Adult:** 80 mg/kg, given in a single dose every third day (intermittent therapy) or 20–30 mg/kg, given in a single daily dose continuously
Resistant chronic **myelocytic leukemia**	**Adult:** 20–30 mg/kg, given in a single daily dose continuously
Primary **squamous cell (epidermoid) carcinomas of the head and neck** (adjunctive therapy)	**Adult:** 80 mg/kg, given in a single dose every third day, beginning at least 1 wk in advance of the start of irradiation and continuing during radiotherapy, as well as indefinitely afterward, if the patient can be strictly monitored and shows no severe or unusual reactions (see WARNINGS/PRECAUTIONS)

CONTRAINDICATIONS

Marked bone marrow depression, manifested by significant leukopenia (WBC count < 2,500/mm³) or thrombocytopenia (platelet count < 100,000/mm³), or severe anemia

ADMINISTRATION/DOSAGE ADJUSTMENTS

Administration of capsules	If the patient is unable to swallow the capsules, the contents may be emptied into a glass of water and taken immediately
Measurement of therapeutic response	Evaluate the response to hydroxyurea after 6 wk; if regression in tumor size or arrest of tumor growth occurs, therapy may be continued indefinitely

WARNINGS/PRECAUTIONS

Bone marrow depression	May occur; perform complete blood tests, including a bone marrow examination if indicated, prior to and repeatedly during hydroxyurea therapy. Determinations of hemoglobin level, total WBC counts, and platelet counts should be made at least once a week. Discontinue therapy if WBC count falls below 2,500/mm³ or platelet count falls below 100,000/mm³. Recheck counts after 3 days and resume therapy when counts rise significantly toward normal values. In rare cases, postponement of concomitant irradiation treatment of head and neck tumors may be indicated. Severe anemia should be corrected with whole blood replacement prior to beginning hydroxyurea treatment; if anemia occurs during therapy, correct with whole blood replacement without interrupting antineoplastic treatment. Because hematopoiesis may be compromised by extensive irradiation or by the use of other antineoplastic agents, use this drug with caution in patients who have recently undergone extensive radiation therapy or chemotherapy with other cytotoxic drugs.
Concomitant irradiation therapy	Mucositis may occur at the irradiated site; although it is usually controllable by such measures as topical anesthetics and oral analgesics, temporary interruption of hydroxyurea therapy or both hydroxurea and irradiation therapy may be indicated in rare cases. Combined therapy may cause an increase in the incidence and severity of side effects of both therapies; severe gastric distress, such as nausea, vomiting, and anorexia, may usually be controlled by temporary interruption of hydroxyurea therapy and, rarely, with the additional interruption of irradiation therapy.[2]
Postirradiation erythema	May be exacerbated in patients who have previously received irradiation therapy
Mutagenicity	Since this drug affects DNA synthesis, potential mutagenic effects must be taken into consideration before administering to patients who may contemplate conception
Erythrocytic abnormalities	May occur, including a self-limited megaloblastic erythropoiesis early in therapy (the morphologic change resembles pernicious anemia, but is not related to vitamin B_{12} or folic acid deficiency), delayed plasma iron clearance, and reduction in the rate of iron utilization by red blood cells
Special risk patients	Use with caution in patients with marked renal dysfunction, and in the elderly, who may require a lower dose regimen; renal and liver function tests should be performed before and repeatedly during therapy

ADVERSE REACTIONS

Hematological	Leukopenia, anemia, thrombocytopenia
Gastrointestinal	Stomatitis, anorexia, nausea, vomiting, diarrhea, constipation
Dermatological	Maculopapular rash, facial erythema
Central nervous system	Drowsiness; headache, dizziness, disorientation, hallucinations, and convulsions (rare)
Renal	Temporary functional impairment; dysuria (rare)
Other	Fever, chills, malaise; alopecia (rare)

DRUG INTERACTIONS

Antigout agents	▽ Hypouricemic effect

HYDREA ■ ONCOVIN

Other myelosuppressive agents, radiotherapy —————— ⇧ Antineoplastic effect

ALTERED LABORATORY VALUES

Blood/serum values —————— ⇧ Uric acid ⇧ BUN ⇧ Creatinine ⇧ Sulfobromophthalein (BSP) retention
⇧ Hepatic enzymes

No clinically significant alterations in urinary values occur at therapeutic dosages

USE IN CHILDREN
Dosage regimens in children have not been established because of the rarity of the indications in the pediatric age group

USE IN PREGNANT AND NURSING WOMEN
Use in women who are or who may become pregnant only if the potential benefits outweigh the possible risks; hydroxyurea has been shown to be teratogenic in animals. Consult manufacturer for use in nursing women.

[1] Dosages should be based on the patient's ideal or actual weight, whichever is less
[2] Adverse reactions observed with combined hydroxyurea and irradiation therapy are similar to those reported for hydroxyurea alone and include primarily bone marrow depression (leukopenia and anemia) and gastric irritation; platelet depression (< 100,000/mm³) occurs rarely. Gastric distress has also been observed with irradiation alone, as well as in combination with hydroxyurea therapy. Although mucositis is attributed to radiation alone, some investigators believe that the more severe cases are due to combination therapy.

MISCELLANEOUS ANTINEOPLASTIC AGENTS

ONCOVIN (vincristine sulfate) Lilly   Rx

Vials: 1 mg/ml (1, 2, 5 ml) for IV use only   **Prefilled syringes:** 1 mg/ml (1, 2 ml) for IV use only

INDICATIONS

Acute leukemia
Hodgkin's disease, non-Hodgkin's malignant lymphomas (lymphocytic, mixed-cell, histiocytic, undifferentiated, nodular, and diffuse types), **rhabdomyosarcoma, neuroblastoma, and Wilms' tumor** when combined with other oncolytic agents

PARENTERAL DOSAGE

Adult: 1.4 mg/m², given IV at weekly intervals
Child (≤ 10 kg or < 1 m²): 0.05 mg/kg, given IV at weekly intervals
Child: (>10 kg or > 1 m²): 2 mg/m², given IV at weekly intervals

CONTRAINDICATIONS

Charcot-Marie-Tooth syndrome (demyelinating form)

ADMINISTRATION/DOSAGE ADJUSTMENTS

Preparation	Exercise extreme care in calculating and administering the required dose; adverse effects are dose-related, and severe reactions can occur in adults given 3 mg/m² and in children under 13 yr of age given 3–4 mg/m². If a vial is used, the required dose should be carefully withdrawn and no additional fluid should be added before or during withdrawal.
Administration	Death will occur if this drug is given intrathecally. Using an intact, free-flowing IV needle or catheter, administer solution directly into a vein or into the tubing of a running IV infusion of glucose or saline. Do not mix with solutions other than normal saline or glucose in water; do not dilute in solutions that can raise or lower the pH outside the range of 3.5–5.5. Injection may be completed in 1 min. To avoid extravasation, which may cause considerable irritation, take particular care in positioning the needle or catheter; if extravasation occurs, discontinue administration immediately, inject hyaluronidase and apply moderate heat at the injection site, and give the remaining portion of the dose in another vein.
Patients with hepatic impairment	Approximately 80% of a dose is excreted by the liver into the bile; liver disease, if sufficiently severe, can affect biliary excretion and cause an increase in the severity of adverse effects. To avoid toxicity in patients with a direct serum bilirubin level of more than 3 mg/dl, reduce dose by 50%. For patients with significantly reduced liver function, give an initial dose of 0.05–1 mg/m² and then increase subsequent doses as tolerated.
Concomitant radiation therapy	Do not administer vincristine to patients receiving radiation therapy through ports that include the liver

COMPENDIUM OF DRUG THERAPY

ONCOVIN

WARNINGS/PRECAUTIONS

Neurotoxicity	Neurological reactions, which are the most troublesome effects of therapy, may become progressively more severe with continued treatment; in a common pattern, sensory impairment and paresthesias appear initially, followed by neuritic pain and then motor difficulties. Impairment of motor function may be limited to paresis or paralysis of the muscles controlled by the cranial nerves (most commonly, the extraocular and laryngeal muscles). Neuritic pain usually lasts less than 7 days and, following a reduction in dosage, may recur with diminished intensity or may not recur at all. Other reactions are usually reversed within 6 wk after treatment has been discontinued, although in some cases they may persist for a prolonged period. Watch for neurotoxic reactions during therapy; clinical evaluation should be based on history and physical examination. Give particular attention to dosage and the risk of neurotoxicity if the patient has a neuromuscular disease or is receiving another potentially neurotoxic drug.
Uric acid nephropathy	To avoid acute hyperuricemia and uric acid nephropathy during induction of remission in acute leukemia, determine serum uric acid level frequently during the first 3–4 wk of therapy, or take appropriate measures to prevent nephropathy
Bone marrow depression	Anemia, leukopenia, and thrombocytopenia may occur, especially when bone marrow function has been impaired; leukopenia usually disappears within 7 days and, following a reduction in dosage, may recur with less severity or may not be evident at all. Obtain a CBC before administration of each dose. If leukopenia or a complicating infection occurs, weigh the risks and benefits before administering the next dose.
Pulmonary reactions	Acute shortness of breath and severe bronchospasm have occurred a few minutes to several hours after injection of a vinca alkaloid, especially when the drug has been used in combination with a mitomycin (pulmonary effects may occur up to 2 wk after administration of mitomycin)
Constipation	Impaction may occur in the upper colon; constipation usually lasts less than 7 days and, following a reduction in dosage, may recur with diminished severity or may not recur at all. If the patient complains of colic, but the rectum is found to be empty, obtain a flat film of the abdomen. Upper-colon impaction may be treated with high enemas and laxatives. A routine prophylactic regimen against constipation is recommended for all patients.
Paralytic ileus	Vincristine may cause paralytic ileus, especially in children; the reaction mimics "surgical abdomen." To treat ileus, temporarily discontinue vincristine administration and provide symptomatic care.
Hair loss	The most common reaction to vincristine is hair loss; during maintenance therapy, the effect may persist or hair may grow back
Urinary retention	Bladder atony due to vincristine may result in urinary retention; if possible, during the first few days after administering a dose, discontinue use of other drugs known to cause urinary retention (particularly drugs that produce this effect in the elderly)
Contamination of the eye	Accidental contamination of the eye can cause severe irritation or, if the drug is delivered under pressure, may produce corneal ulceration. Avoid contamination; if it occurs, treat immediately by washing the eye thoroughly.
CNS leukemia	Combination therapy may be necessary for the treatment of CNS leukemia since the amount of vincristine crossing the blood-brain barrier does not appear to be sufficient for effective therapy; do not administer vincristine intrathecally
Carcinogenicity	Use of vincristine in combination with carcinogenic drugs has produced malignancies; whether vincristine contributed to this effect has not been determined. A limited study has shown no evidence of carcinogenicity in rats and mice given the drug intraperitoneally.
Mutagenicity	No conclusive evidence of mutagenicity has been demonstrated in laboratory tests
Impairment of fertility	Use of vincristine in combination with other drugs may produce azoospermia and amenorrhea; recovery may occur many months after completion of therapy or not at all. If a prepubertal child undergoes treatment, azoospermia and amenorrhea may occur at the time of puberty, but are much less likely to be permanent.

ADVERSE REACTIONS

Central nervous system	Neuritic pain; mild or severe pain in the jaw, pharynx, parotid glands, bones, back, limbs, or muscles; sensory loss, paresthesias, difficulty in walking, slapping gait, loss of deep-tendon reflexes, foot drop, ataxia, muscle atrophy, paresis or paralysis of muscles controlled by cranial nerves; convulsions (often accompanied by hypertension), postictal coma (in children)
Ophthalmic	Optic atrophy and blindness, transient cortical blindness
Hematological	Leukopenia, thrombocytopenia, anemia
Gastrointestinal	Constipation, abdominal cramps, weight loss, nausea, vomiting, oral ulceration, diarrhea, paralytic ileus, intestinal necrosis and/or perforation, anorexia
Genitourinary	Polyuria, dysuria, urinary retention
Cardiovascular	Hypertension, hypotension

ONCOVIN ■ PLATINOL

Pulmonary	Acute shortness of breath, severe bronchospasm
Dermatological	Alopecia, rash
Other	Fever, headache; inappropriate ADH syndrome (rare)

OVERDOSAGE

Signs and symptoms	See ADVERSE REACTIONS
Treatment	Administer 100 mg leucovorin IV q3h for 24 h and then q6h for at least 48 h. Institute supportive measures, as needed, including restriction of fluid intake, administration of a loop diuretic and anticonvulsants, and use of enemas or cathartics to prevent ileus (decompression of the GI tract may be necessary in severe cases). Monitor ECG and blood pressure and obtain daily blood counts to determine transfusion requirements.

DRUG INTERACTIONS

Asparaginase	⇩ Hepatic clearance of vincristine; give vincristine 12–24 h prior to administration of asparaginase
Mitomycin	⇧ Risk of pulmonary reactions
Anticholinergic drugs, antihistamines, other agents associated with urinary retention	⇧ Risk of urinary retention; see WARNINGS/PRECAUTIONS
Digoxin	⇩ Bioavailability of digoxin

ALTERED LABORATORY VALUES

Blood/serum values	⇧ Potassium ⇧ Uric acid
Urinary values	⇧ Uric acid

USE IN CHILDREN

See INDICATIONS, PARENTERAL DOSAGE, and ADMINISTRATION/DOSAGE ADJUSTMENTS; children under 13 yr of age have died after receiving 10 times the recommended dose. Several cases of convulsions and postictal coma have been seen in children.

USE IN PREGNANT AND NURSING WOMEN

Pregnancy Category D: vincristine is teratogenic and embryotoxic in several animal species, including primates. Caution women of childbearing potential against becoming pregnant during therapy; apprise women who are or who become pregnant while taking this drug of the potential risks to the fetus. It is not known whether vincristine is excreted in human milk; patients should not nurse during therapy.

MISCELLANEOUS ANTINEOPLASTIC AGENTS

PLATINOL (cisplatin) Bristol-Myers Oncology   Rx

Vials: 10, 50 mg (1 mg/ml after reconstitution) for IV use only

INDICATIONS	PARENTERAL DOSAGE
Palliative treatment of **metastatic testicular tumors**	Adult: 20 mg/m², given in a single daily IV dose for 5 consecutive days every 3 wk for 3 courses, in combination with bleomycin sulfate and vinblastine sulfate
Palliative treatment of **metastatic ovarian tumors**	Adult: 50 mg/m², given in a single daily IV dose once every 3 wk, in combination with doxorubicin hydrochloride, or 100 mg/m², given alone in a single IV dose once every 4 wk as secondary therapy for patients refractory to standard chemotherapy and who have not been previously treated with cisplatin
Palliative treatment of **advanced bladder cancer**	Adult: 50–70 mg/m², given in a single IV dose once every 3–4 wk, depending upon the extent of prior exposure to radiotherapy and/or chemotherapy; if patient has been heavily pretreated, give 50 mg/m² in a single IV dose once every 4 wk

CONTRAINDICATIONS

Preexisting renal impairment	History of allergy to cisplatin or other platinum-containing compounds	Myelosuppression
Hearing impairment		

ADMINISTRATION/DOSAGE ADJUSTMENTS

Intravenous administration	Reconstitute with Sterile Water for Injection USP, using 10 ml for the 10-mg vial or 50 ml for the 50-mg vial; dilute the reconstituted solution with 2 liters of 5% dextrose in 0.45% or 0.3% sodium chloride containing 37.5 g mannitol and infuse over a period of 6–8 h. Do not use needles or IV infusion sets containing aluminum parts that may come in contact with the drug solution; aluminum reacts with cisplatin to form a precipitate.

COMPENDIUM OF DRUG THERAPY

PLATINOL

Hydration of patient	Infuse 1–2 liters of fluid for 8–12 h prior to administration of cisplatin, and maintain adequate hydration and urinary output for 24 h after administration of the drug

WARNINGS/PRECAUTIONS

Patient monitoring	Monitor renal function and perform audiometric testing before initiating therapy and prior to administering subsequent doses of cisplatin (see below); blood counts should be obtained weekly and liver and neurological function tests periodically
Renal effects	Cumulative nephrotoxicity may be manifested by elevation in BUN, serum creatinine, and/or serum uric acid level or by reduction in creatinine clearance, generally during the 2nd wk after dosing; toxicity is dose-related, becomes more prolonged and severe with repeated courses, and is potentiated by aminoglycoside antibiotics. Measure serum creatinine, BUN, creatinine clearance, and magnesium, potassium, and calcium levels before initiating therapy and prior to each course; do not administer if serum creatinine > 1.5 mg/dl and/or BUN > 25 mg/dl.
Myelosuppressive effects	Myelosuppression may occur in 25–30% of patients and is dose-related; obtain peripheral blood counts weekly and do not administer if platelet count $< 100,000/mm^3$ or WBC count $< 4,000/mm^3$
Ototoxicity	Tinnitus and/or high-frequency hearing loss (4,000–8,000 Hz) may occur in one or both ears; hearing loss tends to become more frequent and severe with repeated doses, particularly in children. Do not administer unless audiometry testing indicates normal auditory acuity.
Ocular toxicity	Optic neuritis, papilledema, and cerebral blindness may occur infrequently at recommended doses. These effects are usually reversed totally or partially after this drug has been discontinued; corticosteroids and mannitol have been used, but effectiveness has not been established. Blurred vision and altered color perception may occur with regimens in which the recommended dose or dosing frequency is exceeded; the change in color perception is characterized by a loss of color discrimination, particularly in the blue-yellow axis, and irregular retinal pigmentation of the macular area on fundoscopic examination.
Nausea and vomiting	May occur in almost all patients, usually within 1–4 h after treatment and lasting up to 24 h; symptoms may persist for up to 1 wk after dosing
Hyperuricemia	May occur approximately as often as increases in BUN and serum creatinine levels; an increase in serum uric acid generally peaks between 3–5 days after treatment and may be controlled with allopurinol
Neurotoxicity	Neuropathy, usual peripheral in nature, may occur after 4–7 mo of therapy, although symptoms have been seen after a single dose. Severe neuropathy, characterized by areflexia, paresthesias in a stocking-glove distribution, or loss of proprioception, vibratory sensation, or motor function, may occur with regimens in which the recommended dose or frequency of dosing is exceeded. In some cases, peripheral neuropathy may be irreversible. To reduce the risk of neurotoxicity, perform a neurological examination regularly (see also warning below concerning ocular toxicity); discontinue this drug at the first sign or symptom of neuropathy.
Skin reactions	May result from accidental contact with powder or solution; wear gloves and handle drug carefully during preparation. If contact with skin or mucosa occurs, wash exposed area thoroughly with soap and water.
Serum electrolyte disturbances	Hypomagnesemia, hypocalcemia, hypokalemia, and hypophosphatemia have been reported, and are probably related to renal tubular damage (see warning, above, regarding renal effects). Tetany has been reported occasionally in patients with hypocalcemia and hypomagnesemia. Usually, normal serum electrolyte levels may be restored by discontinuing cisplatin therapy and administering supplemental electrolytes.
Anaphylactoid-like reactions	Facial edema, wheezing, tachycardia, and hypotension may occur within a few minutes of drug administration; reaction may be controlled with IV epinephrine, corticosteroids, or antihistamines

ADVERSE REACTIONS

Gastrointestinal	Nausea, vomiting, anorexia
Renal	Nephrotoxicity, renal tubular damage
Otic	Tinnitus, high-frequency hearing loss
Ophthalmic	Optic neuritis, papilledema, and cerebral blindness (at recommended dosages); blurred vision and altered color perception (at higher dosages)
Hematological	Leukopenia, thrombocytopenia, anemia
Neurological	Neuropathy (see WARNINGS/PRECAUTIONS), loss of taste sensation, seizures
Allergic	Anaphylactoid-like reactions (see WARNING/PRECAUTIONS)
Other	Cardiac abnormalities

OVERDOSAGE

Signs and symptoms	See ADVERSE REACTIONS
Treatment	Discontinue medication; treat symptomatically and institute supportive measures, as required

PLATINOL ■ VEPESID

DRUG INTERACTIONS

Aminoglycoside antibiotics	↑ Risk of nephrotoxicity

ALTERED LABORATORY VALUES

Blood/serum values	↑ BUN ↑ Creatinine ↑ Uric acid ↑ SGOT ↓ Magnesium ↓ Calcium ↓ Potassium ↓ Phosphate

No clinically significant alterations in urinary values occur at therapeutic dosages

---

USE IN CHILDREN
Consult manufacturer

USE IN PREGNANT AND NURSING WOMEN
Safety for use during pregnancy has not been established. It is not known whether cisplatin is excreted in human milk. Because many drugs are excreted in breast milk and because of the potential for serious adverse reactions in nursing infants, patient should not nurse if use of this drug is deemed essential.

MISCELLANEOUS ANTINEOPLASTIC AGENTS

VEPESID (etoposide) Bristol-Myers Oncology Rx

Vials: 100 mg (5 ml) for IV use only

INDICATIONS

Refractory testicular tumors, when used with other chemotherapeutic agents in patients who have already received appropriate surgical, chemical, and radiation therapy

Small-cell lung cancer, when used with other chemotherapeutic agents

PARENTERAL DOSAGE

Adult: 50–100 mg/m²/day IV, given on days 1–5, or 100 mg/m²/day IV, given on days 1, 3, and 5, every 3–4 wk with other appropriate therapy after adequate recovery from any toxicity

Adult: 35 mg/m²/day IV, given for 4 days, to 50 mg/m²/day IV, given for 5 days, every 3–4 wk with other appropriate therapy after adequate recovery from any toxicity

CONTRAINDICATIONS

Hypersensitivity to etoposide

ADMINISTRATION/DOSAGE ADJUSTMENTS

Preparation of IV solution	Dilute solution with 5% dextrose injection USP or 0.9% sodium chloride injection USP to give a final concentration of 0.2 or 0.4 mg/ml; solution is stable for 48–96 h. Avoid contact of solution with skin or mucosa; if accidental contact occurs, thoroughly wash affected area immediately with soap and water
Administration of IV solution	Administer by slow IV infusion over a period of 30–60 min; do not administer by rapid IV injection (see WARNINGS/PRECAUTIONS)

WARNINGS/PRECAUTIONS

Anaphylactic reactions	An anaphylactic reaction manifested by chills, fever, tachycardia, bronchospasm, dyspnea, and hypotension may occur; terminate infusion immediately and administer pressor agents, corticosteroids, antihistamines, or volume expanders, as needed
Hypotension	Temporary hypotension not associated with cardiac toxicity or ECG changes has been reported following rapid IV administration; no delayed hypotension has been reported. If hypotension occurs, discontinue the infusion and administer fluid replacement and other supportive measures, as needed. To avoid a recurrence, reduce the rate of administration when restarting the infusion.
Myelosuppressive effects	Myelosuppression is frequent (see ADVERSE REACTIONS) and dose-limiting. Following administration of etoposide, the granulocyte count reaches a nadir in 7–14 days and the platelet count in 9–16 days; bone marrow recovery is usually complete by day 20, and no cumulative toxicity has been reported. Determine the platelet, WBC, and differential count, as well as hemoglobin level, upon initiating therapy and before each subsequent dose. Because severe bone marrow suppression with consequent infection or bleeding may occur, patients should be monitored frequently both during and after each course. If the platelet count falls below 50,000/mm³ or the absolute neutrophil count falls below 500/mm³, withhold further therapy until sufficient recovery occurs.
Carcinogenicity	No clinical or laboratory studies have been performed to evaluate the carcinogenic potential of this drug; etoposide may be carcinogenic in humans

COMPENDIUM OF DRUG THERAPY

VEPESID

Mutagenicity	Etoposide has induced chromosome aberrations in embryonic mouse cells; treatment of pregnant SPF rats with 1.2 mg/kg/day IV resulted in a prenatal mortality of 92%, and 50% of implanted fetuses were abnormal

ADVERSE REACTIONS

Frequent reactions (incidence ≥ 1%) are printed in *italics*

Hematological	*Leukopenia (60%), severe leukopenia (< 1,000 WBC/mm³) (7%), thrombocytopenia (28%), severe thrombocytopenia (< 50,000 platelets/mm³) (4%)*
Gastrointestinal	*Nausea and vomiting (31%), anorexia (13%), diarrhea (13%), liver toxicity (3%)*, stomatitis
Dermatological	*Reversible alopecia, sometimes progressing to total baldness (20%)*, rash (rare); radiation recall dermatitis (one case)
Cardiovascular	*Temporary hypotension (2%)*; hypertension (rare)
Hypersensitivity	*Anaphylactic-like reaction characterized by chills, fever, tachycardia, bronchospasm, hypotension, and dyspnea (2%)*
Neurological	*Somnolence and fatigue (3%)*, peripheral neuropathy (rare)
Other	Aftertaste (rare)

DRUG INTERACTIONS

Other myelosuppressive agents, radiotherapy	⇧ Myelosuppression; reduce dosage, if necessary
Live virus vaccines	⇧ Risk of viral infection; use with caution
Cisplatin	Possible synergistic effect ⇩ Elimination of etoposide

ALTERED LABORATORY VALUES

Blood/serum values	⇧ Bilirubin ⇧ SGOT ⇧ Alkaline phosphatase

No clinically significant alterations in urinary values have occurred at therapeutic dosages

USE IN CHILDREN

Safety and effectiveness for use in children have not been established

USE IN PREGNANT AND NURSING WOMEN

Pregnancy Category D: etoposide is teratogenic and embryocidal in rats and mice at doses of 1–3% of the recommended clinical dose based on body surface area; the drug has caused decreased fetal weight and fetal abnormalities, including major skeletal abnormalities, exencephaly, encephalocele, and anophthalmia in SPF rats given 0.4 and 1.2 mg/kg and a significant increase in retarded ossification at a dose of 0.13 mg/kg, the lowest dose tested. Dose-related embryotoxicity, cranial abnormalities, and major skeletal malformations were also observed in Swiss-Albino mice. No adequate, well-controlled studies have been performed in pregnant women; because of the potential for abnormalities, patients who are or who become pregnant during therapy should be apprised of the risk involved. It is not known whether etoposide is excreted in human milk; because many drugs are excreted in human milk and the potential for serious adverse effects, a decision should be made whether to stop nursing or discontinue use in nursing mothers.

[1] Incidence figures given in this section are based on published reports and include data on 1,393 patients. In Bristol-sponsored studies, comprising 148 patients, the incidence of leukopenia was 91%; severe leukopenia (< 1,000 WBC/mm³), 17%; thrombocytopenia, 41%; severe thrombocytopenia (< 50,000 platelets/mm³), 20%; nausea and vomiting, 32%; anorexia, 10%; diarrhea, 1%; stomatitis, 1%; alopecia, 8%; hypotension, 1%; anaphylactic-like reactions, 0.7%; peripheral neuropathy, 0.7%; and somnolence and fatigue, 3%.

Chapter 29

Antiulcer/Antireflux/Antispasmodic Agents

Antiulcer/Antireflux Agents — 1130

CARAFATE (Marion) — 1130
Sucralfate Rx

PEPCID (Merck Sharp & Dohme) — 1131
Famotidine Rx

PEPCID I.V. (Merck Sharp & Dohme) — 1131
Famotidine Rx

REGLAN (Robins) — 1132
Metoclopramide hydrochloride Rx

TAGAMET (Smith Kline & French) — 1135
Cimetidine Rx

ZANTAC 150 (Glaxo) — 1137
Ranitidine hydrochloride Rx

ZANTAC 300 (Glaxo) — 1137
Ranitidine hydrochloride Rx

ZANTAC Injection (Glaxo) — 1137
Ranitidine hydrochloride Rx

Antispasmodics — 1138

BELLADENAL (Sandoz Pharmaceuticals) — 1138
Belladonna alkaloids and phenobarbital Rx

BELLADENAL-S (Sandoz Pharmaceuticals) — 1138
Belladonna alkaloids and phenobarbital Rx

BELLERGAL-S (Sandoz Pharmaceuticals) — 1139
Phenobarbital, ergotamine tartrate, and belladonna alkaloids Rx

BENTYL (Lakeside) — 1141
Dicyclomine hydrochloride Rx

DONNATAL (Robins) — 1142
Phenobarbital, hyoscyamine sulfate, atropine sulfate, and hyoscine hydrobromide Rx

KINESED (Stuart) — 1144
Phenobarbital, hyoscyamine sulfate, atropine sulfate, and scopolamine hydrobromide Rx

LEVSIN (Kremers-Urban) — 1145
Hyoscyamine sulfate Rx

LEVSIN Injection (Kremers-Urban) — 1145
Hyoscyamine sulfate Rx

LEVSINEX (Kremers-Urban) — 1146
Hyoscyamine sulfate Rx

LIBRAX (Roche) — 1147
Chlordiazepoxide hydrochloride and clidinium bromide Rx

PATHIBAMATE (Lederle) — 1148
Tridihexethyl chloride and meprobamate Rx

PRO-BANTHĪNE (Searle) — 1150
Propantheline bromide Rx

Other Antispasmodics — 1128

ANASPAZ (Ascher) — 1128
L-Hyoscyamine sulfate Rx

ANTRENYL (CIBA) — 1128
Oxyphenonium bromide Rx

ANTROCOL (Poythress) — 1128
Atropine sulfate and phenobarbital Rx

Atropine sulfate Rx — 1128

BANTHINE (Searle) — 1128
Methantheline bromide Rx

BARBIDONNA (Wallace) — 1128
Phenobarbital, hyoscyamine sulfate, atropine sulfate, and scopolamine hydrobromide Rx

BELAP (Lemmon) — 1128
Phenobarbital and belladonna extract Rx

Belladonna tincture Rx — 1128

BELLAFOLINE (Sandoz Pharmaceuticals) — 1128
Levorotatory alkaloids of belladonna Rx

BUTIBEL (Wallace) — 1128
Belladonna extract and butabarbital sodium Rx

CANTIL (Merrell Dow) — 1128
Mepenzolate bromide Rx

CHARDONNA-2 (Kremers-Urban) — 1129
Belladonna extract and phenobarbital Rx

DARBID (Smith Kline & French) — 1129
Isopropamide iodide Rx

DARICON (Beecham) — 1129
Oxyphencyclimine hydrochloride Rx

HYBEPHEN (Beecham) — 1129
Atropine sulfate, scopolamine hydrobromide, hyoscyamine sulfate, and phenobarbital Rx

PAMINE (Upjohn) — 1129
Methscopolamine bromide Rx

PATHILON (Lederle) — 1129
Tridihexethyl chloride Rx

QUARZAN (Roche) — 1129
Clidinium bromide Rx

ROBINUL (Robins) — 1129
Glycopyrrolate Rx

ROBINUL Forte (Robins) — 1129
Glycopyrrolate Rx

Scopolamine hydrobromide Rx — 1129

VALPIN 50 (Du Pont) — 1129
Anisotropine methylbromide Rx

VISTRAX (Pfizer) — 1129
Oxyphencyclimine hydrochloride and hydroxyzine hydrochloride Rx

continued

COMPENDIUM OF DRUG THERAPY

OTHER ANTISPASMODICS

DRUG	HOW SUPPLIED	USUAL DOSAGE[1]
ANASPAZ (Ascher) L-Hyoscyamine sulfate *Rx*	**Tablets:** 0.125 mg	**Adult:** 0.125–0.25 mg, given orally or sublingually tid or qid to start
ANTRENYL (CIBA) Oxyphenonium bromide *Rx*	**Tablets:** 5 mg	**Adult:** 10 mg qid for several days
ANTROCOL (Poythress) Atropine sulfate and phenobarbital *Rx*	**Tablets:** 0.195 mg atropine sulfate and 16 mg phenobarbital **Capsules:** 0.195 mg atropine sulfate and 16 mg phenobarbital **Elixir (per milliliter):** 0.039 mg atropine sulfate, 3 mg phenobarbital, and 20% alcohol (1, 8 fl oz, 1 pt) *citrus flavored*	**Adult:** 1–2 tabs or caps or 5–10 ml (1–2 tsp) tid or qid, as needed **Child:** 0.5 ml/15 lb q4–6h, as needed
Atropine sulfate *Rx*	**Tablets:** 0.4 mg **Tablets (soluble):** 0.3, 0.4, 0.6 mg **Ampuls:** 0.4 mg/ml (0.5, 1 ml) **Prefilled syringes:** 0.05 mg/ml (5 ml), 0.1 mg/ml (5, 10 ml), 0.5 mg/ml (5 ml), 1 mg/ml (10 ml) **Vials:** 0.3 mg/ml (1 ml), 0.4 mg/ml (0.5, 1, 20, 30 ml), 0.5 mg/ml (1, 30 ml), 1 mg/ml (1 ml), 1.2 mg/ml (1 ml)	**Adult:** 0.3–1.2 mg PO q4–6h; 0.4–0.6 mg IM, IV, or SC q4–6h **Child:** 0.01 mg/kg, up to 0.4 mg, PO or SC q4–6h or, alternatively, 0.3 mg/m^2 PO or SC
BANTHINE (Searle) Methantheline bromide *Rx*	**Tablets:** 50 mg	**Adult:** for peptic ulcer, 50 or 100 mg q6h, to start; for maintenance, 25 or 50 mg q6h; for uninhibited hypertonic neurogenic bladder, 50–100 mg qid to start, thereafter, adjusting dosage to patient need **Infant (< 1 mo):** 12.5 mg bid, followed by 12.5 mg tid **Infant (1–12 mo):** 12.5 mg qid, followed by 25 mg qid **Child (> 1 yr):** 12.5–50 mg qid
BARBIDONNA (Wallace) Phenobarbital, hyoscyamine sulfate, atropine sulfate, and scopolamine hydrobromide *Rx*	**Tablets:** 16 mg phenobarbital, 0.1286 mg hyoscyamine sulfate, 0.025 mg atropine sulfate, and 0.0074 mg scopolamine hydrobromide (Barbidonna Tablets); 32 mg phenobarbital, 0.1286 mg hyoscyamine sulfate, 0.025 mg atropine sulfate, and 0.0074 mg scopolamine hydrobromide (Barbidonna No. 2 Tablets) **Elixir (per 5 ml):** 21.6 mg phenobarbital, 0.174 mg hyoscyamine sulfate, 0.034 mg atropine sulfate, and 0.01 mg scopolamine hydrobromide (1 pt) *apricot flavored*	**Adult:** 1–2 tabs, 1 No. 2 tab tid, or 5–10 ml (1–2 tsp) tid **Child:** 1/2–1 tab or 2.5–5 ml (1/2–1 tsp) tid
BELAP (Lemmon) Phenobarbital and belladonna extract *Rx*	**Tablets:** 16.2 mg phenobarbital and 10.8 mg belladonna extract	**Adult:** 1–2 tabs tid or qid
Belladonna tincture *Rx*	**Liquid:** 30 mg/100 ml (120 ml, 1 pt, 1 gal)	**Adult:** 0.6–1.0 ml tid or qid **Child:** 0.03 ml/kg tid
BELLAFOLINE (Sandoz Pharmaceuticals) Levorotatory alkaloids of belladonna *Rx*	**Tablets:** 0.25 mg **Ampuls:** 0.5 mg/ml (1 ml)	**Adult:** 0.25–0.5 mg PO tid or 0.5–1.0 ml SC 1–2 times/day **Child (> 6 yr):** 0.125–0.25 mg PO tid, according to age
BUTIBEL (Wallace) Belladonna extract and butabarbital sodium *Rx*	**Tablets:** 15 mg belladonna extract and 15 mg butabarbital sodium **Elixir (per 5 ml):** 15 mg belladonna extract, 15 mg butabarbital sodium, and 7% alcohol (1 pt)	**Adult:** 1–2 tabs or 5–10 ml (1–2 tsp) qid **Child (< 6 yr):** 1.25–2.5 ml (1/4–1/2 tsp) qid; adjust dosage according to age and weight **Child (≥ 6 yr):** 2.5 ml (1/2 tsp) qid
CANTIL (Merrell Dow) Mepenzolate bromide *Rx*	**Tablets:** 25 mg	**Adult:** 25–50 mg tid, with meals, plus 25–50 mg at bedtime

[1] Where pediatric dosages are not given, consult manufacturer

OTHER ANTISPASMODICS continued

DRUG	HOW SUPPLIED	USUAL DOSAGE[1]
CHARDONNA-2 (Kremers-Urban) Belladonna extract and phenobarbital *Rx*	**Tablets:** 15 mg belladonna extract and 15 mg phenobarbital	**Adult:** 1–2 tabs tid or qid
DARBID (Smith Kline & French) Isopropamide iodide *Rx*	**Tablets:** 5 mg	**Adult:** 5 mg q12h to start; adjust dosage according to response; for severe symptoms, 10 mg bid or more **Child ($\geq$ 12 yr):** same as adult
DARICON (Beecham) Oxyphencyclimine hydrochloride *Rx*	**Tablets:** 10 mg	**Adult:** 10 mg bid, preferably given in the morning and at bedtime **Child ($\geq$ 12 yr):** same as adult
HYBEPHEN (Beecham) Atropine sulfate, scopolamine hydrobromide, hyoscyamine sulfate, and phenobarbital *Rx*	**Tablets:** 0.0233 mg atropine sulfate, 0.0094 mg scopolamine hydrobromide, 0.1277 mg hyoscyamine sulfate, and 15 mg phenobarbital	**Adult:** 1–2 tabs tid or qid, as needed
PAMINE (Upjohn) Methscopolamine bromide *Rx*	**Tablets:** 2.5 mg	**Adult:** 2.5 mg 30 min before meals and 2.5–5 mg at bedtime; for severe symptoms, 5 mg 30 min before meals and 5 mg at bedtime
PATHILON (Lederle) Tridihexethyl chloride *Rx*	**Tablets:** 25 mg	**Adult:** 25 mg tid before meals plus 50 mg at bedtime to start; for maintenance, 10 mg tid to 75 mg qid
QUARZAN (Roche) Clidinium bromide *Rx*	**Capsules:** 2.5, 5 mg	**Adult:** 2.5–5 mg tid or qid, given before meals and at bedtime, up to 20 mg/day
ROBINUL (Robins) Glycopyrrolate *Rx*	**Tablets:** 1 mg **Vials:** 0.2 mg/ml (1, 2, 5, 20 ml)	**Adult:** 1 mg PO in the morning and early afternoon plus 1–2 mg at bedtime (for maintenance, 1 mg bid); 0.1–0.2 mg IM or IV tid or qid q4h
ROBINUL Forte (Robins) Glycopyrrolate *Rx*	**Tablets:** 2 mg	**Adult:** 2 mg bid or tid at equally spaced intervals
Scopolamine hydrobromide *Rx*	**Tablets (soluble):** 0.4, 0.6 mg **Ampuls:** 0.4 mg/ml (0.5, 1 ml) **Vials:** 0.3 mg/ml (1 ml), 0.4 mg/ml (1 ml), 1 mg/ml (1 ml)	**Adult:** 0.4–0.8 mg PO tid or qid; 0.3–0.6 mg IM, IV, or SC **Child:** 6 g/kg or 0.2 mg/m2 IM, IV, or SC
VALPIN 50 (Du Pont) Anisotropine methylbromide *Rx*	**Tablets:** 50 mg	**Adult:** 50 mg tid
VISTRAX (Pfizer) Oxyphencyclimine hydrochloride and hydroxyzine hydrochloride *Rx*	**Tablets:** 5 mg oxyphencyclimine hydrochloride and 25 mg hydroxyzine hydrochloride (No. 5); 10 mg oxyphencyclimine hydrochloride and 25 mg hydroxyzine hydrochloride (No. 10)	**Adult:** 1 No. 5 or No. 10 tab bid or tid

[1] Where pediatric dosages are not given, consult manufacturer

CARAFATE

ANTIULCER/ANTIREFLUX AGENTS

CARAFATE (sucralfate) Marion   Rx
Tablets: 1 g

INDICATIONS	**ORAL DOSAGE**
Short-term (up to 8 wk) treatment of **duodenal ulcer**	**Adult:** 1 g qid, given on an empty stomach

CONTRAINDICATIONS

None known

ADMINISTRATION/DOSAGE ADJUSTMENTS

Duration of therapy	Although healing may occur in 1–2 wk, continue treatment for 4–8 wk unless healing has been shown by x-ray or endoscopic examination
Concomitant antacid therapy	Antacids may be prescribed as needed for relief of pain, but should not be taken within ½ h before or after administering sucralfate

WARNINGS/PRECAUTIONS

Recurrence of duodenal ulcer	Although short-term treatment with sucralfate can result in complete ulcer healing, it should not be expected to alter the post-healing frequency or severity of duodenal ulcers
Carcinogenicity, mutagenicity	Chronic (24 mo) oral toxicity studies in mice and rats at 12 times the usual human dose have shown no evidence of tumorigenicity; mutagenicity studies have not been done

ADVERSE REACTIONS[1]   Frequent reactions (incidence ≥ 1%) are printed in *italics*

Gastrointestinal	*Constipation (2.2%)* or diarrhea, nausea, gastric discomfort, indigestion
Central nervous system and musculoskeletal	Back pain, dizziness, sleepiness, vertigo
Dermatological	Rash, pruritus
Other	Dry mouth

OVERDOSAGE

In acute oral toxicity studies in animals given up to 12 g/kg, no lethal dose could be found; there has been no experience with overdosage in humans

DRUG INTERACTIONS

Tetracycline, phenytoin, digoxin, cimetidine	▽ Bioavailability of tetracycline, phenytoin, digoxin, and cimetidine, based on animal studies[2]

ALTERED LABORATORY VALUES

No clinically significant alterations in blood/serum or urinary values occur at therapeutic dosages

---

USE IN CHILDREN

Safety and effectiveness for use in children have not been established

USE IN PREGNANT AND NURSING WOMEN

Pregnancy Category B: use during pregnancy only if clearly needed. Reproduction studies in mice, rats, and rabbits at doses up to 50 times the human dose have shown no evidence of fetal harm; however, no adequate, well-controlled studies have been done in pregnant women. Rats given doses of up to 38 times the human dose revealed no evidence of impaired fertility. It is not known whether this drug is excreted in human milk; use with caution in nursing women.

---

[1] Minor adverse reactions were reported in 121 (4.7%) of over 2,500 patients treated with sucralfate in clinical trials
[2] In animals, simultaneous administration of sucralfate reduces the bioavailability of these drugs, presumably by binding them in the GI tract; separating the administration of these drugs by 2 h restores their normal bioavailability. Although the clinical importance of these studies has not yet been determined, separate administration should be considered whenever drug bioavailability is of critical importance.

PEPCID

ANTIULCER/ANTIREFLUX AGENTS

PEPCID (famotidine) Merck Sharp & Dohme — Rx
Tablets: 20, 40 mg

PEPCID I.V. (famotidine) Merck Sharp & Dohme — Rx
Vials: 10 mg/ml (2, 4 ml) for IV use only

INDICATIONS	ORAL DOSAGE	PARENTERAL DOSAGE
Active duodenal ulcer	Adult: 40 mg at bedtime or 20 mg bid	Adult: 20 mg IV q12h
Maintenance therapy after healing of acute duodenal ulcer	Adult: 20 mg at bedtime	—
Pathological hypersecretory conditions (eg, Zollinger-Ellison syndrome and multiple endocrine adenomas)	Adult: 20 mg q6h to start; adjust dosage as needed and continue treatment as long as clinically indicated. Some patients may require higher initial doses, up to 160 mg q6h.	Adult: 20 mg IV q12h

CONTRAINDICATIONS
Hypersensitivity to any component

ADMINISTRATION/DOSAGE ADJUSTMENTS

Intravenous injection	Dilute 20 mg (2 ml) of famotidine in 0.9% sodium chloride injection or other compatible IV solution (eg, 5% or 10% dextrose injection, lactated Ringer's injection, 5% sodium bicarbonate injection) to a total volume of 5 or 10 ml, and inject over a period of not less than 2 min
Intravenous infusion	Dilute 20 mg (2 ml) of famotidine with 100 ml of 5% dextrose injection or other compatible IV solution (see solutions, above, that may be used for IV injection), and administer over a period of 15–30 min
Concomitant antacid therapy	Antacids may be given, as needed, for the relief of pain
Duration of therapy for duodenal ulcer	Healing of active duodenal ulcers occurs in most patients within 4 wk; there is rarely any reason to continue famotidine therapy at full therapeutic dosage (40 mg/day) for longer than 6–8 wk. In clinical studies, healing occurred in 32% of patients after 2 wk of therapy, 70% of patients after 4 wk, and 83% of patients after 8 wk. Controlled studies of maintenance therapy have not been extended beyond 1 yr.
Elderly patients	No dosage adjustment for age is necessary (but see "patients with renal impairment," below)
Patients with renal impairment	The elimination half-life of famotidine may exceed 20 h in patients with severe renal insufficiency (creatinine clearance < 10 ml/min) and may reach approximately 24 h in anuric patients. To avoid excess accumulation of famotidine in these patients, reduce dose to 20 mg at bedtime, or prolong the dosing interval to 36–48 h, depending upon patient response.

WARNINGS/PRECAUTIONS

Gastric malignancy	A symptomatic response to famotidine therapy does not preclude the presence of gastric malignancy
Carcinogenicity, mutagenicity	No evidence of carcinogenic potential was found in a 106-wk study in rats and in a 92-wk study in mice fed up to 2,000 mg/kg/day (2,500 times the recommended human dose for active duodenal ulcer) of famotidine. No evidence of mutagenicity was observed in the Ames test using *Salmonella typhimurium* and *Escherichia coli* (with or without rat liver enzyme activation at concentrations up to 10,000 μg/plate) or in in vivo studies in mice (micronucleus test and chromosomal aberration test).
Effect on fertility	No adverse effect on fertility or reproductive performance was found in studies with rats fed up to 2,000 mg/kg/day (2,500 times the recommended human dose for active duodenal ulcer) or given IV doses of up to 200 mg/kg/day of famotidine

ADVERSE REACTIONS[1]

	Frequent reactions (incidence ≥ 1%) are printed in *italics*
Central nervous system	*Headache (4.7%), dizziness (1.3%)*
Gastrointestinal	*Diarrhea (1.7%), constipation (1.2%)*
Local	Transient irritation at injection site (with IV use)

OVERDOSAGE

Signs and symptoms	See ADVERSE REACTIONS
Treatment	Employ the usual measures to empty the stomach; treat symptomatically and supportively

COMPENDIUM OF DRUG THERAPY

PEPCID ■ REGLAN

DRUG INTERACTIONS

No clinically significant drug interactions have been identified

ALTERED LABORATORY VALUES

No clinically significant alterations in blood/serum or urinary values have been reported at therapeutic dosages

USE IN CHILDREN

Safety and effectiveness for use in children have not been established

USE IN PREGNANT AND NURSING WOMEN

Pregnancy Category B: sporadic abortions have occurred in rabbits displaying a marked decrease in food intake at oral doses of 200 mg/kg/day or higher; however, no evidence of impaired fertility or fetal harm have been found in reproductive studies in rats and rabbits fed up to 2,000 and 500 mg/kg/day, respectively, of famotidine, or in other studies in which IV doses of up to 200 mg/kg/day were given. No adequate, well-controlled studies have been performed in pregnant women; use during pregnancy only if clearly needed. Famotidine is secreted in the breast milk of rats; transient growth depression has been observed in young rats suckling from mothers treated with at least 600 times the usual human dose of the drug. It is not known whether famotidine is excreted in human milk; because many drugs are excreted in human milk, patients should not nurse during therapy.

[1] Reactions for which no causal relationship has been established include fever, asthenia, fatigue, palpitations, nausea, vomiting, abdominal discomfort, anorexia, dry mouth, liver enzyme abnormalities, thrombocytopenia, orbital edema, conjunctival injection, musculoskeletal pain, arthralgia, paresthesias; grand mal seizure (one report); psychic disturbances, including depression, anxiety, decreased libido, and hallucinations (one report); insomnia, somnolence, bronchospasm, alopecia, acne, pruritus, rash, dry skin, flushing, tinnitus, and taste disorder

ANTIULCER/ANTIREFLUX AGENTS

REGLAN (metoclopramide hydrochloride) Robins   Rx

Tablets: 10 mg **Syrup (per 5 ml):** 5 mg (10 ml; 1 pt) *sugar-free* **Ampuls:** 5 mg/ml (2, 10 ml) **Vials:** 5 mg/ml (2, 10, 30 ml)

INDICATIONS	ORAL DOSAGE	PARENTERAL DOSAGE
Gastroesophageal reflux, when conventional therapy is ineffective	**Adult:** for symptomatic relief, 10–15 mg qid, 30 min before each meal and at bedtime, for 4–12 wk; if symptoms only occur at certain times of the day (eg, after the evening meal), consider giving a single dose of up to 20 mg only before each of those times rather than using the drug throughout the day. For treatment of esophageal lesions, give 15 mg qid for up to 12 wk; monitor therapy endoscopically.	—
Symptomatic relief of acute and recurrent **diabetic gastroparesis (diabetic gastric stasis)**	**Adult:** 10 mg 30 min before each meal and at bedtime for 2–8 wk, as needed; reinstitute therapy at earliest sign of recurrence	**Adult:** for severe symptoms, 10 mg IM or IV 30 min before each meal and at bedtime for up to 10 days; switch to oral therapy when symptoms subside
Prevention of nausea and vomiting associated with emetogenic cancer chemotherapy	—	**Adult:** 1 mg/kg, given by slow IV infusion 30 min before administering the antineoplastic agent, then q2h for 2 doses, and finally q3h for 3 doses; if highly emetogenic drugs such as cisplatin and dacarbazine are used, increase the first 2 doses to 2 mg/kg
Facilitation of small bowel intubation if tube has not passed the pylorus with conventional maneuvers in 10 min **Facilitation of radiological examination** of stomach and/or small intestine in cases where delayed gastric emptying interferes with examination		**Adult:** 10 mg IV **Child (< 6 yr):** 0.1 mg/kg IV **Child (6–14 yr):** 2.5–5 mg IV

CONTRAINDICATIONS

Conditions in which stimulation of GI motility may be hazardous (eg, GI hemorrhage and mechanical obstruction or perforation)	Epilepsy Use of drugs likely to cause extrapyramidal reactions	Pheochromocytoma Hypersensitivity or intolerance to metoclopramide

ADMINISTRATION/DOSAGE ADJUSTMENTS

Treatment of gastroesophageal reflux	The principal effect of metoclopramide is on symptoms of postprandial and daytime heartburn, with less observed effect on nocturnal symptoms
Symptomatic relief of gastroparesis	The usual manifestations of delayed gastric emptying may respond to therapy within different time intervals: relief of nausea occurs early and continues to improve over a 3-wk period; relief of vomiting and anorexia may precede relief of abdominal fullness by 1 wk or more
Intravenous administration	Inject doses of 10 mg or less, undiluted, over a period of 1–2 min; avoid rapid administration, which may evoke intense anxiety and restlessness initially and then cause drowsiness. To administer doses exceeding 10 mg, dilute the drug in 50 ml of a parenteral solution, preferably 0.9% sodium chloride injection, and then give by infusion over a period of at least 15 min. Ringer's injection, lactated Ringer's injection, and 5% dextrose in water or in 0.45% sodium chloride can be used as alternative diluents; do not freeze preparations diluted with 5% dextrose in water. Prepared solutions exposed to light should be used within 24 h. For information on compatibility, see DRUG INTERACTIONS and package insert.
Patients with renal impairment	If creatinine clearance is less than 40 ml/min, begin treatment at 50% of the usual dosage; since only a small amount of the drug is removed by hemodialysis and continuous peritoneal dialysis, a dosage adjustment to compensate for losses due to dialysis is unlikely to be necessary

WARNINGS/PRECAUTIONS

Tardive dyskinesia	Metoclopramide can cause tardive dyskinesia, a potentially irreversible syndrome characterized by involuntary choreoathetoid movements of the tongue, face, mouth, lips, jaw, trunk, and/or extremities. Protrusion of the tongue, puffing of the cheeks, puckering of the mouth, chewing movements, and other manifestations may become evident during treatment, upon dosage reduction, or after the drug is discontinued. The likelihood that tardive dyskinesia will develop or become irreversible increases with duration of treatment and total cumulative dose; however, even relatively brief use of low doses can cause it. Although this reaction appears to occur most often in the elderly, especially among older women, it is impossible to use this information to predict, before therapy is started, which patients are likely to develop the syndrome. Bear in mind that metoclopramide can itself mask signs of the disorder. There is no known treatment for tardive dyskinesia; however, after discontinuation, some or all manifestations may disappear spontaneously. Although metoclopramide can suppress these manifestations, the drug should not be used for this purpose since the effects of suppression on the long-term course of the disorder are not known.
Dystonia	At a dosage of 30–40 mg/day, acute dystonic reactions occur in approximately 0.2% of patients, with effects more commonly seen in children and young adults than in others; at doses of 1–2 mg/kg, the frequency is 2% among patients over 30–35 yr of age and 25% or higher among younger adults and children. Dystonic reactions are usually seen within 24–48 h after starting treatment; they are characterized by involuntary movements of the limbs, facial grimacing, torticollis, oculogyric crisis, rhythmic protrusion of the tongue, bulbar type of speech, trismus, opisthotonus (tetanus-like reactions), or, in rare cases, stridor or dyspnea. To control symptoms, inject 50 mg of diphenhydramine or 1–2 mg of benztropine IM.
Pseudoparkinsonism, akathisia	Parkinsonian-like symptoms, including bradykinesia, tremor, cogwheel rigidity, and mask-like facies, can first occur within 6 mo after starting treatment or, occasionally, after a longer period; effects generally subside within 2–3 mo after discontinuation of therapy. Akathisia, characterized by anxiety, agitation, jitteriness, insomnia, pacing, foot tapping, and inability to sit still, can also result from therapy; reaction may disappear spontaneously or upon reduction in dosage.
Drowsiness, dizziness	Caution ambulatory patients about driving or engaging in other potentially hazardous activities requiring mental alertness or physical coordination; drowsiness occurs in approximately 10% of patients given 10 mg qid and in approximately 70% of patients given doses of 1–2 mg/kg
Hypertensive crisis	A clinical study has shown that IV administration precipitates the release of catecholamines in patients with hypertension; use metoclopramide with caution in these patients
Depression	A temporal association between metoclopramide and depression has been reported
Diabetic patients	Metoclopramide influences the delivery of food to the intestines and, hence, the rate of absorption; patients dependent upon insulin may require an adjustment in insulin dosage or timing of administration
Carcinogenicity	Metoclopramide causes an increase in serum prolactin levels which persists during chronic administration and may be important in patients with previously detected breast cancer. Although endocrine disturbances have been reported with prolactin-elevating drugs, no association has been shown between chronic administration of these drugs and mammary tumorigenesis; the available evidence is considered too limited to be conclusive at this time.
Mutagenicity	No evidence of mutagenicity has been detected in the Ames test

ADVERSE REACTIONS

Central nervous system	Restlessness, drowsiness, fatigue, lassitude, insomnia, headache, confusion, dizziness, depression, extrapyramidal reactions (dystonia, pseudoparkinsonism, akathisia, tardive dyskinesia), convulsive seizures[1]; hallucinations (rare)
Gastrointestinal	Nausea; diarrhea and other intestinal disturbances
Cardiovascular	Hypotension, hypertension; transient flushing of face and upper body (with high IV doses); supraventricular tachycardia (one case)
Endocrinological	Galactorrhea, amenorrhea, gynecomastia, impotence, fluid retention
Renal	Urinary frequency, incontinence
Hematological	Neutropenia,[1] leukopenia,[1] agranulocytosis[1]
Hypersensitivity	Rash, urticaria, and bronchospasm (especially in patients with a history of asthma); angioneurotic edema, including glossal and laryngeal edema (rare)
Other	Visual disturbances, porphyria; neuroleptic malignant syndrome, a potentially fatal syndrome characterized by hyperthermia, altered consciousness, muscular rigidity, and autonomic dysfunction (rare)

OVERDOSAGE

Signs and symptoms	Drowsiness, disorientation, extrapyramidal reactions; methemoglobinemia (in neonates given 1–2 mg/kg/day IM for 3 days or longer)
Treatment	Discontinue medication. Administer anticholinergic or antiparkinson drugs or antihistamines with anticholinergic properties to control extrapyramidal reactions, if needed. Symptoms are self-limited and usually disappear within 24 h. To reverse methemoglobinemia, administer methylene blue IV. Dialysis is unlikely to be effective, since neither hemodialysis nor peritoneal dialysis removes a significant amount of the drug.

DRUG INTERACTIONS

Phenothiazines, other drugs likely to cause extrapyramidal reactions	△ Extrapyramidal effects; do not use metoclopramide with other drugs likely to produce extrapyramidal effects
MAO inhibitors	Hypertensive crisis; use metoclopramide with caution, if at all, in patients receiving MAO inhibitors
Anticholinergic agents	▽ GI motility
Narcotic analgesics	▽ GI motility △ CNS depression
Alcohol, sedative-hypnotics, tranquilizers	△ CNS depression
Apomorphine	▽ Central and peripheral effects of apomorphine
Drugs absorbed from stomach (eg, digoxin)	▽ Absorption
Drugs absorbed from small intestine (eg, acetaminophen, tetracycline, levodopa, ethanol)	△ Absorption
Cephalolithin, chloramphenicol, sodium bicarbonate	Physical incompatibility in solution; do not mix with metoclopramide

ALTERED LABORATORY VALUES

Blood/serum values	△ Prolactin △ Aldosterone (transient)

No clinically significant alterations in urinary values occur at therapeutic dosages

---

USE IN CHILDREN

Metoclopramide can be used in children to facilitate small bowel intubation or radiological examination; for dosage recommendations, see PARENTERAL DOSAGE. Extrapyramidal reactions occur more frequently in children; see warning, above, concerning these reactions.

USE IN PREGNANT AND NURSING WOMEN

Pregnancy Category B: use during pregnancy only if clearly needed. Reproductive studies in rats, mice, and rabbits at doses ranging up to 12–250 times the human dose have shown no evidence of impaired fertility or significant fetal harm. No adequate, well-controlled studies have been done in pregnant women. Metoclopramide is excreted in human milk; use with caution in nursing mothers.

---

[1] No clearcut causal relationship has been established

TAGAMET

ANTIULCER/ANTIREFLUX AGENTS

TAGAMET (cimetidine) Smith Kline & French   Rx

Tablets: 200, 300, 400, 800 mg **Liquid (per 5 ml):** 300 mg[1] (5 ml, 8 fl oz) **Vials:** 300 mg/2 ml (2, 8 ml)
Prefilled syringes: 300 mg/2 ml (2 ml) **Plastic containers:** 6 mg/ml (50 ml) for IV infusion only

INDICATIONS	ORAL DOSAGE	PARENTERAL DOSAGE
Active duodenal ulcer	Adult: 800 mg at bedtime	Adult: 300 mg IM or IV q6h
Maintenance therapy after healing of acute duodenal ulcer	Adult: 400 mg at bedtime	—
Active benign gastric ulcer	Adult: 300 mg qid, with meals and at bedtime, for up to 8 wk	Adult: same as above
Pathological hypersecretory conditions (eg, Zollinger-Ellison syndrome, systemic mastocytosis, and multiple adenomas)	Adult: 300 mg qid, with meals and at bedtime, as long as clinically indicated; some patients may require higher or more frequent doses, up to 2,400 mg/day	Adult: same as above

CONTRAINDICATIONS

None known

ADMINISTRATION/DOSAGE ADJUSTMENTS

Intravenous injection	Dilute 300 mg of cimetidine in 0.9% sodium chloride injection or other compatible IV solution (eg, 5% or 10% dextrose injection, lactated Ringer's solution, 5% sodium bicarbonate injection, etc) to a total volume of 20 ml and inject over a period of not less than 2 min (cardiac arrhythmias and hypotension have occurred, in rare instances, after rapid IV injection)
Intermittent intravenous infusion	Dilute 300 mg of cimetidine in at least 50 ml of 5% dextrose injection or other compatible IV solution (see solutions, above, that may be used for IV injection) or use premixed cimetidine solution; administer over a period of 15–20 min. Some patients may require more frequent dosing, up to 2,400 mg/day.
Use of plastic containers	After removing overwrap, check for minute leaks in container by squeezing it firmly; if leaks are found, discard solution. Do not connect containers in series; residual air drawn from the primary container before administration of the fluid from the secondary container is complete could cause air embolism.
Concomitant antacid therapy	For active duodenal ulcers, antacids should be given as needed for relief of pain; however, simultaneous administration is not recommended (see DRUG INTERACTIONS)
Duration of therapy for duodenal ulcer	Although healing of duodenal ulcers often occurs during the first 1–2 wk of therapy, treatment should be continued for at least 4 wk unless endoscopic examination demonstrates healing. If healing is not seen or symptoms persist after 4 wk of treatment, give the drug for another 2–4 wk; there is rarely any reason to continue cimetidine therapy at therapeutic (ie, nonmaintenance) dosages for more than 6–8 wk. In clinical studies, healing occurred in 80% of patients after 4 wk of therapy, 89% of patients after 6 wk, and 94% of patients after 8 wk. Maintenance therapy has been continued for periods of up to 5 yr.
Administration of 1,600 mg/day for duodenal ulcer	There is some evidence suggesting that administration of 1,600 mg at bedtime, rather than 800 mg, produces more rapid healing in patients who have an duodenal ulcer larger than 1 cm and also smoke one or more packs of cigarettes per day; administration of this larger dose may be an appropriate option when it is important to ensure that healing in these patients occurs within 4 wk
Patients with severely impaired renal function	Although experience is limited, such patients may be given 300 mg q12h orally or by IV injection; if necessary, the dosage frequency may be increased to q8h or further, with caution. If liver function is also impaired, a further reduction in dosage may be necessary. For patients on hemodialysis, schedule the dose to coincide with the end of a dialysis period.

WARNINGS/PRECAUTIONS

Gynecomastia	Has been observed in 4% of patients treated for pathological hypersecretory states and 0.3–1.0% of other patients. The condition, which is seen after 1 mo or more of treatment, may be related to a mild antiandrogenic effect manifested in animals by a reduction in prostate and seminal vesicle weights without impairment of fertility or mating performance.
Impotence	Reversible impotence has been reported in patients with pathological hypersecretory conditions who received cimetidine, particularly at high dosages, for at least 12 mo; however, no significant difference in the incidence of impotence has been observed in large-scale surveillance studies in which patients were given regular dosages

TAGAMET

Effect on male fertility	Cimetidine has been shown to have no effect on human spermatogenesis, sperm count, motility, morphology, or fertilization capacity in vitro
Carcinogenicity	A small increase in the incidence of benign Leydig-cell tumors has been observed in rats treated with 150, 378, and 950 mg/kg/day (9–56 times the recommended human dose) of cimetidine; in a subsequent study, however, only the higher doses caused a significant increase in tumor incidence and only in aged rats
Mental confusion	May occur, especially in elderly and/or severely ill patients; the condition generally clears within 48 h of discontinuing therapy
Gastric malignancy	May be present, despite symptomatic or clinical response to cimetidine therapy
Hepatic reactions	Reversible hepatic reactions, with cholestatic or with cholestatic and hepatocellular features, can occur in rare cases; because these reactions are exclusively or predominantly cholestatic in nature, severe parenchymal injury is considered highly unlikely

ADVERSE REACTIONS

Frequent reactions (incidence $\geq$ 1%) are printed in *italics*

Central nervous system and neuromuscular	*Dizziness, somnolence,* confusion, headache; reversible arthralgia and myalgia (rare); exacerbation of joint symptoms
Gastrointestinal	*Mild and transient diarrhea;* hepatic reactions (cholestatic or cholestatic-hepatocellular) and pancreatitis (rare); periportal hepatic fibrosis (one case)
Dermatological	*Rash*
Hematological	Neutropenia and agranulocytosis (generally with concomitant use of agents known to produce neutropenia), thrombocytopenia, and aplastic anemia (rare)
Other	Gynecomastia and reversible impotence (see WARNINGS/PRECAUTIONS); interstitial nephritis, urinary retention, allergic reactions including hypersensitivity vasculitis, and fever (rare); pain at injection site following IM injection

OVERDOSAGE

Signs and symptoms	Potential respiratory failure and tachycardia (experience with gross overdosage in humans is limited; in the few reported cases, doses of up to 10 g have not been associated with untoward effects)
Treatment	Induce emesis or use gastric lavage, followed by activated charcoal. Monitor patient and provide supportive therapy, as needed. For respiratory failure and tachycardia, provide assisted respiration and administer a beta-blocking agent, such as propranolol.

DRUG INTERACTIONS

Antacids	▽ Absorption of cimetidine
Coumarin anticoagulants	△ Serum anticoagulant level and half-life; monitor prothrombin time closely and adjust anticoagulant dosage as needed
Phenytoin, chlordiazepoxide, diazepam, propranolol, lidocaine, theophylline, and other drugs that undergo hepatic metabolism	△ Serum level and half-life of metabolized drug; monitor serum level and clinical response and adjust dosage as needed when starting or stopping concomitant cimetidine therapy

ALTERED LABORATORY VALUES

Blood/serum values	△ Creatinine △ SGOT △ SGPT

No clinically significant alterations in urinary values occur at therapeutic dosages

---

USE IN CHILDREN

Not recommended for use in children under 16 yr of age unless anticipated benefits of therapy outweigh the potential risks. In a few instances, dosages of 20–40 mg/kg/day have been used.

USE IN PREGNANT AND NURSING WOMEN

Cimetidine crosses the placental barrier in laboratory animals and should not be used in women of childbearing potential or pregnant women unless the expected benefits outweigh the potential risks. Evidence of harm to the fetus has not been observed in animals given 9–56 times the full therapeutic dose; however, clinical studies have not been performed. Cimetidine is excreted in human milk; as a rule, nursing should not be attempted while a patient is taking a drug.

---

[1] Contains 2.8% alcohol
[2] Polymyositis has been reported; however, a causal relationship has not been established

ZANTAC

ANTIULCER/ANTIREFLUX AGENTS

ZANTAC 150 (ranitidine hydrochloride) Glaxo — Rx
Tablets: 150 mg

ZANTAC 300 (ranitidine hydrochloride) Glaxo — Rx
Tablets: 300 mg

ZANTAC Injection (ranitidine hydrochloride) Glaxo — Rx
Vials: 25 mg/ml (2, 10 ml)

INDICATIONS	ORAL DOSAGE	PARENTERAL DOSAGE
Active duodenal ulcer	Adult: 150 mg bid or 300 mg at bedtime for up to 8 wk (usual duration of therapy: 4 wk)	Adult: 50 mg IM or IV q6–8h
Maintenance therapy after healing of acute duodenal ulcer	Adult: 150 mg at bedtime	Adult: 50 mg IM or IV q6–8h
Active benign gastric ulcer	Adult: 150 mg bid for up to 6 wk	Adult: 50 mg IM or IV q6–8h
Pathological hypersecretory conditions (eg, Zollinger-Ellison syndrome, systemic mastocytosis)	Adult: 150 mg bid for as long as clinically indicated; some patients may require up to 6 g/day	Adult: 50 mg IM or IV q6–8h
Gastroesophageal reflux disease	Adult: 150 mg bid	Adult: 50 mg IM or IV q6–8h

CONTRAINDICATIONS
Hypersensitivity to ranitidine

ADMINISTRATION/DOSAGE ADJUSTMENTS

Intravenous injection	Dilute 50 mg of ranitidine in 0.9% sodium chloride injection or another compatible IV solution (eg, 5% or 10% dextrose injection, lactated Ringer's solution, 5% sodium bicarbonate injection) to a total volume of 20 ml, and inject over a period of at least 5 min
Intermittent IV administration	Dilute 50 mg of ranitidine in 100 ml of 5% dextrose injection or another compatible IV solution (see solutions, above, that may be used for IV injection), and administer over a period of 15–20 min. If necessary, the 50-mg dose may be given more frequently than q6h; however, the dosage generally should not exceed 400 mg/day.
Patients with renal impairment	Ranitidine is eliminated primarily by the kidneys. For patients whose creatinine clearance is less than 50 ml/min, give 150 mg orally q24h or 50 mg IM or IV q18–24h to start. The frequency of administration may be cautiously increased, if necessary, up to q12h or more often. For patients on hemodialysis, schedule the dose to coincide with the end of a dialysis period.
Concomitant antacid therapy	Antacids should be given as needed for the relief of pain
Treatment of gastroesophageal reflux disease	Symptomatic relief of gastroesophageal reflux disease commonly occurs within 1–2 wk; treatment for more than 6 wk has not been studied

WARNINGS/PRECAUTIONS

Patients with hepatic impairment	Use with caution in patients with hepatic impairment because ranitidine is metabolized in the liver. If the IV dosage equals or exceeds 400 mg/day for 5 days or longer, check the SGPT level daily, beginning on the fifth day, since elevation of this level may occur.
Elderly patients	Agitation, confusion, depression, and hallucinations have occurred predominantly in severely ill elderly patients
Gastric malignancy	A symptomatic response to ranitidine therapy does not preclude the presence of gastric malignancy
Carcinogenicity, mutagenicity	No carcinogenic or tumorigenic effects have been detected in lifetime studies on rats and rabbits given up to 2,000 mg/kg/day. Standard tests with *E coli* and *Salmonella* and a dominant lethal assay with male rats who were fed single doses of 1,000 mg/kg have shown no evidence of mutagenicity.
Effect on fertility	No clinically significant effect on gonadal function has been reported; rats and rabbits given up to 160 times the human dose have shown no evidence of impaired fertility

ADVERSE REACTIONS

Central nervous system and neuromuscular	Headache; malaise, dizziness, somnolence, insomnia, vertigo, confusion, agitation, depression, hallucinations, and arthralgia (rare)
Cardiovascular	Tachycardia, bradycardia, and premature ventricular contractions (rare)
Gastrointestinal	Hepatitis, constipation, diarrhea, nausea, vomiting, abdominal discomfort and/or pain
Hematological	Leukopenia, granulocytopenia, thrombocytopenia, and pancytopenia (rare)

ZANTAC ■ BELLADENAL

Dermatological	Rash, including rare cases suggestive of mild erythema multiforme; alopecia (rare)
Hypersensitivity	Bronchospasm, fever, rash, and eosinophilia (rare)
Other	Gynecomastia, impotence, loss of libido, pain at IM injection site, local burning or itching with IV use

OVERDOSAGE

Signs and symptoms	Muscular tremors, vomiting, and rapid respiration have been seen in animals given 225 mg/kg/day; no cases of human overdosage have been reported
Treatment	Employ the usual measures to empty the stomach; treat symptomatically and supportively

DRUG INTERACTIONS

No clinically significant drug interactions have been identified

ALTERED LABORATORY VALUES

Blood/serum values	△ Creatinine ▽ WBC ▽ RBC ▽ Platelets
Urinary values	+ Protein (with Multistix test); use sulfosalicylic acid test

USE IN CHILDREN
Safety and effectiveness for use in children have not been established

USE IN PREGNANT AND NURSING WOMEN
Pregnancy Category B: use during pregnancy only if clearly needed. Reproduction studies in rats and rabbits given up to 160 times the human dose have shown no evidence of harm to the fetus; however, no adequate, well-controlled studies have been performed in pregnant women. Ranitidine is excreted in human milk; use with caution in nursing mothers.

ANTISPASMODICS

BELLADENAL (belladonna alkaloids and phenobarbital) Sandoz Pharmaceuticals Rx
Tablets: 0.25 mg belladonna alkaloids and 50 mg phenobarbital

BELLADENAL-S (belladonna alkaloids and phenobarbital) Sandoz Pharmaceuticals Rx
Tablets (sustained release): 0.25 mg belladonna alkaloids and 50 mg phenobarbital

INDICATIONS

Peptic ulcer (adjunctive therapy)[1]
Irritable bowel syndrome
(irritable colon, spastic colon, mucous colitis)[1]
Acute enterocolitis[1]

ORAL DOSAGE

Adult: 2–4 Belladenal tabs/day, given in 4–16 divided doses, or 1 Belladenal-S tab bid (AM and PM)
Child: 1/4–1/2 Belladenal tab 1–4 times/day, depending upon age

CONTRAINDICATIONS

Glaucoma	Hypersensitivity to belladonna alkaloids or phenobarbital	Advanced hepatic or renal disease
Increased intraocular pressure		

WARNINGS/PRECAUTIONS

Special-risk patients	Use with caution in the elderly
Drug dependence	Psychic and/or physical dependence and tolerance may develop following prolonged use of high doses of barbiturates
Tartrazine sensitivity	Presence of FD&C Yellow No. 5 (tartrazine) in sustained-release form may cause allergic-type reactions, including bronchial asthma, in susceptible individuals

ADVERSE REACTIONS

Central nervous system	Drowsiness
Gastrointestinal	Dry mouth
Ophthalmic	Blurred vision
Cardiovascular	Flushing
Genitourinary	Urinary retention

BELLADENAL ■ BELLERGAL-S

OVERDOSAGE

Signs and symptoms — *Belladonna alkaloid-related effects:* dry mouth and throat, blurred vision, urinary retention, CNS excitation, restlessness, confusion, delirium, convulsions, stupor, and coma, leading to death; *phenobarbital-related effects:* drowsiness, confusion, coma, respiratory depression, hypotension, shock.

Treatment — Induce emesis or perform gastric lavage to empty stomach; administer activated charcoal. Maintain adequate pulmonary ventilation, correct hypotension, and control convulsions, if present. Force diuresis, alkalinize urine, and use catheterization to prevent urinary retention. Maintain body temperature. Hemodialysis or peritoneal dialysis may be useful.

DRUG INTERACTIONS

Alcohol, tranquilizers, sedative-hypnotics, and other CNS depressants	△ CNS depression
Coumarin anticoagulants	▽ Anticoagulant effect
Amantadine	△ Atropine-like effects △ CNS depression
Antihistamines, antimuscarinics	△ Atropine-like effects △ CNS depression
Haloperidol, phenothiazines	△ Atropine-like effects △ CNS depression ▽ Antipsychotic effects
Antacids, antidiarrheal suspensions	▽ Belladonna alkaloid effects ▽ Barbiturate effects
Corticosteroids	▽ Corticosteroid effects
Digitalis, digitoxin	▽ Digitalis or digitoxin effects
Griseofulvin	▽ Griseofulvin effects
Tetracyclines, particularly doxycycline	▽ Antimicrobial effect
Anticonvulsants	Change in pattern of epileptiform seizures
MAO inhibitors	△ Atropine-like effects △ CNS effects
Tricyclic antidepressants	△ Atropine-like effects ▽ Antidepressant effect

ALTERED LABORATORY VALUES

Blood/serum values — △ Sulfobromophthalein retention ▽ Bilirubin

No clinically significant alterations in urinary values occur at therapeutic dosages

---

USE IN CHILDREN
See INDICATIONS and ORAL DOSAGE; the sustained-release form is not indicated for use in children.

USE IN PREGNANT AND NURSING WOMEN
Safety for use in pregnant or nursing women has not been established.

---

[1] Possibly effective

ANTISPASMODICS

BELLERGAL-S (phenobarbital, ergotamine tartrate, and belladonna alkaloids) Sandoz Pharmaceuticals Rx

Tablets (sustained release): 40 mg phenobarbital, 0.6 mg ergotamine tartrate, and 0.2 mg belladonna alkaloids

INDICATIONS

Menopausal disorders (hot flushes, sweats, restlessness, insomnia)
Cardiovascular disorders (palpitations, tachycardia, chest oppression, vasomotor disturbances)
Gastrointestinal disorders (hypermotility, hypersecretion, nervous stomach, diarrhea, constipation)
Recurrent, throbbing headache

ORAL DOSAGE

Adult: 1 tab bid, in the morning and evening, not to exceed 16 tabs/wk

COMPENDIUM OF DRUG THERAPY

BELLERGAL-S

CONTRAINDICATIONS

Pregnancy	Hypertension	Hypersensitivity to phenobarbital, ergotamine tartrate, or belladonna alkaloids
Breast-feeding	Impaired hepatic or renal function	
Peripheral vascular disease	Sepsis	Phenobarbital-induced restlessness or excitement
Coronary artery disease	Dopamine therapy	
Manifest or latent porphyria	Glaucoma	

WARNINGS/PRECAUTIONS

Peripheral vascular complications	May develop in patients sensitive to ergotamine; use caution if large doses or prolonged therapy is contemplated and advise patient to report numbness or tingling of the extremities, claudication, or other symptoms of peripheral vasoconstriction
Other special-risk patients	Use with caution in patients with bronchial asthma or obstructive uropathy
Drug dependence	Psychic and/or physical dependence and tolerance may develop following prolonged use of high doses of barbiturates
Tartrazine sensitivity	Presence of FD&C Yellow No. 5 (tartrazine) in sustained-release tablets may cause allergic-type reactions, including bronchial asthma, in susceptible individuals
Carcinogenicity	The long-term carcinogenic potential of this drug has not been investigated

ADVERSE REACTIONS

Central nervous system	Drowsiness, tingling and other paresthesias of the extremities
Ophthalmic	Blurred vision
Cardiovascular	Flushing, palpitations, tachycardia
Gastrointestinal	Dry mouth, decreased GI motility
Genitourinary	Urinary retention
Other	Decreased sweating

OVERDOSAGE

Signs and symptoms	*Phenobarbital-related effects:* drowsiness, confusion, coma, respiratory depression, hypotension, shock; *ergotamine-related effects:* vomiting, numbness, tingling, pain and cyanosis of extremities with diminished or absent peripheral pulses, hypertension or hypotension, drowsiness, stupor, coma, convulsions, shock; *belladonna alkaloid-related effects:* dry mouth and throat, blurred vision, urinary retention, CNS excitation, restlessness, confusion, delirium, convulsions, stupor, and coma leading to death
Treatment	Use gastric lavage and other measures to limit intestinal absorption. Maintain an open airway and adequate pulmonary ventilation. Institute symptomatic and supportive therapy, as needed, including control of blood pressure and body temperature. Parenteral administration of cholinesterase inhibitors may be necessary to counter anticholinergic effects. If vasospasm occurs, administer a peripheral vasodilator.

DRUG INTERACTIONS

Alcohol, tranquilizers, sedative-hypnotics, and other CNS depressants	△ CNS depression
Coumarin anticoagulants	▽ Anticoagulant effect
Amantadine	△ Atropine-like effects △ CNS depression
Antihistamines, antimuscarinics	△ Atropine-like effects △ CNS depression
Haloperidol, phenothiazines	△ Atropine-like effects △ CNS depression ▽ Antipsychotic effects
Antacids, antidiarrheal suspensions	▽ Belladonna alkaloid effects ▽ Barbiturate effects
Corticosteroids	▽ Corticosteroid effects
Digitalis, digitoxin	▽ Digitalis or digitoxin effects
Anticonvulsants	Change in pattern of epileptiform seizures
MAO inhibitors	△ Atropine-like effects △ CNS effects
Tricyclic antidepressants	△ Atropine-like effects ▽ Antidepressant effect
Dopamine	△ Risk of ischemic vasoconstriction
Doxycycline	△ Metabolism of doxycycline
Griseofulvin	△ Metabolism of griseofulvin
Beta-adrenergic blockers	△ Vasoconstriction (variable)
Quinidine	△ Metabolism of quinidine
Estrogen	△ Metabolism of estrogen ▽ Contraceptive effectiveness
Phenytoin	△ Metabolism of phenytoin (variable)

BELLERGAL-S ■ BENTYL

Sodium valproate, valproic acid	⇩ Metabolism of phenobarbital

ALTERED LABORATORY VALUES

Blood/serum values	⇧ Sulfobromophthalein (BSP) retention ⇩ Bilirubin

No clinically significant alterations in urinary values occur at therapeutic dosages

---

USE IN CHILDREN
Safety and effectiveness for use in children have not been established

USE IN PREGNANT AND NURSING WOMEN
Pregnancy Category X: contraindicated for use in pregnant women due to the potential uterotonic effects of ergot alkaloids. Contraindicated for use in nursing mothers due to inhibition of prolactin secretion.

ANTISPASMODICS

BENTYL (dicyclomine hydrochloride) Lakeside   Rx

Capsules: 10 mg **Tablets:** 20 mg **Syrup (per 5 ml):** 10 mg (1 pt) **Ampuls:** 10 mg/ml (2 ml) **Vials:** 10 mg/ml (10 ml) **Prefilled syringes:** 10 mg/ml (2 ml)

INDICATIONS
Irritable bowel syndrome (irritable colon, spastic colon, mucous colitis)

ORAL DOSAGE
Adult: 20 mg qid to start, followed during the first week, if drug is tolerated and increase is necessary, by 40 mg qid; administration should be discontinued if the initial dosage is not tolerated or if a favorable response is not obtained within 2 wk. Safety for use over periods exceeding 2 wk has not been established.

PARENTERAL DOSAGE
Adult: 20 mg IM qid for up to 2 days; switch to oral form as soon as possible

CONTRAINDICATIONS

Infants <6 mo	Intestinal atony in elderly or debilitated patients	Toxic megacolon complicating ulcerative colitis
Obstructive uropathy		
Obstructive GI tract disease (eg, achalasia, pyloroduodenal stenosis)	Unstable cardiovascular status in cases of acute hemorrhage	Myasthenia gravis
		Glaucoma
Paralytic ileus	Severe ulcerative colitis	

WARNINGS/PRECAUTIONS

Drowsiness, blurred vision	Caution patients to avoid driving or other potentially hazardous activities requiring full mental alertness if they experience sedation or blurred vision
Anticholinergic psychosis	Patients sensitive to anticholinergic drugs may experience anticholinergic psychosis. CNS signs and symptoms include confusion, disorientation, short-term memory loss, hallucinations, dysarthria, ataxia, coma, euphoria, decreased anxiety, fatigue, insomnia, agitation and mannerisms, and inappropriate affect. These signs and symptoms usually disappear within 12–24 h after discontinuing dicyclomine.
Ulcerative colitis	Large doses may suppress intestinal motility and lead to paralytic ileus or precipitate or aggravate toxic megacolon
Special-risk patients	Use with caution in patients with prostatic hypertrophy, autonomic neuropathy, hepatic or renal disease, hyperthyroidism, coronary heart disease, congestive heart failure, cardiac arrhythmias, tachycardia (atropine-like drugs may increase heart rate), hypertension, or hiatal hernia associated with reflux esophagitis
Biliary tract disease complications	Drug may be ineffective
Fever and heat stroke	May occur in high environmental temperatures as a result of decreased sweating
Incomplete intestinal obstruction	May be manifested by diarrhea, especially in ileostomy or colostomy patients; use of this drug may be harmful under these circumstances

ADVERSE REACTIONS

Gastrointestinal	Dry mouth, nausea, vomiting, constipation
Genitourinary	Urinary hesitancy and retention, impotence
Central nervous system	Headache, nervousness, drowsiness, weakness, dizziness, insomnia, confusion and/or excitement (especially in the elderly), temporary light-headedness (with parenteral use only)

BENTYL ■ DONNATAL

Cardiovascular	Palpitations, tachycardia
Ophthalmic	Blurred vision, mydriasis, cycloplegia, increased ocular tension
Dermatological	Urticaria
Other	Loss of sense of taste, allergic or idiosyncratic reactions (including anaphylaxis), bloated feeling, anaphoresis, local irritation at injection site, lactation suppression

OVERDOSAGE

Signs and symptoms	Headache, nausea, vomiting, blurred vision, mydriasis, hot, dry skin, dizziness, dry mouth, labored swallowing, CNS stimulation, curare-like effects
Treatment	Induce emesis or perform gastric lavage to empty stomach; administer activated charcoal. A barbiturate may be given orally or IM to provide sedation. If indicated, parenteral cholinergic agents (eg, bethanechol chloride) may be administered.

DRUG INTERACTIONS

No clinically significant drug interactions have been identified

ALTERED LABORATORY VALUES

No clinically significant alterations in blood/serum or urinary values occur at therapeutic dosages

USE IN CHILDREN

Safety and effectiveness for use in children have not been adequately established. Respiratory problems (breathing difficulty, shortness of breath, breathlessness, respiratory collapse, apnea, asphyxia), seizures, syncope, pulse-rate fluctuations, muscular hypotonia, and coma have been seen in infants who received dicyclomine during the first 3 mo of life; in some cases, these reactions have occurred within minutes after the syrup was ingested and have persisted for 20–30 min. A few infants 3 mo of age or younger who had been given dicyclomine syrup have died; excessively high serum dicyclomine levels have been associated with two of the deaths. No causal relationship between these reactions and dicyclomine has been established; nevertheless, use in infants under 6 mo of age is contraindicated.

USE IN PREGNANT AND NURSING WOMEN

Consult manufacturer for use in pregnant women. Dicyclomine may inhibit lactation in nursing mothers.

ANTISPASMODICS

DONNATAL (phenobarbital, hyoscyamine sulfate, atropine sulfate, and hyoscine hydrobromide) Robins Rx

Capsules: 16.2 mg phenobarbital, 0.1037 mg hyoscyamine sulfate, 0.0194 mg atropine sulfate, and 0.0065 mg hyoscine hydrobromide **Tablets:** 16.2 mg phenobarbital, 0.1037 mg hyoscyamine sulfate, 0.0194 mg atropine sulfate, and 0.0065 mg hyoscine hydrobromide **No. 2 tablets:** 32.4 mg phenobarbital and the same amount of belladonna alkaloids as regular Donnatal tablets **Tablets (sustained release):** 48.6 mg phenobarbital, 0.3111 mg hyoscyamine sulfate, 0.0582 mg atropine sulfate, and 0.0195 mg hyoscine hydrobromide (Donnatal Extentabs) **Elixir (per 5 ml):** 16.2 mg phenobarbital, 0.1037 mg hyoscyamine sulfate, 0.0194 mg atropine sulfate, and 0.0065 mg hyoscine hydrobromide[1] (5 ml, 4 fl oz, 1 pt, 1 gal) *citrus-flavored*

INDICATIONS

Duodenal ulcer[2]
Irritable bowel syndrome (irritable colon, spastic colon, mucous colitis)[2]
Acute enterocolitis[2]

ORAL DOSAGE

Adult: 1–2 Donnatal caps or tabs tid or qid, 5–10 ml (1–2 tsp) of the elixir tid or qid, 1–2 Donnatal No. 2 tabs tid, or 1 Donnatal Extentab q12h or, if indicated, q8h
Child (10 lb): 0.5 ml q4h or 0.75 ml q6h to start
Child (20 lb): 1 ml q4h or 1.5 ml q6h to start
Child (30 lb): 1.5 ml q4h or 2 ml q6h to start
Child (50 lb): 2.5 ml (1/2 tsp) q4h or 3.75 ml (3/4 tsp) q6h to start
Child (75 lb): 3.75 ml (3/4 tsp) q4h or 5 ml (1 tsp) q6h to start
Child (100 lb): 5 ml (1 tsp) q4h or 7.5 ml (1 1/2 tsp) q6h to start

DONNATAL

CONTRAINDICATIONS

Hypersensitivity to any component	Obstructive GI tract disease	Paralytic ileus
Glaucoma	Obstructive uropathy	Myasthenia gravis
Acute intermittent porphyria	Hiatal hernia associated with reflux esophagitis	Intestinal atony in elderly or debilitated patients
Unstable cardiovascular status in cases of acute hemorrhage	Severe ulcerative colitis, especially if complicated by toxic megacolon	Phenobarbital-induced restlessness or excitement

WARNINGS/PRECAUTIONS

Drowsiness, blurred vision	Caution patients not to drive or engage in potentially hazardous activities requiring full mental alertness if sedation or blurred vision occurs
Fever and heat stroke	May occur in high environmental temperatures as a result of decreased sweating
Incomplete intestinal obstruction	May be manifested by diarrhea, especially in ileostomy or colostomy patients; use of this drug may be harmful under these circumstances
Delayed gastric emptying (antral stasis)	May occur, possibly complicating management of gastric ulcer
Impaired hepatic function	Administer with caution; give small doses to start
Special-risk patients	Use with caution in patients with autonomic neuropathy, hepatic or renal disease, hyperthyroidism, coronary heart disease, congestive heart failure, cardiac arrhythmias, tachycardia, or hypertension
Elderly patients	May experience excitement, agitation, drowsiness, and other untoward effects from even small doses
Drug dependence	Psychic and/or physical dependence on barbiturates and tolerance may develop, especially in addiction-prone individuals
Abrupt withdrawal	May produce delirium or convulsions in patients habituated to barbiturates
Carcinogenicity	The long-term carcinogenic potential of this drug has not been investigated

ADVERSE REACTIONS

Gastrointestinal	Dry mouth, loss of taste sense, nausea, vomiting, constipation, bloated feeling
Genitourinary	Urinary hesitancy and retention
Ophthalmic	Blurred vision, mydriasis, cycloplegia, increased ocular tension
Cardiovascular	Tachycardia, palpitation
Central nervous system	Headache, nervousness, drowsiness, weakness, dizziness, insomnia, excitement, agitation; delirium and convulsions[3]
Hypersensitivity or idiosyncrasy	Anaphylaxis, urticaria, other dermal manifestations
Other	Impotence, suppression of lactation, musculoskeletal pain, decreased sweating

OVERDOSAGE

Signs and symptoms	Headache, nausea, vomiting, blurred vision, dilated pupils, hot and dry skin, dizziness, dryness of the mouth, difficulty in swallowing, and CNS stimulation
Treatment	Induce emesis or perform gastric lavage to empty stomach; administer activated charcoal. Treat symptomatically and institute supportive measures, as needed. If indicated, administer a parenteral cholinergic agent, eg, physostigmine salicylate or bethanechol chloride.

DRUG INTERACTIONS

Alcohol, tranquilizers, sedative-hypnotics, and other CNS depressants	△ CNS depression
Coumarin anticoagulants	▽ Anticoagulant effect
Amantadine	△ Atropine-like effects △ CNS depression
Antihistamines, antimuscarinics	△ Atropine-like effects △ CNS depression
Haloperidol, phenothiazines	△ Atropine-like effects △ CNS depression ▽ Antipsychotic effects
Antacids, antidiarrheal suspensions	▽ Belladonna alkaloid effects ▽ Barbiturate effects
Corticosteroids	▽ Corticosteroid effects
Digitalis, digitoxin	▽ Digitalis or digitoxin effects
Griseofulvin	▽ Griseofulvin effects
Tetracyclines, particularly doxycycline	▽ Antimicrobial effect
Anticonvulsants	Change in pattern of epileptiform seizures
MAO inhibitors	△ Atropine-like effects △ CNS effects

DONNATAL ■ KINESED

| Tricyclic antidepressants | △ Atropine-like effects ▽ Antidepressant effect |

ALTERED LABORATORY VALUES

| Blood/serum values | △ Sulfobromophthalein (BSP) retention ▽ Bilirubin |

No clinically significant alterations in urinary values occur at therapeutic dosages

USE IN CHILDREN
See INDICATIONS and ORAL DOSAGE

USE IN PREGNANT AND NURSING WOMEN
Pregnancy Category C: use during pregnancy only if clearly needed. It is not known what effect, if any, this drug may have on fetal development or reproductive capacity. It is also not known whether Donnatal is excreted in human milk; use with caution in nursing mothers. Donnatal No. 2 tablets should not be used in pregnant women, nursing mothers, and women of childbearing age unless the expected benefits outweigh the potential hazards.

[1] Contains 23% alcohol
[2] Possibly effective as adjunctive therapy; there is no conclusive evidence that anticholinergic/antispasmodic drugs promote duodenal ulcer healing, decrease recurrences, or prevent ulcer complications
[3] If drug is withdrawn abruptly from patients habituated to barbiturates

ANTISPASMODICS

KINESED (phenobarbital, hyoscyamine sulfate, atropine sulfate, and scopolamine hydrobromide) Stuart — Rx

Chewable tablets: 16 mg phenobarbital, 0.1 mg hyoscyamine sulfate, 0.02 mg atropine sulfate, and 0.007 mg scopolamine hydrobromide *fruit-flavored*

INDICATIONS
Duodenal ulcer[1]
Irritable bowel syndrome (irritable colon, spastic colon, mucous colitis)[1]
Acute enterocolitis[1]

ORAL DOSAGE
Adult: 1–2 tabs, chewed or swallowed with liquid, tid or qid
Child (2–12 yr): ½–1 tab, chewed or swallowed with liquid, tid or qid

CONTRAINDICATIONS

Hypersensitivity to any component	Obstructive GI tract disease	Paralytic ileus
Glaucoma	Obstructive uropathy	Myasthenia gravis
Acute intermittent porphyria	Hiatal hernia associated with reflux esophagitis	Intestinal atony in elderly or debilitated patients
Unstable cardiovascular status in cases of acute hemorrhage	Severe ulcerative colitis, especially if complicated by toxic megacolon	Phenobarbital-induced restlessness or excitement

WARNINGS/PRECAUTIONS

Drowsiness, blurred vision	Caution patients not to drive or engage in potentially hazardous activities requiring full mental alertness if sedation or blurred vision occurs
Fever and heat stroke	May occur in high environmental temperatures as a result of decreased sweating
Incomplete intestinal obstruction	May be manifested by diarrhea, especially in ileostomy or colostomy patients; use of this drug may be harmful under these circumstances
Delayed gastric emptying (antral stasis)	May occur, possibly complicating management of gastric ulcer
Impaired hepatic function	Administer with caution; give small doses to start
Special-risk patients	Use with caution in patients with autonomic neuropathy, hepatic or renal disease, hyperthyroidism, coronary heart disease, congestive heart failure, cardiac arrhythmias, tachycardia, or hypertension
Elderly patients	May experience excitement, agitation, drowsiness, and other untoward effects from even small doses
Drug dependence	Psychic and/or physical dependence on barbiturates and tolerance may develop, especially in addiction-prone individuals
Abrupt withdrawal	May produce delirium or convulsions in patients habituated to barbiturates
Carcinogenicity	No long-term studies have been done in animals to evaluate the carcinogenic potential of this drug

ADVERSE REACTIONS

| Gastrointestinal | Dry mouth, loss of taste sense, nausea, vomiting, constipation, bloated feeling |

KINESED ■ LEVSIN

Genitourinary	Urinary hesitancy and retention
Ophthalmic	Blurred vision, mydriasis, cycloplegia, increased ocular tension
Cardiovascular	Tachycardia, palpitation
Central nervous system	Headache, nervousness, drowsiness, weakness, dizziness, insomnia, excitement, agitation; delirium and convulsions[2]
Hypersensitivity or idiosyncrasy	Anaphylaxis, urticaria, other dermal manifestations
Other	Impotence, suppression of lactation, decreased sweating

OVERDOSAGE

Signs and symptoms	*Phenobarbital-related effects:* drowsiness, confusion, coma, respiratory depression, hypotension, shock; *belladonna alkaloid-related effects:* dry mouth and throat, blurred vision, urinary retention, CNS excitation, restlessness, confusion, delirium, convulsions, stupor, and coma, leading to death
Treatment	Induce emesis or perform gastric lavage to empty stomach; administer activated charcoal. Maintain adequate pulmonary ventilation, correct hypotension, and control convulsions, if present. Force diuresis, alkalinize urine, and use catheterization to prevent urinary retention. Maintain body temperature. Hemodialysis or peritoneal dialysis may be useful.

DRUG INTERACTIONS

Alcohol, tranquilizers, sedative-hypnotics, and other CNS depressants	△ CNS depression
Coumarin anticoagulants	▽ Anticoagulant effect
Amantadine	△ Atropine-like effects △ CNS depression
Antihistamines, antimuscarinics	△ Atropine-like effects △ CNS depression
Haloperidol, phenothiazines	△ Atropine-like effects △ CNS depression ▽ Antipsychotic effects
Antacids, antidiarrheal suspensions	▽ Belladonna alkaloid effects ▽ Barbiturate effects
Corticosteroids	▽ Corticosteroid effects
Digitalis, digitoxin	▽ Digitalis or digitoxin effects
Griseofulvin	▽ Griseofulvin effects
Tetracyclines, particularly doxycycline	▽ Antimicrobial effect
Anticonvulsants	Change in pattern of epileptiform seizures
MAO inhibitors	△ Atropine-like effects △ CNS effects
Tricyclic antidepressants	△ Atropine-like effects ▽ Antidepressant effect

ALTERED LABORATORY VALUES

Blood/serum values	△ Sulfobromophthalein (BSP) retention ▽ Bilirubin

No clinically significant alterations in urinary values occur at therapeutic dosages

---

USE IN CHILDREN

See INDICATIONS and ORAL DOSAGE

USE IN PREGNANT AND NURSING WOMEN

Pregnancy Category C: use during pregnancy only if clearly needed. It is not known what effect, if any, this drug may have on fetal development or reproductive capacity. Because belladonna alkaloids are excreted in human milk, use with caution in nursing mothers.

---

[1] Possibly effective as adjunctive therapy; there is no conclusive evidence that anticholinergic/antispasmodic drugs promote duodenal ulcer healing, decrease recurrences, or prevent ulcer complications
[2] If drug is withdrawn abruptly from patients habituated to barbiturates

---

ANTISPASMODICS

LEVSIN (hyoscyamine sulfate) Kremers-Urban   Rx
Tablets: 0.125 mg   **Elixir (per 5 ml):** 0.125 mg[1] (1 pt) *orange flavored*   **Drops (per ml):** 0.125 mg[2] (15 ml) *orange flavored*

LEVSINEX (hyoscyamine sulfate) Kremers-Urban   Rx
Capsules (sustained release): 0.375 mg

INDICATIONS

Pylorospasm
Infant colic
Peptic ulcer and diverticulitis (adjunctive therapy)
Disorders of intestinal dysfunction, such as irritable bowel syndrome and mild dysentery (adjunctive therapy)
Cystitis (adjunctive therapy)
Biliary and renal colic (with narcotic analgesics)
Acute rhinitis
Parkinsonism

ORAL DOSAGE

Adult: 1–2 tabs or 5–10 ml (1–2 tsp) of the elixir tid or qid, 1–2 ml of the drops q4h, or 1 cap q12h; if necessary, 1 cap may be given q8h or 2 caps may be administered q12h
Infant (5 lb): 3 drops q4h
Infant (7.5 lb): 4 drops q4h
Infant (10 lb): 6 drops or 0.5–0.75 ml of the elixir q4h
Infant (15 lb): 7 drops q4h
Infant (20 lb): 9 drops or 1.25–2 ml of the elixir q4h
Infant (30 lb): 2.5 ml (1/2 tsp) of the elixir q4h
Child (50 lb): 3.75–5 ml (3/4–1 tsp) of the elixir q4h
Child (75-80 lb): 5–7.5 ml (1–1 1/2 tsp) of the elixir q4h
Child (1-10 yr): 0.5–1 ml of the drops q4h

LEVSIN Injection (hyoscyamine sulfate) Kremers-Urban   Rx

Ampuls: 0.5 mg/ml (1 ml)   **Vials:** 0.5 mg/ml (10 ml)

INDICATIONS[3]

Peptic ulcer (adjunctive therapy)	**PARENTERAL DOSAGE** **Adult:** 0.25–0.5 mg SC, IM, or IV tid or qid at 4-h intervals; for some patients, administration once or twice daily may be sufficient
Hypotonic duodenography	**Adult:** 0.25–0.5 mg SC, IM, or IV, given 5–10 min before the procedure
Preanesthetic medication	**Adult:** 5 µg/kg SC, IM, or IV, given either 30–60 min before induction of anesthesia or when other preanesthetic drugs are given
Prevention of bradycardia and excessive secretions during general anesthesia	**Adult:** 1.25 mg IV, as needed
Prevention of bradycardia and excessive secretions during reversal of neuromuscular blockade	**Adult:** 0.2 mg of hyoscyamine, IV, per mg of neostigmine (or the equivalent amount of physostigmine or pyridostigmine)

CONTRAINDICATIONS

Glaucoma	Obstructive GI tract disease	Myasthenia gravis
Obstructive uropathy	Paralytic ileus	Ulcerative colitis associated with toxic megacolon
Unstable cardiovascular status in cases of acute hemorrhage	Intestinal atony in elderly or debilitated patients	Severe ulcerative colitis

ADMINISTRATION/DOSAGE ADJUSTMENTS

Administration of tablets	The tablets can either be swallowed or taken sublingually

WARNINGS/PRECAUTIONS

Fever and heat stroke	At high temperatures, fever and heat stroke may occur as a result of decreased sweating
Drowsiness, blurred vision	Caution patients experiencing drowsiness or blurred vision during therapy not to drive or engage in other potentially hazardous activities requiring mental alertness
Incomplete-intestinal obstruction	Diarrhea may be an early sign of incomplete intestinal obstruction, especially in ileostomy or colostomy patients; use of this drug in a patient with incomplete obstruction is inappropriate and possibly harmful
Special-risk patients	Use with caution in patients with hiatal hernia associated with reflux esophagitis and in those with autonomic neuropathy, hyperthyroidism, coronary artery disease, congestive heart failure, cardiac arrhythmias, or hypertension; investigate any tachycardia before using hyoscyamine since it may increase the heart rate. Exercise caution when giving injectable form to patients with asthma.

ADVERSE REACTIONS

Central nervous system	Headache, nervousness, drowsiness, weakness
Ophthalmic	Blurred vision, mydriasis, cycloplegia, increased intraocular tension
Cardiovascular	Tachycardia, palpitations
Genitourinary	Urinary hesitancy and retention
Dermatological	Urticaria, other dermatological reactions
Hypersensitivity	Allergic reactions, drug idiosyncracy
Other	Dry mouth, suppression of lactation, decreased sweating

OVERDOSAGE

Signs and symptoms	Headache, nausea, vomiting, blurred vision, mydriasis, hot and dry skin, dizziness, dry mouth, and difficulty in swallowing
Treatment	Perform gastric lavage immediately; administer 0.5–2 mg of IV physostigmine, as often as needed, up to a total of 5 mg. Treat fever with alcohol sponging or icepacks. Treat prominent excitement with 2% sodium thiopental solution, given by slow IV infusion, or with 100–200 ml of 2% chloral hydrate solution, given by rectal infusion. If paralysis of the respiratory muscles occurs, institute artificial respiration.

DRUG INTERACTIONS

Cyclopropane	Ventricular arrhythmias (with IV hyoscyamine); exercise caution during anesthesia and administer hyoscyamine in small fractional doses
Phenothiazines	△ Pharmacologic effect of hyoscyamine ▽ Antipsychotic effect of phenothiazine
Haloperidol	▽ Antipsychotic effect of haloperidol
Atenolol	△ Bioavailability of atenolol
Digoxin	△ Serum level of oral digoxin

LEVSIN ■ LIBRAX

Levodopa	▽ Serum levodopa level
Cimetidine	▽ Serum cimetidine level
Thiazide diuretics	△ Bioavailability of thiazide-type diuretic

ALTERED LABORATORY VALUES

No clinically significant alterations in blood/serum or urinary values occur at therapeutic dosages

USE IN CHILDREN	USE IN PREGNANT AND NURSING WOMEN
See INDICATIONS and ORAL DOSAGE	No teratogenic effects have been demonstrated in mice, rats, and dogs; however, IV administration of hyoscyamine during pregnancy may produce tachycardia in the fetus. Traces of hyoscyamine appear in breast milk. The drug may also inhibit lactation.

[1] Contains 20% alcohol
[2] Contains 5% alcohol
[3] Levsin injection may also be used to reduce pain and hypersecretion associated with pancreatitis, reverse partial heart block associated with vagal activity (in certain cases), treat anticholinesterase poisoning, relieve symptoms of biliary or renal colic (when used with narcotic analgesics), and facilitate radiography of the kidneys

---

ANTISPASMODICS

LIBRAX (chlordiazepoxide hydrochloride and clidinium bromide) Roche Rx

Capsules: 5 mg chlordiazepoxide hydrochloride and 2.5 mg clidinium bromide

INDICATIONS	ORAL DOSAGE
Peptic ulcer (adjunctive therapy)[1] **Irritable bowel syndrome** (irritable colon, spastic colon, mucous colitis)[1] **Acute enterocolitis**[1]	**Adult:** 1–2 caps tid or qid, before meals and at bedtime

CONTRAINDICATIONS

Glaucoma	Bladder-neck obstruction	Hypersensitivity to chlordiazepoxide or clidinium
Prostatic hypertrophy		

ADMINISTRATION/DOSAGE ADJUSTMENTS

Discontinuation of therapy	Withdraw gradually following prolonged high dosages; sudden withdrawal may produce anorexia, anxiety, insomnia, vomiting, ataxia, tremors, muscle twitching, confusion, and (rarely) convulsive seizures

WARNINGS/PRECAUTIONS

Drowsiness, confusion	Caution patients against engaging in potentially hazardous activities requiring full mental alertness and that alcohol and other CNS depressants may cause further CNS depression
Paradoxical reactions	Excitement, stimulation, or acute rage may occur in psychiatric patients
Patients with impaired renal or hepatic function	Administer with caution and observe for signs of excessive drug accumulation
Drug dependence	Psychic and/or physical dependence and tolerance may develop, especially in addiction-prone individuals

ADVERSE REACTIONS

Central nervous system and neuromuscular	Drowsiness, confusion, EEG changes, extrapyramidal symptoms
Gastrointestinal	Nausea, constipation, dry mouth
Cardiovascular	Ataxia, edema, syncope
Ophthalmic	Blurred vision
Dermatological	Skin eruptions
Endocrinological	Minor menstrual irregularities, lactation suppression, increased or decreased libido
Hematological	Blood dyscrasias, including agranulocytosis
Hepatic	Jaundice, functional impairment
Genitourinary	Urinary hesitancy

LIBRAX ■ PATHIBAMATE

OVERDOSAGE

Signs and symptoms	*Toxic effects primarily attributable to clidinium bromide:* dry mouth, blurred vision, urinary hesitancy, constipation; *chlordiazepoxide-related effects:* somnolence, confusion, coma, diminished reflexes, cardiac and respiratory depression
Treatment	Employ suppportive measures, along with gastric lavage. Administer 0.5–2.0 mg physostigmine at a rate of not more than 1 mg/min. For recurring arrhythmias, convulsions, or deep coma, repeat in 1- to 4-mg doses. Administer IV fluids and maintain adequate airway. For hypotension, use norepinephrine or metaraminol. Dialysis is of limited value. Do not use barbiturates to combat excitation.

DRUG INTERACTIONS

Alcohol, tranquilizers, sedative-hypnotics, and other CNS depressants	⌂ CNS depression
Tricyclic antidepressants	⌂ Antidepressant effect

ALTERED LABORATORY VALUES

No clinically significant alterations in blood/serum or urinary values occur at therapeutic dosages

---

USE IN CHILDREN
Consult manufacturer

USE IN PREGNANT AND NURSING WOMEN
Use of antianxiety agents during early pregnancy should almost always be avoided. An increased risk of congenital malformations during the first trimester has been associated with minor tranquilizers, including chlordiazepoxide. Clidinium component may inhibit lactation; patient should stop nursing if drug is prescribed.

---

[1] Possibly effective

ANTISPASMODICS

PATHIBAMATE (tridihexethyl chloride and meprobamate) Lederle   Rx

Tablets: 25 mg tridihexethyl chloride and 200 mg meprobamate (Pathibamate-200); 25 mg tridihexethyl chloride and 400 mg meprobamate (Pathibamate-400)

INDICATIONS

Peptic ulcer (adjunctive therapy)[1]
Irritable bowel syndrome (irritable colon, spastic colon, mucous colitis, functional GI disturbances)[1]

ORAL DOSAGE

Adult: 1 Pathibamate-400 tab tid, with meals, plus 2 Pathibamate-400 tabs at bedtime; for greater anticholinergic effect, 2 Pathibamate-200 tabs tid, with meals, plus 2 Pathibamate-200 tabs at bedtime

CONTRAINDICATIONS

Age <12 yr	Acute intermittent porphyria	Allergic or idiosyncratic reactions to meprobamate, tridihexethyl chloride, or related compounds
Obstructive uropathy (eg, urinary bladder neck obstructions due to prostatic hypertrophy)	Unstable cardiovascular status in cases of acute hemorrhage	
	Myasthenia gravis	Severe ulcerative colitis
Obstructive disease of the GI tract	Intestinal atony in elderly or debilitated patients	Toxic megacolon complicating ulcerative colitis
Glaucoma		

ADMINISTRATION/DOSAGE ADJUSTMENTS

Discontinuation of therapy	Withdraw drug gradually over a 1- to 2-wk period following prolonged high dosages; sudden withdrawal may produce anorexia, anxiety, insomnia, vomiting, ataxia, tremors, muscle twitching, confusion, and (rarely) convulsive seizures; alternatively, substitute a short-acting barbiturate, then gradually withdraw medication

WARNINGS/PRECAUTIONS

Mental and/or physical impairment	Caution patients against driving or engaging in potentially hazardous activities requiring full mental alertness, particularly if they experience drowsiness or blurred vision while taking this drug
Oversedation	Use lowest effective dose in elderly or debilitated patients
Potentially suicidal patients	Should not have access to large quantities of meprobamate-containing compounds; prescribe smallest amount feasible at any one time
Patients with impaired renal or hepatic function	Administer with caution and observe for signs of excessive drug accumulation
Seizures	May be precipitated in epileptic patients

PATHIBAMATE

Toxic megacolon	May be precipitated or aggravated in patients with ulcerative colitis
Heat and fever stroke	May occur in high environmental temperatures as a result of decreased sweating
Incomplete intestinal obstruction	May be manifested by diarrhea, especially in ileostomy or colostomy patients; use of this drug may be harmful under these circumstances
Special-risk patients	Use with caution in patients with autonomic neuropathy, hepatic or renal disease, early evidence of ileus (as in peritonitis), hyperthyroidism, coronary heart disease, congestive heart failure, cardiac arrhythmias, hypertension, nonobstructing prostatic hypertrophy, or hiatal hernia associated with reflux esophagitis
Gastric ulcer	Gastric emptying time may be delayed, complicating treatment by producing antral stasis
Biliary tract disease complications	Drug may be ineffective
Drug dependence	Psychic and/or physical dependence and tolerance may develop, especially in addiction-prone individuals
Curare-like action	May occur with overdosage

ADVERSE REACTIONS

Cardiovascular	Tachycardia, palpitations, various forms of arrhythmia, transient ECG changes, syncope, hypotensive crises (one fatal case)
Central nervous system	Headache, nervousness, drowsiness, weakness, dizziness, insomnia, some degree of mental confusion and/or excitement (especially in elderly patients), slurred speech, vertigo, paresthesias, euphoria, overstimulation, paradoxical excitement, fast EEG activity
Gastrointestinal	Dry mouth, nausea, vomiting, constipation, diarrhea
Ophthalmic	Blurred vision, mydriasis, cycloplegia, increased ocular tension, impairment of visual accommodation
Endocrinological	Suppression of lactation
Hematological	Agranulocytosis, aplastic anemia, thrombocytopenic purpura (rare)
Genitourinary	Urinary hesitancy and retention
Allergic or idiosyncratic	*Mild:* itchy, urticarial or erythematous maculopapular rash (generalized or confined to groin), leukopenia, acute nonthrombocytopenic purpura, petechiae, ecchymoses, eosinophilia, peripheral edema, adenopathy, fever, fixed drug eruption with cross-reaction to carisoprodol and cross-sensitivity between meprobamate/mebutamate and meprobamate/carbromal; *severe (rare):* hyperpyrexia, chills, angioneurotic edema, bronchospasm, oliguria, anuria, anaphylaxis, erythema multiforme, exfoliative dermatitis, stomatitis, proctitis, Stevens-Johnson syndrome, bullous dermatitis
Other	Loss of sense of taste, impotence, bloated feeling, exacerbation of porphyric symptoms, decreased sweating

OVERDOSAGE

Signs and symptoms	*Toxic effects primarily attributable to tridihexethyl chloride:* dry mouth, labored swallowing, thirst, blurred vision, photophobia, flushed, hot, dry skin, rash, hyperthermia, palpitations, tachycardia, weak pulse, hypertension, urinary urgency with difficult micturition, abdominal distention, restlessness, confusion, delirium, and other signs of acute organic psychoses; *meprobamate-related effects:* drowsiness, lethargy, stupor, ataxia, coma, shock, vasomotor and respiratory collapse, leading to death; meprobamate blood levels of 3–10 mg/dl usually correspond to mild to moderate symptoms (stupor or light coma) and 10–20 mg/dl with deeper coma, requiring more intensive treatment
Treatment	Administer supportive measures, along with gastric lavage, followed by activated charcoal. For compromised respiration or blood pressure, cautiously administer respiratory assistance, CNS stimulants, and pressor agents, as indicated. Diuresis, osmotic (mannitol) diuresis, peritoneal dialysis, or hemodialysis may be successful. Monitor urinary output to avoid overhydration. Incomplete gastric emptying and delayed absorption can lead to relapse and death.

DRUG INTERACTIONS

Alcohol, tranquilizers, sedative-hypnotics, and other CNS depressants	⇧ CNS depression
Digoxin	⇧ Serum digoxin level
MAO inhibitors, tricyclic antidepressants	⇧ CNS depression ⇧ Antidepressant effect

ALTERED LABORATORY VALUES

Urinary values	⇧ 17-Ketosteroids, 17-ketogenic steroids, and 17-hydroxycorticosteroids (methodologic interference)

PATHIBAMATE ■ PRO-BANTHĪNE

No clinically significant alterations in blood/serum values occur at therapeutic dosages

USE IN CHILDREN
Contraindicated for use in children under 12 yr of age

USE IN PREGNANT AND NURSING WOMEN
Use of antianxiety agents during early pregnancy should almost always be avoided. An increased risk of congenital malformations during the first trimester has been associated with minor tranquilizers, including meprobamate. Meprobamate crosses the placental barrier and appears in umbilical cord blood at or near maternal plasma levels. Meprobamate also appears in breast milk at concentrations 2–4 times that of maternal plasma; patient probably should stop nursing if drug is prescribed.

[1] Possibly effective

ANTISPASMODICS

PRO-BANTHĪNE (propantheline bromide) Searle   Rx
Tablets: 7.5, 15 mg

INDICATIONS
Peptic ulcer (adjunctive therapy)

ORAL DOSAGE
Adult: 15 mg 1/2 h before meals plus 30 mg at bedtime (75 mg/day) to start

CONTRAINDICATIONS
Glaucoma	Intestinal atony (in elderly or debilitated patients)	Unstable cardiovascular status in cases of acute hemorrhage
Obstructive uropathy (eg, bladder-neck obstruction due to prostatic hypertrophy)	Severe ulcerative colitis	Toxic megacolon exacerbating ulcerative colitis
Obstructive GI disease (eg, achalasia, pyloroduodenal stenosis, paralytic ileus)	Myasthenia gravis	

ADMINISTRATION/DOSAGE ADJUSTMENTS
Mild cases, elderly or small patients	Reduce dosage to 7.5 mg tid

WARNINGS/PRECAUTIONS
Drowsiness, blurred vision	Caution patients about driving or engaging in potentially hazardous activities requiring full mental alertness
Ulcerative colitis	Large doses may suppress intestinal motility and lead to paralytic ileus or precipitate or aggravate toxic megacolon
Special-risk patients	Use with caution in the elderly and in those with autonomic neuropathy, hepatic or renal disease, hyperthyroidism, coronary heart disease, congestive heart failure, cardiac tachyarrhythmias, hypertension, or hiatal hernia associated with reflux esophagitis
Fever and heat stroke	May occur in high environmental temperatures as a result of decreased sweating
Incomplete intestinal obstruction	May be manifested by diarrhea, especially in ileostomy or colostomy patients; therapy may be harmful under these circumstances
Carcinogenicity, mutagenicity, effect on fertility	No long-term studies have been done to evaluate the carcinogenic or mutagenic potential of this drug or its effect on fertility

ADVERSE REACTIONS
Gastrointestinal	Dry mouth, nausea, vomiting, constipation, bloated feeling
Genitourinary	Urinary hesitancy and retention, impotence
Central nervous system	Headache, nervousness, confusion, drowsiness, weakness, dizziness, insomnia
Cardiovascular	Palpitations, tachycardia
Ophthalmic	Blurred vision, mydriasis, cycloplegia, increased ocular tension
Other	Dry mouth, ageusia, anaphoresis, suppression of lactation, allergic or idiosyncratic reactions (anaphylaxis; urticaria and other dermatological reactions)

OVERDOSAGE
Signs and symptoms	Intensification of usual side effects, CNS disturbances (restlessness, excitement, psychotic behavior), circulatory changes (flushing, decrease in blood pressure, circulatory failure), respiratory failure, curare-like effects, and coma

PRO-BANTHĪNE

Treatment	Induce emesis or perform gastric lavage immediately, administer 0.5–2 mg of physostigmine IV as often as needed (up to a total of 5 mg), and monitor vital signs. For excessive excitement, slowly inject 2% thiopental sodium IV, or, alternatively, give diazepam (5–10 mg IV or 10 mg IM). If respiratory paralysis occurs, institute mechanical respiration. To treat fever, apply a cooling blanket or alcohol.

DRUG INTERACTIONS

Other oral medications	Delayed absorption of other oral medications
Other anticholinergic drugs (including belladonna alkaloids), narcotic analgesics (eg, meperidine), psychotropic drugs (eg, tricyclic antidepressants), antihistamines, phenothiazines, type 1 antiarrhythmic drugs	⇧ Anticholinergic effects
Corticosteroids	⇧ Intraocular pressure
Digoxin	⇧ Serum digoxin level (with slow-dissolving tablets); use liquid or rapid-dissolving preparation

ALTERED LABORATORY VALUES

No clinically significant alterations in blood/serum or urinary values occur at therapeutic dosages

---

USE IN CHILDREN

Safety and effectiveness for use in children have not been established

USE IN PREGNANT AND NURSING WOMEN

Pregnancy Category C: no reproduction studies have been done to determine whether propantheline can cause harm to the fetus or affect reproductive capacity; use during pregnancy only if clearly needed. Propantheline can suppress lactation; it is not known whether this drug is excreted in human milk. Use with caution in nursing mothers.

Chapter 30

Bronchodilators/Antiasthmatic Agents

Inhalant Bronchodilators/Antiasthmatic Agents — 1156

AEROBID (Forest) — 1156
Flunisolide *Rx*

ALUPENT Inhalant Solution (Boehringer Ingelheim) — 1157
Metaproterenol sulfate *Rx*

ALUPENT Metered Dose Inhaler (Boehringer Ingelheim) — 1158
Metaproterenol sulfate *Rx*

ARM-A-MED Isoetharine Hydrochloride (Armour) — 1158
Isoetharine hydrochloride *Rx*

AZMACORT (Rorer) — 1159
Triamcinolone acetonide *Rx*

BELCOVENT (Glaxo) — 1161
Beclomethasone dipropionate *Rx*

BRETHAIRE (Geigy) — 1162
Terbutaline sulfate *Rx*

BRONKOMETER (Winthrop-Breon) — 1163
Isoetharine mesylate *Rx*

BRONKOSOL (Winthrop-Breon) — 1163
Isoetharine hydrochloride *Rx*

DUO-MEDIHALER (Riker) — 1164
Isoproterenol hydrochloride and phenylephrine bitartrate *Rx*

INTAL Capsules (Fisons) — 1165
Cromolyn sodium *Rx*

INTAL Inhaler (Fisons) — 1166
Cromolyn sodium *Rx*

INTAL Nebulizer Solution (Fisons) — 1165
Cromolyn sodium *Rx*

ISUPREL MISTOMETER (Winthrop-Breon) — 1167
Isoproterenol hydrochloride *Rx*

MEDIHALER-ISO (Riker) — 1168
Isoproterenol sulfate *Rx*

METAPREL Inhalant Solution (Sandoz Pharmaceuticals) — 1169
Metaproterenol sulfate *Rx*

METAPREL Metered Dose Inhaler (Sandoz Pharmaceuticals) — 1169
Metaproterenol sulfate *Rx*

MUCOMYST (Bristol) — 1170
Acetylcysteine *Rx*

PROVENTIL Inhaler (Schering) — 1172
Albuterol *Rx*

RESPIHALER DECADRON Phosphate (Merck Sharp & Dohme) — 1173
Dexamethasone sodium phosphate *Rx*

TORNALATE (Winthrop-Breon) — 1175
Bitolterol mesylate *Rx*

VANCERIL Inhaler (Schering) — 1176
Beclomethasone dipropionate *Rx*

VENTOLIN Inhaler (Glaxo) — 1177
Albuterol *Rx*

Systemic Bronchodilators/Antiasthmatic Agents — 1178

ADRENALIN (Parke-Davis) — 1178
Epinephrine hydrochloride *Rx*

ALUPENT (Boehringer Ingelheim) — 1180
Metaproterenol sulfate *Rx*

AMINOPHYLLIN (Searle) — 1181
Aminophylline *Rx*

BRETHINE (Geigy) — 1182
Terbutaline sulfate *Rx*

BRICANYL (Lakeside) — 1183
Terbutaline sulfate *Rx*

BRONDECON (Parke-Davis) — 1184
Oxtriphylline and guaifenesin *Rx*

BRONKODYL (Winthrop-Breon) — 1185
Theophylline, anhydrous *Rx*

CHOLEDYL (Parke-Davis) — 1188
Oxtriphylline *Rx*

CHOLEDYL SA (Parke-Davis) — 1188
Oxtriphylline *Rx*

CONSTANT-T (Geigy) — 1190
Theophylline, anhydrous *Rx*

DURAPHYL (Forest) — 1192
Theophylline, anhydrous *Rx*

ELIXOPHYLLIN (Forest) — 1194
Theophylline, anhydrous *Rx*

ELIXOPHYLLIN SR (Forest) — 1194
Theophylline, anhydrous *Rx*

LUFYLLIN (Wallace) — 1196
Dyphylline *Rx*

MARAX (Roerig) — 1197
Ephedrine sulfate, theophylline, and hydroxyzine hydrochloride *Rx*

MARAX-DF (Roerig) — 1197
Ephedrine sulfate, theophylline, and hydroxyzine hydrochloride *Rx*

METAPREL (Sandoz Pharmaceuticals) — 1199
Metaproterenol sulfate *Rx*

PROVENTIL (Schering) — 1199
Albuterol sulfate *Rx*

PROVENTIL Syrup (Schering) — 1200
Albuterol sulfate *Rx*

QUADRINAL (Knoll) — 1201
Ephedrine hydrochloride, phenobarbital, theophylline calcium salicylate, and potassium iodide *Rx*

QUIBRON and QUIBRON-300 (Bristol) — 1204
Theophylline and guaifenesin *Rx*

QUIBRON-T (Bristol) — 1204
Theophylline, anhydrous *Rx*

QUIBRON-T/SR (Bristol) Theophylline, anhydrous *Rx*	1204
RESPBID (Boehringer Ingelheim) Theophylline, anhydrous *Rx*	1206
SLO-BID (Rorer) Theophylline, anhydrous *Rx*	1208
SLO-PHYLLIN (Rorer) Theophylline, anhydrous *Rx*	1208
SOMOPHYLLIN (Fisons) Aminophylline, anhydrous *Rx*	1211
SOMOPHYLLIN Rectal Solution (Fisons) Aminophylline, anhydrous *Rx*	1211
SOMOPHYLLIN-CRT (Fisons) Theophylline, anhydrous *Rx*	1212
SOMOPHYLLIN-DF (Fisons) Aminophylline, anhydrous *Rx*	1211
SOMOPHYLLIN-T (Fisons) Theophylline, anhydrous *Rx*	1211
TEDRAL (Warner-Lambert) Theophylline, ephedrine hydrochloride, and phenobarbital *OTC*	1214
TEDRAL SA (Parke-Davis) Theophylline, ephedrine hydrochloride, and phenobarbital *Rx*	1214
THEO-24 (Searle) Theophylline, anhydrous *Rx*	1215
THEOBID (Glaxo) Theophylline, anhydrous *Rx*	1218
THEOBID Jr. (Glaxo) Theophylline, anhydrous *Rx*	1218
THEO-DUR (Key) Theophylline, anhydrous *Rx*	1220
THEO-DUR Sprinkle (Key) Theophylline, anhydrous *Rx*	1220
THEOLAIR (Riker) Theophylline, anhydrous *Rx*	1222
THEOLAIR-SR (Riker) Theophylline, anhydrous *Rx*	1222
THEOPHYL-SR (McNeil Pharmaceutical) Theophylline, anhydrous *Rx*	1225
UNIPHYL (Purdue Frederick) Theophylline, anhydrous *Rx*	1227
VENTOLIN (Glaxo) Albuterol sulfate *Rx*	1229
VENTOLIN Syrup (Glaxo) Albuterol sulfate *Rx*	1229

Other Inhalant Bronchodilators/ Antiasthmatic Agents 1154

AEROLONE (Lilly) Isoproterenol hydrochloride *Rx*	1154
BRONKAID Mist (Winthrop-Breon) Epinephrine *OTC*	1154
MEDIHALER-EPI (Riker) Epinephrine bitartrate *OTC*	1154
PRIMATENE Mist (Whitehall) Epinephrine *OTC*	1154
PRIMATENE Mist Suspension (Whitehall) Epinephrine bitartrate *OTC*	1154

Other Systemic Bronchodilators/ Antiasthmatic Agents 1154

AMINOPHYLLIN Injection (Searle) Aminophylline *Rx*	1154
ASBRON G (Sandoz Pharmaceuticals) Theophylline sodium glycinate and guaifenesin *Rx*	1154
BRONKEPHRINE (Winthrop-Breon) Ethylnorepinephrine hydrochloride *Rx*	1154
BRONKOLIXIR (Winthrop-Breon) Ephedrine sulfate, guaifenesin, theophylline, and phenobarbital *Rx*	1154
DILOR-G (Savage) Dyphylline and guaifenesin *Rx*	1154
ISUPREL (Winthrop-Breon) Isoproterenol hydrochloride *Rx*	1154
LUFYLLIN-EPG (Wallace) Dyphylline, guaifenesin, ephedrine hydrochloride, and phenobarbital *Rx*	1155
LUFYLLIN-GG (Wallace) Dyphylline and guaifenesin *Rx*	1155
MUDRANE-2 (Poythress) Potassium iodide and aminophylline *Rx*	1155
MUDRANE GG (Poythress) Theophylline or aminophylline, ephedrine hydrochloride, phenobarbital, and guaifenesin *Rx*	1155
MUDRANE GG-2 (Poythress) Aminophylline and guaifenesin *Rx*	1155
PRIMATENE (Whitehall) Theophylline, ephedrine hydrochloride, and either phenobarbital (P formula) or pyrilamine maleate (M formula[2]) *OTC*	1155
QUIBRON PLUS (Mead Johnson) Theophylline, guaifenesin, ephedrine hydrochloride, and butabarbital *Rx*	1155
SLO-PHYLLIN GG (Rorer) Theophylline and guaifenesin *Rx*	1155
SUS-PHRINE (Berlex) Epinephrine *Rx*	1155
SYNOPHYLATE (Central) Theophylline sodium glycinate *Rx*	1155
THEO-ORGANIDIN (Wallace) Theophylline and iodinated glycerol *Rx*	1155

continued

COMPENDIUM OF DRUG THERAPY

OTHER INHALANT BRONCHODILATORS/ANTIASTHMATIC AGENTS

DRUG	HOW SUPPLIED	USUAL DOSAGE[1]
AEROLONE (Lilly) Isoproterenol hydrochloride *Rx*	Solution for aerosol nebulization: 2.5 mg/ml (1 fl oz)	Adult: 6–12 inhalations per course, repeated if necessary at 15-min intervals up to 3 times, not to exceed 8 courses/24 h
BRONKAID Mist (Winthrop-Breon) Epinephrine *OTC*	Metered-dose inhaler: 0.25 mg/inhalation (16.7, 25 g)	Adult and child (> 6 yr): 1 inhalation to start, repeated once after 1 min, if necessary; treatment may be repeated not less than 4 h later
MEDIHALER-EPI (Riker) Epinephrine bitartrate *OTC*	Metered-dose inhaler: 0.3 mg/inhalation (15 ml)	Adult: 1 inhalation to start, repeated after at least 1 min, if necessary
PRIMATENE Mist (Whitehall) Epinephrine *OTC*	Metered-dose inhaler: 0.2 mg/inhalation (15 ml)	Adult: 1 inhalation to start, repeated once after 1 min, if necessary; repeat after not less than 4 h, if needed
PRIMATENE Mist Suspension (Whitehall) Epinephrine bitartrate *OTC*	Metered-dose inhaler: 0.16 mg epinephrine/inhalation (10 ml)	Adult: 1 inhalation to start, repeated once after 1 min, if necessary; repeat after not less than 4 h, if needed

[1] Where pediatric dosages are not given, consult manufacturer

OTHER SYSTEMIC BRONCHODILATORS/ANTIASTHMATIC AGENTS

DRUG	HOW SUPPLIED	USUAL DOSAGE[1]
AMINOPHYLLIN Injection (Searle) Aminophylline *Rx*	Ampuls: 25 mg/ml (10, 20 ml)	Adult nonsmoker: 6 mg/kg IV (preferably by infusion) to start, followed by 0.7 mg/kg/h for the next 12 h and then 0.5 mg/kg/h Infant and child (6 mo to 9 yr): 6 mg/kg IV (preferably by infusion) to start, followed by 1.2 mg/kg/h for the next 12 h and then 1.0 mg/kg/h Child (9–16 yr) and young adult smoker: 6 mg/kg IV (preferably by infusion) to start, followed by 1.0 mg/kg/h for the next 12 h and then 0.8 mg/kg/h
ASBRON G (Sandoz Pharmaceuticals) Theophylline sodium glycinate and guaifenesin *Rx*	Tablets: 300 mg theophylline sodium glycinate and 100 mg guaifenesin Elixir (per 15 ml): 300 mg theophylline sodium glycinate and 100 mg guaifenesin (1 pt)	Adult: 1–2 tabs or 15–30 ml (1–2 tbsp) tid or qid Child (1–3 yr): 2.5–5 ml (½–1 tsp) tid or qid Child (3–6 yr): 5–7.5 ml (1–1½ tsp) tid or qid Child (6–12 yr): 10–15 ml (2–3 tsp) tid or qid
BRONKEPHRINE (Winthrop-Breon) Ethylnorepinephrine hydrochloride *Rx*	Ampuls: 2 mg/ml (1 ml)	Adult: 0.5–1 ml SC or IM, depending upon the severity of the attack Child: 0.1–0.5 ml SC or IM; adjust dosage according to age and weight
BRONKOLIXIR (Winthrop-Breon) Ephedrine sulfate, guaifenesin, theophylline, and phenobarbital *Rx*	Elixir (per 5 ml): 12 mg ephedrine sulfate, 50 mg guaifenesin, 15 mg theophylline, and 4 mg phenobarbital (1 pt)	Adult: 10 ml (2 tsp) q3–4h for up to 4 doses/day Child (6–12 yr): 5 ml (1 tsp) q3–4h for up to 4 doses/day
DILOR-G (Savage) Dyphylline and guaifenesin *Rx*	Tablets: 200 mg dyphylline and 200 mg guaifenesin Liquid (per 5 ml): 100 mg dyphylline and 100 mg guaifenesin (1 pt, 1 gal)	Adult: 1 tab or 5–10 ml (1–2 tsp) tid or qid Child (> 6 yr): 2–3 mg/lb/day given in divided doses
ISUPREL (Winthrop-Breon) Isoproterenol hydrochloride *Rx*	Sublingual tablets: 10, 15 mg Ampuls: 0.2 mg/ml (1, 5 ml)	Adult: for pulmonary conditions with bronchospasm, 10 mg sublingually, or up to 15 mg qid or 20 mg tid, if needed; for bronchospasm during anesthesia, 0.01–0.02 mg IV to start, repeated if necessary Child: for pulmonary conditions with bronchospasm, 5–10 mg sublingually, or up to 30 mg/day, if needed

[1] Where pediatric dosages are not given, consult manufacturer

OTHER SYSTEMIC BRONCHODILATORS/ANTIASTHMATIC AGENTS continued

DRUG	HOW SUPPLIED	USUAL DOSAGE[1]
LUFYLLIN-EPG (Wallace) Dyphylline, guaifenesin, ephedrine hydrochloride, and phenobarbital *Rx*	**Tablets:** 100 mg dyphylline, 200 mg guaifenesin, 16 mg ephedrine hydrochloride, and 16 mg phenobarbital **Elixir (per 10 ml):** 100 mg dyphylline, 200 mg guaifenesin, 16 mg ephedrine hydrochloride, and 16 mg phenobarbital (1 pt) *fruit flavored*	**Adult:** 1–2 tabs or 10–20 ml (2–4 tsp) q6h
LUFYLLIN-GG (Wallace) Dyphylline and guaifenesin *Rx*	**Tablets:** 200 mg dyphylline and 200 mg guaifenesin **Elixir (per 15 ml):** 100 mg dyphylline and 100 mg guaifenesin (1 pt, 1 gal) *wine flavored*	**Adult:** 1 tab or 30 ml (2 tbsp) qid **Child ($>$ 6 yr):** ½–1 tab or 15–30 ml (1–2 tbsp) tid or qid
MUDRANE-2 (Poythress) Potassium iodide and aminophylline *Rx*	**Tablets:** 195 mg potassium iodide and 130 mg aminophylline	**Adult:** 1 tab, with a full glass of water, tid or qid, as needed **Child:** ½ tab, with a full glass of water, tid or qid, as needed
MUDRANE GG (Poythress) Theophylline or aminophylline, ephedrine hydrochloride, phenobarbital, and guaifenesin *Rx*	**Tablets:** 130 mg aminophylline, 16 mg ephedrine hydrochloride, 8 mg phenobarbital, and 100 mg guaifenesin **Elixir (per 5 ml):** 20 mg theophylline, 4 mg ephedrine hydrochloride, 2.5 mg phenobarbital, and 26 mg guaifenesin (1 pt, ½ gal)	**Adult:** 1 tab or 15 ml (1 tbsp), with a full glass of water, tid or qid, as needed **Child:** 1 ml (⅕ tsp)/10 lb, with water, tid or qid
MUDRANE GG-2 (Poythress) Aminophylline and guaifenesin *Rx*	**Tablets:** 130 mg aminophylline and 100 mg guaifenesin	**Adult:** 1 tab, with a full glass of water, tid or qid, as needed **Child:** ½ tab, with a full glass of water, tid or qid, as needed
PRIMATENE (Whitehall) Theophylline, ephedrine hydrochloride, and either phenobarbital (P formula) or pyrilamine maleate (M formula[2]) *OTC*	**Tablets:** 130 mg theophylline, 24 mg ephedrine hydrochloride, and either 8 mg phenobarbital or 16.6 mg pyrilamine maleate	**Adult:** 1–2 tabs to start, followed by 1 tab q4h, as needed, up to 6 tabs/24 h **Child (6–12 yr):** ½–1 tab to start, followed by ½ tab q4h, as needed, up to 3 tabs/24 h
QUIBRON PLUS (Mead Johnson) Theophylline, guaifenesin, ephedrine hydrochloride, and butabarbital *Rx*	**Capsules:** 150 mg theophylline, 100 mg guaifenesin, 25 mg ephedrine hydrochloride, and 20 mg butabarbital **Elixir (per 15 ml):** 150 mg theophylline, 100 mg guaifenesin, 25 mg ephedrine hydrochloride, and 20 mg butabarbital (1 pt)	**Adult:** 1–2 caps or 15–30 ml (1–2 tbsp) bid or tid **Child ($<$ 8 yr):** up to 2.5 ml (½ tsp)/10 lb bid or tid **Child (8–12 yr):** 1 cap or 15 ml (1 tbsp) bid or tid
SLO-PHYLLIN GG (Rorer) Theophylline and guaifenesin *Rx*	**Capsules:** 150 mg theophylline and 90 mg guaifenesin **Syrup (per 15 ml):** 150 mg theophylline and 90 mg guaifenesin (1 pt) *lemon/vanilla flavored*	**Adult and child:** see the dosage recommendations for Slo-Phyllin in the main part of this chapter
SUS-PHRINE (Berlex) Epinephrine *Rx*	**Ampuls:** 5 mg/ml (0.3 ml) **Vials:** 5 mg/ml (5 ml)	**Adult:** 0.5–1.5 mg SC, repeated as necessary at intervals not less than 6 h apart **Infant and child (1 mo to 12 yr):** 0.025 mg/kg SC, up to 0.75 mg for children weighing $\leq$ 30 kg, repeated as necessary at intervals not less than 6 h apart
SYNOPHYLATE (Central) Theophylline sodium glycinate *Rx*	**Elixir (per 15 ml):** 330 mg (1 pt, 1 gal)	**Adult:** 15–30 ml (1–2 tbsp) q6–8h, preferably after meals **Child (1–3 yr):** 2.5–5 ml (½–1 tsp) q6–8h, preferably after meals **Child (3–6 yr):** 5–7.5 ml (1–1½ tsp) q6–8h, preferably after meals **Child (6–12 yr):** 10–15 ml (2–3 tsp) q6–8h, preferably after meals

[1] Where pediatric dosages are not given, consult manufacturer
[2] M formula is available only in those states that prohibit OTC marketing of phenobarbital

INHALANT BRONCHODILATORS/ ANTIASTHMATIC AGENTS

AEROBID (flunisolide) Forest   Rx
Metered-dose oral inhaler: 250 µg/inhalation

INDICATIONS	**INHALANT DOSAGE**
Chronic bronchial asthma	**Adult:** 2 inhalations bid (morning and evening) to start; maximum dosage, 4 inhalations bid
	Child (6–15 yr): 2 inhalations bid (morning and evening); use at a higher dosage has not been studied

CONTRAINDICATIONS	
Hypersensitivity to any component	Acute asthma (when used as *primary* therapy)

ADMINISTRATION/DOSAGE ADJUSTMENTS

Selection of patients — This preparation is intended for the relief of bronchial asthma in patients requiring chronic corticosteroid therapy; this group includes both patients who are already receiving systemic steroids and those who are not adequately controlled by bronchodilators or other nonsteroidal medications but have not been given steroids because of concern over their potential side effects. It is not intended for patients who require systemic corticosteroids infrequently.

Patients receiving systemic corticosteroids — Use of this inhaler may permit either replacement of the systemic corticosteroid or a significant reduction in its dosage. Assuming that the patient's asthma is reasonably stable, begin use without changing the patient's usual systemic maintenance dose. Wait about 1 wk and then reduce the systemic dosage; depending on how the patient responds, a second reduction may be made 1 or 2 wk later, followed by further gradual reductions over the ensuing weeks. Do not decrease the dosage at any one time by more than the equivalent of 2.5 mg of prednisone (see warning, below, regarding withdrawal of systemic corticosteroids).

Patients *not* receiving systemic corticosteroids — An improvement in pulmonary function may be anticipated within 1–4 wk after therapy is started in patients who respond to this preparation

Concomitant use of inhalant bronchodilators — An inhalant bronchodilator may be needed in addition to this preparation to control asthmatic symptoms. To ensure penetration of the steroid into the bronchial tree, advise patients to use the bronchodilator before they take this medication. If an aerosol bronchodilator is used, caution the patient to wait several minutes after using it before inhaling this drug; this will reduce the risk of fluorocarbon toxicity resulting from inhaling the propellants in each preparation.

WARNINGS/PRECAUTIONS

Acute asthmatic episodes — This preparation is not a substitute for a bronchodilator and should not be used as the primary drug for treating status asthmaticus or other acute asthmatic episodes requiring intensive measures. Caution patients to report immediately the occurrence of asthmatic episodes that do not respond to use of a bronchodilator; such patients may require systemic corticosteroid therapy to tide them over these periods.

Withdrawal of systemic corticosteroid therapy — Watch carefully for signs of adrenal insufficiency, such as hypotension and weight loss, in patients experiencing arthralgia, myalgia, lassitude, depression, or other steroid withdrawal symptoms (musculoskeletal reactions have been reported in 35% of patients). If evidence of adrenal insufficiency is seen, temporarily increase the systemic steroid dosage and then withdraw the steroid more slowly. Recovery of normal hypothalamic-pituitary-adrenal (HPA) function usually takes several months, but can take up to a year. Until normal HPA function returns, trauma, surgery, or infection (particularly gastroenteritis or other conditions associated with acute electrolyte losses) may precipitate potentially fatal adrenal insufficiency, since this preparation does not provide a systemic amount of steroid sufficient to cope with stress in patients with HPA dysfunction. (To assess the risk of stress-induced adrenal insufficiency, periodically perform routine tests of adrenocortical function, including measurement of the early morning resting cortisol level.) Severe, potentially fatal asthmatic attacks may also occur if the previous oral corticosteroid dosage significantly exceeded the equivalent of 10 mg/day of prednisone. During periods of stress or severe asthmatic attacks, resume systemic steroid therapy in large doses; patients at risk should carry a warning card indicating that they may need such therapy during these periods. Withdrawal of systemic corticosteroid therapy may also unmask such allergic conditions as rhinitis, conjunctivitis, and eczema.

Systemic absorption — Watch carefully for any evidence of a systemic effect. Exercise caution when beginning administration; during chronic therapy, periodically evaluate HPA function if a patient requires 8 inhalations/day. During periods of stress (such as surgery), check particularly for signs of adrenal insufficiency.

Upper respiratory tract infections — Infections due to *Candida albicans* or *Aspergillus niger* have been detected in 3–9% of patients, usually in the mouth and throat and occasionally in the larynx; these infections may necessitate antifungal therapy or discontinuation of this preparation. To prevent infection, patients should be instructed to rinse their mouths after inhalation of each dose.

AEROBID ■ ALUPENT Inhalant Solution and Metered Dose Inhaler

Pulmonary effects	Pulmonary infiltration with eosinophilia may develop during therapy as a reaction to this preparation or, in some cases, may be unmasked as a result of withdrawal of a systemic corticosteroid. The potential effects of this preparation on tuberculosis or other pulmonary infections have not been assessed.
Long-term use	The long-term effects of therapy are not known; potential risks, such as growth inhibition and reduction of immunologic response, have not been evaluated
Carcinogenicity	An increase in pulmonary adenomas has been seen in Swiss-derived mice given flunisolide for 22 mo; this increase fell within the range of spontaneous adenomas characteristic of this species
Effect on fertility	Some evidence of impaired fertility has been seen in female rats following administration at a high dosage (200 µg/kg/day)

ADVERSE REACTIONS

Frequent reactions (incidence ≥ 1%) are printed in *italics*

Respiratory	*Upper respiratory tract infections (25%); sore throat (20%); cold symptoms and nasal congestion (15%); candidal infections in the mouth and throat, chest congestion, cough, hoarseness, rhinitis, rhinorrhea, sneezing, sputum, wheezing, and sinus congestion, drainage, infection, or inflammation (3–9%); dry throat, glossitis, oral irritation, pharyngitis, phlegm, throat irritation, bronchitis, tightness in the chest, dyspnea, epistaxis, stuffiness in the head, laryngitis, nasal irritation, pleurisy, pneumonia, and sinus discomfort (1–3%);* shortness of breath
Gastrointestinal	*Nausea and/or vomiting (25%); diarrhea and upset stomach (10%); abdominal pain and heartburn (3–9%); constipation, dyspepsia, and gas (1–3%);* abdominal fullness
Central nervous system	*Headache (25%); unpleasant taste (10%); dizziness, irritability, nervousness, shakiness, anosmia, ageusia, and decreased appetite (3–9%); anxiety, depression, faintness, fatigue, hypoactivity, hyperactivity, insomnia, moodiness, numbness, vertigo, and increased appetite (1–3%)*
Ophthalmic	*Blurred vision, eye discomfort, and eye infection (1–3%)*
Otic	*Ear infection (3–9%), earache (1–3%)*
Cardiovascular	*Palpitations (3–9%); hypertension and tachycardia (1–3%)*
Dermatological	*Eczema, pruritus, and rash (3–9%); acne, hives, and urticaria (1–3%)*
Other	*Flu (10%); chest pain, edema, fever, and menstrual disturbances (3–9%); chills, weight gain, malaise, peripheral edema, diaphoresis, weakness, capillary fragility, and enlarged lymph nodes (1–3%)*

OVERDOSAGE

Signs and symptoms	Suppression of HPA function
Treatment	Gradually reduce dosage of this preparation

DRUG INTERACTIONS

Prednisone (alternate-day oral therapy)	⇧ Suppression of HPA function; combination therapy is generally not recommended

ALTERED LABORATORY VALUES

Blood/serum values	⇩ Cortisol
Urinary values	⇩ Cortisol ⇩ 17-Hydroxycorticosteroids

USE IN CHILDREN

See INDICATIONS and INHALANT DOSAGE; available data do not warrant use in children under 6 yr of age. During chronic therapy, watch for suppression of HPA function and inhibition of bone growth.

USE IN PREGNANT AND NURSING WOMEN

Pregnancy Category C: fetotoxic and teratogenic effects have been seen in rabbits given 40 µg/kg/day and in rats given 200 µg/kg/day; no adequate, well-controlled studies have been done in pregnant women. Use during pregnancy only if the expected benefit justifies the potential risk to the fetus. It is not known whether flunisolide is excreted in human milk, but it is known that other corticosteroids are excreted; use with caution in nursing mothers.

VEHICLE/BASE
Metered-dose inhaler: trichloromonofluoromethane, dichlorodifluoromethane, dichlorotetrafluoroethane, and sorbitan trioleate

---

INHALANT BRONCHODILATORS/ANTIASTHMATIC AGENTS

ALUPENT Inhalant Solution (metaproterenol sulfate) Boehringer Ingelheim   Rx

Solution: 0.6% (2.5 ml), 5% (10, 30 ml) for inhalation only

INDICATIONS

Bronchial asthma
Reversible bronchospasm associated with bronchitis and emphysema

INHALANT DOSAGE

Adult: for administration by hand bulb nebulizer, 10 inhalations (range: 5–15 inhalations) of undiluted 5% solution per treatment; for administration by IPPB, 2.5 ml (1 vial) of undiluted 0.6% solution per single dose or 0.3 ml (range: 0.2–0.3 ml) of 5% solution, diluted in 2.5 ml of saline or other diluent, per treatment

ALUPENT Inhalant Solution and Metered Dose Inhaler ■ ARM-A-MED

ALUPENT Metered Dose Inhaler (metaproterenol sulfate) Boehringer Ingelheim Rx

Metered-dose inhaler: 0.65 mg/inhalation

INDICATIONS	**INHALANT DOSAGE**
Same as Alupent Inhalant Solution	**Adult:** 2–3 inhalations q3–4h, up to 12 inhalations/day if needed

CONTRAINDICATIONS

Cardiac arrhythmias associated with tachycardia

ADMINISTRATION/DOSAGE ADJUSTMENTS

Inhalant solution	Repeated administration of the inhalant solution more often than q4h is usually unnecessary for acute bronchospastic attacks; for chronic bronchospastic disease, administer tid or qid

WARNINGS/PRECAUTIONS

Excessive use	May be dangerous; cardiac arrest and fatalities have occurred. Repeated excessive administration may lead to paradoxical bronchoconstriction.
Lack of therapeutic response	Advise patient to report any failure to respond to usual doses
Additional sympathomimetic agents	Use with extreme care; allow sufficient time before administering another sympathomimetic agent
Special-risk patients	Use with great caution in patients with hypertension, coronary artery disease, congestive heart failure, hyperthyroidism, diabetes, or hypersensitivity to sympathomimetic amines
Carcinogenicity, mutagenicity, effect on fertility	Long-term studies in mice and rats to evaluate the carcinogenic potential of this drug have not been completed; the mutagenic potential of this drug and its effect on fertility have not been studied

ADVERSE REACTIONS

The most frequent reactions, regardless of incidence, are printed in *italics*

Cardiovascular	*Tachycardia (14%)*, hypertension, palpitations
Central nervous system	*Nervousness (14%), tremor (5%)*
Gastrointestinal	*Nausea (2%)*, vomiting, bad taste

OVERDOSAGE

Signs and symptoms	Excessive beta-adrenergic stimulation (see ADVERSE REACTIONS)
Treatment	Reduce dosage and/or frequency of administration

DRUG INTERACTIONS

Sympathomimetic bronchodilators	⇧ Adrenergic effects
Nonselective beta blockers	⇩ Bronchodilation

ALTERED LABORATORY VALUES

No clinically significant alterations in blood/serum or urinary values occur at therapeutic dosages

---

USE IN CHILDREN

These preparations are not recommended for use in children under 12 yr of age

USE IN PREGNANT AND NURSING WOMEN

Pregnancy Category C: use during pregnancy only if expected benefit of therapy justifies the potential fetal risk. Teratogenicity and embryocidal effects have been observed in rabbits at oral doses of 100 mg/kg (620 times the human inhalation dose). These effects have not occurred in mice, rats, or rabbits given oral doses of 50 mg/kg (310 times the human inhalation dose). No adequate, well-controlled studies have been done in pregnant women. It is not known whether metoproterenol is excreted in human milk; use with caution in nursing women because many drugs are excreted in human milk.

INHALANT BRONCHODILATORS/ANTIASTHMATIC AGENTS

ARM-A-MED Isoetharine Hydrochloride Armour Rx

Solution: 0.062% (4 ml), 0.125% (4 ml), 0.167% (3 ml), 0.2% (2.5 ml), 0.25% (2 ml)

INDICATIONS	**INHALANT DOSAGE**
Bronchial asthma **Reversible bronchospasm** associated with bronchitis and emphysema	**Adult:** for administration by IPPB or oxygen aerosolization, 2 ml of a 0.25% solution, 2.5 ml of a 0.2% solution, 3 ml of a 0.167% solution, or 4 ml of a 0.125% or 0.062% solution; allow an interval between doses of at least 4 h, except when treating severe conditions that require more frequent use

ARM-A-MED ■ AZMACORT

CONTRAINDICATIONS

Hypersensitivity to any component

ADMINISTRATION/DOSAGE ADJUSTMENTS

Oxygen aerosolization	Administer each dose over a period of 15–20 min, with oxygen flow adjusted to deliver 4–6 liters/min; the solution may be administered simultaneously with other therapeutic agents (eg, antibiotics, wetting agents)
IPPB	An inspiratory flow rate of 15 liters/min and a cycling pressure of 15 cm H_2O are generally recommended; however, in some instances, an inspiratory flow rate of 6–30 liters/min, a cycling pressure of 10–15 cm H_2O, and further dilution of the solution may be necessary

WARNINGS/PRECAUTIONS

Excessive aerosol use	Loss of effectiveness, severe paradoxical airway resistance, and cardiac arrest may result from excessive use of an adrenergic aerosol; if severe paradoxical airway resistance develops, discontinue use immediately and institute alternative therapy
Special-risk patients	Adjust dosage carefully in patients with hyperthyroidism, hypertension, acute coronary artery disease, cardiac asthma, limited cardiac reserve, or sensitivity to sympathomimetic amines
Carcinogenicity, mutagenicity, effect on fertility	No long-term studies have been done to evaluate carcinogenic or mutagenic potential of this drug or its effect on fertility

ADVERSE REACTIONS[1]

Central nervous system	Headache, anxiety, tension, restlessness, insomnia, weakness, dizziness, excitement, tremor
Cardiovascular	Tachycardia, palpitations, changes in blood pressure
Gastrointestinal	Nausea

OVERDOSAGE

Signs and symptoms	Tachycardia, palpitations, nausea, headache, epinephrine-like reactions
Treatment	Discontinue use immediately; treat symptomatically and institute supportive measures, as required. It is not known whether isoetharine can be removed from the blood by dialysis.

DRUG INTERACTIONS

Epinephrine and other sympathomimetic agents	Excessive tachycardia; isoetharine and other sympathomimetic agents may be given alternately, but not concomitantly
Nonselective beta blockers	▽ Bronchodilation

ALTERED LABORATORY VALUES

No clinically significant alterations in blood/serum or urinary values occur at therapeutic dosages

---

USE IN CHILDREN

Safety and effectiveness for use in children have not been established

USE IN PREGNANT AND NURSING WOMEN

Pregnancy Category C: no studies have been done to determine whether isoetharine can affect reproductive capacity or cause harm to the fetus; use during pregnancy only if the expected benefit outweighs the potential risk to the fetus. It is not known whether this drug is excreted in human milk; because many drugs are excreted in human milk, use with caution in nursing mothers.

---

[1] Isoetharine is relatively free of adverse effects at therapeutic dosages; the reactions listed in this section are associated with too frequent use

---

INHALANT BRONCHODILATORS/ANTIASTHMATIC AGENTS

AZMACORT (triamcinolone acetonide) Rorer   Rx

Metered-dose oral inhaler: 100 μg/inhalation

INDICATIONS	INHALANT DOSAGE
Chronic bronchial asthma	**Adult:** usual dosage, 2 inhalations tid or qid; for more severe asthma, 12–16 inhalations/day, given in 3–4 doses, to start, followed by a reduction in dosage. For maintenance in some patients, administration twice-daily may be sufficient. **Child (6–12 yr):** 1–2 inhalations tid or qid; maximum dosage, 12 inhalations/day

AZMACORT

CONTRAINDICATIONS

Hypersensitivity to any component	Acute asthma (when used as *primary* therapy)

ADMINISTRATION/DOSAGE ADJUSTMENTS

Selection of patients	This preparation is intended for the relief of bronchial asthma in patients requiring chronic corticosteroid therapy; this group includes both patients who are already receiving systemic steroids and those who are not adequately controlled by bronchodilators or other nonsteroidal medications but have not been given steroids because of concern over their potential side effects. It is not intended for patients who require systemic corticosteroids infrequently.
Patients receiving systemic corticosteroids	Use of this inhaler may permit either replacement of the systemic corticosteroid or a significant reduction in its dosage. Assuming that the patient's asthma is reasonably stable, begin use without changing the patient's usual systemic maintenance dose. Wait about 1 wk and then reduce the systemic dosage; depending on how the patient responds, a second reduction may be made 1 or 2 wk later, followed by further gradual reductions over the ensuing weeks. Do not decrease the dosage at any one time by more than the equivalent of 2.5 mg of prednisone (see warning, below, regarding withdrawal of systemic corticosteroids).
Patients *not* receiving systemic corticosteroids	An improvement in pulmonary function may be anticipated within 1–2 wk after therapy is started in patients who respond to this preparation
Dosage delivery	To ensure reliable delivery of the medication, caution patients not to use an individual aerosol canister more than 240 times (approximately 1 mo when used at a dosage of 2 inhalations qid)
Concomitant use of inhalant bronchodilators	An inhalant bronchodilator may be needed in addition to this preparation to control asthmatic symptoms. To ensure penetration of the steroid into the bronchial tree, advise patients to use the bronchodilator before they take this medication. If an aerosol bronchodilator is used, caution the patient to wait several minutes after using it before inhaling this drug; this will reduce the risk of fluorocarbon toxicity resulting from inhaling the propellants in each preparation.

WARNINGS/PRECAUTIONS

Acute asthmatic episodes	This preparation is not a substitute for a bronchodilator and should not be used as the primary drug for treating status asthmaticus or other acute asthmatic episodes requiring intensive measures. Caution patients to report immediately the occurrence of asthmatic episodes that do not respond to use of a bronchodilator; such patients may require systemic corticosteroid therapy to tide them over these periods.
Withdrawal of systemic corticosteroid therapy	Watch carefully for signs of adrenal insufficiency, such as hypotension and weight loss, in patients experiencing arthralgia, myalgia, lassitude, depression, or other steroid withdrawal symptoms. If evidence of adrenal insufficiency is seen, temporarily increase the systemic steroid dosage and then withdraw the steroid more slowly. Recovery of normal hypothalamic-pituitary-adrenal (HPA) function usually takes several months, but can take a year or more if large oral steroid doses were given for a prolonged period. Until normal HPA function returns, trauma, surgery, or infection (particularly gastroenteritis or other conditions associated with acute electrolyte losses) may precipitate potentially fatal adrenal insufficiency, since this preparation does not provide a systemic amount of steroid sufficient to cope with stress in patients with HPA dysfunction. Severe, potentially fatal asthmatic attacks may also occur if the previous oral corticosteroid dosage significantly exceeded the equivalent of 10 mg/day of prednisone. During periods of stress or severe asthmatic attacks, resume systemic steroid therapy in large doses; patients at risk should carry a warning card indicating that they may need such therapy during these periods. Withdrawal of systemic corticosteroid therapy may also unmask such allergic conditions as rhinitis, conjunctivitis, and eczema.
Systemic absorption	Suppression of HPA function has been seen in some patients who used this preparation for as briefly as 6–12 wk. During therapy, watch carefully for evidence of a systemic reaction, and, during periods of stress (such as surgery), check particularly for signs of adrenal insufficiency.
Upper respiratory tract infections	Oral and pharyngeal infections due to *Candida albicans* have been seen in 2.5% of patients; these infections may disappear spontaneously or may necessitate antifungal therapy or discontinuation of this preparation. At each patient visit, examine the mouth and pharynx. Patients should be instructed to practice good oral hygiene, including rinsing the mouth after inhalation of each dose.
Pulmonary infections	The potential effects of this preparation on tuberculosis and other pulmonary infections have not been assessed; some signs of a pulmonary infection may be masked during therapy
Long-term use	Although no long-term effects have reported following use of this preparation for 2 yr or longer, potential risks, such as growth inhibition and reduction of immunologic response, have not been evaluated

ADVERSE REACTIONS[1]

Respiratory	Oral candidiasis, hoarseness, dry or irritated throat, dry mouth, cough, increased wheezing

AZMACORT ■ BECLOVENT

Other	Facial edema, suppression of HPA function

OVERDOSAGE

Signs and symptoms	Suppression of HPA function
Treatment	Gradually reduce dosage of this preparation

DRUG INTERACTIONS

Prednisone (alternate-day therapy)	△ Suppression of HPA function; combination therapy is generally not recommended

ALTERED LABORATORY VALUES

Blood/serum values	▽ Cortisol
Urinary values	▽ Cortisol ▽ 17-Hydroxycorticosteroids

USE IN CHILDREN

See INDICATIONS and INHALANT DOSAGE; available data do not warrant use in children under 6 yr of age. During therapy, watch for evidence of growth suppression.

USE IN PREGNANT AND NURSING WOMEN

Pregnancy Category D: embryotoxicity, fetotoxicity, and teratogenic reactions, including cleft palate, internal hydrocephaly, and axial skeletal defects, have been seen in rats and rabbits given the maximum recommended human dose by aerosol inhalation. No adverse reactions on the human fetus have been reported following parenteral or topical use of triamcinolone acetonide during pregnancy; however, well-controlled studies in pregnant women have not been done with this preparation. Use during pregnancy only if the expected benefit clearly justifies the potential risk to the fetus. Infants whose mothers received substantial doses during pregnancy should be carefully observed for hypoadrenalism. It is not known whether triamcinolone is excreted in human milk; because of the potential for tumorigenicity, this drug should not be given to patients who elect to breast-feed.

VEHICLE/BASE
Metered-dose inhaler: dichlorodifluoromethane and 1% dehydrated alcohol

[1] Pulmonary infiltration accompanied by eosinophilia has occurred with use of other inhalant corticosteroids

---

INHALANT BRONCHODILATORS/ ANTIASTHMATIC AGENTS

BECLOVENT (beclomethasone dipropionate) Glaxo   Rx

Metered-dose oral inhaler: 42 µg/inhalation

INDICATIONS

Bronchial asthma requiring chronic corticosteroid therapy

INHALANT DOSAGE

Adult: 2 inhalations tid or qid, or up to 20 inhalations/24 h, if needed
Child (6–12 yr): 1–2 inhalations tid or qid, or up to 10 inhalations/24 h, if needed

CONTRAINDICATIONS

Primary treatment of status asthmaticus or other acute asthmatic episodes requiring intensive measures	Hypersensitivity to beclomethasone or other components

ADMINISTRATION/DOSAGE ADJUSTMENTS

Patients with severe asthma (adults)	Initiate therapy with 12–16 inhalations/day and adjust dosage downward according to response
Concomitant use of inhalant bronchodilators	Use of bronchodilator before inhaler administration of beclomethasone enhances penetration of beclomethasone into bronchial tree. Allow several minutes to elapse before using beclomethasone inhaler to avoid toxicity from fluorocarbon propellants in both drugs.
Patients receiving systemic corticosteroids	Initially, use inhaler concurrently with usual dosage of systemic steroid. After 1 wk, *gradually* withdraw systemic steroid by reducing daily or alternate-day dose. Depending on response, continue gradually to withdraw systemic steroid by reducing dosage every 1–2 wk. Decrements generally should not exceed 2.5 mg of prednisone or its equivalent.
Patients experiencing steroid withdrawal symptoms (eg, joint or muscle pain, lassitude, depression)	Continue use of inhaler and observe patient closely for objective signs of adrenal insufficiency (eg, hypotension, weight loss); if signs appear, increase dose of systemic steroid temporarily and taper dosage more gradually

COMPENDIUM OF DRUG THERAPY

BECLOVENT ■ BRETHAIRE

Exacerbation of asthma	Give short course of systemic steroid therapy; taper dosage gradually as symptoms subside

WARNINGS/PRECAUTIONS

Deaths due to adrenal insufficiency	Have occurred in asthmatic patients during and after transfer from systemic corticosteroids to beclomethasone inhaler therapy
Recovery of hypothalamic-pituitary-adrenal (HPA) function	Requires many months after withdrawal from systemic corticosteroids; during this HPA-suppressed period, signs and symptoms of adrenal insufficiency may appear in the presence of trauma, surgery, or infection, especially gastroenteritis
Stress periods or severe asthma attacks	Patients withdrawn from systemic steroids should immediately resume large doses of corticosteroids; these patients should carry a warning card indicating their need of supplementary systemic steroid therapy in case of stress or severe asthma attack
Assessing risk of adrenal insufficiency	Tests of adrenocortical function should be performed periodically, including measurement of early-morning resting cortisol levels
Fungal infections (*Candida albicans, Aspergillus niger*)	Frequently occur in mouth and pharynx and occasionally in larynx; up to 75% of patients may have positive oral *Candida* cultures. Antifungal treatment and discontinuation of inhaler therapy may be necessary.
Episodes of asthma unresponsive to treatment	Patients should report immediately any such episode during treatment; systemic corticosteroid therapy may be needed
Allergic reactions	In rare cases, beclomethasone inhaler therapy may precipitate immediate or delayed hypersensitivity reactions (see ADVERSE REACTIONS). Transfer from systemic corticosteroids to the inhaler may unmask previously suppressed allergic conditions such as rhinitis, conjunctivitis, and eczema. Pulmonary infiltrates with eosinophilia may result from inhaler therapy or, in some cases, may be manifested following transfer from systemic steroids.
Systemic steroid withdrawal symptoms	May occur during withdrawal from oral corticosteroid therapy (see ADMINISTRATION/DOSAGE ADJUSTMENTS)

ADVERSE REACTIONS[1]

Endocrinological	Suppression of hypothalamic-pituitary-adrenal function
Hypersensitivity	Urticaria, angioedema, rash, and bronchospasm (rare)
Other	Hoarseness, dry mouth

OVERDOSAGE

Signs and symptoms	See WARNINGS/PRECAUTIONS
Treatment	Discontinue medication; reinstitute systemic steroid therapy, if needed

DRUG INTERACTIONS

No clinically significant drug interactions have been identified

ALTERED LABORATORY VALUES

No clinically significant alterations in blood/serum or urinary values occur at therapeutic dosages

---

USE IN CHILDREN

See INDICATIONS and INHALANT DOSAGE; not recommended for use in children under 6 yr of age

USE IN PREGNANT AND NURSING WOMEN

Safety for use in pregnant or nursing women has not been established. Glucocorticoids, including beclomethasone, are known teratogens in rodent species. Infants born to mothers who received substantial corticosteroid dosages during pregnancy should be carefully observed for hypoadrenalism. Glucocorticoids are excreted in human milk.

---

[1] Long-term effects in humans are unknown

INHALANT BRONCHODILATORS/ANTIASTHMATIC AGENTS

BRETHAIRE (terbutaline sulfate) Geigy   Rx

Metered-dose oral inhaler: 200 µg/inhalation

INDICATIONS

Bronchospasm associated with reversible obstructive airway disease

INHALANT DOSAGE

Adult: 2 inhalations, separated by a 1-min interval, q4–6h
Child (≥ 12 yr): same as adult

BRETHAIRE ■ BRONKOMETER/BRONKOSOL

CONTRAINDICATIONS

Hypersensitivity to any component

WARNINGS/PRECAUTIONS

Paradoxical bronchospasm	Discontinue use immediately if bronchospasm occurs after inhalation
Excessive use	Caution patients to adhere strictly to the recommended dosage; fatalities have been associated with excessive use of sympathomimetic inhalers
Special-risk patients	Use with caution in patients with cardiovascular disorders (including coronary artery insufficiency and hypertension), hyperthyroidism, diabetes mellitus, or unusual sensitivity to sympathomimetic amines. Large IV doses of terbutaline have been reported to exacerbate diabetes and ketoacidosis.
Tolerance with continuous use	Some studies have shown that continued use results in a decrease in therapeutic response; however, in some patients, effectiveness has been demonstrated after 14 wk of continuous administration
Carcinogenicity, mutagenicity, effect on fertility	Increases in the incidence of ovarian cysts and mesovarial leiomyomas and hyperplasia have been seen in rats fed terbutaline for 2 yr; a 21-mo oral study in mice has shown no evidence of carcinogenicity. Mutagenicity tests have not been done with this drug. No adverse effect on fertility has been demonstrated in an oral study with rats.

ADVERSE REACTIONS

Frequent reactions (incidence ≥ 1%) are printed in *italics*

Cardiovascular	*Arrhythmias (4%), tachycardia (3%)*, increased blood pressure, angina; ECG changes, including sinus pause, premature atrial contractions, AV block, premature ventricular contractions, depression of ST-T segment, T-wave inversion, sinus bradycardia, atrial escape beat with aberrant conduction
Respiratory	Dyspnea, wheezing, drying or irritation of oropharynx
Central nervous system	*Headache (< 10%); tremor, nervousness, and drowsiness (< 5%);* vertigo, stimulation, insomnia, unusual taste
Gastrointestinal	*Nausea and other digestive disorders (< 10%),* vomiting

OVERDOSAGE

Signs and symptoms	See ADVERSE REACTIONS
Treatment	Provide symptomatic treatment; institute other measures as needed

DRUG INTERACTIONS

Other inhalant sympathomimetic bronchodilators, epinephrine, MAO inhibitors, tricyclic antidepressants	△ Sympathomimetic effects; this preparation should not be used in patients receiving other inhalant sympathomimetic bronchodilators or epinephrine and should be used with caution in patients receiving MAO inhibitors or tricyclic antidepressants
Beta-adrenergic blockers	▽ Pharmacologic effects of both drugs

ALTERED LABORATORY VALUES

No clinically significant alterations in blood/serum or urinary values occur at therapeutic dosages

---

USE IN CHILDREN

Safety and effectiveness for use in children under 12 yr of age have not been established

USE IN PREGNANT AND NURSING WOMEN

Pregnancy Category B: reproduction studies in rats and rabbits given up to 1,042 times the human dose have shown no evidence of impaired fertility or harm to the fetus. High IV doses of terbutaline have been reported to inhibit uterine contractions; this effect is extremely unlikely to occur with inhalant use. Use this preparation during pregnancy only if clearly needed; do not use for tocolysis. It is not known whether terbutaline is excreted in human milk; use with caution in nursing mothers.

VEHICLE/BASE
Metered-dose inhaler: trichloromonofluoromethane, dichlorodifluoromethane, dichlorotetrafluoroethane, and sorbitan trioleate

---

**INHALANT BRONCHODILATORS/
ANTIASTHMATIC AGENTS**

BRONKOMETER (isoetharine mesylate) Winthrop-Breon   Rx

Metered-dose inhaler: 340 μg/inhalation

INDICATIONS

Bronchial asthma
Reversible bronchospasm associated with bronchitis and emphysema

INHALANT DOSAGE

Adult: 1–2 inhalations, generally not more often than q4h. If a dose is not sufficiently effective 1 min after administration, a second dose may be given at that time. In severe cases, administration more frequently than q4h may be necessary.

COMPENDIUM OF DRUG THERAPY

BRONKOSOL (isoetharine hydrochloride) Winthrop-Breon Rx

Solution: 1% (10, 30 ml)

INDICATIONS	
Same as Bronkometer	
INHALANT DOSAGE	
	Adult: for administration by hand-bulb nebulizer, 4 inhalations (range: 3–7 inhalations); for administration by oxygen aerosolization or IPPB, 0.5 ml (range: with oxygen, 0.25–0.5 ml; with IPPB, 0.25–1 ml). Allow an interval between doses of at least 4 h, except when treating severe conditions that require more frequent use.

CONTRAINDICATIONS

Hypersensitivity to isoetharine or other components

ADMINISTRATION/DOSAGE ADJUSTMENTS

Dilution of solution	The solution should be diluted 1 : 3 with saline or another diluent before being administered by oxygen aerosolization or IPPB
Oxygen aerosolization	Administer each dose over a period of 15–20 min, with oxygen flow adjusted to deliver 4–6 liters/min
IPPB	An inspiratory flow rate of 15 liters/min and a cycling pressure of 15 cm H_2O are generally recommended; however, in some instances, an inspiratory flow rate of 6–30 liters/min, a cycling pressure of 10–15 cm H_2O, and further dilution of the solution may be necessary

WARNINGS/PRECAUTIONS

Excessive aerosol use	Loss of effectiveness, severe paradoxical airway resistance, and cardiac arrest may result from excessive use of an adrenergic aerosol; if severe paradoxical airway resistance develops, discontinue use immediately and institute alternative therapy
Special-risk patients	Adjust dosage carefully in patients with hyperthyroidism, hypertension, acute coronary artery disease, cardiac asthma, limited cardiac reserve, or sensitivity to sympathomimetic amines

ADVERSE REACTIONS[1]

Central nervous system	Headache, anxiety, tension, restlessness, insomnia, weakness, dizziness, excitement, tremor
Cardiovascular	Tachycardia, palpitations, changes in blood pressure
Gastrointestinal	Nausea

OVERDOSAGE

Signs and symptoms	Tachycardia, palpitations, nausea, headache, changes in blood pressure, anxiety, tension, restlessness, insomnia, tremor, weakness, dizziness, excitement
Treatment	Discontinue medication; treat symptomatically and institute supportive measures, as required

DRUG INTERACTIONS

Epinephrine and other sympathomimetic agents	Excessive tachycardia; isoetharine and other sympathomimetic agents may be given alternately, but should not be administered concomitantly
Nonselective beta blockers	▽ Bronchodilation

ALTERED LABORATORY VALUES

No clinically significant alterations in blood/serum or urinary values occur at therapeutic dosages

---

USE IN CHILDREN	**USE IN PREGNANT AND NURSING WOMEN**
Consult manufacturer	Safety for use in pregnant or nursing women has not been established, although there has been no evidence of teratogenicity

---

[1] Isoetharine is relatively free of adverse effects at therapeutic dosages; the reactions listed in this section are associated with too frequent use

---

INHALANT BRONCHODILATORS/ANTIASTHMATIC AGENTS

DUO-MEDIHALER (isoproterenol hydrochloride and phenylephrine bitartrate) Riker Rx

Metered-dose inhaler: 0.16 mg isoproterenol hydrochloride and 0.24 mg phenylephrine bitartrate per dose

INDICATIONS

Bronchospasm associated with acute and chronic bronchial asthma, pulmonary emphysema, bronchitis, and bronchiectasis

INHALANT DOSAGE

Adult: for acute episodes, 1 inhalation to start, repeated after 2–5 min, if necessary, not to exceed 2 inhalations at any one time or 6 inhalations/h during any 24-h period; for maintenance, 1–2 inhalations 4–6 times/day
Child: same as above

DUO-MEDIHALER ■ INTAL

CONTRAINDICATIONS

Hypersensitivity to either component	Preexisting cardiac arrhythmias associated with tachycardia

WARNINGS/PRECAUTIONS

Excessive use	May lead to loss of effectiveness; discontinue medication immediately if severe paradoxical airway resistance develops and institute alternative therapy; cardiac arrest and death have also occurred
Special-risk patients	Use with caution in patients with cardiovascular disorders (including coronary insufficiency), diabetes, or hyperthyroidism and in patients sensitive to sympathomimetic amines
Concurrent use of epinephrine	May result in serious arrhythmias; however, if desired, both drugs may be alternated, provided that at least 4 h have elapsed between doses

ADVERSE REACTIONS

Essentially none at therapeutic dosages

OVERDOSAGE

Signs and symptoms	*Isoproterenol-related effects:* palpitations, tachycardia, tremulousness, flushing, anginal-type pain, nausea, dizziness, weakness, sweating; *phenylephrine-related effects:* cardiac irregularities, CNS disturbances, reflex bradycardia
Treatment	Discontinue medication; treat symptomatically and institute supportive measures, as required

DRUG INTERACTIONS

Epinephrine	⇧ Cardiac stimulation and risk of arrhythmias

ALTERED LABORATORY VALUES

No clinically significant alterations in blood/serum or urinary values occur at therapeutic dosages

---

USE IN CHILDREN

See INDICATIONS and dosage recommendations (the lower dosage should be used); any child who is old enough to effectively coordinate his or her respiration to the aerosol device may use this product

USE IN PREGNANT AND NURSING WOMEN

Safety for use in pregnant or nursing mothers has not been established, although there has been no evidence of teratogenicity

---

INHALANT BRONCHODILATORS/ANTIASTHMATIC AGENTS

INTAL Capsules (cromolyn sodium) Fisons   Rx

Capsules: 20 mg,[1] for inhalation only

INDICATIONS	INHALANT DOSAGE
Management of **bronchial asthma**	Adult and child ($\geq$ 2 yr): 20 mg qid at regular intervals to start, using a Spinhaler turbo-inhaler for administration
Prevention of **acute bronchospasm** owing to exercise, aspirin, cold dry air, environmental agents (eg, toluene diisocyanate, pollutants, animal dander), or other causes	Adult and child ($\geq$ 2 yr): 20 mg shortly before the precipitating activity or exposure to the precipitating factor, using a Spinhaler turbo-inhaler for administration

INTAL Nebulizer Solution (cromolyn sodium) Fisons   Rx

Ampuls: 20 mg (2 ml), for inhalation only

INDICATIONS	INHALANT DOSAGE
Management of **bronchial asthma**	Adult and child ($\geq$ 2 yr): 20 mg qid at regular intervals, using a power-operated nebulizer for administration
Prevention of **exercise-induced bronchospasm**	Adult and child ($\geq$ 2 yr): 20 mg within 1 h before exercise, using a power-operated nebulizer for administration

INTAL Inhaler (cromolyn sodium) Fisons Rx

Metered-dose oral inhaler: 800 μg per inhalation (8.1, 14.2 g)

INDICATIONS	INHALANT DOSAGE
Management of **bronchial asthma**	Adult and child ($\geq$ 5 yr): 2 inhalations qid, given at regular intervals (see ADMINISTRATION/DOSAGE ADJUSTMENTS)
Prevention of **acute bronchospasm** owing to exercise, cold dry air, environmental agents (eg, toluene diisocyanate, pollutants, animal dander), or other causes	Adult and child ($\geq$ 5 yr): 2 inhalations within 10–15 min, but not more than 60 min, before exposure to precipitating factor

CONTRAINDICATIONS

Hypersensitivity to cromolyn or other components

Hypersensitivity to lactose (capsules only)

ADMINISTRATION/DOSAGE ADJUSTMENTS

Administration of nebulizer solution and capsules	The solution should be administered by a means of a power-operated nebulizer that has an adequate flow rate and a suitable face mask; a hand-operated nebulizer should not be used. To empty the contents of the capsule, several deep inhalations may be necessary; it is normal for a light dusting of powder to remain. If the patient experiences difficulty in emptying the capsule, determine whether directions for use of the Spinhaler have been carefully followed. At least once every week, the Spinhaler should be washed in warm water and then dried thoroughly.
Patients with renal or hepatic impairment	Decrease dosage in patients with renal or hepatic impairment
Starting treatment of chronic asthma	When the acute episode has been controlled, the airway has been cleared, and the patient is able to inhale adequately, cromolyn may be given; clinical effect is usually evident within 2–4 wk
Patients receiving nonsteroidal antiasthmatic agents	Maintain use of other nonsteroidal antiasthmatic agents when beginning treatment of chronic asthma with cromolyn; if a clinical response to cromolyn is seen and asthma is well-controlled, dosage of the other agents may be gradually reduced
Patients receiving corticosteroids	Maintain steroidal antiasthmatic regimen when beginning treatment with cromolyn. If symptoms improve, try to reduce the dosage of the corticosteroid. If improvement is not seen, a reduction may nonetheless be possible and an attempt to decrease the dosage may be made. To avoid exacerbation of asthma, reduce dosage of the corticosteroid slowly and monitor clinical response carefully. Prolonged corticosteroid therapy frequently causes HPA-axis suppression, which may persist even after gradual discontinuation. If a significant stress (eg, severe asthmatic attack, surgery, trauma, severe illness) occurs during concomitant therapy, consider increasing the dosage of the corticosteroid; if such a stress occurs within 1–2 yr after termination of steroid therapy, consider resuming use. A temporary increase in steroid dosage may also be necessary during concomitant therapy if respiratory function becomes impaired (eg, if severe exacerbation of asthma occurs). Exercise great care and provide continued close supervision when discontinuing cromolyn after the drug has permitted termination or a reduced dosage of the corticosteroid; severe asthma may suddenly recur and necessitate not only immediate treatment, but also reintroduction or increased dosage of the corticosteroid.
Reduction in dosage	If asthma has been controlled and other agents are required only occasionally or have been eliminated, the frequency of administration may be reduced from qid to tid or bid. To avoid exacerbation of asthma, reduce dosage gradually. If asthmatic condition deteriorates in a patient receiving less than 4 doses/day, an increase in dosage and introduction or more frequent use of symptomatic medications may be necessary.

WARNINGS/PRECAUTIONS

Status asthmaticus	Do not use cromolyn for treatment of status asthmaticus
Bronchospasm	Cromolyn can cause bronchospasm, which, on rare occasions, may be very severe; if bronchospasm cannot be controlled by prior administration of bronchodilators, discontinue use
Cough, wheezing	The powder in the capsules causes transient cough in 20% of patients and mild wheezing in 4% of patients; the solution produces cough occasionally. In some cases, cough and irritation of the throat can be prevented if mouth is rinsed or water is drunk immediately before and/or after use of the Spinhaler.
Anaphylaxis	Severe anaphylactic reactions may occur following administration of cromolyn sodium
Eosinophilic pneumonia	If the patient develops eosinophilic pneumonia or pulmonary infiltrates with eosinophilia, discontinue use of the metered-dose inhaler
Patients with exercise-induced bronchospasm	Use of the metered-dose inhaler may be effective in relieving bronchospasm in some, but not all, of these patients

INTAL ■ ISUPREL MISTOMETER

Use in patients with impaired renal or hepatic function	Because cromolyn is excreted via the biliary and renal routes, decrease the dosage or discontinue use in patients with renal or hepatic dysfunction
Special-risk patients	Use the metered-dose inhaler with caution in patients with coronary artery disease or a history of cardiac arrhythmias because of the type of propellants contained in this preparation
Carcinogenicity, mutagenicity, effect on fertility	No cromolyn-induced neoplastic effects have been detected in rats following SC administration for 18 mo or in mice and hamsters following intraperitoneal administration for 12 mo. No evidence of chromosomal damage or cytotoxicity has been found in mutagenicity tests. Reproduction studies in animals have shown no evidence of impaired fertility.

ADVERSE REACTIONS[2]

The most frequent reactions, regardless of incidence, are printed in *italics*

With use of capsules and solution

Respiratory	*Bronchospasm, wheezing, cough, nasal congestion;* laryngeal edema (rare)
Central nervous system	Dizziness, headache
Dermatological	Rash, urticaria, angioedema
Genitourinary	Dysuria, urinary frequency
Gastrointestinal	Nausea
Other	Joint swelling and pain, lacrimation, swollen parotid glands; inhalation of gelatin particles, mouthpiece, or propeller (with use of capsules and Spinhaler)

With use of inhaler

Gastrointestinal	*Bad taste, nausea*
Respiratory	*Throat irritation or dryness, cough, wheeze;* pulmonary infiltrates with eosinophilia
Hypersensitivity	Anaphylaxis, angioedema, rash, urticaria
Central nervous system	Dizziness, headache
Genitourinary	Dysuria, urinary frequency
Other	Joint swelling and pain, lacrimation, swollen parotid glands, substernal burning, myopathy

OVERDOSAGE
No clinical signs or symptoms have been seen with overdosage; in studies with mammals, it has not been possible to attain an inhalant dose comparable to the toxic parenteral or oral dose

DRUG INTERACTIONS
See USE IN PREGNANT AND NURSING WOMEN

ALTERED LABORATORY VALUES
No clinically significant alterations in blood/serum or urinary values occur at therapeutic dosages

USE IN CHILDREN
See INDICATIONS and INHALANT DOSAGE; safety and effectiveness of capsules and nebulizer solution have not been established for use in children under 2 yr of age. Safety and effectiveness of the metered-dose inhaler have not been established for use in children under 5 yr of age; for younger children unable to use the Spinhaler or metered-dose inhaler, use the nebulizer solution. Cromolyn may cause adverse effects that could become apparent only after many years; use over a prolonged period in children only if the expected benefit outweighs the potential risk to the child.

USE IN PREGNANT AND NURSING WOMEN
Pregnancy Category B: reproduction studies in mice, rats, and rabbits injected with up to 338 times the human dose have shown no evidence of fetal malformations; an increase in resorptions and a decrease in fetal weight have been seen only at dosages that produced maternal toxicity. In mice, the frequency of resorptions and major fetal malformations associated with SC injection of isoproterenol (at 90 times the human dose) has been increased by the simultaneous SC administration of cromolyn (at 338 times the human dose). No adequate, well-controlled studies have been done in pregnant women; use during pregnancy only if clearly needed. It is not known whether cromolyn is excreted in human milk; use with caution in nursing mothers.

[1] Capsules also contain 20 mg of lactose (see CONTRAINDICATIONS)
[2] Reactions associated with use of the capsules or solution for which a causal relationship has not been established include anaphylaxis, nephrosis, periarteritic vasculitis, pericarditis, peripheral neuritis, pulmonary infiltrates with eosinophilia, polymyositis, exfoliative dermatitis, hemoptysis, anemia, myalgia, hoarseness, photodermatitis, and vertigo; reactions associated with use of the metered-dose inhaler for which a causal relationship has not been established include anemia, exfoliative dermatitis, hemoptysis, hoarseness, myalgia, nephrosis, periarteritic vasculitis, pericarditis, peripheral neuritis, photodermatitis, sneezing, drowsiness, nasal itching, nasal bleeding, nasal burning, serum sickness, stomachache, polymyositis, vertigo, and liver disease

---

INHALANT BRONCHODILATORS/ANTIASTHMATIC AGENTS

ISUPREL MISTOMETER (isoproterenol hydrochloride) Winthrop-Breon   Rx
Metered-dose inhaler: 0.131 mg/inhalation

INDICATIONS
Bronchospasm associated with acute and chronic bronchial asthma, pulmonary emphysema, bronchitis, and bronchiectasis

INHALANT DOSAGE
Adult: for acute episodes, 1 inhalation to start, repeated after 1 min, if necessary, not to exceed 5 doses/day; for chronic conditions, 1–2 inhalations not less than 3–4 h apart
Child: same as adult

ISUPREL MISTOMETER ■ MEDIHALER-ISO

CONTRAINDICATIONS
Preexisting cardiac arrhythmias associated with tachycardia

WARNINGS/PRECAUTIONS

Excessive use	May lead to loss of effectiveness; discontinue medication immediately if severe paradoxical airway resistance develops and institute alternative therapy; cardiac arrest and death have also occurred
Special-risk patients	Use with caution in patients with cardiovascular disorders (including coronary insufficiency), diabetes, hyperthyroidism, or sensitivity to sympathomimetic agents
Status asthmaticus, abnormal blood-gas tensions	Relief of bronchospasm may not be accompanied by improved vital capacity and blood-gas tensions; oxygen-mixture administration and ventilatory assistance are necessary
Concurrent use of epinephrine	May result in serious arrhythmias; however, if desired, both drugs may be alternated, provided that at least 4 h have elapsed between doses

ADVERSE REACTIONS

Respiratory	Throat irritation

OVERDOSAGE

Signs and symptoms	Tachycardia, palpitations, nervousness, nausea, vomiting; rarely: headache, flushing of skin, tremor, dizziness, weakness, sweating, precordial distress, anginal-type pain
Treatment	Discontinue medication; treat symptomatically and institute supportive measures, as required

DRUG INTERACTIONS

Epinephrine	△ Cardiac activity and risk of arrhythmias
Nonselective beta blockers	▽ Bronchodilation

ALTERED LABORATORY VALUES
No clinically significant alterations in blood/serum or urinary values occur at therapeutic dosages

---

USE IN CHILDREN
See INDICATIONS and INHALANT DOSAGE

USE IN PREGNANT AND NURSING WOMEN
Safety for use in pregnant or nursing women has not been established, although there has been no evidence of teratogenicity

---

INHALANT BRONCHODILATORS/ANTIASTHMATIC AGENTS

MEDIHALER-ISO (isoproterenol sulfate) Riker   Rx
Metered-dose inhaler: 0.08 mg/inhalation

INDICATIONS
Bronchospasm associated with acute and chronic bronchial asthma, pulmonary emphysema, bronchitis, and bronchiectasis

INHALANT DOSAGE
Adult: for acute episodes, 1 inhalation to start, repeated after 2–5 min, if necessary, not to exceed 2 inhalations at any one time or 6 inhalations/h during any 24-h period; for maintenance, 1–2 inhalations 4–6 times/day
Child: same as adult

CONTRAINDICATIONS
Preexisting cardiac arrhythmias associated with tachycardia

WARNINGS/PRECAUTIONS

Excessive use	May lead to loss of effectiveness; discontinue medication immediately if severe paradoxical airway resistance develops and institute alternative therapy; cardiac arrest and death have also occurred
Special-risk patients	Use with great caution in patients with cardiovascular disorders (including coronary insufficiency and hypertension), hyperthyroidism, diabetes, or sensitivity to sympathomimetic amines
Concurrent use of epinephrine	May result in serious arrhythmias; however, if desired, both drugs may be alternated, provided that at least 4 h have elapsed between doses

ADVERSE REACTIONS
Essentially none at therapeutic dosages

OVERDOSAGE

Signs and symptoms	Tachycardia with resultant coronary insufficiency, palpitations, vertigo, nausea, tremors, headache, insomnia, central excitation, blood-pressure changes

MEDIHALER-ISO ■ METAPREL Inhalant Solution and Metered Dose Inhaler

| Treatment | Discontinue medication; treat symptomatically and institute supportive measures, as required |

DRUG INTERACTIONS

| Epinephrine | △ Cardiac activity and risk of arrhythmias |
| Nonselective beta blockers | ▽ Bronchodilation |

ALTERED LABORATORY VALUES

No clinically significant alterations in blood/serum or urinary values occur at therapeutic dosages

---

USE IN CHILDREN

See INDICATIONS and dosage recommendations (the lower dosage should be used); any child who is old enough to effectively coordinate his or her respiration to the aerosol device may use this product

USE IN PREGNANT AND NURSING WOMEN

Safety for use in pregnant or nursing women has not been established, although there has been no evidence of teratogenicity

---

INHALANT BRONCHODILATORS / ANTIASTHMATIC AGENTS

METAPREL Inhalant Solution (metaproterenol sulfate) Sandoz Pharmaceuticals Rx

Solution: 5% (10 ml)

INDICATIONS	INHALANT DOSAGE
Bronchial asthma **Reversible bronchospasm** associated with bronchitis and emphysema	**Adult:** 5–15 inhalations (usually 10) of undiluted solution, given in a single dose via hand nebulizer, or 0.2–0.3 ml (usually 0.3 ml), diluted in approximately 2.5 ml of saline solution or other diluent and administered in a single dose by IPPB

METAPREL Metered Dose Inhaler (metaproterenol sulfate) Sandoz Pharmaceuticals Rx

Metered-dose inhaler: 0.65 mg/inhalation

INDICATIONS	INHALANT DOSAGE
Same as Metaprel Inhalant Solution	**Adult:** 2–3 inhalations q3–4h, up to 12 inhalations/day if needed

CONTRAINDICATIONS

Hypersensitivity to metaproterenol sulfate

Cardiac arrhythmias associated with tachycardia

ADMINISTRATION/DOSAGE ADJUSTMENTS

| Dosage frequency | Repeated administration of the inhalant solution more often than q4h is usually unnecessary for acute bronchospastic attacks; for chronic bronchospastic disease, administer tid or qid |

WARNINGS/PRECAUTIONS

Excessive use	May be dangerous; cardiac arrest and fatalities have occurred. Repeated excessive administration may lead to paradoxical bronchoconstriction.
Lack of therapeutic response	Advise patient to report any failure to respond to usual doses
Special-risk patients	Use with great caution in patients with hypertension, coronary artery disease, congestive heart failure, hyperthyroidism, diabetes, or sensitivity to sympathomimetic amines

ADVERSE REACTIONS

Frequent reactions (incidence ≥ 1%) are printed in *italics*

Cardiovascular	*Tachycardia (14.3%)*, hypertension, palpitations
Central nervous system	*Nervousness (14.3%)*, *tremor (5.0%)*
Gastrointestinal	*Nausea (2.0%)*, vomiting, bad taste

OVERDOSAGE

| Signs and symptoms | Excessive beta-adrenergic stimulation (see ADVERSE REACTIONS) |
| Treatment | Reduce dosage and/or frequency of administration |

METAPREL Inhalant Solution and Metered Dose Inhaler ■ MUCOMYST

DRUG INTERACTIONS

Sympathomimetic agents	△ Adrenergic effects; allow sufficient time to elapse between use of metaproterenol and administration of other sympathomimetic agents. If metaproterenol is given in combination with another adrenergic agent, exercise extreme care.
Nonselective beta blockers	▽ Bronchodilation

ALTERED LABORATORY VALUES
No clinically significant alterations in blood/serum or urinary values occur at therapeutic dosages

USE IN CHILDREN
Not recommended for use in children under 12 yr of age

USE IN PREGNANT AND NURSING WOMEN
Pregnancy Category C: use during pregnancy only if expected benefit of therapy justifies the potential fetal risk. Teratogenicity and embryocidal effects have been observed in rabbits at oral doses of 100 mg/kg (620 times the human inhalation dose). These effects have not occurred in mice, rats, or rabbits given oral doses of 50 mg/kg (310 times the human inhalation dose). No adequate, well-controlled studies have been done in pregnant women. No information is available on excretion of metaproterenol in human milk; use with caution in nursing mothers.

INHALANT BRONCHODILATORS/ ANTIASTHMATIC AGENTS

MUCOMYST (acetylcysteine) Bristol   Rx
Vials: 10% (Mucomyst-10) (4, 10, 30 ml), 20% (4, 10, 30 ml)

INDICATIONS	INHALANT DOSAGE	INTRATRACHEAL DOSAGE
Abnormal, viscid, or inspissated mucous secretions associated with or resulting from bronchopulmonary disease, cystic fibrosis, surgery, anesthesia, post-traumatic chest conditions, atelectasis, tracheostomy, and similar conditions	**Adult and child:** for nebulization into a face mask, mouth piece, or tracheostomy, 1–10 ml of the 20% solution or 2–20 ml of the 10% solution q2-6h (usual dosage: 3–5 ml of the 20% solution or 6–10 ml of the 10% solution tid or qid); for nebulization into a tent or Croupette, use a sufficient volume of the 10% or 20% solution (up to 300 ml) to maintain a very heavy mist for the desired period	**Adult and child:** for direct instillation, 1–2 ml of the 10% or 20% solution given as frequently as once every hour; for instillation in the routine care of patients with a tracheostomy, 1–2 ml of the 10% or 20% solution q1–4h; for instillation into a particular bronchopulmonary segment with an intratracheal catheter, 2–5 ml of the 20% solution; for instillation with a percutaneous intratracheal catheter, 1–2 ml of the 20% solution or 2–4 ml of the 10% solution q1–4h
Abnormal, viscid, or inspissated mucous secretions that may interfere with diagnostic bronchial studies, eg, bronchograms, bronchospirometry, and bronchial wedge catheterization	**Adult and child:** 1–2 ml of the 20% solution or 2–4 ml of the 10% solution given by nebulization 2–3 times before the procedure	**Adult and child:** 1–2 ml of the 20% solution or 2–4 ml of the 10% solution instilled 2–3 times before the procedure
Prevention or reduction of hepatotoxicity associated with **acetaminophen overdose**	**ORAL DOSAGE** **Adult and child:** 140 mg/kg, given as a loading dose within 24 h of ingestion, followed by 70 mg/kg, starting 4 h after the loading dose and repeated q4h for 17 doses (unless the serum acetaminophen level indicates minimal risk of hepatotoxicity [see table in ADMINISTRATION/DOSAGE ADJUSTMENTS])	

CONTRAINDICATIONS
Hypersensitivity to acetylcysteine (when used as a mucolytic agent)

ADMINISTRATION/DOSAGE ADJUSTMENTS
When used as a mucolytic agent

Preparation of solution	The 20% solution may be diluted with sterile normal saline or sterile water for injection USP; the 10% solution may be used undiluted. Do not mix either solution with amphotericin B, tetracycline, oxytetracycline, chlortetracycline, ampicillin, erythromycin lactobionate, iodized oil, trypsin, chymotrypsin, or hydrogen peroxide. After a vial is opened, the solution may turn light purple; this change will not significantly affect the safety or effectiveness of the drug. Unused portions should be stored under refrigeration and used within 96 h.
Nebulizing equipment	For aerosol administration, use a conventional mechanical nebulizer made of plastic or glass that produces a high proportion of particles less than 10 μ in diameter; the parts that come into contact with the solution may contain plain or anodized aluminum, chromed metal, tantalum, sterling silver, or stainless steel, but should not contain any other material (especially rubber, iron, or copper). Although hand bulbs may also be used, they are not recommended for routine administration, since their output is generally too low and, in some cases, the particles they produce are too large. For delivery of the solution, compressed tank air or an air compressor is recommended (oxygen may also be used, but with caution in patients with severe respiratory disease and CO_2 retention). To provide a warm mist, add the solution to a separate unheated nebulizer that is attached to an apparatus containing a heated nebulizer; do not place the solution directly into the chamber of a heated nebulizer. Nebulizing equipment should be cleaned immediately after use to avoid accumulation of residues that may clog the fine orifices or corrode the metal parts.

MUCOMYST

Prolonged nebulization	Delivery of the drug may be impeded during prolonged nebulization because of an increase in concentration of the solution as the solvent evaporates; after 75% of the initial volume of solution has been given, dilute the remaining volume 1 : 1 with sterile water for injection USP

When used as an antidote

Initial treatment of acetaminophen overdose	Promptly empty stomach by performing gastric lavage or inducing emesis with syrup of ipecac (15–30 ml for children, 30–45 ml for adults). Give ipecac with copious quantities of water; if emesis does not occur within 20 min, repeat the dose. Activated charcoal may be given if acetaminophen has been ingested with certain other drugs, but should be removed by lavage prior to administration of acetylcysteine. Avoid forced diuresis or use of diuretics when treating acetaminophen overdose.
Preparation of acetylcysteine	Dilute the 20% solution 1 : 4 with cola, Fresca, or other soft drink (water may be used as a diluent for administration by gastric tube or Miller-Abbott tube); use the solution within 1 h of preparation
Administration	Start treatment as soon as possible; each dose should be given orally. If vomiting occurs within 1 h of administration, repeat the dose. If the patient persistently fails to retain the antidote after oral administration, the diluted solution may be given by duodenal intubation.
Laboratory testing	Measure the serum level of *unconjugated* acetaminophen as early as possible, but no sooner than 4 h after an acute overdose; when possible, this should be done by gas-liquid or high-pressure liquid chromatography, although a colorimetric assay may also be used. Do not wait for laboratory results to become available before starting acetylcysteine. If the serum level equals or exceeds the value listed in the table below (or if the serum level cannot be obtained), continue giving the entire 18-dose course; if the serum level is less than the value listed below, administration can be stopped.

Time after ingestion (h)	Plasma acetaminophen level (μg/ml)	Time after ingestion (h)	Plasma acetaminophen level (μg/ml)
4.0	150.0	14.0	25.5
4.5	135.0	15.0	21.5
5.0	125.0	16.0	18.0
6.0	105.0	17.0	15.0
7.0	88.0	18.0	12.5
8.0	74.0	19.0	10.5
9.0	62.0	20.0	8.8
10.0	52.0	21.0	7.4
11.0	46.0	22.0	6.3
12.0	36.0	23.0	5.2
13.0	30.5	24.0	4.4

To monitor hepatic and renal function and electrolyte and fluid balance, determine the prothrombin time, SGOT and SGPT levels, and serum concentrations of bilirubin, creatinine, BUN, glucose, and electrolytes q24h. If the prothrombin time exceeds 1.5 times the control value, give vitamin K_1; if the prothrombin time exceeds 3 times the control value, give fresh frozen plasma. Institute appropriate measures to treat hypoglycemia and electrolyte and fluid imbalance.

WARNINGS/PRECAUTIONS

When used as a mucolytic agent

Airway obstruction	Acetylcysteine may block the airway by causing an increase in the volume of liquefied bronchial secretions. If local accumulation cannot be removed by coughing, provide mechanical suction; if a large mechanical block develops (owing to local accumulation or the presence of a foreign body), clear the airway by endotracheal aspiration, with or without bronchoscopy.
Bronchospasm	Carefully monitor asthmatic patients; if bronchospasm occurs, immediately discontinue acetylcysteine and administer a bronchodilator
Odor, stickiness	A slight transient odor may be detected when beginning administration; stickiness may develop with use of a face mask, but can be easily removed with water

When used as an antidote

Hypersensitivity	If generalized urticaria or other allergic reactions occur, discontinue acetylcysteine unless the drug is essential and the reaction can be controlled
Encephalopathy	Acetylcysteine can theoretically exacerbate hepatic failure; if encephalopathy owing to hepatic failure becomes evident, the drug should be discontinued
Upper GI reactions	Acetylcysteine can exacerbate acetaminophen-induced vomiting; the benefit of preventing or lessening hepatic injury should be weighed against the risk of inducing GI bleeding before administering acetylcysteine to patients susceptible to upper GI hemorrhage (eg, patients with peptic ulcers or esophageal varices)

MUCOMYST ■ PROVENTIL Inhaler

ADVERSE REACTIONS

When used as a mucolytic agent

Respiratory	Bronchospasm, rhinorrhea
Other	Stomatitis, nausea, sensitivity, sensitization

When used as an antidote

Gastrointestinal	Nausea, vomiting, other GI reactions
Hypersensitivity	Rash with or without mild fever (rare)

DRUG INTERACTIONS

Activated charcoal	▽ Bioavailability of oral acetylcysteine
Amphotericin B, tetracycline, oxytetracycline, chlortetracycline, ampicillin, erythromycin lactobionate, iodized oil, trypsin, chymotrypsin, hydrogen peroxide	Physical incompatibility (with mucolytic solutions of acetylcysteine)

ALTERED LABORATORY VALUES

No clinically significant alterations in blood/serum or urinary values occur at therapeutic dosages

---

USE IN CHILDREN
See INDICATIONS and dosage recommendations

USE IN PREGNANT AND NURSING WOMEN
Consult manufacturer

INHALANT BRONCHODILATORS/ ANTIASTHMATIC AGENTS

PROVENTIL Inhaler (albuterol) Schering   Rx

Metered-dose inhaler: 90 µg/inhalation (17 g)

INDICATIONS	INHALANT DOSAGE
Management of **bronchospasm** associated with reversible obstructive airway disease	**Adult:** for treatment of acute episodes of bronchospasm or prevention of asthmatic symptoms, 2 inhalations q4-6h, as needed (some patients may require only 1 inhalation q4h); for maintenance therapy or prevention of exacerbation of bronchospasm, 2 inhalations qid **Child ($\geq$ 12 yr):** same as adult
Prevention of **exercise-induced bronchospasm**	**Adult:** 2 inhalations 15 min before exercise **Child ($\geq$ 12 yr):** same as adult

CONTRAINDICATIONS

Hypersensitivity to any component

WARNINGS/PRECAUTIONS

Paradoxical bronchospasm	May occur; discontinue use immediately and institute alternative therapy
Excessive use	Caution patient not to use inhaler more often than q4h or exceed 2 inhalations at a time; excessive use of inhalant sympathomimetics may lead unexpectedly to the development of severe status asthmaticus and subsequent hypoxia, cardiac arrest, and death
Special-risk patients	Although at recommended dosages albuterol has less effect than isoproterenol on the cardiovascular system, it should be used with caution in patients with cardiovascular disorders (including coronary insufficiency and hypertension), hyperthyroidism, or diabetes mellitus and in patients who are unusually sensitive to the actions of sympathomimetic amines or who are being treated concurrently with MAO inhibitors or tricyclic antidepressants (see DRUG INTERACTIONS)
Preexisting diabetes and ketoacidosis	Are reportedly aggravated by large IV doses of albuterol; relevance to use of inhaler at recommended dosage is unknown, since the aerosol dose is much lower than the doses given IV

ADVERSE REACTIONS

Frequent reactions (incidence $\geq$ 1%) are printed in *italics*

Cardiovascular	*Tachycardia (10%), palpitations (< 10%), increased blood pressure (< 5%)*, hypertension, angina

COMPENDIUM OF DRUG THERAPY

PROVENTIL Inhaler ■ RESPIHALER DECADRON Phosphate

Central nervous system	*Tremor (< 15%), nervousness (< 10%), dizziness (5%)*, vertigo, stimulation, insomnia, headache
Gastrointestinal	*Nausea (< 15%), heartburn (< 5%)*, vomiting
Respiratory	Bronchospasm (rare)
Dermatological	Urticaria, angioedema, and rash (rare)
Oropharyngeal	Unusual taste sensation, drying or irritation of oropharynx; oropharyngeal edema (rare)

OVERDOSAGE

Signs and symptoms	Angina, hypertension, intensification of other adverse effects seen at therapeutic doses, cardiac arrest
Treatment	Discontinue medication immediately; judicious use of a cardioselective beta blocker (eg, metoprolol) may reverse the effects of albuterol, but at the risk of inducing an asthmatic attack. Do not use dialysis.

DRUG INTERACTIONS

Other sympathomimetic aerosol bronchodilators	△ Risk of toxicity; do not use concomitantly
Other adrenergic drugs; MAO inhibitors, tricyclic antidepressants	△ Risk of sympathomimetic toxicity; exercise caution
Beta-adrenergic blocking agents	▽ Pharmacologic effects of both drugs

ALTERED LABORATORY VALUES

No clinically significant alterations in blood/serum or urinary values occur at therapeutic dosages

---

USE IN CHILDREN

Safety and effectiveness have not been established for use in children under 12 yr of age

USE IN PREGNANT AND NURSING WOMEN

Pregnancy Category C: use during pregnancy only when expected benefit outweighs potential risk to the fetus. Albuterol is teratogenic in mice at doses 14 times the human dose. No adequate, well-controlled studies have been done in pregnant women. High IV doses inhibit uterine contractions, but this is extremely unlikely to result from aerosol use. It is not known whether albuterol is excreted in human milk; because of the potential for tumorigenicity shown in animal studies, a decision should be made to discontinue nursing or use of the drug.

INHALANT BRONCHODILATORS/ANTIASTHMATIC AGENTS

RESPIHALER DECADRON Phosphate (dexamethasone sodium phosphate) Merck Sharp & Dohme   Rx

Metered-dose oral inhaler: 0.1 mg/inhalation

INDICATIONS

Bronchial asthma and related corticosteroid-responsive bronchospastic states intractable to an adequate trial of conventional therapy

INHALANT DOSAGE

Adult: 3 inhalations tid or qid, not to exceed 3 inhalations/dose or 12 inhalations/day
Child: 2 inhalations tid or qid, not to exceed 2 inhalations/dose or 8 inhalations/day

CONTRAINDICATIONS

Persistently positive *Candida albicans* sputum cultures	Systemic fungal infections	Hypersensitivity to any component

ADMINISTRATION/DOSAGE ADJUSTMENTS

Selection of patients	Consider use only for (1) patients not on corticosteroid therapy who have not responded adequately to other treatment and (2) patients on systemic steroid therapy in an attempt to reduce or eliminate systemic administration
Concomitant use of systemic corticosteroids	Reduce or eliminate systemic corticosteroids before reducing Respihaler dosage; to avoid withdrawal symptoms, reduce systemic steroid therapy gradually

WARNINGS/PRECAUTIONS

Unwarranted uses	Not recommended for the treatment of occasional, mild, isolated asthmatic attacks responsive to epinephrine, isoproterenol, aminophylline, or other drugs, or for severe status asthmaticus requiring intensive measures

RESPIHALER DECADRON Phosphate

Laryngeal and pharyngeal fungal infections	May occur on rare occasions; discontinue medication and institute antifungal therapy
Systemic absorption	Although low, may lead to adrenal suppression or other systemic effects
Patients subjected to unusual stress	Require increased dosage of rapidly acting corticosteroids before, during, and after emotionally or physically stressful situations
Infection	Clinical signs may be masked, new infections may appear, resistance may be decreased, and infections may be difficult to localize; false-negative results may be obtained with nitroblue-tetrazolium test for bacterial infection
Latent amebiasis	May be activated; before instituting therapy, rule out latent or active amebiasis in any patient with unexplained diarrhea or who has spent time in the tropics
Ocular damage	Prolonged use may produce posterior subcapsular cataracts and glaucoma, with possible damage to optic nerves, and may enhance development of secondary fungal or viral ocular infections
Dietary salt restriction and potassium supplementation	May be necessary to combat blood-pressure elevation, salt and water retention, and increased potassium excretion with average- and high-dose therapy
Immunization procedures	The expected serum antibody response to inactivated viral or bacterial vaccines may not be obtained in patients receiving immunosuppressive doses; such patients must not be given live virus vaccines, including smallpox vaccine
Latent tuberculosis or tuberculin reactivity	Observe patient closely, since reactivation of the disease may occur during prolonged therapy; employ antituberculous chemoprophylactic measures
Secondary adrenocortical insufficiency	May be minimized by gradual dosage reduction; since insufficiency may persist for months, reinstitute corticosteroid therapy in any stressful situation during this period, and administer salt and/or a mineralocorticoid concurrently to correct impaired mineralocorticoid secretion
Withdrawal symptoms	Including fever, myalgia, arthralgia, and malaise, may occur when drug is withdrawn following prolonged therapy, even in the absence of adrenal insufficiency
Hypothyroidism, hepatic cirrhosis	May enhance effects of dexamethasone
Corneal perforation	May occur in patients with ocular herpes simplex; use with caution
Special-risk patients	Use with caution in patients with nonspecific ulcerative colitis if impending perforation, abscess, or other pyogenic infection is likely, as well as in patients with diverticulitis, fresh intestinal anastomoses, active or latent peptic ulcer, renal insufficiency, hypertension, osteoporosis, or myasthenia gravis. In patients receiving large doses, signs of peritoneal irritation following GI perforation may be minimal or absent.
Psychic derangements	May appear, ranging from euphoria, insomnia, mood swings, personality changes, and severe depression to frank psychotic manifestations; existing emotional instability or psychotic tendencies may be aggravated
Concomitant use with aspirin	Use with caution in patients with hypoprothrombinemia during therapy
Concomitant use with oral anticoagulants	Check prothrombin time frequently; anticoagulant effect may be increased or decreased
Concomitant use with potassium-depleting diuretics	Monitor serum potassium level periodically; risk of hypokalemia is increased
Fertility	Motility and number of spermatozoa may be increased or decreased

ADVERSE REACTIONS

Respiratory	Throat irritation, hoarseness, cough, laryngeal and pharyngeal fungal infections
Fluid and electrolyte disturbances	Sodium retention, fluid retention, congestive heart failure in susceptible patients, loss of potassium, hypokalemic alkalosis, hypertension
Musculoskeletal	Muscle weakness, steroid myopathy, loss of muscle mass, osteoporosis, vertebral compression fractures, aseptic necrosis of femoral and humeral heads, pathological fracture of long bones, tendon rupture
Gastrointestinal	Peptic ulcer with possible perforation and hemorrhage, pancreatitis, abdominal distention, ulcerative esophagitis, increased appetite, nausea; perforation of the large and small bowel (particularly in patients with inflammatory bowel disease)
Dermatological	Impaired wound healing, thin fragile skin, petechiae and ecchymoses, erythema, increased sweating, suppressed reaction to skin tests, allergic dermatitis, urticaria, angioneurotic edema
Neurological	Convulsions, increased intracranial pressure with papilledema (pseudotumor cerebri), vertigo, headache, psychic disturbances
Endocrinological	Menstrual irregularities, Cushingoid state, growth suppression in children, secondary adrenocortical and pituitary unresponsiveness, decreased carbohydrate tolerance, latent diabetes mellitus, increased insulin or oral hypoglycemic requirements
Ophthalmic	Posterior subcapsular cataracts, increased intraocular pressure, glaucoma, exophthalmos

RESPIHALER DECADRON Phosphate ■ TORNALATE

Metabolic	Negative nitrogen balance, weight gain
Other	Hypersensitivity reactions, thromboembolism, malaise

OVERDOSAGE

Signs and symptoms	See ADVERSE REACTIONS
Treatment	Discontinue medication; treat symptomatically and institute supportive measures, as required

DRUG INTERACTIONS

Insulin, oral hypoglycemics	△ Hypoglycemic effect
Phenytoin, phenobarbital, ephedrine, rifampin	△ Metabolic clearance of dexamethasone ▽ Steroid blood level and physiological activity
Oral anticoagulants	△ or ▽ Prothrombin time
Potassium-depleting diuretics	△ Risk of hypokalemia
Cardiac glycosides	△ Risk of arrhythmias or digitalis toxicity secondary to hypokalemia
Skin-test antigens	▽ Reactivity
Immunizations	▽ Antibody response

ALTERED LABORATORY VALUES

Blood/serum values	△ Glucose △ Cholesterol △ Sodium △ Potassium ▽ Calcium ▽ PBI ▽ Thyroxine (T_4) ▽ ^{131}I thyroid uptake ▽ Uric acid
Urinary values	△ Glucose △ Potassium △ Calcium △ Uric acid ▽ 17-Hydroxycorticosteroids (17-OHCS) ▽ 17-Ketosteroids

USE IN CHILDREN

Growth and development should be carefully observed in infants and children on prolonged therapy

USE IN PREGNANT AND NURSING WOMEN

Safety for use during pregnancy has not been established. Infants born of mothers who have received substantial doses of corticosteroids during pregnancy should be carefully observed for signs of hypoadrenalism. Corticosteroids appear in breast milk and may suppress growth, interfere with endogenous corticosteroid production, or cause other untoward effects. Patient should stop nursing if drug is prescribed.

INHALANT BRONCHODILATORS/ ANTIASTHMATIC AGENTS

TORNALATE (bitolterol mesylate) Winthrop-Breon Rx

Metered-dose oral inhaler: 370 µg/inhalation

INDICATIONS

Bronchial asthma
Reversible bronchospasm

INHALANT DOSAGE

Adult: for prevention of bronchospasm, 2 inhalations q8h; for relief of bronchospasm, 2 or, if necessary, 3 inhalations. Do not exceed 3 inhalations q6h or 2 inhalations q4h. Allow at least 1–3 min between each inhalation.
Child (> 12 yr): same as adult

CONTRAINDICATIONS

Hypersensitivity to any component

WARNINGS/PRECAUTIONS

Paradoxical bronchospasm, hypersensitivity	Discontinue use immediately and institute appropriate measures if paradoxical bronchospasm or an immediate-type hypersensitivity reaction occurs
Excessive use	Caution patients to adhere strictly to the recommended dosage and to avoid excessive use
Special-risk patients	Use with caution in patients with diabetes mellitus, hyperthyroidism, or a cardiovascular disease such as hypertension, arrhythmia, or ischemic heart disease; beta-adrenergic agonists may cause an increase in heart rate as well as other cardiotoxic effects and may produce a significant change in blood pressure. Caution should also be exercised in patients with convulsive disorders or sensitivity to beta-adrenergic agonists.

TORNALATE ■ VANCERIL Inhaler

Carcinogenicity, mutagenicity, effect on fertility	No evidence of tumorigenicity has been seen in rats fed 23 or 114 times the maximum daily human inhalation dose for 2 yr or in mice fed up to 568 times this dose for 18 mo. The Ames test and the mouse lymphoma assay have shown no results indicating mutagenicity. No significant effect on fertility has been observed in rats at doses of up to 364 times the maximum daily human inhalation dose.

ADVERSE REACTIONS[1]

Frequent reactions (incidence ≥ 1%) are printed in *italics*

Central nervous system	*Tremors (14%), nervousness (5%), headache (4%), dizziness (3%), light-headedness (3%);* insomnia, hyperkinesia
Cardiovascular	*Palpitations (3%), chest discomfort (1%);* tachycardia; premature ventricular contractions and flushing (rare)
Respiratory	*Coughing (4%),* bronchospasm, dyspnea, chest tightness
Other	*Throat irritation (5%), nausea (3%)*

OVERDOSAGE

Signs and symptoms	See ADVERSE REACTIONS
Treatment	Institute supportive therapy; consider judicious use of a cardioselective beta-adrenergic blocker, bearing in mind the potential risk of profound bronchospasm

DRUG INTERACTIONS

Other inhalant beta-adrenergic bronchodilators	⇧ Sympathomimetic effects; this preparation should not be used with other inhalant beta-adrenergic bronchodilators
Theophylline, corticosteroids	⇧ Bronchodilation

ALTERED LABORATORY VALUES

No clinically significant alterations in blood/serum or urinary values occur at therapeutic dosages

USE IN CHILDREN

Safety and effectiveness for use in children 12 yr of age or younger have not been established

USE IN PREGNANT AND NURSING WOMEN

Pregnancy Category C: an increase in cleft palate has been detected in mice with SC administration of 23, 114, and 227 times the maximum daily human inhalation dose; no teratogenic effects have been seen in mice fed up to 284 times this dose or in rats and rabbits fed up to 557 times this dose. Use during pregnancy only if the expected benefit justifies the potential risk to the fetus. It is not known whether bitolterol or its active metabolite, colterol, is excreted in human milk; use with caution in nursing mothers.

VEHICLE/BASE

Metered-dose inhaler: 38% alcohol, dichlorodifluoromethane, dichlorotetrafluoroethane, ascorbic acid, saccharin, and menthol

[1] Reactions that occur rarely and for which a causal relationship has not been established include proteinuria, elevation of SGOT level, and decreases in platelet and WBC counts

---

INHALANT BRONCHODILATORS/ ANTIASTHMATIC AGENTS

VANCERIL Inhaler (beclomethasone dipropionate) Schering   Rx

Metered-dose inhaler: 42 µg/inhalation

INDICATIONS

Bronchial asthma requiring chronic corticosteroid therapy

INHALANT DOSAGE

Adult: 2 inhalations tid or qid, or up to 20 inhalations/24 h, if needed
Child (6–12 yr): 1–2 inhalations tid or qid, or up to 10 inhalations/24 h, if needed

CONTRAINDICATIONS

Primary treatment of status asthmaticus or other acute asthmatic episodes requiring intensive measures

Hypersensitivity to beclomethasone or other components

ADMINISTRATION/DOSAGE ADJUSTMENTS

Patients with severe asthma (adults)	Initiate therapy with 12–16 inhalations/day and adjust dosage downward according to response

VANCERIL Inhaler ■ VENTOLIN Inhaler

Concomitant use of inhalant bronchodilators	Use of bronchodilator before inhaler administration of beclomethasone enhances penetration of beclomethasone into bronchial tree. Allow several minutes to elapse before using beclomethasone inhaler to avoid toxicity from fluorocarbon propellants in both drugs.
Patients receiving systemic corticosteroids	Initially, use inhaler concurrently with usual dosage of systemic steroid. After 1 wk, *gradually* withdraw systemic steroid by reducing daily or alternate-day dose. Depending on response, continue gradually to withdraw systemic steroid by reducing dosage every 1–2 wk. Decrements generally should not exceed 2.5 mg of prednisone or its equivalent.
Patients experiencing steroid withdrawal symptoms (eg, joint or muscle pain, lassitude, depression)	Continue use of inhaler and observe patient closely for objective signs of adrenal insufficiency (eg, hypotension, weight loss); if signs appear, increase dose of systemic steroid temporarily and taper dosage more gradually
Exacerbation of asthma	Give short course of systemic steroid therapy; taper dosage gradually as symptoms subside

WARNINGS/PRECAUTIONS

Deaths due to adrenal insufficiency	Have occurred in asthmatic patients during and after transfer from systemic corticosteroids to beclomethasone inhaler therapy
Recovery of hypothalamic-pituitary-adrenal (HPA) function	Requires many months after withdrawal from systemic corticosteroids; during this HPA-suppressed period, signs and symptoms of adrenal insufficiency may appear in the presence of trauma, surgery, or infection, especially gastroenteritis
Stress periods or severe asthma attacks	Patients withdrawn from systemic steroids should immediately resume large doses of corticosteroids; these patients should carry a warning card indicating their need of supplementary systemic steroid therapy in case of stress or severe asthma attack
Assessing risk of adrenal insufficiency	Tests of adrenocortical function should be performed peridiocally, including measurement of early-morning resting cortisol levels
Fungal infections (*Candida albicans, Aspergillus niger*)	Frequently occur in mouth and pharynx and occasionally in larynx; up to 75% of patients may have positive oral *Candida* cultures. Antifungal treatment and discontinuation of inhaler therapy may be necessary.
Episodes of asthma unresponsive to treatment	Patients should report immediately any such episode during treatment; systemic corticosteroid therapy may be needed
Allergic reactions	In rare cases, beclomethasone inhaler therapy may precipitate immediate or delayed hypersensitivity reactions (see ADVERSE REACTIONS). Transfer from systemic corticosteroids to the inhaler may unmask previously suppressed allergic conditions such as rhinitis, conjunctivitis, and eczema. Pulmonary infiltrates with eosinophilia may result from inhaler therapy or, in some cases, may be manifested following transfer from systemic steroids.
Systemic steroid withdrawal symptoms	May occur during withdrawal from oral corticosteroid therapy (see ADMINISTRATION/DOSAGE ADJUSTMENTS)

ADVERSE REACTIONS[1]

Endocrinological	Suppression of hypothalamic-pituitary-adrenal function
Hypersensitivity	Urticaria, angiodema, rash, and bronchospasm (rare)
Other	Hoarseness, dry mouth; rash (rare)

OVERDOSAGE

Signs and symptoms	See WARNINGS/PRECAUTIONS
Treatment	Discontinue medication; reinstitute systemic steroid therapy, if needed

DRUG INTERACTIONS
No clinically significant drug interactions have been identified

ALTERED LABORATORY VALUES
No clinically significant alterations in blood/serum or urinary values occur at therapeutic dosages

---

USE IN CHILDREN

See INDICATIONS and INHALANT DOSAGE; not recommended for use in children under 6 yr of age

USE IN PREGNANT AND NURSING WOMEN

Safety for use in pregnant or nursing women has not been established. Glucocorticoids, including beclomethasone, are known teratogens in rodent species. Infants born to mothers who received substantial corticosteroid dosages during pregnancy should be carefully observed for hypoadrenalism. Glucocorticoids are excreted in human milk.

---

[1] Long-term effects in humans are unknown

INHALANT BRONCHODILATORS/ANTIASTHMATIC AGENTS

VENTOLIN Inhaler (albuterol) Glaxo Rx
Metered-dose inhaler: 90 µg/inhalation (17 g)

INDICATIONS

Management of **bronchospasm** associated with reversible obstructive airway disease

INHALANT DOSAGE

Adult: 2 inhalations q4–6h, as needed; some patients may require only 1 inhalation q4h
Child ($\geq$ 12 yr): same as adult

VENTOLIN Inhaler ■ ADRENALIN

| Prevention of **exercise-induced bronchospasm** | **Adult:** 2 inhalations 15 min before exercise
Child (≥ 12 yr): same as adult |

CONTRAINDICATIONS
Hypersensitivity to any component

WARNINGS/PRECAUTIONS

Paradoxical bronchospasm	May occur; discontinue use immediately and institute alternative therapy
Excessive use	Caution patient not to use inhaler more often than q4h or exceed 2 inhalations at a time; excessive use of inhalant sympathomimetics may lead unexpectedly to the development of severe status asthmaticus and subsequent hypoxia, cardiac arrest, and death
Special-risk patients	Although at recommended dosages albuterol has less effect than isoproterenol on the cardiovascular system, it should be used with caution in patients with cardiovascular disorders (including coronary insufficiency and hypertension), hyperthyroidism, or diabetes mellitus and in patients who are unusually sensitive to the actions of sympathomimetic amines or who are being treated concurrently with MAO inhibitors or tricyclic antidepressants (see DRUG INTERACTIONS)
Preexisting diabetes and ketoacidosis	Are reportedly aggravated by large IV doses of albuterol; relevance to use of inhaler at recommended dosage is unknown, since the aerosol dose is much lower than the doses given IV

ADVERSE REACTIONS
Frequent reactions (incidence ≥ 1%) are printed in *italics*

Cardiovascular	*Tachycardia (10%), palpitations (< 10%), increased blood pressure (< 5%),* hypertension, angina
Central nervous system	*Tremor (< 15%), nervousness (< 10%), dizziness (< 5%),* vertigo, stimulation, insomnia, headache
Gastrointestinal	*Nausea (< 15%), heartburn (< 5%),* vomiting
Oropharyngeal	Unusual taste sensation, drying or irritation of oropharynx

OVERDOSAGE

Signs and symptoms	See ADVERSE REACTIONS; anginal pain; hypertension
Treatment	Discontinue medication immediately; judicious use of a cardioselective beta blocker (eg, metoprolol) may reverse the effects of albuterol, but at the risk of inducing an asthmatic attack. Do not use dialysis.

DRUG INTERACTIONS

Epinephrine, other sympathomimetic aerosol bronchodilators	△ Sympathomimetic effects and risk of toxicity; do not use concomitantly
MAO inhibitors, tricyclic antidepressants	△ Cardiovascular effects of albuterol; use with caution
Beta-adrenergic blocking agents	▽ Pharmacologic effects of both drugs

ALTERED LABORATORY VALUES
No clinically significant alterations in blood/serum or urinary values occur at therapeutic dosages

---

USE IN CHILDREN

Safety and effectiveness have not been established for use in children under 12 yr of age

---

USE IN PREGNANT AND NURSING WOMEN

Pregnancy Category C: use during pregnancy only when expected benefit outweighs potential risk to the fetus. Albuterol is teratogenic in mice at doses 14 times the human dose. No adequate, well-controlled studies have been done in pregnant women. High IV doses inhibit uterine contractions, but this is extremely unlikely to result from aerosol use. It is not known whether albuterol is excreted in human milk; because of the potential for tumorigenicity shown in animal studies, a decision should be made to discontinue nursing or use of the drug.

SYSTEMIC BRONCHODILATORS/ANTIASTHMATIC AGENTS

ADRENALIN (epinephrine hydrochloride) Parke-Davis   Rx

Ampuls: 1 mg/ml (1 ml)   **Vials:** 1 mg/ml (30 ml)

INDICATIONS	**PARENTERAL DOSAGE**[1]
Bronchial asthma; bronchospasm; angioedema, urticaria, and other **hypersensitivity reactions** to drugs or other allergens	**Adult:** 0.2–0.5 mg SC, repeated every 20 min to 4 h, as needed; in severe cases, up to 1 mg/dose may be given **Child:** 0.01 mg/kg or 0.3 mg/m² SC q4h, as needed; in severe cases, up to 0.5 mg/dose may be given

COMPENDIUM OF DRUG THERAPY

ADRENALIN

Anaphylactic shock	**Adult:** 0.2–0.5 mg SC or IM, repeated every 10–15 min, as needed; in severe cases, up to 1 mg/dose may be given **Child:** 0.01 mg/kg or 0.3 mg/m² SC, repeated every 15 min for two doses, then q4h, as needed; in severe cases, up to 0.5 mg/dose may be given
Cardiopulmonary resuscitation, when electrical or electromechanical methods fail	**Adult:** 0.5 mg (0.5 ml diluted to 10 ml with Sodium Chloride Injection USP) IV or intracardially, repeated every 5 min, as needed; follow intracardial administration with external cardiac massage to permit drug to enter coronary circulation **Child:** 0.005–0.01 mg/kg or 0.15–0.3 mg/m², administered as in adults
Vasopression and syncope due to complete heart block or carotid sinus hypersensitivity	**Adult:** 0.5 mg SC or IM, followed by 0.025–0.05 mg IV every 5–15 min, as needed; alternatively, 0.1–0.25 mg by slow IV injection or 0.01–0.1 µg/kg/min by IV infusion **Child:** 0.3 mg IM or IV, repeated every 15 min for 3–4 doses, if needed, or 0.01–0.1 µg/kg/min by IV infusion
Prolongation of action of intraspinal anesthetics	**Adult:** 0.2–0.4 mg (0.2–0.4 ml of 1:1,000 solution in ampuls only) added to anesthetic spinal fluid mixture **Child:** same as adult
Prolongation of action of local anesthetics	**Adult:** 0.1–0.2 mg (0.1–0.2 ml) added to local anesthetic solution to a final concentration of 1:100,000 to 1:20,000 **Child:** same as adult

CONTRAINDICATIONS

Narrow angle (congestive) glaucoma	Coronary insufficiency	Shock
General anesthesia with halogenated hydrocarbons or cyclopropane	Cardiac dilatation	Organic brain damage
Local anesthesia of fingers or toes	Labor	

ADMINISTRATION/DOSAGE ADJUSTMENTS

Route of administration	The SC route is generally the preferred route, where a choice is indicated; if the drug is given IM, avoid the buttocks

WARNINGS/PRECAUTIONS

Pulmonary edema	May occur due to peripheral constriction and cardiac stimulation and can be fatal
Special-risk patients	Use with caution in elderly patients and those with cardiovascular disease, hypertension, diabetes, hyperthyroidism, or psychoneurosis; use with extreme caution in patients with long-standing bronchial asthma and emphysema who have degenerative heart disease
Anginal pain	May occur in patients with coronary insufficiency
Cerebrovascular hemorrhage	May occur with overdosage or inadvertent IV administration
Storage of solution	Protect from light; do not use if solution is brown or contains a precipitate

ADVERSE REACTIONS

Central nervous system	Anxiety, headache, fear (especially in hyperthyroid patients)
Cardiovascular	Palpitations (especially in hyperthyroid patients)
Local	Necrosis
Other	Epinephrine-fastness (with prolonged use)

OVERDOSAGE

Signs and symptoms	Cerebrovascular hemorrhage due to sharp rise in blood pressure; pulmonary edema resulting from peripheral constriction and cardiac stimulation
Treatment	Counteract excessive pressor effects with rapidly acting vasodilators, such as nitrites or alpha-adrenergic blocking agents

DRUG INTERACTIONS

Other sympathomimetics	⌂ Pressor effect and toxicity
Alpha-adrenergic blocking agents	Antagonism of vasoconstrictor effect of epinephrine
Beta-adrenergic blocking agents	Antagonism of cardiac stimulating and bronchodilating effects of epinephrine
Ergot alkaloids	Severe hypertension
Cyclopropane and halogenated hydrocarbon anesthetics, digitalis glycosides, mercurial diuretics	⌂ Risk of cardiac arrythmias
Tricyclic antidepressants, some antihistamines, thyroid hormones	⌂ Cardiac and cardiovascular effects of epinephrine

COMPENDIUM OF DRUG THERAPY

ADRENALIN ■ ALUPENT

Phenothiazines —————————— Severe hypotension

ALTERED LABORATORY VALUES

Blood/serum values —————————— ⇧ Glucose

No clinically significant alterations in urinary values occur at therapeutic dosages

USE IN CHILDREN
See INDICATIONS and PARENTERAL DOSAGE

USE IN PREGNANT AND NURSING WOMEN
Pregnancy Category C: use during pregnancy only if the expected benefit justifies the potential risk to the fetus. Teratogenic effects have been found in rats at doses approximately 25 times the human dose. No adequate, well-controlled studies have been done in pregnant women. Consult manufacturer for use in nursing mothers.

[1] Manufacturer's recommendations, supplemented, where appropriate, by dosage information from *AMA Drug Evaluations, 4th Ed* (American Medical Association, Chicago), *American Hospital Formulary Service* (American Society of Hospital Pharmacists, Washington, DC), and *United States Pharmacopeia Dispensing Information, 1982* (United States Pharmacopeial Convention, Inc, Rockville, Md); consult manufacturer for details regarding the use of epinephrine as a hemostat, nasal decongestant, uterine-muscle relaxant, and ophthalmologic agent

---

SYSTEMIC BRONCHODILATORS/ ANTIASTHMATIC AGENTS

ALUPENT (metaproterenol sulfate) Boehringer Ingelheim   Rx
Tablets: 10, 20 mg **Syrup (per 5 ml):** 10 mg (16 fl oz) *cherry-flavored*

INDICATIONS
Bronchial asthma
Reversible bronchospasm associated with bronchitis and emphysema

ORAL DOSAGE
Adult: 20 mg or 10 ml (2 tsp) tid or qid
Child (6–9 yr or < 60 lb): 10 mg or 5 ml (1 tsp) tid or qid
Child (> 9 yr or > 60 lb): 20 mg or 10 ml (2 tsp) tid or qid

CONTRAINDICATIONS
Cardiac arrhythmias associated with tachycardia

WARNINGS/PRECAUTIONS
Excessive use —————————— May be dangerous; cardiac arrest and fatalities have occurred. Repeated excessive administration may lead to paradoxical bronchoconstriction.

Lack of therapeutic response —————————— Advise patient to report any failure to respond to usual doses

Additional sympathomimetic agents —————————— Use with extreme caution; allow sufficient time before administering another sympathomimetic agent

Special-risk patients —————————— Use with great caution in patients with hypertension, coronary artery disease, congestive heart failure, hyperthyroidism, diabetes, or hypersensitivity to sympathomimetic amines

Carcinogenicity, mutagenicity, effect on fertility —————————— Long-term studies in mice and rats to evaluate the carcinogenic potential of this drug have not been completed; the mutagenic potential of this drug and its effect on fertility have not been studied

ADVERSE REACTIONS
The most frequent reactions, regardless of incidence, are printed in *italics*

Cardiovascular —————————— *Tachycardia (14%)*, hypertension, palpitations

Central nervous system —————————— *Nervousness (14%)*, *tremor (5%)*

Gastrointestinal —————————— *Nausea (2%)*, vomiting, bad taste

OVERDOSAGE
Signs and symptoms —————————— Excessive beta-adrenergic stimulation (see ADVERSE REACTIONS)

Treatment —————————— Reduce dosage and/or frequency of administration

DRUG INTERACTIONS
Sympathomimetic bronchodilators —————————— ⇧ Adrenergic effects

Nonselective beta-adrenergic blockers —————————— ⇩ Bronchodilation

ALTERED LABORATORY VALUES

No clinically significant alterations in blood/serum or urinary values occur at therapeutic dosages

USE IN CHILDREN

The tablets are not recommended for use in children under 6 yr of age. Limited experience with use of the syrup in children under 6 yr of age suggests a dosage of approximately 1.3–2.6 mg/kg/day.

USE IN PREGNANT AND NURSING WOMEN

Pregnancy Category C: use during pregnancy only if the expected benefit justifies the potential risk to the fetus. Teratogenic and embryocidal effects have been observed in rabbits at 62 times the human oral dose; however, these effects did not occur in rabbits, mice, or rats at 31 times the human oral dose. There are no adequate, well-controlled studies in pregnant women. It is not known whether metaproterenol is excreted in human milk. Use with caution in nursing mothers because many drugs are excreted in human milk.

SYSTEMIC BRONCHODILATORS/ANTIASTHMATIC AGENTS

AMINOPHYLLIN (aminophylline) Searle   Rx

Tablets: 100, 200 mg[1]

INDICATIONS

Asthma
Reversible bronchospasm associated with chronic bronchitis and emphysema

ORAL DOSAGE

Adult: 600–1,600 mg/day, given in 3–4 divided doses
Child: 12 mg/kg/24 h, given in 4 divided doses

CONTRAINDICATIONS

Hypersensitivity to aminophylline or theophylline | Current use of other xanthine medications | Active peptic ulcer disease

ADMINISTRATION/DOSAGE ADJUSTMENTS

Use of serum theophylline levels — Adjust dosage to maintain serum theophylline level between 10 and 20 μg/ml; levels > 20 μg/ml may produce toxicity

WARNINGS/PRECAUTIONS

Patients with congestive heart failure — Use with caution; serum theophylline levels may persist for prolonged periods after drug is discontinued

Peptic ulcer — May be exacerbated in patients with a history of peptic ulcer; use with caution. Chronic administration of high doses may result in GI irritation

Other special-risk patients — Use with caution in patients with severe cardiac disease, hypertension, hyperthyroidism, or acute myocardial injury

ADVERSE REACTIONS

Gastrointestinal — Nausea, vomiting; anorexia, GI distress, bitter aftertaste, dyspepsia, heavy feeling in the stomach

Central nervous system — Dizziness, vertigo, light-headedness, headache, nervousness, insomnia, agitation

Cardiovascular — Palpitations, tachycardia, flushing, extrasystoles

Respiratory — Tachypnea

Dermatological — Urticaria

OVERDOSAGE

Signs and symptoms — *Gastrointestinal:* nausea, vomiting, epigastric pain, hematemesis, and diarrhea. *Central nervous system:* in addition to ADVERSE REACTIONS listed above, hyperreflexia, fasciculations, and clonic and tonic convulsions. *Cardiovascular:* palpitations, tachycardia, flushing, extrasystoles, marked hypotension, and circulatory failure. *Respiratory:* tachypnea and respiratory arrest. *Renal:* albuminuria, microhematuria, and increased excretion of renal tubular cells. *Other:* syncope, collapse, fever, and dehydration.

Treatment — Discontinue drug immediately; perform gastric lavage and administer emetic medication following acute overdosage. Avoid use of sympathomimetic drugs. Administer fluids, oxygen, and other supportive measures to prevent hypotension, overcome dehydration, and correct acid/base imbalance. Control seizures with short-acting barbiturates, IV diazepam (0.1–0.3 mg/kg, up to 10 mg), or phenytoin. For hyperthermia, use a cooling blanket or give sponge baths, as needed. If respiratory depression occurs, maintain patent airway and institute artificial respiration. Monitor serum theophylline levels until they fall below 20 μg/ml.

AMINOPHYLLIN ■ BRETHINE

DRUG INTERACTIONS

Other xanthine derivatives	△ Risk of toxicity; do not administer concurrently
Lithium	△ Lithium excretion
Propranolol	Antagonism of pharmacologic effects of propranolol ▽ Bronchodilation
Cimetidine, clindamycin, erythromycin, lincomycin, troleandomycin	△ Theophylline serum level
Furosemide	△ Diuresis
Reserpine	Tachycardia
Chlordiazepoxide	Fatty acid metabolism
Ephedrine and possibly other sympathomimetic agents	△ Risk of toxicity

ALTERED LABORATORY VALUES

Blood/serum values	△ Glucose △ Uric acid (with Bittner and colorimetric methods) △ Bilirubin (with diazo tablet method)
Urinary values	△ Albumin △ Catecholamines

USE IN CHILDREN

See INDICATIONS and ORAL DOSAGE; some children may be unusually sensitive to aminophylline

USE IN PREGNANT AND NURSING WOMEN

Safety for use during pregnancy has not been established; use only if the expected benefit justifies the potential risk to the mother or fetus. Aminophylline is excreted in human milk; irritability in nursing infants has been reported.[1] Institute an alternative form of infant feeding if use of this drug is deemed essential.

[1] Yurchak AM, Jusko WJ: *Pediatrics* 57:518, 1976

[1] Each 100-mg tablet contains 79 mg of anhydrous theophylline; each 200-mg tablet contains 158 mg of anhydrous theophylline

---

SYSTEMIC BRONCHODILATORS/ANTIASTHMATIC AGENTS

BRETHINE (terbutaline sulfate) Geigy   Rx

Tablets: 2.5, 5 mg   **Ampuls:** 1 mg/ml (2 ml) for SC use only

INDICATIONS	ORAL DOSAGE	PARENTERAL DOSAGE
Bronchial asthma **Reversible bronchospasm** associated with bronchitis and emphysema	**Adult:** 5 mg tid (~ q6h) during waking hours, up to 15 mg/24 h **Adolescent (12–15 yr):** 2.5 mg tid during waking hours, up to 7.5 mg/24 h	**Adult:** 0.25 mg, injected SC into the lateral deltoid area; a second dose may be given after 15–30 min, if needed, but do not administer more than a total of 0.5 mg over a 4-h period

CONTRAINDICATIONS

Hypersensitivity to sympathomimetic amines

ADMINISTRATION/DOSAGE ADJUSTMENTS

Management of side effects	If side effects are particularly disturbing, reduce oral dosage to 2.5 mg tid
Preparation of other dosage forms	Use of the SC injection for preparing other dosage forms (eg, IV infusion) is inappropriate; sterility and accurate dosing cannot be assured unless the ampuls are used only as directed (see PARENTERAL DOSAGE)

WARNINGS/PRECAUTIONS

Special-risk patients	Use with caution in patients with diabetes, hypertension, hyperthyroidism, or a history of seizures and in cardiac patients, especially when arrhythmias are present. Large IV doses have been reported to exacerbate diabetes and ketoacidosis.
Concomitant use with other sympathomimetics	Because the combined cardiovascular effect of two sympathomimetics may be deleterious, concomitant use is not recommended; however, patients receiving chronic oral terbutaline therapy may use an aerosol-type sympathomimetic bronchodilator to relieve acute bronchospasm
Carcinogenicity, mutagenicity	Oral administration of 500, 5,000, and 20,000 times the human SC dose for 18 mo had no tumorigenic effect in NMRI mice; mutagenicity studies have not been done

ADVERSE REACTIONS

Frequent reactions (incidence ≥ 1%) are printed in *italics*

With oral use

Cardiovascular	Increase in heart rate, palpitations

BRETHINE ■ BRICANYL

Central nervous system	*Nervousness, tremor,* headache, drowsiness
Gastrointestinal	Nausea, vomiting
Other	Sweating, muscle cramps

With SC use

Cardiovascular	*Increase in heart rate, palpitations*
Central nervous system	*Nervousness, tremor, dizziness,* headache, anxiety
Gastrointestinal	Nausea, vomiting
Other	Muscle cramps

OVERDOSAGE

Signs and symptoms	Excessive beta-adrenergic stimulation (see ADVERSE REACTIONS)
Treatment	*For oral overdosage:* If patient is alert, induce emesis, followed by gastric lavage. If patient is unconscious, use a cuffed endotracheal tube to secure airway before starting gastric lavage; do not induce emesis. Instill a slurry of activated charcoal. *For parenteral overdosage:* Treat symptomatically. In either case, provide cardiac and respiratory support, as needed, and maintain respiratory exchange. Monitor patient until asymptomatic.

DRUG INTERACTIONS

Other sympathomimetic agents	⇧ Sympathomimetic effect

ALTERED LABORATORY VALUES

No clinically significant alterations in blood/serum or urinary values occur at therapeutic dosages

USE IN CHILDREN

See INDICATIONS and ORAL DOSAGE; not recommended for use in children under 12 yr of age because of insufficient clinical data

USE IN PREGNANT AND NURSING WOMEN

Tablets: Safety for use during pregnancy has not been established; however, no adverse effects on fetal development have been observed in animals. *Ampuls:* Pregnancy Category B: use during pregnancy only if clearly needed. Reproduction studies in mice and rats given up to 1,000 times the human dose have shown no evidence of impaired fertility or harm to the fetus; however, no adequate, well-controlled studies have been done in pregnant women. Serious adverse reactions may occur following parenteral administration to women in labor; these effects include increased heart rate in the fetus, hypoglycemia in the neonate, and transient hypokalemia, transient hyperglycemia, increased heart rate, and pulmonary edema in the mother. Do not use terbutaline for tocolysis.

SYSTEMIC BRONCHODILATORS/ ANTIASTHMATIC AGENTS

BRICANYL (terbutaline sulfate) Lakeside   Rx

Tablets: 2.5, 5 mg **Ampuls:** 1 mg/ml (2 ml) for SC use only

INDICATIONS	ORAL DOSAGE	PARENTERAL DOSAGE
Bronchial asthma **Reversible bronchospasm** associated with bronchitis and emphysema	**Adult:** 5 mg q6h during waking hours, up to 15 mg/24 h **Adolescent (12–15 yr):** 2.5 mg tid during waking hours, up to 7.5 mg/24 h	**Adult:** 0.25 mg, injected SC into the lateral deltoid area; a second dose may be given after 15–30 min, if needed, but do not administer more than a total of 0.5 mg over 4 h

CONTRAINDICATIONS

Hypersensitivity to sympathomimetic amines

ADMINISTRATION/DOSAGE ADJUSTMENTS

Management of side effects	If side effects are particularly disturbing, reduce oral dosage to 2.5 mg tid
Preparation of other dosage forms	Use of the SC injection for preparing other dosage forms (eg, IV infusion) is inappropriate; sterility and accurate dosing cannot be assured unless the ampuls are used only as directed (see PARENTERAL DOSAGE)

WARNINGS/PRECAUTIONS

Special-risk patients	Use with caution in patients with diabetes, hypertension, hyperthyroidism, or a history of seizures, and in cardiac patients, especially when arrhythmias are present

BRICANYL ■ BRONDECON

Concomitant use with other sympathomimetics	Because the combined cardiovascular effect of two sympathomimetics may be deleterious, concomitant use is not recommended; however, patients receiving chronic oral terbutaline therapy may use an aerosol-type sympathomimetic bronchodilator to relieve acute bronchospasm

ADVERSE REACTIONS

Frequent reactions (incidence ≥ 1%) are printed in *italics*

With oral use

Cardiovascular	Increase in heart rate, palpitations
Central nervous system	*Nervousness, tremor,* headache, drowsiness
Gastrointestinal	Nausea, vomiting
Other	Sweating, muscle cramps

With SC use

Cardiovascular	*Increase in heart rate, palpitations*
Central nervous system	*Nervousness, tremor, dizziness,* headache, anxiety
Gastrointestinal	Nausea, vomiting
Other	Muscle cramps

OVERDOSAGE

Signs and symptoms	Symptoms of excessive beta-adrenergic stimulation (see ADVERSE REACTIONS)
Treatment	*For oral overdosage:* If patient is alert, induce emesis, followed by gastric lavage. If patient is unconscious, use a cuffed endotracheal tube to secure airway before starting gastric lavage; do not induce emesis. Instill a slurry of activated charcoal. *For parenteral overdosage:* Treat symptomatically. In either case, provide cardiac and respiratory support, as needed, and maintain respiratory exchange. Monitor patient until asymptomatic.

DRUG INTERACTIONS

Other sympathomimetic agents	⇧ Sympathomimetic effect

ALTERED LABORATORY VALUES

No clinically significant alterations in blood/serum or urinary values occur at therapeutic dosages

USE IN CHILDREN

See INDICATIONS and ORAL DOSAGE; not recommended for use in children under 12 yr of age because of insufficient clinical data

USE IN PREGNANT AND NURSING WOMEN

Safety for use during pregnancy has not been established; however, no adverse effects on fetal development have been observed in animals. Serious adverse reactions have been reported following parenteral administration to women in labor; these effects have included transient hypokalemia and pulmonary edema in the mother and hypoglycemia in both the mother and neonate. Terbutaline, like other drugs, should not be used in pregnant or nursing women unless the expected therapeutic benefit outweighs the potential risk to the mother and child.

SYSTEMIC BRONCHODILATORS/ANTIASTHMATIC AGENTS

BRONDECON (oxtriphylline and guaifenesin) Parke-Davis Rx

Tablets: 200 mg oxtriphylline and 100 mg guaifenesin **Elixir (per 5 ml):** 100 mg oxtriphylline and 50 mg guaifenesin[1] (8, 16 fl oz) cherry flavored

INDICATIONS	ORAL DOSAGE
Bronchitis, bronchial asthma, asthmatic bronchitis, pulmonary emphysema, and other chronic obstructive pulmonary diseases (adjunctive therapy)	Adult: 1 tab or 10 ml (2 tsp) qid; adjust dosage as needed Child (2–12 yr): 5 ml (1 tsp)/60 lb qid; adjust dosage as needed

CONTRAINDICATIONS

None known

WARNINGS/PRECAUTIONS

Concurrent use of other xanthine-containing preparations	May lead to adverse reactions, particularly CNS stimulation in children

BRONDECON ■ BRONKODYL

ADVERSE REACTIONS

Gastrointestinal	Gastric distress
Cardiovascular	Palpitations
Central nervous system	Stimulation

OVERDOSAGE

Signs and symptoms — *Cardiovascular:* precordial pain, tachycardia, ventricular and other arrhythmias, hypotension, and, in extreme cases, severe shock, cardiovascular collapse, and death. *Gastrointestinal:* abdominal pain, nausea, persistent vomiting, and hematemesis. *Central nervous system:* headache, dizziness, restlessness, irritability, tremors, hyperactivity, and agitation, followed, in severe cases, by convulsions, drowsiness, coma, and death.

Treatment — If patient is conscious and seizures have occurred, induce emesis and administer a cathartic and activated charcoal. If patient is convulsing establish an airway and administer oxygen and IV diazepam (0.1–0.3 mg/kg, up to 10 mg). If patient is comatose following the occurrence of seizures, intubate immediately, using an endotracheal tube with an inflated cuff, and perform gastric lavage; introduce the cathartic and activated charcoal through a large-bore gastric lavage tube. Monitor vital signs, maintain blood pressure, and provide adequate hydration. Treat hypotension and shock by appropriate fluid replacement, avoiding the use of vasopressors, if possible. In general, oxtriphylline is metabolized sufficiently rapidly to preclude any additional benefit from dialysis; however, dialysis may be useful in the presence of congestive heart failure or hepatic dysfunction. Serial monitoring of the serum theophylline level is helpful in following the patient's course and in guiding further management.

DRUG INTERACTIONS

Other xanthine derivatives	△ Risk of toxicity; do not administer concurrently
Lithium	△ Lithium excretion
Propranolol	Antagonism of pharmacologic effects of propranolol ▽ Bronchodilation
Cimetidine, clindamycin, erythromycin, lincomycin, troleandomycin	△ Theophylline serum level
Furosemide	△ Diuresis
Reserpine	Tachycardia
Chlordiazepoxide	Fatty acid mobilization
Ephedrine and possibly other sympathomimetic bronchodilators	△ Risk of toxicity

ALTERED LABORATORY VALUES

Blood/serum values	△ Glucose △ Uric acid (with Bittner and colorimetric methods) △ Bilirubin (with diazo tablet method)
Urinary values	△ Albumin △ Catecholamines △ 5-HIAA (with nitrosonaphthol reagent method) △ VMA (with colorimetric methods)

USE IN CHILDREN

See INDICATIONS and ORAL DOSAGE; consult manufacturer for use in children under 2 yr of age

USE IN PREGNANT AND NURSING WOMEN

Consult manufacturer for use in pregnant or nursing women

---

[1] Contains 20% alcohol

SYSTEMIC BRONCHODILATORS/ANTIASTHMATIC AGENTS

BRONKODYL (theophylline, anhydrous) Winthrop-Breon   Rx

Capsules: 100, 200 mg

INDICATIONS

Acute, reversible bronchospasm associated with bronchial asthma, chronic bronchitis, and emphysema

ORAL DOSAGE[1]

Adult, nonsmoker: 6 mg/kg to start, followed by 3 mg/kg q6h for the next 12 h and then q8h for maintenance

Infant and child (6 mo to 9 yr): 6 mg/kg to start, followed by 4 mg/kg q4h for the next 12 h and then q6h for maintenance

Child (9–16 yr) and young adult smoker: 6 mg/kg to start, followed by 3 mg/kg q4h for the next 12 h and then q6h for maintenance

COMPENDIUM OF DRUG THERAPY

BRONKODYL

Chronic, reversible bronchospasm associated with bronchial asthma, chronic bronchitis, and emphysema	**Adult and child:** 16 mg/kg/day or 400 mg/day, whichever is less, given in 3–4 divided doses q6–8h to start, followed, if needed and tolerated, by an approximately 25% increase in dosage every 2–3 days, up to 24 mg/kg/day for children under 9 yr of age, 20 mg/kg/day for children 9–12 yr of age, 18 mg/kg/day for adolescents 12–16 yr of age, and 13 mg/kg/day or 900 mg/day, whichever is less, for patients over 16 yr of age (exceed maximum dosages only when serum levels are being measured); children generally require doses q6h

CONTRAINDICATIONS

Hypersensitivity to theophylline or other xanthine derivatives

ADMINISTRATION/DOSAGE ADJUSTMENTS

Dosage adjustment with measurement of serum levels	Monitoring of serum theophylline levels is recommended, particularly for titration of dosage. Check the peak serum level 1–2 h after the last dose; medication must have been taken at typical intervals, with no missed or added doses, for a period of 48 h prior to measurement. (Serum levels that are measured spectrophotometrically without prior chromatographic isolation may be falsely elevated when coffee, tea, acetaminophen, chocolate, or cola beverages have also been ingested.) Adjust dosage to maintain serum levels of 10–20 µg/ml; the risk of toxicity is significantly increased at higher levels, and, in some patients (eg, those with reduced theophylline clearance), toxic reactions may develop at serum concentrations of 15–20 µg/ml. If the peak level in patients with normal theophylline clearance is between 5 and 7.5 µg/ml, increase the total daily dose by 25%; if between 7.5 and 10 µg/ml, increase the daily dose by 25% and, if symptoms recur at the end of a dosing interval, administer more frequently; if between 20 and 25 µg/ml, reduce the daily dose by 10%; if between 25 and 30 µg/ml, omit the next dose and reduce the daily dose by 25%; if over 30 µg/ml, omit the next 2 doses and reduce the daily dose by 50%. Recheck serum levels after dosage adjustment and then every 6–12 mo thereafter. *Do not attempt to maintain any dosage that is not tolerated.* Patients should be instructed to omit the next dose if they experience adverse effects and to reduce the subsequent dosage when they resume therapy after the reactions have disappeared. Exercise caution when titrating dosage for younger children who cannot complain of minor adverse reactions.
Acute symptoms in patients currently receiving theophylline	Determine (where possible) the time, amount, route, and form of the patient's last dose. If it is not possible to obtain the patient's serum theophylline level quickly and there is sufficient respiratory distress to warrant a small risk, a loading dose may be given, based on the principle that each 0.5 mg/kg of theophylline administered in a rapidly absorbed form will increase the serum drug level by 1 µg/ml. Thus, if the patient is not already experiencing toxicity, a loading dose of 2.5 mg/kg (which will increase the serum level by 5 µg/ml) is unlikely to produce dangerous side effects. During therapy, closely watch for evidence of toxicity.
Patients with reduced theophylline clearance	To avoid toxic reactions in neonates, patients over 55 yr of age (especially men), and patients with renal or hepatic impairment, influenza, alcoholism, chronic lung disease, cor pulmonale, or cardiac failure, reduce the initial dosage and monitor serum theophylline levels. For acute symptoms requiring rapid theophyllinization, give older patients and patients with cor pulmonale 6 mg/kg to start, followed by 2 mg/kg q6h for the next 12 h and then, for maintenance, 2 mg/kg q8h; patients with hepatic failure or congestive heart failure should be given 6 mg/kg to start, followed by 2 mg/kg q8h for the next 12 h and then, for maintenance, 1–2 mg/kg q12h.
Cigarette smokers	Smoking 1–2 packs/day has been shown to decrease the serum half-life of theophylline; consequently, smokers may require larger or more frequent doses than nonsmokers. This effect may persist for 3 mo to 2 yr after the individual has ceased smoking.
Management of GI reactions	Gastric irritation may be prevented by giving medication with food; although absorption may be slower, it is still complete

WARNINGS/PRECAUTIONS

Status asthmaticus	Concomitant parenteral therapy and close monitoring (preferably in an intensive-care unit) are frequently necessary for the optimal management of this medical emergency
Arrhythmia	Theophylline may precipitate or exacerbate arrhythmia; any significant change in cardiac rate or rhythm warrants monitoring and further investigation. Use with caution in patients with severe cardiac disease, acute myocardial injury, or hyperthyroidism. Theophylline toxicity may be masked in patients with tachycardia.
Gastric irritation	Theophylline occasionally may cause local irritation of the GI tract, although GI symptoms are more commonly centrally mediated and associated with serum levels over 20 µg/ml; use with caution in patients with a history of peptic ulcer
Special-risk patients	Use with caution in neonates, the elderly (especially men), and patients with renal or hepatic impairment, chronic lung disease, severe cardiac disease, hypertension, acute myocardial injury, congestive heart failure, cor pulmonale, severe hypoxemia, a history of peptic ulcer, hyperthyroidism, influenza, or alcoholism (see "patients with reduced theophylline clearance" in the ADMINISTRATION/DOSAGE ADJUSTMENTS section); use with particular caution in patients with congestive heart failure because clearance in such patients is very slow
Morphine, curare	These drugs can stimulate histamine release and depress respiration; administer them with caution or, if possible, avoid their use

BRONKODYL

Carcinogenicity, mutagenicity, effect on fertility	No long-term studies have been performed to evaluate the carcinogenic and mutagenic potential of xanthine derivatives or their effect on fertility

ADVERSE REACTIONS

Gastrointestinal	Nausea, vomiting, epigastric pain, hematemesis, diarrhea
Central nervous system and neuromuscular	Headache, irritability, restlessness, insomnia, reflex hyperexcitability, muscle twitching, clonic and tonic generalized convulsions
Cardiovascular	Palpitations, tachycardia, extrasystoles, flushing, hypotension, circulatory failure, ventricular arrhythmias
Respiratory	Tachypnea
Renal	Albuminuria, increased excretion of renal tubule cells and red blood cells, potentiation of diuresis
Other	Hyperglycemia, inappropriate antidiuretic hormone secretion syndrome, rash

OVERDOSAGE

Signs and symptoms	See ADVERSE REACTIONS; ventricular arrhythmias or convulsions may be the first signs of toxicity, although in up to 50% of patients less severe signs of overdosage (eg, nausea, restlessness) occur initially
Treatment	If patient is conscious and seizures have not occurred, induce emesis and administer a cathartic and activated charcoal. If patient is convulsing, establish an airway and administer oxygen and IV diazepam (0.1–0.3 mg/kg, up to 10 mg). If patient is comatose following the occurrence of seizures, intubate immediately, using an endotracheal tube with an inflated cuff, and perform gastric lavage; introduce the cathartic and activated charcoal through a large-bore gastric lavage tube. Monitor vital signs, maintain blood pressure, and provide adequate hydration. Treat hypotension and shock by appropriate fluid replacement, avoiding the use of vasopressors, if possible. In general, the drug is metabolized sufficiently rapidly to preclude any additional benefit from dialysis; however, dialysis may be useful in the presence of congestive heart failure or hepatic dysfunction. Charcoal hemoperfusion may be necessary if serum levels exceed 50 μg/ml. Serial monitoring of the serum theophylline level is helpful in following the patient's course and in guiding further management.

DRUG INTERACTIONS

Other xanthine derivatives	△ Risk of theophylline toxicity; do not administer other xanthine derivatives concomitantly
Cimetidine, erythromycin, troleandomycin, influenza virus vaccine	△ Serum theophylline level; reduce the initial dosage of theophylline and monitor serum level
Ephedrine, other sympathomimetic agents	△ Risk of theophylline and sympathomimetic toxicity
Lithium	▽ Serum lithium level
Propranolol	▽ Pharmacologic effects of propranolol and theophylline
Phenytoin	▽ Serum levels of theophylline and phenytoin
Furosemide	△ Diuresis
Reserpine	Tachycardia
Chlordiazepoxide	Fatty acid mobilization

ALTERED LABORATORY VALUES

Blood/serum values	△ Glucose △ Uric acid (with Bittner and colorimetric methods) △ Bilirubin (with diazo tablet method)
Urinary values	△ Albumin △ Catecholamines

USE IN CHILDREN

See INDICATIONS and ORAL DOSAGE; clearance occurs more rapidly in children over 6 mo of age than in adults. Administration to infants under 6 mo of age is not recommended because clearance varies markedly until the age of 6 mo.

USE IN PREGNANT AND NURSING WOMEN

Pregnancy Category C: reproduction studies have not been done; it is not known whether theophylline can cause harm to the fetus or affect reproductive capacity. Use during pregnancy only if clearly needed. Theophylline is excreted in human milk and may cause adverse reactions in nursing infants; use with caution in nursing mothers.

[1] When calculating dosages on the basis of weight, use the lean (or ideal) body weight, rather than the patient's actual weight (theophylline is not taken up by fatty tissue)

SYSTEMIC BRONCHODILATORS/ ANTIASTHMATIC AGENTS

CHOLEDYL (oxtriphylline) Parke-Davis   Rx

Tablets: 100, 200 mg **Elixir (per 5 ml):** 100 mg[1] (16 fl oz) *sherry-flavored* **Pediatric syrup (per 5 ml):** 50 mg (16 fl oz) *vanilla/mint-flavored*

CHOLEDYL SA (oxtriphylline) Parke-Davis   Rx

Tablets (sustained release): 400, 600 mg

INDICATIONS

Acute bronchial asthma
Reversible bronchospasm associated with chronic bronchitis and emphysema

Chronic asthma

ORAL DOSAGE[2]

Adult, nonsmoker: 9.4 mg/kg to start, followed by 4.7 mg/kg q6h for the next 12 h and then q8h for maintenance
Infant and child (6 mo to 9 yr): 9.4 mg/kg to start, followed by 6.2 mg/kg q4h for the next 12 h and then q6h for maintenance
Child (9–16 yr) and young adult smoker: 9.4 mg/kg to start, followed by 4.7 mg/kg q4h for the next 12 h and then q6h for maintenance

Adult: 25 mg/kg/day or 625 mg/day, whichever is less, given in 3–4 divided doses q6–8h to start, followed, if needed and tolerated, by an approximately 25% increase in dosage every 2–3 days, up to 20 mg/kg/day or 1,400 mg/day, whichever is less
Infant and child (< 9 yr): 25 mg/kg/day or 625 mg/day, whichever is less, given in 3–4 divided doses q6–8h to start, followed, if needed and tolerated, by an approximately 25% increase in dosage every 2–3 days, up to 37.5 mg/kg/day
Child (9–12 yr): 25 mg/kg/day or 625 mg/day, whichever is less, given in 3–4 divided doses q6–8h to start, followed, if needed and tolerated, by an approximately 25% increase in dosage every 2–3 days, up to 31 mg/kg/day
Adolescent (12–16 yr): 25 mg/kg/day or 625 mg/day, whichever is less, given in 3–4 divided doses q6–8h to start, followed, if needed and tolerated, by an approximately 25% increase in dosage every 2–3 days, up to 28 mg/kg/day

NOTE: Current official labeling for Choledyl Tablets and Elixir recommends a dosage of 200 mg or 10 ml qid for adults and 5 ml/60 lb qid for children 2–12 yr of age; no contraindications are specified, but prescribers are cautioned that concomitant use of other xanthine-containing preparations may lead to adverse reactions and that gastric distress, palpitations, and CNS stimulation have been reported. The information presented here is based on the current package labeling of Choledyl SA and Choledyl Pediatric Syrup and may be used as a guide to initiating Choledyl therapy with the tablets or elixir, in determining maintenance dosage requirements, and in recognizing and managing overdosage situations. For further information, consult the manufacturer.

CONTRAINDICATIONS

Hypersensitivity to theophylline or oxtriphylline

ADMINISTRATION/DOSAGE ADJUSTMENTS

Use of serum theophylline levels	Monitoring of serum drug levels is recommended, particularly if the maximal dosages given above for chronic therapy are maintained or exceeded. Adjust dosage to maintain serum theophylline level between 10 and 20 µg/ml; levels above 20 µg/ml may produce toxicity. Check serum level 1–1½ h (pediatric syrup) or 1–2 h (sustained-release tablets) after last dose; medication must have been taken at typical intervals, with no missed or added doses, for a period of 48 h prior to measurement. Do not attempt to maintain any dose that is not tolerated. In increasing the dosage, instruct the patient not to take a subsequent dose if side effects develop and to resume taking the drug at a lower dose only after untoward reactions have disappeared.
Patients currently receiving theophylline products	Determine (where possible) the time, amount, route, and form of the patient's last dose. If it is not possible to obtain the patient's serum theophylline level quickly and there is sufficient respiratory distress to warrant a small risk, a loading dose may be given based on the principle that each 0.8 mg/kg of oxtriphylline administered in a rapidly absorbed form will increase the serum theophylline level by 1 µg/ml. Thus, if the patient is not already experiencing toxicity, a loading dose of 4 mg/kg (which will increase the serum theophylline level by 5 µg/ml) is unlikely to produce dangerous side effects.
Dosing intervals in children	Because of the rapid elimination of theophylline in children, dosing q6h is generally necessary; children (and adults requiring higher than average doses) may benefit from use of sustained-release preparations, which may allow longer dosing intervals and/or less fluctuation in serum theophylline levels during chronic therapy
Use of sustained-release tablets	A non-sustained-release form of oxtriphylline should be used for initial dosage titration and to establish maintenance dosage requirements; therapy may then be switched to sustained-release tablets to provide smoother steady-state serum levels and the convenience of twice-daily dosing. If the total daily maintenance dosage requirement is approximately 800 mg, substitute one 400-mg Choledyl SA tablet q12h; for patients requiring approximately 1,200 mg/day, substitute one 600-mg Choledyl SA tablet q12h.
Older patients and patients with cor pulmonale	For acute asthmatic symptoms requiring rapid theophyllinization, give 9.4 mg/kg to start, followed by 3.1 mg/kg q6h for the next 12 h and then q8h for maintenance
Patients with congestive heart failure or hepatic failure	For acute asthmatic symptoms requiring rapid theophyllinization, give 9.4 mg/kg to start, followed by 3.1 mg/kg q8h for the next 12 h and then 1.6–3.1 mg/kg q12h for maintenance

CHOLEDYL

Management of GI reactions	Gastric irritation may be prevented by giving medication with food; although absorption may be slower, it is still complete
Concomitant bronchodilator therapy	Reduce dosage of oxtriphylline when administered concomitantly with other bronchodilating agents, such as beta-adrenergic receptor agonists

WARNINGS/PRECAUTIONS

Treatment of status asthmaticus	Optimal management of this medical emergency frequently requires additional medication, including corticosteroids, if patient is not responding quickly to bronchodilators alone
Gastric irritation	Theophylline products occasionally may cause local irritation of the GI tract, although GI symptoms are more commonly centrally mediated and associated with serum levels over 20 µg/ml; use with caution in patients with a history of peptic ulcer
Patients with cardiac disease	Use with caution in patients with severe cardiac disease, acute myocardial injury, or cor pulmonale; exercise great caution in giving this drug to patients with congestive heart failure, since theophylline clearance may be particularly slow. Preexisting arrhythmias may worsen during theophylline therapy.
Other special-risk patients	Use with caution in patients with severe hypoxemia, hypertension, hyperthyroidism, or liver disease, persons over 55 yr of age (especially men), and neonates; careful reduction of dosage and serum level monitoring are particularly important in patients likely to have decreased theophylline clearance rates, including elderly and/or debilitated patients and patients with acute hypoxia, cardiac decompensation, hepatic dysfunction, or renal failure
Cigarette smokers	Smoking 1–2 packs/day has been shown to decrease the serum half-life of theophylline; consequently, smokers may require larger doses than nonsmokers. This effect may persist for 3 mo to 2 yr after the individual has ceased smoking.
Concomitant drug therapy	Morphine, curare, and stilbamidine should be used with caution in patients with airflow obstruction, since they depress respiration, stimulate histamine release, and may induce asthmatic attacks (see also DRUG INTERACTIONS) if possible, use an alternative drug

ADVERSE REACTIONS

Gastrointestinal	Nausea, vomiting, epigastric pain, hematemesis, diarrhea
Central nervous system and neuromuscular	Headache, irritability, restlessness, insomnia, reflex hyperexcitability, muscle twitching, clonic and tonic generalized convulsions
Cardiovascular	Palpitations, tachycardia, extrasystoles, flushing, hypotension, circulatory failure, life-threatening ventricular arrhythmias
Respiratory	Tachypnea
Renal	Albuminuria, increased excretion of renal tubule cells and red blood cells, potentiation of diuresis
Metabolic and endocrinological	Hyperglycemia, inappropriate antidiuretic hormone secretion syndrome

OVERDOSAGE

Signs and symptoms[3]	*Cardiovascular:* precordial pain, tachycardia, ventricular and other arrhythmias, hypotension, and, in extreme cases, severe shock, cardiovascular collapse, and death. *Gastrointestinal:* abdominal pain, nausea, persistent vomiting, and hematemesis. *Central nervous system:* headache, dizziness, restlessness, irritability, tremors, hyperactivity, and agitation, followed, in severe cases, by convulsions, drowsiness, coma, and death.
Treatment	If patient is conscious and seizures have not occurred, induce emesis and administer a cathartic and activated charcoal. If patient is convulsing, establish an airway and administer oxygen and IV diazepam (0.1–0.3 mg/kg, up to 10 mg). If patient is comatose following the occurrence of seizures, intubate immediately, using an endotracheal tube with an inflated cuff, and perform gastric lavage; introduce the cathartic and activated charcoal through a large-bore gastric lavage tube. Monitor vital signs, maintain blood pressure, and provide adequate hydration. Treat hypotension and shock by appropriate fluid replacement, avoiding the use of vasopressors, if possible. In general, the drug is metabolized sufficiently rapidly to preclude any additional benefit from dialysis; however, dialysis may be useful in the presence of congestive heart failure or hepatic dysfunction. Serial monitoring of the serum theophylline level is helpful in following the patient's course and in guiding further management.

DRUG INTERACTIONS

Other xanthine derivatives	△ Risk of toxicity; do not administer concurrently
Lithium	△ Lithium excretion
Propranolol	Antagonism of pharmacologic effects of propranolol ▽ Bronchodilation
Cimetidine, clindamycin, erythromycin, lincomycin, troleandomycin	△ Theophylline serum level
Furosemide	△ Diuresis

COMPENDIUM OF DRUG THERAPY

CHOLEDYL ■ CONSTANT-T

Reserpine	Tachycardia
Chlordiazepoxide	Fatty acid mobilization
Ephedrine and possibly other sympathomimetic bronchodilators	⚠ Risk of toxicity

ALTERED LABORATORY VALUES

Blood/serum values	⚠ Glucose ⚠ Uric acid (with Bittner and colorimetric methods) ⚠ Bilirubin (with diazo tablet method)
Urinary values	⚠ Albumin ⚠ Catecholamines

USE IN CHILDREN

See INDICATIONS and ORAL DOSAGE. Children may exhibit marked sensitivity to CNS stimulation. Use with caution in neonates, owing to reduced theophylline clearance rate.

USE IN PREGNANT AND NURSING WOMEN

Safety for use in pregnant or nursing women has not been established in regard to possible adverse effects on fetal or neonatal development. Consequently, these products should not be used in pregnant or nursing women unless the anticipated benefits of therapy outweigh the possible risks.

---

[1] Contains 20% alcohol
[2] When calculating dosages on the basis of weight, use the lean (or ideal) body weight, rather than the patient's actual weight (theophylline is not taken up by fatty tissue)
[3] Serious toxicity may occur suddenly and may or may not be preceded by minor adverse effects, such as nausea, vomiting, or restlessness; in some patients, convulsions, tachycardia, or ventricular arrhythmias may be the first sign of toxicity

---

SYSTEMIC BRONCHODILATORS/ ANTIASTHMATIC AGENTS

CONSTANT-T (theophylline, anhydrous) Geigy   Rx

Tablets (sustained release): 200, 300 mg

INDICATIONS

Asthma
Reversible bronchospasm associated with chronic bronchitis and emphysema

ORAL DOSAGE

Adult: 200 mg q12h to start, followed after 3 days by 300 mg q12h, if needed and tolerated
Child (15–20 kg): 100 mg q12h to start, followed after 3 days by 150 mg q12h, if needed and tolerated
Child (20–25 kg): 150 mg q12h to start, followed after 3 days by 200 mg q12h, if needed and tolerated
Child (25–35 kg): 200 mg q12h to start, followed after 3 days by 250 mg q12h, if needed and tolerated
Child (> 35 kg): same as adult

CONTRAINDICATIONS

Hypersensitivity to theophylline or other xanthine derivatives

Current use of other xanthine medications

ADMINISTRATION/DOSAGE ADJUSTMENTS

Use of serum theophylline levels	If the desired response is not achieved with the maximum dosages given above and there are no adverse reactions after 3 days, increase the dosage to the following minimum dosages requiring measurement of the serum theophylline concentration: for children weighing 15–20 kg, 200 mg q12h; 20–30 kg, 250 mg q12h; 30–35 kg, 300 mg q12h; 35–40 kg, 350 mg q12h; over 40 kg and for adults, 400 mg q12h. Check the serum level 3–8 h after a dose when no doses have been missed or added for at least 3 days. If the serum theophylline concentration is 5–7.5 µg/ml: increase dose by 25% to the nearest 50 mg q12h and recheck the serum level for guidance in making further adjustments; 7.5–10 µg/ml: increase dose by 25% to the nearest 50 mg q12h (if symptoms occur repeatedly at the end of a dosing interval, divide the total daily dose into 3 parts and administer q8h); 10–20 µg/ml: maintain dose, if tolerated, and recheck serum level at 6- to 12-mo intervals (some patients may require finer dosage adjustments); 20–25 µg/ml: decrease dose by 50 mg q12h; 25–30 µg/ml: skip next dose and decrease subsequent doses by 25% to the nearest 50 mg q12h; over 30 µg/ml: skip next 2 doses, decrease subsequent doses by 50% to the nearest 50 mg q12h, and recheck the serum theophylline level.

WARNINGS/PRECAUTIONS

Gastric irritation	Theophylline occasionally may cause local irritation of the GI tract, although GI symptoms are more commonly centrally mediated and associated with serum levels over 20 µg/ml; use with caution in patients with a history of peptic ulcer

CONSTANT-T

Patients with cardiac disease	Use with caution in patients with severe cardiac disease, acute myocardial infarction, or cor pulmonale; exercise great caution in giving this drug to patients with congestive heart failure, since theophylline clearance may be particularly slow. Preexisting arrhythmias may worsen during theophylline therapy.
Other special-risk patients	Use with caution in patients with hypertension, hyperthyroidism, severe hypoxemia, chronic obstructive lung disease, renal insufficiency, or hepatic disease and in patients older than 55 yr of age, particularly men
Food-drug interaction	Administration of some or all controlled-release theophylline products with food may affect absorption and result in altered serum values, especially when high serum levels are maintained or single doses exceeding 900 mg or 13 mg/kg are given; it is not known whether the bioavailability of this preparation is influenced by food

ADVERSE REACTIONS

Gastrointestinal	Nausea, vomiting, epigastric pain, hematemesis, diarrhea
Central nervous system and neuromuscular	Headache, irritability, restlessness, insomnia, reflex hyperexcitability, muscle twitching, clonic and tonic generalized convulsions
Cardiovascular	Palpitations, tachycardia, extrasystoles, flushing, hypotension, circulatory failure, life-threatening ventricular arrhythmias
Respiratory	Tachypnea
Renal	Albuminuria, increased excretion of renal tubule cells and red blood cells, potentiation of diuresis
Metabolic and endocrinological	Hyperglycemia, inappropriate antidiuretic hormone secretion syndrome

OVERDOSAGE

Signs and symptoms[1]	*Cardiovascular:* precordial pain, tachycardia, ventricular and other arrhythmias, hypotension, and, in extreme cases, severe shock, cardiovascular collapse, and death. *Gastrointestinal:* abdominal pain, nausea, persistent vomiting, and hematemesis. *Central nervous system:* headache, dizziness, restlessness, irritability, tremors, hyperactivity, and agitation, followed, in severe cases, by convulsions, drowsiness, coma, and death
Treatment	If patient is conscious and seizures have not occurred, induce emesis and administer a cathartic and activated charcoal. If patient is convulsing, establish an airway and administer oxygen and IV diazepam (0.1–0.3 mg/kg, up to 10 mg). If patient is comatose following the occurrence of seizures, intubate immediately, using an endotracheal tube with an inflated cuff, and perform gastric lavage; introduce the cathartic and activated charcoal through a large-bore gastric lavage tube. Monitor vital signs, maintain blood pressure, and provide adequate hydration. Treat hypotension and shock by appropriate fluid replacement, avoiding the use of vasopressors, if possible. In general, the drug is metabolized sufficiently rapidly to preclude any additional benefit from dialysis; however, dialysis may be useful in the presence of congestive heart failure or hepatic dysfunction. Serial monitoring of the serum theophylline level is helpful in following the patient's course and in guiding further management.

DRUG INTERACTIONS

Other xanthine derivatives	△ Risk of toxicity; do not administer concurrently
Lithium	△ Lithium excretion
Propranolol	Antagonism of pharmacologic effects of propranolol ▽ Bronchodilation
Cimetidine, clindamycin erythromycin, lincomycin, troleandomycin	△ Theophylline serum level
Furosemide	△ Diuresis
Reserpine	Tachycardia
Chlordiazepoxide	Fatty acid mobilization
Ephedrine and possibly other sympathomimetic bronchodilators	△ Risk of toxicity

ALTERED LABORATORY VALUES

Blood/serum values	△ Glucose △ Uric acid (with Bittner and colorimetric methods) △ Bilirubin (with diazo tablet method)
Urinary values	△ Albumin △ Catecholamines

USE IN CHILDREN

See INDICATIONS and ORAL DOSAGE

USE IN PREGNANT AND NURSING WOMEN

Safety for use during pregnancy has not been established; there is no evidence, however, that this drug can adversely affect fetal development. The risk of uncontrolled asthma should be weighed in deciding whether to administer theophylline to a pregnant woman. An insignificant amount of theophylline is excreted in breast milk; use with caution in nursing mothers.

---

[1] Early signs of toxicity (eg, nausea and restlessness) may precede the onset of convulsions in up to 50% of patients; however, in some cases ventricular arrhythmias and seizures may be the first signs of toxicity

SYSTEMIC BRONCHODILATORS/ ANTIASTHMATIC AGENTS

DURAPHYL (theophylline, anhydrous) Forest   Rx
Tablets (controlled release): 100, 200, 300 mg

INDICATIONS
Chronic, reversible bronchospasm associated with bronchial asthma, chronic bronchitis, and emphysema

ORAL DOSAGE[1]
Adult and child ($\geq$ 6 yr): for patients currently receiving theophylline, one half the total daily dose q12h to start. For patients not currently receiving theophylline, titrate dosage with an immediate- or controlled-release product that permits small increases in dosage and then switch to the controlled-release tablets. Do not exceed, without measurement of serum levels, 24 mg/kg/day for children under 9 yr of age, 20 mg/kg/day for children 9–12 yr of age, 18 mg/kg/day for adolescents 12–16 yr of age, or 13 mg/kg/day or 900 mg/day, whichever is less, for patients over 16 yr of age. Tablets should not be crushed or chewed.

CONTRAINDICATIONS
Hypersensitivity to theophylline

ADMINISTRATION/DOSAGE ADJUSTMENTS

Administration with food — Administration of some or all controlled-release theophylline products with food may affect absorption and result in altered serum values, especially when high serum levels are maintained or single doses exceeding 900 mg or 13 mg/kg are given; it is not known whether the bioavailability of Duraphyl tablets is influenced by food.

Dosage adjustment with measurement of serum levels — Monitoring of serum theophylline levels is recommended, particularly for titration of dosage. Check the peak serum level 4 h after the last dose; medication must have been taken at typical intervals, with no missed or added doses, for a period of 48 h prior to measurement. (Serum levels that are measured spectrophotometrically without prior chromatographic isolation may be falsely elevated when coffee, tea, acetaminophen, chocolate, or cola beverages have also been ingested.) Adjust dosage to maintain serum levels of 10–20 μg/ml; the risk of toxicity is significantly increased at higher levels, and, in some patients (eg, those with reduced theophylline clearance), toxic reactions may develop at serum concentrations of 15–20 μg/ml. If the peak level in patients with normal theophylline clearance is between 5 and 7.5 μg/ml, increase the total daily dose by 25%; if between 7.5 and 10 μg/ml, increase the daily dose by 25% and, if symptoms recur at the end of a dosing interval, administer q8h; if between 20 and 25 μg/ml, reduce the daily dose by 10%; if between 25 and 30 μg/ml, omit the next dose and reduce the daily dose by 25%; if over 30 μg/ml, omit the next 2 doses and reduce the daily dose by 50%. Recheck serum levels after dosage adjustment and then every 6–12 mo thereafter. *Do not attempt to maintain any dosage that is not tolerated.* Patients should be instructed to omit the next dose if they experience adverse effects and to reduce the subsequent dosage when they resume therapy after the reactions have disappeared. Exercise caution when titrating dosage for younger children who cannot complain of minor adverse reactions.

Patients with reduced theophylline clearance — To avoid toxic reactions in neonates, patients over 55 yr of age (especially men), and patients with renal or hepatic impairment, influenza, alcoholism, chronic lung disease, cor pulmonale, or cardiac failure, reduce the initial dosage and monitor serum theophylline levels

Patients with rapid theophylline clearance — Children, smokers, and some nonsmoking adults are likely to require administration of this product q8h (smokers may alternatively need higher doses). The effect of smoking on theophylline clearance may persist for 3 mo to 2 yr after the individual has ceased smoking. To determine whether theophylline is rapidly cleared in an individual patient, look for undesirably low trough serum levels or for a recurrence of symptoms at the end of a dosing interval.

WARNINGS/PRECAUTIONS

Arrhythmia — Theophylline may precipitate or exacerbate arrhythmia; any significant change in cardiac rate or rhythm warrants monitoring and further investigation. Use with caution in patients with severe cardiac disease, acute myocardial injury, or hyperthyroidism. Theophylline toxicity may be masked in patients with tachycardia.

Gastric irritation — Theophylline occasionally may cause local irritation of the GI tract, although GI symptoms are more commonly centrally mediated and associated with serum levels over 20 μg/ml; use with caution in patients with a history of peptic ulcer

Special-risk patients — Use with caution in neonates, the elderly (especially men), and patients with renal or hepatic impairment, chronic lung disease, severe cardiac disease, hypertension, acute myocardial injury, congestive heart failure, cor pulmonale, severe hypoxemia, a history of peptic ulcer, hyperthyroidism, influenza, or alcoholism (see "patients with reduced theophylline clearance" in the ADMINISTRATION/DOSAGE ADJUSTMENTS section); use with particular caution in patients with congestive heart failure because clearance in such patients is very slow

Morphine, curare — These drugs can stimulate histamine release and depress respiration; administer them with caution or, if possible, avoid their use

Acute bronchospasm — This product is not indicated for the treatment of acute bronchospastic episodes; for rapid symptomatic relief, use an immediate-release or IV theophylline preparation or other bronchodilators. If status asthmaticus occurs, administer parenteral therapy and closely monitor the patient (preferably in an intensive-care unit).

DURAPHYL

Carcinogenicity, mutagenicity, effect on fertility	No long-term studies have been performed to evaluate the carcinogenic and mutagenic potential of xanthine derivatives or their effect on fertility

ADVERSE REACTIONS

Gastrointestinal	Nausea, vomiting, epigastric pain, hematemesis, diarrhea
Central nervous system and neuromuscular	Headache, irritability, restlessness, insomnia, reflex hyperexcitability, muscle twitching, clonic and tonic generalized convulsions
Cardiovascular	Palpitations, tachycardia, extrasystoles, flushing, hypotension, circulatory failure, ventricular arrhythmias
Respiratory	Tachypnea
Renal	Albuminuria, increased excretion of renal tubule cells and red blood cells, potentiation of diuresis
Other	Hyperglycemia, inappropriate ADH syndrome, rash

OVERDOSAGE

Signs and symptoms	See ADVERSE REACTIONS; ventricular arrhythmias or convulsions may be the first signs of toxicity, although in up to 50% of patients less severe signs of overdosage (eg, nausea, restlessness) occur initially
Treatment	If patient is conscious and seizures have not occurred, induce emesis and administer a cathartic and activated charcoal. If patient is convulsing, establish an airway and administer oxygen and IV diazepam (0.1–0.3 mg/kg, up to 10 mg). If patient is comatose following the occurrence of seizures, intubate immediately, using an endotracheal tube with an inflated cuff, and perform gastric lavage; introduce the cathartic and activated charcoal through a large-bore gastric lavage tube. Monitor vital signs, maintain blood pressure, and provide adequate hydration. Treat hypotension and shock by appropriate fluid replacement, avoiding the use of vasopressors, if possible. In general, the drug is metabolized sufficiently rapidly to preclude any additional benefit from dialysis; however, dialysis may be useful in the presence of congestive heart failure or hepatic dysfunction. Charcoal hemoperfusion may be necessary if serum levels exceed 50 μg/ml. Serial monitoring of the serum theophylline level is helpful in following the patient's course and in guiding further management.

DRUG INTERACTIONS

Other xanthine derivatives	△ Risk of theophylline toxicity; do not administer other xanthine derivatives concomitantly
Cimetidine, erythromycin, troleandomycin, influenza virus vaccine	△ Serum theophylline level; reduce the initial dosage of theophylline and monitor serum level
Ephedrine, other sympathomimetic agents	△ Risk of theophylline and sympathomimetic toxicity
Lithium	▽ Serum lithium level
Propranolol	▽ Pharmacologic effects of propranolol and theophylline
Phenytoin	▽ Serum levels of theophylline and phenytoin
Furosemide	△ Diuresis
Reserpine	Tachycardia
Chlordiazepoxide	Fatty acid mobilization

ALTERED LABORATORY VALUES

Blood/serum values	△ Glucose △ Uric acid (with Bittner and colorimetric methods) △ Bilirubin (with diazo tablet method)
Urinary values	△ Albumin △ Catecholamines

USE IN CHILDREN

See INDICATIONS, ORAL DOSAGE, and ADMINISTRATION/DOSAGE ADJUSTMENTS; safety and effectiveness for use in children under 6 yr of age have not been established

USE IN PREGNANT AND NURSING WOMEN

Pregnancy Category C: reproduction studies have not been done; it is not known whether theophylline can cause harm to the fetus or affect reproductive capacity. Use during pregnancy only if clearly needed. Theophylline is excreted in human milk and may cause adverse reactions in nursing infants; use with caution in nursing mothers.

[1] When calculating dosages on the basis of weight, use the lean (or ideal) body weight, rather than the patient's actual weight (theophylline is not taken up by fatty tissue)

ELIXOPHYLLIN

SYSTEMIC BRONCHODILATORS/ANTIASTHMATIC AGENTS

ELIXOPHYLLIN (theophylline, anhydrous) Forest — Rx
Capsules: 100, 200 mg **Elixir (per 15 ml):** 80 mg[1] (473, 946, 3,785 ml)

INDICATIONS	ORAL DOSAGE[2]
Acute, reversible bronchospasm associated with bronchial asthma, chronic bronchitis, and emphysema	**Adult, nonsmoker:** 6 mg/kg to start, followed by 3 mg/kg q6h for the next 12 h and then q8h for maintenance **Infant and child (6 mo to 9 yr):** 6 mg/kg to start, followed by 4 mg/kg q4h for the next 12 h and then q6h for maintenance **Child (9–16 yr) and young adult smoker:** 6 mg/kg to start, followed by 3 mg/kg q4h for the next 12 h and then q6h for maintenance
Chronic, reversible bronchospasm associated with bronchial asthma, chronic bronchitis, and emphysema	**Adult and child:** 16 mg/kg/day or 400 mg/day, whichever is less, given in 3–4 divided doses q6–8h to start, followed, if needed and tolerated, by an approximately 25% increase in dosage every 2–3 days, 24 mg/kg/day for children under 9 yr of age, 20 mg/kg/day for children 9–12 yr of age, 18 mg/kg/day for adolescents 12–16 yr of age, and 13 mg/kg/day or 900 mg/day, whichever is less, for patients over 16 yr of age

ELIXOPHYLLIN SR (theophylline, anhydrous) Forest — Rx
Capsules (sustained release): 125, 250 mg

INDICATIONS	ORAL DOSAGE[2]
Chronic, reversible bronchospasm associated with bronchial asthma, chronic bronchitis, the emphysema	**Adult and child (≥ 6 yr):** titrate dosage with an immediate-release product and then switch to the sustained-release capsules, giving one-half the total daily dose q12h; for children, smokers, and other patients with rapid theophylline clearance, it may be necessary to administer one-third the total daily dose q8h. If serum level cannot be measured, do not exceed 24 mg/kg/day for children 6–9 yr of age, 20 mg/kg/day for children 9–12 yr of age, 18 mg/kg/day for adolescents 12–16 yr of age, and 13 mg/kg/day or 900 mg/day, whichever is less, for patients over 16 yr of age.

CONTRAINDICATIONS
Hypersensitivity to theophylline or other components

ADMINISTRATION/DOSAGE ADJUSTMENTS

Food-drug interaction	Administration of some or all controlled-release theophylline products with food may affect absorption and result in altered serum values, especially when high serum levels are maintained or single doses exceeding 900 mg or 13 mg/kg are given; it is not known whether the bioavailability of Elixophyllin SR capsules is influenced by food
Dosage adjustment with measurement of serum levels	Monitoring of serum theophylline levels is recommended, particularly for titration of dosage. Check the peak serum level 1–2 h after the last dose if the elixir or immediate-release capsules are used and 4–6 h after the last dose if the sustained-release capsules are used; medication must have been taken at typical intervals, with no missed or added doses, for a period of 48 h prior to measurement. Serum levels that are measured spectrophotometrically without prior chromatographic isolation are falsely high when coffee, tea, acetaminophen, chocolate, or cola beverages have also been ingested. Adjust dosage to maintain serum levels of 10–20 µg/ml; the risk of toxicity is significantly increased at higher levels, and, in some patients (eg, those with reduced theophylline clearance), toxic reactions may develop at serum concentrations of 15–20 µg/ml. If the peak level in patients with normal theophylline clearance is between 5 and 7.5 µg/ml, increase the total daily dose by 25%; if between 7.5 and 10 µg/ml, increase the daily dose by 25% and, if symptoms recur at the end of a dosing interval, administer more frequently; if between 20 and 25 µg/ml, reduce the daily dose by 10%; if between 25 and 30 µg/ml, omit the next dose and reduce the daily dose by 25%; if over 30 µg/ml, omit the next 2 doses and reduce the daily dose by 50%. Recheck serum levels after dosage adjustment and then every 6–12 mo thereafter. *Do not attempt to maintain any dosage that is not tolerated.* Patients should be instructed to omit the next dose if they experience adverse effects and to reduce the subsequent dosage when they resume therapy after the reactions have disappeared. Exercise caution when titrating dosage for younger children who cannot complain of minor adverse reactions.
Acute symptoms in patients currently receiving theophylline	Determine (where possible) the time, amount, route, and form of the patient's last dose. If it is not possible to obtain the patient's serum theophylline level quickly and there is sufficient respiratory distress to warrant a small risk, a loading dose may be given based on the principle that each 0.5 mg/kg of theophylline administered in a rapidly absorbed form will increase the serum drug level by 1 µg/ml. Thus, if the patient is not already experiencing toxicity, a loading dose of 2.5 mg/kg (which will increase the serum level by 5 µg/ml) is unlikely to produce dangerous side effects.
Patients with reduced theophylline clearance	To avoid toxic reactions in neonates, patients over 55 yr of age (especially men), and patients with renal or hepatic impairment, influenza, alcoholism, chronic lung disease, cor pulmonale, or cardiac failure, reduce the initial dosage and monitor serum theophylline levels. For acute symptoms requiring rapid theophyllinization, give older patients and patients with cor pulmonale 6 mg/kg to start, followed by 2 mg/kg q6h for the next 12 h and then, for maintenance, 2 mg/kg q8h; patients with congestive heart failure should be given 6 mg/kg to start, followed by 2 mg/kg q8h for the next 16 h and then, for maintenance, 1–2 mg/kg q12h.

ELIXOPHYLLIN

Patients with rapid theophylline clearance	Children, smokers, and some nonsmoking adults generally require administration of the immediate-release preparations q6h and are likely to require dosing of the sustained-release capsules q8h (smokers may, alternatively, need larger doses). The effect of smoking on theophylline clearance may persist for 3 mo to 2 yr after the individual has ceased smoking. To determine whether theophylline is rapidly cleared in an individual patient, look for undesirably low trough serum levels or for a recurrence of symptoms at the end of a dosing interval.

WARNINGS/PRECAUTIONS

Status asthmaticus	Concomitant parenteral therapy and close monitoring (preferably in an intensive-care unit) are frequently necessary for the optimal management of this medical emergency
Arrhythmia	Theophylline may precipitate or exacerbate arrhythmia; any significant change in cardiac rate or rhythm warrants monitoring and further investigation. Use with caution in patients with severe cardiac disease, acute myocardial injury, or hyperthyroidism. Theophylline toxicity may be masked in patients with tachycardia.
Gastric irritation	Theophylline occasionally may cause local irritation of the GI tract, although GI symptoms are more commonly centrally mediated and associated with serum levels over 20 $\mu g/ml$; use with caution in patients with a history of peptic ulcer
Special-risk patients	Use with caution in neonates, the elderly (especially men), and patients with renal or hepatic impairment, chronic lung disease, severe cardiac disease, hypertension, acute myocardial injury, congestive heart failure, cor pulmonale, severe hypoxemia, a history of peptic ulcer, hyperthyroidism, influenza, or alcoholism (see "patients with reduced theophylline clearance" in the ADMINISTRATION/DOSAGE ADJUSTMENTS section); use with particular caution in patients with congestive heart failure because clearance in such patients is very slow
Carcinogenicity, mutagenicity, effect on fertility	No long-term studies have been performed to evaluate the carcinogenic and mutagenic potential of xanthine derivatives or their effect on fertility

ADVERSE REACTIONS

Gastrointestinal	Nausea, vomiting, epigastric pain, hematemesis, diarrhea
Central nervous system and neuromuscular	Headache, irritability, restlessness, insomnia, reflex hyperexcitability, muscle twitching, clonic and tonic generalized convulsions
Cardiovascular	Palpitations, tachycardia, extrasystoles, flushing, hypotension, circulatory failure, ventricular arrhythmias
Respiratory	Tachypnea
Renal	Albuminuria, increased excretion of renal tubule cells and red blood cells, potentiation of diuresis
Other	Hyperglycemia, inappropriate antidiuretic hormone secretion syndrome, rash

OVERDOSAGE

Signs and symptoms	See ADVERSE REACTIONS; ventricular arrhythmias or convulsions may be the first signs of toxicity, although in up to 50% of patients less severe signs of overdosage (eg, nausea, restlessness) occur initially
Treatment	If patient is conscious and seizures have not occurred, induce emesis and administer a cathartic (especially if sustained-release capsules have been ingested) and activated charcoal. If patient is convulsing, establish an airway and administer oxygen and IV diazepam (0.1–0.3 mg/kg, up to 10 mg). If patient is comatose following the occurrence of seizures, intubate immediately, using an endotracheal tube with an inflated cuff, and perform gastric lavage; introduce the cathartic and activated charcoal through a large-bore gastric lavage tube. Monitor vital signs, maintain blood pressure, and provide adequate hydration. Treat hypotension and shock by appropriate fluid replacement, avoiding the use of vasopressors, if possible. Dialysis may be useful in the presence of congestive heart failure or hepatic dysfunction. Charcoal hemoperfusion may be necessary if serum levels exceed 50 $\mu g/ml$. Serial monitoring of the serum theophylline level is helpful in following the patient's course and in guiding further management.

DRUG INTERACTIONS

Other xanthine derivatives	△ Risk of theophylline toxicity; do not administer other xanthine derivatives concomitantly
Cimetidine, erythromycin, troleandomycin, influenza virus vaccine	△ Serum theophylline level; reduce the initial dosage of theophylline and monitor serum level
Ephedrine, other sympathomimetic agents	△ Risk of theophylline and sympathomimetic toxicity
Lithium	▽ Serum lithium level
Propranolol	▽ Pharmacologic effects of propranolol and theophylline
Phenytoin	▽ Serum levels of theophylline and phenytoin
Furosemide	△ Diuresis

ELIXOPHYLLIN ■ LUFYLLIN

Reserpine	Tachycardia
Chlordiazepoxide	Fatty acid mobilization

ALTERED LABORATORY VALUES

Blood/serum values	⇧ Glucose ⇧ Uric acid (with Bittner and colorimetric methods) ⇧ Bilirubin (with diazo tablet method)
Urinary values	⇧ Albumin ⇧ Catecholamines

USE IN CHILDREN

See INDICATIONS and ORAL DOSAGE; clearance occurs more rapidly in children over 6 mo of age than in adults. Administration to infants under 6 mo of age is not recommended because clearance varies markedly until the age of 6 mo; do not administer the sustained-release capsules to children under 6 yr of age.

USE IN PREGNANT AND NURSING WOMEN

Pregnancy Category C: reproduction studies have not been done; it is not known whether theophylline can cause harm to the fetus or affect reproductive capacity. Use during pregnancy only if clearly needed. Theophylline is excreted in human milk and may cause adverse reactions in nursing infants; use with caution in nursing mothers.

---

[1] The elixir contains 20% alcohol
[2] When calculating dosages on the basis of weight, use the lean (or ideal) body weight, rather than the patient's actual weight (theophylline is not taken up by fatty tissue)

SYSTEMIC BRONCHODILATORS/ANTIASTHMATIC AGENTS

LUFYLLIN (dyphylline) Wallace   Rx

Tablets: 200 mg (Lufyllin), 400 mg (Lufyllin-400) **Elixir (per 15 ml):** 100 mg[1] (1 pt, 1 gal) **Ampuls:** 250 mg/ml (2 ml) for IM use only

INDICATIONS	ORAL DOSAGE	PARENTERAL DOSAGE
Acute, reversible bronchospasm associated with bronchial asthma, chronic bronchitis, and emphysema	**Adult:** 200–400 mg (2–4 tbsp elixir) or up to 15 mg/kg (tablets) q6h, as needed and tolerated	**Adult:** 500 mg IM to start, followed, if needed and tolerated, by 250–500 mg IM q2–6h; maximum dosage: 15 mg/kg q6h

CONTRAINDICATIONS

Hypersensitivity to dyphylline or other xanthine derivatives

WARNINGS/PRECAUTIONS

Toxicity	To reduce the risk of adverse reactions, avoid excessive dosage; serum levels cannot be used to predict clinical response because therapeutic and toxic levels have not been determined
Patients with renal impairment	The clearance of dyphylline is reduced in patients with impaired renal function; the serum half-life in anuric patients may be 3–4 times longer than normal (the half-life in normal individuals after oral administration is approximately 2 h). Adjust dosage to an appropriate level.
Other special-risk patients	Use with caution in patients with severe cardiac disease, hypertension, hyperthyroidism, acute myocardial injury, or peptic ulcer
Status asthmaticus, neonatal apnea	Do not use dyphylline for the management of these serious medical emergencies
Carcinogenicity, mutagenicity, effect on fertility	No studies have been done to evaluate the carcinogenic or mutagenic potential of dyphylline or its effect on fertility

ADVERSE REACTIONS[2]

Gastrointestinal	Nausea, vomiting, epigastric pain, hematemesis, diarrhea
Central nervous system	Headache, irritability, restlessness, insomnia, hyperexcitability, agitation, muscle twitching, clonic and tonic generalized convulsions
Cardiovascular	Palpitations, tachycardia, extrasystoles, flushing, hypotension, circulatory failure, ventricular arrhythmias
Respiratory	Tachypnea
Renal	Albuminuria, gross and microscopic hematuria, diuresis
Other	Hyperglycemia, inappropriate ADH syndrome

OVERDOSAGE[3]

Signs and symptoms	See ADVERSE REACTIONS; ventricular arrhythmias or convulsions may be the first signs of toxicity, although in up to 50% of patients less severe signs of overdosage (eg, nausea, restlessness) occur initially
Treatment	If patient is conscious and seizures have not occurred, induce emesis or perform gastric lavage, and then administer activated charcoal and a cathartic. If patient is convulsing, establish an airway and administer oxygen and IV diazepam (0.1–0.3 mg/kg, up to 10 mg). If patient is comatose following the occurrence of seizures, intubate immediately, using an endotracheal tube with an inflated cuff, and perform gastric lavage; introduce the cathartic and activated charcoal through a large-bore gastric lavage tube. Monitor vital signs, maintain blood pressure, and provide adequate hydration. Treat hypotension and shock by appropriate fluid replacement, avoiding the use of vasopressors, if possible. Hemodialysis of dyphylline may be helpful when toxicity is severe or when general supportive and symptomatic measures are not sufficient.

DRUG INTERACTIONS

Other xanthine derivatives	△	Risk of xanthine toxicity
Ephedrine, other sympathomimetic agents	△	Risk of dyphylline and sympathomimetic toxicity
Probenecid	△	Serum dyphylline half-life
Lithium	▽	Serum lithium level
Propranolol	▽	Pharmacologic effects of propranolol and dyphylline

ALTERED LABORATORY VALUES

No clinically significant alterations in blood/serum or urinary values have been reported at therapeutic dosages

USE IN CHILDREN

Safety and effectiveness for use in children have not been established

USE IN PREGNANT AND NURSING WOMEN

Pregnancy Category C: reproduction studies have not been done; it is not known whether dyphylline can cause harm to the fetus or affect reproductive capacity. Use during pregnancy only if clearly needed. The concentration of dyphylline in human milk is approximately twice the maternal serum level; use with caution in nursing mothers.

[1] Contains 20% alcohol
[2] Includes reactions common to xanthine derivatives in general
[3] Overdosage of dyphylline has not been reported; the information in this section is based primarily on experience with theophylline overdosage

---

SYSTEMIC BRONCHODILATORS/ANTIASTHMATIC AGENTS

MARAX (ephedrine sulfate, theophylline, and hydroxyzine hydrochloride) Roerig   Rx

Tablets: 25 mg ephedrine sulfate, 130 mg theophylline, and 10 mg hydroxyzine hydrochloride

MARAX-DF (ephedrine sulfate, theophylline, and hydroxyzine hydrochloride) Roerig   Rx

Syrup (per 5 ml): 6.25 mg ephedrine sulfate, 32.5 mg theophylline, and 2.5 mg hydroxyzine hydrochloride[1] (1 pt, 1 gal)

INDICATIONS

Bronchospastic disorders[2]

ORAL DOSAGE

Adult: 1 tab bid to qid, allowing at least 4 h between doses
Child (2–5 yr): 2.5–5 ml (½ to 1 tsp) tid or qid
Child (> 5 yr): ½ tab bid to qid, allowing at least 4 h between doses, or 5 ml (1 tsp) tid or qid

CONTRAINDICATIONS

Early pregnancy	Cardiovascular disease	Hyperthyroidism
Hypersensitivity to any component	Hypertension	

ADMINISTRATION/DOSAGE ADJUSTMENTS

Adults sensitive to ephedrine	Give one half the usual adult dose
Bedtime dosage	Some patients may be adequately controlled with ½–1 tab at bedtime

MARAX

Gastric irritation	Upper abdominal discomfort, nausea, and vomiting often occur when theophylline is taken on an empty stomach; advise patient to take medication after meals to minimize irritation

WARNINGS/PRECAUTIONS

Drowsiness	May occur; caution patients against driving or operating dangerous machinery while taking this drug and that it may increase the effects of alcohol
Tolerance	May occur after several weeks of taking ephedrine 3 or more times daily
Special-risk patients	Use with caution in elderly men or in those with prostatic hypertrophy

ADVERSE REACTIONS

Central nervous system and neuromuscular	Excitation, tremulousness, insomnia, nervousness, vertigo, headache, drowsiness; involuntary motor activity, unsteady gait, and weakness (with extremely high doses)
Cardiovascular	Palpitations, tachycardia, precordial pain, arrhythmias, cardiac stimulation
Gastrointestinal	Gastric irritation, upper abdominal discomfort, nausea, vomiting
Genitourinary	Vesical sphincter spasm and resultant urinary hesitation, acute urinary retention, diuresis
Other	Sweating, warmth, dry mouth and throat

OVERDOSAGE

Signs and symptoms	*Cardiovascular:* precordial pain, tachycardia, ventricular and other arrhythmias, hypotension, and, in extreme cases, severe shock, cardiovascular collapse, and death. *Gastrointestinal:* abdominal pain, nausea, persistent vomiting, and hematemesis. *Central nervous system:* headache, dizziness, restlessness, irritability, tremors, hyperactivity, and agitation, followed, in severe cases, by convulsions, drowsiness, coma, and death.
Treatment	If patient is conscious and seizures have not occurred, induce emesis and administer a cathartic and activated charcoal. If patient is convulsing, establish an airway and administer oxygen and IV diazepam (0.1–0.3 mg/kg, up to 10 mg). If patient is comatose following the occurrence of seizures, intubate immediately, using an endotracheal tube with an inflated cuff, and perform gastric lavage; introduce the cathartic and activated charcoal through a large-bore gastric lavage tube. Monitor vital signs, maintain blood pressure, and provide adequate hydration. Treat hypotension and shock by appropriate fluid replacement, avoiding the use of vasopressors, if possible. In general, the drug is metabolized sufficiently rapidly to preclude any additional benefit from dialysis; however, dialysis may be useful in the presence of congestive heart failure or hepatic dysfunction. Serial monitoring of the serum theophylline level is helpful in following the patient's course and in guiding further management.

DRUG INTERACTIONS

Other xanthine derivatives	△ Risk of toxicity; do not administer concurrently
Lithium	△ Lithium excretion due to theophylline component
Propranolol	Antagonism by theophylline component of propranolol effect ▽ Bronchodilation
Erythromycin, clindamycin, lincomycin, troleandomycin	△ Theophylline serum level
Furosemide	△ Diuresis due to theophylline component
Reserpine	Tachycardia due to theophylline component ▽ Pressor effect of ephedrine component
Chlordiazepoxide	Fatty acid mobilization due to interaction with theophylline component
Digitalis glycosides, anesthetics	Cardiac arrhythmias due to ephedrine component
Ergonovine, methylergonovine, oxytocin	Hypertension due to ephedrine component
Guanethidine	▽ Hypotensive effect due to ephedrine component
MAO inhibitors	△ Pressor effect of ephedrine component
Other sympathomimetic agents	△ Sympathomimetic effects of ephedrine component or other sympathomimetics
Tricyclic antidepressants	▽ Pressor effect of ephedrine component
Alcohol, tranquilizers, sedative-hypnotics, and other CNS depressants	△ CNS depression; reduce dosage of other CNS depressants accordingly

ALTERED LABORATORY VALUES

Blood/serum values	△ Glucose △ Uric acid (with Bittner and colorimetric methods) △ Bilirubin (with diazo tablet method)
Urinary values	△ Albumin △ Catecholamines △ 17-Hydroxycorticosteroids

MARAX ■ PROVENTIL

USE IN CHILDREN	USE IN PREGNANT AND NURSING WOMEN
See INDICATIONS and ORAL DOSAGE; not recommended for use in children under 2 yr of age	Contraindicated for use during early pregnancy; consult manufacturer for use during later pregnancy. It is not known whether all of the components of this preparation are excreted in human milk; do not use in nursing mothers.

[1] Contains 5% alcohol
[2] Possibly effective

SYSTEMIC BRONCHODILATORS/ ANTIASTHMATIC AGENTS

METAPREL (metaproterenol sulfate) Sandoz Pharmaceuticals — Rx
Tablets: 10, 20 mg Syrup (per 5 ml): 10 mg (16 fl oz) *cherry flavored*

INDICATIONS	ORAL DOSAGE
Bronchial asthma **Reversible bronchospasm** associated with bronchitis and emphysema	**Adult:** 20 mg or 10 ml (2 tsp) tid or qid **Child (6–9 yr or < 60 lb):** 10 mg or 5 ml (1 tsp) tid or qid **Child (≥ 9 yr or > 60 lb):** 20 mg or 10 ml (2 tsp) tid or qid

CONTRAINDICATIONS	
Hypersensitivity to metaproterenol sulfate	Cardiac arrhythmias associated with tachycardia

WARNINGS/PRECAUTIONS	
Paradoxical bronchoconstriction	Has occurred with excessive use of other sympathomimetic agents; advise patient to report any failure to respond to usual doses
Special-risk patients	Use with great caution in patients with hypertension, coronary artery disease, congestive heart failure, hyperthyroidism, diabetes, or hypersensitivity to sympathomimetic amines

ADVERSE REACTIONS	
Cardiovascular	Tachycardia, hypertension, palpitations
Central nervous system	Nervousness, tremor
Gastrointestinal	Nausea, vomiting

OVERDOSAGE	
Signs and symptoms	Excessive beta-adrenergic stimulation (see ADVERSE REACTIONS)
Treatment	Discontinue medication; treat symptomatically

DRUG INTERACTIONS	
Sympathomimetic agents	△ Adrenergic effects; allow sufficient time to elapse between use of metaproterenol and administration of other sympathomimetic agents. If metaproterenol is given in combination with another adrenergic agent, exercise extreme care.
Nonselective beta-adrenergic blockers	▽ Bronchodilation

ALTERED LABORATORY VALUES
No clinically significant alterations in blood/serum or urinary values occur at therapeutic dosages

USE IN CHILDREN	USE IN PREGNANT AND NURSING WOMEN
See INDICATIONS and ORAL DOSAGE. Limited experience with use of the syrup in children under 6 yr of age suggests a dosage of approximately 1.3–2.6 mg/kg/day. The tablet form is currently not recommended for use in this age group.	Safety for use during pregnancy has not been established; use with caution and only after weighing the expected therapeutic benefit against the possible risk to the fetus. Studies in mice, rats, and rabbits have shown no evidence of teratogenicity at doses up to 31 times the recommended human oral dose; higher doses, however, have resulted in fetal loss and teratogenicity in rabbits. There are no adequate, well-controlled studies in pregnant women. It is not known whether metaproterenol is excreted in human milk; because many drugs are excreted in breast milk, use with caution in nursing mothers.

SYSTEMIC BRONCHODILATORS/ ANTIASTHMATIC AGENTS

PROVENTIL (albuterol sulfate) Schering — Rx
Tablets: 2, 4 mg albuterol[1]

INDICATIONS	ORAL DOSAGE
Bronchospasm associated with reversible obstructive airway disease	**Adult:** 2–4 mg tid or qid to start, followed, if necessary, by careful, gradual increases in dosage; maximum level: 8 mg qid **Child (6–12 yr):** 2 mg tid or qid, followed, if necessary, by careful, gradual increases in dosage; maximum level: 24 mg/day, given in divided doses **Child (≥ 12 yr):** same as adult

COMPENDIUM OF DRUG THERAPY

PROVENTIL Syrup (albuterol sulfate) Schering   Rx

Syrup (per 5 ml): 2 mg albuterol[1] (16 fl oz) *strawberry flavored*

INDICATIONS

Bronchospasm associated with reversible obstructive airway disease

ORAL DOSAGE

Adult: 2–4 mg (5–10 ml) tid or qid to start, followed, if necessary, by careful, gradual increases in dosage; maximum level: 8 mg (20 ml) qid

Child (2–6 yr): 0.1 mg/kg, up to 2 mg (5 ml), tid to start, followed, if necessary, by careful, gradual increases in dosage; maximum level: 0.2 mg/kg, up to 4 mg (10 ml), tid

Child (6–14 yr): 2 mg (5 ml) tid or qid to start, followed, if necessary, by careful, gradual increases in dosage; maximum level: 24 mg (60 ml)/day, given in divided doses

Child ($>$ 14 yr): same as adult

CONTRAINDICATIONS

Hypersensitivity to any component

ADMINISTRATION/DOSAGE ADJUSTMENTS

Elderly or unusually sensitive patients	Elderly patients or those with a history of unusual sensitivity to beta-adrenergic stimulating agents should be given 2 mg tid or qid to start, followed, if necessary, by gradual increases up to 8 mg tid or qid
Management of side effects	If adverse reactions, which are generally transient, occur, it is usually not necessary to discontinue use; in some cases, however, the dosage may be temporarily reduced, and then, after the reaction has subsided, gradually increased

WARNINGS/PRECAUTIONS

Sympathomimetic effects	At recommended dosages, albuterol usually has minimal effects on the cardiovascular system; however, this drug can occasionally cause cardiovascular and CNS effects common to all sympathomimetic agents. Discontinue use if such sympathomimetic effects occur; use with caution in patients with cardiovascular disorders (including coronary insufficiency and hypertension), hyperthyroidism, diabetes mellitus, or unusual sensitivity to sympathomimetic amines, and with extreme caution in patients receiving MAO inhibitors or tricyclic antidepressants (see DRUG INTERACTIONS).
Use with other sympathomimetic bronchodilators	Concomitant use with other *oral* sympathomimetic agents is not recommended; however, concomitant use of an *aerosol* in a judicious, individualized manner (ie, not given on a routine or regular basis) may be considered
Reactions with IV albuterol	Intravenous administration of albuterol has caused a decrease (usually transient) in the serum potassium level; large IV doses have exacerbated diabetes mellitus and ketoacidosis. The relevance of these findings to oral use is not known.
Carcinogenicity, mutagenicity	A significant, dose-related increase in the incidence of benign leiomyomas of the mesovarium has been reported in a 2-yr study of rats given 3, 16, and 78 times the maximum adult human dose (2, 9, and 46 times the maximum oral dose for children weighing 21 kg); in another study, concurrent use of propranolol blocked this effect. No evidence of tumorigenicity has been observed in mice after 18 mo of treatment or in a lifetime study in hamsters. Mutagenic effects have not been detected.

ADVERSE REACTIONS

Frequent reactions (incidence $\geq$ 1%) are printed in *italics*

With use of tablets

Central nervous system	*Nervousness and tremor (20%); headache (7%); insomnia, weakness, and dizziness (2%);* drowsiness, restlessness, irritability, vertigo, stimulation
Cardiovascular	*Tachycardia and palpitations (5%);* flushing, chest discomfort, hypertension, angina
Gastrointestinal	*Nausea (2%),* vomiting
Other	*Muscle cramps (3%),* difficulty in urination, unusual taste sensation, drying or irritation of oropharynx

With use of syrup in children 2–6 yr of age

Central nervous system	*Excitement (20%), nervousness (15%), hyperkinesia (4%), insomnia (2%), emotional lability and fatigue (1%),* vertigo, stimulation
Cardiovascular	*Tachycardia (2%),* hypertension, angina
Gastrointestinal	*GI symptoms (2%), anorexia (1%),* vomiting
Other	*Pallor and conjunctivitis (1%),* unusual taste sensation, drying or irritation of oropharynx

With use of syrup in older children and adults

Central nervous system	*Tremor (10%), nervousness and shakiness (9%), headache (4%), dizziness (3%), hyperactivity and excitement (2%), sleeplessness and irritable behavior (1%),* disturbed sleep, weakness, vertigo, stimulation
Cardiovascular	*Tachycardia (1%),* palpitations, chest pain, hypertension, angina
Gastrointestinal	*Increased appetite (3%),* stomach ache, epigastric pain, vomiting

PROVENTIL ■ QUADRINAL

| Other | *Epistaxis (1%)*, muscle spasm, cough, mydriasis, sweating, unusual taste sensation, drying or irritation of oropharynx |

OVERDOSAGE

| Signs and symptoms | Angina, hypertension, hypokalemia |
| Treatment | A cardioselective beta-adrenergic blocker, such as metaprolol, may be used judiciously; keep in mind the risk of inducing an asthmatic attack |

DRUG INTERACTIONS

Other sympathomimetic agents (including epinephrine)	△ Sympathomimetic effects and risk of toxicity (see WARNINGS/PRECAUTIONS)
MAO inhibitors, tricyclic antidepressants	△ Cardiovascular effects of albuterol (see WARNINGS/PRECAUTIONS)
Beta-adrenergic blocking agents	▽ Pharmacologic effects of both drugs

ALTERED LABORATORY VALUES

No clinically significant alterations in blood/serum or urinary values occur at therapeutic dosages

USE IN CHILDREN

Safety and effectiveness of tablets for use in children under 6 yr of age have not been established; safety and effectiveness of syrup for use in children under 2 yr of age have not yet been adequately demonstrated. Bear in mind that certain adverse reactions occur more frequently in children 2–6 yr of age than in older children (see ADVERSE REACTIONS).

USE IN PREGNANT AND NURSING WOMEN

Pregnancy Category C: albuterol has been shown to be teratogenic in mice, causing cleft palate when given SC at 40% of the maximum human adult oral dose; cranioschisis has been seen in rabbits at 78 times the maximum human adult oral dose. Delay in preterm labor has occurred in clinical use. Administer this drug cautiously during pregnancy and only if the expected benefit clearly justifies the potential risks to the fetus. Reproduction studies in rats have shown no evidence of impaired fertility. It is not known whether albuterol is excreted in human milk; because of the potential for tumorigenicity shown in animal studies, a decision should be made to discontinue nursing or use of the drug.

[1] As the sulfate salt

SYSTEMIC BRONCHODILATORS/ANTIASTHMATIC AGENTS

QUADRINAL (ephedrine hydrochloride, phenobarbital, theophylline calcium salicylate, and potassium iodide) Knoll   Rx

Tablets: 24 mg ephedrine hydrochloride, 24 mg phenobarbital, 130 mg theophylline calcium salicylate, and 320 mg potassium iodide

INDICATIONS

Chronic respiratory disease, such as bronchial asthma, chronic bronchitis, and pulmonary emphysema, in which tenacious mucus and bronchospasm are dominant symptoms

ORAL DOSAGE

Adult: 1 tab tid or qid; for severe bronchospasm, 1½ tabs tid or qid
Child (< 6 yr): decrease the dose for older children proportionately
Child (6–12 yr): ½ tab tid

CONTRAINDICATIONS

| Sensitivity to theophylline, potassium iodide, ephedrine, or other sympathomimetics, or barbiturates | Current use of other xanthine medications | Thyroid enlargement or goiter |
| | | Pregnancy |

ADMINISTRATION/DOSAGE ADJUSTMENTS

Nighttime relief	Patients over 12 yr of age may be given an additional 1 tab at bedtime, if needed
Frequency of administration	To maintain stable "around-the-clock" blood levels of theophylline in children, dosing q6h is generally necessary; because adults eliminate theophylline more slowly, administration at intervals up to 8 h apart may be satisfactory
Monitoring of therapy	Pulmonary function measurements before and after treatment will permit an objective assessment of the patient's response to this drug; measurement of serum theophylline levels is recommended to assure maximal therapeutic benefit without incurring excessive risk (toxicity increases in incidence at levels above 20 µg/ml)

QUADRINAL

WARNINGS/PRECAUTIONS

Reye's syndrome — This product contains theophylline calcium salicylate; salicylates have been associated with the development of Reye's syndrome in children and teenagers having chicken pox or flu

Gastrointestinal irritation — The theophylline component in this drug may cause local irritation, although GI symptoms are more commonly centrally mediated and associated with serum theophylline levels above 20 µg/ml

Acne — May be aggravated in adolescents and adults, due to potassium iodide component

Elderly patients — May be more sensitive to the effects of ephedrine

Patients with cardiac disease — Use with caution in patients with severe cardiac disease, acute myocardial injury, or cor pulmonale; exercise great caution in giving this drug to patients with congestive heart failure, since theophylline clearance may be particularly slow. Preexisting arrhythmias may worsen during theophylline therapy.

Other special-risk patients — Theophylline clearance rate is decreased in neonates, alcoholics, persons over 55 yr of age (especially men), patients with chronic obstructive pulmonary disease or prolonged high fever, and patients receiving certain antibiotics (see DRUG INTERACTIONS); use with caution. Theophylline should also be used with caution in patients with hypertension, hyperthyroidism, severe hypoxia, or peptic ulcer. In addition, ephedrine should be used with caution in patients with diabetes mellitus, predisposition to glaucoma, or prostatic hypertrophy, and phenobarbital should be used with caution in patients with a history of drug abuse, hyperkinesis, uncontrolled pain, or a history of porphyria.

Iodism — May result from chronic ingestion of iodides; initial symptoms may include an unpleasant brassy taste, a burning sensation in the mouth and throat, soreness of the teeth and gums, increased salivation, coryza, sneezing, irritation of the eyes with swelling of the eyelids, headache, cough, skin lesions, diarrhea, gastric irritation, anorexia, fever, and depression. Discontinue medication and institute supportive measures, as needed. Administer abundant fluids and sodium chloride to hasten iodide elimination; in severe cases, mannitol may be given to force diuresis.

Cigarette smokers — Smoking 1–2 packs/day has been shown to decrease the serum half-life of theophylline; consequently, smokers may require larger doses than nonsmokers. This effect may persist for 3 mo to 2 yr after the individual has ceased smoking.

Concomitant drug therapy — Morphine, curare, and stilbamidine should be used with caution in patients with airflow obstruction, since they depress respiration, stimulate histamine release, and may induce asthmatic attacks (see also DRUG INTERACTIONS) if possible, use an alternative drug

Drug dependence — Psychic and/or physical dependence may develop, especially in addiction-prone individuals

ADVERSE REACTIONS

Gastrointestinal — Nausea, vomiting, epigastric pain, hematemesis, diarrhea, loss of appetite

Central nervous system and neuromuscular — Headache, irritability, nervousness, restlessness, insomnia, reflex hyperexcitability, trembling, muscle twitching, clonic and tonic generalized convulsions, dizziness, lightheadedness, mental confusion, depression, excitement, tiredness, weakness

Cardiovascular — Palpitations, irregular heartbeat, tachycardia, extrasystoles, flushing, hypotension, circulatory failure, ventricular arrhythmias, bradycardia, pallor, feeling of warmth

Respiratory — Tachypnea, dyspnea, wheezing, tightness in the chest

Renal — Albuminuria, increased excretion of renal tubule cells and red blood cells, potentiation of diuresis, dysuria, difficult urination

Metabolic and endocrinological — Hyperglycemia, inappropriate antidiuretic hormone secretion syndrome, thyroid adenoma, goiter, myxedema

Dermatological and hypersensitivity — Rash, urticaria, yellowing of eyes and skin, angioneurotic edema, cutaneous and mucosal hemorrhages, sore throat, fever, arthralgia, lymph-node enlargement, eosinophilia

Other — Diaphoresis; swelling of eyelids, face, and lips; unusual bleeding or bruising

OVERDOSAGE

Signs and symptoms[1] — *Cardiovascular:* precordial pain, tachycardia, ventricular and other arrhythmias, hypotension, and, in extreme cases, severe shock, cardiovascular collapse, and death. *Gastrointestinal:* abdominal pain, nausea, persistent vomiting, and hematemesis. *Central nervous system:* headache, dizziness, restlessness, irritability, tremors, hyperactivity, and agitation, followed, in severe cases, by convulsions, drowsiness, coma, and death.

Treatment — If patient is conscious and seizures have not occurred, induce emesis and administer a cathartic and activated charcoal. If patient is convulsing, establish an airway and administer oxygen and IV diazepam (0.1–0.3 mg/kg, up to 10 mg). If patient is comatose following the occurrence of seizures, intubate immediately, using an endotracheal tube with an inflated cuff, and perform gastric lavage; introduce the cathartic and activated charcoal through a large-bore gastric lavage tube. Monitor vital signs, maintain blood pressure, and provide adequate hydration. Treat hypotension and shock by appropriate fluid replacement, avoiding the use of vasopressors, if possible. In general, the drug is metabolized sufficiently rapidly to preclude any additional benefit from dialysis; however, dialysis may be useful in the presence of congestive heart failure or hepatic dysfunction. Serial monitoring of the serum theophylline level is helpful in following the patient's course and in guiding further management.

QUADRINAL

DRUG INTERACTIONS

Other xanthine derivatives	△ Risk of toxicity; do not administer concurrently
Lithium	△ Lithium excretion due to theophylline component △ Hypothyroid and goiterogenic effects of potassium iodide
Propranolol	Antagonism by theophylline component of pharmacologic effects of propranolol ▽ Bronchodilation
Cimetidine, clindamycin, erythromycin, lincomycin, troleandomycin	△ Theophylline serum level
Furosemide	△ Diuresis due to theophylline component
Reserpine	Tachycardia due to theophylline component ▽ Pressor effect of ephedrine component
Chlordiazepoxide	Fatty acid mobilization due to interaction with theophylline component
Digitalis glycosides, anesthetics	Cardiac arrhythmias due to ephedrine component
Ergonovine, methylergonovine, oxytocin	Hypertension due to ephedrine component
Guanethidine	▽ Hypotensive effect due to ephedrine component
MAO inhibitors	△ Pressor effect of ephedrine component and CNS depressant effect of phenobarbital component
Other sympathomimetic agents	△ Sympathomimetic effects of ephedrine component or other sympathomimetics
Tricyclic antidepressants	▽ Pressor effect of ephedrine component
Alcohol, general anesthetics, and other CNS depressants	△ CNS depression due to phenobarbital component
Oral anticoagulants	▽ Anticoagulant effect due to phenobarbital component
Corticosteroids, digitalis, digitoxin, doxycycline, tricyclic antidepressants, griseofulvin, phenytoin	▽ Pharmacologic effect due to phenobarbital component

ALTERED LABORATORY VALUES

Blood/serum values	△ Glucose △ Uric acid (with Bittner and colorimetric methods) △ Bilirubin (with diazo tablet method) △ Potassium
Urinary values	△ Albumin △ Catecholamines

USE IN CHILDREN

Indicated for short-term use in children (see ORAL DOSAGE); if used chronically because other expectorants are ineffective, observe for signs of thyroid enlargement and worsening of acne

USE IN PREGNANT AND NURSING WOMEN

Pregnancy Category X: contraindicated during pregnancy. If patient becomes pregnant while taking this drug, she should be advised of the potential risk to the fetus. The iodide in this drug may cause fetal harm when administered to pregnant women; goiter has developed in infants whose mothers received iodide-containing medications during pregnancy, and a few neonates have died from tracheal obstruction due to congenital goiters. Use of barbiturates during pregnancy may cause physical dependence, with resulting withdrawal symptoms in the neonate; may cause birth defects; may be associated with neonatal hemorrhage, due to reduction in levels of vitamin K-dependent clotting factors in the neonate; and may cause respiratory depression in neonates. Patients who have taken this preparation during pregnancy or become pregnant while taking it should be apprised of the potential hazard to the fetus. Because of the potential for serious adverse effects in nursing infants, a decision should be made to either discontinue use of this drug or stop nursing.

[1] Early signs of toxicity (eg, nausea and restlessness) may appear in up to 50% of patients prior to the onset of convulsions; however, in some cases, ventricular arrhythmias or seizures may be the first signs of toxicity

SYSTEMIC BRONCHODILATORS/ ANTIASTHMATIC AGENTS

QUIBRON and QUIBRON-300 (theophylline and guaifenesin) Bristol — Rx

Capsules: 150 mg theophylline and 90 mg guaifenesin (Quibron); 300 mg theophylline and 180 mg guaifenesin (Quibron-300)
Liquid (per 15 ml): 150 mg theophylline and 90 mg guaifenesin (1 pt)

INDICATIONS
Bronchospasm associated with such conditions as bronchial asthma, chronic bronchitis, and pulmonary emphysema

ORAL DOSAGE[1]
Adult: 16 mg/kg/day or 400 mg/day, whichever is less, given in 3–4 divided doses q6–8h to start, followed, if needed and tolerated, by not more than a 25% increase in dosage every 2–3 days, up to 13 mg/kg/day or 900 mg/day, whichever is less (usual dosage: 150–300 mg q6–8h)

Infant and child (< 9 yr): 16 mg/kg/day or 400 mg/day, whichever is less, given in 3–4 divided doses q6–8h to start, followed, if needed and tolerated, by not more than a 25% increase in dosage every 2–3 days, up to 24 mg/kg/day or 900 mg/day, whichever is less (usual dosage: 4–6 mg/kg q6–8h)

Child (9–12 yr): 16 mg/kg/day or 400 mg/day, whichever is less, given in 3–4 divided doses q6–8h to start, followed, if needed and tolerated, by not more than a 25% increase in dosage every 2–3 days, up to 20 mg/kg/day or 900 mg/day, whichever is less (usual dosage: 4–5 mg/kg q6–8h)

Adolescent (12–16 yr): 16 mg/kg/day or 400 mg/day, whichever is less, given in 3–4 divided doses q6–8h to start, followed, if needed and tolerated, by not more than a 25% increase in dosage every 2–3 days, up to 18 mg/kg/day or 900 mg/day, whichever is less

QUIBRON-T (theophylline, anhydrous) Bristol — Rx

Tablets: 300 mg

INDICATIONS
Acute bronchial asthma
Reversible bronchospasm associated with chronic bronchitis and pulmonary emphysema

Chronic asthma

ORAL DOSAGE[1]
Adult, nonsmoker: 6 mg/kg to start, followed by 3 mg/kg q6h for the next 12 h and then q8h for maintenance
Infant and child (6 mo to 9 yr): 6 mg/kg to start, followed by 4 mg/kg q4h for the next 12 h and then q6h for maintenance
Child (9–16 yr) and young adult: 6 mg/kg to start, followed by 3 mg/kg q4h for the next 12 h and then q6h for maintenance

Adult: 16 mg/kg/day or 400 mg/day, whichever is less, given in 3–4 divided doses q6–8h to start, followed, if needed and tolerated, by not more than a 25% increase in dosage every 2–3 days, up to 13 mg/kg/day or 900 mg/day, whichever is less

Infant and child (< 9 yr): 16 mg/kg/day or 400 mg/day, whichever is less, given in 3–4 divided doses q6–8h to start, followed, if needed and tolerated, by not more than a 25% increase in dosage every 2–3 days, up to 24 mg/kg/day

Child (9–12 yr): 16 mg/kg/day or 400 mg/day, whichever is less, given in 3–4 divided doses q6–8h to start, followed, if needed and tolerated, by not more than a 25% increase in dosage every 2–3 days, up to 20 mg/kg/day

Adolescent (12–16 yr): 16 mg/kg/day or 400 mg/day, whichever is less, given in 3–4 divided doses q6–8h to start, followed, if needed and tolerated, by not more than a 25% increase in dosage every 2–3 days, up to 18 mg/kg/day

QUIBRON-T/SR (theophylline, anhydrous) Bristol — Rx

Tablets (sustained release): 300 mg

INDICATIONS
Same as Quibron and Quibron-300

ORAL DOSAGE[1]
Adult: 200 mg q12h to start, followed, if needed and tolerated, by not more than a 25% increase in dosage every 2–3 days, up to 13 mg/kg/day or 900 mg/day, whichever is less
Child (< 9 yr): 100 mg q12h to start, followed, if needed and tolerated, by not more than a 25% increase in dosage every 2–3 days, up to 24 mg/kg/day
Child (9–12 yr): 150 mg q12h to start, followed, if needed and tolerated, by not more than a 25% increase in dosage every 2–3 days, up to 20 mg/kg/day
Adolescent (12–16 yr): 200 mg q12h to start, followed, if needed and tolerated, by not more than a 25% increase in dosage every 2–3 days, up to 18 mg/kg/day

CONTRAINDICATIONS
Hypersensitivity to guaifenesin, theophylline, or other xanthine derivatives

Current use of other xanthine medications

ADMINISTRATION/DOSAGE ADJUSTMENTS
Use of serum theophylline levels — Monitoring of serum drug levels is highly recommended, particularly if the maximal dosages given above are exceeded. Adjust dosage to maintain a serum theophylline level between 10 and 20 $\mu g/ml$ (although 5–10 $\mu g/ml$ may be effective in some patients); levels above 20 $\mu g/ml$ may produce toxicity. Check serum level approximately 2 h after last dose if immediate-release preparations have been used or 4–5 h after last dose of sustained-release tablets; medication must have been taken at typical intervals, with no missed or added doses, for a period of 72 h prior to measurement. Do not attempt to maintain any dose that is not tolerated.

QUIBRON

Patients currently receiving theophylline products	Determine (where possible) the time, amount, route, and form of the patient's last dose. If it is not possible to obtain the patient's serum theophylline level quickly and there is sufficient respiratory distress to warrant a small risk, a loading dose may be given based on the principle that each 0.5 mg/kg of theophylline administered in a rapidly absorbed form will increase the serum drug level by 1 µg/ml. Thus, if the patient is not already experiencing toxicity, a loading dose of 2.5 mg/kg (which will increase the serum level by 5 µg/ml) is unlikely to produce dangerous side effects.
Use of Quibron-300 capsules	When higher theophylline dosages are required for adults, 1 cap may be given q6–8h after dosage has been raised to achieve therapeutic serum levels
Dosing intervals	Because of the more rapid elimination of theophylline in children and some adults (eg, heavy smokers), dosing of Quibron-T q6h is generally necessary, and dosing of Quibron-T/SR more frequently than q12h may be required in such patients
Older patients and patients with cor pulmonale	For acute asthmatic symptoms requiring rapid theophyllinization, use Quibron-T: give 6 mg/kg to start, followed by 2 mg/kg q6h for the next 12 h and then q8h for maintenance
Patients with congestive heart failure or hepatic failure	For acute asthmatic symptoms requiring rapid theophyllinization, use Quibron-T: give 6 mg/kg to start, followed by 2 mg/kg q8h for the next 12 h and then 1–2 mg/kg q12h for maintenance
Use of sustained-release tablets	Caution patients not to chew or crush tablets; sustained-release dosage form is not indicated for conditions requiring rapid theophyllinization (eg, status asthmaticus)
Management of GI reactions	Gastric irritation may be prevented by giving medication with food; although absorption may be slower, it is still complete

WARNINGS/PRECAUTIONS

Patients with cardiac disease	Use with caution in patients with severe cardiac disease, acute myocardial injury, or cor pulmonale; exercise particular caution in giving this drug to patients with congestive heart failure, since theophylline clearance may be particularly slow. Preexisting arrhythmias may worsen during theophylline therapy.
Other special-risk patients	Use with caution in patients with severe hypoxemia, hypertension, hyperthyroidism, hepatic impairment, or a history of peptic ulcer, persons over 55 yr of age (especially men), and alcoholics
Cigarette smokers	Smoking has been shown to decrease the serum half-life of theophylline

ADVERSE REACTIONS

Gastrointestinal	Nausea, vomiting, epigastric pain, hematemesis, diarrhea
Central nervous system and neuromuscular	Headache, irritability, restlessness, insomnia, reflex hyperexcitability, muscle twitching, clonic and tonic generalized convulsions
Cardiovascular	Palpitations, tachycardia, extrasystoles, flushing, hypotension, circulatory failure, ventricular arrhythmias
Respiratory	Tachypnea
Genitourinary	Albuminuria, increased excretion of renal tubule cells and red blood cells, diuresis
Other	Hyperglycemia, inappropriate antidiuretic hormone secretion syndrome

OVERDOSAGE

Signs and symptoms[2]	*Cardiovascular:* precordial pain, tachycardia, ventricular and other arrhythmias, hypotension, and, in extreme cases, severe shock, cardiovascular collapse, and death. *Gastrointestinal:* abdominal pain, nausea, persistent vomiting, and hematemesis. *Central nervous system:* headache, dizziness, restlessness, irritability, tremors, hyperactivity, and agitation, followed, in severe cases, by convulsions, drowsiness, coma, and death.
Treatment	If patient is conscious and seizures have not occurred, induce emesis and administer a cathartic (especially if sustained-release tablets have been ingested) and activated charcoal. If patient is convulsing, establish an airway and administer oxygen and IV diazepam (0.1–0.3 mg/kg, up to 10 mg). If patient is comatose following the occurrence of seizures, intubate immediately, using an endotracheal tube with an inflated cuff, and perform gastric lavage; introduce the cathartic and activated charcoal through a large-bore gastric lavage tube. Monitor vital signs, maintain blood pressure, and provide adequate hydration. Treat hypotension and shock by appropriate fluid replacement, avoiding the use of vasopressors, if possible. In general, the drug is metabolized sufficiently rapidly to preclude any additional benefit from dialysis; however, dialysis may be useful in the presence of congestive heart failure or hepatic dysfunction. Serial monitoring of the serum theophylline level is helpful in following the patient's course and in guiding further management.

DRUG INTERACTIONS

Other xanthine derivatives	△ Risk of toxicity; do not administer concurrently
Lithium	△ Lithium excretion
Propranolol	Antagonism of pharmacologic effects of propranolol ▽ Bronchodilation

QUIBRON ■ RESPBID

Cimetidine, clindamycin, erythromycin, lincomycin, troleandomycin	⇧ Theophylline serum level
Furosemide	⇧ Diuresis
Reserpine	Tachycardia
Chlordiazepoxide	Fatty acid mobilization
Ephedrine and possibly other sympathomimetic bronchodilators	⇧ Risk of toxicity

ALTERED LABORATORY VALUES

Blood/serum values	⇧ Prothrombin activity ⇧ Coagulation factor V ⇧ Glucose ⇧ Uric acid (with Bittner and colorimetric methods) ⇧ Bilirubin (with diazo tablet method)
Urinary values	⇧ Albumin ⇧ Catecholamines ⇧ 5-HIAA (with nitrosonaphthol reagent method)[3] ⇧ VMA (with colorimetric methods)[3]

USE IN CHILDREN
See INDICATIONS and ORAL DOSAGE

USE IN PREGNANT AND NURSING WOMEN
Pregnancy Category C: use during pregnancy only if clearly indicated. Animal reproduction studies have not been done. It is not known what effect, if any, this drug may have on human fetal development or reproductive capacity, or whether use at parturition can affect the fetus, prolong labor, or increase the possibility of forceps delivery or other obstetric intervention. Theophylline is reportedly excreted in human milk and to have caused irritability in a nursing infant; because of the potential for serious adverse reactions, a decision should be made to either discontinue use of the drug or stop nursing.

[1] When calculating dosages on the basis of weight, use the lean (or ideal) body weight, rather than the patient's actual weight (theophylline is not taken up by fatty tissue); for Quibron and Quibron-300, theophylline dosages are provided
[2] Serious toxicity may or may not be preceded by less serious side effects, such as nausea, irritability, or restlessness
[3] For Quibron and Quibron-300 only (both contain guaifenesin)

SYSTEMIC BRONCHODILATORS/ANTIASTHMATIC AGENTS

RESPBID (theophylline, anhydrous) Boehringer Ingelheim Rx
Tablets (sustained release): 250, 500 mg

INDICATIONS
Chronic, reversible bronchospasm associated with bronchial asthma, chronic bronchitis, and emphysema

ORAL DOSAGE[1]
Adult and child ($\geq$ 6 yr): 16 mg/kg/day, given in 2–3 divided doses q8–12h to start, followed, if needed and tolerated, by an approximately 25% increase in dosage every 2–3 days; for patients currently receiving theophylline, give one-half the established total daily dose q12h to start. Do not exceed, without measurement of serum level, 24 mg/kg/day for children 6–9 yr of age, 20 mg/kg/day for children 9–12 yr of age, 18 mg/kg/day for adolescents 12–16 yr of age, and 13 mg/kg/day or 900 mg/day, whichever is less, for patients over 16 yr of age. Tablets should be swallowed whole, not chewed or crushed.

CONTRAINDICATIONS
Hypersensitivity to theophylline

ADMINISTRATION/DOSAGE ADJUSTMENTS

Administration with food	Administration of some or all controlled-release theophylline products with food may affect absorption and result in altered serum values, especially when high serum levels are maintained or single doses exceeding 900 mg or 13 mg/kg are given; it is not known whether the bioavailability of Respbid tablets is influenced by food.
Dosage adjustment with measurement of serum level	Monitoring of serum theophylline level is recommended, particularly for titration of dosage. Check the peak serum level 4–6 h after the last dose; medication must have been taken at typical intervals, with no missed or added doses, for a period of 48 h prior to measurement. (Serum levels that are measured spectrophotometrically without prior chromatographic isolation may be falsely elevated when coffee, tea, acetaminophen, chocolate, or cola beverages have also been ingested.) Adjust dosage to maintain serum levels of 10–20 µg/ml; the risk of toxicity is significantly increased at higher levels, and, in some patients (eg, those with reduced theophylline clearance), toxic reactions may develop at serum concentrations of 15–20 µg/ml. If the peak serum level in patients with normal theophylline clearance is between 5 and 7.5 µg/ml, increase the total daily dose by 25%; if between 7.5 and 10 µg/ml, increase the daily dose by 25% and, if symptoms recur at the end of a dosing interval, administer more frequently; if between 20 and 25 µg/ml, reduce the daily dose by 10%; if between 25 and 30 µg/ml, omit the next dose and reduce the daily dose by 25%; if over 30 µg/ml, omit the next 2 doses and reduce the daily dose by 50%. Recheck the serum level after each dosage adjustment and then, once the maintenance dosage has been established, every 6–12 mo thereafter. *Do not attempt to maintain any dosage that is not tolerated.* Patients should be instructed to omit the next dose if they experience adverse effects and to resume therapy at a previously tolerated dosage once the reactions have disappeared.

RESPBID

Patients with reduced theophylline clearance	To avoid toxic reactions in neonates, patients over 55 yr of age (especially men), and patients with renal or hepatic impairment, influenza, alcoholism, chronic lung disease, cor pulmonale, or cardiac failure, reduce the initial dosage and monitor serum theophylline levels
Patients with rapid theophylline clearance	Children, smokers, and some nonsmoking adults are likely to require dosing q8h (smokers may, alternatively, need larger doses). The effect of smoking on theophylline clearance may persist for 3 mo to 2 yr after the individual has ceased smoking. To determine whether theophylline is rapidly cleared in an individual patient, look for undesirably low trough serum levels or for a recurrence of symptoms at the end of a dosing interval.

WARNINGS/PRECAUTIONS

Arrhythmia	Theophylline may precipitate or exacerbate arrhythmia; any significant change in cardiac rate or rhythm warrants monitoring and further investigation. Use with caution in patients with severe cardiac disease, acute myocardial injury, or hyperthyroidism. Theophylline toxicity may be masked in patients with tachycardia.
Gastric irritation	Theophylline occasionally may cause local irritation of the GI tract, although GI symptoms are more commonly centrally mediated and associated with serum levels over 20 μg/ml; use with caution in patients with a history of peptic ulcer
Special-risk patients	Use with caution in neonates, the elderly (especially men), and patients with renal or hepatic impairment, chronic lung disease, severe cardiac disease, hypertension, acute myocardial injury, congestive heart failure, cor pulmonale, severe hypoxemia, a history of peptic ulcer, hyperthyroidism, influenza, or alcoholism (see "patients with reduced theophylline clearance" in the ADMINISTRATION/DOSAGE ADJUSTMENTS section); use with particular caution in patients with congestive heart failure because clearance in such patients is frequently very slow
Morphine, curare	Since morphine and curare can stimulate histamine release and depress respiration, they should be given with caution, or, if possible, their use should be avoided
Acute bronchospasm	Do not use this product for treatment of acute bronchospasm. To provide rapid symptomatic relief, use an immediate-release or IV theophylline preparation or another bronchodilator. For status asthmaticus, it is frequently necessary to institute parenteral therapy and then closely monitor the patient (preferably in an intensive-care unit).
Carcinogenicity, mutagenicity, effect on fertility	No long-term studies have been performed to evaluate the carcinogenic and mutagenic potential of xanthine derivatives or their effect on fertility

ADVERSE REACTIONS

Gastrointestinal	Nausea, vomiting, epigastric pain, hematemesis, diarrhea
Central nervous system and neuromuscular	Headache, irritability, restlessness, insomnia, reflex hyperexcitability, muscle twitching, clonic and tonic generalized convulsions
Cardiovascular	Palpitations, tachycardia, extrasystoles, flushing, hypotension, circulatory failure, ventricular arrhythmias
Respiratory	Tachypnea
Renal	Albuminuria, increased excretion of renal tubule cells and red blood cells, potentiation of diuresis
Other	Hyperglycemia, inappropriate ADH syndrome

OVERDOSAGE

Signs and symptoms	See ADVERSE REACTIONS; ventricular arrhythmias or convulsions may be the first signs of toxicity, although in up to 50% of patients less severe signs of overdosage (eg, nausea, restlessness) occur initially
Treatment	If patient is conscious and seizures have not occurred, induce emesis and administer a cathartic and activated charcoal. If patient is convulsing, establish an airway and administer oxygen and IV diazepam (0.1–0.3 mg/kg, up to 10 mg). If patient is comatose following the occurrence of seizures, intubate immediately, using an endotracheal tube with an inflated cuff, and perform gastric lavage; introduce the cathartic and activated charcoal through a large-bore gastric lavage tube. Monitor vital signs, maintain blood pressure, and provide adequate hydration. Treat hypotension and shock by appropriate fluid replacement, avoiding the use of vasopressors, if possible (sympathomimetic drugs may precipitate cardiac arrhythmia). In general, the drug is metabolized sufficiently rapidly to preclude any additional benefit from dialysis; however, dialysis may be useful in the presence of congestive heart failure or hepatic dysfunction. Charcoal hemoperfusion may be necessary if serum levels are very high. Serial monitoring of the serum theophylline level is helpful in following the patient's course and in guiding further management.

DRUG INTERACTIONS

Other xanthine derivatives	◇ Risk of theophylline toxicity; do not administer other xanthine derivatives concomitantly. Caution patients against eating large quantities of chocolate and drinking large amounts of caffeine-containing liquids, such as coffee, tea, cocoa, or cola beverages, during therapy.

COMPENDIUM OF DRUG THERAPY

Cimetidine, erythromycin, troleandomycin, influenza virus vaccine	△ Serum theophylline level; reduce the initial dosage of theophylline and monitor serum levels
Ephedrine, other sympathomimetic agents	△ Risk of theophylline and sympathomimetic toxicity; exercise particular caution if patients with cardiac arrhythmias are given theophylline in combination with sympathomimetic agents
Lithium	▽ Serum lithium level
Propranolol	▽ Pharmacologic effects of propranolol and theophylline
Phenytoin	▽ Serum levels of theophylline and phenytoin
Furosemide	△ Diuresis
Reserpine	Tachycardia
Chlordiazepoxide	Fatty acid mobilization

ALTERED LABORATORY VALUES

Blood/serum values	△ Glucose △ Uric acid (with Bittner and colorimetric methods) △ Bilirubin (with diazo tablet method)
Urinary values	△ Albumin △ Catecholamines

USE IN CHILDREN

See INDICATIONS, ORAL DOSAGE, and ADMINISTRATION/DOSAGE ADJUSTMENTS; use in children under 6 yr of age is not recommended. To titrate dosage for children weighing less than 25 kg, use a liquid preparation, since it permits small increments in dosage. Exercise caution when adjusting dosage for young children who cannot complain of minor adverse reactions.

USE IN PREGNANT AND NURSING WOMEN

Pregnancy Category C: reproduction studies have not been performed; it is not known whether theophylline can cause harm to the fetus or affect reproductive capacity. Use during pregnancy only if clearly needed. Theophylline is excreted in human milk and may cause adverse reactions in infants; use with caution in nursing mothers.

[1] When calculating dosages on the basis of weight, use the lean (or ideal) body weight, rather than the patient's actual weight (theophylline is not taken up by fatty tissue)

SYSTEMIC BRONCHODILATORS/ANTIASTHMATIC AGENTS

SLO-BID (theophylline, anhydrous) Rorer — Rx

Capsules (sustained release): 50, 100, 200, 300 mg

INDICATIONS

Chronic, reversible bronchospasm associated with bronchial asthma, chronic bronchitis, and emphysema

ORAL DOSAGE[1]

Adult and child: 16 mg/kg/day or 400 mg/day, whichever is less, given in 2–3 divided doses q8–12h to start, followed, if needed and tolerated, by an approximately 25% increase in dosage every 3 days; do not exceed, without measurement of serum levels, 24 mg/kg/day for children 6-9 yr of age, 20 mg/kg/day for children 9-12 yr of age, 18 mg/kg/day for adolescents 12–16 yr of age, and 13 mg/kg/day or 900 mg/day, whichever is less, for patients over 16 yr of age

SLO-PHYLLIN (theophylline, anhydrous) Rorer — Rx

Tablets: 100, 200 mg **Syrup (per 15 ml):** 80 mg (15 ml, 4 fl oz, 1 pt, 1 gal) *sugar-free* **Capsules (sustained release):** 60, 125, 250 mg

INDICATIONS

Acute, reversible bronchospasm associated with bronchial asthma, chronic bronchitis, and emphysema

ORAL DOSAGE[1]

Adult, nonsmoker: 6 mg/kg to start, followed by 3 mg/kg q6h for the next 12 h and then q8h for maintenance; do not exceed 900 mg/day without measurement of serum level

Infant and child (6 mo to 9 yr): 6 mg/kg to start, followed by 4 mg/kg q4h for the next 12 h and then q6h for maintenance

Child (9–16 yr) and young adult smoker: 6 mg/kg to start, followed by 3 mg/kg q4h for the next 12 h and then q6h for maintenance

SLO-BID/SLO-PHYLLIN

Chronic, reversible bronchospasm associated with bronchial asthma, chronic bronchitis, and emphysema

Adult and child: 16 mg/kg/day or 400 mg/day, whichever is less, given in 3–4 divided doses q6–8h (if tablets or syrup is used) or 2–3 divided doses q8–12h (if capsules are used) to start, followed, if needed and tolerated, by an approximately 25% increase in dosage every 2–3 days (if tablets or syrup is used) or every 3 days (if capsules are used); do not exceed, without measurement of serum levels, 24 mg/kg/day for children 6 mo to 9 yr of age, 20 mg/kg/day for children 9–12 yr of age, 18 mg/kg/day for adolescents 12–16 yr of age, and 13 mg/kg/day or 900 mg/day, whichever is less, for patients over 16 yr of age

CONTRAINDICATIONS

Hypersensitivity to theophylline

ADMINISTRATION/DOSAGE ADJUSTMENTS

Administration with food — The tablets and syrup can be given with food to prevent some gastric irritation; absorption is slower, but still complete. Administration of some or all controlled-release theophylline products with food may affect absorption and result in altered serum values, especially when high serum levels are maintained or single doses exceeding 900 mg or 13 mg/kg are given; it is not known whether the bioavailability of Slo-Bid or Slo-Phyllin capsules is influenced by food. For patients who have difficulty swallowing Slo-Phyllin capsules and who require dosing q8h, the contents of the capsules can be sprinkled on a spoonful of soft food such as applesauce (the food should not be hot). Such patients should be instructed to swallow the food-theophylline mixture immediately without chewing it and then drink a glass of cool water or juice; they should not consume this mixture at mealtime.

Starting chronic therapy — To titrate dosage for patients who weigh 25 kg or more and who are not currently receiving theophylline, use the capsules or, preferably, an immediate-release product such as the tablets or syrup; children weighing less than 25 kg should be started on the syrup. To switch patients from an immediate-release preparation to the capsules, give one-third the established total daily dose q8h or one-half the dose q12h.

Dosage adjustment with measurement of serum levels — Monitoring of serum theophylline levels is recommended, particularly when the dosage exceeds 300 mg/day for children weighing 15–20 kg, 400 mg/day for children weighing 20–25 kg, 500 mg/day for children weighing 25–35 kg, or 600 mg/day for patients weighing over 35 kg. Check the peak serum level 1–2 h after the last dose if the syrup or tablets are used, 4 h after the last dose if Slo-Phyllin capsules are used, and 5 h after the last dose if Slo-Bid capsules are used; medication must have been taken at typical intervals, with no missed or added doses, for a period of 48 h prior to measurement. (Serum levels that are measured spectrophotometrically without prior chromatographic isolation may be falsely elevated when coffee, tea, acetaminophen, chocolate, or cola beverages have also been ingested.) Adjust dosage to maintain serum levels of 10–20 µg/ml; the risk of toxicity is significantly increased at higher levels, and, in some patients (eg, those with reduced theophylline clearance), toxic reactions may develop at serum concentrations of 15–20 µg/ml. If the peak serum level in patients with normal theophylline clearance is between 5 and 7.5 µg/ml, increase the total daily dose by 25%; if between 7.5 and 10 µg/ml, increase the daily dose by 25% and, if symptoms recur at the end of a dosing interval, administer more frequently (Slo-Bid capsules can be given in 3 divided doses q8h); if between 20 and 25 µg/ml, reduce the daily dose by 10%; if between 25 and 30 µg/ml, omit the next dose and reduce the daily dose by 25%; if over 30 µg/ml, omit the next 2 doses and reduce the daily dose by 50%. Recheck serum levels after dosage adjustment and then every 6–12 mo thereafter. *Do not attempt to maintain any dosage that is not tolerated.* Patients should be instructed to omit the next dose if they experience adverse effects and to reduce the subsequent dosage when they resume therapy after the reactions have disappeared.

Acute symptoms in patients currently receiving theophylline — Determine (where possible) the time, amount, route, and form of the patient's last dose. If it is not possible to obtain the patient's serum theophylline level quickly and there is sufficient respiratory distress to warrant a small risk, a loading dose may be given, based on the principle that each 0.5 mg/kg of theophylline administered in a rapidly absorbed form will increase the serum drug level by 1 µg/ml. Thus, if the patient is not already experiencing toxicity, a loading dose of 2.5 mg/kg (which will increase the serum level by 5 µg/ml) is unlikely to produce dangerous side effects.

Use of sustained-release capsules — To provide longer dosing intervals or less fluctuation in serum levels during chronic therapy, administer sustained-release capsules; do not use for acute symptoms requiring rapid theophyllinization

Patients with reduced theophylline clearance — To avoid toxic reactions in neonates, patients over 55 yr of age (especially men), and patients with renal or hepatic impairment, influenza, alcoholism, chronic lung disease, cor pulmonale, or cardiac failure, reduce the initial dosage and monitor serum theophylline levels. For acute symptoms requiring rapid theophyllinization, give older patients and patients with cor pulmonale 6 mg/kg to start, followed by 2 mg/kg q6h for the next 12 h and, thereafter, 2 mg/kg q8h for maintenance; patients with congestive heart failure should be given 6 mg/kg to start, followed by 2 mg/kg q8h for the next 16 h and, thereafter, 1–2 mg/kg q12h for maintenance.

SLO-BID/SLO-PHYLLIN

Patients with rapid theophylline clearance	Children, smokers, and some nonsmoking adults generally require administration of the syrup or tablets q6h and are likely to require dosing of the Slo-Phyllin capsules q8h (smokers may, alternatively, need larger doses). The effect of smoking on theophylline clearance may persist for 3 mo to 2 yr after the individual has ceased smoking. To determine whether theophylline is rapidly cleared in an individual patient, look for undesirably low trough serum levels or for a recurrence of symptoms at the end of a dosing interval.

WARNINGS/PRECAUTIONS

Status asthmaticus	Concomitant parenteral therapy and close monitoring (preferably in an intensive-care unit) are frequently necessary for the optimal management of this medical emergency
Arrhythmia	Theophylline may precipitate or exacerbate arrhythmia; any significant change in cardiac rate or rhythm warrants monitoring and further investigation. Use with caution in patients with severe cardiac disease, acute myocardial injury, or hyperthyroidism. Theophylline toxicity may be masked in patients with tachycardia.
Gastric irritation	Theophylline occasionally may cause local irritation of the GI tract, although GI symptoms are more commonly centrally mediated and associated with serum levels over 20 $\mu g/ml$; use with caution in patients with a history of peptic ulcer
Special-risk patients	Use with caution in neonates, the elderly (especially men), and patients with renal or hepatic impairment, chronic lung disease, severe cardiac disease, hypertension, acute myocardial injury, congestive heart failure, cor pulmonale, severe hypoxemia, a history of peptic ulcer, hyperthyroidism, influenza, or alcoholism (see "patients with reduced theophylline clearance" in the ADMINISTRATION/DOSAGE ADJUSTMENTS section); use with particular caution in patients with congestive heart failure because clearance in such patients is frequently very slow
Morphine, curare	Since morphine and curare can stimulate histamine release and depress respiration, they should be given with caution, or, if possible, their use should be avoided
Carcinogenicity, mutagenicity, effect on fertility	No long-term studies have been performed to evaluate the carcinogenic and mutagenic potential of xanthine derivatives or their effect on fertility

ADVERSE REACTIONS

Gastrointestinal	Nausea, vomiting, epigastric pain, hematemesis, diarrhea
Central nervous system and neuromuscular	Headache, irritability, restlessness, insomnia, reflex hyperexcitability, muscle twitching, clonic and tonic generalized convulsions
Cardiovascular	Palpitations, tachycardia, extrasystoles, flushing, hypotension, circulatory failure, ventricular arrhythmias
Respiratory	Tachypnea
Renal	Albuminuria, increased excretion of renal tubule cells and red blood cells, potentiation of diuresis
Other	Hyperglycemia, inappropriate antidiuretic hormone secretion syndrome, rash

OVERDOSAGE

Signs and symptoms	See ADVERSE REACTIONS; ventricular arrhythmias or convulsions may be the first signs of toxicity, although in up to 50% of patients less severe signs of overdosage (eg, nausea, restlessness) occur initially.
Treatment	If patient is conscious and seizures have not occurred, induce emesis and administer a cathartic (especially if sustained-release capsules have been ingested) and activated charcoal. If patient is convulsing, establish an airway and administer oxygen and IV diazepam (0.1–0.3 mg/kg, up to 10 mg). If patient is comatose following the occurrence of seizures, intubate immediately, using an endotracheal tube with an inflated cuff, and perform gastric lavage; introduce the cathartic and activated charcoal through a large-bore gastric lavage tube. Monitor vital signs, maintain blood pressure, and provide adequate hydration. Treat hypotension and shock by appropriate fluid replacement, avoiding the use of vasopressors, if possible. In general, the drug is metabolized sufficiently rapidly to preclude any additional benefit from dialysis; however, dialysis may be useful in the presence of congestive heart failure or hepatic dysfunction. Charcoal hemoperfusion may be necessary if serum levels exceed 50 $\mu g/ml$. Serial monitoring of the serum theophylline level is helpful in following the patient's course and in guiding further management.

DRUG INTERACTIONS

Other xanthine derivatives	△ Risk of theophylline toxicity; do not administer other xanthine derivatives concomitantly
Cimetidine, erythromycin, troleandomycin, influenza virus vaccine	△ Serum theophylline level; reduce the initial dosage of theophylline and monitor serum levels
Ephedrine, other sympathomimetic agents	△ Risk of theophylline and sympathomimetic toxicity
Lithium	▽ Serum lithium level

SLO-BID/SLO-PHYLLIN ■ SOMOPHYLLIN

Propranolol	▽ Pharmacologic effects of propranolol and theophylline
Phenytoin	▽ Serum levels of theophylline and phenytoin
Furosemide	△ Diuresis
Reserpine	Tachycardia
Chlordiazepoxide	Fatty acid mobilization

ALTERED LABORATORY VALUES

Blood/serum values	△ Glucose △ Uric acid (with Bittner and colorimetric methods) △ Bilirubin (with diazo tablet method)
Urinary values	△ Albumin △ Catecholamines

USE IN CHILDREN
See INDICATIONS, ORAL DOSAGE, and ADMINISTRATION/DOSAGE ADJUSTMENTS; use of tablets or syrup in children under 6 mo of age is not recommended because theophylline metabolism varies markedly in such patients. Safety and effectiveness of the capsules for use in children under 6 yr of age have not been established. Since the syrup permits small increments in dosage, it should be used to titrate dosage if a child requires chronic therapy and weighs under 25 kg. Exercise caution when adjusting dosage for younger children who cannot complain of minor adverse reactions.

USE IN PREGNANT AND NURSING WOMEN
Pregnancy Category C: reproduction studies have not been done; it is not known whether theophylline can cause harm to the fetus or affect reproductive capacity. Use during pregnancy only if clearly needed. Theophylline is excreted in human milk and may cause adverse reactions in nursing infants; use with caution in nursing mothers.

[1] When calculating dosages on the basis of weight, use the lean (or ideal) body weight, rather than the patient's actual weight (theophylline is not taken up by fatty tissue)

SYSTEMIC BRONCHODILATORS/ANTIASTHMATIC AGENTS

SOMOPHYLLIN (aminophylline, anhydrous) Fisons Rx
Liquid (per 5 ml): aminophylline equivalent to 90 mg theophylline (8, 32 fl oz) *raspberry flavored*

SOMOPHYLLIN-DF (aminophylline, anhydrous) Fisons Rx
Liquid (per 5 ml): aminophylline equivalent to 90 mg theophylline (8 fl oz) *raspberry flavored, dye free*

SOMOPHYLLIN Rectal Solution (aminophylline, anhydrous) Fisons Rx
Enema (per 5 ml): aminophylline equivalent to 255 mg theophylline (3, 5 fl oz)

SOMOPHYLLIN-T (theophylline, anhydrous) Fisons Rx
Capsules: 100, 200, 250 mg

INDICATIONS

Acute reversible bronchospasm associated with bronchial asthma, chronic bronchitis, and emphysema

Chronic, reversible bronchospasm associated with bronchial asthma, chronic bronchitis, and emphysema

ORAL AND RECTAL DOSAGE[1]

Adult, nonsmoker: 6 mg/kg to start, followed by 3 mg/kg q6h for the next 12 h and then q8h for maintenance
Infant and child (6 mo to 9 yr): 6 mg/kg to start, followed by 4 mg/kg q4h for the next 12 h and then q6h for maintenance
Child (9–16 yr) and young adult smoker: 6 mg/kg to start, followed by 3 mg/kg q4h for the next 12 h and then q6h for maintenance

Adult and child: 16 mg/kg/day or 400 mg/day, whichever is less, given in 3–4 divided doses q6–8h to start, followed, if needed and tolerated, by an approximately 25% increase in dosage every 2–3 days; do not exceed, without measurement of serum levels, 24 mg/kg/day for children 6 mo to 9 yr of age, 20 mg/kg/day for children 9–12 yr of age, 18 mg/kg/day for adolescents 12–16 yr of age, and 13 mg/kg/day or 900 mg/day, whichever is less, for patients over 16 yr of age

COMPENDIUM OF DRUG THERAPY

SOMOPHYLLIN

SOMOPHYLLIN-CRT (theophylline, anhydrous) Fisons Rx

Capsules (sustained release): 100, 200, 250, 300 mg

INDICATIONS

Chronic, reversible bronchospasm associated with bronchial asthma, chronic bronchitis, and emphysema

ORAL DOSAGE[1]

Adult and child ($\geq$ 6 yr): for patients currently receiving theophylline, one half the total daily dose q12h to start. For patients not currently receiving theophylline, use an immediate-release product to titrate dosage and then switch to the controlled-release capsules. Do not exceed, without measurement of serum levels, 24 mg/kg/day for children 6–9 yr of age, 20 mg/kg/day for children 9–12 yr of age, 18 mg/kg/day for adolescents 12–16 yr of age, or 13 mg/kg/day or 900 mg/day, whichever is less, for patients over 16 yr of age. Capsules should not be crushed or chewed.

CONTRAINDICATIONS

Hypersensitivity to theophylline or other components[2]

ADMINISTRATION/DOSAGE ADJUSTMENTS

Administration with food	The immediate-release oral preparations can be given with food to prevent some gastric irritation; absorption is slower, but is still complete. Administration of some or all controlled-release theophylline products with food may affect absorption and result in altered serum values, especially when high serum levels are maintained or single doses exceeding 900 mg or 13 mg/kg are given; it is not known whether the bioavailability of Somophyllin-CRT capsules is influenced by food.
Dosage adjustment with measurement of serum level	Monitoring of serum theophylline levels is recommended, particularly for titration of dosage. Check the peak serum level approximately 2 h after the last dose if the rectal solution is used, 1–2 h after the last dose if one of the immediate-release, oral preparations is used, or 4–6 h after the last dose if the controlled-release capsules are used; medication must have been taken at typical intervals, with no missed or added doses, for a period of 48 h prior to measurement. (Serum levels that are measured spectrophotometrically without prior chromatographic isolation may be falsely elevated when coffee, tea, acetaminophen, chocolate, or cola beverages have also been ingested.) Adjust dosage to maintain serum levels of 10–20 μg/ml; the risk of toxicity is significantly increased at higher levels, and, if theophylline clearance is reduced, toxic reactions may even develop at serum concentrations of 15–20 μg/ml. If the peak serum level in patients with normal theophylline clearance is between 5 and 7.5 μg/ml, increase the total daily dose by 25%; if between 7.5 and 10 μg/ml, increase the daily dose by 25% and, if symptoms recur at the end of a dosing interval, administer more frequently; if between 20 and 25 μg/ml, reduce the daily dose by 10%; if between 25 and 30 μg/ml, omit the next dose and reduce the daily dose by 25%; if over 30 μg/ml, omit the next 2 doses and reduce the daily dose by 50%. Recheck the serum level after each dosage adjustment and then, once the maintenance dosage has been established, every 6–12 mo thereafter. *Do not attempt to maintain any dosage that is not tolerated.* Patients should be instructed to omit the next dose if they experience adverse effects and to resume therapy at a previously tolerated dosage once the reactions have disappeared.
Acute symptoms in patients currently receiving theophylline products	Determine (where possible) the time, amount, route, and form of the patient's last dose. If it is not possible to obtain the patient's serum theophylline level quickly and there is sufficient respiratory distress to warrant a small risk, a loading dose may be given based on the principle that each 0.5 mg/kg of theophylline administered in a rapidly absorbed form will increase the serum drug level by 1 μg/ml. Thus, if the patient is not already experiencing toxicity, a loading dose of 2.5 mg/kg (which will increase the serum level by 5 μg/ml) is unlikely to produce dangerous side effects.
Use of sustained-release capsules	To provide longer dosing intervals or less fluctuation in serum levels during chronic therapy, administer sustained-release capsules; do not use for acute symptoms requiring rapid theophyllinization
Patient with reduced theophylline clearance	To avoid toxic reactions due to increased serum levels in neonates, patients over 55 yr of age (especially men), and patients with renal or hepatic impairment, influenza, alcoholism, chronic lung disease, cor pulmonale, or cardiac failure, reduce the initial dosage and monitor serum theophylline levels. For acute symptoms requiring rapid theophyllinization, give older patients and patients with cor pulmonale 6 mg/kg to start, followed by 2 mg/kg q6h for the next 12 h and then, for maintenance, 2 mg/kg q8h, and give patients with congestive heart failure 6 mg/kg to start, followed by 2 mg/kg q8h for the next 6 h and then, for maintenance, 1–2 mg/kg q12h.
Patients with rapid theophylline clearance	Children, smokers, and some nonsmoking adults generally require administration of the immediate-release products q6h and are likely to require dosing of the controlled-release capsules q8h (smokers may, alternatively, need larger doses). The effect of smoking on theophylline clearance may persist for 3 mo to 2 yr after the individual has ceased smoking. To determine whether theophylline is rapidly cleared in an individual patient, look for undesirably low trough serum levels or for a recurrence of symptoms at the end of a dosing interval.

WARNINGS/PRECAUTIONS

Acute bronchospasm	To provide rapid symptomatic relief, use one of the immediate-release products, preferably the oral liquid rather than the rectal solution; do not treat acute bronchospasm with the controlled-release capsules. For status asthmaticus, it is frequently necessary to institute parenteral therapy and then closely monitor the patient (preferably in an intensive-care unit).

SOMOPHYLLIN

Arrhythmia	Theophylline may precipitate or exacerbate arrhythmia; any significant change in cardiac rate or rhythm warrants monitoring and further investigation. Use with caution in patients with severe cardiac disease, acute myocardial injury, or hyperthyroidism. Theophylline toxicity may be masked in patients with tachycardia.
Gastric irritation	Theophylline occasionally may cause local irritation of the GI tract, although GI symptoms are more commonly centrally mediated and associated with serum levels over 20 µg/ml; use with caution in patients with a history of peptic ulcer
Special-risk patients	Use with caution in neonates, the elderly (especially men), and patients with renal or hepatic impairment, chronic lung disease, severe cardiac disease, hypertension, acute myocardial injury, congestive heart failure, cor pulmonale, severe hypoxemia, a history of peptic ulcer, hyperthyroidism, influenza, or alcoholism (see "patients with reduced theophylline clearance" in the ADMINISTRATION/DOSAGE ADJUSTMENTS section); use with particular caution in patients with congestive heart failure because clearance in such patients is frequently very slow
Morphine, curare	Since morphine and curare can stimulate histamine release and depress respiration, they should be given with caution, or, if possible, their use should be avoided
Carcinogenicity, mutagenicity, effect on fertility	No long-term studies have been performed to evaluate the carcinogenic and mutagenic potential of xanthine derivatives or their effect on fertility

ADVERSE REACTIONS

Gastrointestinal	Nausea, vomiting, epigastric pain, hematemesis, diarrhea
Central nervous system and neuromuscular	Headache, irritability, restlessness, insomnia, reflex hyperexcitability, muscle twitching, clonic and tonic generalized convulsions
Cardiovascular	Palpitations, tachycardia, extrasystoles, flushing, hypotension, circulatory failure, ventricular arrhythmias
Respiratory	Tachypnea
Renal	Albuminuria, increased excretion of renal tubule cells and red blood cells, potentiation of diuresis
Metabolic and endocrinological	Hyperglycemia, inappropriate ADH syndrome, rash

OVERDOSAGE

Signs and symptoms	See ADVERSE REACTIONS; ventricular arrhythmias or convulsions may be the first signs of toxicity, although in up to 50% of patients less severe signs of overdosage (eg, nausea, restlessness) occur initially
Treatment	If patient is conscious and seizures have not occurred, induce emesis and administer a cathartic (especially if controlled-release capsules have been ingested) and activated charcoal. If patient is convulsing, establish an airway and administer oxygen and IV diazepam (0.1–0.3 mg/kg, up to 10 mg). If patient is comatose following the occurrence of seizures, intubate immediately, using an endotracheal tube with an inflated cuff, and perform gastric lavage; introduce the cathartic and activated charcoal through a large-bore gastric lavage tube. Monitor vital signs, maintain blood pressure, and provide adequate hydration. Treat hypotension and shock by appropriate fluid replacement, avoiding the use of vasopressors, if possible. In general, the drug is metabolized sufficiently rapidly to preclude any additional benefit from dialysis; however, dialysis may be useful in the presence of congestive heart failure or hepatic dysfunction. Charcoal hemoperfusion may be necessary if serum levels exceed 50 µg/ml. Serial monitoring of the serum theophylline level is helpful in following the patient's course and in guiding further management.

DRUG INTERACTIONS

Other xanthine derivatives	△ Risk of theophylline toxicity; do not administer other xanthine derivatives concomitantly
Cimetidine, erythromycin, troleandomycin, influenza virus vaccine	△ Serum theophylline level; reduce the initial dosage of theophylline and monitor serum levels
Ephedrine, other sympathomimetic agents	△ Risk of theophylline and sympathomimetic toxicity
Lithium	▽ Serum lithium level
Propranolol	▽ Pharmacologic effects of propranolol and theophylline
Furosemide	△ Diuresis
Reserpine	Tachycardia
Chlordiazepoxide	Fatty acid mobilization
Phenytoin	▽ Phenytoin serum level

ALTERED LABORATORY VALUES

Blood/serum values	△ Glucose △ Uric acid (with Bittner and colorimetric methods) △ Bilirubin (with diazo tablet method)

SOMOPHYLLIN ■ TEDRAL

Urinary values —————————————————— ⇧ Albumin   ⇧ Catecholamines

USE IN CHILDREN	USE IN PREGNANT AND NURSING WOMEN
See INDICATIONS, ORAL DOSAGE, and ADMINISTRATION/DOSAGE ADJUSTMENTS; use of the immediate-release products in children under 6 mo of age is not recommended because theophylline metabolism varies markedly in such patients. Safety and effectiveness of the controlled-release capsules for use in children under 6 yr of age have not been established. Exercise caution when adjusting dosage for younger children who cannot complain of minor adverse reactions.	Pregnancy Category C: reproduction studies have not been done; it is not known whether theophylline can cause harm to the fetus or affect reproductive capacity. Use during pregnancy only if clearly needed. Theophylline is excreted in human milk and may cause adverse reactions in nursing infants; use with caution in nursing mothers.

[1] When calculating dosages on the basis of weight, use the lean (or ideal) body weight, rather than the patient's actual weight (theophylline is not taken up by fatty tissue)
[2] Rectal solution and oral liquids contain ethylenediamine

SYSTEMIC BRONCHODILATORS/ANTIASTHMATIC AGENTS

TEDRAL (theophylline, ephedrine hydrochloride, and phenobarbital) Warner-Lambert   OTC
Tablets: 130 mg theophylline, 24 mg ephedrine hydrochloride, and 8 mg phenobarbital   **Suspension (per 5 ml):** 65 mg theophylline, 12 mg ephedrine hydrochloride, and 4 mg phenobarbital (8, 16 fl oz) *licorice-flavored*   **Elixir (per 5 ml):** 32.5 mg theophylline, 6 mg ephedrine hydrochloride, and 2 mg phenobarbital[1] (16 fl oz) *cherry-flavored*

TEDRAL SA (theophylline, ephedrine hydrochloride, and phenobarbital) Parke-Davis   Rx
Tablets (sustained release): 180 mg theophylline, 48 mg ephedrine hydrochloride, and 25 mg phenobarbital

INDICATIONS	**ORAL DOSAGE**
Bronchial asthma, asthmatic bronchitis, and other bronchospastic disorders	**Adult:** 1–2 Tedral tabs, 10–20 ml (2–4 tsp) of the suspension, or 15–30 ml (1–2 tbsp) of the elixir q4h, or 1 Tedral SA (sustained action) tab upon arising and a 2nd tab 12 h later **Child:** 5 ml (1 tsp) of the suspension or 10 ml (2 tsp) of the elixir per 60 lb q4–6h; alternatively, children weighing over 60 lb may be given ½–1 Tedral tab q4h
CONTRAINDICATIONS	
Hypersensitivity to any component	Porphyria
WARNINGS/PRECAUTIONS	
Drug dependence	Psychic and/or physical dependence and tolerance to barbiturates may develop
Drowsiness	May occur
Special-risk patients	Use with caution in patients with cardiovascular disease, severe hypertension, hyperthyroidism, prostatic hypertrophy, or glaucoma
ADVERSE REACTIONS	
Gastrointestinal	Mild epigastric distress
Cardiovascular	Palpitations
Central nervous system	Tremulousness, insomnia, stimulation
Genitourinary	Difficult micturition
OVERDOSAGE	
Signs and symptoms	Palpitations, tachycardia, tremulousness, flushing, anginal-type pain, nausea, dizziness, weakness, sweating, cardiac irregularities, CNS disturbances, reflex bradycardia, respiratory depression, ataxia, miosis, decreased urine formation, hypothermia, shock
Treatment	Empty stomach by gastric lavage, followed by activated charcoal. Maintain patent airway and provide assisted ventilation, as needed. Maintain body temperature. Treat symptomatically and institute supportive measures, as required.
DRUG INTERACTIONS	
Other xanthine derivatives	⇧ Risk of toxicity; do not administer concurrently

TEDRAL ■ THEO-24

Lithium	△ Lithium excretion due to theophylline component
Propranolol	Antagonism by theophylline component of pharmacologic effects of propranolol ▽ Bronchodilation
Cimetidine, clindamycin, erythromycin, lincomycin, troleandomycin	△ Theophylline serum level
Furosemide	△ Diuresis due to theophylline component
Reserpine	Tachycardia due to theophylline component ▽ Pressor effect of ephedrine component
Chlordiazepoxide	Fatty acid mobilization due to interaction with theophylline component
Digitalis glycosides, anesthetics	Cardiac arrhythmias due to ephedrine component
Ergonovine, methylergonovine, oxytocin	Hypertension due to ephedrine component
Guanethidine	▽ Hypotensive effect due to ephedrine component
MAO inhibitors	△ Pressor effect of ephedrine component and CNS depressant effect of phenobarbital component
Other sympathomimetic agents	△ Sympathomimetic effects of ephedrine component or other sympathomimetics
Tricyclic antidepressants	▽ Pressor effect of ephedrine component
Alcohol, general anesthetics, and other CNS depressants	△ CNS depression due to phenobarbital component
Oral anticoagulants	▽ Anticoagulant effect due to phenobarbital component
Corticosteroids, digitalis, digitoxin, doxycycline, tricyclic antidepressants, griseofulvin, phenytoin	▽ Pharmacologic effect due to phenobarbital component

ALTERED LABORATORY VALUES

Blood/serum values	△ Glucose △ Uric acid (with Bittner and colorimetric methods) △ Bilirubin (with diazo tablet method)
Urinary values	△ Albumin △ Catecholamines

USE IN CHILDREN
See INDICATIONS and ORAL DOSAGE. The suspension and elixir formulations should be used with extreme caution in children under 2 yr of age. Dosage of sustained-release formulation has not been established for children under 12 yr of age.

USE IN PREGNANT AND NURSING WOMEN
Consult manufacturer

[1] Contains 15% alcohol

SYSTEMIC BRONCHODILATORS/ANTIASTHMATIC AGENTS

THEO-24 (theophylline, anhydrous) Searle   Rx
Capsules (controlled release): 100, 200, 300 mg

INDICATIONS
Chronic asthma
Reversible bronchospasm associated with chronic bronchitis and emphysema

ORAL DOSAGE[1]
Adult: 400 mg once daily to start, followed, if needed and tolerated, by an increase of 100 mg/day every 3–5 days, up to 900 mg/day or 13 mg/kg/day, whichever is less
Child (30–35 kg): 300 mg once daily to start, followed, if needed and tolerated, by an increase of 100 mg/day every 3–5 days, up to 900 mg/day or 13 mg/kg/day, whichever is less
Child ($\geq$ 35 kg): same as adult

CONTRAINDICATIONS
Hypersensitivity to theophylline

THEO-24

ADMINISTRATION/DOSAGE ADJUSTMENTS

Timing of administration	Instruct the patient to take this preparation in the morning at approximately the same time each day; do not use at night because studies have shown that administration at nighttime, after the evening meal, results in delayed peak and early trough serum levels. If twice-daily administration is necessary, give the second dose before the evening meal, 10–12 h after the morning dose. Administration within 1 h before a high-fat meal may produce an increase in absorption and the peak serum level and, in some cases, may enhance the risk of toxicity. Patients who require a dosage equal to or exceeding 900 mg/day or 13 mg/kg/day (whichever is less) should be instructed to avoid eating a high-fat breakfast or to wait at least 1 h after taking the drug before beginning such a meal; patients who cannot comply should be placed on a twice-daily regimen. Closely observe patients who are receiving single daily doses of less than 900 mg.
Patients with rapid theophylline clearance	In some patients (eg, children, adolescents, smokers), bronchospasm may occur repeatedly, especially at the end of a 24-h interval, or the peak-trough difference may be wider than desired; twice-daily administration may be advisable for such patients (see "timing of administration," above)
Patients with reduced theophylline clearance	To avoid toxic reactions due to increased serum levels in neonates, patients over 55 yr of age (especially men), and patients with renal or hepatic impairment, influenza or other viral infections, alcoholism, chronic lung disease, cor pulmonale, or cardiac failure, reduce the initial dosage and monitor serum theophylline levels
Patients currently receiving theophylline	To transfer patients to this product, administer the established total daily dose as a single dose in the morning; however, do not exceed 900 mg/day or 13 mg/kg/day (whichever is less) to start. Check serum theophylline levels before and immediately after the transfer; administration of this preparation once daily may produce a wider peak-trough difference. Adjust dosage, if necessary, on the basis of the serum level.
Dosage adjustment with measurement of serum levels	Monitoring of serum theophylline levels is highly recommended. Optimal response, determined by improvement in symptomatic response and pulmonary function, often occurs at serum levels of 10–20 µg/ml, but may be obtained at lower levels. Although some patients may require serum levels above 20 µg/ml, the risk of toxicity is increased at these higher levels; if theophylline clearance is reduced because of disease or concomitant drug therapy, toxic reactions may occur even at the upper level of the 10- to 20-µg/ml range. Check the peak level 12 h after the morning dose and the trough level 24 h after that dose; medication must have been taken at 24-h intervals, with no missed or added doses, for a period of 72 h prior to measurement. Serum levels that are measured spectrophotometrically without prior chromatographic isolation are falsely high when coffee, tea, acetaminophen, chocolate, or cola beverages have also been ingested. If serum levels in patients with normal theophylline clearance exceed 30 µg/ml, omit the next dose and decrease the daily dose by 50%; if between 25 and 30 µg/ml, omit the next dose and decrease the daily dose by 25%; and if between 20 and 25 µg/ml, reduce the daily dose by 10%. Recheck serum levels 3 days after the dosage adjustment. If the initial serum level is too low, increase the daily dose by 100–200 mg or 25% every 3 days; recheck serum levels at appropriate intervals or at the end of the dosage adjustment period. *Do not attempt to maintain any dosage that is not tolerated.* After the maintenance dosage has been established, serum levels should be measured every 6–12 mo and whenever theophylline clearance is altered.
Dosage adjustment without measurement of serum levels	See ORAL DOSAGE; if adverse reactions occur during titration of dosage, omit the next dose or decrease the daily dose by 25%

WARNINGS/PRECAUTIONS

Arrhythmia	Theophylline may precipitate or exacerbate arrhythmia; any significant change in cardiac rate or rhythm warrants monitoring and further investigation. Use with caution in patients with severe cardiac disease, acute myocardial injury, or hyperthyroidism. Theophylline toxicity may be masked in patients with tachycardia.
Gastric irritation	Theophylline occasionally may cause local irritation of the GI tract, although GI symptoms are more commonly centrally mediated and associated with serum levels over 20 µg/ml; use with caution in patients with a history of peptic ulcer to avoid exacerbation of the disease
Special-risk patients	Use with caution in neonates, the elderly (especially men), and patients with renal or hepatic impairment, chronic lung disease, severe cardiac disease, hypertension, acute myocardial injury, congestive heart failure, cor pulmonale, severe hypoxemia, hyperthyroidism, influenza or other viral infections, or alcoholism (see "patients with reduced theophylline clearance" in the ADMINISTRATION/DOSAGE ADJUSTMENTS section); use with particular caution in patients with congestive heart failure because clearance in such patients is very slow
Convulsions	Theophylline may lower the seizure threshold; convulsions may occur if serum levels exceed 30 µg/ml
Acute bronchospasm	This product is not indicated for the treatment of acute bronchospastic episodes; for rapid symptomatic relief, use an immediate-release or IV theophylline preparation or other bronchodilators. If status asthmaticus occurs, administer parenteral therapy and closely monitor the patient (preferably in an intensive-care unit).

THEO-24

| Carcinogenicity, mutagenicity, effect on fertility | Theophylline has been shown to be mutagenic in *Escherichia coli* and other lower organisms and to produce chromosome breakage in cultured mouse cells and human lymphocytes; however, no mutagenic activity has been seen in a dominant lethal test with mice. Long-term animal studies to evaluate the carcinogenic or mutagenic potential of this drug or its effect on fertility have not been done. |

ADVERSE REACTIONS

Gastrointestinal	Nausea, vomiting, epigastric pain, hematemesis, diarrhea
Central nervous system	Headache, irritability, restlessness, insomnia, reflex hyperexcitability, muscle twitching, clonic and tonic generalized convulsions, coma
Cardiovascular	Palpitations, tachycardia, extrasystoles, flushing, hypotension, circulatory failure, ventricular arrhythmia
Respiratory	Tachypnea
Renal	Albuminuria, microhematuria, potentiation of diuresis
Other	Hyperglycemia, inappropriate ADH syndrome

OVERDOSAGE

| Signs and symptoms | See ADVERSE REACTIONS; the first signs of toxicity may be ventricular arrhythmias or convulsions rather than less severe reactions, such as persistent nausea and vomiting |
| Treatment | If patient is conscious and seizures have not occurred, induce emesis or perform gastric lavage, and then administer activated charcoal and a cathartic. If patient is convulsing, establish an airway and administer oxygen and IV diazepam (0.1–0.3 mg/kg, up to a total of 10 mg). If patient is comatose following the occurrence of seizures, intubate immediately, using an endotracheal tube with an inflated cuff, and perform gastric lavage; introduce the cathartic and activated charcoal through a large-bore gastric lavage tube. Monitor vital signs, maintain blood pressure, and provide adequate hydration. Treat hypotension and shock by appropriate fluid replacement, avoiding the use of vasopressors, if possible. In general, the drug is metabolized sufficiently rapidly to preclude any additional benefit from dialysis; however, dialysis may be useful in the presence of congestive heart failure or hepatic dysfunction. Charcoal hemoperfusion may be necessary if serum levels exceed 50 µg/ml. Serial monitoring of the serum theophylline level is helpful in following the patient's course and in guiding further management. |

DRUG INTERACTIONS

Other xanthine derivatives	△ Risk of theophylline toxicity; do not administer other xanthine derivatives concomitantly
Cimetidine, ranitidine, erythromycin, troleandomycin, influenza virus vaccine, oral contraceptives, allopurinol	△ Serum theophylline level; carefully watch for signs of toxicity and, if necessary, reduce theophylline dosage
Ephedrine, other sympathomimetic agents	△ Risk of theophylline and sympathomimetic toxicity
Phenobarbital, phenytoin, rifampin	△ Theophylline clearance; increase theophylline dosage, if necessary
Lithium	▽ Serum lithium level
Propranolol	▽ Pharmacologic effects of propranolol and theophylline
Furosemide	△ Diuresis
Reserpine	Tachycardia
Chlordiazepoxide	Fatty acid mobilization

ALTERED LABORATORY VALUES

| Blood/serum values | △ Glucose △ Uric acid (with Bittner and colorimetric methods) △ Bilirubin (with diazo tablet method) |
| Urinary values | △ Albumin △ Catecholamines |

USE IN CHILDREN

See INDICATIONS and ORAL DOSAGE; safety and effectiveness for use in children under 12 yr of age have not been established

USE IN PREGNANT AND NURSING WOMEN

Pregnancy Category C: limited animal studies have shown teratogenic activity in mice and rats; it is not known whether theophylline can cause harm to the fetus when administered to a pregnant woman or can affect reproductive capacity. Use during pregnancy only if clearly needed. Theophylline is excreted in human milk and may cause adverse reactions in infants; use with caution in nursing mothers.

[1] When calculating dosages on the basis of weight, use the lean (or ideal) body weight, rather than the patient's actual weight (theophylline is not taken up by fatty tissue)

SYSTEMIC BRONCHODILATORS/ ANTIASTHMATIC AGENTS

THEOBID (theophylline, anhydrous) Glaxo — Rx
Capsules (sustained release): 260 mg

THEOBID Jr. (theophylline, anhydrous) Glaxo — Rx
Capsules (sustained release): 130 mg

INDICATIONS	**ORAL DOSAGE**[1]
Chronic, reversible bronchospasm associated with bronchial asthma, chronic bronchitis, and emphysema	Adult and child ($\geq$ 6 yr): titrate dosage with an immediate-release product and then switch to the sustained-release capsules, giving one-half the total daily dose q12h; do not exceed, without measurement of serum level, 24 mg/kg/day for children 6–9 yr of age, 20 mg/kg/day for children 9–12 yr of age, 18 mg/kg/day for adolescents 12–16 yr of age, and 13 mg/kg/day or 900 mg/day, whichever is less, for patients over 16 yr of age

CONTRAINDICATIONS
Hypersensitivity to theophylline

ADMINISTRATION/DOSAGE ADJUSTMENTS

Administration with food	Administration of some or all controlled-release theophylline products with food may affect absorption and result in altered serum values, especially when high serum levels are maintained or single doses exceeding 900 mg or 13 mg/kg are given; it is not known whether the bioavailability of Theobid or Theobid Jr. capsules is influenced by food
Dosage adjustment with measurement of serum level	Monitoring of serum theophylline level is recommended, particularly for titration of dosage. Check the peak serum level 4 h after the last dose; medication must have been taken at typical intervals, with no missed or added doses, for a period of 48 h prior to measurement. (Serum levels that are measured spectrophotometrically without prior chromatographic isolation may be falsely elevated when coffee, tea, acetaminophen, chocolate, or cola beverages have also been ingested.) Adjust dosage to maintain serum levels of 10–20 µg/ml; the risk of toxicity is significantly increased at higher levels, and, in some patients (eg, those with reduced theophylline clearance), toxic reactions may develop at serum concentrations of 15–20 µg/ml. If the peak serum level in patients with normal theophylline clearance is between 5 and 7.5 µg/ml, increase the total daily dose by 25%; if between 7.5 and 10 µg/ml, increase the daily dose by 25% and, if symptoms recur at the end of a dosing interval, administer in 3 divided doses q8h; if between 20 and 25 µg/ml, reduce the daily dose by 10%; if between 25 and 30 µg/ml, omit the next dose and reduce the daily dose by 25%; if over 30 µg/ml, omit the next 2 doses and reduce the daily dose by 50%. Recheck the serum level after each dosage adjustment and then, once the maintenance dosage has been established, every 6–12 mo thereafter. *Do not attempt to maintain any dosage that is not tolerated.* Patients should be instructed to omit the next dose if they experience adverse effects and to resume therapy at a previously tolerated dosage once the reactions have disappeared.
Patients with reduced theophylline clearance	To avoid toxic reactions in neonates, patients over 55 yr of age (especially men), and patients with renal or hepatic impairment, influenza, alcoholism, chronic lung disease, cor pulmonale, or cardiac failure, reduce the initial dosage and monitor serum theophylline levels
Patients with rapid theophylline clearance	Children, smokers, and some nonsmoking adults are likely to require dosing q8h (smokers may, alternatively, need larger doses). The effect of smoking on theophylline clearance may persist for 3 mo to 2 yr after the individual has ceased smoking. To determine whether theophylline is rapidly cleared in an individual patient, look for undesirably low trough serum levels or for a recurrence of symptoms at the end of a dosing interval.

WARNINGS/PRECAUTIONS

Arrhythmia	Theophylline may precipitate or exacerbate arrhythmia; any significant change in cardiac rate or rhythm warrants monitoring and further investigation. Use with caution in patients with severe cardiac disease, acute myocardial injury, or hyperthyroidism. Theophylline toxicity may be masked in patients with tachycardia.
Gastric irritation	Theophylline occasionally may cause local irritation of the GI tract, although GI symptoms are more commonly centrally mediated and associated with serum levels over 20 µg/ml; use with caution in patients with a history of peptic ulcer
Special-risk patients	Use with caution in neonates, the elderly (especially men), and patients with renal or hepatic impairment, chronic lung disease, severe cardiac disease, hypertension, acute myocardial injury, congestive heart failure, cor pulmonale, severe hypoxemia, a history of peptic ulcer, hyperthyroidism, influenza, or alcoholism (see "patients with reduced theophylline clearance" in the ADMINISTRATION/DOSAGE ADJUSTMENTS section); use with particular caution in patients with congestive heart failure because clearance in such patients is frequently very slow

THEOBID

Morphine, curare	Since morphine and curare can stimulate histamine release and depress respiration, they should be given with caution, or, if possible, their use should be avoided.
Acute bronchospasm	Do not use this product for treatment of acute bronchospasm. To provide rapid symptomatic relief, use an immediate-release or IV theophylline preparation or another bronchodilator. For status asthmaticus, it is frequently necessary to institute parenteral therapy and then closely monitor the patient (preferably in an intensive-care unit).
Carcinogenicity, mutagenicity, effect on fertility	No long-term studies have been performed to evaluate the carcinogenic and mutagenic potential of xanthine derivatives or their effect on fertility

ADVERSE REACTIONS

Gastrointestinal	Nausea, vomiting, epigastric pain, hematemesis, diarrhea
Central nervous system and neuromuscular	Headache, irritability, restlessness, insomnia, reflex hyperexcitability, muscle twitching, clonic and tonic generalized convulsions
Cardiovascular	Palpitations, tachycardia, extrasystoles, flushing, hypotension, circulatory failure, ventricular arrhythmias
Respiratory	Tachypnea
Renal	Albuminuria, increased excretion of renal tubule cells and red blood cells, potentiation of diuresis
Other	Hyperglycemia, inappropriate ADH syndrome, rash

OVERDOSAGE

Signs and symptoms	See ADVERSE REACTIONS; ventricular arrhythmias or convulsions may be the first signs of toxicity, although in up to 50% of patients less severe signs of overdosage (eg, nausea, restlessness) occur initially
Treatment	If patient is conscious and seizures have not occurred, induce emesis and administer a cathartic and activated charcoal. If patient is convulsing, establish an airway and administer oxygen and IV diazepam (0.1–0.3 mg/kg, up to 10 mg). If patient is comatose following the occurrence of seizures, intubate immediately, using an endotracheal tube with an inflated cuff, and perform gastric lavage; introduce the cathartic and activated charcoal through a large-bore gastric lavage tube. Monitor vital signs, maintain blood pressure, and provide adequate hydration. Treat hypotension and shock by appropriate fluid replacement, avoiding the use of vasopressors, if possible (sympathomimetic drugs may precipitate cardiac arrhythmia). In general, the drug is metabolized sufficiently rapidly to preclude any additional benefit from dialysis; however, dialysis may be useful in the presence of congestive heart failure or hepatic dysfunction. Charcoal hemoperfusion may be necessary if serum levels exceed 50 µg/ml. Serial monitoring of the serum theophylline level is helpful in following the patient's course and in guiding further management.

DRUG INTERACTIONS

Other xanthine derivatives	△ Risk of theophylline toxicity; do not administer other xanthine derivatives concomitantly
Cimetidine, erythromycin, troleandomycin, influenza virus vaccine	△ Serum theophylline level; reduce the initial dosage of theophylline and monitor serum levels
Ephedrine, other sympathomimetic agents	△ Risk of theophylline and sympathomimetic toxicity
Lithium	▽ Serum lithium level
Propranolol	▽ Pharmacologic effects of propranolol and theophylline
Phenytoin	▽ Serum levels of theophylline and phenytoin
Furosemide	△ Diuresis
Reserpine	Tachycardia
Chlordiazepoxide	Fatty acid mobilization

ALTERED LABORATORY VALUES

Blood/serum values	△ Glucose △ Uric acid (with Bittner and colorimetric methods) △ Bilirubin (with diazo tablet method)
Urinary values	△ Albumin △ Catecholamines

USE IN CHILDREN

See INDICATIONS, ORAL DOSAGE, and ADMINISTRATIVE/DOSAGE ADJUSTMENTS; exercise caution when adjusting dosage for young children who cannot complain of minor adverse reactions. Safety and effectiveness for use in children under 6 yr of age have not been established.

USE IN PREGNANT AND NURSING WOMEN

Pregnancy Category C: reproduction studies have not been performed; it is not known whether theophylline can cause harm to the fetus or affect reproductive capacity. Use during pregnancy only if clearly needed. Theophylline is excreted in human milk and may cause adverse reactions in infants; use with caution in nursing mothers.

---

[1] When calculating dosages on the basis of weight, use the lean (or ideal) body weight, rather than the patient's actual weight (theophylline is not taken up by fatty tissue)

SYSTEMIC BRONCHODILATORS/ ANTIASTHMATIC AGENTS

THEO-DUR (theophylline, anhydrous) Key Rx

Tablets (sustained action): 100, 200, 300 mg

INDICATIONS

Chronic, reversible bronchospasm associated with bronchial asthma, chronic bronchitis, and emphysema

ORAL DOSAGE[1]

Adult and child ($\geq$ 6 yr): 200 mg q12h to start, followed, if needed and tolerated, by an approximately 25% increase in dosage every 3 days; for patients currently receiving theophylline, give one half the established total daily dose q12h to start. Do not exceed, without measurement of serum level, 500 mg/24 h for children weighing 25–35 kg, 600 mg/24 h for children or adults weighing 35–70 kg, or 900 mg/24 h for adults weighing over 70 kg.

THEO-DUR Sprinkle (theophylline, anhydrous) Key Rx

Capsules (sustained action): 50, 75, 125, 200 mg

INDICATIONS

Chronic, reversible bronchospasm associated with bronchial asthma, chronic bronchitis, and emphysema

ORAL DOSAGE[1]

Adult and child ($\geq$ 6 yr): 16 mg/kg/day or 400 mg/day, whichever is less, given in 2 divided doses q12h to start, followed, if needed and tolerated, by an approximately 25% increase in dosage every 3 days; for patients currently receiving theophylline, give one-half the established total daily dose q12h to start. Do not exceed, without measurement of serum level, 24 mg/kg/day for children 6–9 yr of age, 20 mg/kg/day for children 9–12 yr of age, 18 mg/kg/day for adolescents 12–16 yr of age, and 13 mg/kg/day or 900 mg/day, whichever is less, for patients over 16 yr of age.

CONTRAINDICATIONS

Hypersensitivity to theophylline

ADMINISTRATION/DOSAGE ADJUSTMENTS

Administration of tablets — Administration of some or all controlled-release theophylline products with food may affect absorption and result in altered serum levels, especially when high serum levels are maintained or single doses exceeding 900 mg or 13 mg/kg are given. A single-dose study has shown that both the rate and extent of absorption of the 200– and 300–mg Theo-Dur tablets are similar following administration under fasting conditions and immediately after a moderately high fat breakfast; it is not known whether the bioavailability of the 100–mg Theo-Dur tablets is affected by food. Tablets should not be crushed or chewed; when given once daily, they must not be split.

Administration of capsules — Instruct the patient to take the capsules at least 1 h before or 2 h after a meal; if compliance with this restriction is difficult, consider changing the frequency of administration from q12h to q8h. Although the capsules may be swallowed whole, they can also be carefully opened and their contents sprinkled on a spoonful of soft food, such as applesauce or pudding (the food should not be hot). After sprinkling the drug, the patient should immediately swallow the mixture (without chewing it) and then drink a glass of cool water or juice. The small amount of food combined with each dose will not affect the bioavailability of the drug. Caution the patient not to subdivide the contents of the capsules.

Dosage adjustment with measurement of serum levels — Monitoring of serum theophylline level is recommended, particularly for titration of dosage. Check the peak serum level 8 h after the last dose if the tablets are used and 5–10 h after the last dose if the capsules are used; medication must have been taken at typical intervals, with no missed or added doses, for a period of at least 48 h prior to measurement. (Serum levels that are measured spectrophotometrically without prior chromatographic isolation may be falsely elevated when coffee, tea, acetaminophen, chocolate, or cola beverages have also been ingested.) Adjust dosage to maintain serum levels of 10–20 µg/ml; the risk of toxicity is significantly increased at higher levels, and, if theophylline clearance is reduced, toxic reactions may even develop at serum concentrations of 15–20 µg/ml. If the peak level in patients with normal theophylline clearance is between 5 and 7.5 µg/ml, increase the total daily dose by 25%; if between 7.5 and 10 µg/ml, increase the daily dose by 25% and, if symptoms recur at the end of a dosing interval, administer more frequently; if between 20 and 25 µg/ml, reduce the daily dose by 10%; if between 25 and 30 µg/ml, omit the next dose and reduce the daily dose by 25%; if over 30 µg/ml, omit the next 2 doses and reduce the daily dose by 50%. Recheck the serum level after each dosage adjustment and then, once the maintenance dosage has been established, every 6–12 mo (or, in some cases, more frequently) thereafter. *Do not attempt to maintain any dosage that is not tolerated.* Patients should be instructed to omit the next dose if they experience adverse effects and to resume therapy at a previously tolerated dosage once the reactions have disappeared.

Once-daily administration of *tablets* — Nonsmoking adults and other patients over 12 yr of age who have low dosage requirements may be given their total daily dose q24h if they respond satisfactorily to bid administration; the tablets should be given during the day, not at night. Monitor the serum theophylline level before and after switching to once-daily dosing because the trough serum level may decrease, particularly in patients with rapid theophylline clearance, and the peak level may increase, especially in patients with reduced clearance. If symptoms recur or toxicity becomes evident, reinstitute bid administration.

THEO-DUR

Patients with rapid theophylline clearance	Children, smokers, and some nonsmoking adults are likely to require dosing q8h (smokers may, alternatively, need larger doses). The effect of smoking on theophylline clearance may persist for 3 mo to 2 yr after the individual has ceased smoking. To determine whether theophylline is rapidly cleared in an individual patient, look for undesirably low trough serum levels or for a recurrence of symptoms at the end of a dosing interval.
Patients with reduced theophylline clearance	To avoid toxic reactions in neonates, patients over 55 yr of age (especially men), and patients with renal or hepatic impairment, influenza, alcoholism, chronic lung disease, cor pulmonale, or cardiac failure, reduce the initial dosage and monitor the serum theophylline level

WARNINGS/PRECAUTIONS

Arrhythmia	Theophylline may precipitate or exacerbate arrhythmia; any significant change in cardiac rate or rhythm warrants monitoring and further investigation. Use with caution in patients with severe cardiac disease, acute myocardial injury, or hyperthyroidism. Theophylline toxicity may be masked in patients with tachycardia.
Gastric irritation	Theophylline occasionally may cause local irritation of the GI tract, although GI symptoms are more commonly centrally mediated and associated with serum levels over 20 μg/ml; use with caution in patients with a history of peptic ulcer
Special-risk patients	Use with caution in neonates, the elderly (especially men), and patients with renal or hepatic impairment, chronic lung disease, severe cardiac disease, hypertension, acute myocardial injury, congestive heart failure, cor pulmonale, severe hypoxemia, a history of peptic ulcer, hyperthyroidism, influenza, or alcoholism (see "patients with reduced theophylline clearance" in the ADMINISTRATION/DOSAGE ADJUSTMENTS section); use with particular caution in patients with congestive heart failure because clearance in such patients is very slow
Morphine, curare	These drugs can stimulate histamine release and depress respiration; administer them with caution or, if possible, avoid their use
Acute bronchospasm	These products are not indicated for the treatment of acute bronchospastic episodes; for rapid symptomatic relief, use an immediate-release or IV theophylline preparation or other bronchodilators. If status asthmaticus occurs, administer parenteral therapy and closely monitor the patient (preferably in an intensive-care unit).
Carcinogenicity, mutagenicity, effect on fertility	No long-term studies have been performed to evaluate the carcinogenic and mutagenic potential of xanthine derivatives or their effect on fertility

ADVERSE REACTIONS

Gastrointestinal	Nausea, vomiting, epigastric pain, hematemesis, diarrhea
Central nervous system and neuromuscular	Headache, irritability, restlessness, insomnia, reflex hyperexcitability, muscle twitching, clonic and tonic generalized convulsions
Cardiovascular	Palpitations, tachycardia, extrasystoles, flushing, hypotension, circulatory failure, ventricular arrhythmias
Respiratory	Tachypnea
Renal	Albuminuria, increased excretion of renal tubule cells and red blood cells, potentiation of diuresis
Other	Rash, hyperglycemia, inappropriate ADH secretion syndrome

OVERDOSAGE

Signs and symptoms	See ADVERSE REACTIONS; ventricular arrhythmias or convulsions may be the first signs of toxicity, although frequently less severe signs of overdosage (eg, nausea, restlessness) occur initially
Treatment	If patient is conscious and seizures have not occurred, induce emesis and administer a cathartic and activated charcoal. If patient is convulsing, establish an airway and administer oxygen and IV diazepam (0.1–0.3 mg/kg, up to 10 mg). If patient is comatose following the occurrence of seizures, intubate immediately, using an endotracheal tube with an inflated cuff, and perform gastric lavage; introduce the cathartic and activated charcoal through a large-bore gastric lavage tube. Monitor vital signs, maintain blood pressure, and provide adequate hydration. Treat hypotension and shock by appropriate fluid replacement, avoiding the use of vasopressors, if possible. In general, the drug is metabolized sufficiently rapidly to preclude any additional benefit from dialysis; however, dialysis may be useful in the presence of congestive heart failure or hepatic dysfunction. Charcoal hemoperfusion may be necessary if serum levels exceed 50 μg/ml. Serial monitoring of the serum theophylline level is helpful in following the patient's course and in guiding further management.

DRUG INTERACTIONS

Other xanthine derivatives	⇧ Risk of theophylline toxicity; do not administer other xanthine derivatives concomitantly
Cimetidine, erythromycin, troleandomycin, influenza virus vaccine	⇧ Serum theophylline level; reduce the initial dosage of theophylline and monitor serum level

Ephedrine, other sympatho-mimetic agents	↑ Risk of theophylline and sympathomimetic toxicity
Lithium	↓ Serum lithium level
Propranolol	↓ Pharmacologic effects of propranolol and theophylline
Phenytoin	↓ Serum levels of theophylline and phenytoin
Furosemide	↑ Diuresis
Reserpine	Tachycardia
Chlordiazepoxide	Fatty acid mobilization

ALTERED LABORATORY VALUES

| Blood/serum values | ↑ Glucose ↑ Uric acid (with Bittner and colorimetric methods) ↑ Bilirubin (with diazo tablet method) |
| Urinary values | ↑ Albumin ↑ Catecholamines |

USE IN CHILDREN
See INDICATIONS, ORAL DOSAGE and ADMINISTRATION/DOSAGE ADJUSTMENTS; the safety and effectiveness of once-daily administration to children under 12 yr of age and of bid or tid administration to children under 6 yr of age have not been established. Use a liquid preparation to titrate dosage for children weighing under 25 kg. Exercise caution when adjusting dosage for younger children who cannot complain of minor adverse reactions.

USE IN PREGNANT AND NURSING WOMEN
Pregnancy Category C: reproduction studies have not been done; it is not known whether theophylline can cause harm to the fetus or affect reproductive capacity. Use during pregnancy only if clearly needed. Theophylline is excreted in human milk and may cause adverse reactions in nursing infants; use with caution in nursing mothers.

[1] When calculating dosages on the basis of weight, use the lean (or ideal) body weight, rather than the patient's actual weight (theophylline is not taken up by fatty tissue)

SYSTEMIC BRONCHODILATORS/ ANTIASTHMATIC AGENTS

THEOLAIR (theophylline, anhydrous) Riker Rx
Tablets: 125, 250 mg **Liquid (per 15 ml):** 80 mg (1 pt)

INDICATIONS
Acute, reversible bronchospasm associated with bronchial asthma, chronic bronchitis, and emphysema

ORAL DOSAGE[1]
Adult, nonsmoker: 6 mg/kg to start, followed by 3 mg/kg q6h for the next 12 h and then either 3 mg/kg q8h or 2.25 mg/kg q6h for maintenance; do not exceed 900 mg/day without measurement of serum level
Infant and child (6 mo to 9 yr): 6 mg/kg to start, followed by 4 mg/kg q4h for the next 12 h and then q6h for maintenance
Child (9–16 yr) and young adult smoker: 6 mg/kg to start, followed by 3 mg/kg q4h for the next 12 h and then q6h for maintenance

Chronic, reversible bronchospasm associated with bronchial asthma, chronic bronchitis, and emphysema

Adult and child: 16 mg/kg/day or 400 mg/day, whichever is less, given in 3–4 divided doses q6–8h to start, followed, if needed and tolerated, by an approximately 25% increase in dosage every 2–3 days; do not exceed, without measurement of serum level, 24 mg/kg/day for children 6 mo to 9 yr of age, 20 mg/kg/day for children 9–12 yr of age, 18 mg/kg/day for adolescents 12–16 yr of age, and 13 mg/kg/day or 900 mg/day, whichever is less, for patients over 16 yr of age

THEOLAIR-SR (theophylline, anhydrous) Riker Rx
Tablets (sustained release): 200, 250, 300, 500 mg

INDICATIONS
Chronic, reversible bronchospasm associated with bronchial asthma, chronic bronchitis, and emphysema

ORAL DOSAGE[1]
Adult and child: 16 mg/kg/day or 400 mg/day, whichever is less, given in 2–3 divided doses q8–12h to start, followed, if needed and tolerated, by an approximately 25% increase in dosage every 2–3 days; for patients currently receiving theophylline, give one-half the established total daily dose q12h to start. Do not exceed, without measurement of serum level, 24 mg/kg/day for children under 9 yr of age, 20 mg/kg/day for children 9–12 yr of age, 18 mg/kg/day for adolescents 12–16 yr of age, and 13 mg/kg/day or 900 mg/day, whichever is less, for patients over 16 yr of age.

THEOLAIR

CONTRAINDICATIONS
Hypersensitivity to theophylline

ADMINISTRATION/DOSAGE ADJUSTMENTS

Administration with food — The liquid and immediate-release tablets can be given with food to prevent some gastric irritation; absorption is slower, but still complete. Administration of some or all controlled-release theophylline products with food may affect absorption and result in altered serum values, especially when high serum levels are maintained or single doses exceeding 900 mg or 13 mg/kg are given; it is not known whether the bioavailability of Theolair-SR is influenced by food.

Dosage adjustment with measurement of serum level — Monitoring of serum theophylline level is recommended, particularly for titration of dosage. Check the peak serum level 1–2 h after the last dose if the liquid or immediate-release tablets are used and 4–6 h after the last dose if the sustained-release tablets are used; medication must have been taken at typical intervals, with no missed or added doses, for a period of 48 h prior to measurement. (Serum levels that are measured spectrophotometrically without prior chromatographic isolation may be falsely elevated when coffee, tea, acetaminophen, chocolate, or cola beverages have also been ingested.) Adjust dosage to maintain serum levels of 10–20 μg/ml; the risk of toxicity is significantly increased at higher levels, and, in some patients (eg, those with reduced theophylline clearance), toxic reactions may develop at serum concentrations of 15–20 μg/ml. If the peak serum level in patients with normal theophylline clearance is between 5 and 7.5 μg/ml, increase the total daily dose by 25%; if between 7.5 and 10 μg/ml, increase the daily dose by 25% and, if symptoms recur at the end of a dosing interval, administer more frequently; if between 20 and 25 μg/ml, reduce the daily dose by 10%; if between 25 and 30 μg/ml, omit the next dose and reduce the daily dose by 25%; if over 30 μg/ml, omit the next 2 doses and reduce the daily dose by 50%. Recheck the serum level after each dosage adjustment and then, once the maintenance dosage has been established, every 6–12 mo thereafter. *Do not attempt to maintain any dosage that is not tolerated.* Patients should be instructed to omit the next dose if they experience adverse effects and to resume therapy at a previously tolerated dosage once the reactions have disappeared.

Acute symptoms in patients currently receiving theophylline — Determine (where possible) the time, amount, route, and form of the patient's last dose. If it is not possible to obtain the patient's serum theophylline level quickly and there is sufficient respiratory distress to warrant a small risk, a loading dose may be given, based on the principle that each 0.5 mg/kg of theophylline administered in a rapidly absorbed form will increase the serum drug level by 1 μg/ml. Thus, if the patient is not already experiencing toxicity, a loading dose of 2.5 mg/kg (which will increase the serum level 5 μg/ml) is unlikely to produce dangerous side effects.

Use of sustained-release tablets — To provide longer dosing intervals or less fluctuation in serum levels during chronic therapy, administer sustained-release tablets; do not use for acute symptoms requiring rapid theophyllinization. Tablets should be swallowed whole, not chewed or crushed.

Patients with reduced theophylline clearance — To avoid toxic reactions in neonates, patients over 55 yr of age (especially men), and patients with renal or hepatic impairment, influenza, alcoholism, chronic lung disease, cor pulmonale, or cardiac failure, reduce the initial dosage and monitor serum theophylline levels. For acute symptoms requiring rapid theophyllinization, give older patients and patients with cor pulmonale 6 mg/kg to start, followed by 2 mg/kg q6h for the next 12 h and, thereafter, either 2 mg/kg q8h or 1.5 mg/kg q6h for maintenance; patients with congestive heart failure should be given 6 mg/kg to start, followed by 2 mg/kg q8h for the next 16 h and, thereafter, 1–2 mg/kg q12h for maintenance.

Patients with rapid theophylline clearance — Children, smokers, and some nonsmoking adults generally require administration of the liquid or immediate-release tablets q6h and are likely to require dosing of the sustained-release tablets q8h (smokers may, alternatively, need larger doses). The effect of smoking on theophylline clearance may persist for 3 mo to 2 yr after the individual has ceased smoking. To determine whether theophylline is rapidly cleared in an individual patient, look for undesirably low trough serum levels or for a recurrence of symptoms at the end of a dosing interval.

WARNINGS/PRECAUTIONS

Status asthmaticus — Concomitant parenteral therapy and close monitoring (preferably in an intensive-care unit) are frequently necessary for the optimal management of this medical emergency

Arrhythmia — Theophylline may precipitate or exacerbate arrhythmia; any significant change in cardiac rate or rhythm warrants monitoring and further investigation. Use with caution in patients with severe cardiac disease, acute myocardial injury, or hyperthyroidism. Theophylline toxicity may be masked in patients with tachycardia.

Gastric irritation — Theophylline occasionally may cause local irritation of the GI tract, although GI symptoms are more commonly centrally mediated and associated with serum levels over 20 μg/ml; use with caution in patients with a history of peptic ulcer

Special-risk patients — Use with caution in neonates, the elderly (especially men), and patients with renal or hepatic impairment, chronic lung disease, severe cardiac disease, hypertension, acute myocardial injury, congestive heart failure, cor pulmonale, severe hypoxemia, a history of peptic ulcer, hyperthyroidism, influenza, or alcoholism (see "patients with reduced theophylline clearance" in the ADMINISTRATION/DOSAGE ADJUSTMENTS section); use with particular caution in patients with congestive heart failure because clearance in such patients is frequently very slow

Morphine, curare — Since morphine and curare can stimulate histamine release and depress respiration, they should be given with caution, or, if possible, their use should be avoided

THEOLAIR

Carcinogenicity, mutagenicity, effect on fertility	No long-term studies have been performed to evaluate the carcinogenic and mutagenic potential of xanthine derivatives or their effect on fertility

ADVERSE REACTIONS

Gastrointestinal	Nausea, vomiting, epigastric pain, hematemesis, diarrhea
Central nervous system and neuromuscular	Headache, irritability, restlessness, insomnia, reflex hyperexcitability, muscle twitching, clonic and tonic generalized convulsions
Cardiovascular	Palpitations, tachycardia, extrasystoles, flushing, hypotension, circulatory failure, ventricular arrhythmias
Respiratory	Tachypnea
Renal	Albuminuria, increased excretion of renal tubule cells and red blood cells, potentiation of diuresis
Other	Hyperglycemia, inappropriate ADH syndrome, rash

OVERDOSAGE

Signs and symptoms	See ADVERSE REACTIONS; ventricular arrhythmias or convulsions may be the first signs of toxicity, although in up to 50% of patients less severe signs of overdosage (eg, nausea, restlessness) occur initially
Treatment	If patient is conscious and seizures have not occurred, induce emesis and administer a cathartic (especially if sustained-release tablets have been ingested) and activated charcoal. If patient is convulsing, establish an airway and administer oxygen and IV diazepam (0.1–0.3 mg/kg, up to 10 mg). If patient is comatose following the occurrence of seizures, intubate immediately, using an endotracheal tube with an inflated cuff, and perform gastric lavage; introduce the cathartic and activated charcoal through a large-bore gastric lavage tube. Monitor vital signs, maintain blood pressure, and provide adequate hydration. Treat hypotension and shock by appropriate fluid replacement, avoiding the use of vasopressors, if possible (sympathomimetic drugs may precipitate cardiac arrhythmia). In general, the drug is metabolized sufficiently rapidly to preclude any additional benefit from dialysis; however, dialysis may be useful in the presence of congestive heart failure or hepatic dysfunction. Charcoal hemoperfusion may be necessary if serum levels are very high. Serial monitoring of the serum theophylline level is helpful in following the patient's course and in guiding further management.

DRUG INTERACTIONS

Other xanthine derivatives	△ Risk of theophylline toxicity; do not administer other xanthine derivatives concomitantly. Caution patients against eating large quantities of chocolate and drinking large amounts of caffeine-containing liquids, such as coffee, tea, cocoa, or cola beverages, during therapy.
Cimetidine, erythromycin, troleandomycin, influenza virus vaccine	△ Serum theophylline level; reduce the initial dosage of theophylline and monitor serum levels
Ephedrine, other sympathomimetic agents	△ Risk of theophylline and sympathomimetic toxicity; exercise particular caution if patients with cardiac arrhythmias are given theophylline in combination with sympathomimetic agents
Lithium	▽ Serum lithium level
Propranolol	▽ Pharmacologic effects of propranolol and theophylline
Phenytoin	▽ Serum levels of theophylline and phenytoin
Furosemide	△ Diuresis
Reserpine	Tachycardia
Chlordiazepoxide	Fatty acid mobilization

ALTERED LABORATORY VALUES

Blood/serum values	△ Glucose △ Uric acid (with Bittner and colorimetric methods) △ Bilirubin (with diazo tablet method)
Urinary values	△ Albumin △ Catecholamines

USE IN CHILDREN

See INDICATIONS, ORAL DOSAGE, and ADMINISTRATION/DOSAGE ADJUSTMENTS; use of liquid or immediate-release tablets in children under 6 mo of age is not recommended because theophylline metabolism varies markedly in such patients. Administration of sustained-release tablets to children under 6 yr of age is also not recommended. Since the liquid permits small increments in dosage, it should be used to titrate dosage if a child requires chronic therapy and weighs under 25 kg. Exercise caution when adjusting dosage for younger children who cannot complain of minor adverse reactions.

USE IN PREGNANT AND NURSING WOMEN

Pregnancy Category C: reproduction studies have not been performed; it is not known whether theophylline can cause harm to the fetus or affect reproductive capacity. Use during pregnancy only if clearly needed. Theophylline is excreted in human milk and may cause adverse reactions in infants; use with caution in nursing mothers.

---

[1] When calculating dosages on the basis of weight, use the lean (or ideal) body weight, rather than the patient's actual weight (theophylline is not taken up by fatty tissue)

SYSTEMIC BRONCHODILATORS/ ANTIASTHMATIC AGENTS

THEOPHYL-SR (theophylline, anhydrous) McNeil Pharmaceutical Rx

Capsules (sustained release): 125, 250 mg

INDICATIONS

Chronic, reversible bronchospasm associated with bronchial asthma, chronic bronchitis, and emphysema

ORAL DOSAGE[1]

Adult and child: for patients currently receiving theophylline, one third the established total daily dose q8h to start; do not exceed, without measurement of serum levels, 24 mg/kg/day for children under 9 yr of age, 20 mg/kg/day for children 9–12 yr of age, 18 mg/kg/day for adolescents 12–16 yr of age, or 13 mg/kg/day or 900 mg/day, whichever is less, for patients over 16 yr of age

CONTRAINDICATIONS

Hypersensitivity to theophylline or other components

ADMINISTRATION/DOSAGE ADJUSTMENTS

Administration with food — Administration of some or all controlled-release theophylline products with food may affect absorption and result in altered serum values, especially when high serum levels are maintained or single doses exceeding 900 mg or 13 mg/kg are given; it is not known whether the bioavailability of Theophyl-SR capsules is influenced by food

Dosage adjustment with measurement of serum level — Monitoring of serum theophylline levels is recommended, particularly for titration of dosage. Check the peak serum level approximately 3.7 h after the last dose; medication must have been taken at typical intervals, with no missed or added doses, for a period of 48 h prior to measurement. (Serum levels that are measured spectrophotometrically without prior chromatographic isolation may be falsely elevated when coffee, tea, acetaminophen, chocolate, or cola beverages have also been ingested.) Adjust dosage to maintain serum levels of 10–20 μg/ml; the risk of toxicity is significantly increased at higher levels, and, if theophylline clearance is reduced, toxic reactions may even develop at serum concentrations of 15–20 μg/ml. If the peak serum level in patients with normal theophylline clearance is between 5 and 7.5 μg/ml, increase the total daily dose by 25%; if between 7.5 and 10 μg/ml, increase the daily dose by 25% and, if symptoms recur at the end of a dosing interval, administer more frequently; if between 20 and 25 μg/ml, reduce the daily dose by 10%; if between 25 and 30 μg/ml, omit the next dose and reduce the daily dose by 25%; if over 30 μg/ml, omit the next 2 doses and reduce the daily dose by 50%. Recheck the serum level after each dosage adjustment and then, once the maintenance dosage has been established, every 6–12 mo thereafter. *Do not attempt to maintain any dosage that is not tolerated.* Patients should be instructed to omit the next dose if they experience adverse effects and to resume therapy at a previously tolerated dosage once the reactions have disappeared.

Patients with reduced theophylline clearance — To avoid toxic reactions due to increased serum levels in neonates, patients over 55 yr of age (especially men), and patients with renal or hepatic impairment, influenza, alcoholism, chronic lung disease, cor pulmonale, or cardiac failure, reduce the initial dosage and monitor serum theophylline levels. For acute symptoms requiring rapid theophyllinization, give older patients and patients with cor pulmonale 6 mg/kg to start, followed by 2 mg/kg q6h for the next 12 h and then, for maintenance, 2 mg/kg q8h, and give patients with hepatic failure or congestive heart failure 6 mg/kg to start, followed by 2 mg/kg q8h for the next 12 h and then, for maintenance, 1–2 mg/kg q12h.

Patients with rapid theophylline clearance — Children, smokers, and some nonsmoking adults are likely to require dosing of the capsules more frequently than q8h (smokers may, alternatively, need larger doses). The effect of smoking on theophylline clearance may persist for 3 mo to 2 yr after the individual has ceased smoking. To determine whether theophylline is rapidly cleared in an individual patient, look for undesirably low trough serum levels or for a recurrence of symptoms at the end of a dosing interval.

WARNINGS/PRECAUTIONS

Status asthmaticus — Concomitant parenteral therapy and close monitoring (preferably in an intensive-care unit) are frequently necessary for the optimal management of this medical emergency

Arrhythmia — Theophylline may precipitate or exacerbate arrhythmia; any significant change in cardiac rate or rhythm warrants monitoring and further investigation. Use with caution in patients with severe cardiac disease, acute myocardial injury, or hyperthyroidism. Theophylline toxicity may be masked in patients with tachycardia.

Gastric irritation — Theophylline occasionally may cause local irritation of the GI tract, although GI symptoms are more commonly centrally mediated and associated with serum levels over 20 μg/ml; use with caution in patients with a history of peptic ulcer

Special-risk patients — Use with caution in neonates, the elderly (especially men), and patients with renal or hepatic impairment, chronic lung disease, severe cardiac disease, hypertension, acute myocardial injury, congestive heart failure, cor pulmonale, severe hypoxemia, a history of peptic ulcer, hyperthyroidism, influenza, or alcoholism (see "patients with reduced theophylline clearance" in the ADMINISTRATION/DOSAGE ADJUSTMENTS section); use with particular caution in patients with congestive heart failure because clearance in such patients is frequently very slow

Morphine, curare	Since morphine and curare can stimulate histamine release and depress respiration, they should be given with caution, or, if possible, their use should be avoided
Carcinogenicity, mutagenicity, effect on fertility	No long-term studies have been performed to evaluate the carcinogenic and mutagenic potential of xanthine derivatives or their effect on fertility

ADVERSE REACTIONS

Gastrointestinal	Nausea, vomiting, epigastric pain, hematemesis, diarrhea
Central nervous system and neuromuscular	Headache, irritability, restlessness, insomnia, reflex hyperexcitability, muscle twitching, clonic and tonic generalized convulsions
Cardiovascular	Palpitations, tachycardia, extrasystoles, flushing, hypotension, circulatory failure, ventricular arrhythmias
Respiratory	Tachypnea
Renal	Albuminuria, increased excretion of renal tubule cells and red blood cells, potentiation of diuresis
Metabolic and endocrinological	Hyperglycemia, inappropriate antidiuretic hormone secretion syndrome, rash

OVERDOSAGE

Signs and symptoms	See ADVERSE REACTIONS; ventricular arrhythmias or convulsions may be the first signs of toxicity, although in up to 50% of patients less severe signs of overdosage (eg, nausea, restlessness) occur initially
Treatment	If patient is conscious and seizures have not occurred, induce emesis and administer a cathartic and activated charcoal. If patient is convulsing, establish an airway and administer oxygen and IV diazepam (0.1–0.3 mg/kg, up to 10 mg). If patient is comatose following the occurrence of seizures, intubate immediately, using an endotracheal tube with an inflated cuff, and perform gastric lavage; introduce the cathartic and activated charcoal through a large-bore gastric lavage tube. Monitor vital signs, maintain blood pressure, and provide adequate hydration. Treat hypotension and shock by appropriate fluid replacement, avoiding the use of vasopressors, if possible. In general, the drug is metabolized sufficiently rapidly to preclude any additional benefit from dialysis; however, dialysis may be useful in the presence of congestive heart failure or hepatic dysfunction. Charcoal hemoperfusion may be necessary if serum levels exceed 50 µg/ml. Serial monitoring of the serum theophylline level is helpful in following the patient's course and in guiding further management.

DRUG INTERACTIONS

Other xanthine derivatives	△ Risk of theophylline toxicity; do not administer other xanthine derivatives concomitantly
Cimetidine, erythromycin, troleandomycin, influenza virus vaccine	△ Serum theophylline level; reduce the initial dosage of theophylline and monitor serum levels
Ephedrine, other sympathomimetic agents	△ Risk of theophylline and sympathomimetic toxicity
Lithium	▽ Serum lithium level
Propranolol	▽ Pharmacologic effects of propranolol and theophylline
Furosemide	△ Diuresis
Reserpine	Tachycardia
Chlordiazepoxide	Fatty acid mobilization
Phenytoin	▽ Phenytoin serum level

ALTERED LABORATORY VALUES

Blood/serum values	△ Glucose △ Uric acid (with Bittner and colorimetric methods) △ Bilirubin (with diazo tablet method)
Urinary values	△ Albumin △ Catecholamines

USE IN CHILDREN

See INDICATIONS, ORAL DOSAGE, and ADMINISTRATION/DOSAGE ADJUSTMENTS; safety and effectiveness for use in children under 6 yr of age have not been established. Exercise caution when adjusting dosage for younger children who cannot complain of minor adverse reactions.

USE IN PREGNANT AND NURSING WOMEN

Pregnancy Category C: reproduction studies have not been done; it is not known whether theophylline can cause harm to the fetus or affect reproductive capacity. Use during pregnancy only if clearly needed. Theophylline is excreted in human milk and may cause adverse reactions in nursing infants; use with caution in nursing mothers.

---

[1] When calculating dosages on the basis of weight, use the lean (or ideal) body weight, rather than the patient's actual weight (theophylline is not taken up by fatty tissue)

UNIPHYL

SYSTEMIC BRONCHODILATORS/ANTIASTHMATIC AGENTS

UNIPHYL (theophylline, anhydrous) Purdue Frederick   Rx

Tablets (controlled release): 200, 400 mg

INDICATIONS

Chronic, reversible bronchospasm associated with asthma, chronic bronchitis, and emphysema

ORAL DOSAGE[1]

Adult: for patients currently receiving theophylline, either use the 200-mg tablets and give one half the total daily dose q12h to start or use the 400-mg tablets and give the total daily dose once daily (q24h) in the morning to start; for patients not currently receiving theophylline, administer one 200-mg tablet q12h to start. Do not exceed 13 mg/kg/day or 900 mg/day, whichever is less, if serum levels are not measured.

Child (6 yr to < 12 yr): for children currently receiving theophylline, use the 200-mg tablets and give one half the total daily dose q12h to start; for children not currently receiving theophylline, administer as an initial dosage one half of a 200-mg tablet q12h if they weigh 15–25 kg or one 200-mg tablet q12h if they weigh over 25 kg

Child (≥ 12 yr): for children currently receiving theophylline, either use the 200-mg tablets and give one half the total daily dose q12h to start or use the 400-mg tablets and give the total daily dose once daily (q24h) in the morning to start; for children not currently receiving theophylline, administer as an initial dosage one half of a 200-mg tablet q12h if they weigh 15–25 kg or one 200-mg tablet q12h if they weigh over 25 kg

CONTRAINDICATIONS

Hypersensitivity to theophylline

ADMINISTRATION/DOSAGE ADJUSTMENTS

Administration — Tablets should be swallowed, not crushed or chewed; the 400-mg tablets should not be broken, even though they are scored

Dosage adjustment — Monitoring of serum theophylline levels is highly recommended, particularly for titration of dosage. Optimal response, determined by improvement in pulmonary function and relief of symptoms, often occurs at serum levels of 10–20 μg/ml, but may be obtained at lower levels. Although some patients may require serum levels above 20 μg/ml, the risk of toxicity is increased at these higher levels; if theophylline clearance is reduced because of disease, age, or concomitant drug therapy, toxic reactions may even occur at the upper level of the 10- to 20-μg/ml range.

To determine serum concentration, check the peak level 8–12 h after the morning dose and the trough level just before the next dose; medication must have been taken at typical intervals, with no missed or added doses, for a period of 72 h prior to measurement. (Serum levels that are measured spectrophotometrically without prior chromatographic isolation may be falsely elevated when coffee, tea, acetaminophen, chocolate, or cola beverages have also been ingested.) Take the first blood sample 4 days after the onset of therapy. If the peak level in patients with normal theophylline clearance is between 5 and 7.5 μg/ml, increase the total daily dose by 25%; if between 7.5 and 10 μg/ml, increase the daily dose by 25% and, if symptoms recur at the end of a dosing interval, administer q8h; if between 20 and 25 μg/ml, reduce the daily dose by 10%; if between 25 and 30 μg/ml, omit the next dose and reduce the daily dose by 25%; if over 30 μg/ml, omit the next 2 doses and reduce the daily dose by 50%. Recheck serum levels after each dosage adjustment. *Do not attempt to maintain any dosage that is not tolerated.* Patients should be instructed to omit the next dose if they experience adverse effects and to reduce the subsequent dosage when they resume therapy after the reactions have disappeared. After the maintenance dosage has been established, serum levels should be measured every 6–12 mo and whenever theophylline clearance is altered.

Exercise caution when titrating dosage for younger children who cannot complain of minor adverse reactions. To adjust dosage for patients who are receiving the 400-mg tablets, switch to a product that allows small changes in dosage and that can be given more frequently than once daily; resume use of the tablets if the titrated dosage equals 400 mg or a multiple of 400 mg.

Patients with rapid theophylline clearance — Cigarette smokers and patients who have recently stopped smoking may require larger doses or more frequent administration (the effect of smoking on theophylline clearance may persist for 3 mo to 2 yr after a patient has ceased smoking). To obtain adequate control of bronchospasm, particularly at the end of a dosing interval, without causing toxicity, it may be necessary to administer the 400-mg tablets to children, smokers, and other patients with rapid clearance q12h rather than once daily.

Patients with reduced theophylline clearance — To avoid toxic reactions due to increased serum levels in neonates, patients over 55 yr of age (especially men), and patients with renal or hepatic impairment, influenza, alcoholism, chronic lung disease, cor pulmonale, or cardiac failure, exercise caution and monitor serum theophylline levels

WARNINGS/PRECAUTIONS

Arrhythmia — Theophylline may precipitate or exacerbate arrhythmia; any significant change in cardiac rate or rhythm warrants monitoring and further investigation. Use with caution in patients with severe cardiac disease, acute myocardial injury, or hyperthyroidism. Theophylline toxicity may be masked in patients with tachycardia.

UNIPHYL

Gastric irritation	Theophylline occasionally may cause local irritation of the GI tract, although GI symptoms are more commonly centrally mediated and associated with serum levels over 20 $\mu g/ml$; use with caution in patients with a history of peptic ulcer to avoid exacerbation of the disease
Special-risk patients	Use with caution in neonates, the elderly (especially men), and patients with renal or hepatic impairment, chronic lung disease, severe cardiac disease, hypertension, acute myocardial injury, congestive heart failure, cor pulmonale, severe hypoxemia, hyperthyroidism, influenza or other viral infections, or alcoholism (see "patients with reduced theophylline clearance" in the ADMINISTRATION/DOSAGE ADJUSTMENTS section); use with particular caution in patients with congestive heart failure because clearance in such patients is very slow
Acute bronchospasm	This product is not indicated for the treatment of acute bronchospastic episodes; for rapid symptomatic relief, use an immediate-release or IV theophylline preparation or other bronchodilators. If status asthmaticus occurs, administer parenteral therapy and closely monitor the patient (preferably in an intensive-care unit).
Carcinogenicity, mutagenicity, effect on fertility	No long-term studies have been performed to evaluate the carcinogenic or mutagenic potential of this drug or its effect on fertility

ADVERSE REACTIONS

Gastrointestinal	Nausea, vomiting, epigastric pain, hematemesis, diarrhea
Central nervous system	Headache, irritability, restlessness, insomnia, reflex hyperexcitability, muscle twitching, clonic and tonic generalized convulsions
Cardiovascular	Palpitations, tachycardia, extrasystoles, flushing, hypotension, circulatory failure, ventricular arrhythmia
Respiratory	Tachypnea
Renal	Albuminuria, microhematuria, potentiation of diuresis
Other	Hyperglycemia, inappropriate ADH syndrome, rash

OVERDOSAGE

Signs and symptoms	See ADVERSE REACTIONS; ventricular arrhythmias or convulsions may be the first signs of toxicity, although less severe signs of overdosage (eg, nausea, restlessness) can occur initially
Treatment	If patient is conscious and seizures have not occurred, induce emesis, and then administer activated charcoal and a cathartic. If patient is convulsing, establish an airway and administer oxygen and IV diazepam (0.1–0.3 mg/kg, up to 10 mg). If patient is comatose following the occurrence of seizures, intubate immediately, using an endotracheal tube with an inflated cuff, and perform gastric lavage; introduce the cathartic and activated charcoal through a large-bore gastric lavage tube. Monitor vital signs, maintain blood pressure, and provide adequate hydration. Treat hypotension and shock by appropriate fluid replacement, avoiding the use of vasopressors, if possible. In general, the drug is metabolized sufficiently rapidly to preclude any additional benefit from dialysis; however, dialysis may be useful in the presence of congestive heart failure or hepatic dysfunction. Charcoal hemoperfusion may be necessary if serum levels exceed 50 $\mu g/ml$. Serial monitoring of the serum theophylline level is helpful in following the patient's course and in guiding further management.

DRUG INTERACTIONS

Other xanthine derivatives	△ Risk of theophylline toxicity; exercise caution if other xanthine derivatives are given concomitantly
Cimetidine, erythromycin, troleandomycin, influenza virus vaccine	△ Serum theophylline level; carefully watch for signs of toxicity and, if necessary, reduce theophylline dosage
Ephedrine, other sympathomimetic agents	△ Risk of theophylline and sympathomimetic toxicity
Lithium	▽ Serum lithium level
Propranolol	▽ Pharmacologic effects of propranolol and theophylline
Furosemide	△ Diuresis
Reserpine	Tachycardia
Chlordiazepoxide	Fatty acid mobilization

ALTERED LABORATORY VALUES

Blood/serum values	△ Glucose △ Uric acid (with Bittner and colorimetric methods) △ Bilirubin (with diazo tablet method)
Urinary values	△ Albumin △ Catecholamines

USE IN CHILDREN

See INDICATIONS, ORAL DOSAGE, and ADMINISTRATION/DOSAGE ADJUSTMENTS; safety and effectiveness for use in children under 6 yr of age (200-mg tablets) or 12 yr of age (400-mg tablets) have not been established

USE IN PREGNANT AND NURSING WOMEN

Pregnancy Category C: reproduction studies have not been performed; it is not known whether theophylline can cause harm to the fetus or affect reproductive capacity. Use during pregnancy only if clearly needed. Theophylline is excreted in human milk and may cause adverse reactions in infants; use with caution in nursing mothers.

---

[1] When calculating dosages on the basis of weight, use the lean (or ideal) body weight, rather than the patient's actual weight (theophylline is not taken up by fatty tissue)

VENTOLIN

SYSTEMIC BRONCHODILATORS/ ANTIASTHMATIC AGENTS

VENTOLIN (albuterol sulfate) Glaxo — Rx

Tablets: 2, 4 mg albuterol[1]

INDICATIONS

Bronchospasm associated with reversible obstructive airway disease

ORAL DOSAGE

Adult: 2–4 mg tid or qid to start, followed, if necessary, by careful, gradual increases in dosage; maximum level: 8 mg qid
Child (6–12 yr): 2 mg tid or qid, followed, if necessary, by careful, gradual increases in dosage; maximum level: 24 mg/day, given in divided doses
Child ($\geq$ 12 yr): same as adult

VENTOLIN Syrup (albuterol sulfate) Glaxo — Rx

Syrup (per 5 ml): 2 mg albuterol[1] (16 fl oz) *strawberry flavored*

INDICATIONS

Bronchospasm associated with reversible obstructive airway disease

ORAL DOSAGE

Adult: 2–4 mg (5–10 ml) tid or qid to start, followed, if necessary, by careful, gradual increases in dosage; maximum level: 8 mg (20 ml) qid
Child (2–6 yr): 0.1 mg/kg, up to 2 mg (5 ml), tid to start, followed, if necessary, by careful, gradual increases in dosage; maximum level: 0.2 mg/kg, up to 4 mg (10 ml), tid
Child (6–14 yr): 2 mg (5 ml) tid or qid to start, followed, if necessary, by careful, gradual increases in dosage; maximum level: 24 mg (60 ml)/day, given in divided doses
Child ($>$ 14 yr): same as adult

CONTRAINDICATIONS

Hypersensitivity to any component

ADMINISTRATION/DOSAGE ADJUSTMENTS

Elderly or unusually sensitive patients — Elderly patients or those with a history of unusual sensitivity to beta-adrenergic stimulating agents should be given 2 mg tid or qid to start, followed, if necessary, by gradual increases up to 8 mg tid or qid

Management of side effects — If adverse reactions, which are generally transient, occur, it is usually not necessary to discontinue use; in some cases, however, the dosage may be temporarily reduced, and then, after the reaction has subsided, gradually increased

WARNINGS/PRECAUTIONS

Sympathomimetic effects — At recommended dosages, albuterol usually has minimal effects on the cardiovascular system; however, this drug can occasionally cause cardiovascular and CNS effects common to all sympathomimetic agents. Discontinue use if such sympathomimetic effects occur; use with caution in patients with cardiovascular disorders (including coronary insufficiency and hypertension), hyperthyroidism, diabetes mellitus, or unusual sensitivity to sympathomimetic amines, and with extreme caution in patients receiving MAO inhibitors or tricyclic antidepressants (see DRUG INTERACTIONS).

Use with other sympathomimetic bronchodilators — Concomitant use with other *oral* sympathomimetic agents is not recommended; however, concomitant use of an *aerosol* in a judicious, individualized manner (ie, not given on a routine or regular basis) may be considered

Reactions with IV albuterol — Intravenous administration of albuterol has caused a decrease (usually transient) in the serum potassium level; large IV doses have exacerbated diabetes mellitus and ketoacidosis. The relevance of these findings to oral use is not known.

Carcinogenicity, mutagenicity — A significant, dose-related increase in the incidence of benign leiomyomas of the mesovarium has been reported in a 2-yr study of rats given 3, 16, and 78 times the maximum adult human dose (2, 9, and 46 times the maximum oral dose for children weighing 21 kg); in another study, concurrent use of propranolol blocked this effect. No evidence of tumorigenicity has been observed in mice after 18 mo of treatment or in a lifetime study in hamsters. Mutagenic effects have not been detected.

ADVERSE REACTIONS

Frequent reactions (incidence $\geq$ 1%) are printed in *italics*

With use of tablets

Central nervous system — *Nervousness and tremor (20%), headache (7%), insomnia, weakness, and dizziness (2%)*, drowsiness, restlessness, irritability, vertigo, stimulation

Cardiovascular — *Tachycardia and palpitations (5%)*, flushing, chest discomfort, hypertension, angina

Gastrointestinal — *Nausea (2%)*, vomiting

Other — *Muscle cramps (3%)*, difficulty in urination, unusual taste sensation, drying or irritation of oropharynx

COMPENDIUM OF DRUG THERAPY

VENTOLIN

With use of syrup in children 2–6 yr of age

Central nervous system	Excitement (20%), nervousness (15%), hyperkinesia (4%), insomnia (2%), emotional lability and fatigue (1%), vertigo, stimulation
Cardiovascular	Tachycardia (2%), hypertension, angina
Gastrointestinal	GI symptoms (2%), anorexia (1%), vomiting
Other	Pallor and conjunctivitis (1%), unusual taste sensation, drying or irritation of oropharynx

With use of syrup in older children and adults

Central nervous system	Tremor (10%), nervousness and shakiness (9%), headache (4%), dizziness (3%), hyperactivity and excitement (2%), sleeplessness and irritable behavior (1%), disturbed sleep, weakness, vertigo, stimulation
Cardiovascular	Tachycardia (1%), palpitations, chest pain, hypertension, angina
Gastrointestinal	Increased appetite (3%), stomachache, epigastric pain, vomiting
Other	Epistaxis (1%), muscle spasm, cough, mydriasis, sweating, unusual taste sensation, drying or irritation of oropharynx

OVERDOSAGE

Signs and symptoms	Angina, hypertension, hypokalemia
Treatment	A cardioselective beta-adrenergic blocker, such as metaprolol, may be used judiciously; keep in mind the risk of inducing an asthmatic attack

DRUG INTERACTIONS

Other sympathomimetic agents (including epinephrine)	△ Sympathomimetic effects and risk of toxicity (see WARNINGS/PRECAUTIONS)
MAO inhibitors, tricyclic antidepressants	△ Cardiovascular effects of albuterol (see WARNINGS/PRECAUTIONS)
Beta-adrenergic blocking agents	▽ Pharmacologic effects of both drugs

ALTERED LABORATORY VALUES

No clinically significant alterations in blood/serum or urinary values occur at therapeutic dosages

---

USE IN CHILDREN

Safety and effectiveness of tablets for use in children under 6 yr of age have not been established; safety and effectiveness of syrup for use in children under 2 yr of age have not yet been adequately demonstrated. Bear in mind that certain adverse reactions occur more frequently in children 2–6 yr of age than in older children (see ADVERSE REACTIONS).

USE IN PREGNANT AND NURSING WOMEN

Pregnancy Category C: albuterol has been shown to be teratogenic in mice, causing cleft palate when given SC at 40% of the maximum adult oral dose; cranioschisis has been seen in rabbits at 78 times the maximum adult oral dose. Delay in preterm labor has occurred in clinical use. Administer this drug cautiously during pregnancy and only if the expected benefit clearly justifies the potential risks to the fetus. Reproduction studies in rats have shown no evidence of impaired fertility. It is not known whether albuterol is excreted in human milk; because of the potential for tumorigenicity shown in animal studies, a decision should be made to discontinue nursing or use of the drug.

---

[1] As the sulfate salt

Chapter 31

Cardiac Agents

Angiotensin-Converting Enzyme Inhibitors — 1232
CAPOTEN (Squibb) — 1232
Captopril *Rx*

Cardiac Glycosides — 1234
CRYSTODIGIN (Lilly) — 1234
Digitoxin *Rx*

LANOXICAPS (Burroughs Wellcome) — 1237
Digoxin *Rx*

LANOXIN (Burroughs Wellcome) — 1237
Digoxin *Rx*

Sympathomimetic Agents — 1241
ARAMINE (Merck Sharp & Dohme) — 1241
Metaraminol bitartrate *Rx*

DOBUTREX (Lilly) — 1242
Dobutamne hydrochloride *Rx*

INTROPIN (Du Pont Critical Care) — 1244
Dopamine hydrochloride *Rx*

ISUPREL (Winthrop-Breon) — 1245
Isoproterenol hydrochloride *Rx*

LEVOPHED (Winthrop-Breon) — 1246
Norephinephrine bitartrate *Rx*

NEO-SYNEPHRINE Injection (Winthrop-Breon) — 1248
Phenylephrine hydrochloride *Rx*

Miscellaneous Inotropic Agents — 1249
INOCOR (Winthrop-Breon) — 1249
Amrinone lactate *Rx*

Other Cardiac Glycosides — 1231
CEDILANID-D (Sandoz Pharmaceuticals) — 1231
Deslanoside *Rx*

Digitalis *Rx* — 1231

OTHER CARDIAC GLYCOSIDES

DRUG	HOW SUPPLIED	USUAL DOSAGE[1]
CEDILANID-D (Sandoz Pharmaceuticals) Deslanoside *Rx*	**Ampuls:** 0.2 mg/ml (2 ml)	**Adult:** for digitalization, 1.6 mg, given IV in a single dose or two 0.8-mg doses, or IM in two 0.8-mg doses at 2 separate sites
Digitalis *Rx*	**Capsules:** 100 mg **Tablets:** 100 mg	**Adult:** 1.2 g, given in equally divided doses q6h; for maintenance, 100–200 mg/day

[1] Where pediatric dosages are not given, consult manufacturer

COMPENDIUM OF DRUG THERAPY

CAPOTEN

ANGIOTENSIN-CONVERTING ENZYME INHIBITORS

CAPOTEN (captopril) Squibb Rx
Tablets: 12.5, 25, 37.5, 50, 100 mg

INDICATIONS
Hypertension in patients with normal renal function

Hypertension in patients with renal impairment who have experienced unacceptable side effects with other antihypertensive drugs or have failed to respond satisfactorily to a combination of other antihypertensive drugs

Heart failure inadequately controlled by conventional diuretic and digitalis therapy

ORAL DOSAGE
Adult: 25 mg bid or tid, administered 1 h before meals, to start; if necessary, increase dosage to 50 mg bid or tid after 1–2 wk. If blood pressure is not satisfactorily controlled after another 1–2 wk, add a thiazide diuretic, beginning with a modest dose (eg, 25 mg/day of hydrochlorothiazide). Increase the dose of the diuretic, as needed, at intervals of 1–2 wk until its maximum antihypertensive dosage is reached. If blood pressure is still not satisfactorily controlled, increase captopril dosage to 100 mg bid or tid and then, if necessary, to 150 mg bid or tid, while continuing the diuretic. Do not exceed 450 mg/day.

Adult: 25 mg tid, administered 1 h before meals, to start, in addition to the usual diuretic and digitalis regimen; if necessary, increase the dosage to 50 mg tid. If heart failure is still not satisfactorily controlled after at least 2 wk, increase the dosage to 100 mg tid or, if necessary, 150 mg tid; usual therapeutic dosage: 50–100 mg tid.

CONTRAINDICATIONS
None known

ADMINISTRATION/DOSAGE ADJUSTMENTS

Initiating therapy for hypertension — Captopril may be used to initiate treatment of hypertension in patients with normal renal function. When planning to give this drug to patients who are currently receiving other antihypertensive agents, discontinue the existing antihypertensive drug regimen (including diuretics) 1 wk before starting captopril, if possible. When captopril is given alone, sodium restriction may be helpful. To avoid excessive hypotension in patients who must continue diuretic therapy, increase salt intake approximately 1 wk before starting captopril, begin with a small dose (6.25 or 12.5 mg), or observe patient for at least 1 h after administering the first dose. Transient hypotension is not a contraindication to further use since this effect should not recur once hypovolemia disappears and blood pressure increases. To begin treatment in patients who require prompt reduction in blood pressure and in patients with severe hypertension (eg, accelerated or malignant hypertension) who cannot interrupt their antihypertensive regimen, discontinue all antihypertensive drugs except diuretics and, under close supervision, promptly substitute captopril; administer the usual starting dosage (25 mg bid or tid) and then, if necessary, increase the daily dose q24h or more frequently, under continuous medical supervision, until a satisfactory response is obtained or the maximum dosage of 450 mg/day is reached. To achieve a satisfactory response, a more potent diuretic, such as furosemide, may be necessary.

Initiating therapy for heart failure — To minimize the risk of hypotension, observe patients closely during the first 2 wk of treatment and whenever the dosage of captopril or the diuretic is increased. For patients who have undergone vigorous diuretic therapy, start with 6.25 or 12.5 mg tid; increase dosage over the next several days, as tolerated, to the usual initial dosage of 25 mg tid.

Patients with significant renal impairment — Reduce initial daily dose; increase dosage in small increments every 1–2 wk, as needed and tolerated. After desired therapeutic effect has been attained, reduce dosage to the minimum effective level. When concomitant diuretic therapy is necessary in a patient with severe renal impairment, use a loop diuretic rather than a thiazide.

WARNINGS/PRECAUTIONS

Neutropenia, agranulocytosis — Captopril has caused myeloid hypoplasia, neutropenia, and agranulocytosis within 3 mo after the start of therapy; oral and systemic infections or other manifestations of agranulocytosis have developed in approximately 50% of patients with neutropenia. On bone marrow examination, erythroid hypoplasia and a decreased number of megakaryocytes have frequently been seen in conjunction with myeloid hypoplasia; in some cases, neutropenia has been accompanied by anemia and thrombocytopenia. Neutropenia has occurred in approximately 0.012% of patients with normal renal function (serum creatinine level <1.6 mg/dl), about 0.2% of patients with renal impairment (serum creatinine level >1.6 mg/dl), and 3.7% of patients with a combination of renal impairment and collagen vascular disease (eg, systemic lupus erythematosus, scleroderma). In over 75% of cases seen during treatment of heart failure, procainamide was given in combination with captopril. Thirteen percent of patients who developed neutropenia while receiving captopril have died; however, almost all of the deaths were associated with one or more of the following complicating factors: serious illness, collagen vascular disease, renal or heart failure, or immunosuppressant therapy.

To reduce the risk of agranulocytosis, instruct all patients to report any sign of infection, such as sore throat or fever. Promptly obtain a WBC count whenever an infection is suspected. If a neutrophil count of less than 1,000/mm^3 is detected, discontinue captopril and closely watch patient; neutropenia generally reverses within 2 wk after termination of therapy. Always assess renal function before beginning therapy. If renal impairment is seen, obtain WBC and differential counts before therapy, every 2 wk during the initial 3-mo period, and then periodically thereafter. In patients who have collagen vascular disease or who are receiving other drugs known to affect leukocytes or the immune response, use with caution and only after weighing benefits and risks, particularly when these patients also have renal impairment.

Proteinuria, nephrotic syndrome	Urinary protein exceeding 1 g/day has been seen in approximately 0.7% of patients; the nephrotic syndrome has developed in about 20% of those with proteinuria. Creatinine and BUN levels were seldom affected. In most cases, proteinuria occurred within 8 mo after the start of therapy and, regardless of whether or not therapy was continued, subsided or disappeared within 6 mo after detection. Instruct patients to report any sign of progressive edema that may indicate proteinuria or the nephrotic syndrome. Patients who had a history of renal disease or who received more than 150 mg/day have accounted for 90% of the cases of proteinuria. If captopril is to be used in these patients, obtain estimates of urinary protein before therapy (or before giving 150 mg/day) and then periodically thereafter; use first morning urine samples for these determinations.
Increases in BUN and creatinine	In some patients with hypertension and renal disease, especially those with severe renal artery stenosis, BUN and serum creatinine levels may increase; if necessary, reduce the dosage of captopril and/or discontinue diuretic therapy since it may not be possible to simultaneously maintain both normal blood pressure and adequate renal perfusion. Although stable increases in BUN and serum creatinine levels of about 20% above normal or baseline may develop in about 20% of patients with heart failure, progressive increases may occur in up to 5% of these patients, generally those with severe renal disease, and necessitate discontinuation of treatment. Transient elevations have also been seen, especially in association with hypovolemia, renovascular hypertension, and rapid control of severe or prolonged hypertension.
Hypotension	Although hypotension rarely occurs during antihypertensive therapy, transient decreases in blood pressure of more than 20% occur in about 50% of patients with heart failure; these episodes, which may occur after the first of several doses, are usually well tolerated, producing either no symptoms or brief, mild light-headedness, but in rare instances may result in arrhythmias or conduction defects; the effects lessen in severity after 1–2 wk and generally disappear within 2 mo. During treatment of heart failure or hypertension, excessive hypotension may occur in patients with severe hyponatremia or hypovolemia, such as those who undergo diuretic therapy (especially if vigorous or instituted recently), have dialysis treatments, or severely restrict their intake of salt; this effect usually occurs within 1 h after the initial dose. If hypotension occurs during therapy, place patient in a supine position and, if necessary, give normal saline by IV infusion. Caution patients that dehydration owing to excessive perspiration, vomiting, or diarrhea may precipitate hypotension. To avoid excessive hypotension, start treatment of heart failure under very close medical supervision. If possible, discontinue diuretic therapy before beginning antihypertensive therapy with captopril; if a diuretic must be used concomitantly, provide close medical supervision when starting treatment. For other appropriate measures, see ADMINISTRATION/DOSAGE ADJUSTMENTS.
Surgery	In patients undergoing major surgery or receiving anesthetics that can cause hypotension, captopril will block a compensatory increase in angiotensin II; if captopril-induced hypotension occurs, correct by volume expansion
Aortic stenosis	Theoretically, patients with aortic stenosis may be at particular risk of decreased coronary perfusion during therapy because of a smaller reduction in afterload
Physical activity	Caution patients with heart failure against rapid increases in physical activity
Rash	Maculopapular or, in rare cases, urticarial rash has been seen in 4–7% of patients, usually during the first 4 wk of therapy; it occurs frequently with pruritus, sometimes with fever and arthralgia, and, in 7–10% of cases, with eosinophilia or a positive ANA test. Rash is usually mild and generally disappears within a few days after reduction of dosage, short-term use of an antihistamine, or termination of therapy.
Impairment of taste	Dysgeusia, seen in 2–4% of patients, is usually reversible even with continued use and generally disappears within 2–3 mo. Weight loss may occur along with dysgeusia.
Concomitant use of other vasodilators	No information is available on the effects of combining captopril with nitroglycerin or other vasodilators in patients with heart failure. If possible, discontinue use of any drug with vasodilator activity before starting captopril; if use of such drugs is resumed, administer them with caution and perhaps at a lower dosage.
Carcinogenicity, effect on fertility	No evidence of carcinogenicity has been seen in mice and rats given 50–1,350 mg/kg/day for 2 yr; studies in rats have shown no adverse effect on fertility
ADVERSE REACTIONS[1]	Frequent reactions (incidence $\geq$ 1%) are printed in *italics*
Cardiovascular	*Hypotension; tachycardia, chest pain, and palpitations (1%);* angina, myocardial infarction, Raynaud's syndrome, congestive heart failure, flushing, pallor
Hematological	Neutropenia, agranulocytosis, anemia, thrombocytopenia, pancytopenia
Dermatological	*Rash (4–7%), pruritus (2%),* pemphigoid-like lesions, photosensitivity; angioedema of the face, mouth, or extremities; laryngeal edema (one case)
Renal	Proteinuria, nephrotic syndrome
Hepatic	Hepatocellular injury and cholestatic jaundice (rare)
Other	*Diminution or loss of taste (2–4%),* weight loss

OVERDOSAGE

Signs and symptoms	Excessive hypotension
Treatment	To restore blood pressure, administer normal saline by IV infusion; captopril may be removed from the blood by hemodialysis

DRUG INTERACTIONS

Diuretics	△ Antihypertensive effect; the combined effect of captopril and thiazide diuretics is additive △ Risk of hypotension (see ADMINISTRATION/DOSAGE ADJUSTMENTS)
Adrenergic blockers, ganglionic blockers	△ Antihypertensive effect; the combined effect of captopril and beta blockers is less than additive △ Risk of hypotension; exercise caution during concomitant therapy
Potassium-sparing diuretics (see also diuretics interaction, above), potassium supplements, potassium-containing salt substitutes	△ Serum potassium level; use potassium supplements or potassium-sparing diuretics with caution and only for documented hypokalemia. Use salt substitutes with caution.
Indomethacin, possibly other nonsteroidal anti-inflammatory agents	▽ Antihypertensive effect, especially in patients with low renin hypertension

ALTERED LABORATORY VALUES

Blood/serum values	△ BUN △ Creatinine △ Potassium, especially in patients with renal impairment
Urinary values	False-positive for acetone

USE IN CHILDREN

Although safety and effectiveness for use in children have not been established, captopril may be given to such patients if other antihypertensive measures have not been effective; in limited experience, captopril has been given at a weight-adjusted adult dosage to children 2 mo to 15 yr of age who had secondary hypertension and varying degrees of renal insufficiency

USE IN PREGNANT AND NURSING WOMEN

Pregnancy Category C: captopril has been shown to be embryocidal in rabbits at 2–70 times the maximum human dose (probably as a result of severe hypotension) and has caused a reduction in neonatal survival in rats at 400 times the recommended human dose; no teratogenic effects have been seen in hamsters, rats, or rabbits following administration of large doses. Captopril crosses the human placenta. Use during pregnancy only if the expected benefit justifies the potential risk to the fetus. The concentration of captopril in human milk is approximately 1% of the maternal serum level. Patients should generally not nurse during therapy; if a patient does nurse, exercise caution.

[1] Reactions for which a causal relationship has not been established include renal insufficiency and failure, polyuria, oliguria, urinary frequency, gastric irritation, abdominal pain, nausea, vomiting, diarrhea, anorexia, constipation, aphthous ulcers, peptic ulcers, dizziness, headache, malaise, fatigue, insomnia, dry mouth, dyspnea, cough, alopecia, and paresthesias

---

CARDIAC GLYCOSIDES

CRYSTODIGIN (digitoxin) Lilly   Rx

Tablets: 0.05, 0.1, 0.15 mg **Ampuls:** 0.2 mg/ml (1 ml)

INDICATIONS

Heart failure
Atrial fibrillation and flutter
Paroxysmal atrial tachycardia

ORAL DOSAGE

Adult: for slow digitalization, 0.2 mg bid for 4 days, followed by maintenance dosage; for rapid digitalization, preferably 0.6 mg to start, followed by 0.4 mg and then 0.2 mg at 4- to 6-h intervals; for maintenance, 0.05–0.3 mg/day (usual maintenance dosage: 0.15 mg/day)

Infant (2 wk to 1 yr): 0.045 mg/kg in 3 or more divided doses at least 6 h apart; for maintenance, give 10% of digitalizing dose

Child (1–2 yr): 0.04 mg/kg in 3 or more divided doses at least 6 h apart; for maintenance, give 10% of digitalizing dose

Child (> 2 yr): 0.03 mg/kg (0.75 mg/m^2) in 3 or more divided doses at least 6 h apart; for maintenance, give 10% of digitalizing dose

PARENTERAL DOSAGE

Adult: 0.6 mg IV (slowly) to start, followed by 0.4 mg 4–6 h later and then 0.2 mg at 4- to 6-h intervals until full therapeutic effect is apparent (average digitalizing dose: 1.2–1.6 mg IV); for maintenance, 0.05–0.3 mg/day IV or switch to oral therapy

Newborn (< 2 wk), premature infant, or infant with renal impairment or myocarditis: 0.022 mg/kg (0.3–0.35 mg/m^2) IV (slowly) in 3 or more divided doses at least 6 h apart; for maintenance, give 10% of digitalizing dose

Infant (2 wk to 1 yr): 0.045 mg/kg IV (slowly) in 3 or more divided doses at least 6 h apart; for maintenance, give 10% of digitalizing dose

Child (1–2 yr): 0.04 mg/kg IV (slowly) in 3 or more divided doses at least 6 h apart; for maintenance, give 10% of digitalizing dose

Child (> 2 yr): 0.03 mg/kg (0.75 mg/m^2) IV (slowly) in 3 or more divided doses at least 6 h apart; for maintenance, give 10% of digitalizing dose

CRYSTODIGIN

CONTRAINDICATIONS

Toxic response or idiosyncratic reaction to any digitalis preparation	Ventricular tachycardia[1]	Hypersensitive carotid sinus syndrome (some cases)[2]
Hypersensitivity to digitoxin	Beriberi heart disease[2]	

ADMINISTRATION/DOSAGE ADJUSTMENTS

Parenteral administration — Use only when oral therapy is contraindicated. The doses given above are for patients who have not received any digitalis preparation for 3 wk; reduce the dose proportionately for partially digitalized patients.

Duration of oral therapy — For *heart failure*, continue treatment after signs and symptoms have been abolished, unless some precipitating factor has been corrected. For *atrial fibrillation*, continue use of digitoxin in adequate doses to maintain the desired ventricular rate and other clinical effects. For *atrial flutter*, continue treatment if heart failure ensues or atrial flutter recurs frequently. For *paroxysmal atrial tachycardia*, continue treatment if heart failure ensues or paroxysms recur frequently.

Serum digitoxin levels — Must be evaluated in conjunction with clinical observations, ECG findings, and results of laboratory tests. The therapeutic serum level ranges from 10 to 35 ng/ml; however, a "therapeutic" serum level for one patient may be excessive or inadequate for another, with approximately 50% of patients showing toxicity at levels exceeding 35 ng/ml.[3]

WARNINGS/PRECAUTIONS

Arrhythmias — May be caused by underlying heart disease or reflect digitalis intoxication; if the latter cannot be excluded, withhold digitoxin temporarily, provided the clinical situation permits

Anorexia, nausea, vomiting — May accompany heart failure or reflect digitalis intoxication; determine the cause of these symptoms before continuing administration of digitoxin

Acute glomerulonephritis — Administer digitoxin with extreme caution, in conjunction with constant ECG monitoring, to patients with heart disease accompanied by acute glomerulonephritis; divided doses, relatively low total doses, and concomitant treatment with reserpine or other antihypertensive drugs may be necessary. Discontinue use of digitoxin in such patients as soon as possible.

Rheumatic carditis — Patients with rheumatic carditis, especially if severe, are unusually sensitive to digitoxin and prone to rhythm disturbances. Relatively low doses may be tried in these patients if heart failure develops; increase the dosage cautiously until a beneficial effect is obtained. If no improvement occurs, discontinue use of digitoxin.

Idiopathic hypertrophic subaortic stenosis (IHSS) — Must be managed with extreme care, since outflow obstruction may increase; digitoxin probably should not be used in patients with IHSS, unless cardiac failure is severe

Progression of heart block — Incomplete AV block may progress to advanced or complete heart block in digitalized patients; heart failure in these patients can usually be managed by other measures and by increasing the heart rate

Chronic atrial fibrillation — Digitoxin may not normalize the ventricular rate in patients with acute or unstable chronic atrial fibrillation, even at serum levels exceeding usual therapeutic concentrations; although such patients may be less susceptible to digitoxin-induced arrhythmias, do not increase the dosage to potentially toxic levels

Myxedema — Delays the excretion of digitoxin, resulting in significantly higher serum levels than in patients with normal thyroid function; reduce dosage accordingly

Elderly patients — Digitalis toxicity is more likely to occur in older than in younger adults because body mass tends to be small and renal function is frequently impaired; exercise caution in giving digitoxin to elderly patients, particularly if coronary artery disease is present

Hepatic impairment — Digitoxin is completely metabolized by the liver; accordingly, smaller doses may be required in patients with impaired liver function

Renal impairment — Digitoxin is partly metabolized to digoxin. Although elimination of digitoxin is independent of renal function, the elimination of digoxin is primarily renal; accordingly, dosages may need to be reduced in patients with renal insufficiency to avoid toxicity.

Potassium depletion — Sensitizes the myocardium to digitalis, increasing the risk of serious arrhythmias, and also tends to diminish the positive inotropic effect of digitoxin. Hypokalemia may result from malnutrition, old age, long-standing heart failure, concomitant use of other drugs (see DRUG INTERACTIONS), hemodialysis, and other therapy. Serum potassium levels may be maintained by administering a potassium-sparing diuretic (spironolactone, triamterene, or amiloride) concomitantly with kaliuretic diuretics (eg, furosemide or thiazides) or by use of oral potassium supplements.

Hypercalcemia — May produce serious arrhythmias in digitalized patients; do not give calcium IV and exercise great caution in giving digitoxin parenterally to patients with hypercalcemia

Special-risk patients — Patients with acute myocardial infarction, severe pulmonary disease, or greatly advanced heart failure may be prone to digitoxin-induced rhythm disturbances. Exercise caution in giving digitoxin to patients with active heart disease (eg, acute myocardial infarction or acute myocarditis), extensive myocardial damage, or conduction defects, and reduce the dosage when necessary. The parenteral route should be used with great caution in the presence of multiple ventricular extrasystoles, carotid sinus hypersensitivity, Adams-Stokes syndrome, or heart block and when patients are still under the influence of prior digitalis therapy. Patients with chronic constrictive pericarditis are likely to respond unfavorably to digitoxin. In patients at great risk, use of a short-acting, rapidly eliminated cardiac glycoside, such as digoxin, may be advisable.

CRYSTODIGIN

Electrical cardioversion	Adjustment of digitoxin dosage may be advisable prior to electrical cardioversion to prevent induction of ventricular arrhythmias

ADVERSE REACTIONS

Cardiovascular	*In adults:* ventricular premature contractions; paroxysmal and nonparoxysmal nodal rhythms; AV dissociation; paroxysmal atrial tachycardia with block; AV block of increasing degree, progressing to complete heart block; *in children:* nodal and atrial systoles; atrial arrhythmias; atrial ectopic rhythms; paroxysmal atrial tachycardia, particularly with AV block; ventricular arrhythmias (rare)
Gastrointestinal	Anorexia, nausea, vomiting, diarrhea, abdominal pain or discomfort
Central nervous system	Headache, weakness, apathy, visual disturbances (blurred or yellow vision), mental depression, confusion, disorientation, delirium
Endocrinological	Gynecomastia

OVERDOSAGE

Signs and symptoms	Anorexia, nausea, vomiting, and CNS disturbances are common signs of toxicity in adults but are rarely conspicuous in infants and children. Excessive slowing of the pulse ($\leq$ 60 beats/min) and almost any kind of arrhythmia may occur, but vary in frequency with age (see ADVERSE REACTIONS). Sinus bradycardia, sinoatrial arrest, and prolongation of the P-R interval are premonitory signs of toxicity in the newborn.
Treatment	Discontinue administration of digitoxin until all signs of toxicity have disappeared. In severe cases, and particularly if hypokalemia is present, administer potassium chloride in divided oral doses totaling 3–6 g (40–80 mEq) for adults and 1–1.5 mEq/kg for children, provided that renal function is normal. If correction of the arrhythmia is urgent and the serum potassium level is low or normal, potassium may be given IV in 5% Dextrose Injection, with careful ECG monitoring. Adults may be given a total of 40–80 mEq (using a concentration of 40 mEq/500 ml) at a rate of up to 20 mEq/h; infants and children may be given approximately 0.5 mEq/kg/h, using a solution dilute enough to avoid local irritation but with care to avoid fluid overload, especially in infants. Additional amounts may be given if the arrhythmia is uncontrolled and the potassium well tolerated. (Potassium should *not* be given, however, to patients with digitalis-induced heart block, unless primarily related to supraventricular tachycardia.) Discontinue the infusion when the desired effect is achieved. Other antiarrhythmic agents that may be tried include lidocaine, procainamide, propranolol, and phenytoin (experimental). Temporary ventricular pacing may be helpful in advanced heart block.

DRUG INTERACTIONS

Potassium-depleting diuretics and corticosteroids, amphotericin B	△ Risk of digitoxin toxicity due to hypokalemia
Calcium, particularly when administered IV; succinylcholine; sympathomimetics	△ Risk of cardiac arrhythmias
Colestipol, cholestyramine	▽ Serum concentration of digitoxin due to impaired absorption
Phenobarbital and other barbiturates, phenytoin, phenylbutazone	▽ Serum concentration of digitoxin due to accelerated hepatic metabolism

ALTERED LABORATORY VALUES

Urinary values	△ 17-Ketogenic steroids (with Zimmerman reaction)

No clinically significant alterations in blood/serum values occur at therapeutic dosages

---

USE IN CHILDREN

See INDICATIONS; dosage must be carefully titrated, and ECG monitoring may be necessary to avoid toxicity if the drug is given IV to newborns. Infants under 1 mo of age have a sharply defined tolerance to digitoxin; premature and immature infants are particularly sensitive and generally require lower doses. Renal function must also be considered.

USE IN PREGNANT AND NURSING WOMEN

Pregnancy Category C: use during pregnancy only when clearly needed. No studies have been done with digitoxin in either animals or pregnant women to determine whether it can cause fetal harm or affect reproductive capacity. No data are available on the effects of this drug on labor or delivery. It is not known whether digitoxin is excreted in human milk; since this remains a possibility, exercise caution in giving it to nursing mothers.

---

[1] The drug may be used, however, if heart failure supervenes after a protracted episode of tachycardia and the patient has not already received digitalis
[2] Contraindications listed by the manufacturer for oral administration only
[3] Gilman AG, Goodman LS, Gilman A (eds): *Goodman and Gilman's The Pharmacological Basis of Therapeutics*, ed 6. New York, Macmillan Publishing Co, Inc, 1980

CARDIAC GLYCOSIDES

LANOXICAPS (digoxin) Burroughs Wellcome   Rx

Capsules: 50, 100, 200 µg

INDICATIONS	ORAL DOSAGE
Heart failure **Atrial fibrillation and flutter** **Paroxysmal atrial tachycardia**	**Adult:** for rapid digitalization, 400–600 µg to start, followed by 100–300 µg at 6- to 8-h intervals until clinical response is adequate (usual loading dose for a 70-kg patient: 600–1,000 µg); for maintenance, see "maintenance dosage for adults" below **Child (2–5 yr):** for rapid digitalization, 25–35 µg/kg, with roughly half given at once and the remainder in fractional doses at 6- to 8-h intervals; for maintenance, give 25–35% of *oral or IV* loading dose daily **Child (5–10 yr):** for rapid digitalization, 15–30 µg/kg, with roughly half given at once and the remainder in fractional doses at 6- to 8-h intervals; for maintenance, give 25–35% of *oral or IV* loading dose daily **Child (> 10 yr):** for rapid digitalization, 8–12 µg/kg, with roughly half given at once and the remainder in fractional doses at 6- to 8-h intervals; for maintenance, give 25–35% of *oral or IV* loading dose daily

LANOXIN (digoxin) Burroughs Wellcome   Rx

Tablets: 125, 250, 500 µg   **Pediatric elixir:** 50 µg/ml[1] (2 fl oz) *lime-flavored*   **Ampuls:** 100 µg/ml (Pediatric Injection) (1 ml), 250 µg/ml (2 ml)

INDICATIONS	ORAL DOSAGE	PARENTERAL DOSAGE
Heart failure **Atrial fibrillation and flutter** **Paroxysmal atrial tachycardia**	**Adult:** for rapid digitalization, 500–750 µg to start, followed by 125–375 µg at 6- to 8-h intervals until clinical response is adequate (usual loading dose for a 70-kg patient: 750–1,250 µg); for maintenance, see "maintenance dosage for adults" below **Premature infant:** for rapid digitalization, 20–30 µg/kg, with roughly half given at once and the remainder in fractional doses at 6- to 8-h intervals; for maintenance, give 20–30% of *oral* loading dose daily **Full-term infant:** for rapid digitalization, 25–35 µg/kg, with roughly half given at once and the remainder in fractional doses at 6- to 8-h intervals; for maintenance, give 25–35% of *oral* loading dose daily **Infant (1–24 mo):** for rapid digitalization, 35–60 µg/kg, with roughly half given at once and the remainder in fractional doses at 6- to 8-h intervals; for maintenance, give 25–35% of *oral* loading dose daily **Child (2–5 yr):** for rapid digitalization, 30–40 µg/kg, with roughly half given at once and the remainder in fractional doses at 6- to 8-h intervals; for maintenance, give 25–35% of *oral* loading dose daily **Child (5–10 yr):** for rapid digitalization, 20–35 µg/kg, with roughly half given at once and the remainder in fractional doses at 6- to 8-h intervals; for maintenance give 25–35% of *oral* loading dose daily **Child (> 10 yr):** for rapid digitalization, 10–15 µg/kg, with roughly half given at once and the remainder in fractional doses at 6- to 8-h intervals; for maintenance, give 25–35% of *oral* loading dose daily	**Adult:** for rapid digitalization, 400–600 µg IV to start, followed by 100–300 µg IV at 4- to 8-h intervals until clinical response is adequate (usual IV loading dose for a 70-kg patient: 600–1,000 µg); for maintenance, see "maintenance dosage for adults" below **Premature infant:** for rapid digitalization, 15–25 µg/kg IV, with roughly half given at once and the remainder in fractional doses at 4- to 8-h intervals; for maintenance, give 20–30% of *IV* loading dose daily **Full-term infant:** for rapid digitalization, 20–30 µg/kg IV, with roughly half given at once and the remainder in fractional doses at 4- to 8-h intervals; for maintenance, give 25–35% of *IV* loading dose daily **Infant (1–24 mo):** for rapid digitalization, 30–50 µg/kg IV, with roughly half given at once and the remainder in fractional doses at 4- to 8-h intervals; for maintenance, give 25–35% of *IV* loading dose daily **Child (2–5 yr):** for rapid digitalization, 25–35 µg/kg IV, with roughly half given at once and the remainder in fractional doses at 4- to 8-h intervals; for maintenance, give 25–35% of *IV* loading dose daily **Child (5–10 yr):** for rapid digitalization, 15–30 µg/kg IV, with roughly half given at once and the remainder in fractional doses at 4- to 8-h intervals; for maintenance, give 25–35% of *IV* loading dose daily **Child (> 10 yr):** for rapid digitalization, 8–12 µg/kg IV, with roughly half given at once and the remainder in fractional doses at 4- to 8-h intervals; for maintenance, give 25–35% of *IV* loading dose daily

CONTRAINDICATIONS		
Untoward reaction sufficient to require discontinuation of other digitalis preparations	Hypersensitivity to digoxin	Ventricular fibrillation

ADMINISTRATION/DOSAGE ADJUSTMENTS

Dosage requirements — The recommended doses given in this chart are average values and may require substantial modification depending upon individual sensitivity and other factors, including (1) the indication for using digoxin (larger doses are often required for adequate control of ventricular rate in atrial flutter or fibrillation), (2) body weight (calculate doses on the basis of lean, or ideal, body weight), (3) renal status (smaller doses are usually required in patients with diminished renal function), (4) age (infants [other than newborns] and children generally require larger doses than adults on the basis of lean body weight or body surface area), and (5) associated conditions, such as concomitant disease states and use of other drugs (see WARNINGS/PRECAUTIONS and DRUG INTERACTIONS). Oral administration with meals that are high in bran may result in reduced GI absorption. In some patients, colonic bacteria convert oral digoxin to inactive metabolites (in 10% of patients who receive the tablets, 40% or more of a single dose is metabolized); use of the capsules, which are rapidly absorbed in the upper GI tract, minimizes this effect.

Initiation of therapy — Digitalization may be accomplished by either (1) administering a loading dose and then calculating the maintenance dose as a percentage of the loading dose or (2) beginning with an appropriate maintenance dose (see tables below) and allowing digoxin body stores to accumulate slowly. Loading doses should be based upon projected peak body stores and administered in several portions, with roughly half given as the first dose; *carefully assess the patient's response to the drug before giving each additional dose.* If maintenance doses are used to initiate therapy, steady-state serum levels will be achieved in approximately 5 half-lives, ie, 1–3 wk depending upon the patient's renal status.

Maintenance dosage for adults — The daily maintenance dose is based upon the percentage of peak body stores (ie, the loading dose) lost each day through renal elimination and may be calculated from the *actual* loading dose and the corrected creatinine clearance rate (CCr), in ml/min/70 kg or 1.73 m^2, by use of the following formula: loading dose $\times$ (14 + CCr/5)/100. To determine the appropriate oral maintenance dose for gradual digitalization of patients with heart failure, use the following tables:

LANOXICAPS

Usual daily maintenance dose (μg) for estimated peak body stores of 10 μg/kg

	Lean body weight (kg)						
CCr[1]	50	60	70	80	90	100	Days[2]
0	50	100	100	100	150	150	22
10	100	100	100	150	150	150	19
20	100	100	150	150	150	200	16
30	100	150	150	150	200	200	14
40	100	150	150	200	200	250	13
50	150	150	200	200	250	250	12
60	150	150	200	200	250	300	11
70	150	200	200	250	250	300	10
80	150	200	200	250	300	300	9
90	150	200	250	250	300	350	8
100	200	200	250	300	300	350	7

[1] Corrected creatinine clearance rate (ml/min/70 kg)
[2] Number of days before steady-state concentration is achieved

LANOXIN Tablets

Usual daily maintenance dose (μg) for estimated peak body stores of 10 μg/kg

	Lean body weight (kg)						
CCr[1]	50	60	70	80	90	100	Days[2]
0	63[3]	125	125	125	188[4]	188	22
10	125	125	125	188	188	188	19
20	125	125	188	188	188	250	16
30	125	188	188	188	250	250	14
40	125	188	188	250	250	250	13
50	188	188	250	250	250	250	12
60	188	188	250	250	250	375	11
70	188	250	250	250	250	375	10
80	188	250	250	250	375	375	9
90	188	250	250	250	375	500	8
100	250	250	250	375	375	500	7

[1] Corrected creatinine clearance rate (ml/min/70 kg)
[2] Number of days before steady-state concentration is achieved
[3] One half of a 125-μg tab or 125 μg every other day
[4] One and one-half 125-μg tabs

If necessary, the CCr may be estimated from the serum creatinine concentration in adult males as (140 − age)/[creatinine]; this value should be reduced by 15% for women. Do not use this formula for estimating the CCr in infants or children.

LANOXICAPS/LANOXIN

Frequency of administration of maintenance doses	Divided daily dosing is recommended for infants and children under 10 yr of age; older children and adults may be given single daily maintenance doses, usually after breakfast. Because the significance of the higher serum levels obtained by once-daily administration of the soft gelatin capsules is not established, divided daily dosing of the capsule form is currently recommended not only for children under 10 yr of age but also for (1) patients requiring 300 µg or more daily, (2) patients with a history of digitalis toxicity or who are likely to become toxic, and (3) patients in whom compliance is not a problem (if it is a problem, single daily dosing may then be appropriate).
Parenteral administration	Use only when need for rapid digitalization is urgent or oral therapy is contraindicated. Digoxin should be administered *slowly* by IV injection over a period of 5 min or longer; rapid infusion may cause systemic and arteriolar constriction. IM injection is extremely painful. If IM route must be used, inject the drug deeply into the muscle and massage afterward; do not give more than 2 ml into a single site. If using a tuberculin syringe to measure minute doses, be careful not to overadminister digoxin; never flush the syringe with the parenteral fluid after the contents are expelled into an indwelling catheter.
Dilution of injectable form	Both the standard and pediatric injection forms can be given undiluted; if dilution is desired, mix the injection form with a 4-fold or greater volume of Sterile Water for Injection, 0.9% Sodium Choride Injection, or 5% Dextrose Injection (use of smaller volumes may result in precipitation). The diluted solution should be used immediately. Do not mix digoxin with other parenteral drugs in the same container or administer it simultaneously with other drugs in the same IV line.
Adjustment of dosage when changing preparations	When switching a patient from an IV loading regimen to oral maintenance therapy, allow for the difference in bioavailability between the different dosage forms; a 100-µg IV dose is approximately equivalent to a 100-µg dose of the capsules but 125 µg of the tablets or elixir
Duration of therapy	For *heart failure,* continue use of digoxin after acute symptoms have been controlled, unless some known precipitating factor has been corrected; however, if therapy is difficult to regulate or if the patient is at great risk of becoming toxic (eg, because of unstable renal function or fluctuating potassium levels), consider cautiously withdrawing the drug (if the drug is withdrawn, monitor the patient regularly for signs of recurrent heart failure). Long-term administration may be required for children who have been digitalized for acute heart failure, unless the cause is transient, and for children with severe congenital heart disease, even after surgery. For *atrial fibrillation,* continue use of digoxin in adequate doses to maintain the desired ventricular rate. For *atrial flutter,* continue treatment if atrial fibrillation persists. For *paroxysmal atrial tachycardia,* continue treatment if heart failure ensues or paroxysms recur frequently; in infants, continue use of digoxin for 3–6 mo after a single episode to prevent recurrence.
Serum digoxin levels	May be helpful in assessing the degree of digitalization and in evaluating the probability of intoxication. Proper interpretation of serum digoxin concentrations must always take into account the observed clinical response; *never use an isolated serum concentration value alone as a basis for adjusting dosage.* The usual therapeutic range is 0.8–2.0 ng/ml in adults; infants and young children may tolerate slightly higher serum levels. Obtain samples at least 6–8 h after the last dose, regardless of the route or dosage form used or, if sampling for assessment of steady-state serum levels, ideally just before the next dose. Once steady-state conditions are achieved, maintenance doses may be adjusted upward or downward in direct proportion to the ratio of the desired versus measured serum concentration, provided the measurement is correct, renal function remains stable, and the needed adjustment is not the result of lack of compliance.

WARNINGS/PRECAUTIONS

Treatment of obesity	Use of digoxin solely for the treatment of obesity is unwarranted and can be dangerous, since potentially fatal arrhythmias and other adverse effects may occur
Anorexia, nausea, vomiting, arrhythmias	May accompany heart failure or reflect digitalis intoxication; determine cause of symptoms before continuing administration. If digitalis intoxication cannot be excluded, withhold digoxin temporarily, provided the clinical situation permits. Measurement of the serum digoxin level may be helpful.
Renal impairment	Decreases excretion of digoxin, increasing the risk of toxicity and its duration; reduce dosage in patients with moderate to severe renal disease (see "maintenance dosage for adults" above). Because of the prolonged serum half-life of digoxin in such patients, more time is needed to achieve steady-state conditions initially and when the dosage is adjusted. Assess renal function periodically by measurement of BUN and/or serum creatinine.
Acute glomerulonephritis	Administer digoxin with extreme caution, and with careful monitoring, to patients with heart failure accompanied by acute glomerulonephritis; relatively low loading and maintenance doses and concomitant antihypertensive therapy may be necessary. Discontinue use of digoxin in such patients as soon as possible.
Hypokalemia	Sensitizes the myocardium to digoxin, increasing the risk of toxicity, even at normal serum digoxin levels. Hypokalemia may result from malnutrition, diarrhea, prolonged vomiting, old age, long-standing heart failure, concomitant use of other drugs (see DRUG INTERACTIONS), dialysis, or mechanical suction of GI secretions. Maintain normal serum levels of potassium during digoxin administration, and avoid rapid changes in serum electrolyte levels. Reserve IV potassium administration for the treatment of digoxin-induced arrhythmias.

Other electrolyte disturbances	Hypercalcemia increases the risk of toxicity; calcium administration, particularly if IV and rapid, may produce serious arrhythmias. Hypomagnesemia also increases the risk of toxicity; institute replacement therapy if serum magnesium levels are low. Hypocalcemia can nullify the effects of digoxin. Monitor serum electrolyte levels periodically.
Thyroid disease	Atrial arrhythmias associated with hypermetabolic states, such as hyperthyroidism, are particularly resistant to digoxin; care must be taken to avoid toxicity if large doses of digoxin are needed (digoxin should not be used alone to treat these arrhythmias). Hypothyroidism reduces digoxin requirements. Patients with compensated thyroid disease respond normally to digoxin.
Electrical cardioversion	A reduction in digoxin dosage prior to cardioversion may be desirable to avoid induction of ventricular arrhythmias; however, the consequences of a rapid increase in ventricular response to atrial fibrillation if digoxin is withheld for 1–2 days should be considered. Elective cardioversion should be delayed if digoxin toxicity is suspected; if this would not be prudent, select a minimal energy level to start and increase the level carefully.
Special-risk patients	Patients with severe carditis (eg, carditis associated with rheumatic fever or viral myocarditis), acute myocardial infarction, or severe pulmonary disease may be particularly sensitive to digoxin-induced rhythm disturbances. Incomplete AV block may progress to advanced or complete heart block, especially in patients with Stokes-Adams attacks. Sinus bradycardia or sinoatrial block may worsen in patients with sinus node disease (sick sinus syndrome). Extremely rapid ventricular rates, and even ventricular fibrillation, may occur in patients with WPW syndrome and atrial fibrillation. Outflow obstruction may worsen in patients with idiopathic hypertrophic subaortic stenosis (IHSS); digoxin probably should not be used in these patients, unless cardiac failure is severe.
Other cardiac conditions	Patients with heart failure resulting from amyloid heart disease or constrictive cardiomyopathies respond poorly to digoxin. Patients with chronic constrictive pericarditis may not only fail to respond but may suffer a further reduction in cardiac output due to slowing of the heart rate by digoxin. Digoxin should not be used to treat sinus tachycardia in the absence of heart failure.
Carcinogenicity	No long-term studies have been done in animals to evaluate the carcinogenic potential of digoxin

ADVERSE REACTIONS

Cardiovascular	*In adults:* unifocal or multiform ventricular premature contractions, especially in bigeminal or trigeminal patterns; ventricular tachycardia; false-positive ST-T changes (with exercise testing); AV dissociation; accelerated junctional (nodal) rhythm; atrial tachycardia, with block; AV block (Wenckebach) of increasing degree, progressing to complete heart block; *in children:* conduction disturbances or supraventricular tachyarrhythmias, including AV block (Wenckebach); atrial tachycardia, with or without block; junctional (nodal) tachycardia; ventricular arrhythmias, including ventricular premature contractions; ventricular tachycardia; sinus bradycardia; other arrhythmias and cardiac conduction abnormalities
Gastrointestinal	Anorexia, nausea, vomiting, diarrhea
Central nervous system	Visual disturbances (blurred or yellow vision), headache, weakness, apathy, psychosis
Endocrinological	Gynecomastia

OVERDOSAGE

Signs and symptoms	Anorexia, nausea, vomiting, and CNS disturbances are common signs of toxicity in adults but are rarely conspicuous in infants and children. Excessive slowing of the pulse ($\leq$ 60 beats/min) and almost any kind of arrhythmia may occur, but vary in frequency with age (see ADVERSE REACTIONS). Sinus bradycardia, sinoatrial arrest, and prolongation of the P-R interval are premonitory signs of toxicity in the newborn.
Treatment	Discontinue administration of digoxin until all signs of toxicity have disappeared; treatment may not be necessary if toxic manifestations are not severe and only occur near the time of peak effect. In severe cases, and particularly if hypokalemia is present, administer potassium chloride in divided oral doses totaling 3–6 g (40–80 mEq) for adults and 1–1.5 mEq/kg for children, provided that renal function is normal. If correction of the arrhythmia is urgent and the serum potassium level is low or normal, potassium may be given IV in 5% dextrose injection, with careful ECG monitoring. Adults may be given a total of 40–80 mEq (using a concentration of 40 mEq/500 ml) at a rate of up to 20 mEq/h; infants and children may be given approximately 0.5 mEq/kg/h, using a solution dilute enough to avoid local irritation but with care to avoid fluid overload, especially in infants. Additional amounts may be given if the arrhythmia is uncontrolled and the potassium well tolerated. (Potassium should *not* be given, however, to patients with digitalis-induced heart block, unless primarily related to supraventricular tachycardia.) Discontinue the infusion when the desired effect is achieved. Other antiarrhythmic agents that may be tried include lidocaine, procainamide, propranolol, and phenytoin (experimental). Temporary ventricular pacing may be helpful in managing advanced heart block. An investigational procedure involving the IV administration of ovine, digoxin-specific, Fab antibody fragments has been used to rapidly reverse potentially life-threatening toxicity unresponsive to conventional measures.

DRUG INTERACTIONS

Potassium-depleting diuretics and corticosteroids, amphotericin B, quinidine	△ Risk of digoxin toxicity
Beta-adrenergic blockers, calcium channel blockers	△ Risk of complete AV block; nevertheless, combination therapy may be useful for control of atrial fibrillation) △ Risk of digoxin toxicity (with verapamil)
Tetracycline, erythromycin	△ Risk of digoxin toxicity if, before antibiotic therapy, colonic bacteria generally convert a portion of an oral dose of digoxin to inactive metabolites; use of the capsules, which are rapidly absorbed in the upper GI tract, significantly reduces this risk
Calcium, particularly when administered IV; succinylcholine; sympathomimetics	△ Risk of cardiac arrhythmias
Antacids, kaolin-pectin antidiarrheal suspensions, sulfasalazine, neomycin, cholestyramine, cyclophosphamide, vincristine, vinblastine, procarbazine, cytarabine, doxorubicin, bleomycin	▽ Serum level of oral digoxin
Propantheline, diphenoxylate	△ Serum level of oral digoxin
Thyroid preparations	△ Dosage requirement for digoxin in hypothyroid patients

ALTERED LABORATORY VALUES

No clinically significant alterations in blood/serum or urinary values occur at therapeutic dosages

USE IN CHILDREN

See INDICATIONS and ADMINISTRATION/DOSAGE ADJUSTMENTS. Newborns vary considerably in their tolerance to digoxin; premature and immature infants are especially sensitive, and dosage must not only be reduced but carefully individualized according to maturity. Beyond the newborn period, children generally require proportionally larger doses, on a mg/kg basis, than adults. The soft gelatin capsules may not be appropriate for young children who require fractional doses and/or frequent dosage adjustment.

USE IN PREGNANT AND NURSING WOMEN

Pregnancy Category C: reproduction studies have not been done; it is not known whether digoxin can cause harm to the fetus or affect reproductive capacity. Use during pregnancy only if clearly needed. Digoxin concentrations in human milk and serum are similar; although the amount present is unlikely to have any pharmacologic effect on the nursing infant, caution should be exercised in giving digoxin to a nursing mother.

[1] Contains 10% alcohol

SYMPATHOMIMETIC AGENTS

ARAMINE (metaraminol bitartrate)   Merck Sharp & Dohme   Rx

Vials: 10 mg/ml (10 ml)

INDICATIONS

Prevention of **acute hypotension due to spinal anesthesia**

Hypotension due to hemorrhage, drug reactions, or surgical complications (adjunctive therapy)

Shock associated with brain damage due to trauma or tumor (adjunctive therapy)

Hypotension due to cardiogenic shock or septicemia (adjunctive therapy)[1]

PARENTERAL DOSAGE

Adult: 2–10 mg (0.2–1.0 ml) IM or SC

Adult: 15–100 mg (1.5–10 ml) in 500 ml of Sodium Chloride Injection or 5% Dextrose Injection, given IV, with infusion rate adjusted to maintain blood pressure at desired level; for severe shock, 0.5–5.0 mg (0.05–0.5 ml) IV to start, followed by IV infusion of 15–100 mg (1.5–10 ml) in 500 ml of Sodium Chloride Injection or 5% Dextrose Injection

CONTRAINDICATIONS

Cyclopropane or halothane anesthesia, unless warranted by clinical circumstances

Hypersensitivity to any component (including sulfites)

ARAMINE ■ DOBUTREX

ADMINISTRATION/DOSAGE ADJUSTMENTS

Patient response	Allow 10 min to elapse before increasing dose if maximum effect is not apparent; response may be poor in patients with coexistent shock and acidosis
Concomitant shock management	Employ blood or fluid replacement when indicated and measures directed at specific cause
Discontinuation of therapy	Observe patient carefully to permit prompt reinitiation of therapy if blood pressure falls too rapidly
Infusion volume	If infusion rate and volume required would provide excessive vasopressor dose, increase recommended infusion volume; infusion volume may also be decreased when necessary
Compatible infusion solutions	Sodium Chloride Injection, 5% Dextrose Injection, Ringer's Injection, Lactated Ringer's Injection, 6% Dextran in Saline, Normosol-R pH 7.4, and Normosol-M in D5-W
Preferred injection sites	Larger veins of antecubital fossa or thigh, particularly in patients with peripheral vascular disease, diabetes, Buerger's disease, or coexistent hypercoagulability

WARNINGS/PRECAUTIONS

Hypersensitivity to sulfites	Sodium bisulfite in the solution may cause severe allergic reactions in certain susceptible individuals, particularly those with asthma
Digitalized patients	Use with caution; ectopic arrhythmic activity may occur
Cirrhotic patients	Use with caution; reduce infusion rate if ventricular extrasystoles appear, and restore electrolytes if diuresis occurs
Other special-risk patients	Use with caution in patients with heart or thyroid disease, hypertension, or diabetes; relapse may occur in patients with a history of malaria
Hypertensive effect	May be prolonged beyond cessation of therapy
Hypovolemia	May occur with extended use, thereby perpetuating shock state; measure central venous pressure to assess adequacy of circulating blood volume, and give blood volume expanders when principal reason for hypotension or shock is decreased circulating volume

ADVERSE REACTIONS

Cardiovascular	Sinus or ventricular tachycardia; arrhythmias (especially in patients with myocardial infarction)
Local	Abscess formation, tissue necrosis, sloughing

OVERDOSAGE

Signs and symptoms	Excessive blood pressure response, leading to acute pulmonary edema, arrhythmias, and cardiac arrest
Treatment	Discontinue use; treat symptomatically and institute supportive measures, as required

DRUG INTERACTIONS

MAO inhibitors, tricyclic antidepressants, guanethidine, parenteral ergot alkaloids	△ Risk of hypertensive crisis
Cyclopropane and halogenated hydrocarbon anesthetics, digitalis, mercurial diuretics	△ Risk of serious cardiac arrhythmias
Atropine	Antagonism of metaraminol-induced reflex bradycardia △ Pressor response
Alpha-adrenergic blocking agents	▽ Pressor response
Beta-adrenergic blocking agents	Antagonism of cardiac-stimulating effect of metaraminol
Diuretics	▽ Vasoconstriction

ALTERED LABORATORY VALUES

No clinically significant alterations in blood/serum or urinary values occur at therapeutic dosages

---

USE IN CHILDREN
Consult manufacturer

USE IN PREGNANT AND NURSING WOMEN
Consult manufacturer for use in pregnant women; no studies have been done regarding the use of this drug in nursing women

---

[1] Probably effective

SYMPATHOMIMETIC AGENTS

DOBUTREX (dobutamine hydrochloride) Lilly   Rx

Vials: 250 mg[1] (20 ml)

INDICATIONS

Short-term treatment of **cardiac decompensation,** when due to depressed contractility resulting from organic heart disease or cardiac surgery

PARENTERAL DOSAGE

Adult: 2.5–10 μg/kg/min or, if necessary, up to 40 μg/kg/min, by continuous IV infusion; in most cases, this drug is given for no more than a few hours

DOBUTREX

CONTRAINDICATIONS

Hypersensitivity to dobutamine | Idiopathic hypertrophic subaortic stenosis

ADMINISTRATION/DOSAGE ADJUSTMENTS

Preparation of solution	Add 10 ml of sterile water for injection or 5% dextrose injection to the vial; if the powder is not completely dissolved, add another 10 ml. Using 5% dextrose injection, 0.9% sodium chloride injection, or sodium lactate injection, dilute the reconstituted solution to a final volume of at least 50 ml; the final volume should be based on the fluid requirements of the patient. Administer diluted solution within 24 h. Do not mix dobutamine with alkaline solutions (eg, 5% sodium bicarbonate injection).
Monitoring of therapy	To reduce the risk of cardiovascular reactions, continuously monitor blood pressure and ECG during therapy. The rate of administration and duration of therapy should be based on heart rate, blood pressure, urine flow, presence of ectopic activity, and, whenever possible, central venous or pulmonary wedge pressure and cardiac output.
Concomitant therapy	According to preliminary studies, use of dobutamine in combination with nitroprusside produces an increase in cardiac output and usually results in a decrease in pulmonary wedge pressure

WARNINGS/PRECAUTIONS

Hypertension, tachycardia	In most patients, dobutamine increases systolic blood pressure by 10–20 mm Hg and heart rate by 5–15 beats/min; systolic pressure is elevated by 50 mm Hg or more in approximately 7.5% of patients, and heart rate is increased by 30 beats/min or more in approximately 10% of patients. A reduction in dosage usually reverses these effects. The risk of an exaggerated pressor response appears to be enhanced in patients with hypertension. For monitoring of therapy, see ADMINISTRATION/DOSAGE ADJUSTMENTS.
Arrhythmia	Dobutamine can precipitate or exacerbate ventricular ectopic activity and, in rare cases, cause ventricular tachycardia; an increase in premature ventricular contractions has been seen in approximately 5% of patients. By facilitating AV conduction, this drug may produce a rapid ventricular response in patients with atrial fibrillation; digitalize these patients before using this drug. For monitoring of therapy, see ADMINISTRATION/DOSAGE ADJUSTMENTS.
Hypersensitivity	Allergic-type reactions, including rash, fever, eosinophilia, and bronchospasm, have been seen occasionally
Hypovolemia	Before beginning therapy, correct hypokalemia by administering a suitable volume-expanding agent
Mechanical obstruction	No improvement may occur in patients with severe valvular aortic stenosis or other marked mechanical obstruction
Beta blockers	Animal studies indicate that dobutamine may not be effective in patients who have recently received a beta blocker
Myocardial infarction	Inotropic agents may intensify myocardial ischemia and increase the size of an infarct; it is not known whether dobutamine has such an effect. There is insufficient clinical experience to establish safety for use after myocardial infarction.

ADVERSE REACTIONS

The most frequent reactions, regardless of incidence, are printed in *italics*

Cardiovascular	*Increases in heart rate, blood pressure, and premature ventricular contractions (> 3%)*; angina, nonspecific chest pain, and palpitations (1–3%)
Other	Nausea, headache, and shortness of breath (1–3%)

OVERDOSAGE

Signs and symptoms	Hypertension, tachycardia
Treatment	Reduce rate of infusion or temporarily discontinue administration

DRUG INTERACTIONS

No clinically significant drug interactions have been identified

ALTERED LABORATORY VALUES

No clinically significant alterations in blood/serum or urinary values occur at therapeutic dosages

---

USE IN CHILDREN

Safety and effectiveness for use in children have not been established

USE IN PREGNANT AND NURSING WOMEN

Reproduction studies in rats and rabbits have shown no evidence of impaired fertility or harm to fetus; use during pregnancy only if the expected benefits clearly outweigh the potential risks. Consult manufacturer for use in nursing mothers.

---

[1] Base equivalent

INTROPIN

SYMPATHOMIMETIC AGENTS

INTROPIN (dopamine hydrochloride) Du Pont Critical Care Rx

Ampuls: 40 mg/ml (5 ml) **Prefilled syringes:** 40 mg/ml, 80 mg/ml, 160 mg/ml (5 ml) **Vials:** 40 mg/ml, 80 mg/ml, 160 mg/ml (5 ml)

INDICATIONS

Hemodynamic imbalances present in the shock syndrome due to myocardial infarction, trauma, endotoxic septicemia, open-heart surgery, renal failure, and chronic cardiac decompensation, as in congestive heart failure

PARENTERAL DOSAGE

Adult: 2–5 µg/kg/min, given by IV drip; for severe cases, 5 µg/kg/min IV to start, followed by gradual increases in dosage at 5–10 µg/kg/min increments up to 20–50 µg/kg/min, as needed; usual maintenance dosage: ≤ 20 µg/kg/min

CONTRAINDICATIONS

Pheochromocytoma | Uncorrected tachyarrhythmias or ventricular fibrillation

ADMINISTRATION/DOSAGE ADJUSTMENTS

Suggested dilution	Transfer contents of one or more ampuls, vials, or syringes by aseptic technique to a 250- or 500-ml bottle of sterile IV solution (Sodium Chloride Injection USP, 5% Dextrose Injection USP, 5% Dextrose and 0.9% Sodium Chloride Injection USP, 5% Dextrose in 0.45% Sodium Chloride Solution, 5% Dextrose in Lactated Ringer's Solution, 1/6 M Sodium Lactate Injection USP, or Lactated Ringer's Injection USP) just prior to administration. Drug is inactivated in alkaline solution; do not add to 5% Sodium Bicarbonate or other alkaline IV solutions.
IV administration	Administer through a suitable intravenous catheter or needle; control the rate of flow in drops/min by IV drip chamber or other suitable metering device. Titrate dosage to the desired hemodynamic and/or renal response.
Advanced circulatory decompensation	Rates > 50 µg/kg/min have been used safely. Monitor urine output frequently and, if necessary, reduce rate of administration if urine flow begins to decrease in the absence of hypotension.
Initiation of therapy	When appropriate, increase blood volume with whole blood or plasma until central venous pressure is 10–15 cm H_2O or pulmonary wedge pressure is 14–18 mm Hg before administering dopamine
Recent MAO inhibitor therapy	Reduce starting dose of dopamine to at least 10% of the usual initial dose
Antidote for peripheral ischemia	To prevent sloughing and necrosis, infiltrate ischemic area with 5–10 mg phentolamine in 10–15 ml of saline as soon as possible after extravasation is noted

WARNINGS/PRECAUTIONS

Hypovolemia	Correct fully, if possible, before administering dopamine
Necrosis	May occur if circulation is compromised; closely monitor patients with a history of occlusive vascular disease (eg, Raynaud's disease, Buerger's disease, arteriosclerosis) for changes in skin color and temperature; if necessary, decrease rate of infusion or discontinue drug (see ADMINISTRATION/DOSAGE ADJUSTMENTS)
Arrhythmogenic potential	Use with extreme caution in patients inhaling cyclopropane or halogenated hydrocarbon anesthetics
Careful monitoring	Urine flow, cardiac output, and blood pressure should be monitored closely during the administration of dopamine
Concomitant or recent MAO inhibitor therapy	Potentiates the effects of dopamine (see ADMINISTRATION/DOSAGE ADJUSTMENTS)
Marked decrease in pulse pressure	May occur; decrease infusion rate and monitor patient for further evidence of predominant vasoconstrictor activity, unless such an effect is desired
Necrosis and sloughing	May occur with extravasation; infuse dopamine into a large vein, preferably an antecubital vein, rather than the small veins in the dorsum of the hand or ankle. Monitor infusion site for free flow (see ADMINISTRATION/DOSAGE ADJUSTMENTS).

ADVERSE REACTIONS

The most frequent reactions, regardless of incidence, are printed in *italics*

Cardiovascular	*Ectopic beats, tachycardia, anginal pain, palpitations, headache, hypotension, vasoconstriction,* bradycardia, widened QRS complex, elevated blood pressure, aberrant conduction
Gastrointestinal	*Nausea, vomiting*
Other	*Dyspnea,* piloerection, azotemia

OVERDOSAGE

Signs and symptoms | Excessive blood pressure, peripheral ischemia

INTROPIN ■ ISUPREL

Treatment — Reduce rate of administration or discontinue use. If necessary, consider using phentolamine.

DRUG INTERACTIONS

MAO inhibitors	⇧ Pressor effect
Cyclopropane and halogenated hydrocarbon anesthetics	⇧ Risk of arrhythmias and hypertension
Phenytoin	Hypotension and bradycardia
Alpha-adrenergic blocking agents	Antagonism of vasoconstrictor effect of dopamine
Beta-adrenergic blocking agents	Antagonism of cardiac effects of dopamine

ALTERED LABORATORY VALUES

Urinary values — ⇧ Sodium

No clinically significant alterations in blood/serum values occur at therapeutic dosages

---

USE IN CHILDREN

The safety and effectiveness of this drug for use in children have not been established

---

USE IN PREGNANT AND NURSING WOMEN

Pregnancy Category C: reproduction studies in animals have shown no evidence of teratogenicity; however, in one study, administration of dopamine to pregnant rats decreased the rate of survival of newborns and increased the potential for cataract formation in the survivors. Use during pregnancy only if the expected benefit justifies the potential risk to the fetus. No studies have been done regarding the safety of using this drug in nursing women.

SYMPATHOMIMETIC AGENTS

ISUPREL (isoproterenol hydrochloride) Winthrop-Breon   Rx

Ampuls: 0.2 mg/ml (1, 5 ml)

INDICATIONS | PARENTERAL DOSAGE

Shock (hypoperfusion syndrome) (adjunctive therapy)

Adult: 0.5–5.0 μg/min (0.25–2.5 ml/min of a 1:500,000 solution) by IV infusion; for advanced stages of shock, infusion rates > 30 μg/min may be used

Cardiac standstill
Carotid sinus hypersensitivity
Adams-Stokes syndrome
Ventricular tachycardia and other ventricular arrhythmias requiring increased inotropic activity for management

Adult: for emergency situations, 0.02–0.06 mg (1–3 ml of a 1:50,000 solution) IV to start, followed by 0.01–0.2 mg (0.5–10 ml of a 1:50,000 solution) IV, or 5 μg/min (1.25 ml/min of a 1:250,000 solution) by IV infusion; alternatively, 0.2 mg (1 ml undiluted) IM or SC to start, followed by 0.02–1 mg (0.1–5 ml undiluted) IM or 0.15–0.2 mg (0.75–1 ml undiluted) SC; in extreme cases, give 0.02 mg (0.1 ml undiluted) intracardially
Child: administer one half the initial adult dosage

Bronchospasm during anesthesia

Adult: 0.01–0.02 mg (0.5–1 ml of a 1:50,000 solution) IV, repeated as necessary

CONTRAINDICATIONS

Tachycardia caused by digitalis intoxication

Preexisting cardiac arrhythmias with tachycardia, except when therapy requires increased inotropic activity

ADMINISTRATION/DOSAGE ADJUSTMENTS

Suggested dilution — For shock, add 1 mg (5 ml) to 500 ml of 5% Dextrose Injection USP (concentrations up to 10 times stronger may be used when infusion volume must be limited). For emergency treatment of cardiac standstill and cardiac arrhythmias, dilute 1 ml of solution as supplied to 10 ml with Sodium Chloride Injection USP or 5% Dextrose Injection USP for direct IV injection or add 2 mg (10 ml) to 500 ml of 5% Dextrose Injection USP for IV infusion. For bronchospasm during anesthesia, dilute 1 ml of solution as supplied to 10 ml with Sodium Chloride Injection USP or 5% Dextrose Injection USP.

Infusion rate in shock — Should be adjusted on the basis of heart rate, central venous pressure, systemic blood pressure, and urine flow; if heart rate exceeds 110 beats/min, consider decreasing the infusion rate or temporarily discontinuing the infusion

Complete heart block following closure of ventricular septal defects — To restore sinus rhythm or maintain an acceptable heart rate above 90–100 beats/min, administer isoproterenol IV in doses ranging from 0.01–0.03 mg (0.5–1.5 ml of a 1:50,000 solution) for infants to 0.04–0.06 mg (2–3 ml) for adults; monitor ECG constantly

ISUPREL ■ LEVOPHED

WARNINGS/PRECAUTIONS

Myocardial work and oxygen consumption	May be increased by IV infusion; these effects may be detrimental to patients who are in cardiogenic shock secondary to coronary artery occlusion and myocardial infarction
Patients with angina pectoris	May experience anginal pain if the cardiac rate increases sharply
Other special-risk patients	Adjust dosage with particular care in patients with coronary insufficiency, diabetes, or hyperthyroidism, and in those sensitive to sympathomimetic amines
Hypovolemia	Should be corrected with suitable volume expanders before treating for shock
Ventricular arrhythmia	May occur with IV infusion for shock if heart rate exceeds 130 beats/min; decrease infusion rate or temporarily discontinue infusion if heart rate exceeds 110 beats/min
Serious arrhythmias	May occur with concomitant use of epinephrine; if necessary, alternate administration of the two drugs, allowing a proper interval between doses

ADVERSE REACTIONS

Cardiovascular	Tachycardia, palpitations; paradoxical Adams-Stokes seizures
Central nervous system	Mild tremors, nervousness, headache
Other	Flushing of the face, sweating; pulmonary edema (one case)

OVERDOSAGE

Signs and symptoms	Slight increase in blood pressure, followed by a marked decrease
Treatment	Institute supportive therapy

DRUG INTERACTIONS

Epinephrine	⇧ Risk of cardiotoxicity
Ergot alkaloids	⇧ Blood pressure
Beta-adrenergic blocking agents	Antagonism of cardiac, vasodilating, and bronchodilating effects of isoproterenol
Cyclopropane and halogenated hydrocarbon anesthetics	⇧ Risk of arrhythmias; use with caution, if at all
Digitalis glycosides, potassium-depleting diuretics, mercurial diuretics	⇧ Risk of arrhythmias

ALTERED LABORATORY VALUES

No clinically significant alterations in blood/serum or urinary values occur at therapeutic dosages

---

USE IN CHILDREN
See INDICATIONS and PARENTERAL DOSAGE

USE IN PREGNANT AND NURSING WOMEN
Administration of isoproterenol during pregnancy has not been associated with teratogenicity; however, it should not be given to a pregnant woman unless the expected therapeutic benefits outweigh the possible hazards. Consult manufacturer for use in nursing mothers.

SYMPATHOMIMETIC AGENTS

LEVOPHED (norepinephrine bitartrate) Winthrop-Breon   Rx

Ampuls: 1 mg/ml (4 ml)

INDICATIONS
Restoration of blood pressure in **acute hypotensive states** (eg, pheochromocytomectomy, sympathectomy, poliomyelitis, spinal anesthesia, myocardial infarction, septicemia, blood transfusion, and drug reactions)
Cardiac arrest and profound hypotension (adjunctive therapy)

PARENTERAL DOSAGE
Adult: 8–12 µg/min (2–3 ml/min of a 1:250 solution) by IV infusion to start, with infusion rate subsequently adjusted to maintain a low-normal blood pressure (80–100 mm Hg systolic); average maintenance dosage: 2–4 µg (0.5–1 ml)/min

LEVOPHED

CONTRAINDICATIONS

Hypotension due to hypovolemia, except in an emergency to maintain perfusion until volume replacement can be instituted

Mesenteric or peripheral vascular thrombosis, except as a life-saving procedure

Hypoxia or hypercarbia

Use of cyclopropane and halothane anesthetics

ADMINISTRATION/DOSAGE ADJUSTMENTS

Suggested dilution	Add contents of ampul to 1,000 ml of 5% dextrose in water or saline; administration in saline alone is not recommended. Whole blood or plasma should be given separately, if indicated.
Volume of infusion fluid	If infusion rate and volume required will result in an excessive dose of norepinephrine, use a more dilute solution; concentrations greater than 4 μg/ml may also be used if required volume of fluid at standard dilution is clinically undesirable
Site of infusion	Administer infusion through a large vein, preferably an antecubital vein, to minimize risk of necrosis of overlying skin; avoid catheter tie-in techniques. Occlusive vascular diseases are more likely in the lower than in the upper extremity; avoid the veins of the legs in patients suffering from such disorders, and in the elderly.
Blood-volume depletion	Should be corrected as fully as possible before administering any vasopressor; in emergencies, norepinephrine may be administered before and concurrently with blood-volume replacement
Duration of therapy	Continue until blood pressure and tissue perfusion are maintained without therapy; avoid abrupt withdrawal. Reduce dosage gradually.
Previously hypertensive patients	Raise blood pressure not higher than 40 mm Hg below the preexisting systolic pressure
Refractory patients	May require doses as high as 68 mg of norepinephrine (17 ampuls)
Antidote for extravasation ischemia	To prevent sloughing and necrosis, infiltrate 5–10 mg phentolamine in 10–15 ml saline into area of extravasation, as soon as possible

WARNINGS/PRECAUTIONS

Concomitant antidepressant therapy	Use with extreme caution in patients receiving MAO inhibitors or tricyclic antidepressants, as severe prolonged hypertension may result
Avoidance of hypertension	To avoid dangerous elevations of blood pressure, monitor blood pressure every 2 min until desired pressure is reached and then every 5 min if administration is to be continued. The rate of flow requires constant attention; never leave patient unattended.
Necrosis and sloughing	Avoid extravasation; check infusion site frequently for free flow. If blanching along the course of the infused vein occurs, change the infusion site at intervals to allow the effects of local vasoconstriction to subside (see ADMINISTRATION/DOSAGE ADJUSTMENTS)
Prolonged administration	May result in plasma volume depletion; replace fluids and electrolytes, as needed. Uncorrected hypovolemia may culminate in hypotension when norepinephrine is withdrawn, or blood pressure may be maintained at the risk of severe peripheral vasoconstriction and diminished blood flow and tissue perfusion.

ADVERSE REACTIONS

Cardiovascular	Bradycardia

OVERDOSAGE

Signs and symptoms	Headache, severe hypertension, reflex bradycardia, increased peripheral resistance, decreased cardiac output
Treatment	Discontinue use; treat symptomatically and institute supportive therapy, as required

DRUG INTERACTIONS

Cyclopropane and halogenated hydrocarbon anesthetics, digitalis, mercurial diuretics	△ Risk of arrhythmias
MAO inhibitors, tricyclic antidepressants	△ Risk of severe, prolonged hypertension
Parenteral ergot alkaloids, guanethidine, methyldopa, diphenhydramine, tripelennamine, dexchlorpheniramine	△ Pressor effect
Alpha-adrenergic blocking agents	Antagonism of pressor response to norepinephrine
Beta-adrenergic blocking agents	Antagonism of cardiostimulating effects of norepinephrine
Atropine	Antagonism of norepinephrine-induced reflex bradycardia △ Pressor response
Diuretics	▽ Arterial responsiveness to norepinephrine

COMPENDIUM OF DRUG THERAPY

LEVOPHED ■ NEO-SYNEPHRINE

ALTERED LABORATORY VALUES

No clinically significant alterations in blood/serum or urinary values occur at therapeutic dosages

USE IN CHILDREN
Not recommended for use in children because pediatric doses have not been established

USE IN PREGNANT AND NURSING WOMEN
Consult manufacturer

SYMPATHOMIMETIC AGENTS

NEO-SYNEPHRINE (phenylephrine hydrochloride) Winthrop-Breon Rx

Ampuls: 10 mg/ml (1 ml) **Cartridge-needle units:** 10 mg/ml (1 ml)

INDICATIONS / PARENTERAL DOSAGE

Indication	Dosage
Mild to moderate hypotension	**Adult:** 1–5 mg SC or IM or 0.1–0.5 mg IV to start, followed by repeated doses of 1–10 mg SC or IM or 0.1–0.5 mg IV, as needed, at intervals of not less than 10–15 min; usual dose: 2–5 mg SC or IM or 0.2 mg IV
Severe hypotension and shock, including drug-related hypotension	**Adult:** 100–180 µg (5–9 ml of 1:50,000 solution) per min to start, followed by 40–60 µg (2–3 ml)/min for maintenance; if prompt initial pressor response is not obtained, add additional amounts of phenylephrine of 10 mg or more to infusion bottle
Prevention and treatment of hypotension during spinal anesthesia	**Adult:** for high anesthetic levels, 3 mg IM or SC 3–4 min before injection of anesthetic; for low anesthetic levels, 2 mg IM or SC 3–4 min before injection of anesthetic; for hypotensive emergencies, 0.2 mg IV to start, increasing subsequent doses by not more than 0.1–0.2 mg over the preceding dose, up to 0.5 mg/dose **Child:** for combatting hypotension during anesthesia, 0.5–1.0 mg/25 lb IM or SC
Prolongation of spinal anesthesia	**Adult:** 2–5 mg added to anesthetic solution
Production of vasoconstriction during regional anesthesia	**Adult:** 1 mg phenylephrine to every 20 ml of local anesthetic solution
Paroxysmal supraventricular tachycardia	**Adult:** up to 0.5 mg IV (within 20–30 s) to start, increasing subsequent doses by not more than 0.1–0.2 mg above the preceding dose, up to 1 mg/dose

CONTRAINDICATIONS

Severe hypertension	Ventricular tachycardia	Hypersensitivity to phenylephrine

ADMINISTRATION/DOSAGE ADJUSTMENTS

Suggested dilution	For intermittent intravenous administration, dilute contents of ampul with 9 ml of Sterile Water for Injection USP; for continuous infusion, add contents of ampul to 500 ml of 5% Dextrose Injection USP or Sodium Chloride Injection USP
Blood-volume depletion	Should be corrected as fully as possible before administering any vasopressor; in emergencies, phenylephrine may be administered before and concurrently with blood-volume replacement
Patients with persistent or untreated severe hypotension or shock	Require higher initial and maintenance doses
Hypotension produced by peripheral adrenergic blocking agents, chlorpromazine, or pheochromocytomectomy	May require intensive therapy
Infusion rate	Adjust rate until desired blood-pressure level is obtained; in some cases, a more potent vasopressor (eg, norepinephrine) may be required

WARNINGS/PRECAUTIONS

Special-risk patients	Use with extreme caution in elderly patients and in those with hyperthyroidism, bradycardia, partial heart block, myocardial disease, or severe arteriosclerosis
Serious arrhythmias	May occur during halothane anesthesia; use with great caution, if at all
Patients receiving MAO inhibitor therapy	Use with great caution; initial dose should be small (see DRUG INTERACTIONS)
Use during induction of labor	Some oxytocic drugs may potentiate the pressor effect of this drug, possibly resulting in severe, persistent hypertension and even rupture of a cerebral blood vessel during the postpartum period
Carcinogenicity, mutagenicity	The carcinogenic and mutagenic potential of this drug have not been evaluated

COMPENDIUM OF DRUG THERAPY

NEO-SYNEPHRINE ■ INOCOR

ADVERSE REACTIONS

Central nervous system	Headache, excitability, restlessness
Cardiovascular	Reflex bradycardia; arrhythmias (rare)

OVERDOSAGE

Signs and symptoms	Ventricular extrasystoles, short paroxysms of ventricular tachycardia, sensation of "fullness" in the head, tingling in the extremities, excessive elevation of blood pressure
Treatment	Discontinue use; for excessive hypertension, administer an alpha-adrenergic blocking agent, such as phentolamine

DRUG INTERACTIONS

Cyclopropane and halogenated hydrocarbon anesthetics	△ Risk of serious cardiac arrhythmias
MAO inhibitors	△ Cardiac and pressor effects
Tricyclic antidepressants	△ Pressor effect
Phenothiazines, alpha-adrenergic blocking agents	▽ Pressor effect
Beta-adrenergic blocking agents	Antagonism of cardiostimulating effects of phenylephrine
Atropine	Antagonism of phenylephrine-induced reflex bradycardia △ Pressor effect
Parenteral ergot alkaloids	Excessive rise in blood pressure
Diuretics	▽ Vasoconstriction

ALTERED LABORATORY VALUES

No clinically significant alterations in blood/serum or urinary values occur at therapeutic dosages

USE IN CHILDREN

See INDICATIONS and PARENTERAL DOSAGE

USE IN PREGNANT AND NURSING WOMEN

Pregnancy Category C: use during pregnancy only if clearly needed. Animal reproduction studies have not been done, nor is it known whether this drug can affect human reproductive capacity or cause fetal harm. If used during labor either to correct hypotension or as a vasoconstrictor with local anesthetics, see the warning, above, regarding certain oxytocics. It is not known whether phenylephrine is excreted in human milk; because many drugs are excreted in milk, this drug should be used with caution in nursing mothers.

MISCELLANEOUS INOTROPIC AGENTS

INOCOR (amrinone lactate) Winthrop-Breon

Rx

Ampuls: 5 mg^1/ml (20 ml)

INDICATIONS

Short-term management of **congestive heart failure**, when conventional measures (digitalis, diuretics, and/or vasodilators) have been inadequate and patient response can be closely monitored

PARENTERAL DOSAGE

Adult: 0.75 mg/kg, given slowly as an IV bolus over a period of 2–3 min, followed by a maintenance infusion of 5–10 µg/kg/min; if necessary, a second bolus dose of 0.75 mg/kg may be given 30 min after the start of therapy. Total daily dose generally should not exceed 10 mg/kg/day; however, in studies with a limited number of patients, up to 18 mg/kg/day has been given when duration of therapy is shortened.

CONTRAINDICATIONS

Hypersensitivity to amrinone lactate or bisulfites

ADMINISTRATION/DOSAGE ADJUSTMENTS

Preparation of solution	The drug may be used as supplied or, alternatively, it may be diluted in normal or half-normal saline to a concentration of 1–3 mg/ml; use diluted solutions within 24 h. To avoid a chemical interaction, do not dilute the drug in a solution containing furosemide or dextrose (glucose). However, since the interaction with glucose occurs slowly over a period of 24 h, the drug may be added directly or through a Y-type apparatus to a running solution that contains glucose. The drug should not be added to IV lines containing furosemide because the interaction with furosemide is immediate.

INOCOR

Expected drug response	A single IV dose of 0.75 mg/kg produces an effect that peaks 10 min after injection and lasts approximately 30 min. The combination of a loading dose and maintenance infusion usually results in a serum level of approximately 3 µg/ml. Within the range of 0.5–7 µg/ml, there is a linear relationship between an increase in the serum level and an increase in the cardiac index; the effects of an increase in the serum level beyond 7 µg/ml are not known.
Duration of therapy	Hemodynamic studies have been limited in most cases to periods of 24 h or less; however, consistent hemodynamic and clinical effects have been seen when treatment exceeded 24 h. Patient response should govern duration of therapy.

WARNINGS/PRECAUTIONS

Valvular disease	In patients with severe aortic or pulmonary valvular disease, amrinone should not be used in place of surgery for relief of the obstruction
Hypertrophic subaortic stenosis	Amrinone may aggravate outflow tract obstruction associated with hypertrophic subaortic stenosis
Increased ventricular rate	In patients with atrial flutter or fibrillation, amrinone may enhance AV conduction slightly and produce an increase in the ventricular rate; these patients should be given digitalis before amrinone therapy
Hypotension	Vasodilation caused by amrinone may result in hypotension. Monitor blood pressure and heart rate; if blood pressure decreases excessively, reduce the rate of infusion or discontinue therapy.
Fluid and electrolyte imbalance	Therapeutic response is adversely affected by fluid or electrolyte imbalance. Correct any fluid or electrolyte imbalance before therapy (see DRUG INTERACTIONS), and carefully monitor renal function and fluid and electrolyte levels during treatment; monitoring of central venous pressure may be valuable. To obtain an adequate response in patients who have undergone vigorous diuretic therapy, it may be necessary to cautiously increase their fluid and electrolyte intake, since cardiac filling pressure (preload) may be inadequate in these patients.
Arrhythmogenicity	Ventricular and supraventricular arrhythmias have occurred during therapy; although amrinone has not been shown to be arrhythmogenic, it may enhance the risk of arrhythmia associated with congestive heart failure
Thrombocytopenia	Reduction in platelet count to less than 100,000/mm³ (or normal limits) is dose-dependent, occurs more commonly following prolonged use, and appears to be due to a decrease in platelet survival time. Check platelet count before therapy and frequently thereafter. Asymptomatic reduction to less than 150,000/mm³ can be reversed within 1 wk of a decrease in dosage; if the dosage is not changed in such a case, the platelet count may stabilize (or even increase) and clinical effects may not occur. Therefore, if the platelet count drops below 150,000/mm³, consider decreasing the daily dose, maintaining the current regimen, or, if the risk exceeds the anticipated benefit, discontinuing therapy.
Hepatotoxicity	Hepatic reactions have occurred in 0.2% of patients. If acute, marked alterations in liver enzyme levels occur in conjunction with clinical signs and symptoms suggesting an idiosyncratic hypersensitivity reaction, therapy should be promptly discontinued; if changes in liver enzyme levels are not marked and clinical manifestations are not seen, weigh risks and benefits and then reduce dosage, discontinue drug, or maintain the current regimen.
Hypersensitivity	Several apparent hypersensitivity reactions have occurred in patients given oral amrinone for approximately 2 wk; one case was characterized by pericarditis, pleuritis, and ascites, a second by myositis, interstitial shadowing on chest x-ray, and an elevated sedimentation rate, and a third by vasculitis, nodular pulmonary densities, hypoxemia, and jaundice. The cause of these reactions is not certain; nevertheless, consider the risk of hypersensitivity reactions during prolonged therapy (see also warning above concerning hepatotoxicity).
Drug accumulation	In patients with compromised renal and hepatic perfusion, the serum level of amrinone may increase during the infusion; for these patients, monitoring of hemodynamic response and serum drug levels may be necessary
Gastrointestinal effects	If severe or debilitating GI reactions occur, weigh risks and benefits; consider reducing dosage or discontinuing use
Myocardial infarction	Use of amrinone during the acute phase following myocardial infarction has not been evaluated in clinical trials and is therefore not recommended
Carcinogenicity, mutagenicity, effect on fertility	An interim, 1-yr evaluation of a study in rats has shown no evidence of tumorigenicity. The mouse micronucleus test (at 7.5–10 times the maximum human dose) and the Chinese hamster ovary assay have demonstrated clastogenic effects and a decrease in polychromatic erythrocytes; however, these findings have not been duplicated in assays using *Salmonella*, mouse lymphoma cells, or human lymphocytes. No evidence of impaired fertility has been seen in rats.

ADVERSE REACTIONS

Frequent reactions (incidence ≥ 1%) are printed in *italics*

Cardiovascular	*Arrhythmia (3%), hypotension (1.3%)*
Hematological	*Thrombocytopenia (2.4%)*

INOCOR

Gastrointestinal	Nausea (1.7%), vomiting, abdominal pain, anorexia
Hepatic	Increased liver enzyme levels, idiosyncratic hypersensitivity reaction
Other	Fever, chest pain, burning at injection site

OVERDOSAGE

Signs and symptoms	Hypotension
Treatment	Reduce dosage or discontinue administration; take general measures to maintain circulatory function

DRUG INTERACTIONS

Diuretics	⇧ Diuresis; a reduction in diuretic dosage may be necessary
Digitalis	⇧ Inotropic effect ⇧ Risk of digitalis toxicity owing to amrinone-induced hypokalemia; correct hypokalemia before or during amrinone therapy
Disopyramide	Excessive hypotension; exercise caution during combination therapy

ALTERED LABORATORY VALUES

No clinically significant alterations in blood/serum or urinary values occur at therapeutic dosages

USE IN CHILDREN

Safety and effectiveness for use in children have not been established

USE IN PREGNANT AND NURSING MOTHERS

Pregnant women: Pregnancy Category C: amrinone has produced skeletal and gross external malformations in New Zealand white rabbits at oral doses of 16 and 50 mg/kg (these doses were toxic for the mother); these results have not been seen in French Hy/Cr rabbits given up to 32 mg/kg/day. In rats, IV administration of 15 mg/kg/day has produced no malformations. Oral administration at 50 mg/kg/day has caused a slight prolongation of gestation in rats; oral administration at 100 mg/kg/day has produced dystocia, which resulted in an increase in stillbirths, a decrease in litter size, and poor pup survival. Use amrinone during pregnancy only if the expected benefit justifies the potential risks. **Nursing mothers:** It is not known whether amrinone is excreted in human milk; use with caution in nursing mothers.

[1] Base equivalent; this product also contains 0.25 mg sodium metabisulfite/ml

Chapter 32

Contraceptives

BREVICON 21-DAY (Syntex) Norethindrone and ethinyl estradiol *Rx*	1255
BREVICON 28-DAY (Syntex) Norethindrone and ethinyl estradiol *Rx*	1255
DEMULEN 1/35-21 (Searle) Ethynodiol diacetate and ethinyl estradiol *Rx*	1257
DEMULEN 1/35-28 (Searle) Ethynodiol diacetate and ethinyl estradiol *Rx*	1257
DEMULEN 1/50-21 (Searle) Ethynodiol diacetate and ethinyl estradiol *Rx*	1260
DEMULEN 1/50-28 (Searle) Ethynodiol diacetate and ethinyl estradiol *Rx*	1260
LEVLEN 21 (Berlex) Levonorgestrel and ethinyl estradiol *Rx*	1263
LEVLEN 28 (Berlex) Levonorgestrel and ethinyl estradiol *Rx*	1263
LOESTRIN 21 1/20 (Parke-Davis) Norethindrone acetate and ethinyl estradiol *Rx*	1265
LOESTRIN Fe 1/20 (Parke-Davis) Norethindrone acetate and ethinyl estradiol; ferrous fumarate *Rx*	1265
LOESTRIN 21 1.5/30 (Parke-Davis) Norethindrone acetate and ethinyl estradiol *Rx*	1265
LOESTRIN Fe 1.5/30 (Parke-Davis) Norethindrone acetate and ethinyl estradiol; ferrous fumarate *Rx*	1265
LO/OVRAL (Wyeth) Norgestrel and ethinyl estradiol *Rx*	1268
LO/OVRAL-28 (Wyeth) Norgestrel and ethinyl estradiol *Rx*	1268
MODICON 21 (Ortho) Norethindrone and ethinyl estradiol *Rx*	1270
MODICON 28 (Ortho) Norethindrone and ethinyl estradiol *Rx*	1270
NORDETTE-21 (Wyeth) Levonorgestrel and ethinyl estradiol *Rx*	1272
NORDETTE-28 (Wyeth) Levonorgestrel and ethinyl estradiol *Rx*	1272
NORINYL 1 + 35 21-DAY (Syntex) Norethindrone and ethinyl estradiol *Rx*	1275
NORINYL 1 + 35 28-DAY (Syntex) Norethindrone and ethinyl estradiol *Rx*	1275
NORINYL 1 + 50 21-DAY (Syntex) Norethindrone and mestranol *Rx*	1277
NORINYL 1 + 50 28-DAY (Syntex) Norethindrone and mestranol *Rx*	1277
NORINYL 1 + 80 21-DAY (Syntex) Norethindrone and mestranol *Rx*	1277
NORINYL 1 + 80 28-DAY (Syntex) Norethindrone and mestranol *Rx*	1277
NORLESTRIN 21 1/50 (Parke-Davis) Norethindrone acetate and ethinyl estradiol *Rx*	1280
NORLESTRIN 28 1/50 (Parke-Davis) Norethindrone acetate and ethinyl estradiol *Rx*	1280
NORLESTRIN Fe 1/50 (Parke-Davis) Norethindrone acetate and ethinyl estradiol; ferrous fumarate *Rx*	1280
NORLESTRIN 21 2.5/50 (Parke-Davis) Norethindrone acetate and ethinyl estradiol *Rx*	1280
NORLESTRIN Fe 2.5/50 (Parke-Davis) Norethindrone acetate and ethinyl estradiol; ferrous fumarate *Rx*	1280
ORTHO-NOVUM 1/35 ☐ 21 (Ortho) Norethindrone and ethinyl estradiol *Rx*	1283
ORTHO-NOVUM 1/35 ☐ 28 (Ortho) Norethindrone and ethinyl estradiol *Rx*	1283
ORTHO-NOVUM 1/50 ☐ 21 (Ortho) Norethindrone and mestranol *Rx*	1285
ORTHO-NOVUM 1/50 ☐ 28 (Ortho) Norethindrone and mestranol *Rx*	1285
ORTHO-NOVUM 1/80 ☐ 21 (Ortho) Norethindrone and mestranol *Rx*	1285
ORTHO-NOVUM 1/80 ☐ 28 (Ortho) Norethindrone and mestranol *Rx*	1285
ORTHO-NOVUM 7/7/7 ☐ 21 (Ortho) Norethindrone and ethinyl estradiol *Rx*	1287
ORTHO-NOVUM 7/7/7 ☐ 28 (Ortho) Norethindrone and ethinyl estradiol *Rx*	1287
ORTHO-NOVUM 10/11 ☐ 21 (Ortho) Norethindrone and ethinyl estradiol *Rx*	1290
ORTHO-NOVUM 10/11 ☐ 28 (Ortho) Norethindrone and ethinyl estradiol *Rx*	1290
OVCON-35 (Mead Johnson) Norethindrone and ethinyl estradiol *Rx*	1292
OVCON-50 (Mead Johnson) Norethindrone and ethinyl estradiol *Rx*	1292
OVRAL (Wyeth) Norgestrel and ethinyl estradiol *Rx*	1295
OVRAL-28 (Wyeth) Norgestrel and ethinyl estradiol *Rx*	1295
OVULEN-21 (Searle) Ethynodiol diacetate and mestranol *Rx*	1297
OVULEN-28 (Searle) Ethynodiol diacetate and mestranol *Rx*	1297
TRI-LEVLEN 21 (Berlex) Levonorgestrel and ethinyl estradiol *Rx*	1300
TRI-LEVLEN 28 (Berlex) Levonorgestrel and ethinyl estradiol *Rx*	1300
TRI-NORINYL 21-DAY (Syntex) Norethindrone and ethinyl estradiol *Rx*	1302
TRI-NORINYL 28-DAY (Syntex) Norethindrone and ethinyl estradiol *Rx*	1302
TRIPHASIL-21 (Wyeth) Levonorgestrel and ethinyl estradiol *Rx*	1305

TRIPHASIL-28 (Wyeth)   1305
Levonorgestrel and ethinyl estradiol *Rx*

Other Contraceptives   1254

Estrogen-Progestin Oral Contraceptives
ENOVID 5 mg (Searle)   1254
Norethynodrel and mestranol *Rx*

ENOVID-E 21 (Searle)   1254
Norethynodrel and mestranol *Rx*

NORINYL 2 mg (Syntex)   1254
Norethindrone and mestranol *Rx*

Progestin-only Oral Contraceptives
MICRONOR (Ortho)   1254
Norethindrone *Rx*

NOR-Q.D. (Syntex)   1254
Norethindrone *Rx*

OVRETTE (Wyeth)   1254
Norgestrel *Rx*

Vaginal Inserts
ENCARE (Thompson)   1254
2.27% Nonoxynol-9 *OTC*

INTERCEPT (Advanced Care Products)   1254
5.56% Nonoxynol-9 *OTC*

SEMICID (Whitehall)   1254
5.56% Nonoxynol-9 *OTC*

Vaginal Creams
CONCEPTROL (Advanced Care Products)   1254
5% Nonoxynol-9 *OTC*

KOROMEX (Schmid)   1254
3.0% Octoxynol *OTC*

ORTHO-CREME (Advanced Care Products)   1254
2% Nonoxynol-9 *OTC*

Vaginal Foams
DELFEN (Advanced Care Products)   1254
12.5% Nonoxynol-9 *OTC*

EMKO (Schering)   1254
8.0% Nonoxynol-9 *OTC*

EMKO BECAUSE (Schering)   1254
8.0% Nonoxynol-9 *OTC*

EMKO PRE-FIL (Schering)   1254
8.0% Nonoxynol-9 *OTC*

KOROMEX (Schmid)   1254
12.5% Nonoxynol-9 *OTC*

Sponges
TODAY (VLI)   1254
1 g Nonoxynol-9 *OTC*

Vaginal Jellies
CONCEPTROL (Advanced Care Products)   1254
4% Nonoxynol-9 *OTC*

GYNOL II (Advanced Care Products)   1254
2% Nonoxynol-9 *OTC*

KOROMEX (Schmid)   1254
3% Nonoxynol-9 *OTC*

KOROMEX Crystal Clear Gel (Schmid)   1254
2% Nonoxynol-9 *OTC*

ORTHO-GYNOL (Advanced Care Products)   1254
1% *p*-Diisobutylphenoxypolyethoxyethanol *OTC*

RAMSES (Schmid)   1254
5% Nonoxynol-9 *OTC*

Diaphragms
KORO-FLEX (Schmid)   1254
Arcing spring *Rx*

KOROMEX (Schmid)   1254
Coil spring *Rx*

ORTHO Diaphragm Kit (Ortho)   1254
Coil spring *Rx*

ORTHO Diaphragm Kit-ALL FLEX (Ortho)   1254
Arcing spring *Rx*

ORTHO-WHITE Diaphragm Kit (Ortho)   1254
Flat spring *Rx*

RAMSES (Schmid)   1254
Coil spring *Rx*

RAMSES BENDEX (Schmid)   1254
Arcing spring *Rx*

Intrauterine Devices
PROGESTASERT (Alza)   1254
Progesterone-bearing *Rx*

COMPENDIUM OF DRUG THERAPY

OTHER CONTRACEPTIVES

DRUG	HOW SUPPLIED	USUAL DOSAGE
Estrogen-Progestin Oral Contraceptives		
ENOVID 5 mg (Searle) Norethynodrel and mestranol *Rx*	**Tablets:** 5 mg norethynodrel and 75 g mestranol	**Adult:** 1 tab q24h for 20 days, beginning on 5th day of menstrual cycle or 8 days after taking last tablet of previous cycle, whichever occurs first
ENOVID-E 21 (Searle) Norethynodrel and mestranol *Rx*	**Tablets:** 2.5 mg norethynodrel and 100 g mestranol	**Adult:** 1 tab q24h for 21 days, beginning on 5th day of menstrual cycle or 8 days after taking last tablet of previous cycle, whichever occurs first
NORINYL 2 mg (Syntex) Norethindrone and mestranol *Rx*	**Tablets:** 2 mg norethindrone and 100 g mestranol	**Adult:** 1 tab q24h for 20 days, beginning on 5th day of menstrual cycle
Progestin-only Oral Contraceptives		
MICRONOR (Ortho) Norethindrone *Rx*	**Tablets:** 0.35 mg	**Adult:** 1 tab/day continuously, beginning on first day of menstruation
NOR-Q.D. (Syntex) Norethindrone *Rx*	**Tablets:** 0.35 mg	**Adult:** 1 tab/day continuously, beginning on first day of menstruation
OVRETTE (Wyeth) Norgestrel *Rx*	**Tablets:** 0.075 mg	**Adult:** 1 tab/day continuously, beginning on first day of menstruation

Vaginal Inserts	Vaginal Foams	Vaginal Jellies
ENCARE (Thompson) 2.27% Nonoxynol-9 *OTC*	**DELFEN** (Advanced Care Products) 12.5% Nonoxynol-9 *OTC*	**CONCEPTROL** (Advanced Care Products) 4% Nonoxynol-9 *OTC*
INTERCEPT (Advanced Care Products) 5.56% Nonoxynol-9 *OTC*	**EMKO** (Schering) 8.0% Nonoxynol-9 *OTC*	**GYNOL II** (Advanced Care Products) 2% Nonoxynol-9 *OTC*
SEMICID (Whitehall) 5.56% Nonoxynol-9 *OTC*	**EMKO BECAUSE** (Schering) 8.0% Nonoxynol-9 *OTC*	**KOROMEX** (Schmid) 3% Nonoxynol-9 *OTC*
Vaginal Creams	**EMKO PRE-FIL** (Schering) 8.0% Nonoxynol-9 *OTC*	**KOROMEX Crystal Clear Gel** (Schmid) 2% Nonoxynol-9 *OTC*
CONCEPTROL (Advanced Care Products) 5% Nonoxynol-9 *OTC*	**KOROMEX** (Schmid) 12.5% Nonoxynol-9 *OTC*	**ORTHO-GYNOL** (Advanced Care Products) 1% *p*-Diisobutylphenoxypolyethoxyethanol *OTC*
KOROMEX (Schmid) 3.0% Octoxynol *OTC*	**Sponges**	
ORTHO-CREME (Advanced Care Products) 2% Nonoxynol-9 *OTC*	**TODAY** (VLI) 1 g Nonoxynol-9 *OTC*	**RAMSES** (Schmid) 5% Nonoxynol-9 *OTC*

Diaphragms		
KORO-FLEX (Schmid) Arcing spring *Rx*	**ORTHO Diaphragm Kit** (Ortho) Coil spring *Rx*	**RAMSES** (Schmid) Coil spring *Rx*
KOROMEX (Schmid) Coil spring *Rx*	**ORTHO Diaphragm Kit-ALL FLEX** (Ortho) Arcing spring *Rx*	**RAMSES BENDEX** (Schmid) Arcing spring *Rx*
	ORTHO-WHITE Diaphragm Kit (Ortho) Flat spring *Rx*	

Intrauterine Devices

PROGESTASERT (Alza) Progesterone-bearing *Rx*

BREVICON

CONTRACEPTIVES

BREVICON 21-DAY (norethindrone and ethinyl estradiol) Syntex — Rx
Tablets: 0.5 mg norethindrone and 35 µg ethinyl estradiol *21-day regimen*

BREVICON 28-DAY (norethindrone and ethinyl estradiol) Syntex — Rx
Tablets: 0.5 mg norethindrone and 35 µg ethinyl estradiol *28-day regimen*

INDICATIONS
Contraception

ORAL DOSAGE
Adult: 1 tab q24h at bedtime for 21 or 28 consecutive days of the menstrual cycle

CONTRAINDICATIONS
- Thrombophlebitis or thromboembolic disorders
- Past history of deep-vein thrombophlebitis or thromboembolic disorders
- Past or present cerebrovascular disease
- Past or present coronary artery disease, including myocardial infarction
- Past or present known or suspected breast cancer
- Past or present known or suspected estrogen-dependent neoplasia
- Undiagnosed abnormal genital bleeding
- Past or present benign or malignant hepatic tumor that developed during the use of oral contraceptives or other estrogen-containing products
- Known or suspected pregnancy

ADMINISTRATION/DOSAGE ADJUSTMENTS

Initiating therapy — First tablet should be taken on the fifth day or first Sunday after the onset of menses or, if menses begins on a Sunday, on that very day. An additional form of contraception should be used during the first week of the initial cycle. Instruct postpartum patients not to initiate oral contraceptive therapy earlier than 2 wk after delivery; patients may start oral contraception immediately after an aborted pregnancy of less than 12 wk gestation, but should not start until 2 wk after an aborted pregnancy of 12 wk gestation or longer.

Subsequent cycles (21-day regimen) — First tablet is taken 8 days after last tablet was taken in preceding cycle

Subsequent cycles (28-day regimen) — First tablet is taken 1 day after last (placebo) tablet was taken in preceding cycle

Missed tablets — If one tablet is missed, it should be taken as soon as it is remembered, with the next tablet taken at the usual time. If two tablets are missed, one of them should be taken as soon as remembered and the other discarded. The remaining tablets should be taken as usual, but an additional form of contraception should be used for the remainder of the cycle. If three or more tablets in a row are missed, the tablet cycle should be discontinued and another form of contraception used until menses has appeared or pregnancy has been excluded.

WARNINGS/PRECAUTIONS

Cigarette smoking — Increases the risk of serious cardiovascular side effects, especially in women over 35 yr of age who smoke 15 or more cigarettes daily; patients who use oral contraceptives should be strongly urged not to smoke

Thromboembolic disease, thrombotic disorders, and other vascular problems — Risk is increased, becoming greater with age (after 30 yr of age) and with the amount of estrogen in the formulation; after use of oral contraceptives is discontinued, the risk of cerebrovascular disease, myocardial infarction, and subarachnoid hemorrhage may persist. Discontinue oral contraception immediately if early signs of thromboembolic disease or thrombotic disorders (eg, thrombophlebitis, pulmonary embolism, cerebrovascular insufficiency, coronary occlusion, or retinal or mesenteric thrombosis) develop or are suspected. The presence of varicose veins may substantially increase the risk of superficial venous thrombosis of the leg.

Postsurgical thromboembolic complications — Risk is increased 4–6 times; if feasible, discontinue oral contraception at least 4 wk before elective surgery associated with an increased risk of thromboembolism or prolonged immobilization

Ocular lesions, including optic neuritis and retinal thrombosis — May occur; discontinue oral contraception in the presence of unexplained gradual or sudden, partial or complete loss of vision; proptosis or diplopia; papilledema; or retinal vascular lesions

Carcinoma — Although several studies have found no overall increase of breast cancer in women taking estrogens or oral contraceptives, the risk may be increased when such use is associated with other risk factors, including benign breast disease (eg, cysts); long-term administration (2–4 yr), particularly in patients under 25 yr of age; prior breast biopsy, or a family history of breast cancer. Closely monitor patients with a strong family history of breast cancer or with breast nodules, fibrocystic disease, or abnormal mammograms. Studies suggest that there is an increased risk of cervical neoplasms associated with longer duration of oral contraceptive use. Investigate all cases of undiagnosed persistent or recurrent abnormal vaginal bleeding for malignancy (see CONTRAINDICATIONS).

Hepatic tumors — May occur and possibly rupture, resulting in intraabdominal hemorrhage and death; investigate all cases of abdominal pain and tenderness, right upper quadrant mass, or shock for liver tumors. The risk of hepatocellular adenoma reportedly increases in women over 30, among users of formulations with high hormonal potency, and with use of oral contraception for more than 4 yr (estimated annual incidence, 3–4/100,000).

BREVICON

Gallbladder disease	Risk increases with duration of oral contraception
Hepatic impairment	Use with caution due to poor steroid hormone metabolism (see CONTRAINDICATIONS)
Jaundice	May recur in patients with a history of jaundice; discontinue oral contraception while cause is investigated
Glucose tolerance	May become impaired; closely monitor patients with latent or active diabetes
Hypertension	May be precipitated or may worsen with oral contraception, particularly with prolonged use and in older patients. Closely monitor patients with a history of hypertension, toxemia, or hypertension during pregnancy; excessive weight gain or fluid retention during the menstrual cycle; preexisting renal disease; or a family history of hypertension or hypertensive complications.
Migraine headache	May develop or worsen; discontinue oral contraception and investigate cause of recurrent, persistent, or severe headaches
Bleeding irregularities, including breakthrough bleeding, spotting, and amenorrhea	May occur, necessitating either a change to a formulation with a higher estrogen content or discontinuation of therapy; higher amounts of estrogen, while potentially useful for minimizing menstrual irregularities, may increase the risk of thromboembolic disease
Mental depression	Risk is increased; discontinue oral contraception if serious depression develops or recurs in patients with a history of depression
Fluid retention	May occur; use with caution in patients with convulsive disorders, migraine, asthma, or cardiac, hepatic, or renal dysfunction
Vitamin deficiencies	May occur, particularly of pyridoxine and folic acid
Intolerance to contact lenses	Patients who wear contact lenses may experience changes in vision or lens tolerance; such changes should be evaluated by an ophthalmologist. It may be necessary to suspend contact lens wear temporarily or permanently.
Chlamydial infections	Infection with *Chlamydia trachomatis* is enhanced by oral contraceptive use
Spotting, breakthrough bleeding	If spotting or breakthrough bleeding occurs, instruct the patient to continue the regimen, but bear in mind the possibility of organic disorder. If abnormal vaginal bleeding persists or recurs, adequate diagnostic measures are indicated to rule out pregnancy or malignancy. Assuming these are excluded, the problem may be corrected by the passage of time or use of another formulation. Preparations with a higher estrogen content should be used only if necessary because of the increased risk of thromboembolic disease.
Failure of withdrawal bleeding	If patient has not adhered to prescribed regimen, pregnancy should be considered after the first missed period and oral contraception withheld until pregnancy has been excluded; if patient has adhered to regimen and misses two consecutive periods, pregnancy should be ruled out before contraceptive regimen is continued. Amenorrhea may occur during therapy and necessitate discontinuation of use.
Postpill amenorrhea and anovulation	May occur, particularly in patients with a history of oligomenorrhea or secondary amenorrhea or in young women who have not established regular menstrual cycles; such patients should be encouraged to use alternative methods of contraception
Infertility	May occur following discontinuation of oral contraception, independent of its duration; diminishes with time but may still be apparent up to 30 mo in parous women and up to 42 mo in nulliparous women

ADVERSE REACTIONS

Frequent reactions (incidence ≥ 1%) are printed in *italics*

Genitourinary	*Breakthrough bleeding, spotting, menstrual irregularities, vaginal candidiasis,* postpill amenorrhea and infertility, dysmenorrhea, altered cervical erosion and secretion, enlargement of uterine leiomyomata, premenstrual-like syndrome, altered libido, cystitis-like syndrome, vaginitis
Cardiovascular	Thrombophlebitis, thrombosis, pulmonary embolism, coronary thrombosis, cerebral thrombosis, cerebral hemorrhage, arterial thromboembolism, Raynaud's disease, hypertension, mesenteric thrombosis, edema, malignant hypertension
Gastrointestinal	*Nausea, vomiting,* gallbladder disease, abdominal cramps, colitis, bloating, change in appetite
Hepatic	Liver tumors, cholestatic jaundice
Metabolic and endocrinological	*Breast enlargement, tenderness, and/or secretion;* carbohydrate intolerance; increase or decrease in weight; hyperlipidemia
Central nervous system and neuromuscular	Migraine, depression, headache, nervousness, dizziness, chorea
Ophthalmic	Optic neuritis, retinal thrombosis, intolerance to contact lenses, altered corneal curvature, cataracts
Allergic and dermatological	Rash, melasma or chloasma, erythema multiforme, erythema nodosum, hirsutism, hair loss, hemorrhagic eruption, porphyria, chilblains

BREVICON ■ DEMULEN 1/35

Other	Congenital abnormalities, prolactin-secreting pituitary tumors, impaired renal function, malignant nephrosclerosis (hemolytic uremic syndrome), acute renal failure

OVERDOSAGE

Signs and symptoms	Nausea, withdrawal bleeding; acute ingestion of large doses by young children has not been associated with serious ill effects
Treatment	Treat symptomatically

DRUG INTERACTIONS

Ampicillin, analgesics, antianxiety agents, antihistamines, antimigraine preparations, barbiturates, chloramphenicol, isoniazid, neomycin, nitrofurantoin, penicillin V, phenylbutazone, phenytoin, primidone, rifampin, sulfonamides, tetracycline, tranquilizers	▽ Contraceptive effect △ Breakthrough bleeding
Antihypertensive agents (eg, guanethidine)	▽ Antihypertensive effect
Oral anticoagulants	▽ Anticoagulant effect
Anticonvulsants	△ Seizure activity
Hypoglycemic agents	▽ Glucose tolerance
Corticosteroids	△ Corticosteroid effects
Cyclosporine	Hepatotoxicity
Tricyclic antidepressants	△ Antidepressant side effects
Benzodiazepines (except lorazepam, oxazepam, and temazepam)	△ Serum benzodiazepine level
Theophylline	△ Serum theophylline level

ALTERED LABORATORY VALUES

Blood/serum values	△ Alkaline phosphatase △ Bilirubin △ Sulfobromophthalein retention △ Prothrombin △ Clotting factors VII, VIII, IX, and X ▽ Antithrombin III △ PBI △ Thyroxine (T_4) ▽ Triiodothyronine (T_3) uptake △ Glucose △ Cortisol △ Transcortin △ Ceruloplasmin △ Triglycerides △ Phospholipids ▽ Folic acid ▽ Pyridoxine
Urinary values	▽ Pregnanediol

USE IN CHILDREN
Not indicated before puberty

USE IN PREGNANT AND NURSING WOMEN
Pregnancy Category X: contraindicated if pregnancy is known or suspected, as serious fetal damage may occur during early pregnancy. Patient should discontinue oral contraception 3 mo before attempting to conceive. Postpartum use may interfere with lactation, causing a decrease in the quantity and quality of breast milk. Patient should use alternative form of contraception until infant is weaned.

CONTRACEPTIVES

DEMULEN 1/35-21 (ethynodiol diacetate and ethinyl estradiol) Searle   Rx
Tablets: 1 mg ethynodiol diacetate and 35 µg ethinyl estradiol *21-day regimen*

DEMULEN 1/35-28 (ethynodiol diacetate and ethinyl estradiol) Searle   Rx
Tablets: 1 mg ethynodiol diacetate and 35 µg ethinyl estradiol *28-day regimen*

INDICATIONS	ORAL DOSAGE
Contraception	**Adult:** 1 tab q24h for 21 or 28 consecutive days of the menstrual cycle

DEMULEN 1/35

CONTRAINDICATIONS

- Thrombophlebitis or thromboembolic disorders
- Past history of deep-vein thrombophlebitis or thromboembolic disorders
- Past of present myocardial infarction
- Past or present coronary artery disease
- Past or present cerebrovascular disease
- Past or present benign or malignant liver tumors that developed during the use of oral contraceptives or other estrogen-containing products
- Known or suspected breast cancer
- Known or suspected estrogen-dependent neoplasia
- Undiagnosed abnormal genital bleeding
- Known or suspected pregnancy

ADMINISTRATION/DOSAGE ADJUSTMENTS

Initiating therapy	First tablet should be taken on the 5th day (Demulen 1/35-21) or 1st Sunday (Demulen 1/35-21, Demulen 1/35-28) after the onset of menses; if menses begins on a Sunday, regimen is started the very same day. An additional form of contraception should be used during the 1st week of the initial cycle.
Subsequent cycles (21-day regimen)	First tablet is taken 8 days after last tablet was taken in preceding cycle
Subsequent cycles (28-day regimen)	First tablet is taken 1 day after last (placebo) tablet was taken in preceding cycle
Missed tablets	If one tablet is missed, it should be taken as soon as it is remembered, with the next tablet taken at the usual time. If two tablets are missed, the dosage should be doubled for the next 2 days. The remaining tablets should be taken as usual, but an additional form of contraception should be used for the remainder of the cycle.

WARNINGS/PRECAUTIONS

Cigarette smoking	Increases the risk of serious cardiovascular side effects, especially in women over 35 yr of age who smoke 15 or more cigarettes daily; patients who use oral contraceptives should be strongly urged not to smoke
Thromboembolic disease, thrombotic disorders, and other vascular problems	Risk is increased, becoming greater with age in women who use oral contraceptives after age 30 and with the amount of estrogen and possibly also of progestin present in the formulation; after use of oral contraceptives is discontinued, the risk may persist. Discontinue oral contraception immediately if early signs of thromboembolic disease or thrombotic disorders (eg, thrombophlebitis, pulmonary embolism, arterial thromboembolism, Raynaud's disease, cerebrovascular insufficiency, coronary artery disease, myocardial infarction, retinal or mesenteric thrombosis) develop or are suspected. The presence of varicose veins may substantially increase the risk of superficial venous thrombosis of the leg.
Postsurgical thromboembolic complications	Risk is increased 4–7 times; if feasible, discontinue oral contraception at least 4 wk before elective surgery or during periods of anticipated prolonged immobilization
Ocular lesions, including optic neuritis and retinal thrombosis	May occur; discontinue oral contraception in the presence of unexplained gradual or sudden, partial or complete loss of vision; proptosis or diplopia; papilledema; or retinal vascular lesions
Carcinoma	Hepatocellular carcinoma has been reported; it is estimated that the risk is increased 7–20 times for women who have used oral contraceptives for 8 or more years. Although several studies have found no overall increase in breast cancer in women taking estrogens or oral contraceptives, the risk may be increased when such use is associated with other risk factors, including benign breast disease (eg, cysts), long-term administration (2–4 yr), prior breast biopsy, family history of breast cancer, or delay in having a first child; closely monitor patients with a strong family history of breast cancer or with breast nodules, fibrocystic disease, recurrent cystic mastitis, abnormal mammograms, or cervical dysplasia. Investigate all cases of undiagnosed persistent or recurrent abnormal vaginal bleeding for malignancy (see CONTRAINDICATIONS).
Hepatic lesions, including benign adenomas	May occur and possibly rupture, resulting in intraabdominal hemorrhage and death; investigate all cases of abdominal pain and tenderness, abdominal mass, or shock for hepatic lesions. The risk of hepatocellular adenoma reportedly increases in women over 30, among users of formulations with high hormonal potency, and with use of oral contraception for more than 4 yr (estimated annual incidence, 3–4/100,000).
Gallbladder disease	Risk increases with duration of oral contraception
Hepatic impairment	Use with caution due to poor steroid hormone metabolism (see CONTRAINDICATIONS)
Jaundice	May recur in patients with a history of jaundice; discontinue oral contraception while cause is investigated. Cholestatic jaundice has been reported after combined use of oral contraceptives and troleandomycin.
Glucose tolerance	May become impaired; closely monitor patients with latent or active diabetes
Hypertension	May be precipitated or may worsen with oral contraception, particularly with prolonged use and in older patients. Closely monitor patients with a history of hypertension, toxemia, hypertension during pregnancy, or excessive weight gain or fluid retention during the menstrual cycle; preexisting renal disease; or a family history of hypertension or hypertensive complications.

Migraine headache	May develop or worsen; discontinue oral contraception and investigate cause of recurrent, persistent, or severe headaches
Mental depression	Risk is increased; discontinue oral contraception if serious depression develops or recurs in patients with a history of depression
Fluid retention	May occur; use with caution in patients with convulsive disorders, migraine, asthma, or cardiac, hepatic, or renal dysfunction
Vitamin deficiencies	May occur, particularly of pyridoxine and folic acid
Spotting, breakthrough bleeding	Spotting and breakthrough bleeding are most likely to occur during the initial cycle and when tablets are missed (particularly if two or more tablets are missed); instruct the patient to continue the regimen, but bear in mind the possibility of organic disorder. If abnormal vaginal bleeding persists or recurs, adequate diagnostic measures are indicated to rule out pregnancy and malignancy. Assuming these are excluded, the problem may be corrected by the passage of time or use of another formulation. Preparations with a higher estrogen content should be used only if necessary because of the increased risk of thromboembolic disease.
Failure of withdrawal bleeding	If patient has not adhered to prescribed regimen, pregnancy should be considered after the first missed period and oral contraception withheld until pregnancy has been excluded; if patient has adhered to regimen and misses two consecutive periods, pregnancy should be ruled out before contraceptive regimen is continued. Amenorrhea may occur during therapy and necessitate discontinuation of use.
Amenorrhea and impaired fertility	After oral contraception has been discontinued, amenorrhea and adverse effects on fertility can occur; amenorrhea may be accompanied by galactorrhea and development of a pituitary tumor. Fertility may be impaired for up to 2.5 yr in parous women aged 25–34 yr and for up to 4 yr in nulliparous women aged 25–29 yr; in nulliparous women aged 30–34 yr, impairment may be evident for up to 6 yr, especially following use of oral contraceptives for 2 or more years. Patients with a history of oligomenorrhea or secondary amenorrhea and young women who have not established regular cycles may tend to remain anovulatory or become amenorrheic following termination of oral contraceptive use and, therefore, should be encouraged to use alternative methods of contraception.
Protection against PID	*Chlamydia trachomatis* appears more frequently in the cervix when women use oral contraceptives; it should not be assumed that these preparations afford protection against pelvic inflammatory disease due to *Chlamydia*
Endocrine and liver-function studies	May be affected (see ALTERED LABORATORY VALUES); repeat any abnormal tests 2 mo after oral contraception is discontinued
Mutagenicity	An increase in lymphocytic chromosomal aberrations has been seen in women receiving oral contraceptives

ADVERSE REACTIONS	Frequent reactions (incidence ≥ 1%) are printed in *italics*
Genitourinary	*Breakthrough bleeding, spotting, menstrual irregularities, vaginal candidiasis,* postpill amenorrhea and infertility, dysmenorrhea, altered cervical erosion and secretion, endocervical hyperplasia, enlargement of uterine leiomyomata, premenstrual-like syndrome, altered libido, cystitis-like syndrome, vaginitis
Cardiovascular	Thrombophlebitis, thrombosis, pulmonary embolism, arterial thromboembolism, Raynaud's disease, myocardial infarction, coronary thrombosis, premature ventricular contractions, thrombotic thrombocytopenic purpura, cerebral thrombosis, cerebral hemorrhage, hypertension (including malignant and pulmonary hypertension), mesenteric thrombosis, edema
Gastrointestinal	*Nausea, vomiting,* gallbladder disease, abdominal cramps, bloating, change in appetite, pancreatitis, colitis, Crohn's disease
Hepatic	Hepatocellular carcinoma, benign adenomas and other hepatic lesions, Budd-Chiari syndrome, cholestatic jaundice, hepatitis
Renal	Impaired renal function, hemolytic uremic syndrome, acute renal failure (sometimes irreversible)
Metabolic and endocrinological	*Breast enlargement, tenderness, and/or secretion;* carbohydrate intolerance; increase or decrease in weight; hyperlipidemia
Central nervous system and neuromuscular	Migraine, depression, headache, nervousness, dizziness, chorea, paresthesia, auditory disturbances, fatigue
Ophthalmic	Optic neuritis, retinal thrombosis, intolerance to contact lenses, altered corneal curvature, cataracts
Allergic and dermatological	Melasma or chloasma, rash, itching, rhinitis, erythema multiforme, erythema nodosum, hirsutism, hair loss, hemorrhagic eruption, porphyria, malignant melanoma, herpes gestationis
Other	Congenital anomalies, prolactin-secreting pituitary tumors, backache, anemia, lupus erythematosus, rheumatoid arthritis, gingivitis, dry socket; endometrial, cervical, and breast carcinoma

DEMULEN 1/35 ■ DEMULEN 1/50

OVERDOSAGE

Signs and symptoms	Nausea, withdrawal bleeding; acute ingestion of large doses by young children has not been associated with serious ill effects
Treatment	Treat symptomatically

DRUG INTERACTIONS

Ampicillin, analgesics, antianxiety agents, antimigraine preparations, barbiturates, chloramphenicol, griseofulvin, isoniazid, neomycin, nitrofurantoin, penicillin V, phenylbutazone, phenytoin, primidone, rifampin, sulfonamides, tetracycline	▽ Contraceptive effect △ Breakthrough bleeding
Antihypertensive agents (eg, guanethidine)	▽ Antihypertensive effect
Oral anticoagulants	▽ Anticoagulant effect
Anticonvulsants	△ Seizure activity
Hypoglycemic agents	▽ Glucose tolerance
Corticosteroids	△ Corticosteroid effects
Tricyclic antidepressants	△ Antidepressant side effects
Diazepam, chlordiazepoxide	△ Serum half-life of benzodiazepines
Troleandomycin	Cholestatic jaundice
Cyclosporine	Hepatotoxicity
Acetaminophen	▽ Serum half-life of acetaminophen
Clofibrate	▽ Hypolipidemic effect
Theophylline	△ Serum half-life of theophylline

ALTERED LABORATORY VALUES

Blood/serum values	△ Alkaline phosphatase △ Bilirubin △ Sulfobromophthalein retention △ Prothrombin △ Clotting factors VII, VIII, IX, and X ▽ Antithrombin III △ PBI △ Thyroxine (T_4) ▽ Triiodothyronine (T_3) uptake △ Glucose △ Cortisol △ Transcortin △ Ceruloplasmin △ Triglycerides △ Phospholipids ▽ Folic acid ▽ Pyridoxine
Urinary values	▽ Pregnanediol

USE IN CHILDREN

Not indicated before puberty

USE IN PREGNANT AND NURSING WOMEN

Pregnancy Category X: contraindicated if pregnancy is known or suspected, as serious fetal damage may occur during early pregnancy. Patient should discontinue oral contraception 3 mo before attempting to conceive. Postpartum use may interfere with lactation, causing a decrease in the quantity and quality of breast milk. Patient should use alternative form of contraception until infant is weaned.

CONTRACEPTIVES

DEMULEN 1/50-21 (ethynodiol diacetate and ethinyl estradiol) Searle   Rx
Tablets: 1 mg ethynodiol diacetate and 50 μg ethinyl estradiol *21-day regimen*

DEMULEN 1/50-28 (ethynodiol diacetate and ethinyl estradiol) Searle   Rx
Tablets: 1 mg ethynodiol diacetate and 50 μg ethinyl estradiol *28-day regimen*

INDICATIONS

Contraception

ORAL DOSAGE

Adult: 1 tab q24h for 21 or 28 consecutive days of the menstrual cycle

CONTRAINDICATIONS

Thrombophlebitis or thromboembolic disorders

Past history of deep-vein thrombophlebitis or thromboembolic disorders

Past or present myocardial infarction

Past or present coronary artery disease

Past or present cerebrovascular disease

Past or present benign or malignant liver tumors that developed during the use of oral contraceptives or other estrogen-containing products

Known or suspected breast cancer

Known or suspected estrogen-dependent neoplasia

Undiagnosed abnormal genital bleeding

Known or suspected pregnancy

DEMULEN 1/50

ADMINISTRATION/DOSAGE ADJUSTMENTS

Initiating therapy	First tablet should be taken on the 5th day (Demulen 1/50-21 only) or 1st Sunday after the onset of menses or on a Sunday that coincides with the onset of menses. An additional form of contraception should be used during the first week of the initial cycle.
Subsequent cycles (21-day regimen)	First tablet is taken 8 days after last tablet was taken in preceding cycle
Subsequent cycles (28-day regimen)	First tablet is taken 1 day after last (placebo) tablet was taken in preceding cycle
Missed tablets	If one tablet is missed, it should be taken as soon as it is remembered, with the next tablet taken at the usual time. If two tablets are missed, the dosage should be doubled for the next 2 days. The remaining tablets should be taken as usual, but an additional form of contraception should be used for the remainder of the cycle.

WARNINGS/PRECAUTIONS

Cigarette smoking	Increases the risk of serious cardiovascular side effects, especially in women over 35 yr of age who smoke 15 or more cigarettes daily; patients who use oral contraceptives should be strongly urged not to smoke
Thromboembolic disease, thrombotic disorders, and other vascular problems	Risk is increased, becoming greater with age in women who use oral contraceptives after age 30 and with the amount of estrogen and possibly also of progestin present in the formulation; after use of oral contraceptives is discontinued, the risk may persist. Discontinue oral contraception immediately if early signs of thromboembolic disease or thrombotic disorders (eg, thrombophlebitis, pulmonary embolism, arterial thromboembolism, Raynaud's disease, cerebrovascular insufficiency, coronary artery disease, myocardial infarction, or retinal or mesenteric thrombosis) develop or are suspected. The presence of varicose veins may substantially increase the risk of superficial venous thrombosis of the leg.
Postsurgical thromboembolic complications	Risk is increased 4–7 times; if feasible, discontinue oral contraception at least 4 wk before elective surgery or during periods of anticipated prolonged immobilization
Ocular lesions, including optic neuritis and retinal thrombosis	May occur; discontinue oral contraception in the presence of unexplained gradual or sudden, partial or complete loss of vision; proptosis or diplopia; papilledema; or retinal vascular lesions
Carcinoma	Hepatocellular carcinoma has been reported; it is estimated that the risk is increased 7–20 times for women who have used oral contraceptives for 8 or more years. Although several studies have found no overall increase in breast cancer in women taking estrogens or oral contraceptives, the risk may be increased when such use is associated with other risk factors, including benign breast disease (eg, cysts), long-term administration (2–4 yr), prior breast biopsy, family history of breast cancer, or delay in having a first child; closely monitor patients with a strong family history of breast cancer or with breast nodules, fibrocystic disease, recurrent cystic mastitis, abnormal mammograms, or cervical dysplasia. Investigate all cases of undiagnosed persistent or recurrent abnormal vaginal bleeding for malignancy (see CONTRAINDICATIONS).
Hepatic lesions, including benign adenomas	May occur and possibly rupture, resulting in intraabdominal hemorrhage and death; investigate all cases of abdominal pain and tenderness, abdominal mass, or shock for hepatic lesions. The risk of hepatocellular adenoma reportedly increases in women over 30, among users of formulations with high hormonal potency, and with use of oral contraception for more than 4 yr (estimated annual incidence, 3–4/100,000).
Gallbladder disease	Risk increases with duration of oral contraception
Hepatic impairment	Use with caution due to poor steroid hormone metabolism (see CONTRAINDICATIONS)
Jaundice	May recur in patients with a history of jaundice; discontinue oral contraception while cause is investigated. Cholestatic jaundice has been reported after combined use of oral contraceptives and troleandomycin.
Glucose tolerance	May become impaired; closely monitor patients with latent or active diabetes
Hypertension	May be precipitated or may worsen with oral contraception, particularly with prolonged use and in older patients. Closely monitor patients with a history of hypertension, toxemia, hypertension during pregnancy, or excessive weight gain or fluid retention during the menstrual cycle; preexisting renal disease; or a family history of hypertension or hypertensive complications.
Migraine headache	May develop or worsen; discontinue oral contraception and investigate cause of recurrent, persistent, or severe headaches
Mental depression	Risk is increased; discontinue oral contraception if serious depression develops or recurs in patients with a history of depression
Fluid retention	May occur; use with caution in patients with convulsive disorders, migraine, asthma, or cardiac, hepatic, or renal dysfunction
Vitamin deficiencies	May occur, particularly of pyridoxine and folic acid
Spotting, breakthrough bleeding	Spotting and breakthrough bleeding are most likely to occur during the initial cycle and when tablets are missed (particularly if two or more tablets are missed); instruct the patient to continue the regimen, but bear in mind the possibility of organic disorder. If abnormal vaginal bleeding persists or recurs, adequate diagnostic measures are indicated to rule out pregnancy and malignancy. Assuming these are excluded, the problem may be corrected by the passage of time or use of another formulation. Preparations with a higher estrogen content should be used only if necessary because of the increased risk of thromboembolic disease.

DEMULEN 1/50

Failure of withdrawal bleeding	If patient has not adhered to prescribed regimen, pregnancy should be considered after the first missed period and oral contraception withheld until pregnancy has been excluded; if patient has adhered to regimen and misses two consecutive periods, pregnancy should be ruled out before contraceptive regimen is continued. Amenorrhea may occur during therapy and necessitate discontinuation of use.
Amenorrhea and impaired fertility	After oral contraception has been discontinued, amenorrhea and adverse effects on fertility can occur; amenorrhea may be accompanied by galactorrhea and development of a pituitary tumor. Fertility may be impaired for up to 2.5 yr in parous women aged 25–34 yr and for up to 4 yr in nulliparous women aged 25–29 yr; in nulliparous women aged 30–34 yr, impairment may be evident for up to 6 yr, especially following use of oral contraceptives for 2 or more years. Patients with a history of oligomenorrhea or secondary amenorrhea and young women who have not established regular cycles may tend to remain anovulatory or become amenorrheic following termination of oral contraceptive use and, therefore, should be encouraged to use alternative methods of contraception.
Protection against PID	*Chlamydia trachomatis* appears more frequently in the cervix when women use oral contraceptives; it should not be assumed that these preparations afford protection against pelvic inflammatory disease due to *Chlamydia*
Endocrine and liver-function studies	May be affected (see ALTERED LABORATORY VALUES); repeat any abnormal tests 2 mo after oral contraception is discontinued
Mutagenicity	An increase in lymphocytic chromosomal aberrations has been seen in women receiving oral contraceptives

ADVERSE REACTIONS

Frequent reactions (incidence ≥ 1%) are printed in *italics*

Genitourinary	*Breakthrough bleeding, spotting, menstrual irregularities, vaginal candidiasis,* postpill amenorrhea and infertility, dysmenorrhea, altered cervical erosion and secretion, endocervical hyperplasia, enlargement of uterine leiomyomata, premenstrual-like syndrome, altered libido, cystitis-like syndrome, vaginitis
Cardiovascular	Thrombophlebitis, thrombosis, pulmonary embolism, arterial thromboembolism, Raynaud's disease, myocardial infarction, coronary thrombosis, premature ventricular contractions, thrombotic thrombocytopenic purpura, cerebral thrombosis, cerebral hemorrhage, hypertension (including malignant and pulmonary hypertension) mesenteric thrombosis, edema
Gastrointestinal	*Nausea, vomiting,* gallbladder disease, abdominal cramps, bloating, change in appetite, pancreatitis, colitis, Crohn's disease
Hepatic	Hepatocellular carcinoma, benign adenomas and other hepatic lesions, Budd-Chiari syndrome, cholestatic jaundice, hepatitis
Renal	Impaired renal function, hemolytic uremic syndrome, acute renal failure (sometimes irreversible)
Metabolic and endocrinological	*Breast enlargement, tenderness, and/or secretion;* carbohydrate intolerance; increase or decrease in weight; hyperlipidemia
Central nervous system and neuromuscular	Migraine, depression, headache, nervousness, dizziness, chorea, paresthesia, auditory disturbances, fatigue
Ophthalmic	Optic neuritis, retinal thrombosis, intolerance to contact lenses, altered corneal curvature, cataracts
Allergic and dermatological	Melasma or chloasma, rash, itching, rhinitis, erythema multiforme, erythema nodosum, hirsutism, hair loss, hemorrhagic eruption, porphyria, malignant melanoma, herpes gestationis
Other	Congenital anomalies, prolactin-secreting pituitary tumors, backache, anemia, lupus erythematosus, rheumatoid arthritis, gingivitis, dry socket; endometrial, cervical, and breast carcinoma

OVERDOSAGE

Signs and symptoms	Nausea, withdrawal bleeding; acute ingestion of large doses by young children has not been associated with serious ill effects
Treatment	Treat symptomatically

DRUG INTERACTIONS

Ampicillin, analgesics, antianxiety agents, antimigraine preparations, barbiturates, chloramphenicol, griseofulvin, isoniazid, neomycin, nitrofurantoin, penicillin V, phenylbutazone, phenytoin, primidone, rifampin, sulfonamides, tetracycline	▽ Contraceptive effect △ Breakthrough bleeding
Antihypertensive agents (eg, guanethidine)	▽ Antihypertensive effect
Oral anticoagulants	▽ Anticoagulant effect

DEMULEN 1/50 ■ LEVLEN

Anticonvulsants	△ Seizure activity
Hypoglycemic agents	▽ Glucose tolerance
Corticosteroids	△ Corticosteroid effects
Tricyclic antidepressants	△ Antidepressant side effects
Diazepam, chlordiazepoxide	△ Serum half-life of benzodiazepines
Troleandomycin	Cholestatic jaundice
Cyclosporine	Hepatotoxicity
Acetaminophen	▽ Serum half-life of acetaminophen
Clofibrate	▽ Hypolipidemic effect
Theophylline	△ Serum half-life of theophylline

ALTERED LABORATORY VALUES

Blood/serum values — △ Alkaline phosphatase △ Bilirubin △ Sulfobromophthalein retention △ Prothrombin △ Clotting factors VII, VIII, IX, and X ▽ Antithrombin III △ PBI △ Thyroxine (T_4) ▽ Triiodothyronine (T_3) uptake △ Glucose △ Cortisol △ Transcortin △ Ceruloplasmin △ Triglycerides △ Phospholipids ▽ Folic acid ▽ Pyridoxine

Urinary values — ▽ Pregnanediol

USE IN CHILDREN

Not indicated before puberty

USE IN PREGNANT AND NURSING WOMEN

Pregnancy Category X: contraindicated if pregnancy is known or suspected, as serious fetal damage may occur during early pregnancy. Patient should discontinue oral contraception 3 mo before attempting to conceive. Postpartum use may interfere with lactation, causing a decrease in the quantity and quality of breast milk. Patient should use alternative form of contraception until infant is weaned.

CONTRACEPTIVES

LEVLEN 21 (levonorgestrel and ethinyl estradiol) Berlex Rx
Tablets: 0.15 mg levonorgestrel and 30 µg ethinyl estradiol *21-day regimen*

LEVLEN 28 (levonorgestrel and ethinyl estradiol) Berlex Rx
Tablets: 0.15 mg levonorgestrel and 30 µg ethinyl estradiol *28-day regimen*

INDICATIONS	ORAL DOSAGE
Contraception	**Adult:** 1 tab q24h for 21 or 28 consecutive days of the menstrual cycle

CONTRAINDICATIONS

Thrombophlebitis or thromboembolic disorders	Known or suspected breast cancer	Known or suspected pregnancy
Past history of deep-vein thrombophlebitis or thromboembolic disorders	Known or suspected estrogen-dependent neoplasia	Benign or malignant liver tumor that developed during the use of oral contraceptives or other estrogen-containing products
Coronary artery disease	Undiagnosed abnormal genital bleeding	
Cerebrovascular disease		

ADMINISTRATION/DOSAGE ADJUSTMENTS

Initiating therapy	First tablet should be taken on the 5th day (Levlen 21) or 1st Sunday (Levlen 28) after the onset of menses; if menses begins on a Sunday, regimen is started the very same day
Subsequent cycles (21-day regimen)	First tablet is taken 8 days after last tablet was taken in preceding cycle
Subsequent cycles (28-day regimen)	First tablet is taken 1 day after last (placebo) tablet was taken in preceding cycle
Missed tablets	If one or two tablets are missed, they should be taken as soon as they are remembered, and an additional form of contraception should be used for 1 wk. If three tablets are missed, the tablet cycle should be discontinued; start the next tablet cycle 8 days after the last tablet was taken (Levlen 21) or on the first Sunday after the last tablet was taken (Levlen 28), and instruct patient to use another form of contraception for the days without tablets and until seven tablets are taken.

LEVLEN

Postpartum administration	For nonnursing mothers, may be started either immediately or after first postpartum examination, regardless of whether spontaneous menstruation has occurred. An additional form of contraception should be used during the first week of the initial cycle.
Monitoring of therapy	A Papanicolaou smear, other appropriate laboratory tests, and a physical examination (with special attention to breasts, abdomen, pelvic organs, and blood pressure) should be done before therapy and then repeated at least annually

WARNINGS/PRECAUTIONS

Cigarette smoking	Increases the risk of serious cardiovascular side effects, especially in women over 35 yr of age who smoke 15 or more cigarettes daily; patients who use oral contraceptives should be strongly urged not to smoke
Thromboembolic disease, thrombotic disorders, and other vascular problems	Risk is increased, becoming greater with age (after 30 yr of age) and with the amount of estrogen present in the formulation; after discontinuation of use, the risk of cerebrovascular disease and myocardial infarction may persist. Discontinue oral contraception immediately if early signs of thromboembolic disease or thrombotic disorders (eg, thrombophlebitis, pulmonary embolism, cerebrovascular insufficiency, coronary occlusion, or retinal or mesenteric thrombosis) develop or are suspected.
Postsurgical thromboembolic complications	Risk is increased 4–6 times; if feasible, discontinue oral contraception at least 4 wk before elective surgery associated with an increased risk of thromboembolism or prolonged immobilization
Ocular lesions, including optic neuritis and retinal thrombosis	May occur; discontinue oral contraception in the presence of unexplained gradual or sudden, partial or complete loss of vision; proptosis or diplopia; papilledema; or retinal vascular lesions
Carcinoma	Closely monitor patients with a strong family history of breast cancer or with breast nodules, fibrocystic disease, or abnormal mammograms; investigate all cases of undiagnosed persistent or recurrent abnormal vaginal bleeding for malignancy (see CONTRAINDICATIONS)
Hepatic tumors, including benign adenomas	May occur and possibly rupture, resulting in intraabdominal hemorrhage and death; investigate all cases of abdominal pain and tenderness, abdominal mass, or shock for hepatic adenoma. The risk reportedly increases among users of formulations with high hormonal potency, and with use of oral contraception for more than 4 yr.
Gallbladder disease	Risk increases with duration of oral contraception
Hepatic impairment	Use with caution due to poor steroid hormone metabolism
Jaundice	May recur in patients with a history of jaundice; discontinue oral contraception while cause is investigated
Glucose tolerance	May become impaired; closely monitor patients with latent or active diabetes
Hypertension	May be precipitated or may worsen with oral contraception, particularly with prolonged use, in older patients, and in patients with a history of hypertension during pregnancy
Migraine headache	May develop or worsen; discontinue oral contraception and investigate cause of recurrent, persistent, or severe headaches
Mental depression	Risk is increased; discontinue oral contraception if serious depression develops or recurs in patients with a history of depression
Fluid retention	May occur; use with caution in patients with convulsive disorders, migraine, asthma, or cardiac, hepatic, or renal dysfunction
Vitamin deficiencies	May occur, particularly of pyridoxine and folic acid
Spotting, breakthrough bleeding	Spotting or breakthrough bleeding may occur when tablets are missed or at other times during therapy; instruct the patient to continue the regimen, but bear in mind the possibility of organic disorder. If abnormal vaginal bleeding persists or recurs, adequate diagnostic measures are indicated to rule out pregnancy or malignancy. Assuming these are excluded, the problem may be corrected by the passage of time or use of another formulation. Preparations with a higher estrogen content should be used only if necessary because of the increased risk of thromboembolic disease.
Failure of withdrawal bleeding	If patient has missed two consecutive periods, pregnancy should be ruled out before contraceptive regimen is continued; if patient has not adhered to prescribed regimen, pregnancy should be considered after the first missed period and oral contraception withheld until pregnancy has been excluded. Amenorrhea may occur during therapy and necessitate discontinuation of use.
Postpill amenorrhea and anovulation	May occur, particularly in patients with a history of oligomenorrhea or secondary amenorrhea or in young women who have not established regular menstrual cycles; such patients should be encouraged to use alternative methods of contraception

ADVERSE REACTIONS

Frequent reactions (incidence ≥ 1%) are printed in *italics*

Genitourinary	*Breakthrough bleeding, spotting, menstrual irregularities, vaginal candidiasis*, postpill amenorrhea and infertility, dysmenorrhea, altered cervical erosion and secretion, enlargement of uterine leiomyomata, premenstrual-like syndrome, altered libido, cystitis-like syndrome, vaginitis

LEVLEN ■ LOESTRIN 1/20/LOESTRIN 1.5/30

Cardiovascular	Thrombophlebitis, pulmonary embolism, coronary thrombosis, cerebral thrombosis, cerebral hemorrhage, hypertension, mesenteric thrombosis, edema
Gastrointestinal	*Nausea, vomiting,* gallbladder disease, abdominal cramps, bloating, change in appetite
Hepatic	Benign hepatomas, cholestatic jaundice
Metabolic and endocrinological	*Breast enlargement, tenderness, and/or secretion;* carbohydrate intolerance; increase or decrease in weight; hyperlipidemia
Central nervous system and neuromuscular	Migraine, depression, headache, nervousness, dizziness, chorea
Ophthalmic	Optic neuritis, retinal thrombosis, intolerance to contact lenses, altered corneal curvature, cataracts
Allergic and dermatological	Rash, melasma or chloasma, erythema multiforme, erythema nodosum, hirsutism, hair loss, hemorrhagic eruption, porphyria
Other	Congenital anomalies, hemolytic uremic syndrome

OVERDOSAGE

Signs and symptoms	Nausea, withdrawal bleeding; acute ingestion of large doses by young children has not been associated with serious ill effects
Treatment	Treat symptomatically

DRUG INTERACTIONS

Ampicillin, analgesics, antianxiety agents, antimigraine agents, barbiturates, chloramphenicol, isoniazid, neomycin, nitrofurantoin, penicillin V, phenylbutazone, phenytoin, primidone, rifampin, sulfonamides, tetracycline	▽ Contraceptive effect △ Breakthrough bleeding
Antihypertensive agents (eg, guanethidine)	▽ Antihypertensive effect
Oral anticoagulants	▽ Anticoagulant effect
Anticonvulsants	△ Seizure activity
Hypoglycemic agents	▽ Glucose tolerance
Corticosteroids	△ Corticosteroid effects
Tricyclic antidepressants	△ Antidepressant side effects

ALTERED LABORATORY VALUES

Blood/serum values	△ Alkaline phosphatase △ Bilirubin △ Sulfobromophthalein retention △ Prothrombin △ Clotting factors VII, VIII, IX, and X ▽ Antithrombin III △ PBI △ Thyroxine (T$_4$) ▽ Triiodothyronine (T$_3$) uptake △ Glucose △ Cortisol △ Transcortin △ Ceruloplasmin △ Triglycerides △ Phospholipids ▽ Folic acid ▽ Pyridoxine
Urinary values	▽ Pregnanediol

USE IN CHILDREN

Not indicated before puberty

USE IN PREGNANT AND NURSING WOMEN

Pregnancy Category X: contraindicated if pregnancy is known or suspected, as serious fetal damage may occur during early pregnancy. Patient should discontinue oral contraception 3 mo before attempting to conceive. Postpartum use may interfere with lactation, causing a decrease in the quantity and quality of breast milk. Because of the potential for adverse reactions in nursing infants from oral contraceptive tablets, patient should either stop nursing or stop use of the drug.

CONTRACEPTIVES

LOESTRIN 21 1/20 (norethindrone acetate and ethinyl estradiol) Parke-Davis   Rx

Tablets: 1 mg norethindrone acetate and 20 µg ethinyl estradiol *21-day regimen*

LOESTRIN Fe 1/20 (norethindrone acetate and ethinyl estradiol; ferrous fumarate) Parke-Davis   Rx

Tablets: 1 mg norethindrone acetate and 20 µg ethinyl estradiol (white); 75 mg ferrous fumarate (brown) *28-day regimen*

LOESTRIN 21 1.5/30 (norethindrone acetate and ethinyl estradiol) Parke-Davis   Rx

Tablets: 1.5 mg norethindrone acetate and 30 µg ethinyl estradiol *21-day regimen*

LOESTRIN Fe 1.5/30 (norethindrone acetate and ethinyl estradiol; ferrous fumarate)   Rx
Parke-Davis

Tablets: 1.5 mg norethindrone acetate and 30 µg ethinyl estradiol (green); 75 mg ferrous fumarate (brown) *28-day regimen*

INDICATIONS	ORAL DOSAGE
Contraception	**Adult:** 1 tab q24h for 21 or 28 consecutive days of the menstrual cycle

COMPENDIUM OF DRUG THERAPY

LOESTRIN 1/20/LOESTRIN 1.5/30

CONTRAINDICATIONS

Thrombophlebitis or thromboembolic disorders	Known or suspected breast cancer	Known or suspected pregnancy
Past history of deep-vein thrombophlebitis or thromboembolic disorders	Known or suspected estrogen-dependent neoplasia	Benign or malignant liver tumor that developed during the use of oral contraceptives or other estrogen-containing products
Coronary artery disease	Undiagnosed abnormal genital bleeding	
Cerebrovascular disease		

ADMINISTRATION/DOSAGE ADJUSTMENTS

Initiating therapy	First tablet should be taken on the 5th day after the onset of menses
Subsequent cycles (21-day regimen)	First tablet is taken 8 days after last tablet was taken in preceding cycle
Subsequent cycles (28-day regimen)	First tablet is taken 1 day after last (placebo) tablet was taken in preceding cycle
Missed tablets	If one tablet is missed, it should be taken as soon as it is remembered or together with the next tablet on the following day. If two tablets are missed, the dosage should be doubled for the next 2 days; an additional form of contraception should be used for 7 consecutive days in patients who are taking Loestrin 1/20 tablets. If three tablets are missed, the tablet cycle should be discontinued and another form of contraception used until the start of the next menstrual period. Instruct the patient to start the next course of tablets 7 days after the last tablet was taken, even if she is still menstruating.

WARNINGS/PRECAUTIONS

Cigarette smoking	Increases the risk of serious cardiovascular side effects, especially in women over 35 yr of age who smoke 15 or more cigarettes daily; patients who use oral contraceptives should be strongly urged not to smoke
Thromboembolic disease, thrombotic disorders, and other vascular problems	Risk is increased, becoming greater with age (after 30 yr of age) and with the amount of estrogen in the formulation; after use of oral contraceptives is discontinued, the risk of cerebrovascular disease, myocardial infarction, and subarachnoid hemorrhage may persist. Discontinue oral contraception immediately if early signs of thromboembolic disease or thrombotic disorders (eg, thrombophlebitis, pulmonary embolism, cerebrovascular insufficiency, coronary occlusion, or retinal or mesenteric thrombosis) develop or are suspected.
Postsurgical thromboembolic complications	Risk is increased 4–6 times; if feasible, discontinue oral contraception at least 4 wk before elective surgery associated with an increased risk of thromboembolism or prolonged immobilization
Ocular lesions, including optic neuritis and retinal thrombosis	May occur; discontinue oral contraception in the presence of unexplained gradual or sudden, partial or complete loss of vision; proptosis or diplopia; papilledema; or retinal vascular lesions
Carcinoma	Closely monitor patients with a strong family history of breast cancer or with breast nodules, fibrocystic disease, or abnormal mammograms; investigate all cases of undiagnosed persistent or recurrent abnormal vaginal bleeding for malignancy (see CONTRAINDICATIONS)
Hepatic tumors, including benign adenomas	May occur and possibly rupture, resulting in intraabdominal hemorrhage and death; investigate all cases of abdominal pain and tenderness, abdominal mass, or shock for hepatic adenoma. The risk reportedly increases among users of formulations with high hormonal potency, and with use of oral contraception for more than 4 yr.
Gallbladder disease	Risk increases with duration of oral contraception
Hepatic impairment	Use with caution due to poor steroid hormone metabolism
Jaundice	May recur in patients with a history of jaundice; discontinue oral contraception while cause is investigated
Glucose tolerance	May become impaired; closely monitor patients with latent or active diabetes
Hypertension	May be precipitated or may worsen with oral contraception, particularly with prolonged use, in older patients, and in patients with a history of hypertension during pregnancy
Migraine headache	May develop or worsen; discontinue oral contraception and investigate cause of recurrent, persistent, or severe headaches
Mental depression	Risk is increased; discontinue oral contraception if serious depression develops or recurs in patients with a history of depression
Fluid retention	May occur; use with caution in patients with convulsive disorders, migraine, asthma, or cardiac, hepatic, or renal dysfunction
Vitamin deficiencies	May occur, particularly of pyridoxine and folic acid
Spotting, breakthrough bleeding	Spotting and breakthrough bleeding are most likely to occur during the initial cycle and when tablets are missed (especially if two or more consecutive tablets are missed); instruct the patient to continue the regimen, but bear in mind the possibility of organic disorder. If unacceptable bleeding patterns are still evident by the third cycle, consider changing to a product with a higher estrogen content; however, such preparations should be given only if necessary because they may increase the risk of thromboembolic disease. If abnormal vaginal bleeding persists or recurs at higher estrogen levels, adequate diagnostic measures are indicated to rule out pregnancy or malignancy. Assuming these are excluded, the problem may be corrected by the passage of time or use of another formulation.

LOESTRIN 1/20/LOESTRIN 1.5/30

Failure of withdrawal bleeding	If patient has missed two consecutive periods, pregnancy should be ruled out before contraceptive regimen is continued; if patient has not adhered to prescribed regimen, pregnancy should be considered after the first missed period and oral contraception withheld until pregnancy has been excluded. Amenorrhea may occur during therapy and necessitate discontinuation of use.
Postpill amenorrhea and anovulation	May occur, particularly in patients with a history of oligomenorrhea or secondary amenorrhea or in young women who have not established regular menstrual cycles; such patients should be encouraged to use alternative methods of contraception

ADVERSE REACTIONS

Frequent reactions (incidence ≥ 1%) are printed in *italics*

Genitourinary	*Breakthrough bleeding, spotting, menstrual irregularities, vaginal candidiasis,* postpill amenorrhea and infertility, dysmenorrhea, altered cervical erosion and secretion, enlargement of uterine leiomyomata, premenstrual-like syndrome, altered libido, cystitis-like syndrome, vaginitis
Cardiovascular	Thrombophlebitis, thrombosis, pulmonary embolism, coronary thrombosis, cerebral thrombosis, cerebral hemorrhage, hypertension, mesenteric thrombosis, edema
Gastrointestinal	*Nausea, vomiting,* gallbladder disease, abdominal cramps, bloating, change in appetite
Hepatic	Benign hepatomas, cholestatic jaundice
Metabolic and endocrinological	*Breast enlargement, tenderness, and/or secretion;* carbohydrate intolerance; increase or decrease in weight; hyperlipidemia
Central nervous system and neuromuscular	Migraine, depression, headache, nervousness, dizziness, chorea
Ophthalmic	Optic neuritis, retinal thrombosis, intolerance to contact lenses, altered corneal curvature, cataracts
Allergic and dermatological	Rash, melasma or chloasma, erythema multiforme, erythema nodosum, hirsutism, hair loss, hemorrhagic eruption, porphyria
Other	Congenital anomalies

OVERDOSAGE

Signs and symptoms	Nausea, withdrawal bleeding; acute ingestion of large doses by young children has not been associated with serious ill effects
Treatment	Treat symptomatically

DRUG INTERACTIONS

Ampicillin, analgesics, antianxiety agents, antimigraine preparations, barbiturates, chloramphenicol, isoniazid, neomycin, nitrofurantoin, penicillin V, phenylbutazone, phenytoin, primidone, rifampin, sulfonamides, tetracycline	▽ Contraceptive effect △ Breakthrough bleeding
Antihypertensive agents (eg, guanethidine)	▽ Antihypertensive effect
Oral anticoagulants	▽ Anticoagulant effect
Anticonvulsants	△ Seizure activity
Hypoglycemic agents	▽ Glucose tolerance
Corticosteroids	△ Corticosteroid effects
Tricyclic antidepressants	△ Antidepressant side effects

ALTERED LABORATORY VALUES

Blood/serum values	△ Alkaline phosphatase △ Bilirubin △ Sulfobromophthalein retention △ Prothrombin △ Clotting factors VII, VIII, IX, and X ▽ Antithrombin III △ PBI △ Thyroxine (T_4) ▽ Triiodothyronine (T_3) uptake △ Glucose △ Cortisol △ Transcortin △ Ceruloplasmin △ Triglycerides △ Phospholipids ▽ Folic acid ▽ Pyridoxine
Urinary values	▽ Pregnanediol

USE IN CHILDREN
Not indicated before puberty

USE IN PREGNANT AND NURSING WOMEN
Pregnancy Category X: contraindicated if pregnancy is known or suspected, as serious fetal damage may occur during early pregnancy. Patient should discontinue oral contraception 3 mo before attempting to conceive. Postpartum use may interfere with lactation, causing a decrease in the quantity and quality of breast milk. Patient should use an alternative form of contraception until infant is weaned.

CONTRACEPTIVES

LO/OVRAL (norgestrel and ethinyl estradiol) Wyeth — Rx

Tablets: 0.3 mg norgestrel and 30 μg ethinyl estradiol *21-day regimen*

LO/OVRAL-28 (norgestrel and ethinyl estradiol) Wyeth — Rx

Tablets: 0.3 mg norgestrel and 30 μg ethinyl estradiol *28-day regimen*

INDICATIONS	ORAL DOSAGE
Contraception	**Adult:** 1 tab q24h for 21 or 28 consecutive days of the menstrual cycle

CONTRAINDICATIONS

- Thrombophlebitis or thromboembolic disorders
- Past history of deep-vein thrombophlebitis or thromboembolic disorders
- Coronary artery disease
- Cerebrovascular disease
- Known or suspected breast cancer
- Known or suspected estrogen-dependent neoplasia
- Undiagnosed abnormal genital bleeding
- Known or suspected pregnancy
- Benign or malignant liver tumor that developed during the use of oral contraceptives or other estrogen-containing products

ADMINISTRATION/DOSAGE ADJUSTMENTS

Initiating therapy	First tablet should be taken on the 5th day (Lo/Ovral) or 1st Sunday (Lo/Ovral-28) after the onset of menses; if menses begins on a Sunday, regimen is started the very same day
Subsequent cycles (21-day regimen)	First tablet is taken 8 days after last tablet was taken in preceding cycle
Subsequent cycles (28-day regimen)	First tablet is taken 1 day after last (placebo) tablet was taken in preceding cycle
Missed tablets	If one or two tablets are missed, they should be taken as soon as they are remembered, and an additional form of contraception should be used for 1 wk. If three tablets are missed, the tablet cycle should be discontinued; start the next tablet cycle 8 days after the last tablet was taken (Lo/Ovral) or on the first Sunday after the last tablet was taken (Lo/Ovral-28), and instruct patient to use another form of contraception for the days without tablets and until seven tablets are taken.
Postpartum administration	For nonnursing mothers, may be started either immediately or after first postpartum examination, regardless of whether spontaneous menstruation has occurred

WARNINGS/PRECAUTIONS

Cigarette smoking	Increases the risk of serious cardiovascular side effects, especially in women over 35 yr of age who smoke 15 or more cigarettes daily; patients who use oral contraceptives should be strongly urged not to smoke
Thromboembolic disease, thrombotic disorders, and other vascular problems	Risk is increased, becoming greater with age (after 30 yr of age) and with the amount of estrogen present in the formulation; after discontinuation of use, the risk of cerebrovascular disease and myocardial infarction may persist. Discontinue oral contraception immediately if early signs of thromboembolic disease or thrombotic disorders (eg, thrombophlebitis, pulmonary embolism, cerebrovascular insufficiency, coronary occlusion, or retinal or mesenteric thrombosis) develop or are suspected.
Postsurgical thromboembolic complications	Risk is increased 4–6 times; if feasible, discontinue oral contraception at least 4 wk before elective surgery associated with an increased risk of thromboembolism or prolonged immobilization
Ocular lesions, including optic neuritis and retinal thrombosis	May occur; discontinue oral contraception in the presence of unexplained gradual or sudden, partial or complete loss of vision; proptosis or diplopia; papilledema; or retinal vascular lesions
Carcinoma	Closely monitor patients with a strong family history of breast cancer or with breast nodules, fibrocystic disease, or abnormal mammograms; investigate all cases of undiagnosed persistent or recurrent abnormal vaginal bleeding for malignancy (see CONTRAINDICATIONS)
Hepatic tumors, including benign adenomas	May occur and possibly rupture, resulting in intraabdominal hemorrhage and death; investigate all cases of abdominal pain and tenderness, abdominal mass, or shock for hepatic adenoma. The risk reportedly increases among users of formulations with high hormonal potency, and with use of oral contraception for more than 4 yr.
Gallbladder disease	Risk increases with duration of oral contraception
Hepatic impairment	Use with caution due to poor steroid hormone metabolism
Jaundice	May recur in patients with a history of jaundice; discontinue oral contraception while cause is investigated
Glucose tolerance	May become impaired; closely monitor patients with latent or active diabetes

LO/OVRAL

Hypertension	May be precipitated or may worsen with oral contraception, particularly with prolonged use in older patients, and in patients with a history of hypertension during pregnancy
Migraine headache	May develop or worsen; discontinue oral contraception and investigate cause of recurrent, persistent, or severe headaches
Mental depression	Risk is increased; discontinue oral contraception if serious depression develops or recurs in patients with a history of depression
Fluid retention	May occur; use with caution in patients with convulsive disorders, migraine, asthma, or cardiac, hepatic, or renal dysfunction
Vitamin deficiencies	May occur, particularly of pyridoxine and folic acid
Spotting, breakthrough bleeding	Spotting or breakthrough bleeding may occur when tablets are missed or at other times during therapy; instruct the patient to continue the regimen, but bear in mind the possibility of organic disorder. If abnormal vaginal bleeding persists or recurs, adequate diagnostic measures are indicated to rule out pregnancy or malignancy. Assuming these are excluded, the problem may be corrected by the passage of time or use of another formulation. Preparations with a higher estrogen content should be used only if necessary because of the increased risk of thromboembolic disease.
Failure of withdrawal bleeding	If patient has missed two consecutive periods, pregnancy should be ruled out before contraceptive regimen is continued; if patient has not adhered to prescribed regimen, pregnancy should be considered after the first missed period and oral contraception withheld until pregnancy has been excluded. Amenorrhea may occur during therapy and necessitate discontinuation of use.
Postpill amenorrhea and anovulation	May occur, particularly in patients with a history of oligomenorrhea or secondary amenorrhea or in young women who have not established regular menstrual cycles; such patients should be encouraged to use alternative methods of contraception

ADVERSE REACTIONS

Frequent reactions (incidence $\geq$ 1%) are printed in *italics*

Genitourinary	*Breakthrough bleeding, spotting, menstrual irregularities, vaginal candidiasis,* postpill amenorrhea and infertility, dysmenorrhea, altered cervical erosion and secretion, enlargement of uterine leiomyomata, premenstrual-like syndrome, altered libido, cystitis-like syndrome, vaginitis
Cardiovascular	Thrombophlebitis, pulmonary embolism, coronary thrombosis, cerebral thrombosis, cerebral hemorrhage, hypertension, mesenteric thrombosis, edema
Gastrointestinal	*Nausea, vomiting,* gallbladder disease, abdominal cramps, bloating, change in appetite
Hepatic	Benign hepatomas, cholestatic jaundice
Metabolic and endocrinological	*Breast enlargement, tenderness, and/or secretion;* carbohydrate intolerance; increase or decrease in weight; hyperlipidemia
Central nervous system and neuromuscular	Migraine, depression, headache, nervousness, dizziness, chorea
Ophthalmic	Optic neuritis, retinal thrombosis, intolerance to contact lenses, altered corneal curvature, cataracts
Allergic and dermatological	Rash, melasma or chloasma, erythema multiforme, erythema nodosum, hirsutism, hair loss, hemorrhagic eruption, porphyria
Other	Congenital anomalies, hemolytic uremic syndrome

OVERDOSAGE

Signs and symptoms	Nausea, withdrawal bleeding; acute ingestion of large doses by young children has not been associated with serious ill effects
Treatment	Treat symptomatically

DRUG INTERACTIONS

Ampicillin, analgesics, antianxiety agents, antimigraine preparations, barbiturates, chloramphenicol, isoniazid, neomycin, nitrofurantoin, penicillin V, phenylbutazone, phenytoin, primidone, rifampin, sulfonamides, tetracycline	▽ Contraceptive effect △ Breakthrough bleeding
Antihypertensive agents (eg, guanethidine)	▽ Antihypertensive effect
Oral anticoagulants	▽ Anticoagulant effect
Anticonvulsants	△ Seizure activity
Hypoglycemic agents	▽ Glucose tolerance
Corticosteroids	△ Corticosteroid effects

LO/OVRAL ■ MODICON

Tricyclic antidepressants	⇧ Antidepressant side effects

ALTERED LABORATORY VALUES

Blood/serum values	⇧ Alkaline phosphatase ⇧ Bilirubin ⇧ Sulfobromophthalein retention ⇧ Prothrombin ⇧ Clotting factors VII, VIII, IX, and X ⇩ Antithrombin III ⇧ PBI ⇧ Thyroxine (T$_4$) ⇩ Triiodothyronine (T$_3$) uptake ⇧ Glucose ⇧ Cortisol ⇧ Transcortin ⇧ Ceruloplasmin ⇧ Triglycerides ⇧ Phospholipids ⇩ Folic acid ⇩ Pyridoxine
Urinary values	⇩ Pregnanediol

USE IN CHILDREN
Not indicated before puberty

USE IN PREGNANT AND NURSING WOMEN
Pregnancy Category X: contraindicated if pregnancy is known or suspected, as serious fetal damage may occur during early pregnancy. Patient should discontinue oral contraception 3 mo before attempting to conceive. Postpartum use may interfere with lactation, causing a decrease in the quantity and quality of breast milk. Patient should use alternative form of contraception until infant is weaned.

CONTRACEPTIVES

MODICON 21 (norethindrone and ethinyl estradiol) Ortho   Rx
Tablets: 0.5 mg norethindrone and 35 µg ethinyl estradiol *21-day regimen*

MODICON 28 (norethindrone and ethinyl estradiol) Ortho   Rx
Tablets: 0.5 mg norethindrone and 35 µg ethinyl estradiol *28-day regimen*

INDICATIONS	ORAL DOSAGE
Contraception	**Adult:** 1 tab q24h for 21 or 28 consecutive days of the menstrual cycle

CONTRAINDICATIONS

Thrombophlebitis or thromboembolic disorders	Known or suspected breast cancer	Pregnancy
Past history of deep-vein thrombophlebitis or thromboembolic disorders	Known or suspected estrogen-dependent neoplasia	Benign or malignant liver tumor that developed during the use of oral contraceptives or other estrogen-containing products
Coronary artery disease	Undiagnosed abnormal genital bleeding	
Cerebrovascular disease		

ADMINISTRATION/DOSAGE ADJUSTMENTS

Initiating therapy	First tablet should be taken on the 5th day (Modicon 21) or 1st Sunday (Modicon 28) after the onset of menses; if menses begins on a Sunday, regimen is started the very same day. Regimen may be started postpartum, bearing in mind the increased risk of thromboembolic disease associated with the postpartum period.
Subsequent cycles (21-day regimen)	First tablet is taken 8 days after last tablet was taken in preceding cycle
Subsequent cycles (28-day regimen)	First tablet is taken 1 day after last (placebo) tablet was taken in preceding cycle
Missed tablets	If more than one tablet is missed, instruct patient to resume taking tablets as soon as remembered, but to use an additional form of contraception for the remainder of the cycle

WARNINGS/PRECAUTIONS

Cigarette smoking	Increases the risk of serious cardiovascular side effects, especially in women over 35 yr of age who smoke 15 or more cigarettes daily; patients who use oral contraceptives should be strongly urged not to smoke
Thromboembolic disease, thrombotic disorders, and other vascular problems	Risk is increased, becoming greater with age and the amount of estrogen present in the formulation, and may persist after discontinuation of use (the degree of residual risk may be related to the duration of use). Discontinue oral contraception immediately if early signs of thromboembolic disease or thrombotic disorders (eg, thrombophlebitis, pulmonary embolism, cerebrovascular insufficiency, coronary occlusion, or retinal or mesenteric thrombosis) develop or are suspected.
Postsurgical thromboembolic complications	Risk is increased 4–6 times; if feasible, discontinue oral contraception at least 4 wk before elective surgery associated with an increased risk of thromboembolism or prolonged immobilization

MODICON

Ocular lesions, including optic neuritis and retinal thrombosis	May occur; discontinue oral contraception in the presence of unexplained gradual or sudden, partial or complete loss of vision; proptosis or diplopia; papilledema; or retinal vascular lesions
Carcinoma	Closely monitor patients with a strong family history of breast cancer or with breast nodules, fibrocystic disease, or abnormal mammograms; investigate all cases of undiagnosed persistent or recurrent abnormal vaginal bleeding for malignancy (see CONTRAINDICATIONS). Hepatocellular carcinoma has been reported rarely; the risk is thought to increase with the duration of oral contraceptive therapy.
Hepatic tumors, including benign adenomas	May occur and possibly rupture, resulting in intraabdominal hemorrhage and death; investigate all cases of abdominal pain and tenderness, abdominal mass, or shock for hepatic tumors. The risk of hepatocellular adenoma reportedly increases in women over 30, among users of formulations with high hormonal potency, and with use of oral contraception for more than 4 yr
Gallbladder disease	Risk increases with duration of oral contraception
Hepatic impairment	Use with caution due to poor steroid hormone metabolism
Jaundice	May recur in patients with a history of jaundice; discontinue oral contraception while cause is investigated
Glucose tolerance	May become impaired; closely monitor patients with latent or active diabetes
Hypertension	May be precipitated or may worsen with oral contraception, particularly with prolonged use, in older patients, and in patients with a history of hypertension during pregnancy
Migraine headache	May develop or worsen; discontinue oral contraception and investigate cause of recurrent, persistent, or severe headaches
Mental depression	Risk is increased; discontinue oral contraception if serious depression develops or recurs in patients with a history of depression
Fluid retention	May occur; use with caution in patients with convulsive disorders, migraine, asthma, or cardiac, hepatic, or renal dysfunction
Vitamin deficiencies	May occur, particularly of pyridoxine and folic acid
Spotting, breakthrough bleeding	If spotting or breakthrough bleeding occurs, the possibility of organic disorder should be borne in mind. If abnormal vaginal bleeding persists or recurs, adequate diagnostic measures are indicated to rule out pregnancy or malignancy. Assuming these are excluded, the problem may be corrected by the passage of time or use of another formulation. Preparations with a higher estrogen content should be used only if necessary because of the increased risk of thromboembolic disease.
Failure of withdrawal bleeding	If patient has not adhered to prescribed regimen, pregnancy should be considered after the first missed period and oral contraception withheld until pregnancy has been excluded; if patient has adhered to regimen and misses two consecutive periods, pregnancy should be ruled out before contraceptive regimen is continued. Amenorrhea may occur during therapy and necessitate discontinuation of use.
Postpill amenorrhea and anovulation	May occur, particularly in patients with a history of oligomenorrhea or secondary amenorrhea or in young women who have not established regular menstrual cycles; such patients should be encouraged to use alternative methods of contraception

ADVERSE REACTIONS

Frequent reactions (incidence $\geq$ 1%) are printed in *italics*

Genitourinary	*Breakthrough bleeding, spotting, menstrual irregularities, vaginal candidiasis,* postpill amenorrhea and infertility, dysmenorrhea, altered cervical erosion and secretion, enlargement of uterine leiomyomata, premenstrual-like syndrome, altered libido, cystitis-like syndrome, vaginitis
Cardiovascular	Thrombophlebitis, pulmonary embolism, coronary thrombosis, cerebral thrombosis, cerebral hemorrhage, hypertension, mesenteric thrombosis, edema
Gastrointestinal	*Nausea, vomiting,* gallbladder disease, abdominal cramps, bloating, change in appetite
Hepatic	Hepatic tumors, cholestatic jaundice
Renal	Impaired renal function, hemolytic uremic syndrome
Metabolic and endocrinological	*Breast enlargement, tenderness, and/or secretion;* carbohydrate intolerance; increase or decrease in weight; hyperlipidemia
Central nervous system and neuromuscular	Migraine, depression, headache, nervousness, dizziness, chorea
Ophthalmic	Optic neuritis, retinal thrombosis, intolerance to contact lenses, altered corneal curvature, cataracts
Allergic and dermatological	Rash, melasma or chloasma, erythema multiforme, erythema nodosum, hirsutism, hair loss, hemorrhagic eruption, porphyria
Other	Congenital anomalies

MODICON ■ NORDETTE

OVERDOSAGE

Signs and symptoms	Nausea, withdrawal bleeding; acute ingestion of large doses by young children has not been associated with serious ill effects
Treatment	Treat symptomatically

DRUG INTERACTIONS

Ampicillin, analgesics, antianxiety agents, antimigraine preparations, barbiturates, chloramphenicol, griseofulvin, isoniazid, neomycin, nitrofurantoin, penicillin V, phenylbutazone, phenytoin, primidone, rifampin, sulfonamides, tetracycline	▽ Contraceptive effect △ Breakthrough bleeding
Antihypertensive agents (eg, guanethidine)	▽ Antihypertensive effect
Oral anticoagulants	▽ Anticoagulant effect
Anticonvulsants	△ Seizure activity
Hypoglycemic agents	▽ Glucose tolerance
Corticosteroids	△ Corticosteroid effect
Tricyclic antidepressants	△ Antidepressant side effects

ALTERED LABORATORY VALUES

Blood/serum values	△ Alkaline phosphatase △ Bilirubin △ Sulfobromophthalein retention △ Prothrombin △ Clotting factors VII, VIII, IX, and X ▽ Antithrombin III △ PBI △ Thyroxine (T_4) ▽ Triiodothyronine (T_3) uptake △ Glucose △ Cortisol △ Transcortin △ Ceruloplasmin △ Triglycerides △ Phospholipids ▽ Folic acid ▽ Pyridoxine
Urinary values	▽ Pregnanediol

USE IN CHILDREN
Not indicated before puberty

USE IN PREGNANT AND NURSING WOMEN
Pregnancy Category X: contraindicated if pregnancy is known or suspected, as serious fetal damage may occur during early pregnancy. If she becomes pregnant while taking this product, she should be apprised of the potential hazard to the fetus. Patient should discontinue oral contraception 3 mo before attempting to conceive. Postpartum use may interfere with lactation, causing a decrease in the quantity and quality of breast milk. The hormonal agents in oral contraceptives are excreted in human milk; because of the potential for tumorigenicity, the patient should use an alternative form of contraception until infant is weaned.

CONTRACEPTIVES

NORDETTE-21 (levonorgestrel and ethinyl estradiol) Wyeth   Rx
Tablets: 0.15 mg levonorgestrel and 30 µg ethinyl estradiol *21-day regimen*

NORDETTE-28 (levonorgestrel and ethinyl estradiol) Wyeth   Rx
Tablets: 0.15 mg levonorgestrel and 30 µg ethinyl estradiol *28-day regimen*

INDICATIONS
Contraception

ORAL DOSAGE
Adult: 1 tab q24h for 21 or 28 consecutive days of the menstrual cycle

CONTRAINDICATIONS

Thrombophlebitis or thromboembolic disorders	Known or suspected breast cancer	Known or suspected pregnancy
Past history of deep-vein thrombophlebitis or thromboembolic disorders	Known or suspected estrogen-dependent neoplasia	Benign or malignant liver tumor that developed during the use of oral contraceptives or other estrogen-containing products
Coronary artery disease	Undiagnosed abnormal genital bleeding	
Cerebrovascular disease		

NORDETTE

ADMINISTRATION/DOSAGE ADJUSTMENTS

Initiating therapy	First tablet should be taken on the 5th day (Nordette-21) or 1st Sunday (Nordette-28) after the onset of menses; if menses begins on a Sunday, regimen is started the very same day
Subsequent cycles (21-day regimen)	First tablet is taken 8 days after last tablet was taken in preceding cycle
Subsequent cycles (28-day regimen)	First tablet is taken 1 day after last (placebo) tablet was taken in preceding cycle
Missed tablets	If one or two tablets are missed, they should be taken as soon as they are remembered, and an additional form of contraception should be used for 1 wk. If three tablets are missed, the tablet cycle should be discontinued; start the next tablet cycle 8 days after the last tablet was taken (Nordette-21) or on the first Sunday after the last tablet was taken (Nordette-28), and instruct patient to use another form of contraception for the days without tablets and until seven tablets are taken.
Postpartum administration	For nonnursing mothers, may be started either immediately or after first postpartum examination, regardless of whether spontaneous menstruation has occurred. An additional form of contraception should be used during the first week of the initial cycle.
Monitoring of therapy	A Papanicolaou smear, other appropriate laboratory tests, and a physical examination (with special attention to breasts, abdomen, pelvic organs, and blood pressure) should be done before therapy and then repeated at least annually

WARNINGS/PRECAUTIONS

Cigarette smoking	Increases the risk of serious cardiovascular side effects, especially in women over 35 yr of age who smoke 15 or more cigarettes daily; patients who use oral contraceptives should be strongly urged not to smoke
Thromboembolic disease, thrombotic disorders, and other vascular problems	Risk is increased, becoming greater with age (after 30 yr of age) and with the amount of estrogen present in the formulation; after discontinuation of use, the risk of cerebrovascular disease and myocardial infarction may persist. Discontinue oral contraception immediately if early signs of thromboembolic disease or thrombotic disorders (eg, thrombophlebitis, pulmonary embolism, cerebrovascular insufficiency, coronary occlusion, or retinal or mesenteric thrombosis) develop or are suspected.
Postsurgical thromboembolic complications	Risk is increased 4–6 times; if feasible, discontinue oral contraception at least 4 wk before elective surgery associated with an increased risk of thromboembolism or prolonged immobilization
Ocular lesions, including optic neuritis and retinal thrombosis	May occur; discontinue oral contraception in the presence of unexplained gradual or sudden, partial or complete loss of vision; proptosis or diplopia; papilledema; or retinal vascular lesions
Carcinoma	Closely monitor patients with a strong family history of breast cancer or with breast nodules, fibrocystic disease, or abnormal mammograms; investigate all cases of undiagnosed persistent or recurrent abnormal vaginal bleeding for malignancy (see CONTRAINDICATIONS)
Hepatic tumors, including benign adenomas	May occur and possibly rupture, resulting in intraabdominal hemorrhage and death; investigate all cases of abdominal pain and tenderness, abdominal mass, or shock for hepatic adenoma. The risk reportedly increases among users of formulations with high hormonal potency, and with use of oral contraception for more than 4 yr.
Gallbladder disease	Risk increases with duration of oral contraception
Hepatic impairment	Use with caution due to poor steroid hormone metabolism
Jaundice	May recur in patients with a history of jaundice; discontinue oral contraception while cause is investigated
Glucose tolerance	May become impaired; closely monitor patients with latent or active diabetes
Hypertension	May be precipitated or may worsen with oral contraception, particularly with prolonged use, in older patients, and in patients with a history of hypertension during pregnancy
Migraine headache	May develop or worsen; discontinue oral contraception and investigate cause of recurrent, persistent, or severe headaches
Mental depression	Risk is increased; discontinue oral contraception if serious depression develops or recurs in patients with a history of depression
Fluid retention	May occur; use with caution in patients with convulsive disorders, migraine, asthma, or cardiac, hepatic, or renal dysfunction
Vitamin deficiencies	May occur, particularly of pyridoxine and folic acid
Spotting, breakthrough bleeding	Spotting or breakthrough bleeding may occur when tablets are missed or at other times during therapy; instruct the patient to continue the regimen, but bear in mind the possibility of organic disorder. If abnormal vaginal bleeding persists or recurs, adequate diagnostic measures are indicated to rule out pregnancy or malignancy. Assuming these are excluded, the problem may be corrected by the passage of time or use of another formulation. Preparations with a higher estrogen content should be used only if necessary because of the increased risk of thromboembolic disease.

NORDETTE

Failure of withdrawal bleeding	If patient has missed two consecutive periods, pregnancy should be ruled out before contraceptive regimen is continued; if patient has not adhered to prescribed regimen, pregnancy should be considered after the first missed period and oral contraception withheld until pregnancy has been excluded. Amenorrhea may occur during therapy and necessitate discontinuation of use.
Postpill amenorrhea and anovulation	May occur, particularly in patients with a history of oligomenorrhea or secondary amenorrhea or in young women who have not established regular menstrual cycles; such patients should be encouraged to use alternative methods of contraception

ADVERSE REACTIONS

Frequent reactions (incidence ≥ 1%) are printed in *italics*

Genitourinary	*Breakthrough bleeding, spotting, menstrual irregularities, vaginal candidiasis,* postpill amenorrhea and infertility, dysmenorrhea; altered cervical erosion and secretion, enlargement of uterine leiomyomata, premenstrual-like syndrome, altered libido, cystitis-like syndrome, vaginitis
Cardiovascular	Thrombophlebitis, pulmonary embolism, coronary thrombosis, cerebral thrombosis, cerebral hemorrhage, hypertension, mesenteric thrombosis, edema
Gastrointestinal	*Nausea, vomiting,* gallbladder disease, abdominal cramps, bloating, change in appetite
Hepatic	Benign hepatomas, cholestatic jaundice
Metabolic and endocrinological	*Breast enlargement, tenderness, and/or secretion;* carbohydrate intolerance; increase or decrease in weight; hyperlipidemia
Central nervous system and neuromuscular	Migraine, depression, headache, nervousness, dizziness, chorea
Ophthalmic	Optic neuritis, retinal thrombosis, intolerance to contact lenses, altered corneal curvature, cataracts
Allergic and dermatological	Rash, melasma or chloasma, erythema multiforme, erythema nodosum, hirsutism, hair loss, hemorrhagic eruption, porphyria
Other	Congenital anomalies, hemolytic uremic syndrome

OVERDOSAGE

Signs and symptoms	Nausea, withdrawal bleeding; acute ingestion of large doses by young children has not been associated with serious ill effects
Treatment	Treat symptomatically

DRUG INTERACTIONS

Ampicillin, analgesics, antianxiety agents, antimigraine agents, barbiturates, chloramphenicol, isoniazid, neomycin, nitrofurantoin, penicillin V, phenylbutazone, phenytoin, primidone, rifampin, sulfonamides, tetracycline	▽ Contraceptive effect △ Breakthrough bleeding
Antihypertensive agents (eg, guanethidine)	▽ Antihypertensive effect
Oral anticoagulants	▽ Anticoagulant effect
Anticonvulsants	△ Seizure activity
Hypoglycemic agents	▽ Glucose tolerance
Corticosteroids	△ Corticosteroid effects
Tricyclic antidepressants	△ Antidepressant side effects

ALTERED LABORATORY VALUES

Blood/serum values	△ Alkaline phosphatase △ Bilirubin △ Sulfobromophthalein retention △ Prothrombin △ Clotting factors VII, VIII, IX, and X ▽ Antithrombin III △ PBI △ Thyroxine (T_4) ▽ Triiodothyronine (T_3) uptake △ Glucose △ Cortisol △ Transcortin △ Ceruloplasmin △ Triglycerides △ Phospholipids ▽ Folic acid ▽ Pyridoxine
Urinary values	▽ Pregnanediol

USE IN CHILDREN

Not indicated before puberty

USE IN PREGNANT AND NURSING WOMEN

Pregnancy Category X: contraindicated if pregnancy is known or suspected, as serious fetal damage may occur during early pregnancy. Patient should discontinue oral contraception 3 mo before attempting to conceive. Postpartum use may interfere with lactation, causing a decrease in the quantity and quality of breast milk. Because of the potential for adverse reactions in nursing infants from oral contraceptive tablets, patient should either stop nursing or stop use of the drug.

CONTRACEPTIVES

NORINYL 1 + 35 21-DAY (norethindrone and ethinyl estradiol) Syntex   Rx
Tablets: 1 mg norethindrone and 35 µg ethinyl estradiol *21-day regimen*

NORINYL 1 + 35 28-DAY (norethindrone and ethinyl estradiol) Syntex   Rx
Tablets: 1 mg norethindrone and 35 µg ethinyl estradiol *28-day regimen*

INDICATIONS	ORAL DOSAGE
Contraception	Adult: 1 tab q24h at bedtime for 21 or 28 consecutive days of the menstrual cycle

CONTRAINDICATIONS

Thrombophlebitis or thromboembolic disorders	Past or present coronary artery disease, including myocardial infarction	Undiagnosed abnormal genital bleeding
Past history of deep-vein thrombophlebitis or thromboembolic disorders	Past or present known or suspected breast cancer	Past or present benign or malignant hepatic tumor that developed during the use of oral contraceptives or other estrogen-containing products
Past or present cerebrovascular disease	Past or present known or suspected estrogen-dependent neoplasia	Known or suspected pregnancy

ADMINISTRATION/DOSAGE ADJUSTMENTS

Initiating therapy	First tablet should be taken on the fifth day or first Sunday after the onset of menses or, if menses begins on a Sunday, on that very day. An additional form of contraception should be used during the first week of the initial cycle. Instruct postpartum patients not to initiate oral contraceptive therapy earlier than 2 wk after delivery; patients may start oral contraception immediately after an aborted pregnancy of less than 12 wk gestation, but should not start until 2 wk after an aborted pregnancy of 12 wk gestation or longer.
Subsequent cycles (21-day regimen)	First tablet is taken 8 days after last tablet was taken in preceding cycle
Subsequent cycles (28-day regimen)	First tablet is taken 1 day after last (placebo) tablet was taken in preceding cycle
Missed tablets	If one tablet is missed, it should be taken as soon as it is remembered, with the next tablet taken at the usual time. If two tablets are missed, one of them should be taken as soon as remembered and the other discarded. The remaining tablets should be taken as usual, but an additional form of contraception should be used for the remainder of the cycle. If three or more tablets in a row are missed, the tablet cycle should be discontinued immediately and another form of contraception used until menses has appeared or pregnancy has been excluded.
Monitoring of therapy	A Papanicolaou smear, other appropriate laboratory tests, and a physical examination (with special attention to breasts, abdomen, pelvic organs, and blood pressure) should be done before therapy and then repeated at least annually

WARNINGS/PRECAUTIONS

Cigarette smoking	Increases the risk of serious cardiovascular side effects, especially in women over 35 yr of age who smoke 15 or more cigarettes daily; patients who use oral contraceptives should be strongly urged not to smoke
Thromboembolic disease, thrombotic disorders, and other vascular problems	Risk is increased, becoming greater with age (after 30 yr of age) and with the amount of estrogen in the formulation; after use of oral contraceptives is discontinued, the risk of cerebrovascular disease, myocardial infarction, and subarachnoid hemorrhage may persist. Discontinue oral contraception immediately if early signs of thromboembolic disease or thrombotic disorders (eg, thrombophlebitis, pulmonary embolism, cerebrovascular insufficiency, coronary occlusion, or retinal or mesenteric thrombosis) develop or are suspected. The presence of varicose veins may substantially increase the risk of superficial venous thrombosis of the leg.
Postsurgical thromboembolic complications	Risk is increased 4–6 times; if feasible, discontinue oral contraception at least 4 wk before elective surgery associated with an increased risk of thromboembolism or prolonged immobilization
Ocular lesions, including optic neuritis and retinal thrombosis	May occur; discontinue oral contraception in the presence of unexplained gradual or sudden, partial or complete loss of vision; proptosis or diplopia; papilledema; or retinal vascular lesions
Carcinoma	Although several studies have found no overall increase of breast cancer in women taking estrogens or oral contraceptives, the risk may be increased when such use is associated with other risk factors, including benign breast disease (eg, cysts); long-term administration (2–4 yr), particularly in patients under 25 yr of age; prior breast biopsy, or a family history of breast cancer. Closely monitor patients with a strong family history of breast cancer or with breast nodules, fibrocystic disease, or abnormal mammograms. Studies suggest that there is an increased risk of cervical neoplasms associated with longer duration of oral contraceptive use. Investigate all cases of undiagnosed persistent or recurrent abnormal vaginal bleeding for malignancy (see CONTRAINDICATIONS).
Hepatic tumors	May occur and possibly rupture, resulting in intraabdominal hemorrhage and death; investigate all cases of abdominal pain and tenderness, right upper quadrant mass, or shock for liver tumors. The risk of hepatocellular adenoma reportedly increases in women over 30, among users of formulations with high hormonal potency, and with use of oral contraception for more than 4 yr (estimated annual incidence, 3–4/100,000).

NORINYL 1 + 35

Gallbladder disease	Risk increases with duration of oral contraception
Hepatic impairment	Use with caution due to poor steroid hormone metabolism (see CONTRAINDICATIONS)
Jaundice	May recur in patients with a history of jaundice; discontinue oral contraception while cause is investigated
Glucose tolerance	May become impaired; closely monitor patients with latent or active diabetes
Hypertension	May be precipitated or may worsen with oral contraception, particularly with prolonged use and in older patients. Closely monitor patients with a history of hypertension, toxemia, hypertension during pregnancy, or excessive weight gain or fluid retention during the menstrual cycle; preexisting renal disease; or a family history of hypertension or hypertensive complications.
Migraine headache	May develop or worsen; discontinue oral contraception and investigate cause of recurrent, persistent, or severe headaches
Bleeding irregularities, including breakthrough bleeding, spotting, and amenorrhea	May occur, necessitating either a change to a formulation with a higher estrogen content or discontinuation of therapy; higher amounts of estrogen, while potentially useful for minimizing menstrual irregularities, may increase the risk of thromboembolic disease
Mental depression	Risk is increased; discontinue oral contraception if serious depression develops or recurs in patients with a history of depression
Fluid retention	May occur; use with caution in patients with convulsive disorders, migraine, asthma, or cardiac, hepatic, or renal dysfunction
Vitamin deficiencies	May occur, particularly of pyridoxine and folic acid
Intolerance to contact lenses	Patients who wear contact lenses may experience changes in vision or lens tolerance; such changes should be evaluated by an ophthalmologist. It may be necessary to suspend contact lens wear temporarily or permanently.
Chlamydial infections	Infection with *Chlamydia trachomatis* is enhanced by oral contraceptive use
Spotting, breakthrough bleeding	If spotting or breakthrough bleeding occurs, instruct the patient to continue the regimen, but bear in mind the possibility of organic disorder. If abnormal vaginal bleeding persists or recurs, adequate diagnostic measures are indicated to rule out pregnancy or malignancy. Assuming these are excluded, the problem may be corrected by the passage of time or use of another formulation. Preparations with a higher estrogen content should be used only if necessary because of the increased risk of thromboembolic disease.
Failure of withdrawal bleeding	If patient has not adhered to prescribed regimen, pregnancy should be considered after the first missed period and oral contraception withheld until pregnancy has been excluded; if patient has adhered to regimen and misses two consecutive periods, pregnancy should be ruled out before contraceptive regimen is continued. Amenorrhea may occur during therapy and necessitate discontinuation of use.
Postpill amenorrhea and anovulation	May occur, particularly in patients with a history of oligomenorrhea or secondary amenorrhea or in young women who have not established regular menstrual cycles; such patients should be encouraged to use alternative methods of contraception
Infertility	May occur following discontinuation of oral contraception, independent of its duration; diminishes with time but may still be apparent up to 30 mo in parous women and up to 42 mo in nulliparous women

ADVERSE REACTIONS	Frequent reactions (incidence $\geq$ 1%) are printed in *italics*
Genitourinary	*Breakthrough bleeding, spotting, menstrual irregularities, vaginal candidiasis,* postpill amenorrhea and infertility, dysmenorrhea, altered cervical erosion and secretion, enlargement of uterine leiomyomata, premenstrual-like syndrome, altered libido, cystitis-like syndrome, vaginitis
Cardiovascular	Thrombophlebitis, thrombosis, pulmonary embolism, coronary thrombosis, cerebral thrombosis, cerebral hemorrhage, arterial thromboembolism, Raynaud's disease, hypertension, malignant hypertension, mesenteric thrombosis, edema
Gastrointestinal	*Nausea, vomiting,* gallbladder disease, abdominal cramps, colitis, bloating, change in appetite
Hepatic	Liver tumors, cholestatic jaundice
Renal	Impaired renal function, acute renal failure
Metabolic and endocrinological	*Breast enlargement, tenderness, and/or secretion;* carbohydrate intolerance; increase or decrease in weight; hyperlipidemia
Central nervous system and neuromuscular	Migraine, depression, headache, nervousness, dizziness, chorea
Ophthalmic	Optic neuritis, retinal thrombosis, intolerance to contact lenses, altered corneal curvature, cataracts
Allergic and dermatological	Rash, melasma or chloasma, erythema multiforme, erythema nodosum, hirsutism, hair loss, hemorrhagic eruption, porphyria, chilblains

NORINYL 1 + 35 ■ NORINYL 1 + 50/NORINYL 1 + 80

Other	Congenital anomalies, prolactin-secreting pituitary tumors, malignant nephrosclerosis (hemolytic uremic syndrome)

OVERDOSAGE

Signs and symptoms	Nausea, withdrawal bleeding; acute ingestion of large doses by young children has not been associated with serious ill effects
Treatment	Treat symptomatically

DRUG INTERACTIONS

Ampicillin, analgesics, antihistamines, antimigraine preparations, barbiturates, chloramphenicol, griseofulvin, isoniazid, neomycin, nitrofurantoin, penicillin V, phenylbutazone, phenytoin, primidone, rifampin, sulfonamides, tetracycline, tranquilizers	▽ Contraceptive effect △ Breakthrough bleeding
Beta blockers	△ Pharmacologic effect of beta blockers
Guanethidine	▽ Antihypertensive effect
Oral anticoagulants	▽ Anticoagulant effect
Anticonvulsants	△ Seizure activity
Hypoglycemic agents	▽ Glucose tolerance
Corticosteroids	△ Corticosteroid effects
Cyclosporine	Hepatotoxicity
Tricyclic antidepressants	△ Antidepressant side effects
Benzodiazepines (except lorazepam, oxazepam, and temazepam)	△ Serum benzodiazepine level
Theophylline	△ Serum theophylline level

ALTERED LABORATORY VALUES

Blood/serum values	△ Alkaline phosphatase △ Bilirubin △ Sulfobromophthalein retention △ Prothrombin △ Clotting factors VII, VIII, IX, and X ▽ Antithrombin III △ PBI △ Thyroxine (T_4) ▽ Triiodothyronine (T_3) uptake △ Glucose △ Cortisol △ Transcortin △ Ceruloplasmin △ Triglycerides △ Phospholipids ▽ Folic acid ▽ Pyridoxine
Urinary values	▽ Pregnanediol

USE IN CHILDREN

Not indicated before puberty

USE IN PREGNANT AND NURSING WOMEN

Pregnancy Category X: contraindicated if pregnancy is known or suspected, as serious fetal damage may occur during early pregnancy. Patient should discontinue oral contraception 3 mo before attempting to conceive. Postpartum use may interfere with lactation, causing a decrease in the quantity and quality of breast milk. Patient should use an alternative form of contraception until infant is weaned.

CONTRACEPTIVES

NORINYL 1 + 50 21-DAY (norethindrone and mestranol) Syntex   Rx

Tablets: 1 mg norethindrone and 50 μg mestranol *21-day regimen*

NORINYL 1 + 50 28-DAY (norethindrone and mestranol) Syntex   Rx

Tablets: 1 mg norethindrone and 50 μg mestranol *28-day regimen*

NORINYL 1 + 80 21-DAY (norethindrone and mestranol) Syntex   Rx

Tablets: 1 mg norethindrone and 80 μg mestranol *21-day regimen*

NORINYL 1 + 80 28-DAY (norethindrone and mestranol) Syntex   Rx

Tablets: 1 mg norethindrone and 80 μg mestranol *28-day regimen*

INDICATIONS	ORAL DOSAGE
Contraception	**Adult:** 1 tab q24h at bedtime for 21 or 28 consecutive days of the menstrual cycle

COMPENDIUM OF DRUG THERAPY

NORINYL 1 + 50/NORINYL 1 + 80

CONTRAINDICATIONS

Thrombophlebitis or thromboembolic disorders	Past or present coronary artery disease, including myocardial infarction	Undiagnosed abnormal genital bleeding
Past history of deep-vein thrombophlebitis or thromboembolic disorders	Past or present known or suspected breast cancer	Past or present benign or malignant hepatic tumor that developed during the use of oral contraceptives or other estrogen-containing products
Past or present cerebrovascular disease	Past or present known or suspected estrogen-dependent neoplasia	Known or suspected pregnancy

ADMINISTRATION/DOSAGE ADJUSTMENTS

Initiating therapy — First tablet should be taken on the fifth day or first Sunday after the onset of menses or, if menses begins on a Sunday, on that very day. An additional form of contraception should be used during the first week of the initial cycle. Instruct postpartum patients not to initiate oral contraceptive therapy earlier than 2 wk after delivery; patients may start oral contraception immediately after an aborted pregnancy of less than 12 wk gestation, but should not start until 2 wk after an aborted pregnancy of 12 wk gestation or longer.

Subsequent cycles (21-day regimen) — First tablet is taken 8 days after last tablet was taken in preceding cycle

Subsequent cycles (28-day regimen) — First tablet is taken 1 day after last (placebo) tablet was taken in preceding cycle

Missed tablets — If one tablet is missed, it should be taken as soon as it is remembered, with the next tablet taken at the usual time. If two tablets are missed, one of them should be taken as soon as remembered and the other discarded. The remaining tablets should be taken as usual, but an additional form of contraception should be used for the remainder of the cycle. If three or more tablets in a row are missed, the tablet cycle should be discontinued immediately and another form of contraception used until menses has appeared or pregnancy has been excluded.

Monitoring of therapy — A Papanicolaou smear, other appropriate laboratory tests, and a physical examination (with special attention to breasts, abdomen, pelvic organs, and blood pressure) should be done before therapy and then repeated at least annually

WARNINGS/PRECAUTIONS

Cigarette smoking — Increases the risk of serious cardiovascular side effects, especially in women over 35 yr of age who smoke 15 or more cigarettes daily; patients who use oral contraceptives should be strongly urged not to smoke

Thromboembolic disease, thrombotic disorders, and other vascular problems — Risk is increased, becoming greater with age (after 30 yr of age) and with the amount of estrogen in the formulation; after use of oral contraceptives is discontinued, the risk of cerebrovascular disease, myocardial infarction, and subarachnoid hemorrhage may persist. Discontinue oral contraception immediately if early signs of thromboembolic disease or thrombotic disorders (eg, thrombophlebitis, pulmonary embolism, cerebrovascular insufficiency, coronary occlusion, or retinal or mesenteric thrombosis) develop or are suspected. The presence of varicose veins may substantially increase the risk of superficial venous thrombosis of the leg.

Postsurgical thromboembolic complications — Risk is increased 4–6 times; if feasible, discontinue oral contraception at least 4 wk before elective surgery associated with an increased risk of thromboembolism or prolonged immobilization

Ocular lesions, including optic neuritis and retinal thrombosis — May occur; discontinue oral contraception in the presence of unexplained gradual or sudden, partial or complete loss of vision; proptosis or diplopia; papilledema; or retinal vascular lesions

Carcinoma — Although several studies have found no overall increase of breast cancer in women taking estrogens or oral contraceptives, the risk may be increased when such use is associated with other risk factors, including benign breast disease (eg, cysts); long-term administration (2–4 yr), particularly in patients under 25 yr of age; prior breast biopsy, or a family history of breast cancer. Closely monitor patients with a strong family history of breast cancer or with breast nodules, fibrocystic disease, or abnormal mammograms. Studies suggest that there is an increased risk of cervical neoplasms associated with longer duration of oral contraceptive use. Investigate all cases of undiagnosed persistent or recurrent abnormal vaginal bleeding for malignancy (see CONTRAINDICATIONS).

Hepatic tumors — May occur and possibly rupture, resulting in intraabdominal hemorrhage and death; investigate all cases of abdominal pain and tenderness, right upper quadrant mass, or shock for liver tumors. The risk of hepatocellular adenoma reportedly increases in women over 30, among users of formulations with high hormonal potency, and with use of oral contraception for more than 4 yr (estimated annual incidence, 3–4/100,000).

Gallbladder disease — Risk increases with duration of oral contraception

Hepatic impairment — Use with caution due to poor steroid hormone metabolism (see CONTRAINDICATIONS)

Jaundice — May recur in patients with a history of jaundice; discontinue oral contraception while cause is investigated

NORINYL 1 + 50/NORINYL 1 + 80

Glucose tolerance	May become impaired; closely monitor patients with latent or active diabetes
Hypertension	May be precipitated or may worsen with oral contraception, particularly with prolonged use and in older patients. Closely monitor patients with a history of hypertension, toxemia, hypertension during pregnancy, or excessive weight gain or fluid retention during the menstrual cycle; preexisting renal disease; or a family history of hypertension or hypertensive complications.
Migraine headache	May develop or worsen; discontinue oral contraception and investigate cause of recurrent, persistent, or severe headaches
Bleeding irregularities, including breakthrough bleeding, spotting, and amenorrhea	May occur, necessitating either a change to a formulation with a higher estrogen content or discontinuation of therapy; higher amounts of estrogen, while potentially useful for minimizing menstrual irregularities, may increase the risk of thromboembolic disease
Mental depression	Risk is increased; discontinue oral contraception if serious depression develops or recurs in patients with a history of depression
Fluid retention	May occur; use with caution in patients with convulsive disorders, migraine, asthma, or cardiac, hepatic, or renal dysfunction
Vitamin deficiencies	May occur, particularly of pyridoxine and folic acid
Intolerance to contact lenses	Patients who wear contact lenses may experience changes in vision or lens tolerance; such changes should be evaluated by an ophthalmologist. It may be necessary to suspend contact lens wear temporarily or permanently.
Chlamydial infections	Infection with *Chlamydia trachomatis* is enhanced by oral contraceptive use
Spotting, breakthrough bleeding	If spotting or breakthrough bleeding occurs, instruct the patient to continue the regimen, but bear in mind the possibility of organic disorder. If abnormal vaginal bleeding persists or recurs, adequate diagnostic measures are indicated to rule out pregnancy or malignancy. Assuming these are excluded, the problem may be corrected by the passage of time or use of another formulation. Preparations with a higher estrogen content should be used only if necessary because of the increased risk of thromboembolic disease.
Failure of withdrawal bleeding	If patient has not adhered to prescribed regimen, pregnancy should be considered after the first missed period and oral contraception withheld until pregnancy has been excluded; if patient has adhered to regimen and misses two consecutive periods, pregnancy should be ruled out before contraceptive regimen is continued. Amenorrhea may occur during therapy and necessitate discontinuation of use.
Postpill amenorrhea and anovulation	May occur, particularly in patients with a history of oligomenorrhea or secondary amenorrhea or in young women who have not established regular menstrual cycles; such patients should be encouraged to use alternative methods of contraception
Infertility	May occur following discontinuation of oral contraception, independent of its duration; diminishes with time but may still be apparent up to 30 mo in parous women and up to 42 mo in nulliparous women

ADVERSE REACTIONS

Frequent reactions (incidence $\geq$ 1%) are printed in *italics*

Genitourinary	*Breakthrough bleeding, spotting, menstrual irregularities, vaginal candidiasis,* postpill amenorrhea and infertility, dysmenorrhea, altered cervical erosion and secretion, enlargement of uterine leiomyomata, premenstrual-like syndrome, altered libido, cystitis-like syndrome, vaginitis
Cardiovascular	Thrombophlebitis, thrombosis, pulmonary embolism, coronary thrombosis, cerebral thrombosis, cerebral hemorrhage, arterial thromboembolism, Raynaud's disease, hypertension, malignant hypertension, mesenteric thrombosis, edema
Gastrointestinal	*Nausea, vomiting,* gallbladder disease, abdominal cramps, colitis, bloating, change in appetite
Hepatic	Liver tumors, cholestatic jaundice
Renal	Impaired renal function, acute renal failure
Metabolic and endocrinological	*Breast enlargement, tenderness, and/or secretion;* carbohydrate intolerance; increase or decrease in weight; hyperlipidemia
Central nervous system and neuromuscular	Migraine, depression, headache, nervousness, dizziness, chorea
Ophthalmic	Optic neuritis, retinal thrombosis, intolerance to contact lenses, altered corneal curvature, cataracts
Allergic and dermatological	Rash, melasma or chloasma, erythema multiforme, erythema nodosum, hirsutism, hair loss, hemorrhagic eruption, porphyria, chilblains
Other	Congenital anomalies, prolactin-secreting pituitary tumors, impaired renal function, malignant nephrosclerosis (hemolytic uremic syndrome)

OVERDOSAGE

Signs and symptoms	Nausea, withdrawal bleeding; acute ingestion of large doses by young children has not been associated with serious ill effects

NORINYL 1 + 50/NORINYL 1 + 80 ■ NORLESTRIN 1/50/NORLESTRIN 2.5/50

Treatment ———————————— Treat symptomatically

DRUG INTERACTIONS

Ampicillin, analgesics, antihistamines, ———— ▽ Contraceptive effect △ Breakthrough bleeding
antimigraine preparations, barbiturates,
chloramphenicol, griseofulvin, isoniazid,
neomycin, nitrofurantoin, penicillin V,
phenylbutazone, phenytoin,
primidone, rifampin, sulfonamides,
tetracycline, tranquilizers

Guanethidine ———————————— ▽ Antihypertensive effect

Beta blockers ———————————— △ Pharmacologic effects of beta blockers

Oral anticoagulants ———————— ▽ Anticoagulant effect

Anticonvulsants —————————— △ Seizure activity

Hypoglycemic agents ———————— ▽ Glucose tolerance

Corticosteroids ——————————— △ Corticosteroid effects

Cyclosporine ———————————— Hepatotoxicity

Tricyclic antidepressants ——————— △ Antidepressant side effects

Benzodiazepines (except lorazepam, ——— △ Serum benzodiazepine level
oxazepam, and temazepam)

Theophylline ———————————— △ Serum theophylline level

ALTERED LABORATORY VALUES

Blood/serum values ————————— △ Alkaline phosphatase △ Bilirubin △ Sulfobromophthalein retention
△ Prothrombin △ Clotting factors VII, VIII, IX, and X ▽ Antithrombin III △ PBI
△ Thyroxine (T_4) ▽ Triiodothyronine (T_3) uptake △ Glucose △ Cortisol
△ Transcortin △ Ceruloplasmin △ Triglycerides △ Phospholipids ▽ Folic
acid ▽ Pyridoxine

Urinary values ———————————— ▽ Pregnanediol

USE IN CHILDREN	USE IN PREGNANT AND NURSING WOMEN
Not indicated before puberty	Pregnancy Category X: contraindicated if pregnancy is known or suspected, as serious fetal damage may occur during early pregnancy. Patient should discontinue oral contraception 3 mo before attempting to conceive. Postpartum use may interfere with lactation, causing a decrease in quantity and quality of breast milk. Patient should use an alternative form of contraception until infant is weaned.

CONTRACEPTIVES

NORLESTRIN 21 **1/50** (norethindrone acetate and ethinyl estradiol) **Parke-Davis** Rx

Tablets: 1 mg norethindrone acetate and 50 μg ethinyl estradiol *21-day regimen*

NORLESTRIN 28 **1/50** (norethindrone acetate and ethinyl estradiol) **Parke-Davis** Rx

Tablets: 1 mg norethindrone acetate and 50 μg ethinyl estradiol *28-day regimen*

NORLESTRIN Fe **1/50** (norethindrone acetate and ethinyl estradiol; ferrous fumarate) Rx
Parke-Davis

Tablets: 1 mg norethindrone acetate and 50 μg ethinyl estradiol (yellow); 75 mg ferrous fumarate (brown) *28-day regimen*

NORLESTRIN 21 **2.5/50** (norethindrone acetate and ethinyl estradiol) **Parke-Davis** Rx

Tablets: 2.5 mg norethindrone acetate and 50 μg ethinyl estradiol *21-day regimen*

NORLESTRIN Fe **2.5/50** (norethindrone acetate and ethinyl estradiol; ferrous fumarate) Rx
Parke-Davis

Tablets: 2.5 mg norethindrone acetate and 50 μg ethinyl estradiol (pink); 75 mg ferrous fumarate (brown) *28-day regimen*

INDICATIONS	ORAL DOSAGE
Contraception	Adult: 1 tab q24h for 21 or 28 consecutive days of the menstrual cycle

NORLESTRIN 1/50 / NORLESTRIN 2.5/50

CONTRAINDICATIONS

Thrombophlebitis or thromboembolic disorders	Known or suspected breast cancer	Known or suspected pregnancy
Past history of deep-vein thrombophlebitis or thromboembolic disorders	Known or suspected estrogen-dependent neoplasia	Benign or malignant liver tumor that developed during the use of oral contraceptives or other estrogen-containing products
Coronary artery disease	Undiagnosed abnormal genital bleeding	
Cerebrovascular disease		

ADMINISTRATION/DOSAGE ADJUSTMENTS

Initiating therapy	First tablet should be taken on the 5th day after the onset of menses
Subsequent cycles (21-day regimen)	First tablet is taken 8 days after last tablet was taken in preceding cycle
Subsequent cycles (28-day regimen)	First tablet is taken 1 day after last (placebo) tablet was taken in preceding cycle
Missed tablets	If one tablet is missed, it should be taken as soon as it is remembered or together with the next tablet on the following day. If two tablets are missed, the dosage should be doubled for the next 2 days. If three tablets are missed, the tablet cycle should be discontinued and another form of contraception used until the start of the next menstrual period. Instruct the patient to start the next course of tablets 7 days after the last tablet was taken, even if she is still menstruating.

WARNINGS/PRECAUTIONS

Cigarette smoking	Increases the risk of serious cardiovascular side effects, especially in women over 35 yr of age who smoke 15 or more cigarettes daily; patients who use oral contraceptives should be strongly urged not to smoke
Thromboembolic disease, thrombotic disorders, and other vascular problems	Risk is increased, becoming greater with age (after 30 yr of age) and with the amount of estrogen in the formulation; after use of oral contraceptives is discontinued, the risk of cerebrovascular disease, myocardial infarction, and subarachnoid hemorrhage may persist. Discontinue oral contraception immediately if early signs of thromboembolic disease or thrombotic disorders (eg, thrombophlebitis, pulmonary embolism, cerebrovascular insufficiency, coronary occlusion, or retinal or mesenteric thrombosis) develop or are suspected.
Postsurgical thromboembolic complications	Risk is increased 4-6 times; if feasible, discontinue oral contraception at least 4 wk before elective surgery associated with an increased risk of thromboembolism or prolonged immobilization
Ocular lesions, including optic neuritis and retinal thrombosis	May occur; discontinue oral contraception in the presence of unexplained gradual or sudden, partial or complete loss of vision; proptosis or diplopia; papilledema; or retinal vascular lesions
Carcinoma	Closely monitor patients with a strong family history of breast cancer or with breast nodules, fibrocystic disease, or abnormal mammograms; investigate all cases of undiagnosed persistent or recurrent abnormal vaginal bleeding for malignancy (see CONTRAINDICATIONS)
Hepatic tumors, including benign adenomas	May occur and possibly rupture, resulting in intraabdominal hemorrhage and death; investigate all cases of abdominal pain and tenderness, abdominal mass, or shock for hepatic adenoma. The risk reportedly increases among users of formulations with high hormonal potency, and with use of oral contraception for more than 4 yr.
Gallbladder disease	Risk increases with duration of oral contraception
Hepatic impairment	Use with caution due to poor steroid hormone metabolism
Jaundice	May recur in patients with a history of jaundice; discontinue oral contraception while cause is investigated
Glucose tolerance	May become impaired; closely monitor patients with latent or active diabetes
Hypertension	May be precipitated or may worsen with oral contraception, particularly with prolonged use, in older patients, and in patients with a history of hypertension during pregnancy
Migraine headache	May develop or worsen; discontinue oral contraception and investigate cause of recurrent, persistent, or severe headaches
Mental depression	Risk is increased; discontinue oral contraception if serious depression develops or recurs in patients with a history of depression
Fluid retention	May occur; use with caution in patients with convulsive disorders, migraine, asthma, or cardiac, hepatic, or renal dysfunction
Vitamin deficiencies	May occur, particularly of pyridoxine and folic acid
Spotting, breakthrough bleeding	If spotting occurs, instruct patient to continue the regimen without interruption. The possibility of spotting or breakthrough bleeding is increased when tablets are missed, particularly if two or more consecutive tablets are not taken. If bleeding occurs, the patient should discontinue use for a period of 4 days and then begin a new tablet cycle on the 5th day. If abnormal vaginal bleeding is not controlled by this method, adequate diagnostic measures are indicated to rule out pregnancy or malignancy. Assuming these are excluded, the problem may be corrected by the passage of time or use of another formulation. Preparations with a higher estrogen content should be used only if necessary because of the increased risk of thromboembolic disease.

NORLESTRIN 1/50/NORLESTRIN 2.5/50

Failure of withdrawal bleeding	If patient has missed two consecutive periods, pregnancy should be ruled out before contraceptive regimen is continued; if patient has not adhered to prescribed regimen, pregnancy should be considered after the first missed period and oral contraception withheld until pregnancy has been excluded. Amenorrhea may occur during therapy and necessitate discontinuation of use.
Postpill amenorrhea and anovulation	May occur, particularly in patients with a history of oligomenorrhea or secondary amenorrhea or in young women who have not established regular menstrual cycles; such patients should be encouraged to use alternative methods of contraception

ADVERSE REACTIONS

Frequent reactions (incidence ≥ 1%) are printed in *italics*

Genitourinary	*Breakthrough bleeding, spotting, menstrual irregularities, vaginal candidiasis,* postpill amenorrhea and infertility, dysmenorrhea, altered cervical erosion and secretion, enlargement of uterine leiomyomata, premenstrual-like syndrome, altered libido, cystitis-like syndrome, vaginitis
Cardiovascular	Thrombophlebitis, pulmonary embolism, coronary thrombosis, cerebral thrombosis, cerebral hemorrhage, hypertension, mesenteric thrombosis, edema
Gastrointestinal	*Nausea, vomiting,* gallbladder disease, abdominal cramps, bloating, change in appetite
Hepatic	Benign hepatomas, cholestatic jaundice
Metabolic and endocrinological	*Breast enlargement, tenderness, and/or secretion;* carbohydrate intolerance; increase or decrease in weight; hyperlipidemia
Central nervous system and neuromuscular	Migraine, depression, headache, nervousness, dizziness, chorea
Ophthalmic	Optic neuritis, retinal thrombosis, intolerance to contact lenses, altered corneal curvature, cataracts
Allergic and dermatological	Rash, melasma or chloasma, erythema multiforme, erythema nodosum, hirsutism, hair loss, hemorrhagic eruption, porphyria
Other	Congenital anomalies

OVERDOSAGE

Signs and symptoms	Nausea, withdrawal bleeding; acute ingestion of large doses by young children has not been associated with serious ill effects
Treatment	Treat symptomatically

DRUG INTERACTIONS

Ampicillin, analgesics, antianxiety agents, antimigraine preparations, barbiturates, chloramphenicol, isoniazid, neomycin, nitrofurantoin, penicillin V, phenylbutazone, phenytoin, primidone, rifampin, sulfonamides, tetracycline	▽ Contraceptive effect △ Breakthrough bleeding
Antihypertensive agents (eg, guanethidine)	▽ Antihypertensive effect
Oral anticoagulants	▽ Anticoagulant effect
Anticonvulsants	△ Seizure activity
Hypoglycemic agents	▽ Glucose tolerance
Corticosteroids	△ Corticosteroid effects
Tricyclic antidepressants	△ Antidepressant side effects

ALTERED LABORATORY VALUES

Blood/serum values	△ Alkaline phosphatase △ Bilirubin △ Sulfobromophthalein retention △ Prothrombin △ Clotting factors VII, VIII, IX, and X ▽ Antithrombin III △ PBI △ Thyroxine (T_4) ▽ Triiodothyronine (T_3) uptake △ Glucose △ Cortisol △ Transcortin △ Ceruloplasmin △ Triglycerides △ Phospholipids ▽ Folic acid ▽ Pyridoxine
Urinary values	▽ Pregnanediol

USE IN CHILDREN

Not indicated before puberty

USE IN PREGNANT AND NURSING WOMEN

Pregnancy Category X: contraindicated if pregnancy is known or suspected, as serious fetal damage may occur during early pregnancy. Patient should discontinue oral contraception 3 mo before attempting to conceive. Postpartum use may interfere with lactation, causing a decrease in the quantity and quality of breast milk. Patient should use an alternative form of contraception until infant is weaned.

CONTRACEPTIVES

ORTHO-NOVUM 1/35 □ 21 (norethindrone and ethinyl estradiol) Ortho — Rx
Tablets: 1 mg norethindrone and 35 μg ethinyl estradiol *21-day regimen*

ORTHO-NOVUM 1/35 □ 28 (norethindrone and ethinyl estradiol) Ortho — Rx
Tablets: 1 mg norethindrone and 35 μg ethinyl estradiol *28-day regimen*

INDICATIONS
Contraception

ORAL DOSAGE
Adult: 1 tab q24h for 21 or 28 consecutive days of the menstrual cycle

CONTRAINDICATIONS
- Thrombophlebitis or thromboembolic disorders
- Past history of deep-vein thrombophlebitis or thromboembolic disorders
- Coronary artery disease
- Cerebrovascular disease
- Known or suspected breast cancer
- Known or suspected estrogen-dependent neoplasia
- Undiagnosed abnormal genital bleeding
- Pregnancy
- Benign or malignant liver tumor that developed during the use of oral contraceptives or other estrogen-containing products

ADMINISTRATION/DOSAGE ADJUSTMENTS

Initiating therapy	First tablet should be taken on the 5th day (21-day regimen) or 1st Sunday (28-day regimen) after the onset of menses; if menses begins on a Sunday, regimen is started the very same day. Regimen may be started postpartum, bearing in mind the increased risk of thromboembolic disease associated with the postpartum period.
Subsequent cycles (21-day regimen)	First tablet is taken 8 days after last tablet was taken in preceding cycle
Subsequent cycles (28-day regimen)	First tablet is taken 1 day after last (placebo) tablet was taken in preceding cycle
Missed tablets	If more than one tablet is missed, instruct patient to resume taking tablets as soon as remembered, but to use an additional form of contraception for the remainder of the cycle

WARNINGS/PRECAUTIONS

Cigarette smoking	Increases the risk of serious cardiovascular side effects, especially in women over 35 yr of age who smoke 15 or more cigarettes daily; patients who use oral contraceptives should be strongly urged not to smoke
Thromboembolic disease, thrombotic disorders, and other vascular problems	Risk is increased, becoming greater with age and the amount of estrogen present in the formulation, and may persist after discontinuation of use (the degree of residual risk may be related to the duration of use). Discontinue oral contraception immediately if early signs of thromboembolic disease or thrombotic disorders (eg, thrombophlebitis, pulmonary embolism, cerebrovascular insufficiency, coronary occlusion, or retinal or mesenteric thrombosis) develop or are suspected.
Postsurgical thromboembolic complications	Risk is increased 4–6 times; if feasible, discontinue oral contraception at least 4 wk before elective surgery associated with an increased risk of thromboembolism or prolonged immobilization
Ocular lesions, including optic neuritis and retinal thrombosis	May occur; discontinue oral contraception in the presence of unexplained gradual or sudden, partial or complete loss of vision; proptosis or diplopia; papilledema; or retinal vascular lesions
Carcinoma	Closely monitor patients with a strong family history of breast cancer or with breast nodules, fibrocystic disease, or abnormal mammograms; investigate all cases of undiagnosed persistent or recurrent abnormal vaginal bleeding for malignancy (see CONTRAINDICATIONS). Hepatocellular carcinoma has been reported rarely; the risk is thought to increase with the duration of oral contraceptive therapy.
Hepatic tumors, including benign adenomas	May occur and possibly rupture, resulting in intraabdominal hemorrhage and death; investigate all cases of abdominal pain and tenderness, abdominal mass, or shock for hepatic tumors. The risk of hepatocellular adenoma reportedly increases in women over 30, among users of formulations with high hormonal potency, and with use of oral contraception for more than 4 yr.
Gallbladder disease	Risk increases with duration of oral contraception
Hepatic impairment	Use with caution due to poor steroid hormone metabolism
Jaundice	May recur in patients with a history of jaundice; discontinue oral contraception while cause is investigated
Glucose tolerance	May become impaired; closely monitor patients with latent or active diabetes
Hypertension	May be precipitated or may worsen with oral contraception, particularly with prolonged use, in older patients and in patients with a history of hypertension during pregnancy
Migraine headache	May develop or worsen; discontinue oral contraception and investigate cause of recurrent, persistent, or severe headaches

ORTHO-NOVUM 1/35

Mental depression	Risk is increased; discontinue oral contraception if serious depression develops or recurs in patients with a history of depression
Fluid retention	May occur; use with caution in patients with convulsive disorders, migraine, asthma, or cardiac, hepatic, or renal dysfunction
Vitamin deficiencies	May occur, particularly of pyridoxine and folic acid
Spotting, breakthrough bleeding	If spotting or breakthrough bleeding occurs, the possibility of organic disorder should be borne in mind. If abnormal vaginal bleeding persists or recurs, adequate diagnostic measures are indicated to rule out pregnancy or malignancy. Assuming these are excluded, the problem may be corrected by the passage of time or use of another formulation. Preparations with a higher estrogen content should be used only if necessary because of the increased risk of thromboembolic disease.
Failure of withdrawal bleeding	If patient has not adhered to prescribed regimen, pregnancy should be considered after the first missed period and oral contraception withheld until pregnancy has been excluded; if patient has adhered to regimen and misses two consecutive periods, pregnancy should be ruled out before regimen is continued. Amenorrhea may occur during therapy and necessitate discontinuation of use.
Postpill amenorrhea and anovulation	May occur, particularly in patients with a history of oligomenorrhea or secondary amenorrhea or in young women who have not established regular menstrual cycles; such patients should be encouraged to use alternative methods of contraception

ADVERSE REACTIONS

Frequent reactions (incidence ≥ 1%) are printed in *italics*

Genitourinary	*Breakthrough bleeding, spotting, menstrual irregularities, vaginal candidiasis,* postpill amenorrhea and infertility, dysmenorrhea, altered cervical erosion and secretion, enlargement of uterine leiomyomata, premenstrual-like syndrome, altered libido, cystitis-like syndrome, vaginitis
Cardiovascular	Thrombophlebitis, pulmonary embolism, coronary thrombosis, cerebral thrombosis, cerebral hemorrhage, hypertension, mesenteric thrombosis, edema
Gastrointestinal	*Nausea, vomiting,* gallbladder disease, abdominal cramps, bloating, change in appetite
Hepatic	Hepatic tumors, cholestatic jaundice
Renal	Impaired renal function, hemolytic uremic syndrome
Metabolic and endocrinological	*Breast enlargement, tenderness, and/or secretion;* carbohydrate intolerance; increase or decrease in weight; hyperlipidemia
Central nervous system and neuromuscular	Migraine, depression, headache, nervousness, dizziness, chorea
Ophthalmic	Optic neuritis, retinal thrombosis, intolerance to contact lenses, altered corneal curvature, cataracts
Allergic and dermatological	Rash, melasma, chloasma, erythema multiforme, erythema nodosum, hirsutism, hair loss, hemorrhagic eruption, porphyria
Other	Congenital anomalies

OVERDOSAGE

Signs and symptoms	Nausea, withdrawal bleeding; acute ingestion of large doses by young children has not been associated with serious ill effects
Treatment	Treat symptomatically

DRUG INTERACTIONS

Ampicillin, analgesics, antianxiety agents, antimigraine preparations, barbiturates, chloramphenicol, griseofulvin, isoniazid, neomycin, nitrofurantoin, penicillin V, phenylbutazone, phenytoin, primidone, rifampin, sulfonamides, tetracycline	▽ Contraceptive effect △ Breakthrough bleeding
Antihypertensive agents (eg, guanethidine)	▽ Antihypertensive effect
Oral anticoagulants	▽ Anticoagulant effect
Anticonvulsants	△ Seizure activity
Hypoglycemic agents	▽ Glucose tolerance
Corticosteroids	△ Corticosteroid effects
Tricyclic antidepressants	△ Antidepressant side effects

ORTHO-NOVUM 1/35 ■ ORTHO-NOVUM 1/50/ORTHO-NOVUM 1/80

ALTERED LABORATORY VALUES

Blood/serum values	△ Alkaline phophatase △ Bilirubin △ Sulfobromophthalein retention △ Prothrombin △ Clotting factors VII, VIII, IX, and X ▽ Antithrombin III △ PBI △ Thyroxine (T_4) ▽ Triiodothyronine (T_3) uptake △ Glucose △ Cortisol △ Transcortin △ Ceruloplasmin △ Triglycerides △ Phospholipids ▽ Folic acid ▽ Pyridoxine
Urinary values	▽ Pregnanediol

USE IN CHILDREN
Not indicated before puberty

USE IN PREGNANT AND NURSING WOMEN
Pregnancy Category X: contraindicated if pregnancy is known or suspected, as serious fetal damage may occur during early pregnancy. If she becomes pregnant while taking this product, she should be apprised of the potential hazard to the fetus. Patient should discontinue oral contraception 3 mo before attempting to conceive. Postpartum use may interfere with lactation, causing a decrease in the quantity and quality of breast milk. The hormonal agents in oral contraceptives are excreted in human milk; because of the potential for tumorigenicity, the patient should use an alternative form of contraception until infant is weaned.

CONTRACEPTIVES

ORTHO-NOVUM 1/50 □ 21 (norethindrone and mestranol) Ortho Rx
Tablets: 1 mg norethindrone and 50 µg mestranol *21-day regimen*

ORTHO-NOVUM 1/50 □ 28 (norethindrone and mestranol) Ortho Rx
Tablets: 1 mg norethindrone and 50 µg mestranol *28-day regimen*

ORTHO-NOVUM 1/80 □ 21 (norethindrone and mestranol) Ortho Rx
Tablets: 1 mg norethindrone and 80 µg mestranol *21-day regimen*

ORTHO-NOVUM 1/80 □ 28 (norethindrone and mestranol) Ortho Rx
Tablets: 1 mg norethindrone and 80 µg mestranol *28-day regimen*

INDICATIONS	ORAL DOSAGE
Contraception	**Adult:** 1 tab q24h for 21 or 28 consecutive days of the menstrual cycle

CONTRAINDICATIONS

Thrombophlebitis or thromboembolic disorders	Known or suspected breast cancer	Pregnancy
Past history of deep-vein thrombophlebitis or thromboembolic disorders	Known or suspected estrogen-dependent neoplasia	Benign or malignant liver tumor that developed during the use of oral contraceptives or other estrogen-containing products
Coronary artery disease	Undiagnosed abnormal genital bleeding	
Cerebrovascular disease		

ADMINISTRATION/DOSAGE ADJUSTMENTS

Initiating therapy	First tablet should be taken on the 5th day (21-day regimen) or 1st Sunday (28-day regimen) after the onset of menses; if menses begins on a Sunday, regimen is started the very same day. Regimen may be started postpartum, bearing in mind the increased risk of thromboembolic disease associated with the postpartum period.
Subsequent cycles (21-day regimen)	First tablet is taken 8 days after last tablet was taken in preceding cycle
Subsequent cycles (28-day regimen)	First tablet is taken 1 day after last (placebo) tablet was taken in preceding cycle
Missed tablets	If more than one tablet is missed, instruct patient to resume taking tablets as soon as remembered, but to use an additional form of contraception for the remainder of the cycle

WARNINGS/PRECAUTIONS

Cigarette smoking	Increases the risk of serious cardiovascular side effects, especially in women over 35 yr of age who smoke 15 or more cigarettes daily; patients who use oral contraceptives should be strongly urged not to smoke

ORTHO-NOVUM 1/50/ORTHO-NOVUM 1/80

Thromboembolic disease, thrombotic disorders, and other vascular problems	Risk is increased, becoming greater with age and the amount of estrogen present in the formulation, and may persist after discontinuation of use (the degree of residual risk may be related to the duration of use). Discontinue oral contraception immediately if early signs of thromboembolic disease or thrombotic disorders (eg, thrombophlebitis, pulmonary embolism, cerebrovascular insufficiency, coronary occlusion, or retinal or mesenteric thrombosis) develop or are suspected.
Postsurgical thromboembolic complications	Risk is increased 4–6 times; if feasible, discontinue oral contraception at least 4 wk before elective surgery associated with an increased risk of thromboembolism or prolonged immobilization
Ocular lesions, including optic neuritis and retinal thrombosis	May occur; discontinue oral contraception in the presence of unexplained gradual or sudden, partial or complete loss of vision; proptosis or diplopia; papilledema; or retinal vascular lesions
Carcinoma	Closely monitor patients with a strong family history of breast cancer or with breast nodules, fibrocystic disease, or abnormal mammograms; investigate all cases of undiagnosed persistent or recurrent abnormal vaginal bleeding for malignancy (see CONTRAINDICATIONS). Hepatocellular carcinoma has been reported rarely; the risk is thought to increase with the duration of oral contraceptive therapy.
Hepatic tumors, including benign adenomas	May occur and possibly rupture, resulting in intraabdominal hemorrhage and death; investigate all cases of abdominal pain and tenderness, abdominal mass, or shock for hepatic tumors. The risk of hepatocellular adenoma reportedly increases in women over 30, among users of formulations with high hormonal potency, and with use of oral contraception for more than 4 yr.
Gallbladder disease	Risk increases with duration of oral contraception
Hepatic impairment	Use with caution due to poor steroid hormone metabolism
Jaundice	May recur in patients with a history of jaundice; discontinue oral contraception while cause is investigated
Glucose tolerance	May become impaired; closely monitor patients with latent or active diabetes
Hypertension	May be precipitated or may worsen with oral contraception, particularly with prolonged use, in older patients, and in patients with a history of hypertension during pregnancy
Migraine headache	May develop or worsen; discontinue oral contraception and investigate cause of recurrent, persistent, or severe headaches
Mental depression	Risk is increased; discontinue oral contraception if serious depression develops or recurs in patients with a history of depression
Fluid retention	May occur; use with caution in patients with convulsive disorders, migraine, asthma, or cardiac, hepatic, or renal dysfunction
Vitamin deficiencies	May occur, particularly of pyridoxine and folic acid
Spotting, breakthrough bleeding	If spotting or breakthrough bleeding occurs, the possibility of organic disorder should be borne in mind. If abnormal vaginal bleeding persists or recurs, adequate diagnostic measures are indicated to rule out pregnancy or malignancy. Assuming these are excluded, the problem may be corrected by the passage of time or use of another formulation. Preparations with a higher estrogen content should be used only if necessary because of the increased risk of thromboembolic disease.
Failure of withdrawal bleeding	If patient has not adhered to prescribed regimen, pregnancy should be considered after the first missed period and oral contraception withheld until pregnancy has been excluded; if patient has adhered to regimen and misses two consecutive periods, pregnancy should be ruled out before contraceptive regimen is continued. Amenorrhea may occur during therapy and necessitate discontinuation of use.
Postpill amenorrhea and anovulation	May occur, particularly in patients with a history of oligomenorrhea or secondary amenorrhea or in young women who have not established regular menstrual cycles; such patients should be encouraged to use alternative methods of contraception

ADVERSE REACTIONS	Frequent reactions (incidence $\geq$ 1%) are printed in *italics*
Genitourinary	*Breakthrough bleeding, spotting, menstrual irregularities, vaginal candidiasis,* postpill amenorrhea and infertility, dysmenorrhea, altered cervical erosion and secretion, enlargement of uterine leiomyomata, premenstrual-like syndrome, altered libido, cystitis-like syndrome, vaginitis
Cardiovascular	Thrombophlebitis, pulmonary embolism, coronary thrombosis, cerebral thrombosis, cerebral hemorrhage, hypertension, mesenteric thrombosis, edema
Gastrointestinal	*Nausea, vomiting,* gallbladder disease, abdominal cramps, bloating, change in appetite
Hepatic	Hepatic tumors, cholestatic jaundice
Renal	Impaired renal function, hemolytic uremic syndrome
Metabolic and endocrinological	*Breast enlargement, tenderness, and/or secretion;* carbohydrate intolerance; increase or decrease in weight; hyperlipidemia

ORTHO-NOVUM 1/50/ORTHO-NOVUM 1/80 ■ ORTHO-NOVUM 7/7/7

Central nervous system and neuromuscular	Migraine, depression, headache, nervousness, dizziness, chorea
Ophthalmic	Optic neuritis, retinal thrombosis, intolerance to contact lenses, altered corneal curvature, cataracts
Allergic and dermatological	Rash, melasma or chloasma, erythema multiforme, erythema nodosum, hirsutism, hair loss, hemorrhagic eruption, porphyria
Other	Congenital anomalies

OVERDOSAGE

Signs and symptoms	Nausea, withdrawal bleeding; acute ingestion of large doses by young children has not been associated with serious ill effects
Treatment	Treat symptomatically

DRUG INTERACTIONS

Ampicillin, analgesics, antianxiety agents, antimigraine preparations, barbiturates, chloramphenicol, griseofulvin, isoniazid, neomycin, nitrofurantoin, penicillin V, phenylbutazone, phenytoin, primidone, rifampin, sulfonamides, tetracycline	▽ Contraceptive effect △ Breakthrough bleeding
Antihypertensive agents (eg, guanethidine)	▽ Antihypertensive effect
Oral anticoagulants	▽ Anticoagulant effect
Anticonvulsants	△ Seizure activity
Hypoglycemic agents	▽ Glucose tolerance
Corticosteroids	△ Corticosteroid effects
Tricyclic antidepressants	△ Antidepressant side effects

ALTERED LABORATORY VALUES

Blood/serum values	△ Alkaline phosphatase △ Bilirubin △ Sulfobromophthalein retention △ Prothrombin △ Clotting factors VII, VIII, IX, and X ▽ Antithrombin III △ PBI △ Thyroxine (T_4) ▽ Triiodothyronine (T_3) uptake △ Glucose △ Cortisol △ Transcortin △ Ceruloplasmin △ Triglycerides △ Phospholipids ▽ Folic acid ▽ Pyridoxine
Urinary values	▽ Pregnanediol

USE IN CHILDREN

Not indicated before puberty

USE IN PREGNANT AND NURSING WOMEN

Pregnancy Category X: contraindicated if pregnancy is known or suspected, as serious fetal damage may occur during early pregnancy. If she becomes pregnant while taking this product, she should be apprised of the potential hazard to the fetus. Patient should discontinue oral contraception 3 mo before attempting to conceive. Postpartum use may interfere with lactation, causing a decrease in the quantity and quality of breast milk. The hormonal agents in oral contraceptives are excreted in human milk; because of the potential for tumorigenicity, the patient should use an alternative form of contraception until infant is weaned.

CONTRACEPTIVES

ORTHO-NOVUM 7/7/7 □ 21 (norethindrone and ethinyl estradiol) Ortho   Rx

Tablets (per dispenser): 7 white tablets containing 0.5 mg norethindrone and 35 μg ethinyl estradiol, 7 light peach tablets containing 0.75 mg norethindrone and 35 μg ethinyl estradiol, and 7 peach tablets containing 1 mg norethindrone and 35 μg ethinyl estradiol *21-day regimen*

ORTHO-NOVUM 7/7/7 □ 28 (norethindrone and ethinyl estradiol) Ortho   Rx

Tablets (per dispenser): 7 white tablets containing 0.5 mg norethindrone and 35 μg ethinyl estradiol, 7 light peach tablets containing 0.75 mg norethindrone and 35 μg ethinyl estradiol, 7 peach tablets containing 1 mg norethindrone and 35 μg ethinyl estradiol, and 7 green tablets containing inert ingredients *28-day regimen*

INDICATIONS	ORAL DOSAGE
Contraception	**Adult:** 1 white tablet q24h for 7 days, followed successively by 1 light peach tablet q24h for 7 days, 1 peach tablet q24h for 7 days, and either no tablets for 7 days (21-day regimen) or 1 green tablet q24h for 7 days (28-day regimen)

ORTHO-NOVUM 7/7/7

CONTRAINDICATIONS

- Thrombophlebitis or thromboembolic disorders
- Past history of deep-vein thrombophlebitis or thromboembolic disorders
- Coronary artery disease
- Cerebrovascular disease
- Known or suspected breast cancer
- Known or suspected estrogen-dependent neoplasia
- Undiagnosed abnormal genital bleeding
- Pregnancy
- Benign or malignant liver tumor that developed during the use of oral contraceptives or other estrogen-containing products

ADMINISTRATION/DOSAGE ADJUSTMENTS

Initiating therapy	First tablet should be taken on the first Sunday after the onset of menses or, if menses begins on a Sunday, on that very day. An additional form of contraception should be used until at least 7 white tablets have been taken. Regimen may be started postpartum, bearing in mind the increased risk of thromboembolic disease associated with the postpartum period.
Subsequent cycles (21-day regimen)	First white tablet is taken 8 days after last tablet was taken in the preceding cycle
Subsequent cycles (28-day regimen)	First white tablet is taken the day after the last green tablet was taken in the preceding cycle
Missed tablets	If more than one tablet is missed, instruct patient to resume taking tablets as soon as remembered, but to use an additional form of contraception for the remainder of the cycle

WARNINGS/PRECAUTIONS

Cigarette smoking	Increases the risk of serious cardiovascular side effects, especially in women over 35 yr of age who smoke 15 or more cigarettes daily; patients who use oral contraceptives should be strongly urged not to smoke
Thromboembolic disease, thrombotic disorders, and other vascular problems	Risk is increased, becoming greater with age and the amount of estrogen present in the formulation, and may persist after discontinuation of use (the degree of residual risk may be related to the duration of use). Discontinue oral contraception immediately if early signs of thromboembolic disease or thrombotic disorders (eg, thrombophlebitis, pulmonary embolism, cerebrovascular insufficiency, coronary occlusion, or retinal or mesenteric thrombosis) develop or are suspected.
Postsurgical thromboembolic complications	Risk is increased 4–6 times; if feasible, discontinue oral contraception at least 4 wk before elective surgery associated with an increased risk of thromboembolism or prolonged immobilization
Ocular lesions, including optic neuritis and retinal thrombosis	May occur; discontinue oral contraception in the presence of unexplained gradual or sudden, partial or complete loss of vision; proptosis or diplopia; papilledema; or retinal vascular lesions
Carcinoma	Closely monitor patients with a strong family history of breast cancer or with breast nodules, fibrocystic disease, or abnormal mammograms; investigate all cases of undiagnosed persistent or recurrent abnormal vaginal bleeding for malignancy (see CONTRAINDICATIONS). Hepatocellular carcinoma has been reported rarely; the risk is thought to increase with the duration of oral contraceptive therapy.
Hepatic tumors, including benign adenomas	May occur and possibly rupture, resulting in intraabdominal hemorrhage and death; investigate all cases of abdominal pain and tenderness, abdominal mass, or shock for hepatic tumors. The risk of hepatocellular adenoma reportedly increases in women over 30, among users of formulations with high hormonal potency, and with use of oral contraception for more than 4 yr.
Gallbladder disease	Risk increases with duration of oral contraception
Hepatic impairment	Use with caution due to poor steroid hormone metabolism
Jaundice	May recur in patients with a history of jaundice; discontinue oral contraception while cause is investigated
Glucose tolerance	May become impaired; closely monitor patients with latent or active diabetes
Hypertension	May be precipitated or may worsen with oral contraception, particularly with prolonged use, in older patients, and in patients with a history of hypertension during pregnancy
Migraine headache	May develop or worsen; discontinue oral contraception and investigate cause of recurrent, persistent, or severe headaches
Mental depression	Risk is increased; discontinue oral contraception if serious depression develops or recurs in patients with a history of depression
Fluid retention	May occur; use with caution in patients with convulsive disorders, migraine, asthma, or cardiac, hepatic, or renal dysfunction
Vitamin deficiencies	May occur, particularly of pyridoxine and folic acid

ORTHO-NOVUM 7/7/7

Spotting, breakthrough bleeding	If spotting or breakthrough bleeding occurs, the possibility of organic disorder should be borne in mind. If abnormal vaginal bleeding persists or recurs, adequate diagnostic measures are indicated to rule out pregnancy or malignancy. Assuming these are excluded, the problem may be corrected by the passage of time or use of another formulation. Preparations with a higher estrogen content should be used only if necessary because of the increased risk of thromboembolic disease.
Failure of withdrawal bleeding	If patient has not adhered to prescribed regimen, pregnancy should be considered after the first missed period and oral contraception withheld until pregnancy has been excluded; if patient has adhered to regimen and misses two consecutive periods, pregnancy should be ruled out before regimen is continued. Amenorrhea may occur during therapy and necessitate discontinuation of use.
Postpill amenorrhea and anovulation	May occur, particularly in patients with a history of oligomenorrhea or secondary amenorrhea or in young women who have not established regular menstrual cycles; such patients should be encouraged to use alternative methods of contraception

ADVERSE REACTIONS

Frequent reactions (incidence ≥ 1%) are printed in *italics*

Genitourinary	*Breakthrough bleeding, spotting, menstrual irregularities, vaginal candidiasis,* postpill amenorrhea and infertility, dysmenorrhea, altered cervical erosion and secretion, enlargement of uterine leiomyomata, premenstrual-like syndrome, altered libido, cystitis-like syndrome, vaginitis
Cardiovascular	Thrombophlebitis, pulmonary embolism, coronary thrombosis, cerebral thrombosis, cerebral hemorrhage, hypertension, mesenteric thrombosis, edema
Gastrointestinal	*Nausea, vomiting,* gallbladder disease, abdominal cramps, bloating, change in appetite
Hepatic	Benign hepatomas, cholestatic jaundice
Renal	Impaired renal function, hemolytic uremic syndrome
Metabolic and endocrinological	*Breast enlargement, tenderness, and/or secretion;* carbohydrate intolerance; increase or decrease in weight; hyperlipidemia
Central nervous system and neuromuscular	Migraine, depression, headache, nervousness, dizziness, chorea
Ophthalmic	Optic neuritis, retinal thrombosis, intolerance to contact lenses, altered corneal curvature, cataracts
Allergic and dermatological	Rash, melasma or chloasma, erythema multiforme, erythema nodosum, hirsutism, hair loss, hemorrhagic eruption, porphyria
Other	Congenital anomalies

OVERDOSAGE

Signs and symptoms	Nausea, withdrawal bleeding; acute ingestion of large doses by young children has not been associated with serious ill effects
Treatment	Treat symptomatically

DRUG INTERACTIONS

Ampicillin, analgesics, antianxiety agents, antimigraine agents, barbiturates, chloramphenicol, griseofulvin, isoniazid, neomycin, nitrofurantoin, penicillin V, phenylbutazone, phenytoin, primidone, rifampin, sulfonamides, tetracycline	▽ Contraceptive effect △ Breakthrough bleeding
Antihypertensive agents (eg, guanethidine)	▽ Antihypertensive effect
Oral anticoagulants	▽ Anticoagulant effect
Anticonvulsants	△ Seizure activity
Hypoglycemic agents	▽ Glucose tolerance
Corticosteroids	△ Corticosteroid effects
Tricyclic antidepressants	△ Antidepressant side effects

ALTERED LABORATORY VALUES

Blood/serum values	△ Alkaline phosphatase △ Bilirubin △ Sulfobromophthalein retention △ Prothrombin △ Clotting factors VII, VIII, IX, and X ▽ Antithrombin III △ PBI △ Thyroxine (T_4) ▽ Triiodothyronine (T_3) uptake △ Glucose △ Cortisol △ Transcortin △ Ceruloplasmin △ Triglycerides △ Phospholipids ▽ Folic acid ▽ Pyridoxine
Urinary values	▽ Pregnanediol

ORTHO-NOVUM 7/7/7 ■ ORTHO-NOVUM 10/11

USE IN CHILDREN	USE IN PREGNANT AND NURSING WOMEN
Not indicated before puberty	Pregnancy Category X: contraindicated during pregnancy, since fetal harm may occur if administered. Patient should discontinue oral contraception 3 mo before attempting to conceive. If she becomes pregnant while taking this product, she should be apprised of the potential hazard to the fetus. Postpartum use may interfere with lactation, causing a decrease in the quantity and quality of breast milk. The hormonal agents in oral contraceptives are excreted in human milk; because of the potential for tumorigenicity, an alternative method of contraception should be used, if possible, until the infant is weaned.

CONTRACEPTIVES

ORTHO-NOVUM 10/11 □ 21 (norethindrone and ethinyl estradiol) Ortho   Rx

Tablets: 10 white tablets containing 0.5 mg norethindrone and 35 µg ethinyl estradiol plus 11 peach tablets containing 1 mg norethindrone and 35 µg ethinyl estradiol *21-day regimen*

ORTHO-NOVUM 10/11 □ 28 (norethindrone and ethinyl estradiol) Ortho   Rx

Tablets: 10 white tablets containing 0.5 mg norethindrone and 35 µg ethinyl estradiol plus 11 peach tablets containing 1 mg norethindrone and 35 µg ethinyl estradiol *28-day regimen*[1]

INDICATIONS	ORAL DOSAGE
Contraception	**Adult:** 1 white tab q24h for 10 days, followed by 1 peach tab q24h for 11 consecutive days of the menstrual cycle

CONTRAINDICATIONS

Thrombophlebitis or thromboembolic disorders	Known or suspected breast cancer	Pregnancy
Past history of deep-vein thrombophlebitis or thromboembolic disorders	Known or suspected estrogen-dependent neoplasia	Benign or malignant liver tumor that developed during the use of oral contraceptives or other estrogen-containing products
Coronary artery disease	Undiagnosed abnormal genital bleeding	
Cerebrovascular disease		

ADMINISTRATION/DOSAGE ADJUSTMENTS

Initiating therapy	First white tablet should be taken on the 1st Sunday after the onset of menses; if menses begins on a Sunday, regimen is started the very same day. Instruct patient to take 1 white tablet daily for 10 consecutive days, followed by 1 peach tablet daily for 11 days and then either nothing for 7 days (21-day regimen) or 1 green (inert) tablet daily for 7 days (28-day regimen). An additional form of contraception should be used until at least 7 white tablets have been taken. Regimen may be started postpartum, bearing in mind the increased risk of thromboembolic disease associated with the postpartum period.
Subsequent cycles (21-day regimen)	First white tablet is taken 8 days after last peach tablet was taken in the preceding cycle
Subsequent cycles (28-day regimen)	First white tablet is taken the day after the last green (inert) tablet was taken in the preceding cycle
Missed tablets	If more than one tablet is missed, instruct patient to resume taking tablets as soon as remembered, but to use an additional form of contraception for the remainder of the cycle

WARNINGS/PRECAUTIONS

Cigarette smoking	Increases the risk of serious cardiovascular side effects, especially in women over 35 yr of age who smoke 15 or more cigarettes daily; patients who use oral contraceptives should be strongly urged not to smoke
Thromboembolic disease, thrombotic disorders, and other vascular problems	Risk is increased, becoming greater with age and the amount of estrogen present in the formulation, and may persist after discontinuation of use (the degree of residual risk may be related to the duration of use). Discontinue oral contraception immediately if early signs of thromboembolic disease or thrombotic disorders (eg, thrombophlebitis, pulmonary embolism, cerebrovascular insufficiency, coronary occlusion, or retinal or mesenteric thrombosis) develop or are suspected.
Postsurgical thromboembolic complications	Risk is increased 4–6 times; if feasible, discontinue oral contraception at least 4 wk before elective surgery associated with an increased risk of thromboembolism or prolonged immobilization

ORTHO-NOVUM 10/11

Ocular lesions, including optic neuritis and retinal thrombosis	May occur; discontinue oral contraception in the presence of unexplained gradual or sudden, partial or complete loss of vision; proptosis or diplopia; papilledema; or retinal vascular lesions
Carcinoma	Closely monitor patients with a strong family history of breast cancer or with breast nodules, fibrocystic disease, or abnormal mammograms; investigate all cases of undiagnosed persistent or recurrent abnormal vaginal bleeding for malignancy (see CONTRAINDICATIONS). Hepatocellular carcinoma has been reported rarely; the risk is thought to increase with the duration of oral contraceptive therapy.
Hepatic tumors, including benign adenomas	May occur and possibly rupture, resulting in intraabdominal hemorrhage and death; investigate all cases of abdominal pain and tenderness, abdominal mass, or shock for hepatic tumors. The risk of hepatocellular adenoma reportedly increases in women over 30, among users of formulations with high hormonal potency, and with use of oral contraception for more than 4 yr.
Gallbladder disease	Risk increases with duration of oral contraception
Hepatic impairment	Use with caution due to poor steroid hormone metabolism
Jaundice	May recur in patients with a history of jaundice; discontinue oral contraception while cause is investigated
Glucose tolerance	May become impaired; closely monitor patients with latent or active diabetes
Hypertension	May be precipitated or may worsen with oral contraception, particularly with prolonged use, in older patients, and in patients with a history of hypertension during pregnancy
Migraine headache	May develop or worsen; discontinue oral contraception and investigate cause of recurrent, persistent, or severe headaches
Mental depression	Risk is increased; discontinue oral contraception if serious depression develops or recurs in patients with a history of depression
Fluid retention	May occur; use with caution in patients with convulsive disorders, migraine, asthma, or cardiac, hepatic, or renal dysfunction
Vitamin deficiencies	May occur, particularly of pyridoxine and folic acid
Spotting, breakthrough bleeding	If spotting or breakthrough bleeding occurs, the possibility of organic disorder should be borne in mind. If abnormal vaginal bleeding persists or recurs, adequate diagnostic measures are indicated to rule out pregnancy or malignancy. Assuming these are excluded, the problem may be corrected by the passage of time or use of another formulation. Preparations with a higher estrogen content should be used only if necessary because of the increased risk of thromboembolic disease.
Failure of withdrawal bleeding	If patient has not adhered to prescribed regimen, pregnancy should be considered after the first missed period and oral contraception withheld until pregnancy has been excluded; if patient has adhered to regimen and misses two consecutive periods, pregnancy should be ruled out before regimen is continued. Amenorrhea may occur during therapy and necessitate discontinuation of use.
Postpill amenorrhea and anovulation	May occur, particularly in patients with a history of oligomenorrhea or secondary amenorrhea or in young women who have not established regular menstrual cycles; such patients should be encouraged to use alternative methods of contraception

ADVERSE REACTIONS

Frequent reactions (incidence $\geq$ 1%) are printed in *italics*

Genitourinary	*Breakthrough bleeding, spotting, menstrual irregularities, vaginal candidiasis,* postpill amenorrhea and infertility, dysmenorrhea, altered cervical erosion and secretion, enlargement of uterine leiomyomata, premenstrual-like syndrome, altered libido, cystitis-like syndrome, vaginitis
Cardiovascular	Thrombophlebitis, pulmonary embolism, coronary thrombosis, cerebral thrombosis, cerebral hemorrhage, hypertension, mesenteric thrombosis, edema
Gastrointestinal	*Nausea, vomiting,* gallbladder disease, abdominal cramps, bloating, change in appetite
Hepatic	Benign hepatomas, cholestatic jaundice
Renal	Impaired renal function, hemolytic uremic syndrome
Metabolic and endocrinological	*Breast enlargement, tenderness, and/or secretion;* carbohydrate intolerance; increase or decrease in weight; hyperlipidemia
Central nervous system and neuromuscular	Migraine, depression, headache, nervousness, dizziness, chorea
Ophthalmic	Optic neuritis, retinal thrombosis, intolerance to contact lenses, altered corneal curvature, cataracts
Allergic and dermatological	Rash, melasma or chloasma, erythema multiforme, erythema nodosum, hirsutism, hair loss, hemorrhagic eruption, porphyria
Other	Congenital anomalies

OVERDOSAGE

Signs and symptoms	Nausea, withdrawal bleeding; acute ingestion of large doses by young children has not been associated with serious ill effects
Treatment	Treat symptomatically

DRUG INTERACTIONS

Ampicillin, analgesics, antianxiety agents, antimigraine agents, barbiturates, chloramphenicol, griseofulvin, isoniazid, neomycin, nitrofurantoin, penicillin V, phenylbutazone, phenytoin, primidone, rifampin, sulfonamides, tetracycline	▽ Contraceptive effect △ Breakthrough bleeding
Antihypertensive agents (eg, guanethidine)	▽ Antihypertensive effect
Oral anticoagulants	▽ Anticoagulant effect
Anticonvulsants	△ Seizure activity
Hypoglycemic agents	▽ Glucose tolerance
Corticosteroids	△ Corticosteroid effects
Tricyclic antidepressants	△ Antidepressant side effects

ALTERED LABORATORY VALUES

Blood/serum values	△ Alkaline phosphatase △ Bilirubin △ Sulfobromophthalein retention △ Prothrombin △ Clotting factors VII, VIII, IX, and X ▽ Antithrombin III △ PBI △ Thyroxine (T_4) ▽ Triiodothyronine (T_3) uptake △ Glucose △ Cortisol △ Transcortin △ Ceruloplasmin △ Triglycerides △ Phospholipids ▽ Folic acid ▽ Pyridoxine
Urinary values	▽ Pregnanediol

USE IN CHILDREN
Not indicated before puberty

USE IN PREGNANT AND NURSING WOMEN
Pregnancy Category X: contraindicated during pregnancy, since fetal harm may occur if administered. Patient should discontinue oral contraception 3 mo before attempting to conceive. If she becomes pregnant while taking this product, she should be apprised of the potential hazard to the fetus. Postpartum use may interfere with lactation, causing a decrease in the quantity and quality of breast milk. The hormonal agents in oral contraceptives are excreted in human milk; because of the potential for tumorigenicity, an alternative method of contraception should be used, if possible, until the infant is weaned.

[1] The 28-day dispenser contains, in addition, 7 green tablets with inert ingredients

---

CONTRACEPTIVES

OVCON-35 (norethindrone and ethinyl estradiol) Mead Johnson   Rx
Tablets: 0.4 mg norethindrone and 35 µg ethinyl estradiol *21- and 28-day regimens*

OVCON-50 (norethindrone and ethinyl estradiol) Mead Johnson   Rx
Tablets: 1 mg norethindrone and 50 µg ethinyl estradiol *21- and 28-day regimens*

INDICATIONS
Contraception

ORAL DOSAGE
Adult: 1 tab q24h, preferably in the evening or at bedtime, for 21 or 28 consecutive days of the menstrual cycle

CONTRAINDICATIONS

Thrombophlebitis or thromboembolic disorders

Past history of deep-vein thrombophlebitis or thromboembolic disorders

Coronary artery disease

Cerebrovascular disease

Known or suspected breast cancer

Known or suspected estrogen-dependent neoplasia

Undiagnosed abnormal genital bleeding

Known or suspected pregnancy

Benign or malignant liver tumor that developed during the use of oral contraceptives or other estrogen-containing products

OVCON

ADMINISTRATION/DOSAGE ADJUSTMENTS

Initiating therapy	First tablet should be taken on the fifth day or first Sunday after the onset of menses or, if menses begins on a Sunday, on that very day. An additional form of contraception should be used during the first week of the initial cycle.
Subsequent cycles (21-day regimen)	First tablet is taken 8 days after last tablet was taken in preceding cycle; if the first tablet is taken more than 7 days after the onset of menses, an additional form of contraception should be used during the first week of the tablet cycle
Subsequent cycles (28-day regimen)	First tablet is taken 1 day after last (placebo) tablet was taken in preceding cycle; if the first tablet is taken more than 7 days after the onset of menses, an additional form of contraception should be used during the first week of the tablet cycle
Missed tablets	If one tablet is missed, it should be taken as soon as it is remembered, with the next tablet taken at the usual time; an additional form of contraception should be used until menses occurs
Monitoring of therapy	A Papanicolaou smear, other appropriate laboratory tests, and a physical examination (with special attention to breasts, abdomen, pelvic organs, and blood pressure) should be done before therapy and then repeated at least annually

WARNINGS/PRECAUTIONS

Cigarette smoking	Increases the risk of serious cardiovascular side effects, especially in women over 35 yr of age who smoke 15 or more cigarettes daily; patients who use oral contraceptives should be strongly urged not to smoke
Thromboembolic disease, thrombotic disorders, and other vascular problems	Risk is increased, becoming greater with age (after 30 yr of age) and with the amount of estrogen in the formulation; after use of oral contraceptives is discontinued, the risk may persist. Discontinue oral contraception immediately if early signs of thromboembolic disease or thrombotic disorders (eg, thrombophlebitis, pulmonary embolism, cerebrovascular insufficiency, coronary occlusion, or retinal or mesenteric thrombosis) develop or are suspected.
Postsurgical thromboembolic complications	Risk is increased 4–6 times; if feasible, discontinue oral contraception at least 4 wk before elective surgery associated with an increased risk of thromboembolism or prolonged immobilization
Ocular lesions, including optic neuritis and retinal thrombosis	May occur; discontinue oral contraception in the presence of unexplained gradual or sudden, partial or complete loss of vision; proptosis or diplopia; papilledema; or retinal vascular lesions
Carcinoma	Closely monitor patients with a strong family history of breast cancer or with breast nodules, fibrocystic disease, or abnormal mammograms; investigate all cases of undiagnosed persistent or recurrent abnormal vaginal bleeding for malignancy (see CONTRAINDICATIONS)
Hepatic lesions, including benign adenomas	May occur and possibly rupture, resulting in intraabdominal hemorrhage and death; investigate all cases of abdominal pain and tenderness, abdominal mass, or shock for hepatic adenoma. The risk reportedly increases among users of formulations with high hormonal potency, and with use of oral contraception for more than 4 yr.
Gallbladder disease	Risk increases with duration of oral contraception
Hepatic impairment	Use with caution due to poor steroid hormone metabolism
Jaundice	May recur in patients with a history of jaundice; discontinue oral contraception while cause is investigated
Glucose tolerance	May become impaired; closely monitor patients with latent or active diabetes
Hypertension	May be precipitated or may worsen with oral contraception, particularly with prolonged use, in older patients, and in patients with a history of hypertension during pregnancy
Migraine headache	May develop or worsen; discontinue oral contraception and investigate cause of recurrent, persistent, or severe headaches
Mental depression	Risk is increased; discontinue oral contraception if serious depression develops or recurs in patients with a history of depression
Fluid retention	May occur; use with caution in patients with convulsive disorders, migraine, asthma, or cardiac, hepatic, or renal dysfunction
Vitamin deficiencies	May occur, particularly of pyridoxine and folic acid
Spotting, breakthrough bleeding	Spotting or breakthrough bleeding may occur when tablets are missed or at other times during therapy; instruct the patient to continue the regimen, but bear in mind the possibility of organic disorder. If abnormal vaginal bleeding persists or recurs, adequate diagnostic measures are indicated to rule out pregnancy or malignancy. Assuming these are excluded, the problem may be corrected by the passage of time or use of another formulation. Preparations with a higher estrogen content should be used only if necessary because of the increased risk of thromboembolic disease.
Failure of withdrawal bleeding	If patient has not adhered to prescribed regimen, pregnancy should be considered after the first missed period and oral contraception withheld until pregnancy has been excluded; if patient has adhered to regimen and misses two consecutive periods, pregnancy should be ruled out before contraceptive regimen is reinstituted. Amenorrhea may occur during therapy and necessitate discontinuation of use.

OVCON

Postpill amenorrhea and anovulation	May occur, particularly in patients with a history of oligomenorrhea or secondary amenorrhea or in young women who have not established regular menstrual cycles; such patients should be encouraged to use alternative methods of contraception

ADVERSE REACTIONS

Frequent reactions (incidence ≥ 1%) are printed in *italics*

Genitourinary	*Breakthrough bleeding, spotting, menstrual irregularities, vaginal candidiasis,* postpill amenorrhea and infertility, dysmenorrhea, altered cervical erosion and secretion, enlargement of uterine leiomyomata, premenstrual-like syndrome, altered libido, cystitis-like syndrome, vaginitis
Cardiovascular	Thrombophlebitis, pulmonary embolism, coronary thrombosis, cerebral thrombosis, cerebral hemorrhage, hypertension, mesenteric thrombosis, edema
Gastrointestinal	*Nausea, vomiting,* gallbladder disease, abdominal cramps, bloating, change in appetite
Hepatic	Benign hepatomas, cholestatic jaundice
Metabolic and endocrinological	*Breast enlargement, tenderness, and/or secretion;* carbohydrate intolerance; increase or decrease in weight; hyperlipidemia
Central nervous system and neuromuscular	Migraine, depression, headache, nervousness, dizziness, chorea
Ophthalmic	Optic neuritis, retinal thrombosis, intolerance to contact lenses, altered corneal curvature, cataracts
Allergic and dermatological	Rash, melasma or chloasma, erythema multiforme, erythema nodosum, hirsutism, hair loss, hemorrhagic eruption, porphyria
Other	Congenital anomalies

OVERDOSAGE

Signs and symptoms	Nausea, withdrawal bleeding; acute ingestion of large doses by young children has not been associated with serious ill effects
Treatment	Treat symptomatically

DRUG INTERACTIONS

Ampicillin, analgesics, antianxiety agents, antimigraine preparations, barbiturates, chloramphenicol, isoniazid, neomycin, nitrofurantoin, penicillin V, phenylbutazone, phenytoin, primidone, rifampin, sulfonamides, tetracycline	▽ Contraceptive effect △ Breakthrough bleeding
Antihypertensive agents (eg, guanethidine)	▽ Antihypertensive effect
Oral anticoagulants	▽ Anticoagulant effect
Anticonvulsants	△ Seizure activity
Hypoglycemic agents	▽ Glucose tolerance
Corticosteroids	△ Corticosteroid effects
Tricyclic antidepressants	△ Antidepressant side effects

ALTERED LABORATORY VALUES

Blood/serum values	△ Alkaline phosphatase △ Bilirubin △ Sulfobromophthalein retention △ Prothrombin △ Clotting factors VII, VIII, IX, and X ▽ Antithrombin III △ PBI △ Thyroxine (T_4) ▽ Triiodothyronine (T_3) uptake △ Glucose △ Cortisol △ Transcortin △ Ceruloplasmin △ Triglycerides △ Phopholipids ▽ Folic acid ▽ Pyridoxine
Urinary values	▽ Pregnanediol

USE IN CHILDREN

Not indicated before puberty

USE IN PREGNANT AND NURSING WOMEN

Pregnancy Category X: contraindicated if pregnancy is known or suspected, as serious fetal damage may occur during pregnancy. Patient should discontinue oral contraception 3 mo before attempting to conceive. Postpartum use may interfere with lactation, causing a decrease in the quantity and quality of breast milk. Patient should use alternative form of contraception until infant is weaned.

OVRAL

CONTRACEPTIVES

OVRAL (norgestrel and ethinyl estradiol) Wyeth — Rx
Tablets: 0.5 mg norgestrel and 50 µg ethinyl estradiol *21-day regimen*

OVRAL-28 (norgestrel and ethinyl estradiol) Wyeth — Rx
Tablets: 0.5 mg norgestrel and 50 µg ethinyl estradiol *28-day regimen*

INDICATIONS	ORAL DOSAGE
Contraception	Adult: 1 tab q24h for 21 or 28 consecutive days of the menstrual cycle

CONTRAINDICATIONS

Thrombophlebitis or thromboembolic disorders	Known or suspected breast cancer	Known or suspected pregnancy
Past history of deep-vein thrombophlebitis or thromboembolic disorders	Known or suspected estrogen-dependent neoplasia	Benign or malignant liver tumor that developed during the use of oral contraceptives or other estrogen-containing products
Coronary artery disease	Undiagnosed abnormal genital bleeding	
Cerebrovascular disease		

ADMINISTRATION/DOSAGE ADJUSTMENTS

Initiating therapy	First tablet should be taken on the 5th day (Ovral) or 1st Sunday (Ovral-28) after the onset of menses; if menses begins on a Sunday, regimen is started the very same day
Subsequent cycles (21-day regimen)	First tablet is taken 8 days after last tablet was taken in preceding cycle
Subsequent cycles (28-day regimen)	First tablet is taken 1 day after last (placebo) tablet was taken in preceding cycle
Missed tablets	If one or two tablets are missed, they should be taken as soon as they are remembered, and an additional form of contraception should be used for 1 wk. If three tablets are missed, the tablet cycle should be discontinued; start the next tablet cycle 8 days after the last tablet was taken (Ovral) or on the first Sunday after the last tablet was taken (Ovral-28), and instruct patient to use another form of contraception for the days without tablets and until seven tablets are taken.
Postpartum administration	For nonnursing mothers, may be started either immediately or after first postpartum examination, regardless of whether spontaneous menstruation has occurred

WARNINGS/PRECAUTIONS

Cigarette smoking	Increases the risk of serious cardiovascular side effects, especially in women over 35 yr of age who smoke 15 or more cigarettes daily; patients who use oral contraceptives should be strongly urged not to smoke
Thromboembolic disease, thrombotic disorders, and other vascular problems	Risk is increased, becoming greater with age (after 30 yr of age) and with the amount of estrogen present in the formulation; after discontinuation of use, the risk of cerebrovascular disease and myocardial infarction may persist. Discontinue oral contraception immediately if early signs of thromboembolic disease or thrombotic disorders (eg, thrombophlebitis, pulmonary embolism, cerebrovascular insufficiency, coronary occlusion, or retinal or mesenteric thrombosis) develop or are suspected.
Postsurgical thromboembolic complications	Risk is increased 4–6 times; if feasible, discontinue oral contraception at least 4 wk before elective surgery associated with an increased risk of thromboembolism or prolonged immobilization
Ocular lesions, including optic neuritis and retinal thrombosis	May occur; discontinue oral contraception in the presence of unexplained gradual or sudden, partial or complete loss of vision; proptosis or diplopia; papilledema; or retinal vascular lesions
Carcinoma	Closely monitor patients with a strong family history of breast cancer or with breast nodules, fibrocystic disease, or abnormal mammograms; investigate all cases of undiagnosed persistent or recurrent abnormal vaginal bleeding for malignancy (see CONTRAINDICATIONS)
Hepatic tumors, including benign adenomas	May occur and possibly rupture, resulting in intraabdominal hemorrhage and death; investigate all cases of abdominal pain and tenderness, abdominal mass, or shock for hepatic adenoma. The risk reportedly increases among users of formulations with high hormonal potency, and with use of oral contraception for more than 4 yr.
Gallbladder disease	Risk increases with duration of oral contraception
Hepatic impairment	Use with caution due to poor steroid hormone metabolism
Jaundice	May recur in patients with a history of jaundice; discontinue oral contraception while cause is investigated
Glucose tolerance	May become impaired; closely monitor patients with latent or active diabetes
Hypertension	May be precipitated or may worsen with oral contraception, particularly with prolonged use, in older patients, and in patients with a history of hypertension during pregnancy

COMPENDIUM OF DRUG THERAPY

OVRAL

Migraine headache	May develop or worsen; discontinue oral contraception and investigate cause of recurrent, persistent, or severe headaches
Mental depression	Risk is increased; discontinue oral contraception if serious depression develops or recurs in patients with a history of depression
Fluid retention	May occur; use with caution in patients with convulsive disorders, migraine, asthma, or cardiac, hepatic, or renal dysfunction
Vitamin deficiencies	May occur, particularly of pyridoxine and folic acid
Spotting, breakthrough bleeding	Spotting or breakthrough bleeding may occur when tablets are missed or at other times during therapy; instruct the patient to continue the regimen, but bear in mind the possibility of organic disorder. If abnormal vaginal bleeding persists or recurs, adequate diagnostic measures are indicated to rule out pregnancy or malignancy. Assuming these are excluded, the problem may be corrected by the passage of time or use of another formulation. Preparations with a higher estrogen content should be used only if necessary because of the increased risk of thromboembolic disease.
Failure of withdrawal bleeding	If patient has missed two consecutive periods, pregnancy should be ruled out before contraceptive regimen is continued; if patient has not adhered to prescribed regimen, pregnancy should be considered after the first missed period and oral contraception withheld until pregnancy has been excluded. Amenorrhea may occur during therapy and necessitate discontinuation of use.
Postpill amenorrhea and anovulation	May occur, particularly in patients with a history of oligomenorrhea or secondary amenorrhea or in young women who have not established regular menstrual cycles; such patients should be encouraged to use alternative methods of contraception

ADVERSE REACTIONS

Frequent reactions (incidence ≥ 1%) are printed in *italics*

Genitourinary	*Breakthrough bleeding, spotting, menstrual irregularities, vaginal candidiasis,* postpill amenorrhea and infertility, dysmenorrhea, altered cervical erosion and secretion, enlargement of uterine leiomyomata, premenstrual-like syndrome, altered libido, cystitis-like syndrome, vaginitis
Cardiovascular	Thrombophlebitis, pulmonary embolism, coronary thrombosis, cerebral thrombosis, cerebral hemorrhage, hypertension, mesenteric thrombosis, edema
Gastrointestinal	*Nausea, vomiting,* gallbladder disease, abdominal cramps, bloating, change in appetite
Hepatic	Benign hepatomas, cholestatic jaundice
Metabolic and endocrinological	*Breast enlargement, tenderness, and/or secretion;* carbohydrate intolerance; increase or decrease in weight; hyperlipidemia
Central nervous system and neuromuscular	Migraine, depression, anxiety, headache, nervousness, dizziness, chorea
Ophthalmic	Optic neuritis, retinal thrombosis, intolerance to contact lenses, altered corneal curvature, cataracts
Allergic and dermatological	Rash, melasma or chloasma, erythema multiforme, erythema nodosum, hirsutism, hair loss, hemorrhagic eruption, porphyria
Other	Congenital anomalies, hemolytic uremic syndrome

OVERDOSAGE

Signs and symptoms	Nausea, withdrawal bleeding; acute ingestion of large doses by young children has not been associated with serious ill effects
Treatment	Treat symptomatically

DRUG INTERACTIONS

Ampicillin, analgesics, antianxiety agents, antimigraine preparations, barbiturates, chloramphenicol, isoniazid, neomycin, nitrofurantoin, penicillin V, phenylbutazone, phenytoin, primidone, rifampin, sulfonamides, tetracycline	▽ Contraceptive effect △ Breakthrough bleeding
Antihypertensive agents (eg, guanethidine)	▽ Antihypertensive effect
Oral anticoagulants	▽ Anticoagulant effect
Anticonvulsants	△ Seizure activity
Hypoglycemic agents	▽ Glucose tolerance
Corticosteroids	△ Corticosteroid effects
Tricyclic antidepressants	△ Antidepressant side effects

ALTERED LABORATORY VALUES

Blood/serum values — △ Alkaline phosphatase △ Bilirubin △ Sulfobromophthalein retention △ Prothrombin △ Clotting factors VII, VIII, IX, and X ▽ Antithrombin III △ PBI △ Thyroxine (T_4) ▽ Triiodothyronine (T_3) uptake △ Glucose △ Cortisol △ Transcortin △ Ceruloplasmin △ Triglycerides △ Phospholipids ▽ Folic acid ▽ Pyridoxine

Urinary values — ▽ Pregnanediol

USE IN CHILDREN
Not indicated before puberty

USE IN PREGNANT AND NURSING WOMEN
Pregnancy Category X: contraindicated if pregnancy is known or suspected, as serious fetal damage may occur during early pregnancy. Patient should discontinue oral contraception 3 mo before attempting to conceive. Postpartum use may interfere with lactation, causing a decrease in the quantity and quality of breast milk. Patient should use alternative form of contraception until infant is weaned.

CONTRACEPTIVES

OVULEN-21 (ethynodiol diacetate and mestranol) Searle — Rx
Tablets: 1 mg ethynodiol diacetate and 100 µg mestranol *21-day regimen*

OVULEN-28 (ethynodiol diacetate and mestranol) Searle — Rx
Tablets: 1 mg ethynodiol diacetate and 100 µg mestranol *28-day regimen*

INDICATIONS	ORAL DOSAGE
Contraception	Adult: 1 tab q24h for 21 or 28 consecutive days of the menstrual cycle

CONTRAINDICATIONS

- Thrombophlebitis or thromboembolic disorders
- Past history of deep-vein thrombophlebitis or thromboembolic disorders
- Past or present myocardial infarction
- Past or present coronary artery disease
- Past or present cerebrovascular disease
- Known or suspected breast cancer
- Known or suspected estrogen-dependent neoplasia
- Undiagnosed abnormal genital bleeding
- Known or suspected pregnancy
- Past or present benign or malignant liver tumors that developed during the use of oral contraceptives or other estrogen-containing products

ADMINISTRATION/DOSAGE ADJUSTMENTS

Initiating therapy — First tablet should be taken on the 5th day (Ovulen-21) or 1st Sunday (Ovulen-28) after the onset of menses; if menses begins on a Sunday, regimen is started the very same day. An additional form of contraception should be used during the 1st week of the initial cycle.

Subsequent cycles (21-day regimen) — First tablet is taken 8 days after last tablet was taken in preceding cycle

Subsequent cycles (28-day regimen) — First tablet is taken 1 day after last (placebo) tablet was taken in preceding cycle

Missed tablets — If one tablet is missed, it should be taken as soon as it is remembered, with the next tablet taken at the usual time. If two tablets are missed, the dosage should be doubled for the next 2 days. The remaining tablets should be taken as usual, but an additional form of contraception should be used for the remainder of the cycle.

Postpartum administration — For nonnursing mothers, may be started (1) immediately after delivery, (2) on first Sunday after delivery, (3) when patient leaves hospital, or (4) after first postpartum examination, regardless of whether spontaneous menstruation has occurred; bear in mind that the risk of thromboembolism is increased during the postpartum period

WARNINGS/PRECAUTIONS

Cigarette smoking — Increases the risk of serious cardiovascular side effects, especially in women over 35 yr of age who smoke 15 or more cigarettes daily; patients who use oral contraceptives should be strongly urged not to smoke

Thromboembolic disease, thrombotic disorders, and other vascular problems — Risk is increased, becoming greater with age in women who use oral contraceptives after age 30 and with the amount of estrogen and possibly also of progestin present in the formulation; after use of oral contraceptives is discontinued, the risk may persist. Discontinue oral contraception immediately if early signs of thromboembolic disease or thrombotic disorders (eg, thrombophlebitis, pulmonary embolism, arterial thromboembolism, Raynaud's disease, cerebrovascular insufficiency, coronary artery disease, myocardial infarction, or retinal or mesenteric thrombosis) develop or are suspected. The presence of varicose veins may substantially increase the risk of superficial venous thrombosis of the leg.

Postsurgical thromboembolic complications	Risk is increased 4–6 times; if feasible, discontinue oral contraception at least 4 wk before elective surgery or during periods of anticipated prolonged immobilization
Ocular lesions, including optic neuritis and retinal thrombosis	May occur; discontinue oral contraception in the presence of unexplained gradual or sudden, partial or complete loss of vision; proptosis or diplopia; papilledema; or retinal vascular lesions
Carcinoma	Hepatocellular carcinoma has been reported; it is estimated that the risk is increased 7–20 times for women who have used oral contraceptives for 8 or more years. Although several studies have found no overall increase in breast cancer in women taking estrogens or oral contraceptives, the risk may be increased when such use is associated with other risk factors, including benign breast disease (eg, cysts), long-term administration (2–4 yr), prior breast biopsy, family history of breast cancer, or delay in having a first child; closely monitor patients with a strong family history of breast cancer or with breast nodules, fibrocystic disease, recurrent cystic mastitis, abnormal mammograms, or cervical dysplasia. Investigate all cases of undiagnosed persistent or recurrent abnormal vaginal bleeding for malignancy (see CONTRAINDICATIONS).
Hepatic lesions, including benign adenomas	May occur and possibly rupture, resulting in intraabdominal hemorrhage and death; investigate all cases of abdominal pain and tenderness, abdominal mass, or shock for hepatic lesions. The risk of hepatocellular adenoma reportedly increases in women over 30, among users of formulations with high hormonal potency, and with use of oral contraception for more than 4 yr (estimated annual incidence, 3–4/100,000).
Gallbladder disease	Risk increases with duration of oral contraception
Hepatic impairment	Use with caution due to poor steroid hormone metabolism (see CONTRAINDICATIONS)
Jaundice	May recur in patients with a history of jaundice; discontinue oral contraception while cause is investigated. Cholestatic jaundice has been reported after combined use of oral contraceptives and troleandomycin.
Glucose tolerance	May become impaired; closely monitor patients with latent or active diabetes
Hypertension	May be precipitated or may worsen with oral contraception, particularly with prolonged use, and in older patients. Closely monitor patients with a history of hypertension, toxemia, hypertension during pregnancy, or excessive weight gain or fluid retention during the menstrual cycle; preexisting renal disease; or a family history of hypertension or hypertensive complications.
Migraine headache	May develop or worsen; discontinue oral contraception and investigate cause of recurrent, persistent, or severe headaches
Mental depression	Risk is increased; discontinue oral contraception if serious depression develops or recurs in patients with a history of depression
Fluid retention	May occur; use with caution in patients with convulsive disorders, migraine, asthma, or cardiac, hepatic, or renal dysfunction
Vitamin deficiencies	May occur, particularly of pyridoxine and folic acid
Spotting, breakthrough bleeding	Spotting and breakthrough bleeding are most likely to occur during the initial cycle and when tablets are missed (particularly if two or more tablets are missed); instruct the patient to continue the regimen, but bear in mind the possibility of organic disorder. If abnormal vaginal bleeding persists or recurs, adequate diagnostic measures are indicated to rule out pregnancy and malignancy. Assuming these are excluded, the problem may be corrected by the passage of time or use of another formulation. Preparations with a higher estrogen content should be used only if necessary because of the increased risk of thromboembolic disease.
Failure of withdrawal bleeding	If patient has not adhered to prescribed regimen, pregnancy should be considered after the first missed period and oral contraception withheld until pregnancy has been excluded; if patient has adhered to regimen and misses two consecutive periods, pregnancy should be ruled out before contraceptive regimen is reinstituted. Amenorrhea may occur during therapy and necessitate discontinuation of use.
Amenorrhea and impaired fertility	After oral contraception has been discontinued, amenorrhea and adverse effects on fertility can occur; amenorrhea may be accompanied by galactorrhea and development of a pituitary tumor. Fertility may be impaired for up to 2.5 yr in parous women aged 25–34 yr and for up to 4 yr in nulliparous women aged 25–29 yr; in nulliparous women aged 30–34 yr, impairment may be evident for up to 6 yr, especially following use of oral contraceptives for 2 or more years. Patients with a history of oligomenorrhea or secondary amenorrhea and young women who have not established regular cycles may tend to remain anovulatory or become amenorrheic following termination of oral contraceptive use and, therefore, should be encouraged to use alternative methods of contraception.
Protection against PID	*Chlamydia trachomatis* appears more frequently in the cervix when women use oral contraceptives; it should not be assumed that these preparations afford protection against pelvic inflammatory disease due to *Chlamydia*
Endocrine and liver-function tests	May be affected (see ALTERED LABORATORY VALUES); repeat any abnormal tests 2 mo after oral contraception is discontinued

OVULEN

Mutagenicity	An increase in lymphocytic chromosomal aberrations has been seen in women receiving oral contraceptives

ADVERSE REACTIONS

Frequent reactions (incidence ≥ 1%) are printed in *italics*

Genitourinary	*Breakthrough bleeding, spotting, menstrual irregularities, vaginal candidiasis,* postpill amenorrhea and infertility, dysmenorrhea, altered cervical erosion and secretion, endocervical hyperplasia, enlargement of uterine leiomyomata, premenstrual-like syndrome, altered libido, cystitis-like syndrome, vaginitis
Cardiovascular	Thrombophlebitis, thrombosis, pulmonary embolism, arterial thromboembolism, Raynaud's disease, myocardial infarction, coronary thrombosis, premature ventricular contractions, thrombotic thrombocytopenic purpura, cerebral thrombosis, cerebral hemorrhage, hypertension (including malignant and pulmonary hypertension), mesenteric thrombosis, edema
Gastrointestinal	*Nausea, vomiting,* gallbladder disease, abdominal cramps, bloating, change in appetite, pancreatitis, colitis, Crohn's disease
Hepatic	Hepatocellular carcinoma, benign adenomas and other hepatic lesions, Budd-Chiari syndrome, cholestatic jaundice, hepatitis
Renal	Impaired renal function, hemolytic uremic syndrome, acute renal failure (sometimes irreversible)
Metabolic and endocrinological	*Breast enlargement, tenderness, and/or secretion;* carbohydrate intolerance; increase or decrease in weight; hyperlipidemia
Central nervous system and neuromuscular	Migraine, depression, headache, nervousness, dizziness, chorea, paresthesia, auditory disturbances, fatigue
Ophthalmic	Optic neuritis, retinal thrombosis, intolerance to contact lenses, altered corneal curvature, cataracts
Allergic and dermatological	Melasma or chloasma, rash, itching, rhinitis, erythema multiforme, erythema nodosum, hirsutism, hair loss, hemorrhagic eruption, porphyria, malignant melanoma, herpes gestationis
Other	Congenital anomalies, prolactin-secreting pituitary tumors, backache, anemia, lupus erythematosus, rheumatoid arthritis, gingivitis, dry socket; endometrial, cervical, and breast carcinoma

OVERDOSAGE

Signs and symptoms	Nausea, withdrawal bleeding; acute ingestion of large doses by young children has not been associated with serious ill effects
Treatment	Treat symptomatically

DRUG INTERACTIONS

Ampicillin, analgesics, antianxiety agents, antimigraine preparations, barbiturates, chloramphenicol, griseofulvin, isoniazid, neomycin, nitrofurantoin, penicillin V, phenylbutazone, phenytoin, primidone, rifampin, sulfonamides, tetracycline	▽ Contraceptive effect △ Breakthrough bleeding
Antihypertensive agents (eg, guanethidine)	▽ Antihypertensive effect
Oral anticoagulants	▽ Anticoagulant effect
Anticonvulsants	△ Seizure activity
Hypoglycemic agents	▽ Glucose tolerance
Corticosteroids	△ Corticosteroid effects
Tricyclic antidepressants	△ Antidepressant side effects
Diazepam, chlordiazepoxide	△ Serum half-life of benzodiazepines
Troleandomycin	Cholestatic jaundice
Cyclosporine	Hepatotoxicity
Acetaminophen	▽ Serum half-life of acetaminophen
Clofibrate	▽ Hypolipidemic effect
Theophylline	△ Serum half-life of theophylline

ALTERED LABORATORY VALUES

Blood/serum values	△ Alkaline phosphatase △ Bilirubin △ Sulfobromophthalein retention △ Prothrombin △ Clotting factors VII, VIII, IX, and X ▽ Antithrombin III △ PBI △ Thyroxine (T_4) ▽ Triiodothyronine (T_3) uptake △ Glucose △ Cortisol △ Transcortin △ Ceruloplasmin △ Triglycerides △ Phospholipids ▽ Folic acid ▽ Pyridoxine

OVULEN ■ TRI-LEVLEN

Urinary values —————————— ▽ Pregnanediol

USE IN CHILDREN
Not indicated before puberty

USE IN PREGNANT AND NURSING WOMEN
Pregnancy Category X: contraindicated if pregnancy is known or suspected, as serious fetal damage may occur during early pregnancy. Patient should discontinue oral contraception 3 mo before attempting to conceive. Postpartum use may interfere with lactation, causing a decrease in the quantity and quality of breast milk. Patient should use alternative form of contraception until infant is weaned.

CONTRACEPTIVES

TRI-LEVLEN 21 (levonorgestrel and ethinyl estradiol) Berlex   Rx

Tablets (per dispenser): 6 brown tablets containing 0.050 mg levonorgestrel and 30 µg ethinyl estradiol, 5 white tablets containing 0.075 mg levonorgestrel and 40 µg ethinyl estradiol, and 10 light-yellow tablets containing 0.125 mg levonorgestrel and 30 µg ethinyl estradiol *21-day regimen*

TRI-LEVLEN 28 (levonorgestrel and ethinyl estradiol) Berlex   Rx

Tablets (per dispenser): 6 brown tablets containing 0.050 mg levonorgestrel and 30 µg ethinyl estradiol, 5 white tablets containing 0.075 mg levonorgestrel and 40 µg ethinyl estradiol, 10 light-yellow tablets containing 0.125 mg levonorgestrel and 30 µg ethinyl estradiol, and 7 light-green tablets containing inert ingredients *28-day regimen*

INDICATIONS	**ORAL DOSAGE**
Contraception	**Adult:** 1 brown tablet q24h for 6 days, followed successively by 1 white tablet q24h for 5 days, 1 light-yellow tablet q24h for 10 days, and either no tablets for 7 days (21-day regimen) or 1 light-green tablet q24h for 7 days (28-day regimen); tablets should preferably be taken after the evening meal or at bedtime

CONTRAINDICATIONS

Thrombophlebitis or thromboembolic disorders	Known or suspected breast cancer	Known or suspected pregnancy
Past history of deep-vein thrombophlebitis or thromboembolic disorders	Known or suspected estrogen-dependent neoplasia	Benign or malignant liver tumor that developed during the use of oral contraceptives or other estrogen-containing products
Coronary artery disease	Undiagnosed abnormal genital bleeding	
Cerebrovascular disease		

ADMINISTRATION/DOSAGE ADJUSTMENTS

Initiating therapy	First tablet should be taken on the first day of the menstrual cycle or, after discontinuation of another oral contraceptive, on the first day of withdrawal bleeding. For postpartum use, the regimen should be started immediately or at the first postpartum examination, regardless of whether spontaneous menstruation has occurred. If the tablets are taken either later than the first day of menstrual bleeding or postpartum, an additional form of contraception should be used for the first week.
Subsequent cycles (21-day regimen)	First brown tablet is taken 8 days after the last light-yellow tablet was taken in the preceding cycle
Subsequent cycles (28-day regimen)	First brown tablet is taken the day after the last light-green tablet was taken in the preceding cycle
Missed tablets	If one or two tablets are missed, they should be taken as soon as they are remembered, and an additional form of contraception should be used for 1 wk. If three tablets are missed, medication should be discontinued until the first day of withdrawal bleeding, at which time a new cycle should be started; another form of contraception should be used for the period without tablets and for the first week after resumption of use.
Monitoring of therapy	A Papanicolaou smear, other appropriate laboratory tests, and a physical examination (with special attention to breasts, abdomen, pelvic organs, and blood pressure) should be done before therapy and then repeated at least annually

WARNINGS/PRECAUTIONS

Cigarette smoking	Increases the risk of serious cardiovascular side effects, especially in women over 35 yr of age who smoke 15 or more cigarettes daily; patients who use oral contraceptives should be strongly urged not to smoke

TRI-LEVLEN

Thromboembolic disease, thrombotic disorders, and other vascular problems	Risk is increased, becoming greater with age (after 30 yr of age) and with the amount of estrogen present in the formulation; after discontinuation of use, the risk of cerebrovascular disease and myocardial infarction may persist. Discontinue oral contraception immediately if early signs of thromboembolic disease or thrombotic disorders (eg, thrombophlebitis, pulmonary embolism, cerebrovascular insufficiency, coronary occlusion, or retinal or mesenteric thrombosis) develop or are suspected.
Postsurgical thromboembolic complications	Risk is increased 4–6 times; if feasible, discontinue oral contraception at least 4 wk before elective surgery associated with an increased risk of thromboembolism or prolonged immobilization
Ocular lesions, including optic neuritis and retinal thrombosis	May occur; discontinue oral contraception in the presence of unexplained gradual or sudden, partial or complete loss of vision; proptosis or diplopia; papilledema; or retinal vascular lesions
Carcinoma	Closely monitor patients with a strong family history of breast cancer or with breast nodules, fibrocystic disease, or abnormal mammograms; investigate all cases of undiagnosed persistent or recurrent abnormal vaginal bleeding for malignancy (see CONTRAINDICATIONS)
Hepatic tumors, including benign adenomas	May occur and possibly rupture, resulting in intraabdominal hemorrhage and death; investigate all cases of abdominal pain and tenderness, abdominal mass, or shock for hepatic adenoma. The risk reportedly increases among users of formulations with high hormonal potency, and with use of oral contraception for more than 4 yr.
Gallbladder disease	Risk increases with duration of oral contraception
Hepatic impairment	Use with caution due to poor steroid hormone metabolism
Jaundice	May recur in patients with a history of jaundice; discontinue oral contraception while cause is investigated
Glucose tolerance	May become impaired; closely monitor patients with latent or active diabetes
Lipid metabolism	An increase in serum triglycerides and total phospholipids has been observed in women taking oral contraceptives; however, three studies performed with this formulation have shown no significant change in lipid metabolism, except for a slight increase in triglyceride levels in one study. The clinical significance of these findings has not been defined.
Hypertension	May be precipitated or may worsen with oral contraception, particularly with prolonged use, in older patients, and in patients with a history of hypertension during pregnancy
Migraine headache	May develop or worsen; discontinue oral contraception and investigate cause of recurrent, persistent, or severe headaches
Mental depression	Risk is increased; discontinue oral contraception if serious depression develops or recurs in patients with a history of depression
Fluid retention	May occur; use with caution in patients with convulsive disorders, migraine, asthma, or cardiac, hepatic, or renal dysfunction
Vitamin deficiencies	May occur, particularly of pyridoxine and folic acid
Spotting, breakthrough bleeding	Spotting or breakthrough bleeding may occur when tablets are missed or at other times during therapy; instruct the patient to continue the regimen, but bear in mind the possibility of organic disorder. If abnormal vaginal bleeding persists or recurs, adequate diagnostic measures are indicated to rule out pregnancy or malignancy. Assuming these are excluded, the problem can be corrected by the passage of time or use of another formulation. Preparations with a higher estrogen content should be used only if necessary because of the increased risk of thromboembolic disease.
Failure of withdrawal bleeding	If patient has missed two consecutive periods, pregnancy should be ruled out before contraceptive regimen is continued; if patient has not adhered to prescribed regimen, pregnancy should be considered after the first missed period and oral contraception withheld until pregnancy has been excluded. Amenorrhea may occur during therapy and necessitate discontinuation of use.
Postpill amenorrhea and anovulation	May occur, particularly in patients with a history of oligomenorrhea or secondary amenorrhea or in young women who have not established regular menstrual cycles; such patients should be encouraged to use alternative methods of contraception
ADVERSE REACTIONS	Frequent reactions (incidence $\geq$ 1%) are printed in *italics*
Genitourinary	*Breakthrough bleeding, spotting, menstrual irregularities, vaginal candidiasis,* postpill amenorrhea and infertility, dysmenorrhea, altered cervical erosion and secretion, enlargement of uterine leiomyomata, premenstrual-like syndrome, altered libido, cystitis-like syndrome, vaginitis
Cardiovascular	Thrombophlebitis, pulmonary embolism, coronary thrombosis, cerebral thrombosis, cerebral hemorrhage, hypertension, mesenteric thrombosis, edema
Gastrointestinal	*Nausea, vomiting,* gallbladder disease, abdominal cramps, bloating, change in appetite
Hepatic	Benign hepatomas, cholestatic jaundice

TRI-LEVLEN ■ TRI-NORINYL

Metabolic and endocrinological	*Breast enlargement, tenderness, and/or secretion;* carbohydrate intolerance; increase or decrease in weight; hyperlipidemia
Central nervous system and neuromuscular	Migraine, depression, anxiety, headache, nervousness, dizziness, chorea
Ophthalmic	Optic neuritis, retinal thrombosis, intolerance to contact lenses, altered corneal curvature, cataracts
Allergic and dermatological	Rash, melasma or chloasma, erythema multiforme, erythema nodosum, hirsutism, hair loss, hemorrhagic eruption, porphyria
Other	Congenital anomalies, hemolytic uremic syndrome

OVERDOSAGE

Signs and symptoms	Nausea, withdrawal bleeding; acute ingestion of large doses by young children has not been associated with serious ill effects
Treatment	Treat symptomatically

DRUG INTERACTIONS

Ampicillin, analgesics, antianxiety agents, antimigraine preparations, barbiturates, chloramphenicol, isoniazid, neomycin, nitrofurantoin, penicillin V, phenylbutazone, phenytoin, primidone, rifampin, sulfonamides, tetracycline	▽ Contraceptive effect △ Breakthrough bleeding
Antihypertensive agents (eg, guanethidine)	▽ Antihypertensive effect
Oral anticoagulants	▽ Anticoagulant effect
Anticonvulsants	△ Seizure activity
Hypoglycemic agents	▽ Glucose tolerance
Corticosteroids	△ Corticosteroid effects
Tricyclic antidepressants	△ Antidepressant side effects

ALTERED LABORATORY VALUES

Blood/serum values	△ Alkaline phosphatase △ Bilirubin △ Sulfobromophthalein retention △ Prothrombin △ Clotting factors VII, VIII, IX, and X ▽ Antithrombin III △ PBI △ Thyroxine (T_4) ▽ Triiodothyronine (T_3) uptake △ Glucose △ Cortisol △ Transcortin △ Ceruloplasmin ▽ Folic acid ▽ Pyridoxine
Urinary values	▽ Pregnanediol

USE IN CHILDREN

Not indicated before puberty

USE IN PREGNANT AND NURSING WOMEN

Pregnancy Category X: contraindicated if pregnancy is known or suspected, as serious fetal damage may occur during early pregnancy. Patient should discontinue oral contraception 3 mo before attempting to conceive. Postpartum use may interfere with lactation, causing a decrease in the quantity and quality of breast milk. Patient should use an alternative form of contraception until infant is weaned.

CONTRACEPTIVES

TRI-NORINYL 21-DAY (norethindrone and ethinyl estradiol) Syntex   Rx

Tablets (per dispenser): 12 blue tablets containing 0.5 mg norethindrone and 35 μg ethinyl estradiol and 9 green tablets containing 1 mg norethindrone and 35 μg ethinyl estradiol *21-day regimen*

TRI-NORINYL 28-DAY (norethindrone and ethinyl estradiol) Syntex   Rx

Tablets (per dispenser): 12 blue tablets containing 0.5 mg norethindrone and 35 μg ethinyl estradiol, 9 green tablets containing 1 mg norethindrone and 35 μg ethinyl estradiol, and 7 orange tablets containing inert ingredients *28-day regimen*

INDICATIONS	ORAL DOSAGE
Contraception	**Adult:** 1 blue tablet q24h for 7 days, followed successively by 1 green tablet q24h for 9 days, 1 blue tablet q24h for 5 days, and either no tablets for 7 days (21-day regimen) or 7 orange tablets q24h for 7 days (28-day regimen); tablets should be taken at bedtime

TRI-NORINYL

CONTRAINDICATIONS

Thrombophlebitis or thromboembolic disorders	Past or present coronary artery disease, including myocardial infarction	Undiagnosed abnormal genital bleeding
Past history of deep-vein thrombophlebitis or thromboembolic disorders	Past or present known or suspected breast cancer	Past or present benign or malignant hepatic tumor that developed during the use of oral contraceptives or other estrogen-containing products
Past or present cerebrovascular disease	Past or present known or suspected estrogen-dependent neoplasia	Known or suspected pregnancy

ADMINISTRATION/DOSAGE ADJUSTMENTS

Initiating therapy	First tablet should be taken on the first Sunday after the onset of menses or, if menses begins on a Sunday, on that very day. An additional form of contraception should be used during the first week of the initial cycle. Instruct postpartum patients not to initiate oral contraceptive therapy earlier than 2 wk after delivery; patients may start oral contraception immediately after an aborted pregnancy of less than 12 wk gestation, but should not start until 2 wk after an aborted pregnancy of 12 wk gestation or longer.
Subsequent cycles (21-day regimen)	First tablet is taken 8 days after the last tablet was taken in the preceding cycle
Subsequent cycles (28-day regimen)	First tablet is taken 1 day after the last orange tablet was taken in the preceding cycle
Missed tablets	If one tablet is missed, it should be taken as soon as it is remembered, with the next tablet taken at the usual time. If two tablets are missed, one of them should be taken as soon as remembered and the other discarded. The remaining tablets should be taken as usual, but an additional form of contraception should be used for the remainder of the cycle. If three or more tablets in a row are missed, the tablet cycle should be discontinued immediately and another form of contraception used until menses has appeared or pregnancy has been excluded.

WARNINGS/PRECAUTIONS

Cigarette smoking	Increases the risk of serious cardiovascular side effects, especially in women over 35 yr of age who smoke 15 or more cigarettes daily; patients who use oral contraceptives should be strongly urged not to smoke
Thromboembolic disease, thrombotic disorders, and other vascular problems	Risk is increased, becoming greater with age (after 30 yr of age) and with the amount of estrogen in the formulation; after use of oral contraceptives is discontinued, the risk of cerebrovascular disease, myocardial infarction, and subarachnoid hemorrhage may persist. Discontinue oral contraception immediately if early signs of thromboembolic disease or thrombotic disorders (eg, thrombophlebitis, pulmonary embolism, cerebrovascular insufficiency, coronary occlusion, or retinal or mesenteric thrombosis) develop or are suspected. The presence of varicose veins may substantially increase the risk of superficial venous thrombosis of the leg.
Postsurgical thromboembolic complications	Risk is increased 4-6 times; if feasible, discontinue oral contraception at least 4 wk before elective surgery associated with an increased risk of thromboembolism or prolonged immobilization
Ocular lesions, including optic neuritis and retinal thrombosis	May occur; discontinue oral contraception in the presence of unexplained gradual or sudden, partial or complete loss of vision; proptosis or diplopia; papilledema; or retinal vascular lesions
Carcinoma	Although several studies have found no overall increase of breast cancer in women taking estrogens or oral contraceptives, the risk may be increased when such use is associated with other risk factors, including benign breast disease (eg, cysts); long-term administration (2-4 yr), particularly in patients under 25 yr of age; prior breast biopsy, or a family history of breast cancer. Closely monitor patients with a strong family history of breast cancer or with breast nodules, fibrocystic disease, or abnormal mammograms. Studies suggest that there is an increased risk of cervical neoplasms associated with longer duration of oral contraceptive use. Investigate all cases of undiagnosed persistent or recurrent abnormal vaginal bleeding for malignancy (see CONTRAINDICATIONS).
Hepatic tumors	May occur and possibly rupture, resulting in intraabdominal hemorrhage and death; investigate all cases of abdominal pain and tenderness, right upper quadrant mass, or shock for liver tumors. The risk of hepatocellular adenoma reportedly increases in women over 30, among users of formulations with high hormonal potency, and with use of oral contraception for more than 4 yr (estimated annual incidence, 3-4/100,000).
Gallbladder disease	Risk increases with duration of oral contraception
Hepatic impairment	Use with caution due to poor steroid hormone metabolism (see CONTRAINDICATIONS)
Jaundice	May recur in patients with a history of jaundice; discontinue oral contraception while cause is investigated
Glucose tolerance	May become impaired; closely monitor patients with latent or active diabetes

COMPENDIUM OF DRUG THERAPY

TRI-NORINYL

Hypertension	May be precipitated or may worsen with oral contraception, particularly with prolonged use and in older patients. Closely monitor patients with a history of hypertension, toxemia, hypertension during pregnancy, or excessive weight gain or fluid retention during the menstrual cycle; preexisting renal disease; or a family history of hypertension or hypertensive complications.
Migraine headache	May develop or worsen; discontinue oral contraception and investigate cause of recurrent, persistent, or severe headaches
Bleeding irregularities, including breakthrough bleeding, spotting, and amenorrhea	May occur, necessitating either a change to a formulation with a higher estrogen content or discontinuation of therapy; higher amounts of estrogen, while potentially useful for minimizing menstrual irregularities, may increase the risk of thromboembolic disease
Mental depression	Risk is increased; discontinue oral contraception if serious depression develops or recurs in patients with a history of depression
Fluid retention	May occur; use with caution in patients with convulsive disorders, migraine, asthma, or cardiac, hepatic, or renal dysfunction
Vitamin deficiencies	May occur, particularly of pyridoxine and folic acid
Intolerance to contact lenses	Patients who wear contact lenses may experience changes in vision or lens tolerance; such changes should be evaluated by an ophthalmologist. It may be necessary to suspend contact lens wear temporarily or permanently.
Spotting, breakthrough bleeding	If spotting or breakthrough bleeding occurs, instruct the patient to continue the regimen, but bear in mind the possibility of organic disorder. If abnormal vaginal bleeding persists or recurs, adequate diagnostic measures are indicated to rule out pregnancy or malignancy. Assuming these are excluded, the problem may be corrected by the passage of time or use of another formulation. Preparations with a higher estrogen content should be used only if necessary because of the increased risk of thromboembolic disease.
Chlamydial infections	Infection with *Chlamydia trachomatis* is enhanced by oral contraceptive use
Failure of withdrawal bleeding	If patient has not adhered to prescribed regimen, pregnancy should be considered after the first missed period and oral contraception withheld until pregnancy has been excluded; if patient has adhered to regimen and misses two consecutive periods, pregnancy should be ruled out before contraceptive regimen is continued. Amenorrhea may occur during therapy and necessitate discontinuation of use.
Postpill amenorrhea and anovulation	May occur, particularly in patients with a history of oligomenorrhea or secondary amenorrhea or in young women who have not established regular menstrual cycles; such patients should be encouraged to use alternative methods of contraception
Infertility	May occur following discontinuation of oral contraception, independent of its duration; diminishes with time but may still be apparent up to 30 mo in parous women and up to 42 mo in nulliparous women

ADVERSE REACTIONS

Frequent reactions (incidence ≥ 1%) are printed in *italics*

Genitourinary	*Breakthrough bleeding, spotting, menstrual irregularities, vaginal candidiasis,* postpill amenorrhea and infertility, dysmenorrhea, altered cervical erosion and secretion, enlargement of uterine leiomyomata, premenstrual-like syndrome, altered libido, cystitis-like syndrome, vaginitis
Cardiovascular	Thrombophlebitis, thrombosis, pulmonary embolism, coronary thrombosis, cerebral thrombosis, cerebral hemorrhage, arterial thromboembolism, Raynaud's disease, hypertension, mesenteric thrombosis, edema, malignant hypertension
Gastrointestinal	*Nausea, vomiting,* gallbladder disease, abdominal cramps, colitis, bloating, change in appetite
Hepatic	Liver tumors, cholestatic jaundice
Metabolic and endocrinological	*Breast enlargement, tenderness, and/or secretion;* carbohydrate intolerance; increase or decrease in weight; hyperlipidemia
Central nervous system and neuromuscular	Migraine, depression, headache, nervousness, dizziness, chorea
Ophthalmic	Optic neuritis, retinal thrombosis, intolerance to contact lenses, altered corneal curvature, cataracts
Allergic and dermatological	Rash, melasma or chloasma, erythema multiforme, erythema nodosum, hirsutism, hair loss, hemorrhagic eruption, porphyria, chilblains
Other	Congenital anomalies, prolactin-secreting pituitary tumors, impaired renal function, malignant nephrosclerosis (hemolytic uremic syndrome), acute renal failure

OVERDOSAGE

Signs and symptoms	Nausea, withdrawal bleeding; acute ingestion of large doses by young children has not been associated with serious ill effects
Treatment	Treat symptomatically

TRI-NORINYL ■ TRIPHASIL

DRUG INTERACTIONS

Ampicillin, analgesics, antianxiety agents, antihistamines, antimigraine preparations, barbiturates, chloramphenicol, isoniazid, neomycin, nitrofurantoin, penicillin V, phenylbutazone, phenytoin, primidone, rifampin, sulfonamides, tetracycline, tranquilizers	▽ Contraceptive effect △ Breakthrough bleeding
Antihypertensive agents (eg, guanethidine)	▽ Antihypertensive effect
Oral anticoagulants	▽ Anticoagulant effect
Anticonvulsants	△ Seizure activity
Hypoglycemic agents	▽ Glucose tolerance
Corticosteroids	△ Corticosteroid effects
Cyclosporine	Hepatotoxicity
Tricyclic antidepressants	△ Antidepressant side effects
Benzodiazepines (except lorazepam, oxazepam, and temazepam)	△ Serum benzodiazepine level
Theophylline	△ Serum theophylline level

ALTERED LABORATORY VALUES

Blood/serum values — △ Alkaline phosphatase △ Bilirubin △ Sulfobromophthalein retention △ Prothrombin △ Clotting factors VII, VIII, IX, and X ▽ Antithrombin III △ PBI △ Thyroxine (T_4) ▽ Triiodothyronine (T_3) uptake △ Glucose △ Cortisol △ Transcortin △ Ceruloplasmin △ Triglycerides △ Phospholipids ▽ Folic acid ▽ Pyridoxine

Urinary values — ▽ Pregnanediol

USE IN CHILDREN
Not indicated before puberty

USE IN PREGNANT AND NURSING WOMEN
Pregnancy Category X: contraindicated if pregnancy is known or suspected, as serious fetal damage may occur during early pregnancy. Patient should discontinue oral contraception 3 mo before attempting to conceive. Postpartum use may interfere with lactation, causing a decrease in the quantity and quality of breast milk. Patient should use an alternative form of contraception until infant is weaned.

CONTRACEPTIVES

TRIPHASIL-21 (levonorgestrel and ethinyl estradiol) Wyeth Rx

Tablets (per dispenser): 6 brown tablets containing 0.050 mg levonorgestrel and 30 μg ethinyl estradiol, 5 white tablets containing 0.075 mg levonorgestrel and 40 μg ethinyl estradiol, and 10 light-yellow tablets containing 0.125 mg levonorgestrel and 30 μg ethinyl estradiol *21-day regimen*

TRIPHASIL-28 (levonorgestrel and ethinyl estradiol) Wyeth Rx

Tablets (per dispenser): 6 brown tablets containing 0.050 mg levonorgestrel and 30 μg ethinyl estradiol, 5 white tablets containing 0.075 mg levonorgestrel and 40 μg ethinyl estradiol, 10 light-yellow tablets containing 0.125 mg levonorgestrel and 30 μg ethinyl estradiol, and 7 light-green tablets containing inert ingredients *28-day regimen*

INDICATIONS
Contraception

ORAL DOSAGE
Adult: 1 brown tablet q24h for 6 days, followed successively by 1 white tablet q24h for 5 days, 1 light-yellow tablet q24h for 10 days, and either no tablets for 7 days (21-day regimen) or 1 light-green tablet q24h for 7 days (28-day regimen); tablets should preferably be taken after the evening meal or at bedtime.

CONTRAINDICATIONS

Thrombophlebitis or thromboembolic disorders

Past history of deep-vein thrombophlebitis or thromboembolic disorders

Coronary artery disease

Cerebrovascular disease

Known or suspected breast cancer

Known or suspected estrogen-dependent neoplasia

Undiagnosed abnormal genital bleeding

Known or suspected pregnancy

Benign or malignant liver tumor that developed during the use of oral contraceptives or other estrogen-containing products

COMPENDIUM OF DRUG THERAPY

TRIPHASIL

ADMINISTRATION/DOSAGE ADJUSTMENTS

Initiating therapy	First tablet should be taken on the first day of the menstrual cycle or, after discontinuation of another oral contraceptive, on the first day of withdrawal bleeding. For postpartum use, the regimen should be started immediately or at the first postpartum examination, regardless of whether spontaneous menstruation has occurred. If the tablets are taken either later than the first day of menstrual bleeding or postpartum, an additional form of contraception should be used for the first week.
Subsequent cycles (21-day regimen)	First brown tablet is taken 8 days after the last light-yellow tablet was taken in the preceding cycle
Subsequent cycles (28-day regimen)	First brown tablet is taken the day after the last light-green tablet was taken in the preceding cycle
Missed tablets	If one or two tablets are missed, they should be taken as soon as they are remembered, and an additional form of contraception should be used for 1 wk. If three tablets are missed, medication should be discontinued until the first day of withdrawal bleeding, at which time a new cycle should be started; another form of contraception should be used for the period without tablets and for the first week after resumption of use.
Monitoring of therapy	A Papanicolaou smear, other appropriate laboratory tests, and a physical examination (with special attention to breasts, abdomen, pelvic organs, and blood pressure) should be done before therapy and then repeated at least annually

WARNINGS/PRECAUTIONS

Cigarette smoking	Increases the risk of serious cardiovascular side effects, especially in women over 35 yr of age who smoke 15 or more cigarettes daily; patients who use oral contraceptives should be strongly urged not to smoke
Thromboembolic disease, thrombotic disorders, and other vascular problems	Risk is increased, becoming greater with age (after 30 yr of age) and with the amount of estrogen present in the formulation; after discontinuation of use, the risk of cerebrovascular disease and myocardial infarction may persist. Discontinue oral contraception immediately if early signs of thromboembolic disease or thrombotic disorders (eg, thrombophlebitis, pulmonary embolism, cerebrovascular insufficiency, coronary occlusion, or retinal or mesenteric thrombosis) develop or are suspected.
Postsurgical thromboembolic complications	Risk is increased 4–6 times; if feasible, discontinue oral contraception at least 4 wk before elective surgery associated with an increased risk of thromboembolism or prolonged immobilization
Ocular lesions, including optic neuritis and retinal thrombosis	May occur; discontinue oral contraception in the presence of unexplained gradual or sudden, partial or complete loss of vision; proptosis or diplopia; papilledema; or retinal vascular lesions
Carcinoma	Closely monitor patients with a strong family history of breast cancer or with breast nodules, fibrocystic disease, or abnormal mammograms; investigate all cases of undiagnosed persistent or recurrent abnormal vaginal bleeding for malignancy (see CONTRAINDICATIONS)
Hepatic tumors, including benign adenomas	May occur and possibly rupture, resulting in intraabdominal hemorrhage and death; investigate all cases of abdominal pain and tenderness, abdominal mass, or shock for hepatic adenoma. The risk reportedly increases among users of formulations with high hormonal potency, and with use of oral contraception for more than 4 yr.
Gallbladder disease	Risk increases with duration of oral contraception
Hepatic impairment	Use with caution due to poor steroid hormone metabolism
Jaundice	May recur in patients with a history of jaundice; discontinue oral contraception while cause is investigated
Glucose tolerance	May become impaired; closely monitor patients with latent or active diabetes
Lipid metabolism	An increase in serum triglycerides and total phospholipids has been observed in women taking oral contraceptives; however, three studies performed with this formulation have shown no significant change in lipid metabolism, except for a slight increase in triglyceride levels in one study. The clinical significance of these findings has not been defined.
Hypertension	May be precipitated or may worsen with oral contraception, particularly with prolonged use, in older patients, and in patients with a history of hypertension during pregnancy
Migraine headache	May develop or worsen; discontinue oral contraception and investigate cause of recurrent, persistent, or severe headaches
Mental depression	Risk is increased; discontinue oral contraception if serious depression develops or recurs in patients with a history of depression
Fluid retention	May occur; use with caution in patients with convulsive disorders, migraine, asthma, or cardiac, hepatic, or renal dysfunction
Vitamin deficiencies	May occur, particularly of pyridoxine and folic acid

TRIPHASIL

Spotting, breakthrough bleeding	Spotting or breakthrough bleeding may occur when tablets are missed or at other times during therapy; instruct the patient to continue the regimen, but bear in mind the possibility of organic disorder. If abnormal vaginal bleeding persists or recurs, adequate diagnostic measures are indicated to rule out pregnancy or malignancy. Assuming these are excluded, the problem may be corrected by the passage of time or use of another formulation. Preparations with a higher estrogen content should be used only if necessary because of the increased risk of thromboembolic disease.
Failure of withdrawal bleeding	If patient has missed two consecutive periods, pregnancy should be ruled out before contraceptive regimen is continued; if patient has not adhered to prescribed regimen, pregnancy should be considered after the first missed period and oral contraception withheld until pregnancy has been excluded. Amenorrhea may occur during therapy and necessitate discontinuation of use.
Postpill amenorrhea and anovulation	May occur, particularly in patients with a history of oligomenorrhea or secondary amenorrhea or in young women who have not established regular menstrual cycles; such patients should be encouraged to use alternative methods of contraception

ADVERSE REACTIONS
Frequent reactions are italicized

Genitourinary	*Breakthrough bleeding, spotting, menstrual irregularities, vaginal candidiasis,* postpill amenorrhea and infertility, dysmenorrhea, altered cervical erosion and secretion, enlargement of uterine leiomyomata, premenstrual-like syndrome, altered libido, cystitis-like syndrome, vaginitis
Cardiovascular	Thrombophlebitis, pulmonary embolism, coronary thrombosis, cerebral thrombosis, cerebral hemorrhage, hypertension, mesenteric thrombosis, edema
Gastrointestinal	*Nausea, vomiting,* gallbladder disease, abdominal cramps, bloating, change in appetite
Hepatic	Benign hepatomas, cholestatic jaundice
Metabolic and endocrinological	*Breast enlargement, tenderness, and/or secretion;* carbohydrate intolerance; increase or decrease in weight, hyperlipidemia
Central nervous system and neuromuscular	Migraine, depression, anxiety, headache, nervousness, dizziness, chorea
Ophthalmic	Optic neuritis, retinal thrombosis, intolerance to contact lenses, altered corneal curvature, cataracts
Allergic and dermatological	Rash, melasma or chloasma, erythema multiforme, erythema nodosum, hirsutism, hair loss, hemorrhagic eruption, porphyria
Other	Congenital anomalies, hemolytic uremic syndrome

OVERDOSAGE

Signs and symptoms	Nausea, withdrawal bleeding; acute ingestion of large doses by young children has not been associated with serious ill effects
Treatment	Treat symptomatically

DRUG INTERACTIONS

Ampicillin, analgesics, antianxiety agents, antimigraine preparations, barbiturates, chloramphenicol, isoniazid, neomycin, nitrofurantoin, penicillin V, phenylbutazone, phenytoin, primidone, rifampin, sulfonamides, tetracycline	▽ Contraceptive effect △ Breakthrough bleeding
Antihypertensive agents (eg, guanethidine)	▽ Antihypertensive effect
Oral anticoagulants	▽ Anticoagulant effect
Anticonvulsants	△ Seizure activity
Hypoglycemic agents	▽ Glucose tolerance
Corticosteroids	△ Corticosteroid effects
Tricyclic antidepressants	△ Antidepressant side effects

ALTERED LABORATORY VALUES

Blood/serum values	△ Alkaline phosphatase △ Bilirubin △ Sulfobromophthalein retention △ Prothrombin △ Clotting factors VII, VIII, IX, and X ▽ Antithrombin III △ PBI △ Thyroxine (T_4) ▽ Triiodothyronine (T_3) uptake △ Glucose △ Cortisol △ Transcortin △ Ceruloplasmin ▽ Folic acid ▽ Pyridoxine
Urinary values	▽ Pregnanediol

TRIPHASIL

USE IN CHILDREN
Not indicated before puberty

USE IN PREGNANT AND NURSING WOMEN
Pregnancy Category X: contraindicated if pregnancy is known or suspected, as serious fetal damage may occur during early pregnancy. Patient should discontinue oral contraception 3 mo before attempting to conceive. Postpartum use may interfere with lactation, causing a decrease in the quantity and quality of breast milk. Patient should use an alternative form of contraception until infant is weaned.

Chapter 33

Corticosteroids

Oral and Injectable Corticosteroids — 1314

ARISTOCORT (Lederle) — 1314
Triamcinolone *Rx*

ARISTOCORT (Lederle) — 1314
Triamcinolone diacetate *Rx*

CELESTONE (Schering) — 1317
Betamethasone *Rx*

CELESTONE Phosphate (Schering) — 1317
Betamethasone sodium phosphate *Rx*

CELESTONE SOLUSPAN (Schering) — 1317
Betamethasone sodium phosphate and betamethasone acetate *Rx*

CORTEF (Upjohn) — 1320
Hydrocortisone *Rx*

CORTEF ACETATE (Upjohn) — 1320
Hydrocortisone acetate suspension *Rx*

CORTEF Oral Suspension (Upjohn) — 1320
Hydrocortisone cypionate *Rx*

Cortisone acetate *Rx* — 1323

DECADRON (Merck Sharp & Dohme) — 1325
Dexamethasone *Rx*

DECADRON Phosphate (Merck Sharp & Dohme) — 1325
Dexamethasone sodium phosphate *Rx*

DECADRON-LA Suspension (Merck Sharp & Dohme) — 1325
Dexamethasone acetate *Rx*

DELTASONE (Upjohn) — 1328
Prednisone *Rx*

DEPO-MEDROL (Upjohn) — 1330
Methylprednisolone acetate suspension *Rx*

KENALOG-10 (Squibb) — 1333
Triamcinolone acetonide *Rx*

KENALOG-40 (Squibb) — 1334
Triamcinolone acetonide *Rx*

MEDROL (Upjohn) — 1330
Methylprednisolone *Rx*

Prednisolone acetate *Rx* — 1337

Prednisolone sodium phosphate *Rx* — 1337

SOLU-CORTEF (Upjohn) — 1320
Hydrocortisone sodium succinate *Rx*

SOLU-MEDROL (Upjohn) — 1330
Methylprednisolone sodium succinate *Rx*

Topical Corticosteroids — 1339

ACLOVATE (Glaxo) — 1339
Alclometasone dipropionate *Rx*

AEROSEB-DEX (Herbert) — 1340
Dexamethasone *Rx*

AEROSEB-HC (Herbert) — 1341
Hydrocortisone *Rx*

ARISTOCORT Cream and Ointment (Lederle) — 1342
Triamcinolone acetonide *Rx*

ARISTOCORT A Cream and Ointment (Lederle) — 1342
Triamcinolone acetonide *Rx*

CARMOL HC (Syntex) — 1343
Hydrocortisone acetate *Rx*

CLODERM (Hermal) — 1344
Clocortolone pivalate *Rx*

CORDRAN (Dista) — 1345
Flurandrenolide *Rx*

CORDRAN SP (Dista) — 1345
Flurandrenolide *Rx*

CORDRAN-N (Dista) — 1347
Flurandrenolide and neomycin sulfate *Rx*

CORT-DOME Cream and Lotion — 1348
(Miles Pharmaceuticals)
Hydrocortisone *Rx*

CORTEF ACETATE Ointment (Upjohn) — 1348
Hydrocortisone acetate *Rx*

CORTISPORIN Cream (Burroughs Wellcome) — 1349
Polymyxin B sulfate, neomycin sulfate, and hydrocortisone acetate *Rx*

CORTISPORIN Ointment (Burroughs Wellcome) — 1350
Polymyxin B sulfate, bacitracin zinc, neomycin sulfate, and hydrocortisone *Rx*

CYCLOCORT (Lederle) — 1351
Amcinonide *Rx*

DECADERM (Merck Sharp & Dohme) — 1352
Dexamethasone *Rx*

DECADRON Phosphate (Merck Sharp & Dohme) — 1352
Dexamethasone sodium phosphate *Rx*

DECASPRAY (Merck Sharp & Dohme) — 1352
Dexamethasone *Rx*

DIPROLENE (Schering) — 1353
Betamethasone dipropionate *Rx*

DIPROSONE (Schering) — 1354
Betamethasone dipropionate *Rx*

FLORONE (Dermik) — 1355
Diflorasone diacetate *Rx*

HALCIDERM (Squibb) — 1356
Halcinonide *Rx*

HALOG (Princeton) — 1357
Halcinonide *Rx*

HALOG-E (Princeton) — 1357
Halcinonide *Rx*

HYTONE (Dermik) — 1358
Hydrocortisone *OTC, Rx*

KENALOG (Squibb) — 1359
Triamcinolone acetonide *Rx*

KENALOG-H (Squibb) — 1359
Triamcinolone acetonide *Rx*

LIDEX (Syntex) — 1360
Fluocinonide *Rx*

LIDEX-E (Syntex) — 1360
Fluocinonide *Rx*

COMPENDIUM OF DRUG THERAPY

Corticosteroids continued

MYCOLOG-II (Squibb)   1361
Nystatin and triamcinolone acetonide *Rx*

NEO-SYNALAR (Syntex)   1362
Neomycin sulfate and fluocinolone acetonide *Rx*

PSORCON (Dermik)   1363
Diflorasone diacetate *Rx*

SYNALAR (Syntex)   1364
Fluocinolone acetonide *Rx*

SYNALAR-HP (Syntex)   1364
Fluocinolone acetonide *Rx*

SYNEMOL (Syntex)   1365
Fluocinolone acetonide *Rx*

TEMOVATE (Glaxo)   1366
Clobetasol propionate *Rx*

TOPICORT (Hoechst-Roussel)   1367
Desoximetasone *Rx*

TOPICORT LP (Hoechst-Roussel)   1367
Desoximetasone *Rx*

TRIDESILON (Miles Pharmaceuticals)   1368
Desonide *Rx*

VALISONE (Schering)   1369
Betamethasone valerate *Rx*

VIOFORM-Hydrocortisone (CIBA)   1370
Clioquinol and hydrocortisone *Rx*

WESTCORT (Westwood)   1371
Hydrocortisone valerate *Rx*

Inhalant Corticosteroids   1372

AEROBID (Forest)   1372
Flunisolide *Rx*

AZMACORT (Rorer)   1374
Triamcinolone acetonide *Rx*

BECLOVENT (Glaxo)   1376
Beclomethasone dipropionate *Rx*

RESPIHALER DECADRON Phosphate   1377
(Merck Sharp & Dohme)
Dexamethasone sodium phosphate *Rx*

VANCERIL Inhaler (Schering)   1379
Beclomethasone dipropionate *Rx*

Nasal Corticosteroids   1380

BECONASE (Glaxo)   1380
Beclomethasone dipropionate *Rx*

NASALIDE (Syntex)   1382
Flunisolide *Rx*

VANCENASE (Syntex)   1383
Beclomethasone dipropionate *Rx*

Rectal Corticosteroids/ Hemorrhoidals   1384

ANUSOL Ointment (Warner-Lambert)   1384
Benzyl benzoate, Peruvian balsam, zinc oxide, and pramoxine hydrochloride *OTC*

ANUSOL Suppositories (Warner-Lambert)   1384
Bismuth subgallate, bismuth resorcin compound, benzyl benzoate, Peruvian balsam, and zinc oxide *OTC*

ANUSOL-HC (Parke-Davis)   1385
Hydrocortisone acetate, bismuth subgallate, bismuth resorcin compound, benzyl benzoate, Peruvian balsam, and zinc oxide *Rx*

CORT-DOME Suppositories (Miles Pharmaceuticals)   1386
Hydrocortisone acetate *Rx*

CORTENEMA (Reid-Rowell)   1386
Hydrocortisone retention enema *Rx*

CORTICAINE Cream (Glaxo)   1388
Hydrocortisone acetate and dibucaine *Rx*

MEDICONE Ointment and Suppositories   1389
(Medicone)
Benzocaine, 8-hydroxyquinoline sulfate, menthol, zinc oxide, and balsam Peru *OTC*

NUPERCAINAL Cream and Ointment (CIBA)   1390
Dibucaine *OTC*

NUPERCAINAL Suppositories (CIBA)   1390
Cocoa butter, zinc oxide, and bismuth subgallate *OTC*

PREPARATION H (Whitehall)   1390
Live yeast cell derivative and shark liver oil *OTC*

PROCTOFOAM-HC (Reed & Carnrick)   1391
Hydrocortisone acetate and pramoxine hydrochloride *Rx*

TRONOLANE (Ross)   1392
Pramoxine hydrochloride *OTC*

TUCKS (Warner-Lambert)   1393
Witch hazel and glycerin *OTC*

TUCKS Cream and Ointment (Warner-Lambert)   1393
Witch hazel *OTC*

Other Oral and Injectable Corticosteroids   1311

A-HYDROCORT (Abbott)   1311
Hydrocortisone sodium succinate *Rx*

A-METHAPRED (Abbott)   1311
Methylprednisolone sodium succinate *Rx*

ARISTOSPAN (Lederle)   1311
Triamcinolone hexacetonide *Rx*

DELTA-CORTEF (Upjohn)   1312
Prednisolone *Rx*

FLORINEF Acetate (Squibb)   1312
Fludrocortisone acetate *Rx*

HALDRONE (Lilly)   1312
Paramethasone acetate *Rx*

HEXADROL (Organon)   1312
Dexamethasone *Rx*

HEXADROL Phosphate Injection (Organon)   1312
Dexamethasone sodium phosphate *Rx*

Other Topical Corticosteroids — 1312

CORTAID (Upjohn) — 1312
Hydrocortisone acetate *OTC*

CORTEF Feminine Itch Cream (Upjohn) — 1312
Hydrocortisone acetate *OTC*

CORTRIL (Pfizer) — 1312
Hydrocortisone *Rx*

DERMOLATE (Schering) — 1312
Hydrocortisone *OTC*

HYDROCORTONE (Merck Sharp & Dohme) — 1313
Hydrocortisone acetate *OTC*

KOMED-HC (Barnes-Hind) — 1313
Hydrocortisone acetate, sodium thiosulfate, salicylic acid, and isopropyl alcohol *Rx*

LIDA-MANTLE-HC — 1313
(Miles Pharmaceuticals)
Hydrocortisone acetate and lidocaine *Rx*

MANTADIL (Burroughs Wellcome) — 1313
Chlorcyclizine hydrochloride and hydrocortisone acetate *Rx*

MAXIFLOR (Herbert) — 1313
Diflorasone diacetate *Rx*

MEDICONE DERMA-HC (Medicone) — 1313
Hydrocortisone acetate, benzocaine, 8-hydroxyquinoline sulfate, ephedrine hydrochloride, menthol, ichthammol, and zinc oxide *Rx*

MEDROL Acetate (Upjohn) — 1313
Methylprednisolone acetate *Rx*

NEO-CORT-DOME (Miles Pharmaceuticals) — 1313
Neomycin sulfate and hydrocortisone *Rx*

NEO-CORTEF (Upjohn) — 1313
Hydrocortisone acetate and neomycin sulfate *Rx*

NeoDECADRON (Merck Sharp & Dohme) — 1313
Dexamethasone sodium phosphate and neomycin sulfate *Rx*

NEO-DELTA-CORTEF (Upjohn) — 1313
Prednisolone acetate and neomycin sulfate *Rx*

NEO-MEDROL (Upjohn) — 1313
Neomycin sulfate and methylprednisolone acetate *Rx*

SYNACORT (Syntex) — 1313
Hydrocortisone *Rx*

UTICORT (Parke-Davis) — 1313
Betamethasone benzoate *Rx*

VYTONE (Dermik) — 1313
Iodoquinol and hydrocortisone *Rx*

OTHER ORAL AND INJECTABLE CORTICOSTEROIDS

DRUG	HOW SUPPLIED	USUAL DOSAGE[1]
A-HYDROCORT (Abbott) Hydrocortisone sodium succinate *Rx*	**Vials:** hydrocortisone sodium succinate equivalent to 100 mg (2 ml), 250 mg (2 ml), 500 mg (4 ml), or 1,000 mg (8 ml) of hydrocortisone	**Adult:** 100–500 mg IV to start, repeated IV or IM at intervals of 2, 4, or 6 h, as determined by patient's response and clinical condition **Infant and child:** adult dosage may be reduced; adjust dosage according to severity of disease and clinical response; minimum dose: 25 mg/day
A-METHAPRED (Abbott) Methylprednisolone sodium succinate *Rx*	**Vials:** methylprednisolone sodium succinate equivalent to 40 mg (1 ml), 125 mg (2 ml), 500 mg (4 ml), or 1,000 mg (8 ml) of methylprednisolone	**Adult:** 10–40 mg IV to start, repeated IV or IM at intervals dictated by patient's response and clinical condition; reduce dosage or discontinue use gradually when administered for more than a few days; when high doses are required, give 30 mg/kg IV over a period of 10–20 min; this dose may be repeated q4–6h until patient's condition stabilizes **Infant and child:** adult dosage may be reduced; adjust dosage according to severity of disease and clinical response; minimum dose: 0.5 mg/kg q24h
ARISTOSPAN (Lederle) Triamcinolone hexacetonide *Rx*	**Vials:** 5 mg/ml (5 ml) for intralesional use; 20 mg/ml (1, 5 ml) for intraarticular use	**Adult:** up to 0.5 mg/in.2 of affected skin, injected intralesionally or sublesionally; 2–20 mg, depending on the size of the joint, the degree of inflammation, and the amount of fluid present, injected intraarticularly at intervals of generally not less than 3 or 4 wk

[1] Where pediatric dosages are not given, consult manufacturer

continued

OTHER ORAL AND INJECTABLE CORTICOSTEROIDS continued

DRUG	HOW SUPPLIED	USUAL DOSAGE[1]
DELTA-CORTEF (Upjohn) Prednisolone *Rx*	**Tablets:** 5 mg	**Adult:** 5–60 mg/day to start, followed by gradual reductions in dosage to lowest level possible consistent with maintaining an adequate clinical response; dosage must be individualized on the basis of the specific disease being treated, its severity, and clinical response
FLORINEF Acetate (Squibb) Fludrocortisone acetate *Rx*	**Tablets:** 0.1 mg	**Adult:** for Addison's disease, 0.1 mg/day in combination with cortisone (10–37.5 mg/day in divided doses) or hydrocortisone (10–30 mg/day in divided doses); some patients may require 0.1 mg 3 times/wk to 0.2 mg/day, depending on disease severity and response to treatment; for salt-losing adrenogenital syndrome, 0.1–0.2 mg/day
HALDRONE (Lilly) Paramethasone acetate *Rx*	**Tablets:** 1, 2 mg	**Adult:** 2–24 mg/day to start, followed by gradual reductions in dosage to lowest level possible consistent with maintaining an adequate clinical response; dosage must be individualized on the basis of the specific disease being treated, its severity, and clinical response
HEXADROL (Organon) Dexamethasone *Rx*	**Tablets:** 0.5, 0.75, 1.5, 4 mg	**Adult:** 0.75–9 mg/day to start, followed by gradual reductions in dosage to lowest level possible consistent with maintaining an adequate clinical response; dosage must be individualized on the basis of the specific disease being treated, its severity, and clinical response
HEXADROL Phosphate Injection (Organon) Dexamethasone sodium phosphate *Rx*	**Prefilled syringes:** 4 mg/ml (1 ml), 10 mg/ml (1 ml), 20 mg/ml (5 ml) **Vials:** 4 mg/ml (1, 5 ml), 10 mg/ml (10 ml), 20 mg/ml (5 ml)	**Adult:** 0.5–9 mg IM or IV to start, followed by gradual reductions in dosage to lowest level possible consistent with maintaining an adequate clinical response; dosage must be individualized on the basis of the specific disease being treated, its severity, and clinical response

[1] Where pediatric dosages are not given, consult manufacturer

OTHER TOPICAL CORTICOSTEROIDS

DRUG	HOW SUPPLIED	USUAL DOSAGE[1]
CORTAID (Upjohn) Hydrocortisone acetate *OTC*	**Cream:** hydrocortisone acetate equivalent to 0.5% hydrocortisone (15, 30 g) **Lotion:** hydrocortisone acetate equivalent to 0.5% hydrocortisone (30, 60 ml) **Ointment:** hydrocortisone acetate equivalent to 0.5% hydrocortisone (15, 30 g) **Spray:** 0.5% hydrocortisone (45 ml)	**Adult:** apply to affected area not more than tid or qid **Child (≥ 2 yr):** same as adult
CORTEF Feminine Itch Cream (Upjohn) Hydrocortisone acetate *OTC*	**Cream:** hydrocortisone acetate equivalent to 0.5% hydrocortisone (½ oz)	**Adult:** apply to affected area up to tid or qid **Child (≥ 2 yr):** same as adult
CORTRIL (Pfizer) Hydrocortisone *Rx*	**Ointment:** 1% (14.2 g)	**Adult:** apply a thin film to affected area tid or qid
DERMOLATE (Schering) Hydrocortisone *OTC*	**Cream:** 0.5% (2, 15, 30 g) **Lotion:** 0.5% (30 ml) **Ointment:** 0.5% (30 g) **Spray:** 0.5% (45 ml)	**Adult:** apply to affected area not more than tid or qid (apply lotion to scalp) **Child (≥ 2 yr):** same as adult

[1] Where pediatric dosages are not given, consult manufacturer

OTHER TOPICAL CORTICOSTEROIDS continued

DRUG	HOW SUPPLIED	USUAL DOSAGE[1]
HYDROCORTONE (Merck Sharp & Dohme) Hydrocortisone acetate *Rx*	**Ointment:** hydrocortisone acetate equivalent to 1% hydrocortisone (15, 30 g)	**Adult:** apply a thin film to affected area tid or qid and rub in lightly
KOMED-HC (Barnes-Hind) Hydrocortisone acetate, sodium thiosulfate, salicylic acid, and isopropyl alcohol *Rx*	**Lotion:** 0.5% hydrocortisone acetate, 8% sodium thiosulfate, 2% salicylic acid, and 25% isopropyl alcohol (52.5 ml)	**Adult:** cleanse skin thoroughly and apply a thin film to washed affected area bid
LIDA-MANTLE-HC (Miles Pharmaceuticals) Hydrocortisone acetate and lidocaine *Rx*	**Cream:** 0.5% hydrocortisone acetate and 3% lidocaine (30 g)	**Adult:** apply a thin film to affected area and rub in lightly
MANTADIL (Burroughs Wellcome) Chlorcyclizine hydrochloride and hydrocortisone acetate *Rx*	**Cream:** 2% chlorcyclizine hydrochloride and 0.5% hydrocortisone acetate (15 g)	**Adult:** apply to affected area 2–5 times/day; if skin condition permits, rub cream in well
MAXIFLOR (Herbert) Diflorasone diacetate *Rx*	**Cream:** 0.05% (15, 30, 60 g) **Ointment:** 0.05% (15, 30, 60 g)	**Adult:** apply a thin film to affected area 1–4 times/day
MEDICONE DERMA-HC (Medicone) Hydrocortisone acetate, benzocaine, 8-hydroxyquinoline sulfate, ephedrine hydrochloride, menthol, ichthammol, and zinc oxide *Rx*	**Ointment (per gram):** 10 mg hydrocortisone acetate, 20 mg benzocaine, 10.5 mg 8-hydroxyquinoline sulfate, 1.1 mg ephedrine hydrochloride, 4.8 mg menthol, 10 mg ichthammol, and 137 mg zinc oxide (7, 20 g)	**Adult:** apply to affected area bid to qid
MEDROL Acetate (Upjohn) Methylprednisolone acetate *Rx*	**Ointment:** 0.25% (7.5, 30, 45 g); 1% (7.5, 30, 45 g)	**Adult:** apply a thin film to affected area 2–4 times/day
NEO-CORT-DOME (Miles Pharmaceuticals) Neomycin sulfate and hydrocortisone *Rx*	**Cream:** neomycin sulfate equivalent to 0.35% neomycin base and 0.5% hydrocortisone (15 g)	**Adult:** apply a thin film to affected area 1–4 times/day
NEO-CORTEF (Upjohn) Hydrocortisone acetate and neomycin sulfate *Rx*	**Cream (per gram):** 1% hydrocortisone acetate and neomycin sulfate equivalent to 3.5 mg neomycin (20 g) **Ointment (per gram):** 0.5% hydrocortisone acetate and neomycin sulfate equivalent to 3.5 mg neomycin (20 g); 1% hydrocortisone acetate and neomycin sulfate equivalent to 3.5 mg neomycin (5, 20 g); 2.5% hydrocortisone acetate and neomycin sulfate equivalent to 3.5 mg neomycin (5, 20 g)	**Adult:** after thorough cleansing, apply a small amount to affected area 1–3 times/day and rub in gently
NeoDECADRON (Merck Sharp & Dohme) Dexamethasone sodium phosphate and neomycin sulfate *Rx*	**Cream:** 0.1% dexamethasone sodium phosphate and neomycin sulfate equivalent to 3.5 mg neomycin (15, 30 g)	**Adult:** apply a thin film to affected area and rub in lightly tid or qid
NEO-DELTA-CORTEF (Upjohn) Prednisolone acetate and neomycin sulfate *Rx*	**Ointment (per gram):** 0.5% prednisolone acetate and neomycin sulfate equivalent to 3.5 mg neomycin (20 g)	**Adult:** apply a small amount to affected area and rub in gently 1–3 times/day
NEO-MEDROL (Upjohn) Neomycin sulfate and methylprednisolone acetate *Rx*	**Lipid base (per gram):** neomycin sulfate equivalent to 3.5 mg neomycin and 0.25% methylprednisolone acetate (7.5, 30, 45 g); neomycin sulfate equivalent to 3.5 mg neomycin and 1% methylprednisolone acetate (7.5, 30 g)	**Adult:** apply a small amount to affected area 1–3 times/day and massage gently
SYNACORT (Syntex) Hydrocortisone *Rx*	**Cream:** 1% (15, 30, 60 g); 2.5% (30 g)	**Adult:** apply a thin film to affected area 2–4 times/day
UTICORT (Parke-Davis) Betamethasone benzoate *Rx*	**Cream:** 0.025% (15, 60 g) **Gel:** 0.025% (15, 60 g) **Lotion:** 0.025% (15, 60 ml) **Ointment:** 0.025% (15, 60 g)	**Adult:** apply a thin film to affected area bid to qid, as needed
VYTONE (Dermik) Iodoquinol and hydrocortisone *Rx*	**Cream:** 1% iodoquinol and 0.5% hydrocortisone (30 g); 1% iodoquinol and 1% hydrocortisone (30 g)	**Adult:** apply to affected area tid or qid

[1] Where pediatric dosages are not given, consult manufacturer

ARISTOCORT

ORAL AND INJECTABLE CORTICOSTEROIDS

ARISTOCORT (triamcinolone) **Lederle** — Rx
Tablets: 1, 2, 4, 8 mg

ARISTOCORT (triamcinolone diacetate) **Lederle** — Rx
Vials: 40 mg/ml (1, 5 ml) (Aristocort Forte) for parenteral use; 25 mg/ml (5 ml) for intralesional use Syrup (per 5 ml): 2 mg (4 fl oz) *cherry-flavored*

INDICATIONS	ORAL DOSAGE	PARENTERAL DOSAGE
Endocrine disorders, including congenital adrenal hyperplasia, nonsuppurative thyroiditis, and hypercalcemia associated with cancer	Adult: 4–48 mg/day to start, followed by gradual reductions in dosage to lowest level consistent with maintaining an adequate clinical response; dosage must be individualized on the basis of the specific disease being treated, its severity, and clinical response	Adult: 3–48 mg in a single weekly IM dose to start, followed by gradual dosage adjustments to the point where adequate, but not necessarily complete, relief of symptoms is obtained
Primary or secondary adrenocortical insufficiency	Adult: 4–12 mg/day in addition to mineralocorticoid therapy	Adult: same as above, as well as preoperatively and in the event of serious trauma or illness
Rheumatic disorders, including psoriatic arthritis, rheumatoid arthritis, juvenile rheumatoid arthritis, ankylosing spondylitis, acute and subacute bursitis, acute nonspecific tenosynovitis, acute gouty arthritis, posttraumatic osteoarthritis, synovitis of osteoarthritis, and epicondylitis (adjunctive, short-term therapy)	Adult: ordinarily, 8–16 mg/day, given in a single morning dose daily or every other day, to start, followed by maintenance doses adjusted to keep symptoms to a tolerable level; some patients may require higher doses or may obtain greater relief on divided doses (bid or qid)	Adult: see ADMINISTRATION/DOSAGE ADJUSTMENTS
Collagen disease, including systemic lupus erythematosus	Adult: 20–32 mg/day to start, followed by maintenance therapy as above; patients with severe symptoms may require 48 mg/day or more and higher daily maintenance doses	Adult: same as above
Acute rheumatic carditis	Adult: 20–60 mg/day to start, followed by maintenance therapy, as above, for at least 6–8 wk (but seldom beyond 3 mo)	
Dermatological diseases, including pemphigus, bullous dermatitis herpetiformis, severe erythema multiforme (Stevens-Johnson syndrome), exfoliative dermatitis, mycosis fungoides, and severe seborrheic dermatitis	Adult: 8–16 mg/day to start, followed by maintenance therapy as above; in these conditions, as well as in certain allergic dermatoses, alternate-day administration is effective and less likely to produce adverse effects	Adult: same as above (see also ADMINISTRATION/DOSAGE ADJUSTMENTS)
Severe psoriasis	Adult: 8–16 mg/day to start, followed by maintenance therapy as above	Adult: same as above
Acute seasonal or perennial allergic rhinitis	Adult: 8–12 mg/day; intractable cases may require high initial and maintenance doses; maintenance therapy should be limited in duration (alternate-day regimen can be used)	Adult: same as above
Bronchial asthma	Adult: 8–16 mg/day; maintenance therapy should be limited in duration (alternate-day regimen can be used)	Adult: same as above
Contact dermatitis, atopic dermatitis	Adult: short courses of 8–16 mg/day (supplementing topical therapy)	Adult: same as above
Serum sickness (adjunctive therapy); **drug hypersensitivity reactions; urticarial transfusion reactions** (IM use only); **acute noninfectious laryngeal edema** (IM use only)	Adult: determine dosage by severity of the disorder, the speed with which the therapeutic response is desired, and the response of the patient to initital therapy	Adult: same as above
Ophthalmic diseases, including allergic conjunctivitis, keratitis, allergic corneal marginal ulcers, herpes zoster ophthalmicus, iritis and iridocyclitis, chorioretinitis, anterior segment inflammation, diffuse posterior uveitis and choroiditis, optic neuritis, and sympathetic ophthalmia	Adult: 12–40 mg/day to start (depending on the severity of the condition, the nature, and degree of involvement of ocular structure), followed by maintenance therapy as above	Adult: same as above
Respiratory diseases, including symptomatic sarcoidosis, Loeffler's syndrome not manageable by other means, berylliosis, fulminating or disseminated pulmonary tuberculosis (with appropriate antituberculous chemotherapy), or aspiration pneumonitis	Adult: 16–48 mg/day to start, followed by maintenance therapy as above	Adult: same as above

ARISTOCORT

Hematological disorders, including idiopathic thrombocytopenic purpura in adults (oral use only), secondary thrombocytopenia in adults, acquired (autoimmune) hemolytic anemia, erythroblastopenia (RBC anemia), and congenital (erythroid) hypoplastic anemia	**Adult:** 16–60 mg/day, followed by lower doses after adequate clinical response is obtained	**Adult:** same as above
Palliative management of **neoplastic diseases,** including leukemias and lymphomas in adult	**Adult:** 16–40 mg/day, or up to 100 mg/day for leukemia, if needed	**Adult:** same as above
Acute **leukemia** of childhood	**Child:** 1–2 mg/kg/day	—
To induce a diuresis or remission of proteinuria in the **nephrotic syndrome,** without uremia, of the idiopathic type or that due to lupus erythematosus	**Adult:** 16–20 mg/day (or up to 48 mg/day, if needed) until diuresis occurs; then continued treatment until maximal or complete chemical and clinical remission occurs; reduce dosage gradually and then discontinue; in less severe cases, as little as 4 mg/day may be adequate for maintenance	**Adult:** same as above
Tuberculosis meningitis with subarachnoid block or impending block (with appropriate antituberculous chemotherapy)	**Adult:** 32–48 mg/day, given in a single daily dose or in divided doses	**Adult:** same as above
Gastrointestinal diseases, including ulcerative colitis and regional enteritis		
Trichinosis associated with neurological or myocardial involvement	Consult manufacturer	Consult manufacturer
Acute exacerbations of **multiple sclerosis**		

CONTRAINDICATIONS

Sensitivity to triamcinolone (for oral use only)	Injection into infected or unstable joints	Systemic fungal infections

ADMINISTRATION/DOSAGE ADJUSTMENTS

Suppression of autogenous pituitary function	May be minimized by administering a single daily dose at or after 8 AM or by use of alternate-day or intermittent dosage regimens if long-term therapy or high doses are needed
Alternate-day regimen	Once minimum effective dose has been established, administer total 48-h dose at 8 AM every other day
Intraarticular or intrasynovial administration	The usual dose varies from 5 to 40 mg, depending on the size of the joint; duration of effect varies from 1 wk to 2 mo. Acutely inflamed joints may require more frequent injections.
Intralesional administration (eg, keloids, lichen planus lesions, psoriatic plaques, ganglia)	The total amount of drug, the concentration, and the number and pattern of injection sites utilized depend on the size of the lesion. No more than 12.5 mg should be injected per injection site or 25 mg per lesion. For many conditions 2–3 injections at intervals of 1–2 wk are sufficient. Injections may be repeated, as needed, but probably no more than 75 mg/wk should be given to any one patient.

WARNINGS/PRECAUTIONS

Patients subjected to unusual stress	Require increased dosage of rapidly acting corticosteroids before, during, and after emotionally or physically stressful situations
Infection	Clinical signs may be masked, new infections may appear, resistance may be decreased, and infections may be difficult to localize
Ocular damage	Prolonged use may produce posterior subcapsular cataracts and glaucoma, with possible damage to optic nerves, and may enhance development of secondary fungal or viral ocular infections
Dietary salt restriction and potassium supplementation	May be necessary to combat blood pressure elevation, salt and water retention, and increased potassium excretion with high-dose therapy
Immunization procedures	Especially against smallpox, should not be undertaken because of possible neurological complications and lack of antibody response
Active tuberculosis	Restrict use to fulminating or disseminated cases, as an adjunct to appropriate antituberculous therapy
Latent tuberculosis or tuberculin reactivity	Observe patient closely, since reactivation of the disease may occur, during prolonged therapy, employ antituberculous chemoprophylactic measures
Secondary adrenocortical insufficiency	May be minimized by gradual dosage reduction; since insufficiency may persist for months, reinstitute corticosteroid therapy in any stressful situation during this period, and administer salt and/or a mineralocorticoid concurrently to correct impaired mineralocorticoid secretion

ARISTOCORT

Hypothyroidism, hepatic cirrhosis	May enhance effects of triamcinolone
Corneal perforation	May occur in patients with ocular herpes simplex; use with caution
Special-risk patients	Use with caution in patients with nonspecific ulcerative colitis if impending perforation, abscess, or other pyogenic infection is likely, as well as in patients with diverticulitis, fresh intestinal anastomoses, active or latent peptic ulcer, renal insufficiency, hypertension, osteoporosis, or myasthenia gravis
Psychic derangements	May appear, ranging from euphoria, insomnia, mood swings, personality changes, and severe depression to frank psychotic manifestations; existing emotional instability or psychotic tendencies may be aggravated
Concomitant use with aspirin	Use with caution in patients with hypoprothrombinemia during therapy
Septic arthritis	May occur with intraarticular injection and require appropriate antimicrobial therapy; observe patient for suggestive symptoms (eg, increased pain, local swelling, further restrictions of joint mobility, fever, malaise) and examine joint fluid microscopically
Anaphylactoid reactions	Have occurred following parenteral corticosteroid administration; take appropriate precautionary measures before injecting triamcinolone diacetate, especially in patients with a history of drug allergy

ADVERSE REACTIONS

Fluid and electrolyte disturbances	Sodium retention, fluid retention, congestive heart failure in susceptible patients, loss of potassium, hypokalemic alkalosis, hypertension
Musculoskeletal	Muscle weakness, steroid myopathy, loss of muscle mass, osteoporosis, vertebral compression fractures, aseptic necrosis of femoral and humeral heads, pathological fracture of long bones
Gastrointestinal	Peptic ulcer with possible perforation and hemorrhage, pancreatitis, abdominal distention, ulcerative esophagitis
Dermatological	Impaired wound healing, thin fragile skin, petechiae and ecchymoses, facial erythema, increased sweating, suppressed reaction to skin tests
Neurological	Convulsions, increased intracranial pressure with papilledema (pseudotumor cerebri), vertigo, headache
Endocrinological	Menstrual irregularities, Cushingoid state, growth suppression in children, secondary adrenocortical and pituitary unresponsiveness, decreased carbohydrate tolerance, latent diabetes mellitus, increased insulin or oral hypoglycemic requirements
Ophthalmic	Posterior subcapsular cataracts, increased intraocular pressure, glaucoma, exophthalmos
Metabolic	Negative nitrogen balance
Hypersensitivity	Anaphylactoid reactions (rare)
Additional reactions to parenteral therapy only	Hyperpigmentation and hypopigmentation, subcutaneous and cutaneous atrophy, sterile abscess, postinjection flare (following intraarticular use), Charcot-like arthropathy, and blindness (rare) associated with intralesional therapy around the face and head

OVERDOSAGE

Signs and symptoms	CNS changes, GI bleeding, hyperglycemia, hypertension, edema
Treatment	Discontinue medication; institute supportive measures, as required

DRUG INTERACTIONS

Insulin, oral hypoglycemics	⇩ Hypoglycemic effect
Phenytoin, phenobarbital, ephedrine, rifampin	⇧ Metabolic clearance of triamcinolone ⇩ Steroid blood level and physiological activity
Oral anticoagulants	⇧ or ⇩ Prothrombin time
Potassium-depleting diuretics	⇧ Risk of hypokalemia
Cardiac glycosides	⇧ Risk of arrhythmias or digitalis toxicity secondary to hypokalemia
Skin test antigens	⇩ Reactivity
Immunizations	⇩ Antibody response

ALTERED LABORATORY VALUES

Blood/serum values	⇧ Glucose ⇧ Cholesterol ⇧ Sodium ⇩ Potassium ⇩ Calcium ⇩ PBI ⇩ Thyroxine (T$_4$) ⇩ ^{131}I thyroid uptake ⇩ Uric acid
Urinary values	⇧ Glucose ⇧ Potassium ⇧ Calcium ⇧ Uric acid ⇩ 17-Hydroxycorticosteroids (17-OHCS) ⇩ 17-Ketosteroids

USE IN CHILDREN

Dosage should be individualized according to severity of disease and patient response. There is no minimum pediatric dosage; the dosage is subject to the same considerations as that of the adult, rather than strict adherence to the ratio indicated by body weight. Growth and development should be carefully observed in infants and children on prolonged therapy.

USE IN PREGNANT AND NURSING WOMEN

Safety for use in pregnant or nursing women has not been established. Infants born of mothers who have received substantial doses of corticosteroids during pregnancy should be carefully observed for signs of hypoadrenalism.

ORAL AND INJECTABLE CORTICOSTEROIDS

CELESTONE (betamethasone) Schering   Rx
Tablets: 0.6 mg **Syrup (per 5 ml):** 0.6 mg[1] (4 fl oz)

CELESTONE Phosphate (betamethasone sodium phosphate) Schering   Rx
Vials (per 1 ml): betamethasone sodium phosphate equivalent to 3 mg betamethasone (5 ml)

CELESTONE SOLUSPAN (betamethasone sodium phosphate and betamethasone acetate) Schering   Rx
Vials (per 1 ml): betamethasone sodium phosphate equivalent to 3 mg betamethasone, and 3 mg betamethasone acetate (5 ml)

INDICATIONS

Endocrine disorders, including primary or secondary adrenocortical insufficiency, congenital adrenal hyperplasia, nonsuppurative thyroiditis, and hypercalcemia associated with cancer (except suspension form), acute adrenocortical insufficiency (except oral form), preoperatively and in the event of serious trauma or illness in patients with known adrenal insufficiency or when adrenocortical reserve is doubtful (except oral form), and shock unresponsive to conventional therapy in patients with known or suspected adrenocortical insufficiency (except oral form)
Rheumatic disorders, including psoriatic arthritis, rheumatoid arthritis, juvenile rheumatoid arthritis, ankylosing spondylitis, acute and subacute bursitis, acute nonspecific tenosynovitis, acute gouty arthritis, posttraumatic osteoarthritis, synovitis of osteoarthritis, and epicondylitis (adjunctive, short-term therapy)
Collagen diseases, including systemic lupus erythematosus and acute rheumatic carditis
Dermatological diseases, including pemphigus, bullous dermatitis herpetiformis, severe erythema multiforme (Stevens-Johnson syndrome), exfoliative dermatitis, mycosis fungoides (except suspension form), severe psoriasis, and severe seborrheic dermatitis
Severe or incapacitating **allergic conditions** intractable to adequate trials of conventional treatment, including seasonal or perennial allergic rhinitis, bronchial asthma, contact dermatitis, atopic dermatitis, serum sickness, drug hypersensitivity reactions, urticarial transfusion reactions (except oral form), and acute noninfectious laryngeal edema (except oral form)
Ophthalmic diseases, including allergic conjunctivitis, keratitis, allergic corneal marginal ulcers, herpes zoster ophthalmicus, iritis and iridocyclitis, chorioretinitis, anterior segment inflammation, diffuse posterior uveitis and choroiditis, optic neuritis, and sympathetic ophthalmia
Respiratory diseases, including symptomatic sarcoidosis, Loeffler's syndrome not manageable by other means (except suspension form), berylliosis, fulminating or disseminated pulmonary tuberculosis (with appropriate antituberculous chemotherapy), and aspiration of pneumonitis
Hematological disorders, including idiopathic thrombocytopenic purpura (oral, IV only) and secondary thrombocytopenia in adults, acquired (autoimmune) hemolytic anemia, erythroblastopenia (RBC anemia) (oral only), and congenital (erythroid) hypoplastic anemia (oral only)
Palliative management of **neoplastic diseases,** including leukemias and lymphomas in adults and acute leukemia of childhood
To induce a diuresis or remission of proteinuria in the **nephrotic syndrome,** without uremia, of the idiopathic type or that due to lupus erythematosus
Gastrointestinal diseases, including ulcerative colitis and regional enteritis
Tuberculous meningitis with subarachnoid block or impending block (with appropriate antituberculous chemotherapy)
Trichinosis associated with neurological or myocardial involvement (except suspension form)

ORAL DOSAGE

Adult: 0.6–7.2 mg/day to start, followed by gradual reductions in dosage to lowest level possible consistent with maintaining an adequate clinical response; dosage must be individualized on the basis of the specific disease being treated, its severity, and clinical response

PARENTERAL DOSAGE

Adult: 0.5–9.0 mg/day IM (Celestone Phosphate, Celestone Soluspan) or IV (Celestone Phosphate only) to start, followed by gradual reductions in dosage to lowest level possible consistent with maintaining an adequate clinical response; dosage must be individualized on the basis of the specific disease being treated, its severity, and clinical response; larger than usual doses may be justified in certain overwhelming, acute, life-threatening situations

CELESTONE

CONTRAINDICATIONS

| Systemic fungal infections | Injection into unstable or previously infected joints |

ADMINISTRATION/DOSAGE ADJUSTMENTS[2]

Intra-articular administration in rheumatoid arthritis and osteoarthritis	Dose of suspension is dependent on joint size, as follows: very large (hip), 1.0–2.0 ml; large, (eg, knee, ankle, shoulder), 1.0 ml; medium (eg, elbow, wrist), 0.5–1.0 ml; small (eg, metacarpophalangeal, interphalangeal, sternoclavicular), 0.25–0.5 ml. Systemic absorption of suspension following intra-articular administration should be considered in determining dosage in patients receiving concomitant oral or parenteral corticosteroids, especially in high doses.
Bursitis	For acute subdeltoid, subacromial, olecranon, and prepatellar bursitis, administer a single 1-ml dose of the suspension directly into the bursa; several intrabursal injections are usually required for recurrent acute bursitis and acute exacerbations of chronic bursitis. Once acute condition is controlled, lower doses may be given intrabursally to treat chronic bursitis.
Tenosynovitis and tendinitis	Inject 1.0 ml of the suspension into affected tendon sheath tree or four times at intervals of 1–2 wk
Ganglia of joint capsules and tendon sheaths	Inject 0.5 ml of the suspension directly into ganglion cysts
Intralesional treatment of dermatologic conditions	Inject 0.2 ml/cm² of the suspension intradermally (not subcutaneously); up to a total of 1.0 ml may be given at weekly intervals
Injections into the foot	Dose of suspension is dependent on disorder and location, as follows: bursitis under heloma durum or heloma molle, 0.25–0.5 ml; bursitis under calcaneal spur or over hallux rigidus or digiti quinti varus, 0.5 ml; tenosynovitis or periostitis of cuboid, 0.5 ml; acute gouty arthritis, 0.5–1.0 ml; injection may be repeated at 3- to 7-day intervals
Concomitant use of local anesthetics	Suspension may be mixed in a syringe with 1 or 2% lidocaine hydrochloride or similar local anesthetic solutions without parabens (avoid diluents containing methylparaben, propylparaben, phenol, etc); do not inject local anesthetics into Celestone Soluspan vial

WARNINGS/PRECAUTIONS

Patients subjected to unusual stress	Require increased dosage of rapidly acting corticosteroids before, during, and after emotionally or physically stressful situations
Infection	Clinical signs may be masked, new infections may appear, resistance may be decreased, and infections may be difficult to localize
Ocular damage	Prolonged use may produce posterior subcapsular cataracts and glaucoma with possible damage to optic nerves, and may enhance development of secondary fungal or viral ocular infections
Dietary salt restriction and potassium supplementation	May be necessary to combat blood pressure elevation, salt and water retention, and increased potassium excretion with average- and high-dose therapy
Immunization procedures	Especially against smallpox, should not be undertaken because of possible neurological complications and lack of antibody response
Active tuberculosis	Restrict use to fulminating or disseminated cases, as an adjunct to appropriate antituberculous therapy
Latent tuberculosis or tuberculin reactivity	Observe patient closely, since reactivation of the disease may occur; during prolonged therapy, employ antituberculous chemoprophylactic measures
Secondary adrenocortical insufficiency	May be minimized by gradual dosage reduction; since insufficiency may persist for months, reinstitute corticosteroid therapy in any stressful situation during this period, and administer salt and/or a mineralocorticoid concurrently to correct impaired mineralocorticoid secretion
Hypothyroidism, hepatic cirrhosis	May enhance effects of betamethasone
Corneal perforation	May occur in patients with ocular herpes simplex; use with caution
Special-risk patients	Use with caution in patients with nonspecific ulcerative colitis if impending perforation, abscess, or other pyogenic infection is likely, as well as in patients with diverticulitis, fresh intestinal anastomoses, active or latent peptic ulcer, renal insufficiency, hypertension, osteoporosis, or myasthenia gravis
Psychic derangements	May appear, ranging from euphoria, insomnia, mood swings, personality changes, and severe depression to frank psychotic manifestations; existing emotional instability or psychotic tendencies may be aggravated
Concomitant use with aspirin	Use with caution in patients with hypoprothrombinemia during therapy
Septic arthritis	May occur with intraarticular injection and require appropriate antimicrobial therapy; observe patients for suggestive symptoms (eg, increased pain, local swelling, further restrictions of joint mobility, fever, malaise) and examine joint fluid microscopically
Anaphylactoid reactions	Have occurred following parenteral corticosteroid administration; take appropriate precautionary measures before injecting betamethasone sodium phosphate, especially in patients with a history of drug allergy
Systemic effects	May occur, in addition to local effects, following intraarticular injection of corticosteroids; systemic effects may also be produced by the soluble component of the suspension form

CELESTONE

ADVERSE REACTIONS

Fluid and electrolyte disturbances	Sodium retention, fluid retention, congestive heart failure in susceptible patients, loss of potassium, hypokalemic alkalosis, hypertension
Musculoskeletal	Muscle weakness, steroid myopathy, loss of muscle mass, osteoporosis, vertebral compression fractures, aseptic necrosis of femoral and humeral heads, pathological fracture of long bones; tendon rupture (with tablets)
Gastrointestinal	Peptic ulcer with possible perforation and hemorrhage, pancreatitis, abdominal distention, ulcerative esophagitis
Dermatological	Impaired wound healing, thin fragile skin, petechiae and ecchymoses, facial erythema, increased sweating, suppressed reaction to skin tests
Neurological	Convulsions, increased intracranial pressure with papilledema (pseudotumor cerebri), vertigo, headache
Endocrinological	Menstrual irregularities, Cushingoid state, growth suppression in children, secondary adrenocortical and pituitary unresponsiveness, decreased carbohydrate tolerance, latent diabetes mellitus, increased insulin or oral hypoglycemic requirements
Ophthalmic	Posterior subcapsular cataracts, increased intraocular pressure, glaucoma, exophthalmos
Metabolic	Negative nitrogen balance
Additional reactions to parenteral therapy only	Hyperpigmentation and hypopigmentation, subcutaneous and cutaneous atrophy, sterile abscess, postinjection flare (following intraarticular use), Charcot-like arthropathy, and blindness (rare) associated with intralesional therapy around face and head

OVERDOSAGE

Signs and symptoms	CNS changes, GI bleeding, hyperglycemia, hypertension, edema
Treatment	Discontinue medication; institute supportive measures, as required

DRUG INTERACTIONS

Insulin, oral hypoglycemics	⇓ Hypoglycemic effects
Phenytoin, phenobarbital, ephedrine, rifampin	⇑ Metabolic clearance of betamethasone ⇓ Steroid blood level and physiological activity
Oral anticoagulants	⇑ or ⇓ Prothrombin time
Potassium-depleting diuretics	⇑ Risk of hypokalemia
Cardiac glycosides	⇑ Risk of arrhythmias or digitalis toxicity secondary to hypokalemia
Skin test antigens	⇓ Reactivity
Immunizations	⇓ Antibody response

ALTERED LABORATORY VALUES

Blood/serum values	⇑ Glucose ⇑ Cholesterol ⇑ Sodium ⇓ Potassium ⇓ Calcium ⇓ PBI ⇓ Thyroxine (T_4) ⇓ ^{131}I thyroid uptake ⇓ Uric acid
Urinary values	⇑ Glucose ⇑ Potassium ⇑ Calcium ⇑ Uric acid ⇓ 17-Hydroxycorticosteroids (17-OHCS) ⇓ 17-Ketosteroids

USE IN CHILDREN

See INDICATIONS and DOSAGE; before prescribing for children, carefully determine whether the particular intended use is appropriate. Growth and development should be carefully observed in infants and children on prolonged therapy.

USE IN PREGNANT AND NURSING WOMEN

Safety for use in pregnant or nursing women has not been established. Infants born of mothers who have received substantial doses of corticosteroids during pregnancy should be carefully observed for signs of hypoadrenalism.

---

[1] Contains less than 1% alcohol
[2] For intraarticular, soft tissue, and intralesional administration of Celestone Phosphate, consult manufacturer

CORTEF

ORAL AND INJECTABLE CORTICOSTEROIDS

CORTEF (hydrocortisone) Upjohn Rx
Tablets: 5, 10, 20 mg

CORTEF ACETATE (hydrocortisone acetate suspension) Upjohn Rx
Vials: 50 mg/ml (5 ml) for local injection only

CORTEF Oral Suspension (hydrocortisone cypionate) Upjohn Rx
Suspension (per 5 ml): hydrocortisone cypionate equivalent to 10 mg hydrocortisone (4 fl oz)

SOLU-CORTEF (hydrocortisone sodium succinate) Upjohn Rx
Vials: 100 mg (2 ml), 250 mg (2 ml), 500 mg (4 ml), 1 g (8 ml)

INDICATIONS

Endocrine disorders, including primary or secondary adrenocortical insufficiency, congenital adrenal hyperplasia, nonsuppurative thyroiditis, hypercalcemia associated with cancer, acute adrenocortical insufficiency (IM, IV only), and preoperatively and in the event of serious trauma or illness in patients with known adrenal insufficiency or when adrenocortical reserve is doubtful (IM, IV only)

Rheumatic disorders, including psoriatic arthritis, rheumatoid arthritis, juvenile rheumatoid arthritis, ankylosing spondylitis, acute and subacute bursitis, acute nonspecific tenosynovitis, acute gouty arthritis, posttraumatic osteoarthritis, synovitis or osteoarthritis, and epicondylitis (for short-term adjunctive treatment of rheumatic disorders and, in selected cases, for low-dosage maintenance therapy of rheumatoid arthritis)

Collagen diseases, including systemic lupus erythematosus, acute rheumatic carditis, and systemic dermatomyositis (polymyositis)

Dermatological diseases, including pemphigus, bullous dermatitis herpetiformis, severe erythema multiforme (Stevens-Johnson syndrome), exfoliative dermatitis, mycosis fungoides, severe psoriasis, and severe seborrheic dermatitis

Severe or incapacitating **allergic conditions** intractable to adequate trials of conventional treatment, including seasonal or perennial allergic rhinitis, bronchial asthma, contact dermatitis, atopic dermatitis, serum sickness, drug hypersensitivity reactions, urticarial transfusion reactions (IM, IV only), and acute noninfectious laryngeal edema (IM, IV only)

Ophthalmic diseases, including allergic conjunctivitis, keratitis, allergic corneal marginal ulcers, herpes zoster ophthalmicus, iritis and iridocyclitis, chorioretinitis, anterior segment inflammation, diffuse posterior uveitis and choroiditis, optic neuritis, and sympathetic ophthalmia

Respiratory diseases, including symptomatic sarcoidosis, Loeffler's syndrome not manageable by other means, berylliosis, fulminating or disseminated pulmonary tuberculosis (with appropriate antituberculous chemotherapy), and aspiration pneumonitis

Hematological disorders, including idiopathic thrombocytopenic purpura (oral, IV only) and secondary thrombocytopenia in adults, acquired (autoimmune) hemolytic anemia, erythroblastopenia (RBC anemia), and congenital (erythroid) hypoplastic anemia

Palliative management of **neoplastic diseases,** including leukemias and lymphomas in adults and acute leukemia of childhood

To induce diuresis or remission of proteinuria in the **nephrotic syndrome,** without uremia, of the idiopathic type or that due to lupus erythematosus

Gastrointestinal diseases, including ulcerative colitis and regional enteritis

Tuberculous meningitis with subarachnoid block or impending block (with appropriate antituberculous chemotherapy)

Trichinosis associated with neurological or myocardial involvement

ORAL DOSAGE

Adult: 20–240 mg/day or 10–120 ml (2–24 tsp)/day to start, followed by gradual reductions in dosage to lowest level possible consistent with maintaining an adequate clinical response; dosage must be individualized on the basis of the specific disease being treated, its severity, and clinical response

PARENTERAL DOSAGE

Adult: 100–500 mg IV, repeated at intervals of 2, 4, or 6 h, as determined by patient's response and clinical condition; dosage must be individualized on the basis of the specific disease being treated, its severity, and clinical response; larger than usual doses may be justified in certain overwhelming, acute, life-threatening situations

CONTRAINDICATIONS

Systemic fungal infections   Injection into previously infected or unstable joints

ADMINISTRATION/DOSAGE ADJUSTMENTS

Severe shock	Therapy is initiated by IV administration of Solu-Cortef over a period of 30 s (eg, 100 mg) to 10 min (eg, 500 mg or more), and should be continued only until patient's condition stabilizes (usually not beyond 48–72 h). Prophylactic antacid therapy may be indicated to prevent peptic ulceration.
Adrenocortical insufficiency	Mineralocorticoid supplementation may be necessary, particularly in infants
Acute exacerbations of multiple sclerosis	Administer 800 mg/day for 1 wk, followed by 320 mg every other day for 1 mo if tablets are used; consult manufacturer for Solu-Cortef dosage
Intraarticular administration in rheumatoid arthritis, synovitis of osteoarthritis, posttraumatic osteoarthritis, and acute gouty arthritis	Dose of suspension depends on joint size, and interval between doses on duration of relief obtained. For the knee, inject 25 mg to start and repeat when symptoms return (every 1–4 wk or longer); subsequent doses may be increased to 37.5 or 50 mg, if needed. For smaller joints, 10–15 mg may suffice. Injections must be made into the synovial space, where the synovial cavity is most superficial and most free of large vessels and nerves.

CORTEF

Local administration for acute and subacute bursitis, epicondylitis, acute nonspecific tenosynovitis	Inject 25–50 mg of the suspension directly into affected site; if needed, dose may be repeated in 3–5 days
Cystic tumor of an aponeurosis or tendon (ganglion)	Inject 10.0–12.5 mg of the suspension directly into the ganglion cyst
Intralesional administration	For keloids, lichen planus, psoriatic plaques, granuloma annulare, lichen simplex chronicus (neurodermatitis), discoid lupus erythematosus, necrobiosis lipoidica diabeticorum, and alopecia areata, inject up to a total of 100 mg of the suspension, depending on the size of the lesion; excessive amounts will cause blanching, which may be followed by a small slough
Preparation of Solu-Cortef solution	Reconstitute solution with diluent supplied or, if 100-mg single-compartment vials are used, with up to 2 ml of bacteriostatic water for injection (for IM or IV injection or IV infusion) or bacteriostatic sodium chloride injection (for IM or IV injection only). For IV infusion, add reconstituted solution to 100–1,000 ml (100-mg solution), 250–1,000 ml (250-mg solution), 500–1,000 ml (500-mg solution), or 1,000 ml (1-g solution) of isotonic saline or 5% dextrose (in water or isotonic saline), and administer within 4 h; if a small volume is desired, add 100–3,000 mg to 50 ml of diluent.

WARNINGS/PRECAUTIONS

Gasping syndrome	Benzyl alcohol, which is contained in the Cortef Acetate and Cortef IM suspensions and in the diluent supplied with the Solu-Cortef vials, has been associated with a gasping syndrome that is fatal in premature infants
Patients subjected to unusual stress	Require increased dosage of rapidly acting corticosteroid before, during, and after emotionally or physically stressful situations
Infection	Clinical signs may be masked, new infections may appear, resistance may be decreased, and infections may be difficult to localize
Ocular damage	Prolonged use may produce posterior subcapsular cataracts and glaucoma, with possible damage to optic nerves, and may enhance development of secondary fungal or viral ocular infections
Dietary salt restriction and potassium supplementation	May be necessary to combat blood pressure elevation, salt and water retention, and increased potassium excretion with average and high-dose therapy
Immunization procedures	Especially against smallpox, should not be undertaken because of possible neurological complications and lack of antibody response
Active tuberculosis	Restrict use to fulminating or disseminated cases, as an adjunct to appropriate antituberculous therapy
Latent tuberculosis or tuberculin reactivity	Observe patient closely, since reactivation of the disease may occur; during prolonged therapy, employ antituberculous chemoprophylactic measures
Secondary adrenocortical insufficiency	May be minimized by gradual dosage reduction; since insufficiency may persist for months, reinstitute corticosteroid therapy in any stressful situation during this period, and administer salt and/or a mineralocortocoid concurrently to correct impaired mineralocorticoid secretion
Hypothyroidism, hepatic cirrhosis	May enhance effects of hydrocortisone
Corneal perforation	May occur in patients with ocular herpes simplex; use with caution
Special-risk patients	Use with caution in patients with nonspecific ulcerative colitis if impending perforation, abscess, or other pyogenic infection is likely, as well as in patients with diverticulitis, fresh intestinal anastomoses, active or latent peptic ulcer, renal insufficiency, hypertension, osteoporosis, or myasthenia gravis
Psychic derangements	May appear, ranging from euphoria, insomnia, mood swings, personality changes, and severe depression to frank psychotic manifestations; existing emotional instability or psychotic tendencies may be aggravated
Concomitant use with aspirin	Use with caution in patients with hypoprothrombinemia
Prolonged therapy	Routine laboratory studies (eg, urinalysis, 2-h postprandial blood sugar, blood pressure, body weight, chest film) should be made at regular intervals; in addition, an upper GI series is suggested in patients with an ulcer history or significant dyspepsia. Withdraw the drug gradually, rather than abruptly, when discontinuing long-term therapy.
Hypernatremia	May occur when high doses of hydrocortisone must be continued beyond 48–72 h (eg, in cases of severe shock); under these circumstances, consider replacing the parenteral form with a corticosteroid that causes little or no sodium retention, such as methylprednisolone sodium succinate
Septic arthritis	May occur with intraarticular injection and require appropriate antimicrobial therapy; observe patient for suggestive symptoms (eg, increased pain, local swelling, further restrictions of joint mobility, fever, malaise) and examine joint fluid microscopically
Anaphylactoid reactions	Have occurred following parenteral corticosteroid administration; take appropriate precautionary measures before injecting hydrocortisone, especially in patients with a history of drug allergy

CORTEF

ADVERSE REACTIONS

Fluid and electrolyte disturbances	Sodium retention, fluid retention, congestive heart failure in susceptible patients, loss of potassium, hypokalemic alkalosis, hypertension
Musculoskeletal	Muscle weakness, steroid myopathy, loss of muscle mass, osteoporosis, vertebral compression fractures, aseptic necrosis of femoral and humeral heads, pathological fracture of long bones
Gastrointestinal	Peptic ulcer with possible perforation and hemorrhage, pancreatitis, abdominal distention, ulcerative esophagitis
Dermatological	Impaired wound healing, thin fragile skin, petechiae and ecchymoses, facial erythema, increased sweating, suppressed reaction to skin tests
Neurological	Convulsions, increased intracranial pressure with papilledema (pseudotumor cerebri), vertigo, headache
Endocrinological	Menstrual irregularities, Cushingoid state, growth suppression in children, secondary adrenocortical and pituitary unresponsiveness, decreased carbohydrate tolerance, latent diabetes mellitus, increased insulin or oral hypoglycemic requirements
Ophthalmic	Posterior subcapsular cataracts, increased intraocular pressure, glaucoma, exophthalmos
Metabolic	Negative nitrogen balance
Additional reactions to parenteral therapy only	Hyperpigmentation or hypopigmentation, subcutaneous and cutaneous atrophy, sterile abscess, postinjection flare (following intraarticular use), Charcot-like arthropathy, blindness (rare) associated with intralesional therapy around the face and head, anaphylactic or other allergic reactions (eg, bronchospasm)

OVERDOSAGE

Signs and symptoms	CNS changes, GI bleeding, hyperglycemia, hypertension, edema
Treatment	Discontinue medication; institute supportive measures, as required

DRUG INTERACTIONS

Insulin, oral hypolgycemics	⇩ Hypoglycemic effect
Phenytoin, phenobarbital, ephedrine, rifampin	⇧ Metabolic clearance of hydrocortisone ⇩ Steroid blood level and physiological activity
Oral anticoagulants	⇧ or ⇩ Prothrombin time
Potassium-depleting diuretics	⇧ Risk of hypokalemia
Cardiac glycosides	⇧ Risk of arrhythmias or digitalis toxicity secondary to hypokalemia
Skin test antigens	⇩ Reactivity
Immunizations	⇩ Antibody response

ALTERED LABORATORY VALUES

Blood/serum values	⇧ Glucose ⇧ Cholesterol ⇧ Sodium ⇧ Potassium ⇩ Calcium ⇩ PBI ⇩ Thyroxine (T_4) ⇩ ^{131}I thyroid uptake ⇩ Uric acid
Urinary values	⇧ Glucose ⇧ Potassium ⇧ Calcium ⇧ Uric acid ⇩ 17-Hydroxycorticosteroids (17-OHCS) ⇩ 17-Ketosteroids

USE IN CHILDREN

Pediatric dosage should be based primarily on the type and severity of the condition to be treated and patient response, rather than on age or body weight, and should not be less than 25 mg/day. In an emergency, the parenteral dosage recommended for adults may be reduced for children (including infants). Growth and development should be carefully observed in infants and children on prolonged therapy.

USE IN PREGNANT AND NURSING WOMEN

Safety for use in pregnant or nursing women has not been established. Infants born of mothers who have received substantial doses of corticosteroids during pregnancy should be carefully observed for signs of hypoadrenalism.

Cortisone

ORAL AND INJECTABLE CORTICOSTEROIDS

Cortisone acetate   Rx

Tablets: 5, 10, 25 mg   **Vials:** 25 mg/ml (10, 20 ml), 50 mg/ml (10 ml)

INDICATIONS

Endocrine disorders, including primary or secondary adrenocortical insufficiency, congenital adrenal hyperplasia, nonsuppurative thyroiditis, hypercalcemia associated with cancer, acute adrenocortical insufficiency (IM only), and preoperatively and in the event of serious trauma or illness in patients with known adrenal insufficiency or when adrenocortical reserve is doubtful (IM only)

Rheumatic disorders, including psoriatic arthritis, rheumatoid arthritis, juvenile rheumatoid arthritis, ankylosing spondylitis, acute and subacute bursitis, acute nonspecific tenosynovitis, acute gouty arthritis, posttraumatic osteoarthritis, synovitis of osteoarthritis, and epicondylitis (adjunctive, short-term therapy)

Collagen diseases, including systemic lupus erythematosus, acute rheumatic carditis, and systemic dermatomyositis (polymyositis) (IM only)

Dermatological diseases, including pemphigus, bullous dermatitis herpetiformis, severe erythema multiforme (Stevens-Johnson syndrome), exfoliative dermatitis, mycosis fungoides, severe psoriasis, and severe seborrheic dermatitis

Severe or incapacitating **allergic conditions** intractable to adequate trials of conventional treatment, including seasonal or perennial allergic rhinitis, bronchial asthma, contact dermatitis, atopic dermatitis, serum sickness, drug hypersensitivity reactions, urticarial transfusion reactions (IM only) and acute noninfectious laryngeal edema (IM only)

Ophthalmic diseases, including allergic conjunctivitis, keratitis, allergic corneal marginal ulcers, herpes zoster ophthalmicus, iritis and iridocyclitis, chorioretinitis, anterior segment inflammation, diffuse posterior uveitis and choroiditis, optic neuritis, and sympathetic ophthalmia

Respiratory diseases, including symptomatic sarcoidosis, Loeffler's syndrome not manageable by other means, berylliosis, fulminating or disseminated pulmonary tuberculosis (with appropriate antituberculous chemotherapy), aspiration pneumonitis

Hematological disorders, including idiopathic thrombocytopenic purpura (oral only), secondary thrombocytopenia in adults, acquired (autoimmune) hemolytic anemia, erythroblastopenia (RBC anemia), and congenital (erythroid) hypoplastic anemia

Palliative management of **neoplastic diseases,** including leukemias and lymphomas in adults and acute leukemia of childhood

To induce diuresis or remission of proteinuria in the **nephrotic syndrome,** without uremia, of the idiopathic type or that due to lupus erythematosus

Gastrointestinal diseases, including ulcerative colitis and regional enteritis

Tuberculous meningitis with subarachnoid block or impending block (with appropriate antituberculous chemotherapy)

Trichinosis associated with neurological or myocardial involvement

ORAL DOSAGE

Adult: 25–300 mg/day to start, followed by gradual reductions in dosage to lowest level possible consistent with maintaining an adequate clinical response; dosage must be individualized on the basis of the specific disease being treated, its severity, and clinical response

PARENTERAL DOSAGE

Adult: 20–300 mg/day IM to start, followed by gradual reductions in dosage to lowest level possible consistent with maintaining an adequate clinical response; dosage must be individualized on the basis of the specific disease being treated, its severity, and clinical response; larger than usual doses may be justified in certain overwhelming, acute, life-threatening situations

CONTRAINDICATIONS

Systemic fungal infections

WARNINGS/PRECAUTIONS

Patients subjected to unusual stress	Require increased dosage of rapidly acting corticosteroids before, during, and after emotionally or physically stressful situations
Infection	Clinical signs may be masked, new infections may appear, resistance may be decreased, and infections may be difficult to localize
Ocular damage	Prolonged use may produce posterior subcapsular cataracts and glaucoma, with possible damage to optic nerves, and may enhance development of secondary fungal viral ocular infections
Dietary salt restriction and potassium supplementation	May be necessary to combat the blood pressure elevation, salt and water retention, and increased potassium excretion with average and high-dose therapy
Immunization procedures	Especially against smallpox, should not be undertaken because of possible neurological complications and lack of antibody response
Active tuberculosis	Restrict use to fulminating or disseminated cases, as an adjunct to appropriate antituberculous therapy
Latent tuberculosis or tuberculin reactivity	Observe patient closely, since reactivation of the disease may occur; during prolonged therapy, employ antituberculous chemoprophylactic measures
Secondary adrenocortical insufficiency	May be minimized by gradual dosage reduction; since insufficiency may persist for months, reinstitute corticosteroid therapy in any stressful situation during this period, and administer salt and/or a mineralocorticoid concurrently to correct impaired mineralocorticoid secretion
Hypothyroidism, hepatic cirrhosis	May enhance effects of cortisone acetate
Corneal perforation	May occur in patients with ocular herpes simplex; use with caution

COMPENDIUM OF DRUG THERAPY

Cortisone

Prolonged therapy	Routine laboratory studies (eg, urinalysis, 2-h postprandial blood sugar, blood pressure, body weight, chest film) should be made at regular intervals; in addition, an upper GI series is suggested in patients with an ulcer history of significant dyspepsia. Withdraw the drug gradually, rather than abruptly, when discontinuing long-term therapy.
Special-risk patients	Use with caution in patients with nonspecific ulcerative colitis if impending perforation, abscess, or other pyogenic infection is likely, as well as in patients with diverticulitis, fresh intestinal anatomoses, active or latent peptic ulcer, renal insufficiency, hypertension, osteoporosis, or myasthenia gravis
Psychic derangements	May appear, ranging from euphoria, insomnia, mood swings, personality changes, and severe depression to frank psychotic manifestations; existing emotional instability or psychotic tendencies may be aggravated
Concomitant use with aspirin	Use with caution in patients with hypoprothrombinemia during therapy
Anaphylactoid reactions	Have occurred following parenteral corticosteroid administration; take appropriate precautionary measures before injecting cortisone acetate, especially in patients with a history of drug allergy

ADVERSE REACTIONS

Fluid and electrolyte disturbances	Sodium retention, fluid retention, congestive heart failure in susceptible patients, loss of potassium, hypokalemic alkalosis, hypertension
Musculoskeletal	Muscle weakness, steroid myopathy, loss of muscle mass, osteoporosis, vertebral compression fractures, aseptic necrosis of femoral and humeral heads, pathological fracture of long bones
Gastrointestinal	Peptic ulcer with possible perforation and hemorrhage, pancreatitis, abdominal distention, ulcerative esophagitis
Dermatological	Impaired wound healing, thin fragile skin, petechiae and ecchymoses, facial erythema, increased sweating, suppressed reaction to skin tests
Neurological	Convulsions, increased intracranial pressure with papilledema (pseudotumor cerebri), vertigo, headache
Endocrinological	Menstrual irregularities, Cushingoid state, growth suppression in children, secondary adrenocortical and pituitary unresponsiveness, decreased carbohydrate tolerance, latent diabetes mellitus, increased insulin or oral hypoglycemic requirements
Ophthalmic	Posterior subcapsular cataracts, increased intraocular pressure, glaucoma, exophthalmos
Metabolic	Negative nitrogen balance
Additional reactions to parenteral therapy only	Hyperpigmentation or hypopigmentation, subcutaneous and cutaneous atrophy, sterile abscess, postinjection flare (following intraarticular use), Charcot-like arthropathy, blindness (rare) associated with intralesional therapy around the face and head

OVERDOSAGE

Signs and symptoms	CNS changes, GI bleeding, hyperglycemia, hypertension, edema
Treatment	Discontinue medication; institute supportive measures, as required

DRUG INTERACTIONS

Insulin, oral hypoglycemics	▽ Hypoglycemic effect
Phenytoin, phenobarbital, ephedrine, rifampin	△ Metabolic clearance of cortisone ▽ Steroid blood level and physiological activity
Oral anticoagulants	△ or ▽ Prothrombin time
Potassium-depleting diuretics	△ Risk of hypokalemia
Cardiac glycosides	△ Risk of arrhythmias or digitalis toxicity secondary to hypokalemia
Skin test antigens	▽ Reactivity
Immunizations	▽ Antibody response

ALTERED LABORATORY VALUES

Blood/serum values	△ Glucose △ Cholesterol △ Sodium ▽ Potassium ▽ Calcium ▽ PBI ▽ Thyroxine (T_4) ▽ ^{131}I thyroid uptake ▽ Uric acid
Urinary values	△ Glucose △ Potassium △ Calcium △ Uric acid ▽ 17-Hydroxycorticosteroids (17-OHCS) ▽ 17-Ketosteroids

---

USE IN CHILDREN

Growth and development should be carefully observed in infants and children on prolonged therapy; consult manufacturer for dosage recommendations

USE IN PREGNANT AND NURSING WOMEN

Safety for use in pregnant or nursing women has not been established. Infants born of mothers who received substantial doses of corticosteroids during pregnancy should be carefully observed for signs of hypoadrenalism.

DECADRON

ORAL AND INJECTABLE CORTICOSTEROIDS

DECADRON (dexamethasone) Merck Sharp & Dohme — Rx
Tablets: 0.25, 0.5, 0.75, 1.5, 4, 6 mg Elixir (per 5 ml): 0.5 mg[1] (100, 237 ml)

DECADRON Phosphate (dexamethasone sodium phosphate) Merck Sharp & Dohme — Rx
Prefilled syringes: 4 mg/ml (1, 2.5 ml) Vials: 4 mg/ml (1, 5, 25 ml); 24 mg/ml (5, 10 ml) for IV use only

INDICATIONS

Endocrine disorders, including primary or secondary adrenocortical insufficiency, congenital adrenal hyperplasia, nonsuppurative thyroiditis, and hypercalcemia associated with cancer

Rheumatic disorders, including psoriatic arthritis, rheumatoid arthritis, juvenile rheumatoid arthritis, ankylosing spondylitis, acute and subacute bursitis, acute nonspecific tenosynovitis, acute gouty arthritis, posttraumatic osteoarthritis, synovitis of osteoarthritis, and epicondylitis (adjunctive, short-term therapy)

Collagen diseases, including systemic lupus erythematosus and acute rheumatic carditis

Dermatological diseases, including pemphigus, bullous dermatitis herpetiformis, severe erythema multiforme (Stevens-Johnson syndrome), exfoliative dermatitis, mycosis fungoides, severe psoriasis, and severe seborrheic dermatitis

Severe or incapacitating **allergic conditions** intractable to adequate trials of conventional treatment, including seasonal or perennial allergic rhinitis, bronchial asthma, contact dermatitis, atopic dermatitis, serum sickness, drug hypersensitivity reactions, urticarial transfusion reactions (IM, IV only), and acute noninfectious laryngeal edema (IM, IV only)

Ophthalmic diseases, including allergic conjunctivitis, keratitis, allergic corneal marginal ulcers, herpes zoster ophthalmicus, iritis and iridocyclitis, chorioretinitis, anterior segment inflammation, diffuse posterior uveitis and choroiditis, optic neuritis, and sympathetic ophthalmia

Respiratory diseases, including symptomatic sarcoidosis, Loeffler's syndrome not manageable by other means, berylliosis, fulminating or disseminated pulmonary tuberculosis (with appropriate antituberculous chemotherapy), and aspiration pneumonitis

Hematological disorders, including idiopathic thrombocytopenic purpura (oral, IV only) and secondary thrombocytopenia in adults, acquired (autoimmune) hemolytic anemia, erythroblastopenia (RBC anemia), and congenital (erythroid) hypoplastic anemia

Palliative management of **neoplastic diseases,** including leukemias and lymphomas in adults and acute leukemia of childhood

To induce a diuresis or remission of proteinuria in the **nephrotic syndrome,** without uremia, of the idiopathic type or that due to lupus erythematosus

Gastrointestinal diseases, including ulcerative colitis and regional enteritis

Tuberculous meningitis with subarachnoid block or impending block (with appropriate antituberculous chemotherapy)

Trichinosis associated with neurological or myocardial involvement

ORAL DOSAGE

Adult: 0.75–9 mg/day to start, followed by gradual reductions in dosage to lowest level possible consistent with maintaining an adequate clinical response; dosage must be individualized on the basis of the specific disease being treated, its severity, and clinical response; smaller doses than these may be sufficient in less severe diseases, while doses higher than 9 mg/day may be required in more severe diseases

PARENTERAL DOSAGE

Adult: 0.5–9 mg/day IM or IV to start, followed by gradual reductions in dosage to lowest level possible consistent with maintaining an adequate clinical response; dosage must be individualized on the basis of the specific disease being treated, its severity, and clinical response; smaller doses than these may be sufficient in less severe diseases, while doses higher than 9 mg/day may be required in more severe diseases. For IV use, inject solution or add to sodium chloride or dextrose injection and give by infusion (use within 24 h after preparation).

DECADRON-LA Suspension (dexamethasone acetate) Merck Sharp & Dohme — Rx
Vials: 8 mg/ml (1, 5 ml)

INDICATIONS
Same as Decadron Phosphate, except for adrenocortical insufficiency, pulmonary tuberculosis, and idiopathic thrombocytopenic purpura in adults

PARENTERAL DOSAGE
Adult: 8–16 mg IM, repeated at 1- to 3-wk intervals, if needed; dosage must be individualized on the basis of the specific disease being treated, its severity, and clinical response; do not inject IV

CONTRAINDICATIONS

Hypersensitivity to any component	Injection into infected or unstable joints	Systemic fungal infections[2]
Hypersensitivity to sulfites (parenteral forms only)		

ADMINISTRATION/DOSAGE ADJUSTMENTS

Unresponsive shock	Suggested regimens include 40 mg IV q2–6h; 1–6 mg/kg as a single IV injection; and 20 mg IV to start, followed by 3 mg/kg/24 h by continuous IV infusion. Treatment should be continued only until patient's condition stabilizes (usually not beyond 48–72 h). Prophylactic antacid therapy may be indicated to prevent peptic ulceration.
Cerebral edema associated with brain tumors, craniotomy, or head injury	Administer 10 mg Decadron Phosphate IV to start, followed by 4 mg IM q6h until symptoms subside; for palliative management, give 2 mg bid or tid, orally or parenterally
Intraarticular, soft tissue, and intralesional administration (keloids, lichen planus lesions, psoriatic plaques, ganglia)	Employ only when the affected joints or areas are limited to one or two sites as follows: large joints (eg, knee), 2–4 mg; small joints (eg, interphalangeal, temporomandibular), 0.8–1.0 mg; bursal, 2–3 mg; tendon sheaths, 0.4–1.0 mg; soft tissue infiltration, 2–6 mg; and ganglia, 1–2 mg. The frequency ranges from once every 3–5 days to once every week for Decadron Phosphate and 1–3 wk for Decadron-LA Suspension.

DECADRON

Dexamethasone suppression tests for Cushing's syndrome	Give 1 mg orally at 11 PM. Draw blood for plasma cortisol determination at 8 AM on the following morning. For greater accuracy, give 0.5 mg orally q6h for 48 h; collect a 24-h urine specimen for determination of 17-hydroxycorticosteroid excretion. To distinguish Cushing's disease from other causes of hypercortisolism, give 2 mg orally q6h for 48 h; collect a 24-h urine specimen for determination of 17-hydroxycorticosteroid excretion.
Acute, self-limiting allergic disorders or acute exacerbations of chronic allergic disorders	Combine parenteral and oral therapy as follows: first day, 4–8 mg Decadron Phosphate IM; second and third days, 3 mg in two divided oral doses; fourth day, 1.5 mg in two divided oral doses; fifth and sixth days, 0.75 mg in a single oral dose; seventh day, no treatment; eighth day, follow up

WARNINGS/PRECAUTIONS

Hypersensitivity to sulfites	Sodium bisulfite in parenteral dosage forms may cause severe allergic reactions in certain susceptible individuals, particularly those with asthma; do not use the injectable forms in patients allergic to sulfites
Patients subjected to unusual stress	Require increased dosage of rapidly acting corticosteroids before, during, and after emotionally or physically stressful situations
Infection	Clinical signs may be masked, new infections may appear, resistance may be decreased, and infections may be difficult to localize; false-negative results may be obtained with nitroblue-tetrazolium test for bacterial infection
Cerebral malaria	The duration of coma may be prolonged and the incidence of pneumonia and gastrointestinal bleeding increased
Latent amebiasis	May be activated; before instituting therapy, rule out latent or active amebiasis in any patient with unexplained diarrhea or who has spent time in the tropics
Ocular damage	Prolonged use may produce posterior subcapsular cataracts and glaucoma with possible damage to optic nerves, and may enhance development of secondary fungal or viral ocular infections
Dietary salt restriction and potassium supplementation	May be necessary to combat blood pressure elevation, salt and water retention, and increased potassium excretion with average- and high-dose therapy
Immunization procedures	The expected serum antibody response to inactivated viral or bacterial vaccines may not be obtained in patients receiving immunosuppressive doses; such patients must not be given live virus vaccines, including smallpox vaccine. Patients receiving corticosteroid replacement therapy (eg, for Addison's disease) may be immunized, however.
Active tuberculosis	Restrict use to fulminating or disseminated cases, as an adjunct to appropriate antituberculous therapy
Latent tuberculosis or tuberculin reactivity	Observe patient closely, since reactivation of the disease may occur; during prolonged therapy, employ antituberculous chemoprophylactic measures
Secondary adrenocortical insufficiency	May be minimized by gradual dosage reduction; since insufficiency may persist for months, reinstitute corticosteroid therapy in any stressful situation during this period, and administer salt and/or a mineralocorticoid concurrently to correct impaired mineralocorticoid secretion
Withdrawal symptoms	Including fever, myalgia, arthralgia, and malaise, may occur when drug is withdrawn following prolonged therapy, even in the absence of adrenal insufficiency
Hypothyroidism, hepatic cirrhosis	May enhance effects of dexamethasone
Corneal perforation	May occur in patients with ocular herpes simplex; use with caution
Special-risk patients	Use with caution in patients with nonspecific ulcerative colitis if impending perforation, abscess, or other pyogenic infection is likely, as well as in patients with diverticulitis, fresh intestinal anastomoses, active or latent peptic ulcer, renal insufficiency, hypertension, osteoporosis, or myasthenia gravis. In patients receiving large doses, signs of peritoneal irritation following GI perforation may be minimal or absent.
Peptic ulcer, with possible perforation and hemorrhage	May occur, especially with large doses; risk may be minimized by administering with meals and taking antacids between meals
Psychic derangements	May appear, ranging from euphoria, insomnia, mood swings, personality changes, and severe depression to frank psychotic manifestations; existing emotional instability or psychotic tendencies may be aggravated
Concomitant use with aspirin	Use with caution in patients with hypoprothrombinemia during therapy
Concomitant use with oral anticoagulants	Check prothrombin time frequently; anticoagulant effect may be increased or decreased
Concomitant use with potassium-depleting diuretics	Monitor serum potassium level periodically; risk of hypokalemia is increased
Suppression tests	May be altered by phenytoin, phenobarbital, ephedrine, and rifampin; interpret with caution
Fertility	Motility and number of spermatozoa may be increased or decreased
Septic arthritis	May occur with intraarticular injection and require appropriate antimicrobial therapy; observe patient for suggestive symptoms (eg, increased pain, local swelling, further restrictions of joint mobility, fever, malaise) and examine joint fluid microscopically

DECADRON

Frequent intraarticular injection	May damage joint tissue
Overuse of joints	Caution patients who experience symptomatic relief against overusing joints as long as inflammatory process remains active
Anaphylactoid reactions	Have occurred following parenteral corticosteroid administration; take appropriate precautionary measures before injecting dexamethasone, especially in patients with a history of drug allergy

ADVERSE REACTIONS

Fluid and electrolyte disturbances	Sodium retention, fluid retention, congestive heart failure in susceptible patients, loss of potassium, hypokalemic alkalosis, hypertension
Musculoskeletal	Muscle weakness, steroid myopathy, loss of muscle mass, osteoporosis, vertebral compression fractures, aseptic necrosis of femoral and humeral heads, pathological fracture of long bones, tendon rupture
Gastrointestinal	Peptic ulcer with possible perforation and hemorrhage, pancreatitis, abdominal distention, ulcerative esophagitis, increased appetite, nausea; perforation of the large and small bowel (particularly in patients with inflammatory bowel disease)
Dermatological	Impaired wound healing, thin fragile skin, petechiae and ecchymoses, facial erythema, increased sweating, suppressed reactions to skin tests, allergic dermatitis, urticaria, angioneurotic edema
Neurological	Convulsions, increased intracranial pressure with papilledema (pseudotumor cerebri), vertigo, headache, psychic disturbances
Endocrinological	Menstrual irregularities, Cushingoid state, growth suppression in children, secondary adrenocortical and pituitary unresponsiveness, decreased carbohydrate tolerance, latent diabetes mellitus, increased insulin or oral hypoglycemic requirements, hirsutism
Ophthalmic	Posterior subcapsular cataracts, increased intraocular pressure, glaucoma, exophthalmos
Metabolic	Negative nitrogen balance, weight gain
Other	Anaphylactoid or hypersensitivity reactions, thromboembolism, malaise
Additional reactions to parenteral therapy only	Hyperpigmentation or hypopigmentation; subcutaneous and cutaneous atrophy; sterile abscess; postinjection flare (following intraarticular use); Charcot-like arthropathy; blindness associated with intralesional therapy around the face and head (rare); burning or tingling, especially in perineal area (with IV use); scarring; induration; inflammation; paresthesia; delayed pain or soreness; muscle twitching, ataxia, hiccoughs, and nystagmus (following use of suspension)

OVERDOSAGE

Signs and symptoms	CNS changes, GI bleeding, hyperglycemia, hypertension, edema
Treatment	Discontinue medication; institute supportive measures, as required

DRUG INTERACTIONS

Insulin, oral hypoglycemics	⇩ Hypoglycemic effect
Phenytoin, phenobarbital, ephedrine, rifampin	⇧ Metabolic clearance of dexamethasone ⇩ Steroid blood level and physiological activity
Oral anticoagulants	⇧ or ⇩ Prothrombin time
Potassium-depleting diuretics	⇧ Risk of hypokalemia
Cardiac glycosides	⇧ Risk of arrhythmias or digitalis toxicity secondary to hypokalemia
Skin test antigens	⇩ Reactivity
Immunizations	⇩ Antibody response

ALTERED LABORATORY VALUES

Blood/serum values	⇧ Glucose ⇧ Cholesterol ⇧ Sodium ⇩ Potassium ⇩ Calcium ⇩ PBI ⇩ Thyroxine (T$_4$) ⇩ ^{131}I thyroid uptake ⇩ Uric acid
Urinary values	⇧ Glucose ⇧ Potassium ⇧ Calcium ⇧ Uric acid ⇩ 17-Hydroxycorticosteroids (17-OHCS) ⇩ 17-Ketosteroids

USE IN CHILDREN

Growth and development should be carefully observed in infants and children on prolonged therapy; consult manufacturer for dosage recommendations for Decadron and Decadron Phosphate. Dosage of Decadron-LA Suspension has not been established in children under 12 yr of age. Use a preservative-free diluent when preparing a solution for administration to full-term or premature neonates.

USE IN PREGNANT AND NURSING WOMEN

Safety for use during pregnancy has not been established. Infants born of mothers who have received substantial doses of corticosteroids during pregnancy should be carefully observed for signs of hypoadrenalism. Corticosteroids appear in breast milk and may suppress growth, interfere with endogenous corticosteroid production, or cause other untoward effects. Patient should stop nursing if drug is prescribed.

[1] Contains 5% alcohol
[2] Unless needed to control drug reactions due to amphotericin B

DELTASONE

ORAL AND INJECTABLE CORTICOSTEROIDS

DELTASONE (prednisone) Upjohn   Rx

Tablets: 2.5, 5, 10, 20, 50 mg

INDICATIONS

Endocrine disorders, including primary or secondary adrenocortical insufficiency, congenital adrenal hyperplasia, nonsuppurative thyroiditis, and hypercalcemia associated with cancer

Rheumatic disorders, including psoriatic arthritis, rheumatoid arthritis, juvenile rheumatoid arthritis, ankylosing spondylitis, acute and subacute bursitis, acute nonspecific tenosynovitis, acute gouty arthritis, posttraumatic osteoarthritis, synovitis of osteoarthritis, and epicondylitis (adjunctive, short-term therapy)

Collagen diseases, including systemic lupus erythematosus, acute rheumatic carditis and systemic dermatomyositis (polymyositis)

Dermatological diseases, including pemphigus, bullous dermatitis herpetiformis, severe erythema multiforme (Stevens-Johnson syndrome), exfoliative dermatitis, mycosis fungoides, severe psoriasis, and severe seborrheic dermatitis

Severe or incapacitating **allergic conditions** intractable to adequate trials of conventional treatment, including seasonal or perennial allergic rhinitis, bronchial asthma, contact dermatitis, atopic dermatitis, serum sickness, and drug hypersensitivity reactions

Ophthalmic diseases, including allergic conjunctivitis, keratitis, allergic corneal marginal ulcers, herpes zoster ophthalmicus, iritis and iridocyclitis, chorioretinitis, anterior segment inflammation, diffuse posterior uveitis and choroiditis, optic neuritis, and sympathetic ophthalmia

Respiratory diseases, including symptomatic sarcoidosis, Loeffler's syndrome not manageable by other means, berylliosis, fulminating or disseminated pulmonary tuberculosis (with appropriate antituberculous chemotherapy), and aspiration pneumonitis

Hematological disorders, including idiopathic thrombocytopenic purpura and secondary thrombocytopenic purpura in adults, acquired (autoimmune) hemolytic anemia, erythroblastopenia (RBC anemia), and congenital (erythroid) hypoplastic anemia

Palliative management of **neoplastic diseases,** including leukemias and lymphomas in adults and acute leukemia of childhood

To induce a diuresis or remission of proteinuria in the **nephrotic syndrome,** without uremia, of the idiopathic type or that due to lupus erythematosus

Gastrointestinal disease, including ulcerative colitis and regional enteritis

Tuberculous meningitis with subarachnoid block or impending block (with appropriate antituberculous chemotherapy)

Trichinosis associated with neurological or myocardial involvement

ORAL DOSAGE

Adult: 5–60 mg/day to start, followed by gradual reductions in dosage to lowest level possible consistent with maintaining an adequate clinical response; dosage must be individualized on the basis of the specific disease being treated, its severity, and clinical response

CONTRAINDICATIONS

Systemic fungal infections

ADMINISTRATION/DOSAGE ADJUSTMENTS

Alternate-day regimen	For patients requiring long-term steroid therapy, twice the usual daily dose may be given every other morning. Continue the initial suppressive dose level until a satisfactory clinical response is obtained (usually 4–10 days for many allergic and collagen diseases). Then change to alternate-day therapy and gradually reduce the dose given every other day, or first reduce the daily dose to the lowest effective level as quickly as possible and then change over to an alternate-day schedule. If an acute flare-up of the disease occurs, return to a full suppressive daily divided dosage regimen for control. Reinstate the alternate-day regimen when control is re-established. If difficulty is encountered in switching patients who have been on a daily regimen for long periods to alternate-day therapy, initially tripling or even quadrupling the daily maintenance dose and giving it every other day may be helpful.
Acute exacerbations of multiple sclerosis	Administer 200 mg/day for 1 wk, followed by 80 mg every other day for 1 mo

WARNINGS/PRECAUTIONS

Patients subjected to unusual stress	Require increased dosage of rapidly acting corticosteroids before, during, and after emotionally or physically stressful situations
Infection	Clinical signs may be masked, new infections may appear, resistance may be decreased, and infections may be difficult to localize
Ocular damage	Prolonged use may produce posterior subcapsular cataracts and glaucoma, with possible damage to optic nerves, and may enhance development of secondary fungal or viral ocular infections
Dietary salt restriction and potassium supplementation	May be necessary to combat blood-pressure elevation, salt and water retention, and increased potassium excretion with average- and high-dose therapy
Immunization procedures	Especially against smallpox, should not be undertaken because of possible neurological complications and lack of antibody response
Active tuberculosis	Restrict use to fulminating or disseminated cases, as an adjunct to appropriate antituberculous therapy

DELTASONE

Latent tuberculosis or tuberculin reactivity	Observe patient closely, since reactivation of the disease may occur; during prolonged therapy, employ antituberculous chemoprophylactic measures
Secondary adrenocortical insufficiency	May be minimized by gradual dosage reduction; since insufficiency may persist for months, reinstitute corticosteroid therapy in any stressful situation during this period, and administer salt and/or a mineralocorticoid concurrently to correct impaired mineralocorticoid secretion
Hypothyroidism, hepatic cirrhosis	May enhance effects of prednisone
Corneal perforation	May occur in patients with ocular herpes simplex; use with caution
Special-risk patients	Use with caution in patients with nonspecific ulcerative colitis if impending perforation, abscess, or other pyogenic infection is likely, as well as in patients with diverticulitis, fresh intestinal anastomoses, active or latent peptic ulcer, renal insufficiency, hypertension, osteoporosis, or myasthenia gravis
Psychic derangements	May appear, ranging from euphoria, insomnia, mood swings, personality changes, and severe depression to frank psychotic manifestations; existing emotional instability or psychotic tendencies may be aggravated
Concomitant use with aspirin	Use with caution in patients with hypoprothrombinemia during therapy

ADVERSE REACTIONS

Fluid and electrolyte disturbances	Sodium retention, fluid retention, congestive heart failure in susceptible patients, loss of potassium, hypokalemic alkalosis, hypertension
Musculoskeletal	Muscle weakness, steroid myopathy, loss of muscle mass, osteoporosis, vertebral compression fractures, aseptic necrosis of femoral and humeral heads, pathological fracture of long bones
Gastrointestinal	Peptic ulcer with possible perforation and hemorrhage, pancreatitis, abdominal distention, ulcerative esophagitis
Dermatological	Impaired wound healing, thin fragile skin, petechiae and ecchymoses, facial erythema, increased sweating, suppressed reaction to skin tests
Neurological	Convulsions, increased intracranial pressure with papilledema (pseudotumor cerebri), vertigo, headache
Endocrinological	Menstrual irregularities, Cushingoid state, growth suppression in children, secondary adrenocortical and pituitary unresponsiveness, decreased carbohydrate tolerance, latent diabetes mellitus, increased insulin or oral hypoglycemic requirements
Ophthalmic	Posterior subcapsular cataracts, increased intraocular pressure, glaucoma, exophthalmos
Metabolic	Negative nitrogen balance
Hypersensitivity	Urticaria, anaphylactic reactions, other allergic reactions

OVERDOSAGE

Signs and symptoms	CNS changes, GI bleeding, hyperglycemia, hypertension, edema
Treatment	Discontinue medication; institute supportive measures, as required

DRUG INTERACTIONS

Insulin, oral hypoglycemics	▽ Hypoglycemic effect
Phenytoin, phenobarbital, ephedrine, rifampin	△ Metabolic clearance of prednisolone ▽ Steroid blood level and physiological activity
Oral anticoagulants	△ or ▽ Prothrombin time
Potassium-depleting diuretics	△ Risk of hypokalemia
Cardiac glycosides	△ Risk of arrhythmias or digitalis toxicity secondary to hypokalemia
Skin test antigens	▽ Reactivity
Immunizations	▽ Antibody response

ALTERED LABORATORY VALUES

Blood/serum values	△ Glucose △ Cholesterol △ Sodium ▽ Potassium ▽ Calcium ▽ PBI ▽ Thyroxine (T_4) ▽ ^{131}I thyroid uptake ▽ Uric acid
Urinary values	△ Glucose △ Potassium △ Calcium △ Uric acid ▽ 17-Hydroxycorticosteroids (17-OHCS) ▽ 17-Ketosteroids

---

USE IN CHILDREN

Growth and development should be carefully observed in infants and children on prolonged therapy; consult manufacturer for dosage recommendations

USE IN PREGNANT AND NURSING WOMEN

Safety for use in pregnant or nursing women has not been established. Infants born of mothers who have received substantial doses of corticosteroids during pregnancy should be carefully observed for signs of hypoadrenalism.

MEDROL

ORAL AND INJECTABLE CORTICOSTEROIDS

DEPO-MEDROL (methylprednisolone acetate suspension) Upjohn — Rx
Prefilled syringes: 80 mg/ml (1 ml) Vials: 20 mg/ml (5 ml), 40 mg/ml (1, 5, 10 ml), 80 mg/ml (1, 5 ml)

MEDROL (methylprednisolone) Upjohn — Rx
Tablets: 2, 4, 8, 16, 24, 32 mg

SOLU-MEDROL (methylprednisolone sodium succinate) Upjohn — Rx
Vials: 40 mg (1 ml), 125 mg (2 ml), 500 mg (8 ml), 1 g (16 ml), 2 g (30.6 ml)

INDICATIONS

Endocrine disorders, including primary or secondary adrenocortical insufficiency, congenital adrenal hyperplasia, nonsuppurative thyroiditis, hypercalcemia associated with cancer, acute adrenocortical insufficiency (IM, IV only), and preoperatively and in the event of serious trauma or illness in patients with known adrenal insufficiency or when adrenocortical reserve is doubtful (IM, IV only)

Rheumatic disorders, including psoriatic arthritis, rheumatoid arthritis, juvenile rheumatoid arthritis, ankylosing spondylitis, acute and subacute bursitis, acute nonspecific tenosynovitis, acute gouty arthritis, posttraumatic osteoarthritis, synovitis of osteoarthritis, and epicondylitis (for short-term adjunctive treatment of rheumatic disorders and, in selected cases, for maintenance therapy of rheumatoid arthritis)

Collagen diseases, including systemic lupus erythematosus, acute rheumatic carditis, and systemic dermatomyositis (polymyositis)

Dermatological diseases, including pemphigus, bullous dermatitis herpetiformis, severe erythema multiforme (Stevens-Johnson syndrome), exfoliative dermatitis, mycosis fungoides, severe psoriasis, and severe seborrheic dermatitis

Severe or incapacitating **allergic conditions** intractable to adequate trials of conventional treatment, including seasonal or perennial allergic rhinitis, bronchial asthma, contact dermatitis, atopic dermatitis, serum sickness, drug hypersensitivity reactions, urticarial transfusion reactions (IM, IV only), and acute noninfectious laryngeal edema (IM, IV only)

Ophthalmic diseases, including allergic conjunctivitis, keratitis, allergic corneal marginal ulcers, herpes zoster ophthalmicus, iritis and iridocyclitis, chorioretinitis, anterior segment inflammation, diffuse posterior uveitis and choroiditis, optic neuritis, and sympathetic ophthalmia

Respiratory diseases, including symptomatic sarcoidosis, Loeffler's syndrome not manageable by other means, berylliosis, fulminating or disseminated pulmonary tuberculosis (with appropriate antituberculous chemotherapy), and aspiration pneumonitis

Hematological disorders, including idiopathic thrombocytopenic purpura in adults (oral, IV only), secondary thrombocytopenia in adults, acquired (autoimmune) hemolytic anemia, erythroblastopenia (RBC anemia), and congenital (erythroid) hypoplastic anemia

Palliative management of **neoplastic diseases,** including leukemias and lymphomas in adults and acute leukemia of childhood

To induce diuresis or remission of proteinuria in the **nephrotic syndrome,** without uremia, of the idiopathic type or that due to lupus erythematosus

Gastrointestinal diseases, including ulcerative colitis and regional enteritis

Tuberculosis meningitis with subarachnoid block or impending block (with appropriate antituberculous chemotherapy)

Trichinosis associated with neurological or myocardial involvement

ORAL DOSAGE

Adult: 4–48 mg/day to start, followed by gradual reductions in dosage to lowest level possible consistent with maintaining an adequate clinical response; dosage must be individualized on the basis of the specific disease being treated, its severity, and clinical response

PARENTERAL DOSAGE

Adult: 4–48 mg of Depo-Medrol, given in a single IM injection q24h, or, for prolonged effect, 7 times the daily oral dose, given in a single IM injection once a week; dosage must be individualized on the basis of disease severity and clinical response; *alternatively,* 10–40 mg of Solu-Medrol, given IV over a period of one to several minutes to start and repeated IV or IM at intervals dictated by patient's response and clinical condition; reduce dosage or discontinue gradually when administered for more than a few days. When high doses are required, give 30 mg/kg of Solu-Medrol IV over a period of 10–20 min; this dose may be repeated q4–6h for 48 h.

CONTRAINDICATIONS

| Systemic fungal infections | Injection into unstable or previously infected joints |

ADMINISTRATION/DOSAGE ADJUSTMENTS

Alternate-day regimen	For patients requiring long-term steroid therapy, twice the usual daily oral dose may be given every other morning. Continue the initial suppressive dose level until a satisfactory clinical response is obtained (usually 4–10 days for many allergic and collagen diseases). Then change to alternate-day therapy and gradually reduce the dose given every other day, or first reduce the daily dose to the lowest effective level as quickly as possible and then change over to an alternate-day schedule. If an acute flare-up of the disease occurs, return to full suppressive daily divided dosage regimen for control. Reinstate the alternate-day regimen when control is reestablished. If difficulty is encountered in switching patients who have been on a daily regimen for long periods to alternate-day therapy, initially tripling or even quadrupling the daily maintenance dose and giving it every other day may be helpful.
Adrenocortical insufficiency	Mineralocorticoid supplementation may be necessary, particularly in infants
Adrenogenital syndrome	As an alternative to daily oral therapy, a single 40-mg IM dose of the suspension injected once every 2 wk may be adequate for control
Systemic treatment of dermatological lesions	When oral therapy is not feasible, 40–120 mg of the suspension may be given in a single IM injection at weekly intervals for 1–4 wk. Relief of acute severe dermatitis due to poison ivy may result within 8–12 h following a single 80- to 120-mg IM dose. For chronic contact dermatitis, repeated IM injections at 5- to 10-day intervals may be required. For seborrheic dermatitis, a single weekly IM injection of 80 mg may be adequate.

MEDROL

Intralesional administration	For keloids, lichen planus, psoriatic plaques, granuloma annulare, lichen simplex chronicus (neurodermatitis), discoid lupus erythematosis, necrobiosis lipoidica diabeticorum, and alopecia areata, inject 20–60 mg of the suspension directly into the lesion. Large lesions may require repeated local injections of 20–40 mg. Excessive amounts will cause blanching, which may be followed by a small slough. Intervals between injections vary with the type of lesion being treated and the duration of improvement produced by the initial injection; usually 1–4 injections are needed.
Allergic conditions	When oral therapy is not feasible in patients with bronchial asthma or allergic rhinitis (hay fever), the suspension may be given in a single IM injection of 80–120 mg. Relief of asthmatic symptoms may result within 6–48 h and persist for several days to 2 wk; relief of coryzal symptoms may be obtained within 6 h and persist for several days to 3 wk.
Systemic treatment of rheumatoid arthritis	As an alternative to daily oral therapy, 40–120 mg of the suspension may be given weekly in a single IM injection
Intraarticular administration in rheumatoid arthritis and osteoarthritis	Dose of suspension is dependent on severity of condition and size of joint, as follows: large (eg, knee, ankle, shoulder), 20–80 mg; medium (eg, elbow, wrist), 10–40 mg; small (eg, metacarpophalangeal, interphalangeal, sternoclavicular, acromioclavicular), 4–10 mg. Injections may be repeated at intervals of 1–5 wk, depending on degree of relief obtained from the initial injection.
Local administration for bursitis, ganglia, tendinitis, tenosynovitis, and epicondylitis	Dose of suspension varies with condition being treated, ranging from 4 to 30 mg per injection; repeated injections may be required in recurrent or chronic conditions. In treating such conditions as tendinitis and tenosynovitis, care should be taken to inject the suspension into the affected tendon sheath, rather than the tendon itself. In treating epicondylitis, the suspension should be infiltrated into the area of greatest tenderness. For ganglia, inject the suspension directly in the ganglion cyst.
Acute exacerbations of multiple sclerosis	Administer 160 mg/day for 1 wk, followed by 64 mg every other day for 1 mo
Unresponsive shock	Solu-Medrol may be given in cases of shock unresponsive to conventional therapy, if adrenocortical insufficiency exists or is suspected, consult manufacturer for dosage recommendations
Intrathecal or IV administration	Of Depo-Medrol is not recommended
Preparation of parenteral solutions	Follow strict aseptic technique when using a Depo-Medrol vial for more than one dose; exercise particular care in withdrawing a dose for intrasynovial administration (eg, use disposable syringes and needles). The preservative prevents the growth of most, but not all, pathogenic agents; thus, if contamination occurs, certain organisms (eg, *Serratia marcescens*) may remain viable and cause injection site infections. Because of possible physical incompatibilities, Depo-Medrol should not be mixed or diluted with other solutions. Use the accompanying diluent or bacteriostatic water for injection with benzyl alcohol to prepare solutions of Solu-Medrol for IM or IV injection (consult manufacturer's labeling for directions); administer solutions within 48 h after preparation. If desired, the prepared solution may be further diluted with Sterile Water for Injection or other suitable diluent or added to 5% dextrose-in-water, isotonic saline solution, or 5% dextrose in isotonic saline solution for IV infusion.

WARNINGS/PRECAUTIONS

Gasping syndrome	Benzyl alcohol, which is contained in the diluent used to reconstitute Solu-Medrol solutions, has been associated with a gasping syndrome that is fatal in premature infants
Patients subjected to unusual stress	Require increased dosage of rapidly acting corticosteroids before, during, and after emotionally or physically stressful situations
Infection	Clinical signs may be masked, new infections may appear, resistance may be decreased, and infections may be difficult to localize
Ocular damage	Prolonged use may produce posterior subcapsular cataracts and glaucoma, with possible damage to optic nerves, and may enhance development of secondary fungal or viral ocular infections
Dietary salt restriction and potassium supplementation	May be necessary to combat blood pressure elevation, salt and water retention, and increased potassium excretion with average- and high-dose therapy
Immunization procedures	Especially against smallpox, should not be undertaken because of possible neurological complications and lack of antibody response
Active tuberculosis	Restrict use to fulminating or disseminated cases, as an adjunct to appropriate antituberculous therapy
Latent tuberculosis or tuberculin reactivity	Observe patient closely, since reactivation of the disease may occur; during prolonged therapy, employ antituberculous chemoprophylactic measures
Secondary adrenocortical insufficiency	May be minimized by gradual dosage reduction; since insufficiency may persist for months, reinstitute corticosteroid therapy in any stressful situation during this period, and administer salt and/or a mineralocorticoid concurrently to correct impaired mineralocorticoid secretion
Hypothyroidism, hepatic cirrhosis	May enhance effects of methylprednisolone

MEDROL

Corneal perforation	May occur in patients with ocular herpes simplex; use with caution
Special-risk patients	Use with caution in patients with nonspecific ulcerative colitis if impending perforation, abscess, or other pyogenic infection is likely, as well as in patients with diverticulitis, fresh intestinal anastomoses, active or latent peptic ulcer, renal insufficiency, hypertension, osteoporosis, or myasthenia gravis
Psychic derangements	May appear, ranging from euphoria, insomnia, mood swings, personality changes, and severe depression to frank psychotic manifestations; existing emotional instability or psychotic tendencies may be aggravated
Concomitant use with aspirin	Use with caution in patients with hypoprothrombinemia
Cardiac arrhythmias, circulatory collapse, and/or cardiac arrest	Have been reported following rapid (< 10 min) administration of large (> 0.5 g) IV doses
Prolonged therapy	Routine laboratory studies (eg, urinalysis, 2-h postprandial blood sugar, blood pressure, body weight, chest film) should be made at regular intervals; in addition, an upper GI series is suggested in patients with an ulcer history or significant dyspepsia. When therapy has been continued for more than a few days, dosage must be reduced gradually.
Dermal and subdermal atrophy	May be minimized by not exceeding recommended doses; administer multiple small injections into lesion area whenever possible. Take precautions against injection or leakage into the dermis. Avoid injection into the deltoid muscle because of a high incidence of subcutaneous atrophy.
Suppression tests	May be altered by phenytoin, phenobarbital, ephedrine, and rifampin; interpret with caution
Septic arthritis	May occur with intraarticular injection and require appropriate antimicrobial therapy; observe patient for suggestive symptoms (eg, increased pain, local swelling, further restrictions of joint mobility, fever, malaise) and examine joint fluid microscopically
Frequent intraarticular administration	May result in joint instability; in selected cases, follow-up x-ray examination to detect deterioration may be advisable
Overuse of joints	Caution patients who experience symptomatic relief against overusing joints as long as inflammatory process remains active
Tartrazine sensitivity	Presence of FD&C Yellow No. 5 (tartrazine) in 24-mg tablets may cause allergic-type reactions, including bronchial asthma, in susceptible individuals
Anaphylactoid reaction (eg, bronchospasm)	Have occurred following parenteral corticosteroid administration; take appropriate precautionary measures before injecting methylprednisolone, especially in patients with a history of drug allergy

ADVERSE REACTIONS

Fluid and electrolyte disturbances	Sodium retention, fluid retention, congestive heart failure in susceptible patients, loss of potassium, hypokalemic alkalosis, hypertension
Musculoskeletal	Muscle weakness, steroid myopathy, loss of muscle mass, osteoporosis, vertebral compression fractures, aseptic necrosis of femoral and humeral heads, pathological fracture of long bones
Gastrointestinal	Peptic ulcer with possible perforation and hemorrhage, pancreatitis, abdominal distention, ulcerative esophagitis
Dermatological	Impaired wound healing, thin fragile skin, petechiae and ecchymoses, facial erythema, increased sweating, suppressed reaction to skin tests
Neurological	Convulsions, increased intracranial pressure with papilledema (pseudotumor cerebri), vertigo, headache
Endocrinological	Menstrual irregularities, Cushingoid state, growth suppression in children, secondary adrenocortical and pituitary unresponsiveness, decreased carbohydrate tolerance, latent diabetes mellitus, increased insulin or oral hypoglycemic requirements
Ophthalmic	Posterior subcapsular cataracts, increased intraocular pressure, glaucoma, exophthalmos
Metabolic	Negative nitrogen balance
Hypersensitivity	Urticaria, anaphylactic reactions, and other allergic reactions
Additional reactions to parenteral therapy only	Hyperpigmentation or hypopigmentation, subcutaneous and cutaneous atrophy, injection site infections (following nonsterile use), sterile abscess, postinjection flare (following intraarticular use), Charcot-like arthropathy, severe arthralgia, blindness (rare) associated with intralesional therapy around the face and head, arachnoiditis (following intrathecal administration), nausea and vomiting, cardiac arrhythmias, hypotension or hypertension, anaphylactic reaction with or without circulatory collapse, cardiac arrest, or bronchospasm

OVERDOSAGE

Signs and symptoms	CNS changes, GI bleeding, hyperglycemia, hypertension, edema

MEDROL ■ KENALOG

Treatment —————————————— Discontinue medication; institute supportive measures, as required

DRUG INTERACTIONS

Insulin, oral hypoglycemics	⇩ Hypoglycemic effect
Phenytoin, phenobarbital, ephedrine, rifampin	⇧ Metabolic clearance of methylprednisolone ⇩ Steroid blood level and physiological activity
Oral anticoagulants	⇧ or ⇩ Prothrombin time
Potassium-depleting diuretics	⇧ Risk of hypokalemia
Cardiac glycosides	⇧ Risk of arrhythmias or digitalis toxicity secondary to hypokalemia
Skin test antigens	⇩ Reactivity
Immunizations	⇩ Antibody response

ALTERED LABORATORY VALUES

Blood/serum values	⇧ Glucose ⇧ Cholesterol ⇧ Sodium ⇩ Potassium ⇩ Calcium ⇩ PBI ⇩ Thyroxine (T₄) ⇩ ¹³¹I thyroid uptake ⇩ Uric acid
Urinary values	⇧ Glucose ⇧ Potassium ⇧ Calcium ⇧ Uric acid ⇩ 17-Hydroxycorticosteroids (17-OHCS) ⇩ 17-Ketosteroids

USE IN CHILDREN

Severity of condition and patient response are more important than age or size in adjusting parenteral dosage for children; consult manufacturer for specific dosage recommendations (minimum Solu-Medrol dosage: 0.5 mg/kg/24 h). Growth and development should be carefully observed in infants and children on prolonged therapy.

USE IN PREGNANT AND NURSING WOMEN

Safety for use in pregnant or nursing women has not been established. Infants born of mothers who received substantial doses of corticosteroids during pregnancy should be carefully observed for signs of hypoadrenalism.

ORAL AND INJECTABLE CORTICOSTEROIDS

KENALOG-10 (triamcinolone acetonide) Squibb   Rx

Vials: 10 mg/ml (5 ml) for local use only

INDICATIONS

Adjunctive, short-term treatment of **synovitis of osteoarthritis, rheumatoid arthritis, acute and subacute bursitis, acute gouty arthritis, epicondylitis, acute nonspecific tenosynovitis, and posttraumatic osteoarthritis**

Keloids, discoid lupus erythematosus, necrobiosis lipoidica diabeticorum, and alopecia areata
Localized hypertrophic, infiltrated, inflammatory lesions of **lichen planus, psoriatic plaques, granuloma annulare, and lichen simplex chronicus** (neurodermatitis)
Cystic tumors of an apnoneurosis or tendon (ganglia)

PARENTERAL DOSAGE

Adult: for intraarticular administration, an initial dose of 2.5–5 mg for smaller joints and 5–15 mg for larger joints; dose depends on the nature of the disease. In the treatment of several joints at one time, a total dose of 20 mg or more has been safely given. To determine the dose for intrabursal administration and injection into the tendon sheath, consult manufacturer.

Adult: for intralesional administration, up to 1 mg per injection site to start, with at least 1 cm between sites; dose may be repeated weekly or less frequently, as needed

KENALOG-40 (triamcinolone acetonide) Squibb   Rx

Vials: 40 mg/ml

INDICATIONS

Nonsuppurative thyroiditis
Adjunctive, short-term treatment of **posttraumatic osteoarthritis, synovitis of osteoarthritis, rheumatoid arthritis, acute and subacute bursitis, epicondylitis, acute nonspecific tenosynovitis, acute gouty arthritis, psoriatic arthritis, ankylosing spondylitis, and juvenile rheumatoid arthritis**
Selected cases of **systemic lupus erythematosus and acute rheumatic carditis**
Pemphigus, severe erythema multiforme (Stevens-Johnson syndrome), exfoliative dermatitis, bullous dermatitis herpetiformis, severe seborrheic dermatitis, and severe psoriasis
Bronchial asthma, contact dermatitis, atopic dermatitis, and seasonal or perennial allergic rhinitis, when these conditions are severe or incapacitating and do not respond to adequate conventional therapy
Severe chronic allergic and inflammatory ophthalmic diseases, such as herpes zoster ophthalmicus, iritis, iridocyclitis, chorioretinitis, diffuse posterior uveitis and choroiditis, optic neuritis, sympathetic ophthalmia, and anterior segment inflammation
Critical periods of **ulcerative colitis and regional enteritis**
Symptomatic sarcoidosis, berylliosis, and aspiration pneumonitis
Acquired (autoimmune) hemolytic anemia
Palliative management of **leukemias and lymphomas** in adults and **acute leukemia** in children
Induction of diuresis or remission of proteinuria in patients with **the nephrotic syndrome,** when this syndrome is nonuremic and either idiopathic or due to lupus erythematosus

Adjunctive, short-term treatment of **synovitis of osteoarthritis, rheumatoid arthritis, acute and subacute bursitis, acute gouty arthritis, epicondylitis, acute nonspecific tenosynovitis, and posttraumatic osteoarthritis**

PARENTERAL DOSAGE

Adult and child (> 12 yr): 60 mg IM to start, followed, as needed, by IM doses of 40–80 mg or, in some cases, as little as 20 mg or less, depending on the disease, initial patient response, and duration of relief. For patients allergic to pollen, a single IM dose of 40–100 mg may provide symptomatic relief throughout the pollen season.
Child (6–12 yr): 40 mg IM to start; dosage should depend more on severity of symptoms than on age or weight

Adult: for intraarticular administration, an initial dose of 2.5–5 mg for smaller joints and 5–15 mg for larger joints; dose depends on the nature of the disease. Symptoms are usually relieved with up to 10 mg in smaller areas and up to 40 mg in larger areas. In the treatment of several joints at one time, a total dose of up to 80 mg has been safely given. To determine dose for intrabursal administration and injection into the tendon sheath, consult manufacturer.

CONTRAINDICATIONS

| Systemic fungal infections | Idiopathic thrombocytopenic purpura (with IM use only) |

ADMINISTRATION/DOSAGE ADJUSTMENTS

Administration — Shake vial before use; if suspension appears granular or clumpy, do not administer it. To avoid settling of the suspension in the syringe, inject the dose without delay once it has been withdrawn from the vial.

Intramuscular administration: Inject dose into the gluteal muscle; use the deltoid muscle only under very unusual circumstances since injection at that site increases the risk of local atrophy. Rotate IM sites when subsequent doses are given. To avoid inadvertent SC injection, which can cause atrophy of SC fat tissue, make sure that each dose is injected deeply into the muscle. The length of the needle should be at least 1.5 in. for normal adults; the minimum length for obese adults may be longer.

Injection into joint, bursa, and tendon sheath: If a joint contains excessive synovial fluid, some, but not all, of the fluid should be aspirated in order to relieve pain and prevent undue dilution of the drug. Avoid overdistention of the joint capsule and deposition of the drug along the needle path since these actions may lead to SC atrophy. Do not inject into unstable or infected joints. Inadvertent injection into soft tissue surrounding a joint may result in systemic reactions and preclude a therapeutic response and therefore should be avoided. When treating acute nonspecific tenosynovitis, make sure that the drug is injected into the tendon sheath rather than the tendon. For epicondylitis (tennis elbow), infiltrate the drug into the area of greatest tenderness. A local anesthetic may be used in conjunction with injection into a joint, bursa, or tendon sheath. The anesthetic should be injected into the surrounding soft tissue before administration of triamcinolone; a small amount of the anesthetic may be instilled into a joint.

Intralesional administration: Using a tuberculin syringe and a 23- to 25-gauge needle, inject the dose directly into the lesion (intradermally or sometimes SC). To relieve injection pain, use ethyl chloride spray. When using this drug at multiple sites, bear in mind that there is a direct relationship between the total volume given at all sites and the risk of systemic absorption.

Monitoring of intraarticular therapy — Overuse of a joint following intraarticular therapy can increase deterioration, and repeated injections may result in joint instability. Follow-up x-rays are advisable for selected patients who have undergone intraarticular therapy, particularly when repeated doses have been given. Caution all patients not to overuse a treated joint.

KENALOG

Intramuscular therapy	Since intramuscular administration produces a sustained or depot effect, it is most commonly instituted after the dosage has been titrated with an oral preparation; for optimal response, dosage should be adjusted after the transition from oral to IM therapy. An IM regimen may be helpful when patients fail to adhere strictly to oral dosage schedules; it is also useful when it is necessary to supplement oral therapy.
Maintenance therapy	Once an adequate response has been obtained, reduce dosage gradually and in small increments to the lowest effective level. Keep patient under supervision during maintenance therapy; dosage adjustments may be necessary because of certain conditions, such as stress, change in response to drug, and remission or progression of the disease. Continue supervision following termination of therapy since acute adrenocortical insufficiency may develop and severe manifestations of the treated disease may suddenly recur at that time.
Prolonged therapy	At regular intervals during prolonged therapy, measure blood pressure and body weight and perform routine laboratory studies such as urinalysis, chest x-ray examination, and a 2-h glucose tolerance test. To reduce the risk of myopathy during prolonged therapy, caution all patients about the critical importance of a liberal intake of protein. Institute an antiulcer regimen, including use of an antacid, when patients with a history of ulcer or significant dyspepsia undergo long-term therapy; perform an upper GI x-ray examination at regular intervals and whenever they report gastric distress.
Decreasing dosage	To minimize the risk of acute adrenocortical insufficiency, reduce dosage gradually rather than abruptly whenever possible.

WARNINGS/PRECAUTIONS

Stress	If unusual stress occurs during therapy, give a rapid-acting corticosteroid before, during, and after the stressful situation; it may also be necessary to increase the dosage of triamcinolone. If a stressful situation such as trauma, surgery, or severe illness occurs in the months after discontinuation of triamcinolone, glucocorticoid therapy should be reinstituted in combination with administration of sodium chloride and/or a mineralocorticoid.
Infection	During therapy, some signs of infection may be masked, new infections may appear, resistance may be decreased, and an infection may be difficult to localize; watch for evidence of intercurrent infection. If an infection is seen, promptly institute vigorous antimicrobial therapy; if possible, discontinue triamcinolone gradually rather than abruptly. Triamcinolone should generally not be given to patients with local or systemic infections; if it is administered to these patients, exercise caution and use in combination with appropriate antimicrobial therapy.
Ocular damage	Prolonged use may cause posterior subcapsular cataracts, glaucoma, and optic nerve damage and may enhance development of secondary fungal or viral infections of the eye. Use with caution in patients with ocular herpes simplex because of possible corneal perforation.
Electrolyte imbalance	Triamcinolone can cause elevation of blood pressure, salt and water retention, and increased potassium and calcium excretion; dietary salt restriction and potassium supplementation may be necessary during therapy. Edema may occur in patients who have renal disease associated with a fixed or decreased GFR.
Gastrointestinal ulceration	Peptic ulcer may recur during therapy; moreover, because corticosteroids may mask GI pain, ulceration may progress and hemorrhage and perforation may be the first detectable manifestations. If patients with a history of peptic ulcer complain of gastric distress, perform an upper GI x-ray examination and, in addition, institute an antiulcer regimen (even if x-ray results are negative). For prolonged use in these patients, see recommendations in ADMINISTRATION/DOSAGE ADJUSTMENTS.
Anaphylactoid reactions	In rare instances, anaphylactoid reactions have occurred after injection of corticosteroids; take appropriate precautionary measures before administration, especially when patients have a history of drug allergy.
Psychological effects	Corticosteroids can cause psychic disturbances, including euphoria, insomnia, mood swings, personality changes, severe depression, and overt psychosis, and may exacerbate preexisting emotional instability or psychotic tendencies
Menstrual irregularities	Caution women past menarche that menstrual irregularities may occur
Hypothyroidism, hepatic cirrhosis	Corticosteroid effects are enhanced in patients with hypothyroidism or hepatic cirrhosis
Special-risk patients	When using in patients with nonspecific ulcerative colitis, exercise caution if there is a possibility of impending perforation, abscess, or other pyogenic infection. Use with caution in patients with diverticulitis, recent intestinal anastomoses, active or latent peptic ulcer, renal insufficiency, hypertension, osteoporosis, acute glomerulonephritis, vaccinia, varicella, exanthema, Cushing's syndrome, antibiotic-resistant infections, diabetes mellitus, congestive heart failure, chronic nephritis, thromboembolic tendencies, thrombophlebitis, convulsive disorders, metastatic carcinoma, or myasthenia gravis. For other special-risk patients, see warnings above.
Septic arthritis	If joint pain increases markedly during local therapy and is accompanied by fever, malaise, local swelling, and further restriction of joint motion, septic arthritis should be suspected and joint fluid should be examined for evidence of infection; if diagnosis is confirmed, discontinue triamcinolone and immediately institute appropriate antimicrobial therapy

KENALOG

Immunization	Vaccination should not be undertaken during therapy, particularly when high corticosteroid doses are being given, because neurological complications may develop and antibody response may fail to occur
Skin tests	Corticosteroids may suppress response to skin tests
Tuberculosis	Corticosteroids may be used as an adjunct to antituberculous therapy, but only for fulminating or disseminated forms of the active disease (see also DRUG INTERACTIONS). When using corticosteroids in patients with latent tuberculosis or tuberculin reactivity, observe patient closely since tuberculosis may be reactivated; during prolonged therapy, institute chemoprophylactic measures.
Inappropriate routes of administration	Do not administer Kenalog-10 IM or IV; do not give Kenalog-40 IV or intradermally. Safety of either preparation for intraturbinal, subconjunctival, subtenon, or retrobulbar administration has not been established.

ADVERSE REACTIONS

Cardiovascular	Sodium and fluid retention, hypertension, congestive heart failure in susceptible patients, cardiac arrhythmias or ECG changes due to hypokalemia, thrombophlebitis, thromboembolism, syncope
Musculoskeletal	Muscle weakness, fatigue, steroid myopathy, loss of muscle mass, osteoporosis, vertebral compression fractures, delayed healing of fractures, aseptic necrosis of femoral and humeral heads, pathologic fractures of long bones, spontaneous fractures
Gastrointestinal	Peptic ulceration, possibly including perforation and hemorrhage; pancreatitis, abdominal distention, ulcerative esophagitis
Dermatological	Impaired wound healing, thin fragile skin, petechiae, ecchymoses, facial erythema, increased sweating, purpura, striae, hirsutism, acneform eruptions, lupus erythematosus-like lesions
Central nervous system	Convulsions, pseudotumor cerebri (usually after therapy), vertigo, headache, insomnia, neuritis, paresthesia, exacerbation of psychiatric conditions
Ophthalmic	Posterior subcapsular cataracts, increased intraocular pressure, glaucoma, exophthalmos; blindness (with intralesional therapy on the head and face)
Endocrinological	Menstrual irregularities, development of cushingoid state, suppression of growth in children, secondary adrenocortical and pituitary insufficiency (particularly with stress), decreased glucose tolerance, manifestations of latent diabetes mellitus
Metabolic	Hypokalemia, hypokalemic alkalosis, hyperglycemia, glycosuria, negative nitrogen balance due to protein catabolism
Local	*With intraarticular administration:* postinjection flare, transient pain, occasional irritation at the injection site, sterile abscess, hyper- and hypopigmentation, Charcot-like arthropathy, and occasional brief increase in joint discomfort; *with intralesional administration:* blindness (with treatment on the face and head), transient local discomfort, sterile abscess, hyper- and hypopigmentation, and SC and cutaneous atrophy (usually transient); *with IM administration:* severe pain, sterile abscess, SC and cutaneous atrophy, hyper- and hypopigmentation, and Charcot-like arthropathy
Other	Necrotizing angiitis, aggravation or masking of infections, anaphylactoid reactions

OVERDOSAGE

Signs and symptoms	Mental disturbances, hyperglycemia, hypertension, edema
Treatment	Induce emesis or perform gastric lavage; institute symptomatic and supportive measures, as needed

DRUG INTERACTIONS

Salicylates, isoniazid	▽ Plasma level of salicylates and isoniazid
Phenytoin, barbiturates, rifampin	▽ Pharmacological effect of corticosteroids
Insulin, sulfonylureas	▽ Control of hyperglycemia; adjustment of hypoglycemic dosage may be necessary
Thiazide-type diuretics, loop diuretics	△ Risk of hypokalemia ▽ Diuretic and natriuretic effects
Potassium-sparing diuretics	▽ Diuretic and natriuretic effects
Cardiac glycosides	△ Risk of digitalis toxicity
Vaccines	▽ Antibody response △ Risk of neurological effects of vaccines △ Risk of viral infection (with live virus vaccines)
Amphotericin B	△ Risk of hypokalemia
Oral anticoagulants	△ Risk of hemorrhage and GI ulceration ▽ Hypoprothrombinemic effect
Anticholinesterase agents	▽ Pharmacologic effect of anticholinesterase agents
Pancuronium, tubocurarine	▽ Neuromuscular blockade

ALTERED LABORATORY VALUES

Blood/serum values	△ Glucose △ Sodium ▽ Potassium ▽ Calcium △ Cholesterol △ Triglycerides ▽ PBI ▽ T_4 ▽ ^{131}I thyroid uptake False-negative nitroblue-tetrazolium test Interference with gonadorelin and protirelin thyroid tests

KENALOG ■ Prednisolone

Urinary values — ↑ Glucose ↓ 17-OHCS ↓ 17-KS

USE IN CHILDREN
See indications and dosage recommendations; do not use Kenalog-40 in children under 6 yr of age. Growth and development should be carefully observed in children undergoing prolonged therapy.

USE IN PREGNANT AND NURSING WOMEN
In animals, corticosteroid doses equivalent to the human pharmacological dose are teratogenic. Safety of triamcinolone for use in pregnant or nursing women has not been established; use only if the expected benefit justifies the potential risks. Infants born of mothers who have received substantial doses of corticosteroids during pregnancy should be carefully observed for signs of hypoadrenalism.

ORAL AND INJECTABLE CORTICOSTEROIDS

Prednisolone Acetate   Rx
Vials: 25 mg/ml (5, 10, 30 ml), 50 mg/ml (10, 30 ml), 100 mg/ml (10 ml)

Prednisolone Sodium Phosphate   Rx
Vials: 22 mg (equivalent to 20 mg prednisolone phosphate)/ml (2, 5, 10 ml)

INDICATIONS

Endocrine disorders, including primary or secondary adrenocortical insufficiency, congenital adrenal hyperplasia, nonsuppurative thyroiditis, hypercalcemia associated with cancer, acute adrenocortical insufficiency, and preoperatively and in the event of serious trauma or illness in patients with known adrenal insufficiency or when adrenocortical reserve is doubtful
Rheumatic disorders, including psoriatic arthritis, rheumatoid arthritis, juvenile rheumatoid arthritis, ankylosing spondylitis, acute and subacute bursitis, acute nonspecific tenosynovitis, acute gouty arthritis, posttraumatic osteoarthritis, synovitis of osteoarthritis, and epicondylitis (adjunctive, short-term therapy)
Collagen diseases, including systemic lupus erythematosus, acute rheumatic carditis, and systemic dermatomyositis (polymyositis)
Dermatological diseases, including pemphigus, bullous dermatitis herpetiformis, severe erythema multiforme (Stevens-Johnson syndrome), exfoliative dermatitis, mycosis fungoides, severe psoriasis, and severe seborrheic dermatitis
Severe or incapacitating **allergic conditions** intractable to adequate trials of conventional treatment, including seasonal or perennial allergic rhinitis, bronchial asthma, contact dermatitis, atopic dermatitis, serum sickness, drug hypersensitivity reactions, urticarial transfusion reactions, and acute noninfectious laryngeal edema
Ophthalmic diseases, including allergic conjunctivitis, keratitis, allergic corneal marginal ulcers, herpes zoster ophthalmicus, iritis and iridocyclitis, chorioretinitis, anterior segment inflammation, diffuse posterior uveitis and choroiditis, optic neuritis, and sympathetic ophthalmia
Respiratory diseases, including symptomatic sarcoidosis, Loeffler's syndrome not manageable by other means, berylliosis, fulminating or disseminated pulmonary tuberculosis (with appropriate antituberculous chemotherapy), and aspiration pneumonitis
Hematological disorders, including idiopathic thrombocytopenic purpura (IV only) and secondary thrombocytopenia in adults, acquired (autoimmune) hemolytic anemia, erythroblastopenia (RBC anemia), and congenital (erythroid) hypoplastic anemia
Palliative management of **neoplastic diseases,** including leukemias and lymphomas in adults and acute leukemia of childhood
To induce diuresis or remission of proteinuria in the **nephrotic syndrome,** without uremia, of the idiopathic type or that due to lupus erythematosus
Gastrointestinal diseases, including ulcerative colitis and regional enteritis
Tuberculous meningitis with subarachnoid block or impending block (with appropriate antituberculous chemotherapy)
Trichinosis associated with neurological or myocardial involvement

Acute exacerbations of **multiple sclerosis**

PARENTERAL DOSAGE[1]
Adult: 4–60 mg/day IM (prednisolone acetate, prednisolone sodium phosphate) or IV (prednisolone sodium phosphate only) to start, followed by gradual reductions in dosage to lowest level possible consistent with maintaining an adequate clinical response; dosage must be individualized on the basis of the specific disease being treated, its severity, and clinical response; larger than usual doses may be justified in certain overwhelming, acute, life-threatening situations

Adult: 200 mg/day IM for 1 wk, followed by 80 mg every other day or 4–8 mg of dexamethasone every other day for 1 mo

CONTRAINDICATIONS
Systemic fungal infections   Injection into unstable or previously infected joints

WARNINGS/PRECAUTIONS
Patients subjected to unusual stress — Require increased dosage of rapidly acting corticosteroids before, during, and after emotionally or physically stressful situations

COMPENDIUM OF DRUG THERAPY

Prednisolone

Infection	Clinical signs may be masked, new infections may appear, resistance may be decreased, and infections may be difficult to localize
Ocular damage	Prolonged use may produce posterior subcapsular cataracts and glaucoma, with possible damage to optic nerves, and may enhance development of secondary fungal or viral ocular infections
Dietary salt restriction and potassium supplementation	May be necessary to combat blood pressure elevation, salt and water retention, and increased potassium excretion with average and high-dose therapy
Immunization procedures	Especially against smallpox, should not be undertaken because of possible neurological complications and lack of antibody response
Active tuberculosis	Restrict use to fulminating or disseminated cases, as an adjunct to appropriate antituberculous therapy
Latent tuberculosis or tuberculin reactivity	Observe patient closely, since reactivation of the disease may occur; during prolonged therapy, employ antituberculous chemoprophylactic measures
Secondary adrenocortical insufficiency	May be minimized by gradual dosage reduction; since insufficiency may persist for months, reinstitute corticosteroid therapy in any stressful situation during this period, and administer salt and/or a mineralocorticoid concurrently to correct impaired mineralocorticoid secretion
Hypothyroidism, hepatic cirrhosis	May enhance effects of prednisolone
Corneal perforation	May occur in patients with ocular herpes simplex; use with caution
Special-risk patients	Use with caution in patients with nonspecific ulcerative colitis if impending perforation, abscess, or other pyogenic infection is likely, as well as in patients with diverticulitis, fresh intestinal anastomoses, active or latent peptic ulcer, renal insufficiency, hypertension, osteoporosis, or myasthenia gravis
Psychic derangements	May appear, ranging from euphoria, insomnia, mood swings, personality changes, and severe depression to frank psychotic manifestations; existing emotional instability or psychotic tendencies may be aggravated
Concomitant use with aspirin	Use with caution in patients with hypoprothrombinemia
Prolonged therapy	Routine laboratory studies (eg, urinalysis, 2-h postprandial blood sugar, blood pressure, body weight, chest film) should be made at regular intervals; in addition, an upper GI series is suggested in patients with an ulcer history or significant dyspepsia. Withdraw the drug gradually, rather than abruptly, when discontinuing long-term therapy.
Septic arthritis	May occur with intraarticular injection and require appropriate antimicrobial therapy; observe patient for suggestive symptoms (eg, increased pain, local swelling, further restrictions of joint mobility, fever, malaise) and examine joint fluid microscopically
Anaphylactoid reactions	Have occurred following parenteral corticosteroid administration; take appropriate precautionary measures before injecting dexamethasone, especially in patients with a history of drug allergy

ADVERSE REACTIONS

Fluid and electrolyte disturbances	Sodium retention, fluid retention, congestive heart failure in susceptible patients, loss of potassium, hypokalemic alkalosis, hypertension, hypotensive or shock-like reactions
Musculoskeletal	Muscle weakness, steroid myopathy, loss of muscle mass, osteoporosis, vertebral compression fractures, aseptic necrosis of femoral and humeral heads, pathological fracture of long bones
Gastrointestinal	Peptic ulcer with possible perforation and hemorrhage, pancreatitis, abdominal distention, ulcerative esophagitis
Dermatological	Impaired wound healing, thin fragile skin, petechiae and ecchymoses, facial erythema, increased sweating, suppressed reaction to skin tests
Neurological	Convulsions, increased intracranial pressure with papilledema (pseudotumor cerebri), vertigo, headache
Endocrinological	Menstrual irregularities, Cushingoid state, growth suppression in children, secondary adrenocortical and pituitary unresponsiveness, decreased carbohydrate tolerance, latent diabetes mellitus, increased insulin or oral hypoglycemic requirments
Ophthalmic	Posterior subcapsular cataracts, increased intraocular pressure, glaucoma, exophthalmos
Metabolic	Negative nitrogen balance
Other	Anaphylactoid or hypersensitivity reactions
Additional reactions to parenteral therapy only	Hyperpigmentation or hypopigmentation, subcutaneous and cutaneous atrophy, sterile abscess, postinjection flare (following intraarticular use), Charcot-like arthropathy, blindness (rare) associated with intralesional therapy around the face and head

OVERDOSAGE

Signs and symptoms	CNS changes, GI bleeding, hyperglycemia, hypertension, edema

Prednisolone ■ ACLOVATE

Treatment —— Discontinue medication; institute supportive measures, as required

DRUG INTERACTIONS

Insulin, oral hypoglycemics	⇩ Hypoglycemic effect	
Phenytoin, phenobarbital, ephedrine, rifampin	⇧ Metabolic clearance of prednisolone	⇩ Steroid blood level and physiological activity
Oral anticoagulants	⇧ or ⇩ Prothrombin time	
Potassium-depleting diuretics	⇧ Risk of hypokalemia	
Cardiac glycosides	⇧ Risk of arrhythmias or digitalis toxicity secondary to hypokalemia	
Skin test antigens	⇩ Reactivity	
Immunizations	⇩ Antibody response	

ALTERED LABORATORY VALUES

Blood/serum values —— ⇧ Glucose ⇧ Cholesterol ⇧ Sodium ⇩ Potassium ⇩ Calcium ⇩ PBI
⇩ Thyroxine (T$_4$) ⇩ ^{131}I thyroid uptake ⇩ Uric acid

Urinary values —— ⇧ Glucose ⇧ Potassium ⇧ Calcium ⇧ Uric acid ⇩ 17-Hydroxycorticosteroids (17-OHCS) ⇩ 17-Ketosteroids

---

USE IN CHILDREN

Growth and development should be carefully observed in infants and children on prolonged therapy; consult manufacturer for dosage recommendations

USE IN PREGNANT AND NURSING WOMEN

Safety for use in pregnant or nursing women has not been established. Infants born of mothers who received substantial doses of corticosteroids during pregnancy should be carefully observed for signs of hypoadrenalism.

---

[1] For intraarticular, soft tissue, and intralesional administration of prednisolone, consult manufacturer

---

TOPICAL CORTICOSTEROIDS

ACLOVATE (alclometasone dipropionate) Glaxo Rx

Cream: 0.05% (15, 45 g) **Ointment:** 0.05% (15, 45 g)

INDICATIONS

Inflammatory and pruritic manifestations of corticosteroid-responsive dermatoses

TOPICAL DOSAGE

Adult and child: apply a thin film to the affected areas and massage gently into the skin bid or tid

CONTRAINDICATIONS

Hypersensitivity to alclometasone, other components, or other corticosteroids

ADMINISTRATION/DOSAGE ADJUSTMENTS

Occlusive dressing technique —— Occlusive dressings may be used for the management of refractory psoriatic lesions and other deep-seated dermatoses such as localized neurodermatitis (lichen simplex chronicus). Follow this procedure: Cover the lesion with a thick layer of cream or ointment, a light gauze dressing, and a pliable plastic film; then seal the edges to the skin and leave in place for 1–4 days. Repeat procedure 3–4 times, as needed.

WARNINGS/PRECAUTIONS

Patient instructions —— Caution patients not to let this preparation come into contact with their eyes. If an occlusive dressing is not used, caution patients not to bandage or otherwise cover the treated area so that it becomes occluded (thus, tight-fitting diapers or plastic pants should not be used on children being treated in the diaper area). Advise patients to report any signs of adverse reactions, especially when an occlusive dressing is used.

Irritation —— Discontinue use and institute appropriate therapy

Dermatological infection —— Discontinue use of any occlusive dressings and institute appropriate antifungal or antibacterial therapy; if infection persists, withhold steroid therapy until infection is adequately controlled

COMPENDIUM OF DRUG THERAPY

ACLOVATE ■ AEROSEB-DEX

Systemic absorption	Reversible hypothalamic-pituitary-adrenal (HPA) axis suppression, Cushing's syndrome, hyperglycemia, and glucosuria may result from systemic absorption following topical application, especially in children (see USE IN CHILDREN). Use over extensive areas, for prolonged periods, or under occlusive dressings increases percutaneous absorption. HPA axis function may be evaluated during therapy by ACTH stimulation or measurement of urinary free cortisol. In clinical studies under exaggerated conditions (eg, application over 30% of the body), alclometasone has produced an approximately 10% decrease in urinary free cortisol and 17-hydroxysteroids, suggesting slight HPA axis suppression.
Carcinogenicity, mutagenicity	Long-term studies have not been done in animals to evaluate the carcinogenic potential of topical corticosteroids; the results of studies to demonstrate mutagenicity of prednisolone have been negative
Effect on fertility	The effect of topical corticosteroids on fertility has not been studied

ADVERSE REACTIONS[1]

With use of the cream

Local	Pruritus (2%); burning, erythema, dryness, irritation, and papular rashes (1%)

With use of the ointment

Local	Pruritus and burning (0.5%); erythema (0.2%)

USE IN CHILDREN

On children, use minimal amount necessary for effective therapy. Children may be more susceptible than adults to HPA axis suppression and Cushing's syndrome because of the larger ratio of surface area to body weight; intracranial hypertension has also been observed in children receiving topical corticosteroids. Chronic therapy may interfere with growth and development.

USE IN PREGNANT AND NURSING WOMEN

Pregnancy Category C: use during pregnancy only if the expected benefit outweighs the potential risk to the fetus. Do not use over extensive areas, in large amounts, or for prolonged periods. In animal studies, systemic corticosteroids have generally been teratogenic at relatively low dosages; the more potent corticosteroids have also been teratogenic when applied to the skin. No adequate, well-controlled studies have been performed in pregnant women. It is not known whether topical corticosteroids are excreted in human milk; although systemic corticosteroids are excreted in quantities unlikely to harm nursing infants, this preparation should be used with caution in nursing mothers.

VEHICLE/BASE
Cream (hydrophilic, emollient): propylene glycol, white petrolatum, cetearyl alcohol, glyceryl stearate, PEG 100 stearate, ceteth-20, monobasic sodium phosphate, chlorocresol, phosphoric acid, and purified water
Ointment: hexylene glycol, white wax, propylene glycol stearate, and white petrolatum

[1] Reactions observed with use of topical corticosteroids include Cushing's syndrome, hyperglycemia, glucosuria, suppression of HPA axis, burning, itching, irritation, dryness, folliculitis, hypertrichosis, acneform eruptions, hypopigmentation, perioral dermatitis, allergic contact dermatitis, maceration of the skin, secondary infection, skin atrophy, striae, and miliaria

---

TOPICAL CORTICOSTEROIDS

AEROSEB-DEX (dexamethasone) Herbert   Rx

Spray: 0.01% (58 g), delivering 0.02 mg of dexamethasone per 1-s application

INDICATIONS

Inflammatory and pruritic manifestations of corticosteroid-responsive dermatoses, especially scalp conditions such as seborrheic dermatitis

TOPICAL DOSAGE

Adult: apply to affected areas bid or tid, depending on severity
Child: use minimal amount necessary for effective therapy (see precaution, below, concerning systemic absorption)

CONTRAINDICATIONS

Hypersensitivity to dexamethasone or other components

ADMINISTRATION/DOSAGE ADJUSTMENTS

Application to scalp	Shampoo and dry scalp. Keeping applicator tube under hair and in contact with scalp, spray for 1–2 s, avoiding forehead and eyes. Massaging is unnecessary.
Application for other dermatoses	Remove applicator tube. Holding can upright, approximately 6 in. from area to be treated, spray for 1–2 s per 4 sq in.

AEROSEB-DEX ■ AEROSEB-HC

WARNINGS/PRECAUTIONS

Patient instructions	Caution patients not to let this preparation come into contact with their eyes; if it is used about the face, the eyes should be covered and inhalation of the spray avoided. Occlusive dressings may be used for the management of psoriasis or other persistent dermatoses. If an occlusive dressing is not indicated, caution patients not to bandage or otherwise cover the treated area so that it becomes occluded (thus tight-fitting diapers or plastic pants should not be used on children being treated in the diaper area). Advise patients to report any signs of adverse reactions, particularly under occlusive dressings.
Irritation	Discontinue use and institute appropriate therapy. Alcohol in product may cause irritation or burning sensation in open lesions.
Dermatological infection	Discontinue use of any occlusive dressings and institute appropriate antifungal or antibacterial therapy; if infection persists, discontinue steroid therapy until a favorable response is obtained
Systemic absorption	Reversible hypothalamic-pituitary-adrenal (HPA) axis suppression, Cushing's syndrome, hyperglycemia, and glucosuria may result from systemic absorption after topical application, particularly in children (see USE IN CHILDREN). Use over extensive areas, for prolonged periods, or of occlusive dressings increases percutaneous absorption. If large doses are applied over extensive areas or are administered using the occlusive dressing technique, evaluate HPA axis function (by ACTH stimulation or measurement of urinary free cortisol) periodically. If HPA axis suppression occurs, discontinue use of this drug, reduce the frequency of application, or administer a less potent steroid. Infrequently, systemic corticosteroids may be needed to treat manifestations of topical steroid withdrawal.
Carcinogenicity, mutagenicity	Long-term studies have not been done in animals to evaluate the carcinogenic potential of topical corticosteroids; the results of studies to demonstrate mutagenicity of prednisolone and hydrocortisone have been negative
Effect on fertility	The effect of topical corticosteroids on fertility has not been studied

ADVERSE REACTIONS[1]

Local	Burning, itching, irritation, dryness, folliculitis, hypertrichosis, acneform eruptions, hypopigmentation, perioral dermatitis, allergic contact dermatitis, maceration, secondary infection, skin atrophy, striae, miliaria

USE IN CHILDREN

Use smallest amount necessary for effective treatment. Children may be more susceptible than adults to HPA axis suppression and Cushing's syndrome because of the larger ratio of surface area to body weight; intracranial hypertension has also been reported in children receiving topical corticosteroids. Chronic therapy may interfere with growth and development.

USE IN PREGNANT AND NURSING WOMEN

Pregnancy Category C: use during pregnancy only if the expected benefit justifies the potential risk to the fetus. Do not use over extensive areas, in large amounts, or for prolonged periods. In animal studies, systemic corticosteroids have generally been teratogenic at relatively low dosages; the more potent corticosteroids have also been teratogenic when applied to the skin. No adequate, well-controlled studies have been done in pregnant women. It is not known whether topical corticosteroids are excreted in human milk; although systemic corticosteroids are excreted in quantities unlikely to harm nursing infants, this preparation should be used with caution in nursing mothers.

VEHICLE/BASE
Spray: 65.1% alcohol and isopropyl myristate, with butane as propellant

[1] Includes reactions common to topical corticosteroids in general

---

TOPICAL CORTICOSTEROIDS

AEROSEB-HC (hydrocortisone) Herbert   Rx

Spray: 0.5% (58 g), delivering 1 mg of hydrocortisone per 1-s application

INDICATIONS

Inflammatory and pruritic manifestations of corticosteroid-responsive dermatoses, especially scalp conditions such as seborrheic dermatitis

TOPICAL DOSAGE

Adult: apply to affected areas bid or tid, depending on severity
Child: use minimal amount necessary for effective therapy (see precaution, below, concerning systemic absorption)

COMPENDIUM OF DRUG THERAPY

AEROSEB-HC ■ ARISTOCORT/ARISTOCORT A Cream and Ointment

CONTRAINDICATIONS	
Hypersensitivity to hydrocortisone or other components	
ADMINISTRATION/DOSAGE ADJUSTMENTS	
Application to scalp	Shampoo and dry scalp. Keeping applicator tube under hair and in contact with scalp, spray for 1–2 s, avoiding forehead and eyes. Massaging is unnecessary.
Application for other dermatoses	Remove applicator tube. Holding can upright, approximately 6 in. from area to be treated, spray for 1–2 s per 4 sq in.
WARNINGS/PRECAUTIONS	
Patient instructions	Caution patients not to let this preparation come into contact with their eyes; if it is used about the face, the eyes should be covered and inhalation of the spray avoided. Occlusive dressings may be used for the management of psoriasis or other persistent dermatoses. If an occlusive dressing is not indicated, caution patients not to bandage or otherwise cover the treated area so that it becomes occluded (thus tight-fitting diapers or plastic pants should not be used on children being treated in the diaper area). Advise patients to report any signs of adverse reactions, particularly under occlusive dressings.
Irritation	Discontinue use and institute appropriate therapy. Alcohol in product may cause irritation or burning sensation in open lesions.
Dermatological infection	Discontinue use of any occlusive dressings and institute appropriate antifungal or antibacterial therapy; if infection persists, discontinue steroid therapy until a favorable response is obtained
Systemic absorption	Reversible hypothalamic-pituitary-adrenal (HPA) axis suppression, Cushing's syndrome, hyperglycemia, and glucosuria may result from systemic absorption after topical application, particularly in children (see USE IN CHILDREN). Use over extensive areas, for prolonged periods, or of occlusive dressings increases percutaneous absorption. If large doses are applied over extensive areas or are administered using the occlusive dressing technique, evaluate HPA axis function (by ACTH stimulation or measurement of urinary free cortisol) periodically. If HPA axis suppression occurs, discontinue use of this drug, reduce the frequency of application, or administer a less potent steroid. Infrequently, systemic corticosteroids may be needed to treat manifestations of topical steroid withdrawal.
Carcinogenicity, mutagenicity	Long-term studies have not been done in animals to evaluate the carcinogenic potential of topical corticosteroids; the results of studies to demonstrate mutagenicity of prednisolone and hydrocortisone have been negative
Effect on fertility	The effect of topical corticosteroids on fertility has not been studied
ADVERSE REACTIONS[1]	
Local	Burning, itching, irritation, dryness, folliculitis, hypertrichosis, acneform eruptions, hypopigmentation, perioral dermatitis, allergic contact dermatitis, maceration, secondary infection, skin atrophy, striae, miliaria

---

USE IN CHILDREN

Use smallest amount necessary for effective treatment. Children may be more susceptible than adults to HPA axis suppression and Cushing's syndrome because of the larger ratio of surface area to body weight; intracranial hypertension has also been reported in children receiving topical corticosteroids. Chronic therapy may interfere with growth and development.

USE IN PREGNANT AND NURSING WOMEN

Pregnancy Category C: use during pregnancy only if the expected benefit justifies the potential risk to the fetus. Do not use over extensive areas, in large amounts, or for prolonged periods. In animal studies, systemic corticosteroids have generally been teratogenic at relatively low dosages; the more potent corticosteroids have also been teratogenic when applied to the skin. No adequate, well-controlled studies have been done in pregnant women. It is not known whether topical corticosteroids are excreted in human milk; although systemic corticosteroids are excreted in quantities unlikely to harm nursing infants, this preparation should be used with caution in nursing mothers.

VEHICLE/BASE
Spray: 64.6% alcohol and isopropyl myristate, with butane as propellant

[1] Includes reactions common to topical corticosteroids in general

---

TOPICAL CORTICOSTEROIDS

ARISTOCORT Cream and Ointment (triamcinolone acetonide) Lederle Rx
Cream: 0.025% (15, 60, 240, 2,380 g), 0.1% (15, 60, 240, 2,380 g), 0.5% (15, 240 g) **Ointment:** 0.1% (15, 60, 240, 2,270 g), 0.5% (15, 240 g)

ARISTOCORT A Cream and Ointment (triamcinolone acetonide) Lederle Rx
Cream: 0.025% (15, 60 g), 0.1% (15, 60, 240 g), 0.5% (15, 240 g) **Ointment:** 0.1% (15, 60 g), 0.5% (15 g)

INDICATIONS	**TOPICAL DOSAGE**
Inflammatory and pruritic manifestations of corticosteroid-responsive dermatoses	**Adult:** apply a thin film to affected areas tid or qid, depending on severity **Child:** use minimal amount necessary for effective therapy (see precaution, below, concerning systemic absorption)

ARISTOCORT/ARISTOCORT A Cream and Ointment ■ CARMOL HC

CONTRAINDICATIONS
Hypersensitivity to triamcinolone or other components

WARNINGS/PRECAUTIONS

Patient instructions	Caution patients not to let these preparations come into contact with their eyes. Occlusive dressings may be used for the management of psoriasis or other persistent dermatoses. If an occlusive dressing is not indicated, caution patients not to bandage or otherwise cover the treated area so that it becomes occluded (thus tight-fitting diapers or plastic pants should not be used on children being treated in the diaper area). Advise patients to report any signs of adverse reactions, particularly under occlusive dressings.
Irritation	Discontinue use and institute appropriate therapy
Dermatological infection	Discontinue use of any occlusive dressings and institute appropriate antifungal or antibacterial therapy; if infection persists, discontinue steroid therapy until a favorable response is obtained
Systemic absorption	Reversible hypothalamic-pituitary-adrenal (HPA) axis suppression, Cushing's syndrome, hyperglycemia, and glucosuria may result from systemic absorption after topical application, particularly in children (see USE IN CHILDREN). Use over extensive areas, for prolonged periods, or of occlusive dressings increases percutaneous absorption. If large doses are applied over extensive areas or are administered using the occlusive dressing technique, evaluate HPA axis function (by ACTH stimulation or measurement of urinary free cortisol) periodically. If HPA axis suppression occurs, discontinue use of this drug, reduce the frequency of application, or administer a less potent steroid. Infrequently, systemic corticosteroids may be needed to treat manifestations of topical steroid withdrawal.
Carcinogenicity, mutagenicity	Long-term studies have not been done in animals to evaluate the carcinogenic potential of topical corticosteroids; the results of studies to demonstrate mutagenicity of prednisolone and hydrocortisone have been negative
Effect on fertility	The effect of topical corticosteroids on fertility has not been studied

ADVERSE REACTIONS[1]

Local	Burning, itching, irritation, dryness, folliculitis, hypertrichosis, acneform eruptions, hypopigmentation, perioral dermatitis, allergic contact dermatitis, maceration, secondary infection, skin atrophy, striae, miliaria

USE IN CHILDREN
Use smallest amount necessary for effective treatment. Children may be more susceptible than adults to HPA axis suppression and Cushing's syndrome because of the larger ratio of surface area to body weight; intracranial hypertension has also been observed in children receiving topical corticosteroids. Chronic therapy may interfere with growth and development.

USE IN PREGNANT AND NURSING WOMEN
Pregnancy Category C: use during pregnancy only if the expected benefit justifies the potential risk to the fetus. Do not use over extensive areas, in large amounts, or for prolonged periods. In animal studies, systemic corticosteroids have generally been teratogenic at relatively low dosages; the more potent corticosteroids have also been teratogenic when applied to the skin. No adequate, well-controlled studies have been done in pregnant women. It is not known whether topical corticosteroids are excreted in human milk; although systemic corticosteroids are excreted in quantities unlikely to harm nursing infants, this preparation should be used with caution in nursing mothers.

VEHICLE/BASE
Aristocort Cream (water-based): mono- and diglycerides, squalane, polysorbate 80, cetyl esters wax, polysorbate 60, stearyl alcohol, Tenox II, and sorbitol solution, with 0.1% sorbic acid and 0.1% potassium sorbate as preservatives
Aristocort Ointment: white petrolatum
Aristocort A Cream (hydrophilic, nonstaining, water-washable, paraben-free, spermaceti-free, light texture and consistency): emulsifying wax, isopropyl palmitate, glycerin, sorbitol solution, lactic acid, 2% benzyl alcohol, and purified water
Aristocort A Ointment: emulsifying wax, white petrolatum, propylene glycol, Tenox II, and lactic acid

[1] Includes reactions common to topical corticosteroids in general

---

TOPICAL CORTICOSTEROIDS

CARMOL HC (hydrocortisone acetate) Syntex   Rx
Cream: 1% (30, 120 g)

INDICATIONS
Inflammatory and pruritic manifestations of corticosteroid-responsive dermatoses

TOPICAL DOSAGE
Adult: apply a thin film to affected areas 2–4 times/day, depending on severity
Child: use minimal amount necessary for effective therapy (see precaution, below, concerning systemic absorption)

COMPENDIUM OF DRUG THERAPY

CONTRAINDICATIONS

Hypersensitivity to hydrocortisone or other components

WARNINGS/PRECAUTIONS

Patient instructions	Caution patients not to let this preparation come into contact with their eyes. Occlusive dressings may be used for the management of psoriasis or other persistent dermatoses. If an occlusive dressing is not indicated, caution patients not to bandage or otherwise cover the treated area so that it becomes occluded (thus tight-fitting diapers or plastic pants should not be used on children being treated in the diaper area). Advise patients to report any signs of adverse reactions, particularly under occlusive dressings.
Irritation	Discontinue use and institute appropriate therapy
Dermatological infection	Discontinue use of any occlusive dressings and institute appropriate antifungal or antibacterial therapy; if infection persists, discontinue steroid therapy until a favorable response is obtained
Systemic absorption	Reversible hypothalamic-pituitary-adrenal (HPA) axis suppression, Cushing's syndrome, hyperglycemia, and glucosuria may result from systemic absorption after topical application, particularly in children (see USE IN CHILDREN). Use over extensive areas, for prolonged periods, or of occlusive dressings increases percutaneous absorption. If large doses are applied over extensive areas or are administered using the occlusive dressing technique, evaluate HPA axis function periodically by ACTH stimulation or measurement of urinary free cortisol. If HPA axis suppression occurs, discontinue use of this drug, reduce the frequency of application, or administer a less potent steroid. Infrequently, systemic corticosteroids may be needed to treat manifestations of topical steroid withdrawal.
Carcinogenicity, mutagenicity	Long-term studies have not been done in animals to evaluate the carcinogenic potential of topical corticosteroids; the results of studies to demonstrate mutagenicity of prednisolone and hydrocortisone have been negative
Effect on fertility	The effect of topical corticosteroids on fertility has not been studied
Sulfite sensitivity	Sodium bisulfite in this product may cause urticaria, pruritus, wheezing, anaphylaxis, or other allergic-type reactions in susceptible patients, such as those with asthma or atopy

ADVERSE REACTIONS[1]

Local	Burning, itching, irritation, dryness, folliculitis, hypertrichosis, acneform eruptions, hypopigmentation, perioral dermatitis, allergic contact dermatitis, maceration, secondary infection, skin atrophy, striae, miliaria

USE IN CHILDREN

Use smallest amount necessary for effective treatment. Children may be more susceptible than adults to HPA axis suppression and Cushing's syndrome because of the larger ratio of surface area to body weight; intracranial hypertension has also been observed in children receiving topical corticosteroids. Chronic therapy may interfere with growth and development.

USE IN PREGNANT AND NURSING WOMEN

Pregnancy Category C: use during pregnancy only if the expected benefit justifies the potential risk to the fetus. Do not use over extensive areas, in large amounts, or for prolonged periods. In animal studies, systemic corticosteroids have generally been teratogenic at relatively low dosages; the more potent corticosteroids have also been teratogenic when applied to the skin. No adequate, well-controlled studies have been done in pregnant women. It is not known whether topical corticosteroids are excreted in human milk; although systemic corticosteroids are excreted in quantities unlikely to harm nursing infants, this preparation should be used with caution in nursing mothers.

VEHICLE/BASE
Cream (water-washable, vanishing): 10% urea, purified water, stearic acid, isopropyl myristate, PPG-26 oleate, isopropyl palmitate, propylene glycol, triethanolamine, cetyl alcohol, carbomer 940, sodium bisulfite, sodium laureth sulfate, edetate disodium, xanthan gum, and hypoallergenic perfume

[1] Includes reactions common to topical corticosteroids in general

---

TOPICAL CORTICOSTEROIDS

CLODERM (clocortolone pivalate) Hermal   Rx

Cream: 0.1% (15, 45 g)

INDICATIONS

Inflammatory and pruritic manifestations of corticosteroid-responsive dermatoses

TOPICAL DOSAGE

Adult: apply sparingly to affected areas tid; rub in gently
Child: use minimal amount necessary for effective therapy (see precaution, below, concerning systemic absorption)

CONTRAINDICATIONS

Hypersensitivity to clocortolone or other components

WARNINGS/PRECAUTIONS

Patient instructions	Caution patients not to let this preparation come into contact with their eyes. Occlusive dressings may be used for the management of psoriasis or other persistent dermatoses. If an occlusive dressing is not indicated, caution patients not to bandage or otherwise cover the treated area so that it becomes occluded (thus tight-fitting diapers or plastic pants should not be used on children being treated in the diaper area). Advise patients to report any signs of adverse reactions, particularly under occlusive dressings.
Irritation	May occur; discontinue use and institute appropriate therapy
Dermatological infection	Discontinue use of any occlusive dressings and institute appropriate antifungal or antibacterial therapy; if infection persists, discontinue steroid therapy until a favorable response is obtained
Systemic absorption	Reversible hypothalamic-pituitary-adrenal (HPA) axis suppression, Cushing's syndrome, hyperglycemia, and glucosuria may result from systemic absorption after topical application, particularly in children (see USE IN CHILDREN). Use over extensive areas, for prolonged periods, or of occlusive dressings increases percutaneous absorption. If large doses are applied over extensive areas or are administered using the occlusive dressing technique, evaluate HPA axis function (by ACTH stimulation or measurement of urinary free cortisol) periodically. If HPA axis suppression occurs, discontinue use of this drug, reduce the frequency of application, or administer a less potent steroid. Infrequently, systemic corticosteroids may be needed to treat manifestations of topical steroid withdrawal.
Carcinogenicity, mutagenicity	Long-term studies have not been done in animals to evaluate the carcinogenic potential of topical corticosteroids; the results of studies to demonstrate mutagenicity of prednisolone and hydrocortisone have been negative
Effect on fertility	The effect of topical corticosteroids on fertility has not been studied

ADVERSE REACTIONS[1]

Local	Burning, itching, irritation, dryness, folliculitis, hypertrichosis, acneform eruptions, hypopigmentation, perioral dermatitis, allergic contact dermatitis, maceration, secondary infection, skin atrophy, striae, miliaria

USE IN CHILDREN

Use smallest amount necessary for effective treatment. Children may be more susceptible than adults to HPA axis suppression and Cushing's syndrome because of the larger ratio of surface area to body weight; intracranial hypertension has also been observed in children receiving topical corticosteroids. Chronic therapy may interfere with growth and development.

USE IN PREGNANT AND NURSING WOMEN

Pregnancy Category C: use during pregnancy only if the expected benefit justifies the potential risk to the fetus. Do not use over extensive areas, in large amounts, or for prolonged periods. In animal studies, systemic corticosteroids have generally been teratogenic at relatively low dosages; the more potent corticosteroids have also been teratogenic when applied to the skin. No adequate, well-controlled studies have been done in pregnant women. It is not known whether topical corticosteroids are excreted in human milk; although systemic corticosteroids are excreted in quantities unlikely to harm nursing infants, this preparation should be used with caution in nursing mothers.

VEHICLE/BASE
Cream (water-washable, emollient): purified water, white petrolatum, mineral oil, stearyl alcohol, polyoxyl 40 stearate, carbomer 943P, edetate disodium, and sodium hydroxide, with methylparaben and propylparaben as preservatives

[1] Includes reactions common to topical corticosteroids in general

---

TOPICAL CORTICOSTEROIDS

CORDRAN (flurandrenolide) Dista   Rx
Lotion: 0.05% (15, 60 ml)   Ointment: 0.025% (30, 60, 225 g), 0.05% (15, 30, 60 225 g)

CORDRAN SP (flurandrenolide) Dista   Rx
Cream: 0.025% (30, 60, 225 g), 0.05% (15, 30, 60, 225 g)

INDICATIONS

Inflammatory and pruritic manifestations of corticosteroid-responsive dermatoses

TOPICAL DOSAGE

Adult: for moist lesions, gently rub a small amount of the cream or lotion into affected area bid or tid; for dry, scaly lesions, apply a thin film of ointment to affected area bid or tid

Child: use minimal amount necessary for effective therapy (see precaution, below, concerning systemic absorption)

CONTRAINDICATIONS

Hypersensitivity to flurandrenolide or other components

ADMINISTRATION/DOSAGE ADJUSTMENTS

Occlusive dressing technique	Remove superficial scales as much as possible by brushing, picking, or rubbing (soaking in a bath will help soften scales and permit easier removal). Rub cream, ointment, or lotion thoroughly into affected area and cover with plastic film. If lotion or cream is used, additional moisture may be provided by placing a slightly dampened cloth or gauze over the lesion before applying film. Seal the edges with tape or a gauze wrapping. Dressing may be changed daily or left in place for 3–4 days in more resistant cases. To prevent relapse, continue treatment for at least a few days after lesions clear.

WARNINGS/PRECAUTIONS

Patient instructions	Caution patients not to let these preparations come into contact with their eyes. Occlusive dressings may be used for the management of psoriasis or other persistent dermatoses, but caution against using any readily flammable plastic film. If an occlusive dressing is not indicated, caution patients not to bandage or otherwise cover the treated area so that it becomes occluded (thus tight-fitting diapers or plastic pants should not be used on children being treated in the diaper area). Advise patients to report any signs of adverse reactions, particularly under occlusive dressings.
Irritation	Discontinue use and institute appropriate therapy
Dermatological infection	Discontinue use of any occlusive dressings and institute appropriate antifungal or antibacterial therapy; if infection persists, discontinue steroid therapy until a favorable response is obtained
Systemic absorption	Reversible hypothalamic-pituitary-adrenal (HPA) axis suppression, Cushing's syndrome, hyperglycemia, and glucosuria may result from systemic absorption after topical application, particularly in children (see USE IN CHILDREN). Use over extensive areas, for prolonged periods, or of occlusive dressings increases percutaneous absorption. If large doses are applied over extensive areas or are administered using the occlusive dressing technique, evaluate HPA axis function (by ACTH stimulation or measurement of urinary free cortisol) periodically. If HPA axis suppression occurs, discontinue use of this drug, reduce the frequency of application, or administer a less potent steroid. Infrequently, systemic corticosteroids may be needed to treat manifestations of topical steroid withdrawal.
Occlusive dressings	Generally, occlusive dressings should not be used on weeping (exudative) lesions; because of the increased risk of secondary infection from resistant staphylococci, use on hospitalized patients should be restricted. Covering large areas of the body may impair thermal homeostasis; discontinue use of the dressing if body temperature rises. Although rare, if miliaria or folliculitis occurs, discontinue use of the dressing and continue treatment by inunction. If sensitivity to the occlusive dressing material occurs, try substituting a different material.
Carcinogenicity, mutagenicity	Long-term studies have not been done in animals to evaluate the carcinogenic potential of topical corticosteroids; the results of studies to demonstrate mutagenicity of prednisolone and hydrocortisone have been negative
Effect on fertility	The effect of topical corticosteroids on fertility has not been studied

ADVERSE REACTIONS[1]

Local	Acneform eruptions, allergic contact dermatitis, burning, dryness, folliculitis, hypertrichosis, hypopigmentation, irritation, itching, perioral dermatitis, maceration, miliaria, secondary infection, skin atrophy, striae

USE IN CHILDREN

Use smallest amount necessary for effective treatment. Children may be more susceptible than adults to HPA axis suppression and Cushing's syndrome because of the larger ratio of surface area to body weight; intracranial hypertension has also been observed in children receiving topical corticosteroids. Chronic therapy may interfere with growth and development.

USE IN PREGNANT AND NURSING WOMEN

Pregnancy Category C: use during pregnancy only if the expected benefit justifies the potential risk to the fetus. Do not use over extensive areas, in large amounts, or for prolonged periods. In animal studies, systemic corticosteroids have generally been teratogenic at relatively low dosages; the more potent corticosteroids have also been teratogenic when applied to the skin. No adequate, well-controlled studies have been done in pregnant women. It is not known whether topical corticosteroids are excreted in human milk; although systemic corticosteroids are excreted in quantities unlikely to harm nursing infants, this preparation should be used with caution in nursing mothers.

VEHICLE/BASE
Cream (emulsion): cetyl alcohol, citric acid, mineral oil, polyoxyl 40 stearate, propylene glycol, sodium citrate, stearic acid, and purified water
Lotion (oil-in-water emulsion): glycerin, cetyl alcohol, stearic acid, glyceryl monostearate, mineral oil, polyoxyl 40 stearate, menthol, benzyl alcohol, and purified water
Ointment: white wax, cetyl alcohol, sorbitan sesquioleate, and white petrolatum

[1] Includes reactions common to topical corticosteroids in general

TOPICAL CORTICOSTEROIDS

CORDRAN-N (flurandrenolide and neomycin sulfate) Dista Rx

Cream (per gram): 0.5 mg (0.05%) flurandrenolide and 5 mg neomycin sulfate (15, 30, 60 g) **Ointment (per gram):** 0.5 mg (0.05%) flurandrenolide and 5 mg neomycin sulfate (15, 30, 60 g)

INDICATIONS	**TOPICAL DOSAGE**
Corticosteroid-responsive dermatoses associated with secondary infection	**Adult:** for moist lesions, gently rub a small amount of the cream into affected area bid or tid; for dry, scaly lesions, apply a thin film of ointment to affected area bid or tid **Child:** use minimal amount necessary for effective therapy (see precaution, below, concerning systemic absorption)

CONTRAINDICATIONS
Hypersensitivity to any component

ADMINISTRATION/DOSAGE ADJUSTMENTS

Occlusive dressing technique	For the management of psoriasis or other persistent dermatoses that are complicated by bacterial infection, an occlusive dressing may be applied. Remove superficial scales as much as possible by brushing, picking, or rubbing (soaking in a bath will help soften scales and permit easier removal). Rub cream or ointment thoroughly into affected area and cover with plastic film. If cream is used, additional moisture may be provided by placing a slightly dampened cloth or gauze over the lesion before applying film. Seal the edges with tape or a gauze wrapping. Dressing may be changed daily or left in place for 3–4 days in more resistant cases. To prevent relapse, continue treatment for at least a few days after lesions clear.

WARNINGS/PRECAUTIONS

Systemic absorption	The neomycin component of this preparation may cause nephrotoxicity and ototoxicity. Therefore, this product should not be used for an extended period, especially since it has not been shown that after 7 days of treatment further use will be more effective than administration of the steroidal component alone; this preparation should also not be applied over a wide area. The steroidal component may also cause systemic reactions; when this product is applied to extensive areas or used under an occlusive dressing, appropriate precautions should be taken, particularly with children.
Irritation	Discontinue use and institute appropriate therapy if irritation occurs
Fungal or yeast infection	Institute additional appropriate therapy and observe patient frequently if superficial fungal or yeast infection occurs
Superinfection	Prolonged use may result in overgrowth of nonsusceptible organisms; take appropriate measures if superinfection occurs
Neomycin sensitivity	Current literature indicates that sensitivity to neomycin has become more common
Occlusive dressings	Generally, occlusive dressings should not be used on weeping (exudative) lesions; because of the increased risk of secondary infection from resistant staphylococci, use on hospitalized patients should be restricted. The occlusive dressing causes an increase in systemic absorption (see warning, above). Covering large areas of the body may impair thermal homeostasis; discontinue use of the dressing if body temperature rises. Although rare, if milaria or folliculitis occurs, discontinue use of the dressing and continue treatment by inunction. If sensitivity to the occlusive dressing material occurs, try substituting a different material. Caution patients against using any readily flammable plastic film.
Ophthalmic application	Caution patients not to let this preparation come into contact with their eyes

ADVERSE REACTIONS[1]

Local	Acneform eruptions, allergic contact dermatitis, burning, dryness, folliculitis, hypertrichosis, hypopigmentation, irritation, itching, perioral dermatitis, maceration, miliaria, secondary infection, skin atrophy, striae
Systemic	Ototoxicity, nephrotoxicity

USE IN CHILDREN	**USE IN PREGNANT AND NURSING WOMEN**
Use smallest amount necessary for effective treatment; take special precautions to limit systemic absorption (see WARNINGS/PRECAUTIONS)	Topical corticosteroids have caused fetal abnormalities in laboratory animals; although no adverse effects on human pregnancy have been reported, safety for use during this time has not been absolutely established. Topical corticosteroids should not be used extensively, in large amounts, or for prolonged periods in pregnant women. Consult manufacturer for use in nursing mothers.

VEHICLE/BASE
Cream: stearic acid, cetyl alcohol, mineral oil, polyoxyl 40 stearate, ethylparaben, glycerin, and purified water
Ointment: white wax, cetyl alcohol, sorbitan sesquioleate, and white petrolatum

[1] Includes reactions common to topical corticosteroids in general

TOPICAL CORTICOSTEROIDS

CORT-DOME Cream and Lotion (hydrocortisone) Miles Pharmaceuticals Rx

Cream: 0.125% (30, 120 g), 0.25% (30, 120, 480 g), 0.5% (15, 30, 120, 480 g), 1% (15, 30, 75 g) Lotion: 0.125% (180 ml), 0.25% (120 ml), 0.5% (15, 30, 120 ml), 1% (15, 30 ml)

INDICATIONS	**TOPICAL DOSAGE**
Inflammatory and pruritic manifestations of corticosteroid-responsive dermatoses	**Adult:** apply a thin film to affected areas 2–4 times/day, depending on severity **Child:** use minimal amount necessary for effective therapy (see precaution, below, concerning systemic absorption)

CONTRAINDICATIONS
Hypersensitivity to hydrocortosone or other components

WARNINGS/PRECAUTIONS

Patient instructions	Caution patients not to let these preparations come into contact with their eyes. Occlusive dressings may be used for the management of psoriasis or other persistent dermatoses. If an occlusive dressing is not indicated, caution patients not to bandage or otherwise cover the treated area so that it becomes occluded (thus tight-fitting diapers or plastic pants should not be used on children being treated in the diaper area). Advise patients to report any signs of adverse reactions, particularly under occlusive dressings.
Irritation	Discontinue use and institute appropriate therapy
Dermatological infection	Discontinue use of any occlusive dressings and institute appropriate antifungal or antibacterial therapy; if infection persists, discontinue steroid therapy until a favorable response is obtained
Systemic absorption	Reversible hypothalamic-pituitary-adrenal (HPA) axis suppression, Cushing's syndrome, hyperglycemia, and glucosuria may result from systemic absorption after topical application, particularly in children (see USE IN CHILDREN). Use over extensive areas, for prolonged periods, or of occlusive dressings increases percutaneous absorption. If large doses are applied over extensive areas or are administered using the occlusive dressing technique, evaluate HPA axis function (by ACTH stimulation or measurement of urinary free cortisol) periodically. If HPA axis suppression occurs, discontinue use of this drug, reduce the frequency of application, or administer a less potent steroid. Infrequently, systemic corticosteroids may be needed to treat manifestations of topical steroid withdrawal.
Carcinogenicity, mutagenicity	Long-term studies have not been done in animals to evaluate the carcinogenic potential of topical corticosteroids; the results of studies to demonstrate mutagenicity of prednisolone and hydrocortisone have been negative
Effect on fertility	The effect of topical corticosteroids on fertility has not been studied

ADVERSE REACTIONS[1]

Local	Burning, itching, irritation, dryness, folliculitis, hypopigmentation, allergic contact dermatitis, secondary infection, acneform eruptions, perioral dermatitis, maceration, skin atrophy, striae, miliaria

USE IN CHILDREN	**USE IN PREGNANT AND NURSING WOMEN**
Use smallest amount necessary for effective treatment. Children may be more susceptible than adults to HPA axis suppression and Cushing's syndrome because of the larger ratio of surface area to body weight; intracranial hypertension has also been observed in children receiving topical corticosteroids. Chronic therapy may interfere with growth and development.	Pregnancy Category C: use during pregnancy only if the expected benefit justifies the potential risk to the fetus. Do not use over extensive areas, in large amounts, or for prolonged periods. In animal studies, systemic corticosteroids have generally been teratogenic at relatively low dosages; the more potent corticosteroids have also been teratogenic when applied to the skin. No adequate, well-controlled studies have been done in pregnant women. It is not known whether topical corticosteroids are excreted in human milk; although systemic corticosteroids are excreted in quantities unlikely to harm nursing infants, this preparation should be used with caution in nursing mothers.

VEHICLE/BASE
Cream 0.125% (emollient): isopropyl myristate, cholesterol, white petrolatum, synthetic beeswax, stearic acid, polyoxyethylene sorbitan monostearate, aluminum sulfate, propylene glycol, calcium acetate, dextrin, perfume, and purified water, with methylparaben and propylparaben as preservatives
Cream 0.25%, 0.5%, 1%: glycerin, sodium lauryl sulfate, calcium acetate, cetyl stearyl alcohol, aluminum sulfate, purified water, synthetic beeswax, white petrolatum, dextrin, and light mineral oil, with methylparaben as preservative
Lotion: glyceryl monostearate, cetyl alcohol, stearyl alcohol, butyl stearate, aluminum acetate, isopropyl myristate, polyoxyethylene sorbitan monolaurate, glycerin, and purified water, with methylparaben and propylparaben as preservatives

[1] Includes reactions common to topical corticosteroids in general

---

TOPICAL CORTICOSTEROIDS

CORTEF ACETATE Ointment (hydrocortisone acetate) Upjohn Rx

Ointment: 1% (20 g), 2.5% (5, 20 g)

INDICATIONS	**TOPICAL DOSAGE**
Inflammatory and pruritic manifestations of corticosteroid-responsive dermatoses	**Adult:** apply a thin film to affected areas 2–4 times/day, depending on severity **Child:** use minimal amount necessary for effective therapy (see precaution, below, concerning systemic absorption)

CORTEF ACETATE Ointment ■ CORTISPORIN Cream

CONTRAINDICATIONS

Hypersensitivity to hydrocortisone or other components

WARNINGS/PRECAUTIONS

Patient instructions	Caution patients not to let this preparation come into contact with their eyes. Occlusive dressings may be used for the management of psoriasis or other persistent dermatoses. If an occlusive dressing is not indicated, caution patients not to bandage or otherwise cover the treated area so that it becomes occluded (thus tight-fitting diapers or plastic pants should not be used on children being treated in the diaper area). Advise patients to report any signs of adverse reactions, particularly under occlusive dressings.
Irritation	Discontinue use and institute appropriate therapy
Dermatological infection	Discontinue use of any occlusive dressings and institute appropriate antifungal or antibacterial therapy; if infection persists, discontinue steroid therapy until a favorable response is obtained
Systemic absorption	Reversible hypothalamic-pituitary-adrenal (HPA) axis suppression, Cushing's syndrome, hyperglycemia, and glucosuria may result from systemic absorption after topical application, particularly in children (see USE IN CHILDREN). Use over extensive areas, for prolonged periods, or of occlusive dressings increases percutaneous absorption. If large doses are applied over extensive areas or are administered using the occlusive dressing technique, evaluate thermal homeostasis and HPA axis function (by ACTH stimulation or measurement of urinary free cortisol) periodically. If HPA axis suppression occurs, discontinue use of this drug, reduce the frequency of application, or administer a less potent steroid. Infrequently, systemic corticosteroids may be needed to treat manifestations of topical steroid withdrawal.
Carcinogenicity, mutagenicity	Long-term studies have not been done in animals to evaluate the carcinogenic potential of topical corticosteroids; the results of studies to demonstrate mutagenicity of prednisolone and hydrocortisone have been negative
Effect on fertility	The effect of topical corticosteroids on fertility has not been studied

ADVERSE REACTIONS[1]

Local	Burning, itching, irritation, dryness, folliculitis, hypertrichosis, acneform eruptions, hypopigmentation, perioral dermatitis, allergic contact dermatitis, maceration, secondary infection, skin atrophy, striae, miliaria

USE IN CHILDREN

Use smallest amount necessary for effective treatment. Children may be more susceptible than adults to HPA axis suppression and Cushing's syndrome because of the larger ratio of surface area to body weight; intracranial hypertension has also been observed in children receiving topical corticosteroids. Chronic therapy may interfere with growth and development.

USE IN PREGNANT AND NURSING WOMEN

Pregnancy Category C: use during pregnancy only if the expected benefit justifies the potential risk to the fetus. Do not use over extensive areas, in large amounts, or for prolonged periods. In animal studies, systemic corticosteroids have generally been teratogenic at relatively low dosages; the more potent corticosteroids have also been teratogenic when applied to the skin. No adequate, well-controlled studies have been done in pregnant women. It is not known whether topical corticosteroids are excreted in human milk; although systemic corticosteroids are excreted in quantities unlikely to harm nursing infants, this preparation should be used with caution in nursing mothers.

VEHICLE/BASE
Ointment: anhydrous lanolin, white petrolatum, and mineral oil

[1] Includes reactions common to topical corticosteroids in general

---

TOPICAL CORTICOSTEROIDS

CORTISPORIN Cream (polymyxin B sulfate, neomycin sulfate, and hydrocortisone acetate) Burroughs Wellcome Rx

Cream (per gram): 10,000 units polymyxin B sulfate, neomycin sulfate equivalent to 3.5 g neomycin, and 5 mg (0.5%) hydrocortisone acetate (7.5 g)

INDICATIONS	TOPICAL DOSAGE
Corticosteroid-responsive dermatoses associated with secondary infection	**Adult:** apply a small amount of cream to affected area 2–4 times/day, as needed; if condition permits, gently rub cream into affected area **Child:** same as adult

CORTISPORIN Cream ■ CORTISPORIN Ointment

CONTRAINDICATIONS

Perforated eardrum (see WARNINGS/PRECAUTIONS)	Viral skin lesions, including herpes simplex, vaccinia, and varicella	Hypersensitivity to any component
Ophthalmic use	Tuberculous or fungal skin lesions	

WARNINGS/PRECAUTIONS

Otic dermatoses or infections	Do not use in the external auditory canal if the eardrum is perforated
Systemic absorption	Prolonged use, application over a wide area of the body, or use of an occlusive dressing may produce nephrotoxicity, ototoxicity, and HPA axis suppression. Do not use this preparation for an extended period of time, especially since it has not been shown that after 7 days of treatment further use will be more effective than administration of the steroidal component alone. Do not apply over a wide area of the body. Take suitable precautions if an occlusive dressing is used.
Local reactions	If erythema, irritation, swelling, or pain persists or increases, discontinue use
Overgrowth of nonsusceptible organisms	Nonsusceptible organisms, including fungi, may proliferate with prolonged use; institute appropriate anti-infective therapy
Systemic corticosteroid therapy	May be required for generalized dermatological conditions
Spread of infection	May be encouraged by use of steroids on infected areas; discontinue treatment and institute appropriate antibacterial therapy
Interference with laboratory tests	An excessive serum hydrocortisone level may cause a reduction in the number of circulating eosinophils or the rate of excretion of 17-OHCS
Carcinogenicity	No evidence of carcinogenicity attributable to oral corticosteroids has been observed in long-term studies in mice, rats, and rabbits

ADVERSE REACTIONS[1]

Local	Allergic contact dermatitis, burning, itching, irritation, dryness, folliculitis, hypertrichosis, acneform eruptions, hypopigmentation, perioral dermatitis, maceration of the skin, secondary infection, skin atrophy, striae, miliaria
Systemic	Ototoxicity and nephrotoxicity

USE IN CHILDREN

See INDICATIONS and TOPICAL DOSAGE; systemic absorption of hydrocortisone in infants and children during prolonged therapy may result in cessation of growth and other signs and symptoms of hyperadrenocorticism

USE IN PREGNANT AND NURSING WOMEN

Pregnancy Category C: topical corticosteroids have been shown to be teratogenic in rabbits at a concentration of 0.5% and in mice at a concentration of 15%. No adequate, well-controlled studies have been done in pregnant women; use during pregnancy only if the expected benefit justifies the potential risk to the fetus. Hydrocortisone appears in human milk following oral administration; since systemic absorption can occur with topical use, exercise caution if the patient is nursing during therapy.

VEHICLE/BASE
Cream: liquid petrolatum, white petrolatum, propylene glycol, polyoxyethylene polyoxypropylene compound, emulsifying wax, purified water, 0.25% methylparaben, and sodium hydroxide or sulfuric acid (to adjust pH)

[1] Includes reactions common to topical corticosteroids in general

---

TOPICAL CORTICOSTEROIDS

CORTISPORIN Ointment (polymyxin B sulfate, bacitracin zinc, neomycin sulfate, and hydrocortisone) Burroughs Wellcome   Rx

Ointment (per gram): 5,000 units polymyxin B sulfate, 400 units bacitracin zinc, 5 mg neomycin sulfate, and 10 mg (1%) hydrocortisone (14.2 g)

INDICATIONS	TOPICAL DOSAGE
Corticosteroid-responsive dermatoses associated with secondary infection	**Adult:** apply a thin film of ointment to affected area 2–4 times/day **Child:** same as adult

CONTRAINDICATIONS	
Hypersensitivity to any component	Perforated eardrum (see WARNINGS/PRECAUTIONS)

ADMINISTRATION/DOSAGE ADJUSTMENTS

Withdrawal of chronic therapy	Decrease frequency of application, until ointment is applied as infrequently as once a week; then discontinue treatment

WARNINGS/PRECAUTIONS

Otic dermatoses or infections	Do not use in the external auditory canal if the eardrum is perforated
Systemic absorption	The neomycin component of this preparation may cause nephrotoxicity and ototoxicity. Therefore, this product should not be used for an extended period, especially since it has not been shown that after 7 days of treatment further use will be more effective than administration of the steroidal component alone; this preparation should also not be applied over a wide area.
Neomycin sensitization	May occur with prolonged use; discontinue medication if low-grade reddening with swelling, dry scaling, and itching occurs or lesion fails to heal
Overgrowth of nonsusceptible organisms	Nonsusceptible organisms, including fungi, may proliferate with prolonged use; institute appropriate anti-infective therapy
Systemic corticosteroid therapy	May be required for generalized dermatological conditions
Spread of infection	May be encouraged by use of steroids on infected areas; discontinue treatment and institute appropriate antibacterial therapy

ADVERSE REACTIONS

Dermatological	Striae, cutaneous sensitization
Other	Ototoxicity, nephrotoxicity

USE IN CHILDREN
See INDICATIONS and TOPICAL DOSAGE

USE IN PREGNANT AND NURSING WOMEN
Safety for use during pregnancy has not been established; use in large amounts, for prolonged periods, or over extensive areas is not recommended. Consult manufacturer for use in nursing mothers.

VEHICLE/BASE
Ointment: white petrolatum

TOPICAL CORTICOSTEROIDS

CYCLOCORT (amcinonide) Lederle   Rx

Cream: 0.1% (15, 30, 60 g)   **Ointment:** 0.1% (15, 30, 60 g)

INDICATIONS
Inflammatory or pruritic manifestations of corticosteroid-responsive dermatoses

TOPICAL DOSAGE
Adult: apply a thin film to affected areas bid (if either cream or ointment is used) or tid (cream only), depending on severity
Child: use minimal amount necessary for effective therapy (see precaution, below, concerning systemic absorption)

CONTRAINDICATIONS
Hypersensitivity to amcinonide or other components

WARNINGS/PRECAUTIONS

Patient instructions	Caution patients not to let this preparation come into contact with their eyes. Occlusive dressings may be used for the management of psoriasis or other persistent dermatoses. If an occlusive dressing is not indicated, caution patients not to bandage or otherwise cover the treated area so that it becomes occluded (thus tight-fitting diapers or plastic pants should not be used on children being treated in the diaper area). Advise patients to report any signs of adverse reactions, particularly under occlusive dressings.
Irritation	Discontinue use and institute appropriate therapy
Dermatological infection	Discontinue use of any occlusive dressings and institute appropriate antifungal or antibacterial therapy; if infection persists, discontinue steroid therapy until a favorable response is obtained

CYCLOCORT ■ DECADERM/DECADRON Phosphate/DECASPRAY

Systemic absorption	Reversible hypothalamic-pituitary-adrenal (HPA) axis suppression, Cushing's syndrome, hyperglycemia, and glucosuria may result from systemic absorption after topical application, particularly in children (see USE IN CHILDREN). Use over extensive areas, for prolonged periods, or of occlusive dressings increases percutaneous absorption. If large doses are applied over extensive areas or are administered using the occlusive dressing technique, evaluate HPA axis function (by ACTH stimulation or measurement of urinary free cortisol) periodically. If HPA axis suppression occurs, discontinue use of this drug, reduce the frequency of application, or administer a less potent steroid. Infrequently, systemic corticosteroids may be needed to treat manifestations of topical steroid withdrawal.
Carcinogenicity, mutagenicity	Long-term studies have not been done in animals to evaluate the carcinogenic potential of topical corticosteroids; the results of studies to demonstrate mutagenicity of prednisolone and hydrocortisone have been negative
Effect on fertility	The effect of topical corticosteroids on fertility has not been studied

ADVERSE REACTIONS[1]

Local	Burning, itching, irritation, dryness, folliculitis, hypertrichosis, acneform eruptions, hypopigmentation, perioral dermatitis, allergic contact dermatitis, maceration, secondary infection, skin atrophy, striae, miliaria

USE IN CHILDREN
Use smallest amount necessary for effective treatment. Children may be more susceptible than adults to HPA axis suppression and Cushing's syndrome because of the larger ratio of surface area to body weight; intracranial hypertension has also been observed in children receiving topical corticosteroids. Chronic therapy may interfere with growth and development.

USE IN PREGNANT AND NURSING WOMEN
Pregnancy Category C: use during pregnancy only if the expected benefit justifies the potential risk to the fetus. Do not use over extensive areas, in large amounts, or for prolonged periods. In animal studies, systemic corticosteroids have generally been teratogenic at relatively low dosages; the more potent corticosteroids have also been teratogenic when applied to the skin. No adequate, well-controlled studies have been done in pregnant women. It is not known whether topical corticosteroids are excreted in human milk; although systemic corticosteroids are excreted in quantities unlikely to harm nursing infants, this preparation should be used with caution in nursing mothers.

VEHICLE/BASE
Cream (hydrophilic): emulsifying wax, isopropyl palmitate, glycerin, sorbitol solution, lactic acid, 2% benzyl alcohol, and purified water
Ointment: white petrolatum, benzyl alcohol, emulsifying wax, and Tenox II

[1] Includes reactions common to topical corticosteroids in general

---

TOPICAL CORTICOSTEROIDS

DECADERM (dexamethasone) Merck Sharp & Dohme   Rx
Gel: 0.1% (30 g)

DECADRON Phosphate (dexamethasone sodium phosphate) Merck Sharp & Dohme   Rx
Cream: 0.1% (15, 30 g)

DECASPRAY (dexamethasone) Merck Sharp & Dohme   Rx
Spray: 0.04% (25 g)

INDICATIONS	**TOPICAL DOSAGE**
Inflammatory and pruritic manifestations of corticosteroid-responsive dermatoses	Adult: apply a thin film of the cream or gel to the affected area or spray each 4-in.² area of the affected surface for 1–2 s tid or qid

CONTRAINDICATIONS
Hypersensitivity to dexamethasone or any component

ADMINISTRATION/DOSAGE ADJUSTMENTS

Aerosol administration	Shake container *gently* once or twice before each use and spray the affected area from about 6 in. away; the container may be held upright or inverted. When a favorable response is obtained, reduce dose gradually and eventually discontinue use. Avoid spraying into the eyes or nose; intentional concentration and inhalation of the contents may be harmful or fatal.

WARNINGS/PRECAUTIONS

Otic use	Confirm that the eardrum is intact. Clean the aural canal thoroughly and sponge dry; with a cotton-tipped applicator, apply a thin coating of the cream or gel to the affected canal area tid or qid
Patient instructions	Caution patients not to let these preparations come into contact with their eyes. Occlusive dressings may be used for the management of psoriasis or other persistent dermatoses. If an occlusive dressing is not indicated, caution patients not to bandage or otherwise cover the treated area so that it becomes occluded (thus tight-fitting diapers or plastic pants should not be used on children being treated in the diaper area). Advise patients to report any signs of adverse reactions, particularly under occlusive dressings.
Irritation	Discontinue use and institute appropriate therapy
Dermatological infection	Discontinue use of any occlusive dressings and institute appropriate antifungal or antibacterial therapy; if infection persists, discontinue steroid therapy until a favorable response is obtained
Ophthalmic reactions	Prolonged use may result in steroid glaucoma; patients with a history of herpes simplex keratitis may experience recurrence following ocular exposure to corticosteroids. Take care when applying near the eyes or on the eyelids, since the drug may enter the eyes.
Sensitivity reactions	Discontinue use if any sensitivity reaction is observed after application of the spray
Systemic absorption	Reversible hypothalamic-pituitary-adrenal (HPA) axis suppression, Cushing's syndrome, hyperglycemia, and glucosuria may result from systemic absorption after topical application, particularly in children (see USE IN CHILDREN). Use over extensive areas, for prolonged periods, or of occlusive dressings increases percutaneous absorption. If large doses are applied over extensive areas or are administered using the occlusive dressing technique, evaluate thermal homeostasis and HPA axis function (by ACTH stimulation or measurement of urinary free cortisol) periodically. If HPA axis suppression occurs, discontinue use of this drug, reduce the frequency of application, or administer a less potent steroid. Infrequently, systemic corticosteroids may be needed to treat manifestations of topical steroid withdrawal.
Carinogenicity, mutagenicity	Long-term studies have not been done in animals to evaluate the carcinogenic potential of topical corticosteroids; the results of studies to demonstrate mutagenicity of prednisolone and hydrocortisone have been negative
Effect on fertility	The effect of topical corticosteroids on fertility has not been studied

ADVERSE REACTIONS[1]

Local	Burning, itching, irritation, dryness, folliculitis, hypertrichosis, acneform eruptions, hypopigmentation, perioral dermatitis, allergic contact dermatitis, maceration, secondary infection, skin atrophy, striae, miliaria

USE IN CHILDREN

Use smallest amount necessary for effective treatment. Children may be more susceptible than adults to HPA axis suppression and Cushing's syndrome because of the larger ratio of surface area to body weight; intracranial hypertension has also been observed in children receiving topical corticosteroids. Chronic therapy may interfere with growth and development.

USE IN PREGNANT AND NURSING WOMEN

Pregnancy Category C: use during pregnancy only if the expected benefit justifies the potential risk to the fetus. Do not use over extensive areas, in large amounts, or for prolonged periods. In animal studies, systemic corticosteroids have generally been teratogenic at relatively low dosages; the more potent corticosteroids have also been teratogenic when applied to the skin. No adequate, well-controlled studies have been done in pregnant women. It is not known whether topical corticosteroids are excreted in human milk; although systemic corticosteroids are excreted in quantities unlikely to harm nursing infants, this preparation should be used with caution in nursing mothers.

VEHICLE/BASE
Decaderm Gel (emollient, anhydrous, lipophilic, hydrophilic, moisture-retentive, vanishing): gelled isopropyl myristate, wool alcohols B.P., refined lanolin alcohol, microcrystalline wax, anhydrous citric acid, anhydrous sodium phosphate dibasic
Decadron Phosphate Cream (greaseless): stearyl alcohol, cetyl alcohol, mineral oil, polyoxyl 40 stearate, sorbitol solution, methyl polysilicone emulsion, creatinine, sodium citrate, disodium edetate, sodium hydroxide, 0.15% methylparaben, 0.1% sorbic acid, and purified water
Decaspray: isopropyl myristate and isobutane

[1] Includes reactions common to topical corticosteroids in general

---

TOPICAL CORTICOSTEROIDS

DIPROLENE (betamethasone dipropionate) Schering   Rx

Cream: 0.05% (15, 45 g)   **Ointment:** 0.05% (15, 45 g)

INDICATIONS

Inflammatory and pruritic manifestations of corticosteroid-responsive dermatoses

TOPICAL DOSAGE

Adult: apply a thin film of cream or ointment to affected areas 1–2 times/day; do not use cream for more than 2 wk or use more than 45 g of cream or ointment weekly

DIPROSONE (betamethasone dipropionate) Schering Rx

Cream: 0.05% (15, 45 g) **Lotion:** 0.05% (20, 60 ml) **Ointment:** 0.05% (15, 45 g) **Spray:** 0.1% (85 g)

INDICATIONS
Inflammatory and pruritic manifestations of corticosteroid-responsive dermatoses

TOPICAL DOSAGE
Adult: apply a thin film of the cream or ointment once daily (bid, if necessary) or a few drops of the lotion bid (morning and at night) to affected areas; massage lotion lightly until it disappears

Child: use smallest effective amount (see precaution, below, concerning systemic absorption)

CONTRAINDICATIONS
Hypersensitivity to betamethasone, other components, or other corticosteroids

ADMINISTRATION/DOSAGE ADJUSTMENTS

Spray application	Direct spray onto affected area from a distance of not less than 6 in. and apply for only 3 s, tid; avoid eyes or other mucous membranes
Occlusive dressings	Do not use these preparations under occlusive dressings

WARNINGS/PRECAUTIONS

Patient instructions	Caution patients not to let these preparations come into contact with their eyes, nor to bandage or otherwise cover the treated area so that it becomes occluded (thus, tight-fitting diapers or plastic pants should not be used on children being treated in the diaper area). Advise patients to report any signs of adverse reactions.
Irritation	Discontinue use and institute appropriate therapy
Dermatological infection	Institute appropriate antifungal or antibacterial therapy; if infection persists, discontinue steroid therapy until a favorable response is achieved
Systemic absorption	Reversible hypothalamic-pituitary-adrenal (HPA) axis suppression, Cushing's syndrome, hyperglycemia, and glucosuria may result from systemic absorption after topical application, particularly in children (see USE IN CHILDREN). Diprolene cream has been shown to suppress the HPA axis at doses as low as 7 g/day. Use of these preparations over extensive areas, for prolonged periods, or under occlusive dressings increases percutaneous absorption. If large doses are applied over extensive areas, evaluate HPA axis function (by ACTH stimulation or measurement of urinary free cortisol) periodically. If HPA axis suppression occurs, discontinue use of this drug, reduce frequency of application, or administer a less potent steroid. Infrequently, systemic corticosteroids may be needed to treat manifestations of topical steroid withdrawal.
Carcinogenicity, mutagenicity	Long-term studies have not been done in animals to evaluate the carcinogenic potential of topical corticosteroids; the results of studies to demonstrate mutagenicity of prednisolone and hydrocortisone have been negative
Effect on fertility	The effect of topical corticosteroids on fertility has not been studied

ADVERSE REACTIONS[1]

Local	Burning, itching, irritation, dryness, folliculitis, hypertrichosis, acneform eruptions, hypopigmentation, perioral dermatitis, allergic contact dermatitis, maceration, secondary infection, skin atrophy, striae, miliaria
Systemic	HPA axis suppression, Cushing's syndrome, hyperglycemia, glucosuria (see WARNINGS/PRECAUTIONS)

USE IN CHILDREN
Use smallest amount necessary for effective treatment; use of Diprolene in children under 12 yr of age is not recommended. Children may be more susceptible than adults to HPA axis suppression and Cushing's syndrome because of the larger ratio of surface area to body weight; intracranial hypertension has also been observed in children receiving topical corticosteroids. Chronic therapy may interfere with growth and development.

USE IN PREGNANT AND NURSING WOMEN
Pregnancy Category C: use during pregnancy only if the expected benefit justifies the potential risk to the fetus. Do not use over extensive areas, in large amounts, or for prolonged periods. In animal studies, systemic corticosteroids have generally been teratogenic at relatively low dosages; the more potent corticosteroids have also been teratogenic when applied to the skin. No adequate, well-controlled studies have been done in pregnant women. It is not known whether topical corticosteroids are excreted in human milk; although systemic corticosteroids are excreted in quantities unlikely to harm nursing infants, this preparation should be used with caution in nursing mothers.

VEHICLE/BASE
Diprolene Cream: propylene glycol, carbomer 940, sodium hydroxide, titanium dioxide, and purified water
Diprolene Ointment: propylene glycol, propylene glycol stearate, white wax, and white petrolatum
Diprosone Cream (hydrophilic, emollient): white petrolatum, ceteareth-30, cetearyl alcohol, phosphoric acid, mineral oil, monobasic sodium phosphate, and purified water, with 4-chlorocresol and propylene glycol as preservatives
Diprosone Lotion: 46.8% isopropyl alcohol, carboxy vinyl polymer, and purified water, with sodium hydroxide to adjust pH to ~ 4.7
Diprosone Ointment: mineral oil and white petrolatum
Diprosone Spray: mineral oil, caprylic/capric triglyceride, and 10% isopropyl alcohol, with propane and isobutane as propellants

[1] Reactions common to topical corticosteroids in general. Folliculitis, erythema, pruritus, and vesiculation have been observed in clinical trials of Diprolene ointment; burning/stinging, dry skin, pruritus, irritation, telangiectasia, erythema, cracking/tightening of the skin, follicular rash, and skin atrophy have been reported in clinical trials of Diprolene cream.

FLORONE

TOPICAL CORTICOSTEROIDS

FLORONE (diflorasone diacetate) Dermik Rx

Cream: 0.05% (15, 30, 60 g)   **Ointment:** 0.05% (15, 30, 60 g)

INDICATIONS	**TOPICAL DOSAGE**
Inflammatory and pruritic manifestations of corticosteroid-responsive dermatoses	Adult: apply a thin film to affected areas 1–4 times/day, depending on severity Child: use minimal amount necessary for effective therapy (see precaution, below, concerning systemic absorption)

CONTRAINDICATIONS

Hypersensitivity to diflorasone or other components

WARNINGS/PRECAUTIONS

Patient instructions	Caution patients not to let these preparations come into contact with their eyes. Occlusive dressings may be used for the management of psoriasis or other persistent dermatoses. If an occlusive dressing is not indicated, caution patients not to bandage or otherwise cover the treated area so that it becomes occluded (thus tight-fitting diapers or plastic pants should not be used on children being treated in the diaper area). Advise patients to report any signs of adverse reactions, particularly under occlusive dressings.
Irritation	Discontinue use and institute appropriate therapy
Dermatological infection	Discontinue use of any occlusive dressings and institute appropriate antifungal or antibacterial therapy; if infection persists, discontinue steroid therapy until a favorable response is obtained
Systemic absorption	Reversible hypothalamic-pituitary-adrenal (HPA) axis suppression, Cushing's syndrome, hyperglycemia, and glucosuria may result from systemic absorption after topical application, particularly in children (see USE IN CHILDREN). Use over extensive areas, for prolonged periods, or of occlusive dressings increases percutaneous absorption. If large doses are applied over extensive areas or are administered using the occlusive dressing technique, evaluate HPA axis function (by ACTH stimulation or measurement of urinary free cortisol) periodically. If HPA axis suppression occurs, discontinue use of this drug, reduce the frequency of application, or administer a less potent steroid. Infrequently, systemic corticosteroids may be needed to treat manifestations of topical steroid withdrawal.
Carcinogenicity, mutagenicity	Long-term studies have not been done in animals to evaluate the carcinogenic potential of topical corticosteroids; the results of studies to demonstrate mutagenicity of prednisolone and hydrocortisone have been negative
Effect on fertility	The effect of topical corticosteroids on fertility has not been studied

ADVERSE REACTIONS[1]

Local	Burning, itching, irritation, dryness, folliculitis, hypertrichosis, acneform eruptions, hypopigmentation, perioral dermatitis, allergic contact dermatitis, maceration, secondary infection, skin atrophy, striae, miliaria

---

USE IN CHILDREN

Use smallest amount necessary for effective treatment. Children may be more susceptible than adults to HPA axis suppression and Cushing's syndrome because of the larger ratio of surface area to body weight; intracranial hypertension has also been observed in children receiving topical corticosteroids. Chronic therapy may interfere with growth and development.

USE IN PREGNANT AND NURSING WOMEN

Pregnancy Category C: use during pregnancy only if the expected benefit justifies the potential risk to the fetus. Do not use over extensive areas, in large amounts, or for prolonged periods. In animal studies, systemic corticosteroids have generally been teratogenic at relatively low dosages; the more potent corticosteroids have also been teratogenic when applied to the skin. No adequate, well-controlled studies have been done in pregnant women. It is not known whether topical corticosteroids are excreted in human milk; although systemic corticosteroids are excreted in quantities unlikely to harm nursing infants, this preparation should be used with caution in nursing mothers.

VEHICLE/BASE
Cream (emulsified, hydrophilic): propylene glycol, stearic acid, polyoxyethylene 20 sorbitan monostearate, sorbitan monostearate and monooleate, sorbic acid, citric acid, and water
Ointment (emollient, occlusive): polyoxypropylene 15-stearyl ether, stearic acid, lanolin alcohol, and white petrolatum

[1] Includes reactions common to topical corticosteroids in general

HALCIDERM

TOPICAL CORTICOSTEROIDS

HALCIDERM (halcinonide) Squibb — Rx
Cream: 0.1% (15, 30, 60 g)

INDICATIONS	**TOPICAL DOSAGE**
Inflammatory and pruritic manifestations of corticosteroid-responsive dermatoses	**Adult:** apply to affected areas 1–3 times/day, rubbing in gently **Child:** use minimal amount necessary for effective therapy (see precaution, below, concerning systemic absorption)

CONTRAINDICATIONS

Hypersensitivity to halcinonide or other components

ADMINISTRATION/DOSAGE ADJUSTMENTS

Occlusive dressing technique	Gently rub a small amount of cream into the lesion until the preparation disappears; reapply the cream, leaving a thin coating on the lesion, cover with plastic film, and seal the edges. If additional moisture is needed, briefly wet the affected area with water immediately before applying the cream or cover the lesion with a dampened cotton cloth before applying the plastic film. Frequency of dressing changes should be determined on an individual basis; reapply medication with each change. If occlusive dressing is used only at night (12-h occlusion), additional cream should be applied, without occlusion, during the day.

WARNINGS/PRECAUTIONS

Patient instructions	Caution patients not to let this preparation come into contact with their eyes. Occlusive dressings may be used for the management or psoriasis or other persistent dermatoses. If an occlusive dressing is not indicated, caution patients not to bandage or otherwise cover the treated area so that it becomes occluded (thus tight-fitting diapers or plastic pants should not be used on children being treated in the diaper area). Advise patients to report any signs of adverse reactions, particularly under occlusive dressings.
Irritation	Discontinue use and institute appropriate therapy; an occasional patient may be sensitive to a particular occlusive dressing material or adhesive, and a substitute may be necessary
Dermatological infection	Discontinue use of any occlusive dressings and institute appropriate antifungal or antibacterial therapy; if infection persists, discontinue steroid therapy until a favorable response is obtained
Systemic absorption	Reversible hypothalamic-pituitary-adrenal (HPA) axis suppression, Cushing's syndrome, hyperglycemia, and glucosuria may result from systemic absorption after topical application, particularly in children (see USE IN CHILDREN). Use over extensive areas, for prolonged periods, or of occlusive dressings increases percutaneous absorption. If large doses are applied over extensive areas or are administered using the occlusive dressing technique, evaluate thermal homeostasis and HPA axis function (by ACTH stimulation or measurement of urinary free cortisol) periodically. If pyrexia or HPA axis suppression occurs, discontinue use of this drug, reduce the frequency of application, administer a less potent steroid, or, when occlusive dressings are necessary, use a sequential approach (ie, occlude only one portion of the body at a time). Infrequently, systemic corticosteroids may be needed to treat manifestations of topical steroid withdrawal.
Carcinogenicity, mutagenicity	Long-term studies have not been done in animals to evaluate the carcinogenic potential of topical corticosteroids; the results of studies to demonstrate mutagenicity of prednisolone and hydrocortisone have been negative
Effect on fertility	The effect of topical corticosteroids on fertility has not been studied

ADVERSE REACTIONS

Local	Burning, itching, irritation, dryness, folliculitis, hypertrichosis, acneform eruptions, hypopigmentation, perioral dermatitis, allergic contact dermatitis, maceration, secondary infection, skin atrophy, striae, and miliaria

USE IN CHILDREN

Use smallest amount necessary for effective treatment. Children may be more susceptible than adults to HPA axis suppression and Cushing's syndrome because of the larger ratio of surface area to body weight; intracranial hypertension has also been observed in children receiving topical corticosteroids. Chronic therapy may interfere with growth and development.

USE IN PREGNANT AND NURSING WOMEN

Pregnancy Category C: use during pregnancy only if the expected benefit justifies the potential risk to the fetus. Do not use over extensive areas, in large amounts, or for prolonged periods. In animal studies, systemic corticosteroids have generally been teratogenic at relatively low dosages; the more potent corticosteroids have also been teratogenic when applied to the skin. No adequate, well-controlled studies have been done in pregnant women. It is not known whether topical corticosteroids are excreted in human milk; although systemic corticosteroids are excreted in quantities unlikely to harm nursing infants, this preparation should be used with caution in nursing mothers.

VEHICLE/BASE
Cream (hydrophilic, vanishing): propylene glycol, dimethicone 350, castor oil, cetearyl alcohol (and) ceteareth-20, propylene glycol stearate, white petrolatum, and purified water

TOPICAL CORTICOSTEROIDS

HALOG (halcinonide) Princeton Rx
Cream: 0.025% (15, 60 g), 0.1% (15, 30, 60, 240 g) Ointment: 0.1% (15, 30, 60, 240 g) Solution: 0.1% (20, 60 ml)

HALOG-E (halcinonide) Princeton Rx
Cream: 0.1% (15, 30, 60 g)

INDICATIONS
Inflammatory and pruritic manifestations of corticosteroid-responsive dermatoses

TOPICAL DOSAGE
Adult: apply Halog cream or solution or a thin film of Halog ointment to affected areas 2–3 times/day, or apply Halog-E cream to affected areas 1–3 times/day; cream should be rubbed in gently after application
Child: use minimal amount necessary for effective therapy (see precaution, below, concerning systemic absorption)

CONTRAINDICATIONS
Hypersensitivity to halcinonide or other components

ADMINISTRATION/DOSAGE ADJUSTMENTS
Occlusive dressing technique	Apply solution or a thin film of ointment to the lesion, cover with plastic film, and seal the edges. Alternatively, gently rub a small amount of cream into the lesion until the preparation disappears; reapply the cream, leaving a thin coating on the lesion, cover with plastic film, and seal the edges. If additional moisture is needed, briefly wet the affected area with water immediately before applying the cream or cover the lesion with a dampened cotton cloth before the plastic film is applied. Frequency of dressing changes should be determined on an individual basis; reapply medication with each change. If occlusive dressing is used only at night (12-h occlusion), additional medication should be applied, without occlusion, during the day.

WARNINGS/PRECAUTIONS
Patient instructions	Caution patients not to let these preparations come into contact with their eyes. Occlusive dressings may be used for the management or psoriasis or other persistent dermatoses. If an occlusive dressing is not indicated, caution patients not to bandage or otherwise cover the treated area so that it becomes occluded (thus tight-fitting diapers or plastic pants should not be used on children being treated in the diaper area). Advise patients to report any signs of adverse reactions, particularly under occlusive dressings.
Irritation	Discontinue use and institute appropriate therapy; an occasional patient may be sensitive to a particular occlusive dressing material or adhesive, and a substitute may be necessary
Dermatological infection	Discontinue use of any occlusive dressings and institute appropriate antifungal or antibacterial therapy; if infection persists, discontinue steroid therapy until a favorable response is obtained
Systemic absorption	Reversible hypothalamic-pituitary-adrenal (HPA) axis suppression, Cushing's syndrome, hyperglycemia, and glucosuria may result from systemic absorption after topical application, particularly in children (see USE IN CHILDREN). Use over extensive areas, for prolonged periods, or of occlusive dressings increases percutaneous absorption. If large doses are applied over extensive areas or are administered using the occlusive dressing technique, evaluate thermal homeostasis and HPA axis function (by ACTH stimulation or measurement of urinary free cortisol) periodically. If pyrexia or HPA axis suppression occurs, discontinue use of this drug, reduce the frequency of application, administer a less potent steroid, or, when occlusive dressings are necessary, use a sequential approach (ie, occlude only one portion of the body at a time). Infrequently, systemic corticosteroids may be needed to treat manifestations of topical steroid withdrawal.
Carcinogenicity, mutagenicity	Long-term studies have not been done in animals to evaluate the carcinogenic potential of topical corticosteroids; the results of studies to demonstrate mutagenicity of prednisolone and hydrocortisone have been negative
Effect on fertility	The effect of topical corticosteroids on fertility has not been studied

ADVERSE REACTIONS[1]
Local	Burning, itching, irritation, dryness, folliculitis, hypertrichosis, acneform eruptions, hypopigmentation, perioral dermatitis, allergic contact dermatitis, maceration, secondary infection, skin atrophy, striae, miliaria

USE IN CHILDREN

Use smallest amount necessary for effective treatment. Children may be more susceptible than adults to HPA axis suppression and Cushing's syndrome because of the larger ratio of surface area to body weight; intracranial hypertension has also been observed in children receiving topical corticosteroids. Chronic therapy may interfere with growth and development.

USE IN PREGNANT AND NURSING WOMEN

Pregnancy Category C: use during pregnancy only if the expected benefit justifies the potential risk to the fetus. Do not use over extensive areas, in large amounts, or for prolonged periods. In animal studies, systemic corticosteroids have generally been teratogenic at relatively low dosages; the more potent corticosteroids have also been teratogenic when applied to the skin. No adequate, well-controlled studies have been done in pregnant women. It is not known whether topical corticosteroids are excreted in human milk; although systemic corticosteroids are excreted in quantities unlikely to harm nursing infants, this preparation should be used with caution in nursing mothers.

VEHICLE/BASE
Halog Cream 0.025%: glyceryl monostearate, cetyl alcohol, cetyl esters wax, polysorbate 60, propylene glycol, dimethicone 350, and purified water
Halog Cream 0.1%: glyceryl monostearate, cetyl alcohol, isopropyl palmitate, dimethicone 350, polysorbate 60, titanium dioxide, propylene glycol, and purified water
Halog-E Cream (hydrophilic, vanishing): propylene glycol, dimethicone 350, castor oil, cetearyl alcohol and ceteareth-20, propylene glycol stearate, white petrolatum, and purified water
Halog Ointment (gel): polyethylene glycol 400, polyethylene glycol 300, polyethylene glycol 1540, polyethylene glycol 6000 distearate, and mineral oil, with butylated hydroxytoluene as a preservative
Halog Solution: edetate disodium, polyethylene glycol 300, and purified water, with butylated hydroxytoluene as an antioxidant

[1] Includes reactions common to topical corticosteroids in general

---

TOPICAL CORTICOSTEROIDS

HYTONE (hydrocortisone) Dermik   OTC
Cream: 0.5% (30 g)

HYTONE (hydrocortisone) Dermik   Rx
Cream: 1% (30, 120 g), 2.5% (30, 60 g)   **Lotion:** 1% (4 fl oz), 2.5% (2 fl oz)   **Ointment:** 1% (30, 120 g), 2.5% (30 g)

INDICATIONS	TOPICAL DOSAGE
Inflammatory and pruritic manifestations of corticosteroid-responsive dermatoses	**Adult:** apply a thin film to affected areas 2–4 times/day, depending on severity **Child:** use minimal amount necessary for effective therapy (see precaution, below, concerning systemic absorption)

CONTRAINDICATIONS
Hypersensitivity to hydrocortisone or other components

WARNINGS/PRECAUTIONS

Patient instructions	Caution patients not to let these preparations come into contact with their eyes. Occlusive dressings may be used for the management of psoriasis or other persistent dermatoses. If an occlusive dressing is not indicated, caution patients not to bandage or otherwise cover the treated area so that it becomes occluded (thus tight-fitting diapers or plastic pants should not be used on children being treated in the diaper area). Advise patients to report any signs of adverse reactions, particularly under occlusive dressings.
Irritation	Discontinue use and institute appropriate therapy
Dermatological infection	Discontinue use of any occlusive dressings and institute appropriate antifungal or antibacterial therapy; if infection persists, discontinue steroid therapy until a favorable response is obtained
Systemic absorption	Reversible hypothalamic-pituitary-adrenal (HPA) axis suppression, Cushing's syndrome, hyperglycemia, and glucosuria may result from systemic absorption after topical application, particularly in children (see USE IN CHILDREN). Use over extensive areas, for prolonged periods, or of occlusive dressings increases percutaneous absorption. If large doses are applied over extensive areas or are administered using the occlusive dressing technique, evaluate HPA axis function (by ACTH stimulation or measurement of urinary free cortisol) periodically. If HPA axis suppression occurs, discontinue use of this drug, reduce the frequency of application, or administer a less potent steroid. Infrequently, systemic corticosteroids may be needed to treat manifestations of topical steroid withdrawal.
Carcinogenicity, mutagenicity	Long-term studies have not been done in animals to evaluate the carcinogenic potential of topical corticosteroids; the results of studies to demonstrate mutagenicity of prednisolone and hydrocortisone have been negative
Effect on fertility	The effect of topical corticosteroids on fertility has not been studied

ADVERSE REACTIONS[1]

Local — Burning, itching, irritation, dryness, folliculitis, hypertrichosis, acneform eruptions, hypopigmentation, perioral dermatitis, allergic contact dermatitis, maceration, secondary infection, skin atrophy, striae, miliaria

USE IN CHILDREN

Use smallest amount necessary for effective treatment. Children may be more susceptible than adults to HPA axis suppression and Cushing's syndrome because of the larger ratio of surface area to body weight; intracranial hypertension has also been observed in children receiving topical corticosteroids. Chronic therapy may interfere with growth and development.

USE IN PREGNANT AND NURSING WOMEN

Pregnancy Category C: use during pregnancy only if the expected benefit justifies the potential risk to the fetus. Do not use over extensive areas, in large amounts, or for prolonged periods. In animal studies, systemic corticosteroids have generally been teratogenic at relatively low dosages; the more potent corticosteroids have also been teratogenic when applied to the skin. No adequate, well-controlled studies have been done in pregnant women. It is not known whether topical corticosteroids are excreted in human milk; although systemic corticosteroids are excreted in quantities unlikely to harm nursing infants, this preparation should be used with caution in nursing mothers.

VEHICLE/BASE
Cream (water-washable): purified water, propylene glycol, glyceryl monostearate, cholesterol and related sterols, isopropyl myristate, polysorbate 60, cetyl alcohol, sorbitan monostearate, polyoxyl 40 stearate, and sorbic acid
Lotion: carbomer 940, propylene glycol, polysorbate 40, propylene glycol stearate, cholesterol and related sterols, isopropyl myristate, sorbitan palmitate, cetyl alcohol, triethanolamine, sorbic acid, simethicone, and purified water
Ointment (emollient): mineral oil, white petrolatum, and sorbitan sesquioleate

[1] Includes reactions common to topical corticosteroids in general

---

TOPICAL CORTICOSTEROIDS

KENALOG (triamcinolone acetonide) Squibb   Rx
Cream: 0.025% (15, 60, 80, 240, 2,380 g), 0.1% (15, 60, 80, 240, 2,380 g), 0.5% (20 g)   **Ointment:** 0.025% (15, 60, 80, 240 g), 0.1% (15, 60, 80 240 g), 0.5% (20 g)   **Lotion:** 0.025% (60 ml), 0.1% (15, 60 ml)   **Spray:** 0.2% (23, 63 g)

KENALOG-H (triamcinolone acetonide) Squibb   Rx
Cream: 0.1% (15, 60 g)

INDICATIONS
Inflammatory and pruritic manifestations of corticosteroid-responsive dermatoses

TOPICAL DOSAGE
Adult: apply cream, lotion, or thin film of ointment to affected areas 2–4 times/day (if 0.025% strength is used) or 2–3 times/day (if 0.1% or 0.5% strength is used); cream and lotion should be rubbed in gently after application
Child: use minimal amount necessary for effective therapy (see precaution, below, concerning systemic absorption)

CONTRAINDICATIONS
Hypersensitivity to triamcinolone or other components

ADMINISTRATION/DOSAGE ADJUSTMENTS

Spray application — Follow directions on aerosol can; preparation may be applied to any part of the body, but if applied to face, care should be taken to avoid contact with eyes or inhalation of spray. Area may also be covered with occlusive dressing (see below). Three or four applications daily are generally adequate.

Occlusive dressing techniques — Apply a thin film of ointment to affected area or spray a small amount on the lesion. Alternatively, gently massage a small amount of cream or lotion into affected area until preparation disappears; reapply cream or lotion, leaving a thin coating. Cover with plastic film and seal the edges. If additional moisture is needed, briefly wet the affected area with water before applying the medication or cover the lesion with a dampened cotton cloth before the plastic film is applied. Frequency of dressing changes should be determined on an individual basis; reapply medication with each change. If occlusive dressing is used only at night (12-h occlusion), additional medication should be applied, without occlusion, during the day.

WARNINGS/PRECAUTIONS

Patient instructions — Caution patients not to let these preparations come into contact with their eyes. Occlusive dressings may be used for the management of psoriasis or other persistent dermatoses. If an occlusive dressing is not indicated, caution patients not to bandage or otherwise cover the treated area so that it becomes occluded (thus tight-fitting diapers or plastic pants should not be used on children being treated in the diaper area). Advise patients to report any signs of adverse reactions, particularly under occlusive dressings.

KENALOG ■ LIDEX

Irritation	Discontinue use and institute appropriate therapy; an occasional patient may be sensitive to a particular occlusive dressing material or adhesive, and a substitute may be necessary
Dermatological infection	Discontinue use of any occlusive dressings and institute appropriate antifungal or antibacterial therapy; if infection persists, discontinue steroid therapy until a favorable response is obtained
Systemic absorption	Reversible hypothalamic-pituitary-adrenal (HPA) axis suppression, Cushing's syndrome, hyperglycemia, and glucosuria may result from systemic absorption after topical application, particularly in children (see USE IN CHILDREN). Use over extensive areas, for prolonged periods, or of occlusive dressings increases percutaneous absorption. If large doses are applied over extensive areas or are administered using the occlusive dressing technique, evaluate thermal homeostasis and HPA axis function (by ACTH stimulation or measurement of urinary free cortisol) periodically. If pyrexia or HPA axis suppression occurs, discontinue use of this drug, reduce the frequency of application, administer a less potent steroid, or, when occlusive dressings are necessary, use a sequential approach (ie, occlude only one portion of the body at a time). Infrequently, systemic corticosteroids may be needed to treat manifestations of topical steroid withdrawal.
Carcinogenicity, mutagenicity	Long-term studies have not been done in animals to evaluate the carcinogenic potential of topical corticosteroids; the results of studies to demonstrate mutagenicity of prednisolone and hydrocortisone have been negative
Effect on fertility	The effect of topical corticosteroids on fertility has not been studied

ADVERSE REACTIONS[1]

Local	Burning, itching, irritation, dryness, folliculitis, hypertrichosis, acneform eruptions, hypopigmentation, perioral dermatitis, allergic contact dermatitis, maceration, secondary infection, skin atrophy, striae, miliaria

USE IN CHILDREN

Use smallest amount necessary for effective treatment. Children may be more susceptible than adults to HPA axis suppression and Cushing's syndrome because of the larger ratio of surface area to body weight; intracranial hypertension has also been observed in children receiving topical corticosteroids. Chronic therapy may interfere with growth and development.

USE IN PREGNANT AND NURSING WOMEN

Pregnancy Category C: use during pregnancy only if the expected benefit justifies the potential risk to the fetus. Do not use over extensive areas, in large amounts, or for prolonged periods. In animal studies, systemic corticosteroids have generally been teratogenic at relatively low dosages; the more potent corticosteroids have also been teratogenic when applied to the skin. No adequate, well-controlled studies have been done in pregnant women. It is not known whether topical corticosteroids are excreted in human milk; although systemic corticosteroids are excreted in quantities unlikely to harm nursing infants, this preparation should be used with caution in nursing mothers.

VEHICLE/BASE
Kenalog Cream (vanishing): propylene glycol, cetearyl alcohol (and) ceteareth-20, white petrolatum, sorbitol solution, glyceryl monostearate, polyethylene glycol monostearate, simethicone, sorbic acid, and purified water
Kenalog-H Cream (vanishing, hydrophilic, water-washable, greaseless, nonstaining, moisturizing, emollient): propylene glycol, dimethicone 350, castor oil, cetearyl alcohol (and) ceteareth-20, propylene glycol stearate, white petrolatum, and purified water
Kenalog Lotion: propylene glycol, cetyl alcohol, stearyl alcohol, sorbitan monopalmitate, polysorbate 20, simethicone, and purified water
Kenalog Ointment (gel): polyethylene and mineral oil
Kenalog Spray: isopropyl palmitate and 10.3% dehydrated alcohol, with isobutane as a propellant

[1] Includes reactions common to topical corticosteroids in general

---

TOPICAL CORTICOSTEROIDS

LIDEX (fluocinonide) Syntex   Rx

Cream: 0.05% (15, 30, 60, 120 g)   **Ointment:** 0.05% (15, 30, 60, 120 g)   **Gel:** 0.05% (15, 30, 60, 120 g)   **Solution:** 0.05% (20, 60 ml)

LIDEX-E (fluocinonide) Syntex   Rx

Cream: 0.05% (15, 30, 60, 120 g)

INDICATIONS

Inflammatory manifestations of corticosteroid-responsive dermatoses

TOPICAL DOSAGE

Adult: apply a thin film to affected areas 2–4 times/day, depending on severity
Child: use minimal amount necessary for effective therapy (see precaution, below, concerning systemic absorption)

CONTRAINDICATIONS

Hypersensitivity to fluocinonide or other components

LIDEX ■ MYCOLOG-II

WARNINGS/PRECAUTIONS

Patient instructions	Caution patients not to let this preparation come into contact with their eyes. If the solution touches the eye and causes severe irritation, the patient should flush the eye immediately with a large volume of water. Occlusive dressings may be used for the management of psoriasis or other persistent dermatoses. If an occlusive dressing is not indicated, caution patients not to bandage or otherwise cover the treated area so that it becomes occluded (thus tight-fitting diapers or plastic pants should not be used on children being treated in the diaper area). Advise patients to report any signs of adverse reactions, particularly under occlusive dressings.
Irritation	Discontinue use and institute appropriate therapy
Dermatological infection	Discontinue use of any occlusive dressings and institute appropriate antifungal or antibacterial therapy; if infection persists, discontinue steroid therapy until a favorable response is obtained
Systemic absorption	Reversible hypothalamic-pituitary-adrenal (HPA) axis suppression, Cushing's syndrome, hyperglycemia, and glucosuria may result from systemic absorption after topical application, particularly in children (see USE IN CHILDREN). Use over extensive areas, for prolonged periods, or of occlusive dressings increases percutaneous absorption. If large doses are applied over extensive areas or are administered using the occlusive dressing technique, evaluate HPA axis function periodically by ACTH stimulation or measurement of urinary free cortisol. If HPA axis suppression occurs, discontinue use of this drug, reduce the frequency of application, or administer a less potent steroid. Infrequently, systemic corticosteroids may be needed to treat manifestations of topical steroid withdrawal.
Carcinogenicity, mutagenicity	Long-term studies have not been done in animals to evaluate the carcinogenic potential of topical corticosteroids; the results of studies to demonstrate mutagenicity of prednisolone and hydrocortisone have been negative
Effect on fertility	The effect of topical corticosteroids on fertility has not been studied

ADVERSE REACTIONS[1]

Local	Burning, itching, irritation, dryness, folliculitis, hypertrichosis, acneform eruptions, hypopigmentation, perioral dermatitis, allergic contact dermatitis, maceration of the skin, secondary infection, skin atrophy, striae, miliaria

USE IN CHILDREN

Use smallest amount necessary for effective treatment. Children may be more susceptible than adults to HPA axis suppression and Cushing's syndrome because of the larger ratio of surface area to body weight; intracranial hypertension has also been observed in children receiving topical corticosteroids. Chronic therapy may interfere with growth and development.

USE IN PREGNANT AND NURSING WOMEN

Pregnancy Category C: use during pregnancy only if the expected benefit justifies the potential risk to the fetus. Do not use over extensive areas, in large amounts, or for prolonged periods. In animal studies, systemic corticosteroids have generally been teratogenic at relatively low dosages; the more potent corticosteroids have also been teratogenic when applied to the skin. No adequate, well-controlled studies have been done in pregnant women. It is not known whether topical corticosteroids are excreted in human milk; although systemic corticosteroids are excreted in quantities unlikely to harm nursing infants, this preparation should be used with caution in nursing mothers.

VEHICLE/BASE
Lidex Cream (greaseless, nonstaining, anhydrous, water-miscible, emollient, hydrophilic): stearyl alcohol, polyethylene glycol 8000, propylene glycol, 1,2,6,-hexanetriol, and citric acid
Lidex Gel (colorless, greaseless, nonstaining, water-miscible): propylene glycol, propyl gallate, disodium edetate, and carbomer 940, with sodium hydroxide and/or hydrochloride acid to adjust pH
Lidex Ointment (occlusive, emollient): Amerchol CAB (mixture of sterols and higher alcohols), white petrolatum, propylene carbonate, and propylene glycol
Lidex Solution: 35% alcohol, diisopropyl adipate, citric acid, and propylene glycol
Lidex-E Cream (water-washable, aqueous, emollient): stearyl alcohol, cetyl alcohol, mineral oil, propylene glycol, sorbitan monostearate, polysorbate 60, citric acid, and purified water

[1] Includes reactions common to topical corticosteroids in general

---

TOPICAL CORTICOSTEROIDS

MYCOLOG-II (nystatin and triamcinolone acetonide) Squibb Rx

Cream (per gram): 100,000 units nystatin and 1 mg triamcinolone acetonide (15, 30, 60, 120 g) **Ointment (per gram):** 100,000 units nystatin and 1 mg triamcinolone acetonide (15, 30, 60, 120 g)

INDICATIONS	TOPICAL DOSAGE
Cutaneous candidiasis	Adult and child ($\geq$ 2 mo): apply cream or a thin film of ointment to affected area bid, in the morning and evening; the cream should be gently and thoroughly massaged into the skin

MYCOLOG-II ■ NEO-SYNALAR

CONTRAINDICATIONS
Hypersensitivity to any component

WARNINGS/PRECAUTIONS

Occlusive dressings	Do not use under occlusive dressings
Patient instructions	Caution patients not to bandage or otherwise cover the treated area so that it becomes occluded; thus tight-fitting diapers or plastic pants should not be used on children being treated in the diaper area, and patients who are undergoing treatment in the inguinal area should apply the preparation sparingly and wear loose-fitting clothing. Warn patients not to let the preparation come into contact with their eyes. Patients should be advised to report any signs of adverse reactions and to take measures to avoid reinfection.
Irritation, other hypersensitivity reactions	Discontinue use and institute appropriate therapy
Lack of response	If signs or symptoms persist after 25 days of treatment, discontinue use; before beginning a second course, repeat appropriate microbiological studies (eg, KOH smears and/or cultures) in order to confirm diagnosis and rule out other pathogens
Systemic absorption	Reversible hypothalamic-pituitary-adrenal (HPA) axis suppression, Cushing's syndrome, hyperglycemia, and glucosuria may result from systemic absorption after topical application, particularly in children (see USE IN CHILDREN). Use over extensive areas, for prolonged periods, or of occlusive dressings increases percutaneous absorption. If large doses are applied over extensive areas, periodically evaluate thermal homeostasis and HPA axis function; ACTH stimulation test and measurement of urinary free cortisol facilitate diagnosis of HPA axis suppression. If pyrexia or HPA axis suppression occurs, discontinue use of this drug, reduce the frequency of application, or administer a less potent steroid. Infrequently, systemic corticosteroids may be needed to treat manifestations of topical steroid withdrawal.
Carcinogenicity, mutagenicity, effect on fertility	No studies have been done to evaluate the carcinogenic or mutagenic potential of this preparation or its effect on fertility

ADVERSE REACTIONS[1]

Local	Acneform eruptions, irritation, burning, itching, dryness, folliculitis, hypertrichosis, hypopigmentation, perioral dermatitis, allergic contact dermatitis, maceration of the skin, secondary infection, skin atrophy, striae, miliaria

USE IN CHILDREN
Use smallest amount necessary for effective treatment. Children may be more susceptible than adults to HPA axis suppression and Cushing's syndrome because of the larger ratio of surface area to body weight; intracranial hypertension has also been reported in children receiving topical corticosteroids. Chronic therapy may interfere with growth and development.

USE IN PREGNANT AND NURSING WOMEN
Pregnancy Category C: in animal studies, systemic corticosteroids have generally been teratogenic at relatively low doses; the more potent corticosteroids have also been shown to be teratogenic when applied to animal skin. Use during pregnancy only if the expected benefit justifies the potential risk to the fetus. Do not use over extensive areas, in large amounts, or for prolonged periods. It is not known whether triamcinolone or nystatin is excreted in human milk; use with caution in nursing mothers.

VEHICLE/BASE
Cream (aqueous, perfumed, vanishing): aluminum hydroxide concentrated wet gel, titanium dioxide, glyceryl monostearate, polyethylene glycol monostearate, simethicone, sorbic acid, propylene glycol, white petrolatum, cetearyl alcohol (and) ceteareth-20, and sorbitol solution
Ointment (gel): mineral oil and polyethylene

[1] Acneform eruptions occurred in 1 of 100 patients during clinical trials; nystatin-induced irritation has been seen in rare cases. Other reactions listed here have been associated with use of topical corticosteroids in general.

TOPICAL CORTICOSTEROIDS

NEO-SYNALAR (neomycin sulfate and fluocinolone acetonide) Syntex — Rx
Cream (per gram): 5 mg (0.5%) neomycin sulfate and 0.25 mg (0.025%) fluocinolone acetonide (15, 30, 60 g)

INDICATIONS
Corticosteroid-responsive dermatoses associated with secondary infection

TOPICAL DOSAGE
Adult: apply a thin film to affected areas 2–4 times/day, depending on severity; occlusive dressings are not recommended
Child: use minimal amount necessary for effective therapy (see precaution, below, concerning systemic absorption); occlusive dressings are not recommended

NEO-SYNALAR ■ PSORCON

CONTRAINDICATIONS

Hypersensitivity to any component	Perforated eardrum (see WARNINGS/PRECAUTIONS)

WARNINGS/PRECAUTIONS

Otic dermatoses or infections	Do not use in the external auditory canal if the eardrum is perforated
Systemic absorption	The neomycin component of this preparation may cause nephrotoxicity and ototoxicity. Therefore, this product should not be used for an extended period, especially since it has not been shown that after 7 days of treatment further use will be more effective than administration of the steroidal component alone; this preparation should also not be applied over a wide area. The steroidal component may cause reversible hypothalamic-pituitary-adrenal (HPA) axis suppression, Cushing's syndrome, hyperglycemia, and glucosuria, particularly in children (see USE IN CHILDREN). Therefore, if large doses are applied over an extensive area, evaluate HPA axis function periodically by ACTH stimulation or by measurement of urinary free cortisol, and, if HPA axis suppression is detected, discontinue administration, reduce frequency of application, or administer a less potent steroid. Infrequently, systemic corticosteroids may be needed to treat manifestations of topical steroid withdrawal.
Patient instructions	Caution patients not to let this preparation come into contact with their eyes. Caution patients not to bandage or otherwise cover the treated area so that it becomes occluded (thus tight-fitting diapers or plastic pants should not be used on children being treated in the diaper area). Advise patients to report any signs of adverse reactions, particularly if an occlusive dressing has been used
Irritation	Discontinue use and institute appropriate therapy
Persistent or severe local infection or systemic infection	Institute appropriate systemic antibacterial therapy based on susceptibility testing
Neomycin sensitivity	Current literature indicates an increase in the prevalence of persons allergic to neomycin
Superinfection	Overgrowth of nonsusceptible organisms may occur with prolonged use
Carcinogenicity, mutagenicity	Long-term studies have not been done in animals to evaluate the carcinogenic potential of topical corticosteroids; the results of studies to demonstrate mutagenicity of prednisolone and hydrocortisone have been negative
Effect on fertility	The effect of topical corticosteroids on fertility has not been studied

ADVERSE REACTIONS[1]

Local	Burning, itching, irritation, dryness, folliculitis, hypertrichosis, acneform eruptions, hypopigmentation, perioral dermatitis, allergic contact dermatitis, maceration of the skin, secondary infection, atrophy, striae, miliaria
Systemic	Ototoxicity, nephrotoxicity

USE IN CHILDREN

Use smallest amount necessary for effective treatment. Children may be more susceptible than adults to HPA axis suppression and Cushing's syndrome because of the larger ratio of surface area to body weight; intracranial hypertension has also been observed in children receiving topical corticosteroids. Chronic therapy may interfere with growth and development.

USE IN PREGNANT AND NURSING WOMEN

Pregnancy Category C: use during pregnancy only if the expected benefit justifies the potential risk to the fetus. Do not use over extensive areas, in large amounts, or for prolonged periods. In animal studies, systemic corticosteroids have generally been teratogenic at relatively low dosages; the more potent corticosteroids have also been teratogenic when applied to the skin. No adequate, well-controlled studies have been done in pregnant women. It is not known whether topical corticosteroids are excreted in human milk; although systemic corticosteroids are excreted in quantities unlikely to harm nursing infants, this preparation should be used with caution in nursing mothers.

VEHICLE/BASE
Cream (water-washable, aqueous): stearic acid, propylene glycol, sorbitan monostearate and monooleate, polysorbate 60, and purified water, with methylparaben and propylparaben as preservatives

[1] Includes reactions common to topical corticosteroids in general

---

TOPICAL CORTICOSTEROIDS

PSORCON (diflorasone diacetate) Dermik Rx

Ointment: 0.05% (15, 30, 60 g)

INDICATIONS	TOPICAL DOSAGE
Inflammatory and pruritic manifestations of corticosteroid-responsive dermatoses	**Adult:** apply a thin film to affected areas 1–3 times/day, depending on severity **Child:** use minimal amount necessary for effective therapy (see precaution, below, concerning systemic absorption)

PSORCON ■ SYNALAR

CONTRAINDICATIONS

Hypersensitivity to diflorasone or other components

WARNINGS/PRECAUTIONS

Patient instructions — Caution patients not to let this preparation come into contact with their eyes. Occlusive dressings may be used for the management of psoriasis or other persistent dermatoses. If an occlusive dressing is not indicated, caution patients not to bandage or otherwise cover the treated area so that it becomes occluded (thus, tight-fitting diapers or plastic pants should not be used on children being treated in the diaper area). Advise patients to report any signs of adverse reactions, particularly under occlusive dressings.

Irritation — Discontinue use and institute appropriate therapy if irritation occurs

Dermatological infection — Discontinue use of any occlusive dressings and institute appropriate antifungal or antibacterial therapy; if infection persists, discontinue steroid therapy until a favorable response is obtained

Systemic absorption — Reversible hypothalamic-pituitary-adrenal (HPA) axis suppression, Cushing's syndrome, hyperglycemia, and glucosuria may result from systemic absorption after topical application, particularly in children (see USE IN CHILDREN). Use over extensive areas, for prolonged periods, or of occlusive dressings increases percutaneous absorption. If large doses are applied over extensive areas or are administered using the occlusive dressing technique, periodically evaluate HPA axis function by ACTH stimulation or measurement of urinary free cortisol. If HPA axis suppression occurs, discontinue use of this drug, reduce the frequency of application, or administer a less potent steroid. Infrequently, systemic corticosteroids may be needed to treat manifestations of topical steroid withdrawal.

Carcinogenicity, mutagenicity — Long-term studies have not been done in animals to evaluate the carcinogenic potential of topical corticosteroids; the results of studies to demonstrate mutagenicity of prednisolone and hydrocortisone have been negative

Effect on fertility — The effect of topical corticosteroids on fertility has not been studied

ADVERSE REACTIONS[1]

Local — Burning, itching, irritation, dryness, folliculitis, hypertrichosis, acneform eruptions, hypopigmentation, perioral dermatitis, allergic contact dermatitis, maceration of the skin, secondary infection, skin atrophy, striae, miliaria

---

USE IN CHILDREN

Use smallest amount necessary for effective treatment. Children may be more susceptible than adults to HPA axis suppression and Cushing's syndrome because of the larger ratio of surface area to body weight; intracranial hypertension has also been observed in children receiving topical corticosteroids. Chronic therapy may interfere with growth and development.

USE IN PREGNANT AND NURSING WOMEN

Pregnancy Category C: use during pregnancy only if the expected benefit justifies the potential risk to the fetus. In animal studies, systemic corticosteroids have generally been teratogenic at relatively low dosages; the more potent corticosteroids have also been teratogenic when applied to the skin. No adequate, well-controlled studies have been done in pregnant women. It is not known whether topical corticosteroids are excreted in human milk; although systemic corticosteroids are excreted in quantities unlikely to harm nursing infants, this preparation should be used with caution in nursing mothers.

VEHICLE/BASE
Ointment: propylene glycol, glyceryl monostearate, and white petrolatum

[1] Includes reactions common to topical corticosteroids in general

---

TOPICAL CORTICOSTEROIDS

SYNALAR (fluocinolone acetonide) Syntex   Rx

Cream: 0.025% (15, 30, 60, 425 g), 0.01% (15, 30, 60, 425 g)   Ointment: 0.025% (15, 30, 60, 120, 425 g)   Solution: 0.01% (20, 60 ml)

SYNALAR-HP (fluocinolone acetonide) Syntex   Rx

Cream: 0.2% (12 g)

INDICATIONS

Inflammatory and pruritic manifestations of corticosteroid-responsive dermatoses

TOPICAL DOSAGE

Adult: apply a thin film to affected areas 2–4 times/day, depending on severity
Child: use minimal amount necessary for effective therapy (see precaution, below, concerning systemic absorption)

SYNALAR ■ SYNEMOL

CONTRAINDICATIONS
Hypersensitivity to fluocinolone or other components

ADMINISTRATION/DOSAGE ADJUSTMENTS

Hirsute sites	Hair should be parted to allow direct contact of the cream or solution with lesion
Maximum dosage	Up to 2 g of the 0.2% cream may be applied daily; use of this preparation for prolonged periods is not recommended

WARNINGS/PRECAUTIONS

Patient instructions	Caution patients not to let this preparation come into contact with their eyes. Occlusive dressings may be used for the management of psoriasis or other persistent dermatoses. If an occlusive dressing is not indicated, caution patients not to bandage or otherwise cover the treated area so that it becomes occluded (thus tight-fitting diapers or plastic pants should not be used on children being treated in the diaper area). Advise patients to report any signs of adverse reactions, particularly under occlusive dressings.
Irritation	Discontinue use and institute appropriate therapy
Dermatological infection	Discontinue use of any occlusive dressings and institute appropriate antifungal or antibacterial therapy; if infection persists, discontinue steroid therapy until a favorable response is obtained
Systemic absorption	Reversible hypothalamic-pituitary-adrenal (HPA) axis suppression, Cushing's syndrome, hyperglycemia, and glucosuria may result from systemic absorption after topical application, particularly in children (see USE IN CHILDREN). Use over extensive areas, for prolonged periods, or of occlusive dressings increases percutaneous absorption. If large doses are applied over extensive areas or are administered using the occlusive dressing technique, evaluate HPA axis function periodically by ACTH stimulation or measurement of urinary free cortisol. If HPA axis suppression occurs, discontinue use of this drug, reduce the frequency of application, or administer a less potent steroid. Infrequently, systemic corticosteroids may be needed to treat manifestations of topical steroid withdrawal.
Carcinogenicity, mutagenicity	Long-term studies have not been done in animals to evaluate the carcinogenic potential of topical corticosteroids; the results of studies to demonstrate mutagenicity of prednisolone and hydrocortisone have been negative
Effect on fertility	The effect of topical corticosteroids on fertility has not been studied

ADVERSE REACTIONS[1]

Local	Burning, itching, irritation, dryness, folliculitis, hypertrichosis, acneform eruptions, hypopigmentation, perioral dermatitis, allergic contact dermatitis, maceration of the skin, secondary infection, skin atrophy, striae, miliaria

USE IN CHILDREN
Use smallest amount necessary for effective treatment. Children may be more susceptible than adults to HPA axis suppression and Cushing's syndrome because of the larger ratio of surface area to body weight; intracranial hypertension has also been observed in children receiving topical corticosteroids. Chronic therapy may interfere with growth and development.

USE IN PREGNANT AND NURSING WOMEN
Pregnancy Category C: use during pregnancy only if the expected benefit justifies the potential risk to the fetus. Do not use over extensive areas, in large amounts, or for prolonged periods. In animal studies, systemic corticosteroids have generally been teratogenic at relatively low dosages; the more potent corticosteroids have also been teratogenic when applied to the skin. No adequate, well-controlled studies have been done in pregnant women. It is not known whether topical corticosteroids are excreted in human milk; although systemic corticosteroids are excreted in quantities unlikely to harm nursing infants, this preparation should be used with caution in nursing mothers.

VEHICLE/BASE
Synalar Cream (water-washable, aqueous): stearyl alcohol, propylene glycol, cetyl alcohol, polyoxyl 20 cetostearyl ether, mineral oil, white wax, simethicone, butylated hydroxytoluene, edetate disodium, citric acid, methylparaben, propylparaben, and purified water
Synalar Ointment: white petrolatum
Synalar Solution (water-washable): propylene glycol and citric acid
Synalar-HP Cream (water-washable, aqueous): stearyl alcohol, cetyl alcohol, mineral oil, propylene glycol, sorbitan monostearate, polysorbate 60, purified water, and citric acid, with methylparaben and propylparaben as preservatives

[1] Includes reactions common to topical corticosteroids in general

---

TOPICAL CORTICOSTEROIDS

SYNEMOL (fluocinolone acetonide) Syntex   Rx
Cream: 0.025% (15, 30, 60, 120 g)

INDICATIONS
Inflammatory and pruritic manifestations of corticosteroid-responsive dermatoses

TOPICAL DOSAGE
Adult: apply a thin film to affected areas 2–4 times/day, depending on severity
Child: use minimal amount necessary for effective therapy (see precaution, below, concerning systemic absorption)

SYNEMOL ■ TEMOVATE

CONTRAINDICATIONS

Hypersensitivity to fluocinolone or other components

ADMINISTRATION/DOSAGE ADJUSTMENTS

Hirsute sites	Hair should be parted to allow direct contact of cream with lesion

WARNINGS/PRECAUTIONS

Patient instructions	Caution patients not to let this preparation come into contact with their eyes. Occlusive dressings may be used for the management of psoriasis or other persistent dermatoses. If an occlusive dressing is not indicated, caution patients not to bandage or otherwise cover the treated area so that it becomes occluded (thus tight-fitting diapers or plastic pants should not be used on children being treated in the diaper area). Advise patients to report any signs of adverse reactions, particularly under occlusive dressings.
Irritation	Discontinue use and institute appropriate therapy
Dermatological infection	Discontinue use of any occlusive dressings and institute appropriate antifungal or antibacterial therapy; if infection persists, discontinue steroid therapy until a favorable response is obtained
Systemic absorption	Reversible hypothalamic-pituitary-adrenal (HPA) axis suppression, Cushing's syndrome, hyperglycemia, and glucosuria may result from systemic absorption after topical application, particularly in children (see USE IN CHILDREN). Use over extensive areas, for prolonged periods, or of occlusive dressings increases percutaneous absorption. If large doses are applied over extensive areas or are administered using the occlusive dressing technique, evaluate thermal homeostasis and HPA axis function (by ACTH stimulation or measurement of urinary free cortisol) periodically. If HPA axis suppression occurs, discontinue use of this drug, reduce the frequency of application, or administer a less potent steroid. Infrequently, systemic corticosteroids may be needed to treat manifestations of topical steroid withdrawal.
Carcinogenicity, mutagenicity	Long-term studies have not been done in animals to evaluate the carcinogenic potential of topical corticosteroids; the results of studies to demonstrate mutagenicity of prednisolone and hydrocortisone have been negative
Effect on fertility	The effect of topical corticosteroids on fertility has not been studied

ADVERSE REACTIONS[1]

Local	Burning, itching, irritation, dryness, folliculitis, hypertrichosis, acneform eruptions, hypopigmentation, perioral dermatitis, allergic contact dermatitis, maceration of the skin, secondary infection, skin atrophy, striae, miliaria

USE IN CHILDREN

Use smallest amount necessary for effective treatment. Children may be more susceptible than adults to HPA axis suppression and Cushing's syndrome because of the larger ratio of surface area to body weight; intracranial hypertension has also been observed in children receiving topical corticosteroids. Chronic therapy may interfere with growth and development.

USE IN PREGNANT AND NURSING WOMEN

Pregnancy Category C: use during pregnancy only if the expected benefit justifies the potential risk to the fetus. Do not use over extensive areas, in large amounts, or for prolonged periods. In animal studies, systemic corticosteroids have generally been teratogenic at relatively low dosages; the more potent corticosteroids have also been teratogenic when applied to the skin. No adequate, well-controlled studies have been done in pregnant women. It is not known whether topical corticosteroids are excreted in human milk; although systemic corticosteroids are excreted in quantities unlikely to harm nursing infants, this preparation should be used with caution in nursing mothers.

VEHICLE/BASE
Cream (water-washable, aqueous, emollient): stearyl alcohol, cetyl alcohol, mineral oil, propylene glycol, sorbitan monostearate, polysorbate 60, purified water, and citric acid

[1] Includes reactions common to topical corticosteroids in general

---

TOPICAL CORTICOSTEROIDS

TEMOVATE (clobetasol propionate) Glaxo Rx

Cream: 0.05% (15, 30 g)   **Ointment:** 0.05% (15, 30 g)

INDICATIONS

Inflammatory and pruritic manifestations of moderate to severe corticosteroid-responsive dermatoses

TOPICAL DOSAGE

Adult and child (>12 yr): gently rub a thin layer into affected areas bid (morning and night); do not apply more than 50 g/wk or use for longer than 2 wk

TEMOVATE ■ TOPICORT

CONTRAINDICATIONS
Hypersensitivity to clobetasol, other components, or other corticosteroids

ADMINISTRATION/DOSAGE ADJUSTMENTS

Occlusive dressings	Do not use this preparation under occlusive dressings

WARNINGS/PRECAUTIONS

Patient instructions	Caution patients not to let this preparation come into contact with their eyes nor to bandage or otherwise cover the treated area so that it becomes occluded (thus, tight-fitting diapers or plastic pants should not be used on children being treated in the diaper area). Advise patients to report any signs of adverse reactions.
Irritation	Discontinue use and institute appropriate therapy
Dermatological infection	Institute appropriate antifungal or antibacterial therapy; if infection persists, withhold steroid therapy until infection is adequately controlled
Systemic absorption	Reversible hypothalamic-pituitary-adrenal (HPA) axis suppression, Cushing's syndrome, hyperglycemia, and glucosuria may result from systemic absorption following topical application, especially in children (see USE IN CHILDREN). Use over extensive areas, for prolonged periods, or under occlusive dressings increases percutaneous absorption. Doses of clobetasol as low as 2 g/day have produced HPA axis suppression. If large doses are applied over extensive areas, periodically evaluate HPA axis function by ACTH stimulation or measurement of urinary free cortisol. If HPA axis suppression occurs, discontinue use of this drug, reduce frequency of application, or administer a less potent steroid. Infrequently, systemic corticosteroids may be needed to treat manifestations of topical steroid withdrawal.
Atrophy	Certain areas of the body, such as the face, groin, and axillae, are more prone to atrophic changes; when treating these areas, examine patient frequently
Rosacea, perioral dermatitis, acne	Do not use these preparations to treat rosacea, perioral dermatitis, or acne
Carcinogenicity, mutagenicity	Long-term studies have not been done in animals to evaluate the carcinogenic potential of topical corticosteroids; the results of studies to demonstrate mutagenicity of prednisolone have been negative
Effect on fertility	The effect of topical corticosteroids on fertility has not been studied

ADVERSE REACTIONS[1]

Local	Burning, stinging, itching, skin atrophy, cracking, and fissures (with use of cream); burning, irritation, itching, stinging, cracking, erythema, folliculitis, numbness of fingers, skin atrophy, and telangiectasia (with use of ointment)
Systemic	Suppression of HPA axis

USE IN CHILDREN

Use of clobetasol in children under 12 yr of age is not recommended. Children may be more susceptible than adults to HPA axis suppression and Cushing's syndrome because of the larger ratio of surface area to body weight; intracranial hypertension has also been observed in children receiving topical corticosteroids. Chronic therapy may interfere with growth and development.

USE IN PREGNANT AND NURSING WOMEN

Pregnancy Category C: use during pregnancy only if the expected benefit outweighs the potential risk to the fetus. Do not use over extensive areas, in large amounts, or for prolonged periods. In animal studies, systemic corticosteroids have generally been teratogenic at relatively low dosages; the more potent corticosteroids have also been teratogenic when applied to the skin. Clobetasol appears to be fairly well absorbed percutaneously; when given SC to mice and rabbits, the drug has been shown to be a relatively potent teratogen. No adequate, well controlled studies have been performed in pregnant women. It is not known whether topical corticosteroids are excreted in human milk; although systemic corticosteroids are excreted in quantities unlikely to harm nursing infants, this preparation should be used with caution in nursing mothers.

VEHICLE BASE
Cream: propylene glycol, glyceryl monostearate, cetostearyl alcohol, glyceryl stearate, PEG 100 stearate, white wax, chlorocresol, sodium citrate, citric acid monohydrate, and purified water
Ointment: propylene glycol, sorbitan sesquioleate, and white petrolatum

[1] Reactions observed with use of topical corticosteroids include Cushing's syndrome, hyperglycemia, glucosuria, suppression of HPA axis, burning, itching, irritation, dryness, folliculitis, hypertrichosis, acneform eruptions, hypopigmentation, perioral dermatitis, allergic contact dermatitis, maceration of the skin, pustular psoriasis (in patients with psoriasis), secondary infection, skin atrophy, striae, and miliaria

---

TOPICAL CORTICOSTEROIDS

TOPICORT (desoximetasone) Hoechst-Roussel   Rx
Cream: 0.25% (15, 60 g; 4 oz)   Gel: 0.05% (15, 60 g)   Ointment: 0.25% (15, 60 g)

TOPICORT LP (desoximetasone) Hoechst-Roussel   Rx
Cream: 0.05% (15, 60 g)

INDICATIONS	**TOPICAL DOSAGE**
Inflammatory and pruritic manifestations of corticosteroid-responsive dermatoses	**Adult:** massage a thin film of cream, gel, or ointment gently into affected areas bid **Child:** use minimal amount necessary for effective therapy (see precaution, below, concerning systemic absorption)

COMPENDIUM OF DRUG THERAPY

TOPICORT ■ TRIDESILON

CONTRAINDICATIONS
Hypersensitivity to desoximetasone or other components

WARNINGS/PRECAUTIONS

Patient instructions	Caution patients not to let this preparation come into contact with their eyes. Occlusive dressings may be used for the management of psoriasis or other persistent dermatoses. If an occlusive dressing is not indicated, caution patients not to bandage or otherwise cover the treated area so that it becomes occluded (thus tight-fitting diapers or plastic pants should not be used on children being treated in the diaper area). Advise patients to report any signs of adverse reactions, particularly under occlusive dressings.
Irritation	Discontinue use and institute appropriate therapy
Dermatological infection	Institute appropriate antifungal or antibacterial therapy; if infection persists, discontinue steroid therapy until a favorable response is achieved
Systemic absorption	Reversible hypothalamic-pituitary-adrenal (HPA) axis suppression, Cushing's syndrome, hyperglycemia, and glucosuria may result from systemic absorption after topical application, particularly in children (see USE IN CHILDREN). Use over extensive areas, for prolonged periods, or under occlusive dressings increases percutaneous absorption. If large doses are applied over extensive areas or are administered using the occlusive dressing technique, evaluate HPA axis function (by ACTH stimulation or measurement of urinary free cortisol) periodically. If HPA axis suppression occurs, discontinue use of this drug, reduce the frequency of application, or administer a less potent steroid. Infrequently, systemic corticosteroids may be needed to treat manifestations of topical steroid withdrawal.
Carcinogenicity, mutagenicity	Long-term studies have not been done in animals to evaluate the carcinogenic potential of topical corticosteroids; the results of studies to demonstrate mutagenicity of prednisolone and hydrocortisone have been negative
Effect on fertility	The effect of topical corticosteroids on fertility has not been studied

ADVERSE REACTIONS[1]

Local	Burning, itching, irritation, dryness, folliculitis, folliculo-pustular lesions, hypertrichosis, acneform eruptions, hypopigmentation, perioral dermatitis, allergic contact dermatitis, maceration, secondary infection, skin atrophy, striae, miliaria, pruritus, erythema, vesiculation

---

USE IN CHILDREN
Use smallest amount necessary for effective treatment. Safety and effectiveness of ointment for use in children under 10 yr of age have not been established. Children may be more susceptible than adults to HPA axis suppression and Cushing's syndrome because of the larger ratio of surface area to body weight; intracranial hypertension has also been observed in children receiving topical corticosteroids. Chronic therapy may interfere with growth and development.

USE IN PREGNANT AND NURSING WOMEN
Pregnancy Category C: use during pregnancy only if the expected benefit justifies the potential risk to the fetus. Do not use over extensive areas, in large amounts, or for prolonged periods. In animal studies, systemic corticosteroids have generally been teratogenic at relatively low dosages; the more potent corticosteroids have also been teratogenic when applied to the skin. Teratogenic and embryotoxic effects have been detected in mice, rats, and rabbits following SC or topical administration of 3–30 times the human dose of the 0.25% cream or ointment (15–150 times the human dose of the 0.05% cream or gel). No adequate, well-controlled studies have been done in pregnant women. It is not known whether topical corticosteroids are excreted in human milk; although systemic corticosteroids are excreted in quantities unlikely to harm nursing infants, this preparation should be used with caution in nursing mothers.

VEHICLE/BASE
Topicort Cream (emollient): Isopropyl myristate, cetylstearyl alcohol, white petrolatum, mineral oil, lanolin alcohol, and purified water
Topicort LP Cream (emollient): same as above plus disodium and lactic acid
Topicort Gel: 20% SD alcohol 40, isopropyl myristate, carbomer 940, trolamine, edetate disodium, docusate sodium, and purified water
Topical Ointment: propylene glycol, sorbitan sesquioleate, fatty alcohol citrate, fatty acid pentaerythritol ester, beeswax, aluminum stearate, citric acid, butylated hydroxyanisole, and white petrolatum

[1] Includes reactions common to topical corticosteroids in general; reactions reported during controlled clinical studies included folliculitis and folliculo-pustular lesions with use of the 0.25% cream; pruritus, erythema, and vesiculation with use of the 0.05% cream; burning with use of either cream; and comedones with the ointment

---

TOPICAL CORTICOSTEROIDS

TRIDESILON (desonide) Miles Pharmaceuticals   Rx
Cream: 0.05% (15, 60, 2,270 g)   **Ointment:** 0.05% (15, 60 g)

INDICATIONS
Inflammatory and pruritic manifestations of corticosteroid-responsive dermatoses

TOPICAL DOSAGE
Adult: apply a thin film to affected areas 2–4 times/day depending on severity
Child: use minimal amount necessary for effective therapy (see precaution, below, concerning systemic absorption)

TRIDESILON ■ VALISONE

CONTRAINDICATIONS
Hypersensitivity to desonide or other components

WARNINGS/PRECAUTIONS

Patient instructions	Caution patients not to let this preparation come into contact with their eyes. Occlusive dressings may be used for the management of psoriasis or other persistent dermatoses. If an occlusive dressing is not indicated, caution patients not to bandage or otherwise cover the treated area so that it becomes occluded (thus tight-fitting diapers or plastic pants should not be used on children being treated in the diaper area). Advise patients to report any signs of adverse reactions, particularly under occlusive dressings.
Irritation	Discontinue use and institute appropriate therapy
Dermatological infection	Discontinue use of any occlusive dressings and institute appropriate antifungal or antibacterial therapy; if infection persists, discontinue steroid therapy until a favorable response is obtained
Systemic absorption	Reversible hypothalamic-pituitary-adrenal (HPA) axis suppression, Cushing's syndrome, hyperglycemia, and glucosuria may result from systemic absorption after topical application, particularly in children (see USE IN CHILDREN). Use over extensive areas, for prolonged periods, or of occlusive dressings increases percutaneous absorption. If large doses are applied over extensive areas or are administered using the occlusive dressing technique, evaluate thermal homeostasis and HPA axis function (by ACTH stimulation or measurement of urinary free cortisol) periodically. If HPA axis suppression occurs, discontinue use of this drug, reduce the frequency of application, or administer a less potent steroid. Infrequently, systemic corticosteroids may be needed to treat manifestations of topical steroid withdrawal.
Carcinogenicity, mutagenicity	Long-term studies have not been done in animals to evaluate the carcinogenic potential of topical corticosteroids; the results of studies to demonstrate mutagenicity of prednisolone and hydrocortisone have been negative
Effect on fertility	The effect of topical corticosteroids on fertility has not been studied

ADVERSE REACTIONS[1]

Local	Burning, itching, irritation, dryness, folliculitis, hypertrichosis, acneform eruptions, hypopigmentation, perioral dermatitis, allergic contact dermatitis, maceration, secondary infection, skin atrophy, striae, miliaria

USE IN CHILDREN
Use smallest amount necessary for effective treatment. Children may be more susceptible than adults to HPA axis suppression and Cushing's syndrome because of the larger ratio of surface area to body weight; intracranial hypertension has also been observed in children receiving topical corticosteroids. Chronic therapy may interfere with growth and development.

USE IN PREGNANT AND NURSING WOMEN
Pregnancy Category C: use during pregnancy only if the expected benefit justifies the potential risk to the fetus. Do not use over extensive areas, in large amounts, or for prolonged periods. In animal studies, systemic corticosteroids have generally been teratogenic at relatively low dosages; the more potent corticosteroids have also been teratogenic when applied to the skin. No adequate, well-controlled studies have been done in pregnant women. It is not known whether topical corticosteroids are excreted in human milk; although systemic corticosteroids are excreted in quantities unlikely to harm nursing infants, this preparation should be used with caution in nursing mothers.

VEHICLE/BASE
Cream: glycerin, sodium lauryl sulfate, aluminum acetate, cetyl stearyl alcohol, synthetic beeswax, white petrolatum, light mineral oil, and purified water, with methylparaben as a preservative; buffered to pH range of normal skin
Ointment: white petrolatum

[1] Includes reactions common to topical corticosteroids in general

TOPICAL CORTICOSTEROIDS

VALISONE (betamethasone valerate) Schering   Rx
Cream: 0.01% (15, 60 g), 0.1% (15, 45, 110, 430 g)   Lotion: 0.1% (20, 60 ml)   Ointment: 0.1% (15, 45 g)

INDICATIONS Inflammatory and pruritic manifestations of corticosteroid-responsive dermatoses	**TOPICAL DOSAGE** Adult: apply a thin film of the cream or ointment to affected area 1–3 times/day; alternatively, apply a few drops of the lotion and massage lightly until the preparation disappears. Use lotion bid (morning and at night) to start, and then once daily when condition improves; for stubborn cases, the dosage may be increased. Child: use smallest effective amount (see precaution, below, concerning systemic absorption)

CONTRAINDICATIONS

Hypersensitivity to betamethasone, other components, or other corticosteroids

WARNINGS/PRECAUTIONS

Patient instructions	Caution patients not to let these preparations come into contact with their eyes. Occlusive dressings may be used for the management of psoriasis or other persistent dermatoses. If an occlusive dressing is not indicated, caution patients not to bandage or otherwise cover the treated area so that it becomes occluded (thus tight-fitting diapers or plastic pants should not be used on children being treated in the diaper area). Advise patients to report any signs of adverse reactions, particularly under occlusive dressings.
Irritation	Discontinue use and institute appropriate therapy
Dermatological infection	Institute appropriate antifungal or antibacterial therapy; if infection persists, discontinue steroid therapy until a favorable response is achieved
Systemic absorption	Reversible hypothalamic-pituitary-adrenal (HPA) axis suppression, Cushing's syndrome, hyperglycemia, and glucosuria may result from systemic absorption after topical application, particularly in children (see USE IN CHILDREN). Use over extensive areas, for prolonged periods, or under occlusive dressings increases percutaneous absorption. If large doses are applied over extensive areas or are administered using the occlusive dressing technique, evaluate HPA axis function (by ACTH stimulation or measurement of urinary free cortisol) periodically. If HPA axis suppression occurs, discontinue use of this drug, reduce the frequency of application, or administer a less potent steroid. Infrequently, systemic corticosteroids may be needed to treat manifestations of topical steroid withdrawal.
Carcinogenicity, mutagenicity	Long-term studies have not been done in animals to evaluate the carcinogenic potential of topical corticosteroids; the results of studies to demonstrate mutagenicity of prednisolone and hydrocortisone have been negative
Effect on fertility	The effect of topical corticosteroids on fertility has not been studied

ADVERSE REACTIONS[1]

Local	Burning, itching, irritation, dryness, folliculitis, hypertrichosis, acneform eruptions, hypopigmentation, perioral dermatitis, allergic contact dermatitis, maceration, secondary infection, skin atrophy, striae, miliaria
Systemic	HPA axis suppression, Cushing's syndrome, hyperglycemia, glucosuria (see WARNINGS/PRECAUTIONS)

USE IN CHILDREN

Use smallest amount necessary for effective treatment. Children may be more susceptible than adults to HPA axis suppression and Cushing's syndrome because of the larger ratio of surface area to body weight; intracranial hypertension has also been observed in children receiving topical corticosteroids. Chronic therapy may interfere with growth and development.

USE IN PREGNANT AND NURSING WOMEN

Pregnancy Category C: use during pregnancy only if the expected benefit justifies the potential risk to the fetus. Do not use over extensive areas, in large amounts, or for prolonged periods. In animal studies, systemic corticosteroids have generally been teratogenic at relatively low dosages; the more potent corticosteroids have also been teratogenic when applied to the skin. No adequate, well-controlled studies have been done in pregnant women. It is not known whether topical corticosteroids are excreted in human milk; although systemic corticosteroids are excreted in quantities unlikely to harm nursing infants, this preparation should be used with caution in nursing mothers.

VEHICLE/BASE
Cream (aqueous, hydrophilic, emollient): mineral oil, white petrolatum, ceteareth-30, cetearyl alcohol, monobasic sodium phosphate, and phosphoric acid, with chlorocresol and propylene glycol as preservatives
Lotion: 47.5% isopropyl alcohol, carbomer 934P, and water, with sodium hydroxide to adjust pH to ~ 4.7
Ointment: mineral oil, white petrolatum, and hydrogenated lanolin

[1] Includes reactions common to topical corticosteroids in general

---

TOPICAL CORTICOSTEROIDS

VIOFORM-Hydrocortisone (clioquinol and hydrocortisone) CIBA Rx

Cream: 3% clioquinol and 1% hydrocortisone (5, 20 g); 3% clioquinol and 0.5% hydrocortisone (14.2, 28.4 g) Ointment: 3% clioquinol and 1% hydrocortisone (20 g); 3% clioquinol and 0.5% hydrocortisone (28.4 g) Lotion: 3% clioquinol and 1% hydrocortisone (15 ml)

INDICATIONS

Acute and chronic dermatoses, including contact or atopic dermatitis, impetiginized eczema, nummular eczema, infantile eczema, endogenous chronic infectious dermatitis, stasis dermatitis, pyoderma, nuchal eczema and chronic eczematoid otitis externa, acne urticata, localied or disseminated neurodermatitis, lichen simplex chronicus, anogenital pruritus (vulvae, scroti, ani), folliculitis, bacterial dermatoses, mycotic dermatoses such as tinea (capitis, cruris, corporis, pedis), moniliasis, and intertrigo[1]

TOPICAL DOSAGE

Adult and child ($>$ 2 yr): apply a thin film of cream, ointment, or lotion to affected areas tid or qid

VIOFORM-Hydrocortisone ■ WESTCORT

CONTRAINDICATIONS

Hypersensitivity to any of the components or related compounds	Most viral skin lesions, including herpes simplex, vaccinia, and varicella	Tuberculosis of the skin
Ophthalmic use	Age < 2 yr	

ADMINISTRATION/DOSAGE ADJUSTMENTS

Selection of appropriate formulation — For moist, weeping lesions, use the cream; for application behind the ears and in intertriginous areas of the body, use the lotion; for dry lesions accompanied by thickening and scaling of the skin, use the ointment; for lesions involving extensive body areas or less severe dermatoses, use the mild cream or mild ointment

WARNINGS/PRECAUTIONS

Irritation — May occur; discontinue medication

Staining — Contact with this preparation may cause staining of skin and fabrics; rarely, discoloration of the hair and nails may occur

Overgrowth of nonsusceptible organisms — Prolonged use may result in proliferation of nonsusceptible organisms, requiring appropriate antiinfective therapy

Systemic infections — Use appropriate systemic antibiotics

Systemic absorption — Increases with extensive treatment, prolonged therapy, or occlusive dressing technique; use with caution, especially in infants and children

Diagnostic interference — Wait at least 1 mo between discontinuation of therapy and performance of thyroid function tests; ferric chloride test for PKU may be false positive if drug is present in diaper or urine

ADVERSE REACTIONS[2]

Local — Rash, hypersensitivity, burning, itching, irritation, dryness, folliculitis, hypertrichosis, acneform eruptions, hypopigmentation, perioral dermatitis, allergic contact dermatitis, maceration, secondary infection, skin atrophy, striae, miliaria

ALTERED LABORATORY VALUES

Urinary values — ⇧ Phenylketones (with ferric chloride test)

No clinically significant alterations in blood/serum values occur at therapeutic dosages

---

USE IN CHILDREN

Safety and effectiveness for use in children have not been established; contraindicated for use in children under 2 yr of age

USE IN PREGNANT AND NURSING WOMEN

Safety for use during pregnancy has not been established; use in large amounts, for prolonged periods, or over extensive areas is not recommended. It is not known whether this drug, when applied topically, is excreted in human milk; use with caution in nursing mothers.

VEHICLE/BASE
Cream (water-washable): stearyl alcohol, cetyl alcohol, stearic acid, petrolatum, sodium lauryl sulfate, glycerin, and water
Ointment: petrolatum
Lotion (water-washable): stearic acid, cetyl alcohol, lanolin, propylene glycol, sorbitan trioleate, polysorbate 60, triethanolamine, perfume Flora, water, methylparaben, and propylparaben

[1] Possibly effective
[2] Includes reactions common to topical corticosteroids in general

---

TOPICAL CORTICOSTEROIDS

WESTCORT (hydrocortisone valerate) Westwood   Rx

Cream: 0.2% (15, 45, 60, 120 g)   **Ointment:** 0.2% (15, 45, 60 g)

INDICATIONS

Inflammatory and pruritic manifestations of corticosteroid-responsive dermatoses

TOPICAL DOSAGE

Adult: apply a thin film to affected areas 2–3 times/day, depending on severity
Child: use minimal amount necessary for effective therapy (see precaution, below, concerning systemic absorption)

CONTRAINDICATIONS

Hypersensitivity to hydrocortisone or other components

WESTCORT ■ AEROBID

WARNINGS/PRECAUTIONS

Patient instructions	Caution patients not to let these preparations come into contact with their eyes. Occlusive dressings may be used for the management of psoriasis or other persistent dermatoses. If an occlusive dressing is not indicated, caution patients not to bandage or otherwise cover the treated area so that it becomes occluded (thus, tight-fitting diapers or plastic pants should not be used on children being treated in the diaper area). Advise patients to report any signs of adverse reactions, particularly under occlusive dressings.
Irritation	Discontinue use and institute appropriate therapy
Dermatological infection	Discontinue use of any occlusive dressings and institute appropriate antifungal or antibacterial therapy; if infection persists, discontinue steroid therapy until a favorable response is obtained
Systemic absorption	Reversible hypothalamic-pituitary-adrenal (HPA) axis suppression, Cushing's syndrome, hyperglycemia, and glucosuria may result from systemic absorption after topical application, particularly in children (see USE IN CHILDREN). Use over extensive areas, for prolonged periods, or of occlusive dressings increases percutaneous absorption. If large doses are applied over extensive areas or are administered using the occlusive dressing technique, evaluate HPA axis function periodically by ACTH stimulation or measurement of urinary free cortisol. If HPA axis suppression occurs, discontinue use of this drug, reduce the frequency of application, or administer a less potent steroid. Infrequently, systemic corticosteroids may be needed to treat manifestations of topical steroid withdrawal.
Carcinogenicity, mutagenicity	Long-term studies have not been done in animals to evaluate the carcinogenic potential of topical corticosteroids; the results of studies to demonstrate mutagenicity of prednisolone and hydrocortisone have been negative
Effect on fertility	The effect of topical corticosteroids on fertility has not been studied

ADVERSE REACTIONS[1]

Local	Burning, itching, irritation, dryness, folliculitis, hypertrichosis, acneform eruptions, hypopigmentation, perioral dermatitis, allergic contact dermatitis, maceration of the skin, secondary infection, skin atrophy, striae, miliaria

USE IN CHILDREN

Use smallest amount necessary for effective treatment. Children may be more susceptible than adults to HPA axis suppression and Cushing's syndrome because of the larger ratio of surface area to body weight; intracranial hypertension has also been observed in children receiving topical corticosteroids. Chronic therapy may interfere with growth and development.

USE IN PREGNANT AND NURSING WOMEN

Pregnancy Category C: use during pregnancy only if the expected benefit justifies the potential risk to the fetus. Do not use over extensive areas, in large amounts, or for prolonged periods. In animal studies, systemic corticosteroids have generally been teratogenic at relatively low dosages; the more potent corticosteroids have also been teratogenic when applied to the skin. No adequate, well-controlled studies have been done in pregnant women. It is not known whether topical corticosteroids are excreted in human milk; although systemic corticosteroids are excreted in quantities unlikely to harm nursing infants, these preparations nevertheless should be used with caution in nursing mothers.

VEHICLE/BASE
Cream (water-washable, emollient): white petrolatum, stearyl alcohol, propylene glycol, amphoteric-9, carbomer 940, dried sodium phosphate, sodium lauryl sulfate, sorbic acid, and water
Ointment (water-washable, emollient): white petrolatum, stearyl alcohol, propylene glycol, sorbic acid, sodium lauryl sulfate, carbomer 934, dried sodium phosphate, mineral oil, steareth-2, steareth-100, and water

[1] Includes reactions common to topical corticosteroids in general

---

INHALANT CORTICOSTEROIDS

AEROBID (flunisolide) Forest   Rx

Metered-dose oral inhaler: 250 μg/inhalation

INDICATIONS	INHALANT DOSAGE
Chronic bronchial asthma	**Adult:** 2 inhalations bid (morning and evening) to start; maximum dosage, 4 inhalations bid **Child (6–15 yr):** 2 inhalations bid (morning and evening); use at a higher dosage has not been studied

AEROBID

CONTRAINDICATIONS

Hypersensitivity to any component

Acute asthma (when used as *primary* therapy)

ADMINISTRATION/DOSAGE ADJUSTMENTS

Selection of patients — This preparation is intended for the relief of bronchial asthma in patients requiring chronic corticosteroid therapy; this group includes both patients who are already receiving systemic steroids and those who are not adequately controlled by bronchodilators or other nonsteroidal medications but have not been given steroids because of concern over their potential side effects. It is not intended for patients who require systemic corticosteroids infrequently.

Patients receiving systemic corticosteroids — Use of this inhaler may permit either replacement of the systemic corticosteroid or a significant reduction in its dosage. Assuming that the patient's asthma is reasonably stable, begin use without changing the patient's usual systemic maintenance dose. Wait about 1 wk and then reduce the systemic dosage; depending on how the patient responds, a second reduction may be made 1 or 2 wk later, followed by further gradual reductions over the ensuing weeks. Do not decrease the dosage at any one time by more than the equivalent of 2.5 mg of prednisone (see warning, below, regarding withdrawal of systemic corticosteroids).

Patients *not* receiving systemic corticosteroids — An improvement in pulmonary function may be anticipated within 1–4 wk after therapy is started in patients who respond to this preparation

Concomitant use of inhalant bronchodilators — An inhalant bronchodilator may be needed in addition to this preparation to control asthmatic symptoms. To ensure penetration of the steroid into the bronchial tree, advise patients to use the bronchodilator before they take this medication. If an aerosol bronchodilator is used, caution the patient to wait several minutes after using it before inhaling this drug; this will reduce the risk of fluorocarbon toxicity resulting from inhaling the propellants in each preparation.

WARNINGS/PRECAUTIONS

Acute asthmatic episodes — This preparation is not a substitute for a bronchodilator and should not be used as the primary drug for treating status asthmaticus or other acute asthmatic episodes requiring intensive measures. Caution patients to report immediately the occurrence of asthmatic episodes that do not respond to use of a bronchodilator; such patients may require systemic corticosteroid therapy to tide them over these periods.

Withdrawal of systemic corticosteroid therapy — Watch carefully for signs of adrenal insufficiency, such as hypotension and weight loss, in patients experiencing arthralgia, myalgia, lassitude, depression, or other steroid withdrawal symptoms (musculoskeletal reactions have been reported in 35% of patients). If evidence of adrenal insufficiency is seen, temporarily increase the systemic steroid dosage and then withdraw the steroid more slowly. Recovery of normal hypothalamic-pituitary-adrenal (HPA) function usually takes several months, but can take up to a year. Until normal HPA function returns, trauma, surgery, or infection (particularly gastroenteritis or other conditions associated with acute electrolyte losses) may precipitate potentially fatal adrenal insufficiency, since this preparation does not provide a systemic amount of steroid sufficient to cope with stress in patients with HPA dysfunction. (To assess the risk of stress-induced adrenal insufficiency, periodically perform routine tests of adrenocortical function, including measurement of the early morning resting cortisol level.) Severe, potentially fatal asthmatic attacks may also occur if the previous oral corticosteroid dosage significantly exceeded the equivalent of 10 mg/day of prednisone. During periods of stress or severe asthmatic attacks, resume systemic steroid therapy in large doses; patients at risk should carry a warning card indicating that they may need such therapy during these periods. Withdrawal of systemic corticosteroid therapy may also unmask such allergic conditions as rhinitis, conjunctivitis, and eczema.

Systemic absorption — Watch carefully for any evidence of a systemic effect. Exercise caution when beginning administration; during chronic therapy, periodically evaluate HPA function if a patient requires 8 inhalations/day. During periods of stress (such as surgery), check particularly for signs of adrenal insufficiency.

Upper respiratory tract infections — Infections due to *Candida albicans* or *Aspergillus niger* have been detected in 3–9% of patients, usually in the mouth and throat and occasionally in the larynx; these infections may necessitate antifungal therapy or discontinuation of this preparation. To prevent infection, patients should be instructed to rinse their mouths after inhalation of each dose.

Pulmonary effects — Pulmonary infiltration with eosinophilia may develop during therapy as a reaction to this preparation or, in some cases, may be unmasked as a result of withdrawal of a systemic corticosteroid. The potential effects of this preparation on tuberculosis or other pulmonary infections have not been assessed.

Long-term use — The long-term effects of therapy are not known; potential risks, such as growth inhibition and reduction of immunologic response, have not been evaluated

Carcinogenicity — An increase in pulmonary adenomas has been seen in Swiss-derived mice given flunisolide for 22 mo; this increase fell within the range of spontaneous adenomas characteristic of this species

AEROBID ■ AZMACORT

Effect on fertility	Some evidence of impaired fertility has been seen in female rats following administration at a high dosage (200 µg/kg/day)

ADVERSE REACTIONS

Frequent reactions (incidence ≥ 1%) are printed in *italics*

Respiratory	*Upper respiratory tract infections (25%); sore throat (20%); cold symptoms and nasal congestion (15%); candidal infections in the mouth and throat, chest congestion, cough, hoarseness, rhinitis, rhinorrhea, sneezing, sputum, wheezing, and sinus congestion, drainage, infection, or inflammation (3–9%);* dry throat, glossitis, oral irritation, pharyngitis, phlegm, throat irritation, bronchitis, tightness in the chest, dyspnea, epistaxis, stuffiness in the head, laryngitis, nasal irritation, pleurisy, pneumonia, and sinus discomfort (1–3%); shortness of breath
Gastrointestinal	*Nausea and/or vomiting (25%); diarrhea and upset stomach (10%); abdominal pain and heartburn (3–9%);* constipation, dyspepsia, and gas (1–3%); abdominal fullness
Central nervous system	*Headache (25%); unpleasant taste (10%); dizziness, irritability, nervousness, shakiness, anosmia, ageusia, and decreased appetite (3–9%);* anxiety, depression, faintness, fatigue, hypoactivity, hyperactivity, insomnia, moodiness, numbness, vertigo, and increased appetite (1–3%)
Ophthalmic	Blurred vision, eye discomfort, and eye infection (1–3%)
Otic	*Ear infection (3–9%),* earache (1–3%)
Cardiovascular	*Palpitations (3–9%);* hypertension and tachycardia (1–3%)
Dermatological	*Eczema, pruritus, and rash (3–9%);* acne, hives, and urticaria (1–3%)
Other	*Flu (10%); chest pain, edema, fever, and menstrual disturbances (3–9%);* chills, weight gain, malaise, peripheral edema, diaphoresis, weakness, capillary fragility, and enlarged lymph nodes (1–3%)

OVERDOSAGE

Signs and symptoms	Suppression of HPA function
Treatment	Gradually reduce dosage of this preparation

DRUG INTERACTIONS

Prednisone (alternate-day oral therapy)	↕ Suppression of HPA function; combination therapy is generally not recommended

ALTERED LABORATORY VALUES

Blood/serum values	▽ Cortisol
Urinary values	▽ Cortisol ▽ 17-Hydroxycorticosteroids

USE IN CHILDREN

See INDICATIONS and INHALANT DOSAGE; available data do not warrant use in children under 6 yr of age. During chronic therapy, watch for suppression of HPA function and inhibition of bone growth.

USE IN PREGNANT AND NURSING WOMEN

Pregnancy Category C: fetotoxic and teratogenic effects have been seen in rabbits given 40 µg/kg/day and in rats given 200 µg/kg/day; no adequate, well-controlled studies have been done in pregnant women. Use during pregnancy only if the expected benefit justifies the potential risk to the fetus. It is not known whether flunisolide is excreted in human milk, but it is known that other corticosteroids are excreted; use with caution in nursing mothers.

VEHICLE/BASE
Metered-dose inhaler: trichloromonofluoromethane, dichlorodifluoromethane, dichlorotetrafluoroethane, and sorbitan trioleate

---

INHALANT CORTICOSTEROIDS

AZMACORT (triamcinolone acetonide) Rorer   Rx

Metered-dose oral inhaler: 100 µg/inhalation

INDICATIONS	INHALANT DOSAGE
Chronic bronchial asthma	**Adult:** usual dosage, 2 inhalations tid or qid; for more severe asthma, 12–16 inhalations/day, given in 3–4 doses, to start, followed by a reduction in dosage. For maintenance in some patients, administration twice-daily may be sufficient. **Child (6–12 yr):** 1–2 inhalations tid or qid; maximum dosage, 12 inhalations/day

AZMACORT

CONTRAINDICATIONS

Hypersensitivity to any component

Acute asthma (when used as *primary* therapy)

ADMINISTRATION/DOSAGE ADJUSTMENTS

Selection of patients — This preparation is intended for the relief of bronchial asthma in patients requiring chronic corticosteroid therapy; this group includes both patients who are already receiving systemic steroids and those who are not adequately controlled by bronchodilators or other nonsteroidal medications but have not been given steroids because of concern over their potential side effects. It is not intended for patients who require systemic corticosteroids infrequently.

Patients receiving systemic corticosteroids — Use of this inhaler may permit either replacement of the systemic corticosteroid or a significant reduction in its dosage. Assuming that the patient's asthma is reasonably stable, begin use without changing the patient's usual systemic maintenance dose. Wait about 1 wk and then reduce the systemic dosage; depending on how the patient responds, a second reduction may be made 1 or 2 wk later, followed by further gradual reductions over the ensuing weeks. Do not decrease the dosage at any one time by more than the equivalent of 2.5 mg of prednisone (see warning, below, regarding withdrawal of systemic corticosteroids).

Patients *not* receiving systemic corticosteroids — An improvement in pulmonary function may be anticipated within 1–2 wk after therapy is started in patients who respond to this preparation

Dosage delivery — To ensure reliable delivery of the medication, caution patients not to use an individual aerosol canister more than 240 times (approximately 1 mo when used at a dosage of 2 inhalations qid)

Concomitant use of inhalant bronchodilators — An inhalant bronchodilator may be needed in addition to this preparation to control asthmatic symptoms. To ensure penetration of the steroid into the bronchial tree, advise patients to use the bronchodilator before they take this medication. If an aerosol bronchodilator is used, caution the patient to wait several minutes after using it before inhaling this drug; this will reduce the risk of fluorocarbon toxicity resulting from inhaling the propellants in each preparation.

WARNINGS/PRECAUTIONS

Acute asthmatic episodes — This preparation is not a substitute for a bronchodilator and should not be used as the primary drug for treating status asthmaticus or other acute asthmatic episodes requiring intensive measures. Caution patients to report immediately the occurrence of asthmatic episodes that do not respond to use of a bronchodilator; such patients may require systemic corticosteroid therapy to tide them over these periods.

Withdrawal of systemic corticosteroid therapy — Watch carefully for signs of adrenal insufficiency, such as hypotension and weight loss, in patients experiencing arthralgia, myalgia, lassitude, depression, or other steroid withdrawal symptoms. If evidence of adrenal insufficiency is seen, temporarily increase the systemic steroid dosage and then withdraw the steroid more slowly. Recovery of normal hypothalamic-pituitary-adrenal (HPA) function usually takes several months, but can take a year or more if large oral steroid doses were given for a prolonged period. Until normal HPA function returns, trauma, surgery, or infection (particularly gastroenteritis or other conditions associated with acute electrolyte losses) may precipitate potentially fatal adrenal insufficiency, since this preparation does not provide a systemic amount of steroid sufficient to cope with stress in patients with HPA dysfunction. Severe, potentially fatal asthmatic attacks may also occur if the previous oral corticosteroid dosage significantly exceeded the equivalent of 10 mg/day of prednisone. During periods of stress or severe asthmatic attacks, resume systemic steroid therapy in large doses; patients at risk should carry a warning card indicating that they may need such therapy during these periods. Withdrawal of systemic corticosteroid therapy may also unmask such allergic conditions as rhinitis, conjunctivitis, and eczema.

Systemic absorption — Suppression of HPA function has been seen in some patients who used this preparation for as briefly as 6–12 wk. During therapy, watch carefully for evidence of a systemic reaction, and, during periods of stress (such as surgery), check particularly for signs of adrenal insufficiency.

Upper respiratory tract infections — Oral and pharyngeal infections due to *Candida albicans* have been seen in 2.5% of patients; these infections may disappear spontaneously or may necessitate antifungal therapy or discontinuation of this preparation. At each patient visit, examine the mouth and pharynx. Patients should be instructed to practice good oral hygiene, including rinsing the mouth after inhalation of each dose.

Pulmonary infections — The potential effects of this preparation on tuberculosis and other pulmonary infections have not been assessed; some signs of a pulmonary infection may be masked during therapy

Long-term use — Although no long-term effects have reported following use of this preparation for 2 yr or longer, potential risks, such as growth inhibition and reduction of immunologic response, have not been evaluated

ADVERSE REACTIONS[1]

Respiratory — Oral candidiasis, hoarseness, dry or irritated throat, dry mouth, cough, increased wheezing

AZMACORT ■ BECLOVENT

| Other | Facial edema, suppression of HPA function |

OVERDOSAGE

| Signs and symptoms | Suppression of HPA function |
| Treatment | Gradually reduce dosage of this preparation |

DRUG INTERACTIONS

| Prednisone (alternate-day therapy) | △ Suppression of HPA function; combination therapy is generally not recommended |

ALTERED LABORATORY VALUES

| Blood/serum values | ▽ Cortisol |
| Urinary values | ▽ Cortisol ▽ 17-Hydroxycorticosteroids |

USE IN CHILDREN

See INDICATIONS and INHALANT DOSAGE; available data do not warrant use in children under 6 yr of age. During therapy, watch for evidence of growth suppression.

USE IN PREGNANT AND NURSING WOMEN

Pregnancy Category D: embryotoxicity, fetotoxicity, and teratogenic reactions, including cleft palate, internal hydrocephaly, and axial skeletal defects, have been seen in rats and rabbits given the maximum recommended human dose by aerosol inhalation. No adverse reactions on the human fetus have been reported following parenteral or topical use of triamcinolone acetonide during pregnancy; however, well-controlled studies in pregnant women have not been done with this preparation. Use during pregnancy only if the expected benefit clearly justifies the potential risk to the fetus. Infants whose mothers received substantial doses during pregnancy should be carefully observed for hypoadrenalism. It is not known whether triamcinolone is excreted in human milk; because of the potential for tumorigenicity, this drug should not be given to patients who elect to breast-feed.

VEHICLE/BASE
Metered-dose inhaler: dichlorodifluoromethane and 1% dehydrated alcohol

[1] Pulmonary infiltration accompanied by eosinophilia has occurred with use of other inhalant corticosteroids

INHALANT CORTICOSTEROIDS

BECLOVENT (beclomethasone dipropionate) Glaxo   Rx

Metered-dose oral inhaler: 42 µg/inhalation

INDICATIONS	INHALANT DOSAGE
Bronchial asthma requiring chronic corticosteroid therapy	**Adult:** 2 inhalations tid or qid, or up to 20 inhalations/24 h, if needed **Child (6–12 yr):** 1–2 inhalations tid or qid, or up to 10 inhalations/24 h, if needed

CONTRAINDICATIONS

| Primary treatment of status asthmaticus or other acute asthmatic episodes requiring intensive measures | Hypersensitivity to beclomethasone or other components |

ADMINISTRATION/DOSAGE ADJUSTMENTS

Patients with severe asthma (adults)	Initiate therapy with 12–16 inhalations/day and adjust dosage downward according to response
Concomitant use of inhalant bronchodilators	Use of bronchodilator before inhaler administration of beclomethasone enhances penetration of beclomethasone into bronchial tree. Allow several minutes to elapse before using beclomethasone inhaler to avoid toxicity from fluorocarbon propellants in both drugs.
Patients receiving systemic corticosteroids	Initially, use inhaler concurrently with usual dosage of systemic steroid. After 1 wk, *gradually* withdraw systemic steroid by reducing daily or alternate-day dose. Depending on response, continue gradually to withdraw systemic steroid by reducing dosage every 1–2 wk. Decrements generally should not exceed 2.5 mg of prednisone or its equivalent.
Patients experiencing steroid withdrawal symptoms (eg, joint or muscle pain, lassitude, depression)	Continue use of inhaler and observe patient closely for objective signs of adrenal insufficiency (eg, hypotension, weight loss); if signs appear, increase dose of systemic steroid temporarily and taper dosage more gradually
Exacerbation of asthma	Give short course of systemic steroid therapy; taper dosage gradually as symptoms subside

BECLOVENT ■ RESPIHALER DECADRON Phosphate

WARNINGS/PRECAUTIONS

Deaths due to adrenal insufficiency	Have occurred in asthmatic patients during and after transfer from systemic corticosteroids to beclomethasone inhaler therapy
Recovery of hypothalamic-pituitary-adrenal (HPA) function	Requires many months after withdrawal from systemic corticosteroids; during this HPA-suppressed period, signs and symptoms of adrenal insufficiency may appear in the presence of trauma, surgery, or infection, especially gastroenteritis
Stress periods or severe asthma attacks	Patients withdrawn from systemic steroids should immediately resume large doses of corticosteroids; these patients should carry a warning card indicating their need of supplementary systemic steroid therapy in case of stress or severe asthma attack
Assessing risk of adrenal insufficiency	Tests of adrenocortical function should be performed periodically, including measurement of early-morning resting cortisol levels
Fungal infections (*Candida albicans, Aspergillus niger*)	Frequently occur in mouth and pharynx and occasionally in larynx; up to 75% of patients may have positive oral *Candida* cultures. Antifungal treatment and discontinuation of inhaler therapy may be necessary.
Episodes of asthma unresponsive to treatment	Patients should report immediately any such episode during treatment; systemic corticosteroid therapy may be needed
Allergic reactions	In rare cases, beclomethasone inhaler therapy may precipitate immediate or delayed hypersensitivity reactions (see ADVERSE REACTIONS). Transfer from systemic corticosteroids to the inhaler may unmask previously suppressed allergic conditions such as rhinitis, conjunctivitis, and eczema. Pulmonary infiltrates with eosinophilia may result from inhaler therapy or, in some cases, may be manifested following transfer from systemic steroids.
Systemic steroid withdrawal symptoms	May occur during withdrawal from oral corticosteroid therapy (see ADMINISTRATION/DOSAGE ADJUSTMENTS)

ADVERSE REACTIONS[1]

Endocrinological	Suppression of hypothalamic-pituitary-adrenal function
Hypersensitivity	Urticaria, angioedema, rash, and bronchospasm (rare)
Other	Hoarseness, dry mouth

OVERDOSAGE

Signs and symptoms	See WARNINGS/PRECAUTIONS
Treatment	Discontinue medication; reinstitute systemic steroid therapy, if needed

DRUG INTERACTIONS

No clinically significant drug interactions have been identified

ALTERED LABORATORY VALUES

No clinically significant alterations in blood/serum or urinary values occur at therapeutic dosages

USE IN CHILDREN

See INDICATIONS and INHALANT DOSAGE; not recommended for use in children under 6 yr of age

USE IN PREGNANT AND NURSING WOMEN

Safety for use in pregnant or nursing women has not been established. Glucocorticoids, including beclomethasone, are known teratogens in rodent species. Infants born to mothers who received substantial corticosteroid dosages during pregnancy should be carefully observed for hypoadrenalism. Glucocorticoids are excreted in human milk.

[1] Long-term effects in humans are unknown

INHALANT CORTICOSTEROIDS

RESPIHALER DECADRON Phosphate (dexamethasone sodium phosphate) Merck Sharp & Dohme Rx

Metered-dose oral inhaler: 0.1 mg/inhalation

INDICATIONS

Bronchial asthma and related corticosteroid-responsive bronchospastic states intractable to an adequate trial of conventional therapy

INHALANT DOSAGE

Adult: 3 inhalations tid or qid, not to exceed 3 inhalations/dose or 12 inhalations/day
Child: 2 inhalations tid or qid, not to exceed 2 inhalations/dose or 8 inhalations/day

RESPIHALER DECADRON Phosphate

CONTRAINDICATIONS

Persistently positive *Candida albicans* sputum cultures	Systemic fungal infections	Hypersensitivity to any component

ADMINISTRATION/DOSAGE ADJUSTMENTS

Selection of patients	Consider use only for (1) patients not on corticosteroid therapy who have not responded adequately to other treatment and (2) patients on systemic steroid therapy in an attempt to reduce or eliminate systemic administration
Concomitant use of systemic corticosteroids	Reduce or eliminate systemic corticosteroids before reducing Respihaler dosage; to avoid withdrawal symptoms, reduce systemic steroid therapy gradually

WARNINGS/PRECAUTIONS

Unwarranted uses	Not recommended for the treatment of occasional, mild, isolated asthmatic attacks responsive to epinephrine, isoproterenol, aminophylline, or other drugs, or for severe status asthmaticus requiring intensive measures
Laryngeal and pharyngeal fungal infections	May occur on rare occasions; discontinue medication and institute antifungal therapy
Systemic absorption	Although low, may lead to adrenal suppression or other systemic effects
Patients subjected to unusual stress	Require increased dosage of rapidly acting corticosteroids before, during, and after emotionally or physically stressful situations
Infection	Clinical signs may be masked, new infections may appear, resistance may be decreased, and infections may be difficult to localize; false-negative results may be obtained with nitroblue-tetrazolium test for bacterial infection
Latent amebiasis	May be activated; before instituting therapy, rule out latent or active amebiasis in any patient with unexplained diarrhea or who has spent time in the tropics
Ocular damage	Prolonged use may produce posterior subcapsular cataracts and glaucoma, with possible damage to optic nerves, and may enhance development of secondary fungal or viral ocular infections
Dietary salt restriction and potassium supplementation	May be necessary to combat blood-pressure elevation, salt and water retention, and increased potassium excretion with average- and high-dose therapy
Immunization procedures	The expected serum antibody response to inactivated viral or bacterial vaccines may not be obtained in patients receiving immunosuppressive doses; such patients must not be given live virus vaccines, including smallpox vaccine
Latent tuberculosis or tuberculin reactivity	Observe patient closely, since reactivation of the disease may occur during prolonged therapy; employ antituberculous chemoprophylactic measures
Secondary adrenocortical insufficiency	May be minimized by gradual dosage reduction; since insufficiency may persist for months, reinstitute corticosteroid therapy in any stressful situation during this period, and administer salt and/or a mineralocorticoid concurrently to correct impaired mineralocorticoid secretion
Withdrawal symptoms	Including fever, myalgia, arthralgia, and malaise, may occur when drug is withdrawn following prolonged therapy, even in the absence of adrenal insufficiency
Hypothyroidism, hepatic cirrhosis	May enhance effects of dexamethasone
Corneal perforation	May occur in patients with ocular herpes simplex; use with caution
Special-risk patients	Use with caution in patients with nonspecific ulcerative colitis if impending perforation, abscess, or other pyogenic infection is likely, as well as in patients with diverticulitis, fresh intestinal anastomoses, active or latent peptic ulcer, renal insufficiency, hypertension, osteoporosis, or myasthenia gravis. In patients receiving large doses, signs of peritoneal irritation following GI perforation may be minimal or absent.
Psychic derangements	May appear, ranging from euphoria, insomnia, mood swings, personality changes, and severe depression to frank psychotic manifestations; existing emotional instability or psychotic tendencies may be aggravated
Concomitant use with aspirin	Use with caution in patients with hypoprothrombinemia during therapy
Concomitant use with oral anticoagulants	Check prothrombin time frequently; anticoagulant effect may be increased or decreased
Concomitant use with potassium-depleting diuretics	Monitor serum potassium level periodically; risk of hypokalemia is increased
Fertility	Motility and number of spermatozoa may be increased or decreased

ADVERSE REACTIONS

Respiratory	Throat irritation, hoarseness, cough, laryngeal and pharyngeal fungal infections
Fluid and electrolyte disturbances	Sodium retention, fluid retention, congestive heart failure in susceptible patients, loss of potassium, hypokalemic alkalosis, hypertension

RESPIHALER DECADRON Phosphate ■ VANCERIL Inhaler

Musculoskeletal	Muscle weakness, steroid myopathy, loss of muscle mass, osteoporosis, vertebral compression fractures, aseptic necrosis of femoral and humeral heads, pathological fracture of long bones, tendon rupture
Gastrointestinal	Peptic ulcer with possible perforation and hemorrhage, pancreatitis, abdominal distention, ulcerative esophagitis, increased appetite, nausea; perforation of the large and small bowel (particularly in patients with inflammatory bowel disease)
Dermatological	Impaired wound healing, thin fragile skin, petechiae and ecchymoses, erythema, increased sweating, suppressed reaction to skin tests, allergic dermatitis, urticaria, angioneurotic edema
Neurological	Convulsions, increased intracranial pressure with papilledema (pseudotumor cerebri), vertigo, headache, psychic disturbances
Endocrinological	Menstrual irregularities, Cushingoid state, growth suppression in children, secondary adrenocortical and pituitary unresponsiveness, decreased carbohydrate tolerance, latent diabetes mellitus, increased insulin or oral hypoglycemic requirements
Ophthalmic	Posterior subcapsular cataracts, increased intraocular pressure, glaucoma, exophthalmos
Metabolic	Negative nitrogen balance, weight gain
Other	Hypersensitivity reactions, thromboembolism, malaise

OVERDOSAGE

Signs and symptoms	See ADVERSE REACTIONS
Treatment	Discontinue medication; treat symptomatically and institute supportive measures, as required

DRUG INTERACTIONS

Insulin, oral hypoglycemics	▽ Hypoglycemic effect
Phenytoin, phenobarbital, ephedrine, rifampin	△ Metabolic clearance of dexamethasone ▽ Steroid blood level and physiological activity
Oral anticoagulants	△ or ▽ Prothrombin time
Potassium-depleting diuretics	△ Risk of hypokalemia
Cardiac glycosides	△ Risk of arrhythmias or digitalis toxicity secondary to hypokalemia
Skin-test antigens	▽ Reactivity
Immunizations	▽ Antibody response

ALTERED LABORATORY VALUES

Blood/serum values	△ Glucose △ Cholesterol △ Sodium △ Potassium ▽ Calcium ▽ PBI ▽ Thyroxine (T$_4$) ▽ ^{131}I thyroid uptake ▽ Uric acid
Urinary values	△ Glucose △ Potassium △ Calcium △ Uric acid ▽ 17-Hydroxycorticosteroids (17-OHCS) ▽ 17-Ketosteroids

USE IN CHILDREN	USE IN PREGNANT AND NURSING WOMEN
Growth and development should be carefully observed in infants and children on prolonged therapy	Safety for use during pregnancy has not been established. Infants born of mothers who have received substantial doses of corticosteroids during pregnancy should be carefully observed for signs of hypoadrenalism. Corticosteroids appear in breast milk and may suppress growth, interfere with endogenous corticosteroid production, or cause other untoward effects. Patient should stop nursing if drug is prescribed.

INHALANT CORTICOSTEROIDS

VANCERIL Inhaler (beclomethasone dipropionate) Schering   Rx

Metered-dose inhaler: 42 µg/inhalation

INDICATIONS

Bronchial asthma requiring chronic corticosteroid therapy

INHALANT DOSAGE

Adult: 2 inhalations tid or qid, or up to 20 inhalations/24 h, if needed
Child (6–12 yr): 1–2 inhalations tid or qid, or up to 10 inhalations/24 h, if needed

CONTRAINDICATIONS

Primary treatment of status asthmaticus or other acute asthmatic episodes requiring intensive measures	Hypersensitivity to beclomethasone or other components

ADMINISTRATION/DOSAGE ADJUSTMENTS

Patients with severe asthma (adults)	Initiate therapy with 12–16 inhalations/day and adjust dosage downward according to response

COMPENDIUM OF DRUG THERAPY

VANCERIL Inhaler ■ BECONASE

Concomitant use of inhalant bronchodilators	Use of bronchodilator before inhaler administration of beclomethasone enhances penetration of beclomethasone into bronchial tree. Allow several minutes to elapse before using beclomethasone inhaler to avoid toxicity from fluorocarbon propellants in both drugs.
Patients receiving systemic corticosteroids	Initially, use inhaler concurrently with usual dosage of systemic steroid. After 1 wk, *gradually* withdraw systemic steroid by reducing daily or alternate-day dose. Depending on response, continue gradually to withdraw systemic steroid by reducing dosage every 1–2 wk. Decrements generally should not exceed 2.5 mg of prednisone or its equivalent.
Patients experiencing steroid withdrawal symptoms (eg, joint or muscle pain, lassitude, depression)	Continue use of inhaler and observe patient closely for objective signs of adrenal insufficiency (eg, hypotension, weight loss); if signs appear, increase dose of systemic steroid temporarily and taper dosage more gradually
Exacerbation of asthma	Give short course of systemic steroid therapy; taper dosage gradually as symptoms subside

WARNINGS/PRECAUTIONS

Deaths due to adrenal insufficiency	Have occurred in asthmatic patients during and after transfer from systemic corticosteroids to beclomethasone inhaler therapy
Recovery of hypothalamic-pituitary-adrenal (HPA) function	Requires many months after withdrawal from systemic corticosteroids; during this HPA-suppressed period, signs and symptoms of adrenal insufficiency may appear in the presence of trauma, surgery, or infection, especially gastroenteritis
Stress periods or severe asthma attacks	Patients withdrawn from systemic steroids should immediately resume large doses of corticosteroids; these patients should carry a warning card indicating their need of supplementary systemic steroid therapy in case of stress or severe asthma attack
Assessing risk of adrenal insufficiency	Tests of adrenocortical function should be performed peridiocally, including measurement of early-morning resting cortisol levels
Fungal infections (*Candida albicans, Aspergillus niger*)	Frequently occur in mouth and pharynx and occasionally in larynx; up to 75% of patients may have positive oral *Candida* cultures. Antifungal treatment and discontinuation of inhaler therapy may be necessary.
Episodes of asthma unresponsive to treatment	Patients should report immediately any such episode during treatment; systemic corticosteroid therapy may be needed
Allergic reactions	In rare cases, beclomethasone inhaler therapy may precipitate immediate or delayed hypersensitivity reactions (see ADVERSE REACTIONS). Transfer from systemic corticosteroids to the inhaler may unmask previously suppressed allergic conditions such as rhinitis, conjunctivitis, and eczema. Pulmonary infiltrates with eosinophilia may result from inhaler therapy or, in some cases, may be manifested following transfer from systemic steroids.
Systemic steroid withdrawal symptoms	May occur during withdrawal from oral corticosteroid therapy (see ADMINISTRATION/DOSAGE ADJUSTMENTS)

ADVERSE REACTIONS[1]

Endocrinological	Suppression of hypothalamic-pituitary-adrenal function
Hypersensitivity	Urticaria, angioedema, rash, and bronchospasm (rare)
Other	Hoarseness, dry mouth; rash (rare)

OVERDOSAGE

Signs and symptoms	See WARNINGS/PRECAUTIONS
Treatment	Discontinue medication; reinstitute systemic steroid therapy, if needed

DRUG INTERACTIONS
No clinically significant drug interactions have been identified

ALTERED LABORATORY VALUES
No clinically significant alterations in blood/serum or urinary values occur at therapeutic dosages

USE IN CHILDREN
See INDICATIONS and INHALANT DOSAGE; not recommended for use in children under 6 yr of age

USE IN PREGNANT AND NURSING WOMEN
Safety for use in pregnant or nursing women has not been established. Glucocorticoids, including beclomethasone, are known teratogens in rodent species. Infants born to mothers who received substantial corticosteroid dosages during pregnancy should be carefully observed for hypoadrenalism. Glucocorticoids are excreted in human milk.

[1] Long-term effects in humans are unknown

NASAL CORTICOSTEROIDS

BECONASE (beclomethasone dipropionate) Glaxo   Rx
Metered-dose nasal inhaler: 42 μg/inhalation

INDICATIONS
Symptomatic relief of **seasonal and perennial rhinitis** in cases poorly responsive to conventional treatment
Prevention of recurrence of **nasal polyps** following surgical removal

INTRANASAL DOSAGE
Adult: 1 inhalation (42 μg) in each nostril 2–4 times/day; for maintenance, up to 1 inhalation in each nostril tid may often suffice
Child ($\geq$ 12 yr): same as adult

BECONASE

CONTRAINDICATIONS

Hypersensitivity to beclomethasone or other components

Untreated localized infection involving the nasal mucosa

ADMINISTRATION/DOSAGE ADJUSTMENTS

Initial trial period — Symptomatic improvement of rhinitis is usually apparent in a few days, but may not occur for as long as 2 wk; discontinue use if significant symptomatic improvement does not occur within 3 wk. Prophylactic treatment of nasal polyps may be necessary for several weeks or more before therapeutic effect can be fully assessed. Excessive nasal mucus or edema of the nasal mucosa may prevent drug from reaching site of intended action; in such cases, use of a nasal vasoconstrictor during the first 2–3 days of therapy is advisable.

WARNINGS/PRECAUTIONS

Transferring patients from systemic corticosteroids — Replacement of systemic corticosteroids with a nasal corticoid may result in adrenal insufficiency, particularly if systemic therapy has been prolonged; in addition, some patients may experience withdrawal symptoms (eg, joint and/or muscular pain, lassitude, and depression). Give careful attention to such patients, especially patients with asthma or other clinical conditions, as a severe exacerbation of their symptoms may occur if systemic therapy is withdrawn too rapidly.

Concurrent use of alternate-day systemic prednisone therapy — Increases the likelihood of hypothalamic-pituitary-adrenal suppression; use with caution if alternate-day therapy is continued for any reason

Systemic absorption — Beclomethasone is absorbed into the circulation; Cushing's syndrome may occur if recommended dosage is exceeded or patient is particularly sensitive. Use of larger-than-recommended doses should be avoided to minimize the potential for systemic side effects and suppression of the hypothalamic-pituitary-adrenal axis.

Recurrence of polyps — After cessation of prophylactic therapy, nasal polyps may recur; likelihood depends on the severity of the disease

Inhibition of wound healing — Avoid use in patients with recent nasal septal ulcers or nasal surgery or trauma, until healing has occurred

Localized candidal infections — Localized infections of the nose and pharynx with *Candida albicans* have occurred rarely in clinical trials; if such an infection develops, institute appropriate antifungal therapy, as needed, or discontinue use of beclomethasone if necessary

Special-risk patients — Use with caution, if at all, in patients with active or latent tuberculous infections of the respiratory tract; untreated fungal, bacterial, or systemic viral infections; or ocular herpes simplex

Long-term therapy — If treatment is continued for several months or longer, examine patient periodically for possible changes in the nasal mucosa

Carcinogenicity, mutagenicity — No evidence of carcinogenicity has been detected in rats treated for a total of 95 wk (13 wk by inhalation and 82 wk orally); mutagenicity studies have not been done

ADVERSE REACTIONS

Frequent reactions (incidence $\geq$ 1%) are printed in *italics*

Local — *Nasal irritation and burning (11%), sneezing attacks immediately following use of inhaler (10%), transient bloody discharge from the nose (2%),* Candida albicans infections of the nose and pharynx, nasal mucosal ulceration (rare); nasal septum perforation (extremely rare)

Hypersensitivity — Immediate and delayed allergic reactions (rare), including urticaria, angioedema, rash, and bronchospasm

OVERDOSAGE

Acute overdosage is unlikely; oral LD_{50} of beclomethasone diproprionate exceeds 1 g/kg

DRUG INTERACTIONS

No clinically significant drug interactions have been identified

ALTERED LABORATORY VALUES

No clinically significant alterations in blood/serum or urinary values occur at therapeutic dosages

---

USE IN CHILDREN

Not recommended for use in children under 12 yr of age

USE IN PREGNANT AND NURSING WOMEN

Pregnancy Category C: use during pregnancy only if anticipated benefit justifies the potential risk to the fetus. Parenteral beclomethasone has been shown to be teratogenic and embryocidal in the mouse and rabbit at doses approximately 10 times the human dose. No teratogenic or embryocidal effects have been seen in the rat when beclomethasone was administered by inhalation at 10 times the human dose or orally at 1,000 times the human dose. No adequate, well-controlled studies have been done in pregnant women; however, hypoadrenalism has been reported in infants of mothers who received corticosteroids during pregnancy. It is not known whether beclomethasone is excreted in human milk. Because other corticoids are excreted, caution should be exercised in prescribing this drug to nursing mothers.

NASAL CORTICOSTEROIDS

NASALIDE (flunisolide) Syntex   Rx

Metered-dose spray bottle: 25 µg/spray (6.25 mg)

INDICATIONS	**INTRANASAL DOSAGE**
Symptomatic relief of **seasonal and perennial rhinitis** when effectiveness of or tolerance to conventional treatment is unsatisfactory	**Adult:** 2 sprays (50 µg) in each nostril bid to start; if needed, increase the dosage to 2 sprays in each nostril tid, or up to 8 sprays in each nostril per day, until desired clinical effect is obtained; thereafter, reduce the maintenance dose to the smallest amount necesssary to control symptoms **Child (6–14 yr):** 1 spray (25 µg) in each nostril tid or 2 sprays (50 µg) in each nostril bid to start, until desired clinical effect is obtained; thereafter, reduce the maintenance dose to the smallest amount necessary to control symptoms
CONTRAINDICATIONS	
Hypersensitivity to flunisolide or other components	Untreated localized infection involving the nasal mucosa
ADMINISTRATION/DOSAGE ADJUSTMENTS	
Initial trial period	Full therapeutic benefit is usually evident within a few days with regular use; however, a longer period may be required for some patients. If no improvement is evident within 3 wk of initiating therapy, discontinue use. Nasal vasoconstrictors or oral antihistamines may be needed until the effects of flunisolide are fully manifested. Advise patient to report if symptoms do not improve, the condition worsens, or sneezing or nasal irritation occurs.
Patients with blocked nasal passages	Should be encouraged to clear their nasal passages of secretions and to use a decongestant just prior to flunisolide administration to ensure adequate penetration of the spray
WARNINGS/PRECAUTIONS	
Transferring patients from systemic corticosteroids	Replacement of systemic corticosteroids with a nasal corticoid may result in adrenal insufficiency, particularly if systemic therapy has been prolonged; in addition, some patients may experience withdrawal symptoms (eg, joint and/or muscular pain, lassitude, and depression). Give careful attention to such patients, especially patients with asthma or other clinical conditions, as a severe exacerbation of their symptoms may occur if systemic therapy is withdrawn too rapidly.
Concurrent use of alternate-day systemic prednisone therapy	Increases the likelihood of hypothalamic-pituitary-adrenal suppression; use with caution if alternate-day therapy is continued for any reason
Systemic absorption	Flunisolide is absorbed into the circulation; use of larger-than-recommended doses should be avoided to minimize the potential for systemic side effects and suppression of the hypothalamic-pituitary-adrenal axis
Inhibition of wound healing	Use with caution if recent nasal septal ulcers or lesions resulting from recurrent epistaxis, nasal surgery, or nasal trauma have not yet healed
Localized candidal infections	Localized infections of the nose and pharynx with *Candida albicans* have occurred rarely in clinical trials; if such an infection develops, institute appropriate antifungal therapy, as needed, or discontinue use of flunisolide if necessary
Special-risk patients	Use with caution, if at all, in patients with active or latent tuberculous infections of the respiratory tract; untreated fungal, bacterial, or systemic viral infections; or ocular herpes simplex
Carcinogenicity	In a 22-mo study in Swiss-derived mice, there was an increase in pulmonary adenomas within the range of spontaneous adenomas previously reported for this strain
ADVERSE REACTIONS[1]	Frequent reactions (incidence ≥ 1%) are printed in *italics*
Local	*Mild, transient nasal burning and stinging (45%);* nasal congestion; sneezing; epistaxis; bloody mucus; nasal irritation; sore throat; nasal septal perforations (rare; causal relationship not established)
Gastrointestinal	Nausea and/or vomiting
Other	Headache, watery eyes, loss of sense of smell and taste
OVERDOSAGE	
Acute overdosage is unlikely; doses up to 4 mg/kg have shown no effect in animals	
DRUG INTERACTIONS	
No clinically significant drug interactions have been identified	
ALTERED LABORATORY VALUES	
No clinically significant alterations in blood/serum or urinary values occur at therapeutic dosages	

NASALIDE ■ VANCENASE

USE IN CHILDREN
See INDICATIONS and INTRANASAL DOSAGE; not recommended for use in children under 6 yr of age, since safety and efficacy have not been established in this age group

USE IN PREGNANT AND NURSING WOMEN
Pregnancy Category C: use during pregnancy only if the expected benefit justifies the potential risk to the fetus. Flunisolide has been shown to be teratogenic in rabbits and rats at doses of 40 and 200 µg/kg/day, respectively, as well as fetotoxic in these species. No adequate, well-controlled studies have been done in pregnant women. Impairment of fertility has been observed in rats receiving high doses of flunisolide (200 µg/kg/day), but not at lower doses (8 and 40 µg/kg/day). It is not known whether flunisolide is excreted in human milk. Because other corticosteroids are excreted in human milk, exercise caution in prescribing this drug to nursing mothers.

[1] Reported in controlled clinical trials and long-term open studies on 595 patients treated with flunisolide; of these patients, 409 were treated for 3 mo or longer, 323 for 6 mo or longer, 259 for 1 yr or longer, and 91 for 2 yr or longer; although systemic corticosteroid side effects were not reported during controlled clinical trials, if recommended doses are exceeded or if individuals are particularly sensitive, symptoms of hypercorticism (Cushing's syndrome) could occur

---

NASAL CORTICOSTEROIDS

VANCENASE (beclomethasone dipropionate) Schering   Rx

Metered-dose nasal inhaler: 42 µg/inhalation

INDICATIONS
Symptomatic relief of **seasonal and perennial rhinitis** in cases poorly responsive to conventional treatment
Prevention of recurrence of **nasal polyps** following surgical removal

INTRANASAL DOSAGE
Adult: 1 inhalation (42 µg) in each nostril 2–4 times/day; for maintenance, up to 1 inhalation in each nostril tid may often suffice
Child (≥ 12 yr): same as adult

CONTRAINDICATIONS
Hypersensitivity to beclomethasone or other components

Untreated localized infection involving the nasal mucosa

ADMINISTRATION/DOSAGE ADJUSTMENTS

Initial trial period	Symptomatic improvement of rhinitis is usually apparent in a few days, but may not occur for as long as 2 wk; discontinue use if significant symptomatic improvement does not occur within 3 wk. Prophylactic treatment of nasal polyps may be necessary for several weeks or more before therapeutic effect can be fully assessed. Excessive nasal mucus or edema of the nasal mucosa may prevent drug from reaching site of intended action; in such cases, use of a nasal vasoconstrictor during the first 2–3 days of therapy is advisable.

WARNINGS/PRECAUTIONS

Transferring patients from systemic corticosteroids	Replacement of systemic corticosteroids with a nasal corticoid may result in adrenal insufficiency, particularly if systemic therapy has been prolonged; in addition, some patients may experience withdrawal symptoms (eg, joint and/or muscular pain, lassitude, and depression). Give careful attention to such patients, especially patients with asthma or other clinical conditions, as a severe exacerbation of their symptoms may occur if systemic therapy is withdrawn too rapidly.
Concurrent use of alternate-day systemic prednisone therapy	Increases the likelihood of hypothalamic-pituitary-adrenal suppression; use with caution if alternate-day therapy is continued for any reason
Systemic absorption	Beclomethasone is absorbed into the circulation; Cushing's syndrome may occur if the recommended dosage is exceeded or the patient is particularly sensitive. Use of larger-than-recommended doses should be avoided to minimize the potential for systemic side effects and suppression of the hypothalamic-pituitary-adrenal axis
Recurrence of polyps	After cessation of prophylactic therapy, nasal polyps may recur; likelihood depends on the severity of the disease
Inhibition of wound healing	Avoid use in patients with recent nasal septal ulcers or nasal surgery or trauma, until healing has occurred
Localized candidal infections	Localized infections of the nose and pharynx with *Candida albicans* have occurred rarely in clinical trials; if such an infection develops, institute appropriate antifungal therapy, as needed, or discontinue use of belcomethasone if necessary
Special-risk patients	Use with caution, if at all, in patients with active or latent tuberculous infections of the respiratory tract; untreated fungal, bacterial, or systemic viral infections; or ocular herpes simplex
Long-term therapy	If treatment is continued for several months or longer, examine patient periodically for possible changes in the nasal mucosa

COMPENDIUM OF DRUG THERAPY

Carcinogenicity, mutagenicity	No evidence of carcinogenicity has been detected in rats treated for a total of 95 wk (13 wk by inhalation and 82 wk orally); mutagenicity studies have not been done

ADVERSE REACTIONS

Frequent reactions (incidence ≥ 1%) are printed in *italics*

Local	*Nasal irritation and burning (11%), sneezing attacks immediately following use of inhaler (10%), transient bloody discharge from the nose (2%), Candida albicans* infections of the nose and pharynx, nasal mucosal ulceration (rare); nasal septum perforation (extremely rare)
Hypersensitivity	Immediate and delayed allergic reactions (rare), including urticaria, angioedema, rash, and bronchospasm

OVERDOSAGE

Acute overdosage is unlikely; oral LD_{50} of beclomethasone dipropionate exceeds 1 g/kg

DRUG INTERACTIONS

No clinically significant drug interactions have been identified

ALTERED LABORATORY VALUES

No clinically significant alterations in blood/serum or urinary values occur at therapeutic dosages

USE IN CHILDREN

Not recommended for use in children under 12 yr of age

USE IN PREGNANT AND NURSING WOMEN

Pregnancy Category C: use during pregnancy only if anticipated benefit justifies the potential risk to the fetus. Parenteral beclomethasone has been shown to be teratogenic and embryocidal in the mouse and rabbit at doses approximately 10 times the human dose. No teratogenic or embryocidal effects have been seen in the rat when beclomethasone was administered by inhalation at 10 times the human dose or orally at 1,000 times the human dose. No adequate, well-controlled studies have been done in pregnant women; however, hypoadrenalism has been reported in infants of mothers who received corticosteroids during pregnancy. It is not known whether beclomethasone is excreted in human milk. Because other corticoids are excreted, caution should be exercised in prescribing this drug to nursing mothers.

RECTAL CORTICOSTEROIDS/HEMORRHOIDALS

ANUSOL Ointment (benzyl benzoate, Peruvian balsam, zinc oxide, and pramoxine hydrochloride) Warner-Lambert   OTC

Ointment (per gram): 12 mg benzyl benzoate, 18 mg Peruvian balsam, 110 mg zinc oxide, and 10 mg pramoxine hydrochloride (1 oz)

ANUSOL Suppositories (bismuth subgallate, bismuth resorcin compound, benzyl benzoate, Peruvian balsam, and zinc oxide) Warner-Lambert   OTC

Rectal suppositories: 2.25% bismuth subgallate, 1.75% bismuth resorcin compound, 1.2% benzyl benzoate, 1.8% Peruvian balsam, and 11.0% zinc oxide

INDICATIONS

Pain and discomfort associated with **external and internal hemorrhoids, proctitis, papillitis, cryptitis, anal fissures, and incomplete fistulas**
Local pain and discomfort following **rectal surgery**
Pruritus ani (ointment only)

RECTAL DOSAGE

Adult: apply ointment q3–4h (or, if needed, q2h) or insert 1 suppository bid (AM and PM) and after each bowel movement

CONTRAINDICATIONS

Hypersensitivity to any component

ADMINISTRATION/DOSAGE ADJUSTMENTS

Use of ointment	For external use, apply freely and rub in gently. For internal use, attach the plastic applicator and insert into the anus, squeezing the tube to deliver the medication.

WARNINGS/PRECAUTIONS

Patient instructions	Caution patient to discontinue use if irritation or rectal bleeding occurs and to report their occurrence

ANUSOL ■ ANUSOL-HC

Staining	If staining from these products occurs, use hand or machine washing with household detergents for removal
Diagnostic considerations	Symptomatic relief resulting from use of these preparations should not delay definitive diagnosis and treatment of the causative condition

ADVERSE REACTIONS

Local	Anal burning (with ointment)
Other	Hypersensitivity reactions (rare)

USE IN CHILDREN
Consult manufacturer

USE IN PREGNANT AND NURSING WOMEN
Consult manufacturer

VEHICLE/BASE
Ointment: dibasic calcium phosphate, kaolin, glyceryl monooleate, glyceryl monostearate, mineral oil, cocoa butter, and polyethylene wax
Rectal suppositories: dibasic calcium phosphate, coconut oil base, hydrogenated fatty acid, FD&C Blue No. 2 Lake, FD&C Red No. 40 Lake, and hydrogenated vegetable oil

---

RECTAL CORTICOSTEROIDS/HEMORRHOIDALS

ANUSOL-HC (hydrocortisone acetate, bismuth subgallate, bismuth resorcin compound, benzyl benzoate, Peruvian balsam, and zinc oxide) **Parke-Davis**   Rx

Cream (per gram): 5.0 mg hydrocortisone acetate, 22.5 mg bismuth subgallate, 17.5 mg bismuth resorcin compound, 12.0 mg benzyl benzoate, 18.0 mg Peruvian balsam, 110.0 mg zinc oxide (1 oz)   **Rectal suppositories:** 10.0 mg hydrocortisone acetate, 2.25% bismuth subgallate, 1.75% bismuth resorcin compound, 1.2% benzyl benzoate, 1.8% Peruvian balsam, 11.0% zinc oxide

INDICATIONS

Symptomatic relief of pain and discomfort in **external and internal hemorrhoids, proctitis, papillitis, cryptitis, anal fissures, incomplete fistulas,** and following **anorectal surgery,** especially when inflammation is present (adjunctive therapy)
Pruritus ani (cream only)

RECTAL DOSAGE

Adult: apply cream tid or qid for 3–6 days or insert 1 suppository bid (AM and PM) for 3–6 days until inflammation subsides

CONTRAINDICATIONS

Hypersensitivity to any component

ADMINISTRATION/DOSAGE ADJUSTMENTS

Use of cream	For external use, apply freely and rub in gently. For internal use, attach the plastic applicator and insert into the anus, squeezing the tube to deliver the medication.

WARNINGS/PRECAUTIONS

Irritation	May occur; discontinue use and institute appropriate therapy
Infection	Institute appropriate antibacterial or antifungal therapy; if favorable response does not occur promptly, discontinue the corticosteroid until the infection is adequately controlled

ADVERSE REACTIONS

Local	Anal irritation

USE IN CHILDREN
Use with caution in children and infants; consult manufacturer for dosage recommendations

USE IN PREGNANT AND NURSING WOMEN
Safety for use during pregnancy has not been established; do not use unnecessarily on extensive areas, in large amounts, or for prolonged periods of time. Consult manufacturer for use in nursing mothers.

VEHICLE/BASE
Cream: propylene glycol, propylparaben, methylparaben, polysorbate 60, sorbitan monostearate, mineral oil, glyceryl stearate, and water
Rectal suppositories: dibasic calcium phosphate and hydrogenated vegetable oil

RECTAL CORTICOSTEROIDS/HEMORRHOIDALS

CORT-DOME Suppositories (hydrocortisone acetate) Miles Pharmaceuticals Rx

Suppositories: 25 mg

INDICATIONS

Inflamed hemorrhoids; postirradiation (factitial) proctitis; chronic ulcerative colitis (adjunctive therapy); **cryptitis; other anorectal inflammatory conditions; pruritus ani**

RECTAL DOSAGE

Adult: 1 suppository inserted in rectum bid (AM and PM) for 2 wk in nonspecific proctitis and up to 6–8 wk in factitial proctitis, depending upon response; for more severe cases insert 1 suppository tid or 2 suppositories bid
Child: same as adult

CONTRAINDICATIONS

Hypersensitivity to hydrocortisone or other components

WARNINGS/PRECAUTIONS

Irritation	Discontinue use and institute appropriate therapy
Infection	Institute appropriate antifungal or antibacterial therapy; if infection persists, discontinue steroid therapy until a favorable response is achieved
Protologic examination	An adequate protologic examination is mandatory prior to use
Carcinogenicity	Long-term studies in animals have not been done to evaluate the carcinogenic potential of corticosteroid suppositories

ADVERSE REACTIONS[1]

Local	Burning, itching, irritation, dryness, folliculitis, hypopigmentation, allergic contact dermatitis, secondary infection

USE IN CHILDREN

Same as adult indications and dosage

USE IN PREGNANT AND NURSING WOMEN

Pregnancy Category C: use during pregnancy only if the expected benefit justifies the potential risk to the fetus. Do not use in large amounts or for prolonged periods. In animal studies, topical corticosteroids have shown evidence of teratogenicity at relatively low dosages. No adequate, well-controlled studies have been done in pregnant women. It is not known whether this drug is excreted in human milk; because many drugs are excreted in human milk and because of the potential for serious adverse reactions in nursing infants, a decision should be made to either discontinue use of this drug or stop nursing.

VEHICLE/BASE
Suppository: monoglyceride

[1] Includes reactions common to rectal corticosteroids in general

---

RECTAL CORTICOSTEROIDS/HEMORRHOIDALS

CORTENEMA (hydrocortisone retention enema) Reid-Rowell Rx

Disposable bottles: 100 mg (60 ml)

INDICATIONS

Ulcerative colitis, especially distal forms (including ulcerative proctitis, ulcerative proctosigmoiditis, and left-sided ulcerative colitis) and in some cases involving the transverse and ascending colon (adjunctive therapy)

RECTAL DOSAGE

Adult: 100 mg nightly for 21 days or until clinical and proctological remission occurs

CONTRAINDICATIONS

Systemic fungal infections

Ileocolostomy during the immediate or early postoperative period

ADMINISTRATION/DOSAGE ADJUSTMENTS

Initial trial period	If clinical or proctologic improvement fails to occur within 2–3 wk of starting treatment, discontinue use. Efficacy cannot be judged solely by symptomatic improvement; sigmoidoscopic examination and x-ray visualization are essential for adequate monitoring of ulcerative colitis. Biopsy is useful for differential diagnosis.

CORTENEMA

Administration	Advise patient to lie on his or her left side during administration and for 30 min afterward, so that the fluid will distribute throughout the left colon. Every effort should be made to retain the enema for at least 1 h, and, preferably, all night; this may be facilitated by prior sedation and/or antidiarrheal medication, especially early in therapy, when the urge to evacuate is great.
Discontinuation of therapy	Difficult cases may require up to 2–3 mo of treatment; if the course of therapy extends beyond 21 days, discontinue gradually by reducing use to every other night for 2–3 wk

WARNINGS/PRECAUTIONS

Severe ulcerative colitis	A delay in needed surgery while awaiting the results of medical treatment can be hazardous
Damage to rectal wall	Can result from careless or improper insertion of enema tip
Patients subjected to unusual stress	Require increased dosage of rapidly acting corticosteroids before, during, and after emotionally or physically stressful situations
Infection	Clinical signs may be masked, new infections may appear, resistance to infection may be decreased, and infections may be difficult to localize
Ocular damage	Prolonged use may produce posterior subcapsular cataracts and glaucoma with possible damage to optic nerves, and may enhance the establishment of secondary fungal or viral ocular infections
Dietary salt restriction and potassium supplementation	May be necessary to combat blood pressure elevation, salt and water retention, and increased potassium excretion with average- and high-dose therapy
Immunization procedures	Especially against smallpox, should not be undertaken because of possible neurological complications and lack of antibody response
Latent tuberculosis or tuberculin reactivity	Observe patient closely, since reactivation of the disease may occur; during prolonged therapy, employ antituberculous chemoprophylactic measures
Special-risk patients	Use with caution if impending perforation, abscess, or other pyogenic infection is likely, as well as in patients with fresh intestinal anastomoses, obstruction, extensive fistulas and sinus tracts, active or latent peptic ulcer, diverticulitis, renal insufficiency, hypertension, osteoporosis, and myasthenia gravis
Prognosis in surgery	May be impaired due to increased hazard of infection; if infection is suspected, administer appropriate therapy, usually in larger than ordinary doses
Secondary adrenocortical insufficiency	May occur with prolonged use; minimize by gradually reducing dosage. Since insufficiency may persist for months, reinstitute corticosteroid therapy in any stressful situation during this period, and administer salt and/or a mineralocorticoid concurrently to correct impaired mineralocorticoid secretion.
Hypothyroidism, hepatic cirrhosis	May enhance effects of corticosteroids
Corenal perforation	May occur in patients with ocular herpes simplex; use with caution
Psychic derangements	May appear, ranging from euphoria, insomnia, mood swings, personality changes and severe depression, to frank psychotic manifestations; existing emotional instability or psychotic tendencies may be aggravated
Concomitant use with aspirin	Exercise caution in patients with hypoprothrombinemia

ADVERSE REACTIONS

Fluid and electrolyte disturbances	Sodium retention, fluid retention, congestive heart failure in susceptible patients, loss of potassium, hypokalemic alkalosis, hypertension
Musculoskeletal	Muscle weakness, steroid myopathy, loss of muscle mass, osteoporosis, vertebral compression fractures, aseptic necrosis of femoral and humeral heads, pathological fracture of long bones
Gastrointestinal	Peptic ulcer with possible perforation and hemorrhage, pancreatitis, abdominal distention, ulcerative esophagitis
Dermatological	Impaired wound healing, thin fragile skin, petechiae and ecchymoses, facial erythema, increased sweating, suppressed reaction to skin tests
Neurological	Convulsions, increased intracranial pressure with papilledema (pseudotumor cerebri), vertigo, headache
Endocrinological	Menstrual irregularities, Cushingoid state, growth suppression in children, secondary adrenocortical and pituitary unresponsiveness, decreased carbohydrate tolerance, latent diabetes mellitus, increased insulin or oral hypoglycemic requirements
Ophthalmic	Posterior subcapsular cataracts, increased intraocular pressure, glaucoma, exophthalmos
Metabolic	Negative nitrogen balance

OVERDOSAGE

Signs and symptoms	CNS changes, GI bleeding, hyperglycemia, hypertension, edema

CORTENEMA ■ CORTICAINE

Treatment	Discontinue medication; institute supportive measures, as required

DRUG INTERACTIONS

Insulin, oral hypoglycemics	▽ Hypoglycemic effects	
Phenytoin, phenobarbital, ephedrine, rifampin	△ Metabolic clearance of hydrocortisone	▽ Steroid blood level and physiological activity
Oral anticoagulants	△ or ▽ Prothrombin time	
Potassium-depleting diuretics	△ Risk of hypokalemia	
Cardiac glycosides	△ Risk of arrhythmias or digitalis toxicity secondary to hypokalemia	
Skin-test antigens	▽ Reactivity	
Immunizations	▽ Antibody response	

ALTERED LABORATORY VALUES

Blood/serum values	△ Glucose △ Cholesterol △ Sodium ▽ Potassium ▽ Calcium ▽ PBI ▽ Thyroxine (T_4) ▽ ^{131}I thyroid uptake ▽ Uric acid
Urinary values	△ Glucose △ Potassium △ Calcium △ Uric acid ▽ 17-Hydroxycorticosteroids (17-OHCS) ▽ 17-Ketosteroids

USE IN CHILDREN

Growth and development should be carefully observed in infants and children on prolonged therapy; pediatric dosages have not been established

USE IN PREGNANT AND NURSING WOMEN

Safety for use during pregnancy has not been established; infants born of mothers who have received substantial doses of corticosteroids during pregnancy should be carefully observed for signs of hypoadrenalism. Studies in nursing women have not been documented. Since use during nursing may result in infant growth suppression, the possible benefits of therapy should be weighed against the potential harm to the infant.

RECTAL CORTICOSTEROIDS/HEMORRHOIDALS

CORTICAINE Cream (hydrocortisone acetate and dibucaine) Glaxo   Rx

Cream: 0.5% hydrocortisone acetate and 0.5% dibucaine (1 oz)

INDICATIONS	TOPICAL DOSAGE	RECTAL DOSAGE
Symptomatic relief of **atopic dermatitis, poison sumac or ivy dermatitis, mild sunburn, minor burns, insect bites, prickly heat, eczema, postanal surgery, diaper rash, intertrigo, pruritus ani,** and **external hemorrhoids**	Adult: apply to affected areas bid to qid for 2 wk	
Symptomatic relief of **internal hemorrhoids, proctitis, papillitis, cryptitis,** and other inflammatory anorectal conditions		Adult: instill cream into rectum bid (morning and evening) and after each bowel movement for 2–6 days

CONTRAINDICATIONS

Hypersensitivity to any component	Local tuberculosis, fungal infections, or viral infections

ADMINISTRATION/DOSAGE ADJUSTMENTS

Rectal instillation	Cleanse the rectal area and dry surface thoroughly. Attach the plastic applicator to the tube and squeeze the tube lightly to fill the applicator with cream. Lubricate the applicator with more cream and then gently insert the tip into the rectum. Squeeze the tube lightly to extrude approximately one applicatorful of cream into the rectum.

WARNINGS/PRECAUTIONS

Pretreatment evaluation	An adequate proctologic examination should precede rectal use of these preparations; do not use if anorectal fistulas or abscesses are present. Topical use for pemphigus and discoid lupus erythematosus is not recommended.
Systemic absorption	Prolonged topical use over extensive areas or under an occlusive dressing may increase systemic absorption and the risk of adverse reactions
Irritation	If irritation occurs, discontinue use and institute appropriate therapy

CORTICAINE ■ MEDICONE

| Secondary bacterial infections | Inflammatory skin conditions complicated by bacterial infections should be treated with an appropriate antibacterial agent; if a favorable response is not obtained promptly, discontinue use of Corticaine until the infection is under control |

ADVERSE REACTIONS[1]

| Local | Burning, itching, irritation, dryness, folliculitis, hypopigmentation, allergic contact dermatitis, secondary infection; hypertrichosis, acneform eruptions, perioral dermatitis, skin maceration, skin atrophy, striae, and miliaria (with cream only) |

USE IN CHILDREN
Safety and effectiveness for use have not been established in children

USE IN PREGNANT AND NURSING WOMEN
Safety for use during pregnancy has not been established. In laboratory animals, topical steroids have shown evidence of teratogenicity, sometimes at relatively low dosages. Do not use these preparations over extensive areas, in large amounts, or for prolonged periods if patient is pregnant. Consult manufacturer for use in nursing mothers.

VEHICLE/BASE
Cream (washable, nongreasy): mixed saturated fatty acid esters, stearyl alcohol, glycerin, polysorbate 40, BHA, BHT, disodium edetate, and purified water, with methylparaben and propylparaben as preservatives

[1] Includes reactions common to topical and rectal corticosteroids in general

---

RECTAL CORTICOSTEROIDS/HEMORRHOIDALS

MEDICONE Ointment and Suppositories (benzocaine, 8-hydroxyquinoline sulfate, menthol, zinc oxide, and balsam Peru) Medicone   OTC

Ointment (per gram): 20 mg benzocaine, 5 mg 8-hydroxyquinoline sulfate, 4 mg menthol, 100 mg zinc oxide, and 12.5 mg balsam Peru (1½ oz) **Rectal suppositories:** 2 g benzocaine, 0.25 g 8-hydroxyquinoline sulfate, 0.143 g menthol, 3 g zinc oxide, and 1 g balsam Peru

INDICATIONS	RECTAL DOSAGE
Temporary relief of pain, burning, and itching of minor **internal and external hemorrhoids and minor anorectal disorders**	**Adult:** apply ointment liberally or insert 1 suppository bid (AM and PM) and after each bowel movement; to help prevent recurrence of symptoms, continue use of suppositories for 10–15 days after discomfort ceases

CONTRAINDICATIONS
Hypersensitivity to any component

ADMINISTRATION/DOSAGE ADJUSTMENTS

External use of ointment	Cover area with gauze
Internal use of ointment	Attach applicator and lubricate tip with a small amount of ointment to ease insertion
Use of suppositories	If the suppository is too soft, refrigerate it for a few minutes before insertion; if the surface of the suppository is too dry or hard, dip the suppository in warm water for 3 s or lubricate the tip with the ointment
Concomitant use of ointment and suppositories	Insert a small amount of the ointment into the rectum before inserting suppository

WARNINGS/PRECAUTIONS

| Patient instructions | Caution patient to discontinue use if rash, irritation, or rectal bleeding develops and to report their occurrence |
| Staining | If clothing or bed linen becomes stained, gently apply brown laundry soap to the discolored area and then rinse thoroughly; do not use detergent |

ADVERSE REACTIONS

| Local | Irritation, rash |

USE IN CHILDREN
Consult manufacturer

USE IN PREGNANT AND NURSING WOMEN
Consult manufacturer

VEHICLE/BASE
Ointment: petrolatum, lanolin, and certified color
Rectal suppositories: cocoa butter, vegetable and petroleum oils, and certified color

NUPERCAINAL ■ PREPARATION H

RECTAL CORTICOSTEROIDS/HEMORRHOIDALS

NUPERCAINAL Cream and Ointment (dibucaine) CIBA — OTC

Cream: 0.5% (1½ oz)   Ointment: 1%, (1, 2 oz)

NUPERCAINAL Suppositories (cocoa butter, zinc oxide, and bismuth subgallate) CIBA — OTC

Rectal suppositories: 2.4 g cocoa butter, 0.25 g zinc oxide, and 0.1 g bismuth subgallate

INDICATIONS / TOPICAL AND RECTAL DOSAGE

Temporary relief of pain (ointment only), itching, burning, and discomfort of **hemorrhoids and other anorectal conditions**
- **Adult:** apply ointment freely bid (AM and PM) and after each bowel movement, or insert 1 suppository after each bowel movement and as needed, up to 6 suppositories/24 h

Temporary relief of pain and itching associated with **sunburn, nonpoisonous insect bites, and minor burns, cuts, and scratches**
- **Adult:** apply cream liberally to affected area and rub in gently or apply ointment gently and, if necessary, cover with a light dressing for protection; do not use more than 1 oz of the ointment per 24 h
- **Child:** same as adult; do not use more than ¼ oz of the ointment per 24 h

CONTRAINDICATIONS

Consult manufacturer

ADMINISTRATION/DOSAGE ADJUSTMENTS

Use of ointment for hemorrhoids — For internal use, attach plastic applicator and insert into the anus, squeezing the tube to deliver the medication; remove applicator from rectum, wipe clean, and apply additional ointment to anal tissues to help relieve symptoms. Detach applicator after each use and wash it with soap and water.

Use of cream — Cream is water-washable; reapply after bathing, swimming, or sweating

Storage of suppositories — To prevent melting, do not store above 86° F

WARNINGS/PRECAUTIONS

Prolonged or extensive use — Not recommended

Poisoning — May occur if these preparations are swallowed; medication should be kept out of the reach of children

Patient instructions — Caution patient to discontinue use if irritation or rectal bleeding occurs and to report their occurrence

ADVERSE REACTIONS

Local — Irritation

USE IN CHILDREN
See INDICATIONS and dosage recommendations

USE IN PREGNANT AND NURSING WOMEN
Consult manufacturer

VEHICLE/BASE
Cream: water-soluble base
Ointment: lanolin, white petrolatum, light mineral oil, and acetone sodium bisulfite
Rectal suppositories: preserved with acetone sodium bisulfite

---

RECTAL CORTICOSTEROIDS/HEMORRHOIDALS

PREPARATION H (live yeast cell derivative and shark liver oil) Whitehall — OTC

Ointment: live yeast cell derivative (equivalent to 2,000 units/oz skin respiratory factor) and 3% shark liver oil (1, 2 oz)
Rectal suppositories: live yeast cell derivative (equivalent to 2,000 units/oz skin respiratory factor) and 3% shark liver oil

INDICATIONS / RECTAL DOSAGE

Temporary relief of pain and itching of **hemorrhoids** and to help reduce swelling of **inflamed hemorrhoidal tissues**
- **Adult:** apply ointment freely or insert 1 suppository 3–5 times/day, especially at night, in the morning, after each bowel movement, and whenever symptoms occur

CONTRAINDICATIONS

Hypersensitivity to any component

ADMINISTRATION/DOSAGE ADJUSTMENTS

Use of ointment — Lubricate applicator before each application and cleanse thoroughly after use

PREPARATION H ■ PROCTOFOAM-HC

Storage of suppositories	Store below 80° F

WARNINGS/PRECAUTIONS

Patient instructions	Caution patient to report if condition persists or bleeding occurs

ADVERSE REACTIONS

Local	Irritation (rare; causal relationship not established)

USE IN CHILDREN

Use according to medical judgment; there are no special precautions concerning use in children

USE IN PREGNANT AND NURSING WOMEN

No adverse reactions have been reported in pregnant or nursing women; there are no special precautions concerning use in these patient groups

---

VEHICLE/BASE
Ointment: petrolatum, beeswax, glycerin, lanolin, lanolin alcohol, mineral oil, paraffin, thyme oil, and phenylmercuric nitrate 1:10,000
Rectal suppositories: cocoa butter, beeswax, glycerin, polyethylene glycol 600 dilaurate, and phenylmercuric nitrate 1:10,000

RECTAL CORTICOSTEROIDS/HEMORRHOIDALS

PROCTOFOAM-HC (hydrocortisone acetate and pramoxine hydrochloride) Reed & Carnrick Rx

Foam: 1% hydrocortisone acetate and 1% pramoxine hydrochloride (10 g)

INDICATIONS	RECTAL DOSAGE
Inflammatory and pruritic manifestations of **corticosteroid-responsive anal dermatoses**	**Adult:** apply to affected areas tid or qid **Child:** use minimal amount necessary for effective therapy (see precaution, below, concerning systemic absorption)

CONTRAINDICATIONS

Hypersensitivity to any component

ADMINISTRATION/DOSAGE ADJUSTMENTS

Rectal use	Shake foam container vigorously before use. Hold container upright and insert into opening of applicator tip with applicator plunger drawn out. Press down slowly on container cap until foam reaches fill line on applicator. Remove filled applicator from container, with some foam remaining on the applicator tip; gently insert tip into the anus. Once in place, push plunger to expel foam. Withdraw the applicator and wash with warm water. *Never* insert the container directly into the anus.
Perianal use	Transfer a small quantity of foam to a tissue and rub in gently
Evaluation of therapy	If condition worsens or, after 2–3 wk, fails to improve, discontinue use

WARNINGS/PRECAUTIONS

Patient instructions	Caution patients not to let this preparation come into contact with their eyes. Advise them to report any signs of adverse reactions.
Irritation	Discontinue use and institute appropriate therapy
Dermatological infection	Institute appropriate antifungal or antibacterial therapy; if infection persists, discontinue steroid therapy until a favorable response is obtained
Systemic absorption	Reversible hypothalamic-pituitary-adrenal (HPA) axis suppression, Cushing's syndrome, hyperglycemia, and glucosuria may result from systemic absorption after topical application, particularly in children (see USE IN CHILDREN). Use over extensive areas, for prolonged periods, or of occlusive dressings increases percutaneous absorption. If large doses are applied over extensive areas or are administered using the occlusive dressing technique, evaluate HPA axis function periodically by ACTH stimulation and measurement of urinary free cortisol. If HPA axis suppression occurs, discontinue use of this drug, reduce the frequency of application, or administer a less potent steroid. Infrequently, systemic corticosteroids may be needed to treat manifestations of topical steroid withdrawal.
Carcinogenicity, mutagenicity	Long-term studies have not been done in animals to evaluate the carcinogenic potential of topical corticosteroids; the results of studies to demonstrate mutagenicity of prednisolone and hydrocortisone have been negative
Effect on fertility	The effect of topical corticosteroids on fertility has not been studied

ADVERSE REACTIONS[1]

Local — Burning, itching, irritation, dryness, folliculitis, hypertrichosis, acneform eruptions, hypopigmentation, perioral dermatitis, allergic contact dermatitis, maceration of the skin, secondary infection, skin atrophy, striae, miliaria

USE IN CHILDREN

Use smallest amount necessary for effective treatment. Children may be more susceptible than adults to HPA axis suppression and Cushing's syndrome because of the larger ratio of surface area to body weight; intracranial hypertension has also been observed in children receiving topical corticosteroids. Chronic therapy may interfere with growth and development.

USE IN PREGNANT AND NURSING WOMEN

Pregnancy Category C: use during pregnancy only if the expected benefit justifies the potential risk to the fetus. Do not use over extensive areas, in large amounts, or for prolonged periods. In animal studies, systemic corticosteroids have generally been teratogenic at relatively low dosages; the more potent corticosteroids have also been teratogenic when applied to the skin. No adequate, well-controlled studies have been done in pregnant women. It is not known whether topical corticosteroids are excreted in human milk; although systemic corticosteroids are excreted in quantities unlikely to harm nursing infants, this preparation should be used with caution in nursing mothers.

VEHICLE/BASE
Foam (hydrophilic): propylene glycol, ethoxylated cetyl and stearyl alcohols, steareth-10, cetyl alcohol, methylparaben, propylparaben, trolamine, and purified water, with dichlorodifluoromethane and dichlorotetrafluoroethane as propellants

[1] Includes reactions common to topical corticosteroids in general

---

RECTAL CORTICOSTEROIDS/HEMORRHOIDALS

TRONALANE (pramoxine hydrochloride) Ross   OTC

Cream: 1% (1, 2 oz)   **Rectal suppositories:** 1%

INDICATIONS
Symptomatic relief of pain, burning, itching, and discomfort due to **hemorrhoids**

TOPICAL DOSAGE
Adult: apply cream liberally to affected area or insert 1 suppository up to 5 times/day, especially in AM and PM and after each bowel movement, or use according to medical judgement
Child (≥12 yr): same as adult

CONTRAINDICATIONS
Consult manufacturer

ADMINISTRATION/DOSAGE ADJUSTMENTS

Intrarectal administration of cream — Remove cap from tube, attach applicator, and remove applicator cover; then squeeze tube to fill applicator and lubricate tip, gently insert applicator into rectum, and squeeze tube again; thoroughly cleanse applicator after use

WARNINGS/PRECAUTIONS

Patient instructions — Patients are cautioned on the package label to consult a physician if bleeding occurs, allergic reactions develop, their condition worsens, or symptoms persist for 7 days

ADVERSE REACTIONS

Local — Allergic reactions

USE IN CHILDREN
Use in children under 12 yr of age according to medical judgment

USE IN PREGNANT AND NURSING WOMEN
Consult manufacturer

VEHICLE/BASE
Cream: beeswax, cetyl alcohol, cetyl esters wax, glycerin, methylparaben, propylparaben, sodium lauryl sulfate, zinc oxide, and water
Suppositories: hydrogenated cocoa glycerides and zinc oxide

RECTAL CORTICOSTEROIDS/HEMORRHOIDALS

TUCKS (witch hazel and glycerin) Warner-Lambert OTC

Premoistened pads: 50% witch hazel and 10% glycerin **Premoistened wipes:** 50% witch hazel and 10% glycerin (Take-Alongs)

INDICATIONS

Temporary relief of discomfort due to **simple hemorrhoids and rectal or vaginal sutures**

Relief of itching, burning, and irritation of **sensitive rectal and outer vaginal surfaces**

Cleansing of perineum and rectal area

Diaper irritation

TOPICAL DOSAGE

Adult: use as a wipe after bowel movements, during menstruation, or after changing sanitary napkin or tampon; to help relieve suture discomfort, apply as a compress to affected area for 10–15 min, as needed, changing the compress every 5 min

Infant: use as a wipe after each bowel movement, as needed

TUCKS Cream and Ointment (witch hazel) Warner-Lambert OTC

Cream: 50% (40 g)   **Ointment:** 50% (40 g)

INDICATIONS

Temporary relief of discomfort due to **hemorrhoids, rectal or outer vaginal irritation and itching, episiotomy, and hemorrhoidectomy**

TOPICAL DOSAGE

Adult: apply to affected area tid or qid; use applicator supplied for rectal instillation, if indicated

CONTRAINDICATIONS

Consult manufacturer

WARNINGS/PRECAUTIONS

Patient instructions — Discontinue use if itching or irritation continues; caution patient to report promptly any signs of rectal bleeding

ADVERSE REACTIONS

Consult manufacturer

USE IN CHILDREN

Premoistened pads may be used to soothe diaper irritation

USE IN PREGNANT AND NURSING WOMEN

Consult manufacturer

VEHICLE/BASE
Cream: arlacel, white petrolatum, anhydrous lanolin, benzethonium chloride, sorbitol solution, polyethylene stearate, cetyl alcohol, and polysorbate
Ointment: arlacel, white petrolatum, anhydrous lanolin, benzethonium chloride, and sorbitol
Premoistened pads and wipes: purified water, citric acid, and sodium citrate, with 0.1% methylparaben and 0.003% benzalkonium chloride as preservatives; buffered to an acid pH

Chapter 34

Cough/Cold/Other Upper Respiratory Medications

Cough/Cold/Other Upper Respiratory Medications	**1401**
Antitussives	**1409**
TESSALON (Du Pont) Benzonatate *Rx*	1409
Antitussive Combinations	**1409**
ACTIFED with Codeine (Burroughs Wellcome) Triprolidine hydrochloride, pseudoephedrine hydrochloride, and codeine phosphate *C-V*	1409
AMBENYL (Forest) Bromodiphenhydramine hydrochloride and codeine phosphate *C-V*	1411
CALCIDRINE (Abbott) Codeine and calcium iodide *C-V*	1412
DILAUDID Cough Syrup (Knoll) Hydromorphone hydrochloride and guaifenesin *C-II*	1413
DIMETANE-DC (Robins) Brompheniramine maleate, phenylpropanolamine hydrochloride, and codeine phosphate *C-V*	1414
DIMETANE-DX (Robins) Brompheniramine maleate, pseudoephedrine hydrochloride, and dextromethorphan hydrobromide *Rx*	1416
HYCODAN (Du Pont) Hydrocodone bitartrate and homatropine methylbromide *C-III*	1417
HYCOMINE Pediatric Syrup (Du Pont) Hydrocodone bitartrate and phenylpropanolamine hydrochloride *C-III*	1418
HYCOMINE Syrup (Du Pont) Hydrocodone bitartrate and phenylpropanolamine hydrochloride *C-III*	1418
NOVAHISTINE DH (Lakeside) Codeine phosphate, pseudoephedrine hydrochloride, and chlorpheniramine maleate *C-V*	1419
NOVAHISTINE Expectorant (Lakeside) Codeine phosphate, pseudoephedrine hydrochloride, and guaifenesin *C-V*	1420
PENNTUSS (Pennwalt) Codeine polistirex and chlorpheniramine polistirex *C-V*	1421
PHENERGAN with Codeine (Wyeth) Promethazine hydrochloride and codeine phosphate *C-V*	1422
PHENERGAN with Dextromethorphan (Wyeth) Promethazine hydrochloride and dextromethorphan hydrobromide *Rx*	1424
PHENERGAN VC with Codeine (Wyeth) Promethazine hydrochloride, phenylephrine hydrochloride, and codeine phosphate *C-V*	1425
ROBITUSSIN A-C (Robins) Guaifenesin and codeine phosphate *C-V*	1428
ROBITUSSIN-DAC (Robins) Guaifenesin, pseudoephedrine hydrochloride, and codeine phosphate *C-V*	1428
RONDEC-DM (Ross) Carbinoxamine maleate, pseudoephedrine hydrochloride, and dextromethorphan hydrobromide *Rx*	1429
RYNA-C (Wallace) Codeine phosphate, pseudoephedrine hydrochloride, and chlorpheniramine maleate *C-V*	1431
RYNA-CX (Wallace) Codeine phosphate, pseudoephedrine hydrochloride, and guaifenesin *C-V*	1432
RYNATUSS (Wallace) Carbetapentane tannate, chlorpheniramine tannate, ephedrine tannate, and phenylephrine tannate *Rx*	1433
Terpin hydrate and codeine elixir *C-V*	1434
TRIAMINIC Expectorant with Codeine (Sandoz Consumer Health Care Group) Codeine phosphate, phenylpropanolamine hydrochloride, and guaifenesin *C-V*	1434
TRIAMINIC Expectorant DH (Sandoz Consumer Health Care Group) Hydrocordone bitartrate, phenylpropanolamine hydrochloride, pheniramine maleate, pyrilamine maleate, and guaifenesin *C-III*	1435
TUSSEND (Merrell Dow) Hydrocordone bitartrate and pseudoephedrine hydrochloride *C-III*	1437
TUSSEND Expectorant (Merrell Dow) Hydrocordone bitartrate, pseudoephedrine hydrochloride, and guaifenesin *C-III*	1438
TUSSIONEX (Pennwalt) Hydrocodone and phenyltoloxamine *C-III*	1439
TUSSI-ORGANIDIN (Wallace) Iodinated glycerol and codeine phosphate *C-V*	1440
TUSSI-ORGANIDIN DM (Wallace) Iodinated glycerol and dextromethorphan hydrobromide *Rx*	1441
TUSS-ORNADE (Smith Kline & French) Caramiphen edisylate and phenylpropanolamine hydrochloride *Rx*	1442
Decongestants/Upper Respiratory Combinations	**1443**
COMHIST (Norwich Eaton) Chlorpheniramine maleate, phenyltoloxamine citrate, and phenylephrine hydrochloride *Rx*	1443
COMHIST LA (Norwich Eaton) Chlorpheniramine maleate, phenyltoloxamine citrate, and phenylephrine hydrochloride *Rx*	1443
DECONAMINE (Berlex) Chlorpheniramine maleate and pseudoephedrine hydrochloride *Rx*	1444

DECONAMINE SR (Berlex)   1444
Chlorpheniramine maleate and pseudoephedrine hydrochloride *Rx*

ENTEX (Norwich Eaton)   1445
Phenylephrine hydrochloride, phenylpropanolamine hydrochloride, and guaifenesin *Rx*

ENTEX LA (Norwich Eaton)   1445
Phenylpropanolamine hydrochloride and guaifenesin *Rx*

NALDECON (Bristol)   1446
Phenylpropanolamine hydrochloride, phenylephrine hydrochloride, phenyltoloxamine citrate, and chlorpheniramine maleate *Rx*

NOVAFED Capsules (Merrell Dow)   1447
Pseudoephedrine hydrochloride *Rx*

NOVAFED Liquid (Merrell Dow)   1447
Pseudoephedrine hydrochloride *OTC*

NOVAFED A Capsules (Merrell Dow)   1448
Pseudoephedrine hydrochloride and chlorpheniramine maleate *Rx*

NOVAFED A Liquid (Merrell Dow)   1448
Pseudoephedrine hydrochloride and chlorpheniramine maleate *OTC*

ORNADE (Smith Kline & French)   1449
Chlorpheniramine maleate and phenylpropanolamine hydrochloride *Rx*

PHENERGAN VC (Wyeth)   1451
Promethazine hydrochloride and phenylephrine hydrochloride *Rx*

RONDEC (Ross)   1453
Carbinoxamine maleate and pseudoephedrine hydrochloride *Rx*

RONDEC-TR (Ross)   1453
Carbinoxamine maleate and pseudoephedrine hydrochloride *Rx*

RU-TUSS (Boots)   1454
Phenylephrine hydrochloride, phenylpropanolamine hydrochloride, chlorpheniramine maleate, hyoscyamine sulfate, atropine sulfate, and scopolamine hydrobromide *Rx*

RYNATAN (Wallace)   1455
Phenylephrine tannate, chlorpheniramine tannate, and pyrilamine tannate *Rx*

SINUBID (Parke-Davis)   1456
Acetaminophen, phenylpropanolamine hydrochloride, and phenyltoloxamine citrate *Rx*

TAVIST-D (Sandoz Pharmaceuticals)   1457
Clemastine fumarate and phenylpropanolamine hydrochloride *Rx*

TRIAMINIC (Sandoz Consumer Health Care Group)   1459
Phenylpropanolamine hydrochloride, pheniramine maleate, and pyrilamine maleate *Rx*

TRIAMINIC TR (Sandoz Consumer Health Care Group)   1459
Phenylpropanolamine hydrochloride, pheniramine maleate, and pyrilamine maleate *Rx*

TRINALIN (Schering)   1460
Azatadine maleate and pseudoephedrine sulfate *Rx*

Expectorants   1462

ORGANIDIN (Wallace)   1462
Iodinated glycerol *Rx*

Other Antitussives/Antitussive Combinations   1396

CHERACOL (Upjohn)   1396
Codeine phosphate and guaifenesin *C-V*

Codeine sulfate *C-II*   1397

COLREX Compound Capsules (Reid-Rowell)   1397
Phenylephrine hydrochloride, chlorpheniramine maleate, codeine phosphate, and acetaminophen *C-III*

COLREX Compound Elixir (Reid-Rowell)   1397
Phenylephrine hydrochloride, chlorpheniramine maleate, codeine phosphate, and acetaminophen *C-V*

CONEX with Codeine (Forest)   1397
Phenylpropanolamine hydrochloride, codeine phosphate, and guaifenesin *C-V*

COPAVIN (Lilly)   1397
Codeine sulfate and papaverine hydrochloride *C-III*

HISTALET DM (Reid-Rowell)   1397
Chlorpheniramine maleate, pseudoephedrine hydrochloride, and dextromethorphan hydrobromide *Rx*

HYCOMINE Compound (Du Pont)   1397
Phenylephrine hydrochloride, chlorpheniramine maleate, hydrocodone bitartrate, acetaminophen, and caffeine *C-III*

HYCOTUSS Expectorant (Du Pont)   1397
Hydrocodone bitartrate and guaifenesin *C-III*

ISOCLOR Expectorant (Fisons)   1397
Codeine phosphate, pseudoephedrine hydrochloride, and guaifenesin *C-V*

NALDECON-CX (Bristol)   1397
Phenylpropanolamine hydrochloride, guaifenesin, and codeine phosphate *C-V*

NUCOFED (Beecham)   1397
Pseudoephedrine hydrochloride and codeine phosphate *C-III*

NUCOFED Expectorant (Beecham)   1397
Codeine phosphate, pseudoephedrine hydrochloride, and guaifenesin *C-III*

NUCOFED Pediatric Expectorant (Beecham)   1398
Codeine phosphate, pseudoephedrine hydrochloride, and guaifenesin *C-V*

PEDIACOF (Winthrop-Breon)   1398
Codeine phosphate, phenylephrine hydrochloride, chlorpheniramine maleate, and potassium iodide *C-V*

PRUNICODEINE (Lilly)   1398
Codeine sulfate and terpin hydrate *C-V*

continued

COMPENDIUM OF DRUG THERAPY   1395

Cough/Cold/Other Upper Respiratory Medications continued

RU-TUSS Expectorant (Boots) 1398
Dextromethorphan hydrobromide, pseudoephedrine hydrochloride, and guaifenesin *Rx*

TUSSAR-2 (Rorer) 1398
Codeine phosphate, carbetapentane citrate, chlorpheniramine maleate, guaifenesin, sodium citrate, and citric acid *C-V*

TUSSAR SF (Rorer) 1398
Codeine phosphate, carbetapentane citrate, chlorpheniramine maleate, guaifenesin, sodium citrate, and citric acid *C-V*

UNPROCO (Reid-Rowell) 1398
Dextromethorphan hydrobromide and guaifenesin *Rx*

Other Decongestants/Upper Respiratory Combinations 1398

DISOPHROL (Schering) 1398
Dexbrompheniramine maleate and pseudoephedrine sulfate *OTC*

FEDAHIST (Rorer) 1398
Pseudoephedrine hydrochloride and chlorpheniramine maleate *Rx*

HISTABID (Glaxo) 1398
Phenylpropanolamine hydrochloride and chlorpheniramine maleate *Rx*

HISTALET (Reid-Rowell) 1398
Chlorpheniramine maleate and pseudoephedrine hydrochloride *Rx*

HISTALET Forte (Reid-Rowell) 1398
Phenylpropanolamine hydrochloride, pyrilamine maleate, chlorpheniramine maleate, and phenylephrine hydrochloride *Rx*

HISTALET X (Reid-Rowell) 1399
Pseudoephedrine hydrochloride and guaifenesin *Rx*

HISTASPAN-D (Rorer) 1399
Chlorpheniramine maleate, phenylephrine hydrochloride, and methscopolamine nitrate *Rx*

HISTASPAN-Plus (Rorer) 1399
Chlorpheniramine maleate and phenylephrine hydrochloride *Rx*

ISOCLOR (Fisons) 1399
Chlorpheniramine maleate and pseudoephedrine hydrochloride *Rx*

NEOTEP (Reid-Rowell) 1399
Phenylephrine hydrochloride and chlorpheniramine maleate *Rx*

NOLAMINE (Carnrick) 1399
Phenindamine tartrate, chlorpheniramine maleate, and phenylpropanolamine hydrochloride *Rx*

PHENERGAN-D (Wyeth) 1399
Pseudoephedrine hydrochloride and promethazine hydrochloride *Rx*

POLARMINE Expectorant (Schering) 1399
Dexchlorpheniramine maleate, pseudoephedrine sulfate, and guaifenesin *Rx*

RHINEX D-LAY (Lemmon) 1399
Phenylpropanolamine hydrochloride, chlorpheniramine maleate, acetaminophen, and salicylamide *Rx*

RU-TUSS with Hydrocodone (Boots) 1399
Hydrocodone bitartrate, phenylephrine hydrochloride, phenylpropanolamine hydrochloride, pheniramine maleate, and pyrilamine maleate *Rx*

RYNATAN (Wallace) 1399
Phenylephrine tannate, chlorpheniramine tannate, and pyrilamine tannate *Rx*

TRIPHED (Lemmon) 1399
Pseudoephedrine hydrochloride and triprolidine hydrochloride *Rx*

TYZINE (Key) 1400
Tetrahydrozoline hydrochloride *Rx*

Other Expectorants/Expectorant Combinations 1400

NORISODRINE with Calcium Iodide (Abbott) 1400
Isoproterenol sulfate and calcium iodide *Rx*

Potassium iodide *Rx* 1400

P-V-TUSSIN Syrup (Reid-Rowell) 1400
Hydrocodone bitartrate, phenylephrine hydrochloride, pyrilamine maleate, chlorpheniramine maleate, phenindamine tartrate, and ammonium chloride *C-III*

P-V-TUSSIN Tablets (Reid-Rowell) 1400
Hydrocodone bitartrate, phenindamine tartrate, and guaifenesin *C-III*

OTHER ANTITUSSIVES/ANTITUSSIVE COMBINATIONS

DRUG	HOW SUPPLIED	USUAL DOSAGE[1]
CHERACOL (Upjohn) Codeine phosphate and guaifenesin *C-V*	**Syrup (per 5 ml):** 10 mg codeine phosphate and 100 mg guaifenesin (4 fl oz)	**Adult:** 10 ml (2 tsp) q4h, as needed **Child (2-6 yr):** 2.5 ml (½ tsp) q4h, as needed **Child (6-12 yr):** 5 ml (1 tsp) q4h, as needed

[1] Where pediatric dosages are not given, consult manufacturer

OTHER ANTITUSSIVES/ANTITUSSIVE COMBINATIONS continued

DRUG	HOW SUPPLIED	USUAL DOSAGE[1]
Codeine sulfate C-II	**Tablets:** 15, 30, 60 mg **Tablets (soluble):** 15, 30, 60 mg	**Adult:** 10–20 mg q4–6h, up to 120 mg/24 h **Child (2–6 yr):** 2.5–5 mg q4–6h, up to 30 mg/24 h **Child (6–12 yr):** 5–10 mg q4–6h, up to 60 mg/24 h
COLREX Compound Capsules (Reid-Rowell) Phenylephrine hydrochloride, chlorpheniramine maleate, codeine phosphate, and acetaminophen C-III	**Capsules:** 10 mg phenylephrine hydrochloride, 2 mg chlorpheniramine maleate, 16 mg codeine phosphate, and 325 mg acetaminophen	**Adult:** 1–2 caps tid or qid
COLREX Compound Elixir (Reid-Rowell) Phenylephrine hydrochloride, chlorpheniramine maleate, codeine phosphate, and acetaminophen C-V	**Elixir (per 5 ml):** 5 mg phenylephrine hydrochloride, 1 mg chlorpheniramine maleate, 8 mg codeine phosphate, and 120 mg acetaminophen (2, 16 fl oz; 1 gal) *sugar-free*	**Adult:** 10–20 ml (2–4 tsp) tid or qid
CONEX with Codeine (Forest) Phenylpropanolamine hydrochloride, codeine phosphate, and guaifenesin C-V	**Syrup (per 5 ml):** 12.5 mg phenylpropanolamine hydrochloride, 10 mg codeine phosphate, and 100 mg guaifenesin (120 ml)	**Adult:** 10 ml (2 tsp) q4–6h
COPAVIN (Lilly) Codeine sulfate and papaverine hydrochloride C-III	**Capsules:** 15 mg codeine sulfate and 15 mg papaverine hydrochloride	**Adult:** 1 cap after meals and 2 caps at bedtime
HISTALET DM (Reid-Rowell) Chlorpheniramine maleate, pseudoephedrine hydrochloride, and dextromethorphan hydrobromide Rx	**Syrup (per 5 ml):** 3 mg chlorpheniramine maleate, 45 mg pseudoephedrine hydrochloride, and 15 mg dextromethorphan hydrobromide (1 pt)	**Adult:** 10 ml (2 tsp) qid **Child (2–6 yr):** 2.5 ml (½ tsp) qid **Child (6–12 yr):** 5 ml (1 tsp) qid
HYCOMINE Compound (Du Pont) Phenylephrine hydrochloride, chlorpheniramine maleate, hydrocodone bitartrate, acetaminophen, and caffeine C-III	**Tablets:** 10 mg phenylephrine hydrochloride, 2 mg chlorpheniramine maleate, 5 mg hydrocodone bitartrate, 250 mg acetaminophen, and 30 mg caffeine	**Adult:** 1 tab qid not more than q4h **Child (2–6 yr):** ½ tab bid, not more than q4h **Child (6–12 yr):** ½ tab qid, not more than q4h
HYCOTUSS Expectorant (Du Pont) Hydrocodone bitartrate and guaifenesin C-III	**Syrup (per 5 ml):** 5 mg hydrocodone bitartrate and 100 mg guaifenesin (1 pt) *butterscotch flavored*	**Adult:** 5 ml (1 tsp) to start, followed by 5–15 ml (1–3 tsp) not more than q4h, after meals and at bedtime, up to 30 ml (6 tsp)/24 h **Child (< 2 yr):** 0.3 mg of hydrocodone/kg/24 h, given in 4 equally divided doses **Child (2–12 yr):** 2.5 ml (½ tsp) to start, followed by 2.5–5 ml (½–1 tsp) not more than q4h, after meals and at bedtime **Child (> 12 yr):** 5 ml (1 tsp) to start, followed by 5–10 ml (1–2 tsp) not more than q4h, after meals and at bedtime
ISOCLOR Expectorant (Fisons) Codeine phosphate, pseudoephedrine hydrochloride, and guaifenesin C-V	**Liquid (per 5 ml):** 10 mg codeine phosphate, 30 mg pseudoephedrine hydrochloride, and 100 mg guaifenesin (16 fl oz)	**Adult:** 10 ml (2 tsp) tid or qid **Child (1–2 yr):** 0.63 ml (⅛ tsp) tid or qid **Child (2–6 yr):** 1.25 ml (¼ tsp) tid or qid **Child (6–12 yr):** 2.5–5 ml (½–1 tsp) tid or qid
NALDECON-CX (Bristol) Phenylpropanolamine hydrochloride, guaifenesin, and codeine phosphate C-V	**Suspension (per 5 ml):** 18 mg phenylpropanolamine hydrochloride, 200 mg guaifenesin, and 10 mg codeine phosphate (4, 16 fl oz)	**Adult:** 10 ml (2 tsp) qid **Child (2–6 yr):** 2.5 ml (½ tsp) qid **Child (6–12 yr):** 5 ml (1 tsp) qid
NUCOFED (Beecham) Pseudoephedrine hydrochloride and codeine phosphate C-III	**Capsules:** 60 mg pseudoephedrine hydrochloride and 20 mg codeine phosphate **Syrup (per 5 ml):** 60 mg pseudoephedrine hydrochloride and 20 mg codeine phosphate (1 pt) *mint flavored*	**Adult:** 1 cap or 5 ml (1 tsp) q6h, up to 4 caps or 20 ml (4 tsp)/24 h **Child (2–6 yr):** 1.25 ml (¼ tsp) q6h, up to 5 ml (1 tsp)/24 h **Child (6–12 yr):** 2.5 ml (½ tsp) q6h, up to 10 ml (2 tsp)/24 h
NUCOFED Expectorant (Beecham) Codeine phosphate, pseudoephedrine hydrochloride, and guaifenesin C-III	**Syrup (per 5 ml):** 20 mg codeine phosphate, 60 mg pseudoephedrine hydrochloride, and 200 mg guaifenesin (1 pt) *wintergreen flavored*	**Adult:** 5 ml (1 tsp) q6h **Child (2–6 yr):** 1.25 ml (¼ tsp) q6h **Child (6–12 yr):** 2.5 ml (½ tsp) q6h

[1] Where pediatric dosages are not given, consult manufacturer

continued

OTHER ANTITUSSIVES/ANTITUSSIVE COMBINATIONS continued

DRUG	HOW SUPPLIED	USUAL DOSAGE[1]
NUCOFED Pediatric Expectorant (Beecham) Codeine phosphate, pseudoephedrine hydrochloride, and guaifenesin *C-V*	**Syrup (per 5 ml):** 10 mg codeine phosphate, 30 mg pseudoephedrine hydrochloride, and 100 mg guaifenesin (1 pt) *strawberry flavored*	**Adult:** 10 ml (2 tsp) q6h **Child (2–6 yr):** 2.5 ml (½ tsp) q6h **Child (6–12 yr):** 5 ml (1 tsp) q6h
PEDIACOF (Winthrop-Breon) Codeine phosphate, phenylephrine hydrochloride, chlorpheniramine maleate, and potassium iodide *C-V*	**Syrup (per 5 ml):** 5 mg codeine phosphate, 2.5 mg phenylephrine hydrochloride, 0.75 mg chlorpheniramine maleate, and 75 mg potassium iodide (1 pt) *raspberry-flavored*	**Infant (6 mo to 1 yr):** 1.25 ml (¼ tsp) q4–6h **Child (1–3 yr):** 2.5–5 ml (½–1 tsp) q4–6h **Child (3–6 yr):** 5–10 ml (1–2 tsp) q4–6h **Child (6–12 yr):** 10 ml (2 tsp) q4–6h
PRUNICODEINE (Lilly) Codeine sulfate and terpin hydrate *C-V*	**Liquid (per 5 ml):** 10 mg codeine sulfate and 29 mg terpin hydrate (1 pt)	**Adult:** 5 ml (1 tsp) q3h
RU-TUSS Expectorant (Boots) Dextromethorphan hydrobromide, pseudoephedrine hydrochloride, and guaifenesin *Rx*	**Liquid (per 5 ml):** 10 mg dextromethorphan hydrobromide, 30 mg pseudoephedrine hydrochloride, and 100 mg guaifenesin (1 pt)	**Adult:** 10 ml (2 tsp) q4–6h **Child (2–6 yr):** 2.5 ml (½ tsp) q4–6h **Child (6–12 yr):** 5 ml (1 tsp) q4–6h
TUSSAR-2 (Rorer) Codeine phosphate, carbetapentane citrate, chlorpheniramine maleate, guaifenesin, sodium citrate, and citric acid *C-V*	**Syrup (per 5 ml):** 10 mg codeine phosphate, 7.5 mg carbetapentane citrate, 2 mg chlorpheniramine maleate, 50 mg guaifenesin, 130 mg sodium citrate, and 20 mg citric acid (1 pt)	**Adult:** 5 ml (1 tsp) tid or qid, as needed, up to 40 ml (8 tsp)/24 h
TUSSAR SF (Rorer) Codeine phosphate, carbetapentane citrate, chlorpheniramine maleate, guaifenesin, sodium citrate, and citric acid *C-V*	**Syrup (per 5 ml):** 10 mg codeine phosphate, 7.5 mg carbetapentane citrate, 2 mg chlorpheniramine maleate, 50 mg guaifenesin, 130 mg sodium citrate, and 20 mg citric acid (1 pt) *sugar-free*	**Adult:** 5 ml (1 tsp) tid or qid, as needed, up to 40 ml (8 tsp)/24 h
UNPROCO (Reid-Rowell) Dextromethorphan hydrobromide and guaifenesin *Rx*	**Capsules:** 30 mg dextromethorphan hydrobromide and 200 mg guaifenesin	**Adult:** 1 cap q4h

[1] Where pediatric dosages are not given, consult manufacturer

OTHER DECONGESTANTS/UPPER RESPIRATORY COMBINATIONS

DRUG	HOW SUPPLIED	USUAL DOSAGE[1]
DISOPHROL (Schering) Dexbrompheniramine maleate and pseudoephedrine sulfate *OTC*	**Tablets:** 2 mg dexbrompheniramine maleate and 60 mg pseudoephedrine sulfate **Tablets (sustained release):** 6 mg dexbrompheniramine maleate and 120 mg pseudoephedrine sulfate	**Adult:** 1 tab q4–6h, up to 4 tabs/24 h or 1 sustained-release tab q12h **Child (6–11 yr):** ½ tab q4–6h, up to 2 tabs/24 h **Child (≥ 12 yr):** same as adult
FEDAHIST (Rorer) Pseudoephedrine hydrochloride and chlorpheniramine maleate *Rx*	**Capsules (timed-release):** 65 mg pseudoephedrine hydrochloride and 10 mg chlorpheniramine maleate **Tablets:** 60 mg pseudoephedrine hydrochloride and 4 mg chlorpheniramine maleate **Syrup (per 5 ml):** 30 mg pseudoephedrine hydrochloride and 2 mg chlorpheniramine maleate (4 fl oz) *grape flavored*	**Adult and child (> 12 yr):** 1 cap bid, 1 tab q6h, or 10 ml (2 tsp) q6h **Child (6–12 yr):** ½ tab or 5 ml (1 tsp) q6h
HISTABID (Glaxo) Phenylpropanolamine hydrochloride and chlorpheniramine maleate *Rx*	**Capsules (sustained release):** 75 mg phenylpropanolamine hydrochloride and 8 mg chlorpheniramine maleate	**Adult:** 1 cap q12h
HISTALET (Reid-Rowell) Chlorpheniramine maleate and pseudoephedrine hydrochloride *Rx*	**Syrup (per 5 ml):** 3 mg chlorpheniramine maleate and 45 mg pseudoephedrine hydrochloride (1 pt)	**Adult:** 10 ml (2 tsp) qid **Child (2–6 yr):** 2.5 ml (½ tsp) qid **Child (6–12 yr):** 5 ml (1 tsp) qid
HISTALET Forte (Reid-Rowell) Phenylpropanolamine hydrochloride, pyrilamine maleate, chlorpheniramine maleate, and phenylephrine hydrochloride *Rx*	**Tablets:** 50 mg phenylpropanolamine hydrochloride, 25 mg pyrilamine maleate, 4 mg chlorpheniramine maleate, and 10 mg phenylephrine hydrochloride	**Adult:** 1 tab bid or tid **Child (6–12 yr):** ½ tab bid or tid

[1] Where pediatric dosages are not given, consult manufacturer

OTHER DECONGESTANTS/UPPER RESPIRATORY COMBINATIONS continued

DRUG	HOW SUPPLIED	USUAL DOSAGE[1]
HISTALET X (Reid-Rowell) Pseudoephedrine hydrochloride and guaifenesin *Rx*	**Tablets:** 120 mg pseudoephedrine hydrochloride and 400 mg guaifenesin **Syrup (per 5 ml):** 45 mg pseudoephedrine hydrochloride and 200 mg guaifenesin (1 pt)	**Adult:** 1 tab q12h or 10 ml (2 tsp) qid **Child (2–6 yr):** 2.5 ml (½ tsp) qid **Child (6–12 yr):** ½ tab q12h or 5 ml (1 tsp) qid **Child (> 12 yr):** same as adult
HISTASPAN-D (Rorer) Chlorpheniramine maleate, phenylephrine hydrochloride, and methscopolamine nitrate *Rx*	**Capsules (sustained release):** 8 mg chlorpheniramine maleate, 20 mg phenylephrine hydrochloride, and 2.5 mg methscopolamine nitrate	**Adult:** 1 cap q12h **Child (> 12 yr):** same as adult
HISTASPAN-Plus (Rorer) Chlorpheniramine maleate and phenylephrine hydrochloride *Rx*	**Capsules (sustained release):** 8 mg chlorpheniramine maleate and 20 mg phenylephrine hydrochloride	**Adult and child (> 12 yr):** 1 cap q12h
ISOCLOR (Fisons) Chlorpheniramine maleate and pseudoephedrine hydrochloride *Rx*	**Capsules (sustained release):** 8 mg chlorpheniramine maleate and 120 mg pseudoephedrine hydrochloride **Tablets:** 4 mg chlorpheniramine maleate and 60 mg pseudoephedrine hydrochloride **Liquid (per 5 ml):** 2 mg chlorpheniramine maleate and 30 mg pseudoephedrine hydrochloride (1, 16 fl oz) *grape flavored*	**Adult:** 1 tab or 10 ml (2 tsp) tid or qid or 1 cap q12h **Child (15–20 lb):** 0.63–1.25 ml (⅛–¼ tsp) tid or qid **Child (20–30 lb):** 1.25–2.5 ml (¼–½ tsp) tid or qid **Child (30–40 lb):** 2.5–3.75 ml (½–¾ tsp) tid or qid **Child (40–50 lb):** 3.75–5 ml (¾–1 tsp) tid or qid **Child (6–12 yr):** 5 ml (1 tsp) tid or qid
NEOTEP (Reid-Rowell) Phenylephrine hydrochloride and chlorpheniramine maleate *Rx*	**Capsules (sustained release):** 21 mg phenylephrine hydrochloride and 9 mg chlorpheniramine maleate	**Adult:** 1 cap q12h
NOLAMINE (Carnrick) Phenindamine tartrate, chlorpheniramine maleate, and phenylpropanolamine hydrochloride *Rx*	**Tablets (timed-release):** 24 mg phenindamine tartrate, 4 mg chlorpheniramine maleate, and 50 mg phenylpropanolamine hydrochloride	**Adult:** 1 tab q8h; for mild cases, 1 tab q10–12h
PHENERGAN-D (Wyeth) Pseudoephedrine hydrochloride and promethazine hydrochloride *Rx*	**Tablets:** 60 mg pseudoephedrine hydrochloride and 6.25 mg promethazine hydrochloride	**Adult:** 1 tab tid or qid, as needed **Child (> 12 yr):** same as adult
POLARAMINE Expectorant (Schering) Dexchlorpheniramine maleate, pseudoephedrine sulfate, and guaifenesin *Rx*	**Syrup (per 5 ml):** 2 mg dexchlorpheniramine maleate, 20 mg pseudoephedrine sulfate, and 100 mg guaifenesin (1 pt)	**Adult:** 5–10 ml (1–2 tsp) tid or qid **Child (2–5 yr):** 1.25–2.5 ml (¼–½ tsp) tid or qid **Child (6–11 yr):** 2.5–5 ml (½–1 tsp) tid or qid
RHINEX D•LAY (Lemmon) Phenylpropanolamine hydrochloride, chlorpheniramine maleate, acetaminophen, and salicylamide *Rx*	**Tablets:** 60 mg phenylpropanolamine hydrochloride, 4 mg chlorpheniramine maleate, 300 mg acetaminophen, and 300 mg salicylamide	**Adult:** 1 tab bid
RU-TUSS with Hydrocodone (Boots) Hydrocodone bitartrate, phenylephrine hydrochloride, phenylpropanolamine hydrochloride, pheniramine maleate, and pyrilamine maleate *Rx*	**Liquid (per 5 ml):** 1.7 mg hydrocodone bitartrate, 5 mg phenylephrine hydrochloride, 3.3 mg phenylpropanolamine hydrochloride, 3.3 mg pheniramine maleate, and 3.3 mg pyrilamine maleate (16 fl oz)	**Adult:** 10 ml (2 tsp) q4–6h **Child (2–6 yr):** 2.5–5 ml (½–1 tsp) q4–6h, up to 5 doses/24 h; adjust dose according to age **Child (6–12 yr):** 5 ml (1 tsp) q4–6h, up to 5 doses/24 h
RYNATAN (Wallace) Phenylephrine tannate, chlorpheniramine tannate, and pyrilamine tannate *Rx*	**Tablets:** 25 mg phenylephrine tannate, 8 mg chlorpheniramine tannate, and 25 mg pyrilamine tannate **Pediatric suspension (per 5 ml):** 5 mg phenylephrine tannate, 2 mg chlorpheniramine tannate, and 12.5 mg pyrilamine tannate (1 pt) *strawberry/currant flavored*	**Adult:** 1–2 tabs q12h **Child (< 2 yr):** titrate dose individually **Child (2–6 yr):** 2.5–5 ml (½–1 tsp) q12h **Child (6–12 yr):** 5–10 ml (1–2 tsp) q12h
TRIPHED (Lemmon) Pseudoephedrine hydrochloride and triprolidine hydrochloride *Rx*	**Capsules (sustained release):** 60 mg pseudoephedrine hydrochloride and 2.5 mg triprolidine hydrochloride	**Adult:** 1 cap q4–8h

[1] Where pediatric dosages are not given, consult manufacturer

continued

OTHER DECONGESTANTS/UPPER RESPIRATORY COMBINATIONS continued

DRUG	HOW SUPPLIED	USUAL DOSAGE[1]
TYZINE (Key) Tetrahydrozoline hydrochloride *Rx*	**Nasal solution:** 0.1% (15, 30 ml; 1 pt) **Pediatric nasal drops:** 0.05% (15 ml)	**Adult:** 2–4 drops (0.1%) in each nostril, as needed, not more than every 3 h **Child (2–6 yr):** 2–3 drops (0.05%) in each nostril, as needed, not more than every 3 h **Child (> 6 yr):** same as adult

[1] Where pediatric dosages are not given, consult manufacturer

OTHER EXPECTORANTS/EXPECTORANT COMBINATIONS

DRUG	HOW SUPPLIED	USUAL DOSAGE[1]
NORISODRINE with Calcium Iodide (Abbott) Isoproterenol sulfate and calcium iodide *Rx*	**Syrup (per 5 ml):** 3 mg isoproterenol sulfate, 150 mg calcium iodide, and 6% alcohol (1 pt)	**Adult and child (> 10 yr):** 5–10 ml (1–2 tsp) to start, followed by 5–10 ml (1–2 tsp) q4–6h, as needed **Child (< 3 yr):** 2.5 ml (½ tsp) to start, followed by 2.5 ml (½ tsp) q4–6h, as needed **Child (3–10 yr):** 2.5–5 ml (½–1 tsp) to start, followed by 2.5–5 ml (½–1 tsp) q4–6h, as needed
Potassium iodide *Rx*	**Tablets (enteric coated):** 300 mg **Liquid (per 15 ml):** 500 mg (15, 500 ml; 1 pt) **Solution:** 1 g/ml (30, 240 ml; 1 pt)	**Adult:** 300–600 mg tid or qid, as needed
P-V-TUSSIN Syrup (Reid-Rowell) Hydrocodone bitartrate, phenylephrine hydrochloride, pyrilamine maleate, chlorpheniramine maleate, phenindamine tartrate, and ammonium chloride *C-III*	**Syrup (per 5 ml):** 2.5 mg hydrocodone bitartrate, 5 mg phenylephrine hydrochloride, 6 mg pyrilamine maleate, 2 mg chlorpheniramine maleate, 5 mg phenindamine tartrate, and 50 mg ammonium chloride (4, 16 fl oz; 1 gal)	**Adult:** 10 ml (2 tsp) q4–6h, up to 4 doses/24 h **Child (1–3 yr):** 2.5 ml (½ tsp) q4–6h, up to 4 doses/24 h **Child (3–6 yr):** 2.5–5 ml (½–1 tsp) q4–6h, up to 4 doses/24 h **Child (6–12 yr):** 5 ml (1 tsp) q4–6h, up to 4 doses/24 h
P-V-TUSSIN Tablets (Reid-Rowell) Hydrocodone bitartrate, phenindamine tartrate, and guaifenesin *C-III*	**Tablets:** 5 mg hydrocodone bitartrate, 25 mg phenindamine tartrate, and 200 mg guaifenesin	**Adult:** 1 tab qid after meals and at bedtime, not more than q4h **Child (6–12 yr):** ½ tab qid after meals and at bedtime, not more than q4h

[1] Where pediatric dosages are not given, consult manufacturer

Composition of Cough/Cold and Other Upper Respiratory Medications

Key: X = present in preparation N = narcotic antitussive
AC = acetaminophen AS = aspirin

	Antihistamine	Antitussive	Decongestant	Expectorant	Analgesic/Antipyretic	Alcohol Content of Liquids and Syrups
ACTIFED Capsules, Tablets, and Syrup (Burroughs Wellcome) OTC	X		X			0%
ACTIFED with Codeine Syrup (Burroughs Wellcome) C-V	X	N	X			4.3%
ACTOL Expectorant Tablets and Syrup (Beecham) OTC		X		X		12.5%
AFRIN Nasal Spray and Drops (Schering) OTC			X			
AFRINOL Tablets (Schering) OTC			X			
ALCONEFRIN Solution (Webcon) OTC			X			
ALKA-SELTZER PLUS Tablets (Miles Laboratories) OTC	X		X		AS	
ALLEREST Capsules, Tablets, and Liquid (Pharmacraft) OTC	X		X			0%
ALLEREST Headache Strength and Sinus Pain Tablets (Pharmacraft) OTC	X		X		AC	
ALLEREST Nasal Spray (Pharmacraft) OTC			X			
AMBENYL Syrup (Forest) C-V	X	N				5%
AMBENYL-D Liquid (Forest) OTC		X	X	X		9.5%
A.R.M. Tablets (SmithKline Consumer Products) OTC	X		X			
BAYER Children's Cold Tablets (Glenbrook) OTC			X		AS	
BAYER Children's Cough Syrup (Glenbrook) OTC		X	X			5%
BENADRYL Decongestant Capsules and Elixir (Warner-Lambert) OTC	X	X	X			5%
BENYLIN Decongestant Liquid (Warner-Lambert) OTC	X		X			5%
BENYLIN Syrup (Warner-Lambert) OTC	X			X		5%
BENYLIN DM Syrup (Warner-Lambert) OTC		X		X		5%
BENYLIN DME Liquid (Warner-Lambert) OTC		X		X		5%
BENZEDREX Inhaler (SmithKline Consumer Products) OTC			X			
BQ Cold Tablets (Bristol-Myers) OTC	X		X		AC	
BREONESIN Capsules (Winthrop Consumer Products) OTC sugar-free				X		
CALCIDRINE Syrup (Abbott) C-V		N		X		6%
CEROSE-DM Expectorant (Wyeth) OTC	X	X	X			0%
CHERACOL Syrup (Upjohn) C-V		N		X		4.75%
CHERACOL D Syrup (Upjohn) OTC		X		X		4.75%
CHERACOL PLUS Syrup (Upjohn) OTC	X	X	X			8%
CHEXIT Tablets (Sandoz Consumer Health Care Group) OTC	X	X	X	X	AC	
CHLOR-TRIMETON Decongestant Tablets (Schering) OTC	X		X			
COLREX Capsules (Reid-Rowell) OTC	X		X		AC	
COLREX Compound Capsules (Reid-Rowell) C-III	X	X	X		AC	
COLREX Compound Elixir (Reid-Rowell) C-V sugar free	X	N	X		AC	9.5%
COLREX Expectorant (Reid-Rowell) OTC sugar-free				X		4.7%
COLREX Syrup (Reid-Rowell) OTC sugar-free	X	X	X			4.5%

continued

COMPENDIUM OF DRUG THERAPY

Composition of Cough/Cold and Other Upper Respiratory Medications continued

Key: X = present in preparation   N = narcotic antitussive
AC = acetaminophen   AS = aspirin

	Antihistamine	Antitussive	Decongestant	Expectorant	Analgesic/Antipyretic	Alcohol Content of Liquids and Syrups
COMHIST Tablets (Norwich Eaton) *Rx*	X		X			
COMHIST LA Capsules (Norwich Eaton) *Rx*	X		X			
COMTREX Caplets, Tablets, and Liquid (Bristol-Myers) *OTC*	X	X	X		AC	20%
COMTREX A/S Tablets (Bristol-Myers) *OTC*	X		X		AC	
CONAR Expectorant (Beecham) *OTC*		X	X	X		0%
CONAR Syrup (Beecham) *OTC sugar-free*		X	X			0%
CONAR-A Tablets (Beecham) *OTC*		X	X	X	AC	
CONEX Syrup (Forest) *OTC*			X	X		0%
CONEX with Codeine Syrup (Forest) *C-V*		N	X	X		0%
CONGESPIRIN Aspirin Free Chewable Tablets (Bristol-Myers) *OTC*			X		AC	
CONGESPIRIN Chewable Tablets (Bristol-Myers) *OTC*			X		AS	
CONGESPIRIN Liquid (Bristol-Myers) *OTC*			X		AC	10%
CONGESPIRIN Syrup (Bristol-Myers) *OTC*		X				0%
CONGESTAC Tablets (SmithKline Consumer Products) *OTC*			X	X		
CONTAC Caplets and Capsules (SmithKline Consumer Products) *OTC*	X		X			
CONTAC Jr. Liquid (SmithKline Consumer Products) *OTC*		X	X		AC	0%
CONTAC Severe Cold Formula Caplets (SmithKline Consumer Products) *OTC*	X		X		AC	
CONTAC Severe Cold Formula Night Strength Liquid (SmithKline Consumer Products) *OTC*	X	X	X		AC	25%
COPAVIN Capsules (Lilly) *C-III*		N				
CO-PYRONIL 2 Capsules and Suspension (Dista) *OTC*	X		X			0%
CORICIDIN Demilets Tablets for Children (Schering) *OTC*	X		X		AC	
CORICIDIN Nasal Mist (Schering) *OTC*			X			
CORICIDIN Sinus Headache Tablets (Schering) *OTC*	X		X		AC	
CORICIDIN Syrup (Schering) *OTC*		X	X	X		<0.5%
CORICIDIN Tablets (Schering) *OTC*	X				AC	
CORICIDIN 'D' Tablets (Schering) *OTC*	X		X		AC	
CORILIN Infant Drops (Schering) *Rx Also contains sodium salicylate*	X					<1%
CORYBAN-D Capsules (Leeming) *OTC Also contains caffeine*	X		X			
CORYBAN-D Syrup (Leeming) *OTC*		X	X	X	AC	7.5%
Children's CoTYLENOL Chewable Tablets and Liquid (McNeil Consumer Products) *OTC*	X		X		AC	0%
CoTYLENOL Caplets and Liquid (McNeil Consumer Products) *OTC*	X	X	X		AC	7%
COVANGESIC Tablets (Wallace) *OTC*			X		AC	
CREMACOAT 1 Liquid (Richardson-Vicks Health Care Products) *OTC*		X				0%
CREMACOAT 2 Liquid (Richardson-Vicks Health Care Products) *OTC*				X		0%

continued

Composition of Cough/Cold and Other Upper Respiratory Medications continued

Key: X = present in preparation N = narcotic antitussive
AC = acetaminophen AS = aspirin

	Antihistamine	Antitussive	Decongestant	Expectorant	Analgesic/Antipyretic	Alcohol Content of Liquids and Syrups
CREMACOAT 3 Liquid (Richardson-Vicks Health Care Products) *OTC*		X	X	X		10%
CREMACOAT 4 Liquid (Richardson-Vicks Health Care Products) *OTC*	X	X	X			10%
DAYCARE Capsules and Liquid (Richardson-Vicks Health Care Products) *OTC*		X	X	X	AC	10%
DECONAMINE Tablets and Syrup (Berlex) *Rx*	X		X			0%
DECONAMINE SR Capsules (Berlex) *Rx*	X		X			
DECONGEST Capsules and Tablets (Thompson) *OTC*	X		X			
DELSYM Syrup (McNeil Consumer Products) *OTC*		X				0%
DEMAZIN Tablets and Syrup (Schering) *OTC*	X		X			7.5%
DILAUDID Syrup (Knoll) *C-II*		N		X		5%
DIMACOL Capsules and Liquid (Robins) *OTC*		X	X	X		4.75%
DIMETANE Decongestant Tablets and Elixir (Robins) *OTC*	X		X			2.3%
DIMETANE-DC Syrup (Robins) *C-V*	X	N	X			0.95%
DIMETANE-DX Syrup (Robins) *Rx*	X	X	X			0.95%
DIMETAPP Tablets and Elixir (Robins) *OTC*	X		X			2.3%
DISOPHROL Tablets (Schering) *OTC*	X		X			
DORCOL Pediatric Cough Syrup (Sandoz Consumer Health Care Group) *OTC*		X	X	X		0%
DORCOL Pediatric Decongestant Liquid (Sandoz Consumer Health Care Group) *OTC*			X			0%
DORCOL Pediatric Liquid Cold Formula (Sandoz Consumer Health Care Group) *OTC*	X		X			0%
DRISTAN Caplets and Tablets (Whitehall) *OTC*	X		X		AC	
DRISTAN Cough Formula Liquid (Whitehall) *OTC*	X	X	X	X		12%
DRISTAN 12 Hour Nasal Decongestant Capsules (Whitehall) *OTC*	X		X			
DRISTAN Long Lasting Nasal and Menthol Nasal Spray (Whitehall) *OTC*			X			
DRISTAN Nasal and Menthol Nasal Spray (Whitehall) *OTC*	X		X			0%
DRISTAN-AF Tablets (Whitehall) *OTC* Also contains caffeine	X		X		AC	
DRIXORAL Syrup and Tablets (Schering) *OTC*	X		X			0%
DUADACIN Capsules (Hoechst-Roussel) *OTC*	X		X		AC	
DURATION Mild Solution (Plough) *OTC*			X			
DURATION Nasal Spray (Plough) *OTC*			X			
ENDECON Tablets (Du Pont) *OTC*			X		AC	
ENTEX Capsules and Liquid (Norwich Eaton) *Rx*			X	X		5%
ENTEX LA Tablets (Norwich Eaton) *Rx*			X	X		
FEDAHIST Capsules, Tablets, and Syrup (Kremers-Urban) *Rx*	X		X			0%
FEDAHIST Expectorant (Kremers-Urban) *OTC*	X		X	X		0%
FEDRAZIL Tablets (Burroughs Wellcome) *OTC*	X		X			

continued

Composition of Cough/Cold and Other Upper Respiratory Medications continued

Key: X = present in preparation   N = narcotic antitussive
AC = acetaminophen   AS = aspirin

	Antihistamine	Antitussive	Decongestant	Expectorant	Analgesic/Antipyretic	Alcohol Content of Liquids and Syrups
FIOGESIC Tablets (Sandoz Pharmaceuticals) *OTC*			X		AS	
FORMULA 44 Discs (Richardson-Vicks Health Care Products) *OTC* Also contains a local anesthetic		X				
FORMULA 44 Syrup (Richardson-Vicks Health Care Products) *OTC*	X	X				10%
FORMULA 44D Syrup (Richardson-Vicks Health Care Products) *OTC*		X	X	X		10%
FORMULA 44M Syrup (Richardson-Vicks Health Care Products) *OTC*		X	X	X	AC	20%
HEAD & CHEST Capsules, Tablets, and Liquid (Richardson-Vicks Health Care Products) *OTC*			X	X		5%
HISTADYL and A.S.A. Capsules (Lilly) *OTC*	X				AS	
HISTADYL E.C. Syrup (Lilly) *C-V*	X	N	X			5%
HISTALET Forte Tablets (Reid-Rowell) *Rx*	X		X			
HISTALET Syrup (Reid-Rowell) *Rx*	X		X			0%
HISTALET DM Syrup (Reid-Rowell) *Rx*	X	X	X			0%
HISTALET X Tablets and Syrup (Reid-Rowell) *Rx*			X	X		15%
HISTASPAN-D Capsules (Rorer) *Rx* Also contains an anticholinergic	X		X			
HISTASPAN-Plus Capsules (Rorer) *Rx*	X		X			
HISTATAPP Elixir (Upsher-Smith) *OTC*	X		X			2.3%
Children's HOLD Lozenges (Beecham) *OTC*		X	X			
HOLD Lozenges (Beecham) *OTC*		X				
HYCODAN Tablets and Syrup (Du Pont) *C-III* Also contains an anticholinergic		N				0%
HYCOMINE Compound Tablets (Du Pont) *C-III* Also contains caffeine	X	N	X		AC	
HYCOMINE Syrup and Pediatric Syrup (Du Pont) *C-III*		N	X			0%
HYCOTUSS Expectorant (Du Pont) *C-III*		N		X		10%
ISOCLOR Capsules, Tablets, and Liquid (Fisons) *Rx*	X		X			0%
ISOCLOR Expectorant (Fisons) *C-V*		N	X	X		5%
MEDIQUELL Chewable Squares (Warner-Lambert) *OTC*		X				
MEDIQUELL Decongestant Chewable Squares (Warner-Lambert) *OTC*		X	X			
NALDECON Tablets, Syrup, Pediatric Syrup, and Drops (Bristol) *Rx*	X		X			0%
NALDECON-CX Liquid (Bristol) *C-V*		N	X	X		0%
NALDECON-DX Adult Liquid (Bristol) *OTC*		X	X	X		0%
NALDECON-DX Pediatric Drops (Bristol) *OTC*		X	X	X		0.6%
NALDECON-DX Pediatric Syrup (Bristol) *OTC*		X	X	X		5%
NALDECON-EX Pediatric Drops (Bristol) *OTC*			X	X		0.6%
NALDECON-EX Pediatric Syrup (Bristol) *OTC*			X	X		5%
NALDEGESIC Tablets (Bristol) *OTC*			X		AC	
NEO-SYNEPHRINE Nasal Spray, Drops, and Jelly (Winthrop Consumer Products) *OTC*			X			

continued

Composition of Cough/Cold and Other Upper Respiratory Medications continued

Key: X = present in preparation   N = narcotic antitussive
AC = acetaminophen   AS = aspirin

	Antihistamine	Antitussive	Decongestant	Expectorant	Analgesic/Antipyretic	Alcohol Content of Liquids and Syrups
NEO-SYNEPHRINE II Long-Acting Nasal Spray and Drops (Winthrop Consumer Products) *OTC*			X			
NEOTEP Capsules (Reid-Rowell) *Rx*	X		X			
NOLAMINE Tablets (Carnrick) *Rx*	X		X			
NORISODRINE with Calcium Iodide Syrup (Abbott) *Rx* Also contains a bronchodilator				X		6%
NŌSTRIL Nasal Spray (Boehringer Ingelheim) *OTC*			X			
NŌSTRILLA Long Acting Nasal Spray (Boehringer Ingelheim) *OTC*			X			
NOVAFED Capsules (Merrell Dow) *Rx*			X			
NOVAFED Liquid (Merrell Dow) *OTC*			X			7.5%
NOVAFED A Capsules (Merrell Dow) *Rx*	X		X			
NOVAFED A Liquid (Merrell Dow) *OTC*	X		X			5%
NOVAHISTINE Cough Liquid (Lakeside) *OTC*		X		X		7.5%
NOVAHISTINE Cough & Cold Liquid (Lakeside) *OTC*	X	X	X			5%
NOVAHISTINE Elixir (Lakeside) *OTC*	X		X			5%
NOVAHISTINE Expectorant (Lakeside) *C-V*		N	X	X		7.5%
NOVAHISTINE DH Liquid (Lakeside) *C-V*	X	N	X			5%
NOVAHISTINE DMX Liquid (Lakeside) *OTC*		X	X	X		10%
NTZ Nasal Spray and Drops (Winthrop Consumer Products) *OTC*			X			
NUCOFED Capsules and Syrup (Beecham) *C-III*		N	X			0%
NUCOFED Expectorant (Beecham) *C-III*		N	X	X		12.5%
NUCOFED Pediatric Expectorant (Beecham) *C-V*		N	X	X		6%
NYQUIL Liquid (Richardson-Vicks Health Care Products) *OTC*	X	X	X		AC	25%
ORGANIDIN Elixir (Wallace) *Rx*				X		21.75%
ORGANIDIN Tablets and Solution (Wallace) *Rx*				X		0%
ORNADE Capsules (Smith Kline & French) *Rx*	X		X			
ORNEX Caplets (SmithKline Consumer Products) *OTC*			X		AC	
ORTHOXICOL Syrup (Upjohn) *OTC*		X	X			0%
OTRIVIN Nasal Spray and Drops (CIBA Consumer) *OTC*			X			
PEDIACARE Infants' Oral Drops (McNeil Consumer Products) *OTC*			X			0%
PEDIACARE 1 Liquid (McNeil Consumer Products) *OTC*		X				0%
PEDIACARE 2 Liquid (McNeil Consumer Products) *OTC*	X		X			0%
PEDIACARE 3 Chewable Tablets and Liquid (McNeil Consumer Products) *OTC*	X	X	X			0%
PEDIACOF Syrup (Winthrop-Breon) *C-V*	X	N	X	X		5%
PENNTUSS Liquid (Pennwalt) *C-V*	X	N				0%
PERTUSSIN AM Liquid (Canaan) *OTC*	X	X	X			9.5%

continued

COMPENDIUM OF DRUG THERAPY

Composition of Cough/Cold and Other Upper Respiratory Medications continued

Key: X = present in preparation   N = narcotic antitussive
AC = acetaminophen   AS = aspirin

	Antihistamine	Antitussive	Decongestant	Expectorant	Analgesic/Antipyretic	Alcohol Content of Liquids and Syrups
PERTUSSIN CS Liquid (Canaan) *OTC*		X		X		8.5%
PERTUSSIN ES Liquid (Canaan) *OTC*		X				9.5%
PERTUSSIN PM Liquid (Canaan) *OTC*	X	X	X		AC	25%
PHENERGAN VC Syrup (Wyeth) *Rx*	X		X			7%
PHENERGAN VC with Codeine Syrup (Wyeth) *C-V*	X	N	X			7%
PHENERGAN with Codeine Syrup (Wyeth) *C-V*	X	N				7%
PHENERGAN with Dextromethorphan Syrup (Wyeth) *Rx*	X	X				7%
PHENERGAN-D Tablets (Wyeth) *Rx*	X		X			
POLARAMINE Expectorant (Schering) *Rx*	X		X	X		7.2%
PRIVINE Nasal Drops and Spray (CIBA) *OTC*			X			
PROPAGEST Tablets (Carnrick) *OTC*			X			
PRUNICODEINE Liquid (Lilly) *C-V*		N		X		25%
P-V-TUSSIN Syrup (Reid-Rowell) *C-III*	X	N	X	X		5%
P-V-TUSSIN Tablets (Reid-Rowell) *C-III*	X	N		X		
PYRROXATE Capsules (Upjohn) *OTC*	X		X		AC	
QUELIDRINE Syrup (Abbott) *OTC*	X	X	X	X		2%
QUELTUSS Tablets (Forest) *OTC*		X		X		
RHINEX D·LAY Tablets (Lemmon) *Rx* Also contains salicylamide	X		X		AC	
ROBITUSSIN NIGHT RELIEF Liquid (Robins) *OTC*	X	X	X		AC	25%
ROBITUSSIN Syrup (Robins) *OTC*				X		3.5%
ROBITUSSIN A-C Syrup (Robins) *C-V*		N		X		3.5%
ROBITUSSIN-CF Liquid (Robins) *OTC*		X	X	X		4.75%
ROBITUSSIN-DAC Syrup (Robins) *C-V*		N	X	X		1.4%
ROBITUSSIN-DM Liquid and Lozenges (Robins) *OTC*		X		X		1.4%
ROBITUSSIN-PE Liquid (Robins) *OTC*			X	X		1.4%
RONDEC Tablets, Syrup, and Drops (Ross) *Rx*	X		X			0%
RONDEC-DM Syrup and Drops (Ross) *Rx*	X	X	X			<0.6%
RONDEC-TR Tablets (Ross) *Rx*	X		X			
RU-TUSS Expectorant (Boots) *C-V*		X	X	X		10%
RU-TUSS Liquid (Boots) *OTC*	X		X			5%
RU-TUSS Tablets (Boots) *Rx* Also contains an anticholinergic	X		X			
RU-TUSS with Hydrocodone Liquid (Boots) *C-III*	X	N	X			5%
RU-TUSS II Capsules (Boots) *Rx*	X		X			
RYNA Liquid (Wallace) *OTC* sugar-free	X		X			0%
RYNA-C Liquid (Wallace) *C-V* sugar-free	X	N	X			0%

continued

Composition of Cough/Cold and Other Upper Respiratory Medications continued

Key: X = present in preparation N = narcotic antitussive
AC = acetaminophen AS = aspirin

Product		Antihistamine	Antitussive	Decongestant	Expectorant	Analgesic/Antipyretic	Alcohol Content of Liquids and Syrups
RYNA-CX Liquid (Wallace) *C-V sugar-free*			N	X	X		0%
RYNATAN Tablets and Pediatric Suspension (Wallace) *Rx*		X		X			0%
RYNATUSS Tablets and Pediatric Suspension (Wallace) *Rx*	Also contains a bronchodilator	X	X	X			0%
SINAREST Nasal Spray (Pharmacraft) *OTC*				X			
SINAREST Tablets (Pharmacraft) *OTC*		X		X		AC	
SINE-AID Caplets and Tablets (McNeil Consumer Products) *OTC*				X		AC	
SINE-OFF Caplets (SmithKline Consumer Products) *OTC*		X		X		AC	
SINE-OFF No Drowsiness Caplets (SmithKline Consumer Products) *OTC*				X		AC	
SINE-OFF Tablets (SmithKline Consumer Products) *OTC*		X		X		AS	
SINEX Nasal Spray (Richardson-Vicks Health Care Products) *OTC*				X			
SINGLET Tablets (Lakeside) *OTC*		X		X		AC	
SINUBID Tablets (Parke-Davis) *Rx*		X		X		AC	
SINULIN Tablets (Carnrick) *OTC Also contains salicylamide and an anticholingergic*		X		X		AC	
SINUTAB Capsules and Tablets (Warner-Lambert) *OTC*		X		X		AC	
SINUTAB II No Drowsiness Capsules and Tablets (Warner-Lambert) *OTC*				X		AC	
SPEC-T Sore Throat/Cough Suppressant Lozenges (Squibb) *OTC*	Also contains a local anesthetic		X				
SPEC-T Sore Throat/Decongestant Lozenges (Squibb) *OTC*	Also contains a local anesthetic			X			
ST. JOSEPH Cold Tablets for Children (Plough) *OTC*				X		AS	
ST. JOSEPH Cough Syrup for Children (Plough) *OTC*			X				0%
SUCRETS Cold Decongestant Lozenges (Beecham) *OTC*				X			
SUCRETS Cough Control Lozenges (Beecham) *OTC*			X				
SUDAFED Capsules, Tablets, and Liquid (Burroughs Wellcome) *OTC*				X			0%
SUDAFED Cough Syrup (Burroughs Wellcome) *OTC*			X	X	X		2.4%
SUDAFED Plus Tablets and Liquid (Burroughs Wellcome) *OTC*		X		X			0%
SUDAFED S.A. Capsules (Burroughs Wellcome) *OTC*				X			
TAVIST-D Tablets (Sandoz Pharmaceuticals) *Rx*		X		X			
Terpin hydrate with codeine elixir (various manufacturers) *C-V*			N		X		40%
Terpin hydrate with dextromethorphan elixir (various manufacturers) *OTC*			X		X		41%
TESSALON Capsules (Du Pont) *Rx*			X				
TRIAMINIC Allergy Tablets, Chewable Tablets, Cold Tablets, and Cold Syrup (Sandoz Consumer Health Care Group) *OTC*		X		X			0%
TRIAMINIC Expectorant (Sandoz Consumer Health Care Group) *OTC*				X	X		5%
TRIAMINIC Expectorant DH (Sandoz Consumer Health Care Group) *C-III*		X	X		X		5%
TRIAMINIC Expectorant with Codeine (Sandoz Consumer Health Care Group) *C-V*			N	X	X		5%
TRIAMINIC Drops (Sandoz Consumer Health Care Group) *Rx*		X		X			0%

continued

Composition of Cough/Cold and Other Upper Respiratory Medications continued

Key: X = present in preparation   N = narcotic antitussive
AC = acetaminophen   AS = aspirin

Medication	Antihistamine	Antitussive	Decongestant	Expectorant	Analgesic/Antipyretic	Alcohol Content of Liquids and Syrups
TRIAMINIC TR Tablets (Sandoz Consumer Health Care Group) Rx	X		X			
TRIAMINIC-12 Tablets (Sandoz Consumer Health Care Group) OTC	X		X			
TRIAMINIC-DM Liquid (Sandoz Consumer Health Care Group) OTC		X	X			0%
TRIAMINICIN Tablets (Sandoz Consumer Health Care Group) OTC	X		X		AC	
TRIAMINICOL Tablets and Syrup (Sandoz Consumer Health Care Group) OTC	X	X	X			0%
TRINALIN Tablets (Schering) Rx	X		X			
TRIND Liquid (Mead Johnson) OTC sugar-free	X		X			5%
TRIND-DM Liquid (Mead Johnson) OTC sugar-free	X	X	X			5%
TRIPHED Tablets (Lemmon) Rx	X		X			
TUSSAGESIC Tablets (Sandoz Consumer Health Care Group) OTC	X	X	X	X	AC	
TUSSAR DM Cough Syrup (Rorer) OTC	X	X	X			0%
TUSSAR SF Cough Syrup (Rorer) C-V sugar-free	X	N		X		12%
TUSSAR-2 Cough Syrup (Rorer) C-V	X	N		X		5%
TUSSEND Expectorant (Merrell Dow) C-III		N	X	X		12.5%
TUSSEND Tablets and Liquid (Merrell Dow) C-III		N	X			5%
TUSSIONEX Capsules, Tablets, and Suspension (Pennwalt) C-III	X	N				0.59%
TUSSI-ORGANIDIN Liquid (Wallace) C-V sugar-free		N		X		0%
TUSSI-ORGANIDIN DM Liquid (Wallace) Rx sugar-free		X		X		0%
TUSS-ORNADE Capsules and Liquid (Smith Kline & French) Rx sugar-free		X	X			5%
TYLENOL Sinus Caplets and Tablets (McNeil Consumer Products) OTC			X		AC	
TYZINE Nasal Drops (Key) Rx			X			
UNPROCO Capsules (Reid-Rowell) Rx		X		X		
URSINUS Tablets (Sandoz Consumer Health Care Group) OTC			X		AS	
VATRONOL Nose Drops (Richardson-Vicks Health Care Products) OTC			X			
VICKS Children's Cough Syrup (Richardson-Vicks Health Care Products) OTC		X		X		0%
VICKS Cough Silencers Lozenges (Richardson-Vicks Health Care Products) OTC Also contains a local anesthetic		X				
VICKS Inhaler (Richardson-Vicks Health Care Products) OTC			X			
VICKS Syrup (Richardson-Vicks Health Care Products) OTC		X		X		5%
VIRO-MED Liquid (Whitehall) OTC		X	X		AC	16.6%
VIRO-MED Tablets (Whitehall) OTC	X	X	X		AC	
4-WAY Cold Tablets (Bristol-Myers) OTC	X		X		AS	
4-WAY Long Acting Nasal Spray (Bristol-Myers) OTC			X			
4-WAY Nasal Spray (Bristol-Myers) OTC	X		X			

ANTITUSSIVES

TESSALON (benzonatate) Du Pont Rx
Capsules: 100 mg

INDICATIONS	**ORAL DOSAGE**
Cough	Adult and child ($>$ 10 yr): 100 mg tid, as needed; maximum dosage: 600 mg/day

CONTRAINDICATIONS

Hypersensitivity to benzonatate or related compounds

WARNINGS/PRECAUTIONS

Oropharyngeal anesthesia	If capsules are chewed or dissolved in the mouth, benzonatate will be released and transient oropharyngeal anesthesia and choking may occur; instruct patients to swallow capsules whole, without chewing them
Carcinogenicity, mutagenicity, effect on fertility	No studies have been conducted to determine the carcinogenic or mutagenic potential of benzonatate or its effect on fertility

ADVERSE REACTIONS

Central nervous system	Sedation, headache, mild dizziness
Gastrointestinal	Constipation, nausea, GI upset
Dermatological	Pruritus, skin eruptions
Other	Nasal congestion, burning in the eyes, vague "chilly" sensation, numbness in the chest, hypersensitivity reactions

OVERDOSAGE

Signs and symptoms	Restlessness and tremors progressing to clonic convulsions and profound postictal depression
Treatment	Induce emesis or perform gastric lavage; then administer copious amounts of activated charcoal as a slurry. Bear in mind that the gag reflex may be so depressed, even in conscious patients, that special measures to prevent aspiration may be necessary. Treat convulsions with a short-acting IV barbiturate. For severe intoxication, provide intensive support of respiratory, cardiovascular, and renal functions. Do not administer CNS stimulants.

ALTERED LABORATORY VALUES

No clinically significant alterations in blood/serum or urinary values occur at therapeutic dosages

DRUG INTERACTIONS

No clinically significant drug interactions have been identified

---

USE IN CHILDREN	**USE IN PREGNANT AND NURSING WOMEN**
See INDICATIONS and ORAL DOSAGE	Pregnancy Category C: reproduction studies have not been performed in animals; it is not known whether benzonatate can cause harm to the fetus or affect reproductive capacity. Use during pregnancy only if clearly needed. It is not known whether this drug is excreted in human milk; use with caution in nursing mothers.

ANTITUSSIVE COMBINATIONS

ACTIFED with Codeine (triprolidine hydrochloride, pseudoephedrine hydrochloride, and codeine phosphate) Burroughs Wellcome C-V

Syrup (per 5 ml): 1.25 mg triprolidine hydrochloride, 30 mg pseudoephedrine hydrochloride, and 10 mg codeine phosphate (1 pt, 1 gal)

INDICATIONS	**ORAL DOSAGE**
Cough and upper respiratory tract reactions, including nasal congestion, associated with allergy or the common cold	Adult: 10 ml (2 tsp) q4–6h, up to 40 ml/24 h Child (2–6 yr): 2.5 ml (1/2 tsp) q4–6h, up to 10 ml/24 h Child (6–12 yr): 5 ml (1 tsp) q4–6h, up to 20 ml/24 h Child ($\geq$ 12 yr): same as adult

ACTIFED with Codeine

CONTRAINDICATIONS

Severe hypertension	Asthma or other lower respiratory tract conditions	Hypersensitivity to codeine or other narcotic drugs, to triprolidine or other structurally related antihistamines, or to pseudoephedrine or other sympathomimetic amines
Severe coronary artery disease		
Full-term or premature neonate	MAO inhibitor therapy	

WARNINGS/PRECAUTIONS

Drowsiness, dizziness	Caution patients about driving or engaging in other potentially hazardous activities requiring mental alertness
Drug dependence	Psychological dependence, tolerance, and physical dependence may result in rare instances from use at high dosages or for prolonged periods; instruct patients to adhere strictly to the recommended dosage and to use this preparation only for short-term treatment
Patients with head injuries or other intracranial lesions	The respiratory depressant effects of this preparation and its capacity to elevate CSF pressure may be markedly exaggerated in patients with head injuries or other intracranial lesions; side effects may also interfere with the clinical evaluation of head injuries
Patients with acute abdominal conditions	Use of this preparation may obscure the diagnosis or clinical course of acute abdominal conditions
Patients sensitive to sympathomimetic decongestants	Do not administer this preparation to patients who cannot tolerate sympathomimetic decongestants, such as phenylephrine, ephedrine, phenylpropanolamine, and epinephrine; manifestations of intolerance include drowsiness, dizziness, weakness, difficulty in breathing, tenseness, muscle tremors, and palpitations
Elderly patients	Dizziness, sedation, and hypotension are more likely to occur in patients aged 60 yr or more; use with caution in such patients
Other special-risk patients	Use with considerable caution in patients with increased intraocular pressure (narrow angle glaucoma), stenosing peptic ulcer, pyloroduodenal obstruction, symptomatic prostatic hypertrophy, bladder neck obstruction, hypertension, diabetes mellitus, ischemic heart disease, or hyperthyroidism and with caution in debilitated patients and patients with severe renal or hepatic impairment, gallstones or gallbladder disease, respiratory impairment, cardiac arrhythmias, or a history of bronchial asthma, prostatic hypertrophy, urethral stricture, peptic ulcer, or glaucoma
Carcinogenicity, mutagenicity, effect on fertility	No adequate studies have been performed to evaluate the carcinogenic or mutagenic potential of this preparation or its effect on fertility

ADVERSE REACTIONS

The most frequent reactions, regardless of incidence, are printed in *italics*

Central nervous system	*Sedation, sleepiness, dizziness, disturbed coordination,* fatigue, confusion, restlessness, excitation, anxiety, nervousness, tremor, irritability, insomnia, euphoria, paresthesias, blurred vision, diplopia, vertigo, tinnitus, acute labyrinthitis, hysteria, neuritis, convulsions, CNS depression, hallucinations
Cardiovascular	Hypotension, headache, palpitations, tachycardia, extrasystoles
Hematological	Hemolytic anemia, thrombocytopenia, agranulocytosis
Gastrointestinal	Epigastric distress, anorexia, nausea, vomiting, diarrhea, constipation
Genitourinary	Urinary frequency, difficult urination, urinary retention, early menses
Respiratory	Thickening of bronchial secretions, tightness in the chest and wheezing, nasal congestion, respiratory depression
Other	*Dry mouth, nose, and throat;* urticaria, drug rash, anaphylactic shock, photosensitivity, diaphoresis, chills

OVERDOSAGE

Signs and symptoms	*CNS:* depressant effects, including sedation, drowsiness, weariness, somnolence, stupor, diminution or loss of sensation, depressed or absent reflexes with a positive Babinski sign, and coma; stimulative effects, including anxiety, tremor, restlessness, insomnia, nervousness, excitement, euphoria, dizziness, hallucinations, convulsions, and delirium; *respiratory:* hyperpnea, cyanosis, pulmonary edema, hypostatic or aspiration pneumonia, respiratory arrest; *cardiovascular:* tachycardia, hypertension, arrhythmias, pallor, flush, hypotension, circulatory collapse; *dermatological:* pruritus, rash, urticaria, cold and clammy skin; *other:* miosis, mydriasis, urinary retention, dry mouth, vomiting, hyperglycemia, severe hypokalemia. In children, acute overdosage is most likely to result in mydriasis, flush, dry mouth, fever, excitation, hallucinations, ataxia, incoordination, athetosis, and tonic-clonic convulsions with postictal depression.
Treatment	Maintain pulmonary function; if necessary, provide an open airway, institute mechanical ventilation, and give oxygen and naloxone. When overdosage is severe, monitor ECG and serum electrolyte levels, and administer, as needed, propranolol and IV potassium; vasopressors may be used to treat hypotension. To control convulsions, carefully administer IV diazepam or a short-acting barbiturate; physostigmine may also be considered if convulsions are centrally mediated. Treat fever with ice packs and cooling sponge baths, not with alcohol. To prevent coma, provide continuous stimulation that arouses, but does not exhaust, the patient; do not use analeptic drugs. Institute measures to remove this preparation within 4 h after ingestion. Induce vomiting, even if it has occurred spontaneously, or, if vomiting is not possible, perform gastric lavage. To avoid aspiration during lavage, especially when treating children, use a cuffed endotracheal tube, and take other appropriate measures. After emesis or lavage, instill charcoal or another suitable agent; a saline cathartic such as milk of magnesia may also be useful.

ACTIFED with Codeine ■ AMBENYL

DRUG INTERACTIONS

Alcohol, tranquilizers, sedative-hypnotics, and other CNS depressants	⬆ CNS depression; instruct patients requiring this preparation not to use other CNS depressants at the same time
MAO inhibitors	Hypertensive crisis; do not use an MAO inhibitor concomitantly
Guanethidine, methyldopa, reserpine	⬇ Antihypertensive effect

ALTERED LABORATORY VALUES

Blood/serum values	⬆ Amylase ⬆ Lipase

No clinically significant alterations in urinary values occur at therapeutic dosages

USE IN CHILDREN
See INDICATIONS and ORAL DOSAGE; use in full-term or premature neonates is contraindicated

USE IN PREGNANT AND NURSING WOMEN
Pregnancy Category C: no evidence of teratogenicity has been detected in rats given up to 150 times the human dose of pseudoephedrine or in rats and rabbits given up to 125 times the human dose of triprolidine or 150 times the human dose of codeine; fetotoxicity, characterized by decreases in body weight, body length, and rate of skeletal ossification, has been seen in rats at maternally toxic doses of pseudoephedrine. Use this preparation during pregnancy only if clearly needed. Small amounts of pseudoephedrine, triprolidine, and codeine are excreted in human milk; because of the potential for serious adverse reactions in nursing infants, patients should not nurse while taking this preparation.

VEHICLE/BASE
Syrup: 4.3% alcohol, 0.1% sodium benzoate, and 0.1% methylparaben

---

ANTITUSSIVE COMBINATIONS

AMBENYL (bromodiphenhydramine hydrochloride and codeine phosphate) Forest C-V

Syrup (per 5 ml): 12.5 mg bromodiphenhydramine hydrochloride and 10 mg codeine phosphate (4 fl oz, 1 pt, 1 gal)

INDICATIONS	ORAL DOSAGE
Cough and upper respiratory tract reactions associated with allergy or the common cold	**Adult:** 5–10 ml (1–2 tsp) q4–6h **Child (6–12 yr):** 2.5–5 ml (½–1 tsp) q6h (maximum permissible dosage of codeine: 1 mg/kg/24 h)

CONTRAINDICATIONS

Asthma or other lower respiratory tract conditions MAO inhibitor therapy	Full-term or premature neonates Breast-feeding	Hypersensitivity to bromodiphenhydramine or other structurally related antihistamines

WARNINGS/PRECAUTIONS

Drowsiness, dizziness	Caution patients about driving or engaging in other potentially hazardous activities requiring mental alertness
Drug dependence	Psychological dependence, tolerance, and physical dependence may result from repeated use
Elderly patients	Dizziness, sedation, and hypotension are more likely to occur in patients aged 60 yr or more
Other special-risk patients	Use with considerable caution in patients with narrow angle glaucoma, stenosing peptic ulcer, pyloroduodenal obstruction, symptomatic prostatic hypertrophy, or bladder neck obstruction and with caution in patients with increased intraocular pressure, hyperthyroidism, cardiovascular disease (including hypertension), or a history of bronchial asthma

ADVERSE REACTIONS

Central nervous system	Drowsiness, confusion, nervousness, restlessness, blurred vision, diplopia, vertigo, headache, insomnia; tingling, heaviness, and weakness in the hands
Gastrointestinal	Nausea, vomiting, diarrhea, constipation, epigastric distress
Respiratory	Nasal congestion, tightness in the chest and wheezing, thickening of bronchial secretions
Cardiovascular	Palpitations, hypotension
Dermatological	Urticaria, drug rash, photosensitivity

AMBENYL ■ CALCIDRINE

Other — Dry mouth, nose, and throat; difficult urination, hemolytic anemia

OVERDOSAGE

Signs and symptoms — CNS stimulation or depression (stimulative effects, including hallucinations and convulsions, are especially likely to occur in children), hypotension, dry mouth, mydriasis, flushing, GI reactions

Treatment — Vasopressors may be used to treat hypotension; do not use analeptic drugs for CNS depression. To remove this preparation, induce vomiting if it has not already occurred; take measures to prevent aspiration, especially in children. When emesis is not possible, perform gastric lavage with 0.9% or 0.45% saline; lavage should generally be done within 3 h after ingestion but may be delayed until a later time if large amounts of milk or cream have previously been consumed. To hasten elimination of this preparation, use a saline cathartic, such as milk of magnesia.

DRUG INTERACTIONS

Alcohol, tranquilizers, sedative-hypnotics, — △ CNS depression
and other CNS depressants

MAO inhibitors — Hypertension, hypotension, restlessness, convulsions, coma; do not use an MAO inhibitor concomitantly

ALTERED LABORATORY VALUES

No clinically significant alterations in blood/serum or urinary values occur at therapeutic dosages

USE IN CHILDREN

See INDICATIONS and ORAL DOSAGE; use in children under 6 yr of age is not recommended

USE IN PREGNANT AND NURSING WOMEN

It is not known whether this preparation can harm fetal development; use in nursing mothers is contraindicated because of the higher risk of antihistaminic reactions in infants

VEHICLE/BASE
Syrup: 5% alcohol

ANTITUSSIVE COMBINATIONS

CALCIDRINE (codeine and calcium iodide) Abbott   C-V

Syrup (per 5 ml): 8.4 mg codeine and 152 mg calcium iodide[1] (4 fl oz, 1 pt)

INDICATIONS	ORAL DOSAGE
Cough Mucus in respiratory tract	Adult: 5–10 ml (1–2 tsp) q4h Child (2–6 yr): 2.5 ml (1/2 tsp) q4h Child (6–10 yr): 2.5–5 ml (1/2–1 tsp) q4h Child (> 10 yr): same as adult

CONTRAINDICATIONS

| Pregnancy, except for short-term use | History of iodism | Hypersensitivity to iodides or codeine |

WARNINGS/PRECAUTIONS

Drug dependence — Psychic and/or physical dependence and tolerance may develop, especially in addiction-prone individuals

Long-term therapy — Evaluate periodically for possible depression of thyroid function

Severe skin eruptions — May occur on rare occasions with prolonged iodide administration and may be fatal

ADVERSE REACTIONS[2]

Dermatological — Acneform skin lesions (see WARNINGS/PRECAUTIONS)
Gastrointestinal — Nausea, vomiting, constipation, metallic taste, gastric distress
Other — Mucous-membrane irritation, salivary gland swelling

OVERDOSAGE

Signs and symptoms — *Codeine-related effects:* respiratory and CNS depression, miosis, coma, fall in blood pressure, hypothermia; *iodide-related effects:* GI irritation, angioedema with laryngeal swelling, shock

CALCIDRINE ■ DILAUDID Cough Syrup

Treatment	Establish a patent airway and institute artificial respiration, if needed. Empty stomach by inducing emesis or gastric lavage, followed by activated charcoal. Treat for shock. Institute general supportive measures, including replacement of fluids and electrolytes, as indicated. For respiratory depression, administer naloxone (0.4 mg for adults, preferably IV), along with attempts at resuscitation.

DRUG INTERACTIONS

Alcohol, tranquilizers, sedative-hypnotics, and other CNS depressants	⇧ CNS depression
Lithium	⇧ Hypothyroid and goitrogenic effects

ALTERED LABORATORY VALUES

Blood/serum values	⇧ PBI ⇩ ^{131}I thyroid uptake
Urinary values	+ Occult blood (with guaiac and benzidine test methods)

USE IN CHILDREN
See INDICATIONS and ORAL DOSAGE

USE IN PREGNANT AND NURSING WOMEN
Pregnancy Category D: contraindicated for long-term use during pregnancy. This preparation can cause harm to the fetus; maternal ingestion of large amounts of iodides is associated with development of fetal goiter and resultant acute respiratory distress in neonates. Iodine is excreted in breast milk; use with caution in nursing mothers.

[1] Contains 6% alcohol
[2] For other possible side effects, see codeine

ANTITUSSIVE COMBINATIONS

DILAUDID Cough Syrup (hydromorphone hydrochloride and guaifenesin) Knoll   C-II

Syrup (per 5 ml): 1 mg hydromorphone hydrochloride and 100 mg guaifenesin[1] (1 pt) *peach-flavored*

INDICATIONS	ORAL DOSAGE	
Cough	Adult: 5 ml (1 tsp) q3–4h	

CONTRAINDICATIONS		
Depressed ventilatory function (chronic obstructive pulmonary disease, cor pulmonale, emphysema, kyphoscoliosis, status asthmaticus)	Intracranial lesion associated with increased intracranial pressure	Hypersensitivity to either component

WARNINGS/PRECAUTIONS

Drug dependence	Psychic and/or physical dependence and tolerance may develop upon repeated administration; however, psychic dependence is unlikely to occur if the cough syrup is used for a short time
Drowsiness	Caution patients about driving or engaging in other potentially hazardous activities requiring mental alertness or physical coordination; if alcohol or other CNS depressants (see DRUG INTERACTIONS) are used concurrently, the dosage of one or all of the agents should be reduced
Respiratory depression	This preparation produces dose-related respiratory depression and may also cause irregular and periodic breathing
Patients with head injuries, other intracranial lesions, or increased intracranial pressure	The respiratory depressant effects of this drug and its capacity to elevate CSF pressure may be markedly exaggerated in such patients; bear in mind that opioid side effects may also interfere with the clinical evaluation of patients with head injuries
Acute abdominal conditions	Diagnosis or clinical course may be obscured
Special-risk patients	Use with caution in elderly or debilitated patients and in patients with impaired renal or hepatic function, hypothyroidism, Addison's disease, prostatic hypertrophy, or urethral stricture
Cough reflex	Is suppressed; use with caution postoperatively or in patients with pulmonary disease
Tartrazine sensitivity	Presence of FD&C Yellow No. 5 (tartrazine) in syrup may cause allergic-type reactions, including bronchial asthma, in susceptible individuals

DILAUDID Cough Syrup ■ DIMETANE-DC

ADVERSE REACTIONS

Central nervous system	Sedation, drowsiness, mental clouding, lethargy, impairment of mental and physical performance, anxiety, fear, dysphoria, dizziness, psychic dependence, mood changes, respiratory depression
Gastrointestinal	Nausea, vomiting, constipation, increased intraluminal pressure (may endanger surgical anastomosis)
Genitourinary	Ureteral spasm, vesical sphincter spasm, urinary retention

OVERDOSAGE

Signs and symptoms	*Hydromorphone-related effects:* respiratory depression, somnolence, stupor, coma, skeletal-muscle flaccidity, cold and clammy skin, bradycardia, hypotension, and, in severe cases, apnea, circulatory collapse, and cardiac arrest, leading to death
Treatment	Give primary attention to reestablishing adequate respiratory exchange through provision of adequate airway and assisted or controlled ventilation; positive-pressure respiration may be desirable if pulmonary edema is present. If respiratory depression is significant, promptly administer naloxone. For adults, give 0.4–2 mg IV (or, if necessary, IM or SC) at intervals of 2–3 min, as needed; for children, give 0.01 mg/kg IV and then, if dose is not adequate, 0.1 mg/kg IV (if IV administration is not feasible, divide each dose and give IM or SC). Keep the patient under constant surveillance since the duration of action of hydromorphone may exceed that of naloxone; if significant respiratory depression recurs, repeat naloxone dose. *Do not use analeptic agents.* Promptly empty stomach by performing gastric lavage or inducing emesis; activated charcoal may also be used to remove hydromorphone. Monitor blood gases, pH, and electrolytes and promptly correct any acid-base or electrolyte abnormalities present (lactic acidosis may require IV sodium bicarbonate for prompt correction). Administer an anticonvulsant in carefully titrated doses if seizures occur. Oxygen, IV fluids, vasopressors, and other supportive measures should be employed, as needed. ECG monitoring is essential since ventricular fibrillation or cardiac arrest can occur.

DRUG INTERACTIONS

Other narcotics, alcohol, general anesthetics, phenothiazines, other tranquilizers, sedative-hypnotics, tricyclic antidepressants, and other CNS depressants	⌂ CNS depression; reduce dosage of one or both agents

ALTERED LABORATORY VALUES

Blood/serum values	⌂ Glucose
Urinary values	⌂ 5-HIAA (with colorimetric interference) ⌂ VMA (colorimetric interference)

USE IN CHILDREN
Safety and efficacy for use in children have not been established

USE IN PREGNANT AND NURSING WOMEN
Pregnancy Category C: use during pregnancy only if the expected benefit justifies the potential risk to the fetus. Teratogenicity has been reported in hamsters at doses 600 times the human dose. No adequate, well-controlled studies have been done in pregnant women. Infants born to mothers taking opioids regularly prior to delivery will be physically dependent and will exhibit withdrawal symptoms. Although the best method of managing neonatal withdrawal signs has not been determined, these reactions have been treated by giving 0.7–1 mg/kg of chlorpromazine q6h, 2 mg/kg of phenobarbital q6h, or 2–4 drops/kg of paregoric q4h initially and then reducing the dosage, as tolerated, over a period of 4–28 days. Infants born to mothers taking this preparation shortly before delivery may experience respiratory depression, especially at higher doses. It is not known whether this preparation is excreted in human milk. Because many drugs are excreted in human milk and because of the potential for serious adverse reactions in nursing infants, patients should not nurse if use of this preparation is deemed essential.

[1] Contains 5% alcohol

ANTITUSSIVE COMBINATIONS

DIMETANE-DC (brompheniramine maleate, phenylpropanolamine hydrochloride, and codeine phosphate) Robins   C-V

Syrup (per 5 ml): 2 mg brompheniramine maleate, 12.5 mg phenylpropanolamine hydrochloride, and 10 mg codeine phosphate (1 pt, 1 gal) *raspberry flavored*

INDICATIONS
Cough and upper respiratory tract reactions, including nasal congestion, associated with allergy or the common cold

ORAL DOSAGE
Adult: 10 ml (2 tsp) q4h
Child (6 mo to 2 yr): use according to medical judgment
Child (2–6 yr): 2.5 (1/2 tsp) q4h
Child (6–12 yr): 5 ml (1 tsp) q4h
Child (≥ 12 yr): same as adult

DIMETANE-DC

CONTRAINDICATIONS

- Asthma or other lower respiratory tract conditions
- MAO inhibitor therapy
- Hypersensitivity to any component
- Severe hypertension
- Severe coronary artery disease
- Full-term or premature neonate
- Breast-feeding

WARNINGS/PRECAUTIONS

Drowsiness, dizziness	Caution patients about driving or engaging in any other potentially hazardous activity requiring mental alertness
Constipation	This preparation may cause or exacerbate constipation
Drug dependence	Psychological dependence, tolerance, and physical dependence may develop with repeated use
Special-risk patients	Use with caution in patients with narrow angle glaucoma, GI obstruction, bladder neck obstruction, diabetes, hypertension, heart disease, thyroid disease, or a history of bronchial asthma
Carcinogenicity, mutagenicity	No long-term studies have been done to evaluate the carcinogenic and mutagenic potential of this preparation

ADVERSE REACTIONS

The most frequent reactions, regardless of incidence, are printed in *italics*

Central nervous system	*Sedation, dizziness,* disturbed coordination, tremor, irritability, insomnia, visual disturbances, weakness, nervousness, convulsions, headache, euphoria, dysphoria
Respiratory	*Thickening of bronchial secretions,* tightness in the chest and wheezing, shortness of breath
Cardiovascular	Hypotension, hypertension, cardiac arrhythmias
Hematological	Hemolytic anemia, thrombocytopenia, agranulocytosis
Gastrointestinal	Epigastric discomfort, anorexia, nausea, vomiting, diarrhea, constipation
Genitourinary	Urinary frequency, difficult urination
Dermatological	Urticaria, drug rash, photosensitivity, pruritus
Other	*Dry mouth, nose, and throat*

OVERDOSAGE

Signs and symptoms	*CNS:* depressant effects, including extreme somnolence, stupor, and coma; stimulative effects, including restlessness, excitement, tremors, hallucinations, delirium, and convulsions (stimulative reactions are especially likely to occur in small children); *respiratory:* depression, apnea; *cardiovascular:* flushing, hypertension, tachycardia, arrhythmia, cardiac arrest, circulatory collapse; *other:* mydriasis, dry mouth, urinary retention
Treatment	Maintain pulmonary function; if necessary, provide an open airway, institute mechanical ventilation, and administer oxygen and naloxone. Give IV fluids and vasopressors, as needed. To treat marked excitement, chloral hydrate or a short-acting barbiturate may be used. Exercise caution when giving stimulants or depressants. To empty the stomach, induce emesis or perform gastric lavage; take precautions against aspiration.

DRUG INTERACTIONS

Alcohol, tranquilizers, sedative-hypnotics, and other CNS depressants	↑ CNS depression
MAO inhibitors	Hypertensive crisis
Guanethidine, methyldopa	↓ Antihypertensive effect

ALTERED LABORATORY VALUES

Blood/serum values	↑ Amylase ↑ Lipase

No clinically significant alterations in urinary values occur at therapeutic dosages

---

USE IN CHILDREN

See INDICATIONS and ORAL DOSAGE; use in full-term or premature neonates is contraindicated.

USE IN PREGNANT AND NURSING WOMEN

Pregnancy Category C: reproduction studies have not been done with this preparation; however, studies in rats and mice given up to 16 times the maximum human dose of brompheniramine have shown no evidence of impaired fertility or harm to the fetus. Use during pregnancy only if clearly needed. Use in nursing mothers is contraindicated because of the potential for serious adverse reactions in nursing infants.

VEHICLE/BASE
Syrup: 0.95% alcohol

COMPENDIUM OF DRUG THERAPY

DIMETANE-DX

ANTITUSSIVE COMBINATIONS

DIMETANE-DX (brompheniramine maleate, pseudoephedrine hydrochloride, and dextromethorphan hydrobromide) Robins   Rx

Syrup (per 5 ml): 2 mg brompheniramine maleate, 30 mg pseudoephedrine hydrochloride, and 10 mg dextromethorphan hydrobromide (1 pt) *butterscotch flavored*

INDICATIONS

Cough and upper respiratory tract reactions, including nasal congestion, associated with allergy or the common cold

ORAL DOSAGE

Adult: 10 ml (2 tsp) q4h
Child (6 mo to 2 yr): use according to medical judgment
Child (2-6 yr): 2.5 ($1/2$ tsp) q4h
Child (6-12 yr): 5 ml (1 tsp) q4h
Child ($\geq$ 12 yr): same as adult

CONTRAINDICATIONS

Asthma or other lower respiratory tract conditions	Severe hypertension	Full-term or premature neonate
MAO inhibitor therapy	Severe coronary artery disease	Breast-feeding
Hypersensitivity to any component		

WARNINGS/PRECAUTIONS

Drowsiness, dizziness	Caution patients about driving or engaging in any other potentially hazardous activity requiring mental alertness
Special-risk patients	Use with caution in patients with narrow angle glaucoma, GI obstruction, bladder neck obstruction, diabetes, hypertension, heart disease, thyroid disease, or a history of bronchial asthma
Carcinogenicity, mutagenicity	No long-term studies have been done to evaluate the carcinogenic and mutagenic potential of this preparation

ADVERSE REACTIONS

The most frequent reactions, regardless of incidence, are printed in *italics*

Central nervous system	*Sedation, dizziness,* disturbed coordination, tremor, irritability, insomnia, visual disturbances, weakness, nervousness, convulsions, headache, euphoria, dysphoria
Respiratory	*Thickening of bronchial secretions,* tightness in the chest and wheezing, shortness of breath
Cardiovascular	Hypotension, hypertension, cardiac arrhythmias, palpitations
Hematological	Hemolytic anemia, thrombocytopenia, agranulocytosis
Gastrointestinal	Epigastric discomfort, anorexia, nausea, vomiting, diarrhea, constipation
Genitourinary	Urinary frequency, difficult urination
Dermatological	Urticaria, drug rash, photosensitivity, pruritus
Other	*Dry mouth, nose, and throat*

OVERDOSAGE

Signs and symptoms	*CNS:* ataxia, nystagmus, opisthotonos; depressant effects, including drowsiness; stimulative effects, including restlessness, excitement, tremors, hallucinations, delirium, and convulsions (stimulative reactions are especially likely to occur in small children); *cardiovascular:* flushing, hypertension, tachycardia, arrhythmia; *other:* mydriasis, dry mouth, urinary retention, fever
Treatment	If patient is alert and is seen within 6 h after ingestion, induce emesis; take precautions against aspiration, especially when the patient is an infant or small child. Gastric lavage may be performed; however, in some cases, tracheostomy may be necessary before lavage. Administer oxygen and IV fluids and take other appropriate supportive measures, as needed. Naloxone may be given to reverse CNS depression; a short-acting IV barbiturate may be used for CNS hyperactivity or convulsive seizures.

DRUG INTERACTIONS

Alcohol, tranquilizers, sedative-hypnotics, and other CNS depressants	△ CNS depression
MAO inhibitors	Hypertensive crisis
Guanethidine, methyldopa	▽ Antihypertensive effect

ALTERED LABORATORY VALUES

No clinically significant alterations in blood/serum or urinary values occur at therapeutic dosages

USE IN CHILDREN
See INDICATIONS and ORAL DOSAGE; use in full-term or premature neonates is contraindicated

USE IN PREGNANT AND NURSING WOMEN
Pregnancy Category C: reproduction studies have not been done with this preparation; however, studies in rats and mice given up to 16 times the maximum human dose of brompheniramine have shown no evidence of impaired fertility or harm to the fetus. Use during pregnancy only if clearly needed. Use in nursing mothers is contraindicated because of the potential for serious adverse reactions in nursing infants.

VEHICLE/BASE
Syrup: 0.95% alcohol

ANTITUSSIVE COMBINATIONS

HYCODAN (hydrocodone bitartrate and homatropine methylbromide) Du Pont C-III

Tablets: 5 mg hydrocodone bitartrate and 1.5 mg homatropine methylbromide **Syrup (per 5 ml):** 5 mg hydrocodone bitartrate and 1.5 mg homatropine methylbromide (1 pt, 1 gal) *wild cherry-flavored*

INDICATIONS
Cough[1]

ORAL DOSAGE
Adult: 1 tab or 5 ml (1 tsp) to start, then up to 3 tabs or 15 ml (1 tbsp) after meals and at bedtime with food (not less than 4 h apart)
Infant (< 2 yr): 1/4 tab or 1.25 ml (1/4 tsp) to start, then continue same dose after meals and at bedtime with food (not less than 4 h apart)
Child (2–12 yr): 1/2 tab or 2.5 ml (1/2 tsp) to start, then up to 1 tab or 5 ml (1 tsp) after meals and at bedtime with food (not less than 4 h apart)
Child (> 12 yr): 1 tab or 5 ml (1 tsp) to start, then up to 2 tabs or 10 ml (2 tsp) after meals and at bedtime with food (not less than 4 h apart)

CONTRAINDICATIONS
Glaucoma — Hypersensitivity to either component

ADMINISTRATION/DOSAGE ADJUSTMENTS
Initiating therapy — Symptomatic treatment of cough should be initiated only when the underlying cause has been identified and appropriate therapy, when available, has been provided, and when the risk of complications resulting from cough suppression is not increased

WARNINGS/PRECAUTIONS
Drug dependence — Psychic and/or physical dependence and tolerance to hydrocodone may develop, especially in addiction-prone individuals

Drowsiness — Caution patients that they should not drive or engage in other activities requiring mental alertness or physical coordination if their faculties become impaired; if alcohol or other CNS depressants (see DRUG INTERACTIONS) are used concurrently, the dosage of one or all of the agents should be reduced

ADVERSE REACTIONS
Gastrointestinal — Nausea, vomiting, constipation

Central nervous system — Sedation

OVERDOSAGE
Signs and symptoms — Respiratory depression, extreme somnolence progressing to stupor or coma, skeletal-muscle flaccidity, cold and clammy skin, occasional bradycardia and hypotension; *severe toxicity:* apnea, circulatory collapse, cardiac arrest, death; ingestion of very large amounts may result in paralytic ileus, blurred vision, dry mouth, pupillary dilatation, urinary retention, and tachycardia

Treatment — Reestablish adequate respiratory exchange. Provide a patent airway and begin assisted or controlled ventilation, if indicated. For respiratory depression, administer naloxone (0.4 mg for adults, preferably IV). Employ oxygen, IV fluids, vasopressors, and other supportive measures, as indicated, including treatment for anticholinergic drug intoxication. Gastric emptying and activated charcoal may be useful.

HYCODAN ■ HYCOMINE

DRUG INTERACTIONS

Alcohol, tranquilizers, sedative-hypnotics, and other CNS depressants	⇧	CNS depression

ALTERED LABORATORY VALUES

No clinically significant alterations in blood/serum or urinary values occur at therapeutic dosages

USE IN CHILDREN	USE IN PREGNANT AND NURSING WOMEN
See INDICATIONS and ORAL DOSAGE	Consult manufacturer

[1] Probably effective

ANTITUSSIVE COMBINATIONS

HYCOMINE Syrup (hydrocodone bitartrate and phenylpropanolamine hydrochloride) Du Pont C-III

Syrup (per 5 ml): 5 mg hydrocodone bitartrate and 25 mg phenylpropanolamine hydrochloride (1 pt, 1 gal) *fruit-flavored*

INDICATIONS	ORAL DOSAGE
Cough and nasal congestion	**Adult:** 5 ml (1 tsp) after meals and at bedtime, not more frequently than q4h, up to 30 ml (6 tsp)/24 h

HYCOMINE Pediatric Syrup (hydrocodone bitartrate and phenylpropanolamine hydrochloride) Du Pont C-III

Pediatric Syrup (per 5 ml): 2.5 mg hydrocodone bitartrate and 12.5 mg phenylpropanolamine hydrochloride (1 pt) *fruit-flavored*

INDICATIONS	ORAL DOSAGE
Cough and nasal congestion	**Child (6–12 yr):** 5 ml (1 tsp) after meals and at bedtime, not more frequently than q4h, up to 30 ml (6 tsp)/24 h

CONTRAINDICATIONS

Cardiac disease	Diabetes	Hyperthyroidism
Hypertension	Depressed ventilatory function	Hypersensitivity to hydrocodone or phenylpropanolamine[1]
Intracranial lesion associated with increased intracranial pressure (see WARNINGS/PRECAUTIONS)	MAO inhibitor therapy (see DRUG INTERACTIONS)	

ADMINISTRATION/DOSAGE ADJUSTMENTS

Initiating therapy	Symptomatic treatment of cough should be initiated only when the underlying cause has been identified and appropriate therapy, when available, has been provided, and when the risk of complications resulting from cough suppression is not increased

WARNINGS/PRECAUTIONS

Drug dependence	Psychic and/or physical dependence and tolerance may develop upon repeated administration; prescribe and administer with the same degree of caution appropriate to the use of other narcotic drugs. Use with special care in emotionally unstable patients and those with a history of drug misuse; closely supervise such patients during long-term therapy.
Drowsiness	Caution patients about driving or engaging in other potentially hazardous activities requiring mental alertness or physical coordination, and about using alcohol or other CNS depressants (see DRUG INTERACTIONS)
Respiratory depression	Overdosage or unusual sensitivity to hydrocodone may cause respiratory depression; for treatment, see OVERDOSAGE
Hypertensive crisis	Use of phenylpropanolamine with MAO inhibitors, indomethacin, beta blockers, or methyldopa can lead to a hypertensive crisis; if such a crisis occurs, use of these drugs should be discontinued, hypotensive therapy initiated, and fever managed by means of external cooling
Diagnosis of underlying disease	The primary disease underlying cough should be ascertained before administering an antitussive so that modification of the cough does not increase the risk of clinical complications, and so that appropriate therapy may be instituted for the underlying disease

HYCOMINE ■ NOVAHISTINE DH

Patients with head injuries or other intracranial lesions	The respiratory depressant effect of hydrocodone and its capacity to elevate CSF pressure may be markedly exaggerated in patients with head injuries, other intracranial lesions, or increased intracranial pressure; the side effects of hydrocodone may also interfere with the clinical evaluation of head injuries
Patients with acute abdominal conditions	Use of hydrocodone may interfere with the diagnosis or subsequent clinical evaluation of acute abdominal conditions
Carcinogenicity	Studies of the carcinogenicity or mutagenicity of these preparations have not been performed

ADVERSE REACTIONS

Respiratory	Respiratory depression
Cardiovascular	Hypertension, orthostatic hypotension, tachycardia, palpitations
Genitourinary	Ureteral spasm, vesical-sphincter spasm, urinary retention
Central nervous system	Sedation, drowsiness, mental clouding, lethargy, impairment of physical and mental performance, anxiety, fear, dysphoria, dizziness, psychic dependence, mood changes
Ophthalmic	Blurred vision
Gastrointestinal	Nausea, vomiting

OVERDOSAGE

Signs and symptoms	*Narcotic effects:* respiratory depression (cyanosis, Cheyne-Stokes respiration, decreased respiratory rate and/or tidal volume), extreme somnolence progressing to stupor or coma, skeletal muscle flaccidity, cold and clammy skin, bradycardia, hypotension; in severe cases, apnea, circulatory collapse, cardiac arrest, and death; *sympathomimetic effects:* tremor, restlessness, hyperreflexia, agitation, hallucinations
Treatment	Give primary attention to reestablishing adequate respiratory exchange through provision of an adequate airway and assisted or controlled ventilation; positive-pressure respiration may be desirable if pulmonary edema is present. If respiratory depression is significant, promptly administer naloxone (adult, 0.4–2 mg; child, 0.01 mg/kg), preferably IV, and repeat at 2- to 3-min intervals until satisfactory breathing is restored. *Do not use analeptic agents.* Oxygen, IV fluids, vasopressors, and other supportive measures should be employed, as needed. Gastric lavage, followed by instillation of activated charcoal, may be useful if performed within 4 h of ingestion.

DRUG INTERACTIONS

Other narcotic drugs, alcohol, sedative-hypnotics, antianxiety agents, phenothiazines, general anesthetics, and other CNS depressants	⇧ CNS depression; reduce dose of one or both agents if used concomitantly or in close succession
MAO inhibitors	⇧ Sympathomimetic effect

ALTERED LABORATORY VALUES

No clinically significant alterations in blood/serum or urinary values occur at therapeutic dosages

USE IN CHILDREN

Safety and effectiveness for use in children under 6 yr of age have not been established

USE IN PREGNANT AND NURSING WOMEN

Pregnancy Category C: use during pregnancy only if clearly needed. Reproduction studies have not been performed in animals; it is not known whether this preparation can harm the fetus or adversely affect reproductive capacity. Physical dependence occurs in infants born to women who have taken opioids regularly prior to delivery. The intensity of the withdrawal syndrome does not always correlate with opioid dosage or duration of opioid use. It is not known whether this preparation is excreted in human milk. Because many drugs are excreted in human milk and because of the potential for serious adverse reactions in nursing infants, a decision should be made to either not nurse or discontinue use of this preparation.

[1] Patients hypersensitive to other opioids or sympathomimetic amines may exhibit cross-sensitivity

ANTITUSSIVE COMBINATIONS

NOVAHISTINE DH (codeine phosphate, pseudoephedrine hydrochloride, and chlorpheniramine maleate) Lakeside   C-V

Liquid (per 5 ml): 10 mg codeine phosphate, 30 mg pseudoephedrine hydrochloride, and 2 mg chlorpheniramine maleate[1] (4 fl oz, 1 pt)

INDICATIONS

Cough associated with minor throat and bronchial irritation or nasal congestion due to colds, sinusitis, and allergic rhinitis
Acute otitis media (adjunctive therapy)
Mild otalgia (adjunctive therapy)

ORAL DOSAGE

Adult and child (≥ 12 yr): 10 ml (2 tsp) q4–6h, up to 40 ml (8 tsp)/day
Infant (< 2 yr): use according to medical judgment
Child (25–50 lb): 1.25–2.5 ml (1/4–1/2 tsp) q4–6h, up to 5–10 ml (1–2 tsp)/day
Child (50–90 lb): 2.5–5 ml (1/2–1 tsp) q4–6h, up to 10–20 ml (2–4 tsp)/day

NOVAHISTINE DH ■ NOVAHISTINE Expectorant

CONTRAINDICATIONS

MAO inhibitor therapy (see DRUG INTERACTIONS)	Severe hypertension	Hypersensitivity or idiosyncratic reaction[2] to any component
Breast-feeding	Severe coronary artery disease	

WARNINGS/PRECAUTIONS

Drug dependence	Psychic and/or physical dependence and tolerance may develop, especially in addiction-prone individuals
Unwarranted uses	Discontinue treatment if cough persists for more than 1 wk, tends to recur, or is accompanied by fever, rash, or headache
Elderly patients	Sympathomimetic side effects are more likely to occur in patients over 60 yr of age
Drowsiness	Caution patients about driving or engaging in other activities requiring mental alertness; if alcohol or other CNS depressants (see DRUG INTERACTIONS) are used concurrently, the dosage of one or all of the agents should be reduced
Respiratory depression	Exceeding the recommended dosage rate may lead to respiratory depression, especially in patients with respiratory disease associated with carbon dioxide retention
Special-risk patients	Use with caution in patients with hypertension, diabetes mellitus, ischemic heart disease, thyroid disease (especially hyperthyroidism), increased intraocular pressure, prostatic hypertrophy, asthma, emphysema, or hyperreactivity to ephedrine

ADVERSE REACTIONS[3]

Gastrointestinal	Nausea, vomiting, constipation, dry mouth, heartburn
Central nervous system	Dizziness, sedation, fear, anxiety, tension, restlessness, tremor, weakness, insomnia, hallucinations, convulsions, CNS depression, anorexia, mild sedation, headache, nervousness
Ophthalmic	Diplopia
Dermatological	Pruritus; dermatitis (very rare)
Cardiovascular	Palpitations, arrhythmias, cardiovascular collapse, pallor, hypotension
Respiratory	Respiratory depression
Genitourinary	Dysuria, polyuria

OVERDOSAGE

Signs and symptoms	Respiratory depression (especially in patients with respiratory disease associated with CO_2 retention), nausea, vomiting, hallucinations, CNS depression, hypotension, cardiovascular collapse, convulsions
Treatment	Empty stomach by gastric lavage or emesis, followed by activated charcoal. For respiratory depression, administer a narcotic antagonist (eg, naloxone).

DRUG INTERACTIONS

Alcohol, tranquilizers, sedative-hypnotics, and other CNS depressants	↑ CNS depression
MAO inhibitors	↑ Sympathomimetic effect
Beta-adrenergic blockers	↓ Antihypertensive effect ↑ Sympathomimetic effect
Methyldopa, mecamylamine, reserpine, *Veratrum* alkaloids	↓ Antihypertensive effect

ALTERED LABORATORY VALUES

No clinically significant alterations in blood/serum or urinary values occur at therapeutic dosages

---

USE IN CHILDREN

See INDICATIONS and ORAL DOSAGE; antihistamines may cause excitability in children

USE IN PREGNANT AND NURSING WOMEN

Safety for use during pregnancy has not been established. Contraindicated for use in nursing mothers because the risk for infants of adverse effects from sympathomimetic amines is higher than usual; codeine is excreted in human milk.

---

[1] Contains 5% alcohol
[2] Insomnia, tremor, weakness, dizziness, and arrhythmias may occur as idiosyncratic responses or as general adverse reactions to sympathomimetic agents
[3] Includes reactions common to sympathomimetic amines in general

---

ANTITUSSIVE COMBINATIONS

NOVAHISTINE Expectorant (codeine phosphate, pseudoephedrine hydrochloride, and guaifenesin) Lakeside   C-V

Liquid (per 5 ml): 10 mg codeine phosphate, 30 mg pseudoephedrine hydrochloride, and 100 mg guaifenesin[1] (4 fl oz, 1 pt)

INDICATIONS

Tenacious pulmonary secretions associated with cough and respiratory congestion

Acute otitis media and **mild otalgia** (adjunctive therapy)

ORAL DOSAGE

Adult: 10 ml (2 tsp) q4–6h, up to 4 doses/24 h
Infant (< 2 yr): use according to medical judgment
Child (25–50 lb): 1.25–2.5 ml (1/4–1/2 tsp) q4–6h, up to 4 doses/24 h
Child (50–90 lb): 2.5–5 ml (1/2–1 tsp) q4–6h, up to 4 doses/24 h

NOVAHISTINE Expectorant ■ PENNTUSS

CONTRAINDICATIONS

Severe hypertension	Severe coronary artery disease	Hypersensitivity or idiosyncratic reaction[2] to any component
MAO inhibitor therapy (see DRUG INTERACTIONS)	Breast-feeding	

WARNINGS/PRECAUTIONS

Drug dependence	Psychic and/or physical dependence and tolerance may develop, especially in addiction-prone individuals
Elderly patients	Adverse reactions to sympathomimetics are more likely to occur in patients over 60 yr of age
Special-risk patients	Use with caution in patients with hypertension, diabetes mellitus, ischemic heart disease, thyroid disease (including hyperthyroidism), increased intraocular pressure, prostatic hypertrophy, asthma, emphysema, or hyperreactivity to ephedrine
Concurrent therapy	If alcohol or other CNS depressants are used concurrently, reduce the dosage of one or all of the agents
Unwarranted use	Discontinue treatment if cough persists for more than 1 wk, tends to recur, or is accompanied by fever, rash, or headache

ADVERSE REACTIONS[3]

Central nervous system and neuromuscular	Dizziness, sedation, fear, anxiety, tension, restlessness, tremor, weakness, insomnia, hallucinations, convulsions, CNS depression
Gastrointestinal	Nausea, vomiting, constipation
Cardiovascular	Palpitations, pallor, arrhythmias, cardiovascular collapse with hypotension
Dermatological	Pruritus
Respiratory	Respiratory difficulty
Genitourinary	Dysuria

OVERDOSAGE

Signs and symptoms	Respiratory depression (especially in patients with respiratory disease associated with CO_2 retention), nausea, vomiting, hallucinations, CNS depression, hypotension, cardiovascular collapse, convulsions
Treatment	Induce emesis or use gastric lavage, followed by activated charcoal, to empty stomach. For respiratory depression, administer a narcotic antagonist (eg, naloxone). Administer oxygen and pressor agents, as needed.

DRUG INTERACTIONS

MAO inhibitors	△ Sympathomimetic effect
Alcohol, tranquilizers, sedative-hypnotics, and other CNS depressants	△ CNS depression
Beta-adrenergic blockers	△ Sympathomimetic effect
Methyldopa, mecamylamine, reserpine, *Veratrum* alkaloids	▽ Antihypertensive effect

ALTERED LABORATORY VALUES

Urinary values	△ 5-HIAA (with colorimetric methods) △ VMA (with colorimetric methods)

No clinically significant alterations in blood/serum values occur at therapeutic dosages

---

USE IN CHILDREN

See INDICATIONS and ORAL DOSAGE

USE IN PREGNANT AND NURSING WOMEN

Safety for use during pregnancy has not been established. Contraindicated for use in nursing mothers because the risk for infants of adverse effects from sympathomimetic amines is higher than usual; codeine is excreted in human milk.

---

[1] Contains 7.5% alcohol
[2] Insomnia, tremor, weakness, dizziness, and arrhythmias may occur as idiosyncratic responses or as general adverse reactions to sympathomimetic agents
[3] Including reactions common to sympathomimetic amines in general

---

ANTITUSSIVE COMBINATIONS

PENNTUSS (codeine polistirex and chlorpheniramine polistirex) Pennwalt   C-V

Controlled-release liquid (per 5 ml): codeine polistirex equivalent to 10 mg codeine and chlorpheniramine polistirex equivalent to 4 mg chlorpheniramine maleate (1 pt)

INDICATIONS

Cough and upper respiratory tract reactions associated with allergy or the common cold

ORAL DOSAGE

Adult: 10–15 ml (2–3 tsp) q12h
Child (6–12 yr): 5 ml (1 tsp) q12h
Child (≥ 12 yr): same as adult

WARNINGS/PRECAUTIONS

Special-risk conditions	Use with caution in patients who are receiving other drugs or who have glaucoma, bronchial asthma, emphysema, chronic pulmonary disease, shortness of breath, dyspnea, or symptomatic prostatic hypertrophy; exercise caution if cough is persistent, chronic, or accompanied by excessive mucus
Drowsiness	Caution patients about driving or engaging in other potentially hazardous activities requiring mental alertness or physical coordination
Excitation, constipation	This product may cause excitation, especially in children; it may also precipitate or aggravate constipation
Drug dependence	Psychological dependence, tolerance, and physical dependence may result from repeated use

OVERDOSAGE

Signs and symptoms	*CNS:* extreme somnolence, skeletal muscle flaccidity, stupor, coma, hyperexcitability, nightmares, convulsions (CNS stimulation is especially likely to occur in children and the elderly); *respiratory:* decrease in respiratory rate and/or tidal volume, Cheyne-Stokes respiration, cyanosis, apnea; *cardiovascular:* flushing, hypotension, bradycardia, cardiac arrest, circulatory collapse; *other:* miosis, mydriasis, dry mouth, cold and clammy skin, GI reactions
Treatment	Empty stomach by inducing emesis or performing gastric lavage. To maintain pulmonary function, establish a patent airway, provide assisted or controlled ventilation, and, for significant respiratory depression, administer naloxone. Correct acidosis and electrolyte losses. To treat severe hypotension, use norepinephrine or phenylephrine, not epinephrine. Diazepam may be given to control convulsions. If fever or pulmonary complications occur, antibiotics may be necessary. Do not give analeptic drugs for CNS depression.

DRUG INTERACTIONS

Alcohol, tranquilizers, sedative hypnotics, and other CNS depressants	△ CNS depression; instruct patients to avoid drinking alcoholic beverages during therapy
MAO inhibitors	△ Anticholinergic effect

ALTERED LABORATORY VALUES

Blood/serum values	△ Amylase △ Lipase

No clinically significant alterations in urinary values occur at therapeutic dosages

---

USE IN CHILDREN
See INDICATIONS and ORAL DOSAGE

USE IN PREGNANT AND NURSING WOMEN
Consult manufacturer

ANTITUSSIVE COMBINATIONS

PHENERGAN with Codeine (promethazine hydrochloride and codeine phosphate) Wyeth C-V

Syrup (per 5 ml): 6.25 mg promethazine hydrochloride and 10 mg codeine phosphate (4, 6, 8 fl oz; 1 pt, 1 gal) *fruit flavored*

INDICATIONS
Cough and upper respiratory tract reactions associated with allergy or the common cold

ORAL DOSAGE
Adult: 5 ml (1 tsp) q4–6h
Child (2–6 yr; 12–18 kg): 1.25–2.5 ml (1/4–1/2 tsp) q4–6h, up to 0.5 ml/kg/24 h
Child (6–12 yr): 2.5–5 ml (1/2–1 tsp) q4–6h

CONTRAINDICATIONS

Hypersensitivity or idiosyncratic reaction to promethazine or other phenothiazines	Asthma or other lower respiratory tract conditions	Hypersensitivity to codeine

WARNINGS/PRECAUTIONS

Productive cough	Do not use this preparation to suppress a productive cough associated with acute febrile illness, chronic respiratory disease, or other disorders. If a cough fails to respond to treatment within 5 days, reevaluate diagnosis instead of increasing the dosage, because coughing may result from an underlying condition such as lower respiratory tract disease or the presence of a foreign body.

PHENERGAN with Codeine

Drowsiness, dizziness, orthostatic hypotension	Caution patients that they may drive or engage in other potentially hazardous activities requiring mental alertness or physical coordination only after it has been established that this preparation does not make them drowsy or dizzy (see also USE IN CHILDREN)
Constipation	This preparation may cause or exacerbate constipation
Photosensitivity, extrapyramidal reactions	Photosensitivity and extrapyramidal reactions such as oculogyric crisis, torticollis, and tongue protrusion have occurred in rare instances; the extrapyramidal reactions have usually resulted from excessive dosage. Instruct patients to report any involuntary muscle movements or unusual sensitivity to sunlight.
Drug dependence	Psychological dependence, tolerance, and physical dependence may occur; closely supervise patients with a history of drug dependence
Patients with head injuries or other intracranial conditions	The respiratory depressant effects of this preparation and its capacity to elevate CSF pressure may be markedly exaggerated in patients with head injuries, other intracranial lesions, or increased intracranial pressure; side effects may also interfere with the clinical evaluation of head injuries
Patients with a history of sleep apnea	Avoid use in patients with a history of sleep apnea
Patients with GI or GU conditions	Use with caution and at a reduced initial dosage in patients who have undergone recent GI or urinary tract surgery or who have acute abdominal disorders, significant hepatic or renal impairment, ulcerative colitis, or prostatic hypertrophy; caution should also be exercised if patients have hepatic impairment, stenosing peptic ulcer, pyloroduodenal obstruction, or bladder neck obstruction. Colonic motility may be increased in patients with chronic colitis, and toxic megacolon may occur in patients with acute ulcerative colitis.
Elderly patients	Use with caution and at a reduced initial dosage in elderly patients
Other special-risk patients	Use with caution and at a reduced initial dosage in debilitated patients and in patients with convulsive disorders, fever, Addison's disease, or hypothyroidism; caution should also be exercised if patients have cardiovascular disease or narrow angle glaucoma
Carcinogenicity, mutagenicity	No long-term studies have been performed in animals to evaluate the carcinogenic potential of this preparation's components; use of codeine in the micronucleus test and promethazine and codeine in the Ames test has produced no evidence of mutagenicity
Effect on fertility	Sperm abnormality assays with codeine have yielded negative results; the effect of promethazine on fertility has not been assessed

ADVERSE REACTIONS

Central nervous system	Sedation, sleepiness, blurred vision, headache, dysphoria, dizziness, light-headedness, euphoria, disorientation, confusion, visual disturbances, hallucinations, weakness, convulsions; extrapyramidal reactions (rare)
Respiratory	Respiratory depression
Cardiovascular	Hypertension, hypotension, tachycardia, bradycardia, palpitations, faintness, syncope
Gastrointestinal	Nausea, vomiting, constipation, biliary tract spasm, cholestatic jaundice
Genitourinary	Oliguria, urinary retention, antidiuretic effect
Hematological	Leukopenia and thrombocytopenia (rare); agranulocytosis (one case)
Dermatological	Rash; photosensitivity (rare)
Hypersensitivity	Flushing, sweating, pruritus, giant urticaria, angioneurotic edema, laryngeal edema
Other	Dry mouth

OVERDOSAGE

Signs and symptoms	*CNS:* extreme somnolence, skeletal muscle flaccidity, stupor, coma, hyperexcitability, nightmares, convulsions (CNS stimulation is especially likely to occur in children and the elderly); *respiratory:* decrease in respiratory rate and/or tidal volume, Cheyne-Stokes respiration, cyanosis, apnea; *cardiovascular:* flushing, hypotension, bradycardia, cardiac arrest, circulatory collapse; *other:* miosis, mydriasis, dry mouth, cold and clammy skin, GI reactions
Treatment	To maintain pulmonary function, establish a patent airway, provide assisted or controlled ventilation, and, for significant respiratory depression, administer naloxone. Correct acidosis and electrolyte losses. To treat severe hypotension, use norepinephrine or phenylephrine, not epinephrine. Diazepam may be given to control convulsions. If fever or pulmonary complications occur, antibiotics may be necessary. Do not give analeptic drugs for CNS depression. Monitor vital signs only in cases of extreme overdosage or individual sensitivity. To remove this preparation from the body, administer activated charcoal or use sodium or magnesium sulfate as a cathartic; limited experience indicates that dialysis is not helpful.

PHENERGAN with Codeine ■ PHENERGAN with Dextromethorphan

DRUG INTERACTIONS

Alcohol, narcotic drugs, sedative-hypnotics (eg, barbiturates), tranquilizers, local anesthetics, and other CNS depressants	△ CNS depression; instruct patients requiring this preparation that other CNS depressants should be avoided or used at a lower dosage (for concomitant use with this preparation, reduce the dosage of a narcotic analgesic by 25–50% and the dosage of a barbiturate by at least 50% △ Risk of convulsions (with concomitant use of narcotic drugs or local anesthetics)
MAO inhibitors	Hypertension, hypotension, restlessness, convulsions, coma; give a small test dose of this preparation to any patient who is receving an MAO inhibitor

ALTERED LABORATORY VALUES

Blood/serum values	△ Amylase △ Lipase △ Glucose
Urinary values	False-positive or false-negative pregnancy test

USE IN CHILDREN

See INDICATIONS and ORAL DOSAGE; do not give to children under 2 yr of age because safety for use in such patients has not been established. Children undergoing treatment should be supervised whenever they ride a bicycle or engage in other potentially hazardous activities requiring mental alertness or physical coordination. Use with caution in young children because respiratory arrest, coma, and death have occurred in such patients following administration of codeine; exercise caution when using in atopic children since histamine may be released.

USE IN PREGNANT AND NURSING WOMEN

Pregnancy Category C: promethazine has been shown to be fetotoxic in rodents; no evidence of teratogenicity has been observed in rats fed 6.25 or 12.5 mg/kg/day. Administration of 120 mg/kg of codeine has caused an increase in resorptions in rats, and a single dose of 100 mg/kg has resulted in delayed ossification in mice; no teratogenic effects have been detected in rats and rabbits given 5–120 mg/kg. Use of this preparation during late pregnancy may cause withdrawal reactions (with regular use) and respiratory depression in a neonate. Inhibition of platelet aggregation may also occur in a neonate if this preparation is taken within 2 wk before delivery. This medication should generally be used during pregnancy only if the expected benefit justifies the potential risk to the fetus or neonate. If a premature delivery is anticipated, do not use during labor because of the risk of respiratory depression. Following use during normal labor, closely observe neonates for signs of respiratory depression; resuscitative measures, including use of naloxone, may be necessary. Small, probably insignificant amounts of codeine may be excreted in human milk; it is not known whether promethazine is excreted in human milk. Use this preparation with caution in nursing mothers.

VEHICLE/BASE
Syrup: 7% alcohol

ANTITUSSIVE COMBINATIONS

PHENERGAN with Dextromethorphan (promethazine hydrochloride and dextromethorphan hydrobromide) Wyeth   Rx

Syrup (per 5 ml): 6.25 mg promethazine hydrochloride and 15 mg dextromethorphan hydrobromide (4, 6 fl oz; 1 pt; 1 gal) *fruit flavored*

INDICATIONS	ORAL DOSAGE
Cough and upper respiratory tract reactions associated with allergy or the common cold	**Adult:** 5 ml (1 tsp) q4–6h **Child (2–6 yr):** 1.25–2.5 ml (¼–½ tsp) q4–6h, up to 10 ml/24 h **Child (6–12 yr):** 2.5–5 ml (½–1 tsp) q4–6h, up to 20 ml/24 h

CONTRAINDICATIONS

Hypersensitivity or idiosyncratic reaction to promethazine or other phenothiazines	Asthma or other lower respiratory tract conditions	MAO inhibitor therapy

WARNINGS/PRECAUTIONS

Drowsiness, dizziness	Caution patients that they may drive or engage in other potentially hazardous activities requiring mental alertness or physical coordination only after it has been established that this preparation does not make them drowsy or dizzy (see also USE IN CHILDREN)
Photosensitivity, extrapyramidal reactions	Photosensitivity and extrapyramidal reactions such as oculogyric crisis, torticollis, and tongue protrusion have occurred in rare instances; the extrapyramidal reactions have usually resulted from excessive dosage. Instruct patients to report any involuntary muscle movements or unusual sensitivity to sunlight.
Drug dependence	Very slight psychological dependence may occur
Patients with a history of sleep apnea	Avoid use in patients with a history of sleep apnea
Patients with GI or GU conditions	Use with caution in patients with hepatic impairment, stenosing peptic ulcer, pyloroduodenal obstruction, symptomatic prostatic hypertrophy, or bladder neck obstruction

PHENERGAN with Dextromethorphan ■ PHENERGAN VC with Codeine

Other special-risk patients	Use with caution in patients who are sedated, debilitated, or confined to a supine position; exercise caution if patients have convulsive disorders, cardiovascular disease, or narrow angle glaucoma
Carcinogenicity, mutagenicity, effect on fertility	No long-term studies have been performed in animals to evaluate the carcinogenic potential of this preparation's components. Use of promethazine in the Ames test has produced no evidence of mutagenicity. The effect of promethazine on fertility has not been assessed.

ADVERSE REACTIONS

Central nervous system	Sedation, sleepiness, drowsiness, blurred vision, dizziness; disorientation, confusion, and extrapyramidal reactions (rare)
Cardiovascular	Hypertension, hypotension
Gastrointestinal	Nausea, vomiting, other GI disturbances, cholestatic jaundice
Hematological	Leukopenia and thrombocytopenia (rare); agranulocytosis (one case)
Dermatological	Rash; photosensitivity (rare)
Other	Dry mouth

OVERDOSAGE

Signs and symptoms	*CNS:* extreme somnolence, stupor, coma, hyperexcitability, confusion, hyperactivity, hallucinations, nightmares, convulsions (CNS stimulation is especially likely to occur in children and the elderly); *respiratory:* decrease in respiratory rate and/or tidal volume; *cardiovascular:* flushing, hypotension; *other:* mydriasis, dry mouth, GI reactions
Treatment	To maintain pulmonary function, establish a patent airway, and provide assisted or controlled ventilation. Correct acidosis and electrolyte losses. To treat severe hypotension, use norepinephrine or phenylephrine, not epinephrine. Diazepam may be given to control convulsions. Do not give analeptic drugs for CNS depression. Monitor vital signs only in cases of extreme overdosage or individual sensitivity. To remove this preparation from the body, administer activated charcoal or use sodium or magnesium sulfate as a cathartic; limited experience indicates that dialysis is not helpful.

DRUG INTERACTIONS

Alcohol, narcotic drugs, sedative-hypnotics (eg, barbiturates), tranquilizers, local anesthetics, and other CNS depressants	⌂ CNS depression; instruct patients requiring this preparation that other CNS depressants should be avoided or used at a lower dosage (for concomitant use with this preparation, reduce the dosage of a narcotic analgesic by 25–50% and the dosage of a barbiturate by at least 50%) ⌂ Risk of convulsions (with concomitant use of narcotic drugs or local anesthetics)
MAO inhibitors	Hypertension, hypotension, restlessness, convulsions, coma; do not use an MAO inhibitor concomitantly

ALTERED LABORATORY VALUES

Blood/serum values	⌂ Glucose
Urinary values	False-positive or false-negative pregnancy test

USE IN CHILDREN

See INDICATIONS and ORAL DOSAGE; do not give to children under 2 yr of age because safety for use in such patients has not been established. Children undergoing treatment should be supervised whenever they ride a bicycle or engage in other potentially hazardous activities requiring mental alertness or physical coordination. Use with caution in atopic children since histamine may be released.

USE IN PREGNANT AND NURSING WOMEN

Pregnancy Category C: promethazine has been shown to be fetotoxic in rodents; no evidence of teratogenicity has been observed in rats fed 6.25 or 12.5 mg/kg/day. Inhibition of platelet aggregation may occur in a neonate if this preparation is taken within 2 wk before delivery. This medication should be used during pregnancy only if the expected benefit justifies the potential risk to the fetus or neonate. It is not known whether promethazine or dextromethorphan is excreted in human milk; use this preparation with caution in nursing mothers.

VEHICLE/BASE
Syrup: 7% alcohol

ANTITUSSIVE COMBINATIONS

PHENERGAN VC with Codeine (promethazine hydrochloride, phenylephrine hydrochloride, and codeine phosphate) Wyeth C-V

Syrup (per 5 ml): 6.25 mg promethazine hydrochloride, 5 mg phenylephrine hydrochloride, and 10 mg codeine phosphate (4, 6, 8 fl oz; 1 pt; 1 gal) *fruit flavored*

INDICATIONS	ORAL DOSAGE
Cough and upper respiratory tract reactions, including nasal congestion, associated with allergy or the common cold	Adult: 5 ml (1 tsp) q4–6h Child (2–6 yr; 12–18 kg): 1.25–2.5 ml (¼–½ tsp) q4–6h, up to 0.5 ml/kg/24 h Child (6–12 yr): 2.5–5 ml (½–1 tsp) q4–6h

COMPENDIUM OF DRUG THERAPY

PHENERGAN VC with Codeine

CONTRAINDICATIONS

Hypersensitivity to codeine or phenylephrine	Asthma or other lower respiratory tract conditions	Peripheral vascular insufficiency
Hypersensitivity or idiosyncratic reaction to promethazine or other phenothiazines	MAO inhibitor therapy	Hypertension

WARNINGS/PRECAUTIONS

Productive cough	Do not use this preparation to suppress a productive cough associated with acute febrile illness, chronic respiratory disease, or other disorders. If a cough fails to respond to treatment within 5 days, reevaluate diagnosis instead of increasing the dosage, because coughing may result from an underlying condition such as lower respiratory tract disease or the presence of a foreign body.
Drowsiness, dizziness, orthostatic hypotension	Caution patients that they may drive or engage in other potentially hazardous activities requiring mental alertness or physical coordination only after it has been established that this preparation does not make them drowsy or dizzy (see also USE IN CHILDREN)
Constipation	This preparation may cause or exacerbate constipation
Photosensitivity, extrapyramidal reactions	Photosensitivity and extrapyramidal reactions, such as oculogyric crisis, torticollis, and tongue protrusion, have occurred in rare instances; the extrapyramidal reactions have usually resulted from excessive dosage. Instruct patients to report any involuntary muscle movements or unusual sensitivity to sunlight.
Drug dependence	Psychological dependence, tolerance, and physical dependence may occur; closely supervise patients with a history of drug dependence
Patients with head injuries or other intracranial conditions	The respiratory depressant effects of this preparation and its capacity to elevate CSF pressure may be markedly exaggerated in patients with head injuries, other intracranial lesions, or increased intracranial pressure; side effects may also interfere with the clinical evaluation of head injuries
Patients with a history of sleep apnea	Avoid use in patients with a history of sleep apnea
Patients with cardiovascular disorders	Use with extreme caution in patients with arteriosclerosis or poor cerebral or coronary circulation because cardiac output may decrease; caution should be exercised if patients have cardiovascular disorders such as heart disease
Patients with GI or GU conditions	Use with caution and at a reduced initial dosage in patients who have undergone recent GI or urinary tract surgery or who have acute abdominal disorders, significant hepatic or renal impairment, ulcerative colitis, or prostatic hypertrophy; caution should also be exercised if patients have hepatic impairment, stenosing peptic ulcer, pyloroduodenal obstruction, or bladder neck obstruction. Colonic motility may be increased in patients with chronic colitis, and toxic megacolon may occur in patients with acute ulcerative colitis. Men with symptomatic prostatic hypertrophy may experience urinary retention.
Elderly patients	Use with extreme caution and at a reduced initial dosage in elderly patients
Other special-risk patients	Use with caution and at a reduced initial dosage in debilitated patients and in patients with convulsive disorders, fever, Addison's disease, or hypothyroidism; caution should also be exercised if patients have other thyroid diseases, diabetes mellitus, or narrow angle glaucoma
Carcinogenicity, mutagenicity	No long-term studies have been performed in animals to evaluate the carcinogenic potential of this preparation's components; an epidemiological study has demonstrated no significant association between phenylephrine and cancer. Use of codeine in the micronucleus test and promethazine and codeine in the Ames test has produced no evidence of mutagenicity; phenylephrine's mutagenic potential has not been studied.
Effect on fertility	Sperm abnormality assays with codeine have yielded negative results; a study of ovum transport in rabbits has shown that phenylephrine does not affect the incidence of pregnancy, but at high doses it significantly reduces the number of implantations. The effect of promethazine on fertility has not been assessed.

ADVERSE REACTIONS

Central nervous system	Sedation, sleepiness, blurred vision, headache, dysphoria, restlessness, anxiety, nervousness, dizziness, light-headedness, euphoria, disorientation, confusion, visual disturbances, hallucinations, weakness, tremor, convulsions; extrapyramidal reactions (rare)
Respiratory	Respiratory depression, respiratory distress
Cardiovascular	Hypertension, hypotension, tachycardia, bradycardia, palpitations, faintness, syncope, precordial pain
Gastrointestinal	Nausea, vomiting, constipation, biliary tract spasm, cholestatic jaundice
Genitourinary	Oliguria, urinary retention, antidiuretic effect
Hematological	Leukopenia and thrombocytopenia (rare), agranulocytosis (one case)

PHENERGAN VC with Codeine

Dermatological	Rash; photosensitivity (rare)
Hypersensitivity	Flushing, sweating, pruritus, giant urticaria, angioneurotic edema, laryngeal edema
Other	Dry mouth

OVERDOSAGE

Signs and symptoms	*CNS:* headache, extreme somnolence, skeletal muscle flaccidity, stupor, coma, hyperexcitability, nightmares, convulsions (CNS stimulation is especially likely to occur in children and the elderly); *respiratory:* decrease in respiratory rate and/or tidal volume, Cheyne-Stokes respiration, cyanosis, apnea; *cardiovascular:* flushing, hypotension, headache, hypertension, cerebral hemorrhage, bradycardia, premature ventricular contractions, paroxysmal ventricular tachycardia, cardiac arrest, circulatory collapse; *other:* miosis, mydriasis, dry mouth, cold and clammy skin, GI reactions (including vomiting)
Treatment	To maintain pulmonary function, establish a patent airway, provide assisted or controlled ventilation, and, for significant respiratory depression, administer naloxone. Correct acidosis and electrolyte losses. To treat severe hypotension, use norepinephrine or phenylephrine, not epinephrine. Diazepam may be given to control convulsions. If fever or pulmonary complications occur, antibiotics may be necessary. Do not give analeptic drugs for CNS depression. Monitor vital signs only in cases of extreme overdosage or individual sensitivity. To remove this preparation from the body, administer activated charcoal or use sodium or magnesium sulfate as a cathartic; limited experience indicates that dialysis is not helpful.

DRUG INTERACTIONS

Alcohol, narcotic drugs, sedative-hypnotics (eg, barbiturates), tranquilizers, and other CNS depressants	△ CNS depression; instruct patients requiring this preparation that other CNS depressants should be avoided or used at a lower dosage (for concomitant use with this preparation, reduce the dosage of a narcotic analgesic by 25–50% and the dosage of a barbiturate by at least 50%) △ Risk of convulsions (with concomitant use of narcotic drugs or local anesthetics)
MAO inhibitors	△ Hypertensive crisis; do not use an MAO inhibitor concomitantly
Tricyclic antidepressants, amphetamines, phenylpropanolamine, ergot alkaloids, atropine	Hypertension; exercise caution if phenylpropanolamine, an amphetamine, or a tricyclic antidepressant is given concomitantly
Phentolamine	▽ Vasopressor response

ALTERED LABORATORY VALUES

Blood/serum values	△ Amylase △ Lipase △ Glucose
Urinary values	False-positive or false-negative pregnancy test

---

USE IN CHILDREN

See INDICATIONS and ORAL DOSAGE; do not give to children under 2 yr of age because safety for use in such patients has not been established. Children undergoing treatment should be supervised whenever they ride a bicycle or engage in other potentially hazardous activities requiring mental alertness or physical coordination. Use with caution in young children because respiratory arrest, coma, and death have occurred in such patients following administration of codeine; exercise caution when using in atopic children since histamine may be released.

USE IN PREGNANT AND NURSING WOMEN

Pregnancy Category C: phenylephrine has caused a decrease in birth weight and may have contributed to perinatal wastage, premature labor, and fetal anomalies in rabbits; this drug has also been associated with ventricular septal defect and aortic arch anomalies in chick embryos. Promethazine has been shown to be fetotoxic in rodents; no evidence of teratogenicity has been observed in rats fed 6.25 or 12.5 mg/kg/day. Administration of 120 mg/kg of codeine has caused an increase in resorptions in rats, and a single dose of 100 mg/kg has resulted in delayed ossification in mice; no teratogenic effects have been detected in rats and rabbits given 5–120 mg/kg. Use of this preparation during late pregnancy may cause anoxia or bradycardia in a fetus and withdrawal reactions (with regular use) and respiratory depression in a neonate. Inhibition of platelet aggregation may also occur in a neonate if this preparation is taken within 2 wk before delivery. This medication should generally be used during pregnancy only if the expected benefit justifies the potential risk to the fetus or neonate. If a premature delivery is anticipated, do not use during labor because of the risk of respiratory depression. Following use during normal labor, closely observe neonates for signs of respiratory depression; resuscitatory measures, including use of naloxone, may be necessary. Small, probably insignificant amounts of codeine may be excreted in human milk; it is not known whether promethazine or phenylephrine is excreted in human milk. Use this preparation with caution in nursing mothers.

VEHICLE/BASE
Syrup: 7% alcohol

ANTITUSSIVE COMBINATIONS

ROBITUSSIN A-C (guaifenesin and codeine phosphate) Robins C-V

Syrup (per 5 ml): 100 mg guaifenesin and 10 mg codeine phosphate[1] (2, 4 fl oz; 1 pt, 1 gal)

INDICATIONS

Cough due to colds, bronchitis, laryngitis, tracheitis, pharyngitis, pertussis, influenza, or measles

ORAL DOSAGE

Adult: 10 ml (2 tsp) q4h, up to 60 ml (12 tsp)/24 h
Child (2–6 yr): 2.5 ml ($\frac{1}{2}$ tsp) q4h, up to 15 ml (3 tsp)/24 h
Child (6–12 yr): 5 ml (1 tsp) q4h, up to 30 ml (6 tsp)/24 h

CONTRAINDICATIONS

Hypersensitivity to any component

WARNINGS/PRECAUTIONS

Drug dependence	Psychic and/or physical dependence and tolerance may develop, especially in addiction-prone individuals
Persistent or chronic cough, or cough accompanied by excessive secretions	Use with caution
Special-risk patients	Use with caution in patients with pulmonary disease or shortness of breath

ADVERSE REACTIONS

Central nervous system	Drowsiness
Gastrointestinal	Nausea, upset, constipation

OVERDOSAGE

Signs and symptoms	*Codeine-related effects:* respiratory depression, somnolence, stupor, coma, skeletal-muscle flaccidity, cold and clammy skin, bradycardia, hypotension, apnea, circulatory collapse, and cardiac arrest, leading to death
Treatment	Reestablish an adequate airway and institute artificial respiration. For respiratory depression, administer a narcotic antagonist (eg, naloxone), along with attempts at resuscitation. Empty stomach by emesis or gastric lavage. Employ supportive measures, as indicated.

DRUG INTERACTIONS

Alcohol, tranquilizers, sedative-hypnotics, and other CNS depressants	△ CNS depression

ALTERED LABORATORY VALUES

Urinary values	△ 5-HIAA (colorimetric interference) △ VMA (colorimetric interference)

No clinically significant alterations in blood/serum values occur at therapeutic dosages

---

USE IN CHILDREN
See INDICATIONS and ORAL DOSAGE; use with caution in children under 2 yr of age or those taking another drug. Consult manufacturer for dosage recommendations.

USE IN PREGNANT AND NURSING WOMEN
Consult manufacturer

---

[1] Contains 3.5% alcohol

ANTITUSSIVE COMBINATIONS

ROBITUSSIN-DAC (guaifenesin, pseudoephedrine hydrochloride, and codeine phosphate) Robins C-V

Syrup (per 5 ml): 100 mg guaifenesin, 30 mg pseudoephedrine hydrochloride, and 10 mg codeine phosphate[1] (1 pt)

INDICATIONS

Cough and nasal congestion associated with colds and inhaled irritants

ORAL DOSAGE

Adult: 5–10 ml (1–2 tsp) q6h, up to 40 ml (8 tsp)/24 h
Child (2–6 yr): 2.5 ml ($\frac{1}{2}$ tsp) q6h, up to 10 ml (2 tsp)/24 h
Child (6–12 yr): 5 ml (1 tsp) q6h, up to 20 ml (4 tsp)/24 h
Child (> 12 yr): same as adult

ROBITUSSIN-DAC ■ RONDEC-DM

CONTRAINDICATIONS

Marked hypertension	MAO inhibitor therapy (see DRUG INTERACTIONS)	Hypersensitivity to any component
Hyperthyroidism		

WARNINGS/PRECAUTIONS

Drug dependence	Psychic and/or physical dependence may occur, especially in addiction-prone individuals
Persistent or chronic cough, or cough accompanied by excessive secretions	Use with caution
Special-risk patients	Use with caution in patients with hypertension, heart disease, diabetes mellitus, chronic pulmonary disease, shortness of breath, prostatic hypertrophy, or glaucoma

ADVERSE REACTIONS

Central nervous system	Agitation, dizziness, insomnia
Gastrointestinal	Nausea, constipation
Cardiovascular	Palpitations

OVERDOSAGE

Signs and symptoms	Nervousness, dizziness, and sleeplessness, progressing to somnolence, respiratory depression, stupor, and coma
Treatment	Induce emesis or use gastric lavage, followed by activated charcoal, to empty stomach. Maintain a patent airway and ventilatory exchange. For respiratory depression, administer a narcotic antagonist (eg, naloxone). Administer oxygen and pressor agents, as needed.

DRUG INTERACTIONS

Alcohol, tranquilizers, sedative-hypnotics, and other CNS depressants	△ CNS depression
MAO inhibitors	△ Sympathomimetic and anticholinergic effects
Methyldopa, mecamylamine, reserpine, *Veratrum* alkaloids	▽ Antihypertensive effect

ALTERED LABORATORY VALUES

Urinary values	△ 5-HIAA (with colorimetric methods) △ VMA (with colorimetric methods)

No clinically significant alterations in blood/serum values occur at therapeutic dosages

---

USE IN CHILDREN

See INDICATIONS and ORAL DOSAGE; use with caution in children under 2 yr of age or those taking another drug. Consult manufacturer for dosage recommendations.

USE IN PREGNANT AND NURSING WOMEN

Consult manufacturer

---

[1] Contains 1.4% alcohol

ANTITUSSIVE COMBINATIONS

RONDEC-DM (carbinoxamine maleate, pseudoephedrine hydrochloride, and dextromethorphan hydrobromide) Ross   Rx

Syrup (per 5 ml): 4 mg carbinoxamine maleate, 60 mg pseudoephedrine hydrochloride, and 15 mg dextromethorphan hydrobromide[1] (4, 16 fl oz) *grape flavored*   **Pediatric drops (per dropperful [1 ml]):** 2 mg carbinoxamine maleate, 25 mg pseudoephedrine hydrochloride, and 4 mg dextromethorphan hydrobromide[1] (30 ml) *grape flavored*

INDICATIONS[2]

Cough, nasal congestion, and other upper respiratory tract reactions associated with allergy or the common cold

ORAL DOSAGE

Adult: 5 ml (1 tsp) qid
Infant (1–3 mo): 0.25 ml (1/4 dropperful) qid
Infant (3–6 mo): 0.5 ml (1/2 dropperful) qid
Infant (6–9 mo): 0.75 ml (3/4 dropperful) qid
Infant (9–18 mo): 1 ml (1 dropperful) qid
Child (18 mo to 6 yr): 2.5 ml (1/2 tsp) qid
Child (≥ 6 yr): same as adult

RONDEC-DM

CONTRAINDICATIONS

Hypersensitivity or idiosyncratic reaction to any component	Narrow angle glaucoma	Asthmatic attack
MAO inhibitor therapy (see DRUG INTERACTIONS)	Urinary retention	Severe hypertension
	Peptic ulcer	Severe coronary artery disease

ADMINISTRATION/DOSAGE ADJUSTMENTS

Mild cough	Less frequent or reduced doses may be adequate

WARNINGS/PRECAUTIONS

Drowsiness	Caution patients about driving or engaging in other activities requiring mental alertness, and to avoid the use of alcohol or other CNS depressants (see DRUG INTERACTIONS)
Special-risk patients	Use with caution in patients over 60 yr of age and in patients with hypertension, ischemic or other heart disease, asthma, hyperthyroidism, increased intraocular pressure, diabetes mellitus, or prostatic hypertrophy

ADVERSE REACTIONS

Cardiovascular	Pallor, increased blood pressure or heart rate, arrhythmias
Central nervous system	Dizziness, sedation, headache, weakness, mild stimulation, nervousness, insomnia, tremor, convulsions, depression, hallucinations, drowsiness; excitability in children (rare)
Gastrointestinal	Nausea, anorexia, dry mouth, heartburn, vomiting, diarrhea, other GI disturbances
Genitourinary	Dysuria, polyuria
Ophthalmic	Diplopia
Respiratory	Difficult breathing

OVERDOSAGE

Signs and symptoms	*Antihistamine-related effects (in small children):* excitation, hallucinations, ataxia, incoordination, tremors, flushing, fever, and in severe cases, convulsions, fixed and dilated pupils, coma, death; *antihistamine-related effects (in adults):* excitement leading to convulsions and postical depression, often preceded by drowsiness and coma; *dextromethorphan-related effects:* respiratory depression; *sympathomimetic-related effects:* dry mouth, metallic taste, anorexia, nausea, vomiting, diarrhea, abdominal cramps, restlessness, dizziness, tremor, hyperactive reflexes, talkativeness, irritability, insomnia, headache, difficulty in micturition, flushing, palpitation, arrhythmias, hypertension leading to hypotension and circulatory collapse
Treatment	Empty stomach, as patient's condition warrants, and administer activated charcoal. Maintain a quiet environment and monitor cardiovascular status. Reduce fever with cool sponging. If dextromethorphan toxicity is suspected, administer naloxone. To reverse anticholinergic symptoms of carbinoxamine, physostigmine may be given. CNS excitation and convulsions may be controlled with sedatives or anticonvulsants. Administer ammonium chloride to increase urinary excretion of pseudoephedrine. Further care is generally symptomatic and supportive. *Do not give stimulants.*

DRUG INTERACTIONS

Alcohol, tricyclic antidepressants, barbiturates, and other CNS depressants	△ CNS depression	
MAO inhibitors	△ Anticholinergic effect of antihistamines	△ Sympathomimetic effects
Beta-adrenergic blockers	△ Sympathomimetic effects	
Methyldopa, mecamylamine, reserpine, and *Veratrum* alkaloids	▽ Antihypertensive effect	
Narcotic antitussives	△ Cough-suppressant action	

ALTERED LABORATORY VALUES

No clinically significant alterations in blood/serum or urinary values occur at therapeutic dosages

USE IN CHILDREN	USE IN PREGNANT AND NURSING WOMEN
See INDICATIONS and ORAL DOSAGE	Pregnancy Category C: use during pregnancy only if clearly needed; safety for use during pregnancy has not been established. Reproduction studies have not been performed in animals; it is not known whether this preparation can adversely affect fetal development or reproductive capacity. Use with caution in nursing mothers.

[1] Contains < 0.6% alcohol
[2] Before prescribing an antitussive, identify and provide appropriate therapy for the underlying cause

---

ANTITUSSIVE COMBINATIONS

RYNA-C (codeine phosphate, pseudoephedrine hydrochloride, and chlorpheniramine maleate) Wallace   C-V

Liquid (per 5 ml): 10 mg codeine phosphate, 30 mg pseudoephedrine hydrochloride, and 2 mg chlorpheniramine maleate[1] (4 fl oz, 1 pt) *cinnamon-flavored, sugar-free*

INDICATIONS
Cough, nasal congestion, sneezing, itchy and watery eyes, and running nose associated with the common cold or allergic rhinitis

ORAL DOSAGE
Adult: 10 ml (2 tsp) q6h, up to 4 doses/24 h
Child (2–5 yr): 2.5 ml (1/2 tsp) q6h, up to 4 doses/24 h
Child (6–12 yr): 5 ml (1 tsp) q6h, up to 4 doses/24 h

CONTRAINDICATIONS
None known

WARNINGS/PRECAUTIONS

Drug dependence	Psychic and/or physical dependence may occur, especially in addiction-prone individuals
Drowsiness	Caution patients not to drive or engage in other activities requiring mental alertness, and not to use alcohol or other CNS depressants (see DRUG INTERACTIONS)
Constipation	May be caused or aggravated by codeine component
Persistent or chronic cough, or cough accompanied by excessive secretions, high fever, rash, or persistent headache	Use with caution; discontinue use if symptoms do not improve within 3 days
Drowsiness	May occur, leading to impaired performance of potentially hazardous activities; caution patients accordingly and about possible additive effect of alcohol
Excitability	May occur, especially in children
Nervousness, dizziness, sleeplessness	May occur at higher than recommended dosage
Special-risk patients	Use with caution in patients with chronic pulmonary disease, shortness of breath, high blood pressure, thyroid disease, diabetes, asthma, glaucoma, or difficulty in urination due to prostatic hypertrophy, and in patients receiving MAO inhibitors (see DRUG INTERACTIONS) or antihypertensive medications

ADVERSE REACTIONS

Gastrointestinal	Constipation
Central nervous system	Excitability, drowsiness

OVERDOSAGE

Signs and symptoms	*Codeine-related effects:* respiratory depression, somnolence, stupor, coma, skeletal-muscle flaccidity, cold and clammy skin, bradycardia, hypotension, apnea, circulatory collapse, and cardiac arrest, leading to death
Treatment	Reestablish an adequate airway and institute artificial respiration. For respiratory depression, administer a narcotic antagonist (eg, naloxone), along with attempts at resuscitation. Empty stomach by emesis or gastric lavage. Employ supportive measures, as indicated.

DRUG INTERACTIONS

MAO inhibitors	⇧ Sympathomimetic and anticholinergic effects

RYNA-C ■ RYNA-CX

| Alcohol, sedative-hypnotics, and other CNS depressants | ⇧ CNS depression |

ALTERED LABORATORY VALUES

No clinically significant alterations in blood/serum or urinary values occur at therapeutic dosages

USE IN CHILDREN

See INDICATIONS and ORAL DOSAGE; use with caution in children under 6 yr of age. Product should not be given indiscriminately to children taking other drugs. Antihistamines may cause excitability in children.

USE IN PREGNANT AND NURSING WOMEN

Consult manufacturer

[1] Contains no alcohol

ANTITUSSIVE COMBINATIONS

RYNA-CX (codeine phosphate, pseudoephedrine hydrochloride, and guaifenesin) Wallace   C-V

Liquid (per 5 ml): 10 mg codeine phosphate, 30 mg pseudoephedrine hydrochloride, and 100 mg guaifenesin[1] (4 fl oz, 1 pt) cherry/vanilla/menthol-flavored, sugar-free

INDICATIONS
Dry, nonproductive cough and nasal congestion

ORAL DOSAGE
Adult: 10 ml (2 tsp) q6h, up to 4 doses/24 h
Child (2–5 yr): 2.5 ml (½ tsp) q6h, up to 4 doses/24 h
Child (6–12 yr): 5 ml (1 tsp) q6h, up to 4 doses/24 h

CONTRAINDICATIONS
None known

WARNINGS/PRECAUTIONS

Drug dependence	Psychic and/or physical dependence may occur, especially in addiction-prone individuals
Constipation	May be caused or aggravated by codeine component
Persistent or chronic cough, or cough accompanied by excessive secretions, high fever, rash, or persistent headache	Use with caution; discontinue use if symptoms do not improve within 3 days
Nervousness, dizziness, sleeplessness	May occur at higher than recommended dosage
Special-risk patients	Use with caution in patients with chronic pulmonary disease, shortness of breath, high blood pressure, thyroid disease, or diabetes and in patients receiving MAO inhibitors (see DRUG INTERACTIONS) or antihypertensive medications

ADVERSE REACTIONS

| Gastrointestinal | Constipation |

OVERDOSAGE

| Signs and symptoms | *Codeine-related effects:* respiratory depression, somnolence, stupor, coma, skeletal-muscle flaccidity, cold and clammy skin, bradycardia, hypotension, apnea, circulatory collapse, and cardiac arrest, leading to death |
| Treatment | Reestablish an adequate airway and institute artificial respiration. For respiratory depression, administer a narcotic antagonist (eg, naloxone), along with attempts at resuscitation. Empty stomach by emesis or gastric lavage. Employ supportive measures, as indicated. |

DRUG INTERACTIONS

| MAO inhibitors | ⇧ Sympathomimetic and anticholinergic effects |

COMPENDIUM OF DRUG THERAPY

ALTERED LABORATORY VALUES

No clinically significant alterations in blood/serum or urinary values occur at therapeutic dosages

USE IN CHILDREN
See INDICATIONS and ORAL DOSAGE; use with caution in children under 2 yr of age. Product should not be given indiscriminately to children taking other drugs.

USE IN PREGNANT AND NURSING WOMEN
Consult manufacturer

1 Contains no alcohol

ANTITUSSIVE COMBINATIONS

RYNATUSS (carbetapentane tannate, chlorpheniramine tannate, ephedrine tannate, and phenylephrine tannate) Wallace — Rx

Tablets: 60 mg carbetapentane tannate, 5 mg chlorpheniramine tannate, 10 mg ephedrine tannate, and 10 mg phenylephrine tannate **Pediatric suspension (per 5 ml):** 30 mg carbetapentane tannate, 4 mg chlorpheniramine tannate, 5 mg ephedrine tannate, and 5 mg phenylephrine tannate (8 fl oz, 1 pt) *strawberry/currant–flavored*

INDICATIONS
Cough due to colds, bronchial asthma, acute and chronic bronchitis, or other respiratory tract conditions

ORAL DOSAGE
Adult: 1–2 tabs q12h
Child (2–6 yr): 2.5–5 ml (1/2–1 tsp) q12h
Child (> 6 yr): 5–10 ml (1–2 tsp) q12h

CONTRAINDICATIONS
Hypersensitivity or idiosyncratic reaction to any component or related compounds

Neonates

Breast-feeding

WARNINGS/PRECAUTIONS
Drowsiness — Caution patients not to drive or engage in other activities requiring mental alertness, and not to use alcohol or other CNS depressants (see DRUG INTERACTIONS)

Special-risk patients — Use with caution in patients with hypertension, cardiovascular disease, hyperthyroidism, diabetes, narrow-angle glaucoma, or prostatic hypertrophy

Elderly patients — Dizziness, sedation, and hypotension are more likely to occur

Tartrazine sensitivity — Presence of FD&C Yellow No. 5 (tartrazine) in suspension form may cause allergic-type reactions, including bronchial asthma, in susceptible individuals

ADVERSE REACTIONS
Gastrointestinal — Various effects

Central nervous system — Drowsiness, mild stimulation or sedation, dizziness, excitation

Cardiovascular — Hypotension

Other — Dryness of mucous membranes

OVERDOSAGE
Signs and symptoms — CNS depression or stimulation, restlessness, convulsions; atropine-like effects; chlorpheniramine overdosage may lead to convulsions and death in young children

Treatment — Induce emesis, taking precautions against aspiration. If gastric lavage is indicated, isotonic or 1/2 isotonic saline solution is preferred. A vasopressor may be used to treat hypotension, if needed. *Do not give stimulants.*

DRUG INTERACTIONS
MAO inhibitors — ⇧ Anticholinergic effects of antihistamines ⇧ Sympathomimetic effects

Alcohol, tranquilizers, sedative-hypnotics, and other CNS depressants — ⇧ CNS depression

ALTERED LABORATORY VALUES

No clinically significant alterations in blood/serum or urinary values occur at therapeutic dosages

USE IN CHILDREN	USE IN PREGNANT AND NURSING WOMEN
See INDICATIONS and ORAL DOSAGE; for use in children under 2 yr of age, titrate dosage individually. Contraindicated for use in neonates. Antihistamines in combination with sympathomimetic agents may cause either mild stimulation or mild sedation.	Pregnancy Category C: use during pregnancy only if clearly needed. Reproduction studies have not been performed in animals; it is not known whether this preparation can adversely affect fetal development or reproductive capacity. Contraindicated for use in nursing mothers.

ANTITUSSIVE COMBINATIONS

Terpin hydrate and codeine elixir   C-V

Elixir (per 5 ml): 85 mg terpin hydrate and 10 mg codeine[1] (5, 60, 120 ml; 1 pt; 1 gal)

INDICATIONS	ORAL DOSAGE
Cough due to colds and minor bronchial irritations	Adult and child ($\geq$ 6 yr): 5 ml (1 tsp) q3–4h

CONTRAINDICATIONS
Hypersensitivity to terpin hydrate or codeine

WARNINGS/PRECAUTIONS

Drug dependence	Psychic and/or physical dependence and tolerance may develop with prolonged use, especially in addiction-prone individuals
CNS depression	Caution patients about driving or engaging in other potentially hazardous activities requiring mental alertness or physical coordination; use with caution in elderly, debilitated, or sedated patients (see also DRUG INTERACTIONS)
Pulmonary impairment	By suppressing the cough reflex and increasing the viscosity of bronchial secretions, codeine may impair pulmonary function in patients who are hypoxic or recovering from surgery or who have a chronic obstructive pulmonary disease such as asthma, emphysema, or bronchitis
Cough due to serious disease	Monitor response of patients who have a high fever or a persistent cough

ADVERSE REACTIONS

Gastrointestinal	Nausea, constipation, epigastric pain, vomiting
Central nervous system	Drowsiness, dizziness; sweating and agitation (rare)
Other	Palpitations, pruritus

OVERDOSAGE

Signs and symptoms	Respiratory depression, miosis, somnolence, stupor, coma, skeletal-muscle flaccidity, cold and clammy skin, bradycardia, hypotension, apnea, circulatory collapse, and cardiac arrest
Treatment	Reestablish an adequate airway and institute artificial respiration. For respiratory depression, administer a narcotic antagonist (eg, naloxone) along with attempts at resuscitation. Empty stomach by emesis or gastric lavage. Employ supportive measures, as indicated.

DRUG INTERACTIONS

Alcohol, tranquilizers, sedative-hypnotics, and other CNS depressants	⇧ CNS depression

ALTERED LABORATORY VALUES
No clinically significant alterations in blood/serum or urinary values occur at therapeutic dosages

USE IN CHILDREN	USE IN PREGNANT AND NURSING WOMEN
See ORAL DOSAGE; exercise caution	Safety for use during pregnancy has not been established. Codeine is excreted in breast milk; patient should stop nursing if drug is prescribed.

[1] Contains approximately 40% alcohol

ANTITUSSIVE COMBINATIONS

TRIAMINIC Expectorant with Codeine (codeine phosphate, phenylpropanolamine hydrochloride, and guaifenesin)   Sandoz Consumer Health Care Group   C-V

Liquid (per 5 ml): 10 mg codeine phosphate, 12.5 mg phenylpropanolamine hydrochloride, and 100 mg guaifenesin[1] (4 fl oz, 1 pt)

INDICATIONS	ORAL DOSAGE
Cough and nasal congestion due to colds	**Adult:** 10 ml (2 tsp) q4h **Infant (3 mo to 2 yr):** 2 drops/kg q4h **Child (2–6 yr):** 2.5 ml (1/2 tsp) q4h **Child (6–12 yr):** 5 ml (1 tsp) q4h

TRIAMINIC Expectorant with Codeine ■ TRIAMINIC Expectorant DH

CONTRAINDICATIONS		
Long-term, continuous use (see warning concerning drug dependence)	Hypersensitivity to any component	MAO inhibitor therapy
	Severe hypertension	Severe coronary artery disease

WARNINGS/PRECAUTIONS

Drug dependence — Psychic and/or physical dependence and tolerance may develop, especially in addiction-prone individuals

Special-risk patients — Use with caution in patients with persistent or chronic cough, hypertension, hyperthyroidism, cardiovascular disease, diabetes, chronic pulmonary disease, or shortness of breath; children and elderly patients may be more susceptible to the effects of codeine, especially the respiratory depressant effects

ADVERSE REACTIONS

Central nervous system — Dizziness, sedation, mild stimulation

Gastrointestinal — Nausea, vomiting, constipation

OVERDOSAGE

Signs and symptoms — *Narcotic effects:* respiratory depression (cyanosis, Cheyne-Stokes respiration, decreased respiratory rate and/or tidal volume), extreme somnolence progressing to stupor or coma, skeletal muscle flaccidity, cold and clammy skin, bradycardia, hypotension; in severe cases, apnea, circulatory collapse, cardiac arrest, and death; *sympathomimetic effects:* tremor, restlessness, hyperreflexia, agitation, hallucinations

Treatment — Give primary attention to reestablishing adequate respiratory exchange through provision of an adequate airway and assisted or controlled ventilation; positive-pressure respiration may be desirable if pulmonary edema is present. If respiratory depression is significant, promptly administer naloxone. For adults, give 0.4–2 mg IV (or, if necessary, IM or SC) at 2- to 3-min intervals, as needed; for children, give 0.01 mg/kg IV, followed, if necessary, by 0.1 mg/kg IV (administer IM or SC in divided doses if IV administration is not feasible). *Do not use analeptic agents.* Oxygen, IV fluids, vasopressors, and other supportive measures should be employed, as needed. To remove drug from GI tract, induce emesis or perform gastric lavage; instillation of activated charcoal may also be considered.

DRUG INTERACTIONS

Alcohol, tranquilizers, sedative-hypnotics, and other CNS depressants — △ CNS depression

MAO inhibitors — △ Sympathomimetic effects

ALTERED LABORATORY VALUES

Urinary values — △ 5-HIAA (with colorimetric methods)   △ VMA (with colorimetric methods)

No clinically significant alterations in blood/serum values occur at therapeutic dosages

---

USE IN CHILDREN	**USE IN PREGNANT AND NURSING WOMEN**
See INDICATIONS and ORAL DOSAGE; use with caution in children taking other drugs	Use with caution in pregnant or nursing patients

[1] Contains 5% alcohol

ANTITUSSIVE COMBINATIONS

TRIAMINIC Expectorant DH (hydrocodone bitartrate, phenylpropanolamine hydrochloride, pheniramine maleate, pyrilamine maleate, and guaifenesin) Sandoz Consumer Health Care Group   C-III

Liquid (per 5 ml): 1.67 mg hydrocodone bitartrate, 12.5 mg phenylpropanolamine hydrochloride, 6.25 mg pheniramine maleate, 6.25 mg pyrilamine maleate, and 100 mg guaifenesin[1] (1 pt)

INDICATIONS	**ORAL DOSAGE**
Cough, nasal congestion, and postnasal drip due to colds, nasal allergies, sinusitis, or rhinitis	Adult: 10 ml (2 tsp) q4h
Severe, prolonged, or refractory cough associated with other respiratory infections	Child (1–6 yr): 2.5 ml (½ tsp) q4h
Allergic rhinitis symptoms, such as sneezing, rhinorrhea, pruritus, and lacrimation	Child (6–12 yr): 5 ml (1 tsp) q4h

COMPENDIUM OF DRUG THERAPY

TRIAMINIC Expectorant DH

CONTRAINDICATIONS

Hypersensitivity to any component	Severe hypertension	MAO inhibitor therapy (see DRUG INTERACTIONS)
Lower respiratory tract conditions	Severe coronary artery disease	
Breast-feeding		

WARNINGS/PRECAUTIONS

Diagnosis of underlying disease	The primary disease underlying cough should be ascertained before administering an antitussive so that modification of the cough does not increase the risk of clinical complications, and so that appropriate therapy may be instituted for the underlying disease
Drug dependence	Psychic and/or physical dependence and tolerance may develop, especially in addiction-prone individuals
Drowsiness	Caution patients about driving or engaging in other activities requiring mental alertness, and about alcohol or other CNS depressants
Elderly patients	Dizziness, sedation, and hypotension occur more frequently in patients over 60 yr of age; overdose of sympathomimetics in this age group may cause hallucinations, convulsions, CNS depression, and death
Other special-risk patients	Use with caution in patients with increased intraocular pressure or narrow-angle glaucoma, stenosing peptic ulcer, pyloroduodenal obstruction, symptomatic prostatic hypertrophy, bladder-neck obstruction, hypertension or other cardiovascular disease, hyperthyroidism, diabetes mellitus, or bronchial asthma
Carcinogenicity, mutagenicity, effect on fertility	The long-term carcinogenic and mutagenic potential of this preparation and its effect on fertility are unknown

ADVERSE REACTIONS

The most frequent reactions, regardless of incidence, are printed in *italics*

Central nervous system	*Sedation, sleepiness, dizziness, disturbed coordination, restlessness, excitation, nervousness, insomnia,* fatigue, confusion, tremor, irritability, euphoria, paresthesias, vertigo, hysteria, neuritis, convulsions, CNS depression, hallucinations
Special senses	Blurred vision, diplopia, tinnitus, acute labyrinthitis
Cardiovascular	Hypotension, headache, palpitations, tachycardia, extrasystoles
Gastrointestinal	*Epigastric distress, nausea, vomiting, constipation,* anorexia, diarrhea
Genitourinary	Urinary frequency, difficult urination, urinary retention, early menses
Hematologic	Hemolytic anemia, thrombocytopenia, agranulocytosis
Respiratory	Thickening of bronchial secretions, tightness of the chest and wheezing, nasal stuffiness
Dermatological and hypersensitivity	Urticaria, drug rash, anaphylactic shock, photosensitivity
Other	Excessive perspiration, chills; dry mouth, nose, and throat

OVERDOSAGE

Signs and symptoms	Coma, pinpoint pupils, and depressed respiration (this triad suggests hydrocodone poisoning); respiratory depression, extreme somnolence progressing to stupor or coma, skeletal muscle flaccidity, cold and clammy skin, bradycardia, hypotension; in severe cases, apnea, circulatory collapse, cardiac arrest, and death; excitation may occur in children in the presence of fever and dehydration
Treatment	Reestablish an adequate airway and institute artificial respiration. For respiratory depression, administer a narcotic antagonist (naloxone, nalorphine, or levallorphan) preferably IV, along with attempts at resuscitation. Keep patient under continued surveillance and administer repeated doses of the antagonist as necessary to maintain adequate respiration. Oxygen, IV fluids, vasopressors, specific treatment for anticholinergic drug intoxication, and other supportive measures may be indicated. Gastric lavage, followed by activated charcoal, may be useful in removing unabsorbed drug.

DRUG INTERACTIONS

Alcohol, tranquilizers, sedative-hypnotics, phenothiazines, MAO inhibitors, tricyclic antidepressants, and other CNS depressants	△ CNS depression
MAO inhibitors	△ Pressor and anticholinergic effects
Methyldopa, guanethidine, mecamylamine, reserpine, *Veratrum* alkaloids	▽ Antihypertensive effect

ALTERED LABORATORY VALUES

Blood/serum values	▽ Uric acid

TRIAMINIC Expectorant DH ■ TUSSEND

Urinary values —————————————— ◊ 5-HIAA ◊ VMA

USE IN CHILDREN
See INDICATIONS and ORAL DOSAGE. This preparation may elicit either mild stimulation or mild sedation; the former is the response most frequently seen in young children.

USE IN PREGNANT AND NURSING WOMEN
Pregnancy Category C: use during pregnancy only if the expected therapeutic benefits outweigh the potential hazards. Animal reproduction studies have not been done, and the safety of using these preparations in pregnant women has not been established with regard to their possible effects on fetal development. Contraindicated for use in nursing mothers because of the higher risk of antihistaminic side effects in premature and full-term infants.

[1] Contains 5% alcohol

ANTITUSSIVE COMBINATIONS

TUSSEND (hydrocodone bitartrate and pseudoephedrine hydrochloride) Merrell Dow   C-III

Tablets: 5 mg hydrocodone bitartrate and 60 mg pseudoephedrine hydrochloride **Liquid (per 5 ml):** 5 mg hydrocodone bitartrate and 60 mg pseudoephedrine hydrochloride[1] (1 pt)

INDICATIONS	**ORAL DOSAGE**
Exhausting cough spasms accompanying **upper-respiratory-tract congestion** due to colds, influenza, bronchitis, or sinusitis	Adult: 1 tab or 5 ml (1 tsp) qid, as needed Child (25–50 lb): 1.25 ml (¼ tsp) qid, as needed Child (50–90 lb): 2.5 ml (½ tsp) qid, as needed Child (> 90 lb): same as for adult

CONTRAINDICATIONS

Hypersensitivity or idiosyncratic reaction[2] to any component or to other sympathomimetic amines or phenanthrene derivatives	Breast-feeding MAO inhibitor therapy (see DRUG INTERACTIONS)	Severe hypertension Severe coronary artery disease

WARNINGS/PRECAUTIONS

Drug dependence	Psychic and/or physical dependence and tolerance may develop, especially in addiction-prone individuals
Drowsiness	Caution patients about driving or engaging in other potentially hazardous activities requiring mental alertness and/or physical coordination, and about using alcohol or other CNS depressants (see DRUG INTERACTIONS)
Elderly patients	Adverse reactions to sympathomimetics are more likely in patients over 60 yr of age
Special-risk patients	Use with extreme caution in patients with severe respiratory impairment or impaired respiratory drive; use with caution in patients with diabetes mellitus, hypertension, ischemic heart disease, hyperthyroidism, increased intraocular pressure, or prostatic hypertrophy, or in those with a history of hyperreactivity to ephedrine

ADVERSE REACTIONS[3]

Gastrointestinal	Upset, nausea, constipation
Central nervous system and neuromuscular	Drowsiness, headache, dizziness, fear, anxiety, tension, restlessness, tremor, weakness, insomnia, hallucinations, convulsions, depression
Cardiovascular	Tachycardia, palpitations, pallor, arrhythmias, cardiovascular collapse with hypotension
Respiratory	Difficult breathing
Genitourinary	Dysuria

OVERDOSAGE

Signs and symptoms	*Hydrocodone-related effects:* CNS depression, cardiovascular depression; *pseudoephedrine-related effects:* CNS stimulation, variable cardiovascular effects; in patients over 60 yr of age, pseudoephedrine overdosage may cause hallucinations, convulsions, CNS depression, and death
Treatment	Reestablish an adequate airway and institute artificial respiration. For respiratory depression, administer a narcotic antagonist (eg, naloxone) along with attempts at resuscitation. Empty stomach by emesis or gastric lavage. Employ supportive measures, as indicated. If patient shows signs of stimulation, treat conservatively. Avoid CNS depressants, if possible, due to potential drug interaction with hydrocodone.

TUSSEND ■ TUSSEND Expectorant

DRUG INTERACTIONS

Pressor amines	△	Blood pressure; use concomitantly with great caution
Alcohol, tranquilizers, sedative-hypnotics, and other CNS depressants	△	CNS depression
MAO inhibitors, beta-adrenergic blockers	△	Sympathomimetic effect
Methyldopa, mecamylamine, reserpine, *Veratrum* alkaloids	▽	Antihypertensive effect

ALTERED LABORATORY VALUES

Blood/serum values — △ SGOT △ SGPT

No clinically significant alterations in urinary values occur at therapeutic dosages

---

USE IN CHILDREN

See INDICATIONS and ORAL DOSAGE

USE IN PREGNANT AND NURSING WOMEN

Pregnancy Category C: use during pregnancy only if clearly needed. Reproduction studies have not been performed in animals; it is not known whether this preparation can adversely affect fetal development or reproductive capacity. Contraindicated for use in nursing mothers, due to the potential for serious adverse reactions in infants from sympathomimetic amines.

---

[1] Contains 5% alcohol
[2] In sensitive patients, small doses of sympathomimetic agents can cause idiosyncratic reactions, including insomnia, tremor, weakness, dizziness, and arrhythmia
[3] Includes reactions common to sympathomimetic amines in general

---

ANTITUSSIVE COMBINATIONS

TUSSEND Expectorant (hydrocodone bitartrate, pseudoephedrine hydrochloride, and guaifenesin) Merrell Dow   C-III

Liquid (per 5 ml): 5 mg hydrocodone bitartrate, 60 mg pseudoephedrine hydrochloride, and 200 mg guaifenesin[1] (1 pt)

INDICATIONS

Cough (nonproductive) accompanying respiratory tract congestion due to colds, influenza, sinusitis, and bronchitis

ORAL DOSAGE

Adult: 5 ml (1 tsp) qid, as needed
Child (25–50 lb): 1.25 ml (1/4 tsp) qid, as needed
Child (50–90 lb): 2.5 ml (1/2 tsp) qid, as needed

CONTRAINDICATIONS

Hypersensitivity or idiosyncratic reaction[2] to any component or to other sympathomimetic amines or phenanthrene derivatives	Breast-feeding	Severe hypertension
	MAO inhibitor therapy (see DRUG INTERACTIONS)	Severe coronary artery disease

WARNINGS/PRECAUTIONS

Drug dependence	Psychic and/or physical dependence and tolerance may develop, especially in addiction-prone individuals
Drowsiness	Caution patients about driving or engaging in other potentially hazardous activities requiring mental alertness and/or physical coordination, and about using alcohol or other CNS depressants (see DRUG INTERACTIONS)
Elderly patients	Sympathomimetic side effects are more likely to occur in patients over 60 yr of age
Special-risk patients	Use with extreme caution in patients with severe respiratory impairment or impaired respiratory drive; use with caution in patients with hypertension, diabetes mellitus, ischemic heart disease, hyperthyroidism, increased intraocular pressure, prostatic hypertrophy, or hypersensitivity to ephedrine (see CONTRAINDICATIONS)

ADVERSE REACTIONS[3]

Gastrointestinal	Upset, nausea, constipation
Central nervous system and neuromuscular	Drowsiness, dizziness, headache, fear, anxiety, tension, restlessness, tremor, weakness, insomnia, hallucinations, convulsions, CNS depression
Cardiovascular	Tachycardia, palpitations, pallor, arrhythmias, cardiovascular collapse with hypotension
Respiratory	Difficult breathing

TUSSEND Expectorant ■ TUSSIONEX

Genitourinary	Dysuria

OVERDOSAGE

Signs and symptoms	*Toxic effects primarily attributable to hydrocodone:* CNS depression, cardiovascular depression; *pseudoephedrine-related effects:* CNS stimulation, variable cardiovascular effects; in patients over 60 yr of age, pseudoephedrine overdosage may cause hallucinations, convulsions, CNS depression, and death
Treatment	Reestablish an adequate airway and institute artificial respiration. For respiratory depression, administer a narcotic antagonist (eg, naloxone) along with attempts at resuscitation. Empty stomach by emesis or gastric lavage. Employ supportive measures, as indicated. If patient shows signs of stimulation, treat conservatively. Avoid CNS depressants, if possible, due to potential drug interaction with hydrocodone.

DRUG INTERACTIONS

Pressor amines	△ Blood pressure; use concomitantly with great caution
Alcohol, tranquilizers, sedative-hypnotics, and other CNS depressants	△ CNS depression
MAO inhibitors, beta-adrenergic blockers	△ Sympathomimetic effect
Methyldopa, mecamylamine, reserpine, *Veratrum* alkaloids	▽ Antihypertensive effect

ALTERED LABORATORY VALUES

Blood/serum values	△ SGOT △ SGPT
Urinary values	△ 5-HIAA (colorimetric interference) △ VMA (colorimetric interference)

USE IN CHILDREN	USE IN PREGNANT AND NURSING WOMEN
See INDICATIONS and ORAL DOSAGE	Pregnancy Category C: use during pregnancy only if clearly needed. Reproduction studies have not been performed in animals; it is not known whether this preparation can adversely affect fetal development or reproductive capacity. Contraindicated for use in nursing mothers, due to the potential for serious adverse reactions in infants from sympathomimetic amines.

[1] Contains 12.5% alcohol
[2] In sensitive patients, small doses of sympathomimetic agents can cause idiosyncratic reactions, including insomnia, tremor, weakness, dizziness, and arrhythmia
[3] Includes reactions common to sympathomimetic amines in general

---

ANTITUSSIVE COMBINATIONS

TUSSIONEX (hydrocodone and phenyltoloxamine) Pennwalt   C-III

Capsules: 5 mg hydrocodone and 10 mg phenyltoloxamine   **Tablets:** 5 mg hydrocodone and 10 mg phenyltoloxamine
Suspension (per 5 ml): 5 mg hydrocodone and 10 mg phenyltoloxamine (16 fl oz, 900 ml)

INDICATIONS	ORAL DOSAGE
Cough (nonproductive)	**Adult:** 1 tab or cap or 5 ml (1 tsp) q8–12h **Infant** (< 1 yr): 1.25 ml (¼ tsp) q12h **Child** (1–5 yr): 2.5 ml (½ tsp) q12h **Child** (6–12 yr): 5 ml (1 tsp) q12h

CONTRAINDICATIONS

Consult manufacturer

WARNINGS/PRECAUTIONS

Drug dependence	Psychic and/or physical dependence and tolerance may develop, especially in addiction-prone individuals

ADVERSE REACTIONS

Gastrointestinal	Mild constipation, nausea
Central nervous system	Drowsiness
Dermatological	Facial pruritus

OVERDOSAGE

Signs and symptoms	Respiratory depression, convulsions (sometimes seen in children), hypothermia

TUSSIONEX ■ TUSSI-ORGANIDIN

Treatment	Immediately empty the stomach. To counteract respiratory depression, use respiratory stimulants. Administer short-acting barbiturates to treat convulsions. Hypothermia can be controlled by the usual supportive methods.

DRUG INTERACTIONS

Alcohol, tranquilizers, sedative-hypnotics, and other CNS depressants	◇	CNS depression

ALTERED LABORATORY VALUES

No clinically significant alterations in blood/serum or urinary values occur at therapeutic dosages

---

USE IN CHILDREN

See INDICATIONS and ORAL DOSAGE. Respiratory depression may be precipitated in children with compromised respiration; young children are especially susceptible to the depressant action of narcotic cough suppressants.

USE IN PREGNANT AND NURSING WOMEN

Pregnancy Category C: use during pregnancy only if clearly needed. Reproduction studies have not been performed in animals; it is not known whether this preparation can harm the fetus or affect reproductive capacity. Physical dependence, with resulting withdrawal signs, has been reported in infants of women who have taken narcotics during pregnancy. When given in therapeutic doses, hydrocodone is excreted in breast milk in trace amounts; use this preparation with caution in nursing mothers.

ANTITUSSIVE COMBINATIONS

TUSSI-ORGANIDIN (iodinated glycerol and codeine phosphate) Wallace   C-V

Liquid (per 5 ml): 30 mg iodinated glycerol and 10 mg codeine phosphate (1 pt, 1 gal)

INDICATIONS	ORAL DOSAGE
Cough (nonproductive) associated with colds, chronic bronchitis, bronchial asthma, tracheobronchitis, or other respiratory tract conditions (eg, laryngitis, pharyngitis, croup, pertussis, and emphysema)	**Adult:** 5–10 ml (1–2 tsp) q4h **Child:** 2.5–5 ml (½–1 tsp) q4h

CONTRAINDICATIONS

Pregnancy	Neonates	Breast-feeding
History of marked sensitivity to inorganic iodides	Hypersensitivity to any component or related compound	

WARNINGS/PRECAUTIONS

Rash	Discontinue use if evidence of hypersensitivity occurs
Iodism	Dermatitis and other reversible manifestations may occur, particularly with prolonged therapy
Drug dependence	Psychic and/or physical dependence and tolerance to codeine may develop, especially in addiction-prone individuals
Flare-up of adolescent acne	May occur
Special-risk patients	Use with caution or avoid use in patients with a history or evidence of thyroid disease
Carcinogenicity, mutagenicity, effect on fertility	No long-term animal studies have been performed to evaluate the carcinogenic or mutagenic potential of this preparation or its effect on fertility

ADVERSE REACTIONS

Central nervous system	Drowsiness, dizziness, miosis
Gastrointestinal	Nausea, vomiting, constipation; GI irritation (rare)
Dermatological	Rash (rare)
Other	Thyroid gland enlargement, acute parotitis, and hypersensitivity (rare)

OVERDOSAGE

Acute overdosage, which has been reported in rare cases, has caused no serious problems

DRUG INTERACTIONS

Lithium	◇	Risk of hypothyroidism

Antithyroid drugs	⇧ Hypothyroid effect

ALTERED LABORATORY VALUES

Blood/serum values	⇧ PBI

No clinically significant alterations in urinary values occur at therapeutic dosages

---

USE IN CHILDREN

See INDICATIONS and ORAL DOSAGE. Children with cystic fibrosis may have an increased susceptibility to the goitrogenic effects of iodides. Contraindicated for use in newborns.

USE IN PREGNANT AND NURSING WOMEN

Pregnancy Category X: contraindicated for use during pregnancy. Use of inorganic iodides during and after the 12th wk of gestation has been reported to induce fetal goiter with the potential for airway obstruction. If patient becomes pregnant while taking this drug, discontinue use and inform patient of the potential risk to the fetus. Contraindicated for use in nursing mothers.

ANTITUSSIVE COMBINATIONS

TUSSI-ORGANIDIN DM (iodinated glycerol and dextromethorphan hydrobromide) Wallace   Rx

Liquid (per 5 ml): 30 mg iodinated glycerol and 10 mg dextromethorphan hydrobromide (1 pt, 1 gal)

INDICATIONS

Cough (nonproductive) associated with colds, chronic bronchitis, bronchial asthma, tracheobronchitis, or other respiratory tract conditions (eg, laryngitis, pharyngitis, croup, pertussis, and emphysema)

ORAL DOSAGE

Adult: 5–10 ml (1–2 tsp) q4h
Child: 2.5–5 ml (½–1 tsp) q4h

CONTRAINDICATIONS

Pregnancy	Neonates	Breast-feeding
History of marked sensitivity to inorganic iodides	Hypersensitivity to any component or related compound	

WARNINGS/PRECAUTIONS

Rash	Discontinue use if evidence of hypersensitivity occurs
Iodism	Dermatitis and other reversible manifestations may occur, particularly with prolonged therapy
Flare-up of adolescent acne	May occur
Special-risk patients	Use with caution or avoid use in patients with a history or evidence of thyroid disease
Carcinogenicity, mutagenicity, effect on fertility	No long-term animal studies have been performed to evaluate the carcinogenic or mutagenic potential of this preparation or its effect on fertility

ADVERSE REACTIONS

Central nervous system	Drowsiness (rare)
Gastrointestinal	GI irritation and other disturbances (rare)
Dermatological	Rash (rare)
Other	Thyroid gland enlargement, acute parotitis, and hypersensitivity (rare)

OVERDOSAGE

Acute overdosage, which has been reported in rare cases, has caused no serious problems

DRUG INTERACTIONS

Lithium	⇧ Risk of hypothyroidism
Antithyroid drugs	⇧ Hypothyroid effect

ALTERED LABORATORY VALUES

Blood/serum values	⇧ PBI

No clinically significant alterations in urinary values occur at therapeutic dosages.

USE IN CHILDREN

See INDICATIONS and ORAL DOSAGE. Children with cystic fibrosis may have an increased susceptibility to the goitrogenic effects of iodides. Contraindicated for use in newborns.

USE IN PREGNANT AND NURSING WOMEN

Pregnancy Category X: contraindicated for use during pregnancy. Use of inorganic iodides during and after the 12th wk of gestation has been reported to induce fetal goiter with the potential for airway obstruction. If patient becomes pregnant while taking this drug, discontinue use and inform patient of the potential risk to the fetus. Contraindicated for use in nursing mothers.

ANTITUSSIVE COMBINATIONS

TUSS-ORNADE (caramiphen edisylate and phenylpropanolamine hydrochloride) Smith Kline & French — Rx

Capsules (sustained release): 40 mg caramiphen edisylate and 75 mg phenylpropanolamine hydrochloride **Liquid (per 5 ml):** 6.7 mg caramiphen edisylate and 12.5 mg phenylpropanolamine hydrochloride[1] (16 fl oz) *fruit-flavored, sugar-free*

INDICATIONS	**ORAL DOSAGE**
Symptomatic relief of **cough and nasal congestion** associated with common colds[2]	**Adult:** 1 cap q12h or 10 ml (2 tsp) q4h, up to 60 ml (12 tsp)/24 h **Child (2–6 yr):** 2.5 ml (½ tsp) q4h, up to 15 ml (3 tsp)/24 h **Child (6–12 yr):** 5 ml (1 tsp) q4h, up to 30 ml (6 tsp)/24 h **Child (> 12 yr):** same as adult

CONTRAINDICATIONS		
Hypersensitivity to either component	Severe hypertension	MAO inhibitor therapy (see DRUG INTERACTIONS)
Bronchial asthma	Coronary artery disease	

WARNINGS/PRECAUTIONS	
Drowsiness	Caution patients about driving or engaging in other activities requiring mental alertness
Special-risk patients	Use with caution in patients with cardiovascular disease, glaucoma, prostatic hypertrophy, thyroid disease, or diabetes or when a productive cough is desirable to remove excessive bronchial secretions
Concomitant use	Caution patient not to take other medications containing phenylpropanolamine or amphetamines simultaneously, and about using alcohol or other CNS depressants (see DRUG INTERACTIONS)

ADVERSE REACTIONS	
Central nervous system	Dizziness, drowsiness, nervousness, insomnia, weakness, irritability, headache, incoordination, tremor, visual disturbances
Gastrointestinal	Nausea, upset, diarrhea, abdominal pain, constipation, anorexia
Cardiovascular, respiratory	Tightness in the chest, angina pain, palpitations, hypertension, hypotension
Genitourinary	Difficulty in urination, dysuria

OVERDOSAGE	
Signs and symptoms	Dryness of mouth, dysphagia, thirst, blurred vision, dilated pupils, photophobia, fever, rapid pulse and respiration, disorientation, dizziness, nausea, fainting, tachycardia, CNS excitation or depression
Treatment	Empty stomach immediately by emesis and gastric lavage. Administer a saline cathartic to hasten evacuation of timed-release pellets. Treat respiratory depression promptly with oxygen. Do not treat respiratory or CNS depression with analeptics that might precipitate convulsions; if convulsions or marked CNS excitement occurs, only short-acting barbiturates or chloral hydrate should be given.

DRUG INTERACTIONS	
Alcohol, tranquilizers, sedative-hypnotics, and other CNS depressants	△ CNS depression
MAO inhibitors	△ Sympathomimetic effects

ALTERED LABORATORY VALUES

No clinically significant alterations in blood/serum or urinary values occur at therapeutic dosages

USE IN CHILDREN
See INDICATIONS and ORAL DOSAGE; do not use sustained-release capsules in children under 12 yr of age, or liquid in children under 15 lb or 6 mo of age

USE IN PREGNANT AND NURSING WOMEN
Use in pregnant women, nursing mothers, or women of childbearing age only if the expected benefits outweigh the potential risks. Safety for use during pregnancy has not been established.

[1] Contains 5% alcohol
[2] A final determination has not been made on the effectiveness of this drug combination in accordance with efficacy requirements of the 1962 Amendments to the Food, Drug and Cosmetic Act.

DECONGESTANTS/UPPER RESPIRATORY COMBINATIONS

COMHIST (chlorpheniramine maleate, phenyltoloxamine citrate, and phenylephrine hydrochloride) Norwich Eaton — Rx

Tablets: 2 mg chlorpheniramine maleate, 25 mg phenyltoloxamine citrate, and 10 mg phenylephrine hydrochloride

COMHIST LA (chlorpheniramine maleate, phenyltoloxamine citrate, and phenylephrine hydrochloride) Norwich Eaton — Rx

Capsules (sustained release): 4 mg chlorpheniramine maleate, 50 mg phenyltoloxamine citrate, and 20 mg phenylephrine hydrochloride

INDICATIONS	**ORAL DOSAGE**
Relief of **rhinorrhea and congestion** associated with seasonal and/or perennial allergic rhinitis and vasomotor rhinitis	Adult: 1–2 tabs q8h or 1 cap q8–12h Child (6–12 yr): 1 tab q8h Child ($\geq$ 12 yr): same as adult

CONTRAINDICATIONS
Hypersensitivity to any component	Narrow angle glaucoma	Asthmatic symptoms
MAO inhibitor therapy (see DRUG INTERACTIONS)	Age < 12 yr for capsules and < 6 yr for tablets	Severe hypertension

WARNINGS/PRECAUTIONS
Drowsiness	Caution patients not to drive or engage in other potentially hazardous activities requiring mental alertness
Special-risk patients	Use with extreme caution in patients with stenosing peptic ulcer, pyloroduodenal obstruction, prostatic hypertrophy, or bladder neck obstruction, and with caution in patients with increased intraocular pressure, cardiovascular disease (including heart disease and hypertension), diabetes mellitus, hyperthyroidism, or a history of bronchial asthma

ADVERSE REACTIONS
Central nervous system	Sedation, dizziness, excitation (especially in children), nervousness, insomnia, blurred vision, convulsions
Gastrointestinal	Epigastric distress, anorexia, nausea, vomiting, diarrhea, constipation
Cardiovascular	Hypotension, headache, palpitations
Respiratory	Thickening of bronchial secretions, tightness in the chest and wheezing, nasal stuffiness
Dermatological	Urticaria, rash
Hematological	Leukopenia, agranulocytosis, thrombocytopenia
Other	Urinary retention or frequency; dry mouth, nose, and throat

OVERDOSAGE
Signs and symptoms	See ADVERSE REACTIONS

Treatment	Treatment should be symptomatic and supportive and, if the sustained-release capsules have been ingested, should be continued for at least 12 h. To remove this product from the GI tract, induce emesis with ipecac syrup or, if the patient is convulsing, comatose, or cannot gag, perform gastric lavage with a large-bore tube; if necessary, administer activated charcoal and a saline cathartic following lavage or emesis.

DRUG INTERACTIONS

Alcohol, tranquilizers, sedative-hypnotics, and other CNS depressants	△ CNS depression
MAO inhibitors	△ Sympathomimetic and anticholinergic effects; do not use MAO inhibitors with this preparation
Methyldopa, guanethidine, mecamylamine, reserpine, *Veratrum* alkaloids	▽ Antihypertensive effect

ALTERED LABORATORY VALUES

No clinically significant alterations in blood/serum or urinary values occur at therapeutic dosages

USE IN CHILDREN
See INDICATIONS and ORAL DOSAGE; tablets are contraindicated for use in children under 6 yr of age and capsules in children under 12

USE IN PREGNANT AND NURSING WOMEN
Pregnancy Category C: reproduction studies have not been done; it is not known whether this preparation can cause harm to the fetus or affect reproductive capacity. Use during pregnancy only if clearly needed. It is not known whether the components of this product are excreted in human milk; patients should not nurse while taking this preparation.

DECONGESTANTS/UPPER RESPIRATORY COMBINATIONS

DECONAMINE (chlorpheniramine maleate and pseudoephedrine hydrochloride) Berlex   Rx

Tablets: 4 mg chlorpheniramine maleate and 60 mg pseudoephedrine hydrochloride **Syrup (per 5 ml):** 2 mg chlorpheniramine maleate and 30 mg pseudoephedrine hydrochloride (473 ml) *grape-flavored*

DECONAMINE SR (chlorpheniramine maleate and pseudoephedrine hydrochloride) Berlex   Rx

Capsules (sustained release): 8 mg chlorpheniramine maleate and 120 mg pseudoephedrine hydrochloride

INDICATIONS	ORAL DOSAGE	
Nasal congestion associated with the common cold, hay fever and other allergies, sinusitis, eustachian tube blockage, and vasomotor and allergic rhinitis	Adult: 1 tab or 5–10 ml (1–2 tsp) tid or qid or 1 cap q12h Child (2–6 yr): 2.5 ml (½ tsp) tid or qid, up to 10 ml (2 tsp)/24 h Child (6–12 yr): 2.5–5 ml (½–1 tsp) tid or qid, up to 20 ml (4 tsp)/24 h Child (> 12 yr): same as adult	

CONTRAINDICATIONS

Severe hypertension	MAO inhibitor therapy (see DRUG INTERACTIONS)	Sensitivity to antihistamines or sympathomimetic amines
Severe coronary artery disease		

WARNINGS/PRECAUTIONS

Cardiovascular collapse, convulsions	Sympathomimetic agents may precipitate cardiovascular collapse accompanied by hypotension or produce convulsions and other manifestations of CNS stimulation
Drowsiness, dizziness	Caution patients about driving or engaging in other potentially hazardous activities requiring mental alertness and/or physical coordination, and about using alcohol or other CNS depressants (see DRUG INTERACTIONS)
Special-risk patients	Use with extreme caution in patients with narrow angle glaucoma, stenosing peptic ulcer, pyloroduodenal or bladder neck obstruction, or symptomatic prostatic hypertrophy and with caution in patients with hypertension, ischemic heart disease, diabetes mellitus, increased intraocular pressure, hyperthyroidism, or bronchial asthma

ADVERSE REACTIONS[1]

Central nervous system	Drowsiness, sedation, dizziness, light-headedness, disturbed coordination, fatigue, weakness, confusion, restlessness, excitation, nervousness, fear, anxiety, tenseness, tremor, irritability, insomnia, euphoria, hallucination, paresthesia, blurred vision, diplopia, vertigo, tinnitus, hysteria, neuritis, convulsions
Cardiovascular	Hypotension, headache, palpitations, arrhythmia (including tachycardia and extrasystole), pallor; cardiovascular collapse with hypotension
Hematological	Hemolytic anemia, thrombocytopenia, agranulocytosis

DECONAMINE ■ ENTEX

Respiratory	Thickening of bronchial secretions, tightness of the chest, wheezing, respiratory difficulty, nasal congestion, dry nose and throat
Gastrointestinal	Epigastric distress, anorexia, nausea, vomiting, diarrhea, constipation
Genitourinary	Frequent urination, dysuria, urinary retention, early menses
Other	Urticaria, drug rash, anaphylactic shock, photosensitivity, excessive perspiration, chills, dry mouth

OVERDOSAGE

Signs and symptoms	CNS stimulation, cardiovascular reactions
Treatment	Remove the drug from the GI tract. Institute supportive measures and symptomatic therapy; signs of stimulation should be treated conservatively. Use vasopressors with great caution.

DRUG INTERACTIONS

Other sympathomimetic drugs, beta-adrenergic blockers	△ Sympathomimetic effect
MAO inhibitors	△ Sympathomimetic effect; hypertensive crisis may occur △ Anticholinergic effect
Alcohol, tranquilizers, sedative-hypnotics, and other CNS depressants	△ CNS depression
Guanethidine, methyldopa, mecamylamine, reserpine, *Veratrum* alkaloids	▽ Antihypertensive effect

ALTERED LABORATORY VALUES

No clinically significant alterations in blood/serum or urinary values occur at therapeutic dosages

---

USE IN CHILDREN

See INDICATIONS and ORAL DOSAGE; use according to medical judgment in children under 2 yr of age. The capsules and tablets should not be given to children under 12 yr of age.

USE IN PREGNANT AND NURSING WOMEN

Pregnancy Category C: reproduction studies have not been performed; it is not known whether this preparation can cause harm to the fetus or affect reproductive capacity. Use during pregnancy only if clearly needed. Pseudoephedrine and chlorpheniramine may be excreted in human milk; because the risk of adverse reactions is higher than usual in infants, patients should not nurse while taking this preparation.

---

[1] Includes reactions common to antihistamines and sympathomimetic amines in general

---

DECONGESTANTS/UPPER RESPIRATORY COMBINATIONS

ENTEX (phenylephrine hydrochloride, phenylpropanolamine hydrochloride, and guaifenesin) Norwich Eaton   Rx

Capsules: 5 mg phenylephrine hydrochloride, 45 mg phenylpropanolamine hydrochloride, and 200 mg guaifenesin   **Liquid (per 5 ml):** 5 mg phenylephrine hydrochloride, 20 mg phenylpropanolamine hydrochloride, and 100 mg guaifenesin[1] (1 pt)

ENTEX LA (phenylpropanolamine hydrochloride and guaifenesin) Norwich Eaton   Rx

Tablets (long acting): 75 mg phenylpropanolamine hydrochloride and 400 mg guaifenesin

INDICATIONS

Symptomatic relief of **sinusitis, bronchitis, pharyngitis, and coryza** associated with nasal congestion and viscous mucus in the lower respiratory tract

ORAL DOSAGE

Adult: 1 cap, with food or fluid, or 10 ml (2 tsp) q6h, or, alternatively, 1 tab q12h; tablets should not be crushed or chewed
Child (2–4 yr): 2.5 ml (½ tsp) q6h
Child (4–6 yr): 5 ml (1 tsp) q6h
Child (6–12 yr): 7.5 ml (1½ tsp) q6h or ½ tab q12h; tablets should not be crushed or chewed
Child (≥12 yr): same as adult

CONTRAINDICATIONS

Hypersensitivity to sympathomimetic agents	MAO inhibitor therapy (see DRUG INTERACTIONS)	Severe hypertension

WARNINGS/PRECAUTIONS

Special-risk patients	Use with caution in patients with hypertension, diabetes mellitus, heart disease, peripheral vascular disease, increased intraocular pressure, hyperthyroidism, or prostatic hypertrophy

ENTEX ■ NALDECON

ADVERSE REACTIONS

Central nervous system	Nervousness, insomnia, restlessness, headache
Gastrointestinal	Gastric irritation, nausea
Genitourinary	Urinary retention in patients with prostatic hypertrophy

OVERDOSAGE

Signs and symptoms	See ADVERSE REACTIONS
Treatment	Treatment should be symptomatic and supportive and, if the tablets have been ingested, should be continued for at least 12 h. To remove this product from the GI tract, induce emesis with ipecac syrup or, if the patient is convulsing, comatose, or cannot gag, perform gastric lavage with a large-bore tube; if necessary, administer activated charcoal and a saline cathartic following lavage or emesis.

DRUG INTERACTIONS

MAO inhibitors, other sympathomimetic drugs	⇧ Sympathomimetic effects; do not use these drugs with this preparation

ALTERED LABORATORY VALUES

Urinary values	⇧ 5-HIAA (colorimetric interference) ⇧ VMA (colorimetric interference)

No clinically significant alterations in blood/serum values occur at therapeutic dosages

---

USE IN CHILDREN

See INDICATIONS and ORAL DOSAGE; do not use capsules in children under 12 yr of age, tablets in children under 6 yr of age, or liquid in children under 2 yr of age

USE IN PREGNANT AND NURSING WOMEN

Pregnancy Category C: reproduction studies have not been done; it is not known whether this preparation can cause harm to the fetus or affect reproductive capacity. Use during pregnancy only if clearly needed. It is not known whether the components of this product are excreted in human milk; patients should not nurse while taking this preparation.

---

[1] Contains 5% alcohol

DECONGESTANTS/UPPER RESPIRATORY COMBINATIONS

NALDECON (phenylpropanolamine hydrochloride, phenylephrine hydrochloride, phenyltoloxamine citrate, and chlorpheniramine maleate) Bristol   Rx

Tablets (sustained-release): 40 mg phenylpropanolamine hydrochloride, 10 mg phenylephrine hydrochloride, 15 mg phenyltoloxamine citrate, and 5 mg chlorpheniramine maleate   **Syrup (per 5 ml):** 20 mg phenylpropanolamine hydrochloride, 5 mg phenylephrine hydrochloride, 7.5 mg phenyltoloxamine citrate, and 2.5 mg chlorpheniramine maleate   **Pediatric syrup (per 5 ml):** 5 mg phenylpropanolamine hydrochloride, 1.25 mg phenylephrine hydrochloride, 2.0 mg phenyltoloxamine citrate, and 0.5 mg chlorpheniramine maleate   **Pediatric drops (per dropperful [1 ml]):** 5 mg phenylpropanolamine hydrochloride, 1.25 mg phenylephrine hydrochloride, 2.0 mg phenyltoloxamine citrate, and 0.5 mg chlorpheniramine maleate

INDICATIONS

Nasal and eustachian tube congestion associated with colds, sinusitis, and acute upper respiratory infections[1]
Symptomatic relief of **allergic and vasomotor rhinitis**

ORAL DOSAGE

Adult: 1 tab tid or 5 ml syrup (1 tsp) q3–4h, up to 4 doses/24 h
Infant (3–6 mo; 12–17 lb): 1/4 ml drops q3–4h, up to 4 doses/24 h
Infant (6–12 mo; 17–24 lb): 1/2 ml drops or 2.5 ml ped syrup (1/2 tsp) q3–4h, up to 4 doses/24 h
Child (1–6 yr; 24–50 lb): 1 ml drops or 5 ml ped syrup (1 tsp) q3–4h, up to 4 doses/24 h
Child (6–12 yr; > 50 lb): 1/2 tab tid or 10 ml (2 tsp) ped syrup or 2.5 ml (1/2 tsp) syrup q3–4h, up to 4 doses/24 h
Child (> 12 yr): same as adult

CONTRAINDICATIONS

Severe hypertension	Asthmatic attack	Narrow angle glaucoma
Severe coronary artery disease	Hypersensitivity or idiosyncratic reaction to sympathomimetic amines or antihistamines	Urinary retention
MAO inhibitor therapy (see DRUG INTERACTIONS)		Peptic ulcer

WARNINGS/PRECAUTIONS

Drowsiness	Caution patients about driving or engaging in other potentially hazardous activities requiring mental alertness or physical coordination, and about using alcohol or other CNS depressants (see DRUG INTERACTIONS)

NALDECON ■ NOVAFED

Special-risk patients	Use judiciously and sparingly in patients with hypertension, cardiovascular disease, ischemic heart disease, diabetes mellitus, increased intraocular pressure, hyperthyroidism, prostatic hypertrophy, hyperreactivity to ephedrine, or history of bronchial asthma (see CONTRAINDICATIONS)

ADVERSE REACTIONS

Central nervous system	Stimulation, headache, dizziness, mild sedation, restlessness, tremor, weakness, pallor, insomnia, hallucinations, convulsions, depression, drowsiness, nervousness
Cardiovascular	Tachycardia, palpitations, arrhythmias, cardiovascular collapse, hypotension
Gastrointestinal	Nausea, vomiting, dry mouth, anorexia, heartburn
Genitourinary	Dysuria, polyuria
Other	Blurred vision, respiratory difficulty; dermatitis (very rare)

OVERDOSAGE

Signs and symptoms	Hypertension, hyperventilation, CNS depression
Treatment	Induce emesis or use gastric lavage to empty stomach. Activated charcoal may be helpful. Treat symptomatically.

DRUG INTERACTIONS

Alcohol, tranquilizers, sedative-hypnotics, and other CNS depressants	△ CNS depression
MAO inhibitors and beta blockers	△ Sympathomimetic effects
Methyldopa, mecamylamine, reserpine, and *Veratrum* alkaloids	▽ Antihypertensive effects

ALTERED LABORATORY VALUES

No clinically significant alterations in blood/serum or urinary values occur at therapeutic dosages

---

USE IN CHILDREN

See INDICATIONS and ORAL DOSAGE

USE IN PREGNANT AND NURSING WOMEN

Pregnancy Category C: use during pregnancy only if clearly needed. Reproduction studies have not been performed in animals; it is not known whether this preparation can adversely affect fetal development or reproductive capacity. Use with caution in nursing mothers, because in infants the risk due to sympathomimetic amines is higher than usual.

---

[1] Decongestants in combination with antihistamines have been used to relieve eustachian tube congestion associated with acute eustachian salpingitis, aerotitis, and serous otitis media

---

DECONGESTANTS/UPPER RESPIRATORY COMBINATIONS

NOVAFED Capsules (pseudoephedrine hydrochloride) Merrell Dow   Rx

Capsules (sustained release): 120 mg

NOVAFED Liquid (pseudoephedrine hydrochloride) Merrell Dow   OTC

Liquid (per 5 ml): 30 mg[1] (4 fl oz)

INDICATIONS

Relief of **nasal and eustachian-tube congestion** associated with the common cold, sinusitis, acute upper-respiratory infections, hay fever, upper-respiratory allergies, acute eustachian salpingitis, aerotitis media, acute otitis media, and serous otitis media

ORAL DOSAGE

Adult: 10 ml (2 tsp) q4–6h, not to exceed 4 doses in any 24-h period; if sustained-release capsules are used, 120 mg q12h
Child (2–5 yr): 2.5 ml (1/2 tsp) q4–6h, not to exceed 4 doses in any 24-h period
Child (6–12 yr): 5 ml (1 tsp) q4–6h, not to exceed 4 doses in any 24-h period

CONTRAINDICATIONS

Breast-feeding	Severe hypertension	Hypersensitivity or idiosyncratic reaction[2] to sympathomimetic amines
MAO inhibitor therapy (see DRUG INTERACTIONS)	Severe coronary artery disease	

NOVAFED ■ NOVAFED A

WARNINGS/PRECAUTIONS

Special-risk patients	Use sparingly and with caution in patients with hypertension, diabetes mellitus, ischemic heart disease, increased intraocular pressure, hyperthyroidism, prostatic hypertrophy, cardiovascular disease, and hyperreactivity to ephedrine
Elderly patients	Adverse reactions to sympathomimetic agents are more likely to occur in patients over 60 yr of age

ADVERSE REACTIONS[3]

Cardiovascular	Tachycardia, palpitations, pallor, arrhythmias; cardiovascular collapse with hypotension
Central nervous system	Headache, dizziness, fear, anxiety, tension, restlessness, tremor, weakness, insomnia, hallucinations, convulsions, CNS depression
Gastrointestinal	Nausea
Other	Respiratory difficulty, dysuria

OVERDOSAGE

Signs and symptoms	See ADVERSE REACTIONS; *in elderly patients:* hallucinations, convulsions, CNS depression
Treatment	Discontinue medication; treat symptomatically and institute supportive measures, as required

DRUG INTERACTIONS

MAO inhibitors, beta blockers	△ Sympathomimetic effect
Guanethidine, methyldopa, mecamylamine, reserpine, *Veratrum* alkaloids	▽ Antihypertensive effect

ALTERED LABORATORY VALUES

No clinically significant alterations in blood/serum or urinary values occur at therapeutic dosages

---

USE IN CHILDREN

See INDICATIONS and ORAL DOSAGE; do not use sustained-release capsules in children under 12 yr of age

USE IN PREGNANT AND NURSING WOMEN

Safety for use during pregnancy has not been established. Contraindicated for use in nursing mothers, because in infants the risk due to sympathomimetic amines is higher than usual.

---

[1] Contains 7.5% alcohol
[2] Insomnia, tremor, weakness, dizziness, and arrhythmias may occur as idiosyncratic responses or as general adverse reactions to sympathomimetic agents
[3] Includes reactions common to sympathomimetic amines in general

---

DECONGESTANTS/UPPER RESPIRATORY COMBINATIONS

NOVAFED A Capsules (pseudoephedrine hydrochloride and chlorpheniramine maleate)   Rx
Merrell Dow

Capsules (sustained release): 120 mg pseudoephedrine hydrochloride and 8 mg chlorpheniramine maleate

NOVAFED A Liquid (pseudoephedrine hydrochloride and chlorpheniramine maleate)   Merrell Dow   OTC

Liquid (per 5 ml): 30 mg pseudoephedrine hydrochloride and 2 mg chlorpheniramine maleate[1] (4 fl oz)

INDICATIONS	ORAL DOSAGE
Relief of **nasal and eustachian-tube congestion** associated with the common cold, sinusitis, acute upper-respiratory infections, hay fever, upper-respiratory allergies, acute eustachian salpingitis, aerotitis media, acute otitis media, and serous otitis media	**Adult:** 1 cap q12h or 10 ml (2 tsp) q4–6h, up to 4 doses/24 h **Child (< 6 yr):** 2.5 ml (½ tsp) q4–6h, up to 4 doses/24 h **Child (6–12 yr):** 5 ml (1 tsp) q4–6h, up to 4 doses/24 h **Child (> 12 yr):** same as adult
Symptomatic relief of **seasonal and perennial allergic rhinitis; vasomotor rhinitis; allergic conjunctivitis** due to inhalant allergens and foods; and mild, uncomplicated **allergic skin manifestations of urticaria and angioedema**	**Adult:** 1 cap q12h

NOVAFED A ■ ORNADE

CONTRAINDICATIONS

Severe hypertension	Narrow-angle glaucoma	Asthmatic attack
Severe coronary artery disease	Breast-feeding	Hypersensitivity or idiosyncratic reaction[2] to sympathomimetic amines or phenanthrene derivatives
Peptic ulcer	MAO inhibitor therapy (see DRUG INTERACTIONS)	
Urinary retention		

WARNINGS/PRECAUTIONS

Drowsiness, disturbed coordination	Caution patients about driving or engaging in other potentially hazardous activities requiring mental alertness and/or physical coordination, and about using alcohol or other CNS depressants (see DRUG INTERACTIONS)
Special-risk patients	Use sparingly and with caution in patients with hypertension, diabetes mellitus, ischemic heart disease, cardiovascular disease, increased intraocular pressure, prostatic hypertrophy, hyperthyroidism, a history of bronchial asthma, or hyperreactivity to ephedrine
Elderly patients	Sympathomimetic effects are more likely to occur in patients over 60 yr of age; demonstrate safe use of short-acting form before giving sustained-release capsules

ADVERSE REACTIONS

Central nervous system	Drowsiness, sedation, headache, dizziness, fear, anxiety, tension, restlessness, nervousness, tremor, weakness, insomnia, hallucinations, convulsions, CNS depression
Cardiovascular	Tachycardia, palpitations, arrhythmias, collapse with hypotension
Gastrointestinal	Dry mouth, nausea, vomiting, anorexia, heartburn
Other	Blurred vision, dysuria, polyuria, difficult breathing, pallor; dermatitis (rare)

OVERDOSAGE

Signs and symptoms	CNS stimulation, variable cardiovascular effects; *in elderly patients:* hallucinations, convulsions, CNS depression, death
Treatment	Induce emesis or use gastric lavage to empty stomach. Activated charcoal may be helpful. Institute supportive measures, as indicated. Treat symptomatically.

DRUG INTERACTIONS

Alcohol, tranquilizers, sedative-hypnotics, and other CNS depressants	⇧ CNS depression
MAO inhibitors, beta blockers	⇧ Sympathomimetic effect
Guanethidine, methyldopa, mecamylamine, reserpine, *Veratrum* alkaloids	⇩ Antihypertensive effect
Pressor amines	⇧ Blood pressure

ALTERED LABORATORY VALUES

No clinically significant alterations in blood/serum or urinary values occur at therapeutic dosages

---

USE IN CHILDREN

See INDICATIONS and ORAL DOSAGE; do not give sustained-release capsules to children under 12 yr of age. Antihistamines may impair mental alertness in children.

USE IN PREGNANT AND NURSING WOMEN

Sustained-release capsules: Pregnancy Category C: use during pregnancy only if clearly needed. Reproduction studies have not been performed in animals; it is not known whether this preparation can adversely affect fetal development or reproductive capacity. *Liquid:* Safety of pseudoephedrine for use during pregnancy has not been established. Both forms of this preparation are contraindicated for use in nursing mothers due to the higher than usual risk for infants from sympathomimetic amines.

---

[1] Contains 5% alcohol
[2] Insomnia, tremor, weakness, dizziness, and arrhythmias may occur as idiosyncratic responses or as general adverse reactions to sympathomimetic agents

---

DECONGESTANTS/UPPER RESPIRATORY COMBINATIONS

ORNADE (chlorpheniramine maleate and phenylpropanolamine hydrochloride) Smith Kline & French Rx

Capsules (sustained release): 12 mg chlorpheniramine maleate and 75 mg phenylpropanolamine hydrochloride

INDICATIONS

Nasal congestion and other symptoms associated with seasonal and perennial allergic rhinitis and vasomotor rhinitis
Runny nose, sneezing, and nasal congestion associated with the common cold

ORAL DOSAGE

Adult: 1 cap q12h
Child (> 12 yr): same as adult

ORNADE

CONTRAINDICATIONS

Hypersensitivity to either component and other antihistamines of similar structure	Coronary artery disease	Bladder-neck obstruction
	MAO inhibitor therapy (see DRUG INTERACTIONS)	Breast-feeding
Severe hypertension		Full-term or premature neonates

WARNINGS/PRECAUTIONS

Drowsiness — Caution patients about driving or engaging in other activities requiring mental alertness, and about using alcohol or other CNS depressants (see DRUG INTERACTIONS)

Special-risk patients — Use with considerable caution in patients with narrow-angle glaucoma, stenosing peptic ulcer, pyloroduodenal obstruction, symptomatic prostatic hypertrophy, or bladder-neck obstruction; use with caution in patients with lower respiratory disease (including asthma), hypertension, cardiovascular disease, hyperthyroidism, increased intraocular pressure, or diabetes

Elderly patients — Dizziness, sedation, and hypotension are more likely in patients over 60 yr of age

Concomitant medication — Caution patients not to take other medications containing phenylpropanolamine or amphetamines simultaneously

Carcinogenicity, mutagenicity — Chlorpheniramine has shown no evidence of carcinogenic potential in a long-term study in rats, nor has there been any evidence of mutagenicity in a battery of mutagenic studies, including the Ames test. The carcinogenic and mutagenic potential of phenylpropanolamine has not been evaluated.

Impairment of fertility — A reduction in fertility was observed in an early study in female rats given 67 times the human dose of chlorpheniramine; however, more recent studies in rabbits and rats given doses up to 50 and 85 times the human dose have shown no reduction in fertility. No studies are available to determine whether phenylpropanolamine impairs fertility.

ADVERSE REACTIONS[1]

Cardiovascular — Anginal pain, extrasystoles, headache, hypertension, hypotension, palpitations, tachycardia

Hematological — Agranulocytosis, hemolytic anemia, leukopenia, thrombocytopenia

Central nervous system — Blurred vision, confusion, convulsions, diplopia, disturbed coordination, dizziness, drowsiness, euphoria, excitation, fatigue, hysteria, insomnia, irritability, acute labyrinthitis, nervousness, neuritis, paresthesia, restlessness, sedation, tinnitus, tremor, vertigo

Gastrointestinal — Abdominal pain, anorexia, constipation, diarrhea, epigastric distress, nausea, vomiting

Genitourinary — Dysuria, early menses, urinary frequency, urinary retention

Respiratory — Thickening of bronchial secretions, tightness of the chest and wheezing, nasal stuffiness

Other — Anaphylactic shock, chills, drug rash; excessive dryness of the mouth, nose, and throat; increased intraocular pressure, excessive perspiration, photosensitivity, urticaria, weakness

OVERDOSAGE

Signs and symptoms — *Antihistaminic effects:* vary from CNS depression (sedation, apnea, diminished mental alertness, cardiovascular collapse) to CNS stimulation (insomnia, hallucinations, tremors, convulsions) to death; dizziness, tinnitus, ataxia, blurred vision, hypotension; CNS stimulation and atropine-like signs and symptoms (dry mouth; fixed, dilated pupils; flushing, hyperthermia, GI disturbances) are particularly likely in children. *Sympathomimetic effects:* giddiness, headache, nausea, vomiting, sweating, thirst, tachycardia, precordial pain, palpitations, difficulty in micturition, muscular weakness and tenseness, anxiety, restlessness, insomnia, delusions, hallucinations, cardiac arrhythmias, circulatory collapse, convulsions, coma, respiratory failure.

Treatment — Induce vomiting even if emesis has spontaneously occurred, preferably with syrup of ipecac (the action of ipecac is facilitated by physical activity and ingestion of 8–12 fl oz of water); however, do not induce vomiting in unconscious patients. If emesis does not occur within 15 min, repeat the dose of ipecac; take care to avoid aspiration, especially in infants and children. Instill an activated charcoal slurry with water to remove any drug remaining in the stomach after inducing emesis. If vomiting is contraindicated, perform gastric lavage with isotonic or 1/2 isotonic saline. Administer saline cathartics (eg, milk of magnesia) to draw water into the bowel and rapidly dilute the bowel content. Treatment is symptomatic and supportive. Vasopressors may be used for hypotension. Short-acting barbiturates, diazepam, or paraldehyde may be administered to control seizures. Treat hyperpyrexia with tepid water sponge baths or a hypothermic blanket. For apnea, provide ventilatory support; *do not use stimulants or analeptics.* Dialysis is of little value.

ORNADE ■ PHENERGAN VC

DRUG INTERACTIONS

Alcohol, tranquilizers, sedative-hypnotics, other CNS depressants	△ CNS depression; caution patient about additive effects
MAO inhibitors	△ Sympathomimetic and anticholinergic effects; do not use concomitantly
Ganglionic blocking agents (eg, mecamylamine)	△ Sympathomimetic effects; do not use concomitantly
Adrenergic blockers (eg, guanethidine and bethanidine)	△ Hypotensive effect; do not use concomitantly
Oral anticoagulants	▽ Anticoagulant effect
Antihistamines	△ CNS depression △ Atropine-like effects
Anticholinergics (eg, trihexyphenidyl), imipramine	△ Risk of xerostomia
Beta-adrenergic blocking agents	▽ Pharmacologic effects of beta-adrenergic blockers
Corticosteroids	▽ Pharmacologic effects of corticosteroids
Norepinephrine	△ Cardiovascular effects of norepinephrine
Phenothiazines	△ CNS depression △ Risk of urinary retention or glaucoma

ALTERED LABORATORY VALUES

No clinically significant alterations in blood/serum or urinary values occur at therapeutic dosages

---

USE IN CHILDREN

See INDICATIONS and ORAL DOSAGE; contraindicated for use in full-term or premature neonates and should not be used in children under 12 yr of age. Antihistamines may diminish mental alertness in children and may produce excitation, particularly in young children.

USE IN PREGNANT AND NURSING WOMEN

Pregnancy Category B: studies in rats given 33 and 67 times the human dose of chlorpheniramine have shown a decrease in postnatal survival of offspring; studies in rabbits and rats at doses up to 50 and 85 times the human dose of chlorpheniramine and studies in rats at doses up to 7 times the human dose of phenylpropanolamine have revealed no evidence of fetal harm. No adequate, well-controlled studies have been performed in pregnant women; use during pregnancy only if clearly needed. Small amounts of antihistamines are excreted in breast milk; this preparation should not be given to nursing mothers because of the higher risk of antihistaminic side effects for infants in general and for neonates in particular.

[1] Includes reactions observed with other antihistamines and sympathomimetic compounds

---

DECONGESTANTS/UPPER RESPIRATORY COMBINATIONS

PHENERGAN VC (promethazine hydrochloride and phenylephrine hydrochloride) Wyeth Rx

Syrup (per 5 ml): 6.25 mg promethazine hydrochloride and 5 mg phenylephrine hydrochloride (4, 6, 8 fl oz; 1 pt; 1 gal) *fruit flavored*

INDICATIONS	ORAL DOSAGE
Upper respiratory tract reactions, including nasal congestion, associated with allergy or the common cold	**Adult:** 5 ml (1 tsp) q4–6h **Child (2–6 yr):** 1.25–2.5 ml (1/4–1/2 tsp) q4–6h **Child (6–12 yr):** 2.5–5 ml (1/2–1 tsp) q4–6h

CONTRAINDICATIONS

Hypersensitivity to phenylephrine	Asthma or other lower respiratory tract conditions	Peripheral vascular insufficiency
Hypersensitivity or idiosyncratic reaction to promethazine or other phenothiazines	MAO inhibitor therapy	Hypertension

WARNINGS/PRECAUTIONS

Drowsiness, dizziness	Caution patients that they may drive or engage in other potentially hazardous activities requiring mental alertness or physical coordination only after it has been established that this preparation does not make them drowsy or dizzy (see also USE IN CHILDREN)
Photosensitivity, extrapyramidal reactions	Photosensitivity and extrapyramidal reactions such as oculogyric crisis, torticollis, and tongue protrusion have occurred in rare instances; the extrapyramidal reactions have usually resulted from excessive dosage. Instruct patients to report any involuntary muscle movements or unusual sensitivity to sunlight.
Patients with a history of sleep apnea	Avoid use in patients with a history of sleep apnea

PHENERGAN VC

Patients with cardiovascular disorders	Use with extreme caution in patients with arteriosclerosis or poor cerebral or coronary circulation because cardiac output may decrease; caution should be exercised if patients have cardiovascular disorders such as heart disease
Patients with GI or GU conditions	Use with caution in patients with hepatic impairment, stenosing peptic ulcer, pyloroduodenal obstruction, symptomatic prostatic hypertrophy, or bladder neck obstruction; urinary retention may occur in men with symptomatic prostatic hypertrophy
Elderly patients	Use with extreme caution in elderly patients
Other special-risk patients	Use with caution in patients with convulsive disorders, thyroid diseases, diabetes mellitus, or narrow angle glaucoma
Carcinogenicity, mutagenicity	No long-term studies have been performed in animals to evaluate the carcinogenic potential of this preparation's components; an epidemiological study has demonstrated no significant association between phenylephrine and cancer. Use of promethazine in the Ames test has produced no evidence of mutagenicity; phenylephrine's mutagenic potential has not been studied.
Effect on fertility	A study of ovum transport in rabbits has shown that phenylephrine does not affect the incidence of pregnancy, but at high doses it significantly reduces the number of implantations; the effect of promethazine on fertility has not been assessed

ADVERSE REACTIONS

Central nervous system	Sedation, sleepiness, blurred vision, restlessness, anxiety, nervousness, dizziness, weakness, tremor; disorientation, confusion, and extrapyramidal reactions (rare)
Respiratory	Respiratory distress
Cardiovascular	Hypertension, hypotension, precordial pain
Gastrointestinal	Nausea, vomiting, cholestatic jaundice
Hematological	Leukopenia and thrombocytopenia (rare); agranulocytosis (one case)
Dermatological	Rash; photosensitivity (rare)
Other	Dry mouth

OVERDOSAGE

Signs and symptoms	*CNS:* headache, extreme somnolence, stupor, coma, hyperexcitability, nightmares, convulsions (CNS stimulation is especially likely to occur in children and the elderly); *respiratory:* decrease in respiratory rate and/or tidal volume; *cardiovascular:* flush, hypotension, headache, hypertension, cerebral hemorrhage, bradycardia, premature ventricular contractions, paroxysmal ventricular tachycardia; *other:* mydriasis, dry mouth, GI reactions (including vomiting)
Treatment	To maintain pulmonary function, establish a patent airway, and provide assisted or controlled ventilation. Correct acidosis and electrolyte losses. To treat severe hypotension, use norepinephrine or phenylephrine, not epinephrine. Diazepam may be given to control convulsions. Do not give analeptic drugs for CNS depression. Monitor vital signs only in cases of extreme overdosage or individual sensitivity. To remove this preparation from the body, administer activated charcoal or use sodium or magnesium sulfate as a cathartic; limited experience indicates that dialysis is not helpful.

DRUG INTERACTIONS

Alcohol, narcotic drugs, sedative-hypnotics (eg, barbiturates), tranquilizers, local anesthetics, and other CNS depressants	△ CNS depression; instruct patients requiring this preparation that other CNS depressants should be avoided or used at a lower dosage (for concomitant use with this preparation, reduce the dosage of a narcotic analgesic by 25–50% and the dosage of a barbiturate by at least 50%) △ Risk of convulsions (with concomitant use of narcotic drugs or local anesthetics)
MAO inhibitors	Hypertensive crisis; do not use an MAO inhibitor concomitantly
Tricyclic antidepressants, amphetamines, phenylpropanolamine, ergot alkaloids, atropine	Hypertension; exercise caution if phenylpropanolamine, an amphetamine, or a tricyclic antidepressant is given concomitantly
Phentolamine	▽ Vasopressor response

ALTERED LABORATORY VALUES

Blood/serum values	△ Glucose
Urinary values	False-positive or false-negative pregnancy test

---

USE IN CHILDREN

See INDICATIONS and ORAL DOSAGE; do not give to children under 2 yr of age because safety for use in such patients has not been established. Children undergoing treatment should be supervised whenever they ride a bicycle or engage in other potentially hazardous activities requiring mental alertness or physical coordination.

USE IN PREGNANT AND NURSING WOMEN

Pregnancy Category C: phenylephrine has caused a decrease in birth weight and may have contributed to perinatal wastage, premature labor, and fetal anomalies in rabbits; this drug has also been associated with ventricular septal defect and aortic arch anomalies in chick embryos. Promethazine has been shown to be fetotoxic in rodents; no evidence of teratogenicity has been observed in rats fed 6.25 or 12.5 mg/kg/day. Use of this preparation during late pregnancy may cause anoxia or bradycardia in a fetus. Inhibition of platelet aggregation may also occur in a neonate if this preparation is taken within 2 wk before delivery. This medication should be used during pregnancy only if the expected benefit justifies the potential risk to the fetus or neonate. It is not known whether promethazine or phenylephrine is excreted in human milk; use this preparation with caution in nursing mothers.

VEHICLE/BASE
Syrup: 7% alcohol

DECONGESTANTS/UPPER RESPIRATORY COMBINATIONS

RONDEC (carbinoxamine maleate and pseudoephedrine hydrochloride) Ross — Rx

Tablets: 4 mg carbinoxamine maleate and 60 mg pseudoephedrine hydrochloride **Pediatric drops (per dropperful [1 ml]):** 2 mg carbinoxamine maleate and 25 mg pseudoephedrine hydrochloride (30 ml) *berry flavored* **Syrup (per 5 ml):** 4 mg carbinoxamine maleate and 60 mg pseudoephedrine hydrochloride (4, 16 fl oz) *berry flavored*

RONDEC-TR (carbinoxamine maleate and pseudoephedrine hydrochloride) Ross — Rx

Tablets (timed release): 8 mg carbinoxamine maleate and 120 mg pseudoephedrine hydrochloride

INDICATIONS	ORAL DOSAGE
Symptomatic relief of seasonal and perennial **allergic rhinitis** and **vasomotor rhinitis**	**Adult:** 1 tab or 5 ml (1 tsp) qid or 1 timed-release tab q12h **Infant (1–3 mo):** ¼ dropperful qid **Infant (3–6 mo):** ½ dropperful qid **Infant (6–9 mo):** ¾ dropperful qid **Infant (9–18 mo):** 1 dropperful qid **Child (18 mo to 6 yr):** 2.5 ml (½ tsp) qid **Child (6–12 yr):** 1 tab or 5 ml (1 tsp) qid **Child ($\geq$ 12 yr):** same as adult

CONTRAINDICATIONS

Hypersensitivity or idiosyncratic reaction to any component	Narrow-angle glaucoma	Asthmatic attack
	Urinary retention	Severe hypertension
MAO inhibitor therapy (see DRUG INTERACTIONS)	Peptic ulcer	Severe coronary artery disease

ADMINISTRATION/DOSAGE ADJUSTMENTS

Mild symptoms or particularly sensitive patients	Less frequent or reduced doses may be adequate

WARNINGS/PRECAUTIONS

Drowsiness	Caution patients about driving or engaging in other activities requiring mental alertness, and that the use of alcohol or other CNS depressants (see DRUG INTERACTIONS) should be avoided
Special-risk patients	Use with caution in patients over 60 yr of age and in patients with hypertension, ischemic or other heart disease, asthma, hyperthyroidism, increased intraocular pressure, diabetes mellitus, or prostatic hypertrophy

ADVERSE REACTIONS

Cardiovascular	Pallor, increased blood pressure or heart rate, arrhythmias
Central nervous system	Dizziness, sedation, headache, weakness, mild stimulation, nervousness, insomnia, tremor, convulsions, hallucinations; excitability in children (rare)
Gastrointestinal	Nausea, anorexia, dry mouth, heartburn, vomiting, diarrhea
Genitourinary	Dysuria, polyuria
Ophthalmic	Diplopia
Respiratory	Difficult breathing

OVERDOSAGE

Signs and symptoms	*Antihistamine-related effects (in small children):* excitation, hallucinations, ataxia, incoordination, tremors, flushing, fever, and in severe cases, convulsions, fixed and dilated pupils, coma, death; *antihistamine-related effects (in adults):* excitement leading to convulsions and postictal depression, often preceded by drowsiness and coma; *sympathomimetic-related effects:* dry mouth, metallic taste, anorexia, nausea, vomiting, diarrhea, abdominal cramps, restlessness, dizziness, tremor, hyperactive reflexes, talkativeness, irritability, insomnia, headache, difficulty in micturition, flushing, palpitation, arrhythmias, hypertension followed by hypotension and circulatory collapse
Treatment	Empty stomach, as patient's condition warrants; administer activated charcoal. Maintain a quiet environment and monitor cardiovascular status. Reduce fever with cool sponging. Support respiration. To reverse anticholinergic symptoms of carbinoxamine, physostigmine may be given. CNS excitation and convulsions may be controlled with sedatives or anticonvulsants. Administer ammonium chloride to increase urinary excretion of pseudoephedrine. Further care is generally symptomatic and supportive. *Do not give stimulants.*

DRUG INTERACTIONS

Alcohol, tranquilizers, sedative-hypnotics, and other CNS depressants	⇧ CNS depression
MAO inhibitors	⇧ Sympathomimetic and anticholinergic effects
Beta-adrenergic blockers	⇧ Sympathomimetic effects

Methyldopa, mecamylamine, reserpine, and *Veratrum* alkaloids	▽ Antihypertensive effect

ALTERED LABORATORY VALUES
No clinically significant alterations in blood/serum or urinary values occur at therapeutic dosages

---

USE IN CHILDREN
See INDICATIONS and ORAL DOSAGE; the timed-release tablets should not be given to children under 12 yr of age

USE IN PREGNANT AND NURSING WOMEN
Pregnancy Category C: use during pregnancy only if clearly needed. Safety for use during pregnancy has not been established. Reproduction studies have not been performed in animals, nor is it known whether these preparations can adversely affect human fetal development or reproductive capacity. Use with caution in nursing mothers.

DECONGESTANTS/UPPER RESPIRATORY COMBINATIONS

RU-TUSS (phenylephrine hydrochloride, phenylpropanolamine hydrochloride, chlorpheniramine maleate, hyoscyamine sulfate, atropine sulfate, and scopolamine hydrobromide) Boots — Rx

Tablets (prolonged action): 25 mg phenylephrine hydrochloride, 50 mg phenylpropanolamine hydrochloride, 8 mg chlorpheniramine maleate, 0.19 mg hyoscyamine sulfate, 0.04 mg atropine sulfate, and 0.01 mg scopolamine hydrobromide

INDICATIONS	ORAL DOSAGE
Upper respiratory tract irritation	**Adult:** 1 tab bid (morning and evening); tablets should be swallowed whole **Child (> 12 yr):** same as adult

CONTRAINDICATIONS

Bronchial asthma	Glaucoma	Age < 12 yr
MAO inhibitor therapy (see DRUG INTERACTIONS)	Hypersensitivity to antihistamines or sympathomimetic amines	Pregnancy

WARNINGS/PRECAUTIONS

Drowsiness	Caution patients against driving or engaging in other potentially hazardous activities that require mental alertness or physical coordination; patients should also be warned about using alcohol or other CNS depressants (see DRUG INTERACTIONS)
Special-risk patients	Use with caution in patients with bladder neck obstruction, peripheral vascular or cardiac disease, hypertension, or hyperthyroidism

ADVERSE REACTIONS

Central nervous system	Drowsiness, lassitude, giddiness, dizziness, tinnitus, headache, incoordination, hyperirritability, nervousness, insomnia
Ophthalmic	Visual disturbances, mydriasis, blurred vision
Cardiovascular	Palpitations, tachycardia, hypotension, hypertension, faintness
Respiratory	Tightness of the chest, thickening of bronchial secretions, dryness of mucous membranes
Gastrointestinal	Anorexia, nausea, vomiting, diarrhea, constipation, epigastric distress
Genitourinary	Frequent urination, dysuria
Hypersensitivity	Rash, urticaria, leukopenia, agranulocytosis, thrombocytopenia
Other	Dry mouth

OVERDOSAGE

Signs and symptoms	Tachypnea, delirium, fever, stupor, coma, respiratory failure; convulsions and death may occur in infants and children
Treatment	Empty stomach; use saline cathartics to hasten evacuation of the medication. Maintain supportive measures and symptomatic therapy for at least 12 h after ingestion.

DRUG INTERACTIONS

MAO inhibitors	△ Sympathomimetic and anticholinergic effects
Alcohol, tranquilizers, sedative-hypnotics, and other CNS depressants	△ CNS depression
Beta-adrenergic blockers	△ Sympathomimetic effect

RU-TUSS ■ RYNATAN

Guanethidine, methyldopa, mecamylamine, reserpine, *Veratrum* alkaloids	▽ Antihypertensive effect
Antimuscarinics, tricyclic antidepressants, amantadine	△ Anticholinergic effect
Haloperidol	▽ Antipsychotic effect
Phenothiazines	▽ Antipsychotic effect ▽ Anticholinergic effect
Antacids, antidiarrheal suspensions	▽ Absorption of belladonna alkaloids

ALTERED LABORATORY VALUES

No clinically significant alterations in blood/serum or urinary values occur at therapeutic dosages

---

USE IN CHILDREN

This preparation is not recommended for children under 12 yr of age

USE IN PREGNANT AND NURSING WOMEN

Administration during pregnancy is contraindicated; for use in nursing mothers, consult manufacturer

---

DECONGESTANTS/UPPER RESPIRATORY COMBINATIONS

RYNATAN (phenylephrine tannate, chlorpheniramine tannate, and pyrilamine tannate) Wallace   Rx

Tablets: 25 mg phenylephrine tannate, 8 mg chlorpheniramine tannate, and 25 mg pyrilamine tannate   **Pediatric suspension (per 5 ml):** 5 mg phenylephrine tannate, 2 mg chlorpheniramine tannate, and 12.5 mg pyrilamine tannate (1 pt) *strawberry-currant flavored*

INDICATIONS
Coryza and nasal congestion associated with the common cold, sinusitis, allergic rhinitis, and other upper respiratory tract conditions

ORAL DOSAGE
Adult: 1–2 tabs q12h
Child (2–6 yr): 2.5–5 ml (1/2–1 tsp) q12h
Child (> 6 yr): 5–10 ml (1–2 tsp) q12h

CONTRAINDICATIONS

Hypersensitivity to any component or related compounds	Neonates	Breast-feeding

WARNINGS/PRECAUTIONS

Drowsiness	Caution patients not to drive or engage in other potentially hazardous activities requiring mental alertness
Special-risk patients	Use with caution in patients with hypertension, cardiovascular disease, hyperthyroidism, diabetes, narrow-angle glaucoma, or prostatic hypertrophy
Elderly patients	Dizziness, sedation, and hypotension are more likely to occur in elderly patients
Carcinogenicity, mutagenicity, effect on fertility	No long-term studies have been done in animals to evaluate the carcinogenic or mutagenic potential of this preparation or its effect on fertility

ADVERSE REACTIONS

Central nervous system	Drowsiness, sedation
Gastrointestinal	Various effects
Other	Dryness of mucous membranes

OVERDOSAGE

Signs and symptoms	CNS depression or stimulation, restlessness, convulsions; atropine-like effects; chlorpheniramine overdosage may lead to convulsions and death in young children
Treatment	Induce emesis, taking precautions against aspiration. If gastric lavage is indicated, isotonic or 1/2 isotonic saline solution is preferred. A vasopressor may be used to treat hypotension, if needed. *Do not give stimulants.*

DRUG INTERACTIONS

MAO inhibitors	△ Anticholinergic and sympathomimetic effects; use this preparation with caution, if at all, in patients receiving MAO inhibitors
Alcohol, tranquilizers, sedative-hypnotics, and other CNS depressants	△ CNS depression; caution patients not to drink alcoholic beverages during therapy

ALTERED LABORATORY VALUES

No clinically significant alterations in blood/serum or urinary values occur at therapeutic dosages

USE IN CHILDREN

See INDICATIONS and ORAL DOSAGE; for use in children under 2 yr of age, titrate dosage individually. Contraindicated for use in neonates. Antihistamines in combination with sympathomimetic agents may cause either mild stimulation or mild sedation.

USE IN PREGNANT AND NURSING WOMEN

Pregnancy Category C: reproduction studies have not been performed in animals; it is not known whether this preparation can adversely affect fetal development or reproductive capacity. Use during pregnancy only if clearly needed. Contraindicated for use in nursing mothers.

DECONGESTANTS/UPPER RESPIRATORY COMBINATIONS

SINUBID (acetaminophen, phenylpropanolamine hydrochloride, and phenyltoloxamine citrate) **Parke-Davis** Rx

Tablets: 600 mg acetaminophen, 100 mg phenylpropanolamine hydrochloride, and 66 mg phenyltoloxamine citrate

INDICATIONS

Nasal congestion, sinusitis, allergic and vasomotor rhinitis, coryza, facial pain and "pressure" of sinusitis, fever

ORAL DOSAGE

Adult: 1 tab q12h

CONTRAINDICATIONS

Hypersensitivity to any component	Idiosyncratic reaction (oversensitivity) to sympathomimetic amines[1]

WARNINGS/PRECAUTIONS

Drowsiness	Caution patients that if they experience drowsiness, they should not drive or engage in other activities requiring mental alertness
Special-risk patients	Use with caution in patients with hypertension, heart disease, diabetes mellitus, chronic renal disease, or thyroid disease
Concomitant medication	Avoid concurrent use of MAO inhibitors or barbiturates, or ingestion of alcoholic beverages
Carcinogenicity, mutagenicity, effect on fertility	No long-term studies have been performed to determine the carcinogenic or mutagenic potential of this product or its effect on fertility

ADVERSE REACTIONS

Central nervous system	Dizziness, headache, anxiety, restlessness, tension, insomnia, tremor, weakness, nervousness, vertigo, drowsiness, disturbed coordination, poor concentration, convulsions
Gastrointestinal	Epigastric distress, nausea, vomiting, diarrhea, intestinal cramps, dry mouth
Ophthalmic	Blurred vision
Respiratory	Dry nose and throat
Cardiovascular	Palpitations, arrhythmias, hypotension
Dermatological	Urticaria, diaphoresis
Genitourinary	Urinary retention

OVERDOSAGE

Signs and symptoms	*Antihistaminic effects:* CNS depression ranging from drowsiness to coma; CNS stimulation ranging from excitement to hallucinations and convulsions (with postictal depression); hypotension and cardiovascular collapse; anticholinergic reactions (dry mouth, mydriasis, flushing, fever); toxic effects are seen within 90–120 min after ingestion. In children, excitement, hallucinations, cyanosis, anticholinergic effects, ataxia, incoordination, muscle twitching, athetosis, tremors, hyperreflexia, and tonic-clonic convulsions may occur initially (convulsions can also occur after mild depression); reactions may be followed by postictal depression and cardiorespiratory arrest. *Sympathomimetic effects:* hypertension, arrhythmias, headache, excitement, psychosis, hostility, muscle twitching, convulsions, diaphoresis, malaise; mydriasis. *Acetaminophen-related effects:* nausea, anorexia, vomiting, abdominal pain, diarrhea, diaphoresis, malaise; hepatotoxicity may not be evident until after 2–4 days.

SINUBID ■ TAVIST-D

Treatment	If patient is conscious, induce vomiting even though it may have occurred spontaneously. If emesis is not possible, perform gastric lavage. Take appropriate precautions against aspiration, especially in children. The airway should be secured with a cuffed endotracheal tube before lavage if the patient is unconscious. After emptying stomach, instill a charcoal slurry or another suitable agent; a saline cathartic such as milk of magnesia may also be helpful. Maintain pulmonary function; if necessary, establish an adequate airway, provide mechanically assisted ventilation, and administer oxygen. Treat hypertension with IV phentolamine. For hypotension, give IV fluids; if great caution is exercised, a vasopressor other than epinephrine may also be used. To control convulsions, carefully administer IV diazepam or a short-acting barbiturate, as needed; physostigmine may also be considered if convulsions are centrally mediated. Treat fever with ice packs and cooling sponge baths, not with alcohol. Do not use CNS stimulants. Administer oral acetylcysteine as soon as possible (no later than 24 h after ingestion); give a loading dose of 140 mg/kg and then, at 4-h intervals, 17 maintenance doses of 70 mg/kg. (Charcoal should be removed before acetylcysteine is given.) Measure the plasma level of unconjugated acetaminophen as early as possible, but no sooner than 4 h after ingestion. Determine prothrombin time, SGOT and SGPT levels, and serum concentrations of bilirubin, creatinine, BUN, glucose, and electrolytes every 24 h. If the prothrombin time exceeds 1.5 times the control value, give vitamin K_1; if the prothrombin time exceeds 3 times this value, give fresh frozen plasma. Institute appropriate measures to treat hypoglycemia and electrolyte and fluid imbalance. Avoid forced diuresis or use of diuretics when treating an acetaminophen overdose. For additional information on use of acetylcysteine and interpretation of the plasma acetaminophen level, see Mucomyst chart.

DRUG INTERACTIONS

Alcohol, tranquilizers, sedative-hypnotics, and other CNS depressants	⇧ CNS depression
MAO inhibitors	⇧ Sympathomimetic and anticholinergic effects

ALTERED LABORATORY VALUES

Blood/serum values	⇩ Glucose (with glucose oxidase/peroxidase tests)
Urinary values	+ 5-HIAA (with nitrosonaphthol reagent test)

USE IN CHILDREN
Do not use this preparation in children under 12 yr of age

USE IN PREGNANT AND NURSING WOMEN
Pregnancy Category C: reproduction studies have not been done with this preparation; whether it can cause harm to the fetus or affect reproductive capacity is not known. Use during pregnancy only if clearly needed. This preparation should not be used by nursing mothers.

[1] Contraindicated if small doses of sympathomimetic amines cause insomnia, dizziness, light-headedness, weakness, tremor, or weakness

---

DECONGESTANTS/UPPER RESPIRATORY COMBINATIONS

TAVIST-D (clemastine fumarate and phenylpropanolamine hydrochloride) Sandoz Pharmaceuticals Rx

Tablets (long-acting): 1.34 mg clemastine fumarate, equivalent to 1 mg clemastine, and 75 mg phenylpropanolamine hydrochloride

INDICATIONS
Symptoms associated with **allergic rhinitis**, including sneezing, rhinorrhea, lacrimation, nasal congestion, and pruritus of the eyes, nose, or throat

ORAL DOSAGE
Adult: 1 tab, swallowed whole, q12h
Child (≥ 12 yr): same as adult

CONTRAINDICATIONS

Hypersensitivity to either component	Lower respiratory tract conditions, including asthma	Severe hypertension
Premature or full-term neonates		Severe coronary artery disease
Breast-feeding	MAO inhibitors (see DRUG INTERACTIONS)	

WARNINGS/PRECAUTIONS

Drowsiness	Caution patients about driving or engaging in other activities requiring mental alertness; advise patients to avoid alcohol and other CNS depressants (see DRUG INTERACTIONS)

TAVIST-D

Elderly patients	Antihistaminic reactions (dizziness, sedation, and hypotension) are more likely to occur in patients 60 yr of age or older
Other special-risk patients	Use with considerable caution in patients with narrow angle glaucoma, stenosing peptic ulcer, pyloroduodenal obstruction, symptomatic prostatic hypertrophy, or bladder neck obstruction and with caution in patients with increased intraocular pressure, diabetes mellitus, cardiovascular disease (including hypertension), hyperthyroidism, or a history of bronchial asthma. Phenylpropanolamine can cause elevated blood pressure and tachyarrhythmias, especially in hyperthyroid patients.
Carcinogenicity, mutagenicity	Carcinogenicity studies have not been performed with Tavist-D; however, in studies with clemastine alone, no evidence of carcinogenesis has been observed in rats given orally 1,500 times the human dose for 2 yr or in mice given orally 3,800 times the human dose for 85 wk. Mutagenicity studies have not been performed.
Effect on fertility	Clemastine alone, given orally to male rats, produced a decrease in mating ability at 933 times the human dose, but not at 466 times the human dose

ADVERSE REACTIONS[1]

Frequent reactions (incidence ≥ 1%) are printed in *italics*

Central nervous system	*Sedation, sleepiness, dizziness, disturbed coordination,* fatigue, confusion, restlessness, excitation, nervousness, tremor, irritability, insomnia, euphoria, paresthesias, blurred vision, diplopia, vertigo, tinnitus, acute labyrinthitis, hysteria, neuritis, convulsions
Gastrointestinal	*Epigastric distress,* anorexia, nausea, vomiting, diarrhea, constipation
Respiratory	*Thickening of bronchial secretions,* tightness of the chest and wheezing, nasal congestion
Cardiovascular	Hypotension, elevated blood pressure, headache, palpitations, tachycardia, extrasystoles, tachyarrhythmias
Hematological	Hemolytic anemia, thrombocytopenia, agranulocytosis
Genitourinary	Urinary frequency, difficult urination, urinary retention, early menses
Other	Urticaria, drug rash, anaphylactic shock, photosensitivity, excessive perspiration, chills; dry mouth, nose, and throat

OVERDOSAGE

Signs and symptoms	*Antihistaminic effects:* vary from CNS depression (sedation, apnea, diminished mental alertness, cyanosis, coma, cardiovascular collapse) to CNS stimulation (insomnia, hallucinations, tremors, or convulsions) to death; also: euphoria, excitement, tachycardia, palpitations, thirst, perspiration, nausea, dizziness, tinnitus, ataxia, blurred vision, and hypertension or hypotension; CNS stimulation and atropine-like signs and symptoms (dry mouth; fixed, dilated pupils; flushing; hyperthermia; gastrointestinal disturbances) are particularly likely in children. *Sympathomimetic effects:* giddiness, headache, nausea, vomiting, sweating, thirst, tachycardia, precordial pain, palpitations, difficulty in micturition, muscular weakness and tenseness, anxiety, restlessness, insomnia, delusions, hallucinations, cardiac arrhythmias, circulatory collapse, convulsions, coma, respiratory failure.
Treatment	If patient is conscious and emesis has not occurred spontaneously, induce vomiting, preferably by giving syrup of ipecac along with milk or water. Take care to avoid aspiration, particularly with infants and children. Instill activated charcoal to remove any drug remaining in the stomach after inducing emesis. If vomiting is contraindicated or, after 20 min, unsuccessful, and ingestion has occurred within 3 h, perform gastric lavage with isotonic or 1/2 isotonic saline solution; lavage may be done even after 3 h, if large amounts of milk or cream have been given earlier. Administer a saline cathartic to rapidly dilute bowel contents. Treatment is symptomatic and supportive. Vasopressors may be used for hypotension. Short-acting barbiturates, diazepam, or paraldehyde may be administered to control seizures. Treat hyperpyrexia with tepid water sponge baths or a hypothermic blanket. For apnea, provide ventilatory support; *do not use stimulants or analeptics.* Dialysis is of little value.

DRUG INTERACTIONS

Alcohol, tranquilizers, sedative-hypnotics, and other CNS depressants	△ CNS depression
MAO inhibitors	△ Sympathomimetic and anticholinergic effects
Methyldopa, mecamylamine, reserpine, *Veratrum* alkaloids	▽ Antihypertensive effect

ALTERED LABORATORY VALUES

No clinically significant alterations in blood/serum or urinary values occur at therapeutic dosages

TAVIST-D ■ TRIAMINIC

USE IN CHILDREN	USE IN PREGNANT AND NURSING WOMEN
Safety and effectiveness for use in children under 12 yr of age have not been established	Pregnancy Category B: use during pregnancy only if clearly needed. Reproduction studies performed in animals given clemastine alone, in oral doses up to 933 (rats) or 560 (rabbits) times the human dose, or a 1:49 combination of clemastine and phenylpropanolamine, in oral doses up to 100 (rats) or 67 (rabbits) times the human dose, have shown no evidence of teratogenicity. The following phenylpropanolamine-related effects have been observed: in rats, impaired maternal weight gain and maternal deaths (at 33 times the human dose), as well as a reduction in fetal weight and a slight increase in preimplantation loss and prenatal deaths (at 100 times the human dose); in rabbits, an increase in maternal deaths (at 20 and 67 times the human dose), as well as maternal weight loss and a slight, within normal limits increase in prenatal deaths (at 67 times the human dose). No adequate, well-controlled studies have been performed in pregnant women. Use of Tavist-D in nursing mothers is contraindicated.

[1] Includes reactions observed with other antihistamines and sympathomimetic compounds

---

DECONGESTANTS/UPPER RESPIRATORY COMBINATIONS

TRIAMINIC (phenylpropanolamine hydrochloride, pheniramine maleate, and pyrilamine maleate) Sandoz Consumer Health Care Group — Rx

Drops (per milliliter): 20 mg phenylpropanolamine hydrochloride, 10 mg pheniramine maleate, and 10 mg pyrilamine maleate (15 ml)

TRIAMINIC TR (phenylpropanolamine hydrochloride, pheniramine maleate, and pyrilamine maleate) Sandoz Consumer Health Care Group — Rx

Tablets (timed release): 50 mg phenylpropanolamine hydrochloride, 25 mg pheniramine maleate, and 25 mg pyrilamine maleate

INDICATIONS	**ORAL DOSAGE**
Nasal congestion and postnasal drip associated with colds, allergies, sinusitis, and rhinitis Symptoms of **allergic rhinitis,** including sneezing, rhinorrhea, pruritus, and lacrimation	Adult: 1 tab tid (in the morning, midafternoon, and at bedtime) Infant and young child: 1 drop/2 lb qid

CONTRAINDICATIONS		
Hypersensitivity to any component	Severe hypertension	MAO inhibitor therapy (see DRUG INTERACTIONS)
Lower respiratory tract conditions	Severe coronary artery disease	
Breast-feeding		

WARNINGS/PRECAUTIONS	
Drowsiness	Caution patients about driving or engaging in other activities requiring mental alertness, and about alcohol or other CNS depressants
Elderly patients	Antihistaminic (dizziness, sedation, and hypotension) and sympathomimetic (eg, confusion, hallucinations, convulsions, CNS depression) side effects are more likely to occur in patients over 60 yr of age
Special-risk patients	Use with caution in patients with increased intraocular pressure or narrow-angle glaucoma, stenosing peptic ulcer, pyloroduodenal obstruction, symptomatic prostatic hypertrophy, bladder-neck obstruction, hypertension or other cardiovascular disease, hyperthyroidism, diabetes mellitus, or bronchial asthma
Carcinogenicity, mutagenicity, effect on fertility	No long-term studies have been done to determine the carcinogenic or mutagenic potential of these preparations or their effect, if any, on fertility

ADVERSE REACTIONS	The most frequent reactions, regardless of incidence, are printed in *italics*
Central nervous system	*Sedation, sleepiness, dizziness, disturbed coordination, restlessness, excitement, nervousness, insomnia,* fatigue, confusion, tremor, irritability, euphoria, paresthesias, blurred vision, diplopia, vertigo, tinnitus, acute labyrinthitis, hysteria, neuritis, convulsions, CNS depression, hallucinations
Cardiovascular	Hypotension, headache, palpitations, tachycardia, extrasystoles
Hematological	Hemolytic anemia, thrombocytopenia, agranulocytosis
Gastrointestinal	*Epigastric distress,* anorexia, nausea, vomiting, diarrhea, constipation

COMPENDIUM OF DRUG THERAPY

Genitourinary	Urinary frequency, difficult urination, urinary retention, early menses
Respiratory	Thickening of bronchial secretions, tightness in the chest and wheezing, nasal stuffiness
Dermatological and hypersensitivity	Urticaria, drug rash, photosensitivity, anaphylactic shock
Other	Dry mouth, nose, and throat; excessive perspiration, chills

OVERDOSAGE

Signs and symptoms	CNS depression or stimulation, atropine-like effects (dry mouth; fixed, dilated pupils; flushing; GI symptoms). Stimulation is particularly likely in children; hallucinations, convulsions, and death may have occurred in infants and children.
Treatment	If patient has not vomited spontaneously, induce emesis; administer activated charcoal if less than 1 h has elapsed. Gastric lavage, using isotonic or half-isotonic saline, is indicated if performed within 3 h of ingestion or later if large amounts of milk or cream were given earlier. Administer a saline cathartic to dilute bowel contents and hasten evacuation. A vasopressor may be given for hypotension. *Do not use stimulants*.

DRUG INTERACTIONS

Alcohol, tranquilizers, sedative-hypnotics, and other CNS depressants	△ CNS depression
MAO inhibitors	△ Sympathomimetic and anticholinergic effects
Methyldopa, guanethidine, mecamylamine, reserpine, *Veratrum* alkaloids	▽ Antihypertensive effect

ALTERED LABORATORY VALUES

No clinically significant alterations in blood/serum or urinary values occur at therapeutic dosages

---

USE IN CHILDREN

See INDICATIONS and ORAL DOSAGE. These preparations may elicit either mild stimulation or mild sedation; the former is most often seen in young children.

USE IN PREGNANT AND NURSING WOMEN

Pregnancy Category C: use during pregnancy only if the expected therapeutic benefits outweigh the potential hazards. Animal reproduction studies have not been done, and the safety of using these preparations in pregnant women has not been established with regard to their possible effects on fetal development. Contraindicated for use in nursing mothers because of the higher risk of antihistaminic side effects in premature and full-term infants.

DECONGESTANTS/UPPER RESPIRATORY COMBINATIONS

TRINALIN (azatadine maleate and pseudoephedrine sulfate) Schering Rx

Tablets (sustained release): 1 mg azatadine maleate and 120 mg pseudoephedrine sulfate

INDICATIONS	ORAL DOSAGE
Upper respiratory mucosal congestion associated with perennial and allergic rhinitis **Nasal and eustachian tube congestion**	Adult: 1 tab bid

CONTRAINDICATIONS

Treatment of lower respiratory tract symptoms, including asthma	Severe hypertension	Hypersensitivity or idiosyncratic reaction to azatadine or pseudoephedrine adrenergic agents,[1] or structurally related compounds
Narrow-angle glaucoma	Severe coronary artery disease	
Urinary retention	Hyperthyroidism	
		MAO inhibitor therapy (see WARNINGS/PRECAUTIONS)

WARNINGS/PRECAUTIONS

MAO inhibitor therapy	Wait at least 10 days after discontinuing use of a MAO inhibitor before initiating therapy with this preparation
Drowsiness, mental impairment	Caution patients not to engage in potentially hazardous activities requiring full mental alertness and that alcohol and other CNS depressants may cause further impairment

TRINALIN

Elderly patients	Antihistaminic (dizziness, sedation, and hypotension) and sympathomimetic (eg, confusion, hallucinations, convulsions, CNS depression) side effects are more likely to occur in patients over 60 yr of age; safe use of a short-acting sympathomimetic should be established before this preparation is prescribed
Atropine-like action	Use with caution in patients with a history of bronchial asthma (see CONTRAINDICATIONS)
Special-risk patients	Use with considerable caution in patients with stenosing peptic ulcer, pyloroduodenal obstruction, urinary bladder obstruction due to symptomatic prostatic hypertrophy, or bladder neck obstruction and with caution in the presence of cardiovascular disease (including hypertension or ischemic heart disease), increased intraocular pressure (see CONTRAINDICATIONS), or diabetes mellitus and in patients taking digitalis or oral anticoagulants (see DRUG INTERACTIONS)
Carcinogenicity, mutagenicity	The carcinogenic and mutagenic potential of this preparation are unknown
Drug dependence	Abuse or dependency has not occurred with azatadine maleate. Abuse of pseudoephedrine has been reported, and, with continued use, tolerance can develop; depression may follow rapid withdrawal of pseudoephedrine.

ADVERSE REACTIONS

Frequent reactions (incidence $\geq$ 1%) are printed in *italics*

Cardiovascular	Hypertension, hypotension, arrhythmias, cardiovascular collapse, headache, palpitations, extrasystoles, tachycardia, angina
Hematological	Hemolytic anemia, hypoplastic anemia, thrombocytopenia, agranulocytosis
Central nervous system	*Sedation, sleepiness, dizziness, disturbed coordination,* vertigo, tinnitus, acute labyrinthitis, fatigue, mydriasis, confusion, restlessness, excitation, nervousness, tension, tremor, irritability, insomnia, euphoria, paresthesias, blurred vision, hysteria, neuritis, convulsions, fear, anxiety, hallucinations, CNS depression, weakness, pallor
Gastrointestinal	*Epigastric distress,* anorexia, nausea, vomiting, diarrhea, constipation, abdominal cramps
Genitourinary	Urinary frequency, urinary retention, dysuria, early menses
Respiratory	*Thickening of bronchial secretions,* tightness in the chest and wheezing, nasal stuffiness, respiratory difficulty
Dermatological and hypersensitivity	Urticaria, drug rash, photosensitivity, anaphylactic shock
Other	Excessive perspiration; chills; dry mouth, nose, and throat

OVERDOSAGE

Signs and symptoms	*Antihistaminic effects:* vary from CNS depression (sedation, apnea, diminished mental alertness, cyanosis, coma, cardiovascular collapse) to CNS stimulation (insomnia, hallucinations, tremors, or convulsions) to death; also: euphoria, excitement, tachycardia, palpitations, thirst, perspiration, nausea, dizziness, tinnitus, ataxia, blurred vision, and hypertension or hypotension; CNS stimulation and atropine-like signs and symptoms (dry mouth; fixed, dilated pupils; flushing; hyperthermia; gastrointestinal disturbances) are particularly likely in children. *Sympathomimetic effects:* giddiness, headache, nausea, vomiting, sweating, thirst, tachycardia, precordial pain, palpitations, difficulty in micturition, muscular weakness and tenseness, anxiety, restlessness, insomnia, delusions, hallucinations, cardiac arrhythmias, circulatory collapse, convulsions, coma, respiratory failure
Treatment	If patient is conscious, induce vomiting (preferably with ipecac), even if emesis has occurred spontaneously. Take care to avoid aspiration, particularly with infants and children. Instill activated charcoal to remove any drug remaining in the stomach after inducing emesis. If vomiting is unsuccessful or contraindicated, perform gastric lavage with isotonic or ½ isotonic saline solution. Administer a saline cathartic to rapidly dilute bowel contents. Treatment is symptomatic and supportive. Vasopressors may be used for hypotension. Short-acting barbiturates, diazepam, or paraldehyde may be administered to control seizures. Treat hyperpyrexia with tepid water sponge baths or a hypothermic blanket. For apnea, provide ventilatory support; *do not use stimulants or analeptics.* Dialysis is of little value.

DRUG INTERACTIONS

MAO inhibitors	⌂ Antihistaminic effects Hypertensive reactions, including hypertensive crises
Alcohol, tricyclic antidepressants, barbiturates, and other CNS depressants	⌂ CNS depression
Oral anticoagulants	▽ Anticoagulant effect
Methyldopa, mecamylamine, reserpine, and *Veratrum* alkaloids	▽ Antihypertensive effect
Beta-adrenergic blockers	⌂ Sympathomimetic effects
Digitalis	⌂ Ectopic pacemaker activity
Antacids	⌂ Rate of absorption of pseudoephedrine

TRINALIN ■ ORGANIDIN

Kaolin ———————————————— ▽ Rate of absorption of pseudoephedrine

ALTERED LABORATORY VALUES

Blood/serum values ———————— Inhibition of creatine phosphokinase MB in vitro (clinical significance unknown)

No clinically significant alterations in urinary values occur at therapeutic dosages

USE IN CHILDREN
Safety and effectiveness for use in children under 12 yr of age have not been established

USE IN PREGNANT AND NURSING WOMEN
Pregnancy Category C: use during pregnancy only if the expected benefits of therapy justify the potential risk to the fetus. Retarded fetal development, increased resorption, and congenital abnormalities have been observed in reproduction studies on rabbits at 12.5, 25, and 5 times the recommended human dose, respectively. No adequate, well-controlled studies have been done in pregnant women; however, antihistamines should not be used during the third trimester because of reports of severe reactions (eg, convulsions) in newborns and premature infants. It is not known whether these drugs are excreted in human milk; because of the potential for serious adverse reactions to antihistamines in infants and, particularly, premature infants, patient should not nurse if use of this preparation is deemed essential.

[1] In sensitive individuals, small doses of adrenergic agents may cause idiosyncratic reactions, including insomnia, tremor, weakness, dizziness, or arrhythmias.

EXPECTORANTS

ORGANIDIN (iodinated glycerol) Wallace   Rx

Tablets: 30 mg **Elixir (per 5 ml):** 60 mg[1] (1 pt, 1 gal) **Solution (per 10 drops):** 30 mg (30 ml)

INDICATIONS
Respiratory tract conditions, including bronchitis, bronchial asthma, pulmonary emphysema, cystic fibrosis, and chronic sinusitis (adjunctive therapy)
Prevention of postoperative atelectasis

ORAL DOSAGE
Adult: 60 mg (2 tabs), 5 ml (1 tsp), or 20 drops (60 mg) qid; tablets must be administered with liquid, and drops must be added to fruit juice or other liquid
Child: up to 30 mg (1 tab), 2.5 ml (1/2 tsp), or 10 drops (30 mg), based on child's weight, qid; tablets must be administered with liquid, and drops must be added to fruit juice or other liquid

CONTRAINDICATIONS
Pregnancy | Neonates | Breast-feeding
History of marked sensitivity to inorganic iodides | Hypersensitivity to any component or related compound |

WARNINGS/PRECAUTIONS
Iodism ———————————————— Discontinue use if dermatitis or other manifestations of hypersensitivity develop
Flare-up of adolescent acne ———— May occur
Special-risk patients ——————— Use with caution or avoid use in patients with history or evidence of thyroid disease

ADVERSE REACTIONS
Gastrointestinal ——————————— Irritation (rare)
Dermatological ——————————— Rash (rare)
Other ———————————————— Thyroid gland enlargement, acute parotitis, and hypersensitivity reactions (rare)

OVERDOSAGE
Signs and symptoms ——————— See ADVERSE REACTIONS
Treatment ———————————— Empty stomach by inducing emesis; treat symptomatically

DRUG INTERACTIONS
Antithyroid drugs ————————— △ Hypothyroid effect
Lithium ——————————————— △ Risk of lithium toxicity

ALTERED LABORATORY VALUES
Blood/serum values ———————— △ PBI ▽ [131]I thyroid uptake

No clinically significant alterations in urinary values occur at therapeutic dosages

1462   COMPENDIUM OF DRUG THERAPY

USE IN CHILDREN

See INDICATIONS and ORAL DOSAGE; children with cystic fibrosis may have an increased susceptibility to the goitrogenic effects of iodides. Contraindicated for use in newborns.

USE IN PREGNANT AND NURSING WOMEN

Pregnancy Category X: contraindicated for use during pregnancy. Use of inorganic iodides during and after the 12th wk of gestation has been reported to induce fetal goiter with the potential for airway obstruction. If patient becomes pregnant while taking this drug, discontinue use and inform patient of the potential risk to the fetus. Contraindicated for use in nursing mothers.

[1] Contains 21.75% alcohol

Chapter 35

Diagnostics

Blood Chemistry Tests — 1467
ACETEST Reagent Tablets (Ames)	1467
AZOSTIX Reagent Strips (Ames)	1467
CHEMSTRIP bG (Boehringer Mannheim Diagnostics)	1467
DEXTROSTIX Reagent Strips (Ames)	1468
GLUCOSTIX Reagent Strips (Ames)	1468
VISIDEX II Reagent Strips (Ames)	1468

Urine Chemistry Tests — 1469
ACETEST Reagent Tablets (Ames)	1469
ALBUSTIX (Ames)	1469
BILI-LABSTIX (Ames)	1469
BILI-LABSTIX SG (Ames)	1469
CLINISTIX (Ames)	1469
COMBISTIX (Ames)	1469
DIASTIX (Ames)	1469
HEMA-COMBISTIX (Ames)	1469
HEMASTIX (Ames)	1469
KETO-DIASTIX (Ames)	1469
KETOSTIX (Ames)	1469
LABSTIX (Ames)	1469
MULTISTIX (Ames)	1469
MULTISTIX SG (Ames)	1470
N-MULTISTIX (Ames)	1470
N-MULTISTIX SG (Ames)	1470
N-URISTIX (Ames)	1470
PHENISTIX (Ames)	1470
URISTIX (Ames)	1470
UROBILISTIX (Ames)	1470
BUMINTEST Reagent Tablets (Ames)	1471
CHEMSTRIP 3 (Boehringer Mannheim Diagnostics)	1472
CHEMSTRIP 4 (Boehringer Mannheim Diagnostics)	1472
CHEMSTRIP 5 (Boehringer Mannheim Diagnostics)	1472
CHEMSTRIP 5L (Boehringer Mannheim Diagnostics)	1472
CHEMSTRIP 6 (Boehringer Mannheim Diagnostics)	1472
CHEMSTRIP 6L (Boehringer Mannheim Diagnostics)	1472
CHEMSTRIP 7 (Boehringer Mannheim Diagnostics)	1472
CHEMSTRIP 7L (Boehringer Mannheim Diagnostics)	1472
CHEMSTRIP 8 (Boehringer Mannheim Diagnostics)	1472
CHEMSTRIP 9 (Boehringer Mannheim Diagnostics)	1472
CHEMSTRIP GP (Boehringer Mannheim Diagnostics)	1472
CHEMSTRIP K (Boehringer Mannheim Diagnostics)	1472
CHEMSTRIP L (Boehringer Mannheim Diagnostics)	1472
CHEMSTRIP LN (Boehringer Mannheim Diagnostics)	1472
CHEMSTRIP uG (Boehringer Mannheim Diagnostics)	1472
CHEMSTRIP uGK (Boehringer Mannheim Diagnostics)	1472
CLINITEST Reagent Tablets (Ames)	1473
ICTOTEST Reagent Tablets (Ames)	1474
TES-TAPE (Lilly)	1474

Fecal Occult Blood Tests — 1474
COLOSCREEN Self Test (CS-T) (Helena Laboratories)	1474
EARLY DETECTOR (Warner-Lambert)	1475
EZ-DETECT (Self-Care Systems)	1475
FLEET DETECATEST (Fleet)	1475
HEMA-CHEK Slide Test (Ames)	1476
HEMATEST Reagent Tablets (Ames)	1476
HEMOCCULT (SmithKline Diagnostics)	1476

Ovulation Tests — 1477
FIRST RESPONSE Ovulation Predictor Test (Tambrands)	1477
OVUSTICK Self-Test (Monoclonal Antibodies)	1478
QTEST Ovulation Test (Clay Adams)[1]	1479

Pregnancy Tests — 1480
βhCG-ROCHE EIA (Roche Diagnostics)	1480
NEO-PLANOTEST DUOCLON Slide (Organon Teknika)	1481
NEO-PREGNOSTICON DUOCLON Tube (Organon Teknika)	1481
β-NEOCEPT 30 (Organon Teknika)	1482
NIMBUS (NMS Pharmaceuticals)	1483
ORTHO β-hCG (Ortho Diagnostic Systems)	1483
PREGNACLONE Slide (Fisher Scientific)	1484
PREGNACLONE Tube (Fisher Scientific)	1485
PREGNAZYME (Wampole Laboratories)	1485
PREGNOLISA (Organon Teknika)	1486

[1]These tests are also available over-the-counter from Becton Dickinson Consumer Products

PREGNOSIS (Roche Diagnostics)	1487
PREGNOSPIA (Organon Teknika)	1488
PREGNOSTICON DRI-DOT (Organon Teknika)	1488
PREGNOSTICON Slide (Organon Teknika)	1489
QTEST Pregnancy Test (Clay Adams)[1]	1490
RAMP (Monoclonal Antibodies)	1491
TESTPACK hCG-Serum (Abbott Laboratories)	1491
TESTPACK hCG-Urine (Abbott Laboratories)	1492
UCG-BETA SLIDE Monoclonal II (Wampole Laboratories)	1492
UCG-BETA STAT (Wampole Laboratories)	1493
UCG-LYPHOTEST (Wampole Laboratories)	1494
UCG-Slide (Wampole Laboratories)	1494

Bacterial Screening Tests — 1495

BACTIGEN Group A Streptococcus (Wampole Laboratories)	1495
BACTIGEN H. Influenzae Type b (Wampole Laboratories)	1495
BACTIGEN N. meningitidis (Wampole Laboratories)	1496
BACTIGEN S. pneumoniae (Wampole Laboratories)	1496
CULTURETTE 10-Minute Group A Strep ID (Marion Scientific)	1497
DETECT-A-STREP (Antibodies Incorporated)	1497
GONODECTEN (United States Packaging Corporation)	1497
INSTA KIT for Group A Strep ID (Mead Johnson Nutritional)	1498
MICROSTIX-Nitrite (Ames)	1498
MICROTRAK Chlamydia trachomatis Direct Specimen Test (Syva)	1498
PATHODX Strep A (Diagnostics Products Corporation)	1499
QTEST Group A Strep Test (Clay Adams)	1499
RAPIDTEST-STREP (SmithKline Diagnostics)	1500
STREPTOZYME (Wampole Laboratories)	1500
TESTPACK Strep A (Abbott Laboratories)	1500

Culture Tests — 1501

BACTURCULT (Wampole Laboratories)	1501
ISOCULT Culture Test for Bacteriuria (SmithKline Diagnostics)	1501
ISOCULT Culture Test for Candida (Monilia) (SmithKline Diagnostics)	1501
ISOCULT Culture Test for Neisseria gonorrhoeae (SmithKline Diagnostics)	1502
ISOCULT Culture Test for Pseudomonas aeruginosa (SmithKline Diagnostics)	1502
ISOCULT Culture Test for Staphylococcus aureus (SmithKline Diagnostics)	1502
ISOCULT Culture Test for Throat Streptococci (SmithKline Diagnostics)	1503
ISOCULT Culture Test for Trichomonas vaginalis (SmithKline Diagnostics)	1503
MICROCULT-GC (Ames)	1503
MICROSTIX-3 (Ames)	1504
MICROSTIX-CANDIDA (Ames)	1504

Mononucleosis Tests — 1504

MONO-DIFF (Wampole Laboratories)	1504
MONO-LATEX (Wampole Laboratories)	1505
MONOSPOT (Ortho Diagnostic Systems)	1505
MONOSTICON (Organon Teknika)	1506
MONOSTICON DRI-DOT (Organon Teknika)	1506
MONO-SURE (Wampole Laboratories)	1506
MONO-TEST (Wampole Laboratories)	1507
MONO-TEST (FTB) (Wampole Laboratories)	1507

Rubella Tests — 1508

RUBACELL II (Abbott Laboratories)	1508
RUBAQUICK (Abbott Laboratories)	1508
VIROGEN Rubella (Wampole Laboratories)	1508

Rheumatoid Factor Tests — 1508

LAtest-RF Kit (Fisher Scientific)	1508
R$_3$-SCREEN TEST (Wampole Laboratories)	1509
RHEUMANOSTICON (Organon Teknika)	1509
RHEUMANOSTICON DRI-DOT (Organon Teknika)	1509
RHEUMATEX (Wampole Laboratories)	1510
RHEUMATON (Wampole Laboratories)	1510

[1] These tests are also available over-the-counter from Becton Dickinson Consumer Products

continued

HOME PREGNANCY TESTS

TEST	METHOD	SENSITIVITY
ADVANCE (Advanced Care Products)	Enzyme immunoassay	150–200 mIU/ml
CLEARBLUE (VLI)	Enzyme immunoassay	50–100 mIU/ml
DAISY 2 (Advanced Care Products)	Hemagglutination inhibition	200 mIU/ml
EPT PLUS (Warner-Lambert)	Gold sol agglutination	150 mIU/ml
FACT (Advanced Care Products)	Hemagglutination inhibition	150–200 mIU/ml
FIRST RESPONSE (Tambrands)	Enzyme immunoassay	50 mIU/ml

BLOOD CHEMISTRY TESTS

ACETEST Reagent Tablets Ames

Intended use	Semiquantitative determination of ketones in urine, serum, plasma, and whole blood
Materials provided	Tablets containing sodium nitroprusside and glycine
Additional materials required	Dropper; clean, white piece of paper
Time for reading	**Urine:** 30 seconds; appearance of purple color at end of this waiting period is positive for ketones **Serum or plasma:** 2 min; appearance of purple color at end of this waiting period is positive for ketones **Whole blood:** 10 min; appearance of purple color at end of this waiting period and after removal of clotted blood from tablet is positive for ketones
Performance characteristics	Test is specific for acetoacetic acid and acetone; sensitivity for acetoacetic acid is 5 mg/dl in urine and 10 mg/dl in serum, plasma, or whole blood
Limitations and precautions	Bromsulfalein, 8-hydroxyquinoline, and very high quantities of phenylketones may produce false-positive results in urine samples; metabolites of levodopa may also give false-positive reactions; improper handling of the tablets to allow moisture absorption will adversely affect test results

BLOOD CHEMISTRY TESTS

AZOSTIX Reagent Strips Ames

Intended use	Semiquantitative determination of blood urea nitrogen
Materials provided	Plastic strip with reagent-impregnated test area; color chart
Additional materials required	Lancet or other finger-puncturing device; wash bottle; watch with second hand
Time for reading	60 seconds (color fades rapidly after this time)
Performance characteristics	Test is specific for blood urea nitrogen within a range of 10–60 mg/dl
Limitations and precautions	Fluoride preservatives may produce erroneously low values; anticoagulants containing ammonium salts may yield erroneously high values; color changes are less distinct at higher BUN levels

BLOOD CHEMISTRY TESTS

CHEMSTRIP bG Boehringer Mannheim Diagnostics

Intended use	Semiquantitative determination of blood glucose
Materials provided	Plastic strip with two reagent-impregnated test areas; color chart
Additional materials required	Lancet or other finger-puncturing device; cotton ball; alcohol swab (optional); timer (stopwatch or a watch with a second hand) or ACCU-CHEK II Blood Glucose Monitor
Time for reading	2 minutes
Performance characteristics	Test is specific for blood glucose over a range of 20–800 mg/dl; correlation coefficient is 0.978, when compared with Beckman Glucose Analyzer; hematocrit values of 30–70% have no significant effect on test results, nor does treatment with heparin, EDTA, or the usual plasma expanders
Limitations and precautions	Venous blood must be analyzed within 30 min of collection to avoid the effects of hemolysis; blood specimens preserved with fluoride cannot be used; dopamine and methyldopa will inhibit the reaction of the test pads at a blood concentration of 10 mg/dl; very low ($<$ 35%) or very high ($>$ 55%) hematocrit values can alter test results; grossly lipemic samples may interfere with the test procedure; the Accu-Check II system is not recommended for use with neonatal blood specimens

BLOOD CHEMISTRY TESTS

DEXTROSTIX Reagent Strips Ames

Intended use	Semiquantitative or quantitative determination of blood glucose
Materials provided	Plastic strip with reagent-impregnated test area; color chart
Additional materials required	Lancet or other finger-puncturing device; wash bottle; lint-free paper towel; watch with second hand; an Ames blood glucose meter is necessary for quantitative determinations
Time for reading	60 seconds for visual reading; less than 2 min for instrument use
Performance characteristics	Test is specific for blood glucose and will react to a concentration as low as 10 mg/dl; when read with the Ames GLUCOMETER Reflectance Photometer, accuracy is under 4 mg/dl at a blood glucose level of 50 mg/dl, under 17 mg/dl at 175 mg/dl, and under 30 mg/dl at 300 mg/dl, with a within-run coefficient of variation of 4.5% at each glucose level
Limitations and precautions	Vitamin C, bilirubin (total), sodium fluoride, uric acid, and a high hematocrit ($>$ 55%) may give erroneously low values, whereas creatinine, sodium salicylate, acetoacetic acid (ketone bodies), beta-hydroxybutyric acid, and a low hematocrit ($<$ 35%) tend to produce falsely high results; color changes are less distinct at higher blood glucose levels; this test is not intended for use with neonatal blood specimens or with serum or plasma

BLOOD CHEMISTRY TESTS

GLUCOSTIX Reagent Strips Ames

Intended use	Semiquantitative or quantitative determination of blood glucose
Materials provided	Plastic strip with two reagent-impregnated test areas; color chart
Additional materials required	Lancet or other finger-puncturing device; lint-free paper towel or facial tissue; watch with second hand; an Ames blood glucose meter (GLUCOMETER II, GLUCOMETER II with Memory, or GLUCOMETER M) is necessary for quantitative determinations
Time for reading	90 seconds for visual reading; timing is performed automatically when an Ames blood glucose monitor is used
Performance characteristics	Test is specific for blood glucose; when read visually, the lower range pad (or test area) measures glucose levels between 20 and 110 mg/dl, while the upper range pad measures between 140 and 800 mg/dl; accuracy of visual readings is 93–98% over a blood glucose range of 70–250 mg/dl
Limitations and precautions	Vitamin C, sodium fluoride, uric acid, and a high hematocrit ($>$ 50%) may give erroneously low values, whereas a low hematocrit ($<$ 35%) tends to cause falsely high results; extremes in operating temperature (above 30°C or below 18°C) may produce incorrect instrument readings; glucose values obtained from specimens with highly elevated cholesterol and/or triglyceride levels should be interpreted with caution; blood specimens preserved with fluoride cannot be used; this test is not intended for use with neonatal blood specimens or with serum or plasma

BLOOD CHEMISTRY TESTS

VISIDEX II Reagent Strips Ames

Intended use	Semiquantitative determination of blood glucose
Materials provided	Plastic strip with two reagent-impregnated test areas; color chart
Additional materials required	Lancet or other finger-puncturing device; facial tissue; watch with second hand
Time for reading	90 seconds
Performance characteristics	Test is specific for blood glucose; the lower range pad (or test area) measures glucose levels between 20 and 110 mg/dl, while the upper range pad measures between 140 and 800 mg/dl; accuracy is 95–99% over a blood glucose range of 70–400 mg/dl

VISIDEX II ■ AMES Reagent Strips for Urinalysis

Limitations and precautions	A high hematocrit (> 55%) may give erroneously low values, whereas a low hematocrit (< 35%) tends to produce falsely high results; blood specimens preserved with fluoride cannot be used; this test is not intended for use with neonatal blood specimens or with serum or plasma

URINE CHEMISTRY TESTS

ACETEST Reagent Tablets Ames

Intended use	Semiquantitative determination of ketones in urine, serum, plasma, and whole blood
Materials provided	Tablets containing sodium nitroprusside and glycine
Additional materials required	Dropper; clean, white piece of paper
Time for reading	**Urine:** 30 seconds; appearance of purple color at end of this waiting period is positive for ketones **Serum or plasma:** 2 min; appearance of purple color at end of this waiting period is positive for ketones **Whole blood:** 10 min; appearance of purple color at end of this waiting period and after removal of clotted blood from tablet is positive for ketones
Performance characteristics	Test is specific for acetoacetic acid and acetone; sensitivity for acetoacetic acid is 5 mg/dl in urine and 10 mg/dl in serum, plasma, or whole blood
Limitations and precautions	Bromsulfalein, 8-hydroxyquinoline, and very high quantities of phenylketones may produce false-positive results in urine samples; metabolites of levodopa may also give false-positive reactions; improper handling of the tablets to allow moisture absorption will adversely affect test results

URINE CHEMISTRY TESTS

ALBUSTIX Ames
Reagent strip for qualitative and semiquantitative determination of urinary protein

BILI-LABSTIX Ames
Reagent strip for qualitative and semiquantitative determination of urinary pH, protein, glucose, ketone, bilirubin, and blood

BILI-LABSTIX SG Ames
Reagent strip for qualitative and semiquantitative determination of urinary specific gravity, pH, protein, glucose, ketone, bilirubin, and blood

CLINISTIX Ames
Reagent strip for qualitative and semiquantitative determination of urinary glucose

COMBISTIX Ames
Reagent strip for qualitative and semiquantitative determination of urinary pH, protein, and glucose

DIASTIX Ames
Reagent strip for qualitative and semiquantitative determination of urinary glucose

HEMA-COMBISTIX Ames
Reagent strip for qualitative and semiquantitative determination of urinary pH, protein, glucose, and blood

HEMASTIX Ames
Reagent strip for qualitative and semiquantitative determination of urinary blood

KETO-DIASTIX Ames
Reagent strip for qualitative and semiquantitative determination of urinary glucose and ketone

KETOSTIX Ames
Reagent strip for qualitative and semiquantitative determination of urinary ketone

LABSTIX Ames
Reagent strip for qualitative and semiquantitative determination of urinary pH, protein, glucose, ketone, and blood

MULTISTIX Ames
Reagent strip for qualitative and semiquantitative determination of urinary pH, protein, glucose, ketone, bilirubin, blood, and urobilinogen

AMES Reagent Strips for Urinalysis

MULTISTIX SG Ames

Reagent strip for qualitative and semiquantitative determination of urinary specific gravity, pH, protein, glucose, ketone, bilirubin, blood, and urobilinogen

N-MULTISTIX Ames

Reagent strip for qualitative and semiquantitative determination of urinary pH, protein, glucose, ketone, bilirubin, blood, nitrite, and urobilinogen

N-MULTISTIX SG Ames

Reagent strip for qualitative and semiquantitative determination of urinary specific gravity, pH, protein, glucose, ketone, bilirubin, blood, nitrite, and urobilinogen

N-URISTIX Ames

Reagent strip for qualitative and semiquantitative determination of urinary protein, glucose, and nitrite

PHENISTIX Ames

Reagent strip for qualitative and semiquantitative determination of urinary phenylketones

URISTIX Ames

Reagent strip for qualitative and semiquantitative determination of urinary protein and glucose

UROBILISTIX Ames

Reagent strip for qualitative and semiquantitative determination of urinary bilinogen

Materials provided	Plastic strip with reagent-impregnated test area(s); color chart
Additional materials required	None (if desired, certain tests may be read instrumentally with an AMES Clinitek 200 Urine Chemistry Analyzer)
Time for reading	**Specific gravity:** 45–60 seconds **pH:** any time up to 1 minute after dipping **Protein:** any time up to 1 minute after dipping **Glucose:** 10 seconds for qualitative results; 30 seconds for quantitative determinations **Ketone:** 15 seconds **Bilirubin:** 20 seconds **Blood:** 40 seconds **Nitrite:** 40 seconds **Urobilinogen:** 45 seconds **Phenylketones:** 30 seconds
Performance characteristics	**Specific gravity:** permits determination of urinary specific gravity between 1.000 and 1.030; test results correlate within 0.005 of values obtained with refractive index method; not affected by nonionic urine constituents (eg, glucose) or by presence of radiopaque dyes **pH:** accurate to within 0.5 pH unit from pH 5 to pH 8.5; not affected by variations in urinary buffer concentrations **Protein:** sensitivity is 20–25 mg/dl for albumin; test is less sensitive to globulins, hemoglobin, Bence-Jones protein, and mucoprotein **Glucose:** sensitivity is 100 mg/dl and is specific for glucose **Ketone:** sensitivity is 5–10 mg/dl; test is specific for acetoacetic acid and will not react with acetone or β-hydroxybutyric acid **Bilirubin:** sensitivity is 0.8 mg/dl **Blood:** sensitivity is 0.015–0.062 mg of hemoglobin/dl (equivalent to 5–20 intact red blood cells/μl) in urine specimens with a specific gravity of 1.005 or less and an ascorbic acid content of 5 mg/dl or less **Nitrite:** sensitivity is 0.06–0.1 mg/dl, which can detect up to 80% of bacterial urinary tract infections after sufficient bladder incubation; test is specific for nitrite **Urobilinogen:** sensitivity is 0.1 Ehrlich unit/dl **Phenylketones:** sensitivity for phenylpyruvic acid is 8 mg/dl; in addition to testing for phenylketones, the test may be used to screen for salicylate intoxication and urinary metabolites of phenothiazines and paraaminosalicylate (PAS)

AMES Reagent Strips for Urinalysis ■ BUMINTEST

Limitations and precautions — **Specific gravity:** the presence of glucose or urea in the urine and highly buffered alkaline urine specimens may produce falsely low readings; moderate amounts of protein (100–750 mg/dl) may cause elevated readings
pH: excess urine remaining on the strip after it is removed from the specimen container may produce falsely low readings
Protein: urine of high specific gravity may produce a "trace" result, even though only a normal amount of protein is present; highly buffered alkaline urine specimens and contamination by chlorhexidine or quaternary ammonium disinfectants may produce false-positive results; a negative result does not rule out the presence of globulins, hemoglobin, Bence-Jones protein, or mucoprotein
Glucose: ascorbic acid concentrations of 50 mg/dl or more and moderately high (40 mg/dl) ketone levels may produce false-negative results with samples containing small amounts of glucose (100 mg/dl); reactivity decreases as the specific gravity of the urine increases; sensitivity may also vary with temperature
Ketone: highly pigmented urine specimens and those containing large amounts of levodopa metabolites, as well as alkaline urine samples with high specific gravities, may read positively ("trace" or less)
Bilirubin: very small amounts of bilirubin (as may be found in the earliest phases of liver disease) may not be detected; bilirubin-derived bile pigments may mask the bilirubin reaction and produce atypical results; metabolites of drugs that color the urine at low pH (eg, phenazopyridine, ethoxazene) may give a false-positive reading; ascorbic acid concentrations of 25 mg/dl or more may produce false-negative results
Blood: sensitivity is decreased by high concentrations of protein, a high specific gravity, and by an ascorbic acid concentration of 5 mg/dl or more; the test is slightly more sensitive to free hemoglobin and myoglobin than to intact erythrocytes; certain oxidizing contaminants, such as sodium hypochlorite (bleach), and microbial peroxidases associated with urinary tract infections may produce false-positive results
Nitrite: non-nitrite-forming bacteria cannot be detected; the urine must be in the bladder for 4 h or more to allow adequate reduction of nitrate to nitrite to occur; sensitivity is decreased by a high specific gravity; an ascorbic acid concentration of 20 mg/dl or more may produce false-negative results with urine specimens containing small amounts of nitrite (0.1 mg/dl or less)
Urobilinogen: interfering substances, such as paraaminosalicylic acid, may cause false-positive results; drugs containing azo dyes (eg, phenazopyridine) may mask the color change; the test cannot be used to determine the total absence of urobilinogen or reliably detect porphobilinogen
Phenylketones: salicylates and large quantities of phenothiazine metabolites may mask the color change or give false-positive results; large amounts of bilirubin may produce a greenish color; other ketones may react if present in the large concentrations associated with severe ketosis; stale ammoniacal urine specimens may give false-negative results

URINE CHEMISTRY TESTS

BUMINTEST Reagent Tablets Ames

Intended use	Qualitative determination of urinary protein
Materials provided	Tablets containing sulfosalicylic acid
Additional materials required	Test tubes; dropper; water
Time for reading	Immediate; presence of turbidity is positive for protein
Performance characteristics	Sensitivity for albumin is 10 mg/dl
Limitations and precautions	X-ray contrast media and metabolites of tolbutamide may produce false-positive results; a highly buffered alkaline urine may yield a false-negative result

CHEMSTRIP Reagent Strips for Urinalysis

URINE CHEMISTRY TESTS

CHEMSTRIP 3 Boehringer Mannheim Diagnostics
Reagent strip for qualitative and semiquantitative determination of urinary pH, protein, and glucose

CHEMSTRIP 4 Boehringer Mannheim Diagnostics
Reagent strip for qualitative and semiquantitative determination of urinary pH, protein, blood, and nitrite

CHEMSTRIP 5 Boehringer Mannheim Diagnostics
Reagent strip for qualitative and semiquantitative determination of urinary pH, protein, glucose, ketones, and blood

CHEMSTRIP 5L Boehringer Mannheim Diagnostics
Reagent strip for qualitative and semiquantitative determination of urinary pH, protein, glucose, ketones, blood, and leukocytes

CHEMSTRIP 6 Boehringer Mannheim Diagnostics
Reagent strip for qualitative and semiquantitative determination of urinary pH, protein, glucose, ketones, bilirubin, and blood

CHEMSTRIP 6L Boehringer Mannheim Diagnostics
Reagent strip for qualitative and semiquantitative determination of urinary pH, protein, glucose, ketones, bilirubin, blood, and leukocytes

CHEMSTRIP 7 Boehringer Mannheim Diagnostics
Reagent strip for qualitative and semiquantitative determination of urinary pH, protein, glucose, ketones, bilirubin, blood, and urobilinogen

CHEMSTRIP 7L Boehringer Mannheim Diagnostics
Reagent strip for qualitative and semiquantitative determination of urinary pH, protein, glucose, ketones, bilirubin, blood, urobilinogen, and leukocytes

CHEMSTRIP 8 Boehringer Mannheim Diagnostics
Reagent strip for qualitative and semiquantitative determination of urinary pH, protein, glucose, ketones, bilirubin, blood, nitrite, and urobilinogen

CHEMSTRIP 9 Boehringer Mannheim Diagnostics
Reagent strip for qualitative and semiquantitative determination of urinary pH, protein, glucose, ketones, bilirubin, blood, nitrite, urobilinogen, and leukocytes

CHEMSTRIP GP Boehringer Mannheim Diagnostics
Reagent strip for qualitative and semiquantitative determination of urinary protein and glucose

CHEMSTRIP K Boehringer Mannheim Diagnostics
Reagent strip for qualitative and semiquantitative determination of urinary ketones

CHEMSTRIP L Boehringer Mannheim Diagnostics
Reagent strip for qualitative and semiquantitative determination of urinary leukocytes

CHEMSTRIP LN Boehringer Mannheim Diagnostics
Reagent strip for qualitative and semiquantitative determination of urinary nitrite and leukocytes

CHEMSTRIP uG Boehringer Mannheim Diagnostics
Reagent strip for qualitative and semiquantitative determination of urinary glucose

CHEMSTRIP uGK Boehringer Mannheim Diagnostics
Reagent strip for qualitative and semiquantitative determination of urinary glucose and ketones

Materials provided — Plastic strip with reagent-impregnated test area(s); color chart

Additional materials required — None

Time for reading — **pH:** any time up to 2 minutes after dipping
Protein: 30–60 seconds
Glucose: 60 seconds
Ketones: 60 seconds
Bilirubin: 30–60 seconds
Blood: 60 seconds
Nitrite: 30 seconds
Urobilinogen: 10–30 seconds
Leukocytes: 1–2 minutes

CHEMSTRIP Reagent Strips for Urinalysis ■ CLINITEST

Performance characteristics	**pH:** accurate to within 0.5 pH unit from pH 5 to pH 9 **Protein:** sensitivity is 6 mg/dl for albumin; test is less sensitive to globulins, hemoglobin, Bence-Jones protein, and mucoprotein **Glucose:** sensitivity is 40 mg/dl (60 mg/dl for Chemstrip uG and uGK) and is specific for glucose; test is unaffected by urinary pH, hemoglobin, or high concentrations of ketone bodies **Ketones:** sensitivity is 9 mg/dl for acetoacetic acid and 70 mg/dl for acetone; test will not react with β-hydroxybutyric acid **Bilirubin:** sensitivity is 0.5 mg/dl; test is unaffected by vitamin B_2 (up to 6 mg/dl), ascorbic acid (up to 60 mg/dl), or nitrite (up to 3 mg/dl) **Blood:** sensitivity is 5 red blood cells/μl or a hemoglobin content corresponding to 10 red blood cells/μl; test is unaffected by reasonable concentrations of ascorbic acid in the urine **Nitrite:** sensitivity is 0.05 mg/dl, which can detect up to 90% of bacterial urinary tract infections in early morning specimens **Urobilinogen:** sensitivity is 0.4 mg/dl **Leukocytes:** sensitivity is 97.2% and specificity 90.1%; test is unaffected by presence of erythrocytes (up to 10,000/μl) or common urinary bacteria
Limitations and precautions	**pH:** there are no known interferences with this test **Protein:** treatment with phenazopyridine, infusion of polyvinylpyrrolidone (blood substitutes), and residues of chlorhexidine or quaternary ammonium disinfectants may produce false-positive results **Glucose:** ascorbic acid concentrations of 40 mg/dl or more may produce falsely lowered glucose values with Chemstrip uG and uGK (the effect of ascorbic acid on glucose determinations is negligible with other Chemstrip products at glucose concentrations of 100 mg/dl or above, so that false-negative results should be rare, even at high concentrations of ascorbic acid); pigmentation (due, for example, to large amounts of bilirubin or nitrofurantoin) may mask the color reaction of Chemstrip uG and uGK; the presence of strongly oxidizing agents in the urine container may produce false-positive readings **Ketones:** phenylketones and phthalein compounds may produce a red-orange or red color change, which, however, can be readily distinguished from the color change produced by ketone bodies **Bilirubin:** large amounts of ascorbic acid in the urine can lower the sensitivity of the test (in doubtful cases, the test should be repeated on urine voided at least 10 h after the last ingestion of vitamin C); elevated urinary nitrite levels (due to urinary tract infections) may lower bilirubin values; medications that color the urine red or turn red in an acid medium (eg, phenazopyridine) may produce a false-positive reading; urobilinogen may affect the color reaction of bilirubin test pad, but not enough to give a positive result **Blood:** urine specimens preserved with formalin may give false-negative readings; urinary concentrations of nitrite exceeding 10 mg/dl (rare in urinary tract infections) delay the test reaction; residues of strongly oxidizing cleaning agents in the urine container can produce false-positive results; urine from menstruating women may test positively **Nitrite:** large amounts of ascorbic acid in the urine can lower the sensitivity of the test; medications that color the urine red or turn red in an acid medium (eg, phenazopyridine) may produce a false-positive reading **Urobilinogen:** treatment with phenazopyridine may cause a false-positive reaction; nitrite concentrations above 5 mg/dl and formalin concentrations exceeding 200 mg/dl may decrease the color change; the test cannot be used to determine the total absence of urobilinogen or reliably detect porphobilinogen **Leukocytes:** specimens that have been collected in containers cleaned with strong oxidizing agents or that have been preserved with formaldehyde should not be used; treatment with cephalexin, gentamicin, or nitrofurantoin, as well as high levels (50 mg/dl or more) of albumin in the urine, may interfere with test results

URINE CHEMISTRY TESTS

CLINITEST Reagent Tablets Ames

Intended use	Quantitative determination of urinary reducing sugars
Materials provided	Copper sulfate tablets, with sodium hydroxide, sodium carbonate, and citric acid
Additional materials required	Test tube; dropper; water
Time for reading	15 seconds
Performance characteristics	The 2-drop method can detect glucose at a level of 0.35 g/dl when testing urine with a specific gravity of 1.010–1.020 and no interfering substances and measures up to 5 g/dl; the 5-drop method can detect glucose at a level of 0.25 g/dl and measures up to 2 g/dl

CLINITEST ■ COLOSCREEN Self Test

Limitations and precautions	Test is not specific for glucose and will react with sufficient quantities of any reducing substance in urine, including other reducing sugars; large quantities of vitamin C, nalidixic acid, cephalosporins, and probenicid may cause false-positive results; the metabolites of some sulfonamides and methapyrilline compounds may interfere with the sensitivity of the 2-drop method at glucose levels below 0.5 g/dl; certain x-ray contrast media may produce false-negative results; a low specific gravity may produce slightly elevated results for glucose; high urinary protein concentrations extend boiling time, increase foaming, and make visual comparison with color chart difficult

URINE CHEMISTRY TESTS

ICTOTEST Reagent Tablets Ames

Intended use	Detection of urinary bilirubin
Materials provided	Tablets containing 2,4-dichlorobenzenediazonium tetrachlorozincate and sulfosalicylic acid; absorbent mats
Additional materials required	Dropper; water; paper towel
Time for reading	60 seconds; presence of blue or purple color on mat at end of this waiting period is positive for bilirubin
Performance characteristics	Sensitivity for urinary bilirubin is 0.05–0.1 mg/dl
Limitations and precautions	Metabolites of phenazopyridine and ethoxazene produce bright red-orange colors that may mask the reaction of small amounts of bilirubin; elevated urobilinogen levels do not mask the reaction of small amounts of bilirubin but produce atypical orange colors; large amounts of chlorpromazine may give a false-positive result

URINE CHEMISTRY TESTS

TES-TAPE Lilly

Intended use	Semiquantitative determination of urinary glucose
Materials provided	Roll of paper tape impregnated with glucose oxidase, horseradish peroxidase, and orthotolidine in plastic tape dispenser; color chart
Additional materials required	None
Time for reading	1–2 min (colors gradually change after 2 min)
Performance characteristics	Test is specific for glucose, with 96% accuracy; sensitivity is 0.5 g/dl
Limitations and precautions	Vitamin C in large doses, dipyrone, gentisic acid (a metabolite of aspirin), homogentisic acid (present in alkaptonuria), meralluride, levodopa, and methyldopa may produce false-negative results (patients who may have these substances in their urine should read the narrow band of color in the moist portion of the tape above the level to which it was dipped into the specimen); ingestion of more than 1.5 g of vitamin C in a single dose is likely to completely block the test 3–7 h afterward; contamination of the tape by glucose from other sources (eg, perspiration, tears, saliva) or a residue of chlorine from toilet bowl cleaners or disinfectants may produce false-positive results

FECAL OCCULT BLOOD TESTS

COLOSCREEN Self Test (CS-T) Helena Laboratories

Intended use	At-home detection of fecal occult blood
Materials provided	Three guaiacol-impregnated test pads with positive and negative control areas (sufficient materials for 3 stool samples)
Additional materials required	None
Time for reading	15–30 seconds (color reaction may fade after this time); presence of red-orange color in any test area is positive for occult blood

COLOSCREEN Self Test ■ FLEET DETECATEST

Performance characteristics	Sensitivity for hemoglobin is 2 mg/dl; according to the manufacturer, the performance of this test is not affected by iron compounds and compares favorably with that of guaiac paper slide tests, while yielding fewer false positives
Limitations and precautions	Medications that can cause GI irritation or occult bleeding (eg, aspirin, anti-inflammatory drugs, reserpine), vitamin C in doses exceeding 250 mg/day, rectal ointments or medications, laxatives containing mineral oil, and red or rare meat should be avoided for 2 days before and throughout test period; the test should not be done if patient is constipated, menstruating, or has bleeding hemorrhoids (diarrhea, however, does not affect test results); toilet bowl cleaners, disinfectants, and deodorizers containing sodium hypochlorite (bleach) or ammonia may cause false-positive results and should be removed from the toilet bowl and tank before testing

FECAL OCCULT BLOOD TESTS

EARLY DETECTOR Warner-Lambert

Intended use	At-home detection of fecal occult blood
Materials provided	Specimen pads with positive and negative control areas; developing solution and tablets (sufficient materials for 3 stool samples)
Additional materials required	None
Time for reading	30–60 seconds (color reaction may fade after 60 seconds); any trace of blue color on or around a stool specimen is positive for occult blood
Performance characteristics	Positive test results are obtained in 2–5% of patients
Limitations and precautions	Medications that can cause GI irritation or occult bleeding (eg, aspirin, anti-inflammatory drugs), vitamin C in doses exceeding 250 mg/day, iron supplements, rectal ointments, red or rare meat, turnips, and horseradish should be avoided for 2 days before and throughout test period; the test should not be done if patient is actively bleeding (eg, hemorrhoids, menstruation)

FECAL OCCULT BLOOD TESTS

EZ-DETECT Self-Care Systems

Intended use	At-home detection of fecal occult blood
Materials provided	Three film-coated, chemically impregnated test pads plus chemicals to check on the efficacy of the reagents in the pads (sufficient materials for 3 stool samples)
Additional materials required	None
Time for reading	2 min; appearance of blue cross on test pad is positive for occult blood
Performance characteristics	Sensitivity for hemoglobin is 2 mg/dl; according to the manufacturer, the test is 100% accurate at this level of hemoglobin and correlates 100% with the results of Hemoccult testing
Limitations and precautions	Medications that can cause GI irritation or occult bleeding (aspirin, indomethacin, phenylbutazone, and other nonsteroidal anti-inflammatory drugs, dipyridamole, and reserpine), cimetidine, vitamin C in doses exceeding 250 mg/day, rectal ointments or medications, red meats, turnips, horseradish, and melons should be avoided for 2 days before and throughout test period; the test should not be done if patient is constipated, menstruating, or has bleeding hemorrhoids; toilet bowl cleaners, disinfectants, and deodorizers should be removed from the toilet bowl and tank before testing

FECAL OCCULT BLOOD TESTS

FLEET DETECATEST Fleet

Intended use	At-home detection of fecal occult blood
Materials provided	Three guaiac-impregnated paper slides with positive control area; stool collection sticks; developing solution (sufficient materials for 3 stool samples)
Additional materials required	None

FLEET DETECATEST ■ HEMOCCULT

Time for reading	60 seconds (color reaction may fade after 4 min); any trace of blue color in test window is positive for occult blood
Performance characteristics	Information not provided in manufacturer's package labeling or patient instructions
Limitations and precautions	Medications that can cause GI irritation or occult bleeding (eg, aspirin, anti-inflammatory drugs, reserpine), vitamin C in doses exceeding 250 mg/day, rectal ointments or medications, red meat, turnips, and horseradish should be avoided for 2 days before and throughout test period; the test should not be done if bleeding hemorrhoids, diarrhea, or constipation is present or patient is menstruating

FECAL OCCULT BLOOD TESTS

HEMA-CHEK Slide Test Ames

Intended use	Detection of fecal occult blood
Materials provided	Guaiac-impregnated paper slides; specimen applicators; developing solution; bovine hemoglobin (5 mg/dl) control (sufficient materials for 100, 300, or 1,000 tests)
Additional materials required	None
Time for reading	Within 30 seconds; any trace of blue color appearing within 30 seconds after adding developer is positive for occult blood
Performance characteristics	Sensitivity is 4 ml of whole blood/100 g of feces, or 6 mg of hemoglobin/g of stool
Limitations and precautions	Medications that can cause GI bleeding (eg, aspirin, phenylbutazone), large doses of vitamin C, iron supplements, red meat, turnips, and horseradish should be avoided for 2 days before and throughout test period; the test should not be done if patient is actively bleeding due to menstruation, hemorrhoids, or other conditions

FECAL OCCULT BLOOD TESTS

HEMATEST Reagent Tablets Ames

Intended use	Detection of fecal occult blood
Materials provided	Test tablets; filter paper (sufficient materials for 100 tests)
Additional materials required	Applicator stick; glass slide or porcelain plate; distilled water; dropper
Time for reading	Within 2 min; any trace of blue color on the filter paper surrounding the tablet within the 2-min reading time is positive for occult blood
Performance characteristics	Sensitivity is 4 ml of whole blood/100 g of feces, or 6 mg of hemoglobin/g of stool
Limitations and precautions	Ingestion of raw or rare meat, dietary peroxidases (eg, horseradish), vitamin C in doses exceeding 500 mg/day, and iron preparations may give false test results and should be avoided prior to testing

FECAL OCCULT BLOOD TESTS

HEMOCCULT SmithKline Diagnostics

Intended use	At-home or in-office detection of fecal occult blood
Materials provided	**Hemoccult slides:** guaiac-impregnated paper slide with positive and negative control areas; specimen applicator; developing solution **Hemoccult II slides:** three guaiac-impregnated paper slides with positive and negative control areas; specimen applicators; developing solution (sufficient materials for 3 stool samples) **Hemoccult tape:** guaiac-impregnated paper tape in plastic tape dispenser; developing solution
Additional materials required	None
Time for reading	Within 60 seconds (color reaction may fade after 2–4 min); any trace of blue color on or around a stool specimen is positive for occult blood

HEMOCCULT ■ FIRST RESPONSE Ovulation Predictor Test

Performance characteristics	Sensitivity is 25 ml of blood or 10 mg of hemoglobin/g of stool; positive test results are obtained in 3–5% of patients, with a false-positive rate of 1–2% for patients receiving adequate preparation
Limitations and precautions	Medications that can cause GI irritation or occult bleeding (eg, aspirin, anti-inflammatory drugs, reserpine), vitamin C in doses exceeding 250 mg/day, iron supplements, rectal ointments, red meat, turnips, horseradish, and melons should be avoided for 2 days before and throughout test period; the test should not be done if hemorrhoids, diarrhea, or constipation is present or patient is menstruating

OVULATION TESTS

FIRST RESPONSE Ovulation Predictor Test Tambrands
Enzyme immunoassay for qualitative determination of the midcycle urinary hLH surge

Performance characteristics	**Specificity:** no false-positive results with 400 mIU/ml of hCG, 500 mIU/ml of FSH, or 50 ng/ml of prolactin
Materials	**Supplied materials:** 6 dipsticks with fins coated with monoclonal antibody to hLH; 6 vials with lyophilized conjugate of enzyme and monoclonal antibody to hLH; 6 vials with enzyme substrate solution; 6 tubes with chromogen solution; 6 disposable droppers; 6 disposable specimen cups; work station; color chart **Storage temperature:** 2–30°C **Additional materials required:** flowing tap water; positive and negative controls
Specimen	A woman should collect first morning specimens for up to 12 consecutive days, with the first day of the schedule based on the length of her cycle (see table below); if a woman's cycle varies monthly by more than a few days, she should determine the first day on the basis of her shortest cycle. If no positive result is seen after a total of 12 days, the test should be started 3 days earlier during the next cycle. Refrigerate specimens that cannot be assayed within 3 h and test them within 12 h.

Number of days in cycle	Day in cycle to begin test	Number of days in cycle	Day in cycle to begin test
18	2	30	14
19	3	31	15
20	4	32	16
21	5	33	17
22	6	34	18
23	7	35	19
24	8	36	20
25	9	37	21
26	10	38	22
27	11	39	23
28	12	40	24
29	13		

Procedure	Allow specimens and reagents to reach room temperature. Add specimen to the vial containing the conjugate, insert dipstick, and mix until powder is dissolved. Incubate mixture and dipstick at room temperature for 15 min; at the beginning of this 15-min period, add chromogen solution to the vial containing the enzyme substrate. After incubation, remove dipstick and wash fins thoroughly with a full-force stream of cold tap water for 15 s; then insert dipstick into the vial containing the substrate and chromogen, incubate at room temperature for 5 min, discard dipstick, and observe results. Match color of the test solution with one of 4 shades of color on the chart and record number (0, 1, 2, or 3) associated with the shade.
Results	**Positive reaction:** (a) shade number 3 or (b) shade number 2, when greater than that of a previous test **Negative reaction:** (a) shade number 0 or 1 or (b) shade number 2, when equal to that of a previous test
Interpretation	(1) Ovulation occurs 20–44 h (mean: 30 h) after onset of the hLH surge. (2) Conditions other than impending ovulation that may be associated with elevated levels of hLH include the following: (a) gonadotropin and clomiphene therapy, (b) ovarian failure, (c) polycystic ovary syndrome, (d) pituitary, hypothalamic, and gonadotropin-producing neoplasia, (e) hyperthyroidism, (f) renal failure, and (g) menopause and postmenopause; before making a diagnosis of ovulation, rule out all of these conditions. (3) Conditions that may be associated with low levels of hLH include the following: (a) use of estrogens, testosterone, danazol, or oral contraceptives, (b) pituitary failure, and (c) certain hypothalamic defects; consider these conditions when evaluating negative results. If these factors are ruled out, repeat the test the following month since approximately 25% of normally menstruating women do not ovulate during every cycle.

OVULATION TESTS

OVUSTICK Self-Test Monoclonal Antibodies

Enzyme immunoassay for qualitative determination of the midcycle urinary hLH surge

Performance characteristics — **Specificity:** false-positive results with elevated hCG levels (see "Interpretation," below); no false-positive results with FSH or TSH; no interference with biological products or commonly used medications
Accuracy: 96%

Materials — **Supplied materials:** 10 dipsticks coated with monoclonal antibody to hLH; 9 tubes with lyophilized conjugate of alkaline phosphatase and monoclonal antibody to hLH (test conjugate); 1 tube with lyophilized conjugate of alkaline phosphatase and monoclonal antibody to hLH *plus* human glycoprotein hormone equivalent to 30–40 mIU/ml of LH (control conjugate); 10 tubes with enzyme substrate and cofactor; 10 dropper vials with buffered saline; 10 disposable specimen cups and lids; dipstick holder; work station; color chart
Storage temperature: 2–30°C
Additional materials required: flowing tap water; negative control

Specimen — A woman should collect a specimen once daily for up to 9 consecutive days, with the first day of the schedule based on the length of her cycle (see table below); if a woman's cycle varies monthly by more than a few days, she should determine the first day on the basis of her shortest cycle. A baseline control test should be done 1 day before the start of urine testing. For optimal detection of the LH surge, the patient should collect a daily specimen between 10 AM and 8 PM; the specimen should be obtained at approximately the same time each day. A first morning specimen should not be used. Since unnecessary dilution of specimens may affect results, instruct the patient to keep her liquid intake fairly constant, urinate at least every 3 h during the day, and avoid excessive liquid intake shortly before the time of collection. Refrigerate specimens that cannot be assayed within 8 h and test them within 24 h; do not freeze them.

Number of days in cycle	Day in cycle to begin test	Number of days in cycle	Day in cycle to begin test
18	2	33	17
19	3	34	18
20	4	35	19
21	5	36	20
22	6	37	21
23	7	38	22
24	8	39	23
25	9	40	24
26–32	10		

Procedure — Allow reagents and specimens to reach room temperature. Reconstitute the test conjugate with supplied buffered saline; then partially fill empty dropper vial with urine and add 10 drops to the test conjugate. (To perform the baseline control test, substitute the control conjugate for the test conjugate and water for urine.) After drops have been added, insert the rounded end of the dipstick into the tube with conjugate, rapidly move the dipstick up and down for 1 min, and then incubate at room temperature for 30 min. After incubation, remove the dipstick and rinse each side for 2–3 sec in a gentle, steady stream of cold water; then insert dipstick in tube containing substrate, incubate at room temperature for 30 min, remove from tube, rinse as before, and observe results immediately. Match color of the dipstick with one of 5 shades of color on the chart and record the number (1, 2, 3, 4, or 5) associated with that shade; if color is deeper than that associated with number 5, identify color as 5+. The shade number for the baseline control should be 2, 3, or 4.

Results — **Positive reaction:** shade number higher than that of baseline control
Negative reaction: shade number equal to or lower than that of baseline control

Interpretation — (1) Ovulation occurs 20–44 h (mean: 30 h) after onset of the hLH surge. (2) Conditions other than impending ovulation that may be associated with elevated levels of hLH include the following: (a) gonadotropin and clomiphene therapy, (b) ovarian failure, (c) polycystic ovary syndrome, (d) pituitary, hypothalamic, and gonadotropin-producing neoplasia, (e) hyperthyroidism, (f) renal failure, and (g) menopause and postmenopause; before making a diagnosis of ovulation, rule out all of these conditions. (3) An elevated hCG level will produce a false-positive result; do not use this test in patients who are pregnant or have other conditions associated with an elevated hCG level. (4) Conditions that may be associated with low levels of hLH include the following: (a) use of estrogens, testosterone, danazol, or oral contraceptives, (b) pituitary failure, and (c) certain hypothalamic defects; consider these conditions when evaluating negative results. If these factors are ruled out, repeat the test the following month since approximately 25% of normally menstruating women do not ovulate during every cycle.

OVULATION TESTS

QTEST Ovulation Test   Clay Adams

Enzyme immunoassay for qualitative determination of the midcycle urinary hLH surge

Performance characteristics — **Specificity:** false-positive results with elevated hCG levels (see "Interpretation," below); no interference with 2,000 mg/dl of albumin or glucose, 1.5 mg/dl of pregnanediol, 1.4 mg/dl of estriol, 1 mg/dl of bilirubin or hemoglobin, or the following chemical compounds: acetaminophen, ascorbic acid, caffeine, ephedrine, gentisic acid, phenothiazines, phenylpropanolamine, and salicylic acid
Accuracy: 97%

Materials — **Supplied materials:** 5 dipsticks with test and reference pads coated with antibody to hLH; 5 tubes with lyophilized conjugate of alkaline phosphatase and monoclonal antibody to hLH; 5 tubes with enzyme substrate solution; 5 disposable droppers; 5 disposable specimen cups and lids; dipstick holder; work station
Storage temperature: < 30°C
Additional materials required: absorbent paper; flowing tap water; positive and negative controls; filter paper or centrifuge

Specimen — A woman with a regular menstrual cycle should collect specimens for a period of 5 consecutive days, with the first day of the schedule based on the length of her cycle (see table below); a woman with a variable cycle should collect specimens for a period of 10 consecutive days, beginning on day 9 or 10 of her cycle. For optimal detection of the LH surge, obtain a first morning specimen and either a midday or evening specimen daily; do not vary the timing of the second daily specimen during the test period (ie, midday on one day, evening on another). Instruct patients to avoid large variations in liquid intake since unnecessary dilution of specimens may affect results. Do not add any chemicals to the urine. If particulate matter is seen, filter or centrifuge specimen or allow precipitate to settle. Refrigerate specimens that cannot be assayed immediately and test them within 1 wk; do not freeze specimens.

Number of days in cycle	Day in cycle to begin test	Number of days in cycle	Day in cycle to begin test
23	8	29	12
24	9	30	13
25	9	31	14
26	10	32	15
27	11	33	16
28	12	34	16

Procedure — Allow specimens and reagents to reach room temperature. Add approximately 0.5 ml of specimen to the tube containing the conjugate, mix vigorously to dissolve the powder, and incubate mixture at room temperature for 5 min; next, insert dipstick pads into mixture, incubate at room temperature for 20 min, and then remove pads and wash them thoroughly with a full-force stream of cold tap water for at least 30 s, until gold-red color disappears. After shaking off excess water, insert pads into tube containing the enzyme substrate solution and incubate at room temperature for 10 min; then place pads between two absorbent paper towels, blot repeatedly until pads are completely dry, and observe results.

Results — **Positive reaction:** color on test pad significantly darker than that of pads from previous tests
Negative reaction: color on test pad not significantly darker than that of pads from previous tests

Interpretation — (1) Ovulation occurs 20–44 h (mean: 30 h) after onset of the hLH surge. (2) Conditions other than impending ovulation that may be associated with elevated levels of hLH include the following: (a) gonadotropin and clomiphene therapy, (b) ovarian failure, (c) polycystic ovary syndrome, (d) pituitary, hypothalamic, and gonadotropin-producing neoplasia, (e) hyperthyroidism, (f) renal failure, and (g) menopause and postmenopause; before making a diagnosis of ovulation, rule out all of these conditions. (3) An elevated hCG level will produce a false-positive result; do not use this test in patients who are pregnant or have other conditions associated with an elevated hCG level. (4) Conditions that may be associated with low levels of hLH include the following: (a) use of estrogens, testosterone, danazol, or oral contraceptives, (b) pituitary failure, and (c) certain hypothalamic defects; consider these conditions when evaluating negative results. If these factors are ruled out, repeat the test the following month since approximately 25% of normally menstruating women do not ovulate during every cycle. (5) The presence of a lighter color on the reference pad provides assurance of a proper procedure. Interference, misuse, or reagent failure may cause the reference pad to be the same color or slightly darker than the test pad; if such results are observed, repeat the test.

Precautions — Sodium azide in the reagents may react with lead and copper plumbing to form highly explosive metal azides; after disposing of reagents, flush drains with a large volume of water.

βhCG-ROCHE EIA

PREGNANCY TESTS

βhCG-ROCHE EIA Roche Diagnostics
Enzyme immunoassay for qualitative and quantitative determination of plasma and serum hCG

Performance characteristics	**Sensitivity:** 25 mIU/ml with qualitative assay; 3–200 mIU/ml (without dilution) with quantitative assay **Specificity:** 0.015% cross-reactivity with 20,000 mIU/ml LH, 0.03% cross-reactivity with 10,000 mIU/ml FSH, and 0.3% cross-reactivity with 1,000 mIU/ml TSH; interfering effects with sodium azide and metals; no interference with EDTA or heparin
Materials	**Supplied materials:** beads coated with monoclonal antibody to carboxyl-terminal amino acid sequence of hCG beta subunit; conjugate of peroxidase and monoclonal antibody to hCG beta subunit; o-phenylenediamine tablets; citrate buffer; 1N sulfuric acid; controls with 0, 10, 25, 50, 100, and 200 mIU/ml hCG; positive control; test tubes; test tube holder; plastic forceps **Storage temperature:** 2–8°C **Additional materials required:** water bath or incubator; metal-free deionized or distilled water; spectrophotometer; pipettes; water dispenser and aspirator or automated bead washer; vortex mixer; absorbent paper
Specimen	Do not test specimens with gross hemolysis. Serum or plasma with EDTA or heparin may be used; however, the dilution effects of anticoagulants should be considered. Specimens that cannot be tested immediately should be refrigerated for up to 48 h or frozen; do not add sodium azide. If the hCG concentration exceeds 200 mIU/ml, but not 20,000 mIU/ml, dilute the specimen 1:10 and 1:100 with the 0-mIU/ml control; if the concentration exceeds 20,000 mIU/ml, prepare a more dilute solution.
Procedure	Allow specimens and reagents to reach room temperature. For the qualitative assay, use the positive control and the 0- and 25-mIU/ml controls; for the quantitative assay, test the controls containing 0–200 mIU/ml. Add 20 ul of the specimen or control and then 250 ul of the conjugate to each test tube; after mixing, remove the basket of beads from the bottle, drain briefly on absorbent paper, and, with tweezers, add 1 bead to each test tube. Next, shake test tube holder, cover tubes, and incubate for 30 min at room temperature (for qualitative assay) or for 55–65 min at 36–38°C (for quantitative assay). Approximately 10 min before the end of the incubation period, dissolve 1 phenylenediamine tablet in 5 ml of citrate buffer. After incubation, aspirate liquid in the test tubes, wash tubes 3 times with 3–5 ml of distilled or deionized water, and then immediately add 250 ul of the phenylenediamine solution. Shake test tube holder and incubate tubes for 29–31 min at room temperature in the dark. After incubation, add 1 ml of sulfuric acid, mix well, and insert into a spectrophotometer set at 492 nm. To calculate the hCG level from results of the quantitative assay, plot an absorbance-concentration curve for the controls and then extrapolate concentration of the sample.
Results	**Positive reaction:** absorbance value more than 20% greater than that of the 25-mIU/ml control **Negative reaction:** absorbance value more than 20% smaller than that of the 25-mIU/ml control
Interpretation	(1) If the qualitative assay results in an absorbance value that is less than or up to 20% greater than that of the 25-mIU/ml control, repeat test after waiting at least 24 h. The hCG level doubles every 1.3–2 days during the early stages of pregnancy. (2) Conditions other than normal pregnancy that may be associated with detectable levels of hCG include the following: (a) molar and ectopic pregnancy, (b) trophoblastic disorders such as choriocarcinoma and hydatiform mole, (c) certain nontrophoblastic neoplasia and certain GI diseases, and (d) delivery or abortion within a few weeks before this test, and (e) injection of hCG at some time before this test; before making a diagnosis of normal pregnancy, rule out all of these conditions.
Precautions	(1) Serum controls are derived from human blood; handle these materials as if they were capable of transmitting hepatitis since negative results from current blood tests do not rule out this risk. (2) Wear gloves while handling reagents and wash hands thoroughly after the test; do not pipette reagents by mouth. Handle phenylenediamine tablets and sulfuric acid with particular care; if contact with skin or mucous membranes occurs, wash immediately with water. (3) Do not expose reagents or tablets to strong light or metal; do not allow phenylenediamine solution to come into contact with any oxidizing agents.

PREGNANCY TESTS

NEO-PLANOTEST DUOCLON Slide Organon Teknika

Latex agglutination slide test for qualitative determination of urinary hCG

Performance characteristics	**Sensitivity:** 500 mIU/ml; can usually detect pregnancy within 1 wk after the time of expected menses **Specificity:** no interference with abnormal amounts of protein, erythrocytes, or hemoglobin or with the following drugs: acetaminophen, aspirin, belladonna, butabarbital, caffeine, chlordiazepoxide, chlorpromazine, codeine, diazepam, diphenoxylate, flurazepam, glutethimide, hydrochlorothiazide, meprobamate, methadone, methyclothiazide, methylphenidate, meperidine, meprobamate, perphenazine, phenobarbital, propoxyphene, pyrrobutamine, and secobarbital **Accuracy:** 98.6%
Materials	**Supplied materials:** latex coated with monoclonal antibodies to hCG and the beta subunit of hCG; lyophilized positive and negative controls; calibrated droppers; pipette-stirrers; glass slide **Storage temperature:** 2–8°C (not necessary to warm to room temperature for test) **Additional materials required:** none
Specimen	For optimal detection of hCG, obtain a first morning specimen and test as soon as possible. Specimens that cannot be assayed immediately should be refrigerated for up to 2 days or frozen for up to 1 yr. It is generally not necessary to filter or centrifuge bloody or turbid specimens.
Procedure	Add 25 μl of the latex reagent and then 50 μl (1 drop) of urine to a circle on the slide; mix latex and urine and spread over entire test area; then gently rock slide for 3 min and observe results. If agglutination is seen before the end of the 3-min period, rocking may be stopped at that time.
Results	**Positive reaction:** any granular clumping (agglutination) within 3 min **Negative reaction:** smooth suspension (no agglutination) after 3 min
Interpretation	(1) This test does not detect hCG at levels below 500 mIU/ml; if results are negative, repeat test in 1–2 days since the hCG level doubles every 1.3–2 days during the early stages of pregnancy. (2) Conditions other than normal pregnancy that may be associated with detectable levels of hCG include the following: (a) molar and ectopic pregnancy, (b) trophoblastic disorders such as choriocarcinoma and hydatiform mole, (c) certain nontrophoblastic neoplasia, (d) delivery a few days to a week before this test, and (e) abortion or injection of hCG at some time before this test; before making a diagnosis of normal pregnancy, rule out all of these conditions. (3) Extremely high hCG levels may produce false-negative reactions; these levels may be seen with certain pregnancies and with disorders such as choriocarcinoma and hydatiform mole.

PREGNANCY TESTS

NEO-PREGNOSTICON DUOCLON Tube Organon Teknika

Hemagglutination tube test for qualitative determination of urinary hCG

Performance characteristics	**Sensitivity:** 75 mIU/ml; can usually detect pregnancy at or before the time of expected menses **Specificity:** no interference with abnormal amounts of protein, erythrocytes, or hemoglobin or with the following drugs: acetaminophen, aspirin, belladonna, butabarbital, chlordiazepoxide, chlorpromazine, codeine, diazepam, diphenoxylate, flurazepam, glutethimide, hydrochlorothiazide, meprobamate, methadone, methyclothiazide, methylphenidate, meperidine, meprobamate, perphenazine, phenobarbital, propoxyphene, pyrrobutamine, and secobarbital **Accuracy:** 99%
Materials	**Supplied materials:** tubes containing lyophilized erythrocytes coated with monoclonal antibodies to hCG and the beta subunit of hCG; lyophilized positive and negative controls; pipette-stirrers; dropper unit **Storage temperature:** 2–8°C **Additional materials required:** mirrored test tube holder; additive-free, sterile deionized or distilled water; Whatman No. 1 filter paper
Specimen	For optimal detection of hCG, obtain a first morning specimen and test as soon as possible. Specimens that cannot be assayed within 4 h should be refrigerated for up to 2 days or frozen for up to 1 yr; bear in mind that even with these storage conditions some hCG may be lost. Filter turbid urine; do not use specimens containing blood, blood components, or excessive bacteria.

NEO-PREGNOSTICON DUOCLON Tube ■ β-NEOCEPT 30

Procedure	Allow reagents and specimens to reach room temperature. Add 500 µl of deionized or distilled water to reagent tube; after gently shaking until reagent is suspended (about 15 s), add 50 µl of urine and again shake for approximately 15 s; allow mixture to incubate for 2 h, undisturbed by heat or vibration, and then observe results.
Results	**Positive reaction:** diffuse yellow-brown sediment (agglutination) after 2 h **Negative reaction:** clearly defined brown ring (no agglutination) within 2 h
Interpretation	(1) This test does not detect hCG at levels below 75 mIU/ml; if results are negative, repeat test in 1–2 days since the hCG level doubles every 1.3–2 days during the early stages of pregnancy. (2) Conditions other than normal pregnancy that may be associated with detectable levels of hCG include the following: (a) molar and ectopic pregnancy, (b) trophoblastic disorders such as choriocarcinoma and hydatiform mole, (c) certain nontrophoblastic neoplasia, (d) delivery a few days to a week before this test, (e) abortion within about a week before this test, and (f) injection of hCG at some time before this test; before making a diagnosis of normal pregnancy, rule out all of these conditions. (3) Extremely high hCG levels may produce false-negative reactions; these levels may be seen with certain pregnancies and with disorders such as choriocarcinoma and hydatiform mole.

PREGNANCY TESTS

β-NEOCEPT 30 Organon Teknika

Hemagglutination-inhibition tube test for qualitative and semiquantitative determination of urinary hCG

Performance characteristics	**Sensitivity:** 150 mIU/ml; can detect pregnancy at or before the time of expected menses **Specificity:** false-positive results with hLH levels seen in women over 40 yr of age (see "Specimen," below); rare interference with large amounts of protein or blood; no interference with a variety of drugs, including methadone and other psychotropic drugs **Accuracy:** 100%
Materials	**Supplied materials:** tubes containing lyophilized antibody to beta subunit of hCG and lyophilized erythrocytes covalently bonded to hCG; lyophilized positive and negative controls; Hepes buffer; serum albumin (for diluent); dropper unit; pipette-stirrers **Storage temperature:** 2–8°C **Additional materials required:** mirrored test tube holder; serological pipettes; distilled water; centrifuge or Whatman No. 4 filter paper
Specimen	For optimal qualitative detection of hCG, obtain a first morning specimen and test as soon as possible; specimens that cannot be assayed immediately should be refrigerated for up to 72 h or frozen for up to 6 mo. If urine is turbid or a precipitate is visible, centrifuge or filter. In women whose gonads have been injured or removed and in women over 40 yr of age, pituitary gonadotropin levels may be sufficiently high to produce a false-positive effect; specimens from such women should be diluted 1:1 with distilled water before the test. No interference has been seen with use of a variety of drugs, including methadone and psychotropic drugs; nevertheless, since these drugs as well as others reportedly interfere with pregnancy tests, obtain specimens when a drug is not being used, if possible. For semiquantitative analysis, collect urine over a 24-h period, beginning with the second morning specimen; if a 24-h collection is not feasible, the first morning specimen may be assayed. To prepare serial dilutions of urine, use a solution consisting of distilled water and albumin.
Procedure	Add 150 µl of diluted buffer and then 50 µl of urine to the reagent tube; after shaking for 1 min, allow mixture to incubate at room temperature for 30 min, undisturbed by vibration or heat, and then observe results. For semiquantitative analysis, first test dilutions of 1:10, 1:100, and 1:500 and then serial dilutions within the appropriate range (eg, dilutions of 1:2–1:9 if positive with undiluted sample and negative with 1:10 sample); to estimate the concentration in IU/ml, multiply the highest dilution showing positive results by 0.15.
Results	**Positive reaction:** clearcut red-brown ring (no agglutination) within 60 min **Negative reaction:** diffuse yellow-brown sediment agglutination), with no ring, after 30 min
Interpretation	(1) This test does not detect hCG at levels below 150 mIU/ml; if results are negative, repeat test in a few days since the hCG level doubles every 1.3–2 days during the early stages of pregnancy. (2) An ill-defined, jagged, or incomplete ring may appear if tubes are jarred; repeat test if these results are seen. (3) Conditions other than normal pregnancy that may be associated with detectable levels of hCG include the following: (a) molar and ectopic pregnancy, (b) trophoblastic disorders such as choriocarcinoma and hydatiform mole, (c) certain nontrophoblastic neoplasia, (d) delivery a few days to a week before this test, (e) abortion within about a week before this test, and (f) injection of hCG at some time before this test; before making a diagnosis of normal pregnancy, rule out all of these conditions.

PREGNANCY TESTS

NIMBUS NMS Pharmaceuticals
Enzyme immunoassay for qualitative determination of urinary and serum hCG

Performance characteristics
- **Sensitivity:** 50 mIU/ml with two 5-min incubation periods; 25 mIU/ml with two 15-min incubation periods
- **Specificity:** no false-positive results with 600 mIU/ml of hLH, 1,000 mIU/ml of hFSH, or 1,000 μIU/ml of hTSH; no interference with abnormal levels of protein, bilirubin, hemoglobin, or ketones; and no interference with the following chemical compounds: acetaminophen, ascorbic acid, aspirin, atropine, caffeine, gentisic acid, methadone, and phenothiazines
- **Accuracy:** 99.2%

Materials
- **Supplied materials:** tubes coated with monoclonal antibody to the alpha subunit of hCG; conjugate of peroxidase and monoclonal antibody to the beta subunit of hCG; urea peroxide (enzyme sybstrate); chromogen; controls with 0, 25, and 50 mIU/ml of hCG; disposable pipettes
- **Storage temperature:** 2–8°C
- **Additional materials required:** absorbent paper; centrifuge

Specimen
For optimal detection of urinary hCG, obtain a first morning specimen and test as soon as possible; do not add a preservative. Centrifuge any urine specimen that appears grossly turbid or has particulate matter. To obtain a serum specimen, collect blood (without adding anticoagulants), allow it to clot, centrifuge, and then test as soon as possible. Do not use a urine or serum specimen that shows gross contamination or hemolysis; serum must also be free of cellular matter and other physical grossness. Urine or serum specimens that cannot be assayed immediately should be refrigerated for up to 24 h; serum specimens may also be frozen.

Procedure
Allow reagents and specimens to reach room temperature. Add 2 drops of the specimen or control to the antibody-coated tubes, swirl tubes briefly to mix, add 2 drops of the conjugate, and again swirl tubes; incubate solution at room temperature for 5 min (if 50-mIU/ml sensitivity is desired) or 15 min (if 25-mIU/ml sensitivity is desired). Next, wash tubes at least 6 times with tap water, add 2 drops of chromogen and then 2 drops of peroxide, and swirl briefly; incubate tubes at room temperature for 5 min (if 50-mIU/ml sensitivity is desired) or 15 min (if 25-mIU/ml sensitivity is desired) and observe results. If the sample contains a high concentration of hCG, do the following before adding the conjugate: incubate the coated tubes and specimen for 5 min at room temperature and then wash tubes once with tap water.

Results
- **Positive reaction:** blue color equal to or deeper than that of the 50- or 25-mIU/ml control
- **Negative reaction:** no color or slightly bluish tinge

Interpretation
(1) If the results are negative or the intensity of color is less than that of the 25- or 50-mIU/ml control, repeat the test in 48–72 h since hCG levels double every 1.3–2 days during the early stages of pregnancy. Bear in mind that *serum* with a bluish tinge less intense than that of the positive controls may also be due to a high rheumatoid factor titer. (2) Conditions other than normal pregnancy that may be associated with detectable levels of hCG include the following: (a) molar and ectopic pregnancy, (b) trophoblastic disorders such as choriocarcinoma and hydatiform mole, (c) certain nontrophoblastic neoplasia, (d) delivery or abortion within a few weeks before this test, and (e) injection of hCG at some time before this test; before making a diagnosis of normal pregnancy, rule out all of these conditions. (3) Extremely high hCG levels, such as those seen in the middle of the first trimester, can cause false-negative results; to avoid this effect, see "Procedure."

Precautions
(1) Serum controls are derived from human blood; handle these materials as if they were capable of transmitting hepatitis or AIDS since negative results from current blood tests do not rule out these risks. (2) Sodium azide in the reagents may react with lead and copper plumbing to form highly explosive metal azides; after disposing of reagents, flush drains with a large volume of water.

PREGNANCY TESTS

ORTHO β-hCG Ortho Diagnostic Systems
Latex agglutination-inhibition slide test for qualitative and semiquantitative determination of urinary hCG

Performance characteristics
- **Sensitivity:** 800 mIU/ml
- **Specificity:** no false-positive results with 10 times the normal peak level of LH or 100 times the normal peak level of FSH; no interference with methadone, urine preservatives, 5 g/dl of albumin, or 20 g/dl of serum
- **Accuracy:** 98.6%

Materials
- **Supplied materials:** hCG covalently bonded to latex; monoclonal antibodies to different portions of the beta subunit of hCG; lyophilized positive and negative controls; disposable pipettes; rubber bulbs for pipettes; wooden mixing sticks; black glass slide
- **Storage temperature:** 2–8°C
- **Additional materials required:** pipette; 0.9% saline; centrifuge

ORTHO β-hCG ■ PREGNACLONE Slide

Specimen	For optimal qualitative detection of hCG, obtain a first morning specimen and test as soon as possible. If the assay cannot be done within 12 h, add 0.01% thimerosal or 0.1% sodium azide to the specimen and refrigerate it for up to 1 wk or freeze it for up to 1 yr. Centrifuge urine that is turbid or bloody; do not use specimens with excessive bacteria. For semiquantitative analysis, collect specimens over a period of 24 h; during this period, pool specimens in a refrigerated container to which 0.01% thimerosal or 0.1% sodium azide has been added. To prepare serial dilutions of urine, use 0.9% saline.
Procedure	Allow reagents and specimens to reach room temperature. Place 1 drop of urine within a circle on the slide; add 1 drop of antibody to the drop of urine, mix, spread over the entire area of the circle, and rotate slide for 30 s. Then add 1 drop of latex to this mixture, rotate slide for 2 min, and observe results. For semiquantitative analysis, test serial two-fold dilutions (ie, 1:2, 1:4, 1:8, etc); to estimate the concentration in IU/ml, multiply the highest dilution showing positive results by 0.8.
Results	**Positive reaction:** smooth milky suspension (no agglutination) after 2 min **Negative reaction:** clumping (agglutination) within 2 min
Interpretation	(1) This test does not detect hCG at levels below 800 mIU/ml; repeat test in 7 days if results are negative or in a few days if results are questionable. The hCG level doubles every 1.3–2 days during the early stages of pregnancy. (2) Conditions other than normal pregnancy that may be associated with detectable levels of hCG include the following: (a) molar and ectopic pregnancy, (b) trophoblastic disorders such as choriocarcinoma and hydatiform mole, (c) certain nontrophoblastic neoplasia, and (d) delivery, abortion, or injection of hCG at some time before this test; before making a diagnosis of normal pregnancy, rule out all of these conditions.
Precautions	Sodium azide in the reagents may react with lead and copper plumbing to form highly explosive metal azides; dispose of reagents by flushing with a large volume of water

PREGNANCY TESTS

PREGNACLONE Slide Fisher Scientific

Latex agglutination-inhibition slide test for qualitative determination of urinary hCG

Performance characteristics	**Sensitivity:** 300–500 mIU/ml; can detect pregnancy within the first week after the time of expected menses **Specificity:** false-positive results with very high levels of hLH; no interference with up to 2 g/dl of albumin **Accuracy:** 98.8%
Materials	**Supplied materials:** hCG-coated latex; monoclonal antibody to beta subunit of hCG; positive and negative controls; disposable pipettes; applicator sticks; glass slide **Storage temperature:** 2–8°C **Additional materials required:** centrifuge
Specimen	For optimal detection of hCG, obtain a first morning specimen and test as soon as possible. Specimens that cannot be assayed immediately should be refrigerated for up to 24 h or frozen. Centrifuge specimens that are unusually cloudy or have a precipitate. Whenever possible, do not use specimens obtained during drug therapy.
Procedure	Allow reagents and specimens to reach room temperature. Add 1 drop of urine and then 1 drop of antibody to a circle on the slide; mix, spread over entire circle, and rotate slide for 1 min; add 1 drop of hCG-coated latex reagent, mix, and spread over entire circle; rotate slide for 1.5 min and then immediately observe results. Do not examine slide with a light source that may heat the reagents.
Results	**Positive reaction:** smooth, milky appearance (no agglutination) after 1.5 min **Negative reaction:** any agglutination within 1.5 min
Interpretation	(1) This test does not detect hCG at levels below 300 mIU/ml; if results are negative, repeat test at a later date since the hCG level doubles every 1.3–2 days during the early stages of pregnancy. (2) Conditions other than normal pregnancy that may be associated with detectable levels of hCG include the following: (a) molar and ectopic pregnancy, (b) trophoblastic disorders such as choriocarcinoma and hydatiform mole, (c) certain nontrophoblastic neoplasia, and (d) delivery, abortion, or injection of hCG at some time before this test; before making a diagnosis of normal pregnancy, rule out all of these conditions. (3) Very high levels of hLH ($>$ 2 IU/ml) may cause false-positive results; exercise caution when interpreting results of samples obtained from menopausal women.
Precautions	Sodium azide in the reagents may react with lead and copper plumbing to form highly explosive metal azides; dispose of reagents by flushing with a large volume of water

PREGNANCY TESTS

PREGNACLONE Tube Fisher Scientific

Latex agglutination-inhibition tube test for qualitative and semiquantitative determination of urinary hCG

Performance characteristics	**Sensitivity:** 200–300 mIU/ml; can detect pregnancy at the time of expected menses or within 1 wk afterwards **Specificity:** false-positive results with hLH levels seen at or after menopause (see "Specimen," below); interfering effects with blood or excessive bacteria; no interference with 50 mg/dl of albumin **Accuracy:** 99.6%
Materials	**Supplied materials:** hCG-coated latex; tubes containing monoclonal antibody to beta subunit of hCG; positive and negative controls **Storage temperature:** 2–8°C (not necessary to warm reagents to room temperature for test) **Additional materials required:** heating block; pipettes; test tube holder; centrifuge or filter paper
Specimen	For optimal qualitative detection of hCG, obtain a first morning specimen and test as soon as possible; specimens that cannot be assayed immediately should be refrigerated for up to 24 h or frozen. If urine is unusually cloudy or a precipitate is visible, centrifuge or filter. Whenever possible, do not use specimens obtained during drug therapy. To avoid false-positive results, do not test urine containing blood or excessive bacteria. In menopausal and postmenopausal women, pituitary gonadotropin levels may be sufficiently high to produce a false-positive effect; if samples from such women produce positive results, repeat test using specimens diluted 1:2 with the negative control or normal urine. For semiquantitative analysis, collect urine over a 24-h period; do not add a preservative to the pooled specimen. Prepare serial dilutions of the specimen with the negative control or normal urine.
Procedure	Add 1 ml of urine and then 1 drop of latex to the tube containing antibody; mix contents and then place tubes in a heating block set at 37°C; after 90 min, observe results. For semiquantitative analysis, test serial two-fold dilutions (ie, 1:2, 1:4, 1:8, etc); to estimate the concentration in IU/ml, multiply the highest dilution showing positive results by 0.25.
Results	**Positive reaction:** smooth suspension (no agglutination) after 90 min **Negative reaction:** any clumping (agglutination) after 90 min
Interpretation	(1) This test does not detect hCG at levels below 200 mIU/ml; repeat test in 1 wk if results are negative or in at least 48 h if results are equivocal or questionable. The hCG level doubles every 1.3–2 days during the early stages of pregnancy. (2) Conditions other than normal pregnancy that may be associated with detectable levels of hCG include the following: (a) molar and ectopic pregnancy, (b) trophoblastic disorders such as choriocarcinoma and hydatiform mole, (c) certain nontrophoblastic neoplasia, (d) delivery or abortion within a week or more before this test, and (e) injection of hCG at some time before this test; before making a diagnosis of normal pregnancy, rule out all of these conditions. (3) False-positive results may occur with specimens obtained from menopausal and postmenopausal women (see "Specimen," above).
Precautions	Sodium azide in the reagents may react with lead or copper plumbing to form highly explosive metal azides; dispose of reagents by flushing with a large volume of water.

PREGNANCY TESTS

PREGNAZYME Wampole Laboratories

Enzyme immunoassay for qualitative determination of urinary and serum hCG

Performance characteristics	**Sensitivity:** 25 mIU/ml with 10-min incubation periods (25-mIU/ml test) and 100 mIU/ml with 5-min incubation periods (100-mIU/ml test); pregnancy can be detected as early as 7–10 days after conception with the 25-mIU/ml test and as early as the time of expected menses with the 100-mIU/ml test **Specificity:** no false-positive results with 1,000 mIU/ml of LH or FSH; interfering effects with hemolysis or lipemia in serum and with excessive bacteria in urine and serum; no interference with acetaminophen, amitriptyline, amphetamine, barbiturates, cannabinoids, cimetidine, cocaine, digoxin, flurazepam, furosemide, haloperidol, imipramine, methadone, opiates, phenytoin, propranolol, or thioridazine **Accuracy:** 99–100%
Materials	**Supplied materials:** tubes coated with monoclonal and polyclonal antibody to hCG and its beta subunit; conjugate of alkaline phosphatase and monoclonal antibody to beta subunit of hCG; phenolphthalein monophosphate (enzyme substrate); controls with 0, 25, and 100 mIU/ml hCG; concentrated saline; reagent droppers; test tube holder; disposable pipettes **Storage temperature:** 2–8°C **Additional materials required:** plastic wash bottle; additive-free distilled or deionized water; absorbent paper; centrifuge

PREGNAZYME ■ PREGNOLISA

Specimen — For optimal detection of urinary hCG, obtain a first morning specimen and test as soon as possible. If urine is turbid or a precipitate is visible, centrifuge or allow particulate matter to settle; do not use urine specimens containing excessive bacteria. For optimal detection of serum hCG, collect blood (without adding anticoagulants), allow it to clot for 20–30 min, centrifuge, and then test as soon as possible. Do not use blood specimens that are contaminated, hemolyzed, turbid, or lipemic. Urine or serum specimens that cannot be assayed immediately should be refrigerated or kept reasonably cool ($< 26°C$) for up to 24 h or frozen. If an extremely high hCG level is suspected, dilute the specimen 1:10 with diluted saline.

Procedure — Allow reagents and specimens to reach room temperature. Add 2 drops of specimen or control and then 2 drops of the conjugate to the bottom of the antibody-coated tubes; after mixing, incubate at room temperature for 5 min (if 100-mIU/ml sensitivity is desired) or for 10 min (if 25-mIU/ml sensitivity is desired). Then wash tubes 4 times with diluted saline, add 0.5 ml of phenolphthalein, mix, incubate at room temperature (as above), and observe results. For spectrophotometric evaluation, insert sample into a spectrophotometer set at 550 nm immediately after the second incubation.

Results — **Positive reaction:** pink or orange color equal to or darker than that of the 25- or 100-mIU/ml control
Negative reaction: yellow or pink color lighter than that of the 25- or 100-mIU/ml control

Interpretation — (1) If results are negative, repeat test after at least 48 h since the hCG level doubles every 1.3–2 days during the early stages of pregnancy. (2) Conditions other than normal pregnancy that may be associated with detectable levels of hCG include the following: (a) molar and ectopic pregnancy, (b) trophoblastic disorders such as choriocarcinoma and hydatiform mole, (c) certain nontrophoblastic neoplasia, (d) delivery or abortion within a few weeks before this test, and (e) injection of hCG at some time before this test; before making a diagnosis of normal pregnancy, rule out all of these conditions. (3) Extremely high hCG levels may attenuate the color reaction or cause false-negative results; these levels may occur with certain pregnancies and with disorders such as choriocarcinoma and hydatiform mole. To avoid this effect, see "Specimen," above. (4) Light positive results may indicate impending spontaneous abortion and therefore necessitate a subsequent test to assure that the hCG level is increasing and pregnancy is progressing normally. (5) Ectopic pregnancy may also be associated with a very low hCG level and therefore, when suspected, may be further evaluated with a quantitative assay.

Precautions — Sodium azide in the reagents may react with lead and copper plumbing to form highly explosive metal azides; dispose of reagents by flushing with a large volume of water

PREGNANCY TESTS

PREGNOLISA Organon Teknika

Enzyme immunoassay for qualitative determination of urinary hCG and qualitative and quantitative determination of plasma and serum hCG

Performance characteristics — **Sensitivity:** 50 mIU/ml with urine assay; 25 mIU/ml with qualitative serum or plasma assay; and 1.5–200 mIU/ml (without dilution) with quantitative serum or plasma assay
Specificity: 0.05% cross-reactivity with 2,000 mIU/ml hLH, 0.07% cross-reactivity with 2,000 mIU/ml hFSH, and 0.39% cross-reactivity with 2,000 µIU/ml hTSH; no interference with plasma or serum containing EDTA or 800 mg/dl hemoglobin; no interference with urine containing a variety of drugs, including methadone and other psychotropic drugs
Accuracy: 97–99.6%

Materials — **Supplied materials:** tubes coated with monoclonal antibody to hCG; lyophilized conjugate of peroxidase and monoclonal antibody to hCG; hydrogen peroxide (enzyme substrate); tetramethylbenzidine (chromogen); serum controls[1] with 0, 25, 50, 100, 200 mIU/ml hCG; urine controls[1] with 0 and 50 mIU/ml hCG; positive serum and urine controls[1]; 1N sulfuric acid[2]; droppers; calibrated tube; pipette-stirrers
Storage temperature: 2–8°C
Additional materials required: deionized water; Whatman No. 4 filter paper or centrifuge; spectrophotometer; pipettes

Specimen — For optimal detection of urinary hCG, obtain a first morning specimen and test as soon as possible; if sediment appears, centrifuge, filter, or allow it to settle. Collect serum or plasma by venipuncture. Specimens that cannot be tested immediately should be refrigerated for up to 48 h or frozen; do not add preservatives.

PREGNOLISA ■ PREGNOSIS

Procedure — Allow specimens and reagents to reach room temperature. For the qualitative assay, use the positive and 0-mIU/ml controls plus either the 50-mIU/ml control (for urine tests) or the 25-mIU/ml control (for serum or plasma tests); for the quantitative assay, use the controls containing 0–200 mIU/ml. Add 200 ul of reconstituted conjugate and then 100 ul of the specimen or control to the bottom of each antibody-coated tube; mix and then incubate at room temperature for 15 min (qualitative assay) or 30 min (quantitative assay). During incubation period, add 100 ul (6 drops) of chromogen to each 10 ml of substrate. After incubation, wash each tube 4 times with deionized water, add 500 ul of the chromogen-substrate mixture, incubate at room temperature for 15 min (qualitative assay) or 30 min (quantitative assay), and observe results. For spectrophotometric evaluation, add 1 ml of sulfuric acid to each tube, mix, and then insert tube into a spectrophotometer set at 450–460 nm. To calculate the hCG level from results of the quantitative assay, plot an absorbance-concentration curve for the controls and then extrapolate the concentration of the sample.

Results — **Positive reaction:** blue color equal to or more intense than that of the 25-mIU/ml serum control or 50-mIU/ml urine control
Negative reaction: no color

Interpretation — (1) If the qualitative assay results in no color or an intensity of color (or absorbance value) less than that of the 25-mIU/ml serum control or 50-mIU/ml urine control, repeat test after waiting at least 48 h. The hCG level doubles every 1.3–2 days during the early stages of pregnancy. (2) Conditions other than normal pregnancy that may be associated with detectable levels of hCG include the following: (a) molar and ectopic pregnancy, (b) trophoblastic disorders such as choriocarcinoma and hydatiform mole, (c) certain nontrophoblastic neoplasia, and (d) delivery or abortion within a few weeks before this test, and (e) injection of hCG at some time before this test; before making a diagnosis of normal pregnancy, rule out all of these conditions.

Precautions — Serum controls are derived from human blood; handle these materials as if they were capable of transmitting hepatitis since negative results from current blood tests do not rule out this risk.

[1] Controls are lyophilized; serum controls with 50–200 mIU/ml (ie, those for quantitative assay) and all urine controls are supplied separately
[2] Stopping solution for quantitative assay; supplied separately

PREGNANCY TESTS

PREGNOSIS Roche Diagnostics

Latex agglutination-inhibition slide test for qualitative and semiquantitative determination of urinary hCG

Performance characteristics — **Sensitivity:** 1,500–2,500 mIU/ml
Specificity: false-positive results with LH levels seen after menopause or hysterectomy or with 100 mg/dl of protein; no interference with hemoglobin
Accuracy: 95.4–100%

Materials — **Supplied materials:** hCG chemically bonded to latex; antibody to hCG; reagent droppers; disposable pipettes; applicator sticks; black glass slide
Storage temperature: 2–8°C
Additional materials required: positive and negative controls

Specimen — For optimal qualitative detection of hCG, obtain a first morning specimen; do not add a preservative. Test as soon as possible; if the assay cannot be done within 12 h, refrigerate specimen for up to 1 wk or, preferably, freeze it for up to 1 yr. Whenever possible, do not use specimens obtained during drug therapy. For semiquantitative analysis, collect specimens over a period of 24 h without adding a preservative; prepare serial dilutions of the specimen with normal urine.

Procedure — Allow reagents and specimens to reach room temperature. Place 1 drop of urine within a circle on the slide; add 1 drop of antibody, mix with urine, and gently rotate slide for 30 s. Then add 1 drop of latex, mix, and spread over the entire circle; rotate slide for 2 min and observe results. For semiquantitative analysis, test serial two-fold dilutions (ie, 1:2, 1:4, 1:8, etc); to estimate the concentration in IU/ml, multiply the highest dilution showing positive results by 2.

Results — **Positive reaction:** smooth milky suspension (no agglutination) after 2 min
Negative reaction: clumping (agglutination) within 2 min

Interpretation — (1) This test does not detect hCG at levels below 1,500 mIU/ml; if results are negative, repeat test in 1–2 wk since the hCG level doubles every 1.3–2 days during the early stages of pregnancy. (2) Repeat test whenever results are doubtful. (3) Conditions other than normal pregnancy that may be associated with detectable levels of hCG include the following: (a) molar and ectopic pregnancy, (b) trophoblastic disorders such as choriocarcinoma and hydatiform mole, (c) certain nontrophoblastic neoplasia, and (d) delivery, abortion, or injection of hCG at some time before this test; before making a diagnosis of normal pregnancy, rule out all of these conditions. (4) In postmenopausal women and those who have undergone hysterectomy, hLH levels may be sufficiently high to produce false-positive results.

PREGNANCY TESTS

Precautions	Sodium azide in the antibody reagent may react with lead and copper plumbing to form highly explosive metal azides; dispose of reagent by flushing with a large volume of water.

PREGNOSPIA Organon Teknika

Gold sol agglutination tube test for qualitative determination of urinary hCG

Performance characteristics	**Sensitivity:** 150 mIU/ml; can usually detect pregnancy at or before the time of expected menses **Specificity:** no false-positive results with LH levels higher than those associated with the midcycle surge; interference with abnormal amounts of protein, erythrocytes, or hemoglobin (in rare cases); no interference with a variety of drugs, including methadone and other psychotropic drugs **Accuracy:** 99%
Materials	**Supplied materials:** lyophilized gold sol particles coated with monoclonal antibodies against hCG and the beta subunit of hCG; lyophilized positive and negative controls; buffer; pipette-stirrers; dropper unit **Storage temperature:** 2–8°C **Additional materials required:** centrifuge or Whatman No. 4 filter paper
Specimen	For optimal detection of hCG, obtain a first morning specimen and test as soon as possible. Specimens that cannot be assayed immediately should be refrigerated for up to 2 days or frozen for up to 1 yr. If urine is turbid or has visible sediment, filter or centrifuge. No interference has been seen with use of a variety of drugs; nevertheless, since drugs reportedly interfere with pregnancy tests, obtain specimens when a drug is not being used, if possible.
Procedure	Allow reagents and specimens to reach room temperature. Add 400 ul of buffer to each vial containing lyophilized gold sol; after shaking vial until sol is suspended (about 15 s), add 100 µl (2 drops) of urine and mix for approximately 30 s; allow mixture to incubate for 30 min and then observe results. A positive reaction may be apparent in less than 30 min. Place vial anywhere during incubation since the test is not affected by vibration or light.
Results	**Positive reaction:** distinct change in color within 30 min **Negative reaction:** no change in color after 30 min
Interpretation	(1) This test does not detect hCG at levels below 150 mIU/ml; if results are negative, repeat test in a few days since the hCG level doubles every 1.3–2 days during the early stages of pregnancy. (2) Conditions other than normal pregnancy that may be associated with detectable levels of hCG include the following: (a) molar and ectopic pregnancy, (b) trophoblastic disorders such as choriocarcinoma and hydatiform mole, (c) certain nontrophoblastic neoplasia, (d) delivery a few days to a week before this test, (e) abortion within about a week before this test, and (f) injection of hCG at some time before this test; before making a diagnosis of normal pregnancy, rule out all of these conditions. (3) Extremely high hCG levels may produce false-negative reactions; these levels may be seen with certain pregnancies and with disorders such as choriocarcinoma and hydatiform mole.

PREGNANCY TESTS

PREGNOSTICON DRI-DOT Organon Teknika

Latex agglutination-inhibition slide test for the qualitative determination of urinary hCG

Performance characteristics	**Sensitivity:** 1,000–2,000 mIU/ml; can usually detect pregnancy 12 days after the time of expected menses and, in some cases, may detect pregnancy as early as 4 days after the time of expected menses **Specificity:** false-positive results with pituitary gonadotropin levels seen in women whose gonads have been injured or removed and in women over 40 yr of age (see "Specimen," below); interfering effects with large amounts of blood or methadone doses exceeding 100 mg/day; possible interfering effects with presence of protein, hemoglobin, or distilled water containing additives **Accuracy:** 97%

PREGNOSTICON DRI-DOT ■ PREGNOSTICON Slide

Materials	**Supplied materials:** antibody to hCG and hCG-coated latex, dried as individual dots on a slide; lyophilized positive and negative controls; pipette-stirrers; dropper bottle; rocker (supplied separately) **Storage temperature:** < 45°C **Additional materials required:** centrifuge
Specimen	For optimal detection of hCG, obtain a first morning specimen and test as soon as possible. Specimens that cannot be assayed immediately should be refrigerated for up to 72 h or frozen for up to 6 mo. Centrifuge excessively turbid urine; do not use bloody specimens. In women whose gonads have been injured or removed and in women over 40 yr of age, pituitary gonadotropin levels may be sufficiently high to produce a false-positive effect; specimens from such women should be diluted 1:1 with additive-free distilled water before the test. Whenever possible, do not use specimens obtained during drug therapy.
Procedure	Place 1 drop of water (tap water or additive-free distilled water) on the green dot containing hCG-coated latex and 1 drop of urine on the colorless dot containing antibody; mix urine and antibody and rock slide for 30 s; then mix latex with urine and antibody, spread over the entire area of the circle, gently rock slide for 2 min, and observe results
Results	**Positive reaction:** green homogenous suspension (no agglutination) after 2 min **Negative reaction:** granular clumping (agglutination) within 2 min
Interpretation	(1) This test does not provide definitive results at hCG levels below 1–2 IU/ml; if no clumping or slight coarseness is seen, repeat test 1–2 wk later (when hCG level will presumably be higher) or use a more sensitive test. (2) Conditions other than normal pregnancy that may be associated with detectable levels of hCG include the following: (a) molar and ectopic pregnancy, (b) trophoblastic disorders such as choriocarcinoma and hydatiform mole, (c) certain nontrophoblastic neoplasia, (d) delivery a few days to a week before this test, (e) abortion within about a week before this test, and (f) injection of hCG at some time before this test; before making a diagnosis of normal pregnancy, rule out all of these conditions. (3) Methadone doses exceeding 100 mg/day can produce a false-positive reaction; if test results are positive and use of methadone is known or suspected, perform a hemagglutination-inhibition test to confirm results. (4) Protein, hemoglobin, and distilled water containing additives may interfere with this test. Use tap water or additive-free distilled water.

PREGNANCY TESTS

PREGNOSTICON Slide Organon Teknika

Latex agglutination-inhibition slide test for the qualitative determination of urinary hCG

Performance characteristics	**Sensitivity:** 1,000–2,000 mIU/ml; can usually detect pregnancy 12 days after the time of expected menses and, in some cases, may detect pregnancy as early as 4 days after the time of expected menses **Specificity:** false-positive results with pituitary gonadotropin levels seen in women whose gonads have been injured or removed and in women over 40 yr of age (see "Specimen," below); interfering effects with large amounts of blood or methadone doses exceeding 140 mg/day; possible interfering effects with presence of protein or hemoglobin **Accuracy:** 96.7%
Materials	**Supplied materials:** antibody to beta subunit of hCG; hCG-coated latex; lyophilized positive and negative controls; pipette-stirrers; black glass slide; rocker (supplied separately) **Storage temperature:** 2–8°C (not necessary to warm to room temperature for test) **Additional materials required:** centrifuge or Whatman No. 4 filter paper
Specimen	For optimal detection of hCG, obtain a first morning specimen and test as soon as possible. Specimens that cannot be assayed immediately should be refrigerated for up to 72 h or frozen for up to 6 mo; do not add a preservative to any specimens. Centrifuge or filter excessively turbid urine; do not use bloody specimens. In women whose gonads have been injured or removed and in women over 40 yr of age, pituitary gonadotropin levels may be sufficiently high to produce a false-positive effect; specimens from such women should be diluted 1:1 with additive-free distilled water before the test. Whenever possible, do not use specimens obtained during drug therapy.
Procedure	Place 1 drop of antibody and then 1 drop of urine within a circle on the slide and mix; add 1 drop of hCG-coated latex to the mixture, mix, and spread over the entire area of the circle; then rock slide for 2 min and observe results
Results	**Positive reaction:** smooth milky suspension (no agglutination) after 2 min **Negative reaction:** granular clumping (agglutination) within 2 min

PREGNOSTICON Slide ■ QTEST Pregnancy Test

Interpretation — (1) This test does not provide definitive results at hCG levels below 1–2 IU/ml; if no clumping or slight coarseness is seen, repeat test 1–2 wk later (when hCG level will presumably be higher) or use a more sensitive test. (2) Conditions other than normal pregnancy that may be associated with detectable levels of hCG include the following: (a) molar and ectopic pregnancy, (b) trophoblastic disorders such as choriocarcinoma and hydatiform mole, (c) certain nontrophoblastic neoplasia, (d) delivery a few days to a week before this test, (e) abortion within about a week before this test, and (f) injection of hCG at some time before this test; before making a diagnosis of normal pregnancy, rule out all of these conditions. (3) Methadone doses exceeding 140 mg/day can produce a false-positive reaction; protein and hemoglobin may interfere with this test.

PREGNANCY TESTS

QTEST Pregnancy Test Clay Adams

Enzyme immunoassay for qualitative determination of urinary and serum hCG

Performance characteristics — **Sensitivity:** 50 mIU/ml when total incubation time is 14.5 min; 500 mIU/ml when total incubation time is 4.5 min; 50-mIU/ml test can detect pregnancy two days before the time of expected menses
Specificity: no false-positive reactions with 500 mIU/ml of hLH, 200 mIU/ml of hFSH, or 500 uIU/ml of hTSH; no interference with 2000 mg/dl of albumin or glucose, 1.5 mg/dl of pregnanediol, 1.4 mg/dl of estriol, 1 mg/dl of bilirubin or hemoglobin, or the following chemical compounds: acetaminophen, ascorbic acid, caffeine, EDTA, ephedrine, gentisic acid, phenothiazines, phenylpropanolamine, or salicylic acid

Materials — **Supplied materials:** dipsticks with test and reference pads coated with antibody to the beta subunit of hCG; tubes with lyophilized conjugate of alkaline phosphatase and monoclonal antibody to the beta subunit of hCG; tubes with enzyme substrate solution; disposable droppers; work station
Storage temperature: < 30°C
Additional materials required: absorbent paper; flowing tap water; positive and negative controls; filter paper or centrifuge

Specimen — For optimal detection of urinary hCG, obtain a first morning specimen; do not add any chemicals to the urine. If particulate matter is seen, filter or centrifuge specimen or allow precipitate to settle. Refrigerate urine specimens that cannot be assayed immediately and test them within 12 h. To obtain a serum specimen, collect blood, allow it to clot, and centrifuge; do not use serum from patients receiving anticoagulants and do not add any chemicals to the specimen. Refrigerate serum specimens that cannot be assayed immediately and test them within 7 days.

Procedure — Allow specimens to reach room temperature. Add sample to the tubes containing the conjugate, swirl tubes to dissolve the powder, and incubate mixture at room temperature for 1 min. Next, insert dipstick pads into mixture and incubate at room temperature for 2.5 min (if 500-mIU/ml sensitivity is desired) or for 5 min (if 50-mIU/ml sensitivity is desired). Remove pads and wash them immediately with a full-force stream of cold tap water for at least 30 s, until gold-red color disappears. After shaking off excess water, insert pads into tubes containing the enzyme substrate and incubate at room temperature for 1 min (if 500-mIU/ml sensitivity is desired) or for up to 8.5 min (if 50-mIU/ml sensitivity is desired); then place pads between two absorbent paper towels, blot repeatedly until pads are completely dry, and observe results. If a distinct color difference is seen before the end of the 8.5-incubation period, the dipstick may be removed at that point.

Results — **Positive reaction:** color on test pad darker than that of the adjacent reference pad
Negative reaction: color on test pad equal to or slightly lighter than that of the adjacent reference pad

Interpretation — (1) If a negative reaction occurs with the 50-mIU/ml test, repeat assay in 48–72 h. If the difference in color of the test and reference pads is greater with a 50 mIU/ml control than with the specimen, repeat test in 48 h. Since the hCG level doubles every 1.3–2 days during the early stages of pregnancy, this second test should enable one to determine whether these negative or ambiguous results occurred because the hCG level was less than 50 mIU/ml. (2) Conditions other than normal pregnancy that may be associated with detectable levels of hCG include the following: (a) molar and ectopic pregnancy, (b) trophoblastic disorders such as choriocarcinoma and hydatiform mole, (c) certain nontrophoblastic neoplasia, and (d) delivery, abortion, or injection of hCG a few days to several weeks before this test; before making a diagnosis of normal pregnancy, rule out all of these conditions.

Precautions — (1) Sodium azide in the reagents may react with lead and copper plumbing to form highly explosive metal azides; after disposing of reagents, flush drains with a large volume of water. (2) For the diagnosis and management of pathologic pregnancies such as threatened abortion and suspected ectopic pregnancy, use a quantitative assay rather than this test.

PREGNANCY TESTS

RAMP Monoclonal Antibodies

Enzyme immunoassay for qualitative determination of urinary hCG

Performance characteristics	**Sensitivity:** 50 mIU/ml; can detect pregnancy as early as 10 days after conception **Specificity:** no false-positive results with 408 mIU/ml of hLH or clinically significant levels of hFSH or hTSH; no interference with 2,000 mg/dl of albumin or glucose, 1.4 mg/dl of estriol or pregnanediol, 1 mg/dl of hemoglobin or bilirubin, or the following chemical compounds: acetaminophen, ascorbic acid, caffeine, EDTA, ephedrine, gentisic acid, methadone, phenothiazines, phenylpropanolamine, and salicyclic acid **Accuracy:** 100%
Materials	**Supplied materials:** matrix pads coated with monoclonal antibody to hCG; conjugate of alkaline phosphatase and monoclonal antibody to beta subunit of hCG; buffered solution; substrate with cofactor; disposable pipettes **Storage temperature:** 2–8°C **Additional materials required:** positive and negative controls, centrifuge
Specimen	For optimal detection of hCG, obtain a first morning specimen. If particulate matter is present, allow it to settle; centrifuge turbid specimens. Test urine as soon as possible; specimens that cannot be assayed within 8 h should be refrigerated for up to 1 wk or frozen.
Procedure	Allow reagents and specimens to reach room temperature. Place 6 drops of urine and then 6 drops of the conjugate on the matrix pad; after waiting 1 min, add 9 drops of buffered solution and then 3 drops of the substrate solution. Wait 2 min and then immediately observe results. Add drops in 3-drop doses; allow each dose to be absorbed before adding the next dose.
Results	**Positive reaction:** blue spot in the center of the matrix pad **Negative reaction:** no blue spot in the center of the matrix pad
Interpretation	(1) If result is negative, repeat test in 48–72 h since the hCG level doubles every 1.3–2 days during the early stages of pregnancy. (2) If color or random specks appear outside the center of the pad, consider results as negative. (3) Conditions other than normal pregnancy that may be associated with detectable levels of hCG include the following: (a) molar and ectopic pregnancy, (b) trophoblastic disorders such as choriocarcinoma and hydatiform mole, (c) certain nontrophoblastic neoplasia, and (d) delivery, abortion, or injection of hCG a few days to several weeks before this test; before making a diagnosis of normal pregnancy, rule out all of these conditions.
Precautions	Sodium azide in the reagents may react with lead and copper plumbing to form highly explosive metal azides; after disposing of reagents, flush drains with a large volume of water

PREGNANCY TESTS

TESTPACK hCG-Serum Abbott Laboratories

Enzyme immunoassay for qualitative determination of serum hCG

Performance characteristics	**Sensitivity:** 25 mIU/ml; can detect pregnancy as early as 4–5 days before the time of expected menses **Specificity:** no false-positive results have been seen with 1,000 μIU/ml of TSH or 1,000 mIU/ml of LH or FSH; no interference with 2,000 mg/dl of triglyceride, 40 mg/dl of bilirubin, or 500 mg/dl of hemoglobin **Accuracy:** 100%
Materials	**Supplied materials:** reaction disk coated with monoclonal antibody to hCG; vial with lyophilized conjugate of alkaline phosphatase and monoclonal antibody to hCG; saline; chromogen; filter inserted in reaction disk; pipettes **Storage temperature:** 2–30°C **Additional materials required:** positive and negative controls, centrifuge
Specimen	Avoid hemolysis when collecting the specimen; centrifuge serum that cannot pass through the reaction disk's filter because of lipemia, turbidity, or presence of precipitate. Test serum as soon as possible; specimens that cannot be assayed immediately should be refrigerated for up to 48 h or frozen.
Procedure	Allow reagents and specimens to reach room temperature. Reconstitute conjugate with the sample, transfer solution to reaction disk's filter, and incubate at room temperature for 2 min; remove filter, wash reaction disk with saline, and add 3 drops of chromogen. Allow color to develop over a period of 2 min, wash disk with saline, and observe results.
Results	**Positive reaction:** plus sign (+) on the reaction disk (even if intensity of color on the two axes differs) **Negative reaction:** minus sign (−) on the reaction disk

Interpretation	(1) If neither a plus nor minus sign is seen, repeat test; absence of these signs indicates improper addition of reagents or deterioration of reagents. (2) Weak positive results obtained during the first days after conception should be reconfirmed by a second test 48 h later since spontaneous abortion can occur. (3) Conditions other than normal pregnancy that may be associated with detectable levels of hCG include the following: (a) molar and ectopic pregnancy, (b) trophoblastic disorders such as choriocarcinoma and hydatiform mole, (c) certain nontrophoblastic neoplasia, (d) delivery or abortion within a few weeks before this test, and (e) injection of hCG at some time before this test; before making a diagnosis of normal pregnancy, rule out all of these conditions.
Precautions	Sodium azide in the reagents may react with lead and copper plumbing to form highly explosive metal azides; after disposing of reagents, flush drains with a large volume of water

PREGNANCY TESTS

TESTPACK hCG-Urine Abbott Laboratories
Enzyme immunoassay for qualitative determination of urinary hCG

Performance characteristics	**Sensitivity:** 50 mIU/ml; can detect pregnancy as early as 4–5 days before the time of expected menses **Specificity:** no false-positive results with 1,000 µIU/ml of TSH or 1,000 mIU/ml of LH or FSH; no interference with 24 mg/dl of hemoglobin, 2,000 mg/dl of protein or glucose, 100 mg/dl of ketones, 2 mg/dl of bilirubin, or the following chemical compounds: acetaminophen, aspirin, ascorbic acid, atropine, caffeine, and gentisic acid **Accuracy:** 100%
Materials	**Supplied materials:** reaction disk coated with monoclonal antibody to hCG; conjugate of alkaline phosphatase and monoclonal antibody to hCG; saline; chromogen; filter inserted in reaction disk; pipettes **Storage temperature:** 2–8°C for conjugate; 2–30°C for other reagents **Additional materials required:** positive and negative controls
Specimen	For optimal detection of hCG, obtain a first morning specimen; if urine is obtained at other times and results are negative, repeat test with a first morning specimen. Test urine as soon as possible; specimens that cannot be assayed immediately should be refrigerated for up to 72 h.
Procedure	Allow reagents and specimens to reach room temperature. Add 5 drops of specimen to the center of the reaction disk's filter; after allowing urine to soak through the filter (about 10 s), add 3 drops of the conjugate and incubate at room temperature for 1 min. Remove filter, wash reaction disk with saline, and add 3 drops of chromogen. Allow color to develop over a period of 2 min, wash disk with saline, and then observe results.
Results	**Positive reaction:** plus sign (+) on the reaction disk (even if intensity of color on the two axes differs) **Negative reaction:** minus sign (−) on the reaction disk
Interpretation	(1) If neither a plus nor minus sign is seen, repeat test; absence of these signs indicates improper addition of reagents or deterioration of reagents. (2) Weak positive results obtained during the first days after conception should be reconfirmed by a second test 48 h later since spontaneous abortion can occur. (3) Conditions other than normal pregnancy that may be associated with detectable levels of hCG include the following: (a) molar and ectopic pregnancy, (b) trophoblastic disorders such as choriocarcinoma and hydatiform mole, (c) certain nontrophoblastic neoplasia, (d) delivery or abortion within a few weeks before this test, and (e) injection of hCG at some time before this test; before making a diagnosis of normal pregnancy, rule out all of these conditions.
Precautions	Sodium azide in the reagents may react with lead and copper plumbing to form highly explosive metal azides; after disposing of reagents, flush drains with a large volume of water

PREGNANCY TESTS

UCG-BETA SLIDE Monoclonal II Wampole Laboratories
Latex agglutination-inhibition slide test for qualitative determination of urinary hCG

Performance characteristics	**Sensitivity:** 500 mIU/ml; can usually detect pregnancy a few days after the time of expected menses **Specificity:** false-positive results with LH levels seen at or after menopause; interference with blood, large amounts of protein, or excessive bacteria **Accuracy:** 99%
Materials	**Supplied materials:** hCG-coated latex; monoclonal antibody to beta subunit of hCG; disposable pipettes; rubber bulbs for pipettes; disposable stirrers; glass slide **Storage temperature:** 2–8°C **Additional materials required:** positive and negative controls; centrifuge or Whatman No. 42 filter paper

UCG-BETA SLIDE Monoclonal II ■ UCG-BETA STAT

Specimen	For optimal detection of hCG, obtain a first morning urine specimen and test as soon as possible. Specimens that cannot be assayed immediately should be refrigerated or kept reasonably cool ($< 30°C$) for up to 24 h or frozen. Whenever possible, do not use specimens obtained during drug therapy. If urine is turbid or a precipitate is visible, centrifuge or filter. To avoid interfering effects, do not use urine containing blood, excessive bacteria, or large amounts of protein.
Procedure	Allow reagents and specimens to reach room temperature. Place 1 drop of antibody within a circle on the slide; add 2 drops of urine directly onto the antibody drop and 1 drop of latex opposite the antibody-urine drop (but within the circle). Mix reagents, spread over circle, gently rock slide 8–20 times/min for 2 min, and then observe results.
Results	**Positive reaction:** opaque suspension (no agglutination) after 2 min **Negative reaction:** clumping (agglutination) within 2 min
Interpretation	(1) This test does not detect hCG at levels below 500 mIU/ml; if results are negative, repeat test in about 7 days since the hCG level doubles every 1.3–2 days during the early stages of pregnancy. (2) Conditions other than normal pregnancy that may be associated with detectable levels of hCG include the following: (a) molar and ectopic pregnancy, (b) trophoblastic disorders such as choriocarcinoma and hydatiform mole, (c) certain nontrophoblastic neoplasia, and (d) delivery, abortion, or injection of hCG at some time before this test; before making a diagnosis of normal pregnancy, rule out all of these conditions. (3) Pituitary gonadotropins such as hLH may cause false-positive results; exercise caution when interpreting results of samples obtained from menopausal and postmenopausal women.
Precautions	Sodium azide in the reagents may react with lead and copper plumbing to form highly explosive metal azides; dispose of reagents by flushing with a large volume of water

PREGNANCY TESTS

UCG-BETA STAT Wampole Laboratories

Hemagglutination-inhibition tube test for qualitative and semiquantitative determination of urinary hCG

Performance characteristics	**Sensitivity:** 200 mIU/ml; can usually detect pregnancy at the time of expected menses **Specificity:** false-positive results with LH levels seen at or after menopause; interfering effects with blood, excessive bacteria, or large amounts of protein **Accuracy:** 98.3%
Materials	**Supplied materials:** tubes containing lyophilized hCG-sensitized erythrocytes and lyophilized antibody to the beta subunit of hCG; buffer; dropper; 100-μl capillary tubes; rubber bulbs **Storage temperature:** cool **Additional materials required:** mirrored test tube holder; positive and negative controls; 0.9% saline or distilled water; centrifuge or Whatman No. 42 filter paper
Specimen	For optimal detection of hCG, obtain a first morning specimen and test as soon as possible; specimens that cannot be assayed immediately should be refrigerated or kept reasonably cool ($< 30°C$) for up to 24 h or frozen. If urine is turbid or a precipitate is visible, centrifuge or filter. To avoid interfering effects, do not use urine containing blood, large amounts of protein, or excessive bacteria. Use of phenothiazines and methadone has produced no significant effect on the UCG-Test, which has liquid reagents similar to those of UCG-Beta Stat; nevertheless, since these drugs as well as others reportedly interfere with pregnancy tests, obtain specimens when a drug is not being used, if possible. For semiquantitative analysis, obtain a 24-h specimen; use 0.9% saline or distilled water to prepare serial dilutions.
Procedure	Allow reagents and specimens to reach room temperature. Add 100 μl of urine and then 2 drops of buffer to the reagent tube; after mixing contents, allow them to incubate undisturbed at room temperature for 60 min and then observe results. For semiquantitative analysis, test serial two-fold dilutions (ie, 1:2, 1:4, 1:8, etc); to estimate the concentration in IU/ml, multiply the highest dilution showing positive results by 0.2.
Results	**Positive reaction:** well-defined ring or doughnut-like pattern (no agglutination) within 60 min **Negative reaction:** mat (agglutination), with no ring, after 60 min
Interpretation	(1) This test does not detect hCG at levels below 200 mIU/ml; if results are negative, repeat test in approximately 7 days since the hCG level doubles every 1.3–2 days during the early stages of pregnancy. (2) An ill-defined, jagged, or incomplete ring may appear if tubes are jarred or urine is not clear; repeat test if these results are seen. (3) Conditions other than normal pregnancy that may be associated with detectable levels of hCG include the following: (a) molar and ectopic pregnancy, (b) trophoblastic disorders such as choriocarcinoma and hydatiform mole, (c) certain nontrophoblastic neoplasia, and (d) delivery, abortion, or injection of hCG at some time before this test; before making a diagnosis of normal pregnancy, rule out all of these conditions. (3) Pituitary gonadotropins such as hLH may cause false-positive results; exercise caution when interpreting results of samples obtained from menopausal and postmenopausal women.

UCG-BETA STAT ∎ UCG-Slide

| Precautions | Sodium azide in the reagents may react with lead and copper plumbing to form highly explosive metal azides; dispose of reagents by flushing with a large volume of water. |

PREGNANCY TESTS

UCG-LYPHOTEST Wampole Laboratories

Hemagglutination-inhibition tube test for qualitative and semiquantitative determination of urinary hCG

Performance characteristics	**Sensitivity:** 500–1,000 mIU/ml; can usually detect pregnancy 12 days after the time of expected menses and, in a few cases, may detect pregnancy as early as 4 days after the time of expected menses **Specificity:** false-positive results with LH levels seen at or after menopause; interfering effects with blood, excessive bacteria, or large amounts of protein **Accuracy:** > 99%
Materials	**Supplied materials:** tubes containing lyophilized hCG-sensitized erythrocytes and lyophilized antibody to hCG; buffer; dropper; 100-μl capillary tubes; rubber bulbs **Storage temperature:** cool **Additional materials required:** mirrored test tube holder; positive and negative controls; 0.9% saline or distilled water; centrifuge or Whatman No. 42 filter paper
Specimen	For optimal detection of hCG, obtain a first morning specimen and test as soon as possible; specimens that cannot be assayed immediately should be refrigerated or kept reasonably cool (< 30°C) for up to 48 h or frozen. If urine is turbid or a precipitate is visible, centrifuge or filter. To avoid interfering effects, do not use urine containing blood, large amounts of protein, or excessive bacteria. Use of phenothiazines and methadone has produced no significant effect on the UCG-Test, which has liquid reagents similar to those of UCG-Lyphotest; nevertheless, since these drugs as well as others reportedly interfere with pregnancy tests, obtain specimens when a drug is not being used, if possible. For semiquantitative estimation, obtain a 24-h specimen; use 0.9% saline or distilled water to prepare serial dilution.
Procedure	Allow reagents and specimens to reach room temperature. Add 100 μl of urine and then 2 drops of buffer to the reagent tube; after mixing contents, allow them to incubate undisturbed at room temperature for 60 min and then observe results. For semiquantitative analysis, test serial two-fold dilutions (ie, 1:2, 1:4, 1:8, etc); to estimate the concentration in IU/ml, multiply the highest dilution showing positive results by 1.
Results	**Positive reaction:** well-defined ring or doughnut-like pattern (no agglutination) within 60 min **Negative reaction:** mat (agglutination), with no ring, after 60 min
Interpretation	(1) This test does not detect hCG at levels below 500–1,000 mIU/ml; if results are negative, repeat test in approximately 7 days since the hCG level doubles every 1.3–2 days during the early stages of pregnancy. (2) An ill-defined, jagged, or incomplete ring may appear if tubes are jarred; repeat test if these results are seen. (3) Conditions other than normal pregnancy that may be associated with detectable levels of hCG include the following: (a) molar and ectopic pregnancy, (b) trophoblastic disorders such as choriocarcinoma and hydatiform mole, (c) certain nontrophoblastic neoplasia, and (d) delivery, abortion, or injection of hCG at some time before this test; before making a diagnosis of normal pregnancy, rule out all of these conditions; before that time, repeat test 7 days later. (4) Pituitary gonadotropins such as hLH may cause false-positive results; exercise caution when interpreting results of samples obtained from menopausal and postmenopausal women.
Precautions	Sodium azide in the reagents may react with lead and copper plumbing to form highly explosive metal azides; dispose of reagents by flushing with a large volume of water.

PREGNANCY TESTS

UCG-Slide Wampole Laboratories

Latex agglutination-inhibition slide test for qualitative determination of urinary hCG

Performance characteristics	**Sensitivity:** 2,000 mIU/ml; can usually detect pregnancy 12 days after the time of expected menses and, in some cases, may detect pregnancy as early as 5 days after time of expected menses **Specificity:** false-positive results with LH levels seen at or after menopause; interference with blood, excessive bacteria, or large amounts of protein **Accuracy:** 97%

UCG-Slide ■ BACTIGEN H. influenzae Type b

Materials	**Supplied materials:** antibody to hCG; hCG-coated latex; disposable pipettes with reusable rubber bulbs; stirrers; glass slide **Storage temperature:** 2–8°C **Additional materials required:** positive and negative controls
Specimen	For optimal detection of hCG, obtain a first morning specimen and test as soon as possible. Specimens that cannot be assayed immediately should be refrigerated or kept reasonably cool ($< 30°C$) for up to 48 h or frozen. Whenever possible, do not use specimens obtained during drug therapy. To avoid interfering effects, do not use urine containing blood, excessive bacteria, or large amounts of protein.
Procedure	Allow reagents and specimens to reach room temperature. Place 1 drop of urine on the slide; add 1 drop of antibody and then 1 drop of hCG-coated latex; after mixing, gently rock slide for 2 min and then immediately observe results.
Results of test	**Positive reaction:** no agglutination after 2 min **Negative reaction:** clumping (agglutination) within 2 min
Interpretation	(1) This test does not detect hCG at levels below 2 IU/ml; if results are negative, repeat test in approximately 7 days since the hCG level doubles every 1.3–2 days during the early stages of pregnancy. (2) Conditions other than normal pregnancy that may be associated with detectable levels of hCG include the following: (a) molar and ectopic pregnancy, (b) trophoblastic disorders such as choriocarcinoma and hydatiform mole, (c) certain nontrophoblastic neoplasia, and (d) delivery, abortion, or injection of hCG at some time before this test; before making a diagnosis of normal pregnancy, rule out all of these conditions. (3) Pituitary gonadotropins such as hLH may cause false-positive results; exercise caution when interpreting results of samples obtained from menopausal and postmenopausal women.
Precautions	Sodium azide in the reagents may react with lead and copper plumbing to form highly explosive metal azides; dispose of reagents by flushing with a large volume of water.

BACTERIAL SCREENING TESTS

BACTIGEN Group A *Streptococcus* Wampole Laboratories

Intended use	Detection of Group A streptococcal antigen in throat swab specimens
Materials provided	Extraction reagents; rabbit anti-Group A streptococcal immunoglobulin-sensitized latex suspension; normal rabbit gamma globulin-sensitized latex suspension (negative control); suspension of nonviable Group A streptococcal cells (positive control); test plate
Additional materials required	Sterile polyester (Dacron) or rayon swabs; 12 × 75 mm test tubes; timer; incandescent lamp (optional)
Time for reading	2 min (entire test can be completed within 10 min)
Performance characteristics	Sensitivity is 87.1% and specificity 98.7%; overall agreement with culture results is 97.4%; positive predictive value is 90.0% and negative predictive value 98.3%
Limitations and precautions	The test cannot distinguish colonized from infected individuals, nor identify individuals colonized or infected with other serogroups or organisms; the use of cotton-tipped or calcium alginate swabs or transport media containing charcoal, agar, or gelatin can decrease the sensitivity of the test and should not be used; the quality of the test depends on the quality of the specimen collected; antigen concentrations at the onset of infection may be below the sensitivity of the test; if symptoms persist or intensify in seronegative patients, additional specimens should be obtained and tested

BACTERIAL SCREENING TESTS

BACTIGEN H. influenzae Type b Wampole Laboratories

Intended use	Detection of *Hemophilus influenza* Type b antigen in cerebrospinal fluid, serum, and urine[1]
Materials provided	Horse anti-*Hemophilus influenzae* Type b globulin-sensitized latex; normal horse globulin-sensitized latex; specimen buffer; specimen absorbent (normal horse and rabbit globulin); positive and negative controls; diluent; serologic test slide
Additional materials required	Serologic slide shaker/rotator; oblique light source over a black background; 0.01-, 0.05-, and 0.1-ml pipettes; 0.45-μ filter (for urine specimens); disposable stirrers; distilled water; test tubes with stoppers; distilled water; centrifuge

BACTIGEN H. influenzae Type b ■ BACTIGEN S. pneumoniae

Time for reading	10 min (entire test can be completed within 22–25 min)
Performance characteristics	Reagent sensitivity is 0.2–1.0 ng of Hemophilus influenzae PRP antigen/ml; clinical sensitivity is 100% for cerebrospinal fluid (CSF), serum, and urine; specificity is 100% for CSF, 99.8% for serum, and 99.6% for urine
Limitations and precautions	Antigen concentration may be below reagent sensitivity at the onset of infection; if symptoms persist or intensify, retesting is indicated; specimens showing gross hemolysis, lipemia, or turbidity may yield incorrect results and should not be used; specimens taken from patients infected with Escherichia coli Type K-100 and Streptococcus pneumoniae Groups 6, 15, 29, and 35 may test positively

[1] Wampole Laboratories also manufactures a combination Bactigen latex agglutination test (Bactigen Meningitis Panel) for simultaneous testing for Hemophilus influenzae Type b, Neisseria meningitidis Groups A/B/C/Y/W135, and Streptococcus pneumoniae antigens in cerebrospinal fluid, serum, or urine. The portion of the test devoted to detecting Hemophilus influenzae Type b antigen is identical to that described here.

BACTERIAL SCREENING TESTS

BACTIGEN N. meningitidis Wampole Laboratories

Intended use	Detection of Neisseria meningitidis Groups A/B/C/Y/W135 antigens in cerebrospinal fluid, serum, and urine[1]
Materials provided	Horse anti-Neisseria meningitidis Group A globulin-sensitized latex; horse anti-N meningitidis Group B globulin-sensitized latex; horse anti-N meningitidis Group C globulin-sensitized latex; horse anti-N meningitidis Group Y globulin-sensitized latex; horse anti-N meningitidis Group W135 globulin-sensitized latex; normal horse globulin-sensitized latex; specimen buffer; specimen absorbent (normal horse and rabbit globulin); positive and negative controls; diluent; serologic test slide
Additional materials required	Serologic slide shaker/rotator; oblique light source over a black background; 0.005-, 0.01-, 0.05-, and 0.15-ml pipettes; 0.45-μ filter (for urine specimens); disposable stirrers; distilled water; test tubes with stoppers; distilled water; centrifuge
Time for reading	10 min (entire test can be completed within 22–25 min)
Performance characteristics	Sensitivity is 20 ng of meningococcal antigen/ml and is significantly greater than that of counterimmunoelectrophoresis (CIE); specificity is 98%; clinical accuracy in detecting N meningitidis antigens in cerebrospinal fluid is 100% in culture-confirmed cases, 72% in cases confirmed by gram-staining, and 56% in unconfirmed cases
Limitations and precautions	Antigen concentration may be below reagent sensitivity at the onset of infection; if symptoms persist or intensify, retesting is indicated; specimens showing gross hemolysis, lipemia, or turbidity may yield incorrect results and should not be used; specimens taken from patients infected with Escherichia coli Type K-1 may test positively

[1] Wampole Laboratories also manufactures a combination Bactigen latex agglutination test (Bactigen Meningitis Panel) for simultaneous testing for Hemophilus influenzae Type b, Neisseria meningitidis Groups A/B/C/Y/W135, and Streptococcus pneumoniae antigens in cerebrospinal fluid, serum, or urine. The portion of the test devoted to detecting N meningitidis Groups A/B/C/YW135 antigens is identical to that described here.

BACTERIAL SCREENING TESTS

BACTIGEN S. pneumoniae Wampole Laboratories

Intended use	Detection of Streptococcus pneumoniae antigens in cerebrospinal fluid, serum, and urine[1]
Materials provided	Rabbit anti-Streptococcus pneumoniae globulin-sensitized latex; normal rabbit globulin-sensitized latex; specimen buffer; specimen absorbent (normal rabbit globulin); positive and negative controls; diluent; serologic test slide
Additional materials required	Serologic slide shaker/rotator; oblique light source over a black background; 0.01-, 0.05-, and 0.1-ml pipettes; 0.45-μ filter (for urine specimens); disposable stirrers; distilled water; test tubes with stoppers; distilled water; centrifuge
Time for reading	10 min (entire test can be completed within 22–25 min)
Performance characteristics	Reagent sensitivity is significantly greater than that of counterimmunoelectrophoresis (CIE), ranging from 0.4 to 25 ng/ml for the 14 pneumococcal antigens associated with 87% of pneumococcal disease cases; the test is most sensitive in testing cerebrospinal fluid (CSF), followed by serum and then urine; specificity is 99.4%; clinical accuracy is 94%, the same as culture testing and significantly greater than that of CIE (56%)

BACTIGEN S. pneumoniae ■ GONODECTEN

Limitations and precautions	Antigen concentration may be below reagent sensitivity at the onset of infection; if symptoms persist or intensify, retesting is indicated; specimens showing gross hemolysis, lipemia, or turbidity may yield incorrect results and should not be used; specimens taken from patients infected with *Hemophilus influenzae* Type b may test positively

[1] Wampole Laboratories also manufactures a combination Bactigen latex agglutination test (Bactigen Meningitis Panel) for simultaneous testing for *Hemophilus influenzae* Type b, *Neisseria meningitidis* Groups A/B/C/Y/W135, and *Streptococcus pneumoniae* antigens in cerebrospinal fluid, serum, or urine. The portion of the test devoted to detecting *Streptococcus pneumoniae* antigens is identical to that described here.

BACTERIAL SCREENING TESTS

CULTURETTE 10-Minute Group A Strep ID Marion Scientific

Intended use	Detection of Group A streptococcal antigen in throat swab specimens
Materials provided	Extraction reagents; rabbit anti-Group A streptococcal polysaccharide-coated latex suspension; nonspecific rabbit antibody-coated latex suspension (negative control); suspension of killed Group A streptococcal cells (positive control); extraction tubes; micropipettes; test plate
Additional materials required	Sterile polyester (Dacron) swabs; glass-marking pencil; high-intensity incandescent light source; slide rotator (recommended); wooden applicator sticks
Time for reading	3 min (entire test can be completed within 10 min)
Performance characteristics	Sensitivity is 95% and specificity 92%; the test can also be used to confirm the identity of Group A streptococci on blood agar plates (suspect colonies should be sampled with a clean wooden applicator stick and handled in the same way as a throat swab)
Limitations and precautions	The test cannot distinguish colonized from infected individuals, nor identify individuals colonized or infected with other serogroups or organisms

---

BACTERIAL SCREENING TESTS

DETECT-A-STREP Antibodies Incorporated

Intended use	Detection of Group A streptococcal antigen in throat swab specimens
Materials provided	Extraction reagents; rabbit anti-Group A streptococcal immunoglobulin-coated latex suspension; normal rabbit gamma globulin-coated latex suspension (negative control); suspension of inactivated Group A streptococcal cells (positive control); test plate
Additional materials required	Sterile polyester (Dacron) or rayon swabs; 12 × 75 mm or 10 × 75 mm test tubes; high-intensity incandescent light source (recommended); slide rotator (recommended)
Time for reading	2–3 min (entire test can be completed within 10 min)
Performance characteristics	Sensitivity is 87.1% and specificity 98.7%; overall agreement with culture results is 97.4%; positive predictive value is 90.0% and negative predictive value 98.3%; the test can also be used for serologic confirmation of suspected colonies of beta-hemolytic streptococci
Limitations and precautions	The test cannot distinguish colonized from infected individuals, nor identify individuals colonized or infected with other serogroups or organisms; the use of cotton-tipped or calcium alginate swabs or transport media containing charcoal, agar, or gelatin can decrease the sensitivity of the test and should not be used; the quality of the test depends on the quality of the specimen collected

---

BACTERIAL SCREENING TESTS

GONODECTEN United States Packaging Corporation

Intended use	Detection of *Neisseria gonorrhoeae* in male urethral exudates
Materials provided	Plastic tube containing frangible glass ampul with normal saline (pH 7.2) and Webril pledget impregnated with reactive agent; sterile swab
Additional materials required	None

GONODECTEN ■ MICROTRAK *Chlamydia trachomatis*

Time for reading	Less than 3 min
Performance characteristics	Sensitivity is 91.9–94.7% and specificity 64.5–74.6%, based on gram staining and/or culture results
Limitations and precautions	The test should not be performed if the patient has urinated within the past hour; iron-containing substances and the unlikely presence of other oxidase-positive organisms, such as *Pseudomonas aeruginosa* and *Mima polymorpha* v. *oxidans,* in the urethral exudate will react with the test reagent, producing a positive test result; if the test is negative in a patient with a urethral discharge, additional tests (eg, gram staining, cultures) should be performed for diagnosis

BACTERIAL SCREENING TESTS

INSTA KIT for Group A Strep ID Mead Johnson Nutritional

Intended use	Detection of Group A streptococcal antigen in throat swab specimens
Materials provided	Extraction reagents; rabbit anti-Group A streptococcal polysaccharide-coated latex suspension; normal rabbit nonspecific antibody-coated latex suspension (negative control); suspension of killed Group A streptococcal cells (positive control); extraction cups; sterile polyester (Dacron) swabs; glass test slide; work station
Additional materials required	Labels for swabs; high-intensity incandescent light source; slide rotator (recommended); timer
Time for reading	3 min (entire test can be completed within 10 min)
Performance characteristics	Sensitivity is 90% and specificity 95%; positive predictive value is 84% and negative predictive value 97%
Limitations and precautions	The test cannot distinguish colonized from infected individuals, nor identify individuals colonized or infected with other serogroups or organisms; the use of cotton-tipped or calcium alginate swabs or transport media containing charcoal, agar, or gelatin can decrease the sensitivity of the test and should not be used; small numbers of group A streptococci due to low-grade infection or poor or improper specimen collection may not be detected

BACTERIAL SCREENING TESTS

MICROSTIX-Nitrite Ames

Intended use	Detection of nitrite-forming organisms in urine
Materials provided	Plastic strip with single reagent-impregnated test area; color chart
Additional materials required	None
Time for reading	30 seconds
Performance characteristics	Sensitivity is up to 80% with a single specimen and as high as 93.6% for enteric gram-negative bacteria when three consecutive first-morning specimens are tested
Limitations and precautions	Patient must be on a normal diet containing sufficient nitrate; non-nitrite-forming bacteria cannot be detected; urine must be in the bladder for 4 h or more to allow adequate reduction of nitrate to occur; sensitivity is decreased by ingestion of large amounts of vitamin C preceding the test and by a specific gravity ≥ 1.020

BACTERIAL SCREENING TESTS

MICROTRAK *Chlamydia trachomatis* Direct Specimen Test Syva

Intended use	Detection of *Chlamydia trachomatis* in urethral and cervical specimens
Materials provided	Specimen reagent containing fluorescein-labeled monoclonal antibodies and counterstain; control slides with two wells (one with mammalian cells and chlamydial elementary bodies, the other with mammalian cells only); mounting fluid with photobleaching inhibitor

MICROTRAK *Chlamydia trachomatis* ■ QTEST

Additional materials required	Microscope slide with 8-mm wells; large and small Dacron-tipped swabs; fixative; transport container; 30-μl micropipette; coverslips; blotting paper; deionized or distilled water; immersion oil; fluorescence microscope (with filter system for fluorescein isothiocyanate)[1]
Time for reading	15 minutes
Performance characteristics	Sensitivity is 91–92% and specificity 98% when compared with immunofluorescent-stained primary cultures and iodine-stained passaged cultures
Limitations and precautions	Optimal performance is dependent on quality of specimen collection and slide-smearing technique; foreign matter may cause irregular fluorescent patterns; positive test results obtained in a population with a low incidence of chlamydial infection (5% or less) should be interpreted with caution

[1] Syva manufactures a Microtrak *Chlamydia trachomatis* Specimen Collection Kit, containing a single-well glass slide, swabs, fixative, a container for transporting the slide to the laboratory, and detailed instructions on specimen collection

---

BACTERIAL SCREENING TESTS

PATHODX Strep A Diagnostics Products Corporation

Intended Use	Detection of Group A streptococcal antigen in throat swab specimens
Materials provided	Extraction reagents; latex suspension sensitized with rabbit anti-Group A streptococcal IgG; control latex suspension sensitized with rabbit anti-Group C streptococcal IgG; control swabs impregnated with inactive Group C streptococci; dispensing bottle; stirring paddles; glass test slide; sterile rayon swabs; transfer pipette; pipette tips; 12 × 75 mm test tubes; test tube rack; black cardboard viewer
Additional materials required	Distilled or deionized water; humidity chamber; forceps (recommended); incandescent lamp on a black surface (recommended); slide rotator (recommended)
Time for reading	4 min (entire test can be completed within 10 min)
Performance characteristics	Sensitivity is 97.3% and specificity 98.6%; overall agreement with culture results is 98.2%; positive predictive value is 96.5% and negative predictive value 98.9%; the test can also be used to type beta-hemolytic streptococcal isolates obtained by conventional culture methods
Limitations and precautions	The test kit should be used as an adjunct to standard culture methods until the user is sufficiently familiar with it to determine if there is a need to continue culture testing; the use of charcoal-impregnated or calcium alginate swabs, Amies' transport media, or transport media containing charcoal can decrease the sensitivity of the test and should be avoided

---

BACTERIAL SCREENING TESTS

QTEST Group A Strep Test Clay Adams

Intended use	Detection of Group A streptococcal antigen in throat swab specimens or culture plate colonies
Materials provided	Extraction reagents; rabbit Group A streptococcal antibody conjugated to bovine alkaline phosphatase; plastic dipstick with pad containing immobilized rabbit anti-Group A streptococcal antibody and reference control pad; enzyme substrate solution; heat-killed Group A streptococcal culture (positive control); sterile throat swabs; 10 × 50 mm test tubes; disposable droppers; work station
Additional materials required	Watch with second hand; flowing tap water; absorbent paper towels
Time for reading	3 min (entire test can be completed within 10 min)
Performance characteristics	**Throat swabs:** sensitivity is 96% and specificity 91%; overall agreement with culture results is 92% **Culture plate colonies:** sensitivity, specificity, and overall accuracy are all 99% or better
Limitations and precautions	The test cannot distinguish colonized from infected individuals, nor identify individuals colonized or infected with other serogroups or organisms; calcium alginate swabs should not be used for throat collections; the effects of charcoal, agar, silica gel, or Amies' transport media have not been established, and their use is not recommended

BACTERIAL SCREENING TESTS

RAPIDTEST-STREP SmithKline Diagnostics

Intended use	Detection of Group A streptococcal antigen in throat swab specimens
Materials provided	Extraction reagents; rabbit anti-Group A streptococcal antibody-coated latex suspension (test latex); normal rabbit gamma globulin-coated latex suspension (control latex); suspension of nonviable Group A streptococcal cells (positive control antigen); polyester (Dacron) throat swabs; extraction tubes; test slide; work station
Additional materials required	Clean, dry test tube or one containing modified Stuart's transport medium for storing specimen swab (if necessary); incandescent lamp; plate rotator; timer
Time for reading	2–3 min (entire test can be completed within 10 min)
Performance characteristics	Sensitivity is 83.5–88.9% and specificity 98.6–98.9%; overall agreement with culture results is 96.4–97.0%; positive predictive value is 80–91% and negative predictive value 97–98.9%
Limitations and precautions	The test cannot distinguish colonized from infected individuals, nor identify individuals colonized or infected with other serogroups or organisms; the use of cotton-tipped or calcium alginate swabs or transport media containing charcoal, agar, or gelatin can decrease the sensitivity of the test and should not be used; the quality of the test depends on the quality and quantity of the specimen collected

BACTERIAL SCREENING TESTS

STREPTOZYME Wampole Laboratories

Intended use	Detection and quantitative determination of antibodies to Group A streptococcal extracellular antigens in serum, plasma, and peripheral blood
Materials provided	Sheep cells sensitized with Group A streptococcal extracellular antigens; positive human control serum; negative human control serum; calibrated capillary tubes and bulbs; mirrored glass slide
Additional materials required	Isotonic saline (0.85% NaCl); disposable stirrers; conventional test tubes; pipettes or syringes with hypodermic needles
Time for reading	2 min (entire test can be completed within 3 min)
Performance characteristics	Accuracy is 95% in detecting antibodies to Group A extracellular antigens in patients with confirmed streptococcal disease, including acute rheumatic fever, acute glomerulonephritis, pharyngitis, and pyoderma; positive results correlate with positive findings from standard serologic tests for a single exoenzyme antibody (eg, ASO, ADNase-B, AH) in 96% of cases
Limitations and precautions	Single determinations of antibodies to Group A extracellular antigens are not as significant as weekly or biweekly serial titrations performed up to 6 wk following streptococcal infection; positive sera should be further diluted to determine the titer

BACTERIAL SCREENING TESTS

TESTPACK Strep A Abbott Laboratories

Intended use	Detection of Group A streptococcal antigen in throat swab specimens
Materials provided	Extraction reagents; rabbit Group A streptococcal antibody-coated reaction discs; anti-Group A streptococcal alkaline phosphatase; guanidine hydrochloride; chromogen; extraction tubes; micropipettes; filters
Additional materials required	Sterile polyester (Dacron) swabs; clock or watch
Time for reading	2 min (entire test can be completed within 10 min)
Performance characteristics	Sensitivity is 95.7% and specificity 96.5%; the test can also be used to confirm the identity of Group A streptococci on blood agar plates that are less than 72 h old (suspect colonies should be sampled with sterile swabs and handled in the same way as a throat swab)

TESTPACK ■ ISOCULT Culture Test for *Candida (Monilia)*

Limitations and precautions	The test cannot distinguish colonized from infected individuals, nor identify individuals colonized or infected with other serogroups or organisms; the use of calcium alginate swabs or semisolid transport media can decrease the sensitivity of the test and should not be used

CULTURE TESTS

BACTURCULT Wampole Laboratories

Intended use	Urine collection, detection, and quantitation of bacteriuria, and presumptive identification of the causative organisms as one of three groups: (1) *Escherichia coli, Citrobacter,* or *Enterobacter;* (2) *Klebsiella, Staphylococcus,* or *Streptococcus;* (3) *Proteus* or *Pseudomonas*
Materials provided	Sterile, disposable culture tubes; transparent counting strips
Additional materials required	Incubator (optional)
Incubation time	18–24 h at 35°–37°C or 32–48 h at room temperature (20°–25°C)
Performance characteristics	Colony count agrees with standard plate method in approximately 90% of cases; identification agrees with conventional biochemical identification in 83% of cases
Limitations and precautions	Antibacterial therapy and urinary acidification may affect test results; color changes may be masked by dyes in urine (eg, azo dyes, methylene blue); mixed infections may not produce conclusive color change

CULTURE TESTS

ISOCULT Culture Test for Bacteriuria SmithKline Diagnostics

Intended use	Detection and quantitation of bacteriuria; differentiation of gram-negative from gram-positive organisms; screening of asymptomatic patients, especially females; test for cure following antibacterial therapy of urinary tract infections
Materials provided	Plastic paddle layered on one side with modified trypticase soy agar and on the other with eosin methylene blue agar with crystal violet; plastic culture tube and collar with tines for streaking specimen; patient ID label; color chart
Additional materials required	Incubator
Incubation time	18–24 h at 35°–37°C
Performance characteristics	Identification of significant infection ($\geq 10^5$ organisms/ml of urine) versus contamination or no growth agrees with standard laboratory methods in 98% of cases
Limitations and precautions	Antibiotic medication prior to specimen collection may affect test results; sufficient time (usually 7–14 days) should be allowed to elapse after anti-infective treatment has been discontinued before testing for cure

CULTURE TESTS

ISOCULT Culture Test for *Candida (Monilia)*[1] SmithKline Diagnostics

Intended use	Detection of *Candida* species in vaginal specimens
Materials provided	Plastic paddle layered on both sides with Canditect medium; plastic culture tube and collar with tines for streaking specimen; patient ID label; organism identification chart
Additional materials required	Sterile swab; incubator
Incubation time	24–48 h at 35°–37°C
Performance characteristics	Accuracy is 97%, comparable to results obtained from parallel cultures run on Sabouraud's medium and superior to those obtained with Nickerson's medium (80% of positive specimens identified); growth of other, non-yeast organisms produces a clear or distinct yellow color in the medium and can be readily distinguished from the white or grayish white colonies of *Candida* on the purple medium

ISOCULT Culture Test for Candida (Monilia) ■ ISOCULT Culture Test for Staphylococcus aureus

Limitations and precautions	Douching or antifungal therapy prior to specimen collection may affect test results; sufficient time (usually 7–14 days) should be allowed to elapse after antifungal therapy is discontinued before testing for cure

[1] SmithKline Diagnostics also manufactures combination Isocult culture tests for simultaneously culturing specimens for Candida and Trichomonas in one of these tests and Candida and Neisseria gonorrhoeae in the other. The portion of these tests devoted to the detection of Candida is identical to the test described here, while the portions devoted to the detection of Trichomonas and N gonorrhoeae are identical to those described for each of these organisms separately.

CULTURE TESTS

ISOCULT Culture Test for *Neisseria gonorrhoeae*[1] SmithKline Diagnostics

Intended use	Detection of Neisseria gonorrhoeae in urethral, endocervical, rectal, and pharyngeal specimens
Materials provided	Plastic paddle layered on both sides with modified Transgrow medium; plastic culture tube and collar with tines for streaking specimen; CO_2-generating tablet; Detect-ase oxidase reagent; patient ID label; organism identification chart; carton and plastic bag for transporting suspected positive cultures to a clinical laboratory; laboratory instruction sheet
Additional materials required	Sterile swab; incubator
Incubation time	24–48 h at 35°–37°C
Performance characteristics	Accuracy is 95% for cervical specimens, compared to 93% positively identified in parallel cultures run on Thayer-Martin medium; 82% for rectal specimens, compared to 87% on Thayer-Martin; and 90% for urethral specimens, compared to 95% on Thayer-Martin or unmodified Transgrow medium
Limitations and precautions	Colonies should be examined 10–20 seconds, and no later than 60 seconds, following application of reagent; douching and antibiotic therapy prior to specimen collection may affect test results; sufficient time (usually 7–14 days) should be allowed to elapse after antibiotic therapy is discontinued before testing for cure; for positive identification, laboratory confirmation (eg, by gram-staining, fluorescent antibody testing, or sugar fermentation) is necessary (particularly for pharyngeal cultures)

[1] SmithKline Diagnostics also manufactures a combination Isocult culture test for simultaneously culturing specimens for Candida and Neisseria gonorrhoeae; the test is intended as an aid to diagnosing candidiasis and gonorrhea in patients with suspected concurrent infection and for screening asymptomatic, sexually active patients. When used to determine whether a patient's gonorrhea has been cured, the test will also help establish whether the anti-infective therapy used to treat the disease has resulted in candidiasis. The portion of the test devoted to the detection of N gonorrhoeae is identical to the test described here, while the portion devoted to the detection of Candida is identical to that described for Candida alone.

CULTURE TESTS

ISOCULT Culture Test for *Pseudomonas aeruginosa* SmithKline Diagnostics

Intended use	Detection of Pseudomonas aeruginosa in burn or wound exudates, sputum, urine, and similar specimens
Materials provided	Plastic paddle layered on both sides with modified cetrimide agar and a color indicator; plastic culture tube and collar with tines for streaking specimen; patient ID label; organism identification chart
Additional materials required	Sterile swab; incubator
Incubation time	18–24 h at 35°–37°C; cultures showing colonies but no color change should be incubated at room temperature for an additional 24–48 h
Performance characteristics	Colonies are deep red; medium turns yellow to blue-green; accuracy is 95%, compared to 81% in parallel cultures run on standard laboratory media
Limitations and precautions	Antibiotic medication, gargles, or topical medication prior to specimen collection may affect test results; results may be obscured if cultures are incubated for more than 24 h

CULTURE TESTS

ISOCULT Culture Test for *Staphylococcus aureus* SmithKline Diagnostics

Intended use	Detection of Staphylococcus aureus in nasopharyngeal specimens, wound exudates, and other specimens from sites suspected of harboring staphylococci

ISOCULT Culture Test for *Staphylococcus aureus* ∎ MICROCULT-GC

Materials provided	Plastic paddle layered on both sides with Vogel and Johnson agar; plastic culture tube and collar with tines for streaking specimen; patient ID label; organism identification chart
Additional materials required	Sterile swab; incubator
Incubation time	24–30 h at 35°–37°C
Performance characteristics	Colonies are black; medium changes from pink to yellow adjacent to growth; accuracy is 93%, compared with 64% in parallel cultures run on standard laboratory media
Limitations and precautions	Antibiotic medication or other antiseptic procedures (eg, topical medication) prior to specimen collection may affect test results; results may be obscured if cultures are incubated for more than 30 h

CULTURE TESTS

ISOCULT Culture Test for Throat Streptococci SmithKline Diagnostics

Intended use	Detection of Group A beta-hemolytic streptococci in throat specimens; identification of carriers among family members or in the general population
Materials provided	Plastic paddle layered on both sides with modified sheep blood agar; plastic culture tube and collar with tines for streaking specimen; CO_2-generating tablet; patient ID label; organism identification chart
Additional materials required	Sterile swab; incubator
Incubation time	18–48 h at 35°–37°C
Performance characteristics	Accuracy is 88% compared with 90% in parallel cultures run on standard laboratory media; although alpha-hemolytic streptococci (primarily *Streptococcus viridans* and *S pneumoniae* and, less often *S fecalis*) can also grow on the medium, their green hemolytic zones are readily distinguishable from the pale yellow zones produced by Group A beta-hemolytic streptococci
Limitations and precautions	Antibiotic medication or use of an antiseptic mouthwash prior to specimen collection may affect test results; sufficient time (usually 7–14 days) should be allowed to elapse after anti-infective treatment has been discontinued before testing for cure

CULTURE TESTS

ISOCULT Culture Test for *Trichomonas vaginalis*[1] SmithKline Diagnostics

Intended use	Detection of *Trichomonas vaginalis* in vaginal or male urethral specimens and in urine sediment obtained by light centrifugation
Materials provided	Perforated plastic paddle for inoculating culture medium; plastic culture tube containing modified trypticase–yeast extract–maltose medium and a pH indicator; patient ID label; organism identification chart
Additional materials required	Sterile swab (or sterile loop for males); incubator
Incubation time	Usually 3–5 days at 35°–37°C; cultures that become turbid but do not show a change in color from blue-green to yellow should be incubated for up to 7 days
Performance characteristics	Accuracy is 98%, compared to 78% obtained with the hanging-drop test; turbid medium may be examined microscopically (100x) directly through the tube at any time during incubation for the presence of motile trichomonads; growth of yeast contaminants in the medium may cause turbidity but does not produce the characteristic color change to a distinct yellow; the absence of both turbidity and a color change at the end of 7 days indicates a negative test
Limitations and precautions	Douching or antiprotozoal therapy prior to specimen collection may affect test results; sufficient time (usually 7–14 days) should be allowed to elapse after antitrichomonal therapy has been discontinued before testing for cure

[1] SmithKline Diagnostics also manufactures a combination Isocult culture test for simultaneously culturing specimens for *Candida* and *Trichomonas;* the test is intended as an aid to differentially diagnosing the symptomatically similar infections produced by these two organisms. The portion of the test devoted to the detection of *Trichomonas* is identical to the test described here, while the portion devoted to the detection of *Candida* is identical to that described for *Candida* alone.

CULTURE TESTS

MICROCULT-GC Ames

Intended use	Detection of *Neisseria gonorrhoeae* in urethral, endocervical, rectal, and pharyngeal specimens

MICROCULT-GC ■ MONO-DIFF

Materials provided	Plastic strip with two impregnated culture areas; rehydration fluid, CO_2-generating tablet; cytochrome oxidase test strip; clear plastic and aluminum foil incubation pouches; patient ID labels; color chart
Additional materials required	Sterile swabs; incubator; gram-staining reagents; microscope
Incubation time	24–28 h at 35°C
Performance characteristics	Accuracy is 97.5% compared with parallel cultures run on conventional Thayer-Martin medium
Limitations and precautions	Culture area may be overgrown by heavy concentrations of Candida and gram-negative rods (eg, Pseudomonas); microscopic identification is essential for identification of gram-negative diplococci; sugar fermentation tests or a fluorescent antibody test is needed for confirmation

CULTURE TESTS

MICROSTIX-3 Ames

Intended use	Detection of nitrite-forming organisms and semiquantitative determination of total bacteria and gram-negative bacteria in urine
Materials provided	Plastic strip with three reagent-impregnated test areas, two of which also contain nutrients for bacterial growth; plastic incubating pouch; color chart; bacterial concentration chart
Additional materials required	Incubator
Incubation time	18–24 h at 35°–37°C
Time for reading	30 seconds for detection of nitrite-forming bacteria
Performance characteristics	Sensitivity is up to 80% with a single specimen and as high as 93.6% for enteric gram-negative bacteria when three consecutive first-morning specimens are tested; the two growth areas will detect growth in the range of 10^2–10^5 (or more) organisms/ml of urine
Limitations and precautions	Patient must be on a normal diet containing sufficient nitrate; non-nitrite-forming bacteria cannot be detected; urine must be in the bladder for 4 h or more to allow adequate reduction of nitrate to occur; sensitivity is decreased by ingestion of large amounts of vitamin C preceding the test and by a specific gravity $\geq$ 1.020; the presence of blood, bilirubin, methylene blue and other abnormal pigments, and drugs containing phenazopyridine may interfere with interpretation of the test; antibacterial therapy should be stopped at least 48 h before test to determine efficacy of treatment

CULTURE TESTS

MICROSTIX-CANDIDA Ames

Intended use	Detection of Candida species in vaginal specimens
Materials provided	Plastic strip with impregnated culture area; water for rehydration; plastic incubation pouch; patient ID label; color identification chart
Additional materials required	Sterile swab; incubator
Incubation time	24 h at 35°–37°C; 72–96 h at room temperature
Performance characteristics	Accuracy is 97% compared with parallel cultures run on Nickerson's agar or Sabouraud's medium; positive results are obtained in half the time required for conventional culture
Limitations and precautions	Antifungal therapy or douching prior to culture may produce false-negative results

MONONUCLEOSIS TESTS

MONO-DIFF Wampole Laboratories

Intended use	Qualitative and quantitative determination of infectious mononucleosis and other heterophile antibodies in serum or plasma

MONO-DIFF ■ MONOSPOT

Materials provided	Horse erythrocytes; horse kidney antigen; beef erythrocyte stroma; human positive control serum; calibrated capillary tubes and bulbs; disposable stirrers; disposable card slides
Additional materials required	Isotonic saline (0.85% NaCl); 0.5- and 1.0-ml graduated pipettes; 12 × 75 mm test tubes
Time for reading	2 min
Performance characteristics	Accuracy, when compared with Davidsohn differential absorption test, is 99%
Limitations and precautions	Infectious mononucleosis heterophile antibodies have been associated with leukemia, Epstein-Barr virus infection, cytomegalovirus infection, Burkitt's lymphoma, rheumatoid arthritis, viral hepatitis, and other disease states; detectable infectious mononucleosis heterophile levels usually develop within 3 wk of infection, but may take as long as 3 mo to develop in some patients or never occur at all; if the initial specimen proves negative in the face of clinical and hematological evidence of infectious mononucleosis, the test should be repeated every few days (continued negative results suggest that some other disease condition is responsible); positive test results may persist for months or years due to the presence of persistent heterophile antibodies (conversely, a confirmed heterophile antibody test may indicate an occult infection)

MONONUCLEOSIS TESTS

MONO-LATEX Wampole Laboratories

Intended use	Qualitative and semiquantitative determination of infectious mononucleosis heterophile antibodies in serum or plasma, as well as serum or plasma derived from fingertip blood
Materials provided	Bovine mononucleosis antigen-sensitized latex suspension; human positive control serum; human negative control serum; calibrated capillary tubes and bulbs; black glass slide; disposable stirrers
Additional materials required	**Qualitative procedure:** timer; serologic slide rocker/rotator (optional); capillary tubes (optional; for collection of fingertip blood); test tubes (optional; for capillary specimen pooling) **Semiquantitative procedure:** 0.1-, 0.5-, and 1.0-ml graduated pipettes or calibrated micropipettor; 12 × 75 mm test tubes
Time for reading	2 min
Performance characteristics	Sensitivity, compared to differential red cell slide test, is 96% and specificity 100% for infectious mononucleosis heterophile antibodies; overall accuracy is 98.4% in differentiating between patients with and without infectious mononucleosis
Limitations and precautions	Specimens containing exceptionally high titers of serum sickness antibodies (uncommon in the US) may produce agglutination; infectious mononucleosis heterophile antibodies have been associated with leukemia, Epstein-Barr virus infection, cytomegalovirus infection, Burkitt's lymphoma, rheumatoid arthritis, viral hepatitis, and other disease states; detectable infectious mononucleosis heterophile levels usually develop within 3 wk of infection, but may take as long as 3 mo to develop in some patients or never occur at all; if the initial specimen proves negative in the face of clinical and hematological evidence of infectious mononucleosis, the test should be repeated with the specimen diluted 1:7 and undiluted; if further testing is desired, additional specimens should be collected and retested every few days (some patients may remain persistently negative); tests that give an inconclusive or weakly positive (finely granular) reaction should be repeated with the specimen diluted 1:7 and undiluted; positive test results may persist for months or years due to the presence of persistent heterophile antibodies (conversely, a confirmed heterophile antibody test may indicate an occult infection)

MONONUCLEOSIS TESTS

MONOSPOT Ortho Diagnostic Systems

Intended use	Qualitative and quantitative determination of infectious mononucleosis heterophile antibodies in serum or plasma
Materials provided	Stabilized horse erythrocytes; guinea pig kidney antigen; beef erythrocyte stroma antigen; human positive control serum; human negative control serum; glass slide; microcapillary pipettes with rubber bulbs; plastic pipettes; wooden applicators
Additional materials required	None

MONOSPOT ■ MONO-SURE

Time for reading	1 min
Performance characteristics	Accuracy is greater than 99%
Limitations and precautions	Only clear, particle-free serum or plasma samples should be used; false-positive results, as well as seronegative infectious mononucleosis, have been reported; because the heterophile antibody response may be delayed, clinical and hematological symptoms of infectious mononucleosis may appear before serologic confirmation is possible; since the clinical symptoms of infectious mononucleosis mimic those of many other diseases, it may be difficult to rule out concomitant infection; infectious mononucleosis may occur simultaneously with hepatitis; persistence of infectious mononucleosis heterophile antibodies after clinical infection has subsided may produce a positive test result

MONONUCLEOSIS TESTS

MONOSTICON Organon Technika

Intended use	Qualitative and quantitative determination of infectious mononucleosis heterophile antibodies in serum, plasma, or whole blood
Materials provided	Horse/sheep erythrocyte stroma antigen; bovine erythrocyte stroma antigen; guinea pig tissue extract; human positive control serum; human negative control serum; Dispenstirs; white background glass slide
Additional materials required	**Qualitative procedure:** lancet or other finger-puncturing device (required for whole-blood testing); high-intensity lamp **Quantitative procedure:** isotonic saline (0.9% NaCl); 13 × 75 mm test tubes; calibrated pipettes for making serial dilutions
Time for reading	2 min
Performance characteristics	Accuracy, when compared with Paul-Bunnell-Davidsohn test, is 98.8%, specificity 99.1%, and sensitivity 98.2%
Limitations and precautions	A negative test result may occur if the antibody response is below the detectable level; antibody titer levels may not correlate with disease severity; both false-positive and false-negative results have been reported

MONONUCLEOSIS TESTS

MONOSTICON DRI-DOT Organon Teknika

Intended use	Qualitative and quantitative determination of infectious mononucleosis heterophile antibodies in serum, plasma, or whole blood
Materials provided	Horse/sheep erythrocyte antigen-treated test slide; guinea pig antigen-treated test slide; human positive control serum; human negative control serum; dropper bottle; Dispenstirs
Additional materials required	**Qualitative procedure:** lancet or other finger-puncturing device and slide holder (required for whole-blood testing) **Quantitative procedure:** isotonic saline (0.9% NaCl); 13 × 75 mm test tubes; calibrated pipettes for making serial dilutions
Time for reading	2 min
Performance characteristics	Accuracy, when compared with Davidsohn differential absorption test, is 97.4%
Limitations and precautions	Infectious mononucleosis heterophile antibodies have been associated with leukemia, Epstein-Barr virus infection, Burkitt's lymphoma, rheumatoid arthritis, and other pathological conditions; both false-positive and false-negative results have been reported

MONONUCLEOSIS TESTS

MONO-SURE Wampole Laboratories

Intended use	Qualitative and quantitative determination of infectious mononucleosis heterophile antibodies in serum or plasma

MONO-SURE ■ MONO-TEST (FTB)

Materials provided	Horse erythrocytes; horse kidney antigen; beef erythrocyte stroma; human positive control serum; human negative control serum; calibrated capillary tubes and bulbs; disposable stirrers; disposable card slides; glass slide
Additional materials required	Isotonic saline (0.85% NaCl)s
Time for reading	1 min
Performance characteristics	Correlation with serum MONO-TEST procedure is 100% (see MONO-TEST chart for sensitivity, specificity, and accuracy of test results)
Limitations and precautions	See MONO-TEST chart or package labeling

MONONUCLEOSIS TESTS

MONO-TEST Wampole Laboratories

Intended use	Qualitative and quantitative determination of infectious mononucleosis heterophile antibodies in serum or plasma
Materials provided	Stabilized horse erythrocytes; human positive control serum; human negative control serum; calibrated capillary tubes and bulbs; glass slide; disposable card slides
Additional materials required	Isotonic saline (0.85% NaCl); disposable stirrers; 0.5- and 1.0-ml graduated pipettes; 12 × 75 mm test tubes
Time for reading	2 min
Performance characteristics	Sensitivity is 98.6% and specificity 99.3% for the infectious mononucleosis heterophile; overall accuracy is 99% in differentiating between patients with and without infectious mononucleosis
Limitations and precautions	Specimens containing exceptionally high titers of serum sickness antibodies (uncommon in the US) may give a positive test result; infectious mononucleosis heterophile antibodies have been associated with leukemia, Epstein-Barr virus infection, cytomegalovirus infection, Burkitt's lymphoma, rheumatoid arthritis, viral hepatitis, and other disease states; detectable infectious mononucleosis heterophile levels usually develop within 3 wk of infection, but may take as long as 3 mo to develop in some patients or never occur at all; if the initial specimen proves negative in the face of clinical and hematological evidence of infectious mononucleosis, the test should be repeated every few days (continued negative results suggest that some other disease condition is responsible); positive test results may persist for months or years due to the presence of persistent heterophile antibodies (conversely, a confirmed heterophile antibody test may indicate an occult infection)

MONONUCLEOSIS TESTS

MONO-TEST (FTB) Wampole Laboratories

Intended use	Qualitative determination of infectious mononucleosis heterophile antibodies in whole blood
Materials provided	Stabilized horse erythrocytes; hemolyzing solution; nonagglutinated (negative reading reference) and agglutinated (positive reading reference) sheep erythrocytes; calibrated capillary tubes and bulbs; frosted glass slide
Additional materials required	Lancet or other finger-puncturing device; disposable stirrers
Time for reading	2 min
Performance characteristics	Correlation with serum MONO-TEST procedure is 100% (see MONO-TEST chart for sensitivity, specificity, and accuracy of test results)
Limitations and precautions	Specimens containing exceptionally high titers of serum sickness antibodies (uncommon in the US) may give a positive test result; infectious mononucleosis heterophile antibodies have been associated with leukemia, Epstein-Barr virus infection, cytomegalovirus infection, Burkitt's lymphoma, rheumatoid arthritis, viral hepatitis, and other disease states; detectable infectious mononucleosis heterophile levels usually develop within 3 wk of infection, but may take as long as 3 mo to develop in some patients or never occur at all; if the initial specimen proves negative in the face of clinical and hematological evidence of infectious mononucleosis, the patient should be monitored over the next several weeks for development of seropositivity (some patients, however, may remain persistently seronegative for infectious mononucleosis antibody)

RUBELLA TESTS

RUBACELL II Abbott Laboratories

Intended use	Detection of rubella virus antibodies in serum
Materials provided	Human erythrocytes coated with rubella virus antigen; positive human control plasma; negative human control plasma; buffer solution; disposable "V" plates; plastic sealers; disposable 25-μl pipette droppers
Additional materials required	Micropipette (10 μl); micropipette tips; test reading mirror
Time for reading	2 h
Performance characteristics	Sensitivity is 100.00% and specificity 99.16%, with an overall agreement between test results of 99.92%, based on passive hemagglutination test
Limitations and precautions	The test cannot be used to determine a recent rubella infection

RUBELLA TESTS

RUBAQUICK Abbott Laboratories

Intended use	Detection of rubella virus antibodies in serum
Materials provided	Human erythrocytes coated with rubella virus antigen; positive human control serum; negative human control serum; disposable test trays; disposable mixing sticks
Additional materials required	Micropipette (20 μl); micropipette tips; platform rotator; light box
Time for reading	15–30 min
Performance characteristics	Sensitivity is 98.43% and specificity 97.60%, with an overall agreement between test results of 98.32%, based on passive hemagglutination test; when compared with hemagglutination-inhibition assay, sensitivity is 100.00% and specificity 99.27%, with an overall agreement between test results of 99.93%; precision and reproducibility are 100%
Limitations and precautions	The test cannot be used to determine a recent rubella infection; a positive test result does not eliminate the possibility of an ongoing rubella infection

RUBELLA TESTS

VIROGEN Rubella Wampole Laboratories

Intended use	Qualitative and quantitative detection of rubella virus antibodies in serum
Materials provided	Rubella virus-sensitized latex; high- and low-titer human rubella virus antisera (positive controls); human serum (negative control); diluent; disposable plates; dispensing cannula
Additional materials required	Serologic shaker/rotator; plate reading tray with magnifying mirror; overhead fluorescent light source; 20-, 50-, and 60-μl micropipettes or adjustable micropipettor; centrifuge
Time for reading	Less than 45 min
Performance characteristics	Sensitivity of qualitative screening procedure is 95.5–99.4% and specificity 99.5–100%, based on hemagglutination-inhibition (HAI) assay; reproducibility of quantitative titration procedure is 100% within ± 1 twofold dilution, compared with HAI assay
Limitations and precautions	Specimens showing gross hemolysis, lipemia, or turbidity may yield incorrect results and should not be used; proper timing of sample collection is critical when determining recent or active rubella infection; the absence of a fourfold rise in titer does not necessarily rule out the possibility of rubella virus exposure and infection; the validity of the test for use with plasma has not been established

RHEUMATOID FACTOR TESTS

LAtest-RF Kit Fisher Scientific

Intended use	Qualitative and quantitative determination of rheumatoid factor in serum

LAtest-RF Kit ■ RHEUMANOSTICON DRI-DOT

Materials provided	Latex particles coated with immune complexes of antigen and rabbit immunoglobulin G; human positive control serum; human negative control serum; buffer solution; disposable pipetting straws; glass slide; applicator sticks
Additional materials required	Serologic test tubes; 1.0-ml serologic pipettes
Time for reading	2 min
Performance characteristics	Sensitivity is 1–2 IU/ml and is claimed by the manufacturer to exceed that of a commercially available sheep cell agglutination test and another commercial latex kit in detecting rheumatoid factor in the sera of patients with definite rheumatoid arthritis and other inflammatory diseases; specificity in normal individuals is 99%
Limitations and precautions	Detectable levels of rheumatoid factor (RF) may occur in patients with diseases or conditions other than rheumatoid arthritis, including cancer, infectious mononucleosis, tuberculosis, syphilis, viral infections, and systemic lupus erythematosus; conversely, certain patients with rheumatoid arthritis may be RF-negative; the results of RF testing cannot be considered diagnostic for the presence or absence of rheumatoid arthritis but should be evaluated along with clinical signs and symptoms

RHEUMATOID FACTOR TESTS

R$_3$-SCREEN TEST Wampole Laboratories

Intended use	Detection of rheumatoid factor activity in serum
Materials provided	Eosin solution; latex solution; normal rabbit serum (positive control); glass slide
Additional materials required	Stirrers; syringe, pipette, or calibrated dropper
Time for reading	3 min
Performance characteristics	Accuracy is 97%, based on comparison with fraction II latex particle method
Limitations and precautions	Specimens showing gross hemolysis, gross lipemia, or turbidity must not be used; the test is not intended for use with plasma; the test is not specific for rheumatoid arthritis and may produce a positive result with sera obtained from patients with systemic lupus erythematosus, subacute bacterial endocarditis, hepatocellular disease (biliary and portal cirrhosis, viral hepatitis), and myeloproliferative disorders (chronic and acute myelogenous leukemia); any serum giving a positive reaction should be tested further with more specific serologic tests

RHEUMATOID FACTOR TESTS

RHEUMANOSTICON Organon Teknika

Intended use	Qualitative and quantitative determination of rheumatoid factor in fingertip blood (slide test) and serum (tube test)
Materials provided	Human gamma globulin-coated latex; buffer; human positive control serum; human negative control serum; Dispenstirs; black background slide
Additional materials required	**Qualitative procedure:** lancet or other finger-puncturing device; high-intensity lamp; pipettes; test tubes; timer **Quantitative procedure:** 12 × 75 mm test tubes; test tube rack; 0.1-, 1.0-, and 2.0-ml pipettes; centrifuge
Time for reading	1 min
Performance characteristics	Sensitivity is 96% and specificity 97.1%
Limitations and precautions	Rheumatoid factor is not always detectable in patients with documented rheumatoid arthritis and, conversely, elevated rheumatoid factor levels may occur in the elderly and in persons with various infections, parasitic diseases, and related connective tissue diseases

RHEUMATOID FACTOR TESTS

RHEUMANOSTICON DRI-DOT Organon Teknika

Intended use	Qualitative and quantitative determination of rheumatoid factor in peripheral blood and serum

RHEUMANOSTICON DRI-DOT ■ RHEUMATON

Materials provided	Disposable test slide containing dried human gamma globulin-coated latex suspension and glycine buffer; buffer concentrate; human positive control serum; human negative control serum; Dispenstirs; dropper bottle
Additional materials required	**Qualitative procedure:** lancet or other finger-puncturing device (for obtaining peripheral blood); 13 × 75 mm test tube; 125-ml flask or other suitable container; high-intensity lamp; pipettes; slide holder (optional); timer **Quantitative procedure:** 12 × 75 mm test tubes; test tube rack; 0.1-, 1.0-, and 2.0-ml pipettes; centrifuge
Time for reading	1 min
Performance characteristics	Sensitivity is 97.0% and specificity 98.8%; overall accuracy is 97.6%
Limitations and precautions	Rheumatoid factor is not specific for rheumatoid arthritis and may be associated with other diseases, including other rheumatic diseases (such as systemic lupus erythematosus and polyarthritis) as well as a variety of chronic inflammatory diseases (tuberculosis, leprosy, syphilis, bacterial endocarditis); rheumatoid factor is also found in a small number of healthy people, and especially in the elderly

RHEUMATOID FACTOR TESTS

RHEUMATEX Wampole Laboratories

Intended use	Qualitative and quantitative determination of rheumatoid factor in serum
Materials provided	Latex particles coated with human immunoglobulin G; concentrated diluent; human positive control serum; human negative control serum; glass slide
Additional materials required	Disposable stirrers; conventional test tubes; distilled water; serologic pipettes
Time for reading	1 min
Performance characteristics	Overall accuracy is 99%, when compared with results of a commercially established latex agglutination test
Limitations and precautions	Specimens showing gross hemolysis, gross lipemia, or turbidity may yield incorrect results and should not be used; serum specimens from approximately 25% of patients with definite rheumatoid arthritis may be negative for rheumatoid factor (RF) (specimens from patients with juvenile rheumatoid arthritis are usually RF-negative); conversely, RF may be detected in the serum of healthy persons (especially the elderly) as well as patients with diseases other than rheumatoid arthritis, including systemic lupus erythematosus, subacute bacterial endocarditis, hepatocellular disease (biliary and portal cirrhosis, viral hepatitis), myeloproliferative disorders (chronic and acute myelogenous leukemia), syphilis, and pulmonary tuberculosis; the strength of the agglutination reaction in the qualitative procedure does not indicate the actual RF titer (weak agglutination reactions may occur with either slightly elevated or markedly elevated RF titers)

RHEUMATOID FACTOR TESTS

RHEUMATON Wampole Laboratories

Intended use	Qualitative and quantitative determination of rheumatoid factor in peripheral blood or serum and synovial fluid
Materials provided	Sheep erythrocytes sensitized with rabbit gamma globulin; human positive control serum; human negative control serum; calibrated capillary tubes with rubber bulbs; glass slide
Additional materials required	Disposable stirrers; distilled water or isotonic saline (0.85% NaCl); 12 × 75 mm test tubes; centrifuge
Time for reading	2 min
Performance characteristics	Accuracy in detecting rheumatoid factor exceeds 95%, based on comparison with median results of other tests for rheumatoid factor; correlation with conventional Waaler-Rose tube procedure is excellent; false-positive rate in serum specimens (diluted 1:10) is 3%; rate of true positives in undiluted serum specimens is 91%

RHEUMATON

Limitations and precautions — Specimens showing gross hemolysis, gross lipemia, or turbidity may yield incorrect results and should not be used; low rheumatoid factor (RF) titers may not be detected if a card slide, rather than a glass slide, is used; specimens from approximately 25% of patients with definite rheumatoid arthritis may be negative for RF (specimens from patients with juvenile rheumatoid arthritis are usually RF-negative); very low RF titers (eg, a specimen that gives a positive test result when tested undiluted but tests negatively when diluted 1:10) may be due to other diseases, including systemic lupus erythematosus, endocarditis, tuberculosis, syphilis, sarcoidosis, viral infections, and diseases affecting the liver, lung, or kidney; serum specimens that have high titers of sheep agglutinins, as encountered in patients with infectious mononucleosis or serum sickness, may also agglutinate the reagent in this test

Chapter 36

Diuretics

Thiazide-Type Diuretics — 1515

DIULO (Searle) — 1515
Metolazone

DIURIL (Merck Sharp & Dohme) — 1516
Chlorothiazide *Rx*

Sodium DIURIL (Merck Sharp & Dohme) — 1516
Chlorothiazide sodium *Rx*

ENDURON (Abbott) — 1518
Methyclothiazide *Rx*

ESIDRIX (CIBA) — 1519
Hydrochlorothiazide *Rx*

HydroDIURIL (Merck Sharp & Dohme) — 1521
Hydrochlorothiazide *Rx*

HYGROTON (Rorer) — 1523
Chlorthalidone *Rx*

ZAROXOLYN (Pennwalt) — 1524
Metolazone *Rx*

Loop Diuretics — 1526

BUMEX (Roche) — 1526
Bumetanide *Rx*

LASIX (Hoechst-Roussel) — 1528
Furosemide *Rx*

Potassium-Sparing Diuretics — 1530

ALDACTONE (Searle) — 1530
Spironolactone *Rx*

DYRENIUM (Smith Kline & French) — 1532
Triamterene *Rx*

MIDAMOR (Merck Sharp & Dohme) — 1534
Amiloride hydrochloride *Rx*

Carbonic Anhydrase Inhibitors — 1536

DIAMOX (Lederle) — 1536
Acetazolamide *Rx*

Diuretic Combinations — 1537

ALDACTAZIDE (Searle) — 1537
Spironolactone and hydrochlorothiazide *Rx*

DYAZIDE (Smith Kline & French) — 1539
Triamterene and hydrochlorothiazide *Rx*

MAXZIDE (Lederle) — 1541
Triamterene and hydrochlorothiazide *Rx*

MODURETIC (Merek Sharp & Dohme) — 1543
Amiloride hydrochloride and hydrochlorothiazide *Rx*

Other Thiazide-Type Diuretics — 1513

ANHYDRON (Lilly) — 1513
Cyclothiazide *Rx*

AQUATENSEN (Wallace) — 1513
Methyclothiazide *Rx*

DIUCARDIN (Ayerst) — 1513
Hydroflumethiazide *Rx*

EXNA (Robins) — 1513
Benzthiazide *Rx*

HYDROMOX (Lederle) — 1513
Quinethazone *Rx*

METAHYDRIN (Merrell Dow) — 1513
Trichlormethiazide *Rx*

NAQUA (Schering) — 1513
Trichlormethiazide *Rx*

NATURETIN (Princeton) — 1513
Bendroflumethiazide *Rx*

RENESE (Pfizer) — 1513
Polythiazide *Rx*

SALURON (Bristol) — 1513
Hydroflumethiazide *Rx*

THALITONE (Boehringer Ingelheim) — 1513
Chlorthalidone *Rx*

Other Loop Diuretics — 1514

EDECRIN (Merck Sharp & Dohme) — 1514
Ethacrynic acid *Rx*

Sodium EDECRIN (Merck Sharp & Dohme) — 1514
Ethacrynate sodium *Rx*

Other Miscellaneous Diuretics — 1514

Mannitol *Rx* — 1514

OSMITROL (Travenol) — 1514
Mannitol *Rx*

UREAPHIL (Abbott) — 1514
Urea *Rx*

OTHER THIAZIDE-TYPE DIURETICS

DRUG	HOW SUPPLIED	USUAL DOSAGE[1]
ANHYDRON (Lilly) Cyclothiazide *Rx*	Tablets: 2 mg	**Adult:** for edema, 1–2 mg once daily in AM, followed by 1–2 mg on alternate days or 2–3 times/wk; for hypertension, 2 mg once daily (or bid or tid, if necessary)
AQUATENSEN (Wallace) Methyclothiazide *Rx*	Tablets: 5 mg	**Adult:** 2.5–5 mg once daily, or up to 10 mg once daily, if necessary
DIUCARDIN (Ayerst) Hydroflumethiazide *Rx*	Tablets: 50 mg	**Adult:** for edema, 50 mg 1–2 times/day to start, followed by 25–200 mg daily, every other day, or 3–5 times/wk for maintenance; for hypertension, 50 mg bid to start, followed by a decrease or increase in dosage (up to 200 mg/day) according to response; for maintenance, 50–100 mg/day (divide doses over 100 mg/day)
EXNA (Robins) Benzthiazide *Rx*	Tablets: 50 mg	**Adult:** for edema, 50–200 mg/day until dry weight is attained, followed by 50–150 mg/day for maintenance (divide doses over 100 mg/day); titrate to minimal effective level; for hypertension, 50–100 mg/day, given in 2 equally divided doses after breakfast and lunch, to start, followed by a decrease to minimal effective dosage level or increase (up to 50 mg qid) for maintenance
HYDROMOX (Lederle) Quinethazone *Rx*	Tablets: 50 mg	**Adult:** 50–100 mg once daily (or up to 200 mg/day, if necessary)
METAHYDRIN (Merrell Dow) Trichlormethiazide *Rx*	Tablets: 2, 4 mg	**Adult:** 2–4 mg 1–2 times/day to start, followed by 2–4 mg once daily for maintenance
NAQUA (Schering) Trichlormethiazide *Rx*	Tablets: 2, 4 mg	**Adult:** for edema, 1–4 mg/day; for hypertension, 2–4 mg/day; titrate to minimal effective dosage level **Child** (> 6 mo): for edema or hypertension, 0.07 mg/kg/24 h or 2 mg/m²/24 h, given in a single dose or 2 equally divided doses
NATURETIN (Princeton) Bendroflumethiazide *Rx*	Tablets: 2.5, 5, 10 mg	**Adult:** for edema, up to 20 mg/day, given in a single dose or 2 equally divided doses, to start, followed by 2.5–5 mg daily, every other day, or 3–5 times/wk for maintenance; for hypertension, 5–20 mg/day to start, followed by 2.5–15 mg/day for maintenance
RENESE (Pfizer) Polythiazide *Rx*	Tablets: 1, 2, 4 mg	**Adult:** for edema, 1–4 mg/day; for hypertension, 2–4 mg/day
SALURON (Bristol) Hydroflumethiazide *Rx*	Tablets: 50 mg	**Adult:** for edema, 25–200 mg/day; for hypertension, 50–100 mg/day
THALITONE (Boehringer Ingelheim) Chlorthalidone *Rx*	Tablets: 25 mg	**Adult:** for hypertension, 25 mg to start, given once daily in the morning with food; if blood pressure response is unsatisfactory, increase dosage to 50 or 100 mg/day or add a second antihypertensive drug; for edema, 50–100 mg/day or 100 mg every other day to start (some patients may require up to 200 mg/day or 150–200 mg every other day); for maintenance therapy of hypertension or edema, adjust dosage according to clinical response

[1] Where pediatric dosages are not given, consult manufacturer

continued

OTHER LOOP DIURETICS

DRUG	HOW SUPPLIED	USUAL DOSAGE[1]
EDECRIN (Merck Sharp & Dohme) Ethacrynic acid *Rx*	**Tablets:** 25, 50 mg	**Adult:** for edema, 50 mg given after a meal on day 1, followed by 50 mg bid after meals on day 2, if necessary, followed by 100 mg in the morning and 50–100 mg after lunch or dinner on day 3, depending on response to morning dose; for maintenance, reduce dosage and frequency of administration, if feasible; for severe refractory edema, 200 mg bid may be required for initial and maintenance dosage **Child:** initial dosage, 25 mg/day; for maintenance, increase dosage by increments of 25 mg until satisfactory response is attained
Sodium EDECRIN (Merck Sharp & Dohme) Ethacrynate sodium *Rx*	**Vials:** ethacrynate sodium equivalent to 50 mg ethacrynic acid	**Adult:** for edema in urgent situations or when oral intake is impractical, 50 mg IV or 0.5–1.0 mg/kg (up to 100 mg IV if need is critical)

[1] Where pediatric dosages are not given, consult manufacturer

OTHER MISCELLANEOUS DIURETICS

DRUG	HOW SUPPLIED	USUAL DOSAGE[1]
Mannitol *Rx*	**Injection:** 5% (1,000 ml), 10% (500, 1,000 ml), 15% (150, 500 ml), 20% (250, 500 ml), 25% (50 ml)	**Adult:** 50–200 g/24 h, given by IV infusion
OSMITROL (Travenol) Mannitol *Rx*	**Injection:** 5% (1,000 ml), 10% (500, 1,000 ml), 15% (150, 500 ml), 20% (250, 500 ml)	**Adult:** 50–100 g/24 h, given by IV infusion
UREAPHIL (Abbott) Urea *Rx*	**Injection:** 40 g/150 ml	**Adult:** 1–1.5 g/kg, up to 120 g/day, administered as a 30% solution by slow IV infusion **Child:** 0.5–1.5 g/kg, up to 120 g/day, administered as a 30% solution by slow IV infusion; for children ≤ 2 yr, as little as 0.1 g/kg may be adequate

[1] Where pediatric dosages are not given, consult manufacturer

THIAZIDE-TYPE DIURETICS

DIULO (metolazone) Searle

Rx

Tablets: 2.5, 5, 10 mg

INDICATIONS	ORAL DOSAGE
Mild to moderate hypertension	Adult: 2.5–5 mg once daily
Edema associated with congestive heart failure	Adult: 5–10 mg once daily
Edema associated with renal disease or dysfunction (including the nephrotic syndrome)	Adult: 5–20 mg once daily

CONTRAINDICATIONS

Anuria	Hepatic coma or pre-coma	Hypersensitivity to metolazone

ADMINISTRATION/DOSAGE ADJUSTMENTS

Paroxysmal nocturnal dyspnea	May occur in patients with congestive heart failure; dosage near upper end of range may help ensure 24-h duration of diuretic and saluretic effects
Combination therapy	Dosage of other antihypertensive agents or diuretics and metolazone should be carefully adjusted, particularly during initial therapy; dosage of other agents, especially ganglionic blockers, should be reduced. Concurrent administration of metolazone and furosemide should be initiated under hospital conditions (see WARNINGS/PRECAUTIONS).
Adjustment of dosage for optimal therapy	Initial dose should be reduced to lowest maintenance level as soon as desired effect is obtained; the time interval may range from days for edematous states to 3–4 wk for hypertension. Dosage adjustment is usually necessary during course of therapy, based on clinical and laboratory evaluations.
Management of side effects	Reduce dosage or discontinue therapy if side effects are moderate or severe (see ADVERSE REACTIONS)

WARNINGS/PRECAUTIONS

Azotemia	May be precipitated in patients with renal disease; if azotemia and oliguria worsen during treatment, discontinue drug
Hyperuricemia and/or gouty attacks	May occur in patients with a history of gout; use with caution
Electrolyte imbalance	In rare cases, initial doses of diuretics have produced severe hyponatremia and/or hypokalemia; if symptoms of severe electrolyte imbalance appear rapidly after onset of therapy, discontinue drug, immediately institute supportive measures, and carefully reevaluate the appropriateness of diuretic therapy. Measure serum and urine electrolytes periodically, especially if patient is vomiting excessively or receiving parenteral fluids. Monitor BUN, uric acid, and glucose levels. Watch for dry mouth, thirst, weakness, lethargy, drowsiness, restlessness, muscle pain or cramps, muscular fatigue, hypotension, oliguria, tachycardia, and GI disturbances.
Hypokalemia	May develop, especially with intensive or prolonged diuresis, concomitant corticosteroid or ACTH therapy, or inadequate electrolyte intake; may require potassium supplementation. Hypokalemia may result in dangerous or fatal arrhythmias in digitalized patients.
Concurrent use of furosemide	May result in unusually large or prolonged effects on volume and electrolytes; if necessary, administer in hospital setting to provide for adequate monitoring
Concurrent use of potassium-sparing diuretics	May potentiate diuresis; dosages of both diuretics should be reduced and potassium supplements discontinued
Patients with severe renal impairment	Use with caution to avoid accumulation, as metolazone is primarily excreted by the kidneys
Chloride deficit and hypochloremic alkalosis	May occur
Dilutional hyponatremia (low-salt syndrome)	May occur in patients with severe edema accompanying cardiac failure or renal disease, especially in hot weather or if dietary salt intake is restricted
Orthostatic hypotension	May occur; symptoms may be potentiated by alcohol, barbiturates, narcotics, or concurrent antihypertensive therapy
Insulin requirements	May increase, decrease, or remain unchanged; latent diabetes may become active
Elective surgery	Discontinue metolazone 3 days before elective surgery; related diuretics (but not metolazone) have increased responsiveness to tubocurarine and decreased arterial responsiveness to norepinephrine
Cross-allergenicity	Theoretically may occur in patients allergic to sulfonamide derivatives, thiazides, or quinethazone

Parathyroid changes with hypercalcemia	Theoretically may occur (reported in rare cases following use of other diuretics)

ADVERSE REACTIONS[1]

Gastrointestinal	Constipation, nausea, vomiting, anorexia, diarrhea, abdominal bloating, epigastric distress, intrahepatic cholestatic jaundice, hepatitis
Central nervous system	Syncope, dizziness, drowsiness, vertigo, headache, paresthesias
Hematological	Leukopenia, aplastic anemia
Cardiovascular	Orthostatic hypotension, excess volume depletion, hemoconcentration, venous thrombosis, palpitations, chest pain
Hypersensitivity	Urticaria, other skin rashes, purpura, necrotizing angiitis (cutaneous vasculitis)
Other	Dry mouth, hypokalemia (symptomatic and asymptomatic), hyponatremia, hypochloremia, hypochloremic alkalosis, hyperuricemia, hyperglycemia, glycosuria, fatigue, muscle cramps or spasms, weakness, restlessness, insomnia, chills, acute gouty attacks, transient blurred vision

OVERDOSAGE

Signs and symptoms	Diuresis; lethargy progressing to coma, with minimal cardiorespiratory depression and with or without significant serum electrolyte changes or dehydration; GI irritation; hypermotility; transient elevation in BUN level
Treatment	Empty stomach by gastric lavage, taking care to avoid aspiration. Monitor serum electrolyte levels and renal function, and institute supportive measures, as required, to maintain hydration, electrolyte balance, respiration, and cardiovascular and renal function. Treat GI effects symptomatically.

DRUG INTERACTIONS

Other antihypertensive agents	△ Antihypertensive effect
Steroids, ACTH	△ Risk of hypokalemia
Lithium	▽ Lithium clearance
Alcohol, barbiturates, narcotic analgesics	△ Risk of orthostatic hypotension

ALTERED LABORATORY VALUES

Blood/serum values	△ Uric acid △ Calcium ▽ Sodium ▽ Potassium ▽ Chloride ▽ Bicarbonate ▽ Phosphate ▽ PBI △ or ▽ Glucose △ BUN △ Creatinine
Urinary values	△ Sodium △ Potassium △ Chloride △ Bicarbonate △ Uric acid △ Phosphate △ Magnesium

USE IN CHILDREN	USE IN PREGNANT AND NURSING WOMEN
Not recommended for use in children	Safety for use during pregnancy has not been established. Metolazone crosses the placental barrier and appears in cord blood. In general, diuretics should not be given to pregnant women except for pathologic edema; however, a short course of metolazone therapy may be appropriate for hypervolemia-dependent edema that is causing extreme discomfort unrelieved by rest. Metolazone is excreted in human milk and may cause fetal or neonatal jaundice, thrombocytopenia, and other possible reactions; patient should stop nursing if drug is prescribed.

[1] Adverse reactions reported with other diuretics, but which, to date, have not been reported with metolazone, include pancreatitis, xanthopsia, agranulocytosis, thrombocytopenia, and photosensitivity; there is a possibility that these may occur in patients taking this drug

---

THIAZIDE-TYPE DIURETICS

DIURIL (chlorothiazide) Merck Sharp & Dohme   Rx
Tablets: 250, 500 mg   **Suspension (per 5 ml):** 250 mg (237 ml)

Sodium DIURIL (chlorothiazide sodium) Merck Sharp & Dohme   Rx
Vials: 0.5 g for IV use only

INDICATIONS
Edema, associated with congestive heart failure, hepatic cirrhosis, corticosteroid and estrogen therapy, or renal dysfunction (adjunctive therapy)

ORAL DOSAGE
Adult: 0.5–1.0 g 1–2 times/day
Infant (< 2 yr): 125–375 mg/day, given in 2 divided doses, according to weight (< 6 mo, up to 15 mg/lb/day; older infants, 10 mg/lb/day)
Child (2–12 yr): 375 mg to 1.0 g/day, given in 2 divided doses, according to weight (10 mg/lb/day)

PARENTERAL DOSAGE
Adult: 0.5–1.0 g IV 1–2 times/day

DIURIL

Hypertension	**Adult:** 0.5–1.0 g, given in single or divided daily doses, to start; adjust dosage according to blood pressure response

CONTRAINDICATIONS

Anuria	Hypersensitivity to chlorothiazide or other sulfonamide derivatives

ADMINISTRATION/DOSAGE ADJUSTMENTS

Refractory hypertension (rare)	Administer up to 2.0 g/day in divided doses
Combination antihypertensive therapy	Dosage of other antihypertensive agents must be reduced when chlorothiazide is added to the regimen to prevent excessive blood pressure drop; further reductions or even discontinuation of other agents may be necessary as blood pressure continues to fall
Intermittent treatment of edema	Administer normal daily oral or IV dose on alternate days or 3–5 days each week to reduce risk of excessive response and resultant electrolyte imbalance
Management of side effects	Reduce dosage or discontinue diuretic therapy if side effects are moderate or severe (see ADVERSE REACTIONS)
Intravenous use	Reserve for patients unable to take drug orally or for emergencies. Extravasation must be avoided; do not give SC or IM or simultaneously with whole blood or derivatives. To prepare, dilute contents of vial with 18 ml of Sterile Water for Injection.

WARNINGS/PRECAUTIONS

Patients with renal impairment	Renal insufficiency may result in excessive drug accumulation (see OVERDOSAGE); if renal impairment progresses, consider withholding or discontinuing diuretic therapy
Azotemia	May be precipitated in patients with renal disease
Electrolyte imbalance	Measure serum and urine electrolytes periodically, especially if patient is vomiting excessively or receiving parenteral fluids. Watch for dry mouth, thirst, weakness, lethargy, drowsiness, restlessness, muscle pain or cramps, muscular fatigue, hypotension, oliguria, tachycardia, and GI disturbances.
Hypokalemia	May develop, especially with brisk diuresis, concomitant corticosteroid or ACTH therapy, interference with adequate oral intake of electrolytes, or in the presence of severe cirrhosis; may be minimized by including potassium-rich foods in diet or, if necessary, with potassium supplements. Hypokalemia may result in digitalis toxicity.
Dilutional hyponatremia	May occur in edematous patients when weather is hot; restrict intake of water. Replace salt only for actual salt depletion or when hyponatremia is life-threatening.
Hepatic coma	May be precipitated by minor changes in fluid and electrolyte balance in patients with hepatic impairment or progressive liver disease; use with caution
Sensitivity reactions	May occur in patients with or without a history of allergy or bronchial asthma
Insulin requirements	May increase, decrease, or remain unchanged; latent diabetes may become active
Hypomagnesemia	May occur
Hyperuricemia or overt gout	May occur in certain patients
Lithium therapy	Renal clearance is reduced, increasing risk of lithium toxicity; coadministration generally should be avoided unless adequate precautions are taken
Systemic lupus erythematosus	May be activated or exacerbated
Postsympathectomy patients	Antihypertensive effect may be enhanced
Parathyroid function tests	Discontinue drug before testing

ADVERSE REACTIONS

Gastrointestinal	Anorexia, gastric irritation, nausea, vomiting, cramping, diarrhea, constipation, intrahepatic cholestatic jaundice, pancreatitis, sialadenitis
Central nervous system	Dizziness, vertigo, paresthesias, headache, weakness, restlessness
Ophthalmic	Xanthopsia, transient blurred vision
Hematological	Leukopenia, agranulocytosis, thrombocytopenia, aplastic anemia, hemolytic anemia
Cardiovascular	Orthostatic hypotension
Hypersensitivity	Purpura, photosensitivity, rash, urticaria, necrotizing angiitis, fever, respiratory distress (including pneumonitis and pulmonary edema), anaphylactic reactions
Other	Hyperglycemia, glycosuria, hyperuricemia, electrolyte imbalance, muscle spasm, hematuria[1]

OVERDOSAGE

Signs and symptoms	Diuresis; lethargy progressing to coma, with minimal cardiorespiratory depression and with or without significant serum electrolyte changes or dehydration; GI irritation; hypermotility; transient elevation in BUN level
Treatment	Empty stomach by gastric lavage, taking care to avoid aspiration. Monitor serum electrolyte levels and renal function, and institute supportive measures, as required, to maintain hydration, electrolyte balance, respiration, and cardiovascular and renal function. Treat GI effects symptomatically.

DIURIL ■ ENDURON

DRUG INTERACTIONS

Other antihypertensive agents	△ Antihypertensive effect
Tubocurarine	△ Skeletal-muscle relaxation
Nonsteroidal anti-inflammatory agents	▽ Diuretic, natriuretic, and antihypertensive effects; observe patient closely during concomitant therapy to ensure that desired therapeutic effect is obtained
Norepinephrine	▽ Vasopressor effect
Steroids, ACTH	△ Risk of hypokalemia
Lithium	▽ Lithium clearance
Alcohol, barbiturates, narcotic analgesics	△ Risk of orthostatic hypotension

ALTERED LABORATORY VALUES

Blood/serum values	△ Uric acid △ Calcium ▽ Magnesium ▽ Sodium ▽ Potassium ▽ Chloride ▽ Bicarbonate ▽ Phosphate ▽ PBI △ or ▽ Glucose
Urinary values	△ Sodium △ Potassium △ Chloride △ Bicarbonate △ Uric acid ▽ Calcium △ Magnesium

---

USE IN CHILDREN

See INDICATIONS and ORAL DOSAGE; IV use in infants and children has been limited and is not recommended

USE IN PREGNANT AND NURSING WOMEN

Safety for use during pregnancy has not been established. Thiazides cross the placental barrier and appear in cord blood. In general, thiazides should not be given to pregnant women except for pathologic edema; however, a short course of diuretic therapy may be appropriate for hypervolemia-dependent edema that is causing extreme discomfort unrelieved by rest. Thiazides are excreted in human milk and may cause fetal or neonatal jaundice, thrombocytopenia, and other possible reactions; patient should stop nursing if drug is prescribed.

[1] One case following IV use

THIAZIDE-TYPE DIURETICS

ENDURON (methyclothiazide) Abbott   Rx

Tablets: 2.5, 5 mg

INDICATIONS

Edema associated with congestive heart failure, hepatic cirrhosis, corticosteroid and estrogen therapy, or renal dysfunction (adjunctive therapy)

Hypertension

ORAL DOSAGE

Adult: 2.5–10 mg once daily

Adult: 2.5–5.0 mg once daily, or up to 10 mg once daily if needed

CONTRAINDICATIONS

Renal decompensation	Hypersensitivity to methyclothiazide or other sulfonamide derivatives

ADMINISTRATION/DOSAGE ADJUSTMENTS

Combination antihypertensive therapy	Other antihypertensive agents should be added gradually; dosage of ganglionic blockers must be reduced by at least 50% to prevent excessive blood pressure drop
Management of side effects	Discontinue diuretic therapy if side effects are severe (see ADVERSE REACTIONS)

WARNINGS/PRECAUTIONS

Patients with renal impairment	Renal insufficiency may result in excessive drug accumulation (see OVERDOSAGE); if renal impairment progresses, consider withholding or discontinuing diuretic therapy
Azotemia	May be precipitated in patients with renal disease
Electrolyte imbalance	Measure serum and urine electrolytes periodically, especially if patient is vomiting excessively or receiving parenteral fluids. Watch for dry mouth, thirst, weakness, lethargy, drowsiness, restlessness, muscle pain or cramps, muscular fatigue, hypotension, oliguria, tachycardia, and GI disturbances.
Hypokalemia	May develop, especially with brisk diuresis, concomitant corticosteroid or ACTH therapy, interference with adequate oral intake of electrolytes, or in the presence of severe cirrhosis; may be minimized by including potassium-rich foods in diet or, if necessary, with potassium supplements. Hypokalemia may result in digitalis toxicity.

ENDURON ■ ESIDRIX

Dilutional hyponatremia	May occur in edematous patients when weather is hot; restrict intake of water. Replace salt only for actual salt depletion or when hyponatremia is life-threatening.
Hepatic coma	May be precipitated by minor changes in fluid and electrolyte balance in patients with hepatic impairment or progressive liver disease; use with caution
Hyperuricemia or overt gout	May occur in certain patients
Sensitivity reactions	May occur in patients with a history of allergy or bronchial asthma
Insulin requirements	May increase, decrease, or remain unchanged; latent diabetes may become active
Systemic lupus erythematosus	May be activated or exacerbated
Postsympathectomy patients	Antihypertensive effect may be enhanced

ADVERSE REACTIONS

Gastrointestinal	Anorexia, gastric irritation, nausea, vomiting, cramping, diarrhea, constipation, intrahepatic cholestatic jaundice, pancreatitis
Central nervous system	Dizziness, vertigo, paresthesias, headache, weakness, restlessness
Ophthalmic	Xanthopsia
hematological	Leukopenia, agranulocytosis, thrombocytopenia, aplastic anemia
Cardiovascular	Orthostatic hypotension

OVERDOSAGE

Signs and symptoms	Electrolyte imbalance, signs of potassium deficiency, confusion, dizziness, muscular weakness, and GI disturbances
Treatment	Institute general supportive measures, as indicated, including fluid and electrolyte replacement

DRUG INTERACTIONS

Other antihypertensive agents	△ Antihypertensive effect
Tubocurarine	△ Skeletal-muscle relaxation
Norepinephrine	▽ Vasopressor effect
Steroids, ACTH	△ Risk of hypokalemia
Lithium	▽ Lithium clearance
Alcohol, barbiturates, narcotic analgesics	△ Risk of orthostatic hypotension

ALTERED LABORATORY VALUES

Blood/serum values	△ Uric acid △ Calcium ▽ Sodium ▽ Potassium ▽ Chloride ▽ Bicarbonate ▽ Phosphate ▽ PBI △ Glucose
Urinary values	△ Sodium △ Potassium △ Chloride △ Bicarbonate △ Uric acid ▽ Calcium

---

USE IN CHILDREN

Safety and effectiveness for use in children have not been established

USE IN PREGNANT AND NURSING WOMEN

Safety for use during pregnancy has not been established. Thiazides cross the placental barrier and appear in cord blood. In general, thiazides should not be given to pregnant women except for pathologic edema; however, a short course of diuretic therapy may be appropriate for hypervolemia-dependent edema that is causing extreme discomfort unrelieved by rest. Thiazides are excreted in human milk and may cause fetal or neonatal jaundice, thrombocytopenia, and other possible reactions; patient should stop nursing if drug is prescribed.

THIAZIDE-TYPE DIURETICS

ESIDRIX (hydrochlorothiazide) CIBA

Rx

Tablets: 25, 50, 100 mg

INDICATIONS
Hypertension

ORAL DOSAGE
Adult: 50–100 mg/day, given as a single morning dose, to start; after 1 wk, dosage may be reduced to 25 mg/day or increased, as needed (in rare cases, up to 200 mg/day, given in divided doses, may be necessary)
Infant (< 2 yr): 12.5–37.5 mg/day, given in 2 divided doses, according to weight (< 6 mo, up to 1.5 mg/lb/day; older infants, 1 mg/lb/day)
Child (2–12 yr): 37.5–100 mg/day to start, given in 2 divided doses, according to weight (1 mg/lb/day)

ESIDRIX

Edema associated with congestive heart failure, hepatic cirrhosis, corticosteroid and estrogen therapy, or renal dysfunction (adjunctive therapy)	**Adult:** 25–200 mg/day for several days or until dry weight is attained, followed by 25–100 mg daily or intermittently, depending upon clinical response (up to 200 mg/day may be necessary in a few cases) **Infant (< 2 yr):** 12.5–37.5 mg/day, given in 2 divided doses, according to weight (< 6 mo, up to 1.5 mg/lb/day; older infants, 1 mg/lb/day) **Child (2–12 yr):** 37.5–100 mg/day, given in 2 divided doses, according to weight (1 mg/lb/day)

CONTRAINDICATIONS

Anuria	Hypersensitivity to hydrochlorothiazide or other sulfonamide derivatives

ADMINISTRATION/DOSAGE ADJUSTMENTS

Management of adverse reactions	Adverse effects can usually be reversed by discontinuing therapy or reducing dosage

WARNINGS/PRECAUTIONS

Azotemia, drug accumulation	In patients with renal impairment, thiazides can precipitate azotemia or accumulate; use with caution in patients with severe renal disease. If renal impairment progresses during therapy, consider interrupting or discontinuing use.
Hepatic coma	Minor changes in fluid and electrolyte balance may precipitate hepatic coma in patients with hepatic impairment or progressive liver disease; use with caution in such patients
Electrolyte disorders	Hypokalemia may occur, especially with brisk diuresis, when severe cirrhosis is present, ACTH or corticosteroids are given concomitantly, or oral intake of electrolytes is inadequate; potassium supplements or potassium-rich foods may be given to avoid or treat hypokalemia. Dilutional hyponatremia may occur in edematous patients when the weather is hot; restrict the intake of water, and administer salt only if hyponatremia is life-threatening or actual salt depletion occurs. For hypochloremia, specific treatment is usually unnecessary, except for certain patients (eg, those with hepatic or renal disease). To prevent electrolyte imbalance, measure serum and urinary electrolyte levels periodically in all patients (these determinations are especially important if excessive vomiting occurs or parenteral fluids are being given); watch for premonitory signs and symptoms of hypokalemia, hyponatremia, and hypochloremic alkalosis, such as dry mouth, thirst, weakness, lethargy, drowsiness, restlessness, muscle pain or cramps, muscular fatigue, hypotension, oliguria, tachycardia, and GI disturbances (eg, nausea and vomiting).
Diabetes	Thiazides may activate latent diabetes or affect insulin requirements
Parathyroid dysfunction	Thiazides decrease calcium excretion. Discontinue therapy before performing parathyroid function tests. Pathological changes in the parathyroid gland, accompanied by hypercalcemia and hypophosphatemia, have occurred in a few patients after prolonged thiazide therapy; however, the common complications of hyperparathyroidism have not been seen.
Other thiazide-related effects	Thiazides may activate or exacerbate systemic lupus erythematosus, cause hyperuricemia or overt gout, precipitate hypersensitivity reactions (especially in patients with a history of allergy or bronchial asthma), or, in postsympathectomy patients, produce an enhanced antihypertensive effect
Carcinogenicity, mutagenicity, effect on fertility	No long-term studies have been performed in animals to evaluate the carcinogenic potential of hydrochlorothiazide; the drug does not appear to be mutagenic and does not seem to affect fertility

ADVERSE REACTIONS

Gastrointestinal	Pancreatitis, intrahepatic cholestatic jaundice, sialadenitis, vomiting, diarrhea, cramping, nausea, gastric irritation, constipation, anorexia
Cardiovascular	Orthostatic hypotension
Central nervous system	Vertigo, dizziness, transient blurred vision, headache, paresthesia, xanthopsia, weakness, restlessness
Musculoskeletal	Muscle spasm
Hematological	Aplastic anemia, agranulocytosis, leukopenia, thrombocytopenia
Hypersensitivity	Necrotizing angiitis, Stevens-Johnson syndrome, purpura, urticaria, rash, photosensitivity
Other	Glycosuria, hyperglycemia, hyperuricemia

OVERDOSAGE

Signs and symptoms	Tachycardia, hypotension, shock, weakness, confusion, dizziness, cramps of the calf muscles, paresthesia, fatigue, impairment of consciousness, nausea, vomiting, thirst, polyuria, oliguria, anuria, hypokalemia, hyponatremia, hypochloremia, alkalosis, increased BUN level (especially in patients with impaired renal function)

ESIDRIX ■ HydroDIURIL

Treatment	Induce vomiting or perform gastric lavage; administer activated charcoal to reduce absorption. To treat hypotension, raise the patient's legs and replace lost fluid and electrolytes. Monitor renal function and fluid and electrolyte balance (especially the serum potassium level) until condition normalizes.

DRUG INTERACTIONS

Other antihypertensive drugs	△ Antihypertensive effect; if necessary, other antihypertensive drugs may be given. However, these drugs should be added cautiously and gradually; reduce the initial dosage of ganglionic blockers by 50%.
Digitalis	△ Risk of digitalis toxicity
Lithium	△ Risk of lithium toxicity
Norepinephrine, other vasopressors	▽ Vasopressor effect; nevertheless, this interaction does not preclude therapeutic use of vasopressors
Corticosteroids, ACTH	△ Risk of hypokalemia
Alcohol, barbiturates, narcotic analgesics	△ Risk of orthostatic hypotension
Tubocurarine, other nondepolarizing skeletal muscle relaxants	△ Skeletal muscle relaxation

ALTERED LABORATORY VALUES

Blood/serum values	▽ Sodium ▽ Potassium △ Calcium ▽ Magnesium ▽ Chloride ▽ Phosphate △ Uric acid ▽ PBI △ Glucose △ Amylase
Urinary values	△ Sodium △ Potassium ▽ Calcium △ Magnesium △ Chloride △ Bicarbonate ▽ Uric acid △ Glucose

---

USE IN CHILDREN

See INDICATIONS and ORAL DOSAGE; safety and effectiveness for use in children have not been established

USE IN PREGNANT AND NURSING WOMEN

Pregnancy Category B: reproduction studies in rats given 62.5 times the maximum human daily dose have shown no evidence of impaired fertility or harm to the fetus; however, thiazides cross the placental barrier and may cause fetal or neonatal jaundice, thrombocytopenia, and other possible reactions. Use during pregnancy only if clearly needed. After appropriate evaluation, thiazides may be used during pregnancy for hypertension or pathological edema; they may also be given in a short course if edema associated with hypovolemia occurs and cannot be relieved by rest. Do not use for toxemia of pregnancy or for edema resulting from restriction of venous return by the expanded uterus. Thiazides are excreted in human milk; patients should not nurse while taking this drug.

THIAZIDE-TYPE DIURETICS

HydroDIURIL (hydrochlorothiazide) Merck Sharp & Dohme Rx

Tablets: 25, 50, 100 mg

INDICATIONS	ORAL DOSAGE
Edema associated with congestive heart failure, hepatic cirrhosis, corticosteroid and estrogen therapy, or renal dysfunction (adjunctive therapy)	**Adult:** 50–100 mg 1–2 times/day **Infant (< 2 yr):** 12.5–37.5 mg/day, given in 2 divided doses, according to weight (< 6 mo, up to 1.5 mg/lb/day; older infants, 1.0 mg/lb/day) **Child (2–12 yr):** 37.5–100 mg/day, given in 2 divided doses, according to weight (1.0 mg/lb/day)
Hypertension	**Adult:** 50–100 mg, given in single or divided daily doses, or up to 200 mg/day in divided doses, if needed

CONTRAINDICATIONS

Anuria	Hypersensitivity to hydrochlorothiazide or other sulfonamide derivatives

ADMINISTRATION/DOSAGE ADJUSTMENTS

Combination antihypertensive therapy	Dosage of other antihypertensive agents must be reduced when hydrochlorothiazide is added to the regimen to prevent an excessive fall in blood pressure
Intermittent treatment of edema	Administer normal daily dose on alternate days or 3–5 days each week to reduce risk of excessive response and resultant electrolyte imbalance
Management of side effects	Reduce dosage or discontinue diuretic therapy if side effects (see ADVERSE REACTIONS) are moderate or severe

HydroDIURIL

WARNINGS/PRECAUTIONS

Patients with renal impairment	Renal insufficiency may result in excessive drug accumulation (see OVERDOSAGE); if renal impairment progresses, consider withholding or discontinuing diuretic therapy
Azotemia	May be precipitated in patients with renal disease
Electrolyte imbalance	Measure serum and urine electrolytes periodically, especially if patient is vomiting excessively or receiving parenteral fluids. Watch for dry mouth, thirst, weakness, lethargy, drowsiness, restlessness, muscle pain or cramps, muscular fatigue, hypotension, oliguria, tachycardia, and GI disturbances.
Hypokalemia	May develop, especially with brisk diuresis, concomitant corticosteroid or ACTH therapy, interference with adequate oral intake of electrolytes, or in the presence of severe cirrhosis; may be minimized by including potassium-rich foods in diet or, if necessary, with potassium supplements. Hypokalemia may result in digitalis toxicity.
Dilutional hyponatremia	May occur in edematous patients when weather is hot; restrict intake of water. Replace salt only for actual salt depletion or when hyponatremia is life-threatening.
Hepatic coma	May be precipitated by minor changes in fluid and electrolyte balance in patients with hepatic impairment or progressive liver disease; use with caution
Hypomagnesemia	May occur
Hyperuricemia or overt gout	May occur in certain patients
Sensitivity reactions	May occur in patients with or without a history of allergy or bronchial asthma
Insulin requirements	May increase, decrease, or remain unchanged; latent diabetes may become active
Lithium therapy	Renal clearance is reduced, increasing risk of lithium toxicity; coadministration generally should be avoided unless adequate precautions are taken
Systemic lupus erythematosus	May be activated or exacerbated
Postsympathectomy patients	Antihypertensive effect may be enhanced
Parathyroid function tests	Discontinue drug before testing

ADVERSE REACTIONS

Gastrointestinal	Anorexia, gastric irritation, nausea, vomiting, cramping, diarrhea, constipation, intrahepatic cholestatic jaundice, pancreatitis, sialadenitis
Central nervous system	Dizziness, vertigo, paresthesias, headache, weakness, restlessness
Ophthalmic	Xanthopsia, transient blurred vision
Hematological	Leukopenia, agranulocytosis, thrombocytopenia, aplastic anemia, hemolytic anemia
Cardiovascular	Orthostatic hypotension
Hypersensitivity	Purpura, photosensitivity, rash, urticaria, necrotizing angiitis, fever, respiratory distress (including pneumonitis), anaphylactic reactions
Other	Hyperglycemia, glycosuria, hyperuricemia, electrolyte imbalance, muscle spasm

OVERDOSAGE

Signs and symptoms	Diuresis; lethargy progressing to coma, with minimal cardiorespiratory depression and with or without significant serum electrolyte changes or dehydration; GI irritation; hypermotility; transient elevation in BUN level
Treatment	Empty stomach by gastric lavage, taking care to avoid aspiration. Monitor serum electrolyte levels and renal function, and institute supportive measures, as required, to maintain hydration, electrolyte balance, respiration, and cardiovascular and renal function. Treat GI effects symptomatically.

DRUG INTERACTIONS

Other antihypertensive agents	△ Antihypertensive effect
Tubocurarine	△ Skeletal-muscle relaxation
Nonsteroidal anti-inflammatory agents	▽ Diuretic, natriuretic, and antihypertensive effects; observe patient closely during concomitant therapy to ensure that desired therapeutic effect is obtained
Norepinephrine	▽ Vasopressor effect
Steroids, ACTH	△ Risk of hypokalemia
Lithium	▽ Lithium clearance
Alcohol, barbiturates, narcotic analgesics	△ Risk of orthostatic hypotension

ALTERED LABORATORY VALUES

Blood/serum values	△ Uric acid △ Calcium ▽ Magnesium ▽ Sodium ▽ Potassium ▽ Chloride ▽ Bicarbonate ▽ Phosphate ▽ PBI △ or ▽ Glucose

HydroDIURIL ■ HYGROTON

Urinary values	△ Sodium △ Potassium △ Chloride △ Bicarbonate △ Uric acid ▽ Calcium △ Magnesium

USE IN CHILDREN
See INDICATIONS and ORAL DOSAGE

USE IN PREGNANT AND NURSING WOMEN
Safety for use during pregnancy has not been established. Thiazides cross the placental barrier and appear in cord blood. In general, thiazides should not be given to pregnant women except for pathologic edema; however, a short course of diuretic therapy may be appropriate for hypervolemia-dependent edema that is causing extreme discomfort unrelieved by rest. Thiazides are excreted in human milk and may cause fetal or neonatal jaundice, thrombocytopenia, and other possible reactions; patient should stop nursing if drug is prescribed.

THIAZIDE-TYPE DIURETICS

HYGROTON (chlorthalidone) Rorer   Rx
Tablets: 25, 50, 100 mg

INDICATIONS
Hypertension

Edema associated with congestive heart failure, hepatic cirrhosis, corticosteroid and estrogen therapy, or renal dysfunction (adjunctive therapy)

ORAL DOSAGE
Adult: 25 mg, given in a single daily dose, preferably with breakfast, to start; if response is inadequate after a suitable trial, increase dosage to 50 mg/day; if response is still inadequate, increase dosage to 100 mg/day or add a second antihypertensive agent. Adjust maintenance dosage to clinical response.

Adult: 50–100 mg, given in a single daily dose, preferably with breakfast, or 100 mg on alternate days, to start (some patients may require up to 150–200 mg once daily or every other day); for maintenance, adjust dosage to clinical response

CONTRAINDICATIONS
Anuria	Hypersensitivity to chlorthalidone or other sulfonamide derivatives

ADMINISTRATION/DOSAGE ADJUSTMENTS
Resistant cases	Increase initial dosage to 150–200 mg on alternate days or up to 200 mg once daily for edema or 100 mg once daily for hypertension
Management of side effects	Reduce dosage or discontinue diuretic therapy if side effects are moderate or severe (see ADVERSE REACTIONS)

WARNINGS/PRECAUTIONS
Patients with renal impairment	Renal insufficiency may result in excessive drug accumulation (see OVERDOSAGE); if renal impairment progresses, consider withholding or discontinuing diuretic therapy
Azotemia	May be precipitated in patients with renal disease
Electrolyte imbalance	Measure serum and urine electrolytes periodically, especially if patient is vomiting excessively or receiving parenteral fluids; drugs such as digitalis may also affect serum electrolytes. Watch for dry mouth, thirst, weakness, lethargy, drowsiness, restlessness, muscle pain or cramps, muscular fatigue, hypotension, oliguria, tachycardia, and GI disturbances.
Hypokalemia	May develop, especially with brisk diuresis, concomitant corticosteroid or ACTH therapy, interference with adequate oral intake of electrolytes, or in the presence of severe cirrhosis; may be minimized by including potassium-rich foods in diet or, if necessary, with potassium supplements. Hypokalemia may result in digitalis toxicity.
Dilutional hyponatremia	May occur in edematous patients when weather is hot; restrict intake of water. Replace salt only for actual salt depletion or when hyponatremia is life-threatening.
Hepatic coma	May be precipitated by minor changes in fluid and electrolyte balance in patients with hepatic impairment or progressive liver disease; use with caution
Hyperuricemia or overt gout	May occur in certain patients
Sensitivity reactions	May occur in patients with a history of allergy or bronchial asthma
Insulin requirements	May increase, decrease, or remain unchanged; latent diabetes may become active
Postsympathectomy patients	Antihypertensive effect may be enhanced

ADVERSE REACTIONS
Gastrointestinal	Anorexia, gastric irritation, nausea, vomiting, cramping, diarrhea, constipation, intrahepatic cholestatic jaundice, pancreatitis

COMPENDIUM OF DRUG THERAPY

HYGROTON ■ ZAROXOLYN

Central nervous system	Dizziness, vertigo, paresthesias, headache, weakness, restlessness
Ophthalmic	Xanthopsia
Hematological	Leukopenia, agranulocytosis, thrombocytopenia, aplastic anemia
Cardiovascular	Orthostatic hypotension
Hypersensitivity	Purpura, photosensitivity, rash, urticaria, necrotizing angiitis, Lyell's syndrome (toxic epidermal necroylsis)
Other	Hyperglycemia, glycosuria, hyperuricemia, muscle spasm, impotence

OVERDOSAGE

Signs and symptoms	Nausea, weakness, dizziness, and disturbance of electrolyte balance
Treatment	Empty stomach by gastric lavage, taking care to avoid aspiration. Monitor serum electrolyte levels and renal function, and institute supportive measures, as required, to maintain hydration, electrolyte balance, respiration, and cardiovascular and renal function. Treat GI effects symptomatically. If necessary, IV dextrose-saline with potassium may be administered with caution.

DRUG INTERACTIONS

Other antihypertensive agents	△ Antihypertensive effect
Tubocurarine	△ Skeletal-muscle relaxation
Norepinephrine	▽ Vasopressor effect
Steroids, ACTH	△ Risk of hypokalemia
Lithium	▽ Lithium clearance
Alcohol, barbiturates, narcotic analgesics	△ Risk of orthostatic hypotension

ALTERED LABORATORY VALUES

Blood/serum values	△ Uric acid △ Calcium ▽ Sodium ▽ Potassium ▽ Chloride ▽ Bicarbonate ▽ Phosphate ▽ PBI △ or ▽ Glucose
Urinary values	△ Sodium △ Potassium △ Chloride △ Bicarbonate △ Uric acid ▽ Calcium

---

USE IN CHILDREN

Safety and effectiveness for use in children have not been established

USE IN PREGNANT AND NURSING WOMEN

Pregnancy Category B: reproduction studies at up to 420 times the human dose have shown no evidence of impaired fertility or harm to the fetus in rats and rabbits; however, thiazides cross the placental barrier and may cause fetal or neonatal jaundice, thrombocytopenia, and other possible reactions. Use chlorthalidone during pregnancy only if clearly needed and expected benefits outweigh possible hazards. After appropriate evaluation, this drug may be used for hypertension or pathological edema in pregnant women; it may also be given in a short course if edema associated with hypervolemia occurs during pregnancy and produces extreme discomfort that cannot be relieved by rest. Do not use for toxemia of pregnancy or for dependent edema resulting from restriction of venous return by uterine expansion. Thiazides are excreted in human milk; patients should not nurse while taking this drug.

THIAZIDE-TYPE DIURETICS

ZAROXOLYN (metolazone) Pennwalt Rx

Tablets: 2.5, 5, 10 mg

INDICATIONS	ORAL DOSAGE
Mild to moderate hypertension	**Adult:** 2.5–5 mg once daily to start
Edema associated with congestive heart failure	**Adult:** 5–10 mg once daily to start
Edema associated with renal disease or dysfunction (including the nephrotic syndrome)	**Adult:** 5–20 mg once daily to start

CONTRAINDICATIONS

Anuria	Hepatic coma or pre-coma	Hypersensitivity to metolazone

ADMINISTRATION/DOSAGE ADJUSTMENTS

Paroxysmal nocturnal dyspnea	May occur in patients with congestive heart failure; dosage near upper end of range may help ensure 24-h duration of diuretic and saluretic effects
Combination therapy	Dosage of other antihypertensive agents or diuretics and metolazone should be carefully adjusted, particularly during initial therapy; dosage of other agents, especially ganglionic blockers, should be reduced. Concurrent administration of metolazone and furosemide should be initiated under hospital conditions (see WARNINGS/PRECAUTIONS).
Adjustment of dosage for optimal therapy	Initial dose should be reduced to lowest maintenance level as soon as desired effect is obtained; the time interval may range from days for edematous states to 3–4 wk for hypertension. Dosage adjustment is usually necessary during course of therapy, based on clinical and laboratory evaluations.
Management of side effects	Reduce dosage or discontinue therapy if side effects are moderate or severe (see ADVERSE REACTIONS)

WARNINGS/PRECAUTIONS

Electrolyte imbalance	In rare cases, the initial doses of diuretics have produced severe hyponatremia and/or hypokalemia; if symptoms of severe electrolyte balance appear rapidly after onset of therapy, discontinue drug, immediately institute supportive measures, and carefully reevaluate the appropriateness of diuretic therapy. Measure serum and urine electrolytes periodically, especially if patient is vomiting excessively or receiving parenteral fluids. Watch for dry mouth, thirst, weakness, lethargy, drowsiness, restlessness, muscle pain or cramps, muscular fatigue, hypotension, oliguria, tachycardia, and GI disturbances.
Hypokalemia	May develop, especially with intensive or prolonged diuresis, concomitant corticosteroid or ACTH therapy, or inadequate electrolyte intake; may require potassium supplementation. Hypokalemia may result in dangerous or fatal arrhythmias in digitalized patients.
Concurrent use of furosemide	May result in unusually large or prolonged effects on volume and electrolytes; if necessary, administer in hospital setting to provide for adequate monitoring
Concurrent use of potassium-sparing diuretics	May potentiate diuresis; dosages of both diuretics should be reduced and potassium supplements discontinued
Dilutional hyponatremia	May occur in patients with severe edema accompanying cardiac failure or renal disease, especially in hot weather, or in those with a low salt intake
Chloride deficit and hypochloremic alkalosis	May occur
Azotemia	May be precipitated or exacerbated; monitor BUN level. If azotemia and oliguria worsen in patients with severe renal disease, the drug should be discontinued.
Drug accumulation	May occur in patients with severe renal impairment; exercise caution
Hyperuricemia, gouty attacks	May occur in patients with history of gout; use with caution and monitor serum uric acid level
Orthostatic hypotension	May occur; symptoms may be potentiated by alcohol, barbiturates, narcotics, or concurrent antihypertensive therapy
Insulin requirements	May change; latent diabetes may become active. Monitor serum glucose level.
Elective surgery	Discontinue metolazone 3 days before elective surgery; related diuretics (but not metolazone) have increased responsiveness to tubocurarine and decreased arterial responsiveness to norepinephrine
Cross-sensitivity	Has not been reported, but theoretically may occur if the patient is allergic to sulfonamide derivatives, thiazides, or quinethazone
Parathyroid changes with hypercalcemia and hypophosphatemia[1]	May occur rarely with diuretics

ADVERSE REACTIONS

Gastrointestinal	Constipation, nausea, vomiting, anorexia, diarrhea, abdominal bloating, epigastric distress, intrahepatic cholestatic jaundice, hepatitis[2]
Central nervous system	Syncope, dizziness, drowsiness, vertigo, headache, paresthesias[2]
Hematological	Leukopenia, aplastic anemia[2]
Cardiovascular	Orthostatic hypotension, excess volume depletion, hemoconcentration, venous thrombosis, palpitations, chest pain
Hypersensitivity	Urticaria and other skin rashes; purpura; necrotizing angiitis (cutaneous vasculitis)
Other	Dry mouth, hypokalemia (symptomatic and asymptomatic), hyponatremia, hypochloremia, hypochloremic alkalosis, hypophosphatemia, hyperuricemia, hyperglycemia, glycosuria, fatigue, muscle cramps or spasm, weakness, restlessness, insomnia, chills, acute gouty attacks, transient blurred vision[2]

OVERDOSAGE

Signs and symptoms	Diuresis; lethargy progressing to coma, with minimal cardiorespiratory depression and with or without significant serum electrolyte changes or dehydration; GI irritation; hypermotility; transient elevation in BUN level
Treatment	Empty stomach by gastric lavage, taking care to avoid aspiration. Monitor serum electrolyte levels and renal function, and institute supportive measures, as required, to maintain hydration, electrolyte balance, respiration, and cardiovascular and renal function. Treat GI effects symptomatically.

DRUG INTERACTIONS

Other antihypertensive agents	⇧ Antihypertensive effect
Steroids, ACTH	⇧ Risk of hypokalemia
Lithium	⇩ Lithium clearance
Alcohol, barbiturates, narcotic analgesics	⇧ Risk of orthostatic hypotension

ALTERED LABORATORY VALUES

Blood/serum values	⇧ Uric acid ⇧ Calcium ⇩ Sodium ⇩ Potassium ⇩ Chloride ⇩ Bicarbonate ⇩ Phosphate ⇩ PBI ⇧ or ⇩ Glucose ⇧ BUN ⇧ Creatinine
Urinary values	⇧ Sodium ⇧ Potassium ⇧ Chloride ⇧ Bicarbonate ⇧ Glucose ⇧ Uric acid ⇧ Phosphate ⇧ Magnesium

---

USE IN CHILDREN

Not recommended for use in children

USE IN PREGNANT AND NURSING WOMEN

Safety for use during pregnancy has not been established. Metolazone crosses the placental barrier and appears in cord blood. In general, diuretics should not be given to pregnant women except for pathologic edema; however, a short course of metolazone therapy may be appropriate for hypervolemia-dependent edema that is causing discomfort unrelieved by rest. Metolazone also appears in breast milk and may cause fetal or neonatal jaundice, thrombocytopenia, and other possible reactions. Patient should stop nursing if drug is prescribed.

---

[1] Not reported to date for metolazone
[2] Adverse reactions reported with other diuretics, but which, to date, have not been reported with metolazone include pancreatitis, xanthopsia, agranulocytosis, thrombocytopenia, and photosensitivity; there is a possibility that these may occur in patients taking this drug

---

LOOP DIURETICS

BUMEX (bumetanide) Roche   Rx

Tablets: 0.5, 1, 2 mg **Ampuls:** 0.25 mg/ml (2 ml) **Vials:** 0.25 mg/ml (2, 4, 10 ml)

INDICATIONS	ORAL DOSAGE	PARENTERAL DOSAGE
Edema associated with congestive heart failure, hepatic disease, and renal disease (including the nephrotic syndrome)	**Adult:** 0.5–2 mg/day, given in a single dose; if necessary, give 1 or 2 more doses each day (but not more than a total of 10 mg/day), with an interval of 4–5 h between doses; for continued control, administer the drug on alternate days or for 3–4 consecutive days followed by a rest period of 1–2 days	**Adult:** 0.5–1 mg, given in a single IV or IM dose, followed, if necessary, by 1 or 2 more IV or IM doses, up to a total of 10 mg/day, with an interval of 2–3 h between doses; switch to oral therapy as soon as possible

CONTRAINDICATIONS

Anuria	Severe electrolyte depletion	Hypersensitivity to bumetanide
Hepatic coma		

ADMINISTRATION/DOSAGE ADJUSTMENTS

Parenteral use	If impaired GI absorption is suspected or oral administration is not practical, bumetanide may be given IV or IM. The parenteral drug product can be diluted with 5% dextrose in water, 0.9% sodium chloride injection, or lactated Ringer's solution; to ensure stability, solutions should be administered within 24 h of preparation. When giving the drug IV, inject slowly, over a period of 1–2 min.
Diuretic effect after oral administration	The onset of diuresis occurs within 30–60 min after oral administration; the duration of action is approximately 4 h with usual doses (1–2 mg) and 4–6 h with higher doses

Patients with hepatic cirrhosis and ascites	Begin therapy in a hospital, because sudden changes in electrolyte balance may precipitate hepatic encephalopathy and coma in such patients. Use small doses initially, and, if necessary, increase dosage very carefully. Monitor electrolyte balance and other vital signs. Use of potassium supplements or spironolactone may prevent hypokalemia and metabolic alkalosis.
Patients allergic to furosemide	Bumetanide may be substituted for furosemide, because cross-sensitivity has rarely been observed; 1 mg of bumetanide has a diuretic potency equivalent to approximately 40 mg of furosemide

WARNINGS/PRECAUTIONS

Patients with progressive renal disease	If the BUN or serum creatinine level markedly increases or oliguria occurs, discontinue use
Excessive dosage	If administration is too frequent or excessive doses are given, profound water loss, electrolyte depletion, dehydration, hypovolemia, and circulatory collapse can occur; vascular thrombosis and embolism are also possible, particularly in elderly patients. Carefully monitor response to therapy (see also OVERDOSAGE).
Changes in electrolyte balance	Bumetanide may cause hypokalemia; serum potassium levels should be measured periodically, and, if necessary, potassium supplements or potassium-sparing diuretics should also be used. Use with caution in patients with potassium-losing nephropathy, certain types of diarrhea, hepatic cirrhosis and ascites, hyperaldosteronism with normal renal function, ventricular arrhythmias, congestive heart failure that is being treated with digitalis, or other conditions for which hypokalemia constitutes an added risk. Intensive therapy may cause significant changes in electrolyte balance, including hypocalcemia (see ALTERED LABORATORY VALUES); periodically measure levels of potassium and other electrolytes in patients who are receiving high doses or undergoing prolonged treatment, especially if these patients are following a low-salt diet.
Ototoxicity	Bumetanide causes ototoxic effects in cats, dogs, and guinea pigs. In these animals, bumetanide is 5–6 times more potent than furosemide as a diuretic, whereas, in humans, it is 40–60 times more potent. Thus, the serum bumetanide level in test animals at which diuresis (accompanied by ototoxicity) occurs is considerably higher than the serum level that is usually achieved during diuretic therapy; it is anticipated that during therapy an ototoxic serum level will rarely be attained. However, ototoxic effects may occur in patients with renal impairment after repeated IV administration, especially if high doses are given. Concomitant use of aminoglycosides and parenteral bumetanide should be avoided, especially in patients with renal impairment, unless the situation is life-threatening.
Hypersensitivity	Patients allergic to sulfonamides may be hypersensitive to bumetanide
Hyperglycemia	Bumetanide may affect glucose metabolism; periodically measure blood glucose levels, especially in patients with active or latent diabetes
Hyperuricemia	Bumetanide elevates serum uric acid levels; asymptomatic cases of hyperuricemia have been reported
Renal effects	Reversible elevation of BUN and serum creatinine levels may occur, especially in patients who are dehydrated or have renal impairment
Blood and liver disorders; idiosyncratic reactions	Blood dyscrasias, liver damage, and idiosyncratic reactions have been reported occasionally in clinical use outside the United States; a causal relationship has not been established. Patients should be observed regularly for the possible development of such reactions.
Carcinogenicity, mutagenicity	An increase in mammary adenomas of questionable significance was detected in female rats fed 60 mg/kg/day, but this finding could not be repeated; tests with various strains of *Salmonella typhimurium* have shown no evidence of mutagenic activity
Effect on fertility	A small, insignificant decrease in pregnancy rate has been observed in rats fed 10–100 mg/kg/day

ADVERSE REACTIONS

The most frequent reactions, regardless of incidence, are printed in *italics*

Central nervous system	*Dizziness (1.1%), headache (0.6%), encephalopathy in patients with liver disease (0.6%),* impaired hearing, vertigo, ear discomfort, fatigue
Musculoskeletal	*Muscle cramps (1.1%),* weakness, arthritic pain, musculoskeletal pain, asterixis
Cardiovascular	*Hypotension (0.8%),* ECG changes, chest pain
Gastrointestinal	*Nausea (0.6%),* abdominal pain, vomiting, upset stomach, diarrhea
Dermatological	Pruritus, hives, rash, itching
Genitourinary	Premature ejaculation, difficulty maintaining an erection
Other	Dehydration, sweating, hyperventilation, dry mouth, renal failure, nipple tenderness

OVERDOSAGE

Signs and symptoms	Acute profound water loss; dehydration; hypovolemia; circulatory collapse; possible vascular thrombosis and embolism; electrolyte depletion, manifested by weakness, dizziness, mental confusion, anorexia, lethargy, vomiting, and cramps

BUMEX ■ LASIX

| Treatment | Replace fluid and electrolyte losses; carefully observe urinary output and electrolyte levels |

DRUG INTERACTIONS

Ototoxic drugs	△ Risk of ototoxicity (see WARNINGS/PRECAUTIONS)
Nephrotoxic drugs	△ Risk of nephrotoxicity; avoid concomitant use
Lithium	△ Risk of lithium toxicity, due to decreased renal clearance of lithium; avoid concomitant use
Probenecid	▽ Diuretic effects of bumetanide; natriuretic and hyperreninemic effects are reduced, because of decreased renal tubular secretion of bumetanide. Avoid concomitant use.
Indomethacin	▽ Diuretic effects of bumetanide; natriuretic and hyperreninemic effects are reduced. Avoid concomitant use.
Antihypertensive drugs	△ Antihypertensive effect; adjust dosage of antihypertensive drugs

ALTERED LABORATORY VALUES

| Blood/serum values | ▽ Sodium ▽ Chloride ▽ Potassium △ Uric acid ▽ Calcium △ Glucose △ BUN △ Creatinine △ Renin Changes in phosphorus, CO_2, bicarbonate, LDH, SGOT, SGPT, alkaline phosphatase, bilirubin (total), cholesterol, protein, and hemoglobin levels and in prothrombin time, hematocrit, WBC, platelet counts, differential counts, and creatinine clearance |
| Urinary values | △ Sodium △ Chloride △ Potassium ▽ Uric acid △ Calcium △ Glucose △ Protein △ Phosphate |

USE IN CHILDREN

Safety and effectiveness for use in children under 18 yr of age have not been established

USE IN PREGNANT AND NURSING WOMEN

Pregnancy Category C: use during pregnancy only if the expected benefit justifies the potential risk to the fetus. Bumetanide is not teratogenic in mice or rats given up to 100 mg/kg/day orally or up to ~ 10 mg/kg/day IV, in rabbits given 0.1 mg/kg/day orally, or in hamsters given 0.5 mg/kg/day orally. This drug is not embryocidal in mice given up to 100 mg/kg/day orally. In rats, a slight embryocidal effect has been observed at an oral dose of 100 mg/kg/day but not at doses of 30–60 mg/kg/day; in rabbits, a dose-related decrease in litter size and an increase in resorption rate have been observed at oral doses of 0.1 and 0.3 mg/kg/day. Maternal weight reduction, accompanied by moderate growth retardation and an increased incidence of delayed sternebral ossification, has been detected in rats given 100 mg/kg/day orally; no such effects have been detected in rats given 30 mg/kg/day. A slightly increased incidence of delayed sternebral ossification also occurred in the offspring of rabbits at an oral dose of 0.3 mg/kg/day; no such effect occurred at an oral dose of 0.03 mg/kg/day. Adverse effects on the fetus have not been reported in clinical use outside the United States and limited investigational use in the United States; however, no adequate, well-controlled studies have been performed in pregnant women. Thus, the possibility of adverse effects should not be ruled out. It is not known whether bumetanide is excreted in human milk; because this possibility remains, patients should not nurse while taking this drug.

LOOP DIURETICS

LASIX (furosemide) Hoechst-Roussel   Rx

Tablets: 20, 40, 80 mg   **Oral solution:** 10 mg/ml[1] (60, 120 ml) *orange flavored*   **Prefilled syringes:** 10 mg/ml (2, 4, 10 ml)
Ampuls: 10 mg/ml (2, 4, 10 ml)   **Vials:** 10 mg/ml (2, 4, 10 ml)

INDICATIONS

Edema associated with congestive heart failure, hepatic cirrhosis, or renal disease (including the nephrotic syndrome)

ORAL DOSAGE

Adult: 20–80 mg to start, followed, if needed, by increments of 20–40 mg q6–8h, up to 600 mg/day, until adequate diuresis ensues; for maintenance, give the titrated dose once or twice daily for 2–4 consecutive days of each week
Infant and child: 2 mg/kg to start, followed, if needed, by increments of 1–2 mg/kg q6–8h, up to 6 mg/kg, until adequate diuresis ensues; for maintenance, reduce the dose to the lowest effective level

PARENTERAL DOSAGE

Adult: 20–40 mg IM or IV (slowly) to start, followed, if needed, by increments of 20 mg q2h until adequate diuresis ensues; for maintenance, the dose finally arrived at may be repeated 1–2 times/day
Infant and child: 1 mg/kg IM or IV (slowly) to start, followed, if needed, by increments of 1 mg/kg q2h, up to 6 mg/kg, until adequate diuresis ensues; for maintenance, reduce dose to lowest effective level

LASIX

Acute pulmonary edema (adjunctive therapy)	—	**Adult:** 40 mg IV (slowly) to start, followed by 80 mg IV (slowly) 1 h later, if needed
Hypertension	**Adult:** 40 mg bid; adjust dosage according to patient response	—

CONTRAINDICATIONS

Anuria	Hypersensitivity to furosemide

ADMINISTRATION/DOSAGE ADJUSTMENTS

Intravenous administration	Inject slowly over a period of 1–2 min. If high parenteral doses are needed, dilute the drug in isotonic saline, lactated Ringer's, or 5% dextrose in water, adjust the pH if necessary, and administer as a controlled IV infusion at a rate not exceeding 4 mg/min. Do not mix furosemide with acidic solutions (pH < 5.5).
Combination antihypertensive therapy	Reduce dosage of other antihypertensive agents by at least 50% as soon as furosemide is added to the regimen to prevent an excessive fall in blood pressure; as blood pressure falls under furosemide's potentiating effect, a further reduction in dosage or discontinuation of other antihypertensive drugs may be required
Management of side effects	Reduce dosage or discontinue therapy if side effects are moderate or severe

WARNINGS/PRECAUTIONS

Monitoring of therapy	Serum electrolytes, CO_2, and BUN should be determined frequently during the first few months of therapy and periodically thereafter; correct any abnormalities, or withdraw drug temporarily. Patients should be observed regularly for the possible development of blood dyscrasias, liver damage, or other idiosyncratic reactions. Careful clinical and laboratory observation is particularly important if dosages exceeding 80 mg/day are given for prolonged periods.
Electrolyte depletion	May occur, especially with high dosages and salt restriction; monitor patients for hyponatremia, hypochloremic alkalosis, and hypokalemia; obtain serum and urine electrolyte determinations regularly, especially if patient is vomiting excessively or receiving parenteral fluids. Watch for dry mouth, thirst, weakness, lethargy, drowsiness, restlessness, muscle pain or cramps, muscular fatigue, hypotension, oliguria, tachycardia, arrhythmia, and GI disturbances.
Hypokalemia	May develop, especially with brisk diuresis, concomitant corticosteroid or ACTH therapy, interference with adequate oral intake of electrolytes, or in the presence of severe cirrhosis; effects may be exaggerated by digitalis. Hypokalemia may be prevented or treated with dietary measures, potassium supplements, or, if necessary, an aldosterone antagonist, such as spironolactone.
Ototoxicity	Furosemide has been reported to cause tinnitus and irreversible hearing impairment, generally when injection is rapid, dosage exceeds the recommended level, patients have severe renal impairment, or ototoxic drugs (such as ethacrynic acid and aminoglycosides) are given concomitantly (see DRUG INTERACTIONS)
Hyperuricemia or overt gout	May occur
Patients with hepatic cirrhosis	Sudden alterations of fluid and electrolyte balance in such patients may precipitate hepatic coma; strict observation is therefore essential. Patients with hepatic cirrhosis and ascites should be hospitalized before initiating furosemide therapy. In cases of hepatic coma and electrolyte depletion, improvement of the basic condition should be evident before the drug is used.
Patients with active or latent diabetes	Blood glucose concentration may be increased and glucose tolerance tests may be altered; check urine and blood glucose levels periodically. Precipitation of diabetes mellitus has been reported rarely in patients receiving furosemide.
Hypocalcemia	May occur and (rarely) lead to tetany; monitor serum calcium concentration periodically
Dehydration	May occur, causing an increase in the BUN level, especially in patients with renal impairment, and possibly resulting in hypovolemia, circulatory collapse, and vascular thrombosis and embolism, particularly in elderly patients
Orthostatic hypotension	May occur and may be aggravated by alcohol, barbiturates, or narcotics; instruct patients who experience orthostatic hypotension to stand up slowly
Concomitant indomethacin therapy	The natriuretic and antihypertensive effects of furosemide may be reduced by indomethacin; plasma renin levels and aldosterone excretion may also be affected by coadministration. Patients receiving both of these drugs should be closely observed to determine if the desired therapeutic effect of furosemide is being achieved.
Severe, progressive renal disease	If increasing azotemia and oliguria occur during treatment, discontinue therapy
Allergic reactions	May occur in patients with sulfonamide sensitivity
Systemic lupus erythematosus	May be activated or exacerbated
Diarrhea	May occur, especially in children, if large doses of the oral solution are given, due to large amount of sorbitol present in the vehicle

ADVERSE REACTIONS

Carcinogenicity, mutagenicity	Studies have not been done to evaluate the carcinogenic or mutagenic potential of this drug; no evidence of impaired fertility has been seen in rats given 8 times the maximum human dose
Gastrointestinal	Anorexia, oral and gastric irritation, nausea, vomiting, cramping, diarrhea, constipation, cholestatic jaundice, pancreatitis
Central nervous system	Dizziness, vertigo, paresthesias, headache, blurred vision, xanthopsia, tinnitus and hearing loss, muscle spasm, weakness, restlessness
Hematological	Anemia, leukopenia, thrombocytopenia; agranulocytosis and aplastic anemia (rare)
Hypersensitivity	Purpura, photosensitivity, rash, pruritus, urticaria, necrotizing angiitis, exfoliative dermatitis, erythema multiforme
Cardiovascular	Orthostatic hypotension
Other	Hyperglycemia, glycosuria, hyperuricemia, urinary bladder spasm, thrombophlebitis, transient pain at IM injection site

OVERDOSAGE

Signs and symptoms	Dehydration, hypovolemia, hypotension, electrolyte imbalance, hypokalemia, hypochloremic alkalosis
Treatment	Replace fluid and electrolyte losses; frequently check blood pressure and serum electrolyte and carbon dioxide levels. If the urinary bladder neck is obstructed, take measures to provide adequate drainage.

DRUG INTERACTIONS

Other antihypertensive agents	△ Antihypertensive effect
Digitalis glycosides	△ Digitalis toxicity
Steroids, ACTH	△ Risk of hypokalemia
Lithium	△ Risk of lithium toxicity; concomitant use should generally be avoided
Aminoglycosides, ethacrynic acid	△ Risk of ototoxicity; do not use concomitantly, except in life-threatening cases
Salicylates	△ Salicylate toxicity
Succinylcholine	△ Muscle relaxation
Tubocurarine	▽ Muscle relaxation
Norepinephrine	▽ Arterial responsiveness
Indomethacin	▽ Diuretic and/or antihypertensive effect of furosemide
Oral hypoglycemics	▽ Hypoglycemic effect
Alcohol, barbiturates, narcotics	△ Risk of orthostatic hypotension

ALTERED LABORATORY VALUES

Blood/serum values	△ Glucose △ BUN △ Uric acid ▽ Sodium ▽ Potassium ▽ Chloride ▽ Calcium ▽ Magnesium
Urinary values	△ Glucose △ Sodium △ Potassium △ Chloride

USE IN CHILDREN
See INDICATIONS and dosage recommendations. Renal calculi, including staghorn stones, have developed in some very premature infants given furosemide IV for edema owing to patent ductus arteriosus and hyaline membrane disease; chlorothiazide has been administered concomitantly to decrease hypercalciuria and dissolve some calculi.

USE IN PREGNANT AND NURSING WOMEN
Pregnancy Category C: use during pregnancy only when expected benefit justifies the potential risk to the mother and fetus. Administration of 2–8 times the maximum recommended human dose to rabbits has resulted in maternal deaths and abortions. No adequate, well-controlled studies have been done in pregnant women. Furosemide is excreted in human milk; use with caution in nursing mothers.

¹ Contains 11.5% alcohol

POTASSIUM-SPARING DIURETICS

ALDACTONE (spironolactone) Searle   Rx

Tablets: 25, 50, 100 mg

INDICATIONS
Edema associated with congestive heart failure, hepatic cirrhosis, or the nephrotic syndrome (adjunctive therapy)

ORAL DOSAGE
Adult: 25–200 mg/day, given in either single or divided daily doses, to start; recommended initial dosage: 100 mg/day
Child: 3.3 mg/kg/day (1.5 mg/lb/day), given in either single or divided daily doses, to start

ALDACTONE

Essential hypertension	**Adult:** 50–100 mg/day, given in either single or divided daily doses, to start, followed by larger or smaller doses until optimal response is achieved
Hypokalemia when oral potassium supplementation or other potassium-sparing regimens are deemed inappropriate or inadequate	**Adult:** 25–100 mg/day
Short-term treatment of **primary hyperaldosteronism** prior to surgery	**Adult:** 100–400 mg/day
Long-term maintenance of patients with discrete **inoperable aldosterone-producing adrenal adenomas** or bilateral micro- or macronodular **adrenal hyperplasia** (idiopathic hyperaldosteronism)	**Adult:** use lowest effective dosage

CONTRAINDICATIONS

Anuria	Significant renal impairment	Hyperkalemia
Acute renal insufficiency		

ADMINISTRATION/DOSAGE ADJUSTMENTS

Initiating therapy	For hypertension, continue initial dosage level for at least 2 wk; for edema, continue initial dosage level for at least 5 days. If response is inadequate, a second diuretic may be added.
Combination therapy	Effects of other diuretics or antihypertensive agents, especially ganglionic-blocking agents, are potentiated; reduce dosage of such agents by at least 50% when spironolactone is added to regimen
Diagnosis of hyperaldosteronism	*Long test:* Administer 400 mg/day for 3–4 wk; correction of hypokalemia and hypertension provides presumptive evidence of primary hyperaldosteronism. *Short test:* Administer 400 mg/day for 4 days; if serum potassium increases during spironolactone administration but drops when drug is discontinued, a presumptive diagnosis of primary hyperaldosteronism should be considered.

WARNINGS/PRECAUTIONS

Hyperkalemia	May occur in patients with impaired renal function or excessive potassium intake; avoid potassium supplements, potassium-rich food, and concomitant use of other potassium-sparing diuretics. Potentially fatal cardiac irregularities may occur. Significant hyperkalemia can be promptly corrected by rapid IV infusion of 20–50% glucose with regular insulin (0.25–0.50 units/g glucose); repeat, as needed; discontinue spironolactone and restrict potassium intake.
Hyponatremia	May be precipitated or may worsen, especially if other diuretics are given simultaneously. Observe patient for such symptoms as dry mouth, thirst, lethargy, and drowsiness; a low serum sodium level confirms the diagnosis.
Gynecomastia	May develop, especially with high dosages or prolonged therapy; usually reverses when drug is withdrawn. Rarely, some breast enlargement may persist.
Fluid and electrolyte imbalances	May develop; carefully evaluate patients for suggestive signs and symptoms
Mild acidosis	May occur during therapy; patients with decompensated hepatic cirrhosis may develop reversible hyperchloremic metabolic acidosis (usually with hyperkalemia), even in the presence of normal renal function
Transient elevation of BUN levels	May occur, especially in patients with preexisting renal impairment
Carcinogenicity, mutagenicity	In rats, spironolactone has caused proliferative effects, including malignant breast tumors, benign thyroid and testicular adenomas, hepatocytomegaly, and hyperplastic hepatic nodules. Breast cancer has been detected in women given spironolactone, but a causal relationship has not been established. Long-term studies in rats have shown an increase in myelocytic leukemia with potassium canrenoate, but not with spironolactone. (Both potassium canrenoate and spironolactone are metabolized to canrenone.) Potassium canrenoate has been mutagenic in several in vitro tests with mammalian cells, but has failed to produce such an effect in an in vivo mammalian system.

ADVERSE REACTIONS

Gastrointestinal	Cramping, diarrhea
Central nervous system	Drowsiness, lethargy, headache, mental confusion, ataxia, drug fever
Dermatological	Maculopapular or erythematous eruptions, urticaria, hirsutism
Hematological	Agranulocytosis
Endocrinological and genitourinary	Gynecomastia, irregular menses, amenorrhea, postmenopausal bleeding, impotence, deepening of voice[1]

OVERDOSAGE

Signs and symptoms	See ADVERSE REACTIONS

ALDACTONE ■ DYRENIUM

| Treatment | Discontinue medication; treat symptomatically and institute supportive measures, as required |

DRUG INTERACTIONS

Other antihypertensive agents	△ Antihypertensive effect
Norepinephrine	▽ Vasopressor effect; exercise caution when using norepinephrine and a general or regional anesthetic in a patient receiving spironolactone
Potassium supplements, other potassium-sparing diuretics	△ Risk of hyperkalemia
Digoxin	△ Risk of digoxin toxicity; carefully monitor serum digoxin level and, if necessary, reduce dosage of digoxin

ALTERED LABORATORY VALUES

| Blood/serum values | △ Digoxin (with RIA) ▽ Sodium △ Potassium ▽ Chloride △ BUN |
| Urinary values | △ Sodium ▽ Potassium △ Chloride |

USE IN CHILDREN

See INDICATIONS and ORAL DOSAGE

USE IN PREGNANT AND NURSING WOMEN

Safety for use during pregnancy has not been established. Spironolactone or its metabolites may cross the placental barrier. In general, diuretics should not be given to pregnant women except for pathologic edema; however, a short course of spironolactone therapy may be appropriate for hypervolemia-dependent edema that is causing extreme discomfort unrelieved by rest. Canrenone, a metabolite of spironolactone, is excreted in breast milk; patient should stop nursing if drug is prescribed.

[1] Breast carcinoma has also been reported, but a causal relationship has not been established

---

POTASSIUM-SPARING DIURETICS

DYRENIUM (triamterene) Smith Kline & French   Rx

Capsules: 50, 100 mg

INDICATIONS

Edema associated with congestive heart failure, hepatic cirrhosis, the nephrotic syndrome, steroid therapy, idiopathic causes, or secondary hyperaldosteronism

ORAL DOSAGE

Adult: 100 mg bid after meals to start, followed, if necessary, by up to 300 mg/day; when using this drug in combination with another diuretic or antihypertensive agent, reduce the initial daily dose of each drug

CONTRAINDICATIONS

Anuria	Severe hepatic disease	Hypersensitivity to triamterene
Severe or progressive renal disease or dysfunction (with the possible exception of nephrosis)	Concomitant use of other potassium-sparing preparations, such as spironolactone, amiloride, or medications containing triamterene (see DRUG INTERACTIONS)	Concomitant use of potassium supplements, potassium-rich diets, or potassium-containing salt substitutes (see DRUG INTERACTIONS)
Elevated serum potassium level		

ADMINISTRATION/DOSAGE ADJUSTMENTS

| Once-daily administration | If this drug is given once daily, it should be administered in the morning in order to minimize the frequency of nocturnal urination |

WARNINGS/PRECAUTIONS

| Hyperkalemia | Triamterene can cause hyperkalemia, which, in rare instances, may result in cardiac abnormalities. Hyperkalemia is more likely to occur if renal function is impaired or large doses are given for a considerable period of time. To avoid hyperkalemia, check BUN and serum potassium levels periodically; exercise particular care when using in elderly patients and those with diabetes or suspected or known renal insufficiency or azotemia. Bear in mind that a decrease in the serum potassium level, when seen during metabolic alkalosis, may result from a shift in the extracellular-intracellular potassium balance rather than from any change in total potassium stores.

If hyperkalemia occurs, discontinue use; if the serum potassium level remains above 6 mEq/liter, carefully monitor response. Obtain an ECG whenever hyperkalemia is seen or suspected; promptly institute treatment if an arrhythmia or widening of the QRS complex is present. For tachyarrhythmia, give 44 mEq of sodium bicarbonate or 10 ml of 10% calcium gluconate or calcium chloride by IV infusion over a period of several minutes; repeat dose, as needed. For asystole, bradycardia, or AV block, provide transvenous pacing. Excessive potassium may be removed by dialysis or administration of sodium polystyrene sulfonate. Glucose and insulin have also been used to treat hyperkalemia. |

DYRENIUM

Rebound kaliuresis	Withdraw drug gradually after intensive or prolonged therapy since it is theoretically possible that abrupt discontinuation under these circumstances may precipitate rebound kaliuresis
Hyponatremia	A low-salt syndrome may occur during therapy if salt intake is restricted
Cardiac failure, renal disease	Triamterene can cause or exacerbate electrolyte disturbances in patients with disorders such as cardiac failure or renal disease
Hypersensitivity	Allergic reactions, including blood dyscrasias and liver damage, have been reported in isolated cases; watch regularly for idiosyncratic reactions
Cirrhosis	Triamterene can cause or exacerbate electrolyte disturbances in patients with cirrhosis. In cirrhotic patients with splenomegaly and depleted folic acid stores, this drug may exacerbate cirrhosis and increase the risk of megaloblastic anemia; when using triamterene in these patients, watch for exacerbation of liver disease and perform blood studies periodically.
Azotemia	Triamterene can cause mild reversible nitrogen retention; this effect is seldom observed when the drug is given every other day. Check BUN level periodically, especially in patients with suspected or confirmed renal insufficiency.
Renal stones	Use with caution in patients with a history of renal stones, since triamterene has been detected in renal calculi
Hyperuricemia	Elevation of serum uric acid level can occur, especially in patients predisposed to gouty arthritis
Metabolic acidosis	Triamterene may deplete alkali reserves and produce metabolic acidosis
Carcinogenicity, mutagenicity, effect on fertility	No studies have been performed to determine the carcinogenic or mutagenic potential of triamterene; studies in rats given up to 30 times the human dose have shown no impairment of fertility

ADVERSE REACTIONS[1]

Metabolic	Hyperkalemia, hypokalemia
Hematological	Thrombocytopenia, megaloblastic anemia
Renal	Azotemia, elevated BUN and creatinine levels, renal stones, acute interstitial nephritis
Gastrointestinal	Jaundice, liver enzyme abnormalities, nausea, vomiting, diarrhea
Central nervous system	Weakness, fatigue, dizziness, headache, dry mouth
Hypersensitivity	Anaphylaxis, rash, photosensitivity

OVERDOSAGE

Signs and symptoms	Electrolyte imbalance (especially hyperkalemia), weakness, hypotension, GI disturbances (eg, nausea and vomiting)
Treatment	Immediately induce emesis and perform gastric lavage; carefully monitor electrolyte levels and fluid balance. Although this drug is 67% protein-bound, dialysis may be of some benefit.

DRUG INTERACTIONS

Lithium	⇧ Risk of lithium toxicity; exercise caution, closely monitor serum lithium levels, and adjust dosage of lithium, if necessary
Indomethacin, other nonsteroidal anti-inflammatory agents	⇧ Risk of acute renal failure; exercise caution
Captopril, amiloride, spironolactone, potassium supplements, potassium-containing medications (eg, penicillin G potassium), low-salt milk, salt substitutes, plasma or whole blood from blood banks	⇧ Risk of hyperkalemia, especially in patients with renal impairment; see CONTRAINDICATIONS
Sulfonylureas, insulin	⇩ Control of hyperglycemia; adjust dosage of hypoglycemic agents as needed ⇧ Risk of severe hyponatremia (with chlorpropamide only)
Antihypertensive drugs (including other diuretics), preanesthetics, anesthetics, nondepolarizing neuromuscular blockers	⇧ Pharmacologic effect of interacting drug

ALTERED LABORATORY VALUES

Blood/serum values	⇧ Glucose ⇧ Magnesium ⇧ Potassium ⇩ Sodium ⇧ Chloride ⇩ Bicarbonate ⇧ Uric acid ⇧ BUN ⇧ Creatinine ⇧ Liver enzymes ⇧ Plasma renin activity (PRA) Interference with fluorescent measurement of quinidine
Urinary values	⇧ Sodium ⇧ Calcium

USE IN CHILDREN

Safety and effectiveness for use in children have not been established. The normal serum potassium level in neonates, 7.7 mEq/liter, is considerably higher than the normal adult level of 3.5–5 mEq/liter.

USE IN PREGNANT AND NURSING WOMEN

Pregnancy Category B: studies in rats given up to 30 times the human dose of triamterene have shown no evidence of harm to the fetus; however, triamterene has been detected in the cord blood of animals and may appear in the cord blood of humans. Adverse reactions seen in adults may occur in utero. Use during pregnancy only if the expected benefits outweigh the potential risks to the fetus. Although this drug is generally used for pathological edema, it may also be given in a short course for edema due to pregnancy-induced hypervolemia when extreme discomfort associated with this form of edema cannot be relieved by rest. Do not use for toxemia of pregnancy or edema caused by uterine restriction of venous return. Triamterene has been detected in animal milk and may be excreted in human milk; patients should not nurse while taking this drug.

[1] All reactions occur rarely ($\leq$ 0.1%)

POTASSIUM-SPARING DIURETICS

MIDAMOR (amiloride hydrochloride) Merck Sharp & Dohme Rx

Tablets: 5 mg

INDICATIONS

Congestive heart failure or hypertension, as adjunctive therapy with kaliuretic diuretics to help restore normal serum potassium levels or to prevent hypokalemia in patients for whom hypokalemia would pose a particular risk (eg, those taking digitalis or those with significant cardiac arrhythmias)

ORAL DOSAGE

Adult: 5 mg/day, with food, to start, followed by 10 mg/day, if needed; if hypokalemia persists, dosage may be increased to 15 mg/day and then to 20 mg/day, with careful monitoring of serum electrolytes

CONTRAINDICATIONS

Hyperkalemia (serum potassium levels > 5.5 mEq/liter)	Potassium supplementation in the form of medication or a potassium-rich diet[1]	Anuria
Therapy with other potassium-conserving agents	Hypersensitivity to amiloride	Acute or chronic renal insufficiency
		Diabetic nephropathy

ADMINISTRATION/DOSAGE ADJUSTMENTS

Use of amiloride as the sole diuretic — Treatment with amiloride alone is rarely warranted; use amiloride alone only when persistent hypokalemia is documented and only with careful dosage titration and close monitoring of serum electrolyte levels; recommended dosage is same as for use as adjunctive therapy (see ORAL DOSAGE, above, and WARNINGS/PRECAUTIONS, below)

Congestive heart failure patients — After an initial diuresis has been achieved, potassium loss may also decrease, and the need for amiloride should be reevaluated; dosage adjustment may be necessary. Maintenance therapy may be intermittent.

WARNINGS/PRECAUTIONS

Hyperkalemia — May occur, particularly if amiloride is used without a kaliuretic diuretic agent or in the elderly or in patients with renal impairment or diabetes mellitus (with or without renal insufficiency); monitor serum potassium levels carefully in any patient receiving this drug, particularly at the start of therapy, at the time of diuretic dosage adjustment, and during any illness that might affect renal function. Warning signs and symptoms include paresthesias, muscular weakness, fatigue, flaccid paralysis of the extremities, bradycardia, shock, and ECG abnormalities. If hyperkalemia occurs, discontinue drug immediately and, if serum potassium level > 6.5 mEq/liter, take measures to reduce it; eg, administer sodium bicarbonate IV or glucose (orally or parenterally) with a rapid-acting insulin preparation, or, if needed, administer a cation exchange resin (eg, sodium polystyrene sulfonate) orally or by enema; persistent hyperkalemia may require dialysis.

Patients with renal impairment — Monitor serum electrolytes, serum creatinine, and BUN frequently in patients with BUN > 30 mg/dl or serum creatinine levels > 1.5 mg/dl

Patients with diabetes mellitus — Avoid use of this drug, if possible; if amiloride is administered, perform careful, frequent monitoring of serum electrolytes, serum creatinine, and BUN. Discontinue use at least 3 days before glucose tolerance testing.

MIDAMOR

Metabolic or respiratory acidosis	May be associated with rapid increases in serum potassium levels; use this drug with caution in severely ill patients in whom metabolic or respiratory acidosis may occur, such as patients with cardiopulmonary disease or poorly controlled diabetes, and monitor acid-base balance frequently
Increased BUN levels	Have occurred, usually in association with vigorous fluid elimination and especially when diuretic therapy was used in seriously ill patients (eg, those who had hepatic cirrhosis with ascites and metabolic alkalosis or those with resistant edema); when amiloride is given with other diuretics to such patients, monitor BUN levels carefully
Electrolyte imbalance	Hyponatremia and hypochloremia may occur when amiloride is used in combination with other diuretics; when such regimens are used in seriously ill patients, monitor serum electrolytes carefully
Hepatic encephalopathy and increased jaundice	Have been reported in association with the use of diuretics, including amiloride, in patients with preexisting severe liver disease
Carcinogenicity, mutagenicity	Amiloride showed no evidence of tumorigenicity when administered to mice for 92 wk at 25 times the maximum human dose, no evidence of carcinogenicity when administered to rats for 104 wk at 15–20 times the maximum human dose, and no evidence of mutagenicity as determined by the Ames test

ADVERSE REACTIONS[2]

Frequent reactions (incidence $\geq$ 1%) are printed in *italics*

Central nervous system	*Headache (3–8%); weakness, fatigue, dizziness, and encephalopathy ($<$ 3%)*; paresthesias, tremors, vertigo, nervousness, confusion, insomnia, decreased libido, depression, and somnolence ($\leq$ 1%)
Cardiovascular	Angina pectoris, orthostatic hypotension, arrhythmia, and palpitation ($\leq$ 1%)
Gastrointestinal	*Nausea/anorexia, diarrhea, and vomiting (3–8%); abdominal pain, gas pain, appetite changes, and constipation ($<$ 3%)*; jaundice, bleeding, abdominal fullness, thirst, heartburn, flatulence, dyspepsia, and dry mouth ($\leq$ 1%)[3]
Metabolic	*Hyperkalemia (10% when used without a kaliuretic diuretic; as low as 1–2% when used with a thiazide diuretic), hypochloremia, and hyponatremia* (see WARNINGS/PRECAUTIONS)
Dermatological	Skin rash, itching, and pruritus ($\leq$ 1%)
Musculoskeletal	*Muscle cramps ($<$ 3%)*, joint pain, leg ache, back pain, chest pain, neck/shoulder ache, and pain in the extremities ($\leq$ 1%)
Respiratory	*Cough and dyspnea ($<$ 3%)*; shortness of breath ($\leq$ 1%)
Genitourinary	*Impotence ($<$ 3%)*; polyuria, dysuria, urinary frequency, and bladder spasms ($\leq$ 1%)
Ophthalmic	Visual disturbances and increased intraocular pressure ($\leq$ 1%)
Other	Nasal congestion, tinnitus, and alopecia ($\leq$ 1%); aplastic anemia and neutropenia (rare; causal relationships not established)

OVERDOSAGE

Signs and symptoms	Dehydration and electrolyte imbalance are likely signs of overdose but have not been observed in clinical use
Treatment	Discontinue medication and empty stomach by emesis or gastric lavage. Treat symptomatically and institute supportive measures, as needed; there is no specific antidote. It is not known whether amiloride is dialyzable. Reduce serum potassium level if hyperkalemia develops (see WARNINGS/PRECAUTIONS).

DRUG INTERACTIONS

Lithium	▽ Renal clearance of lithium △ Risk of lithium toxicity
Potassium supplements, other potassium-sparing diuretics	△ Risk of hyperkalemia
Nonsteroidal anti-inflammatory agents	▽ Diuretic, natriuretic, and antihypertensive effects; observe patient closely during concomitant therapy to ensure that desired therapeutic effect is obtained
Indomethacin	△ Serum potassium levels; consider potential effects on potassium kinetics and renal function during concomitant therapy

ALTERED LABORATORY VALUES

Blood/serum values	△ Potassium △ BUN ▽ Sodium ▽ Chloride Abnormal liver function tests (rare; causal relationship not established)
Urinary values	▽ Potassium △ Sodium △ Chloride

USE IN CHILDREN

Safety and effectiveness for use in children have not been established

USE IN PREGNANT AND NURSING WOMEN

Pregnancy Category B: use during pregnancy only if clearly needed. Although there are no adequate, well-controlled studies in pregnant women, studies in rabbits and mice (given 20 and 25 times the maximum human dose, respectively) showed no evidence of fetal harm, and studies in rats (at 20 times the maximum human dose) showed no evidence of impaired fertility; however, a decrease in pup survival and growth was observed in rats following intrauterine exposure to amiloride. It is not known whether amiloride is excreted in human milk; because of the potential for serious adverse effects in nursing infants, either the mother should stop nursing or the drug should be discontinued.

---

[1] Except in severe and/or refractory cases, along with careful monitoring of the serum potassium level
[2] Based on clinical studies in the United States (837 amiloride-treated patients)
[3] Activation of a probable preexisting peptic ulcer has also been reported, but a causal relationship has not been established

DIAMOX

CARBONIC ANHYDRASE INHIBITORS

DIAMOX (acetazolamide) Lederle   Rx

Capsules (sustained release): 500 mg   **Tablets:** 125, 250 mg   **Vials:** 500 mg

INDICATIONS	ORAL DOSAGE	PARENTERAL DOSAGE
Chronic simple (open-angle) glaucoma (adjunctive therapy)	Adult: if capsules are used, 500 mg bid (AM and PM); if tablets are used, 250 mg to 1 g/24 h (divide daily doses > 250 mg)	Adult: 250 mg to 1 g/24 h IV (divide daily doses > 250 mg)
Secondary glaucoma (adjunctive therapy) and preoperatively for **acute angle-closure glaucoma**, where surgery is delayed in order to lower intraocular pressure	Adult: if capsules are used, 500 mg bid (AM and PM); if tablets are used, 250 mg q4h, or 500 mg to start, followed by 125 or 250 mg q4h; for short-term use, 250 mg bid may be sufficient	Adult: 250 mg IV q4h, or 500 mg IV to start, followed by 125 or 250 mg IV q4h; for short-term use, 250 mg bid may be sufficient
Edema associated with congestive heart failure (adjunctive therapy)	Adult: 250–375 mg (5 mg/kg) in a single morning dose to start, followed by 250–375 mg every other day or daily for 2 days at a time, alternating with a day of rest	Adult: 250–375 mg (5 mg/kg) IV in a single morning dose to start, followed by 250–375 mg IV every other day or daily for 2 days at a time, alternating with a day of rest
Drug-induced edema (adjunctive therapy)	Adult: 250–375 mg (5 mg/kg) every other day or daily for 2 days at a time, alternating with a day of rest	Adult: 250–375 mg (5 mg/kg) IV every other day or daily for 2 days at a time, alternating with a day of rest
Centrencephalic epilepsy (petit mal, unlocalized seizures; adjunctive therapy)	Adult: 8–30 mg/kg/day in divided doses; optimum dosage: 375 mg/day to 1 g/day in divided doses Child: same as adult	Adult: 8–30 mg/kg/day IV in divided doses; optimum dosage: 375 mg/day to 1 g/day IV in divided doses Child: same as adult
Prevention or amelioration of **acute mountain sickness** in climbers who are very susceptible or who are attempting a rapid ascent	Adult: 500–1,000 mg/day, in divided doses, beginning 24–48 h before ascent and continuing while at high altitude for 48 h or as long as needed; for rapid ascent, give 1,000 mg/day	

CONTRAINDICATIONS

Pregnancy	Marked kidney disease or dysfunction	Hyperchloremic acidosis
Hyponatremia	Marked liver disease or dysfunction	Chronic, noncongestive angle-closure glaucoma (prolonged therapy only)
Hypokalemia	Suprarenal gland failure	

ADMINISTRATION/DOSAGE ADJUSTMENTS

Use of sustained-release capsules	If glaucoma is not adequately controlled by the capsules, switch to the tablets or parenteral solution, which are given more frequently. The capsules are not indicated for treatment of edema or epilepsy.
Parenteral use	Intramuscular administration is painful because of the high pH; direct IV injection is recommended. Reconstitute contents of vial with at least 5 ml of sterile water for injection prior to use; the reconstituted solution is stable for 1 wk if refrigerated, but preferably should be used within 24 h of reconstitution.
Combination therapy for angle-closure glaucoma	Acetazolamide may be given with miotics or mydriatics, as needed
Combination anticonvulsant therapy	Initiate acetazolamide therapy at 250 mg/day, while maintaining dosage of existing anticonvulsant medications, followed by a gradual increase in the dosage of acetazolamide to the level recommended above

WARNINGS/PRECAUTIONS

Excessive dosage	May decrease diuresis and cause drowsiness or paresthesia; do not exceed recommended dosage (however, very high doses have been given with other diuretics to secure diuresis in certain cases of completely refractory heart failure)
Sulfonamide-related effects	Fever, crystalluria, renal stones, severe rash (including Stevens-Johnson syndrome and toxic epidermal necrolysis), and blood dyscrasias (including bone marrow depression, thrombocytopenic purpura, hemolytic anemia, leukopenia, pancytopenia, and agranulocytosis) can occur with use of sulfonamides. Watch for early signs and symptoms; determine CBC and platelet count regularly during therapy (obtain baseline counts before starting treatment). If significant changes in blood counts are seen or other early manifestations are detected, administration should be discontinued and appropriate therapy instituted.
Acidosis	May be precipitated or exacerbated in patients with impaired alveolar ventilation due to pulmonary obstruction or emphysema; long-term therapy may also produce acidosis, which can usually be corrected by administration of bicarbonate

Severe mountain sickness — If high-altitude pulmonary or cerebral edema occurs during rapid ascent, the climber should promptly descend; use of this drug does not obviate the need for such a measure

ADVERSE REACTIONS

Central nervous system and neuromuscular — Paresthesias (particularly a "tingling" sensation in the extremities), drowsiness, confusion, flaccid paralysis, convulsions

Renal — Polyuria, hematuria, glycosuria

Dermatological — Urticaria

Other — Fever, decreased appetite, acidosis (with long-term therapy), transient myopia, hepatic insufficiency, melena; photosensitivity (rare)

OVERDOSAGE

Signs and symptoms — See ADVERSE REACTIONS

Treatment — Discontinue medication; treat symptomatically and institute general supportive measures, as indicated

DRUG INTERACTIONS

Other diuretics — △ Diuretic effect and risk of hypokalemia

Lithium — △ Excretion, resulting in diminished pharmacologic activity of interacting drug

Aspirin (high doses) — Anorexia, tachypnea, lethargy, and coma; exercise caution during concomitant therapy

Amphetamines, ephedrine, pseudoephedrine, quinidine — ▽ Excretion, resulting in enhanced pharmacologic activity and/or prolonged duration of action of interacting drug

Methenamine — Inactivation of antimicrobial effect

Insulin, oral hypoglycemics — ▽ Hypoglycemic effect

Digitalis glycosides — △ Risk of cardiotoxicity due to hypokalemia

Amphotericin B, corticosteroids — △ Risk of severe hypokalemia

Phenytoin — △ Osteopenia

Primidone — ▽ Anticonvulsant effect

ALTERED LABORATORY VALUES

Blood/serum values — ▽ Sodium △ Chloride ▽ Bicarbonate △ Ammonia △ Bilirubin △ Uric acid ▽ Potassium ▽ ^{131}I thyroid uptake (in euthyroid and hyperthyroid patients only) △ Glucose (in prediabetic and diabetic patients)

Urinary values — △ Sodium △ Potassium ▽ Chloride △ Bicarbonate △ Phosphate ▽ Citrate ▽ Uric acid ▽ Ammonia △ Urobilinogen △ Glucose (in prediabetic and diabetic patients) + Protein (with bromophenol blue reagent, sulfosalicylic acid, heat and acetic acid, or nitric acid ring test methods) + 17-OHCS (with modified Glenn-Nelson technique)

USE IN CHILDREN
See INDICATIONS and dosage recommendations

USE IN PREGNANT AND NURSING WOMEN
Contraindicated during pregnancy, especially during the first trimester, unless expected benefits outweigh potential risk to the fetus. Acetazolamide has been shown to be embryocidal and teratogenic in rats and mice at doses exceeding 10 times the recommended human dose; however, there is no evidence of these effects in human beings. Consult manufacturer for use in nursing mothers.

DIURETIC COMBINATIONS

ALDACTAZIDE (spironolactone and hydrochlorothiazide) Searle   Rx

Tablets: 25 mg spironolactone and 25 mg hydrochlorothiazide; 50 mg spironolactone and 50 mg hydrochlorothiazide

INDICATIONS
Edema associated with congestive heart failure, hepatic cirrhosis, or the nephrotic syndrome (adjunctive therapy)

ORAL DOSAGE
Adult: 25–200 mg/day of each component (see WARNINGS/PRECAUTIONS), given in a single daily dose or divided; usual maintenance dosage: 100 mg/day of each component; additional spironolactone or hydrochlorothiazide may be administered, if necessary

Child: 0.75–1.5 mg spironolactone/lb/day (1.65–3.3 mg/kg/day) (see WARNINGS/PRECAUTIONS)

ALDACTAZIDE

Essential hypertension, when other measures are deemed inadequate or inappropriate	**Adult:** 50–100 mg/day of each component (see WARNINGS/PRECAUTIONS), given in a single daily dose or divided
Diuretic-induced hypokalemia in hypertensive patients, when other measures are deemed inappropriate	

CONTRAINDICATIONS

Anuria	Hyperkalemia	Hypersensitivity to hydrochlorothiazide or other sulfonamide derivatives
Acute renal insufficiency	Acute or severe hepatic failure (relative)	
Significant renal impairment		

WARNINGS/PRECAUTIONS

Fixed combination	Not indicated for initial therapy of edema or hypertension; dosages of component drugs must be individually titrated and then periodically reviewed, as conditions warrant
Hyperkalemia	May occur in patients with impaired renal function or excessive potassium intake; avoid potassium supplements, potassium-rich food, and concomitant use of other potassium-sparing diuretics. Potentially fatal cardiac irregularities may occur. Significant hyperkalemia can be promptly corrected by rapid IV infusion of 20–50% glucose with regular insulin (0.25–0.50 units/g glucose); repeat, as needed.
Electrolyte imbalance	Measure serum and urine electrolytes periodically, especially if patient is vomiting excessively or receiving parenteral fluids. Watch for dry mouth, thirst, weakness, lethargy, drowsiness, restlessness, muscle pain or cramps, muscular fatigue, hypotension, oliguria, tachycardia, and GI disturbances.
Hypokalemia	May develop, especially with brisk diuresis, concomitant loop diuretic, corticosteroid, or ACTH therapy, or interference with adequate oral intake of electrolytes; hypokalemia may result in digitalis cardiotoxicity at previously tolerated dosage levels
Dilutional hyponatremia	May be precipitated, especially if other diuretics are given simultaneously. Observe patient for tell-tale signs (dry mouth, thirst, lethargy, drowsiness); a low serum sodium level confirms diagnosis. Rarely, a true low-salt syndrome may develop, signaled by progressive mental confusion resembling that of hepatic coma; discontinue drug and administer sodium.
Gynecomastia	May develop, especially with high dosages or prolonged therapy; usually reverses when drug is withdrawn. Rarely, some breast enlargement may persist.
Hyperuricemia, gout, decreased glucose tolerance	May develop, due to thiazide-induced changes in metabolism of uric acid and carbohydrates; abnormal glucose metabolism may develop in latent diabetics or may worsen in diabetics
Postsympathectomy patients	Antihypertensive effect may be enhanced
Transient elevation of BUN levels	May occur; progressive rise in BUN suggests preexisting renal impairment
Parathyroid changes with hypercalcemia and hypophosphatemia	May occur with prolonged therapy
Systemic lupus erythematosus	May be activated or exacerbated
Reversible hyperchloremic metabolic acidosis (usually with hyperkalemia)	May develop in patients with decompensated hepatic cirrhosis, even in the presence of normal renal function
Carcinogenicity, mutagenicity	In rats, spironolactone has caused proliferative effects, including malignant breast tumors, benign thyroid and testicular adenomas, hepatocytomegaly, and hyperplastic hepatic nodules. Breast cancer has been detected in women given spironolactone, but a causal relationship has not been established. Long-term studies in rats have shown an increase in myelocytic leukemia with potassium canrenoate, but not with spironolactone. (Both potassium canrenoate and spironolactone are metabolized to canrenone.) Potassium canrenoate has been mutagenic in several in vitro tests with mammalian cells, but has failed to produce such an effect in an in vivo mammalian system.

ADVERSE REACTIONS

Gastrointestinal	Cramping, diarrhea, anorexia, nausea, vomiting, acute pancreatitis, jaundice
Central nervous system and neuromuscular	Drowsiness, lethargy, headache, mental confusion, dizziness, vertigo, paresthesias, ataxia, muscle spasm, weakness, restlessness
Ophthalmic	Xanthopsia, photosensitivity
Endocrine, genitourinary	Gynecomastia, impotence, irregular menses, amenorrhea, postmenopausal bleeding, deepening of voice[1]
Hematological	Purpura, thrombocytopenia, leukopenia, agranulocytosis, aplastic anemia
Cardiovascular	Orthostatic hypotension
Dermatological and hypersensitivity	Maculopapular or erythematous eruptions, pruritus, purpura, photosensitivity, urticaria, necrotizing angiitis, drug fever, erythema multiforme, hirsutism

ALDACTAZIDE ■ DYAZIDE

OVERDOSAGE

Signs and symptoms	Hyperkalemia, cardiac irregularities
Treatment	Discontinue drug; hyperkalemia can be promptly corrected by rapid IV infusion of 20–50% glucose with regular insulin (0.25–0.5 units/g glucose); repeat, as needed

DRUG INTERACTIONS

Other antihypertensive agents	△ Antihypertensive effect
Tubocurarine	△ Skeletal-muscle relaxation
Norepinephrine	▽ Vasopressor effect; exercise caution when using norepinephrine and a general or regional anesthetic in a patient receiving spironolactone
Steroids, ACTH	△ Risk of hypokalemia
Potassium supplements, other potassium-sparing diuretics	△ Risk of hyperkalemia
Digoxin	△ Risk of digoxin toxicity; carefully monitor serum digoxin level and, if necessary, reduce dosage of digoxin

ALTERED LABORATORY VALUES

Blood/serum values	△ Digoxin (with RIA) △ Uric acid △ Calcium ▽ Sodium △ Potassium ▽ Chloride △ BUN ▽ Bicarbonate ▽ Phosphate ▽ PBI △ or ▽ Glucose
Urinary values	△ Sodium ▽ Potassium △ Chloride △ Bicarbonate △ Uric acid ▽ Calcium

USE IN CHILDREN

See INDICATIONS and ORAL DOSAGE

USE IN PREGNANT AND NURSING WOMEN

Safety for use during pregnancy has not been established. Thiazides cross the placental barrier and appear in cord blood, and spironolactone may do so as well. In general, diuretics should not be given to pregnant women except for pathologic edema; however, a short course of diuretic therapy may be appropriate for hypervolemia-dependent edema that is causing extreme discomfort unrelieved by rest. Canrenone, a metabolite of spironolactone, and hydrochlorothiazide are excreted in human milk; use of this drug may cause fetal or neonatal jaundice, thrombocytopenia, and other possible reactions. Patient should stop nursing if drug is prescribed.

[1] Breast carcinoma has also been reported, but a causal relationship has not been established

---

DIURETIC COMBINATIONS

DYAZIDE (triamterene and hydrochlorothiazide) Smith Kline & French Rx

Capsules: 50 mg triamterene and 25 mg hydrochlorothiazide

INDICATIONS

Edema associated with congestive heart failure, hepatic cirrhosis, the nephrotic syndrome, corticosteroid and estrogen therapy, or idiopathic edema (adjunctive therapy)
Hypertension

ORAL DOSAGE

Adult: 1–2 caps bid after meals, up to 4 caps/day, if needed (see WARNINGS/PRECAUTIONS); some patients may be maintained on 1 cap once daily or every other day

CONTRAINDICATIONS

Anuria or progressive renal dysfunction, including increasing oliguria and azotemia

Therapy with other potassium-sparing diuretics

Preexisting hyperkalemia or hyperkalemia developing during therapy

Progressive hepatic dysfunction

Hypersensitivity to triamterene, hydrochlorothiazide, or other sulfonamide derivatives

ADMINISTRATION/DOSAGE ADJUSTMENTS

Combination antihypertensive therapy	If indicated, other antihypertensive agents may be added cautiously to regimen. Additions should be gradual; reduce starting dosage by at least 50%, particularly of ganglionic or peripheral adrenergic blockers, to prevent an excessive fall in blood pressure. Potassium supplementation should be discontinued unless triamterene component fails to compensate for potassium loss.

COMPENDIUM OF DRUG THERAPY

DYAZIDE

WARNINGS/PRECAUTIONS

Fixed combination	Not indicated for initial therapy of edema or hypertension; dosages of component drugs must be individually titrated and then periodically reviewed, as conditions warrant. Theoretically, a patient transferred to this preparation may show an increase in blood pressure, fluid retention, or an increase in serum potassium levels due to the 50% reduction in bioavailability of the hydrochlorothiazide component; however, in clinical practice, such conditions have not been commonly observed.
Hyperkalemia	May occur, especially in the severely ill, in those with small urine volumes ($<$ 1 liter/day), or in elderly or diabetic patients with known or suspected renal insufficiency; acute transient hyperkalemia has occurred during IV glucose-tolerance testing of triamterene-treated diabetics
Potassium supplementation	Should not be used concurrently unless hypokalemia develops or potassium intake is markedly impaired. If supplementation is needed, avoid potassium in tablet form: small-bowel lesions may occur with potassium tablets.
Electrolyte imbalance	May occur and can be intensified by concomitant therapy with amphotericin B, corticosteroids, or ACTH. Measure serum electrolytes and urine periodically, especially if patient is vomiting excessively or receiving parenteral fluids. Watch for dry mouth, thirst, weakness, lethargy, drowsiness, restlessness, muscle pain or cramps, muscular fatigue, hypotension, oliguria, tachycardia, and GI disturbances.
Hypokalemia	May occur rarely and may result in cardiotoxicity in patients being treated with digitalis; institute corrective measures (eg, potassium supplementation, an increased dosage of triamterene, and increased dietary potassium) with caution and frequent serum potassium determinations. If potassium level rises excessively, discontinue corrective measures immediately and substitute a thiazide alone for Dyazide until serum potassium level normalizes.
Azotemia	Reversible azotemia, characterized by elevation of the serum creatinine and/or BUN level, may occur; the azotemia results from reduction in the GFR or depletion of intravascular fluid volume rather than from renal toxicity and seldom develops with alternate-day therapy. If azotemia progresses, discontinue use (see CONTRAINDICATIONS). Periodic BUN and creatinine determinations are advisable, especially in the elderly and in those with suspected or confirmed renal insufficiency.
Renal stones	Triamterene has been detected in renal stones; use with caution in patients with a history of stone formation
Drug accumulation	This preparation may accumulate in patients with renal impairment
Hepatic coma	May be precipitated, possibly as a result of potassium depletion, in patients with severe liver disease; use with caution. Observe patient for signs of impending coma (eg, confusion, drowsiness, tremor); if mental confusion persists, withhold the drug for a few days. Other factors which might precipitate this condition include blood in the GI tract or preexisting potassium depletion.
Hyperuricemia or overt gout	May occur or be precipitated in certain patients
Blood dyscrasias, liver damage, other idiosyncratic reactions	May occur; monitor patients regularly
Insulin requirements	May increase, decrease, or remain unchanged; latent diabetes may become active
Apparent megaloblastosis	Cirrhotic patients with splenomegaly have marked hematological variations. Periodic blood studies should be performed; apparent megaloblastosis may be due to depletion of folic acid stores by folic acid antagonistic effect of drug.
Postsympathectomy patients	Antihypertensive effect may be enhanced
Metabolic acidosis	May occur due to depletion of alkali reserve
Quinidine serum-level determinations	Fluorescent measurement may be disturbed, owing to similarity of spectra of triamterene and quinidine; discontinue use of triamterene before measuring quinidine serum level
Concomitant therapy	Lithium generally should not be given concomitantly because diuretics reduce its renal clearance and increase the risk of toxicity; exercise caution if ACE inhibitors or nonsteroidal anti-inflammatory agents (especially indomethacin) are administered with triamterene (see DRUG INTERACTIONS)
Dilutional hyponatremia	May occur in edematous patients in hot weather; restrict water intake. Replace salt only for actual salt depletion or when hyponatremia is life-threatening.
Sensitivity reactions	May occur in patients with or without a history of allergy or bronchial asthma
Systemic lupus erythematosus	May be activated or exacerbated by hydrochlorothiazide component
Parathyroid function tests	Discontinue drug before testing parathyroid function; pathologic changes, with hypercalcemia and hypophosphatemia, may occur occasionally with prolonged use of thiazides

ADVERSE REACTIONS

Central nervous system	Weakness, dizziness, headache, paresthesias, vertigo
Ophthalmic	Xanthopsia, transient blurred vision

Gastrointestinal	Dry mouth, nausea and vomiting,[1] diarrhea, jaundice, pancreatitis, constipation, sialadenitis, other GI disturbances
Dermatological and hypersensitivity	Anaphylaxis, rash, urticaria, photosensitivity, purpura, necrotizing vasculitis, other skin conditions
Other	Muscle cramps, respiratory distress (including pneumonitis and pulmonary edema), renal stones; acute interstitial nephritis (rare)[2]

OVERDOSAGE

Signs and symptoms	Polyuria, nausea, vomiting, weakness, lassitude, fever, flushed face, hyperactive deep-tendon reflexes
Treatment	Discontinue medication; immediately empty stomach by emesis or gastric lavage. Maintain fluid and electrolyte balance; treat hypotension with pressor agents, such as norepinephrine. If hyperkalemia develops, discontinue drug and any potassium supplementation; substitute a thiazide alone, and obtain an ECG. Absence of arrhythmia or of widening of QRS complex indicates steps taken are sufficient; *widened QRS or arrhythmia in presence of hyperkalemia necessitates prompt additional therapy.* For tachyarrhythmia: give 44 mEq sodium bicarbonate or 10 ml of 10% calcium gluconate or calcium chloride IV over several minutes; for asystole, bradycardia, or AV block: also institute transvenous pacing, and repeat, as needed. Dialysis may be helpful in removing triamterene, even though it is largely protein-bound. In addition, dialysis or oral or rectal administration of sodium polystyrene sulfonate may be used to help remove excess potassium; infusion of glucose and insulin also may be used to treat hyperkalemia.

DRUG INTERACTIONS

Other antihypertensive agents	△ Antihypertensive effect
Spironolactone, amiloride, potassium salts, ACE inhibitors	△ Risk of hyperkalemia
Amphotericin B, ACTH, corticosteroids	△ Electrolyte imbalance, particularly hypokalemia
Oral anticoagulants	▽ Anticoagulant effect; adjust dosage accordingly
Tubocurarine	△ Skeletal-muscle relaxation
Norepinephrine	▽ Vasopressor effect
Lithium	▽ Lithium clearance
Indomethacin	Acute renal failure
Alcohol, barbiturates, narcotic analgesics	△ Risk of orthostatic hypotension

ALTERED LABORATORY VALUES

Blood/serum values	△ Uric acid △ Calcium ▽ Sodium △ Potassium ▽ Chloride △ Creatinine △ BUN △ or ▽ Glucose ▽ Folic acid ▽ PBI
Urinary values	△ Sodium ▽ Potassium △ Chloride △ Bicarbonate △ Uric acid ▽ Calcium △ Folic acid △ Glucose

USE IN CHILDREN

Safety and effectiveness for use in children have not been established

USE IN PREGNANT AND NURSING WOMEN

Safety for use during pregnancy has not been established. Thiazides cross the placental barrier and appear in cord blood. In rare instances, newborns whose mothers received thiazides during pregnancy developed thrombocytopenia, jaundice, or pancreatitis. In general, thiazides should not be given to pregnant women except for pathologic edema; however, a short course of diuretic therapy may be appropriate for hypervolemia-dependent edema that is causing extreme discomfort unrelieved by rest. Thiazides, and possibly triamterene as well, are excreted in human milk; patient should stop nursing if drug is prescribed.

[1] May indicate electrolyte imbalance; other nausea preventable by giving drug with meals
[2] Impotence has been reported, rarely, but a causal relationship has not been established

---

DIURETIC COMBINATIONS

MAXZIDE (triamterene and hydrochlorothiazide) Lederle   Rx
Tablets: 75 mg triamterene and 50 mg hydrochlorothiazide

INDICATIONS
Edema
Hypertension

ORAL DOSAGE
Adult: for hypokalemic patients receiving 50 mg/day of hydrochlorothiazide, as well as patients who require a thiazide diuretic but cannot risk hypokalemia (eg, because of concurrent digitalization or a history of arrhythmia), 1 tab/day (alone or with another antihypertensive agent); for patients receiving 50–100 mg/day of hydrochlorothiazide and 100–200 mg/day of triamterene in less bioavailable formulations, substitute 1 tab/day. A twofold increase in absorption of hydrochlorothiazide and triamterene will occur when patients are switched from less bioavailable formulations containing 25 mg of hydrochlorothiazide and 50 mg of triamterene to one-half of a Maxzide tablet (25 mg hydrochlorothiazide and 37.5 mg triamterene).

MAXZIDE

CONTRAINDICATIONS

Anuria, renal insufficiency, or significant renal impairment

Hypersensitivity to triamterene, hydrochlorothiazide, or other sulfonamide derivatives

Serum potassium level > 5.5 mEq/liter

Antikaliuretic therapy with potassium-sparing agents

Potassium supplements, potassium-containing salt substitutes, or potassium-enriched diets

WARNINGS/PRECAUTIONS

Hyperkalemia — The serum potassium level may exceed 5.5 mEq/liter during therapy, particularly in patients who are elderly or severely ill or who have renal impairment or diabetes; if hyperkalemia is not treated, death may occur. Frequently check the serum potassium level, especially when initiating therapy with this preparation, changing dosages, switching from less bioavailable formulations, or using this product in patients with disorders that affect renal function. Measure serum potassium and other electrolyte levels at frequent intervals in patients with mild renal impairment or with diabetes; in general, use in diabetic patients should be avoided (even when renal impairment is not evident). Since acidosis may be associated with hyperkalemia, frequently evaluate acid-base balance and serum electrolyte levels in severely ill patients who may be susceptible to respiratory or metabolic acidosis; use in such patients should generally be avoided.

If premonitory signs and symptoms of hyperkalemia, such as paresthesias, muscular weakness, fatigue, flaccid paralysis of the extremities, bradycardia, and shock, are observed during therapy, obtain an ECG and check the serum potassium level; it is important to determine the serum level because mild hyperkalemia may not be manifested by ECG changes. To treat hyperkalemia, immediately substitute a thiazide diuretic for this preparation, and, if the serum level exceeds 6.5 mEq/liter, take additional measures, including infusion of calcium chloride or sodium bicarbonate, oral or parenteral administration of glucose with a rapid-acting insulin preparation, and rectal or oral administration of a cation-exchange resin, such as sodium polystyrene sulfonate; if hyperkalemia persists, dialysis may be necessary.

Other electrolyte disorders — Dilutional hyponatremia may occur in edematous patients when the weather is hot; restrict the intake of water, and administer salt only if hyponatremia is life-threatening or actual salt depletion occurs. For hypochloremic alkalosis, specific treatment is usually unnecessary, except for certain patients (eg, those with hepatic or renal disease). Hypomagnesemia can also occur during therapy. Thiazides may cause hypokalemia and increase the risk of digitalis toxicity, expecially with brisk diuresis, if their use is prolonged; severe cirrhosis is present; ACTH, amphotericin B, or corticosteroids are given concomitantly; or oral intake of electrolytes is inadequate. (However, triamterene usually prevents thiazide-induced hypokalemia.) To avoid a fluid and electrolyte imbalance, measure serum and urinary electrolyte levels at appropriate intervals in all patients (these determinations are especially important and therefore should be done frequently if vomiting occurs or parenteral fluids are being given); watch for premonitory signs and symptoms, such as dry mouth, thirst, weakness, lethargy, drowsiness, restlessness, muscle pain or cramps, muscular fatigue, hypotension, oliguria, tachycardia, and GI disturbances (eg, nausea and vomiting).

Drug accumulation — Because of increased serum levels of hydrochlorothiazide and the active metabolite of triamterene, the risk of hyperkalemia and other reactions may be enhanced in patients who are elderly or have renal impairment

Azotemia — Elevation of BUN and/or serum creatinine levels may occur, probably owing to reduction of intravascular volume or glomerular filtration rate. Periodically measure BUN and serum creatinine levels, especially in patients who are elderly or when renal or hepatic impairment is known or suspected; if an increase in azotemia is detected, use of this preparation should be discontinued.

Renal stones — Triamterene has been detected in renal stones; use with caution in patients with a history of renal lithiasis

Megaloblastosis — Triamterene, a weak folic acid antagonist, may induce megaloblastosis in patients with reduced folic acid levels; perform blood studies periodically in such patients.

Hepatic coma — Minor changes in fluid and electrolyte balance may precipitate hepatic coma in patients with hepatic impairment or progressive liver disease; use with caution in such patients

Diabetes — Thiazides may activate latent diabetes or affect the insulin requirements of diabetic patients

Parathyroid dysfunction — Thiazides decrease calcium excretion. Discontinue therapy before performing parathyroid function tests. Pathological changes in the parathyroid gland, accompanied by hypercalcemia and hypophosphatemia, have occurred in a few patients after prolonged thiazide therapy; however, the common complications of hyperparathyroidism have not been seen.

Other thiazide-related effects — Thiazides may activate or exacerbate systemic lupus erythematosus, cause hyperuricemia or overt gout, or precipitate hypersensitivity reactions (even in patients without a history of allergy)

ADVERSE REACTIONS[1]

Gastrointestinal	Nausea, vomiting, diarrhea, constipation
Central nervous system	Drowsiness, fatigue, insomnia, muscle cramps and weakness, headache, appetite disturbances, dizziness, depression, anxiety
Other	Shortness of breath, chest pain, decreased sexual performance, dry mouth, urine discoloration

OVERDOSAGE

Signs and symptoms	Hyperkalemia, hypokalemia, hypochloremia, hyponatremia, dehydration, hypotension, nausea, vomiting, GI irritation, weakness, lethargy, coma
Treatment	Induce emesis or perform gastric lavage. Monitor serum electrolyte levels and fluid balance. Institute supportive measures, as needed, to maintain fluid and electrolyte balance and renal and cardiorespiratory function.

DRUG INTERACTIONS

Beta blockers, other antihypertensive drugs	△ Antihypertensive effect; if necessary, adjust dosage of antihypertensive drug used in combination with this preparation
Lithium	△ Risk of lithium toxicity; lithium generally should not be given with this preparation
Indomethacin, other nonsteroidal anti-inflammatory drugs	△ Risk of acute renal failure; exercise caution during concomitant therapy
Angiotensin-converting enzyme inhibitors	△ Risk of hyperkalemia; exercise caution during concomitant therapy
Norepinephrine, other vasopressors	▽ Vasopressor effect (however, this interaction does not preclude therapeutic use of vasopressors)
Tubocurarine, other nondepolarizing skeletal muscle relaxants	△ Skeletal muscle relaxation

ALTERED LABORATORY VALUES

Blood/serum values	△ Quinidine (with fluorometric assay) △ BUN △ Creatinine ▽ Sodium △ or ▽ Potassium △ Calcium ▽ Magnesium ▽ Chloride ▽ Phosphate △ Uric acid ▽ PBI △ or ▽ Glucose
Urinary values	△ Sodium △ or ▽ Potassium ▽ Calcium △ Magnesium △ Chloride △ Bicarbonate ▽ Uric acid △ or ▽ Glucose

---

USE IN CHILDREN

Safety and effectiveness for use in children have not been established

USE IN PREGNANT AND NURSING WOMEN

Pregnancy Category C: no reproduction studies in animals or pregnant women have been done with this preparation. Since adverse reactions, including jaundice, thrombocytopenia, and pancreatitis, may occur in a fetus or neonate following administration of thiazides during pregnancy, this preparation should not be used unless the expected benefit justifies the potential risk to the fetus. During pregnancy, this preparation can be administered not only for hypertension and pathological edema, but also, if given in a short course, for extreme discomfort that results from hypovolemic edema and that does not respond to rest. Do not use for toxemia of pregnancy or for dependent edema resulting from restriction of venous return by the expanded uterus. Thiazides are excreted in breast milk; patients should not nurse while taking this preparation.

---

[1] Reactions associated with use of an individual component of this preparation, but not with use of the combination product, include anorexia, gastric irritation, abdominal cramps, intrahepatic cholestatic jaundice, pancreatitis, sialadenitis, vertigo, paresthesias, xanthopsia, leukopenia, agranulocytosis, thrombocytopenia, aplastic anemia, hemolytic anemia, megaloblastosis, orthostatic hypotension, anaphylaxis, purpura, photosensitivity, rash, urticaria, vasculitis, cutaneous vasculitis, fever, respiratory distress (including pneumonitis), hyperglycemia, glycosuria, hyperuricemia, restlessness, and transient blurred vision

---

DIURETIC COMBINATIONS

MODURETIC (amiloride hydrochloride and hydrochlorothiazide) Merck Sharp & Dohme Rx

Tablets: 5 mg amiloride hydrochloride and 50 mg hydrochlorothiazide

INDICATIONS

Hypertension or congestive heart failure in patients who develop hypokalemia when thiazides or other kaliuretic agents are used alone, or for whom it is clinically important to maintain normal serum potassium levels (eg, those taking digitalis or those with significant cardiac arrhythmias), alone or as adjunctive therapy

ORAL DOSAGE

Adult: 1 tab/day, with food, to start, followed by 2 tabs/day, if needed, given in a single dose or divided. Once an initial diuresis is achieved, dosage adjustment may be necessary; maintenance therapy may be intermittent.

MODURETIC

CONTRAINDICATIONS

Hyperkalemia (serum potassium levels > 5.5 mEq/liter)

Hypersensitivity to amiloride, hydrochlorothiazide, or other sulfonamide-derived drugs

Concurrent potassium supplementation in the form of medication or a potassium-rich diet[1]

Concurrent therapy with other potassium-conserving agents

Anuria

Acute or chronic renal insufficiency

Diabetic nephropathy

WARNINGS/PRECAUTIONS

Fixed combination	This drug is not indicated for initial therapy of edema or hypertension, except in patients in whom the development of hypokalemia cannot be risked
Hyperkalemia	May occur, particularly in patients with renal impairment or diabetes mellitus (with or without renal insufficiency); monitor serum potassium levels carefully in any patient receiving this drug, particularly at the start of therapy, at the time of diuretic dosage adjustment, and during any illness that might affect renal function. Warning signs and symptoms include paresthesias, muscular weakness, fatigue, flaccid paralysis of the extremities, bradycardia, shock, and ECG abnormalities. If hyperkalemia occurs, discontinue use immediately and, if serum potassium level > 6.5 mEq/liter, take measures to reduce it, eg, administer sodium bicarbonate IV or glucose (orally or parenterally) with a rapid-acting insulin preparation, or, if needed, administer a cation exchange resin (eg, sodium polystyrene sulfonate) orally or by enema; persistent hyperkalemia may require dialysis.
Hypokalemia	May develop during thiazide therapy, especially with brisk diuresis, severe cirrhosis, concomitant corticosteroid or ACTH therapy, prolonged therapy, or interference with adequate oral electrolyte intake; hypokalemia can sensitize or exaggerate the heart's response to the toxic effects of digitalis
Carcinogenicity, mutagenicity	Amiloride showed no evidence of tumorigenicity when administered to mice for 92 wk at 25 times the maximum human dose, no evidence of carcinogenicity when administered to rats for 104 wk at 15–20 times the maximum human dose, and no evidence of mutagenicity as determined by the Ames test
Increased BUN levels	Have occurred, usually in association with vigorous fluid elimination and especially when diuretic therapy was used in seriously ill patients (eg, those who had hepatic cirrhosis with ascites and metabolic alkalosis or those with resistant edema); when this agent is given to such patients, monitor BUN levels carefully
Patients with renal impairment	Diuretics may precipitate azotemia, and cumulative effects of the components of this drug may develop. If used in patients with BUN > 30 mg/dl or serum creatinine level > 1.5 mg/dl, perform careful, frequent monitoring of serum electrolytes, serum creatinine, and BUN; if renal impairment becomes evident, discontinue use.
Patients with diabetes mellitus	Avoid use of this drug, if possible; hyperkalemia may develop, insulin requirements may be increased or decreased (or unchanged), and latent diabetes mellitus may become manifest. If drug is administered, perform careful, frequent monitoring of serum electrolytes, serum creatinine, and BUN. Discontinue use at least 3 days before glucose tolerance testing.
Systemic lupus erythematosus	May be activated or exacerbated
Sensitivity reactions	May occur in patients with or without a history of allergy or bronchial asthma
Electrolyte imbalance	Measure serum and urine electrolytes periodically, especially if patient is vomiting excessively or receiving parenteral fluids. Watch for dry mouth, thirst, weakness, lethargy, drowsiness, restlessness, muscle pain or cramps, muscular fatigue, hypotension, oliguria, tachycardia, and GI disturbances.
Hypochloremia	May occur but is usually mild and does not usually require specific therapy
Dilutional hyponatremia	May occur in edematous patients in hot weather; appropriate therapy is water restriction, rather than salt administration (except in rare cases, when the hyponatremia is life-threatening)
Hepatic encephalopathy and increased jaundice	Have been reported in association with the use of diuretic agents, including amiloride and hydrochlorothiazide, in patients with preexisting severe liver disease
Hypomagnesemia	May occur; however, bear in mind that the amiloride component of this preparation decreases the enhanced urinary excretion of magnesium caused by the thiazide component
Hyperuricemia	May occur or acute gout may be precipitated in certain patients on thiazide therapy
Parathyroid changes with hypercalcemia and hypophosphatemia	Have been reported in a few patients on prolonged thiazide therapy; however, the common complications of hyperparathyroidism have not been observed
Metabolic or respiratory acidosis	May be associated with rapid increases in serum potassium levels; use this drug with caution in severely ill patients in whom metabolic or respiratory acidosis may occur, such as patients with cardiopulmonary disease or poorly controlled diabetes, and monitor acid-base balance frequently

MODURETIC

ADVERSE REACTIONS

Frequent reactions (incidence ≥ 1%) are printed in *italics*

Central nervous system	*Headache, weakness, and dizziness (3–8%); fatigue/tiredness (1–3%)*, malaise, paresthesia/numbness, stupor, vertigo, insomnia, nervousness, depression, sleepiness, confusion, encephalopathy, tremors, restlessness
Cardiovascular	*Arrhythmia (1–3%)*, tachycardia, digitalis toxicity, orthostatic hypotension, angina pectoris, flush, palpitations, syncope
Digestive	*Nausea/anorexia (3–8%), diarrhea and gastrointestinal or abdominal pain (1–3%)*; constipation, bleeding, appetite changes, abdominal fullness, hiccups, thirst, vomiting, flatulence, bad taste sensation, abnormal liver function, activation of probable preexisting peptic ulcer, heartburn, dyspepsia, dry mouth, cramping, gastric irritation, jaundice, pancreatitis, sialadenitis
Metabolic	*Hyperkalemia (1–2% in patients without renal impairment or diabetes mellitus)*, gout, dehydration, glycosuria, hyperglycemia, hyperuricemia, electrolyte imbalance
Dermatological	*Rash (3–8%), pruritus (1–3%)*, itching, alopecia
Musculoskeletal	*Leg ache (1–3%)*; muscle cramps/spasm, joint pain, back pain, neck/shoulder ache, pain in the extremities
Respiratory	*Dyspnea (1–3%)*, nasal congestion, cough, shortness of breath
Genitourinary	Nocturia, dysuria, incontinence, impotence, decreased libido, polyuria, urinary frequency, bladder spasms, renal dysfunction (including renal failure)
Hematological	Aplastic anemia, neutropenia, agranulocytosis, hemolytic anemia, leukopenia, thrombocytopenia
Ophthalmic	Visual disturbances, increased intraocular pressure, transient blurred vision, xanthopsia
Hypersensitivity	Purpura, photosensitivity, urticaria, necrotizing angiitis, fever, respiratory distress (including pneumonitis and pulmonary edema), anaphylactic reactions
Other	Tinnitus, chest pain

OVERDOSAGE

Signs and symptoms	Dehydration and electrolyte imbalance are likely signs of overdose but have not been observed in clinical use
Treatment	Discontinue medication and empty stomach by emesis or gastric lavage. Treat symptomatically and institute supportive measures, as needed; there is no specific antidote. It is not known whether this drug is dialyzable. Reduce serum potassium levels if hyperkalemia develops (see WARNINGS/PRECAUTIONS).

DRUG INTERACTIONS

Other antihypertensive agents	△ Antihypertensive effect
Lithium	▽ Renal clearance of lithium △ Risk of lithium toxicity
Tubocurarine	△ Skeletal muscle relaxation
Nonsteroidal anti-inflammatory agents	▽ Diuretic, natriuretic, and antihypertensive effects; observe patient closely during concomitant therapy to ensure that desired therapeutic effect is obtained
Indomethacin	△ Serum potassium levels; consider potential effects on potassium kinetics and renal function during concomitant therapy
Corticosteroids, ACTH	△ Risk of hypokalemia

ALTERED LABORATORY VALUES

Blood/serum values	▽ PBI △ BUN △ Calcium ▽ Magnesium ▽ Phosphate △ or ▽ Potassium ▽ Sodium ▽ Chloride △ Uric acid ▽ Bicarbonate
Urinary values	▽ Calcium △ Magnesium △ or ▽ Potassium △ Sodium △ Chloride △ Bicarbonate △ Uric acid

USE IN CHILDREN

Safety and effectiveness for use in children have not been established

USE IN PREGNANT AND NURSING WOMEN

Pregnancy Category B: potential benefits of therapy must be weighed against possible fetal risk. Although there are no adequate, well-controlled studies of the effects of this combination agent in pregnant women, studies in rabbits and mice (given up to 25 times the maximum human dose) showed no evidence of fetal harm and studies in rats (at up to 25 times the maximum human dose) showed no evidence of impaired fertility; however, a decrease in body weight was observed in rat pups. Thiazides cross the placental barrier and may pose hazards to the fetus, including neonatal jaundice and thrombocytopenia. Hydrochlorothiazide is excreted in human milk; whether amiloride is also excreted in human milk is not known. Because of the potential for serious adverse effects in the nursing infant, either the mother should stop nursing or the drug should be discontinued.

[1] Except in severe and/or refractory cases of hypokalemia, along with careful monitoring of the serum potassium level

Chapter 37

Hormones

Androgens — 1550
DANOCRINE (Winthrop-Breon) — 1550
Danazol *Rx*

DEPO-Testosterone (Upjohn) — 1551
Testosterone cypionate *Rx*

HALOTESTIN (Upjohn) — 1553
Fluoxymesterone *Rx*

Estrogens — 1554
Diethylstilbestrol *Rx* — 1554

ESTRACE (Mead Johnson) — 1556
Estradiol *Rx*

ESTRACE Vaginal Cream (Mead Johnson) — 1556
Estradiol *Rx*

ESTRADERM (CIBA) — 1558
Estradiol *Rx*

ESTROVIS (Parke-Davis) — 1560
Quinestrol *Rx*

OGEN (Abbott) — 1562
Estropipate *Rx*

OGEN Vaginal Cream (Abbott) — 1562
Estropipate *Rx*

ORTHO Dienestrol Cream (Ortho) — 1564
Dienestrol *Rx*

PREMARIN (Ayerst) — 1566
Conjugated estrogens *Rx*

PREMARIN Vaginal Cream (Ayerst) — 1567
Conjugated estrogens *Rx*

TACE (Merrell Dow) — 1569
Chlorotrianisene *Rx*

Progestins — 1570
NORLUTATE (Parke-Davis) — 1570
Norethindrone acetate *Rx*

NORLUTIN (Parke-Davis) — 1570
Norethindrone *Rx*

PROVERA (Upjohn) — 1572
Medroxyprogesterone acetate *Rx*

Fertility Inducers — 1573
CLOMID (Merrell Dow) — 1573
Clomiphene citrate *Rx*

PARLODEL (Sandoz Pharmaceuticals) — 1574
Bromocriptine mesylate *Rx*

PERGONAL (Serono) — 1577
Menotropins *Rx*

PROFASI HP (Serono) — 1579
Chorionic gonadotropin, human (HCG) *Rx*

SEROPHENE (Serono) — 1580
Clomiphene citrate *Rx*

Prolactin Inhibitors — 1581
PARLODEL (Sandoz Pharmaceuticals) — 1581
Bromocriptine mesylate *Rx*

Growth Hormones — 1584
PROTROPIN (Genentech) — 1584
Somatrem *Rx*

Thyroid Hormones — 1585
ARMOUR Thyroid (Rorer) — 1585
Thyroid *Rx*

CYTOMEL (Smith Kline & French) — 1587
Liothyronine sodium *Rx*

EUTHROID (Parke-Davis) — 1590
Liotrix *Rx*

LEVOTHROID (Rorer) — 1591
T_4 thyroxine sodium *Rx*

LEVOTHROID Injection (Rorer) — 1591
T_4 thyroxine sodium *Rx*

PROLOID (Parke-Davis) — 1593
Thyroglobulin *Rx*

SYNTHROID (Flint) — 1594
Levothyroxine sodium *Rx*

THYROLAR (Rorer) — 1596
T_3 / T_4 liotrix *Rx*

Other Androgens — 1547
ANDROID (Brown) — 1547
Methyltestosterone *Rx*

DELATESTRYL (Squibb) — 1547
Testosterone enanthate *Rx*

METANDREN (CIBA) — 1547
Methyltestosterone *Rx*

ORA-TESTRYL (Squibb) — 1547
Fluoxymesterone *Rx*

ORETON Methyl (Schering) — 1548
Methyltestosterone *Rx*

Other Estrogens — 1548
DELESTROGEN (Squibb) — 1548
Estradiol valerate *Rx*

DEPO-ESTRADIOL (Upjohn) — 1548
Estradiol cypionate *Rx*

DV Cream (Merrell Dow) — 1548
Dienestrol *Rx*

ENOVID 10 mg (Searle) — 1548
Norethynodrel and mestranol *Rx*

ESTINYL (Schering) — 1548
Ethinyl estradiol *Rx*

MENEST (Beecham) Esterified estrogens Rx	1548
MENRIUM (Roche) Chlordiazepoxide and esterified estrogens Rx	1549
MILPREM (Wallace) Meprobamate and conjugated estrogens Rx	1549
PMB (Ayerst) Meprobamate and conjugated estrogens Rx	1549
Other Progestins	**1549**
AMEN (Carnrick) Medroxyprogesterone acetate Rx	1549
AYGESTIN (Ayerst) Norethindrone acetate Rx	1549
DEPO-PROVERA (Upjohn) Medroxyprogesterone acetate Rx	1549

OTHER ANDROGENS

DRUG	HOW SUPPLIED	USUAL DOSAGE[1]
ANDROID (Brown) Methyltestosterone Rx	**Tablets:** 10, 25 mg **Buccal tablets:** 5 mg	**Adult (male):** for primary or hypogonadotropic hypogonadism (congenital or acquired) or stimulation of puberty, 10–50 mg/day orally or 5–25 mg/day buccally **Adult (female):** for postpartum breast pain and engorgement, 80 mg/day orally or 40 mg/day buccally for 3–5 days; for breast cancer, 50–200 mg/day orally or 25–100 mg/day buccally
DELATESTRYL (Squibb) Testosterone enanthate Rx	**Vials:** 200 mg/ml (5 ml) **Disposable syringes:** 200 mg/ml (1 ml)	**Adult (male):** for hypogonadism, 50–400 mg IM every 2–4 wk; for stimulation of puberty, 50–200 mg IM every 2–4 wk **Adult (female):** for breast cancer, 200–400 mg IM every 2–4 wk
METANDREN (CIBA) Methyltestosterone Rx	**Tablets:** 10, 25 mg **Buccal tablets:** 5, 10 mg	**Adult (male):** for hypogonadism, climacteric symptoms, or impotence, 10–40 mg/day orally or 5–20 mg/day buccally; for postpubertal cryptorchidism, 30 mg/day orally or 15 mg/day buccally **Adult (female):** for postpartum breast pain and engorgement, 80 mg/day orally or 40 mg/day buccally for 3–5 days; for breast cancer, 200 mg/day orally or 100 mg/day buccally
ORA-TESTRYL (Squibb) Fluoxymesterone Rx	**Tablets:** 5 mg	**Adult (male):** for hypogonadism, 5–20 mg/day (usual dose: 10 mg/day); for stimulation of puberty, 2.5–20 mg/day (usual dose: 2.5–10 mg/day) **Adult (female):** for postpartum breast pain and engorgement, 2.5 mg to start, followed by 5–10 mg/day given in divided doses for 4–5 days; for breast cancer, 10–40 mg/day given in divided doses

continued

COMPENDIUM OF DRUG THERAPY

1547

OTHER ANDROGENS continued

DRUG	HOW SUPPLIED	USUAL DOSAGE[1]
ORETON Methyl (Schering) Methyltestosterone *Rx*	**Tablets:** 10, 25 mg **Buccal tablets:** 10 mg	**Adult (male):** for primary or hypogonadotropic hypogonadism (congenital or acquired) or stimulation of puberty, 10–50 mg/day orally or 5–25 mg/day buccally **Adult (female):** for postpartum breast pain and engorgement, 80 mg/day orally or 40 mg/day buccally for 3–5 days; for breast cancer, 50–200 mg/day orally or 25–100 mg/day buccally

OTHER ESTROGENS

DRUG	HOW SUPPLIED	USUAL DOSAGE
DELESTROGEN (Squibb) Estradiol valerate *Rx*	**Vials:** 10 mg/ml (5 ml), 20 mg/ml (5 ml), 40 mg/ml (5 ml) **Disposable syringes:** 20 mg/ml (1 ml)	**Adult:** for moderate to severe menopausal vasomotor symptoms, atrophic vaginitis, kraurosis vulvae, female hypogonadism or castration, or primary ovarian failure, 10–20 mg IM every 4 wk; for prevention of postpartum breast engorgement, 10–25 mg IM, given in a single dose at the end of the first stage of labor; for prostatic cancer, 30 mg or more IM every 1–2 wk
DEPO-ESTRADIOL (Upjohn) Estradiol cypionate *Rx*	**Vials:** 1 mg/ml (10 ml), 5 mg/ml (5 ml)	**Adult:** for moderate to severe menopausal vasomotor symptoms, 1–5 mg IM every 3–4 wk; for female hypogonadism, 1.5–2 mg IM once a month
DV Cream (Merrell Dow) Dienestrol *Rx*	**Cream:** 0.01% (3 oz)	**Adult:** 1 applicatorful 1–2 times/day for 1 or 2 wk, followed by ½ the initial dosage or 1 applicatorful every other day for an additional 1–2 wk; for maintenance, 1 applicatorful 1–3 times/wk
ENOVID 10 mg (Searle) Norethynodrel and mestranol *Rx*	**Tablets:** 9.85 mg norethynodrel and 0.15 mg mestranol	**Adult:** for endometriosis, 5–10 mg/day for 2 wk, beginning on 5th day of menstrual cycle, followed by increments of 5–10 mg at 2-wk intervals, up to 20 mg/day for 6–9 mo; for hypermenorrhea, 20–30 mg/day until bleeding is controlled, followed by 10 mg/day through 24th day of cycle
ESTINYL (Schering) Ethinyl estradiol *Rx*	**Tablets:** 0.02, 0.05, 0.5 mg	**Adult:** for moderate to severe menopausal vasomotor symptoms, 0.02–0.05 mg/day in 28-day cycles with 3 wk on and 1 wk off; some patients may require less or more (up to 0.05 mg tid) depending on severity; for female hypogonadism, 0.05 mg 1–3 times/day for 2 wk followed by a 2-wk course on progesterone; for prostatic cancer, 0.15–2.0 mg/day; for postmenopausal breast cancer, 1 mg tid
MENEST (Beecham) Esterified estrogens *Rx*	**Tablets:** 0.3, 0.625, 1.25, 2.5 mg	**Adult:** for moderate to severe menopausal vasomotor symptoms, 1.25 mg/day and for atrophic vaginitis or kraurosis vulvae, 0.3–1.25 mg/day, in 28-day cycles with 3 wk on and 1 wk off; for female hypogonadism, 2.5–7.5 mg/day, given in divided doses, for 20 days, followed by a rest period of 10 days; for female castration and primary ovarian failure, 1.25 mg/day, cyclically; for prostatic cancer, 1.25–2.5 mg tid; for male and postmenopausal breast cancer, 10 mg tid for 3 mo

OTHER ESTROGENS continued

DRUG	HOW SUPPLIED	USUAL DOSAGE
MENRIUM (Roche) Chlordiazepoxide and esterified estrogens *Rx*	**Tablets:** 5 mg chlordiazepoxide and 0.2 mg esterified estrogens (Menrium 5-2); 5 mg chlordiazepoxide and 0.4 mg esterified estrogens (Menrium 5-4); 10 mg chlordiazepoxide and 0.4 mg esterified estrogens (Menrium 10-4)	**Adult:** for menopausal syndrome or climacteric symptoms accompanied by anxiety and tension, 1 Menrium 5-2 tab tid in 28-day cycles with 3 wk on and 1 wk off; for more severe vasomotor manifestations, 1 Menrium 5-4 tab tid in 28-day cycles with 3 wk on and 1 wk off; for pronounced anxiety and tension and marked vasomotor complaints, 1 Menrium 10-4 tab tid in 28-day cycles with 3 wk on and 1 wk off
MILPREM (Wallace) Meprobamate and conjugated estrogens *Rx*	**Tablets:** 200 mg meprobamate and 0.45 mg conjugated estrogens (Milprem-200); 400 mg meprobamate and 0.45 mg conjugated estrogens (Milprem-400)	**Adult:** for moderate to severe menopausal vasomotor symptoms, atrophic vaginitis, or kraurosis vulvae accompanied by anxiety and tension, 1 Milprem-200 or Milprem-400 tab tid in 28-day cycles with 3 wk on and 1 wk off; adjust dosage as needed, up to 2,400 mg of meprobamate/day
PMB (Ayerst) Meprobamate and conjugated estrogens *Rx*	**Tablets:** 200 mg meprobamate and 0.45 mg conjugated estrogens (PMB 200); 400 mg meprobamate and 0.45 mg conjugated estrogens (PMB 400)	**Adult:** for moderate to severe menopausal vasomotor symptoms accompanied by anxiety and tension, 1 PMB 200 or PMB 400 tab tid in 28-day cycles with 3 wk on and 1 wk off; adjust dosage as needed, up to 6 PMB 200 or 4 PMB 400 tabs/day

OTHER PROGESTINS

DRUG	HOW SUPPLIED	USUAL DOSAGE
AMEN (Carnrick) Medroxyprogesterone acetate *Rx*	**Tablets:** 10 mg	**Adult:** for secondary amenorrhea, 10 mg/day for 10 days; for abnormal uterine bleeding due to hormonal imbalance in the absence of organic pathology, 10 mg/day for 10 days, from the 16th day of cycle
AYGESTIN (Ayerst) Norethindrone acetate *Rx*	**Tablets:** 5 mg	**Adult:** for secondary amenorrhea or abnormal uterine bleeding due to hormonal imbalance in the absence of organic pathology, 2.5–10 mg/day for 5–10 days during the second half of the theoretical menstrual cycle; for endometriosis, 5 mg/day for 2 wk, followed by an increase in dosage of 2.5 mg/day every 2 wk until level equals 15 mg/day; endometriosis therapy may be continued for 6–9 mo or until annoying breakthrough bleeding demands temporary suspension
DEPO-PROVERA (Upjohn) Medroxyprogesterone acetate *Rx*	**Prefilled syringes:** 400 mg/ml (1 ml) **Vials:** 100 mg/ml (5 ml), 400 mg/ml (2.5, 10 ml)	**Adult:** for adjunctive or palliative treatment of advanced, inoperable endometrial or renal carcinoma, 400–1,000 mg IM once weekly to start; for maintenance, 400 mg IM once monthly may be sufficient if disease appears to be stabilized

COMPENDIUM OF DRUG THERAPY

ANDROGENS

DANOCRINE (danazol) Winthrop-Breon Rx
Capsules: 50, 100, 200 mg

INDICATIONS	ORAL DOSAGE
Endometriosis amenable to hormonal management	**Adult:** for mild cases, 100–200 mg bid to start (adjust subsequent dosage depending upon patient response); for moderate to severe cases, 400 mg bid to start, followed (depending upon patient response) by a gradual reduction in dosage to a level sufficient to maintain amenorrhea
Fibrocystic breast disease	**Adult:** 50–200 mg bid for 2–6 mo; treatment may be reinstituted if symptoms recur after therapy is terminated
Hereditary angioedema, including cutaneous, abdominal, and laryngeal angioedema	**Adult:** 200 mg bid or tid to start, followed, after an initial satisfactory response is obtained, by a reduction in dosage of up to 50% at 1- to 3-mo intervals (or longer if indicated by frequency of attacks prior to treatment); monitor patient closely, particularly if there is a history of airway involvement. If an attack occurs, increase daily dosage by up to 200 mg.

CONTRAINDICATIONS

Pregnancy	Undiagnosed abnormal genital bleeding	Markedly impaired hepatic, renal, or cardiac function
Breast-feeding		

ADMINISTRATION/DOSAGE ADJUSTMENTS

Initiating therapy of endometriosis and fibrocystic breast disease	Begin therapy during menstruation, unless appropriate tests have been performed to rule out pregnancy
Duration of therapy for endometriosis	Continue therapy uninterrupted for at least 3–6 mo; if necessary, the drug may be given for up to 9 mo without interruption. If symptoms recur after treatment has been discontinued, it may be reinstituted.

WARNINGS/PRECAUTIONS

Breast carcinoma	Must be excluded before initiating treatment of fibrocystic breast disease or if any nodule persists or enlarges during therapy
Virilization	Monitor patient closely for signs of virilization (see ADVERSE REACTIONS); some androgenic effects may not be reversible even when therapy is stopped
Hepatic dysfunction	May occur in the form of elevated serum liver enzymes and/or jaundice, especially with dosages of 400 mg/day or more; perform liver function tests periodically and observe patient for clinical signs of hepatic impairment
Cholestatic jaundice, peliosis hepatitis	Have occurred following long-term therapy with chemically related steroids; attempt periodically to determine lowest dose that will provide adequate protection. If treatment was started during an exacerbation of angioneurotic edema due to trauma, stress, or other causes, consider decreasing or withdrawing therapy.
Fluid retention	May occur; patients with epilepsy, migraine, or cardiac or renal dysfunction should be closely observed
Suppression of ovulation	May not occur at the dosage recommended for fibrocystic breast disease; caution patients to use a nonhormonal method of contraception
Testicular atrophy	May occur; check semen for volume, vicosity, sperm count, and motility every 3–4 mo, especially if patient is an adolescent
Effects on lipoproteins	A decrease in the plasma HDL level and a possible increase in the LDL level have been observed during therapy; the clinical significance of these findings is not known

ADVERSE REACTIONS[1]

Dermatological	Acne, mild hirsutism, oily skin or hair
Endocrinological and metabolic	Decrease in breast size, deepening of the voice, edema, weight gain; irregular menstrual pattern and amenorrhea (dose-related)
Genitourinary	Vaginitis, including itching, dryness, burning, and vaginal bleeding; clitoral hypertrophy or testicular atrophy (rare)
Central nervous system	Nervousness and emotional lability
Hepatic	Elevated serum liver enzyme levels, jaundice
Other	Flushing, sweating

OVERDOSAGE
There have been no reports of acute overdosage in humans

DRUG INTERACTIONS

Oral anticoagulants	⇧ Prothrombin time

ALTERED LABORATORY VALUES

Blood/serum values —————————————— ▽ FSH ▽ LH △ C4 △ Liver enzymes

No clinically significant alterations in urinary values occur at therapeutic dosages

USE IN CHILDREN
Consult manufacturer

USE IN PREGNANT AND NURSING WOMEN
Contraindicated during pregnancy and for use in nursing mothers. If patient becomes pregnant during treatment, medication should be discontinued; continuing treatment may cause virilization of the female fetus (which, to date, has been limited to clitoral hypertrophy and lateral fusion of the external genitalia). Patients who become pregnant while taking danazol should be apprised of the potential risk to the fetus.

[1] Reactions for which no causal relationship has been established include urticaria, nasal congestion, headache, dizziness, depression, fatigue, sleep disorders, tremor, paresthesias, visual disturbances, anxiety, changes in appetite, chills, Guillain-Barre syndrome, gastroenteritis, nausea, vomiting, constipation, pancreatitis, muscle cramps or spasms, joint lockup, joint swelling; pain in the back, neck, or extremities; carpal tunnel syndrome, hematuria, prolonged posttherapy amenorrhea, thrombocytopenia, eosinophilia, leukocytosis, rashes (maculopapular, vesicular, papular, purpuric, petechial), hair loss, sun sensitivity, Stevens-Johnson syndrome, abnormal glucose tolerance test, increased insulin requirements in diabetic patients, changes in libido, elevated blood pressure, cataracts, bleeding gums, fever, pelvic pain, and nipple discharge

---

ANDROGENS

DEPO-Testosterone (testosterone cypionate) Upjohn   Rx

Vials: 50 mg/ml[1] (10 ml), 100 mg/ml (1, 10 ml), 200 mg/ml (1, 10 ml) for IM use only

INDICATIONS

Primary hypogonadism caused by orchidectomy or by testicular failure owing to cryptorchidism, bilateral torsion, orchitis, or vanishing testis syndrome

Hypogonadotropic hypogonadism caused by idiopathic gonadotropin or luteinizing hormone-releasing hormone deficiency or by hypothalamic or pituitary injury owing to tumors, trauma, or radiation

PARENTERAL DOSAGE

Adult: for replacement therapy, 50–400 mg IM every 2–4 wk

CONTRAINDICATIONS

Serious cardiac, hepatic, or renal disease	Breast cancer in men	Pregnancy
Hypersensitivity to testosterone	Prostate cancer	

ADMINISTRATION/DOSAGE ADJUSTMENTS

Administration	Inject dose deeply in the gluteal muscle
Induction of puberty in hypogonadal patients	Various regimens have been recommended for induction of puberty in hypogonadal patients. According to some experts, one should use a low dose initially, gradually increase it as puberty progresses, and then maintain or reduce it after puberty; according to others, one should use a higher dose to induce pubertal changes and a lower dose for maintenance after puberty. When determining the initial dose and subsequent adjustments, take into account both the chronological and skeletal ages of the patient.
Use of testosterone propionate	Testosterone cypionate should not be used interchangeably with testosterone propionate since the duration of action for the two drugs is different

WARNINGS/PRECAUTIONS

Hypercalcemia	Testosterone may cause hypercalcemia in immobilized patients; caution patients to report nausea or vomiting. If hypercalcemia is detected, drug should be discontinued.
Hepatotoxicity	Androgens can cause cholestatic jaundice and, after prolonged, high-dose therapy, can produce peliosis hepatis, a potentially life-threatening reaction. Caution patients to report any change in skin color.
Edema	Androgens cause salt and water retention; caution patients to report ankle swelling. Edema, either alone or with congestive heart failure, may be a serious complication of therapy in patients with cardiac, renal, or hepatic disease; do not use this drug in patients who have a serious form of one of these diseases.
Gynecomastia	During treatment of hypogonadism, gynecomastia may develop and occasionally may persist

DEPO-Testosterone

Reduction in mature height	By accelerating bone maturation in children without producing a proportionate increase in linear growth, androgens can prevent children from reaching their potential height at maturity; the younger the child, the greater this risk. Use of testosterone in children is not recommended. Exercise caution when treating delayed puberty in healthy adolescents; to monitor bone maturation, assess bone age of the wrist and hand every 6 mo.
Priapism, urethral obstruction	Androgens can cause excessive sexual stimulation or priapism; instruct patient to report persistent or too frequent penile erections. In patients with benign prostatic hypertrophy, androgens can precipitate acute urethral obstruction. If priapism, excessive sexual stimulation, or urethral obstruction occurs, therapy should be stopped; if treatment is resumed, the drug should be given at a lower dosage.
Polycythemia	During long-term therapy, periodically check hemoglobin level and hematocrit for evidence of polycythemia
Carcinogenicity	Prolonged, high-dose androgen therapy has been associated with hepatic adenoma and hepatocellular carcinoma; withdrawal of the drug has not always produced regression of the cancer. In elderly patients, androgens may enhance the risk of prostatic hypertrophy and prostate cancer (evidence is not conclusive). Implantation of testosterone in mice has resulted in cervical-uterine tumors, including some that metastasized. In rats, testosterone has increased the number of tumors and decreased the degree of differentiation of chemically-induced carcinomas of the liver. There is suggestive evidence that SC injection of testosterone can enhance the risk of hepatoma in some strains of female mice.
Impairment of fertility	Administration for a prolonged period or at an excessive dosage may cause oligospermia. If reaction occurs, therapy should be stopped; if treatment is resumed, the drug should be given at a lower dosage.

ADVERSE REACTIONS

Genitourinary	Priapism, frequent penile erections, change in libido, oligospermia
Dermatological	Hirsutism, male-patterned alopecia, seborrhea, acne
Gastrointestinal	Nausea
Hepatic	Cholestatic jaundice, abnormal liver function tests; hepatocellular carcinoma and peliosis hepatis (rare)
Hematological	Suppression of clotting factors II, V, VII, and X; polycythemia
Central nervous system	Headache, anxiety, depression, generalized paresthesia
Hypersensitivity	Anaphylactoid reactions, skin reactions
Local	Inflammation and pain at injection site
Other	Gynecomastia; retention of sodium, chloride, potassium, calcium, inorganic phosphates, and water

OVERDOSAGE

Acute overdosage has not been reported

DRUG INTERACTIONS

Oral anticoagulants	△ Risk of bleeding; a reduction in anticoagulant dosage may be necessary
Oxyphenbutazone	△ Serum oxyphenbutazone level
Insulin	△ Risk of hypoglycemia; a reduction in insulin dosage may be necessary

ALTERED LABORATORY VALUES

Blood/serum values	△ Cholesterol ▽ Total T_4 △ RT_3U △ RT_4U △ Sodium △ Chloride △ Potassium △ Calcium △ Phosphates
Urinary values	▽ Sodium ▽ Chloride ▽ Potassium ▽ Calcium ▽ Phosphates

USE IN CHILDREN

Use in children is not recommended; see warning above concerning reduction in height. Benzyl alcohol, the preservative used in the 100 and 200 mg/ml solutions, has been associated with a fatal gasping syndrome seen in premature neonates.

USE IN PREGNANT AND NURSING WOMEN

Pregnancy Category X: androgens are teratogenic; use in women who are or may become pregnant is contraindicated. Administration to nursing mothers is not recommended.

[1] Contains 5.4 mg/ml chlorobutanol as a preservative; this component may be habit-forming

ANDROGENS

HALOTESTIN (fluoxymesterone) Upjohn   Rx

Tablets: 2, 5, 10 mg

INDICATIONS

Primary hypogonadism caused by orchidectomy or by testicular failure owing to cryptorchidism, bilateral torsion, orchitis, or vanishing testis syndrome

Hypogonadotropic hypogonadism caused by idiopathic gonadotropin or luteinizing hormone-releasing hormone deficiency or by hypothalamic or pituitary injury owing to tumors, trauma, or radiation

Delayed puberty in male adolescents, when the disorder has been definitely established and is not just a familial trait

Recurrent breast cancer that has responded to oophorectomy or, alternatively, that is seen 1–5 yr after menopause and is androgen-responsive

ORAL DOSAGE

Adult: for replacement therapy, 5–20 mg/day, given once daily or in 3–4 divided doses, to start

Adolescent: give a low daily dose, once daily or in 3–4 divided doses, to start. Carefully titrate dosage; do not administer for more than 4–6 mo.

Adult: for palliative therapy, 10–40 mg/day, given in 3–4 divided doses for 2–3 mo

CONTRAINDICATIONS

Serious cardiac, hepatic, or renal disease

Hypersensitivity to fluoxymesterone

Breast cancer in men

Prostate cancer

Pregnancy

WARNINGS/PRECAUTIONS

Hypercalcemia — Fluoxymesterone may cause hypercalcemia in patients who have breast cancer or are immobilized. Caution patients to report nausea or vomiting; during breast cancer therapy, check urinary and serum calcium levels frequently. If hypercalcemia occurs, the drug should be discontinued.

Hepatotoxicity — Alkylated androgens can cause cholestatic hepatitis or jaundice and, after prolonged, high-dose therapy, can produce peliosis hepatis, a potentially life-threatening reaction. Caution patients to report any change in skin color; perform liver function tests periodically. If jaundice or hepatitis is detected, the drug should be discontinued; these reactions are reversible.

Edema — Androgens cause salt and water retention; caution patients to report ankle swelling. Edema, either alone or with congestive heart failure, may be a serious complication of therapy in patients with cardiac, renal, or hepatic disease; do not use this drug in patients who have a serious form of one of these diseases.

Gynecomastia — During treatment of hypogonadism, gynecomastia may develop and occasionally may persist

Reduction in mature height — By accelerating bone maturation in children without producing a proportionate increase in linear growth, androgens can prevent children from reaching their potential height at maturity. Use very cautiously when treating delayed puberty; every 6 mo, obtain x-rays of the wrist and hand and assess bone age.

Priapism, urethral obstruction — In male patients, androgens can cause excessive sexual stimulation or priapism. Instruct patients to report persistent or too frequent penile erections; priapism is a sign of excessive dosage. In patients with benign prostatic hypertrophy, androgens can precipitate acute urethral obstruction. If priapism, excessive sexual stimulation, or urethral obstruction occurs, therapy should be stopped; if treatment is resumed, the drug should be given at a lower dosage.

Virilization — During breast cancer therapy, watch for signs of virilization; reaction occurs commonly at high dosages. Instruct patients to report hoarseness, deepening of the voice, clitoral enlargement, or an increase in facial hair. A decision may be made to tolerate some virilization during treatment; however, bear in mind that to prevent irreversible effects, drug must be discontinued when mild signs are detected.

Acne, menstrual irregularities — Instruct women to report acne or any change in their menstrual period

Polycythemia — During long-term therapy, periodically check hemoglobin level and hematocrit for evidence of polycythemia

Carcinogenicity — Prolonged, high-dose androgen therapy has been associated with hepatic adenoma and hepatocellular carcinoma; withdrawal of the drug has not always produced regression of the cancer. In elderly patients, androgens may enhance the risk of prostatic hypertrophy and prostate cancer (evidence is not conclusive). Implantation of testosterone in mice has resulted in cervical-uterine tumors, including some that metastasized. In rats, testosterone has increased the number of tumors and decreased the degree of differentiation of chemically-induced carcinomas of the liver. There is suggestive evidence that SC injection of testosterone can enhance the risk of hepatoma in some strains of female mice.

HALOTESTIN ■ Diethylstilbestrol

Impairment of fertility	Administration for a prolonged period or at an excessive dosage may cause oligospermia. If reaction occurs, therapy should be stopped; if treatment is resumed, drug should be given at a lower dosage.
Tartrazine sensitivity	Presence of FD&C Yellow No. 5 (tartrazine) in tablets may cause allergic-type reactions, including bronchial asthma, in susceptible patients such as those hypersensitive to aspirin

ADVERSE REACTIONS

Genitourinary	Priapism, frequent penile erections, change in libido, oligospermia, menstrual irregularities (including amenorrhea)
Dermatological	Hirsutism, male-patterned alopecia, seborrhea, acne
Gastrointestinal	Nausea
Hepatic	Cholestatic jaundice, abnormal liver function tests; hepatocellular carcinoma and peliosis hepatis (rare)
Hematological	Suppression of clotting factors II, V, VII, and X; polycythemia
Central nervous system	Headache, anxiety, depression, generalized paresthesia
Hypersensitivity	Anaphylactoid reactions, skin reactions
Other	Virilization and inhibition of gonadotropin secretion in women, gynecomastia; retention of sodium, chloride, potassium, calcium, inorganic phosphates, and water

OVERDOSAGE

Acute overdosage has not been reported

DRUG INTERACTIONS

Oral anticoagulants	△ Risk of bleeding; a reduction in anticoagulant dosage may be necessary
Oxyphenbutazone	△ Serum oxyphenbutazone level
Insulin	△ Risk of hypoglycemia; a reduction in insulin dosage may be necessary

ALTERED LABORATORY VALUES

Blood/serum values	△ Cholesterol ▽ Total T_4 △ RT_3U △ RT_4U △ Sodium △ Chloride △ Potassium △ Calcium △ Phosphates
Urinary values	▽ Sodium ▽ Chloride ▽ Potassium ▽ Calcium ▽ Phosphates

USE IN CHILDREN
Use very cautiously in children; see warning above concerning reduction in height

USE IN PREGNANT AND NURSING WOMEN
Pregnancy Category X: androgens can cause virilization of the external genitalia of the female fetus; use in pregnant women is contraindicated. Administration to nursing mothers is not recommended.

ESTROGENS

Diethylstilbestrol   Rx

Tablets: 0.1, 0.25, 0.5, 1, 5 mg   **Tablets (enteric coated):** 0.1, 0.25, 0.5, 1, 5 mg

INDICATIONS

Moderate to severe **menopausal vasomotor symptoms**
Atrophic vaginitis
Kraurosis vulvae
Female hypogonadism
Female castration
Primary ovarian failure

ORAL DOSAGE

Adult: 0.2–0.5 mg/day, given in 28-day cycles with 3 wk on and 1 wk off; atrophic vaginitis may require up to 2 mg/day for several years of cyclic therapy

Palliation of inoperable, progressing, metastatic **breast cancer** in appropriately selected men and postmenopausal women

Adult: 15 mg/day

Palliation of inoperable, progressing **prostatic carcinoma**

Adult: 1–3 mg/day to start; for advanced cases, increase dosage as needed; usual maintenance dosage: 1 mg/day

CONTRAINDICATIONS

Known or suspected breast cancer (except when used in the treatment of metastatic disease)

Known or suspected estrogen-dependent neoplasia

Known or suspected pregnancy

History of thrombophlebitis, thrombosis, or thromboembolism associated with prior use of estrogen (except when used in the treatment of breast or prostatic malignancy)

Active thrombophlebitis or thromboembolic disorders

Undiagnosed abnormal genital bleeding

Diethylstilbestrol

ADMINISTRATION/DOSAGE ADJUSTMENTS

Pretreatment physical examination	Obtain a complete medical and family history before initiating estrogen therapy (see WARNINGS/PRECAUTIONS). Special attention during the physical examination should be given to blood pressure, breasts, abdomen, and pelvic organs; obtain a Papanicolaou smear.
Duration of postmenopausal therapy	For vasomotor symptoms, atrophic vaginitis, and kraurosis vulvae, attempt to discontinue or taper medication at intervals of 3–6 mo

WARNINGS/PRECAUTIONS

Malignant neoplasms	May occur with prolonged use; use with caution and closely monitor patients with a family history of breast cancer or with breast nodules, fibrocystic disease, or abnormal mammograms. Risk of endometrial carcinoma in postmenopausal women increases with duration of estrogen therapy and dose; provide close clinical surveillance and investigate all cases of undiagnosed, persistent, or recurrent abnormal vaginal bleeding for malignancy (see CONTRAINDICATIONS).
Gallbladder disease	Risk is increased 2–3 times in postmenopausal women treated with estrogens
Thromboembolic disease, thrombotic disorders, and other vascular problems	Risk is increased with dose; if feasible, discontinue medication at least 4 wk before elective surgery associated with an increased risk of thromboembolism or possibly requiring prolonged immobilization. Use with caution in patients with cerebrovascular or coronary artery disease and only when clearly needed. Large doses of estrogen (eg, 5 mg/day) have been shown to increase the risk of nonfatal myocardial infarction, pulmonary embolism, and thrombophlebitis in men.
Benign hepatic adenoma	Has occurred with use of estrogen-containing oral contraceptives, at times rupturing and resulting in intraabdominal hemorrhage and death, and should be considered in all cases of abdominal pain and tenderness, abdominal mass, or hypovolemic shock
Hepatocellular carcinoma	Has occurred with use of estrogen-containing oral contraceptives
Hypertension	Has occurred with use of estrogen-containing oral contraceptives and may occur with menopausal use of estrogens; monitor blood pressure during therapy, especially if high doses are used
Impaired glucose tolerance	Has been observed with use of estrogen-containing oral contraceptives; closely monitor patients with diabetes
Severe hypercalcemia	May develop in patients with breast cancer and bone metastases; discontinue medication and institute appropriate measures to reduce the serum calcium level
Fluid retention	May occur; use with caution in patients with convulsive disorders, migraine, asthma, or cardiac or renal dysfunction
Excessive estrogenic stimulation	May be manifested by abnormal or excessive uterine bleeding, mastodynia, or other reactions
Mental depression	Has occurred with use of oral contraceptives; as it is unclear whether this is due to the estrogenic or progestogenic component, patients with a history of mental depression should be monitored closely during estrogen therapy
Uterine leiomyomata	May increase in size
Altered cytology	Advise pathologist of estrogen therapy when submitting relevant specimens
Jaundice	Has recurred in patients with a history of jaundice with the use of estrogen-containing oral contraceptives; if jaundice develops with estrogen therapy, discontinue medication while cause is investigated
Special-risk patients	Use with caution in patients with hepatic impairment, renal insufficiency, or metabolic bone disease associated with hypercalcemia

ADVERSE REACTIONS[1]

Genitourinary	Breakthrough bleeding, spotting, change in menstrual flow, dysmenorrhea, premenstrual-like syndrome, amenorrhea during and after treatment, increase in size of uterine fibromyomata, vaginal candidiasis, change in cervical erosion and in degree of cervical secretion, cystitis-like syndrome
Endocrinological	Breast tenderness, enlargement, and secretion; altered libido
Gastrointestinal	Nausea, vomiting, abdominal cramps, bloating, cholestatic jaundice
Dermatological	Persistent chloasma or melasma, erythema multiforme, erythema nodosum, hemorrhagic eruption, loss of scalp hair, hirsutism
Ophthalmic	Steepening of corneal curvature, intolerance to contact lenses
Central nervous system	Headache, migraine, dizziness, mental depression, chorea
Other	Weight gain or loss, reduced carbohydrate tolerance, aggravation of porphyria, edema

OVERDOSAGE

Signs and symptoms	Nausea, withdrawal bleeding (see ADVERSE REACTIONS)

Diethylstilbestrol ■ ESTRACE

Treatment	Discontinue medication

DRUG INTERACTIONS

Oral anticoagulants	▽ Anticoagulant effect
Tricyclic antidepressants	△ Antidepressant side effects

ALTERED LABORATORY VALUES

Blood/serum values	△ Alkaline phosphatase △ Bilirubin △ Sulfobromophthalein retention △ Prothrombin △ Clotting factors VII, VIII, IX, and X ▽ Antithrombin III △ PBI △ Thyroxine (T₄) ▽ Triiodothyronine (T₃) uptake △ Glucose △ Cortisol △ Transcortin △ Ceruloplasmin △ Triglycerides △ Phospholipids ▽ Folic acid ▽ Pyridoxine
Urinary values	▽ Pregnanediol

USE IN CHILDREN

May cause premature epiphyseal closure; use with caution in young patients in whom bone growth is incomplete

USE IN PREGNANT AND NURSING WOMEN

Pregnancy Category X: contraindicated if pregnancy is known or suspected, as use of exogenous ovarian hormones during early pregnancy may cause serious fetal harm. Intrauterine exposure to these hormones, even for very brief periods, may increase the risk of congenital anomalies, including congenital heart defects and limb reduction defects. In addition, exposure in utero to diethylstilbestrol (and possibly other estrogens as well) has been shown to increase the risk of vaginal or cervical cancer developing in later life. Women who have taken this drug during pregnancy or who become pregnant while taking it should be apprised of the potential risks to the fetus and the advisability of continuing the pregnancy. Since many drugs are excreted in human milk, patients who are nursing should not be given this drug unless it is clearly needed.

[1] See WARNINGS/PRECAUTIONS regarding induction of neoplasia and increased incidence of gallbladder and thromboembolic disease

---

ESTROGENS

ESTRACE (estradiol) Mead Johnson   Rx

Tablets: 1, 2 mg

INDICATIONS	ORAL DOSAGE
Moderate to severe **menopausal vasomotor symptoms** **Atrophic vaginitis** **Kraurosis vulvae** **Female hypogonadism** **Female castration** **Primary ovarian failure**	Adult: 1–2 mg/day, given in 28-day cycles with 3 wk on and 1 wk off; adjust dosage, as necessary, to control presenting symptoms
Palliation of inoperable, progressing, metastatic **breast cancer** in appropriately selected men and postmenopausal women	Adult: 10 mg tid for a minimum of 3 mo
Palliation of inoperable, progressing **prostatic carcinoma**	Adult: 1–2 mg tid

ESTRACE Vaginal Cream (estradiol) Mead Johnson   Rx

Vaginal cream: 0.01% (42.5 g)

INDICATIONS	INTRAVAGINAL AND TOPICAL DOSAGE
Atrophic vaginitis **Kraurosis vulvae**	Adult: 2–4 g/day, given for 1–2 wk, followed by a gradual reduction to 1–2 g/day, given for 1–2 wk; for maintenance, 1 g may be given 1–3 times/wk. Administer cream in 28-day cycles with 3 wk on and 1 wk off.

CONTRAINDICATIONS

Known or suspected breast cancer (except when used in the treatment of metastatic disease)	History of thrombophlebitis, thrombosis, or thromboembolism associated with prior use of estrogen (except when used in the treatment of breast or prostatic malignancy)	Active thrombophlebitis or thromboembolic disorders
Known or suspected estrogen-dependent neoplasia		Undiagnosed abnormal genital bleeding
Known or suspected pregnancy		

ESTRACE

ADMINISTRATION/DOSAGE ADJUSTMENTS

Pretreatment physical examination	Obtain a complete medical and family history before initiating estrogen therapy (see WARNINGS/PRECAUTIONS). Special attention during the physical examination should be given to blood pressure, breasts, abdomen, and pelvic organs; obtain a Papanicolaou smear.
Duration of therapy	For vasomotor symptoms, atrophic vaginitis, and kraurosis vulvae, attempt to discontinue or taper medication at intervals of 3–6 mo

WARNINGS/PRECAUTIONS

Carcinogenicity	The risk of endometrial carcinoma in postmenopausal women is increased by prolonged use of estrogen; the degree of risk depends on the duration of treatment and the dose. Closely observe patients during therapy, and investigate for malignancy any case of persistent or recurrent abnormal vaginal bleeding that is undiagnosed. One study has suggested that estrogen enhances the risk of breast cancer in postmenopausal women; use with caution in patients with a strong family history of breast cancer or with breast nodules, fibrocystic disease, or abnormal mammograms. Hepatocellular carcinoma has been associated with use of estrogen-containing oral contraceptives, but a causal relationship has not been established. Long-term administration of estrogen has been found to produce carcinomas of the breast, vagina, cervix, and liver in animals.
Gallbladder disease	Risk is increased 2–3 times in postmenopausal women treated with estrogens
Thromboembolic disease, thrombotic disorders, and other vascular problems	Risk is increased with dose; if feasible, discontinue medication at least 4 wk before elective surgery associated with an increased risk of thromboembolism or during periods of prolonged immobilization. Use with caution in patients with cerebrovascular or coronary artery disease and only when clearly needed. Large doses of estrogen (eg, 5 mg/day) have been shown to increase the risk of nonfatal myocardial infarction, pulmonary embolism, and thrombophlebitis in men.
Benign tumors	Uterine leiomyomata may increase in size during therapy; benign hepatic adenomas have occurred with use of estrogen-containing oral contraceptives, at times rupturing and resulting in intraabdominal hemorrhage and death, and should be considered in all cases of abdominal pain and tenderness, abdominal mass, or hypovolemic shock
Hypertension	Has occurred with use of estrogen-containing oral contraceptives and may occur with menopausal use of estrogens; monitor blood pressure during therapy, especially if high doses are used
Impaired glucose tolerance	Has been observed with use of estrogen-containing oral contraceptives; closely monitor patients with diabetes
Severe hypercalcemia	May develop in patients with breast cancer and bone metastases; discontinue medication and institute appropriate measures to reduce the serum calcium level
Fluid retention	May occur; use with caution in patients with convulsive disorders, migraine, asthma, or cardiac or renal dysfunction
Excessive estrogenic stimulation	May be manifested by abnormal or excessive uterine bleeding, mastodynia, and other reactions
Mental depression	Has occurred with use of oral contraceptives; as it is unclear whether this is due to the estrogenic or progestogenic component, patients with a history of mental depression should be monitored closely during estrogen therapy
Altered cytology	Advise the pathologist of estrogen therapy when submitting relevant specimens
Jaundice	Has recurred with the use of estrogen-containing oral contraceptives in patients with a history of jaundice; if jaundice develops with estrogen therapy, discontinue medication while cause is investigated
Special-risk patients	Use with caution in patients with hepatic impairment, renal insufficiency, or metabolic bone disease associated with hypercalcemia
Tartrazine sensitivity	Presence of FD&C Yellow No. 5 (tartrazine) in 2-mg tablets may cause allergic-type reactions, including bronchial asthma, in susceptible individuals

ADVERSE REACTIONS[1]

Genitourinary	Breakthrough bleeding, spotting, change in menstrual flow, dysmenorrhea, premenstrual-like syndrome, amenorrhea during and after treatment, increase in size of uterine fibromyomata, vaginal candidiasis, change in cervical erosion and in degree of cervical secretion, cystitis-like syndrome
Endocrinological	Breast tenderness, enlargement, and secretion; altered libido
Gastrointestinal	Nausea, vomiting, abdominal cramps, bloating, cholestatic jaundice
Dermatological	Persistent chloasma or melasma, erythema multiforme, erythema nodosum, hemorrhagic eruption, loss of scalp hair, hirsutism
Ophthalmic	Steepening of corneal curvature, intolerance to contact lenses
Central nervous system	Headache, migraine, dizziness, mental depression, chorea

ESTRACE ■ ESTRADERM

| Other | Weight gain or loss, reduced carbohydrate tolerance, aggravation of porphyria, edema |

OVERDOSAGE

| Signs and symptoms | Nausea, withdrawal bleeding (see ADVERSE REACTIONS) |
| Treatment | Discontinue medication |

DRUG INTERACTIONS

| Oral anticoagulants | ▽ Anticoagulant effect |
| Tricyclic antidepressants | △ Antidepressant side effects |

ALTERED LABORATORY VALUES

| Blood/serum values | △ Alkaline phosphatase △ Bilirubin △ Sulfobromophthalein retention △ Prothrombin △ Clotting factors VII, VIII, IX, and X ▽ Antithrombin III △ PBI △ Thyroxine (T_4) ▽ Triiodothyronine (T_3) uptake △ Glucose △ Cortisol △ Transcortin △ Ceruloplasmin △ Triglycerides △ Phospholipids ▽ Folic acid ▽ Pyridoxine |
| Urinary values | ▽ Pregnanediol |

USE IN CHILDREN

May cause premature epiphyseal closure; use with caution in young patients in whom bone growth is incomplete

USE IN PREGNANT AND NURSING WOMEN

Pregnancy Category X: contraindicated if pregnancy is known or suspected, as use of exogenous ovarian hormones during early pregnancy may cause serious fetal harm. Intrauterine exposure to these hormones, even for very brief periods, may increase the risk of congenital anomalies, including congenital heart defects and limb reduction defects. In addition, exposure in utero to diethylstilbestrol (and possibly other estrogens as well) has been shown to increase the risk of vaginal or cervical cancer developing in later life. Women who have taken this drug during pregnancy or who become pregnant while taking it should be apprised of the potential risks to the fetus and the advisability of continuing the pregnancy. Since many drugs are excreted in human milk, patients who are nursing should not be given this drug unless it is clearly needed.

VEHICLE/BASE
Cream (nonliquefying): propylene glycol, stearyl alcohol, white ceresin wax, glyceryl monostearate, hydroxypropyl methylcellulose, sodium lauryl sulfate, methylparaben, disodium edetate, t-butylhydroquinone, and purified water

[1] See WARNINGS/PRECAUTIONS regarding induction of neoplasia and increased incidence of gallbladder and thromboembolic disease

---

ESTROGENS

ESTRADERM (estradiol) CIBA Rx

Transdermal drug delivery system: 0.05 mg/24 h (10 cm²), 0.1 mg/24 h (20 cm²)

INDICATIONS

Moderate to severe **menopausal vasomotor symptoms**
Female hypogonadism
Female castration
Primary ovarian failure
Atrophic conditions caused by deficient endogenous estrogen production, including **atrophic vaginitis** and **kraurosis vulvae**

TRANSCUTANEOUS DOSAGE

Adult: initially apply a 10-cm² system twice weekly to any clean, dry area of the skin on the trunk of the body, preferably the abdomen, that is not oily, damaged, or irritated; *avoid application to the breasts or the waistline.* Administer on a cyclic schedule (eg, 3 wk on therapy and 1 wk off), especially when the patient has not undergone a hysterectomy. Rotate the sites of application, leaving at least 1 wk between applications to a particular site.

CONTRAINDICATIONS

Known or suspected breast cancer	History of thrombophlebitis, thrombosis, or thromboembolism associated with prior use of estrogen	Active thrombophlebitis or thromboembolic disorders
Known or suspected estrogen-dependent neoplasia		Undiagnosed abnormal genital bleeding
Known or suspected pregnancy		

ESTRADERM

ADMINISTRATION/DOSAGE ADJUSTMENTS

Application	Apply the system immediately after opening the pouch and removing the protective liner; press the system firmly in place for about 10 s, making sure that good contact is made with the skin, especially around the edges. Should a system fall off, it may be reapplied or, if necessary, a new system may be used; continue the original treatment schedule.
Switching from oral estrogen	For women currently taking oral estrogen, initiate transdermal treatment 1 wk after withdrawal of oral therapy or sooner if symptoms reappear before the week's end
Dosage titration	Use the lowest effective dose to relieve symptoms
Duration of therapy	Attempt to discontinue or taper therapy at intervals of 3–6 mo
Patient monitoring	A Papanicolaou smear and a physical examination (with special attention to breasts, abdomen, pelvic organs, and blood pressure) should be done before therapy and then repeated at least annually
Concomitant progestin therapy	The addition of a progestin for 7 or more days (according to some studies, at least 12–13 days) during each cycle of estrogen replacement therapy may lower the incidence of endometrial hyperplasia (see WARNINGS/PRECAUTIONS); however, whether this addition will provide protection against endometrial carcinoma has not been clearly established. Although possible additional risks (eg, adverse effects on carbohydrate and lipid metabolism) may result from addition of a progestin, the choice of a particular progestin and dosage may minimize the risk.

WARNINGS/PRECAUTIONS

Carcinogenicity	The risk of endometrial carcinoma is increased by prolonged use ($>$ 1 yr) of estrogen; the degree of risk depends on the duration of treatment and the dose. Closely observe patients during therapy, and investigate for malignancy any case of persistent or recurrent abnormal vaginal bleeding that is undiagnosed. One study has suggested that estrogen enhances the risk of breast cancer in postmenopausal women; use with caution in patients with a strong family history of breast cancer or with breast nodules, fibrocystic disease, or abnormal mammograms. Hepatocellular carcinoma has been associated with use of estrogen-containing oral contraceptives, but a causal relationship has not been established. Long-term administration of estrogen has been found to produce carcinomas of the breast, vagina, cervix, and liver in animals.
Gallbladder disease	The risk of gallbladder disease is increased 2–3 times in postmenopausal women treated with oral estrogens
Thromboembolic disease, thrombotic disorders, and other vascular problems	The risk of thromboembolic disease, thrombotic disorders, and other vascular problems is increased with dose; if feasible, discontinue medication at least 4 wk before elective surgery associated with an increased risk of thromboembolism or during periods of prolonged immobilization. Use with caution in patients with cerebrovascular or coronary artery disease and only when clearly needed. Large doses of conjugated estrogens (5 mg/day) have been shown to increase the risk of nonfatal myocardial infarction, pulmonary embolism, and thrombophlebitis in men.
Benign tumors	Uterine leiomyomata may increase in size during prolonged therapy; discontinue use until a cause is established. Benign hepatic adenomas have occurred with use of estrogen-containing oral contraceptives, at times rupturing and resulting in intraabdominal hemorrhage and death, and should be considered in all cases of abdominal pain and tenderness, abdominal mass, or hypovolemic shock.
Hypertension	Elevated blood pressure has occurred with use of estrogen-containing oral contraceptives and may occur with menopausal use of estrogen; monitor blood pressure during therapy, especially if high doses are used
Glucose tolerance	Impaired glucose tolerance has been observed with use of estrogen-containing oral contraceptives; closely monitor patients with diabetes
Severe hypercalcemia	Patients with breast cancer and bone metastases may develop severe hypercalcemia; discontinue medication and institute appropriate measures to reduce the serum calcium level
Fluid retention	Estrogens may cause some degree of fluid retention; use with caution in patients with convulsive disorders, migraine, asthma, or in those with cardiac or renal dysfunction
Excessive estrogenic stimulation	Some patients may develop signs of excessive estrogenic stimulation, manifested by abnormal or excessive uterine bleeding, mastodynia, or other reactions; reduce dosage accordingly
Endometrial hyperplasia	Prolonged estrogen use may increase the risk of endometrial hyperplasia; use with caution in patients who have or have had endometriosis
Mental depression	Use of oral contraceptives has been associated with mental depression; as it is unclear whether this is due to the estrogenic or progestogenic component, patients with a history of mental depression should be monitored closely during estrogen therapy
Altered cytology	Advise the pathologist of estrogen therapy when submitting relevant specimens
Jaundice	Use of estrogen-containing oral contraceptives has been associated with a recurrence of jaundice in patients with a history of jaundice during pregnancy; if jaundice develops during estrogen therapy, discontinue use while the cause is investigated

ESTRADERM ■ ESTROVIS

Special-risk patients	Use with caution in patients with hepatic impairment, renal insufficiency, or metabolic bone disease associated with hypercalcemia

ADVERSE REACTIONS[1]

The most frequent reactions, regardless of incidence, are printed in *italics*

Genitourinary	Breakthrough bleeding, spotting, change in menstrual flow, increased size of uterine fibromyomata, change in cervical erosion and in degree of cervical secretion
Endocrinological	Breast tenderness and enlargement, altered libido
Dermatological	*Redness and irritation at the application site (17%)*
Gastrointestinal	Nausea, vomiting, abdominal cramps, bloating, cholestatic jaundice
Ophthalmic	Steepening of corneal curvature, intolerance to contact lenses
Central nervous system	Headache, migraine, dizziness
Other	Change in weight, edema

OVERDOSAGE

Signs and symptoms	Nausea, withdrawal bleeding
Treatment	Discontinue medication; treat symptomatically

DRUG INTERACTIONS

Oral anticoagulants	▽ Anticoagulant effect
Tricyclic antidepressants	△ Antidepressant side effects

ALTERED LABORATORY VALUES

Blood/serum values	△ Alkaline phosphatase △ Bilirubin △ Sulfobromophthalein retention △ Prothrombin time △ Clotting factors VII, VIII, IX, and X ▽ Antithrombin III △ Cortisol △ Transcortin △ Ceruloplasmin △ Triglycerides △ Phospholipids ▽ Folic acid ▽ Pyridoxine
Urinary values	▽ Pregnandiol

USE IN CHILDREN

Not indicated for use in children

USE IN PREGNANT AND NURSING WOMEN

Pregnancy Category X: contraindicated if pregnancy is known or suspected, as use of exogenous ovarian hormones during early pregnancy may cause serious fetal harm. Intrauterine exposure to these hormones, even for very brief periods, may increase the risk of congenital anomalies, including congenital heart defects and limb reduction defects. In addition, exposure in utero to diethylstilbestrol (and possibly other estrogens as well) has been shown to increase the risk of vaginal or cervical cancer developing in later life. Women who have taken this drug during pregnancy or who become pregnant while taking it should be apprised of the potential risks to the fetus and the advisability of continuing the pregnancy. It is not known whether this drug is excreted in human milk; because of the potential for serious adverse effects in nursing infants, women should not nurse during therapy.

[1] See WARNINGS/PRECAUTIONS regarding induction of neoplasia and increased incidence of gallbladder and thromboembolic disease

---

ESTROGENS

ESTROVIS (quinestrol) Parke-Davis   Rx

Tablets: 100 μg

INDICATIONS

Moderate to severe vasomotor symptoms associated with the menopause
Atrophic vaginitis
Kraurosis vulvae
Female hypogonadism
Female castration
Primary ovarian failure

ORAL DOSAGE

Adult: 100 μg/day, given in a single daily dose for 7 consecutive days, followed 2 wk after initiating therapy by 100 μg/wk for maintenance; if therapeutic response is not optimal or a greater response is desired, increase maintenance dosage to 200 μg/wk

ESTROVIS

CONTRAINDICATIONS

Known or suspected breast cancer (except when used in the treatment of metastatic disease)

Known or suspected estrogen-dependent neoplasia

Known or suspected pregnancy

History of thrombophlebitis, thrombosis, or thromboembolism associated with prior use of estrogen (except when used in the treatment of breast or prostatic malignancy)

Active thrombophlebitis or thromboembolic disorders

Undiagnosed abnormal genital bleeding

ADMINISTRATION/DOSAGE ADJUSTMENTS

Pretreatment physical examination	Obtain a complete medical and family history before initiating estrogen therapy (see WARNINGS/PRECAUTIONS). Special attention during the physical examination should be given to blood pressure, breasts, abdomen, and pelvic organs; obtain a Papanicolaou smear.
Duration of postmenopausal therapy	For vasomotor symptoms, atrophic vaginitis, and kraurosis vulvae, attempt to discontinue or taper medication at intervals of 3–6 mo

WARNINGS/PRECAUTIONS

Malignant neoplasms	May occur with prolonged use; use with caution and closely monitor patients with a family history of breast cancer or with breast nodules, fibrocystic disease, or abnormal mammograms. Risk of endometrial carcinoma in postmenopausal women increases with duration of estrogen therapy and dose; provide close clinical surveillance and investigate all cases of undiagnosed, persistent, or recurrent abnormal vaginal bleeding for malignancy (see CONTRAINDICATIONS).
Gallbladder disease	Risk is increased 2–3 times in postmenopausal women treated with estrogens
Thromboembolic disease, thrombotic disorders, and other vascular problems	Risk is increased with dose; if feasible, discontinue medication at least 4 wk before elective surgery associated with an increased risk of thromboembolism or during periods of prolonged immobilization. Use with caution in patients with cerebrovascular or coronary artery disease and only when clearly needed. Large doses of estrogen (eg, 5 mg/day) have been shown to increase the risk of nonfatal myocardial infarction, pulmonary embolism, and thrombophlebitis in men.
Benign hepatic adenoma	Has occurred with use of estrogen-containing oral contraceptives, at times rupturing and resulting in intraabdominal hemorrhage and death, and should be considered in all cases of abdominal pain and tenderness, abdominal mass, or hypovolemic shock
Hepatocellular carcinoma	Has occurred with use of estrogen-containing oral contraceptives
Hypertension	Has occurred with use of estrogen-containing oral contraceptives and may occur with menopausal use of estrogens; monitor blood pressure during therapy, especially if high doses are used
Impaired glucose tolerance	Has been observed with use of estrogen-containing oral contraceptives; closely monitor patients with diabetes
Severe hypercalcemia	May develop in patients with breast cancer and bone metastases; discontinue medication and institute appropriate measures to reduce the serum calcium level
Fluid retention	May occur; use with caution in patients with convulsive disorders, migraine, asthma, or cardiac or renal dysfunction
Excessive estrogen stimulation	May be manifested by abnormal or excessive uterine bleeding, mastodynia, or other reactions; reduce dosage accordingly
Mental depression	Has occurred with use of oral contraceptives; as it is unclear whether this is due to the estrogenic or progestogenic component, patients with a history of mental depression should be monitored closely during estrogen therapy
Uterine leiomyomata	May increase in size
Altered cytology	Advise the pathologist of estrogen therapy when submitting relevant specimens
Jaundice	Has recurred with use of estrogen-containing oral contraceptives in patients with a history of jaundice; if jaundice develops with estrogen therapy, discontinue medication while cause is investigated
Special-risk patients	Use with caution in patients with hepatic impairment, renal insufficiency, or metabolic bone disease associated with hypercalcemia

ADVERSE REACTIONS[1]

Genitourinary	Breakthrough bleeding, spotting, change in menstrual flow, dysmenorrhea, premenstrual-like syndrome, amenorrhea during and after treatment, increased size of uterine fibromyomata, vaginal candidiasis, change in cervical erosion and in degree of cervical secretion, cystitis-like syndrome
Endocrinological	Breast tenderness, enlargement, and secretion; altered libido
Gastrointestinal	Nausea, vomiting, abdominal cramps, bloating, cholestatic jaundice
Dermatological	Persistent chloasma or melasma, erythema multiforme, erythema nodosum, hemorrhagic eruption, loss of scalp hair, hirsutism

ESTROVIS ■ OGEN

Ophthalmic	Steepening of corneal curvature, intolerance to contact lenses
Central nervous system	Headache, migraine, dizziness, mental depression, chorea
Other	Weight gain or loss, reduced carbohydrate tolerance, aggravation of porphyria, edema

OVERDOSAGE

Signs and symptoms	Nausea, withdrawal bleeding (see ADVERSE REACTIONS)
Treatment	Discontinue medication

DRUG INTERACTIONS

Oral anticoagulants	▽ Anticoagulant effect
Tricyclic antidepressants	△ Antidepressant side effects

ALTERED LABORATORY VALUES

Blood/serum values	△ Alkaline phosphatase △ Bilirubin △ Sulfobromophthalein retention △ Prothrombin △ Clotting factors VII, VIII, IX, and X ▽ Antithrombin III △ PBI △ Thyroxine (T₄) ▽ Triiodothyronine (T₃) uptake ▽ Glucose △ Cortisol △ Transcortin △ Ceruloplasmin △ Triglycerides △ Phospholipids ▽ Folic acid ▽ Pyridoxine
Urinary values	▽ Pregnanediol

USE IN CHILDREN

May cause premature epiphyseal closure; use with caution in young patients in whom bone growth is incomplete.

USE IN PREGNANT AND NURSING WOMEN

Pregnancy Category X: contraindicated if pregnancy is known or suspected, as use of exogenous ovarian hormones during early pregnancy may cause serious fetal harm. Intrauterine exposure to these hormones, even for very brief periods, may increase the risk of congenital anomalies, including congenital heart defects and limb reduction defects. In addition, exposure in utero to diethylstilbestrol (and possibly other estrogens as well) has been shown to increase the risk of vaginal or cervical cancer developing in later life. Women who have taken this drug during pregnancy or who become pregnant while taking it should be apprised of the potential risks to the fetus and the advisability of continuing the pregnancy. Since many drugs are excreted in human milk, patients who are nursing should not be given this drug unless it is clearly needed.

[1] See WARNINGS/PRECAUTIONS regarding induction of neoplasia and increased incidence of gallbladder and thromboembolic disease

ESTROGENS

OGEN (estropipate) Abbott Rx

Tablets: 0.75 mg (Ogen .625), 1.5 mg (Ogen 1.25), 3 mg (Ogen 2.5), 6 mg (Ogen 5)

INDICATIONS	ORAL DOSAGE
Moderate to severe **menopausal vasomotor symptoms**	**Adult:** 0.75–6 mg/day, given in 28-day cycles with 3 wk on and 1 wk off, starting on the 5th day of bleeding if the patient is menstruating or arbitrarily if the patient has not menstruated for at least 2 mo
Atrophic vaginitis **Kraurosis vulvae**	**Adult:** 0.75–6 mg/day, given in 28-day cycles with 3 wk on and 1 wk off
Female hypogonadism	**Adult:** 1.5–9 mg/day, given in cycles of 29–31 days, with 3 wk on and 8–10 days off; bleeding does not occur by the end of rest period, repeat cycle at the same dosage. The number of cycles necessary to produce bleeding may vary. If satisfactory withdrawal bleeding does not occur, add an oral progestin during the 3rd wk of cycle.
Female castration **Primary ovarian failure**	**Adult:** 1.5–9 mg/day, given in cycles of 29–31 days, with 3 wk on and 8–10 days off

OGEN Vaginal Cream (estropipate) Abbott Rx

Vaginal cream: 0.15% (42.5 g)

INDICATIONS	INTRAVAGINAL DOSAGE
Atrophic vaginitis or kraurosis vulvae	**Adult:** 2–4 g/day, applied in 28-day cycles with 3 wk on and 1 wk off

CONTRAINDICATIONS

Known or suspected breast cancer	History of thrombophlebitis, thrombosis, or thromboembolism associated with prior use of estrogen	Active thrombophlebitis or thromboembolic disorders
Known or suspected estrogen-dependent neoplasia		Undiagnosed abnormal genital bleeding
Pregnancy	Hypersensitivity to any component of the cream	

ADMINISTRATION/DOSAGE ADJUSTMENTS

Pretreatment physical examination	Obtain a complete medical and family history before initiating estrogen therapy. Special attention should be given to blood pressure, breasts, abdomen, and pelvic organs; obtain a Papanicolaou smear.
Duration of postmenopausal therapy	For vasomotor symptoms, atrophic vaginitis, and kraurosis vulvae, attempt to discontinue or taper medication at intervals of 3–6 mo

WARNINGS/PRECAUTIONS

Carcinogenicity	The risk of endometrial carcinoma in postmenopausal women is increased by prolonged use (> 1 yr) of estrogen; the degree of risk depends on the duration of treatment and the dose. Closely observe patients during therapy, and investigate for malignancy any case of persistent or recurrent abnormal vaginal bleeding that is undiagnosed. A few retrospective studies have suggested that estrogen enhances the risk of breast cancer in postmenopausal women; use with caution in patients with a strong family history of breast cancer or with breast nodules, fibrocystic disease, or abnormal mammograms, and periodically perform a careful breast examination. Hepatocellular carcinoma has been associated with use of estrogen-containing oral contraceptives, but a causal relationship has not been established. Long-term administration of estrogen has been found to produce carcinomas of the breast, vagina, cervix, and liver in animals.
Gallbladder disease	Risk is increased 2–3 times in postmenopausal women treated with estrogens
Thromboembolic disease, thrombotic disorders, and other vascular problems	Risk is increased with dose; if feasible, discontinue medication at least 4 wk before elective surgery associated with an increased risk of thromboembolic disease or during periods of prolonged immobilization. Use with caution in patients with cerebrovascular or coronary artery disease and only when clearly needed. Large doses of estrogen (eg, 5 mg/day) have been shown to increase the risk of nonfatal myocardial infarction, pulmonary embolism, and thrombophlebitis in men.
Benign tumors	Uterine leiomyomata may increase in size during therapy; benign hepatic adenomas have occurred with use of estrogen-containing oral contraceptives, at times rupturing and resulting in intraabdominal hemorrhage and death, and should be considered in all cases of abdominal pain and tenderness, abdominal mass, or hypovolemic shock
Hypertension	Has occurred with use of estrogen-containing oral contraceptives and may occur with menopausal use of estrogens; monitor blood pressure during therapy, especially if high doses are used
Impaired glucose tolerance	Has been observed with use of estrogen-containing oral contraceptives; closely monitor patients with diabetes and, if necessary, adjust insulin dosage
Severe hypercalcemia	May develop in patients with breast cancer and bone metastases; discontinue medication and institute appropriate measures to reduce the serum calcium level
Fluid retention	May occur; use with caution in patients with convulsive disorders, migraine, asthma, or cardiac, or renal dysfunction
Excessive estrogenic stimulation	May be manifested by abnormal or excessive uterine bleeding, mastodynia, or other reactions
Mental depression	Has occurred with use of oral contraceptives; as it is unclear whether this is due to the estrogenic or progestogenic component, patients with a history of mental depression should be monitored closely during estrogen therapy
Altered cytology	Advise the pathologist of estrogen therapy when submitting relevant specimens
Jaundice	Has recurred with the use of estrogen-containing oral contraceptives in patients with a history of jaundice; if jaundice develops with estrogen therapy, discontinue medication while cause is investigated
Special-risk patients	Use with caution in patients with hepatic impairment, renal insufficiency, or metabolic bone disease associated with hypercalcemia

ADVERSE REACTIONS

Genitourinary	Increased size of uterine fibromyomata, vaginal candidiasis, cystitis-like syndrome, dysmenorrhea, amenorrhea during and after treatment, change in cervical erosion and degree of cervical secretion, breakthrough bleeding, spotting, change in menstrual flow, premenstrual-like syndrome
Endocrinological	Breast tenderness, enlargement, and secretion; altered libido
Gastrointestinal	Cholestatic jaundice, vomiting, nausea, abdominal cramps, bloating

OGEN ■ ORTHO Dienestrol Cream

Dermatological	Hemorrhagic eruption, erythema nodosum, erythema multiforme, hirsutism, persistent chloasma or melasma, loss of scalp hair; local irritation (particularly when cream is applied to inflamed area)
Ophthalmic	Steepening of corneal curvature, intolerance to contact lenses
Central nervous system	Chorea, mental depression, migraine, dizziness, headache
Other	Aggravation of porphyria, edema, reduced carbohydrate tolerance, weight gain or loss

OVERDOSAGE

Signs and symptoms	Nausea, withdrawal bleeding (see ADVERSE REACTIONS)
Treatment	Discontinue medication

DRUG INTERACTIONS

Oral anticoagulants	▽ Anticoagulant effect
Rifampin, carbamazepine, phenobarbital, phenytoin, primidone, and other hepatic enzyme-inducing drugs	▽ Pharmacologic effects of estrogen
Broad-spectrum antibiotics that profoundly affect intestinal flora	▽ Absorption of oral estrogen

ALTERED LABORATORY VALUES

Blood/serum values	△ Alkaline phosphatase △ Bilirubin △ Sulfobromophthalein retention △ Prothrombin △ Clotting factors VII, VIII, IX, and X ▽ Antithrombin III △ PBI △ Thyroxine (T_4) ▽ Triiodothyronine (T_3) uptake △ Glucose △ Cortisol △ Transcortin △ Ceruloplasmin △ Triglycerides △ Phospholipids ▽ Folic acid ▽ Pyridoxine
Urinary values	▽ Pregnanediol

USE IN CHILDREN

May cause premature epiphyseal closure; use with caution in young patients in whom bone growth is incomplete

USE IN PREGNANT AND NURSING WOMEN

Pregnancy Category X: contraindicated for use in women who are or may become pregnant because use of exogenous ovarian hormones during early pregnancy may cause serious fetal harm. Intrauterine exposure to these hormones, even for very brief periods, may increase the risk of congenital anomalies, including congenital heart defects and limb reduction defects. In addition, exposure in utero to diethylstilbestrol (and possibly other estrogens as well) has been shown to increase the risk of vaginal or cervical cancer developing in later life. Women who have taken this drug during pregnancy or who become pregnant while taking it should be apprised of the potential risks to the fetus and the advisability of continuing the pregnancy. Estrogens are excreted in human milk; use with caution in nursing mothers.

VEHICLE/BASE
Cream: glycerin, mineral oil, glyceryl monostearate, polyethylene glycol ether complex of higher fatty alcohols, cetyl alcohol, anhydrous lanolin, sodium biphosphate, cis-N-(3-chloroallyl) hexaminium chloride, propylparaben, methylparaben, piperazine hexahydrate, citric acid, and water

---

ESTROGENS

ORTHO Dienestrol Cream (dienestrol) Ortho Rx

Vaginal cream: 0.01% (78 g)

INDICATIONS

Atrophic vaginitis
Kraurosis vulvae

INTRAVAGINAL DOSAGE

Adult: 1–2 applicatorsful/day for 1–2 wk, followed by a gradual reduction in dosage to ½–1 applicatorful/day for 1–2 wk, then repeat cycle; usual maintenance dosage: 1 applicatorful 1–3 times/wk

CONTRAINDICATIONS

Known or suspected breast cancer

Known or suspected estrogen-dependent neoplasia

Pregnancy

History of thrombophlebitis, thrombosis, or thromboembolism associated with prior use of estrogen

Active thrombophlebitis or thromboembolic disorders

Undiagnosed abnormal genital bleeding

ORTHO Dienestrol Cream

ADMINISTRATION/DOSAGE ADJUSTMENTS

Pretreatment physical examination	Obtain a complete medical and family history before initiating estrogen therapy (see WARNINGS/PRECAUTIONS). Special attention during the physical examination should be given to blood pressure, breasts, abdomen, and pelvic organs; obtain a Papanicolaou smear.
Duration of therapy	Attempt to discontinue or taper medication at intervals of 3–6 mo
Concomitant progestin therapy	The addition of a progestin for 7 or more days (according to some studies, at least 12–13 days) during each cycle of estrogen replacement therapy may lower the incidence of endometrial hyperplasia (see WARNINGS/PRECAUTIONS); however, whether this addition will provide protection against endometrial carcinoma has not been clearly established. Although possible additional risks (eg, adverse effects on carbohydrate and lipid metabolism) may result from addition of a progestin, the choice of a particular progestin and dosage may minimize the risk.

WARNINGS/PRECAUTIONS

Carcinogenicity	The risk of endometrial carcinoma in postmenopausal women is increased by prolonged use (> 1 yr) of estrogen; the degree of risk depends on the duration of treatment and the dose. Closely observe patients during therapy, and investigate for malignancy any case of persistent or recurrent abnormal vaginal bleeding that is undiagnosed. One study has suggested that estrogen enhances the risk of breast cancer in postmenopausal women; use with caution in patients with a strong family history of breast cancer or with breast nodules, fibrocystic disease, or abnormal mammograms, and periodically perform a careful breast examination. Hepatocellular carcinoma has been associated with use of estrogen-containing oral contraceptives, but a causal relationship has not been established. Long-term administration of estrogen has been found to produce carcinomas of the breast, vagina, cervix, and liver in animals.
Gallbladder disease	Risk is increased 2–3 times in postmenopausal women treated with estrogens
Thromboembolic disease, thrombotic disorders, and other vascular problems	Risk is increased with dose; if feasible, discontinue medication at least 4 wk before elective surgery associated with an increased risk of thromboembolism or during periods of prolonged immobilization. Use with caution in patients with cerebrovascular or coronary artery disease and only when clearly needed. Large doses of estrogen (eg, 5 mg/day) have been shown to increase the risk of nonfatal myocardial infarction, pulmonary embolism, and thrombophlebitis in men.
Benign tumors	Uterine leiomyomata may increase in size during therapy; benign hepatic adenomas have occurred with use of estrogen-containing oral contraceptives, at times rupturing and resulting in intraabdominal hemorrhage and death, and should be considered in all cases of abdominal pain and tenderness, abdominal mass, or hypovolemic shock.
Hypertension	Has occurred with use of estrogen-containing oral contraceptives and may occur with menopausal use of estrogen; monitor blood pressure during therapy, especially if high doses are used
Impaired glucose tolerance	Has been observed with use of estrogen-containing oral contraceptives; closely monitor patients with diabetes
Severe hypercalcemia	May develop in patients with breast cancer and bone metastases; discontinue medication and institute appropriate measures to reduce the serum calcium level
Fluid retention	May occur; use with caution in patients with convulsive disorders, migraine, asthma, or cardiac or renal dysfunction
Excessive estrogenic stimulation	May be manifested by abnormal or excessive uterine bleeding, mastodynia, or other reactions
Mental depression	Has occurred with use of oral contraceptives; as it is unclear whether this is due to the estrogenic or progestogenic component, patients with a history of mental depression should be monitored closely during estrogen therapy
Altered cytology	Advise the pathologist of estrogen therapy when submitting relevant specimens
Jaundice	Has recurred with the use of estrogen-containing oral contraceptives in patients with a history of jaundice; if jaundice develops with estrogen therapy, discontinue medication while cause is investigated
Special-risk patients	Use with caution in patients with hepatic impairment, renal insufficiency, or metabolic bone disease associated with hypercalcemia

ADVERSE REACTIONS[1]

Genitourinary	Breakthrough bleeding, spotting, change in menstrual flow, dysmenorrhea, premenstrual-like syndrome, amenorrhea during and after treatment, increased size of uterine fibromyomata, vaginal candidiasis, change in cervical erosion and in degree of cervical secretion, cystitis-like syndrome
Endocrinological	Breast tenderness, enlargement, and secretion; altered libido
Gastrointestinal	Nausea, vomiting, abdominal cramps, bloating, cholestatic jaundice

ORTHO Dienestrol Cream ■ PREMARIN

Dermatological	Persistent chloasma or melasma, erythema multiforme, erythema nodosum, hemorrhagic eruption, loss of scalp hair, hirsutism
Ophthalmic	Steepening of corneal curvature, intolerance to contact lenses
Central nervous system	Headache, migraine, dizziness, mental depression, chorea
Other	Weight gain or loss, reduced carbohydrate tolerance, aggravation of porphyria, edema

DRUG INTERACTIONS

Oral anticoagulants	▽ Anticoagulant effect
Tricyclic antidepressants	△ Antidepressant side effects

ALTERED LABORATORY VALUES

Blood/serum values	△ Alkaline phosphatase △ Bilirubin △ Sulfobromophthalein retention △ Prothrombin △ Clotting factors VII, VIII, IX, and X ▽ Antithrombin III △ PBI △ Thyroxine (T_4) ▽ Triiodothyronine (T_3) uptake △ Glucose △ Cortisol △ Transcortin △ Ceruloplasmin △ Triglycerides △ Phospholipids ▽ Folic acid ▽ Pyridoxine
Urinary values	▽ Pregnanediol

USE IN CHILDREN
May cause premature epiphyseal closure; use with caution in young patients in whom bone growth is incomplete

USE IN PREGNANT AND NURSING WOMEN
Pregnancy Category X: contraindicated for use in women in who are or may become pregnant because administration of exogenous ovarian hormones during early pregnancy may cause serious fetal harm. Intrauterine exposure to these hormones, even for very brief periods, may increase the risk of congenital anomalies, including congenital heart defects and limb reduction defects. In addition, exposure in utero to diethylstilbestrol (and possibly other estrogens as well) has been shown to increase the risk of vaginal or cervical cancer developing in later life. Women who have taken this drug during pregnancy or who become pregnant while taking it should be apprised of the potential risks to the fetus and the advisability of continuing the pregnancy. It is not known whether dienestrol is excreted in human milk; use with caution in nursing mothers.

VEHICLE/BASE
Cream: glyceryl monostearate, peanut oil, glycerin, benzoic and glutamic acid, butylated hydroxyanisole, citric acid, sodium hydroxide, and water

[1] See WARNINGS/PRECAUTIONS regarding induction of neoplasia and increased incidence of gallbladder and thromboembolic disease

ESTROGENS

PREMARIN (conjugated estrogens) Ayerst   Rx

Tablets: 0.3, 0.625, 0.9, 1.25, 2.5 mg

INDICATIONS	ORAL DOSAGE
Moderate to severe **menopausal vasomotor symptoms**	**Adult:** 1.25 mg/day, given in 28-day cycles with 3 wk on and 1 wk off, starting on the 5th day of bleeding if the patient is menstruating or arbitrarily if the patient has not menstruated for at least 2 mo
Atrophic vaginitis **Kraurosis vulvae**	**Adult:** 0.3–1.25 mg/day, given in 28-day cycles with 3 wk on and 1 wk off
Female hypogonadism	**Adult:** 2.5–7.5 mg/day, given in divided doses for 20 days, followed by a 10-day, drug-free rest period; if bleeding occurs before the end of the 10-day rest period, add an oral progestin during the last 5 days of the next cycle
Female castration and primary ovarian failure	**Adult:** 1.25 mg/day, given in 28-day cycles with 3 wk on and 1 wk off; adjust dosage in accordance with patient response
Palliation of inoperable, progressing, metastatic **breast cancer** in appropriately selected men and postmenopausal women	**Adult:** 10 mg tid for at least 3 mo
Palliation of inoperable, progressing **prostatic carcinoma**	**Adult:** 1.25–2.5 mg tid
Postpartum breast engorgement	**Adult:** 3.75 mg q4h for 5 doses, or 1.25 mg q4h for 5 days

PREMARIN

Osteoporosis due to estrogen deficiency, when used in conjunction with other therapeutic measures, such as diet, calcium, and physiotherapy

Adult: 0.625 mg/day, given in 28-day cycles with 3 wk on and 1 wk off

PREMARIN Vaginal Cream (conjugated estrogens) Ayerst   Rx

Vaginal cream: 0.0625% (42.5 g)

INDICATIONS	INTRAVAGINAL AND TOPICAL DOSAGE
Atrophic vaginitis or kraurosis vulvae	Adult: 2–4 g/day, given in 28-day cycles with 3 wk on and 1 wk off

CONTRAINDICATIONS

Known or suspected breast cancer (except when used in the treatment of metastatic disease)	History of thrombophlebitis, thrombosis, or thromboembolism associated with prior use of estrogen (except when used in the treatment of breast or breast or prostatic malignancy)	Active thrombophlebitis or thromboembolic disorders
Known or suspected estrogen-dependent neoplasia		Undiagnosed abnormal genital bleeding
Known or suspected pregnancy	Hypersensitivity to any component of the cream	

ADMINISTRATION/DOSAGE ADJUSTMENTS

Monitoring of therapy	A Papanicolaou smear and a physical examination (with special attention to breasts, abdomen, pelvic organs, and blood pressure) should be done before therapy and then repeated at least annually
Duration of postmenopausal therapy	For vasomotor symptoms, atrophic vaginitis, and kraurosis vulvae, attempt to discontinue or taper medication at intervals of 3–6 mo
Osteoporosis	This product may be used in postmenopausal women with evidence of loss or deficiency in bone mass to retard further bone loss and osteoporosis due to estrogen deficiency. Although there is evidence that the rate of bone loss can be reduced in postmenopausal women, substantial evidence is lacking that estrogens decrease the incidence of osteoporotic bone fractures. Women who have had an early surgical menopause (oophorectomy) appear to be at increased risk for developing osteoporosis; women who have undergone a hysterectomy have a more favorable benefit/risk ratio for prophylactic osteoporosis therapy, because they have no risk of endometrial carcinoma.
Concomitant progestin therapy	The addition of a progestin for 7 or more days (according to some studies, for 10–13 days) to an estrogen replacement cycle may lower the incidence of endometrial hyperplasia (see WARNINGS/PRECAUTIONS); however, whether this addition will provide protection against endometrial carcinoma has not been clearly established. Although possible additional risks (eg, adverse effects on carbohydrate and lipid metabolism) may result from addition of a progestin, the choice of a particular progestin and dosage may minimize the risk.

WARNINGS/PRECAUTIONS

Carcinogenicity	The risk of endometrial carcinoma in postmenopausal women is increased by prolonged use ($>$ 1 yr) of estrogen; the degree of risk depends on the duration of treatment and the dose. Closely observe patients during therapy, and investigate for malignancy any case of persistent or recurrent abnormal vaginal bleeding that is undiagnosed. Hepatocellular carcinoma has been associated with use of estrogen-containing oral contraceptives, but a causal relationship has not been established. Long-term administration of estrogen has been found to produce carcinomas of the breast, vagina, cervix, and liver in animals; however, a recent large, case-controlled study indicated no increased risk of breast cancer in postmenopausal women undergoing therapy with conjugated estrogens.
Gallbladder disease	Risk is increased 2–3 times in postmenopausal women treated with estrogens
Thromboembolic disease, thrombotic disorders, and other vascular problems	Risk is increased with dose; if feasible, discontinue medication at least 4 wk before elective surgery associated with an increased risk of thromboembolism or during periods of prolonged immobilization. Use with caution in patients with cerebrovascular or coronary artery disease and only when clearly needed. Large doses of estrogen (eg, 5 mg/day) have been shown to increase the risk of nonfatal myocardial infarction, pulmonary embolism, and thrombophlebitis in men.
Benign tumors	Uterine leiomyomata may increase in size during therapy; benign hepatic adenomas have occurred with use of estrogen-containing oral contraceptives, at times rupturing and resulting in intraabdominal hemorrhage and death, and should be considered in all cases of abdominal pain and tenderness, abdominal mass, or hypovolemic shock
Hypertension	Has occurred with use of estrogen-containing oral contraceptives and may occur with menopausal use of estrogen; monitor blood pressure during therapy, especially if high doses are used
Impaired glucose tolerance	Has been observed with use of estrogen-containing oral contraceptives; closely monitor patients with diabetes

PREMARIN

Severe hypercalcemia	May develop in patients with breast cancer and bone metastases; discontinue medication and institute appropriate measures to reduce the serum calcium level
Fluid retention	May occur; use with caution in patients with convulsive disorders, migraine, asthma, or in those with cardiac or renal dysfunction
Excessive estrogenic stimulation	May be manifested by abnormal or excessive uterine bleeding, mastodynia, or other reactions; reduce dosage accordingly
Endometrial hyperplasia	May occur with prolonged use
Mental depression	Has occurred with use of oral contraceptives; as it is unclear whether this is due to the estrogenic or progestogenic component, patients with a history of mental depression should be monitored closely during estrogen therapy
Altered cytology	Advise the pathologist of estrogen therapy when submitting relevant specimens
Jaundice	Has recurred with the use of estrogen-containing oral contraceptives in patients with a history of jaundice; if jaundice develops with estrogen therapy, discontinue medication while cause is investigated
Special-risk patients	Use with caution in patients with hepatic impairment, renal insufficiency, or metabolic bone disease associated with hypercalcemia

ADVERSE REACTIONS[1]

Genitourinary	Breakthrough bleeding, spotting, change in menstrual flow, dysmenorrhea, premenstrual-like syndrome, amenorrhea during and after treatment, increased size of uterine fibromyomata, vaginal candidiasis, change in cervical erosion and in degree of cervical secretion, cystitis-like syndrome
Endocrinological	Breast tenderness, enlargement, and secretion; altered libido
Gastrointestinal	Nausea, vomiting, abdominal cramps, bloating, cholestatic jaundice
Dermatological	Persistent chloasma or melasma, erythema multiforme, erythema nodosum, hemorrhagic eruption, loss of scalp hair, hirsutism
Ophthalmic	Steepening of corneal curvature, intolerance to contact lenses
Central nervous system	Headache, migraine, dizziness, mental depression, chorea
Other	Weight gain or loss, reduced carbohydrate tolerance, aggravation of porphyria, edema

OVERDOSAGE

Signs and symptoms	Nausea, withdrawal bleeding (see ADVERSE REACTIONS)
Treatment	Discontinue medication; treat symptomatically

DRUG INTERACTIONS

Oral anticoagulants	▽ Anticoagulant effect
Tricyclic antidepressants	△ Antidepressant side effects

ALTERED LABORATORY VALUES

Blood/serum values	△ Alkaline phosphatase △ Bilirubin △ Sulfobromophthalein retention △ Prothrombin △ Clotting factors VII, VIII, IX, and X ▽ Antithrombin III △ PBI △ Thyroxine (T_4) ▽ Triiodothyronine (T_3) uptake △ Glucose △ Cortisol △ Transcortin △ Ceruloplasmin △ Triglycerides △ Phospholipids ▽ Folic acid ▽ Pyridoxine
Urinary values	▽ Pregnanediol

USE IN CHILDREN

Safety and effectiveness for use in children have not been established. Estrogens may cause premature epiphyseal closure; use with caution in young patients in whom bone growth is incomplete.

USE IN PREGNANT AND NURSING WOMEN

Pregnancy Category X: contraindicated if pregnancy is known or suspected, as use of exogenous ovarian hormones during early pregnancy may cause serious fetal harm. Intrauterine exposure to these hormones, even for very brief periods, may increase the risk of congenital anomalies, including congenital heart defects and limb reduction defects. In addition, exposure in utero to diethylstilbestrol (and possibly other estrogens as well) has been shown to increase the risk of vaginal or cervical cancer developing in later life. Women who have taken this drug during pregnancy or who become pregnant while taking it should be apprised of the potential risks to the fetus and the advisability of continuing the pregnancy. It is not known whether this drug is excreted in human milk; because of the potential for serious adverse effects in nursing infants, women should not nurse during therapy.

VEHICLE/BASE
Cream (nonliquefying): cetyl esters wax, cetyl alcohol, white wax, glyceryl monostearate, propylene glycol monostearate, methyl stearate, phenylethyl alcohol, sodium lauryl sulfate, glycerin, and mineral oil

[1] See WARNINGS/PRECAUTIONS regarding induction of neoplasia and increased incidence of gallbladder and thromboembolic disease

ESTROGENS

TACE (chlorotrianisene) Merrell Dow Rx
Capsules: 12, 25, 72 mg

INDICATIONS	ORAL DOSAGE
Postpartum breast engorgement	Adult: 12 mg qid for 7 days, 50 mg q6h for 6 doses, or 72 mg bid for 2 days; administer the first dose within 8 h after delivery
Palliation of inoperable, progressing **prostatic carcinoma**	Adult: 12–25 mg/day
Moderate to severe **menopausal vasomotor symptoms**	Adult: 12–25 mg/day for 30 days, followed by repeated courses, as necessary
Atrophic vaginitis / Kraurosis vulvae	Adult: 12–25 mg/day for 30–60 days
Female hypogonadism	Adult: 12–25 mg/day in 21-day cycles; if desired, give 100 mg IM progesterone immediately after the cycle or add an oral progestin during the last 5 days of the cycle; begin the next course on the 5th day of induced uterine bleeding

CONTRAINDICATIONS

- Known or suspected breast cancer (except when used in the treatment of metastatic disease)
- Known or suspected estrogen-dependent neoplasia
- Known or suspected pregnancy
- History of thrombophlebitis, thrombosis, or thromboembolism associated with prior use of estrogen (except when used in the treatment of breast or prostatic malignancy)
- Active thrombophlebitis or thromboembolic disorders
- Undiagnosed abnormal genital bleeding

ADMINISTRATION/DOSAGE ADJUSTMENTS

Pretreatment physical examination	Obtain a complete medical and family history before initiating estrogen therapy (see WARNINGS/PRECAUTIONS). Special attention during the physical examination should be given to blood pressure, breasts, abdomen, and pelvic organs; obtain a Papanicolaou smear.
Duration of postmenopausal therapy	For vasomotor symptoms, atrophic vaginitis, and kraurosis vulvae, attempt to discontinue or taper medication at intervals of 3–6 mo

WARNINGS/PRECAUTIONS

Malignant neoplasms	May occur with prolonged use; use with caution and closely monitor patients with a family history of breast cancer or with breast nodules, fibrocystic disease, or abnormal mammograms. Risk of endometrial carcinoma in postmenopausal women increases with duration of estrogen therapy and dose; provide close clinical surveillance and investigate all cases of undiagnosed, persistent, or recurrent abnormal vaginal bleeding for malignancy (see CONTRAINDICATIONS).
Gallbladder disease	Risk is increased 2–3 times in postmenopausal women treated with estrogens
Thromboembolic disease, thrombotic disorders, and other vascular problems	Risk is increased with dose; if feasible, discontinue medication at least 4 wk before elective surgery associated with an increased risk of thromboembolism or during periods of prolonged immobilization. Use with caution in patients with cerebrovascular or coronary artery disease and only when clearly needed. Large doses of estrogen (eg, 5 mg/day) have been shown to increase the risk of nonfatal myocardial infarction, pulmonary embolism, and thrombophlebitis in men.
Benign hepatic adenoma	Has occurred with use of estrogen-containing oral contraceptives, at times rupturing and resulting in intraabdominal hemorrhage and death, and should be considered in all cases of abdominal pain and tenderness, abdominal mass, or hypovolemic shock
Hepatocellular carcinoma	Has occurred with use of estrogen-containing oral contraceptives
Hypertension	Has occurred with use of estrogen-containing oral contraceptives and may occur with menopausal use of estrogens; monitor blood pressure during therapy, especially if high doses are used
Impaired glucose tolerance	Has been observed with use of estrogen-containing oral contraceptives; closely monitor patients with diabetes
Severe hypercalcemia	May develop in patients with breast cancer and bone metastases; discontinue medication and institute appropriate measures to reduce the serum calcium level
Fluid retention	May occur; use with caution in patients with convulsive disorders, migraine, asthma, or cardiac or renal dysfunction
Excessive estrogen stimulation	May be manifested by abnormal or excessive uterine bleeding, mastodynia, or other reactions; reduce dosage accordingly
Mental depression	Has occurred with use of oral contraceptives; as it is unclear whether this is due to the estrogenic or progestogenic component, patients with a history of mental depression should be monitored closely during estrogen therapy

Uterine leiomyomata	May increase in size
Altered cytology	Advise the pathologist of estrogen therapy when submitting relevant specimens
Jaundice	Has recurred with use of estrogen-containing oral contraceptives in patients with a history of jaundice; if jaundice develops with estrogen therapy, discontinue medication while cause is investigated
Special-risk patients	Use with caution in patients with hepatic impairment, renal insufficiency, or metabolic bone disease associated with hypercalcemia
Tartrazine sensitivity	Presence of FD&C Yellow No. 5 (tartrazine) may cause allergic-type reactions, including bronchial asthma, in susceptible individuals

ADVERSE REACTIONS[1]

Genitourinary	Breakthrough bleeding, spotting, change in menstrual flow, dysmenorrhea, premenstrual-like syndrome, amenorrhea during and after treatment, increased size of uterine fibromyomata, vaginal candidiasis, change in cervical erosion and in degree of cervical secretion, cystitis-like syndrome
Endocrinological	Breast tenderness, enlargement, and secretion; altered libido and/or potency
Gastrointestinal	Nausea, vomiting, abdominal cramps, bloating, cholestatic jaundice
Dermatological	Persistent chloasma or melasma, erythema multiforme, erythema nodosum, hemorrhagic eruption, loss of scalp hair, hirsutism, urticaria
Ophthalmic	Steepening of corneal curvature, intolerance to contact lenses
Central nervous system	Headache, migraine, dizziness, mental depression, chorea
Other	Weight gain or loss, reduced carbohydrate tolerance, aggravation of porphyria

OVERDOSAGE

Signs and symptoms	Nausea, withdrawal bleeding (see ADVERSE REACTIONS)
Treatment	Discontinue medication

DRUG INTERACTIONS

Oral anticoagulants	▽ Anticoagulant effect
Tricyclic antidepressants	△ Antidepressant side effects

ALTERED LABORATORY VALUES

Blood/serum values	△ Alkaline phosphatase △ Bilirubin △ Sulfobromophthalein retention △ Prothrombin △ Clotting factors VII, VIII, IX, and X ▽ Antithrombin III △ PBI △ Thyroxine (T_4) ▽ Triiodothyronine (T_3) uptake △ Glucose △ Cortisol △ Transcortin △ Ceruloplasmin △ Triglycerides △ Phospholipids ▽ Folic acid ▽ Pyridoxine
Urinary values	▽ Pregnanediol

USE IN CHILDREN

May cause premature epiphyseal closure; use with caution in young patients in whom bone growth is incomplete.

USE IN PREGNANT AND NURSING WOMEN

Pregnancy Category X: contraindicated if pregnancy is known or suspected, as use of exogenous ovarian hormones during early pregnancy may cause serious fetal harm. Intrauterine exposure to these hormones, even for very brief periods, may increase the risk of congenital anomalies, including congenital heart defects and limb reduction defects. In addition, exposure in utero to diethylstilbestrol (and possibly other estrogens as well) has been shown to increase the risk of vaginal or cervical cancer developing in later life. Women who have taken this drug during pregnancy or who become pregnant while taking it should be apprised of the potential risks to the fetus and the advisability of continuing the pregnancy. Since many drugs are excreted in human milk, patients who are nursing should not be given this drug unless it is clearly needed.

[1] See WARNINGS/PRECAUTIONS regarding induction of neoplasia and increased incidence of gallbladder and thromboembolic disease

---

PROGESTINS

NORLUTIN (norethindrone) Parke-Davis   Rx
Tablets: 5 mg

NORLUTATE (norethindrone acetate) Parke-Davis   Rx
Tablets: 5 mg

INDICATIONS	ORAL DOSAGE
Amenorrhea **Abnormal uterine bleeding** due to hormonal imbalance in the absence of organic pathology (eg, fibroids or uterine cancer)	**Adult:** 5–20 mg/day of Norlutin or 2.5–10 mg/day of Norlutate on days 5–25 of menstrual cycle

NORLUTIN

Endometriosis	**Adult:** 10 mg/day of Norlutin or 5 mg/day of Norlutate to start, followed after 2 wk by increments of 5 mg/day of Norlutin or 2.5 mg/day of Norlutate every 2 wk, up to 30 mg/day of Norlutin or 15 mg/day of Norlutate; therapy may be continued at this level for 6–9 mo or until annoying breakthrough bleeding demands temporary suspension

CONTRAINDICATIONS

Past or present thrombophlebitis, thromboembolic disorders, or cerebral apoplexy

Known or suspected breast carcinoma

Undiagnosed vaginal bleeding

Missed abortion

Diagnosis of pregnancy

WARNINGS/PRECAUTIONS

Pretreatment physical examination	Should include examination of the breasts and pelvic organs as well as a Papanicolaou smear
Thrombotic disorders	May occur; follow patient closely for early signs of thrombophlebitis or pulmonary embolism
Visual impairment	Discontinue medication until cause of sudden complete or partial loss of vision, proptosis, diplopia, or migraine can be investigated; do not reinitiate therapy if papilledema or retinal vascular lesions are found
Mammary nodules	Have developed in medroxyprogesterone-treated dogs; clinical relevance has not been established
Fluid retention	May occur; use with caution in patients with epilepsy, migraine, asthma, or cardiac or renal dysfunction
Mental depression	May be exacerbated; closely monitor patients with a history of psychic depression. Discontinue medication if depression becomes severe.
Impaired glucose tolerance	Has been observed with use of estrogen-progestin combination drugs; closely monitor patients with diabetes
Abnormal vaginal bleeding	Consider nonfunctional causes; take adequate diagnostic measures
Hepatic impairment	May cause drug accumulation; use with caution
Prolonged use	Long-term effect on pituitary, ovarian, adrenal, hepatic, or uterine function has not been established
Onset of climacteric	May be masked
Altered cytology	Advise the pathologist of progestin therapy when submitting relevant specimens

ADVERSE REACTIONS[1]

Genitourinary	Breakthrough bleeding, spotting, change in menstrual flow, amenorrhea, changes in cervical erosion and cervical secretions, premenstrual-like syndrome, cystitis-like syndrome
Metabolic and endocrinological	Edema, weight gain or loss
Dermatological	Rash (allergic) with or without pruritus, melasma or chloasma, alopecia, hirsutism, erythema multiforme, erythema nodosum, hemorrhagic eruption
Thromboembolic	Thrombophlebitis, pulmonary embolism, cerebral thrombosis and embolism
Central nervous system	Headache, nervousness, dizziness, fatigue, backache, mental depression
Other	Cholestatic jaundice, rise in blood pressure in susceptible individuals, changes in libido, changes in appetite

OVERDOSAGE

Signs and symptoms	See ADVERSE REACTIONS
Treatment	Discontinue medication; treat symptomatically

DRUG INTERACTIONS

No clinically significant drug interactions have been identified

ALTERED LABORATORY VALUES

Blood/serum values	△ Bilirubin △ SGOT △ SGPT △ Sulfobromophthalein (BSP) retention △ Clotting factors VII, VIII, IX, and X △ PBI △ Butanol-extractable PBI ▽ Triiodothyronine (T_3) uptake
Urinary values	▽ Pregnanediol

USE IN CHILDREN

Consult manufacturer

USE IN PREGNANT AND NURSING WOMEN

Not recommended for use during the first 4 mo of pregnancy, as intrauterine exposure to exogenous sex hormones, even for very brief periods, may increase the risk of congenital anomalies, including congenital heart defects and limb reduction defects. In addition, masculinization of female fetuses may occur. Patients who have taken this drug during the first 4 mo of pregnancy or who become pregnant while taking it should be apprised of the potential risk to the fetus. Progestins are excreted in human milk; effect on nursing infant has not been determined.

---

[1] Includes reactions observed in patients taking estrogen-progestin combinations; neuro-ocular lesions (eg, retinal thrombosis and optic neuritis) have also been reported, but a causal relationship has not been established

PROGESTINS

PROVERA (medroxyprogesterone acetate) Upjohn Rx

Tablets: 2.5, 5, 10 mg

INDICATIONS

Secondary amenorrhea

Abnormal uterine bleeding due to hormonal imbalance in the absence of organic pathology (eg, fibroids or uterine cancer)

ORAL DOSAGE

Adult: 5–10 mg/day for 5–10 days; to induce optimum secretory transformation of an adequately primed endometrium, 10 mg/day for 10 days, beginning at any time; withdrawal bleeding usually occurs within 3–7 days after discontinuing therapy

Adult: 5–10 mg/day for 5–10 days, beginning on the 16th or 21st day of menstrual cycle; to induce optimum secretory transformation of an adequately primed endometrium, 10 mg/day for 10 days, beginning on the 16th day of menstrual cycle; withdrawal bleeding usually occurs within 3–7 days after discontinuing therapy

CONTRAINDICATIONS

Past or present thrombophlebitis, thromboembolic disorders, or cerebral apoplexy

Hepatic dysfunction or disease

Known or suspected malignancy of breast or genital organs

Undiagnosed vaginal bleeding

Missed abortion

Hypersensitivity to medroxyprogesterone

Diagnosis of pregnancy

WARNINGS/PRECAUTIONS

Pretreatment physical examination	Should include examination of the breasts and pelvic organs as well as a Papanicolaou smear
Thrombotic disorders	May occur; discontinue medication immediately at earliest manifestations or suspicion of thrombophlebitis, cerebrovascular disorders, pulmonary embolism, or retinal thrombosis
Visual impairment	Discontinue medication until cause of sudden complete or partial visual loss, proptosis, diplopia, or migraine can be investigated; do not reinitiate therapy if papilledema or retinal vascular lesions are found
Mammary nodules	Have appeared in medroxyprogesterone-treated dogs, including some breast malignancies with metastases; clinical relevance has not been established
Fluid retention	May occur; use with caution in patients with epilepsy, migraine, asthma, or cardiac or renal dysfunction
Mental depression	May be exacerbated; closely monitor patients with a history of psychic depression; discontinue medication if depression becomes severe
Impaired glucose tolerance	Has been observed with use of estrogen-progestin combination drugs; closely monitor patients with diabetes
Abnormal vaginal bleeding	Consider nonfunctional causes; take adequate diagnostic measures
Prolonged use	Long-term effect on pituitary, ovarian, adrenal, hepatic, or uterine function has not been established
Onset of climacteric	May be masked
Altered cytology	Advise the pathologist of progestin therapy when submitting relevant specimens

ADVERSE REACTIONS[1]

Cardiovascular	Thrombotic disorders, including thrombophlebitis, pulmonary embolism, and cerebral thrombosis and embolism; edema, increased blood pressure
Central nervous system	Insomnia, somnolence, fatigue, depression, headache, nervousness, dizziness, backache
Genitourinary	Breakthrough bleeding, spotting, altered menstrual flow, amenorrhea, changes in cervical erosion and cervical secretions, premenstrual-like syndrome, cystitis-like syndrome, change in libido
Dermatological	Urticaria, pruritus, edema, generalized rash, acne, alopecia, hirsutism, erythema multiforme, erythema nodosum, hemorrhagic eruption
Other	Anaphylaxis, anaphylactoid reactions, pyrexia, cholestatic jaundice, nausea, change in weight, change in appetite; breast tenderness and galactorrhea (rare)

OVERDOSAGE

Signs and symptoms	See ADVERSE REACTIONS
Treatment	Discontinue medication; treat symptomatically

DRUG INTERACTIONS

No clinically significant drug interactions have been identified

ALTERED LABORATORY VALUES

Blood/serum values — △ Bilirubin △ SGOT △ SGPT △ Sulfobromophthalein retention △ Clotting factors VII, VIII, IX, and X △ PBI △ Butanol-extractable PBI ▽ Triiodothyronine (T_3) uptake

| Urinary values | ▽ Pregnanediol |

USE IN CHILDREN	USE IN PREGNANT AND NURSING WOMEN
Consult manufacturer	Not recommended for use during the first 4 mo of pregnancy, as intrauterine exposure to exogenous sex hormones, even for very brief periods, may increase the risk of congenital anomalies, including congenital heart defects and limb reduction defects. Patients who have taken this drug during the first 4 mo of pregnancy or who become pregnant while taking it should be apprised of the potential risk to the fetus. Progestins are excreted in human milk; effect on nursing infant has not been determined.

[1] Includes reactions observed in patients taking estrogen-progestin combinations; neuro-ocular lesions (eg, retinal thrombosis and optic neuritis) have also been reported, but a causal relationship has not been established

FERTILITY INDUCERS

CLOMID (clomiphene citrate) Merrell Dow   Rx
Tablets: 50 mg

INDICATIONS	ORAL DOSAGE
Induction of ovulation in patients with secondary anovulatory infertility	**Adult:** 50 mg/day for 5 days, beginning on or about the 5th day of the menstrual cycle if spontaneous uterine bleeding occurs or progesterone-induced bleeding is planned, or at any time if there has been no recent history of bleeding; repeat course up to two more times if ovulation, but not conception, occurs during the first cycle

CONTRAINDICATIONS

Abnormal bleeding of undetermined origin	Hepatic disease or history of hepatic dysfunction	Pregnancy
Ovarian cysts		

ADMINISTRATION/DOSAGE ADJUSTMENTS

Pretreatment evaluation	Clomiphene should be used only in patients with evidence of good estrogen function (as estimated by vaginal smears, endometrial biopsy, urinary assay, or progesterone-induced bleeding), potent and fertile partners, and normal adrenal, thyroid, and liver function. Do not give to patients with primary pituitary or ovarian failure, ovarian cysts, abnormal uterine bleeding, or endometrial carcinoma (do not overlook neoplastic lesions; obtain an endometrial biopsy in older patients). Perform a complete pelvic examination before each course of treatment.
Lack of response to initial course of therapy	If ovulation does not occur following 50 mg/day, increase dosage during next course to 100 mg/day for 5 days, beginning as early as 30 days after previous course; if ovulation, but not conception, occurs at this dosage, course may be repeated once
Patients with unusual sensitivity to pituitary gonadotropins	Reduce dosage or duration of treatment course (see WARNINGS/PRECAUTIONS)

WARNINGS/PRECAUTIONS

Visual symptoms	Blurring and other visual disturbances (see ADVERSE REACTIONS) may occur, depending on dose; discontinue use and perform a complete ophthalmological evaluation. Caution patients that performance of potentially hazardous activities may be impaired if vision is affected, particularly under variable lighting.
Ovarian overstimulation	Abnormal ovarian enlargement and cyst formation, possibly accompanied by pain, may occur, especially in patients with polycystic ovary syndrome; to reduce the hazard, the lowest dose consistent with expectation of good results should be used. Maximal enlargement of the ovary, whether physiological or abnormal, does not occur until several days after discontinuation of therapy; patients who complain of pelvic pain after clomiphene treatment should be carefully examined. If ovarian enlargement does occur, stop treatment until the ovaries have returned to pretreatment size, and reduce the dosage or duration of the next course; manage cystic enlargement conservatively, unless a surgical indication for laparotomy exists.
Inadvertent use during early pregnancy	May be avoided by recording the basal body temperature throughout all treatment cycles and by observing patient carefully to determine whether ovulation has occurred; if basal body temperature following clomiphene treatment is biphasic and is not followed by menses, examine patient for an ovarian cyst and perform a pregnancy test. Delay the next course of therapy until it is determined that the patient is not pregnant.

CLOMID ■ PARLODEL

Multiple pregnancy	The prospective parents should be advised of the frequency and potential hazards of multiple pregnancy before starting treatment; of the pregnancies reported following the use of clomiphene in clinical trials, 6.9% resulted in twins and 0.93% in more than two infants

ADVERSE REACTIONS[1]

	Frequent reactions (incidence ≥ 1%) are printed in *italics*
Cardiovascular	*Vasomotor flushes (10.4%)*
Gastrointestinal	*Abdominal or pelvic discomfort (including distention, bloating, pain, or soreness) (5.5%), nausea and vomiting (2.2%)*, increased appetite, acute abdomen, constipation, diarrhea
Endocrinological	*Ovarian enlargement and cyst formation (13.6%), breast discomfort (2.1%)*, menorrhagia, intermenstrual spotting, dryness of the vaginal mucosa
Ophthalmic	Phosphenes, blurred vision, diplopia, scotomata, afterimages, photophobia, lights, floaters, waves, other visual complaints[2]; electroretinographic changes, objectively defined scotomata
Central nervous system	*Headache (1.3%)*, dizziness, light-headedness, vertigo, nervous tension, insomnia, fatigue, depression
Genitourinary	Increased urinary frequency and/or volume
Dermatological	Dermatitis, rash, hair loss, dry hair
Congenital anomalies[3]	Congenital heart lesions, Down's syndrome, clubfoot, congenital gut lesions, hypospadias, microcephaly, harelip, cleft palate, congenital hip, hemangioma, undescended testes, polydactyly, conjoined twins with teratomatous malformation, patent ductus arteriosus, amaurosis, arteriovenous fistula, inguinal hernia, umbilical hernia, syndactyly, pectus excavatum, myopathy, dermoid cyst of scalp, omphalocele, spina bifida occulta, ichthyosis, persistent lingual frenulum, multiple somatic defects
Other	Weight gain or loss, cholestatic jaundice (one case), ascites (two cases)

OVERDOSAGE

Signs and symptoms	See WARNINGS/PRECAUTIONS and ADVERSE REACTIONS
Treatment	Discontinue use; treat symptomatically and institute supportive measures, as needed

DRUG INTERACTIONS

No clinically significant drug interactions have been identified

ALTERED LABORATORY VALUES

Blood/serum values	⇧ Sulfobromophthalein (BSP) retention ⇧ FSH ⇧ LH ⇧ Desmosterol ⇧ Transcortin ⇧ Thyroxine ⇧ Sex hormone-binding globulin ⇧ Thyroxine-binding globulin
Urinary values	⇧ FSH ⇧ LH ⇧ Estrogen

USE IN CHILDREN

Not indicated for use in children

USE IN PREGNANT AND NURSING WOMEN

Contraindicated for use during pregnancy (see WARNINGS/PRECAUTIONS). Not indicated for use in nursing mothers.

---

[1] Adverse effects appear to be dose-dependent
[2] Other reactions for which a causal relationship has not been established include posterior capsular cataract, detachment of posterior vitreous, spasm of retinal arteriole, thrombosis of temporal arteries of retina, and hydatidiform mole
[3] Congenital anomalies were reported in 2.4% (58/2,369) of births following clomiphene use; the cumulative rate does not exceed that observed in the general population

---

FERTILITY INDUCERS

PARLODEL (bromocriptine mesylate)   Sandoz Pharmaceuticals   Rx

Capsules: 5 mg   **Tablets:** 2.5 mg

INDICATIONS	ORAL DOSAGE
Hyperprolactinemic disorders, including amenorrhea, galactorrhea, hypogonadism (infertility), and prolactin-secreting adenomas	Adult: 1.25–2.5 mg/day to start, followed, as tolerated, by an increase in dosage of 2.5 mg/day every 3–7 days, until an optimal response is achieved; therapeutic dosage is usually 5–7.5 mg/day, but may range from 2.5–15 mg/day. To manage adverse reactions, temporarily reduce dosage to 1.25 mg bid or tid.
Prevention of physiological lactation after parturition, stillbirth, or abortion	Adult: 2.5 mg bid for 14 days or, if necessary, up to 21 days (dosage range: 2.5–7.5 mg/day); begin administration after vital signs have stabilized, but not sooner than 4 h after delivery

PARLODEL

Acromegaly	**Adult:** 1.25–2.5 mg/day, given at bedtime with food for 3 days, followed, as tolerated, by an increase in dosage of 1.25–2.5 mg/day every 3–7 days until optimal response or a maximum of 100 mg/day is achieved; usual dosage: 20–30 mg/day
Idiopathic or postencephalitic Parkinson's disease, as an adjunct to levodopa (alone or with a peripheral decarboxylase inhibitor, such as carbidopa)	**Adult:** 1.25 mg bid to start, followed, as needed, by an increase in dosage of 2.5 mg/day every 14–28 days until optimal response or a maximum of 100 mg/day is achieved. If possible, maintain dosage of levodopa while titrating dosage of bromocriptine; if dosage of levodopa is subsequently reduced, retitrate dosage of bromocriptine.

CONTRAINDICATIONS
Sensitivity to ergot alkaloids

ADMINISTRATION/DOSAGE ADJUSTMENTS

Administration	Give each dose with food
Use of contraceptives and pregnancy tests	Bromocriptine can restore fertility, which may not only be undesirable, but may also pose the following two risks: (1) the drug may subsequently affect fetal development if pregnancy is not detected at the time of conception (see USE IN PREGNANT AND NURSING WOMEN) and (2) the hormonal changes during pregnancy may cause optic nerve compression if the woman has a prolactin-secreting macroadenoma (see WARNINGS/PRECAUTIONS). Instruct women who do not wish to become pregnant to use a contraceptive, other than an oral contraceptive, as long as they are undergoing treatment. To avoid prolonged in utero exposure in the event of an unsuspected pregnancy, instruct women seeking to become pregnant to use such a contraceptive during the period of amenorrhea. Test for pregnancy in all patients at least every 4 wk during the period of amenorrhea and, after a normal ovulatory cycle has been restored, whenever menstruation does not occur within 3 days of the expected date. Discontinue therapy any time pregnancy is suspected.
Amenorrhea, galactorrhea	In patients with amenorrhea, menses is usually seen after 6–8 wk of therapy; however, response may vary from a few days to up to 8 mo. Control of galactorrhea depends on the degree of mammary stimulation prior to therapy. A reduction in secretion of at least 75% usually occurs after 8–12 wk of therapy; however, galactorrhea may fail to respond even after 12 mo of treatment.
Prolactinomas	Bromocriptine may be given alone to treat prolactin-secreting adenomas or, alternatively, may be used to reduce the size of macroadenomas prior to adenectomy. It is not known whether drug therapy or surgery is the more effective treatment for patients experiencing loss of visual field; if loss progresses rapidly, the appropriate form of therapy should be decided after a neurosurgeon has examined the patient. Caution patients that discontinuation of drug therapy usually results in rapid regrowth of macroadenomas and recurrence of symptoms.
Acromegaly	When used alone or in conjunction with surgery or radiotherapy, bromocriptine reduces the serum growth hormone level by at least 50% in approximately one-half of patients; however, a normal serum level is usually not attained. After each adjustment in dosage, reevaluate diagnosis and then evaluate clinical response and check serum level; if no significant reduction in the serum level occurs after a brief trial, either continue to titrate dosage or terminate administration. Once a maintenance dosage has been established, monitor clinical response and serum level monthly and then at periodic intervals. If a patient has undergone radiotherapy, use of the drug should be interrupted annually for a period of 4–8 wk to assess the relative effects of radiation and drug treatment, since the full therapeutic effect of radiotherapy may not occur until after several years; if signs or symptoms recur or the serum level increases, consider resuming therapy.
Parkinson's disease	Bromocriptine can enhance therapeutic response in patients receiving levodopa and may also permit a reduction in the maintenance dose when these patients experience adverse effects such as dyskinesia and "on-off" phenomenon; bear in mind that safety and effectiveness of bromocriptine for use as an antiparkinson agent for more than 2 yr have not been established. When titrating dosage of bromocriptine, assess therapeutic response every 2 wk. During chronic therapy, check renal, hepatic, cardiovascular, and hematopoietic functions periodically.

WARNINGS/PRECAUTIONS

Dizziness, drowsiness, syncope	Caution all patients that their ability to drive, operate machinery, or engage in other activities requiring rapid and precise response may be impaired during therapy
Renal, hepatic disease	Safety and effectiveness for use in patients with renal or hepatic disease have not been established
Compression of the optic nerve	Hormonal changes during pregnancy can cause expansion of prolactin-secreting adenomas and result in compression of the optic or other cranial nerves. Although compression usually disappears after delivery, emergency surgery may be necessary in some cases. Bromocriptine has reportedly caused improvement of visual field symptoms owing to nerve compression; however, safety for use during pregnancy has not been established. To reduce the risk of nerve compression, carefully assess the pituitary gland and look for evidence of a prolactin-secreting adenoma before beginning treatment of hyperprolactinemic disorders such as hypogonadism and amenorrhea since these disorders may be due to a pituitary adenoma. Avoid pregnancy, when possible (see ADMINISTRATION/DOSAGE ADJUSTMENTS). If or when the patient becomes pregnant, watch closely for signs and symptoms that may indicate enlargement of a known or previously undetected adenoma.

PARLODEL

CSF rhinorrhea	In rare instances, bromocriptine may cause CSF rhinorrhea in patients who have macroadenomas that extend into the sphenoid sinus or who have undergone transsphenoidal surgery or pituitary radiotherapy; caution these patients to report any persistent watery nasal discharge
Effects on blood pressure	Bromocriptine can cause symptomatic hypotension, particularly when given postpartum; in 28% of patients who received this drug for prevention of lactation, systolic pressure decreased by more than 20 mm Hg and diastolic pressure declined by more than 10 mm Hg. In rare instances, postpartum use may precipitate hypertension in patients who have toxemia or are receiving other drugs, including other ergot alkaloids, that can increase blood pressure. Do not begin postpartum administration until vital signs have stabilized (wait at least 4 h after delivery); exercise particular caution if a patient has toxemia or has received within the preceding 24-h period a drug that can affect blood pressure. Monitor blood pressure periodically, especially during the first few days of therapy, and exercise caution if patient is taking other medications that are known to lower blood pressure.
Rebound lactation	Discontinuing bromocriptine following use for prevention of lactation results in mild to moderate breast engorgement, congestion, or secretion in 18–40% of patients
Digital vasospasm	In some acromegalic patients receiving bromocriptine, digital vasospasm may occur following exposure to the cold; reaction can be prevented by keeping the fingers warm and reversed by lowering the dosage
Peptic ulcers	In acromegalic patients, severe GI bleeding, sometimes followed by death, has occurred as a result of peptic ulcers; however, no evidence has shown that bromocriptine affects the incidence of peptic ulcers. Nevertheless, during therapy, thoroughly investigate any sign or symptom suggestive of peptic ulcer.
Tumor expansion	Possible expansion of growth hormone secreting tumors has been seen in a few acromegalic patients; since the natural course of these tumors is not known, any acromegalic patient should be carefully observed and, if evidence of tumor expansion is detected, therapy should be discontinued
Confusion and mental disturbances	May occur in Parkinson's disease patients receiving high doses; since these patients may manifest mild degrees of dementia, use bromocriptine with caution
Pulmonary reactions	In a few patients receiving 20–100 mg/day for 6–36 mo, bromocriptine has produced pulmonary infiltrates, pleural effusion, and thickening of the pleura; these effects were slowly reversed following discontinuation of therapy
Hallucinations, confusion	Bromocriptine has caused visual hallucinations in patients with acromegaly and visual and auditory hallucinations in patients with Parkinson's disease; in rare instances, hallucinations have persisted for several weeks after discontinuation of high-dose antiparkinson therapy. If hallucinations occur, reduce dosage or, if necessary, discontinue bromocriptine. High doses of bromocriptine can produce confusion and other CNS disturbances; exercise caution during antiparkinson therapy.
Arrhythmia	During antiparkinson therapy, exercise caution if the patient has a history of myocardial infarction and a residual arrhythmia

ADVERSE REACTIONS Frequent reactions (incidence ≥ 1%) are printed in *italics*

When used to treat hyperprolactinemic disorders

Gastrointestinal	*Nausea (49%), vomiting (5%), abdominal cramps (4%), constipation and diarrhea (3%)*
Central nervous system	*Headache (19%), dizziness (17%), fatigue (7%), light-headedness (5%), drowsiness (3%)*, CSF rhinorrhea (rare)
Other	*Nasal congestion (3%)*, slight hypotension

When used to prevent physiological lactation

Gastrointestinal	*Nausea (7%), vomiting (3%)*, abdominal cramps and diarrhea (0.4%)
Central nervous system	*Headache (10%), dizziness (8%), fatigue (1%)*
Cardiovascular	*Hypotension (28%)*, syncope (0.7%); hypertension, cerebrovascular accident, and seizures (rare)

When used to treat acromegaly

Gastrointestinal	*Nausea (18%), constipation (14%), anorexia and dyspepsia (4%), vomiting (2%)*, GI bleeding (< 2%)
Central nervous system	*Drowsiness/tiredness (3%), dizziness and headache (< 2%)*, alcohol potentiation, faintness, light-headedness, decreased sleep requirement, visual hallucinations, lassitude, vertigo, paresthesia, sluggishness, delusional psychosis, paranoia, insomnia, heavy headedness
Cardiovascular	*Orthostatic hypotension (6%), digital vasospasm (3%)*, syncope and exacerbation of Raynaud's syndrome (< 2%), vasovagal attack, arrhythmia, ventricular tachycardia, bradycardia, reduced tolerance to cold, tingling of ears, facial pallor, muscle cramps
Other	*Dry mouth/nasal congestion (4%)*, hair loss, shortness of breath

When used as an adjunct to levodopa in Parkinson's disease

Gastrointestinal	*Nausea, vomiting, abdominal discomfort, constipation*, anorexia, dry mouth, dysphagia

PARLODEL ■ PERGONAL

Central nervous system	*Abnormal involuntary movements, hallucinations, confusion, "on-off" phenomenon, dizziness, drowsiness, faintness/fainting, asthenia, visual disturbance, ataxia, insomnia, depression, vertigo,* anxiety, blepharospasm, epileptiform seizure, fatigue, headache, lethargy, nervousness, nightmares, paresthesia
Cardiovascular	*Hypotension,* pedal and ankle edema, erythromelalgia, signs and symptoms of ergotism (eg, tingling of the fingers, cold feet, numbness, muscle cramps of the feet and legs, exacerbation of Raynaud's syndrome; rare)
Dermatological	Mottling, rash
Genitourinary	Urinary frequency, incontinence, or retention
Other	*Shortness of breath,* nasal congestion

OVERDOSAGE

Signs and symptoms	See ADVERSE REACTIONS
Treatment	Discontinue medication; treat symptomatically and institute supportive measures, as required

DRUG INTERACTIONS

Diuretics, antihypertensive agents	△ Risk of hypotension; exercise caution
Dopamine antagonists (eg, phenothiazines, haloperidol)	▽ Therapeutic effect of bromocriptine, especially in patients undergoing treatment of macroadenomas
Estrogens, progestins (including oral contraceptives)	▽ Antiamenorrheic effect of bromocriptine

ALTERED LABORATORY VALUES

Blood/serum values	▽ Prolactin ▽ Growth hormone △ BUN △ SGOT △ SGPT △ GGPT △ Creatine phosphokinase △ Alkaline phosphatase △ Uric acid

No clinically significant alterations in urinary values occur at therapeutic dosages

---

USE IN CHILDREN

Safety and effectiveness for use in children under 15 yr of age have not been established

USE IN PREGNANT AND NURSING WOMEN

Pregnant women: Congenital malformations have been seen in 3.3% of infants born to women who received this drug during pregnancy; spontaneous abortions have occurred in 11% of pregnancies during which this drug was used. Although these frequencies do not exceed those generally reported for the population at large, safety for use during pregnancy has not been established. Women who wish to become pregnant should use a contraceptive, other than an oral contraceptive, during the period of amenorrhea (see ADMINISTRATION/DOSAGE ADJUSTMENTS). Bromocriptine has been used during pregnancy to treat optic nerve compression and visual field defects associated with macroadenomas (see WARNINGS/PRECAUTIONS). **Nursing mothers:** Since bromocriptine inhibits lactation, it should not be administered to women who elect to breast-feed.

FERTILITY INDUCERS

PERGONAL (menotropins) Serono   Rx

Ampuls: 75 IU follicle-stimulating hormone (FSH) and 75 IU luteinizing hormone (LH); 150 IU FSH and 150 IU LH

INDICATIONS

Induction of ovulation in patients with anovulatory infertility due to pituitary dysfunction

Stimulation of spermatogenesis in patients with primary hypogonadotropic hypogonadism due to prepuberal hypophysectomy or a congenital factor, or with secondary hypogonadotropic hypogonadism due to hypophysectomy, craniopharyngioma, cerebral aneurysm, or chromophobe adenoma

PARENTERAL DOSAGE

Adult: 75 IU each of FSH and LH daily by IM injection for 7–12 days, followed, when sufficient follicular maturation has occurred, by 5,000–10,000 USP units human chorionic gonadotropin (HCG) 1 day after the last dose. If there are signs of ovulation, but pregnancy does not ensue, repeat the same course at least twice before increasing the dosage to 150 IU each of FSH and LH daily. If necessary, repeat the higher-dosage course twice.

Adult: 5,000 USP units HCG 3 times/wk for 4–6 mo, until adequate masculinization and normal serum testosterone levels are achieved, followed for 4 mo by 75 IU each of FSH and LH 3 times/wk by IM injection plus 2,000 USP units HCG 2 times/wk. If increased spermatogenesis does not occur, continue concomitant regimen with the daily dose of menotropins either unchanged or increased to 150 IU each of FSH and LH

CONTRAINDICATIONS

Women

Elevated gonadotropin levels indicating primary ovarian failure

Thyroid and adrenal dysfunction

Infertility not caused by anovulation

Pregnancy

Organic intracranial lesion (eg, pituitary tumor)

Abnormal bleeding of undetermined origin

Ovarian cysts or enlargement not due to polycystic ovary syndrome

Men

Normal gonadotropin levels indicating normal pituitary function, or elevated levels indicating primary testicular failure

Infertility not caused by hypogonadotropic hypogonadism

COMPENDIUM OF DRUG THERAPY

ADMINISTRATION/DOSAGE ADJUSTMENTS

Pretreatment evaluation — **Women:** Document anovulation; rule out endometrial carcinoma (particularly in older patients), uterine and tubal pathology, primary ovarian failure, and early pregnancy; evaluate the male partner's fertility potential. **Men:** Document lack of normal pituitary function (suitable patients have low testosterone levels, low or absent gonadotropin levels, and underdeveloped secondary sex characteristics or decreased masculinization).

Monitoring of therapy — Follicular growth and development may be monitored by ultrasonography, increases in serum and 24-h urinary estrogen levels, and changes in vaginal and cervical smears; when examining cervical mucus, note volume, appearance, and Spinnbarkeit and look for ferning. For confirmation of ovulation, watch for the following: (1) increases in basal body temperature and urinary pregnanediol level, (2) change in the cervical mucus from a fern pattern to a cellular pattern, (3) vaginal cytology characteristic of the luteal phase, and (4) menstruation after the shift in basal body temperature.

Timing of intercourse — Beginning on the day before HCG administration, the couple should be encouraged to have intercourse daily until ovulation becomes evident

Preparation of parenteral solution and IM administration — Reconstitute with sterile saline solution, using 1–2 ml per ampul; administer IM immediately, and discard any unused reconstituted material

WARNINGS/PRECAUTIONS

Ovarian overstimulation — Mild to moderate uncomplicated ovarian enlargement, possibly with abdominal distension and/or pain, occurs in ~ 20% of patients and generally regresses without treatment in 2–3 wk. The hyperstimulation syndrome occurs in ~ 0.4% of patients given the recommended dose; this syndrome, characterized by sudden ovarian enlargement and ascites and sometimes accompanied by pain and/or pleural effusion, develops rapidly over a period of 3–4 days, generally within the first 2 wk following treatment. Excessive ovarian stimulation is most evident 7–10 days after ovulation. During therapy and the 2-wk period after HCG administration, examine all patients at least every other day for signs of overstimulation and perform appropriate tests and procedures (see "Monitoring of therapy," above). If the ovaries become abnormally enlarged or abdominal pain occurs, stop therapy; for treatment of the hyperstimulation syndrome, see OVERDOSAGE.

Hemoperitoneum — During therapy, hemoperitoneum from ruptured ovarian cysts can occur, usually as a result of pelvic examination. If bleeding necessitates surgery, perform partial resection of the enlarged ovary or ovaries. To lessen the danger of hemoperitoneum, instruct patients with significant postovulatory ovarian enlargement not to engage in intercourse.

Multiple births — Before beginning treatment of anovulation, advise patients of the frequency[1] and potential hazards of multiple births; 15% of deliveries have involved twins (93% of which were viable), and 5% of deliveries have involved three or more conceptuses (of which only 20% were viable)

Arterial thromboembolism — In four women, arterial thromboembolism developed after treatment with menotropins and HCG; two of these women died

Birth defects — In clinical studies of menotropins in infertile women, birth defects were seen in 1.7% of completed pregnancies, but these defects were not considered to be drug-related.[2] A single instance of infant death due to hydrocephalus and cardiac anomalies has subsequently been reported. Birth defects have also been seen following use of menotropins and HCG in men.[3]

Fever — Febrile reactions occasionally occur; it is not clear whether they are pyrogenic responses or possible allergic reactions

Carcinogenicity — No long-term studies have been done to determine the carcinogenic potential of this preparation

ADVERSE REACTIONS

Frequent reactions (incidence ≥ 1%) are printed in *italics*

Women

Genitourinary — *Mild to moderate uncomplicated ovarian enlargement, possibly with abdominal distension and/or pain (~ 20%);* hyperstimulation syndrome: sudden ovarian enlargement and ascites, possibly with pain and/or pleural effusion; hemoperitoneum resulting from ruptured ovarian cysts; ectopic pregnancy

Local — Pain, rash, swelling, irritation

Other — Fever, arterial thromboembolism, birth defects

Men

Hematological — Erythrocytosis (one case)

Other — Gynecomastia

OVERDOSAGE

Signs and symptoms — Hyperstimulation syndrome (see ADVERSE REACTIONS)

Treatment — Stop therapy, hospitalize patient, and determine if hemoconcentration associated with fluid loss into the abdominal cavity has occurred by evaluating fluid intake and output, weight, hematocrit, serum and urinary electrolytes, and urine specific gravity daily or more often, if necessary. Treat symptomatically with bed rest, fluid and electrolyte replacement, and analgesics, as needed. *Do not remove ascitic fluid.*

PERGONAL ■ PROFASI HP

DRUG INTERACTIONS

No clinically significant drug interactions have been identified

ALTERED LABORATORY VALUES

Blood/serum values	⇧ Estrogen		
Urinary values	⇧ Estrogen	⇧ Estriol	⇧ Pregnanediol

USE IN CHILDREN
Not indicated for use in children

USE IN PREGNANT AND NURSING WOMEN
Pregnant women: Pregnancy Category X: this preparation may cause harm to the fetus; do not use during pregnancy. Women who inadvertently receive this preparation during pregnancy should be apprised of the potential hazard to the fetus. **Nursing mothers:** It is not known whether this preparation is excreted in human milk; use with caution in nursing mothers.

[1] Frequency of multiple births (by diagnosis): primary amenorrhea, 25%; secondary amenorrhea, 28%; secondary amenorrhea with galactorrhea, 41%; polycystic ovaries, 17%; anovulatory cycles, 14%; other, 2%
[2] The following congenital anomalies have been observed in clinical studies: imperforate anus, sigmoid colon aplasia, third-degree hypospadias, cecovesicle fistula, bifid scrotum, meningocele, bilateral internal tibial torsion, right metatarsus adductus, possible heart lesions, supernumerary digit, bladder exstrophy, and Down's syndrome; abortions occurred in 25% of pregnancies
[3] Among 160 pregnancies resulting from the use of this drug and HCG in men, there were three congenital anomalies at birth (esophageal atresia, unilateral cryptorchidism, and inguinal hernia), seven spontaneous abortions, and one ectopic pregnancy

FERTILITY INDUCERS

PROFASI HP (chorionic gonadotropin, human [HCG]) Serono   Rx

Vials: 5,000 USP units, 10,000 USP units (= International Units [IU]) (10 ml) for IM use only

INDICATIONS	PARENTERAL DOSAGE
Prepuberal cryptorchism not due to anatomical obstruction	**Child:** 4,000 IU, given IM 3 times/wk for 3 wk; 5,000 IU, given IM every other day for 4 doses; 500–1,000 IU, given IM for 15 doses over a period of 6 wk; or 500 IU, given IM 3 times/wk for 4–6 wk, followed 1 mo later, if necessary, by a second course using 1,000 IU/injection
Male hypogonadotropic hypogonadism secondary to pituitary (luteinizing hormone) deficiency	**Adult:** 500–1,000 IU, given IM 3 times/wk for 3 wk and then 2 times/wk for an additional 3 wk, or 4,000 IU, given IM 3 times/wk for 6–9 mo, followed by 2,000 IU, given IM 3 times/wk for an additional 3 mo
Stimulation of spermatogenesis in patients with primary hypogonadotropic hypogonadism due to prepuberal hypophysectomy or a congenital factor, or with secondary hypogonadotropic hypogonadism due to hypophysectomy, craniopharyngioma, cerebral aneurysm, or chromophobe adenoma	**Adult:** 5,000 IU, given IM 3 times/wk for 4–6 mo (until adequate masculinization and normal serum testosterone levels are achieved), followed by 2,000 IU, given IM 2 times/wk with 1 ampul of menotropins 3 times/wk for 4 mo; if increased spermatogenesis does not occur, continue concomitant regimen with either the same dosage of menotropins or 2 ampuls 3 times/wk
Induction of ovulation in patients with anovulatory infertility due to secondary causes	**Adult:** 5,000–10,000 IU, given IM 1 day after the last dose of menotropins

CONTRAINDICATIONS

Prostatic carcinoma or other androgen-dependent neoplasms	Hypersensitivity to HCG	Precocious puberty

ADMINISTRATION/DOSAGE ADJUSTMENTS

Treatment of cryptorchism	Therapy is usually instituted in children 4–9 yr of age. Testicular descent usually reverses when HCG is discontinued, although in some cases the descent is permanent. Since HCG is thought to be effective in patients in whom descent would otherwise occur at puberty, therapy may help predict whether orchiopexy will eventually be necessary.
Reconstitution of parenteral solution	Withdraw sterile air from lyophilized vial and inject into diluent vial. Remove 10 ml of Bacteriostatic Water for Injection from diluent vial, add to lyophilized vial, and agitate gently. Refrigerate solution after reconstitution, and use within 60 days.
Use of menotropins and HCG	See appropriate information on use of menotropins before beginning concomitant or sequential therapy

COMPENDIUM OF DRUG THERAPY

PROFASI HP ■ SEROPHENE

WARNINGS/PRECAUTIONS

Androgenic effects	Discontinue treatment of cryptorchidism if signs of precocious puberty occur, since HCG induces androgen secretion
Treatment of obesity	HCG is ineffective as an adjunct in obesity management programs; it has no known effect on appetite, hunger, body fat distribution, or fat mobilization
Special-risk patients	Use with caution in patients with cardiac or renal disease, epilepsy, migraine, or asthma, since androgens may cause fluid retention and edema

ADVERSE REACTIONS

Central nervous system	Headache, irritability, restlessness, depression, fatigue
Other	Edema, precocious puberty, gynecomastia, pain at injection site

OVERDOSAGE

There have been no reports of acute overdosage in humans

DRUG INTERACTIONS

No clinically significant drug interactions have been identified

ALTERED LABORATORY VALUES

Urinary values	False-positive pregnancy tests 17-Ketosteroids 17-Hydroxycorticosteroids

No clinically significant alterations in blood/serum values occur at therapeutic dosages

---

USE IN CHILDREN

See INDICATIONS and PARENTERAL DOSAGE

USE IN PREGNANT AND NURSING WOMEN

Not indicated for use in pregnant or nursing women

FERTILITY INDUCERS

SEROPHENE (clomiphene citrate) Serono Rx

Tablets: 50 mg

INDICATIONS	ORAL DOSAGE
Induction of ovulation in patients with secondary anovulatory infertility	**Adult:** 50 mg/day for 5 days, beginning on or about the 5th day of the menstrual cycle if spontaneous uterine bleeding occurs or progesterone-induced bleeding is planned, or at any time if there has been no recent history of bleeding; repeat course up to two more times if ovulation, but not conception, occurs during the first cycle

CONTRAINDICATIONS

Abnormal uterine bleeding	Hepatic disease or history of hepatic dysfunction	Pregnancy
Ovarian cysts		

ADMINISTRATION/DOSAGE ADJUSTMENTS

Pretreatment evaluation	Clomiphene should be used only in patients with evidence of normal estrogen function (as estimated by vaginal smears, endometrial biopsy, urinary assay, or progesterone-induced bleeding), potent and fertile partners, and normal adrenal, thyroid, and liver function. Do not give to patients with primary pituitary or ovarian failure, ovarian cysts, abnormal uterine bleeding, or endometrial carcinoma (do not overlook neoplastic lesions; obtain an endometrial biopsy in older patients). Perform a complete pelvic examination before each course of treatment.
Lack of response to initial course of therapy	If ovulation does not occur following 50 mg/day, increase dosage during next course to 100 mg/day for 5 days, beginning as early as 30 days after previous course; if ovulation, but not conception, occurs at this dosage, course may be repeated once
Patients with unusual sensitivity to pituitary gonadotropins	Reduce dosage or duration of treatment course (see WARNINGS/PRECAUTIONS)

WARNINGS/PRECAUTIONS

Visual symptoms	Blurring and other visual disturbances (see ADVERSE REACTIONS) may occur, depending on dose; discontinue use and perform a complete ophthalmological evaluation. Caution patients that performance of potentially hazardous activities may be impaired if vision is affected, particularly under variable lighting.

SEROPHENE ■ PARLODEL

Ovarian overstimulation	Abnormal ovarian enlargement and cyst formation, possibly accompanied by pain, may occur, especially in patients with polycystic ovary syndrome; to reduce the hazard, the lowest dose consistent with expectation of good results should be used. Maximal enlargement of the ovary, whether physiological or abnormal, does not occur until several days after discontinuation of therapy; patients who complain of pelvic pain after clomiphene treatment should be carefully examined. If ovarian enlargement does occur, stop treatment until the ovaries have returned to pretreatment size, and reduce the dosage or duration of the next course; manage cystic enlargement conservatively, unless a strong indication for laparotomy exists.
Inadvertent use during early pregnancy	May be avoided by recording the basal body temperature throughout all treatment cycles and by observing patient carefully to determine whether ovulation has occurred; if basal body temperature following clomiphene treatment is biphasic and is not followed by menses, examine patient for an ovarian cyst and perform a pregnancy test. Delay the next course of therapy until it is determined that the patient is not pregnant.
Mulitple pregnancy	The prospective parents should be advised of the frequency and potential hazards of multiple pregnancy before starting treatment; of the pregnancies reported following the use of clomiphene, 10% resulted in twins and < 1% in more than two infants

ADVERSE REACTIONS[1]

Frequent reactions (incidence ≥ 1%) are printed in *italics*

Genitourinary	*Ovarian enlargement and cyst formation (14%)*, increased urination, abnormal uterine bleeding; prolongation of the luteal phase (with higher dosages or prolonged use)
Cardiovascular	*Vasomotor flushes (11%)*
Gastrointestinal	*Abdominal discomfort (7.4%), nausea and vomiting (2.1%)*
Central nervous system	*Nervousness and insomnia (1.9%), headache (1%), dizziness and light-headedness (1%)*, depression, fatigue
Ophthalmic	*Visual symptoms (1.6%)*, including blurred vision, spots, or flashes (scintillating scotomata); electroretinographic changes, objectively defined scotomata
Dermatological	Urticaria, allergic dermatitis, reversible hair loss
Congenital anomalies[2]	Down's syndrome (six cases); extrophia, club foot, tibial torsion, blocked tear duct, and hemangioma (one case each)
Other	*Breast tenderness (2.1%)*, weight gain

OVERDOSAGE

Signs and symptoms	See WARNINGS/PRECAUTIONS and ADVERSE REACTIONS
Treatment	Discontinue use; treat symptomatically and institute supportive measures, as needed

DRUG INTERACTIONS

No clinically significant drug interactions have been identified

ALTERED LABORATORY VALUES

Blood/serum values	△ Sulfobromophthalein (BSP) retention △ FSH △ LH △ Desmosterol △ Transcortin △ Thyroxine △ Sex hormone-binding globulin △ Thyroxine-binding globulin
Urinary values	△ FSH △ LH △ Estrogen

USE IN CHILDREN

Not indicated for use in children

USE IN PREGNANT AND NURSING WOMEN

Contraindicated for use during pregnancy (see WARNINGS/PRECAUTIONS). Not indicated for use in nursing mothers.

---

[1] Adverse effects appear to be dose-dependent
[2] Congenital anomalies were reported in 2.5% (45/1,803) of births following clomiphene use; the cumulative rate does not exceed that observed in the general population

---

PROLACTIN INHIBITORS

PARLODEL (bromocriptine mesylate) Sandoz Pharmaceuticals Rx

Capsules: 5 mg **Tablets:** 2.5 mg

INDICATIONS

Hyperprolactinemic disorders, including amenorrhea, galactorrhea, hypogonadism (infertility), and prolactin-secreting adenomas

Prevention of physiological lactation after parturition, stillbirth, or abortion

ORAL DOSAGE

Adult: 1.25–2.5 mg/day to start, followed, as tolerated, by an increase in dosage of 2.5 mg/day every 3–7 days, until an optimal response is achieved; therapeutic dosage is usually 5–7.5 mg/day, but may range from 2.5–15 mg/day. To manage adverse reactions, temporarily reduce dosage to 1.25 mg bid or tid.

Adult: 2.5 mg bid for 14 days or, if necessary, up to 21 days (dosage range: 2.5–7.5 mg/day); begin administration after vital signs have stabilized, but not sooner than 4 h after delivery

COMPENDIUM OF DRUG THERAPY

PARLODEL

Acromegaly	**Adult:** 1.25–2.5 mg/day, given at bedtime with food for 3 days, followed, as tolerated, by an increase in dosage of 1.25–2.5 mg/day every 3–7 days until optimal response or a maximum of 100 mg/day is achieved; usual dosage: 20–30 mg/day
Idiopathic or postencephalitic Parkinson's disease, as an adjunct to levodopa (alone or with a peripheral decarboxylase inhibitor, such as carbidopa)	**Adult:** 1.25 mg bid to start, followed, as needed, by an increase in dosage of 2.5 mg/day every 14–28 days until optimal response or a maximum of 100 mg/day is achieved. If possible, maintain dosage of levodopa while titrating dosage of bromocriptine; if dosage of levodopa is subsequently reduced, retitrate dosage of bromocriptine.

CONTRAINDICATIONS
Sensitivity to ergot alkaloids

ADMINISTRATION/DOSAGE ADJUSTMENTS

Administration	Give each dose with food
Use of contraceptives and pregnancy tests	Bromocriptine can restore fertility, which may not only be undesirable, but may also pose the following two risks: (1) the drug may subsequently affect fetal development if pregnancy is not detected at the time of conception (see USE IN PREGNANT AND NURSING WOMEN) and (2) the hormonal changes during pregnancy may cause optic nerve compression if the woman has a prolactin-secreting macroadenoma (see WARNINGS/PRECAUTIONS). Instruct women who do not wish to become pregnant to use a contraceptive, other than an oral contraceptive, as long as they are undergoing treatment. To avoid prolonged in utero exposure in the event of an unsuspected pregnancy, instruct women seeking to become pregnant to use such a contraceptive during the period of amenorrhea. Test for pregnancy in all patients at least every 4 wk during the period of amenorrhea and, after a normal ovulatory cycle has been restored, whenever menstruation does not occur within 3 days of the expected date. Discontinue therapy any time pregnancy is suspected.
Amenorrhea, galactorrhea	In patients with amenorrhea, menses is usually seen after 6–8 wk of therapy; however, response may vary from a few days to up to 8 mo. Control of galactorrhea depends on the degree of mammary stimulation prior to therapy. A reduction in secretion of at least 75% usually occurs after 8–12 wk of therapy; however, galactorrhea may fail to respond even after 12 mo of treatment.
Prolactinomas	Bromocriptine may be given alone to treat prolactin-secreting adenomas or, alternatively, may be used to reduce the size of macroadenomas prior to adenectomy. It is not known whether drug therapy or surgery is the more effective treatment for patients experiencing loss of visual field; if loss progresses rapidly, the appropriate form of therapy should be decided after a neurosurgeon has examined the patient. Caution patients that discontinuation of drug therapy usually results in rapid regrowth of macroadenomas and recurrence of symptoms.
Acromegaly	When used alone or in conjunction with surgery or radiotherapy, bromocriptine reduces the serum growth hormone level by at least 50% in approximately one-half of patients; however, a normal serum level is usually not attained. After each adjustment in dosage, reevaluate diagnosis and then evaluate clinical response and check serum level; if no significant reduction in the serum level occurs after a brief trial, either continue to titrate dosage or terminate administration. Once a maintenance dosage has been established, monitor clinical response and serum level monthly and then at periodic intervals. If a patient has undergone radiotherapy, use of the drug should be interrupted annually for a period of 4–8 wk to assess the relative effects of radiation and drug treatment, since the full therapeutic effect of radiotherapy may not occur until after several years; if signs or symptoms recur or the serum level increases, consider resuming therapy.
Parkinson's disease	Bromocriptine can enhance therapeutic response in patients receiving levodopa and may also permit a reduction in the maintenance dose when these patients experience adverse effects such as dyskinesia and "on-off" phenomenon; bear in mind that safety and effectiveness of bromocriptine for use as an antiparkinson agent for more than 2 yr have not been established. When titrating dosage of bromocriptine, assess therapeutic response every 2 wk. During chronic therapy, check renal, hepatic, cardiovascular, and hematopoietic functions periodically.

WARNINGS/PRECAUTIONS

Dizziness, drowsiness, syncope	Caution all patients that their ability to drive, operate machinery, or engage in other activities requiring rapid and precise response may be impaired during therapy
Renal, hepatic disease	Safety and effectiveness for use in patients with renal or hepatic disease have not been established
Compression of the optic nerve	Hormonal changes during pregnancy can cause expansion of prolactin-secreting adenomas and result in compression of the optic or other cranial nerves. Although compression usually disappears after delivery, emergency surgery may be necessary in some cases. Bromocriptine has reportedly caused improvement of visual field symptoms owing to nerve compression; however, safety for use during pregnancy has not been established. To reduce the risk of nerve compression, carefully assess the pituitary gland and look for evidence of a prolactin-secreting adenoma before beginning treatment of hyperprolactinemic disorders such as hypogonadism and amenorrhea since these disorders may be due to a pituitary adenoma. Avoid pregnancy, when possible (see ADMINISTRATION/DOSAGE ADJUSTMENTS). If or when the patient becomes pregnant, watch closely for signs and symptoms that may indicate enlargement of a known or previously undetected adenoma.

PARLODEL

CSF rhinorrhea	In rare instances, bromocriptine may cause CSF rhinorrhea in patients who have macroadenomas that extend into the sphenoid sinus or who have undergone transsphenoidal surgery or pituitary radiotherapy; caution these patients to report any persistent watery nasal discharge
Effects on blood pressure	Bromocriptine can cause symptomatic hypotension, particularly when given postpartum; in 28% of patients who received this drug for prevention of lactation, systolic pressure decreased by more than 20 mm Hg and diastolic pressure declined by more than 10 mm Hg. In rare instances, postpartum use may precipitate hypertension in patients who have toxemia or are receiving other drugs, including other ergot alkaloids, that can increase blood pressure. Do not begin postpartum administration until vital signs have stabilized (wait at least 4 h after delivery); exercise particular caution if a patient has toxemia or has received within the preceding 24-h period a drug that can affect blood pressure. Monitor blood pressure periodically, especially during the first few days of therapy, and exercise caution if patient is taking other medications that are known to lower blood pressure.
Rebound lactation	Discontinuing bromocriptine following use for prevention of lactation results in mild to moderate breast engorgement, congestion, or secretion in 18–40% of patients
Digital vasospasm	In some acromegalic patients receiving bromocriptine, digital vasospasm may occur following exposure to the cold; reaction can be prevented by keeping the fingers warm and reversed by lowering the dosage
Peptic ulcers	In acromegalic patients, severe GI bleeding, sometimes followed by death, has occurred as a result of peptic ulcers; however, no evidence has shown that bromocriptine affects the incidence of peptic ulcers. Nevertheless, during therapy, thoroughly investigate any sign or symptom suggestive of peptic ulcer.
Tumor expansion	Possible expansion of growth hormone secreting tumors has been seen in a few acromegalic patients; since the natural course of these tumors is not known, any acromegalic patient should be carefully observed and, if evidence of tumor expansion is detected, therapy should be discontinued
Confusion and mental disturbances	May occur in Parkinson's disease patients receiving high doses; since these patients may manifest mild degrees of dementia, use bromocriptine with caution
Pulmonary reactions	In a few patients receiving 20–100 mg/day for 6–36 mo, bromocriptine has produced pulmonary infiltrates, pleural effusion, and thickening of the pleura; these effects were slowly reversed following discontinuation of therapy
Hallucinations, confusion	Bromocriptine has caused visual hallucinations in patients with acromegaly and visual and auditory hallucinations in patients with Parkinson's disease; in rare instances, hallucinations have persisted for several weeks after discontinuation of high-dose antiparkinson therapy. If hallucinations occur, reduce dosage or, if necessary, discontinue bromocriptine. High doses of bromocriptine can produce confusion and other CNS disturbances; exercise caution during antiparkinson therapy.
Arrhythmia	During antiparkinson therapy, exercise caution if the patient has a history of myocardial infarction and a residual arrhythmia

ADVERSE REACTIONS

Frequent reactions (incidence $\geq$ 1%) are printed in *italics*

When used to treat hyperprolactinemic disorders

Gastrointestinal	*Nausea (49%), vomiting (5%), abdominal cramps (4%), constipation and diarrhea (3%)*
Central nervous system	*Headache (19%), dizziness (17%), fatigue (7%), light-headedness (5%), drowsiness (3%)*, CSF rhinorrhea (rare)
Other	*Nasal congestion (3%)*, slight hypotension

When used to prevent physiological lactation

Gastrointestinal	*Nausea (7%), vomiting (3%)*, abdominal cramps and diarrhea (0.4%)
Central nervous system	*Headache (10%), dizziness (8%), fatigue (1%)*
Cardiovascular	*Hypotension (28%)*, syncope (0.7%); hypertension, cerebrovascular accident, and seizures (rare)

When used to treat acromegaly

Gastrointestinal	*Nausea (18%), constipation (14%), anorexia and dyspepsia (4%), vomiting (2%)*, GI bleeding (< 2%)
Central nervous system	*Drowsiness/tiredness (3%)*, dizziness and headache (< 2%), alcohol potentiation, faintness, light-headedness, decreased sleep requirement, visual hallucinations, lassitude, vertigo, paresthesia, sluggishness, delusional psychosis, paranoia, insomnia, heavy headedness
Cardiovascular	*Orthostatic hypotension (6%), digital vasospasm (3%)*, syncope and exacerbation of Raynaud's syndrome (< 2%), vasovagal attack, arrhythmia, ventricular tachycardia, bradycardia, reduced tolerance to cold, tingling of ears, facial pallor, muscle cramps
Other	*Dry mouth/nasal congestion (4%)*, hair loss, shortness of breath

When used as an adjunct to levodopa in Parkinson's disease

PARLODEL ■ PROTROPIN

Gastrointestinal	*Nausea, vomiting, abdominal discomfort, constipation,* anorexia, dry mouth, dysphagia
Central nervous system	*Abnormal involuntary movements, hallucinations, confusion, "on-off" phenomenon, dizziness, drowsiness, faintness/fainting, asthenia, visual disturbance, ataxia, insomnia, depression, vertigo,* anxiety, blepharospasm, epileptiform seizure, fatigue, headache, lethargy, nervousness, nightmares, paresthesia
Cardiovascular	*Hypotension,* pedal and ankle edema, erythromelalgia, signs and symptoms of ergotism (eg, tingling of the fingers, cold feet, numbness, muscle cramps of the feet and legs, exacerbation of Raynaud's syndrome; rare)
Dermatological	Mottling, rash
Genitourinary	Urinary frequency, incontinence, or retention
Other	*Shortness of breath,* nasal congestion

OVERDOSAGE

Signs and symptoms	See ADVERSE REACTIONS
Treatment	Discontinue medication; treat symptomatically and institute supportive measures, as required

DRUG INTERACTIONS

Diuretics, antihypertensive agents	△ Risk of hypotension; exercise caution
Dopamine antagonists (eg, phenothiazines, haloperidol)	▽ Therapeutic effect of bromocriptine, especially in patients undergoing treatment of macroadenomas
Estrogens, progestins (including oral contraceptives)	▽ Antiamenorrheic effect of bromocriptine

ALTERED LABORATORY VALUES

Blood/serum values	▽ Prolactin ▽ Growth hormone △ BUN △ SGOT △ SGPT △ GGPT △ Creatine phosphokinase △ Alkaline phosphatase △ Uric acid

No clinically significant alterations in urinary values occur at therapeutic dosages

---

USE IN CHILDREN

Safety and effectiveness for use in children under 15 yr of age have not been established

USE IN PREGNANT AND NURSING WOMEN

Pregnant women: Congenital malformations have been seen in 3.3% of infants born to women who received this drug during pregnancy; spontaneous abortions have occurred in 11% of pregnancies during which this drug was used. Although these frequencies do not exceed those generally reported for the population at large, safety for use during pregnancy has not been established. Women who wish to become pregnant should use a contraceptive, other than an oral contraceptive, during the period of amenorrhea (see ADMINISTRATION/DOSAGE ADJUSTMENTS). Bromocriptine has been used during pregnancy to treat optic nerve compression and visual field defects associated with macroadenomas (see WARNINGS/PRECAUTIONS). **Nursing mothers:** Since bromocriptine inhibits lactation, it should not be administered to women who elect to breast-feed.

GROWTH HORMONES

PROTROPIN (somatrem) Genentech Rx

Vials: 5 mg

INDICATIONS

Growth failure due to lack of endogenous growth hormone secretion[1]

PARENTERAL DOSAGE

Child: 0.1 mg/kg IM, given 3 times/wk

CONTRAINDICATIONS

Progression of underlying intracranial lesions (see WARNINGS/PRECAUTIONS)	Hypersensitivity to benzyl alcohol (see WARNINGS/PRECAUTIONS)	Patients with closed epiphyses

ADMINISTRATION/DOSAGE ADJUSTMENTS

Dosage titration	Titrate dosage individually according to patient needs; because of the potential for adverse effects, do not exceed recommended dosage

PROTROPIN ■ ARMOUR Thyroid

Reconstitution of solution	Remove 1–5 ml of bacteriostatic water for injection USP (supplied); add to contents of vial, aiming the stream of liquid towards the glass wall. Gently swirl vial until contents are completely dissolved and solution is clear; any solution that is cloudy immediately after reconstitution or refrigeration must not be used. Do not shake vial since solution can then become cloudy. Occasionally, small, colorless particles that do not affect use may appear after refrigeration. Use only one dose per vial; do not reuse solution.

WARNINGS/PRECAUTIONS

Benzyl alcohol toxicity	The benzyl alcohol preservative in the supplied bacteriostatic water for injection USP has been associated with toxicity in newborns; for use in newborns, reconstitute lyophilized powder with water for injection USP
Intracranial lesions	Patients with growth hormone deficiency secondary to an intracranial lesion should be examined frequently for progression or recurrence of the underlying disease; lesions should be inactive and antitumor therapy completed before initiating therapy with somatrem. Discontinue therapy if tumor growth recurs.
Insulin resistance	Somatrem may induce a state of insulin resistance; observe patient for evidence of glucose intolerance
Concomitant glucocorticoid therapy	The growth-promoting effect of somatrem may be inhibited by glucocorticoid therapy; carefully adjust glucocorticoid dosage in patients with coexisting ACTH deficiency to avoid growth inhibition
Hypothyroidism	Somatrem may induce hypothyroidism, which, in turn, may prevent optimal response to the drug; perform periodic thyroid function tests and treat deficiencies with thyroid hormone, where indicated
Slipped capital femoral epiphysis	Dislocation of capital femoral epiphysis may occur during therapy; watch for development of a limp and be alert to complaints of hip and knee pain
Antibody proliferation	Persistent IgG-class antibodies to growth hormone have developed in approximately 30% of patients treated with somatrem, primarily children who had not previously been treated with exogenous growth hormone. Generally, these antibodies are not neutralizing and do not interfere with the growth response to somatrem. Perform tests for antibodies to human growth hormone in patients who fail to respond to therapy.
Hypersensitivity	A systemic allergic reaction may occur during therapy
Histopathologic effects	Microscopic examination of the kidneys, pituitary gland, lungs, liver, and pancreas of monkeys treated with somatrem has revealed no evidence of treatment-related toxicity

ADVERSE REACTIONS

Immunological	Antibody proliferation to growth hormone (see WARNINGS/PRECAUTIONS)

DRUG INTERACTIONS

Insulin	▽ Physiologic effect of insulin
Glucocorticosteroids	▽ Growth response to somatrem; adjust glucocorticoid dosage accordingly

ALTERED LABORATORY VALUES

Blood/serum values	▽ BUN △ Phosphate
Urinary values	△ Calcium △ Hydroxyproline

USE IN CHILDREN

See INDICATIONS and PARENTERAL DOSAGE; supplied diluent should not be used when treating newborns (see WARNINGS/PRECAUTIONS)

USE IN PREGNANT AND NURSING WOMEN

This drug is not indicated for use in pregnant or nursing women

---

[1] Somatrem is indicated only for the long-term treatment of growth failure caused by inadequate growth hormone secretion; other causes of short stature should be ruled out before starting treatment

---

THYROID HORMONES

ARMOUR Thyroid (thyroid) Rorer   Rx

Tablets: 15, 30, 60, 90, 120, 180, 240, 300 mg

INDICATIONS[1]
Hypothyroidism

ORAL DOSAGE
Adult: 30 mg/day to start, followed, as needed and tolerated, by an increase in dosage of 15 mg/day every 2–3 wk; usual dosage: 60–120 mg/day. Lack of response at 180 mg/day suggests noncompliance or malabsorption.

ARMOUR Thyroid

Congenital hypothyroidism	Infant (0–6 mo): 15–30 mg/day (4.8–6 mg/kg/day) Infant (6–12 mo): 30–45 mg/day (3.6–4.8 mg/kg/day) Child (1–5 yr): 45–60 mg/day (3–3.6 mg/kg/day) Child (6–12 yr): 60–90 mg/day (2.4–3 mg/kg/day) Child ($>$ 12 yr): 90 mg/day (1.2–1.8 mg/kg/day)

CONTRAINDICATIONS

Apparent hypersensitivity to any component — Adrenocortical insufficiency — Thyrotoxicosis

ADMINISTRATION/DOSAGE ADJUSTMENTS

Patients with cardiovascular disease, elderly patients	Give 15–30 mg/day to start if the patient is elderly or has a cardiovascular disease
Patients with long-standing myxedema	Give 15 mg/day to start if the patient has long-standing myxedema; exercise extreme caution if myxedema is accompanied by cardiovascular impairment
Monitoring of therapy	To evaluate thyroid hormone replacement therapy, periodically assess clinical response and appropriate laboratory values, including serum levels of TSH, total T_4, and free T_4; the first assessment should be done within 4 wk after starting treatment. Determination of free T_4 level is particularly warranted when the total T_4 level is low and the TSH level is normal. Bear in mind that in infants TSH secretion is relatively insensitive to thyroid hormone and therefore may not be a reliable indication of therapeutic response. If the serum concentration of thyroxine-binding globulin (TBG) is altered, the free T_4 level, rather than the total serum T_4 level, should be measured. The TBG level is increased by pregnancy, infectious hepatitis, and the use of estrogens or estrogen-containing oral contraceptives; the TBG level is decreased by nephrosis, acromegaly, and the use of androgens or corticosteroids. Familial hypo- and hyperthyroxine-binding globulinemia have also been described. Medicinal or dietary iodine reduces uptake of radioactive iodine. The persistence of clinical and laboratory evidence of hypothyroidism despite adequate dosage indicates poor compliance, malabsorption, excessive fecal loss, or inactivity of the preparation (intracellular resistance to thyroid hormone is quite rare).
Duration of therapy	Thyroid hormone replacement therapy is generally continued for life except in cases of transient hypothyroidism, which are usually associated with thyroiditis

WARNINGS/PRECAUTIONS

Obesity, infertility	In euthyroid patients, doses within the range of normal hormonal requirements are ineffective for weight reduction and higher doses may produce serious or even life-threatening toxicity, particularly when given with sympathomimetic amines; use of thyroid hormones for obesity is unjustified. Thyroid hormone therapy for infertility unaccompanied by hypothyroidism is also unjustified.
Subacute thyroiditis	Thyroid hormones should not be used for transient hypothyroidism occurring during the recovery phase of subacute thyroiditis
Toxicity	Caution patients to report immediately any signs or symptoms of overdosage. If toxicity occurs during therapy, reduce the dosage or, alternatively, discontinue administration temporarily and then resume use at a lower dosage. In normal individuals, hypothalamic-pituitary-thyroid function is fully restored in 6–8 wk after suppression. When performing the thyroid suppression test, exercise caution if thyroid gland autonomy is strongly suspected, since the effects of exogenous and endogenous hormone stimulation are additive.
Cardiovascular disease	Thyroid hormone therapy can exacerbate cardiovascular disease. Exercise great caution if a cardiovascular disorder, especially coronary artery disease, is suspected; consider elderly patients in general to be at increased risk since they are more likely to have occult heart disease. For patients with known or suspected cardiovascular disease, dosage should be reduced initially (see ADMINISTRATION/DOSAGE ADJUSTMENTS) and then whenever the disease is exacerbated.
Adrenocortical insufficiency	Thyroid hormone therapy can exacerbate symptoms of adrenocortical insufficiency; any such insufficiency should be corrected before the start of therapy, and, during treatment, measures used to control the disorder should be adjusted as needed
Diabetes	Thyroid hormone therapy can exacerbate signs and symptoms of diabetes mellitus or insipidus; closely monitor urinary glucose level during treatment (see also DRUG INTERACTIONS)
Carcinogenicity, mutagenicity, effect on fertility	An apparent association between prolonged thyroid hormone therapy and breast cancer has not been confirmed and therefore should not serve as a reason for discontinuing treatment; no long-term studies have been performed to evaluate the carcinogenic potential of thyroid hormone therapy. Long-term studies of mutagenicity and effects of exogenous thyroid hormones on fertility have also not been done.

ADVERSE REACTIONS

Hyperthyroidism

OVERDOSAGE

Signs and symptoms	Headache, irritability, nervousness, sweating, tachycardia, increased bowel motility, menstrual irregularities, occurrence or exacerbation of angina and cardiac failure, shock, thyroid storm

ARMOUR Thyroid ■ CYTOMEL

Treatment — Induce vomiting if further GI absorption can be reasonably prevented and coma, convulsions, and loss of the gagging reflex have not occurred. Maintain respiratory function, using oxygen, if necessary. Give cardiac glycosides for congestive heart failure and beta blockers, especially propranolol, for signs and symptoms associated with increased sympathomimetic activity. Institute appropriate measures, as needed, to control fever, hypoglycemia, and fluid loss.

DRUG INTERACTIONS

Oral anticoagulants — △ Anticoagulant effect with shift from hypothyroid to euthyroid state. Any patient receiving an oral anticoagulant should be watched very closely when thyroid hormone replacement therapy is started; the prothrombin time should be determined frequently throughout the course of combination therapy. A reduction in anticoagulant dosage will probably be necessary at least at the beginning of replacement therapy.

Insulin, sulfonylureas — Hyperglycemia; a patient receiving insulin or a sulfonylurea should be watched closely when thyroid hormone replacement therapy is started and, if necessary, the dosage of the antidiabetic agent should be increased

Cholestyramine — ▽ Absorption of thyroid hormone; separate administration of cholestyramine and thyroid hormone by 4–5 h

Estrogens (including oral contraceptives) — ▽ Free (unbound) thyroid hormone when thyroid gland is not functioning; an increase in the dosage of thyroid hormone may be necessary during concomitant therapy, but only if thyroid gland function is inadequate and the decrease in the free hormone level, which results from an estrogen-induced increase in the serum thyroxine-binding globulin level, cannot be reversed by a compensatory increase in hormonal output

Cardiac glycosides — ▽ Pharmacologic effect of cardiac glycosides with shift from hypothyroid to euthyroid state; increase dosage of cardiac glycosides during thyroid hormone replacement therapy

Tricyclic antidepressants — △ Pharmacologic effects of tricyclic antidepressants and thyroid hormone (transient cardiac arrhythmias have occurred)

Ketamine — Hypertension and tachycardia; exercise caution when using ketamine in a patient receiving thyroid hormone and be prepared to treat hypertension

Norepinephrine, epinephrine — △ Risk of coronary artery insufficiency, especially in a patient with coronary artery disease; any patient receiving thyroid hormone should be carefully observed after injection of a catecholamine

ALTERED LABORATORY VALUES

Blood/serum values — △ Glucose △ T_4 ▽ PBI
Urinary values — + Glucose

USE IN CHILDREN

Since congenital hypothyroidism occurs relatively frequently (1:4,000), the serum level of T_4 and/or TSH should be determined routinely in neonates; treatment should be started immediately after diagnosis (see ORAL DOSAGE). Administration of thyroid hormone is generally maintained for life. However, if transient hypothyroidism is suspected, therapy can be withdrawn after the age of 3 yr for a period of 2–8 wk; if a normal TSH level is maintained during this period, administration of thyroid hormone may be permanently discontinued. Bear in mind that excessive doses of thyroid hormone may produce craniosynostosis in infants. Partial loss of hair may occur in children during the first few months of therapy, but this condition usually reverses with continued treatment.

USE IN PREGNANT AND NURSING WOMEN

Pregnancy Category A: no adverse effect on fetal development has resulted from use of thyroid hormones in pregnant women (these hormones do not readily cross the placental barrier); thyroid hormone replacement therapy should not be discontinued during pregnancy. Use free hormone levels to assess therapy since thyroxine-binding globulin levels are increased during pregnancy. Minimal amounts of thyroid hormone are excreted in human milk; use with caution in nursing mothers, even though these hormones are not associated with any serious adverse reactions.

[1] As a TSH suppressant, thyroid hormone can be used to prevent or treat euthyroid goiter, subacute thyroiditis, or Hashimoto's disease or, in conjunction with radioactive iodine, to produce regression of metastases from follicular and papillary carcinoma; the drug can also be used diagnostically at a suppressive dosage to show thyroid gland autonomy in patients with Graves' ophthalmopathy or to evaluate patients who exhibit clinical signs of mild hyperthyroidism despite normal laboratory values

---

THYROID HORMONES

CYTOMEL (liothyronine sodium) Smith Kline & French   Rx
Tablets: 5, 25, 50 µg

INDICATIONS
Mild hypothyroidism

ORAL DOSAGE
Adult: 25 µg/day to start, followed, as needed, by an increase in dosage of 12.5–25 µg/day every 1–2 wk; maintenance dosage is usually 25–75 µg/day, but may be less than 25 µg/day or as high as 100 µg/day
Child: 5 µg/day, to start, followed, as needed, by an increase in dosage of 5 µg/day every 1–2 wk

CYTOMEL

Myxedema	**Adult:** 5 μg/day, followed, as needed, by an increase in dosage of 5–10 μg/day every 1–2 wk and then, once 25 μg/day is reached, by an increase in dosage of 12.5–25 μg/day every 1–2 wk; usual maintenance dosage: 50–100 μg/day
Simple (nontoxic) goiter	**Adult:** 5 μg/day, followed, as needed, by an increase in dosage of 5–10 μg/day every 1–2 wk and then, once 25 μg/day is reached, by an increase in dosage of 12.5–25 μg/day every 1–2 wk; usual maintenance dosage: 75 μg/day **Child:** 5 μg/day to start, followed, as needed, by an increase in dosage of 5 μg/day every 1–2 wk
Congenital hypothyroidism	**Child:** 5 μg/day, followed, as needed, by an increase in dosage of 5 μg/day every 3–4 days; for maintenance, children may require 20 μg/day at a few months of age, 50 μg/day at 1 yr of age, and the full adult dosage when over 3 yr of age
Thyroid suppression test	**Adult and child:** 75–100 μg/day for 7 days, with radioactive iodine uptake determined before and after the course

CONTRAINDICATIONS

Apparent hypersensitivity to any component	Adrenocortical insufficiency	Thyrotoxicosis

ADMINISTRATION/DOSAGE ADJUSTMENTS

Timing of administration	Give tablets once daily
Patients with cardiovascular disease, elderly patients	Give 5 μg/day to start; increase dosage, as needed and tolerated, by not more than 5 μg/day every 2 wk. Bear in mind that liothyronine has a relatively rapid onset of action.
Switching from other thyroid drugs	After levothyroxine, thyroglobulin, or thyroid has been discontinued, begin administration of liothyronine; dosage should be low to start and then gradually increased. When selecting the initial dosage, bear in mind that liothyronine has a rapid onset of action and that the effects of the other thyroid drug may persist for several weeks after withdrawal.
Thyroid suppression tests	When given in doses that exceed the amount secreted by the thyroid gland and that are capable of suppressing production of TSH, thyroid hormone can be used to show thyroid gland autonomy in patients with Graves' ophthalmopathy or to evaluate patients who exhibit clinical signs of mild hyperthyroidism despite normal laboratory values. If radioactive iodine uptake decreases by 50% or more after administration of suppressive doses, thyroid gland autonomy and hyperthyroidism can be ruled out.
Monitoring of therapy	Thyroid hormone replacement therapy should be evaluated periodically on the basis of clinical response and changes in the serum TSH level and other appropriate laboratory values; do not use serum T_4 values to assess effectiveness of treatment. Bear in mind that in infants TSH secretion is relatively insensitive to thyroid hormone and therefore may not be a reliable indication of therapeutic response. If the serum concentration of thyroxine-binding globulin (TBG) is altered, the free T_3 level, rather than the total serum T_3 level, should be measured. The TBG level is increased by pregnancy, infectious hepatitis, and the use of estrogens or estrogen-containing oral contraceptives; the TBG level is decreased by nephrosis, acromegaly, and the use of androgens or corticosteroids. Familial hypo- and hyperthyroxine-binding globulinemia have also been described. Medicinal or dietary iodine reduces uptake of radioactive iodine. The persistence of clinical and laboratory evidence of hypothyroidism despite adequate dosage indicates poor compliance, malabsorption, excessive fecal loss, or inactivity of the preparation (intracellular resistance to thyroid hormone is quite rare).
Duration of therapy	Thyroid hormone replacement therapy is generally continued for life except in cases of transient hypothyroidism, which are usually associated with thyroiditis
Liothyronine vs levothyroxine	Liothyronine may be preferred to levothyroxine when impaired peripheral conversion of T_4 to T_3 is suspected. Liothyronine may also be preferred for patients who undergo periodic radioisotope scanning procedures. The shorter half-life of liothyronine allows more abrupt discontinuation before the procedure, and the more rapid onset of action provides quicker resumption of therapeutic effect after the procedure; as a result, duration of hypothyroidism before and after the scan may be shorter. For replacement therapy in patients who may be particularly susceptible to adverse reactions, liothyronine offers the advantages of more rapid dosage adjustment and quicker control of toxicity; however, these advantages tend to be counterbalanced by the wide swings in the serum T_3 level following administration and the possibility of more severe cardiovascular reactions.

WARNINGS/PRECAUTIONS

Obesity, infertility	In euthyroid patients, doses within the range of normal hormonal requirements are ineffective for weight reduction and higher doses may produce serious or even life-threatening toxicity, particularly when given with sympathomimetic amines; use of thyroid hormones for obesity is unjustified. Thyroid hormone therapy for infertility unaccompanied by hypothyroidism is also unjustified.
Subacute thyroiditis	Thyroid hormones should not be used for transient hypothyroidism occurring during the recovery phase of subacute thyroiditis
Nephrosis, hypogonadism	Rule out nephrosis and morphologic hypogonadism before starting thyroid hormone therapy

CYTOMEL

Toxicity	In rare cases, use of thyroid hormones may precipitate or exacerbate hyperthyroidism. Caution patients to report immediately any signs or symptoms of overdosage. If toxicity occurs during therapy, reduce the dosage or, alternatively, discontinue administration temporarily and then resume use at a lower dosage. In normal individuals, hypothalamic-pituitary-thyroid function is fully restored in 6–8 wk after suppression. When performing the thyroid suppression test, exercise caution if thyroid gland autonomy is strongly suspected, since the effects of exogenous and endogenous hormone stimulation are additive.
Cardiovascular disease	Thyroid hormone therapy can exacerbate cardiovascular disease. Exercise great caution if a cardiovascular disorder, especially coronary artery disease, is suspected; consider elderly patients in general to be at increased risk since they are more likely to have occult heart disease. For patients with known or suspected cardiovascular disease, dosage should be reduced initially (see ADMINISTRATION/DOSAGE ADJUSTMENTS) and then whenever the disease is exacerbated.
Adrenocortical insufficiency	Treatment of severe, prolonged hypothyroidism with thyroid hormone can precipitate adrenocortical insufficiency; to avoid this reaction, concomitant administration of a corticosteroid may be necessary. Thyroid hormone therapy can also exacerbate symptoms of adrenocortical insufficiency; any such insufficiency should be corrected before the start of therapy, and, during treatment, measures used to control the disorder should be adjusted as needed.
Diabetes	Thyroid hormone therapy can exacerbate signs and symptoms of diabetes mellitus or insipidus; closely monitor urinary glucose level during treatment (see also DRUG INTERACTIONS)
Carcinogenicity, mutagenicity, effect on fertility	An apparent association between prolonged thyroid hormone therapy and breast cancer has not been confirmed and therefore should not serve as a reason for discontinuing treatment; no long-term studies have been performed to evaluate the carcinogenic potential of thyroid hormone therapy. Long-term studies of mutagenicity and effects of exogenous thyroid hormones on fertility have also not been done.

ADVERSE REACTIONS

Hyperthyroidism; allergic skin reactions (rare)

OVERDOSAGE

Signs and symptoms	Headache, irritability, nervousness, sweating, tachycardia, increased bowel motility, menstrual irregularities, occurrence or exacerbation of angina and cardiac failure, shock, thyroid storm
Treatment	Induce vomiting if further GI absorption can be reasonably prevented and coma, convulsions, and loss of the gagging reflex have not occurred. Maintain respiratory function, using oxygen, if necessary. Give cardiac glycosides for congestive heart failure and beta blockers, especially propranolol, for signs and symptoms associated with increased sympathomimetic activity. Institute appropriate measures, as needed, to control fever, hypoglycemia, and fluid loss.

DRUG INTERACTIONS

Oral anticoagulants	△ Anticoagulant effect with shift from hypothyroid to euthyroid state. Any patient receiving an oral anticoagulant should be watched very closely when thyroid hormone replacement therapy is started; the prothrombin time should be determined frequently throughout the course of combination therapy. A reduction in anticoagulant dosage will probably be necessary at least at the beginning of replacement therapy.
Insulin, sulfonylureas	Hyperglycemia; a patient receiving insulin or a sulfonylurea should be watched closely when thyroid hormone replacement therapy is started and, if necessary, the dosage of the antidiabetic agent should be increased
Cholestyramine	▽ Absorption of thyroid hormone; separate administration of cholestyramine and thyroid hormone by 4–5 h
Estrogens (including oral contraceptives)	▽ Free (unbound) thyroid hormone when thyroid gland is not functioning; an increase in the dosage of thyroid hormone may be necessary during concomitant therapy, but only if thyroid gland function is inadequate and the decrease in the free hormone level, which results from an estrogen-induced increase in the serum thyroxine-binding globulin level, cannot be reversed by a compensatory increase in hormonal output
Cardiac glycosides	▽ Pharmacologic effect of cardiac glycosides with shift from hypothyroid to euthyroid state; increase dosage of cardiac glycosides during thyroid hormone replacement therapy △ Risk of cardiac glycoside toxicity
Tricyclic antidepressants	△ Pharmacologic effects of tricyclic antidepressants and thyroid hormone (transient cardiac arrhythmias have occurred)
Ketamine	Hypertension and tachycardia; exercise caution when using ketamine in a patient receiving thyroid hormone and be prepared to treat hypertension
Norepinephrine, epinephrine	△ Risk of coronary artery insufficiency, especially in a patient with coronary artery disease; any patient receiving thyroid hormone should be carefully observed after injection of a catecholamine

CYTOMEL ■ EUTHROID

ALTERED LABORATORY VALUES

Blood/serum values — △ Glucose ▽ T_4 ▽ PBI

Urinary values — + Glucose

USE IN CHILDREN

Since congenital hypothyroidism occurs relatively frequently (1:4,000), the serum level of T_4 and/or TSH should be determined routinely in neonates; treatment should be started immediately after diagnosis (See ORAL DOSAGE). Administration of thyroid hormone is generally maintained for life. However, if transient hypothyroidism is suspected, therapy can be withdrawn after the age of 3 yr for a period of 2–8 wk; if a normal TSH level is maintained during this period, administration of thyroid hormone may be permanently discontinued. Bear in mind that excessive doses of thyroid hormone may produce craniosynostosis in infants. Partial loss of hair may occur in children during the first few months of therapy, but this condition usually reverses with continued treatment.

USE IN PREGNANT AND NURSING WOMEN

Pregnancy Category A: no adverse effect on fetal development has resulted from use of thyroid hormones in pregnant women (these hormones do not readily cross the placental barrier); thyroid hormone replacement therapy should not be discontinued during pregnancy. Use free hormone levels to assess therapy since thyroxine-binding globulin levels are increased during pregnancy. Minimal amounts of thyroid hormone are excreted in human milk; use with caution in nursing mothers, even though these hormones are not associated with any serious adverse reactions.

THYROID HORMONES

EUTHROID (liotrix) Parke-Davis Rx

Tablets: 30 μg levothyroxine sodium (T_4) and 7.5 μg liothyronine sodium (T_3) (Euthroid-½); 60 μg T_4 and 15 μg T_3 (Euthroid-1); 120 μg T_4 and 30 μg T_3 (Euthroid-2); 180 μg T_4 and 45 μg T_3 (Euthroid-3)

INDICATIONS

Hypothyroidism, including myxedema and cretinism
Simple (nontoxic) goiter
Subacute or chronic **thyroiditis**, including Hashimoto's disease
Goiter prophylaxis in patients receiving thiouracil derivatives
Intolerance to thyroid preparations of animal origin

ORAL DOSAGE

Adult: start at low daily doses, followed by gradual increases every 2 wk until desired clinical response is obtained; usual maintenance dosage: 1 Euthroid-1, -2, or -3 tab/day

Child: same as adult; eventual maintenance dosage may be higher than in adults

CONTRAINDICATIONS

Hypersensitivity to synthetic levothyroxine or liothyronine

Uncorrected adrenal insufficiency

Acute myocardial infarction

Nephrosis

Morphological hypogonadism

ADMINISTRATION/DOSAGE ADJUSTMENTS

Patients with cardiovascular disease — Use only if clearly indicated; start with 1 Euthroid-½ or Euthroid-1 tab/day and increase dosage by the same amount at 2-wk intervals, as needed

WARNINGS/PRECAUTIONS

Patients with coronary artery disease — May experience cardiac arrhythmias while undergoing surgery and should be carefully monitored

Adrenal insufficiency (Addison's disease) — May coexist as a result of hypopituitarism and should be corrected with corticosteroids before instituting thyroid therapy

Patients with severe hypothyroidism or myxedema — May be unusually sensitive to thyroid hormones; initiate therapy at very low dosage levels and increase dosage gradually

Diabetic patients — Diabetics may require higher doses of insulin or oral hypoglycemic agents; if thyroid hormone dosage is decreased, insulin or oral hypoglycemic dosage may need to be decreased to avoid hypoglycemia

Concomitant anticoagulant therapy — Prothrombin time may be altered; monitor patient closely

EUTHROID ■ LEVOTHROID

| Tartrazine sensitivity | Presence of FD&C Yellow No. 5 (tartrazine) in Euthroid-½, -1, and -3 tablets may cause allergic-type reactions, including bronchial asthma, in susceptible individuals |

ADVERSE REACTIONS

Cardiovascular	Cardiac arrhythmias, angina pectoris
Central nervous system	Nervousness
Metabolic	Menstrual irregularities

OVERDOSAGE

| Signs and symptoms | Headache, instability, nervousness, sweating, tachycardia, unusual bowel motility, angina pectoris, congestive heart failure, shock; massive overdosage may produce symptoms of thyroid storm |
| Treatment | Discontinue medication for several days and reinstitute therapy at a lower dosage. For acute poisoning, induce emesis or use gastric lavage to empty stomach. For tachycardia and arrhythmias, administer propranolol. Institute supportive measures, as indicated. Treatment of unrecognized adrenal insufficiency should be considered. |

DRUG INTERACTIONS

Oral anticoagulants	△ Anticoagulant effect
Insulin, oral hypoglycemics	▽ Hypoglycemic effect
Ketamine	△ Blood pressure and heart rate
Phenytoin	△ Thyroxine blood level
Cholestyramine	▽ Absorption of liotrix
Tricyclic antidepressants	△ Antidepressant effect

ALTERED LABORATORY VALUES

Blood/serum values — △ Glucose ▽ Cholesterol ▽ TSH ▽ ^{131}I thyroid uptake

No clinically significant alterations in urinary values occur at therapeutic dosages

---

USE IN CHILDREN
See INDICATIONS

USE IN PREGNANT AND NURSING WOMEN
Consult manufacturer

THYROID HORMONES

LEVOTHROID (T$_4$ thyroxine sodium) Rorer   Rx

Tablets: 25, 50, 75, 100, 125, 150, 175, 200, 300 μg

INDICATIONS[1]

Hypothyroidism
Nontoxic goiter

ORAL DOSAGE

Adult: 50 μg/day to start, followed by increases of 50 μg/day every 2–4 wk until patient is euthyroid or symptoms preclude further dosage increases; patients with no complicating endocrine or cardiovascular disease may be started immediately on full maintenance dosage (usually 100–200 μg/day)

Cretinism
Severe hypothyroidism

Child: 25–50 μg/day to start, followed by increases of 50–100 μg/day every 2 wk until patient is euthyroid and laboratory values are in the normal range; usual maintenance dosage in growing children may be as high as 300–400 μg/day

LEVOTHROID Injection (T$_4$ thyroxine sodium) Rorer   Rx

Vials: 200, 500 μg[2] (6 ml)

INDICATIONS

Myxedema coma

PARENTERAL DOSAGE

Adult: 200–500 μg IV, followed in 24 h by 100–200 μg IV

CONTRAINDICATIONS

Acute myocardial infarction   Uncorrected adrenal insufficiency   Thyrotoxicosis

Hypersensitivity to any component[2] (injection only)

LEVOTHROID

ADMINISTRATION/DOSAGE ADJUSTMENTS

Adult patients with myxedema or hypothyroidism complicated by angina	Initiate therapy with 25 µg/day and increase the dosage gradually in increments of 25–50 µg/day at 2- to 4-wk intervals, depending upon clinical response
Concomitant use of cholestyramine	Give oral thyroxine 4–5 h before or after administration of cholestyramine (see DRUG INTERACTIONS)
Myxedema coma	For treatment of myxedema coma, administer corticosteroids as well as thyroxine, correct electrolyte disturbances, and control possible infection; switch to oral replacement therapy as soon as situation permits. Normal serum T_4 levels may be attained in 24 h followed in 3 days by a 3-fold increase in the serum T_3 level. Before using thyroxine in patients with severe cardiac disease, weigh the risk of a rapid increase in metabolism against the danger of prolonging the severely hypothyroid state; a smaller initial dose may be necessary for these patients.
Preparation of IV solution	To reconstitute the IV solution, add 2 ml of 0.9% sodium chloride injection USP to the 200-µg vial or 5 ml to the 500-µg vial; do not use bacteriostatic sodium chloride injection USP

WARNINGS/PRECAUTIONS

Treatment of obesity and infertility	Normal thyroid-replacement doses are ineffective for weight reduction or treatment of infertility in euthyroid patients; higher doses may produce serious or even life-threatening toxicity, particularly when given with sympathomimetic amines
Patients with adrenal cortical insufficiency	The signs and symptoms of adrenal cortical insufficiency are exacerbated by exogenous thyroxine; correct this disorder before beginning therapy
Patients with cardiovascular disease (including hypertension)	Use in patients with acute myocardial infarction is contraindicated; administer with caution to other patients with cardiovascular disease. Reduce dosage if chest pain or other manifestations of aggravated disease develop. Concomitant use of epinephrine or other catecholamines may precipitate an episode of coronary artery insufficiency in patients with coronary artery disease; carefully observe such patients if they are given catecholamines.
Diabetic patients	Closely monitor urinary glucose levels during therapy. Diabetics may require higher doses of insulin or oral hypoglycemic agents; if thyroid hormone dosage is decreased, insulin or oral hypoglycemic dosage may need to be decreased as well to avoid hypoglycemia.
Concomitant anticoagulant therapy	Reduce dosage of coumarin anticoagulants by one third when initiating thyroid therapy; measure prothrombin time frequently during treatment, and, if necessary, adjust anticoagulant dosage
Concomitant use of estrogen	A patient with a nonfunctioning thyroid gland may require a higher thyroxine dosage if estrogen or estrogen-containing oral contraceptives are given concomitantly; such an adjustment is not necessary in patients with adequate thyroid gland function because the decrease in the free thyroxine level, which results from an estrogen-induced increase in the serum thyroxine-binding globulin (TBG) level, is followed by a compensatory increase in thyroxine output
Monitoring of therapy	Response to thyroid replacement therapy may be followed by clinical evaluation and measurement of serum thyroxine (T_4), triiodothyronine (T_3), and thyroid stimulating hormone (TSH) levels, free thyroxine index, and other tests of thyroid function. If the serum concentration of thyroxine-binding globulin (TBG) is altered, the free thyroxine level should be measured; the TBG level is affected by genetic factors (hyper- and hypothyroxine-binding globulinemia); increased by pregnancy, infectious hepatitis, and the use of estrogens and estrogen-containing oral contraceptives; and decreased by nephrosis, acromegaly, and the use of corticosteroids or androgens. Salicylates inhibit binding of thyroxine by thyroid-binding prealbumin. Exogenous iodine interferes with the measurement of radioactive iodine uptake. Caution patients to report any sign or symptom of hyperthyroidism. Hypothyroidism can persist, despite adequate dosage, as a result of poor compliance, malabsorption, excessive fecal loss, or inactivity of the preparation (intracellular resistance to thyroxine is quite rare).
Lactose intolerance	Patients who are sensitive to lactose may be unable to tolerate thyroxine tablets, since lactose is used in their manufacture
Carcinogenicity, mutagenicity, effect on fertility	An apparent association between prolonged thyroid therapy and breast cancer has not been confirmed; no long-term studies have been performed to evaluate the carcinogenic potential of this preparation. Long-term studies of mutagenicity and effect on fertility have not been done.

ADVERSE REACTIONS

Central nervous system	Nervousness, tremor, headache, insomnia
Cardiovascular	Palpitations, tachycardia, cardiac arrhythmias, angina pectoris
Metabolic	Weight loss, diaphoresis, heat intolerance, fever
Gastrointestinal	Diarrhea, abdominal cramps

LEVOTHROID ■ PROLOID

OVERDOSAGE

Signs and symptoms	See ADVERSE REACTIONS; elevation of serum T_4 and T_3 levels and free thyroxine index; in severe cases, cardiac failure and death resulting from arrhythmia or failure
Treatment	Discontinue medication for several days and reinstitute therapy at a lower dosage. For acute poisoning, induce emesis or use gastric lavage to empty stomach. Maintain respiratory function; if necessary, administer oxygen. For congestive heart failure, administer cardiac glycosides; for tachycardia and arrhythmias, administer propranolol. Institute supportive measures, as indicated. Treatment of unrecognized adrenal insufficiency should be considered.

DRUG INTERACTIONS

Oral anticoagulants	△	Anticoagulant effect
Insulin, oral hypoglycemics	▽	Hypoglycemic effect
Ketamine	△	Blood pressure and heart rate
Phenytoin	△	Thyroxine blood level
Cholestyramine	▽	Absorption of thyroxine
Tricyclic antidepressants	△	Antidepressant effect

ALTERED LABORATORY VALUES

Blood/serum values — △ Glucose △ PBI ▽ Cholesterol ▽ TSH ▽ ^{131}I thyroid uptake ▽ Uric acid

No clinically significant alterations in urinary values occur at therapeutic dosages

---

USE IN CHILDREN

See INDICATIONS and ORAL DOSAGE. To prevent developmental deficiency, diagnose and initiate treatment of cretinism as soon as possible after birth; screening tests for serum T_4 and TSH will identify newborns at risk. Partial loss of hair may occur in children during the first few months of therapy; this effect is usually transient and, as treatment continues, generally reversible.

USE IN PREGNANT AND NURSING WOMEN

Pregnancy Category A: no adverse effect on fetal development has resulted from use of thyroid hormones in pregnant women (these hormones do not readily cross the placental barrier); replacement therapy in hypothyroid women should not be discontinued during pregnancy. Use free thyroxine levels to evaluate therapy, since thyroxine-binding globulin levels are increased during pregnancy. Minimal amounts of thyroid hormones are excreted in human milk; use with caution in nursing mothers, even though these hormones are not associated with any serious adverse reactions.

---

[1] Thyroid hormones may also be used for the treatment of simple nonendemic goiter and chronic lymphocytic thyroiditis and for TSH suppression tests and may be used with antithyroid drugs in the treatment of thyrotoxicosis to prevent goitrogenesis and hypothyroidism, especially during pregnancy; consult manufacturer for details
[2] Each vial contains 15 mg of mannitol

THYROID HORMONES

PROLOID (thyroglobulin) Parke-Davis Rx

Tablets: 32, 65, 100, 130, 200 mg (½, 1, 1½, 2, 3 gr, respectively)

INDICATIONS	ORAL DOSAGE
Myxedema Hypothyroidism Simple (nontoxic) goiter Cretinism	Adult: give a small amount to start, followed by gradual increases every 1–2 wk until desired clinical response is obtained; usual maintenance dosage: 32–200 mg (½–3 gr)/day

CONTRAINDICATIONS

Uncorrected adrenal insufficiency	Morphological hypogonadism	Nephrosis

ADMINISTRATION/DOSAGE ADJUSTMENTS

Patients with cardiovascular disease	Administer 32–65 mg (½–1 gr) to start, followed by increases of 32–65 mg every 2 wk; use only if thyroid replacement therapy is clearly indicated

WARNINGS/PRECAUTIONS

Treatment of obesity	Normal thyroid-replacement doses are ineffective for weight reduction in euthyroid patients; higher doses may produce serious or even life-threatening toxicity, particularly when given with sympathomimetic amines
Adrenal insufficiency (Addison's disease)	May coexist as a result of hypopituitarism and should be corrected with corticosteroids before instituting thyroid therapy

PROLOID ■ SYNTHROID

| Myxedematous patients | May be unusually sensitive to thyroid preparations; initiate therapy at very low dosage levels and increase dosage gradually |

ADVERSE REACTIONS

Cardiovascular	Cardiac arrhythmias, angina pectoris
Central nervous system	Nervousness
Other	Menstrual irregularities

OVERDOSAGE

| Signs and symptoms | Headache, instability, nervousness, sweating, tachycardia, unusual bowel motility, angina pectoris, congestive heart failure, shock; massive overdosage may produce symptoms of thyroid storm |
| Treatment | Discontinue medication for several days and reinstitute therapy at a lower dosage. For acute poisoning, induce emesis or use gastric lavage to empty stomach. For tachycardia and arrhythmias, administer propranolol. Institute supportive measures, as indicated. Treatment of unrecognized adrenal insufficiency should be considered. |

DRUG INTERACTIONS

Oral anticoagulants	△ Anticoagulant effect
Insulin, oral hypoglycemics	▽ Hypoglycemic effect
Ketamine	△ Blood pressure and heart rate
Phenytoin	△ Thyroxine blood level
Cholestyramine	▽ Absorption of thyroglobulin
Tricyclic antidepressants	△ Antidepressant effect

ALTERED LABORATORY VALUES

| Blood/serum values | △ Glucose △ PBI ▽ Cholesterol ▽ TSH ▽ ^{131}I thyroid uptake |

No clinically significant alterations in urinary values occur at therapeutic dosages

---

USE IN CHILDREN
Consult manufacturer

USE IN PREGNANT AND NURSING WOMEN
Consult manufacturer

THYROID HORMONES

SYNTHROID (levothyroxine sodium) Flint   Rx

Tablets: 25, 50, 75, 100, 125, 150, 200, 300 µg **Vials:** 100, 200, 500 µg (10 ml)

INDICATIONS	ORAL DOSAGE	PARENTERAL DOSAGE
Reduced or absent thyroid function	**Adult:** 25–87.5 µg/day to start, followed by a gradual increase in dosage over a period of 2–3 wk until desired clinical response is obtained; usual maintenance dosage: 100–200 µg/day **Infant (0–1 yr):** 9 µg/kg/day, given in a single daily dose **Child (1–5 yr):** 6 µg/kg/day, given in a single daily dose **Child (6–10 yr):** 4 µg/kg/day, given in a single daily dose **Child (11–20 yr):** 3 µg/kg/day, given in a single daily dose	**Adult:** when oral administration is precluded for long periods, give one half the previously established oral dosage IM or IV; adjust subsequent dosage as needed, with patient under close observation **Child:** same as adult
Myxedema coma or stupor, without concomitant severe heart disease		**Adult:** 200–500 µg IV to start, followed, if needed, by an additional 100–300 µg, or more, on the following day; for maintenance, give 50–100 µg/day IM or IV until oral doses can be tolerated

CONTRAINDICATIONS

| Acute myocardial infarction | Uncorrected adrenal insufficiency | Thyrotoxicosis |

SYNTHROID

ADMINISTRATION/DOSAGE ADJUSTMENTS

Reconstitution of parenteral solution	Immediately before use, reconstitute with 5 ml of 0.9% Sodium Chloride Injection USP or Bacteriostatic Sodium Chloride Injection USP with Benzyl Alcohol only and shake the vial to ensure complete mixing; *do not add the reconstituted solution to other IV fluids.* For myxedema coma or stupor, use the 500-µg vial to prepare a solution of 100 µg/ml. Discard any unused portion.
Elderly patients with long-standing disease and evidence of myxedematous infiltration and cardiovascular dysfunction	Initiate oral therapy with as little as 25 µg/day and increase the dosage in increments of 25 µg/day at 3- to 4-wk intervals, as needed and tolerated

WARNINGS/PRECAUTIONS

Treatment of obesity	Normal thyroid-replacement doses are ineffective for weight reduction in euthyroid patients; higher doses may produce serious or even life-threatening toxicity, particularly when given with sympathomimetic amines
Patients with cardiovascular disease	For patients with myxedema coma or stupor, weigh the risks and benefits of replacement therapy, and consider using smaller IV doses; for other patients, start with a lower dosage, and follow gradually with small increments. Partial restoration of thyroid function is advisable if euthyroidism will impose metabolic demands that, because of compromised cardiovascular capacity, cannot be tolerated.
Patients with concomitant endocrine disorders	Thyroid therapy may unmask symptoms of concomitant endocrine disorders, such as diabetes mellitus, adrenal insufficiency, hypopituitarism, and diabetes insipidus, requiring an adjustment in the corrective measures aimed at these conditions
Refractory cases	If patient fails to respond adequately to daily oral doses of 400 µg or more, reconsider the diagnosis of hypothyroidism and explore the possibility of impaired absorption of levothyroxine from the GI tract or poor compliance with the prescribed regimen
Laboratory monitoring of therapy	Although appropriate laboratory tests are helpful in monitoring thyroid-replacement therapy, dosage should be based primarily on clinical impressions of the patient's well-being. In treating hypothyroidism in children, the maintenance dosage generally should be adjusted to obtain within several weeks of therapy normal values of the free thyroxine (FT_4) index and serum T_3, T_4, and TSH levels; the patient's clinical status is most important, however, since some patients may be clinically euthyroid despite an elevated T_4 level. If the cause is congenital, normalization of the FT_4 index is usually considered sufficient, since serum TSH levels may remain elevated for the first 2–3 yr of life, despite therapy.
Tartrazine sensitivity	Presence of FD&C Yellow No. 5 (tartrazine) in 100- and 300-µg tablets may cause allergic-type reactions, including bronchial asthma, in susceptible individuals

ADVERSE REACTIONS

Central nervous system	Nervousness, tremor, headache, insomnia
Cardiovascular	Palpitations, tachycardia, cardiac arrhythmias, angina pectoris
Gastrointestinal	Diarrhea, abdominal cramps
Metabolic	Weight loss, diaphoresis, heat intolerance, fever

OVERDOSAGE

Signs and symptoms	See ADVERSE REACTIONS
Treatment	Discontinue medication for several days and reinstitute therapy at a lower dosage. For acute poisoning, induce emesis or use gastric lavage to empty stomach. For tachycardia and arrhythmias, administer propranolol. Institute supportive measures, as indicated. Treatment of unrecognized adrenal insufficiency should be considered.

DRUG INTERACTIONS

Oral anticoagulants	△ Anticoagulant effect; readjust anticoagulant dosage, as needed
Insulin, oral hypoglycemics	▽ Hypoglycemic effect
Ketamine	△ Blood pressure and heart rate
Phenytoin	△ Thyroxine blood level
Cholestyramine	▽ Absorption of levothyroxine
Tricyclic antidepressants	△ Antidepressant effect

ALTERED LABORATORY VALUES

Blood/serum values	△ Glucose △ PBI ▽ Cholesterol ▽ TSH ▽ ^{131}I thyroid uptake ▽ Uric acid

No clinically significant alterations in urinary values occur at therapeutic dosages

USE IN CHILDREN	USE IN PREGNANT AND NURSING WOMEN
See INDICATIONS and ORAL DOSAGE	Treatment of hypothyroidism may be continued or initiated while a patient is pregnant or nursing. Confirm a diagnosis of hypothyroidism during pregnancy by evaluating serum T_3 and TSH levels.

THYROID HORMONES

THYROLAR (T_3/T_4 liotrix) Rorer   Rx

Tablets: 12.5 µg T_4 and 3.1 µg T_3 (Thyrolar-1/4), 25 µg T_4 and 6.25 µg T_3 (Thyrolar-1/2), 50 µg T_4 and 12.5 µg T_3 (Thyrolar-1), 100 µg T_4 and 25 µg T_3 (Thyrolar-2), 150 µg T_4 and 37.5 µg T_3 (Thyrolar-3)

INDICATIONS[1]

Hypothyroidism

ORAL DOSAGE

Adult: 25 µg T_4 and 6.25 µg T_3 (1 Thyrolar-1/2 tab) daily to start, followed, as needed and tolerated, by an increase in the daily dose of 12.5 µg T_4 and 3.1 µg T_3 every 2–3 wk; usual daily dose: 50–100 µg T_4 and 12.5–25 µg T_3. Lack of response at a daily dose of 150 µg T_4 and 37.5 µg T_3 (1 Thyrolar-3 tab/day) suggests noncompliance or malabsorption.

Congenital hypothyroidism

Infant (0–6 mo): 12.5–25 µg T_4 and 3.1–6.25 µg T_3 daily
Infant (6–12 mo): 25–37.5 µg T_4 and 6.25–9.35 µg T_3 daily
Child (1–5 yr): 37.5–50 µg T_4 and 9.35–12.5 µg T_3 daily
Child (6–12 yr): 50–75 µg T_4 and 12.5–18.75 µg T_3 daily
Child (> 12 yr): > 75 µg T_4 and > 18.75 µg T_3 daily

CONTRAINDICATIONS

Apparent hypersensitivity to any component	Adrenocortical insufficiency	Thyrotoxicosis

ADMINISTRATION/DOSAGE ADJUSTMENTS

Patients with cardiovascular disease, elderly patients	Give 12.5–25 µg T_4 and 3.1–6.25 µg T_3 (1 Thyrolar-1/4 or 1 Thyrolar-1/2 tab) daily to start if the patient is elderly or has a cardiovascular disease
Patients with long-standing myxedema	Give 12.5 µg T_4 and 3.1 µg T_3 (1 Thyrolar-1/4 tab) daily to start if the patient has long-standing myxedema; exercise extreme caution if myxedema is accompanied by cardiovascular impairment
Monitoring of therapy	To evaluate thyroid hormone replacement therapy, periodically assess clinical response and appropriate laboratory values, including serum levels of TSH, total T_4, and free T_4; the first assessment should be done within 4 wk after starting treatment. Determination of free T_4 level is particularly warranted when the total T_4 level is low and the TSH level is normal. Bear in mind that in infants TSH secretion is relatively insensitive to thyroid hormone and therefore may not be a reliable indication of therapeutic response. If the serum concentration of thyroxine-binding globulin (TBG) is altered, the free T_4 level, rather than the total serum T_4 level, should be measured. The TBG level is increased by pregnancy, infectious hepatitis, and the use of estrogens or estrogen-containing oral contraceptives; the TBG level is decreased by nephrosis, acromegaly, and the use of androgens or corticosteroids. Familial hypo- and hyperthyroxine-binding globulinemia have also been described. Medicinal or dietary iodine reduces uptake of radioactive iodine. The persistence of clinical and laboratory evidence of hypothyroidism despite adequate dosage indicates poor compliance, malabsorption, excessive fecal loss, or inactivity of the preparation (intracellular resistance to thyroid hormone is quite rare).
Duration of therapy	Thyroid hormone replacement therapy is generally continued for life except in cases of transient hypothyroidism, which are usually associated with thyroiditis

WARNINGS/PRECAUTIONS

Obesity, infertility	In euthyroid patients, doses within the range of normal hormonal requirements are ineffective for weight reduction and higher doses may produce serious or even life-threatening toxicity, particularly when given with sympathomimetic amines; use of thyroid hormones for obesity is unjustified. Thyroid hormone therapy for infertility unaccompanied by hypothyroidism is also unjustified.
Subacute thyroiditis	Thyroid hormones should not be used for transient hypothyroidism occurring during the recovery phase of subacute thyroiditis
Toxicity	Caution patients to report immediately any signs or symptoms of overdosage. If toxicity occurs during therapy, reduce the dosage or, alternatively, discontinue administration temporarily and then resume use at a lower dosage. In normal individuals hypothalamic-pituitary-thyroid function is fully restored in 6–8 wk after suppression. When performing the thyroid suppression test, exercise caution if thyroid gland autonomy is strongly suspected, since the effects of exogenous and endogenous hormone stimulation are additive.

Cardiovascular disease	Thyroid hormone therapy can exacerbate cardiovascular disease. Exercise great caution if a cardiovascular coronary disorder, especially coronary artery disease, is suspected; consider elderly patients in general to be at increased risk since they are more likely to have occult heart disease. For patients with known or suspected cardiovascular disease, dosage should be reduced initially (see ADMINISTRATION/DOSAGE ADJUSTMENTS) and then whenever the disease is exacerbated.
Adrenocortical insufficiency	Thyroid hormone therapy can exacerbate symptoms of adrenocortical insufficiency; any such insufficiency should be corrected before the start of therapy, and, during treatment, measures used to control the disorder should be adjusted as needed
Diabetes	Thyroid hormone therapy can exacerbate signs and symptoms of diabetes mellitus or insipidus; closely monitor urinary glucose level during treatment (see also DRUG INTERACTIONS)
Carcinogenicity, mutagenicity, effect on fertility	An apparent association between prolonged thyroid hormone therapy and breast cancer has not been confirmed and therefore should not serve as a reason for discontinuing treatment; no long-term studies have been performed to evaluate the carcinogenic potential of thyroid hormone therapy. Long-term studies of mutagenicity and effects of exogenous thyroid hormones on fertility have also not been done.

ADVERSE REACTIONS

Hyperthyroidism

OVERDOSAGE

Signs and symptoms	Headache, irritability, nervousness, sweating, tachycardia, increased bowel motility, menstrual irregularities, occurrence or exacerbation of angina and cardiac failure, shock, thyroid storm
Treatment	Induce vomiting if further GI absorption can be reasonably prevented and coma, convulsions, and loss of the gagging reflex have not occurred. Maintain respiratory function, using oxygen, if necessary. Give cardiac glycosides for congestive heart failure and beta blockers, especially propranolol, for signs and symptoms associated with increased sympathomimetic activity. Institute appropriate measures, as needed, to control fever, hypoglycemia, and fluid loss.

DRUG INTERACTIONS

Oral anticoagulants	△ Anticoagulant effect with shift from hypothyroid to euthyroid state. Any patient receiving an oral anticoagulant should be watched very closely when thyroid hormone replacement therapy is started; the prothrombin time should be determined frequently throughout the course of combination therapy. A reduction in anticoagulant dosage will probably be necessary at least at the beginning of replacement therapy.
Insulin, sulfonylureas	Hyperglycemia; a patient receiving insulin or a sulfonylurea should be watched closely when thyroid hormone replacement therapy is started and, if necessary, the dosage of the antidiabetic agent should be increased
Cholestyramine	▽ Absorption of thyroid hormone; separate administration of cholestyramine and thyroid hormone by 4–5 h
Estrogens (including oral contraceptives)	▽ Free (unbound) thyroid hormone when thyroid gland is not functioning; an increase in the dosage of thyroid hormone may be necessary during concomitant therapy, but only if thyroid gland function is inadequate and the decrease in the free hormone level, which results from an estrogen-induced increase in the serum thyroxine-binding globulin level, cannot be reversed by a compensatory increase in hormonal output
Cardiac glycosides	▽ Pharmacologic effect of cardiac glycosides with shift from hypothyroid to euthyroid state; increase dosage of cardiac glycosides during thyroid hormone replacement therapy
Tricyclic antidepressants	△ Pharmacologic effects of tricyclic antidepressants and thyroid hormone (transient cardiac arrhythmias have occurred)
Ketamine	Hypertension and tachycardia; exercise caution when using ketamine in a patient receiving thyroid hormone and be prepared to treat hypertension
Norepinephrine, epinephrine	△ Risk of coronary artery insufficiency, especially in a patient with coronary artery disease; any patient receiving thyroid hormone should be carefully observed after injection of a catecholamine

ALTERED LABORATORY VALUES

Blood/serum values	△ Glucose ▽ T_4 ▽ PBI
Urinary values	+ Glucose

USE IN CHILDREN

Since congenital hypothyroidism occurs relatively frequently (1:4,000), the serum level of T_4 and/or TSH should be determined routinely in neonates; treatment should be started immediately after diagnosis (see ORAL DOSAGE). Administration of thyroid hormone is generally maintained for life. However, if transient hypothyrodism is suspected, therapy can be withdrawn after the age of 3 yr for a period of 2–8 wk; if a normal TSH level is maintained during this period, administration of thyroid hormone may be permanently discontinued. Bear in mind that excessive doses of thyroid hormone may produce craniosynostosis in infants. Partial loss of hair may occur in children during the first few months of therapy, but this condition usually reverses with continued treatment.

USE IN PREGNANT AND NURSING WOMEN

Pregnancy Category A: no adverse effect on fetal development has resulted from use of thyroid hormones in pregnant women (these hormones do not readily cross the placental barrier); thyroid hormone replacement therapy should not be discontinued during pregnancy. Use free hormone levels to assess therapy since thyroxine-binding globulin levels are increased during pregnancy. Minimal amounts of thyroid hormone are excreted in human milk; use with caution in nursing mothers, even though these hormones are not associated with any serious adverse reactions.

---

[1] As a TSH suppressant, thyroid hormone can be used to prevent or treat euthyroid goiter, subacute thyroiditis, or Hashimoto's disease or, in conjunction with radioactive iodine, to produce regression of metastases from follicular and papillary carcinoma; the drug can also be used diagnostically at a suppressant dosage to show thyroid gland autonomy in patients with Graves' ophthalmopathy or to evaluate patients who exhibit clinical signs of mild hyperthyroidism despite normal laboratory values

Chapter 38

Hypoglycemic Agents

Insulin	**1600**
HUMULIN BR (Lilly) Human insulin *OTC*	1600
HUMULIN L (Lilly) Human insulin *OTC*	1601
HUMULIN N (Lilly) Human insulin *OTC*	1600
HUMULIN R (Lilly) Human insulin *OTC*	1600
Lente ILETIN I (Lilly) Beef and pork insulin *OTC*	1601
NPH ILETIN I (Lilly) Beef and pork insulin *OTC*	1601
Protamine, Zinc & ILETIN I (Lilly) Beef and pork insulin *OTC*	1601
Regular ILETIN I (Lilly) Beef and pork insulin *OTC*	1600
Semilente ILETIN I (Lilly) Beef and pork insulin *OTC*	1600
Ultralente ILETIN I (Lilly) Beef and pork insulin *OTC*	1601
Lente ILETIN II (Lilly) Purified beef insulin *OTC*	1601
Lente ILETIN II (Lilly) Purified pork insulin *OTC*	1601
NPH ILETIN II (Lilly) Purified beef insulin *OTC*	1601
NPH ILETIN II (Lilly) Purified pork insulin *OTC*	1601
Protamine, Zinc & ILETIN II (Lilly) Purified beef insulin *OTC*	1601
Protamine, Zinc & ILETIN II (Lilly) Purified pork insulin *OTC*	1601
Regular ILETIN II (Lilly) Purified beef insulin *OTC*	1600
Regular ILETIN II (Lilly) Purified pork insulin *OTC*	1600
Regular (Concentrated) ILETIN II (Lilly) Purified pork insulin *Rx*	1602
INSULATARD NPH (Nordisk-USA) Purified pork insulin *OTC*	1600
INSULATARD NPH Human (Nordisk-USA) Human insulin *OTC*	1601
Lente Insulin (Squibb-Novo) Beef insulin *OTC*	1601
Lente Purified Insulin (Squibb-Novo) Purified pork insulin *OTC*	1601
NPH Insulin (Squibb-Novo) Beef insulin *OTC*	1601
NPH Purified Insulin (Squibb-Novo) Purified pork insulin *OTC*	1601
Regular Insulin (Squibb-Novo) Pork insulin *OTC*	1600
Regular Purified Insulin (Squibb-Novo) Purified pork insulin *OTC*	1600
Semilente Insulin (Squibb-Novo) Beef insulin *OTC*	1600
Semilente Purified Insulin (Squibb-Novo) Purified pork insulin *OTC*	1600
Ultralente Insulin (Squibb-Novo) Beef insulin *OTC*	1601
Ultralente Purified Insulin (Squibb-Novo) Purified beef insulin *OTC*	1602
MIXTARD (Nordisk-USA) Purified pork insulin *OTC*	1600
NOVOLIN 70/30 (Squibb-Novo) Human insulin *OTC*	1600
NOVOLIN L (Squibb-Novo) Human insulin *OTC*	1601
NOVOLIN N (Squibb-Novo) Human insulin *OTC*	1601
NOVOLIN R (Squibb-Novo) Human insulin *OTC*	1600
VELOSULIN (Nordisk-USA) Purified pork insulin *OTC*	1600
VELOSULIN Human (Nordisk-USA) Human insulin *OTC*	1600
Oral Hypoglycemic Agents	**1603**
DIAβETA (Hoechst-Roussel) Glyburide *Rx*	1603
DIABINESE (Pfizer) Chlorpropamide *Rx*	1605
GLUCOTROL (Roerig) Glipizide *Rx*	1607
MICRONASE (Upjohn) Glyburide *Rx*	1609
ORINASE (Upjohn) Tolbutamide *Rx*	1611
TOLINASE (Upjohn) Tolazamide *Rx*	1612

COMPENDIUM OF DRUG THERAPY

1599

Insulin

INSULIN

Regular Insulin   Onset: 1/2–1 h   Peak: 2–4 h   Duration: 5–7 h

HUMULIN BR (human insulin) Lilly   OTC
Vials: 100 units/ml (10 ml) for use in external infusion pumps only

HUMULIN R (human insulin) Lilly   OTC
Vials: 100 units/ml (10 ml)

Regular ILETIN I (beef and pork insulin) Lilly   OTC
Vials: 40, 100 units/ml (10 ml)

Regular ILETIN II (purified beef insulin) Lilly   OTC
Vials: 100 units/ml (10 ml)

Regular ILETIN II (purified pork insulin) Lilly   OTC
Vials: 100 units/ml (10 ml)

Regular Insulin (pork insulin) Squibb-Novo   OTC
Vials: 100 units/ml (10 ml)

Regular Purified Insulin (purified pork insulin) Squibb-Novo   OTC
Vials: 100 units/ml (10 ml)

NOVOLIN R (human insulin) Squibb-Novo   OTC
Vials: 100 units/ml (10 ml)

VELOSULIN (purified pork insulin) Nordisk-USA   OTC
Vials: 100 units/ml (10 ml)

VELOSULIN Human (human insulin) Nordisk-USA   OTC
Vials: 100 units/ml (10 ml)

Prompt Insulin Zinc Suspension   Onset: 1–3 h   Peak: 2–8 h   Duration: 12–16 h

Semilente ILETIN I (beef and pork insulin) Lilly   OTC
Vials: 40, 100 units/ml (10 ml)

Semilente Insulin (beef insulin) Squibb-Novo   OTC
Vials: 100 units/ml (10 ml)

Semilente Purified Insulin (purified pork insulin) Squibb-Novo   OTC
Vials: 100 units/ml (10 ml)

Isophane Insulin Suspension and Regular Insulin   Onset: 1/2 h   Peak: 4–8 h   Duration: 24 h

MIXTARD (purified pork insulin) Nordisk-USA   OTC
Vials: 100 units (70% NPH insulin and 30% regular insulin) per milliliter (10 ml)

NOVOLIN 70/30 (human insulin) Squibb-Novo   OTC
Vials: 100 units (70% NPH insulin and 30% regular insulin) per milliliter (10 ml)

Isophane Insulin Suspension (NPH)   Onset: 3–4 h   Peak: 6–12 h   Duration: 24–28 h

HUMULIN N (human insulin) Lilly   OTC
Vials: 100 units/ml (10 ml)

INSULATARD NPH (purified pork insulin) Nordisk-USA   OTC
Vials: 100 units/ml (10 ml)

Insulin

INSULATARD NPH Human (human insulin) Nordisk-USA — OTC
Vials: 100 units/ml (10 ml)

NOVOLIN N (human insulin) Squibb-Novo — OTC
Vials: 100 units/ml (10 ml)

NPH ILETIN I (beef and pork insulin) Lilly — OTC
Vials: 40, 100 units/ml (10 ml)

NPH ILETIN II (purified beef insulin) Lilly — OTC
Vials: 100 units/ml (10 ml)

NPH ILETIN II (purified pork insulin) Lilly — OTC
Vials: 100 units/ml (10 ml)

NPH Insulin (beef insulin) Squibb-Novo — OTC
Vials: 100 units/ml (10 ml)

NPH Purified Insulin (purified pork insulin) Squibb-Novo — OTC
Vials: 100 units/ml (10 ml)

Insulin Zinc Suspension   Onset: 1–3 h   Peak: 8–12 h   Duration: 24–28 h

HUMULIN L (human insulin) Lilly — OTC
Vials: 100 units/ml (10 ml)

Lente ILETIN I (beef and pork insulin) Lilly — OTC
Vials: 40, 100 units/ml (10 ml)

Lente ILETIN II (purified beef insulin) Lilly — OTC
Vials: 100 units/ml (10 ml)

Lente ILETIN II (purified pork insulin) Lilly — OTC
Vials: 100 units/ml (10 ml)

Lente Insulin (beef insulin) Squibb-Novo — OTC
Vials: 100 units/ml (10 ml)

Lente Purified Insulin (purified pork insulin) Squibb-Novo — OTC
Vials: 100 units/ml (10 ml)

NOVOLIN L (human insulin) Squibb-Novo — OTC
Vials: 100 units/ml (10 ml)

Protamine Zinc Insulin (PZI)   Onset: 4–6 h   Peak: 14–24 h   Duration: 36 h

Protamine, Zinc & ILETIN I (beef and pork insulin) Lilly — OTC
Vials: 40, 100 units/ml (10 ml)

Protamine, Zinc & ILETIN II (purified beef insulin) Lilly — OTC
Vials: 100 units/ml (10 ml)

Protamine, Zinc & ILETIN II (purified pork insulin) Lilly — OTC
Vials: 100 units/ml (10 ml)

Extended Insulin Zinc Suspension   Onset: 4–6 h   Peak: 18–24 h   Duration: 36 h

Ultralente ILETIN I (beef and pork insulin) Lilly — OTC
Vials: 40, 100 units/ml (10 ml)

Ultralente Insulin (beef insulin) Squibb-Novo — OTC
Vials: 100 units/ml (10 ml)

Insulin

Ultralente Purified Insulin (purified beef insulin) Squibb-Novo OTC

Vials: 100 units/ml (10 ml)

INDICATIONS	PARENTERAL DOSAGE
Diabetes mellitus not controllable by diet alone	Adult and child: dosage and timing of SC administration must be determined individually under direct and continuous medical supervision (for diabetic acidosis and coma, IM and/or IV injection of regular insulin may be necessary)

Regular (Concentrated) ILETIN II (purified pork insulin) Lilly Rx

Vials: 500 units/ml (20 ml)

INDICATIONS	PARENTERAL DOSAGE
Diabetes mellitus, especially in patients who require more than 200 units/day of insulin	Adult and child: administer 1–3 doses/day SC or IM (IV injection may precipitate allergic or anaphylactoid reactions). Closely observe patients during initial use of this preparation; if insulin resistance has resulted from antibodies to beef insulin, the daily dose may be only a fraction of the previous dose of beef insulin. After several weeks or months of high-dosage therapy, patients may regain insulin responsiveness and dosage can then be reduced.

CONTRAINDICATIONS
Hypersensitivity to any component

ADMINISTRATION/DOSAGE ADJUSTMENTS

Change of insulin preparation	Any change in refinement, purity, strength, brand, type, or source should be done with caution and may require a change in dosage; the need for dosage adjustment may occur with the first dose or over a period of several weeks. When switching patients of normal weight from beef insulin or pork and beef insulin to either Velosulin Human or Insulatard NPH Human, it may be prudent to reduce the dosage by 5–10%.
Combination insulin therapy	Lente, semilente, and ultralente insulins may be mixed with one another in any proportion but must not be mixed with any other modified insulin preparations. Regular (crystalline) insulin may be mixed with NPH or lente insulins in any proportion. Regular insulin may be mixed with protamine zinc insulin (PZI), but the excess free protamine content combines with the regular insulin to produce varying durations of action. Do not mix Humulin BR with any other insulin.
Human insulins	Humulin is synthesized by a strain of *E coli* that has been genetically altered by the addition of the human gene for insulin production; Novolin, Velosulin Human, and Insulatard NPH Human are derived by enzymatic alteration of pork insulin. Humulin BR, buffered regular insulin, has been tested only in Cardiac Pacemakers No. 9100 and No. 9200 infusion pumps; insulin in the reservoir of these devices was changed every 24 h during clinical studies.
Insulin administration during hyperalimentation	Adding insulin directly to IV hyperalimentation solutions provides significantly less insulin to the patient; use SC route or a separate IV line
Catheter obstruction	Catheters used with infusion pumps may become clogged with insulin crystals, especially during menses; if obstruction occurs, change the administration set more frequently or minimize direct contact of the catheter with the skin

WARNINGS/PRECAUTIONS

Insulin requirements	May increase in the presence of high fever, obesity, hyperthyroidism, severe infection, diabetic ketoacidosis, trauma, or surgery and may decrease in the presence of impaired hepatic or renal function, hypothyroidism, nausea, or vomiting. Perform periodic ophthalmologic examinations for early vascular and visual changes and instruct patient to test urine frequently for excess glucose and ketones.
Insulin reaction and shock	May occur due to excessive dosage, delaying or skipping meals, excessive exercise or work just prior to meals, infection or illness (especially with diarrhea or vomiting), or change in patient's insulin requirements (see above). Initial symptoms, which may include fatigue, nervousness, confusion, trembling, rapid heartbeat, nausea, and cold sweats, occur suddenly and may be corrected by drinking a glass of milk or orange juice or eating sugar or a sugar-sweetened product. Symptoms of more severe reactions include shallow breathing and pallor. When using regular (concentrated) insulin, measure dosage with extreme caution to avoid irreversible insulin shock; deep secondary hypoglycemic reactions may develop 18–24 h after the original injection.
Diabetic acidosis and coma	May occur due to omission or reduction of insulin dose, significantly increased food consumption, or development of fever or infection. Initial symptoms, including drowsiness, flushed face, thirst, and loss of appetite, usually occur gradually over hours or days. Symptoms of more severe reactions include heavy breathing and rapid pulse.
Local reactions	Red, swollen, itchy skin may occur at the injection site due to improper injection, sensitivity to cleansing solution, or allergy to insulin
Severe allergic reactions	Insulin may produce severe hypersensitivity reactions such as generalized urticaria, dyspnea, and wheezing; with continued use, these reactions may progress to anaphylaxis. If a severe allergic reaction develops, discontinue administration and institute appropriate therapy; a desensitization regimen may permit resumption of use. Patients who have experienced a severe allergic reaction should be given another preparation only after a skin test has been performed.

Insulin ■ DIAβETA

Diet	Must be low in refined carbohydrates and provide appropriate caloric distribution in meals and snacks

ADVERSE REACTIONS

Hypersensitivity	Erythema, edema, or pruritus at injection site; generalized urticaria, angioedema, shortness of breath, rapid pulse, diaphoresis, decreased blood pressure, anaphylaxis
Gastrointestinal	Nausea
Central nervous system	Fatigue, nervousness, trembling, drowsiness, coma
Cardiovascular	Increased heart rate, pallor, flushed face
Respiratory	Shallow or heavy breathing
Other	Cold sweat, thirst, loss of appetite

OVERDOSAGE

Signs and symptoms	Fatigue, nervousness, trembling, increased heart rate, nausea, cold sweat, shallow breathing, pallor, shock
Treatment	Administer carbohydrate immediately; for more severe hypoglycemic reactions, give 10–20 g glucose IV promptly; carefully monitor electrolytes and treat symptomatically

DRUG INTERACTIONS

Alcohol, anabolic steroids, disopyramide, guanethidine, MAO inhibitors, oral hypoglycemics, fenfluramine, salicylates (large doses)	△ Risk of hypoglycemia
Corticosteroids, dextrothyroxine, epinephrine, oral contraceptives, ethacrynic acid, furosemide, phenytoin, sympathomimetics, thiazides or thiazide-like diuretics, thyroid hormones	△ Risk of hyperglycemia
Nonselective beta blockers	△ Duration of insulin-induced hypoglycemia Hypertension and marked bradycardia during insulin-induced hypoglycemic episode; to diagnose hypoglycemia during concomitant therapy, look for diaphoresis rather than tachycardia

ALTERED LABORATORY VALUES

Blood/serum values	▽ Glucose ▽ Potassium
Urinary values	▽ Glucose

USE IN CHILDREN

See INDICATIONS and PARENTERAL DOSAGE

USE IN PREGNANT AND NURSING WOMEN

Consult manufacturer for use in pregnant or nursing women. Insulin requirements of pregnant diabetic patients are often increased, especially during the second and third trimesters.

ORAL HYPOGLYCEMIC AGENTS

DIAβETA (glyburide) Hoechst-Roussel   Rx

Tablets: 1.25, 2.5, 5 mg

INDICATIONS

Noninsulin-dependent (type II) diabetes mellitus that cannot be adequately controlled by dietary measures alone (adjunctive therapy)

ORAL DOSAGE

Adult: 2.5–5 mg/day to start; for more sensitive patients, give 1.25 mg/day to start; for patients receiving other sulfonylureas or less than 20 units/day of insulin, substitute 2.5–5 mg/day of glyburide to start; for patients receiving 20–40 units/day of insulin, substitute 5 mg/day of glyburide to start. Increase dosage weekly, as needed, by increments of up to 2.5 mg/day; do not exceed 20 mg/day. For patients receiving more than 40 units/day of insulin, give 5 mg/day of glyburide and reduce the insulin dosage by 50% to start; then, increase the glyburide dosage every 2–10 days by increments of 1.25–2.5 mg/day (maximum dosage: 20 mg/day) and decrease the insulin dosage gradually.

CONTRAINDICATIONS

Hypersensitivity to glyburide	Diabetic ketoacidosis

COMPENDIUM OF DRUG THERAPY

DIAβETA

ADMINISTRATION/DOSAGE ADJUSTMENTS

Timing of administration	Glyburide should generally be given once daily with breakfast; however, for some patients, particularly those who require more than 10 mg/day, twice-daily administration may produce a more satisfactory response
Switching from other sulfonylureas	A 5-mg dose of glyburide has approximately the same hypoglycemic effect as 1–1.5 g of tolbutamide, 500–750 mg of acetohexamide, and 250–375 mg of chlorpropamide or tolazamide. Exercise particular care during the first 2 wk of therapy if a patient has been switched from chlorpropamide, a long-acting drug, because hypoglycemia may occur.
Monitoring of therapy	Urinary glucose tests should be performed frequently; for titration of dosage and periodic evaluation of therapeutic response, the blood glucose level must also be checked (determination of the glycosylated hemoglobin level may also be helpful). If an unsatisfactory hypoglycemic response is detected during therapy and persists despite adjustment of dosage and compliance with dietary measures, glyburide should be discontinued; the effectiveness of this drug diminishes in many patients over time, possibly owing to a decrease in responsiveness or an increase in the severity of diabetes. When insulin and glyburide are given concomitantly during the initial transition period, urinary glucose and acetone tests should be done at least 3 times/day; if glycosuria and persistent acetonuria are detected, the initial insulin dosage should be reinstituted and glyburide should be discontinued.
Short-term use	For patients whose diabetes is usually well controlled by dietary measures, short-term use may be sufficient to treat transient episodes of hyperglycemia that do not respond adequately to dietary management alone

WARNINGS/PRECAUTIONS

Cardiovascular risk	The use of sulfonylureas has been associated with an increase in cardiovascular mortality. In a controversial prospective clinical study conducted by the University Group Diabetes Program,[1] administration of 1.5 g/day of tolbutamide for 5–8 yr increased cardiovascular mortality 2½ times. A significant increase in overall mortality was not observed, possibly because the clinical trial was discontinued prematurely.
Hypoglycemia	Severe hypoglycemia is more likely to occur in patients who are elderly, debilitated, or malnourished; who have renal, hepatic, adrenal, or pituitary impairment; who are using other hypoglycemic drugs or alcohol; or who have undergone severe or prolonged exercise. Exercise caution when titrating dosage for patients who are particularly susceptible to hypoglycemia; for treatment of hypoglycemia, see OVERDOSAGE. In elderly patients and patients receiving beta-adrenergic blockers, the signs and symptoms of hypoglycemia may be masked.
Hyperglycemia	Fever, trauma, infection, surgery, or other types of stress may precipitate hyperglycemia during therapy and necessitate use of insulin in place of glyburide
Gastrointestinal reactions	Consider reducing the dosage if GI disturbances occur, since these reactions tend to be dose-related
Jaundice, allergic skin reactions	Discontinue use if cholestatic jaundice occurs or allergic skin reactions persist
Asymptomatic patients	When considering use in asymptomatic patients, bear in mind that control of the serum glucose level has not been definitely shown to prevent the long-term cardiovascular and neural complications of diabetes
Diet and exercise	Caution patients about the importance of adhering to a dietary regimen and a regular exercise program; this drug should not be considered a substitute for dietary restraint or exercise
Carcinogenicity, mutagenicity	No carcinogenic effects have been detected in rats given up to 300 mg/kg/day for 18 mo; the Ames test and the DNA damage/alkaline elution assay have shown no evidence of mutagenicity

ADVERSE REACTIONS[2]

Frequent reactions (incidence ≥ 1%) are printed in *italics*

Gastrointestinal	*Gastrointestinal disturbances (1.8%), including nausea, epigastric fullness, and heartburn;* cholestatic jaundice (rare)
Dermatological	*Allergic skin reactions (1.5%), including pruritus, erythema, urticaria, and morbilliform or maculopapular eruptions;* porphyria cutanea tarda, photosensitivity
Hematological	Leukopenia, agranulocytosis, thrombocytopenia, hemolytic anemia, aplastic anemia, pancytopenia
Other	*Hypoglycemia;* disulfiram-like reactions (very rare)

OVERDOSAGE

Signs and symptoms	Hypoglycemic reactions
Treatment	For mild hypoglycemic symptoms, administer glucose orally and adjust dosage and/or meal patterns; patient response should be closely monitored. Patients who have severe hypoglycemic reactions associated with coma, seizures, or other neurological effects should be hospitalized immediately. To treat hypoglycemic coma, administer 50% glucose by rapid IV injection and then give a 10% glucose solution by continuous IV infusion at a rate that will maintain the serum glucose level above 100 mg/dl; closely monitor patient response for at least 24–48 h because hypoglycemia may recur.

DIAβETA ■ DIABINESE

DRUG INTERACTIONS

Other sulfonylureas, insulin, salicylates and other nonsteroidal anti-inflammatory drugs, sulfonamides, chloramphenicol, probenecid, oral anticoagulants, MAO inhibitors, beta-adrenergic blockers	Hypoglycemia; watch closely for hypoglycemia during combination therapy and for hyperglycemia when concomitant use is discontinued
Thiazides and other diuretics, corticosteroids, thyroid hormones, estrogens, oral contraceptives, phenothiazines, phenytoin, nicotinic acid, sympathomimetic drugs, calcium channel blockers, isoniazid	Hyperglycemia; watch closely for hyperglycemia during combination therapy and for hypoglycemia when concomitant use is discontinued
Alcohol	Hypoglycemia Disulfiram-like reactions (very rare)
Oral miconazole (not approved for use in the US)	Severe hypoglycemia (whether other forms of miconazole similarly interact is currently unknown)

ALTERED LABORATORY VALUES

Blood/serum values	▽ Glucose
Urinary values	▽ Glucose

USE IN CHILDREN

Safety and effectiveness for use in children have not been established

USE IN PREGNANT AND NURSING WOMEN

Pregnancy Category B: reproduction studies in rats and rabbits given up to 500 times the human dose have shown no evidence of impaired fertility or harm to the fetus; however, no adequate, well-controlled studies have been done in pregnant women. Prolonged, severe hypoglycemia has occurred in neonates whose mothers received a sulfonylurea at the time of delivery. Glyburide should be administered during pregnancy only if clearly needed; many experts recommend the use of insulin for control of hyperglycemia in pregnant women. If glyburide is given during the third trimester, administration should be discontinued at least 2 wk before the expected delivery date. Although it is not known whether glyburide is excreted in human milk, other sulfonylureas have been detected in human milk; because of the potential for hypoglycemia in nursing infants, patients should not nurse while taking this drug. Insulin therapy should be considered for patients who do wish to nurse.

[1] *Diabetes* 19 (suppl 2):747–830 (1970)
[2] Includes reactions common to sulfonylureas in general

ORAL HYPOGLYCEMIC AGENTS

DIABINESE (chlorpropamide) Pfizer   Rx

Tablets: 100, 250 mg

INDICATIONS

Noninsulin-dependent (type II) diabetes mellitus that cannot be adequately controlled by dietary measures alone (adjunctive therapy)

ORAL DOSAGE

Adult: 250 mg/day to start; for elderly patients, give 100–125 mg/day to start; for patients receiving another sulfonylurea or up to 40 units/day of insulin, substitute 250 mg/day to start. For patients receiving more than 40 units/day, give 250 mg/day and reduce the insulin dosage by 50% to start. Subsequent reductions in the insulin dosage can be made after the first few days of therapy; for some patients, hospitalization during the transition period may be advisable. To achieve an optimal response in any patient, increase or decrease dosage, as needed, by 50–125 mg/day, allowing 5–7 days to elapse between the start of therapy and the first change in dosage and 3–5 days to elapse between each adjustment. If 500 mg/day does not result in control of hyperglycemia, it is unlikely that a higher dosage will be effective; dosage should not exceed 750 mg/day.

CONTRAINDICATIONS

Hypersensitivity to chlorpropamide	Diabetic ketoacidosis

ADMINISTRATION/DOSAGE ADJUSTMENTS

Timing of administration	Chlorpropamide should generally be given once daily with breakfast

DIABINESE

Monitoring of therapy	Urinary glucose tests should be performed frequently; for titration of dosage and periodic evaluation of therapeutic response, the blood glucose level must also be checked (determination of the glycosylated hemoglobin level may also be helpful). If an unsatisfactory hypoglycemic response is detected during therapy and persists despite adjustment of dosage and compliance with dietary measures, chlorpropamide should be discontinued; the effectiveness of this drug diminishes in many patients over time, possibly owing to a decrease in responsiveness or an increase in the severity of diabetes. When insulin and chlorpropamide are given concomitantly during the initial transition period, urinary glucose and acetone tests should be done at least 3 times/day; if glycosuria and persistent acetonuria are detected, the initial insulin dosage should be reinstituted and chlorpropamide should be discontinued.
Short-term use	For patients whose diabetes is usually well controlled by dietary measures, short-term use may be sufficient to treat transient episodes of hyperglycemia that do not respond adequately to dietary management alone

WARNINGS/PRECAUTIONS

Cardiovascular risk	The use of sulfonylureas has been reported to be associated with an increase in cardiovascular mortality. In a controversial prospective clinical study conducted by the University Group Diabetes Program,[1] administration of 1.5 g/day of tolbutamide for 5–8 yr increased cardiovascular mortality 2½ times. A significant increase in overall mortality was not observed, possibly because the clinical trial was discontinued prematurely.
Hypoglycemia	Severe hypoglycemia is more likely to occur in patients who are elderly, debilitated, or malnourished; who have renal, hepatic, adrenal, or pituitary impairment; who are using other hypoglycemic drugs or alcohol; or who have undergone severe or prolonged exercise. Exercise caution when titrating dosage for patients who are particularly susceptible to hypoglycemia; for treatment of hypoglycemia, see OVERDOSAGE. In elderly patients and patients receiving beta-adrenergic blockers, the signs and symptoms of hypoglycemia may be masked.
Hyperglycemia	Fever, trauma, infection, surgery, or other types of stress may precipitate hyperglycemia during therapy and necessitate use of insulin in place of chlorpropamide
Gastrointestinal reactions	Consider reducing or dividing the daily dose if GI disturbances occur, since these reactions are dose-related
Jaundice, allergic skin reactions	Discontinue use if cholestatic jaundice occurs or allergic skin reactions persist
Asymptomatic patients	When considering use in asymptomatic patients, bear in mind that control of the serum glucose level has not been definitely shown to prevent the long-term cardiovascular and neural complications of diabetes
Diet and exercise	Caution patients about the importance of adhering to a dietary regimen and a regular exercise program; this drug should not be considered a substitute for dietary restraint or exercise
Effect on fertility	Suppression of spermatogenesis has been seen in rats given up to 125 mg/kg for 6–12 mo

ADVERSE REACTIONS[2]

Frequent reactions (incidence ≥ 1%) are printed in *italics*

Gastrointestinal	*Nausea (< 5%); diarrhea, vomiting, anorexia, and hunger (< 2%);* proctocolitis, other GI disturbances, hepatic porphyria; cholestatic jaundice (rare)
Dermatological	*Pruritus (< 3%); other allergic skin reactions (1%), including urticaria and maculopapular eruptions;* porphyria cutanea tarda, photosensitivity; skin eruptions, progressing in rare cases to erythema multiforme and exfoliative dermatitis
Hematological	Leukopenia, agranulocytosis, thrombocytopenia, hemolytic anemia, aplastic anemia, pancytopenia; eosinophilia
Other	*Hypoglycemia,* disulfiram-like reactions; inappropriate ADH secretion syndrome (rare)

OVERDOSAGE

Signs and symptoms	Hypoglycemic reactions
Treatment	For mild hypoglycemic symptoms, administer glucose orally, adjust dosage, and give meals at more frequent intervals. Patients who have severe hypoglycemic reactions associated with coma, seizures, or other neurological effects should be hospitalized immediately. To treat hypoglycemic coma, administer 50% glucose by rapid IV injection and then give 10% glucose by continuous IV infusion at a rate that will maintain the serum glucose level above 100 mg/dl. To avoid recurrence of mild or severe hypoglycemia, closely monitor patient response for at least 3–5 days.

DRUG INTERACTIONS

Other sulfonylureas, insulin, salicylates and other nonsteroidal anti-inflammatory drugs, sulfonamides, chloramphenicol, probenecid, oral anticoagulants, MAO inhibitors, beta-adrenergic blockers	Hypoglycemia; watch closely for hypoglycemia during combination therapy and for hyperglycemia when concomitant use is discontinued

DIABINESE ■ GLUCOTROL

Thiazides and other diuretics, corticosteroids, thyroid hormones, estrogens, oral contraceptives, phenothiazines, phenytoin, nicotinic acid, sympathomimetic drugs, calcium channel blockers, isoniazid	Hyperglycemia; watch closely for hyperglycemia during combination therapy and for hypoglycemia when concomitant use is discontinued
Alcohol	Hypoglycemia Disulfiram-like reactions
Barbiturates	⌂ Pharmacologic effects of barbiturates; exercise caution during concomitant therapy

ALTERED LABORATORY VALUES

Blood/serum values	▽ Glucose
Urinary values	▽ Glucose

USE IN CHILDREN

Safety and effectiveness for use in children have not been established

USE IN PREGNANT AND NURSING WOMEN

Pregnancy Category C: no reproduction studies have been done in animals or pregnant women. Prolonged, severe hypoglycemia has occurred in neonates whose mothers received a sulfonylurea at the time of delivery. Chlorpropamide should be administered during pregnancy only if clearly needed; many experts recommend the use of insulin for control of hyperglycemia in pregnant women. If chlorpropamide is given during the third trimester, administration should be discontinued at least 1 mo before the expected delivery date. Chlorpropamide is excreted in human milk; because of the potential for hypoglycemia in nursing infants, patients should not nurse while taking this drug. Insulin therapy should be considered for patients who do wish to nurse.

[1] *Diabetes* 19(suppl 2):747–830, 1970
[2] Includes reactions common to sulfonylureas in general

ORAL HYPOGLYCEMIC AGENTS

GLUCOTROL (glipizide) Roerig   Rx
Tablets: 5, 10 mg

INDICATIONS

Noninsulin-dependent (type II) diabetes mellitus that cannot be adequately controlled by dietary measures alone (adjunctive therapy)

ORAL DOSAGE

Adult: 5 mg/day to start; for elderly patients and patients with hepatic disease, give 2.5 mg/day to start; for patients receiving another sulfonylurea or up to 20 units/day of insulin, substitute 5 mg/day of glipizide to start; for patients receiving more than 20 units/day, give 5 mg/day of glipizide and reduce the insulin dosage by 50% to start. Increase glipizide dosage, as needed, by increments of 2.5–5 mg/day, allowing several days between each adjustment; do not exceed 40 mg/day. The insulin dosage for patients who were initially receiving more than 20 units/day should be gradually reduced after being decreased by 50%.

CONTRAINDICATIONS

Hypersensitivity to glipizide	Diabetic ketoacidosis

ADMINISTRATION/DOSAGE ADJUSTMENTS

Timing of administration	Glipizide should be given 30 min before a meal. A daily dose of 15 mg or less should generally be administered before breakfast; however, if the response is unsatisfactory, the dose may be divided. A daily dose that exceeds 15 mg should ordinarily be divided, and each dose given before a meal of adequate caloric content.
Switching from chlorpropamide	During the first 1–2 wk after discontinuation of chlorpropamide, watch carefully for hypoglycemia
Switching from insulin	Hospitalization may be advisable when insulin and glyburide are given concomitantly during the initial transition period, particularly if a patient has been receiving more than 40 units/day of insulin
Monitoring of therapy	Urinary glucose tests should be performed frequently; for titration of dosage and periodic evaluation of therapeutic response, the blood glucose level must also be checked (determination of the glycosylated hemoglobin level may also be helpful). If an unsatisfactory hypoglycemic response is detected during therapy and persists despite adjustment of dosage and compliance with dietary measures, glipizide should be discontinued; the effectiveness of this drug diminishes in many patients over time, possibly owing to a decrease in responsiveness or an increase in the severity of diabetes. When insulin and glipizide are given concomitantly during the initial transition period, urinary glucose and acetone tests should be done at least 3 times/day; if glycosuria and persistent acetonuria are detected, the initial insulin dosage should be reinstituted and glipizide should be discontinued.

GLUCOTROL

Short-term use	For patients whose diabetes is usually well controlled by dietary measures, short-term use may be sufficient to treat transient episodes of hyperglycemia that do not respond adequately to dietary management alone

WARNINGS/PRECAUTIONS

Cardiovascular risk	The use of sulfonylureas has been associated with an increase in cardiovascular mortality. In a controversial prospective clinical study conducted by the University Group Diabetes Program,[1] administration of 1.5 g/day of tolbutamide for 5–8 yr increased cardiovascular mortality 2½ times. A significant increase in overall mortality was not observed, possibly because the clinical trial was discontinued prematurely.
Hypoglycemia	Severe hypoglycemia is more likely to occur in patients who are elderly, debilitated, or malnourished; who have renal, hepatic, adrenal, or pituitary impairment; who are using other hypoglycemic drugs or alcohol; or who have undergone severe or prolonged exercise. In patients with renal or hepatic impairment, hypoglycemia may also be prolonged. Exercise caution when titrating dosage for patients who are particularly susceptible to hypoglycemia; for treatment of hypoglycemia, see OVERDOSAGE. In elderly patients and patients receiving beta-adrenergic blockers, the signs and symptoms of hypoglycemia may be masked.
Hyperglycemia	Fever, trauma, infection, surgery, or other types of stress may precipitate hyperglycemia during therapy and necessitate use of insulin in place of glipizide
Gastrointestinal reactions	Consider reducing or dividing the daily dose if GI disturbances occur, since these reactions are dose-related
Jaundice, allergic skin reactions	Discontinue use if cholestatic jaundice occurs or allergic skin reactions persist
Asymptomatic patients	When considering use in asymptomatic patients, bear in mind that control of the serum glucose level has not been definitely shown to prevent the long-term cardiovascular and neural complications of diabetes
Diet and exercise	Caution patients about the importance of adhering to a dietary regimen and a regular exercise program; this drug should not be considered a substitute for dietary restraint or exercise
Carcinogenicity, mutagenicity, effect on fertility	No carcinogenic effects have been seen in rats and mice following long-term administration of up to 75 times the maximum human dose; no evidence of mutagenicity has been detected in bacterial and in vivo tests; and no adverse effect on fertility has been observed in rats given up to 75 times the human dose

ADVERSE REACTIONS[2]

Frequent reactions (incidence ≥ 1%) are printed in *italics*

Central nervous system	*Dizziness, drowsiness, and headache (2%)*
Gastrointestinal	*Nausea and diarrhea (1.4%); constipation and gastralgia (1%)*; cholestatic jaundice (rare)
Dermatological	*Allergic skin reactions (1.4%), including erythema, morbilliform or maculopapular eruptions, urticaria, pruritus, and eczema*; porphyria cutanea tarda, photosensitivity
Hematological	Leukopenia, agranulocytosis, thrombocytopenia, hemolytic anemia, aplastic anemia, pancytopenia
Endocrinological	Hyponatremia, inappropriate ADH secretion syndrome
Other	*Hypoglycemia*, hepatic porphyria; disulfiram-like reactions (very rare)

OVERDOSAGE

Signs and symptoms	Hypoglycemic reactions
Treatment	For mild hypoglycemic symptoms, administer glucose orally and adjust dosage and/or meal patterns; patient response should be closely monitored. Patients who have severe hypoglycemic reactions associated with coma, seizures, or other neurological effects should be hospitalized immediately. To treat hypoglycemic coma, administer 50% glucose by rapid IV injection and then give a 10% glucose solution by continuous IV infusion at a rate that will maintain the serum glucose level above 100 mg/dl; closely monitor patient response for at least 24–48 h because hypoglycemia may recur. The serum half-life of glipizide in patients with hepatic impairment is prolonged and, because this drug binds extensively to proteins, is probably not affected by dialysis.

DRUG INTERACTIONS

Other sulfonylureas, insulin, salicylates and other nonsteroidal anti-inflammatory drugs, sulfonamides, chloramphenicol, probenecid, oral anticoagulants, MAO inhibitors, beta-adrenergic blockers	Hypoglycemia; watch closely for hypoglycemia during combination therapy and for hyperglycemia when concomitant use is discontinued
Thiazides and other diuretics, corticosteroids, thyroid hormones, estrogens, oral contraceptives, phenothiazines, phenytoin, nicotinic acid, sympathomimetic drugs, calcium channel blockers, isoniazid	Hyperglycemia; watch closely for hyperglycemia during combination therapy and for hypoglycemia when concomitant use is discontinued

| Alcohol | Hypoglycemia Disulfiram-like reactions (very rare) |
| Oral miconazole (not approved for use in the US) | Severe hypoglycemia (whether other forms of miconazole similarly interact is currently unknown) |

ALTERED LABORATORY VALUES

| Blood/serum values | ▽ Glucose △ Alkaline phosphatase △SGOT △ LDH △ BUN △ Creatinine |
| Urinary values | ▽ Glucose |

USE IN CHILDREN

Safety and effectiveness for use in children have not been established

USE IN PREGNANT AND NURSING WOMEN

Pregnancy Category C: no teratogenic effects have been found in rats and rabbits, but mild fetotoxicity has occurred in rats given 5–50 mg/kg; no adequate, well-controlled studies have been done in pregnant women. Prolonged, severe hypoglycemia has occurred in neonates whose mothers received a sulfonylurea at the time of delivery. Glipizide should be administered during pregnancy only if the expected benefit justifies the potential risk to the fetus; many experts recommend the use of insulin for control of hyperglycemia in pregnant women. If glipizide is given during the third trimester, administration should be discontinued at least 1 mo before the expected delivery date. Although it is not known whether glipizide is excreted in human milk, other sulfonylureas have been detected in human milk; because of the potential for hypoglycemia in nursing infants, patients should not nurse while taking this drug. Insulin therapy should be considered for patients who do wish to nurse.

[1] *Diabetes* 19 (suppl 2):747–830 (1970)
[2] Includes reactions common to sulfonylureas in general

ORAL HYPOGLYCEMIC AGENTS

MICRONASE (glyburide) Upjohn   Rx

Tablets: 1.25, 2.5, 5 mg

INDICATIONS

Noninsulin-dependent (type II) diabetes mellitus that cannot be adequately controlled by dietary measures alone (adjunctive therapy)

ORAL DOSAGE

Adult: 2.5–5 mg/day to start; for more sensitive patients, give 1.25 mg/day to start; for patients receiving other sulfonylureas or less than 20 units/day of insulin, substitute 2.5–5 mg/day of glyburide to start; for patients receiving 20–40 units/day of insulin, substitute 5 mg/day of glyburide to start. Increase dosage weekly, as needed, by increments of up to 2.5 mg/day; do not exceed 20 mg/day. For patients receiving more than 40 units/day of insulin, give 5 mg/day of glyburide and reduce the insulin dosage by 50% to start; then, increase the glyburide dosage every 2–10 days by increments of 1.25–2.5 mg/day (maximum dosage: 20 mg/day) and decrease the insulin dosage gradually.

CONTRAINDICATIONS

| Insulin-dependent (type I) diabetes mellitus (sole therapy) | Hypersensitivity to glyburide | Diabetic ketoacidosis |

ADMINISTRATION/DOSAGE ADJUSTMENTS

Timing of administration	Glyburide should generally be given once daily with breakfast; however, for some patients, particularly those who require more than 10 mg/day, twice-daily administration may produce a more satisfactory response
Switching from other sulfonylureas	A 5-mg dose of glyburide has approximately the same hypoglycemic effect as 1–1.5 g of tolbutamide, 500–750 mg of acetohexamide, and 250–375 mg of chlorpropamide or tolazamide. Exercise particular care during the first 2 wk of therapy if a patient has been switched from chlorpropamide, a long-acting drug, because hypoglycemia may occur.
Monitoring of therapy	Urinary glucose tests should be performed frequently; for titration of dosage and periodic evaluation of therapeutic response, the blood glucose level must also be checked (determination of the glycosylated hemoglobin level may also be helpful). If an unsatisfactory hypoglycemic response is detected during therapy and persists despite adjustment of dosage and compliance with dietary measures, glyburide should be discontinued; the effectiveness of this drug diminishes in many patients over time, possibly owing to a decrease in responsiveness or an increase in the severity of diabetes. When insulin and glyburide are given concomitantly during the initial transition period, urinary glucose and acetone tests should be done at least 3 times/day; if glycosuria and persistent acetonuria are detected, the initial insulin dosage should be reinstituted and glyburide should be discontinued.

MICRONASE

Short-term use	For patients whose diabetes is usually well controlled by dietary measures, short-term use may be sufficient to treat transient episodes of hyperglycemia that do not respond adequately to dietary management alone

WARNINGS/PRECAUTIONS

Cardiovascular risk	The use of sulfonylureas has been reported to be associated with an increase in cardiovascular mortality. In a controversial prospective clinical study conducted by the University Group Diabetes Program,[1] administration of 1.5 g/day of tolbutamide for 5–8 yr increased cardiovascular mortality 2½ times. A significant increase in overall mortality was not observed, possibly because the clinical trial was discontinued prematurely.
Hypoglycemia	Severe hypoglycemia is more likely to occur in patients who are elderly, debilitated, or malnourished; who have renal, hepatic, adrenal, or pituitary impairment; who are using other hypoglycemic drugs or alcohol; or who have undergone severe or prolonged exercise. Exercise caution when titrating dosage for patients who are particularly susceptible to hypoglycemia; for treatment of hypoglycemia, see OVERDOSAGE. In elderly patients and patients receiving beta-adrenergic blockers, the signs and symptoms of hypoglycemia may be masked.
Hyperglycemia	Fever, trauma, infection, surgery, or other types of stress may precipitate hyperglycemia during therapy and necessitate use of insulin in place of glyburide
Gastrointestinal reactions	Consider reducing the dosage if GI disturbances occur, since these reactions tend to be dose-related
Jaundice, allergic skin reactions	Discontinue use if cholestatic jaundice occurs or allergic skin reactions persist
Asymptomatic patients	When considering use in asymptomatic patients, bear in mind that control of the serum glucose level has not been definitely shown to prevent the long-term cardiovascular and neural complications of diabetes
Diet and exercise	Caution patients about the importance of adhering to a dietary regimen and a regular exercise program; this drug should not be considered a substitute for dietary restraint or exercise
Carcinogenicity, mutagenicity	No carcinogenic effects have been detected in rats given up to 300 mg/kg/day for 18 mo; the Ames test and the DNA damage/alkaline elution assay have shown no evidence of mutagenicity

ADVERSE REACTIONS[2]

Frequent reactions (incidence ≥ 1%) are printed in *italics*

Gastrointestinal	*Gastrointestinal disturbances (1.8%), including nausea, epigastric fullness, and heartburn;* cholestatic jaundice (rare)
Dermatological	*Allergic skin reactions (1.5%), including pruritus, erythema, urticaria, and morbilliform or maculopapular eruptions;* porphyria cutanea tarda, photosensitivity
Hematological	Leukopenia, agranulocytosis, thrombocytopenia, hemolytic anemia, aplastic anemia, pancytopenia
Other	*Hypoglycemia;* disulfiram-like reactions (very rare)

OVERDOSAGE

Signs and symptoms	Hypoglycemic reactions
Treatment	For mild hypoglycemic symptoms, administer glucose orally and adjust dosage and/or meal patterns; patient response should be closely monitored. Patients who have severe hypoglycemic reactions associated with coma, seizures, or other neurological effects should be hospitalized immediately. To treat hypoglycemic coma, administer 50% glucose by rapid IV injection and then give a 10% glucose solution by continuous IV infusion at a rate that will maintain the blood glucose level above 100 mg/dl; closely monitor patient response for at least 24–48 h because hypoglycemia may recur.

DRUG INTERACTIONS

Other sulfonylureas, insulin, salicylates and other nonsteroidal anti-inflammatory drugs, sulfonamides, chloramphenicol, probenecid, oral anticoagulants, MAO inhibitors, beta-adrenergic blockers	Hypoglycemia; watch closely for hypoglycemia during combination therapy and for hyperglycemia when concomitant use is discontinued
Thiazides and other diuretics, corticosteroids, thyroid hormones, estrogens, oral contraceptives, phenothiazines, phenytoin, nicotinic acid, sympathomimetic drugs, calcium channel blockers, isoniazid	Hyperglycemia; watch closely for hyperglycemia during combination therapy and for hypoglycemia when concomitant use is discontinued
Alcohol	Hypoglycemia Disulfiram-like reactions (very rare)
Oral miconazole (not approved for use in the US)	Severe hypoglycemia (whether other forms of miconazole similarly interact is currently unknown)

ALTERED LABORATORY VALUES

Blood/serum values — ⇩ Glucose
Urinary values — ⇩ Glucose

USE IN CHILDREN

Safety and effectiveness for use in children have not been established

USE IN PREGNANT AND NURSING WOMEN

Pregnancy Category B: reproduction studies in rats and rabbits given up to 500 times the human dose have shown no evidence of impaired fertility or harm to the fetus; however, no adequate, well-controlled studies have been done in pregnant women. Prolonged, severe hypoglycemia has occurred in neonates whose mothers received a sulfonylurea at the time of delivery. Glyburide should be administered during pregnancy only if clearly needed; many experts recommend the use of insulin for control of hyperglycemia in pregnant women. If glyburide is given during the third trimester, administration should be discontinued at least 2 wk before the expected delivery date. Although it is not known whether glyburide is excreted in human milk, other sulfonylureas have been detected in human milk; because of the potential for hypoglycemia in nursing infants, patients should not nurse while taking this drug. Insulin therapy should be considered for patients who do wish to nurse.

[1] *Diabetes* 19 (suppl 2):747–830 (1970)
[2] Includes reactions common to sulfonylureas in general

ORAL HYPOGLYCEMIC AGENTS

ORINASE (tolbutamide) Upjohn   Rx

Tablets: 250, 500 mg

INDICATIONS

Noninsulin-dependent (type II) diabetes mellitus that cannot be adequately controlled by dietary measures alone (adjunctive therapy)

ORAL DOSAGE

Adult: 1–2 g/day to start; for maintenance, 0.25–2 g/day or, in exceptional cases, up to 3 g/day. Substitute tolbutamide directly for other sulfonylureas or for 20 units/day or less of insulin. For patients receiving 20–40 units/day of insulin, start tolbutamide and, at the same time, reduce the insulin dosage daily, beginning with a decrease of 30–50%. For patients receiving more than 40 units/day of insulin, start tolbutamide and, at the same time, carefully reduce the insulin dosage, beginning with a decrease of 20%; for these patients, hospitalization during the transition period may occasionally be advisable.

CONTRAINDICATIONS

Insulin-dependent (type I) diabetes mellitus (sole therapy) | Hypersensitivity to tolbutamide | Diabetic ketoacidosis

ADMINISTRATION/DOSAGE ADJUSTMENTS

Timing of administration — Administer the total daily dose either as a single dose in the morning or in divided doses; GI disturbances may be avoided if the dose is divided

Monitoring of therapy — Urinary glucose tests should be performed frequently; for titration of dosage and periodic evaluation of therapeutic response, the blood glucose level must also be checked (determination of the glycosylated hemoglobin level may also be helpful). During the first 2 wk of therapy, exercise particular care and watch for hypoglycemia if a patient has been switched from chlorpropamide. If an unsatisfactory hypoglycemic response is detected during therapy and persists despite adjustment of dosage and compliance with dietary measures, tolbutamide should be discontinued; the effectiveness of this drug diminishes in many patients over time, possibly owing to a decrease in responsiveness or an increase in the severity of diabetes. When insulin and tolbutamide are given concomitantly during the initial transition period, urinary glucose and acetone tests should be done at least 3 times/day; if glycosuria and persistent acetonuria are detected, the initial insulin dosage should be reinstituted and tolbutamide should be discontinued.

Short-term use — For patients whose diabetes is usually well controlled by dietary measures, short-term use may be sufficient to treat transient episodes of hyperglycemia that do not respond adequately to dietary management alone

WARNINGS/PRECAUTIONS

Cardiovascular risk — The use of sulfonylureas has been reported to be associated with an increase in cardiovascular mortality. In a controversial prospective clinical study conducted by the University Group Diabetes Program,[1] administration of 1.5 g/day of tolbutamide for 5–8 yr increased cardiovascular mortality 2½ times. A significant increase in overall mortality was not observed, possibly because the clinical trial was discontinued prematurely.

Hypoglycemia — Severe hypoglycemia is more likely to occur in patients who are elderly, debilitated, or malnourished; who have renal, hepatic, adrenal, or pituitary impairment; who are using other hypoglycemic drugs or alcohol; or who have undergone severe or prolonged exercise. Exercise caution when titrating dosage for patients who are particularly susceptible to hypoglycemia; for treatment of hypoglycemia, see OVERDOSAGE. In elderly patients and patients receiving beta-adrenergic blockers, the signs and symptoms of hypoglycemia may be masked.

ORINASE

Hyperglycemia	Fever, trauma, infection, surgery, or other types of stress may precipitate hyperglycemia during therapy and necessitate use of insulin in place of tolbutamide
Gastrointestinal reactions	Consider reducing or dividing the daily dose if GI disturbances occur, since these reactions tend to be dose-related
Jaundice, allergic skin reactions	Discontinue use if cholestatic jaundice occurs or allergic skin reactions persist
Asymptomatic patients	When considering use in asymptomatic patients, bear in mind that control of the serum glucose level has not been definitely shown to prevent the long-term cardiovascular and neural complications of diabetes
Diet and exercise	Caution patients about the importance of adhering to a dietary regimen and a regular exercise program; this drug should not be considered a substitute for dietary restraint or exercise
Carcinogenicity, mutagenicity	No carcinogenic effects have been detected in rats and mice fed tolbutamide for 78 wk; the Ames test has shown no evidence of mutagenicity

ADVERSE REACTIONS[2]
Frequent reactions (incidence $\geq$ 1%) are printed in *italics*

Gastrointestinal	*Gastrointestinal disturbances (1.4%), including nausea, epigastric fullness, and heartburn;* hepatic porphyria; cholestatic jaundice (rare)
Dermatological	*Allergic skin reactions (1.1%), including pruritus, erythema, urticaria, and morbilliform or maculopapular eruptions;* porphyria cutanea tarda, photosensitivity
Hematological	Leukopenia, agranulocytosis, thrombocytopenia, hemolytic anemia, aplastic anemia, pancytopenia
Other	*Hypoglycemia;* disulfiram-like reactions, headache, taste alterations

OVERDOSAGE

Signs and symptoms	Hypoglycemic reactions
Treatment	For mild hypoglycemic symptoms, administer glucose orally and adjust dosage and/or meal patterns; patient response should be closely monitored. Patients who have severe hypoglycemic reactions associated with coma, seizures, or other neurological effects should be hospitalized immediately. To treat hypoglycemic coma, administer 50% glucose by rapid IV injection and then give a 10% glucose solution by continuous IV infusion at a rate that will maintain the blood glucose level above 100 mg/dl; closely monitor patient response for at least 24–48 h because hypoglycemia may recur.

DRUG INTERACTIONS

Other sulfonylureas, insulin, salicylates and other nonsteroidal anti-inflammatory drugs, sulfonamides, chloramphenicol, probenecid, oral anticoagulants, MAO inhibitors, beta-adrenergic blockers	Hypoglycemia; watch closely for hypoglycemia during combination therapy and for hyperglycemia when concomitant use is discontinued
Thiazides and other diuretics, corticosteroids, thyroid hormones, estrogens, oral contraceptives, phenothiazines, phenytoin, nicotinic acid, sympathomimetic drugs, calcium channel blockers, isoniazid	Hyperglycemia; watch closely for hyperglycemia during combination therapy and for hypoglycemia when concomitant use is discontinued
Alcohol	Hypoglycemia Disulfiram-like reactions
Oral miconazole (not approved for use in the US)	Severe hypoglycemia (whether other forms of miconazole similarly interact is currently unknown)

ALTERED LABORATORY VALUES

Blood/serum values	▽ Glucose
Urinary values	▽ Glucose + Albumin (with heat and acetic acid test)

USE IN CHILDREN

Safety and effectiveness for use in children have not been established

USE IN PREGNANT AND NURSING WOMEN

Pregnancy Category C: teratogenicity has been shown in rats (at 25–100 times the human dose) but not in rabbits; in some studies with rats, ocular and bony abnormalities and an increase in the mortality of offspring have been seen following the use of high doses. No adequate, well-controlled studies have been done in pregnant women. Prolonged, severe hypoglycemia has occurred in neonates whose mothers received a sulfonylurea at the time of delivery. Tolbutamide should not be administered during pregnancy; use in women of childbearing age, particularly those who are likely to become pregnant during therapy, should be seriously considered in light of the potential risks of this drug. Many experts recommend the use of insulin for control of hyperglycemia in pregnant women. If tolbutamide is given during the third trimester, administration should be discontinued at least 2 wk before the expected delivery date. Although it is not known whether tolbutamide is excreted in human milk, other sulfonylureas have been detected in human milk; because of the potential for hypoglycemia in nursing infants, patients should not nurse while taking this drug. Insulin therapy should be considered for patients who do wish to nurse.

---

[1] *Diabetes* 19(suppl 2):747–830, 1970
[2] Includes reactions common to sulfonylureas in general

ORAL HYPOGLYCEMIC AGENTS

TOLINASE (tolazamide) Upjohn   Rx
Tablets: 100, 250, 500 mg

INDICATIONS	ORAL DOSAGE
Noninsulin-dependent (type II) diabetes mellitus that cannot be adequately controlled by dietary measures alone (adjunctive therapy)	**Adult:** for patients who have a fasting serum glucose level of less than 200 mg/dl or who are malnourished, underweight, elderly, or not eating properly, 100 mg/day to start; for patients whose glucose level exceeds 200 mg/dl, 250 mg/day to start. For patients receiving other sulfonylureas: substitute 100 mg/day of tolazamide to start if the tolbutamide dosage is less than 1 g/day or 250 mg/day to start if the tolbutamide dosage equals or exceeds 1 g/day; a 100-mg dose of tolazamide has approximately the same hypoglycemic effect as 250 mg of acetohexamide, and a 250-mg dose has approximately the same effect as 250 mg of chlorpropamide. For patients receiving insulin: substitute 100 mg/day of tolazamide to start if the insulin dosage is less than 20 units/day or 250 mg/day to start if the insulin dosage equals 20–40 units/day; if the dosage exceeds 40 units/day, given 250 mg/day of tolazamide and reduce the insulin dosage by 50% to start. To achieve an optimal response in any patient, increase the dosage, as needed, in increments of 100–125 mg/day, allowing between adjustments either 1 wk or, if more than 40 units/day of insulin was originally given, a shorter period; do not exceed 1 g/day.

CONTRAINDICATIONS

Insulin-dependent (type I) diabetes mellitus (sole therapy)	Hypersensitivity to tolazamide	Diabetic ketoacidosis

ADMINISTRATION/DOSAGE ADJUSTMENTS

Timing of administration	Tolazamide should be administered once daily with breakfast if the daily dose is 500 mg or less; a higher daily dose may be given in 2 divided doses
Monitoring of therapy	Urinary glucose tests should be performed frequently; for titration of dosage and periodic evaluation of therapeutic response, the blood glucose level must also be checked (determination of the glycosylated hemoglobin level may also be helpful). During the first 1–2 wk of therapy, exercise particular care and watch for hypoglycemia if a patient has been switched from chlorpropamide. If an unsatisfactory hypoglycemic response is detected during therapy and persists despite adjustment of dosage and compliance with dietary measures, tolazamide should be discontinued; the effectiveness of this drug diminishes in many patients over time, possibly owing to a decrease in responsiveness or an increase in the severity of diabetes. When insulin and tolazamide are given concomitantly during the initial transition period, urinary glucose and acetone tests should be done at least 3 times/day; if glycosuria and persistent acetonuria are detected, the initial insulin dosage should be reinstituted and tolazamide should be discontinued.
Short-term use	For patients whose diabetes is usually well controlled by dietary measures, short-term use may be sufficient to treat transient episodes of hyperglycemia that do not respond adequately to dietary management alone

WARNINGS/PRECAUTIONS

Cardiovascular risk	The use of sulfonylureas has been reported to be associated with an increase in cardiovascular mortality. In a controversial prospective clinical study conducted by the University Group Diabetes Program,[1] administration of 1.5 g/day of tolbutamide for 5–8 yr increased cardiovascular mortality 2½ times. A significant increase in overall mortality was not observed, possibly because the clinical trial was discontinued prematurely.
Hypoglycemia	Severe hypoglycemia is more likely to occur in patients who are elderly, debilitated, or malnourished; who have renal, hepatic, adrenal, or pituitary impairment; who are using other hypoglycemic drugs or alcohol; or who have undergone severe or prolonged exercise. Exercise caution when titrating dosage for patients who are particulary susceptible to hypoglycemia; for treatment of hypoglycemia, see OVERDOSAGE. In elderly patients and patients receiving beta-adrenergic blockers, the signs and symptoms of hypoglycemia may be masked.
Hyperglycemia	Fever, trauma, infection, surgery, or other types of stress may precipitate hyperglycemia during therapy and necessitate use of insulin in place of tolazamide
Gastrointestinal reactions	Consider reducing the dosage if GI disturbances occur, since these reactions tend to be dose-related
Jaundice, allergic skin reactions	Discontinue use if cholestatic jaundice occurs or allergic skin reactions persist
Asymptomatic patients	When considering use in asymptomatic patients, bear in mind that control of the serum glucose level has not been definitely shown to prevent the long-term cardiovascular and neural complications of diabetes
Diet and exercise	Caution patients about the importance of adhering to a dietary regimen and a regular exercise program; this drug should not be considered a substitute for dietary restraint or exercise

TOLINASE

Carcinogenicity	No evidence of carcinogenicity has been detected in rats and mice given tolazamide for 103 wk

ADVERSE REACTIONS[2]

Frequent reactions (incidence ≥ 1%) are printed in *italics*

Gastrointestinal	*Gastrointestinal disturbances (1%), including nausea, epigastric fullness, and heartburn;* hepatic porphyria; cholestatic jaundice (rare)
Dermatological	Allergic skin reactions, including pruritus, erythema, urticaria, and morbilliform or maculopapular eruptions; porphyria cutanea tarda, photosensitivity
Hematological	Leukopenia, agranulocytosis, thrombocytopenia, hemolytic anemia, aplastic anemia, pancytopenia
Other	*Hypoglycemia;* disulfiram-like reactions (very rare)

OVERDOSAGE

Signs and symptoms	Hypoglycemic reactions
Treatment	For mild hypoglycemic symptoms, administer glucose orally and adjust dosage and/or meal patterns; patient response should be closely monitored. Patients who have severe hypoglycemic reactions associated with coma, seizures, or other neurological effects should be hospitalized immediately. To treat hypoglycemic coma, administer 50% glucose by rapid IV injection and then give a 10% glucose solution by continuous IV infusion at a rate that will maintain the blood glucose level above 100 mg/dl; closely monitor patient response for at least 24–48 h because hypoglycemia may recur.

DRUG INTERACTIONS

Other sulfonylureas, insulin, salicylates and other nonsteroidal anti-inflammatory drugs, sulfonamides, chloramphenicol, probenecid, oral anticoagulants, MAO inhibitors, beta-adrenergic blockers	Hypoglycemia; watch closely for hypoglycemia during combination therapy and for hyperglycemia when concomitant use is discontinued
Thiazides and other diuretics, corticosteroids, thyroid hormones, estrogens, oral contraceptives, phenothiazines, phenytoin, nicotinic acid, sympathomimetic drugs, calcium channel blockers, isoniazid	Hyperglycemia; watch closely for hyperglycemia during combination therapy and for hypoglycemia when concomitant use is discontinued
Alcohol	Hypoglycemia Disulfiram-like reactions (very rare)
Oral miconazole (not approved for use in the US)	Severe hypoglycemia (whether other forms of miconazole similarly interact is currently unknown)

ALTERED LABORATORY VALUES

Blood/serum values	▽ Glucose
Urinary values	▽ Glucose

USE IN CHILDREN

Safety and effectiveness for use in children have not been established

---

USE IN PREGNANT AND NURSING WOMEN

Pregnancy Category C: a decrease in litter size has been seen in rats given 10 times the human dose; no adequate, well-controlled studies have been done in pregnant women. Prolonged, severe hypoglycemia has occurred in neonates whose mothers received a sulfonylurea at the time of delivery. Tolazamide should not be administered during pregnancy; use in women of childbearing age, particularly those who are likely to become pregnant during therapy, should be seriously considered in light of the potential risks of this drug. Many experts recommend the use of insulin for control of hyperglycemia in pregnant women. If tolazamide is given during the third trimester, administration should be discontinued at least 2 wk before the expected delivery date. Although it is not known whether tolazamide is excreted in human milk, other sulfonylureas have been detected in human milk; because of the potential for hypoglycemia in nursing infants, patients should not nurse while taking this drug. Insulin therapy should be considered for patients who do wish to nurse.

---

[1] *Diabetes* 19(suppl 2):747–830, 1970
[2] Reactions common to sulfonylureas in general have been included in this section. Weakness, fatigue, dizziness, vertigo, malaise, and headache have occurred with use of tolazamide, but a causal relationship has not been established.

Chapter 39

Hypolipidemic Agents

ATROMID-S (Ayerst) Clofibrate Rx	1616
CHOLOXIN (Flint) Dextrothyroxine sodium Rx	1617
COLESTID (Upjohn) Colestipol hydrochloride Rx	1618
LOPID (Parke-Davis) Gemfibrozil Rx	1620
LORELCO (Merrell Dow) Probucol Rx	1621
NICOLAR (Rorer) Niacin Rx	1622
QUESTRAN (Bristol) Cholestyramine Rx	1623

COMPENDIUM OF DRUG THERAPY

HYPOLIPIDEMIC AGENTS

ATROMID-S (clofibrate) Ayerst Rx
Capsules: 500 mg

INDICATIONS	ORAL DOSAGE
Primary dysbetalipoproteinemia (type III hyperlipidemia) **Hypertriglyceridemia** (types IV and V hyperlipidemia)	**Adult:** 2 g/day, given in divided doses; some patients may require smaller daily doses

CONTRAINDICATIONS
Pregnancy | Significant hepatic or renal dysfunction | Primary biliary cirrhosis
Breast-feeding

WARNINGS/PRECAUTIONS

Selection of patients	Clofibrate is indicated for patients with primary dysbetalipoproteinemia (type III hyperlipidemia) who have not responded adequately to diet and may be considered for adults with very high serum triglyceride levels ($>$ 750 mg/dl) in whom abdominal pain and pancreatitis are likely and who present a clearly defined risk of developing coronary heart disease due to severe hypercholesterolemia (eg, individuals with familial hypercholesterolemia starting in childhood) that has not responded adequately to dietary management and more effective cholesterol-lowering agents. Clofibrate is not effective for type I hyperlipidemia and generally has little effect on elevated serum cholesterol levels; its administration does not diminish the importance of adherence to an appropriate diet and physical exercise. Prior to initiating therapy, contributory causes (eg, hypothyroidism or diabetes) should be looked for and treated.
Cardiovascular morbidity and mortality	There is no substantial evidence that clofibrate exerts a beneficial effect on cardiovascular mortality or reduces the incidence of fatal myocardial infarction; an increased incidence of cardiac arrhythmias, intermittent claudication, definite or suspected thromboembolism, and angina has been reported in patients treated with clofibrate
Carcinogenicity	The risk of malignancy may be increased, contributing to the increased incidence of noncardiovascular deaths among clofibrate users reported in one large clinical trial; hepatic tumorigenicity has been demonstrated in rodents receiving high doses for prolonged periods
Biliary disease	Risk of cholelithiasis and cholecystitis requiring surgery is increased twofold; perform appropriate diagnostic tests if signs and symptoms of biliary disease occur
Adjunctive therapy	Attempt to control serum lipids by appropriate dietary measures, weight reduction, control of diabetes mellitus, etc, before instituting clofibrate therapy
Serum lipid values	Determine that the patient has significantly elevated serum lipid levels before initiating therapy. Obtain frequent determinations of serum lipids during the first few months of therapy and periodic determinations thereafter. Discontinue medication after 3 mo if lipid response is inadequate, unless patient has xanthoma tuberosum and is responding to therapy. Perform subsequent determinations to detect a paradoxical rise in serum cholesterol or triglyceride levels. Clofibrate does not alter seasonal variations in serum cholesterol levels. Elevated serum triglycerides are generally reduced to a greater extent than elevated serum cholesterol, although both may be lowered substantially in type III hyperlipidemia.
Hepatic impairment	May occur; obtain frequent serum transaminase determinations and perform other liver-function tests and hepatic biopsy, if necessary. Discontinue medication if tests reveal excessive abnormality. Use with caution in patients with past jaundice or hepatic disease.
Flu-like symptoms	May occur, including muscle ache, soreness, and cramping; distinguish this from actual viral and/or bacterial infections
Patients with a history of peptic ulcer disease	Reactivation of peptic ulcer may occur; use with caution
Leukopenia, anemia	May occur; obtain complete blood counts periodically
Concomitant anticoagulant therapy	May lead to bleeding complications; reduce anticoagulant dosage by about 50%; obtain frequent prothrombin determinations until prothrombin level has been definitely stabilized
Discontinuation of therapy	Continue the patient on an appropriate hypolipidemic diet; monitor serum lipids until stabilized

ADVERSE REACTIONS

Gastrointestinal	Nausea, vomiting, loose stools, dyspepsia, flatulence, bloating, abdominal distress, hepatomegaly, gallstones, stomatitis, gastritis[1]
Dermatological	Rash, alopecia, urticaria, dry skin, brittle hair, pruritus
Musculoskeletal	Muscle cramping, aching, and weakness; arthralgia "flu-like" symptoms[1]

ATROMID-S ■ CHOLOXIN

Central nervous system	Headache, dizziness, fatigue, drowsiness, weakness[1]
Hematological	Leukopenia, anemia, eosinophilia[1]
Cardiovascular	Increased or decreased angina, arrhythmias, swelling and phlebitis at site of xanthomas
Genitourinary	Impotence, decreased libido, dysuria, hematuria, proteinuria, decreased urine output
Other	Weight gain, polyphagia[1]

OVERDOSAGE

Signs and symptoms	See ADVERSE REACTIONS
Treatment	Discontinue medication; treat symptomatically and institute supportive measures, as required

DRUG INTERACTIONS

Oral anticoagulants	△ Prothrombin time
Furosemide	Muscular pain, stiffness, and diuresis

ALTERED LABORATORY VALUES

Blood/serum values	△ SGOT △ SGPT △ Sulfobromophthalein retention △ Thymol turbidity △ Creatine phosphokinase △ Beta-lipoprotein ▽ Fibrinogen
Urinary values	△ Protein

USE IN CHILDREN
The safety and effectiveness of this drug for use in children have not been established

USE IN PREGNANT AND NURSING WOMEN
Contraindicated for use in pregnant and nursing women. Withdraw medication several months before conception. Strict birth control must be exercised by women of childbearing potential.

[1] Other reactions for which a causal relationship has not been established include peptic ulcer and GI bleeding, rheumatoid arthritis, tremors, blurred vision, thrombocytopenic purpura, systemic lupus erythematosus, and gynecomastia

---

HYPOLIPIDEMIC AGENTS

CHOLOXIN (dextrothyroxine sodium) Flint   Rx

Tablets: 1, 2, 4, 6 mg

INDICATIONS
Hypercholesterolemia, as an adjunct to diet and other measures in euthyroid patients with no known evidence of organic heart disease

ORAL DOSAGE
Adult: 1–2 mg/day to start, followed by increases of 1–2 mg/day at not less than monthly intervals, up to 4–8 mg/day
Child: 0.05 mg/kg/day to start, followed by increases of up to 0.05 mg/kg/day at monthly intervals, up to 4 mg/day, if needed

CONTRAINDICATIONS

Pregnancy	Hypertensive states (other than mild, labile systolic hypertension)	History of iodism
Breast-feeding		
Known organic heart disease (see WARNINGS/PRECAUTIONS)	Advanced liver or kidney disease	

WARNINGS/PRECAUTIONS

Patients with organic heart disease	This drug should not be given to euthyroid patients with angina pectoris, a history of myocardial infarction, cardiac arrhythmias, tachycardia, rheumatic heart disease, or congestive heart failure, or decompensated or borderline compensated cardiac status
Cardiovascular morbidity and mortality	It has not been established whether drug-induced lowering of serum cholesterol or lipid levels has a beneficial or detrimental effect (or no effect) on morbidity or mortality due to atherosclerosis or coronary heart disease
Obesity	Doses within the range of daily hormonal requirements are ineffective for weight reduction in euthyroid patients, but larger doses may produce serious or life-threatening toxicity, particularly when given in combination with sympathomimetic amines
Anticoagulant effect	May be potentiated by concomitant therapy; reduce anticoagulant dosage by one third when initiating dextrothyroxine therapy; readjust dosage on the basis of prothrombin time and observe patient at least weekly during the first few weeks of treatment. Consider withdrawal of dextrothyroxine 2 wk prior to surgery if the use of anticoagulants during surgery is contemplated.

CHOLOXIN ■ COLESTID

Concomitant thyroid therapy	Hypothyroid patients are more sensitive to thyroactive drugs than euthyroid patients; adjust dosage accordingly
Coronary insufficiency	May be precipitated by injection of epinephrine and enhanced by dextrothyroxine in patients with coronary-artery disease; use with caution
Cardiac arrhythmias	May occur during surgery. Discontinue use 2 wk before elective surgery; if this is impossible or inadvisable, careful observation is essential.
Diabetic patients	Dextrothyroxine may increase blood sugar levels, with a resultant increase in insulin or oral hypoglycemic requirements
Patients with hepatic or renal impairment	Use with caution
Increased serum thyroxine values (10–25 μg/dl)	Indicate absorption and transport of dextrothyroxine; do not interpret these values as hypermetabolism or use them for dosage titration
Iodism	Discontinue use if manifestations appear
Tartrazine sensitivity	Presence of FD&C Yellow No. 5 (tartrazine) in 2- and 6-mg tablets may cause allergic-type reactions, including bronchial asthma, in susceptible individuals

ADVERSE REACTIONS

Gastrointestinal	Dyspepsia, nausea, vomiting, constipation, diarrhea, anorexia, gallstones[1]
Cardiovascular	Angina pectoris, palpitations, extrasystoles, ectopic beats, supraventricular tachycardia, ECG evidence of myocardial ischemia, cardiac enlargement, peripheral edema, worsened peripheral vascular disease[1]
Central nervous system and neuromuscular	Insomnia, nervousness, tremor, headache, tinnitus, dizziness, malaise, fatigue, psychic changes, paresthesia, muscle pain, altered sensorium
Ophthalmic	Visual disturbances, exophthalmos, retinopathy
Dermatological	Alopecia, rash, itching
Genitourinary	Diuresis, menstrual irregularities, increased or decreased libido
Other	Increased metabolism, weight loss, lid lag, sweating, flushing, hyperthermia, hoarseness

OVERDOSAGE

Signs and symptoms	See ADVERSE REACTIONS
Treatment	Discontinue medication; institute supportive measures, as required

DRUG INTERACTIONS

Oral anticoagulants	△ Prothrombin time
Catecholamines	△ Risk of coronary insufficiency

ALTERED LABORATORY VALUES

Blood/serum values	△ Thyroxine

No clinically significant alterations in urinary values occur at therapeutic dosages

---

USE IN CHILDREN

See INDICATIONS and ORAL DOSAGE; continued therapy (over 1 yr) is recommended only if a significant serum cholesterol-lowering effect is observed

USE IN PREGNANT AND NURSING WOMEN

Contraindicated for use during pregnancy and in nursing mothers; however, reproduction studies in two animal species have shown no evidence of teratogenicity. This drug may be given to women of childbearing age who exercise strict birth-control procedures.

---

[1] Other reactions for which a causal relationship has not been established include cholestatic jaundice (one case) and myocardial infarction

---

HYPOLIPIDEMIC AGENTS

COLESTID (colestipol hydrochloride) Upjohn Rx

Granules: 5 g/packet or level scoopful (5-g packets, 500-g bottles)

INDICATIONS	ORAL DOSAGE
Primary hypercholesterolemia (adjunctive therapy)	**Adult:** 15–30 g/day, given in divided doses bid to qid

COLESTID

CONTRAINDICATIONS

Hypersensitivity to any component

ADMINISTRATION/DOSAGE ADJUSTMENTS

Oral administration	*Colestipol resin should never be taken in dry form.* Caution patient to mix the granules with at least 3 fl oz of water or other liquid, such as orange juice, tomato juice, milk, or a carbonated beverage; since colestipol will not dissolve in such liquids, the glass should be rinsed with a small amount of additional beverage to ensure that all the medication is taken. The granules may also be mixed with milk in hot or cold breakfast cereal, added to highly fluid soups, or taken with pulpy fruits, such as crushed pineapple, pears, peaches, or fruit cocktail. To minimize interference with the absorption of other drugs, advise patient to take other medications at least 1 h before or 4 h after taking colestipol.

WARNINGS/PRECAUTIONS

Cardiovascular morbidity and mortality	It has not been established whether drug-induced lowering of serum cholesterol or triglyceride levels has a beneficial or detrimental effect (or no effect) on morbidity or mortality due to atherosclerosis, including coronary heart disease
Adjunctive therapy	Determine the type of hyperlipoproteinemia and attempt to control serum cholesterol by dietary measures, weight reduction, and treatment of any underlying disorder which might be the cause of hypercholesterolemia before instituting colestipol therapy
Vitamin deficiency	May result from interference with the absorption of fat-soluble vitamins, such as A, D, and K; consider giving supplemental vitamin A and D if colestipol therapy is prolonged. Hypoprothrombinemia resulting in an increased bleeding tendency may occur during chronic therapy due to vitamin K deficiency. If necessary, administer parenteral vitamin K_1; recurrences may be prevented by oral administration of vitamin K_1.
Serum cholesterol and triglyceride levels	A baseline should be established before initiating colestipol therapy, and during therapy levels should be measured periodically to detect significant changes. Discontinue medication if cholesterol level fails to fall or if a significant rise in the serum triglyceride level occurs.
Constipation	May occur or worsen; reduce dosage or, if necessary, discontinue use to prevent fecal impaction and aggravated hemorrhoids; particular care should be taken to avert constipation in patients with symptomatic coronary artery disease
Hypothyroidism	Theoretically may occur, especially in patients with limited thyroid reserve
Concomitant oral medication	Colestipol can delay or reduce the absorption of many drugs, and, therefore, the interval between its administration and that of other oral medication should be as long as possible (see ADMINISTRATION/DOSAGE ADJUSTMENTS); discontinuing colestipol could pose a hazard to health if a potentially toxic drug that is significantly bound to the resin had been titrated to a maintenance dose during concomitant therapy.

ADVERSE REACTIONS[1]

Frequent reactions (incidence $\geq$ 1%) are printed in *italics*

Gastrointestinal	*Constipation, sometimes accompanied by fecal impaction or aggravated hemorrhoids (10%); abdominal discomfort (pain and distention), belching, flatulence, nausea, vomiting, and diarrhea (1–3%);* anorexia
Hypersensitivity	Urticaria, dermatitis
Musculoskeletal	Muscle and joint pains, arthritis
Central nervous system	Headache, dizziness, fatigue, weakness, anxiety, vertigo, drowsiness
Other	Shortness of breath

OVERDOSAGE

Signs and symptoms	Gastrointestinal obstruction
Treatment	Treat according to location and degree of obstruction and status of gut motility

DRUG INTERACTIONS

Chlorthiazide, tetracycline, penicillin G	▽ Absorption
Digitalis preparations	▽ Absorption (not clearly established)

ALTERED LABORATORY VALUES

Blood/serum values	▽ Cholestrol ▽ Beta-lipoprotein/low-density lipoprotein ▽ Vitamins A, D, and K △ SGOT △ Alkaline phosphatase △ Phosphorus △ Chloride △ Sodium ▽ Potassium △ Triglycerides (with long-term use)

No clinically significant alterations in urinary values occur at therapeutic dosages

COLESTID ■ LOPID

USE IN CHILDREN	USE IN PREGNANT AND NURSING WOMEN
Safety and effectiveness for use in children have not been established	Safety for use during pregnancy has not been established; the use of colestipol in pregnant or nursing women, as well as those of childbearing age, requires weighing the potential benefits of drug therapy against the possible hazards to mother and child.

[1] Other adverse reactions for which a causal relationship has not been established include peptic ulceration, gastrointestinal irritation and bleeding, cholecystitis, and cholelithiasis; asthma and wheezing have not been observed in colestipol-treated patients but have been noted with other cholesterol-lowering agents

---

HYPOLIPIDEMIC AGENTS

LOPID (gemfibrozil) Parke-Davis   Rx

Capsules: 300 mg

INDICATIONS

Hypertriglyceridemia (type IV hyperlipidemia)

ORAL DOSAGE

Adult: 600 mg bid, taken 30 min before the morning and evening meals; some patients can be adequately treated with 900 mg/day, while a few may require 1,500 mg/day for satisfactory results

CONTRAINDICATIONS

Hepatic dysfunction, including primary biliary cirrhosis

Severe renal dysfunction

Preexisting gallbladder disease (see WARNINGS/PRECAUTIONS)

Hypersensitivity to gemfibrozil

WARNINGS/PRECAUTIONS

Selection of patients	Reserve for patients with very high serum triglyceride levels ($>$ 750 mg/dl) in whom abdominal pain and pancreatitis are likely and who present a clearly defined risk of developing coronary heart disease due to severe hypercholesterolemia (eg, individuals with familial hypercholesterolemia starting in childhood) that has not responded adequately to dietary management and more effective cholesterol-lowering agents. Gemfibrozil is not effective for type I hyperlipidemia and generally has little effect on elevated serum cholesterol levels; its administration does not diminish the importance of adherence to an appropriate diet and physical exercise. Prior to initiating therapy, contributory causes (eg, hypothyroidism or diabetes) should be looked for and treated.
Cholelithiasis	May result from increased cholesterol excretion into the bile; perform gallbladder studies if cholelithiasis is suspected, and discontinue therapy if gallstones are found. A twofold increase in cholelithiasis and cholecystitis requiring surgery has been reported in patients treated with clofibrate, which is chemically, pharmacologically, and clinically similar to gemfibrozil.
Serum lipid response	Determine serum lipid levels prior to initiating therapy and periodically thereafter; discontinue use of gemfibrozil after 3 mo if a significant improvement in serum lipid values is not obtained
Concomitant anticoagulant therapy	Reduce anticoagulant dosage to maintain desired prothrombin time and prevent bleeding complications; monitor prothrombin time frequently until it stabilizes
Laboratory monitoring during long-term therapy	Periodic blood counts are advisable during the first 12 mo of therapy; perform liver function studies periodically and discontinue use of gemfibrozil if elevations in hepatic enzyme levels (see ALTERED LABORATORY VALUES) persist
Carcinogenicity	A statistically significant increase in benign liver nodules and hepatic carcinomas has been observed in male rats at 10 times the human dose but not at the human dose level or in female rats or male or female mice; male rats have also shown a dose-dependent increase in Leydig cell tumors. Proliferation of hepatic peroxisomes has been demonstrated in rat and human liver.

ADVERSE REACTIONS[1]

Frequent reactions (incidence $\geq$ 1%) are printed in *italics*

Gastrointestinal	*Abdominal pain (6.0%), epigastric pain (4.9%), diarrhea (4.8%), nausea (4.0%), vomiting (1.6%), flatulence (1.1%)*[2]
Dermatological	Rash, dermatitis, pruritus, urticaria
Central nervous system	Headache, dizziness, blurred vision[2]
Hematological	Anemia, eosinophilia, leukopenia, transient decreases in hemoglobin level and hematocrit
Other	Painful extremities[2]

OVERDOSAGE

The effects of an acute overdosage of this drug are unknown

DRUG INTERACTIONS

Oral anticoagulants	◊ Risk of hypoprothrombinemia; use with caution to prevent bleeding complications

ALTERED LABORATORY VALUES

Blood/serum values	▽ Potassium ◊ SGOT ◊ SGPT ◊ Alkaline phosphatase ◊ Lactic dehydrogenase ◊ Creatine phosphokinase

No clinically significant alterations in urinary values occur at therapeutic dosages

---

USE IN CHILDREN

The safety and effectiveness of this drug for use in children have not been established

USE IN PREGNANT AND NURSING WOMEN

Pregnancy Category B: use during pregnancy only when the expected therapeutic benefit clearly outweighs the potential risk to the patient or fetus. Reproduction studies in rats at 3 and 9 times the human dose and in rabbits at 2 and 6.7 times the human dose have shown no evidence of impaired fertility or fetal harm, except for reduced birth rates at the higher dose levels. A reversible, dose-dependent decrease in male fertility has been observed in rats given 3 and 10 times the human dose for 10 wk; the effect was not heritable. No studies have been done in pregnant women. Because of the potential for tumorigenicity shown in male rats, nursing should not be attempted if use of the drug is continued.

---

[1] Reactions reported during controlled clinical trials involving 805 patients, 245 of whom received gemfibrozil for at least 1 yr
[2] Other reactions for which a causal relationship has not been established include dry mouth, constipation, anorexia, gas pain, dyspepsia, vertigo, insomnia, paresthesia, tinnitus, back pain, arthralgia, muscle cramps, myalgia, swollen joints, fatigue, malaise, syncope, and an increased incidence of bacterial and viral infections

---

HYPOLIPIDEMIC AGENTS

LORELCO (probucol) Merrell Dow   Rx

Tablets: 250 mg

INDICATIONS	ORAL DOSAGE
Primary hypercholesterolemia Combined hypercholesterolemia and hypertriglyceridemia	**Adult:** 500 mg bid with morning and evening meals

CONTRAINDICATIONS

Hypersensitivity to probucol

WARNINGS/PRECAUTIONS

Selection of patients	Probucol may be considered for patients with primary hypercholesterolemia (elevated low-density lipoproteins) who have not responded adequately to dietary management, weight reduction, and control of diabetes mellitus; it may also be useful in lowering elevated cholesterol levels in patients with combined hypercholesterolemia and hypertriglyceridemia, but not if the latter is the primary concern. Its administration does not diminish the importance of adherence to an appropriate diet and physical exercise. Prior to initiating therapy, contributory causes (eg, hypothyroidism or diabetes) should be looked for and treated.
Cardiovascular morbidity and mortality	It has not been established whether drug-induced lowering of serum cholesterol or triglyceride levels or alteration of HDL-cholesterol levels has any effect on morbidity or mortality due to coronary heart disease
Myocardial effects	Fatalities, preceded by marked (30–50%) prolongation of the Q-T interval and syncope, have occurred in probucol-treated monkeys placed on an atherogenic diet; however, no adverse effects were observed in monkeys that received a normal, low-fat diet and were treated continuously for 8 yr with probucol at doses 3–30 times the human dose or when, in another study, the administration of this drug and feeding of an atherogenic diet were separated in time. Studies in beagles have shown that probucol sensitizes the canine myocardium to epinephrine, resulting in ventricular fibrillation; this effect, however, has so far been seen only in dogs. Although Q-T prolongation can occur in patients being treated with probucol, there have been no reports of arrhythmias. Nevertheless, patients should be advised to adhere to a low-cholesterol, low-fat diet throughout treatment, and an ECG should be obtained prior to therapy, 6 mo later, and then after 1 yr. If after correction for rate the Q-T interval shows marked prolongation, reconsider the advisability of continuing therapy. *Probucol should not be given to patients with evidence of recent or progressive myocardial damage or findings suggesting ventricular arrhythmias.* Although no increase in ectopy has been associated with clinical use of probucol, patients who have unexplained syncopal episodes while taking this drug should be examined electrocardiographically.

LORELCO ■ NICOLAR

Serum lipid levels	Should be determined before starting therapy and then repeated during the first few months of treatment and periodically thereafter; if the serum cholesterol level has not decreased satisfactorily within the first 3–4 mo, discontinue use
Abnormal laboratory values	Certain laboratory test results (see ALTERED LABORATORY VALUES) may exceed the normal range during therapy; if abnormal levels persist or worsen, clinical signs consistent with abnormal findings develop, or secondary systemic manifestations occur, probucol should be discontinued
Carcinogenicity, mutagenicity, effect on fertility	No evidence of carcinogenicity has been detected in rats given probucol for 2 yr; studies in rats have not demonstrated mutagenicity or impairment of fertility

ADVERSE REACTIONS

Gastrointestinal	Diarrhea, loose stools, flatulence, abnormal pain, nausea, vomiting, indigestion, bleeding, anorexia
Neurological	Headache, dizziness, paresthesias, insomnia, tinnitus, peripheral neuritis
Ophthalmic	Conjunctivitis, tearing, blurred vision
Hematological	Eosinophilia, low hemoglobin and/or hematocrit, thrombocytopenia
Dermatological	Rash, pruritus, ecchymosis, petechiae, hyperhidrosis, fetid sweat
Genitourinary	Impotence, nocturia
Other	Prolongation of the Q-T interval, enlargement of multinodular goiter, diminished sense of taste and smell, angioneurotic edema; an idiosyncratic reaction characterized by dizziness, palpitations, syncope, nausea, vomiting, and chest pain

OVERDOSAGE

Signs and symptoms	Loose stools, flatulence
Treatment	Empty stomach; treat symptomatically and institute supportive measures, as needed. Probucol cannot be removed by dialysis.

DRUG INTERACTIONS

Clofibrate	⇩ Serum HDL-cholesterol level; do not use probucol in combination with clofibrate

ALTERED LABORATORY VALUES

Blood/serum values	⇧ SGOT ⇧ SGPT ⇧ Alkaline phosphatase ⇧ Bilirubin ⇧ Creatine phosphokinase ⇧ Uric acid ⇧ BUN ⇧ Glucose

No clinically significant alterations in urinary values occur at therapeutic dosages

---

USE IN CHILDREN
The safety and effectiveness of this drug for use in children have not been established

USE IN PREGNANT AND NURSING WOMEN
Pregnancy Category B: reproduction studies in rats and rabbits given up to 50 times the human dose have shown no evidence of impaired fertility or harm to the fetus; however, no adequate, well-controlled studies have been done in pregnant women. Use during pregnancy only if clearly needed. Patients who wish to become pregnant should wait at least 6 mo after the drug is withdrawn because of its persistence in the body; an effective birth-control measure should be used during this period. It is not known whether probucol is excreted in human milk; this is likely, however, since the drug is excreted in the breast milk of animals. Breast-feeding is not recommended during therapy.

HYPOLIPIDEMIC AGENTS

NICOLAR (niacin) Rorer Rx
Tablets: 500 mg

INDICATIONS	ORAL DOSAGE
Significant hyperlipidemia (elevated cholesterol and/or triglycerides) in patients unresponsive to diet and weight loss (adjunctive therapy)	**Adult:** 1–2 g tid, given with or following meals

CONTRAINDICATIONS

Hepatic dysfunction	Active acute peptic ulcer

ADMINISTRATION/DOSAGE ADJUSTMENTS

Initiation of therapy	Because flushing, pruritus, and GI distress occur frequently, begin therapy with small doses and slowly increase dose according to patient response; usual maximum dosage: 8 g/day

WARNINGS/PRECAUTIONS

Special-risk patients	Patients with gallbladder disease or a past history of jaundice, liver disease, or peptic ulcer should be observed closely during therapy; monitor liver function frequently after starting this drug, until it is ascertained that liver function is not adversely affected
Diabetic patients	Closely observe diabetic or potential diabetic patients to detect decreased glucose tolerance; monitor blood glucose upon initiation of therapy and periodically thereafter, adjusting diet and/or instituting hypoglycemic therapy, as necessary
Hyperuricemia	Elevated uric acid levels have been reported; use with caution in patients predisposed to gout
Cardiovascular morbidity and mortality	It has not been established whether drug-induced lowering of serum cholesterol or triglyceride levels has a beneficial or detrimental effect, or any effect at all, on morbidity or mortality due to atherosclerosis, including coronary heart disease
Tartrazine sensitivity	The presence of FD&C Yellow No. 5 (tartrazine) in this product may cause allergic-type reactions, including bronchial asthma, in susceptible individuals

ADVERSE REACTIONS

Central nervous system	Transient headache
Cardiovascular	Severe generalized flushing; hypotension
Dermatological	Dryness of the skin, keratosis nigricans, pruritus
Metabolic	Decreased glucose tolerance, hyperuricemia
Gastrointestinal	Activation of peptic ulcer, various GI disorders, abnormal hepatic function tests, jaundice
Other	Toxic amblyopia

OVERDOSAGE

Signs and symptoms	See ADVERSE REACTIONS
Treatment	Discontinue therapy and institute supportive measures, as needed

DRUG INTERACTIONS

Ganglionic blocking agents	⇧ Risk of postural hypotension
Insulin, oral sulfonylureas	⇧ or ⇩ Glucose; adjust dosage of hypoglycemic drug and diet accordingly

ALTERED LABORATORY VALUES

Blood/serum values	⇧ Uric acid ⇧ Glucose ⇧ Bilirubin ⇧ SGOT ⇧ SGPT ⇧ LDH ⇩ Albumin
Urinary values	⇧ Glucose False-positive glucose tests (with Benedict's reagent) ⇧ Catecholamines (with fluorometric methods)

USE IN CHILDREN

Safety and effectiveness for use in children have not been established

USE IN PREGNANT AND NURSING WOMEN

Although fetal abnormalities have not been reported with niacin, its use as a hypolipidemic agent requires high dosages, and reproduction studies have not been done. The potential benefits of using this drug in women who are pregnant or nursing should be weighed against the possible hazards to the mother and child.

HYPOLIPIDEMIC AGENTS

QUESTRAN (cholestyramine) Bristol   Rx

Powder (per packet or level scoopful): 4 g[1]

INDICATIONS	ORAL DOSAGE
Primary **hypercholesterolemia**, alone or associated with hypertriglyceridemia (adjunctive therapy) Reduction in risk of **coronary artery disease** in hypercholesterolemic patients[2] (adjunctive therapy)	**Adult:** 4 g (1 packet or level scoopful) 1–6 times/day in combination with an appropriate dietary regimen
Pruritus associated with partial biliary obstruction	**Adult:** 4 g (1 packet or level scoopful) 1–6 times/day

QUESTRAN

CONTRAINDICATIONS

Hypersensitivity to cholestyramine	Complete biliary obstruction

ADMINISTRATION/DOSAGE ADJUSTMENTS

Administration	Mix 1 scoopful or the contents of 1 packet with at least 2–6 fl oz of water or any other noncarbonated beverage; alternatively, mix with highly fluid soups or with moist, pulpy fruit preparations, such as applesauce and crushed pineapple. Stir until consistency is uniform. Do not administer this product in dry form. Patients should be well-hydrated during therapy.

WARNINGS/PRECAUTIONS

Hypercholesterolemia	Before instituting cholestyramine therapy, attempt to control serum cholesterol by dietary measures, weight reduction, and treatment of any underlying disorder (eg, hypothyroidism, diabetes mellitus, nephrotic syndrome, dysproteinemias, obstructive liver disease) that might be the cause of hypercholesterolemia
Serum cholesterol levels	Should be measured frequently during the first few months of therapy and periodically thereafter; a favorable trend in cholesterol reduction should be evident during the first month of treatment. If adequate reduction in the serum level is not attained, therapy should be discontinued.
Triglyceride levels	Should be measured periodically to detect any significant change
Vitamin deficiency	May result from altered absorption of fat-soluble vitamins (such as A, D, and K) with long-term therapy; provide daily vitamin A and D supplements in water-miscible or parenteral form. For increased bleeding due to hypoprothrombinemia, administer vitamin K_1 parenterally; prevent recurrences by administering the oral form.
Folic acid absorption	May be reduced; consider folic acid supplementation for these patients
Concurrent medication	Absorption may be impeded; patient should take other medications at least 1 h before or 4–6 h after cholestyramine
Hyperchloremic acidosis	May occur after prolonged use, especially in smaller and younger patients
Constipation	May occur or worsen, especially with high doses and in patients over 60 yr of age, and result in fecal impaction or aggravation of hemorrhoids; for some patients, it may be necessary to reduce the dosage temporarily or discontinue treatment. All possible measures should be taken to prevent severe constipation in patients with symptomatic coronary artery disease.
Tartrazine sensitivity	Presence of FD&C Yellow No. 5 (tartrazine) in powder may cause allergic-type reactions, including bronchial asthma, in susceptible individuals
Carcinogenicity	Cholestyramine has been found to cause an increase in the incidence of intestinal tumors in rats and has been associated, in a large-scale, long-term study, with a somewhat higher incidence of alimentary system cancers; further investigation is now being planned to clarify the results of the clinical study

ADVERSE REACTIONS[3]

The most frequent reactions, regardless of incidence, are printed in *italics*

Gastrointestinal	*Constipation*, fecal impaction, aggravation of hemorrhoids, abdominal discomfort, flatulence, nausea, vomiting, diarrhea, heartburn, anorexia, indigestion, steatorrhea; biliary colic (one case)
Dermatological	Rash and irritation of skin, tongue, and perianal area
Hematological	Bleeding tendencies due to hypoprothrombinemia (vitamin K deficiency)
Metabolic	Vitamin A and D deficiency, hyperchloremic acidosis in children, osteoporosis

OVERDOSAGE

Signs and symptoms	Gastrointestinal obstruction
Treatment	Discontinue medication; treat symptomatically, according to location and degree of obstruction and the presence or absence of normal gut motility

DRUG INTERACTIONS

Phenylbutazone, warfarin, chlorothiazide, propranolol, tetracycline, penicillin G, phenobarbital, thyroid preparations, digitalis, other medications	⇩ Rate and/or extent of absorption

ALTERED LABORATORY VALUES

Blood/serum values	⇧ Triglycerides ⇩ Bile acids ⇩ Beta-lipoprotein/low-density lipoprotein ⇩ Cholesterol ⇩ Vitamins A, D, and K

No clinically significant alterations in urinary values occur at therapeutic dosages

USE IN CHILDREN

Because of limited experience, a practical dosage schedule has not been established for infants and children; in calculating pediatric dosages, bear in mind that 100 mg of powder contains 44.4 mg of anhydrous cholestyramine resin. The effects of long-term administration, as well as the drug's ability to maintain lowered cholesterol levels in pediatric patients, are unknown.

USE IN PREGNANT AND NURSING WOMEN

Administration of cholestyramine in the recommended dosage during pregnancy is unlikely to have any adverse effect on the fetus, because the drug is not absorbed systemically. However, no adequate, well-controlled studies have been done in pregnant women, and interference with absorption of fat-soluble vitamins may be detrimental, even if supplements are given. Use with caution in nursing mothers; maternal vitamin malabsorption may have a harmful effect on nursing infants.

---

[1] Each packet or level scoopful contains 9 g of powder and 4 g of anhydrous cholestyramine resin

[2] In a 7-yr study (JAMA 251:351–374, 1984), use of cholestyramine and a modest cholesterol-reducing diet in men aged 35–59 yr who had serum cholesterol levels above 265 mg/dl and no previous history of heart disease has been shown to reduce the combined incidence of nonfatal myocardial infarction and coronary artery disease death by 19% (from 8.6% in the placebo-controlled group to 7% in the group receiving cholestyramine). According to the study, the reduction in coronary risk was dose-dependent and was greatest in patients given 20–24 g/day of cholestyramine resin.

[3] Other reactions for which a causal relationship has not been established include biliary tract calcification, rectal bleeding, black stools, hemorrhoidal bleeding, bleeding from known duodenal ulcer, dysphagia, hiccups, ulcer attack, sour taste, pancreatitis, rectal pain, diverticulitis, decreased prothrombin time, ecchymosis, anemia, urticaria, asthma, wheezing, shortness of breath, backache, muscle and joint pains, arthritis, headache, anxiety, vertigo, dizziness, fatigue, tinnitus, syncope, drowsiness, femoral nerve pain, paresthesia, uveitis, hematuria, dysuria, burnt odor to urine, diuresis, weight loss, weight gain, increased libido, swollen glands, edema, and dental bleeding

Chapter 40

Laxatives/Stool Softeners

CHRONULAC (Merrell Dow)   1629
Lactulose *Rx*

CITRUCEL (Lakeside)   1629
Methylcellulose *OTC*

COLACE (Mead Johnson)   1630
Docusate sodium *OTC*

DIALOSE (Stuart)   1630
Docusate potassium *OTC*

DIALOSE Plus (Stuart)   1631
Docusate potassium and casanthranol *OTC*

DORBANTYL (3M)   1631
Danthron and docusate sodium *OTC*

DORBANTYL Forte (3M)   1631
Danthron and docusate sodium *OTC*

DOXIDAN (Hoechst-Roussel)   1632
Docusate calcium and danthron *OTC*

DOXINATE (Hoechst-Roussel)   1632
Docusate sodium *OTC*

DULCOLAX (Boehringer Ingelheim)   1633
Bisacodyl *OTC*

EFFER-SYLLIUM (Stuart)   1634
Psyllium *OTC*

EX-LAX (Sandoz Consumer Health Care Group)   1635
Yellow phenolphthalein *OTC*

Extra Gentle EX-LAX (Sandoz Consumer Health Care Group)   1635
Docusate sodium and yellow phenolphthalein *OTC*

FLEET Enema (Fleet)   1635
Sodium phosphate and sodium biphosphate *OTC*

Glycerin suppositories   1636
Glycerin and sodium stearate *OTC*

METAMUCIL (Procter & Gamble)   1637
Psyllium *OTC*

Instant Fiber Mix METAMUCIL (Procter & Gamble)   1637
Psyllium *OTC*

MITROLAN (Robins)   1638
Calcium polycarbophil *OTC*

MODANE (Adria)   1638
Danthron *OTC*

PERDIEM (Rorer)   1639
Psyllium and senna *OTC*

PERDIEM Plain (Rorer)   1640
Psyllium *OTC*

PERI-COLACE (Mead Johnson)   1641
Casanthranol and docusate sodium *OTC*

PHILLIPS' Milk of Magnesia (Glenbrook)   1642
Magnesium hydroxide *OTC*

REGUTOL (Plough)   1643
Docusate sodium *OTC*

SENOKOT (Purdue Frederick)   1643
Senna *OTC*

SURFAK (Hoechst-Roussel)   1644
Docusate calcium *OTC*

Other Laxatives/Stool Softeners   1627

AGORAL (Warner-Lambert)   1627
Mineral oil and phenolphthalein *OTC*

AGORAL Plain (Warner-Lambert)   1627
Mineral oil *OTC*

CAROID Laxative Tablets (Mentholatum)   1627
Cascara sagrada extract and phenolphthalein *OTC*

CLYSODRAST (Armour)   1627
Bisacodyl tannex *Rx*

COLOGEL (Lilly)   1627
Methylcellulose *OTC*

CORRECTOL Liquid (Plough)   1627
Yellow phenolphthalein *OTC*

CORRECTOL Powder (Plough)   1627
Psyllium *OTC*

CORRECTOL Tablets (Plough)   1627
Yellow phenolphthalein and docusate sodium *OTC*

DECHOLIN (Miles Pharmaceuticals)   1627
Dehydrocholic acid *OTC*

FLEET Bisacodyl Enema (Fleet)   1627
Bisacodyl *OTC*

FLEET Mineral Oil Enema (Fleet)   1627
Mineral oil *OTC*

GENTLE NATURE (Sandoz Consumer Health Care Group)   1627
Sennosides *OTC*

KASOF (Stuart)   1627
Docusate potassium *OTC*

LAXCAPS (Glenbrook)   1627
Phenolphthalein and docusate sodium *OTC*

MALTSUPEX (Wallace)   1628
Malt soup extract *OTC*

Mineral oil *OTC*   1628

MODANE Plus (Adria)   1628
Danthron and docusate sodium *OTC*

NATURACIL (Mead Johnson)   1628
Psyllium *OTC*

PHOSPHO-SODA (Fleet)   1628
Sodium phosphate and sodium biphosphate *OTC*

SENOKAP DSS (Purdue Frederick)   1628
Senna concentrate and docusate sodium *OTC*

SENOKOT-S (Purdue Frederick)   1628
Senna concentrate and docusate sodium *OTC*

X-PREP (Gray)   1628
Senna extract *OTC*

OTHER LAXATIVES/STOOL SOFTENERS

DRUG	HOW SUPPLIED	USUAL DOSAGE[1]
AGORAL (Warner-Lambert) Mineral oil and phenolphthalein *OTC*	**Emulsion (per 15 ml):** 4.2 g mineral oil and 0.2 g phenolphthalein (8, 16 fl oz) *marshmallow flavored;* (16 fl oz) *raspberry flavored*	**Adult:** 7.5–15 ml (1/2–1 tbsp) at bedtime **Child (> 6 yr):** 5–10 ml (1–2 tsp) at bedtime
AGORAL Plain (Warner-Lambert) Mineral oil *OTC*	**Emulsion (per 15 ml):** 4.2 g mineral oil (16 fl oz)	**Adult:** 15–30 ml (1–2 tbsp) at bedtime **Child (> 6 yr):** 10–20 ml (2–4 tsp) at bedtime
CAROID Laxative Tablets (Mentholatum) Cascara sagrada extract and phenolphthalein *OTC*	**Tablets:** 50 mg cascara sagrada extract and 32.4 mg phenolphthalein	**Adult:** 2 tabs 2 h after breakfast and at bedtime, with 2 glasses of water; reduce dosage gradually
CLYSODRAST (Armour) Bisacodyl tannex *Rx*	**Packet:** 1.5 mg bisacodyl complexed with 2.5 g tannic acid per packet	**Adult:** for cleansing enema, 1 packet in 1 liter of warm water; for barium enema, 1–2 packets in 1 liter of barium suspension; total dosage for one colonic examination should not exceed 3 packets; cumulative dosage should not exceed 4 packets/72 h
COLOGEL (Lilly) Methylcellulose *OTC*	**Liquid (per 5 ml):** 450 mg (16 fl oz) *lemon flavored*	**Adult:** 5–20 ml (1–4 tsp) with 8 fl oz water tid after meals
CORRECTOL Liquid (Plough) Yellow phenolphthalein *OTC*	**Liquid (per 15 ml):** 65 mg yellow phenolphthalein (8, 16 fl oz)	**Adult:** 15–30 ml (1–2 tbsp)/day, as needed, taken at bedtime or upon arising **Child (> 6 yr):** 15 ml (1 tbsp)/day, as needed
CORRECTOL Powder (Plough) Psyllium *OTC*	**Powder:** 3.5 g/rounded tsp (11 oz) *natural, apple, and orange flavored*	**Adult:** 3.5 g stirred into 8 fl oz of water, juice, or other liquid, followed by a further 8 fl oz of liquid, 1–3 times/day, for 2–3 days
CORRECTOL Tablets (Plough) Yellow phenolphthalein and docusate sodium *OTC*	**Tablets:** 65 mg yellow phenolphthalein and 100 mg docusate sodium	**Adult:** 1–2 tabs/day, as needed, taken at bedtime or upon arising **Child (> 6 yr):** 1 tab/day, as needed
DECHOLIN (Miles Pharmaceuticals) Dehydrocholic acid *OTC*	**Tablets:** 250 mg	**Adult and child (> 12 yr):** 250–500 mg tid
FLEET Bisacodyl Enema (Fleet) Bisacodyl *OTC*	**Enema:** 10 mg bisacodyl per 30 ml (delivered dose) (1 1/4 fl oz)	**Adult:** 30 ml (delivered dose) **Child (> 2 yr):** same as adult
FLEET Mineral Oil Enema (Fleet) Mineral oil *OTC*	**Enema:** 118 ml (delivered dose) (4 1/2 fl oz)	**Adult:** 118 ml (delivered dose) **Child (≥ 2 yr):** 1/4–1/2 adult dose
GENTLE NATURE (Sandoz Consumer Health Care Group) Sennosides *OTC*	**Tablets:** 20 mg	**Adult:** 20–40 mg/day with water, preferably at bedtime **Child (> 6 yr):** 20 mg/day with water, preferably at bedtime
KASOF (Stuart) Docusate potassium *OTC*	**Capsules:** 240 mg	**Adult:** 240 mg/day, taken with a glass of water, for several days or until bowel movements are normal
LAXCAPS (Glenbrook) Phenolphthalein and docusate sodium *OTC*	**Capsules:** 90 mg phenolphthalein and 83 mg docusate sodium	**Adult:** 1–2 caps/day with 8 fl oz water

[1] Where pediatric dosages are not given, consult manufacturer

continued

OTHER LAXATIVES/STOOL SOFTENERS continued

DRUG	HOW SUPPLIED	USUAL DOSAGE[1]
MALTSUPEX (Wallace) Malt soup extract *OTC*	**Tablets:** 750 mg **Powder:** 16 g/0.56 oz (1 tbsp) (8, 16 oz) **Liquid (per ½ fl oz):** 16 g (1 tbsp) (8, 16 fl oz)	**Adult:** 4 tabs with 8 fl oz of water qid to start, then adjust dosage as needed, or 2 tbsp bid for 3–4 days, followed by 1–2 tbsp at bedtime, as needed; each dose should be followed by 8 fl oz of water **Infant (> 1 mo):** *bottle-fed:* ½–2 tbsp/day added to total daily formula or 1–2 tsp/feeding; for prevention of constipation, 1–2 tsp/day added to total daily formula or 1 tsp added to every second feeding; *breast-fed:* 1–2 tsp in 2–4 fl oz of water or fruit juice 1–2 times/day **Child:** 1–2 tbsp in 8 fl oz of liquid 1–2 times/day
Mineral oil *OTC*	**Liquid:** 30 ml; 8, 16, 32 fl oz; 1, 5 gal	**Adult:** 15–30 ml (3–6 tsp) at bedtime **Child:** 5–15 ml (1–3 tsp) at bedtime
MODANE Plus (Adria) Danthron and docusate sodium *OTC*	**Tablets:** 50 mg danthron and 100 mg of docusate sodium	**Adult and child (> 12 yr):** 1 tab/day
NATURACIL (Mead Johnson) Psyllium *OTC*	**Chewable pieces:** 1.7 g *chocolate flavored*	**Adult:** 2 pieces 1–3 times/day with 8 fl oz of liquid **Child (6–12 yr):** 1 piece 1–3 times/day with 8 fl oz of liquid
PHOSPHO-SODA (Fleet) Sodium phosphate and sodium biphosphate *OTC*	**Solution (per 5 ml):** 0.9 g sodium phosphate and 2.4 g sodium biphosphate (1.5, 3, 8 fl oz) *regular and ginger-lemon flavored*	**Adult:** 20 ml (4 tsp) mixed with 4 fl oz of cold water and followed by 8 fl oz of water upon arising, at least 30 min before a meal, or at bedtime **Child (5–10 yr):** 5 ml (1 tsp), diluted and administered as above **Child (≥ 10 yr):** 10 ml (2 tsp), diluted and administered as above
SENOKAP DSS (Purdue Frederick) Senna concentrate and docusate sodium *OTC*	**Capsules:** 163 mg senna concentrate and 50 mg docusate sodium	**Adult:** 1–2 caps at bedtime with 8 fl oz of water
SENOKOT-S (Purdue Frederick) Senna concentrate and docusate sodium *OTC*	**Tablets:** 187 mg senna concentrate and 50 mg docusate sodium	**Adult:** 2 tabs at bedtime or up to 4 tabs bid, if needed **Child (> 60 lb):** 1 tab at bedtime or up to 2 tabs bid, if needed
X-PREP (Gray) Senna extract *OTC*	**Liquid:** 75 ml senna extract (2½ fl oz)	**Adult:** 75 ml taken between 2 and 4 PM on day prior to diagnostic bowel procedure

[1] Where pediatric dosages are not given, consult manufacturer

LAXATIVES/STOOL SOFTENERS

CHRONULAC (lactulose) Merrell Dow Rx

Syrup (per 15 ml): 10 g (30 ml; 8 fl oz; 1 qt)

INDICATIONS	ORAL DOSAGE
Constipation	**Adult:** 15–30 ml (1–2 tbsp)/day, with water, milk, or juice, if desired; up to 60 ml/day, if needed

CONTRAINDICATIONS

Low-galactose diet

ADMINISTRATION/DOSAGE ADJUSTMENTS

Onset of action	Up to 24–48 h may be required to produce a normal bowel movement

WARNINGS/PRECAUTIONS

Elderly, debilitated patients	Measure serum electrolytes periodically if drug is prescribed for more than 6 mo
Diabetics	Use with caution since drug contains galactose (< 2.2 g/15 ml) and lactose (< 1.2 g/15 ml)
Patients undergoing proctoscopy or colonoscopy	As a cautionary measure, patients who may be required to undergo electrocautery procedures during proctoscopy or colonoscopy should have a thorough bowel cleansing with a nonfermentable solution, because the combination of an electric spark and significant concentrations of hydrogen gas may result in an explosive reaction

ADVERSE REACTIONS

Gastrointestinal	Flatulence, cramps, nausea

OVERDOSAGE

Signs and symptoms	Diarrhea, abdominal cramps
Treatment	Discontinue medication

DRUG INTERACTIONS

No clinically significant drug interactions have been identified

ALTERED LABORATORY VALUES

No clinically significant alterations in blood/serum or urinary values occur at therapeutic dosages

---

USE IN CHILDREN

Safety and effectiveness have not been established for use in children

USE IN PREGNANT AND NURSING WOMEN

No data are available on what effect, if any, administration to pregnant women may have on the mother or fetus; studies in laboratory animals have shown no evidence of teratogenicity. Use during pregnancy only if potential benefits outweigh possible risks. No data exist on excretion in breast milk or effects in nursing infants.

LAXATIVES/STOOL SOFTENERS

CITRUCEL (methylcellulose) Lakeside OTC

Powder (per heaping tbsp): 2 g (16, 30 oz) *orange flavored*

INDICATIONS	ORAL DOSAGE
Constipation	**Adult and child ($\geq$ 12 yr):** 1 heaping tbsp, given 1–3 times/day in 8 fl oz of cold water **Child (6–12 yr):** 1 level tsp, given 3–4 times/day in 4 fl oz of cold water

CONTRAINDICATIONS

Intestinal obstruction	Fecal impaction

ADMINISTRATION/DOSAGE ADJUSTMENTS

Therapeutic response	A bowel movement is usually produced within 12–72 h after ingestion; optimal response may not be evident until after 2–3 days of use

CITRUCEL ■ DIALOSE

WARNINGS/PRECAUTIONS

Drug dependence	Laxative dependence and loss of normal bowel function may develop with frequent or prolonged use
Patient instructions	Instruct patients not to use this product on their own if abdominal pain, nausea, or vomiting are present or a change in bowel habits has occurred suddenly and then persisted for 2 wk; caution patients to discontinue use if rectal bleeding is seen or no bowel movement occurs (these responses should be reported)
Sugar content	60 kcal/tbsp

DRUG INTERACTIONS

Salicylates, cardiac glycosides, nitrofurantoin	▽ Bioavailability of these drugs

---

USE IN CHILDREN
See INDICATIONS and ORAL DOSAGE

USE IN PREGNANT AND NURSING WOMEN
Consult manufacturer

LAXATIVES/STOOL SOFTENERS

COLACE (docusate sodium) Mead Johnson — OTC
Capsules: 50, 100 mg   Liquid: 10 mg/ml (30 ml, 16 fl oz)   Syrup (per 5 ml): 20 mg[1] (8, 16 fl oz)

INDICATIONS
Constipation due to hard stools
Painful **anorectal conditions**
Cardiac and other conditions in which difficult or painful defecation is to be avoided and peristaltic stimulation is contraindicated

ORAL DOSAGE
Adult: 50–200 mg/day
Infant and child (< 3 yr): 10–40 mg/day
Child (3–6 yr): 20–60 mg/day
Child (6–12 yr): 40–120 mg/day

CONTRAINDICATIONS
None known

ADMINISTRATION/DOSAGE ADJUSTMENTS

Initiation of therapy	Use higher dose
Onset of action	Usually apparent 1–3 days after first dose
Administration of liquid dosage form	To mask the bitter taste, administer the liquid with ½ glass of milk or fruit juice or in infant formula
Enema	Add 50–100 mg (5–10 ml of liquid form) to retention or flushing enema

WARNINGS/PRECAUTIONS
None reported by manufacturer

ADVERSE REACTIONS

Gastrointestinal, oropharyngeal	Bitter taste, throat irritation, and nausea (primarily associated with use of syrup and liquid)
Dermatological	Rash

OVERDOSAGE
Product is not absorbed; no toxic effects have been observed in clinical use

DRUG INTERACTIONS
No clinically significant drug interactions have been identified

ALTERED LABORATORY VALUES
No clinically significant alterations in blood/serum or urinary values occur at therapeutic dosages

---

USE IN CHILDREN
See INDICATIONS and ORAL DOSAGE

USE IN PREGNANT AND NURSING WOMEN
May safely be administered to pregnant or nursing women

---

[1] Contains not more than 1% alcohol

LAXATIVES/STOOL SOFTENERS

DIALOSE (docusate potassium) Stuart — OTC
Capsules: 100 mg

INDICATIONS
Softening of hard stools or prevention of their formation

ORAL DOSAGE
Adult: 100 mg with 8 fl oz water 1–3 times/day
Child (< 6 yr): use according to medical judgment
Child (> 6 yr): 100 mg with 8 fl oz of water at bedtime

USE IN CHILDREN	USE IN PREGNANT AND NURSING WOMEN
See INDICATIONS and ORAL DOSAGE	Consult manufacturer

LAXATIVES/STOOL SOFTENERS

DIALOSE Plus (docusate potassium and casanthranol) Stuart   OTC

Capsules: 100 mg docusate potassium and 30 mg casanthranol

INDICATIONS	ORAL DOSAGE
Constipation associated with hardness, lack of moisture in intestinal contents, or decreased intestinal motility	**Adult:** 1 cap with 8 fl oz water bid to start; then adjust dosage as needed **Child:** use according to medical judgment

CONTRAINDICATIONS

Abdominal pain, nausea, or vomiting

WARNINGS/PRECAUTIONS

Drug dependence	Laxative dependence and loss of normal bowel function may develop with frequent or prolonged use

ADVERSE REACTIONS

Consult manufacturer

OVERDOSAGE

Product is not absorbed; no toxic effects have been observed in clinical use

DRUG INTERACTIONS

No clinically significant drug interactions have been identified

ALTERED LABORATORY VALUES

No clinically significant alterations in blood/serum or urinary values occur at therapeutic dosages

USE IN CHILDREN	USE IN PREGNANT AND NURSING WOMEN
Use according to medical judgment	Consult manufacturer

LAXATIVES/STOOL SOFTENERS

DORBANTYL (danthron and docusate sodium) 3M   OTC

Capsules: 25 mg danthron and 50 mg docusate sodium

DORBANTYL Forte (danthron and docusate sodium) 3M   OTC

Capsules: 50 mg danthron and 100 mg docusate sodium

INDICATIONS	ORAL DOSAGE
Constipation (occasional)	**Adult:** 2 Dorbantyl caps or 1 Dorbantyl Forte cap at bedtime; repeat if needed **Child (6–12 yr):** 1 Dorbantyl cap at bedtime; repeat if needed

CONTRAINDICATIONS

Abdominal pain, nausea, or vomiting

WARNINGS/PRECAUTIONS

Drug dependence	Laxative dependence and loss of normal bowel function may develop with frequent or prolonged use
Urine discoloration	May occur
Tartrazine sensitivity	Presence of FD&C Yellow No. 5 (tartrazine) in capsules may cause allergic-type reactions, including bronchial asthma, in susceptible individuals

DORBANTYL ■ DOXINATE

ADVERSE REACTIONS

Dermatological — Rash (occasional)

OVERDOSAGE

Product is not absorbed; no toxic effects have been observed in clinical use

DRUG INTERACTIONS

No clinically significant drug interactions have been identified

ALTERED LABORATORY VALUES

No clinically significant alterations in blood/serum or urinary values occur at therapeutic dosages

USE IN CHILDREN	USE IN PREGNANT AND NURSING WOMEN
See INDICATIONS and ORAL DOSAGE	Consult manufacturer

LAXATIVES/STOOL SOFTENERS

DOXIDAN (docusate calcium and danthron) Hoechst-Roussel — OTC

Capsules: 60 mg docusate calcium and 50 mg danthron[1]

INDICATIONS	ORAL DOSAGE
Chronic functional constipation in geriatric, inactive, obstetric, and postsurgical patients **Bowel evacuation** in preparation for barium enema prior to x-ray examination of colon	**Adult:** 1–2 caps/day at bedtime **Child (6–12 yr):** 1 cap/day at bedtime

CONTRAINDICATIONS

Abdominal pain, nausea, or vomiting

ADMINISTRATION/DOSAGE ADJUSTMENTS

Onset of action — Usually apparent in 8–12 h
Duration of therapy — Maintain dosage for 2–3 days or until bowel movements return to normal

WARNINGS/PRECAUTIONS

Drug dependence — Laxative dependence and loss of normal bowel function may develop with frequent or prolonged use

Urine discoloration — Pink or orange color may appear in alkaline urine; reaction is harmless

ADVERSE REACTIONS

Gastrointestinal — Cramps

OVERDOSAGE

Product is not absorbed; no toxic effects have been observed in clinical use

DRUG INTERACTIONS

No clinically significant drug interactions have been identified

ALTERED LABORATORY VALUES

No clinically significant alterations in blood/serum or urinary values occur at therapeutic dosages

USE IN CHILDREN	USE IN PREGNANT AND NURSING WOMEN
See INDICATIONS and ORAL DOSAGE	See INDICATIONS for use in pregnancy. Use with caution in nursing mothers.

[1] Contains up to 1.5% alcohol

LAXATIVES/STOOL SOFTENERS

DOXINATE (docusate sodium) Hoechst-Roussel — OTC

Capsules: 240 mg **Solution:** 50 mg/ml[1] (60 ml, 1 gal)

INDICATIONS	ORAL DOSAGE
Constipation (temporary)	**Adult:** 240 mg or 2.5–5 ml (½–1 tsp) once daily **Child (3–6 yr):** 1–2 ml once daily **Child (> 6 yr):** 2.5–5 ml (½–1 tsp) once daily

DOXINATE ■ DULCOLAX

ADMINISTRATION/DOSAGE ADJUSTMENTS

Administration of solution	Give solution with milk, fruit juice, or formula
Duration of therapy	Continue use for several days or until bowel movements are normal

USE IN CHILDREN
See INDICATIONS and ORAL DOSAGE

USE IN PREGNANT AND NURSING WOMEN
Consult manufacturer

[1] Contains 5% alcohol

LAXATIVES/STOOL SOFTENERS

DULCOLAX (bisacodyl) Boehringer Ingelheim
Tablets (enteric coated): 5 mg **Suppositories:** 10 mg

OTC

INDICATIONS
Acute or chronic constipation
Bowel preparation prior to surgery, abdominal radiography, or special procedures

ORAL DOSAGE
Adult: for use as a laxative, 10–15 mg at bedtime or before breakfast (usual dosage, 10 mg); for more complete bowel evacuation, up to 30 mg may be given at once
Child: 5–10 mg, depending on age and severity of constipation, at bedtime or before breakfast

RECTAL DOSAGE
Adult: 1 suppository when bowel movement is required
Infant and child ($<$ 2 yr): 1/2 suppository when bowel movement is required
Child ($\geq$ 2 yr): same as adult

CONTRAINDICATIONS
Acute surgical abdomen

ADMINISTRATION/DOSAGE ADJUSTMENTS

Administration of tablets	Tablets should be taken whole, not chewed or crushed (see also DRUG INTERACTIONS, below)
Use of suppositories	The suppository should be retained against the bowel wall for 15–20 min; advise patient that the suppository should be pushed higher if an urge to evacuate immediately occurs. The suppository tip may be coated with petroleum jelly if fissures or hemorrhoids exist. If the suppository softens, it may be held under cold water, unwrapped, for 1–2 min.
Constipation	The tablets will generally produce one or two soft, formed stools overnight when taken at bedtime or within 6 h when taken before breakfast; the suppositories are usually effective within 15 min to 1 h after insertion
Bowel retraining	To restore normal bowel hygiene, gradually lengthen the interval between doses as colonic tone improves; rebound constipation does not occur with this preparation
Preoperative bowel preparation	Administer up to 6 tablets the night before surgery and a suppository in the morning; although this regimen will replace the usual enema preparation prior to abdominal surgery or other surgery requiring general anesthesia, it cannot substitute for the colonic irrigations usually given prior to colon surgery
Preparation for radiography	Administer up to 6 tablets the night before (such doses may result in several loose, unformed stools) and a suppository in the morning; if a barium enema will be given, caution the patient not to eat after taking the tablets and administer the suppository 1–2 h before the examination
Preparation for sigmoidoscopy or proctoscopy	A single suppository is usually adequate for unscheduled examinations; if the examination is scheduled in advance, use of up to 6 tablets the night before and a suppository in the morning will almost always result in adequate preparation
Colostomies	Administration of the tablets the night before or insertion of a suppository into the colostomy opening in the morning will expedite and often obviate the need for irrigations

WARNINGS/PRECAUTIONS

Drug dependence	Laxative dependence and loss of normal bowel function may result from frequent or continued use
Pain, nausea, vomiting	Patients should be cautioned not to use this product, unless otherwise directed, if abdominal pain, nausea, or vomiting is present
Tartrazine sensitivity	Presence of FD&C Yellow No. 5 (tartrazine) in tablets may cause allergic-type reactions, including bronchial asthma, in susceptible individuals

DULCOLAX ■ EFFER-SYLLIUM

ADVERSE REACTIONS

Gastrointestinal	Abdominal cramps

OVERDOSAGE

Product is not absorbed; no toxic effects have been observed in clinical use

DRUG INTERACTIONS

Antacids, milk	Gastric or duodenal irritation owing to enhanced dissolution of enteric coating; tablets should not be taken within 1 h of ingestion of milk or antacids

ALTERED LABORATORY VALUES

No clinically significant alterations in blood/serum or urinary values occur at therapeutic dosages

---

USE IN CHILDREN

See INDICATIONS and dosage recommendations; the tablets should not be given to a child who is too young to swallow them whole

USE IN PREGNANT AND NURSING WOMEN

Either dosage form can safely be given for constipation during pregnancy without risking uterine stimulation. During delivery, the suppositories may be used instead of an enema, provided that they are given at least 2 h before the onset of the second stage of labor. Either dosage form may safely be used by nursing mothers.

LAXATIVES/STOOL SOFTENERS

EFFER-SYLLIUM (psyllium) Stuart   OTC

Effervescent powder (per rounded tsp or packet): 3 g (7-g packets; 9-, 16-oz bottles) *lemon-lime flavored*

INDICATIONS

Chronic **constipation**
Constipation associated with **irritable bowel syndrome and anorectal disorders**

ORAL DOSAGE

Adult: 1 rounded tsp or 1 packet, given in 8 fl oz of water 1–3 times/day
Child (< 6 yr): use according to medical judgment
Child (≥ 6 yr): 1 level tsp or one half of a packet, given in 4 fl oz of water at bedtime

CONTRAINDICATIONS

Undiagnosed intestinal pain	Intestinal obstruction	Fecal impaction

ADMINISTRATION/DOSAGE ADJUSTMENTS

Preparation	Place powder in a glass, add water, stir, and administer; to avoid caking, always use a dry spoon when removing powder from the bottle
Therapeutic response	Optimal response may not be evident until after several days

WARNINGS/PRECAUTIONS

Obstruction, impaction	If passage of a psyllium bolus through the alimentary tract is temporarily impeded, obstruction or impaction may occur, and, in the intestinal tract, the bolus may become inspissated. The use of psyllium may be hazardous when any section of the alimentary lumen is abnormally narrowed (see CONTRAINDICATIONS). Inspissation should not occur in the normal lumen if psyllium is given with at least one glass of liquid.
Allergic reactions	Caution patients who are hypersensitive to psyllium powder to avoid inhalation of this product (allergic reactions, such as wheezing, may otherwise occur)
Drug dependence	Laxative dependence and loss of normal bowel function may develop with frequent or prolonged use
Sodium content	< 5 mg/rounded tsp

DRUG INTERACTIONS

Salicylates, cardiac glycosides, nitrofurantoin	▽ Bioavailability of these drugs

---

USE IN CHILDREN

See INDICATIONS and ORAL DOSAGE

USE IN PREGNANT AND NURSING WOMEN

Consult manufacturer

LAXATIVES/STOOL SOFTENERS

EX-LAX (yellow phenolphthalein) Sandoz Consumer Health Care Group   OTC

Tablets: 90 mg   **Chewable tablets:** 90 mg *chocolate flavored*

INDICATIONS	ORAL DOSAGE
Short-term relief of **constipation**	Adult: 1–2 tabs with 8 fl oz water or 1–2 chewable tabs, preferably at bedtime; adjust dosage as needed Child ($>$ 6 yr): 1 tab with 8 fl oz of water or ½–1 chewable tab, preferably at bedtime

Extra Gentle EX-LAX (docusate sodium and yellow phenolphthalein) Sandoz Consumer Health Care Group   OTC

Tablets: 75 mg docusate sodium and 65 mg yellow phenolphthalein

INDICATIONS	ORAL DOSAGE
Short-term relief of **constipation**	Adult: 1–2 tabs with 8 fl oz of water, preferably at bedtime Child ($>$ 6 yr): 1 tab with 8 fl oz of water, preferably at bedtime

CONTRAINDICATIONS

Abdominal pain, nausea, or vomiting

ADMINISTRATION/DOSAGE ADJUSTMENTS

Constipation resistant to initial therapy —— Adult dose may be increased slightly and administered the following day

WARNINGS/PRECAUTIONS

Drug dependence —————————— Laxative dependence and loss of normal bowel function may develop with frequent or prolonged use

Skin rash ————————————————— May appear; discontinue use of this and any other medication containing phenolphthalein

ADVERSE REACTIONS

Dermatological ——————————— Rash (see WARNINGS/PRECAUTIONS)

OVERDOSAGE

Signs and symptoms ——————— Abdominal cramps

Treatment ——————————————— Discontinue medication

DRUG INTERACTIONS

No clinically significant drug interactions have been identified

ALTERED LABORATORY VALUES

No clinically significant alterations in blood/serum or urinary values occur at therapeutic dosages

USE IN CHILDREN	USE IN PREGNANT AND NURSING WOMEN
See INDICATIONS and ORAL DOSAGE	May safely be administered to pregnant or nursing women

---

LAXATIVES/STOOL SOFTENERS

FLEET Enema (sodium phosphate and sodium biphosphate) Fleet   OTC

Solution (per 118 ml): 7 g sodium phosphate and 19 g sodium biphosphate (2¼, 4½ fl oz)

INDICATIONS	RECTAL DOSAGE
Constipation, including that due to fecal or barium impaction, during pregnancy, and pre- and postnatally **Bowel evacuation** as routine enema, in preparation for rectal examination, for preoperative cleansing, and for general postoperative care	Adult: 4 fl oz Child ($\geq$ 2 yr): 2 fl oz

COMPENDIUM OF DRUG THERAPY

FLEET Enema ■ Glycerin Suppositories

CONTRAINDICATIONS

Nausea, vomiting, or abdominal pain

Congenital megacolon or congestive heart failure (hypernatremic dehydration may occur)

ADMINISTRATION/DOSAGE ADJUSTMENTS

Administration of enema — The enema should be gently and carefully inserted into the rectum under steady pressure, with the tip pointing toward the navel; squeeze the bottle until nearly all the liquid is expelled. Discontinue the procedure if resistance is encountered upon insertion or administration; forcing can cause perforation and/or abrasion of the rectum. Patient should lie on left side with left knee slightly bent and right leg drawn up, or in knee-chest position; after administration of the enema, the patient should maintain this position until the urge to evacuate is strong (usually 2–5 min)

WARNINGS/PRECAUTIONS

Patient instructions — The package labeling warns patients not to use a laxative product for more than 1 wk, unless otherwise directed; frequent or prolonged use may result in dependence. If rectal bleeding or failure to have a bowel movement occurs after laxative use, it should be discontinued and a physician consulted. Patients should also contact a physician if there is a sudden change in bowel habits persisting over 2 wk (see also CONTRAINDICATIONS).

Dehydration — Because of the high sodium content of this preparation (4.4 g/118 ml dose), there is a risk of acute elevation of serum sodium levels and consequent dehydration, especially in children with megacolon; additional fluids by mouth are recommended where appropriate

Special-risk patients — Use with caution in patients with renal impairment or a colostomy; hypernatremia and acidosis may occur in such patients, as well as hypocalcemia and hyperphosphatemia, which may also result from prolonged use; immediately administer appropriate fluid replacement therapy to correct electrolyte imbalances, and carefully monitor calcium and phosphorous levels

ADVERSE REACTIONS

None reported by manufacturer

OVERDOSAGE

No toxic effects have been observed in clinical use

DRUG INTERACTIONS

No clinically significant drug interactions have been identified

ALTERED LABORATORY VALUES

No clinically significant alterations in blood/serum or urinary values occur at therapeutic dosages

---

USE IN CHILDREN

See INDICATIONS and RECTAL DOSAGE. Do not use in children under 2 yr of age. For children aged 2–12 yr, use the pediatric size bottle only (2¼ fl oz); give careful consideration to the use of enemas in general in children, and use this preparation with caution in children of any age.

USE IN PREGNANT AND NURSING WOMEN

See INDICATIONS and RECTAL DOSAGE

LAXATIVES/STOOL SOFTENERS

Glycerin Suppositories (glycerin and sodium stearate) OTC

Rectal suppositories: 85% glycerin and 10% sodium stearate   **Infant rectal suppositories:** 85% glycerin and 10% sodium stearate

INDICATIONS

Constipation

RECTAL DOSAGE

Adult: insert 1 suppository and retain for 15 min
Infant and child: insert 1 infant or regular suppository and retain for 15 min

CONTRAINDICATIONS

None reported

Glycerin Suppositories ■ METAMUCIL

WARNINGS/PRECAUTIONS
None reported

ADVERSE REACTIONS
None reported

USE IN CHILDREN	USE IN PREGNANT AND NURSING WOMEN
See INDICATIONS and RECTAL DOSAGE	Consult manufacturer

LAXATIVES/STOOL SOFTENERS

METAMUCIL (psyllium) Procter & Gamble OTC

Powder: 3.4 g per rounded tsp or packet (7-, 14-, 21-oz containers; single-dose packets) *regular flavored*, (3.7-, 7.4-, 11.1-oz containers; single-dose packets) *regular flavored and sugar-free*, (3.7-, 7.4-, 11.1-oz containers) *orange flavored and sugar-free*; 3.4 g per rounded tbsp (7-, 14-, 21-oz containers) *orange flavored, strawberry flavored*

Instant Fiber Mix METAMUCIL (psyllium) Procter & Gamble OTC

Effervescent powder (per packet): 3.4 g (single-dose packets) *lemon-lime flavored and sugar-free, orange flavored and sugar-free*

INDICATIONS
Chronic **constipation**
Constipation associated with **irritable bowel syndrome, duodenal ulcer, diverticular disease, hemorrhoids, pregnancy, convalescence, and advanced age**

ORAL DOSAGE
Adult: 3.4 g, given 1–3 times/day in 8 fl oz of cool water (regular-flavored Metamucil may also be mixed with milk, fruit juice, or other suitable liquids); give an additional 8 fl oz of liquid after each dose

CONTRAINDICATIONS
Intestinal obstruction — Fecal impaction

ADMINISTRATION/DOSAGE ADJUSTMENTS
Therapeutic response — Optimal response may not be evident until after 2–3 days

WARNINGS/PRECAUTIONS

Obstruction, impaction — If passage of a psyllium bolus through the alimentary tract is temporarily impeded, obstruction or impaction may occur, and, in the intestinal tract, the bolus may become inspissated. The use of psyllium may be hazardous when any section of the alimentary lumen is abnormally narrowed (see CONTRAINDICATIONS). Inspissation should not occur in the normal lumen if psyllium is given with at least one glass of liquid.

Drug dependence — Laxative dependence and loss of normal bowel function may develop with frequent or prolonged use

Hypersensitivity — Allergic reactions may occur in patients who are hypersensitive to psyllium powder

Sodium content — Regular-flavored Metamucil or regular-flavored, sugar-free Metamucil: < 10 mg/rounded tsp or packet; orange- or strawberry-flavored Metamucil: < 10 mg/rounded tbsp; orange-flavored, sugar-free Metamucil: < 10 mg/rounded tsp; lemon-lime- or orange-flavored, sugar-free Instant Fiber Mix Metamucil: 1 mg/packet

Carbohydrate content — Regular-flavored Metamucil: 3.5 g of dextrose (14 kcal)/rounded tsp or packet; regular-flavored, sugar-free Metamucil: 1 kcal/rounded tsp or packet; orange- or strawberry-flavored Metamucil: 7.1 g of sucrose (30 kcal)/rounded tbsp; orange-flavored, sugar-free Metamucil: 2 kcal/rounded tsp; lemon-lime- or orange-flavored, sugar-free Instant Fiber Mix Metamucil: < 1 kcal/packet

Phenylalanine content — Regular-flavored, sugar-free Metamucil: 6 mg/rounded tsp or packet; orange-flavored, sugar-free Metamucil: 30 mg/rounded tsp; lemon-lime- or orange-flavored, sugar-free Instant Fiber Mix Metamucil: 27 mg/packet

DRUG INTERACTIONS
Salicylates, cardiac glycosides, nitrofurantoin — ▽ Bioavailability of these drugs

METAMUCIL ■ MODANE

USE IN CHILDREN	USE IN PREGNANT AND NURSING WOMEN
Consult manufacturer	See INDICATIONS and ORAL DOSAGE for use during pregnancy; consult manufacturer for use in nursing mothers

LAXATIVES/STOOL SOFTENERS

MITROLAN (calcium polycarbophil) Robins — OTC

Chewable tablets: calcium polycarbophil equivalent to 500 mg polycarbophil *citrus/vanilla flavored*

INDICATIONS	ORAL DOSAGE
Constipation or diarrhea	**Adult:** 2 tabs qid or as needed, up to 12 tabs/24 h, to be chewed before swallowing **Child (3–5 yr):** 1 tab bid or as needed, up to 3 tabs/24 h, to be chewed before swallowing **Child (6–11 yr):** 1 tab tid or as needed, up to 6 tabs/24 h, to be chewed before swallowing

CONTRAINDICATIONS
Gastrointestinal obstruction

ADMINISTRATION/DOSAGE ADJUSTMENTS

Acute diarrhea	If necessary, repeat dose every 1/2 h, without exceeding maximum daily dosage
Laxative use	Each dose should be taken with 8 fl oz of liquid
Avoidance of abdominal fullness	Give smaller doses at more frequent, equally spaced intervals

WARNINGS/PRECAUTIONS

Self-medication for constipation	Package label cautions patients to consult a physician before using this product if there has been a sudden change in bowel habits that has persisted over a period of 2 wk, to discontinue use and seek medical attention if taking this product has had no effect after 1 wk, and not to use it, unless directed by a physician, if abdominal pain, nausea, or vomiting is present
Self-medication for diarrhea	Package label cautions patients against using this product for more than 2 days, in the presence of a high fever, or in children under 3 yr of age, unless directed by a physician; patients are also advised to seek medical attention if diarrhea is accompanied by a high fever

ADVERSE REACTIONS

Gastrointestinal	Abdominal fullness (see ADMINISTRATION/DOSAGE ADJUSTMENTS)

OVERDOSAGE
Product is not absorbed; no toxic effects have been observed in clinical use

DRUG INTERACTIONS

Tetracycline	▽ Absorption of tetracycline; do not use concomitantly

ALTERED LABORATORY VALUES
No clinically significant alterations in blood/serum or urinary values occur at therapeutic dosages

USE IN CHILDREN	USE IN PREGNANT AND NURSING WOMEN
See INDICATIONS and ORAL DOSAGE	Caution should be exercised before prescribing this product for pregnant or nursing patients

LAXATIVES/STOOL SOFTENERS

MODANE (danthron) Adria — OTC

Tablets: 37.5 mg (Modane Mild Tablets), 75 mg (Modane Tablets)   **Liquid (per 5 ml):** 37.5 mg[1] (1 pt)

INDICATIONS	ORAL DOSAGE
Constipation, including constipation in geriatric, cardiac, surgical, and postpartum patients **Drug-induced constipation**	**Adult:** 37.5–75 mg or 5–10 ml (1–2 tsp) with evening meal **Child (6–12 yr):** 37.5 mg or 5 ml (1 tsp) with evening meal

MODANE ■ PERDIEM

CONTRAINDICATIONS

Abdominal pain, nausea, vomiting, or other signs and symptoms of appendicitis

ADMINISTRATION/DOSAGE ADJUSTMENTS

Onset of action	A soft or semifluid stool is passed 6–8 h after administration
Hypersensitive, diet-restricted, or bedfast adults	Administer 37.5 mg or 5 ml (1 tsp) with evening meal

WARNINGS/PRECAUTIONS

Drug dependence	Laxative dependence and loss of normal bowel function may develop with frequent or prolonged use
Urine discoloration	Urine may appear pink, while alkaline urine may turn pink-red, red-violet, or red-brown; effect is harmless
Concurrent hypokalemia	May impair drug effectiveness
Carcinogenicity, mutagenicity	Long-term studies to evaluate the carcinogenic potential of this drug have not been done, nor have any studies been conducted to determine its mutagenic potential

ADVERSE REACTIONS

Gastrointestinal	Excessive bowel activity (gripping, diarrhea, nausea, vomiting)
Central nervous system	Weakness, dizziness
Other	Perianal irritation, palpitations, sweating; transient brownish mucosal staining (with prolonged use)[2]

OVERDOSAGE

Signs and symptoms	Excessive bowel activity (see ADVERSE REACTIONS)
Treatment	Discontinue medication; treat symptomatically if effects are prolonged

DRUG INTERACTIONS

Docusate sodium, potassium, or calcium	△ Intestinal absorption and/or hepatic cell uptake of danthron

ALTERED LABORATORY VALUES

No clinically significant alterations in blood/serum or urinary values occur at therapeutic dosages

---

USE IN CHILDREN

See INDICATIONS and ORAL DOSAGE; in general, stimulant cathartics should seldom be used in children

USE IN PREGNANT AND NURSING WOMEN

Pregnancy Category C: use during pregnancy only if clearly needed. Animal reproduction studies have not been done, nor are the effects of danthron on human reproductive capacity or fetal development known. Danthron is excreted in human milk, and increased bowel activity has been reported in infants nursed by women taking this drug; use with caution in nursing mothers.

---

[1] Contains 5% alcohol
[2] A suspected allergic reaction, characterized by facial swelling, redness, and discomfort, has also been reported

---

LAXATIVES/STOOL SOFTENERS

PERDIEM (psyllium and senna) Rorer OTC

Granules (per rounded tsp): 3.25 mg psyllium and 0.74 mg senna (6, 100, 250 g)

INDICATIONS

Constipation

ORAL DOSAGE

Adult: 1–2 rounded tsp, given in the evening and/or before breakfast; if 2-tsp dose is given initially, reduce it to 1 tsp when this preparation takes effect
Child (7–11 yr): 1 rounded tsp, given in the evening and/or before breakfast
Child ($\geq$ 12 yr): same as adult

CONTRAINDICATIONS

Undiagnosed abdominal pain	Esophageal narrowing	Hypersensitivity to psyllium
Intestinal obstruction	Fecal impaction	Dysphagia

ADMINISTRATION/DOSAGE ADJUSTMENTS

Oral administration	Wet mouth with a cool liquid, place a full or partial teaspoon of granules on the tongue, and wash down; repeat until entire dose has been swallowed. Granules should not be chewed. Give each dose with at least 8 fl oz of a cool liquid; an additional amount would be helpful.

PERDIEM ■ PERDIEM Plain

Therapeutic response	Onset of action generally occurs after 24 h; in resistant cases, optimal response may not be evident until after 36–48 h
Obstinate cases	Dosage may be increased, as needed, up to 2 rounded tsp q6h
Patients dependent on strong cathartics	Administer up to 2 rounded tsp of Perdiem in the morning and evening along with half the usual dose of the cathartic; discontinue use of the cathartic as soon as possible, and reduce the dosage of Perdiem when bowel tone shows less laxative dependence
Colostomy patients	Administer 1–2 rounded tsp in the evening
Patients with cardiovascular disease; inactive or bedridden patients	Administer 1 rounded tsp 1–2 times/day

WARNINGS/PRECAUTIONS

Obstruction, impaction	If passage of a psyllium bolus through the alimentary tract is temporarily impeded, obstruction or impaction may occur, and, in the intestinal tract, the bolus may become inspissated. The use of this preparation may be hazardous when any section of the alimentary lumen is abnormally narrowed (see CONTRAINDICATIONS). Instruct patients to take each dose with at least 8 fl oz of cool liquid and to report immediately any symptom of esophageal obstruction, including chest pain or pressure, regurgitation, and difficulty in swallowing.
Allergic reactions	In rare cases, psyllium can precipitate severe allergic reactions; discontinue use if an allergic reaction occurs. Administration to patients who are hypersensitive to psyllium is contraindicated.
Drug dependence	Laxative dependence and loss of normal bowel function may develop with frequent or prolonged use
Sodium content	1.7 mg/rounded tsp
Caloric content	4 kcal/rounded tsp

DRUG INTERACTIONS

Salicylates, cardiac glycosides, nitrofurantoin	▽ Bioavailability of these drugs

---

USE IN CHILDREN
See INDICATIONS and ORAL DOSAGE

USE IN PREGNANT AND NURSING WOMEN
Consult manufacturer for use in pregnant women and nursing mothers

---

LAXATIVES/STOOL SOFTENERS

PERDIEM Plain (psyllium) Rorer   OTC

Granules (per rounded tsp): 4.03 g (6, 100, 250 g) *mint flavored*

INDICATIONS

Simple, chronic, and spastic **constipation**
Constipation associated with **irritable bowel syndrome, diverticular disease, hemorrhoids, anal fissures, convalescence, pregnancy, advanced age, and low-fiber diets**

ORAL DOSAGE

Adult: 1–2 rounded tsp, given in the evening and/or before breakfast
Child (7–11 yr): 1 rounded tsp, given in the evening and/or before breakfast
Child (≥ 12 yr): same as adult

CONTRAINDICATIONS

Undiagnosed abdominal pain	Esophageal narrowing	Hypersensitivity to psyllium
Intestinal obstruction	Fecal impaction	Dysphagia

ADMINISTRATION/DOSAGE ADJUSTMENTS

Oral administration	Wet mouth with a cool liquid, place a full or partial teaspoon of granules on the tongue, and wash down; repeat until entire dose has been swallowed. Granules should not be chewed. Give each dose with at least 8 fl oz of a cool liquid; an additional amount would be helpful.
Therapeutic response	Onset of action generally occurs after 24 h; in resistant cases, optimal response may not be evident until after 48–72 h
Obstinate cases	Dosage may be increased, as needed, up to 2 rounded tsp q6h
Pregnant patients	Administer 1–2 rounded tsp each evening

PERDIEM Plain ■ PERI-COLACE

Inactive or bedridden patients — Administer 1 rounded tsp 1–2 times/day

WARNINGS/PRECAUTIONS

Obstruction, impaction	If passage of a psyllium bolus through the alimentary tract is temporarily impeded, obstruction or impaction may occur, and, in the intestinal tract, the bolus may become inspissated. The use of psyllium may be hazardous when any section of the alimentary lumen is abnormally narrowed (see CONTRAINDICATIONS). Instruct patients to take each dose with at least 8 fl oz of cool liquid and to report immediately any symptom of esophageal obstruction, including chest pain or pressure, regurgitation, and difficulty in swallowing.
Allergic reactions	In rare cases, psyllium can precipitate severe allergic reactions; discontinue use if an allergic reaction occurs. Administration to patients who are hypersensitive to psyllium is contraindicated.
Drug dependence	Laxative dependence and loss of normal bowel function may develop with frequent or prolonged *unsupervised* use
Sodium content	1.7 mg/rounded tsp
Caloric content	4 kcal/rounded tsp

DRUG INTERACTIONS

Salicylates, cardiac glycosides, nitrofurantoin	▽ Bioavailability of these drugs

USE IN CHILDREN
See INDICATIONS and ORAL DOSAGE

USE IN PREGNANT AND NURSING WOMEN
See ADMINISTRATION/DOSAGE ADJUSTMENTS for use during pregnancy; consult manufacturer for use in nursing mothers

---

LAXATIVES/STOOL SOFTENERS

PERI-COLACE (casanthranol and docusate sodium) Mead Johnson   OTC

Capsules: 30 mg casanthranol and 100 mg docusate sodium **Syrup (per 15 ml):** 30 mg casanthranol and 60 mg docusate sodium[1] (8, 16 fl oz) *root beer-flavored*

INDICATIONS
Constipation

ORAL DOSAGE
Adult: 1–2 caps or 15–30 ml (1–2 tbsp) at bedtime, or as needed
Child: 5–15 ml (1–3 tsp) at bedtime, or as needed

CONTRAINDICATIONS
Abdominal pain, nausea, or vomiting

ADMINISTRATION/DOSAGE ADJUSTMENTS

Onset of action	Usually apparent within 8–12 h after administration
Severe cases	Dosage may be increased to 2 caps or 2 tbsp bid, or 3 caps at bedtime

WARNINGS/PRECAUTIONS

Drug dependence	Laxative dependence and loss of normal bowel function may develop with frequent or prolonged use

ADVERSE REACTIONS

Gastrointestinal	Nausea, cramps, discomfort, diarrhea
Dermatological	Rash

OVERDOSAGE

Signs and symptoms	See ADVERSE REACTIONS
Treatment	Treat symptomatically; empty stomach by gastric lavage if large amounts have been ingested

COMPENDIUM OF DRUG THERAPY

DRUG INTERACTIONS

No clinically significant drug interactions have been identified

ALTERED LABORATORY VALUES

No clinically significant alterations in blood/serum or urinary values occur at therapeutic dosages

USE IN CHILDREN	USE IN PREGNANT AND NURSING WOMEN
See INDICATIONS and ORAL DOSAGE	Consult manufacturer

[1] Contains 10% alcohol

LAXATIVES/STOOL SOFTENERS

PHILLIPS' Milk of Magnesia (magnesium hydroxide) Glenbrook OTC

Chewable tablets: 311 mg **Suspension (per 5 ml):** 405 mg (4, 12, 26 fl oz) *regular and mint flavored*

INDICATIONS	ORAL DOSAGE
Occasional constipation	Adult and child (> 12 yr): 6–8 tabs, chewed thoroughly, or 30–60 ml (2–4 tbsp); give preferably before bedtime and follow with 8 fl oz of water Child (2–5 yr): 1–2 tabs, chewed thoroughly, or 5–15 ml (1–3 tsp); give preferably before bedtime and follow with 8 fl oz of water Child (6–11 yr): 3–4 tabs, chewed thoroughly, or 15–30 ml (1–2 tbsp); give preferably before bedtime and follow with 8 fl oz of water
Acid indigestion, sour stomach, and heartburn	Adult: 2–4 tabs, chewed thoroughly, or 5–15 ml (1–3 tsp) with a little water, up to qid Child (7–14 yr): 1 tab, chewed thoroughly, up to qid

CONTRAINDICATIONS

Abdominal pain, nausea, or vomiting
Renal disease
Change in bowel habits persisting for over 2 wk
Rectal bleeding

WARNINGS/PRECAUTIONS

Patient instructions for use as a laxative	The package labeling cautions patients that unless otherwise directed by a physician, they should follow the dosage recommendations and should not use these products for longer than 1 wk; the patient is also advised to discontinue use and consult a physician if no bowel movement results from use (onset of laxative effect is usually 30 min to 6 h)
Patient instructions for use as an antacid	The package labeling cautions patients that unless otherwise directed by a physician, they should not exceed the maximum dosage recommendations or use these products for longer than 2 wk; the patient is also advised that a laxative effect may result from use
Dependency	Habitual use of laxatives may result in dependency

ADVERSE REACTIONS

Consult manufacturer

OVERDOSAGE

Signs and symptoms	Muscle weakness, hypotension, ECG changes, sedation, and confusion, followed, in severe cases, by depression of deep-tendon reflexes, respiratory paralysis, and complete heart block
Treatment	Discontinue use of medication, institute supportive measures, as required, and treat symptomatically. Administer furosemide, ethacrynic acid, or ammonium chloride to force diuresis of magnesium. IV calcium salts may be helpful in reversing respiratory effects.

DRUG INTERACTIONS

Tetracycline — ▽ Tetracycline absorption

ALTERED LABORATORY VALUES
No clinically significant alterations in blood/serum or urinary values occur at therapeutic dosages

---

USE IN CHILDREN	USE IN PREGNANT AND NURSING WOMEN
See INDICATIONS and ORAL DOSAGE	The package labeling cautions pregnant and nursing women to consult a health professional before using this product

---

LAXATIVES/STOOL SOFTENERS

REGUTOL (docusate sodium) Plough   OTC
Tablets: 100 mg

INDICATIONS
Constipation

ORAL DOSAGE
Adult: 100–300 mg/day, as needed
Child (2–12 yr): 100 mg/day, as needed
Child (> 12 yr): same as adult

CONTRAINDICATIONS
None known

ADMINISTRATION/DOSAGE ADJUSTMENTS
Onset of action —————————————— The full therapeutic effect usually occurs 1–3 days after initial administration

WARNINGS/PRECAUTIONS
Consult manufacturer

ADVERSE REACTIONS
Consult manufacturer

OVERDOSAGE
Product is not absorbed; no toxic effects have been observed in clinical use

DRUG INTERACTIONS
No clinically significant drug interactions have been identified

ALTERED LABORATORY VALUES
No clinically significant alterations in blood/serum or urinary values occur at therapeutic dosages

---

USE IN CHILDREN	USE IN PREGNANT AND NURSING WOMEN
See INDICATIONS and ORAL DOSAGE	Consult manufacturer

LAXATIVES/STOOL SOFTENERS

SENOKOT (senna) Purdue Frederick   OTC
Tablets: 187 mg   **Granules:** 326 mg/tsp (2, 6, 12 oz) *cocoa-flavored*   **Syrup (per 5 ml):** 218 mg[1] (2, 8 fl oz)   **Suppositories:** 652 mg

INDICATIONS
Functional constipation

ORAL DOSAGE
Adult: 2 tabs, 1 level tsp granules, or 10–15 ml (2–3 tsp) syrup at bedtime, up to 4 tabs, 2 level tsp granules, or 15 ml (3 tsp) syrup bid
Infant (1 mo to 1 yr): 1.25–2.5 ml (1/4–1/2 tsp) syrup at bedtime or up to 2.5 ml (1/2 tsp) syrup bid
Child (1–5 yr): 2.5–5 ml (1/2–1 tsp) syrup at bedtime or up to 5 ml (1 tsp) syrup bid
Child (5–15 yr): 5–10 ml (1–2 tsp) syrup at bedtime or up to 10 ml (2 tsp) syrup bid, or (if child weighs > 60 lb) 1 tab or 1/2 level tsp granules at bedtime or up to 2 tabs or 1 level tsp granules bid

RECTAL DOSAGE
Adult: for evacuation, 1 suppository; for refractory cases, repeat 2 h later
Child (> 60 lb): for evacuation, 1/2 suppository; for refractory cases, repeat 2 h later

SENOKOT ■ SURFAK

CONTRAINDICATIONS

Acute surgical abdomen

ADMINISTRATION/DOSAGE ADJUSTMENTS

Onset of action	Usually apparent within 8–10 h after administration of tablets or granules and 1/2–2 h following insertion of the suppositories
Elderly, debilitated, or pregnant patients	Administer 1/2 the initial adult dosage
Refractory constipation	If comfortable bowel movement is not achieved by the second day when using the syrup, tablets, or granules, daily dosage should be decreased or increased in increments of 1/2 the starting dose, until optimum dosage is established

WARNINGS/PRECAUTIONS

Consult manufacturer

ADVERSE REACTIONS

Consult manufacturer

OVERDOSAGE

Product is not absorbed; no toxic effects have been observed in clinical use

DRUG INTERACTIONS

No clinically significant drug interactions have been identified

ALTERED LABORATORY VALUES

No clinically significant alterations in blood/serum or urinary values occur at therapeutic dosages

---

USE IN CHILDREN

See INDICATIONS and ORAL DOSAGE

USE IN PREGNANT AND NURSING WOMEN

See ADMINISTRATION/DOSAGE ADJUSTMENTS for use in pregnant women. Consult manufacturer use in nursing mothers.

---

[1] Contains 7% alcohol

LAXATIVES/STOOL SOFTENERS

SURFAK (docusate calcium) Hoechst-Roussel — OTC

Capsules: 50, 240 mg[1]

INDICATIONS	**ORAL DOSAGE**
Constipation	**Adult:** 240 mg/day for several days or until bowel movements are normal; for mild cases, 50–150 mg/day **Child (> 6 yr):** 50–150 mg/day for several days or until bowel movements are normal

CONTRAINDICATIONS

None known

WARNINGS/PRECAUTIONS

Consult manufacturer

ADVERSE REACTIONS

Gastrointestinal	Cramps (mild)

OVERDOSAGE

Signs and symptoms	Cramps
Treatment	Reduce dosage; discontinue use if cramps persist

SURFAK

DRUG INTERACTIONS
No clinically significant drug interactions have been identified

ALTERED LABORATORY VALUES
No clinically significant alterations in blood/serum or urinary values occur at therapeutic dosages

---

USE IN CHILDREN
See INDICATIONS and ORAL DOSAGE

USE IN PREGNANT AND NURSING WOMEN
May safely be administered to pregnant or nursing women

---

[1] Each 50-mg capsule contains up to 1.3% alcohol, and each 240-mg capsule contains up to 3% alcohol

Chapter 41

Major Tranquilizers

Antimanic Agents — 1647

CIBALITH-S (CIBA) — 1647
Lithium citrate *Rx*

ESKALITH (Smith Kline & French) — 1648
Lithium carbonate *Rx*

ESKALITH CR (Smith Kline & French) — 1648
Lithium carbonate *Rx*

Lithium carbonate (Roxane) *Rx* — 1651

Lithium citrate (Roxane) *Rx* — 1651

LITHOBID (CIBA) — 1647
Lithium carbonate *Rx*

LITHONATE (Reid-Rowell) — 1652
Lithium carbonate *Rx*

LITHOTABS (Reid-Rowell) — 1652
Lithium carbonate *Rx*

Butyrophenones — 1654

HALDOL (McNeil Pharmaceutical) — 1654
Haloperidol *Rx*

HALDOL Decanoate (McNeil Pharmaceutical) — 1655
Haloperidol decanoate *Rx*

Dibenzoxazepines — 1657

LOXITANE (Lederle) — 1657
Loxapine succinate *Rx*

LOXITANE C (Lederle) — 1657
Loxapine hydrochloride *Rx*

LOXITANE IM (Lederle) — 1657
Loxapine hydrochloride *Rx*

Dihydroindolones — 1659

MOBAN (Du Pont) — 1659
Molindone hydrochloride *Rx*

Phenothiazines — 1661

COMPAZINE (Smith Kline & French) — 1661
Prochlorperazine *Rx*

MELLARIL (Sandoz Pharmaceuticals) — 1665
Thioridazine hydrochloride *Rx*

MELLARIL-S (Sandoz Pharmaceuticals) — 1665
Thioridazine *Rx*

PERMITIL (Schering) — 1666
Fluphenazine hydrochloride *Rx*

PROLIXIN (Princeton) — 1669
Fluphenazine hydrochloride *Rx*

PROLIXIN Decanoate (Princeton) — 1669
Fluphenazine decanoate *Rx*

PROLIXIN Enanthate (Princeton) — 1670
Fluphenazine enanthate *Rx*

SERENTIL (Boehringer Ingelheim) — 1672
Mesoridazine besylate *Rx*

SPARINE (Wyeth) — 1674
Promazine hydrochloride *Rx*

STELAZINE (Smith Kline & French) — 1676
Trifluoperazine hydrochloride *Rx*

THORAZINE (Smith Kline & French) — 1680
Chlorpromazine hydrochloride *Rx*

TINDAL (Schering) — 1684
Acetophenazine maleate *Rx*

TRILAFON (Schering) — 1687
Perphenazine *Rx*

VESPRIN (Princeton) — 1690
Triflupromazine hydrochloride *Rx*

Thioxanthenes — 1692

NAVANE (Roerig) — 1692
Thiothixene *Rx*

TARACTAN (Roche) — 1694
Chlorprothixene *Rx*

Other Major Tranquilizers — 1646

LITHANE (Miles Pharmaceuticals) — 1646
Lithium carbonate *Rx*

ORAP (McNeil Pharmaceutical) — 1646
Pimozide *Rx*

OTHER MAJOR TRANQUILIZERS

DRUG	HOW SUPPLIED	USUAL DOSAGE[1]
LITHANE (Miles Pharmaceuticals) Lithium carbonate *Rx*	Tablets: 300 mg	**Adult:** 600 mg tid during acute phase of mania, followed by 300 mg tid or qid for long-term control
ORAP (McNeil Pharmaceutical) Pimozide *Rx*	Tablets: 2 mg	**Adult:** for Tourette's syndrome, 1–2 mg/day, given in divided doses, to start; for maintenance, up to 0.2 mg/kg/day or 10 mg/day, whichever is less

[1] Where pediatric dosages are not given, consult manufacturer

CIBALITH-S/LITHOBID

ANTIMANIC AGENTS

CIBALITH-S (lithium citrate) CIBA   Rx

Syrup (per 5 ml): 8 mEq lithium, equivalent to the amount of lithium contained in 300 mg lithium carbonate (480 ml) *raspberry-flavored, sugar-free*

LITHOBID (lithium carbonate) CIBA   Rx

Tablets (slow release): 300 mg

INDICATIONS	ORAL DOSAGE
Manic episodes of manic-depressive illness	**Adult:** for acute episodes, 10 ml (2 tsp) tid or 900 mg bid or 600 mg tid; for long-term control, 5 ml (1 tsp) tid or qid 900–1,200 mg/day, given in 2–3 divided doses

CONTRAINDICATIONS

See "special-risk patients" under WARNINGS/PRECAUTIONS

ADMINISTRATION/DOSAGE ADJUSTMENTS

Administration of tablets	Slow-release tablets must be swallowed whole, not crushed or chewed
Use of serum lithium levels to adjust dosage	During acute manic episodes, determine the serum lithium level twice a week; blood samples should be drawn immediately prior to the next dose (ie, 8–12 h after the previous dose). Adjust the dosage to maintain a serum level between 1.0 and 1.5 mEq/liter, and continue monitoring the serum level twice a week until the serum level and patient's clinical condition stabilize. For long-term control, adjust the dosage to maintain a serum level between 0.6 and 1.2 mEq/liter, and measure the serum level at least once every 2 mo. Any adjustment in dosage must take into account the clinical response to the drug, as well as the serum lithium level; elderly patients, in particular, often respond to lower dosages and may show signs of toxicity at serum levels tolerated by other patients.

WARNINGS/PRECAUTIONS

Special-risk patients	In patients with significant renal or cardiovascular disease, severe debilitation or dehydration, or sodium depletion, and in those receiving diuretics, use only if the psychiatric indication is life-threatening and if the patient fails to respond to other measures; in such instances, hospitalize patient and use with extreme caution (including daily serum lithium determinations)
Morphological changes in the kidneys	Have been reported with lithium; the relationship between these changes and renal function has not been established
Lithium toxicity	May occur at doses close to therapeutic levels; instruct outpatients (and their families) to discontinue use of lithium if diarrhea, vomiting, tremors, mild ataxia, drowsiness, or muscular weakness occurs and to contact their physician
Pseudotumor cerebri	Lithium use has been associated with pseudotumor cerebri (increased intracranial pressure and papilledema), which, if undetected, may result in enlargement of the blind spot, constriction of visual fields, and eventual blindness due to optic atrophy; discontinue use if this syndrome occurs and it is clinically feasible to stop the drug
Mental and/or physical impairment	Caution patients about driving or engaging in other activities requiring alertness
Sodium depletion	May occur; patient must maintain a normal diet, including salt, and an adequate fluid intake (2,500–3,000 ml/day), at least during initial stabilization period. Supplemental fluid and salt should be given if protracted sweating or diarrhea occurs.
Concomitant infection with elevated temperatures	May necessitate temporary dosage reduction or cessation of medication
Thyroid dysfunction	Lithium has caused hypothyroidism and, in rare instances, paradoxical hyperthyroidism; in some cases, these effects have persisted after discontinuation of therapy. If hypothyroidism occurs during therapy, thyroid hormone may be given. Carefully monitor thyroid function in patients with hypothyroidism.
Lithium tolerance	May decrease when manic symptoms subside

ADVERSE REACTIONS

Central nervous system and neuromuscular	Fine hand tremor, drowsiness, muscular weakness, incoordination, tremor, muscle hyperirritability (fasciculations, twitching, clonic movements of whole limbs), ataxia, choreoathetotic movements, hyperactive deep-tendon reflexes, blackout spells, epileptiform seizures, slurred speech, dizziness, vertigo, somnolence, psychomotor retardation, restlessness, confusion, stupor, coma, EEG changes, fatigue, lethargy, headache, tendency to sleep, worsening of organic brain syndromes, tinnitus, giddiness
Genitourinary	Polyuria, incontinence, albuminuria, oliguria, glycosuria
Cardiovascular	Arrhythmia, hypotension, peripheral circulatory collapse, ECG changes
Autonomic nervous system	Blurred vision, dry mouth
Gastrointestinal	Nausea, diarrhea, vomiting, fecal incontinence, anorexia, metallic taste

CIBALITH-S/LITHOBID ■ ESKALITH

Metabolic and endocrinological	Euthyroid goiter and/or hypothyroidism (including myxedema); diffuse nontoxic goiter, with or without hypothyroidism; transient hyperglycemia; hyperthyroidism (rare)
Dermatological	Drying and thinning of hair, alopecia, anesthesia of skin, chronic folliculitis, exacerbation of psoriasis, xerosis cutis, pruritus with or without rash, ulcers
Other	General discomfort, transient scotomata, dehydration, thirst, leukocytosis, weight changes, edematous swelling of ankles or wrists; painful discoloration of fingers and toes, accompanied by coldness of the extremities (one case)

OVERDOSAGE

Signs and symptoms	Diarrhea, vomiting, drowsiness, muscular weakness, lack of coordination, ataxia, giddiness, tinnitus (see ADVERSE REACTIONS); serum lithium levels above 3.0 mEq/liter may produce a complex clinical picture, involving multiple organs and organ systems
Treatment	In mild cases, reduce dosage or discontinue therapy and resume in 24–48 h at lower dosage. In severe cases, empty stomach by gastric lavage. Correct fluid and electrolyte imbalance. Regulate kidney function. Increase lithium excretion with urea, mannitol, or aminophylline. For severe toxicity, employ hemodialysis. Maintain adequate respiration. Infection prophylaxis and regular chest x-rays are essential.

DRUG INTERACTIONS

Other neuroleptic drugs	Encephalopathic syndrome, characterized by weakness, lethargy, fever, tremulousness, confusion, extrapyramidal symptoms, leukocytosis, and elevated levels of plasma glucose, BUN, and plasma enzymes; this syndrome, similar or identical to NMS, may result in irreversible brain damage. During combination therapy, watch closely for premonitory evidence of neurological toxicity; if early signs of neurotoxicity are seen, promptly discontinue use.
Chlorpromazine, possibly other phenothiazines	↓ Plasma level of phenothiazine Encephalopathic syndrome (see interaction, above)
Carbamazepine	↑ Risk of neurotoxicity Encephalopathic syndrome (see interaction, above)
Diuretics, especially thiazides	↑ Risk of lithium toxicity; closely monitor plasma lithium level and, if necessary, adjust lithium dosage
Neuromuscular blockers	↑ Neuromuscular blockade; exercise caution
Nonsteroidal anti-inflammatory agents, especially piroxicam and indomethacin	↑ Risk of lithium toxicity; monitor plasma lithium level more frequently during combination therapy
Theophylline and other xanthines, acetazolamide, urea, alkalinizing agents (eg, sodium bicarbonate)	↓ Plasma lithium level
Iodide	Hypothyroidism
Norepinephrine	↓ Vasopressor effect

ALTERED LABORATORY VALUES

Blood/serum values	↑ ^{131}I uptake ↓ Triiodothyronine (T_3) uptake ↓ Thyroxine (T_4) uptake
Urinary values	↑ Glucose ↑ Albumin ↑ VMA

USE IN CHILDREN

Not recommended for use in children under 12 yr of age; the safety and effectiveness of lithium in this age group are unknown

USE IN PREGNANT AND NURSING WOMEN

Not recommended for use during pregnancy, especially during the first trimester, unless the potential benefits of therapy outweigh the possible hazard to the fetus. Lithium is excreted in human milk; nursing should not be undertaken during lithium therapy except in rare circumstances.

ANTIMANIC AGENTS

ESKALITH (lithium carbonate) Smith Kline & French   Rx
Capsules: 300 mg   **Tablets:** 300 mg

ESKALITH CR (lithium carbonate) Smith Kline & French   Rx
Tablets (controlled release): 450 mg

INDICATIONS	ORAL DOSAGE
Manic episodes of manic-depressive illness	Adult: for acute episodes, 1,800 mg/day, given in divided doses; for long-term control, 900–1,200 mg/day, given in divided doses

ESKALITH

CONTRAINDICATIONS

See "special-risk patients" under WARNINGS/PRECAUTIONS

ADMINISTRATION/DOSAGE ADJUSTMENTS

Frequency of administration — The immediate-release capsules and tablets are usually given tid or qid; the controlled-release tablets are usually given bid (approximately q12h)

Use of serum lithium levels to adjust dosage — During acute manic episodes, determine the serum lithium level twice a week; blood samples should be drawn immediately prior to the next dose (ie, 8–12 h after the previous dose). Adjust the dosage to maintain a serum level between 1.0 and 1.5 mEq/liter, and continue monitoring the serum level twice a week until the serum level and patient's clinical condition stabilize. For long-term control, adjust the dosage to maintain a serum level between 0.6 and 1.2 mEq/liter, and measure the serum level at least once every 2 mo. Any adjustment in dosage must take into account the clinical response to the drug, as well as the serum lithium level; elderly patients, in particular, often respond to lower dosages and may show signs of toxicity at serum levels tolerated by younger patients.

Switching patients from immediate-release preparations to controlled-release tablets — When possible, give the same total daily dose. If the previous daily dose is not a multiple of 450 mg, initiate therapy with Eskalith CR at the dose nearest to, but below, the original daily dose (eg, a patient who had been maintained on 1,500 mg/day should be started on 1,350 mg/day). If the 2 doses are unequal, give the larger dose in the evening (eg, 450 mg in the morning and 900 mg at night); if desired, however, the total daily dose may be given in 3 equally divided doses. Monitor treatment every 1–2 wk and adjust the dosage, as needed, until stable, satisfactory serum levels and clinical status are achieved. When patients require closer dosage titration than 450-mg steps will allow, an immediate-release preparation of lithium should be used.

WARNINGS/PRECAUTIONS

Special-risk patients — In patients with significant renal or cardiovascular disease, severe debilitation or dehydration, or sodium depletion, use only if the psychiatric indication is life-threatening and if the patient fails to respond to other measures; in such instances, hospitalize patient and use with extreme caution (including daily serum lithium determinations)

Renal function — Chronic therapy may diminish renal concentrating ability and may result in nephrogenic diabetes insipidus with polyuria and polydipsia. Morphological changes, including glomerular and interstitial nephrosis and nephron atrophy, have also occurred during chronic therapy, although the relationship between these changes and renal function and their association with the use of lithium have not been established. Assess kidney function prior to starting therapy and periodically thereafter by routine urinalysis and other tests of tubular and glomerular function; if renal function suddenly or progressively changes, even within the normal range, reevaluate the need for continued lithium therapy. Patients presenting with nephrogenic diabetes insipidus should be carefully managed to avoid dehydration and resulting lithium retention and toxicity.

Lithium toxicity — May occur at doses close to therapeutic levels; instruct outpatients (and their families) to discontinue use of lithium if diarrhea, vomiting, tremors, mild ataxia, drowsiness, or muscular weakness occurs and to contact their physician

Pseudotumor cerebri — Lithium use has been associated with pseudotumor cerebri (increased intracranial pressure and papilledema), which, if undetected, may result in enlargement of the blind spot, constriction of visual fields, and eventual blindness due to optic atrophy; discontinue use if this syndrome occurs and it is clinically feasible to stop the drug

Mental impairment, reflex-slowing — Performance of potentially hazardous activities may be impaired; caution patients accordingly

Sodium depletion — May occur; patient must maintain a normal diet, including salt, and an adequate fluid intake (2,500–3,000 ml/day), at least during initial stabilization period. If protracted sweating or diarrhea occurs, supplemental fluid and salt should be given under careful supervision and lithium intake should be reduced or discontinued until condition is corrected.

Concomitant infection with elevated temperatures — May necessitate temporary dosage reduction or cessation of medication

Thyroid dysfunction — Lithium has caused hypothyroidism and, in rare instances, paradoxical hyperthyroidism; in some cases, these effects persisted after discontinuation of therapy. If hypothyroidism occurs during therapy, thyroid hormone may be given. Carefully monitor thyroid function in patients with hypothyroidism.

Lithium tolerance — Decreases when manic symptoms subside

ADVERSE REACTIONS

Central nervous system and neuromuscular — Fine hand tremor, drowsiness, muscular weakness, incoordination, tremor, muscle hyperirritability (fasciculations, twitching, clonic movements of whole limbs), hypertonicity, ataxia, choreoathetotic movements, hyperactive deep-tendon reflexes, extrapyramidal symptoms, acute dystonia, cogwheel rigidity, blackout spells, epileptiform seizures, slurred speech, dizziness, vertigo, downbeat nystagmus, somnolence, psychomotor retardation, restlessness, confusion, stupor, coma, pseudotumor cerebri, EEG changes, fatigue, lethargy, headache, tendency to sleep, worsening of organic brain syndromes, tinnitus, giddiness, tongue movements, tics, hallucinations, poor memory, slowed intellectual functioning, startled response, dysgeusia/taste distortion, metallic/salty taste, thirst

ESKALITH

Genitourinary	Albuminuria, oliguria, nephrogenic diabetes insipidus (with polyuria, thirst, and polydipsia) incontinence, glycosuria, decreased creatinine clearance, impotence/sexual dysfunction
Cardiovascular	Arrhythmia, hypotension, peripheral circulatory collapse, bradycardia, sinus node dysfunction with severe bradycardia (possibly resulting in syncope), ECG changes
Autonomic nervous system	Blurred vision, dry mouth
Gastrointestinal	Nausea, diarrhea, vomiting, fecal incontinence, anorexia, gastritis, salivary gland swelling, abdominal pain, excessive salivation, flatulence, indigestion
Metabolic and endocrinological	Euthyroid goiter and/or hypothyroidism (including myxedema); diffuse nontoxic goiter, with or without hypothyroidism; transient hyperglycemia; hypercalcemia; hyperparathyroidism; hyperthyroidism (rare)
Dermatological	Drying and thinning of hair, alopecia, anesthesia of skin, chronic folliculitis, psoriasis, exacerbation of psoriasis, itching, xerosis cutis, pruritus with or without rash, ulcers, angioedema
Other	General discomfort, transient scotomata, dehydration, leukocytosis, weight changes, edematous swelling of ankles or wrists, swollen lips, tightness in the chest, swollen and/or painful joints, fever, polyarthralgia, hypertoxicity, dental caries; painful discoloration of fingers and toes, accompanied by coldness of the extremities (rare)

OVERDOSAGE

Signs and symptoms	Diarrhea, vomiting, drowsiness, muscular weakness, lack of coordination, ataxia, giddiness, tinnitus, blurred vision, polyuria; serum lithium levels above 3.0 mEq/liter may produce a complex clinical picture, involving multiple organs and organ systems
Treatment	In mild cases, reduce dosage or discontinue therapy and resume in 24–48 h at lower dosage. In severe cases, empty stomach by gastric lavage. Correct fluid and electrolyte imbalance. Regulate kidney function. Increase lithium excretion with urea, mannitol, or aminophylline. For severe toxicity, employ hemodialysis. Maintain adequate respiration. Infection prophylaxis and regular chest x-rays are essential.

DRUG INTERACTIONS

Other neuroleptic drugs	Encephalopathic syndrome, characterized by weakness, lethargy, fever, tremulousness, confusion, extrapyramidal symptoms, leukocytosis, and elevated levels of plasma glucose, BUN, and plasma enzymes; this syndrome, similar or identical to NMS, may result in irreversible brain damage. During combination therapy, watch closely for premonitory evidence of neurological toxicity; if early signs of neurotoxicity are seen, promptly discontinue use.
Chlorpromazine, possibly other phenothiazines	⇩ Plasma level of phenothiazine Encephalopathic syndrome (see interaction, above)
Carbamazepine	⇧ Risk of neurotoxicity Encephalopathic syndrome (see interaction, above)
Diuretics, especially thiazides	⇧ Risk of lithium toxicity; closely monitor plasma lithium level and, if necessary, adjust lithium dosage
Neuromuscular blockers	⇧ Neuromuscular blockade; exercise caution
Nonsteroidal anti-inflammatory agents, especially piroxicam and indomethacin	⇧ Risk of lithium toxicity; monitor plasma lithium level more frequently during combination therapy
Theophylline and other xanthines, acetazolamide, urea, alkalinizing agents (eg, sodium bicarbonate)	⇩ Plasma lithium level
Iodide	Hypothyroidism
Norepinephrine	⇩ Vasopressor effect

ALTERED LABORATORY VALUES

Blood/serum values	⇧ ^{131}I uptake ⇩ Triiodothyronine (T_3) uptake ⇩ Thyroxine (T_4) uptake
Urinary values	⇧ Glucose ⇧ Albumin ⇧ VMA

USE IN CHILDREN

Not recommended for use in children under 12 yr of age; the safety and effectiveness of lithium in this age group are unknown. Ingestion of 300 mg of lithium carbonate by a 15-kg child has resulted in transient acute dystonia and hyperreflexia.

USE IN PREGNANT AND NURSING WOMEN

An increased incidence of cardiac and other anomalies, especially Ebstein's anomaly, has been associated with lithium therapy in pregnant women; women of childbearing potential and pregnant women should be apprised of the potential hazard to the fetus. Lithium is excreted in human milk; nursing should not be undertaken during lithium therapy except in rare circumstances.

Lithium

ANTIMANIC AGENTS

Lithium carbonate Roxane   Rx
Capsules: 300 mg   **Tablets:** 300 mg

Lithium citrate Roxane   Rx
Syrup (per 5 ml): 8 mEq lithium, equivalent to the amount of lithium contained in 300 mg lithium carbonate[1] (5, 10, 500 ml)

INDICATIONS	ORAL DOSAGE
Manic episodes of manic-depressive illness	**Adult:** for acute episodes, 600 mg or 10 ml (2 tsp) tid; for long-term control, 300 mg or 5 ml (1 tsp) tid or qid

CONTRAINDICATIONS
See "special-risk patients" under WARNINGS/PRECAUTIONS

ADMINISTRATION/DOSAGE ADJUSTMENTS

Use if serum lithium levels to adjust dosage	During acute manic episodes, determine the serum lithium level twice a week; blood samples should be drawn immediately prior to the next dose (ie, 8–12 h after the previous dose). Adjust the dosage to maintain a serum level between 1.0 and 1.5 mEq/liter, and continue monitoring the serum level twice a week until the serum level and patient's clinical condition stabilize. For long-term control, adjust the dosage to maintain a serum level between 0.6 and 1.2 mEq/liter, and measure the serum level at least once every 2 mo. Any adjustment in dosage must take into account the clinical response to the drug, as well as the serum lithium level; elderly patients, in particular, often respond to lower dosages and may show signs of toxicity at serum levels tolerated by other patients.

WARNINGS/PRECAUTIONS

Special-risk patients	In patients with significant renal or cardiovascular disease, severe debilitation or dehydration, or sodium depletion, and in those receiving diuretics, use only if the psychiatric indication is life-threatening and if the patient fails to respond to other measures; in such instances, hospitalize patient and use with extreme caution (including daily serum lithium determinations)
Renal function	Chronic therapy may diminish renal concentrating ability and may result in nephrogenic diabetes insipidus with polyuria and polydipsia. Morphological changes, including glomerular and interstitial nephrosis and nephron atrophy, have also occurred during chronic therapy, although the relationship between these changes and renal function and their association with the use of lithium have not been established. Assess kidney function prior to starting therapy and periodically thereafter by routine urinalysis and other tests of tubular and glomerular function; if renal function suddenly or progressively changes, even within the normal range, reevaluate the need for continued lithium therapy. Patients presenting with nephrogenic diabetes insipidus should be carefully managed to avoid dehydration and resulting lithium retention and toxicity.
Concomitant use of haloperidol or other antipsychotics	May be associated with an encephalopathic syndrome characterized by weakness, lethargy, fever, tremulousness, confusion, extrapyramidal symptoms, leukocytosis, and elevated serum enzymes, BUN, and FBS, followed by irreversible brain damage. Although a causal relationship has not been established, patients should be monitored closely for early evidence of neurological toxicity and concomitant therapy discontinued promptly if such signs appear.
Lithium toxicity	May occur at doses close to therapeutic levels; instruct outpatients and their families to discontinue use of lithium if diarrhea, vomiting, tremors, mild ataxia, drowsiness, or muscular weakness occurs and to contact their physician
Pseudomotor cerebri	Lithium use has been associated with pseudotumor cerebri (increased intracranial pressure and papilledema), which, if undetected, may result in enlargement of the blind spot, constriction of visual fields, and eventual blindness due to optic atrophy; discontinue use if this syndrome occurs and it is clinically feasible to stop the drug
Neuromuscular blocking agents	Should be used with caution in patients receiving lithium (see DRUG INTERACTIONS)
Mental and/or physical impairment	Caution patients about driving or engaging in other activities requiring alertness
Sodium depletion	May occur; patient must maintain a normal diet, including salt, and an adequate fluid intake (2,500–3,000 ml/day), at least during initial stabilization period. Supplemental fluid and salt should be given if protracted sweating or diarrhea occurs.
Concomitant infection with elevated temperatures	May necessitate temporary dosage reduction or suspending of medication
Hypothyroid patients	Monitor thyroid function and administer supplemental thyroid therapy, if necessary
Lithium tolerance	May decrease when manic symptoms subside

COMPENDIUM OF DRUG THERAPY

Lithium ■ LITHONATE/LITHOTABS

ADVERSE REACTIONS

Central nervous system and neuromuscular	Fine hand tremor, drowsiness, muscular weakness, incoordination, tremor, muscle hyperirritability (fasciculations, twitching, clonic movements of whole limbs), ataxia, choreoathetotic movements, hyperactive deep-tendon reflexes, blackout spells, epileptiform seizures, slurred speech, dizziness, vertigo, somnolence, psychomotor retardation, restlessness, confusion, stupor, coma, pseudotumor cerebri, EEG changes, fatigue, lethargy, headache, tendency to sleep, worsening of organic brain syndromes, tinnitus, giddiness
Genitourinary	Polyuria, incontinence, albuminuria, oliguria, glycosuria
Cardiovascular	Arrhythmia, hypotension, peripheral circulatory collapse, ECG changes
Autonomic nervous system	Blurred vision, dry mouth
Gastrointestinal	Nausea, diarrhea, vomiting, fecal incontinence, anorexia, metallic taste
Metabolic and endocrinological	Euthyroid goiter and/or hypothyroidism (including myxedema); diffuse nontoxic goiter, with or without hypothyroidism; transient hyperglycemia; hyperthyroidism (rare)
Dermatological	Drying and thinning of hair, alopecia, anesthesia of skin, chronic folliculitis, exacerbation of psoriasis, xerosis cutis, pruritus with or without rash, ulcers
Other	General discomfort, transient scotomata, dehydration, thirst, leukocytosis, weight changes, edematous swelling of ankles or wrists; painful discoloration of the fingers and toes, accompanied by coldness of the extremities (one case)

OVERDOSAGE

Signs and symptoms	Diarrhea, vomiting, drowsiness, muscular weakness, lack of coordination, ataxia, giddiness, tinnitus (see ADVERSE REACTIONS); serum lithium levels above 3.0 mEq/liter may produce a complex clinical picture, involving multiple organs and organ systems
Treatment	In mild cases, reduce dosage or discontinue therapy and resume in 24–48 h at lower dosage. In severe cases, empty stomach by gastric lavage. Correct fluid and electrolyte imbalance. Regulate kidney function. Increase lithium excretion with urea, mannitol, or aminophylline. For severe toxicity, employ hemodialysis. Maintain adequate respiration. Infection prophylaxis and regular chest x-rays are essential.

DRUG INTERACTIONS

Neuromuscular blocking agents	⇧ Neuromuscular blocking effect
Methylxanthines, sodium bicarbonate	⇧ Lithium clearance
Chlorpromazine	⇩ Serum chlorpromazine levels
Diuretics (especially thiazides)	⇩ Lithium clearance
Iodide	Hypothyroidism
Norepinephrine	⇩ Pressor effects
Haloperidol	Neurotoxicity (causal relationship not established)
Indomethacin, possibly other nonsteroidal anti-inflammatory agents	⇧ Serum lithium levels

ALTERED LABORATORY VALUES

Blood/serum values	⇧ ^{131}I uptake ⇩ Triiodothyronine (T_3) uptake ⇩ Thyroxine (T_4) uptake
Urinary values	⇧ Glucose ⇧ Albumin ⇧ VMA

USE IN CHILDREN

Not recommended for use in children under 12 yr of age; the safety and effectiveness of lithium in this age group are unknown

USE IN PREGNANT AND NURSING WOMEN

Pregnancy Category D: lithium may cause fetal harm if administered during pregnancy. An increased incidence of cardiac and other anomalies, especially Ebstein's anomaly, has been associated with lithium therapy in pregnant women. Patients receiving lithium during pregnancy or who become pregnant while taking lithium should be apprised of the potential hazard to the fetus. If possible, discontinue use of lithium during at least the first trimester, unless doing so would seriously endanger the mother. Lithium is excreted in human milk; nursing should not be undertaken during lithium therapy except in rare circumstances.

[1] Contains 0.3% alcohol

ANTIMANIC AGENTS

LITHONATE (lithium carbonate) Reid-Rowell   Rx
Capsules: 300 mg

LITHOTABS (lithium carbonate) Reid-Rowell   Rx
Tablets: 300 mg

INDICATIONS	ORAL DOSAGE
Manic episodes of manic-depressive illness	Adult: for acute episodes, 600 mg tid; for long-term control, 300 mg tid or qid

LITHONATE/LITHOTABS

CONTRAINDICATIONS

See "special-risk patients" under WARNINGS/PRECAUTIONS

ADMINISTRATION/DOSAGE ADJUSTMENTS

Use of serum lithium levels to adjust dosage	During acute manic episodes, determine the serum lithium level twice a week; blood samples should be drawn immediately prior to the next dose (ie, 8–12 h after the previous dose). Adjust the dosage to maintain a serum level between 1.0 and 1.5 mEq/liter, and continue monitoring the serum level twice a week until the serum level and patient's clinical condition stabilize. For long-term control, adjust the dosage to maintain a serum level between 0.6 and 1.2 mEq/liter, and measure the serum level at least once every 2 mo. Any adjustment in dosage must take into account the clinical response to the drug, as well as the serum lithium level; elderly patients, in particular, often respond to lower dosages and may show signs of toxicity at serum levels tolerated by other patients.

WARNINGS/PRECAUTIONS

Special-risk patients	In patients with significant renal or cardiovascular disease, severe debilitation or dehydration, or sodium depletion, and in those receiving diuretics, use only if the psychiatric indication is life-threatening and if the patient fails to respond to other measures; in such instances, hospitalize patient and use with extreme caution (including daily serum lithium determinations)
Morphological changes in the kidneys	Have been reported with lithium; the relationship between these changes and renal function has not been established
Lithium toxicity	May occur at doses close to therapeutic levels; instruct outpatients (and their families) to discontinue use of lithium if diarrhea, vomiting, tremors, mild ataxia, drowsiness, or muscular weakness occurs and to contact their physician
Pseudotumor cerebri	Lithium use has been associated with pseudotumor cerebri (increased intracranial pressure and papilledema), which, if undetected, may result in enlargement of the blind spot, constriction of visual fields, and eventual blindness due to optic atrophy; discontinue use if this syndrome occurs and it is clinically feasible to stop the drug
Mental and/or physical impairment	Caution patients about driving or engaging in other activities requiring alertness
Sodium depletion	May occur; patient must maintain a normal diet, including salt, and an adequate fluid intake (2,500–3,000 ml/day), at least during initial stabilization period. Supplemental fluid and salt should be given if protracted sweating or diarrhea occurs.
Concomitant infection with elevated temperatures	May necessitate temporary dosage reduction or cessation of medication
Thyroid dysfunction	Lithium has caused hypothyroidism and, in rare instances, paradoxical hyperthyroidism; in some cases, these effects persisted after discontinuation of therapy. If hypothyroidism occurs during therapy, thyroid hormone may be given. Carefully monitor thyroid function in patients with hypothyroidism.
Lithium tolerance	May decrease when manic symptoms subside

ADVERSE REACTIONS

Central nervous system and neuromuscular	Fine hand tremor, drowsiness, muscular weakness, incoordination, tremor, muscle hyperirritability (fasciculations, twitching, clonic movements of whole limbs), ataxia, choreoathetotic movements, hyperactive deep-tendon reflexes, blackout spells, epileptiform seizures, slurred speech, dizziness, vertigo, somnolence, psychomotor retardation, restlessness, confusion, stupor, coma, acute dystonia, downbeat nystagmus, pseudotumor cerebri, EEG changes, fatigue, lethargy, headache, tendency to sleep, worsening of organic brain syndromes, tinnitus, giddiness
Genitourinary	Polyuria, incontinence, albuminuria, oliguria, glycosuria
Cardiovascular	Arrhythmia, hypotension, peripheral circulatory collapse, ECG changes
Autonomic nervous system	Blurred vision, dry mouth
Gastrointestinal	Nausea, diarrhea, vomiting, fecal incontinence, anorexia, metallic taste
Metabolic and endocrinological	Euthyroid goiter and/or hypothyroidism (including myxedema); diffuse nontoxic goiter, with or without hypothyroidism; transient hyperglycemia; hyperthyroidism (rare)
Dermatological	Drying and thinning of hair, alopecia, anesthesia of skin, chronic folliculitis, exacerbation of psoriasis, xerosis cutis, pruritus with or without rash, ulcers
Other	General discomfort, transient scotomata, dehydration, thirst, leukocytosis, weight changes, edematous swelling of ankles or wrists; painful discoloration of the fingers and toes, accompanied by coldness of the extremities (one case)

OVERDOSAGE

Signs and symptoms	Diarrhea, vomiting, drowsiness, muscular weakness, lack of coordination, ataxia, giddiness, tinnitus (see ADVERSE REACTIONS); serum lithium levels above 3.0 mEq/liter may produce a complex clinical picture, involving multiple organs and organ systems
Treatment	In mild cases, reduce dosage or discontinue therapy and resume in 24–48 h at lower dosage. In severe cases, empty stomach by gastric lavage. Correct fluid and electrolyte imbalance. Regulate kidney function. Increase lithium excretion with urea, mannitol, or aminophylline. For severe toxicity, employ hemodialysis. Maintain adequate respiration. Infection prophylaxis and regular chest x-rays are essential.

LITHONATE/LITHOTABS ■ HALDOL

DRUG INTERACTIONS

Other neuroleptic drugs	Encephalopathic syndrome, characterized by weakness, lethargy, fever, tremulousness, confusion, extrapyramidal symptoms, leukocytosis, and elevated levels of plasma glucose, BUN, and plasma enzymes; this syndrome, similar or identical to NMS, may result in irreversible brain damage. During combination therapy, watch closely for premonitory evidence of neurological toxicity; if early signs of neurotoxicity are seen, promptly discontinue use.
Chlorpromazine, possibly other phenothiazines	⇩ Plasma level of phenothiazine Encephalopathic syndrome (see interaction, above)
Carbamazepine	⇧ Risk of neurotoxicity Encephalopathic syndrome (see interaction, above)
Diuretics, especially thiazides	⇧ Risk of lithium toxicity; closely monitor plasma lithium level and, if necessary, adjust lithium dosage
Neuromuscular blockers	⇧ Neuromuscular blockade; exercise caution
Nonsteroidal anti-inflammatory agents, especially piroxicam and indomethacin	⇧ Risk of lithium toxicity; monitor plasma lithium level more frequently during combination therapy
Theophylline and other xanthines, acetazolamide, urea, alkalinizing agents (eg, sodium bicarbonate)	⇩ Plasma lithium level
Iodide	Hypothyroidism
Norepinephrine	⇩ Vasopressor effect

ALTERED LABORATORY VALUES

Blood/serum values	⇧ ^{131}I uptake ⇩ Triiodothyronine (T_3) uptake ⇩ Thyroxine (T_4) uptake
Urinary values	⇧ Glucose ⇧ Albumin ⇧ VMA

USE IN CHILDREN

Not recommended for use in children under 12 yr of age; the safety and effectiveness of lithium in this age group are unknown. Ingestion of 300 mg of lithium carbonate by a 15-kg child has resulted in transient acute dystonia and hyperreflexia.

USE IN PREGNANT AND NURSING WOMEN

Not recommended for use during pregnancy, especially during the first trimester, unless the potential benefits of therapy outweigh the possible hazard to the fetus. Lithium is excreted in human milk; nursing should not be undertaken during lithium therapy except in rare circumstances.

BUTYROPHENONES

HALDOL (haloperidol) McNeil Pharmaceutical   Rx

Tablets: 0.5, 1, 2, 5, 10, 20 mg **Concentrate:** 2 mg haloperidol[1] per ml (15, 120 ml) **Ampuls:** 5 mg haloperidol[1] per ml (1 ml)
Vials: 5 mg haloperidol[1] per ml (10 ml) **Prefilled syringes:** 5 mg haloperidol[1] per ml (1 ml)

INDICATIONS

Manifestations of **pyschotic disorders**
Gilles de la Tourette's syndrome
Severe behavioral problems, characterized by combative, explosive hyperexplosivity, when these problems occur in children and do not respond to psychotherapy or drugs other than antipsychotics
Hyperactivity (excessive motor activity) accompanied by a **conduct disorder,** characterized by impulsiveness, inattentiveness, aggressiveness, mood changes, or poor tolerance of frustration, when this condition occurs in children, does not respond to psychotherapy or drugs other than antipsychotics, and can be treated in a short period

ORAL DOSAGE

Adult: 0.5–2.0 mg bid or tid to start or, for severe, chronic, or resistant symptoms, 3–5 mg bid or tid to start, followed, if necessary, by up to 100 mg/day; for maintenance therapy, reduce dosage to lowest effective level
Child (3–12 yr; 15–40 kg): 0.5 mg/day, given in divided doses (bid or tid), to start, followed, if necessary, by 0.5-mg increments in dosage every 5–7 days until desired therapeutic effect is obtained (usual dosage for psychotic disorders, 0.05–0.15 mg/kg/day[2]; for nonpsychotic behavioral disorders and Gilles de la Tourette's syndrome, 0.05–0.075 mg/kg/day); for maintenance, reduce dosage to lowest effective level

PARENTERAL DOSAGE

Adult: for prompt control of moderately severe to very severe symptoms, 2–5 mg IM q1–8h, as needed; switch to oral form as soon as possible

HALDOL Decanoate (haloperidol decanoate) McNeil Pharmaceutical Rx

Ampuls: 50 mg of haloperidol[3] per ml (1 ml)

INDICATIONS

Manifestations of **psychotic disorders** in patients requiring prolonged parenteral antipsychotic therapy (eg, chronic schizophrenics)

PARENTERAL DOSAGE

Adult: 10–15 times the previous daily dose of oral haloperidol, up to 100 mg, to start, administered by deep IM injection into the gluteal region using a 2 in.-long, 21-gauge needle; the recommended interval between doses is 4 wk. Maximum volume per injection site: 3 ml.

CONTRAINDICATIONS

| Severe toxic CNS depression or comatose states | Parkinson's disease | Hypersensitivity to haloperidol |

ADMINISTRATION/DOSAGE ADJUSTMENTS

Initial dosage — Base the initial dosage on the patient's age, severity of illness, response to other antipsychotic drugs, and any concomitant medication or disease. For elderly or debilitated patients, give a lower initial dose of the long-acting form and adjust dosage gradually; when using the short-acting forms in these patients, limit the initial dosage to 0.5–2.0 mg bid or tid and adjust dosage gradually, as needed, for optimal response.

Adjustment of dosage — Closely monitor patients during the initial period of dose adjustment because of the risk of overdosage or the reappearance of psychotic symptoms before the next injection; during dose adjustment or periods of exacerbation of psychotic symptoms, the long-acting form may be supplemented with the short-acting forms of haloperidol. Although the long-acting form is often effective when administered at monthly intervals, variation in patient response may indicate adjustment of the dosing interval as well as the dose.

Switching from parenteral therapy to oral therapy — As soon as possible, switch to oral therapy. The parenteral dose given in the preceding 24-h period may be used as an initial estimate of the daily dose required for oral administration. Give the first oral dose 12–24 h after the last parenteral dose, depending upon the patient's condition. During the first few days after the changeover, monitor clinical signs and symptoms periodically for therapeutic efficacy and adverse effects, and, if necessary, adjust dosage.

Prolonged high-dose therapy — The safety of prolonged use of haloperidol in dosages above 100 mg/day has not been established; clinical experience with the long-acting form in monthly doses greater than 300 mg has been limited

WARNINGS/PRECAUTIONS

Tardive dyskinesia — Antipsychotic drugs can cause tardive dyskinesia, a potentially irreversible syndrome characterized by involuntary choreoathetoid movements of the tongue, face, mouth, lips, jaw, trunk, and/or extremities. Protrusion of the tongue, puffing of the cheeks, puckering of the mouth, chewing movements, and other manifestations may become evident during treatment, upon dosage reduction, or after the drug is discontinued. The likelihood that tardive dyskinesia will develop or become irreversible increases with duration of treatment and total cumulative dose; however, even relatively brief use of low doses can cause it. Although this reaction appears to occur most often in the elderly, especially among older women, it is impossible to use this information to predict, before therapy is started, which patients are likely to develop the syndrome.

In general, reserve chronic therapy for patients who respond to antipsychotics and who cannot undergo another, equally effective form of treatment that is potentially less harmful. Use the lowest effective dosage, keep the duration of therapy as short as possible, and periodically reassess the need for the drug. Watch carefully for manifestations of tardive dyskinesia; fine vermicular movements of the tongue reportedly may be an early sign. However, do not forget that neuroleptic therapy can itself mask the signs and symptoms of tardive dyskinesia. If evidence of the syndrome is seen, consider terminating use of the drug, bearing in mind that some patients may require continued antipsychotic treatment despite the development of dyskinesia. There is no known treatment for tardive dyskinesia; however, after discontinuation, some or all manifestations of this syndrome may disappear spontaneously.

Other extrapyramidal reactions — Extrapyramidal reactions other than tardive dyskinesia occur frequently, especially during the first few days of treatment. Although most cases are characterized by mild to moderately severe pseudoparkinsonism, other reactions, including dystonias and akathisia, do occur and often are more severe. Extrapyramidal effects are generally dose-related and can usually be alleviated by a reduction in dosage; however, severe reactions have been seen at relatively low dosages. Antiparkinson drugs such as benztropine or trihexyphenidyl may be necessary for control of reactions; if effects persist, withdrawal of the drug may be required.

Convulsions — Haloperidol can lower the convulsive threshold; use with caution in patients who are receiving anticonvulsants and in those who have EEG abnormalities or a history of seizures

Concomitant lithium therapy — May result in an encephalopathic syndrome characterized by weakness, lethargy, fever, tremulousness and confusion, extrapyramidal symptoms, leukocytosis, and elevated serum enzymes, BUN, and FBS, followed by irreversible brain damage. Although a causal relationship has not been established, patients should be monitored closely for early evidence of neurological toxicity and concomitant therapy discontinued promptly if such signs appear.

HALDOL

Bronchopneumonia	May occur; monitor patients, especially the elderly, and initiate remedial therapy promptly if signs of dehydration, hemoconcentration, or reduced pulmonary ventilation develop
Mental and/or physical impairment	Caution ambulatory patients that their ability to drive or perform other potentially hazardous activities may be impaired, and to avoid alcohol, since it may cause further CNS depression and hypotension when used with this drug
Patients with severe cardiovascular disorders	Haloperidol may cause transient hypotension and/or precipitate anginal pain; use with caution. If hypotension occurs and use of a vasopressor is warranted, administer metaraminol, phenylephrine, or norepinephrine; *do not use epinephrine.*
Patients receiving anticoagulants	Haloperidol has, in one instance, interfered with the action of phenindione; use with caution
Patients receiving antiparkinson agents	To avoid extrapyramidal symptoms, it may be necessary to continue required antiparkinson medication after haloperidol is discontinued because of different excretion rates; the anticholinergic action of antiparkinson agents should also be kept in mind when treating patients who may be affected by an increase in intraocular pressure
Patients with manic-depressive illness	Haloperidol may cause a rapid mood swing to depression when used to control manic episodes in patients with cyclic disorders
Patients with thyrotoxicosis	Haloperidol may cause severe neurotoxicity, characterized by rigidity and an inability to walk or talk, in such patients
Other special-risk patients	Use with caution in patients with known allergies or a history of allergic reactions to drugs
Abrupt discontinuation of therapy	May produce transient dyskinesias; withdraw haloperidol gradually
Neuroleptic malignant syndrome	Haloperidol can cause the neuroleptic malignant syndrome (NMS), a potentially fatal reaction whose cardinal features are hyperpyrexia, muscle rigidity, mental changes (including catatonia), and irregular pulse or blood pressure; other manifestations of NMS include rhabdomyolysis, elevated serum CPK level, myoglobinuria, and acute renal failure. If NMS occurs, institute intensive symptomatic therapy and immediately discontinue the drug.
Carcinogenicity	Chronic use of antipsychotic drugs causes a persistent elevation of the serum prolactin level, an effect that may be of potential importance if the patient has prolactin-dependent breast cancer. In 18-mo studies with female mice, haloperidol has produced increases in tumors found throughout the body and mammary neoplasia in particular at 5 times the maximum initial human dosage and has caused an increase in pituitary neoplasia at the same dosage; however, no increase in the incidence of neoplasia has been shown in rats fed up to 20 times the usual human daily dose for 24 mo. Endocrine disturbances have been seen in humans. Although no clinical or epidemiological studies have shown an association between chronic antipsychotic therapy and mammary tumorigenesis, the available evidence is considered too limited to be conclusive at this time.
Tartrazine sensitivity	Presence of FD&C Yellow No. 5 (tartrazine) in 1-, 5-, and 10-mg tablets may cause allergic-type reactions, including bronchial asthma, in susceptible individuals

ADVERSE REACTIONS[4]

Central nervous system	Extrapyramidal reactions, including pseudoparkinsonism, motor restlessness, dystonia, tardive dystonia, akathisia, hyperreflexia, opisthotonos, oculogyric crisis, and tardive dyskinesia; insomnia, restlessness, anxiety, euphoria, agitation, drowsiness, depression, lethargy, headache, confusion, vertigo, grand mal seizures, and exacerbation of psychotic symptoms, including hallucinations and catatonic-like states
Ophthalmic	Cataracts, retinopathy, visual disturbances
Cardiovascular	Tachycardia, hypotension, hypertension, ECG changes
Hematological	Leukopenia, leukocytosis, minimal decrease in red-blood-cell counts, anemia, lymphomonocytosis; agranulocytosis (rare)
Dermatological	Maculopapular and acneform skin reactions, photosensitivity, alopecia; local tissue reactions (with use of haloperidol decanoate)
Endocrinological	Lactation, breast engorgement, mastalgia, menstrual irregularities, gynecomastia, impotence, increased libido, hyperglycemia, hypoglycemia, hyponatremia
Gastrointestinal	Anorexia, constipation, diarrhea, hypersalivation, dyspepsia, nausea, vomiting
Autonomic nervous system	Dry mouth, blurred vision, urinary retention, diaphoresis, priapism
Hepatic	Impaired function, jaundice
Respiratory	Laryngospasm, bronchospasm, increased depth of respiration
Other	Hyperpyrexia, heat stroke, neuroleptic malignant syndrome

OVERDOSAGE

Signs and symptoms	Severe extrapyramidal reactions (muscular weakness or rigidity and tremor), hypotension, sedation, coma, respiratory depression (see ADVERSE REACTIONS)

HALDOL ■ LOXITANE

Treatment	Empty stomach by emesis or gastric lavage, followed by administration of activated charcoal. Institute supportive measures, as required. Establish a patent airway using an oropharyngeal airway or endotracheal tube or, in prolonged cases of coma, by tracheostomy. For respiratory depression, employ artificial respiration and a mechanical respirator. Combat hypotension and circulatory collapse with IV fluids, plasma, or concentrated albumin and vasopressor agents, such as metaraminol, phenylephrine, or norepinephrine. *Do not use epinephrine.* For severe extrapyramidal symptoms, administer antiparkinson medication for several weeks and then withdraw very cautiously, as extrapyramidal symptoms may reemerge.

DRUG INTERACTIONS

Alcohol	Severe hypotension △ Alcohol intoxication
CNS depressants	△ CNS depression
Anticonvulsants	▽ Convulsion threshold
Epinephrine	Severe hypotension
Antihypertensives	Excessive hypotension
Antimuscarinics	△ Intraocular pressure ▽ Effect of haloperidol in schizophrenic patients
Amphetamines	▽ Amphetamine effect
Lithium	△ Risk of encephalopathic syndrome, characterized by weakness, lethargy, fever, tremulousness, confusion, extrapyramidal symptoms, leukocytes, elevated serum enzymes, BUN, and FBS, followed by irreversible brain damage; discontinue use and closely monitor patients on combined therapy if early signs of neurological toxicity appear

ALTERED LABORATORY VALUES

No clinically significant alterations in blood/serum or urinary values occur at therapeutic dosages

USE IN CHILDREN

See INDICATIONS and ORAL DOSAGE. Not recommended for use in children under 3 yr of age. The safety and effectiveness of IM administration and use of the long-acting form in children have not been established.

USE IN PREGNANT AND NURSING WOMEN

Pregnancy Category C: rodents given up to 3 times the maximum human dose have shown an increase in resorption, fetal mortality, and pup mortality; cleft palate has been observed in the offspring of mice receiving oral haloperidol at doses 15 times the usual maximum human dose. There are two reports of neonatal limb malformations during maternal use of haloperidol along with other drugs with suspected teratogenic potential during the first trimester of pregnancy; however, no causal relationship has been established. No adequate, well-controlled studies have been done in pregnant women; use during pregnancy only if the expected benefit justifies the potential risk to the fetus. Nursing is not advisable during haloperidol therapy.

[1] As the lactate salt
[2] Severely disturbed, psychotic children may require higher dosages. There is little evidence that therapeutic effectiveness in children with nonpsychotic behavioral disorders is further enhanced by dosages exceeding 6 mg/day.
[3] As the decanoate ester
[4] Sudden, unexpected death has also been reported, but a causal relationship has not been established; decreases in the serum cholesterol level, with or without cutaneous and ocular changes, have been associated with drugs chemically related to haloperidol

---

DIBENZOXAZEPINES

LOXITANE (loxapine succinate) Lederle   Rx
Capsules: 5, 10, 25, 50 mg

LOXITANE C (loxapine hydrochloride) Lederle   Rx
Concentrate: 25 mg/ml (120 ml)

LOXITANE IM (loxapine hydrochloride) Lederle   Rx
Ampuls: 50 mg/ml (1 ml) for IM use only   **Vials:** 50 mg/ml (10 ml) for IM use only

INDICATIONS	ORAL DOSAGE	PARENTERAL DOSAGE
Manifestations of **psychotic disorders**	**Adult:** 10 mg bid to start, followed by a rapid increase in dosage over 7–10 days, up to 250 mg/day, until symptoms are controlled; usual dosage: 60–100 mg/day, given in divided doses 2–4 times/day; for severe symptoms, up to 50 mg/day to start. Mix concentrate with orange or grapefruit juice just before administration.	**Adult:** 12.5–50 mg IM (*not IV*) q4–6h or longer, adjusted according to patient response (many patients respond satisfactorily to bid dosing); replace with oral medication once acute symptoms are controlled and patient is able to take medication orally, usually within 5 days

LOXITANE

CONTRAINDICATIONS

| Hypersensitivity to loxapine | Drug-induced CNS depression | Comatose states |

WARNINGS/PRECAUTIONS

Tardive dyskinesia — Neuroleptic drugs can cause tardive dyskinesia, a potentially irreversible syndrome characterized by involuntary choreoathetoid movements of the tongue, face, mouth, lips, jaw, trunk, and/or extremities. Protrusion of the tongue, puffing of the cheeks, puckering of the mouth, chewing movements, and other manifestations may become evident during treatment, upon dosage reduction, or after the drug is discontinued. The likelihood that tardive dyskinesia will develop or become irreversible increases with duration of treatment and total cumulative dose; however, even relatively brief use of low doses can cause it. Although this reaction appears to occur most often in the elderly, especially among older women, it is impossible to use this information to predict, before therapy is started, which patients are likely to develop the syndrome.

In general, reserve chronic therapy for patients who respond to neuroleptics and who cannot undergo another, equally effective form of treatment that is potentially less harmful. Use the lowest effective dosage, keep the duration of therapy as short as possible, and periodically reassess the need for the drug. Watch carefully for manifestations of tardive dyskinesia; fine vermicular movements of the tongue reportedly may be an early sign. However, do not forget that neuroleptic therapy can itself mask the signs and symptoms of tardive dyskinesia. If evidence of the syndrome is seen, consider terminating use of the drug, bearing in mind that some patients may require continued neuroleptic treatment despite the development of dyskinesia. There is no known treatment for tardive dyskinesia; however, after discontinuation, some or all manifestations of this syndrome may disappear spontaneously.

Other extrapyramidal reactions — To control akathisia and parkinson-like symptoms, reduce dosage or use an antiparkinson drug; for dystonias and dyskinesias other tardive dyskinesia, institute appropriate drug therapy and, if necessary, reduce dosage of loxapine or temporarily discontinue use of the drug

Intramuscular therapy — Extrapyramidal reactions may occur slightly more frequently with IM use than with oral therapy, possibly as a result of the higher serum level following injection

Mental and/or physical impairment — Caution ambulatory patients that their ability to drive or engage in other activities requiring alertness may be impaired, and that use of alcohol or other CNS depressants may cause further impairment

Seizures — May occur in epileptic patients despite anticonvulsant therapy; use with extreme caution in patients with a history of convulsive disorders

Antiemetic effect — May mask signs and symptoms of overdosage of other drugs and such conditions as intestinal obstruction and brain tumor

Patients with cardiovascular disease — Loxapine may increase the pulse rate and/or cause transient hypotension; use with caution

Other special-risk patients — Use with caution in patients with glaucoma or a tendency toward urinary retention, particularly with concomitant anticholinergic antiparkinson agents

Ocular changes — Have occurred during prolonged therapy with other antipsychotics; monitor patients for pigmentary retinopathy and lenticular pigmentation

Carcinogenicity — Chronic therapy may cause a persistent elevation of serum prolactin levels, which may be of importance in patients with previously detected breast cancer (one third of human breast cancers are prolactin-dependent in vitro). Although endocrine disturbances have been reported, no association between chronic neuroleptic administration and mammary tumorigenesis has been demonstrated. No neoplastic changes have been seen in rats after chronic oral administration of up to twice the human dose of loxapine; however, the available evidence is considered too limited to be conclusive at this time.

Mutagenicity — No evidence of mutagenicity has been observed in microbial assays or in the mouse micronucleus test

Effect on fertility — No effect on fertility has been detected in rabbits or dogs given oral or IM doses up to twice the human dose or in male rats that were given oral doses within the human therapeutic range. However, persistent diestrus and failure to copulate have been seen in female rats who were fed doses within the human therapeutic range before mating, and pregnancy occurred less frequently in female mice who were fed twice the human dose from 5 days after copulation until late gestation. These reactions resulted, though, from doses at least 40 times the level that is pharmacologically effective in these species.

ADVERSE REACTIONS

Frequent reactions (incidence $\geq$ 1%) are printed in *italics*

Central nervous system and neuromuscular — *Rigidity (27%), tremor (22%), akathisia (20%), dystonia (7%), drowsiness (11%), insomnia, confusion, excessive salivation, dizziness, parkinsonism,* agitation, tension, seizures, akinesia, dyskinesia (including tardive dyskinesia), slurred speech, shuffling gait, weakness, paresthesia, numbness, headache, neuroleptic malignant syndrome

Gastrointestinal — *Nausea,* vomiting, paralytic ileus, constipation

Cardiovascular	*Tachycardia,* hypotension (including orthostatic hypotension), syncope, flushing, hypertension
Endocrinological	Galactorrhea, amenorrhea, gynecomastia, menstrual irregularity
Respiratory	Nasal congestion, dyspnea
Hematological	Agranulocytosis, thrombocytopenia, and leukopenia (rare)
Dermatological	Rash and alopecia (rare)
Other	*Blurred vision, dry mouth,* urinary retention, hyperpyrexia, weight changes, ptosis, polydipsia[1]

OVERDOSAGE

Signs and symptoms	Varies from mild CNS and cardiovascular depression to profound hypotension, respiratory depression, and unconsciousness; extrapyramidal symptoms, convulsions, and renal failure may also occur
Treatment	Empty stomach by gastric lavage. Maintain patent airway. *Do not induce emesis.* Treat severe extrapyramidal symptoms with antiparkinson drugs or diphenhydramine, and initiate standard anticonvulsant therapy, if indicated. Avoid use of convulsion-inducing stimulants (eg, picrotoxin or pentylenetetrazol). Employ standard measures for circulatory shock. Restrict use of vasoconstrictors to norepinephrine and phenylephrine; *do not use epinephrine.* Extended dialysis is likely to be beneficial. Additional supportive measures include oxygen and IV fluids.

DRUG INTERACTIONS

Epinephrine	Severe hypotension
Alcohol, anesthetics, barbiturates, narcotics, and other CNS depressants	⬆ CNS depression
Antidepressants	⬆ Serum antidepressant level; adjust antidepressant dosage, if necessary

ALTERED LABORATORY VALUES

Blood/serum values	⬆ Liver enzymes

No clinically significant alterations in urinary values occur at therapeutic dosages

USE IN CHILDREN

Not recommended for use in children under 16 yr of age because studies have not been done in pediatric patients

USE IN PREGNANT AND NURSING WOMEN

Pregnancy Category C: no teratogenic effects have been observed in mice, rats, rabbits, or dogs given oral or IM doses up to twice the maximum recommended human dose. Fetotoxicity (increased resorptions, decreased fetal weight) has been demonstrated in mice and rats given doses within the human therapeutic range, but has not been shown in rabbits or dogs given oral or IM doses up to twice the human dose; these reactions resulted from doses at least 50 times the level that is pharmacologically effective in these species. Renal papillary abnormalities have occurred in the offspring of rats who were given 0.6 and 1.8 mg/kg (usual human doses) from the middle of pregnancy until birth. No adequate, well-controlled studies have been performed in pregnant women; use during pregnancy only if the expected benefits justify the potential risk to the fetus. Loxapine has been detected in the milk of lactating dogs; however, it is not known whether this drug is excreted in human milk. If possible, avoid use in nursing mothers.

[1] Other reactions for which a causal relationship has not been established include jaundice and hepatitis

---

DIHYDROINDOLONES

MOBAN (molindone hydrochloride) Du Pont Rx

Tablets: 5, 10, 25, 50, 100 mg **Concentrate:** 20 mg/ml (120 ml)

INDICATIONS

Manifestations of **psychotic disorders**

ORAL DOSAGE

Adult: 50–75 mg/day to start, followed in 3–4 days by an increase to 100 mg/day and then, if necessary, by further increases, up to 225 mg/day; for maintenance, 5–15 mg tid or qid in mild conditions, 10–25 mg tid or qid in moderate conditions, or up to 225 mg/day in severe conditions

CONTRAINDICATIONS

Severe drug-induced CNS depression	Comatose states	Hypersensitivity to molindone

MOBAN

ADMINISTRATION/DOSAGE ADJUSTMENTS

Elderly or debilitated patients	Initiate therapy at a lower dosage

WARNINGS/PRECAUTIONS

Tardive dyskinesia	Neuroleptic drugs can cause tardive dyskinesia, a potentially irreversible syndrome characterized by involuntary choreoathetoid movements of the tongue, face, mouth, lips, jaw, trunk, and/or extremities. Protrusion of the tongue, puffing of the cheeks, puckering of the mouth, chewing movements, and other manifestations may become evident during treatment, upon dosage reduction, or after the drug is discontinued. The likelihood that tardive dyskinesia will develop or become irreversible increases with duration of treatment and total cumulative dose; however, even relatively brief use of low doses can cause it. Although this reaction appears to occur most often in the elderly, especially among older women, it is impossible to use this information to predict, before therapy is started, which patients are likely to develop the syndrome. In general, reserve chronic therapy for patients who respond to neuroleptics and who cannot undergo another, equally effective form of treatment that is potentially less harmful. Use the lowest effective dosage, keep the duration of therapy as short as possible, and periodically reassess the need for the drug. Watch carefully for manifestations of tardive dyskinesia; fine vermicular movements of the tongue reportedly may be an early sign. However, do not forget that neuroleptic therapy can itself mask the signs and symptoms of tardive dyskinesia. If evidence of the syndrome is seen, consider terminating use of the drug, bearing in mind that some patients may require continued neuroleptic treatment despite the development of dyskinesia. There is no known treatment for tardive dyskinesia; however, after discontinuation, some or all manifestations of this syndrome may disappear spontaneously.
Drowsiness	Caution patients not to drive or engage in other activities requiring mental alertness until their response to molindone has been established
Increased activity	May occur; use with caution in patients in whom increased activity may be harmful
Convulsive seizures	May occur, although molindone does not lower the seizure threshold in experimental animals to the degree noted with more sedating antipsychotic drugs
Antiemetic action	May mask signs and symptoms of intestinal obstruction or brain damage
Patients with previously detected breast cancer	Use with caution, as chronic therapy may cause a persistent elevation of serum prolactin levels, which may be of importance in patients with prolactin-dependent breast cancers. Although endocrine disturbances have been reported, no association between chronic neuroleptic administration and mammary tumorigenesis has been demonstrated; the avaliable evidence is considered too limited to be conclusive at this time.
Dystonic syndrome	Prolonged abnormal contractions of muscle groups may occur, albeit infrequently; if symptoms develop, reduce antipsychotic dosage, add a synthetic antiparkinson agent other than levodopa to the regimen, and/or administer small doses of sedatives
Sulfite sensitivity	Sodium metabisulfite in this product may cause urticaria, pruritus, wheezing, anaphylaxis, or other allergic-type reactions in susceptible patients, such as those with asthma or atopy

ADVERSE REACTIONS

Central nervous system	Drowsiness; depression; hyperactivity; euphoria; extrapyramidal symptoms, including akathisia, parkinson syndrome (akinesia, characterized by rigidity, immobility, reduction of voluntary movements, and tremor), dystonia, and tardive dyskinesia
Autonomic nervous system	Blurred vision, tachycardia, nausea, dry mouth, salivation, urinary retention, constipation
Hematological	Leukopenia and leukocytosis (rare)
Hepatic	Abnormal liver function values
Metabolic and endocrinological	Amenorrhea, resumption of menses in previously amenorrheic women, insignificant changes in thyroid function, heavy menses, galactorrhea, gynecomastia, increased libido, weight changes
Cardiovascular	Hypotension and transient nonspecific ECG changes (rare)
Dermatological	Rash

OVERDOSAGE

Signs and symptoms	See ADVERSE REACTIONS
Treatment	Treat symptomatically and institute supportive measures, as required. Empty stomach by gastric lavage. Treat extrapyramidal symptoms with diphenhydramine, amantadine, or a synthetic anticholinergic antiparkinson agent. Forced diuresis, peritoneal dialysis, or renal dialysis would not significantly increase the rate of removal of unmetabolized molindone from the body. Emesis is contraindicated in comatose patients.

DRUG INTERACTIONS

No clinically significant drug interactions have been reported with molindone; however, tablets contain calcium sulfate (as an excipient), which may interfere with the absorption of phenytoin sodium and tetracyclines

ALTERED LABORATORY VALUES

Blood/serum values —————————— Abnormal liver function tests

No clinically significant alterations in urinary values occur at therapeutic dosages

USE IN CHILDREN

Not recommended for use in children under 12 yr of age; the safety and effectiveness of this drug have not been established in children

USE IN PREGNANT AND NURSING WOMEN

Studies in pregnant patients have not been carried out; animal reproduction studies have shown no evidence of teratogenicity. Data are not available on the content of molindone in breast milk.

PHENOTHIAZINES

COMPAZINE (prochlorperazine) Smith Kline & French   Rx

Capsules (sustained release): 10, 15, 30 mg **Tablets:** 5, 10, 25 mg **Syrup (per 5 ml):** 5 mg (4 fl oz) *fruit flavored* **Ampuls:** 5 mg/ml (2 ml) **Vials:** 5 mg/ml (10 ml) **Prefilled syringes:** 5 mg/ml (2 ml) **Rectal suppositories:** 2.5, 5, 25 mg

INDICATIONS	ORAL DOSAGE	PARENTERAL DOSAGE
Severe nausea and vomiting	**Adult:** 5–10 mg tid or qid or, if sustained-release capsules are used, 15 mg on arising or 10 mg q12h **Child (20–29 lb):** 2.5 mg 1–2 times/day, up to 7.5 mg/day **Child (30–39 lb):** 2.5 mg bid or tid, up to 10 mg/day **Child (40–85 lb):** 2.5 mg tid or 5 mg bid, up to 15 mg/day	**Adult:** 5–10 mg IM to start, repeated q3–4h, as needed, up to 40 mg/day. For preoperative use, give 5–10 mg IM 1–2 h before induction of anesthesia (if necessary, dose may be repeated after 30 min); alternatively, give either 5–10 mg by IV injection or 20 mg by IV infusion 15–30 min before induction of anesthesia. To control acute reactions during or after surgery, administer 5–10 mg by IM or IV injection (if necessary, dose may be repeated once). **Child:** 0.06 mg/lb IM
Manifestations of **psychotic disorders**	**Adult:** for office patients and outpatients, 5–10 mg tid or qid; for hospitalized or otherwise closely supervised patients, 10 mg tid or qid to start, followed, if necessary, by small increases in dosage every 2–3 days, up to 50–75 mg/day or, in more severe cases, up to 100–150 mg/day **Child (2–12 yr):** 2.5 mg bid or tid, up to 10 mg on 1st day, followed by increases in dosage up to 20 mg/day (2–5 yr) or 25 mg/day (6–12 yr), as needed	**Adult:** for severe cases, 10–20 mg IM to start, repeated q2–4h (in resistant cases, every hour) as needed; for prolonged therapy, 10–20 mg IM q4–6h **Child (< 12 yr):** 0.06 mg/lb IM
Generalized **nonpsychotic anxiety**[1]	**Adult:** 5 mg tid or qid or, if sustained-release capsules are used, 15 mg on arising or 10 mg q12h; do not exceed 20 mg/day or administer for more than 12 wk	—

CONTRAINDICATIONS

Age < 2 yr or weight < 20 lb
Use in pediatric surgery

Presence of large amounts of CNS depressants

Coma

ADMINISTRATION/DOSAGE ADJUSTMENTS

Initial dosage titration —————— Adjust dosage according to individual response and severity of the condition; begin with the lowest recommended dose

Parenteral administration —————— Administer IM by injecting solution deeply into the upper outer quadrant of the buttock; because of local irritation, SC administration is inadvisable. For IV injection, dilute dose in an isotonic solution or give undiluted; rate of administration should not exceed 5 mg/min (do not give as a bolus). For IV infusion, dilute 20 mg in at least 1 liter of isotonic solution and then add to the primary IV solution. Do not mix prochlorperazine with other drugs; do not dilute the contents of the ampuls with any solution that contains parabens.

COMPAZINE

Rectal dosage	For severe nausea and vomiting in adults, give 25 mg bid. For children, rectal dosages are the same as oral dosages.
Elderly, emaciated, or debilitated patients	Increase dosage more gradually if the patient is elderly, emaciated, or debilitated; for most elderly patients, a dosage in the lower range is sufficient. Carefully monitor clinical response of elderly patients since they appear to be more susceptible to hypotension and extrapyramidal reactions; elderly patients with brain damage are especially susceptible to extrapyramidal effects.
Monitoring of long-term therapy	Periodically evaluate patients with a history of long-term neuroleptic treatment in order to determine whether the maintenance dosage can be reduced or therapy discontinued; watch for tardive dyskinesia, ocular changes, and skin pigmentation during prolonged use

WARNINGS/PRECAUTIONS

Tardive dyskinesia	Neuroleptic drugs can cause tardive dyskinesia, a potentially irreversible syndrome characterized by involuntary choreoathetoid movements of the tongue, face, mouth, lips, jaw, trunk, and/or extremities. Protrusion of the tongue, puffing of the cheeks, puckering of the mouth, chewing movements, and other manifestations may become evident during treatment, upon dosage reduction, or after the drug is discontinued. The likelihood that tardive dyskinesia will develop or become irreversible increases with duration of treatment and total cumulative dose; however, even relatively brief use of low doses can cause it. Although this reaction appears to occur most often in the elderly, especially among older women, it is impossible to use this information to predict, before therapy is started, which patients are likely to develop the syndrome.

In general, reserve chronic therapy for patients who respond to neuroleptics and who cannot undergo another, equally effective form of treatment that is potentially less harmful. Use the lowest effective dosage, keep the duration of therapy as short as possible, and periodically reassess the need for the drug. Watch carefully for manifestations of tardive dyskinesia; fine vermicular movements of the tongue reportedly may be an early sign. However, do not forget that neuroleptic therapy can itself mask the signs and symptoms of tardive dyskinesia. If evidence of the syndrome is seen, consider terminating use of the drug, bearing in mind that some patients may require continued neuroleptic treatment despite the development of dyskinesia. There is no known treatment for tardive dyskinesia; however, after discontinuation, some or all manifestations of this syndrome may disappear spontaneously. |
Dystonias	To control dystonias, discontinue neuroleptic therapy and take the following measures: for mild cases, provide reassurance or give a barbiturate; for moderate cases, use a barbiturate; for more severe cases, administer an antiparkinson agent other than levodopa; for children, provide reassurance and give either a barbiturate or parenteral diphenhydramine. If antiparkinson agents or diphenhydramine fail to reverse signs and symptoms, reevaluate diagnosis. Appropriate supportive measures, such as those needed to maintain adequate hydration and a patent airway, should be instituted as required. Dystonias usually subside within a few hours and almost always within 24–48 h after the drug has been discontinued. If treatment is resumed, administer at a lower dosage.
Akathisia	Symptoms of akathisia often disappear spontaneously; if they become too troublesome, reduce dosage or give a barbiturate. Wait until effects subside before increasing dosage. At times, drug-induced symptoms of akathisia may resemble psychotic or neurotic manifestations seen before therapy.
Pseudoparkinsonism	In most cases, pseudoparkinsonism can be controlled by concomitant use of an antiparkinson agent other than levodopa; occasionally, it is necessary to reduce the dosage of prochlorperazine or discontinue the drug. Administration of antiparkinson drugs for a period ranging from a few weeks to 2–3 mo is generally sufficient; clinical response should be evaluated before continuing therapy for a longer period. Reassurance and sedation are also important in the treatment of pseudoparkinsonism.
Convulsions	Phenothiazines can precipitate petit or grand mal convulsions, particularly in patients with EEG abnormalities or a history of such disorders
Cross-sensitivity	Do not use prochlorperazine in patients with a history of hypersensitivity to a phenothiazine unless potential benefits outweigh possible risks; see also warnings below concerning hepatotoxicity and blood dyscrasias
Hepatotoxicity	Cholestatic jaundice has occurred. If fever with grippe-like symptoms occurs, perform appropriate liver tests; if an abnormality is detected, stop treatment. Do not give prochlorperazine to patients with a history of phenothiazine-induced jaundice unless the potential benefits outweigh the possible risks. Since this drug is potentially hepatotoxic, use in children or adolescents with signs or symptoms suggesting Reye's syndrome should be avoided. Fatty changes have been detected in the livers of patients who died during treatment; however, no causal relationship has been established.
Blood dyscrasias	Agranulocytosis and leukopenia can occur during therapy. Caution patients to report the sudden appearance of sore throat or other signs or symptoms of infection; if signs of infection are seen and WBC and differential counts are depressed, stop therapy and institute appropriate measures. Do not give prochlorperazine to patients with bone marrow depression or a history of phenothiazine-induced blood dyscrasias unless the potential benefits outweigh the possible risks.

COMPAZINE

Hypotension	Prochlorperazine can cause hypotension. In patients with mitral insufficiency or pheochromocytoma, certain phenothiazines have produced severe hypotension. To minimize risk of hypotension, keep all patients lying down and under observation for at least 30 min after the initial injection. Exercise caution when giving prochlorperazine parenterally or in large doses to patients with cardiovascular dysfunction. If hypotension occurs, place patient in a head-low position with the legs raised; if a vasopressor is needed, use norepinephrine or phenylephrine, not epinephrine.
Masking of nonpsychotic conditions	Extrapyramidal symptoms associated with prochlorperazine may be confused with the neurological manifestations of an undiagnosed primary disease such as Reye's syndrome or another encephalopathy; antiemetic effect may mask nausea and vomiting associated with intestinal obstruction, brain tumor, Reye's syndrome, or toxicity of antineoplastic agents or other drugs
Drowsiness	Caution patients about driving and engaging in other activities requiring mental alertness; drowsiness may occur, especially during the first few days of therapy
Sedation, coma	Deep sleep and coma have occurred, usually as a result of overdosage
Contact dermatitis	To prevent contact dermatitis, avoid getting injectable solution on hands or clothing
Glaucoma	Prochlorperazine may exacerbate glaucoma; use with caution in patients with glaucoma
Extreme heat	Phenothiazines may affect thermal homeostasis; use with caution in patients who will be exposed to extreme heat
Aspiration of vomitus	During postsurgical recovery, aspiration of vomitus has occurred in a few patients given prochlorperazine; bear in mind this risk even though no causal relationship has been established
Sudden death	Patients taking phenothiazines have occasionally died suddenly; in some cases, death appeared to result from cardiac arrest or from asphyxia due to failure of the cough reflex
Abrupt withdrawal	Nausea, vomiting, dizziness, and tremulousness may occur following abrupt discontinuation of high-dose therapy
Carcinogenicity	Chronic use of neuroleptic drugs causes a persistent elevation of the serum prolactin level, an effect that may be of potential importance if the patient has prolactin-dependent breast cancer. Chronic administration has produced an increase in mammary neoplasia in rodents, and endocrine disturbances have been seen in humans; although no clinical or epidemiological studies have shown an association between chronic neuroleptic therapy and mammary tumorigenesis, the available evidence is considered too limited to be conclusive at this time.

ADVERSE REACTIONS[2]

Central nervous system	Drowsiness, dystonias (spasm of neck muscles, torticollis, extensor rigidity of back muscles, opisthotonos, carpopedal spasm, trismus, swallowing difficulty, oculogyric crisis, protrusion of the tongue), akathisia (agitation, jitteriness, insomnia), pseudoparkinsonism (mask-like facies, drooling, tremors, pill-rolling motion, cogwheel rigidity, shuffling gait), tardive dyskinesia, tardive dystonia, hyperreflexia, dyskinesia, reactivation of psychosis, catatonic-like states, grand mal and petit mal seizures, cerebral edema, CSF protein abnormalities, coma
Ophthalmic	Blurred vision, miosis, mydriasis, pigmentary retinopathy; corneal and lenticular deposits and epithelial keratopathy (with prolonged use of substantial doses)
Cardiovascular	Hypotension, dizziness, headache, ECG changes (especially distortions of Q and T waves), cardiac arrest, peripheral edema
Hematological	Agranulocytosis, eosinophilia, leukopenia, hemolytic anemia, aplastic anemia, thrombocytopenic purpura, pancytopenia
Gastrointestinal	Jaundice, biliary stasis, nausea, constipation, obstipation, adynamic ileus, atonic colon
Genitourinary	Priapism, ejaculatory disorders/impotence, urinary retention
Endocrinological	Hyperglycemia, hypoglycemia, glucosuria, lactation, galactorrhea, amenorrhea, menstrual irregularities, gynecomastia
Dermatological	Hypersensitivity reactions (see below); skin pigmentation (with prolonged use of substantial doses)
Hypersensitivity	Jaundice, blood dyscrasias, asthma, laryngeal edema, angioneurotic edema, anaphylactoid reactions, urticaria, pruritus, erythema, eczema, photosensitivity, contact dermatitis, exfoliative dermatitis
Other	Dry mouth, nasal congestion, mild fever (with large IM doses), hyperthermia (especially with exposure to extreme heat), hyperpyrexia, increased appetite, weight gain, systemic lupus erythematosus-like syndrome, enhanced effect of organophosphorous insecticides; neuroleptic malignant syndrome, a potentially fatal reaction characterized by hyperthermia, altered consciousness, muscular rigidity, and autonomic dysfunction

COMPAZINE

OVERDOSAGE

Signs and symptoms	Extrapyramidal effects (see ADVERSE REACTIONS), CNS depression, deep sleep, coma, agitation, restlessness, convulsions, fever, hypotension, dry mouth, ileus
Treatment	Empty stomach by gastric lavage, repeated several times. *Do not induce emesis.* For respiratory depression, administer oxygen and, if needed, perform a tracheostomy, and assist ventilation. For extrapyramidal reactions, keep patient under observation and maintain open airway. Treat extrapyramidal symptoms with antiparkinson drugs (except levodopa), barbiturates, or diphenhydramine. For hypotension, employ standard measures. If a vasoconstrictor is indicated, use norepinephrine or phenylephrine; other pressor agents may lower blood pressure further. Use saline cathartics to hasten evacuation of pellets that have not already released medication. Continue supportive therapy as long as overdosage symptoms remain.

DRUG INTERACTIONS

Other CNS depressants, including alcohol	△ CNS depression
Anticonvulsants	△ Risk of convulsions; adjustment of anticonvulsant dosage may be necessary △ Pharmacologic effect of phenytoin
Metrizamide	△ Risk of convulsions; discontinue use of prochlorperazine at least 48 h before administration of metrizamide for myelography and wait at least 24 h after the procedure before resuming use. Do not use prochlorperazine before or after myelography for control of nausea and vomiting.
Anticholinergic drugs	△ Anticholinergic effects ▽ Antipsychotic effect
Epinephrine	Severe hypotension
Guanethidine	▽ Antihypertensive effect
Thiazide diuretics	△ Orthostatic hypotensive effect
Propranolol	△ Pharmacologic effects of propranolol and prochlorperazine
Amphetamines	▽ Antipsychotic effect ▽ Anorectic effect
Phenmetrazine	▽ Anorectic effect
Lithium	△ Risk of acute encephalopathy and extrapyramidal reactions ▽ Serum prochlorperazine level △ Renal clearance of lithium
Tricyclic antidepressants	△ Serum level of tricyclic antidepressants and prochlorperazine ▽ Antipsychotic effect
Oral anticoagulants	▽ Anticoagulant effect

ALTERED LABORATORY VALUES

Blood/serum values	△ SGOT △ SGPT △ LDH △ Alkaline phosphatase △ Bilirubin △ Prolactin △ or ▽ Glucose
Urinary values	▽ VMA + Glucose + PKU + Pregnancy (with immunologic pregnancy tests) + Bilirubin (with reagent test strips) △ Urobilinogen (with Ehrlich's reagent test) ▽ 5-HIAA (with nitrosonaphthol reagent test) Interference with determination of catecholamines (with Pisano method), 17-KS (with Haltorff-Koch modification of Zimmerman reaction), and 17-OHCS (with modified Glenn-Nelson technique)

USE IN CHILDREN

See INDICATIONS and dosage recommendations; contraindicated for use in pediatric surgery or children under 2 yr of age. Drug should not be used for conditions in which pediatric dosages have not been established. In children, an IM dose may be effective for up to 12 h. Children appear to be more susceptible to extrapyramidal reactions than adults, even at moderate doses; children who are dehydrated or who have an acute illness such as chicken pox, CNS infection, measles, or gastroenteritis are especially susceptible to these reactions, particularly to dystonias, and therefore must be closely supervised during therapy. If a child experiences an extrapyramidal reaction, discontinue use and do not reinstitute treatment at a later time. Avoid use in children or adolescents with signs or symptoms suggesting Reye's syndrome.

USE IN PREGNANT AND NURSING WOMEN

Jaundice, prolonged extrapyramidal signs, and hyper- and hyporeflexia have been seen in neonates born to mothers who received phenothiazines during pregnancy. Safety for use during pregnancy has not been established; use during pregnancy is not recommended except in serious and intractable cases of severe nausea and vomiting when the potential benefits outweigh possible hazards. If neuromuscular (extrapyramidal) reactions occur in pregnant patients, discontinue therapy and do not reinstitute treatment with prochlorperazine. Phenothiazines are excreted in human milk.

---

[1] For most patients, prochlorperazine is not the initial treatment of choice because certain risks associated with its use are not shared by common alternatives, such as benzodiazepines. It has not been established that this drug is effective in the treatment of anxiety or anxiety-like signs associated with nonpsychotic conditions (eg, physical illness, organic mental conditions, agitated depression, character pathology) other than generalized anxiety disorder.

MELLARIL

PHENOTHIAZINES

MELLARIL (thioridazine hydrochloride) Sandoz Pharmaceuticals Rx
Tablets: 10, 15, 25, 50, 100, 150, 200 mg Concentrate: 30 mg/ml[1] (4 fl oz), 100 mg/ml[2] (4 fl oz)

MELLARIL-S (thioridazine) Sandoz Pharmaceuticals Rx
Suspension (per 5 ml): 25, 100 mg (1 pt) *buttermint-flavored*

INDICATIONS

Manifestations of **psychotic disorders**

Short-term treatment of **moderate to marked depression accompanied by anxiety** in adult patients

Agitation, anxiety, depressed mood, tension, sleep disturbances, fears, and other symptoms in geriatric patients

Severe behavioral problems, marked by combativeness and/or explosive hyperexcitable behavior, in children

Short-term treatment of hyperactive children with **excessive motor activity accompanied by conduct disorders**

ORAL DOSAGE

Adult: 50–100 mg tid to start, followed by a gradual increase, up to 800 mg/day, if necessary (usual dosage: 200–800 mg/day, given in 2–4 divided doses); for maintenance, reduce dosage gradually to lowest effective level

Adult: 10 mg bid to qid for mild cases, or up to 50 mg tid or qid for more severe cases; usual starting dosage, 25 mg tid

Child (2–12 yr): 10 mg bid or tid to start; for severe symptoms, 25 mg bid or tid to start, followed by larger doses until optimum response is obtained or maximum dosage (3 mg/kg/day) is reached

CONTRAINDICATIONS

Extreme hypotensive or hypertensive heart disease

Severe CNS depression

Comatose states

WARNINGS/PRECAUTIONS

Tardive dyskinesia — Neuroleptic drugs can cause tardive dyskinesia, a potentially irreversible syndrome characterized by involuntary choreoathetoid movements of the tongue, face, mouth, lips, jaw, trunk, and/or extremities. Protrusion of the tongue, puffing of the cheeks, puckering of the mouth, chewing movements, and other manifestations may become evident during treatment, upon dosage reduction, or after the drug is discontinued. The likelihood that tardive dyskinesia will develop or become irreversible increases with duration of treatment and total cumulative dose; however, even relatively brief use of low doses can cause it. Although this reaction appears to occur most often in the elderly, especially among older women, it is impossible to use this information to predict, before therapy is started, which patients are likely to develop the syndrome.

In general, reserve chronic therapy for patients who respond to neuroleptics and who cannot undergo another, equally effective form of treatment that is potentially less harmful. Use the lowest effective dosage, keep the duration of therapy as short as possible, and periodically reassess the need for the drug. Since neuroleptic therapy can mask the signs of tardive dyskinesia, reduce the dosage periodically (if clinically feasible); if signs of dyskinesia appear, consider terminating use of the drug, bearing in mind that some patients may require continued neuroleptic treatment despite the development of dyskinesia. There is no known treatment for tardive dyskinesia; however, after discontinuation, some or all manifestations of this syndrome may disappear spontaneously.

Hypersensitivity to phenothiazines — Use with caution in patients with past history of blood dyscrasias or jaundice or similar reactions to phenothiazines

Pigmentary retinopathy — May occur with larger than recommended doses; symptoms include diminished visual acuity, brownish coloring of vision, impaired night vision, and pigment deposits

Leukopenia and/or agranulocytosis — May occur infrequently

Convulsive seizures — May occur; patients taking anticonvulsant medication should continue their regimens

Orthostatic hypotension — Occurs more often in female patients

Mental and/or physical impairment — Drowsiness may occur during therapy, especially when large doses are given at an early stage; this effect tends to subside with continued use or a reduction in dosage. Administer with caution and increase dosage gradually if patients will be engaging in activities requiring full mental alertness.

Elderly patients — May have less tolerance for phenothiazines and may be more likely to develop agranulocytosis and leukopenia than younger patients

Patients with previously detected breast cancer — Use with caution, as chronic therapy may cause a persistent elevation of serum prolactin levels, which may be of importance in patients with prolactin-dependent breast cancers. Although endocrine disturbances have been reported, no association between chronic neuroleptic administration and mammary tumorigenesis has been demonstrated; the available evidence is considered too limited to be conclusive at this time.

High-dose therapy — Daily dosages of 300 mg or more should be reserved for severe neuropsychiatric conditions

MELLARIL ■ PERMITIL

ADVERSE REACTIONS[3]

Central nervous system	Drowsiness; pseudoparkinsonism and other extrapyramidal symptoms; nocturnal confusion, hyperactivity, lethargy, psychotic reactions, restlessness, and headache (extremely rare)
Autonomic nervous system	Dry mouth, blurred vision, constipation, nausea, vomiting, diarrhea, nasal stuffiness, pallor
Endocrinological	Galactorrhea, breast engorgement, amenorrhea, inhibition of ejaculation, peripheral edema
Dermatological	Dermatitis, urticarial skin eruptions; photosensitivity (extremely rare)
Cardiovascular	ECG changes (Q-T prolongation, lowering and inversion of the T-wave, bifid T- or U-wave)
Other	Parotid swelling (rare)

OVERDOSAGE

Signs and symptoms	See ADVERSE REACTIONS
Treatment	Discontinue medication; treat symptomatically and institute supportive measures, as required. Restrict use of vasoconstrictors to norepinephrine and phenylephrine; *do not use epinephrine.*

DRUG INTERACTIONS

Alcohol, anesthetics, barbiturates, narcotics, and other CNS depressants	△ CNS depression
Anticonvulsants	▽ Convulsion threshold
Epinephrine	Severe hypotension
Guanethidine	▽ Antihypertensive effect
Antimuscarinics	△ Atropine-like effect ▽ Thioridazine plasma level
Amphetamines	▽ Amphetamine effect
Antacids containing aluminum and/or magnesium ions	▽ Absorption of thioridazine
MAO inhibitors, tricyclic antidepressants	△ Sedation and antimuscarinic effects

ALTERED LABORATORY VALUES

Urinary values	False-positive or false-negative pregnancy tests △ Bilirubin (false elevation)

No clinically significant alterations in blood/serum values occur at therapeutic dosages

USE IN CHILDREN

See INDICATIONS and ORAL DOSAGE; not intended for use in children under 2 yr of age

USE IN PREGNANT AND NURSING WOMEN

Safety for use during pregnancy has not been established. Although reproduction studies in animals and clinical experience to date have shown no evidence of teratogenicity, thioridazine should be used in pregnant women only when the therapeutic benefits outweigh the possible risks to the mother and fetus. Thioridazine is excreted in human milk.

[1] Contains 3.0% alcohol
[2] Contains 4.2% alcohol
[3] Various other side effects common to phenothiazines in general may occur but have not been specifically reported with thioridazine

PHENOTHIAZINES

PERMITIL (fluphenazine hydrochloride) Schering   Rx

Tablets: 2.5, 5, 10 mg   **Concentrate:** 5 mg/ml[1] (118 ml)

INDICATIONS

Manifestations of **psychotic disorders**

ORAL DOSAGE

Adult: 0.5–10 mg/day, given in divided doses; dosages exceeding 3 mg/day are rarely needed; for maintenance, reduce dosage gradually to lowest effective level

PERMITIL

CONTRAINDICATIONS

- Coma or severe obtundation
- Blood dyscrasias
- Bone-marrow depression
- Hypersensitivity to fluphenazine or related compounds
- Known or suspected subcortical brain damage, with or without hypothalamic damage
- Use of CNS depressants in large doses
- Liver damage

ADMINISTRATION/DOSAGE ADJUSTMENTS

Elderly, debilitated, or adolescent patients	Initiate therapy at reduced dosages
Patients with acute psychosis	Rapid dosage increases may be necessary; however, such patients may respond to doses lower than those required by patients with chronic psychosis
Outpatients	Should receive smaller doses than closely supervised hospitalized patients
Dilution of concentrate	Dilute with water, saline, Seven-Up, homogenized milk, carbonated orange drink, or pineapple, apricot, prune, orange, V-8, tomato, or grapefruit juice; do not mix with beverages containing caffeine (coffee, cola), tannics (tea), or pectinates (apple juice), since physical incompatability may result

WARNINGS/PRECAUTIONS

Tardive dyskinesia	Neuroleptic drugs can cause tardive dyskinesia, a potentially irreversible syndrome characterized by involuntary choreoathetoid movements of the tongue, face, mouth, lips, jaw, trunk, and/or extremities. Protrusion of the tongue, puffing of the cheeks, puckering of the mouth, chewing movements, and other manifestations may become evident during treatment, upon dosage reduction, or after the drug is discontinued. The likelihood that tardive dyskinesia will develop or become irreversible increases with duration of treatment and total cumulative dose; however, even relatively brief use of low doses can cause it. Although this reaction appears to occur most often in the elderly, especially among older women, it is impossible to use this information to predict, before therapy is started, which patients are likely to develop the syndrome. In general, reserve chronic therapy for patients who respond to neuroleptics and who cannot undergo another, equally effective form of treatment that is potentially less harmful. Use the lowest effective dosage, keep the duration of therapy as short as possible, and periodically reassess the need for the drug. Watch carefully for manifestations of tardive dyskinesia; fine vermicular movements of the tongue reportedly may be an early sign. However, do not forget that neuroleptic therapy can itself mask the signs and symptoms of tardive dyskinesia. If evidence of the syndrome is seen, consider terminating use of the drug, bearing in mind that some patients may require continued neuroleptic treatment despite the development of dyskinesia. There is no known treatment for tardive dyskinesia; however, after discontinuation, some or all manifestations of this syndrome may disappear spontaneously.
Other extrapyramidal effects	Extrapyramidal reactions other than tardive dyskinesia can usually be controlled by a reduction in dosage, use of an antiparkinson agent such as benztropine, or a combination of both approaches
Severe, acute hypotension	May occur, especially in patients with mitral insufficiency or pheochromocytoma
Rebound hypertension	May occur in patients with pheochromocytoma
Convulsive threshold	May be lowered in alcohol withdrawal and in patients with convulsive disorders; use fluphenazine with caution and maintain adequate concomitant anticonvulsant therapy
Psychic depression	Use with caution
Drowsiness	May occur, particularly during the 1st or 2nd week; if troublesome, reduce dosage
Mental and/or physical impairment	Caution patients that their ability to drive or engage in other potentially hazardous activities may be impaired
Concurrent administration of CNS depressants	Use opiates, analgesics, antihistamines, barbiturates, and other CNS depressants with caution and at reduced dosages; advise patient to avoid use of alcohol, as response to alcohol may be heightened and additive effects and hypotension may occur
Potentially suicidal patients	Should not have access to large quantities of fluphenazine
Antiemetic effect	May mask signs and symptoms of overdosage of other drugs and such conditions as brain tumors and intestinal obstruction
Adynamic ileus	May occur and, if severe, can result in complications and death; provide close supervision, as patient may fail to seek treatment
Rise in body temperature	May suggest intolerance; if not otherwise explained, discontinue use
Surgical patients	Monitor patients requiring high doses closely for hypotensive phenomena; if necessary, reduce the amount if anesthetic or CNS depressant used
Cross-sensitivity	Use with caution in patients who have previously exhibited severe adverse reactions to other phenothiazines

PERMITIL

Special-risk patients	Use with caution in patients with diminished renal function, respiratory impairment due to acute pulmonary infections, or chronic respiratory disorders (eg, severe asthma or emphysema), in those receiving atropine-like drugs, and in those exposed to extreme heat or phosphorous insecticides
Hepatic and renal function	Should be checked periodically; discontinue use if hepatic abnormalities occur or BUN level rises
Abrupt discontinuation of therapy	May produce gastritis, nausea, vomiting, dizziness, and tremulousness; continue concomitant antiparkinson therapy for several weeks after fluphenazine is withdrawn
Prolonged therapy	May lead to liver damage, corneal and lenticular deposits, and irreversible dyskinesias
Photosensitivity	May occur; caution patients to avoid undue exposure to sunlight
Sudden death	Has occasionally occurred with phenothiazine therapy, and in some instances was attributable to cardiac arrest or asphyxia due to failure of the cough reflex
Blood dyscrasias	May occur; observe patient closely, especially during the 4th to 10th weeks of therapy (when most cases of agranulocytosis have occurred), for the sudden appearance of sore throat or infection. Monitor WBC count and differential; if count is significantly depressed, discontinue use of drug and institute appropriate therapy.
Patients with previously detected breast cancer	Use with caution, as chronic therapy may cause a persistent elevation of serum prolactin levels, which may be of importance in patients with prolactin-dependent breast cancers. Although endocrine disturbances have been reported, no association between chronic neuroleptic administration and mammary tumorigenesis has been demonstrated; the available evidence is considered too limited to be conclusive at this time.
Tartrazine sensitivity	Presence of FD&C Yellow No. 5 (tartrazine) in 0.25-mg tablets may cause allergic-type reactions, including bronchial asthma, in susceptible individuals

ADVERSE REACTIONS[2]

Central nervous system	Extrapyramidal reactions (opisthotonos, trismus, torticollis, retrocollis, aching and numbness of the limbs, motor restlessness, oculogyric crisis, hyperreflexia, dystonia, including protrusion, discoloration, aching and rounding of the tongue, tonic spasm of the masticatory muscles, tight feeling in the throat, slurred speech, dysphagia, akathisia, dyskinesia, parkinsonism, ataxia, persistent tardive dyskinesia), cerebral edema, abnormal CSF proteins, drowsiness (especially during 1st or 2nd wk of therapy), convulsive seizures, headache, paradoxical exacerbation of psychotic symptoms, catatonic-like states, paranoid reactions, lethargy, paradoxical excitement, restlessness, hyperactivity, nocturnal confusion, bizarre dreams, insomnia
Autonomic nervous system	Dry mouth or salivation, nausea, vomiting, diarrhea, anorexia, constipation, obstipation, fecal impaction, urinary retention, urinary frequency or incontinence, bladder paralysis, polyuria, nasal congestion, pallor, adynamic ileus, miosis, mydriasis, blurred vision, glaucoma, perspiration, hypertension, hypotension, change in pulse rate
Allergic	Urticaria, erythema, eczema, exfoliative dermatitis, pruritus, photosensitivity, asthma, fever, anaphylactoid reactions, laryngeal edema, angioneurotic edema, contact dermatitis; cerebral edema and circulatory collapse leading to death (very rare)
Metabolic and endocrinological	Lactation, galactorrhea, moderate breast engorgement in females and gynecomastia in males on large doses, disturbances in the menstrual cycle, amenorrhea, changes in libido, inhibition of ejaculation, syndrome of inappropriate ADH secretion, hyperglycemia, hypoglycemia, glycosuria
Cardiovascular	Postural hypotension, tachycardia (especially with sudden marked increase in dosage), bradycardia, cardiac arrest, faintness, dizziness, shock-like condition, nonspecific ECG changes
Hematological	Agranulocytosis, eosinophilia, leukopenia, hemolytic anemia, thrombocytopenic purpura, pancytopenia
Hepatic	Biliary stasis, jaundice
Dermatological	Pigmentation of the skin
Ophthalmic	Deposition of fine particulate matter in the cornea and lens, progressing in more severe cases to star-shaped lenticular opacities; epithelial keratopathies; pigmentary retinopathy
Other	Peripheral edema, parotid swelling (rare), hyperpyrexia, systemic lupus erythematosus-like syndrome, increases in appetite and weight, photophobia, polyphagia, muscle weakness; neuroleptic malignant syndrome, a potentially fatal reaction characterized by hyperthermia, autonomic disturbances, and severe extrapyramidal dysfunction (muscular rigidity followed by stupor or coma)

OVERDOSAGE

Signs and symptoms	See ADVERSE REACTIONS

PERMITIL ■ PROLIXIN

Treatment — Induce emesis with ipecac syrup, taking precautions against aspiration, especially in infants and children. Follow with activated charcoal and, if vomiting is unsuccessful, gastric lavage. Do not induce vomiting if patient is unconscious. Saline cathartics may be helpful. Treat circulatory shock or metabolic acidosis with standard measures. Maintain an open airway and adequate fluid intake. Regulate body temperature. Treat hyperthermia with total-body ice-packing and antipyretics. Treat cardiac arrhythmias with neostigmine, pyridostigmine, or propranolol. Consider digitalis for cardiac failure. Monitor cardiac function for at least 5 days. For hypotension, administer norepinephrine; *do not use epinephrine.* To control convulsions, use an inhalation anesthetic, diazepam, or paraldehyde. For acute parkinson-like symptoms, administer benztropine mesylate or diphenhydramine. When treating CNS depression, avoid convulsion-producing stimulants (eg, picrotoxin, pentylenetetrazol). Dialysis is not useful. Signs of arousal may not occur for 48 h.

DRUG INTERACTIONS

Alcohol, anesthetics, barbiturates, narcotics, and other CNS depressants	△ CNS depression
Anticonvulsants	▽ Convulsion threshold
Epinephrine	Severe hypotension
Guanethidine	▽ Antihypertensive effect
Antimuscarinics	△ Atropine-like effect
Amphetamines	▽ Amphetamine effect
Antacids containing aluminum or magnesium ions	▽ Absorption of fluphenazine
Levodopa	▽ Antiparkinson effect
MAO inhibitors, tricyclic antidepressants	△ Sedation and antimuscarinic effects

ALTERED LABORATORY VALUES

Blood/serum values	△ or ▽ Glucose △ PBI
Urinary values	△ Glucose △ Bilirubin (false elevation)

USE IN CHILDREN
Not recommended for use in children; the safety and effectiveness of this drug in children have not been established

USE IN PREGNANT AND NURSING WOMEN
Safety for use in pregnant or nursing women has not been established

[1] Contains 1% alcohol
[2] These reactions are common to phenothiazines in general and may not necessarily occur with fluphenazine

PHENOTHIAZINES

PROLIXIN (fluphenazine hydrochloride) Princeton Rx

Tablets: 1, 2.5, 5, 10 mg **Elixir (per 5 ml):** 2.5 mg[1] (60 ml, 1 pt) *orange flavored* **Concentrate:** 5 mg/ml[1] (120 ml) **Vials:** 2.5 mg/ml (10 ml) for IM use only

INDICATIONS	ORAL DOSAGE	PARENTERAL DOSAGE
Manifestations of **psychotic disorders**	**Adult:** 2.5–10.0 mg/day, given in divided doses q6–8h to start, followed by up to 20 mg/day, if needed; thereafter, reduce dosage gradually to 1.0–5.0 mg/day for maintenance	**Adult:** 1.25 mg IM to start, followed by 2.5–10.0 mg/day, given in divided doses q6–8h; switch to oral therapy for maintenance (an equivalent oral dose is 2–3 times the parenteral dose)

PROLIXIN Decanoate (fluphenazine decanoate) Princeton Rx

Vials: 25 mg/ml (5 ml) **Prefilled syringes:** 25 mg/ml (1 ml)

INDICATIONS	PARENTERAL DOSAGE
Manifestations of **psychotic disorders** in patients requiring prolonged parenteral neuroleptic therapy	**Adult:** 12.5–25 mg SC or IM to start, followed, if necessary, by up to 100 mg SC or IM; increase the dose cautiously in 12.5-mg increments if more than 50 mg is needed. Adjust the dosing interval according to clinical response; a single dose may be effective for up to 4–6 wk.

PROLIXIN Enanthate (fluphenazine enanthate) Princeton Rx

Vials: 25 mg/ml (5 ml)

INDICATIONS

Manifestations of **psychotic disorders** in patients requiring prolonged parenteral neuroleptic therapy

PARENTERAL DOSAGE

Adult: 25 mg SC or IM every 2 wk to start. The dose may be increased, if necessary, up to 100 mg SC or IM; however, titrate the dose cautiously in 12.5-mg increments if more than 50 mg is needed. Adjust the dosing interval according to clinical response (usual interval: 1–3 wk).

CONTRAINDICATIONS

Known or suspected subcortical brain damage

Severe CNS depression

Comatose states

Use of hypnotics in large doses

Blood dyscrasias

Hypersensitivity to fluphenazine

Hepatic disease

ADMINISTRATION/DOSAGE ADJUSTMENTS

Dilution of concentrate	Add desired dose of concentrate to at least 60 ml of diluent just before administration; suggested diluents include tomato or fruit juice, milk, or uncaffeinated soft drinks (beverages containing caffeine [coffee, cola], tannics [tea], or pectinates [apple juice] should not be used because of potential incompatability)
Elderly patients	Administer 1.0–2.5 mg/day orally to start; adjust dosage according to patient response
Severely disturbed or inadequately controlled patients	If necessary, increase oral dosage up to 40 mg/day until symptoms are satisfactorily controlled; the safety of prolonged administration of such dosages has not been determined in controlled clinical trials
Severely agitated patients	Initiate therapy with parenteral fluphenazine hydrochloride or other rapid-acting phenothiazine. If necessary, dosages exceeding 10.0 mg/day may be given with caution. When acute symptoms subside, switch to oral therapy or substitute 25 mg of fluphenazine decanoate or enanthate; adjust subsequent dosage as needed.
Poor-risk patients	Patients with known hypersensitivity to phenothiazines or who may be expected to have undue reactions should be started on fluphenazine hydrochloride, with caution. Once the effects of fluphenazine therapy and dosage are established, an equivalent dose of fluphenazine decanoate or enanthate may be given; adjust subsequent dosage as needed.
Initial therapy in patients with no history of taking phenothiazines	Begin with the shorter-acting form before administering fluphenazine decanoate or enanthate to determine patient response and to establish appropriate dosage
Dosage conversions between short- and long-acting forms	Although exact conversion is not possible, 12.5 mg of fluphenazine decanoate every 3 wk is approximately equivalent to 10 mg/day of oral fluphenazine hydrochloride. Exercise particular caution in switching from the hydrochloride to fluphenazine enanthate, since dosage comparability is unknown.
Parenteral administration of long-acting forms	For SC or IM administration of fluphenazine decanoate or enanthate, use a dry syringe and needle of at least 21 gauge

WARNINGS/PRECAUTIONS

Tardive dyskinesia	Neuroleptic drugs can cause tardive dyskinesia, a potentially irreversible syndrome characterized by involuntary choreoathetoid movements of the tongue, face, mouth, lips, jaw, trunk, and/or extremities. Protrusion of the tongue, puffing of the cheeks, puckering of the mouth, chewing movements, and other manifestations may become evident during treatment, upon dosage reduction, or after the drug is discontinued. The likelihood that tardive dyskinesia will develop or become irreversible increases with duration of treatment and total cumulative dose; however, even relatively brief use of low doses can cause it. Although this reaction appears to occur most often in the elderly, especially among older women, it is impossible to use this information to predict, before therapy is started, which patients are likely to develop the syndrome.
	In general, reserve chronic therapy for patients who respond to neuroleptics and who cannot undergo another, equally effective form of treatment that is potentially less harmful. Use the lowest effective dosage, keep the duration of therapy as short as possible, and periodically reassess the need for the drug. Since neuroleptic therapy can mask the signs of tardive dyskinesia, reduce the dosage periodically (if clinically feasible); if signs of dyskinesia appear, consider terminating use of the drug, bearing in mind that some patients may require continued neuroleptic treatment despite the development of dyskinesia. There is no known treatment for tardive dyskinesia; however, after discontinuation, some or all manifestations of this syndrome may disappear spontaneously.
Other extrapyramidal reactions	Caution patients not only concerning tardive dyskinesia, but also about other extrapyramidal reactions. Use of an antiparkinson agent (eg, benztropine) and a reduction in dosage are usually effective for control of extrapyramidal reactions other than tardive dyskinesia. Reassurance is also important.

PROLIXIN

Convulsions	Grand mal convulsions have been seen during therapy. Sudden death has also occurred; previous brain damage or seizures may increase this risk. Exercise caution when patients have a history of convulsive disorders; avoid use of high doses in patients who have such disorders.
Autonomic reactions	To control autonomic reactions, reduce dosage or temporarily withdraw the drug
Neuroleptic malignant syndrome	Neuroleptic drugs can on rare occasions cause the neuroleptic malignant syndrome (NMS), a potentially fatal reaction characterized by hyperthermia, muscular rigidity, labile blood pressure, tachycardia, diaphoresis, akinesia, and altered consciousness (including, at a later stage, stupor and coma); other manifestations include leukocytosis, elevated CPK, liver function abnormalities, and acute renal failure. If NMS occurs, immediately discontinue the drug and institute vigorous symptomatic treatment.
Cross-sensitivity	Use with caution in patients with a history of phenothiazine-related hypersensitivity reactions (eg, jaundice, dermatoses)
Hepatotoxicity	Cholestatic jaundice may occur, especially during the first months of therapy. Check hepatic function periodically; if jaundice develops, treatment should be discontinued. Abnormal liver function values, including an increase in cephalin flocculation, have been detected during therapy even when no clinical evidence of liver damage was apparent.
Hypotension	Patients with pheochromocytoma, cerebrovascular or renal insufficiency, or a severe cardiac-reserve deficiency such as mitral insufficiency appear to be especially susceptible to phenothiazine-induced hypotension and therefore should be closely observed when the drug is administered. During surgery, patients who have received large doses should be carefully watched since hypotension may occur at that time. If severe hypotension is seen, immediately give norepinephrine; do not use epinephrine (see DRUG INTERACTIONS).
Blood dyscrasias	Agranulocytosis and other hematological reactions may occur during therapy; obtain routine blood counts periodically. If WBC count is depressed and soreness of the mouth, gums, or throat or any other sign or symptom of upper respiratory tract infection is detected, discontinue drug and institute appropriate measures immediately.
Ophthalmic reactions	Phenothiazines can cause pigmentary retinopathy and, with long-term use, produce lenticular and corneal opacities
Drowsiness	Caution ambulatory patients that their ability to drive or perform other activities requiring mental alertness or physical coordination may be impaired; if necessary, reduce dosage to control drowsiness
Pneumonia	Watch for "silent" pneumonias
Renal function	Check renal function periodically during prolonged therapy; if BUN level becomes abnormal, treatment should be discontinued
Extreme heat, insecticides	Use with caution in patients exposed to extreme heat or organophosphorous insecticides
Abrupt withdrawal	Gastritis, nausea, vomiting, dizziness, and tremulousness may occur following abrupt discontinuation of high-dose therapy; these reactions may be minimized if antiparkinson therapy is continued for several weeks after withdrawal
Carcinogenicity	Chronic use of neuroleptic drugs causes a persistent elevation of the serum prolactin level, an effect that may be of potential importance if the patient has prolactin-dependent breast cancer. Chronic administration has produced an increase in mammary neoplasia in rodents, and endocrine disturbances have been seen in humans; although no clinical or epidemiological studies have shown an association between chronic neuroleptic therapy and mammary tumorigenesis, the available evidence is considered too limited to be conclusive at this time.
Tartrazine sensitivity	Presence of FD&C Yellow No. 5 (tartrazine) in 2.5-, 5-, and 10-mg tablets may cause allergic-type reactions, including bronchial asthma, in certain susceptible individuals, such as those hypersensitive to aspirin

ADVERSE REACTIONS[2]

Central nervous system	Drowsiness, lethargy; extrapyramidal reactions, including pseudoparkinsonism, dystonia, dyskinesia, akathisia, oculogyric crisis, opisthotonos, hyperreflexia, and tardive dyskinesia; catatonic-like states (at a dosage far above recommended level), restlessness, excitement, bizarre dreams, reactivation or aggravation of psychosis, CSF protein abnormalities, cerebral edema, EEG changes
Ophthalmic	Blurred vision, glaucoma, pigmentary retinopathy; with prolonged use, corneal and lenticular deposits
Cardiovascular	Hypotension, hypertension, headache, fluctuations in blood pressure, tachycardia, ECG changes, cardiac arrest, peripheral edema
Hematological	Agranulocytosis, leukopenia, pancytopenia, thrombocytopenic and nonthrombocytopenic purpura, eosinophilia
Gastrointestinal	Cholestatic jaundice, anorexia, nausea, constipation, fecal impaction, paralytic ileus
Genitourinary	Impotence, increased libido (in women), polyuria, bladder paralysis

PROLIXIN ■ SERENTIL

Endocrinological	Lactation, menstrual irregularities, gynecomastia
Dermatological	Hypersensitivity reactions (see below); with prolonged use, skin pigmentation
Hypersensitivity	Pruritus, erythema, urticaria, seborrhea, photosensitivity, eczema, exfoliative dermatitis, asthma, laryngeal edema, angioneurotic edema, anaphylactoid reactions
Other	Dry mouth, nasal congestion, salivation, perspiration, hyperthermia (with exposure to extreme heat), weight change, enhanced effect of organophosphorous insecticides, systemic lupus erythematosus-like syndrome; muscle rigidity, sometimes accompanied by hyperthermia (with fluphenazine decanoate)

OVERDOSAGE

Signs and symptoms	See ADVERSE REACTIONS
Treatment	Discontinue medication; treat symptomatically and institute supportive measures, as required. Combat hypotension with norepinephrine. *Do not use epinephrine.*

DRUG INTERACTIONS

Other CNS depressants, including alcohol	↑ CNS depression; a reduction in the dosage of CNS depressants used with fluphenazine may be necessary
Anticonvulsants	↑ Risk of convulsions ↑ Pharmacologic effect of phenytoin
Metrizamide	↑ Risk of convulsions; discontinue use of fluphenazine at least 48 h before administration of metrizamide for myelography and wait at least 24 h after the procedure before resuming use. Do not use fluphenazine before or after myelography for control of nausea and vomiting.
Anticholinergic drugs	↑ Anticholinergic effects ↓ Antipsychotic effect
Epinephrine	Severe hypotension
Guanethidine	↓ Antihypertensive effect
Propranolol	↑ Pharmacologic effects of propranolol and fluphenazine
Amphetamines	↓ Antipsychotic effect ↓ Anorectic effect
Phenmetrazine	↓ Anorectic effect
Lithium	↑ Risk of acute encephalopathy and extrapyramidal reactions ↓ Serum fluphenazine level ↑ Renal clearance of lithium
Tricyclic antidepressants	↑ Serum level of tricyclic antidepressants and fluphenazine ↓ Antipsychotic effect
Oral anticoagulants	↓ Anticoagulant effect

ALTERED LABORATORY VALUES

Blood/serum values	↑ SGOT ↑ SGPT ↑ LDH ↑ Alkaline phosphatase ↑ Bilirubin ↑ Cephalin flocculation ↑ Prolactin
Urinary values	↓ VMA + Pregnancy (with immunologic pregnancy tests) + Bilirubin (with reagent test strips) ↑ Urobilinogen (with Ehrlich's reagent test) ↓ 5-HIAA (with nitrosonaphthol reagent test) Interference with determination of catecholamines (with Pisano method), 17-KS (with Haltorff-Koch modification of Zimmerman reaction), and 17-OHCS (with modified Glenn-Nelson technique)

USE IN CHILDREN
Safety and effectiveness for use in children have not been established

USE IN PREGNANT AND NURSING WOMEN
Safety for use during pregnancy has not been established; weigh potential benefits against possible risks before using in pregnant women. Consult manufacturer for use in nursing mothers.

[1] Contains 14% alcohol
[2] Sudden, inexplicable death has occurred in patients taking phenothiazines; autopsy findings have usually revealed intramyocardial lesions, aspirated gastric contents, or evidence of acute fulminating pneumonia or pneumonitis. In several cases, psychosis suddenly recurred shortly before death. Previous brain damage or seizures may be predisposing factors (see warning above concerning convulsions).

PHENOTHIAZINES

SERENTIL (mesoridazine besylate) Boehringer Ingelheim   Rx

Tablets: 10, 25, 50, 100 mg   **Concentrate:** 25 mg/ml[1] (4 fl oz)   **Ampuls:** 25 mg/ml (1 ml)

INDICATIONS	ORAL DOSAGE	PARENTERAL DOSAGE
Manifestations of **schizophrenia**	**Adult:** 50 mg tid to start, followed by 100–400 mg/day	**Adult:** 25 mg IM to start; repeat dose in 30–60 min, if needed; usual maintenance dosage, 25–200 mg/day

SERENTIL

Behavioral problems in mental deficiency and chronic brain syndrome	**Adult:** 25 mg tid to start, followed by 75–300 mg/day	**Adult:** same as above
Alcoholism	**Adult:** 25 mg bid to start, followed by 50–200 mg/day	**Adult:** same as above
Psychoneurotic manifestations	**Adult:** 10 mg tid to start, followed by 30–150 mg/day	**Adult:** same as above

CONTRAINDICATIONS

Hypersensitivity to mesoridazine	Severe CNS depression	Comatose states

ADMINISTRATION/DOSAGE ADJUSTMENTS

Maintenance regimen	When maximum effect is achieved, reduce dosage to lowest effective level
Dilution of concentrate	May be done with distilled water, acidified tap water, orange juice, or grape juice; dilute just before administration

WARNINGS/PRECAUTIONS

Tardive dyskinesia	Neuroleptic drugs can cause tardive dyskinesia, a potentially irreversible syndrome characterized by involuntary choreoathetoid movements of the tongue, face, mouth, lips, jaw, trunk, and/or extremities. Protrusion of the tongue, puffing of the cheeks, puckering of the mouth, chewing movements, and other manifestations may become evident during treatment, upon dosage reduction, or after the drug is discontinued. The likelihood that tardive dyskinesia will develop or become irreversible increases with duration of treatment and total cumulative dose; however, even relatively brief use of low doses can cause it. Although this reaction appears to occur most often in the elderly, especially among older women, it is impossible to use this information to predict, before therapy is started, which patients are likely to develop the syndrome.
	In general, reserve chronic therapy for patients who respond to neuroleptics and who cannot undergo another, equally effective form of treatment that is potentially less harmful. Use the lowest effective dosage, keep the duration of therapy as short as possible, and periodically reassess the need for the drug. Since neuroleptic therapy can mask the signs of tardive dyskinesia, reduce the dosage periodically (if clinically feasible); if signs of dyskinesia appear, consider terminating use of the drug, bearing in mind that some patients may require continued neuroleptic treatment despite the development of dyskinesia. There is no known treatment for tardive dyskinesia; however, after discontinuation, some or all manifestations of this syndrome may disappear spontaneously.
Mental and/or physical impairment	Administer with caution and increase dosage gradually if patient will be engaging in activities requiring full mental alertness, such as driving
Ocular changes	Have occurred with other drugs of this class
Leukopenia and/or agranulocytosis	May occur with mesoridazine therapy
Convulsive seizures	May occur; maintain adequate concomitant anticonvulsant medication in patients with seizure disorders
Hypotension	May occur following parenteral administration; reserve for bedridden or acute ambulatory patients. Keep patient recumbent for at least 1/2 h after injection.
Special-risk patients	Use with caution in patients exposed to organophosphorus insecticides or atropine or related drugs
Patients with previously detected breast cancer	Use with caution, as chronic therapy may cause a persistent elevation of serum prolactin levels, which may be of importance in patients with prolactin-dependent breast cancers. Although endocrine disturbances have been reported, no association between chronic neuroleptic administration and mammary tumorigenesis has been demonstrated; the available evidence is considered too limited to be conclusive at this time.

ADVERSE REACTIONS[2]

Central nervous system	Drowsiness, dizziness, Parkinson's syndrome, weakness, tremor, restlessness, ataxia, dystonia, faintness, rigidity, slurring, akathisia, opisthotonos
Cardiovascular	Hypotension, tachycardia, ECG changes
Gastrointestinal	Nausea, vomiting
Dermatological	Itching, rash, hypertrophic papillae of tongue, angioneurotic edema
Genitourinary	Inhibited ejaculation, impotence, enuresis, incontinence
Autonomic nervous system	Dry mouth, nasal congestion, photophobia, blurred vision, constipation

OVERDOSAGE

Signs and symptoms	See ADVERSE REACTIONS
Treatment	Discontinue medication, treat symptomatically, and institute supportive measures, as required

DRUG INTERACTIONS

Alcohol, anesthetics, barbiturates, narcotics, and other CNS depressants	⇧ CNS depression

SERENTIL ■ SPARINE

Anticonvulsants	▽ Convulsion threshold
Epinephrine	Severe hypotension
Guanethidine	▽ Antihypertensive effect
Antimuscarinics	△ Atropine-like effect
Amphetamines	▽ Amphetamine effect
Antacids containing aluminum or magnesium ions	▽ Absorption of mesoridazine
MAO inhibitors, tricyclic antidepressants	△ Sedation and antimuscarinic effects

ALTERED LABORATORY VALUES

Urinary values	False-positive or false-negative pregnancy tests △ Bilirubin (false elevation)

No clinically significant alterations in blood/serum values occur at therapeutic dosages

USE IN CHILDREN
Not recommended for use in children under 12 yr of age because conditions for the safe use of this drug in children have not been established

USE IN PREGNANT AND NURSING WOMEN
Safety for use during pregnancy has not been established; use only when the anticipated therapeutic benefits outweigh the possible hazards.

¹ Contains 0.61% alcohol
² Other side effects common to phenothiazines in general should be considered, but have not been specifically reported with mesoridazine

---

PHENOTHIAZINES

SPARINE (promazine hydrochloride) Wyeth   Rx

Tablets: 25, 50, 100 mg **Syrup (per 5 ml):** 10 mg (120 ml) **Cartridge-needle units:** 50 mg/ml (1, 2 ml)
Vials: 25 mg/ml (10 ml); 50 mg/ml (2, 10 ml)

INDICATIONS	ORAL DOSAGE	PARENTERAL DOSAGE
Manifestations of **psychotic disorders**	**Adult:** 10–200 mg q4–6h, up to 1,000 mg/day, depending on patient response **Child (> 12 yr):** for acute episodes, 10–25 mg q4–6h	**Adult:** for severe agitation, 50–150 mg IM to start, followed after 30 min by additional doses up to a total of 300 mg, if necessary; once desired control is obtained, 10–200 mg IM q4–6h, up to 1,000 mg/day, depending on patient response

CONTRAINDICATIONS

Bone marrow depression	Comatose states induced by CNS depressants	Hypersensitivity to promazine
Intraarterial injection		

ADMINISTRATION/DOSAGE ADJUSTMENTS

Acutely inebriated patients	Do not give more than 50 mg to start, to ensure that depressant effect of alcohol is not enhanced
Parenteral administration	Patient should be kept recumbent after injection to avoid postural hypotension
Intravenous administration	May result in spasm of digital vessels and gangrene; not recommended for outpatients or office-based patients or for routine use in hospitalized patients. Inject slowly in a concentration no greater than 25 mg/ml. Avoid extravasation.
Use of syrup	The syrup may be diluted in an appropriate citrus- or chocolate-flavored liquid
Concomitant use of CNS depressants	Reduce dosage of narcotics and barbiturates by 50–75% when used concomitantly

WARNINGS/PRECAUTIONS

Tardive dyskinesia	Neuroleptic drugs can cause tardive dyskinesia, a potentially irreversible syndrome characterized by involuntary choreoathetoid movements of the tongue, face, mouth, lips, jaw, trunk, and/or extremities. Protrusion of the tongue, puffing of the cheeks, puckering of the mouth, chewing movements, and other manifestations may become evident during treatment, upon dosage reduction, or after the drug is discontinued. The likelihood that tardive dyskinesia will develop or become irreversible increases with duration of treatment and total cumulative dose; however, even relatively brief use of low doses can cause it. Although this reaction appears to occur most often in the elderly, especially among older women, it is impossible to use this information to predict, before therapy is started, which patients are likely to develop the syndrome. In general, reserve chronic therapy for patients who respond to neuroleptics and who cannot undergo another, equally effective form of treatment that is potentially less harmful. Use the lowest effective dosage, keep the duration of therapy as short as possible, and periodically reassess the need for the drug. Watch carefully for manifestations of tardive dyskinesia; fine vermicular movements of the tongue reportedly may be an early sign. However, do not forget that neuroleptic therapy can itself mask the signs and symptoms of tardive dyskinesia. If evidence of the syndrome is seen, consider terminating use of the drug, bearing in mind that some patients may require continued neuroleptic treatment despite the development by dyskinesia. There is no known treatment for tardive dyskinesia; however, after discontinuation, some or all manifestations of this syndrome may disappear spontaneously.

SPARINE

Other extrapyramidal reactions	Pseudoparkinsonism, dysarthria, and dyskinesia can occur with use of large doses. To manage reactions, reduce dosage or give an antiparkison agent; if effects are severe, promazine should be discontinued.
Hepatotoxicity	Drug-induced jaundice, a hypersensitivity reaction with clinical characteristics of infectious hepatitis and laboratory features of obstructive jaundice, has in most cases been seen during the early weeks of therapy; the reaction is generally reversible, but may be chronic. Although there is no conclusive evidence that patients with hepatic disease are particularly susceptible to jaundice, use with caution in such patients.
Blood dyscrasias	Agranulocytosis and other hematological reactions can occur during therapy. Watch closely for evidence of agranulocytosis between the fourth and tenth week of therapy since the disease is most likely to occur at that time; if sore throat or other signs of infection suddenly appear and the WBC and differential counts are significantly depressed, stop therapy and institute appropriate measures.
Hypotension	Transient orthostatic hypotension has occurred in a few patients, usually following the first parenteral dose and especially when the first dose is given by rapid IV administration. Hypotensive effects usually disappear, but occasionally may be severe and prolonged, producing a shock-like condition. In rare cases (eg, when the patient is an alcoholic), it may be necessary to lower the dosage or discontinue the drug. To reduce the risk associated with parenteral use, keep the patient under observation and preferably recumbent for a short time after the initial dose; exercise caution if the patient has cerebral arteriosclerosis, coronary artery disease, severe hypotension, or any other condition that can be exacerbated by a decrease in blood pressure. If hypotension occurs during therapy, place the patient in a head-low position with the legs raised; administration of oxygen may also be advisable. If a vasopressor is needed, use norepinephrine, not epinephrine (see DRUG INTERACTIONS).
Seizures	Use only when absolutely necessary in patients with a history of epilepsy; administer adequate concomitant anticonvulsant therapy
Mental and/or physical impairment	Caution ambulatory patients that their ability to drive or perform other potentially hazardous activities may be impaired, especially during the first few days of therapy, and to avoid alcohol, since it may cause further CNS depression and hypotension when used with this drug. Drowsiness usually disappears with continued use or a reduction in dosage.
Endocrinological reactions	A reduction in dosage or withdrawal of the drug may be necessary if breast engorgement, lactation, amenorrhea, or gynecomastia occurs
Autonomic effects	Dry mouth and other autonomic effects may occur, especially with prolonged use of large oral doses
Contact dermatitis	To prevent contact dermatitis, instruct persons hypersensitive to phenothiazines to exercise caution when handling the drug
Respiratory depression	Use with caution in patients with respiratory impairment due to acute pulmonary infections or chronic respiratory disorders, such as asthma or emphysema
Potentiation of atropine, heat, and insecticides	Use with caution in patients receiving anticholinergic drugs and in those exposed to extreme heat or organophosphorous insecticides
Antiemetic effect	May mask signs and symptoms of overdosage of other drugs or such conditions as gastrointestinal obstruction
Abrupt discontinuation	May cause temporary nausea, vomiting, dizziness, and tremulousness in patients on prolonged high-dose therapy; continue concomitant antiparkinson therapy for several weeks after the phenothiazine is withdrawn to reduce these symptoms
Photosensitivity	May occur; caution patients to avoid undue exposure to sunlight
Sudden death	Has occasionally occurred with phenothiazine therapy and, in some instances, was attributable to cardiac arrest or asphyxia due to failure of the cough reflex
Tartrazine sensitivity	Presence of FD&C Yellow No. 5 (tartrazine) in 25-mg tablets and syrup may cause allergic-type reactions, including bronchial asthma, in susceptible individuals

ADVERSE REACTIONS[1]

Central nervous system	Drowsiness, extrapyramidal symptoms (pseudoparkinsonism, dysarthria, dyskinetic disturbances, tardive dyskinesia), paradoxical exacerbation of psychotic symptoms, cerebral edema, abnormal CSF proteins, convulsive seizures
Cardiovascular	Postural hypotension, nonspecific ECG changes
Hematological	Agranulocytosis, eosinophilia, leukopenia, hemolytic anemia, thrombocytopenic purpura, pancytopenia
Allergic	Dermatitis, dry skin, edema, mild urticaria, photosensitivity, systemic lupus erythematosus-like syndrome
Metabolic and endocrinological	Lactation and moderate breast engorgement in females, gynecomastia in males, amenorrhea, hyperglycemia, hypoglycemia, glycosuria, false-positive pregnancy tests
Autonomic nervous system	Dry mouth, nasal congestion, constipation, adynamic ileus, miosis, mydriasis
Other	Mild fever (with large IM doses), increased appetite, weight change (usually gain), ocular changes, changes in skin pigmentation, jaundice

OVERDOSAGE

Signs and symptoms — Extreme somnolence accompanied by slight changes in blood pressure, respiration, and pulse; or mild to moderate drop in blood pressure with or without loss of consciousness, accompanied by slow and regular respiration and strong but increased pulse; or severe hypotension, possibly accompanied by weakness, cyanosis, perspiration, rapid thready pulse, and respiratory depression

Treatment — Treat symptomatically and institute supportive measures, as required. Employ early gastric lavage and intestinal purges. Do not use centrally acting emetics. Combat hypotension with norepinephrine. Apply pressure bandages to lower limbs. Administer oxygen and IV fluids, if indicated. *Do not use epinephrine.* Dialysis is not helpful. Manage extrapyramidal symptoms with anticholinergic antiparkinson agents. *Do not use levodopa.* Avoid stimulants that may cause convulsions (eg, picrotoxin and pentylenetetrazol).

DRUG INTERACTIONS

Alcohol, anesthetics, barbiturates, narcotics, and other CNS depressants	△ CNS depression
Anticonvulsants	▽ Convulsion threshold
Epinephrine	Severe hypotension
Guanethidine	▽ Antihypertensive effect
Antimuscarinics	△ Atropine-like effect
Amphetamines	▽ Amphetamine effect
Antacids containing aluminum or magnesium ions	▽ Absorption of promazine
Levodopa	▽ Antiparkinson effect
MAO inhibitors, tricyclic antidepressants	△ Sedation and antimuscarinic effects

ALTERED LABORATORY VALUES

Blood/serum values	△ or ▽ Glucose
Urinary values	△ Glucose △ Bilirubin (false elevation)

USE IN CHILDREN
Not recommended for use in children under 12 yr of age

USE IN PREGNANT AND NURSING WOMEN
Safety for use in pregnant or nursing women has not been established; hyperreflexia has been seen in neonates born to mothers who received a phenothiazine during pregnancy. Use only if the expected therapeutic benefits outweigh the possible hazards.

[1] Includes reactions common to phenothiazines in general which should be considered when prescribing promazine

---

PHENOTHIAZINES

STELAZINE (trifluoperazine hydrochloride) Smith Kline & French   Rx

Tablets: 1, 2, 5, 10 mg **Concentrate:** 10 mg/ml (2 fl oz) *banana-vanilla flavored* **Vials:** 2 mg/ml (10 ml) for IM use only

INDICATIONS	ORAL DOSAGE	PARENTERAL DOSAGE
Manifestations of **psychotic disorders**	**Adult:** 2–5 mg bid to start or, if these patients are small or emaciated, 2 mg bid to start, followed in either case, if needed and tolerated, by up to 40 mg/day or more (usual maintenance dosage, 15–20 mg/day) **Child (6–12 yr):** for hospitalized or otherwise closely supervised patients, 1 mg 1–2 times/day to start, followed, if needed and tolerated, by up to 15 mg/day (older psychotic children with severe symptoms may require higher dosages)	**Adult:** for prompt control of severe symptoms, 1–2 mg IM (deeply) q4–6h, as needed, up to a total of 10 mg/24 h (in very exceptional cases, higher daily doses may be given) **Child (6–12 yr):** for prompt control of severe symptoms, 1 mg IM (deeply) 1–2 times/day
Generalized **nonpsychotic anxiety**[1]	**Adult:** 1–2 mg bid; do not exceed 6 mg/day or administer for more than 12 wk	

STELAZINE

CONTRAINDICATIONS

Severe CNS depression	Bone marrow depression	Liver damage
Comatose states	Blood dyscrasias	

ADMINISTRATION/DOSAGE ADJUSTMENTS

Frequency of administration — Because of the long duration of action of this drug, it may be given orally bid or even once daily; the parenteral form should not be given more frequently than q4h to avoid accumulation

Antipsychotic oral therapy — Titrate dosage over a period of 2–3 wk; for maintenance, reduce dosage gradually to the lowest effective level once optimal response has been achieved

Elderly, emaciated, or debilitated patients — Increase dosage more gradually if the patient is elderly, emaciated, or debilitated; for most elderly patients, a dosage in the lower range is sufficient. Carefully monitor clinical response of elderly patients since they appear to be more susceptible to hypotension and extrapyramidal reactions; elderly patients with brain damage are especially susceptible to extrapyramidal effects.

Preparation of oral concentrate — Add concentrate to 60 ml or more of diluent just before administration; suggested diluents include juice, milk, simple syrup, orange syrup, carbonated beverages, coffee, tea, water, or semi-solid foods (eg, soups, puddings)

Monitoring of long-term therapy — Periodically evaluate patients with a history of long-term neuroleptic treatment in order to determine whether the maintenance dosage can be reduced or therapy discontinued; watch for tardive dyskinesia, ocular changes, and skin pigmentation during prolonged use

WARNINGS/PRECAUTIONS

Tardive dyskinesia — Neuroleptic drugs can cause tardive dyskinesia, a potentially irreversible syndrome characterized by involuntary choreoathetoid movements of the tongue, face, mouth, lips, jaw, trunk, and/or extremities. Protrusion of the tongue, puffing of the cheeks, puckering of the mouth, chewing movements, and other manifestations may become evident during treatment, upon dosage reduction, or after the drug is discontinued. The likelihood that tardive dyskinesia will develop or become irreversible increases with duration of treatment and total cumulative dose; however, even relatively brief use of low doses can cause it. Although this reaction appears to occur most often in the elderly, especially among older women, it is impossible to use this information to predict, before therapy is started, which patients are likely to develop the syndrome.

In general, reserve chronic therapy for patients who respond to neuroleptics and who cannot undergo another, equally effective form of treatment that is potentially less harmful. Use the lowest effective dosage, keep the duration of therapy as short as possible, and periodically reassess the need for the drug. Watch carefully for manifestations of tardive dyskinesia; fine vermicular movements of the tongue reportedly may be an early sign. However, do not forget that neuroleptic therapy can itself mask the signs and symptoms of tardive dyskinesia. If evidence of the syndrome is seen, consider terminating use of the drug, bearing in mind that some patients may require continued neuroleptic treatment despite the development of dyskinesia. There is no known treatment for tardive dyskinesia; however, after discontinuation, some or all manifestations of this syndrome may disappear spontaneously.

Dystonias — To control dystonias, discontinue neuroleptic therapy and take the following measures: for mild cases, provide reassurance or give a barbiturate; for moderate cases, use a barbiturate; for more severe cases, administer an antiparkinson agent other than levodopa; for children, provide reassurance and give either a barbiturate or parenteral diphenhydramine. If antiparkinson agents or diphenhydramine fail to reverse signs and symptoms, reevaluate diagnosis. Appropriate supportive measures, such as those needed to maintain adequate hydration and a patent airway, should be instituted as required. Dystonias usually subside within a few hours and almost always within 24–48 h after the drug has been discontinued. If treatment is resumed, administer at a lower dosage.

Akathisia — Symptoms of akathisia often disappear spontaneously; if they become too troublesome, reduce dosage or give a barbiturate. Wait until effects subside before increasing dosage. At times, drug-induced symptoms of akathisia may resemble psychotic or neurotic manifestations seen before therapy.

Pseudoparkinsonism — In most cases, pseudoparkinsonism can be controlled by concomitant use of an antiparkinson agent other than levodopa; occasionally, it is necessary to reduce the dosage of trifluoperazine or discontinue the drug. Administration of antiparkinson drugs for a period ranging from a few weeks to 2–3 mo is generally sufficient; clinical response should be evaluated before continuing therapy for a longer period. Reassurance and sedation are also important in the treatment of pseudoparkinsonism.

Convulsions — Phenothiazines can precipitate petit or grand mal convulsions, particularly in patients with EEG abnormalities or a history of such disorders

Cross-sensitivity — Do not use trifluoperazine in patients with a history of hypersensitivity to a phenothiazine unless potential benefits outweigh possible risks; see also warnings below concerning hepatotoxicity, blood dyscrasias, and contact dermatitis

STELAZINE

Hepatotoxicity	Trifluoperazine can cause liver damage, including cholestatic jaundice. If fever with grippe-like symptoms occurs, perform appropriate liver tests; if an abnormality is detected, stop treatment. Do not give trifluoperazine to patients with a history of phenothiazine-induced jaundice unless the potential benefits outweigh the possible risks; administration to patients with liver damage is contraindicated.
Blood dyscrasias	Agranulocytosis and pancytopenia can occur during therapy. Caution patients to report the sudden appearance of sore throat or other signs or symptoms of infection; if signs of infection are seen and WBC and differential counts are depressed, stop therapy and institute appropriate measures. Thrombocytopenia and anemia have also been associated with trifluoperazine. Do not give this drug to patients with a history of phenothiazine-induced blood dyscrasias unless the potential benefits outweigh the possible risks; use in patients with blood dyscrasias or bone marrow depression is contraindicated.
Hypotension	Trifluoperazine can cause hypotension; in patients with mitral insufficiency or pheochromocytoma, certain phenothiazines have produced severe hypotension. To minimize risk of hypotension, keep all patients lying down and under observation for at least 30 min after the initial injection. Avoid giving trifluoperazine parenterally or in large doses to patients with cardiovascular dysfunction. If hypotension occurs, place patient in a head-low position with the legs raised; if a vasopressor is needed, use norepinephrine or phenylephrine, not epinephrine.
Angina	By stimulating physical activity, trifluoperazine may exacerbate angina. Carefully observe patients with angina; if an untoward reaction occurs, the drug should be discontinued.
Retinopathy	Certain phenothiazines have been associated with retinopathy; if ophthalmoscopic examination or visual field studies reveal retinal changes, therapy should be discontinued
Severe CNS or vasomotor symptoms	Prolonged use at high dosages may precipitate severe CNS or vasomotor symptoms
Masking of nonpsychotic conditions	Antiemetic effect of trifluoperazine may mask nausea and vomiting associated with intestinal obstruction, brain tumor, Reye's syndrome, or toxicity of antineoplastic agents or other drugs
Drowsiness	Caution patients about driving and engaging in other activities requiring mental alertness; drowsiness may occur, especially during the first few days of therapy
Glaucoma	Trifluoperazine may exacerbate glaucoma; use with caution in patients with glaucoma
Extreme heat	Phenothiazines may affect thermal homeostasis; use with caution in patients who will be exposed to extreme heat
Contact dermatitis	Persons hypersensitive to phenothiazines should avoid direct contact of solution with hands or clothing
Sudden death	Patients taking phenothiazines have occasionally died suddenly; in some cases, death appeared to result from cardiac arrest or from asphyxia due to failure of the cough reflex
Abrupt withdrawal	Nausea, vomiting, dizziness, and tremulousness may occur following abrupt discontinuation of high-dose therapy
Carcinogenicity	Chronic use of neuroleptic drugs causes a persistent elevation of the serum prolactin level, an effect that may be of potential importance if the patient has prolactin-dependent breast cancer. Chronic administration has produced an increase in mammary neoplasia in rodents, and endocrine disturbances have been seen in humans; although no clinical or epidemiological studies have shown an association between chronic neuroleptic therapy and mammary tumorigenesis, the available evidence is considered too limited to be conclusive at this time.

ADVERSE REACTIONS

Central nervous system	Drowsiness, fatigue, muscle weakness, dystonias (spasm of neck muscles, torticollis, extensor rigidity of back muscles, opisthotonos, carpopedal spasm, trismus, swallowing difficulty, oculogyric crisis, protrusion of the tongue), akathisia (agitation, jitteriness, insomnia), pseudoparkinsonism (mask-like facies, drooling, tremors, pillrolling motion, cogwheel rigidity, shuffling gait), tardive dyskinesia, tardive dystonia, hyperreflexia, dyskinesia, reactivation of psychosis, catatonic-like states, grand mal and petit mal seizures, cerebral edema, CSF protein abnormalities
Ophthalmic	Blurred vision, miosis, mydriasis, pigmentary retinopathy; corneal and lenticular deposits and epithelial keratopathy (with prolonged use of substantial doses)
Cardiovascular	Hypotension, dizziness, headache, ECG changes (especially distortions of Q and T waves), cardiac arrest, peripheral edema
Hematological	Agranulocytosis, eosinophilia, leukopenia, hemolytic anemia, aplastic anemia, thrombocytopenic purpura, pancytopenia
Gastrointestinal	Jaundice, biliary stasis, anorexia, nausea, constipation, obstipation, adynamic ileus, atonic colon
Genitourinary	Priapism, ejaculatory disorders/impotence, urinary retention

STELAZINE

Endocrinological	Hyperglycemia, hypoglycemia, glycosuria, lactation, galactorrhea, amenorrhea, menstrual irregularities, gynecomastia
Dermatological	Rash, hypersensitivity reactions (see below); skin pigmentation (with prolonged use of substantial doses)
Hypersensitivity	Jaundice, blood dyscrasias, asthma, laryngeal edema, angioneurotic edema, anaphylactoid reactions, urticaria, pruritus, erythema, eczema, photosensitivity, exfoliative dermatitis
Other	Dry mouth, nasal congestion, mild fever (with large IM doses), hyperthermia (especially with exposure to extreme heat), hyperpyrexia, increased appetite, weight gain, systemic lupus erythematosus-like syndrome, enhanced effect of organophosphorous insecticides; neuroleptic malignant syndrome, a potentially fatal reaction characterized by hyperthermia, altered consciousness, muscular rigidity, and autonomic dysfunction

OVERDOSAGE

Signs and symptoms	CNS depression, somnolence, coma, hypotension, extrapyramidal symptoms, agitation, restlessness, convulsions, fever, dry mouth, ileus
Treatment	Empty stomach by gastric lavage. Maintain patent airway. *Do not induce emesis.* Treat extrapyramidal symptoms with antiparkinson drugs (except levodopa), barbiturates, or diphenhydramine. Avoid use of convulsion-inducing stimulants (eg, picrotoxin or pentylenetetrazol). Employ standard measures for circulatory shock. Restrict use of vasoconstrictors to norepinephrine and phenylephrine; *do not use epinephrine.* Dialysis is not helpful.

DRUG INTERACTIONS

Other CNS depressants, including alcohol	△ CNS depression
Anticonvulsants	△ Risk of convulsions; adjustment of anticonvulsant dosage may be necessary △ Pharmacologic effect of phenytoin
Metrizamide	△ Risk of convulsions; discontinue use of trifluoperazine at least 48 h before administration of metrizamide for myelography and wait at least 24 h after the procedure before resuming use. Do not use trifluoperazine before or after myelography for control of nausea and vomiting.
Anticholinergic drugs	△ Anticholinergic effects ▽ Antipsychotic effect
Epinephrine	Severe hypotension
Guanethidine	▽ Antihypertensive effect
Thiazide diuretics	△ Orthostatic hypotensive effect
Propranolol	△ Pharmacologic effects of propranolol and trifluoperazine
Amphetamines	▽ Antipsychotic effect ▽ Anorectic effect
Phenmetrazine	▽ Anorectic effect
Lithium	△ Risk of acute encephalopathy and extrapyramidal reactions ▽ Serum trifluoperazine level △ Renal clearance of lithium
Tricyclic antidepressants	△ Serum level of tricyclic antidepressants and trifluoperazine ▽ Antipsychotic effect
Oral anticoagulants	▽ Anticoagulant effect

ALTERED LABORATORY VALUES

Blood/serum values	△ SGOT △ SGPT △ LDH △ Alkaline phosphatase △ Bilirubin △ Prolactin △ or ▽ Glucose
Urinary values	▽ VMA + Glucose + PKU + Pregnancy (with immunologic pregnancy tests) + Bilirubin (with reagent test strips) △ Urobilinogen (with Ehrlich's reagent test) ▽ 5-HIAA (with nitrosonaphthol reagent test) Interference with determination of catecholamines (with Pisano method), 17-KS (with Haltorff-Koch modification of Zimmerman reaction), and 17-OHCS (with modified Glenn-Nelson technique)

USE IN CHILDREN

See INDICATIONS and dosage recommendations; if a child experiences an extrapyramidal reaction, discontinue use and do not reinstitute treatment at a later time

USE IN PREGNANT AND NURSING WOMEN

Jaundice, prolonged extrapyramidal signs, and hyper- and hyporeflexia have been seen in neonates born to mothers who received phenothiazines during pregnancy. Studies in rats given over 600 times the human dose of trifluoperazine have shown an increase in malformations; decreases in litter size and body weight were also seen in these studies, but have been attributed to maternal toxicity. No adverse effect on fetal development has been observed in rabbits given 700 times the human dose or in monkeys given 25 times the human dose. Use during pregnancy only if essential and only if the potential benefits clearly outweigh the possible risks. Phenothiazines are excreted in human milk.

---

[1] For most patients, trifluoperazine is not the initial treatment of choice because certain risks associated with its use are not shared by common alternatives such as the benzodiazepines. It has not been established that this drug is effective in the treatment of anxiety or anxiety-like signs associated with conditions such as physical illness, organic mental disorders, agitated depression, or character pathology.

THORAZINE

PHENOTHIAZINES

THORAZINE (chlorpromazine hydrochloride) Smith Kline & French — Rx

Capsules (sustained release): 30, 75, 150, 200, 300 mg **Tablets:** 10, 25, 50, 100, 200 mg **Concentrate:** 30 mg/ml (4 fl oz, 1 gal), 100 mg/ml (8 fl oz) **Syrup (per 5 ml):** 10 mg (4 fl oz) **Ampuls:** 25 mg/ml (1, 2 ml) **Vials:** 25 mg/ml (10 ml) **Rectal suppositories:** 25, 100 mg

INDICATIONS	ORAL DOSAGE	PARENTERAL DOSAGE
Manifestations of **psychotic disorders** **Manic episodes** of manic-depressive illness **Nonpsychotic anxiety**[1]	**Adult:** for excessive anxiety, tension, and agitation, 30–75 mg/day (10 mg, tid or qid, or 25 mg, bid or tid); for more severe symptoms in outpatients and office patients, 25 mg tid for 1–2 days, followed, as needed, by semiweekly increases in dosage of 20–50 mg/day (usual effective dosage: 200–800 mg/day); for more severe symptoms in hospitalized patients, 25 mg tid to start, followed by a gradual increase in dosage (usual effective dosage: 400 mg/day). When treating nonpsychotic anxiety, do not exceed 100 mg/day or administer for more than 12 wk.	**Adult:** for severe symptoms in outpatients and office patients, 25 mg IM for 1 or, if necessary, 2 doses (with 1 h between doses), followed by 25–50 mg orally tid; for acute agitation, mania, or disturbance in hospitalized patients, 25 mg IM, followed, if necessary, by 25–50 mg IM 1 h later, a subsequent gradual increase in the IM dose over a period of several days (up to 400 mg q4–6h in exceptionally severe cases), and then, when the patient becomes quiet and cooperative, further titration of dosage with oral preparations
Manifestations of psychotic disorders Disproportionately severe **explosive hyperexcitability or combativeness** **Conduct disorders,** associated with **hyperactivity** and characterized by impulsiveness, inattention, aggressiveness, mood lability, or poor frustration tolerance (short-term use only)	**Child:** 0.25 mg/lb q4–6h; for severe behavioral disorders or psychoses, younger hospitalized patients may need 50–100 mg/day and older hospitalized patients may require 200 mg/day or more. There is little evidence that dosages exceeding 500 mg/day further improve the behavior of severely disturbed, mentally retarded patients.	**Child:** (< 5 yr or ≤ 50 lb): 0.25 mg/lb IM q6–8h, up to 40 mg/day **Child (5–12 yr or 50–100 lb):** 0.25 mg/lb IM q6–8h, up to 75 mg/day, except in unmanageable cases
Preoperative restlessness and apprehension	**Adult:** 25–50 mg 2–3 h before surgery **Child:** 0.25 mg/lb 2–3 h before surgery	**Adult:** 12.5–25 mg IM 1–2 h before surgery **Child:** 0.25 mg/lb IM 1–2 h before surgery
Postoperative medication	**Adult:** 10–25 mg q4–6h, as needed **Child:** 0.25 mg/lb q4–6h, as needed	**Adult:** 12.5–25 mg IM; repeat in 1 h, if needed and if no hypotension occurs **Child:** 0.25 mg/lb IM; repeat in 1 h, if needed and if no hypotension occurs
Nausea and vomiting	**Adult:** 10–25 mg q4–6h, as needed; increase dosage, if necessary **Child:** 0.25 mg/lb q4–6h	**Adult:** 25 mg IM to start; if no hypotension occurs, 25–50 mg q3–4h, as needed, until vomiting ceases; follow with oral regimen **Child (< 5 yr or < 50 lb):** 0.25 mg/lb IM q6–8h, up to 40 mg/day, if needed **Child (5–12 yr or 50–100 lb):** 0.25 mg/lb IM q6–8h, up to 75 mg/day, except in severe cases
Nausea and vomiting during surgery	—	**Adult:** 12.5 mg IM; repeat in ½ h, if needed and if no hypotension occurs; alternative regimen: 2 mg/fractional IV injection every 2 min, up to 25 mg; dilute to 1 mg/ml for IV administration **Child:** 0.125 mg/lb IM; repeat in ½ h if needed and if no hypotension occurs; alternative regimen: 1 mg/fractional IV injection every 2 min, up to 0.125 mg/lb; dilute to 1 mg/ml for IV administration
Intractable hiccups	**Adult:** 25–50 mg tid or qid; if symptoms persist for 2–3 days, switch to IM use	**Adult:** 25–50 mg IM, followed, if necessary, by 25–50 mg, given by slow IV infusion in 500–1,000 ml of saline while patient is lying in bed (closely monitor blood pressure)
Acute intermittent porphyria	**Adult:** 25–50 mg tid or qid	**Adult:** 25 mg IM tid or qid until patient can take oral therapy
Tetanus (adjunctive therapy)	—	**Adult:** 25–50 mg IM tid or qid; alternative regimen: 25–50 mg IV (1 mg/min); dilute to at least 1 mg/ml for IV administration **Child:** 0.25 mg/lb IM or IV (0.5 mg/min) q6–8h, up to 40 mg/day (for children ≤ 50 lb) or 75 mg/day (for children 50–100 lb), except in severe cases; dilute to at least 1 mg/ml for IV administration

THORAZINE

CONTRAINDICATIONS

Coma	Presence of large amounts of CNS depressants

ADMINISTRATION/DOSAGE ADJUSTMENTS

Parenteral administration	Reserve for bedfast patients and acute ambulatory cases; keep patient lying down for at least ½ h after injection to minimize hypotensive effects. Preferred route is IM; however, IV route may be used during surgery and for tetanus and intractable hiccups. SC administration is not recommended. Intramuscular injections should be given slowly and deeply in upper outer quadrant of buttock. If irritation is a problem, dilute solution with saline or 2% procaine; do not mix with other agents in the syringe.
Rectal use	For nausea and vomiting in adults, insert one 100-mg suppository q6–8h, as needed; in some patients, dosage may be halved. For nausea and vomiting and manifestations of psychiatric disorders in children, administer 0.5 mg/lb q6–8h, as needed (eg, if child is 20–30 lb, use half a 25-mg suppository).
Dilution and storage of concentrate	Immediately prior to use, dilute desired dose of concentrate with 60 ml (2 fl oz) or more of fruit or tomato juice, milk, coffee, tea, water, carbonated beverage, simple syrup, orange syrup, or semisolid food (eg, soup, pudding). Protect concentrate from light and dispense in amber bottles; refrigeration is unnecessary.
Psychiatric regimens	Increase dosage gradually until symptoms are controlled; maximum improvement may take weeks or even months. Continue optimum dosage for 2 wk, then gradually reduce to lowest effective level for maintenance. Therapeutic response is usually not enhanced by exceeding 1 g/day for extended periods.
Elderly, emaciated, or debilitated patients	Increase dosage more gradually if the patient is elderly, emaciated, or debilitated; for most elderly patients, a dosage in the lower range is sufficient. Carefully monitor clinical response of elderly patients since they appear to be more susceptible to hypotension and extrapyramidal reactions.
Monitoring of long-term therapy	Periodically evaluate patients with a history of long-term neuroleptic treatment in order to determine whether the maintenance dosage can be reduced or therapy discontinued; watch for tardive dyskinesia, ocular changes, and skin pigmentation during prolonged use (see warnings below)

WARNINGS/PRECAUTIONS

Tardive dyskinesia	Neuroleptic drugs can cause tardive dyskinesia, a potentially irreversible syndrome characterized by involuntary choreoathetoid movements of the tongue, face, mouth, lips, jaw, trunk, and/or extremities. Protrusion of the tongue, puffing of the cheeks, puckering of the mouth, chewing movements, and other manifestations may become evident during treatment, upon dosage reduction, or after the drug is discontinued. The likelihood that tardive dyskinesia will develop or become irreversible increases with duration of treatment and total cumulative dose; however, even relatively brief use of low doses can cause it. Although this reaction appears to occur most often in the elderly, especially among older women, it is impossible to use this information to predict, before therapy is started, which patients are likely to develop the syndrome. In general, reserve chronic therapy for patients who respond to neuroleptics and who cannot undergo another, equally effective form of treatment that is potentially less harmful. Use the lowest effective dosage, keep the duration of therapy as short as possible, and periodically reassess the need for the drug. Watch carefully for manifestations of tardive dyskinesia; fine vermicular movements of the tongue reportedly may be an early sign. However, do not forget that neuroleptic therapy can itself mask the signs and symptoms of tardive dyskinesia. If evidence of the syndrome is seen, consider terminating use of the drug, bearing in mind that some patients may require continued neuroleptic treatment despite the development of dyskinesia. There is no known treatment for tardive dyskinesia; however, after discontinuation, some or all manifestations of this syndrome may disappear spontaneously.
Dystonias	To control dystonias, discontinue neuroleptic therapy and take the following measures: for mild cases, provide reassurance or give a barbiturate; for moderate cases, use a barbiturate; for more severe cases, administer an antiparkinson agent other than levodopa; for children, provide reassurance and give either a barbiturate or parenteral diphenhydramine. If antiparkinson agents or diphenhydramine fail to reverse signs and symptoms, reevaluate diagnosis. Appropriate supportive measures, such as those needed to maintain adequate hydration and a patent airway, should be instituted as required. Dystonias usually subside within a few hours and almost always within 24–48 h after the drug has been discontinued. If treatment is resumed, administer at a lower dosage.
Akathisia	Symptoms of akathisia often disappear spontaneously; if they become too troublesome, reduce dosage or give a barbiturate. Wait until effects subside before increasing dosage. At times, drug-induced symptoms of akathisia may resemble psychotic or neurotic manifestations seen before therapy.
Pseudoparkinsonism	In most cases, pseudoparkinsonism can be controlled by concomitant use of an antiparkinson agent other than levodopa; occasionally, it is necessary to reduce the dosage of chlorpromazine or discontinue the drug. Administration of antiparkinson drugs for a period ranging from a few weeks to 2–3 mo is generally sufficient; clinical response should be evaluated before continuing therapy for a longer period.
Cross-sensitivity	Do not use chlorpromazine in patients with a history of hypersensitivity to a phenothiazine unless potential benefits outweigh possible risks; see also warnings below concerning hepatotoxicity and blood dyscrasias

THORAZINE

Hepatotoxicity	Drug-induced jaundice, a hypersensitivity reaction with clinical characteristics of infectious hepatitis and laboratory features of obstructive jaundice, has been seen in most cases between the second and fourth weeks of therapy; the reaction is generally reversible, but may be chronic. Do not give chlorpromazine to patients with a history of phenothiazine-induced jaundice unless the potential benefits outweigh the possible risks. Although there is no conclusive evidence that patients with hepatic disease are particularly susceptible to jaundice, use with caution in such patients. If fever with grippe-like symptoms occurs, perform appropriate liver tests; if an abnormality is detected, stop treatment. Since this drug is potentially hepatotoxic, use in children or adolescents with signs or symptoms suggesting Reye's syndrome should be avoided. Abnormal values associated with extrahepatic obstruction may be similar to those seen with drug-induced jaundice; confirm diagnosis of extrahepatic obstruction before performing exploratory laparotomy.
Blood dyscrasias	Agranulocytosis and other hematological reactions can occur during therapy; caution patients to report the sudden appearance of sore throat or other signs or symptoms of infection. Watch closely for evidence of agranulocytosis between the fourth and tenth week of therapy since the disease is most likely to occur at that time; if signs of infection are seen and WBC and differential counts are depressed, stop therapy and institute appropriate measures. Do not give chlorpromazine to patients with bone marrow depression or a history of phenothiazine-induced blood dyscrasias unless the potential benefits outweigh the possible risks.
Hypotension	The first parenteral dose may produce orthostatic hypotension, simple tachycardia, momentary faintness, and dizziness; these effects occasionally occur after subsequent injections and, in rare cases, following the first oral dose. Hypotensive effects usually disappear within 30–120 min, but occasionally may be severe and prolonged, causing a shock-like condition. Severe hypotension has occurred in patients with pheochromocytoma or mitral insufficiency. To minimize the risk of hypotension, keep all patients recumbent and under observation for at least 30 min after the initial injection. Exercise caution when giving this drug to patients with cardiovascular disease. If hypotension occurs, place patient in a head-low position with the legs raised; if a vasopressor is needed, use norepinephrine or phenylephrine, not epinephrine (see DRUG INTERACTIONS).
Ocular effects, skin pigmentation	Use of substantial doses for a prolonged period may cause ocular changes and skin pigmentation. Administration of 300 mg or more daily for 2 yr or longer has caused deposition of fine particulate matter in the lens and cornea and, in more severe cases, star-shaped lenticular opacities and visual impairment; epithelial keratopathy and pigmentary retinopathy have also been detected. Changes in skin pigment, seen primarily in women given 500–1,500 mg/day for 3 yr or longer, range from an almost imperceptible darkening to a slate-gray color (sometimes with a violet hue). Following discontinuation of the drug, skin pigmentation may fade and eye lesions may regress. Although the cause of the ophthalmic and dermatological effects is not clear, dosage, duration of use, and exposure to sunlight appear to be the most significant factors. During long-term therapy at moderate-to-high dosage levels, perform ophthalmological examinations periodically. If ocular changes or skin pigmentation is observed during treatment, weigh benefits of continued use against possible risks and then determine whether or not to maintain the current regimen, reduce the dosage, or discontinue the drug.
Masking of nonpsychotic conditions	Extrapyramidal symptoms associated with chlorpromazine may be confused with the neurological manifestations of an undiagnosed primary disease such as Reye's syndrome or another encephalopathy; antiemetic effect may mask nausea and vomiting associated with intestinal obstruction, brain tumor, Reye's syndrome, or toxicity of antineoplastic agents or other drugs
Drowsiness	Caution patients about driving and engaging in other activities requiring mental alertness. Drowsiness may occur, especially during the first or second week of therapy, but usually disappears after this period; if drowsiness is troublesome, reduce dosage.
Cerebral dysfunction	In patients with a history of cirrhotic encephalopathy, chlorpromazine can cause abnormal slowing of the EEG and impairment of cerebral function
Convulsions	Petit mal and grand mal seizures have occurred, especially in patients with EEG abnormalities or a history of such disorders
Respiratory impairment	Use with caution in patients (especially children) with chronic respiratory disorders, such as emphysema, severe asthma, and acute respiratory infections, since this drug is a CNS depressant
Photosensitivity	Instruct patients to avoid undue exposure to the sun
Contact dermatitis	To prevent contact dermatitis, use rubber gloves when handling liquid dosage forms and avoid getting solution on clothing
Swelling of breasts, lactation	Moderate breast engorgement and lactation may occur in women with use of large doses; if reaction persists, reduce dosage or discontinue drug
Hyperthermia, glaucoma	Chlorpromazine may cause hyperthermia or exacerbate glaucoma; use with caution in patients who are exposed to extreme heat or who have glaucoma
Insecticides	Use with caution in patients exposed to organophosphorous insecticides
Aspiration of vomitus	Chlorpromazine suppresses the cough reflex and thus may increase the risk that vomitus will be aspirated

THORAZINE

Abrupt withdrawal	Gastritis, nausea, vomiting, dizziness, and tremulousness may occur following abrupt discontinuation of high-dose therapy; to minimize risk, reduce dosage gradually or continue antiparkinson therapy for several weeks after withdrawal
Carcinogenicity	Chronic use of neuroleptic drugs causes a persistent elevation of the serum prolactin level, an effect that may be of potential importance if the patient has prolactin-dependent breast cancer. Chronic administration has produced an increase in mammary neoplasia in rodents, and endocrine disturbances have been seen in humans; although no clinical or epidemiological studies have shown an association between chronic neuroleptic therapy and mammary tumorigenesis, the available evidence is considered too limited to be conclusive at this time.
Tartrazine sensitivity	Presence of FD&C Yellow No. 5 (tartrazine) in tablets may cause allergic-type reactions, including bronchial asthma, in certain susceptible individuals, such as those hypersensitive to aspirin

ADVERSE REACTIONS[2]

Central nervous system	Drowsiness, dystonias (spasm of neck muscles, acute reversible torticollis, extensor rigidity of back muscles, opisthotonos, carpopedal spasm, trismus, swallowing difficulty, oculogyric crisis, protrusion of the tongue), akathisia (agitation, jitteriness, insomnia), pseudoparkinsonism (mask-like facies, drooling, tremors, pill-rolling motion, cogwheel rigidity, shuffling gait), tardive dyskinesia, tardive dystonia, psychotic symptoms, catatonic-like states, convulsive seizures, cerebral edema, CSF protein abnormalities
Ophthalmic	Miosis, mydriasis, corneal and lenticular changes, visual impairment, epithelial keratopathy, pigmentary retinopathy
Cardiovascular	Orthostatic hypotension, tachycardia, dizziness, syncope, shock, ECG changes (especially distortions of Q and T waves), peripheral edema
Hematological	Agranulocytosis, eosinophilia, leukopenia, hemolytic anemia, aplastic anemia, thrombocytopenic purpura, pancytopenia
Gastrointestinal	Jaundice, nausea, obstipation, constipation, adynamic ileus, atonic colon
Genitourinary	Priapism, urinary retention, ejaculatory disorders/impotence
Endocrinological	Lactation, breast engorgement (in women), amenorrhea, gynecomastia, hyperglycemia, hypoglycemia, glycosuria
Dermatological	Skin pigmentation, hypersensitivity reactions (see below)
Hypersensitivity	Jaundice, blood dyscrasias, urticaria, photosensitivity, exfoliative dermatitis, contact dermatitis, asthma, laryngeal edema, angioneurotic edema, anaphylactoid reactions
Other	Dry mouth, nasal congestion, mild fever (with large IM doses), hyperpyrexia, increased appetite, weight gain, systemic lupus erythematosus–like syndrome; neuroleptic malignant syndrome, a potentially fatal reaction characterized by hyperthermia, altered consciousness, muscular rigidity, and autonomic dysfunction

OVERDOSAGE

Signs and symptoms	CNS depression, somnolence, coma, hypotension, extrapyramidal symptoms, agitation, restlessness, convulsions, fever, dry mouth, ileus, ECG changes, cardiac arrhythmias
Treatment	Empty stomach by gastric lavage. Maintain a patent airway. *Do not induce emesis.* Treat extrapyramidal symptoms with antiparkinson drugs (except levodopa), barbiturates, or diphenhydramine; exercise caution to avoid increasing respiratory depression. Avoid use of convulsion-inducing stimulants (eg, picrotoxin or pentylenetetrazol). Employ standard measures for circulatory shock. If a vasoconstrictor is needed, use norepinephrine or phenylephrine; *do not use epinephrine.* Dialysis is not helpful. Use saline cathartics to hasten the evacuation of sustained-release pellets.

DRUG INTERACTIONS

Other CNS depressants, including alcohol	⇧ CNS depression; before starting chlorpromazine, discontinue other CNS depressants unless this drug is being used to permit a reduction in their dosage. Use of other CNS depressants may be resumed at a later time, with dosage initially at a low level and then increased as needed. The dosage requirement of CNS depressants used in combination with chlorpromazine is 50–75% less than their usual level. Do not give large amounts of CNS depressants in combination with chlorpromazine; avoid concomitant use of alcohol.
Anticonvulsants	⇧ Risk of convulsions; when patients are receiving anticonvulsants, dosage of chlorpromazine should be kept low initially and then increased as needed. Adjustment of anticonvulsant dosage may also be necessary. ⇧ Pharmacologic effect of phenytoin
Metrizamide	⇧ Risk of convulsions; discontinue use of chlorpromazine at least 48 h before administration of metrizamide for myelography and wait at least 24 h after the procedure before resuming use. Do not use chlorpromazine before or after myelography for control of nausea and vomiting.
Anticholinergic drugs	⇧ Anticholinergic effects; exercise caution during combination therapy ⇩ Antipsychotic effect

THORAZINE ■ TINDAL

Epinephrine	Severe hypotension
Guanethidine	⇩ Antihypertensive effect
Propranolol	⇧ Pharmacologic effects of propranolol and chlorpromazine
Amphetamines	⇩ Antipsychotic effect ⇩ Anorectic effect
Phenmetrazine	⇩ Anorectic effect
Lithium	⇧ Risk of acute encephalopathy and extrapyramidal reactions ⇩ Serum chlorpromazine level ⇧ Renal clearance of lithium
Tricyclic antidepressants	⇧ Serum level of tricyclic antidepressants and chlorpromazine ⇩ Antipsychotic effect
Oral anticoagulants	⇩ Anticoagulant effect
Thiazide-type diuretics	⇧ Risk of orthostatic hypotension

ALTERED LABORATORY VALUES

Blood/serum values	⇧ SGOT ⇧ SGPT ⇧ LDH ⇧ Alkaline phosphatase ⇧ Bilirubin ⇧ Prolactin ⇧ or ⇩ Glucose
Urinary values	⇧ Glucose ⇩ VMA + Pregnancy (with immunologic pregnancy tests) + PKU + Bilirubin (with reagent test strips) ⇧ Urobilinogen (with Ehrlich's reagent test) ⇩ 5-HIAA (with nitrosonaphthol reagent test) Interference with determination of catecholamines (with Pisano method), 17-KS (with Haltorff-Koch modification of Zimmerman reaction), and 17-OHCS (with modified Glenn-Nelson technique)

USE IN CHILDREN

See INDICATIONS and dosage recommendations; not generally recommended for use in children under 6 mo of age or for conditions in which children's dosages have not been established. After IM administration, the duration of activity may last up to 12 h. If a child experiences dystonia, discontinue use and do not reinstitute treatment at a later time. Avoid use in children or adolescents with signs or symptoms suggesting Reye's syndrome.

USE IN PREGNANT AND NURSING WOMEN

Safety for use during pregnancy has not been established; prolonged jaundice, extrapyramidal signs, and hyperreflexia have occurred in neonates born to mothers who received phenothiazines, and embryotoxicity, increased neonatal mortality, and evidence of possible neurological damage have been seen in reproduction studies with rodents. Use during pregnancy only if essential and only if potential benefits clearly outweigh possible hazards. If a pregnant women experiences dystonia, discontinue use and do not reinstitute treatment at a later time. Chlorpromazine is excreted in human milk.

[1] Possibly effective; for most patients, chlorpromazine is not the initial treatment of choice because certain risks associated with its use are not shared by common alternatives, such as benzodiazepines
[2] Sudden death has occasionally occurred in patients taking phenothiazines; in some cases, death appeared to result from cardiac arrest or from asphyxia due to failure of the cough reflex

---

PHENOTHIAZINES

TINDAL (acetophenazine maleate) Schering   Rx

Tablets: 20 mg

INDICATIONS	ORAL DOSAGE
Manifestations of **psychotic disorders**	**Adult:** 40–80 mg/day (usually 20 mg tid); for hospitalized patients with severe schizophrenia, 80–120 mg/day, given in divided doses, or up to 400–600 mg/day, given in divided doses, if needed

CONTRAINDICATIONS

Hypersensitivity to acetophenazine or related compounds	Coma or severe obtundation	Use of CNS depressants in large doses
Known or suspected subcortical brain damage, with or without hypothalamic damage	Blood dyscrasias	Liver damage
	Bone marrow depression	

ADMINISTRATION/DOSAGE ADJUSTMENTS

Adolescent, elderly, or debilitated patients	Initiate therapy at reduced dosages
Patients who have difficulty sleeping	Give the last tablet 1 h before bedtime

TINDAL

Acutely ill patients	May respond to lower doses than chronically ill patients but require a rapid increase in dosage

WARNINGS/PRECAUTIONS

Tardive dyskinesia	Neuroleptic drugs can cause tardive dyskinesia, a potentially irreversible syndrome characterized by involuntary choreoathetoid movements of the tongue, face, mouth, lips, jaw, trunk, and/or extremities. Protrusion of the tongue, puffing of the cheeks, puckering of the mouth, chewing movements, and other manifestations may become evident during treatment, upon dosage reduction, or after the drug is discontinued. The likelihood that tardive dyskinesia will develop or become irreversible increases with duration of treatment and total cumulative dose; however, even relatively brief use of low doses can cause it. Although this reaction appears to occur most often in the elderly, especially among older women, it is impossible to use this information to predict, before therapy is started, which patients are likely to develop the syndrome. In general, reserve chronic therapy for patients who respond to neuroleptics and who cannot undergo another, equally effective form of treatment that is potentially less harmful. Use the lowest effective dosage, keep the duration of therapy as short as possible, and periodically reassess the need for the drug. Watch carefully for manifestations of tardive dyskinesia; fine vermicular movements of the tongue reportedly may be an early sign. However, do not forget that neuroleptic therapy can itself mask the signs and symptoms of tardive dyskinesia. If evidence of the syndrome is seen, consider terminating use of the drug, bearing in mind that some patients may require continued neuroleptic treatment despite the development of dyskinesia. There is no known treatment for tardive dyskinesia; however, after discontinuation, some or all manifestations of this syndrome may disappear spontaneously.
Other extrapyramidal effects	Extrapyramidal reactions other than tardive dyskinesia can usually be controlled by a reduction in dosage, use of an antiparkinson agent such as benztropine, or a combination of both approaches
Severe, acute hypotension	May occur, especially in patients with mitral insufficiency or pheochromocytoma
Rebound hypertension	May occur in patients with pheochromocytoma
Convulsive threshold	May be lowered in alcohol withdrawal and in patients with convulsive disorders; use acetophenazine with caution and maintain adequate concomitant anticonvulsant therapy
Psychic depression	Use with caution
Drowsiness	May occur, particularly during the 1st or 2nd week; if troublesome, reduce dosage
Mental and/or physical impairment	Caution patients that their ability to drive or perform other potentially hazardous activities may be impaired
Concurrent administration of CNS depressants	Use opiates, analgesics, antihistamines, barbiturates, and other CNS depressants with caution and at reduced dosages; advise patient to avoid use of alcohol, as response to alcohol may be heightened and additive effects and hypotension may occur
Potentially suicidal patients	Should not have access to large quantities of acetophenazine
Antiemetic effect	May mask signs and symptoms of overdosage of other drugs and such conditions as brain tumors and intestinal obstruction
Adynamic ileus	May occur and, if severe, can result in complications and death, provide close supervision, as patient may fail to seek treatment
Rise in body temperature	May suggest intolerance; if not otherwise explained, discontinue use
Surgical patients	Monitor patients requiring high doses closely for hypotensive phenomena; if necessary, reduce the amount of anesthetic or CNS depressant used
Cross-sensitivity	Use with caution in patients who have previously exhibited severe adverse reactions to other phenothiazines
Special-risk patients	Use with caution in patients with diminished renal function, respiratory impairment due to acute pulmonary infections, or chronic respiratory disorders (eg, severe asthma or emphysema), in those receiving atropine-like drugs, and in those exposed to extreme heat or phosphorous insecticides
Hepatic and renal function	Should be checked periodically; discontinue use if hepatic abnormalities occur or BUN level rises
Abrupt discontinuation of therapy	May produce gastritis, nausea, vomiting, dizziness, and tremulousness; continue concomitant antiparkinson therapy for several weeks after acetophenazine is withdrawn
Prolonged therapy	May lead to liver damage, corneal and lenticular deposits, and irreversible dyskinesias
Photosensitivity	May occur; caution patients to avoid undue exposure to sunlight
Sudden death	Has occasionally occurred with phenothiazine therapy and, in some instances, was attributable to cardiac arrest or asphyxia due to failure of the cough reflex
Blood dyscrasias	May occur; observe patient closely, especially during the 4th to 10th weeks of therapy (when most cases of agranulocytosis have occurred), for the sudden appearance of sore throat or infection. Monitor WBC count and differential; if count is significantly depressed, discontinue use of drug and institute appropriate therapy.

ADVERSE REACTIONS[1]

Central nervous system	Extrapyramidal reactions (opisthotonos, trismus, torticollis, retrocollis, aching and numbness of the limbs, motor restlessness, oculogyric crisis, hyperreflexia, dystonia, including protrusion, discoloration, aching and rounding of the tongue, tonic spasm of the masticatory muscles, tight feeling in the throat, slurred speech, dysphagia, akathisia, dyskinesia, parkinsonism, ataxia, persistent tardive dyskinesia), cerebral edema, abnormal CSF proteins, drowsiness (especially during 1st or 2nd wk of therapy), convulsive seizures, headache, paradoxical exacerbation of psychotic symptoms, catatonic-like states, paranoid reactions, lethargy, paradoxical excitement, restlessness, hyperactivity, nocturnal confusion, bizarre dreams, insomnia
Autonomic nervous system	Dry mouth or salivation, nausea, vomiting, diarrhea, anorexia, constipation, obstipation, fecal impaction, urinary retention, urinary frequency or incontinence, bladder paralysis, polyuria, nasal congestion, pallor, adynamic ileus, miosis, mydriasis, blurred vision, glaucoma, perspiration, hypertension, hypotension, change in pulse rate
Allergic	Urticaria, erythema, eczema, exfoliative dermatitis, pruritus, photosensitivity, asthma, fever, anaphylactoid reactions, laryngeal edema, angioneurotic edema, contact dermatitis; cerebral edema and circulatory collapse leading to death (very rare)
Metabolic and endocrinological	Lactation, galactorrhea, moderate breast engorgement in females and gynecomastia in males on large doses, disturbances in the menstrual cycle, amenorrhea, changes in libido, inhibition of ejaculation, syndrome of inappropriate ADH secretion, hyperglycemia, hypoglycemia, glycosuria
Cardiovascular	Postural hypotension, tachycardia (especially with sudden marked increase in dosage), bradycardia, cardiac arrest, faintness, dizziness, shock-like condition, nonspecific ECG changes
Hematological	Agranulocytosis, eosinophilia, leukopenia, hemolytic anemia, thrombocytopenic purpura, pancytopenia
Hepatic	Biliary stasis, jaundice
Dermatological	Pigmentation of the skin
Ophthalmic	Deposition of fine particulate matter in the cornea and lens, progressing in more severe cases to star-shaped lenticular opacities; epithelial keratopathies; pigmentary retinopathy
Other	Peripheral edema, parotid swelling (rare), hyperpyrexia, systemic lupus erythematosus-like syndrome, increases in appetite and weight, photophobia, polyphagia, muscle weakness; neuroleptic malignant syndrome, a potentially fatal reaction characterized by hyperthermia, autonomic disturbances, and severe extrapyramidal dysfunction (muscular rigidity followed by stupor or coma)

OVERDOSAGE

Signs and symptoms	See ADVERSE REACTIONS
Treatment	Induce emesis with ipecac syrup, taking precautions against aspiration, especially in infants and children. Follow with activated charcoal, and if vomiting is unsuccessful, gastric lavage. Do not induce vomiting if patient is unconscious. Saline cathartics may be helpful. Treat circulatory shock or metabolic acidosis with standard measures. Maintain an open airway and adequate fluid intake. Regulate body temperature. Treat hyperthermia with total-body ice-packing and antipyretics. Treat cardiac arrhythmias with neostigmine, pyridostigmine, or propranolol. Consider digitalis for cardiac failure. Monitor cardiac function for at least 5 days. For hypotension, administer norepinephrine; *do not use epinephrine.* To control convulsions, use an inhalation anesthetic, diazepam, or paraldehyde. For acute parkinson-like symptoms, administer benztropine mesylate or diphenhydramine. When treating CNS depression, avoid convulsion-producing stimulants (eg, picrotoxin, pentylenetetrazol). Dialysis is not useful. Signs of arousal may not occur for 48 h.

DRUG INTERACTIONS

Alcohol, anesthetics, barbiturates, narcotics, and other CNS depressants	↑ CNS depression
Anticonvulsants	↓ Convulsion threshold
Epinephrine	Severe hypotension
Guanethidine	↓ Antihypertensive effect
Antimuscarinics	↑ Atropine-like effect

Patients with previously detected breast cancer — Use with caution, as chronic therapy may cause a persistent elevation of serum prolactin levels, which may be of importance in patients with prolactin-dependent breast cancers. Although endocrine disturbances have been reported, no association between chronic neuroleptic administration and mammary tumorigenesis has been demonstrated; the available evidence is considered too limited to be conclusive at this time.

TINDAL ■ TRILAFON

Amphetamines	▽ Amphetamine effect
Antacids containing aluminum or magnesium ions	▽ Absorption of acetophenazine
Levodopa	▽ Antiparkinson effect
MAO inhibitors, tricyclic antidepressants	△ Sedation and antimuscarinic effects

ALTERED LABORATORY VALUES

Blood/serum values	△ or ▽ Glucose
Urinary values	△ Glucose △ Bilirubin (false elevation) △ PBI

USE IN CHILDREN

Not recommended for use in children; the safety and effectiveness of this drug have not been established in children

USE IN PREGNANT AND NURSING WOMEN

Safety for use in pregnant or nursing women has not been established

---

[1] These reactions are common to phenothiazines in general and may not necessarily occur with acetophenazine

---

PHENOTHIAZINES

TRILAFON (perphenazine) Schering   Rx

Tablets: 2, 4, 8, 16 mg   **Tablets (sustained release):** 8 mg   **Concentrate (per 5 ml):** 16 mg[1] (4 fl oz)   **Ampuls:** 5 mg/ml (1 ml)

INDICATIONS	ORAL DOSAGE	PARENTERAL DOSAGE
Manifestations of **psychotic disorders**	Adult: 4–8 mg tid to start, followed by minimum effective dosage; if sustained-release tablets are used, 8–16 mg bid to start, followed by minimum effective dosage. For hospitalized patients, 8–16 mg bid to qid; if sustained-release tablets are used, 8–32 mg bid (avoid dosages > 64 mg/day).	Adult: 5–10 mg IM (deeply), repeated as necessary q6h, up to 15 mg/day for ambulatory patients and 30 mg/day for hospitalized patients; a higher dosage may be needed when patient is transferred to oral therapy Child (> 12 yr): use lowest adult dosage
Severe nausea and vomiting	Adult: 8–24 mg/day, given in divided doses; if sustained-release tablets are used, 8–16 mg bid	Adult: 5–10 mg IM (deeply) Child (> 12 yr): use lowest adult dosage

CONTRAINDICATIONS

Hypersensitivity to perphenazine or related compounds	Coma or severe obtundation	Use of CNS depressants in large doses
Known or suspected subcortical brain damage, with or without hypothalamic damage	Blood dyscrasias Bone marrow depression	Liver damage

ADMINISTRATION/DOSAGE ADJUSTMENTS

Intravenous administration	Doses up to 5 mg may be given IV to recumbent, hospitalized adult patients by slow drip infusion or fractional injection (the former is preferable for surgical patients). For fractional injection, dilute the solution in isotonic saline to a final concentration of 0.5 mg/ml and administer not more than 1 mg at intervals of not less than 1–2 min. Use the IV route with particular caution and only when absolutely necessary to control severe vomiting, intractable hiccups, or acute conditions (eg, violent retching during surgery). Make sure that appropriate means for the management of hypotension and extrapyramidal reactions are available; blood pressure and pulse should be monitored continuously during IV administration
Dilution of concentrate	Dilute each 5 ml (1 tsp) of concentrate with approximately 60 ml (2 fl oz) of water, saline, Seven-Up, homogenized milk, carbonated orange drink, or pineapple, apricot, prune, orange, V-8, tomato, or grapefruit juice; do not mix with beverages containing caffeine (coffee, cola), tannics (tea), or pectinates (apple juice), since physical incompatibility may result

TRILAFON

WARNINGS/PRECAUTIONS

Tardive dyskinesia	Neuroleptic drugs can cause tardive dyskinesia, a potentially irreversible syndrome characterized by involuntary choreoathetoid movements of the tongue, face, mouth, lips, jaw, trunk, and/or extremities. Protrusion of the tongue, puffing of the cheeks, puckering of the mouth, chewing movements, and other manifestations may become evident during treatment, upon dosage reduction, or after the drug is discontinued. The likelihood that tardive dyskinesia will develop or become irreversible increases with duration of treatment and total cumulative dose; however, even relatively brief use of low doses can cause it. Although this reaction appears to occur most often in the elderly, especially among older women, it is impossible to use this information to predict, before therapy is started, which patients are likely to develop the syndrome. In general, reserve chronic therapy for patients who respond to neuroleptics and who cannot undergo another, equally effective form of treatment that is potentially less harmful. Use the lowest effective dosage, keep the duration of therapy as short as possible, and periodically reassess the need for the drug. Watch carefully for manifestations of tardive dyskinesia; fine vermicular movements of the tongue reportedly may be an early sign. However, do not forget that neuroleptic therapy can itself mask the signs and symptoms of tardive dyskinesia. If evidence of the syndrome is seen, consider terminating use of the drug, bearing in mind that some patients may require continued neuroleptic treatment despite the development of dyskinesia. There is no known treatment for tardive dyskinesia; however, after discontinuation, some or all manifestations of this syndrome may disappear spontaneously.
Other extrapyramidal effects	Extrapyramidal reactions other than tardive dyskinesia can usually be controlled by a reduction in dosage, use of an antiparkinson agent such as benztropine, or a combination of both approaches
Severe, acute hypotension	May occur, especially in patients with mitral insufficiency or pheochromocytoma
Rebound hypertension	May occur in patients with pheochromocytoma
Convulsive threshold	May be lowered in alcohol withdrawal and in patients with convulsive disorders; use perphenazine with caution and maintain adequate concomitant anticonvulsant therapy
Psychic depression	Use with caution
Drowsiness	May occur, particularly during the 1st or 2nd week; if troublesome, reduce dosage
Mental and/or physical impairment	Caution patients that their ability to drive or perform other potentially hazardous activities may be impaired
Concurrent administration of CNS depressants	Use opiates, analgesics, antihistamines, barbiturates, and other CNS depressants with caution and at reduced dosages; advise patient to avoid use of alcohol, as response to alcohol may be heightened and additive effects and hypotension may occur
Potentially suicidal patients	Should not have access to large quantities of perphenazine
Antiemetic effect	May mask signs and symptoms of overdosage of other drugs and such conditions as brain tumors and intestinal obstruction
Adynamic ileus	May occur and, if severe, can result in complications and death; provide close supervision, as patient may fail to seek treatment
Rise in body temperature	May suggest intolerance; if not otherwise explained, discontinue use
Surgical patients	Monitor patients requiring high doses closely for hypotensive phenomena; if necessary, reduce the amount of anesthetic or CNS depressant used
Cross-sensitivity	Use with caution in patients who have previously exhibited severe adverse reactions to other phenothiazines
Special-risk patients	Use with caution in patients with diminished renal function, respiratory impairment due to acute pulmonary infections, or chronic respiratory disorders (eg, severe asthma or emphysema), in those receiving atropine-like drugs, and in those exposed to extreme heat or phosphorous insecticides
Hepatic and renal function	Should be checked periodically; discontinue use if hepatic abnormalities occur or BUN level rises
Abrupt discontinuation of therapy	May produce gastritis, nausea, vomiting, dizziness, and tremulousness; continue concomitant antiparkinson therapy for several weeks after perphenazine is withdrawn
Prolonged therapy	May lead to liver damage, corneal and lenticular deposits, and irreversible dyskinesias
Photosensitivity	May occur; caution patients to avoid undue exposure to sunlight
Sudden death	Has occasionally occurred with phenothiazine therapy, and in some instances was attributable to cardiac arrest or asphyxia due to failure of the cough reflex
Blood dyscrasias	May occur; observe patient closely, especially during the 4th to 10th weeks of therapy (when most cases of agranulocytosis have occurred), for the sudden appearance of sore throat or infection. Monitor WBC count and differential; if count is significantly depressed, discontinue use of drug and institute appropriate therapy.
Patients with previously detected breast cancer	Use with caution, as chronic therapy may cause a persistent elevation of serum prolactin levels, which may be of importance in patients with prolactin-dependent breast cancers. Although endocrine disturbances have been reported, no association between chronic neuroleptic administration and mammary tumorigenesis has been demonstrated; the available evidence is considered too limited to be conclusive at this time.

TRILAFON

ADVERSE REACTIONS[2]

Central nervous system	Extrapyramidal reactions (opisthotonos, trismus, torticollis, retrocollis, aching and numbness of the limbs, motor restlessness, oculogyric crisis, hyperreflexia, dystonia, including protrusion, discoloration, aching and rounding of the tongue, tonic spasm of the masticatory muscles, tight feeling in the throat, slurred speech, dysphagia, akathisia, dyskinesia, parkinsonism, ataxia, persistent tardive dyskinesia), cerebral edema, abnormal CSF proteins, drowsiness (especially during 1st and 2nd wk of therapy), convulsive seizures, headache, paradoxical exacerbation of psychotic symptoms, catatonic-like states, paranoid reactions, lethargy, paradoxical excitement, restlessness, hyperactivity, nocturnal confusion, bizarre dreams, insomnia
Autonomic nervous system	Dry mouth or salivation, nausea, vomiting, diarrhea, anorexia, constipation, obstipation, fecal impaction, urinary retention, urinary frequency or incontinence, bladder paralysis, polyuria, nasal congestion, pallor, adynamic ileus, miosis, mydriasis, blurred vision, glaucoma, perspiration, hypertension, hypotension, change in pulse rate
Allergic	Urticaria, erythema, eczema, exfoliative dermatitis, pruritus, photosensitivity, asthma, fever, anaphylactoid reactions, laryngeal edema, and angioneurotic edema, contact dermatitis; cerebral edema and circulatory collapse leading to death (very rare)
Metabolic and endocrinological	Lactation, galactorrhea, moderate breast engorgement in females and gynecomastia in males on large doses, disturbances in the menstrual cycle, amenorrhea, changes in libido, inhibition of ejaculation, syndrome of inappropriate ADH secretion, hyperglycemia, hypoglycemia, glycosuria
Cardiovascular	Postural hypotension, tachycardia (especially with sudden marked increase in dosage), bradycardia, cardiac arrest, faintness, dizziness, shock-like condition, nonspecific ECG changes
Hematological	Agranulocytosis, eosinophilia, leukopenia, hemolytic anemia, thrombocytopenic purpura, pancytopenia
Hepatic	Biliary stasis, jaundice
Dermatological	Pigmentation of the skin
Ophthalmic	Deposition of fine particulate matter in the cornea and lens, progression in more severe cases to star-shaped lenticular opacities; epithelial keratopathies; pigmentary retinopathy
Other	Peripheral edema, parotid swelling (rare), hyperpyrexia, systemic lupus erythematosus-like syndrome, increases in appetite and weight, photophobia, polyphagia, muscle weakness; neuroleptic malignant syndrome, a potentially fatal reaction characterized by hyperthermia, autonomic disturbances, and severe extrapyramidal dysfunction (muscular rigidity followed by stupor or coma)

OVERDOSAGE

Signs and symptoms	See ADVERSE REACTIONS
Treatment	Induce emesis with ipecac syrup, taking precautions against aspiration, especially in infants and children. Follow with activated charcoal and, if vomiting is unsuccessful, gastric lavage. Do not induce vomiting if patient is unconscious. Saline cathartics may be helpful. Treat circulatory shock or metabolic acidosis with standard measures. Maintain an open airway and adequate fluid intake. Regulate body temperature. Treat hyperthermia with total-body ice-packing and antipyretics. Treat cardiac arrhythmias with neostigmine, pyridostigmine, or propranolol. Consider digitalis for cardiac failure. Monitor cardiac function for at least 5 days. For hypotension, administer norepinephrine; *do not use epinephrine*. To control convulsions, use an inhalation anesthetic, diazepam, or paraldehyde. For acute parkinson-like symptoms, administer benztropine mesylate or diphenhydramine. When treating CNS depression, avoid convulsion-producing stimulants (eg, picrotoxin, pentylenetetrazol). Dialysis is not useful. Signs of arousal may not occur for 48 h.

DRUG INTERACTIONS

Alcohol, anesthetics, barbiturates, narcotics, and other CNS depressants	△ CNS depression
Anticonvulsants	▽ Convulsion threshold
Epinephrine	Severe hypotension
Guanethidine	▽ Antihypertensive effect
Antimuscarinics	△ Atropine-like effect
Amphetamines	▽ Amphetamine effect
Antacids containing aluminum and/or magnesium ions	▽ Absorption of perphenazine
MAO inhibitors, tricyclic antidepressants	△ Sedation and antimuscarinic effects

ALTERED LABORATORY VALUES

Blood/serum values	△ PBI △ Glucose
Urinary values	False-positive or false-negative pregnancy tests △ Bilirubin (false elevation)

USE IN CHILDREN	USE IN PREGNANT AND NURSING WOMEN
Not recommended for use in children under 12 yr of age	Safety for use in pregnant or nursing women has not been established

[1] Contains < 0.1% alcohol
[2] These reactions are common to phenothiazines in general and may not necessarily occur with perphenazine

PHENOTHIAZINES

VESPRIN (triflupromazine hydrochloride) Princeton — Rx

Tablets: 10, 25, 50 mg **Vials:** 10, 20 mg/ml

INDICATIONS	ORAL DOSAGE	PARENTERAL DOSAGE
Manifestations of **psychotic disorders,** excluding depressive reactions	**Adult:** 100 mg to start, up to 150 mg/day; for maintenance, 30–150 mg/day **Child (2½–12 yr):** 2 mg/kg, up to 150 mg/day, given in divided doses	**Adult:** 60 mg IM, up to 150 mg/day, until symptoms are controlled **Child (2½–12 yr):** 0.2–0.25 mg/kg IM, up to 10 mg/day
Severe nausea and vomiting	**Adult:** 20–30 mg/day **Child (2½–12 yr):** 0.2 mg/kg, up to 10 mg/day in 3 divided doses	**Adult:** 1 mg IV, up to 3 mg/day, or 5–15 mg IM as a single dose repeated q4h, up to 60 mg/day **Child (2½–12 yr):** 0.2–0.25 mg/kg IM, up to 10 mg/day

CONTRAINDICATIONS		
Known or suspected subcortical brain damage, with or without hypothalamic damage	Use of hypnotics in high doses	Blood dyscrasias
	Hepatic damage	Comatose states
Severe CNS depression		

ADMINISTRATION/DOSAGE ADJUSTMENTS

Elderly or debilitated patients — For severe nausea and vomiting, give 2.5 mg IM, up to 15 mg/day

WARNINGS/PRECAUTIONS

Tardive dyskinesia — Neuroleptic drugs can cause tardive dyskinesia, a potentially irreversible syndrome characterized by involuntary choreoathetoid movements of the tongue, face, mouth, lips, jaw, trunk, and/or extremities. Protrusion of the tongue, puffing of the cheeks, puckering of the mouth, chewing movements, and other manifestations may become evident during treatment, upon dosage reduction, or after the drug is discontinued. The likelihood that tardive dyskinesia will develop or become irreversible increases with duration of treatment and total cumulative dose; however, even relatively brief use of low doses can cause it. Although this reaction appears to occur most often in the elderly, especially among older women, it is impossible to use this information to predict, before therapy is started, which patients are likely to develop the syndrome.

In general, reserve chronic therapy for patients who respond to neuroleptics and who cannot undergo another, equally effective form of treatment that is potentially less harmful. Use the lowest effective dosage, keep the duration of therapy as short as possible, and periodically reassess the need for the drug. Since neuroleptic therapy can mask the signs of tardive dyskinesia, reduce the dosage periodically (if clinically feasible); if signs of dyskinesia appear, consider terminating use of the drug, bearing in mind that some patients may require continued neuroleptic treatment despite the development of dyskinesia. There is no known treatment for tardive dyskinesia; however, after discontinuation, some or all manifestations of this syndrome may disappear spontaneously.

Other extrapyramidal reactions — Caution patients not only concerning tardive dyskinesia, but also about other extrapyramidal reactions. Use of an antiparkinson agent (eg, benztropine) and a reduction in dosage are usually effective for control of extrapyramidal reactions other than tardive dyskinesia. Reassurance is also important.

Convulsions — Grand mal convulsions have been seen during therapy. Sudden death has also occurred; previous brain damage or seizures may increase this risk. Exercise caution when patients have a history of convulsive disorders; avoid use of high doses in patients who have such disorders.

Autonomic reactions — To control autonomic reactions, reduce dosage or temporarily withdraw the drug

VESPRIN

Cross-sensitivity	Use with caution in patients with either a history of phenothiazine-related hypersensitivity reactions (eg, jaundice, dermatoses) or a history of idiosyncratic reactions to central acting drugs
Hepatotoxicity	Cholestatic jaundice or biliary stasis may occur, especially during the first months of therapy. Check hepatic function periodically; if jaundice develops, treatment should be discontinued. Since triflupromazine is potentially hepatotoxic, use in children or adolescents with signs or symptoms suggesting Reye's syndrome should be avoided. Abnormal liver function values, including an increase in cephalin flocculation, have been detected during therapy even when no clinical evidence of liver damage was apparent.
Hypotension	Patients with pheochromocytoma, cerebrovascular or renal insufficiency, or a severe cardiac-reserve deficiency such as mitral insufficiency appear to be especially susceptible to phenothiazine-induced hypotension and therefore should be closely observed when the drug is administered. During surgery, patients who have received large doses should be carefully watched since hypotension may occur at that time. Triflupromazine should generally not be used before spinal anesthesia. If severe hypotension is seen, immediately give norepinephrine or phenylephrine; do not use epinephrine (see DRUG INTERACTIONS). To avoid postural hypotension following parenteral administration, keep patient under close supervision and, if necessary, in a recumbent position.
Blood dyscrasias	Agranulocytosis and other hematological reactions may occur during therapy; obtain routine blood counts periodically. If WBC count is depressed and soreness of the mouth, gums, or throat or any other sign or symptom of upper respiratory tract infection is detected, discontinue drug and institute appropriate measures immediately.
Masking of nonpsychotic conditions	Extrapyramidal symptoms associated with triflupromazine may be confused with the neurological manifestations of an undiagnosed primary disease such as Reye's syndrome or another encephalopathy; antiemetic effect may mask nausea and vomiting associated with intestinal obstruction, brain tumor, Reye's syndrome, or toxicity of antineoplastic agents or other drugs
Drowsiness	Caution ambulatory patients that their ability to drive or perform other activities requiring mental alertness or physical coordination may be impaired; if necessary, reduce dosage to control drowsiness
Pneumonia	Watch for "silent" pneumonias
Renal function	Check renal function periodically during prolonged therapy; if BUN level becomes abnormal, treatment should be discontinued
Carcinogenicity	Chronic use of neuroleptic drugs causes a persistent elevation of the serum prolactin level, an effect that may be of potential importance if the patient has prolactin-dependent breast cancer. Chronic administration has produced an increase in mammary neoplasia in rodents, and endocrine disturbances have been seen in humans; although no clinical or epidemiological studies have shown an association between chronic neuroleptic therapy and mammary tumorigenesis, the available evidence is considered too limited to be conclusive at this time.
Tartrazine sensitivity	Presence of FD&C Yellow No. 5 (tartrazine) in 25- and 50-mg tablets may cause allergic-type reactions, including bronchial asthma, in certain susceptible individuals, such as those hypersensitive to aspirin

ADVERSE REACTIONS[1]

Central nervous system	Drowsiness, lethargy; extrapyramidal reactions, including pseudoparkinsonism, dystonia, dyskinesia, akathisia, oculogyric crisis, opisthotonos, hyperreflexia, and tardive dyskinesia; catatonic-like states (at dosage far above recommended level), restlessness, excitement, bizarre dreams, reactivation or aggravation of psychosis, CSF protein abnormalities, cerebral edema, EEG changes
Ophthalmic	Blurred vision, glaucoma, pigmentary retinopathy; with prolonged use, corneal and lenticular deposits
Cardiovascular	Hypotension, hypertension, headache, fluctuations in blood pressure, tachycardia, ECG changes, cardiac arrest, peripheral edema
Hematological	Agranulocytosis, leukopenia, pancytopenia, thrombocytopenic and nonthrombocytopenic purpura, eosinophilia
Gastrointestinal	Cholestatic jaundice, biliary stasis, anorexia, nausea, constipation, fecal impaction, paralytic ileus
Genitourinary	Impotence, increased libido (in women), polyuria, bladder paralysis
Endocrinological	Lactation, menstrual irregularities, gynecomastia
Dermatological	Hypersensitivity reactions (see below); with prolonged use, skin pigmentation
Hypersensitivity	Pruritus, erythema, urticaria, seborrhea, photosensitivity, eczema, exfoliative dermatitis, asthma, laryngeal edema, angioneurotic edema, anaphylactoid reactions
Other	Dry mouth, nasal congestion, salivation, perspiration, hyperthermia (with exposure to extreme heat), weight change, enhanced effect of organophosphorous insecticides, systemic lupus erythematosus-like syndrome

OVERDOSAGE

Signs and symptoms	See ADVERSE REACTIONS
Treatment	Discontinue medication; treat symptomatically and institute supportive measures, as required. Combat hypotension with norepinephrine. *Do not use epinephrine.* Treat extrapyramidal reactions with antiparkinson agents other than levodopa (such as benztropine mesylate).

DRUG INTERACTIONS

Other CNS depressants, including alcohol	△ CNS depression; a reduction in the dosage of CNS depressants used with triflupromazine may be necessary
Anticonvulsants	△ Risk of convulsions △ Pharmacologic effect of phenytoin
Metrizamide	△ Risk of convulsions; discontinue use of triflupromazine at least 48 h before administration of metrizamide for myelography and wait at least 24 h after the procedure before resuming use. Do not use triflupromazine before or after myelography for control of nausea and vomiting.
Anticholinergic drugs	△ Anticholinergic effects ▽ Antipsychotic effect
Epinephrine	Severe hypotension
Guanethidine	▽ Antihypertensive effect
Propranolol	△ Pharmacologic effects of propranolol and triflupromazine
Amphetamines	▽ Antipsychotic effect ▽ Anorectic effect
Phenmetrazine	▽ Anorectic effect
Lithium	△ Risk of acute encephalopathy and extrapyramidal reactions ▽ Serum triflupromazine level △ Renal clearance of lithium
Tricyclic antidepressants	△ Serum level of tricyclic antidepressants and triflupromazine ▽ Antipsychotic effect
Oral anticoagulants	▽ Anticoagulant effect

ALTERED LABORATORY VALUES

Blood/serum values	△ SGOT △ SGPT △ LDH △ Alkaline phosphatase △ Bilirubin △ Cephalin flocculation △ Prolactin
Urinary values	▽ VMA + Pregnancy (with immunologic pregnancy tests) + Bilirubin (with reagent test strips) △ Urobilinogen (with Ehrlich's reagent test) ▽ 5-HIAA (with nitrosonaphthol reagent test) Interference with determination of catecholamines (with Pisano method), 17-KS (with Haltorff-Koch modification of Zimmerman reaction), and 17-OHCS (with modified Glenn-Nelson technique)

USE IN CHILDREN

See INDICATIONS and dosage recommendations; not recommended for use in children under 2½ yr of age or for conditions in which pediatric dosages have not been established. Avoid use in children or adolescents with signs or symptoms suggesting Reye's syndrome. In children, an IM dose may be effective for up to 12 h.

USE IN PREGNANT AND NURSING WOMEN

Safety for use during pregnancy have not been established; weigh potential benefits against possible risks before using in pregnant women. Consult manufacturer for use in nursing mothers.

---

[1] Sudden, inexplicable death has occurred in patients taking phenothiazines; autopsy findings have usually revealed intramyocardial lesions, aspirated gastric contents, or evidence of acute fulminating pneumonia or pneumonitis. In several cases, psychosis suddenly recurred shortly before death. Previous brain damage or seizures may be predisposing factors (see warning above concerning convulsions).

THIOXANTHENES

NAVANE (thiothixene) Roerig   Rx

Capsules: 1, 2, 5, 10, 20 mg   **Concentrate:** 5 mg/ml[1] (30, 120 ml)   **Vials:** 2 mg/ml (Navane Intramuscular Solution; 2 ml); 5 mg/ml after reconstitution (Navane Intramuscular for Injection)

INDICATIONS	ORAL DOSAGE	PARENTERAL DOSAGE
Manifestations of **psychotic disorders**	**Adult:** 2 mg tid to start, followed by up to 15 mg/day, if needed; for severe symptoms, 5 mg bid to start, followed by up to 60 mg/day[2]; optimal maintenance dosage, 20–30 mg/day (some patients may be maintained on single daily doses)	**Adult:** 4 mg IM bid to qid, followed by up to 30 mg/day; usual dosage, 16–20 mg/day (switch to oral medication as soon as possible)

NAVANE

CONTRAINDICATIONS

Hypersensitivity to thiothixene	Blood dyscrasias	Comatose states
CNS depression	Circulatory collapse	

ADMINISTRATION/DOSAGE ADJUSTMENTS

Reconstitution of Navane Intramuscular for Injection	To prepare the solution for injection, add 2.2 ml of sterile water for injection to the contents of the vial; the reconstituted solution may be kept at room temperature for up to 48 h before it must be discarded
Intramuscular administration	Parenteral therapy should be reserved for patients who are unable or unwilling to take oral medication and for rapid control and treatment of acute behavioral symptoms. To help prevent inadvertent intravascular injection, aspirate before administration; then, inject deeply into a relatively large muscle, preferably the gluteus maximus or a midlateral thigh muscle. Use the deltoid area only if it is well developed and only if caution is exercised to avoid radial nerve injury; do not inject into the lower or middle third of the upper arm.

WARNINGS/PRECAUTIONS

Tardive dyskinesia	Neuroleptic drugs can cause tardive dyskinesia, a potentially irreversible syndrome characterized by involuntary choreoathetoid movements of the tongue, face, mouth, lips, jaw, trunk, and/or extremities. Protrusion of the tongue, puffing of the cheeks, puckering of the mouth, chewing movements, and other manifestations may become evident during treatment, upon dosage reduction, or after the drug is discontinued. The likelihood that tardive dyskinesia will develop or become irreversible increases with duration of treatment and total cumulative dose; however, even relatively brief use of low doses can cause it. Although this reaction appears to occur most often in the elderly, especially among older women, it is impossible to use this information to predict, before therapy is started, which patients are likely to develop the syndrome. In general, reserve chronic therapy for patients who respond to neuroleptics and who cannot undergo another, equally effective form of treatment that is potentially less harmful. Use the lowest effective dosage, keep the duration of therapy as short as possible, and periodically reassess the need for the drug. Watch carefully for manifestations of tardive dyskinesia; fine vermicular movements of the tongue reportedly may be an early sign. However, do not forget that neuroleptic therapy can itself mask the signs and symptoms of tardive dyskinesia. If evidence of the syndrome is seen, consider terminating use of the drug, bearing in mind that some patients may require continued neuroleptic treatment despite the development of dyskinesia. There is no known treatment for tardive dyskinesia; however, after discontinuation, some or all manifestations of this syndrome may disappear spontaneously.
Other extrapyramidal effects	Management of extrapyramidal reactions such as pseudoparkinsonism, akathisia, and dystonia depends on the nature of the reaction. Acute symptoms may require use of a parenteral antiparkinson agent, whereas more slowly emerging symptoms may be controlled by a reduction in dosage, use of an oral antiparkinson agent, or a combination of both approaches.
Mental and/or physical impairment	Caution ambulatory patients that their ability to drive or perform other potentially hazardous activities may be impaired, especially during the first few days of therapy, and that use of alcohol or other CNS depressants with this drug may have additive effects, including possibly hypotension
Antiemetic action	May mask signs and symptoms of overdosage of other drugs or such conditions as intestinal obstruction and brain tumor
Special-risk patients	Use with caution in patients with cardiovascular disease or glaucoma (with IM use), in those receiving atropine or similar drugs and CNS depressants other than anticonvulsants, and in those exposed to extreme heat
Convulsions	May occur; use with extreme caution in patients with a history of convulsive disorders or those in a state of alcohol withdrawal; do not reduce dosage of concomitant anticonvulsant therapy
Ocular changes	May occur; monitor patients for pigmentary retinopathy and lenticular pigmentation
Photosensitivity	May occur; advise patients to avoid undue exposure to sunlight
Radial nerve injury	May result from IM injection into deltoid muscle; use the deltoid region with extreme caution and only if it is well developed (see ADMINISTRATION/DOSAGE ADJUSTMENTS)
Blood dyscrasias	Agranulocytosis, pancytopenia, and thrombocytopenic purpura have occurred with related drugs
Hepatic damage	Jaundice and biliary stasis have occurred with related drugs
Sudden death	Has occasionally occurred with phenothiazine therapy and, in some instances, was attributable to cardiac arrest or asphyxia due to failure of cough reflex
Patients with previously detected breast cancer	Use with caution, as chronic therapy may cause a persistent elevation of serum prolactin levels, which may be of importance in patients with prolactin-dependent breast cancers. Although endocrine disturbances have been reported, no association between chronic neuroleptic administration and mammary tumorigenesis has been demonstrated; the available evidence is considered too limited to be conclusive at this time.

NAVANE ■ TARACTAN

ADVERSE REACTIONS[3]

Central nervous system	Drowsiness, sedation, restlessness, agitation, insomnia, seizures, paradoxical exacerbation of psychotic symptoms, cerebral edema, CSF abnormalities; extrapyramidal symptoms, including pseudoparkinsonism, akathisia, and dystonia, persistent tardive dyskinesia, weakness, fatigue
Cardiovascular	Tachycardia, hypotension, lightheadedness, syncope, nonspecific ECG changes
Hematological	Leukopenia, leukocytosis
Allergic	Rash, pruritus, urticaria, photosensitivity; anaphylaxis (rare)
Endocrinological	Lactation, breast enlargement, amenorrhea
Autonomic nervous system	Dry mouth, blurred vision, nasal congestion, constipation, diaphoresis, increased salivation, impotence
Other	Hyperpyrexia, anorexia, nausea, vomiting, diarrhea, increased appetite and weight gain, polydipsia, peripheral edema

OVERDOSAGE

Signs and symptoms	Muscular twitching, drowsiness, dizziness, CNS depression, rigidity, weakness, torticollis, tremor, salivation, dysphagia, hypotension, disturbance of gait, coma
Treatment	Empty stomach by gastric lavage. Maintain patent airway. Treat extrapyramidal symptoms with antiparkinson drugs. Avoid use of convulsion-inducing stimulants (eg, picrotoxin or pentylenetetrazol). Employ standard measures for circulatory shock, including the use of IV fluids. Restrict use of vasoconstrictors to norepinephrine and phenylephrine; *do not use epinephrine*. Peritoneal dialysis or hemodialysis is not helpful.

DRUG INTERACTIONS

Alcohol, anesthetics, barbiturates, narcotics, and other CNS depressants	△ CNS depression
Anticonvulsants	▽ Convulsion threshold
Epinephrine	Severe hypotension
Guanethidine	▽ Antihypertensive effect
Antimuscarinics	△ Atropine-like effect
Amphetamines	▽ Amphetamine effect
Antacids containing aluminum or magnesium ions	▽ Absorption of thiothixene
MAO inhibitors, tricyclic antidepressants	△ Sedation and antimuscarinic effects

ALTERED LABORATORY VALUES

Blood/serum values	△ Alkaline phosphatase △ SGOT △ SGPT ▽ Uric acid

No clinically significant alterations in urinary values occur at therapeutic dosages

---

USE IN CHILDREN

Not recommended for use in children under 12 yr of age because conditions for the safe use of this drug in children have not been established

USE IN PREGNANT AND NURSING WOMEN

Safety for use during pregnancy has not been established. Animal reproduction studies have not demonstrated teratogenicity, but some decrease in conception rate and litter size and an increase in resorption rate were observed in rats and rabbits. Hyperreflexia has occurred in infants of mothers receiving structurally related drugs. Use with caution in nursing mothers; it is not known whether thiothixene is excreted in human milk.

---

[1] Contains 7.0% alcohol
[2] Dosages exceeding 60 mg/day rarely increase the beneficial response to this drug
[3] Various other side effects common to phenothiazines in general may occur but have not been specifically reported with thiothixene, which is structurally related to these compounds

---

THIOXANTHENES

TARACTAN (chlorprothixene) Roche Rx

Tablets: 10, 25, 50, 100 mg **Concentrate (per 5 ml):** 100 mg[1] (1 pt) *fruit-flavored* **Ampuls:** 12.5 mg/ml[2] (2 ml)

INDICATIONS	ORAL DOSAGE	PARENTERAL DOSAGE
Manifestations of **psychotic disorders**	**Adult:** 25–50 mg tid or qid to start, followed by increases in dosage, as needed (dosages exceeding 600 mg/day are rarely necessary); for elderly or debilitated patients, give 10–25 mg tid or qid to start **Child (> 6 yr):** 10–25 mg tid or qid	**Adult:** 25–50 mg IM up to 3–4 times/day

TARACTAN

CONTRAINDICATIONS

| Coma due to CNS depressants | Circulatory collapse | Hypersensitivity to chlorprothixene |

ADMINISTRATION/DOSAGE ADJUSTMENTS

Parenteral use	To avoid postural hypotension, inject the drug with the patient in a seated or recumbent position; if hypotension occurs, observe patient until symptoms disappear. Switch gradually from parenteral to oral therapy once acute agitation has been controlled; give oral and parenteral doses alternately on the same day and then give oral doses alone.
Dilution of oral concentrate	Give concentrate as supplied or dilute in milk, water, fruit juice, coffee, or a carbonated beverage

WARNINGS/PRECAUTIONS

Tardive dyskinesia	Neuroleptic drugs can cause tardive dyskinesia, a potentially irreversible syndrome characterized by involuntary choreoathetoid movements of the tongue, face, mouth, lips, jaw, trunk, and/or extremities. Protrusion of the tongue, puffing of the cheeks, puckering of the mouth, chewing movements, and other manifestations may become evident during treatment, upon dosage reduction, or after the drug is discontinued. The likelihood that tardive dyskinesia will develop or become irreversible increases with duration of treatment and total cumulative dose; however, even relatively brief use of low doses can cause it. Although this reaction appears to occur most often in the elderly, especially among older women, it is impossible to use this information to predict, before therapy is started, which patients are likely to develop the syndrome. In general, reserve chronic therapy for patients who respond to neuroleptics and who cannot undergo another, equally effective form of treatment that is potentially less harmful. Use the lowest effective dosage, keep the duration of therapy as short as possible, and periodically reassess the need for the drug. Since neuroleptic therapy can mask the signs of tardive dyskinesia, reduce the dosage periodically (if clinically feasible); if signs of dyskinesia appear, consider terminating use of the drug, bearing in mind that some patients may require continued neuroleptic treatment despite the development of dyskinesia. There is no known treatment for tardive dyskinesia; however, after discontinuation, some or all manifestations of this syndrome may disappear spontaneously.
Dystonias	Control dystonias by giving either diphenhydramine or an anticholinergic antiparkinson agent parenterally
Akathisia	Constant motor restlessness (akathisia) due to this drug is often confused with agitation associated with psychosis; asking patients if they have the ability to stop moving may permit one to make a distinction. To treat akathisia, temporarily reduce dosage until symptoms subside.
Pseudoparkinsonism	To alleviate symptoms of pseudoparkinsonism, first reduce dosage; if symptoms are not adequately controlled, administer benztropine, biperiden, procyclidine, trihexyphenidyl, or amantadine. Antiparkinson therapy should be evaluated periodically to determine whether it is still necessary.
Convulsions, ECT	Chlorprothixene can cause convulsions, particularly in patients with EEG abnormalities; use with caution in patients with a history of epilepsy. Give chlorprothixene in combination with electroconvulsive therapy (ECT) only when essential, since this drug may increase the hazards of ECT.
Drowsiness	Lethargy and drowsiness occur frequently, are dose-related, and usually disappear with continued use. Closely supervise patients, particularly at higher dosages; to control sedation, reduce dosage. Caution all patients about driving and engaging in other potentially hazardous activities requiring mental alertness or physical coordination.
Hypotension, tachycardia	Chlorprothixene commonly produces orthostatic hypotension; if a vasopressor is required, use norepinephrine or metaraminol, not epinephrine. This drug also causes tachycardia, especially with a sudden and marked increase in dosage. Use with caution in patients with cardiovascular disease.
Blood dyscrasias	In very rare cases, agranulocytosis or other hematological disorders may occur during therapy; if signs of blood dyscrasia are seen, discontinue use immediately and institute appropriate treatment
Photosensitivity	Instruct patients to avoid undue exposure to the sun
Hyperpyrexia	Use with caution in patients exposed to extreme heat
Respiratory impairment	If respiratory function is impaired because of an acute pulmonary infection or a chronic respiratory disorder such as severe asthma or emphysema, exercise caution
Insecticides	Use with caution in patients exposed to organophosphorous insecticides
Depressed patients	Take appropriate precautions when using chlorprothixene in depressed patients; protective measures may be necessary, since these patients may have suicidal tendencies
Abrupt withdrawal	Gastritis, nausea, vomiting, dizziness, and tremulousness may occur following abrupt discontinuation of high-dose therapy
Prolonged use	Watch for liver damage, thyroid function abnormalities, pigmentary retinopathy, lenticular and corneal deposits, and irreversible dyskinesia during prolonged therapy

TARACTAN

Combination psychotropic therapy	Chlorprothixene may augment or interfere with the absorption, metabolism, or therapeutic activity of other psychotropic drugs, and these drugs may, in turn, have a similar effect on chlorprothixene (see DRUG INTERACTIONS)
Carcinogenicity	Chronic use of neuroleptic drugs causes a persistent elevation of the plasma prolactin level, an effect that may be of potential importance if the patient has prolactin-dependent breast cancer. Chronic administration has produced an increase in mammary neoplasia in rodents, and endocrine disturbances have been seen in humans; although no clinical or epidemiological studies have shown an association between chronic neuroleptic therapy and mammary tumorigenesis, the available evidence is considered too limited to be conclusive at this time.
Tartrazine sensitivity	Presence of FD&C Yellow No. 5 (tartrazine) in tablets may cause allergic-type reactions, including bronchial asthma, in certain susceptible individuals, such as those hypersensitive to aspirin

ADVERSE REACTIONS[3]

Central nervous system	Drowsiness, dystonias (acute torticollis, opisthotonos, carpopedal spasm, trismus, dysphagia, respiratory difficulty, oculogyric crisis, protrusion of the tongue), akathisia, pseudoparkinsonism (generalized increase in muscle tone, cogwheel rigidity, tremor, bradyphrenia, bradykinesia, masked facies, drooling, difficulty initiating movements, lack of associated movements, micrographia), tardive dyskinesia, insomnia, hyperactivity, stimulation, convulsions, ataxia, headache, exacerbation of psychotic symptoms, weakness
Ophthalmic	Visual and ocular changes
Cardiovascular	Orthostatic hypotension, tachycardia, dizziness, ECG changes (especially nonspecific distortions of Q and T waves)
Hematological	Agranulocytosis, eosinophilia, leukopenia, hemolytic anemia, thrombocytopenic purpura, pancytopenia
Gastrointestinal	Jaundice, constipation, upset stomach
Endocrinological	Galactorrhea, increased libido
Dermatological	Dermatitis, urticaria, photosensitivity
Other	Dry mouth, nasal congestion, excessive weight gain, excessive thirst, hyperpyrexia

OVERDOSAGE

Signs and symptoms	Drowsiness, coma, respiratory depression, hypotension, tachycardia, fever, and miosis, followed during recovery by convulsions, hyperactivity, and hematuria; hypotension may occur several hours after the overdose and persist for 2–3 days
Treatment	Empty stomach by gastric lavage. Institute measures to maintain respiratory function. Treat hypotension with IV fluids and, if severe, with norepinephrine or metaraminol; *do not use epinephrine.* The judicious use of amobarbital sodium is recommended for convulsions. Caffeine and sodium benzoate injection or ethamivan may be used to reverse prolonged coma; however, bear in mind that these preparations may precipitate a convulsion.

DRUG INTERACTIONS

Other CNS depressants, including alcohol	⇧ CNS depression; reduce dosage of barbiturates and narcotic drugs given in combination with chlorprothixene. Caution patients about the risks of consuming alcohol during therapy.
Anticonvulsants	⇧ Risk of convulsions; adjust anticonvulsant dosage ⇧ Pharmacologic effect of phenytoin
Metrizamide	⇧ Risk of convulsions; discontinue use of chlorthixene at least 48 h before administration of metrizamide for myelography and wait at least 24 h after the procedure before resuming use. Do not use chlorprothixene before or after myelography for control of nausea and vomiting.
Anticholinergic drugs	⇧ Anticholinergic effects; exercise caution during combination therapy ⇩ Antipsychotic effect
Epinephrine	Severe hypotension
Guanethidine	⇩ Antihypertensive effect
Propranolol	⇧ Pharmacologic effects of propranolol and chlorprothixene
Amphetamines	⇩ Antipsychotic effect ⇩ Anorectic effect
Phenmetrazine	⇩ Anorectic effect
Lithium	⇧ Risk of acute encephalopathy and extrapyramidal reactions ⇩ Plasma chlorprothixene level ⇧ Renal clearance of lithium
Tricyclic antidepressants	⇧ Plasma level of tricyclic antidepressants and chlorprothixene ⇩ Antipsychotic effect

TARACTAN

Oral anticoagulants	▽ Anticoagulant effect

ALTERED LABORATORY VALUES

Blood/serum values	△ SGOT △ SGPT △ LDH △ Alkaline phosphatase △ Bilirubin △ Prolactin
Urinary values	▽ VMA + Pregnancy (with immunologic pregnancy tests) + Bilirubin (with reagent test strips) △ Urobilinogen (with Ehrlich's reagent test) ▽ 5-HIAA (with nitrosonaphthol reagent test) Interference with determination of catecholamines (with Pisano method), 17-KS (with Haltorff Koch modification of Zimmerman reaction), and 17-OHCS (with modified Glenn-Nelson technique)

USE IN CHILDREN

See INDICATIONS and ORAL DOSAGE; safety and effectiveness for oral use in children under 6 yr of age and for parenteral use in children under 12 yr of age have not been established

USE IN PREGNANT AND NURSING WOMEN

Pregnant women: Safety for use in pregnant women has not been established. Reproduction studies with rats have shown the following: (1) an increase in stillborn fetuses and decreases in rate of conception, number of implantation sites, number of live fetuses per litter, and mean fetal body weight at 12 mg/kg and (2) an increase in resorptions at 24 mg/kg. Use in women who may become pregnant only if the expected benefits justify the possible risks. **Nursing mothers:** Safety for use in nursing mothers has not been established.

[1] As the lactate and hydrochloride salts
[2] As the hydrochloride salt
[3] The effects associated with phenothiazines should be considered before beginning therapy since these drugs are structurally related to chlorprothixene; the following reactions have been seen with phenothiazines but have not been reported for chlorprothixene: hyperreflexia, CSF protein abnormalities, cerebral edema; enhanced response to CNS depressants, atropine, extreme heat, and organophosphorous insecticides; obstipation, adynamic ileus, inhibition of ejaculation, cardiac arrest, bradycardia, faintness, biliary stasis, gynecomastia, menstrual irregularities, moderate breast engorgement, hyperglycemia, hypoglycemia, glycosuria, pruritus, erythema, eczema, exfoliative dermatitis, asthma, laryngeal edema, angioneurotic edema, anaphylactoid reactions, enlargement of the parotid gland, catatonic-like states, peripheral edema, systemic lupus erythematosus-like syndrome, pigmentary retinopathy, skin pigmentation, epithelial keratopathy, and lenticular and corneal deposits. Occasionally, patients receiving phenothiazines have suddenly died; although in some cases death appeared to result from cardiac arrest or from asphyxia due to failure of the cough reflex, there was insufficient evidence to establish that it was drug-related.

Chapter 42

Muscle Relaxants

Muscle Relaxants — 1699

DANTRIUM (Norwich Eaton) — 1699
Dantrolene sodium *Rx*

FLEXERIL (Merck Sharp & Dohme) — 1700
Cyclobenzaprine hydrochloride *Rx*

LIORESAL (Geigy) — 1701
Baclofen *Rx*

MAOLATE (Upjohn) — 1703
Chlorphenesin carbamate *Rx*

NORFLEX (Riker) — 1703
Orphenadrine citrate *Rx*

PARAFLEX (McNeil Pharmaceutical) — 1704
Chlorzoxazone *Rx*

QUINAMM (Merrell Dow) — 1705
Quinine sulfate *Rx*

ROBAXIN (Robins) — 1707
Methocarbamol *Rx*

SKELAXIN (Carnrick) — 1708
Metaxalone *Rx*

SOMA (Wallace) — 1708
Carisoprodol *Rx*

VALIUM (Roche) — 1709
Diazepam *C-IV*

VALRELEASE (Roche) — 1710
Diazepam *C-IV*

Muscle Relaxants with Analgesics — 1712

NORGESIC (Riker) — 1712
Orphenadrine citrate, aspirin, and caffeine *Rx*

NORGESIC Forte (Riker) — 1712
Orphenadrine citrate, aspirin, and caffeine *Rx*

PARAFON FORTE (McNeil Pharmaceutical) — 1714
Chlorzoxazone and acetaminophen *Rx*

ROBAXISAL (Robins) — 1715
Methocarbamol and aspirin *Rx*

SOMA Compound (Wallace) — 1716
Carisoprodol and aspirin *Rx*

SOMA Compound with Codeine (Wallace) — 1717
Carisoprodol, aspirin, and codeine phosphate *C-III*

MUSCLE RELAXANTS

DANTRIUM (dantrolene sodium) Norwich Eaton   Rx

Capsules: 25, 50, 100 mg

INDICATIONS	**ORAL DOSAGE**
Spasticity resulting from upper motor neuron disorders (eg, spinal cord injury, stroke, cerebral palsy, and multiple sclerosis)	**Adult:** 25 mg once daily to start; increase to 25 mg bid to qid, followed by 25-mg increments at 4- to 7-day intervals, up to 100 mg bid to qid, as needed **Child (5–12 yr):** 0.5 mg/kg bid to start; increase to 0.5 mg/kg tid or qid, followed by increments of 0.5 mg/kg at 4- to 7-day intervals, up to 3 mg/kg bid to qid, as needed, but not more than 100 mg qid
Prevention or attenuation of **malignant hyperthermia** in susceptible patients who require **anesthesia or surgery**	**Adult:** 4–8 mg/kg/day, given in 3–4 divided doses for 1–2 days before procedure; administer final dose, with a minimum of water, approximately 3–4 h before procedure
Prevention of **recurrence of malignant hyperthermia**	**Adult:** 4–8 mg/kg/day, given in 4 divided doses for 1–3 days after a hyperthermic crisis
CONTRAINDICATIONS	
Active hepatic disease (eg, hepatitis and cirrhosis)	Spasticity utilized to sustain upright posture and balance in locomotion or to obtain or maintain increased function
Breast-feeding	
ADMINISTRATION/DOSAGE ADJUSTMENTS	
Chronic spasticity	Dosage must be individually titrated; use lowest dose compatible with optimal response. Maintain each dosage level for 4 to 7 days to determine response. Do not increase dosage beyond level at which patient received maximal benefit without adverse effects (dose may have to be reduced to this level). If benefits are not evident within 45 days, stop therapy because of potential for liver damage (see WARNINGS/PRECAUTIONS).
Malignant hyperthermia	Adjust dosage to avoid incapacitation or excessive GI irritation (including nausea and vomiting); skeletal muscle weakness and sedation (sleepiness or drowsiness) often occur at recommended dosages
WARNINGS/PRECAUTIONS	
Hepatic dysfunction or injury	May occur, sometimes fatally. Overt hepatitis can occur at any time during therapy but is most frequently observed between the 3rd and 12th months. If clinical signs of hepatitis appear, accompanied by abnormal liver function tests or jaundice, treatment should be discontinued. Risk of liver damage is greater in females and in patients over 35 yr of age (see also DRUG INTERACTIONS). Liver function studies should be performed at appropriate intervals. If results are abnormal, therapy should be reevaluated and the possibility of discontinuing therapy considered. If therapy is stopped, reinstitution should be attempted only after clinical and laboratory abnormalities have returned to normal. The patient should be hospitalized and closely monitored.
Mental impairment	Caution patients not to drive or participate in potentially hazardous activities; exercise caution in prescribing tranquilizers to patients taking this drug
Photosensitivity	May occur; caution patients about exposure to sunlight
Diarrhea	May be severe and necessitate temporary withdrawal of therapy; if diarrhea recurs upon reinstitution of therapy, discontinue use of dantrolene permanently
Special-risk patients	Use with caution in patients with preexisting liver disease or dysfunction, pulmonary function impairment (particularly obstructive pulmonary disease), or with severely impaired cardiac function owing to myocardial disease
ADVERSE REACTIONS	The most frequent reactions, regardless of incidence, are printed in *italics*
Central nervous system and neuromuscular	*Drowsiness, dizziness, weakness, malaise, fatigue,* speech disturbances, seizures, headache, light-headedness, taste alterations, insomnia, mental depression, confusion, increased nervousness, myalgia, backache
Ophthalmic	Visual disturbances, diplopia
Cardiovascular	Tachycardia, erratic blood pressure, phlebitis
Respiratory	Feeling of suffocation
Gastrointestinal	*Diarrhea,* constipation, GI bleeding, anorexia, difficulty in swallowing, gastric irritation, abdominal cramps
Hepatic	Hepatitis
Genitourinary	Increased urinary frequency, crystalluria, hematuria, difficult erection, urinary incontinence and/or nocturia, difficult urination and/or urinary retention
Dermatological	Abnormal hair growth, acne-like rash, pruritus, urticaria, eczematoid eruption, sweating, photosensitivity

DANTRIUM ■ FLEXERIL

Hypersensitivity	Pleural effusion with pericarditis
Other	Chills, fever

OVERDOSAGE

Signs and symptoms	See ADVERSE REACTIONS
Treatment	Generally supportive; immediately empty stomach by gastric lavage. Maintain adequate airway; resuscitation equipment should be readily available. Administer IV fluids to maintain adequate urine output and to prevent crystalluria. Monitor ECG and observe patient closely. Value of dialysis is unknown.

DRUG INTERACTIONS

Estrogens	△ Hepatotoxicity, especially in women over 35 yr of age
Alcohol, sedative-hypnotics, tranquilizers, and other CNS depressants	△ CNS depression

ALTERED LABORATORY VALUES

Blood/serum values	△ Alkaline phosphatase △ SGOT △ SGPT △ Bilirubin (total)

No clinically significant alterations in urinary values occur at therapeutic dosages

---

USE IN CHILDREN
See INDICATIONS and ORAL DOSAGE; the long-term safety of this drug for use in children under 5 yr of age has not been established

USE IN PREGNANT AND NURSING WOMEN
Safety for use during pregnancy has not been established. Dantrolene should not be used in nursing mothers.

MUSCLE RELAXANTS

FLEXERIL (cyclobenzaprine hydrochloride) Merck Sharp & Dohme   Rx

Tablets: 10 mg

INDICATIONS	ORAL DOSAGE
Muscle spasm associated with acute, painful musculoskeletal conditions (adjunctive therapy)	**Adult:** 20–60 mg/day, given in divided doses for not more than 2–3 wk; usual therapeutic dosage, 10 mg tid

CONTRAINDICATIONS

Hyperthyroidism	MAO inhibitor therapy (see WARNINGS/PRECAUTIONS)	Hypersensitivity to cyclobenzaprine
Cardiovascular conditions (see WARNINGS/PRECAUTIONS)		

WARNINGS/PRECAUTIONS

Patients with cardiovascular conditions	Cyclobenzaprine should not be given during the acute recovery phase following myocardial infarction or to patients with arrhythmias, heart block, conduction disturbances, or congestive heart failure
MAO inhibitor therapy	Do not give this drug concomitantly with MAO inhibitors or within 14 days of discontinuation of their use
Mental and/or physical impairment	Caution patients that their ability to drive or perform other potentially hazardous activities may be impaired
Special-risk patients	Use with caution in patients with narrow-angle glaucoma, increased intraocular pressure, urinary retention, or those taking anticholinergic medication
Abrupt termination of therapy	May produce nausea, headache, and malaise after prolonged administration
Potentially suicidal patients	Deaths by deliberate or accidental overdosage have occurred with this class of drug
Carcinogenicity, mutagenicity	Rats given approximately 5–40 times the maximum human dose for up to 67 wk developed pale and occasionally enlarged livers, as well as dose-related hepatocyte vacuolation with lipidosis. Two other studies on rats and mice demonstrated no neoplastic effects of this drug.

FLEXERIL ■ LIORESAL

ADVERSE REACTIONS[1]	Frequent reactions (incidence ≥ 1%) are printed in *italics*
Central nervous system	*Drowsiness (16–39%); dizziness (3–11%); fatigue/tiredness, asthenia, headache, nervousness, and confusion (1–3%);* ataxia, vertigo, dysarthria, paresthesia, tremors, hypertonia, convulsions, muscle twitching, disorientation, insomnia, depressed mood, abnormal sensations, anxiety, agitation, abnormal thinking and dreaming, hallucinations, excitement, tinnitus
Cardiovascular	Tachycardia, arrhythmia, vasodilation, palpitation, hypotension
Digestive	*Dry mouth (7–27%); nausea, constipation, dyspepsia, and unpleasant taste (1–3%);* ageusia, vomiting, anorexia, diarrhea, gastrointestinal pain, gastritis, thirst, flatulence, edema of the tongue, abnormal liver function; hepatitis, jaundice, and cholestasis (rare)
Dermatological	Sweating, rash, urticaria
Genitourinary	Urinary frequency and/or retention
Other	*Blurred vision (1–3%),* syncope, facial edema, malaise, local weakness
OVERDOSAGE	
Signs and symptoms	Temporary confusion, disturbed concentration, transient visual hallucinations, agitation, hyperactive reflexes, muscle rigidity, and vomiting or hyperpyrexia, in addition to any of the previously noted ADVERSE REACTIONS. Overdosage may also cause drowsiness, hypothermia, tachycardia, and other cardiac-rhythm abnormalities, such as bundle-branch block, ECG evidence of impaired conduction, and congestive heart failure, as well as dilated pupils, convulsions, severe hypotension, stupor, and coma.
Treatment	Institute symptomatic and supportive therapy. Empty stomach quickly by emesis and then use gastric lavage; may be followed by administration of 20–30 g activated charcoal q4–6h for first 24–48 h. Monitor ECG and cardiac function closely. Maintain an open airway, adequate fluid intake, and body temperature. Administer 1–3 mg physostigmine salicylate IV and repeat as needed, especially if life-threatening signs recur or persist. (Physostigmine should not be used routinely, however, since it may itself be toxic.) Use standard measures to manage circulatory shock and metabolic acidosis. Treat arrhythmias with neostigmine, pyridostigmine, or propranolol. Consider use of a short-acting digitalis preparation when there are signs of cardiac failure; monitor cardiac function closely for at least 5 days. Use anticonvulsants to control seizures. Dialysis is probably not helpful.
DRUG INTERACTIONS	
MAO inhibitors	Hyperpyretic crisis, severe convulsions, and death have occurred
Anticholinergic medication	△ Anticholinergic effect
Alcohol, tranquilizers, sedative-hypnotics, and other CNS depressants	△ CNS depression
Guanethidine, clonidine	▽ Antihypertensive effect
ALTERED LABORATORY VALUES	
No clinically significant alterations in blood/serum or urinary values occur at therapeutic dosages	

USE IN CHILDREN

The safety and effectiveness of this drug for use in children under 15 yr of age have not been established

USE IN PREGNANT AND NURSING WOMEN

Pregnancy Category B: use this drug during pregnancy only if clearly needed. Reproduction studies performed in mice, rats, and rabbits have revealed no evidence of impaired fertility or harm to the fetus due to cyclobenzaprine; however, there have been no adequate, well-controlled studies in pregnant women. It is not known whether this drug is excreted in human milk; because some tricyclic antidepressants, to which this drug is closely related, are excreted in human milk, caution should be exercised when cyclobenzaprine is administered to a nursing woman.

[1] Other reactions, which have not been associated by a causal relationship with cyclobenzaprine or which have occurred with other tricyclic drugs, include chest pain, edema, hypertension, myocardial infarction, heart block, stroke, paralytic ileus, tongue discoloration, stomatitis, parotid swelling, inappropriate ADH syndrome, purpura, bone marrow depression, leukopenia, eosinophilia, thrombocytopenia, changes in serum glucose level, weight gain or loss, myalgia, changes in libido, abnormal gait, delusions, peripheral neuropathy, Bell's palsy, altered EEG patterns, extrapyramidal symptoms, dyspnea, pruritus, photosensitization, alopecia, impaired urination, dilatation of urinary tract, impotence, testicular swelling, gynecomastia, breast enlargement, and galactorrhea

---

MUSCLE RELAXANTS

LIORESAL (baclofen) Geigy   Rx
Tablets: 10, 20 mg

INDICATIONS	**ORAL DOSAGE**
Spasticity associated with multiple sclerosis **Spinal cord injuries and diseases**	**Adult:** 5 mg tid for 3 days to start, followed by 10 mg tid for 3 days, 15 mg tid for 3 days, 20 mg tid for 3 days, and gradual increases thereafter, as necessary, up to 80 mg/day (20 mg qid); usual therapeutic dosage, 40–80 mg/day

LIORESAL

CONTRAINDICATIONS
Hypersensitivity to baclofen

WARNINGS/PRECAUTIONS

Abrupt withdrawal of therapy	Has precipitated hallucinations; reduce dose slowly when discontinuing drug, except when adverse reactions are serious
Patients with renal impairment	Baclofen is primarily excreted unchanged through the kidneys; use with caution and, if necessary, reduce dosage
Stroke patients	Have shown poor tolerance to the drug and do not appear to benefit from its use
Sedation	Caution patients about driving or other potentially hazardous activities, and about using alcohol or other CNS depressants (see DRUG INTERACTIONS)
Epilepsy	Deterioration in seizure control and EEG patterns has been reported; patients with epilepsy should be monitored clinically and electroencephalographically at regular intervals
Ovarian cysts, adrenal effects	A dose-related increase in the incidence of ovarian cysts and a less marked increase in enlarged and/or hemorrhagic adrenal glands have been observed in female rats during chronic therapy with baclofen. Ovarian cysts have been detected by palpation in about 4% of multiple sclerosis patients treated with baclofen for up to 1 yr (such cysts occur spontaneously in approximately 1–5% of the normal female population); in most cases, these cysts disappeared spontaneously while treatment was continued.
Special-risk patients	Use with caution when spasticity is utilized to sustain upright posture and balance in locomotion or to obtain increased function

ADVERSE REACTIONS
Frequent reactions (incidence ≥ 1%) are printed in *italics*

Central nervous system	*Transient drowsiness (10–63%), dizziness (5–15%), weakness (5–15%), confusion (1–11%), headache (4–8%), fatigue (2–4%), insomnia (2–7%)*, euphoria, excitement, depression, hallucinations, paresthesias, tinnitus, slurred speech, ataxia, epileptic seizures, syncope, dysarthria
Cardiovascular	*Hypotension (0–9%)*, dyspnea, palpitations, chest pain
Ophthalmic	Blurred vision, nystagmus, strabismus, miosis, mydriasis, diplopia
Gastrointestinal	*Nausea (4–12%), constipation (2–6%)*, dry mouth, taste disorders, anorexia, abdominal pain, vomiting, diarrhea, positive test for occult blood in stool
Genitourinary	*Urinary frequency (2–6%)*, enuresis, urinary retention, dysuria, nocturia, hematuria, ejaculatory inhibition, impotence
Musculoskeletal	Muscle pain, coordination disorders, rigidity, tremor, dystonia
Dermatological	Rash, pruritus
Respiratory	Nasal congestion
Other	Ankle edema, excessive perspiration, weight gain

OVERDOSAGE

Signs and symptoms	Vomiting, muscular hypotonia, drowsiness, accommodation disorders, coma, respiratory depression, seizures
Treatment	*Alert patient:* Empty stomach promptly by induced emesis, followed by gastric lavage. *Obtunded patient:* Do not induce emesis. Secure airway with a curved endotracheal tube before beginning lavage. Maintain adequate respiratory exchange. *Do not use respiratory stimulants.*

DRUG INTERACTIONS

Alcohol, tranquilizers, sedative-hypnotics, and other CNS depressants	⇧ CNS depression

ALTERED LABORATORY VALUES

Blood/serum values	⇧ Alkaline phosphatase ⇧ SGOT ⇧ Glucose

No clinically significant alterations in urinary values occur at therapeutic dosages

USE IN CHILDREN
Not recommended for use in children under 12 yr of age; the safety of using this drug in children has not been established

USE IN PREGNANT AND NURSING WOMEN
Use in pregnant women only if the expected benefit clearly justifies the potential risk to the fetus. Baclofen has been found to increase the incidence of omphalocele (ventral hernia) and incomplete sternebral ossification in fetuses of rats given approximately 13 times the maximal human dose; an increased incidence of unossified phalangeal nuclei of forelimbs and hindlimbs has also been reported in fetuses of rabbits given 7 times the maximal human dose. Teratogenic effects have not been observed in mice; however, reductions in mean fetal weight followed by delays in skeletal ossification occurred when dams were given 17 or 34 times the human daily dose. No studies have been done in pregnant women. It is not known whether baclofen is excreted in human milk; because many drugs are excreted in milk, patients should not nurse if use of this drug is essential.

MUSCLE RELAXANTS

MAOLATE (chlorphenesin carbamate) Upjohn   Rx

Tablets: 400 mg

INDICATIONS	ORAL DOSAGE
Acute, painful musculoskeletal conditions (adjunctive therapy)	Adult: 800 mg tid until desired effect has been achieved, followed by 400 mg qid or less, as needed

CONTRAINDICATIONS
Hypersensitivity to chlorphenesin

WARNINGS/PRECAUTIONS

Mental and/or physical impairment	Caution patients that their ability to drive or perform other potentially hazardous activities may be impaired
Patients with liver disease or impaired hepatic function	Use with caution
Hypersensitivity reactions	Anaphylaxis, drug fever, skin rash, or other allergic phenomena may occur; discontinue medication should these reactions develop
Tartrazine sensitivity	Presence of FD&C Yellow No. 5 (tartrazine) in tablets may cause allergic-type reactions, including bronchial asthma, in susceptible individuals
Long-term safety	Safety of administration for more than 8 wk has not been established

ADVERSE REACTIONS

Central nervous system and neuromuscular	Drowsiness, dizziness, confusion, paradoxical stimulation (including insomnia, increased nervousness, and headache)[1]
Gastrointestinal	Nausea, epigastric distress[2]
Hematological	Leukopenia, thrombocytopenia, agranulocytosis, pancytopenia
Allergic	Anaphylactoid reactions, drug fever, possibly other allergic phenomena

OVERDOSAGE

Signs and symptoms	Nausea, drowsiness
Treatment	Induce emesis or perform gastric lavage to empty stomach and administer a saline cathartic. Remainder of therapy is mostly supportive.

DRUG INTERACTIONS
No clinically significant drug interactions have been observed

ALTERED LABORATORY VALUES
No clinically significant alterations in blood/serum or urinary values occur at therapeutic dosages

---

USE IN CHILDREN

Not recommended for use in children because the safety and effectiveness of this drug have not been established in pediatric patients

USE IN PREGNANT AND NURSING WOMEN

Use in pregnant or nursing women is not recommended unless the potential therapeutic benefits outweigh the possible hazards. Adequate reproduction studies have not been done with this drug in animals.

---

[1] Can usually be controlled by dose reduction
[2] Two cases of GI bleeding have also been reported, but a causal relationship has not been established

---

MUSCLE RELAXANTS

NORFLEX (orphenadrine citrate) Riker   Rx

Tablets (sustained release): 100 mg   **Ampuls:** 30 mg/ml (2 ml)

INDICATIONS	ORAL DOSAGE	PARENTERAL DOSAGE
Discomfort associated with acute, painful musculoskeletal conditions (adjunctive therapy)	Adult: 100 mg bid (AM and PM)	Adult: 60 mg IM or IV q12h, as needed; for maintenance, switch to oral therapy, beginning 12 h after last parenteral dose

CONTRAINDICATIONS

Glaucoma	Prostatic hypertrophy	Myasthenia gravis
Achalasia	Bladder-neck obstruction	Hypersensitivity to orphenadrine
Pyloric or duodenal obstruction	Stenosing peptic ulcer	

NORFLEX ■ PARAFLEX

ADMINISTRATION/DOSAGE ADJUSTMENTS

Intravenous administration	Inject the drug over a period of approximately 5 min while the patient is lying down; wait 5–10 min and then help the patient to sit up

WARNINGS/PRECAUTIONS

Mental and/or physical impairment	Caution patients that their ability to drive or perform other potentially hazardous activities may be impaired; advise patients not to consume alcohol
Special-risk patients	Use with caution in patients with tachycardia, cardiac decompensation, coronary insufficiency, or cardiac arrhythmias
Management of adverse effects	To control mild reactions, reduce dosage
Long-term therapy	Safety of long-term treatment has not been established; periodically check blood, urinary, and liver function values during prolonged use
Carcinogenicity, mutagenicity, effect on fertility	No studies have been done to evaluate the carcinogenic or mutagenic potential of orphenadrine or its effect, if any, on fertility

ADVERSE REACTIONS

Cardiovascular	Tachycardia, palpitations, transient syncope
Central nervous system	Weakness, headache, dizziness, drowsiness, confusion (in the elderly), hallucinations, agitation, tremor
Ophthalmic	Blurred vision, mydriasis, increased intraocular pressure
Gastrointestinal	Vomiting, nausea, constipation, gastric irritation
Genitourinary	Urinary hesitancy or retention
Hypersensitivity	Urticaria, pruritus, and other skin reactions (rare); anaphylaxis following parenteral use (rare)
Other	Dry mouth[1]

OVERDOSAGE

Signs and symptoms	Dry mouth, blurred vision, urinary retention, tachycardia, confusion, paralytic ileus, and, in severe cases, deep coma, tonic and clonic seizures, shock, respiratory arrest, serious cardiac arrhythmias, and death
Treatment	Institute supportive therapy and maintain a patent airway. Induce emesis and, if necessary, perform gastric lavage, followed by activated charcoal, to empty stomach. Monitor vital signs and fluid and electrolyte balance. Hemodialysis or peritoneal dialysis may not be helpful because rapid distribution results in extremely low serum levels (less than 0.04 mg/dl).

DRUG INTERACTIONS

Other anticholinergic agents	◊ Anticholinergic effect
Alcohol, general anesthetics, and other CNS depressants	◊ CNS depression
MAO inhibitors, tricyclic antidepressants	◊ CNS depression ◊ Antidepressant effect
Propoxyphene	Tremors, mental confusion, and anxiety (reported in a few patients)

ALTERED LABORATORY VALUES

No clinically significant alterations in blood/serum or urinary values occur at therapeutic dosages

---

USE IN CHILDREN

Safety and effectiveness for use in children have not been established

USE IN PREGNANT AND NURSING WOMEN

Pregnancy Category C: degenerative changes in the urinary bladder have been detected in rats (5% of pups) at 5 times the daily human dose (however, this abnormality was not observed in a subsequent study at 12 times the daily human dose). No adequate, well-controlled studies have been performed in pregnant women; use during pregnancy only if the expected benefits justify the potential risk to the fetus. It is not known whether orphenadrine is excreted in human milk; use with caution in nursing mothers.

---

[1] Aplastic anemia has also been reported (rarely), but a causal relationship has not been established

---

MUSCLE RELAXANTS

PARAFLEX (chlorzoxazone) McNeil Pharmaceutical   Rx

Tablets: 250 mg

INDICATIONS

Acute, painful musculoskeletal conditions (adjunctive therapy)

ORAL DOSAGE

Adult: 500 mg tid or qid to start, followed by an increase in dosage to 750 mg tid or qid, if necessary; usual maintenance dosage, 250 mg tid or qid
Child: 125–500 mg tid or qid, according to age and weight

PARAFLEX ■ QUINAMM

CONTRAINDICATIONS
Hypersensitivity to chlorzoxazone

WARNINGS/PRECAUTIONS
Liver dysfunction	Discontinue use if any suggestive signs or symptoms develop
Patients with allergies	Use with caution in patients with allergies or a history of drug allergy; discontinue use if urticaria, redness, itching, or other sensitivity reactions occur

ADVERSE REACTIONS
Gastrointestinal	Occasional GI disturbances; bleeding (rare)
Central nervous system	Drowsiness, dizziness, light-headedness, malaise, overstimulation
Allergic	Skin rashes, petechiae, ecchymoses, angioneurotic edema, and anaphylactic reactions (rare)
Hepatic	Liver damage (approximately 36 cases)

OVERDOSAGE
Signs and symptoms	Gastrointestinal disturbances, such as nausea, vomiting, or diarrhea; drowsiness; dizziness; light-headedness; headache; malaise or sluggishness, followed by marked loss of muscle tone; decreased or absent deep-tendon reflexes; respiratory depression, with rapid, irregular breathing and intercostal and substernal retraction; reduction in blood pressure
Treatment	Empty stomach by inducing emesis or by gastric lavage, followed by administration of activated charcoal. Institute supportive measures, as needed. For respiratory depression, secure an open airway by use of an oropharyngeal airway or endotracheal tube; administer oxygen and, if necessary, artificial respiration. *Do not use cholinergic agents or analeptics.* Treat hypotension by administering dextran, plasma, concentrated albumin, or a vasopressor (eg, norepinephrine).

DRUG INTERACTIONS
Alcohol, general anesthetics, other CNS depressants	△ CNS depression
MAO inhibitors, tricyclic antidepressants	△ CNS depression △ Antidepressant effect

ALTERED LABORATORY VALUES
Urinary values	Discoloration (orange, purple-red)

No clinically significant alterations in blood/serum values occur at therapeutic dosages

---

USE IN CHILDREN
See INDICATIONS and ORAL DOSAGE; tablets may be crushed and mixed with food or a suitable vehicle for administration

USE IN PREGNANT AND NURSING WOMEN
Safety for use during pregnancy has not been established. Consult manufacturer for use in nursing mothers.

MUSCLE RELAXANTS

QUINAMM (quinine sulfate) Merrell Dow   Rx
Tablets: 260 mg

INDICATIONS
Nocturnal recumbency leg cramps

ORAL DOSAGE
Adult: 260 mg at bedtime; if necessary, increase dosage to 520 mg nightly, with 1 tab taken after dinner and the 2nd tab upon retiring

CONTRAINDICATIONS
Pregnancy	Hypersensitivity to quinine	G6PD deficiency
History of thrombocytopenic purpura due to quinine	Tinnitus	Optic neuritis
History of blackwater fever		

WARNINGS/PRECAUTIONS
Thrombocytopenic purpura	May follow administration to highly sensitive individuals; recovery usually occurs after drug is discontinued and appropriate therapy is given

COMPENDIUM OF DRUG THERAPY

QUINAMM

Cinchonism	May occur after repeated use or with overdosage. Mild cases are characterized by ringing in the ears, headache, nausea, and slightly disturbed vision; with continued medication or after ingestion of large single doses, however, patients may manifest additional GI and CNS reactions, as well as cardiovascular and cutaneous signs and symptoms (see ADVERSE REACTIONS). If any of these reactions occur, discontinue use of the drug and institute appropriate supportive measures (see also treatment of OVERDOSAGE).
Hypersensitivity	Discontinue use of the drug if cutaneous flushing, pruritus, skin rash, fever, gastric distress, dyspnea, ringing in the ears, and/or visual impairment occurs, especially with small doses; rarely, hemoglobinuria and asthma may occur as idiosyncratic reactions to quinine
Patients with atrial fibrillation	Administer this drug with the same degree of caution appropriate to the use of quinidine
Drug dependence	Tolerance, abuse, or dependence has not been reported in patients taking quinine
Carcinogenicity, mutagenicity	Long-term studies in rats have shown no evidence of carcinogenicity. An increase in the exchange of genetic material between sister chromatids has been observed in mice; studies have shown an increase in chromatid breaks in two strains of inbred mice, and the micronucleus test has produced positive findings in one of the inbred strains. No evidence of mutagenicity has been detected in Chinese hamsters. Results of *Salmonella* tests have been positive when mammalian liver homogenate has been added.

ADVERSE REACTIONS

Hematological	Acute hemolysis, thrombocytopenic purpura, agranulocytosis, hypoprothrombinemia
Central nervous system	Visual disturbances, including blurred vision with scotomata, photophobia, diplopia, diminished visual fields, and disturbed color vision; tinnitus, deafness, vertigo, headache, nausea, vomiting, fever, apprehension, restlessness, confusion, syncope
Dermatological and hypersensitivity	Urticarial rashes, papular or scarlatinal rash, pruritus, flushing, sweating, occasional facial edema
Gastrointestinal	Nausea and vomiting (may be CNS-related), epigastric pain, hepatitis
Other	Asthmatic and/or anginal symptoms

OVERDOSAGE

Signs and symptoms	Tinnitus, impaired hearing, dizziness, rash, intestinal cramping, headache, fever, vomiting, apprehension, confusion, convulsions, blindness (followed by partial recovery of vision); see also ADVERSE REACTIONS
Treatment	Empty stomach by inducing emesis or by gastric lavage; administer activated charcoal. Institute measures to support and maintain blood pressure, adequate ventilation, and renal function. Administer IV fluids, as needed, to maintain fluid and electrolyte balance. Urinary acidifiers may be used to promote renal excretion of the drug; in the presence of hemoglobinuria, however, acidification of the urine may augment renal blockade. Hemodialysis and/or hemoperfusion procedures may also be useful in eliminating the drug. Angioedema or asthma may require the use of epinephrine, corticosteroids, and/or antihistamines. IV vasodilators may be useful for toxic amaurosis; stellate block has also proved helpful for quinine-related blindness. Residual visual impairment may respond to vasodilators.

DRUG INTERACTIONS

Aluminum-containing antacids	▽ Rate or extent of absorption of quinine
Oral anticoagulants	△ Anticoagulant effect
Neuromuscular blocking agents (especially pancuronium, succinyl-choline, and tubocurarine)	△ Neuromuscular blockade, possibly resulting in respiratory difficulties
Urinary alkalinizers (eg, acetazolamide and sodium bicarbonate)	△ Quinine blood level, possibly resulting in toxicity
Digoxin, digitoxin	△ Serum digoxin or digitoxin level; periodically measure digoxin or digitoxin level during concomitant therapy

ALTERED LABORATORY VALUES

Urinary values	△ 17-Hydroxycorticosteroids (with Reddy, Jenkins, and Thorn method) △ 17-Ketogenic steroids (with Zimmermann method)

No clinically significant alterations in blood/serum values occur at therapeutic dosages

---

USE IN CHILDREN
Consult manufacturer

USE IN PREGNANT AND NURSING WOMEN
Pregnancy Category X: contraindicated for use in women who are or who may become pregnant, because of the risk of fetal harm. Teratogenic effects have been observed in rabbits and guinea pigs, but not in mice, rats, dogs, or monkeys. Congenital malformations have occurred in humans, mainly following the use of large doses (up to 30 g) for attempted abortions; reported defects have included limb anomalies, deafness associated with auditory nerve hypoplasia, visceral defects, and visual changes. Quinine is excreted in breast milk in small amounts; use with caution in nursing mothers.

MUSCLE RELAXANTS

ROBAXIN (methocarbamol) Robins   Rx

Tablets: 500 mg, 750 mg (Robaxin-750)   **Vials:** 100 mg/ml (10 ml)

INDICATIONS	ORAL DOSAGE	PARENTERAL DOSAGE
Acute, painful musculoskeletal conditions (adjunctive therapy)	Adult: 1.5 g qid for 48–72 h, followed by 750 mg q4h, 1 g qid, or 1.5 g tid; for severe conditions, 8 g/day may be given for the first 48–72 h	Adult: 1–3 g/day IM or IV for up to 3 days; if condition persists, course may be repeated after a drug-free interval of 48 h. Switch to oral form as soon as possible
Tetanus (adjunctive therapy)	Adult: up to 24 g/day; tablets should be crushed, suspended in water or saline, and then given through a nasogastric tube	Adult: 1–3 g IV q6h until a nasogastric tube can be inserted (see ORAL DOSAGE); for each dose, give 1–2 g by direct IV injection, and, if necessary, 1–2 g by IV infusion, but do not exceed 3 g total Child: 15 mg/kg or more IV q6h

CONTRAINDICATIONS

Hypersensitivity to methocarbamol   Known or suspected renal pathology (injectable form only)

ADMINISTRATION/DOSAGE ADJUSTMENTS

Intramuscular use — Inject not more than 5 ml into each buttock; repeat, if necessary, q8h

Intravenous use — For IV infusion, dilute the solution with 0.9% sodium chloride injection or 5% dextrose injection to a final concentration of not less than 0.4 mg/ml. For direct IV injection, administer the supplied solution at a rate not exceeding 300 mg (3 ml)/min; take appropriate care to avoid vascular extravasation of the hypertonic solution, which could result in thrombophlebitis. The patient should be recumbent during the injection and for at least 10–15 min afterward.

WARNINGS/PRECAUTIONS

Epileptic patients — Use injectable form with caution in suspected or known epileptic subjects; convulsive seizures have occurred during IV administration

Extravasation — Must be avoided since injectable form is hypertonic; thrombophlebitis and sloughing at injection site have been reported

Concomitant use of CNS depressants — Caution patients that combined use of alcohol or other CNS depressants may cause additional CNS depression

ADVERSE REACTIONS

Central nervous system and neuromuscular — Dizziness, light-headedness, drowsiness, headache; vertigo, fainting, mild muscular incoordination, and convulsions (injectable form only)

Gastrointestinal — Nausea; GI upset and metallic taste (injectable form only)

Cardiovascular — Flushing, syncope, hypotension, and bradycardia (injectable form only)

Ophthalmic — Blurred vision; nystagmus and diplopia (injectable form only)

Hypersensitivity — Urticaria, pruritus, rash, fever, conjunctivitis with nasal congestion; anaphylactic reaction (injectable form only)

Other — Thrombophlebitis (injectable form only), pain and sloughing at injection site

OVERDOSAGE

Signs and symptoms — See ADVERSE REACTIONS

Treatment — Methocarbamol is excreted via the kidney within 24 h; therapy is largely supportive

DRUG INTERACTIONS

Alcohol, tranquilizers, sedative-hypnotics, and other CNS depressants — ⇧ CNS depression

ALTERED LABORATORY VALUES

Urinary values — ⇧ 5-HIAA (color interference)   ⇧ VMA (color interference)

No clinically significant alterations in blood/serum values occur at therapeutic dosages

---

USE IN CHILDREN

Safety and effectiveness for use in children under 12 yr of age have not been established except for tetanus

USE IN PREGNANT AND NURSING WOMEN

Safety for use during pregnancy had not been established; use only if the expected therapeutic benefits outweigh the possible hazards. It is not known whether methocarbamol is excreted in human milk; because many drugs are excreted in milk, nursing is not advisable.

MUSCLE RELAXANTS

SKELAXIN (metaxalone) Carnrick Rx

Tablets: 400 mg

INDICATIONS	**ORAL DOSAGE**
Acute, painful musculoskeletal conditions (adjunctive therapy)	**Adult:** 800 mg tid or qid **Adolescent (> 12 yr):** same as adult

CONTRAINDICATIONS

Known tendency to drug-induced, hemolytic, or other anemias	Significantly impaired renal or hepatic function	Hypersensitivity to metaxalone

WARNINGS/PRECAUTIONS

Elevations in cephalin flocculation tests	May occur without concurrent changes in other liver-function parameters. Use with extreme caution in patients with preexisting liver damage; perform serial liver function studies, as required.

ADVERSE REACTIONS

Gastrointestinal	Nausea, vomiting, upset
Central nervous system	Drowsiness, dizziness, nervousness, headache, irritability
Dermatological	Light rash with or without pruritus
Hematological	Leukopenia, hemolytic anemia
Hepatic	Jaundice

OVERDOSAGE

Signs and symptoms	No documented case of major toxicity has been reported. In rats and mice, progressive sedation, hypnosis, and respiratory failure were noted as the dosage increased. In dogs, higher doses produced an emetic action.
Treatment	Employ gastric lavage and supportive therapy, as required

DRUG INTERACTIONS

Alcohol	⇧ Sedative effect

ALTERED LABORATORY VALUES

Urinary values	⇧ Glucose (with Benedict's solution)

No clinically significant alterations in blood/serum values occur at therapeutic dosages

---

USE IN CHILDREN

The safety and effectiveness of this drug for use in children under 12 yr of age have not been established

USE IN PREGNANT AND NURSING WOMEN

Pregnant women: Reproduction studies in rats have revealed no evidence of impaired fertility or fetal harm. While there have been no reports of fetal injury resulting from clinical use of this drug, this does not preclude the possibility of infrequent or subtle damage to the human fetus. This drug should not be used in pregnant women (especially those at an early stage of pregnancy) or in women who may become pregnant unless the potential benefits outweigh the possible hazards to the fetus.
Nursing Mothers: It is not known whether metaxalone is excreted in human milk; because many drugs are excreted in milk, nursing is not advisable.

MUSCLE RELAXANTS

SOMA (carisoprodol) Wallace Rx

Tablets: 350 mg

INDICATIONS	**ORAL DOSAGE**
Acute, painful musculoskeletal conditions (adjunctive therapy)	**Adult:** 350 mg tid and at bedtime

CONTRAINDICATIONS

Acute intermittent porphyria	Allergic or idiosyncratic reaction to carisoprodol or related compounds, such as meprobamate, mebutamate, or tybamate

SOMA ■ VALIUM/VALRELEASE

WARNINGS/PRECAUTIONS

Idiosyncratic reactions	On very rare occasions such reactions have been reported within minutes or hours of the first dose, including extreme weakness, transient quadriplegia, dizziness, ataxia, temporary loss of vision, diplopia, mydriasis, dysarthria, agitation, euphoria, confusion, and disorientation. Symptoms usually subside over the course of the next several hours. Supportive and symptomatic therapy, including hospitalization, may be necessary (see ADVERSE REACTIONS).
Drug dependence	Mild withdrawal symptoms (abdominal cramps, insomnia, chills, headache, and nausea) have followed abrupt cessation of therapy with doses of 100 mg/kg/day; use with caution in addiction-prone individuals
Mental and/or physical impairment	Caution patients that their ability to drive or perform other potentially hazardous activities may be impaired
Patients with compromised hepatic or renal function	Carisoprodol is metabolized by the liver and excreted by the kidney; watch for signs of excessive drug accumulation (see OVERDOSAGE)

ADVERSE REACTIONS[1]

Central nervous system and neuromuscular	Drowsiness, dizziness, vertigo, ataxia, tremor, agitation, irritability, headache, depression, syncope, insomnia
Allergic or idiosyncratic[2]	Skin rash, erythema multiforme, pruritus, eosinophilia, fixed-drug eruption, asthmatic episodes, fever, weakness, dizziness, angioneurotic edema, smarting eyes, hypotension, anaphylactic shock
Cardiovascular	Tachycardia, postural hypotension, facial flushing
Gastrointestinal	Nausea, vomiting, hiccups, epigastric distress

OVERDOSAGE

Signs and symptoms	Stupor, coma, shock, respiratory depression, and (very rarely) death
Treatment	Induce emesis or perform gastric lavage to empty stomach, and administer activated charcoal. Should respiration or blood pressure become compromised, administer respiratory assistance and pressor agents cautiously, as indicated. Careful monitoring of urinary output is necessary, and caution should be taken to avoid overhydration. Observe for possible relapse due to incomplete gastric emptying and delayed absorption.

DRUG INTERACTIONS

Alcohol, tranquilizers, sedative-hypnotics, and other CNS depressants	⇧ CNS depression

ALTERED LABORATORY VALUES

No clinically significant alterations in blood/serum or urinary values occur at therapeutic dosages

---

USE IN CHILDREN

Not recommended for use in children under 12 yr of age because of limited clinical experience

USE IN PREGNANT AND NURSING WOMEN

Safety for use in pregnant or nursing women has not been established; use only if the expected therapeutic benefits outweigh the possible hazards.

---

[1] Leukopenia has also been reported, but a causal relationship has not been established
[2] Discontinue drug and institute symptomatic therapy, including use of epinephrine, antihistamines, and, in severe cases, corticosteroids; consider allergic reactions to excipients in all cases

---

MUSCLE RELAXANTS

VALIUM (diazepam) Roche

C-IV

Tablets: 2, 5, 10 mg **Ampuls:** 5 mg/ml (2 ml) **Prefilled syringes:** 5 mg/ml (2 ml) **Vials:** 5 mg/ml (10 ml)

INDICATIONS	ORAL DOSAGE	PARENTERAL DOSAGE
Anxiety disorders and short-term relief of **symptoms of anxiety**[1]	**Adult:** 2–10 mg bid to qid, depending upon severity	**Adult:** 2–10 mg IM or IV to start; repeat 3–4 h later, if needed
Acute alcohol withdrawal syndrome	**Adult:** 10 mg tid or qid over initial 24 h; then 5 mg tid or qid, as needed	**Adult:** 10 mg IM or IV to start, then 5–10 mg 3–4 h later, if needed
Preoperative medication		**Adult:** 10 mg IM (preferred) before surgery

COMPENDIUM OF DRUG THERAPY

VALIUM/VALRELEASE

Indication	Oral	Parenteral
Skeletal muscle spasm due to reflex spasm secondary to muscle or joint inflammation, trauma, or other local pathology (adjunctive therapy) **Spasticity due to upper motor neuron disorders,** such as cerebral palsy and paraplegia (adjunctive therapy) **Athetosis** (adjunctive therapy) **Stiff-man syndrome** (adjunctive therapy)	**Adult:** 2–10 mg tid or qid **Child (> 6 mo):** 1–2.5 mg tid or qid to start; increase gradually, as needed	**Adult:** 5–10 mg IM or IV to start; repeat 3–4 h later, if needed
Tetanus (adjunctive therapy)	—	**Adult:** same as for muscle spasm, except that larger doses may be needed **Child (1 mo to 5 yr):** 1–2 mg IM or IV (slowly); repeat q3–4h, as needed **Child (> 5 yr):** 5–10 mg IM or IV (slowly); repeat q3–4h, as needed
Convulsive disorders (adjunctive therapy)	**Adult:** 2–10 mg bid to qid **Child (> 6 mo):** 1–2.5 mg tid or qid to start; increase gradually, as needed	—
Status epilepticus **Severe recurrent convulsive seizures**	—	**Adult:** 5–10 mg IM or IV (preferred), slowly, every 10–15 min, up to 30 mg; repeat 2–4 h later, if needed **Child (1 mo to 5 yr):** 0.2–0.5 mg IM or IV (preferred), slowly, every 2–5 min, up to 5 mg; repeat 2–4 h later, if needed **Child (> 5 yr):** 1 mg IM or IV (preferred), slowly, every 2–5 min, up to 10 mg; repeat 2–4 h later, if needed
Endoscopic procedures (adjunctive therapy)	—	**Adult:** 5–10 mg IM 30 min prior to procedure or 10–20 mg, or less, IV (preferred), slowly, just prior to procedure
Cardioversion (adjunctive therapy)	—	**Adult:** 5–15 mg IV within 5–10 min before procedure

VALRELEASE (diazepam) Roche

C-IV

Capsules (slow release): 15 mg

INDICATIONS

Anxiety disorders and short-term relief of **symptoms of anxiety**[1]
Skeletal muscle spasm due to reflex spasm secondary to muscle or joint inflammation, trauma, or other local pathology (adjunctive therapy)
Spasticity due to upper motor neuron disorders, such as cerebral palsy and paraplegia (adjunctive therapy)
Athetosis (adjunctive therapy)
Stiff-man syndrome (adjunctive therapy)
Convulsive disorders (adjunctive therapy)

Acute alcohol withdrawal syndrome

ORAL DOSAGE

Adult: 15–30 mg once daily, depending upon severity
Child (> 6 mo): 15 mg once daily if 5 mg tid is the optimum dosage of the tablet form

Adult: 30 mg for the initial 24 h, followed by 15 mg once daily, as needed

CONTRAINDICATIONS

Hypersensitivity to diazepam

Acute narrow-angle glaucoma

Open-angle glaucoma (unless patient is receiving appropriate antiglaucoma therapy)

Depression of vital signs in patients undergoing acute alcohol intoxication

Shock or coma (for parenteral use only)

ADMINISTRATION/DOSAGE ADJUSTMENTS

Elderly and/or debilitated patients	To preclude ataxia or oversedation, start with 2–2.5 mg 1–2 times/day orally and increase the dosage gradually; if the optimum dosage is 5 mg tid, slow-release capsules may be substituted in a dosage of 15 mg once daily. When using the injectable form, start with 2–5 mg and then increase the dosage gradually (see WARNINGS/PRECAUTIONS).
Intravenous use	May result in venous thrombosis, phlebitis, local irritation, swelling, and (rarely) vascular impairment. Administer solution slowly, no faster than 5 mg (1 ml)/min, *into large veins only;* carefully avoid intraarterial administration or extravasation. Do not mix or dilute with other drugs or solutions. If direct IV administration is not possible, slow injection through infusion tubing as close as possible to vein insertion (since diazepam is sparingly soluble) may be substituted.
Concomitant therapy with narcotic analgesics	Reduce narcotic dosage by a least one third and administer in small increments

VALIUM/VALRELEASE

Long-term use (> 4 mo)	Effectiveness for prolonged use as an antianxiety agent has not been tested in systematic clinical studies; reassess need for continued therapy periodically

WARNINGS/PRECAUTIONS

Psychosis	Diazepam is of no value in psychotic patients
Mental impairment, reflex-slowing	Caution patients not to engage in potentially hazardous activities requiring full mental alertness and that alcohol and other CNS depressants may cause further impairment
Drug dependence	Psychic and/or physical dependence may develop, especially in addiction-prone individuals
Abrupt discontinuation of therapy	May precipitate barbiturate-like withdrawal symptoms, including convulsions, tremor, abdominal and muscle cramps, vomiting, and sweating; milder withdrawal symptoms have also been observed infrequently following abrupt discontinuation of several months of continuous benzodiazepine therapy, generally when higher therapeutic doses have been used. Taper dosage gradually after extended treatment.
Potentially suicidal patients	Should not have access to large quantities of diazepam; prescribe smallest amount feasible
Apnea and/or cardiac arrest	May occur in the elderly or gravely ill or in patients with limited pulmonary reserve when parenteral route (particularly IV) is used; risk of apnea is increased by concomitant use of CNS depressants (see DRUG INTERACTIONS)
Convulsive disorders	May increase frequency and/or severity of grand mal seizures. Dosages of standard anticonvulsants may have to be increased. Abrupt withdrawal may also be associated temporarily with increased seizure activity. The parenteral form should be used with extreme caution in patients with chronic lung disease or unstable cardiovascular status.
Hepatic or renal impairment	Monitor patient closely to avoid excessive drug accumulation (see OVERDOSAGE)
Prolonged therapy	Blood counts and liver-function tests should be performed periodically

ADVERSE REACTIONS

Frequent reactions (incidence ≥ 1%) are printed in *italics*

Central nervous system and neuromuscular	*Drowsiness, fatigue, ataxia,* confusion, depression, dysarthria, headache, hypoactivity, slurred speech, syncope, tremor, vertigo, acute hyperexcitability, anxiety, hallucinations, increased muscle spasticity, insomnia, rage, sleep disturbances, stimulation, EEG changes, muscular weakness (with parenteral use)
Cardiovascular	Bradycardia, cardiovascular collapse, hypotension, cardiac arrest
Gastrointestinal	Constipation, nausea, hiccoughs, salivary changes
Hepatic	Jaundice
Genitourinary	Incontinence, urinary retention
Ophthalmic	Blurred vision, diplopia, nystagmus
Respiratory	Coughing, depressed respiration, dyspnea, hyperventilation, laryngospasm, throat or chest pain (during peroral endoscopy)
Dermatological	Urticaria, skin rash
Hematological	Neutropenia
Other	*Venous thrombosis and phlebitis at injection site,* changes in libido

OVERDOSAGE

Signs and symptoms	Somnolence, confusion, coma, diminished reflexes, hypotension
Treatment	Empty stomach immediately by gastric lavage. Monitor respiration, pulse, and blood pressure. Employ general supportive measures, as needed. Administer IV fluids and maintain adequate airway. Hypotension may be combated with levarterenol or metaraminol. Dialysis is of limited value.

DRUG INTERACTIONS

Alcohol, narcotic analgesics, sedative-hypnotics, and other CNS depressants	△ CNS depression △ Hypotension (with parenteral use) △ Muscular weakness (with parenteral use)
MAO inhibitors and other antidepressants	△ CNS effects
Cimetidine	▽ Clearance of diazepam

ALTERED LABORATORY VALUES

No clinically significant alterations in blood/serum or urinary values occur at therapeutic dosages

USE IN CHILDREN

See INDICATIONS and ORAL DOSAGE. When using the injectable form, give not more than 0.25 mg/kg over a 3-min period; the initial dose may be safely repeated after 15–30 min. Oral diazepam is not indicated for use in infants under 6 mo of age. Consult manufacturer for use of the injectable form in newborns (< 30 days of age); prolonged CNS depression has been observed in neonates.

USE IN PREGNANT AND NURSING WOMEN

Use of antianxiety agents during early pregnancy should almost always be avoided. Although diazepam has not been sufficiently studied to determine conclusively its effects during pregnancy, an increased risk of congenital malformations during the first trimester has been associated with minor tranquilizers (meprobamate, diazepam, and chlordiazepoxide). Patient should stop breast-feeding if drug is prescribed; lethargy, weight loss, and hyperbilirubinemia in nursing infants have been reported.[1]

[1] Erkkola R, Kanto J: *Lancet* 1:542, 1972; Patrick MJ, Tilstone WJ; *Lancet* 1:542, 1972; Takyi BE: *J Hosp Pharm* 28:317, 1970

[1] Anxiety or tension associated with the stress of everyday life usually does not require treatment with an antianxiety agent

MUSCLE RELAXANTS WITH ANALGESICS

NORGESIC (orphenadrine citrate, aspirin, and caffeine) Riker — Rx

Tablets: 25 mg orphenadrine citrate, 385 mg aspirin, and 30 mg caffeine

NORGESIC Forte (orphenadrine citrate, aspirin, and caffeine) Riker — Rx

Tablets: 50 mg orphenadrine citrate, 770 mg aspirin, and 60 mg caffeine

INDICATIONS

Discomfort and mild to moderate pain associated with acute musculoskeletal disorders (adjunctive therapy)

ORAL DOSAGE

Adult: 1–2 Norgesic tabs or ½–1 Norgesic Forte tab tid or qid

CONTRAINDICATIONS

Glaucoma	Prostatic hypertrophy	Hypersensitivity to orphenadrine, aspirin, or caffeine
Achalasia	Bladder-neck obstruction	
Pyloric or duodenal obstruction	Myasthenia gravis	

WARNINGS/PRECAUTIONS

Mental and/or physical impairment	Caution patients that their ability to drive or perform other potentially hazardous activities may be impaired; advise patients not to consume alcohol
Reye's syndrome	Some studies have suggested that salicylates may increase the risk of Reye's syndrome; do not use this preparation in patients with chicken pox, influenza, or influenza-like signs and symptoms since these patients are susceptible to this syndrome
Special-risk patients	Use with extreme caution in patients with peptic ulcers or coagulation abnormalities
Patients with nasal polyps	Hypersensitivity to aspirin, manifested by urticaria, bronchospasm, or anaphylaxis, is more likely to occur in patients with nasal polyps
Management of adverse effects	To control mild reactions, reduce dosage
Long-term therapy	Safety of long-term treatment with Norgesic Forte has not been established; periodically check liver function, hematological, and urinary values during prolonged use
Carcinogenicity, mutagenicity	Aspirin and caffeine have been shown to be noncarcinogenic; studies to determine the carcinogenic potential of orphenadrine have not been done. Caffeine is generally considered to be nonmutagenic; aspirin and orphenadrine have not been tested for mutagenicity
Effect on fertility	Caffeine does not impair fertility in rats; the effect of aspirin and orphenadrine on fertility has not been studied

ADVERSE REACTIONS

Cardiovascular	Tachycardia, palpitations, syncope
Central nervous system	Weakness, headache, dizziness, light-headedness, drowsiness, confusion (in the elderly), mild excitation, hallucinations
Ophthalmic	Blurred vision, mydriasis, increased intraocular pressure

NORGESIC

Gastrointestinal	Vomiting, nausea, constipation; hemorrhage (rare)
Genitourinary	Urinary hesitancy or retention
Hypersensitivity	Urticaria, pruritus, and other skin reactions
Other	Dry mouth[1]

OVERDOSAGE

Signs and symptoms — *Aspirin-related effects:* rapid and deep breathing, hyperventilation, nausea, vomiting, vertigo, tinnitus, flushing, sweating, thirst, headache, drowsiness, diarrhea, and tachycardia, followed by fever, hemorrhage, dehydration, excitement, confusion, convulsions, vasomotor depression, coma, respiratory failure, and respiratory alkalosis progressing to respiratory and metabolic acidosis (primarily in children); *caffeine-related effects:* insomnia, restlessness, tremor, delirium, tachycardia, extrasystoles; *orphenadrine-related effects:* dry mouth, blurred vision, urinary retention, tachycardia, confusion, paralytic ileus and, in severe cases, deep coma, tonic and clonic seizures, shock, respiratory arrest, serious cardiac arrhythmias, and death

Treatment — If less than 4 h have elapsed since ingestion, induce emesis or perform gastric lavage, followed by activated charcoal, to remove any remaining drug from the stomach. Initial therapy should be directed at reducing hyperthermia by external sponging with tepid water, correcting dehydration by appropriate IV fluid replacement, and maintaining adequate cardiorespiratory and renal function. In moderately severe cases of salicylate poisoning, cautiously administer sodium bicarbonate IV in sufficient quantity, if possible, to maintain an alkaline diuresis; intermittent peritoneal dialysis may also be helpful. In severe cases, hemodialysis should be seriously considered. Potassium should be added to the repair solution to compensate for potassium losses once urine formation is deemed adequate. Glucose may be provided to correct ketosis and hypoglycemia. Plasma transfusion may be beneficial if shock intervenes. Hemorrhagic phenomena may necessitate whole-blood transfusions and use of phytonadione (vitamin K$_1$). Do not administer barbiturates to treat excitement or convulsions.

DRUG INTERACTIONS

Alcohol	△ CNS depression △ Risk of GI ulceration
Anticoagulants	△ Risk of bleeding
Phenylbutazone, oxyphenbutazone	△ Risk of GI ulceration
Corticosteroids	▽ Aspirin plasma levels △ Risk of GI ulceration
Probenecid, sulfinpyrazone	▽ Uricosuria
Spironolactone	▽ Diuretic effect
Methotrexate	△ Methotrexate plasma level and risk of toxicity
Tolbutamide, chlorpropamide, tolazamide, acetohexamide	△ Hypoglycemic effect
Other anticholinergic agents	△ Anticholinergic effect
Theophylline, other methylxanthines	△ Methylxanthine effects
Propoxyphene	Tremors, mental confusion, and anxiety (reported in a few patients)

ALTERED LABORATORY VALUES

Blood/serum values	△ Prothrombin time △ Uric acid (with low doses) ▽ Uric acid (with high doses) ▽ Thyroxine (T$_4$) ▽ Thyroid-stimulating hormone
Urinary values	△ Glucose (with Clinitest tablets)

USE IN CHILDREN

Do not use in children under 12 yr of age; safety and effectiveness for use in this age group have not been established

USE IN PREGNANT AND NURSING WOMEN

Pregnancy Category C: aspirin has been shown to be teratogenic and embryocidal in rats at 3–4 times, but not at twice, the usual human dose; chronic or excessive use of aspirin may cause prolonged gestation and labor, delivery problems, reduced birth weight, neonatal anemia, maternal and neonatal bleeding complications, and increased perinatal mortality. Degenerative changes in the urinary bladder have been detected in rats (5% of pups) at 5 times the daily human dose of orphenadrine (however, this abnormality was not observed in a subsequent study at 12 times the daily human dose). Caffeine is generally not considered to be teratogenic; daily administration of an amount of caffeine equivalent to 20 cups of coffee has not resulted in teratogenic effects. No adequate, well-controlled studies have been performed in pregnant women; use this preparation during pregnancy only if the expected benefits justify the potential risk to the fetus. It is not known whether orphenadrine is excreted in human milk; the concentration of salicylic acid and caffeine in human milk is approximately equal to maternal blood levels. Use this preparation with caution in nursing mothers.

---

[1] One case of aplastic anemia has been reported; however, a causal relationship has not been established

MUSCLE RELAXANTS WITH ANALGESICS

PARAFON FORTE (chlorzoxazone and acetaminophen) McNeil Pharmaceutical   Rx

Tablets: 250 mg chlorzoxazone and 300 mg acetaminophen

INDICATIONS
Acute, painful musculoskeletal conditions (adjunctive therapy)[1]

ORAL DOSAGE
Adult: 2 tabs qid

CONTRAINDICATIONS
Hypersensitivity to chlorzoxazone or acetaminophen

WARNINGS/PRECAUTIONS

Liver dysfunction	Discontinue use if signs or symptoms occur
Patients with allergies	Use with caution in patients with allergies or history of drug allergy; discontinue use if urticaria, redness, or itching occurs
Tartrazine sensitivity	Presence of FD&C Yellow No. 5 (tartrazine) in tablets may cause allergic-type reactions, including bronchial asthma, in susceptible individuals
Sulfite sensitivity	Sodium metabisulfite in this product may cause urticaria, pruritus, wheezing, anaphylaxis, or other allergic-type reactions in susceptible patients, such as those with asthma or atopy

ADVERSE REACTIONS

Gastrointestinal	Occasional GI disturbances, bleeding
Hepatic	Liver damage
Central nervous system	Drowsiness, dizziness, light-headedness, malaise, overstimulation
Dermatological	Rash, petechiae, ecchymoses
Hypersensitivity	Angioneurotic edema, anaphylactic reactions

OVERDOSAGE

Signs and symptoms	*Acetaminophen-related effects:* nausea, vomiting, diaphoresis, and general malaise; clinical and laboratory evidence of hepatotoxicity (vomiting; right upper quadrant tenderness; increased SGOT, SGPT, serum bilirubin, and prothrombin time; and possible hypoglycemia) may not be apparent until 48–72 h after ingestion; *chlorzoxazone-related effects:* gastrointestinal disturbances, such as nausea, vomiting, or diarrhea; drowsiness; dizziness; light-headedness; headache; malaise or sluggishness, followed by marked loss of muscle tone; decreased or absent deep-tendon reflexes; respiratory depression, with rapid, irregular breathing and intercostal and substernal retraction; reduction in blood pressure
Treatment	Remove stomach contents promptly by inducing emesis or by gastric lavage, followed by activated charcoal. If respiration is depressed, secure an open airway by use of an oropharyngeal airway or endotracheal tube; administer oxygen and, if necessary, artificial respiration. *Do not use cholinergic agents or analeptics.* Treat hypotension by administering dextran, plasma, concentrated albumin, or a vasopressor (eg, norepinephrine). Administer oral acetylcysteine as soon as possible (no later than 24 h after ingestion); give a loading dose of 140 mg/kg and then, at 4-h intervals, 17 maintenance doses of 70 mg/kg. (Activated charcoal, if used, should be removed before acetylcysteine is given.) Measure the plasma level of unconjugated acetaminophen as early as possible, but no sooner than 4 h after ingestion. Determine prothrombin time, SGOT and SGPT levels, and serum concentrations of bilirubin, creatinine, BUN, glucose, and electrolytes every 24 h. If the prothrombin time exceeds 1.5 times the control value, give vitamin K_1; if the prothrombin time exceeds 3 times this value, give fresh frozen plasma. Institute appropriate measures to treat hypoglycemia and electrolyte and fluid imbalance. Avoid forced diuresis or use of diuretics when treating an acetaminophen overdose. For additional information on use of acetylcysteine and interpretation of the plasma acetaminophen level, see Mucomyst chart and contact the Rocky Mountain Poison Center (800-525-6115).

DRUG INTERACTIONS

CNS depressants, including alcohol	⇧ CNS depression

ALTERED LABORATORY VALUES

Blood/serum values	Glucose (with glucose oxidase/peroxidase test)
Urinary values	Discoloration of urine + 5-HIAA (with nitrosonaphthal reagent test)

USE IN CHILDREN	USE IN PREGNANT AND NURSING WOMEN
Safety and effectiveness for use in children have not been established	Safety for use during pregnancy has not been established. Consult manufacturer for use in nursing mothers.

[1] Probably effective

MUSCLE RELAXANTS WITH ANALGESICS

ROBAXISAL (methocarbamol and aspirin) Robins Rx
Tablets: 400 mg methocarbamol and 325 mg aspirin

INDICATIONS	ORAL DOSAGE
Acute painful musculoskeletal conditions (adjunctive therapy)	Adult: 2 tabs qid; for severe conditions in patients able to tolerate salicylates, 3 tabs qid for 1–3 days

CONTRAINDICATIONS[1]
Hypersensitivity to methocarbamol or aspirin

WARNINGS/PRECAUTIONS

Gastritis, peptic ulcer	May be exacerbated by aspirin component
Mental and/or physical impairment	Caution patients not to drive or perform other potentially hazardous activities until their response to this product has been determined, and that use of alcohol and other CNS depressants during therapy may cause additional CNS depression

ADVERSE REACTIONS
Frequent reactions (incidence ≥ 1%) are printed in *italics*

Gastrointestinal[2]	*Nausea (4–5%)*, gastritis, gastric erosion, vomiting, constipation, diarrhea
Central nervous system	*Dizziness or light-headedness (4–5%)*, drowsiness, headache
Ophthalmic	Blurred vision
Hypersensitivity	Angioedema, asthma, rash, pruritus, urticaria
Other	Fever

OVERDOSAGE

Signs and symptoms	*Toxic effects primarily attributable to aspirin:* rapid and deep breathing, hyperventilation, nausea, vomiting, vertigo, tinnitus, flushing, sweating, thirst, headache, drowsiness, diarrhea, tachycardia; *late symptoms:* fever, hemorrhage, excitement, confusion, convulsions, vasomotor depression, coma, respiratory failure, and respiratory alkalosis followed by respiratory and metabolic acidosis (primarily in children)
Treatment	If less than 4 h have elapsed since ingestion, induce emesis or perform gastric lavage, followed by activated characoal, to remove any remaining drug from the stomach. Initial therapy should be directed at reducing hyperthermia by external sponging with tepid water, correcting dehydration by appropriate IV fluid replacement, and maintaining adequate cardiorespiratory and renal function. In moderately severe cases of salicylate poisoning, cautiously administer sodium bicarbonate IV in sufficient quantity, if possible, to maintain an alkaline diuresis; intermittent peritoneal dialysis may also be helpful. In severe cases, hemodialysis should be seriously considered. Potassium should be added to the repair solution to compensate for potassium losses once urine formation is deemed adequate. Glucose may be provided to correct ketosis and hypoglycemia. Plasma transfusion may be beneficial if shock intervenes. Hemorrhagic phenomena may necessitate whole-blood transfusions and phytonadione (vitamin K$_1$). Do not administer barbiturates to treat excitement or convulsions.

DRUG INTERACTIONS

Anticoagulants	⇧ Risk of bleeding
Alcohol, corticosteroids, phenylbutazone, oxyphenbutazone	⇧ Risk of GI ulceration
Probenecid, sulfinpyrazone	⇩ Uricosuria
Spironolactone	⇩ Diuretic effect
Methotrexate	⇧ Methotrexate plasma level and risk of toxicity

ALTERED LABORATORY VALUES

Blood/serum values — ⇧ Prothrombin time   ⇧ Uric acid (with low doses)   ⇩ Uric acid (with high doses)
⇩ Thyroxine (T₄)   ⇩ Thyroid-stimulating hormone

Urinary values — ⇧ Glucose (with Clinitest tablets)   ⇧ 5-HIAA (color interference)   ⇧ VMA (color interference)

USE IN CHILDREN
Safety and effectiveness have not been established for use in children under 12 yr of age

USE IN PREGNANT AND NURSING WOMEN
Safety for use during pregnancy has not been established. Moderate amounts of aspirin are excreted in human milk and may interfere with platelet function or decrease prothrombin levels in the infant, resulting in an increased risk of bleeding. Risk appears to be minimal if drug is taken by the mother just after nursing and if the infant has adequate stores of vitamin K. It is not known whether methocarbamol is also excreted in human milk.

1 For other possible contraindications, see aspirin
2 May be minimized by taking drug with meals

MUSCLE RELAXANTS WITH ANALGESICS

SOMA Compound (carisoprodol and aspirin) Wallace — Rx

Tablets: 200 mg carisoprodol and 325 mg aspirin

INDICATIONS	**ORAL DOSAGE**
Pain, muscle spasm, and limited mobility associated with acute musculoskeletal conditions (adjunctive therapy)	Adult: 1–2 tabs qid

CONTRAINDICATIONS

Allergic or idiosyncratic reaction to carisoprodol, aspirin, or related compounds   Acute intermittent porphyria   Bleeding disorders

WARNINGS/PRECAUTIONS

Idiosyncratic reactions — These very rare reactions (see ADVERSE REACTIONS) generally occur within the period of the first to fourth dose in patients who have never received carisoprodol; symptoms usually subside within a few hours. If idiosyncratic reactions occur, discontinue use and institute appropriate therapy, including administration of epinephrine, antihistamines, and, in severe cases, corticosteroids.

Allergic reactions — Discontinue use and treat symptomatically if allergic reactions occur; in evaluating these reactions, also consider allergy to excipients

Drug dependence — Dependence owing to carisoprodol may occur in rare cases; use with caution in addiction-prone patients. No significant reactions have been precipitated by withdrawal of this preparation; however, abrupt cessation of carisoprodol, given at a dosage of 100 mg/kg/day (5 times the recommended dosage), has resulted in mild abstinence symptoms, including abdominal cramps, insomnia, chills, headache, and nausea.

Mental and/or physical impairment — Caution patients that their ability to drive or perform other potentially hazardous activities may be impaired

Special-risk patients — Use with caution in patients with a history of gastritis or peptic ulcer; to avoid excessive accumulation of this preparation, use with caution in elderly or debilitated patients and in patients with renal or hepatic impairment

Carcinogenicity, mutagenicity, effect on fertility — No long-term studies of the carcinogenic and mutagenic potential or the effect on fertility of this preparation have been done

ADVERSE REACTIONS[1]

Central nervous system and neuromuscular — Drowsiness, dizziness, vertigo, ataxia; tremor, agitation, irritability, headache, depression, syncope, and insomnia (rare)

Cardiovascular — Tachycardia, postural hypotension, facial flushing

Gastrointestinal — Nausea, vomiting, epigastric distress, hiccups, gastritis, occult bleeding, constipation, diarrhea, gastric erosion

Allergic — Dermatological reactions, including rash, erythema multiforme, pruritus, fixed drug eruptions, urticaria, edema, and angioneurotic edema; respiratory tract reactions, ranging from rhinorrhea and shortness of breath to severe asthma; eosinophilia

SOMA Compound ■ SOMA Compound with Codeine

Idiosyncratic	Extreme weakness, transient quadriplegia, dizziness, ataxia, temporary loss of vision, diplopia, mydriasis, dysarthria, agitation, euphoria, confusion, disorientation, asthmatic attacks, fever, angioneurotic edema, smarting eyes, hypotension, anaphylactoid shock

OVERDOSAGE

Signs and symptoms	*Aspirin-related effects:* hyperpnea, nausea, vomiting, vertigo, tinnitus, flushing, sweating, thirst, headache, drowsiness, diarrhea, and tachycardia, progressing to hyperthermia, dehydration, pulmonary edema, hemorrhage, acid-base disturbances, restlessness, confusion, convulsions, vasomotor depression, coma, and respiratory failure; *carisoprodol-related effects:* stupor, coma, shock, respiratory depression
Treatment	If less than 4 h have elapsed since ingestion, induce emesis or perform gastric lavage, followed by activated charcoal, to remove any remaining drug from the stomach. Initial therapy should be directed at reducing hyperthermia by external sponging with tepid water, correcting dehydration by appropriate IV fluid replacement, and maintaining adequate cardiorespiratory and renal function. In moderately severe cases of salicylate poisoning, cautiously administer sodium bicarbonate IV in sufficient quantity, if possible, to maintain an alkaline diuresis; carefully monitor urinary output and avoid overhydration. Hemodialysis, peritoneal dialysis, and diuretics (including mannitol) may be useful in removing carisoprodol. In severe cases of salicylate poisoning, hemodialysis should be seriously considered. Potassium should be added to the repair solution to compensate for potassium losses once urine formation is deemed adequate. Glucose may be provided to correct ketosis and hypoglycemia. Plasma transfusion may be beneficial if shock intervenes. Hemorrhagic phenomena may necessitate whole-blood transfusions and phytonadione (vitamin K$_1$). Do not administer barbiturates to treat excitement or convulsions.

DRUG INTERACTIONS

Alcohol	△ CNS depression; exercise appropriate caution
	△ Risk of GI ulceration; caution patients with a predisposition to GI bleeding
Tranquilizers, sedative-hypnotics, and other CNS depressants	△ CNS depression; exercise appropriate caution
Anticoagulants	△ Risk of bleeding; use with caution in patients receiving anticoagulants
Probenecid, sulfinpyrazone	▽ Uricosuria; caution patients with gout or arthritis that dosage adjustment or discontinuation of uricosuric agent may be necessary
Sulfonylureas	△ Hypoglycemic effect; caution patients with diabetes that dosage adjustment or discontinuation of hypoglycemic agent may be necessary
Methotrexate	△ Risk of methotrexate toxicity
Antacids, other urinary alkalinizers, corticosteroids	▽ Serum level of aspirin component
Ammonium chloride, other urinary acidifiers	△ Serum level of aspirin component

ALTERED LABORATORY VALUES

Blood/serum values	△ Prothrombin time △ Uric acid (with low doses) ▽ Uric acid (with high doses) ▽ Thyroxine (T$_4$) ▽ Thyroid-stimulating hormone
Urinary values	△ Glucose (with Clinitest tablets)

USE IN CHILDREN

Safety and effectiveness for use in children under 12 yr of age have not been established

USE IN PREGNANT AND NURSING WOMEN

Pregnancy Category C: reproduction studies in rodents have shown aspirin to be teratogenic and, if given at a level considerably greater than the usual human dose, embryocidal; however, an increased incidence of congenital abnormalities has not been seen in the children of women who took aspirin during pregnancy. Use of aspirin near term or before delivery may prolong delivery and cause maternal, fetal, or neonatal bleeding. No adequate reproduction studies of Soma Compound have been performed in animals. It is not known whether this preparation can cause harm to the fetus or affect reproductive capacity; use during pregnancy only if clearly needed. The concentration of carisoprodol in human milk is 2–4 times the maternal plasma level; moderate amounts of aspirin are excreted in human milk and may increase the risk of bleeding in nursing infants. Because of the potential for serious adverse reactions, patients should not nurse while taking this preparation.

---

[1] Leukopenia and pancytopenia have been reported in very rare cases; however, a causal relationship has not been established

---

MUSCLE RELAXANTS WITH ANALGESICS

SOMA Compound with Codeine (carisoprodol, aspirin, and codeine phosphate) Wallace   C-III

Tablets: 200 mg carisoprodol, 325 mg aspirin, and 16 mg codeine phosphate

INDICATIONS	ORAL DOSAGE
Pain, muscle spasm, and limited mobility associated with acute musculoskeletal conditions (adjunctive therapy)	Adult: 1–2 tabs qid

SOMA Compound with Codeine

CONTRAINDICATIONS

Allergic or idiosyncratic reaction to carisoprodol, aspirin, codeine, or related compounds

Acute intermittent porphyria

Bleeding disorders

WARNINGS/PRECAUTIONS

Idiosyncratic reactions — These very rare reactions (see ADVERSE REACTIONS) generally occur within the period of the first to fourth dose in patients who have never received carisoprodol; symptoms usually subside within a few hours. If idiosyncratic reactions occur, discontinue use and institute appropriate therapy, including administration of epinephrine, antihistamines, and, in severe cases, corticosteroids.

Allergic reactions — Discontinue use and treat symptomatically if allergic reactions occur; in evaluating these reactions, also consider allergy to excipients

Drug dependence — Dependence owing to carisoprodol and codeine may occur in rare cases; use with caution in addiction-prone patients. No significant reactions have been precipitated by withdrawal of this preparation; however, abrupt cessation of carisoprodol, given at a dosage of 100 mg/kg/day (5 times the recommended dosage), has resulted in mild abstinence symptoms, including abdominal cramps, insomnia, chills, headache, and nausea.

Mental and/or physical impairment — Caution patients that their ability to drive or perform other potentially hazardous activities may be impaired

Special-risk patients — Use with caution in patients with a history of gastritis or peptic ulcer; to avoid excessive accumulation of this preparation, use with caution in elderly or debilitated patients and in patients with renal or hepatic impairment

Carcinogenicity, mutagenicity, effect on fertility — No long-term studies of the carcinogenic and mutagenic potential or the effect on fertility of this preparation have been done

ADVERSE REACTIONS[1]

Central nervous system and neuromuscular — Drowsiness, sedation, dizziness, vertigo, ataxia; tremor, agitation, irritability, headache, depression, syncope, and insomnia (rare)

Ophthalmic — Miosis

Cardiovascular — Tachycardia, postural hypotension, facial flushing

Gastrointestinal — Nausea, vomiting, epigastric distress, hiccups, gastritis, occult bleeding, constipation, diarrhea, gastric erosion

Allergic — Dermatological reactions, including rash, erythema multiforme, pruritus, fixed drug eruptions, urticaria, edema, and angioneurotic edema; respiratory tract reactions, ranging from rhinorrhea and shortness of breath to severe asthma; eosinophilia

Idiosyncratic — Extreme weakness, transient quadriplegia, dizziness, ataxia, temporary loss of vision, diplopia, mydriasis, dysarthria, agitation, euphoria, confusion, disorientation, asthmatic attacks, fever, angioneurotic edema, smarting eyes, hypotension, anaphylactoid shock

OVERDOSAGE

Signs and symptoms — *Codeine-related effects:* respiratory depression, miosis, extreme somnolence progressing to stupor or coma, skeletal-muscle flaccidity, cold and clammy skin, bradycardia, hypotension, and, in severe cases, apnea, circulatory collapse, and cardiac arrest; *aspirin-related effects:* hyperpnea, nausea, vomiting, vertigo, tinnitus, flushing, sweating, thirst, headache, drowsiness, diarrhea, and tachycardia, progressing to hyperthermia, dehydration, pulmonary edema, hemorrhage, acid-base disturbances, restlessness, confusion, convulsions, vasomotor depression, coma, and respiratory failure; *carisoprodol-related effects:* stupor, coma, shock, respiratory depression

Treatment — Give primary attention to reestablishing adequate respiratory exchange through provision of an adequate airway and assisted or controlled ventilation; positive-pressure respiration may be desirable if pulmonary edema is present. If respiratory depression is significant, promptly administer naloxone (adult, 0.4 mg; child, 0.01 mg/kg), preferably IV, and repeat at 2- to 3-min intervals until satisfactory breathing is restored. *Do not use analeptic agents.* Oxygen, IV fluids, vasopressors, and other supportive measures should be employed, as needed. Gastric lavage, followed by instillation of activated charcoal, may be used if performed within 4 h of ingestion. In moderately severe cases of salicylate poisoning, cautiously administer sodium bicarbonate IV in sufficient quantity, if possible, to maintain an alkaline diuresis; carefully monitor urinary output and avoid overhydration. Hemodialysis, peritoneal dialysis, and diuretics (including mannitol) may be useful in removing carisoprodol. In severe cases of salicylate poisoning, hemodialysis should be seriously considered. Hyperthermia, particularly in children, and dehydration require prompt correction. Hemorrhagic phenomena may necessitate whole-blood transfusions and phytonadione (vitamin K_1). Do not use barbiturates to treat excitement or convulsions.

SOMA Compound with Codeine

DRUG INTERACTIONS

Alcohol	⇧ CNS depression; exercise appropriate caution
	⇧ Risk of GI ulceration; caution patients with a predisposition to GI bleeding
Tranquilizers, sedative-hypnotics, and other CNS depressants	⇧ CNS depression; exercise appropriate caution
Anticoagulants	⇧ Risk of bleeding; use with caution in patients receiving anticoagulants
Probenecid, sulfinpyrazone	⇩ Uricosuria; caution patients with gout or arthritis that dosage adjustment or discontinuation of uricosuric agent may be necessary
Sulfonylureas	⇧ Hypoglycemic effect; caution patients with diabetes that dosage adjustment or discontinuation of hypoglycemic agent may be necessary
Methotrexate	⇧ Risk of methotrexate toxicity
Antacids, other urinary alkalinizers, corticosteroids	⇩ Serum level of aspirin component
Ammonium chloride, other urinary acidifiers	⇧ Serum level of aspirin component

ALTERED LABORATORY VALUES

Blood/serum values	⇧ Amylase ⇧ Lipase ⇧ Prothrombin time ⇧ Uric acid (with low doses)
	⇩ Uric acid (with high doses) ⇩ Thyroxine (T$_4$) ⇩ Thyroid-stimulating hormone
Urinary values	⇧ Glucose (with Clinitest tablets)

USE IN CHILDREN

Safety and effectiveness for use in children under 12 yr of age have not been established

USE IN PREGNANT AND NURSING WOMEN

Pregnancy Category C: reproduction studies in rodents have shown aspirin to be teratogenic and, if given at a level considerably greater than the usual human dose, embryocidal; however, an increased incidence of congenital abnormalities has not been seen in the children of women who took aspirin during pregnancy. Use of aspirin near term or before delivery may prolong delivery and cause maternal, fetal, or neonatal bleeding. No adequate reproduction studies of Soma Compound with Codeine have been performed in animals. It is not known whether this preparation can cause harm to the fetus or affect reproductive capacity; use during pregnancy only if clearly needed. The concentration of carisoprodol in human milk is 2–4 times the maternal plasma level; moderate amounts of aspirin are excreted in human milk and may increase the risk of bleeding in nursing infants. Because of the potential for serious adverse reactions, patients should not nurse while taking this preparation.

[1] Leukopenia and pancytopenia have been reported in very rare cases; however, a causal relationship has not been established

Chapter 43

Ophthalmic/Otic Preparations

Antiglaucoma Agents/Miotics — 1722

BETAGAN (Allergan) — 1722
Levobunolol hydrochloride *Rx*

BETOPTIC (Alcon) — 1723
Betaxolol hydrochloride *Rx*

DIAMOX (Lederle) — 1724
Acetazolamide *Rx*

EPIFRIN Ophthalmic Solution (Allergan) — 1726
Levo-epinephrine hydrochloride *Rx*

OCUSERT Ocular Therapeutic System (Alza) — 1727
Pilocarpine *Rx*

P_1E_1, P_2E_1, P_3E_1, P_4E_1, and P_6E_1 Ophthalmic Solutions (Alcon) — 1729
Pilocarpine hydrochloride and epinephrine bitartrate *Rx*

PHOSPHOLINE IODIDE Ophthalmic Solution (Ayerst) — 1730
Echothiophate iodide *Rx*

PILOPINE HS Ophthalmic Gel (Alcon) — 1732
Pilocarpine hydrochloride *Rx*

PROPINE Ophthalmic Solution (Allergan) — 1733
Dipivefrin hydrochloride *Rx*

TIMOPTIC (Merck Sharp & Dohme) — 1734
Timolol maleate *Rx*

Mydriatics/Cycloplegics — 1736

CYCLOGYL Ophthalmic Solution (Alcon) — 1736
Cyclopentolate hydrochloride *Rx*

MYDRIACYL Ophthalmic Solution (Alcon) — 1737
Tropicamide *Rx*

Ophthalmic Anti-Infectives — 1738

BLEPH-10 Ophthalmic Ointment and Solution (Allergan) — 1738
Sulfacetamide sodium *Rx*

BLEPHAMIDE Ophthalmic Suspension (Allergan) — 1739
Sulfacetamide sodium and prednisolone acetate *Rx*

BLEPHAMIDE S.O.P. Ophthalmic Ointment (Allergan) — 1739
Sulfacetamide sodium and prednisolone acetate *Rx*

CHLOROMYXIN Ophthalmic Ointment (Parke-Davis) — 1742
Chloramphenicol and polymyxin B sulfate *Rx*

CORTISPORIN Ophthalmic Ointment (Burroughs Wellcome) — 1740
Polymyxin B sulfate, bacitracin zinc, neomycin sulfate, and hydrocortisone *Rx*

CORTISPORIN Ophthalmic Suspension (Burroughs Wellcome) — 1741
Polymyxin B sulfate, neomycin sulfate, and hydrocortisone *Rx*

GARAMYCIN Ophthalmic Ointment and Solution (Schering) — 1743
Gentamicin sulfate *Rx*

GENTACIDIN Ophthalmic Ointment and Solution (CooperVision) — 1744
Gentamicin sulfate *Rx*

ILOTYCIN Ophthalmic Ointment (Dista) — 1744
Erythromycin *Rx*

MAXITROL Ophthalmic Ointment and Suspension (Alcon) — 1745
Dexamethasone, neomycin sulfate, and polymyxin B sulfate *Rx*

NEODECADRON Sterile Ophthalmic Ointment and Suspension (Merck Sharp & Dohme) — 1746
Neomycin sulfate and dexamethasone sodium phosphate *Rx*

NEOSPORIN Ophthalmic Ointment (Burroughs Wellcome) — 1748
Polymyxin B sulfate, bacitracin zinc, and neomycin sulfate *Rx*

NEOSPORIN Ophthalmic Solution (Burroughs Wellcome) — 1748
Polymyxin B sulfate, neomycin sulfate and gramicidin *Rx*

POLY-PRED Ophthalmic Suspension (Allergan) — 1748
Prednisolone acetate, neomycin sulfate, and polymyxin B sulfate *Rx*

Sodium SULAMYD Ophthalmic Ointment and Solution (Schering) — 1749
Sulfacetamide sodium *Rx*

TOBREX Ophthalmic Ointment and Solution (Alcon) — 1750
Tobramycin *Rx*

VASOCIDIN Ophthalmic Ointment (CooperVision) — 1751
Sulfacetamide sodium and prednisolone acetate *Rx*

VASOCIDIN Ophthalmic Solution (CooperVision) — 1752
Sulfacetamide sodium and prednisolone sodium phosphate *Rx*

VIROPTIC Ophthalmic Solution (Burroughs Wellcome) — 1754
Trifluridine *Rx*

Ophthalmic Corticosteroids — 1755

DECADRON Phosphate Ophthalmic Ointment (Merck Sharp & Dohme) — 1755
Dexamethasone sodium phosphate *Rx*

DECADRON Phosphate Ophthalmic Solution (Merck Sharp & Dohme) — 1755
Dexamethasone sodium phosphate *Rx*

FLUOR-OP Ophthalmic Suspension (CooperVision) — 1756
Fluorometholone *Rx*

FML Ophthalmic Ointment and Suspension (Allergan) — 1757
Fluorometholone *Rx*

FML Forte Ophthalmic Suspension (Allergan) Fluorometholone *Rx*	1757
INFLAMASE 1/8% Ophthalmic Solution (CooperVision) Prednisolone sodium phosphate *Rx*	1758
INFLAMASE Forte 1% Ophthalmic Solution (CooperVision) Prednisolone sodium phosphate *Rx*	1758

Ophthalmic Decongestants/ Antiallergic Agents — 1759

NAPHCON-A Ophthalmic Solution (Alcon) Naphazoline hydrochloride and pheniramine maleate *Rx*	1759
NEO-SYNEPHRINE Ophthalmic Solution (Winthrop-Breon) Phenylephrine hydrochloride *Rx*	1760
OPTICROM 4% Ophthalmic Solution (Fisons) Cromolyn sodium *Rx*	1762
VASOCON-A (CooperVision) Naphazoline hydrochloride and antazoline phosphate *Rx*	1762

Otic Analgesics/Anesthetics — 1763

AMERICAINE-Otic (Du Pont Critical Care) Benzocaine *Rx*	1763
AURALGAN Otic Solution (Ayerst) Antipyrine and benzocaine *Rx*	1764
TYMPAGESIC Otic Solution (Adria) Phenylephrine hydrochloride, antipyrine, and benzocaine *Rx*	1764

Otic Anti-Infectives — 1765

CHLOROMYCETIN Otic (Parke-Davis) Chloramphenicol *Rx*	1765
COLY-MYCIN S Otic (Parke-Davis) Colistin sulfate, neomycin sulfate, thonzonium bromide, and hydrocortisone acetate *Rx*	1766
CORTISPORIN Otic Solution (Burroughs Wellcome) Polymyxin B sulfate, neomycin sulfate, and hydrocortisone *Rx*	1767
CORTISPORIN Otic Suspension (Burroughs Wellcome) Polymyxin B sulfate, neomycin sulfate, and hydrocortisone *Rx*	1767
Otic TRIDESILON Solution (Miles Pharmaceuticals) Desonide and acetic acid *Rx*	1768
OTOBIOTIC Otic Solution (Schering) Polymyxin B sulfate and hydrocortisone *Rx*	1769
VōSoL Otic Solution (Wallace) Acetic acid *Rx*	1769
VōSoL HC Otic Solution (Wallace) Hydrocortisone and acetic acid *Rx*	1770

Cerumen Softeners — 1770

CERUMENEX (Purdue Frederick) Triethanolamine polypeptide oleate-condensate *Rx*	1770
DEBROX (Marion) Carbamide peroxide *OTC*	1771
MURINE Ear Drops (Ross) Carbamide peroxide *OTC*	1772
MURINE Ear Wax Removal System (Ross) Carbamide peroxide *OTC*	1772

ANTIGLAUCOMA AGENTS/MIOTICS

BETAGAN (levobunolol hydrochloride) Allergan   Rx

Solution: 0.5% (5, 10 ml)

INDICATIONS
Elevated intraocular pressure in patients with chronic open-angle glaucoma or ocular hypertension

TOPICAL DOSAGE
Adult: 1 drop instilled into the affected eye(s) 1–2 times/day

CONTRAINDICATIONS
Bronchial asthma or a history of bronchial asthma

Severe chronic obstructive pulmonary disease

Sinus bradycardia

Second- or third-degree AV block

Overt cardiac failure (see WARNINGS/PRECAUTIONS)

Cardiogenic shock

Hypersensitivity to any component

ADMINISTRATION/DOSAGE ADJUSTMENTS
Concomitant therapy	If response is not satisfactory at recommended dosage, miotics, sympathomimetics (eg, dipivefrin), or carbonic anhydrase inhibitors may be given concomitantly. When treating angle-closure glaucoma, use levobunolol in combination with a miotic because the beta blocker has little, if any, effect on pupil size.

WARNINGS/PRECAUTIONS
Cardiac failure	Beta blockade can cause or exacerbate cardiac failure. Administration of levobunolol to patients with no history of cardiac failure should be discontinued at the first sign or symptom of this reaction; use of this drug in patients with overt cardiac failure is contraindicated.
Patients with bronchospastic disease	Levobunolol is specifically contraindicated for use in patients with bronchial asthma or a history of bronchial asthma; use with caution in patients with diminished pulmonary function, nonallergic bronchospasm (eg, chronic bronchitis, emphysema), or a history of nonallergic bronchospasm.
Major surgery	By impairing cardiac responsiveness to reflex beta-adrenergic stimuli, beta blockade may increase the risks associated with general anesthesia and precipitate severe, protracted hypotension. Gradual withdrawal before elective surgery may be an appropriate measure; however, bear in mind that the necessity or desirability of discontinuing use before major surgery is controversial. If necessary, the effects of beta blockade may be reversed during surgery by adequate doses of beta-adrenergic agonists such as isoproterenol, dopamine, dobutamine, or norepinephrine.
Diabetes and hypoglycemia	Use with caution in patients susceptible to spontaneous hypoglycemia and in diabetic patients (especially labile diabetics) who are taking insulin or sulfonylureas. Beta blockade may mask certain signs and symptoms of acute hypoglycemia.
Thyrotoxicosis	If thyrotoxicosis is suspected, abrupt withdrawal should be avoided since it may precipitate a thyroid storm. Certain signs of hyperthyroidism (eg, tachycardia) may be masked by beta blockade.
Myasthenia	Beta blockade may exacerbate certain myasthenic signs and symptoms (eg, diplopia, ptosis, generalized weakness)
Decreased corneal sensitivity	Prolonged use may cause decreased corneal sensitivity
Hypersensitivity	Use with caution in patients hypersensitive to other beta blockers
Carcinogenicity, mutagenicity	An increase in benign leiomyomas has been shown in female mice fed 14,000 times the human topical dose throughout their lifetime, and an increase in benign hepatomas has been demonstrated in male rats fed 12,800 times the human topical dose for 2 yr. No evidence of mutagenicity has been seen in mammalian or microbiological assays.
Effect on fertility	Administration to rats of up to 1,800 times the human topical dose has not caused any adverse effect on fertility

ADVERSE REACTIONS[1]
The most frequent reactions, regardless of incidence, are printed in *italics*

Ophthalmic	*Transient ocular burning and stinging (25%), blepharoconjunctivitis (5%);* decreased corneal sensitivity; iridocyclitis (rare)
Cardiovascular	Decreases in heart rate and blood pressure
Central nervous system	Headache, transient ataxia, dizziness, and lethargy (rare)
Dermatological	Urticaria and pruritus (rare)

OVERDOSAGE
Signs and symptoms	Symptomatic bradycardia, hypotension, bronchospasm, acute cardiac failure

BETAGAN ■ BETOPTIC

Treatment	Flush eyes with water or normal saline; if drug is accidentally ingested, empty stomach by gastric lavage. For symptomatic bradycardia, administer atropine sulfate (0.25–2 mg IV). If bradycardia persists, cautiously give IV isoproterenol; in refractory cases, consider using a transvenous cardiac pacemaker. To reverse hypotension, administer a sympathomimetic amine (eg, dopamine, dobutamine, or norepinephrine); in refractory cases, try glucagon. For bronchospasm, give isoproterenol and, if necessary, aminophylline. To treat acute cardiac failure, administer digitalis, diuretics, and oxygen immediately; for refractory cases, give IV aminophylline and then, if necessary, glucagon. Correct second- or third-degree heart block by using isoproterenol or a transvenous cardiac pacemaker.

DRUG INTERACTIONS

Systemic beta blockers	⬆ Pharmacological effects of beta blockade
Epinephrine	Mydriasis
Reserpine, other catecholamine-depleting drugs	⬆ Risk of hypotension or marked bradycardia (vertigo, syncope, or orthostatic hypotension may occur); closely observe patients during concomitant therapy

ALTERED LABORATORY VALUES

No clinically significant alterations in blood/serum or urinary values occur at therapeutic dosages

USE IN CHILDREN

Safety and effectiveness for use in children have not been established

USE IN PREGNANT AND NURSING WOMEN

Pregnancy Category C: fetotoxicity, characterized by an increase in resorption sites, has been observed in rabbits at 200 and 700 times the human topical dose; however, reproduction studies in rats at up to 1,800 times the human topical dose have shown no evidence of fetotoxicity or teratogenicity. Results from the studies in rats as well as from studies with other beta blockers suggest that rabbits may be a particularly sensitive species. Nevertheless, use during pregnancy only if the expected benefits outweigh the potential risk to the fetus. It is not known whether this drug is excreted in human milk; because systemic beta blockers and topical timolol are excreted in human milk, use with caution in nursing mothers.

VEHICLE/BASE
Solution: **1.4% polyvinyl alcohol, 0.004% benzalkonium chloride, edetate disodium, sodium metabisulfite, dibasic sodium phosphate, monobasic potassium phosphate, sodium chloride, purified water, and hydrochloric acid or sodium hydroxide (to adjust pH)**

[1] Reactions associated with other nonselective topical beta blockers include arrhythmias, syncope, heart block, cerebrovascular accident, cerebral ischemia, congestive heart failure, palpitation, nausea, depression, allergic skin reactions (including localized and generalized rash), bronchospasm (mainly in patients with bronchospastic disease), respiratory failure, keratitis, blepharoptosis, visual disturbances (including refractive changes and diplopia), and ptosis

---

ANTIGLAUCOMA AGENTS/MIOTICS

BETOPTIC (betaxolol hydrochloride) Alcon   Rx

Solution: 0.5% (2.5, 5, 10, 15 ml)

INDICATIONS

Elevated intraocular pressure in patients with ocular hypertension and chronic open-angle glaucoma

TOPICAL DOSAGE

Adult: 1 drop instilled into the affected eye(s) bid

CONTRAINDICATIONS

Sinus bradycardia	Cardiogenic shock	Hypersensitivity to any component
Second- or third-degree AV block	Overt cardiac failure	

ADMINISTRATION/DOSAGE ADJUSTMENTS

Concomitant therapy	If response is not satisfactory using 1 drop bid, pilocarpine or other miotics, epinephrine, or systemic carbonic anhydrase inhibitors may be given concomitantly; mydriasis has been reported occasionally after concomitant use with epinephrine
Transferring patients from other antiglaucoma agents	On day 1, continue other agent and add 1 drop of betaxolol in the affected eye(s) bid; on day 2, discontinue previously used agent and continue treatment with betaxolol. To transfer patients from several agents, discontinue one agent at a time at intervals of not less than 1 wk.

WARNINGS/PRECAUTIONS

Cardiac failure	Use with caution in patients with a history of cardiac failure; discontinue use at the first signs of cardiac failure
Concurrent administration of oral beta-blocking agents	Monitor patient for possible additive effects on either intraocular pressure or the systemic effects of beta-adrenergic blockade

COMPENDIUM OF DRUG THERAPY

BETOPTIC ■ DIAMOX

Pulmonary disease	Use with caution in patients with severe reactive airway disease, as well as in those with excessive restriction of pulmonary function
Patients undergoing anesthesia and major surgery	Beta blockage may augment the risks; gradual withdrawal of beta blockers prior to elective surgery should be considered
Diabetes and hypoglycemia	Use with caution in patients subject to spontaneous hypoglycemia and in diabetic patients (especially labile diabetics) who are taking insulin or oral hypoglycemic agents; beta blockade may mask the signs and symptoms of acute hypoglycemia
Thyrotoxicosis	Clinical signs of hyperthyroidism (eg, tachycardia) may be masked; manage patients suspected of developing thyrotoxicosis carefully to avoid abrupt withdrawal of beta blockade, which may precipitate thyroid storm
Patients with angle-closure glaucoma	Since the immediate treatment objective is to reopen the angle, use a miotic concomitantly with betaxolol
Prolonged use	As with other antiglaucoma agents, diminished responsiveness to betaxolol after protracted therapy has been reported; however, no significant difference in mean intraocular pressure after initial stabilization has been observed over a period of 2 yr
Carcinogenicity, mutagenicity	Betaxolol has demonstrated no carcinogenic effect in mice; the drug has also been shown to be nonmutagenic in a variety of in vitro and in vivo bacterial and mammalian cell assays

ADVERSE REACTIONS

Ophthalmic	Discomfort of short duration (25%), occasional tearing; decreased corneal sensitivity, erythema, itching, corneal punctate staining, keratitis, anisocoria, and photophobia (rare)
Systemic	Insomnia and depressive neuroses (rare)

OVERDOSAGE

Signs and symptoms	Bradycardia, hypotension, acute cardiac failure
Treatment	For topical overdose, flush eye(s) with warm tap water. In cases of accidental ingestion, empty stomach by gastric lavage. For symptomatic bradycardia, administer atropine sulfate (0.25–2 mg IV) to induce vagal blockage; if bradycardia persists, give IV isoproterenol cautiously and, in refractory cases, consider using a transvenous cardiac pacemaker. For hypotension, administer a sympathomimetic amine (eg, dopamine, dobutamine, or norepinephrine); in refractory cases, try glucagon HCl. For acute cardiac failure, institute treatment with digitalis, diuretics, and oxygen immediately; in refractory cases, try IV aminophylline, followed, if necessary, by glucagon HCl. For second- or third-degree heart block, use isoproterenol or a transvenous cardiac pacemaker. Hemodialysis may or may not be helpful in removing the drug from the circulation.

DRUG INTERACTIONS

Propranolol and other beta-adrenergic blockers	⇧ Systemic effects of beta blockade ⇩ Intraocular pressure
Epinephrine	Mydriasis
Reserpine, other catecholamine-depleting drugs	Hypotension and/or bradycardia
Pilocarpine and other topical miotics; topical epinephrine; acetazolamide and other systemic carbonic anhydrase inhibitors	⇩ Intraocular pressure

ALTERED LABORATORY VALUES

No clinically significant alterations in blood/serum or urinary values occur at therapeutic dosages

USE IN CHILDREN

Safety and effectiveness for use in children have not been established

USE IN PREGNANT AND NURSING WOMEN

Pregnancy Category C: use during pregnancy only if the anticipated benefit of treatment exceeds the potential fetal risk. Drug-related postimplantation fetal loss was observed in rabbits and rats at oral doses exceeding 12 mg/kg and 128 mg/kg, respectively. Although teratogenic effects have not been seen in rodents, no adequate, well-controlled studies have been done in pregnant women. It is not known if betaxolol is excreted in human milk; because many drugs are, use with caution in nursing women.

VEHICLE/BASE
Solution: 0.01% benzalkonium chloride, edetate disodium, sodium chloride, hydrochloric acid and/or sodium hydroxide (to adjust pH), and purified water

---

ANTIGLAUCOMA AGENTS/MIOTICS

DIAMOX (acetazolamide) Lederle   Rx

Capsules (sustained release): 500 mg   **Tablets:** 125, 250 mg   **Vials:** 500 mg

INDICATIONS	ORAL DOSAGE	PARENTERAL DOSAGE
Chronic simple (open-angle) glaucoma (adjunctive therapy)	Adult: if capsules are used, 500 mg bid (AM and PM); if tablets are used, 250 mg to 1 g/24 h (divide daily doses > 250 mg)	Adult: 250 mg to 1 g/24 h IV (divide daily doses > 250 mg)

DIAMOX

Secondary glaucoma (adjunctive therapy) and preoperatively for acute angle-closure glaucoma, where surgery is delayed in order to lower intraocular pressure	**Adult:** if capsules are used, 500 mg bid (AM and PM); if tablets are used, 250 mg q4h, or 500 mg to start, followed by 125 or 250 mg q4h; for short-term use, 250 mg bid may be sufficient	**Adult:** 250 mg IV q4h, or 500 mg IV to start, followed by 125 or 250 mg IV q4h; for short-term use, 250 mg bid may be sufficient
Edema associated with congestive heart failure (adjunctive therapy)	**Adult:** 250–375 mg (5 mg/kg) in a single morning dose to start, followed by 250–375 mg every other day or daily for 2 days at a time, alternating with a day of rest	**Adult:** 250–375 mg (5 mg/kg) IV in a single morning dose to start, followed by 250–375 mg IV every other day or daily for 2 days at a time, alternating with a day of rest
Drug-induced edema (adjunctive therapy)	**Adult:** 250–375 mg (5 mg/kg) every other day or daily for 2 days at a time, alternating with a day of rest	**Adult:** 250–375 mg (5 mg/kg) IV every other day or daily for 2 days at a time, alternating with a day of rest
Centrencephalic epilepsy (petit mal, unlocalized seizures; adjunctive therapy)	**Adult:** 8–30 mg/kg/day in divided doses; optimum dosage: 375 mg/day to 1 g/day in divided doses **Child:** same as adult	**Adult:** 8–30 mg/kg/day IV in divided doses; optimum dosage: 375 mg/day to 1 g/day IV in divided doses **Child:** same as adult
Prevention or amelioration of acute mountain sickness in climbers who are very susceptible or who are attempting a rapid ascent	**Adult:** 500–1,000 mg/day, in divided doses, beginning 24–48 h before ascent and continuing while at high altitude for 48 h or as long as needed; for rapid ascent, give 1,000 mg/day	

CONTRAINDICATIONS

Pregnancy	Marked kidney disease or dysfunction	Hyperchloremic acidosis
Hyponatremia	Marked liver disease or dysfunction	Chronic, noncongestive angle-closure glaucoma (prolonged therapy only)
Hypokalemia	Suprarenal gland failure	

ADMINISTRATION/DOSAGE ADJUSTMENTS

Use of sustained-release capsules	If glaucoma is not adequately controlled by the capsules, switch to the tablets or parenteral solution, which are given more frequently. The capsules are not indicated for treatment of edema or epilepsy.
Parenteral use	Intramuscular administration is painful because of the high pH; direct IV injection is recommended. Reconstitute contents of vial with at least 5 ml of sterile water for injection prior to use; the reconstituted solution is stable for 1 wk if refrigerated, but preferably should be used within 24 h of reconstitution.
Combination therapy for angle-closure glaucoma	Acetazolamide may be given with miotics or mydriatics, as needed
Combination anticonvulsant therapy	Initiate acetazolamide therapy at 250 mg/day, while maintaining dosage of existing anticonvulsant medications, followed by a gradual increase in the dosage of acetazolamide to the level recommended above

WARNINGS/PRECAUTIONS

Excessive dosage	May decrease diuresis and cause drowsiness or paresthesia; do not exceed recommended dosage (however, very high doses have been given with other diuretics to secure diuresis in certain cases of completely refractory heart failure)
Sulfonamide-related effects	Fever, crystalluria, renal stones, severe rash (including Stevens-Johnson syndrome and toxic epidermal necrolysis), and blood dyscrasias (including bone marrow depression, thrombocytopenic purpura, hemolytic anemia, leukopenia, pancytopenia, and agranulocytosis) can occur with use of sulfonamides. Watch for early signs and symptoms; determine CBC and platelet count regularly during therapy (obtain baseline counts before starting treatment). If significant changes in blood counts are seen or other early manifestations are detected, administration should be discontinued and appropriate therapy instituted.
Acidosis	May be precipitated or exacerbated in patients with impaired alveolar ventilation due to pulmonary obstruction or emphysema; long-term therapy may also produce acidosis, which can usually be corrected by administration of bicarbonate
Severe mountain sickness	If high-altitude pulmonary or cerebral edema occurs during rapid ascent, the climber should promptly descend; use of this drug does not obviate the need for such a measure

ADVERSE REACTIONS

Central nervous system and neuromuscular	Paresthesias (particularly a "tingling" sensation in the extremities), drowsiness, confusion, flaccid paralysis, convulsions
Renal	Polyuria, hematuria, glycosuria
Dermatological	Urticaria

DIAMOX ■ EPIFRIN

Other	Fever, decreased appetite, acidosis (with long-term therapy), transient myopia, hepatic insufficiency, melena; photosensitivity (rare)

OVERDOSAGE

Signs and symptoms	See ADVERSE REACTIONS
Treatment	Discontinue medication; treat symptomatically and institute general supportive measures, as indicated

DRUG INTERACTIONS

Other diuretics	△ Diuretic effect and risk of hypokalemia
Lithium	△ Excretion, resulting in diminished pharmacologic activity of interacting drug
Aspirin (high doses)	Anorexia, tachypnea, lethargy, and coma; exercise caution during concomitant therapy
Amphetamines, ephedrine, pseudoephedrine, quinidine	▽ Excretion, resulting in enhanced pharmacologic activity and/or prolonged duration of action of interacting drug
Methenamine	Inactivation of antimicrobial effect
Insulin, oral hypoglycemics	▽ Hypoglycemic effect
Digitalis glycosides	△ Risk of cardiotoxicity due to hypokalemia
Amphotericin B, corticosteroids	△ Risk of severe hypokalemia
Phenytoin	△ Osteopenia
Primidone	▽ Anticonvulsant effect

ALTERED LABORATORY VALUES

Blood/serum values	▽ Sodium △ Chloride ▽ Bicarbonate △ Ammonia △ Bilirubin △ Uric acid ▽ Potassium ▽ ^{131}I thyroid uptake (in euthyroid and hyperthyroid patients only) △ Glucose (in prediabetic and diabetic patients)
Urinary values	△ Sodium △ Potassium △ Chloride △ Bicarbonate △ Phosphate ▽ Citrate ▽ Uric acid △ Ammonia △ Urobilinogen △ Glucose (in prediabetic and diabetic patients) + Protein (with bromophenol blue reagent, sulfosalicylic acid, heat and acetic acid, or nitric acid ring test methods) + 17-OHCS (with modified Glenn-Nelson technique)

USE IN CHILDREN

See INDICATIONS and dosage recommendations

USE IN PREGNANT AND NURSING WOMEN

Contraindicated during pregnancy, especially during the first trimester, unless expected benefits outweigh potential risk to the fetus. Acetazolamide has been shown to be embryocidal and teratogenic in rats and mice at doses exceeding 10 times the recommended human dose; however, there is no evidence of these effects in human beings. Consult manufacturer for use in nursing mothers.

ANTIGLAUCOMA AGENTS/MIOTICS

EPIFRIN Ophthalmic Solution (levo-epinephrine hydrochloride) Allergan   Rx

Solution: levo-epinephrine hydrochloride equivalent to 0.25% (15 ml), 0.5% (15 ml), 1.0% (15 ml) and 2.0% (15 ml) epinephrine

INDICATIONS	**TOPICAL DOSAGE**
Chronic simple glaucoma	**Adult:** 1 drop instilled into the affected eye(s) 1–2 times/day

CONTRAINDICATIONS

Attack of narrow-angle glaucoma (pupillary dilation may trigger an acute attack)

ADMINISTRATION/DOSAGE ADJUSTMENTS

Dosage titration	The dosage (choice of strength) should be adjusted to the individual patient
Administration	This product is for topical use only; do not administer as an injection

WARNINGS/PRECAUTIONS

Patients with a narrow angle	Use this preparation with caution in patients with a narrow angle, as pupillary dilation may trigger an acute attack of narrow-angle glaucoma
Aphakic patients	Epinephrine has been known to produce reversible macular edema in some aphakic patients and, therefore, should be used with caution in these individuals

EPIFRIN ■ OCUSERT

Other special-risk patients	Use with caution in patients with hypertension or coronary artery disease
Discomfort upon instillation	Epinephrine in any form is relatively uncomfortable when administered; discomfort lessens with lower concentrations
Carcinogenicity, mutagenicity, effect on fertility	No studies have been conducted to evaluate the carcinogenic or mutagenic potential of this drug or its effect, if any, on fertility

ADVERSE REACTIONS

Ophthalmic	Eye pain or ache, browache, headache, conjunctival hyperemia, allergic lid reactions, adrenochrome deposits in the conjunctiva and cornea (after prolonged use); reversible macular edema in aphakic patients

OVERDOSAGE

Signs and symptoms	Hypertension, tachycardia, extrasystoles, premature ventricular contractions, pulmonary edema, occipital headaches, pallor, trembling, palpitations, faintness, diaphoresis
Treatment	Institute appropriate supportive measures. Hypertension may be treated, if necessary, with an injectable vasodilator, with a rapid-acting alpha-adrenergic blocker, such as phentolamine, or with trimethophan; if antihypertensive therapy results in prolonged hypotension, a vasopressor such as norepinephrine may be given. For pulmonary edema that interferes with respiration, administer a rapid-acting alpha-adrenergic blocker and/or provide intermittent positive-pressure respiration. To control arrhythmias, use a beta-adrenergic blocker, such as propranolol.

DRUG INTERACTIONS

Miotics, carbonic anhydrase inhibitors	△ Lowering of intraocular pressure
Cyclopropane, halogenated general anesthetics, digitalis	Arrhythmias
Tricyclic antidepressants, diphenhydramine, tripelennamine, dexchlorpheniramine	△ Cardiovascular effects of epinephrine

USE IN CHILDREN
Safety and effectiveness for use in children have not been established

USE IN PREGNANT AND NURSING WOMEN
Pregnancy Category C: use during pregnancy only if clearly needed. Animal reproduction studies have not been conducted with this drug, and it is not known whether epinephrine can cause fetal harm when administered to a pregnant woman or affect reproductive capacity. Specific guidelines for use in nursing women are not available; use according to medical judgment.

VEHICLE/BASE
Solution: benzalkonium chloride, sodium metabisulfite, edetate disodium, sodium chloride (in 0.25% strength only), and purified water

---

ANTIGLAUCOMA AGENTS/MIOTICS

OCUSERT Ocular Therapeutic System (pilocarpine) Alza   Rx

Ocular therapeutic system: 20 µg/hr (Pilo-20), 40 µg/hr (Pilo-40)

INDICATIONS
Control of intraocular pressure in patients responsive to pilocarpine

TOPICAL DOSAGE
Adult: insert 1 Pilo-20 or Pilo-40 system into the conjunctival cul-de-sac at bedtime, replacing the unit every 7 days

CONTRAINDICATIONS
Conditions where miosis is undesirable, such as glaucoma associated with acute inflammatory disease of the anterior segment and glaucoma occurring or persisting after extracapsular cataract extraction where posterior synechiae may occur

ADMINISTRATION/DOSAGE ADJUSTMENTS

Placement and removal	Instructions for placement and removal of the Ocusert system are provided in a patient package insert; the patient's ability to follow these instructions should be reviewed during the first visit after therapy is started. Because pilocarpine may induce myopia, advise the patient to insert the system at bedtime. Hands should be thoroughly washed, and if a displaced unit comes into contact with a contaminated surface, it should be rinsed with cool tap water before replacing it in the eye. The system should be discarded if it has been obviously contaminated. During the initial adaptation period, the unit may slip out of the eye and onto the cheek; the patient is usually aware of this occurrence and can easily replace the unit. If retention is a problem, the system may be worn in the upper conjunctival cul-de-sac, and, if possible, the system should be moved to the upper conjunctival cul-de-sac before the patient retires. Instruct the patient to check the eye for the presence of the Ocusert system before going to sleep and upon arising.

OCUSERT

Dosage titration	Therapy may be initiated with the Pilo-20 system, irrespective of the strength of pilocarpine solution that the patient previously required, or with the Pilo-40 system, depending on the patient's age, family history, and disease status or progression. Evaluate intraocular pressure during the first week of therapy and thereafter according to medical judgment. If pressure reduction is satisfactory with Pilo-20, continue its use. If a greater reduction of intraocular pressure is indicated, transfer the patient to the Pilo-40 system.
Concomitant therapy	If necessary, epinephrine, timolol, or a carbonic anhydrase inhibitor may be used with this system for the treatment of glaucoma (see WARNINGS/PRECAUTIONS)
Follow-up	After a satisfactory therapeutic regimen has been established, the frequency of follow-up should be determined according to the rate of patient progress

WARNINGS/PRECAUTIONS

Concomitant therapy	Systemic reactions, in rare instances severe, associated with increased absorption of autonomic drugs, such as epinephrine, have been observed in combination therapy with Ocusert. The release rate of pilocarpine from this system is not influenced by carbonic anhydrase inhibitors, ophthalmic epinephrine, fluorescein, or ophthalmic anesthetic, antibiotic, or anti-inflammatory solutions. Mild bulbar conjunctival edema, which is frequently associated with ophthalmic epinephrine, is not influenced by Ocusert. When intense miosis is desired in certain ocular conditions, the use of pilocarpine drops should be considered.
Special-risk patients	Patients with acute infectious conjunctivitis or keratitis should be given special consideration and evaluation prior to the use of this system. Safety of this system in patients with retinal detachment and filtration blebs has not been established. Use with particular caution in young myopic patients.
Defective systems	Damaged or deformed Ocusert systems should not be used or allowed to remain in the eye; systems believed to be associated with an unanticipated increase in drug action should be removed and replaced with a new system
Hypersensitivity	True allergic reactions may occur rarely; discontinue therapy
Irritation	Conjunctival irritation, including mild erythema with or without a slight increase in mucous secretion may occur; these effects usually lessen or disappear during the first week of therapy. Irritation may indicate cessation of therapy, according to medical judgment.

ADVERSE REACTIONS

Ophthalmic	Ciliary spasm, irritation, allergic reactions, angle closure, retinal detachment; sudden increase in pilocarpine effects (rare)

OVERDOSAGE

Signs and symptoms	*Gastrointestinal:* nausea, vomiting, diarrhea, abdominal pain, intestinal cramps (GI reactions are the most common toxic effects); *respiratory:* bronchospasm, cyanosis, increase in bronchial secretions, nasal congestion, rhinorrhea, respiratory paralysis; *central nervous system:* vertigo, tremors, muscle weakness, paresthesias, excitation, depression, confusion, ataxia, seizures, coma; *cardiovascular:* pallor, hypotension, syncope, bradycardia, arrhythmias, hypertension, cardiovascular collapse; *other:* excessive salivation, lacrimation, diaphoresis, incontinence
Treatment	Maintain adequate respiratory function; tracheostomy, bronchial aspiration, postural drainage, mechanically assisted ventilation, and oxygen may be necessary. To control muscarinic reactions, administer atropine parenterally as needed (usually at intervals of 3–60 min) for 24–48 h. The adult dose ranges from 0.4 mg to 4 mg; during the first 24 h, a total dose of up to 50 mg may be necessary. Give children 0.04–0.08 mg/kg every 5 min IV or every 15 min IM; the total dose should not exceed 4 mg. If cyanosis occurs, use atropine with caution since ventricular fibrillation may be precipitated. For seizures that cannot be controlled by atropine, consider giving a short-acting barbiturate.

DRUG INTERACTIONS

Epinephrine and timolol (topical forms); carbonic anhydrase inhibitors	△ Lowering of intraocular pressure
Demecarium, echothiophate, isofluorophate, physostigmine	▽ Pharmacologic effect of pilocarpine

---

USE IN CHILDREN

Safety and effectiveness for use in children have not been established; use according to medical judgment

USE IN PREGNANT AND NURSING WOMEN

Specific guidelines are not available; use according to medical judgment

ANTIGLAUCOMA AGENTS/MIOTICS

P_1E_1, P_2E_1, P_3E_1, P_4E_1, and P_6E_1 Ophthalmic Solutions (pilocarpine hydrochloride and epinephrine bitartrate) Alcon   Rx

Solution: 1% pilocarpine hydrochloride and 1% epinephrine bitartrate (P_1E_1); 2% pilocarpine hydrochloride and 1% epinephrine bitartrate (P_2E_1); 3% pilocarpine hydrochloride and 1% epinephrine bitartrate (P_3E_1); 4% pilocarpine hydrochloride and 1% epinephrine bitartrate (P_4E_1); 6% pilocarpine hydrochloride and 1% epinephrine bitartrate (P_6E_1) (15 ml)

INDICATIONS

Reduction of intraocular pressure in open-angle glaucoma

TOPICAL DOSAGE

Adult: 1 drop instilled into the affected eye(s) 1–4 times daily

CONTRAINDICATIONS

Conditions where miosis is undesirable, such as acute iritis	Concomitant wearing of soft contact lenses	Hypersensitivity to any component
Narrow-angle or pupillary block glaucoma		

ADMINISTRATION/DOSAGE ADJUSTMENTS

Administration	This product is intended for topical use only; do not administer orally or parenterally
Patients with heavily pigmented irides	Individuals with heavily pigmented irides may require larger doses

WARNINGS/PRECAUTIONS

General anesthesia	Discontinue use prior to general anesthesia with anesthetics that sensitize the myocardium to adrenergics
Special-risk patients	These preparations should be used with caution in patients with unverified glaucoma, hypertension, diabetes, hyperthyroidism, cardiac disease, or cerebral arteriosclerosis
Ocular inflammation	Synechiae with seclusion or occlusion of the pupil may occur
Maculopathy	These products may produce maculopathy in aphakic patients; discontinue use at first sign of maculopathy
Patient instructions	If irritation occurs and persists, pilocarpine should be discontinued and the condition reported

ADVERSE REACTIONS[1]

Ophthalmic	Ocular pain or ache, headache, conjunctival hyperemia, allergic lid reactions; innocuous adrenochrome deposits in the palpebral conjunctiva and cornea, lens opacity (after prolonged use), stinging or burning after application; retinal detachment (rare)
Other	Palpitation, tachycardia, perspiration, and occipital headache (rare)

OVERDOSAGE

Signs and symptoms	*Gastrointestinal:* nausea, vomiting, diarrhea, abdominal pain, intestinal cramps (GI reactions are the most common toxic effects); *respiratory:* bronchospasm, cyanosis, increase in bronchial secretions, nasal congestion, rhinorrhea, respiratory paralysis; *central nervous system:* occipital headaches, faintness, vertigo, tremors, muscle weakness, paresthesias, excitation, depression, confusion, ataxia, seizures, coma; *cardiovascular:* pallor, hypotension, syncope, bradycardia, palpitations, arrhythmias, hypertension, cardiovascular collapse; *other:* excessive salivation, lacrimation, diaphoresis, incontinence, pulmonary edema
Treatment	*Pilocarpine-related effects:* Maintain adequate respiratory function; tracheostomy, bronchial aspiration, postural drainage, mechanically assisted ventilation, and oxygen may be necessary. To control muscarinic reactions, administer atropine parenterally as needed (usually at intervals of 3–60 min) for 24–48 h. The adult dose ranges from 0.4 mg to 4 mg; during the first 24 h, a total dose of up to 50 mg may be necessary. Give children 0.04–0.08 mg/kg every 5 min IV or every 15 min IM; the total dose should not exceed 4 mg. If cyanosis occurs, use atropine with caution since ventricular fibrillation may be precipitated. For seizures that cannot be controlled by atropine, consider giving a short-acting barbiturate. *Epinephrine-related effects:* Institute appropriate supportive measures. Hypertension may be treated, if necessary, with an injectable vasodilator, with a rapid-acting alpha-adrenergic blocker, such as phentolamine, or with trimethophan; if antihypertensive therapy results in prolonged hypotension, a vasopressor such as norepinephrine may be given. For pulmonary edema that interferes with respiration, administer a rapid-acting alpha-adrenergic blocker and/or provide intermittent positive-pressure respiration. To control arrhythmias, use a beta-adrenergic blocker, such as propranolol.

DRUG INTERACTIONS

Miotics, carbonic anhydrase inhibitors, timolol	⇩ Lowering of intraocular pressure

P₁E₁/P₂E₁/P₃E₁/P₄E₁/P₆E₁ ■ PHOSPHOLINE IODIDE

Cyclopropane, halogenated general anesthetics, digitalis	Arrhythmias
Demecarium, echothiophate, isofluorophate, physostigmine	▽ Pharmacologic effect of pilocarpine component
Tricyclic antidepressants, diphenhydramine, tripelennamine, dexchlorpheniramine	△ Cardiovascular effects of epinephrine component

USE IN CHILDREN
Safety and effectiveness for use in children have not been established; use according to medical judgment

USE IN PREGNANT AND NURSING WOMEN
Specific guidelines are not available; use according to medical judgment

VEHICLE/BASE
Solution: 0.01% benzalkonium chloride, chlorobutanol, methylcellulose, polyethylene glycol, edetate disodium, sodium bisulfite, dried sodium phosphate, sodium hydroxide and/or hydrochloric acid (to adjust pH), and purified water

[1] As with all miotics, rare cases of retinal detachment have been reported in susceptible individuals

---

ANTIGLAUCOMA AGENTS/MIOTICS

PHOSPHOLINE IODIDE Ophthalmic Solution (echothiophate iodide) Ayerst   Rx

Solution: 0.03% (1.5 mg), 0.06% (3 mg), 0.125% (6.25 mg), or 0.25% (12.5 mg) after reconstitution

INDICATIONS
Chronic simple (open-angle) glaucoma, when diurnal pressure variations cannot be satisfactorily controlled with pilocarpine
Glaucoma following cataract surgery
Accommodative esotropia (convergent strabismus)

TOPICAL DOSAGE
Adult and child: 1 drop of a 0.03% solution instilled into the conjunctival sac of each eye bid, in the morning and at bedtime; if this dosage proves inadequate after a brief trial period, epinephrine and a carbonic anhydrase inhibitor may be added or, if necessary, a higher-strength solution may be used (do not increase the frequency of instillation)

Adult and child: for diagnosis and initial therapy, 1 drop of a 0.125% solution instilled into the conjunctival sac of each eye once daily, at bedtime, for 2–3 wk (a favorable response may begin within a few hours); after this initial trial period, the dosage may be reduced to 1 drop of a 0.125% solution every other day or to 1 drop of a 0.06% solution daily (as treatment progresses, these dosages can be gradually lowered; some patients may be adequately treated with the 0.03% solution)

CONTRAINDICATIONS
Active uveal inflammation   Most cases of angle-closure glaucoma   Hypersensitivity to any component

ADMINISTRATION/DOSAGE ADJUSTMENTS

Diurnal regulation of intraocular tension	Evaluations of intraocular tension should be made at different times of the day so that inadequate control may be more readily detected; if acceptable tension is not maintained, a change in therapy is indicated. To maintain a smooth diurnal tension curve, two daily doses are preferable to one, although a satisfactory response may be achieved by giving one dose daily or every other day.
Timing of administration	The daily dose or one of the two daily doses should be given just before the patient retires, to avoid any inconvenience caused by the miosis
Minimization of systemic absorption	Caution the patient to exert digital pressure on the inner canthus for 1–2 min after instilling this medication to minimize drainage into the nose and throat; excess solution around the eye should be removed with a tissue, and any medication on the hands should be rinsed off
Duration of therapy for accommodative esotropia	There is no definite limit to the duration of treatment as long as the drug is well tolerated; however, if deviation recurs when the drug is gradually withdrawn after 1–2 yr of therapy, surgery should be considered. As with other miotics, tolerance may occasionally develop after prolonged use; a rest period will restore the original effectiveness of the drug.

WARNINGS/PRECAUTIONS

"Tonometric glaucoma"	This drug is not recommended for use in treating ocular hypertension in the absence of other evidence of disease
Pretreatment examination	Gonioscopy should be performed before therapy with this drug is initiated to ensure that the angle of the eye is open

PHOSPHOLINE IODIDE

Concomitant drug therapy	Succinylcholine should be administered with great caution, if at all, before or during general anesthesia in patients receiving this medication, because of the potential for cardiovascular or respiratory collapse; in addition, exercise caution in using this drug to treat glaucoma in patients undergoing therapy with systemic anticholinesterase drugs for myasthenia gravis, because of possible additive effects
Systemic reactions	Discontinue therapy temporarily if salivation, urinary incontinence, diarrhea, profuse sweating, muscle weakness, respiratory difficulties, or cardiac irregularities occur (see also OVERDOSAGE)
Exposure to pesticides	Exposure to carbamate or organophosphate-type insecticides may cause additive systemic effects due to absorption of the pesticide through the skin or respiratory tract; it may be helpful for patients subject to such exposure (eg, professional gardeners, farmers, and chemical workers) to wear respiratory masks and to wash and change clothes frequently
Ophthalmic surgery	Echothiophate should not be used prior to ophthalmic surgery except as a considered risk, as hyphema may occur during surgery
Patients with quiescent uveitis or a history of uveitis	Intense, persistent miosis and ciliary muscle contraction may occur if this drug is used; echothiophate should be used only with great caution in patients with latent iritis or uveitis
Other special-risk patients	Use this drug with extreme caution, if at all, in patients with a history of retinal detachment and in patients with marked vagotonia, bronchial asthma, spastic GI disturbances, peptic ulcer, pronounced bradycardia and hypotension, recent myocardial infarction, epilepsy, parkinsonism, or other disorders that may respond adversely to the vagotonic effects of echothiophate
Iris cysts	Iris cysts may form, especially in children, and may enlarge to obscure vision if treatment is continued. The cysts usually shrink upon discontinuation of therapy or reduction in strength or dosage frequency; rarely, they may rupture or break free into the aqueous. Patients undergoing therapy for accommodative esotropia should be examined regularly for such cysts.
Lens opacities	Patients undergoing treatment with this drug for glaucoma may develop lens opacities; similar changes have been observed in experiments with normal monkeys. Routine examinations should be performed.
Increase in intraocular pressure	A paradoxical increase in intraocular pressure may occur following instillation of this drug; for relief, administer a sympathomimetic mydriatic such as phenylephrine

ADVERSE REACTIONS

Ophthalmic	Stinging, burning, lacrimation, lid muscle twitching, conjunctival and ciliary redness, browache, induced myopia with visual blurring (activation of latent iritis or uveitis; iris cysts, conjunctival thickening and obstruction of nasolacrimal canals (with prolonged therapy), lens opacities (in patients being treated for glaucoma), paradoxical increase in intraocular pressure[1]

OVERDOSAGE

Signs and symptoms	*Gastrointestinal:* nausea, vomiting, diarrhea, abdominal pain, intestinal cramps (GI reactions are the most common toxic effects); *respiratory:* bronchospasm, cyanosis, increase in bronchial secretions, nasal congestion, rhinorrhea, respiratory paralysis; *central nervous system:* vertigo, tremors, muscle weakness, paresthesias, excitation, depression, confusion, ataxia, seizures, coma; *cardiovascular:* pallor, hypotension, syncope, bradycardia, arrhythmias, hypertension, cardiovascular collapse; *other:* excessive salivation, lacrimation, diaphoresis, incontinence
Treatment	Maintain adequate respiratory function; tracheostomy, bronchial aspiration, postural drainage, mechanically assisted ventilation, and oxygen may be necessary. To control muscarinic reactions, administer atropine parenterally as needed (usually at intervals of 3–60 min) for 24–48 h. The adult dose ranges from 0.4 mg to 4 mg; during the first 24 h, a total dose of up to 50 mg may be necessary. Give children 0.04–0.08 mg/kg every 5 min IV or every 15 min IM; the total dose should not exceed 4 mg. If cyanosis occurs, use atropine with caution since ventricular fibrillation may be precipitated. For seizures that cannot be controlled by atropine, consider giving a short-acting barbiturate. To reverse nicotinic effects such as muscular paralysis, IV pralidoxime may be used.

DRUG INTERACTIONS

Other anticholinesterase agents (including pesticides)	△ Anticholinesterase effects
Succinylcholine	△ Pharmacologic effects of succinylcholine (prolonged apnea, cardiovascular collapse)
Cyclopropane, halothane	△ Pharmacologic effects of cyclopropane and halothane
Epinephrine and timolol (topical forms); carbonic anhydrase inhibitors	△ Lowering of intraocular pressure
Pilocarpine	▽ Pharmacologic effect of echothiophate

PHOSPHOLINE IODIDE ■ PILOPINE HS

Physostigmine	▽ Pharmacologic effect of echothiophate

ALTERED LABORATORY VALUES

Blood/serum values	▽ Cholinesterase

No clinically significant alterations in urinary values occur at therapeutic dosages

---

USE IN CHILDREN
See INDICATIONS and TOPICAL DOSAGE

USE IN PREGNANT AND NURSING WOMEN
The safety of using anticholinesterase medications during pregnancy has not been established; it is not known whether this drug effects the fetus or neonatal respiration. Specific guidelines for use in nursing women are not available; use according to medical judgment.

VEHICLE/BASE
Solution (reconstituted): 0.5% chlorobutanol, 1.2% mannitol, 0.06% boric acid, 0.026% exsiccated sodium phosphate, and sodium hydroxide or acetic acid (to adjust pH)

[1] Retinal detachment has also been reported in a few cases; however, a causal relationship has not been established

---

ANTIGLAUCOMA AGENTS/MIOTICS

PILOPINE HS Ophthalmic Gel (pilocarpine hydrochloride) Alcon   Rx

Gel: 4% (5 g)

INDICATIONS	TOPICAL DOSAGE
Control of intraocular pressure	**Adult and child:** apply a ½-in. ribbon into the lower conjunctival sac of the affected eye(s) once daily at bedtime; for selected conditions, more frequent applications may be needed

CONTRAINDICATIONS

Conditions where miosis is undesirable, such as acute iritis	Hypersensitivity to any component

ADMINISTRATION/DOSAGE ADJUSTMENTS

Concomitant therapy	This preparation may be used in combination with other miotics, beta-adrenergic blockers, carbonic anhydrase inhibitors, sympathomimetics, or hyperosmotic agents for the treatment of glaucoma

WARNINGS/PRECAUTIONS

Impairment of night vision	Advise patient that miosis usually causes difficulty in dark adaptation and that caution should be exercised while driving at night or performing other hazardous activities in poor illumination
Adverse effects	Systemic reactions following topical application of pilocarpine are extremely rare; ocular reactions usually occur during initiation of therapy and will not persist with continued use

ADVERSE REACTIONS[1]

Ophthalmic	Lacrimation, burning or discomfort, ciliary spasm, conjunctival vascular congestion, temporal or supraorbital headache, superficial keratitis, induced myopia (especially in younger patients); reduced visual acuity in poor illumination and in individuals with lens opacity; lens opacities (with prolonged use); subtle corneal granularity (in 10% of patients); retinal detachment (rare; especially in young myopic patients)

OVERDOSAGE

Signs and symptoms	*Gastrointestinal:* nausea, vomiting, diarrhea, abdominal pain, intestinal cramps (GI reactions are the most common toxic effects); *respiratory:* bronchospasm, cyanosis, increase in bronchial secretions, nasal congestion, rhinorrhea, respiratory paralysis; *central nervous system:* vertigo, tremors, muscle weakness, paresthesias, excitation, depression, confusion, ataxia, seizures, coma; *cardiovascular:* pallor, hypotension, syncope, bradycardia, arrhythmias, hypertension, cardiovascular collapse; *other:* excessive salivation, lacrimation, diaphoresis, incontinence

Treatment	Maintain adequate respiratory function; tracheostomy, bronchial aspiration, postural drainage, mechanically assisted ventilation, and oxygen may be necessary. To control muscarinic reactions, administer atropine parenterally as needed (usually at intervals of 3-60 min) for 24-48 h. the adult dose ranges from 0.4 mg to 4 mg; during the first 24 h, a total dose of up to 50 mg may be necessary. Give children 0.04-0.08 mg/kg every 5 min IV or every 15 min IM; the total dose should not exceed 4 mg. If cyanosis occurs, use atropine with caution since ventricular fibrillation may be precipitated. For seizures that cannot be controlled by atropine, consider giving a short-acting barbiturate.

DRUG INTERACTIONS

Epinephrine and timolol (topical forms), carbonic anhydrase inhibitors	△ Lowering of intraocular pressure
Demecarium, echothiophate, isofluorophate, physostigmine	▽ Pharmacologic effect of pilocarpine

USE IN CHILDREN	USE IN PREGNANT AND NURSING WOMEN
See INDICATIONS and TOPICAL DOSAGE	Specific guidelines are not available; use according to medical judgment

VEHICLE/BASE
Gel: 0.008% benzalkonium chloride, carbopol 940, edetate disodium, hydrochloric acid and/or sodium hydroxide (to adjust pH), and purified water

[1] The incidence of corneal granularity during testing with other therapies including pilocarpine drops, timolol, or epinephrine was the same as reported with pilocarpine gel

---

ANTIGLAUCOMA AGENTS/MIOTICS

PROPINE Ophthalmic Solution (dipivefrin hydrochloride) Allergan   Rx

Solution: 0.1% (5, 10, 15 ml)

INDICATIONS	TOPICAL DOSAGE
Reduction of intraocular pressure in chronic open-angle glaucoma	Adult: 1 drop instilled into the eye(s) q12h

CONTRAINDICATIONS

Narrow angle (pupillary dilatation may precipitate angle-closure glaucoma)	Hypersensitivity to any component

ADMINISTRATION/DOSAGE ADJUSTMENTS

Replacement of other antiglaucoma therapy	When transferring patients to dipivefrin from antiglaucoma agents other than epinephrine, continue the previous medication on the first day and add 1 drop of dipivefrin into each eye q12h; on the following day, discontinue the first medication and continue therapy with dipivefrin. When transferring patients from conventional epinephrine therapy, simply discontinue the epinephrine medication and continue therapy with dipivefrin.
Concomitant or supplemental therapy	For patients with difficult to control conditions, dipivefrin may be added to a dosage regimen with other agents such as pilocarpine, carbachol, echothiophate iodide, or acetazolamide. Instill 1 drop of dipivefrin into each eye q12h.
Administration	This product is for topical use only; do not administer as an injection

WARNINGS/PRECAUTIONS

Aphakic patients	Macular edema has been reported in up to 30% of aphakic patients treated with epinephrine, the active metabolite of dipivefrin; generally, discontinuation of the medication has resulted in reversal of the maculopathy
Animal studies	Studies performed in rabbits have shown a dose-related incidence of meibomian gland retention cysts following topical administration of both dipivefrin hydrochloride and epinephrine

ADVERSE REACTIONS

The most frequent reactions, regardless of incidence, are printed in *italics*

Ophthalmic	*Injection (6.5%), burning and stinging (6%)*, adrenochrome deposits in the conjunctiva and cornea
Cardiovascular	Tachycardia, arrhythmias, hypertension

OVERDOSAGE

Signs and symptoms	Hypertension, tachycardia, extrasystoles, premature ventricular contractions, pulmonary edema, occipital headaches, pallor, trembling, palpitations, faintness, diaphoresis
Treatment	Institute appropriate supportive measures. Hypertension may be treated, if necessary, with an injectable vasodilator, with a rapid-acting alpha-adrenergic blocker, such as phentolamine, or with trimethophan; if antihypertensive therapy results in prolonged hypotension, a vasopressor such as norepinephrine may be given. For pulmonary edema that interferes with respiration, administer a rapid-acting alpha-adrenergic blocker and/or provide intermittent positive-pressure respiration. To control arrhythmias, use a beta-adrenergic blocker, such as propranolol.

DRUG INTERACTIONS

Miotics, carbonic anhydrase inhibitors	⇧ Lowering of intraocular pressure
Cyclopropane, halogenated general anesthetics, digitalis	Arrhythmias
Tricyclic antidepressants, diphenhydramine, tripelennamine, dexchlorpheniramine	⇧ Cardiovascular effects of epinephrine

USE IN CHILDREN

Studies have not been performed to determine the safety and effectiveness of this preparation in children

USE IN PREGNANT AND NURSING WOMEN

Pregnancy Category B: this drug should be used during pregnancy only if clearly needed; rats and rabbits given daily oral doses of up to 10 mg/kg (5 mg/kg in teratogenicity studies) have shown no evidence of impaired fertility or fetal harm. However, there have been no adequate, well-controlled studies in pregnant women. It is not known whether dipivefrin is excreted in human milk; because many drugs are excreted in human milk, use with caution in nursing women.

VEHICLE/BASE
Solution: 0.004% benzalkonium chloride, edetate sodium, mannitol, sodium chloride, sodium metabisulfite, hydrochloric acid (to adjust pH), and purified water

---

ANTIGLAUCOMA AGENTS/MIOTICS

TIMOPTIC (timolol maleate) Merck Sharp & Dohme Rx

Solution: 0.25%, 0.5% (2.5, 5, 10, 15 ml)

INDICATIONS

Elevated intraocular pressure in patients with chronic open-angle glaucoma or aphakic glaucoma, in selected patients with secondary glaucoma, and in other patients with pressure elevation sufficient to require reduction[1]

TOPICAL DOSAGE

Adult: 1 drop of the 0.25% solution instilled into the affected eye(s) bid to start, followed by 1 drop of the 0.5% solution in the affected eye(s) bid, if needed; for maintenance, 1 drop (0.25% or 0.5%) in the affected eye(s) once daily

CONTRAINDICATIONS

Bronchial asthma or a history of bronchial asthma	Second- or third-degree AV block	Cardiogenic shock
Severe chronic obstructive pulmonary disease	Overt cardiac failure (see WARNINGS/PRECAUTIONS)	Hypersensitivity to any component
Sinus bradycardia		

ADMINISTRATION/DOSAGE ADJUSTMENTS

Concomitant therapy	If response is not satisfactory with 1 drop of the 0.5% solution bid, pilocarpine or other miotics, epinephrine, and/or systemic carbonic anhydrase inhibitors may be given concomitantly; mydriasis has been reported occasionally after concomitant use with epinephrine
Transferring patients from other antiglaucoma agents	On day 1, continue other agent and add 1 drop of 0.25% timolol in the affected eye(s) bid; on day 2, discontinue previously used agent and adjust timolol dosage, as needed, using up to 1 drop of the 0.5% solution in the affected eye(s) bid. To transfer patients from several agents, discontinue one agent at a time, as above, at intervals of usually not less than 1 wk.

TIMOPTIC

WARNINGS/PRECAUTIONS

Cardiac failure	May be precipitated by further or continued depression of myocardial contractility; discontinue use if cardiac failure persists despite adequate digitalization and diuretic therapy. In cases of well-compensated congestive heart failure, use with caution.
Pulmonary disease	Since this preparation can block catecholamine-dependent bronchodilation, it is contraindicated for use in patients with bronchial asthma, a history of bronchial asthma, or severe nonasthmatic chronic obstructive pulmonary disease (COPD) and it is to be used with caution and only if necessary in patients with nonasthmatic bronchospastic disease, a history of such a disorder, or mild-to-moderate nonasthmatic COPD
Patients undergoing anesthesia and major surgery	Beta blockade may augment the risks; gradual withdrawal of beta blockers prior to elective surgery is recommended by some authorities. If necessary, the effects of beta blockade may be reversed during surgery by sufficient doses of such beta-adrenergic agonists as isoproterenol, dobutamine, or norepinephrine.
Diabetes and hypoglycemia	Use with caution in patients subject to spontaneous hypoglycemia and in diabetic patients (especially labile diabetics) who are taking insulin or oral hypoglycemic agents; beta blockade may mask the signs and symptoms of acute hypoglycemia
Thyrotoxicosis	Clinical signs of hyperthyroidism (eg, tachycardia) may be masked; manage patients suspected of developing thyrotoxicosis carefully to avoid abrupt withdrawal of beta blockade, which might precipitate a thyroid storm
Muscle weakness	Beta blockade can cause certain myasthenic signs and symptoms (eg, diplopia, ptosis, generalized weakness) and, in rare cases, may exacerbate myasthenia
Cerebrovascular insufficiency	Since beta blockers affect blood pressure and heart rate, they should be used with caution in patients with cerebrovascular insufficiency; if signs or symptoms suggesting reduced cerebral blood flow are noted, consider alternative therapy
Concurrent use of oral beta-blocking agents	Monitor patient for possible additive effects on either intraocular pressure or the systemic effects of beta-adrenergic blockade
Patients with angle-closure glaucoma	Since the immediate treatment objective to reopen the angle, use a miotic concomitantly with timolol
Carcinogenicity, mutagenicity	A 2-yr study in male rats showed a statistically significant increase in adrenal pheochromocytomas at 300 times the maximum recommended human oral dose (1 mg/kg/day), and a lifetime study in female mice showed a statistically significant increase in the overall incidence of neoplasms (including benign and malignant pulmonary tumors, benign uterine polyps, and mammary adenocarcinomas associated with increased serum prolactin levels) at 500 mg/kg/day. Results of various mutagenicity studies were negative.
Impairment of fertility	Administration of timolol at doses up to 150 times the maximum recommended human oral dose had no adverse effect on the fertility of male or female rats

ADVERSE REACTIONS[2]

Ophthalmic	Ocular irritation (including conjunctivitis), blepharitis, keratitis, blepharoptosis, decreased corneal sensitivity, visual disturbances (including refractive changes), diplopia, ptosis
Cardiovascular	Bradycardia, arrhythmia, hypotension, syncope, heart block, cerebral vascular accident, cerebral ischemia, cardiac failure, palpitation, cardiac arrest
Digestive	Nausea, diarrhea
Central nervous system	Headache, dizziness, depression, asthenia, exacerbation of myasthenia gravis, paresthesia
Respiratory	Bronchospasm (primarily in patients with preexisting bronchospastic disease), respiratory failure, dyspnea, nasal congestion, chest pain
Endocrine	Hypoglycemia (masked symptoms in insulin-dependent diabetics)
Dermatological	Hypersensitivity (including localized and generalized rash), urticaria

OVERDOSAGE

Signs and symptoms	Symptomatic bradycardia, hypotension, bronchospasm, and acute cardiac failure, based on the anticipated effects of excessive beta blockade
Treatment	Discontinue medication. Empty stomach by gastric lavage. For symptomatic bradycardia, administer atropine sulfate (0.25–2 mg IV) to induce vagal blockade; if bradycardia persists, give IV isoproterenol cautiously and, in refractory cases, consider using a transvenous cardiac pacemaker. For hypotension, administer a sympathomimetic amine (eg, dopamine, dobutamine, or norepinephrine); in refractory cases, try glucagon HCl. For bronchospasm, give isoproterenol and possibly also aminophylline. For acute cardiac failure, institute treatment with digitalis, diuretics, and oxygen immediately; in refractory cases, try IV aminophylline, followed, if necessary, by glucagon HCl. For second- or third-degree heart block, use isoproterenol or a transvenous cardiac pacemaker. Hemodialysis may or may not be helpful in removing the drug from the circulation.

DRUG INTERACTIONS

Calcium antagonists	Hypotension (with oral antagonists, especially nifedipine), left ventricular failure (with oral antagonists, especially verapamil and diltiazem), AV conduction disturbances (with oral or IV antagonists, especially verapamil and diltiazem). Although timolol can be given with an oral calcium antagonist if heart function is normal, concomitant use should be avoided if heart function is impaired. Exercise caution when administering an IV antagonist with timolol.
Propranolol and other beta-adrenergic blockers	△ Systemic effects of beta blockade ▽ Intraocular pressure
Epinephrine	Mydriasis
Reserpine, other catecholamine-depleting drugs	Hypotension and/or marked bradycardia
Pilocarpine and other topical miotics; topical epinephrine; acetazolamide and other systemic carbonic anhydrase inhibitors	▽ Intraocular pressure

ALTERED LABORATORY VALUES

No clinically significant alterations in blood/serum or urinary values occur at therapeutic dosages

USE IN CHILDREN

Safety and effectiveness for use in children have not been established

USE IN PREGNANT AND NURSING WOMEN

Pregnancy Category C: use during pregnancy only if the anticipated benefit of treatment exceeds the potential fetal risk. An increase in fetal resorption has been observed in mice and rabbits at 1,000 and 100 times the maximum recommended human dose, respectively. While teratogenic effects have not been seen in rodents at doses up to 50 times the maximum recommended human dose, no adequate, well-controlled studies have been done in pregnant women. Because of the potential for serious adverse effects in nursing infants, a decision should be made to either discontinue nursing or discontinue use of this drug, taking into account its importance to the mother.

[1] Clinical trials have also shown that in patients who respond adequately to multiple antiglaucoma agents, the addition of timolol may produce a further reduction in intraocular pressure
[2] Other reactions reported with this drug and for which a causal relationship has not been established include fatigue, hypertension, pulmonary edema, worsening of angina pectoris, dyspepsia, anorexia, dry mouth; confusion, hallucinations, anxiety, disorientation, nervousness, somnolence, and other psychic disturbances; alopecia; aphakic cystoid macular edema; retroperitoneal fibrosis, and impotence. Other reactions reported in clinical experience with oral timolol, and may be considered potential effects of ophthalmic timolol, include extremity pain, decreased exercise tolerance, weight loss; worsening of arterial insufficiency, sinoatrial block, Raynaud's phenomenon, vasodilatation; gastrointestinal pain, hepatomegaly, vomiting, diarrhea; nonthrombocytopenic purpura; hyperglycemia, hypoglycemia; pruritus, skin irritation, increased pigmentation, sweating, cold hands and feet; arthralgia, claudication; vertigo, local weakness; decreased libido, nightmares, insomnia, nervousness, diminished concentration; nonfatal pulmonary edema, rales, cough, bronchial obstruction; tinnitus, dry eyes; and urinary difficulties. Other reactions associated with beta blocker therapy but not observed with timolol include reversible mental depression, progressing to catatonia; an acute reversible syndrome characterized by temporal and spatial disorientation, short-term memory loss, emotional lability, slightly cloudy sensorium, and decreased performance on neuropsychometric tests; mesenteric arterial thrombosis, ischemic colitis; agranulocytosis, thrombocytopenic purpura; erythematous rash, fever combined with aching and sore throat, laryngospasm, respiratory distress; and Peyronie's disease.

MYDRIATICS/CYCLOPLEGICS

CYCLOGYL Ophthalmic Solution (cyclopentolate hydrochloride) Alcon Rx

Solution: 0.5%, 1%, 2% (2, 5, 15 ml)

INDICATIONS	TOPICAL DOSAGE
Mydriasis and cycloplegia	**Adult:** 1 drop instilled into each eye, followed by a second drop in 5 min **Infant:** 1 drop of the 0.5% solution instilled into each eye **Child:** 1 drop of the 0.5%, 1%, or 2% solution instilled into each eye, followed in 5 min with a second application of the 0.5% or 1% solution if needed; pretreatment with cyclopentolate on the day before examination is usually not necessary

CONTRAINDICATIONS

Narrow-angle glaucoma or anatomical narrow angle	Hypersensitivity to any component

WARNINGS/PRECAUTIONS

Systemic absorption	Central nervous system disturbances may occur, especially in younger patients and with use of the stronger solutions. Premature and small infants are particularly prone to the CNS and cardiopulmonary side effects of cyclopentolate; very young infants should not be given any solution strength greater than 0.5%. To avoid excessive systemic absorption after instillation, compress the lacrimal sac by digital pressure for 1 min (2–3 min in small infants, who should also be observed closely for 30 min following administration).

CYCLOGYL ■ MYDRIACYL

Patient instructions	Caution patients not to drive or engage in other potentially hazardous activities while their pupils are dilated and to protect their eyes from bright illumination. Care should be taken not to get the preparation into a child's mouth when an adult is administering cyclopentolate, and both the child's and adult's hands should be washed after administration.
Special-risk patients	Use with caution in the elderly and in other patients who might have increased intraocular pressure; to avoid inducing angle-closure glaucoma, estimate the angle of the anterior chamber of the eye before administering this preparation

ADVERSE REACTIONS

Ophthalmic	Increased intraocular pressure
Central nervous system	Psychotic reactions and behavioral disturbances in children (especially with the 2% concentration), including ataxia, incoherent speech, restlessness, hallucinations, hyperactivity, seizures, disorientation of time and place, failure to recognize people
Cardiovascular	Tachycardia, vasodilation
Other	Hyperpyrexia, urinary retention, diminished gastrointestinal motility; decreased secretion in salivary and sweat glands, pharnyx, bronchii, and nasal passages; coma, medullary paralysis, and death

OVERDOSAGE

Signs and symptoms	Flushing, dry skin, blurred vision, rapid heartbeat, fever, dry mouth, slurred speech, abdominal distention (in infants), mental confusion, drowsiness, weakness, incoordination, hypotension, respiratory depression
Treatment	Institute appropriate measures for maintenance of adequate respiratory function. For shock, give fluids and take other standard measures. To treat fever, sponge with tepid water, apply cold packs, or use a mechanical cooling device. Diazepam may be given to control acute psychotic symptoms (do not use phenothiazines). To avoid urinary retention in a comatose patient, perform urinary catheterization. To manage severe toxicity when supportive measures are not sufficient, administer physostigmine salicylate IV. For adults, inject 0.5–2 mg every 20 min until a response occurs or cholinergic reactions are seen; after anticholinergic symptoms have been controlled, additional doses of 1–4 mg can be administered whenever symptoms recur (usually every 30–60 min). For children, inject up to 0.5 mg every 5–10 min until a response occurs, cholinergic reactions are detected, or a total dose of 2 mg is administered. Injection rate in adults should not exceed 1 mg/min; a pediatric dose should be administered very slowly over a period of at least 1 min.

DRUG INTERACTIONS

No clinically significant drug interactions have been identified

---

USE IN CHILDREN

See TOPICAL DOSAGE and WARNINGS/PRECAUTIONS

USE IN PREGNANT AND NURSING WOMEN

Specific guidelines have not been established; use according to medical judgment

---

VEHICLE/BASE
Solution: 0.01% benzalkonium chloride, boric acid, edetate disodium, potassium chloride (except 2% concentration), sodium carbonate and/or hydrochloric acid (to adjust pH), and purified water

---

MYDRIATICS/CYCLOPLEGICS

MYDRIACYL Ophthalmic Solution (tropicamide) Alcon Rx

Solution: 0.5, 1.0% (15 ml)

INDICATIONS

Mydriasis and cycloplegia in diagnostic procedures
Mydriasis of short duration in some pre- and postoperative states

TOPICAL DOSAGE

Adult: for refraction studies, instill 1 drop of the 1.0% solution into each eye and repeat in 5 min (if patient is not seen within 20–30 min, an additional drop may be given); for funduscopy, instill 1 drop of the 0.5% solution 15–20 min prior to examination of the fundus

CONTRAINDICATIONS

Narrow-angle glaucoma

Hypersensitivity to any component

MYDRIACYL ■ BLEPH-10

WARNINGS/PRECAUTIONS

Systemic absorption	Central nervous system disturbances, which may be dangerous to infants and children, may occur; the possibility of psychotic reaction and behavioral disturbance as a result of hypersensitivity to anticholinergic drugs should be considered. To avoid excessive systemic absorption, compress the lacrimal sac by digital pressure for 1 min after instillation of tropicamide.
Use precautions	Caution patients not to drive or engage in other potentially hazardous activities while their pupils are dilated and to protect their eyes from bright illumination. Care should also be taken not to get the preparation into a child's mouth when an adult is administering tropicamide, and both the child's and adult's hands should be washed after administration.
Special-risk patients	Use with caution in the elderly and in other patients who might have increased intraocular pressure; to avoid inducing angle-closure glaucoma, estimate the angle of the anterior chamber of the eye before administering this preparation

ADVERSE REACTIONS

Ophthalmic	Increased intraocular pressure, transient stinging, photophobia with or without corneal staining, blurred vision
Other	Psychotic reactions, behavioral disturbances, and cardiorespiratory collapse (in children); dryness of the mouth; tachycardia; headache; parasympathetic stimulation; allergic reaction

OVERDOSAGE

Signs and symptoms	Flushing, dry skin, blurred vision, rapid heartbeat, fever, dry mouth, slurred speech, abdominal distention (in infants), mental confusion, drowsiness, weakness, incoordination, hypotension, respiratory depression
Treatment	Institute appropriate measures for maintenance of adequate respiratory function. For shock, give fluids and take other standard measures. To treat fever, sponge with tepid water, apply cold packs, or use a mechanical cooling device. Diazepam may be given to control acute psychotic symptoms (do not use phenothiazines). To avoid urinary retention in a comatose patient, perform urinary catheterization. To manage severe toxicity when supportive measures are not sufficient, administer physostigmine salicylate IV. For adults, inject 0.5–2 mg every 20 min until a response occurs or cholinergic reactions are seen; after anticholinergic symptoms have been controlled, additional doses of 1–4 mg can be administered whenever symptoms recur (usually every 30–60 min). For children, inject up to 0.5 mg every 5–10 min until a response occurs, cholinergic reactions are detected, or a total dose of 2 mg is administered. Injection rate in adults should not exceed 1 mg/min; a pediatric dose should be administered very slowly over a period of at least 1 min.

DRUG INTERACTIONS

No clinically significant drug interactions have been identified

---

USE IN CHILDREN

See INDICATIONS and TOPICAL DOSAGE; infants and small children are particularly susceptible to the CNS effects of this drug (see WARNINGS/PRECAUTIONS)

USE IN PREGNANT AND NURSING WOMEN

No reproductive studies have been performed in animals with this drug, and it is not known whether tropicamide affects fertility or causes fetal damage in humans. Specific guidelines for use in nursing women are not available; use according to medical judgment.

VEHICLE/BASE
Solution: 0.01% benzalkonium chloride, sodium chloride, edetate disodium, hydrochloric acid and/or sodium hydroxide (to adjust pH), and purified water

---

OPHTHALMIC ANTI-INFECTIVES

BLEPH-10 Ophthalmic Ointment and Solution (sulfacetamide sodium) Allergan Rx

Ointment: 10% (3.5 g)   Solution: 10% (5, 15 ml)

INDICATIONS	TOPICAL DOSAGE
Conjunctivitis, corneal ulcer, and other superficial ocular infections caused by susceptible organisms[1]	**Adult and child:** apply a small amount of ointment in the conjunctival sac qid and again at bedtime or instill 1 drop into the lower conjunctival sac q2–3h during the day and less often at night

BLEPH-10 ■ BLEPHAMIDE

CONTRAINDICATIONS

Hypersensitivity to any component

WARNINGS/PRECAUTIONS

Overgrowth of nonsusceptible organisms	Nonsusceptible organisms, including fungi, may proliferate during treatment
Purulent exudates	These preparations may be inactivated by the *para*-aminobenzoic acid present in purulent exudates
Corneal healing	Use of the ophthalmic ointment may retard corneal wound healing
Discoloration of solution	Do not use if solution is discolored (dark brown); protect from light and excessive heat
Hypersensitivity	Sensitization to sulfacetamide, and cross-sensitivity between sulfonamides, may occur; discontinue use if signs of sensitivity or other untoward reactions occur

ADVERSE REACTIONS

Ophthalmic	Allergic sensitization, secondary infection

DRUG INTERACTIONS

Silver nitrate, mild silver protein	Incompatible with sulfacetamide; do not administer concurrently
Tetracaine	▽ Antibacterial activity of sulfacetamide

USE IN CHILDREN
See indications and dosage recommendations

USE IN PREGNANT AND NURSING WOMEN
Specific guidelines are not available; use according to medical judgment

VEHICLE/BASE
Ointment: 0.0008% phenylmercuric acetate, white petrolatum, mineral oil, and nonionic lanolin derivatives
Solution: 1.4% polyvinyl alcohol (Liquifilm), 0.005% thimerosal, polysorbate 80, sodium thiosulfate, potassium phosphate monobasic, edetate disodium, sodium phosphate dibasic (anhydrous), hydrochloric acid (to adjust pH), and purified water

[1] A significant percentage of staphylococcal isolates are resistant to sulfonamides

---

OPHTHALMIC ANTI-INFECTIVES

BLEPHAMIDE Ophthalmic Suspension (sulfacetamide sodium and prednisolone acetate) Allergan   Rx

Suspension: 10% sulfacetamide sodium and 0.2% prednisolone acetate (2.5, 5, 10 ml)

BLEPHAMIDE S.O.P. Ophthalmic Ointment (sulfacetamide sodium and prednisolone acetate) Allergan   Rx

Ointment: 10% sulfacetamide sodium and 0.2% prednisolone acetate (3.5 g)

INDICATIONS[1]

Steroid-responsive inflammatory ophthalmic conditions, such as those of the palpebral and bulbar conjuctiva, cornea, and anterior segment of the globe
Chronic anterior uveitis
Corneal injury from chemical, radiation, or thermal burns or from penetration of foreign bodies

TOPICAL DOSAGE

Adult and child: instill 1 drop of the solution into the eye or drop it onto the lid bid to qid, depending on severity, or apply a small amount of the ointment into the conjunctival sac tid or qid and once or twice at night

CONTRAINDICATIONS

Epithelial herpes simplex keratitis (dendritic keratitis)

Vaccinia, varicella, and many other viral diseases of the cornea and conjunctiva

Mycobacterial infections of the eye

Fungal diseases of the eye

Following uncomplicated removal of a corneal foreign body

Hypersensitivity to any component

COMPENDIUM OF DRUG THERAPY

ADMINISTRATION/DOSAGE ADJUSTMENTS

Instillation — Early or acute stages of blepharitis usually respond best when the solution is instilled directly into the eye, with the excess spread over the eyelids; if the lesions are confined to the lids, apply the solution directly to the lesion sites. Instruct patient to wash hand thoroughly, tilt head back, and instill 1 drop into the eye or onto the lid. With the eye closed, the excess medication should be spread along the full length of both the upper and lower lids and allowed to dry completely (4–5 min). Once or twice a day the medication should be washed off and then reapplied.

WARNINGS/PRECAUTIONS

Resistance to sulfa drugs — A significant percentage of staphylococcal strains are totally resistant to sulfonamides

Initial prescription — Do not prescribe more than 20 ml of the suspension or 8 g of the ointment until the patient can be examined with the aid of magnification, such as slit-lamp microscopy, and, where appropriate, fluorescein staining

Prolonged use — Protracted ophthalmic use of these preparations may result in glaucoma, optic nerve damage, and visual acuity and field defects; check intraocular pressure frequently if used for 10 days or longer. Chronic therapy may also cause posterior subcapsular cataracts and promote secondary ocular infections; fungal invasion of the cornea should be suspected in any case of persistent corneal ulceration.

Concomitant infections — Topical steroid therapy may mask or enhance untreated acute, purulent infections of the eye and may exacerbate bacterial and fungal ocular infections

Diseases causing corneal or scleral thinning — Perforation of the globe has been associated with topical steroid use in patients with diseases that cause corneal or scleral thinning

Herpetic keratitis — Use with great caution in the treatment of herpes simplex

ADVERSE REACTIONS

Ophthalmic — Elevation of intraocular pressure, possibly developing into glaucoma; infrequent optic nerve damage, posterior subcapsular cataract formation, delayed wound healing, secondary infections

Other — Allergic sensitization

DRUG INTERACTIONS

Silver nitrate, mild silver protein — Incompatible with sulfacetamide; do not administer concurrently

Tetracaine — ▽ Antibacterial activity of sulfacetamide

USE IN CHILDREN

See indications and dosage recommendations; do not use longer than absolutely necessary, since prolonged therapy increases the risk of adrenal suppression in children 2 yr of age or younger

USE IN PREGNANT AND NURSING WOMEN

The safety of intensive or prolonged topical steroid therapy during pregnancy has not been established. Specific guidelines are not available for use in nursing women; use according to medical judgment.

VEHICLE/BASE
Suspension: 1.4% polyvinyl alcohol (Liquifilm), benzalkonium chloride, polysorbate 80, edetate disodium, sodium phosphate, monobasic potassium phosphate, sodium thiosulfate, hydrochloric acid and/or sodium hydroxide (to adjust pH), and purified water
Ointment: 0.0008% phenylmercuric acetate, mineral oil, white petrolatum, and nonionic lanolin derivatives

[1] The use of an anti-infective steroid combination is indicated in those conditions where the risk of infection is high or it is anticipated that there are potentially dangerous numbers of bacteria present in the eye; the anti-infective component in this preparation is effective against the following pathogens: *Escherichia coli, Staphylococcus aureus, Streptococcus viridans, S pneumoniae, Pseudomonas* sp, *Hemophilus influenzae, Klebsiella* sp, and *Enterobacter* sp; it does not provide adequate coverage against *Neisseria* sp and *Serratia marcescens*. A significant percentage of staphylococcal isolates are completely resistant to sulfonamides.

OPHTHALMIC ANTI-INFECTIVES

CORTISPORIN Ophthalmic Ointment (polymyxin B sulfate, bacitracin zinc, neomycin sulfate, and hydrocortisone) Burroughs Wellcome — Rx

Ointment (per gram): 10,000 units polymyxin B sulfate, 400 units bacitracin zinc, neomycin sulfate equivalent to 0.35% neomycin base, and 10 mg (1%) hydrocortisone (1/8 oz)

INDICATIONS[1]

Steroid-responsive inflammatory ophthalmic conditions, such as those of the palpebral and bulbar conjunctiva, cornea, and anterior segment of the globe
Chronic anterior uveitis
Corneal injury from chemical, radiation, or thermal burns, or from penetration of foreign bodies

TOPICAL DOSAGE

Adult and child: apply the ointment into the affected eye q3–4h, depending upon the severity of the infection

CORTISPORIN Ointment ■ CORTISPORIN Suspension

CONTRAINDICATIONS

Epithelial herpes simplex keratitis (dendritic keratitis)	Mycobacterial infections of the eye	Following uncomplicated removal of a corneal foreign body
	Fungal diseases of the eye	
Vaccinia, varicella, and many other viral diseases of the cornea and conjunctiva		Hypersensitivity to any component

ADMINISTRATION/DOSAGE ADJUSTMENTS

Chronic conditions	Withdraw treatment by decreasing the frequency of applications, until the dosage is as infrequent as once a week

WARNINGS/PRECAUTIONS

Initial prescription	Do not prescribe more than 8 g until the patient can be examined with the aid of magnification, such as slit-lamp microscopy, and, where appropriate, fluorescein staining
Prolonged use	Protracted use of this preparation may result in glaucoma, optic nerve damage, and visual acuity and field defects; check intraocular pressure frequently if used for 10 days or longer. Chronic therapy may also cause posterior subcapsular cataracts and promote secondary ocular infections; fungal invasion of the cornea should be suspected in any case of persistent corneal ulceration.
Concomitant infections	Topical steroid therapy may mask or enhance untreated acute, purulent infections of the eye and may exacerbate ocular infections
Diseases causing corneal or scleral thinning	Perforation of the globe has been associated with topical steroid use in patients with diseases that cause corneal or scleral thinning
Herpetic keratitis	Use with great caution in the treatment of herpes simplex
Hypersensitivity	Topical application of neomycin sulfate may cause cutaneous sensitization. The exact incidence of hypersensitivity reactions—primarily skin rash—is not known. Sensitization is manifested usually by itching, reddening, and edema of the conjunctiva and eyelid, or simply as failure to heal; during long-term therapy with neomycin, the patient should be periodically examined for such signs and advised to discontinue the medication if they should appear. These symptoms quickly disappear upon withdrawal of the drug, and medications containing neomycin should be avoided for the patient thereafter. Allergic cross-sensitization may prevent the future use of any or all of the following antibiotics: kanomycin, paromomycin, streptomycin, and possibly gentamicin.

ADVERSE REACTIONS

Ophthalmic	Elevation of intraocular pressure, possibly developing into glaucoma, and, infrequently, optic nerve damage; posterior subcapsular cataract formation; delayed wound healing; secondary ocular infections
Other	Allergic sensitization

DRUG INTERACTIONS

No clinically significant drug interactions have been identified

---

USE IN CHILDREN

See indications and dosage recommendations; do not use longer than absolutely necessary, since prolonged therapy increases the risk of adrenal suppression in children 2 yr or age or younger

USE IN PREGNANT AND NURSING WOMEN

Pregnancy Category C: topical administration of corticosteroids has been shown to be teratogenic in mice and rabbits; however, there have been no adequate, well-controlled studies in pregnant women. This preparation should be used during pregnancy only if the expected benefit to the mother outweighs the potential risk to the fetus. Because hydrocortisone is excreted in human milk and systemic absorption may occur following topical application of this steroid, exercise caution in prescribing this preparation to nursing women.

VEHICLE/BASE
Ointment: white petrolatum

[1] The use of an anti-infective steroid combination is indicated in those conditions where the risk of infection is high or it is anticipated that there are potentially dangerous numbers of bacteria present in the eye; the anti-infective components in this preparation are effective against the following pathogens: *Staphylococcus aureus*, streptococci (including *Streptococcus pneumoniae*), *Escherichia coli*, *Hemophilus influenzae*, *Klebsiella* sp, *Enterobacter* sp, *Neisseria* sp, and *Pseudomonas aeruginosa*; it does not provide adequate coverage against *Serratia marcescens*

OPHTHALMIC ANTI-INFECTIVES

CORTISPORIN Ophthalmic Suspension (polymyxin B sulfate, neomycin sulfate, and hydrocortisone) Burroughs Wellcome Rx

Suspension (per milliliter): 10,000 units polymyxin B sulfate, neomycin sulfate equivalent to 0.35% neomycin base, and 10 mg (1%) hydrocortisone (7.5 ml)

INDICATIONS[1]

Steroid-responsive inflammatory ophthalmic conditions, such as those of the palpebral and bulbar conjunctiva, cornea, and anterior segment of the globe
Chronic anterior uveitis
Corneal injury from chemical, radiation, or thermal burns, or from penetration of foreign bodies

TOPICAL DOSAGE

Adult and child: 1 drop instilled into the affected eye q3–4h, or more frequently, depending upon the severity of the condition

COMPENDIUM OF DRUG THERAPY

CONTRAINDICATIONS

Epithelial herpes simplex keratitis (dendritic keratitis)

Vaccinia, varicella, and many other viral diseases of the cornea and conjunctiva

Mycobacterial infections of the eye

Fungal diseases of the eye

Following uncomplicated removal of a corneal foreign body

Hypersensitivity to any component

WARNINGS/PRECAUTIONS

Initial prescription	Do not prescribe more than 20 ml until the patient can be examined with the aid of magnification, such as slit-lamp microscopy, and, where appropriate, fluorescein staining
Prolonged use	Protracted use of this preparation may result in glaucoma, optic nerve damage, and visual acuity and field defects; check intraocular pressure frequently if used for 10 days or longer. Chronic therapy may also cause posterior subcapsular cataracts and promote secondary ocular infections; fungal invasion of the cornea should be suspected in any case of persistent corneal ulceration.
Concomitant infections	Topical steroid therapy may mask or enhance untreated acute, purulent infections of the eye and may exacerbate fungal ocular infections
Corneal or scleral perforation	Perforation of the globe has been associated with topical steroid use in patients with diseases that cause corneal or scleral thinning
Herpetic keratitis	Use with great caution in the treatment of herpes simplex
Hypersensitivity	Topical application of neomycin sulfate may cause cutaneous sensitization. The exact incidence of hypersensitivity reactions—primarily skin rash—is not known. Sensitization is manifested usually by itching, reddening, and edema of the conjunctiva and eyelid, or simply as failure to heal; during long-term therapy with neomycin, the patient should be periodically examined for such signs and advised to discontinue the medication if they should appear. These symptoms quickly disappear upon withdrawal of the drug, and medications containing neomycin should be avoided for the patient thereafter. Allergic cross-sensitization may prevent the future use of any or all of the following antibiotics: kanomycin, paromomycin, streptomycin, and possibly gentamicin.
Carcinogenicity	Long-term animal studies have demonstrated no carcinogenic effects from oral administration of corticosteroids
Contamination	The patient should be advised to avoid contaminating the dropper with material from the eyes, fingers, or other sources

ADVERSE REACTIONS

Ophthalmic	Localized hypersensitivity including itching, swelling, and conjunctival erythema; irritation upon instillation; elevation of intraocular pressure, possibly developing into glaucoma and, infrequently, optic nerve damage; posterior subcapsular cataract formation; delayed wound healing; secondary infections, especially fungal infections of the cornea, with prolonged use

DRUG INTERACTIONS

No clinically significant drug interactions have been identified

USE IN CHILDREN

See indications and dosage recommendations; do not use longer than absolutely necessary, since prolonged therapy increases the risk of adrenal suppression in children 2 yr of age or younger

USE IN PREGNANT AND NURSING WOMEN

Pregnancy Category C: topical administration of corticosteroids has been shown to be teratogenic in mice and rabbits; however, there have been no adequate, well-controlled studies in pregnant women. This preparation should be used during pregnancy only if the expected benefit to the mother outweighs the potential risk to the fetus. Because hydrocortisone is excreted in human milk and systemic absorption may occur following topical application of this steroid, exercise caution in prescribing this preparation to nursing women.

VEHICLE/BASE
Suspension: cetyl alcohol, glyceryl monostearate, mineral oil, polyoxyl 40 stearate, propylene glycol, 0.001% thimerosal, sulfuric acid (to adjust pH), and water for injection

[1] The use of an anti-infective steroid combination is indicated in those conditions where the risk of infection is high or it is anticipated that there are potentially dangerous numbers of bacteria present in the eye; the anti-infective components in this preparation are effective against the following pathogens: *Staphylococcus aureus, Escherichia coli, Hemophilus influenzae, Klebsiella* sp, *Enterobacter* sp, *Neisseria* sp, and *Pseudomonas aeruginosa*; it does not provide adequate coverage against *Serratia marcescens* or streptococci (including *Streptococcus pneumoniae*)

OPHTHALMIC ANTI-INFECTIVES

CHLOROMYXIN Ophthalmic Ointment (chloramphenicol and polymyxin B sulfate) Parke-Davis Rx

Ointment: 1% chloramphenicol and 10,000 units/g polymyxin B sulfate (3.5 g)

INDICATIONS

Superficial ocular infections involving the conjunctiva and/or cornea caused by susceptible organisms

TOPICAL DOSAGE

Adult and child: apply a small amount of ointment to the lower conjunctival sac q3h (or more often if needed) day and night for the first 48 h; thereafter, the interval between applications may be lengthened

CHLOROMYXIN ■ GARAMYCIN Ophthalmic Ointment and Solution

CONTRAINDICATIONS

Hypersensitivity to any component

ADMINISTRATION/DOSAGE ADJUSTMENTS

Duration of treatment	Continue treatment for at least 48 h after the eye appears normal
Concomitant therapy	Unless the infection is very superficial, topical therapy should be supplemented with a suitable systemic antibiotic regimen; however, the total daily dose of polymyxin from both topical and systemic administration should not exceed 2.5 mg (25,000 units)/kg

WARNINGS/PRECAUTIONS

Blood dyscrasias	Bone marrow hypoplasia, including aplastic anemia and death, has been reported following local application of chloramphenicol
Overgrowth of nonsusceptible organisms	Nonsusceptible organisms, including fungi, may proliferate with prolonged use; if new infections develop, discontinue use and institute appropriate measures

ADVERSE REACTIONS

Systemic	Bone marrow hypoplasia (see WARNINGS/PRECAUTIONS)

DRUG INTERACTIONS

No clinically significant drug interactions have been identified

---

USE IN CHILDREN

See indications and dosage recommendations

USE IN PREGNANT AND NURSING WOMEN

Specific guidelines are not available; use according to medical judgment

---

VEHICLE/BASE
Ointment: liquid petrolatum and polyethylene

OPHTHALMIC ANTI-INFECTIVES

GARAMYCIN Ophthalmic Ointment and Solution (gentamicin sulfate) Schering Rx

Ointment: gentamicin sulfate equivalent to 0.3% gentamicin (3.5 g) **Solution:** gentamicin sulfate equivalent to 0.3% gentamicin (5 ml)

INDICATIONS

Infections of the external eye and its adnexa, including conjunctivitis, keratitis and keratoconjunctivitis, corneal ulcers, blepharitis and blepharoconjunctivitis, acute meibomianitis, and dacryocystitis, caused by susceptible organisms

TOPICAL DOSAGE

Adult and child ($\geq$ 6 yr): instill 1 drop into affected eye q4h or apply a small amount of ointment to the affected eye bid or tid; for severe infections, up to 2 drops every hour may be used

CONTRAINDICATIONS

Hypersensitivity to any component

WARNINGS/PRECAUTIONS

Inappropriate methods of administration	Never inject solution subconjunctivally or introduce directly into the anterior chamber of the eye
Overgrowth of nonsusceptible organisms	Nonsusceptible organisms, including fungi, may proliferate with prolonged use; if new infections develop, discontinue use and institute appropriate therapy
Hypersensitivity	Discontinue use and institute appropriate therapy if signs of irritation or hypersensitivity occur
Corneal healing	Use of the ophthalmic ointment may retard corneal wound healing

ADVERSE REACTIONS

Ophthalmic	Transient irritation (with use of solution); occasional burning or stinging (with use of ointment)

GARAMYCIN Ophthalmic Ointment and Solution ■ ILOTYCIN

DRUG INTERACTIONS
No clinically significant drug interactions have been identified

USE IN CHILDREN	USE IN PREGNANT AND NURSING WOMEN
Safety and effectiveness have not been established for use in children under 6 yr of age	Safety for use during pregnancy has not been established; use only if clearly needed. Aminoglycosides cross the placental barrier. Total irreversible bilateral congenital deafness has been reported in children whose mothers received streptomycin during pregnancy. However, serious side effects have not been reported in pregnant women given other aminoglycosides. Trace amounts of gentamicin are excreted in human milk; use with caution in nursing mothers. However, no adverse effect was observed in animal pups nursed by dams receiving gentamicin.

VEHICLE/BASE
Ointment: white petrolatum, methylparaben, propylparaben
Solution: disodium phosphate, monosodium phosphate, sodium chloride, and benzalkonium chloride

---

OPHTHALMIC ANTI-INFECTIVES

GENTACIDIN Ophthalmic Ointment and Solution (gentamicin sulfate) CooperVision   Rx

Ointment: gentamicin sulfate equivalent to 0.3% gentamicin (3.5 g)   Solution: gentamicin sulfate equivalent to 0.3% gentamicin (5 ml)

INDICATIONS
Infections of the external eye and its adnexa, including conjunctivitis, keratitis and keratoconjunctivitis, corneal ulcers, blepharitis and blepharoconjunctivitis, acute meibomianitis, and dacryocystitis, caused by susceptible organisms[1]

TOPICAL DOSAGE
Adult and child: instill 1 drop into affected eye q4h or apply a small amount of ointment to the affected eye bid or tid; for severe infections, up to 2 drops every hour may be used

CONTRAINDICATIONS
Hypersensitivity to any component

WARNINGS/PRECAUTIONS

Inappropriate methods of administration	Never inject solution subconjunctivally or introduce directly into the anterior chamber of the eye
Overgrowth of nonsusceptible organisms	Nonsusceptible organisms, including fungi, may proliferate with prolonged use; if new infections develop, discontinue use and institute appropriate therapy
Adverse reactions	Discontinue use and institute appropriate therapy if signs of irritation or hypersensitivity occur
Corneal healing	Use of the ophthalmic ointment may retard corneal wound healing

ADVERSE REACTIONS

Ophthalmic	Transient irritation (with use of solution); occasional burning or stinging (with use of ointment)

DRUG INTERACTIONS
No clinically significant drug interactions have been identified

USE IN CHILDREN	USE IN PREGNANT AND NURSING WOMEN
See indications and dosage recommendations	Safety for use during pregnancy has not been established; use only if clearly needed. Aminoglycosides cross the placental barrier. Total irreversible bilateral congenital deafness has been reported in children whose mothers received streptomycin during pregnancy. However, serious side effects have not been reported in pregnant women given other aminoglycosides. Trace amounts of gentamicin are excreted in human milk; use with caution in nursing mothers. However, no adverse effect was observed in animal pups nursed by dams receiving gentamicin.

VEHICLE/BASE
Ointment: white petrolatum and mineral oil
Solution: dried sodium phosphate, monobasic sodium phosphate, sodium chloride, benzalkonium chloride, and purified water

[1] Gentamicin sulfate is effective against the following pathogens: coagulase-positive and coagulase-negative staphylococci (including certain penicillin-resistant strains), Group A beta-hemolytic and nonhemolytic streptococci, *Diplococcus pneumoniae*, *Pseudomonas aeruginosa*, indole-positive and indole-negative *Proteus* sp, *Escherichia coli* (Friedlander's bacillus), *Hemophilus influenzae* and *H aegyptius* (Koch-Weeks bacillus), *Aerobacter aerogenes*, *Moraxella lacunata*, and *Neisseria* sp, including *N gonorrhoeae*

OPHTHALMIC ANTI-INFECTIVES

ILOTYCIN Ophthalmic Ointment (erythromycin) Dista   Rx

Ointment: 0.5% (3.5 g)

INDICATIONS
Superficial ocular infections involving the conjunctiva and/or cornea caused by susceptible organisms

TOPICAL DOSAGE
Adult and child: apply directly to the infected structure once daily or more often, depending on the severity of the infection

ILOTYCIN ■ MAXITROL

Prophylaxis of **ophthalmia neonatorum** due to *Neisseria gonorrhoeae* or *Chlamydia trachomatis* | **Infant:** instill a ribbon of ointment approximately 0.5–1 cm in length into each conjunctival sac

CONTRAINDICATIONS

Hypersensitivity to erythromycin

ADMINISTRATION/DOSAGE ADJUSTMENTS

Prevention of neonatal conjunctivitis — Use a new tube of ointment for each infant, and do not flush the ointment from the eye after instillation. Infants born to mothers with clinically apparent gonorrhea should also be given a single IM or IV injection of aqueous crystalline penicillin G in a dose of 50,000 units for term infants and 20,000 units for low-birth-weight infants

WARNINGS/PRECAUTIONS

Overgrowth of nonsusceptible organisms — Nonsusceptible organisms may proliferate; if superinfection occurs, discontinue use and institute appropriate therapy

Hypersensitivity — Discontinue use if signs of hypersensitivity occur

ADVERSE REACTIONS

Ophthalmic — Sensitivity reactions (rare)

DRUG INTERACTIONS

No clinically significant drug interactions have been identified

---

USE IN CHILDREN
See indications and dosage recommendations

USE IN PREGNANT AND NURSING WOMEN
Specific guidelines are not available; use according to medical judgment

---

VEHICLE/BASE
Ointment: mineral oil and white petrolatum

OPHTHALMIC ANTI-INFECTIVES

MAXITROL Ophthalmic Ointment and Suspension (dexamethasone, neomycin sulfate, and polymyxin B sulfate) Alcon ℞

Ointment (per gram): 1 mg (0.1%) dexamethasone, neomycin sulfate equivalent to 0.35% neomycin, and 10,000 units polymyxin B sulfate (3.5 g) **Suspension (per milliliter):** 1 mg (0.1%) dexamethasone, neomycin sulfate equivalent to 0.35% neomycin, and 10,000 units polymyxin B sulfate (5 ml)

INDICATIONS

Steroid-responsive inflammatory ophthalmic conditions of the palpebral and bulbar conjunctiva, cornea, and anterior segment of the globe
Chronic anterior uveitis
Corneal injury from chemical, radiation, or thermal burns, or from penetration of foreign bodies

TOPICAL DOSAGE

Adult and child: apply a small amount of ointment into the conjunctival sac(s) up to 3–4 times/day or instill 1 drop into the conjunctival sac(s) up to 4–6 times/day for mild conditions or hourly for severe conditions, tapering the dosage as the inflammation subsides; the ointment may also be used adjunctively with the drops at bedtime to provide prolonged contact with the affected eye(s)

CONTRAINDICATIONS

Epithelial herpes simplex keratitis (dendritic keratitis)

Vaccinia, varicella, and many other viral diseases of the cornea and conjunctiva

Mycobacterial infections of the eye

Fungal infections of the eye

Following uncomplicated removal of a corneal foreign body

Hypersensitivity to any component

WARNINGS/PRECAUTIONS

Initial prescription — Do not prescribe more than 20 ml or 8 g until the patient can be examined with the aid of magnification, such as by slit-lamp microscopy, and, where appropriate, fluorescein staining

MAXITROL ■ NEODECADRON

Prolonged use	Protracted use of these preparations may result in glaucoma, optic nerve damage, and visual acuity and field defects; check intraocular pressure frequently if used for 10 days or longer. Chronic therapy may also cause posterior subcapsular cataracts and promote secondary ocular infections; fungal invasion of the cornea should be suspected in any case of persistent corneal ulceration (see CONTRAINDICATIONS).
Concomitant infections	Topical steroid therapy may mask or enhance untreated acute, purulent infections of the eye and may exacerbate bacterial or fungal ocular infections (see CONTRAINDICATIONS)
Stromal herpetic keratitis	Use with great caution when treating herpes simplex keratitis involving the stroma; frequent slit-lamp microscopy examinations are mandatory
Diseases causing corneal or scleral thinning	Perforation of the globe has occurred with topical steroid use in patients with diseases that cause corneal or scleral thinning
Hypersensitivity	The neomycin sulfate component in this preparation may cause cutaneous sensitization

ADVERSE REACTIONS

Ophthalmic	Elevation of intraocular pressure, possibly developing into glaucoma and, infrequently, optic nerve damage; posterior subcapsular cataract formation; delayed wound healing; secondary ocular infections
Other	Allergic sensitization

DRUG INTERACTIONS

No clinically significant drug interactions have been identified

---

USE IN CHILDREN

See indications and dosage recommendations; do not use longer than absolutely necessary, since prolonged therapy increases the risk of adrenal suppression in children 2 yr of age or younger

USE IN PREGNANT AND NURSING WOMEN

The safety of intensive or prolonged topical steroid therapy during pregnancy has not been established. Specific guidelines are not available for use in nursing women; use according to medical judgment.

VEHICLE/BASE
Ointment: white petrolatum and anhydrous liquid lanolin, 0.05% methylparaben, and 0.01% propylparaben
Suspension: 0.004% benzalkonium chloride, 0.5% hydroxypropyl methylcellulose, sodium chloride, polysorbate 20, hydrochloric acid and/or sodium hydroxide, and purified water

[1] The use of an anti-infective steroid combination is indicated in those conditions where the risk of infection is high or it is anticipated that there are potentially dangerous numbers of bacteria present in the eye; the anti-infective components in this preparation are effective against the following pathogens: *Staphylococcus aureus, Escherichia coli, Hemophilus influenzae, Klebsiella* sp, *Enterobacter* sp, *Neisseria* sp, and *Pseudonomas aeruginosa*; it does not provide adequate coverage effective against *Serratia marescens* and streptococci (including *Streptococcus pneumoniae*)

OPHTHALMIC ANTI-INFECTIVES

NEODECADRON Sterile Ophthalmic Ointment and Solution (neomycin sulfate and dexamethasone sodium phosphate) Merck Sharp & Dohme   Rx

Ointment: dexamethasone sodium phosphate equivalent to 0.05% dexamethasone phosphate and neomycin sulfate equivalent to 0.35% mg neomycin base (3.5 g) Solution: dexamethasone sodium phosphate equivalent to 0.1% dexamethasone phosphate and neomycin sulfate equivalent to 0.35% mg neomycin base (5 ml)

INDICATIONS[1]

Steroid-responsive inflammatory ophthalmic conditions, such as those of the palpebral and bulbar conjunctiva, cornea, and anterior segment of the globe
Chronic anterior uveitis
Corneal injury from chemical, radiation, or thermal burns, or from penetration of foreign bodies

TOPICAL DOSAGE

Adult and child: apply a thin coating of the ointment tid or qid or instill 1 drop of the solution into the conjunctival sac every hour during the day and q2h at night to start; once a favorable response is obtained, reduce the dosage of the ointment to bid and of the solution to 1 drop q4h; later, dosage may be reduced to one daily application of ointment, if symptoms permit, or 1 drop of solution tid or qid

NEODECADRON

CONTRAINDICATIONS

- Epithelial herpes simplex keratitis (dendritic keratitis)
- Acute, infectious vaccinia, varicella, and many other viral diseases of the cornea and conjunctiva
- Mycobacterial infections of the eye
- Fungal diseases of the eye
- Following uncomplicated removal of a corneal foreign body
- Hypersensitivity to any component, including sulfite-containing compounds

ADMINISTRATION/DOSAGE ADJUSTMENTS

Duration of therapy	Treatment duration varies according to the type of lesion, and may range from a few days to several wk, depending on patient response. Relapses, which occur more commonly in chronic than in acute conditions, can usually be controlled by topical steroid therapy.
Choice of dosage form	The ointment may be the treatment form of choice when an eye pad is used, or when it is desirable to have the active ingredients of a preparation in contact with the ocular tissues for longer periods

WARNINGS/PRECAUTIONS

Initial prescription	Do not prescribe more than 8 g of the ointment or 20 ml of the solution until the patient can be examined with the aid of magnification, such as slit-lamp microscopy, and, where appropriate, fluorescein staining
Corneal or scleral thinning	Perforation of the globe has been associated with topical steroid use in patients with diseases that cause corneal or scleral thinning
Concomitant infections	Topical steroid therapy may mask or enhance untreated acute, purulent infections of the eye and may exacerbate bacterial or fungal ocular infections of the cornea; acute, purulent infections of the eye may be masked or enhanced by topical steroid therapy
Herpetic keratitis	Use with great caution in the presence of herpetic keratitis; periodic slit-lamp microscopy is recommended
Prolonged use	Protracted ophthalmic use of these preparations may result in glaucoma, optic nerve damage, and visual acuity and field defects; check intraocular pressure frequently if used for 10 days or longer. Chronic therapy may also cause posterior subcapsular cataracts and promote secondary ocular infections; fungal invasion of the cornea should be suspected in any case of persistent corneal ulceration.
Hypersensitivity	The neomycin sulfate component in this preparation may cause cutaneous sensitization; discontinue therapy if symptoms occur. The solution contains sodium bisulfite; sulfites have reportedly caused severe allergic reactions in susceptible individuals, particularly asthmatics.

ADVERSE REACTIONS

Ophthalmic	Elevation of intraocular pressure, possibly developing into glaucoma and, infrequently, optic nerve damage; posterior subcapsular cataract formation; delayed wound healing; secondary ocular infections
Other	Allergic sensitization

DRUG INTERACTIONS

No clinically significant drug interactions have been identified

USE IN CHILDREN

See indications and dosage recommendations; do not use longer than absolutely necessary, since prolonged therapy increases the risk of adrenal suppression in children 2 yr of age or younger

USE IN PREGNANT AND NURSING WOMEN

The safety of intensive or prolonged topical steroid therapy during pregnancy has not been established. Specific guidelines are not available for use in nursing women; use according to medical judgment.

VEHICLE/BASE
Ointment: white petrolatum and mineral oil
Solution: creatinine, sodium citrate, sodium borate, polysorbate 80, disodium edetate, hydrochloric acid (to adjust pH), water for injection, 0.02% benzalkonium chloride, and 0.1% sodium bisulfite

---

[1] The use of an anti-infective steroid combination is indicated in those conditions where the risk of infection is high or it is anticipated that there are potentially dangerous numbers of bacteria present in the eye; the anti-infective component in this preparation is effective against the following pathogens: *Staphylococcus aureus*, *Escherichia coli*, *Hemophilus influenzae*, *Klebsiella* sp, *Enterobacter* sp, and *Neisseria* sp; it does not provide adequate coverage against *Pseudomonas aeruginosa*, *Serratia marcescens*, or streptococci (including *Streptococcus pneumoniae*)

OPHTHALMIC ANTI-INFECTIVES

NEOSPORIN Ophthalmic Ointment (polymyxin B sulfate, bacitracin zinc, and neomycin sulfate) Burroughs Wellcome Rx

Ointment (per gram): 10,000 units polymyxin B sulfate, 400 units bacitracin zinc, and neomycin sulfate equivalent to 3.5 mg neomycin base (3.5 g)

NEOSPORIN Ophthalmic Solution (polymyxin B sulfate, neomycin sulfate, and gramicidin) Burroughs Wellcome Rx

Solution (per milliliter): 10,000 units polymyxin B sulfate, neomycin sulfate equivalent to 1.75 mg neomycin base, and 0.025 mg gramicidin (10 ml)

INDICATIONS
Short-term treatment of **superficial external ocular infections** caused by susceptible organisms[1]

TOPICAL DOSAGE
Adult and child: apply the ointment q3–4h depending on the severity of the infection, or instill 1 drop into the affected eye bid to qid or more frequently, as needed, for 7–10 days; for acute infections, instill 1 drop every 15–30 min to start, followed by a gradual reduction in frequency of administration as improvement occurs

CONTRAINDICATIONS
Hypersensitivity to any component

WARNINGS/PRECAUTIONS

Overgrowth of nonsusceptible organisms — Nonsusceptible organisms, including fungi, may proliferate with prolonged use; if new infections develop, discontinue use and institute appropriate therapy

Hypersensitivity — Topical application of neomycin sulfate may cause cutaneous sensitization. The exact incidence of hypersensitivity reactions—primarily skin rash—is not known. Sensitization is manifested usually by itching, reddening, and edema of the conjunctiva and eyelid, or simply as failure to heal; during long-term therapy with neomycin, the patient should be periodically examined for such signs and advised to discontinue the medication if they should appear. These symptoms quickly disappear upon withdrawal of the drug, and medications containing neomycin should be avoided for the patient thereafter. Allergic cross-sensitization may prevent the future use of any or all of the following antibiotics: kanomycin, paromomycin, streptomycin, and possibly gentamicin.

Contamination — The patient should be advised to avoid contaminating the dropper with material from the eyes, fingers, or other sources

ADVERSE REACTIONS

Ophthalmic — Cutaneous and conjunctival sensitization, including itching, reddening, and edema of the conjunctiva and eyelid

DRUG INTERACTIONS
No clinically significant drug interactions have been identified

USE IN CHILDREN
See indications and dosage recommendations

USE IN PREGNANT AND NURSING WOMEN
Specific guidelines are not available; use according to medical judgment

VEHICLE/BASE
Ointment: white petrolatum
Solution: 0.5% alcohol, 0.001% thimerosal, propylene glycol, polyoxyethylene polyoxypropylene compound, sodium chloride, and water for injection

[1] The anti-infective components of this preparation are effective against the following pathogens: *Staphylococcus aureus*, streptococci (including *Streptococcus pneumoniae*), *Escherichia coli*, *Hemophilus influenzae*, *Klebsiella* sp, *Enterobacter* sp, *Neisseria* sp, and *Pseudomonas aeruginosa*; it does not provide adequate coverage against *Serratia marcescens*

OPHTHALMIC ANTI-INFECTIVES

POLY-PRED Ophthalmic Suspension (prednisolone acetate, neomycin sulfate, and polymyxin B sulfate) Allergan Rx

Suspension (per milliliter): 0.5% prednisolone acetate, 0.5% neomycin sulfate equivalent to 0.35% neomycin base, and 10,000 units polymyxin B sulfate (5, 10 ml)

INDICATIONS[1]
Steroid-responsive inflammatory ophthalmic conditions, such as those of the palpebral and bulbar conjunctiva, cornea, and anterior segment of the globe
Chronic anterior uveitis
Corneal injury from chemical, radiation, or thermal burns, or from penetration of foreign bodies

TOPICAL DOSAGE
Adult and child: 1 drop q3–4h or more frequently, as needed; acute infections may require administration every 30 min, followed by a reduction in frequency as the condition is brought under control; to treat the lid, instill 1 drop into the eye q3–4h, close the eye, and rub the excess onto the lid and lid margins

POLY-PRED ■ Sodium SULAMYD

CONTRAINDICATIONS

Epithelial herpes simplex keratitis (dendritic keratitis)

Vaccinia, varicella, and many other viral diseases of the cornea and conjunctiva

Mycobacterial infections of the eye

Fungal diseases of the eye

Following uncomplicated removal of a corneal foreign body

Hypersensitivity to any component

WARNINGS/PRECAUTIONS

Initial prescription	Do not prescribe more than 20 ml or refill the prescription until the patient can be examined with the aid of magnification such as slit-lamp microscopy, and, where appropriate, fluorescein staining
Prolonged use	Protracted use of this preparation may result in glaucoma, optic nerve damage, and visual acuity and field defects; check intraocular pressure frequently if used for 10 days or longer. Chronic therapy may also cause posterior subcapsular cataracts and promote secondary ocular infections; fungal invasion of the cornea should be suspected in any case of persistent corneal ulceration.
Concomitant infections	Topical steroid therapy may mask or enhance untreated acute, purulent infections of the eye and may exacerbate fungal ocular infections of the cornea
Diseases causing corneal or scleral thinning	Perforation of the globe has been associated with topical steroid use in patients with diseases that cause corneal or scleral thinning
Herpetic keratitis	Topical steroids should be used with great caution in the treatment of herpes simplex
Hypersensitivity	The neomycin sulfate component of this preparation may cause cutaneous sensitization; the exact incidence is unknown

ADVERSE REACTIONS

Ophthalmic	Elevation of intraocular pressure, possibly developing into glaucoma and, infrequently, optic nerve damage; posterior subcapsular cataract formation; delayed wound healing; secondary ocular infections
Other	Allergic sensitization

DRUG INTERACTIONS

No clinically significant drug interactions have been identified

---

USE IN CHILDREN

See indications and dosage recommendations; do not use longer than absolutely necessary, since prolonged therapy increases the risk of adrenal suppression in children 2 yr of age or younger

USE IN PREGNANT AND NURSING WOMEN

The safety of intensive or prolonged topical steroid therapy during pregnancy has not been established. Specific guidelines are not available for use in nursing women; use according to medical judgment.

VEHICLE/BASE
Suspension: 1.4% polyvinyl alcohol (Liquifilm), 0.001% thimerosal, polysorbate 80, propylene glycol, sodium acetate, and purified water

[1] The use of an anti-infective steroid combination is indicated in those conditions where the risk of infection is high or it is anticipated that there are potentially dangerous numbers of bacteria present in the eye; the anti-infective components in this preparation are effective against the following pathogens: *Staphylococcus aureus, Escherichia coli, Hemophilus influenzae, Klebsiella* sp, *Enterobacter* sp, *Neisseria* sp, and *Pseudomonas aeruginosa*; it does not provide adequate coverage against *Serratia marcescens* and streptococci (including *Streptococcus pneumoniae*)

OPHTHALMIC ANTI-INFECTIVES

Sodium SULAMYD Ophthalmic Ointment and Solution (sulfacetamide sodium) Schering   Rx

Ointment: 10% (3.5 g)   **Solution:** 10% (5 ml), 30% (15 ml)

INDICATIONS

Conjunctivitis, corneal ulcer, and other superficial ocular infections caused by susceptible organisms

Trachoma (as an adjunct to systemic sulfonamide therapy)

TOPICAL DOSAGE

Adult and child: instill 1 drop of the 30% solution into the lower conjunctival sac q2h or less frequently, depending on the severity of the infection, or 1 drop of the 10% solution into the lower conjunctival sac q2–3h during the day and less often at night; alternatively, apply a small amount of the ointment qid and again at bedtime (the ointment may also be used adjunctively with either of the solution forms)

Adult and child: 2 drops of the 30% solution q2h

Sodium SULAMYD ■ TOBREX

CONTRAINDICATIONS

Hypersensitivity to sulfonamides or any component

WARNINGS/PRECAUTIONS

Overgrowth of nonsusceptible organisms	Nonsusceptible organisms, including fungi, may proliferate during treatment
Purulent exudates	These preparations may be inactivated by the *para*-aminobenzoic acid present in purulent exudates
Corneal healing	Use of the ophthalmic ointment may retard corneal wound healing
Hypersensitivity	Sensitization may recur when a sulfonamide is readministered, regardless of the route of administration, and patients who are hypersensitive to one sulfonamide may be allergic to other sulfonamides as well; discontinue use of these preparations if signs of hypersensitivity or other untoward reactions develop during therapy

ADVERSE REACTIONS

Ophthalmic	Transient local irritation; stinging and burning
Hypersensitivity	Stevens-Johnson syndrome (one case); local hypersensitivity progressing to a fatal syndrome resembling systemic lupus erythematosus (one case)

DRUG INTERACTIONS

Silver nitrate, mild silver protein	Incompatible with sulfacetamide; do not administer concurrently
Tetracaine	▽ Antibacterial activity of sulfacetamide

USE IN CHILDREN
See indications and dosage recommendations

USE IN PREGNANT AND NURSING WOMEN
Specific guidelines are not available; use according to medical judgment

VEHICLE/BASE
10% Ointment: 0.05% methylparaben, 0.01% propylparaben, 0.025% benzalkonium chloride, sorbitan monolaurate, petrolatum, and water
10% Solution: 0.31% sodium thiosulfate, 0.5% methylcellulose, 0.05% methylparaben, 0.01% propylparaben, and monobasic sodium phosphate
30% Solution: 0.15% sodium thiosulfate, 0.05% methylparaben, 0.01% propylparaben, and monobasic sodium phosphate

---

OPHTHALMIC ANTI-INFECTIVES

TOBREX Ophthalmic Ointment and Solution (tobramycin) Alcon   Rx

Ointment: 0.3% (3.5 g)   **Solution:** 0.3% (5 ml)

INDICATIONS

External infections of the eye and its adnexa caused by susceptible organisms[1]

TOPICAL DOSAGE

Adult and child: for mild to moderate infections, apply a 1/2 in. ribbon of ointment to infected eye bid or tid or instill 1 drop into the infected eye q4h; for severe infections, apply a 1/2 in. ribbon of ointment to the infected eye q3–4h or instill 2 drops of the solution every hour until improvement occurs, then reduce dosage before discontinuation

CONTRAINDICATIONS

Hypersensitivity to any component

WARNINGS/PRECAUTIONS

Monitoring of therapy	Bacterial monitoring should be performed during therapy to determine response to treatment
Concomitant therapy	Monitor total serum concentration if tobramycin is administered concomitantly with systemic aminoglycoside antibiotics
Overgrowth of nonsusceptible organisms	Nonsusceptible organisms, including fungi, may proliferate with prolonged use; if superinfection occurs, institute appropriate therapy
Hypersensitivity	Discontinue use if signs of hypersensitivity occur
Corneal healing	Use of the ophthalmic ointment may retard corneal wound healing
Direct injection	The solution is intended for topical use only and should never be injected into the eye

TOBREX ■ VASOCIDIN Ophthalmic Ointment

ADVERSE REACTIONS

Frequent reactions (incidence ≥ 1%) are printed in *italics*

Ophthalmic — *Lid itching and swelling and conjunctival erythema (~ 3%)*[2]

OVERDOSAGE

Signs and symptoms — Punctate keratitis, erythema, increased lacrimation, edema, lid itching

Treatment — Discontinue use; treat symptomatically

DRUG INTERACTIONS

No clinically significant drug interactions have been identified

ALTERED LABORATORY VALUES

No clinically significant alterations in blood/serum or urinary values occur at therapeutic dosages

---

USE IN CHILDREN

See indications and dosage recommendations

USE IN PREGNANT AND NURSING WOMEN

Pregnancy Category B: use during pregnancy only if clearly needed. Reproduction studies in animals at doses up to 33 times the normal human systemic dose have shown no evidence of impaired fertility or fetal harm. No adequate, well-controlled studies have been done in pregnant women. Considering the potential for adverse reactions in nursing infants, a decision should be made either to discontinue nursing or discontinue the drug, taking into account its importance to the mother.

VEHICLE/BASE
Ointment: mineral oil, petrolatum, and 0.5% chlorobutanol
Solution: boric acid, sodium sulfate, sodium chloride, tyloxapol, sodium hydroxide and/or sulfuric acid (to adjust pH), 0.01% benzalkonium chloride, and purified water

[1] Tobramycin is effective against staphylococci (including *S aureus* and *S epidermidis* [coagulase-positive and -negative], including penicillin-resistant strains), streptococci (including some Group-A beta-hemolytic species, some nonhemolytic species, and some *Streptococcus pneumoniae* strains), *Pseudomonas aeruginosa, Escherichia coli, Klebsiella pneumoniae, Enterobacter aerogenes, Proteus mirabilis* (indole-negative) and indole-positive *Proteus* sp, *Hemophilus influenzae* and *H aegyptius, Moraxella lacunata, Acinetobacter calcoaceticus (Herellea vaginacola),* and some *Neisseria* sp; although resistant bacterial strains to tobramyin have not yet emerged, bacterial resistance may develop after prolonged use
[2] Other adverse reactions have not been reported from topical use of these preparations; however, if systemic aminoglycoside therapy is given concomitantly, monitor the total serum aminoglycoside concentration

---

OPHTHALMIC ANTI-INFECTIVES

VASOCIDIN Ophthalmic Ointment (sulfacetamide sodium and prednisolone acetate) CooperVision

Rx

Ointment: 10% sulfacetamide sodium and 0.5% prednisolone acetate (3.5 g)

INDICATIONS[1]

Steroid-responsive inflammatory ophthalmic conditions, such as those of the palpebral and bulbar conjuctiva, cornea, and anterior segment of the globe
Chronic anterior uveitis
Corneal injury from chemical, radiation, or thermal burns or from penetration of foreign bodies

TOPICAL DOSAGE

Adult and child: apply a small amount 3–4 times during the day and 1–2 times at night

CONTRAINDICATIONS

Epithelial herpes simplex keratitis (dendritic keratitis)

Vaccinia, varicella, and most other viral diseases of the cornea and conjunctiva

Mycobacterial infections of the eye

Fungal diseases of the eye

Following uncomplicated removal of a corneal foreign body

Known or suspected hypersensitivity to any component or to other sulfonamides or corticosteroids

ADMINISTRATION/DOSAGE ADJUSTMENTS

Duration of therapy — Do not discontinue treatment prematurely; in chronic conditions, withdraw treatment by gradually increasing the interval between applications

WARNINGS/PRECAUTIONS

Bacterial susceptibility — A significant percentage of staphyloccocal strains are totally resistant to sulfonamides

Initial prescription — Do not prescribe more than 8 g until the patient can be examined with the aid of magnification, such as slit-lamp microscopy, and, where appropriate, fluorescein staining

VASOCIDIN Ophthalmic Ointment ■ VASOCIDIN Ophthalmic Solution

Diseases causing corneal or scleral thinning	Perforation of the globe has been associated with topical steroid use in patients with diseases that cause corneal or scleral thinning
Herpetic keratitis	Topical steroids should be used with great caution in the treatment of herpes simplex
Prolonged use	Protracted use of these preparations may result in glaucoma, optic nerve damage, and visual acuity and field defects; check intraocular pressure frequently if used for 10 days or longer. Chronic therapy may also cause posterior subcapsular cataracts and promote secondary ocular infections; fungal invasion of the cornea should be suspected in any case of persistent corneal ulceration.
Concomitant infections	Topical steroid therapy may mask or enhance untreated acute, purulent infections of the eye and may exacerbate bacterial or fungal ocular infections
Hypersensitivity	Sensitization may recur when a sulfonamide is readministered, regardless of the route of administration; cross-sensitivity may also occur among different sulfonamides and different corticosteroids. Sulfonamides have been known to cause Steven's-Johnson syndrome and systemic lupus erythematosus in hypersensitive individuals (see ADVERSE REACTIONS). Discontinue use of this preparation if signs of hypersensitivity or other adverse reactions occur.
Corneal healing	Use of an ophthalmic ointment may retard corneal healing

ADVERSE REACTIONS

Ophthalmic	Irritation, elevation of intraocular pressure, possibly developing into glaucoma and infrequent optic nerve damage, posterior subcapsular cataract formation, delayed wound healing, secondary ocular infections, acute anterior uveitis, perforation of the globe, mydriasis, loss of accommodation, ptosis
Other	Allergic sensitization; Stevens-Johnson syndrome (one case), local hypersensitivity reaction progressing to a fatal syndrome resembling systemic lupus erythematosus (one case)

DRUG INTERACTIONS

Silver nitrate, mild silver protein	Incompatible with sulfacetamide; do not administer concurrently
Tetracaine	▽ Antibacterial activity of sulfacetamide

USE IN CHILDREN
See indications and dosage recommendations; do not use longer than absolutely necessary, since prolonged therapy increases the risk of adrenal suppression in children 2 yr of age or younger

USE IN PREGNANT AND NURSING WOMEN
The safety of intensive or prolonged topical steroid therapy during pregnancy has not been established. Specific guidelines are not available for use in nursing women; use according to medical judgment.

VEHICLE/BASE
Ointment: white petrolatum and mineral oil

[1] The use of an anti-infective steroid combination is indicated in those conditions where the risk of infection is high or it is anticipated that there are potentially dangerous numbers of bacteria present in the eye; the anti-infective component in this preparation is effective against the following pathogens: *Escherichia coli, Staphylococcus aureus, Streptococcus viridans, S pneumoniae, Pseudomonas* sp, *Hemophilus influenzae, Klebsiella* sp, and *Enterobacter* sp; it does not provide adequate coverage against *Neisseria* sp and *Serratia marcescens*. A significant percentage of staphylococcal isolates are completely resistant to sulfonamides.

OPHTHALMIC ANTI-INFECTIVES

VASOCIDIN Ophthalmic Solution (sulfacetamide sodium and prednisolone sodium phosphate) CooperVision Rx

Solution: 10% sulfacetamide sodium and prednisolone sodium phosphate equivalent to 0.23% prednisolone phosphate (5, 10 ml)

INDICATIONS[1]

Steroid-responsive inflammatory ophthalmic conditions, such as those of the palpebral and bulbar conjunctiva, cornea, and anterior segment of the globe
Chronic anterior uveitis
Corneal injury from chemical, radiation, or thermal burns or from penetration of foreign bodies

TOPICAL DOSAGE

Adult and child ($\geq$ 6 yr): 2 drops instilled into the eye(s) 4–6 times/day for mild infections and every hour for severe infections, tapering the dosage to discontinuation as the inflammation subsides

VASOCIDIN Ophthalmic Solution

CONTRAINDICATIONS

Acute epithelial herpes simplex keratitis (dendritic keratitis)	Following uncomplicated removal of a corneal foreign body	Fungal diseases of the eye
Vaccinia, varicella, and many other viral diseases of the cornea and conjunctiva	Mycobacterial infections of the eye	Known or suspected hypersensitivity to any component, mercury, or other sulfonamides or corticosteroids

ADMINISTRATION/DOSAGE ADJUSTMENTS

Duration of therapy — Treatment duration varies according to the type and severity of the infection and should be adjusted according to the individual patient's response; do not discontinue therapy prematurely. In chronic conditions, withdraw treatment by gradually increasing the intervals between applications.

WARNINGS/PRECAUTIONS

Bacterial susceptibility — A significant percentage of staphyloccocal strains are totally resistant to sulfonamides. If signs or symptoms of the infection persist or recur, eyelid cultures and tests may be indicated to determine the susceptibility of the causative organisms to this preparation. If it is suspected that the infection is caused by organisms that are not susceptible to sulfonamides, supplement therapy with a suitable antibiotic regimen; if a prompt favorable response is not seen, discontinue medication and institute appropriate treatment.

Initial prescription — Do not prescribe more than 20 ml until the patient can be examined with the aid of magnification, such as slit-lamp microscopy, and, where appropriate, fluorescein staining

Diseases causing corneal or scleral thinning — Perforation of the globe has been associated with topical steroid use in patients with diseases that cause corneal or scleral thinning

Herpetic keratitis — Use with great caution and observe patient closely; in patients with a history of herpetic infection of the cornea, reactivation may occur

Prolonged use — Protracted use of these preparations may result in glaucoma, optic nerve damage, and visual acuity and field defects; check intraocular pressure frequently if used for 10 days or longer. Use with caution in patients with glaucoma. Chronic therapy may also cause posterior subcapsular cataracts and promote secondary ocular infections; fungal invasion of the cornea should be suspected in any case of persistent corneal ulceration.

Patients susceptible to increased intraocular pressure — Patients who are particularly susceptible to increased intraocular pressure include those with a family history of open-angle glaucoma, those who exhibit a high degree of myopia, and those with diabetes mellitus

Concomitant infections — Topical steroid therapy may mask or enhance untreated acute, purulent infections of the eye and may exacerbate bacterial or fungal ocular infections. The *para*-aminobenzoic acid in purulent exudates may reduce the effectiveness of sulfonamides.

Hypersensitivity — Sensitization may recur when a sulfonamide is readministered, regardless of the route of administration; cross-sensitivity may also occur among different sulfonamides and different corticosteroids. Sulfonamides have been known to cause Stevens-Johnson syndrome and systemic lupus erythematosus in hypersensitive individuals. Discontinue use of this preparation if signs of hypersensitivity or other adverse reactions occur.

Uveitis — Acute anterior uveitis may occur in susceptible individuals, primarily blacks

Concomitant therapy — In deep-seated infections, such as endophthalmitis or panophthalmitis, or when there is threat of systemic infection, specific systemic antibiotic therapy should be instituted, using local treatment as adjunctive therapy, if desired. This medication is incompatible with silver preparations.

Patient instructions — Advise patient to discontinue use if inflammation or pain persists for longer than 48 h or if it worsens; the patient should also be warned not to touch the dropper tip to the eye

Carcinogenicity, mutagenicity — No long-term studies have been performed to determine the carcinogenic potential of either prednisolone or sulfacetamide; chromosomal nondisjunction has been detected in yeast cells (*Saccharomyces cerevisiae*) following application of sulfacetamide sodium, but the relevance of this finding to humans is unknown. Mutagenicity studies conducted with prednisolone have been negative.

Impairment of fertility — Long-term administration of high oral doses of prednisolone to dogs has blocked onset of estrus; oral doses of another glucocorticoid have caused a decrease in fertility in rats

Overdosage — Acute overdosage in humans will probably not lead to life-threatening situations. Oral doses of prednisolone exceeding 5 g/kg have not been fatal in rats; the oral LD_{50} of sulfacetamide in mice is 16.5 g/kg.

ADVERSE REACTIONS

Ophthalmic — Stinging, burning, irritation, elevation of intraocular pressure, possibly developing into glaucoma, and infrequent optic nerve damage, posterior subcapsular cataract formation, delayed wound healing, secondary ocular infections, anterior uveitis, perforation of the globe; mydriasis, loss of accommodation, ptosis; increased incidence of filtering blebs following cataract surgery

VASOCIDIN Ophthalmic Solution ■ VIROPTIC

Hypersensitivity	Allergic sensitization; Stevens-Johnson syndrome, systemic lupus erythematosus (including death in one case), exfoliative dermatitis, toxic epidermal necrolysis, and photosensitivity (rare)
Other	Systemic hypercorticoidism (rare)

DRUG INTERACTIONS

Silver nitrate, mild silver protein	Incompatible with sulfacetamide; do not administer concurrently
Tetracaine	▽ Antibacterial activity of sulfacetamide

USE IN CHILDREN

See INDICATIONS and TOPICAL DOSAGE; the safety and effectiveness of this preparation for children under 6 yr of age have not been established

USE IN PREGNANT AND NURSING WOMEN

Pregnancy Category C: use during pregnancy only if the potential benefits outweigh the possible risks to the fetus. Prednisolone has been shown to be teratogenic in animals; fetuses of mice who received multiples of the therapeutic dose in the eyes in 1 ml drops given 5 times/day have shown an increased incidence of cleft palate. No adequate, well-controlled studies have been done in pregnant women receiving corticosteroids. Animal reproduction studies have not been done with sulfacetamide sodium, and it is not known whether it can cause fetal harm when administered to a pregnant woman. Very small amounts of prednisolone appear in human milk after ophthalmic administration; use with caution in nursing women.

VEHICLE/BASE
Solution: edetate disodium, poloxamer 407, boric acid, 0.01% thimerosal, hydrochloric acid and/or sodium hydroxide (to adjust pH), and purified water

[1] The use of an anti-infective steroid combination is indicated in those conditions where the risk of infection is high or it is anticipated that there are potentially dangerous numbers of bacteria present in the eye; the anti-infective components in this preparation are effective against the following pathogens: *Staphylococcus aureus, Streptococcus pneumoniae,* viridans streptococci, *Pseudomonas* sp, *Hemophilus influenzae, Klebsiella* sp, *Enterobacter* sp, and *Escherichia coli;* it does not provide adequate coverage against *Neisseria* sp and *Serratia marcescens.* This preparation is not effective in treating mustard gas keratitis or Sjorgen's keratoconjunctivitis.

OPHTHALMIC ANTI-INFECTIVES

VIROPTIC Ophthalmic Solution (trifluridine) Burroughs Wellcome Rx

Solution: 1% (7.5 ml)

INDICATIONS

Acute keratoconjunctivitis and recurrent epithelial keratitis due to herpes simplex virus types 1 and 2[1]
Epithelial keratitis that is resistant to idoxuridine or when toxic or hypersensitivity reactions to idoxuridine preclude its use

TOPICAL DOSAGE

Adult and child: 1 drop q2h during waking hours, up to 9 doses/day, until re-epithelialization is complete; continue treatment for an additional 7 days after re-epithelialization has occurred at a level of 1 drop q4h during waking hours for a minimum of 5 doses/day

CONTRAINDICATIONS

Hypersensitivity or chemical intolerance to trifluridine

ADMINISTRATION/DOSAGE ADJUSTMENTS

Duration of therapy	If there are no signs of improvement after 7 days or if complete re-epithelialization has not occurred by 14 days, other forms of therapy should be considered; because of potential ocular toxicity, continuous therapy with trifluridine for more than 21 days should be avoided
Concomitant therapy	The following drugs have been administered topically in combination with trifluridine with no apparent adverse interaction: *antibiotics:* chloramphenicol, erythromycin, polymyxin B sulfate, bacitracin, gentamicin sulfate, tetracycline hydrochloride, sodium sulfacetamide, neomycin sulfate; *corticosteroids:* dexamethasone, dexamethasone sodium phosphate, prednisolone acetate, prednisolone sodium phosphate, hydrocortisone, fluorometholone; *other ophthalmic drugs:* atropine sulfate, scopolamine hydrobromide, naphazoline hydrochloride, cyclopentolate hydrochloride, homatropine hydrobromide, pilocarpine, epinephrine hydrochloride, and sodium chloride

WARNINGS/PRECAUTIONS

Diagnostic confirmation	This preparation should be prescribed only for those patients in whom a clinical diagnosis of herpetic keratitis has been established
Excessive application	Do not exceed the recommended dosage and frequency of administration given above; acute overdosage resulting from a single excessive ocular instillation is unlikely, however, because any excess solution should be quickly expelled from the conjunctival sac

VIROPTIC ■ DECADRON Phosphate

Irritation upon administration	Mild local irritation of the cornea and conjunctiva may occur upon instillation of trifluridine, but it is usually transient
Carcinogenicity, mutagenicity	Trifluridine has been shown to produce mutagenic effects, DNA damage, and cell transformation in vitro and acts as a clastogen in *Vicia faba* cells; although the significance of these effects is not fully understood, there is a possibility that genetic damage could occur in humans. The carcinogenic potential of trifluridine is presently unknown but is being evaluated in rodents.

ADVERSE REACTIONS

Frequent reactions (incidence ≥ 1%) are printed in *italics*

Ophthalmic	*Mild, transient burning or stinging upon instillation (4.6%), palpebral edema (2.8%),* superficial punctate keratopathy, epithelial keratopathy, hypersensitivity reactions, stromal edema, irritation, keratitis sicca, hyperemia, increased intraocular pressure

DRUG INTERACTIONS

No clinically significant drug interactions have been identified

USE IN CHILDREN

See indications and dosage recommendations

USE IN PREGNANT AND NURSING WOMEN

This drug should be used in pregnant women only if the potential therapeutic benefit justifies the potential risk to the fetus. Trifluridine was found to be teratogenic when injected directly into the yolk sac of developing chick embryos, and drug-induced fetal toxicity due to delayed ossification of portions of the skeletal system was observed in rats and rabbits given 2.5 mg/kg/day. No teratogenic effects were evidenced in rabbits who received topical applications of this preparation in the eyes on days 6–18 of pregnancy, or in rats and rabbits who received up to 5.0 mg/kg/day SC. Based on these findings, it is unlikely that trifluridine would cause embryonic or fetal damage when administered in the recommended ophthalmic dosage to pregnant women; a safe dose, however, has not been established for the human embryo or fetus. Do not use this drug in nursing women unless the potential benefit outweighs the possible risk. It is unlikely, however, that trifluridine is excreted in human milk, due to the relatively small dosage, its dilution in body fluids, and its extremely short half-life (~ 12 min).

VEHICLE/BASE
Solution: acetic acid, sodium acetate, sodium chloride, and 0.001% thimerosal

[1] The effectiveness of trifluridine in treating stromal keratitis and uveitis due to herpes simplex virus or ophthalmic infections caused by vaccinia virus or adenovirus has not been established. This preparation is not effective in the prophylaxis of herpes simplex virus keratoconjunctivitis and epithelial keratitis, or against bacterial, fungal, or chlamydial infections of the cornea or nonviral trophic lesions. Viral resistance to trifluridine has not been documented but may exist.

OPHTHALMIC CORTICOSTEROIDS

DECADRON Phosphate Ophthalmic Ointment (dexamethasone sodium phosphate) Merck Sharp & Dohme   Rx

Ointment: dexamethasone sodium phosphate equivalent to 0.05% dexamethasone phosphate (3.5 g)

INDICATIONS

Steroid-responsive inflammation of the palpebral and bulbar conjunctiva, cornea, and anterior segment of the globe, including allergic conjunctivitis, acne rosacea, superficial punctate keratitis, herpes zoster keratitis, iritis, cyclitis, and selected infective conjunctivitis

Corneal injury caused by chemical or thermal burns or by penetration of foreign bodies

TOPICAL DOSAGE

Adult: apply a thin film tid or qid to start; when a favorable response is obtained, reduce dosage to bid and later to once a day, if sufficient to control symptoms

DECADRON Phosphate Ophthalmic Solution (dexamethasone sodium phosphate) Merck Sharp & Dohme   Rx

Solution: dexamethasone sodium phosphate equivalent to 0.1% dexamethasone phosphate (5 ml)

INDICATIONS

Steroid-responsive inflammation of the palpebral and bulbar conjunctiva, cornea, and anterior segment of the globe, including allergic conjunctivitis, acne rosacea, superficial punctate keratitis, herpes zoster keratitis, iritis, cyclitis, and selected infective conjunctivitis

Corneal injury caused by chemical or thermal burns or by penetration of foreign bodies

TOPICAL DOSAGE

Adult: instill 1 drop every hour during the day and q2h at night to start; when a favorable response is obtained, reduce dosage to 1 drop q4h and later to 1 drop tid or qid, if sufficient to control symptoms

COMPENDIUM OF DRUG THERAPY

DECADRON Phosphate ■ FLUOR-OP

Steroid-responsive inflammation of the external auditory meatus

Adult: after thoroughly cleaning and drying the aural canal, instill 3–4 drops bid or tid; when a favorable response is obtained, reduce dosage gradually and eventually discontinue use. Alternatively, pack the aural canal with a gauze wick saturated with the solution; keep the wick moist with the solution and remove it after 12–24 h, repeating as needed.

CONTRAINDICATIONS

Epithelial herpes simplex keratitis (dendritic keratitis)

Fungal diseases of the eye or ear

Vaccinia, varicella, and most other viral diseases of the cornea and conjunctiva during acute, infectious stages

Tympanic membrane perforation

Mycobacterial infection of the eye

Hypersensitivity to any component, including sulfite-containing compounds

ADMINISTRATION/DOSAGE ADJUSTMENTS

Choice of dosage form — The ointment form is particularly convenient when an eye pad will be used, and provides longer contact with the eye

Duration of therapy — Treatment duration varies with the type of lesion and may range from a few days to several weeks, depending on patient response (see warning, below, regarding prolonged use); relapses, which are more common in chronic active lesions than in self-limited conditions, usually respond to retreatment

WARNINGS/PRECAUTIONS

Prolonged use — Protracted ophthalmic use of these preparations may result in ocular hypertension and/or glaucoma, optic nerve damage, visual acuity and field defects, and posterior subcapsular cataract formation; check intraocular pressure frequently if used for 10 days or longer. Chronic therapy may cause suppression of the host response and increase the risk of secondary infection; the possibility of persistent fungal infection of the cornea should be considered after long-term use.

Concomitant infections — Topical steroid therapy may mask or enhance untreated acute, purulent infections of the eye or ear

Herpes simplex — Use with great caution when treating herpes simplex other than epithelial herpes simplex keratitis; periodic slit-lamp examinations are essential

Diseases causing corneal or scleral thinning — Perforation of the globe has occurred with topical steroid use in patients with diseases that cause corneal or scleral thinning

Hypersensitivity — The solution contains sodium bisulfite; sulfites have reportedly caused severe allergic reactions in susceptible individuals, particularly asthmatics

Carcinogenicity, effect on fertility — No long-term studies have been performed to determine the carcinogenic potential of this drug or its effect on fertility

ADVERSE REACTIONS

Ophthalmic — Glaucoma with optic nerve damage, visual acuity and field defects, posterior subcapsular cataract formation, secondary ocular infection, perforation of the globe; stinging or burning after instillation, filtering blebs following cataract surgery (rare)

DRUG INTERACTIONS

No clinically significant drug interactions have been identified

USE IN CHILDREN

Safety and effectiveness for use in children have not been established

USE IN PREGNANT AND NURSING WOMEN

Pregnancy Category C: dexamethasone has been shown to be teratogenic in mice and rabbits following topical ophthalmic application at doses greater than the therapeutic dose; fetal resorptions and cleft palate have occurred in mice given corticosteroids, and fetal resorptions and multiple abnormalities involving the head, ears, limbs, and palate have occurred in rabbits. No adequate, well-controlled studies have been performed in pregnant women; use during pregnancy only if the expected benefit outweighs the potential risk. Infants born of mothers who have received substantial doses of corticosteroids during pregnancy should be observed carefully for signs of hypoadrenalism. Topical corticosteroids are absorbed systemically; patients should not nurse during therapy.

VEHICLE/BASE
Ointment: white petrolatum and mineral oil
Solution: 0.1% sodium bisulfite, 0.25% phenylethanol, 0.02% benzalkonium chloride, creatinine, sodium citrate, sodium borate, polysorbate 80, disodium edetate, hydrochloric acid (to adjust pH), and water for injection

---

OPHTHALMIC CORTICOSTEROIDS

FLUOR-OP Ophthalmic Suspension (fluorometholone) CooperVision   Rx

Suspension: 0.1% (5, 10, 15 ml)

INDICATIONS

Corticosteroid-responsive inflammation of the palpebral and bulbar conjunctiva, cornea, and anterior segment of the globe

TOPICAL DOSAGE

Adult and child: 1 drop instilled into the eye(s) bid to qid (in severe cases, administer 2 drops every hour for the first 24–48 h); do not discontinue treatment prematurely

FLUOR-OP ■ FML

CONTRAINDICATIONS

Acute superficial herpes simplex keratitis	Vaccinia, varicella, and most other viral diseases of the cornea and conjunctiva	Hypersensitivity to any component
Fungal diseases of the eye	Tuberculosis of the eye	

WARNINGS/PRECAUTIONS

Prolonged use	Protracted use of this preparation may result in glaucoma, optic nerve damage, and visual acuity and field defects; check intraocular pressure frequently. Chronic therapy may also cause posterior subcapsular cataracts and promote secondary ocular infections; fungal invasion of the cornea must be suspected in any case of persistent corneal ulceration.
Concomitant infections	Topical steroid therapy may mask or enhance untreated acute, purulent infections of the eye
Stromal herpetic keratitis	Use with great caution when treating herpes simplex keratitis involving the stroma; frequent slit-lamp examinations are mandatory
Diseases causing corneal or scleral thinning	Perforation of the globe has occurred with topical steroid use in patients with diseases that cause corneal or scleral thinning

ADVERSE REACTIONS

Ophthalmic	Glaucoma and optic nerve damage; loss of visual acuity; visual field defects; posterior subcapsular cataract formation; secondary ocular infections; perforation of the globe

DRUG INTERACTIONS

No clinically significant drug interactions have been identified

---

USE IN CHILDREN

Safety and effectiveness have not been established in children 2 yr of age and younger

USE IN PREGNANT AND NURSING WOMEN

Safety and effectiveness for use in pregnant and nursing women have not been established

---

VEHICLE/BASE
Suspension: 1.4% polyvinyl alcohol, 0.004% benzalkonium chloride, edetate disodium, sodium chloride, sodium phosphate monobasic (monohydrate), sodium phosphate dibasic (anhydrous), polysorbate 80, sodium hydroxide (to adjust pH), and purified water

---

OPHTHALMIC CORTICOSTEROIDS

FML Ophthalmic Ointment and Suspension (fluorometholone) Allergan   Rx
Ointment: 0.1% (3.5 g) Suspension: 0.1% (5, 10, 15 ml)

FML Forte Ophthalmic Suspension (fluorometholone) Allergan   Rx
Suspension: 0.25% (5, 10, 15 ml)

INDICATIONS

Corticosteroid-responsive inflammation of the palpebral and bulbar conjunctiva, cornea, and anterior segment of the globe

TOPICAL DOSAGE

Adult and child: 1 drop instilled into the eye(s) bid to qid, or apply a small amount of ointment into the conjunctival sac(s) up to tid (in severe cases, administer 1 drop of the 0.25% suspension more frequently or 2 drops of the 0.1% suspension every hour or apply ointment q4h for the first 24–48 h); do not discontinue treatment prematurely

CONTRAINDICATIONS

Epithelial herpes simplex keratitis (dendritic keratitis)	Vaccinia, varicella, and other viral diseases of the cornea and conjunctiva	Hypersensitivity to any component
Fungal diseases of the eye	Tuberculosis of the eye	

ADMINISTRATION/DOSAGE ADJUSTMENTS

Persistent inflammation	If inflammation persists after 2 wk of therapy, reevaluate patient's condition

WARNINGS/PRECAUTIONS

Prolonged use	Protracted use of this preparation may result in glaucoma, optic nerve damage, and visual acuity and field defects; check intraocular pressure frequently. Chronic therapy may also cause posterior subcapsular cataracts and promote secondary ocular infections; fungal invasion of the cornea should be suspected in any case of persistent corneal ulceration.

FML ■ INFLAMASE/INFLAMASE FORTE

Concomitant infections	Topical steroid therapy may mask or enhance untreated acute, purulent infections of the eye
Stromal herpetic keratitis	Use with great caution when treating herpes simplex keratitis involving the stroma; frequent slit-lamp examinations are mandatory
Diseases causing corneal or scleral thinning	Perforation of the globe has occurred with topical steroid use in patients with diseases that cause corneal or scleral thinning
Corneal healing	Use of an ophthalmic ointment may retard corneal healing
Carcinogenicity, mutagenicity, effect on fertility	No studies have been done with these preparations to evaluate their carcinogenic or mutagenic potential or their effect, if any, on fertility

ADVERSE REACTIONS[1]

Ophthalmic	Elevation of intraocular pressure with possible development of glaucoma and optic nerve damage; loss of visual acuity; visual field defects; posterior subcapsular cataract formation; delayed wound healing, conjunctival erythema; secondary ocular infections; perforation of the globe (rare)

DRUG INTERACTIONS

No clinically significant drug interactions have been identified

---

USE IN CHILDREN

Safety and effectiveness of the 0.1% suspension have not been established in children 2 yr of age and younger; safety and effectiveness of the 0.25% suspension have not been established in children

USE IN PREGNANT AND NURSING WOMEN

Pregnancy Category C: fluorometholone has been shown to be embryocidal and teratogenic in rabbits given doses approximating the usual human dose and above. Fluorometholone caused a significant dose-related increase in fetal abnormalities and fetal loss when applied ocularly to both eyes of pregnant rabbits at various dosage levels on days 6–18 of gestation. However, no adequate, well-controlled studies have been done in pregnant women. Use during pregnancy only if the expected benefit outweighs the potential risk to the fetus. Specific guidelines are not available for use in nursing women; use according to medical judgment.

VEHICLE/BASE
FML Ointment: 0.0008% phenylmercuric acetate, white petrolatum, mineral oil, and petrolatum (and) lanolin alcohol
FML Suspension: 1.4% polyvinyl alcohol (Liquifilm), benzalkonium chloride, edetate disodium, sodium chloride, sodium phosphate monobasic (monohydrate), sodium phosphate dibasic (anhydrous), polysorbate 80, sodium hydroxide (to adjust pH), and purified water
FML Forte Suspension: 1.4% polyvinyl alcohol (Liquifilm), 0.005% benzalkonium chloride, edetate disodium, sodium chloride, sodium biphosphate, sodium phosphate, polysorbate 80, sodium hydroxide (to adjust pH), and purified water

[1] Includes reactions associated with topical corticosteroids in general

---

OPHTHALMIC CORTICOSTEROIDS

INFLAMASE 1/8% Ophthalmic Solution (prednisolone sodium phosphate) CooperVision   Rx

Solution: 0.125% prednisolone sodium phosphate, equivalent to 0.11% prednisolone (5, 10 ml)

INFLAMASE Forte 1% Ophthalmic Solution (prednisolone sodium phosphate) CooperVision   Rx

Solution (per milliliter): 1% prednisolone sodium phosphate, equivalent to 0.9% prednisolone (5, 10 ml)

INDICATIONS[1]

Steroid-responsive inflammation of the palpebral and bulbar conjunctiva, cornea, and anterior segment of the globe, including allergic conjunctivitis, acne rosacea, superficial punctate keratitis, herpes zoster keratitis, iritis, cyclitis, and selected infective conjunctivitis
Corneal injury caused by chemical, radiation, or thermal burns, or by penetration of foreign bodies

TOPICAL DOSAGE

Adult: 1 drop instilled up to every hour during the day and q2h at night to start, depending on severity of symptoms; when a favorable response is obtained, reduce dosage to 1 drop q4h and, later, 1 drop tid or qid if sufficient to control symptoms

CONTRAINDICATIONS

Acute, superficial herpes simplex keratitis

Fungal diseases of the eye

Acute, infectious stages of vaccinia, varicella, and most other viral diseases of the cornea and conjunctiva

Tuberculosis of the eye

Following uncomplicated removal of a superficial corneal foreign body

Hypersensitivity to any component

INFLAMASE/INFLAMASE FORTE ■ NAPHCON-A

ADMINISTRATION/DOSAGE ADJUSTMENTS

Systemic therapy — In some stubborn cases of anterior segment eye disease, or when the deeper ocular structures are involved, systemic adrenocortical hormone therapy may be necessary

Duration of therapy — Duration of treatment varies with the type of lesion and may extend from a few days to several weeks, depending on therapeutic response; relapses tend to be more common in chronic conditions than self-limiting conditions and usually respond to treatment

WARNINGS/PRECAUTIONS

Prolonged use — Protracted ophthalmic use of these preparations may result in increased intraocular pressure and/or glaucoma, optic nerve damage, and visual acuity and field defects; check intraocular pressure frequently. Chronic therapy may also cause posterior subcapsular cataracts and promote secondary ocular infections; fungal invasion of the cornea should be suspected in any case of persistent corneal ulceration.

Concomitant infections — Topical steroid therapy may mask or enhance untreated acute, purulent infections of the eye; if infection is present, institute appropriate antimicrobial therapy. Viral, bacterial, or fungal corneal infections may be exacerbated by topical steroid therapy.

Stromal herpetic keratitis — Use with great caution when treating herpes simplex keratitis involving the stroma; frequent slit-lamp examinations are mandatory

Diseases causing corneal or scleral thinning — Perforation of the globe has occurred with topical steroid use in patients with diseases that cause corneal or scleral thinning

Patient instructions — Advise the patient to discontinue use and report back if irritation persists or develops; the patient should also be instructed not to touch the dropper tip to the eyelids or surrounding area to avoid contamination of the tip or solution and to keep bottle tightly closed, away from light, and at room temperature

ADVERSE REACTIONS

Ophthalmic — Glaucoma with optic nerve damage, visual acuity and field defects, posterior subcapsular cataract formation, secondary ocular infection from pathogens, including herpes simplex and fungi; perforation of the globe

DRUG INTERACTIONS

No clinically significant drug interactions have been identified

---

USE IN CHILDREN

Safety and effectiveness for use in children have not been established; do not use longer than absolutely necessary, since prolonged therapy increases the risk of adrenal suppression in children 2 yr of age and younger

USE IN PREGNANT AND NURSING WOMEN

Pregnancy Category C: reproduction studies have not been done in animals, nor is it known whether prednisolone can cause harm to the fetus when administered to a pregnant woman or affect reproductive capacity. Use during pregnancy only if clearly needed. Specific guidelines are not available for use in nursing women; use according to medical judgment.

VEHICLE/BASE
Solution: edetate disodium, benzalkonium chloride, biphosphate, anhydrous sodium phosphate, sodium chloride, and purified water

[1] These drugs are not effective in treating mustard gas keratitis and Sjorgen's keratoconjunctivitis

---

OPHTHALMIC DECONGESTANTS/ANTIALLERGIC AGENTS

NAPHCON-A Ophthalmic Solution (naphazoline hydrochloride and pheniramine maleate) Alcon Rx

Solution: 0.025% naphazoline hydrochloride and 0.3% pheniramine maleate (5, 15 ml)

INDICATIONS

Ocular irritation and/or congestion[1]
Allergic or inflammatory ocular conditions[1]

TOPICAL DOSAGE

Adult: 1 drop instilled into the eye(s) up to q3-4h, as needed

CONTRAINDICATIONS

Hypersensitivity to any component

WARNINGS/PRECAUTIONS

Patients receiving MAO inhibitors — Concomitant therapy with an MAO inhibitor may result in a severe hypertensive crisis

NAPHCON-A ■ NEO-SYNEPHRINE

Other special-risk patients	Use with caution in elderly patients with severe cardiac disease, including cardiac arrhythmias; patients with poorly controlled hypertension; and those with diabetes, especially patients with a tendency toward diabetic ketoacidosis.

ADVERSE REACTIONS

Ophthalmic	Mydriasis, increased intraocular pressure
Systemic	Hypertension, cardiac irregularities, hyperglycemia

DRUG INTERACTIONS

MAO inhibitors	Severe hypertensive crisis

USE IN CHILDREN
CNS depression leading to coma and marked hypothermia may occur if this drug is used in infants or children

USE IN PREGNANT AND NURSING WOMEN
Specific guidelines are not available; use according to medical judgment

---

VEHICLE/BASE
Solution: 0.01% benzalkonium chloride, boric acid, sodium borate, edetate disodium, sodium chloride, sodium hydroxide and/or hydrochloric acid (to adjust pH), and purified water

[1] Possibly effective

OPHTHALMIC DECONGESTANTS/ANTIALLERGIC AGENTS

NEO-SYNEPHRINE Ophthalmic Solution (phenylephrine hydrochloride) Winthrop-Breon   Rx

Low surface tension solution: 2.5% (15 ml), 10% (5 ml)   Viscous solution: 10% (5 ml)

INDICATIONS	TOPICAL DOSAGE
Mydriasis and vasoconstriction	**Adult:** 1 drop of the 10% solution, followed, if necessary, by a second dose 1 h later (see "use of topical anesthetics," below)
Posterior synechiae associated with uveitis	**Adult:** to free recently formed synechiae, apply 1 drop of the 10% solution to the upper surface of the cornea, followed, if necessary, by a second dose the next day; between doses, apply hot compresses for 5–10 min tid, with 1 drop of a 1% or 2% atropine sulfate solution before and after each compress application
Increased intraocular pressure associated with wide-angle glaucoma	**Adult:** for temporary reduction of intraocular pressure, 1 drop of the 10% solution to the upper surface of the cornea; repeat dose as needed
Intraocular surgery	**Adult:** to produce mydriasis, 1 drop of the 2.5% or 10% solution 30–60 min prior to surgery (see "use of topical anesthetics," below)
Refraction studies	**Adult:** 1 drop of the 2.5% solution in each eye; instill 1 drop of an appropriate cycloplegic (atropine, homatropine, or a combination of homatropine and cocaine) 5 min before and 10 min after application of phenylephrine. Alternatively, administer the 2.5% solution and the cycloplegic in a single dose (a more concentrated cycloplegic solution may be necessary). Perform the examination 50–60 min after the last dose. **Child:** 1 drop of the 2.5% solution in each eye; instill 1 drop of 1% atropine sulfate 10–15 min before and 5–10 min after application of phenylephrine. Alternatively, administer the 2.5% solution and atropine in a single dose (a more concentrated atropine solution may be necessary). Perform the examination 1–2 h after the last dose.
Ophthalmoscopic examination	**Adult:** 1 drop of the 2.5% solution in each eye 15–30 min prior to examination
Diagnostic procedures	**Adult:** for the provocative test for narrow-angle glaucoma when latent increased intraocular pressure is suspected, use the 2.5% solution; a rise in pressure of 3–5 mm Hg suggests the presence of narrow-angle glaucoma (negative findings do not, however, rule out glaucoma due to other causes). For the shadow test (retinoscopy), use the 2.5% solution alone to produce mydriasis without cycloplegia. For the blanching test, apply 1–2 drops of the 2.5% solution to the injected eye and examine the eye for perilimbal blanching 5 min later; if blanching occurs, the congestion is probably superficial and not due to iritis.

CONTRAINDICATIONS

Narrow-angle glaucoma	Administration to infants (10% solution only)	Aneurysm (10% solution only)
Hypersensitivity to any component		

ADMINISTRATION/DOSAGE ADJUSTMENTS

Use of topical anesthetics	To prevent pain and consequent dilution of the phenylephrine solution by lacrimation, apply 1 drop of a suitable topical anesthetic a few minutes before instilling 10% phenylephrine (phenylephrine is incompatible with butacaine)
Concomitant use of miotics	In patients with wide-angle glaucoma, phenylephrine may be given in combination with a miotic to improve visual acuity; phenylephrine enlarges the small field produced by miosis, but does not interfere with the effect of the miotic on intraocular pressure

WARNINGS/PRECAUTIONS

Cardiovascular reactions	A systemic vasopressor response may occur when the recommended dosage is exceeded, lacrimation is suppressed (as during anesthesia), or the eye or its adnexa are subjected to stress (eg, by disease, trauma, or surgery). Serious, potentially fatal reactions, including ventricular arrhythmias, myocardial infarction, and significant blood-pressure elevation, may result in rare instances from use of the 10% solution (these reactions usually have occurred in elderly patients with preexisting cardiovascular disease). Administer the 10% solution with caution to elderly patients, children with low body weights, and patients with insulin-dependent diabetes, hyperthyroidism, or cardiovascular disease (including hypertension and generalized arteriosclerosis); the blood pressure of these patients, as well as other patients who manifest cardiovascular symptoms in response to the solution, should be carefully monitored. The hypertensive effects of phenylephrine may be treated with an alpha-adrenergic blocker, such as phentolamine (5–10 mg, given IV and repeated as necessary).
Elderly patients	Serious cardiovascular reactions have occurred after use of the 10% solution (see warning above). Transient pigment floaters, which may resemble microscopic hyphema or signs of anterior uveitis, may develop in the aqueous humor 30–45 min after instillation. Rebound miosis and a reduction in mydriasis (with a second dose) may occur the day after this drug is used; this may be important when mydriasis is required prior to retinal detachment or cataract surgery.
Patients with wide-angle glaucoma	Mydriatics are generally contraindicated in patients with glaucoma because they may occasionally increase intraocular pressure. However, when vasoconstriction of intrinsic vessels may lower intraocular pressure or when temporary dilatation of the pupil may free adhesions or improve visual acuity, the benefits for patients with wide-angle glaucoma may temporarily outweigh the risks.
Patients with uveitis	The hyperemic response to uveal infection may be opposed by phenylephrine-induced vasoconstriction
Patients receiving MAO inhibitors	To avoid enhancement of the pressor effects of phenylephrine, adjust dosage and provide careful supervision when this drug is given with an MAO inhibitor or within 21 days after use of an MAO inhibitor has been discontinued
Carcinogenicity, mutagenicity, effect on fertility	No long-term studies have been done in animals to determine the carcinogenic or mutagenic potential of this drug or its effect on fertility

ADVERSE REACTIONS

Ophthalmic	Increased intraocular pressure; transient pigment floaters resembling microscopic hyphema or signs of anterior uveitis, rebound miosis, reduction in mydriasis (in elderly patients)
Systemic	Ventricular arrhythmias, myocardial infarction, hypertension (rare; with 10% solution)

OVERDOSAGE

Signs and symptoms	Ventricular arrhythmias, myocardial infarction, hypertension (rare)
Treatment	To treat hypertensive effects, administer an alpha-adrenergic blocker, such as 5–10 mg phentolamine, given IV and repeated as needed

DRUG INTERACTIONS

MAO inhibitors, tricyclic antidepressants, propranolol, reserpine, guanethidine, methyldopa, atropine-like drugs	⇧ Vasopressor effects of phenylephrine (see warning above regarding MAO inhibitors)
Beta blockers	Acute hypertension Ruptured congenital cerebral aneurysm (one case)

USE IN CHILDREN

See INDICATIONS and TOPICAL DOSAGE; use of the 10% solution is contraindicated in infants

USE IN PREGNANT AND NURSING WOMEN

Pregnancy Category C: reproduction studies have not been done in animals; it is not known whether phenylephrine can cause harm to the fetus or affect reproductive capacity. Use during pregnancy only if clearly needed. It is not known whether phenylephrine is excreted in human milk; because many drugs are, use with caution in nursing women.

VEHICLE/BASE
Low surface tension solution (2.5%): sodium phosphate, sodium biphosphate, boric acid, benzalkonium chloride 1:7,500, and phosphoric acid or sodium hydroxide (to adjust pH)
Low surface tension solution (10%): sodium phosphate, sodium biphosphate, benzalkonium chloride 1:10,000, and phosphoric acid or sodium hydroxide (to adjust pH)
Viscous solution: sodium phosphate, sodium biphosphate, methylcellulose, benzalkonium chloride 1:10,000, and phosphoric acid or sodium hydroxide (to adjust pH)

OPHTHALMIC DECONGESTANTS/ANTIALLERGIC AGENTS

OPTICROM 4% Ophthalmic Solution (cromolyn sodium) Fisons Rx

Solution: 4% (10 ml)

INDICATIONS

Vernal keratoconjunctivitis, vernal conjunctivitis, giant papillary conjunctivitis, vernal keratitis, and allergic keratoconjunctivitis

TOPICAL DOSAGE

Adult and child ($\geq$ 4 yr): 1–2 drops instilled into each eye 4–6 times/day at regular intervals

CONTRAINDICATIONS

Hypersensitivity to cromolyn sodium or any other component

Wearing of soft contact lenses (due to benzalkonium chloride preservative)

ADMINISTRATION/DOSAGE ADJUSTMENTS

Duration of therapy	Symptomatic response (decreased itching, tearing, redness, and discharge) usually occurs within a few days; however, therapy for up to 6 wk is sometimes needed. Once symptomatic improvement has been established, continue therapy for as long as is needed to sustain improvement.
Concomitant therapy	If needed, corticosteroids may be given concomitantly

WARNINGS/PRECAUTIONS

Soft contact lenses	As with all preparations containing benzalkonium chloride, this solution should not be used while soft contact lenses are worn; patient can resume wearing soft lenses a few hours after the drug is discontinued
Transient stinging or burning	Following application, some transient stinging or burning may be experienced
Carcinogenicity, mutagenicity, effect on fertility	Long-term SC or intraperitoneal administration of cromolyn had no effect on the incidence of neoplasia in mice, hamsters, and rats. No evidence of chromosomal damage or cytotoxicity has been found in mutagenicity tests. Reproduction studies in animals have shown no evidence of impaired fertility.
Patient instructions	To avoid contamination, advise patient to discard the bottle and any remaining contents 4 wk after the blister pack is opened

ADVERSE REACTIONS

The most frequent reaction is italicized

Ophthalmic	*Transient stinging or burning,* conjunctival injection, watery or itchy eyes, dryness around the eye, puffiness, irritation, styes

OVERDOSAGE

Cromolyn is poorly absorbed; in normal volunteers, approximately 0.03% of a dose is absorbed systematically after ophthalmic administration

DRUG INTERACTIONS

No clinically significant drug interactions have been identified

---

USE IN CHILDREN

See INDICATIONS and TOPICAL DOSAGE; safety and effectiveness have not been established in children under 4 yr of age

USE IN PREGNANT AND NURSING WOMEN

Pregnancy Category B: reproduction studies in mice, rats, and rabbits injected with up to 338 times the human dose have shown no evidence of fetal malformations; an increase in resorptions and a decrease in fetal weight have been observed only at dosages that produced maternal toxicity. No adequate, well-controlled studies have been performed in pregnant women; use during pregnancy only if clearly needed. It is not known whether cromolyn is excreted in human milk; use with caution in nursing mothers.

VEHICLE/BASE
Solution: 0.4% phenylethyl alcohol, 0.01% benzalkonium chloride, 0.01% EDTA, and purified water

---

OPHTHALMIC DECONGESTANTS/ANTIALLERGIC AGENTS

VASOCON-A Ophthalmic Solution (naphazoline hydrochloride and antazoline phosphate) CooperVision Rx

Solution: 0.05% naphazoline hydrochloride and 0.5% antazoline phosphate (15 ml)

INDICATIONS

Ocular irritation and/or congestion[1]
Allergic, inflammatory, or infectious ocular conditions[1]

TOPICAL DOSAGE

Adult: 1 drop instilled into the eye(s) up to q3–4h, as needed

VASOCON-A ■ AMERICAINE-Otic

CONTRAINDICATIONS

| Anatomically narrow angle or narrow-angle glaucoma | Wearing of contact lenses | Hypersensitivity to any component |

WARNINGS/PRECAUTIONS

Patients receiving MAO inhibitor therapy	Concomitant therapy with an MAO inhibitor may result in a severe hypertensive crisis
Other special-risk patients	Use with caution in patients with hypertension, cardiac irregularities, hyperglycemia (diabetes), hyperthyroidism; eye disease, infection, or injury; and in conjunction with other medications
CNS depression	Use of this preparation may cause CNS depression leading to coma and marked hypothermia in children, especially infants
Patient instructions	Advise patient to report severe eye pain, headache, rapid change in direct or peripheral vision, sudden appearance of floating spots, acute eye redness, pain on exposure to light, or double vision; the patient should also be advised that overuse of this product may produce increased ocular redness and irritation
Contamination	To prevent contamination, avoid touching dropper tip to eyelid or any other surface; keep bottle tightly closed when not in use and protect from light
Carcinogenicity, mutagenicity, effect on fertility	No long-term studies have been done in animals with either naphazoline or antazoline to determine their carcinogenic or mutagenic potential or their effect on fertility

ADVERSE REACTIONS

| Ophthalmic | Mydriasis, increased or decreased intraocular pressure; mild, transient stinging, burning, tearing, diffuse epithelial haze |
| Systemic | Hypertension, cardiac irregularities, hyperglycemia, hypothermia, lightheadedness, weakness, nausea, nervousness, anaphylactic reaction (rare); drowsiness; coma (in children) |

DRUG INTERACTIONS

| MAO inhibitors | Severe hypertensive crisis |

USE IN CHILDREN

Safety and effectiveness for use in children have not been established; CNS depression leading to coma and marked hypothermia may occur if this drug is used in children, especially infants

---

USE IN PREGNANT AND NURSING WOMEN

Pregnancy Category C: reproduction studies have not been done in animals with either component of this preparation, nor is it known whether administration of naphazoline or antazoline, either alone or in combination, to a pregnant woman can cause harm to the fetus or affect reproductive capacity. Use during pregnancy only when clearly needed. It is also not known whether either component is excreted in human milk; because many drugs are, use with caution in nursing women.

VEHICLE/BASE
Solution: polyethylene glycol 8000, sodium chloride, polyvinyl alcohol, edetate disodium, purified water, 0.01% benzalkonium chloride, and sodium hydroxide and/or hydrochloric acid (to adjust pH)

[1] Possibly effective

OTIC ANALGESICS/ANESTHETICS

AMERICAINE-Otic (benzocaine) Du Pont Critical Care   Rx
Drops: 20% (½ fl oz)

INDICATIONS

Pain and pruritus of acute congestive and serous otitis media, acute swimmer's ear, and otitis externa

TOPICAL DOSAGE

Adult: instill 4–5 drops of warm solution along side of ear canal (to prevent air pocket) and insert cotton pledget in meatus; patient should be laid on side with affected ear up and should remain in this position for about 10 min after instillation of drops; may be repeated q1–2h, if needed
Child (1–12 yr): same as adult

CONTRAINDICATIONS

Age < 1 yr

WARNINGS/PRECAUTIONS

| Local reactions | If sensitivity occurs, discontinue medication |

COMPENDIUM OF DRUG THERAPY

AMERICAINE-Otic ■ TYMPAGESIC Otic Solution

| Fulminating middle-ear infection | Symptoms may be masked by indiscriminate use of anesthetic ear drops |

ADVERSE REACTIONS
None reported by manufacturer

USE IN CHILDREN
Same as adult indications and dosage; contraindicated for use in infants under 1 yr of age

USE IN PREGNANT AND NURSING WOMEN
No clinically significant problems have occurred from use of this drug in pregnant or nursing women

VEHICLE/BASE
Drops: 1% glycerin, polyethylene glycol-300, and 0.1% benzethonium chloride

---

OTIC ANALGESICS/ANESTHETICS

AURALGAN Otic Solution (antipyrine and benzocaine) Ayerst Rx

Drops (per milliliter): 54 mg antipyrine and 14 mg benzocaine (10 ml)

INDICATIONS
Pain and inflammation of acute congestive and serous otitis media
As an adjunct to systemic antibiotics for resolution of **acute otitis media**

Removal of cerumen

TOPICAL DOSAGE
Adult: instill solution, permitting it to run along wall of ear canal until filled, and insert cotton pledget moistened with solution into meatus; repeat q1–2h until pain and congestion are relieved
Child: same as adult

Adult: instill solution and insert cotton pledget moistened with solution into meatus tid for 2–3 days; after cerumen is removed, instill solution and insert a moistened cotton pledget into meatus to dry out canal and relieve discomfort
Child: same as adult

CONTRAINDICATIONS
| Spontaneous perforation or discharge | Hypersensitivity to any component or related substances |

WARNINGS/PRECAUTIONS
| Carcinogenicity, mutagenicity | No long-term studies have been conducted in either animals or man to determine the carcinogenicity or mutagenicity of this preparation |

ADVERSE REACTIONS
Consult manufacturer

USE IN CHILDREN
Same as adult indications and dosage

USE IN PREGNANT AND NURSING WOMEN
Pregnancy Category C: use during pregnancy only when clearly needed. Animal reproduction studies have not been done, nor are the effects of this drug on human reproductive capacity or fetal development known. It is also not known whether this drug is excreted in human milk; use with caution in nursing mothers.

VEHICLE/BASE
Drops: glycerin and oxyquinoline sulfate

OTIC ANALGESICS/ANESTHETICS

TYMPAGESIC Otic Solution (phenylephrine hydrochloride, antipyrine, and benzocaine) Adria Rx

Drops: 0.25% phenylephrine hydrochloride, 5% antipyrine, and 5% benzocaine (13 ml)

INDICATIONS
Pain in the external auditory canal
As an adjunct to systemic antibiotics for **acute otitis media**

TOPICAL DOSAGE
Adult: using the dropper, instill solution into the external ear canal until it is filled, then plug the meatus with a solution-moistened cotton pledget; repeat q2–4h, if needed, until pain is relieved

TYMPAGESIC Otic Solution ■ CHLOROMYCETIN Otic

CONTRAINDICATIONS

Hypersensitivity to any component[1] | Perforated tympanic membrane | Ear discharge

WARNINGS/PRECAUTIONS

Systemic reactions — May occur; phenylephrine may cause blanching and a feeling of coolness in the skin, while benzocaine and antipyrine may produce CNS stimulation with nausea and vomiting, as well as allergic and idiosyncratic reactions. Such reactions, however, are unlikely because of minimal absorption from the ear drum and external ear canal.

Special-risk patients — Use with caution in the elderly and in patients with hypertension, increased intraocular pressure, diabetes mellitus, ischemic heart disease, hyperthyroidism, and prostatic hypertrophy

Carcinogenicity, mutagenicity — No studies have been done to evaluate the carcinogenic or mutagenic potential of this drug

ADVERSE REACTIONS

Central nervous system — Restlessness, anxiety, nervousness, weakness, headache, dizziness, tinnitus

Gastrointestinal — Nausea, vomiting

Hypersensitivity — Rash, urticaria, edema; contact dermatitis characterized by erythema and pruritus, which may progress to vesiculation and oozing

Cardiovascular — Elevation in blood pressure, pallor

Other — Chills, agranulocytosis

OVERDOSAGE

Signs and symptoms — *Phenylephrine-related effects:* hypertension, headache, vomiting, palpitations; *benzocaine-related effects:* yawning, restlessness, excitement, nausea, vomiting; *antipyrine-related effects:* giddiness, tremor, sweating, skin eruptions

Treatment — Treat symptomatically; if ingestion of a bottle or more of the drug is recent, or if there is food present in the stomach, induction of emesis with ipecac syrup, gastric emptying and lavage, and administration of activated charcoal may be advisable

DRUG INTERACTIONS

MAO inhibitors, beta-adrenergic blockers — △ Sympathomimetic effects

Sulfonamides — ▽ Antibacterial activity

ALTERED LABORATORY VALUES

No clinically significant alterations in blood/serum or urinary values occur at therapeutic dosages

---

USE IN CHILDREN

Safety and effectiveness for use in children under 12 yr of age have not been established

USE IN PREGNANT AND NURSING WOMEN

Pregnancy Category C: use during pregnancy only if clearly needed. Animal reproduction studies have not been performed with this drug, nor is it known whether it can affect reproductive capacity or cause fetal harm in humans. It is not known whether this drug is excreted in human milk; because many drugs are excreted in human milk, use with caution in nursing women.

VEHICLE/BASE
Drops: propylene glycol

[1] Cross-sensitivity between "caine" anesthetics has been reported

---

OTIC ANTI-INFECTIVES

CHLOROMYCETIN Otic (chloramphenicol) Parke-Davis   Rx

Drops: 0.5% (15 ml)

INDICATIONS

Superficial infections of the external auditory canal caused by susceptible organisms, including susceptible strains of *Staphylococcus aureus, Escherichia coli, Hemophilus influenzae, Pseudomonas aeruginosa, Aerobacter aerogenes, Klebsiella pneumoniae,* and *Proteus*

TOPICAL DOSAGE

Adult: instill 2–3 drops into the ear tid

COMPENDIUM OF DRUG THERAPY

CHLOROMYCETIN Otic ■ COLY-MYCIN S Otic

CONTRAINDICATIONS
Sensitivity to any component

WARNINGS/PRECAUTIONS

Systemic absorption	May occur; bone marrow hypoplasia, including aplastic anemia and death, has been reported following local application of chloramphenicol. Chloramphenicol should not be used when less potentially dangerous agents would be expected to provide effective treatment.
Overgrowth of nonsusceptible organisms	Nonsusceptible organisms, including fungi, may proliferate during treatment; discontinue use and institute appropriate therapeutic measures
Supplemental therapy	Appropriate systemic therapy should supplement topical therapy in all serious infections
Ototoxicity	The possibility of ototoxicity must be considered if this product is allowed to enter the middle ear

ADVERSE REACTIONS

Local	Local irritation with itching or burning, angioneurotic edema, urticaria, vesicular and maculopapular dermatitis
Systemic	Bone marrow hypoplasia (see WARNINGS/PRECAUTIONS)

USE IN CHILDREN
Consult manufacturer

USE IN PREGNANT AND NURSING WOMEN
Consult manufacturer

VEHICLE/BASE
Drops: propylene glycol

OTIC ANTI-INFECTIVES

COLY-MYCIN S Otic (colistin sulfate, neomycin sulfate, thonzonium bromide, and hydrocortisone acetate) Parke-Davis   Rx

Drops (per milliliter): colistin sulfate equivalent to 3 mg colistin base, neomycin sulfate equivalent to 3.3 mg neomycin base, 0.5 mg thonzonium bromide, and 10 mg (1%) hydrocortisone acetate (5, 10 ml)

INDICATIONS
Superficial bacterial infections of the external auditory canal caused by susceptible organisms, notably *Pseudomonas aeruginosa, Escherichia coli, Klebsiella-Aerobacter, Staphylococcus aureus,* and *Proteus*
Mastoidectomy and fenestration cavity infections caused by susceptible organisms

TOPICAL DOSAGE
Adult: instill 5 drops into the affected ear tid or qid for no more than 10 days
Child: instill 4 drops into the affected ear tid or qid for no more than 10 days

CONTRAINDICATIONS

Hypersensitivity to any component	Herpes simplex infections	Vaccinia or varicella

ADMINISTRATION/DOSAGE ADJUSTMENTS

Instillation of drops	Thoroughly cleanse and dry external auditory canal with a sterile cotton applicator. Drops should be instilled, using the calibrated dropper supplied, with patient lying down and affected ear turned upward; this position should be maintained for 5 min after instillation. Repeat, if necessary, for opposite ear.
Alternative technique using a cotton wick	Thoroughly cleanse and dry external auditory canal with a sterile cotton applicator. Insert a cotton wick saturated with medication into the ear canal; add more suspension q4h to keep wick moist. Replace wick at least once every 24 h.

WARNINGS/PRECAUTIONS

Loss of antibiotic potency	Caution patients who prefer to warm the medication before use to avoid heating it above body temperature
Overgrowth of nonsusceptible organisms	Nonsusceptible organisms, including fungi, may proliferate during treatment; if infection does not improve after 1 wk, repeat culture and susceptibility tests to determine whether therapy should be changed
Local reactions	If sensitization or irritation occurs, discontinue medication promptly

COLY-MYCIN S Otic ■ CORTISPORIN Otic Solution and Suspension

Ototoxicity	May occur; use with caution in patients with a perforated eardrum or long-standing chronic otitis media
Allergic cross-reactions	May occur, thus precluding future use of kanamycin, paromomycin, streptomycin, and possibly gentamicin

ADVERSE REACTIONS

Local	Cutaneous sensitization

USE IN CHILDREN
See INDICATIONS

USE IN PREGNANT AND NURSING WOMEN
Consult manufacturer

VEHICLE/BASE
Drops: polysorbate 80, acetic acid, sodium acetate, thimerosal, and water

---

OTIC ANTI-INFECTIVES

CORTISPORIN Otic Solution (polymyxin B sulfate, neomycin sulfate, and hydrocortisone) Burroughs Wellcome — Rx

Solution (per milliliter): 10,000 units polymyxin B sulfate, 5 mg neomycin sulfate, and 10 mg hydrocortisone (10 ml)

INDICATIONS
Superficial bacterial infections of the external auditory canal caused by susceptible organisms

TOPICAL DOSAGE
Adult: instill 4 drops into affected ear(s) tid or qid
Infant and child: instill 3 drops into affected ear(s) tid or qid

CORTISPORIN Otic Suspension (polymyxin B sulfate, neomycin sulfate, and hydrocortisone) Burroughs Wellcome — Rx

Suspension (per milliliter): 10,000 units polymyxin B sulfate, 5 mg neomycin sulfate, and 10 mg hydrocortisone (10 ml)

INDICATIONS
Superficial bacterial infections of the external auditory canal caused by susceptible organisms
Infections of mastoidectomy and fenestration cavities caused by susceptible organisms

TOPICAL DOSAGE
Adult: instill 4 drops into affected ear(s) tid or qid
Infant and child: instill 3 drops into affected ear(s) tid or qid

CONTRAINDICATIONS

Hypersensitivity to any component	Herpes simplex infections	Vaccinia or varicella

ADMINISTRATION/DOSAGE ADJUSTMENTS

Instillation	Thoroughly clean auditory canal; patient should lie with affected ear upward and maintain position for 5 min after drops are instilled. Caution patient to avoid contaminating dropper. If preferred, a saturated cotton wick may be used. Moisten wick every 4 h and replace after 24 h.
Duration of treatment	Do not administer for longer than 10 days

WARNINGS/PRECAUTIONS

Loss of antibiotic potency	Caution patients who prefer to warm the medication before use to avoid heating it above body temperature
Overgrowth of nonsusceptible organisms	Nonsusceptible organisms, including fungi, may proliferate with prolonged use; if infection does not improve after 1 wk, repeat cultures and susceptibility tests to determine whether therapy should be changed
Neomycin sensitization	May occur with prolonged use, especially during treatment of chronic dermatoses; discontinue medication if low-grade reddening with swelling, dry scaling, or itching occurs, and do not use neomycin-containing products thereafter
Allergic cross-reactions	May occur and may preclude future administration of kanamycin, paromomycin, streptomycin, and possibly gentamicin
Ototoxicity	May occur; use solution with caution when integrity of tympanic membrane is in question. Use suspension with caution in cases of perforated eardrum and in long-standing cases of chronic otitis media.

CORTISPORIN Otic Solution and Suspension ■ Otic TRIDESILON

ADVERSE REACTIONS

Local — Stinging and burning if drug reaches middle ear (with use of solution); cutaneous sensitization (due to neomycin component)

USE IN CHILDREN
See INDICATIONS and TOPICAL DOSAGE

USE IN PREGNANT AND NURSING WOMEN
Consult manufacturer

VEHICLE/BASE
Solution: cupric sulfate, glycerin, hydrochloric acid, propylene glycol, water, and 0.1% potassium metabisulfite
Suspension: cetyl alcohol, propylene glycol, polysorbate 80, purified water, and 0.01% thimerosal

---

OTIC ANTI-INFECTIVES

Otic TRIDESILON Solution (desonide and acetic acid) Miles Pharmaceuticals Rx

Solution: 0.05% desonide and 2% acetic acid (10 ml)

INDICATIONS
Superficial infections, accompanied by inflammation, of the external auditory canal caused by susceptible organisms

TOPICAL DOSAGE
Adult: instill 3–4 drops into the affected ear tid or qid
Child: use smallest effective amount (see warning, below, concerning systemic absorption)

CONTRAINDICATIONS
Hypersensitivity to any component — Perforated tympanic membrane (see WARNINGS/PRECAUTIONS)

ADMINISTRATION/DOSAGE ADJUSTMENTS

Instillation of drops — Carefully remove all cerumen and debris from the auditory canal prior to instillation to permit contact of solution with infected surfaces

Alternative technique using a wick — Insert a gauze or cotton wick saturated with medication into the ear canal; keep wick moist by adding further solution, as needed

WARNINGS/PRECAUTIONS

Perforated tympanic membrane — A perforated tympanic membrane is frequently considered a contraindication to the use of external ear canal medication

Patient instructions — Caution patients not to let solution come into contact with the eyes

Irritation — Discontinue use and institute appropriate therapy

Infection — If infection persists or new infection develops, institute appropriate therapy; if a favorable response is not obtained promptly, discontinue steroid therapy until the infection is adequately controlled

Systemic absorption — Reversible hypothalamic-pituitary-adrenal (HPA) axis suppression, Cushing's syndrome, hyperglycemia, and glucosuria may result from systemic absorption after topical application, particularly in children (see USE IN CHILDREN). Use over extensive areas, for prolonged periods, or of occlusive dressings increases percutaneous absorption. Evaluate HPA axis function by ACTH stimulation or measurement of urinary free cortisol.

Carcinogenicity, mutagenicity — Long-term studies have not been done in animals to evaluate the carcinogenic potential of topical corticosteroids; the results of studies to demonstrate mutagenicity of prednisolone and hydrocortisone have been negative

Effect on fertility — The effect of topical corticosteroids on fertility has not been studied

ADVERSE REACTIONS[1]

Local — Burning, itching, irritation, dryness, folliculitis, hypertrichosis, hypopigmentation, allergic contact dermatitis, maceration of the skin, secondary infection, skin atrophy

USE IN CHILDREN
Use smallest amount necessary for effective treatment. Children may be more susceptible than adults to HPA axis suppression and Cushing's syndrome because of the larger ratio of surface area to body weight; intracranial hypertension has also been observed in children receiving topical corticosteroids. Chronic therapy may interfere with growth and development.

USE IN PREGNANT AND NURSING WOMEN
Pregnancy Category C: use during pregnancy only if the expected benefit justifies the potential risk to the fetus. Do not use over extensive areas, in large amounts, or for prolonged periods. In animal studies, systemic corticosteroids have generally been teratogenic at relatively low dosages; the more potent corticosteroids have also been teratogenic when applied to the skin. No adequate, well-controlled studies have been done in pregnant women. It is not known whether topical corticosteroids are excreted in human milk; although systemic corticosteroids are excreted in quantities unlikely to harm nursing infants, this preparation should be used with caution in nursing mothers.

VEHICLE/BASE
Solution: propylene glycol, sodium acetate, citric acid, and purified water

[1] Includes reactions common to otic use of topical corticosteroids in general

OTOBIOTIC ■ VōSoL Otic Solution

OTIC ANTI-INFECTIVES

OTOBIOTIC Otic Solution (polymyxin B sulfate and hydrocortisone) Schering   Rx

Solution (per milliliter): 10,000 units polymyxin B sulfate and 5 mg hydrocortisone (15 ml)

INDICATIONS	TOPICAL DOSAGE
Superficial bacterial infections of the external auditory canals caused by susceptible organisms	**Adult:** instill 4 drops into affected ear tid or qid **Infant and child:** instill 3 drops into affected ear tid or qid

CONTRAINDICATIONS

Hypersensitivity to any component	Herpes simplex infections	Vaccinia or varicella
Fungal diseases of the ear	Perforated tympanic membrane	

ADMINISTRATION/DOSAGE ADJUSTMENTS

Instillation	Thoroughly clean and dry auditory canal; patient should lie with affected ear upward and maintain position for 5 min after drops are instilled. Repeat, if necessary, for the opposite ear. Instruct patient to keep dropper from touching the affected area, fingers, or any other surface.
Duration of treatment	Do not administer for longer than 10 days

WARNINGS/PRECAUTIONS

Loss of antibiotic potency	Caution patients who prefer to warm the medication before use to avoid heating it above body temperature
Overgrowth of nonsusceptible organisms	Nonsusceptible organisms, including fungi, may proliferate with prolonged use; if infection does not improve after 1 wk, repeat cultures and susceptibility tests to determine whether therapy should be changed
Hypersensitivity	Discontinue treatment promptly if sensitization or irritation occurs

ADVERSE REACTIONS

Local	Sensitization, irritation

USE IN CHILDREN	USE IN PREGNANT AND NURSING WOMEN
See INDICATIONS and TOPICAL DOSAGE	Consult manufacturer

VEHICLE/BASE
Solution: propylene glycol, glycerin, edetate disodium, sodium bisulfite, anhydrous sodium sulfite, sulfuric acid, and purified water

---

OTIC ANTI-INFECTIVES

VōSoL Otic Solution (acetic acid) Wallace   Rx

Drops: 2% (15, 30 ml)

INDICATIONS	TOPICAL DOSAGE
Superficial infections of the external auditory canal caused by susceptible organisms	**Adult and child:** saturate a cotton wick and place in the ear canal (if desired, the wick may also be saturated after insertion); keep wick moist by adding 3–5 drops q4–6h; after 24 h (or longer), remove wick and instill 5 drops tid or qid, for as long as needed

CONTRAINDICATIONS

Hypersensitivity to any component	Perforated tympanic membrane (see WARNINGS/PRECAUTIONS)

ADMINISTRATION/DOSAGE ADJUSTMENTS

Instillation of drops	Carefully remove all cerumen and debris from the auditory canal prior to insertion of wick to permit direct contact of solution with infected surfaces

WARNINGS/PRECAUTIONS

Perforated tympanic membrane	A perforated tympanic membrane is frequently considered a contraindication to the use of any external ear canal medication; avoid use or use with caution in patients with perforated ear drums

COMPENDIUM OF DRUG THERAPY

VōSoL Otic Solution ■ CERUMENEX

| Local reactions | If sensitization or irritation occurs, discontinue medication promptly |

ADVERSE REACTIONS

| Local | Irritation (very rare) |

USE IN CHILDREN
See INDICATIONS and TOPICAL DOSAGE

USE IN PREGNANT AND NURSING WOMEN
Consult manufacturer

VEHICLE/BASE
Drops (nonaqueous): 3% propylene glycol diacetate, 0.02% benzethonium chloride, and 0.015% sodium acetate

---

OTIC ANTI-INFECTIVES

VōSoL HC Otic Solution (hydrocortisone and acetic acid) Wallace — Rx

Drops: 1% hydrocortisone and 2% acetic acid (10 ml)

INDICATIONS	TOPICAL DOSAGE
Superficial infections, complicated by inflammation, of the external auditory canal caused by susceptible organisms	Adult and child: saturate a cotton wick and place in the ear canal (if desired, the wick may also be saturated after insertion); keep wick moist by adding 3–5 drops q4–6h; after 24 h (or longer), remove wick and instill 5 drops tid or qid, for as long as needed

CONTRAINDICATIONS

Hypersensitivity to any component
Herpes simplex infections
Perforated tympanic membrane (see WARNINGS/PRECAUTIONS)
Vaccinia or varicella

ADMINISTRATION/DOSAGE ADJUSTMENTS

| Instillation of drops | Carefully remove all cerumen and debris from the auditory canal prior to insertion of wick to permit direct contact of solution with infected surfaces |

WARNINGS/PRECAUTIONS

| Perforated tympanic membrane | A perforated tympanic membrane is frequently considered a contraindication to the use of any external ear canal medication; avoid use or use with caution in patients with perforated ear drums |
| Local reactions | If sensitization or irritation occurs, discontinue medication promptly |

ADVERSE REACTIONS

| Local | Irritation (very rare) |

USE IN CHILDREN
See INDICATIONS and TOPICAL DOSAGE

USE IN PREGNANT AND NURSING WOMEN
Consult manufacturer

VEHICLE/BASE
Drops (nonaqueous): 3% propylene glycol diacetate, 0.02% benzethonium chloride, 0.015% sodium acetate, and 0.2% citric acid

---

CERUMEN SOFTENERS

CERUMENEX (triethanolamine polypeptide oleate-condensate) Purdue Frederick — Rx

Drops: 10% triethanolamine polypeptide oleate-condensate (6, 12 ml)

INDICATIONS	TOPICAL DOSAGE
Removal of cerumen Removal of impacted cerumen prior to ear examination, otologic therapy, or audiometry	Adult: fill ear canal with solution with patient's head tilted at a 45° angle, and insert a cotton plug for 30 min; *gently* flush ear with lukewarm water, using a soft rubber bulb syringe; for unusually hard impactions, procedure may be repeated Child: same as adult

CERUMENEX ■ DEBROX

CONTRAINDICATIONS

Previous untoward reaction to triethanolamine polypeptide oleate-condensate	Positive patch test (see WARNINGS/PRECAUTIONS)	Perforated ear drum or otitis media (relative contraindication)

WARNINGS/PRECAUTIONS

Dermatological idiosyncrasies or history of allergic reactions	Use with extreme caution in known cases of idiosyncratic or allergic skin reactions. In doubtful cases, perform a patch test by placing a drop of solution on the flexor surface of the arm or forearm and covering it with a small bandage strip; a positive reaction 24 h later indicates probability of an allergic reaction following instillation in ear (see CONTRAINDICATIONS)
Duration of exposure	Ear canal should not be exposed to solution for more than 15–30 min
Contact with periaural skin	Should be avoided; if such undue exposure occurs, wash area with soap and water
External otitis	Use with caution
Local reactions	Occur in 1% of patients; reaction generally lasts for 2–10 days and clears with no residual complications. Treatment in mild cases is symptomatic and may include anti-inflammatory agents, when indicated.
Patient instructions	Advise patients not to exceed time of exposure, not to use drops more frequently than directed, and to discontinue use and consult physician if adverse reaction occurs

ADVERSE REACTIONS

Frequent reactions (incidence ≥ 1%) are printed in *italics*

Local	*Dermatitis, ranging from mild erythema and pruritus of external canal to a severe eczematoid reaction involving external ear and periauricular tissue (1%)*

USE IN CHILDREN
Same as adult indications and dosage

USE IN PREGNANT AND NURSING WOMEN
Consult manufacturer

VEHICLE/BASE
Drops: propylene glycol and 0.5% chlorbutanol

CERUMEN SOFTENERS

DEBROX (carbamide peroxide) Marion   OTC
Drops: 6.5% (½, 1 fl oz)

INDICATIONS
Removal of cerumen

TOPICAL DOSAGE
Adult: instill 5–10 drops into ear canal, with patient's head tilted to the side, and allow drops to remain in ear for several minutes; repeat bid for up to 4 days, if needed. Any remaining wax may be removed by flushing with warm water, using a soft rubber bulb ear syringe; avoid excessive pressure
Child: use according to medical judgment

CONTRAINDICATIONS
None known

WARNINGS/PRECAUTIONS

Duration of use	This product should not be used for more than 4 consecutive days; package label cautions patients to consult a physician if excessive ear wax remains after use
Precautions regarding patient self-medication	Package label cautions patients against using this product, unless directed by a physician, after ear surgery, if there is drainage or a discharge from the ear or pain, irritation, or rash in the ear, if the eardrum is injured or perforated, or if dizziness is present
Eye irritant	Use with caution to avoid contact of solution with eyes

COMPENDIUM OF DRUG THERAPY

DEBROX ■ MURINE

ADVERSE REACTIONS
None reported by manufacturer

USE IN CHILDREN	USE IN PREGNANT AND NURSING WOMEN
Use according to medical judgment in children under 12 yr of age	There are no restrictions on use in pregnant or nursing women

VEHICLE/BASE
Drops: citric acid, glycerin, propylene glycol, sodium stannate, water, and other ingredients

---

CERUMEN SOFTENERS

MURINE Ear Drops (carbamide peroxide) Ross — OTC
Drops: 6.5% (0.5 fl oz)

MURINE Ear Wax Removal System (carbamide peroxide) Ross — OTC
Drops: 6.5% (0.5 fl oz), packaged with a 1.0 fl oz soft rubber bulb ear washer

INDICATIONS
Removal of cerumen

TOPICAL DOSAGE
Adult: to remove cerumen, instill 5–10 drops into the affected ear bid for up to 4 consecutive days. Administer with the head in a tilted position and with the tip of the bottle *outside* the ear canal. After each instillation, keep the head tilted or place cotton in the ear, since the solution should remain in the ear for several minutes; to remove the softened wax, place the bulb ear washer (supplied with the wax removal system) at the edge of the ear canal, and gently flush the ear with warm water.
Child (>12 yr): same as adult

CONTRAINDICATIONS
Perforated ear drum

WARNINGS/PRECAUTIONS
Patient instructions — Caution patient not to use this product without medical supervision if irritation, rash, dizziness, or ear pain or drainage is present or develops during treatment. Instruct patient to avoid contact with the eyes; if contact occurs, patient should flush the eyes immediately with water and report the accident.

ADVERSE REACTIONS
Consult manufacturer

USE IN CHILDREN	USE IN PREGNANT AND NURSING WOMEN
Use according to medical judgment in children under 12 yr of age	Consult manufacturer

VEHICLE/BASE
Drops: 6.3% alcohol, glycerin, polysorbate 20, and other ingredients

Chapter 44

Potassium Supplements

KAOCHLOR 10% Liquid (Adria) Potassium chloride Rx	1774
KAOCHLOR-EFF (Adria) Potassium chloride, potassium citrate, potassium bicarbonate, and betaine hydrochloride Rx	1774
KAOCHLOR S-F 10% Liquid (Adria) Potassium chloride Rx	1774
KAON (Adria) Potassium gluconate Rx	1775
KAON-CL (Adria) Potassium chloride Rx	1776
KAON CL-10 (Adria) Potassium chloride Rx	1776
KAON-CL 20% (Adria) Potassium chloride Rx	1776
KAY CIEL (Forest) Potassium chloride Rx	1778
K-DUR (Key) Potassium chloride Rx	1779
K-LOR (Abbott) Potassium chloride Rx	1780
KLORVESS 10% Liquid (Sandoz Pharmaceuticals) Potassium chloride Rx	1781
KLORVESS Effervescent Tablets and Granules (Sandoz Pharmaceuticals) Potassium chloride, potassium bicarbonate, and L-lysine monohydrochloride Rx	1781
KLOTRIX (Mead Johnson) Potassium chloride Rx	1782
K-LYTE Effervescent Tablets (Bristol) Potassium bicarbonate Rx	1784
K-LYTE/CL and K-LYTE/CL 50 Effervescent Tablets (Bristol) Potassium chloride, potassium bicarbonate, and L-lysine monohydrochloride Rx	1784
K-LYTE/CL Powder (Bristol) Potassium chloride Rx	1784
K-LYTE DS Effervescent Tablets (Bristol) Potassium bicarbonate and potassium citrate Rx	1784
K·TAB (Abbott) Potassium chloride Rx	1785
MICRO-K (Robins) Potassium chloride Rx	1786
SLOW-K (CIBA) Potassium chloride Rx	1788
TEN-K (Geigy) Potassium chloride Rx	1789

Other Potassium Supplements 1773

Bi-K (Rorer) Potassium gluconate and potassium citrate Rx	1773
KOLYUM (Pennwalt) Potassium gluconate and potassium chloride Rx	1773
TRIKATES (Lilly) Potassium acetate, potassium bicarbonate, and potassium citrate Rx	1773
TWIN-K (Boots) Potassium gluconate and potassium citrate Rx	1773
TWIN-K-Cl (Boots) Potassium gluconate, potassium citrate, and ammonium chloride Rx	1773

OTHER POTASSIUM SUPPLEMENTS

DRUG	HOW SUPPLIED	USUAL DOSAGE[1]
Bi-K (Rorer) Potassium gluconate and potassium citrate Rx	**Liquid (per 15 ml):** 20 mEq potassium (1 pt) *sugar-free*	**Adult:** 15 ml (1 tbsp) in 6–8 fl oz of water or fruit juice, bid to qid (40–80 mEq/day)
KOLYUM (Pennwalt) Potassium gluconate and potassium chloride Rx	**Powder:** 20 mEq potassium and 3.4 mEq chloride per 5-g packet *cherry flavored, sugar-free* **Liquid (per 15 ml):** 20 mEq potassium and 3.4 mEq chloride (1 pt, 1 gal) *cherry flavored, sugar-free*	**Adult:** 15 ml (1 tbsp) in 30 ml (1 fl oz) or more of water or 5 g in 3–4 fl oz of cool water bid (40 mEq/day)
TRIKATES (Lilly) Potassium acetate, potassium bicarbonate, and potassium citrate Rx	**Liquid (per 5 ml):** 15 mEq potassium (1 pt, 1 gal) *sugar-free*	**Adult:** 5 ml (1 tsp), diluted with a glass of tomato juice, orange juice, or other suitable vehicle, tid or qid, after meals (45–60 mEq/day)
TWIN-K (Boots) Potassium gluconate and potassium citrate Rx	**Liquid (per 15 ml):** 20 mEq potassium (1 pt) *sugar-free*	**Adult:** 15 ml (1 tbsp) in 8 fl oz of water or fruit juice, bid to qid (40–80 mEq/day)
TWIN-K-Cl (Boots) Potassium gluconate, potassium citrate, and ammonium chloride Rx	**Liquid (per 15 ml):** 15 mEq potassium and 4 mEq chloride (1 pt) *sugar-free*	**Adult:** 15 ml (1 tbsp) in 8 fl oz of water or fruit juice, bid to qid (30–60 mEq/day)

[1] Where pediatric dosages are not given, consult manufacturer

COMPENDIUM OF DRUG THERAPY

KAOCHLOR

POTASSIUM SUPPLEMENTS

KAOCHLOR 10% Liquid (potassium chloride) Adria — Rx

Liquid (per 15 ml): 1.5 g (20 mEq)[1] (1 pt)

KAOCHLOR-EFF (potassium chloride, potassium citrate, potassium bicarbonate, and betaine hydrochloride) Adria — Rx

Effervescent tablets: 0.60 g potassium chloride, 0.22 g potassium citrate, 1.00 g potassium bicarbonate, and 1.84 g betaine hydrochloride (20 mEq each of potassium and chloride) *sugar-free*

KAOCHLOR S-F 10% Liquid (potassium chloride) Adria — Rx

Liquid (per 15 ml): 1.5 g (20 mEq)[1] (4 fl oz, 1 pt) *sugar-free*

INDICATIONS

Hypokalemia with or without metabolic alkalosis; **digitalis intoxication; hypokalemic familial periodic paralysis; hypokalemia secondary to diuretic therapy** of essential hypertension, when dietary supplementation alone is inadequate

Prevention of potassium depletion, when dietary potassium intake is inadequate in patients receiving digitalis and diuretics (for congestive heart failure) or diuretics alone (for hepatic cirrhosis with ascites) and in patients with hyperaldosteronism and normal renal function, potassium-wasting nephropathies, or certain diarrheal states

ORAL DOSAGE

Adult: 15 ml (1 tbsp) or 1 tab, diluted or dissolved in 3 fl oz or more of water or other liquid, 2–5 times/day (40–100 mEq/day)

Adult: 15 ml (1 tbsp) or 1 tab, diluted or dissolved in 3 fl oz or more of water or other liquid, once daily (20 mEq/day)

CONTRAINDICATIONS

Hyperkalemia (further elevation of serum potassium level may produce cardiac arrest)

WARNINGS/PRECAUTIONS

Chronic renal disease or impaired potassium excretion	Asymptomatic hyperkalemia may rapidly develop, leading to cardiac arrest and death; carefully monitor serum potassium level and adjust dosage as needed
Concomitant metabolic acidosis	Should be treated with an alkalinizing potassium salt, such as potassium bicarbonate, citrate, acetate, or gluconate
Total body potassium stores	May not be accurately reflected by serum potassium levels; monitor acid-base status, serum electrolytes, ECG, and clinical status, particularly in patients with cardiac or renal disease or in the presence of acidosis
Tartrazine sensitivity	Presence of FD&C Yellow No. 5 (tartrazine) in Kaochlor 10% Liquid (not S-F) and Kaochlor-EFF may cause allergic-type reactions, including bronchial asthma, in susceptible individuals

ADVERSE REACTIONS

Gastrointestinal	Nausea, vomiting, diarrhea, abdominal discomfort, obstruction, bleeding, perforation
Other	Hyperkalemia

OVERDOSAGE

Signs and symptoms	Hyperkalemia, ECG changes (peaked T waves, ST-segment depression, loss of P wave, prolongation of Q-T interval, widening and slurring of QRS complex), paresthesias of the extremities, muscle weakness, heaviness, flaccid paralysis, listlessness, mental confusion, peripheral vascular collapse with fall in blood pressure, cardiac arrhythmias, and heart block
Treatment	Discontinue medication and eliminate potassium-rich foods and drugs and use of potassium-sparing diuretics. Administer over a period of 1 h 300–500 ml of 10% dextrose containing 10–20 units of insulin per liter of solution. Correct acidosis, if present, with IV sodium bicarbonate. Use of sodium or ammonium cation exchange resins, hemodialysis, and/or peritoneal dialysis may be needed (ammonium compounds should not be used in patients with hepatic cirrhosis). If patient is receiving digitalis, too rapid lowering of the serum potassium level may result in digitalis toxicity.

DRUG INTERACTIONS

Blood from blood bank, potassium-sparing diuretics, low-salt milk, potassium-containing medications, salt substitutes	⇧ Serum potassium level

Sodium cycle exchange resins, glucose-insulin infusions, sodium bicarbonate, laxatives	▽ Serum potassium level

ALTERED LABORATORY VALUES

Blood/serum values	△ Potassium
Urinary values	△ Potassium

USE IN CHILDREN
Safety and effectiveness for use in children have not been established

USE IN PREGNANT AND NURSING WOMEN
Pregnancy Category C: use during pregnancy only if clearly needed. Animal reproduction studies have not been done, nor is it known whether these preparations can affect human fetal development or reproductive capacity. It is also not known whether they are excreted in human milk; use with caution in nursing mothers.

[1] Contains 5% alcohol

POTASSIUM SUPPLEMENTS

KAON (potassium gluconate) Adria   Rx
Tablets: 5 mEq   **Elixir (per 15 ml):** 20 mEq[1] *(1 pt, 1 gal) grape flavored, sugar-free; (1 pt) lemon-lime flavored, sugar-free*

INDICATIONS
Treatment of **hypokalemia, digitalis intoxication, and hypokalemic familial periodic paralysis**

Prevention of **hypokalemia,** when dietary intake of potassium is inadequate, in patients receiving digitalis and diuretics for congestive heart failure and in patients with hepatic cirrhosis and ascites, hyperaldosteronism (and normal renal function), potassium-losing nephropathy, or certain diarrheal states

ORAL DOSAGE
Adult: 40–100 mEq/day or more; the usual dosage of the tablets is 10 mEq qid (after meals and at bedtime), and the usual dosage of the elixir is 20 mEq bid (morning and evening). Use tablets only in patients who cannot tolerate liquid potassium preparations or refuse or find it difficult to take these preparations.

Adult: 20 mEq/day; use tablets only in patients who cannot tolerate liquid potassium preparations or refuse or find it difficult to take these preparations

CONTRAINDICATIONS
Hyperkalemia (see WARNINGS/PRECAUTIONS)	Conditions that can arrest or delay passage of the tablets through the GI tract

ADMINISTRATION/DOSAGE ADJUSTMENTS
Administration	Tell the patient to dilute each 15-ml dose of the elixir in at least 1 fl oz of water or other liquid; instruct the patient to take the tablets, with a full glass of water or other liquid, during or immediately after meals or a snack
GI irritation	To manage nausea, vomiting, abdominal discomfort, and diarrhea, reduce the dose, give it with meals, or dilute it further
Interpretation of plasma potassium level	The relationship between total body stores of potassium and the plasma potassium level is affected by changes in the acid-base balance: acute alkalosis can cause hypokalemia in the absence of a deficit in total body potassium, whereas acute acidosis can produce a normal plasma level in the presence of such a deficit. Artifactual elevation of the plasma level can occur if the patient's fist is repeatedly clenched before the blood sample is drawn.
Monitoring of therapy	Check the plasma potassium level regularly. During treatment of hypokalemia, carefully monitor other plasma electrolyte levels, the acid-base balance, clinical response, and the ECG, especially in patients with acidosis or cardiac or renal disease.
Diuretic-induced hypokalemia	Consider giving potassium supplements to patients receiving diuretics for uncomplicated essential hypertension only if hypokalemia occurs during therapy and cannot be adequately controlled by changes in diet
Hypochloremic alkalosis	For hypokalemia associated with hypochloremic alkalosis, administration of chloride as well as potassium may be necessary, especially for patients on a low-salt diet; to provide both potassium and chloride, use potassium chloride rather than this product or, alternatively, give this product with a chloride supplement

WARNINGS/PRECAUTIONS
Hyperkalemia	Administration of potassium to patients with chronic renal disease or other disorders associated with impaired potassium excretion may cause hyperkalemia and precipitate cardiac arrest, which may be fatal. The resulting increase in potassium may also complicate the following conditions: chronic renal failure, systemic acidosis (eg, diabetic acidosis), adrenal insufficiency, acute dehydration, or disorders associated with extensive tissue breakdown (eg, severe burns). Hyperkalemia is usually asymptomatic and its only manifestations may be an increased plasma potassium level and characteristic ECG changes (peaking of T waves, loss of P wave, depression of S-T segment, and prolongation of the Q-T interval); muscle paralysis and cardiovascular collapse are late signs. Potentially fatal effects can develop rapidly. To avoid hyperkalemia, monitor the plasma potassium level with particular care when giving this product to patients with impaired potassium excretion and adjust dosage as needed. Do not give this product to patients receiving potassium-sparing diuretics. For treatment of hyperkalemia, see OVERDOSAGE.

KAON ■ KAON-CL

Gastrointestinal toxicity	Potassium tablets have caused fatal GI stenosis, ulceration, and bleeding; these effects have resulted from a high, localized concentration of potassium ion in the GI tract. The frequency of small-bowel lesions with Kaon tablets is less than 2 per million patient-years. Instruct patients to report immediately tarry stools or any other evidence of GI bleeding. If severe vomiting, abdominal pain, distention, or GI bleeding occurs, discontinue use immediately and consider the possibility of GI obstruction or perforation.
Carcinogenicity, mutagenicity, effect on fertility	No studies have been done to evaluate the carcinogenic or mutagenic potential of potassium supplements or their effect on fertility
Tartrazine sensitivity	Presence of FD&C Yellow No. 5 (tartrazine) in lemon-lime flavored elixir may cause allergic-type reactions, including bronchial asthma, in susceptible patients such as those hypersensitive to aspirin

ADVERSE REACTIONS

Gastrointestinal	Nausea, vomiting, abdominal discomfort, diarrhea; GI obstruction, bleeding, and perforation (with tablets only)
Other	Hyperkalemia

OVERDOSAGE

Signs and symptoms	Hyperkalemia (see WARNINGS/PRECAUTIONS)
Treatment	Discontinue use of potassium-containing drugs and food. Administer a solution of 10% dextrose containing 10–20 units of insulin per liter at a rate of 300–500 ml/h. Correct acidosis, if present, with IV sodium bicarbonate. Administer sodium polystyrene sulfonate and perform hemodialysis or peritoneal dialysis, as needed. When treating hyperkalemia in patients who are receiving digitalis, exercise caution; digitalis toxicity can occur if the plasma potassium level is reduced too rapidly.

DRUG INTERACTIONS

Potassium-sparing diuretics	Severe hyperkalemia; do not use potassium-sparing diuretics in combination with this product
Captopril, enalapril, potassium-rich foods (including salt substitutes and low-salt milk)	⇧ Plasma potassium level; exercise caution

ALTERED LABORATORY VALUES

Blood/serum values	⇧ Potassium
Urinary values	⇧ Potassium

USE IN CHILDREN

Safety and effectiveness for use in children have not been established

---

USE IN PREGNANT AND NURSING WOMEN

Pregnant women: Pregnancy Category C: it is not known whether this preparation can cause harm to the fetus or affect reproductive capacity; reproduction studies have not been done in animals. Use during pregnancy only if clearly needed. **Nursing mothers:** It is not known whether this product is excreted in human milk; use with caution in nursing mothers.

---

[1] Contains 5% alcohol

POTASSIUM SUPPLEMENTS

KAON-CL (potassium chloride) Adria — Rx

Tablets (controlled release): 500 mg (6.67 mEq)

KAON CL-10 (potassium chloride) Adria — Rx

Tablets (controlled release): 750 mg (10 mEq)

KAON-CL 20% (potassium chloride) Adria — Rx

Liquid (per 15 ml): 3 g (40 mEq)[1] (1 pt) *sugar-free*

INDICATIONS

Hypokalemia with or without metabolic alkalosis; **digitalis intoxication; hypokalemic familial periodic paralysis; hypokalemia secondary to diuretic therapy** of essential hypertension, when dietary supplementation alone is inadequate

ORAL DOSAGE

Adult: 2–5 Kaon-Cl tabs, with a glass of water or other liquid, tid (40–100 mEq/day); 2–5 Kaon Cl-10 tabs, with a glass of water or other liquid, bid (40–100 mEq/day); or 15 ml (1 tbsp) of Kaon-Cl 20%, diluted in at least 6 fl oz of water or other liquid, 1–2 times/day (40–80 mEq/day); some patients may require higher doses

COMPENDIUM OF DRUG THERAPY

KAON-CL

Prevention of potassium depletion, when dietary potassium intake is inadequate in patients receiving digitalis and diuretics (for congestive heart failure) or diuretics alone (for hepatic cirrhosis with ascites) and in patients with hyperaldosteronism and normal renal function, potassium-wasting nephropathies, or certain diarrheal states

Adult: 1 Kaon-Cl tab, with a glass of water or other liquid, tid, 1 Kaon Cl-10 tab, with a glass of water or other liquid, bid, or 7.5 ml (½ tbsp) of Kaon-Cl 20%, diluted in at least 6 fl oz of water or other liquid, once daily (20 mEq/day)

CONTRAINDICATIONS

Hyperkalemia (further elevation of serum potassium level may produce cardiac arrest)

Esophageal compression due to left-atrial enlargement (esophageal ulceration may occur)

GI motility problems or obstruction (see WARNINGS/PRECAUTIONS)

ADMINISTRATION/DOSAGE ADJUSTMENTS

GI irritation — Nausea, vomiting, abdominal discomfort, and diarrhea may occur; caution patient to follow directions for diluting Kaon-Cl 20%

WARNINGS/PRECAUTIONS

Chronic renal disease or impaired potassium excretion — Asymptomatic hyperkalemia may develop, leading to cardiac arrest and death; carefully monitor serum potassium level and adjust dosage as needed

GI obstruction, hemorrhage, or perforation — Stenotic and/or ulcerative small-bowel lesions and death may occur with tablets because of a high local concentration of potassium ion near the bowel wall; discontinue medication immediately if severe vomiting, abdominal pain, distention, or GI bleeding occurs. Use a liquid preparation for potassium supplementation if tablet passage through the GI tract is likely to be delayed or arrested. Use of slow-release tablets should be reserved for patients who cannot tolerate or refuse to take liquid or effervescent preparations or when a compliance problem exists.

Concomitant metabolic acidosis — Should be treated with an alkalinizing potassium salt, such as potassium bicarbonate, citrate, acetate, or gluconate

Total body potassium stores — May not be accurately reflected by serum potassium levels; monitor acid-base status, serum electrolytes, ECG, and clinical status, particularly in patients with cardiac or renal disease or in the presence of acidosis

Tartrazine sensitivity — Presence of FD&C Yellow No. 5 (tartrazine) in Kaon-Cl tablets may cause allergic-type reactions, including bronchial asthma, in susceptible individuals

ADVERSE REACTIONS

Gastrointestinal — Nausea, vomiting, abdominal discomfort, diarrhea, obstruction, bleeding, perforation

Other — Hyperkalemia

OVERDOSAGE

Signs and symptoms — Hyperkalemia, ECG changes (peaked T waves, ST-segment depression, loss of P wave, prolongation of Q-T interval, widening and slurring of QRS complex), paresthesias of the extremities, muscle weakness, heaviness, flaccid paralysis, listlessness, mental confusion, peripheral vascular collapse with fall in blood pressure, cardiac arrhythmias, and heart block

Treatment — Discontinue medication and eliminate potassium-rich foods and drugs and use of potassium-sparing diuretics. Administer over a period of 1 h 300–500 ml of 10% dextrose containing 10–20 units of insulin per liter of solution. Correct acidosis, if present, with IV sodium bicarbonate. Use of sodium or ammonium cation exchange resins, hemodialysis, and/or peritoneal dialysis may be needed (ammonium compounds should not be used in patients with hepatic cirrhosis). If patient is receiving digitalis, too rapid lowering of the serum potassium level may result in digitalis toxicity.

DRUG INTERACTIONS

Blood from blood bank, potassium-sparing diuretics, low-salt milk, potassium-containing medications, salt substitutes — ⇧ Serum potassium level

Sodium cycle exchange resins, glucose-insulin infusions, sodium bicarbonate, laxatives — ⇩ Serum potassium level

ALTERED LABORATORY VALUES

Blood/serum values — ⇧ Potassium

Urinary values — ⇧ Potassium

COMPENDIUM OF DRUG THERAPY

KAON-CL ■ KAY CIEL

USE IN CHILDREN
Elixir: Safety and effectiveness for use in children have not been established; *tablets:* consult manufacturer

USE IN PREGNANT AND NURSING WOMEN
Elixir: Pregnancy Category C: use during pregnancy only if clearly needed. Animal reproduction studies have not been done, nor is it known whether this preparation can affect human fetal development or reproductive capacity. It is also not known whether it is excreted in human milk; use with caution in nursing mothers. *Tablets:* consult manufacturer.

[1] Contains 5% alcohol

POTASSIUM SUPPLEMENTS

KAY CIEL (potassium chloride) Forest   Rx

Solution (per 15 ml): 1.5 g (20 mEq)[1] (118, 473, 3,785 ml) *sugar-free*   **Powder:** 1.5 g (20 mEq) per packet *sugar-free*

INDICATIONS
Prevention and treatment of **potassium deficiency** caused by thiazide diuretic or corticosteroid therapy, digitalis intoxication, low dietary intake of potassium, or as a result of vomiting or diarrhea, or for correction of associated hypochloremic alkalosis

ORAL DOSAGE
Adult: 15 ml (1 tbsp) or 1.5 g (1 packet), diluted or dissolved in 4 fl oz of cold water or fruit juice, bid, preferably after meals (40 mEq/day)

CONTRAINDICATIONS
Impaired renal function	Dehydration	Hyperkalemia
Untreated Addison's disease	Heat cramps	

WARNINGS/PRECAUTIONS
Monitoring of therapy	Potassium supplementation should be done with caution, with dosage adjusted to meet individual requirements; frequently check patient's clinical status and periodically monitor ECG and/or serum potassium level, especially in the presence of cardiac disease
Hypokalemia	Frequently associated hypochloremic alkalosis should be corrected
GI injury	Caution patients to adhere to dilution instructions to avoid injury

ADVERSE REACTIONS
Gastrointestinal	Nausea, vomiting, abdominal discomfort, diarrhea

OVERDOSAGE
Signs and symptoms	Hyperkalemia, ECG changes (peaked T waves, ST-segment depression, loss of P wave, prolongation of Q-T interval, widening and slurring of QRS complex), paresthesias of the extremities, muscle weakness, heaviness, flaccid paralysis, listlessness, mental confusion, peripheral vascular collapse with fall in blood pressure, cardiac arrhythmias, and heart block
Treatment	Discontinue medication and eliminate potassium-rich foods and drugs and use of potassium-sparing diuretics. Administer over a period of 1 h 300–500 ml of 10% dextrose containing 10–20 units of insulin per liter of solution. Correct acidosis, if present, with IV sodium bicarbonate. Use of sodium or ammonium cation exchange resins, hemodialysis, and/or peritoneal dialysis may be needed (ammonium compounds should not be used in patients with hepatic cirrhosis). If patient is receiving digitalis, too rapid lowering of the serum potassium level may result in digitalis toxicity.

DRUG INTERACTIONS
Blood from blood bank, potassium-sparing diuretics, low-salt milk, potassium-containing medications, salt substitutes	⇧ Serum potassium level
Sodium cycle exchange resins, glucose-insulin infusions, sodium bicarbonate, laxatives	⇩ Serum potassium level

ALTERED LABORATORY VALUES
Blood/serum values	⇧ Potassium

KAY CIEL ■ K-DUR

Urinary values ──────────────── ⬦ Potassium

USE IN CHILDREN	USE IN PREGNANT AND NURSING WOMEN
Consult manufacturer	Consult manufacturer

¹ Contains 4% alcohol

POTASSIUM SUPPLEMENTS

K-DUR (potassium chloride) Key Rx

Tablets (sustained release): 10 mEq (K-Dur 10), 20 mEq (K-Dur 20)

INDICATIONS

Treatment of **hypokalemia, digitalis intoxication, and hypokalemic familial periodic paralysis** in patients who cannot tolerate liquid potassium preparations or refuse or find it difficult to take these preparations

Prevention of **hypokalemia** in patients receiving digitalis and diuretics for congestive heart failure and in patients with hepatic cirrhosis and ascites, hyperaldosteronism (and normal renal function), potassium-losing nephropathy, or certain diarrheal states, but only when dietary intake of potassium is inadequate and these patients cannot tolerate liquid potassium preparations or refuse or find it difficult to take these preparations

ORAL DOSAGE

Adult: 40–100 mEq/day or more, given in 2 or more divided doses (no single dose should exceed 20 mEq)

Adult: 20 mEq/day

CONTRAINDICATIONS

Hyperkalemia (see WARNINGS/PRECAUTIONS) Conditions that can arrest or delay passage of the tablets through the GI tract

ADMINISTRATION/DOSAGE ADJUSTMENTS

Administration	Instruct the patient to take the tablets with a glass of water or another liquid and to swallow tablets whole without crushing, chewing, or sucking them; the patient should report any difficulty swallowing the tablets or any tendency for the tablets to stick in the throat
GI irritation	To manage nausea, vomiting, abdominal discomfort, and diarrhea, reduce the dose or give it with meals
Interpretation of plasma potassium level	The relationship between total body stores of potassium and the plasma potassium level is affected by changes in the acid-base balance: acute alkalosis can cause hypokalemia in the absence of a deficit in total body potassium, whereas acute acidosis can produce a normal plasma level in the presence of such a deficit
Monitoring of therapy	Check the plasma potassium level regularly. During treatment of hypokalemia, carefully monitor other plasma electrolyte levels, the acid-base balance, clinical response, and the ECG, especially in patients with acidosis or cardiac or renal disease
Diuretic-induced hypokalemia	Consider giving potassium supplements to patients receiving diuretics for uncomplicated essential hypertension only if hypokalemia occurs during therapy and cannot be adequately controlled by changes in diet
Metabolic acidosis	For treatment of hypokalemia associated with metabolic acidosis, use an alkalinizing potassium salt (eg, potassium citrate, potassium gluconate) rather than this product

WARNINGS/PRECAUTIONS

Hyperkalemia Administration of potassium to patients with chronic renal disease or other disorders associated with impaired potassium excretion may cause hyperkalemia and precipitate cardiac arrest, which may be fatal. The resulting increase in potassium may also complicate the following conditions: chronic renal failure, systemic acidosis (eg, diabetic acidosis), adrenal insufficiency, acute dehydration, or disorders associated with extensive tissue breakdown (eg, severe burns). Hyperkalemia is usually asymptomatic and its only manifestations may be an increased plasma potassium level and characteristic ECG changes (peaking of T waves, loss of P wave, depression of S-T segment, and prolongation of the Q-T interval); muscle paralysis and cardiovascular collapse are late signs. Potentially fatal effects can develop rapidly. To avoid hyperkalemia, monitor the plasma potassium level with particular care when giving this product to patients with impaired potassium excretion and adjust dosage as needed. Do not give this product to patients receiving potassium-sparing diuretics. For treatment of hyperkalemia, see OVERDOSAGE.

COMPENDIUM OF DRUG THERAPY

K-DUR ■ K-LOR

Gastrointestinal toxicity	Potassium chloride tablets have produced fatal GI bleeding, stenosis, and ulceration resulting from a high, localized concentration of potassium ion in the vicinity of the GI mucosa and consequent damage to the GI wall. GI ulceration and bleeding have also been reported with slow-release potassium chloride preparations. This product contains polymeric-coated crystals that rapidly disperse following disintegration of the tablet; the coating provides for a controlled release of potassium. Whether this design minimizes the risk of GI lesions is not currently known, since the frequency of lesions resulting from use of this product has not been established. Instruct patients to report immediately tarry stools or any other evidence of GI bleeding. If severe vomiting, abdominal pain, distention, or GI bleeding occurs, discontinue use immediately and consider the possibility of obstruction or perforation.
Esophageal ulcers	In certain patients with esophageal compression owing to an enlarged left atrium, wax matrix potassium preparations have produced esophageal ulceration (K-Dur is not formulated with a wax matrix)
Carcinogenicity	No long-term studies have been done to evaluate the carcinogenic potential of potassium chloride

ADVERSE REACTIONS

Gastrointestinal	Nausea, vomiting, abdominal discomfort, diarrhea; GI obstruction, bleeding, ulceration, and perforation
Other	Hyperkalemia; rash (rare)

OVERDOSAGE

Signs and symptoms	Hyperkalemia (see WARNINGS/PRECAUTIONS)
Treatment	Discontinue use of potassium-containing drugs and food. Administer a solution of 10% dextrose containing 10–20 units of insulin per liter at a rate of 300–500 ml/h. Correct acidosis, if present, with IV sodium bicarbonate. Administer sodium polystyrene sulfonate and perform hemodialysis or peritoneal dialysis, as needed. When treating hyperkalemia in patients who are receiving digitalis, exercise caution; digitalis toxicity can occur if the plasma potassium level is reduced too rapidly.

DRUG INTERACTIONS

Potassium-sparing diuretics	Severe hyperkalemia; do not use potassium-sparing diuretics in combination with this product
Captopril, enalapril, potassium-rich foods (including salt substitutes and low-salt milk)	△ Plasma potassium level

ALTERED LABORATORY VALUES

Blood/serum values	△ Potassium
Urinary values	△ Potassium

USE IN CHILDREN

Safety and effectiveness for use in children have not been established

---

USE IN PREGNANT AND NURSING WOMEN

Pregnant women: Pregnancy Category C: it is not known whether this preparation can cause harm to the fetus or affect reproductive capacity; reproduction studies have not been done in animals. Use during pregnancy only if clearly needed. **Nursing mothers:** Administration of potassium chloride should have little or no effect on potassium levels in human milk as long as total body stores of potassium are not excessive.

POTASSIUM SUPPLEMENTS

K-LOR (potassium chloride) Abbott   Rx

Powder: 1.125 g (15 mEq), 1.5 g (20 mEq) per packet

INDICATIONS

Hypokalemia with or without metabolic alkalosis; **digitalis intoxication; hypokalemic familial periodic paralysis; hypokalemia secondary to diuretic therapy** of essential hypertension, when dietary supplementation alone is inadequate; **prevention of potassium depletion** when dietary potassium intake is inadequate in patients receiving digitalis and diuretics (for congestive heart failure) or diuretics alone (for hepatic cirrhosis with ascites) and in patients with hyperaldosteronism and normal renal function, potassium-wasting nephropathies, or certain diarrheal states

ORAL DOSAGE

Adult: 1 K-Lor 15-mEq packet, dissolved in 3 fl oz or more of cold water or juice, 2–5 times/day after meals (30–75 mEq/day) or 1 K-Lor 20-mEq packet, dissolved in 4 fl oz or more of cold water or juice, 1–4 times/day after meals (20–80 mEq/day)

K-LOR ■ KLORVESS

CONTRAINDICATIONS

Hyperkalemia (see WARNINGS/PRECAUTIONS)	Use of potassium-sparing diuretics (may produce severe hyperkalemia)	Hypokalemia with metabolic acidosis (see WARNINGS/PRECAUTIONS)
Hypersensitivity to any component		

WARNINGS/PRECAUTIONS

Hyperkalemia	Further elevation of serum potassium level may produce cardiac arrest; hyperkalemia may complicate chronic renal failure, systemic acidosis (eg, diabetic acidosis), acute dehydration, extensive tissue breakdown (eg, as in severe burns), and adrenal insufficiency
Hypokalemia with metabolic acidosis	Substitute an alkalinizing potassium salt, such as potassium bicarbonate, citrate, acetate, or gluconate
Chronic renal disease or impaired potassium excretion	Asymptomatic hyperkalemia may develop, leading to cardiac arrest and death; carefully monitor serum potassium level and adjust dosage as needed
Total body potassium stores	May not be accurately reflected by serum potassium levels; monitor acid-base status, serum electrolytes, ECG, and clinical status, particularly in patients with cardiac or renal disease or in the presence of acidosis

ADVERSE REACTIONS

Gastrointestinal	Nausea, vomiting, abdominal discomfort, diarrhea
Other	Hyperkalemia, skin rash (rare)

OVERDOSAGE

Signs and symptoms	Hyperkalemia, ECG changes (peaked T waves, ST-segment depression, loss of P wave, prolongation of Q-T interval, widening and slurring of QRS complex), paresthesias of the extremities, muscle weakness, heaviness, flaccid paralysis, listlessness, mental confusion, peripheral vascular collapse with fall in blood pressure, cardiac arrhythmias, and heart block
Treatment	Discontinue medication and eliminate potassium-rich foods and drugs and use of potassium-sparing diuretics. Administer over a period of 1 h 300–500 ml of 10–25% dextrose containing 10–20 units of insulin per liter of solution. Correct acidosis, if present, with IV sodium bicarbonate. Use of sodium or ammonium cation exchange resins, hemodialysis, and/or peritoneal dialysis may be needed (ammonium compounds should not be used in patients with hepatic cirrhosis). If patient is receiving digitalis, too rapid lowering of the serum potassium level may result in digitalis toxicity.

DRUG INTERACTIONS

Blood from blood bank, potassium-sparing diuretics, low-salt milk, potassium-containing medications, salt substitutes	△ Serum potassium level
Sodium cycle exchange resins, glucose-insulin infusions, sodium bicarbonate, laxatives	▽ Serum potassium level

ALTERED LABORATORY VALUES

Blood/serum values	△ Potassium
Urinary values	△ Potassium

USE IN CHILDREN

Safety and effectiveness for use in children have not been established

USE IN PREGNANT AND NURSING WOMEN

Not expected to cause fetal harm when given in dosages that do not result in hyperkalemia. It is presumed that potassium chloride is excreted in human milk; use with caution in nursing mothers.

POTASSIUM SUPPLEMENTS

KLORVESS 10% Liquid (potassium chloride) Sandoz Pharmaceuticals Rx

Liquid (per 15 ml): 1.5 g (20 mEq)[1] (1 pt) *cherry and pit-flavored*

KLORVESS Effervescent Tablets and Granules (potassium chloride, potassium bicarbonate, and L-lysine monohydrochloride) Sandoz Pharmaceuticals Rx

Tablets: 1.125 g potassium chloride, 0.5 g potassium bicarbonate, and 0.913 g L-lysine monohydrochloride (20 mEq each of potassium and chloride) *sugar-free* **Granules:** 1.125 g potassium chloride, 0.5 g potassium bicarbonate, and 0.913 g L-lysine monohydrochloride (20 mEq each of potassium and chloride) per packet *sugar-free*

INDICATIONS

Prevention and treatment of **potassium depletion and hypokalemic-hypochloremic alkalosis**

ORAL DOSAGE

Adult: 15 ml (1 tbsp), completely diluted in 3–4 fl oz of cold water, or 1 packet or tablet, completely dissolved in 3–4 fl oz of cold water, fruit juice, or other liquid, 2–4 times/day (40–80 mEq/day); prepared solutions should be ingested slowly with or immediately after meals

CONTRAINDICATIONS

Severe renal impairment with azotemia or oliguria	Acute dehydration	Hyperkalemia
Untreated Addison's disease	Heat cramps	Use of aldosterone-inhibiting or potassium-sparing diuretics
Familial periodic paralysis		

WARNINGS/PRECAUTIONS

GI irritation	Caution patient to adhere to dilution instructions to avoid injury
Monitoring of therapy	Since the extent of potassium deficiency cannot be determined accurately, use with caution and periodically monitor patient's clinical status, serum electrolytes, and ECG, particularly if the patient has cardiac disease or is receiving digitalis

ADVERSE REACTIONS

Gastrointestinal	Nausea, vomiting, abdominal discomfort, diarrhea
Other	Hyperkalemia

OVERDOSAGE

Signs and symptoms	Hyperkalemia, ECG changes (peaked T waves, ST-segment depression, loss of P wave, prolongation of Q-T interval, widening and slurring of QRS complex), paresthesias of the extremities, muscle weakness, heaviness, flaccid paralysis, listlessness, mental confusion, peripheral vascular collapse with fall in blood pressure, cardiac arrhythmias, and heart block
Treatment	Discontinue medication and eliminate potassium-rich foods and drugs and use of potassium-sparing diuretics. Administer over a period of 1 h 300–500 ml of 10–25% dextrose containing 10–20 units of insulin per liter of solution. Correct acidosis, if present, with IV sodium bicarbonate. Use of sodium or ammonium cation exchange resins, hemodialysis, and/or peritoneal dialysis may be needed (ammonium compounds should not be used in patients with hepatic cirrhosis). If patient is receiving digitalis, too rapid lowering of the serum potassium level may result in digitalis toxicity.

DRUG INTERACTIONS

Blood from blood bank, potassium-sparing diuretics, low-salt milk, potassium-containing medications, salt substitutes	⇧ Serum potassium level
Sodium cycle exchange resins, glucose-insulin infusions, sodium bicarbonate, laxatives	⇩ Serum potassium level

ALTERED LABORATORY VALUES

Blood/serum values	⇧ Potassium
Urinary values	⇧ Potassium

USE IN CHILDREN

Not indicated for use in children

USE IN PREGNANT AND NURSING WOMEN

There are no contraindications regarding use of these preparations in pregnant or nursing women

---

[1] Contains 0.75% alcohol

POTASSIUM SUPPLEMENTS

KLOTRIX (potassium chloride) Mead Johnson   Rx

Tablets (slow release): 750 mg (10 mEq)

INDICATIONS

Hypokalemia with or without metabolic alkalosis; **digitalis intoxication; hypokalemic familial periodic paralysis; hypokalemia secondary to diuretic therapy** of essential hypertension, when dietary supplementation alone is inadequate

Prevention of potassium depletion when dietary potassium intake is inadequate in patients receiving digitalis and diuretics (for congestive heart failure) or diuretics alone (for hepatic cirrhosis with ascites) and in patients with hyperaldosteronism and normal renal function, potassium-wasting nephropathies, or certain diarrheal states

ORAL DOSAGE

Adult: 4–8 tabs (40–80 mEq)/day; tablets must be swallowed whole and never crushed or chewed

Adult: 2 tabs (20 mEq)/day; tablets must be swallowed whole and never crushed or chewed

KLOTRIX

CONTRAINDICATIONS

Hyperkalemia (further elevation of serum potassium level may produce cardiac arrest)

Esophageal compression due to left-atrial enlargement (esophageal ulceration may occur)

GI motility problems or obstruction (see WARNINGS/PRECAUTIONS)

ADMINISTRATION/DOSAGE ADJUSTMENTS

GI irritation	Nausea, vomiting, abdominal discomfort, and diarrhea may occur; reduce dose or instruct patient to take dose with meals

WARNINGS/PRECAUTIONS

Chronic renal disease or impaired potassium excretion	Asymptomatic hyperkalemia may develop, leading to cardiac arrest and death; carefully monitor serum potassium level and adjust dosage as needed
GI obstruction, hemorrhage, or perforation	Stenotic and/or ulcerative small-bowel lesions and death may occur because of a high local concentration of potassium ion near the bowel wall; discontinue medication immediately if severe vomiting, abdominal pain, distention, or GI bleeding occurs. Use a liquid preparation for potassium supplementation if tablet passage through the GI tract is likely to be delayed or arrested. Use of slow-release tablets should be reserved for patients who cannot tolerate or refuse to take liquid or effervescent preparations or when some other compliance problem exists.
Concomitant metabolic acidosis	Should be treated with an alkalinizing potassium salt, such as potassium bicarbonate, citrate, acetate, or gluconate
Total body potassium stores	May not be accurately reflected by serum potassium levels; monitor acid-base status, serum electrolytes, ECG, and clinical status, particularly in patients with cardiac or renal disease or in the presence of acidosis

ADVERSE REACTIONS

Gastrointestinal	Nausea, vomiting, abdominal discomfort, diarrhea, obstruction, bleeding, ulceration, perforation (see WARNINGS/PRECAUTIONS)
Other	Hyperkalemia, skin rash (rare)

OVERDOSAGE

Signs and symptoms	Hyperkalemia, ECG changes (peaked T waves, ST-segment depression, loss of P wave, prolongation of Q-T interval, widening and slurring of QRS complex), paresthesias of the extremities, muscle weakness, heaviness, flaccid paralysis, listlessness, mental confusion, peripheral vascular collapse with fall in blood pressure, cardiac arrhythmias, and heart block
Treatment	Discontinue medication and eliminate potassium-rich foods and drugs and use of potassium-sparing diuretics. Administer over a period of 1 h 300–500 ml of 10% dextrose containing 10–20 units of insulin per liter of solution. Correct acidosis, if present, with IV sodium bicarbonate. Use of sodium or ammonium cation exchange resins, hemodialysis, and/or peritoneal dialysis may be needed (ammonium compounds should not be used in patients with hepatic cirrhosis). If patient is receiving digitalis, too rapid lowering of the serum potassium level may result in digitalis toxicity.

DRUG INTERACTIONS

Blood from blood bank, potassium-sparing diuretics, low-salt milk, potassium-containing medications, salt substitutes	△ Serum potassium level
Sodium cycle exchange resins, glucose-insulin infusions, sodium bicarbonate, laxatives	▽ Serum potassium level

ALTERED LABORATORY VALUES

Blood/serum values	△ Potassium
Urinary values	△ Potassium

USE IN CHILDREN

Safety and effectiveness for use in children have not been established

USE IN PREGNANT AND NURSING WOMEN

Use of this drug in pregnant women is not expected to cause fetal harm unless administered in doses which would result in hyperkalemia. It is not known whether this drug is excreted in human milk. Because many drugs are so excreted and because of the risk of hyperkalemia, the patient should not nurse if use of the drug is deemed essential.

POTASSIUM SUPPLEMENTS

K-LYTE Effervescent Tablets (potassium bicarbonate) Bristol   Rx

Effervescent tablets: 2.5 g[1] (25 mEq) *lime- or orange-flavored*

K-LYTE DS Effervescent Tablets (potassium bicarbonate and potassium citrate) Bristol   Rx

Effervescent tablets: 2.5 g potassium bicarbonate and 2.7 g potassium citrate[1] (50 mEq) *lime- or orange-flavored*

INDICATIONS

Prevention and treatment of **potassium deficiency** caused by thiazide diuretics, corticosteroids, vomiting or diarrhea, or low dietary intake of potassium; **digitalis intoxication**

ORAL DOSAGE

Adult: 1 K-Lyte tab, completely dissolved in 3–4 fl oz of cold or ice water, bid to qid, or 1 K-Lyte DS tab, completely dissolved in 6–8 fl oz of cold or ice water, 1–2 times/day, sipped slowly (5–10 min) with meals (50–100 mEq/day)

K-LYTE/CL and K-LYTE/CL 50 Effervescent Tablets (potassium chloride, potassium bicarbonate, and L-lysine monohydrochloride) Bristol   Rx

Effervescent tablets: 1.5 g potassium chloride, 0.5 g potassium bicarbonate, and 0.91 g L-lysine monohydrochloride[1] (25 mEq each of potassium and chloride) (K-Lyte/Cl); 2.24 g potassium chloride, 2 g potassium bicarbonate, and 3.65 g L-lysine monohydrochloride[1] (50 mEq each of potassium and chloride) (K-Lyte/Cl 50) *citrus- or fruit punch-flavored*

K-LYTE/CL Powder (potassium chloride) Bristol   Rx

Powder: 1.86 g/measured scoop (25 mEq) *fruit punch-flavored*

INDICATIONS

Prevention and treatment of **potassium deficiency** caused by thiazide diuretics, corticosteroids, vomiting or diarrhea, or low dietary intake of potassium; **digitalis intoxication**
Hypokalemia accompanied by metabolic alkalosis and hypochloremia

ORAL DOSAGE

Adult: 1 K-Lyte/Cl tab, completely dissolved in 3–4 fl oz of cold or ice water, or 25 mEq of powder (1 scoop), completely dissolved in 6 fl oz of cold or ice water, bid to qid, or 1 K-Lyte/Cl 50 tab, completely dissolved in 6–8 fl oz of cold or ice water, 1–2 times/day, sipped slowly (5–10 min) with meals (50–100 mEq/day)

CONTRAINDICATIONS

Hyperkalemia (see WARNINGS/PRECAUTIONS)

Use with potassium-sparing diuretics (severe hyperkalemia may occur)

WARNINGS/PRECAUTIONS

Monitoring of therapy	Since the degree of potassium deficiency may be difficult to determine accurately, use with caution, adjust dosage to individual requirements, and frequently monitor patient's clinical status, ECG, serum potassium level, and acid-base balance
GI irritation	Caution patients to dissolve each dose completely, as indicated (see ORAL DOSAGE)
Hyperkalemia	Further elevation of serum potassium level may produce cardiac arrest; hyperkalemia may complicate chronic renal failure, systemic acidosis (eg, diabetic acidosis), acute dehydration, extensive tissue breakdown (eg, as in severe burns), and adrenal insufficiency
Chronic renal disease or impaired potassium excretion	Asymptomatic hyperkalemia may develop, leading to cardiac arrest and death; carefully monitor serum potassium level and adjust dosage as needed

ADVERSE REACTIONS

Gastrointestinal	Nausea, vomiting, diarrhea, abdominal discomfort
Other	Hyperkalemia (rare)

OVERDOSAGE

Signs and symptoms	Hyperkalemia, ECG changes (peaked T waves, ST-segment depression, loss of P wave, prolongation of Q-T interval, widening and slurring of QRS complex), paresthesias of the extremities, muscle weakness, heaviness, flaccid paralysis, listlessness, mental confusion, peripheral vascular collapse with fall in blood pressure, cardiac arrhythmias, and heart block
Treatment	Discontinue medication and eliminate potassium-rich foods and drugs and use of potassium-sparing diuretics. Administer over a period of 1 h 300–500 ml of 10% dextrose containing 10–20 units of insulin per liter of solution. Correct acidosis, if present, with IV sodium bicarbonate. Use of sodium or ammonium cation exchange resins, hemodialysis, and/or peritoneal dialysis may be needed (ammonium compounds should not be used in patients with hepatic cirrhosis). If patient is receiving digitalis, too rapid lowering of the serum potassium level may result in digitalis toxicity.

K-LYTE ■ K·TAB

DRUG INTERACTIONS

Blood from blood bank, potassium-sparing diuretics, low-salt milk, potassium-containing medications, salt substitutes	△	Serum potassium level
Sodium cycle exchange resins, glucose-insulin infusions, sodium bicarbonate, laxatives	▽	Serum potassium level

ALTERED LABORATORY VALUES

Blood/serum values	△	Potassium
Urinary values	△	Potassium

USE IN CHILDREN

Safety and effectiveness for use in children have not been established

USE IN PREGNANT AND NURSING WOMEN

Pregnancy Category C: use during pregnancy only if clearly needed. Animal reproduction studies have not been done, nor is it known whether these preparations can affect human fetal development or reproductive capacity. It is also not known whether they are excreted in human milk. Because many drugs are excreted in human milk, and because of the potential risk of hyperkalemia in the infant, patient should stop nursing if use of these preparations is essential.

[1] Tablets also contain citric acid (2.1 g, K-Lyte and K-Lyte DS; 0.55 g, K-Lyte/Cl; 1 g, K-Lyte/Cl 50)

POTASSIUM SUPPLEMENTS

K·TAB (potassium chloride) Abbott   Rx

Tablets (extended release): 750 mg (10 mEq)

INDICATIONS

Hypokalemia with or without metabolic alkalosis; **digitalis intoxication; hypokalemic familial periodic paralysis; hypokalemia secondary to diuretic therapy** of essential hypertension, when dietary supplementation alone is inadequate

Prevention of potassium depletion, when dietary potassium intake is inadequate, in patients receiving digitalis and diuretics (for congestive heart failure) or diuretics alone (for hepatic cirrhosis with ascites) and in patients with hyperaldosteronism and normal renal function, potassium-wasting nephropathies, or certain diarrheal states

ORAL DOSAGE

Adult: 2–8 tabs (20–80 mEq)/day; tablets must be swallowed whole and not crushed or chewed

Adult: consult manufacturer

CONTRAINDICATIONS

Hyperkalemia (see WARNINGS/PRECAUTIONS)	Esophageal compression due to left-atrial enlargement	Hypersensitivity to any component
Concomitant metabolic acidosis (see WARNINGS/PRECAUTIONS)	Conditions that can arrest or delay passage of the tablets through the GI tract	

ADMINISTRATION/DOSAGE ADJUSTMENTS

GI irritation	To manage nausea, vomiting, abdominal discomfort, and diarrhea, reduce the dose or give it with meals
Interpretation of plasma potassium level	The relationship between total body stores of potassium and the plasma potassium level is affected by changes in the acid-base balance; acute alkalosis can cause hypokalemia in the absence of a deficit in total body potassium, whereas acute acidosis can produce a normal plasma level in the presence of such a deficit
Monitoring of therapy	Check the plasma potassium level regularly. During treatment of hypokalemia, carefully monitor other plasma electrolyte levels, the acid-base balance, clinical response, and the ECG, especially in patients with acidosis or cardiac or renal disease
Diuretic-induced hypokalemia	Consider giving potassium supplements to patients receiving diuretics for uncomplicated essential hypertension only if hypokalemia occurs during therapy and cannot be adequately controlled by changes in diet
Metabolic acidosis	For treatment of hypokalemia associated with metabolic acidosis, use an alkalinizing potassium salt (eg, potassium citrate, potassium gluconate) rather than this product

K·TAB ■ MICRO-K

WARNINGS/PRECAUTIONS

Hyperkalemia — Administration of potassium to patients with chronic renal disease or other disorders associated with impaired potassium excretion may cause hyperkalemia and precipitate cardiac arrest, which may be fatal. The resulting increase in potassium may also complicate the following conditions: cardiac disease, chronic renal failure, systemic acidosis (eg, diabetic acidosis), adrenal insufficiency, acute dehydration, or disorders associated with extensive tissue breakdown (eg, severe burns). Hyperkalemia is usually asymptomatic, and its only manifestations may be an increased plasma potassium level and characteristic ECG changes (peaking of T waves, loss of P wave, depression of S–T segment, and prolongation of the Q–T interval); muscle paralysis and cardiovascular collapse are late signs. Potentially fatal effects can develop rapidly. To avoid hyperkalemia, monitor the plasma potassium level with particular care when giving this product to patients with impaired potassium excretion and adjust dosage as needed. Do not give this product to patients receiving potassium-sparing diuretics. For treatment of hyperkalemia, see OVERDOSAGE.

Gastrointestinal toxicity — Potassium chloride tablets have produced fatal GI bleeding, stenosis, and ulceration resulting from a high, localized concentration of potassium ion in the vicinity of the GI mucosa and consequent damage to the GI wall. GI ulceration and bleeding have also been reported with slow-release potassium chloride preparations. The frequency of GI lesions with wax-matrix tablets is approximately 1 per 100,000 patient-years. Instruct all patients to report immediately tarry stools or any other evidence of GI bleeding. If severe vomiting, abdominal pain, distention, or GI bleeding occurs, discontinue use immediately and consider the possibility of GI obstruction or perforation.

Esophageal ulcers — This preparation can cause esophageal ulceration in patients with esophageal compression owing to an enlarged left atrium; use is contraindicated in these patients

Carcinogenicity — No long-term studies have been done to evaluate the carcinogenic potential of potassium chloride

ADVERSE REACTIONS

Gastrointestinal — Nausea, vomiting, abdominal discomfort, diarrhea; GI obstruction, bleeding, ulceration, and perforation

Other — Hyperkalemia, skin rash (rare)

OVERDOSAGE

Signs and symptoms — Hyperkalemia (see WARNINGS/PRECAUTIONS)

Treatment — Discontinue use of potassium-containing drugs and food. Administer a solution of 10% dextrose containing 10–20 units of insulin per liter at a rate of 300–500 ml/h. Correct acidosis, if present, with IV sodium bicarbonate. Administer sodium polystyrene sulfonate and perform hemodialysis or peritoneal dialysis, as needed. When treating hyperkalemia in patients who are receiving digitalis, exercise caution; digitalis toxicity can occur if the plasma potassium level is reduced too rapidly.

DRUG INTERACTIONS

Potassium-sparing diuretics — Severe hyperkalemia; do not use potassium-sparing diuretics in combination with this product

Captopril, enalapril, potassium-rich foods (including salt substitutes and low-salt milk) — △ Plasma potassium level

ALTERED LABORATORY VALUES

Blood/serum values — △ Potassium
Urinary values — △ Potassium

USE IN CHILDREN

Safety and effectiveness for use in children have not been established

USE IN PREGNANT AND NURSING WOMEN

Pregnant women: Not expected to cause fetal harm when given in dosages that do not result in hyperkalemia. **Nursing women:** It is presumed that potassium chloride is excreted in human milk; use with caution in nursing mothers.

POTASSIUM SUPPLEMENTS

MICRO-K (potassium chloride) Robins   Rx

Capsules (controlled release): 600 mg (8 mEq) (Micro-K), 750 mg (10 mEq) (Micro-K 10)

INDICATIONS

Hypokalemia with or without metabolic alkalosis; **digitalis intoxication**; **hypokalemic familial periodic paralysis**; **hypokalemia secondary to diuretic therapy** of essential hypertension, when dietary supplementation alone is inadequate

ORAL DOSAGE

Adult: 40–100 mEq/day (5–12 8-mEq caps/day or 4–10 10-mEq caps/day)
Child: use according to medical judgment

MICRO-K

Prevention of potassium depletion, when dietary potassium intake is inadequate, in patients receiving digitalis and diuretics (for congestive heart failure) or diuretics alone (for hepatic cirrhosis with ascites) and in patients with hyperaldosteronism and normal renal function, potassium-wasting nephropathies, or certain diarrheal states	**Adult:** 16–24 mEq/day (2–3 8-mEq caps/day or 2 10–mEq caps/day) **Child:** use according to medical judgment

CONTRAINDICATIONS

Hyperkalemia (see WARNINGS/PRECAUTIONS)	Conditions that arrest or delay passage of the capsules through the GI tract

ADMINISTRATION/DOSAGE ADJUSTMENTS

Frequency of administration	Up to 2 caps/day may be given in a single daily dose; divide larger daily doses into 2 or more doses
Administration	Instruct the patient to take the capsules with a glass of water or other liquid; patients experiencing difficulty in swallowing the capsules whole may sprinkle the contents onto a spoonful of soft food
GI irritation	To manage nausea, vomiting, abdominal discomfort, and diarrhea, reduce the dose or give it with meals
Interpretation of plasma potassium level	The relationship between total body stores of potassium and the plasma potassium level is affected by changes in the acid-base balance; acute alkalosis can cause hypokalemia in the absence of a deficit in total body potassium, whereas acute acidosis can produce a normal plasma level in the presence of such a deficit
Monitoring of therapy	Check the plasma potassium level regularly. During treatment of hypokalemia, carefully monitor other plasma electrolyte levels, the acid-base balance, clinical response, and the ECG, especially in patients with acidosis or cardiac or renal disease
Diuretic-induced hypokalemia	Consider giving potassium supplements to patients receiving diuretics for uncomplicated essential hypertension only if hypokalemia occurs during therapy and cannot be adequately controlled by changes in diet
Metabolic acidosis	For treatment of hypokalemia associated with metabolic acidosis, use an alkalinizing potassium salt (eg, potassium citrate, potassium gluconate) rather than this product

WARNINGS/PRECAUTIONS

Hyperkalemia	Administration of potassium to patients with chronic renal disease or other disorders associated with impaired potassium excretion may cause hyperkalemia and precipitate cardiac arrest, which may be fatal. The resulting increase in potassium may also complicate the following conditions: chronic renal failure, systemic acidosis (eg, diabetic acidosis), adrenal insufficiency, acute dehydration, or disorders associated with extensive tissue breakdown (eg, severe burns). Hyperkalemia is usually asymptomatic, and its only manifestations may be an increased plasma potassium level and characteristic ECG changes (peaking of T waves, loss of P wave, depression of S–T segment, and prolongation of the Q–T interval); muscle paralysis and cardiovascular collapse are late signs. Potentially fatal effects can develop rapidly. To avoid hyperkalemia, monitor the plasma potassium level with particular care when giving this product to patients with impaired potassium excretion and adjust dosage as needed. Do not give this product to patients receiving potassium-sparing diuretics. For treatment of hyperkalemia, see OVERDOSAGE.
Gastrointestinal toxicity	Potassium chloride tablets have produced fatal GI bleeding, stenosis, and ulceration resulting from a high, localized concentration of potassium ion in the vicinity of the GI mucosa and consequent damage to the GI wall. GI ulceration and bleeding have also been reported with slow-release potassium chloride preparations. This product contains polymeric-coated microcapsules that rapidly disperse following dissolution of the hard-gelatin capsule; the coating provides for a controlled release of potassium over a period of 8–10 h. Whether this design minimizes the risk of GI lesions is not currently known, since the frequency of lesions resulting from use of this product has not been established. Instruct patients to report immediately tarry stools or any other evidence of GI bleeding. If severe vomiting, abdominal pain, distention, or GI bleeding occurs, discontinue use immediately and consider the possibility of obstruction or perforation.
Esophageal ulcers	In certain patients with esophageal compression owing to an enlarged left atrium, wax matrix potassium preparations have produced esophageal ulceration (Micro-K is not formulated with a wax matrix)

ADVERSE REACTIONS

Gastrointestinal	Nausea, vomiting, abdominal discomfort, diarrhea; GI obstruction, bleeding, ulceration, and perforation (see WARNINGS/PRECAUTIONS)
Other	Hyperkalemia; skin rash (rare)

OVERDOSAGE

Signs and symptoms	Hyperkalemia (see WARNINGS/PRECAUTIONS)
Treatment	Discontinue use of potassium-containing drugs and food. Administer a solution of 10% dextrose containing 10–20 units of insulin per liter at a rate of 300–500 ml/h. Correct acidosis, if present, with IV sodium bicarbonate. Administer sodium polystyrene sulfonate and perform hemodialysis or peritoneal dialysis, as needed. When treating hyperkalemia in patients who are receiving digitalis, exercise caution; digitalis toxicity can occur if the plasma potassium level is reduced too rapidly.

DRUG INTERACTIONS

Potassium-sparing diuretics	Severe hyperkalemia; do not use potassium-sparing diuretics in combination with this product
Captopril, enalapril, potassium-rich foods (including salt substitutes and low-salt milk)	⇧ Plasma potassium level

ALTERED LABORATORY VALUES

Blood/serum values	⇧ Potassium
Urinary values	⇧ Potassium

USE IN CHILDREN
Use according to medical judgment

USE IN PREGNANT AND NURSING WOMEN
Consult manufacturer

POTASSIUM SUPPLEMENTS

SLOW-K (potassium chloride) CIBA   Rx

Tablets (slow release): 8 mEq

INDICATIONS

Treatment of **hypokalemia, digitalis intoxication, and hypokalemic familial periodic paralysis** in patients who cannot tolerate liquid potassium preparations or refuse or find it difficult to take these preparations

Prevention of **hypokalemia** in patients receiving digitalis and diuretics for congestive heart failure and in patients with hepatic cirrhosis and ascites, hyperaldosteronism (and normal renal function), potassium-losing nephropathy, or certain diarrheal states, but only when dietary intake of potassium is inadequate and these patients cannot tolerate liquid potassium preparations or refuse or find it difficult to take these preparations

ORAL DOSAGE

Adult: 40–100 mEq/day or more; if a large number of tablets is required daily, administer in divided doses

Adult: 20 mEq/day

CONTRAINDICATIONS

Hyperkalemia (see WARNINGS/PRECAUTIONS)	Conditions that can arrest or delay passage of the tablets through the GI tract	Esophageal compression owing to an enlarged left atrium

ADMINISTRATION/DOSAGE ADJUSTMENTS

Administration	Instruct the patient to take the tablets with a glass of water or another liquid and to swallow tablets whole without crushing, chewing, or sucking them; the patient should report any difficulty swallowing the tablets or any tendency for the tablets to stick in the throat
GI irritation	To manage nausea, vomiting, abdominal discomfort, and diarrhea, reduce the dose or give it with meals
Interpretation of plasma potassium level	The relationship between total body stores of potassium and the plasma potassium level is affected by changes in the acid-base balance: acute alkalosis can cause hypokalemia in the absence of a deficit in total body stores, while acute acidosis can produce a normal plasma level in the presence of such a deficit
Monitoring of therapy	Check the plasma potassium level regularly. During treatment of hypokalemia, carefully monitor other plasma electrolyte levels, the acid-base balance, clinical response, and the ECG, especially in patients with acidosis or cardiac or renal disease
Diuretic-induced hypokalemia	Consider giving potassium supplements to patients receiving diuretics for uncomplicated essential hypertension only if hypokalemia occurs during therapy and cannot be adequately controlled by changes in diet

SLOW-K ■ TEN-K

Metabolic acidosis	For treatment of hypokalemia associated with metabolic acidosis, use an alkalinizing potassium salt (eg, potassium citrate, potassium gluconate) rather than this product

WARNINGS/PRECAUTIONS

Hyperkalemia	Administration of potassium to patients with chronic renal disease or other disorders associated with impaired potassium excretion may cause hyperkalemia and precipitate cardiac arrest, which may be fatal. The resulting increase in potassium may also complicate the following conditions: chronic renal failure, systemic acidosis (eg, diabetic acidosis), adrenal insufficiency, acute dehydration, or disorders associated with extensive tissue breakdown (eg, severe burns). Hyperkalemia is usually asymptomatic, and its only manifestations may be an increased plasma potassium level and characteristic ECG changes (peaking of T waves, loss of P wave, depression of S–T segment, and prolongation of the Q–T interval); muscle paralysis and cardiovascular collapse are late signs. Potentially fatal effects can develop rapidly. To avoid hyperkalemia, monitor the plasma potassium level with particular care when giving this product to patients with impaired potassium excretion and adjust dosage as needed. Do not give this product to patients receiving potassium-sparing diuretics. For treatment of hyperkalemia, see OVERDOSAGE.
Gastrointestinal toxicity	Potassium chloride tablets have produced fatal GI bleeding, stenosis, and ulceration resulting from a high, localized concentration of potassium ion in the vicinity of the GI mucosa and consequent damage to the GI wall. GI ulceration and bleeding have also been reported with slow-release potassium chloride preparations. The frequency of GI lesions with wax-matrix tablets is approximately 1 per 100,000 patient-years. Instruct all patients to report immediately tarry stools or any other evidence of GI bleeding. If severe vomiting, abdominal pain, distention, or GI bleeding occurs, discontinue use immediately and consider the possibility of GI obstruction or perforation.
Esophageal ulcers	This preparation can cause esophageal ulceration in patients with esophageal compression owing to an enlarged left atrium; use is contradindicated in these patients
Carcinogenicity	No long-term studies have been done to evaluate the carcinogenic potential of potassium chloride

ADVERSE REACTIONS

Gastrointestinal	Nausea, vomiting, abdominal discomfort, diarrhea; GI obstruction, bleeding, ulceration, and perforation
Other	Hyperkalemia; rash (rare)

OVERDOSAGE

Signs and symptoms	Hyperkalemia (see WARNINGS/PRECAUTIONS)
Treatment	Discontinue use of potassium-containing drugs and food. Administer a solution of 10% dextrose containing 10–20 units of insulin per liter at a rate of 300–500 ml/h. Correct acidosis, if present, with IV sodium bicarbonate. Administer sodium polystyrene sulfonate and perform hemodialysis or peritoneal dialysis, as needed. When treating hyperkalemia in patients who are receiving digitalis, exercise caution; digitalis toxicity can occur if the plasma potassium level is reduced too rapidly.

DRUG INTERACTIONS

Potassium-sparing diuretics	Severe hyperkalemia; do not use potassium-sparing diuretics in combination with this product
Captopril, enalapril, potassium-rich foods (including salt substitutes and low-salt milk)	⌂ Plasma potassium level

ALTERED LABORATORY VALUES

Blood/serum values	⌂ Potassium
Urinary values	⌂ Potassium

USE IN CHILDREN

Safety and effectiveness for use in children have not been established

---

USE IN PREGNANT AND NURSING WOMEN

Pregnant women: Pregnancy Category C: it is not known whether this preparation can cause harm to the fetus or affect reproductive capacity; reproduction studies have not been done in animals. Use during pregnancy only if clearly needed. **Nursing mothers:** It is not known whether administration of this product will affect the potassium level in human milk; use with caution in nursing mothers.

POTASSIUM SUPPLEMENTS

TEN-K (potassium chloride) Geigy   Rx
Tablets (controlled release): 10 mEq

INDICATIONS

Treatment of **hypokalemia, digitalis intoxication,** and **hypokalemic familial periodic paralysis** in patients who cannot tolerate liquid potassium preparations or refuse or find it difficult to take these preparations

ORAL DOSAGE

Adult: 40–100 mEq/day or more, given in 2 or more divided doses; no single dose should exceed 20 mEq

COMPENDIUM OF DRUG THERAPY

TEN-K

Prevention of **hypokalemia** in patients receiving digitalis and diuretics for congestive heart failure and in patients with hepatic cirrhosis and ascites, hyperaldosteronism (and normal renal function), potassium-losing nephropathy, or certain diarrheal states, but only when dietary intake of potassium is inadequate and these patients cannot tolerate liquid potassium preparations or refuse or find it difficult to take these preparations

Adult: 20–30 mEq/day; no single dose should exceed 20 mEq

CONTRAINDICATIONS

Hyperkalemia (see WARNINGS/PRECAUTIONS)	Conditions that can arrest or delay passage of the tablets through the GI tract

ADMINISTRATION/DOSAGE ADJUSTMENTS

Administration	Instruct the patient to take the tablets with a glass of water or other liquid; patients experiencing difficulty in swallowing the tablets whole may break them in half or crush them
GI irritation	To manage nausea, vomiting, abdominal discomfort, and diarrhea, reduce the dose or give it with meals
Interpretation of plasma potassium level	The relationship between total body stores of potassium and the plasma potassium level is affected by changes in the acid-base balance; acute alkalosis can cause hypokalemia in the absence of a deficit in total body potassium, whereas acute acidosis can produce a normal plasma level in the presence of such a deficit
Monitoring of therapy	Check the plasma potassium level regularly. During treatment of hypokalemia, carefully monitor other plasma electrolyte levels, the acid-base balance, clinical response, and the ECG, especially in patients with acidosis or cardiac or renal disease
Diuretic-induced hypokalemia	Consider giving potassium supplements to patients receiving diuretics for uncomplicated essential hypertension only if hypokalemia occurs during therapy and cannot be adequately controlled by changes in diet
Metabolic acidosis	For treatment of hypokalemia associated with metabolic acidosis, use an alkalinizing potassium salt (eg, potassium citrate, potassium gluconate) rather than this product

WARNINGS/PRECAUTIONS

Hyperkalemia	Administration of potassium to patients with chronic renal disease or other disorders associated with impaired potassium excretion may cause hyperkalemia and precipitate cardiac arrest, which may be fatal. The resulting increase in potassium may also complicate the following conditions: chronic renal failure, systemic acidosis (eg, diabetic acidosis), adrenal insufficiency, acute dehydration, or disorders associated with extensive tissue breakdown (eg, severe burns). Hyperkalemia is usually asymptomatic, and its only manifestations may be an increased plasma potassium level and characteristic ECG changes (peaking of T waves, loss of P wave, depression of S-T segment, and prolongation of the Q-T interval); muscle paralysis and cardiovascular collapse are late signs. Potentially fatal effects can develop rapidly. To avoid hyperkalemia, monitor the plasma potassium level with particular care when giving this product to patients with impaired potassium excretion and adjust dosage as needed. Do not give this product to patients receiving potassium-sparing diuretics. For treatment of hyperkalemia, see OVERDOSAGE.
Gastrointestinal toxicity	Potassium chloride tablets have produced fatal GI bleeding, stenosis, and ulceration resulting from a high, localized concentration of potassium ion in the vicinity of the GI mucosa and consequent damage to the GI wall. GI ulceration and bleeding have also been reported with slow-release potassium chloride preparations. This product contains polymeric-coated crystals that rapidly disperse following disintegration of the tablet; the coating provides for a controlled release of potassium over a period of 8–10 h. Whether this design minimizes the risk of GI lesions is not currently known, since the frequency of lesions resulting from use of this product has not been established. Instruct patients to report immediately tarry stools or any other evidence of GI bleeding. If severe vomiting, abdominal pain, distention, or GI bleeding occurs, discontinue use immediately and consider the possibility of obstruction or perforation.
Esophageal ulcers	In certain patients with esophageal compression owing to an enlarged left atrium, wax matrix potassium preparations have produced esophageal ulceration (Ten-K is not formulated with a wax matrix)
Carcinogenicity	No long-term studies have been done to evaluate the carcinogenic potential of potassium chloride

ADVERSE REACTIONS

Gastrointestinal	Nausea, vomiting, abdominal discomfort, diarrhea; GI obstruction, bleeding, ulceration, and perforation
Other	Hyperkalemia; rash (rare)

OVERDOSAGE

Signs and symptoms	Hyperkalemia (see WARNINGS/PRECAUTIONS)
Treatment	Discontinue use of potassium-containing drugs and food. Administer a solution of 10% dextrose containing 10–20 units of insulin per liter at a rate of 300–500 ml/h. Correct acidosis, if present, with IV sodium bicarbonate. Administer sodium polystyrene sulfonate and perform hemodialysis or peritoneal dialysis, as needed. When treating hyperkalemia in patients who are receiving digitalis, exercise caution; digitalis toxicity can occur if the plasma potassium level is reduced too rapidly.

TEN-K

DRUG INTERACTIONS

Potassium-sparing diuretics	Severe hyperkalemia; do not use potassium-sparing diuretics in combination with this product
Captopril, enalapril, potassium-rich foods (including salt substitutes and low-salt milk)	⇧ Plasma potassium level

ALTERED LABORATORY VALUES

Blood/serum values	⇧ Potassium
Urinary values	⇧ Potassium

USE IN CHILDREN

Safety and effectiveness for use in children have not been established

---

USE IN PREGNANT AND NURSING WOMEN

Pregnant women: Pregnancy Category C: it is not known whether this preparation can cause harm to the fetus or affect reproductive capacity; reproduction studies have not been done in animals. Use during pregnancy only if clearly needed. **Nursing mothers:** It is not known whether administration of this product will affect the potassium level in human milk; use with caution in nursing mothers.

Chapter 45

Sedatives/Hypnotics

Barbiturates	**1793**
AMYTAL (Lilly) Amobarbital C-II	1793
AMYTAL Sodium (Lilly) Amobarbital sodium C-II	1793
BUTICAPS (Wallace) Sodium butabarbital C-III	1794
BUTISOL Sodium (Wallace) Sodium butabarbital C-III	1794
LOTUSATE (Winthrop-Breon) Talbutal C-III	1796
MEBARAL (Winthrop-Breon) Mephobarbital C-IV	1797
NEMBUTAL Elixir (Abbott) Pentobarbital C-II	1799
NEMBUTAL Sodium Capsules and Solution (Abbott) Pentobarbital sodium C-II	1799
NEMBUTAL Sodium Suppositories (Abbott) Pentobarbital sodium C-III	1800
Phenobarbital C-IV	1802
Phenobarbital sodium C-IV	1802
SECONAL Sodium Capsules (Lilly) Secobarbital sodium C-II	1804
SECONAL Sodium Injection (Lilly) Secobarbital sodium C-II	1804
SECONAL Sodium Suppositories (Lilly) Secobarbital sodium C-III	1804
TUINAL (Lilly) Secobarbital sodium and amobarbital sodium C-II	1806

Nonbarbiturates	**1807**
DALMANE (Roche) Flurazepam hydrochloride C-IV	1807
DORIDEN (Rorer) Glutethimide C-III	1808
HALCION (Upjohn) Triazolam C-IV	1810
NOCTEC (Squibb) Chloral hydrate C-IV	1811
NOLUDAR (Roche) Methyprylon C-III	1813
NOLUDAR 300 (Roche) Methyprylon C-III	1813
PLACIDYL (Abbott) Ethchlorvynol C-IV	1814
RESTORIL (Sandoz Pharmaceuticals) Temazepam C-IV	1815
VALMID (Dista) Ethinamate C-IV	1816
VERSED (Roche) Midazolam hydrochloride C-IV	1817
Other Sedatives/Hypnotics	**1792**
ALURATE (Roche) Aprobarbital C-III	1792

OTHER SEDATIVES/HYPNOTICS

DRUG	HOW SUPPLIED	USUAL DOSAGE[1]
ALURATE (Roche) Aprobarbital C-III	**Elixir (per 5 ml):** 40 mg (16 fl oz)	**Adult:** for sedation, 5 ml (1 tsp) tid; for mild insomnia, 5–10 ml (1–2 tsp) at bedtime; for severe insomnia, 10–20 ml (2–4 tsp) at bedtime

[1] Where pediatric dosages are not given, consult manufacturer

BARBITURATES

AMYTAL (amobarbital) Lilly C-II
Tablets: 30, 50, 100 mg

INDICATIONS	ORAL DOSAGE
Daytime sedation	Adult: 15–120 mg 2–4 times/day; usual sedative dosage, 30–50 mg bid or tid
Insomnia Preanesthetic sedation	Adult: 100–200 mg; higher doses may be given if needed

AMYTAL Sodium (amobarbital sodium) Lilly C-II
Capsules: 65, 200 mg **Vials:** 250, 500 mg

INDICATIONS	ORAL DOSAGE	PARENTERAL DOSAGE
Insomnia	Adult: 65–200 mg at bedtime	—
Preanesthetic sedation	Adult: 200 mg 1–2 h prior to surgery	—
Labor	Adult: 200–400 mg to start, followed by 200–400 mg q1-3h, if needed, up to a total of 1,000 mg	—
Convulsive seizures, including seizures due to chorea, eclampsia, meningitis, tetanus, procaine or cocaine reactions, and strychnine or picrotoxin poisoning Epileptiform seizures Catatonic, negativistic, or manic reactions Narcoanalysis Narcotherapy Diagnosis of schizophrenia	—	Adult: 65–500 mg IM or IV, up to 500 mg IM or 1 g IV, as needed Child (6–12 yr): 65–500 mg IM or IV, as needed

CONTRAINDICATIONS

Hypersensitivity to barbiturates	History of manifest or latent porphyria	Severe hepatic impairment
Respiratory disease accompanied by dyspnea or obstruction	Prior addiction to sedative-hypnotics	Acute or chronic pain

ADMINISTRATION/DOSAGE ADJUSTMENTS

Preparation of parenteral solution	Dilute contents of ampul with Sterile Water for Injection; ordinarily, a 10% solution is used for IV administration and a 20% solution for IM injection. Discard solution if drug does not dissolve completely within 5 min of mixing with diluent or if a precipitate forms after the solution clears. Inject within 30 min of opening the ampul. Do not use drug supplied in capsules for injection.
Intramuscular administration	Inject deeply into a large muscle mass, such as the gluteus maximus; to preclude irritation, give no more than 5 ml at any one site
Intravenous administration	Administer slowly ($\leq$ 1 ml/min); overly rapid IV administration may result in apnea and/or hypotension

WARNINGS/PRECAUTIONS

Patients with hepatic impairment	Use with caution to avoid excessive accumulation
Elderly or debilitated patients	May experience marked excitement or CNS depression; use with caution
Patients with borderline hypoadrenal function	Systemic effects of both endogenous and exogenous hydrocortisone may be diminished; use with caution
Mental and/or physical impairment	Caution patients that their ability to drive or perform other potentially hazardous activities may be impaired
Overdosage	Excessive doses, either alone or in combination with other CNS depressants, may result in toxicity and death; warn patients not to exceed recommended dosage and to limit alcohol intake, and that the concomitant use of other CNS depressants can cause additional CNS depression. Use with caution in patients who have a history of emotional disturbances or suicidal ideation.
Drug dependence	Psychic and/or physical dependence and tolerance may develop, especially in addiction-prone individuals; abrupt discontinuation after chronic use of large doses may result in withdrawal reactions, including delirium, convulsions, and death

ADVERSE REACTIONS

Central nervous system	Residual sedation ("hangover"), drowsiness; lethargy and headache (with oral use); idiosyncratic excitement and pain (with parenteral use)
Respiratory	Depression, apnea; laryngospasm (with parenteral use)

AMYTAL ■ BUTICAPS/BUTISOL

Cardiovascular	Circulatory collapse; vasodilation and hypotension (with rapid IV injection)
Hypersensitivity	Allergic reactions, skin eruptions
Gastrointestinal	Nausea, vomiting
Other	Postoperative atelectasis (with parenteral use)

OVERDOSAGE

Signs and symptoms	Early hypothermia followed by fever, sluggish or absent reflexes, respiratory depression, circulatory collapse, pulmonary edema, and coma
Treatment	Empty stomach by gastric lavage and institute general supportive measures, as needed, including IV fluid replacement and maintenance of blood pressure, body temperature, and adequate respiratory exchange. Dialysis may be helpful. Antibiotics may be required to control pulmonary complications.

DRUG INTERACTIONS

Alcohol, antihistamines, tranquilizers, and other CNS depressants	△ CNS depression
Oral anticoagulants	▽ Prothrombin time
Corticosteroids	▽ Corticosteroid effects
Digitalis, digitoxin	▽ Cardiac glycoside effects
Doxycycline	▽ Anti-infective effect
Tricyclic antidepressants	▽ Antidepressant effect
Griseofulvin	▽ Griseofulvin absorption
MAO inhibitors	△ Antidepressant or barbiturate effects

ALTERED LABORATORY VALUES

Blood/serum values	▽ Bilirubin

No clinically significant alterations in urinary values occur at therapeutic dosages

---

USE IN CHILDREN

See INDICATIONS for use of parenteral form; the safety and effectiveness of oral administration have not been established in children

USE IN PREGNANT AND NURSING WOMEN

Pregnancy Category B: use during pregnancy only if clearly needed. Animal reproduction studies have shown no evidence of impaired fertility or fetal harm; however, no adequate, well-controlled studies have been done in pregnant women. Neonatal depression may occur following use during labor. Administer with caution to nursing mothers.

BARBITURATES

BUTICAPS (sodium butabarbital) Wallace C-III
Capsules: 15, 30 mg

BUTISOL Sodium (sodium butabarbital) Wallace C-III
Tablets: 15, 30, 50, 100 mg Elixir (per 5 ml): 30 mg[1] (1 pt, 1 gal)

INDICATIONS	ORAL DOSAGE
Daytime sedation	Adult: 15–30 mg tid or qid
Short-term (up to 2 wk) treatment of insomnia	Adult: 50–100 mg at bedtime
Preanesthetic medication	Adult: 50–100 mg 60–90 min before surgery Child: 2–6 mg/kg, up to 100 mg, 60–90 min before surgery

CONTRAINDICATIONS

Sensitivity to barbiturates	History of manifest or latent porphyria

WARNINGS/PRECAUTIONS

Drug dependence	Psychic and/or physical dependence and tolerance may develop with continued use; abrupt cessation after chronic use of large doses may precipitate withdrawal reactions, including delirium, convulsions, and death. Instruct patients to adhere strictly to the dosage regimen. Use with caution, if at all, in mentally depressed patients and patients with suicidal tendencies or a history of drug abuse.

Excitement	In some patients, barbiturates repeatedly produce excitement rather than depression
Elderly or debilitated patients	Reduce dosage, since such patients may be more sensitive to barbiturates, and may respond to usual doses with marked excitement, depression, or confusion
Patients with acute or chronic pain	Use with caution because paradoxical excitement may be induced or important symptoms masked; however, use as a sedative after surgery or as an adjunct to cancer chemotherapy is well established
Patients with hepatic or renal impairment	Reduce initial dosage. Use with caution in patients with hepatic damage, since butabarbital is almost entirely metabolized in the liver before it is excreted. Barbiturates should not be given to patients with premonitory signs of hepatic coma.
Ambulatory patients	Caution patients that their performance of potentially hazardous activities may be impaired while taking barbiturates, and that concurrent use with other CNS depressants (see DRUG INTERACTIONS) may cause increased CNS depression; instruct patients not to consume alcohol while taking this drug
Long-term therapy	Periodic laboratory evaluations, including tests of renal, hepatic, and hematopoietic function, should be performed during prolonged therapy
Carcinogenicity, mutagenicity	No long-term studies have been done in animals to evaluate the carcinogenic or mutagenic potential of this drug
Effect on fertility	No studies have been done to determine the effects of this drug on fertility
Tartrazine sensitivity	Presence of FD&C Yellow No. 5 (tartrazine) in elixir, 30- and 50-mg tablets, and 30-mg capsules may cause allergic-type reactions, including bronchial asthma, in susceptible individuals

ADVERSE REACTIONS[2]

	Frequent reactions (incidence $\geq$ 1%) are printed in *italics*
Central nervous system	*Somnolence (1–3%)*, agitation, confusion, hyperkinesia, ataxia, CNS depression, nightmares, nervousness, psychiatric disturbance, hallucinations, insomnia, anxiety, dizziness, thinking abnormality
Respiratory	Hypoventilation, apnea
Cardiovascular	Bradycardia, hypotension, syncope
Gastrointestinal	Nausea, vomiting, constipation
Other	Headache, hypersensitivity reactions (angioedema, skin rashes, exfoliative dermatitis), fever, hepatic damage

OVERDOSAGE

Signs and symptoms	Respiratory and CNS depression, possibly progressing to Cheyne-Stokes respiration, absent reflexes, slight miosis (in severe cases, paralytic dilation may occur), oliguria, tachycardia, hypotension, hypothermia, coma, and, in severe cases, apnea, circulatory collapse, respiratory arrest, and death
Treatment	Maintain an adequate airway, assist ventilation, and administer oxygen, as needed. Induce emesis if patient is conscious, taking care to avoid pulmonary aspiration; if emesis is contraindicated, perform gastric lavage with a cuffed endotracheal tube and with the patient in a face-down position. Activated charcoal, followed by a saline cathartic, may be administered after emesis or lavage. Monitor vital signs and fluid balance. Treat shock with fluids and other standard measures. If renal function is normal, force diuresis to help eliminate drug. Dialysis may be helpful in patients who are anuric, in shock, or severely intoxicated. For pulmonary complications, administer antibiotics.

DRUG INTERACTIONS

Alcohol, antihistamines, tranquilizers, and other CNS depressants	△ CNS depression
Oral anticoagulants	▽ Prothrombin time
Corticosteroids	▽ Corticosteroid effects
Digitalis, digitoxin	▽ Cardiac glycoside effects
Doxycycline	▽ Anti-infective effect
Griseofulvin	▽ Griseofulvin absorption
Tricyclic antidepressants	▽ Antidepressant effect
MAO inhibitors	△ Antidepressant or barbiturate effects

ALTERED LABORATORY VALUES

Blood/serum values	▽ Bilirubin

No clinically significant alterations in urinary values occur at therapeutic dosages

USE IN CHILDREN	USE IN PREGNANT AND NURSING WOMEN
See INDICATIONS and ORAL DOSAGE	Pregnancy Category D: barbiturates can cause harm to the fetus, and patients who use this drug during pregnancy or who become pregnant while taking it should be apprised of the potential hazards. Retrospective, case-controlled studies have suggested a connection between maternal barbiturate use and an increased incidence of fetal abnormalities. Long-term exposure to barbiturates in utero (eg, throughout the last trimester) can result in neonatal dependence on barbiturates and withdrawal reactions, including hyperirritability and seizures, 0–14 days after birth. Hypnotic doses do not significantly impair uterine activity; however, administration of barbiturates during labor and delivery may cause respiratory depression in newborns, especially premature infants, and resuscitation equipment should be available. Because small amounts of some barbiturates have been detected in human milk, this drug should be used with caution in nursing mothers.

[1] Contains 7% alcohol
[2] These reactions have been reported in hospitalized patients, who may be less aware than fully ambulatory patients of some of the milder adverse effects of barbiturates; the incidence of such effects, therefore, may be somewhat higher in fully ambulatory patients

BARBITURATES

LOTUSATE (talbutal) Winthrop-Breon C-III
Tablets: 120 mg

INDICATIONS	ORAL DOSAGE
Insomnia	**Adult:** 120 mg, taken 15–30 min before retiring

CONTRAINDICATIONS	
Sensitivity to barbiturates	History of manifest or latent porphyria

ADMINISTRATION/DOSAGE ADJUSTMENTS	
Persistent insomnia	Administration for more than 2 wk is not recommended, because barbiturates appear to lose their effectiveness as hypnotics if used continuously for longer periods
Special-risk patients	Reduce dosage in elderly or debilitated patients and patients with hepatic or renal impairment (see WARNINGS/PRECAUTIONS)

WARNINGS/PRECAUTIONS	
Drug dependence	Psychic and/or physical dependence and tolerance may develop with continued use. Instruct patients to adhere strictly to the dosage regimen. Use with caution, if at all, in mentally depressed patients and patients with suicidal tendencies or a history of drug abuse.
Excitement	In some patients, barbiturates repeatedly produce excitement rather than depression
Elderly or debilitated patients	Reduce dosage, since such patients may be more sensitive to barbiturates, and may respond to usual doses with marked excitement, depression, or confusion
Patients with hepatic or renal impairment	Reduce initial dosage and use with caution in patients with hepatic damage. Barbiturates should not be given to patients with premonitory signs of hepatic coma.
Mental and/or physical impairment	Caution patients that their performance of potentially hazardous activities may be impaired while taking barbiturates, and that concurrent use with other CNS depressants (see DRUG INTERACTIONS) may cause increased CNS depression; instruct patients not to consume alcohol while taking this drug
Carcinogenicity	Lifetime administration of the related drug phenobarbital sodium has caused benign and malignant liver-cell tumors in mice and benign liver-cell tumors in aged rats

ADVERSE REACTIONS[1]	
Central nervous system	Agitation, confusion, hyperkinesia, ataxia, CNS depression, nightmares, nervousness, psychiatric disturbance, hallucinations, insomnia, anxiety, dizziness, thinking abnormality
Respiratory	Hypoventilation, apnea
Cardiovascular	Bradycardia, hypotension, syncope
Gastrointestinal	Nausea, vomiting, constipation
Other	Headache, injection site reactions, hypersensitivity reactions (angioedema, skin rashes, exfoliative dermatitis), fever

OVERDOSAGE

Signs and symptoms	Respiratory and CNS depression, possibly progressing to Cheyne-Stokes respiration, absent reflexes, slight miosis (in severe cases, paralytic dilation may occur), oliguria, tachycardia, hypotension, hypothermia, coma, and, in severe cases, apnea, circulatory collapse, respiratory arrest, and death
Treatment	Maintain an adequate airway, assist ventilation, and administer oxygen, as needed. Empty stomach by gastric lavage, taking care to avoid pulmonary aspiration. Monitor vital signs and fluid balance. Treat shock with fluids and other standard measures. If renal function is normal, force diuresis to help eliminate drug. Dialysis may be helpful in patients who are anuric, in shock, or severely intoxicated. For pulmonary complications, administer antibiotics.

DRUG INTERACTIONS

Alcohol, antihistamines, tranquilizers, and other CNS depressants	△ CNS depression
Oral anticoagulants	▽ Prothrombin time
Corticosteroids	▽ Corticosteroid effects
Digitalis, digitoxin	▽ Cardiac glycoside effects
Doxycycline	▽ Anti-infective effect
Griseofulvin	▽ Griseofulvin absorption
Tricyclic antidepressants	▽ Antidepressant effect
MAO inhibitors	△ Antidepressant or barbiturate effects

ALTERED LABORATORY VALUES

Blood/serum values	▽ Bilirubin

No clinically significant alterations in urinary values occur at therapeutic dosages

USE IN CHILDREN

Not recommended for use in children under 15 yr of age; the safety and effectiveness of this drug have not been established in persons under this age

USE IN PREGNANT AND NURSING WOMEN

Pregnancy Category D: barbiturates can cause harm to the fetus, and patients who use this drug during pregnancy or who become pregnant while taking it should be apprised of the potential hazards. Barbiturates readily cross the placental barrier and, following parenteral administration, can attain concentrations in fetal blood approaching those in the maternal circulation. They are distributed in all fetal tissues, reaching the highest concentration in the placenta, liver, and brain. Retrospective, case-controlled studies have suggested a connection between maternal barbiturate use and an increased incidence of fetal abnormalities; prenatal exposure to barbiturates has also been linked to an increased risk of brain tumors. Long-term exposure to barbiturates in utero (eg, throughout the last trimester) can result in neonatal dependence on barbiturates and withdrawal reactions, including hyperirritability and seizures, 0–14 days after birth. Although hypnotic doses do not significantly impair uterine activity, full anesthetic doses given during labor decrease the force and frequency of uterine contractions. Administration of barbiturates during labor and delivery, however, may cause respiratory depression in newborns, especially premature infants, and resuscitation equipment should be available. Because small amounts of barbiturates have been detected in human milk, this drug should be used with caution in nursing mothers.

[1] Reactions observed in patients taking barbiturates in general

BARBITURATES

MEBARAL (mephobarbital) Winthrop-Breon C-IV

Tablets: 32, 50, 100 mg

INDICATIONS	ORAL DOSAGE
Sedation for the relief of anxiety, tension, and apprehension	Adult: 32–100 mg (optimally, 50 mg) tid or qid Child: 16–32 mg tid or qid
Grand mal and petit mal seizures	Adult: 400–600 mg/day Child (< 5 yr): 16–32 mg tid or qid Child (> 5 yr): 32–64 mg tid or qid

MEBARAL

CONTRAINDICATIONS

Hypersensitivity to barbiturates	History of manifest or latent porphyria

ADMINISTRATION/DOSAGE ADJUSTMENTS

Special-risk patients	Reduce dosage in elderly or debilitated patients and patients with hepatic or renal impairment (see WARNINGS/PRECAUTIONS
Initiating anticonvulsant therapy	Start with small doses, and gradually titrate dosage upward over a period of 4–5 days until optimal dosage level is obtained (see ORAL DOSAGE). In patients receiving other anticonvulsants, gradually increase the dosage of mephobarbital while tapering the dosage of other agents.
Maintenance anticonvulsant therapy	Gradually reduce the dosage of mephobarbital over a period of 4–5 days to the lowest effective level
Combination anticonvulsant therapy	Mephobarbital may be alternated with phenobarbital or given concurrently (for adults, give 200–300 mg/day of mephobarbital combined with 50–100 mg/day of phenobarbital); when used in combination with phenytoin in adults, give 600 mg/day of mephobarbital and reduce the dosage of phenytoin to 230 mg/day
Timing of administration in epileptic patients	For nocturnal seizures, dosage should be taken at night; for diurnal seizures, dosage should be taken during the day

WARNINGS/PRECAUTIONS

Drug dependence	Psychic and/or physical dependence and tolerance may develop, especially after prolonged use of high doses. Instruct patients to adhere strictly to the dosage regimen. Use with caution, if at all, in mentally depressed patients and patients with suicidal tendencies or a history of drug abuse.
Excitement	In some patients, barbiturates repeatedly produce excitement rather than depression
Mental and/or physical impairment	Caution patients that their performance of potentially hazardous activities may be impaired while taking barbiturates, and that concurrent use with other CNS depressants (see DRUG INTERACTIONS) may cause increased CNS depression; instruct patients not to consume alcohol while taking this drug
Long-term therapy	Periodic laboratory evaluations, including tests of renal, hepatic, and hematopoietic function, should be performed during prolonged therapy
Elderly or debilitated patients	Reduce dosage, since such patients may be more sensitive to barbiturates, and may respond to usual doses with marked excitement, depression, or confusion
Patients with acute or chronic pain	Use with caution because paradoxical excitement may be induced or important symptoms masked; however, use as a sedative after surgery or as an adjunct to cancer chemotherapy is well established
Patients with hepatic or renal impairment	Reduce initial dosage and use with caution in patients with hepatic damage. Barbiturates should not be given to patients with premonitory signs of hepatic coma.
Abrupt discontinuation of therapy	May produce withdrawal symptoms after chronic use of high doses, resulting in tremors, weakness, insomnia, convulsions, and delirium. In epileptic patients, abrupt cessation of therapeutic doses may precipitate status epilepticus. Dosage should be gradually reduced over a period of 4–5 days.
Vitamin D deficiency	Vitamin D requirements may be increased; rickets and osteomalacia have occurred rarely following prolonged use of barbiturates
Other special-risk patients	Use with caution and adjust dosage carefully in patients with impaired hepatic, renal, cardiac, or respiratory function, and in patients with myasthenia gravis or myxedema
Status epilepticus	May be precipitated if treatment of epilesy is suddenly discontinued; reduce the dosage of mephobarbital gradually over a period of 4–5 days
Carcinogenicity	Lifetime administration of phenobarbital sodium has caused benign and malignant liver-cell tumors in mice and benign liver-cell tumors in aged rats; phenobarbital is the major metabolite of mephobarbital

ADVERSE REACTIONS[1]

Frequent reactions (incidence ≥ 1%) are printed in *italics*

Central nervous system	*Somnolence (1–3%)*, agitation, confusion, hyperkinesia, ataxia, CNS depression, nightmares, nervousness, psychiatric disturbance, hallucinations, insomnia, anxiety, dizziness, thinking abnormality
Respiratory	Hypoventilation, apnea
Cardiovascular	Bradycardia, hypotension, syncope
Gastrointestinal	Nausea, vomiting, constipation
Other	Headache, injection site reactions, hypersensitivity reactions (angioedema, skin rashes, exfoliative dermatitis), fever, hepatic damage, megaloblastic anemia (following chronic phenobarbital use)

MEBARAL ■ NEMBUTAL

OVERDOSAGE

Signs and symptoms	Respiratory and CNS depression, possibly progressing to Cheyne-Stokes respiration, absent reflexes, slight miosis (in severe cases, paralytic dilation may occur), oliguria, tachycardia, hypotension, hypothermia, coma, and, in severe cases, apnea, circulatory collapse, respiratory arrest, and death
Treatment	Maintain an adequate airway, assist ventilation, and administer oxygen, as needed. Empty stomach by gastric lavage, taking care to avoid pulmonary aspiration. Monitor vital signs and fluid balance. Treat shock with fluids and other standard measures. If renal function is normal, force diuresis and alkalinize urine to help eliminate drug. Dialysis may be helpful in patients who are anuric, in shock, or severely intoxicated. For pulmonary complications, administer antibiotics.

DRUG INTERACTIONS

Alcohol, antihistamines, tranquilizers, and other CNS depressants	△ CNS depression
Oral anticoagulants	▽ Prothrombin time
Corticosteroids	▽ Corticosteroid effects
Digitalis, digitoxin	▽ Cardiac glycoside effects
Doxycycline	▽ Anti-infective effect
Griseofulvin	▽ Griseofulvin absorption
Tricyclic antidepressants	▽ Antidepressant effect
MAO inhibitors	△ Antidepressant or barbiturate effects

ALTERED LABORATORY VALUES

Blood/serum values	▽ Bilirubin

No clinically significant alterations in urinary values occur at therapeutic dosages

USE IN CHILDREN
See INDICATIONS and dosage recommendations

USE IN PREGNANT AND NURSING WOMEN
Pregnancy Category D: barbiturates can cause harm to the fetus, and patients who use this drug during pregnancy or who become pregnant while taking it should be apprised of the potential hazards. Barbiturates readily cross the placental barrier and, following parenteral administration, can attain concentrations in fetal blood approaching those in the maternal circulation. They are distributed in all fetal tissues, reaching the highest concentration in the placenta, liver, and brain. Retrospective, case-controlled studies have suggested a connection between maternal barbiturate use and an increased incidence of fetal abnormalities; prenatal exposure to barbiturates has also been linked to an increased risk of brain tumors. Long-term exposure to barbiturates in utero (eg, throughout the last trimester) can result in neonatal dependence on barbiturates and withdrawal reactions, including hyperirritability and seizures, 0–14 days after birth. Although hypnotic doses do not significantly impair uterine activity, full anesthetic doses given during labor decrease the force and frequency of uterine contractions. Administration of barbiturates during labor and delivery, however, may cause respiratory depression in newborns, especially premature infants, and resuscitation equipment should be available. Neonatal coagulation defects, which have been observed in infants following exposure to anticonvulsants in utero, may be prevented by administering vitamin K_1 to the mother before delivery or to the infant at birth. Because small amounts of barbiturates have been detected in human milk, this drug should be used with caution in nursing mothers.

[1] These reactions have been reported in hospitalized patients, who may be less aware than fully ambulatory patients of some of the milder adverse effects of barbiturates; the incidence of such effects, therefore, may be somewhat higher in fully ambulatory patients

---

BARBITURATES

NEMBUTAL Elixir (pentobarbital) Abbott   C-II
Elixir (per 5 ml): pentobarbital equivalent to 20 mg pentobarbital sodium[1] (1 pt, 1 gal)

NEMBUTAL Sodium Capsules and Solution (pentobarbital sodium) Abbott   C-II
Capsules: 50, 100 mg   Ampuls: 50 mg/ml (2 ml)   Vials: 50 mg/ml (20, 50 ml)

INDICATIONS	ORAL DOSAGE	PARENTERAL DOSAGE
Daytime sedation Short-term (up to 2 wk) treatment of **insomnia** **Preanesthetic medication** Control of **acute convulsive episodes,** including those associated with status epilepticus, cholera, eclampsia, meningitis, tetanus, and toxic reactions to strychnine and local anesthetics (parenteral use only)	**Adult:** for use as a sedative, 5 ml (1 tsp) tid or qid; for use as a hypnotic, 25 ml (5 tsp) or 100 mg at bedtime **Child:** preoperatively, 2–6 mg/kg/24 h, up to 100 mg/day, depending upon age, weight, and desired degree of sedation; for use as a hypnotic, adjust dosage according to age and weight	**Adult:** 150–200 mg, given in a single IM injection, or 100 mg/70 kg IV to start, followed, if necessary, by additional small IV doses, up to a total of 200–500 mg IV **Child:** 2–6 mg/kg, up to 100 mg, given in a single IM injection, or administer IV, using a proportionate reduction of the adult IV dose

COMPENDIUM OF DRUG THERAPY

NEMBUTAL Sodium Suppositories (pentobarbital sodium) Abbott   C-III

Suppositories: 30, 60, 120, 200 mg

INDICATIONS

Daytime sedation
Short-term (up to 2 wk) treatment of **insomnia**

RECTAL DOSAGE

Adult (average to above-average weight): for use as a hypnotic, one 120-mg or one 200-mg suppository; for use as a sedative, reduce dose appropriately
Child (2 mo to 1 yr; 10–20 lb): for use as a hypnotic, one 30-mg suppository
Child (1–4 yr; 20–40 lb): for use as a hypnotic, one 30-mg or one 60-mg suppository
Child (5–12 yr; 40–80 lb): for use as a hypnotic, one 60-mg suppository; for use as a sedative, reduce dose appropriately
Child (12–14 yr; 80–110 lb): for use as a hypnotic, one 60-mg or one 120-mg suppository; for use as a sedative, reduce dose appropriately

CONTRAINDICATIONS

Sensitivity to barbiturates

History of manifest or latent porphyria

ADMINISTRATION/DOSAGE ADJUSTMENTS

Parenteral therapy	Parenteral routes should be used only if oral administration is impossible or impractical. Since parenteral solutions are highly alkaline, exercise extreme caution to avoid extravascular or intraarterial injection. Any complaint of pain warrants stopping the injection.
Intramuscular administration	Intramuscular injection should be made deeply into a large muscle mass; to avoid possible tissue irritation, inject not more than 5 ml into any one site. Monitor vital signs after IM injection of hypnotic doses.
Intravenous administration	Use the IV route when prompt action is essential or when other routes are not feasible because of unconsciousness or patient resistance. Inject slowly ($\leq$ 50 mg/min), using fractional doses; wait at least 1 min after each dose to determine its full effect. Too rapid administration may cause vasodilation and decreased blood pressure, respiratory depression, apnea, and/or laryngospasm. During IV administration, monitor blood pressure, respiration, and cardiac function, and have equipment for resuscitation and artificial ventilation on hand.
Rectal administration	Use the rectal route when oral or parenteral routes are undesirable. Suppositories should not be divided.
Anticonvulsant use	Anesthetic doses are required for controlling seizures in emergencies; to avoid compounding the postictal depression that may occur, use the smallest effective dose. Inject slowly, and allow time for the drug to penetrate the blood-brain barrier and for the anticonvulsant effect to develop before administering a second dose.
Discontinuation of therapy	Reduce hypnotic doses gradually after regular use (eg, decrease the daily dose by one therapeutic dose every 5 or 6 days), since drug-withdrawal insomnia, increased dreaming, and nightmares may accompany abrupt cessation. Gradual discontinuation is essential after prolonged use by patients dependent on barbiturates since withdrawal manifestations (including delirium, convulsions, and possibly death) may otherwise result.

WARNINGS/PRECAUTIONS

Drug dependence	Psychic and/or physical dependence and tolerance may develop, especially after prolonged use of high doses. Instruct patients to adhere strictly to the dosage regimen. Use with caution, if at all, in mentally depressed patients and patients with suicidal tendencies or a history of drug abuse.
Excitement	In some patients, barbiturates repeatedly produce excitement rather than depression
Elderly or debilitated patients	Reduce dosage, since such patients may be more sensitive to barbiturates, and may respond to usual doses with marked excitement, depression, or confusion
Patients with acute or chronic pain	Use with caution because paradoxical excitement may be induced or important symptoms masked; however, use as a sedative after surgery or as an adjunct to cancer chemotherapy is well established
Patients with hepatic or renal impairment	Reduce initial dosage. Use with caution in patients with hepatic damage, since pentobarbital is almost entirely metabolized in the liver before it is excreted. Barbiturates should not be given to patients with premonitory signs of hepatic coma.
Ambulatory patients	Caution patients that their performance of potentially hazardous activities may be impaired while taking barbiturates, and that concurrent use with other CNS depressants (see DRUG INTERACTIONS) may cause increased CNS depression; instruct patients not to consume alcohol while taking this drug
Long-term therapy	Periodic laboratory evaluations, including tests of renal, hepatic, and hematopoietic function, should be performed during prolonged therapy
Tartrazine sensitivity	Presence of FD&C Yellow No. 5 (tartrazine) in the 100-mg capsules may cause allergic-type reactions, including bronchial asthma, in susceptible individuals
Carcinogenicity	Adequate data on the long-term potential for carcinogenicity have not been reported

NEMBUTAL

ADVERSE REACTIONS[2]

Frequent reactions (incidence ≥ 1%) are printed in *italics*

Central nervous system	*Somnolence (1–3%)*, agitation, confusion, hyperkinesia, ataxia, CNS depression, nightmares, nervousness, psychiatric disturbance, hallucinations, insomnia, anxiety, dizziness, thinking abnormality
Respiratory	Hypoventilation, apnea
Cardiovascular	Bradycardia, hypotension, syncope
Gastrointestinal	Nausea, vomiting, constipation
Other	Headache, injection site reactions, hypersensitivity reactions (angioedema, skin rashes, exfoliative dermatitis), fever, hepatic damage

OVERDOSAGE

Signs and symptoms	Respiratory and CNS depression, possibly progressing to Cheyne-Stokes respiration, absent reflexes, slight miosis (in severe cases, paralytic dilation may occur), oliguria, tachycardia, hypotension, hypothermia, coma, and, in severe cases, apnea, circulatory collapse, respiratory arrest, and death
Treatment	Maintain an adequate airway, assist ventilation, and administer oxygen, as needed. If patient is conscious, empty stomach by emesis and administer 30 mg of activated charcoal; if emesis is contraindicated, perform gastric lavage and instill activated charcoal. Take measures to prevent pulmonary aspiration during emesis; use a cuffed endotracheal tube for lavage. Administer a saline cathartic. Monitor vital signs and fluid balance. Treat shock with fluids and other standard measures. If renal function is normal, force diuresis to help eliminate drug. Dialysis may be helpful in patients who are anuric, in shock, or severely intoxicated. For pulmonary complications, administer antibiotics.

DRUG INTERACTIONS

Alcohol, antihistamines, tranquilizers, and other CNS depressants	△ CNS depression
Oral anticoagulants	▽ Prothrombin time
Corticosteroids	▽ Corticosteroid effects
Digitalis, digitoxin	▽ Cardiac glycoside effects
Doxycycline	▽ Anti-infective effect
Griseofulvin	▽ Griseofulvin absorption
Tricyclic antidepressants	▽ Antidepressant effect
MAO inhibitors	△ Antidepressant or barbiturate effects
Valproic acid	△ Barbiturate effects

ALTERED LABORATORY VALUES

Blood/serum values	▽ Bilirubin

No clinically significant alterations in urinary values occur at therapeutic dosages

---

USE IN CHILDREN

See INDICATIONS and dosage recommendations

USE IN PREGNANT AND NURSING WOMEN

Pregnancy Category D: barbiturates can cause harm to the fetus, and patients who use this drug during pregnancy or who become pregnant while taking it should be apprised of the potential hazards. Barbiturates readily cross the placental barrier and, following parenteral administration, can attain concentrations in fetal blood approaching those in the maternal circulation. They are distributed in all fetal tissues, reaching the highest concentration in the placenta, liver, and brain. Retrospective, case-controlled studies have suggested a connection between maternal barbiturate use and an increased incidence of fetal abnormalities; prenatal exposure to barbiturates has also been linked to an increased risk of brain tumors. Long-term exposure to barbiturates in utero (eg, throughout the last trimester) can result in neonatal dependence on barbiturates and withdrawal reactions, including hyperirritability and seizures, 0–14 days after birth. Although hypnotic doses do not significantly impair uterine activity, full anesthetic doses given during labor decrease the force and frequency of uterine contractions. Administration of barbiturates during labor and delivery, however, may cause respiratory depression in newborns, especially premature infants, and resuscitation equipment should be available. Because small amounts of barbiturates have been detected in human milk, this drug should be used with caution in nursing mothers.

VEHICLE/BASE
Suppositories: semisynthetic glycerides and other ingredients

[1] Contains 18% alcohol
[2] These reactions have been reported in hospitalized patients, who may be less aware than fully ambulatory patients of some of the milder adverse effects of barbiturates; the incidence of such effects, therefore, may be somewhat higher in fully ambulatory patients

BARBITURATES

Phenobarbital C-IV
Capsules: 16 mg **Capsules (sustained release):** 65 mg **Drops:** 16 mg/ml **Elixir (per 5 ml):** 20 mg **Tablets:** 8, 15, 16, 30, 32, 65, 100 mg

Phenobarbital sodium C-IV
Ampuls: 65 mg/ml (2 ml), 130 mg/ml (1 ml), 163 mg/ml (2 ml) **Vials:** 65, 120, 130, 325 mg **Cartridge-needle units:** 30 mg/ml (1 ml) **Prefilled syringes:** 65 mg/ml (1 ml), 130 mg/ml (1 ml)

INDICATIONS	ORAL DOSAGE	PARENTERAL DOSAGE
Daytime sedation	**Adult:** 30–120 mg/day, given in 2–3 divided doses; if sustained-release capsules are used, 65 mg bid (AM and PM) **Child:** 2 mg/kg or 60 mg/m² tid	**Adult:** 30–120 mg/day IM or IV, given in 2–3 divided doses
Preanesthetic medication	**Child:** 1–3 mg/kg	**Adult:** 100–200 mg IM 60–90 min before surgery **Child:** 16–100 mg or 1–3 mg/kg IM 60–90 min before surgery
Short-term (up to 2 wk) treatment of **insomnia**	**Adult:** 100–320 mg at bedtime **Child:** individualize dosage according to age and weight	**Adult:** 100–320 mg IM or IV at bedtime **Child:** 3–5 mg/kg IM or IV
Long-term treatment of **generalized tonic-clonic and cortical focal seizures**	**Adult:** 50–100 mg bid or tid **Child:** 3–5 mg/kg/day or 125 mg/m²/day given as a single dose at bedtime or divided	—
Control of **acute convulsive episodes**, including those associated with status epilepticus, cholera, eclampsia, meningitis, tetanus, and toxic reactions to strychnine and local anesthetics	—	**Adult:** for status epilepticus, 200–320 mg IV, repeated after 6 h, if needed **Child:** for status epilepticus, 15–20 mg/kg IV, given over a period of 10–15 min

CONTRAINDICATIONS
Sensitivity to barbiturates   History of manifest or latent porphyria

ADMINISTRATION/DOSAGE ADJUSTMENTS

Parenteral therapy	Parenteral routes should be used only if oral administration is impossible or impractical. Since parenteral solutions are highly alkaline, exercise extreme caution to avoid extravascular or intraarterial injection. Any complaint of pain warrants stopping the injection.
Intramuscular administration	Intramuscular injection should be made deeply into a large muscle mass; to avoid possible tissue irritation, inject not more than 5 ml into any one site. Monitor vital signs after IM injection of hypnotic doses.
Intravenous administration	Use the IV route when prompt action is essential or when other routes are not feasible because of unconsciousness or patient resistance. Inject slowly ($\leq$ 60 mg/min), using fractional doses (however, in the treatment of status epilepticus, use a full anticonvulsant dose initially). Wait after each dose to determine its full effect; it may take 15 min or longer before peak levels in the brain are attained. Too rapid administration may cause vasodilation and decreased blood pressure, respiratory depression, apnea, and/or laryngospasm. During IV administration, monitor blood pressure, respiration, and cardiac function, and have equipment for resuscitation and artificial ventilation on hand.
Anticonvulsant use	Subhypnotic, oral doses of phenobarbital are effective in long-term anticonvulsant therapy. Adjust dosage to achieve a serum phenobarbital level of 10–25 µg/ml; children may require higher per-kilogram dosages than adults to achieve therapeutic serum levels. For acute convulsant episodes, use the smallest effective dose to avoid compounding the postictal depression that may occur. Inject slowly, and allow time for the drug to penetrate the blood-brain barrier.
Discontinuation of therapy	Reduce hypnotic doses gradually after regular use (eg, decrease the daily dose by one therapeutic dose every 5 or 6 days), since drug-withdrawal insomnia, increased dreaming, and nightmares may accompany abrupt cessation. Gradual discontinuation is essential after prolonged use by patients dependent on barbiturates, since withdrawal manifestations (including delirium, convulsions, and possibly death) may otherwise result.

WARNINGS/PRECAUTIONS

Drug dependence	Psychic and/or physical dependence and tolerance may develop, especially after prolonged use of high doses. Instruct patients to adhere strictly to the dosage regimen. Use with caution, if at all, in mentally depressed patients and patients with suicidal tendencies or a history of drug abuse.
Excitement	In some patients, barbiturates repeatedly produce excitement rather than depression
Elderly or debilitated patients	Reduce dosage, since such patients may be more sensitive to barbiturates, and may respond to usual doses with marked excitement, depression, or confusion
Patients with acute or chronic pain	Use with caution because paradoxical excitement may be induced or important symptoms masked; however, use as a sedative after surgery or as an adjunct to cancer chemotherapy is well established

Phenobarbital

Patients with hepatic or renal impairment	Reduce initial dosage; approximately 25–50% of a phenobarbital dose is excreted unchanged. Use with caution in patients with hepatic damage; barbiturates should not be given to patients with premonitory signs of hepatic coma.
Ambulatory patients	Caution patients that their performance of potentially hazardous activities may be impaired while taking barbiturates, and that concurrent use with other CNS depressants (see DRUG INTERACTIONS) may cause increased CNS depression; instruct patients not to consume alcohol while taking this drug
Long-term therapy	Periodic laboratory evaluations, including tests of renal, hepatic, and hematopoietic function, should be performed during prolonged therapy
Treatment and prophylaxis of febrile seizures	Phenobarbital has been used in the treatment and prophylaxis of febrile seizures; however, it has not been established that prevention of febrile seizures can influence the subsequent development of epilepsy
Carcinogenicity	Lifetime administration of phenobarbital sodium has caused benign and malignant liver-cell tumors in mice and benign liver-cell tumors in rats

ADVERSE REACTIONS[1]

Frequent reactions (incidence ≥ 1%) are printed in *italics*

Central nervous system	*Somnolence (1–3%)*, agitation, confusion, hyperkinesia, ataxia, CNS depression, nightmares, nervousness, psychiatric disturbance, hallucinations, insomnia, anxiety, dizziness, thinking abnormality
Respiratory	Hypoventilation, apnea
Cardiovascular	Bradycardia, hypotension, syncope
Gastrointestinal	Nausea, vomiting, constipation
Other	Headache, injection site reactions, hypersensitivity reactions (angioedema, skin rashes, exfoliative dermatitis), fever, hepatic damage, megaloblastic anemia (following chronic use)

OVERDOSAGE

Signs and symptoms	Respiratory and CNS depression, possibly progressing to Cheyne-Stokes respiration, absent reflexes, slight miosis (in severe cases, paralytic dilation may occur), oliguria, tachycardia, hypotension, hypothermia, coma, and, in severe cases, apnea, circulatory collapse, respiratory arrest, and death
Treatment	Maintain an adequate airway, assist ventilation, and administer oxygen, as needed. Empty stomach by gastric lavage, taking care to avoid pulmonary aspiration. Monitor vital signs and fluid balance. Treat shock with fluids and other standard measures. If renal function is normal, force diuresis and alkalinize urine to help eliminate drug. Dialysis may be helpful in patients who are anuric, in shock, or severely intoxicated. For pulmonary complications, administer antibiotics.

DRUG INTERACTIONS

Alcohol, antihistamines, tranquilizers, and other CNS depressants	△ CNS depression
Oral anticoagulants	▽ Prothrombin time
Corticosteroids	▽ Corticosteroid effects
Digitalis, digitoxin	▽ Cardiac glycoside effects
Doxycycline	▽ Anti-infective effect
Griseofulvin	▽ Griseofulvin absorption
Tricyclic antidepressants	▽ Antidepressant effect
MAO inhibitors	△ Antidepressant or barbiturate effects

ALTERED LABORATORY VALUES

Blood/serum values	▽ Bilirubin

No clinically significant alterations in urinary values occur at therapeutic dosages

---

USE IN CHILDREN

See INDICATIONS and dosage recommendations

USE IN PREGNANT AND NURSING WOMEN

Pregnancy Category D: barbiturates can cause harm to the fetus, and patients who use this drug during pregnancy or who become pregnant while taking it should be apprised of the potential hazards. Barbiturates readily cross the placental barrier and, following parenteral administration, can attain concentrations in fetal blood approaching those in the maternal circulation. They are distributed in all fetal tissues, reaching the highest concentration in the placenta, liver, and brain. Retrospective, case-controlled studies have suggested a connection between maternal barbiturate use and an increased incidence of fetal abnormalities; prenatal exposure to barbiturates has also been linked to an increased risk of brain tumors. Long-term exposure to barbiturates in utero (eg, throughout the last trimester) can result in neonatal dependence on barbiturates and withdrawal reactions, including hyperirritability and seizures, 0–14 days after birth. Although hypnotic doses do not significantly impair uterine activity, full anesthetic doses given during labor decrease the force and frequency of uterine contractions. Administration of barbiturates during labor and delivery, however, may cause respiratory depression in newborns, especially premature infants, and resuscitation equipment should be available. Because small amounts of barbiturates have been detected in human milk, this drug should be used with caution in nursing mothers.

---

[1] These reactions have been reported in hospitalized patients, who may be less aware than fully ambulatory patients of some of the milder adverse effects of barbiturates; the incidence of such effects, therefore, may be somewhat higher in fully ambulatory patients

SECONAL Sodium

BARBITURATES

SECONAL Sodium Capsules (secobarbital sodium) Lilly   C-II
Capsules: 50, 100 mg

INDICATIONS	ORAL DOSAGE
Insomnia	**Adult:** 100 mg at bedtime for up to 2 wk
Preanesthetic medication	**Adult:** 200–300 mg 1–2 h before surgery **Child:** 2–6 mg/kg, up to 100 mg, 1–2 h before surgery

SECONAL Sodium Injection (secobarbital sodium) Lilly   C-II
Vials: 50 mg/ml (20 ml)

INDICATIONS	PARENTERAL DOSAGE	RECTAL DOSAGE
Preanesthetic medication	**Adult:** for general, spinal, or regional anesthesia or for intubation procedures, up to 250 mg IV (usual dosage for spinal or regional anesthesia: 50–100 mg); if the desired degree of hypnosis is not attained after use of 250 mg, give a small quantity of meperidine. For dental nerve block, administer 100–150 mg IV.	**Child (< 40 kg):** for ear, nose, and throat procedures, 5 mg/kg of a 1–1.5% solution **Child (≥ 40 kg):** for ear, nose, and throat procedures, 4 mg/kg of a 1–1.5% solution
Preoperative sedation	**Adult:** 2.2 mg/kg, up to 100 mg, IM 10–15 min before a dental procedure; for lighter sedation, reduce dose to 1.1–1.6 mg/kg **Child:** same as adult	—
Convulsions associated with tetanus	**Adult:** 5.5 mg/kg IM or IV q3–4h, as needed	—

SECONAL Sodium Suppositories (secobarbital sodium) Lilly   C-III
Suppositories: 200 mg

INDICATIONS	RECTAL DOSAGE
Sedative-hypnotic use	**Adult:** 120–200 mg for up to 2 wk

CONTRAINDICATIONS

Hypersensitivity to barbiturates	History of addiction to a sedative-hypnotic	Significant cardiac disease (vials only)
History of manifest or latent porphyria	Marked hepatic impairment	Obstetrical delivery (vials only)
Respiratory disease associated with dyspnea or obstruction	Acute or chronic pain	Renal impairment (vials only)

ADMINISTRATION/DOSAGE ADJUSTMENTS

Use of vials — For IV or IM administration, the solution may be used as supplied or diluted with sterile water for injection, 0.9% sodium chloride injection, or Ringer's injection. The rate of IV injection should not exceed 50 mg/15 s; respiratory depression, apnea, laryngospasm, or vasodilation with hypotension may occur if IV administration is too rapid. If the IM route is used, inject deeply into a large muscle, and do not give more than 5 ml (regardless of dilution) at any one site; after IM injection of large hypnotic doses, observe patient for 20–30 min, since excessive narcosis may occur. For rectal administration to children, the solution should be diluted with lukewarm water to a concentration of 1–1.5% and then given after a cleansing enema; atropine may be administered concomitantly to dry respiratory-tract secretions. After rectal administration, children should be observed for 15–20 min.

WARNINGS/PRECAUTIONS

Drug dependence — Psychic and/or physical dependence and tolerance may develop with continued use. Administration of more than 400 mg/day for 90 days can produce physical dependence; use of 600–800 mg/day for at least 35 days, when followed by abrupt discontinuation, can result in withdrawal seizures. (A barbiturate addict usually takes 1.5 g/day.) Symptoms of dependence are similar to those of chronic alcoholism; withdrawal reactions range in severity from anxiety, muscle twitching, and dizziness to convulsions, delirium, and death. To avoid dependence, limit each prescription to an amount required until the next appointment, warn patients not to increase the dosage on their own, and use with caution, if at all, in patients with a history of drug abuse. To treat dependence, cautiously and gradually reduce the dosage of secobarbital or a substituted drug. The specific method of withdrawal may vary. In one regimen, phenobarbital is given orally 3–4 times/day as a substitute for the total daily dose of secobarbital (30 mg/day of phenobarbital for each 100–200 mg/day of secobarbital). Once the patient is stabilized, the dosage is reduced daily by 10%. In a modification of this regimen, up to 600 mg/day of phenobarbital is substituted; however, if withdrawal reactions occur on the first day of treatment, an additional 200–300 mg of phenobarbital is given IM as a loading dose. Once the patient is stabilized, the dosage is reduced daily by 30 mg.

SECONAL Sodium

Depressed or suicidal patients	Use with caution, if at all, in patients who are mentally depressed or who have suicidal tendencies
Elderly or debilitated patients	Reduce dosage for elderly or debilitated patients, since these patients may be more sensitive to barbiturates and may respond to usual doses with marked excitement, depression, or confusion
Patients with hepatic or renal impairment	Reduce the dosage for patients with decreased hepatic function, and do not use in patients with marked hepatic impairment, since secobarbital is metabolized in the liver. Reduce the dosage of the capsules and suppositories for patients with renal impairment; do not administer the solution contained in the vials to such patients because the polyethylene glycol vehicle may irritate the kidneys.
Patients with borderline hypoadrenal function	Secobarbital may diminish the systemic effects of cortisol and exogenous hydrocortisone; use secobarbital with caution in patients with borderline hypoadrenal function
Drowsiness	Caution patients that their ability to drive or perform other potentially hazardous activities may be impaired. If secobarbital has been used in an office procedure, the patient should be discharged in the company of another person.
Paradoxical response	In some patients, barbiturates repeatedly produce excitement rather than depression
Long-term therapy	Periodic laboratory evaluations, including tests of renal, hepatic, and hematopoietic function, should be performed during prolonged therapy

ADVERSE REACTIONS[1]

The most frequent reaction is italicized

Central nervous system	*Somnolence (1–3%)*, agitation, confusion, hyperkinesia, ataxia, CNS depression, nightmares, nervousness, psychiatric disturbance, hallucinations, insomnia, anxiety, dizziness, thinking abnormality
Respiratory	Hypoventilation, apnea
Cardiovascular	Bradycardia, hypotension, syncope
Gastrointestinal	Nausea, vomiting, constipation
Other	Headache, injection site reactions, hypersensitivity reactions (angioedema, skin rashes, exfoliative dermatitis), fever, hepatic damage

OVERDOSAGE

Signs and symptoms	Respiratory and CNS depression, possibly progressing to Cheyne-Stokes respiration, absent reflexes, slight miosis (in severe cases, paralytic dilation may occur), oliguria, tachycardia, hypotension, hypothermia, coma, and, in severe cases, apnea, circulatory collapse, respiratory arrest, and death. A flat EEG, which may be observed following extreme overdosage, does not indicate death; cessation of electric activity in the brain can be fully reversed if hypoxic damage has not occurred.
Treatment	Maintain an adequate airway, assist ventilation, and administer oxygen, as needed. Induce emesis if patient is conscious, taking care to avoid pulmonary aspiration; if emesis is contraindicated, perform gastric lavage with a cuffed endotracheal tube and with the patient in a face-down position. Activated charcoal, followed by a saline cathartic, may be administered after emesis or lavage. Monitor vital signs and fluid balance. Treat shock with fluids and other standard measures. If renal function is normal, force diuresis to help eliminate drug. Dialysis may be helpful in patients who are anuric, in shock, or severely intoxicated. For pulmonary complications, administer antibiotics. To prevent hypostatic pneumonia, decubiti, aspiration, and other complications, roll patient from side to side every 30 min and take other appropriate measures.

DRUG INTERACTIONS

Alcohol, antihistamines, tranquilizers, and other CNS depressants	△ CNS depression; instruct patients not to consume alcohol during therapy, and warn them about using other CNS depressants in combination with secobarbital
Oral anticoagulants	▽ Prothrombin time; during concomitant therapy, check the prothrombin time more frequently
Corticosteroids	▽ Corticosteroid effects
Digitalis, digitoxin	▽ Cardiac glycoside effects
Doxycycline	▽ Anti-infective effect
Griseofulvin	▽ Griseofulvin absorption
Tricyclic antidepressants	▽ Antidepressant effect
MAO inhibitors	△ Antidepressant or barbiturate effects

ALTERED LABORATORY VALUES

Blood/serum values	▽ Bilirubin

No clinically significant alterations in urinary values occur at therapeutic dosages

SECONAL Sodium ■ TUINAL

USE IN CHILDREN
See INDICATIONS and dosage recommendations

USE IN PREGNANT AND NURSING WOMEN
Pregnancy Category D: barbiturates can cause harm to the fetus, and patients who use this drug during pregnancy or who become pregnant while taking it should be apprised of the potential hazards. Retrospective, case-controlled studies have suggested a connection between maternal barbiturate use and an increased incidence of fetal abnormalities. Exposure to barbiturates in utero throughout the last trimester can result in neonatal dependence and in withdrawal reactions, including hyperirritability and seizures, 0–14 days after birth; phenobarbital may be used to treat dependence (3–10 mg/kg/day is given until withdrawal reactions cease, and then the dosage is decreased gradually over a period of 2 wk). Full anesthetic doses of barbiturates decrease the force and frequency of uterine contractions; however, hypnotic doses do not significantly impair uterine activity. Administration of barbiturates during labor and delivery may cause respiratory depression in newborns, especially premature infants, and resuscitation equipment should be available. Because small amounts of some barbiturates have been detected in human milk, this drug should be used with caution in nursing mothers.

[1] These reactions have been reported in hospitalized patients, who may be less aware than fully ambulatory patients of some of the milder adverse effects of barbiturates; the incidence of such effects, therefore, may be somewhat higher in fully ambulatory patients

BARBITURATES

TUINAL (secobarbital sodium and amobarbital sodium) Lilly   C-II

Capsules: 25 mg secobarbital sodium and 25 mg amobarbital sodium; 50 mg secobarbital sodium and 50 mg amobarbital sodium; 100 mg secobarbital sodium and 100 mg amobarbital sodium

INDICATIONS
Insomnia
Preanesthetic sedation

ORAL DOSAGE
Adult: 50–200 mg at bedtime or 1 h before surgery

CONTRAINDICATIONS
Hypersensitivity to barbiturates	History of manifest or latent porphyria	Marked hepatic impairment
Respiratory disease associated with dyspnea or obstruction	Acute or chronic pain	Previous addiction to sedative-hypnotics

ADMINISTRATION/DOSAGE ADJUSTMENTS
Persistent insomnia	Allow a drug-free interval of 1 wk or more to elapse before considering retreatment
Duration of therapy	Prolonged use is not recommended, since this drug has not been shown to be effective for more than 2 wk; for chronic insomnia, attempt alternative, nonpharmacologic therapy

WARNINGS/PRECAUTIONS
Mental and/or physical impairment	Caution patients that their ability to drive or perform other potentially hazardous activities may be impaired
Patients with hepatic impairment	Use with caution to avoid excessive accumulation
Elderly or debilitated patients	May experience marked excitement or depression; use with caution
Patients with borderline hypoadrenal function	Effects of cortisol may be diminished; use with caution
Drug dependence	Psychic and/or physical dependence and tolerance may develop, especially in addiction-prone individuals; abrupt discontinuation after chronic use of large dosages may result in withdrawal reactions, including delirium, convulsions, and death
Hypersensitivity reactions	May occur, especially in patients with asthma, urticaria, or angioneurotic edema

ADVERSE REACTIONS
Central nervous system	Residual sedation ("hangover"), drowsiness, lethargy, headache
Respiratory	Depression, apnea
Cardiovascular	Circulatory collapse
Allergic	Hypersensitivity reactions, skin eruptions
Gastrointestinal	Nausea, vomiting

OVERDOSAGE

Signs and symptoms	Early hypothermia followed by fever, sluggish or absent reflexes, respiratory depression, gradual appearance of circulatory collapse, pulmonary edema, and coma
Treatment	Empty stomach by gastric lavage. Institute symptomatic and supportive therapy. Administer IV fluids. Maintain adequate respiratory exchange, blood pressure, and body temperature. Dialysis may be helpful. Antibiotics may be required for pulmonary complications.

DRUG INTERACTIONS

Alcohol, antihistamines, tranquilizers, and other CNS depressants	△ CNS depression
Oral anticoagulants	▽ Prothrombin time
Corticosteroids	▽ Corticosteroid effects
Digitalis, digitoxin	▽ Cardiac glycoside effects
Doxycycline	▽ Anti-infective effect
Griseofulvin	▽ Griseofulvin absorption
Tricyclic antidepressants	▽ Antidepressant effect
MAO inhibitors	△ Antidepressant or barbiturate effects

ALTERED LABORATORY VALUES

Blood/serum values	▽ Bilirubin (in neonates, patients with congenital nonhemolytic unconjugated hyperbilirubinemia, and epileptics)

No clinically significant alterations in urinary values occur at therapeutic dosages

---

USE IN CHILDREN
Safety and effectiveness have not been established for use in children

USE IN PREGNANT AND NURSING WOMEN
Pregnancy Category B: use during pregnancy only when clearly needed. Animal reproduction studies have shown no evidence of impaired fertility or fetal harm; however, no adequate, well-controlled studies have been done in pregnant women. Neonatal depression may occur following use during labor. Administer with caution to nursing mothers.

NONBARBITURATES

DALMANE (flurazepam hydrochloride) Roche   C-IV

Capsules: 15, 30 mg

INDICATIONS	ORAL DOSAGE
Insomnia	Adult: 15–30 mg at bedtime

CONTRAINDICATIONS	
Hypersensitivity to flurazepam	Pregnancy

ADMINISTRATION/DOSAGE ADJUSTMENTS

Elderly and/or debilitated patients	Initiate therapy with 15 mg flurazepam until individual response is determined
Persistent insomnia	Prolonged use is usually not indicated and should only be undertaken concomitantly with appropriate evaluation; effectiveness lasts for at least 28 consecutive nights of drug administration

WARNINGS/PRECAUTIONS

Mental impairment	Caution patients about engaging in hazardous activities requiring full mental alertness after ingesting this drug and that their performance of such activities may also be impaired the following day. Patients should also be warned that alcohol and other CNS depressants (see DRUG INTERACTIONS) may have a combined additive effect with flurazepam, and that this may occur if alcoholic beverages are consumed the following day if flurazepam was taken the night before for sedation; the potential for this interaction continues for several days after flurazepam has been discontinued.
Potentially suicidal patients	Use with caution and appropriate safeguards in severely depressed patients and in any patient with signs or symptoms of latent depression
Elderly or debilitated patients	The risk of oversedation, dizziness, confusion, and/or ataxia increases substantially with larger doses in these patients (see ADMINISTRATION/DOSAGE ADJUSTMENTS)

DALMANE ■ DORIDEN

Other special-risk patients	Use with caution in patients with impaired hepatic or renal function or chronic pulmonary insufficiency; caution must also be exercised in giving this drug to patients who are addiction-prone or otherwise likely to increase the dosage on their own
Withdrawal reactions	In rare cases, abrupt discontinuation following continuous use for several months or longer, generally at higher therapeutic levels, has precipitated withdrawal reactions similar to those seen with other benzodiazepines as well as alcohol and barbiturates; therapy should generally be discontinued gradually after prolonged administration, especially when excessive doses have been given

ADVERSE REACTIONS

Central nervous system	Dizziness, drowsiness, light-headedness, staggering, ataxia, falling, headache, nervousness, talkativeness, apprehension, irritability, weakness; euphoria, depression, slurred speech, confusion, restlessness, hallucinations, and paradoxical excitement, stimulation, and hyperactivity (rare)
Ophthalmic	Difficulty focusing, blurred vision, and burning eyes (rare)
Gastrointestinal	Heartburn, upset stomach, nausea, vomiting, diarrhea, constipation, abdominal pain; dry mouth, bitter taste, excessive salivation, and anorexia (rare)
Cardiovascular	Palpitations, chest pain; faintness, hypotension, and shortness of breath (rare)
Hematological	Leukopenia and granulocytopenia (rare)
Dermatological	Pruritus and rash (rare)
Other	Genitourinary complaints; sweating, flushes, and body and joint pains (rare)

OVERDOSAGE

Signs and symptoms	Somnolence, severe sedation, lethargy, ataxia, disorientation, confusion, hypotension, coma
Treatment	Empty stomach immediately by gastric lavage. Maintain an adequate airway, and administer IV fluids, as needed. Monitor respiration, pulse, and blood pressure. Treat hypotension with norepinephrine or metaraminol. If excitation occurs, do not use barbiturates. The value of dialysis is unknown.

DRUG INTERACTIONS

Alcohol, antihistamines, tranquilizers, and other CNS depressants	△ CNS depression

ALTERED LABORATORY VALUES

Blood/serum values	△ SGOT △ SGPT △ Bilirubin (total and direct) △ Alkaline phosphatase

No clinically significant alterations in urinary values occur at therapeutic dosages

---

USE IN CHILDREN

Not recommended for use in children under 15 yr of age; this drug has not been studied clinically in children

USE IN PREGNANT AND NURSING WOMEN

Contraindicated in pregnant women. Benzodiazepines may cause fetal harm when administered during pregnancy. Patients likely to become pregnant while taking this drug should be apprised of the potential hazard and instructed to discontinue use of flurazepam before attempting to conceive. Neonatal depression has been reported following maternal use of this drug prior to delivery. Benzodiazepines are excreted in human milk; use with caution in nursing mothers.

NONBARBITURATES

DORIDEN (glutethimide) Rorer   C-III

Tablets: 0.25, 0.5 g

INDICATIONS	ORAL DOSAGE
Insomnia	**Adult:** 0.25–0.5 g at bedtime for not more than 3–7 consecutive nights

CONTRAINDICATIONS

Hypersensitivity to glutethimide	Porphyria

DORIDEN

ADMINISTRATION/DOSAGE ADJUSTMENTS

Elderly or debilitated patients	To avoid oversedation, limit initial dosage to 0.5 g at bedtime
Persistent insomnia	Allow a drug-free interval of 1 wk or more to elapse before considering retreatment and attempt to find an alternative, nonpharmacologic means of treating chronic insomnia

WARNINGS/PRECAUTIONS

Mental impairment, disturbed coordination	Caution patients against driving or performing potentially hazardous activities while taking this drug and that alcohol and other CNS depressants may cause further impairment of their abilities
Drug dependence	Psychic and/or physical dependence may develop, especially in addiction-prone individuals; each prescription should generally be limited to an amount sufficient for 1 wk. Abrupt discontinuation following chronic overdosage can precipitate withdrawal reactions, including nervousness, anxiety, nausea, abdominal discomfort, dysphagia, chills, tremors, numbness of the extremities, delirium, and convulsions; to control reactions, administer glutethimide again or give pentobarbital. To discontinue use in dependent patients, reduce the dosage gradually over a period of days or weeks, carefully watching the patient.
Rash	Discontinue use if generalized skin rash occurs
Carcinogenicity	No studies have been done in animals to evaluate the carcinogenic potential of this drug

ADVERSE REACTIONS

Frequent reactions (incidence $\geq$ 1%) are printed in *italics*

Dermatological	*Rash (8.6%)*
Central nervous system	*Residual sedation ("hangover"; 1.1%), drowsiness (1%)*, vertigo, headache, depression, dizziness, ataxia, confusion, light-headedness, euphoria, memory impairment, slurred speech, tinnitus; paradoxical excitation and blurred vision (rare)
Gastrointestinal	*Nausea (2.7%)*, indigestion, vomiting
Other	Edema, nocturnal diaphoresis, dry mouth; acute hypersensitivity reactions, porphyria, and blood dyscrasias, including thrombocytopenic purpura, aplastic anemia, and leukopenia (rare)

OVERDOSAGE

Signs and symptoms	CNS depression, coma, hypothermia, fever, depressed or lost deep-tendon reflexes, depressed or lost corneal and pupillary reflexes, mydriasis, depressed or absent pain response, inadequate ventilation, cyanosis, sudden apnea (especially with gastric lavage or endotracheal intubation), diminished or absent peristalsis, severe hypotension, tonic muscular spasms, twitching, convulsions. The threshold serum level for severe toxicity is generally 3 mg/dl, but may be higher in tolerant patients. For proper assessment of toxicity, obtain serial determinations of the serum level; a single measurement is not useful because significant amounts of the drug may be sequestered in adipose tissue or the GI tract.
Treatment	Maintain cardiopulmonary function; if necessary, perform a tracheostomy, use mechanical ventilation, and give plasma volume expanders (use vasopressors only if absolutely essential). Monitor vital signs; watch the ECG for arrhythmias. If coma is prolonged, maintain urine output, but do not cause overhydration, which can increase the risk of pulmonary or cerebral edema; use appropriate antibiotics to treat infection. To remove the drug, induce emesis (if patient is fully conscious) and perform lavage. For gastric lavage, use a 1:1 mixture of castor oil and water (leave 50 ml of castor oil in the stomach as a cathartic); for intestinal lavage, use 100–250 ml of 20–40% sorbitol or mannitol. To prevent aspiration of gastric contents, insert a cuffed endotracheal tube. Exercise caution during lavage, intubation, tracheostomy, or other procedures because manipulation may precipitate apnea. If emesis and lavage are not possible and the patient is fully conscious, absorption can be delayed by giving aqueous charcoal, flour or cornstarch suspension, or 1 pt of water, milk, or fruit juice (induce emesis or perform lavage as soon as possible). For severe toxicity characterized by grade III or grade IV coma or accompanied by renal impairment, pulmonary edema, heart failure, circulatory collapse, significant hepatic disease, major metabolic disturbance, or uremia, consider hemodialysis with pure food-grade soybean oil or, for reportedly more effective removal, hemoperfusion with microencapsulated charcoal or Amberlite XAD-2 resin. Hemodialysis or hemoperfusion should be continued for at least 2 h after patient has regained consciousness; if either of these techniques is discontinued at an earlier time, significant amounts of the drug may be released from adipose tissue, causing a secondary increase in the serum level and a recurrence of coma.

DRUG INTERACTIONS

Alcohol, antihistamines, tranquilizers, and other CNS depressants	△ CNS depression
Coumarin anticoagulants	▽ Prothrombin time

COMPENDIUM OF DRUG THERAPY

ALTERED LABORATORY VALUES

No clinically significant alterations in blood/serum or urinary values occur at therapeutic dosages

USE IN CHILDREN
Not recommended for use in children; the safety and effectiveness of this drug have not been established by clinical trials in pediatric populations

USE IN PREGNANT AND NURSING WOMEN
Pregnancy Category C: animal reproduction studies have not been done, nor is it known whether this drug can cause harm to the fetus when administered to a pregnant woman or can affect reproductive capacity in humans. Newborn infants of mothers who are dependent on glutethimide may exhibit withdrawal reactions. Use during pregnancy only if clearly needed. Because of the potential for serious adverse reactions in nursing infants, nursing is inadvisable while the patient is taking this drug.

NONBARBITURATES

HALCION (triazolam) Upjohn   C-IV
Tablets: 0.125, 0.25, 0.5 mg

INDICATIONS	**ORAL DOSAGE**
Short-term treatment of **insomnia**	**Adult:** 0.25–0.5 mg or, for selected patients, 0.125 mg, given at bedtime
CONTRAINDICATIONS	
Pregnancy	Hypersensitivity to triazolam or other benzodiazepines
ADMINISTRATION/DOSAGE ADJUSTMENTS	
Elderly, debilitated patients	Administer 0.125 mg at bedtime to start; usual therapeutic dose, 0.125–0.25 mg
WARNINGS/PRECAUTIONS	
Mental impairment	Caution patients not to exceed the recommended dosage, because even a 2-mg dose can cause somnolence, confusion, and other manifestations of overdosage; patients should also be advised not to drive or engage in other potentially hazardous activities requiring complete mental alertness (unless it is apparent that this drug does not affect their performance) and not to consume alcohol during treatment (see DRUG INTERACTIONS)
Drug dependence	Psychic and/or physical dependence may occur, especially in addiction-prone patients, who should be under careful surveillance while receiving triazolam. The quantity of tablets indicated in a single prescription should not exceed a 1-mo supply; repeat prescriptions should only be given to patients under medical supervision.
Termination of therapy	Caution patients that they may experience increased difficulty in falling asleep or staying asleep (rebound insomnia) on the first or second night after discontinuing treatment. Abrupt discontinuation of benzodiazepine drugs has resulted in barbiturate-like withdrawal reactions, ranging from mild dysphoria to a major syndrome characterized by abdominal and muscle cramps, vomiting, sweating, tremor, and convulsions. Discontinue therapy gradually in patients with a history of seizures.
Paradoxical reactions	Discontinue therapy if paradoxical reactions (see ADVERSE REACTIONS) or other adverse behavioral effects occur
Depressed patients	A suicidal propensity can be present in such patients; use with caution, and take appropriate protective measures
Other special-risk patients	Use with caution in patients with renal or hepatic impairment or with chronic pulmonary insufficiency
Laboratory testing	Significant abnormalities have not been observed in clinical trials of triazolam, and laboratory tests are usually unnecessary; if treatment is protracted, however, periodic blood counts, urinalyses, and blood chemistry tests are advisable
Carcinogenicity	No evidence of carcinogenicity has been detected in mice given up to 4,000 times the human dose for 24 mo
ADVERSE REACTIONS[1]	Frequent reactions (incidence ≥ 1%) are printed in *italics*
Central nervous system	*Drowsiness, headache, dizziness, nervousness, light-headedness, and coordination disorders/ataxia;* euphoria, tiredness, confusional states/memory impairment (including anterograde amnesia), cramps/pain, depression, and visual disturbances (0.5–0.9%); paradoxical reactions (including stimulation, agitation, increased muscle spasticity, hallucinations, sleep disturbances, and insomnia), dreaming/nightmares, paresthesia, tinnitus, dysesthesia, and weakness (< 0.5%); minor changes in EEG activity (clinical significance not known)

HALCION ■ NOCTEC

Gastrointestinal	*Nausea/vomiting;* constipation and diarrhea (< 0.5%)
Cardiovascular	Tachycardia (0.5–0.9%)
Other	Taste alterations, dry mouth, dermatitis/allergy, and congestion (< 0.5%); death due to hepatic failure (reported in a patient who was also taking diuretics)

OVERDOSAGE

Signs and symptoms	Somnolence, confusion, impaired coordination, and slurred speech, progressing, in severe cases, to coma
Treatment	Empty stomach immediately by gastric lavage. Monitor respiration, pulse, and blood pressure, and employ general supportive measures, as needed (IV fluids may be given). Maintain an adequate airway. If cardiopulmonary collapse occurs, use positive pressure, mechanical ventilation to reestablish an adequate respiratory exchange, and administer norepinephrine or metaraminol by IV infusion to combat hypotension. Hemodialysis and forced diuresis are probably of little value.

DRUG INTERACTIONS

Alcohol, sedative-hypnotics, anticonvulsants, antihistamines, and other CNS depressants	↕ CNS depression; caution patients accordingly
Cimetidine	↕ Serum triazolam level

ALTERED LABORATORY VALUES

No clinically significant alterations in blood/serum or urinary values occur at therapeutic dosages

---

USE IN CHILDREN

Safety and effectiveness for use in patients under 18 yr of age have not been established

USE IN PREGNANT AND NURSING WOMEN

Pregnancy Category X: contraindicated for use during pregnancy, because benzodiazepines may cause harm to the fetus. An increased risk of congenital malformations has been associated with the use of diazepam and chlordiazepoxide during the first trimester. The possibility that a woman of childbearing potential may be pregnant at the time of therapy should be considered; patients likely to become pregnant should be apprised of the potential risk to the fetus and instructed to discontinue use before becoming pregnant. Withdrawal reactions have occurred in neonates of mothers who used benzodiazepines during the last weeks of pregnancy; neonatal flaccidity has also been observed in one instance. Use of triazolam in nursing mothers is not recommended, because triazolam and its metabolites are excreted in the milk of rats (studies in women have not been performed).

[1] Adverse reactions not observed with the use of triazolam but reported with the use of other benzodiazepines include dystonia, irritability, anorexia, fatigue, sedation, slurred speech, jaundice, pruritus, dysarthria, changes in libido, menstrual irregularities, incontinence, and urinary retention

---

NONBARBITURATES

NOCTEC (chloral hydrate) Squibb   C-IV

Capsules: 250, 500 mg **Syrup (per 5 ml):** 500 mg (473 ml)

INDICATIONS

Nocturnal sedation
Preoperative sedation
Postoperative medication, as an adjunct to opiates and analgesics

ORAL DOSAGE

Adult: for sedation, 250 mg tid after meals; for use as a hypnotic, 500 mg to 1 g 15–30 min before bedtime or 30 min before surgery; maximum dosage: 2 g/day
Child: for sedation, 25 mg/kg/day, up to 500 mg/day, given in single or divided doses; for use as a hypnotic, 50 mg/kg/day, up to 1 g/day, given in single or divided doses

CONTRAINDICATIONS

Marked hepatic or renal impairment	Idiosyncratic reaction or hypersensitivity to chloral hydrate	Gastritis
Severe cardiac disease		

ADMINISTRATION/DOSAGE ADJUSTMENTS

Administration with fluids	Chloral hydrate is a gastric irritant; capsules should be swallowed whole with a full glass (8 fl oz) of water or fruit juice; syrup should be diluted in half a glass (4 fl oz) of water, fruit juice, or ginger ale

NOCTEC

WARNINGS/PRECAUTIONS

Drug dependence	Psychic and/or physical dependence and tolerance may develop with prolonged use of higher than usual therapeutic dosages, especially in addiction-prone individuals; caution patients accordingly. Sudden withdrawal of this drug from patients who have become dependent on it may result in tremor, anxiety, hallucinations, delirium, and death; withdrawal should be undertaken in a hospital with the same supportive management appropriate for barbiturate withdrawal.
Chronic chloral hydrate intoxication	Gastritis is common; skin eruptions and parenchymatous renal injury may also occur
Drowsiness	Caution patients about driving or performing other potentially hazardous activities after taking this drug and to avoid alcohol and other CNS depressants. Do not administer to patients who have ingested significant amounts of alcohol within the preceding 24 h.
Abrupt withdrawal of therapy	May result in CNS excitation with tremor, anxiety, hallucinations, or delirium, which may be fatal; caution patients accordingly
Patients with severe cardiac disease	Large doses should be avoided (see CONTRAINDICATIONS)
Concomitant use with oral anticoagulants	May stimulate hepatic metabolism of coumarin anticoagulants, thereby reducing their effectiveness, and may also potentiate the hypoprothrombinemic effects of coumarin anticoagulants; monitor prothrombin time closely and adjust anticoagulant dosage, as needed, both during therapy and after discontinuing chloral hydrate
Concomitant use with IV furosemide	May produce sweating, hot flashes, and variable blood pressure, including hypertension, due to a hypermetabolic state caused by displacement of thyroid hormone from its bound state
Acute intermittent porphyria	May be precipitated; use with caution in susceptible patients
Carcinogenicity, mutagenicity	Long-term studies in animals have not been done

ADVERSE REACTIONS

Central nervous system	Somnambulism, disorientation, incoherence, paranoia; residual sedation ("hangover"), excitement, tolerance, addiction, delirium, drowsiness, staggering gait, ataxia, light-headedness, vertigo, dizziness, nightmares, malaise, confusion, hallucinations, and headache (rare)
Hematological	Leukopenia, eosinophilia
Allergic	Skin rash, including hives, erythema, eczematoid dermatitis, urticaria, scarlatiniform exanthems
Gastrointestinal	Gastric irritation, nausea, vomiting, flatulence, diarrhea, unpleasant taste
Other	Idiosyncratic syndrome and ketonuria (rare)

OVERDOSAGE

Signs and symptoms	Hypothermia, pinpoint pupils, decreased blood pressure, comatose state, slow or rapid and shallow breathing, vomiting, gastric necrosis; if patient survives, icterus due to hepatic damage and albuminuria from renal irritation may appear
Treatment	Empty stomach by inducing emesis or by gastric lavage. Employ supportive measures, as needed. Hemodialysis may be helpful.

DRUG INTERACTIONS

Alcohol, antihistamines, tranquilizers, and other CNS depressants	△ CNS depression; reduce dosage of chloral hydrate
Coumarin anticoagulants	△ or ▽ Prothrombin time

ALTERED LABORATORY VALUES

Urinary values	△ Glucose (with Benedict's solution or copper sulfate test) △ Catecholamines (with fluorometric tests) △ 17-Hydroxycorticosteroids (with Reddy, Jenkins, and Thorn procedure) △ Ketones (rare)

No clinically significant alterations in blood/serum values occur at therapeutic dosages

---

USE IN CHILDREN
See INDICATIONS and ORAL DOSAGE

USE IN PREGNANT AND NURSING WOMEN
Pregnancy Category C: use during pregnancy only when clearly needed. Chloral hydrate crosses the placental barrier, and chronic use during pregnancy may cause withdrawal symptoms in the neonate. It is not known what effect, if any, this drug may have on reproductive capacity. Chloral hydrate is excreted in human milk; use by nursing mothers may cause sedation in the infant.

NONBARBITURATES

NOLUDAR (methyprylon) Roche   C-III
Tablets: 50, 200 mg

NOLUDAR 300 (methyprylon) Roche   C-III
Capsules: 300 mg

INDICATIONS	**ORAL DOSAGE**
Insomnia	Adult: 200–400 mg at bedtime Child (> 12 yr): 50 mg at bedtime to start, followed, if necessary, by up to 200 mg at bedtime

CONTRAINDICATIONS

Hypersensitivity to methyprylon

ADMINISTRATION/DOSAGE ADJUSTMENTS

Persistent insomnia	Prolonged use is usually not indicated and should only be undertaken concomitantly with appropriate evaluation; effectiveness lasts for at least 7 consecutive nights of drug administration

WARNINGS/PRECAUTIONS

Mental impairment	Caution patients not to drive or engage in other potentially hazardous activities requiring full mental alertness soon after they have taken this drug and that alcohol and other CNS depressants (see DRUG INTERACTIONS) may have a combined additive effect
Special-risk patients	Use with caution in patients with hepatic or renal disorders or porphyria
Repeated or prolonged use	Perform blood counts periodically (see ADVERSE REACTIONS)
Drug dependence	Psychic and/or physical dependence and tolerance may develop, especially in addiction-prone individuals; withdrawal reactions tend to resemble those associated with barbiturate withdrawal and should be treated similarly
Carcinogenicity, mutagenicity	No adequate studies of carcinogenicity and mutagenicity have been performed
Effect on fertility	No adverse effects on reproduction have been detected in rats given 5 and 50 mg/kg/day

ADVERSE REACTIONS

Central nervous system	Convulsions, hallucinations, ataxia, EEG changes, pyrexia, morning drowsiness, headache, dizziness, vertigo, paradoxical excitation, anxiety, depression, nightmares, dreaming; acute brain syndrome and confusion (especially in elderly patients)
Ophthalmic	Diplopia, blurred vision
Hematological	Aplastic anemia, thrombocytopenic purpura, neutropenia
Cardiovascular	Hypotension, syncope
Gastrointestinal	Esophagitis, vomiting, nausea, diarrhea, constipation
Dermatological	Pruritus, rash
Other	Generalized allergic reactions, hangover

OVERDOSAGE

Signs and symptoms	Somnolence, confusion, coma, shock, miosis, respiratory depression, hypotension, tachycardia, edema, hepatic impairment, excitation, convulsions; serum drug levels of 3–6 mg/dl have been associated with serious toxic manifestations, and deaths have occurred at serum levels of 5.3–114 mg/dl. One fatality resulted from the ingestion of 6 g.
Treatment	Empty stomach immediately by gastric lavage, taking care to prevent pulmonary aspiration. Maintain an adequate airway, and administer appropriate IV fluids, as needed. Combat hypotension with norepinephrine, metaraminol, or other accepted antihypotensive measures. Hemodialysis may be useful, particularly if an adequate urinary output cannot be maintained and supportive measures are insufficient. For excitation and convulsions, use barbiturates with great caution.

DRUG INTERACTIONS

Alcohol, antihistamines, tranquilizers, and other CNS depressants	↿ CNS depression

ALTERED LABORATORY VALUES

Blood/serum levels	↿ Hepatic microsomal enzymes

USE IN CHILDREN

Safety and effectiveness for use in children under 12 yr of age have not been established; use of the drug in this age group is not recommended. The effective dosage in older children varies greatly.

USE IN PREGNANT AND NURSING WOMEN

Pregnancy Category B: use during pregnancy only if clearly needed. Reproduction studies performed in rats and rabbits given ~ 9 times the maximum human dose have shown no evidence of teratogenic effects. An increased incidence of resorptions has been observed in rabbits given 50 mg/kg/day. No adequate, well-controlled studies have been conducted in pregnant women. It is not known whether methyprylon is excreted in human milk; use with caution in nursing mothers because many drugs are excreted in human milk.

NONBARBITURATES

PLACIDYL (ethchlorvynol) Abbott   C-IV

Capsules: 200, 500, 750 mg

INDICATIONS

Insomnia

ORAL DOSAGE

Adult: 500 mg at bedtime; if response is inadequate or patient is being switched from another hypnotic, 750 mg at bedtime; if insomnia is unusually severe, up to 1 g at bedtime. A course of therapy should not exceed 1 wk.

CONTRAINDICATIONS

Hypersensitivity to ethchlorvynol	Porphyria

ADMINISTRATION/DOSAGE ADJUSTMENTS

Persistent insomnia	Allow a drug-free interval of 1 wk or more to elapse and further evaluate patient before prescribing a second course
Early morning awakening	A single dose of 200 mg may be given to reinstitute sleep
Elderly and/or debilitated individuals	Use the smallest effective dose

WARNINGS/PRECAUTIONS

Drug dependence	Psychic and/or physical dependence and tolerance may develop with prolonged use; severe withdrawal reactions, including convulsions, delirium, schizoid reactions, perceptual distortions, memory loss, ataxia, insomnia, slurred speech, unusual anxiety, irritability, agitation, tremors, anorexia, nausea, vomiting, weakness, dizziness, diaphoresis, muscle twitching, and weight loss, may occur as late as 9 days after abrupt discontinuation if ethchlorvynol has been used for a prolonged period. To prevent drug dependence, avoid long-term use, caution patients not to increase the dosage on their own, and prescribe the smallest feasible amount for addiction-prone patients.
Dizziness	Caution patients that their ability to drive or perform other potentially hazardous activities may be impaired and that alcohol and other CNS depressants may cause further impairment
Mentally depressed patients	Prescribe the smallest feasible amount for mentally depressed patients, even if suicidal tendencies are not evident
Patients with acute or chronic pain	Administer ethchlorvynol only if insomnia persists after pain is controlled with analgesics
Other special-risk patients	Use with caution in the elderly and/or debilitated and in patients with hepatic or renal impairment
Idiosyncratic behavior	Patients who behave unpredictably or exhibit paradoxical restlessness or excitement in response to alcohol or barbiturates may react similarly to ethchlorvynol
Transient giddiness and ataxia	May result from especially rapid absorption; these reactions may be controlled in some cases by taking the drug with food
Tartrazine sensitivity	Presence of FD&C Yellow No. 5 (tartrazine) in 750-mg capsules may cause allergic-type reactions, including bronchial asthma, in susceptible individuals
Carcinogenicity	A small, but significant, increase in total lung tumors has been observed in female mice fed 7 times the maximum human dose for 22–24 mo; no evidence of carcinogenicity has been detected in rats given 5–15 times the maximum human dose for up to 2 yr

ADVERSE REACTIONS

Neurological	Dizziness, facial numbness, ataxia, giddiness

PLACIDYL ■ RESTORIL

Gastrointestinal	Vomiting, gastric upset, nausea, aftertaste
Hematological	Thrombocytopenia; fatal immune thrombocytopenia (one case)
Hypersensitivity	Cholestatic jaundice, urticaria, rash
Idiosyncratic	Syncope without marked hypotension, profound muscular weakness, hysteria, marked excitement, prolonged hypnosis, mild stimulation
Other	Blurred vision, hypotension; mild, residual sedation ("hangover")

OVERDOSAGE

Signs and symptoms	*Acute toxicity:* prolonged deep coma, severe respiratory depression, hypothermia, hypotension, bradycardia, nystagmus, pancytopenia, death; *Chronic toxicity:* incoordination, tremors, ataxia, confusion, slurred speech, hyperreflexia, diplopia, muscle weakness, amblyopia, scotoma, nystagmus, peripheral neuropathy
Treatment	*Acute toxicity:* Empty stomach immediately by gastric lavage. (In the unconscious patient, precede lavage by tracheal intubation with a cuffed tube.) Assist ventilation, monitor vital signs, and control blood pressure. Hemoperfusion using the Amberlite column technique is reportedly the most effective method of managing acute overdosage of this drug. Hemodialysis or peritoneal dialysis may be of value. Forced diuresis may also be useful. The magnitude of an overdose cannot be reliably determined by measurement of the serum ethchlorvynol level because large amounts of the drug are taken up by adipose tissue. *Chronic toxicity:* Reduce dosage gradually over a period of days or weeks. For psychotic symptoms, add a phenothiazine compound to the regimen. Provide supportive care as indicated. *Withdrawal symptoms:* Readminister ethchlorvynol or give phenobarbital at the level of chronic toxicity that existed before abrupt discontinuation. Treat chronic toxicity as stated above.

DRUG INTERACTIONS

Alcohol, tranquilizers, other CNS depressants, MAO inhibitors	△ CNS depression
Coumarin anticoagulants	▽ Prothrombin time
Tricyclic antidepressants	Transient delirium

ALTERED LABORATORY VALUES

No clinically significant alterations in blood/serum or urinary values occur at therapeutic dosages

USE IN CHILDREN

Not recommended for use in children; the safety and effectiveness of this drug have not been established in pediatric populations

USE IN PREGNANT AND NURSING WOMEN

Pregnancy Category C: an increase in stillbirths and a decrease in surviving progeny have been demonstrated in rats given 40 mg/kg/day; no adequate, well-controlled studies have been performed in pregnant women. Therefore, use of ethchlorvynol during the first two trimesters of pregnancy is not recommended. Administration during the third trimester may lead to CNS depression and transient withdrawal reactions (eg, episodic jitteriness, hyperactivity, restlessness, irritability, disturbed sleep, hunger) in neonates. It is not known whether ethchlorvynol is excreted in human milk; because of the potential for serious adverse reactions in nursing infants, patients should not nurse while taking this drug.

NONBARBITURATES

RESTORIL (temazepam) Sandoz Pharmaceuticals C-IV

Capsules: 15, 30 mg

INDICATIONS	ORAL DOSAGE
Insomnia	**Adult:** 15–30 mg at bedtime

CONTRAINDICATIONS

Pregnancy

ADMINISTRATION/DOSAGE ADJUSTMENTS

Elderly or debilitated patients	Initiate therapy with 15 mg at bedtime; adjust subsequent dose according to clinical response

WARNINGS/PRECAUTIONS

Elderly or debilitated patients	The risk of oversedation, dizziness, confusion, and/or ataxia increases substantially with larger doses in these patients (see ADMINISTRATION/DOSAGE ADJUSTMENTS)

COMPENDIUM OF DRUG THERAPY

RESTORIL ■ VALMID

Potentially suicidal patients	Use with caution and with appropriate safeguards in patients with severe or latent depression
Mental impairment	Caution patients not to drive or perform other potentially hazardous activities after taking this drug and that alcohol and other CNS depressants may cause further impairment
Nocturnal sleep disturbances	May be experienced during first or second night after discontinuing temazepam
Patients with renal or hepatic impairment	Use with caution and observe patient for signs of drug accumulation
Abnormal liver-function tests, blood dyscrasias	Have been reported in patients taking benzodiazepines
Drug dependence	Psychic and/or physical dependence may develop, especially in addiction-prone individuals
Abrupt discontinuation of therapy	Barbiturate-like withdrawal symptoms, including convulsions, have occurred in patients receiving excessive doses of benzodiazepines over extended periods; milder withdrawal symptoms have occurred infrequently following abrupt withdrawal of continuous benzodiazepine therapy, generally at higher therapeutic levels, for at least several months
Persistent insomnia	Prolonged use is generally not necessary or recommended; in sleep laboratory studies, temazepam has been employed for sleep maintenance for up to 35 consecutive nights

ADVERSE REACTIONS

Frequent reactions (incidence ≥ 1%) are printed in *italics*

Central nervous system	*Drowsiness (17%); dizziness (7%); lethargy (5%); confusion, euphoria, and relaxed feeling (2–3%); weakness (1–2%);* tremor; ataxia; lack of concentration; loss of equilibrium; falling; rarely, hallucinations, horizontal nystagmus, and paradoxical reactions (excitement, stimulation, hyperactivity)
Cardiovascular	Palpitations
Gastrointestinal	*Anorexia and diarrhea (1–2%)*

OVERDOSAGE

Signs and symptoms	Somnolence, confusion, coma, diminished or absent reflexes, respiratory depression, hypotension
Treatment	If patient is conscious, induce emesis or perform gastric lavage to empty stomach; if patient is unconscious, use a cuffed endotracheal tube to prevent pulmonary aspiration. Maintain adequate pulmonary ventilation. Hypotension may require use of pressor agents. Administer IV fluids to promote diuresis. Dialysis is of undetermined value. If excitation occurs, do not give barbiturates.

DRUG INTERACTIONS

Alcohol, antihistamines, tranquilizers, and other CNS depressants	△ CNS depression

ALTERED LABORATORY VALUES

No clinically significant alterations in blood/serum or urinary values occur at therapeutic dosages

USE IN CHILDREN

Safety and effectiveness for use in children under 18 yr of age have not been established

USE IN PREGNANT AND NURSING WOMEN

Pregnancy Category X: contraindicated during pregnancy. An increased risk of congenital malformations has been associated with use of benzodiazepine anxiolytics (diazepam and chlordiazepoxide) during the first trimester. Transplacental distribution of therapeutic doses of a benzodiazepine hypnotic during the last weeks of pregnancy has resulted in neonatal CNS depression. Increased nursing mortality has been reported in rats and rabbits treated with temazepam. Patients likely to become pregnant while taking this drug should be apprised of the potential hazard and cautioned to discontinue use of temazepam before attempting to conceive. It is not known whether this drug is excreted in human milk; use with caution in nursing mothers.

NONBARBITURATES

VALMID (ethinamate) Dista C-IV

Capsules: 500 mg

INDICATIONS	ORAL DOSAGE
Insomnia	**Adult:** 500–1,000 mg 20 min before bedtime

VALMID ■ VERSED

CONTRAINDICATIONS
Hypersensitivity to ethinamate

ADMINISTRATION/DOSAGE ADJUSTMENTS

Elderly or debilitated patients	Limit dosage to 500 mg/day to avoid oversedation, dizziness, confusion, and/or ataxia
Persistent insomnia	Prolonged use is not recommended, since this drug has not been shown to be effective for more than 7 days; allow a drug-free interval of 1 wk or more to elapse before considering retreatment and attempt to find an alternative, nonpharmacologic means of treating chronic insomnia
Abrupt withdrawal	May precipitate a typical abstinence syndrome and convulsions in physically dependent patients; hospitalize patient and reduce addictive daily dose by 500–1,000 mg every 2–3 days

WARNINGS/PRECAUTIONS

Mental impairment	Caution patients against driving or performing other potentially hazardous activities shortly after ingesting this drug and that alcohol and other CNS depressants may cause further impairment
Depressed patients	Use with caution in patients who are severely depressed or in whom there is any evidence of latent depression, particularly if patient is potentially suicidal
Drug dependence	Psychic and/or physical dependence may develop with prolonged use of higher than recommended dosages, especially in addiction-prone individuals

ADVERSE REACTIONS

Hematological	Thrombocytopenic purpura (rare)
Central nervous system	Paradoxical excitement in children
Gastrointestinal	Mild GI symptoms
Dermatological	Rash
Other	Idiosyncratic reaction with fever (rare)

OVERDOSAGE

Signs and symptoms	CNS and respiratory depression
Treatment	Empty stomach by gastric lavage. Institute symptomatic and supportive therapy. Administer IV fluids. Maintain adequate respiratory exchange, blood pressure, and body temperature. Dialysis may be helpful. Antibiotics may be required for pulmonary complications.

DRUG INTERACTIONS

Alcohol, antihistamines, tranquilizers, and CNS depressants	⇧ CNS depression
MAO inhibitors, tricyclic antidepressants	⇧ Antidepressant effect and/or sedation

ALTERED LABORATORY VALUES

Urinary values	⇧ 17-Ketosteroids (with modified Zimmerman reaction) ⇧ 17-Hydroxycorticosteroids (with Porter-Silber test)

No clinically significant alterations in blood/serum values occur at therapeutic dosages

---

USE IN CHILDREN
Not recommended for use in children under 15 yr of age; the safety and effectiveness of this drug have not been established in pediatric populations

USE IN PREGNANT AND NURSING WOMEN
Pregnancy Category C: use during pregnancy only if clearly needed. Animal reproduction studies have not been done, nor has it been determined whether this drug can affect human reproductive capacity or cause harm to the fetus when administered to a pregnant woman. It is not known whether ethinamate is excreted in human milk; use with caution in nursing mothers because many drugs are excreted in human milk.

NONBARBITURATES

VERSED (midazolam hydrochloride) Roche C-IV
Vials: 5 mg midazolam/ml (1, 2, 5, 10 ml) **Prefilled syringes:** 5 mg midazolam/ml (2 ml)

INDICATIONS
Induction of sleepiness or drowsiness and relief of apprehension before surgery
Impairment of memory of perioperative events

PARENTERAL DOSAGE
Adult: 0.07–0.08 mg/kg IM approximately 1 h before surgery

COMPENDIUM OF DRUG THERAPY

VERSED

Conscious sedation before short diagnostic or endoscopic procedures, such as bronchoscopy, gastroscopy, cystoscopy, coronary angiography, and cardiac catheterization	**Adult:** 2–2.5 mg (0.035 mg/kg) IV to start, followed by small increments in dosage until speech begins to become slurred (usual *total* dose: 0.1–0.15 mg/kg, administered over a period of 2–3 min); additional doses in increments of 25% of the initial dose may be given to maintain the desired level of sedation
Induction of general anesthesia (before administration of other anesthetics)	**Adult (< 55 yr):** for induction in patients who have received a preoperative sedative or narcotic, 0.15–0.35 mg/kg IV (usual dose: 0.25 mg/kg); for induction in patients who have *not* received a preoperative sedative or narcotic, 0.3–0.35 mg/kg IV, followed, if necessary, by additional doses in increments of 25% of the initial dose, up to a total of 0.6 mg/kg
	Adult (> 55 yr): for induction in surgical patients who are good risks (ASA Category I or II) and have received a preoperative sedative or narcotic, 0.2 mg/kg IV; for induction in patients who have *not* received a preoperative sedative or narcotic, 0.3 mg/kg IV
	Adult with severe systemic disease or other debility: for induction in patients who have received a preoperative sedative or narcotic, as little as 0.15 mg/kg IV in some cases; for induction in patients who have *not* received a preoperative sedative or narcotic, 0.2–0.25 mg/kg IV or, in some cases, as little as 0.15 mg/kg IV
Maintenance of anesthesia during *short* surgical procedures, when used in conjunction with oxygen and nitrous oxide (balanced anesthesia)	**Adult:** approximately 25% of the induction dose, given IV whenever signs of lightening of anesthesia are seen

CONTRAINDICATIONS

Hypersensitivity to midazolam	Acute narrow angle glaucoma

ADMINISTRATION/DOSAGE ADJUSTMENTS

Intramuscular use	Inject dose deeply into a large muscle mass. Onset is within 15 min after IM injection; peak effect occurs 30–60 min after administration. If the patient is elderly or debilitated, reduce the dose. Midazolam can be given with atropine or scopolamine and with reduced doses of a narcotic.
Endoscopic and diagnostic procedures	Although a *total* dose of 0.1–0.15 mg/kg is generally adequate, up to 0.2 mg/kg may be required, especially if a narcotic drug is not given concomitantly. For debilitated patients and those 60 yr of age or older, reduce the dose by 25–30%. In these patients, the risk of drowsiness or respiratory depression may be increased if the dose exceeds 0.15 mg/kg. Narcotic premedication results in less variability in response and is recommended for bronchoscopy; bear in mind that in conscious sedation studies hypotension has occurred more frequently in patients premedicated with a narcotic drug. If a narcotic is used concomitantly, the dosage of midazolam should be reduced by 25–30%. To avoid respiratory depression and apnea, inject each dose of midazolam slowly. The onset of action occurs within 3–5 min, the exact time depending on the total dose and whether or not a narcotic drug is given concomitantly. To reduce the risk of cough and laryngospasm during peroral endoscopy, use a topical anesthetic and, in addition, ensure that these reactions can be treated once they occur.
Induction of anesthesia	Administer the initial dose over a period of 20–30 s; allow 2 min to elapse before valuating the effect of this drug. Individual response to midazolam is variable, especially when preoperative narcotic medication is not used. Induction may be completed, when necessary, with additional doses of midazolam or with administration of a volatile liquid inhalational anesthetic. If the total dose of midazolam is large (up to 0.6 mg/kg), postoperative recovery may be delayed. In clinical studies, the following were used in conjunction with midazolam: morphine (up to 0.15 mg/kg IM), meperidine (up to 1 mg/kg IM), fentanyl (1.5–2.0 µg/kg IV), fentanyl and droperidol (0.02 ml/kg IM), hydroxyzine pamoate (100 mg orally), and secobarbital sodium (200 mg orally). Administer premedications, except fentanyl, 1 h before induction; administer fentanyl approximately 5 min before anticipated induction time.
Maintenance of anesthesia	Administration of an effective narcotic drug is recommended before surgery if midazolam is to be used for maintenance of anesthesia
Intraarterial injection, extravasation	Take extreme care to avoid intraarterial injection and extravasation
Compatibility with other products	Midazolam may be mixed with morphine sulfate, meperidine, atropine sulfate, or scopolamine in the same syringe and is compatible with 5% dextrose in water, 0.9% sodium chloride, and lactated Ringer's solution

WARNINGS/PRECAUTIONS

Respiratory depression	Intravenous doses can depress respiration and cause apnea. Before IV administration, make sure that oxygen, resuscitative equipment, and trained personnel are available for immediate support of ventilation and maintenance of a patent airway. Use with caution in patients with chronic obstructive pulmonary disease, since they are unusually sensitive to the respiratory depressant effect of this drug.
Fluctuations in vital signs	Midazolam can cause hypotension, alter the heart rate, and depress pulmonary function. The occurrence and severity of these reactions are affected by intubation, instrumentation, concomitant therapy, and the degree of anesthesia. Do not use this drug in patients who are in shock, coma, or a state of acute alcohol intoxication accompanied by depression of vital signs. Bear in mind that this drug does not reverse the increase in intracranial pressure associated with succinylcholine and does not affect the changes in circulatory function associated with both succinylcholine and pancuronium; midazolam also does not blunt the increases in intracranial pressure, heart rate, and blood pressure seen with endotracheal intubation under light general anesthesia.

VERSED

Elderly and debilitated patients	Reduce the dosage for elderly and debilitated patients (see PARENTERAL DOSAGE and ADMINISTRATION/DOSAGE ADJUSTMENTS); when midazolam is used in these patients, the possibility of a profound and/or prolonged effect should be considered
Glaucoma	In patients without ophthalmic disease, midazolam has produced a moderate decrease in intraocular pressure following induction of anesthesia; however, use of this drug in patients with glaucoma has not been studied. Administer to patients with open angle glaucoma only if they are undergoing appropriate treatment; do not use in patients with acute narrow angle glaucoma
Renal failure	In patients with chronic renal failure, the elimination half-life, total body clearance, and volume of distribution is increased 1.5 to 2 fold
Congestive heart failure	In patients with congestive heart failure, the elimination half-life and volume of distribution is increased 2 to 3 fold
Ambulatory patients	Caution patients not to drive or engage in other activities requiring complete mental alertness until the effects of the drug (eg, drowsiness) have subsided or until the day after anesthesia and surgery, whichever is longer
Physical dependence	Midazolam has produced mild to moderate physical dependence in cynomolgus monkeys after 5–10 wk of administration; available data suggest that the abuse potential of this drug is at least equivalent to that of diazepam
Carcinogenicity, mutagenicity, effect on fertility	A marked increase in hepatic tumors has been observed in female mice and a small increase in benign thyroid follicular cell tumors has been detected in male rats following oral administration of midazolam maleate at 80 mg/kg/day for 2 yr; no increase in tumors has occurred at 9 mg/kg/day (25 times a human dose of 0.35 mg/kg). Midazolam showed no mutagenic activity in *Salmonella typhimurium*, Chinese hamster lung cells, human lymphocytes, or the mouse micronucleus test. No evidence of impaired fertility has been seen in male and female rats given up to 3.5 mg/kg.

ADVERSE REACTIONS[1]

Frequent reactions (incidence $\geq$ 1%) are printed in *italics*

Respiratory	*Decreased tidal volume and/or respiratory rate (23.3% with IV use, 10.8% with IM use), apnea,*[2] laryngospasm, bronchospasm, dyspnea, hyperventilation, wheezing, shallow breathing, airway obstruction, tachypnea
Cardiovascular	*Changes in blood pressure and heart rate,* bigeminy, premature ventricular contractions, vasovagal episode, tachycardia, nodal rhythm; transient fall in blood pressure of more than 50% during induction (0.2%)
Central nervous system	*Hiccoughs (3.9% with IV use only), oversedation (1.6% with IV use only), headache (1.5% with IV use, 1.3% with IM use), coughing (1.3% with IV use only), drowsiness (1.2% with IV use only),* retrograde amnesia, euphoria, confusion, argumentativeness, nervousness, agitation, anxiety, grogginess, restlessness, emergence delirium or agitation, prolonged emergence from anesthesia, dreaming during emergence, sleep disturbance, insomnia, nightmares, tonic/clonic movements, muscle tremor, involuntary movements, athetoid movements, ataxia, dizziness, dysphoria, slurred speech, dysphonia, paresthesia, lightheadedness, loss of balance
Ophthalmic	Blurred vision, diplopia, nystagmus, miosis, cyclic movements of eyelids, visual disturbance, difficulty focusing eyes
Gastrointestinal	*Nausea (2.8% with IV use only), vomiting (2.6% with IV use only),* acid taste, excessive salivation, retching
Dermatological	Urticaria, rash, pruritus
Local	*Tenderness (5.6% with IV use only), pain during IV injection (5%), pain at IM site (3.7%), erythema (2.6% with IV use, 0.5% with IM use), induration (1.7% with IV use, 0.5% with IM use),* phlebitis (0.4% with IV use only), muscle stiffness (0.3% with IM use only), urticaria-like reaction, swelling, burning, warmth, coldness
Other	Yawning, lethargy, chills, weakness, toothache, faint feeling, hematoma, blockage of ears

OVERDOSAGE

Signs and symptoms	Sedation, somnolence, confusion, impaired coordination, diminished reflexes, coma, changes in vital signs
Treatment	Monitor respiration, pulse rate, and blood pressure, and employ general supportive measures. Attention should be given to maintaining a patent airway and support of ventilation. An IV infusion should be started. Hypotension may be treated by IV fluid therapy, repositioning the patient, judicious use of vasopressors (if indicated), and other appropriate countermeasures. It is not known whether peritoneal dialysis, hemodialysis, or forced diuresis would have any benefit in treating midazolam overdosage.

DRUG INTERACTIONS

CNS depressants (including alcohol and preanesthetics)	△ Pharmacological effects of midazolam; see PARENTERAL DOSAGE and ADMINISTRATION/DOSAGE ADJUSTMENTS
Thiopental	△ Hypnotic effect of thiopental; if midazolam is given IM as a preanesthetic, reduce dosage of thiopental by approximately 15%
Halothane	△ Anesthetic effect; if midazolam is used for induction, it may be necessary to reduce the dosage of halothane

VERSED

ALTERED LABORATORY VALUES

No clinically significant alterations in blood/serum or urinary values occur at therapeutic dosages

USE IN CHILDREN

Safety and effectiveness for children under 18 yr of age have not been established

USE IN PREGNANT AND NURSING WOMEN

Pregnant women: Pregnancy Category D: several studies have suggested an increased risk of congenital malformations following the use of certain benzodiazepines (diazepam and chlordiazepoxide) during pregnancy; although no evidence of teratogenicity has been seen in rats and rabbits injected with 1.75 and 3.5 mg/kg of midazolam maleate, the drug should be considered a potential teratogen because it is a benzodiazepine and because it has been detected in human cord blood. Pregnant women should be apprised of the potential hazard to the fetus. The use of midazolam in obstetrics has not been evaluated in clinical studies. Because it crosses the placenta and because other benzodiazepines given in the last weeks of pregnancy have resulted in neonatal CNS depression, midazolam is not recommended for obstetrical use. **Nursing mothers:** It is not known whether midazolam is excreted in human milk; use with caution in nursing mothers.

[1] Reactions shown in normal typeface (except muscle stiffness) have been reported mainly following IV administration
[2] In clinical trials, 246/1,073 (22.9%) of patients experienced apnea when midazolam was given for induction of anesthesia, but only 5/512 (1%) when the drug was given for conscious sedation; the overall incidence of apnea following IV administration was 15.4% (263/1,709 patients)

Chapter 46

Urinary Anti-Infectives/Other Urinary Agents

Urinary Anti-Infectives — 1823

AZO GANTANOL (Roche) — 1823
Sulfamethoxazole and phenazopyridine hydrochloride *Rx*

AZO GANTRISIN (Roche) — 1824
Sulfisoxazole and phenazopyridine hydrochloride *Rx*

BACTRIM (Roche) — 1826
Trimethoprim and sulfamethoxazole *Rx*

BACTRIM DS (Roche) — 1826
Trimethoprim and sulfamethoxazole *Rx*

BACTRIM I.V. Infusion (Roche) — 1828
Trimethoprim and sulfamethoxazole *Rx*

CINOBAC (Dista) — 1830
Cinoxacin *Rx*

COACTIN (Roche) — 1831
Amdinocillin *Rx*

FURADANTIN (Norwich Eaton) — 1832
Nitrofurantoin *Rx*

GEOCILLIN (Roerig) — 1834
Carbenicillin indanyl sodium *Rx*

HIPREX (Merrell Dow) — 1834
Methenamine hippurate *Rx*

MACRODANTIN (Norwich Eaton) — 1835
Nitrofurantoin macrocrystals *Rx*

MANDELAMINE (Parke-Davis) — 1837
Methenamine mandelate *Rx*

NegGram (Winthrop-Breon) — 1837
Nalidixic acid *Rx*

NOROXIN (Merck Sharp & Dohme) — 1839
Norfloxacin *Rx*

PROLOPRIM (Burroughs Wellcome) — 1840
Trimethoprim *Rx*

SEPTRA (Burroughs Wellcome) — 1841
Trimethoprim and sulfamethoxazole *Rx*

SEPTRA DS (Burroughs Wellcome) — 1841
Trimethoprim and sulfamethoxazole *Rx*

SEPTRA I.V. Infusion (Burroughs Wellcome) — 1843
Trimethoprim and sulfamethoxazole *Rx*

TRIMPEX (Roche) — 1845
Trimethoprim *Rx*

URISED (Webcon) — 1847
Methenamine, methylene blue, phenyl salicylate, benzoic acid, atropine sulfate, and hysocyamine *Rx*

Urinary Analgesics — 1848

PYRIDIUM (Parke-Davis) — 1848
Phenazopyridine hydrochloride *Rx*

PYRIDIUM Plus (Parke-Davis) — 1849
Phenazopyridine hydrochloride, hyoscyamine hydrobromide, and butabarbial *Rx*

Urinary Antispasmodics — 1850

CYSTOSPAZ (Webcon) — 1850
Hyoscyamine *Rx*

CYSTOSPAZ-M (Webcon) — 1850
Hyoscyamine sulfate *Rx*

DITROPAN (Marion) — 1851
Oxybutynin chloride *Rx*

URISPAS (Smith Kline & French) — 1852
Flavoxate hydrochloride *Rx*

Parasympathomimetics — 1853

DUVOID (Norwich Eaton) — 1853
Bethanechol chloride *Rx*

URECHOLINE (Merck Sharp & Dohme) — 1854
Bethanechol chloride *Rx*

Other Urinary Anti-Infectives — 1822

COMOXOL (Squibb) — 1822
Sulfamethoxazole and trimethoprim *Rx*

COTRIM (Lemmon) — 1822
Sulfamethoxazole and trimethoprim *Rx*

THIOSULFIL-A (Ayerst) — 1822
Sulfamethizole and phenazopyridine hydrochloride *Rx*

UROBIOTIC-250 (Roerig) — 1822
Oxytetracycline hydrochloride, sulfamethizole, and phenazopyridine hydrochloride *Rx*

COMPENDIUM OF DRUG THERAPY

OTHER URINARY ANTI-INFECTIVES

DRUG	HOW SUPPLIED	USUAL DOSAGE[1]
COMOXOL (Squibb) Sulfamethoxazole and trimethoprim *Rx*	**Tablets:** 400 mg sulfamethoxazole and 80 mg trimethoprim (Comoxol 400/80); 800 mg sulfamethoxazole and 160 mg trimethoprim (Comoxol 800/160)	**Adult:** 2 Comoxol 400/80 tabs or 1 Comoxol 800/160 tab q12h for 10–14 days **Child ($\geq$ 2 mo):** 4 mg/kg trimethoprim and 20 mg/kg sulfamethoxazole q12h for 10 days
COTRIM (Lemmon) Sulfamethoxazole and trimethoprim *Rx*	**Tablets:** 400 mg sulfamethoxazole and 80 mg trimethoprim (Cotrim); 800 mg sulfamethoxazole and 160 mg trimethoprim (Cotrim DS)	**Adult:** 2 Cotrim tabs or 1 Cotrim DS tab q12h for 10–14 days **Child ($\geq$ 2 mo):** 4 mg/kg trimethoprim and 20 mg/kg sulfamethoxazole q12h for 10 days
THIOSULFIL-A (Ayerst) Sulfamethizole and phenazopyridine hydrochloride *Rx*	**Tablets:** 0.25 g sulfamethizole and 50 mg phenazopyridine hydrochloride (Thiosulfil-A); 0.5 g sulfamethizole and 50 mg phenazopyridine hydrochloride (Thiosulfil-A Forte)	**Adult:** 2–4 Thiosulfil-A tabs or 2 Thiosulfil-A Forte tabs, tid or qid for 2 days
UROBIOTIC-250 (Roerig) Oxytetracycline hydrochloride, sulfamethizole, and phenazopyridine hydrochloride *Rx*	**Capsules:** oxytetracycline hydrochloride equivalent to 250 mg oxytetracycline, 250 mg sulfamethizole, and 50 mg phenazopyridine hydrochloride	**Adult:** 1 cap qid (2 caps qid in resistant cases), 1 h before or 2 h after meals, for at least 7 days or until bacteriologically cured

[1] Where pediatric dosages are not given, consult manufacturer

AZO GANTANOL

URINARY ANTI-INFECTIVES

AZO GANTANOL (sulfamethoxazole and phenazopyridine hydrochloride) Roche   Rx

Tablets: 0.5 g sulfamethoxazole and 100 mg phenazopyridine hydrochloride

INDICATIONS	ORAL DOSAGE
Uncomplicated urinary tract infections caused by susceptible strains of *Escherichia coli*, *Klebsiella*, *Enterobacter*, *Staphylococcus aureus*, *Proteus mirabilis*, and *P vulgaris*, when symptomatic relief of pain, burning, or urgency is needed during the initial 2 days of therapy	Adult: 4 tabs to start, followed by 2 tabs bid (AM and PM) for up to 2 days; continue treatment beyond 2 days with sulfamethoxazole alone

CONTRAINDICATIONS

Pregnancy at term	Hypersensitivity to sulfonamides	Glomerulonephritis
Breast-feeding	Uremia	Pyelonephritis of pregnancy with GI disturbances
Age < 12 yr	Severe hepatitis	

ADMINISTRATION/DOSAGE ADJUSTMENTS

Therapeutic blood sulfonamide levels	For most infections, 5–15 mg/dl; for serious infections, 12–15 mg/dl; blood levels > 20 mg/dl increase the probability of adverse reactions. Blood levels should be measured in patients with serious infections.

WARNINGS/PRECAUTIONS

In vitro sulfonamide sensitivity tests	May not be reliable; coordinate test results with bacteriological and clinical responses
Blood dyscrasias	May occur and can be fatal (see ADVERSE REACTIONS); obtain CBC frequently and watch for early signs (eg, sore throat, fever, pallor, purpura, jaundice) of serious blood disorders
Hypersensitivity reactions	May occur and can be fatal (see ADVERSE REACTIONS); use with caution in patients allergic to some goitrogens, diuretics, and oral hypoglycemic agents
Hepatic toxicity	Fatalities resulting from hepatocellular necrosis have occurred in patients taking sulfonamides
Renal effects	Crystalluria, urolithiasis, and other renal complications have occurred in patients taking sulfonamides; caution patients to maintain an adequate fluid intake and perform a urinalysis, including a careful microscopic examination, frequently during therapy
Special-risk patients	Use with caution in patients with impaired renal or hepatic function, severe allergy, bronchial asthma, G6PD deficiency (hemolysis may occur), or porphyria[1]
Urine discoloration	Inform patients that their urine may turn reddish-orange (due to excretion of phenazopyridine) soon after they take this medication
Carcinogenicity	Long-term administration of sulfonamides has been associated with thyroid malignancies in rats. Prolonged administration of phenazopyridine has induced intestinal tumors in rats and liver tumors in mice; although phenazopyridine has not been linked with human neoplasia, there have been no adequate epidemiological studies.

ADVERSE REACTIONS

Hematological	Agranulocytosis, aplastic anemia, thrombocytopenia, leukopenia, hemolytic anemia, purpura, hypoprothrombinemia, methemoglobinemia
Allergic	Erythema multiforme (Stevens-Johnson syndrome), generalized skin eruptions, epidermal necrolysis, urticaria, serum sickness, pruritus, exfoliative dermatitis, anaphylactoid reactions, periorbital edema, conjunctival and scleral injection, photosensitization, arthralgia, allergic myocarditis
Gastrointestinal	Nausea, vomiting, abdominal pain, hepatitis, hepatocellular necrosis, diarrhea, anorexia, pancreatitis, stomatitis
Central nervous system	Headache, peripheral neuritis, mental depression, convulsions, ataxia, hallucinations, tinnitus, vertigo, insomnia
Renal	Toxic nephrosis with oliguria and anuria, crystalluria, urinary calculi; diuresis (rare)
Endocrinological	Goiter and hypoglycemia (rare)
Other	Drug fever, chills, periarteritis nodosa, lupus erythematosus phenomena

OVERDOSAGE

Signs and symptoms	See ADVERSE REACTIONS
Treatment	Discontinue use of drug; treat symptomatically

AZO GANTANOL ■ AZO GANTRISIN

DRUG INTERACTIONS

Para-aminobenzoic acid	⇩ Bacteriostatic effect of sulfamethoxazole
Oral anticoagulants, oral hypoglycemics, methotrexate, phenytoin, thiopental	Pharmacologic effects increased or prolonged ⇧ Risk of toxicity
Methenamine	⇧ Risk of crystalluria
Methotrexate	⇧ Methotrexate serum level

ALTERED LABORATORY VALUES

Blood/serum values	⇩ PBI ⇩ ^{131}I thyroid uptake
Urinary values	⇧ Glucose (with Clinitest tablets) ⇧ Protein (with sulfosalicylic acid method)

USE IN CHILDREN
Contraindicated for use in children under 12 yr of age

USE IN PREGNANT AND NURSING WOMEN
Safety for use during pregnancy has not been established (sulfonamides cross the placental barrier); administration at term is contraindicated. A significant increase in the incidence of cleft palate and other bony abnormalities has been detected in the offspring of rats and mice fed certain sulfonamides in large amounts (7–25 times the human therapeutic dose); however, the teratogenic potential of most sulfonamides has not been thoroughly studied in animals or humans. Use in nursing mothers is contraindicated; sulfonamides are excreted in breast milk and may cause kernicterus.

[1] 1983 USP Dispensing Information. Rockville, Md., United States Pharmacopeial Convention, Inc., 1982, vol 1

URINARY ANTI-INFECTIVES

AZO GANTRISIN (sulfisoxazole and phenazopyridine hydrochloride) Roche   Rx

Tablets: 0.5 g sulfisoxazole and 50 mg phenazopyridine hydrochloride

INDICATIONS
Initial episodes of uncomplicated urinary tract infections, when associated with **pain, burning, or urgency** and caused by susceptible strains of *Escherichia coli, Klebsiella, Enterobacter, Proteus mirabilis, P vulgaris,* and *Staphylococcus aureus*

ORAL DOSAGE
Adult: 4–6 tabs to start, followed by 2 tabs qid for up 2 days; for treatment beyond 2 days, use sulfisoxazole alone

CONTRAINDICATIONS

Pregnancy at term	Sensitivity to either component	Glomerulonephritis
Breast-feeding	Uremia	Pyelonephritis of pregnancy with GI disturbances
Age < 12 yr	Severe hepatitis	

ADMINISTRATION/DOSAGE ADJUSTMENTS

Therapeutic blood sulfonamide levels	For most infections, 5–15 mg/dl; for serious infections, 12–15 mg/dl; blood levels > 20 mg/dl increase the probability of adverse reactions. Blood levels should be measured in patients with serious infections.

WARNINGS/PRECAUTIONS

Group A streptococcal infections	Sulfonamides will neither eradicate the causative organism nor prevent complications
In vitro sulfonamide sensitivity tests	May not be reliable; coordinate test results with bacteriological and clinical responses
Blood dyscrasias	May occur and can be fatal (see ADVERSE REACTIONS). Obtain blood counts regularly if therapy continues for more than 2 wk; watch for early signs (eg, sore throat, fever, pallor, purpura, jaundice) of serious blood disorders.
Hypersensitivity reactions	May occur and can be fatal (see ADVERSE REACTIONS); use with caution in patients allergic to some goitrogens, diuretics, and oral hypoglycemic agents
Hepatic toxicity	Fatalities resulting from hepatocellular necrosis have occurred in patients taking sulfonamides

AZO GANTRISIN

Renal effects	Crystalluria, urolithiasis, and other renal complications have occurred in patients taking sulfonamides; caution patients to maintain an adequate fluid intake, and perform a urinalysis, including a careful microscopic examination, frequently during therapy
Urine discoloration	Inform patients that their urine may turn reddish-orange (due to excretion of phenazopyridine) soon after they take this medication
Special-risk patients	Use with caution in patients with impaired renal or hepatic function, severe allergy, bronchial asthma, G6PD deficiency (hemolysis may occur), or porphyria[1]
Carcinogenicity, mutagenicity	After long-term administration, sulfonamides have caused thyroid malignancies in rats, and phenazopyridine has induced large intestine neoplasia in rats and hepatic neoplasia in mice; no studies have been done to evaluate the mutagenic potential of this preparation's components
Effect on fertility	Administration of 800 mg/kg/day of sulfisoxazole had no effect on mating behavior, conception rate, or fertility index in rats; administration of 50 mg/kg/day of phenazopyridine also had no effect on fertility in rats

ADVERSE REACTIONS

Hematological	Leukopenia, agranulocytosis, aplastic anemia, thrombocytopenia, purpura, hemolytic anemia, anemia, eosinophilia, clotting disorders (including hypoprothrombinemia and hypofibrinogenemia), sulfhemoglobinemia, methemoglobinemia
Allergic	Anaphylaxis, generalized allergic reactions, angioneurotic edema, arteritis, vasculitis, myocarditis, serum sickness, conjunctival and scleral injection, periarteritis nodosa, systemic lupus erythematosus
Gastrointestinal	Nausea, vomiting, abdominal pain, anorexia, diarrhea, glossitis, stomatitis, flatulence, salivary gland enlargement, GI hemorrhage, pseudomembranous enterocolitis, melena, pancreatitis, hepatic dysfunction, jaundice, hepatocellular necrosis
Cardiovascular	Flushing, tachycardia, palpitations, syncope, cyanosis
Central nervous system and neuromuscular	Headache, dizziness, peripheral neuritis, paresthesia, convulsions, tinnitus, vertigo, ataxia, intracranial hypertension, psychosis, hallucinations, disorientation, depression, anxiety, drowsiness, weakness, fatigue, lassitude, rigors, hearing loss, insomnia, arthralgia, chest pain, myalgia
Renal	Crystalluria, hematuria, nephritis and toxic nephrosis with oliguria and anuria, acute renal failure, urinary retention; diuresis (rare)
Endocrinological	Goiter and hypoglycemia (rare)
Dermatological	Rash, urticaria, pruritus, erythema multiforme, Stevens-Johnson syndrome, toxic epidermal necrolysis, exfoliative dermatitis, photosensitivity
Other	Edema (including periorbital edema), pyrexia, pneumonitis

OVERDOSAGE

Signs and symptoms	Anorexia, colic, nausea, vomiting, dizziness, drowsiness, unconsciousness, pyrexia, hematuria, crystalluria, blood dyscrasias, jaundice, cyanosis, methemoglobinemia
Treatment	Empty stomach by emesis or gastric lavage. Force oral fluids; if urine output is low and renal function normal, administer IV fluids. Monitor blood counts and appropriate blood chemistries, including electrolytes. If patient becomes cyanotic, methemoglobinemia is a possibility and, if present, should be treated with 1% methylene blue, given IV. Institute specific therapy if a blood dyscrasia or jaundice occurs.

DRUG INTERACTIONS

Para-aminobenzoic acid	▽ Bacteriostatic effect of sulfisoxazole
Oral anticoagulants, oral hypoglycemics, methotrexate, phenytoin thiopental	Pharmacologic effects increased or prolonged △ Risk of toxicity
Methenamine	△ Risk of crystalluria
Methotrexate	△ Methotrexate serum level

ALTERED LABORATORY VALUES

Blood/serum values	△ BUN △ Creatinine ▽ PBI ▽ [131]I thyroid uptake Altered liver function test results in patients with hepatitis
Urinary values	△ Glucose (with Clinitest tablets) △ Protein (with sulfosalicylic acid method)

USE IN CHILDREN

Contraindicated for use in children under 12 yr of age

USE IN PREGNANT AND NURSING WOMEN

Pregnancy Category C: use during pregnancy only if the anticipated therapeutic benefit justifies the potential risk to the fetus. There are no adequate or well-controlled studies of this drug combination in either laboratory animals or pregnant women; consequently, it is not known whether it can affect human reproductive capacity or cause harm to the human fetus. Teratogenicity studies of sulfisoxazole alone have produced conflicting results in animals. Treatment of pregnant rats with phenazopyridine (50 mg/kg/day) did not give rise to congenital malformations. However, this drug is contraindicated in pregnant women at term and in nursing mothers because sulfonamides cross the placental barrier, are excreted in human milk, and may cause kernicterus.

---

[1] *1984 USP Dispensing Information.* Rockville, Md., United States Pharmacopeial Convention, Inc., 1983, vol 1

BACTRIM

URINARY ANTI-INFECTIVES

BACTRIM (trimethoprim and sulfamethoxazole) Roche — Rx

Tablets: 80 mg trimethoprim and 400 mg sulfamethoxazole **Suspension (per 5 ml):** 40 mg trimethoprim and 200 mg sulfamethoxazole[1] (16 fl oz) *fruit/licorice-flavored* **Pediatric suspension (per 5 ml):** 40 mg trimethoprim and 200 mg sulfamethoxazole[1] (100 ml, 16 fl oz) *cherry-flavored*

BACTRIM DS (trimethoprim and sulfamethoxazole) Roche — Rx

Tablets: 160 mg trimethoprim and 800 mg sulfamethoxazole

INDICATIONS	ORAL DOSAGE
Urinary tract infections caused by susceptible strains of *Escherichia coli*, *Klebsiella*, *Enterobacter*, *Morganella morganii*, *Proteus mirabilis*, and *P vulgaris* [2]	**Adult:** 2 Bactrim tabs, 1 Bactrim DS tab, or 20 ml (4 tsp) q12h for 10–14 days **Child (≥ 2 mo):** 4 mg/kg trimethoprim and 20 mg/kg sulfamethoxazole q12h for 10 days, as follows: **Child (10 kg):** 5 ml (1 tsp) q12h for 10 days **Child (20 kg):** 1 Bactrim tab or 10 ml (2 tsp) q12h for 10 days **Child (30 kg):** 1½ Bactrim tabs or 15 ml (3 tsp) q12h for 10 days **Child (40 kg):** 2 Bactrim tabs, 1 Bactrim DS tab, or 20 ml (4 tsp) q12h for 10 days
Acute otitis media caused by susceptible strains of *Hemophilus influenzae* or *Streptococcus pneumoniae*[3]	**Child (≥ 2 mo):** same as pediatric dosages above
Acute exacerbations of chronic bronchitis caused by susceptible strains of *Hemophilus influenzae* or *Streptococcus pneumoniae*[4]	**Adult:** same as adult dosage above for 14 days
Enteritis caused by susceptible strains of *Shigella flexneri* and *S sonnei*	**Adult:** same as adult dosage above for 5 days **Child (≥ 2 mo):** same as pediatric dosages above for 5 days
Pneumocystis carinii pneumonitis	**Adult:** 5 mg/kg trimethoprim and 25 mg/kg sulfamethoxazole q6h for 14 days **Child (≥ 2 mo):** same as adult, as follows: **Child (8 kg):** 5 ml (1 tsp) q6h for 14 days **Child (16 kg):** 1 Bactrim tab or 10 ml (2 tsp) q6h for 14 days **Child (24 kg):** 1½ Bactrim tabs or 15 ml (3 tsp) q6h for 14 days **Child (32 kg):** 2 Bactrim tabs, 1 Bactrim DS tab, or 20 ml (4 tsp) q6h for 14 days

CONTRAINDICATIONS

Pregnancy at term	Age < 2 mo	Megaloblastic anemia due to folate deficiency
Breast-feeding	Hypersensitivity to trimethoprim or sulfonamides	

ADMINISTRATION/DOSAGE ADJUSTMENTS

Patients with renal impairment	Follow the usual dosage regimen if creatinine clearance (Ccr) > 30 ml/min. Administer half the usual dosage if Ccr = 15–30 ml/min. Use is not recommended if Ccr < 15 ml/min.

WARNINGS/PRECAUTIONS

Group A beta-hemolytic streptococcal pharyngitis	Sulfonamides have no place in the treatment of such infections, as they will neither eradicate the causative organism from the tonsillopharyngeal area nor prevent complications
Life-threatening reactions	Severe, potentially fatal reactions, including Stevens-Johnson syndrome, toxic epidermal necrolysis, fulminant hepatic necrosis, and serious blood dyscrasias (eg, agranulocytosis, aplastic anemia) have occurred on rare occasions in patients receiving sulfonamides. These drugs have caused hemolytic anemia in patients with G6PD deficiency. The risk of severe adverse reactions may be increased in elderly patients, particularly when these patients are receiving other drugs (see DRUG INTERACTIONS) or they have renal or hepatic impairment or another complicating condition; the most frequent serious adverse effects seen in elderly patients are severe skin reactions, generalized bone marrow depression, and thrombocytopenia.
	When using this preparation, obtain a CBC frequently and watch for early clinical signs such as rash, sore throat, fever, pallor, purpura, and jaundice; *discontinue administration at the first sign of skin rash or any adverse reaction.*
Bone marrow depression	High doses or prolonged use may cause bone marrow depression and, as a result, produce thrombocytopenia, leukopenia, and/or megaloplastic anemia; if signs of bone marrow depression appear, give 5-15 mg/day of leucovorin until normal hematopoiesis is restored
Cross-sensitivity	Patients allergic to acetazolamide, thiazide-type diuretics, sulfonylureas, or certain goitrogens may also be hypersensitive to this preparation
Renal effects	Crystalluria, urolithiasis, and other renal complications have occurred in patients taking sulfonamides. Caution patients to maintain an adequate fluid intake; urinalysis, including careful microscopic examination, and renal function tests should be performed during therapy, particularly when a patient has renal impairment.

BACTRIM

Special-risk patients	Use with caution in elderly patients and those with renal or hepatic impairment, possible folate deficiency, severe allergies, bronchial asthma, or G6PD deficiency. Among the conditions that may be associated with folate deficiency are malnutrition, malabsorption syndrome, chronic alcoholism, advanced age, and anticonvulsant therapy.
AIDS	Patients with AIDS may not tolerate or respond to this preparation in the same manner as other patients; the frequency of adverse effects, particularly rash, fever, and leukopenia, has been reported to be greatly increased in AIDS patients who were undergoing treatment of *Pneumocystis carinii* pneumonia
Carcinogenicity	No long-term studies have been done in animals to evaluate the oncogenic potential of this drug
Mutagenicity	Although bacterial mutagenicity studies have not been done with this preparation, trimethoprim alone has shown no mutagenic potential in the Ames assay, and no chromosomal abnormalities have been detected in human leukocytes cultured in vitro with either component alone or in combination or in leukocytes from treated patients
Effect on fertility	No adverse effects on fertility or general reproductive performance have been observed in rats given oral dosages as high as 70 mg/kg/day of trimethoprim plus 350 mg/kg/day of sulfamethoxazole

ADVERSE REACTIONS

Hematological	Agranulocytosis, aplastic anemia, thrombocytopenia, leukopenia, neutropenia, hemolytic anemia, megaloblastic anemia, hypoprothrombinemia, methemoglobinemia, eosinophilia
Gastrointestinal	Hepatitis (including cholestatic jaundice and fulminant hepatic necrosis), elevation of serum transaminase and bilirubin levels, pseudomembranous enterocolitis, pancreatitis, stomatitis, glossitis, nausea, vomiting, abdominal pain, diarrhea, anorexia
Genitourinary	Renal failure, interstitial nephritis, elevation of BUN and serum creatinine levels, toxic nephrosis with oliguria and anuria, crystalluria
Central nervous system	Aseptic meningitis, convulsions, peripheral neuritis, ataxia, vertigo, tinnitus, headache, hallucinations, depression, apathy, nervousness, weakness, fatigue, insomnia
Endocrinological	Diuresis, hypoglycemia
Musculoskeletal	Arthralgia, myalgia
Hypersensitivity	Stevens-Johnson syndrome, toxic epidermal necrolysis, anaphylaxis, allergic myocarditis, erythema multiforme, exfoliative dermatitis, angioedema, drug fever, chills, Henoch-Schoenlein purpura, serum sickness-like syndrome, generalized allergic reactions, generalized skin eruptions, photosensitivity, conjunctival and scleral injection, pruritus, urticaria, rash, periarteritis nodosa, systemic lupus erythematosus

OVERDOSAGE

Signs and symptoms	Anorexia, colic, nausea, vomiting, dizziness, headache, drowsiness, mental depression, confusion, unconsciousness, pyrexia, hematuria, crystalluria, bone marrow depression, other blood dyscrasias, jaundice
Treatment	Induce emesis or perform gastric lavage. To enhance renal elimination, acidify urine and institute forced diuresis; if urine output is low and renal function is normal, administer IV fluids. Monitor blood counts and electrolyte balance. Institute specific therapy if jaundice or a significant blood dyscrasia occurs. Peritoneal dialysis is not useful, and hemodialysis only moderately effective, in removing the components of this preparation.

DRUG INTERACTIONS

Diuretics (especially thiazides)	△ Risk of thrombocytopenic purpura in elderly patients
Warfarin	△ Prothrombin time; if this preparation is given during warfarin therapy, recheck prothrombin time
Phenytoin	△ Serum half-life of phenytoin; watch for evidence of phenytoin toxicity during combination therapy
Methotrexate	△ Serum level of methotrexate

ALTERED LABORATORY VALUES

Blood/serum values	△ Methotrexate (with competitive binding protein assay using dihydrofolate reductase) △ BUN △ Creatinine (especially with Jaffé test) △ Bilirubin △ SGOT △ SGPT ▽ PBI ▽ [131]I thyroid uptake

No clinically significant alterations in urinary values occur at therapeutic dosages

---

USE IN CHILDREN

See INDICATIONS and ORAL DOSAGE. Data on the safety of repeated use in children under 2 yr of age are limited; contraindicated for infants under 2 mo of age.

USE IN PREGNANT AND NURSING WOMEN

Pregnancy Category C: use during pregnancy only if expected benefit justifies the potential fetal risk, since the drug may interfere with folic acid metabolism. Teratogenic effects (mainly cleft palate) have been observed in rats and increased fetal loss has been observed in rats and rabbits at doses several times the recommended human dose. Although no large, well-controlled studies have been done in pregnant women, two limited studies have shown no increase in congenital abnormalities. The drug is contraindicated at term and for use in nursing mothers because sulfonamides cross the placental barrier, are excreted in human milk, and may cause kernicterus.

---

[1] Contains 0.3% alcohol
[2] Initial episodes of uncomplicated infections should be treated with a single, effective antibacterial agent, rather than a combination
[3] Not indicated for prophylaxis or prolonged administration
[4] When in the physician's judgment this preparation offers some advantage over the use of a single antimicrobial agent

URINARY ANTI-INFECTIVES

BACTRIM I.V. Infusion (trimethoprim and sulfamethoxazole) Roche — Rx

Ampuls (per 5 ml): 80 mg trimethoprim and 400 mg sulfamethoxazole (5 ml) for IV infusion only   **Vials (per 5 ml):** 80 mg trimethoprim and 400 mg sulfamethoxazole (5, 10, 30 ml) for IV infusion only

INDICATIONS

Pneumocystis carinii pneumonitis

Severe or complicated **urinary tract infections** caused by susceptible strains of *Escherichia coli*, *Klebsiella*, *Enterobacter*, *Morganella morganii*, and *Proteus*, when oral administration is not feasible or when the organism is not susceptible to single urinary anti-infectives alone
Enteritis caused by susceptible strains of *Shigella flexneri* and *S sonnei*

PARENTERAL DOSAGE[1]

Adult: 15–20 mg/kg/day, given in 3 or 4 equally divided doses via IV infusion q6–8h
Child: same as adult

Adult: 8–10 mg/kg/day, up to 960 mg/day, given in 2–4 equally divided doses via IV infusion q6–12h
Child: same as adult

CONTRAINDICATIONS

Pregnancy at term	Hypersensitivity to trimethoprim or sulfonamides	Documented megaloblastic anemia due to folate deficiency
Breast-feeding	Age ≤ 2 mo	

ADMINISTRATION/DOSAGE ADJUSTMENTS

Preparation of infusion — Dilute each 5 ml of the preparation in 125 ml of 5% dextrose-in-water and use within 6 h; do not refrigerate. If fluid restriction is desired, dilute in 100 ml and use within 4 h or dilute in 75 ml and use within 2 h. Do not mix with other drugs or solutions in the same container. The contents of the 30 ml vial must be used within 48 h after withdrawal of the initial dose.

Intravenous administration — Administer slowly by IV drip over a period of 60–90 min; avoid rapid infusion or bolus injection

Local irritation and inflammation — May occur, due to extravascular infiltration of the infusion; discontinue infusion and restart at another site

Susceptibility tests — Cultures and appropriate microbiological tests should be performed to determine susceptibility; therapy may be started, however, before the results of these tests are available

Duration of therapy — Pneumonitis due to *Pneumocystis carinii* and severe urinary tract infections should be treated for up to 14 days and shigellosis for up to 5 days

Patients with renal impairment — Follow the usual dosage regimen if creatinine clearance (Ccr) > 30 ml/min. Administer half the usual dosage if Ccr = 15–30 ml/min; use is not recommended if Ccr < 15 ml/min.

WARNINGS/PRECAUTIONS

Streptococcal pharyngitis — Should not be treated with this drug, as it may fail to eliminate group A beta-hemolytic streptococci from the tonsillopharyngeal area

Life-threatening reactions — Severe, potentially fatal reactions, including Stevens-Johnson syndrome, toxic epidermal necrolysis, fulminant hepatic necrosis, and serious blood dyscrasias (eg, agranulocytosis, aplastic anemia) have occurred on rare occasions in patients receiving sulfonamides. These drugs have caused hemolytic anemia in patients with G6PD deficiency. The risk of severe adverse reactions may be increased in elderly patients, particularly when these patients are receiving other drugs (see DRUG INTERACTIONS) or they have renal or hepatic impairment or another complicating condition; the most frequent serious adverse effects seen in elderly patients are severe skin reactions, generalized bone marrow depression, and thrombocytopenia.

When using this preparation, obtain a CBC frequently and watch for early clinical signs such as rash, sore throat, fever, pallor, purpura, and jaundice; *discontinue administration at the first sign of skin rash or any adverse reaction.*

Bone marrow depression — High doses or prolonged use may cause bone marrow depression and, as a result, produce thrombocytopenia, leukopenia, and/or megaloblastic anemia; if signs of bone marrow depression appear, give 5–15 mg/day of leucovorin until normal hematopoiesis is restored

Cross-sensitivity — Patients allergic to acetazolamide, thiazide-type diuretics, sulfonylureas, or certain goitrogens may also be hypersensitive to this preparation

Renal effects — Crystalluria, urolithiasis, and other renal complications have occurred in patients taking sulfonamides. Caution patients to maintain an adequate fluid intake; urinalysis, including careful microscopic examination, and renal function tests should be performed during therapy, particularly when a patient has renal impairment.

BACTRIM I.V. Infusion

Special-risk patients	Use with caution in elderly patients and those with renal or hepatic impairment, possible folate deficiency, severe allergies, bronchial asthma, or G6PD deficiency. Among the conditions that may be associated with folate deficiency are malnutrition, malabsorption syndrome, chronic alcoholism, advanced age, and anticonvulsant therapy.
AIDS	Patients with AIDS may not tolerate or respond to this preparation in the same manner as other patients; the frequency of adverse effects, particularly rash, fever, and leukopenia, has been reported to be greatly increased in AIDS patients who were undergoing treatment of *Pneumocystis carinii* pneumonia
Sulfite sensitivity	Sodium metabisulfite in this product may cause urticaria, pruritus, wheezing, anaphylaxis, or other allergic-type reactions in susceptible patients, such as those with asthma or atopy
Carcinogenicity	No long-term studies have been done in animals to evaluate the oncogenic potential of this drug
Mutagenicity	Although bacterial mutagenicity studies have not been done with this preparation, trimethoprim alone has shown no mutagenic potential in the Ames assay, and no chromosomal abnormalities have been detected in human leukocytes cultured in vitro with either component alone or in combination or in leukocytes from treated patients
Effect on fertility	No adverse effects on fertility or general reproductive performance have been observed in rats given oral dosages as high as 70 mg/kg/day of trimethoprim plus 350 mg/kg/day of sulfamethoxazole

ADVERSE REACTIONS

Hematological	Agranulocytosis, aplastic anemia, thrombocytopenia, leukopenia, neutropenia, hemolytic anemia, megaloblastic anemia, hypoprothrombinemia, methemoglobinemia, eosinophilia
Gastrointestinal	Hepatitis (including cholestatic jaundice and fulminant hepatic necrosis), elevation of serum transaminase and bilirubin levels, pseudomembranous enterocolitis, pancreatitis, stomatitis, glossitis, nausea, vomiting, abdominal pain, diarrhea, anorexia
Genitourinary	Renal failure, interstitial nephritis, elevation of BUN and serum creatinine levels, toxic nephrosis with oliguria and anuria, crystalluria
Central nervous system	Aseptic meningitis, convulsions, peripheral neuritis, ataxia, vertigo, tinnitus, headache, hallucinations, depression, apathy, nervousness, weakness, fatigue, insomnia
Endocrinological	Diuresis, hypoglycemia
Musculoskeletal	Arthralgia, myalgia
Hypersensitivity	Stevens-Johnson syndrome, toxic epidermal necrolysis, anaphylaxis, allergic myocarditis, erythema multiforme, exfoliative dermatitis, angioedema, drug fever, chills, Henoch-Schoenlein purpura, serum sickness-like syndrome, generalized allergic reactions, generalized skin eruptions, photosensitivity, conjunctival and scleral injection, pruritus, urticaria, rash, periarteritis nodosa, systemic lupus erythematosus

OVERDOSAGE

Signs and symptoms	Anorexia, colic, nausea, vomiting, dizziness, headache, drowsiness, mental depression, confusion, unconsciousness, pyrexia, hematuria, crystalluria, bone marrow depression, other blood dyscrasias, jaundice
Treatment	To enhance renal elimination, acidify the urine and institute forced diuresis; if output is low and renal function is normal, administer IV fluids. Monitor blood counts and electrolyte balance. Institute specific therapy if jaundice or a significant blood dyscrasia occurs. Peritoneal dialysis is not useful and hemodialysis is only moderately effective in removing the components of this preparation.

DRUG INTERACTIONS

Diuretics (especially thiazides)	⇧ Risk of thrombocytopenic purpura in elderly patients
Warfarin	⇧ Prothrombin time; if this preparation is given during warfarin therapy, recheck prothrombin time
Phenytoin	⇧ Serum half-life of phenytoin; watch for evidence of phenytoin toxicity during combination therapy
Methotrexate	⇧ Serum level of methotrexate

ALTERED LABORATORY VALUES

Blood/serum values	⇧ Methotrexate (with competitive binding protein assay using dihydrofolate reductase) ⇧ BUN ⇧ Creatinine (especially with Jaffé test) ⇧ Bilirubin ⇧ SGOT ⇧ SGPT

No clinically significant alterations in urinary values occur at therapeutic dosages

USE IN CHILDREN

Same as adult indications and dosage; contraindicated for use in infants under 2 mo of age

USE IN PREGNANT AND NURSING WOMEN

Pregnancy Category C: use during pregnancy only if expected benefit justifies the potential fetal risk, since the drug may interfere with folic acid metabolism. Teratogenic effects (mainly cleft palate) have been observed in rats and increased fetal loss has been observed in rats and rabbits at doses several times the recommended human dose. Although no large, well-controlled studies have been done in pregnant women, two limited studies have shown no increase in congenital abnormalities. The drug is contraindicated at term and for use in nursing mothers because sulfonamides cross the placental barrier, are excreted in human milk, and may cause kernicterus.

[1] Dosage is based on trimethoprim component

URINARY ANTI-INFECTIVES

CINOBAC (cinoxacin) Dista   Rx

Capsules: 250, 500 mg

INDICATIONS
Initial and recurrent urinary tract infections caused by susceptible strains of *Escherichia coli*, *Proteus mirabilis*, *P vulgaris*, *Klebsiella*, and *Enterobacter*

ORAL DOSAGE
Adult: 500 mg bid or 250 mg qid for 7–14 days

CONTRAINDICATIONS
Hypersensitivity to cinoxacin

ADMINISTRATION/DOSAGE ADJUSTMENTS

Cultures and susceptibility tests	Should be initiated prior to and, when clinically indicated, during therapy
Patients with renal impairment	Administer 500 mg to start, followed by 250 mg tid if creatinine clearance rate (CCr) = 50–80 ml/min/1.73 m² (mild impairment), 250 mg bid if CCr = 20–49 ml/min/1.73 m² (moderate impairment), or 250 mg once daily if CCr < 20 ml/min/1.73 m² (marked impairment). If necessary, creatinine clearance may be calculated from the serum creatinine concentration by use of the following formula: CCr (in males) = [patient's weight (*kg*) × (140 − patient's age)]/[72 × creatinine concentration (*mg/dl*)]; for females, multiply the value obtained by this formula by 0.9.

WARNINGS/PRECAUTIONS

Anuric patients	Not recommended for use in anuric patients, as elimination is primarily renal
Special-risk patients	Use with caution in patients with a history of hepatic disease; lower dosage in patients with reduced renal function (see ADMINISTRATION/DOSAGE ADJUSTMENTS)
Cross-resistance	Organisms resistant to nalidixic acid and oxolinic acid may also be resistant to cinoxacin

ADVERSE REACTIONS[1]
Frequent reactions (incidence ≥ 1%) are printed in *italics*

Central nervous system[2]	*Headache and dizziness (1%)*
Gastrointestinal	*Nausea (< 3%)*; anorexia, vomiting, abdominal cramps, and *diarrhea (1%)*
Hematological	Thrombocytopenia (rare)
Hypersensitivity	*Rash, urticaria, pruritus, and edema (< 3%)*; anaphylactoid reactions (rare)

OVERDOSAGE

Signs and symptoms	See ADVERSE REACTIONS
Treatment	Discontinue medication and treat symptomatically, if necessary

DRUG INTERACTIONS
No clinically significant drug interactions have been identified

ALTERED LABORATORY VALUES

Blood/serum values	⇧ BUN ⇧ SGOT ⇧ SGPT ⇧ Creatinine ⇧ Alkaline phosphatase

No clinically significant alterations in urinary values occur at therapeutic dosages

USE IN CHILDREN	USE IN PREGNANT AND NURSING WOMEN
Not recommended for use in prepubertal children, since arthropathy has been demonstrated in immature animals	Pregnancy Category B: not recommended for use during pregnancy since the drug causes arthropathy in immature animals. Excretion in human breast milk unknown; patient should stop nursing if drug is prescribed.

[1] Other reactions (all reversible) occurring with pharmacologically related drugs include: restlessness, nervousness, overbrightness of lights, change in color perception, difficulty in focusing, decrease in visual acuity, double vision, abdominal pain, weakness, constipation, angioedema, erythema and bullae, feelings of disorientation or agitation or acute anxiety, palpitation, soreness of the gums, drowsiness, joint stiffness, swelling of the extremities, metallic taste, toxic psychosis or convulsions (rare), reduction in hematocrit/hemoglobin, and eosinophilia

[2] Other reactions for which a causal relationship has not been established include insomnia, tingling sensation, perineal burning, photophobia, and tinnitus

---

URINARY ANTI-INFECTIVES

COACTIN (amdinocillin) Roche Rx

Vials: 0.5, 1 g

INDICATIONS

Urinary tract infections caused by susceptible strains of *Escherichia coli*, *Klebsiella* (including *K pneumoniae*), and *Enterobacter*

Bacteremia associated with severe urinary tract infections caused by susceptible strains of *Escherichia coli*

PARENTERAL DOSAGE

Adult: for serious infections, 10 mg/kg, given IV either q4h if used alone or q6h if used in combination with another beta-lactam antibiotic; for less serious infections, drug can also be given by IM injection

CONTRAINDICATIONS

Hypersensitivity to penicillins

ADMINISTRATION/DOSAGE ADJUSTMENTS

Intramuscular administration	To reconstitute solution, add 2.2 ml of sterile water for injection USP or 0.9% sodium chloride injection USP to the 500-mg vial or 4.4 ml to the 1-g vial and then shake well. Before administration, aspirate to help prevent inadvertent intravascular injection. The solution should be injected well within the body of a relatively large muscle, such as the gluteus maximus.
Intravenous administration	To prepare the solution, add 4.8 ml of sterile water for injection USP to the 500-mg vial or 9.6 ml to the 1-g vial; then shake well, withdraw the contents of the vial, and dilute with 5% dextrose injection USP to a final volume of 50 ml. The reconstituted solution can also be diluted with other appropriate solutions (see package insert), and the final concentration can vary from 5 to 100 mg/ml. Administer each dose over a period of 15–30 min by infusion; when using a Y-type set or piggyback arrangement, temporarily discontinue administration of any other solution (amdinocillin should not be mixed with other drugs).
Duration of therapy	Administration should generally be continued for at least 2 days after signs and symptoms of infection have disappeared; duration of therapy is usually 7–10 days, but may be longer if the infection is complicated
Combination therapy	For the treatment of more severe urinary tract infections, the synergistic combination of amdinocillin and another beta-lactam antibiotic may be considered
Patients with renal impairment	If the creatinine clearance is less than 30 ml/min, the dosage should be limited to 10 mg/kg tid or qid

WARNINGS/PRECAUTIONS

Hypersensitivity	Serious, occasionally fatal anaphylactic reactions have occurred in patients receiving penicillin; use with caution in patients with a history of allergy, particularly if they have demonstrated hypersensitivity to a number of substances. If an allergic reaction occurs, amdinocillin should be discontinued; for the treatment of serious reactions, give epinephrine, oxygen, and IV corticosteroids and take appropriate measures (eg, intubation) to ensure adequate pulmonary function.
Prolonged therapy	Evaluate hematopoietic, renal, and hepatic function periodically during long-term therapy; bear in mind that superinfection may occur with prolonged use
Effect on fertility	No evidence of impaired fertility has been seen in rats given daily up to 7.5 times the recommended human dose

COACTIN ■ FURADANTIN

ADVERSE REACTIONS

Frequent reactions (incidence ≥ 1%) are printed in *italics*

Hematological	*Eosinophilia and thrombocytosis (5%); anemia, neutropenia, and leukopenia (1%);* thrombocytopenia
Hepatic	*Elevated SGOT and serum alkaline phosphatase levels (5%),* elevated SGPT and serum bilirubin levels
Gastrointestinal	*Diarrhea and nausea (1%),* vomiting
Central nervous system	*Dizziness (1%),* drowsiness, lethargy
Dermatological	*Allergic rash (1%),* pruritus, urticaria
Other	*Thrombophlebitis (1%),* tenderness and/or pain at injection site, elevated blood pressure, vaginitis

OVERDOSAGE

Signs and symptoms	Neuromuscular hypersensitivity, convulsive seizures
Treatment	If it is necessary to enhance removal of the drug from the blood, hemodialysis can be performed

DRUG INTERACTIONS

Other beta-lactam antibiotics	△ Bactericidal effect
Probenecid	△ Serum amdinocillin level

ALTERED LABORATORY VALUES

Blood/serum values	△ SGOT △ Alkaline phosphatase

No clinically significant alterations in urinary values occur at therapeutic dosages

---

USE IN CHILDREN

Safety and effectiveness for use in children under 12 yr of age have not been established

USE IN PREGNANT AND NURSING WOMEN

Pregnancy Category B: reproduction studies in rats and mice given up to 7.5 times the recommended human dose have shown no evidence of harm to the fetus; however, no adequate, well-controlled studies have been done in pregnant women. Low concentrations of amdinocillin are found in cord blood and amniotic fluid. Use during pregnancy only if clearly needed. In limited, single-dose studies, amdinocillin has not been detected in human milk; use with caution in nursing mothers.

URINARY ANTI-INFECTIVES

FURADANTIN (nitrofurantoin) Norwich Eaton Rx

Tablets: 50, 100 mg **Suspension (per 5 ml):** 25 mg (60, 470 ml)

INDICATIONS

Urinary tract infections caused by susceptible strains of *Escherichia coli*, enterococci, and *Staphylococcus aureus*,[1] and certain susceptible strains of *Klebsiella, Enterobacter,* and *Proteus*

ORAL DOSAGE

Adult: for uncomplicated infections, 50 mg qid; for other infections, 50–100 mg qid
Child: 5–7 mg/kg/24 h in 4 divided doses

CONTRAINDICATIONS

Pregnancy at term	Significantly impaired renal function (creatinine clearance rate < 40 ml/min)	Anuria or oliguria
Age < 1 mo		Hypersensitivity to nitrofurantoin

ADMINISTRATION/DOSAGE ADJUSTMENTS

Cultures and susceptibility tests	Should be obtained prior to and during therapy
Oral administration	Give each dose with food; if GI reactions occur, reduce dosage
Minimum duration of therapy	Continue treatment for 1 wk and at least 3 days after urine becomes sterile; re-evaluate patient if infection persists
Long-term prophylactic therapy	Reduce adult dosage to 50–100 mg/day, given at bedtime, and pediatric dosage to as low as 1 mg/kg/24 h, given in a single dose or 2 divided doses. Hypersensitivity reactions may occur during long-term therapy (see WARNINGS/PRECAUTIONS).

FURADANTIN

WARNINGS/PRECAUTIONS

Hypersensitivity reactions	Hepatitis or pulmonary reactions may occur and can be fatal (hepatitis, including chronic active hepatitis, and cholestatic jaundice have been reported rarely); if these hypersensitivity reactions occur, discontinue the drug immediately and take appropriate measures. Closely observe patients undergoing long-term therapy, and periodically evaluate their liver function; the onset of chronic pulmonary reactions (diffuse interstitial pneumonitis and/or pulmonary fibrosis) and chronic active hepatitis can be insidious.
Hemolytic anemia of the primaquine-sensitivity type	May be induced in patients with G6PD deficiency; discontinue therapy if hemolysis is detected
Superinfection	May occur, caused by *Pseudomonas* species or other resistant organisms; limited to genitourinary tract
Severe or irreversible peripheral neuropathy	May occur and can be fatal; administer with caution to patients with renal impairment (Ccr < 40 ml/min), anemia, diabetes mellitus, electrolyte imbalance, vitamin B deficiency, or debilitating disease
Carcinogenicity, mutagenicity	Nitrofurantoin has shown no carcinogenic potential when fed to female Holtzman rats at levels of 0.3% for up to 44.5 wk or when fed to female Sprague-Dawley rats at levels of 0.1–0.187% for 75 wk. In vitro studies using *Escherichia coli*, *Salmonella typhimium*, and *Aspergillus nidulans* suggest that nitrofurantoin is a weak mutagen; however, the results of a dominant lethal assay in the mouse were negative.
Impairment of fertility	Temporary, reversible spermatogenic arrest has occurred in rats given high doses of nitrofurantoin; doses ≥ 10 mg/kg in healthy human males may produce slight to moderate spermatogenic arrest, with a decrease in sperm count, in certain unpredictable instances

ADVERSE REACTIONS[2]

The most frequent reactions, regardless of incidence, are printed in *italics*

Gastrointestinal	*Anorexia, nausea, vomiting,* abdominal pain, diarrhea
Dermatological	Maculopapular, erythematous, or eczematous eruption; pruritus, urticaria, rash, angioedema; exfoliative dermatitis and erythema multiforme, including Stevens-Johnson syndrome (rare)
Hematological	Hemolytic anemia, granulocytopenia, agranulocytosis, thrombocytopenia, leukopenia, eosinophilia, G6PD deficiency anemia, megaloblastic anemia; aplastic anemia (rare)
Central nervous system	Peripheral neuropathy
Acute hypersensitivity[3]	Fever, chills, chills and fever, cough, chest pain, dyspnea, pulmonary infiltration with consolidation or pleural effusion on x-ray, eosinophilia
Chronic hypersensitivity[4]	Malaise, dyspnea on exertion, cough, altered pulmonary function, diffuse interstitial pneumonitis and/or pulmonary fibrosis, fever (rarely prominent)
Other hypersensitivity reactions	Lupus-like syndrome associated with pulmonary reactions, anaphylaxis, drug fever, arthralgia, myalgia, sialadenitis, pancreatitis; hepatitis, including chronic active hepatitis (rare)
Other	Transient alopecia, genitourinary superinfection

OVERDOSAGE

Signs and symptoms	Vomiting
Treatment	Induce emesis if vomiting does not occur spontaneously. Maintain a high fluid intake to promote urinary excretion of the drug.

DRUG INTERACTIONS

Nalidixic acid	▽ Antimicrobial effect of nalidixic acid
Magnesium trisilicate	▽ Absorption of nitrofurantoin
Probenecid, sulfinpyrazone	△ Nitrofurantoin serum level and/or toxicity ▽ Urinary level of nitrofurantoin

ALTERED LABORATORY VALUES

Urinary values	△ Glucose (with Clinitest tablets)

No clinically significant alterations in blood/serum values occur at therapeutic dosages

---

USE IN CHILDREN

See INDICATIONS; adjust dosage according to body weight. Contraindicated for use in infants under 1 mo of age because of the risk of hemolytic anemia due to glutathione instability

USE IN PREGNANT AND NURSING WOMEN

Contraindicated at term; use during pregnancy only if the expected benefit outweighs the potential risk to the fetus. Trace amounts of nitrofurantoin are excreted in human milk; use with caution in nursing women, especially if the infant is known or suspected to have G6PD deficiency.

---

[1] Not indicated for associated cortical renal or perinephric abscesses
[2] Reactions for which no causal relationship has been established include nystagmus, dizziness, headache, and drowsiness
[3] Usually occurs within the first week of treatment and is reversible with cessation of therapy; if drug is not withdrawn, symptoms may worsen
[4] More likely to occur after the first 6 mo of continuous treatment; permanent impairment of pulmonary function may remain even after drug is discontinued, particularly when reaction is not recognized early

URINARY ANTI-INFECTIVES

GEOCILLIN (carbenicillin indanyl sodium) Roerig Rx

Tablets: carbenicillin indanyl sodium equivalent to 382 mg carbenicillin

INDICATIONS	ORAL DOSAGE
Urinary tract infections and asymptomatic bacteriuria caused by susceptible strains of *Escherichia coli, Proteus mirabilis, P morgani, P rettgeri, P vulgaris,* and *Enterobacter*	**Adult:** 1–2 tabs qid
Urinary tract infections caused by susceptible strains of *Pseudomonas* and *Streptococcus fecalis*	**Adult:** 2 tabs qid
Prostatitis caused by susceptible strains of *Escherichia coli, Proteus mirabilis, Enterobacter,* and *Streptococcus fecalis*	

CONTRAINDICATIONS
Hypersensitivity to penicillins

WARNINGS/PRECAUTIONS

Hypersensitivity	Serious and occasionally fatal anaphylactoid reactions may occur, most likely in patients with a history of sensitivity to multiple allergens, and may necessitate immediate emergency treatment with epinephrine, oxygen, IV corticosteroids, and airway management, including intubation; use with caution in patients who have experienced allergic reactions to cephalosporins
Long-term therapy	Perform blood, renal, and hepatic studies periodically
Superinfection	Overgrowth of nonsusceptible organisms may occur
Renal impairment	Patients with severe impairment (creatinine clearance < 10 ml/min) will not achieve therapeutic urine levels of carbenicillin

ADVERSE REACTIONS

Gastrointestinal	Nausea, vomiting, diarrhea, flatulence, dry mouth, furry tongue, abdominal cramps
Hypersensitivity	Skin rash, urticaria, pruritus
Hematological	Anemia, thrombocytopenia, leukopenia, neutropenia, eosinophilia
Other	Vaginitis

OVERDOSAGE

Signs and symptoms	See ADVERSE REACTIONS
Treatment	Discontinue medication; treat symptomatically

DRUG INTERACTIONS

Probenecid	△ Carbenicillin blood level and/or toxicity ▽ Urine level

ALTERED LABORATORY VALUES

Blood/serum values	△ SGOT △ SGPT

No clinically significant alterations in urinary values occur at therapeutic dosages

---

USE IN CHILDREN
Safety for use in children has not been established

USE IN PREGNANT AND NURSING WOMEN
Safety for use during pregnancy has not been established. Carbenicillin is excreted in human milk; use with caution in nursing mothers.

URINARY ANTI-INFECTIVES

HIPREX (methenamine hippurate) Merrell Dow Rx

Tablets: 1 g

INDICATIONS	ORAL DOSAGE
Prophylaxis or suppression of frequently recurring urinary tract infections following eradication of acute infection by other appropriate antimicrobial agents	**Adult:** 1 g bid (AM and PM) **Child (6–12 yr):** 0.5–1.0 g bid (AM and PM)

HIPREX ■ MACRODANTIN

CONTRAINDICATIONS

Renal insufficiency	Severe dehydration	Sulfonamide therapy
Severe hepatic insufficiency		

WARNINGS/PRECAUTIONS

High-dosage therapy (8 g/day for 3–4 wk)	May lead to bladder irritation, painful and frequent micturition, albuminuria, and gross hematuria
Urine acidity	Should be maintained, especially in treating infections due to urea-splitting organisms, such as *Proteus* and strains of *Pseudomonas;* restrict alkalinizing foods and medications, and provide supplemental acidifying medications, if necessary
Elevated serum transaminase levels	Perform liver-function studies periodically, especially in patients with liver dysfunction
Urine cultures	Should be obtained periodically to monitor efficacy of regimen
Tartrazine sensitivity	Presence of FD&C Yellow No. 5 (tartrazine) in tablets may cause allergic-type reactions, including bronchial asthma, in susceptible individuals

ADVERSE REACTIONS

Gastrointestinal	Nausea, upset stomach
Genitourinary	Dysuria
Dermatological	Rash

DRUG INTERACTIONS

Urinary alkalinizing agents, antacids, carbonic anhydrase inhibitors, thiazide diuretics	▽ Antibacterial effectiveness
Sulfonamides	△ Risk of crystalluria

ALTERED LABORATORY VALUES

Blood/serum values	△ SGOT △ SGPT (see WARNINGS/PRECAUTIONS)
Urinary values	△ Catecholamines (with fluorometric methods) △ 17-OHCS (with Reddy method) ▽ Estriol (with acid hydrolysis method) ▽ 5-HIAA (with nitrosonaphthol reagent test)

USE IN CHILDREN
See INDICATIONS and ORAL DOSAGE

USE IN PREGNANT AND NURSING WOMEN
Safety for use during early pregnancy has not been established; the drug appears to be safe for use during the third trimester. Methenamine is excreted in human milk, but amount is not sufficient to affect nursing infant.[1]

[1] Illingworth RS: *Practitioner* 171:533–538, 1953; Speika N: *Br J Obstet Gynaecol* (formerly *J Obstet Gynaecol Br Commonw*) 54:426–431, 1947

URINARY ANTI-INFECTIVES

MACRODANTIN (nitrofurantoin macrocrystals) Norwich Eaton   Rx

Capsules: 25, 50, 100 mg

INDICATIONS
Urinary tract infections caused by susceptible strains of *Escherichia coli*, enterococci, and *Staphylococcus aureus*,[1] and certain susceptible strains of *Klebsiella*, *Enterobacter*, and *Proteus*

ORAL DOSAGE
Adult: for uncomplicated infections, 50 mg qid; for other infections, 50–100 mg qid
Child: 5–7 mg/kg/24 h in 4 divided doses

CONTRAINDICATIONS

Pregnancy at term	Significantly impaired renal function (creatinine clearance rate < 40 ml/min)	Anuria or oliguria
Age < 1 mo		Hypersensitivity to nitrofurantoin

ADMINISTRATION/DOSAGE ADJUSTMENTS

Cultures and susceptibility tests	Should be obtained prior to and during therapy
Oral administration	Give each dose with food; if GI reactions occur, reduce dosage
Minimum duration of therapy	Continue treatment for 1 wk and at least 3 days after urine becomes sterile; re-evaluate patient if infection persists
Long-term prophylactic therapy	Reduce adult dosage to 50–100 mg/day, given at bedtime, and pediatric dosage to as low as 1 mg/kg/24 h, given in a single dose or 2 divided doses. Hypersensitivity reactions may occur during long-term therapy (see WARNINGS/PRECAUTIONS).

WARNINGS/PRECAUTIONS

Hypersensitivity reactions	Hepatitis or pulmonary reactions may occur and can be fatal (hepatitis, including chronic active hepatitis, and cholestatic jaundice has been reported rarely); if these hypersensitivity reactions occur, discontinue the drug immediately and take appropriate measures. Closely observe patients undergoing long-term therapy, and periodically evaluate their liver function; the onset of chronic pulmonary reactions (diffuse interstitial pneumonitis and/or pulmonary fibrosis) and chronic active hepatitis can be insidious.
Hemolytic anemia of the primaquine-sensitivity type	May be induced in patients with G6PD deficiency; discontinue therapy if hemolysis is detected
Superinfection	May occur, caused by *Pseudomonas* species or other resistant organisms; limited to genitourinary tract
Severe or irreversible peripheral neuropathy	May occur and can be fatal; administer with caution to patients with renal impairment (Ccr < 40 ml/min), anemia, diabetes mellitus, electrolyte imbalance, vitamin B deficiency, or debilitating disease
Carcinogenicity, mutagenicity	Nitrofurantoin has shown no carcinogenic potential when fed to female Holtzman rats at levels of 0.3% for up to 44.5 wk or when fed to female Sprague-Dawley rats at levels of 0.1–0.187% for 75 wk. In vitro studies using *Escherichia coli*, *Salmonella typhimium*, and *Aspergillus nidulans* suggest that nitrofurantoin is a weak mutagen; however, the results of a dominant lethal assay in the mouse were negative.
Impairment of fertility	Temporary, reversible spermatogenic arrest has occurred in rats given high doses of nitrofurantoin; doses ≥ 10 mg/kg in healthy human males may produce slight to moderate spermatogenic arrest, with a decrease in sperm count, in certain unpredictable instances

ADVERSE REACTIONS[2]

The most frequent reactions, regardless of incidence, are printed in *italics*

Gastrointestinal	*Anorexia, nausea, vomiting,* abdominal pain, diarrhea
Dermatological	Maculopapular, erythematous, or eczematous eruption; pruritus, urticaria, rash, angioedema; exfoliative dermatitis and erythema multiforme, including Stevens-Johnson syndrome (rare)
Hematological	Hemolytic anemia, granulocytopenia, agranulocytosis, thrombocytopenia, leukopenia, eosinophilia, G6PD deficiency anemia, megaloblastic anemia; aplastic anemia (rare)
Central nervous system	Peripheral neuropathy
Acute hypersensitivity[3]	Fever, chills, chills and fever, cough, chest pain, dyspnea, pulmonary infiltration with consolidation or pleural effusion on x-ray, eosinophilia
Chronic hypersensitivity[4]	Malaise, dyspnea on exertion, cough, altered pulmonary function, diffuse interstitial pneumonitis and/or pulmonary fibrosis, fever (rarely prominent)
Other hypersensitivity reactions	Lupus-like syndrome associated with pulmonary reactions, anaphylaxis, drug fever, arthralgia, myalgia, sialadenitis, pancreatitis; hepatitis, including chronic active hepatitis (rare)
Other	Transient alopecia, genitourinary superinfection

OVERDOSAGE

Signs and symptoms	Vomiting
Treatment	Induce emesis if vomiting does not occur spontaneously. Maintain a high fluid intake to promote urinary excretion of the drug.

DRUG INTERACTIONS

Nalidixic acid	▽ Antimicrobial effect of nalidixic acid
Magnesium trisilicate	▽ Absorption of nitrofurantoin
Probenecid, sulfinpyrazone	△ Nitrofurantoin serum level and/or toxicity ▽ Urinary level of nitrofurantoin

ALTERED LABORATORY VALUES

Urinary values	△ Glucose (with Clinitest tablets)

No clinically significant alterations in blood/serum values occur at therapeutic dosages

---

USE IN CHILDREN

See INDICATIONS; adjust dosage according to body weight. Contraindicated for use in infants under 1 mo of age because of the risk of hemolytic anemia due to glutathione instability

USE IN PREGNANT AND NURSING WOMEN

Contraindicated at term; use during pregnancy only if the expected benefit outweighs the potential risk to the fetus. Trace amounts of the nitrofurantoin are excreted in human milk; use with caution in nursing women, especially if the infant is known or suspected to have a G6PD deficiency.

---

[1] Not indicated for associated cortical renal or perinephric abscesses
[2] Reactions for which no causal relationship has been established include nystagmus, dizziness, headache, and drowsiness
[3] Usually occurs within the first week of treatment and is reversible with cessation of therapy; if drug is not withdrawn, symptoms may worsen
[4] More likely to occur after the first 6 mo of continuous treatment; permanent impairment of pulmonary function may remain even after drug is discontinued, particularly when reaction is not recognized early

URINARY ANTI-INFECTIVES

MANDELAMINE (methenamine mandelate) Parke-Davis   Rx
Tablets: 0.5, 1.0 g   **Granules:** 0.5, 1.0 g *orange flavored*   **Suspension (per 5 ml):** 250 mg (16 fl oz) *coconut flavored*, 500 mg (Mandelamine Forte) (8, 16 fl oz) *cherry flavored*

INDICATIONS
Suppression or elimination of **bacteria associated with pyelonephritis, cystitis, and other chronic urinary tract infections**
Infected residual urine accompanying neurological disease

ORAL DOSAGE
Adult: 1 g qid after each meal and at bedtime
Child (< 6 yr): 0.25 g/30 lb qid
Child (6–12 yr): 0.5 g qid after each meal and at bedtime

CONTRAINDICATIONS
Renal insufficiency   Hypersensitivity to methenamine

ADMINISTRATION/DOSAGE ADJUSTMENTS
Acidification	To maintain the urine pH of 5.5 or less that is required for maximum efficacy, restrict the intake of alkalinizing foods and medications and, if necessary, administer supplemental acidifying agents. Use of methenamine is not recommended for conditions in which acidification is contraindicated or unattainable (eg, infections caused by some urea-splitting bacteria)
Use of granules	Dissolve contents of the packet in 2–4 fl oz of water immediately before use

WARNINGS/PRECAUTIONS
Dysuria	May occur, especially at dosages higher than those recommended above; control by reducing dosage and the acidification
Elderly and/or debilitated patients	Administer suspension formulas with caution to avoid inducing lipid pneumonia

ADVERSE REACTIONS
Gastrointestinal	GI disturbance
Dermatological	Rash
Genitourinary	Microscopic hematuria; gross hematuria (rare)

OVERDOSAGE
Signs and symptoms	See ADVERSE REACTIONS
Treatment	Discontinue medication; treat symptomatically

DRUG INTERACTIONS
Urinary alkalinizing agents, antacids, carbonic anhydrase inhibitors, thiazide diuretics	▽ Antibacterial effectiveness
Sulfamethizole	△ Risk of crystalluria; do not administer sulfamethizole concomitantly

ALTERED LABORATORY VALUES
Urinary values   △ Catecholamines (with fluorometric methods)   △ VMA (with fluorometric methods)   △ 17-OHCS (with Porter-Silber method)   ▽ Estriol (with acid hydrolysis method)   ▽ 5-HIAA (with nitrosonaphthol reagent test)

No clinically significant alterations in blood/serum values occur at therapeutic dosages

USE IN CHILDREN
See INDICATIONS and ORAL DOSAGE

USE IN PREGNANT AND NURSING WOMEN
Pregnancy Category C: reproduction studies have not been performed in animals or humans; reports of use in pregnant women have not shown an increased risk of teratogenicity. It is not known whether methenamine can cause harm to the fetus or affect reproductive capacity; use during pregnancy only if clearly needed. Methenamine is excreted in human milk, but amount is not sufficient to affect nursing infant.[1]

[1] Illingworth RS: *Practitioner* 171:533–538, 1953; Speika N: *Br J Obstet Gynaecol* (formerly *J Obstet Gynaecol Br Commonw*) 54:426–431, 1947

URINARY ANTI-INFECTIVES

NegGram (nalidixic acid) Winthrop-Breon   Rx
Tablets: 250, 500, 1,000 mg   **Suspension (per 5 ml):** 250 mg (16 fl oz) *raspberry-flavored*

INDICATIONS
Urinary tract infections caused by susceptible Gram-negative microorganisms, including most *Proteus* strains, *Klebsiella*, *Enterobacter*, and *Escherichia coli*

ORAL DOSAGE
Adult: 1 g qid for 1–2 wk, followed by 2 g/day for prolonged therapy
Child: 55 mg/kg/day in 4 divided doses for 1–2 wk, followed by 33 mg/kg/day for prolonged therapy

NegGram

CONTRAINDICATIONS

Age < 3 mo	Hypersensitivity to nalidixic acid	History of convulsive disorders

ADMINISTRATION/DOSAGE ADJUSTMENTS

Susceptibility tests	Should be performed with 30-μg disc prior to therapy, as well as during treatment if warranted by the clinical response
Bacterial resistance	May emerge within 48 h after start of therapy; repeat cultures and sensitivity tests and institute appropriate anti-infective therapy

WARNINGS/PRECAUTIONS

Prolonged therapy	Perform blood counts and renal- and liver-function tests periodically if treatment continues for longer than 2 wk
Special-risk patients	Use with caution in patients with liver disease, epilepsy, severe cerebral arteriosclerosis, or severe renal failure
Photosensitivity	Avoid undue exposure to direct sunlight; discontinue therapy if photosensitivity occurs. Bullae may continue to appear with successive exposures to sunlight or with mild skin trauma for up to 3 mo after discontinuation of drug.
Underdosage during initial therapy	May lead to emergence of bacterial resistance
CNS toxicity (rare)	Brief convulsions, increased intracranial pressure, and toxic psychosis may occur, especially in infants, children, and elderly patients (usually from overdosage) and in patients with predisposing factors. Discontinue therapy and institute appropriate corrective measures; diagnostic procedures involving risk to the patient should be undertaken only if CNS symptoms do not rapidly disappear within 48 h.
Cross-resistance	May occur with oxolinic acid

ADVERSE REACTIONS

Central nervous system	Drowsiness, weakness, headache, dizziness, vertigo, toxic psychosis, brief convulsions, 6th cranial nerve palsy; paresthesia (rare)
Ophthalmic	Reversible visual disturbances, including overbrightness of lights, change in color perception, difficulty in focusing, decreased acuity, double vision
Gastrointestinal	Abdominal pain, nausea, vomiting, diarrhea; cholestasis (rare)
Allergic	Rash, pruritus, urticaria, angioedema, eosinophilia, arthralgia with joint stiffness and swelling, anaphylaxis, photosensitivity reactions, including erythema and bullae
Metabolic	Acidosis (rare)
Hematological	Thrombocytopenia, leukopenia, hemolytic anemia, and G6PD deficiency (rare)

OVERDOSAGE

Signs and symptoms	Toxic psychosis, convulsions, increased intracranial pressure, metabolic acidosis, vomiting, nausea, lethargy
Treatment	Drug is rapidly excreted. If overdosage is noted early, empty stomach contents by gastric lavage. Employ supportive measures, and administer IV fluids. Provide assisted ventilation, if needed. For severe toxicity, anticonvulsant therapy may be indicated.

DRUG INTERACTIONS

Oral anticoagulants	△ Anticoagulant effect
Nitrofurantoin	▽ Antimicrobial effect of nalidixic acid

ALTERED LABORATORY VALUES

Urinary values	△ Glucose (with Clinitest tablets) △ 17-Ketosteroids (with Zimmerman method)

No clinically significant alterations in blood/serum values occur at therapeutic dosages

---

USE IN CHILDREN

See INDICATIONS; adjust dosage according to body weight. Contraindicated in children under 3 mo of age; reversible increased intracranial pressure, with bulging anterior fontanels, papilledema, and headache, has been reported in infants and children receiving therapeutic doses. Erosions of the cartilage in weight-bearing joints and other signs of arthropathy have been observed in immature animals treated with nalidixic acid and related drugs; although no such joint lesions have been reported in humans, use with caution in prepubertal children until significance of this finding is clarified.

USE IN PREGNANT AND NURSING WOMEN

Pregnant women: Safety for use during the first trimester of pregnancy has not been established. A theoretical risk exists that exposure to maternal nalidixic acid in utero may result in significant neonatal blood levels of the drug immediately following delivery; use with caution in obstetric patients in the days prior to delivery, and advise patients to discontinue use at the first sign of labor. **Nursing mothers:** Insignificant amounts (4 μg/ml) of nalidixic acid are excreted in human milk when the drug is taken in the recommended dosage. A single case of hemolytic anemia has been reported in a nursing infant with normal G6PD activity whose mother was receiving nalidixic acid for severe pyelonephritis.[1] The mother was uremic, and it is possible that a reduction in maternal excretion of the drug raised the serum level and, hence, the amount excreted in her milk. The infant fully recovered after breastfeeding was discontinued.

[1] Belton EM, Jones RV: *Lancet* 2:691, 1965

URINARY ANTI-INFECTIVES

NOROXIN (norfloxacin) Merck Sharp & Dohme
Tablets: 400 mg

Rx

INDICATIONS
Urinary tract infections caused by susceptible strains of *Escherichia coli*, *Klebsiella pneumoniae*, *Enterobacter cloacae*, *Proteus mirabilis*, indole-positive *Proteus* (including *P vulgaris*, *Providencia rettgeri*, and *Morganella morganii*), *Pseudomonas aeruginosa*, *Citrobacter freundii*, *Staphylococcus aureus*, *S epidermidis*, and Group D streptococci

ORAL DOSAGE
Adult: 400 mg bid, given with a full glass of water

CONTRAINDICATIONS
Hypersensitivity to norfloxacin or quinolone antibacterials (eg, nalidixic acid, cinoxacin)

ADMINISTRATION/DOSAGE ADJUSTMENTS

Duration of therapy	For uncomplicated infections, continue therapy for 7–10 days; for complicated infections, continue treatment for 10–21 days
Timing of administration	Administer 1 h before or 2 h after meals for maximum absorption
Cultures and susceptibility tests	Perform culture and susceptibility testing prior to initiating treatment and, when clinically indicated, during therapy
Elderly patients	No dosage adjustment for age is necessary, provided the creatinine clearance (Ccr) exceeds 30 ml/min (see below)
Patients with renal impairment	Reduce dosage to 400 mg once daily if the creatinine clearance (Ccr) < 30 ml/min. If necessary, Ccr may be calculated from the serum creatinine concentration by use of the following formula: Ccr (in males) = [patient's weight (kg) × (140 − patient's age)]/[72 × creatinine concentration (mg/dl)]; for females, multiply the quotient by 0.85.

WARNINGS/PRECAUTIONS

Crystalluria	Needle-shaped crystals have been found in the urine of volunteers taking daily doses of 800 or 1,600 mg of norfloxacin or placebo; although crystalluria is not expected at the recommended dosage, do not exceed the daily recommended dose and advise patients to drink sufficient fluids to ensure proper hydration and adequate urinary output
Dizziness, light-headedness	Norfloxacin may cause dizziness or light-headedness; caution patients not to drive or engage in other potentially hazardous activities requiring mental alertness and coordination until they know how they react to this drug
Special-risk patients	Use with caution in patients with known factors that predispose to seizures; reduce dosage in patients with impaired renal function (see ADMINISTRATION/DOSAGE ADJUSTMENTS)
Carcinogenicity	No evidence of carcinogenicity has been found in rats receiving norfloxacin in oral doses 8–9 times the usual human dose for 96 wk
Mutagenicity	No mutagenic potential has been detected in the dominant lethal test in mice, the Ames microbial mutagen test, Chinese hamster fibroblasts, or the V-79 mammalian cell assay, nor have chromosomal aberrations been seen in hamsters or rats at doses 30–60 times the usual human dose; although norfloxacin was weakly positive in the Rec-assay for DNA repair, all other tests for mutagenicity have been negative
Effect on fertility	No adverse effect on fertility has been found in male or female mice receiving up to 33 times the usual human dose

ADVERSE REACTIONS[1]
Frequent reactions (incidence ≥ 1%) are printed in *italics*

Gastrointestinal	*Nausea (2.8%)*, abdominal pain, dyspepsia, constipation, flatulence, heartburn, diarrhea, vomiting
Hepatic	*Elevated SGOT and SGPT levels (1.8%), increased serum alkaline phosphatase level (1.4%)*; increased BUN, serum creatinine, and LDH levels
Central nervous system	*Headache (2.7%), dizziness (1.8%)*, fatigue, somnolence, depression, insomnia
Dermatological	Rash, erythema
Hematological	*Eosinophilia (1.8%), decreased WBC or neutrophil count (1.2%)*, decreased hematocrit
Other	Fever

OVERDOSAGE

Signs and symptoms	See ADVERSE REACTIONS
Treatment	Induce emesis or perform gastric lavage to evacuate stomach. Observe patient carefully and maintain adequate hydration; supply symptomatic and supportive treatment, as needed.

NOROXIN ■ PROLOPRIM

DRUG INTERACTIONS

Probenecid	⇩ Urinary excretion of norfloxacin
Nitrofurantoin	⇩ Antibacterial effect of norfloxacin; do not use concomitantly
Antacids	⇩ Pharmacologic effect of norfloxacin; advise patients not to take antacids concomitantly or within 2 h after taking norfloxacin

ALTERED LABORATORY VALUES

Blood/serum levels — ⇧ SGOT ⇧ SGPT ⇧ Alkaline phosphatase ⇧ BUN ⇧ Creatinine ⇧ LDH

No clinically significant alterations in urinary values occur at therapeutic dosages

---

USE IN CHILDREN

Because norfloxacin causes arthropathy in immature animals, it should not be given to children

USE IN PREGNANT AND NURSING WOMEN

Pregnant women: Pregnancy Category C: norfloxacin has produced embryonic loss in monkeys given 10 times the maximum human daily dose; however, no teratogenic effect has been found in rats, rabbits, mice, or monkeys given 6–50 times the human dose. No adequate well-controlled studies have been performed in pregnant women. Because norfloxacin can produce arthropathy in immature animals, it should not be given to pregnant women. **Nursing mothers:** It is not known whether norfloxacin is excreted in human milk; however, other quinolone antibacterial agents have been detected in human milk. Because of this, and given the potential for serious adverse reactions in nursing infants, women who require this drug should not nurse.

---

[1] Other reactions occurring with pharmacologically related drugs include visual disturbances

---

URINARY ANTI-INFECTIVES

PROLOPRIM (trimethoprim) Burroughs Wellcome   Rx

Tablets: 100, 200 mg

INDICATIONS

Initial episodes of uncomplicated urinary tract infections caused by susceptible strains of *Escherichia coli*, *Proteus mirabilis*, *Klebsiella pneumoniae*, *Enterobacter*, and coagulase-negative *Staphylococcus*, including *S saprophyticus*

ORAL DOSAGE

Adult: 100 mg q12h or 200 mg q24h, each for 10 days

CONTRAINDICATIONS

Hypersensitivity to trimethoprim — Established megaloblastic anemia due to folate deficiency

ADMINISTRATION/DOSAGE ADJUSTMENTS

Cultures and susceptibility tests	Should be performed to determine bacterial susceptibility to trimethoprim, although therapy may be initiated prior to test results
Patients with renal impairment	Reduce dosage to 50 mg q12h if creatinine clearance rate (CCr) = 15–30 ml/min; do not administer if CCr < 15 ml/min

WARNINGS/PRECAUTIONS

Blood dyscrasias	May occur rarely, especially with high doses and/or prolonged therapy. Obtain CBC if early signs develop (eg, sore throat, fever, pallor, or purpura). If signs of bone marrow depression (thrombocytopenia, leukopenia, and/or megaloblastic anemia) are present, discontinue therapy and administer leucovorin, 3–6 mg/day IM, for 3 days or until hematopoiesis is normal.
Suspected folate deficiency	Use with caution; concomitant administration of folates does not interfere with antibacterial action
Patients with hepatic or renal impairment	Use with caution if hepatic or renal insufficiency is present (see ADMINISTRATION/DOSAGE ADJUSTMENTS)

ADVERSE REACTIONS

Frequent reactions (incidence ≥ 1%) are printed in *italics*

Dermatological	*Mild-to-moderate maculopapular, morbilliform rash (2.9–6.7%); pruritus*; exfoliative dermatitis
Gastrointestinal	Epigastric distress, nausea, vomiting, glossitis

PROLOPRIM ■ SEPTRA

Hematological	Thrombocytopenia, leukopenia, neutropenia, megaloblastic anemia, methemoglobinemia
Other	Fever

OVERDOSAGE

Signs and symptoms	Nausea, vomiting, dizziness, headache, mental depression, confusion, bone marrow depression (manifested as thrombocytopenia, leukopenia, megaloblastic anemia)
Treatment	Evacuate stomach by gastric lavage and institute general supportive measures. Acidify urine to increase renal elimination. Peritoneal dialysis is ineffective and hemodialysis only moderately effective.

DRUG INTERACTIONS

No clinically significant drug interactions have been identified

ALTERED LABORATORY VALUES

Blood/serum values — ⬆ SGOT ⬆ SGPT ⬆ Bilirubin ⬆ BUN ⬆ Creatinine

No clinically significant alterations in urinary values occur at therapeutic dosages

---

USE IN CHILDREN

Safety for use in infants under 2 mo of age has not been established; effectiveness has not been established in children under 12 yr of age

USE IN PREGNANT AND NURSING WOMEN

Pregnancy Category C. Teratogenicity has been shown in rats at doses 40 times human dose; in rabbits, doses 6 times human dose have been associated with an increase in fetal loss. Human studies have been inconclusive. Trimethoprim may interfere with folic acid metabolism and appears in breast milk. Use during pregnancy or lactation with caution, and only if potential benefit outweighs risk to fetus or nursing infant.

URINARY ANTI-INFECTIVES

SEPTRA (trimethoprim and sulfamethoxazole) Burroughs Wellcome — Rx

Tablets: 80 mg trimethoprim and 400 mg sulfamethoxazole **Suspension (per 5 ml):** 40 mg trimethoprim and 200 mg sulfamethoxazole[1] (100, 473 ml) *cherry-flavored*

SEPTRA DS (trimethoprim and sulfamethoxazole) Burroughs Wellcome — Rx

Tablets: 160 mg trimethoprim and 800 mg sulfamethoxazole

INDICATIONS / ORAL DOSAGE

Urinary tract infections caused by susceptible strains of *Escherichia coli*, *Klebsiella*, *Enterobacter*, *Morganella morganii*, *Proteus mirabilis*, and *P vulgaris*[2]

Adult: 2 Septra tabs, 1 Septra DS tab, or 20 ml (4 tsp) q12h for 10–14 days
Child (≥ 2 mo): 4 mg/kg trimethoprim and 20 mg/kg sulfamethoxazole q12h for 10 days, as follows:
Child (10 kg): 5 ml (1 tsp) q12h for 10 days
Child (20 kg): 1 Septra tab or 10 ml (2 tsp) q12h for 10 days
Child (30 kg): 1½ Septra tabs or 15 ml (3 tsp) q12h for 10 days
Child (≥ 40 kg): 2 Septra tabs, 1 Septra DS tab, or 20 ml (4 tsp) q12h for 10 days

Acute otitis media caused by susceptible strains of *Hemophilus influenzae* or *Streptococcus pneumoniae*[3]

Child (≥ 2 mo): same as pediatric dosages above

Acute exacerbations of chronic bronchitis caused by susceptible strains of *Hemophilus influenzae* or *Streptococcus pneumoniae*[4]

Adult: same as adult dosage above for 14 days

Enteritis caused by susceptible strains of *Shigella flexneri* and *S sonnei*

Adult: same as above for 5 days
Child (≥ 2 mo): same as above for 5 days

Pneumocystis carinii pneumonitis

Adult: 5 mg/kg trimethoprim and 25 mg/kg sulfamethoxazole q6h for 14 days
Child (≥ 2 mo): same as adult, as follows:
Child (8 kg): 5 ml (1 tsp) q6h for 14 days
Child (16 kg): 1 Septra tab or 10 ml (2 tsp) q6h for 14 days
Child (24 kg): 1½ Septra tabs or 15 ml (3 tsp) q6h for 14 days
Child (≥ 32 kg): 2 Septra tabs, 1 Septra DS tab, or 20 ml (4 tsp) q6h for 14 days

SEPTRA

CONTRAINDICATIONS

Pregnancy at term	Breast-feeding	Megaloblastic anemia due to folate deficiency
Age < 2 mo	Hypersensitivity to trimethoprim or sulfonamides	

ADMINISTRATION/DOSAGE ADJUSTMENTS

Patients with renal impairment	Follow the usual dosage regimen if creatinine clearance (Ccr) > 30 ml/min. Administer half the usual dosage if Ccr = 15–30 ml/min. Use is not recommended if Ccr < 15 ml/min.

WARNINGS/PRECAUTIONS

Group A beta-hemolytic streptococcal pharyngitis	Sulfonamides have no place in the treatment of such infections, as they will neither eradicate the causative organism from the tonsillopharyngeal area nor prevent complications
Life-threatening reactions	Severe, potentially fatal reactions, including Stevens-Johnson syndrome, toxic epidermal necrolysis, fulminant hepatic necrosis, and serious blood dyscrasias (eg, agranulocytosis, aplastic anemia) have occurred on rare occasions in patients receiving sulfonamides. These drugs have caused hemolytic anemia in patients with G6PD deficiency. The risk of severe adverse reactions may be increased in elderly patients, particularly when these patients are receiving other drugs (see DRUG INTERACTIONS) or they have renal or hepatic impairment or another complicating condition; the most frequent serious adverse effects seen in elderly patients are severe skin reactions, generalized bone marrow depression, and thrombocytopenia. When using this preparation, obtain a CBC frequently and watch for early clinical signs such as rash, sore throat, fever, pallor, purpura, and jaundice; *discontinue administration at the first sign of skin rash or any adverse reaction*
Bone marrow depression	High doses or prolonged use may cause bone marrow depression and, as a result, produce thrombocytopenia, leukopenia, and/or megaloplastic anemia; if signs of bone marrow depression appear, give 5–15 mg/day of leucovorin until normal hematopoiesis is restored
Cross-sensitivity	Patients allergic to acetazolamide, thiazide-type diuretics, sulfonylureas, or certain goitrogens may also be hypersensitive to this preparation
Renal effects	Crystalluria, urolithiasis, and other renal complications have occurred in patients taking sulfonamides. Caution patients to maintain an adequate fluid intake; urinalysis, including careful microscopic examination, and renal function tests should be performed during therapy, particularly when a patient has renal impairment.
Special-risk patients	Use with caution in elderly patients and those with renal or hepatic impairment, possible folate deficiency, severe allergies, bronchial asthma, or G6PD deficiency. Among the conditions that may be associated with folate deficiency are malnutrition, malabsorption syndrome, chronic alcoholism, advanced age, and anticonvulsant therapy.
AIDS	Patients with AIDS may not tolerate or respond to this preparation in the same manner as other patients; the frequency of adverse effects, particularly rash, fever, and leukopenia, has been reported to be greatly increased in AIDS patients who were undergoing treatment of *Pneumocystis carinii* pneumonia
Carcinogenicity	No long-term studies have been done in animals to evaluate the oncogenic potential of this drug
Mutagenicity	Although bacterial mutagenicity studies have not been done with this preparation, trimethoprim alone has shown no mutagenic potential in the Ames assay, and no chromosomal abnormalities have been detected in human leukocytes cultured in vitro with either component alone or in combination or in leukocytes from treated patients
Effect on fertility	No adverse effects on fertility or general reproductive performance have been observed in rats given oral dosages as high as 70 mg/kg/day of trimethoprim plus 350 mg/kg/day of sulfamethoxazole

ADVERSE REACTIONS

Hematological	Agranulocytosis, aplastic anemia, thrombocytopenia, leukopenia, neutropenia, hemolytic anemia, megaloblastic anemia, hypoprothrombinemia, methemoglobinemia, eosinophilia
Gastrointestinal	Hepatitis (including cholestatic jaundice and fulminant hepatic necrosis), elevation of serum transaminase and bilirubin levels, pseudomembranous enterocolitis, pancreatitis, stomatitis, glossitis, nausea, vomiting, abdominal pain, diarrhea, anorexia
Genitourinary	Renal failure, interstitial nephritis, elevation of BUN and serum creatinine levels, toxic nephrosis with oliguria and anuria, crystalluria
Central nervous system	Aseptic meningitis, convulsions, peripheral neuritis, ataxia, vertigo, tinnitus, headache, hallucinations, depression, apathy, nervousness, weakness, fatigue, insomnia
Endocrinological	Diuresis, hypoglycemia
Musculoskeletal	Arthralgia, myalgia

SEPTRA ■ SEPTRA I.V. Infusion

Hypersensitivity	Stevens-Johnson syndrome, toxic epidermal necrolysis, anaphylaxis, allergic myocarditis, erythema multiforme, exfoliative dermatitis, angioedema, drug fever, chills, Henoch-Schoenlein purpura, serum sickness-like syndrome, generalized allergic reactions, generalized skin eruptions, photosensitivity, conjunctival and scleral injection, pruritus, urticaria, rash, periarteritis nodosa, systemic lupus erythematosus

OVERDOSAGE

Signs and symptoms	Anorexia, colic, nausea, vomiting, dizziness, headache, drowsiness, mental depression, confusion, unconsciousness, pyrexia, hematuria, crystalluria, bone marrow depression, other blood dyscrasias, jaundice
Treatment	Induce emesis or perform gastric lavage. To enhance renal elimination, acidify urine and institute forced diuresis; if urine output is low and renal function is normal, administer IV fluids. Monitor blood counts and electrolyte balance. Institute specific therapy if jaundice or a significant blood dyscrasia occurs. Peritoneal dialysis is not useful and hemodialysis is only moderately effective in removing the components of this preparation.

DRUG INTERACTIONS

Diuretics (especially thiazides)	△ Risk of thrombocytopenic purpura in elderly patients
Warfarin	△ Prothrombin time; if this preparation is given during warfarin therapy, recheck prothrombin time
Phenytoin	△ Serum half-life of phenytoin; watch for evidence of phenytoin toxicity during combination therapy
Methotrexate	△ Serum level of methotrexate

ALTERED LABORATORY VALUES

Blood/serum values	△ Methotrexate (with competitive binding protein assay using dihydrofolate reductase) △ BUN △ Creatinine (especially with Jaffé test) △ Bilirubin △ SGOT △ SGPT ▽ PBI ▽ ^{131}I thyroid uptake

No clinically significant alterations in urinary values occur at therapeutic dosages

---

USE IN CHILDREN

See INDICATIONS and ORAL DOSAGE. Data on the safety of repeated use in children under 2 yr of age are limited; contraindicated for infants under 2 mo of age.

USE IN PREGNANT AND NURSING WOMEN

Pregnancy Category C: use during pregnancy only if expected benefit justifies the potential fetal risk, since the drug may interfere with folic acid metabolism. Teratogenic effects (mainly cleft palate) have been observed in rats and increased fetal loss has been observed in rats and rabbits at doses several times the recommended human dose. Although no large, well-controlled studies have been done in pregnant women, two limited studies have shown no increase in congenital abnormalities. The drug is contraindicated at term and for use in nursing mothers because sulfonamides cross the placental barrier, are excreted in human milk, and may cause kernicterus.

---

[1] Contains 0.26% alcohol
[2] Initial episodes of uncomplicated infections should be treated with a single, effective antibacterial agent, rather than a combination
[3] Not indicated for prophylaxis or prolonged administration
[4] When in the physician's judgment this preparation offers some advantage over the use of a single antimicrobial agent

---

URINARY ANTI-INFECTIVES

SEPTRA I.V. Infusion (trimethoprim and sulfamethoxazole) Burroughs Wellcome   Rx

Ampuls (per 5 ml): 80 mg trimethoprim and 400 mg sulfamethoxazole (5 ml) for IV infusion only   **Vials (per 5 ml):** 80 mg trimethoprim and 400 mg sulfamethoxazole (5, 10, 20 ml) for IV infusion only

INDICATIONS

Pneumocystis carinii **pneumonitis**

Severe or complicated **urinary tract infections** caused by susceptible strains of *Escherichia coli*, *Klebsiella*, *Enterobacter*, *Morganella morganii*, and *Proteus* when oral administration is not feasible or when the organism is not susceptible to single urinary anti-infectives alone
Enteritis caused by susceptible strains of *Shigella flexneri* and *S sonnei*

PARENTERAL DOSAGE[1]

Adult: 15–20 mg/kg/day, given in 3–4 equally divided doses via IV infusion q6–8h
Child: same as adult

Adult: 8–10 mg/kg/day, up to 960 mg/day, given in 2–4 equally divided doses via IV infusion q6–12h
Child: same as adult

SEPTRA I.V. Infusion

CONTRAINDICATIONS

Pregnancy at term
Breast-feeding
Age < 2 mo

Hypersensitivity to trimethoprim or sulfonamides

Documented megaloblastic anemia due to folate deficiency

ADMINISTRATION/DOSAGE ADJUSTMENTS

Preparation of infusion	Dilute each 5 ml of the preparation in 125 ml of 5% dextrose-in-water and use within 6 h; do not refrigerate. If fluid restriction is desired, dilute in 100 ml and use within 4 h or dilute in 75 ml and use within 2 h. Do not mix with other drugs or solutions in the same container. The contents of the 20-ml vial must be used within 48 h after withdrawal of the initial dose.
Intravenous administration	Administer slowly by IV drip over a period of 60–90 min; avoid rapid infusion or bolus injection
Local irritation and inflammation	May occur, due to extravascular infiltration of the infusion; discontinue infusion and restart at another site
Susceptibility tests	Cultures and appropriate microbiological tests should be performed to determine susceptibility; therapy may be initiated, however, before the results of these tests are available
Duration of therapy	Pneumonitis due to *Pneumocystis carinii* and severe urinary tract infections should be treated for up to 14 days and shigellosis for up to 5 days
Patients with renal impairment	Follow the usual dosage regimen if creatinine clearance (Ccr) > 30 ml/min. Administer half the usual dosage if Ccr = 15–30 ml/min; use is not recommended if Ccr < 15 ml/min.

WARNINGS/PRECAUTIONS

Streptococcal pharyngitis	Should not be treated with this drug, as it may fail to eliminate group A beta-hemolytic streptococci from the tonsillopharyngeal area
Life-threatening reactions	Severe, potentially fatal reactions, including Stevens-Johnson syndrome, toxic epidermal necrolysis, fulminant hepatic necrosis, and serious blood dyscrasias (eg, agranulocytosis, aplastic anemia) have occurred on rare occasions in patients receiving sulfonamides. These drugs have caused hemolytic anemia in patients with G6PD deficiency. The risk of severe adverse reactions may be increased in elderly patients, particularly when these patients are receiving other drugs (see DRUG INTERACTIONS) or they have renal or hepatic impairment or another complicating condition; the most frequent serious adverse effects seen in elderly patients are severe skin reactions, generalized bone marrow depression, and thrombocytopenia. When using this preparation, obtain a CBC frequently and watch for early clinical signs such as rash, sore throat, fever, pallor, purpura, and jaundice; *discontinue administration at the first sign of skin rash or any adverse reaction*
Bone marrow depression	High doses or prolonged use may cause bone marrow depression and, as a result, produce thrombocytopenia, leukopenia, and/or megaloblastic anemia; if signs of bone marrow depression appear, give 5–15 mg/day of leucovorin until normal hematopoiesis is restored.
Cross-sensitivity	Patients allergic to acetazolamide, thiazide-type diuretics, sulfonylureas, or certain goitrogens may also be hypersensitive to this preparation
Renal effects	Crystalluria, urolithiasis, and other renal complications have occurred in patients taking sulfonamides. Caution patients to maintain an adequate fluid intake; urinalysis, including careful microscopic examination, and renal function tests should be performed during therapy, particularly when a patient has renal impairment.
Special-risk patients	Use with caution in elderly patients and those with renal or hepatic impairment, possible folate deficiency, severe allergies, bronchial asthma, or G6PD deficiency. Among the conditions that may be associated with folate deficiency are malnutrition, malabsorption syndrome, chronic alcoholism, advanced age, and anticonvulsant therapy.
AIDS	Patients with AIDS may not tolerate or respond to this preparation in the same manner as other patients; the frequency of adverse effects, particularly rash, fever, and leukopenia, has been reported to be greatly increased in AIDS patients who were undergoing treatment of *Pneumocystis carinii* pneumonia
Sulfite sensitivity	Sodium metabisulfite in this product may cause urticaria, pruritus, wheezing, anaphylaxis, or other allergic-type reactions in susceptible patients, such as those with asthma or atopy
Carcinogenicity	No long-term studies have been done in animals to evaluate the oncogenic potential of this drug
Mutagenicity	Although bacterial mutagenicity studies have not been done with this preparation, trimethoprim alone has shown no mutagenic potential in the Ames assay, and no chromosomal abnormalities have been detected in human leukocytes cultured in vitro with either component alone or in combination or in leukocytes from treated patients

SEPTRA I.V. Infusion ■ TRIMPEX

Effect on fertility	No adverse effects on fertility or general reproductive performance have been observed in rats given oral dosages as high as 70 mg/kg/day of trimethoprim plus 350 mg/kg/day of sulfamethoxazole

ADVERSE REACTIONS

Hematological	Agranulocytosis, aplastic anemia, thrombocytopenia, leukopenia, neutropenia, hemolytic anemia, megaloblastic anemia, hypoprothrombinemia, methemoglobinemia, eosinophilia
Gastrointestinal	Hepatitis (including cholestatic jaundice and fulminant hepatic necrosis), elevation of serum transaminase and bilirubin levels, pseudomembranous enterocolitis, pancreatitis, stomatitis, glossitis, nausea, vomiting, abdominal pain, diarrhea, anorexia
Genitourinary	Renal failure, interstitial nephritis, elevation of BUN and serum creatinine levels, toxic nephrosis with oliguria and anuria, crystalluria
Central nervous system	Aseptic meningitis, convulsions, peripheral neuritis, ataxia, vertigo, tinnitus, headache, hallucinations, depression, apathy, nervousness, weakness, fatigue, insomnia
Endocrinological	Diuresis, hypoglycemia
Musculoskeletal	Arthralgia, myalgia
Hypersensitivity	Stevens-Johnson syndrome, toxic epidermal necrolysis, anaphylaxis, allergic myocarditis, erythema multiform, exfoliative dermatitis, angiodema, drug fever, chills, Henoch-Schoenlein purpura, serum sickness-like syndrome, generalized allergic reactions, generalized skin eruptions, photosensitivity, conjunctival and scleral injection, pruritus, urticaria, rash, periarteritis nodosa, systemic lupus erythematosus

OVERDOSAGE

Signs and symptoms	Anorexia, colic, nausea, vomiting, dizziness, headache, drowsiness, mental depression, confusion, unconsciousness, pyrexia, hematuria, crystalluria, bone marrow depression, other blood dyscrasias, jaundice
Treatment	To enhance renal elimination, acidify urine and institute forced diuresis; if urine output is low and renal function is normal, administer IV fluids. Monitor blood counts and electrolyte balance. Institute specific therapy if jaundice or a significant blood dyscrasia occurs. Peritoneal dialysis is not useful and hemodialysis is only moderately effective in removing the components of this preparation.

DRUG INTERACTIONS

Diuretics (especially thiazides)	△ Risk of thrombocytopenic purpura in elderly patients
Warfarin	△ Prothrombin time; if this preparation is given during warfarin therapy, recheck prothrombin time
Phenytoin	△ Serum half-life of phenytoin; watch for evidence of phenytoin toxicity during combination therapy
Methotrexate	△ Serum level of methotrexate

ALTERED LABORATORY VALUES

Blood/serum values	△ Methotrexate (with competitive binding protein assay using dihydrofolate reductase) △ BUN △ Creatinine (especially with Jaffé test) △ Bilirubin △ SGOT △ SGPT ▽ PBI ▽ ^{131}I thyroid uptake ▽ Glucose (rare)

No clinically significant alterations in urinary values occur at therapeutic dosages

---

USE IN CHILDREN

Same as adult indications and dosage; contraindicated for use in infants under 2 mo of age

USE IN PREGNANT AND NURSING WOMEN

Pregnancy Category C: use during pregnancy only if expected benefit justifies the potential fetal risk, since the drug may interfere with the folic acid metabolism. Teratogenic effects (mainly cleft palate) have been observed in rats and increased fetal loss has been observed in rats and rabbits at doses several times the recommended human dose. Although no large, well-controlled studies have been done in pregnant women, two limited studies have shown no increase in congenital abnormalities. The drug is contraindicated at term and for use in nursing mothers because sulfonamides cross the placental barrier, are excreted in human milk, and may cause kernicterus.

---

[1] Dosage is based on the trimethoprim component

URINARY ANTI-INFECTIVES

TRIMPEX (trimethoprim) Roche

Tablets: 100 mg

Rx

INDICATIONS

Initial episodes of uncomplicated urinary tract infections caused by susceptible strains of *Escherichia coli*, *Proteus mirabilis*, *Klebsiella pneumoniae*, *Enterobacter*, and coagulase-negative *Staphylococcus*, including *S saprophyticus*

ORAL DOSAGE

Adult: 100 mg q12h or 200 mg q24h, each for 10 days

TRIMPEX

CONTRAINDICATIONS

Hypersensitivity to trimethoprim	Established megaloblastic anemia due to folate deficiency

ADMINISTRATION/DOSAGE ADJUSTMENTS

Cultures and susceptibility tests	Should be performed to determine bacterial susceptibility to trimethoprim, although therapy may be initiated prior to test results
Patients with renal impairment	Reduce dosage to 50 mg q12h if creatinine clearance rate (CCr) = 15–30 ml/min; do not administer if CCr < 15 ml/min

WARNINGS/PRECAUTIONS

Blood dyscrasias	May occur rarely, especially with high doses and/or prolonged therapy. Obtain CBC if early signs develop (eg, sore throat, fever, pallor, or purpura). If signs of bone marrow depression (thrombocytopenia, leukopenia, and/or megaloblastic anemia) are present, discontinue therapy and administer leucovorin, 3–6 mg/day IM, for 3 days or until hematopoiesis is normal.
Suspected folate deficiency	Use with caution; concomitant administration of folates does not interfere with antibacterial action
Patients with hepatic or renal impairment	Use with caution if hepatic or renal insufficiency is present (see ADMINISTRATION/DOSAGE ADJUSTMENTS)
Carcinogenicity, mutagenicity, effect on fertility	No long-term studies have been done to evaluate the carcinogenic potential of trimethoprim. The Ames test and human leukocyte cultures have shown no evidence of mutagenicity or chromosomal damage. No adverse effects on fertility or general reproductive performance have been seen in male rats fed up to 70 mg/kg/day or in female rats fed up to 14 mg/kg/day.

ADVERSE REACTIONS

Frequent reactions (incidence ≥ 1%) are printed in *italics*

Dermatological	*Mild-to-moderate maculopapular, morbilliform rash (2.9–6.7%); pruritus;* exfoliative dermatitis
Gastrointestinal	Epigastric distress, nausea, vomiting, glossitis
Hematological	Thrombocytopenia, leukopenia, neutropenia, megaloblastic anemia, methemoglobinemia
Other	Fever

OVERDOSAGE

Signs and symptoms	Nausea, vomiting, dizziness, headache, mental depression, confusion, bone marrow depression (manifested as thrombocytopenia, leukopenia, megaloblastic anemia)
Treatment	Evacuate stomach by gastric lavage and institute general supportive measures. Acidify urine to increase renal elimination. Peritoneal dialysis is ineffective and hemodialysis only moderately effective.

DRUG INTERACTIONS

Phenytoin	△ Serum level of phenytoin

ALTERED LABORATORY VALUES

Blood/serum values	△ SGOT △ SGPT △ Bilirubin △ BUN △ Creatinine (physiological reaction; interference with Jaffé's test) ▽ Methotrexate (with competitive binding protein assay)

No clinically significant alterations in urinary values occur at therapeutic dosages

---

USE IN CHILDREN

Safety for use in infants under 2 mo of age has not been established; effectiveness has not been established in children under 12 yr of age

USE IN PREGNANT AND NURSING WOMEN

Pregnancy Category C: teratogenicity has been shown in rats given 40 times the human dose, and embryotoxicity has been shown in rabbits given 6 times the human dose; oral administration of 70 mg/kg/day to rats from the last trimester to the time of weaning has resulted in no adverse effects on gestation or pup survival and growth. Small retrospective surveys of pregnant women have provided no evidence that trimethoprim increases the risk of congenital abnormalities; however, no large, well-controlled studies have been done. Trimethoprim is excreted in human milk. Because this drug may interfere with folic acid metabolism, use during pregnancy only if the expected benefits outweigh the potential risks to the fetus, and use with caution in nursing mothers.

URISED

URINARY ANTI-INFECTIVES

URISED (methenamine, methylene blue, phenyl salicylate, benzoic acid, atropine sulfate, and hyoscyamine) Webcon   Rx

Tablets: 40.8 mg methenamine, 5.4 mg methylene blue, 18.1 mg phenyl salicylate, 4.5 mg benzoic acid, 0.03 mg atropine sulfate, and 0.03 mg hyoscyamine

INDICATIONS

Lower urinary tract discomfort caused by hypermotility due to inflammation or diagnostic procedures

Cystitis, urethritis, and trigonitis caused by organisms that produce or maintain an acid urine and are susceptible to formaldehyde

ORAL DOSAGE

Adult: 2 tabs qid, followed by liberal fluid intake
Child ($\geq$ 12 yr): reduce dosage in proportion to body weight and age

CONTRAINDICATIONS

Urinary bladder-neck obstruction	Glaucoma	Hypersensitivity to any component
Pyloric or duodenal obstruction	Cardiospasm	Sulfonamide therapy

WARNINGS/PRECAUTIONS

Monitoring of therapy	Bacteriological studies may be helpful in evaluating response to therapy
Drug-food interactions	Caution patients to restrict their intake of foods that produce an alkaline urine (see also DRUG INTERACTIONS)
Special-risk patients	Use with caution in patients with cardiac disease or a history of idiosyncratic reactions to atropine-like compounds
Discoloration of urine and feces	Caution patients that their urine will turn blue to blue-green and that their feces may be discolored as a result of excretion of methylene blue
Management of side effects	Decrease the dosage if pronounced dryness of the mouth, flushing, or difficulty in initiating micturition occurs; discontinue use immediately if a rapid pulse, dizziness, or blurred vision occurs
Carcinogenicity	No long-term studies have been done to evaluate the carcinogenic potential of this drug

ADVERSE REACTIONS

Gastrointestinal	Dry mouth
Genitourinary	Difficulty in initiating micturition; acute urinary retention in patients with prostatic hypertrophy
Central nervous system	Blurred vision, dizziness
Cardiovascular	Rapid pulse, flushing

OVERDOSAGE

Signs and symptoms	Hot, dry, flushed skin; dryness of mucous membranes, dilatation of pupils, hyperpyrexia, tachycardia, palpitations, elevated blood pressure, coma, circulatory collapse, death from respiratory failure
Treatment	Induce emesis or perform gastric lavage to empty stomach. Instill activated charcoal. In severe cases, administer 1–4 mg physostigmine salicylate IV (slowly) and repeat as needed if life-threatening signs recur or persist. Maintain an open airway and adequate pulmonary ventilation; reduce fever by external cooling, and institute additional supportive measures, as required.

DRUG INTERACTIONS

Other antimuscarinics, amantadine, antihistamines, haloperidol, phenothiazines, MAO inhibitors, tricyclic antidepressants	⇧ Atropine-like effects
Urinary alkalinizing agents, antacids, carbonic anhydrase inhibitors, thiazide diuretics	⇩ Antibacterial effectiveness
Sulfonamides	Formation of insoluble precipitates with formaldehyde (the urinary metabolite of methenamine) in the urine; do not use concomitantly

ALTERED LABORATORY VALUES

Urinary values	⇧ Catecholamines (with fluorometric methods) ⇧ 17-OHCS (with Reddy method) ⇩ Estriol (with acid hydrolysis method) ⇩ 5-HIAA (with nitrosonaphthol reagent test)

URISED ■ PYRIDIUM

No clinically significant alterations in blood/serum values occur at therapeutic dosages

USE IN CHILDREN
See INDICATIONS and ORAL DOSAGE; not indicated for use in children under 12 yr of age

USE IN PREGNANT AND NURSING WOMEN
Pregnancy Category C: use during pregnancy only if clearly needed. Reproduction studies have not been done in animals, nor has it been determined whether this drug can affect human reproductive capacity or cause harm to the human fetus. It is not known whether this drug is excreted in human milk; because many drugs are excreted in human milk, use with caution in nursing mothers.

URINARY ANALGESICS

PYRIDIUM (phenazopyridine hydrochloride) Parke-Davis Rx

Tablets: 100, 200 mg

INDICATIONS	**ORAL DOSAGE**
Symptomatic relief of **pain, burning, urgency, frequency, and other discomfort** associated with irritation of the lower urinary tract mucosa	**Adult:** 200 mg tid after meals; do not administer for more than 2 days if a urinary tract anti-infective is given concomitantly

CONTRAINDICATIONS

Renal impairment	Hypersensitivity to phenazopyridine

WARNINGS/PRECAUTIONS

Drug accumulation	If renal function is impaired, drug may accumulate. Do not use in patients with renal impairment; bear in mind that elderly patients commonly have renal dysfunction. If accumulation occurs during therapy, discontinue use. Yellowing of the skin or sclera during therapy may indicate accumulation.
Urine discoloration	Caution patients that urine may appear reddish-orange and may stain fabric
Carcinogenicity	Long-term administration of phenazopyridine has caused neoplasia in the large intestines of rats and the livers of mice; although no association between phenazopyridine and human neoplasia has been reported, adequate epidemiological studies have not been done

ADVERSE REACTIONS

Central nervous system	Headache
Dermatological	Rash
Gastrointestinal	GI disturbances
Hematological	Methemoglobinemia, hemolytic anemia
Other	Renal and hepatic toxicity

OVERDOSAGE

Signs and symptoms	Methemoglobinemia, cyanosis, oxidative Heinz body hemolytic anemia, degmacytes (G6PD deficiency may increase the risk of hemolysis), renal and hepatic impairment or failure
Treatment	To reduce methemoglobinemia, administer 1–2 mg/kg of methylene blue IV or 100–200 mg of ascorbic acid orally

DRUG INTERACTIONS

No clinically significant drug interactions have been identified

ALTERED LABORATORY VALUES

Urinary values	Interference with: BSP PSP Glucose (with glucose oxidase tests) Bilirubin (with foam, talc-disk-Fouchet-spot, and Franklin's tablet-Fouchet tests) Urobilinogen (with Ehrlich's test) Ketone (with sodium nitroprusside and Gerhardt ferric chloride tests) Protein (with reagent test strips and nitric acid ring test) 17-Hydroxycorticosteroid (with modified Glenn-Nelson method) 17-Ketosteroid (with Haltorff-Koch modification of the Zimmerman reaction) Porphyrins (with spectrophotometric tests) Urinalysis (with spectrometric or color-based methods)

No clinically significant alterations in blood/serum values occur at therapeutic dosages

PYRIDIUM ∎ PYRIDIUM Plus

USE IN CHILDREN	USE IN PREGNANT AND NURSING WOMEN
Consult manufacturer	Pregnancy Category B: reproduction studies in rats given up to 50 mg/kg/day have shown no evidence of impaired fertility or harm to the fetus; use during pregnancy only if clearly needed. It is not known whether this drug is excreted in human milk.

URINARY ANALGESICS

PYRIDIUM Plus (phenazopyridine hydrochloride, hyoscyamine hydrobromide, and butabarbital) Parke-Davis Rx

Tablets: 150 mg phenazopyridine hydrochloride, 0.3 mg hyoscyamine hydrobromide, and 15 mg butabarbital

INDICATIONS	ORAL DOSAGE
Symptomatic relief of **pain, burning, urgency, frequency, and dysuria** associated with irritation of the lower urinary tract mucosa, especially when accompanied by detrusor muscle spasm and apprehension	**Adult:** 1 tab qid, after meals and at bedtime; do not administer for more than 2 days if a urinary tract anti-infective is given concomitantly

CONTRAINDICATIONS

| Renal or hepatic impairment | Glaucoma | Hypersensitivity to any component |
| Porphyria | Bladder neck obstruction | |

WARNINGS/PRECAUTIONS

Drug accumulation	If renal function is impaired, drug may accumulate. Do not use in patients with renal impairment; bear in mind that elderly patients commonly have renal dysfunction. If accumulation occurs during therapy, discontinue use. Yellowing of the skin or sclera during therapy may indicate phenazopyridine accumulation.
Drowsiness, dizziness	Caution patients about driving or operating machinery
Urine discoloration	Caution patients that urine may appear reddish-orange and may stain fabric
Drug dependence	Psychic and/or physical dependence and tolerance to the butabarbital component may occur
Carcinogenicity	Long-term administration of phenazopyridine has caused neoplasia in the large intestines of rats and the livers of mice; although no association between phenazopyridine and human neoplasia has been reported, adequate epidemiological studies have not been done

ADVERSE REACTIONS

The most frequent reactions, regardless of incidence, are printed in *italics*

Central nervous system	*Drowsiness and dizziness* ($>$ 33%), blurred vision
Gastrointestinal	GI disturbances
Hematological	Methemoglobinemia, hemolytic anemia
Other	*Dry mouth* ($>$ 33%), barbiturate reactions, renal and hepatic toxicity

OVERDOSAGE

| Signs and symptoms | Methemoglobinemia, cyanosis, respiratory depression, oxidative Heinz body hemolytic anemia, degmacytes (G6PD deficiency may increase the risk of hemolysis), renal and hepatic impairment or failure, sedation, mydriasis, blurred vision, rapid pulse, increased intraocular pressure, dry mouth, disorientation, delirium; hot, dry, red skin; fever, convulsions, coma |
| Treatment | To remove drug from the GI tract, induce emesis or perform gastric lavage and then administer an activated charcoal slurry. Institute supportive measures, as needed. Reduce methemoglobinemia by administering 1–2 mg/kg of methylene blue IV or 100–200 mg of ascorbic acid orally. For atropinic reactions, physostigmine may be given in slow IV doses of 0.2 mg (for children) or 0.5–2 mg (for adults) every 5 min, as needed, up to a total of 2 mg (for children) or 6 mg (for adults) every 30 min. |

DRUG INTERACTIONS

| Alcohol | ⌂ Sedation |

PYRIDIUM Plus ■ CYSTOSPAZ

Oral anticoagulants, corticosteroids, oral contraceptives, doxycycline, griseofulvin, quinidine, propranolol, metoprolol, antiobesity agents	⇩ Pharmacologic effect of interacting drug	
Phenothiazines	⇧ Pharmacologic effect of hyoscyamine component	⇩ Antipsychotic effect of phenothiazines
Haloperidol	⇩ Antipsychotic effect of haloperidol	
Atenolol	⇧ Bioavailability of atenolol	
Digoxin	⇧ Serum level of oral digoxin	
Levodopa	⇩ Serum levodopa level	
Cimetidine	⇩ Serum cimetidine level	
Thiazide diuretics	⇧ Bioavailability of thiazide diuretics	
Methoxyflurane	⇧ Risk of nephrotoxicity	

ALTERED LABORATORY VALUES

Urinary values — Interference with: BSP PSP Glucose (with glucose oxidase tests) Bilirubin (with foam, talc-disk-Fouchet-spot, and Franklin's tablet-Fouchet tests) Urobilinogen (with Ehrlich's test) Ketone (with sodium nitroprusside and Gerhardt ferric chloride tests) Protein (with reagent test strips and nitric acid ring test) 17-Hydroxycorticosteroid (with modified Glenn-Nelson method) 17-Ketosteroid (with Haltorff-Koch modification of the Zimmerman reaction) Porphyrins (with spectrophotometric tests) Urinalysis (with spectrometric or color-based methods)

No clinically significant alterations in blood/serum values occur at therapeutic dosages

USE IN CHILDREN
Consult manufacturer

USE IN PREGNANT AND NURSING WOMEN
Pregnancy Category C: reproduction studies have not been done with this preparation; it is not known whether it can cause harm to the fetus or affect reproductive capacity. Use during pregnancy only if clearly needed. It is also not known whether this preparation is excreted in human milk.

URINARY ANTISPASMODICS

CYSTOSPAZ (hyoscyamine) Webcon — Rx
Tablets: 150 µg

CYSTOSPAZ-M (hyoscyamine sulfate) Webcon — Rx
Capsules (timed release): 375 µg

INDICATIONS	ORAL DOSAGE
Lower urinary tract hypermotility	Adult: 1–2 tabs (150–300 µg) up to qid or 1 cap (375 µg) q12h Child (≤ 12 yr): reduce dosage in proportion to age and weight

CONTRAINDICATIONS

Glaucoma	Duodenal obstruction	Hypersensitivity to hyoscyamine
Urinary bladder neck or pyloric obstruction	Cardiospasm	

WARNINGS/PRECAUTIONS

Tachycardia, dizziness, blurred vision	Discontinue use immediately if rapid pulse, dizziness, or blurred vision occurs
Slight dryness of the mouth	May occur as a result of parasympathomimetic blockade; caution patient accordingly
Special-risk patients	Use with caution in patients with known idiosyncratic reactions to atropine-like compounds and in the presence of cardiac disease
Acute urinary retention	May be precipitated in patients with prostatic hypertrophy

ADVERSE REACTIONS

Central nervous system	Drowsiness, dizziness
Cardiovascular	Rapid pulse
Gastrointestinal	Dry mouth, constipation

CYSTOSPAZ ■ DITROPAN

Genitourinary	Urinary retention (in patients with prostatic hypertrophy)
Ophthalmic	Photophobia, blurred vision

OVERDOSAGE

Signs and symptoms	Severe dryness of the mouth, nose, and throat; hot, flushed, dry skin; hyperpyrexia (especially in children), difficulty or inability to swallow, difficult speech, mydriasis, restlessness, garrulity, marked tremors, convulsions, respiratory failure, death; ingestion of 0.6–1 mg (approximately 4–7 tabs or 2–3 caps) may elicit toxic symptoms in adults, with doses of 1–2 mg producing more profound toxicity
Treatment	Induce emesis or perform gastric lavage to empty stomach. Instill activated charcoal. In severe cases, administer 1–4 mg physostigmine salicylate IV (slowly) and repeat as needed if life-threatening signs recur or persist. Treat convulsions with diazepam. Maintain an open airway and adequate pulmonary ventilation; reduce fever by external cooling, and institute additional supportive measures, as required.

DRUG INTERACTIONS

Amantadine, antihistamines, other antimuscarinics, haloperidol, MAO inhibitors, phenothiazines, tricyclic antidepressants	△ Atropine-like effects of hyoscyamine
Antacids, antidiarrheal agents	▽ Absorption of hyoscyamine

ALTERED LABORATORY VALUES

No clinically significant alterations in blood/serum or urinary values occur at therapeutic dosages

---

USE IN CHILDREN	USE IN PREGNANT AND NURSING WOMEN
See INDICATIONS and ORAL DOSAGE	Pregnancy Category C: no adequate, well-controlled studies have been conducted in either laboratory animals or pregnant women to determine effect, if any, on fetal development or reproductive capacity; use during pregnancy only if clearly needed. It is not known whether hyoscyamine is excreted in human milk; use with caution in nursing mothers.

URINARY ANTISPASMODICS

DITROPAN (oxybutynin chloride) Marion   Rx

Tablets: 5 mg   **Syrup (per 5 ml):** 5 mg (473 ml)

INDICATIONS	ORAL DOSAGE
Voiding symptoms associated with uninhibited or reflex neurogenic bladder	**Adult:** 5 mg or 5 ml (1 tsp) bid or tid or, if necessary, qid **Child (> 5 yr):** 5 mg or 5 ml (1 tsp) bid or, if necessary, tid

CONTRAINDICATIONS

Glaucoma	Partial or complete GI-tract obstruction	Paralytic ileus
Intestinal atony in elderly or debilitated patients	Megacolon	Toxic megacolon complicating ulcerative colitis
	Severe colitis	
Unstable cardiovascular status in acute hemorrhage	Myasthenia gravis	Obstructive uropathy

WARNINGS/PRECAUTIONS

Drowsiness, blurred vision	Caution patients about driving or engaging in other potentially hazardous activities while taking this drug
Ulcerative colitis	Large doses may suppress intestinal motility and lead to paralytic ileus or precipitate or aggravate toxic megacolon
Special-risk patients	Use with caution in the elderly and in those with autonomic neuropathy, hepatic or renal disease, hyperthyroidism, coronary heart disease, congestive heart failure, cardiac arrhythmias, hypertension, tachycardia, prostatic hypertrophy, or hiatal hernia associated with reflux esophagitis
Fever and heat stroke	May occur in high environmental temperatures as a result of decreased sweating
Incomplete intestinal obstruction	May be manifested by diarrhea, especially in ileostomy or colostomy patients; therapy may be harmful under these circumstances

ADVERSE REACTIONS

Gastrointestinal	Dry mouth, nausea, vomiting, constipation, bloating
Genitourinary	Urinary hesitancy and retention, impotence
Dermatological	Decreased sweating
Ophthalmic	Blurred vision, pupillary dilatation, increased ocular tension, cycloplegia
Cardiovascular	Tachycardia, palpitations
Central nervous system	Drowsiness, weakness, dizziness, insomnia
Endocrinological	Suppression of lactation
Allergic	Urticaria and other dermatoses

OVERDOSAGE

Signs and symptoms	Intensification of usual side effects, CNS disturbances (restlessness, excitement, psychotic behavior), circulatory changes (flushing, decrease in blood pressure, circulatory failure), respiratory failure, curare-like effects (neuromuscular blockade, leading to muscle weakness and possible paralysis), coma
Treatment	Immediately empty stomach by gastric lavage; inject physostigmine, 0.5–2.0 mg IV, up to 5 mg as needed. Treat fever symptomatically (ice, alcohol). Manage excessive excitement with 2% sodium thiopental IV (slowly) or 100–200 ml of 2% chloral hydrate via rectal infusion. For paralysis of respiratory muscles, institute artificial respiration.

DRUG INTERACTIONS

Digoxin	⇧ Serum digoxin level
Belladonna alkaloids, anticholinergic agents, phenothiazines, tricyclic antidepressants, quinidine, antihistamines, procainamide	⇧ Cholinergic blockade

ALTERED LABORATORY VALUES

No clinically significant alterations in blood/serum or urinary values occur at therapeutic dosages

---

USE IN CHILDREN

See INDICATIONS and ORAL DOSAGE; the safety and effectiveness of this drug for use in children under 5 yr of age have not been established

USE IN PREGNANT AND NURSING WOMEN

Use during pregnancy only if the probable clinical benefits outweigh the possible hazards. Reproduction studies in animals have shown no definite evidence of impaired fertility or fetal harm; however, the safety of administering this drug to women who are or who may become pregnant has not been established. Consult manufacturer for use in nursing mothers.

URINARY ANTISPASMODICS

URISPAS (flavoxate hydrochloride) Smith Kline & French Rx

Tablets: 100 mg

INDICATIONS

Symptomatic relief of **dysuria, urgency, nocturia, suprapubic pain, frequency,** and **incontinence** associated with cystitis, prostatitis, urethritis, and urethrocystitis/urethrotrigonitis

ORAL DOSAGE

Adult: 100–200 mg tid or qid, followed by a reduction in dosage as symptoms improve

CONTRAINDICATIONS

Pyloric or duodenal obstruction	Obstructive intestinal lesions or ileus	Obstructive uropathy of the lower urinary tract
GI hemorrhage	Achalasia	

WARNINGS/PRECAUTIONS

Suspected glaucoma	Use with caution
Drowsiness, blurred vision	Caution patients not to drive, operate machinery, or participate in other activities requiring alertness if these side effects develop
Carcinogenicity, mutagenicity	No studies have been done to determine the carcinogenic or mutagenic potential of flavoxate

ADVERSE REACTIONS

Gastrointestinal	Dry mouth, nausea, vomiting
Genitourinary	Dysuria
Hematological	Eosinophilia, leukopenia (one case)
Central nervous system	Headache, nervousness, vertigo, confusion (especially in the elderly), drowsiness
Cardiovascular	Palpitations, tachycardia
Ophthalmic	Blurred vision, increased ocular tension, disturbance in eye accommodation
Hypersensitivity	Urticaria, other dermatoses, eosinophilia, hyperpyrexia

OVERDOSAGE

There has been no overdosage experience with this drug; it is not known whether flavoxate can be removed by dialysis

DRUG INTERACTIONS

Digoxin	↑ Serum digoxin level
Belladonna alkaloids, anticholinergic agents, phenothiazines, tricyclic antidepressants, quinidine, antihistamines, procainamide	↑ Cholinergic blockade

ALTERED LABORATORY VALUES

No clinically significant alterations in blood/serum or urinary values occur at therapeutic dosages

USE IN CHILDREN

Not recommended for use in children under 12 yr of age because the safety and effectiveness of using this drug in this age group have not been established

USE IN PREGNANT AND NURSING WOMEN

Pregnancy Category B: reproduction studies in rats and rabbits given up to 34 times the human dose have shown no evidence of impaired fertility or harm to the fetus; however, no well-controlled studies have been done in pregnant women. Use during pregnancy only if clearly needed. It is not known whether this drug is excreted in human milk; use with caution in nursing mothers.

PARASYMPATHOMIMETICS

DUVOID (bethanechol chloride) Norwich Eaton   Rx

Tablets: 10, 25, 50 mg

INDICATIONS

Acute postoperative and postpartum nonobstructive urinary retention
Urinary retention associated with neurogenic bladder

ORAL DOSAGE

Adult: 10–50 mg tid or qid; determine the minimum effective dose by giving 5–10 mg at 1-h intervals, up to a total of 50 mg. To minimize nausea and vomiting, administer when patient's stomach is empty.

CONTRAINDICATIONS

Mechanical obstruction of the GI or urinary tracts

Peptic ulcer

Marked vagotonia

Coronary occlusion

Vasomotor instability

Coronary artery disease

Conditions where integrity of gastrointestinal or bladder wall is questionable

Acute inflammatory conditions of the GI tract

Active or latent asthma

Bradycardia

Hypotension

Spastic GI disturbances

Peritonitis

Hyperthyroidism

Parkinsonism

Epilepsy

WARNINGS/PRECAUTIONS

Asthma, substernal pressure or pain	Asthmatic attacks may be precipitated, especially in susceptible patients (see CONTRAINDICATIONS). Substernal pressure or pain may occur as a result of bronchoconstriction or esophageal spasm (it is not known which of these reactions is the specific cause).
Fall in blood pressure	The risk of myocardial hypoxia must be considered if blood pressure decreases markedly. In patients with hypertension, the pressure may fall precipitously.
Reflux infection	May result when bacteruria is present if the sphincter fails to relax as bethanechol contracts the bladder, forcing urine up the ureter into the kidney pelvis

DUVOID ■ URECHOLINE

Concomitant use of ganglionic blocking agents	May result in a critical fall in blood pressure, usually preceded by severe abdominal symptoms; use bethanechol with caution

ADVERSE REACTIONS

Cardiovascular	Decreased blood pressure; transient syncope with cardiac arrest, transient complete heart block, and orthostatic hypotension (with large doses); atrial fibrillation (in hyperthyroid patients)
Gastrointestinal	Involuntary defecation (with large doses), vomiting, colic, abdominal cramps, diarrhea, nausea, belching, salivation, borborygmi
Respiratory	Asthmatic attacks; dyspnea (with large doses)
Other	Headache, facial flushing, substernal pressure or pain, malaise; urinary urgency (with large doses)

OVERDOSAGE

Signs and symptoms	See ADVERSE REACTIONS
Treatment	Maintain a patent airway and adequate respiratory exchange; administer atropine sulfate (doses of 0.6–1.2 mg) by IM, slow IV, or SC injection

DRUG INTERACTIONS

Quinidine, procainamide, atropine	⇩ Cholinergic effect
Cholinergic drugs, especially cholinesterase inhibitors	⇧ Cholinergic effect
Ganglionic blocking agents	⇧ Risk of critical fall in blood pressure

ALTERED LABORATORY VALUES

Blood/serum values	⇧ Amylase ⇧ Lipase ⇧ Bilirubin ⇧ SGOT ⇧ Sulfobromophthalein retention time

No clinically significant alterations in urinary values occur at therapeutic dosages

---

USE IN CHILDREN

Safety and effectiveness for use in children under 8 yr of age have not been established

USE IN PREGNANT AND NURSING WOMEN

Pregnancy Category C: reproduction studies have not been performed. It is not known whether bethanechol can cause harm to the fetus or affect reproductive capacity; use during pregnancy only if clearly needed. It is also not known whether this drug is excreted in human milk; use with caution in nursing mothers.

PARASYMPATHOMIMETICS

URECHOLINE (bethanechol chloride) Merck Sharp & Dohme   Rx

Tablets: 5, 10, 25, 50 mg **Vials:** 5 mg/ml (1 ml) for SC use only

INDICATIONS	ORAL DOSAGE	PARENTERAL DOSAGE
Acute postoperative and postpartum nonobstructive urinary retention Urinary retention associated with neurogenic atony of the bladder	**Adult:** give 5 or 10 mg at hourly intervals until a satisfactory response occurs or a cumulative dose of 50 mg is reached (usual dose: 10–50 mg); administer titrated total dose tid or qid	**Adult:** give 2.5 mg SC at intervals of 15–30 min until a satisfactory response occurs, a disturbing reaction is seen, or a cumulative dose of 10 mg is reached (usual dose: 5 mg); administer titrated dose tid or qid. However, if titrated dose is 7.5 or 10 mg, give 2.5–5 mg tid or qid initially, and then, once it is established that the lower doses are inadequate, give a larger dose tid or qid; bear in mind that severe reactions can occur with doses of 7.5 or 10 mg.

CONTRAINDICATIONS

Hypersensitivity to bethanechol	Hyperthyroidism	Peptic ulcer
Latent or active bronchial asthma	Pronounced bradycardia or hypotension	Vasomotor instability
Coronary artery disease	Epilepsy	Parkinsonism
Conditions where strength or integrity of GI or bladder wall is questionable	Mechanical obstruction of intestinal or urinary tract	Conditions where increased muscular activity of GI tract or urinary bladder may be harmful
Bladder neck obstruction	Spastic GI disturbances	
Marked vagotonia	Peritonitis	Acute GI inflammatory lesions

URECHOLINE

ADMINISTRATION/DOSAGE ADJUSTMENTS

Oral administration	To avoid nausea and vomiting, give tablets 1 h before or 2 h after meals
Use of atropine	After SC administration, a syringe containing atropine should always be available for treatment of toxicity; peak muscarinic effects are usually seen 15–30 min after SC injection

WARNINGS/PRECAUTIONS

Cholinergic toxicity	Violent manifestations of cholinergic overstimulation such as circulatory collapse, decreased blood pressure, abdominal cramps, bloody diarrhea, shock, and cardiac arrest are likely to occur following IM or IV administration, and, in rare instances, may result from SC injection, overdosage, or hypersensitivity. Never give this drug IM or IV. Adverse reactions rarely occur following oral administration.
Reflux infection	If the urinary sphincter fails to relax as bethanechol contracts the bladder, and urine containing bacteria is forced up the ureter into the renal pelvis, reflux infection may result
Decrease in blood pressure	Caution patients that they may experience dizziness, light-headedness, or fainting, especially when they get up from a supine or sitting position
Carcinogenicity, mutagenicity, effect on fertility	No long-term studies have been done to evaluate the carcinogenic or mutagenic potential of this drug or its effect on fertility

ADVERSE REACTIONS

Gastrointestinal	Abdominal cramps or discomfort, colicky pain, nausea, belching, diarrhea, borborgymi
Central nervous system	Headache, malaise
Ophthalmic	Lacrimation, miosis
Cardiovascular	Decreased blood pressure with reflex tachycardia, vasomotor response
Dermatological	Flushing and feeling of warmth, sensation of heat about the face, sweating
Respiratory	Bronchial constriction, asthmatic attacks
Other	Urinary urgency, salivation

OVERDOSAGE

Signs and symptoms	Abdominal discomfort, salivation, flushing ("hot feeling"), sweating, nausea, and vomiting are early signs
Treatment	Give 0.6 mg of atropine to adults and 0.01 mg/kg to children up to 12 yr of age; repeat dose q2h, as needed and tolerated. Subcutaneous administration of atropine is preferred except in emergencies when the drug can be administered IV.

DRUG INTERACTIONS

Ganglionic blocking agents	Critical fall in blood pressure; severe abdominal symptoms usually precede reaction. Exercise caution during combination therapy.
Quinidine, procainamide	▽ Cholinergic effect and possible antagonism of bethanechol
Cholinergic drugs, especially cholinesterase inhibitors	△ Cholinergic effect
Atropine sulfate	Antagonism of pharmacologic effect of bethanechol

ALTERED LABORATORY VALUES

Blood/serum values	△ Amylase △ Lipase △ Bilirubin △ Aspartate aminotransferase △ Sulfobromophthalein (BSP) retention time

No clinically significant alterations in urinary values occur at therapeutic dosages

---

USE IN CHILDREN

Safety and effectiveness for use in children have not been established

USE IN PREGNANT AND NURSING WOMEN

Pregnancy Category C: reproduction studies have not been performed. It is not known whether this drug can cause harm to the fetus or affect reproductive capacity; use during pregnancy only if clearly needed. It is also not known whether this drug is excreted in human milk; because many drugs are excreted in human milk and because of the potential for serious adverse reactions in the infant, a decision should be made to discontinue either nursing or drug therapy.

Chapter 47

Vitamins/Minerals/Infant Formulas/Nutritionals

Multivitamins/Multivitamins with Minerals	1857	**Prenatal Vitamins with Minerals**	1866
B-Complex Vitamins/B-Complex with C Vitamins	1859	**Calcium Supplements**	1867
Hematinics	1861	**Nutritionals**	1868
Pediatric Vitamins	1863	**Infant Formulas**	1871

This chapter's design allows you to compare the active ingredients of a wide variety of vitamin and mineral supplements, infant formulas, and nutritional products. The chart format makes any similarities and differences between products self-evident and lists the relative quantities of each component. The products are arranged alphabetically within the categories above; if you are unsure of exactly which category a product falls under, consult the index at the front of this book.

Across the top of each table are the US Recommended Daily Allowances (USRDA) of vitamins and minerals for various age groups. The quantities listed for each product reflect the amount supplied when taken as recommended by the manufacturer (generally, one capsule or tablet per day). As with any pharmaceutical product, it must be stressed that these products should be used according to the package labeling, unless otherwise recommended by a health-care professional. At the foot of each table is a key explaining the abbreviations used within the product descriptions.

A multivitamin product in this chapter is defined as one having at least vitamins A, D, E, and C, and some or all of the B vitamins. Niacin and niacinamide are considered interchangeable; they are designated in the table as vitamin B_3. Pantothenic acid and calcium pantothenate are also considered equivalent. The presence of dexpanthenol in a product is indicated by a footnote. The quantity of each mineral is given for the elemental form of the mineral (that is, the amount of mineral actually supplied by the product) and not the salt. Unusual or rare components are listed separately in the column headed "OTHER INGREDIENTS."

Multivitamins/Multivitamins with Minerals

		VITAMINS[1]													MINERALS											
	Form	A IU	D IU	E IU	C mg	B₁ mg	B₂ mg	B₃ mg	B₆ mg	B₁₂ µg	FA µg	BT µg	PA mg	Ca mg	P mg	Mg mg	Fe mg	Zn mg	Cu mg	I µg	Mn mg	Cr µg	Mo µg	Se µg	OTHER INGREDIENTS
---	---	---	---	---	---	---	---	---	---	---	---	---	---	---	---	---	---	---	---	---	---	---	---	---	---
USRDA (children ≥ 4 yr and adults)	–	5,000	400	30	60	1.5	1.7	20	2	6	400	300	10	1,000	1,000	400	18	15	2	150	4	–	–	–	–
BEROCCA Parenteral Nutrition (Roche) Rx	Inj	3,300	200	10	100	3	3.6	40	4	5	400	60	15	–	–	–	–	–	–	–	–	–	–	–	–
BEROCCA Plus (Roche) Rx	Tabs	5,000	–	30	500	20	20	100	25	50	800	150	25	–	–	50	27	22.5	3	–	5	100	–	–	–
	Tabs	5,000	–	30	500	20	20	100	25	50	800	150	25	–	–	50	27	22.5	3	–	5	100	–	–	–
CENTRUM (Lederle) OTC	Tabs	5,000	400	30	90	2.25	2.6	20	3	9	400	45	10	162	125	100	27	15	2	150	5	25	25	25	Vit K₁ (25 µg), K (30 mg), Cl (27.2 mg)
CLUVISOL (Ayerst) OTC	Caps	10,000	400	0.5	150	10	5	50	0.5	2.5	–	–	–	120	–	3	15	0.6	–	–	0.5	–	–	–	d-Panthenol (1 mg)
CLUVISOL 130 (Ayerst) OTC	Tabs	10,000	400	0.5	150	10	5	50	0.5	2.5	–	–	–	120	–	3	15	0.6	–	–	0.5	–	–	–	d-Panthenol (1 mg)
CLUVISOL Syrup (Ayerst) OTC	Liq	2,500	400	–	15	1	1	5	0.6	2	–	–	–	–	–	3	–	0.5	–	–	0.5	–	–	–	d-Panthenol (3 mg)
DAYALETS (Abbott) OTC	Tabs	5,000	400	30	60	1.5	1.7	20	2	6	400	–	–	–	–	–	–	–	–	–	–	–	–	–	–
DAYALETS + Iron (Abbott) OTC	Tabs	5,000	400	30	60	1.5	1.7	20	2	6	400	–	–	–	–	–	18	–	–	–	–	–	–	–	–
ELDEC (Parke-Davis) Rx	Caps	1,667	–	10	66.7	10	0.87	16.7	0.67	2	330	–	10[2]	66.7	–	–	16.7	–	–	50	–	–	–	–	–
FEMIRON Multi-Vitamins and Iron (Beecham) OTC	Tabs	5,000	400	15	60	1.5	1.7	20	2	6	400	–	–	–	–	–	20	–	–	–	–	–	–	–	–
GERIPLEX-FS (Warner-Lambert) OTC	Caps	5,000	–	5	50	5	5	15	–	2	–	–	–	80	–	–	6	0.45	1	–	1	–	–	–	Choline (20 mg), Aspergillus enzymes (2.5 gr), docusate sodium (100 mg), K (7.7 mg), Cl (7 mg)
GERITOL COMPLETE (Beecham) OTC	Tabs	5,000	400	30	60	1.5	1.7	20	2	6	400	300	10	162	125	100	50	15	2	150	7.5	15	–	15	Vit K (50 µg), K (37.5 mg), Cl (34 mg), Ni (5 µg), Si (10 µg), Sn (10 µg), V (10 µg)
GEVRAL (Lederle) OTC	Tabs	5,000	–	30	60	1.5	1.7	20	2	6	400	–	–	162	125	100	18	–	–	150	–	–	–	–	–
GEVRAL T (Lederle) OTC	Tabs	5,000	400	45	90	2.25	2.6	30	3	9	400	–	–	162	125	100	27	22.5	1.5	225	–	–	–	–	–
HEPICEBRIN (Lilly) OTC	Tabs	5,000	400	–	75	2	3	20	–	–	–	–	–	–	–	–	–	–	–	–	–	–	–	–	–
HOMICEBRIN (Lilly) OTC	Liq	2,500	400	–	60	1	1.2	10	0.8	3	–	–	–	–	–	–	–	–	–	–	–	–	–	–	Alcohol (5%)
MI-CEBRIN (Dista) OTC	Tabs	10,000	400	5.5	100	10	5	30	1.7	3	–	–	10	–	–	5	15	1.5	1	150	1	–	–	–	–
MI-CEBRIN T (Dista) OTC	Tabs	10,000	400	5.5	150	15	10	100	2	7.5	–	–	10	–	–	5	15	1.5	1	150	1	–	–	–	–

[1] B = niacin; FA = folic acid; BT = biotin; PA = pantothenic acid or calcium pantothenate
[2] Given as dexpanthenol

Multivitamins/Multivitamins with Minerals continued

				VITAMINS[1]											MINERALS										
	Form	A IU	D IU	E IU	C mg	B$_1$ mg	B$_2$ mg	B$_3$ mg	B$_6$ mg	B$_{12}$ μg	FA μg	BT μg	PA mg	Ca mg	P mg	Mg mg	Fe mg	Zn mg	Cu mg	I μg	Mn mg	Cr μg	Mo μg	Se μg	OTHER INGREDIENTS
USRDA (children ≥ 4 yr and adults)	–	5,000	400	30	60	1.5	1.7	20	2	6	400	300	10	1,000	1,000	400	18	15	2	150	4	–	–	–	–
MULTICEBRIN (Lilly) OTC	Tabs	10,000	400	6.6	75	3	3	25	1.2	3	–	–	5	–	–	–	–	–	–	–	–	–	–	–	–
M.V.I.-12 (Armour) Rx	Inj	3,300	200	10	100	3	3.6	40	4	5	400	60	15	–	–	–	–	–	–	–	–	–	–	–	Mannitol (375 mg)
M.V.I. Pediatric (Armour) Rx	Inj	2,300	400	7	80	1.2	1.4	17	1	1	140	20	5	–	–	–	–	–	–	–	–	–	–	–	Vit K$_1$ (200 μg), mannitol (375 mg)
MYADEC (Warner-Lambert) OTC	Tabs	9,000	400	30	90	10	10	20	5	10	400	45	20	70	54	100	30	15	3	150	7.5	15	15	15	Vit K (25 μg), K (8 mg)
ONE-A-DAY Essential (Miles Laboratories) OTC	Tabs	5,000	400	30	60	1.5	1.7	20	2	6	400	–	10	–	–	–	–	–	–	–	–	–	–	–	–
ONE-A-DAY Maximum Formula (Miles Laboratories) OTC	Tabs	5,000	400	30	60	1.5	1.7	20	2	6	400	30	10	129.6	100	100	18	15	2	150	2.5	10	10	10	Vit K (50 μg), K (37.5 mg), Cl (34 mg)
ONE-A-DAY Plus Extra C (Miles Laboratories) OTC	Tabs	5,000	400	30	300	1.5	1.7	20	2	6	400	–	10	–	–	–	–	–	–	–	–	–	–	–	–
OPTILETS-500 (Abbott) OTC	Tabs	10,000	400	30	500	15	10	100	5	12	–	–	20	–	–	–	–	–	–	–	–	–	–	–	–
OPTILETS-M-500 (Abbott) OTC	Tabs	10,000	400	30	500	15	10	100	5	12	–	–	20	–	–	80	20	1.5	2	150	1	–	–	–	–
SIGTAB (Upjohn) OTC	Tabs	5,000	400	15	333	10.3	10	100	6	18	400	–	20	–	–	–	–	–	–	–	–	–	–	–	–
SPARTUS (Lederle) OTC	Tabs	3,000	300	30	300	7.5	8.5	100	10	30	400	45	25	162	75	100	27	15	2	150	5	25	25	25	K (40 mg), Cl (36.3 mg)
SPARTUS + Iron (Lederle) OTC	Tabs	3,000	300	30	300	7.5	8.5	100	10	30	400	45	25	162	75	100	27	15	2	150	5	25	25	25	K (40 mg), Cl (36.3 mg)
STRESSGARD (Miles Laboratories) OTC	Tabs	5,000	400	30	600	15	10	100	5	12	400	–	20	–	–	–	18	15	2	–	–	–	–	–	–
STUART FORMULA (Stuart) OTC	Tabs	5,000	400	15	60	1.5	1.7	20	2	6	400	–	–	160	125	100	18	–	–	150	–	–	–	–	–
THERACEBRIN (Lilly) Rx	Caps	25,000	1,500	19	150	15	10	150	2.5	10	–	–	20	–	–	–	–	–	–	–	–	–	–	–	–
THERAGRAN (Squibb) OTC	Tabs	5,500	400	30	120	3	3.4	30	3	9	400	15	10	–	–	–	–	–	–	–	–	–	–	–	–
THERAGRAN Liquid (Squibb) OTC	Liq	10,000	400	–	200	10	10	100	4.1	5	–	–	21.4	–	–	–	–	–	–	–	–	–	–	–	–
THERAGRAN-M (Squibb) OTC	Tabs	5,500	400	30	120	3	3.4	30	3	9	400	15	10	40	–	100	27	15	2	150	5	15	15	10	K (7.5 mg), Cl (7.5 mg)
TYCOPAN (Lilly) Rx	Caps	20,000	1,000	22	200	10	8	60	10	15	450	160	60	–	–	–	–	–	–	–	–	–	–	–	Inositol (160 mg), choline (160 mg), aminobenzoic acid (33 mg), lipoic acid (300 μg)
UNICAP (Upjohn) OTC	Caps Tabs	5,000	400	15	60	1.5	1.7	20	2	6	400	–	–	–	–	–	–	–	–	–	–	–	–	–	–

[1] B$_3$ = niacin; FA = folic acid; BT = biotin; PA = pantothenic acid or calcium pantothenate
[2] Given as dexpanthenol

Multivitamins / Multivitamins with Minerals continued

	Form	A IU	D IU	E IU	C mg	B₁ mg	B₂ mg	B₃ mg	B₆ mg	B₁₂ μg	FA μg	BT μg	PA mg	Ca mg	P mg	Mg mg	Fe mg	Zn mg	Cu mg	I μg	Mn mg	Cr μg	Mo μg	Se μg	OTHER INGREDIENTS
USRDA (children ≥ 4 yr and adults)	–	5,000	400	30	60	1.5	1.7	20	2	6	400	300	10	1,000	1,000	400	18	15	2	150	4	–	–	–	–
UNICAP M (Upjohn) OTC	Tabs	5,000	400	30	60	1.5	1.7	20	2	6	400	–	10	60	45	–	18	15	2	150	1	–	–	–	–
UNICAP Plus Iron (Upjohn) OTC	Tabs	5,000	400	15	60	1.5	1.7	20	2	6	400	–	10	–	–	–	18	–	–	–	–	–	–	–	K (5 mg)
UNICAP Senior (Upjohn) OTC	Tabs	5,000	200	15	60	1.2	1.4	16	2.2	3	400	–	10	100	77	30	10	15	2	150	1	–	–	–	–
UNICAP T Stress Formula (Upjohn) OTC	Tabs	5,000	400	30	500	10	10	100	6	18	400	–	25	–	–	–	18	15	2	150	1	–	–	10	K (5 mg)
VICON FORTE (Glaxo) Rx	Caps	8,000	–	50	150	10	5	25	2	10	1,000	–	10	–	–	10	–	20	–	–	2	–	–	–	–
VICON Plus (Glaxo) OTC	Caps	4,000	–	50	150	10	5	25	2	–	–	–	10	–	–	10	–	20	–	–	2	–	–	–	–
VIGRAN (Squibb) OTC	Tabs	5,000	400	30	60	1.5	1.7	20	2	6	400	–	–	–	–	–	–	–	–	–	–	–	–	–	–
VITA-KAPS (Abbott) OTC	Caps	5,000	400	–	50	3	2.5	20	1	3	–	–	–	–	–	–	–	–	–	–	–	–	–	–	–
VITAKAPS-M (Abbott) OTC	Tabs	5,000	400	–	50	3	2.5	20	1	3	–	–	–	–	–	–	10	7.5	1	150	1	–	–	–	–
VI-ZAC (Glaxo) OTC	Caps	5,000	–	50	500	–	–	–	–	–	–	–	–	–	–	–	–	20	–	–	–	–	–	–	–
WITHIN (Miles Laboratories) OTC	Tabs	5,000	400	30	60	1.5	1.7	20	2	6	400	–	10	300	–	–	27	–	–	–	–	–	–	–	–
ZYMACAP (Upjohn) OTC	Caps	5,000	400	15	90	2.25	2.6	30	3	9	400	–	15	–	–	–	–	–	–	–	–	–	–	–	–

¹ B₃ = niacin; FA = folic acid; BT = biotin; PA = pantothenic acid or calcium pantothenate
² Given as dexpanthenol

B-Complex Vitamins / B-Complex with C Vitamins

	Form	A IU	D IU	E IU	C mg	B₁ mg	B₂ mg	B₃ mg	B₆ mg	B₁₂ μg	FA μg	BT μg	PA mg	Ca mg	P mg	Mg mg	Fe mg	Zn mg	Cu mg	I μg	Mn mg	Cr μg	Mo μg	Se μg	OTHER INGREDIENTS
USRDA (children ≥ 4 yr and adults)	–	5,000	400	30	60	1.5	1.7	20	2	6	400	300	10	1,000	1,000	400	18	15	2	150	4	–	–	–	–
ALLBEE C-800 (Robins) OTC	Tabs	–	–	45	800	15	17	100	25	12	–	–	25	–	–	–	–	–	–	–	–	–	–	–	–
ALLBEE C-800 plus Iron (Robins) OTC	Tabs	–	–	45	800	15	17	100	25	12	400	–	25	–	–	–	27	–	–	–	–	–	–	–	–
ALLBEE with C (Robins) OTC	Caps	–	–	–	300	15	10.2	50	5	–	–	–	10	–	–	–	–	–	–	–	–	–	–	–	–
ALLBEE-T (Robins) OTC	Tabs	–	–	–	500	15.5	10	100	8.2	5	–	–	23	–	–	–	–	–	–	–	–	–	–	–	–
BECOTIN (Dista) OTC	Caps	–	–	–	–	10	10	50	4.1	1	–	–	25	–	–	–	–	–	–	–	–	–	–	–	–
BECOTIN with Vitamin C (Dista) OTC	Caps	–	–	–	150	10	10	50	4.1	1	–	–	25	–	–	–	–	–	–	–	–	–	–	–	–
BECOTIN-T (Dista) OTC	Tabs	–	–	–	300	15	10	100	5	4	–	–	20	–	–	–	–	–	–	–	–	–	–	–	–
BEMINAL 500 (Ayerst) OTC	Tabs	–	–	–	500	25	12.5	100	10	5	–	–	20	–	–	–	–	–	–	–	–	–	–	–	–
BEMINAL Forte (Ayerst) OTC	Caps	–	–	–	250	25	12.5	50	3	2.5	–	–	10	–	–	–	–	–	–	–	–	–	–	–	–
BEMINAL STRESS PLUS with Iron (Ayerst) OTC	Tabs	–	–	45	787	25	12.5	100	10	25	400	–	20	–	–	–	27	–	–	–	–	–	–	–	–
BEMINAL STRESS PLUS with Zinc (Ayerst) OTC	Tabs	–	–	45	787	25	12.5	100	10	25	–	–	20	–	–	–	–	36	–	–	–	–	–	–	–
BEROCCA (Roche) Rx	Tabs	–	–	–	500	15	15	100	4	5	500	–	18	–	–	–	–	–	–	–	–	–	–	–	–

¹ B₃ = niacin; FA = folic acid; BT = biotin; PA = pantothenic acid or calcium pantothenate

B-Complex Vitamins/B-Complex with C Vitamins continued

					VITAMINS[1]												MINERALS							
	Form	A IU	D IU	E IU	C mg	B₁ mg	B₂ mg	B₃ mg	B₆ mg	B₁₂ μg	FA μg	BT μg	PA mg	Ca mg	P mg	Mg mg	Fe mg	Zn mg	Cu mg	I μg	Mn mg	Cr μg	Mo μg	Se μg	OTHER INGREDIENTS
USRDA (children ≥ 4 yr and adults)	—	5,000	400	30	60	1.5	1.7	20	2	6	400	300	10	1,000	1,000	400	18	15	2	150	4	—	—	—	—
CEBENASE (Upjohn) Rx	Tabs	—	—	—	150	10	10	75	2.5	—	—	—	10	—	—	—	—	—	—	—	—	—	—	—	Vit B₁₂ with intrinsic factor concentrate [intrinase] (0.17 NF units)
CEFOL (Abbott) Rx	Tabs	—	—	30	750	15	10	100	5	6	500	—	20	—	—	—	—	—	—	—	—	—	—	—	—
GERIPLEX FS Liquid (Warner-Lambert) OTC	Liq	—	—	—	—	1.2	1.7	15	1	5	—	—	—	—	—	—	15	—	—	—	—	—	—	—	Pluronic F-68 (200 mg), alcohol (18%)
GERITOL High Potency Iron & Vitamin Tonic (Beecham) OTC	Liq	—	—	—	—	2.5	2.5	50	0.5	0.75	—	—	—	—	—	—	50	—	—	—	—	—	—	—	Panthenol (2 mg), methionine (25 mg), choline (50 mg)
GERIX (Abbott) OTC	Liq	—	—	—	—	3	3	50	0.8	3	—	—	—	—	—	—	15	—	—	—	—	—	—	—	Alcohol (20%)
GEVRABON (Lederle) OTC	Liq	—	—	—	—	5	2.5	50	1	1	—	—	10	—	—	2	15	2	—	100	2	—	—	—	Choline (100 mg)
LAROBEC (Roche) Rx	Tabs	—	—	—	500	15	15	100	—	5	500	—	18	—	—	—	—	—	—	—	—	—	—	—	—
LEDERPLEX (Lederle) OTC	Caps Liq	—	—	—	—	2.25	2.6	30	3	9	—	—	15	—	—	—	—	—	—	—	—	—	—	—	—
OREXIN (Stuart) OTC	Tabs	—	—	—	—	10	—	—	5	25	—	—	—	—	—	—	—	—	—	—	—	—	—	—	—
PROBEC-T (Stuart) OTC	Tabs	—	—	—	600	15	10	100	5	5	—	—	20	—	—	—	—	—	—	—	—	—	—	—	—
STRESSCAPS (Lederle) OTC	Caps	—	—	—	300	10	10	100	2	6	—	—	20	—	—	—	—	—	—	—	—	—	—	—	—
STRESSTABS 600 (Lederle) OTC	Tabs	—	—	30	600	15	10	100	5	12	400	45	20	—	—	—	—	—	—	—	—	—	—	—	—
STRESSTABS 600 + Iron (Lederle) OTC	Tabs	—	—	30	600	15	10	100	5	12	400	45	20	—	—	—	27	—	—	—	—	—	—	—	—
STRESSTABS 600 + Zinc (Lederle) OTC	Tabs	—	—	30	600	15	10	100	5	12	400	45	20	—	—	—	—	23.9	3	—	—	—	—	—	—
SURBEX (Abbott) OTC	Tabs	—	—	—	—	6	6	30	2.5	5	—	—	10	—	—	—	—	—	—	—	—	—	—	—	—
SURBEX with C (Abbott) OTC	Tabs	—	—	—	250	6	6	30	2.5	5	—	—	10	—	—	—	—	—	—	—	—	—	—	—	—
SURBEX-750 with Iron (Abbott) OTC	Tabs	—	—	30	750	15	15	100	25	12	400	—	20	—	—	—	27	—	—	—	—	—	—	—	—
SURBEX-750 with Zinc (Abbott) OTC	Tabs	—	—	30	750	15	15	100	20	12	400	—	20	—	—	—	—	22.5	—	—	—	—	—	—	—
SURBEX-T (Abbott) OTC	Tabs	—	—	—	500	15	10	100	5	10	—	—	20	—	—	—	—	—	—	—	—	—	—	—	—
THERA-COMBEX H-P (Warner-Lambert) OTC	Caps	—	—	—	500	25	15	100	10	5	—	—	—	—	—	—	—	—	—	—	—	—	—	—	*dl*-Panthenol (20 mg)
THERAGRAN Stress Formula (Squibb) OTC	Tabs	—	—	30	600	15	15	100	25	12	400	45	20	—	—	—	27	—	—	—	—	—	—	—	—
TRI-B-PLEX (Anabolic) OTC	Caps	—	—	—	—	100	40	200	50	25	400	300	100	—	—	—	—	—	—	—	—	—	—	—	—
TROPH-IRON (SmithKline Consumer Products) OTC	Liq	—	—	—	—	10	—	—	—	25	—	—	—	—	—	—	20	—	—	—	—	—	—	—	—

[1] B₃ = niacin; FA = folic acid; BT = biotin; PA = pantothenic acid or calcium pantothenate

B-Complex Vitamins / B-Complex with C Vitamins continued

	Form	VITAMINS[1]												MINERALS										OTHER INGREDIENTS
		A IU	D IU	E IU	C mg	B$_1$ mg	B$_2$ mg	B$_3$ mg	B$_6$ mg	B$_{12}$ μg	FA μg	BT μg	PA mg	Ca mg	P mg	Mg mg	Fe mg	Zn mg	Cu mg	I μg	Mn mg	Cr μg	Mo μg	Se μg	
USRDA (children ≥ 4 yr and adults)	—	5,000	400	30	60	1.5	1.7	20	2	6	400	300	10	1,000	1,000	400	18	15	2	150	4	—	—	—	—
TROPHITE (SmithKline Consumer Products) OTC	Liq Tabs	—	—	—	—	10	—	—	—	25	—	—	—	—	—	—	—	—	—	—	—	—	—	—	—
VICON-C (Glaxo) OTC	Caps	—	—	—	300	20	10	100	5	—	—	—	20	—	—	70	—	80	—	—	—	—	—	—	—
Z-BEC (Robins) OTC	Tabs	—	—	45	600	15	10.2	100	10	6	—	—	25	—	—	—	—	22.5	—	—	—	—	—	—	—

[1] B$_3$ = niacin; FA = folic acid; BT = biotin; PA = pantothenic acid or calcium pantothenate

Hematinics

	Form	VITAMINS[1]												MINERALS										OTHER INGREDIENTS
		A IU	D IU	E IU	C mg	B$_1$ mg	B$_2$ mg	B$_3$ mg	B$_6$ mg	B$_{12}$ μg	FA μg	BT μg	PA mg	Ca mg	P mg	Mg mg	Fe mg	Zn mg	Cu mg	I μg	Mn mg	Cr μg	Mo μg	Se μg	
USRDA (children ≥ 4 yr and adults)	—	5,000	400	30	60	1.5	1.7	20	2	6	400	300	10	1,000	1,000	400	18	15	2	150	4	—	—	—	—
FEMIRON (Beecham) OTC	Tabs	—	—	—	—	—	—	—	—	—	—	—	—	—	—	—	20	—	—	—	—	—	—	—	—
FEOSOL (SmithKline Consumer Products) OTC	Caps	—	—	—	—	—	—	—	—	—	—	—	—	—	—	—	50	—	—	—	—	—	—	—	—
FEOSOL (SmithKline Consumer Products) OTC	Tabs	—	—	—	—	—	—	—	—	—	—	—	—	—	—	—	65	—	—	—	—	—	—	—	—
FEOSOL Elixir (SmithKline Consumer Products) OTC	Liq	—	—	—	—	—	—	—	—	—	—	—	—	—	—	—	44	—	—	—	—	—	—	—	Alcohol (5%)
FERANCEE (Stuart) OTC	Tabs	—	—	—	150	—	—	—	—	—	—	—	—	—	—	—	67	—	—	—	—	—	—	—	—
FERANCEE-HP (Stuart) OTC	Tabs	—	—	—	600	—	—	—	—	—	—	—	—	—	—	—	110	—	—	—	—	—	—	—	—
FERGON (Winthrop Consumer Products) OTC	Tabs	—	—	—	—	—	—	—	—	—	—	—	—	—	—	—	36	—	—	—	—	—	—	—	—
FERGON Plus (Winthrop Consumer Products) Rx	Tabs	—	—	—	75	—	—	—	—	0.5 unit	—	—	—	—	—	—	60	—	—	—	—	—	—	—	—
FERMALOX (Rorer) OTC	Tabs	—	—	—	—	—	—	—	—	—	—	—	—	—	—	—	40	—	—	—	—	—	—	—	Magnesium-aluminum hydroxide (200 mg)
FERO-FOLIC-500 (Abbott) Rx	Tabs	—	—	—	500	—	—	—	—	—	800	—	—	—	—	—	105	—	—	—	—	—	—	—	—
FERO-GRAD-500 (Abbott) OTC	Tabs	—	—	—	500	—	—	—	—	—	—	—	—	—	—	—	105	—	—	—	—	—	—	—	—
FERO-GRADUMET (Abbott) OTC	Tabs	—	—	—	—	—	—	—	—	—	—	—	—	—	—	—	105	—	—	—	—	—	—	—	—
FERRO-SEQUELS (Lederle) OTC	Caps	—	—	—	—	—	—	—	—	—	—	—	—	—	—	—	50	—	—	—	—	—	—	—	Docusate sodium (100 mg)

[1] B$_3$ = niacin; FA = folic acid; BT = biotin; PA = pantothenic acid or pantothenate
[2] Given as dexpanthenol

COMPENDIUM OF DRUG THERAPY

Hematinics continued

	Form	VITAMINS[1]													MINERALS										OTHER INGREDIENTS
		A IU	D IU	E IU	C mg	B₁ mg	B₂ mg	B₃ mg	B₆ mg	B₁₂ μg	FA μg	BT μg	PA mg	Ca mg	P mg	Mg mg	Fe mg	Zn mg	Cu mg	I μg	Mn mg	Cr μg	Mo μg	Se μg	
USRDA (children ≥ 4 yr and adults)	–	5,000	400	30	60	1.5	1.7	20	2	6	400	300	10	1,000	1,000	400	18	15	2	150	4	–	–	–	–
HEPTUNA Plus (Roerig) Rx	Caps	–	–	–	150	3.1	2	15	1.6	5	–	–	0.9	37.4	29	2	100	–	1	50	0.03	–	200	–	Desiccated liver (50 mg), intrinsic factor concentrate (25 mg), K (1.7 mg)
IBERET (Abbott) OTC	Tabs	–	–	–	150	6	6	30	5	25	–	–	10	–	–	–	105	–	–	–	–	–	–	–	–
IBERET-500 (Abbott) OTC	Tabs	–	–	–	500	6	6	30	5	25	–	–	10	–	–	–	105	–	–	–	–	–	–	–	–
IBERET Liquid (Abbott) OTC	Liq	–	–	–	37.5	1.5	1.5	7.5	1.25	6.25	–	–	2.5[2]	–	–	–	26.25	–	–	–	–	–	–	–	–
IBERET-500 Liquid (Abbott) OTC	Liq	–	–	–	125	1.5	1.5	7.5	1.25	6.25	–	–	2.5[2]	–	–	–	26.25	–	–	–	–	–	–	–	–
IBERET-FOLIC-500 (Abbott) Rx	Tabs	–	–	–	500	6	6	30	5	25	800	–	10	–	–	–	105	–	–	–	–	–	–	–	–
IMFERON (Merrell Dow) Rx	Inj	–	–	–	–	–	–	–	–	–	–	–	–	–	–	–	50	–	–	–	–	–	–	–	–
INCREMIN with Iron (Lederle) OTC	Liq	–	–	–	–	10	–	–	5	25	–	–	–	–	–	–	30	–	–	–	–	–	–	–	Lysine (300 mg), sorbitol (3.5 g), alcohol (0.75%)
IRCON-FA (Key) Rx	Tabs	–	–	–	–	–	–	–	–	–	1,000	–	–	–	–	–	82	–	–	–	–	–	–	–	–
MOL-IRON (Schering) OTC	Tabs	–	–	–	–	–	–	–	–	–	–	–	–	–	–	–	39	–	–	–	–	–	–	–	–
MOL-IRON with Vitamin C (Schering) OTC	Tabs	–	–	–	75	–	–	–	–	–	–	–	–	–	–	–	39	–	–	–	–	–	–	–	–
PERIHEMIN (Lederle) Rx	Caps	–	–	–	50	–	–	–	–	5	330	–	–	–	–	–	55	–	–	–	–	–	–	–	Intrinsic factor concentrate (25 mg)
PERITINIC (Lederle) Rx	Tabs	–	–	–	200	7.5	7.5	30	7.5	50	50	–	15	–	–	–	100	–	–	–	–	–	–	–	Docusate sodium (100 mg)
PRONEMIA (Lederle) Rx	Caps	–	–	–	150	–	–	–	–	15	1,000	–	–	–	–	–	115	–	–	–	–	–	–	–	Intrinsic factor concentrate (75 mg)
SIMRON (Merrell Dow) OTC	Caps	–	–	–	–	–	–	–	–	–	–	–	–	–	–	–	10	–	–	–	–	–	–	–	–
SIMRON PLUS (Merrell Dow) OTC	Caps	–	–	–	50	–	–	–	1	3.33	100	–	–	–	–	–	10	–	–	–	–	–	–	–	–
SLOW FE (CIBA) OTC	Tabs	–	–	–	–	–	–	–	–	–	–	–	–	–	–	–	50	–	–	–	–	–	–	–	–
STUARTINIC (Stuart) OTC	Tabs	–	–	–	500	6	6	20	1	25	–	–	10	–	–	–	100	–	–	–	–	–	–	–	–
TABRON (Parke-Davis) Rx	Tabs	–	–	30	500	6	6	30	5	25	1,000	–	10	–	–	–	100	–	–	–	–	–	–	–	Docusate sodium (50 mg)
THERAGRAN HEMATINIC (Squibb) Rx	Tabs	8,333	133	5	100	3.3	3.3	33.3	3.3	50	330	–	11.7	–	–	41.7	66.7	–	0.67	–	–	–	–	–	–

[1] B₃ = niacin; FA = folic acid; BT = biotin; PA = pantothenic acid or pantothenate
[2] Given as dexpanthenol

Hematinics continued

	Form	VITAMINS[1] A IU	D IU	E IU	C mg	B₁ mg	B₂ mg	B₃ mg	B₆ mg	B₁₂ μg	FA μg	BT μg	PA mg	MINERALS Ca mg	P mg	Mg mg	Fe mg	Zn mg	Cu mg	I μg	Mn mg	Cr μg	Mo μg	Se μg	OTHER INGREDIENTS
USRDA (children ≥ 4 yr and adults)	—	5,000	400	30	60	1.5	1.7	20	2	6	400	300	10	1,000	1,000	400	18	15	2	150	4	—	—	—	—
TriHEMIC 600 (Lederle) Rx	Tabs	—	—	30	600	—	—	—	—	25	1,000	—	—	—	—	—	115	—	—	—	—	—	—	—	Docusate sodium (50 mg), intrinsic factor concentrate (75 mg)
TRINSICON (Glaxo) Rx	Caps	—	—	—	75	—	—	—	—	15	500	—	—	—	—	—	110	—	—	—	—	—	—	—	Intrinsic factor concentrate (240 mg)
TRINSICON M (Glaxo) Rx	Caps	—	—	—	75	—	—	—	—	15	—	—	—	—	—	—	110	—	—	—	—	—	—	—	Intrinsic factor concentrate (240 mg)
VITRON-C (Fisons) OTC	Tabs	—	—	—	125	—	—	—	—	—	—	—	—	—	—	—	66	—	—	—	—	—	—	—	—
VITRON-C-PLUS (Fisons) OTC	Tabs	—	—	—	250	—	—	—	—	—	—	—	—	—	—	—	131	—	—	—	—	—	—	—	—

[1] B₃ = niacin; FA = folic acid; BT = biotin; PA = pantothenic acid or pantothenate
[2] Given as dexpanthenol

Pediatric Vitamins

	Form	VITAMINS[1] A IU	D IU	E IU	C mg	B₁ mg	B₂ mg	B₃ mg	B₆ mg	B₁₂ μg	FA μg	BT μg	PA mg	MINERALS Ca mg	P mg	Mg mg	Fe mg	Zn mg	Cu mg	I μg	Mn mg	Cr μg	Mo μg	Se μg	OTHER INGREDIENTS
USRDA (infants)	—	1,500	400	5	35	0.5	0.6	8	0.4	2	100	150	3	600	500	70	15	5	0.6	45	—	—	—	—	—
USRDA (children < 4 yr)	—	2,500	400	10	40	0.7	0.8	9	0.7	3	200	150	5	800	800	200	10	8	1	70	—	—	—	—	—
USRDA (children ≥ 4 yr and adults)	—	5,000	400	30	60	1.5	1.7	20	2	6	400	300	10	1,000	1,000	400	18	15	2	150	4	—	—	—	—
ABDEC (Warner-Lambert) OTC	Drps	1,500	400	5	35	0.5	0.6	8	0.4	2	—	50	3	—	—	—	—	—	—	—	—	—	—	—	—
ALDEFLOR Chewable (Upjohn) Rx	Tabs	4,000	400	—	75	2	2	18	1	2	—	—	5	—	—	—	—	—	—	—	—	—	—	—	Fluoride (0.5 mg)
	Tabs	4,000	400	—	75	2	2	18	1	2	—	—	5	—	—	—	—	—	—	—	—	—	—	—	Fluoride (1 mg)
ALDEFLOR Drops (Upjohn) Rx	Drps	2,000	400	—	50	—	—	—	1	—	—	—	—	—	—	—	—	—	—	—	—	—	—	—	Fluoride (0.5 mg)
ALDEFLOR M (Upjohn) Rx	Tabs	6,000	400	—	100	1.5	2.5	20	10	2	100	—	10	250	—	—	30	—	—	—	—	—	—	—	Fluoride (1 mg)
BUGS BUNNY (Miles Laboratories) OTC	Tabs	2,500	400	15	60	1.05	1.2	13.5	1.05	4.5	300	—	—	—	—	—	—	—	—	—	—	—	—	—	—
BUGS BUNNY plus Iron (Miles Laboratories) OTC	Tabs	2,500	400	15	60	1.05	1.2	13.5	1.05	4.5	300	—	—	—	—	—	15	—	—	—	—	—	—	—	—
BUGS BUNNY + Minerals (Miles Laboratories) OTC	Tabs	5,000	400	30	60	1.5	1.7	20	2	6	400	40	10	100	100	20	18	15	2	150	—	—	—	—	—
BUGS BUNNY with Extra C (Miles Laboratories) OTC	Tabs	2,500	400	15	250	1.05	1.2	13.5	1.05	4.5	300	—	—	—	—	—	—	—	—	—	—	—	—	—	—

[1] B₃ = niacin; FA = folic acid; BT = biotin; PA = pantothenic acid or pantothenate
[2] Given as dexpanthenol

Pediatric Vitamins continued

	Form	VITAMINS[1] A IU	D IU	E IU	C mg	B₁ mg	B₂ mg	B₃ mg	B₆ mg	B₁₂ μg	FA μg	BT μg	PA mg	MINERALS Ca mg	P mg	Mg mg	Fe mg	Zn mg	Cu mg	I μg	Mn mg	Cr μg	Mo μg	Se μg	OTHER INGREDIENTS
USRDA (infants)	–	1,500	400	5	35	0.5	0.6	8	0.4	2	100	150	3	600	500	70	15	5	0.6	45	–	–	–	–	–
USRDA (children < 4 yr)	–	2,500	400	10	40	0.7	0.8	9	0.7	3	200	150	5	800	800	200	10	8	1	70	–	–	–	–	–
USRDA (children ≥ 4 yr and adults)	–	5,000	400	30	60	1.5	1.7	20	2	6	400	300	10	1,000	1,000	400	18	15	2	150	4	–	–	–	–
CENTRUM, Jr. (Lederle) *OTC*	Tabs	5,000	400	30	60	1.5	1.7	20	2	6	400	45	10	108	50	40	18	15	2	150	1	20	20	–	Vit K₁ (6 μg)
CENTRUM, Jr. + Extra C (Lederle) *OTC*	Tabs	5,000	400	30	300	1.5	1.7	20	2	6	400	45	10	108	50	40	18	15	2	150	1	20	20	–	Vit K₁ (10 μg)
CENTRUM, Jr. + Extra Calcium (Lederle) *OTC*	Tabs	5,000	400	30	60	1.5	1.7	20	2	6	400	45	10	160	50	40	18	15	2	150	1	20	20	–	Vit K₁ (10 μg)
CENTRUM, Jr. + Iron (Lederle) *OTC*	Tabs	5,000	400	30	60	1.5	1.7	20	2	6	400	45	10	108	50	40	18	15	2	150	1	20	20	–	Vit K₁ (10 μg)
CE-VI-SOL (Mead Johnson) *OTC*	Drps	–	–	–	35	–	–	–	–	–	–	–	–	–	–	–	–	–	–	–	–	–	–	–	Alcohol (5%)
FLINTSTONES (Miles Laboratories) *OTC*	Tabs	2,500	400	15	60	1.05	1.2	13.5	1.05	4.5	300	–	–	–	–	–	–	–	–	–	–	–	–	–	–
FLINTSTONES Complete (Miles Laboratories) *OTC*	Tabs	5,000	400	30	60	1.5	1.7	20	2	6	400	40	10	100	100	20	18	15	2	150	–	–	–	–	–
FLINTSTONES plus Extra C (Miles Laboratories) *OTC*	Tabs	2,500	400	15	250	1.05	1.2	13.5	1.05	4.5	300	–	–	–	–	–	–	–	–	–	–	–	–	–	–
FLINTSTONES plus Iron (Miles Laboratories) *OTC*	Tabs	2,500	400	15	60	1.05	1.2	13.5	1.05	4.5	300	–	–	–	–	–	15	–	–	–	–	–	–	–	–
LURIDE (Colgate-Hoyt) *Rx*	Drps	–	–	–	–	–	–	–	–	–	–	–	–	–	–	–	–	–	–	–	–	–	–	–	Fluoride (0.125 mg)
LURIDE 0.25 mg F (Colgate-Hoyt) *Rx*	Tabs	–	–	–	–	–	–	–	–	–	–	–	–	–	–	–	–	–	–	–	–	–	–	–	Fluoride (0.25 mg)
LURIDE 0.5 mg F Chewable (Colgate-Hoyt) *Rx*	Tabs	–	–	–	–	–	–	–	–	–	–	–	–	–	–	–	–	–	–	–	–	–	–	–	Fluoride (0.5 mg)
LURIDE 1.0 mg F (Colgate-Hoyt) *Rx*	Tabs	–	–	–	–	–	–	–	–	–	–	–	–	–	–	–	–	–	–	–	–	–	–	–	Fluoride (1 mg)
LURIDE-SF 1.0 mg F (Colgate-Hoyt) *Rx*	Tabs	–	–	–	–	–	–	–	–	–	–	–	–	–	–	–	–	–	–	–	–	–	–	–	Fluoride (1 mg)
MULVIDREN-F (Stuart) *Rx*	Tabs	4,000	400	–	75	2	2	10	1.2	3	–	–	3	–	–	–	–	–	–	–	–	–	–	–	Fluoride (1 mg)
POLY-VI-FLOR 0.25 mg (Mead Johnson) *Rx*	Drps	1,500	400	5	35	0.5	0.6	8	0.4	2	–	–	–	–	–	–	–	–	–	–	–	–	–	–	Fluoride (0.25 mg)
POLY-VI-FLOR 0.5 mg (Mead Johnson) *Rx*	Drps	1,500	400	5	35	0.5	0.6	8	0.4	2	–	–	–	–	–	–	–	–	–	–	–	–	–	–	Fluoride (0.5 mg)
POLY-VI-FLOR 0.5 mg (Mead Johnson) *Rx*	Tabs	2,500	400	15	60	1.05	1.2	13.5	1.05	4.5	300	–	–	–	–	–	–	–	–	–	–	–	–	–	Fluoride (0.5 mg)
POLY-VI-FLOR 1.0 mg (Mead Johnson) *Rx*	Tabs	2,500	400	15	60	1.05	1.2	13.5	1.05	4.5	300	–	–	–	–	–	–	–	–	–	–	–	–	–	Fluoride (1 mg)
POLY-VI-FLOR 0.25 mg with Iron (Mead Johnson) *Rx*	Drps	1,500	400	5	35	0.5	0.6	8	0.4	–	–	–	–	–	–	–	10	–	–	–	–	–	–	–	Fluoride (0.25 mg)
POLY-VI-FLOR 0.5 mg with Iron (Mead Johnson) *Rx*	Drps	1,500	400	5	35	0.5	0.6	8	0.4	–	–	–	–	–	–	–	10	–	–	–	–	–	–	–	Fluoride (0.5 mg)
POLY-VI-FLOR 0.5 mg with Iron (Mead Johnson) *Rx*	Tabs	2,500	400	15	60	1.05	1.2	13.5	1.05	4.5	300	–	–	–	–	–	12	10	1	–	–	–	–	–	Fluoride (0.5 mg)

[1] B₃ = niacin; FA = folic acid; BT = biotin; PA = pantothenic acid or pantothenate
[2] Given as dexpanthenol

Pediatric Vitamins continued

	Form	VITAMINS[1] A IU	D IU	E IU	C mg	B₁ mg	B₂ mg	B₃ mg	B₆ mg	B₁₂ μg	FA μg	BT μg	PA mg	MINERALS Ca mg	P mg	Mg mg	Fe mg	Zn mg	Cu mg	I μg	Mn mg	Cr μg	Mo μg	Se μg	OTHER INGREDIENTS
USRDA (infants)	—	1,500	400	5	35	0.5	0.6	8	0.4	2	100	150	3	600	500	70	15	5	0.6	45	—	—	—	—	—
USRDA (children < 4 yr)	—	2,500	400	10	40	0.7	0.8	9	0.7	3	200	150	5	800	800	200	10	8	1	70	—	—	—	—	—
USRDA (children ≥ 4 yr and adults)	—	5,000	400	30	60	1.5	1.7	20	2	6	400	300	10	1,000	1,000	400	18	15	2	150	4	—	—	—	—
POLY-VI-FLOR 1.0 mg with Iron (Mead Johnson) Rx	Tabs	2,500	400	15	60	1.05	1.2	13.5	1.05	4.5	300	—	—	—	—	—	12	10	1	—	—	—	—	—	Fluoride (1 mg)
POLY-VI-SOL (Mead Johnson) OTC	Drps	1,500	400	5	35	0.5	0.6	8	0.4	2	—	—	—	—	—	—	—	—	—	—	—	—	—	—	—
POLY-VI-SOL (Mead Johnson) OTC	Tabs	2,500	400	15	60	1.05	1.2	13.5	1.05	4.5	300	—	—	—	—	—	—	—	—	—	—	—	—	—	—
POLY-VI-SOL with Iron (Mead Johnson) OTC	Drps	1,500	400	5	35	0.5	0.6	8	0.4	—	—	—	—	—	—	—	10	—	—	—	—	—	—	—	—
POLY-VI-SOL with Iron and Zinc (Mead Johnson) OTC	Tabs	2,500	400	15	60	1.05	1.2	13.5	1.05	4.5	300	—	—	—	—	—	12	8	—	—	—	—	—	—	—
SMURF (Mead Johnson) OTC	Tabs	2,500	400	15	60	1.05	1.2	13.5	1.05	4.5	300	—	—	—	—	—	—	—	—	—	—	—	—	—	—
SMURF with Iron and Zinc (Mead Johnson) OTC	Tabs	2,500	400	15	60	1.05	1.2	13.5	1.05	4.5	300	—	—	—	—	—	12	8	—	—	—	—	—	—	—
TRI-VI-FLOR 0.25 mg (Mead Johnson) Rx	Drps	1,500	400	—	35	—	—	—	—	—	—	—	—	—	—	—	—	—	—	—	—	—	—	—	Fluoride (0.25 mg)
TRI-VI-FLOR 0.5 mg (Mead Johnson) Rx	Drps	1,500	400	—	35	—	—	—	—	—	—	—	—	—	—	—	—	—	—	—	—	—	—	—	Fluoride (0.5 mg)
TRI-VI-FLOR 1.0 mg (Mead Johnson) Rx	Tabs	2,500	400	—	60	—	—	—	—	—	—	—	—	—	—	—	—	—	—	—	—	—	—	—	Fluoride (1.0 mg)
TRI-VI-FLOR 0.25 mg with Iron (Mead Johnson) Rx	Drps	1,500	400	—	35	—	—	—	—	—	—	—	—	—	—	—	10	—	—	—	—	—	—	—	Fluoride (0.25 mg)
TRI-VI-SOL (Mead Johnson) OTC	Drps	1,500	400	—	35	—	—	—	—	—	—	—	—	—	—	—	—	—	—	—	—	—	—	—	—
TRI-VI-SOL with Iron (Mead Johnson) OTC	Drps	1,500	400	—	35	—	—	—	—	—	—	—	—	—	—	—	10	—	—	—	—	—	—	—	—
UNICAP Jr Chewable (Upjohn) OTC	Tabs	5,000	400	15	60	1.5	1.7	20	2	6	400	—	—	—	—	—	—	—	—	—	—	—	—	—	—
VI-DAYLIN ADC Drops (Ross) OTC	Drps	1,500	400	—	35	0.5	0.6	8	0.4	—	—	—	—	—	—	—	—	—	—	—	—	—	—	—	—
VI-DAYLIN Chewable (Ross) OTC	Tabs	2,500	400	15	60	1.05	1.2	13.5	1.05	4.5	300	—	—	—	—	—	—	—	—	—	—	—	—	—	—
VI-DAYLIN Drops (Ross) OTC	Drps	1,500	400	5	35	0.5	0.6	8	0.4	1.5	—	—	—	—	—	—	—	—	—	—	—	—	—	—	—
VI-DAYLIN Liquid (Ross) OTC	Liq	2,500	400	15	60	1.05	1.2	13.5	1.05	4.5	—	—	—	—	—	—	—	—	—	—	—	—	—	—	—
VI-DAYLIN ADC + Iron Drops (Ross) OTC	Drps	1,500	400	—	35	—	—	—	—	—	—	—	—	—	—	—	10	—	—	—	—	—	—	—	—
VI-DAYLIN + Iron Chewable (Ross) OTC	Tabs	2,500	400	15	60	1.05	1.2	13.5	1.05	4.5	300	—	—	—	—	—	12	—	—	—	—	—	—	—	—
VI-DAYLIN + Iron Drops (Ross) OTC	Drps	1,500	400	5	35	0.5	0.6	8	0.4	1.5	—	—	—	—	—	—	10	—	—	—	—	—	—	—	—
VI-DAYLIN + Iron Liquid (Ross) OTC	Liq	2,500	400	15	60	1.05	1.2	13.5	1.05	4.5	—	—	—	—	—	—	10	—	—	—	—	—	—	—	—
VI-DAYLIN/F ADC Drops (Ross) Rx	Drps	1,500	400	—	35	—	—	—	—	—	—	—	—	—	—	—	—	—	—	—	—	—	—	—	Fluoride (0.25 mg)
VI-DAYLIN/F Chewable (Ross) Rx	Tabs	2,500	400	15	60	1.05	1.2	13.5	1.05	4.5	300	—	—	—	—	—	—	—	—	—	—	—	—	—	Fluoride (1 mg)

[1] B₃ = niacin; FA = folic acid; BT = biotin; PA = pantothenic acid or pantothenate
[2] Given as dexpanthenol

Pediatric Vitamins continued

	Form	A IU	D IU	E IU	C mg	B₁ mg	B₂ mg	B₃ mg	B₆ mg	B₁₂ µg	FA µg	BT µg	PA mg	Ca mg	P mg	Mg mg	Fe mg	Zn mg	Cu mg	I µg	Mn mg	Cr µg	Mo µg	Se µg	OTHER INGREDIENTS
USRDA *(infants)*	—	1,500	400	5	35	0.5	0.6	8	0.4	2	100	150	3	600	500	70	15	5	0.6	45	—	—	—	—	—
USRDA *(children < 4 yr)*	—	2,500	400	10	40	0.7	0.8	9	0.7	3	200	150	5	800	800	200	10	8	1	70	—	—	—	—	—
USRDA *(children ≥ 4 yr and adults)*	—	5,000	400	30	60	1.5	1.7	20	2	6	400	300	10	1,000	1,000	400	18	15	2	150	4	—	—	—	—
VI-DAYLIN/F Drops (Ross) Rx	Drps	1,500	400	5	35	0.5	0.6	8	0.4	—	—	—	—	—	—	—	—	—	—	—	—	—	—	—	Fluoride (0.25 mg)
VI-DAYLIN/F ADC + Iron Drops (Ross) Rx	Drps	1,500	400	—	35	—	—	—	—	—	—	—	—	—	—	—	10	—	—	—	—	—	—	—	Fluoride (0.25 mg)
VI-DAYLIN/F + Iron Chewable (Ross) Rx	Tabs	2,500	400	15	60	1.05	1.2	13.5	1.05	4.5	300	—	—	—	—	—	12	—	—	—	—	—	—	—	Fluoride (1 mg)
VI-DAYLIN/F + Iron Drops (Ross) Rx	Drps	1,500	400	5	35	0.5	0.6	8	0.4	—	—	—	—	—	—	—	10	—	—	—	—	—	—	—	Fluoride (0.25 mg)
VI-PENTA Infant Drops (Roche) OTC	Drps	5,000	400	2	50	—	—	—	—	—	—	—	—	—	—	—	—	—	—	—	—	—	—	—	—
VI-PENTA Multivitamin Drops (Roche) OTC	Drps	5,000	400	2	50	1	1	10	1	3	—	30	10[2]	—	—	—	—	—	—	—	—	—	—	—	—
VI-PENTA F Chewable (Roche) Rx	Tabs	5,000	400	2	60	1.2	1.5	10	1	3	—	40	9	—	—	—	—	—	—	—	—	—	—	—	Fluoride (1 mg)
VI-PENTA F Infant Drops (Roche) Rx	Drps	5,000	400	2	50	—	—	—	—	—	—	—	—	—	—	—	—	—	—	—	—	—	—	—	Fluoride (0.5 mg)
VI-PENTA F Multivitamin Drops (Roche) Rx	Drps	5,000	400	2	50	1	1	10	0.8	—	—	30	10[2]	—	—	—	—	—	—	—	—	—	—	—	Fluoride (0.5 mg)

[1] B₃ = niacin; FA = folic acid; BT = biotin; PA = pantothenic acid or pantothenate
[2] Given as dexpanthenol

Prenatal Vitamins with Minerals

	Form	A IU	D IU	E IU	C mg	B₁ mg	B₂ mg	B₃ mg	B₆ mg	B₁₂ µg	FA µg	BT µg	PA mg	Ca mg	P mg	Mg mg	Fe mg	Zn mg	Cu mg	I µg	Mn mg	Cr µg	Mo µg	Se µg	OTHER INGREDIENTS
USRDA *for pregnant or lactating women*	—	8,000	400	30	60	1.7	2	20	2.5	8	800	300	10	1,300	1,300	450	18	15	2	150	—	—	—	—	—
EN-CEBRIN (Lilly) OTC	Caps	4,000	400	—	50	3	2	10	1.7	5	—	—	5	250	—	5	30	1.5	1	150	1	—	—	—	—
EN-CEBRIN F (Lilly) Rx	Caps	4,000	400	—	50	3	2	10	2	5	1,000	—	5	250	—	5	30	1.5	1	150	1	—	—	—	—
FILIBON (Lederle) OTC	Tabs	5,000	400	30	60	1.5	1.7	20	2	6	400	—	—	125	—	100	18	—	—	150	—	—	—	—	—
FILIBON F.A. (Lederle) Rx	Tabs	8,000	400	30	60	1.7	2	20	4	8	1,000	—	—	250	—	100	45	—	—	150	—	—	—	—	—
FILIBON Forte (Lederle) Rx	Tabs	8,000	400	45	90	2	2.5	30	3	12	1,000	—	—	300	—	100	45	—	—	200	—	—	—	—	—
MATERNA 1•60 (Lederle) Rx	Tabs	8,000	400	30	100	3	3.4	20	10	12	1,000	30	10	250	—	25	60	25	2	150	5	25	25	—	—
NATABEC (Warner-Lambert) OTC	Caps	4,000	400	—	50	3	2	10	3	5	—	—	—	240	—	—	30	—	—	—	—	—	—	—	—
NATABEC Rx (Parke-Davis) Rx	Caps	4,000	400	—	50	3	2	10	3	5	1,000	—	—	240	—	—	30	—	—	—	—	—	—	—	—
NATABEC with Fluoride (Parke-Davis) Rx	Caps	4,000	400	—	50	3	2	10	3	5	—	—	—	240	—	—	30	—	—	—	—	—	—	—	Fluoride (2.2 mg)
NATAFORT (Parke-Davis) Rx	Tabs	6,000	400	30	120	3	2	20	15	6	1,000	—	—	350	—	100	65	25	—	150	—	—	—	—	—
NATALINS (Mead Johnson) OTC	Tabs	8,000	400	30	90	1.7	2	20	4	8	800	—	—	200	—	100	45	—	—	150	—	—	—	—	—
NATALINS Rx (Mead Johnson) Rx	Tabs	8,000	400	30	90	2.55	3	20	10	8	1,000	50	15	200	—	100	60	15	2	150	—	—	—	—	—

[1] B₃ = niacin; FA = folic acid; BT = biotin; PA = pantothenic acid or pantothenate

Prenatal Vitamins with Minerals continued

	Form	VITAMINS[1]												MINERALS									
		A IU	D IU	E IU	C mg	B₁ mg	B₂ mg	B₃ mg	B₆ mg	B₁₂ µg	FA µg	BT µg	PA mg	Ca mg	P mg	Mg mg	Fe mg	Zn mg	Cu mg	I µg	Mn mg	Cr µg	Mo µg	Se µg	OTHER INGREDIENTS
USRDA for pregnant or lactating women	–	8,000	400	30	60	1.7	2	20	2.5	8	800	300	10	1,300	1,300	450	18	15	2	150	–	–	–	–	–
PRAMET FA (Ross) Rx	Tabs	4,000	400	–	100	3	2	10	5	3	1,000	–	0.92	250	–	–	60	–	0.15	100	–	–	–	–	–
PRAMILET FA (Ross) Rx	Tabs	4,000	400	–	60	3	2	10	3	3	1,000	–	1	250	–	10	40	0.09	0.15	100	–	–	–	–	–
STUART PRENATAL (Stuart) OTC	Tabs	8,000	400	30	60	1.7	2	20	4	8	800	–	–	200	–	100	60	25	–	150	–	–	–	–	–
STUARTNATAL 1+1 (Stuart) Rx	Tabs	8,000	400	30	90	2.55	3	20	10	12	1,000	–	–	200	–	100	65	25	–	150	–	–	–	–	–

[1] B₃ = niacin; FA = folic acid; BT = biotin; PA = pantothenic acid or pantothenate

Calcium Supplements

	Form	VITAMINS[1]												MINERALS									
		A IU	D IU	E IU	C mg	B₁ mg	B₂ mg	B₃ mg	B₆ mg	B₁₂ µg	FA µg	BT µg	PA mg	Ca mg	P mg	Mg mg	Fe mg	Zn mg	Cu mg	I µg	Mn mg	Cr µg	Mo µg	Se µg	OTHER INGREDIENTS
USRDA (children < 4 yr)	–	2,500	400	10	40	0.7	0.8	9	0.7	3	200	150	5	800	500	200	10	8	1	70	–	–	–	–	–
USRDA (children ≥ 4 yr and adults)	–	5,000	400	30	60	1.5	1.7	20	2	6	400	300	10	1,000	1,000	400	18	15	2	150	4	–	–	–	–
ALKA-MINTS Chewable Antacid (Miles Laboratories) OTC	Tabs	–	–	–	–	–	–	–	–	–	–	–	–	340	–	–	–	–	–	–	–	–	–	–	–
AVAIL (Norcliff Thayer) OTC	Tabs	5,000	400	30	90	2.25	2.55	20	3	9	400	–	–	400	–	100	18	22.5	–	150	–	15	–	15	–
BIOCAL Chewable (Miles Laboratories) OTC	Tabs	–	–	–	–	–	–	–	–	–	–	–	–	250	–	–	–	–	–	–	–	–	–	–	–
BIOCAL Swallowable (Miles Laboratories) OTC	Tabs	–	–	–	–	–	–	–	–	–	–	–	–	500	–	–	–	–	–	–	–	–	–	–	–
CALEL-D (Rorer) OTC	Tabs	–	200	–	–	–	–	–	–	–	–	–	–	500	–	–	–	–	–	–	–	–	–	–	–
CAL SUP 300 Chewable (3M) OTC	Tabs	–	–	–	–	–	–	–	–	–	–	–	–	300	–	–	–	–	–	–	–	–	–	–	–
CAL SUP 600 (3M) OTC	Tabs	–	200	–	–	–	–	–	–	–	–	–	–	600	–	–	–	–	–	–	–	–	–	–	–
CAL SUP 600 Plus (3M) OTC	Tabs	–	200	–	30	–	–	–	–	–	–	–	–	600	–	–	–	–	–	–	–	–	–	–	–
CAL SUP Instant 1000 (3M) OTC	Pwdr	–	400	–	60	–	–	–	–	–	–	–	–	1,000	–	–	–	–	–	–	–	–	–	–	–
CALTRATE 600 (Lederle) OTC	Tabs	–	–	–	–	–	–	–	–	–	–	–	–	600	–	–	–	–	–	–	–	–	–	–	–
CALTRATE 600 + Vitamin D (Lederle) OTC	Tabs	–	125	–	–	–	–	–	–	–	–	–	–	600	–	–	–	–	–	–	–	–	–	–	–
CALTRATE 600 + Iron and Vitamin D (Lederle) OTC	Tabs	–	125	–	–	–	–	–	–	–	–	–	–	600	–	–	18	–	–	–	–	–	–	–	–
DICAL-D (Abbott) OTC	Caps	–	399	–	–	–	–	–	–	–	–	–	–	350	270	–	–	–	–	–	–	–	–	–	–
DICAL-D Wafers (Abbott) OTC	Wfrs	–	200	–	–	–	–	–	–	–	–	–	–	232	18	–	–	–	–	–	–	–	–	–	–
DIOSTATE D (Upjohn) OTC	Tabs	–	133	–	–	–	–	–	–	–	–	–	–	114	88	–	–	–	–	–	–	–	–	–	–
NEO-CALGLUCON (Sandoz Pharmaceuticals) OTC	Liq	–	–	–	–	–	–	–	–	–	–	–	–	115[2] 345[3]	–	–	–	–	–	–	–	–	–	–	–

[1] B₃ = niacin; FA = folic acid; BT = biotin; PA = pantothenic acid or pantothenate
[2] Teaspoonful dose for children
[3] Tablespoonful dose for adults

Calcium Supplements continued

	Form	VITAMINS[1] A IU	D IU	E IU	C mg	B$_1$ mg	B$_2$ mg	B$_3$ mg	B$_6$ mg	B$_{12}$ µg	FA µg	BT µg	PA mg	MINERALS Ca mg	P mg	Mg mg	Fe mg	Zn mg	Cu mg	I µg	Mn mg	K mg	Na mg	Cl mg	Cr µg	Mo µg	Se µg	OTHER INGREDIENTS
USRDA (children < 4 yr)	—	2,500	400	10	40	0.7	0.8	9	0.7	3	200	150	5	800	500	200	10	8	1	70	—	—	—	—	—	—	—	—
USRDA (children ≥ 4 yr and adults)	—	5,000	400	30	60	1.5	1.7	20	2	6	400	300	10	1,000	1,000	400	18	15	2	150	4	—	—	—	—	—	—	—
OS-CAL 250 (Marion) OTC	Tabs	—	125	—	—	—	—	—	—	—	—	—	—	250	—	—	—	—	—	—	—	—	—	—	—	—	—	—
OS-CAL 500 (Marion) OTC	Tabs	—	—	—	—	—	—	—	—	—	—	—	—	500	—	—	—	—	—	—	—	—	—	—	—	—	—	—
OS-CAL Forte (Marion) OTC	Tabs	1,668	125	0.8	50	1.7	1.7	15	2	1.6	—	—	—	250	—	1.6	5	0.5	—	—	0.3	—	—	—	—	—	—	—
OS-CAL Plus (Marion) OTC	Tabs	1,666	125	—	33	0.5	0.66	3.33	0.5	—	—	—	—	250	—	—	16.6	0.75	—	—	0.75	—	—	—	—	—	—	—
POSTURE (Ayerst) OTC	Tabs	—	—	—	—	—	—	—	—	—	—	—	—	300	—	—	—	—	—	—	—	—	—	—	—	—	—	—
POSTURE-D (Ayerst) OTC	Tabs	—	125	—	—	—	—	—	—	—	—	—	—	600	—	—	—	—	—	—	—	—	—	—	—	—	—	—
SUPLICAL (Warner-Lambert) OTC	Tabs	—	—	—	—	—	—	—	—	—	—	—	—	1,200	—	—	—	—	—	—	—	—	—	—	—	—	—	—
SUPLICAL Chewable (Warner-Lambert) OTC	Tabs	—	—	—	—	—	—	—	—	—	—	—	—	600	—	—	—	—	—	—	—	—	—	—	—	—	—	—
THERACAL Chewable (Warner-Lambert) OTC	Tabs	—	—	—	—	—	—	—	—	—	—	—	—	334	—	—	—	—	—	—	—	—	—	—	—	—	—	—
TUMS (Norcliff Thayer) OTC	Tabs	—	—	—	—	—	—	—	—	—	—	—	—	200	—	—	—	—	—	—	—	—	—	—	—	—	—	—
TUMS E-X (Norcliff Thayer) OTC	Tabs	—	—	—	—	—	—	—	—	—	—	—	—	300	—	—	—	—	—	—	—	—	—	—	—	—	—	—

[1] B$_3$ = niacin; FA = folic acid; BT = biotin; PA = pantothenic acid or pantothenate
[2] Teaspoonful dose for children
[3] Tablespoonful dose for adults

Nutritionals[1]

	Form	VITAMINS[2] A IU	D IU	E IU	C mg	B$_1$ mg	B$_2$ mg	B$_3$ mg	B$_6$ mg	B$_{12}$ µg	FA µg	BT µg	PA mg	MINERALS Ca mg	P mg	Mg mg	Fe mg	Zn mg	Cu mg	I µg	Mn mg	K mg	Na mg	Cl mg	Cr µg	Mo µg	Se µg	OTHER INGREDIENTS
USRDA (children ≥ 4 yr and adults)	—	5,000	400	30	60	1.5	1.7	20	2	6	400	300	10	1,000	1,000	400	18	15	2	150	4	—	—	—	—	—	—	—
CRITICARE HN (Mead Johnson) OTC Protein: 9 g Fat: 0.8 g Carbohydrate: 52.5 g	Liq	625	50	9.4	38	0.48	0.54	6.2	0.6	1.9	50	38	3.1	125	125	50	2.2	2.5	0.25	19	0.6	310	150	250	Vit K$_1$ (31 µg), choline (62 mg)
ENRICH (Ross) OTC Protein: 9.4 g Fat: 8.8 g Carbohydrate: 38.3 g	Liq	850	68	7.7	51	0.4	0.4	5.1	0.5	1.6	102	77	2.6	170	170	68	3	3.8	0.34	26	0.9	370	200	340	Vit K$_1$ (12 µg), choline (102 mg)
ENSURE (Ross) OTC Protein: 8.8 g Fat: 8.8 g Carbohydrate: 34.3 g	Liq	625	50	5.6	38	0.4	0.4	5	0.5	1.5	50	38	1.3	125	125	50	2.3	2.8	0.25	19	0.6	370	200	340	Vit K$_1$ (9 µg), choline (75 mg)
ENSURE HN (Ross) OTC Protein: 10.5 g Fat: 8.4 g Carbohydrate: 33.4 g	Liq	893	72	8.1	54	0.4	0.5	5.4	0.5	1.7	108	81	2.7	179	179	72	3.2	4	0.36	27	0.9	370	220	340	Vit K$_1$ (13 µg), choline (107 mg)

[1] Values given are amounts per serving
[2] B$_3$ = niacin; FA = folic acid; BT = biotin; PA = pantothenic acid or calcium pantothenate

Nutritionals[1] continued

	Form	A IU	D IU	E IU	C mg	B$_1$ mg	B$_2$ mg	B$_3$ mg	B$_6$ mg	B$_{12}$ µg	FA µg	BT µg	PA mg	Ca mg	P mg	Mg mg	Fe mg	Zn mg	Cu mg	I µg	Mn mg	K mg	Na mg	Cl mg	OTHER INGREDIENTS
USRDA (children ≥ 4 yr and adults)	—	5,000	400	30	60	1.5	1.7	20	2	6	400	300	10	1,000	1,000	400	18	15	2	150	4	—	—	—	—
ENSURE PLUS (Ross) *OTC* Protein: 13 g Fat: 12.6 g Carbohydrate: 47.3 g	Liq	834	67	7.5	50	0.5	0.6	6.8	0.7	2	134	100	3.3	167	167	67	3	3.8	0.34	25	0.8	500	270	470	Vit K$_1$ (12 µg), choline (100 mg)
ENSURE PLUS HN (Ross) *OTC* Protein: 14.8 g Fat: 11.8 g Carbohydrate: 47.3 g	Liq	1,250	100	11.3	75	0.75	0.85	10	1	3	200	150	5	250	250	100	4.5	5.6	0.5	38	1.3	430	280	380	Vit K$_1$ (18 µg), choline (150 mg)
ENSURE PUDDING (Ross) *OTC* Protein: 6.8 g Fat: 9.7 g Carbohydrate: 34 g	Pdng	850	68	7.7	15.4	0.26	0.29	3.4	0.34	1.1	68	51	1.7	200	200	68	3.1	3.8	0.34	60	0.85	330	240	220	Vit K$_1$ (12 µg), choline (25 mg)
GEVRAL Protein (Lederle) *OTC* Protein: 15.6 g Fat: 0.52 g Carbohydrate: 7.05 g	Pdwr	2,167	217	4.3	22	2.2	2.2	6.5	0.22	0.87	—	—	2.2	267	52.8	0.4	4.3	0.22	0.4	40	0.4	13	50	—	Choline (21 mg), inositol (22 mg), lysine (1.1 g)
ISOCAL (Mead Johnson) *OTC* Protein: 8.1 g Fat: 10.5 g Carbohydrate: 31.5 g	Liq	625	50	9.4	38	0.48	0.54	6.2	0.6	1.9	50	38	3.1	150	125	50	2.2	2.5	0.25	19	0.6	310	125	250	Vit K$_1$ (31 µg), choline (62 mg)
ISOCAL HCN (Mead Johnson) *OTC* Protein: 17.7 g Fat: 24.2 g Carbohydrate: 47.3 g	Liq	1,180	95	17.7	71	0.9	1.02	11.8	1.18	3.5	95	71	5.9	240	240	95	4.3	7.1	0.71	35	0.8	400	190	280	Vit K$_1$ (59 µg), choline (118 mg)
OSMOLITE (Ross) *OTC* Protein: 8.8 g Fat: 9.1 g Carbohydrate: 34.3 g	Liq	625	50	5.6	37.5	0.38	0.43	5	0.5	1.5	100	75	2.5	125	125	50	2.3	2.82	0.25	19	0.6	240	150	200	Vit K$_1$ (9 µg), choline (75 mg)
OSMOLITE HN (Ross) *OTC* Protein: 10.5 g Fat: 8.7 g Carbohydrate: 33.4 g	Liq	893	72	8.1	53.6	0.41	0.46	5.4	0.5	1.7	108	81	2.7	179	179	71.5	3.2	4	0.36	27	0.9	370	220	340	Vit K$_1$ (13 µg), choline (107 mg)
PORTAGEN (Mead Johnson) *OTC* Protein: 8.5 g Fat: 11.45 g Carbohydrate: 27.5 g	Pwdr	1,875	188	7.5	20	0.38	0.45	5	0.5	1.5	37.5	18.8	2.5	225	169	50	4.5	2.3	0.4	17.5	0.3	300	113	206	Vit K$_1$ (37.5 µg), choline (31 mg)
PRECISION HIGH NITROGEN DIET (Sandoz Nutrition) *OTC* Protein: 12.5 g Fat: 0.36 g Carbohydrate: 62 g	Pwdr	500	40	3	9	0.23	0.26	2	0.3	0.6	40	30	1	100	100	40	1.8	1.5	0.2	15	0.4	260	280	340	Vit K$_1$ (10 µg), choline (10 mg), Cr (15 µg), Mo (30 µg), Se (17.5 µg)
PRECISION ISOTONIC DIET (Sandoz Nutrition) *OTC* Protein: 7.5 g Fat: 7.8 g Carbohydrate: 37.5 g	Pwdr	833	67	5	15	0.37	0.43	3.3	0.5	1	70	50	1.7	170	170	67	3	2.5	0.3	25	0.67	250	200	270	Vit K$_1$ (17 µg), choline (17 mg), Cr (25 µg), Mo (50 µg), Se (17 µg)

[1] Values given are amounts per serving
[2] B$_3$ = niacin; FA = folic acid; BT = biotin; PA = pantothenic acid or calcium pantothenate

Nutritionals[1] continued

	Form	VITAMINS[2]												MINERALS										OTHER INGREDIENTS
		A IU	D IU	E IU	C mg	B₁ mg	B₂ mg	B₃ mg	B₆ mg	B₁₂ μg	FA μg	BT μg	PA mg	Ca mg	P mg	Mg mg	Fe mg	Zn mg	Cu mg	I μg	Mn mg	K mg	Na mg	Cl mg	
USRDA (children ≥ 4 yr and adults)	—	5,000	400	30	60	1.5	1.7	20	2	6	400	300	10	1,000	1,000	400	18	15	2	150	4	—	—	—	
PRECISION LR DIET (Sandoz Nutrition) *OTC* **Protein:** 7.5 g **Fat:** 0.45 g **Carbohydrate:** 71 g	Pwdr	833	67	5	15	0.37	0.43	3.3	0.5	1	70	50	1.7	170	170	67	3	2.5	0.33	25	0.67	250	200	320	Vit K₁ (17 μg), choline (17 mg), Cr (25 μg), Mo (50 μg), Se (17 μg)
PULMOCARE (Ross) *OTC* **Protein:** 14.8 g **Fat:** 21.8 g **Carbohydrate:** 25 g	Liq	1,250	100	11.3	75	0.75	0.85	10	1	3	200	150	5	250	250	100	4.5	5.6	0.5	37.5	1.25	450	310	400	Vit K₁ (18 μg), choline (150 mg)
ROSS SLD (Ross) *OTC* **Protein:** 7.5 g **Fat:** 0.1 g **Carbohydrate:** 27.3 g	Liq	834	67	7.5	15	0.39	0.43	5	0.5	1.5	100	75	2.5	167	167	67	3	3.8	0.3	25	0.84	167	167	200	Vit K₁ (6 μg), choline (75 mg)
SUSTACAL HC (Mead Johnson) *OTC* **Protein:** 14.4 g **Fat:** 13.6 g **Carbohydrate:** 45 g	Liq	1,000	80	6	18	0.45	0.6	6	0.6	1.8	120	90	3	200	200	80	3.6	3	0.4	30	0.6	350	200	300	Vit K₁ (50 μg), choline (50 mg)
SUSTACAL Liquid (Mead Johnson) *OTC* **Protein:** 14.5 g **Fat:** 5.5 g **Carbohydrate:** 33.1 g	Liq	1,110	89	6.7	13.3	0.33	0.4	4.7	0.5	1.3	89	67	2.3	240	220	90	4	3.3	0.5	33	0.7	490	220	370	Vit K₁ (56 μg), choline (56 mg)
SUSTACAL Powder (Mead Johnson) *OTC* **Protein:** 20.5 g **Fat:** 9.2 g **Carbohydrate:** 48 g	Pwdr	1,290	33	10	20	0.4	0.2	6.8	0.6	1	133	93	2.7	290	250	105	6	4	0.7	40	1	560	190	220	—
SUSTACAL Pudding (Mead Johnson) *OTC* **Protein:** 6.8 g **Fat:** 9.5 g **Carbohydrate:** 32 g	Pdng	750	60	4.5	9	0.23	0.3	3	0.3	0.9	60	50	1.5	220	220	60	2.7	2.2	0.3	22	0.7	320	120	200	—
SUSTAGEN (Mead Johnson) *OTC* **Protein:** 23.5 g **Fat:** 3.5 g **Carbohydrate:** 66.4 g	Pwdr	1,114	89	10	67	0.85	0.95	11	1.1	3.3	89	70	5.5	710	530	89	4	4.4	0.4	33	1.1	710	225	605	Vit K₁ (60 μg), choline (110 mg)
TRAUMA-AID HBC (American McGaw) *OTC* **Protein:** 28 g **Fat:** 6.2 g **Carbohydrate:** 83 g	Pwdr	833	67	10	17	0.25	0.3	3.3	0.3	1	67	50	1.7	200	200	67	3	3.3	0.3	25	0.67	583	267	417	Vit K₁ (25 μg), choline (70 mg), Cr (8.3 μg), Mo (25 μg), Se (25 μg)
TRAUMACAL (Mead Johnson) *OTC* **Protein:** 19.5 g **Fat:** 16.2 g **Carbohydrate:** 33.7 g	Liq	590	47	8.9	35	0.45	0.5	5.9	0.6	1.8	47	35	3	177	177	47	2.1	3.5	0.4	18	0.6	330	280	380	Vit K₁ (30 μg), choline (59 mg)
TwoCal HN (Ross) *OTC* **Protein:** 19.8 g **Fat:** 21.5 g **Carbohydrate:** 51.4 g	Liq	1,250	100	11.3	75	0.6	0.7	8	0.8	2.4	160	120	4	250	250	100	4.5	5.6	0.5	38	1.3	550	250	370	Vit K₁ (18 μg), choline (150 mg)
VITAL High Nitrogen (Ross) *OTC* **Protein:** 12.5 g **Fat:** 3.25 g **Carbohydrate:** 55.4 g	Pwdr	1,000	80	9	60	0.6	0.7	8	0.8	2.4	160	120	4	200	200	80	3.6	4.5	0.4	30	1	400	140	270	Vit K₁ (14 μg), choline (120 mg)

[1] Values given are amounts per serving
[2] B₃ = niacin; FA = folic acid; BT = biotin; PA = pantothenic acid or calcium pantothenate

Nutritionals[1] continued

VITAMINS[2] / MINERALS

	Form	A IU	D IU	E IU	C mg	B₁ mg	B₂ mg	B₃ mg	B₆ mg	B₁₂ μg	FA μg	BT μg	PA mg	Ca mg	P mg	Mg mg	Fe mg	Zn mg	Cu mg	I μg	Mn mg	K mg	Na mg	Cl mg	OTHER INGREDIENTS
USRDA (children ≥ 4 yr and adults)	—	5,000	400	30	60	1.5	1.7	20	2	6	400	300	10	1,000	1,000	400	18	15	2	150	4	—	—	—	
HIGH NITROGEN VIVONEX (Norwich Eaton) *OTC* **Protein:** 13.3 g **Fat:** 0.26 g **Carbohydrate:** 61.1 g	Pwdr	500	40	3	6	0.15	0.17	2	0.2	0.6	40	30	1	100	100	40	1.8	1.5	0.2	15	0.3	352	156	245	Vit K₁ (6.7 μg), choline (74 mg), Cr (5 μg), Mo (15 μg), Se (15 μg)
STANDARD VIVONEX (Norwich Eaton) *OTC* **Protein:** 6.18 g **Fat:** 0.44 g **Carbohydrate:** 67.9 g	Pwdr	833	67	5	10	0.25	0.28	3.3	0.3	1	67	50	1.7	167	167	67	3	2.5	0.3	25	0.5	211	84	130	Vit K₁ (11.2 μg), choline (12.3 mg), Cr (8.3 μg), Mo (25 μg), Se (25 μg)
VIVONEX T.E.N. (Norwich Eaton) *OTC* **Protein:** 11.46 g **Fat:** 0.83 g **Carbohydrate:** 61.67 g	Pwdr	750	60	4.5	18	0.45	0.5	6	0.6	1.8	60	90	3	150	150	60	2.7	3	0.3	22.5	0.3	—	—	—	Vit K₁ (6.7 μg), choline (22.1 mg), Cr (5 μg), Mo (15 μg), Se (15 μg)

[1] Values given are amounts per serving
[2] B₃ = niacin; FA = folic acid; BT = biotin; PA = pantothenic acid or calcium pantothenate

Infant Formulas

VITAMINS[1] / MINERALS

	Form[2]	A IU	D IU	E IU	C mg	B₁ mg	B₂ mg	B₃ mg	B₆ mg	B₁₂ μg	FA μg	BT μg	PA mg	Ca mg	P mg	Mg mg	Fe mg	Zn mg	Cu mg	I μg	Mn mg	K mg	Na mg	Cl mg	OTHER INGREDIENTS
USRDA for infants	—	1,500	400	5	35	0.5	0.6	8	0.4	2	100	150	3	600	500	70	15	5	0.6	45	—	—	—	—	
ADVANCE (Ross) *OTC* **Protein:** 18.8 g **Fat:** 25.4 g **Carbohydrate:** 51.9 g	Conc	2,032	380	18.8	45.6	0.71	0.86	9.4	0.56	2.5	96.3	—	3.8	477	366	61	9.1	4.6	0.6	55	0.03	864	188	483	Vit K₁ (51 μg)
ENFAMIL (Mead Johnson) *OTC* **Protein:** 14.4 g **Fat:** 36 g **Carbohydrate:** 66 g	Conc Pwdr Nurs	2,000	400	20	52	0.5	1	8	0.4	1.5	100	15	3	440	300	50	1	5	0.6	65	0.1	690	175	400	Vit K₁ (55 μg), choline (106 mg), inositol (32 mg)
ENFAMIL with Iron (Mead Johnson) *OTC* **Protein:** 14.4 g **Fat:** 36 g **Carbohydrate:** 66 g	Conc Pwdr Nurs	2,000	400	20	52	0.5	1	8	0.4	1.5	100	15	3	440	300	50	12	5	0.6	65	0.1	690	175	400	Vit K₁ (55 μg), choline (100 mg), inositol (30 mg)
ISOMIL (Ross) *OTC* **Protein:** 17 g **Fat:** 34.6 g **Carbohydrate:** 64.6 g	Conc Pwdr Nurs	1,920	384	19.2	57.6	0.4	0.6	9	0.4	3	96	28.8	4.8	672	480	48	11.5	4.8	0.5	96	0.2	896	300	416	Vit K₁ (96 μg), choline (51 mg), inositol (32 mg)

[1] B₃ = niacin; FA = folic acid; BT = biotin; PA = pantothenic acid or calcium pantothenate
[2] Values given are amounts per quart (standard dilution)
[3] Varies depending upon the quantity of carbohydrate and water added; if no carbohydrate is used, a 1:1 dilution with water provides approximately 12 kcal/fl oz

COMPENDIUM OF DRUG THERAPY

Infant Formulas continued

	Form[2]	**VITAMINS**[1]												**MINERALS**										**OTHER INGREDIENTS**
		A IU	D IU	E IU	C mg	B₁ mg	B₂ mg	B₃ mg	B₆ mg	B₁₂ µg	FA µg	BT µg	PA mg	Ca	P	Mg mg	Fe mg	Zn mg	Cu mg	I µg	Mn mg	K mg	Na mg	Cl mg	
USRDA for infants	—	1,500	400	5	35	0.5	0.6	8	0.4	2	100	150	3	600	500	70	15	5	0.6	45	—	—	—	—	
ISOMIL SF (Ross) *OTC* Protein: 18.9 g Fat: 34.1 g Carbohydrate: 64.6 g	Conc Nurs	1,920	384	19.2	57.6	0.4	0.6	9	0.4	3	96	28.8	4.8	672	480	48	11.5	4.8	0.5	96	0.2	736	300	563	Vit K₁ (96 µg), choline (51 mg), inositol (32 mg)
I-SOYALAC (Loma Linda) *OTC* Protein: 20 g Fat: 35 g Carbohydrate: 65 g	Conc Nurs	2,000	400	15	75	0.6	0.6	8	0.55	2	150	50	3	650	450	70	12	5	0.75	50	0.3	750	270	500	Vit K (50 µg), choline (125 mg), inositol (110 mg)
LOFENALAC (Mead Johnson) *OTC* Protein: 21 g Fat: 25 g Carbohydrate: 83 g	Pwdr	1,600	400	10	52	0.5	0.6	8	0.4	2	100	50	3	600	450	70	12	4	0.6	45	1	650	300	450	Vit K₁ (100 µg), choline (85 mg), inositol (30 mg)
NURSOY (Wyeth) *OTC* Protein: 20.2 g Fat: 34.6 g Carbohydrate: 66 g	Conc Nurs	2,500	400	9	55	0.67	1	9.5	0.4	2	50	35	3	600	420	65	12	3.5	0.45	65	0.2	700	190	355	Vit K₁ (100 µg), choline (85 mg), inositol (26 mg)
NUTRAMIGEN (Mead Johnson) *OTC* Protein: 18 g Fat: 25 g Carbohydrate: 86 g	Pwdr	2,000	400	20	52	0.5	0.6	8	0.4	2	100	50	3	600	400	70	12	5	0.6	45	0.2	700	300	550	Vit K₁ (100 µg), choline (85 mg), inositol (30 mg)
PREGESTIMIL (Mead Johnson) *OTC* Protein: 18 g Fat: 26 g Carbohydrate: 86 g	Pwdr	2,000	400	15	52	0.5	0.6	8	0.4	2	100	50	3	600	400	70	12	4	0.6	45	0.2	700	300	550	Vit K₁ (100 µg), choline (85 mg), inositol (30 mg)
PROSOBEE (Mead Johnson) *OTC* Protein: 19.2 g Fat: 34 g Carbohydrate: 64 g	Pwdr	2,000	400	20	52	0.5	0.6	8	0.4	2	100	50	3	600	475	70	12	5	0.6	65	0.16	780	230	530	Vit K₁ (100 µg), choline (50 mg), inositol (30 mg)
RCF (Ross) *OTC* Protein: 18.9 g Fat: 33.9 g Carbohydrate:[3]	Conc	1,920	384	19.2	57.6	0.4	0.6	9	0.4	3	96	28.8	5	672	480	4.8	1.4	5	0.5	96	0.2	736	300	563	Vit K₁ (96 µg), choline (51 mg), inositol (32 mg)
SIMILAC (Ross) *OTC* Protein: 14.2 g Fat: 34.4 g Carbohydrate: 68.5 g	Conc Pwdr Nurs	1,920	384	19.2	58	0.64	0.96	6.7	0.4	1.6	96	—	2.9	480	371	38.4	1.4	4.8	0.6	96	0.03	768	205	480	Vit K₁ (51 µg)
SIMILAC PM 60/40 (Ross) *OTC* Protein: 14.2 g Fat: 35.8 g Carbohydrate: 65.3 g	Pwdr	1,920	384	16	58	0.64	0.96	6.7	0.4	1.6	96	29	2.9	358	179	38.4	0.03	4.8	0.6	38.4	0.03	550	205	378	Vit K₁ (51 µg), choline (77 mg), inositol (153 mg)
SIMILAC with Iron (Ross) *OTC* Protein: 14.2 g Fat: 34.4 g Carbohydrate: 68.5 g	Conc Pwdr Nurs	1,920	384	19.2	58	0.64	0.96	6.7	0.4	1.6	96	—	2.9	480	371	38.4	11.5	4.8	0.6	96	0.03	768	205	480	Vit K₁ (51 µg)
SMA (Wyeth) *OTC* Protein: 14.4 g Fat: 34.6 g Carbohydrate: 69.1 g	Conc Pwdr Nurs	2,500	400	9	55	0.67	1	9.5	0.4	1	50	14	2	420	312	50	12	3.5	0.45	65	0.15	530	142	355	Vit K₁ (55 µg), choline (100 mg)
SOYALAC (Loma Linda) *OTC* Protein: 20 g Fat: 35 g Carbohydrate: 65 g	Conc Pwdr Nurs	2,000	400	15	75	0.5	0.6	8	0.45	2	150	60	3	600	350	75	12	5	0.5	50	1	750	280	420	Vit K (50 µg), choline (100 mg), inositol (100 mg)

[1] B₃ = niacin; FA = folic acid; BT = biotin; PA = pantothenic acid or calcium pantothenate
[2] Values given are amounts per quart (standard dilution)
[3] Varies depending upon the quantity of carbohydrate and water added; if no carbohydrate is used, a 1 : 1 dilution with water provides approximately 12 kcal/fl oz

Glossary

accommodation • Adjustment of the eye to variations in distance
achalasia • Inability of the esophagus to relax during swallowing
acidosis • Abnormal acidity of the blood, serum, and/or tissue fluids
acne rosacea • A chronic skin condition affecting the nose, cheeks, and forehead and characterized by redness, swelling, and pimple formation
acne vulgaris • Simple, uncomplicated acne
acneform • Resembling acne
acromegaly • Chronic disease caused by excessive growth hormone and characterized by overgrowth of bone and connective tissue, resulting in enlargement of the hands, feet, face, and head
activated charcoal • Finely ground charcoal used to reduce stomach acid, absorb harmful substances, and remove various poisons from the stomach
acute • Having a rapid onset and short course
adenitis • Inflammation of a gland or lymph node
adenocarcinoma • A form of cancer arising from glandular tissue
adenoma • A benign tumor developing in glandular or secreting tissue
adenopathy • Any disease of a gland, especially when accompanied by swelling and enlargement of the lymph nodes
adhesion • An abnormal joining of the one organ to another with fibrous tissue
adiadochokinesis • Inability to perform rapidly alternating movements
adipose • Fatty
adjuvant • Administered to enhance the effectiveness of a treatment
adrenergic • Pertaining to nerve cells or fibers of the autonomic nervous system that use norepinephrine to transmit nerve impulses
adrenocorticotrophic hormone (ACTH) • A hormone secreted by the pituitary gland that influences the growth and functioning of the adrenal cortex
adventitious • Accidental, acquired, or foreign; occurring in unusual places
adynamic ileus • Obstruction of the ileum of the small intestine due to inadequate muscular activity
aerobic • Requiring air or free oxygen to live

aerophagia • Gulping of air
afebrile • Without fever
aggregation • Cluster
agonist • A substance that can combine with receptors on various target organs to initiate drug actions
agranulocytosis • A condition characterized by fever, chills, weakness, mouth ulcers, and greatly increased susceptibility to infection
akathisia • A condition characterized by frequent changes in position, inability to sit still, and floor pacing
akinesia • Slowness of movement
akinetic seizure • A type of epilepsy marked by a sudden loss of consciousness, resulting in head nodding, body slumping, and a violent fall
albumin • An important protein found in plasma
alkaline phosphatase • An enzyme produced by the liver that participates in several metabolic processes, including bone formation
alkalosis • Abnormal alkalinity of the blood, serum, and/or tissue fluids
allergen • Any substance that produces an allergic reaction on or within the body
allergy • An inappropriate, harmful response of the immune system to normally harmless factors
alopecia • Loss of hair
alveolitis • Inflammation of an air sac within the lung
Alzheimer's disease • A geriatric condition characterized by progressive loss of memory and thinking processes
amblyopia • Partial loss of sight
ambulatory • Able to walk about
amebiasis • A diarrheal disease caused by infestation with an amebic parasite
amenorrhea • Absence of menstruation
amnesia • Loss of memory
amniotic fluid • The fluid surrounding the fetus
ampul • A sealed glass container meant to hold sterile preparations that are to be injected or infused into the body
amylase • One of a group of enzymes that break down starch to sugar
anabolic • Pertaining to the conversion of nutritive matter to living substance
anaerobic • Pertaining to a type of bacteria that can live only in the absence of oxygen
analeptic agent • A drug that can stimulate the central nervous system

analgesic • A drug that relieves pain

anaphylaxis • A sudden, exaggerated allergic reaction to a foreign substance that may lead to severe breathing difficulty, shock, loss of consciousness, and, possibly, death

anastomosis • Intermingling of fibers from two nerves or two blood vessels

androgen • A hormone that promotes the development and maintenance of male sexual characteristics, such as deepening of the voice and beard growth

anemia • Abnormally low concentration of circulating red blood cells

anesthesia • Local or general loss of sensation brought on by use of drugs, hypnosis, or acupuncture

anesthetic • A drug that causes local or general loss of sensation

angiitis • Inflammation of an artery

angina • Severe, constricting pain

angina pectoris • Severe chest pain that may radiate to the left shoulder and down the arm

angioedema • An acute, painless swelling of the hands, face, feet, genitals, or other organs

angioma • A swelling or tumor due to a rapid increase in cell growth

angioneurotic edema • Swelling due to disease or injury of the nerves supplying blood vessels

anhidrosis • Absence of sweating

anisocoria • Unequal pupil diameter

ankylosing spondylitis • A progressive arthritic condition affecting young men, characterized by fusion and deformity of the spinal column and hip

anogenital • Pertaining to the area of the anus and genitals

anomaly • Abnormality

anorectic • A drug that causes loss of appetite

anorexia • Diminished appetite

antacid • A drug that relieves stomach acidity

antagonist • A substance that resists or prevents the action of another substance

antepartum • Before birth

anterograde • Pertaining to events that follow the onset of a condition

anterolateral • Located in front and to the side

anthelmintic • A drug that kills worms

anthrax • An acute infectious disease of cattle and sheep that can be transmitted to man

anti-infective agent • A drug that prevents or treats infection

anti-inflammatory agent • A drug that relieves pain, swelling, heat, and redness of tissue

antianginal agent • A drug that relieves or prevents severe, constricting chest pain

antiarrhythmic agent • A drug that controls or corrects abnormal heart rhythms

antibiotic • A drug that limits the multiplication of bacteria by interfering with their normal growth (bacteriostatic) or by killing them (bactericidal)

antibody • Protein molecules produced and stored by certain types of blood cells in response to stimulation by certain substances (allergens)

anticholinergic agent • A drug that blocks the actions of the neurotransmitter acetylcholine

anticholinesterase agent • A drug that blocks an enzyme that breaks down acetylcholine, thereby prolonging or potentiating its actions

anticoagulant • A drug that prevents or slows down the clotting of blood

anticonvulsant • A drug that prevents or treats convulsions (seizures)

antidepressant • A drug that treats depression

antidote • Any agent that prevents or counteracts the action of a poison or an overdose of a drug

antiemetic • A drug that relieves or prevents nausea and vomiting

antifibrinolytic agent • A drug that stops bleeding by inhibiting the digestion of fibrin, a factor involved in blood clotting

antiflatulent • A drug that relieves or prevents intestinal gas

antifungal agent • A drug that kills or inhibits the growth of disease-producing fungi

antigenemia • Presence of a substance causing an allergic response in the blood

antihistamine • A drug that prevents, counteracts, or diminishes allergic reactions, including tearing of the eyes, sneezing, itching, and laryngeal swelling

antihypertensive agent • A drug that treats high blood pressure

antimanic agent • A drug used to treat a mental disorder characterized by mental and physical hyperactivity, disorganized behavior, and elevated mood

antimetabolite • A drug used to treat cancer

antimicrobial agent • A drug that kills or inhibits the growth of microorganisms

antimigraine agent • A drug used to treat recurrent painful headaches that are often accompanied by nausea and vomiting

antinauseant • A drug that relieves or prevents nausea

antineoplastic agent • A drug that inhibits or destroys cancer cells

antinuclear antibody (ANA) • Component of the immune system that attacks the parts of a cell's nucleus, particularly the genetic protein DNA; a positive reading of ANA in the blood indicates the presence of certain arthritic disorders

antiparkinson agent • A drug that diminishes the signs and symptoms of parkinsonism

antiplatelet agent • A drug that inhibits the aggregation of blood platelets at bleeding sites

antipruritic agent • A drug that relieves or prevents itching

antipsychotic agent • A drug that treats psychoses, fundamental mental derangements characterized by defective or lost contact with reality

antipyretic • A drug that reduces fever and the symptoms of fever (discomfort, chills, etc.)

antireflux agent • A drug that prevents the contents of the stomach from flowing back to the esophagus

antiseptic • An agent that inhibits or stops bacterial growth

antispasmodic agent • A drug that relieves or prevents intestinal or genitourinary smooth muscle spasms

antitussive • A drug that decreases or relieves coughing

antiviral agent • A drug that destroys viruses or prevents their replication

anuria • Suppression of urinary output

anxiolytic agent • A drug that relieves anxiety

aorta • The large vessel leading from the left ventricle of the heart that distributes oxygenated blood to the body

aortic stenosis • Narrowing of the aorta or its parts

aphagia • Inability to swallow

aphakic • Deprived of a lens

aphonia • Loss of speech

aphthous • Pertaining to white, painful mouth ulcers

aplastic anemia • Abnormally low concentration of circulating red blood cells due to depression or destruction of the bone marrow

apnea • Absence of breathing

arachnoiditis • Inflammation of the membranes covering the spinal cord and the brain

arrhythmia • Abnormal heart rhythm

arrhythmogenic • Producing abnormal heartbeats

arteritis • Inflammation of an artery

arthralgia • Joint pain

ascariasis • Roundworm infestation

ascites • Excess fluid in the abdominal cavity

aseptic • Absence of microorganisms; sterile

aspergillosis • A primary or secondary fungal infection of the lung caused by inhalation of spores and that may involve other organs and tissues

aspermatogenesis • Cessation of sperm production

asphyxia • Deficiency of oxygen and accumulation of carbon dioxide, usually due to impaired respiration and leading to loss of consciousness

aspiration • Drawing of foreign substances into the lungs with the breath

asplenia • Absence of the spleen

assay • Test or analysis of a substance

asterixis • A movement disturbance characterized by flapping movements of the outstretched hands

asthenia • Weakness

asthma • A disease characterized by narrowing of the lung air passages, resulting in an inability to breathe normally

astrocytoma • A benign tumor involving nerve cells attached to the blood vessels of the brain and spinal cord

asymptomatic • Pertaining to the absence of clinical symptoms

asystole • Absence of heartbeats

ataractic • Tranquilizing

ataxia • Inability to coordinate voluntary muscular movements

atelectasis • Collapse or incomplete expansion of the lungs

atherosclerosis • A condition characterized by a buildup of cholesterol, fatty acids, and other substances along the inner walls of blood vessels, restricting the flow of blood through the arteries

athetosis • Continual slow, writhing, involuntary movements of the fingers and hands and, occasionally, other parts of the body

atopic • An increased susceptibility to allergic diseases, especially hay fever, asthma, hives, and eczema

atresia • Closure or lack of an adequate opening or canal

atrial • Pertaining to the two upper chambers of the heart

atrial fibrillation • An abnormal heartbeat characterized by rapid, irregular electrical impulses within the atria and weak contractions

atrial flutter • An abnormal heart rhythm due to excitation of the upper chamber of the heart, resulting in an extremely fast heart rate

atrioventricular (AV) • Pertaining to the upper and lower chambers of the heart

atrium • One of the upper chambers of the heart that receives blood from the body or pulmonary veins

atrophic vaginitis • Breaking down of the mucous membranes of the vagina, usually after menopause

atrophy • Shrinking or wasting of tissue

attention deficit disorder • A syndrome seen in children of average to above-average intelligence, characterized by hyperactivity, a short attention span, and impairments in perception, memory, language, and conceptualization

attenuated virus • A virus that has been weakened by heat, chemicals, or other means so that it can no longer cause disease
audiometric • Pertaining to the testing of hearing acuity
autoimmune disease • A condition in which the body's immune system produces factors that react against the person's own tissue
autologous • Derived from the same organism
autonomic • Involuntary; not under conscious control
AV block • Slowing or stoppage of electrical transmission from the upper to the lower chambers of the heart
AV conduction time • The time interval required for an electrical impulse to travel from the upper to the lower chambers of the heart
AV node • A mass of nervous tissue located below the right atrium that conducts electrical impulses from the upper to the lower chambers of the heart
azoospermia • Absence of live sperm in semen
azotemia • An excessive level of nitrogen and its compounds in the blood
bacteremia • The presence of bacteria in the blood
bacteriostatic • Stopping or hindering bacterial growth
ballism • Swinging, jerky, or flinging movements of the legs and arms
basophil • A type of white blood cell
bejel • An infectious disease that occurs mainly in Middle Eastern children
Bell's palsy • Paralysis or weakness of the muscles supplied by the facial nerve
benign • Harmless
beriberi • A disease of the heart and peripheral nerves caused by nutritional deficiency, mainly of vitamin B$_1$
berylliosis • An acute form of pneumonia caused by inhaling beryllium
bid • Twice a day
bile • A fluid produced by the liver and secreted into the small intestine, where it aids in the digestion of fats, increases peristalsis, and alkalinizes the intestinal contents
biliary stasis • Abnormal stoppage of bile flow in capillaries and ducts
bilirubin • A red bile pigment that, when present in large amounts in the blood or urine, may indicate excessive red blood cell destruction or obstructive jaundice
bioavailability • Amount of a nutrient or drug that can be absorbed and become available to the body in an active state
biopsy • Surgical removal of tissue for microscopic examination
black hairy tongue • The presence of a brown, furlike patch on the back of the tongue
blastomycosis • Any disease caused by yeastlike microorganisms
bleb • Collection of blood or serum in the skin
blepharism • Eyelid spasm
blepharitis • Inflammation of the eyelids
blepharoconjunctivitis • Inflammation of both the eyelids and the mucous membrane covering the upper part of the eyeball
blepharoptosis • Drooping of the upper eyelid
blepharospasm • Eyelid spasm caused by a foreign body or inflammatory condition
bolus • A large pill or volume of drug solution given all at once
bone marrow • A soft tissue within the bones that produces blood cells and new bone tissue
borborygmus • The rumbling noise caused by gas rumbling through intestinal liquid
bovine • Pertaining to or derived from cattle
brachial • Pertaining to an arm or a structure resembling an arm
bradycardia • Abnormally slow heartbeat
bradykinesia • Slowness of voluntary movement
breakthrough bleeding • Prolonged, excessive bleeding caused by the breakdown and elimination of the uterine lining during the normally nonbleeding phase of the menstrual cycle
Bromsulphalein (BSP) • A diagnostic agent used to evaluate liver function
bronchial • Pertaining to the air passages in the lungs
bronchodilator • A drug that widens the air passages of the lungs
bronchoscopy • Direct visual examination of the interior of the bronchi
bronchospasm • Contraction of the smooth muscle lining the walls of the air passages, choking off the supply of air to the lungs
bruit • Murmur or other sound related to circulation
bruxism • Grinding or gnashing of the teeth
buccal • Pertaining to the cheek
Buerger's disease • A disease of young and middle-aged tobacco smokers characterized by clotting and inflammation of the arteries and veins of the extremities
bulla • A large blister within or beneath the skin that is filled with lymph or serum
bullous dermatitis • Skin inflammation characterized by large blisters within or beneath the skin
BUN • Blood urea nitrogen, used as a measure of kidney function
bundle-branch block • Delayed or blocked conduction through the conductive tissue of the heart, causing one ventricle to contract before the other

calculus • A stone in the kidney or gallbladder
callus • The hard bony tissue that develops between and around the ends of a fractured bone
cancellous • Having a veiny or spongy structure
candidiasis • Yeast infection
carcinogenic • Capable of causing cancer
carcinoma • A tumor or cancerous growth
cardiac • Pertaining to the heart
cardiac aneurysm • Ballooning of a weakened part of the heart wall
cardiac catheterization • Insertion of a long flexible tube into the heart via a peripheral artery or vein for diagnostic or therapeutic reasons
cardiac output • The blood volume (in liters) ejected by the left ventricle per minute
cardiac tamponade • Compression of the heart by fluid within the sac holding the heart
cardiogenic • Originating in the heart
cardiomegaly • Enlargement of the heart
cardiomyopathy • Disease affecting the heart muscles
cardiopathy • Disease or disorder of the heart
cardioplegia • Paralysis of the heart muscle resulting from direct trauma, a blow, or the action of a drug
cardiopulmonary • Pertaining to the heart and respiratory system
cardiostenosis • Constriction of the heart
cardiotonic • Capable of increasing the strength of contraction of heart muscle
cardiovascular • Pertaining to the heart and blood vessels
cardioversion • Electrical stimulation applied directly to the heart for the purpose of converting an abnormal rhythm to a normal heartbeat
carditis • Inflammation of the heart
carpopedal spasm • Muscle spasm of the hands and feet or of the thumbs and the big toes, often associated with tetanus
cataract • Clouding or opacity of the eye's lens or its capsule, resulting in dimming or blurring of vision
catarrh • Inflammation of the mucous membranes, especially concerning the air passages
catatonia • A type of schizophrenia characterized by profound withdrawal and motor inhibition, alternating with bouts of marked excitement and frenzied activity
catecholamine • A type of sympathomimetic agent that imitates the action of the sympathetic nervous system
cathartic • A drug that causes evacuation of the bowels
CBC • Complete blood count, including red blood cells, white blood cells, and platelets
cellulitis • Inflammation of the connective tissue beneath the skin due to infection
central nervous system • The brain, spinal cord, olfactory bulb, and optic nerve
central venous pressure (CVP) • The pressure representing the filling pressure of the right ventricle of the heart, used to monitor the replacement of fluids in shock or severe burns
cerebral • Pertaining to the brain
cerebrospinal fluid (CSF) • The fluid surrounding and protecting the brain and spinal cord
cerebrovascular Pertaining to the blood vessels or blood supply to the brain
cerebrovascular accident • Condition resulting from blood leakage or clotting of the blood vessels of the brain, characterized by loss of consciousness, seizures, and partial paralysis
cerumen • The waxy substance lining the external ear canal
cervicitis • Inflammation of the lower part of the uterus extending into the vagina
cesarean section • Delivery of a fetus through an opening made in the abdomen and uterus
chancroid • A soft chancre, sore, or ulcer
Charcot-like arthropathy • A type of joint disease characterized by irregular deformities and joint instability
cheilitis • Inflammation of the lips
chemotherapy • Prevention or treatment of disease using chemical agents
Cheyne-Stokes respiration • Periodic breathing characterized by periods of quick breathing alternating with nonbreathing intervals
chiasma • Crossing of the eyes
cholangitis • Inflammation of the biliary ducts
cholecystitis • Inflammation of the gallbladder
cholelithiasis • Presence of gravelly mineral deposits (gallstones) in the gallbladder or in a bile duct
cholestasis • Slowing or stoppage of the flow of bile from the gallbladder
cholestatic hepatitis • Inflammation of the liver caused by blockage of the bile ducts by a changed, thick type of bile
cholestatic jaundice • Yellowing of the eyes and skin caused by blockage of the bile ducts
cholinergic duct • A drug that imitates the actions of acetylcholine
chorea • Continual, involuntary, jerky movements of the limbs, neck, and/or facial muscles
choreiform • Resembling the jerky, involuntary movements of chorea
choreoathetoid • Having the features of both chorea and athetosis
chorion • The outermost fetal membrane

chorioretinitis • Inflammation of the choroid and retina of the eye

chromatography • A laboratory procedure used to detect minute quantities of various substances, such as drugs and poisons

chromosome • One of the 46 such structures in the human cell nucleus that carry the genes that are passed on from one generation to the next

chronic • Lasting a long time

cinchonism • Quinine toxicity, characterized by diminished appetite, nausea, vomiting, diarrhea, dizziness, ringing in the ears, headache, and visual disturbances

cirrhosis • Progressive disease of the liver associated with interference of blood flow into the liver and frequently resulting in yellowing of the skin

claudication • Limping

cleft lip • Splitting of the upper lip and occasionally the palate

clonic • Marked by alternate contracting and relaxing of muscles

coagulation • Change from a fluid to a semisolid state

coarctation • Narrowing of a blood vessel

coccidioidomycosis • A fungal infection or disease acquired by inhalation of spores and common in the southwestern United States, Mexico, and some areas of South America

cochlear • Pertaining to the essential organ of hearing within the inner ear

colic • Abdominal pain caused by smooth muscle spasms of the intestine

colitis • Inflammation of the colon

coma • A state of profound unconsciousness from which one cannot be aroused, even by powerful stimulation

compensatory • Making up for a loss

conception • Fertilization of an egg by a sperm

concomitant • Simultaneous

congener • A substance related to another by function, origin, or nature

congenital • Existing before or at birth

congestion • Abnormal accumulation of fluid within the vessels of an organ

congestive heart failure • Circulatory congestion resulting from heart failure

conjunctiva • The delicate membrane lining the interior of the eyelids and the front of the eyeball

conjunctivitis • Inflammation of the conjunctiva

constipation • A condition in which the bowels are evacuated with great difficulty or at long intervals

contact dermatitis • Inflammation of the skin resulting from contact with an irritating substance

contraceptive • A drug or appliance that prevents conception

convulsion • Involuntary muscle spasm

Coombs' test • A blood test for detecting antibodies to red blood cells

copious • Great amounts

cor pulmonale • Overgrowth of the right ventricle of the heart due to lung disease

cornea • The transparent outer layer of the eyeball in front of the lens

corneal opacity • Clouding of the cornea

coronary artery • Blood vessel supplying oxygen to heart muscle

coronary occlusion • Blockage of a coronary artery

coronary stenosis • Narrowing of a coronary artery

coronary thrombosis • Formation of a clot in a coronary artery

cortical • Pertaining to the layer of gray matter over most of the brain

corticosteroid • A drug that has the properties characteristic of the hormones of the adrenal cortex

cranial • Pertaining to the head or skull

craniosynostosis • Premature fusing of the cranial bones at or shortly after birth

creatine phosphokinase (CPK) • An enzyme found in heart and skeletal muscles, used to diagnose heart attacks and certain muscle diseases

creatinine clearance rate (Ccr) • A measurement of kidney function

cretinism • Deficiency of thyroid hormone present at birth, characterized by a large protruding tongue, dry skin, protruding abdomen, mental retardation, and dwarfism

cryoglobulinemia • A disease caused by the presence of an abnormal protein in the blood, resulting in restricted blood flow through areas of the body exposed to cold

cryptitis • Inflammation of a small sac or glandular cavity

cryptococcosis • A fungal infection involving the lungs, bones, or skin that can cause primary meningitis when it involves the central nervous system

cryptorchism (cryptorchidism) • Failure of the testes to descend

crystalluria • Presence of crystals in the urine

culture • Growth of microorganisms or tissue cells in an artificial medium

Cushing's syndrome • A condition caused by excessive adrenocortical hormone stimulation and characterized, in part, by obesity of the face and trunk, weakness, easy fatigability, hypertension, bone loss, and glucose intolerance

cutaneous • Pertaining to the skin
cyanosis • A dark bluish or purplish coloring of the skin due to lack of oxygen in the blood
cycloplegia • Paralysis of the eye muscles
cycloplegic • A drug that causes temporary paralysis of the muscles of the eye lens
cylindruria • Presence of casts in the urine
cyst • A nodule usually filled with fluid, gas, or semisolid material
cystitis • Inflammation of the urinary bladder
cytotoxic • Harmful to living cells
dacrocystitis • Inflammation of the lacrimal sac of the eye
debilitated • Weakened
decompensation • Failure to compensate for stress
decubital ulcer • Bed sore
decubitus • Recumbent; horizontal
decubitus position • Lying down horizontally
defibrillation • Regulation of rapid, unsynchronized heartbeats
dehiscence • To split open
delirium • A disordered mental state characterized by confusion, disorientation, hallucinations, delusions, and unusual alertness
delirium tremens • A form of acute intoxication caused by alcohol withdrawal, characterized by tremor, sweating, restlessness, anxiety, confusion, and hallucinations
deltoid muscle • The triangular-shaped muscle covering the shoulder joint
depersonalization • Loss of the sense of one's individuality, reality, or identity
dermatitis • Inflammation of the skin
dermatographism • A form of hives in which stroking or scratching the skin with a fingernail or dull instrument causes a raised welt or wheal to appear
dermatological • Pertaining to the skin
dermatomyositis • A condition characterized by skin rash and progressive muscle weakness
dermatosis • Any disease of the skin
desquamation • Shedding of the outer layer of the skin
diabetes insipidus • A disorder of the pituitary gland characterized by a progressive increase in urination and excessive thirst
diabetes mellitus • A disease characterized by decreased production of insulin or number of insulin receptors and, consequently, impaired carbohydrate metabolism
dialysis • The separation of dissolved substances from one another by taking advantage of differences in their capacity to diffuse through a porous membrane
diaphoresis • Perspiration
diaphragm • A device worn by a female to prevent conception; the chief muscle of respiration
diarrhea • A symptom of gastrointestinal disease characterized by frequent, watery stools
diastolic pressure • The minimum pressure exerted on the walls of an artery when the ventricles of the heart relax and fill with blood
diathesis • A condition or tendency present in the body that increases susceptibility to an abnormality or disease
dicrotic • Pertaining to a secondary pressure wave leading from the descending portion of a main wave
digitalization • Administration of drugs derived from digitalis to strengthen and regulate the heart
dilatation • Enlargement or stretching
dilation • The process of being enlarged or stretched
diluent • A fluid used to dilute the strength of a solution or drug
diplopia • Double vision
discitis • Inflammation of a disk
disseminated • Scattered
dissolution • Separation of a compound placed in a solvent to form a solution
distal • Remote; situated far from the point of origin; near the end
distention • Stretched; widened
diuresis • Excretion of urine
diuretic • A drug that promotes urinary excretion
diurnal • Occurring during daytime; recurring once every 24 hours
diverticulitis • Inflammation of a pouch or sac in the wall of the intestine
DTP • Diphtheria-tetanus-pertussis
dura mater • Fibrous membrane covering the brain and spinal cord
dysarthria • Stammering or stuttering due to speech-muscle impairment
dyscrasia • Abnormal state or condition of the body
dysentery • Inflammation of the intestine, characterized by frequent watery stools (often tinged with blood or mucus), straining, abdominal pain, fever, and dehydration
dysesthesia • Impairment of the senses, especially touch
dysgalactia • Loss or impairment of milk secretion
dysgeusia • Abnormal or impaired taste
dyskinesia • Abnormal or disordered movements
dysmenorrhea • Difficult or painful menstruation
dysmetria • Inability to control the range of muscular movements, especially of the hands
dyspareunia • Painful or difficult sexual

intercourse
dyspepsia • Indigestion
dysphagia • Difficulty in swallowing
dysphasia • Impaired speech
dysphonia • Impairment of the voice
dysphoria • Unpleasant or uncomfortable feeling
dyspnea • Shortness of breath
dystocia • Difficult childbirth
dystonia • Disordered or absent muscle tone
dysuria • Painful or burning urination
ecchymosis • A purplish skin patch caused by release of blood into the skin
ECG (EKG) • Electrocardiogram, a test to record the electrical activity of the heart
echolalia • Purposeless, involuntary repetition of the words uttered by another person, often seen in schizophrenia
eclampsia • A condition occurring in the second half of pregnancy, characterized by high blood pressure, protein in the urine, swelling, salt retention, convulsions, and sometimes coma
ectopic • Out of place
eczema • A noncontagious, itching, inflammatory skin disease
edema • Accumulation of fluids resulting in swelling, particularly of the ankles
EEG • Electroencephalogram, a test to record the electrical activity of the brain
effusion • Pouring or spreading out of a fluid into a body cavity or tissue
electroconvulsive therapy (ECT) • The use of electrical current to produce convulsions or unconsciousness in the treatment of psychotic or, particularly, severely depressed patients
electrolyte • A compound that breaks up into charged particles (ions) when put into solution and can conduct an electric current, such as in plasma and other body fluids
embolism • Blockage of a blood vessel by a clot
embryocidal • Fatal to an embryo
embryotoxic • Harmful to a developing embryo
emesis • Vomiting
emetic • A drug used to induce vomiting
emetogenic • Causing vomiting
encephalitis • Inflammation of the brain
encephalopathy • Any disease of the brain
endocarditis • Inflammation of the membrane lining the interior of the heart and valves
endocrinological • Hormonal
endogenous • Due to an internal cause or condition
endoscopy • A diagnostic procedure involving insertion of an instrument into a body cavity for visual examination
endotracheal intubation • An emergency procedure in which a tube is passed into the windpipe to facilitate ventilation
enteric • Pertaining to the intestines
enteritis • Inflammation of the intestine, especially the small intestine
enterobiasis • Pinworm infestation
enterocolitis • Inflammation of the small and large intestines
enuresis • Bedwetting
eosinophil • A type of white blood cell
eosinophilia • Abnormally low concentration of eosinophils in the blood
ependymoma • A central nervous system tumor with cells resembling those lining the central canal of the brain and spinal cord
epicondylitis • Inflammation of the rounded part of the joint
epidemiological • Pertaining to the study of the incidence and distribution of disease in different population groups
epigastric • Pertaining to the upper and middle part of the abdominal surface
epilepsy • A brain disorder characterized by transient episodes of abnormal movement, sensations, or thoughts, with or without unconsciousness and convulsive movements
epileptiform • Resembling epilepsy
epiphysis • The end of a long bone that develops separately from the shaft and is connected to it early on by a layer of cartilage
epistaxis • Nosebleed
epithelial keratopathy • Degeneration of the covering of the cornea
ergotism • Ergot intoxication, characterized by vomiting, stomach cramps, convulsions, numbness, psychotic behavior, and possibly gangrene
erosion • Surface destruction of an area by inflammation or trauma
eructation • Belching
eruption • The sudden appearance of skin lesions, such as hives
erythema • Redness
erythema multiforme (Stevens-Johnson syndrome) • An acute, inflammatory disease characterized by red marks on the neck, face, legs, and the back of the hands, forearms, and feet
erythema nodosum • A skin eruption characterized by tender elevations, usually on the lower extremities, and often associated with joint pain
erythrasma • A skin disease affecting the groin, characterized by red or brown, sharply defined, raised patches
erythrocytes • Red blood cells
erythroid • Reddish
erythromelalgia • Dilation of the blood vessels

beneath the skin of the feet, and sometimes hands, resulting in redness, mottling, changes in skin temperature, and pain
esophagitis • Inflammation of the esophagus
esotropia • Eye condition in which one eye fixes on an object and the other moves inward
estrogen • A hormone produced in the ovaries that is essential for normal reproduction and development of female secondary sex characteristics
etiology • The cause or origin of a disease; the study of disease causes
euphoria • Feeling of well-being that may be exaggerated
euthyroidism • Normal thyroid function
eutocia • Normal childbirth
exacerbation • An increase in the severity of a disease or in its signs or symptoms
excoriation • Abrasion of a skin area
exfoliative dermatitis • Extensive, abnormal skin peeling, including hair loss
exogenous • Due to an external cause
expectorant • A drug that causes ejection of matter from the lungs and air passages
extrapyramidal • Pertaining to the extrapyramidal system in the brain, stimulation of which produces tremors, muscular rigidity, and abnormal or uncoordinated movements
extrasystole • Heart contraction arising from a site other than the normal pacemaker in the atrium
extravasation • The passing of blood from a vein or artery into the surrounding tissues following rupture of the blood-vessel wall
facies • Appearance of the face
fasciculation • Uncoordinated skeletal muscle contraction in which muscle groups supplied by the same nerve contract together
fasciotomy • Cutting of a tissue under the skin or between muscle layers
febrile • Feverish
fetal • Pertaining to a growing fetus within the womb
fetid • Having a foul odor
fetotoxic • Harmful to the fetus
fibrillation • Uncoordinated muscle contractions, commonly of the heart muscle, characterized by a very rapid, unsynchronized, and unproductive heartbeat
fibromyomata • A benign tumor consisting of cancerous smooth muscle cells
fibroplasia • Growth of fibrous connective tissue, as in the healing of a wound
fibrosarcoma • A malignant tumor consisting of cancerous connective tissue cells
fissure • Crack in the skin or an ulcer in a mucous membrane

fistula • An abnormal connection from a hollow organ to the surface or from one organ to another
flaccid • Soft, flabby, relaxed
flank • The fleshy part on the side of the abdomen, between the ribs and the hip
flare • Red area spreading outward from an infected site; sudden worsening of an arthritic condition
flatulence • Excessive amounts of gas in the stomach and intestine
flatus • Intestinal gas
flora • The bacteria and fungi inhabiting an area of the body
flutter • Quick, irregular motion
focal seizure • A type of epilepsy often associated with irritation of a localized area of the brain and usually occurring without loss of consciousness
follicle-stimulating hormone (FSH) • A hormone that stimulates egg development in the female ovary and sperm development in the testes
folliculitis • Inflammation of a small secretory sac or cavity from which a hair grows
frank • Clinically obvious
frontal • Pertaining to the forehead or to the anterior part of an organ or body
fulminant • Sudden, severe, and rapid in course
fulminating • Becoming rapidly worse
fundus • The bottom or lowest part of an organ
funduscopy • Examination of the interior of the eye
furfur • Dandruff
furunculosis • A condition in which multiple boils rapidly form
fusospirochetosis • A bacterial infection
galactorrhea • Excessive or spontaneous flow of milk
galacturia • Milkiness of the urine
ganglionic blocker • A drug that blocks the transmission of nerve impulses at the level of the ganglions, used to reduce blood pressure
gangrene • Death of a body part due to disease, lack of blood supply, or injury
gastrocolitis • Inflammation of the stomach and colon
gastroenteritis • Inflammation of the lining of the stomach and intestines
gastroesophageal reflux • Regurgitation of stomach acid into the esophagus
gastrointestinal tract • The mouth, oral cavity, esophagus, stomach, duodenum, small intestine, colon, and rectum
gastroparesis • Prolonged retention of food in the stomach resulting from impaired gastric motility
genitalia • The male or female reproductive organs

genitourinary • Pertaining to the genitals and the urinary organs
gestation • Pregnancy
Gilles de la Tourette syndrome • Severe habit spasm beginning in late childhood and adolescence and characterized by tics, repeating of words, obscene talk, and other compulsive acts
gingival hyperplasia • Overgrowth of gum tissue around a tooth
glaucoma • Disease of the eye resulting in increased pressure within the eye
glioma • Tumor of the special supporting tissue of the central nervous system
globe • Eyeball
glomerulonephritis • A type of kidney disease characterized by blood, protein, and casts in the urine, nitrogen retention, edema, and hypertension
glossitis • Inflammation of the tongue
glottis • The vocal cords and the space between them
gluteus maximus • The largest muscle of the buttock
glycosuria • The presence of sugar in the urine
goiter • Enlargement of the thyroid gland
goitrogen • A substance that produces enlargement of the thyroid gland
gonadotropin • A hormone that stimulates the ovaries or testes
gout • Recurrent attacks of acute arthritis, commonly of the big toe, caused by increased uric acid in the blood
grand mal seizure • An epileptic seizure characterized by loss of consciousness, convulsions, dilated pupils, and skin discoloration, followed by muscle spasm, upward eye rotation, frothing at the mouth, and sudden loss of urine
granulation • Formation of grains or granules
granulocyte • A type of white blood cell
granulocytopenia • Abnormally low concentration of granulocytes in the blood
granuloma inguinale • Ulcer of the groin
Guillain-Barré syndrome • Acute paralysis of the limb, trunk, and skull muscles of unknown cause
guttate • Resembling a drop
guttural • Pertaining to the throat
gynecomastia • Excessive development of male mammary glands, sometimes resulting in milk excretion
h • Hour(s)
halitosis • A foul odor coming from the mouth
hematemesis • Vomiting of blood
hematinic • A drug that increases the hemoglobin content of red blood cells
hematocrit • The percentage of the whole blood volume occupied by red blood cells
hematological • Pertaining to the blood or circulatory system
hematoma • A confined mass of clotted blood resulting from a break in a blood-vessel wall
hematopoietic • Pertaining to blood cell formation
hematuria • Blood in the urine
hemeralopia • Day blindness
hemiparesis • Muscle weakness on one side of the body
hemodialysis • The removal of harmful substances from the blood by filtration outside the body
hemodynamic • Pertaining to blood movement
hemoglobin • A pigment present in red blood cells that is capable of reversibly binding oxygen
hemoglobinuria • The presence of hemoglobin in the urine
hemolytic anemia • Abnormally low concentration of circulating red blood cells due to destruction (lysis)
hemopathy • Any disease of the blood
hemoptysis • Spitting of blood from the windpipe or lungs
hemorheologic agent • A drug that improves the rate of blood flow in capillaries by increasing the flexibility of red blood cells
hemostatic agent • A drug that stops bleeding or hemorrhaging
hepatic • Pertaining to the liver
hepatocellular • Pertaining to liver cells
hepatoma • A liver tumor
hepatomegaly • Enlargement of the liver
hepatotoxic • Harmful to the liver
herniated • Pertaining to the protrusion of a structure or part through the wall of tissues containing it
herpes simplex • An acute viral infection characterized by cold sores or fever blisters around the mouth (type 1) and by painful sores and blisters on the genitals, thighs, and buttocks (type 2)
herpes zoster • An acute viral infection characterized by a self-limited eruption of groups of blisters on one side of the body following the course of a nerve
heterotopic • Occurring in an abnormal location
hirsutism • Unusual or excessive hair growth
histoplasmosis • A fungal infection that may range from a mild respiratory infection to a severe disease characterized by fever, anemia, swelling of the liver and spleen, leukopenia, lung scarring, and gastrointestinal ulceration
Hodgkin's disease • A cancerous growth of the lymph glands
homeostasis • The state of balance in organic

function and cellular and fluid composition maintained in the healthy body
human chorionic gonadotropins (hCG) • Hormone present in the blood and urine of pregnant women that is detectable with pregnancy tests
hydatidiform • Resembling a cyst formed by tapeworm larvae
hydroxyproline • An amino acid, one of the building blocks of protein
hyperaldosteronism • Excessive secretion of aldosterone, resulting in muscle weakness, frequent urination, high blood pressure, low blood potassium, and alkalosis
hyperalgesia • Extreme sensitivity to pain
hyperalimentation • The administration or consumption of nutrients beyond the body's immediate needs
hypercalcemia • Excessive calcium in the blood
hypercapnia • Excessive carbon dioxide in the blood
hyperglycemia • Excessive glucose in the blood
hyperkalemia • Excessive concentration of potassium in the blood
hyperkinesia • Excessive movement
hyperlipidemia • Excessive concentration of lipids (fats) in the blood
hyperostosis • A general increase in the bulk of bone
hyperparathyroidism • Excessive secretion of parathyroid hormone, resulting in abnormal calcium and phosphorus metabolism
hyperphosphatemia • Excessive phosphates in the blood
hyperplasia • An increase in the number of cells in a tissue or organ, excluding tumors
hyperpnea • Increase in respiratory depth and rate
hyperpyrexia • High fever
hyperreflexia • Excessive reflex activity
hypersomnia • Excessive sleepiness
hypertension • High blood pressure
hyperthermia • High body temperature
hypertrichosis • Excessive hair growth
hypertriglyceridemia • Excessive triglycerides in the blood
hyperuricemia • Excessive concentration of uric acid in the urine
hyperventilation • Abnormally rapid, deep breathing
hypervitaminosis • Condition resulting from overconsumption of a vitamin
hypesthesia (hypoesthesia) • Decreased sensitivity to stimulation
hyphema • Blood in the anterior chamber of the eye between the cornea and the lens
hypnotic • A drug that induces sleep
hypoadrenal • Decreased adrenal-gland function
hypoaldosteronism • Deficient secretion of aldosterone, resulting in excessive water excretion, dehydration, decreased blood volume, hypotension, and circulatory collapse
hypoalimentation • Deficient or inadequate food intake
hypocalcemia • Deficient calcium in the blood
hypocapnia • Deficient carbon dioxide in the blood
hypochloremia • Deficient chloride in the blood
hypoglycemia • Deficient glucose in the blood
hypoglycemic agent • A drug that lowers the concentration of glucose in the blood
hypogonadism • Deficient ovarian or testicular function
hypohidrosis • Deficient perspiration
hypokalemia • Deficient potassium in the blood
hypokinesia • Decreased muscular movement
hypolipidemic agent • A drug that lowers the concentration of fats in the blood
hypomagnesemia • Deficient magnesium in the blood
hypomania • A mild form of manic-depressive illness, characterized by rapid fluctuations between happiness and irritation, energy, euphoria, impatience, and occasional depression
hyponatremia • Deficient sodium in the blood
hypophosphatemia • Deficient phosphates in the blood
hypoplasia • Defective or incomplete development of an organ or body part
hypopnea • Abnormally slow or shallow breathing
hypoprothrombinemia • Deficient prothrombin in the blood
hyposthenuria • Constant secretion of urine with low specific gravity, primarily seen in chronic hepatitis
hypotension • Low blood pressure
hypothalamic • Pertaining to the hypothalamus, which is primarily involved with autonomic and hormonal regulation
hypothermia • Low body temperature
hypothyroidism • Condition resulting from a deficiency of thyroid hormone
hypovolemia • Low or decreased blood volume
hypoxia • Deficient oxygen in blood or tissue
iatrogenic • Induced by medical treatment
ichthyosis • A skin disease characterized by dry, scaly skin
icterus • Yellowing of the skin
idiopathic • Primary; spontaneous; not arising from another disease or condition
idiosyncratic • Pertaining to any peculiar or special characteristic of an individual
ileitis • Inflammation of the ileum, the third

portion of the small intestine
iliac • Pertaining to part of the pelvic bone
IM • Intramuscular (within a muscle)
immunocompromised • Having deficient defenses against infection because of chemotherapy or an inborn or acquired disorder
immunodeficiency • Any deficiency of the immune response to a foreign protein
immunogenic • Ability to stimulate the immune system; specifically, to produce antibodies
immunosuppressant • A drug that inhibits or blocks the immune response
impetigo • A bacterial skin disease characterized by blisters that erupt and rupture to form yellow crusts
impotence • Inability to achieve an erection
in utero • Within the uterus
in vitro • Pertaining to a reaction observed in a test tube or culture dish
in vivo • Pertaining to a reaction observed in a living organism
incontinence • Inability to control excretion of urine and feces
incoordination • Inability to coordinate or bring together various muscular movements in a harmonious fashion
induction • The period from when an anesthetic is first given to when a patient loses consciousness and the desired level of anesthesia is obtained
induration • Hardening of a tissue or part
infarction • Sudden lack of arterial or venous blood that produces tissue death
infection • Multiplication of microorganisms within the body
infestation • Invasion of animal parasites (such as lice) that live on the surface of a host or in the immediate environment
inflammation • Pain, swelling, heat, and redness of tissue
infusion • The slow injection of a solution into a vein or tissue
inguinal • Pertaining to the groin region
inhalation therapy • The administration of a drug directly into the respiratory system by being inhaled through the nose and/or mouth
inhibitory • Causing a reduction in response to stimulation
inotropic • Changing the force of heart-muscle contractions
insomnia • Inability to sleep
inspissated • Thickened by absorption or evaporation
insulin • A hormone secreted by the pancreas that helps to regulate the breakdown of carbohydrates and fats; deficiency causes diabetes mellitus

intermittent • Occuring at intervals
intermittent claudication • Cramping and weakness of the legs, particularly the calves, brought on by walking and relieved with rest
interstitial • Pertaining to the spaces in a tissue or between body parts
intertriginous • Pertaining to a reddish skin condition produced by friction of adjacent parts
intoxication • Poisoning by a drug, serum, alcohol, or any harmful substance
intraabdominal • Within the cavity of the abdomen
intraarterial • Within an artery
intraarticular • Within a joint
intrabursal • Within a bursa, the capsule surrounding a joint
intracardiac • Within the heart
intracellular • Within a cell
intracholedochal • Within the common bile duct
intracranial • Within the skull
intralesional • Within a lesion or damaged tissue
intramucosal • Within a mucous membrane
intramuscular (IM) • Within a muscle
intraocular • Within the globe of the eye
intrapartum • During labor and childbirth
intraperitoneal • Within the abdominal cavity
intrathecal • Within the subarachnoid space of the spine
intratracheal • Within the windpipe
intravenous (IV) • Within a vein
involuntary muscle • Muscle not consciously controlled by a person, such as intestinal muscle
iritis • Inflammation of the iris of the eye
ischemia • Lack of blood supply to a tissue
isotonic • Pertaining to a solution which causes neither swelling nor shrinkage of the cells bathed in it
IV • Intravenous (within a vein)
jaundice • Yellowing of the skin due to an increased concentration of bile pigments
jejunitis • Inflammation of the middle portion of the small intestine between the duodenum and the ileum
kaliuresis • Increased excretion of potassium in the urine
keloid • An overgrowth of fibrous scar tissue
keratitis • Inflammation of the cornea
keratoconjunctivitis • Inflammation of the cornea and the conjunctiva
kernicterus • Pigmentation of the gray matter in the brain with bilirubin
ketoacidosis • A condition occasionally seen in diabetics and characterized by metabolic acidosis and the presence of ketone bodies in the blood
kg • Kilogram(s)

kraurosis vulvae • Itching, wearing away, and dryness of the external female genitalia
kyphoscoliosis • Curvature of the spine accompanied by formation of a hump
labile • Capable of being altered or modified
labyrinthitis • Inflammation of the canals and cavities that make up the inner ear
lacrimation • Tearing of the eyes
lactation • Production of milk
laparotomy • Direct visual examination of the abdominal organs
laryngospasm • Spasmodic closure of the vocal cords and the space between them
lassitude • Tiredness
lavage • Washing out of a cavity or organ with great amounts of water
laxative • A drug that causes evacuation of the bowels
LDH • Lactic acid dehydrogenase, the enzyme that transforms lactic acid to pyruvic acid; used in the diagnosis of heart attacks
lenticular opacity • Shading of the crystalline lens of the eye
lethargy • Drowsiness or stupor
leukocyte • A white blood cell
leukocytosis • Abnormally high number of circulating white blood cells
leukopenia • Abnormally low concentration of circulating white blood cells
libido • Sexual drive
lichen planus • A skin disease characterized by flat, shiny eruptions that often combine to form patches on the wrist, legs, penis, and inside of the cheek
ligament • A band of tough connective tissue connecting the ends of two bones together
lipid • A fat or fatlike substance
lipoprotein • A complex or compound made up of a lipid and a protein
listeriosis • An infection primarily affecting cattle and sheep that, when transmitted to man, causes meningitis, diarrhea, fever, circulatory collapse, and other serious problems; fatal when transmitted to a developing fetus
lithiasis • The formation of gallstones or kidney stones
loading dose • The initial dosage given to raise the plasma level of a drug into the therapeutic range
lobar • Pertaining to a rounded part or projection of an organ
lower respiratory tract • The trachea (or windpipe), bronchi, bronchioles, and alveoli
lumbago • Pain in the middle and lower back
lumbar • Pertaining to the part of the back and sides between the ribs and the pelvis
luteinizing hormone (LH) • Hormone responsible for preparing an egg for maturation and its release from the ovary
lymph • A clear, yellowish fluid containing small white blood cells (lymphocytes) and composed of tissue fluid that is being returned to the blood through the lymphatic vessels
lymphadenopathy • Any disease of the lymph nodes
lymphoma • Any cancerous tumor of the lymph nodes
lyophilized • Freeze dried
maceration • Softening of a tissue or solid by immersion in a liquid
macrocephaly • Congenital condition characterized by an abnormally large head
macrocyte • An abnormally large red blood cell
macrocytosis • Presence of abnormally large red blood cells in the blood
maculopapular rash • A spotty, elevated skin rash
maculopathy • Any disease affecting the macula, the point of clearest vision on the retina
malignant • Dangerous to health or life; tending to become progressively worse; resistant to treatment
mast cell • A connective tissue cell from which histamine is released during an allergic reaction
mast-cell stabilizer • A drug that prevents allergic symptoms by stabilizing the outer membrane of mast cells, thereby blocking the release of histamine
mastoid • Shaped like a breast
maternotoxic • Harmful to the mother
maxillary • Pertaining to the upper jaw bone
meatus • Opening or passage
megaloblastic anemia • A type of anemia characterized by the presence of large, immature red blood cells in the bone marrow and abnormally large red blood cells in the bloodstream
meibomianitis • Inflammation of the oil glands of the eyelids
melanoma • A malignant skin tumor
melena • Discharge of black stools colored by blood
meningitis • Inflammation of the brain or spinal chord
menometrorrhagia • Excessive menstrual bleeding and irregular bleeding at other times
menses • Menstrual period
mesenteric • Pertaining to the connective tissue that attaches the folds of the small intestine to the abdominal wall
metabolite • The product of an enzyme reaction in the body
metastasis • Migration of a disease from one area to another via the blood vessels or lymph

channels
methemoglobin • A form of hemoglobin that can not bind reversibly with oxygen
methemoglobinemia • Excess of methemoglobin in the blood
methemoglobinuria • Presence of methemoglobin in the urine
mg • Milligram(s)
microcephaly • Congenital condition characterized by an abnormally small head
micturition • Urination
migraine • Recurrent vascular headache often associated with nausea, vomiting, and disturbances of the senses, movement, and mood
miliaria • An acute inflammatory disease of the sweat glands characterized by blistering of the skin and a prickling or tingling sensation
miosis • Contraction of the pupil
miotic • A drug that constricts the pupil of the eye
mitral valve insufficiency • Defect in the mitral valve that allows blood to flow backward from the left ventricle to the left atrium of the heart
ml • Milliliter(s)
monilia • Yeast infection
monocyte • A type of white blood cell
monocytosis • An increase in the number of monocytes in the blood
morbidity • The number of reported cases of a disease occurring in a given population over a period of time; the rate of illness
morbilliform rash • A skin rash resembling measles
moribund • Dying
Moro reflex • The startle reflex exhibited by normal infants from birth through the first few months of life
mortality • The number of reported deaths occurring in a given population over a period of time; the death rate
mottling • Varied coloration with no discernible pattern
mountain sickness • Altitude sickness
mucocutaneous • Pertaining to mucous membranes and the skin
mucolytic • Dissolving, dispersing, or liquefying mucus
murine • Pertaining to mice
mutagenic • Capable of altering genes
myalgia • Muscular pain
myasthenia gravis • A progressive disease characterized by skeletal muscle weakness and abnormal fatigability, which may become severe enough to produce paralysis
mycosis • An infection or disease caused by a fungus
mycotic • Pertaining to fungi

mydriatic • A drug that widens the pupil
myelitis • Inflammation of the spinal cord
myelography • An x-ray examination of the spinal canal following the introduction of a contrast medium
myeloma • A malignant cancer originating in the bone marrow and causing widespread skeletal destruction and collapse of the backbone
myelopathy • Pertaining to disease of the spinal cord or the tissues surrounding it
myelosuppression • Inhibition of the blood-forming function of the bone marrow
myocardial infarction • Death of heart muscle tissue resulting from a lack of blood flow in the arteries surrounding the heart
myocarditis • Inflammation of the heart muscle
myoclonic seizure • A type of epilepsy characterized by very abrupt, irregular muscle contractions
myoclonus • Very abrupt, shocklike muscle contractions having an irregular rhythm and strength
myofacial • Pertaining to the facial muscles
myopathy • Disease or abnormality of muscular tissue
myopia • Nearsightedness
myositis • Inflammation of skeletal muscle
myxadenitis • Inflammation of a mucous gland
myxedema • Hypothyroidism caused by removal or malfunctioning of the thyroid gland, characterized by swelling, dryness and loss of hair, hoarseness, reduced body temperature, muscular weakness, and abnormal reflexes
nadir • Lowest point or level
narcoanalysis • Form of psychotherapy involving slow administration of a barbiturate into a vein to release suppressed or repressed thoughts
narcolepsy • Sleep disorder characterized by sudden attacks of sleep
narcosis • State of stupor, unconsciousness, or arrested activity produced by drugs
narrow-angle glaucoma • Opaquing of the lens and increased pressure within the eyeball caused by a band of fibers blocking the angular space between the cornea and the iris, resulting in extreme eye pain and sudden vision loss
nasopharyngeal • Pertaining to the nose and pharynx
nasopharyngeal carriage • Population of the nasal passages and pharynx with disease-producing microorganisms in the absence of clinical infection
natriuretic • Promoting the excretion of abnormal amounts of sodium into the urine
nebulizer • An inhalation device which breaks

up a solution into fine droplets for delivery into the lungs

necrobiosis lipoidica diabeticorum • A skin disease characterized by wasting of connective tissue, accumulation of fatty white cells, and multiple yellowish to reddish patches on the limbs

necrosis • Death or destruction of living tissue resulting from loss of blood supply or severe injury

necrotizing • Causing the death of living tissue

neonate • Newborn less than one month old

neoplasm • A tumor; an abnormal, uncontrolled, or progressive growth of new cells or tissue

neoplastic • Pertaining to an abnormal, uncontrolled, or progressive growth of new cells or tissue; cancerous

nephritis • A disease of the kidney characterized by inflammation and degeneration of kidney tissue and formation of fibrous tissue

nephrocalcinosis • Condition characterized by accumulation of calcium phosphate in the kidney tubules, resulting in disturbed kidney function

nephrogenic • Having the ability to produce kidney tissue

nephron • The essential functional unit of the kidney, consisting of the glomerular capsule, the capillary loops inside the capsule, and the attached tubules

nephropathy • Any disease of the kidney

nephrosclerosis • Hardening of the kidney arteries and arterioles

nephrotic syndrome (nephrosis) • Condition characterized by massive swelling due to accumulation of fluids, increased protein and decreased albumin in the urine, and susceptibility to infectious complications

nephrotoxic • Harmful or destructive to the kidney

neuralgia • Severe, sharp, stabbing pain along the course of a nerve of usually brief duration

neuritis • Inflammation of nerve tissue

neuroblastoma • Malignant tumor consisting of cancerous nerve cells and usually arising in the nerves responsible for involuntary functions

neurodermatitis • A skin condition characterized by local, itchy, inflamed, leathery patches and presumed to be caused by emotional factors

neurogenic bladder • Dysfunction of the urinary bladder due to a disease of the central or peripheral nervous system

neuroleptic • A drug that decreases psychotic behavior; a major tranquilizer

neuroleptic malignant syndrome • A potentially fatal syndrome characterized by high fever, muscle rigidity, irregular pulse or blood pressure, protein in the urine, and acute kidney failure

neurologic • Pertaining to the nervous system

neuromuscular blockade • Inhibition of transmission of nerve impulses at the junction of a nerve with a muscle, producing paralysis

neuropathy • Any disease of the nervous system

neurosis • One of two major types of emotional disorders, usually characterized by anxiety and some impairment of thinking and judgment

neurotoxic • Harmful to the nervous system

neutropenia • An abnormally low concentration of neutrophils in the blood

neutrophil • A mature white blood cell

nitrogen balance • Difference between the nitrogen excreted from the body and the nitrogen taken in, excluding the nitrogen inhaled and exhaled during respiration

nocardiosis • A pus-producing, abscess-forming infection of the lungs that may spread to other sites in the body, especially the brain

nocturia • Urination at night

nocturnal • Occurring at night

nodule • A small cluster of cells that is detectable by touch

nonsteroidal anti-inflammatory agent • Any drug used for the treatment of arthritis that does not have a structure similar to that of corticosteroids

normochromic anemia • A condition characterized by an abnormally low concentration of red blood cells, in which the amount of hemoglobin is normal

normocytic anemia • A condition characterized by an abnormally low concentration of red blood cells of normal size but with a proportionate decrease in hemoglobin

normotensive • Pertaining to or having normal blood pressure

nummular dermatitis • A skin condition characterized by blisters and scabs that form coin-shaped patches on the feet and legs

nystagmus • A rapid, involuntary, oscillatory movement of the eyes

obesity • An abnormal increase in body fat

obstetric • Pertaining to pregnancy and childbirth

obstipation • Stubborn constipation

obstructive jaundice • Yellowing of the skin resulting from blocking of the flow of bile into the small intestine

obstructive uropathy • Blocking of the bladder neck due to an increase in size of the prostate gland

obtund • Blunt or to make dull
occipital • Pertaining to back of the head
occlusive coronary episode • Blockage of an artery supplying the heart
occlusive dressing • A wrapping that seals a wound from contact with air or bacteria
occult blood • Blood not visible in body products, such as feces, but detectable with use of laboratory tests
ocular • Pertaining to the eye
oculogyric • Pertaining to the movements of the eyeball
oculogyric crisis • A condition in which the eyeballs become fixed in one position for minutes or hours
oculomotor • Pertaining to eyeball movement or the nerve that arises from the midbrain and supplies most muscles of the eye
oligomenorrhea • Scanty menstruation
oligospermia • Scarcity of sperm in semen
oliguria • Decreased excretion of urine
omphalocele • Protrusion of part of the intestine into the umbilical cord
oncogenic • Pertaining to tumor formation
onycholysis • Loosening of a fingernail or toenail
ophthalmia neonatorium • Any acute, pus-filled inflammation of the eye membranes occurring during the first 10 days of life, usually caused by a vaginal infection
ophthalmic • Pertaining to the eye
opisthotonus • A type of spasm in which the head and heels are bent backward and the body is bowed forward
optic atrophy • Reduction in size of the optic nerve
optic neuritis • Inflammation of the optic nerve
oral • Pertaining to the mouth
orchitis • Inflammation of the testis
organic • Pertaining to an organ or organs
organogenesis • The development and growth of the organs during fetal life
orthostatic hypotension • A decrease in blood pressure caused by sitting up or standing
osteoarthritis • A chronic joint disease characterized by the breaking down of cartilage and the overgrowth of bone
osteolysis • Breaking down or dissolution of bone due to bone calcium loss
osteomalacia • Softening of bones due to a deficiency in vitamin D and calcium, resulting in pain, tenderness, muscular weakness, and loss of appetite and weight
osteopenia • Any decrease in bone mass below normal levels
osteoporosis • A condition mainly affecting postmenopausal women, characterized by a thinning and weakening of the bones, back pain, and curvature of the spine
otic • Pertaining to the ear
otitis externa • Inflammation of the outer ear
otitis media • Inflammation of the middle ear
ototoxic • Harmful to the ear, especially the parts supplied by nerves
ovarian • Pertaining to the ovaries
ovine • Pertaining to or derived from sheep
ovulation • Maturation and discharge of an egg from the ovary
oxytocic agent • A drug that hastens childbirth by stimulating uterine contractions
P wave • Portion of an ECG that denotes excitation of the atrium
Paget's disease • A progressive bone disease characterized by accelerated growth and dissolution of bone tissue; a type of breast cancer involving the nipple, the area surrounding the nipple, and the larger breast ducts
palliative • Relieving or soothing the signs or symptoms of a disease without curing it
palpebral • Pertaining to the eyelid
palpitation • Abnormally rapid heart rate, characterized by fluttering or throbbing within the chest
pancreatitis • Inflammation of the pancreas
pancytopenia • A reduction in the numbers of red blood cells, white blood cells, and platelets in the blood
Papanicolaou smear • A diagnostic test to determine malignant and premalignant conditions of the female genital tract by microscopic examination of vaginal cell scrapings
papilledema • Swelling of the optic disk, the area of the retina that adjoins the optic nerve
papular • Pimple-like
papulovesicular lesion • Injury characterized by pimples and small blisters on the skin
paracoccidioidomycosis • A chronic fungal skin disease characterized by inflamed elevations of the skin and mucous membranes, which may involve the lymph nodes and internal organs
paradoxical • Different than or opposite to that expected
paralysis agitans • A condition that may be drug-induced and is characterized by rhythmic tremors, poor movement, rigid muscles, and reduced or absent postural reflexes
paralytic (adynamic) ileus • Failure of peristalsis in the intestine, resulting in obstruction
paranoia • A condition characterized by delusions of persecution or grandeur
parasite • An animal or plant that lives, grows, and feeds on or inside another living organism
parasympathetic nervous system • A part of the autonomic (involuntary) nervous system

parasympathetic agent • A drug that imitates the actions of the parasympathetic nervous system

parathyroid hormone • Hormone secreted by the parathyroid gland that regulates calcium and phosphorus levels in the blood

parenchyma • The essential or functional tissue of an organ

parenteral • Introduction of substances through means other than through the gastrointestinal system or the lungs

paresthesia • An abnormal burning, tingling, or prickling sensation

parkinsonism • A condition that is sometimes drug induced and is characterized by rhythmic tremors, poor movement, rigid muscles, and a reduction in or loss of postural reflexes

paronychia • A pus-filled inflammation bordering a nail

parotid gland • Salivary gland in front of and below the ear

parotitis • Inflammation of either the parotid gland or the lymph node overlying it

paroxysmal tachycardia • A condition characterized by recurrent episodes of rapid heartbeats that begin and end abruptly

parturition • Process of giving birth

patent • Open or exposed

patent ductus arteriosus • An abnormality present at birth in which the channel between the left pulmonary artery and the aorta persists after birth

pathogen • Disease-producing agent

pathological • Pertaining to a disease

pectus excavation • Deformity of the breastbone and adjacent supportive tissue and the front part of the ribs, resulting in a depression of the lower chest

pedal • Pertaining to the feet

pediculicide • A drug that kills lice

pediculosis capitis • Head lice

pediculosis corporis • Body lice

pediculosis pubis • Crab lice

pemphigoid-type reaction • A condition resembling a skin disease and characterized by successive groups of blisters

penicillinase • A bacterial enzyme that destroys penicillin before it can kill the bacterium

penile • Pertaining to the penis

peptic esophagitis • Inflammation of the esophagus due to acid flowing back from the stomach

peptic ulcer • A marked loss of tissue in areas of the digestive tract exposed to acidic gastric juices, particularly the lower esophagus, stomach, and the first portion of the duodenum

percutaneous • Administered or performed through the skin

perfusion • The introduction of a fluid into an organ or tissue via its blood supply, primarily through injection into a vein

periarteritis nodosum • A disease characterized by inflammation of the external lining of small and medium-sized arteries

pericardiocentesis • Puncture of the pericardium

pericarditis • Inflammation of the pericardium

perioperative • The period immediately before, during, and after a surgical operation or procedure

perioral • Around the mouth

periorbital edema • Swelling around the bony cavity containing the eyeball

peripheral neuropathy • Numbness, burning, prickling, and tingling of the limbs

peristalsis • Wave of contractions within the digestive tract, enabling the contents to be pushed forward

peritoneal dialysis • Introduction and removal of dialyzing fluid into the sac lining the abdominal cavity to remove soluble substances and water from the body

peritoneum • The smooth, transparent membrane lining the abdominal cavity and surrounding the organs within

peritonitis • Inflammation of the peritoneum

pernicious anemia • Abnormally low concentration of circulating red blood cells resulting from inadequate absorption of vitamin B_{12}

peroral • Formed or passed through the mouth

petechiae • Tiny skin spots, ranging in size from a pinpoint to a pinhead, caused by the rupture of blood vessels beneath the skin

petit mal seizure • An epileptic convulsion characterized by a sudden lapse of consciousness, a blank stare, and, sometimes, blinking, lip smacking, and hand movements

Peyronie's disease • A condition characterized by the development of dense fibrous tissue surrounding the erectile tissues of the penis, causing deformity and painful erection

pH   Measurement of the degree of acidity or alkalinity of a solution

phalanges • Bones of the fingers or toes

pharmacokinetics • Study of the uptake, distribution, biotransformation, and elimination of drugs in the body

pharmacologic • Pertaining to the properties and actions of a drug

pharyngitis • Inflammation of the pharynx

phenylketonuria • A congenital metabolic disorder characterized by mental retardation, epilepsy, light coloring, eczema, and a mousy odor

pheochromocytoma • A tumor of the adrenal gland that can cause extremely high blood pressure

phlebitis • Inflammation of a vein and clot formation, accompanied by stiffness, pain, and swelling, usually in the legs

photometer • An instrument for measuring the intensity of light

photophobia • An abnormal intolerance, sensitivity, or fear of light

photosensitivity • An abnormal increase in sensitivity of the skin to ultraviolet radiation

pigmentary retinopathy • An eye disease characterized by a progressive breakdown of the pigmented cells in the inner layers of the retina, resulting in eventual blindness

pilomotor • Causing movement of the hair

pinta • A contagious skin disease characterized by skin patches of various colors

pipette • A calibrated glass or plastic tube used to measure or transfer specific quantities of liquid

pituitary gland • A small gland at the base of the brain that secretes hormones important for normal body functioning

placenta • The organ to which the embryo or fetus is attached by the umbilical cord to the maternal uterus; it is responsible for the exchange of nutrients and waste products, as well as hormones needed to maintain the uterine lining

plantar • Pertaining to the sole of the foot

plasma • The portion of blood remaining after the blood cells are removed

platelet • Thrombocyte; a flattened spherical or oval body in the blood that aids in blood clotting

platelet count • The number of platelets in a cubic millimeter of blood

pleura • The delicate membrane surrounding the lung and lining the internal surface of the chest cavity

pleurisy • Inflammation of the pleura

pneumonitis • Inflammation of the lungs

pollakiuria • Abnormally frequent urination

polyarthralgia • Simultaneous pain in many joints

polycystic • Containing or made up of many cysts

polycythemia • A condition characterized by an increased number of immature and mature red blood cells

polydactyly • The existence of more than the usual number of fingers on the hands and feet

polydipsia • Excessive thirst

polymyalgia rheumatica • A condition in the elderly characterized by joint and muscle pain and stiffness

polymyositis • Simultaneous inflammation of many muscles

polyneuritis • Simultaneous inflammation of many nerves

polyp • A protruding growth from a mucous membrane

polyphagia • Excessive eating

polyradiculoneuropathy • Guillain-Barré syndrome; acute lower paralysis of unknown cause

polyuria • Excessive excretion of urine

porcine • Pertaining to or derived from pigs

porphobilinogen • A derivative of the pigment in red blood cells that is excreted in the urine in certain forms of porphyria

porphyria • A rare inherited disease affecting the liver, digestive system, central nervous system, and skin

postauricular skin • The skin behind the ear

postencephalitic • Taking place as a consequence of or following an episode of brain inflammation (encephalitis)

posterior subcapsular cataract • Clouding or opacity beneath the back of the capsule of the eye

postictal • Following a seizure

postinjection flare • Prolonged, widespread flushing of the skin following the administration of an injectable substance

postpartum • After birth

postpill amenorrhea • Absence of menstruation for at least three months after use of oral contraceptive pills is discontinued

postprandial • After a meal

postsympathectomy • Following surgical removal of part of the autonomic or sympathetic nervous system

postural hypotension • A decrease in blood pressure upon arising or standing

precordial distress • Pain or discomfort in the region of the heart and lower chest

preeclampsia • A condition occurring in the second half of pregnancy and characterized by an acute rise in blood pressure, swelling, and the presence of protein in the urine

pregnancy category • A designation established by the Food and Drug Administration to indicate the relative risk a drug holds for causing malformations in a fetus

premonitory sign • Early manifestations of an impending disease, before specific symptoms begin

prepuberal • Prior to sexual maturation

pressor • Producing a rise in blood pressure

priapism • An abnormal, persistent, painful erection of the penis unrelated to sexual desire

Prinzmetal's syndrome • A form of severe, constricting chest pain occurring while one is asleep or resting
proctitis • Inflammation of the anus or rectum
progesterone • A hormone secreted by the ovary that is essential for implantation of the fertilized egg in the uterus; its cessation at the end of the menstrual cycle initiates menstruation
progestogen (progestin) • Any substance or drug that imitates the action of progesterone
prolactin • A hormone produced by the pituitary gland that promotes milk production
prolactin inhibitor • A drug that inhibits secretion of milk
prophylaxis • A measure or measures taken to prevent the development or spread of disease
proptosis • Falling downward or forward
prostaglandin • A natural, biologically active substance affecting the nervous system, circulation, female reproductive organs, and metabolism
prostate gland • The gland surrounding the neck of the bladder and base of the male urethra and which secretes a milky fluid that makes up approximately 40% of semen
prostatic hypertrophy • Increase in the size of the prostate gland
prostatitis • Inflammation of the prostate gland
prosthetic arthroplasty • The surgical replacement of a nonfunctional arthritic joint with an artificial joint
prostration • Loss of strength
protein binding • Chemical binding of a drug to albumin or other blood proteins; only the portion of drug that is "free" in the plasma (that is, the unbound portion) is pharmacologically active
proteinuria • The presence of protein in the urine
prothrombin • A substance in plasma that is converted to thrombin, a factor involved in blood clotting
prothrombin time • Interval required for clot formation
protopsis • Protrusion of the eye
proximal • Near; situated close to the point of origin
pruritus • Itching
pseudomembranous colitis • A syndrome usually caused by the postsurgical use of antibiotics and characterized by severe diarrhea, pain and swelling of the abdomen, and circulatory collapse
pseudoparkinsonism • Resembling the signs and symptoms of Parkinson's disease
pseudotumor cerebri • A condition simulating the presence of a brain tumor, probably due to a congestion of blood or swelling of the brain
psittacosis • An infection carried by parrots that, when transmitted to humans, causes headache, nausea, constipation, fever, and symptoms of bronchopneumonia
psoriasiform • Resembling psoriasis
psoriasis • A chronic skin condition characterized by scaly, reddish patches
psychometric tests • Intelligence tests
psychomotor • Pertaining to muscular movement directly proceeding from mental activity
psychosis • Fundamental mental derangement characterized by a defective or lost contact with reality
psychotropic • Pertaining to an effect on the psyche or mind
ptosis • Drooping of an eyelid; slipping of an organ or part
PTT • Partial thromboplastin time; a measurement of the blood's ability to clot
puberal (pubertal) • Pertaining to the period of sexual maturation, characterized, in boys, by deepening of the voice and the discharge of semen and, in girls, by the onset of menstruation
puerperal • Pertaining to or following childbirth
pulmonary • Pertaining to the lungs
pulmonary edema • Escape of fluid into the air sacs and tissues of the lungs, producing a severe shortage of breath
pulmonary fibrosis • A condition characterized by the formation of fibrous connective tissue in the lungs
pulmonary infiltration • Accumulation of foreign material in lung tissue and air sacs
pulsate • To beat or throb
punctate • Dotted
purpura • A condition caused by rupture of minute blood vessels under the skin or within the mucous membranes lining body canals and cavities
purulent exudate • Pus
pustule • A pus-filled pimple or blister, surrounded by inflamed skin
pyelonephritis • Infection and inflammation of the kidney
pylorus • The opening of the stomach into the duodenum, or upper part of the small intestine
pyoderma • Any pus-producing skin injury
pyogenic • Producing pus
pyrexia • Fever
pyrogenic • Capable of inducing fever
pyrosis • Heartburn
qid • Four times a day
QRS interval • The portion of an electrocardiogram that denotes excitation of the ventricles

quadriceps femoris fibrosis • Increases in the fibrous tissue of the quadriceps muscle of the thigh

qualitative • Pertaining to the presence or absence of an element or constituent in a substance

quantitative • Pertaining to the amount of an element or constituent in a substance

radioactive • Pertaining to the spontaneous decay or disintegration of atomic matter and emission of radiant energy

radiogram • X-ray photograph; roentgenogram

radioimmunoassay (RIA) • The quantitative determination of antigen or antibody in a laboratory sample by introducing a radioactively labeled substance that will bind to it and then measuring the radioactivity of the bound complex

radiotherapy • Treatment of disease with X-rays or rays from a radioactive substance, such as radium or cobalt 60

rat-bite fever • An infectious disease caused by a rodent bite and characterized by a bluish-red rash, fever, and muscular pain

Raynaud's phenomenon • A vascular condition caused by cold or emotion, characterized by intermittent pallor or redness and pain in the fingers or toes, and sometimes both

reactive depression • Depression caused by an external situation that is relieved when that situation is removed

reagent • A substance used to detect another substance by chemical, microscopic, or other means, or that converts one substance into another by a chemical reaction

receptor • A sensory nerve terminal; a molecular structure on or within a cell that can combine with a drug or other substance to alter cell function

recombinant • Pertaining to the receipt of genetic material from different sources

reconstitute • To restore a substance to its original form after it has been altered for storage or preservation, such as by freeze drying

red-cell aplasia • Defective production of red blood cells

reflux esophagitis • Inflammation of the esophagus due to regurgitation of the contents of the stomach

refractory • Resistant to treatment or stimulation

regional (block) anesthesia • Numbing of a region of the body by injection of an anesthetic solution into and around the nerve endings supplying the area

regurgitate • Vomit

renal • Pertaining to the kidney

renal colic • Pain in any part of the kidney system

renin • A kidney enzyme involved in the regulation of blood pressure and production of the hormone aldosterone

resorption • Disappearance of a fetus, tissue, or fluid from the body by absorption back into the body and eventual elimination

respiratory acidosis • A condition caused by excessive retention of carbon dioxide in the body, resulting in a decrease in blood pH

respiratory alkalosis • A condition caused by excessive loss of carbon dioxide from the body, resulting in an increase in blood pH

respiratory depression • Lessened or decreased breathing

respiratory tract • The cavities and passages through which air enters and leaves the body

resuscitation • A measure or measures used to restore breathing or the heartbeat

reticulocyte • An immature red blood cell

retinoblastoma • A malignant tumor of the sensory portion of the retina

retinopathy • Any of various noninflammatory disorders of the retina, including some that are major causes of blindness

retinoscopy • Method of evaluating the refraction of the eye by observing how the eye reacts to a beam of light

retrobulbar • Behind the eyeball

retrocollis • Spasm of the muscles behind the neck, causing the head to draw back

retrograde • Movement opposite the normal or previous direction

retrosternal • Located or occurring behind the breastbone

Reye's syndrome • A rare, acute, and often fatal brain disease of childhood, accompanied by fatty breakdown of the liver and kidneys and often preceded by influenza or other viral infection

rhabdomyolysis • Disintegration of skeletal muscle, accompanied by the excretion of muscle protein in the urine

rheumatic fever • A disease resulting from a streptococcal infection and characterized by fever, pain, joint swelling, and inflammation of the heart, valves, and blood vessels

rheumatism • A general term pertaining to diseases of muscle, tendon, joint, bone, or nerve that result in inflammation and are characterized by pain and stiffness

rheumatoid arthritis • A chronic disease of the joints, characterized by inflammation, pain, limitation of motion, and deformity

rheumatoid factor • A protein present in the blood of most patients with rheumatoid arthritis and detectable in serum tests

rhinitis • Inflammation of the mucous membranes of the nose
rhinorrhea • Running nose
Ringer's solution (injection) • An intravenous solution used as a diluent for some injections and as a fluid and electrolyte replenisher
rouleau formation • A column of red blood cells stacked like a roll of coins
rubella • German measles; an acute, highly contagious disease characterized by rash, fever, and enlargement of the lymph nodes; if contracted during early pregnancy, rubella may cause fetal malformations
SA node • Sinoatrial node; a network of specialized heart-muscle fibers that acts as the dominant pacemaker of the heart
saline • A solution of sodium chloride; salty or saltlike
saline cathartic • A salt solution used to evacuate the bowels by causing retention of water in the intestine and increasing the fluidity of the intestinal contents
salpingitis • Inflammation of the auditory or uterine tube
sanguineous • Pertaining to or containing blood
sarcoidosis • A chronic disease of unknown origin characterized by the formation of granular elevations in the lymph nodes, lungs, bones, skin, liver, spleen, and heart
SC • Subcutaneous (under the skin)
scabicide • A drug that kills scabies mites
scarlatiniform • Resembling scarlet fever
schizophrenia • A psychotic disorder characterized by delusions, hallucinations, withdrawal of interest from other people and the outside world, and disturbances in mood, behavior, and intellect
scintillating scotomata • A sensation of bright, flickering, zig-zag flashes before the eyes
sclera • The tough, white outer layer of the eyeball
scleral injection • Widening of the blood vessels in the tough outer layer of the eyeball
sclerosis • Hardening of the nerves or arteries
scoliosis • A condition characterized by curvature of the spine toward one side of the body
scotoma • A "blind" spot in the visual field surrounded by areas of normal or near-normal vision
seborrhea • A skin disorder characterized by excessive production of sebum (the fatty skin-lubricating substance secreted by the sebaceous glands in the skin) and scale or crust formation
sedative • A drug that produces a calming effect and drowsiness

seizure • A fit, convulsion, or epileptic attack
seminiferous tubules • Any of the microscopic channels of the testes where sperm are produced or transported
senile • Pertaining to, caused by, or characteristic of old age
senile dementia • A chronic, progressive mental disease of the elderly, characterized by failing memory and loss of other intellectual functions
sensitivity • In diagnostic tests, the degree to which a test can detect the substance being investigated or diagnose a condition in a group of patients
sensorium • Pertaining to a patient's consciousness or mental clarity
sepsis • A severe toxic condition resulting from the spread of bacteria or their poisonous products from an infection site
septicemia • Blood poisoning; invasion of the blood by bacteria or other microorganisms from an infection site
seroconversion • Measure or degree of immunity produced by a vaccine
serology • The laboratory discipline concerned with the preparation, use, and immunologic properties of the fluid portion of the blood
serous • Pertaining to blood serum
serum • A clear, watery fluid that moistens the surface of membranes or is released by inflammation; the fluid portion of the blood remaining after the blood cells and fibrin are removed
serum half-life • Time required for the serum concentration of a drug to fall by one half
serum sickness • A strong allergic reaction following a relatively large injection of serum, characterized by hives, swelling, swollen lymph nodes, joint pains, high fever, and loss of strength
SGOT • Serum glutamic oxaloacetic transaminase, an enzyme released by tissue injury; elevated SGOT levels may indicate a heart attack, liver disease, or other disorders
SGPT • Serum glutamic pyruvic transaminase, a liver enzyme; increased SGPT levels may indicate liver disease or functional impairment of the liver
shigellosis • A bacterial infection of the colon characterized by abdominal cramps, fever, and frequent passing of bloody stools or of fluids consisting of blood and mucus
shock • A condition caused by poor return of blood to the heart and reduction in cardiac output, characterized by low blood pressure, reduced urinary output, a weak pulse, increased heart rate, and pallor
sialadenitis • Inflammation of a salivary gland
sick sinus syndrome • A complex disturbance

of the normal heartbeat characterized by episodes of excessive bradycardia or alternating bradycardia and tachycardia

sigmoid colon • The S-shaped part of the colon

sinoatrial (SA) node • A small bundle of specialized pacemaker cells in the right atrium, the firing of which generates the impulses that stimulate and pace the heart

sinus arrest • Stoppage of the pacemaker activity of the sinoatrial node

sinus bradycardia • Sinus rhythm of less than 60 beats per minute

sinus rhythm • The normal heart rhythm established by impulses originating in the sinoatrial node

Sjogren's syndrome • A condition seen in menopausal women characterized by drying of the mucous membranes, swelling of the salivary glands, and multiple painful joints

skeletal muscle • A muscle attached between two bones for the purpose of movement; voluntary muscle

smallpox • Variola; a severe, contagious, but now virtually extinct, viral infection characterized by a high fever and the eruption of blisters over most of the body

smooth muscle • Muscle tissue found in the walls of organs, ducts, bronchioles, and blood vessels; involuntary muscle

sodium metabisulfite • A preservative used in many solid and liquid drug preparations that can cause allergic-type reactions in susceptible individuals

solar keratosis • Sharply outlined, red or flesh-colored, wartlike growth caused by excessive sun exposure

solubilization • Capability of being dissolved

solution • A homogeneous mixture of a solid or solids in a liquid

somatic • Pertaining to the body, as distinct from the genes

somnambulism • Sleepwalking

somnolence • Sleepiness

spasticity • State of increased muscle tone with exaggerated tendon reflexes

specificity • In diagnostic tests, the degree to which a test can distinguish the substance being investigated from other substances or rule out the condition being tested for

spectrophotometer • Apparatus for estimating the quantity of coloring matter in a solution by measuring light absorption

spermatozoa • Mature male sex cells; sperm

spider telangiectasis • Network of a small group of widened capillaries forming dark red, wartlike spots on the skin surface

spina bifida cystica • An abnormality present at birth, characterized by defective closure of the bones surrounding the spinal cord with the spinal cord

spina bifida occulta • An abnormality present at birth characterized by defective closure of the bones surrounding the spinal cord but without protrusion of the spinal cord and its membranes

splenectomy • Surgical removal of the spleen

splenomegaly • Enlargement of the spleen

sporotrichosis • A fungal infection characterized by skin elevations and abscesses in the superficial lymph nodes, skin, and the tissues beneath the skin

spotting • Small amounts of blood from the vagina discharged usually between menstrual periods

sputum • Saliva, mucus, or pus expelled from the body by spitting

squamous cell carcinoma • A type of skin cancer in which the skin cells are reduced to thin, flat plates resembling fish scales

stasis dermatitis • A skin condition involving part or all of the lower leg and characterized by swelling, pigmentation, and, often, ulceration

status asthmaticus • Severe and protracted asthma, characterized by shortness of breath to the point of exhaustion and collapse that is unresponsive to usual treatment

status epilepticus • A severe form of epilepsy in which convulsions occur frequently and consciousness is not regained between seizures

steatorrhea • Excessive amounts of fat in the feces

stellate lenticular opacity • A star-shaped opaque spot on the lens of the eye

stenosing • Narrowing of a duct or canal

sternum • Breastbone

steroid hormone • A type of hormone produced by the adrenal cortex, ovaries, and testes

steroid myopathy • Muscle weakness caused by prolonged or excessive use of corticosteroids

Stevens-Johnson syndrome • An acute, inflammatory disease characterized by red marks on the neck, face, legs, and the back of the hands, forearms, and feet; erythema multiforme

stiff-man syndrome • A progressive fluctuating stiffness of the spinal column and limb muscles

Stokes-Adams syndrome • Condition caused by heart block and characterized by sudden fainting attacks

stomatitis • Inflammation of the soft mouth tissues

strabismus • Squinting

striae • Stripes or streaks distinguished by color, elevation, or texture

stridor • A harsh, high-pitched sound coming from the respiratory tract
stroma • The supporting tissue of an organ
stupor • Partial or complete unconsciousness
subarachnoid • Beneath the membrane covering the brain and spinal cord
subcortical • Beneath the layer of gray matter making up most of the brain
sublingual • Beneath the tongue
submucosal • Beneath a mucous membrane
substernal • Beneath the breastbone
substrate • The substance that an enzyme acts upon
sulfhemoglobinemia • A condition in which a greenish substance derived from hemoglobin appears in the blood
sulfobromophthalein • Chemical used in certain tests of liver function
superinfection • Development of a second infection in addition to the original one
suprapubic • Above the pubic bone
supraventricular • Above the ventricles
suspension • A dispersion of solid particles in a liquid
swab • A small, cotton-tipped stick used to clean wounds, clear mucus, take cultures, or apply drugs to the skin surface
swimmer's ear • Inflammation of the external ear canal, often seen in swimmers
sympathectomy • Removal of a portion of the nervous system responsible for involuntary actions
sympathetic nervous system • The part of the autonomic (involuntary) nervous system that decreases gastrointestinal secretions and motility, increases the heart rate and blood pressure, and widens the air passages and pupils
sympathetic ophthalmia • A granular inflammation of the pigmented area of an uninjured eye occurring a few weeks after damage to the area of the other eye had occurred
sympatholytic agent • A drug that can inhibit or block the actions of the sympathetic nervous system
sympathomimetic agent • A drug that imitates the actions of the sympathetic nervous system
syncope • Fainting or swooning
syndactyly • Webbed fingers or toes
synechia • Adhesion of the iris to the cornea or lens of the eye
synostosis • Union of bones or bony material making up a joint
synovial fluid • A transparent, sticky, lubricating fluid secreted by joint membranes
synovitis • Inflammation of the synovial membrane of a joint

syphilis • A sexually transmitted disease that can also be passed on to a newborn baby by its mother
systemic • Pertaining to the body as a whole or to the general circulation
systemic lupus erythematosus (SLE) • A disease characterized by joint pain and stiffness, a butterfly-shaped rash on the face, sun sensitivity, mouth ulcers, hair loss, and a variety of bodily signs and symptoms
systole • Contraction of the heart that forces blood onward
systolic pressure • The peak pressure exerted on the walls of the arteries when the ventricles contract
T wave • Portion of an electrocardiogram that denotes recovery of the ventricles
tachyarrhythmia • A disturbance in heart rhythm resulting in a rate greater than 100 beats per minute
tachycardia • Abnormally fast heartbeat
tachypnea • Abnormally rapid breathing rate
tamponade • Compression of the heart by the fluid surrounding it
tardive dyskinesia • A potentially irreversible condition characterized by involuntary movements of the tongue, face, mouth, lips, jaws, trunk, and/or extremities
tartrazine • FD&C Yellow No. 5, a bright-yellow dye used in medicines and which may cause allergic-type reactions in susceptible individuals, especially people who are allergic to aspirin
taste perversion • Deviation from normal taste sensation
tbsp • Tablespoon(s)
telangiectasia • An elevated, dark-red, wartlike spot resulting from the widening of small blood vessels beneath the surface
temporal arteritis • A chronic vascular disease of the elderly that affects the arteries that supply blood to the head and brain and causes inflammation, headache, chewing difficulties, weakness, weight loss, and fever
tendinitis • Inflammation of a tendon
tendon • A bundle of tough connective tissue attaching a muscle to a bone
tenesmus • Painful, unproductive straining to empty the bowel or bladder
tenosynovitis • Inflammation of the bundle of connective tissue attached to a muscle and its sheath
teratogenic • Capable of causing birth defects
testicular • Pertaining to the testes
testosterone • The principal male sex hormone secreted by the testes
tetanus • An infectious disease characterized by extreme body stiffness, painful contractions of

COMPENDIUM OF DRUG THERAPY

voluntary muscles, and generalized convulsions

tetany • An abnormal condition characterized by intermittent numbness and cramps, twitching of the limbs, spasms in the windpipe, bizarre behavior, loss of consciousness, and convulsions

theophyllinization • Control of certain respiratory diseases characterized by bronchospasm with the drug theophylline or a theophylline-like agent

therapeutic • Pertaining to the remedies used to treat a disease or disorder

thoracic • Pertaining to the chest

thrombocytopenia • An abnormally low concentration of platelets in the blood

thrombocytopenic purpura • A condition characterized by leakage of blood into the skin, coupled with a reduction in platelet count

thrombocytosis • An excessive number of platelets in the blood

thromboembolism • Blockage of a blood vessel by a dislodged blood clot (thrombus) or portion of a blood clot

thrombolytic agent • A drug that dissolves blood clots

thrombopenia • Abnormally low concentration of platelets in the blood

thrombophlebitis • Inflammation of a vein associated with formation of a clot

thrombosis • Formation, development, or presence of a clot

thrombus • A clot that frequently blocks a blood vessel at the point of formation

thrush • Candidiasis; a fungal disease characterized by white patches in the mouth

thyroid gland • A gland lying at the base of the neck, in front of the windpipe

thyroid hormone • A generic term for two hormones, throxine and triiodothyronine, that influence growth and energy production

thyroid stimulating hormone (TSH) • A hormone produced by the anterior pituitary gland that stimulates hormone production by the thyroid gland

thyroid storm • An acute, sudden, intense overactivity of the thyroid gland, resulting in an extremely rapid heartbeat, muscle weakness, coma, and eventual death if left untreated

thyroiditis • Inflammation of the thyroid gland

thyrotoxicosis • Poisoning caused by excessive quantities of thyroid hormone

tic • A habitual, repetitious movement or series of movements that a person is aware of but performs to relieve tension

tid • Three times a day

tidal volume • The amount of air moved by a single breath at any level of activity

tinea capitis • Fungus infection of the scalp; ringworm

tinea corporis • Fungus infection affecting nonhairy areas of the body

tinea cruris • Fungus infection of the groin and the area between the anus and genitalia

tinea manuum • Fungus infection of the hand

tinea pedis • Fungus infection of the foot; athlete's foot

tinea unguium • Fungus infection of the nails

tinea versicolor • Fungus infection of the skin, usually in the trunk region, that results in brownish patches

tinnitus • Ringing in the ears

titer • The strength of a substance or concentration of a solution

titrate • The process of increasing or decreasing the dose of a drug until the desired effect is obtained

tolerance • Loss of responsiveness to a given dose of a drug, particularly after continuous use; ability to receive a particular dose without showing side effects

tonic • Pertaining to the contracting phase of a muscle spasm

tophaceous gout • A prominent, sandy, gritty deposit of sodium urate in the tissues affected by gout

topical • Pertaining to the surface of the body

torsade de pointes • A sharp increase in the rate of contraction of the ventricles

torticollis • A spasmodic contraction of the neck muscles, resulting in limited movement of the head and a twisted position

torulosis • A fungal infection that mainly affects the central nervous system and primarily causes meningitis, but which may also involve the lungs, bones, and skin

Tourette's syndrome • See Gilles de la Tourette syndrome

toxemia • A condition in which the blood contains poisonous products from body cells or microorganisms

toxic epidermal necrolysis • A condition characterized by a sudden high fever and large, soft blisters on the skin or mucous membranes

toxic megacolon • An abnormally large or widened colon accompanied by chronic recurrent ulceration and possibly resulting in perforation

toxin • Poison produced by some higher plants, animals, and bacteria that the body reacts to by producing antibodies

toxoid • A bacterial toxin, or poison, that has been weakened by heat or chemical treatment but has retained its ability to induce antibodies against it

toxoplasmosis • A disease caused by protozoa that affects the brain, liver, spleen, and other

organs
tracheitis • Inflammation of the trachea or windpipe
tracheostomy • A surgically created opening into the trachea through the neck, usually performed to insert a tube to facilitate ventilation
trachoma • An infectious disease of the conjunctiva and cornea of the eye
transaminase • A type of enzyme produced mainly by the liver and involved in the biotransformation of amino acids, the building blocks of proteins
transcutaneous • Passing or entering through the skin
transdermal • Through the skin
transient ischemic attack (TIA) • Temporary loss of neurological function resulting from impaired blood flow to the brain, characterized by dim vision, muscle weakness and numbness on one side of the body, and dizziness and thick speech
tremulousness • Trembling, quivering
trichinosis • A disease caused by ingestion of uncooked pork, resulting in worm infestation and characterized by nausea, fever, diarrhea, stiffness, and swelling of the face and muscles
trichomonad • A type of protozoan that moves with a whiplike tail
trichomonal vaginitis • A protozoan infection characterized by inflammation and itching of the vagina and vulva and a white, frothy discharge
trichuriasis • Whipworm infection
trigeminal neuralgia A sharp, severe pain along the course of a facial nerve
triglyceride A fatty compound produced by the liver, essential for the proper metabolism of fatty foods
trigonitis • Inflammation of a triangular area on the inner surface of the urinary bladder
trimester • The initial, middle, or last three months of pregnancy
trismus • Spasms of the jaw muscles
trophoblastic • Pertaining to the embryonic layer of cells that attach to the wall of the uterus for nourishment
tsp • Teaspoon(s)
tuberculin • A preparation injected into the skin to determine if a person is sensitive to the bacteria that cause tuberculosis
tuberculosis • A chronic infectious disease primarily involving the lungs and characterized by fever, weight loss, cough, chest pain, and blood- and pus-filled phlegm
tularemia • A rare infection transmitted to man from rodents by the deer fly and characterized by symptoms similar to those of plague and undulant fever
tumorigenic • Giving rise to tumors
turbid • Cloudy
turgid • Swollen
tympanic membrane • Eardrum
typhoid fever • An acute infection characterized by fever, headache, cough, abnormal pulse, reduced numbers of white blood cells, live bacteria in the blood, and rose-colored skin spots
ulcerative colitis • A chronic, recurrent ulceration of the colon characterized by cramping abdominal pain, rectal bleeding, and loose excretion of blood, pus, and feces
ultrasound • A diagnostic technique in which sound waves are transmitted through body tissues, and echoes reflected off objects in the body are transformed into photographic images
umbilical hernia • Protrusion of part of the intestine at the navel
uncinariasis • Hookworm infection
unctuous • Greasy or oily
upper respiratory tract • The nasal and oral cavities, pharynx, and larynx
urate • Salt of uric acid
uremia • A biochemical disorder associated with kidney failure and characterized by increased blood nitrogen, acidosis, anemia, and other abnormalities
ureter • A long, narrow tube that carries urine from a kidney to the urinary bladder
urethra • The tube leading from the kidney through which urine is transported to the outside
urethral stricture • Narrowing of the urethra due to inflammation or instrumentation
urethritis • Inflammation of the urethra
uric acid • A product of the breakdown of proteins present in the blood and urine
uricosuria • Excretion of uric acid in the urine
uricosuric agent • A drug that promotes the excretion of uric acid in the urine
urinalysis • Examination of the urine involving chemical, physical, and microscopic tests
urinary hesitancy • Inability to pass urine, even when an urge is present
urinary tract • The urinary passage, including the kidneys, ureters, bladder, and urethra
urobilinogen • A substance formed from the bile pigment by the action of intestinal bacteria and which is then converted to a brown pigment
urolithiasis • Formation of or presence of urinary stones
uropathy • Any disease involving the urinary tract
urticaria • Hives
uterine leiomyomata • A benign fibroid tumor

of the uterus
uterotonic • Increased muscle tone of the uterus
uveitis • Inflammation of the entire pigmented area of the eye, consisting of the iris, ciliary body, and choroid
vaccine • A substance that contains a weakened or killed virus or bacterium that stimulates the body to produce antibodies against subsequent infection by that factor
vaccinia • An acute viral disease caused by smallpox vaccination
vagal • Pertaining to the vagus nerve
vaginitis • Inflammation of the vagina
vagolytic • Pertaining to or resembling the interruption of electrical impulses in the vagus nerve
vagospastic reaction • A spasm of the blood vessels, resulting in a decreased diameter and increased blood pressure
Valsalva maneuver • Forcible exhalation of breath while holding the throat closed, which increases chest pressure and impedes the return of blood to the heart
varicella zoster • Chickenpox
vasculitis • Inflammation of a blood vessel
vasoconstriction • Narrowing of blood vessels
vasoconstrictor • A drug or nerve that narrows blood vessels, thereby raising blood pressure
vasodilation • Widening of blood vessels
vasodilator • A drug or nerve that widens blood vessels, thereby lowering blood pressure
vasomotor • Pertaining to the widening or constriction of blood vessels as a result of smooth-muscle action in the vessel walls
vasomotor rhinitis • Congestion of the mucous membranes of the nose in the absence of infection or allergy
vasopressor • A substance that constricts the smooth muscles of blood vessels, thereby raising blood pressure
vasospasm • A sudden constriction of a blood vessel
vasovagal episode • Excessive activity of the vagus nerve, resulting in anxiety, pallor, slow heartbeat, low blood pressure, sweating, nausea, labored breathing, and fainting
vehicle • The medium (cream, ointment, solution, etc) containing the drug
venipuncture • Intentional puncture of a vein with a blade or blood-collecting device
ventilation • The exchange of air between the lungs and the atmosphere
ventricle • The lower chamber of the heart, which receives blood from the atrium and pumps it into the arteries
ventricular • Pertaining to the lower two chambers of the heart

ventricular trigeminy • The occurrence in the ventricles of three heartbeats in rapid succession
vermicular • Wormlike
vertebra • One of the 33 bones forming the spinal (vertebral) column
vertigo • Dizziness
vesiculobullous • Having small and large water-filled blisters
vesiculobullous reaction • A skin reaction characterized by both small and large blisters
vestibular • Pertaining to the part of the inner ear concerned with maintaining balance
vibriosis • An infectious disease that primarily affects cattle, sheep, and goats but, when transmitted to humans, may cause fever, sweating, weakness, and generalized aching
Vincent's infection • A noncontagious infection of the mucous membranes of the mouth characterized by ulceration and the formation of a false membrane
virilization • The development of certain male sex characteristics in a female, such as enlargement of the clitoris, growth of facial and body hair, and deepening of the voice
viscera • The internal organs, especially the abdominal organs
visual acuity • Clarity of central vision
vital capacity • The volume of air that can be expelled from the lungs by breathing out with the greatest force after inhaling fully
VMA • Vanillylmandelic acid, the measurement of which in urine is used as a test for pheochromocytoma
voluntary muscle • Muscle that is under conscious control, such as that of the limbs; skeletal muscle
vulva • The female external genital organs
vulvovaginitis • Inflammation of the vulva and vagina
WBC • White blood cell
wedge pressure • An indirect determination of the pressure in the left atrium by measuring the pressure in the lung capillaries during cardiac catheterization
Wenckebach phenomenon • A form of second-degree atrioventricular block characterized by progressive prolongation of the P-R interval
wheezing • Whistling or sighing, often audible only with a stethoscope
whole blood • Blood containing all of its elements
Wilms' tumor • A malignant mixed kidney tumor usually seen in infants and children
Wilson's disease • A heritable disorder associated with the abnormal breakdown of copper

withdrawal symptoms • Physical and psychological disturbances brought on by discontinuation of a drug, generally after prolonged use

Wolff-Parkinson-White syndrome • A heart disorder characterized by accelerated impulse conduction between the upper and lower chambers of the heart and abnormal excitation of the lower chamber

xanthoma • A yellowish mass of fat-filled cells situated in the tissue beneath the skin surface, often around tendons

xanthopsia • Yellow vision, a condition in which various objects look yellow

yaws • An infectious tropical disease characterized by crusted, granular ulcers that can spread from the extremities to the whole body, especially the face and limbs

yellow atrophy • Acute, localized death of liver tissue due to hepatitis

Zollinger-Ellison syndrome • A condition characterized by excessive stomach secretions and acidity, severe peptic ulceration, and increased growth of pancreatic islet cells